GOODMAN and GILMAN's

The Pharmacological Basis of Therapeutics

GOODMAN and GILMAN's

The Pharmacological Basis of Therapeutics

EIGHTH EDITION

McGRAW-HILL, INC.
Health Professions Division
New York St. Louis San Francisco Auckland Bogotá Caracas
Lisbon London Madrid Mexico Milan Montreal New Delhi Paris
San Juan Singapore Sydney Tokyo Toronto

Goodman and Gilman's The Pharmacological Basis of Therapeutics

34567890 RMTRMT 9876542

ISBN 0-07-105270-4

Library of Congress Cataloging-in-Publication Data

Goodman and Gilman's the pharmacological basis of therapeutics.

Includes bibliographical references.
Includes index.
ISBN 0-07-105270-4
1. Pharmacology 2. Chemotherapy. I. Goodman, Louis Sanford, 1906- II. Gilman, Alfred, 1908-
III. Gilman, Alfred Goodman, 1941-
IV. Title: Pharmacological basis of therapeutics.
[DNLM: 1. Drug Therapy. 2. Pharmacology. QV 4 G6532]
RM300.G644 1991 615′.7 90-7660

ERRATUM

Goodman and Gilman's

The Pharmacological Basis of Therapeutics, 8/e

The copyright date on page iv is incorrectly printed as 1993.
The book was published and copyrighted in 1990.

PREFACE TO THE EIGHTH EDITION

THIS eighth edition of *Goodman and Gilman's The Pharmacological Basis of Therapeutics* marks its fiftieth anniversary. Comparison of the volumes provides a remarkable view of the accelerating pace of acquisition of pharmacological knowledge during the last half of the twentieth century. The first edition was widely proclaimed to have provided the naissance of the teaching and practice of pharmacology; one is now amazed to recall its three chapters on the chemotherapy of syphilis and four chapters that described the newly discovered sulfonamides. There is no mention of antibiotics, cancer chemotherapy, or psychopharmacology, to list but a few examples. The eighth edition reflects the full impact of modern biology on pharmacology and therapeutics: novel drugs produced by recombinant DNA technology, detailed knowledge of the structure and function of dozens of receptors, major progress toward the goals of rational and facile drug design, and improved treatment from appreciation of the importance of the interplay between pharmacodynamics and pharmacokinetics. Despite such extraordinary change, the three objectives that have guided the writing of this book through a half century remain intact. These are stated in the Preface to the First Edition, which is reprinted herein. Adherence to these objectives has encouraged widespread and successful use of this textbook by students and practitioners of medicine, pharmacology, and other health professions.

While those familiar with previous editions of this textbook will immediately recognize the organization of the present volume, there have been important changes in its structure, in addition to extensive revision. The section on General Principles (Section I) has been expanded and now includes a chapter on Principles of Toxicology. Several chapters in the important section on Autonomic Pharmacology are newly authored, and every chapter in this section reflects the extraordinary amount of new information on cholinergic and adrenergic receptors that has accrued during the past five years. Entirely new sections include those on drugs that affect gastrointestinal function, immunosuppressive agents, and dermatopharmacology. Newly organized chapters include those about autacoids and the drug therapy of inflammation; renin, angiotensin, and the converting enzyme inhibitors; antiviral agents; antifungal agents; hematopoietic agents; and sedatives and hypnotics. More than 50 newly marketed drugs and many investigational agents are discussed; a few of the more important examples include erythropoietin, lovastatin, zidovudine (AZT), and alteplase (tissue plasminogen activator). The appendix of pharmacokinetic data now includes 243 drug entries.

Most of the contributors to the seventh edition were able and anxious to participate in the current undertaking, and we are pleased with their loyalty. Despite this, revision and reorganization afford us the opportunity to welcome over two dozen new authors to the textbook. They are an outstanding group and this eighth edition amply reflects their knowledge. Two new editors also made a significant impact on this volume—Alan S. Nies and Palmer Taylor. Happily, Theodore Rall again dedicated himself completely to the editorial task.

In addition to the editors and contributors, four other individuals played a vital role in the production of this edition. Wendy Deaner was, for the third time, our primary editorial assistant; we have been sustained by her intelligence, organization, and energy. Michele Ferguson reviewed all sections of the text on pharmaceutical preparations and dosage; she was exhaustive in her efforts to insure accuracy of this information. Jane Rall and Kathryn Gilman accepted two joyless tasks with remarkable cheer—marriage to a textbook and compilation of all of the bibliographies; we thank them.

Of course, the passage of time brings unwelcome change as well. Alfred Gilman died just prior to initiation of work on the seventh edition. This eighth edition is the first to be produced without the participation of Louis Goodman—the book's creator and original coauthor. We miss his superb scientific judgment, beautiful writing style, and sense of humor. He was a particularly effective teacher as I took over responsibility for the textbook during the fifth and sixth editions. He provided constant encouragement with praise, effective criticism by example, and, always, packets of reprints from his enormous collection when a section required editorial input. I became particularly proud of my middle name, acquired as a tribute to a friend and colleague when the first edition and I were born nearly simultaneously. There would have been no G&G without Louis Goodman, and pharmacology would have been much diminished. This edition is dedicated to its founder.

ALFRED GOODMAN GILMAN

Dallas, Texas
April, 1990

PREFACE TO THE FIRST EDITION

THREE objectives have guided the writing of this book—the correlation of pharmacology with related medical sciences, the reinterpretation of the actions and uses of drugs from the viewpoint of important advances in medicine, and the placing of emphasis on the applications of pharmacodynamics to therapeutics.

Although pharmacology is a basic medical science in its own right, it borrows freely from and contributes generously to the subject matter and technics of many medical disciplines, clinical as well as preclinical. Therefore, the correlation of strictly pharmacological information with medicine as a whole is essential for a proper presentation of pharmacology to students and physicians. Furthermore, the reinterpretation of the actions and uses of well-established therapeutic agents in the light of recent advances in the medical sciences is as important a function of a modern textbook of pharmacology as is the description of new drugs. In many instances these new interpretations necessitate radical departures from accepted but outworn concepts of the actions of drugs. Lastly, the emphasis throughout the book, as indicated in its title, has been clinical. This is mandatory because medical students must be taught pharmacology from the standpoint of the actions and uses of drugs in the prevention and treatment of disease. To the student, pharmacological data per se are valueless unless he is able to apply his information in the practice of medicine. This book has also been written for the practicing physician, to whom it offers an opportunity to keep abreast of recent advances in therapeutics and to acquire the basic principles necessary for the rational use of drugs in his daily practice.

The criteria for the selection of bibliographic references require comment. It is obviously unwise, if not impossible, to document every fact included in the text. Preference has therefore been given to articles of a review nature, to the literature on new drugs, and to original contributions in controversial fields. In most instances, only the more recent investigations have been cited. In order to encourage free use of the bibliography, references are chiefly to the available literature in the English language.

The authors are greatly indebted to their many colleagues at the Yale University School of Medicine for their generous help and criticism. In particular they are deeply grateful to Professor Henry Gray Barbour, whose constant encouragement and advice have been invaluable.

LOUIS S. GOODMAN
ALFRED GILMAN

New Haven, Connecticut
November 20, 1940

CONTRIBUTORS

Baldessarini, Ross J., M.D. Professor of Psychiatry and in Neuroscience, Harvard Medical School; Director, Laboratories for Psychiatric Research, Mailman Research Center, McLean Hospital, Belmont, Massachusetts

Benet, Leslie Z., Ph.D., D.Pharm.(Hon.) Professor and Chairman, Department of Pharmacy, School of Pharmacy, University of California, San Francisco, California

Bennett, John E., M.D. Head, Clinical Mycology, Laboratory of Clinical Investigation, National Institute of Allergy and Infectious Diseases, Bethesda, Maryland

Bickers, David R., M.D. Professor and Chairman, Department of Dermatology, Case Western Reserve University School of Medicine, University Hospitals of Cleveland, Cleveland, Ohio

Bigger, J. Thomas, Jr., M.D. Professor of Medicine and Pharmacology, and Director of Cardiology, Columbia University College of Physicians and Surgeons, New York, New York

Bloom, Floyd E., M.D. Chairman, Department of Neuropharmacology, Research Institute of Scripps Clinic, La Jolla, California

Brown, Joan Heller, Ph.D. Associate Professor of Pharmacology, University of California, San Diego, La Jolla, California

Brown, Michael S., M.D., D.Sc.(Hon.) Paul J. Thomas Professor of Genetics and Medicine, University of Texas Southwestern Medical Center, Dallas, Texas

Broze, George J., Jr., M.D. Associate Professor of Medicine, Washington University School of Medicine, St. Louis, Missouri

Brunton, Laurence L., Ph.D. Associate Professor of Pharmacology and Medicine, University of California, San Diego, School of Medicine, La Jolla, California

Calabresi, Paul, M.D. Professor and Chairman of Medicine, Brown University; Physician-in-Chief, Roger Williams General Hospital, Providence, Rhode Island

Campbell, William B., Ph.D. Professor of Pharmacology, University of Texas Southwestern Medical Center, Dallas, Texas

Cedarbaum, Jesse M., M.D. Program Director, Clinical Research, Regeneron Pharmaceuticals, Inc., Tarrytown, New York; Clinical Associate Professor of Neurology, Cornell University Medical College, New York, New York

Chabner, Bruce A., M.D. Director, Division of Cancer Treatment, National Cancer Institute, National Institutes of Health, Bethesda, Maryland

Chren, Mary-Margaret, M.D. Senior Instructor of Dermatology, Case Western Reserve University School of Medicine, University Hospitals of Cleveland, Cleveland, Ohio

Coulston, Ann M., M.S., R.D. Research Dietitian, Stanford University Hospital; Lecturer, Department of Medicine, Stanford University School of Medicine, Stanford, California

Douglas, R. Gordon, Jr., M.D. Senior Vice President, Medical and Scientific Affairs, Merck Sharp and Dohme International, Rahway, New Jersey; Clinical Professor of Medicine, Cornell University Medical College, New York, New York

Eckenhoff, Roderic G., M.D. Assistant Professor of Anesthesia, University of Pennsylvania School of Medicine, Philadelphia, Pennsylvania

Garrison, James C., Ph.D. Professor of Pharmacology, University of Virginia School of Medicine, Charlottesville, Virginia

Gerber, John G., M.D. Professor of Medicine and Pharmacology, University of Colorado School of Medicine, Denver, Colorado

Goldstein, Joseph L., M.D., D.Sc.(Hon.) Paul J. Thomas Professor and Chairman, Department of Molecular Genetics, University of Texas Southwestern Medical Center, Dallas, Texas

Greene, Nicholas M., M.D. Professor Emeritus of Anesthesiology, Yale University School of Medicine, New Haven, Connecticut

Handschumacher, Robert E., Ph.D. Professor of Pharmacology, Yale University School of Medicine, New Haven, Connecticut

Haynes, Robert C., M.D., Ph.D. Professor of Pharmacology, University of Virginia School of Medicine, Charlottesville, Virginia

Hays, Richard M., M.D. Professor of Medicine, Albert Einstein College of Medicine of Yeshiva University, Bronx, New York

Hillman, Robert S., M.D. Professor of Medicine, University of Vermont College of Medicine, Burlington, Vermont; Chief of Medicine, Maine Medical Center, Portland, Maine

Hoffman, Brian B., M.D. Associate Professor of Medicine, Stanford University School of Medicine and Veterans Administration Medical Center, Palo Alto, California

Hoffman, Brian F., M.D. David Hosack Professor of Pharmacology, Columbia University College of Physicians and Surgeons, New York, New York

Insel, Paul A., M.D. Professor of Pharmacology and Medicine, University of California, San Diego, La Jolla, California

Jaffe, Jerome H., M.D. Clinical Professor of Psychiatry, University of Connecticut School of Medicine, Farmington, Connecticut

Kahn, C. Ronald, M.D. Research Director, Joslin Diabetes Center, Harvard Medical School, Boston, Massachusetts

Kapusnik-Uner, Joan E., Pharm. D. Assistant Clinical Professor, Division of Clinical Pharmacy, School of Pharmacy, University of California, San Francisco, California

Kennedy, Sean K., M.D. Associate Professor of Anesthesia, University of Pennsylvania School of Medicine, Philadelphia, Pennsylvania

Klaassen, Curtis D., Ph.D. Professor of Pharmacology and Toxicology, University of Kansas Medical Center, Kansas City, Kansas

Kuret, Jeffrey A., Ph.D. Senior Staff Investigator, Cold Spring Harbor Laboratory, Cold Spring Harbor, New York

Lefkowitz, Robert J., M.D. Investigator, Howard Hughes Medical Institute, James B. Duke Professor of Medicine and Professor of Biochemistry, Duke University Medical Center, Durham, North Carolina

Longnecker, David E., M.D. Robert Dunning Dripps Professor and Chairman, Department of Anesthesia, University of Pennsylvania School of Medicine, Philadelphia, Pennsylvania

Majerus, Philip W., M.D. Professor of Medicine and Biochemistry, Washington University School of Medicine, St. Louis, Missouri

Mandell, Gerald L., M.D. Professor of Medicine, and Head, Division of Infectious Diseases and Owen R. Cheatham Professor of Sciences, University of Virginia School of Medicine, Charlottesville, Virginia

Marcus, Robert, M.D. Director, Aging Study Unit, Geriatrics Research, Education and Clinical Center, Veterans Administration Medical Center, Palo Alto, California; Professor of Medicine, Stanford University School of Medicine, Stanford, California

Marshall, Bryan E., M.D., F.R.C.P. Horatio C. Wood Professor of Anesthesia, University of Pennsylvania School of Medicine, Philadelphia, Pennsylvania

Martin, William R., M.D. Professor and Chairman of Pharmacology, University of Kentucky College of Medicine, Lexington, Kentucky

Miletich, Joseph P., M.D., Ph.D. Associate Professor of Medicine and Biochemistry, Washington University School of Medicine, St. Louis, Missouri

Mitchell, Jerry R., M.D., Ph.D. President, Upjohn Laboratories, Kalamazoo, Michigan

Mudge, Gilbert H., M.D. Emeritus Professor of Pharmacology and Medicine, Dartmouth Medical School, Hanover, New Hampshire

Murad, Ferid, M.D., Ph.D. Vice President for Research and Development, Pharmaceutical Products, Abbott Laboratories, Abbott Park, Illinois; Professor, Department of Pharmacology, Northwestern University School of Medicine, Chicago, Illinois

Nies, Alan S., M.D. Professor of Medicine and Pharmacology, and Head, Division of Clinical Pharmacology, University of Colorado School of Medicine, Denver, Colorado

Peach, Michael J., Ph.D. Professor of Pharmacology, University of Virginia School of Medicine, Charlottesville, Virginia

Rall, Theodore W., Ph.D., D.Med.(Hon.) Professor of Pharmacology, University of Virginia School of Medicine, Charlottesville, Virginia

Ritchie, J. Murdoch, Ph.D., D.Sc., F.R.S. Eugene Higgins Professor of Pharmacology, Yale University School of Medicine, New Haven, Connecticut

Ross, Elliott M., Ph.D. Professor of Pharmacology, University of Texas Southwestern Medical Center, Dallas, Texas

Sande, Merle A., M.D. Professor and Vice-Chairman, Department of Medicine, University of California, San Francisco School of Medicine; Chief, Medical Service, San Francisco General Hospital, San Francisco, California

Schleifer, Leonard S., M.D., Ph.D. President, Regeneron Pharmaceuticals, Inc., Tarrytown, New York; Clinical Assistant Professor of Neurology, Cornell University Medical College, New York, New York

Shechter, Yoram, Ph.D. Associate Professor, Department of Hormone Research, The Weizmann Institute of Science, Rehovot, Israel

Sheiner, Lewis B., M.D. Professor of Laboratory Medicine, Medicine, and Pharmacy, Schools of Medicine and Pharmacy, University of California, San Francisco, California

Taylor, Palmer, Ph.D. Professor and Chairman, Department of Pharmacology, University of California, San Diego, La Jolla, California

Tollefsen, Douglas M., M.D., Ph.D. Associate Professor of Medicine and Biochemistry, Washington University School of Medicine, St. Louis, Missouri

Webster, Leslie T., Jr., M.D., Sc.D.(Hon.) John H. Hord Professor and Chairman of Pharmacology and Professor of Medicine, Case Western Reserve University School of Medicine, Cleveland, Ohio

Weiner, Irwin M., M.D. Professor of Pharmacology, State University of New York, Upstate Medical Center, Syracuse, New York

Williams, Roger L., M.D. Associate Professor of Medicine and Pharmacy, Schools of Medicine and Pharmacy, University of California, San Francisco, California

Wilson, Jean D., M.D. Professor of Internal Medicine, University of Texas Southwestern Medical Center, Dallas, Texas

CONTENTS

SECTION
III

Drugs Acting on the Central Nervous System

SECTION
IV

Autacoids; Drug Therapy of Inflammation

SECTION
V

Water, Salts, and Ions

SECTION
VI

Drugs Affecting Renal Function and Electrolyte Metabolism

SECTION
VII

Cardiovascular Drugs

SECTION
VIII

Drugs Affecting Gastrointestinal Function

SECTION
IX

Drugs Affecting Uterine Motility

SECTION
X

Chemotherapy of Parasitic Infections

SECTION
XI

Chemotherapy of Microbial Diseases

SECTION
XII

Chemotherapy of Neoplastic Diseases

SECTION
XIII

Drugs Used for Immunosuppression

SECTION
XIV

Drugs Acting on the Blood and the Blood-Forming Organs

SECTION
XV

Hormones and Hormone Antagonists

GOODMAN and GILMAN's

The Pharmacological Basis of Therapeutics

SECTION

I

General Principles

INTRODUCTION

Leslie Z. Benet, Jerry R. Mitchell, and Lewis B. Sheiner

In its entirety, *pharmacology* embraces the knowledge of the history, source, physical and chemical properties, compounding, biochemical and physiological effects, mechanisms of action, absorption, distribution, biotransformation and excretion, and therapeutic and other uses of drugs. Since a *drug* is broadly defined as any chemical agent that affects processes of living, the subject of pharmacology is obviously quite extensive.

For the clinician and the student of health sciences, however, the scope of pharmacology is less expansive than indicated by the above definitions. The clinician is interested primarily in drugs that are useful in the prevention, diagnosis, and treatment of human disease. Study of the pharmacology of these drugs can be reasonably limited to aspects that provide the basis for their rational clinical use. Secondarily, the clinician is also concerned with chemical agents that are not used in therapy but are commonly responsible for household and industrial poisoning as well as environmental pollution. Study of these substances is justifiably restricted to the general principles of prevention, recognition, and treatment of such toxicity or pollution. Finally, all health professionals share in the responsibility to help resolve the continuing sociological problem of the abuse of drugs.

The basic pharmacological concepts summarized in this section apply to the characterization, evaluation, and comparison of all drugs. A clear understanding and appreciation of these principles is essential for the subsequent study of the individual drugs. The relationship between the dose of a drug given to a patient and the utility of that drug in treating the patient's disease is described by two basic areas of pharmacology: *pharmacokinetics* and *pharmacodynamics*. Operationally, these terms may be defined as what the body does to the drug (pharmacokinetics) and what the drug does to the body (pharmacodynamics).

Pharmacokinetics (Chapter 1) deals with the *absorption, distribution, biotransformation,* and *excretion* of drugs. These factors, coupled with dosage, determine the concentration of a drug at its sites of action and, hence, the intensity of its effects as a function of time. Many basic principles of biochemistry and enzymology and the physical and chemical principles that govern the active and passive transfer and the distribution of substances across biological membranes are readily applied to the understanding of this important aspect of pharmacology.

The study of the biochemical and physiological *effects* of drugs and their *mechanisms of action* is termed *pharmacodynamics* (Chapter 2). As a border science, pharmacodynamics borrows freely from both the subject matter and the experimental techniques of physiology, biochemistry, cellular and molecular biology, microbiology, immunology, genetics, and pathology. It is unique mainly in that attention is focused on the characteristics of drugs. As the name implies, the subject is a dynamic one. The student who attempts merely to memorize the pharmacodynamic properties of drugs is forgoing one of the best opportunities for correlating the entire field of preclinical medicine. For example, the actions and effects of the saluretic agents can be fully understood only in terms of the basic principles of renal physiology and of the pathogenesis of edema. Conversely, great insight into normal and abnormal renal physiology can be gained by the study of the pharmacokinetics and pharmacodynamics of the saluretic agents.

The clinician is understandably interested mainly in the effects of drugs in man. This emphasis on *clinical pharmacology* is justified, since the effects of drugs are often characterized by significant interspecies variation, and since they may be further modified by disease. In addition, some drug effects, such as those on mood and behavior, can be adequately studied only in man. However, technical, legal, and ethical considerations limit pharmacological evaluation in man, and the choice of drugs must be based in part on their pharmacological evaluation in animals. Consequently, some knowledge of animal pharmacology and comparative pharmacology is helpful in deciding the extent to which claims for a drug based upon studies in animals can be reasonably extrapolated to man.

Toxicology (Chapter 3) is the aspect of pharmacology that deals with the adverse effects of drugs. It is concerned not only with drugs used in therapy but also with the many other chemicals that may be responsible for household, environmental, or industrial intoxication. The adverse effects of the pharmacological agents employed in therapy are properly considered an integral part of their total pharmacology. The toxic effects of other chemicals is such an extensive subject that the clinician must usually confine his attention to the general principles applicable to the prevention, recognition, and treatment of drug poisonings of any cause.

Pharmacotherapeutics (Chapter 4) deals with the use of drugs in the prevention and treatment of disease. Many drugs stimulate or depress biochemical or physiological function in man in a sufficiently reproducible manner to provide relief of symptoms or, ideally, to alter favorably the course of disease. Conversely, chemotherapeutic agents are useful in therapy because they have only minimal effects on man but can destroy or eliminate pathogenic cells or organisms.

Whether a drug is useful for therapy is crucially dependent upon its ability to produce its desired effects only with tolerable undesired effects. Thus, from the standpoint of the clinician interested in the therapeutic uses of a drug, the selectivity of its effects is one of its most important characteristics. Drug therapy is rationally based upon the correlation of the actions and effects of drugs with the physiological, biochemical, microbiological, immunological, and behavioral aspects of disease. In addition, disease may modify the pharmacokinetic properties of a drug by alteration of its absorption into the systemic circulation and/or its disposition.

CHAPTER

1 PHARMACOKINETICS: THE DYNAMICS OF DRUG ABSORPTION, DISTRIBUTION, AND ELIMINATION

Leslie Z. Benet, Jerry R. Mitchell, and Lewis B. Sheiner

To produce its characteristic effects, a drug must be present in appropriate concentrations at its sites of action. Although obviously a function of the amount of drug administered, the concentrations attained also depend upon the extent and rate of its absorption, distribution, binding or localization in tissues, biotransformation, and excretion. These factors are depicted in Figure 1–1.

PHYSICOCHEMICAL FACTORS IN TRANSFER OF DRUGS ACROSS MEMBRANES

The absorption, distribution, biotransformation, and excretion of a drug all involve its passage across cell membranes. It is essential, therefore, to consider the mechanisms by which drugs cross membranes and the physicochemical properties of molecules and membranes that influence this transfer. Important characteristics of a drug are its molecular size and shape, solubility at the site of its absorption, degree of ionization, and relative lipid solubility of its ionized and nonionized forms.

When a drug permeates a cell, it must obviously traverse the cellular plasma membrane. Other barriers to drug movement may be a single layer of cells (intestinal epithelium) or several layers of cells (skin). Despite these structural differences, the diffusion and transport of drugs across these various boundaries have many common characteristics, since drugs in general pass through cells rather than between

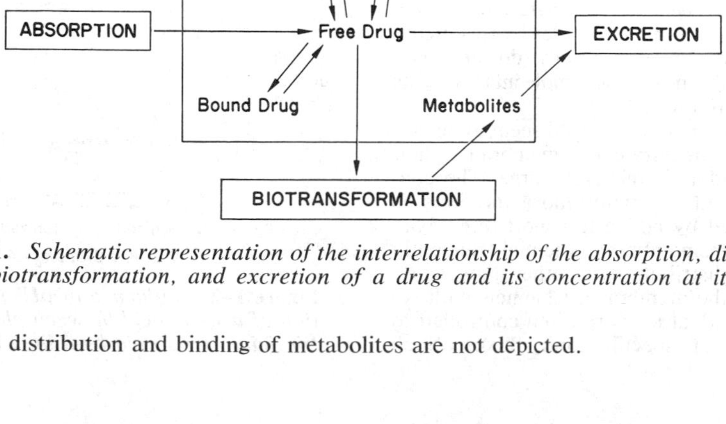

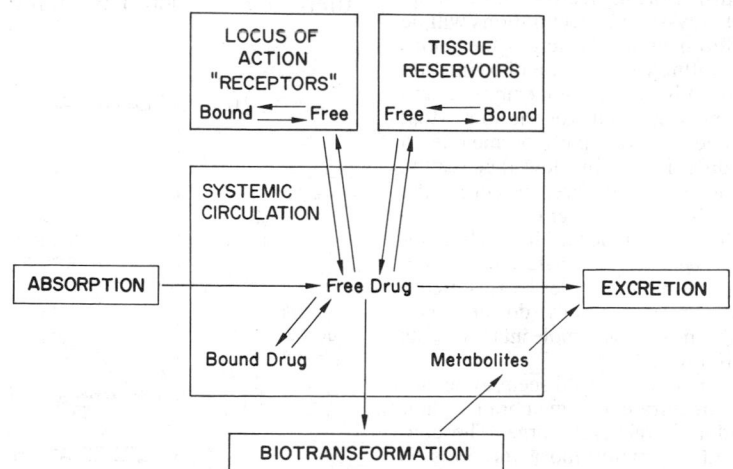

Figure 1–1. *Schematic representation of the interrelationship of the absorption, distribution, binding, biotransformation, and excretion of a drug and its concentration at its locus of action.*

Possible distribution and binding of metabolites are not depicted.

them. The plasma membrane thus represents the common barrier.

Cell Membranes. Initially, cell membranes were hypothesized to consist of a thin layer of lipid-like material interspersed with minute water-filled channels. Subsequent studies suggested that the plasma membrane consisted of a bilayer of amphipathic lipids, with their hydrocarbon chains oriented inward to form a continuous hydrophobic phase and their hydrophilic heads oriented outward. This hypothesis has been broadened to a more dynamic fluid-mosaic model, where globular protein molecules penetrate into either side of or entirely through a fluid phospholipid bilayer (Singer and Nicolson, 1972). Individual lipid molecules in the bilayer can move laterally, endowing the membrane with fluidity, flexibility, high electrical resistance, and relative impermeability to highly polar molecules. However, it is also appreciated that complexes of intrinsic membrane proteins and lipids can form either hydrophilic or hydrophobic channels that allow transport of molecules with different characteristics.

Passive Processes. Drugs cross membranes either by passive processes or by mechanisms involving the active participation of components of the membrane. In the former, the drug molecule usually penetrates by passive diffusion along a concentration gradient by virtue of its solubility in the lipid bilayer. Such transfer is directly proportional to the magnitude of the concentration gradient across the membrane and the lipid:water partition coefficient of the drug. The greater the partition coefficient, the higher is the concentration of drug in the membrane and the faster is its diffusion. After a steady state is attained, the concentration of the free drug is the same on both sides of the membrane, if the drug is a nonelectrolyte. For ionic compounds, the steady-state concentrations will be dependent on differences in pH across the membrane, which may influence the state of ionization of the molecule on each side of the membrane, and on the electrochemical gradient for the ion. Most biological membranes are relatively permeable to water, either by diffusion or by flow that results from hydrostatic or osmotic differences across the membrane. Such bulk flow of water can carry with it small, water-soluble substances. Most cell membranes permit passage only of water, urea, and other small, water-soluble molecules by this mechanism. Such substances generally do not pass through cell membranes if their molecular weights are greater than 100 to 200.

While most inorganic ions would seem to be sufficiently small to penetrate the membrane, their hydrated ionic radius is relatively large. The concentration gradient of many inorganic ions is largely determined by active transport (*e.g.*, Na^+ and K^+). The transmembrane potential frequently determines the distribution of other ions (*e.g.*, chloride) across the membrane. Channels with selectivity for individual ions are often controlled to allow regulation of specific ionic fluxes. Such mechanisms are of obvious importance in the generation of action potentials in nerve and muscle (*see* Chapter 5) and in transmembrane signaling events (*see* Chapter 2).

Weak Electrolytes and Influence of pH. Most drugs are weak acids or bases that are present in solution as both the nonionized and ionized species. The nonionized molecules are usually lipid soluble and can diffuse across the cell membrane. In contrast, the ionized molecules are usually unable to penetrate the lipid membrane because of their low lipid solubility.

Therefore, the transmembrane distribution of a weak electrolyte is usually determined by its pK_a and the pH gradient across the membrane. To illustrate the effect of pH on distribution of drugs, the partitioning of a weak acid ($pK_a = 4.4$) between plasma (pH = 7.4) and gastric juice (pH = 1.4) is depicted in Figure 1–2. It is assumed that the gastric mucosal membrane behaves as a simple lipid barrier that is permeable only to the lipid-soluble, nonionized form of the acid. The ratio of nonionized to ionized drug at each pH is easily calculated from the Henderson–Hasselbalch equation. Thus, in plasma, the ratio of nonionized to ionized drug is 1:1000; in gastric juice, the ratio is 1:0.001. These values are given in brackets in Figure 1–2. The total concentration ratio between the plasma and the gastric juice would therefore be 1000:1 if such a system came

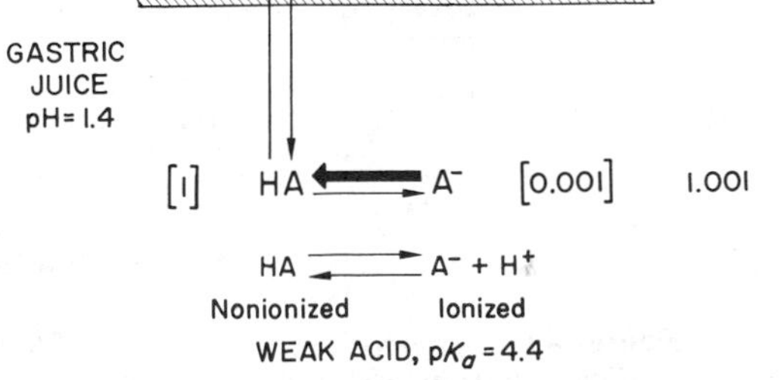

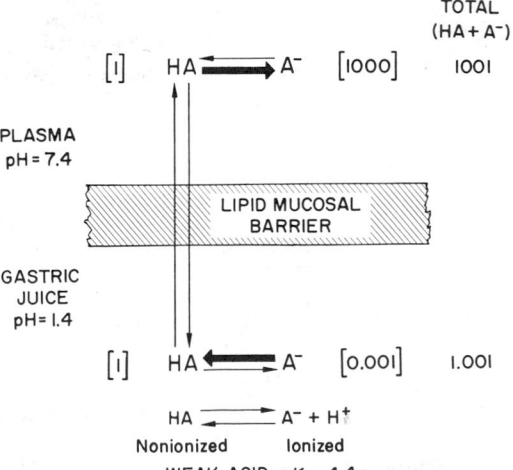

Figure 1–2. *Influence of pH on the distribution of a weak acid between plasma and gastric juice, separated by a lipid barrier.*

to a steady state. For a weak base with a pK_a of 4.4 ($BH^+ \rightleftharpoons B + H^+$), the ratio would be reversed, as would the thick horizontal arrows in Figure 1–2, which indicate the predominant species at each pH. These considerations have obvious implications for the absorption and excretion of drugs, as will be discussed more specifically below. The establishment of concentration gradients of weak electrolytes across membranes with a pH gradient is a purely physical process and does not require an active transport system. All that is necessary is a membrane preferentially permeable to one form of the weak electrolyte and a pH gradient across the membrane. The establishment of the pH gradient is, however, an active process.

Bulk flow through intercellular pores is the major mechanism of passage of drugs across most capillary endothelial membranes, with the important exception of the central nervous system (CNS) (*see* below). These intercellular gaps are sufficiently large that diffusion across most capillaries is limited by blood flow and not by the lipid solubility of drugs or pH gradients. This is an important factor in filtration across glomerular membranes in the kidney (*see* below). Tight junctions are characteristic of capillaries of the CNS and a variety of epithelia. Intercellular diffusion is consequently limited. Pinocytosis, the formation and movement of vesicles across cell membranes, has been implicated in drug absorption. However, the quantitative significance of pinocytosis is questionable.

Carrier-Mediated Membrane Transport. While passive diffusion through the bilayer is dominant in the absorption and distribution of most drugs, more active and selective mechanisms can play important roles. Active transport of some drugs occurs across neuronal membranes, the choroid plexus, renal tubular cells, and hepatocytes. The characteristics of active transport—selectivity, competitive inhibition by congeners, a requirement for energy, saturability, and movement against an electrochemical gradient—may be important in the mechanism of action of drugs that are subject to active transport or that interfere with the active transport of natural metabolites or neurotransmitters. The term *facilitated diffusion* describes a carrier-mediated transport process to which there is no input of energy, and movement of the substance in question thus cannot occur against an electrochemical gradient. Such mechanisms, which may also be highly selective for specific conformational structures of drugs, are necessary for the transport of endogenous compounds whose rate of movement across biological membranes by simple diffusion would otherwise be too slow.

DRUG ABSORPTION, BIOAVAILABILITY, AND ROUTES OF ADMINISTRATION

Absorption describes the rate at which a drug leaves its site of administration and the extent to which this occurs. However, the clinician is primarily concerned with a parameter designated as *bioavailability,* rather than absorption. Bioavailability is a term used to indicate the extent to which a drug reaches its site of action *or* a biological fluid from which the drug has access to its site of action. For example, a drug that is absorbed from the stomach and intestine must first pass through the liver before it reaches the systemic circulation. If the drug is metabolized in the liver or excreted in the bile, some of the active drug will be inactivated or diverted before it can reach the general circulation and be distributed to its sites of action. If the metabolic or excretory capacity of the liver for the agent in question is great, bioavailability will be substantially decreased (the so-called first-pass effect). This decrease in availability is a function of the anatomical site from which absorption takes place; other anatomical, physiological, and pathological factors can influence bioavailability (*see* below), and the choice of the route of drug administration must be based on an understanding of these conditions. Moreover, factors that modify the absorption of a drug can change its bioavailability.

Factors That Modify Absorption. Many variables, in addition to the physicochemical factors that affect transport across membranes, influence the absorption of drugs. Absorption, regardless of the site, is dependent upon drug solubility. Drugs given in aqueous solution are more rapidly absorbed than those given in oily solution, suspension, or solid form because they mix more readily with the aqueous phase at the absorptive site. For those given in solid form, the rate of dissolution may be the limiting factor in their absorption. Local conditions at the site of absorption alter solubility, particularly in the gastrointestinal tract. Aspirin, which is relatively insoluble in acidic gastric contents, is a common example of such a drug. The concentration of a drug influences its rate of absorption. Drugs ingested or injected in solutions of high concentration are absorbed more rapidly than are drugs in solutions of low concentration. The circulation to the site of absorption also affects drug absorption. Increased blood flow, brought about by massage or local application of heat, enhances the rate of drug absorption; decreased blood flow, produced by vasoconstrictor agents, shock, or other disease factors, can slow absorption. The area of the absorbing surface to which a drug is exposed is one of the more important determinants of the rate of drug absorption. Drugs are absorbed very rapidly from large surface areas such as the pulmonary alveolar epithelium, the intestinal mucosa, or, in a few cases after extensive application, the skin. The absorbing surface is determined largely by the route of administration. Each of these factors separately or in conjunction with one another may have profound effects on the efficacy and toxicity of a drug.

Enteral (Oral) vs. Parenteral Administration. Often there is a choice of the route by which a therapeutic agent may be given, and a knowledge of the advantages and disadvantages of the different routes of administration is then of primary importance. Some characteristics of the major routes employed for systemic drug effect are compared in Table 1–1.

Oral ingestion is the most common method of drug administration. It is also the safest, most convenient, and most economical. Disadvantages to the oral route include the incapability to absorb some drugs because of their physical characteristics (*e.g.*, polarity), emesis as a result of irritation to the gastrointestinal mucosa, destruction of some drugs by digestive enzymes or low gastric pH, irregularities in absorption or propulsion in the presence of food or other drugs, and necessity for cooperation on the part of the patient. In addition, drugs in the gastrointestinal tract may be metabolized by the enzymes of the mu-

Table 1–1. SOME CHARACTERISTICS OF COMMON ROUTES OF DRUG ADMINISTRATION *

ROUTE	ABSORPTION PATTERN	SPECIAL UTILITY	LIMITATIONS AND PRECAUTIONS
Intravenous	Absorption circumvented Potentially immediate effects	Valuable for emergency use Permits titration of dosage Suitable for large volumes and for irritating substances, when diluted	Increased risk of adverse effects Must inject solutions *slowly*, as a rule Not suitable for oily solutions or insoluble substances
Subcutaneous	Prompt, from aqueous solution Slow and sustained, from repository preparations	Suitable for some insoluble suspensions and for implantation of solid pellets	Not suitable for large volumes Possible pain or necrosis from irritating substances
Intramuscular	Prompt, from aqueous solution Slow and sustained, from repository preparations	Suitable for moderate volumes, oily vehicles, and some irritating substances	Precluded during anticoagulant medication May interfere with interpretation of certain diagnostic tests (*e.g.*, creatine kinase)
Oral ingestion	Variable; depends upon many factors (*see* text)	Most convenient and economical; usually more safe	Requires patient cooperation Availability potentially erratic and incomplete for drugs that are poorly soluble, slowly absorbed, unstable, or extensively metabolized by the liver

* *See* text for more complete discussion and for other routes.

cosa, the intestinal flora, or the liver before they gain access to the general circulation.

The parenteral injection of drugs has certain distinct advantages over oral administration. In some instances, parenteral administration is essential for the drug to be absorbed in active form. Availability is usually more rapid and more predictable than when a drug is given by mouth. The effective dose can therefore be more accurately selected. In emergency therapy, parenteral administration is particularly serviceable. If a patient is unconscious, uncooperative, or unable to retain anything given by mouth, parenteral therapy may be a necessity. The injection of drugs also has its disadvantages. Asepsis must be maintained, an intravascular injection may occur when it is not intended, pain may accompany the injection, and it is sometimes difficult for a patient to perform the injection himself if self-medication is necessary. Expense is another consideration.

Oral Ingestion. Absorption from the gastrointestinal tract is governed by factors that are generally applicable, such as surface area for absorption, blood flow to the site of absorption, the physical state of the drug, and its concentration at the site of absorption. Since most drug absorption from the gastrointestinal tract occurs via passive processes, absorption is favored when the drug is in the nonionized and more lipophilic form. Thus, one might expect the absorption of weak acids to be optimal in the acidic environment of the stomach, whereas absorption of bases might be favored in the relatively alkaline small intestine. However, it is an oversimplification to extrapolate the pH-partition concept presented in Figure 1–2 to a comparison of two different biological membranes, such as the epithelia of the stomach and the intestine. The stomach is lined by a thick, mucus-covered membrane with a small surface area and high electrical resistance. The primary function of the stomach is digestive. In contrast, the epithelium of the intestine has an extremely large surface area; it is thin, it has low electrical resistance, and its primary function is to facilitate the absorption of nutrients. Thus, any factor that accelerates gastric emptying will be likely to increase the rate of drug absorption, while any factor that delays gastric emptying will probably have the opposite effect, regardless of the characteristics of the drug. The experimental data available from the classical work of Brodie (1964) and more recent studies (Prescott and Nimmo, 1981) are all consistent with the following conclusion: the nonionized form of a drug will be absorbed more rapidly than the ionized form at any particular site in the gastrointestinal tract. However, the rate of absorption of a drug from the intestine will be greater than that from the stomach even if the drug is predominantly ionized in the intestine and largely nonionized in the stomach.

Drugs that are destroyed by gastric juice or that cause gastric irritation are sometimes administered in dosage forms with a coating that prevents dissolution in the acidic gastric contents. However, some enteric-coated preparations of a drug also may resist dissolution in the intestine, and very little of the drug may be absorbed.

Controlled-Release Preparations. The rate of absorption of a drug administered as a tablet or other solid oral-dosage form is partly dependent upon its rate of dissolution in the gastrointestinal fluids. This factor is the basis for the so-called controlled-release, timed-release, sustained-release, or prolonged-action pharmaceutical preparations that are designed to produce slow, uniform absorption of the drug for 8 hours or longer. Potential advantages of such preparations are reduction in the frequency of administration of the drug as compared with conventional dosage forms (possibly with improved compliance by the patient), maintenance of a therapeutic effect overnight, and decreased incidence and/or intensity of undesired effects by elimination of the peaks in drug concentration that often occur after administration of immediate-release dosage forms.

Many controlled-release preparations fulfill these theoretical expectations. However, the clinician must be aware of some drawbacks of these products. Generally, interpatient variability in terms of the systemic concentration of the drug that is achieved is greater for controlled-release as compared with immediate-release dosage forms. During repeated drug administration, trough drug concentrations resulting from controlled-release dosage forms may not be different from those observed with immediate-release preparations, although the time interval between trough concentrations is greater for a well-designed controlled-release product. It is possible that the dosage form may fail, and "dose-dumping" with resultant toxicity can occur, since the total dose of drug ingested at one time may be several times the amount contained in the conventional preparation. Controlled-release dosage forms are most appropriate for drugs with short half-lives (less than 4 hours). So-called controlled-release dosage forms are sometimes developed for drugs with long half-lives (greater than 12 hours). These usually more expensive products should not be prescribed unless specific advantages have been demonstrated.

Sublingual Administration. Absorption from the oral mucosa has special significance for certain drugs, despite the fact that the surface area available is small. For example, nitroglycerin is effective when retained sublingually because it is nonionic and has a very high lipid solubility. Thus, the drug is absorbed very rapidly. Nitroglycerin is also very potent; relatively few molecules need to be absorbed to produce the therapeutic effect. Since venous drainage from the mouth is to the superior vena cava, the drug is also protected from rapid first-pass metabolism by the liver. Hepatic first-pass metabolism is sufficient to prevent the appearance of any active nitroglycerin in the systemic circulation if the conventional tablet is swallowed.

Rectal Administration. The rectal route is often useful when oral ingestion is precluded by vomiting or when the patient is unconscious. Approximately 50% of the drug that is absorbed from the rectum will bypass the liver; the potential for hepatic first-pass metabolism is thus less than that for an oral dose. However, rectal absorption is often irregular and incomplete, and many drugs cause irritation of the rectal mucosa.

Parenteral Injection. The major routes of parenteral administration are intravenous, subcutaneous, and intramuscular. Absorption from subcutaneous and intramuscular sites occurs by simple diffusion along the gradient from drug depot to plasma. The rate is limited by the area of the absorbing capillary membranes and by the solubility of the substance in the interstitial fluid. Relatively large aqueous channels in the endothelial membrane account for the indiscriminate diffusion of molecules regardless of their lipid solubility. Larger molecules, such as proteins, slowly gain access to the circulation by way of lymphatic channels.

Drugs administered into the systemic circulation by any route, excluding the intra-arterial, are subject to possible first-pass elimination in the lung prior to distribution to the rest of the body. The lungs serve as a temporary clearing site for a number of agents, especially drugs that are weak bases and are predominantly nonionized at the blood pH, apparently by their partition into lipid. The lungs also serve as a filter for particulate matter that may be given intravenously, and, of course, they provide a route of elimination for volatile substances.

Intravenous. The factors concerned in absorption are circumvented by intravenous injection of drugs in aqueous solution, and the desired concentration of a drug in blood is obtained with an accuracy and immediacy not possible by any other procedure. In some instances, as in the induction of surgical anesthesia by a barbiturate, the dose of a drug is not predetermined but is adjusted to the response of the patient. Also, certain irritating solutions can be given only in this manner, since the blood vessel walls are relatively insensitive and the drug, if injected slowly, is greatly diluted by the blood.

As there are assets to the use of this route of administration, so are there liabilities. Unfavorable reactions are likely to occur, since high concentrations of drug may be attained rapidly in both plasma and tissues. Once the drug is injected there is no retreat. Repeated intravenous injections are dependent upon the ability to maintain a patent vein. Drugs in an oily vehicle or those that precipitate blood constituents or hemolyze erythrocytes should not be given by this route. Intravenous injection must usually be performed slowly and with constant monitoring of the responses of the patient.

Subcutaneous. Injection of a drug into a subcutaneous site is often used. It can be used only for drugs that are not irritating to tissue; otherwise, severe pain, necrosis, and slough may occur. The rate of absorption following subcutaneous injection of a drug is often sufficiently constant and slow to provide a sustained effect. Moreover, it may be varied intentionally. For example, the rate of absorption of a suspension of insoluble insulin is slow compared with that of a soluble preparation of the hormone. The incorporation of a vasoconstrictor agent in a solution of a drug to be injected subcutaneously also retards absorption. Absorption of drugs implanted under the skin in a solid pellet form occurs slowly over a period of weeks or months; some hormones are effectively administered in this manner.

Intramuscular. Drugs in aqueous solution are absorbed quite rapidly after intramuscular injection, depending upon the rate of blood flow to the injection site. Joggers who inject insulin into their thigh may experience a precipitous drop in blood sugar that is not seen following injection into the arm or abdominal wall, since running markedly increases blood flow to the leg. Generally, the rate of absorption following injection of an aqueous preparation into the deltoid or vastus lateralis is faster than when the injection is made into the gluteus maximus. The rate is particularly slower for females after injection into the gluteus maximus. This has been attributed to the different distribution of subcutaneous fat in males and females, since fat is relatively poorly perfused. Very obese or emaciated patients may exhibit unusual patterns of absorption following intramuscular or subcutaneous injection. Very slow, constant absorption from the intramuscular site results if the drug is injected in solution in oil or suspended in various other repository vehicles. Penicillin is often administered in this manner. Substances too irritating to be injected subcutaneously may sometimes be given intramuscularly.

Intra-arterial. Occasionally a drug is injected directly into an artery to localize its effect in a particular tissue or organ. However, this practice usually has dubious therapeutic value. Diagnostic agents are sometimes administered by this route. Intra-arterial injection requires great care and should be reserved for experts. The first-pass and cleansing effects of the lung are not available when drugs are given by this route.

Intrathecal. The blood–brain barrier and the blood–cerebrospinal fluid barrier often preclude or slow the entrance of drugs into the CNS. Therefore, when local and rapid effects of drugs on the meninges or cerebrospinal axis are desired, as in spinal anesthesia or acute CNS infections, drugs are sometimes injected directly into the spinal subarachnoid space.

Intraperitoneal. The peritoneal cavity offers a large absorbing surface from which drugs enter the circulation rapidly, but primarily by way of the portal vein; first-pass hepatic losses are thus possible. Intraperitoneal injection is a common laboratory procedure, but it is seldom employed clinically. The dangers of producing infection and adhesions are too great to warrant the routine use of this route in man.

Pulmonary Absorption. Gaseous and volatile drugs may be inhaled and absorbed through the pulmonary epithelium and mucous membranes of the respiratory tract. Access to the circulation is rapid by this route, because the surface area is large. The principles governing absorption and excretion of the anesthetic gases and vapors are discussed in Chapter 13.

In addition, solutions of drugs can be atomized and the fine droplets in air (aerosol) inhaled. Advantages are the almost instantaneous absorption of a drug into the blood, avoidance of hepatic first-pass loss, and, in the case of pulmonary disease, local application of the drug at the desired site of action. For example, β-adrenergic agonists can be given in this manner for the treatment of bronchial asthma. The main disadvantages are poor ability to regulate the dose, cumbersomeness of the methods of administration, and the fact that many gaseous and volatile drugs produce irritation of the pulmonary epithelium.

Pulmonary absorption is an important route of entry of certain drugs of abuse and of toxic environmental substances of varied composition and physical states (*see* Section XVIII). Both local and systemic reactions to allergens may occur subsequent to inhalation.

Topical Application. *Mucous Membranes.* Drugs are applied to the mucous membranes of the conjunctiva, nasopharynx, oropharynx, vagina, colon, urethra, and urinary bladder primarily for their local effects. Occasionally, as in the application of antidiuretic hormone to the nasal mucosa, systemic absorption is the goal. Absorption through mucous membranes occurs readily. In fact, local anesthetics applied for local effect may sometimes be absorbed so rapidly that they produce systemic toxicity.

Skin. Few drugs readily penetrate the intact skin. Absorption of those that do is proportional to the surface area over which they are applied and to their lipid solubility, since the epidermis behaves as a lipid barrier. The dermis, however, is freely permeable to many solutes; consequently, systemic absorption of drugs occurs much more readily through abraded, burned, or denuded skin. Inflammation and other conditions that increase cutaneous blood flow also enhance absorption. Toxic effects are sometimes produced by absorption through the skin of highly lipid-soluble substances (*e.g.*, a lipid-soluble insecticide in an organic solvent). Absorption through the skin can be enhanced by suspending the drug in an oily vehicle and rubbing the resulting preparation into the skin. This method of administration is known as inunction. Because hydrated skin is more permeable than dry skin, the dosage form may be modified or an occlusive dressing may be used to facilitate absorption. Controlled-release topical patches are recent innovations. A patch containing scopolamine, placed behind the ear where body temperature and blood flow enhance absorption, releases sufficient drug to the systemic circulation to protect the wearer from motion sickness. Patches containing nitroglycerin are used to provide sustained delivery of a drug that is subject to extensive first-pass metabolism after oral administration (*see* Ridout *et al.*, 1988).

Eye. Topically applied ophthalmic drugs are used primarily for their local effects. Systemic absorption that results from drainage through the nasolacrimal canal is usually undesirable. In addition, drug that is absorbed after such drainage is not subject to first-pass hepatic elimination. Unwanted systemic pharmacological effects may occur for this reason when β-adrenergic antagonists are administered as ophthalmic drops. Local effects usually require absorption of the drug through the cornea; corneal infection or trauma may thus result in more rapid absorption. Ophthalmic delivery systems that provide prolonged duration of action (*e.g.*, suspensions and ointments) are useful additions to ophthalmic therapy. Ocular inserts, developed more recently, provide continuous delivery of low amounts of drug. Very little is lost through drainage; hence, systemic side effects are minimized.

Bioequivalence. Drug products are considered to be pharmaceutical equivalents if they contain the same active ingredients and are identical in strength or concentration, dosage form, and route of administration. Two pharmaceutically equivalent drug products are considered to be bioequivalent when the rates and extents of bioavailability of the active ingredient in the two products are not significantly different under suitable test conditions. In the past, dosage forms of a drug from different manufacturers and even different lots of preparations from a single manufacturer sometimes differed in their bioavailability. Such differences were seen primarily among oral dosage forms of poorly soluble, slowly absorbed drugs. They result from differences in crystal form, particle size, or other physical characteristics of the drug that are not rigidly controlled in formulation and manufacture of the preparations. These factors affect disintegration of the dosage form and dissolution of the drug and hence the rate and extent of drug absorption.

The potential nonequivalence of different drug preparations is a matter of concern. Strengthened regulatory requirements over the past few years have resulted in significantly fewer documented cases of nonequivalence between approved drug products. However, since equivalence of measured systemic concentrations of active drug and known metabolites is not necessarily proof of therapeutic equivalence, some clinicians prefer to maintain certain "fragile" patients on a single manufacturer's product. The significance of possible nonequivalence of drug preparations is further discussed in connection with drug nomenclature and the choice of drug name in writing prescription orders (*see* Appendix I).

DISTRIBUTION OF DRUGS

After a drug is absorbed or injected into the bloodstream, it may be distributed into interstitial and cellular fluids. Patterns of drug distribution reflect certain physiological factors and physicochemical properties of drugs. An initial phase of distribution may be distinguished that reflects cardiac output and regional blood flow. Heart, liver, kidney, brain, and other well perfused organs receive most of the drug during the first few minutes after absorption. Delivery of drug to muscle, most viscera, skin, and fat is slower, and these tissues may require several minutes to several hours before steady state is attained. A second phase of drug distribution may therefore be distinguished; this is also limited by blood flow, and it involves a far larger fraction of the body mass than does the first phase. Superimposed on patterns of distribution of blood flow are factors that determine the rate at which drugs diffuse into tissues. Diffusion into the interstitial compartment occurs rapidly because of the highly permeable nature of capillary endothelial membranes (except in the brain). Lipid-insoluble drugs that permeate membranes poorly are restricted in their distribution and hence in their potential sites of action. Distribution may also be limited by drug binding to plasma proteins, particularly albumin for acidic drugs and α_1-acid glycoprotein for basic drugs. An agent that is extensively and strongly bound has limited access to cellular sites of action, and it may be metabolized and eliminated slowly. Drugs may accumulate in tissues in higher concentrations than would be expected from diffusion equilibria as a result of pH gradients, binding to intracellular constituents, or partitioning into lipid.

Drug that has accumulated in a given tissue may serve as a reservoir that prolongs drug action in that same tissue or at a distant site reached through the circulation. An example that illustrates many of these factors is the use of the intravenous anesthetic thiopental, a highly lipid-soluble drug. Because blood flow to the brain is so high, the drug reaches its maximal concentration in brain within a minute after it is injected intravenously. After injection is concluded, the plasma concentration falls as thiopental diffuses into other tissues, such as muscle. The concentration of the drug in brain follows that of the plasma, because there is little binding of the drug to brain constituents. Thus, onset of anesthesia is rapid, but so is its termination. Both are directly related to the concentration of drug in the brain. A third phase of distribution for this drug is due to the slow, blood-flow–limited uptake by fat. With administration of successive doses of thiopental, accumulation of drug takes place in fat and other tissues that can store large amounts of the compound. These can become reservoirs for the maintenance of the plasma concentration, and, therefore the brain concentration, at or above the threshold required for anesthesia. Thus, a drug that is short acting because of rapid redistribution to sites at which the agent has no pharmacological action can become long acting when these storage sites are "filled" and termination of the drug's action becomes dependent on biotransformation and excretion (*see* Benet, 1978).

Since the difference in pH between intracellular and extracellular fluids is small (7.0 vs. 7.4), this factor can result in only a relatively small concentration gradient of drug across the plasma membrane. Weak bases are concentrated slightly inside of cells, while the concentration of weak acids is slightly lower in the cells than in extracellular fluids. Lowering the pH of extracellular fluid increases the intracellular concentration of weak acids and decreases that of weak bases, provided that the intracellular pH does not also change and that the pH change does not simultaneously affect the binding, biotransformation, or excretion of the drug. Elevating the pH produces the opposite effects (*see* Figure 1–2).

Central Nervous System and Cerebrospinal Fluid. The distribution of drugs to the CNS from the bloodstream is unique, mainly in that entry of drugs into the cerebrospinal fluid and extracellular space of the CNS is restricted. The restriction is similar to that across the gastrointestinal epithelium. Endothelial cells of the brain capillaries differ from their counterparts in most tissues by the absence of intercellular pores and pinocytotic vesicles. Tight junctions predominate, and aqueous bulk flow is thus severely restricted. This is not unique to the CNS capillaries (tight junctions appear in many muscle capillaries as well). It is likely that the unique arrangement of pericapillary glial cells also contributes to the slow diffusion of organic acids and bases into the CNS. The drug molecules probably must traverse not only endothelial but also perivascular cell membranes before reaching neurons or other target cells in the CNS. Cerebral blood flow is the only limitation to permeation of the CNS by highly lipid-soluble drugs. With increasing polarity the rate of diffusion of drugs into the CNS is proportional to the lipid solubility of the nonionized species. Strongly ionized agents such as quaternary amines are normally unable to enter the CNS from the circulation.

In addition, organic ions are extruded from the cerebrospinal fluid into blood at the choroid plexus by transport processes similar to those in the renal tubule. Lipid-soluble substances leave the brain by diffusion through the capillaries and the blood–choroid plexus boundary. Drugs and endogenous metabolites, regardless of lipid solubility and molecular size, also exit with bulk flow of the cerebrospinal fluid through the arachnoid villi.

The blood–brain barrier is adaptive in that exclusion of drugs and other foreign agents such as penicillin or tubocurarine protects the CNS against severely toxic effects. However, the barrier is neither absolute nor invariable. Very large doses of penicillin may produce seizures; meningeal or encephalic inflammation increases the local permeability. Maneuvers to increase permeability of the blood–brain barrier are potentially important to enhance the efficacy of chemotherapeutic agents that are used to treat infections or tumors localized in the brain.

Drug Reservoirs. As mentioned, the body compartments in which a drug accumulates are potential reservoirs for the drug. If stored drug is in equilibrium with that in plasma and is released as the plasma concentration declines, a concentration of the drug in plasma and at its locus of action is sustained, and pharmacological effects of the drug are prolonged. However, if the reservoir for the drug has a large capacity and fills rapidly, it so alters the distribution of the drug that larger quantities of the drug are required initially to provide a therapeutically effective concentration in the target organ.

Plasma Proteins. Many drugs are bound to plasma proteins, mostly to plasma albumin for acidic drugs and to α_1-acid glycoprotein for basic drugs; binding to other plasma proteins generally occurs to a much smaller extent. The binding is usually reversible; covalent binding of reactive drugs such as alkylating agents occurs occasionally.

The fraction of total drug in plasma that is bound is determined by the drug concentration, its affinity for the binding sites, and the number of binding sites. Simple mass-action equations are used to describe the free and bound concentrations (*see* Chapter 2). At low concentrations of drug (less than the plasma protein–binding dissociation constant), the fraction bound is a function of the concentration of binding sites and the dissociation constant. At high drug concentrations (greater than the dissociation constant), the fraction bound is a function of the number of binding sites and the drug concentration. Therefore, statements that a given drug is bound to a specified extent apply only over a limited range of concentrations. The percentage values listed in Appendix II refer only to the therapeutic range of concentrations for each drug.

Binding of a drug to plasma proteins limits its concentration in tissues and at its locus of action, since only unbound drug is in equilibrium across membranes. Binding also limits glomerular filtration of the drug, since this process does not immediately change the concentration of free drug in the plasma (water is also filtered). However, plasma protein binding does *not* generally limit renal tubular secretion or biotransformation, since these processes lower the free drug concentration, and this is rapidly followed by dissociation of the drug–protein complex. If a drug is avidly transported or metabolized and its clearance, calculated on the basis of unbound drug, exceeds organ plasma flow, binding of the drug to plasma protein may be viewed as a transport mechanism that fosters drug elimination by delivering drug to sites for elimination.

Since binding of drugs to plasma proteins is rather nonselective, many drugs with similar physicochemical characteristics can compete with each other and with endogenous substances for these binding sites. For example, displacement of unconjugated bilirubin from binding to albumin by the sulfonamides and other organic anions is known to increase the risk of bilirubin encephalopathy in the newborn, and drug toxicity has sometimes been attributed to similar competition between drugs for binding sites. Such interactions are often more complex than generally stated. Since drug displaced from plasma protein will redistribute into its full potential volume of distribution, the concentration of free drug in plasma and tissues after redistribution may be increased only slightly. The interaction may also involve altered elimination of the drug. Risk of adverse effect is greatest if the displaced drug has a limited volume of distribution, if the competition extends to the drug bound in tissues, if elimination of the drug is also reduced, or if the displacing drug is administered in high dosage by rapid intravenous injection. Competition of drugs for plasma protein-binding sites may also cause misinterpretation of measured concentrations of drugs in plasma, since most assays do not distinguish free from bound drug.

Cellular Reservoirs. Many drugs accumulate in muscle and other cells in higher concentrations than in the extracellular fluids. If the intracellular concentration is high and if the binding is reversible, the tissue involved may represent a sizable drug reservoir, particularly if the tissue represents a large fraction of body mass. For example, during long-term administration of the antimalarial agent quinacrine, the concentration of the drug in liver may be several thousand times that in plasma. Accumulation in cells may be the result of active transport or, more commonly, binding. Tissue binding of drugs usually occurs to proteins, phospholipids, or nucleoproteins and is generally reversible.

Fat as a Reservoir. Many lipid-soluble drugs are stored by physical solution in the neutral fat. In obese persons, the fat content of the body may be as high as 50%, and even in starvation it constitutes 10% of body weight; hence, fat can serve as an important reservoir for lipid-soluble drugs. For example, as much as 70% of the highly lipid-soluble barbiturate thiopental may be present in body fat 3 hours after administration. However, fat is a rather stable reservoir because it has a relatively low blood flow.

Bone. The tetracycline antibiotics (and other divalent-metal-ion chelating agents) and heavy metals may accumulate in bone by adsorption onto the bone-crystal surface and eventual incorporation into the crystal lattice. Bone can become a reservoir for the slow release of toxic agents such as lead or radium into the blood. Their effects can thus persist long after exposure has ceased. Local destruction of the bone medulla may also lead to reduced blood flow and prolongation of the reservoir effect, since the toxic agent becomes sealed off from the circulation; this may further enhance the direct local damage to the bone. A vicious cycle results whereby the greater the exposure to the toxic agent the slower is its rate of elimination.

Transcellular Reservoirs. Drugs also cross epithelial cells and may accumulate in the transcellular fluids. The major transcellular reservoir is the gastrointestinal tract. Weak bases are passively concentrated in the stomach from the blood, because of the large pH differential between the two fluids, and some drugs are secreted in the bile in an active form or as a conjugate that can be hydrolyzed in the intestine. In these cases, and when an orally administered drug is slowly absorbed, the gastrointestinal tract serves as a drug reservoir.

Other transcellular fluids, including cerebrospinal fluid, aqueous humor, endolymph, and joint fluids, do not generally accumulate significant total amounts of drugs.

Redistribution. Termination of drug effect is usually by biotransformation and excretion, but it may also result from redistribution of the drug from its site of action into other tissues or sites. Redistribution is a factor in terminating drug effect primarily when a highly lipid-soluble drug that acts on the brain or cardiovascular system is administered rapidly by intravenous injection or by inhalation. The factors involved in redistribution of drugs have been discussed above.

Placental Transfer of Drugs. The potential transfer of drugs across the placenta is important, since drugs may cause congenital anomalies. Administered immediately before delivery, they may also have adverse effects on the neonate. Drugs cross the placenta primarily by simple diffusion. Lipid-soluble, nonionized drugs readily enter the fetal blood from the maternal circulation. Penetration is least with drugs possessing a high degree of dissociation or low lipid solubility. The view that the placenta is a barrier to drugs is inaccurate. A more appropriate approximation is that the fetus is to at least some extent exposed to essentially all drugs taken by the mother.

BIOTRANSFORMATION OF DRUGS

The physicochemical properties of drug molecules that permit rapid passage across cellular membranes during absorption and distribution also impair subsequent excretion. For example, after filtration at the renal glomerulus most lipid-soluble drugs largely escape excretion from the body because they are readily reabsorbed from the filtrate by diffusion through the renal tubular cells. Thus, the enzymatic biotransformation of drugs to more polar and less lipid-soluble metabolites enhances their excretion and reduces their volume of distribution. Such biotransformation relieves the burden of foreign chemicals and is critical for the survival of the organism. Studies of the genes that encode the enzymes of biotransformation have led to the view that they evolved millions of years ago as a mechanism for removal of natural constituents of foods, such as flavones, terpenes, steroids, and alkaloids. (For excellent summaries of drug biotransformation, *see* Goldstein *et al.,* 1974; Lee *et al.,* 1977; Jacqz *et al.,* 1986; Nebert and Gonzalez, 1987.)

Enzymes Responsible for Biotransformation. The enzyme systems responsible for the biotransformation of many drugs are located in the smooth endoplasmic reticulum of the liver (operationally designated the microsomal fraction). These enzymes also are present in other organs, such as the kidney, lung, and gastrointestinal epithelium, although in smaller quantities. Drugs absorbed from the intestine may thus be subject to the first-pass effect. This represents the combined action of hepatic and gastrointestinal epithelial enzymes, which can at times prevent effective concentrations of active drug from reaching the systemic circulation after oral administration, as discussed above.

The chemical reactions of enzymatic biotransformation are classified as either phase-I or phase-II reactions. Phase-I reactions convert the parent drug to a more polar metabolite by oxidation, reduction, or hydrolysis. The resulting metabolite may be pharmacologically inactive, less active, or occasionally more active than the parent molecule. When the metabolite itself is the active drug, the parent compound is said to be a *prodrug* (*e.g.,* enalapril). Phase-II reactions, which are also called conjugation or synthetic reactions, involve coupling the drug or frequently its polar metabolite with an endogenous substrate, such as glucuronate, sulfate, acetate, or an amino acid.

Various biotransformations involving phase-I and phase-II reactions are illustrated schematically in Table 1–2. The ability of these systems to handle highly diverse chemical structures is noteworthy. Many reactions occur concurrently or consecutively, such that the parent drug is converted to several metabolites; phase-I metabolism followed by conjugation (phase-II) is particularly active in the liver, although the kidney, gastrointestinal tract, lung, and plasma also contribute.

Oxidation. The hepatic endoplasmic reticulum contains an important group of oxidative enzymes called *monooxygenases* that require both a reducing agent, nicotinamide adenine dinucleotide phosphate (NADPH), and molecular (atmospheric) oxygen. The biotransformations catalyzed by the monooxygenases include N- and

Table 1–2. DRUG BIOTRANSFORMATION RECTIONS

	EXAMPLE
I. *Oxidative Reactions*	
(1) N- and O-Dealkylation	
$RNHCH_3 \xrightarrow{[O]} [RNHCH_2OH] \longrightarrow RNH_2 + CH_2O$	Desipramine
$ROCH_3 \xrightarrow{[O]} [ROCH_2OH] \longrightarrow ROH + CH_2O$	Phenacetin
(2) Side-Chain (Aliphatic) and Aromatic Hydroxylation	
$RCH_2CH_3 \xrightarrow{[O]} RCH(OH)CH_3$	Phenobarbital
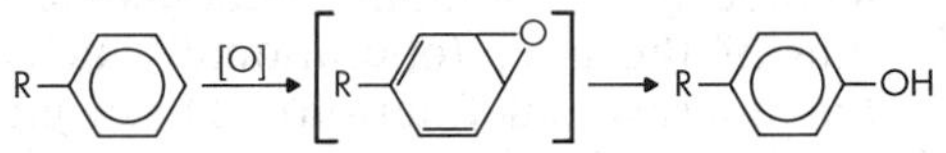	Phenytoin
(3) N-Oxidation	
$R_3N \xrightarrow[H^+]{[O]} [R_3N—OH]^+ \longrightarrow R_3N \rightarrow O + H^+$	Guanethidine
(4) Sulfoxide Formation	
$RSR' \xrightarrow[H^+]{[O]} [R—S(OH)—R']^+ \longrightarrow RS(=O)R' + H^+$	Chlorpromazine
(5) Deamination of Amines	
$R_2CHNH_2 \xrightarrow{[O]} [R_2C(OH)—NH_2] \longrightarrow R_2CO + NH_3$	Amphetamine
(6) Desulfuration	
$R_2CS \xrightarrow{[O]} R_2CO$	Thiobarbital
II. *Hydrolysis of Esters and Amides*	
$RC(=O)OR' \longrightarrow RCOOH + R'OH$	Procaine
$RC(=O)NR' \longrightarrow RCOOH + R'NH_2$	Lidocaine

Table 1–2. DRUG BIOTRANSFORMATION REACTIONS (Continued)

	EXAMPLE
III. *Reduction*	
(1) Azo Reduction	
$RN{=}NR' \longrightarrow RNH_2 + R'NH_2$	Prontosil
(2) Nitro Reduction	
$RNO_2 \longrightarrow RNH_2$	Chloramphenicol
IV. *Conjugation Reactions*	
(1) Glucuronidation (Ether and Ester)	
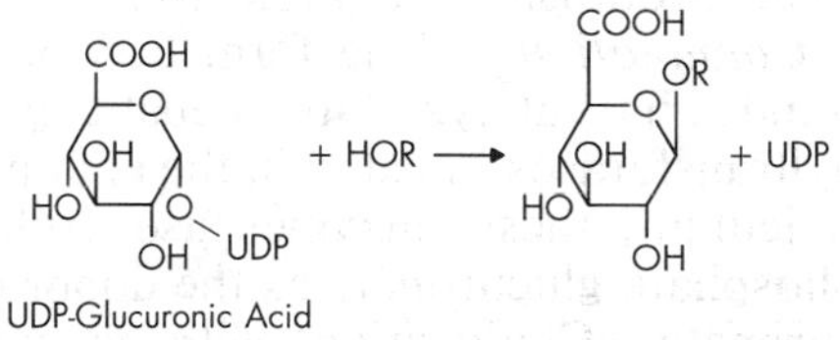	Acetaminophen
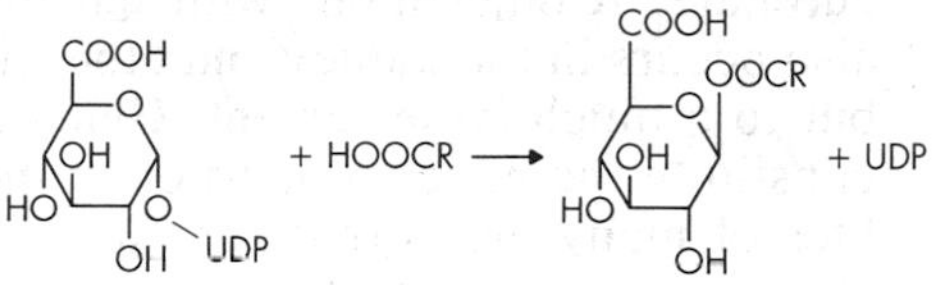	Naproxen
(2) Acetylation	
$RNH_2 + CH_3\overset{\overset{O}{\|}}{C}SCoA \longrightarrow RNH\overset{\overset{O}{\|}}{C}CH_3 + CoA{-}SH$ Acetyl CoA	Isoniazid
(3) Conjugation with Glycine	
$RCOOH \longrightarrow R\overset{\overset{O}{\|}}{C}SCoA + NH_2CH_2COOH \longrightarrow R\overset{\overset{O}{\|}}{C}NHCH_2COOH + CoA{-}SH$	Salicylic acid
(4) Conjugation with Sulfate	
ROH + 3′-phosphoadenosine 5′-phosphosulfate $\longrightarrow RO\underset{\underset{O}{\|}}{\overset{\overset{O}{\|}}{S}}OH$ + 3′-phosphoadenosine 5′-phosphate	Steroids
(5) O-, S-, and N-Methylation	
R—XH + S-adenosylmethionine $\longrightarrow$ R—X—CH_3 + S-adenosylhomocysteine (X = O, S, N)	Norepinephrine

O-dealkylation, aromatic ring and side chain hydroxylation, sulfoxide formation, N-oxidation, N-hydroxylation, deamination of primary and secondary amines, and the replacement of a sulfur by an oxygen atom (desulfuration). Examples are given in Table 1–2.

The key step in these oxidative reactions is the insertion of one atom of molecular oxygen into the substrate, often producing an unstable intermediate (indicated by the bracketed structures in Table 1–2), that breaks down to yield the final product. These intermediates may be highly reactive chemically (*see* below). In quantitative terms, most oxidative reactions are carried out by a large family of isozymes called cytochromes P_{450} (Figure 1–3). The cytochrome P_{450} proteins are embedded in the lipid bilayer of the smooth endoplasmic reticulum. An important associated protein, NADPH–cytochrome P_{450} oxidoreductase, is also attached to this lipid bilayer in a stoichiometry of about ten P_{450} molecules to one reductase. A drug substrate initially binds to oxidized (Fe^{3+}) cytochrome P_{450} (Figure 1–3). The resulting drug-cytochrome complex is reduced by the reductase, and the reduced complex then combines with molecular oxygen. A second electron and two hydrogen ions are acquired from the donor system, and the subsequent products are oxidized metabolite and water, with regeneration of the oxidized cytochrome P_{450}. As mentioned, the cytochromes P_{450} are the dominant phase-I oxidative system, although oxidation by amine oxidases, several heme peroxidases, prostaglandin H synthase, xanthine oxidase, and alcohol and aldehyde dehydrogenases are also important.

Hydrolysis. Esters such as procaine (*see* Table 1–2) are hydrolyzed by a variety of nonspecific esterases in liver, plasma, the gastrointestinal tract, and other tissues. Hydrolysis of amides, such as lidocaine, occurs primarily in the liver. Proteases and peptidases in plasma, erythrocytes, and many other tissues are involved in the biotransformation of polypeptide drugs. With the marked interest in the therapeutic application of proteins and peptides, these enzymatic reactions have assumed greater importance. Delivery of such drugs across biological membranes requires the inhibition of these enzymes or the masking of their substrates.

Reduction. Enzymes in the endoplasmic reticulum and cytosol of liver and other tissues can catalyze the reduction of nitro groups (*e.g.,* chloramphenicol) and the cleavage and reduction of an azo linkage (*e.g.,* prontosil) (*see* Table 1–2).

Conjugations. The formation of glucuronides is catalyzed by hepatic glucuronyltransferases, located in the endoplasmic reticulum; these enzymes use uridine diphosphate-glucuronate as the donor of glucuronate. Conjugation with glucuronate also occurs in the kidney and other tissues, but to a much lesser extent. Glucuronides constitute the major proportion of metabolites of many drugs that contain a phenol, alcohol, or carboxylate group (*see* Table 1–2). They are generally inactive and are rapidly secreted into the urine and bile by an anion transport system. However, concentrations of some glucuronides in plasma may approach those of the parent compound. Glucuronides formed from carboxylic acids (*i.e.,* ester glucuronides) are readily hydrolyzed back to the parent compound (both enzymatically and spontaneously). Glucuronides formed from phe-

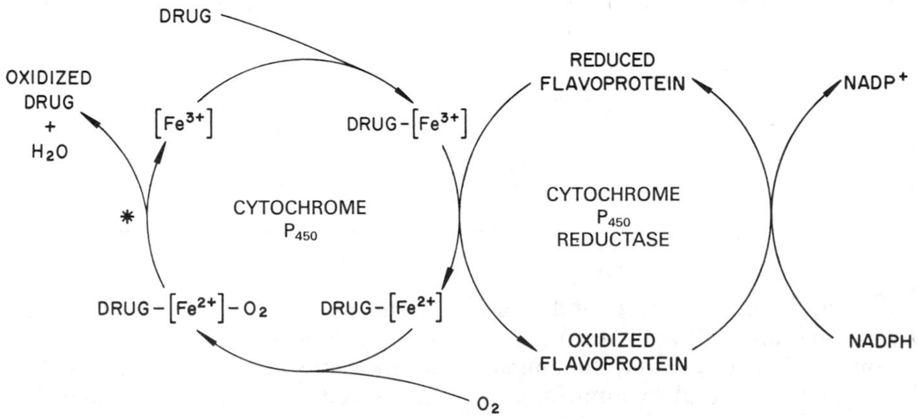

* Denotes contribution of a second electron and two hydrogen ions from NADH–flavoprotein–cytochrome b_5 or from NADPH–flavoprotein.

Figure 1–3. *Major components of the hepatic cytochrome P_{450} monooxygenase system.*

nols or alcohols (*i.e.*, ether glucuronides) are stable chemically. However, both types of glucuronide can be hydrolyzed enzymatically in the intestine following biliary excretion, with subsequent reabsorption of the liberated drug. This enterohepatic cycling may prolong the action of the drug.

Conjugation of aromatic primary amines or hydrazines with acetic acid (using acetyl coenzyme A as the acetyl donor) involves several N-acetyl transferases. Examples include many sulfonamides and drugs such as isoniazid, hydralazine, and procainamide. Aromatic carboxylic acids, such as salicylic acid, are often inactivated by conjugation with glycine. Other reactions include conjugation of phenolic compounds (including steroids) with sulfate and O-, S-, and N-methylation of amines and phenols (*e.g.*, epinephrine). Conjugation with the nucleophilic sulfhydryl-containing tripeptide, glutathione, is not usually quantitatively significant (and is not shown in Table 1–2). However, it contributes to inactivation of unstable and potentially toxic intermediates produced during some biotransformation reactions and thus is important (*see* below).

Factors That Modify Biotransformation. Studies of biotransformation in experimental animals have shown a large number of genetic, environmental, and physiological factors that affect the metabolic fate of a drug. In man, the most important factors are genetically determined polymorphisms in drug oxidations and conjugations; environmental influences, including concomitant use of other drugs that induce or inhibit drug-metabolizing enzymes; and the presence of liver disease, often with severe malnutrition.

At least ten families of cytochrome P_{450} genes are now known to constitute the P_{450} gene superfamily (*see* Nebert and Gonzalez, 1987). The ancestral cytochrome P_{450} gene was probably present more than 1.5 billion years ago. It is believed that some of the P_{450} gene families evolved and diverged because of exposure of organisms to plant metabolites and decayed plant products; this has led to the remarkable overlap of substrate specificities of the P_{450} enzymes. Numerous examples are known of drugs that are good substrates for the enzymes encoded by two or more P_{450} gene families that diverged so long ago as to be unlinked chromosomally. It is speculated that P_{450}s in certain other families are more closely related to the earliest P_{450} and carry out critical metabolic transformations of endogenous substances including steroid biosynthesis and fatty acid catabolism.

At this time the basis of genetic polymorphism, the number of cytochrome P_{450} isozymes, the extent of microheterogeneity of these isozymes, and the mechanisms that regulate gene expression have not been examined in sufficient detail for complete delineation (*see* Bridges, 1987). However, two major types of P_{450} enzyme inducers have been identified—aromatic hydrocarbons and agents that resemble phenobarbital. A number of other inducers of individual isozymes also have been detected (*e.g.*, ethanol, rifampin, dexamethasone, clofibrate). Inducers of the phenobarbital type enhance accumulation of biotransforming enzymes in selected organs (liver, intestine), whereas the aromatic hydrocarbons induce enzymes in most tissues. Moreover, just as subsets of P_{450} enzymes are induced by various chemicals, subsets of glucuronyltransferases and other enzymes are also induced by these same agents.

In man, inhibition of the P_{450} enzymes also occurs commonly after exposure to two drugs, cimetidine and ethanol. In addition, competitive inhibition between the many substrates for the enzymes of biotransformation is readily demonstrated *in vitro*. Such interactions are not usually of practical significance *in vivo*. This is not unexpected, since the inactivation of most drugs *in vivo* exhibits first-order rather than zero-order kinetics; that is, the activity of the enzymes is usually not rate limiting. Drug concentrations are commonly well below those necessary to saturate metabolizing enzymes, and competition between substrates is minimized under these conditions. An important corollary, however, is that significant mutual inhibition of drug metabolism is to be expected for drugs that normally exhibit saturable inactivation kinetics. For example, dicumarol inhibits the metabolism of phenytoin and can increase the incidence and severity of side effects of phenytoin, such as ataxia and drowsiness.

Reduction in the rate of drug metabolism may also occur when biotransformation is so rapid that hepatic blood flow is the rate-limiting factor. Hepatic blood flow may decrease acutely after β-adrenergic blockade, and this can affect the rate of metabolism of drugs that are cleared from the plasma at very high rates (*e.g.*, lidocaine). Certain drugs can inhibit the activity of cytochrome P_{450} irreversibly because of covalent interaction with a reactive intermediate generated by the enzyme.

Biotransformation in the Fetus and Neonate. The activities of the hepatic biotransformation enzymes are low in the neonate, particularly in premature babies. Reduced conjugating activity contributes to hyperbilirubinemia and the risk of bilirubin-induced encephalopathy. It is also the basis for the increased toxicity in the neonate of drugs such as chloramphenicol and certain opioids. A poorly developed blood–brain barrier, weak biotransformation activity, and immature mechanisms for excretion combine to make the fetus and neonate very vulnerable to toxic effects of drugs. The capacity for biotransformation increases during the early months of postnatal life, although the pattern for different enzymes is variable. Cytochrome P_{450} enzymes are usually near adult activities after a few months, whereas phase-II enzymes develop more slowly.

Biotransformation in the Elderly. It is more difficult to generalize about the effect of advanced age on the biotransformation of drugs; the elderly are in many ways a more heterogeneous group than the very young. Because of wide differences in the rates of deterioration of enzyme systems and organs of elimination with age, it is impossible to make blanket recommendations for adjustments of dosage in the elderly. Although the metabolism of some drugs (*e.g.*, quinidine) may be decreased, there are no changes in rates of metabolic clearance of most drugs with age. However, because of the heterogeneity of the elderly population, a small subset of patients may experience alterations in biotransformation, and they may not be identified by studies conducted in healthy, elderly normal volunteers.

Relationship of Biotransformation to Drug Toxicity. Reference was made above to the formation of unstable and potentially toxic metabolites as the result of biotransformation of drugs. Oxidation can cause the formation of highly reactive compounds that normally have such a transient existence that they exert no biological action. Two examples of formation and inactivation of such substances are shown in Figure 1–4. As long as the terminal hydroxylation or conjugation keeps pace, accumulation of reactive intermediates does not occur. However, when induction occurs or when very large amounts of drug are present, oxidation by cytochrome P_{450} is accelerated. Since glutathione is in limited supply in liver and kidney and can be depleted, the drug epoxide or quinone may reach a sufficient concentration to react with nucleophilic cell constituents rather than with glutathione. Hepatic or renal necrosis results. The discovery that the availability of glutathione determines the threshold for the toxic response has led to attempts to use thiols (*e.g.*, N-acetylcysteine) to treat poisoning by drugs such as acetaminophen.

EXCRETION OF DRUGS

Drugs are eliminated from the body either unchanged or as metabolites. Excretory organs, the lung excluded, eliminate polar compounds more efficiently than substances with high lipid solubility. Lipid-soluble drugs are thus not readily eliminated until they are metabolized to more polar compounds.

The kidney is the most important organ for elimination of drugs and their metabolites. Substances excreted in the feces are mainly unabsorbed orally ingested drugs or metabolites excreted in the bile and not reabsorbed from the intestinal tract. Excretion of drugs in breast milk is important not because of the amounts eliminated but because the excreted drugs are potential sources of unwanted pharmacological effects in the nursing infant. Pulmonary excretion is important mainly for the elimination of anesthetic gases and vapors (*see* Chapter 13); occasionally, small quantities of other drugs or metabolites are excreted by this route.

Renal Excretion. Excretion of drugs and metabolites in the urine involves three processes: glomerular filtration, active tubular secretion, and passive tubular reabsorption.

The amount of drug entering the tubular lumen by filtration is dependent on its fractional plasma protein binding and glomerular filtration rate. In the proximal renal tubule, certain organic anions and cations are added to the glomerular filtrate by active, carrier-mediated tubular secretion. Many organic acids (such as penicillin) and metabolites (such as glucuronides) are transported by the system that secretes naturally occurring substances such as uric acid; organic bases, such as tetraethylammonium,

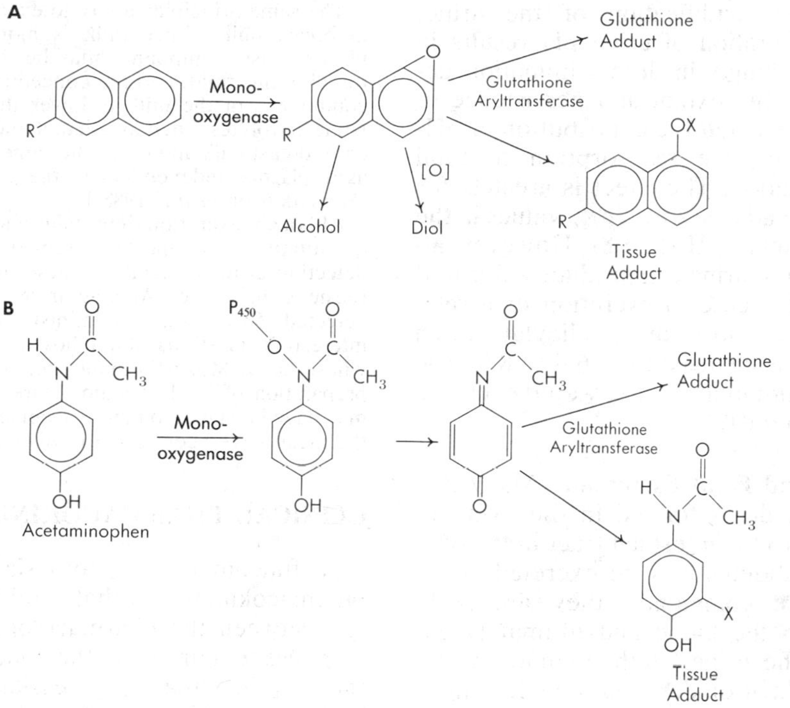

Figure 1–4. *Formation of reactive intermediates during the metabolism of drugs and environmental substances.*

A. A compound with an aromatic ring susceptible to hydroxylation may be metabolized to an arene oxide (epoxide) that can be converted spontaneously to the monoalcohol. The epoxide also can be converted enzymatically to a ''diol'' or can react with glutathione. The latter compound is eventually excreted as a mercapturic acid derivative. When concentrations of compounds such as glutathione are limiting, reaction can occur with macromolecular constituents of tissues.

B. Acetaminophen may be converted to a quinone type of reactive intermediate that is rapidly transformed to a mercapturate when the concentration of glutathione is not limiting. (The major route of acetaminophen metabolism is to an O-glucuronide.) X represents a tissue site of covalent reaction.

are transported by a separate system that secretes choline, histamine, and other endogenous bases.

Both carrier systems are relatively nonselective, and organic ions of similar charge compete for transport. Both transport systems can also be bidirectional, and at least some drugs are both secreted and actively reabsorbed. However, transport of most exogenous ions is predominantly secretory. The outstanding example of the bidirectional tubular transport of an endogenous organic acid is uric acid. The characteristics of tubular transport systems for organic compounds are described in detail in Chapter 30.

In the proximal and distal tubules, the nonionized forms of weak acids and bases undergo net passive reabsorption. The concentration gradient for back-diffusion is created by the reabsorption of water with Na^+ and other inorganic ions. Since the tubular cells are less permeable to the ionized forms of weak electrolytes, passive reabsorption of these substances is pH dependent. When the tubular urine is made more alkaline, weak acids are excreted more rapidly, primarily because they are more ionized and passive reabsorption is decreased. When the tubular urine is made more acidic, the excretion of weak acids is reduced. Alkalinization and acidification of the urine have the opposite effects on the excretion of weak bases. In the treatment of drug poisoning, the excretion of some drugs can be hastened by appropriate alkalinization or acidification of the urine. Whether alteration of urine pH results in significant change in drug elimination depends upon the extent and persistence of the pH change and the contribution of pH-dependent passive reabsorption to total drug elimination. The effect is greatest for weak acids and bases with pK_a values in the range of urinary pH (5 to 8). However, alkalinization of urine can produce a fourfold to sixfold increase in excretion of a relatively strong acid such as salicylate when urinary pH is changed from 6.4 to 8.0. The fraction of nonionized drug would decrease from 1% to 0.04%.

Biliary and Fecal Excretion. Many metabolites of drugs formed in the liver are excreted into the intestinal tract in the bile. These metabolites may be excreted in the feces; more commonly, they are reabsorbed into the blood and ultimately excreted in the urine. Both organic anions, including glucuronides, and organic cations are actively transported into bile by carrier systems similar to those that transport these substances across the renal tubule. Both transport systems are nonselective, and ions of like charge may compete for transport. Steroids and related substances are transported into bile by a third carrier system. The effectiveness of the liver as an excretory organ for glucuronide conjugates is very much limited by their enzymatic hydrolysis after the bile is mixed with the contents of the small intestine, and the parent drug can be reabsorbed from the intestine. Thus, such compounds may undergo extensive biliary cycling with eventual excretion by the kidney.

Excretion by Other Routes. Excretion of drugs into sweat, saliva, and tears is quantitatively unimportant. Elimination by these routes is dependent mainly upon diffusion of the nonionized, lipid-soluble form of drugs through the epithelial cells of the glands and is pH dependent. Reabsorption of the nonionized drug from the primary secretion probably also occurs in the ducts of the glands, and active secretion of drugs across the ducts of the gland may also occur. Drugs excreted in the saliva enter the mouth, where they are usually swallowed. The concentration of some drugs in saliva parallels that in plasma. Saliva may therefore be a useful biological fluid in which to determine drug concentrations when it is difficult or inconvenient to obtain blood.

The same principles apply to excretion of drugs in breast milk. Since milk is more acidic than plasma, basic compounds may be slightly concentrated in this fluid, and the concentration of acidic compounds in the milk is lower than in plasma. Nonelectrolytes, such as ethanol and urea, readily enter breast milk and reach the same concentration as in plasma, independent of the pH of the milk. (*See* Atkinson *et al.*, 1988.)

Although excretion into hair and skin is also quantitatively unimportant, sensitive methods of detection of toxic metals in these tissues have forensic significance. Arsenic in Napoleon's hair, detected 150 years after administration, has raised interesting questions about how he died, and by whose hand. Mozart's manic behavior during the preparation of his last major work, the *Requiem*, may have been due to mercury poisoning; traces of the metal have been found in his hair.

CLINICAL PHARMACOKINETICS

A fundamental hypothesis of clinical pharmacokinetics is that a relationship exists between the pharmacological or toxic response to a drug and the concentration of the drug in a readily accessible site in the body (*e.g.*, blood). This hypothesis has been documented for many drugs (*see* Appendix II), although it is apparent for some drugs that no clear or simple relationship has been found between pharmacological effect and concentration in plasma. In most cases, as depicted in Figure 1–1, the concentration of drug in the systemic circulation will be related to the concentration of drug at its sites of action. The pharmacological effect that results may be the clinical effect desired, a toxic effect, or, in some cases, an effect unrelated to efficacy or toxicity. Clinical pharmacokinetics attempts to provide both a more quantitative relationship between dose and effect and the framework with which to interpret measurements of concentrations of drugs in biological fluids. The importance of pharmacokinetics in patient care rests on the improvement in efficacy that can be attained by attention to its principles when dosage regimens are chosen and modified.

The various physiological and pathophysiological variables that dictate adjustment of dosage in individual patients often do so as a result of modification of pharmacokinetic parameters. The three most important parameters are *clearance*, a measure of the body's ability to eliminate drug;

volume of distribution, a measure of the apparent space in the body available to contain the drug; and *bioavailability,* the fraction of drug absorbed as such into the systemic circulation. Of lesser importance are the *rates* of availability and distribution of the agent.

CLEARANCE

Clearance is the most important concept to be considered when a rational regimen for long-term drug administration is to be designed. The clinician usually wants to maintain steady-state concentrations of a drug within a known therapeutic range (*see* Appendix II). Assuming complete bioavailability, the steady state will be achieved when the rate of drug elimination equals the rate of drug administration:

$$\text{Dosing rate} = CL \cdot C_{ss} \qquad (1)$$

where CL is clearance and C_{ss} is the steady-state concentration of drug. Thus, if the desired steady-state concentration of drug in plasma or blood is known, the rate of clearance of drug by the patient will dictate the rate at which the drug should be administered.

The concept of clearance is extremely useful in clinical pharmacokinetics because clearance of a given drug is usually constant over the range of concentrations encountered clinically. This is true because systems for elimination of drugs are not usually saturated and, thus, the *absolute* rate of elimination of the drug is essentially a linear function of its concentration in plasma. A synonymous statement is that the elimination of most drugs follows first-order kinetics—a constant *fraction* of drug is eliminated per unit of time. If mechanisms for elimination of a given drug become saturated, the kinetics become zero-order—a constant *amount* of drug is eliminated per unit of time. Under such a circumstance, clearance becomes variable. Principles of drug clearance are similar to those of renal physiology, where, for example, creatinine clearance is defined as the rate of elimination of creatinine in the urine relative to its concentration in plasma. At the simplest level, clearance of a drug is the rate of elimination by all routes normalized to the concentration of drug C in some biological fluid:

$$CL = \text{Rate of elimination}/C \qquad (2)$$

It is important to note that clearance does not indicate how much drug is being removed but, rather, the volume of biological fluid such as blood or plasma that would have to be completely freed of drug to account for the elimination. Clearance is expressed as a volume per unit of time. Clearance is usually further defined as blood clearance (CL_b), plasma clearance (CL_p), or clearance based on the concentration of unbound or free drug (CL_u), depending on the concentration measured (C_b, C_p, or C_u). (For additional discussion of clearance concepts, *see* Benet *et al.*, 1984.)

Clearance by means of various organs of elimination is additive. Elimination of drug may occur as a result of processes that occur in the kidney, liver, and other organs. Division of the rate of elimination by each organ by a concentration of drug (*e.g.*, plasma concentration) will yield the respective clearance by that organ. Added together, these separate clearances will equal total systemic clearance:

$$CL_{renal} + CL_{hepatic} + CL_{other} = CL_{systemic} \qquad (3)$$

Other routes of elimination could include that in saliva or sweat, partition into the gut, and metabolism at other sites.

Total systemic clearance may be determined at steady state by using equation 1. For a single dose of a drug with complete bioavailability and first-order kinetics of elimination, total systemic clearance may be determined from mass balance and the integration of equation 2 over time.

$$CL = \text{Dose}/AUC \qquad (4)$$

where AUC is the total area under the curve that describes the concentration of drug in the systemic circulation as a function of time (from zero to infinity).

Examples. In Appendix II, the plasma clearance for cephalexin is reported as $4.3 \text{ ml} \cdot \text{min}^{-1} \cdot \text{kg}^{-1}$, with 91% of the drug excreted unchanged in the urine. For a 70-kg man, the total body clearance from plasma would be 300 ml/min, with renal clearance accounting for 91% of this elimination. In other words, the kidney is able to excrete cephalexin at a rate such that approximately 273 ml of plasma would be freed of drug per minute. Because clearance is usually assumed to remain constant in a stable patient, the total rate of elimination of cephalexin will depend on the concentration of drug in the plasma (equation 2). Propranolol is cleared at a rate of 12 ml · min^{-1} · kg^{-1} (or 840 ml/min in a 70-kg man), almost exclusively by the liver. Thus, the liver is able to remove the amount of drug contained in 840 ml of plasma per minute. Of the drugs listed in Appendix II, one of the highest values of plasma clearance is that for labetalol—1750 ml/min; this value exceeds the rate of plasma (and blood) flow to the liver, the dominant organ for elimination of this drug. However, because labetalol partitions readily into red blood cells ($C_{rbc}/C_p = 1.8$), the amount of drug delivered to the excretory organ is considerably higher than suspected from measurement of its concentration in plasma. The relationship between plasma and blood clearance at steady state is given by:

$$\frac{CL_p}{CL_b} = \frac{C_b}{C_p} = 1 + H\left(\frac{C_{rbc}}{C_p} - 1\right) \qquad (5)$$

One may solve for labetalol clearance from blood by substituting the red blood cell to plasma concentration ratio and the average value for the hematocrit ($H = 0.45$). Clearance of labetalol, when measured in terms of its concentration in blood, is actually 1290 ml/min, a more reasonable value. Thus the plasma clearance may assume values that are not "physiological." A drug with an extremely low concentration in plasma that is concentrated in erythrocytes (*e.g.*, mecamylamine) can show a plasma clearance of tens of liters per minute. However, if the concentration in blood is used to define clearance, the maximal clearance possible is equal to the sum of blood flows to the various organs of elimination.

As mentioned, clearance of most drugs is constant over the range of concentration in plasma or blood that is encountered in clinical settings. This means that elimination is not saturated and the rate of elimination of drug is directly proportional to its concentration (equation 2). For drugs that exhibit saturable or dose-dependent elimination, clearance will vary with the concentration of drug, often according to the following equation:

$$\text{Total plasma clearance} = V_m/(K_m + C_p) \qquad (6)$$

where K_m represents the plasma concentration at which half of the maximal rate of elimination is reached (in units of mass/volume) and V_m is equal to the maximal rate of elimination (in units of mass/time). This equation is entirely analogous to the Michaelis–Menten equation for enzyme kinetics. Design of dosage regimens for such drugs is more complex (*see* below).

A further definition of clearance is useful for understanding the effects of pathological and physiological variables on drug elimination, particularly with respect to an individual organ. The rate of elimination of a drug by an individual organ can be defined in terms of the blood flow to the organ and the concentration of drug in the blood. The rate of presentation of drug to the organ is the product of blood flow (Q) and the arterial drug concentration (C_A), and the rate of exit of drug from the organ is the product of blood flow and the venous drug concentration (C_V). The difference between these rates at steady state is the rate of drug elimination:

$$\begin{aligned}\text{Rate of elimination} &= Q \cdot C_A - Q \cdot C_V \\ &= Q(C_A - C_V)\end{aligned} \qquad (7)$$

Division of equation 7 by the concentration of drug that enters the organ of elimination, C_A, yields an expression for clearance of the drug by the organ in question:

$$CL_{organ} = Q\left(\frac{C_A - C_V}{C_A}\right) = Q \cdot E \qquad (8)$$

The expression $(C_A - C_V)/C_A$ in equation 8 can be referred to as the extraction ratio for the drug (E).

Hepatic Clearance. The concepts developed in equation 8 have important implications for drugs that are eliminated by the liver. Consider a drug that is efficiently removed from the blood by hepatic processes—biotransformation and/or excretion of unchanged drug into the bile. In this instance, the concentration of drug in the blood leaving the liver will be low, the extraction ratio will approach unity, and the clearance of the drug from blood will become limited by hepatic blood flow. Drugs that are cleared efficiently by the liver (*e.g.*, drugs in Appendix II with clearances greater than 6 ml · min^{-1} · kg^{-1}, such as chlorpromazine, diltiazem, imipramine, lidocaine, morphine, and propranolol) are restricted in their rate of elimination not by intrahepatic processes but by the rate at which they can be transported in the blood to hepatic sites of elimination.

Additional complexities have also been considered. For example, the equations presented above do not account for drug binding to components of blood and tissues, nor do they permit an estimation of the intrinsic ability of the liver or kidney to eliminate a drug in the absence of limitations imposed by blood flow. Extensions of the relationships of equation 8 to include expressions for protein binding and intrinsic clearance have been proposed for a number of models of hepatic elimination (*see* Roberts *et al.*, 1988). All of these models indicate that when the capacity of the eliminating organ to metabolize the drug is large in comparison with the rate of presentation of drug, the clearance will approximate the organ blood flow. In contrast, when the metabolic capability is small in comparison to the rate of drug presentation, the clearance will be proportional to the unbound fraction of drug in blood and the intrinsic clearance. Appreciation of these concepts allows one to understand a number of possibly puzzling experimental results. For example, enzyme induction or hepatic disease may change the rate of drug metabolism in an isolated hepatic microsomal enzyme system but not change clearance in the whole animal. For a drug with a high extraction ratio, clearance is limited by blood flow, and changes in the intrinsic clearance due to enzyme induction or hepatic disease should have little effect. Similarly, for drugs with high extraction ratios, changes in protein binding due to disease or competitive binding interactions should have little effect on clearance. In contrast, changes in intrinsic clearance and protein binding will affect the clearance of drugs with low extraction ratios but changes in blood flow should have little effect.

Renal Clearance. Renal clearance of a drug results in its appearance as such in the urine; changes in the pharmacokinetic properties of drugs due to renal disease may also be explained in terms of clearance concepts. However, the complications that relate to filtration, active secretion, and reabsorption must be considered. The rate of filtration of a drug depends on the volume of fluid that is filtered in the glomerulus and the unbound concentration of drug in plasma, since drug bound to protein is not filtered. The rate of secretion of drug by the kidney will depend on the binding of drug to the proteins involved in active transport relative to that bound to plasma proteins, the degree of saturation of these carriers, the rate of transfer of the drug across the tubular membrane, and the rate of delivery of the drug to the secretory site. The influences of changes in protein binding, blood flow, and the number of functional nephrons are analogous to the examples given above for hepatic elimination.

DISTRIBUTION

Volume of Distribution. Volume is a second fundamental parameter that is useful in discussing processes of drug disposition. The volume of distribution (V) relates the amount of drug in the body to the concentration of drug (C) in the blood or plasma, depending upon the fluid measured. This volume does not necessarily refer to an identifiable physiological volume, but merely to the fluid volume that would be required to contain all of the drug in the body at the same concentration as in the blood or plasma:

$$V = \text{Amount of drug in body}/C \qquad (9)$$

The plasma volume of a normal 70-kg man is 3 liters, blood volume is about 5.5 liters, extracellular fluid volume outside the plasma is 12 liters, and the volume of total body water is approximately 42 liters. However, many drugs exhibit volumes of distribution far in excess of these values. For example, if 500 μg of digoxin were in the body of a 70-kg subject, a plasma concentration of approximately 0.7 ng/ml would be observed. Dividing the amount of drug in the body by the plasma concentration yields a volume of distribution for digoxin of about 700 liters, or a value ten times greater than the total body volume of a 70-kg man. In fact, digoxin, which is relatively hydrophobic, distributes preferentially to muscle and adipose tissue and to its specific receptors, leaving a very small amount of drug in the plasma. For drugs that are extensively bound to plasma proteins but that are not bound to tissue components, the volume of distribution will approach that of the plasma volume. In contrast, certain drugs have high volumes of distribution even though most of the drug in the circulation is bound to albumin, because these drugs are also sequestered elsewhere.

The volume of distribution may vary widely depending on the pK_a of the drug, the degree of binding to plasma proteins, the partition coefficient of the drug in fat, the degree of binding to other tissues, and so forth. As might be expected, the volume of distribution for a given drug can change as a function of the patient's age, gender, disease, and body composition.

Several volume terms are commonly used to describe drug distribution, and they have been derived in a number of ways. The volume of distribution defined in equation 9 considers the body as a single homogeneous compartment (Figure 1–1). In this one-compartment model, all drug administration occurs directly into the central compartment and distribution of drug is instantaneous throughout volume (V). Clearance of drug from this compartment occurs in a first-order fashion, as defined in equation 2; that is, the amount of drug eliminated per unit time depends on the amount (concentration) of drug in the body compartment. Figure 1–5, *A* and equation 10 describe the decline of plasma concentration with time for a drug introduced into this compartment.

$$C = (\text{Dose}/V) \cdot exp(-kt) \qquad (10)$$

where k is the rate constant for elimination of the drug from the compartment. This rate constant is inversely related to the half-life of the drug ($k = 0.693/t_{1/2}$).

For most drugs the idealized one-compartment model discussed above does not describe the entire time course of the plasma concentration. That is, certain tissue reservoirs can be distinguished from the central compartment, and the drug concentration appears to decay in a manner that can be described by multiple exponential terms (*see* Figure 1–5, *B*).

Rate of Drug Distribution. The multiple exponential decay observed for a drug that is eliminated from the body with first-order kinetics results from differences in the rates at which the drug equilibrates with tissue reservoirs. The rate of equilibration will depend upon the ratio of the perfusion of the tissue to the partition of drug into the tissue. In

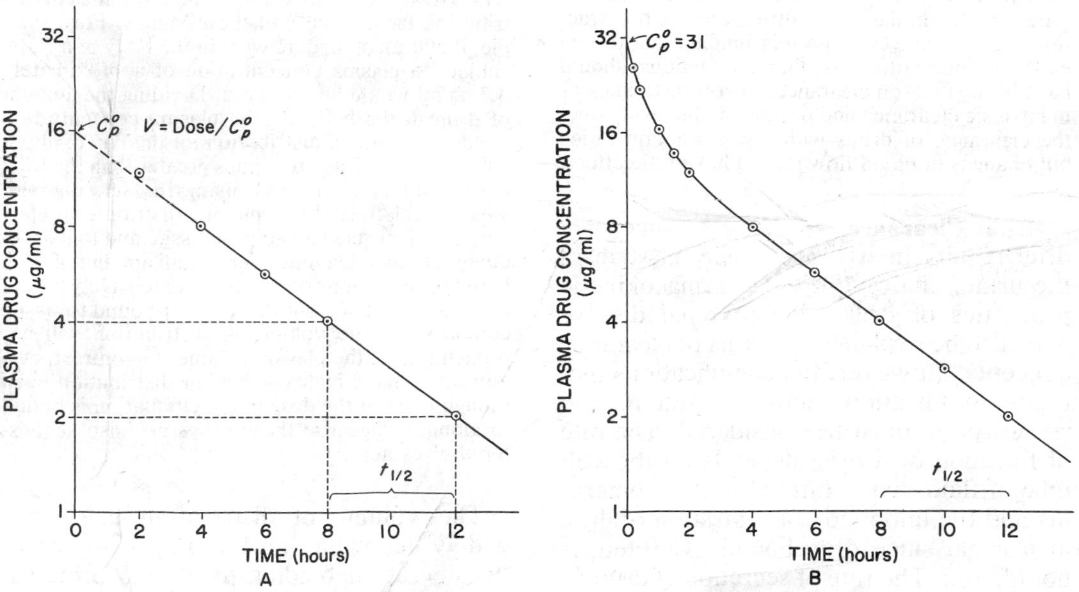

Figure 1–5. *Plasma concentration–time curves following intravenous administration of a drug (500 mg) to a 70-kg man.*

A. In this example, drug concentrations are measured in plasma 2 hours after the dose is administered. The semilogarithmic plot of plasma concentration versus time appears to indicate that the drug is eliminated from a single compartment by a first-order process (equation 10) with a half-life of 4 hours ($k = 0.693/t_{1/2} = 0.173$ hr^{-1}). The volume of distribution (V) may be determined from the value of C_p obtained by extrapolation to $t = 0$ ($C_p^o = 16$ μg/ml). Volume of distribution (equation 9) for the one-compartment model is 31.3 liters or 0.45 liter/kg (V = dose/C_p^o). The clearance for this drug is 92 ml/min; for a one-compartment model, $CL = k \cdot V$.

B. Sampling before 2 hours indicates that, in fact, the drug follows multiexponential kinetics. The terminal disposition half-life is 4 hours, clearance is 103 ml/min (equation 4), V_{area} is 28 liters (equation 11), and V_{ss} is 25.4 liters (equation 12). The initial or "central" distribution volume for the drug (V_1 = dose/C_p^o) is 16.1 liters. The example chosen indicates that multicompartment kinetics may be overlooked when sampling at early times is neglected. In this particular case, there is only a 10% error in the estimate of clearance when the multicompartment characteristics are ignored. However, for many drugs multicompartment kinetics may be observed for significant periods of time, and failure to consider the distribution phase can lead to significant errors in estimates of clearance and in predictions of the appropriate dosage.

many cases, groups of tissues with similar perfusion/partition ratios all equilibrate at essentially the same rate, such that only one apparent phase of distribution (rapid initial fall of concentration, as in Figure 1–5, *B*) is seen. It is as though the drug starts in a "central" volume, which consists of plasma and tissue reservoirs that are in rapid equilibrium with it, and distributes to a "final" volume, at which point concentrations in plasma decrease in a log-linear fashion at rate k (*see* Figure 1–5, *B*).

If the pattern or ratio of blood flows to various tissues changes within an individual or differs between individuals, rates of drug distribution to tissues will also change. However, changes in blood flow may also cause some tissues that were originally in the "central" volume to equilibrate sufficiently more slowly so as to appear only in the "final" volume. This means that central volumes will appear to vary with disease states that cause altered regional blood flow. After an intravenous bolus dose, drug concentrations in plasma may be higher in individuals with poor perfusion (*e.g.*, shock) than they would be if perfusion were better. These higher systemic concentrations may, in turn, cause higher concentrations (and greater effects) in tissues such as brain and heart whose usually high perfusion has not been reduced by the altered hemodynamic state. Thus, the effect of a drug at various sites of action can be variable, depending on perfusion of these sites.

Multicompartment Volume Terms. Two different terms have been used to describe the volume of distribution for drugs that follow multiple exponential decay. The first, designated V_{area}, is calculated as the ratio of clearance to the rate of decline of concentration during the elimination (final) phase of the logarithmic concentration versus time curve:

$$V_{area} = \frac{CL}{k} = \frac{\text{Dose}}{k \cdot AUC} \tag{11}$$

The calculation of this parameter is straightforward, and the volume term may be determined after administration of drug by intravenous or enteral routes (where the dose used must be corrected for bioavailability). However, another multicompartment volume of distribution may be more useful, especially when the effect of disease states on pharmacokinetics is to be determined. The volume of distribution at steady state (V_{ss}) represents the volume in which a drug would appear to be distributed during steady state if the drug existed throughout that volume at the same concentration as that in the measured fluid (plasma or blood). This volume can be determined by the use of areas, as described by Benet and Galeazzi (1979):

$$V_{ss} = (\text{Dose}_{iv})(AUMC)/AUC^2 \tag{12}$$

where $AUMC$ is the area under the first moment of the curve that describes the time course of the plasma or blood concentration, that is, the area under the curve of the product of time t and plasma or blood concentration C over the time span zero to infinity.

Although V_{area} is a convenient and easily calculated parameter, it varies when the rate constant for drug elimination changes, even when there has been no change in the distribution space. This is because the terminal rate of decline of the concentration of drug in blood or plasma depends not only on clearance but also on the rates of distribution of drug between the central and final volumes. V_{ss} does not suffer from this disadvantage (*see* Benet *et al.*, 1984).

HALF-LIFE

The half-life ($t_{1/2}$) is the time it takes for the plasma concentration or the amount of drug in the body to be reduced by 50%. For the simplest case, the one-compartment model (Figure 1–5, *A*), half-life may be determined readily and used to make decisions about drug dosage. However, as indicated in Figure 1–5, *B*, drug concentrations in plasma often follow a multiexponential pattern of decline; two or more half-life terms may thus be calculated.

In the past, the half-life that was usually reported corresponded to the terminal log-linear phase of elimination. However, as greater analytical sensitivity has been achieved, the lower concentrations measured appeared to yield longer and longer terminal half-lives. For example, a terminal half-life of 53 hours is observed for gentamicin (versus the 2-to-3-hour value in Appendix II), and biliary cycling is probably responsible for the 120-hour terminal value for indomethacin (as compared with the 2.4-hour half-life listed in Appendix II). The relevance of a particular half-life may be defined in terms of the fraction of the clearance and volume of distribution that is related to each half-life and whether plasma concentrations or amounts of drug in the body are best related to measures of response (*see* Benet, 1984). The single half-life values given for each drug in Appendix II are chosen to represent the most clinically relevant half-life.

Early studies of pharmacokinetic properties of drugs in disease were compromised by their reliance on half-life as the sole measure of alterations of drug disposition. Only recently has it been appreciated that half-life is a derived parameter that changes as a function of both clearance and volume of distribution. A useful approximate relationship between the clinically relevant half-life, clearance, and volume of distribution is given by:

$$t_{1/2} \cong 0.693 \cdot V/CL \tag{13}$$

Clearance is the measure of the body's ability to eliminate a drug. However, the organs of elimination can only clear drug from the blood or plasma with which they are in direct contact. As clearance decreases, due to a disease process, for example, half-life would be expected to increase. However, this reciprocal relationship is exact only when the disease does not change the volume of distribution. For example, the half-life of diazepam increases with increasing age; however, it is not clearance that changes as a function of age, but the volume of distribution (Klotz *et al.*, 1975). Similarly, changes in protein binding of the drug may affect its clearance as well as its volume of distribution, leading to unpredictable changes in half-life as a function of disease. The half-life of tolbutamide, for example, decreases in patients with acute viral hepatitis, exactly the opposite from what one might expect. The disease appears to modify protein binding in both plasma and tissues, causing no change in volume of distribution but an increase in total clearance because higher concentrations of free drug are present (Williams *et al.*, 1977).

Although it can be a poor index of drug elimination, half-life does provide a good indication of the time required to reach steady state after a dosage regimen is initiated (*i.e.*, four half-lives to reach approximately 94% of a new steady state), the time for a drug to be removed from the body, and a means to estimate the appropriate dosing interval (*see* below).

Steady State. Equation 1 indicates that a steady-state concentration will eventually be achieved when a drug is administered at a constant rate. At this point, drug elimination (the product of clearance and concentration; equation 2) will equal the rate of drug availability. This concept also extends to intermittent dosage (*e.g.*, 250 mg of drug every 8 hours). During each interdose interval, the concentration of drug rises and falls. At steady state, the entire cycle is repeated identically in each interval. Equation 1 still applies for intermittent dosing, but it now describes the average drug concentration during an interdose interval. Steady-state dosing is illustrated in Figure 1–6.

EXTENT AND RATE OF AVAILABILITY

Bioavailability. It is important to distinguish between the rate and extent of drug absorption and the amount that ultimately reaches the systemic circulation, as discussed above. The amount of the drug that reaches the systemic circulation can be expressed as a fraction of the dose F, which is often called bioavailability. Reasons for incomplete absorption have been discussed above. Also, as noted previously, if the drug is metabolized in the liver or excreted in bile, some of the active drug absorbed from the gastrointestinal tract will be inactivated by the liver before it can reach the general circulation and be distributed to its sites of action.

Knowing the extraction ratio (E) for a drug across the liver (*see* equation 8), it is possible to predict the maximum oral availability (F_{max}), assuming hepatic elimination follows first-order processes:

$$F_{max} = 1 - E = 1 - (CL_{\text{hepatic}}/Q_{\text{hepatic}}) \qquad (14)$$

Thus, if the hepatic blood clearance for the drug is large relative to hepatic blood flow, the extent of availability will be low when it is given orally (*e.g.*, lidocaine). This decrease in availability is a function of the physiological site from which absorption takes place, and no modification of dosage form will improve the availability under conditions of linear kinetics.

When drugs are administered by a route that is subject to first-pass loss, the equations presented previously that contain the terms *dose* or *dosing rate* (equations 1, 4, 10, and 11) must also include the bioavailability term F such that the available dose or dosing rate is used. For example, equation 1 is modified to:

$$F \cdot \text{Dosing rate} = CL \cdot C_{ss} \qquad (15)$$

Rate of Absorption. Although the rate of drug absorption does not, in general, influence the average steady-state concentration of the drug in plasma, it may still influence drug therapy. If a drug is absorbed very rapidly (*e.g.*, a dose given as an intravenous bolus) and has a small central vol-

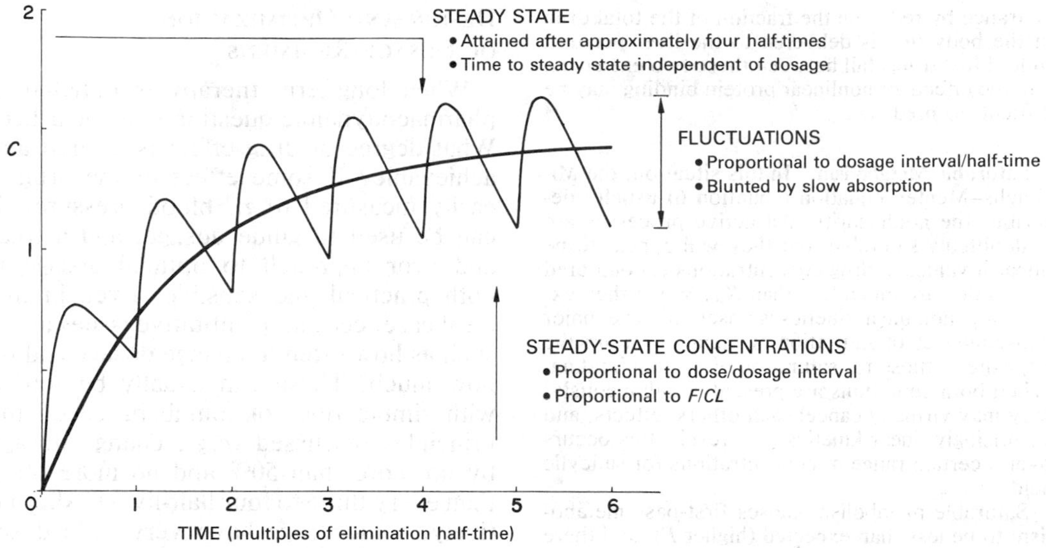

Figure 1–6. *Fundamental pharmacokinetic relationships for repeated administration of drugs.*

Light line is the pattern of drug accumulation during repeated administration of a drug at intervals equal to its elimination half-time, when drug absorption is ten times as rapid as elimination. As the relative rate of absorption increases, the concentration maxima approach 2 and the minima approach 1 during the steady state. Heavy line depicts the pattern during administration of equivalent dosage by continuous intravenous infusion. Curves are based upon the one-compartment model.

Average concentration ($\bar{C}_{ss}$) when the steady state is attained during intermittent drug administration:

$$\bar{C}_{ss} = \frac{F \cdot \text{dose}}{CL \cdot T}$$

where F = fractional bioavailability of the dose and T = dosage interval (time). By substitution of infusion rate for $F \cdot \text{dose}/T$, the formula is equivalent to equation 1 and provides the concentration maintained at steady state during continuous intravenous infusion.

ume, the concentration of drug will be high initially. It will then fall as the drug is distributed to its final (larger) volume (*see* Figure 1–5, *B*). If the same drug is absorbed more slowly (*e.g.*, by slow infusion), it will be distributed while it is being given, and peak concentrations will be lower and will occur later. A given drug may act to produce both desirable and undesirable effects at several sites in the body, and the rates of distribution of drug to these sites may not be the same. The relative intensities of these different effects of a drug may thus vary transiently when its rate of administration is changed.

NONLINEAR PHARMACOKINETICS

Nonlinearity in pharmacokinetics (*i.e.*, changes in such parameters as clearance, volume of distribution, and half-life as a function of dose or concentration of drug) is usually due to saturation of protein binding, hepatic metabolism, or active renal transport of the drug.

Saturable Protein Binding. As the molar concentration of drug increases, the unbound fraction must eventually also increase (as all binding sites become saturated). This usually occurs only when drug concentrations in plasma are in the range of tens to hundreds of micrograms per milliliter. For a drug that is metabolized by the liver with a low extraction ratio, saturation of plasma protein binding will cause both V and clearance to increase as drug concentrations increase; half-life may thus remain constant (*see* equation 13). For such a drug, C_{ss} will not increase linearly as the rate of drug administration is increased. For drugs that are cleared with high extraction ratios, C_{ss} can remain linearly proportional to the rate of drug administration. In this case, hepatic clearance would not change, and the increase in V would increase the half-time of disappearance by reducing the fraction of the total drug in the body that is delivered to the liver per unit time. Most drugs fall between these two extremes, and the effects of nonlinear protein binding may be difficult to predict.

Saturable Metabolism. In this situation, the Michaelis–Menten equation (equation 6) usually describes the nonlinearity. All active processes are undoubtedly saturable, but they will appear to be linear if values of drug concentrations encountered in practice are much less than K_m. When they exceed K_m, nonlinear kinetics is observed. The major consequences of saturation of metabolism are the opposite of those for saturation of protein binding. When both conditions are present simultaneously, they may virtually cancel each others' effects, and surprisingly linear kinetics may result; this occurs over a certain range of concentrations for salicylic acid.

Saturable metabolism causes first-pass metabolism to be less than expected (higher *F*), and there is a greater fractional increase in C_{ss} than the corresponding fractional increase in the rate of drug administration. The latter can be seen most easily by substituting equation 6 into equation 1 and solving for the steady-state concentration:

$$C_{ss} = \frac{\text{Dosing rate} \cdot K_m}{V_m - \text{Dosing rate}} \qquad (16)$$

As the dosing rate approaches the maximal elimination rate (V_m), the denominator of equation 16 approaches zero and C_{ss} increases disproportionately. Fortunately, saturation of metabolism should have no effect on the volume of distribution; thus, as clearance decreases, the apparent half-life for elimination increases and the approach to the (disproportionate) new steady state is slow. However, the concept of "four half-lives to steady state" is not applicable for drugs with nonlinear metabolism in the usual range of clinical concentrations.

Phenytoin provides an example of a drug for which metabolism becomes saturated in the therapeutic range of concentrations (*see* Appendix II). K_m is typically near the lower end of the therapeutic range (K_m = 5 to 10 mg per liter). For some individuals, especially children, K_m may be as low as 1 mg per liter. If, for such an individual, the target concentration is 15 mg per liter and this is attained at a dosing rate of 300 mg per day, then, from equation 16, V_m equals 320 mg per day. For such a patient, a dose 10% less than optimal (*i.e.*, 270 mg per day) will produce a C_{ss} of 5 mg per liter, well below the desired value. In contrast, a dose 10% greater than optimal (330 mg per day) will exceed metabolic capacity (by 10 mg per day) and cause a long and slow but unending climb in concentration until toxicity occurs. Dosage cannot be controlled so precisely (less than 10% error). Therefore, for those patients in whom the target concentration for phenytoin is more than tenfold greater than the K_m, alternating inefficacious therapy and toxicity is almost unavoidable.

Design and Optimization of Dosage Regimens

When long-term therapy is initiated, a pharmacodynamic question must be asked: What degree of drug effect is desired and achievable? If some effect of the drug is easily measured (*e.g.*, blood pressure), it can be used to guide dosage, and a trial-and-error approach to optimal dosage is both practical and sensible. Even in this ideal case, certain quantitative issues arise, such as how often to change dosage and by how much. These can usually be settled with simple rules of thumb based on the principles discussed (*e.g.*, change dosage by no more than 50% and no more often than every three to four half-lives). Alternatively, some drugs have very little dose-related toxicity, and maximum efficacy is usually desired. For these drugs, doses well in excess of the average required will both ensure efficacy (if this is possible) and prolong drug action. Such a "maximal dose" strategy is typically used for penicillins and most β-adrenergic blocking agents.

Target Level. For some drugs, the effects are difficult to measure (or the drug is given for prophylaxis), toxicity and lack of efficacy are both potential dangers, and/or the therapeutic index is narrow. In these circumstances doses must be titrated carefully, and a target-level strategy is reasonable. A desired (target) steady-state concentration of the drug (usually in plasma) is chosen, and a dosage is computed that is expected to achieve this value. Drug concentrations are subsequently measured, and dosage is adjusted if necessary to approximate the target more closely (*see also* Chapter 4).

To apply the target-level strategy, the therapeutic objective must be defined in terms of a desirable range for the C_{ss}, often called the therapeutic range. For drugs for which this can be done, such as theophylline and digoxin, the lower limit of the therapeutic range appears to be approximately equal to the drug concentration that produces about half of the greatest possible therapeutic effect. The upper limit of the therapeutic range (for drugs with such a limit) is fixed by toxicity, not by efficacy.

In general, the upper limit of the therapeutic range is such that no more than 5 to 10% of patients will experience a toxic effect. For some drugs, this may mean that the upper limit of the range is no more than twice the lower limit. Of course, these figures can be highly variable, and some patients may benefit greatly from drug concentrations that exceed the therapeutic range while others may suffer significant toxicity at much lower values. Barring more specific information, however, the target is usually chosen as the center of the therapeutic range.

Maintenance Dose. In most clinical situations, drugs are administered in a series of repetitive doses or as a continuous infusion in order to maintain a steady-state concentration of drug in plasma within a given therapeutic range. Thus, calculation of the appropriate maintenance dosage is a primary goal. To maintain the chosen steady-state or target concentration, the rate of drug administration is adjusted such that the rate of input equals the rate of loss. This relationship was defined previously in equations 1 and 15 and is expressed here in terms of the desired target concentration:

$$\text{Dosing rate} = \text{Target} \cdot CL/F \tag{17}$$

If the clinician chooses the desired concentration of drug in plasma and knows the clearance and availability for that drug in a particular patient, the appropriate dose and dosing interval can be calculated.

Example. A steady-state plasma concentration of theophylline of 15 mg per liter is desired to relieve acute bronchial asthma in a 68-kg patient. If the patient does not smoke and is otherwise normal except for the asthmatic condition, one can use the mean clearance given in Appendix II, that is, $0.65\ \text{ml} \cdot \text{min}^{-1} \cdot \text{kg}^{-1}$. Because the drug is to be given as an intravenous infusion, $F = 1$:

$$\begin{aligned}\text{Dosing rate} &= \text{Target} \cdot CL/F\\ &= 15\ \mu\text{g/ml} \cdot 0.65\ \text{ml} \cdot \text{min}^{-1} \cdot \text{kg}^{-1}\\ &= 9.75\ \mu\text{g} \cdot \text{min}^{-1} \cdot \text{kg}^{-1}\\ &= 40\ \text{mg/hr for a 68-kg patient}\end{aligned}$$

Since almost all intravenous preparations of theophylline are available as the ethylenediamine salt (aminophylline), which contains 85% theophylline, the infusion rate will be 47 mg per hour of aminophylline [(40 mg per hour)/(0.85)].

Dosing Interval for Intermittent Dosage. In general, marked fluctuations in drug concentrations between doses are not beneficial. If absorption and distribution were instantaneous, fluctuation of drug concentrations between doses would be governed entirely by the drug's elimination half-life. If the dosing interval (T) was chosen to be equal to the half-life, then the total fluctuation would be twofold; this is usually a tolerable variation.

Pharmacodynamic considerations modify this. If a drug is relatively nontoxic, such that concentrations many times that necessary for therapy can easily be tolerated, the maximal dose strategy can be used and the dosing interval can be much longer than the elimination half-life (for convenience). The half-life of penicillin G is less than 1 hour, but it is often given in very large doses every 6 or 12 hours.

For some drugs with a narrow therapeutic range, it may be important to estimate the maximal and minimal concentrations that will occur for a particular dosing interval. The minimal steady-state concentration $C_{ss,min}$ may be reasonably determined by the use of equation 18:

$$C_{ss}, min = \frac{F \cdot \text{dose}/V_{ss}}{1 - exp(-kT)} \cdot exp(-kT) \tag{18}$$

where k equals 0.693 divided by the clinically relevant plasma half-life and T is the dosing interval. The term $exp(-kT)$ is, in fact, the fraction of the last dose (corrected for bioavailability) that remains in the body at the end of a dosing interval.

For drugs that follow multiexponential kinetics and that are administered orally, the estimation of the maximal steady-state concentration $C_{ss,max}$ involves a complicated set of exponential constants for distribution and absorption. If these terms are ignored for multiple oral dosing, one may easily predict a maximal steady-state concentration by omitting the $exp(-kT)$ term in the numerator of equation 18 (*see* equation 19, below). Because of the approximation, the predicted maximal concentration from equation 19 will be greater than that actually observed.

Example. When the acute asthmatic attack in the patient discussed above is relieved, the clinician might want to maintain the plasma concentration of theophylline at 15 mg per liter, with oral dosage at intervals of 6, 8, or 12 hours. The correct rate of drug administration, independent of consideration of the dosing interval, is 40 mg per hour for this patient, as calculated above, since the availability of theophylline from an oral dose is 100%. Thus, the appropriate intermittent doses would be 240 mg every 6 hours, 320 mg every 8 hours, or 480 mg every 12 hours. All of these regimens would yield the same average concentration of 15 mg per liter, but different maximal and minimal concentrations would obtain. For a 12-hour dosing interval, the following maximal and minimal concentrations would be predicted:

$$C_{ss,max} = \frac{F \cdot dose/V_{ss}}{1 - exp(-kT)} = \frac{480 \text{ mg/34 liters}}{0.65} = 22 \text{ mg/liter} \quad (19)$$

$$C_{ss,min} = C_{ss,max} \cdot exp(-kT) = (21.7 \text{ mg/liter}) \cdot (0.35) = 7.6 \text{ mg/liter} \quad (20)$$

The calculations in equations 19 and 20 were performed assuming oral doses of 480 mg every 12 hours of a drug with a half-life of 8 hours ($k = 0.693/8$ hr $= 0.0866$ hr^{-1}), a volume of distribution of 0.5 liter/kg ($V_{ss} = 34$ liters for a 68-kg patient), and an oral availability of 1. Since the predicted minimal concentration, 7.6 mg per liter, falls below the suggested effective concentration and the predicted maximal concentration is above that suggested to avoid toxicity (*see* Appendix II), the choice of a 12-hour dosing interval is probably inappropriate. A more appropriate choice would be 320 mg every 8 hours or 240 mg every 6 hours; for $T = 6$ hr, $C_{ss,max} = 17$ mg per liter; $C_{ss,min} = 10$ mg per liter. Of course the clinician must balance the problem of compliance with regimens that involve frequent dosage against the problem of periods when the patient may be subjected to concentrations of the drug that could be too high or too low.

Loading Dose. The "loading dose" is one or a series of doses that may be given at the onset of therapy with the aim of achieving the target concentration rapidly. The appropriate magnitude for the loading dose is:

$$\text{Loading dose} = \text{Target } C_p \cdot V_{ss}/F \quad (21)$$

A loading dose may be desirable if the time required to attain steady state by the administration of drug at a constant rate (four elimination half-lives) is long relative to the temporal demands of the condition being treated. For example, the half-life of lidocaine is usually more than 1 hour. Arrhythmias encountered after myocardial infarction may obviously be life threatening, and one cannot wait 4 to 6 hours to achieve a therapeutic concentration of lidocaine by infusion of the drug at the rate required to maintain this concentration. Hence, use of a loading dose of lidocaine in the coronary care unit is standard.

The use of a loading dose also has significant disadvantages. First, the particularly sensitive individual may be exposed abruptly to a toxic concentration of a drug. Moreover, if the drug involved has a long half-life, it will take a long time for the concentration to fall if the level achieved was excessive. Loading doses tend to be large, and they are often given parenterally and rapidly; this can be particularly dangerous if toxic effects occur as a result of actions of the drug at sites that are in rapid equilibrium with plasma.

Individualizing Dosage. To design a rational dosage regimen, the clinician must know F, CL, V_{ss}, and $t_{1/2}$, and have some knowledge about rates of absorption and distribution of the drug. Moreover, one must judge what variations in these parameters might be expected in a particular patient. Usual values for the important parameters and appropriate adjustments that may be necessitated by disease or other factors are presented in Appendix II. There is, however, unpredictable variation between normal individuals; for many drugs, one standard deviation in the values observed for F, CL, and V_{ss} is about 20%, 50%, and 30%, respectively. This means that 95% of the time the C_{ss} that is achieved will be between 35% and 270% of the target; this is an unacceptably wide range for a drug with a low therapeutic index. If values of C_p are measured, one can estimate values of F, CL, and V_{ss} directly, and this permits more precise adjustment of a dosage regimen. Such measurement and adjustment are appropriate for many drugs with low therapeutic indices (*e.g.*, cardiac glycosides, antiarrhythmic agents, anticonvulsants, theophylline, and others).

THERAPEUTIC DRUG MONITORING

The major use of measured concentrations of drugs (at steady state) is to refine the estimate of CL/F for the patient being treated (using equation 15 as rearranged below):

$$CL/F \text{ (patient)} = \text{Dosing rate}/C_{ss} \text{ (measured)} \quad (22)$$

The new estimate of CL/F can be used in equation 17 to adjust the maintenance dose to achieve the desired target concentration.

Certain practical details and pitfalls related to therapeutic drug monitoring should be kept in mind. The first of these concerns the time of sampling for measurement of the drug concentration. If intermittent dosing is used, when during a dosing interval should samples be taken? It is necessary to distinguish between two possible uses of measured drug concentrations in order to understand the possible answers. A concentration of drug measured in a sample taken at virtually any time during the dosing interval will provide information that may aid in the assessment of drug toxicity. This is one type of therapeutic drug monitoring. It should be stressed, however, that such use of a measured concentration of drug is fraught with difficulties because of interindividual variability in sensitivity to the drug. When there is a question of toxicity, the drug concentration can be no more than just one of many items that serve to inform the clinician.

Changes in the effects of drugs may be delayed relative to changes in plasma concentration because of a slow rate of distribution or pharmacodynamic factors. Concentrations of digoxin, for example, regularly exceed 2 ng/ml (a potentially toxic value) shortly after an oral dose, yet these peak concentrations do not cause toxicity; indeed, they occur well before peak effects. Thus, concentrations of drugs in samples obtained shortly after administration can be uninformative or even misleading.

When concentrations of drugs are used for purposes of adjusting dosage regimens, samples obtained shortly after administration of a dose are almost invariably misleading. The point of sampling during supposed steady state is to modify one's estimate of *CL/F* and thus one's choice of dosage. Early postabsorptive concentrations do not reflect clearance; they are determined primarily by the rate of absorption, the central (rather than the steady-state) volume of distribution, and the rate of distribution, all of which are pharmacokinetic features of virtually no relevance in choosing the long-term maintenance dosage. When the goal of measurement is adjustment of dosage, the sample should be taken well after the previous dose—as a rule of thumb just before the next planned dose, when the concentration is at its minimum. There is an exception to this approach: some drugs are nearly completely eliminated between doses and act only during the initial portion of each dosing interval. If, for such drugs, it is questionable whether efficacious concentrations are being achieved, a sample taken shortly after a dose may be helpful. Yet, if another concern is that low clearance (as in renal failure) may cause accumulation of drug, concentrations measured just before the next dose will reveal such accumulation and are considerably more useful for this purpose than is knowledge of the maximal concentration. For such drugs, determination of both maximal and minimal concentrations is thus recommended.

A second important aspect of the timing of sampling is its relationship to the beginning of the maintenance dosage regimen. When constant dosage is given, steady state is reached only after four half-lives have passed. If a sample is obtained too soon after dosage is begun, it will not accurately reflect clearance. Yet, for toxic drugs, if one waits until steady state is ensured, the damage may have been done. Some simple guidelines can be offered. When it is important to maintain careful control of concentrations, one may take the first sample after two half-lives (as calculated and expected for the patient), assuming no loading dose has been given. If the concentration already exceeds 90% of the eventual expected mean steady-state concentration, the dosage rate should be halved, another sample obtained in another two (supposed) half-lives, and the dosage halved again if this sample exceeds the target. If the first concentration is not too high, one proceeds with the initial rate of dosage; even if the concentration is lower than expected, one can usually await the attainment of steady state in another two estimated half-lives and then proceed to adjust dosage as described above.

If dosage is intermittent, there is a third concern with the time at which samples are obtained for determination of drug concentrations. If the sample has been obtained just prior to the next dose, as recommended, concentration will be a minimal value, not the mean. However, as discussed above, the estimated mean concentration may be calculated by using equation 15.

If a drug follows first-order kinetics, the average, minimum, and maximum concentrations at steady state are linearly related to dose and dosing rate (*see* equations 15, 18, and 19). Therefore, the ratio between the measured and the desired concentrations can be used to adjust the dose:

$$\frac{C_{ss}(\text{measured})}{C_{ss}(\text{desired})} = \frac{\text{Dose(previous)}}{\text{Dose(new)}} \tag{23}$$

Finally, for some drugs that are particularly difficult to manage, computer programs may be useful for the design of dosage regimens. Such programs, which take into account measured drug concentrations and individual factors such as those listed in Appendix II, are becoming increasingly available (see Sheiner *et al.*, 1972; Vozeh and Steimer, 1985).

General References

Goldstein, A.; Aronow, L.; and Kalman, S. M. *Principles of Drug Action: The Basis of Pharmacology*, 2nd ed. John Wiley & Sons, Inc., New York, **1974.**

Melmon, K. L., and Morrelli, H. F. (eds.). *Clinical Pharmacology: Basic Principles in Therapeutics*, 2nd ed. Macmillan Publishing Co., New York, **1978.**

Speight, T. M. (ed.). *Avery's Drug Treatment*, 3rd ed. Williams and Wilkins Co., Baltimore, **1987.**

Absorption, Distribution, Biotransformation, and Excretion

Atkinson, H. C.; Begg, E. J.; and Darlow, B. A. Drugs in human milk: clinical pharmacokinetic considerations. *Clin. Pharmacokinet.*, **1988**, *14*, 217–240.

Bridges, J. W. Metabolism and molecular interactions related to toxicity. In, *Mechanisms of Cell Injury: Implications for Human Health*. (Fowler, B. A., ed.) John Wiley & Sons, Inc., New York, **1987**, pp. 353–382.

Brodie, B. B. Physicochemical factors in drug absorption. In, *Absorption and Distribution of Drugs*. (Binns, T. B., ed.) The Williams & Wilkins Co., Baltimore, **1964**, pp. 16–48.

Jacqz, E.; Hall, S. D.; and Branch, R. A. Genetically determined polymorphisms in drug oxidation. *Hepatology*, **1986**, *6*, 1020–1032.

Lee, D. H. K.; Falk, H. L.; Murphy, S. D.; and Geiger, S. R. (eds.). *Reactions to Environmental Agents. Handbook of Physiology,* Sect. 9. American Physiological Society, Bethesda, **1977.** (*See* especially Chapters 12 to 34 for absorption, distribution, and excretion of foreign agents.)

Mitchell, J. R., and Horning, M. G. (eds.). *Drug Metabolism and Drug Toxicity.* Raven Press, New York, **1984.**

Nebert, D. W., and Gonzalez, F. J. P_{450} genes: structure, evolution and regulation. *Annu. Rev. Biochem.,* **1987,** *56,* 945–993.

Prescott, L. F., and Nimmo, W. S. (eds.). *Drug Absorption.* ADIS Press, New York, **1981.**

Ridout, G.; Santus, G. C.; and Guy, R. H. Pharmacokinetic considerations in the use of new transdermal formulations. *Clin. Pharmacokinet.,* **1988,** *15,* 114–131.

Singer, S. J., and Nicolson, G. L. The fluid-mosaic model of the structure of membranes. *Science,* **1972,** *175,* 720–731.

Symposium. (Various authors.) Clinical implications of drug-protein binding. (Levy, R., and Shand, D., eds.) *Clin. Pharmacokinet.,* **1984,** *9,* Suppl. 1, 1–104.

Tillement, J.-P., and Lindenlaub, E. (eds.). *Protein Binding and Drug Transport.* F. K. Schattauer Verlag, Stuttgart, **1986.**

Pharmacokinetic Principles

Benet, L. Z. Effect of route of administration and distribution on drug action. *J. Pharmacokinet. Biopharm.,* **1978,** *6,* 559–585.

———. Pharmacokinetic parameters: which are necessary to define a drug substance? *Eur. J. Resp. Dis.* [*Suppl. 134*], **1984,** *65,* 45–61.

Benet, L. Z., and Galeazzi, R. L. Noncompartmental determination of the steady-state volume of distribution. *J. Pharm. Sci.,* **1979,** *68,* 1971–1974.

Benet, L. Z.; Massoud, N.; and Gambertoglio, J. G. (eds.). *Pharmacokinetic Basis for Drug Treatment.* Raven Press, New York, **1984.**

Evans, W. E.; Schentag, J. J.; and Jusko, W. J. (eds.). *Applied Pharmacokinetics: Principles of Therapeutic Drug Monitoring,* 2nd ed. Applied Therapeutics, Inc., Spokane, WA, **1986.**

Gibaldi, M., and Perrier, D. *Pharmacokinetics,* 2nd ed. Marcel Dekker, Inc., New York, **1982.**

Klotz, U.; Avant, G. R.; Hoyumpa, A.; Schenker, S.; and Wilkinson, G. R. The effects of age and liver disease on the disposition and elimination of diazepam in adult man. *J. Clin. Invest.,* **1975,** *55,* 347–359.

Roberts, M. S.; Donaldson, J. D.; and Rowland, M. Models of hepatic elimination: comparison of stochastic models to describe residence time distributions and to predict the influence of drug distribution, enzyme heterogeneity, and systemic recycling on hepatic elimination. *J. Pharmacokinet. Biopharm.,* **1988,** *16,* 41–83.

Rowland, M., and Tozer, T. N. *Clinical Pharmacokinetics: Concepts and Applications,* 2nd ed. Lea & Febiger, Philadelphia, **1989.**

Sheiner, L. B.; Rosenberg, B.; and Melmon, K. L. Modelling of individual pharmacokinetics for computer-aided drug dosage. *Comput. Biomed. Res.,* **1972,** *5,* 441–459.

Vozeh, S., and Steimer, J.-L. Feedback control methods for drug dosage optimization: concepts, classification and clinical application. *Clin. Pharmacokinet.,* **1985,** *10,* 457–476.

Williams, R. L.; Blaschke, T. F.; Meffin, P. J.; Melmon, K. L.; and Rowland, M. Influence of acute viral hepatitis on disposition and plasma binding of tolbutamide. *Clin. Pharmacol. Ther.,* **1977,** *21,* 301–309.

CHAPTER

2 PHARMACODYNAMICS: MECHANISMS OF DRUG ACTION AND THE RELATIONSHIP BETWEEN DRUG CONCENTRATION AND EFFECT

Elliott M. Ross

Pharmacodynamics can be defined as the study of the biochemical and physiological effects of drugs and their mechanisms of action. The latter aspect of the subject is perhaps the most fundamental challenge to the investigator in pharmacology, and information derived from such study is of basic utility to the clinician. The objectives of the analysis of drug action are to identify the primary action (as distinguished from describing resultant effects), to delineate the chemical or physical interactions between drug and cell, and to characterize the full sequence and scope of actions and effects. Such a complete analysis provides the basis for both the rational therapeutic use of a drug and the design of new and superior therapeutic agents. Basic research in pharmacodynamics also provides fundamental insight into biochemical and physiological regulation.

MECHANISMS OF DRUG ACTION

The effects of most drugs result from their interaction with macromolecular components of the organism. Such interaction alters the function of the pertinent component and thereby initiates the biochemical and physiological changes that are characteristic of the response to the drug. This concept—now obvious—had its origins in the experimental work of Ehrlich and Langley during the late nineteenth and early twentieth centuries. Ehrlich was struck by the high degree of chemical specificity for the antiparasitic and toxic effects of a variety of synthetic organic chemicals. Langley noted the ability of the South American arrow poison, curare, to inhibit the contraction of skeletal muscles caused by nicotine; however, the tissue remained responsive to direct electrical stimulation. The terms *receptive substance* and, more simply, *receptor* were coined to denote the component of the organism with which the chemical agent was presumed to interact.

The statement that the receptor for a drug can be any functional macromolecular component of the organism has several fundamental corollaries. One is that a drug is potentially capable of altering the rate at which any bodily function proceeds. Another is that drugs do not create effects but merely modulate ongoing function; a drug cannot impart a new function to a cell. Although gene therapy may soon challenge this principle, it remains valid for the immediate future.

Whereas any functional macromolecular component of the organism may serve operationally as a drug receptor, a particularly important group of drug receptors are proteins that normally serve as receptors for endogenous regulatory ligands (*e.g.*, hormones, neurotransmitters). Many drugs act on such physiological receptors. Those that mimic the effects of the endogenous regulatory compound are termed *agonists*. Other compounds may bind to the receptor but have no intrinsic regulatory activity; the result of such binding may be interference with the effect of an agonist. Compounds that are themselves devoid of intrinsic regulatory activity but cause effects by inhibition of the action of an agonist (*e.g.*, by competition for agonist binding sites) are termed *antagonists*.

Drug Receptors

Chemical Properties. At least from a numerical standpoint, the proteins of the cell form the most important class of drug receptors. Obvious examples are the natural physiological receptors mentioned above, the enzymes of crucial metabolic or regulatory pathways (*e.g.*, dihydrofolate reductase, acetylcholinesterase), proteins involved in transport processes (*e.g.*, Na^+,K^+-ATPase), or proteins that serve structural roles (*e.g.*, tubulin). Specific binding properties of other cellular constituents can also be exploited. Thus, nucleic acids are important drug receptors, particularly for chemotherapeutic approaches to the control of malignancy.

The binding of drugs to receptors can involve all known types of interactions—ionic, hydrogen, hydrophobic, van der Waals, and covalent. In most interactions between drugs and receptors it is likely that bonds of multiple types are important. If binding is covalent, the duration of drug action is frequently, but not necessarily, prolonged. Noncovalent interactions of high affinity may also appear to be essentially irreversible.

Structure–Activity Relationship. Both the affinity of a drug for its receptor and its intrinsic activity are intimately related to its chemical structure. The relationship is frequently quite stringent. Relatively minor modifications in the drug molecule, including such subtle changes as stereoisomerism, may result in major changes in pharmacological properties. Exploitation of structure–activity relationships has on many occasions led to the synthesis of valuable therapeutic agents. Because changes in molecular configuration need not alter all actions and effects of a drug equally, it is sometimes possible to develop a congener with a more favorable ratio of therapeutic to toxic effects, enhanced selectivity among different cells or tissues, or more acceptable secondary characteristics than those of the parent drug. Therapeutically useful antagonists of hormones or neurotransmitters have been developed by chemical modification of the structure of the physiological agonist. Minor modifications of structure can also have profound effects on the pharmacokinetic properties of drugs.

Given adequate information about both the molecular structures and the pharmacological activities of a relatively large group of congeners, it should be possible to identify those properties that are required for optimal action at the receptor—size, shape, the position and orientation of charged groups or hydrogen bond donors, and so on. Although this goal is rarely approached in practice, recent advances in computational chemistry and structural analysis of organic compounds have given new impetus to the quantitation of structure–activity relationships and drug design. Molecular modeling of drug binding sites has been used to predict the placement of functional groups in the drug molecule to enhance activity or selectivity or to alter pharmacokinetic properties. This practice is a sharp departure from the traditional quasi-random synthesis and screening of congeners. More exciting are recent advances in using the structures of receptors, determined at atomic resolution by X-ray crystallography, for the initial design of ligands. To date, this approach has been restricted to soluble drug receptors, generally enzymes. However, the ability to clone and express DNA molecules that encode less abundant regulatory proteins and increasing success in the crystallization of membrane-bound proteins hold great promise for drug design based on a detailed knowledge of the drug binding site and the effect of drug binding on receptor structure (*see* Marshall, 1987).

Cellular Sites of Drug Action. The sites at which a drug acts and the extent of its action are determined by the localization and functional capacity of the specific receptors with which the drug interacts and the concentration of drug to which the receptor is exposed. Selective localization of drug action is therefore not necessarily dependent upon selective distribution of the drug. If a drug acts on a receptor that serves functions common to most cells, its effects will be widespread. If the function is a vital one, the drug will be particularly difficult or dangerous to use. Nevertheless, such a drug may be clinically important. Digitalis glycosides, important in the treatment of heart failure, are potent inhibitors of an ion transport process that is vital to most cells. As such, they can cause widespread toxicity, and their margin of safety is dangerously low. Other examples could be cited, particularly in the area of cancer chemotherapy.

If a drug interacts with receptors that are unique to only a few types of differentiated cells, its effects are more specific. The hypothetical ideal drug would cause its therapeutic effect by virtue of such types of action. Side effects would be minimized, but toxicity might not be. If the differentiated function were a vital one, this type of drug could also be very dangerous. Some of the most lethal chemical agents known (*e.g.*, botulinus toxin) show such specificity and toxicity. Note also that even if the primary action of a drug is localized, the physiologic effects of the drug may be widespread.

RECEPTORS FOR PHYSIOLOGICAL REGULATORY MOLECULES

In the discussion above, the term *receptor* has been used operationally to denote any cellular macromolecule to which a drug binds to initiate its effects. The functional properties of the receptors that have been used as examples are evident. In addition, however, there exist groups of cellular proteins whose normal function is to act as receptors for endogenous regulatory ligands—particularly hormones, neurotransmitters, and autacoids (*see* Cold Spring Harbor Symposium, 1988). The function of such physiological receptors, many of which are components of the plasma membrane, consists of binding the appropriate ligand and propagating its regulatory signal in the target cell, either by virtue of a direct intracellular effect or by promoting the synthesis or release of another intracellular regulatory molecule, known as a *second messenger*.

Identification of the two functions of a receptor, ligand binding and message propagation, led to speculation on the existence of functional domains within the receptor: a *ligand-binding domain* and an *effector domain*. The evolution of different receptors for diverse ligands that act by similar biochemical mechanisms, on the one hand, and of multiple receptors for a single ligand that act by unrelated mechanisms, on the other, supports this concept. Indeed, elucidation of the structure of a well-characterized receptor often allows the identification of these specialized domains within the primary amino acid sequence or the three-dimensional structure of the protein.

In some cases, an individual receptor molecule may interact with closely associated cellular proteins in order to generate its effect; this constitutes a *receptor–effector system*. A particularly well-characterized example of such a system is the hormone-sensitive adenylyl cyclase system. Here, receptors regulate the activity of the enzyme adenylyl cyclase, the effector that synthesizes the second messenger adenosine 3′,5′-monophosphate (cyclic AMP). This system is complex, in that two separate guanine nucleotide–binding regulatory proteins (G proteins) act as intermediaries between receptors and the enzyme. One serves to transduce stimulatory signals, while the other is involved with inhibitory events (*see* below).

Receptors (and their associated effector and coupling proteins) also act as integrators of extracellular information as they coordinate signals from multiple ligands with each other and with the metabolic activities of the cell (*see* below). This integrative function is particularly evident when one considers that the different receptors for scores of chemically unrelated ligands utilize relatively few biochemical mechanisms to exert their regulatory functions, and that even these few pathways may share common elements.

Physiological Receptors: Structural and Functional Families. The last decade has witnessed both a vast extension and a coalescence of our knowledge of the structures, mechanisms of action, and biochemical functions of physiological receptors. Members of the various classes of receptors and many of the other proteins that are involved in biological signal transduction have been purified. The mechanism of action of most of these molecules is now understood in considerable detail. Molecular cloning has provided amino acid sequences for dozens of receptors, permitted their expression and study in genetically defined backgrounds, and allowed a detailed analysis of structure–function relationships of signaling proteins through site-directed mutagenesis.

Receptors for physiological regulatory molecules fall into a few families—probably fewer than ten—that share homologous structures and common mechanisms of action (Figure 2–1). The idea that a receptor has two domains has advanced to understanding of the structure of common effector domains for numerous receptors and at least a rudimentary understanding of

A

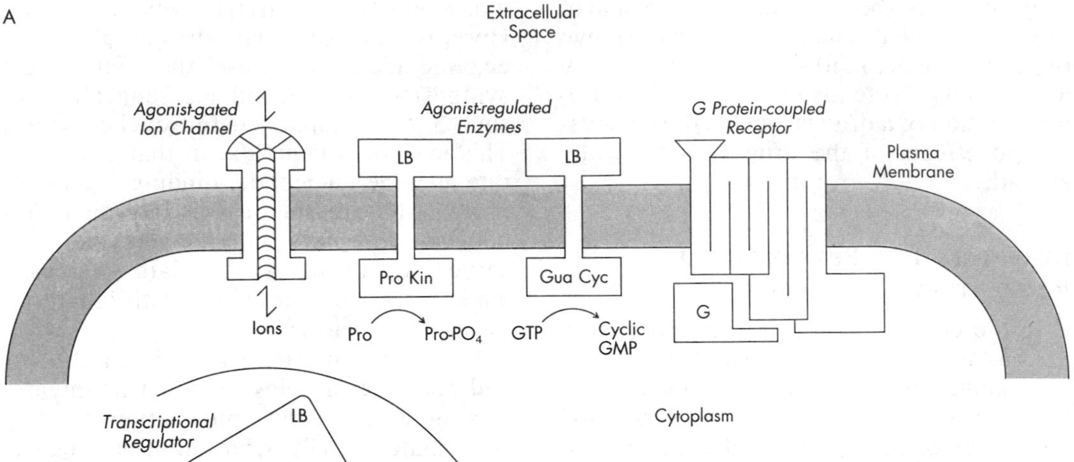

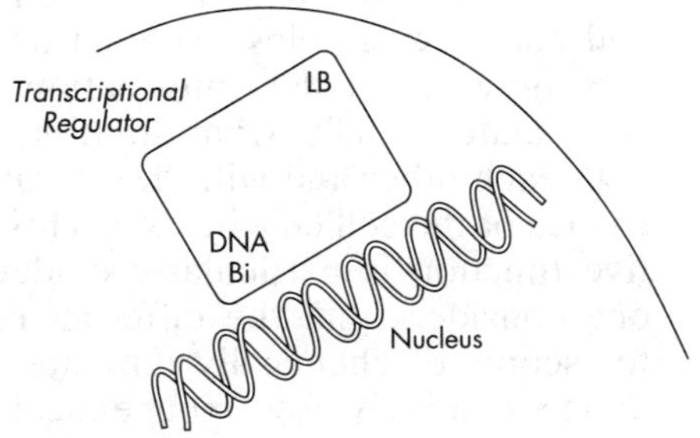

B

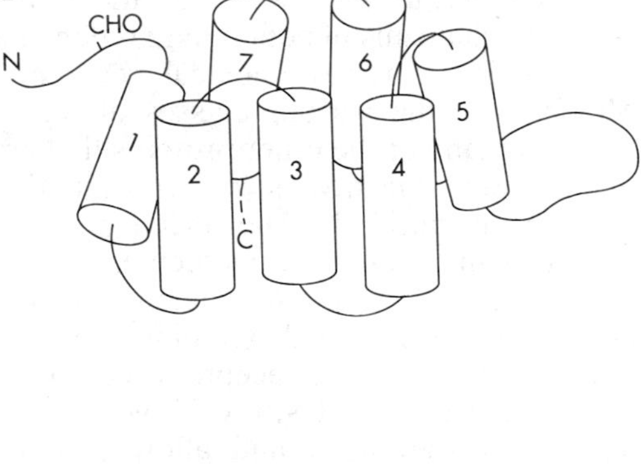

Figure 2–1. *Structural motifs of physiological receptors.*

A. The individual classes of physiological receptors are built from definable functional domains. The agonist-gated ion channels, shown at the left, are composed of several subunits (each of which may contain many membrane-spanning sequences) that are arrayed around the central channel. (For a more detailed model of such a receptor, *see* Figure 9–1, page 168. Voltage-gated ion channels are related molecules; *see* Figure 15–1, page 314, and Figure 15–2, page 315.) Catalytic receptors that function as protein kinases (Pro Kin) or guanylyl cyclases (Gua Cyc) have presumably globular catalytic domains on the cytoplasmic face of the plasma membrane, separated from their ligand binding (LB) domains by a single membrane-spanning polypeptide sequence. The ligand-binding site of the G protein–coupled receptors apparently lies within a bundle of seven membrane spanning helices, to which the G protein binds on the intracellular face of the receptor (*see* Figure 2–1, *B*). Although the nuclear receptors that regulate the transcription of DNA are soluble proteins with a single subunit, their carboxyl-terminal ligand binding domains are structurally separable from their regulatory DNA-binding domains (DNA Bi).

B. G protein–coupled receptors are thought to fold as seven membrane-spanning helices (cylinders numbered 1 to 7) with the glycosylated (CHO) amino terminus outside the cell. The actual spatial positioning of the helices is speculative. Ligands such as β-adrenergic and muscarinic agonists appear to bind within the bundle of helices, such that an agonist can induce a conformational change on the receptor's cytoplasmic face (bottom of figure). (From Ross, 1989; © Cell Press.)

some of the structures that form ligand binding domains. The small number of mechanisms and structural formats has profound implications both for the integration of signals from receptors for diverse ligands and for the regulation of receptors and receptor–effector systems by the target cell. (For more detailed discussions of individual receptors, *see* Cold Spring Harbor Symposium, 1988.)

Receptors for steroid hormones, thyroid hormone, vitamin D, and the retinoids form one of the better understood families (Evans, 1988). These receptors are soluble DNA-binding proteins that regulate the transcription of specific genes. They provide striking examples of conservation of structure and mechanism, in part because they are assembled as three largely independent domains. The region nearest the carboxyl terminus binds hormone and serves a negative regulatory role; that is, removal of this domain leaves a constitutively active fragment that may be nearly as effective at regulating transcription as is the intact hormone-liganded receptor. Hormone binding presumably also relieves this inhibitory constraint. The central region of the receptor mediates binding to specific sites on nuclear DNA to activate or inhibit transcription of the nearby gene. These regulatory sites in DNA are likewise receptor-specific: the sequence of a "glucocorticoid-responsive element," with only slight variation, is associated with each glucocorticoid-responsive gene. The function of the amino-terminal region of the receptor is less well defined, but its loss decreases the receptor's regulatory activity. The DNA-binding receptors form a homologous family, sharing quite similar amino acid sequences in their DNA-binding domains, less similarity in their hormone-binding domains, and negligible similarity at their amino termini. The activity of each domain is stereotyped and largely independent, a phenomenon best demonstrated by the construction of chimeric receptors. If the hormone-binding domain of one receptor is fused genetically to the DNA-binding regulatory domain of another, the resultant chimera will bind and be controlled by the ligand of one "parent" and will bind to and regulate the genes typically controlled by the other.

Receptors for peptide hormones that regulate growth, differentiation, and development (and in some cases acute metabolic activity) are frequently protein kinases that act by phosphorylating target proteins on tyrosine residues (Yarden and Ullrich, 1988). It is often difficult to identify and study these targets, which may be enzymes (including other kinases), regulatory proteins, or structural proteins, but phosphorylation is assumed to alter their individual activities. This family includes the receptors for insulin, epidermal growth factor, platelet-derived growth factor, and certain lymphokines. These receptors are also assembled from definable domains that are distinguished in part by their location relative to the plasma membrane. The extracellular, hormone-binding domain is connected to an intracellular protein kinase catalytic domain by a relatively short sequence of hydrophobic amino acid residues that cross the plasma membrane. Hormone binding domains and catalytic domains that have been expressed separately retain their distinct activities. Because of the homology among the protein kinase domains in this family, active chimeric receptors have been constructed from different intracellular (catalytic) and extracellular (hormone binding) regions; these chimeras display specificity for hormones and substrates that reflects their parentage.

The domain structure just described for the tyrosine protein kinases is varied in other receptors to utilize other signaling outputs. In one receptor for atrial natriuretic peptide, the intracellular domain is not a protein kinase, but rather a guanylyl cyclase that synthesizes the second messenger cyclic GMP (Chinkers *et al.*, 1989). Although other receptors with guanylyl cyclase activity have not yet been identified in mammals, several serve as pheromone receptors in invertebrates. There may be other variations on this transmembrane topology. A protein tyrosine phosphatase described recently has an extracellular domain with a sequence reminiscent of cellular adhesion molecules (Charbonneau *et al.*, 1989). The receptor for nerve growth factor, which is oriented similarly across the membrane, has an intracellular domain of unknown function.

Receptors for several neurotransmitters form ion-selective channels in the plasma membrane and convey their signals by altering the cell's membrane potential or ionic composition. This group includes the nicotinic cholinergic receptor, the gamma-aminobutyrate type A receptor, and receptors for glutamate, aspartate, and glycine (*see* Chapters 5, 9, and 12). They are all multi-subunit proteins that span the plasma membrane many times to form the channel. They display some similarity of amino acid sequence, but they do not have easily identifiable structural domains. It is not yet clear how binding of transmitter to the channel's extracellular face causes the channel to open.

A large number of receptors in the plasma membrane regulate distinct effector proteins through the mediation of a group of GTP binding proteins known as G proteins (Ross, 1989). Receptors for biogenic amines, eicosanoids, and many peptide hormones all utilize G protein–coupled receptors. Receptors in this group act by facilitating the binding of GTP to specific G proteins. GTP binding activates the G protein, such that it in turn can regulate the activity of specific effectors. The effectors include enzymes such as adenylyl cyclase and phospholipases C and A_2; channels that are specific for Ca^{2+}, K^+, or Na^+; and certain transport proteins. An individual cell may express five or more G proteins; each of these may respond to several different receptors and regulate several different effectors with a characteristic pattern of selectivities. G protein–linked receptors and the G proteins themselves both constitute families of homologous proteins. The receptors are hydrophobic molecules that span the plasma membrane in seven α-helical segments; they interact with G proteins at their cytoplasmic face. The hormone binding site evidently consists of a pocket formed within the bundle of membrane-spanning helices. By using chimeras and other genetic and biochemical techniques, it has been possible to define a specific region that is responsible for regulation and selectivity among the different G proteins.

The G proteins are bound to the inner face of the plasma membrane. They are heterotrimeric molecules (subunits are designated α, β, and γ), and their classification is based on the identity of their distinct α subunit. These polypeptides have highly homologous guanine nucleotide binding domains, and they are thought to have distinct domains for interactions with receptors and effectors. When the system is inactive, GDP is bound to the α subunit (Figure 2–2). An agonist–receptor complex facilitates GTP binding to α in part by promoting the dissociation of this GDP. Binding of GTP activates the α subunit, and α-GTP is then thought to dissociate from βγ and interact with a membrane-bound effector. Termination of signal transmission results from hydrolysis of GTP to GDP by a GTPase that is intrinsic to the α subunit. Thus, G proteins serve as regulated molecular switches in transmembrane signaling systems. The switch is turned on by the receptor; it turns itself off within a few seconds—a time sufficient for considerable amplification of signal transmission (*see* Gilman, 1987, 1989).

If a cell has several receptors that regulate a common effector or that utilize a common transducer, many individual extracellular signals can be integrated to yield a cumulative intracellular signal. G protein–coupled receptor–effector systems provide impressive examples of such integration, as well as the ability to direct a signal to divergent cellular effectors (Figure 2–3). It is not unusual for several receptors in an individual cell to activate a single G protein; several agonists may stimulate adenylyl cyclase through a single G protein known as G_s. One receptor can also regulate more than one G protein; an individual muscarinic receptor can cause the inhibition of adenylyl cyclase and the activation of phospholipase C by interactions with at least two different G proteins. Similarly, one G protein can regulate several effectors (the same G protein that activates adenylyl cyclase also activates a Ca^{2+} channel), and one effector can respond to multiple G proteins (phospholipase Cs are activated by at least two different G proteins in response to distinct groups of receptors). Thus, the receptor–G protein–effector systems are complex networks of convergent and divergent interactions that permit extraordinarily versatile regulation of cell function.

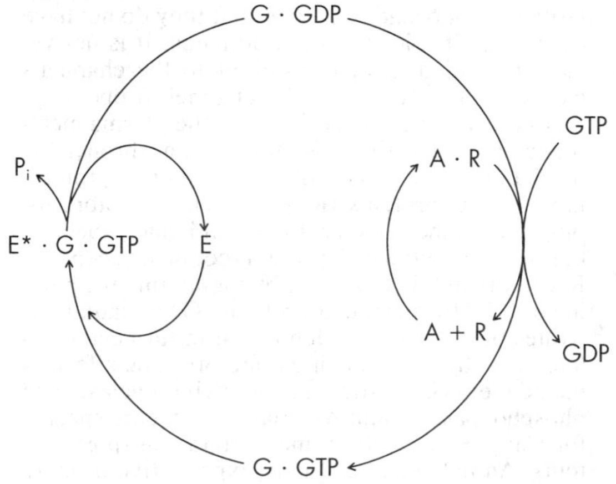

Figure 2–2. *The regulatory cycles involved in G protein–mediated signal transduction.*

A = agonist; R = receptor; G = G protein; E = effector; E* = activated effector. *See* the text for a detailed description.

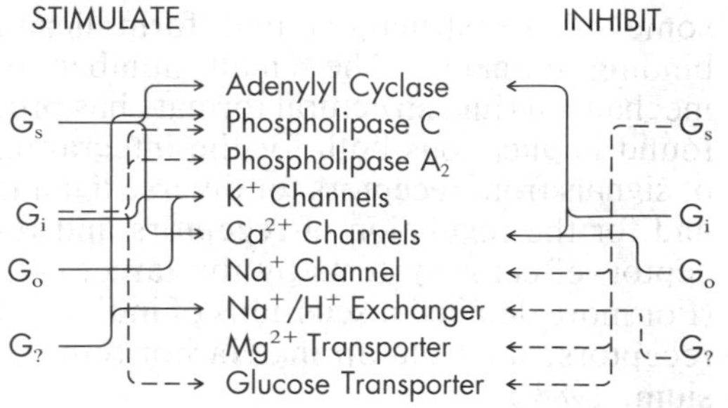

Figure 2–3. *The G protein–effector regulatory network.*

G proteins convey stimulatory and inhibitory signals to several effector proteins. In some cases, the G protein that controls a specific effector has not been identified ($G_?$). In others (Ca^{2+} channels and K^+ channels), isoforms of the effector may be differentially sensitive to different G proteins. Relatively well-characterized pathways are shown with solid lines; less well-defined pathways are indicated with dashed lines. This diagram underestimates the complexity of the network.

Cytoplasmic Second Messengers. Physiological signals are also integrated within the cell as a result of interactions between second messenger pathways (Figure 2–4). There are relatively few recognized cytoplasmic second messengers. Thus, their synthesis or release often results from activation of many pathways. Second messengers influence each other both directly, by altering the other's metabolism, and indirectly, by sharing intracellular targets. This superficially confusing pattern of regulatory pathways allows the cell to respond to agonists, singly or in combinations, with an integrated array of cytoplasmic second messengers and responses.

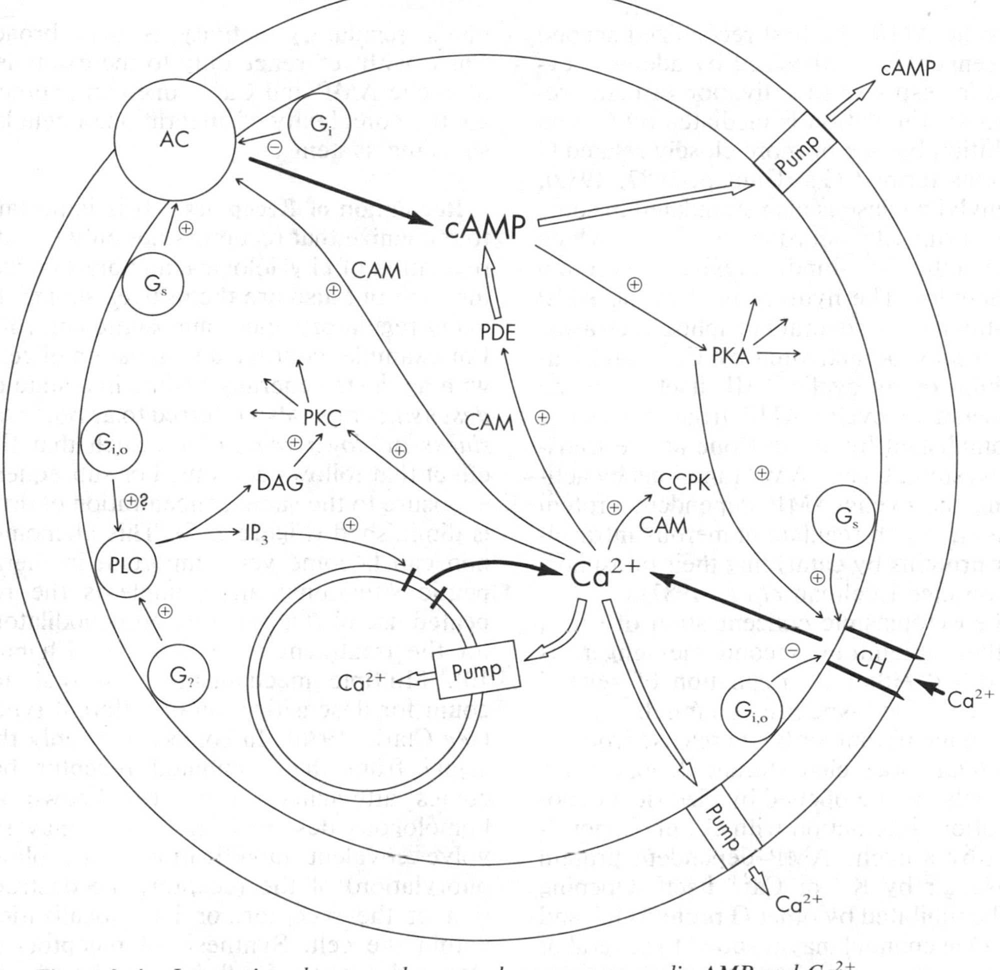

Figure 2–4. *Interactions between the second messengers cyclic AMP and Ca^{2+}.*

The second messengers cyclic AMP and Ca^{2+} regulate cell function through parallel and highly interactive pathways. In this diagram, single arrows indicate regulation (either activation [+] or inhibition [−]), bold arrows indicate synthesis or entry of messenger, and open arrows indicate degradation or loss of messenger.

Ca^{2+} enters the cytoplasm both from outside the cell (via several types of Ca^{2+}-specific channels [CH]) and from intracellular organellar storage depots. Cyclic AMP (cAMP) is synthesized from ATP by the enzyme adenylyl cyclase (AC) in the plasma membrane. Adenylyl cyclase is activated by the G protein G_s, which, in myocardial plasma membranes, activates Ca^{2+} channels as well. These channels are also activated by phosphorylation, which is catalyzed by the cyclic AMP–dependent protein kinase (PKA). Adenylyl cyclase is inhibited by G_i, and some neuronal Ca^{2+} channels are also inhibited by G_i or G_o. In addition, neuronal adenylyl cyclase is stimulated by Ca^{2+} when the ion is bound to a cytoplasmic Ca^{2+} binding–regulatory protein, calmodulin (CAM). Release of Ca^{2+} from organellar stores is mediated by inositol trisphosphate (IP_3), the product of the phospholipase C (PLC)–catalyzed hydrolysis of phosphatidylinositol bisphosphate. Ca^{2+} and diacylglycerol (DAG), the other product of the phospholipase C reaction, combine to activate protein kinase C (PKC).

Cyclic AMP is hydrolyzed by several phosphodiesterases (PDE), one of which is activated by Ca^{2+} plus calmodulin, and cyclic AMP is actively excreted from some cells by a specific pump. Ca^{2+} is removed from the cytoplasm by pumps in the plasma membrane and intracellular organelles.

Cyclic AMP acts exclusively through cyclic AMP–dependent protein kinase to phosphorylate enzymes (including other protein kinases) and proteins involved in transport and structure. Ca^{2+} regulates its many targets through protein kinase C, calmodulin (which activates a distinct protein kinase, CCPK), and other Ca^{2+}-binding proteins. This figure is an oversimplification of an extraordinarily complex regulatory network.

Cyclic AMP, the first recognized second messenger, is synthesized by adenylyl cyclase in response to activation of many receptors; stimulation is mediated by G_s and inhibition by one or more closely related G proteins termed G_is (Gilman, 1987, 1989). Adenylyl cyclase is also stimulated in some cells, primarily neurons, by Ca^{2+}, which acts via the Ca^{2+}-binding regulatory protein calmodulin. The hydrolysis of cyclic AMP is catalyzed by several phosphodiesterases, which may be activated by Ca^{2+} and calmodulin or by cyclic AMP itself, and the extrusion of cyclic AMP from the cell is accomplished by at least one active transport system. Cyclic AMP functions by activating the cyclic AMP–dependent protein kinases, which regulate numerous intracellular proteins by catalyzing their phosphorylation (*see* Edelman *et al.,* 1987).

The cytoplasmic concentration of Ca^{2+}, another ubiquitous second messenger, is controlled either by regulation of several different Ca^{2+}-specific channels in the plasma membrane or by its release from intracellular organellar storage depots. Ca^{2+} channels can be opened by electrical depolarization, interaction with G_s, phosphorylation by a cyclic AMP–dependent protein kinase, or by K^+ or Ca^{2+} itself. Opening can be inhibited by other G proteins (G_i and G_o). One channel may respond to several of these inputs.

Release of Ca^{2+} from intracellular depots is mediated by yet another second messenger, inositol 1,4,5-trisphosphate (IP_3). IP_3 is the product of the hydrolysis of the membrane lipid phosphatidylinositol 4,5-bisphosphate; this reaction is catalyzed by a phospholipase C (*see* Berridge, 1987). The relevant enzyme is itself regulated by at least two different G proteins, neither of which has been identified. Ca^{2+} regulates cellular activity by interaction with several protein mediators, but the salient examples are protein kinase C and calmodulin. Protein kinase C, like the cyclic AMP–dependent protein kinase, has many substrates, including several proteins that are involved in other signaling systems. The activation of protein kinase C by Ca^{2+} is potentiated by diacylglycerol, the other product of the phospholipase C reaction that liberates IP_3. The scope of calmodulin's regulatory activity is also broad. Thus, with reference only to the examples of cyclic AMP and Ca^{2+}, one can appreciate the complexity of integration of cellular signaling systems.

Regulation of Receptors. It is important to recognize that receptors not only initiate regulation of physiological and biochemical function but also are themselves subject to many regulatory and homeostatic controls. For example, continued stimulation of cells with agonists generally results in a state of *desensitization* (also referred to as *refractoriness* or *down regulation*), such that the effect that follows continued or subsequent exposure to the same concentration of drug is diminished (Figure 2–5). This phenomenon can become very important in therapeutic situations; an example is the repeated use of β-adrenergic bronchodilators for the treatment of asthma (*see* Chapter 10). Multiple mechanisms exist that account for desensitization of different types (*see* Clark, 1986). In some cases, only the signal from the stimulated receptor becomes attenuated, a process known as homologous desensitization. This may involve covalent modification (*e.g.,* phosphorylation) of the receptor, the destruction of the receptor, or its relocalization within the cell. Synthesis of receptors is also subject to feedback regulation. In other situations, receptors for different hormones that act on a single signaling pathway may become less effective. Such heterologous desensitization may result either from modification of each receptor by a common feedback mechanism or from effects exerted at some common point in the effector pathway distal to the receptor itself.

Predictably, hyperreactivity or supersensitivity to receptor agonists is also frequently observed to follow reduction in the chronic level of receptor stimulation. Situations of this type can result from the long-term administration of antagonists such as propranolol (*see* Chapter 11). In at least some cases supersensitivity may result from the synthesis of additional receptors.

Diseases Resulting from Receptor Malfunction. In addition to variability among individuals in their

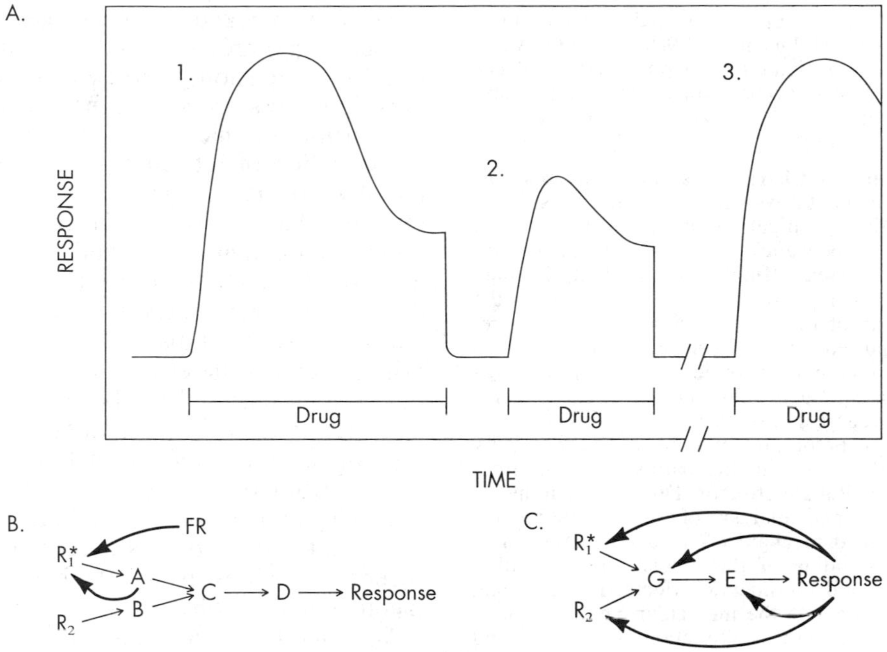

Figure 2–5. *Desensitization in response to an agonist.*

A. (1) Upon exposure to an agonist, the initial response usually peaks and then decreases to approach some tonic level, elevated but below the maximum. (2) If the drug is removed for a brief period, the state of desensitization is maintained. (3) Removal of the drug for a more extended period allows the cell to "reset" its capacity to respond. *B* and *C*. Desensitization may be homologous (*B*), that is, acting only on the stimulated receptor, or heterologous (*C*), acting on several receptors or on a pathway that is common to many receptors. Single arrows in *B* and *C* show the primary response pathway, while bold arrows show the feedback mechanisms that cause desensitization. Mechanisms for homologous desensitization must arise from a pathway that is unique to a single receptor or from a feedback regulator (FR) that can specifically detect the agonist-liganded form of the receptor (R*). For example, the receptors coupled to G proteins can be phosphorylated by protein kinases that act selectively on the agonist-liganded form (*see* Benovic *et al.*, 1989). Heterologous desensitization can potentially arise from any point on a common pathway and regulate any upstream event, as shown for a G protein–regulated pathway.

responses to drugs (Chapter 4), several definable diseases arise from disorders in receptors or receptor–effector systems. The loss of a receptor in a highly specialized signaling system may cause a relatively limited phenotypic disorder, such as the genetic deficiency of the androgen receptor in the testicular feminization syndrome (Griffin and Wilson, 1989). Deficiencies of more widely used signaling systems have a broader spectrum of effects, as are seen in myasthenia gravis or some forms of insulin-resistant diabetes mellitus, which result from autoimmune depletion of nicotinic cholinergic receptors (Chapter 7) or insulin receptors (Chapter 61), respectively. A lesion in a component of a signaling pathway that is used by many receptors can cause a generalized endocrinopathy. Heterozygous deficiency of G_s, the G protein that activates adenylyl cyclase in all cells, causes multiple endocrine disorders; the disease is termed pseudohypoparathyroidism type 1a (Spiegel, 1989). Homozygous deficiency in G_s would presumably be lethal.

The expression of aberrant or ectopic receptors, effectors, or coupling proteins can potentially lead to supersensitivity, subsensitivity, or other untoward responses. Among the most interesting and significant events is the appearance of aberrant receptors as products of oncogenes, which transform otherwise normal cells into malignant cells. Virtually any type of signaling system may have oncogenic potential. The *erb*A oncogene product is an altered form of a receptor for thyroid hormone, constitutively active because of the loss of its ligand binding domain (Evans, 1988). The *ros* and *erb*B oncogene products are activated, uncontrolled forms of the receptors for insulin and epidermal growth factor, both known to enhance cellular proliferation (Yarden and Ullrich, 1988). The *mas* oncogene product (Young *et al.*, 1986) is a G protein–coupled receptor, probably the receptor for a peptide hormone. Although the metabolic explanation for its oncogenic activity is uncertain, a receptor for 5-hydroxytryptamine (5-HT_{1c}) is also oncogenic when expressed at high concentrations in certain cells (Julius *et al.*, 1989). Even G_s, when constitutively activated by a point mutation, has been identified as an oncogene in certain pituitary tumors (Landis *et al.*, 1989).

Detection and Characterization of Receptors by Ligand-Binding Assays. Much of the success in the identification, purification, and characterization of receptors reflects the development of radioactive ligands with great affinity and specificity for individual receptors. Use of such ligands permits the direct study of the drug-binding properties of receptors and reduces the need to rely on inferences derived from the measurement of distal physiological responses. Such inferences are treacherous if the observed response lies many steps removed from the receptor and may be compromised by changes at any site in the pathway leading from receptor to ultimate effector. Direct measurements of receptors and analysis of their ligand-binding properties and mechanisms of action have led to our understanding of the mechanisms of pathophysiology and therapeutic effects. For example, we now appreciate the molecular causes of many diseases of receptor malfunction (*see* above) and can deal with them more effectively. Ligand-binding studies at the light and electron microscopic levels with preparations from the central nervous system can localize receptors and, by inference, specific synapses. This ability facilitates the mapping of pathways of neurotransmission and understanding their organization. Furthermore, ligand-binding assays for many individual receptors are requisite for their purification and molecular characterization. Again, one may not be able to rely on the response that is characteristic of the drug–receptor complex for assay during receptor purification, because other components of the system necessary for the response may be lost. The ultimate goal of this type of research is to analyze the molecular events that are responsible for the interactions between the essential components of the system. Studies of this kind will allow a detailed definition of the differences between subtypes of receptors (*e.g.*, nicotinic and muscarinic receptors for acetylcholine) and an understanding of how receptors function and are regulated.

Classification of Receptors and Drug Effects. Drug receptors have traditionally been identified and classified primarily on the basis of the effect and relative potency of selective agonists and antagonists—the structure–activity relationship (*see* Molinoff *et al.*, 1981). For example, the effects of acetylcholine that are mimicked by the alkaloid muscarine and that are selectively antagonized by atropine are termed *muscarinic effects*. Other effects of acetylcholine that are mimicked by nicotine and that are not readily antagonized by atropine but are selectively blocked by other agents (*e.g.*, tubocurarine) are described as *nicotinic effects*. By extension, these two types of cholinergic effects are said to be mediated by muscarinic or nicotinic receptors. Such classification of receptors results in an internally consistent scheme that supports the view that two types of receptor are involved. Although it frequently contributes little to delineation of the mechanism of drug action, such categorization does provide a convenient basis for summarizing drug effects. If the effects and receptors in the various tissues have been classified, a statement that a drug activates a specified type of receptor is a succinct summary of its spectrum of effects and of the agents that will antagonize it. Similarly, a statement that a drug blocks a certain type of receptor specifies the agents that it will antagonize and at what sites.

Significance of Receptor Subtypes. As the diversity and selectivity of drugs have increased, it has become clear that multiple subtypes of receptors exist within many previously defined classes of receptors. Moreover, molecular cloning frequently reveals the presence of several closely related subtypes of receptors where only a single species was thought to exist. Knowledge of receptor subtypes is of interest to the researcher and of utility to the clinician who desires to manipulate them. In the case of the nicotinic cholinergic receptor, referred to above, there are distinct differences in the ligand-binding and functional properties between the receptors that are found in the ganglia of the autonomic nervous system and those at the somatic neuromuscular junction. This difference is exploited for therapeutic benefit. Thus, antagonists that act preferentially at the nicotinic receptors in ganglia can be used to control blood pressure; they do not, happily, paralyze skeletal muscle. Tubocurarine and related agents constitute the converse example, and their ability to antagonize the action of acetylcholine is relatively well confined to the receptor sites at the neuromuscular junction. These subtypes of the nicotinic receptor or, for example, the subtypes of the β-adrenergic receptor for catecholamines (*e.g.*, β_1 in the heart, β_2 in the bronchi) are conceptually analogous to tissue-specific isozymes of an enzyme. In these instances, the mechanisms of action of the subtypes are largely identical, but they presumably fulfill important tissue-specific functions, either in their differential sensitivity to endogenous ligands or in their intracellular effects. Different receptor subtypes may also be found within a single tissue at different stages of growth and development, again presumably reflecting altered needs of the organism. With the application of molecular cloning techniques to the analysis of the multiplicity of receptors and to their structures, new subtypes of previously well known receptors are being discovered at a rapid pace; exploitation of this knowledge for therapy is being pursued actively.

Subtypes of some classes of receptors (*e.g.*, α_1- and α_2-adrenergic or M_1- and M_2-muscarinic) also display fundamental differences in their biochemical regulatory activities. Such differences allow an agonist to evoke unique responses in specific cells or tissues. When a tissue or cell expresses more than a single subtype of receptor or when only insufficiently selective drugs are available, identification of the specific signal that is generated by an individual receptor may require approaches such as expression of the cloned gene for the receptor in a well-studied cellular background.

Regardless of their mechanistic meaning (or lack thereof), schemes of receptor classification have facilitated the development of a number of therapeutic agents that have selectivity for specific types or subtypes of receptors. Such drug development has allowed the clinician to utilize more fully the therapeutic efficacy of these compounds, while limiting the frequency or intensity of unwanted effects.

Actions of Drugs Not Mediated by Receptors

If one restricts the definition of receptors to *macro*molecules, then several drugs may be said not to act by virtue of combination with receptors. Certain drugs may interact specifically with small molecules or ions that are normally or abnormally found in the body. The chelating agents, which bind a variety of metal cations, are an excellent example (*see* Chapter 66). Chelators are available that show a remarkable degree of preference for specific ionic species—even among divalent cations. Thus, the affinity of ethylenediaminetetraacetate (EDTA) is ten orders of magnitude greater for Pb^{2+} than it is for Ba^{2+}, Sr^{2+}, or Mg^{2+}. A less specific but still gratifying example is the therapeutic neutralization of gastric acid by a base (antacid).

Certain drugs that are structural analogs of normal biological chemicals may be incorporated into cellular components and thereby alter their function. This property has been termed a "counterfeit incorporation mechanism" (*see* Pratt and Taylor, 1990). It has been particularly useful with analogs of pyrimidines and purines that can be incorporated into nucleic acids, yielding drugs that have clinical utility in cancer and viral chemotherapy (*see* Chapters 51 and 52).

Additionally, there is a group of agents that act more by virtue of their colligative effects than by more classical chemical mechanisms. A hint of this type of mechanism is provided by a lack of requirement for highly specific chemical structure. Stereoisomers or close congeners of such drugs would not be expected to differ in their potency or efficacy. For example, certain relatively benign compounds, such as mannitol, can be administered in quantities sufficient to increase the osmolarity of various body fluids, and thereby cause appropriate changes in the distribution of water (*see* Chapter 28). Depending on the agent and route of administration, this effect can be exploited to promote diuresis, catharsis, expansion of circulating volume in the vascular compartment, or reduction of cerebral edema. The volatile general anesthetic agents interact with membranes to depress excitability. They appear to act colligatively as solutes in the lipid bilayer of the membrane. Their diversity of structure is consistent with such a mechanism; their individual potencies correlate best with their oil:water partition coefficients.

QUANTITATION OF DRUG-RECEPTOR INTERACTIONS

As early as 1878, even before he coined the term *receptive substance*, Langley suggested that drug–cell combinations, and hence the actions and effects of drugs, were probably governed by the law of mass action. This view was extensively developed by A. J. Clark in the 1920s, and it remains basic to most theories of drug action (*see* Clark, 1933). Thus, the quantitative analysis of drug action borrows freely from theory developed for ligand-binding reactions and for enzyme–substrate interaction, and there is obvious coalescence when the effect of a drug results from a direct interaction with an enzyme.

When one attempts to extend analysis of drug–receptor interactions beyond the initial reaction—the binding of drug to receptor—important questions arise as to the relationship between the concentration of drug–receptor complex and the magnitude of the effect that is observed. In the classical receptor theory developed by Clark, it was assumed that the effect of a drug is proportional to the fraction of receptors occupied by drug, and that maximal effect results when all receptors are occupied. While these assumptions are probably true in some cases, exceptions are common, particularly when the pathway leading from receptor to effect is complex (*e.g.*, drug–receptor interaction → → alteration of cardiac contractility). However, the simplifying assumption has often served as a useful point of departure.

Molecular studies of how purified receptors regulate their cellular targets have actually reinforced Clark's initial simple model. Furthermore, many instances in which the proportionality between agonist binding and physiological response is not maintained can now be reconciled quantitatively. Thus, although the pursuit of mechanism via the mathematical description of dose–response relationships has usually produced more heat than light, the basic descriptive concepts are frequently instructive and help to provide an appreciation of how the concentration of a drug at its target organ determines the therapeutic response. It also provides a clear conceptual foundation for understanding the effects of antagonists. (*See* Limbird, 1986, for further discussion.)

Quantitative Descriptions of Drug Action. If one assumes that an agonist drug interacts reversibly with its receptor and that the resultant effect is proportional to the number of receptors occupied, the following reaction scheme can be written:

$$\text{Drug }(D) + \text{Receptor }(R) \underset{k_2}{\overset{k_1}{\rightleftharpoons}} DR \longrightarrow \text{Effect} \qquad (1)$$

The relationship between effect and the concentration of free drug can be described simply for this model as:

$$\text{Effect} = \frac{\text{Maximal Effect }[D]}{K_D + [D]} \qquad (2)$$

where $[D]$ is the concentration of free drug and K_D (equal to k_2/k_1) is the dissociation constant for the drug–receptor complex. The fraction of receptors that is occupied by drug is equal to $[D]/(K_D + [D])$. This equation describes a simple rectangular hyperbola and is analogous to the Michaelis–Menten equation that is used to describe the interaction of enzyme and substrate. There is no effect at $[D] = 0$; the effect is half-maximal when $[D] = K_D$, that is, when half the receptors are occupied; the maximal effect is approached asymptotically as $[D]$ increases above K_D (Figure 2–6, *A*). The scheme defines the drug's *potency*—that is, the dependency of its effect on its concentration—as being equal to its *affinity* for the receptor—that is, the dependency of binding on concentration. The concentration of the drug at which it is half-maximally effective, its EC_{50}, is equal to its K_D, the equilibrium dissociation constant. K_D has units of concentration and defines the concentration at which the receptor is half-maximally saturated.

It is frequently convenient to plot the magnitude of effect versus log $[D]$, because a wide range of drug concentrations is easily displayed and the potency of different drugs can be readily compared. In this case, the result is the familiar sigmoidal log dose–effect curve, probably the most intuitively helpful graphical display of drug action (Figure 2–6, *B*).

Linear forms of equation (2) are frequently encountered and were commonly used for quantita-

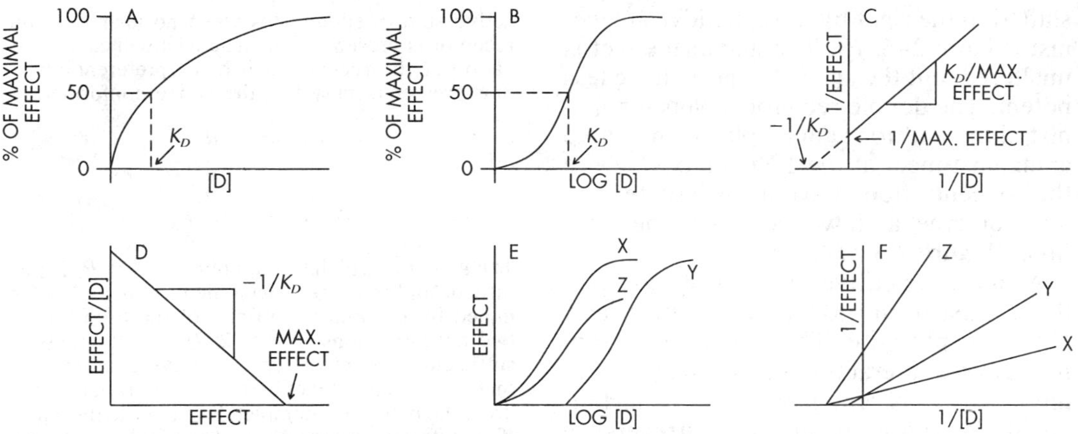

Figure 2–6. *Different representations of dose–effect curves.*

A. The ideal relationship between the concentration of a drug [D] and the magnitude of response to it. When plotted on a linear scale, a typical hyperbolic curve results.

B. A sigmoidal dose–effect curve results when the magnitude of effect observed is plotted versus the logarithm of the drug concentration.

C and *D.* A double-reciprocal plot (*C*) and a Scatchard or Eadie–Hofstee type of plot (*D*) of the concentration dependence of drug effect (*see* text for explanation).

E and *F.* Representative log dose–effect curves (*E*) and double-reciprocal plots (*F*).

Curves X and Y. Two agonists with similar efficacy but differing in potency (X more potent than Y) *or* an agonist in the absence (X) and presence (Y) of a competitive antagonist.

Curves X and Z. Two agonists with similar potency but differing in efficacy (full agonist, X, and partial agonist, Z) *or* an agonist in the absence (X) and presence (Z) of a noncompetitive antagonist.

tive analysis of data before the ready availability of computers. One linearization is obtained by taking the reciprocal of both sides of the expression and constructing the equivalent of the Lineweaver–Burk plot:

$$\frac{1}{\text{Effect}} = \frac{K_D}{\text{Max. Effect } [D]} + \frac{1}{\text{Max. Effect}} \qquad (3)$$

A plot of 1/Effect versus $1/[D]$ yields a straight line that intersects the Y-axis at 1/(Max. Effect) and the X-axis at $-1/K_D$. Its slope is equal to K_D/(Max. Effect) (Figure 2–6, *C*). Another common linearization, analogous to Scatchard or Eadie–Hofstee plots, is based on the equation:

$$\frac{\text{Effect}}{[D]} = -\left(\frac{1}{K_D}\right) \cdot \frac{\text{Effect} + \text{Max. Effect}}{K_D} \qquad (4)$$

Thus, a graph of Effect/$[D]$ versus Effect yields a line with a slope of $-1/K_D$ that intersects the X-axis at (Max. Effect) (Figure 2–6, *D*). Values for K_D and for the maximal effect can be readily estimated from such graphs. Additional numerical and graphic analytical methods are discussed by Segel (1984) and by Limbird (1986). Although these linearizations are not recommended as primary tools for the quantitative analysis of pharmacodynamic data, they can be useful as aids for recognizing nonideal behavior, which may appear as nonlinear plots. Numerous software systems designed specifically to analyze pharmacodynamic data are available for quantitative studies.

As stated above, certain drugs, termed *antagonists,* interact with the receptor or with other components of the effector mechanism to inhibit the action of an agonist, while initiating no effect themselves. If the inhibition can be overcome by increasing the concentration of the agonist, ultimately achieving the same maximal effect, the antagonist is said to be *competitive* or *surmountable*. This type of inhibition is commonly observed with antagonists that bind reversibly at the receptor site. (A somewhat similar situation would also result from reversible or irreversible interaction of the antagonist at other sites so that the affinity of the receptor for the agonist is decreased. This is, however, more appropriately referred to as negative cooperativity between the two drugs than as competitive antagonism.)

Because the maximal effect can still be achieved if sufficient agonist is used, the log dose–effect curve for the agonist is shifted to the right by a competitive antagonist (Figure 2–6, *E*). The maximal effect is unaltered, but the agonist appears to be less potent. The double reciprocal plots for agonist alone and for agonist plus competitive antagonist meet at the 1/Effect axis, where the concentration of agonist is infinite. The lines diverge at lower agonist concentrations (Figure 2–6, *F*).

A noncompetitive antagonist prevents the agonist from producing any effect at a given receptor site. This could result from irreversible interaction of the antagonist at any site to prevent binding of agonist. It could also follow reversible or irreversible interaction with any component of the system so as to decrease the effect of the binding of agonist. Intuitively, these results may be conceptualized as *removal* of receptor or of the system's capacity to respond. The maximal effect possible is reduced, but agonist can act normally at receptor–effector units that are not so influenced. The affinity of the agonist for the receptor and its potency are thus unaltered. The log dose–effect curves show unaltered potency and reduced efficacy (Figure 2–6, *E*). The double reciprocal plot shows intersection of the lines for agonist and for antagonist plus agonist on the $1/[D]$ axis at $-1/K_D$ (the affinity is unaltered). The maximal effect is different (Figure 2–6, *F*).

Antagonists may thus be classified as acting reversibly or irreversibly. If the antagonist binds at the active site for the agonist, reversible antagonists will be competitive and irreversible antagonists will be noncompetitive. If binding is elsewhere, however, these simple rules do not hold, and any combination is possible.

If two drugs bind to the same receptor at the same site, why can one be an agonist and the other produce no effect—acting as an antagonist because of its presence? This question lies at the heart of the biophysics of protein structure and protein–ligand interactions. Its answer is still only incompletely known. The literature on the kinetics, thermodynamics, and structural bases of ligand-induced conformational changes in proteins is vast. However, the following model may help to conceptualize a working answer to this question.

Consider a receptor that can exist in two conformations: active (*a*) or inactive (*i*). These might correspond to the open and closed states of an ion channel or the active and inactive forms of an enzyme. If these states are in equilibrium and the inactive state predominates when no ligand for the receptor is present, then an agonist will cause activation of the receptor if it binds preferentially to (has greater affinity for) the active conformation.

$$\begin{array}{ccc} R_i & \rightleftharpoons & R_a \\ \upharpoonleft\downharpoonright & & \upharpoonleft\downharpoonright \\ D \cdot R_i & \rightleftharpoons & D \cdot R_a \end{array}$$

The *extent* to which the equilibrium $R_i \rightleftharpoons R_a$ is perturbed, and thus the magnitude of effect, is determined by the *relative* affinity of the drug for the two conformations (Figure 2–7). A full agonist is sufficiently selective for the active conformation that, at a maximally effective concentration, it will drive the receptor "completely" to the active state. If a different but perhaps structurally analogous compound binds to the same site on R but with only slightly greater affinity for R_a than for R_i, the magnitude of effect observed may be less, despite the presence of maximally effective concentrations of the agent. A drug that displays such intermediate effectiveness is referred to as a *partial agonist*. (Partial agonists are not hypothetical; they are quite common.) It then follows that an agent that has equal affinity for R_i and R_a will not alter the preexisting equilibrium. Such a compound will have no activity as an agonist but, when bound,

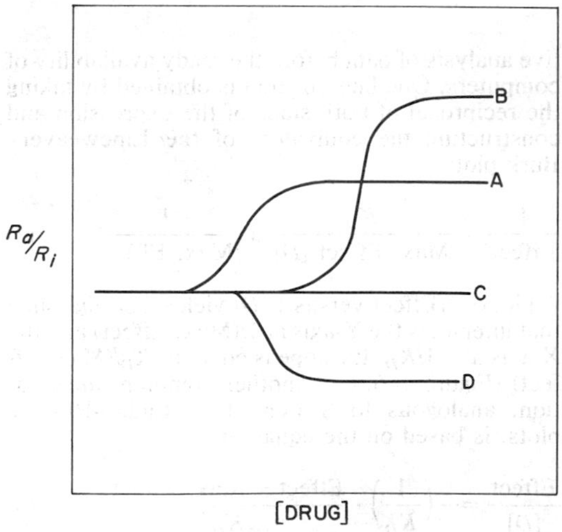

Figure 2–7. *Effects of drugs on the relative concentrations of two hypothetical forms of a receptor,* R_a *and* R_i*, that are in equilibrium* ($R_i \rightleftharpoons R_a$).

Drugs A through D all bind to both forms of the receptor but with differing absolute and relative affinities. For drug A, affinity (*K*) for $R_a > R_i$ and binding affinity is relatively high; for drug B, *K* for $R_a \gg R_i$, but binding affinity is relatively poor; for drug C, *K* for $R_a = R_i$ (or *K* for $R_a = R_i = 0$); for drug D, *K* for $R_a < R_i$. (*See* text for additional explanation.)

will act as an antagonist because it blocks the ability of an agonist to bind and alter the equilibrium and, thus, to produce a response. (A drug with preferential affinity for R_i will actually produce an effect opposite to that of an agonist, and a few examples of so-called *inverse agonists* or superantagonists are known [*see* Chapter 17]. However, if the *preexisting* equilibrium lies far in the direction of R_i this may be difficult to observe and the agent will be difficult to distinguish from the simple antagonist just described.) Finally, a partial agonist can also act as an antagonist. When it binds to the receptor (and produces a submaximal response), it also occupies the drug binding site competitively with respect to a full agonist. A greater concentration of a full agonist will be required to produce a maximal effect because of this competition.

It is obvious that something different from a simple receptor-occupancy theory has now been invoked, in that antagonists and partial agonists occupy receptors fully but do not produce maximal effects. Again, this is a question of how the binding of a ligand influences protein conformation. At a purely descriptive level, however, one can adequately modify the simple occupancy model by imposing a new factor called *intrinsic activity* or *efficacy* to distinguish drugs that bind to the same receptor site but do not produce equal effects. Simplistically, the efficacy of a full agonist can be set equal to 1, that of an antagonist to 0, and that of a partial agonist to a value between 0 and 1. Fractional effect is then equal to the product of fractional occupancy of the receptor and the fractional efficacy. The action of partial agonists can also be described adequately using other, equally *ad hoc*, correction factors derived from the conformational equilibrium model described above.

It should be noted at this point that the use of the word *efficacy* can, at times, be confusing. While an antagonist has no efficacy in this sense as an initiator of an action that leads to a sequence of effects, it may have great therapeutic efficacy when used as an antagonist.

Even if the proximal molecular action of an agonist at a receptor site is proportional to its efficacy and to the number of receptor sites occupied, additional complications frequently impede the meaningful quantitative interpretation of the dose dependence of effect. This is particularly true when the drug–receptor interaction is but one event in a complex sequence of reactions that ultimately result in the observed effect. For example, while occupancy of a certain minimal number of receptors by an agonist may cause a proportional response, a later step in the pathway may become limiting at some greater level of stimulation. Further receptor occupancy can then produce no additional effect. Thus, a plot of the drug's effect versus log concentration will lie to the left of a plot of fractional binding; potency will be greater than predicted by affinity (Figure 2–8). This situation, in which a maximal apparent effect is achieved when a relatively small fraction of receptors is occupied, is referred to by the term *spare receptors*. In at least some of these cases, a certain number of receptors can be lost (*e.g.*, with an irreversible antagonist) without diminution of the maximal observable response. Note that the existence of spare receptors does not necessarily imply a molecular excess of receptors over effector or transducer proteins. Spare receptors are frequently encountered whenever a receptor acts catalytically rather than stoichiometrically. In the case of the receptors that are tyrosine protein kinases, a few agonist-liganded receptors may be sufficiently active to maintain the phosphorylation of a greater number of substrate protein molecules. Similarly, a single G protein–coupled receptor can maintain the activation of hundreds of G protein molecules. Conversely, if a drug acts to inhibit a step in a reaction sequence, the ultimate consequences of receptor occupation will be visible only when the step inhibited is or becomes the limiting step. It may be necessary to occupy the majority of the receptors before any change in function is observed. The drug's potency would then be less than its affinity for its site of action (*see* Figure 2–8).

Still other situations have required consideration of the possibility that certain receptors may have multiple drug binding sites, either identical or distinct. These sites may not act independently, and drug attachment at one point may alter the affinity for binding or reaction characteristics of agonists or antagonists at other locations. The potentiative actions of GABA and benzodiazepines (Chapter 17)

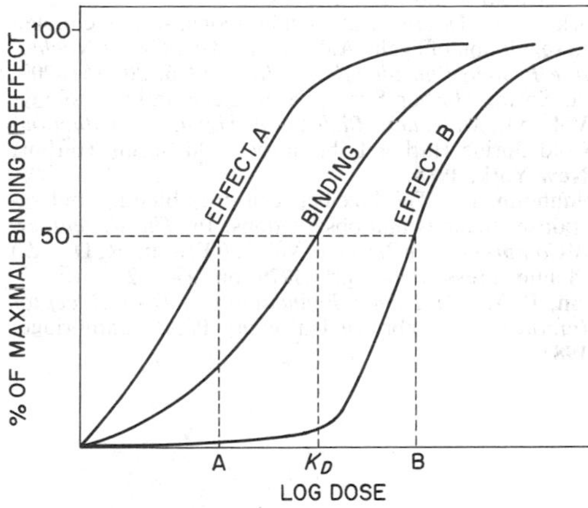

Figure 2–8. *Anomalous relationships between receptor occupation and response to a drug.*

The middle curve, labeled *binding*, depicts the occupation of receptor by increasing concentrations of drug. Hypothetical dose–effect curve (*A*) is seen if maximal response results from less than maximal receptor occupation (spare receptors). Dose–effect curve (*B*) is seen if a significant fraction of receptors must be occupied before noticeable response to the drug occurs. The concentration of drug required to produce a half-maximal effect (*A* or *B*) thus bears a complex relationship to the dissociation constant of the drug–receptor complex (K_D).

or of two acetylcholine molecules at two sites on the nicotinic receptor (Chapter 9) are examples of such interactions. It should be pointed out that increasingly involved receptor theories may be required when a pharmacological response bears an indirect relationship to the proximal action of the receptor. Mathematical models can be derived to describe systems of arbitrary complexity, but it is often more productive and satisfying to analyze the individual steps in the receptor–response pathway at a molecular level.

Benovic, J. L.; DeBlasi, A.; Stone, W. C.; Caron, M. G.; and Lefkowitz, R. J. *β*-Adrenergic receptor kinase: primary structure delineates a multigene family. *Science*, **1989**, *246*, 235–240.

Berridge, M. J. Inositol trisphosphate and diacylglycerol: two interacting second messengers. *Annu. Rev. Biochem.*, **1987**, *56*, 159–193.

Charbonneau, H.; Tonks, N. K.; Kumar, S.; Diltz, C. D.; Harrylock, M.; Cool, D. E.; Krebs, E. G.; Fischer, E. H.; and Walsh, K. A. Human placenta protein-tyrosine-phosphatase: amino acid sequence and relationship to a family of receptor-like proteins. *Proc. Natl. Acad. Sci. U.S.A.*, **1989**, *86*, 5252–5256.

Chinkers, M.; Garbers, D. L.; Chang, M.-S.; Lowe, D. G.; Chin, H.; Goeddel, D. V.; and Schulz, S. A membrane form of guanylate cyclase is an atrial natriuretic peptide receptor. *Nature*, **1989**, *338*, 78–83.

Clark, A. J. *The Mode of Action of Drugs on Cells.* E. Arnold & Co., London, **1933.**

Clark, R. B. Desensitization of hormonal stimuli coupled to regulation of cyclic AMP levels. *Adv. Cyclic Nucleotide Protein Phosphorylation Res.*, **1986**, *20*, 151–209.

Cold Spring Harbor Symposia on Quantitative Biology. Vol. 53, *Molecular Biology of Signal Transduction.* Cold Spring Harbor Laboratory, Cold Spring Harbor, New York, **1988.**

Colquhoun, D. The link between drug binding and response: theories and observations. In, *The Receptors: A Comprehensive Treatise*, Vol. 1. (O'Brien, R. D., ed.) Plenum Press, New York, **1979**, pp. 93–142.

Dean, P. M. *Molecular Foundations of Drug-Receptor Interaction.* Cambridge University Press, Cambridge, **1987.**

Edelman, A. M.; Blumenthal, D. K.; and Krebs, E. G. Protein serine/threonine kinases. *Annu. Rev. Biochem.*, **1987**, *56*, 567–613.

Evans, R. M. The steroid and thyroid hormone receptor superfamily. *Science*, **1988**, *240*, 889–895.

Gilman, A. G. G proteins: transducers of receptor-generated signals. *Annu. Rev. Biochem.*, **1987**, *56*, 615–649.

———. G proteins and regulation of adenylyl cyclase. *J.A.M.A.*, **1989**, *262*, 1819–1825.

Griffin, J. E., and Wilson, J. D. The androgen resistance syndromes. In, *The Metabolic Basis of Inherited Disease*, 6th ed. (Scriver, C. R.; Beaudet, A. L.; Sly, W. L.; and Valle, D.; eds.) McGraw-Hill Book Company, New York, **1989**, pp. 1919–1944.

Julius, D.; Livelli, T. J.; Jessell, T. M.; and Axel, R. Ectopic expression of the serotonin 1c receptor and the triggering of malignant transformation. *Science*, **1989**, *244*, 1057–1062.

Landis, C. A.; Masters, S. B.; Spada, A.; Pace, A. M.; Bourne, H. R.; and Valler, L. GTPase inhibiting mutations activate the α chain of G_s and stimulate adenylyl cyclase in human pituitary tumors. *Nature*, **1989**, *340*, 692–696.

Limbird, L. E. *Cell Surface Receptors: A Short Course on Theory and Methods.* Martinus Nijhoff, Boston, **1986.**

Marshall, G. R. Computer-aided drug design. *Annu. Rev. Pharmacol. Toxicol.*, **1987**, *27*, 193–213.

Molinoff, P. B.; Wolfe, B. B.; and Weiland, G. A. Quantitative analysis of drug-receptor interactions. II. Determination of the properties of receptor subtypes. *Life Sci.*, **1981**, *29*, 427–443.

Pratt, W. B., and Taylor, P. *Principles of Drug Action*, 3rd ed. Churchill Livingstone, Inc., New York, **1990.**

Ross, E. M. Signal sorting and amplification through G protein-coupled receptors. *Neuron*, **1989**, *3*, 141–142.

Segel, I. H. *Enzyme Kinetics*, 2nd ed. John Wiley & Sons, Inc., New York, **1984.**

Spiegel, A. M. Pseudohypoparathyroidism. In, *The Metabolic Basis of Inherited Disease*, 6th ed. (Scriver, C. R.; Beaudet, A. L.; Sly, W. L.; and Valle, D.; eds.) McGraw-Hill Book Company, New York, **1989**, pp. 2013–2027.

Yarden, Y., and Ullrich, A. Growth factor receptor tyrosine kinases. *Annu. Rev. Biochem.*, **1988**, *57*, 443–478.

Young, D.; Waitches, G.; Birchmeier, C.; Fasano, O.; and Wigler, M. Isolation and characterization of a new cellular oncogene encoding a protein with multiple potential transmembrane domains. *Cell*, **1986**, *45*, 711–719.

CHAPTER

3 PRINCIPLES OF TOXICOLOGY

Curtis D. Klaassen

Toxicology is the science of the adverse effects of chemicals on living organisms. The discipline is often divided into several major areas. The *descriptive toxicologist* performs toxicity tests (described below) to obtain information that can be used to evaluate the risk that exposure to a chemical poses to man and the environment. The *mechanistic toxicologist* attempts to determine how chemicals exert deleterious effects on living organisms. Such studies are essential for the development of tests for the prediction of risks, to facilitate the search for safer chemicals, and for rational treatment of the manifestations of toxicity. The *regulatory toxicologist* judges if a drug or other chemical has a low enough risk to justify making it available for its intended purpose. The Food and Drug Administration (FDA) regulates drugs, medical devices, cosmetics, and food additives in interstate commerce. For food additives, the FDA attempts to determine the acceptable daily intake (ADI) that can be consumed over an entire lifetime without any appreciable risk. The Environmental Protection Agency (EPA) is responsible for regulation of pesticides, toxic chemicals, hazardous wastes, and toxic pollutants in water and air. The Occupational Safety and Health Administration (OSHA) determines whether employers are providing working conditions that are safe for employees. Employers must keep the concentration of each chemical in the air of the workplace below a threshold limit value. The Consumer Products Safety Commission regulates all articles sold for use in homes, in schools, or for recreation, except those products regulated by the FDA and the EPA.

Two specialized areas of toxicology are particularly important for medicine. *Forensic toxicology,* which combines analytical chemistry and fundamental toxicology, is concerned with the medicolegal aspects of the use of chemicals that are harmful to animals and man. Forensic toxicologists assist in postmortem investigations to establish the cause or circumstances of death. *Clinical toxicology* focuses on diseases that are caused by or are uniquely associated with toxic substances. Clinical toxicologists treat patients who are poisoned by drugs and other chemicals and develop new techniques for the diagnosis and treatment of such intoxications.

The physician must evaluate the possibility that a patient's signs and symptoms might be caused by toxic chemicals present in the environment or administered as therapeutic agents. Many of the adverse effects of drugs mimic symptoms of disease. Appreciation of the principles of toxicology is necessary for the recognition and management of such problems.

DOSE-EFFECT RELATIONSHIP

Evaluation of the dose-response or the dose-effect relationship is crucially important to toxicologists (*see* Chapters 2 and 4). There is both a graded dose-response relationship in an *individual* and a quantal dose-response relationship in the *population.* Graded doses of a drug given to an individual usually result in a greater magnitude of response as the dose is increased. In a quantal dose-effect relationship, the percentage of the population affected increases as the dose is raised; the relationship is quantal in that the effect is specified to be either present or absent in a given individual. This quantal dose-effect phenomenon is extremely important in toxicology and is used to determine the *median lethal dose* (LD_{50}) of drugs and other chemicals.

The LD_{50} is determined experimentally. The chemical is usually administered to mice or rats (orally or intraperitoneally) at several doses (usually four or five) in the lethal range (*see* Figure 4–3). To linearize such data, the response (deaths) can be converted to units of *deviation from the mean*, or *probits* (from the contraction of *probability units*). The probit designates the deviation from the median; a probit of 5 corresponds to a 50% response, and, because each probit equals one standard deviation, a probit of 4 equals 16% and a probit of 6 equals 84% (Klaassen, 1985). A plot of percent of population responding, in probit units, against log dose yields a straight line (Figure 3–1). The LD_{50} is determined by drawing a vertical line from the point where the probit unit = 5 (50% mortality). The slope of the dose-effect is also important. The LD_{50} for both compounds depicted in Figure 3–1 is the same (10 mg/kg). However, the slopes of the dose-response curves are quite different. At a dose equal to one half of the LD_{50} (5 mg/kg), less than 5% of the animals exposed to compound B would die, but 30% of the animals given compound A would die.

The quantal or "all-or-none" response is not limited to lethality. Similar dose-effect curves can be constructed for any effect produced by chemicals.

TOXIC OR SAFE VERSUS RISK OR HAZARD

There obviously are marked differences in the LD_{50} of various chemicals. Some result in death at doses of a fraction of a microgram (LD_{50} for botulinus toxin = 10 pg/kg); others may be relatively harmless in doses of several grams or more.

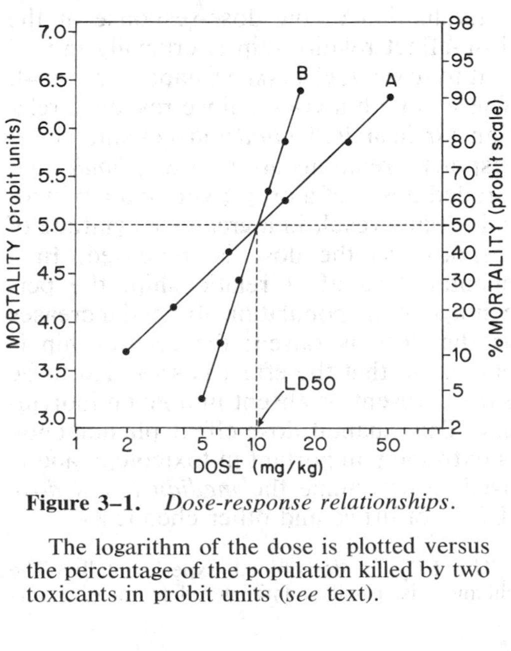

Figure 3–1. *Dose-response relationships.*

The logarithm of the dose is plotted versus the percentage of the population killed by two toxicants in probit units (*see* text).

While categories of toxicity that are of some practicality have been devised, based on the amount required to produce death, it often is not easy to distinguish between toxic and nontoxic chemicals. Paracelsus (1493–1541) noted that "All substances are poisons; there is none which is not a poison. The right dose differentiates a poison and a remedy." Although society wants the toxicologist to categorize all chemicals as either safe or toxic, this is not possible. The real concern is the *risk* or *hazard* associated with use of the chemical, not whether a chemical is toxic or safe. In the assessment of risk one must also consider the harmful effects of the chemical accrued directly or indirectly through adverse effects on the environment when used in the quantity and in the manner proposed. Depending on the use and disposition of a chemical, a very toxic compound may ultimately be less harmful than a relatively nontoxic one.

At present there is much concern about the risk from exposure to chemicals that have produced cancer in laboratory animals. For most of these chemicals it is not known if they also produce cancer in man. The regulatory agencies take one of two approaches to potential chemical carcinogens. For food additives, the FDA must enforce the Delany Amendment, which provides that no substance that produces cancer in man or laboratory animals should be added to our diet in any amount. In the regulation of environmental carcinogens, the EPA attempts to limit lifetime exposure such that the incidence of cancer due to the chemical would be no more than one in a million people. To determine the daily allowable exposure, mathematical models are used to extrapolate doses of chemicals that produce a particular incidence of tumors in laboratory animals (often in the range of 10 to 20%) to those that should produce cancer in no more than one person in a million. The models used are conservative and are thought to provide adequate protection from undue risks from exposure to potential carcinogens.

Acute versus Chronic Exposure. Effects of acute exposure to a chemical often differ from those that follow subacute or chronic exposure. Acute exposure occurs when a dose is delivered as a single event. Chronic exposure is likely to be to small quantities of a substance over a long period of time, which often results in the slow accumulation of the compound in the body. Evaluation of *cumulative* toxic effects is receiving increased attention because of chronic exposure to low concentrations of various natural and synthetic chemical substances in the environment.

Spectrum of Undesired Effects

The spectrum of undesired effects of chemicals may be broad and ill defined. In therapeutics, a drug typically produces numerous effects, but usually only one is sought as the primary goal of treatment; most of the other effects are referred to as *undesirable* or *side effects* of that drug for that therapeutic indication. Mechanistic categorization of such effects is a necessary prelude to avoidance of them or, if they occur, to rational and successful management of them.

Toxic Reactions. Toxic effects of drugs may be classified as pharmacological, pathological, or genotoxic (alterations of DNA), and their incidence and seriousness are related, at least over some range, to the concentration of the toxic chemical in the body. An example of a pharmacological toxicity is excessive depression of the central nervous system (CNS) by barbiturates; an example of a pathological effect is hepatic injury produced by acetaminophen; an example of a genotoxic effect is a neoplasm produced by a nitrogen mustard. If the concentration of chemical in the tissues does not exceed a critical level, the effects will usually be reversible. The pharmacological effects usually disappear when the concentration of chemical in the tissues is decreased by excretion from the body. Pathological and genotoxic effects may be repaired. If these effects are severe, death may ensue within a short time; if more subtle damage to DNA is not repaired, cancer may appear in a few months or years in laboratory animals or in a decade or more in man.

Many chemicals are not toxic themselves but are activated by biotransformation into toxic metabolites. The toxic response is then dependent on the balance of the rate at which the toxic metabolite is produced and destroyed.

Phototoxic and Photoallergic Reactions. Many chemicals are activated to toxic metabolites by enzymatic biotransformation. However, some chemicals can be activated in the skin by ultraviolet and/or visible radiation. In photoallergy, radiation absorbed by the drug, such as a sulfonamide, results in its conversion to a product that is a more potent allergen than the parent compound. The clinical manifestations may range from acute urticarial reactions, which develop a few minutes after exposure to sunlight, to eczematous or papular lesions, which appear after 24 hours or more. Phototoxic reactions to drugs, in contrast to photoallergic ones, do not have an immunological component. Drugs, either absorbed locally into the skin or reaching the skin through the systemic circulation, may be the object of photochemical reactions within the skin; this can lead directly either to chemically induced photosensitivity reactions or to enhancement of the usual effects of sunlight. Tetracyclines, sulfonamides, chlorpromazine, and nalidixic acid are examples of phototoxic chemicals; they are generally innocuous to skin if not exposed to light.

Local versus Systemic Toxicity. Local toxicity is the effect that occurs at the site of first contact between the biological system and the toxicant. Local effects can be caused by ingestion of caustic substances or inhalation of irritant materials. Systemic toxicity requires absorption and distribution of the toxicant; most substances, with the exception of highly reactive chemical species, produce such toxic effects. The two categories are not mutually exclusive. Tetraethyllead, for example, injures skin at the site of contact and is absorbed into the circulation to affect the CNS.

Most systemic toxicants affect one or a few organs predominantly. The target organ of toxicity is not necessarily the site of accumulation of the chemical. For example, lead is concentrated in bone, but its primary toxic action is on soft tissues; DDT (chlorophenothane) is concentrated in adipose tissue but produces no known toxic effects there.

The CNS is most frequently involved in systemic toxicity. Many compounds with prominent effects elsewhere also affect the brain. Next in order of frequency of involvement in systemic toxicity are the circulatory system; the blood and hematopoietic system; visceral organs such as liver, kidney, and lung; and the skin. Muscle and bone are least often affected. With substances that have a predominant local effect, the frequency of tissue reaction depends largely on the portal of entry (skin, gastrointestinal tract, or respiratory tract).

Reversible and Irreversible Toxic Effects. The effects of drugs on man must, whenever possible, be reversible; otherwise the drugs would be prohibitively toxic. If a chemical produces injury to a tissue, the capacity of the tissue to regenerate or recover will largely determine the reversibility of the effect. Injuries to a tissue such as liver, which has a high capacity to regenerate, are usually reversible; injury to the CNS is largely irreversible because the highly differentiated neurons of the brain cannot divide and regenerate.

Delayed Toxicity. Most toxic effects of drugs occur at a predictable (usually short) time after administration. However, such is not always the case. For example, aplastic anemia caused by chloramphenicol may appear weeks after the drug has been discontinued. Carcinogenic effects of chemicals usually have a long latency period, and often 20 to 30 years must pass before tumors are observed. Such delayed effects obviously cannot be assessed during any reasonable period of initial evaluation of a chemical; there is an urgent need for reliably predictive, short-term tests for such toxicity as well as for systematic surveillance of the long-term effects of marketed drugs and other chemicals (*see* Chapter 4).

Chemical carcinogenesis is a multistep process. Most carcinogens are themselves unreactive (*procarcinogens* or *proximate carcinogens*) but are converted to *primary* or *ultimate carcinogens* in the body. The cytochrome P_{450}-dependent monooxygenases of the endoplasmic reticulum often convert the proximate carcinogens to reactive electron-deficient intermediates (electrophils). These reactive intermediates can interact with electron-rich (nucleophilic) centers in DNA to produce a mutation. Such interaction of the ultimate carcinogen with DNA in a cell is thought to be the initial step in chemical carcinogenesis. The DNA may revert to normal if DNA repair mechanisms operate successfully; if not, the transformed cell may grow into a tumor that becomes apparent clinically. A *cocarcinogen* or *promoter* is not a carcinogen by itself, but it potentiates the effects of a carcinogen. Promotion involves facilitation of the growth and development of so-called dormant or latent tumor cells. The time from initiation to the development of a tumor probably depends on the presence of such promoters; for many human tumors the latent period is 15 to 45 years.

Allergic Reactions. *Chemical allergy* is an adverse reaction that results from previous sensitization to a particular chemical or to one that is structurally similar. Such reactions are mediated by the immune system. The terms *hypersensitivity* and *drug allergy* are often used to describe the allergic state.

For a low-molecular-weight chemical to cause an allergic reaction, it or its metabolic product usually acts as a hapten, combining with an endogenous protein to form an antigenic complex. Such antigens induce the synthesis of antibodies, usually after a latent period of at least 1 or 2 weeks. Subsequent exposure of the organism to the chemical results in an antigen–antibody interaction that provokes the typical manifestations of allergy. Dose-response relationships are usually not apparent for the provocation of allergic reactions.

Allergic responses have been divided into four general categories, based on the mechanism of immunological involvement (Coombs and Gell, 1975). Type-I, or anaphylactic, reactions in man are mediated by IgE antibodies. The Fc portion of IgE can bind to receptors on mast cells and basophils. If the Fab portion of the antibody molecule then binds antigen, various mediators (histamine, leukotrienes, prostaglandins) are released and cause vasodilatation, edema, and an inflammatory response. The main targets of this type of reaction are the gastrointestinal tract (food allergies), the skin (urticaria and atopic dermatitis), the respiratory system (rhinitis and asthma), and the vasculature (anaphylactic shock). These responses tend to occur quickly after challenge with an antigen to which the individual has been sensitized and are termed *immediate hypersensitivity reactions*.

Type-II, or cytolytic, reactions are mediated by both IgG and IgM antibodies and are usually attributed to their ability to activate complement. The major target tissues are the cells in the circulatory system. Examples of this phenomenon include penicillin-induced hemolytic anemia, methyldopa-induced autoimmune hemolytic anemia, quinidine-induced thrombocytopenic purpura, sulfonamide-induced granulocytopenia, and hydralazine- or procainamide-induced systemic lupus erythematosus. Fortunately, these autoimmune reactions to drugs usually subside within several months after removal of the offending agent.

Type-III, or Arthus, reactions are predominantly mediated by IgG; the mechanism involves the generation of antigen–antibody complexes that subsequently fix complement. The complexes are deposited in the vascular endothelium, where a destructive inflammatory response called serum sickness occurs. This is in contrast to the type-II reaction, in which the inflammatory response is induced by antibodies directed against tissue antigens. The clinical symptoms of serum sickness include urticarial skin eruptions, arthralgia or arthritis, lymphadenopathy, and fever. These reactions usually last for 6 to 12 days and then subside after the offending agent is eliminated. Several drugs, such as sulfonamides, penicillins, certain anticonvulsants, and iodides, can induce serum sickness. Stevens–Johnson syndrome, such as that caused by sulfonamides, is a more severe form of immune vasculitis. Symptoms of this reaction include erythema multiforme, arthritis, nephritis, CNS abnormalities, and myocarditis.

Type-IV, or delayed-hypersensitivity, reactions are mediated by sensitized T lymphocytes and macrophages. When sensitized cells come in contact with antigen, an inflammatory reaction is generated by the production of lymphokines and the subsequent influx of neutrophils and macrophages. An example of type-IV or delayed hypersensitivity is the contact dermatitis caused by poison ivy.

Idiosyncratic Reactions. *Idiosyncrasy* is defined as a genetically determined abnormal reactivity to a chemical (Goldstein *et al.*, 1974). The observed response is qualitatively similar in all individuals, but it may take the form of extreme sensitivity to low doses or extreme insensitivity to high doses of the agent. For example, many black males (about 10%) develop a serious hemolytic anemia when they receive primaquine. Such individuals have a deficiency of erythrocytic glucose-6-phosphate dehydrogenase (*see* Chapter 41). Genetically determined resistance to the anticoagulant action of warfarin is due to an alteration in the receptor for the drug (*see* Chapter 55).

Interactions between Chemicals. The existence of numerous toxicants requires consideration of their potential interactions (*see also* Chapters 1, 2, and 4). Concurrent exposures may alter rates of absorption, change the degree of protein binding, or alter the rates of biotransformation or excretion of one or both interacting compounds. The response to combined toxicants may thus be equal to, greater than, or less than the sum of the effects of the individual agents.

Numerous terms describe pharmacological and toxicological interactions. An *additive* effect describes the combined effect of two chemicals that is equal to the sum of the effect of each agent given alone; the additive effect is the most common. A *synergistic* effect is one in which the combined effect of two chemicals is greater than the sum of the effect of each agent given alone. For example, both carbon tetrachloride and ethanol are hepatotoxins, but together they produce much more injury to the liver than expected from the mathematical sum of their individual effects. *Potentiation* is the increased effect of a toxic agent acting simultaneously with a nontoxic one. Isopropanol alone, for example, is not hepatotoxic; however, it greatly increases the hepatotoxicity of carbon tetrachloride. *Antagonism* is the interference of one chemical with the action of another. An antagonistic agent is often desirable as an antidote. *Functional* or *physiological antagonism* occurs when two chemicals produce opposite effects on the same physiological function. For example, this principle is applied to the ability of an intravenous infusion of dopamine to maintain perfusion of vital organs during certain severe intoxications characterized by marked hypotension. *Chemical antagonism* or *inactivation* is a reaction between two chemicals to neutralize their effects. For example, dimercaprol (BAL) chelates with various metals to decrease their toxicity. *Dispositional antagonism* is the alteration of the disposition of a substance (its absorption, biotransformation, distribution, or excretion) so that less of the agent reaches the target organ or its persistence there is reduced (*see* below). *Antagonism* at the *receptor* for the chemical entails the blockade of the effect of an agonist with an appropriate antagonist that competes for the same site. For example, the antagonist naloxone is used to treat the respiratory-depressant effects of opioids.

DESCRIPTIVE TOXICITY TESTS IN ANIMALS

Two main principles underlie all descriptive toxicity tests that are performed in animals. First, effects of chemicals produced in laboratory animals, when properly qualified, apply to toxicity in man. When calculated on the basis of dose per unit of body surface, toxic effects in man are usually encountered in the same range of concentrations as are those in experimental animals. On the basis of body weight, man is generally more vulnerable than experimental animals. Such information is used to select dosages for clinical trials of candidate therapeutic agents and to attempt to set limits on permissible exposure to environmental toxicants.

The second main principle is that exposure of experimental animals to toxic agents in high doses is a necessary and valid method to discover possible hazards to humans who are exposed to much lower doses. This principle is based on the quantal dose-response concept. As a matter of practicality, the number of animals used in experiments on toxic materials will usually be small compared with the size of human populations potentially at risk. For example, 0.01% incidence of a serious toxic effect (such as cancer) represents 25,000 people in a population of 250 million. Such an incidence is unacceptably high. Yet, detecting an incidence of 0.01% experimentally would probably require a minimum of 30,000 animals. To estimate risk at low dosage, large doses must be given to relatively small groups. The validity of the necessary extrapolation is clearly a crucial question.

Chemicals are first tested for toxicity by estimation of the LD_{50} in two animal species by two routes of administration; one of these is the expected route of exposure. The number of animals that die in a 14-day period after a single dose is tabulated. The animals are also examined for signs of intoxication, lethargy, behavioral modification, and morbidity.

The chemical is next tested for toxicity by subacute exposure, usually for 90 days. The subacute study is most often performed in two species by the route of intended use or exposure, and at least three doses are employed. A variety of parameters are monitored during this period, and at the end of the study organs and tissues are examined by a pathologist.

Long-term or chronic studies are carried out in animals at the same time that clinical trials are undertaken (*see* Chapter 4). The length of exposure depends somewhat on the intended clinical use. If the drug would normally be used for short periods under medical supervision, as would an antimicrobial agent, a chronic exposure of animals for 6 months might suffice. If the drug would be used in man for longer periods, a study of chronic use for 2 years might be required.

Study of chronic exposure is often used to determine the carcinogenic potential of chemicals. These studies are usually performed in rats and mice and cover the average lifetime of the species. Other tests are designed to evaluate teratogenicity (congenital malformations), perinatal and postnatal toxicity, and effects on fertility. Teratogenicity studies are usually performed by administering the drug to pregnant rats and rabbits during the period of organogenesis. In addition, drugs are often tested for *mutagenic* potential. The most popular such test currently available, the reverse mutation test developed by Ames and colleagues (Ames *et al.*, 1975), uses a strain of *Salmonella typhimurium* that has a mutant gene for the enzyme phosphoribosyl adenosine triphosphate (ATP) synthetase. This enzyme is required for histidine synthesis, and the bacterial strain is unable to grow in a histidine-deficient medium unless a reverse mutation is induced. Because many chemicals are not mutagenic or carcinogenic unless activated by the endoplasmic reticulum, rat hepatic microsomes are usually added to the medium containing the mutant bacteria and the drug. The Ames test is rapid and sensitive. However, its usefulness for the prediction of the carcinogenic potential of chemicals for man is controversial, and the subject continues to receive considerable attention.

INCIDENCE OF ACUTE POISONING

The true incidence of poisoning in the United States is not known, but, in 1987, over 1 million cases were voluntarily reported to the American Association of Poison Control Centers. The number of real or potential poisonings is probably at least fivefold greater than the number reported.

Deaths in the United States due to poisoning number over 400 per year. The incidence of poisoning in children (under 5 years of age) has decreased dramatically over the past 3 decades. For example, there were no childhood deaths due to aspirin in 1987, compared to about 140 deaths per year in the early 1960s. This favorable trend is probably due to safety packaging of aspirin, prescription drugs, drain cleaners, turpentine, and other household chemicals; improved medical training and care; and increased public awareness of potential poisons. The substances most frequently involved in human poison exposures are shown in Table 3–1. Three of the four categories of substances most frequently responsible for human poisoning are not drugs. Children under 6 years of age account for 65 to 85% of the poisoning in these three categories. Children between 1 and 2 years of age have the highest incidence of accidental poisoning. Fortunately, most of the substances available to these young children are not highly toxic and their accessibility accounts for the high frequency of their involvement in poisonings.

While most drugs are not frequently involved in human poisoning, the top five categories of substances that produce deaths are drugs (Table 3–2). Most of the people who die from poisoning are adults, and the deaths often result from intentional rather than accidental exposure.

Table 3–1. SUBSTANCES MOST FREQUENTLY INVOLVED IN HUMAN POISON EXPOSURES

SUBSTANCE	NO.	%*
Cleaning substances	114,888	9.4
Analgesics	111,148	9.1
Cosmetics	94,349	7.7
Plants	88,251	7.2
Cough and cold preparations	62,240	5.1
Hydrocarbons	46,186	3.8
Bites/envenomations	43,971	3.6
Topicals	41,411	3.4
Foreign bodies	40,290	3.3
Pesticides (includes rodenticides)	37,856	3.1
Food poisoning	37,571	3.1
Sedative/hypnotics/antipsychotics	36,851	3.0
Antimicrobials	35,698	2.9
Chemicals	35,365	2.9
Alcohols	31,533	2.6
Vitamins	31,366	2.6

* Percentages are based on total number of known ingested substances (1,221,855) rather than the total number of human exposures cases. (From Litovitz *et al.*, 1988. Courtesy of the *American Journal of Emergency Medicine.*)

Table 3–2. CATEGORIES WITH LARGEST NUMBERS OF DEATHS

CATEGORY	NO.	% OF ALL EXPOSURES IN CATEGORY
Antidepressants	105	0.649
Analgesics	93	0.083
Stimulants and street drugs	54	0.337
Cardiovascular drugs	52	0.372
Sedative/hypnotics	48	0.130
Gases and fumes	36	0.250
Chemicals	23	0.065
Alcohols/glycols	19	0.060
Asthma therapies	16	0.204
Cleaning substances	14	0.012
Hydrocarbons	13	0.028

(From Litovitz *et al.*, 1988. Courtesy of the *American Journal of Emergency Medicine.*)

MAJOR SOURCES OF INFORMATION ON TOXICOLOGY

Pharmacology textbooks are a good source of information on treatment of poisoning by drugs, but they usually say little about other chemicals. Additional information on drugs and other chemicals can be found in various books on poisoning. (*See* Haddad and Winchester, 1983; Klaassen *et al.,* 1985; Goldfrank *et al.,* 1986; Ellenhorn and Barceloux, 1988.)

An extremely useful source of information on the treatment of acute poisoning by commercial products is *Clinical Toxicology of Commercial Products* by Gosselin and associates (1984). This book contains seven major sections. One section lists over 17,500 trade names of products that might be ingested accidentally or suicidally. It lists the manufacturer and ingredients of each commercial product and notes components believed responsible for harmful effects. A popular computerized system for information on toxic substances is POISINDEX (Micromedex, Inc., Denver, Colo.).

There are about 120 poison control centers in the United States, coordinated and served by the Food and Drug Administration's Poisoning Surveillance and Epidemiology Branch, and there are 36 regional poison control centers designated by the American Association of Poison Control Centers. These centers are a valuable source of information that can be obtained by telephone.

PREVENTION AND TREATMENT OF POISONING

Many acute poisonings could be prevented if physicians provided and parents accepted common-sense instructions about the storage of drugs and other chemicals. These are so widely publicized that they need not be repeated here.

For clinical purposes all toxic agents can be divided into two classes: those for which a specific treatment and antidote exists and those for which there is no specific treatment. For the vast majority of drugs and other chemicals, there is no specific treatment, and symptomatic medical care that supports vital functions is the only approach.

Supportive therapy, as in other medical emergencies, is the most important aspect of the treatment of drug poisoning. The adage, "Treat the patient, not the poison," remains the most basic and important principle of clinical toxicology. Maintenance of respiration and circulation takes precedence. Serial measurement and charting of vital signs and important reflexes help to judge progress of intoxication, response to therapy, and the need for additional treatment. This usually requires hospitalization. The classification in Table 3–3 is often used to indicate the severity of CNS intoxication. Treatment with large doses of stimulants and sedatives can often cause more harm than the poison. Chemical antidotes should be used judiciously; heroic measures are seldom necessary.

Treatment of acute poisoning must be prompt. The first goal is to keep the concentration of poison in the crucial tissues as low as possible by preventing absorption and enhancing elimination. The second goal is to combat the pharmacological and toxicological effects at the effector sites.

Table 3–3. SIGNS AND SYMPTOMS OF CNS INTOXICATION

DEGREE OF SEVERITY	CHARACTERISTICS
	Depressants
0	Asleep, but can be aroused and can answer questions
I	Semicomatose, withdraws from painful stimuli, reflexes intact
II	Comatose, does not withdraw from painful stimuli, no respiratory or circulatory depression, most reflexes intact
III	Comatose, most or all reflexes absent, but without depression of respiration or circulation
IV	Comatose, reflexes absent, respiratory depression with cyanosis or circulatory failure and shock or both
	Stimulants
I	Restlessness, irritability, insomnia, tremor, hyperreflexia, sweating, mydriasis, flushing
II	Confusion, hyperactivity, hypertension, tachypnea, tachycardia, extrasystoles, sweating, mydriasis, flushing, mild hyperpyrexia
III	Delirium, mania, self-injury, marked hypertension, tachycardia, arrhythmias, hyperpyrexia
IV	As in III, plus convulsions, coma, and circulatory collapse

PREVENTION OF FURTHER ABSORPTION OF POISON

Emesis. Although emesis is indicated after poisoning by oral ingestion of most chemicals, it is contraindicated in certain situations: (1) If the patient has ingested a corrosive poison, such as strong acids or alkalis (*e.g.*, drain cleaners), emesis increases the likelihood of gastric perforation and further necrosis of the esophagus. (2) If the patient is comatose or in a state of stupor or delirium, emesis may cause aspiration of the gastric contents. (3) If the patient has ingested a CNS stimulant, further stimulation associated with vomiting may precipitate convulsions. (4) If the patient has ingested a petroleum distillate (*e.g.*, kerosene, gasoline, or petroleum-based liquid furniture polish), regurgitated hydrocarbons can be aspirated readily and cause chemical pneumonitis (Ervin, 1983). However, emesis should be considered if the solution that is ingested contains potentially dangerous compounds, such as pesticides.

There are marked differences in the capabilities of various petroleum distillates to produce hydrocarbon pneumonia, which is an acute, hemorrhagic necrotizing process. In general, the ability of various hydrocarbons to produce pneumonitis is inversely proportional to the viscosity of the agent: if the viscosity is high, as with oils and greases, the risk is limited; if viscosity is low, as with mineral seal oil found in liquid furniture polishes, the risk of aspiration is high.

Vomiting can be induced mechanically by stroking the posterior pharynx. However, this technique is not as effective as the administration of ipecac or apomorphine.

Ipecac. The most useful household emetic is syrup of ipecac (not ipecac fluid extract, which is 14 times more potent and may cause fatalities). It is available in 0.5- and 1-fluid ounce containers (approximately 15 and 30 ml), which may be purchased without prescription. The drug can be given orally, but it takes 15 to 30 minutes to produce emesis; this compares favorably with the time usually required for adequate gastric lavage. The oral dose is 15 ml in children from 6 months to 12 years of age and 30 ml in older children and adults. Since emesis may not occur if the stomach is empty, the administration of ipecac should be followed by a drink of water.

Ipecac acts as an emetic because of its local irritant effect on the enteric tract and its effect on the chemoreceptor trigger zone (CTZ) in the area postrema of the medulla. Syrup of ipecac may be effective even when antiemetic drugs (such as phenothiazines) have been ingested (Thoman and Verhulst, 1966), presumably due to its direct irritant action on the gastrointestinal tract. Charcoal should not be administered with ipecac, because charcoal can adsorb the ipecac and reduce the emetic effect. Ipecac can produce toxic effects on the heart because of its content of emetine (*see* Chapter 42), but this is usually not a problem with the dose used for emesis (Manno and Manno, 1977). If emesis does not occur, ipecac should be removed by gastric lavage. Chronic abuse of ipecac for weight reduction can result in cardiomyopathy, ventricular fibrillation, and death.

Apomorphine. Apomorphine stimulates the CTZ and causes emesis. The drug is unstable in solution and must be prepared just prior to use and thus is often not readily available. Additionally, apomorphine is not effective orally and must be given parenterally, usually by the subcutaneous route—6 mg for adults and 0.06 mg/kg for children (Goldfrank, 1982). However, this can be an advantage over ipecac in that it can be administered to an uncooperative patient and produces vomiting in 3 to 5 minutes. Because apomorphine is a respiratory depressant, it should not be used if the patient has been poisoned by a CNS depressant or if the patient's respiration is slow and labored. Respiratory depression and emesis produced by apomorphine can be reversed by an opioid antagonist such as naloxone, but this usually is not necessary.

Gastric Lavage. Gastric lavage is accomplished by inserting a tube into the stomach and washing the stomach with water, normal saline, or one-half normal saline to remove the unabsorbed poison. The procedure should be performed as soon as possible, but only if vital functions are adequate or supportive procedures have been implemented. Lavage may be useful for as long as 6 hours after ingestion of a poison and, if gastric emptying has been delayed, lavage may be useful for as long as 24 hours after ingestion. The contraindications to this procedure are generally the same as for emesis. Unlike emesis, gastric lavage can be used for patients who are hysterical, comatose, or otherwise uncooperative.

The only equipment needed for gastric lavage is a tube and a large syringe. The tube should be as large as possible so that the wash solution, food, and the poison (whether in the form of a capsule, pill, or liquid) will flow freely, and lavage can be accomplished quickly. A 36-French tube or larger should be used in adults and a 24-French tube or larger in children. Orogastric lavage is preferred over nasogastric, because a larger tube can be employed. To prevent aspiration, an endotracheal tube with an inflatable cuff should be positioned before lavage is initiated if the patient is comatose, having seizures, or has lost the gag reflex. During gastric lavage the patient should be placed on his left side, due to the anatomical asymmetry of the stomach, with the head hanging face down over the edge of the examining table. If possible, the foot of the table should be elevated. This technique minimizes chances of aspiration (Arena, 1979).

The contents of the stomach should be aspirated with an irrigating syringe and saved for chemical analysis. The stomach may then be washed with saline solution. Saline solution is safer than water in young children because of the risk of water intoxication, manifested by tonic and clonic seizures and coma (Arena, 1975). Only small volumes (120 to 300 ml) of lavage solution should be instilled into the stomach at one time so that the poison is not pushed into the intestine. Lavage should be repeated until the returns are clear, which usually requires 10 to 12 washings and a total of 1.5 to 4 liters of lavage fluid. When the lavage is complete, the stomach may be left empty or an antidote may be instilled through the tube. If no specific antidote is known for the poison, an aqueous suspension of activated charcoal and a cathartic is often given.

Chemical Adsorption. Activated charcoal avidly adsorbs drugs and chemicals on the surfaces of the charcoal particles, thereby preventing absorption and toxicity. The effectiveness of charcoal is dependent on the time since the ingestion and on the dose of charcoal; one should attempt to achieve a charcoal:drug ratio of at least 10:1. Activated charcoal can also interrupt the enterohepatic circulation of drugs and enhance the net rate of diffusion of the chemical from the body into the gastrointestinal tract (Levy, 1982). The use of serial doses of activated charcoal (15 to 20 g every 2 to 4 hours) has been shown to enhance the elimination of theophylline and phenobarbital (Berg *et al.*, 1982; Berlinger *et al.*, 1983).

Activated charcoal is usually prepared as a mixture of at least 50 g (about 10 heaping tablespoons) in a glass of water. The mixture is then administered either orally or via a gastric tube. Because most poisons do not appear to desorb from the charcoal if it is present in excess, the adsorbed poison need not be removed from the gastrointestinal tract. As mentioned, activated charcoal should not be used simultaneously with ipecac. Charcoal may also adsorb and decrease the effectiveness of specific antidotes.

Activated charcoal must be distinguished from the so-called universal antidote, which consists of two parts burned toast (not activated charcoal), one part tannic acid (strong tea), and one part magnesium oxide. In practice, the universal antidote is ineffective.

As mentioned, the presence of an adsorbent in the intestine may interrupt enterohepatic circulation of a toxicant, thus enhancing its excretion. Activated charcoal is useful in interrupting the enterohepatic circulation of drugs such as tricyclic antidepressants and glutethimide. Poisoning by methylmercury can be treated with a nonabsorbable polythiol resin, which binds mercury excreted into the bile (*see* Chapter 66). Cholestyramine hastens the elimination of cardiac glycosides by a similar mechanism (*see* Chapter 34).

Chemical Inactivation. Antidotes can change the chemical nature of a poison by rendering it less toxic or by preventing its absorption. Formaldehyde poisoning can be treated with ammonia to form hexamethylenetetramine (Goldstein *et al.*, 1974); sodium formaldehyde sulfoxylate can convert mercuric ion to the less soluble metallic mercury (Gosselin *et al.*, 1984); and sodium bicarbonate converts ferrous iron to ferrous carbonate, which is poorly absorbed. However, these techniques are seldom used today because valuable time may be lost. Emetics and gastric lavage are rapid and effective.

In the past, neutralization was the usual treatment of poisoning with acids or bases. Vinegar, orange juice, or lemon juice have often been used for the patient who has ingested alkali, and various antacids have often been advocated for treatment of acid burns. The use of neutralizing agents is controversial, because this may produce excessive heat. Carbon dioxide gas produced from bicarbonates used to treat oral poisoning with acids can cause gastric distention and even perforation. The treatment of choice for ingestion of either acids or alkalis is dilution with water or milk. Similarly, burns produced by acid or alkali on the skin should be treated with copious amounts of water.

Purgation. The rationale for using an osmotic cathartic is to minimize absorption by hastening the passage of the toxicant through the gastrointestinal tract. Few, if any, controlled clinical data are available on the effectiveness of cathartics in the treatment of poisoning. Cathartics are generally considered harmless unless the poison has injured the gastrointestinal tract. Cathartics are indicated after the ingestion of enteric-coated tablets, when the time after ingestion is greater than 1 hour, and for poisoning by volatile hydrocarbons (Rumack and Lovejoy, 1985). Preferred agents are sodium sulfate, magnesium sulfate, or sorbitol, which act promptly and usually have minimal toxicity. However, magnesium sulfate should be used cautiously in patients with renal failure or those likely to develop renal dysfunction, and Na^+-containing cathartics should be avoided in patients with congestive heart failure.

Inhalation and Dermal Exposure to Poisons. When a poison has been inhaled, the first priority is to remove the patient from the source of exposure. Similarly, the skin should be thoroughly washed with water if it has come in contact with a poison. Contaminated clothing should be removed. Initial treatment of all types of chemical injuries to the eye must be rapid; thorough irrigation of the eye with water for 15 minutes should be performed immediately.

ENHANCED BIOTRANSFORMATION AND EXCRETION OF THE POISON

Biotransformation. Once a chemical has been absorbed, procedures can sometimes be employed to enhance its rate of elimination. Many drugs are metabolized by the cytochrome P_{450} system in the endoplasmic reticulum of the liver, and components of this system can be induced by a number of compounds (*see* Chapter 1). However, induction of these oxidative enzymes is too slow (days) to be valuable in the treatment of acute poisoning by most chemical agents.

Many chemicals are toxic because they are biotransformed into more toxic chemicals. Thus, inhibition of biotransformation should decrease the toxicity of such drugs. For example, ethanol is used to inhibit the conversion of methanol to its highly toxic metabolite, formic acid, by alcohol dehydrogenase (*see* Chapter 67). Acetaminophen is converted by the cytochrome P_{450} system to an electrophilic metabolite that is detoxified by glutathione, a cellular nucleophil. Acetaminophen does not cause hepatotoxicity until glutathione is depleted, whereupon the reactive metabolite binds to essential macromolecular constituents of the hepatocyte, resulting in cell death. The liver can be protected by maintenance of the concentration of glutathione, and this can be accomplished by the administration of N-acetylcysteine (Black, 1980; *see* Chapter 26).

Some drugs are detoxified by conjugation with glucuronic acid or sulfate before elimination from the body, and the availability of the endogenous cosubstrates for conjugation may limit the rate of elimination; such is the case in the detoxication of acetaminophen (Hjelle *et al.*, 1985). When methods become available to replete these compounds, an additional mechanism will be available to treat poisoning. Similarly, detoxication of cyanide by conversion to thiocyanate can be accelerated by the administration of thiosulfate (*see* Chapter 67).

Biliary Excretion. The liver excretes many drugs and other foreign chemicals into bile, but little is known about efficient ways to enhance biliary excretion of xenobiotics for the treatment of acute poisoning. Inducers of microsomal enzyme activity enhance biliary excretion of some xenobiotics, but the effect is slow in onset. Eventually, the procedure may be useful to enhance the elimination of certain compounds with long biological half-lives (Klaassen and Watkins, 1984).

Urinary Excretion. Drugs and poisons are excreted into the urine by glomerular filtration and active tubular secretion (*see* Chapter 1); they can be reabsorbed into the blood if they are in a lipid-soluble form that will penetrate the tubule or if there is an active mechanism for their transport.

There are no methods known to accelerate the active transport of poisons into urine, and enhancement of glomerular filtration is not a practical means to facilitate elimination of toxicants. However, passive reabsorption from the tubular lumen can be altered. Diuretics decrease reabsorption by decreasing the concentration gradient of the drug from the lumen to the tubular cell and by increasing flow through the tubule. Furosemide is used most often, but osmotic diuretics are also employed (*see* Chapter 28). Forced diuresis should be used with caution, especially in patients with renal, cardiac, or pulmonary complications.

Nonionized compounds are reabsorbed far more rapidly than ionized, polar molecules; therefore a shift from the nonionized to the ionized species of the toxicant by alteration of the pH of the tubular fluid may hasten elimination (*see* Chapter 1). Acidic compounds such as phenobarbital and salicylates are cleared much more rapidly in alkaline than in acidic urine. The effect of increasing urine flow and alkalinization of urine on the clearance of phenobarbital is shown in Figure 3–2. Intravenous sodium bicarbonate is used to alkalinize the urine. Renal excretion of basic drugs such as amphetamine can be enhanced by acidification of the urine. This can be accomplished by the administration of ammonium chloride or ascorbic acid. Urinary excretion of an acidic compound is particularly sensitive to changes in urinary pH if its pK_a is within the range of 3.0 to 7.5; for bases the corresponding range is 7.5 to 10.5.

Dialysis. Hemodialysis or hemoperfusion usually has limited use in the treatment of intoxication with chemicals. However, under certain circumstances, such procedures can be lifesaving. The utility of dialysis depends on the amount of poison in the blood relative to the total body burden. Thus, if a poison has a large volume of distribution, as is the case for the tricyclic antidepressants, the plasma will contain too little of the compound for effective removal

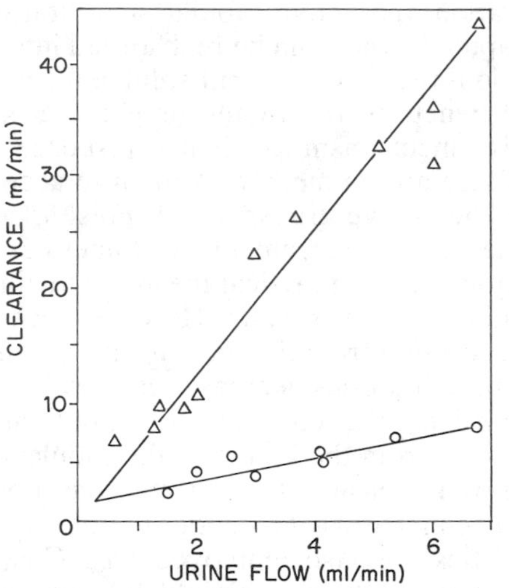

Figure 3–2. *Renal clearance of phenobarbital in the dog as it is related to urinary pH and the rate of urine flow.*

The values designated by circles are from experiments in which diuresis was induced by administration of water orally or Na_2SO_4 intravenously and the urinary pH was below 7.0. The values designated by triangles are from experiments in which $NaHCO_3$ was administered intravenously and in which the urinary pH was 7.8 to 8.0. (After Waddell and Butler, 1957. Courtesy of *Journal of Clinical Investigation.*)

by dialysis. Extensive binding of the compound to plasma proteins impairs dialysis greatly. The kinetics of elimination of a toxicant by dialysis is also dependent on the rate of dissociation of the compound from binding sites in tissues, and, for some chemicals, this may be slow.

Although peritoneal dialysis requires a minimum of personnel and can be started as soon as the patient is admitted to the hospital, it is too inefficient to be of value for the treatment of acute intoxications. Hemodialysis (extracorporeal dialysis) is much more effective than peritoneal dialysis and may be essential in a few life-threatening intoxications, such as with methanol, ethylene glycol, and salicylates. Passage of blood through a column of charcoal or adsorbent resin (hemoperfusion) is a technique for the extracorporeal removal of a poison (Winchester, 1983). Because of the high adsorptive capacity and affinity of the material in the column, some chemicals that are bound to plasma proteins can be removed. The principal side effect of hemoperfusion is depletion of platelets.

Antagonism or Chemical Inactivation of an Absorbed Poison

Functional and pharmacological antagonism of the effects of absorbed toxicants has been discussed above. If a patient is poisoned with a compound that acts as an agonist at a receptor for which a specific blocking agent is available, administration of the antagonist may be highly effective. Functional antagonism is also a cornerstone of treatment in that support of the patient's vital functions is imperative. However, drugs that stimulate antagonistic physiological mechanisms may be of little clinical value and may even decrease the incidence of survival. It is often difficult to titrate the effect of one drug against another when the two act on opposing systems. An example of such difficulty is the use of CNS stimulants to attempt to reverse respiratory depression. Convulsions are a typical complication of such therapy, and mechanical support of respiration is much preferred. In addition, the duration of action of the poison and the antidote may differ, sometimes leading to poisoning with the antidote.

Specific chemical antagonists of a toxicant are valuable but unfortunately rare. Chelating agents with high selectivity for certain metallic ions provide such examples (*see* Chapter 66). Antibodies offer the potential for the production of specific antidotes for a host of common poisons and for drugs that are frequently abused or misused. A notable example of such success is the use of purified digoxin-specific Fab fragments of antibodies in the treatment of potentially fatal cases of poisoning with digoxin (Smith *et al.*, 1982). The development of human monoclonal antibodies directed against specific toxins has significant potential.

Ames, B. N.; McCann, J.; and Yamasaki, E. Methods for detecting carcinogens and mutagens with the *Salmonella*/mammalian microsome mutagenicity test. *Mutat. Res.*, **1975**, *31*, 347–364.

Berg, M. J.; Berlinger, W. G.; Goldberg, J. J.; Spector, R.; and Johnson, G. F. Acceleration of the body clearance of phenobarbital by oral activated charcoal. *N. Engl. J. Med.*, **1982**, *307*, 642–644.

Berlinger, W. G.; Spector, R.; Goldberg, M. J.; Johnson, G. F.; Quee, C. K.; and Berg, M. J. Enhancement of theophylline clearance by oral activated charcoal. *Clin. Pharmacol. Ther.*, **1983**, *33*, 351–354.

Black, M. Acetaminophen hepatotoxicity. *Gastroenterology*, **1980**, *78*, 382–392.

Hjelle, J. J.; Hazelton, G. A.; and Klaassen, C. D. Acetaminophen decreases adenosine 3′-phosphate 5′-phosphosulfate and uridine diphosphoglucuronic acid in liver. *Drug Metab. Dispos.*, **1985**, *13*, 35–41.

Levy, G. Gastrointestinal clearance of drugs with activated charcoal. *N. Engl. J. Med.*, **1982**, *307*, 676–677.

Litovitz, T. L.; Schmitz, B. F.; Matyunas, N.; and Margin, T. G. 1987 Annual Report of the American Association of Poison Control Centers National Data Collection System. *Am. J. Emerg. Med.*, **1988**, *6*, 479–515.

Smith, T. W.; Butler, V. P., Jr.; Haber, E.; Fozzard, H.; Marcus, F. I.; Bremner, W. F.; Schulman, I. C.; and Phillips, A. Treatment of life-threatening digitalis intoxication with digoxin-specific Fab antibody fragments. *N. Engl. J. Med.*, **1982**, *307*, 1357–1362.

Thoman, M. E., and Verhulst, H. L. Ipecac syrup in antiemetic ingestion. *J.A.M.A.*, **1966**, *196*, 433–434.

Waddell, W. J., and Butler, T. C. The distribution and excretion of phenobarbital. *J. Clin. Invest.*, **1957**, *36*, 1217–1226.

Monographs and Reviews

Arena, J. M. Poisoning and its treatment. In, *Pediatric Therapy*, 5th ed. (Shirkey, H. C., ed.) C. V. Mosby Co., St. Louis, **1975**, pp. 101–136.

———. *Poisoning: Toxicology, Symptoms, Treatments*, 4th ed. Charles C Thomas, Springfield, Ill., **1979**.

Coombs, R. R. A., and Gell, P. G. H. Classification of allergic reactions responsible for clinical hypersensitivity and disease. In, *Clinical Aspects of Immunology*. (Gell, P. G. H.; Coombs, R. R. A.; and Lachmann, P. J.; eds.) Blackwell Scientific Publications, Oxford, **1975**, p. 761.

Ellenhorn, M. J., and Barceloux, D. G. *Medical Toxicology*. Elsevier-North Holland, Inc., New York, **1988**.

Ervin, M. E. Petroleum distillates and turpentine. In, *Clinical Management of Poisoning and Drug Overdose*. (Haddad, L. M., and Winchester, J. F., eds.) W. B. Saunders Co., Philadelphia, **1983**, pp. 771–779.

Goldfrank, L. R. *Toxicologic Emergencies*. Appleton-Century-Crofts, New York, **1982**.

Goldfrank, L. R.; Flomenbaum, N. E.; Lesin, N. A.; Weisman, R. S.; Howland, M. A.; and Keelberg, A. G. *Goldfrank's Toxicologic Emergencies*, 3rd ed. Appleton-Century-Crofts, East Norwalk, Conn., **1986**.

Goldstein, A.; Aronow, L.; and Kalman, S. M. *Principles of Drug Action: The Basis of Pharmacology*, 2nd ed. John Wiley & Sons, Inc., New York, **1974**.

Gosselin, R. E.; Smith, R. P.; and Hodge, H. C. *Clinical Toxicology of Commercial Products*, 5th ed. The Williams & Wilkins Co., Baltimore, **1984**.

Haddad, L. M., and Winchester, J. F. (eds.). *Clinical Management of Poisoning and Drug Overdose*. W. B. Saunders Co., Philadelphia, **1983**.

Klaassen, C. D. Principles of toxicology. In, *Casarett and Doull's Toxicology: The Basic Science of Poisons*, 3rd ed. (Klaassen, C. D.; Amdur, M.; and Doull, J.; eds.) Macmillan Publishing Co., New York, **1985**.

Klaassen, C. D.; Amdur, M. O.; and Doull, J. (eds.). *Casarett and Doull's Toxicology: The Basic Science of Poisons*, 3rd ed. Macmillan Publishing Co., New York, **1985**.

Klaassen, C. D., and Watkins, J. B., III. Mechanisms of bile formation, hepatic uptake, and biliary excretion. *Pharmacol. Rev.*, **1984**, *36*, 1–67.

Manno, B. R., and Manno, J. E. Toxicology of ipecac: a review. *Clin. Toxicol.*, **1977**, *10*, 221–242.

Rumack, B. H., and Lovejoy, F. H., Jr. Clinical toxicology. In, *Casarett and Doull's Toxicology: The Basic Science of Poisons*, 3rd ed. (Klaassen, C. D.; Amdur, M. O.; and Doull, J.; eds.) Macmillan Publishing Co., New York, **1985**.

Winchester, J. F. Active methods for detoxification: oral sorbents, forced diuresis, hemoperfusion, and hemodialysis. In, *Clinical Management of Poisoning and Drug Overdose*. (Haddad, L. M., and Winchester, J. F., eds.) W. B. Saunders Co., Philadelphia, **1983**, pp. 154–169.

CHAPTER

4 PRINCIPLES OF THERAPEUTICS

Alan S. Nies

THERAPY AS A SCIENCE

Over a century ago Claude Bernard formalized criteria for gathering valid information in experimental medicine. However, application of these criteria to therapeutics and to the process of making decisions about therapeutics has, until recently, been slow and inconsistent. At a time when the diagnostic aspects of medicine had become scientifically sophisticated, therapeutic decisions were often made on the basis of impressions and traditions. Historically, the absence of accurate data on the effects of drugs in man was due in large part to ethical standards of human experimentation. "Experimentation" in human beings was precluded, and it was not generally conceded that every treatment by any physician should be designed and in some sense recorded as an experiment.

Although there must always be ethical concern about experimentation in man, principles have been defined, and there are no longer ethical restraints on the gathering of either experimental or observational data on the efficacy and toxicity of drugs in adults. Furthermore, it should now be considered absolutely unethical to use the *art* as opposed to the *science* of therapeutics on any patient who directly (the adult or child) or indirectly (the fetus) receives drugs for therapeutic purposes. Observational (nonexperimental) techniques that can greatly add to our knowledge of the effects of drugs can be applied to all populations (Sheiner and Benet, 1985; Whiting *et al.*, 1986). The fact that such observational techniques have largely been applied in a nonsystematic fashion has led us to rely on a relative paucity of information about many drugs. Therapeutics must now be dominated by objective evaluation of an adequate base of factual knowledge.

Conceptual Barriers to Therapeutics as a Science. The most important barrier that inhibited the development of therapeutics as a science seems to have been the belief that multiple variables in diseases and in the effects of drugs are uncontrollable. If this were true, the scientific method would not be applicable to the study of pharmacotherapy. In fact, therapeutics is the aspect of patient care that is most amenable to the acquisition of useful data, since it involves an intervention and provides an opportunity to observe a response. It is now appreciated that clinical phenomena can be defined, described, and quantified with some precision. The approach to complex clinical data has been artfully discussed by Feinstein (1983).

Another barrier to the realization of therapeutics as a science was overreliance on traditional diagnostic labels for disease. This encouraged the physician to think of a disease as static rather than dynamic, to view patients with the same "label" as a homogeneous rather than a heterogeneous population, and to consider a disease as an entity even when information about pathogenesis was not available. If diseases are not considered to be dynamic, "standard" therapies in "standard" doses will be the order of the day; decisions will be reflexive. Needed instead is an attitude that makes the physician responsible for recognition of and compensation for changes that occur in pathophysiology as the underlying process evolves. For example, the term *myocardial infarction* refers to localized destruction of myocardial cells caused by interruption of the blood supply; however, decisions about therapy must take into account a variety of autonomic, hemodynamic, and electrophysiological variables that change as a function of time, size, and location of the infarction. Failure to take all such variables into account while planning a therapeutic maneuver may result in ineffective therapy in some patients while exposing others to avoidable toxicity. If groups of patients are in reality heterogeneous and receive alternative treatments, true differences in efficacy or toxicity between therapies may go unrecognized. A diagnosis or label of a disease or syndrome usually indicates a spectrum of possible causes and outcomes. Therapeutic experiments that fail to match groups for the known variables that affect prognosis yield uninterpretable data.

A third conceptual barrier was the incorrect notion that data derived empirically are useless because they are not generated by application of the scientific method. Empiricism is often defined as the practice of medicine founded on mere experience, without the aid of science or a knowledge of principles. The connotations of this definition are misleading; empirical observations need not be scientifically unsound. In fact, concepts of therapeutics have been greatly advanced by the clinical observer who makes careful and controlled observations on the outcome of a therapeutic intervention. The results, even when the mechanisms of disease and their interactions with the effects of drugs are not understood, are nevertheless often crucial to appropriate therapeutic decisions. Frequently, the initial suggestion that a drug may be efficacious in one condition arises from careful, empirical observations that are made while the drug is being used for another purpose. Examples of valid empirical observations that have resulted in new uses of drugs include the use of penicillamine to treat arthritis, lidocaine to treat cardiac arrhythmias, and propranolol and clonidine to treat hypertension. Conversely, empiricism, when not coupled with appropriate observational methods and statistical techniques, often results in findings that are inadequate or invalid.

Clinical Trials. Application of the scientific method to experimental therapeutics is exemplified by a well-designed and well-executed clinical trial. Clinical trials form the basis for therapeutic decisions by all physicians, and it is therefore essential that they be able to evaluate the results and conclusions of such trials critically. To maximize the likelihood that useful information will result from the experiment, the objectives of the study must be defined, homogeneous populations of patients must be selected, appropriate control groups must be found, meaningful and sensitive indices of drug effects must be chosen for observation, and the observations must be converted into data and then into valid conclusions (Feinstein, 1977). The *sine qua non* of any clinical trial is its controls. Many different types of controls may be used, and the term *controlled study* is not synonymous with *randomized double-blind technique*. Selection of a proper control group is as critical to the eventual utility of an experiment as the selection of the experimental group. Although the randomized, double-blind controlled trial is the most effective design for distributing bias and unknown variables between the "treatment" and the "control" groups, it is not necessarily the optimal design for all studies. It may be impossible to use this design to study disorders that occur rarely, disorders in patients who cannot, by regulation or ethics or both, be studied (*e.g.*, children, women of childbearing age, fetuses, or some patients with psychiatric diseases), or disorders with a uniformly fatal outcome (*e.g.*, rabies, where historical controls can be used).

There are several requirements in the design of clinical trials to test the relative effects of alternative therapies. (1) *Specific outcomes* of therapy that are clinically relevant and quantifiable must be measured. (2) The *accuracy of diagnosis* and the *severity of the disease* must be comparable in the groups being contrasted; otherwise, false-positive and false-negative errors may occur. (3) The *dosages* of the drugs must be chosen and individualized in a manner that allows relative efficacy to be compared at equivalent toxicities or allows relative toxicities to be compared at equivalent efficacies. (4) *Placebo effects*, which occur in a large percentage of patients, can confound many studies—particularly those that involve subjective responses; controls must take this into account. However, subjective assessments are important in determining whether a therapy improves the patient's well-being. In fact, quality of life can be assessed by the experimental subject and can be objectively tabulated and incorporated into evaluation of a therapy (Williams, 1987). (5) *Compliance* with the experimental regimens should be assessed before subjects are assigned to experimental or control groups. The drug-taking behavior of the subjects should be reassessed during the course of the trial. Noncompliance, even if randomly distributed between both groups, may cause falsely low estimates of the true potential benefits or toxicity of a particular treatment. (6) *Sample size* should be estimated prior to beginning a clinical trial and must be taken into account in interpreting the results of the trial. Depending upon such factors as the overall prognosis of the disease and the anticipated improvement in outcome or toxicity from the new treatment, very large numbers of subjects may be needed; otherwise, the possibility of a false-negative result is high (*i.e.*, no statistically significant differences between the two treatments will be found, even though differences actually exist) (Young *et al.*, 1983; Simon, 1986). (7) *Ethical considerations* may be major determinants of the types of controls that can be used and must be evaluated explicitly (Rosner, 1987; Rothman, 1987). For example, in therapeutic trials that involve life-threatening diseases for which there is already an effective therapy, the use of a placebo is unethical, and new treatments must be compared with "standard" therapies.

The results of clinical trials of new therapeutic agents or of old agents for new indications may have severe limitations in terms of what can be expected of drugs when they are used in an office practice. The selection of the patients for experimental trials usually eliminates those with coexisting diseases, and such trials usually assess the effect of only one or two drugs, not the many that might be given to or taken by the same patient under the care of a physician. Clinical trials are usually performed with relatively small numbers of patients for periods of time that may be shorter than are necessary in practice, and compliance may be better controlled than it can be in practice. These factors lead to several inescapable conclusions:

1) Even if the result of a valid clinical trial of a drug is thoroughly understood, the physician can only develop a hypothesis about what the drug might do to a particular patient, and there can be no assurance that what occurred in other patients will be seen. In effect, the physician uses the results of a clinical trial to establish an experiment in each patient. The detection of anticipated and unanticipated effects and the determination of whether or not they are due to the drug(s) being used are important responsibilities of the physician during the supervision of a therapeutic regimen. If an effect of a drug is not seen in a clinical trial, it may still be revealed in the setting of clinical practice. About one half or more of both useful and adverse effects of drugs that were not recognized in the initial formal trials were subsequently discovered and reported by practicing physicians.

2) If an anticipated effect of a drug has not occurred in a patient, this does not mean that the effect cannot occur in that patient or in others. Many factors in the individual patient may contribute to lack of efficacy of a drug. They include, for example, misdiagnosis, poor compliance by the patient to the regimen, poor choice of dosage or dosage intervals, coincidental development of an undiagnosed separate illness that influences the outcome, the use of other agents that interact with primary drugs to nullify or alter their effects, undetected genetic or environmental variables that modify the disease or the pharmacological actions of the drug, or unknown therapy by another physician who is caring for the same patient. Of equal importance, even when a regimen appears to be efficacious and innocuous, a physician should not attribute all improvement to the therapeutic regimen chosen, nor should a physician assume that a deteriorating condition reflects only the natural course of the disease. Similarly, if an anticipated untoward or toxic effect is not seen in a particular patient, it can still occur in others. Physicians who use only their own experience with a drug to make decisions about its use unduly expose their patients to unjustifiable risk or unrealized efficacy. For example, simply because a doctor has not seen a case of chloramphenicol-induced aplastic anemia in his own practice does not mean that such a disaster may not occur; the drug should still be used for the proper indications.

3) Rational therapy is therapy based on the use of observations that have been evaluated critically. It is no less crucial to have a scientific approach to the treatment of an individual patient than to use this approach when investigating drugs in a research setting. In both instances, it is the patient who benefits. Such an approach can be formalized in the practice setting by performing randomized, controlled trials in individual patients who have stable clinical symptomatology. With this strategy a specific ther-

apy of uncertain efficacy can be compared with a placebo or alternative therapy in a double-blind design with well-defined end points that are tailored to the individual patient. The outcome of such a trial is immediately relevant to the particular patient, although it may not apply to all other patients (Guyatt *et al.*, 1986).

INDIVIDUALIZATION OF DRUG THERAPY

As has been implied above, therapy as a science does not apply simply to the evaluation and testing of new, investigational drugs in animals and man. It applies with equal importance to the treatment of each patient as an individual. Therapists of every type have long recognized and acknowledged that individual patients show wide variability in response to the same drug or treatment method. Progress has been made in identifying the sources of variability (Vesell, 1986). Important factors are presented in Figure 4–1; the basic principles that underlie these sources of variability have been presented in Chapters 1 and 2.

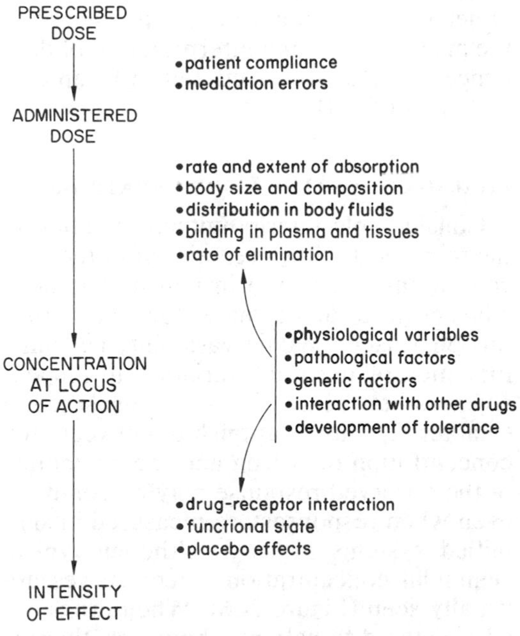

Figure 4–1. *Factors that determine the relationship between prescribed drug dosage and drug effect.* (Modified from Koch-Weser, 1972.)

The following discussion relates to the strategies that have been developed to deal with variability in the clinical setting. (*See also* Appendix II.)

PHARMACOKINETIC CONSIDERATIONS

Interpatient and intrapatient variation in disposition of a drug must be taken into account in choosing a drug regimen. For a given drug, there may be wide variation in its pharmacokinetic properties among individuals. For some drugs, this variability may account for one half or more of the total variation in eventual response. The relative importance of the many factors that contribute to these differences depends in part on the drug itself and on its usual route of elimination. Drugs that are excreted primarily unchanged by the kidney tend to have smaller differences in disposition among patients with similar renal function than do drugs that are inactivated by metabolism. Of drugs that are extensively metabolized, those with high metabolic clearance and large first-pass elimination have marked differences in bioavailability, whereas those with slower biotransformation tend to have the largest variation in elimination rates between individuals. Studies in identical and nonidentical twins have revealed that genotype is a very important determinant of differences in the rates of metabolism (Penno and Vesell, 1983). For many drugs, physiological and pathological variations in organ function are major determinants of their rate of disposition. For example, the clearance of digoxin and gentamicin is related to the rate of glomerular filtration, whereas that of lidocaine and propranolol is primarily dependent on the rate of hepatic blood flow. The effect of aging and diseases that involve the kidneys or liver is to impair elimination and to increase the variability in the disposition of drugs. In such settings, measurements of concentrations of drugs in biological fluids can be used to assist in the individualization of drug therapy (Spector *et al.*, 1988). Since old age and renal or hepatic diseases may also affect the responsiveness of target tissues (*e.g.*, the brain), the physician should be alert to the possibility of a shift in the range of therapeutic concentrations

A test should not be performed simply because an assay is available. More assays of drugs are available than are generally useful. Determinations of concentrations of drug in blood, serum, or plasma are particularly useful when well-defined criteria are fulfilled. (1) There must be a demonstrated relationship between the concentration of the drug in plasma and the eventual therapeutic effect that is desired and/or the toxic effect that must be avoided. (2) There should be substantial interpatient variability in disposition of the drug (and small intrapatient variation). Otherwise, concentrations of drug in plasma could be predicted adequately from dose alone. (3) It should be difficult to monitor intended or unintended effects of the drug. Whenever clinical effects or minor toxicity are easily measured (*e.g.*, the effect of a drug on blood pressure), such assessments should be preferred in the decision to make any necessary adjustment of dosage of the drug. However, the effects of some drugs in certain settings are not easily monitored. For example, the effect of Li^+ on manic–depressive psychosis may be delayed and difficult to quantify. For some drugs, the initial manifestation of toxicity may be serious (*e.g.*, digitalis-induced arrhythmias or theophylline-induced seizures). The same concepts apply to a number of agents used for cancer chemotherapy. Other drugs (*e.g.*, antiarrhythmic agents) produce toxic effects that mimic symptoms or signs of the disease being treated. Many drugs are used for prophylaxis of an intermittent, potentially dangerous event; examples include anticonvulsants and antiarrhythmic agents. In each of these situations, titration of drug dosage may be aided by measurements of concentrations of the drug in blood. (4) The concentration of drug required to produce therapeutic effects should be close to the value that causes substantial toxicity (*see* below). If this circumstance does not apply, patients could simply be given the largest dose known to be necessary to treat a disorder, as is commonly done with penicillin. However, if there is an overlap in the concentration–response relationship for desirable and undesirable effects of the drug, as is true for theophylline, determinations of concentration of drug in plasma may allow the dose to be optimized. All four of the above-described criteria should be met if the measurement of drug concentrations is to be of significant value in the adjustment of dosage. Knowledge of concentrations of drugs in plasma or urine is also particularly useful for detection of therapeutic failures that are due to lack of patient compliance with a medical regimen or for identification of patients with unexpected extremes in the rate of drug disposition.

Assay of drugs to assist the physician in achieving a desired concentration of drug in blood or plasma (*i.e.*, "targeting" the dose) is an example of the use of an *intermediate end point of therapy*. An intermediate end point is defined as a specific goal of treatment that is used in place of the ultimate clinical goal, which may be difficult to assess. The concept of intermediate end points, including concentrations of drugs, as a guide to individualization of therapy can also be applied in other ways; one is to provide an indication for a change in the choice of drug therapy. Measurements of concentrations of drugs in plasma and/or measurements of one or more pharmacological effects of the drug can provide an indication of probable lack of efficacy. Other issues of importance with regard to the measurement and interpretation of drug concentrations are discussed in Chapter 1 and Appendix II.

PHARMACODYNAMIC CONSIDERATIONS

Considerable interindividual variation in the response to drugs remains after the concentration of the drug in plasma has been adjusted to a target value; for some drugs this pharmacodynamic variability accounts for much of the total variation in responsiveness between patients. As discussed in Chapter 2, the relationship between the concentration of a drug and the magnitude of the observed response may be complex, even when responses are measured in simplified systems *in vitro*, although typical sigmoidal concentration–effect curves are usually seen (Figure 2–6). When drugs are administered to patients, however, there is no single characteristic relationship between the drug concentration in plasma and the measured effect; the concentration–

effect curve may be concave upward, concave downward, linear, or sigmoid. Moreover, the concentration–effect relationship may be distorted if the response being measured is a composite of several effects, such as the change in blood pressure produced by a combination of cardiac, vascular, and reflex effects. However, such a composite concentration–effect curve can often be resolved into simpler curves for each of its components. These simplified concentration–effect relationships, regardless of their exact shape, can be viewed as having four characteristic variables: potency, slope, maximal efficacy, and individual variation. These are illustrated in Figure 4–2 for the common sigmoid log dose–effect curve.

Potency. The location of the concentration–effect curve along the *concentration axis* is an expression of the potency of a drug. Although often related to the dose of a drug required to produce an effect, potency is more properly related to the concentration of the drug in plasma in order to approximate more closely the situation in isolated systems *in vitro* and to avoid the complicating factors of pharmacokinetic variables. Although potency obviously affects drug dosage, potency *per se* is relatively unimportant in the clinical use of drugs as long as the required dose can be given conveniently. There is no justification for the view that more potent drugs are superior therapeutic agents. However, if

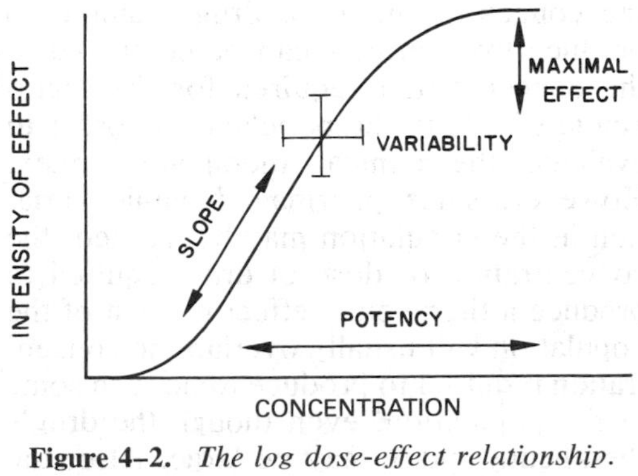

Figure 4–2. *The log dose-effect relationship.*

Representative log dose-effect curve, illustrating its four characterizing variables (*see* text for explanation).

the drug is to be administered by transdermal absorption, a highly potent drug is required, since the capacity of the skin to absorb drugs is limited.

Maximal Efficacy. The maximal effect that can be produced by a drug is its *maximal efficacy* or, simply, *efficacy*. As discussed in Chapter 2, maximal efficacy is determined by the properties of the drug and its receptor–effector system and is reflected in the plateau of the concentration–effect curve. In clinical use, however, a drug's dosage may be limited by undesired effects, and the true maximal efficacy of the drug may not be achievable. Efficacy of a drug is clearly a major characteristic—of much more clinical importance than is potency; furthermore, the two properties are not related and should not be confused. For instance, although some thiazide diuretics have similar or greater potency than the loop diuretic furosemide, the maximal efficacy of furosemide is considerably greater.

Slope. The slope of the concentration–effect curve reflects the mechanism of action of a drug, including the shape of the curve that describes drug binding to its receptor (*see* Chapter 2). The steepness of the curve dictates the range of doses that are useful for achieving a clinical effect. Aside from this fact, the slope of the concentration–effect curve has more theoretical than practical usefulness.

Biological Variability. Different individuals vary in the magnitude of their response to the same concentration of a single drug or to similar drugs when the appropriate correction has been made for differences in potency, maximal efficacy, and slope. In fact, a single individual may not always respond in the same way to the same concentration of drug. A concentration–effect curve applies only to a single individual at one time or to an average individual. The intersecting brackets in Figure 4–2 indicate that an effect of varying intensity will occur in different individuals at a specified concentration of a drug or that a range of concentrations is required to produce an effect of specified intensity in all of the patients.

Specific terms are used to refer to individuals who are unusually sensitive or resistant to a drug and to describe those in whom the drug produces a qualitatively different effect. The mechanisms of these unusual effects are described in general in this chapter and are discussed for individual drugs throughout this textbook. If a drug produces an effect at a very low dosage, the individual is said to be *hyperreactive*. (*Hypersensitivity* usually refers to effects associated with drug allergy, and *supersensitivity* is used to describe the increased sensitivity that results from denervation or long-term treatment with a receptor antagonist.) Individuals who are resistant to drug effect are said to be *hyporeactive*. *Tolerance* connotes hyporeactivity acquired as a result of exposure to the drug, and if tolerance develops rapidly, it is called *tachyphylaxis*. *Idiosyncrasy* is a term that describes an unusual effect of the drug, irrespective of intensity or dosage, that occurs in a small percentage of the population. However, because this term is often confused with drug allergy and because it conveys no useful information, it should probably be abandoned in favor of simple descriptions of the effect and terms that refer to the underlying mechanisms, which are often genetic or immunological.

Attempts have been made to define and measure individual "sensitivity" to drugs in the clinical setting, and progress has been made in understanding some of the determinants of sensitivity to drugs that act at specific receptors. For example, responsiveness to β-adrenergic receptor agonists may change because of disease (*e.g.*, thyrotoxicosis) or because of prior administration of either β-adrenergic agonists or antagonists that can cause changes in the concentration of the β-adrenergic receptor and/or coupling of the receptor to its effector systems (Bristow *et al.*, 1982; Stiles *et al.*, 1984). Resistance of tumors to the antineoplastic agent methotrexate may occur because of gene amplification and subsequent synthesis of large quantities of the receptor for the cytotoxic action of this drug, dihydrofolate reductase (Brown *et al.*, 1983). Receptors are not static components of the cell; they are in a dynamic state that is influenced by both endogenous and exogenous factors (*see* Chapters 2 and 5).

Concentration–Percent Curve. The concentration of a drug that produces a specified effect in a single patient is termed the *individual effective concentration*. This is a *quantal* response, since the defined effect is either present or absent. Individual effective concentrations are usually lognormally distributed, which means that a normal variation curve is the result of plotting the logarithms of the concentration against the frequency of patients achieving the defined effect (Figure 4–3A). A cumulative frequency distribution of individuals achieving the defined effect as a function of drug concentration is the *concentration–percent curve* or the *quantal concentration–effect curve*. This curve resembles the sigmoid shape of the graded concentration–effect curve discussed above (Figure 4–2), but the slope of the concentration–percent curve is an expression of the pharmacodynamic variability in the population rather than an expression of the concentration range from a threshold to a maximal effect in the individual patient.

The dose of a drug required to produce a specified effect in 50% of the population is the *median effective dose*, abbreviated as the ED_{50} (Figure 4–3B). In preclinical studies of drugs, the *median lethal dose*, as determined in experimental animals, is abbreviated as LD_{50}. The ratio of the LD_{50} to the ED_{50} is an indication of the *therapeutic index*, which is a statement of how *selective* the drug is in producing its desired effects. In clinical studies, the dose, or preferably the concentration, of a drug required to produce toxic effects can be compared to the concentration required for the therapeutic effects in the population in order to evaluate the clinical therapeutic index. However, since pharmacodynamic variation in the population may be marked, the concentration or dose of drug required to produce a therapeutic effect in most of the population will usually overlap the concentration required to produce toxicity in some of the population, even though the drug's therapeutic index may be large. Also, the concentration–percent curves for efficacy and toxicity need not be parallel, adding yet

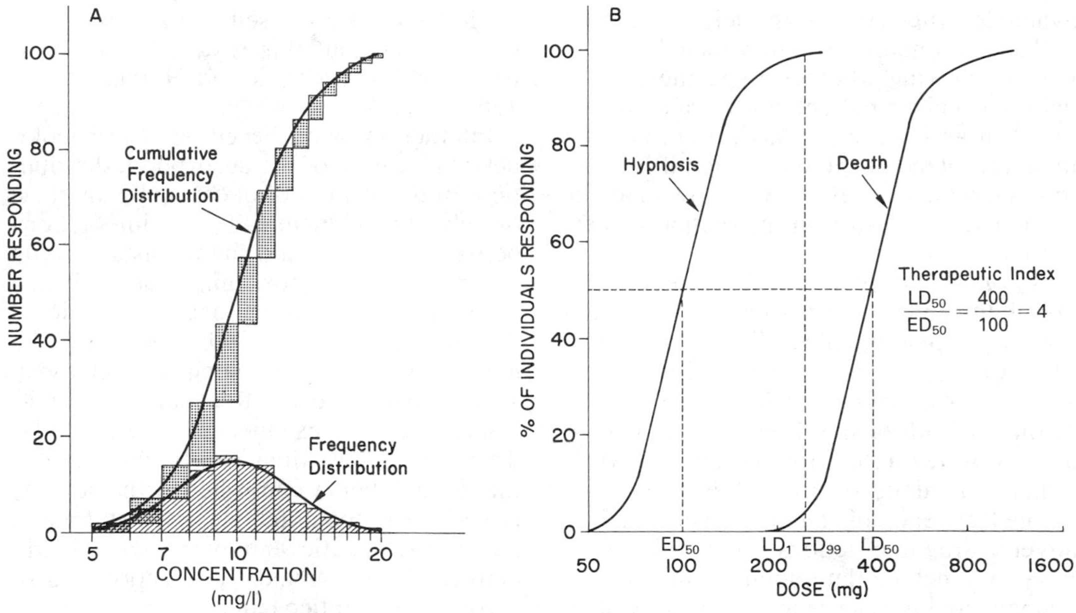

Figure 4–3. *Frequency distribution curves and quantal dose-effect curves.*

A. An experiment was performed on 100 subjects and the effective concentration to produce a quantal response was determined for each individual. The number of subjects who required each dose is plotted, giving a lognormal frequency distribution (bars with diagonal lines). The stippled bars demonstrate that the normal frequency distribution, when summated, yields the cumulative frequency distribution—a sigmoidal curve that is a quantal concentration–effect curve.

B. Quantal Dose-Effect Curves. Animals were injected with varying doses of a sedative–hypnotic, and the responses determined and plotted (*see* text for additional explanation).

another complexity to the determination of the therapeutic index in patients. Finally, *no drug produces a single effect*, and, depending on the effect being measured, the therapeutic index for a drug will vary. For example, much less codeine is required for cough suppression than for control of pain in 50% of the population, and thus the margin of safety, selectivity, or therapeutic index of codeine is much greater as an antitussive than as an analgesic.

OTHER FACTORS THAT AFFECT THERAPEUTIC OUTCOME

The variation in pharmacokinetic and pharmacodynamic parameters that accounts for much of the need to individualize therapy has been discussed. Other factors, listed in Figure 4–1, should also be considered as potential determinants of success or failure of therapy. The following presentation serves as an introduction to these subjects, some of which are also discussed elsewhere in this textbook.

Drug–Drug Interactions. The use of several drugs is often essential to obtain a desired therapeutic objective or to treat coexisting diseases. Examples abound, and the choice of drugs to be employed concurrently can be based on sound pharmacological principles. In the treatment of hypertension, a single drug is effective in only a modest percentage of patients. In the treatment of heart failure, the concurrent use of a diuretic with a vasodilator and/or a cardiac glycoside is often essential to achieve an adequate cardiac output and to keep the patient free from edema. Multiple-drug therapy is the norm in cancer chemotherapy and for the treatment of certain infectious diseases. The goals in these cases are usually to improve efficacy and to delay the emergence of malignant cells or of microorganisms that are resistant to the effects of available drugs. When physicians use several drugs concurrently, they face the problem of knowing whether a specific combination in a given patient has the potential to result in an interaction, and, if so, how to take advantage of the interaction if it leads to improvement in efficacy or how to avoid the consequences of an interaction if they are adverse.

A *potential drug interaction* refers to the possibility that one drug may alter the intensity of pharmacological effects of another drug given concurrently. The net result may be enhanced or diminished effects of one or both of the drugs or the appearance of a new effect that is not seen with either drug alone.

The frequency of significant beneficial or adverse drug interactions is unknown. Surveys that include data obtained *in vitro,* in animals, and in case reports tend to predict a frequency of interactions that is higher than actually occurs. While such reports have contributed to skepticism about the overall importance of drug interactions, there certainly are a number of potential interactions of clinical importance, and the physician must be alert to the possibility of their occurrence (McInnes and Brodie, 1988). Estimates of the incidence of clinical drug–drug interactions range from 3 to 5% in patients taking a few drugs to 20% in patients who are receiving 10 to 20 drugs. Because most hospitalized patients receive at least six drugs, the scope of the problem is clearly significant (Steel *et al.,* 1981). Recognition of beneficial effects and recognition and prevention of adverse drug interactions require a thorough knowledge of the intended and possible effects of drugs that are prescribed, a mental set to attribute unusual events to drugs rather than to disease, and adequate observation of the patient. Automated monitoring of prescription orders in the hospital or outpatient pharmacy may decrease the physician's need to memorize potential interactions. Nevertheless, knowledge of likely mechanisms of drug interactions is the only way the clinician can be prepared to analyze new findings systematically. It is incumbent upon the physician to be familiar with the basic principles of drug–drug interactions in planning a therapeutic regimen. Such reactions are discussed for individual drugs throughout this textbook. (*See also* Hansten, 1985; Rizack and Hillman, 1987; Tatro, 1988.)

Interactions may be either pharmacokinetic (alteration of the absorption, distribution, or disposition of one drug by another) or pharmacodynamic (*e.g.,* interactions between agonists and antagonists at drug receptors). The most important adverse drug–drug interactions occur with drugs that have easily recognizable toxicity and a low therapeutic index, such that relatively small changes in drug effect can have significant adverse consequences. Additionally, drug–drug interactions can be important if the disease being controlled with the drug is serious or potentially fatal if untreated and if therapeutic end points are clearly defined. Thus, major interactions have involved oral anticoagulants, oral hypoglycemics, antibiotics, antiepileptics, antiarrhythmics, and cardiac glycosides.

Pharmacokinetic Drug Interactions. Drugs may interact at any point during their absorption, distribution, metabolism, or excretion; the result may be an increase or decrease in the concentration of drug at the site of action. Since individuals vary in their rate of disposition of any given drug, the magnitude of an interaction that alters pharmacokinetic parameters is not always predictable, but can be very significant.

The delivery of drug into the circulation may be altered by physicochemical interactions that occur prior to absorption. For example, drugs may interact in an intravenous solution to produce an insoluble precipitate that may or may not be obvious. In the gut, drugs may chelate with metal ions or adsorb to medicinal resins. Thus, Ca^{2+} and other metallic cations contained in antacids are chelated by tetracycline, and the complex is not absorbed. Cholestyramine adsorbs and inhibits the absorption of thyroxine, cardiac glycosides, warfarin, corticosteroids, and probably other drugs. The rate and sometimes the extent of absorption can be affected by drugs that reduce gastric motility, but this is usually of little clinical consequence. Interactions within the gut may be indirect and complex. Antibiotics that alter the gastrointestinal flora can reduce the rate of bacterial synthesis of vitamin K such that the effect of oral anticoagulants, which compete with vitamin K, will be enhanced. If a drug is metabolized by the gastrointestinal microorganisms, antibiotic therapy may result in an increase in the absorption of the drug, as has been demonstrated for some patients receiving digoxin (Lindenbaum *et al.,* 1981).

Many drugs are extensively bound to plasma albumin (acidic drugs) or α_1-acid glycoprotein (basic drugs). In general, only unbound drug is free to exert an effect or to be distributed to the tissues. Thus, displacement of one drug from its binding site by another might be expected to result in a change in drug effects. Although such binding/displacement interactions occur, they are rarely of clinical significance. This is because the displaced drug distributes rapidly into the tissues; the larger the apparent volume of distribution of the drug, the less is the rise in the concentration of free drug in the plasma. Furthermore, following the displacement, more free drug is available for metabolism and excretion. Thus, the body's clearance processes eventually reduce the free drug concentration to that which existed prior to the drug-displacement interaction. As a result, the effect of such an interaction is usually small, transient, and frequently unrecognized. However, the relationship of free drug to the total (bound plus free) drug is changed, and the interpretation of plasma drug assays that measure total drug concentration must be altered.

A few drugs are actively transported to their site of action. For instance, the antihypertensive drugs guanethidine and guanadrel cause inhibition of sympathetic function after being transported into adrenergic neurons by the norepinephrine uptake mechanism. Inhibition of this neuronal uptake system by tricyclic antidepressants and some sympathomimetic amines will inhibit the sympathetic blockade and reduce the antihypertensive effects of guanethidine and guanadrel.

Interactions involving drug metabolism can increase or decrease the amount of drug available for action by inhibition or induction of metabolism, respectively. Inhibition of metabolism is usually more predictable than induction, which is influenced by genetic differences between patients. Examples of drugs that inhibit the metabolism of others include inhibitors of some isozymes of cytochrome P_{450} (cimetidine, amiodarone, phenylbutazone, isoniazid, sodium valproate, and erythromycin), xanthine oxidase (allopurinol), and monoamine oxidase (MAO) inhibitors. Drugs that accelerate the metabolism of other agents include barbiturates, rifampin, phenytoin, carbamazepine, chronic smoking, and certain chlorinated hydrocarbons. The effects of enzyme induction are most obvious when drugs are given orally, because all of the absorbed compound must pass through the liver prior to reaching the systemic circulation. Therefore, even for drugs that have a systemic clearance that is mainly dependent on hepatic blood flow (*e.g.*, propranolol), the amount of drug that escapes metabolism on the first pass will be influenced by enzyme induction. Examples of drugs that are affected by enzyme inducers are oral anticoagulants, quinidine, corticosteroids, low-dose estrogen contraceptives, theophylline, mexiletine, methadone, and some β-adrenergic blocking agents.

The ability of one drug to inhibit the renal excretion of another is dependent on an interaction at active transport sites. Many of the reported interactions occur at the anion transport site, where, for example, probenecid inhibits the excretion of penicillin to cause the desirable effects of elevated plasma concentrations of the antibiotic and a longer half-life. Similarly, the renal elimination of methotrexate is inhibited by probenecid, salicylates, and phenylbutazone, but in this case methotrexate toxicity may result from the interaction. Interactions at the transport site for basic drugs include the inhibition of excretion of procainamide by cimetidine and amiodarone. An interaction at an unknown tubular site causes inhibition of the excretion of digoxin by quinidine, verapamil, and amiodarone. Finally, the excretion of Li^+ can be affected by drugs that alter the ability of the proximal renal tubule to reabsorb Na^+. Thus, clearance of Li^+ is reduced and concentrations of Li^+ in plasma are increased by diuretics that cause volume depletion and by nonsteroidal antiinflammatory drugs that enhance proximal tubular reabsorption of Na^+.

Pharmacodynamic Interactions. There are numerous examples of drugs that interact at a common receptor site or that have additive or inhibitory effects due to actions at different sites in an organ. Such interactions are described throughout this textbook. Frequently overlooked is the multiplicity of effects of many drugs. Thus, phenothiazines are effective α-adrenergic antagonists; many antihistamines and tricyclic antidepressants are potent inhibitors of muscarinic receptors. These "minor" actions of drugs may be the cause of drug interactions.

Other interactions of an apparently pharmacodynamic nature are poorly understood or are mediated indirectly. Halogenated hydrocarbons, including many general anesthetics, sensitize the myocardium to the arrhythmogenic actions of catecholamines. This effect may result from an action on the pathway that leads from adrenergic receptor to effector, but the details are unclear. The striking interaction between meperidine and monoamine oxidase inhibitors to produce seizures and hyperpyrexia may be related to excessive amounts of an excitatory neurotransmitter, but the mechanism has not been elucidated.

One drug may alter the normal internal milieu, thereby augmenting or diminishing the effect of another agent. A well-known example of such an interaction is the enhancement of the toxic effects of digoxin as a result of diuretic-induced hypokalemia.

Summary. Drug–drug interactions are only one of the many factors discussed in this chapter that can alter the patient's response to therapy. The major task of the physician is to determine if an interaction has occurred and the magnitude of its effect. When unexpected effects are seen, a drug interaction should be suspected. Careful drug histories are important because patients may take over-the-counter drugs, may take drugs prescribed by another physician, or may take drugs prescribed for another patient. Care must be exercised when major changes are made in a drug regimen, and drugs that are not necessary should be discontinued. When an interaction is discovered, the interacting drugs may often be used effectively with adjustment of dosage or other therapeutic modifications.

Fixed-Dose Combinations. The concomitant use of two or more drugs adds to the complexity of individualization of drug therapy. The dose of each drug should be adjusted to achieve optimal benefit. Thus, patient compliance is essential, yet more difficult to achieve. To obviate the latter problem many fixed-dose drug combinations are marketed. The use of such combinations is advantageous only if the ratio of the fixed doses corresponds to the needs of the individual patient.

In the United States, a fixed-dose combination of drugs must be approved by the Food and Drug Administration (FDA) before it can be marketed, even though the individual drugs are available for concurrent use. To be approved, certain conditions must be met. The two drugs must act to achieve a better therapeutic response than either drug alone (*e.g.*, many antihypertensive drug combinations); or one drug must act to reduce the incidence of adverse effects caused by the other (*e.g.*, a diuretic that promotes the urinary excretion of K^+ combined with a K^+-sparing diuretic).

Placebo Effects. The net effect of drug therapy is the sum of the pharmacological effects of the drug and the nonspecific placebo effects associated with the therapeutic effort. Although identified specifically with administration of an inert substance in the guise of medication, placebo effects are associated with the taking of any drug, active as well as inert.

Placebo effects result from the physician–patient relationship, the significance of the therapeutic effort to the patient, and the mental set imparted by the therapeutic setting and by the physician. They vary significantly in different individuals and in any one patient at different times. Placebo effects are commonly manifested as alterations of mood, other subjective effects, and objective effects that are under autonomic or voluntary control. They may be favorable or unfavorable relative to the therapeutic objectives. Exploited to advantage, placebo effects can significantly supplement pharmacological effects and can represent the difference between success and failure of therapy (Brody, 1982).

A placebo (in this context, better termed *dummy medication*) is an indispensable element of the controlled clinical trial. In contrast, a placebo has only a limited role in the routine practice of medicine. Although the inert medication may be an effective vehicle for a placebo effect, the physician–patient relationship is generally preferable. Relief or lack of relief of symptoms upon administration of a placebo is not a reliable basis for determining whether the symptoms have a "psychogenic" or "somatic" origin.

Tolerance. Tolerance may be acquired to the effects of many drugs, especially the opioids, various central nervous system (CNS) depressants, and organic nitrates. When this occurs, *cross-tolerance* may develop to the effects of pharmacologically related drugs, particularly those acting at the same receptor site, and drug dosage must be increased to maintain a given therapeutic effect. Since tolerance does not usually develop equally to all effects of a drug, the therapeutic index may decrease. However, there are also examples of the development of tolerance to the undesired effects of a drug and a resultant increase in its therapeutic index (*e.g.*, tolerance to sedation produced by phenobarbital when used as an anticonvulsant).

The mechanisms involved in the development of tolerance are only partially understood. In animals, tolerance often occurs as the result of induced synthesis of the hepatic microsomal enzymes involved in drug biotransformation; the possible significance of this *drug-disposition* or *pharmacokinetic tolerance* during chronic medication in man is an area of continuing investigation. The most important factor in the development of tolerance to the opioids, barbiturates, ethanol, and organic nitrates is some type of cellular adaptation referred to as *pharmaco-*

dynamic tolerance; multiple mechanisms are involved. Tachyphylaxis, such as that to histamine-releasing agents and to the sympathomimetic amines that act indirectly by releasing norepinephrine, has been attributed to depletion of available mediator, but other mechanisms may also contribute. The subject of tolerance is discussed in more detail in Chapter 22.

Genetic Factors. Genetic factors are the major determinants of the normal variability of drug effects and are responsible for a number of striking quantitative and qualitative differences in pharmacological activity (Vesell, 1986). Many of the genetically determined *quantitative* differences in drug response are due to polygenic influences on drug metabolism, which result in a more or less normal distribution of rates of drug clearance across the population. Recently, however, there has been an increasing number of drugs whose metabolic clearances segregate into distinct groups because the drug biotransformation is controlled by a single gene.

Metabolic processes that are under monogenic control include (1) N-acetyltransferase-catalyzed N-acetylation of isoniazid, procainamide, hydralazine, dapsone, sulfamethazine, sulfasalazine, and some potential carcinogenic amines (Horai and Ishizaki, 1987); (2) cytochrome P_{450}-catalyzed oxidation of several β-adrenergic receptor blocking agents, encainide, propafenone, tricyclic antidepressants, phenformin, and dextromethorphan (Clark, 1985; Gonzalez, *et al.*, 1988); (3) several methyltransferase-catalyzed methylations of thiopurines (mercaptopurine, thioguanine, and azathioprine), aliphatic thiol-containing drugs (captopril and penicillamine), catecholamines, and possibly histamine (Weinshilboum, 1988); and (4) plasma cholinesterase-catalyzed hydrolysis of succinylcholine. The quantitative differences in drug response in patients with these genetically determined differences in drug metabolism are due to greater or lesser amounts of active compound in the body, whether this be the parent drug or an active metabolite.

Genetically determined *qualitative* differences in drug effect occur when a known minor toxic property of a drug assumes an exaggerated importance due to a genetic defect in the ability to avoid the toxicity. For example, individuals who are deficient in glucose-6-phosphate dehydrogenase activity are unable to cope with the oxidative stress produced by some drugs, resulting in drug-induced hemolysis.

The objectives of *pharmacogenetics* include not only identification of differences in drug effects that have a genetic basis but also development of simple methods by which susceptible individuals can be recognized before the drug is administered.

APPROACH TO INDIVIDUALIZATION

After it has been determined that pharmacotherapy is necessary to modify the symptoms or outcome of a disease, the therapist is faced with two types of decisions: the first is qualitative (the initial choice of a specific drug) and the second quantitative (the initial dosage regimen). Optimal treatment will result only when the physician is aware of the sources of variation in response to drugs, and when the dosage regimen is designed on the basis of the best available data about the diagnosis, severity and stage of the disease, presence of concurrent diseases or drug treatment, and predefined goals of acceptable efficacy and limits of acceptable toxicity. If objectively assessable expectations of drug therapy are not set before therapy is initiated, therapy is likely to be ineffective and continued longer than necessary, unless an obvious adverse effect occurs.

In most clinical settings, the decision about the choice of drug is substantially influenced by the confidence the physician has in the accuracy of his diagnosis and estimates of the extent and severity of disease. Based on the best available information, the physician must decide on an initial drug from a group of reasonable alternatives. The extent of this evaluation is itself dependent on many factors, including a cost–benefit analysis of diagnostic tests, and this must be based on the availability and specificity of alternative therapies (Pauker and Kassirer, 1987). The initial dosage regimen is determined by estimation, if possible, of the pharmacokinetic properties of the drug in the individual patient. The estimate must be based on an appreciation of the variables that are most likely to affect the disposition of the particular drug. These variables have been discussed above (*see* Figure 4–1 and Appendix II). Subsequent adjustments may be aided in some instances by measurement of drug concentrations but must ultimately be based on whether the regimen is efficacious, either without adverse effects or at an acceptable level of toxicity.

It has been stated above that every therapeutic plan is and should be treated as an experiment. As such, most of the considerations that were specified in the discussion of clinical trials must be applied to individual patients. Of utmost importance is the definition of specific goals of treatment and the means to assess whether these goals are being achieved. Whenever possible, the objective end point should be related as closely as possible to the clinical goals of therapy (*e.g.*, shrinkage of a tumor or eradication of an infection). Many clinical goals are, however, difficult to assess (*e.g.*, the prevention of cardiovascular complications associated with hypertension and diabetes). In such cases it is necessary to set intermediate end points to therapy, such as a reduction in blood pressure or the concentration of glucose in plasma. These intermediate end points are based on demonstrated or assumed correlations with the ultimate clinical benefit. In many cases, such as reduction of the concentration of cholesterol in plasma by drugs or the elimination of asymptomatic ventricular arrhythmias, the link between the intermediate goal and the ultimate goal is controversial.

Certain general considerations apply to the individualization of a drug regimen and the concept of intermediate end points. The value or utility of the regimen obviously needs to be assessed at intervals during the course of therapy. The utility of a regimen can be defined as the benefit it produces plus the dangers of not treating the disease minus the sum of the adverse effects of therapy. Another common expression of the usefulness of a regimen is its ratio of risks to benefits (representing a balance between the efficacious and toxic effects of the drug). A definitive evaluation of the utility of a drug is not easy; nevertheless, some sense of the value of a regimen must be established in the minds of the physician and the patient. Knowledge of the usefulness of a given regimen may be a critical determinant of protracted compliance by the patient to a long-term regimen or logical discontinuation by the physician of a marginally efficacious and risky therapy. It must be remembered that the physician, the patient, and the patient's family may have disparate opinions of the utility of a therapeutic regimen. In one study of antihypertensive therapy where all patients were judged to be improved by the physician, only 48% of the patients considered themselves improved and 8% felt worse. Relatives thought that only 1% of the patients were improved and that 99% had evidence of adverse effects of therapy (Jachuck *et al.*, 1982).

DRUG REGULATION AND DEVELOPMENT

DRUG REGULATION

The history of drug regulation in the United States reflects the growing involvement of governments in most countries to ensure some degree of efficacy and safety in marketed medicinal agents. The first act, the Federal Food and Drug Act of 1906, was concerned with the interstate transport of adulterated or misbranded foods and drugs. There were no obligations to establish drug efficacy and safety. The federal act was amended in 1938, following the deaths of about 100 children that resulted from the marketing of a solution of sulfanilamide in diethylene glycol, an excellent but highly toxic solvent. The amended act, the enforcement of which was entrusted to the FDA, was primarily concerned with the truthful labeling and safety of drugs. Toxicity studies were required, as well as approval of a new drug application (NDA), before a drug could be promoted and distributed. However, no proof of efficacy was required, and extravagant claims for therapeutic indications were commonly made. Drugs could go from the laboratory to clinical testing without approval by the FDA.

In this relatively relaxed atmosphere, research in basic and clinical pharmacology burgeoned in both industrial and academic laboratories. The result was a flow of new drugs, called "wonder drugs" by the lay press, for the treatment of both infectious and organic disease. Because efficacy was not rigorously defined, a number of therapeutic claims could not be supported by data. The risk-to-benefit ratio was seldom mentioned, but it emerged in dramatic fashion early in the 1960s. At that time thalidomide, a hypnotic with no obvious advantage over other drugs in its class, was introduced in the European market. After a short period, it became apparent that the incidence of a relatively rare birth defect, phocomelia, was increasing. It soon reached epidemic proportions, and retrospective epidemiological research firmly established the causative agent to be thalidomide taken early in the course of pregnancy. The reaction to the dramatic demonstration of the teratogenicity of a needless drug was worldwide. In the United States it resulted in the Harris–Kefauver Amendments to the Food, Drug, and Cosmetic Act in 1962.

The Harris–Kefauver Amendments are sound legislation. They require sufficient pharmacological and toxicological research in animals before a drug can be tested in man. The data from such studies must be submitted to the FDA in the form of an application for an investigational new drug (IND) before clinical studies can begin. Three phases of clinical testing (*see* below) have evolved to provide the data that are used to support a new drug application. For drugs introduced after 1962, proof of efficacy is required, as is documentation of relative safety in terms of the risk-to-benefit ratio for the disease entity to be treated. The 1962 amendments also required manufacturers to provide data to support the claims of efficacy for all drugs marketed between 1938 and 1962.

The provisions of the Harris–Kefauver amendments have greatly increased the time and the cost required to market a new drug. Moreover, although the law requires action on the part of the FDA within a period of 6 months, an NDA may be returned to the applicant for additional basic or clinical research, so that the period actually required for approval of an NDA is on the order of 2 to 3 years. The total time of drug development from the time of filing of an IND application to final approval averages 8 to 9 years (Kaitin *et al.*, 1987). The result has been an increase in the inherent tension that exists between the FDA, which is motivated to protect the public health, and the drug developers, who are motivated to market effective and profitable drug products. Additionally, medical practitioners have criticized the FDA for delaying the approval of new drugs, whereas some consumer groups demand the recall of drugs that may play an important part in the therapeutic regimen of appropriately selected patients. In this climate, the FDA has the difficult task of balancing the requirement to ensure the safety of new drugs with the needs of society for useful medications to be made available in a timely manner. This dilemma has been brought into sharp focus recently by the demands of patients with acquired immunodeficiency syndrome (AIDS) for new and effective therapies. In response to the needs of patients with AIDS and other life-threatening illnesses, the FDA is moving on several fronts (Young *et al.*, 1988). First, the FDA has initiated new "treatment" IND regulations that allow patients with life-threatening diseases for which there is no satisfactory alternative treatment to receive drugs for therapy prior to general marketing if there is limited evidence of drug efficacy without unreasonable toxicity (Figure 4–4). Second, the agency has established a priority review system for potentially useful AIDS-related drugs to assure that the review process is expedited. Finally, the FDA is attempting to be involved more actively in drug development in order to facilitate the approval of drugs designed to treat life-threatening and severely debilitating diseases. By working with the pharmaceutical industry throughout the period of clinical drug development instead of involving themselves only at the end of this process, the FDA hopes to reduce the time from submission of an IND application to the approval of an NDA. This streamlining process will be accomplished by the interactive design of well-planned, focused clinical studies. Sufficient data should then be available earlier in the development process to allow a risk–benefit analysis and a possible decision for approval. In some cases this system may reduce or obviate the need for phase-3 testing prior to approval. Coupled with this expedited development process will be the requirement, when appropriate, for postmarketing studies to answer remaining issues of risks, benefits, and optimal uses of the drug (*Federal Register,* 1988). This new initiative by the FDA is based on the assumption that society is more willing to accept unknown risks from drugs used to treat life-threatening or debilitating diseases. As long as the patient's safety can be reasonably ensured, the new plans to accelerate the drug-development process should prove beneficial to patients with such illnesses.

A seemingly contradictory directive to the FDA is also contained in the Food, Drug, and Cosmetic Act—that is, the FDA cannot interfere with the practice of medicine. Thus, once the efficacy of a new agent has been proven in the context of acceptable toxicity, the drug can be marketed. The physician is then allowed to determine its most appropriate use. However, physicians must realize that new drugs are inherently more risky because of the relatively small amount of data about their effects. Yet there is no practical way to increase knowledge about a drug before it is marketed. A systematic method for postmarketing surveillance is an indispensable requirement for early optimization of drug use.

Before a drug can be marketed, a package insert for use by physicians must be prepared. This is a cooperative effort between the FDA and the pharmaceutical company. The insert usually contains basic pharmacological information, as well as essential clinical information in regard to approved indications, contraindications, precautions, warnings, adverse reactions, usual dosage, and available preparations. Promotional materials cannot deviate from information contained in the insert.

DRUG DEVELOPMENT

Except for concern about the so-called drug lag (Kennedy, 1978) and governmental interference with the practice of medicine, the average physician has not considered it important to understand the process of drug development. Yet an appreciation of this process is necessary if the therapist wishes to have the ability to estimate the risk-to-benefit ratio of a drug and to realize the limitations of the data that support the efficacy and safety of a marketed product.

By the time an IND application has been initiated and a drug reaches the stage of testing in man, its pharmacokinetic, pharmacodynamic, and toxic properties have been evaluated *in vitro* and in several species of animals in accordance with regulations and guidelines published by the FDA. Although the value of many requirements for

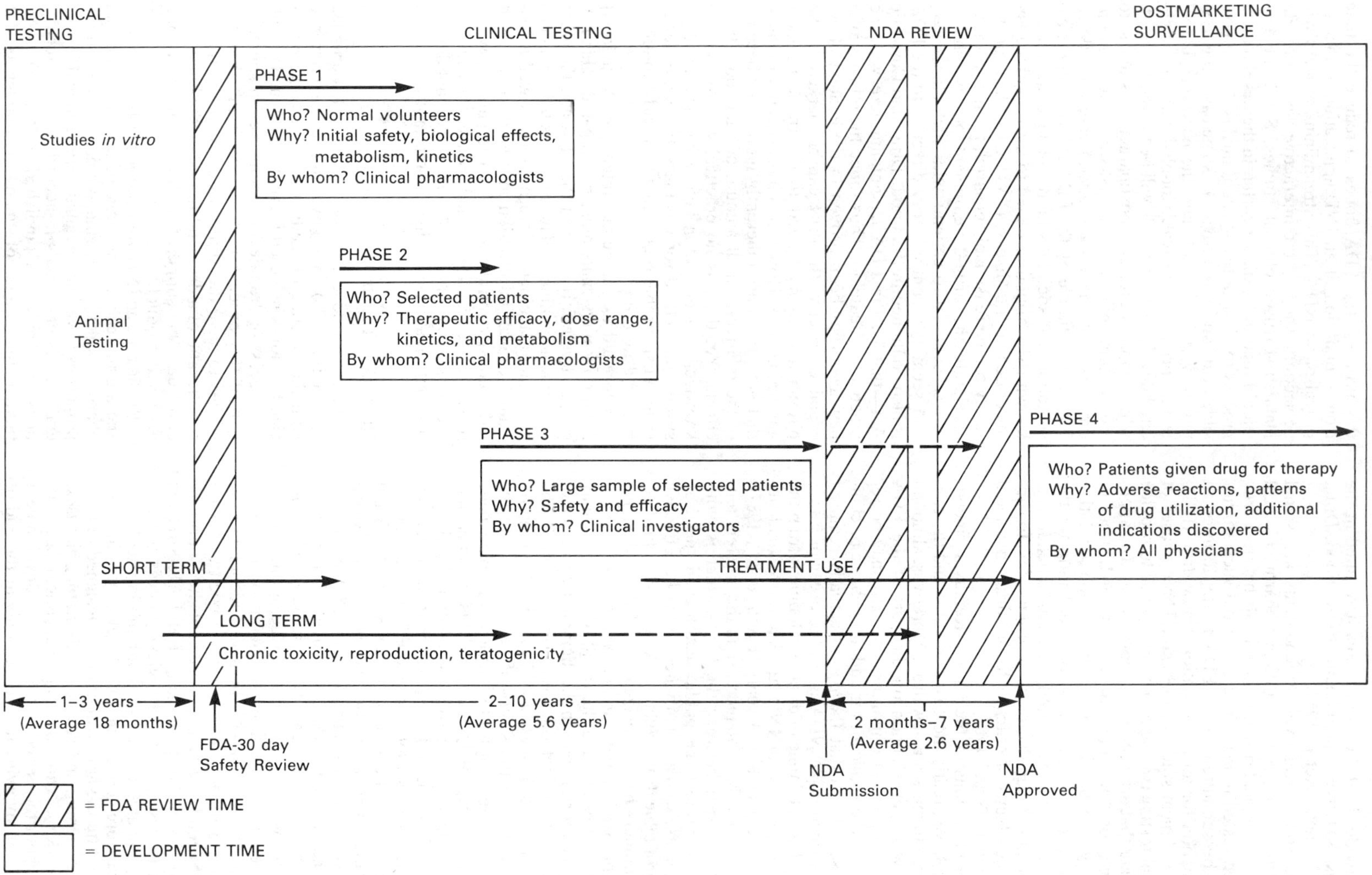

Figure 4–4. *The phases of drug development in the United States.* (Sources: Smith, 1978; Kaitin *et al.*, 1987; Young *et al.*, 1988.)

preclinical testing is self-evident, such as those that screen for direct toxicity to organs and characterize dose-related effects, the value of others is controversial, particularly because of the well-known interspecies variation in the effects of drugs. Interestingly, although many of the preclinical tests have not been convincingly shown to predict effects that are eventually observed in man, the risk of cautious testing of a new drug is surprisingly low.

Trials of drugs in man in the United States are generally conducted in three phases that must be completed before an NDA can be submitted to the FDA for review; these are outlined in Figure 4–4. Although assessment of risk is a major objective of such testing, this is far more difficult than is the determination of whether a drug is efficacious for a selected clinical condition. Usually about 500 to 3000 carefully selected patients receive a new drug during phase-3 clinical trials. At most, only a few hundred are treated for more than 3 to 6 months, regardless of the likely duration of therapy that will be required in practice. Thus, the most profound and overt risks that occur almost immediately after the drug is given can be detected in a phase-3 study, if these occur more often than once per 100 administrations. Risks that are medically important but delayed or less frequent than 1 in 1000 administrations may not be revealed prior to marketing. It is thus obvious that a number of unanticipated adverse and beneficial effects of drugs are only detectable after the drug is used broadly. The same can be more convincingly stated about most of the effects of drugs on children or the fetus, where premarketing experimental studies are restricted. It is for these reasons that many countries, including the United States, have established systematic methods for the surveillance of the effects of drugs after they have been approved for distribution (Joint Commission on Prescription Drug Use, 1980; Venning, 1983; Strom, 1987a; *see also* below).

ADVERSE DRUG REACTIONS AND DRUG TOXICITY

Any drug, no matter how trivial its therapeutic actions, has the potential to do harm. Adverse reactions are a cost of modern medical therapy. Although the mandate of the FDA is to ensure that drugs are safe and effective, both of these terms are relative. The anticipated benefit from any therapeutic decision must be balanced by the potential risks. Patients, to a greater extent than physicians, are unaware of the limitations of the premarketing phase of drug development in defining even relatively common risks of new drugs. Since only a few thousand patients are exposed to experimental drugs in more or less controlled and well-defined circumstances during drug development, adverse drug effects that occur as frequently as 1 in 1000 patients may not be detected prior to marketing. Postmarketing surveillance of drug usage is thus imperative to detect infrequent but significant adverse effects.

Several strategies exist to detect adverse reactions after marketing of a drug, but debate continues about the most efficient and effective method. Formal approaches for estimation of the magnitude of an adverse drug effect are the follow-up or "cohort" study of patients who are receiving a particular drug and the "case–control" study, where the potential for a drug to cause a particular disease is assessed. Cohort studies can estimate the incidence of an adverse reaction, but they cannot, for practical reasons, discover rare events. To have any significant advantage over the premarketing studies, a cohort study must follow at least 10,000 patients who are receiving the drug in order to detect with 95% confidence one event that occurs at a rate of 1 in 3300, and the event can be attributed to the drug only if it does not occur spontaneously in the control population. If the adverse event occurs spontaneously in the control population, substantially more patients and controls must be followed to establish the drug as the cause of the event (Rawlins, 1984; Strom, 1987a). Case–control studies, on the other hand, can discover rare drug-induced events. However, it may be difficult to establish the appropriate control group (Feinstein and Horwitz, 1988), and a case–control study cannot establish the incidence of an adverse drug effect. Furthermore, the suspicion of a drug as a causative factor in a disease must be the impetus for the initiation of such case–control studies.

The magnitude of the problem of adverse reactions to marketed drugs is difficult to quantify. It has been estimated that 3 to 5% of all hospitalizations can be attributed to adverse drug reactions, resulting in 300,000 hospitalizations annually in the United States. Once hospitalized, patients have about a 30% chance of an untoward event related to drug therapy, and the risk attributable to each course of drug therapy is about 5%. The chance of a life-threatening drug reaction is about 3% per patient in the hospital and about 0.4% per each course of therapy (Jick, 1984). On a university medical service where severely ill patients and patients with complicated courses of disease are treated, adverse reactions to drugs were found to be the most common cause of iatrogenic disease (Steel *et al.*, 1981).

Because of the shortcomings of both cohort and case–control studies, other approaches must be used. Spontaneous reporting of adverse reactions has proven to be an effective way to generate an early signal that a drug may be causing an adverse event (Rawlins, 1988; Rossi *et al.*, 1988). It is the only practical way to detect rare events, events that occur after prolonged use of drug, adverse effects that are delayed in appearance, and many drug–drug interactions (Edlavitch, 1988). In the past few years considerable effort has gone into improving the reporting system in the United States, and the number of reports has increased recently (Faich *et al.*, 1988). Still, the voluntary reporting system in the United States is deficient when compared with the legally mandated systems of the United Kingdom, Canada, New Zealand, Denmark, and Sweden (Rogers *et al.*, 1988). Most physicians feel that detecting adverse reactions is a professional obligation, but relatively few actually report such reactions. Over 40% of physicians are not aware that the FDA has a reporting system for adverse drug reactions, even though the system has been repeatedly publicized in major medical journals.

The most important spontaneous reports are those that describe serious reactions, whether they have been described previously or not. Reports on newly marketed drugs are the most significant, even though the physician may not be able to attribute a causal role to a particular drug. The major use of this system is to provide early warning signals of unexpected adverse effects that can then be investigated by more formal techniques. However, the system also serves to monitor changes in the nature or frequency of adverse drug reactions due to aging of the population, changes in the disease itself, or the introduction of new, concurrent therapies. The primary sources for the reports are responsible, alert physicians; other potentially useful sources are nurses, pharmacists, and students in these disciplines. In addition, hospital based pharmacy and therapeutics committees and quality assurance committees frequently are charged with monitoring adverse drug reactions in hospitalized patients, and reports from these committees should be forwarded to the FDA (Edlavitch, 1988). The simple, one-page forms for reporting are now readily available as the last page of the *Physicians' Desk Reference* and *AMA Drug Evaluations* and are mailed to all physicians at least yearly as part of the FDA "Drug Bulletin." Additionally, physicians may contact the pharmaceutical manufacturer and/or write to the Office of Epidemiology and Biostatistics (HFN-700), Center for Drug Evaluation and Research, Food and Drug Administration, Parklawn Building, Rockville, MD 20857 (Faich *et al.*, 1988).

As with drug interactions, classification of adverse effects of drugs according to information about their causes provides a framework for the transfer of principles to the clinical setting. Such classification appears in Chapter 3. In addition, the clinician obviously also needs to know the frequencies and types of untoward effects caused by each individual drug prescribed; such information is presented throughout this textbook.

GUIDE TO THE "THERAPEUTIC JUNGLE"

The flood of new drugs in recent years has provided many dramatic improvements in therapy, but it has also created a number of problems of equal magnitude. Not the least of these is the "therapeutic jungle," the term used to refer to the combination of the overwhelming number of drugs, the confusion over nomenclature, and the associated uncertainty of the status of many of these drugs. A reduction in the marketing of close congeners and drug mixtures and an improvement in the quality of advertising are important ingredients in the remedy for the "therapeutic jungle." However, physicians can also contribute to the remedy by employing nonproprietary rather than proprietary names whenever appropriate, by using prototypes both as an instructional device and in clinical practice, by adopting a properly critical attitude toward new drugs, and by knowing and making use of reliable sources of pharmacological information. Most important, they should develop a "way of thinking about drugs" based upon pharmacological principles.

Drug Nomenclature. The existence of many names for each drug, even when reduced to a minimum, has led to a lamentable and confusing situation in drug nomenclature. In addition to its formal *chemical* name, a new drug is usually assigned a *code* name by the pharmaceutical manufacturer. If the drug appears promising and the manufacturer wishes to place it on the market, a *United States Adopted Name* (USAN) is selected by the USAN Council, which is jointly sponsored by the American Medical Association, the American Pharmaceutical Association, and the United States Pharmacopeial Convention, Inc. This *nonproprietary* name is often referred to as the *generic* name. This term has become entrenched, but by definition it should be more properly reserved to designate a chemical or pharmacological class of drugs, such as sulfonamides or sympathomimetics. If the drug is eventually admitted to *The United States Pharmacopeia* (*see* below), the USAN becomes the *official* name. However, the nonproprietary name and the official name of an older drug may differ. Subsequently, the drug will also be assigned a *proprietary* name or *trademark* by the manufacturer. If the drug is marketed by more than one company, it may have several proprietary names. If mixtures of the drug with other agents are marketed, each such mixture may also have a separate proprietary name.

There is increasing worldwide adoption of the same name for each therapeutic substance. For newer drugs, the USAN is usually adopted for the nonproprietary name in other countries, but this is not true for older drugs. International agreement on drug names is mediated through the World Health Organization and the pertinent health agencies of the cooperating countries.

One area of continued confusion and ambiguity is the designation of the stereochemical composition in the name of a drug. The nonproprietary names usually give no indication of the drug's stereochemistry, except for a few drugs such as levodopa and dextroamphetamine. Even the chemical names cited by the USAN Council are often ambiguous. Physicians and other medical scientists are frequently ignorant about drug stereoisomerism and are likely to remain so until the system of nonproprietary nomenclature incorporates stereoisomeric information (Gal, 1988).

The nonproprietary or official name of a drug should be used whenever possible, and such a practice has been adopted in this textbook. The use of the nonproprietary name is clearly less confusing when the drug is available under multiple proprietary names and when the nonproprietary name more readily identifies the drug with its pharmacological class. The best argument for the proprietary name is that it is frequently more easily pronounced and remembered as a result of advertising. For purposes of identification, representative proprietary names, designated by SMALLCAP TYPE, appear throughout the text in chapter sections dealing with preparations as well as in the index. This list is far from complete, since the number of proprietary names for a single drug may be large and since proprietary names differ from country to country.

The Drug Price Competition and Patent Term Restoration Act of 1984 allows more generic versions of brand-name drugs to be approved for marketing. When the physician prescribes drugs, the question arises as to whether the nonproprietary name or a proprietary name should be employed. In practically all states, a pharmacist may substitute a preparation that is equivalent unless the physician indicates "no substitution" on the prescription. Likewise, if the nonproprietary name of a drug is employed, the physician can specify the manufacturer. In view of the discussion above on the individualization of drug therapy, it is understandable why a physician who has carefully adjusted the dose of a drug to a patient's individual requirements for chronic therapy may be reluctant to surrender control over the source of the drug that the patient receives (Strom, 1987b).

Based on a number of considerations, such as the frequency of use of a drug that is only available from a single manufacturer, the cost of filling a prescription, and the mark-up of the pharmacist, it appears as though the overall savings to society of prescribing the least expensive nonproprietary preparation is about 5% (*see* Trout and Lee, 1981). Of course, savings in individual situations can be very much greater. On the other hand, the lower wholesale cost of the nonproprietary preparation is sometimes not passed on to the consumer (Bloom *et al.,* 1986). More importantly, prescribing by nonproprietary name could result in the patient receiving a preparation of inferior quality or of uncertain bioavailability, and therapeutic failures due to decreased bioavailability have been reported (Strom, 1987b). To address this issue, the FDA has established standards for bioavailability and compiled information about the interchangeability of drug products; unfortunately, data on therapeutic equivalence based on clinical studies do not exist for most of these products (*Approved Prescription Drug Products with Therapeutic Evaluations,* 1987). In spite of this limitation, potential cost savings to the individual patient and simplification of the "therapeutic jungle" dictate that nonproprietary names be used when prescribing, except for drugs with a low therapeutic index and known differences in bioavailability among marketed products (*Medical Letter,* 1986).

Use of Prototypes. It is obviously crucial for the physician to be thoroughly familiar with the pharmacological properties of a drug before it is administered. It follows that the patient will benefit if the physician avoids the temptation to choose from many different drugs for the patient's regimen. A physician's needs for therapeutic agents can usually be satisfied by thorough knowledge of one or two drugs in each therapeutic category. Inevitably, a small number of drugs can be used more effectively. When the clinical setting calls for a drug that the physician uses infrequently, he or she should feel obligated to learn about its effects, to use great caution in its administration, and to apply appropriate procedures in monitoring its effects.

For teaching purposes in this textbook, the confusion created by the welter of similar drugs is reduced by restricting major attention to prototypes in each pharmacological class. Focusing on the representative drugs results in better characterization of a class as a whole, and thereby permits sharper recognition of the occasional member that possesses unique properties. A teaching prototype is often the agent most likely to be employed in clinical use, but this is not always true. A particular drug may be retained as the prototype, even though a new congener is clinically superior, either because more is known about the older drug or because it is more illustrative for the entire class of agents.

Attitude toward New Drugs. A reasonable attitude toward new drugs is summarized by the adage that advises the physician to be "neither the first to use a new drug nor the last to discard the old." Only a minor fraction of new drugs represents a significant therapeutic advance. The limitation of information about toxicity and efficacy at the time of release of a drug has been emphasized above, and this is particularly pertinent to comparisons with older agents in the same therapeutic class. Nevertheless, the important advances in therapeutics in the last 50 years emphasize the obligation to keep abreast of significant advances in pharmacotherapy.

SOURCES OF DRUG INFORMATION

The physician's need for objective, concise, and well-organized information on drugs is obvious. Among the available sources are textbooks of pharmacology and therapeutics, leading medical journals, drug compendia, professional seminars and meetings, and advertising. Despite this cornucopia of information, responsible medical spokesmen insist that most practicing physicians are unable to extract the objective and unbiased data required for the practice of rational therapeutics (*see* Task Force, 1969).

Depending on their aim and scope, pharmacology textbooks provide (in varying proportions) basic pharmacological principles, critical appraisal of useful categories of therapeutic agents, and detailed descriptions of individual drugs or prototypes that serve as standards of reference for assessing new drugs. In addition, pharmacodynamics and pathological physiology are correlated. Therapeutics is considered in virtually all textbooks of medicine, but often superficially. For obvious reasons, textbooks cannot contain information on the most recently introduced drugs.

The source of information described as most often used by physicians in an industry survey is the *Physicians' Desk Reference* (PDR). The brand-name manufacturers whose products appear support this book. No comparative data on efficacy, safety, or cost are included. The information is identical to that contained in drug package inserts, which are largely based on the results of phase-3 testing; its primary value is thus in learning what indications for use of a drug have been approved by the FDA.

There are, however, several inexpensive, unbiased sources of information on the clinical uses of drugs that are preferable to the industry-supported PDR. All recognize that the physician's legitimate use of a drug in a particular patient is not limited by FDA-approved labeling in the package insert. *The United States Pharmacopeia Dispensing Information* (USPDI), first published in 1980, comes in two volumes. One, *Drug Information for the Health Care Provider,* consists of drug monographs that contain practical, clinically significant information aimed at minimizing the risks and enhancing the benefits of drugs. Monographs are developed by USP staff and are reviewed by advisory panels and other reviewers. The *Advice for the Patient* volume is intended to reinforce, in lay language, the oral consultation provided by the therapist, and this may be provided to the patient in written form. It is planned that the volumes will be published frequently. The *American Hospital Formulary Service* (AHFS), published by the American Society of Hospital Pharmacists, is a collection of monographs that are kept current by periodic supplements. The monographs are written on a single drug; there are also general discussions of drugs that are included in a defined class. *AMA Drug Evaluations,* compiled by the American Medical Association Department of Drugs in cooperation with the American Society for Clinical Pharmacology and Therapeutics, includes general information on the use of drugs in special settings (*e.g.,* pediatrics, geriatrics, renal insufficiency, *etc.*) and reflects the consensus of a panel on the effective clinical use of therapeutic agents. *Facts and Comparisons* (Olin, 1988), published by a division of J. B. Lippincott Company, is also organized by pharmacological classes and is updated monthly. Information in monographs is presented in a standard format and incorporates FDA-approved information, which is supplemented with current data obtained from the biomedical literature. A useful feature is the comprehensive list of preparations with a "Cost Index," an index of the average wholesale price for equivalent quantities of similar or identical drugs.

Industry promotion, in the form of direct-mail brochures, journal advertising, displays, professional courtesies, or the detail person or pharmaceutical representative, is intended to be persuasive rather than educational. The pharmaceutical industry cannot, should not, and indeed does not purport to be responsible for the education of physicians in the use of drugs.

Over 1500 medical journals are published regularly in the United States. However, of the two to three dozen medical publications with circulations in excess of 70,000 copies, the great majority are sent to physicians free of charge and paid for by the industry. In addition, special supplements of some peer-reviewed journals are entirely supported by a single drug manufacturer whose product is prominently featured and favorably described. Objective journals, which are not supported by drug manufacturers, include *Clinical Pharmacology and Therapeutics,* which is devoted to original articles that evaluate the actions and effects of drugs in man, and *Drugs,* which publishes timely reviews of individual drugs and drug classes. The *New England Journal of Medicine, Annals of Internal Medicine, Journal of the American Medical Association, Archives of Internal Medicine, British Medical Journal, Lancet,* and *Postgraduate Medicine* offer timely therapeutic reports and reviews. Three publications deserve special emphasis here because they exemplify effective attempts to provide objective drug information in easily assimilable form.

These are *The Medical Letter, Clin-Alert,* and *Rational Drug Therapy. The Medical Letter* provides summaries of scientific reports and consultants' evaluations of the safety, efficacy, and rationale for use of a drug. *Clin-Alert* consists mainly of abstracts from the literature on drugs. *Rational Drug Therapy* presents a monthly review article on groups of drugs or on the management of specific conditions.

The United States Pharmacopeia (USP) and *The National Formulary* (NF) were recognized as "official compendia" by the Federal Food and Drug Act of 1906. The approved therapeutic agents used in medical practice in the United States are described and defined with respect to source, chemistry, physical properties, tests for identity and purity, assay, and storage. The two official compendia are now published in a single volume.

Bloom, B. S.; Wierz, D. J.; and Pauley, M. D. Cost and price of comparable branded and generic pharmaceuticals. *J.A.M.A.*, **1986**, *256*, 2523–2530.

Bristow, M. R.; Ginsburg, R.; Minobe, W.; Cubicciotti, R. S.; Sageman, W. S.; Lurie, K.; Billingham, M. E.; Harrison, D. C.; and Stinson, E. B. Decreased catecholamine sensitivity and β-adrenergic-receptor density in failing human hearts. *N. Engl. J. Med.*, **1982**, *307*, 205–211.

Faich, G. A.; Dreis, M.; and Tomita, D. National adverse drug reaction surveillance 1986. *Arch. Intern. Med.*, **1988**, *148*, 785–787.

Feinstein, A. R. An additional basic science for clinical medicine. *Ann. Intern. Med.*, **1983**, *99*, 393–397, 544–550, 705–712, 843–848.

Gonzalez, F. J.; Skoda, R. C.; Kimura, S.; Umeno, M.; Zanger, U. M.; Nebert, D. W.; Gelboin, H. V.; Hardwick, J. P.; and Meyer, U. A. Characterization of the common genetic defect in humans deficient in debrisoquine metabolism. *Nature*, **1988**, *331*, 442–446.

Guyatt, G.; Sackett, D.; Taylor, D. W.; Chong, J.; Roberts, R.; and Pugsley, S. Determining optimal therapy—randomized trials in individual patients. *N. Engl. J. Med.*, **1986**, *314*, 889–892.

Jachuck, S. J.; Brierley, H.; Jachuck, S.; and Wilcox, P. M. The effect of hypotensive drugs on the quality of life. *J. R. Coll. Gen. Pract.*, **1982**, *32*, 103–105.

Kaitin, K. I.; Richard, B. W.; and Lasagna, L. Trends in drug development: the 1985–86 new drug approvals. *J. Clin. Pharmacol.*, **1987**, *27*, 542–548.

Kennedy, D. A calm look at "drug lag." *J.A.M.A.*, **1978**, *239*, 423–426.

Lindenbaum, J.; Rund, D. G.; Butler, V. P.; Tse-Eng, D.; and Saha, J. R. Inactivation of digoxin by the gut flora: reversal by antibiotic therapy. *N. Engl. J. Med.*, **1981**, *305*, 789–794.

Penno, M. B., and Vesell, E. S. Monogenic control of variations in antipyrine metabolite formation. *J. Clin. Invest.*, **1983**, *71*, 1698–1709.

Rawlins, M. D. Spontaneous reporting of adverse drug reactions. *Br. J. Clin. Pharmacol.*, **1988**, *26*, 1–5, 7–11.

Rogers, A. S.; Israel, E.; Smith, C. R.; Levine, D.; McBean, A. M.; Valente, C.; and Faich, G. Physician knowledge, attitudes, and behavior related to reporting adverse drug events. *Arch. Intern. Med.*, **1988**, *148*, 1596–1600.

Rossi, A. C.; Bosco, L.; Faich, G. A.; Tanner, A.; and Temple, R. The importance of adverse reaction reporting by physicians. *J.A.M.A.*, **1988**, *259*, 1203–1204.

Simon, R. Confidence intervals for reporting results of clinical trials. *Ann. Intern. Med.*, **1986**, *105*, 429–435.

Steel, K.; Gertman, P. M.; Cresienze, C.; and Anderson, J. Iatrogenic illness on a general medical service at a university hospital. *N. Engl. J. Med.*, **1981**, *304*, 638–642.

Young, F. E.; Norris, J. A.; Levitt, J. A.; and Nightingale, S. L. The FDA's new procedures for the use of investigational drugs in treatment. *J.A.M.A.*, **1988**, *259*, 2267–2270.

Young, M. J.; Bresnitz, E. A.; and Strom, B. L. Sample size nomograms for interpreting negative clinical studies. *Ann. Intern. Med.*, **1983**, *99*, 248–251.

Monographs and Reviews

AMA Drug Evaluations, 6th ed. American Medical Association, Chicago, **1986**.

American Hospital Formulary Service. American Society of Hospital Pharmacists, Bethesda, Md., **1987**.

Approved Prescription Drug Products with Therapeutic Evaluations, 7th ed. Department of Health and Human Services, Public Health Service, Food and Drug Administration, Center for Drugs and Biologics, Rockville, Md., **1987**.

Brody, H. The lie that heals: the ethics of giving placebos. *Ann. Intern. Med.*, **1982**, *97*, 112–118.

Brown, P. C.; Johnston, R. N.; and Schimke, R. T. Approaches to the study of mechanisms of selective gene amplification in cultured mammalian cells. In, *Gene Studies in Regulation and Development*. Alan R. Liss, Inc., New York, **1983**, pp. 197–212.

Clark, D. W. J. Genetically determined variability in acetylation and oxidation. Therapeutic implications. *Drugs*, **1985**, *29*, 342–375.

Edlavitch, S. A. Adverse drug event reporting. Improving the low U.S. reporting rates. *Arch. Intern. Med.*, **1988**, *148*, 1499–1503.

Federal Register. **1988**, *53*, 41516–41524.

Feinstein, A. R. *Clinical Biostatistics*. C. V. Mosby Co., St. Louis, **1977**.

Feinstein, A. R., and Horwitz, R. I. Choosing cases and controls: the clinical epidemiology of "clinical investigation." *J. Clin. Invest.*, **1988**, *81*, 1–5.

Gal, J. Stereoisomerism and drug nomenclature. *Clin. Pharmacol. Ther.*, **1988**, *44*, 251–253.

Hansten, P. D. *Drug Interactions*, 5th ed. Lea & Febiger, Philadelphia, **1985**.

Horai, Y., and Ishizaki, T. Pharmacogenetics and its clinical implications: *N*-acetylation polymorphism. *Ration. Drug Ther.*, **1987**, *21*, 1–7.

Jick, H. Adverse drug reactions: the magnitude of the problem. *J. Allergy Clin. Immunol.*, **1984**, *74*, 555–557.

Joint Commission on Prescription Drug Use. *The Final Report of the Joint Commission on Prescription Drug Use, Inc.*, U.S. Government Printing Office, Washington, D.C., **1980**.

Koch-Weser, J. Serum drug concentrations as therapeutic guides. *N. Engl. J. Med.*, **1972**, *287*, 227–231.

McInnes, G. T., and Brodie, M. J. Drug interactions that matter. A critical reappraisal. *Drugs*, **1988**, *36*, 83–110.

Medical Letter. Generic drugs. **1986**, *28*, 1–4.

Olin, B. R. (ed.). *Facts and Comparisons*. Facts and Comparisons, Division of J. B. Lippincott Co., St. Louis, **1988**.

Pauker, S. G., and Kassirer, J. P. Decision analysis. *N. Engl. J. Med.*, **1987**, *316*, 250–258.

Rawlins, M. D. Postmarketing surveillance of adverse reactions to drugs. *Br. Med. J. [Clin. Res.]*, **1984**, *288*, 879–880.

Rizack, M. A., and Hillman, C. D. M. *Handbook of Adverse Drug Interactions*. The Medical Letter, New York, **1987.**

Rosner, F. The ethics of randomized clinical trials. *Am. J. Med.*, **1987**, *82*, 283–290.

Rothman, D. J. Ethics and human experimentation: Henry Beecher revisited. *N. Engl. J. Med.*, **1987**, *317*, 1195–1199.

Sheiner, L. B., and Benet, L. Z. Premarketing observational studies of population pharmacokinetics of new drugs. *Clin. Pharmacol. Ther.*, **1985**, *38*, 481–486.

Smith, W. M. Drug choice in disease states. In, *Clinical Pharmacology: Basic Principles in Therapeutics*, 2nd ed. (Melmon, K. L., and Morrelli, H. F., eds.) Macmillan Publishing Co., New York, **1978**, pp. 3–24.

Spector, R.; Park, G. D.; and Vesell, E. S. Therapeutic drug monitoring. *Clin. Pharmacol. Ther.*, **1988**, *43*, 345–353.

Stiles, G. L.; Caron, M. G.; and Lefkowitz, R. J. β-Adrenergic receptors: biochemical mechanisms of physiological regulation. *Physiol. Rev.*, **1984**, *64*, 661–743.

Strom, B. L. The promise of pharmacoepidemiology. *Annu. Rev. Pharmacol. Toxicol.*, **1987a**, *27*, 71–86.

———. Generic drug substitution revisited. *N. Engl. J. Med.*, **1987b**, *316*, 1456–1462.

Task Force on Prescription Drugs. *Final Report*. Department of Health, Education and Welfare, U.S. Government Printing Office, Washington, D.C., **1969.**

Tatro, D. S. (ed.). *Drug Interaction Facts*. Facts and Comparisons, Division of J. B. Lippincott Co., St. Louis, **1988.**

Trout, M. E., and Lee, A. M. Generic substitution: a boon or a bane to the physician and the consumer? In, *Drug Therapeutics: Concepts for Physicians*. (Melmon, K. L., ed.) Elsevier North-Holland, Inc., New York, **1981.**

The United States Pharmacopeia, 22nd rev., and *The National Formulary*, 17th ed. The United States Pharmacopeial Convention, Inc. Mack Printing Co., Easton, Pa., **1990.**

The United States Pharmacopeia Dispensing Information. The United States Pharmacopeial Convention, Inc. Mack Printing Co., Easton, Pa., **1988.**

Venning, G. R. Identification of adverse reactions to new drugs. *Br. Med. J. [Clin. Res.]*, **1983**, *286*, 199–202, 289–292, 365–368, 458–460, 544–547.

Vesell, E. S. Pharmacogenetic Approaches to the Prediction of Drug Response. In, *Genetic and Biological Markers in Drug Abuse and Alcoholism*. (Braude, M. C., and Chao, H. M., eds.) National Institute on Drug Abuse Research Monograph Series No. 66. Department of Health and Human Services, U. S. Government Printing Office, Washington, D. C., **1986**, pp. 25–40.

Weinshilboum, R. Pharmacogenetics of methylation: relationship to drug metabolism. *Clin. Biochem.*, **1988**, *21*, 201–210.

Whiting, B.; Kelman, A. W.; and Grevel, J. Population pharmacokinetics. Theory and clinical application. *Clin. Pharmacokinet.*, **1986**, *11*, 387–401.

Williams, G. H. Quality of life and its impact on hypertensive patients. *Am. J. Med.*, **1987**, *82*, 98–105.

SECTION

II

Drugs Acting at Synaptic and Neuroeffector Junctional Sites

CHAPTER

5 NEUROHUMORAL TRANSMISSION: THE AUTONOMIC AND SOMATIC MOTOR NERVOUS SYSTEMS

Robert J. Lefkowitz, Brian B. Hoffman, and Palmer Taylor

The theory of neurohumoral transmission received direct experimental validation over 80 years ago (*see* von Euler, 1981), and extensive investigation during the ensuing years led to its general acceptance. Nerves transmit their impulses across most synapses and neuroeffector junctions by means of specific chemical agents known as *neurohumoral transmitters* or, more simply, *neurotransmitters*. The actions of the so-called autonomic drugs that affect smooth muscle, cardiac muscle, and gland cells can be understood and classified in terms of their mimicking or modifying the actions of the neurotransmitters released by the autonomic fibers at either ganglia or effector cells.

Most of the general principles concerning the physiology and pharmacology of the peripheral autonomic nervous system and its effector organs also apply with certain modifications to the neuromuscular junction of skeletal muscle, and in a more limited sense to the central nervous system (CNS). In fact, the study of neurotransmission in the CNS has benefited greatly from the delineation of this process in the periphery (*see* Chapter 12).

A clear understanding of the anatomy and physiology of the autonomic nervous system is essential to a study of the pharmacology of the autonomic drugs. The actions of an autonomic agent on various organs of the body can often be predicted if the responses to nerve impulses that reach the organs are known.

ANATOMY AND GENERAL FUNCTIONS OF THE AUTONOMIC AND SOMATIC MOTOR NERVOUS SYSTEMS

The autonomic nervous system is also called the visceral, vegetative, or involuntary nervous system. In the periphery, its representation consists of nerves, ganglia, and plexuses that provide the innervation to the heart, blood vessels, glands, other visceral organs, and smooth muscles. It is therefore widely distributed throughout the body and regulates autonomic functions, which occur without conscious control.

Differences between Autonomic and Somatic Nerves. The efferent nerves of the involuntary system supply all innervated structures of the body except skeletal muscle, which is served by somatic nerves. The most distal synaptic junctions in the autonomic reflex arc occur in ganglia that are entirely outside the cerebrospinal axis. These ganglia are small but complex structures that contain axodendritic synapses between the preganglionic and postganglionic neurons. Somatic nerves contain no peripheral ganglia, and the synapses are located entirely within the cerebrospinal axis. Many autonomic nerves form extensive peripheral plexuses, whereas such networks are absent from the somatic system. While motor nerves to skeletal muscles are myelinated, postganglionic autonomic nerves are generally nonmyelinated. When the cerebrospinal nerves are interrupted, the skeletal muscles that they innervate are completely paralyzed and undergo atrophy, whereas smooth muscles and glands generally show some level of spontaneous activity independent of intact innervation.

Visceral Afferent Fibers. The afferent fibers from visceral structures are the first link in the reflex arcs of the autonomic system. With certain exceptions, such as local axon reflexes, most visceral reflexes are mediated through the CNS. The afferent fibers are, for the most part, nonmyelinated fibers and are carried into the cerebrospinal axis by the vagus, pelvic, splanchnic, and other autonomic nerves. For example, about four fifths of the fibers in the vagus are sensory. Other autonomic afferents from blood vessels in skeletal muscles and from certain integumental structures are carried in the somatic nerves. The cell bodies of visceral afferent fibers lie in the dorsal root ganglia of the spinal nerves and in the corresponding sensory ganglia of certain cranial nerves, such as the nodose ganglion of the vagus. The efferent link of the autonomic reflex arc is discussed in the following sections.

The autonomic afferent fibers are concerned with the mediation of visceral sensation (including pain and referred pain); with vasomotor, respiratory, and viscerosomatic reflexes; and with the regulation of interrelated visceral activities. An example of an autonomic afferent system is that arising from the pressoreceptive endings in the carotid sinus and the aortic arch and from the chemoreceptor cells in the carotid and aortic bodies; this system is important in the reflex control of blood pressure, heart rate, and respiration, and its afferent fibers pass in the glossopharyngeal and vagus nerves to the medulla oblongata in the brainstem.

The neurohumoral agents that mediate transmission from sensory fibers have not been established unequivocally. However, substance P is present in afferent sensory fibers, in the dorsal root ganglia, and in the dorsal horn of the spinal cord, and this peptide is a leading candidate for the neurotransmitter that functions in the passage of nociceptive stimuli from the periphery to the spinal cord and higher structures (Jessell, 1983; Pernow, 1983). Other neuroactive peptides, including somatostatin, vasoactive intestinal polypeptide (VIP), and cholecystokinin, have also been found in sensory neurons (Hökfelt *et al.,* 1989), and one or more such peptides may play a role in the transmission of afferent impulses from autonomic structures. Enkephalins, present in interneurons in the dorsal spinal cord (within an area termed the substantia gelatinosa), have antinociceptive effects that appear to be brought about by presynaptic and postsynaptic actions to inhibit the release of substance P and diminish the activity of cells that project from the spinal cord to higher centers in the CNS (Duggan and North, 1983).

Central Autonomic Connections. There are probably no purely autonomic or somatic centers of integration, and extensive overlap occurs. Somatic responses are always accompanied by visceral responses and vice versa. Autonomic reflexes can be elicited at the level of the spinal cord. They are clearly demonstrable in the spinal animal, including man, and are manifested by sweating, blood pressure alterations, vasomotor responses to temperature changes, and reflex emptying of the urinary bladder, rectum, and seminal vesicles. Extensive central ramifications of the autonomic nervous system exist above the level of the spinal cord. For example, the integration of the control of blood pressure and respiration in the medulla oblongata is well known. The hypothalamus is generally regarded as the principal locus of integration of the entire autonomic system and is concerned with the regulation of body temperature, water balance, carbohydrate and fat metabolism, blood pressure, emotions, sleep, and sexual reflexes, although higher centers, including the cerebral cortex, also contribute crucially to these processes. Stimulation of the hypothalamus activates highly organized neuronal systems that induce a variety of integrated functions in the organism, including autonomic responses; these neuronal systems involve the cortex, the limbic system, and other structures in the brain (Morgane, 1981). The hypothalamic nuclei that lie posteriorly and laterally are sympathetic in their main connections, while parasympathetic functions are evidently integrated by the midline nuclei in the region of the tuber cinereum and by nuclei lying anteriorly. The baroreceptor reflex is mediated via neural connections in the posteromedial hypothalamus, which originate in an ascending polysynaptic pathway from the nucleus of the solitary tract (Mancia and Zanchetti, 1981). The neostriatum is also involved in the regulation of certain autonomic functions, as indicated clinically by the autonomic disturbances accompanying lesions in this region. The cortex provides another suprasegmental level of integration for autonomic, sensory, and motor functions. The limbic system, which includes the olfactory lobe, hippocampal formation, and the pyriform lobe, is also important in the integration of emotional state and pain sensations with motor and visceral activities.

The actions of autonomic drugs on CNS transmission, although not fully understood, are often prominent and may overshadow the peripheral effects (*e.g.*, scopolamine, dextroamphetamine, di*iso*propyl phosphorofluoridate, *etc.*). Likewise, many centrally acting drugs may exert important visceral effects (*e.g.*, phenothiazines, barbiturates, morphine, *etc.*) (*see* Chapter 12).

Divisions of the Peripheral Autonomic System. On the efferent or motor side, the autonomic nervous system consists of two large divisions: (1) the *sympathetic* or *thoracolumbar* outflow and (2) the *parasympathetic* or *craniosacral* outflow. A brief outline of those anatomical features necessary for an understanding of the actions of autonomic drugs is given here.

The arrangement of the principal parts of the peripheral autonomic nervous system is presented schematically in Figure 5–1. As will be discussed, the neurotransmitter of all preganglionic autonomic fibers, all postganglionic parasympathetic fibers, and a few postganglionic sympathetic fibers is *acetylcholine* (ACh); these so-called *cholinergic fibers* are depicted in blue. The *adrenergic fibers,* shown in red, comprise the majority of the postganglionic sympathetic fibers; here the transmitter is *norepinephrine* (*noradrenaline, levarterenol*). As mentioned, the transmitter(s) of the *primary afferent fibers,* shown in green, has not been identified conclusively. Substance P and perhaps glutamate are prime candidates, since both are present in high concentrations in the dorsal regions of the spinal cord. The terms *cholinergic* and *adrenergic* were proposed originally by Dale to describe neurons that liberate ACh and norepinephrine, respectively. Subsequently, Dale (1954) suggested the terms *cholinoceptive* and *adrenoceptive* to denote postjunctional sites that are acted upon by the respective transmitters, but the terms *cholinergic receptor* and *adrenergic receptor* have been generally adopted.

Sympathetic Nervous System. The cells that give rise to the preganglionic fibers of this division lie mainly in the intermediolateral columns of the spinal cord and extend from the first thoracic to the second or third lumbar segment. The axons from these cells are carried in the anterior nerve roots and synapse with neurons lying in sympathetic ganglia outside the cerebrospinal axis. The sympathetic ganglia are found in three locations: paravertebral, prevertebral, and terminal.

The paravertebral sympathetic ganglia consist of 22 pairs that lie on either side of the vertebral column to form the lateral chains. The ganglia are connected to each other by nerve trunks and to the spinal nerves by rami communicantes. The white rami are restricted to the segments of the thoracolumbar outflow; they carry the preganglionic myelinated fibers that exit from the spinal cord by way of the anterior spinal roots. The gray rami arise from the ganglia and carry postganglionic fibers back to the spinal nerves for distribution to sweat glands and pilomotor muscles, and to blood vessels of skeletal muscle and skin. The prevertebral ganglia lie in the abdomen and the pelvis near the ventral surface of the bony vertebral column, and consist mainly of the celiac (solar), superior mesenteric, aorticorenal, and inferior mesenteric ganglia. The terminal ganglia are few in number, lie near the organs that they innervate, and consist especially of ganglia connected with the urinary bladder and rectum. In addition to the above ganglia, there are small intermediate ganglia, especially in the thoracolumbar region, that lie outside the conventional vertebral chain. They are variable in number and location, but are usually in close proximity to the communicating rami and to the anterior spinal nerve roots.

Preganglionic fibers issuing from the spinal cord may synapse with the neurons of more than one sympathetic ganglion. Their principal ganglia of termination need not correspond to the original level from which the preganglionic fiber exits the spinal cord. Many of the preganglionic fibers from the fifth to the last thoracic segment pass through the paravertebral ganglia and form the splanchnic nerves. Most of the splanchnic nerve fibers do not synapse until they reach the celiac ganglion; others directly innervate the adrenal medulla (*see* below).

Postganglionic fibers arising from sympathetic ganglia innervate the visceral structures of the thorax, abdomen, head, and neck. The trunk and the limbs are supplied by means of sympathetic fibers in spinal nerves, as previously described. The prevertebral ganglia contain cell bodies, the axons of which innervate the glands and the smooth muscles of the abdominal and the pelvic viscera. Many of the upper thoracic sympathetic fibers from the vertebral ganglia form terminal plexuses, such as the cardiac, esophageal, and pulmonary. The sympathetic distribution to the head and the neck (vasomotor, pupillodilator, secretory, and pilomotor) is by way of the cervical sympathetic chain and its three ganglia. All postganglionic fibers in this chain arise from cell bodies located in these three ganglia; all preganglionic fibers arise from the upper thoracic segments of the spinal cord, there being no sympathetic fibers that leave the CNS above the first thoracic level.

The adrenal medulla and other chromaffin tissue are embryologically and anatomically homologous to sympathetic ganglia; all are derived from the neural crest. The adrenal medulla differs from sympathetic ganglia in that the principal catecholamine that is released in man and many other species is epinephrine (adrenaline). The chromaffin cells in the adrenal medulla are innervated by typical preganglionic fibers.

Parasympathetic Nervous System. This system consists of preganglionic fibers that originate in three areas of the CNS and their postganglionic connections. The regions of central origin are the midbrain, the medulla oblongata, and the sacral part of the spinal cord. The midbrain or tectal outflow consists of fibers arising from the Edinger–Westphal nucleus of the third cranial nerve and going to the ciliary ganglion in the orbit. The medullary outflow consists of the parasympathetic components of the seventh, ninth, and tenth cranial nerves. The fibers in the seventh cranial, or facial, nerve form the chorda tympani, which innervates the ganglia lying on the submaxillary and sublingual glands. They also form the greater superficial petrosal nerve, which innervates the sphenopalatine ganglion. The ninth cranial, or glossopharyngeal, autonomic components innervate the otic ganglion. Postganglionic parasympathetic fibers from these ganglia supply the sphincter of the iris, the ciliary muscle, the salivary and lacrimal glands, and the mucous glands of the nose, mouth, and pharynx. These fibers also include vasodilator nerves to the organs mentioned. The tenth cranial, or vagus, nerve arises in the medulla and contains preganglionic fibers, most of which do not synapse until they reach the many small ganglia lying directly on or in the viscera of the thorax and abdomen. In the intestinal wall, the vagal fibers terminate around ganglion cells in the plexuses of Auerbach and Meissner. The preganglionic fibers are thus very long and the postganglionic fibers quite short. The vagus nerve in addition carries a far greater number of afferent fibers (but apparently not pain fibers) from the viscera into the medulla; the cell bodies of these fibers lie mainly in the nodose ganglion.

The parasympathetic sacral outflow consists of axons that arise from cells in the second, third, and fourth segments of the sacral cord and proceed as preganglionic fibers to form the pelvic nerves (nervi erigentes). They synapse in terminal ganglia lying near or within the bladder, rectum, and sexual organs. The vagal and sacral outflows provide motor and secretory fibers to thoracic, abdominal, and pelvic organs, as indicated in Figure 5–1.

Differences Between Sympathetic, Parasympathetic, and Motor Nerves. The sympathetic system is distributed to effectors throughout the body, whereas the parasympathetic distribution is much more limited. Furthermore, the sympathetic fibers ramify to a much greater extent. A preganglionic sympathetic fiber may traverse a considerable distance of the sympathetic chain and pass through several ganglia before it finally synapses with a postganglionic neuron; also, its terminals make contact with a large number of postganglionic neurons. In some ganglia, the ratio of preganglionic axons to ganglion cells may be 1:20 or more. In this manner, a diffuse discharge of the sympathetic system is possible. In addition, synaptic innervation overlaps, so that one ganglion cell may be supplied by several preganglionic fibers.

The parasympathetic system, by contrast, has its terminal ganglia very near to or within the organs innervated and thus can be more circumscribed in its influences. In some organs a 1:1 relationship between the number of preganglionic and postganglionic fibers has been suggested, but the ratio of preganglionic vagal fibers to ganglion cells in Auerbach's plexus has been estimated as 1:8000. Hence, this distinction between the two systems does not apply to all sites.

The cell bodies of somatic motoneurons are in the ventral horn of the spinal cord; the axon divides into many branches, each of which innervates a single muscle fiber, so that more than 100 muscle fibers may be supplied by one motoneuron to form a motor unit. At each neuromuscular junction, or motor end-plate, the axonal terminal loses its myelin sheath and forms a terminal arborization that lies in apposition to a specialized surface of the muscle membrane. Mitochondria and a collection of synaptic vesicles are concentrated at the nerve terminal.

Details of Innervation. The terminations of the postganglionic autonomic fibers in smooth muscle and glands form a rich plexus, or terminal reticulum. The terminal reticulum (sometimes called the autonomic ground plexis) consists of the final ramifications of the postganglionic sympathetic (adrenergic), parasympathetic (cholinergic), and visceral afferent fibers, all of which are enclosed within a frequently interrupted sheath of satellite or Schwann cells. At these interruptions, varicosities packed with vesicles are seen in the efferent fibers. Such varicosities occur repeatedly along the course of the ramifications of the axon. Apparently the distance between the nerve varicosities and smooth muscle fibers varies widely, ranging from 200 Å in the vas deferens to 10,000 Å in certain blood vessels (Gabella, 1981).

"Protoplasmic bridges" occur between the smooth muscle fibers themselves at points of contact between their plasma membranes. They are believed to permit the direct conduction of impulses from cell to cell without the need for chemical transmission. These structures have been variously termed nexuses, caveolae, or tight junctions, and they enable the smooth muscle fibers to function as a unit or syncytium.

Sympathetic ganglia are extremely complex, both anatomically and pharmacologically (*see* Chapter 9). The preganglionic fibers lose their myelin sheaths, and divide repeatedly into a vast number of end fibers with diameters ranging from 0.1 to 0.3 μm; except at points of synaptic contact, they retain their satellite-cell sheaths. The vast majority of synapses are axodendritic. Apparently, a given axonal terminal may synapse with one or more dendritic processes at several points.

Responses of Effector Organs to Autonomic Nerve Impulses. A clear understanding of the response of the various effector organs to autonomic nerve impulses makes it possible to anticipate the actions of drugs that mimic or inhibit the actions of these nerves. In most instances, the sympathetic and parasympathetic systems can be viewed as physiological antagonists. If one system inhibits a certain function, the other usually augments that function. Most viscera are innervated by both divisions of the autonomic nervous system, and the level of activity at any one moment represents the integration of influences of the two components. Despite the conventional concept of antagonism between the two portions of the autonomic nervous system, their activities on specific structures may be either different and independent or integrated and interdependent. For example, the effects of sympathetic and parasympathetic stimulation of the heart and the iris follow a highly integrated pattern of antagonism. Their actions on male sexual organs are complementary and are integrated to promote sexual function. The control of peripheral vascular resistance is primarily, but not exclusively, due to sympathetic control of arteriolar resistance. The effects of stimulating the sympathetic (adrenergic) and parasympathetic (cholinergic) nerves to various organs, visceral structures, and effector cells are summarized in Table 5–1.

General Functions of the Autonomic Nervous System. The integrating action of the autonomic nervous system is of vital importance for the well-being of the organism. In general, the autonomic nervous system regulates the activities of structures that are not under voluntary control and that, as a rule, function below the level of consciousness. Thus, respiration, circulation, digestion, body temperature, metabolism, sweating, and the secretions of certain endocrine glands are regulated, in part or entirely, by the autonomic nervous system. As Claude Bernard (1878–1879) and Cannon (1929, 1932) emphasized, the constancy of the internal environment of the organism is to a large extent controlled by the vegetative, or autonomic, nervous system.

The sympathetic and parasympathetic systems have contrasting functions in regulating the internal environment. The sympathetic system and its associated adrenal medulla are not essential to life in a controlled environment. Under circumstances of stress, however, the lack of the sympathoadrenal functions becomes evident. Body temperature cannot be regulated when environmental temperature varies; the concentration of glucose in blood does not rise in response to urgent need; compensatory vascular responses to hemorrhage, oxygen deprivation, excitement, and exercise are lacking; resistance to fatigue is lessened; sympathetic components of instinctive reactions to fright and danger are lost; and other serious deficiencies in the protective forces of the body are discernible.

The sympathetic system is normally active continuously; the degree of activity varies from moment to moment and from organ to organ. In this manner, adjustments to a constantly changing environment are accomplished. The sympathoadrenal system can also discharge as a unit. This occurs especially during rage and fright, when sympathetically innervated structures over the entire body are affected simultaneously. Heart rate is accelerated; blood pressure rises; red blood cells are poured into the circulation from the spleen (in certain species); blood flow is shifted from the skin and splanchnic region to the skeletal muscles; blood glucose rises; the bronchioles and pupils dilate; and, on the whole, the organism is better prepared for "fight or flight." Many of these effects result primarily from, or are reinforced by, the actions of epinephrine, secreted by the adrenal medulla (*see* below).

Table 5–1. RESPONSES OF EFFECTOR ORGANS TO AUTONOMIC NERVE IMPULSES

EFFECTOR ORGANS	ADRENERGIC IMPULSES [1]		CHOLINERGIC IMPULSES [1]
	Receptor Type [2]	*Responses* [3]	*Responses* [3]
Eye			
Radial muscle, iris	α_1	Contraction (mydriasis) ++	—
Sphincter muscle, iris		—	Contraction (miosis) +++
Ciliary muscle	β_2	Relaxation for far vision +	Contraction for near vision +++
Heart [4]			
SA node	β_1	Increase in heart rate ++	Decrease in heart rate; vagal arrest +++
Atria	β_1	Increase in contractility and conduction velocity ++	Decrease in contractility, and shortened AP duration ++
AV node	β_1	Increase in automaticity and conduction velocity ++	Decrease in conduction velocity; AV block +++
His–Purkinje system	β_1	Increase in automaticity and conduction velocity +++	Little effect
Ventricles	β_1	Increase in contractility, conduction velocity, automaticity, and rate of idioventricular pacemakers +++	Slight decrease in contractility claimed by some
Arterioles			
Coronary	$\alpha_1, \alpha_2; \beta_2$	Constriction +; dilatation [5] ++	Constriction +
Skin and mucosa	α_1, α_2	Constriction +++	Dilatation [6]
Skeletal muscle	$\alpha; \beta_2$	Constriction ++; dilatation [5,7] ++	Dilatation [8] +
Cerebral	α_1	Constriction (slight)	Dilatation [6]
Pulmonary	$\alpha_1; \beta_2$	Constriction +; dilatation [5]	Dilatation [6]
Abdominal viscera	$\alpha_1; \beta_2$	Constriction +++; dilatation [7] +	—
Salivary glands	α_1, α_2	Constriction +++	Dilatation ++
Renal	$\alpha_1, \alpha_2; \beta_1, \beta_2$	Constriction +++; dilatation [7] +	—
Veins (Systemic)	$\alpha_1; \beta_2$	Constriction ++; dilatation ++	—
Lung			
Tracheal and bronchial muscle	β_2	Relaxation +	Contraction ++
Bronchial glands	$\alpha_1; \beta_2$	Decreased secretion; increased secretion	Stimulation +++
Stomach			
Motility and tone	$\alpha_1, \alpha_2; \beta_2$	Decrease (usually) [9] +	Increase +++
Sphincters	α_1	Contraction (usually) +	Relaxation (usually) +
Secretion		Inhibition (?)	Stimulation +++
Intestine			
Motility and tone	$\alpha_1, \alpha_2; \beta_1, \beta_2$	Decrease [9] +	Increase +++
Sphincters	α_1	Contraction (usually) +	Relaxation (usually) +
Secretion	α_2	Inhibition	Stimulation ++
Gallbladder and Ducts	β_2	Relaxation +	Contraction +
Kidney			
Renin secretion	$\alpha_1; \beta_1$	Decrease +; increase ++	—
Urinary Bladder			
Detrusor	β_2	Relaxation (usually) +	Contraction +++
Trigone and sphincter	α_1	Contraction ++	Relaxation ++
Ureter			
Motility and tone	α_1	Increase	Increase (?)
Uterus	$\alpha_1; \beta_2$	Pregnant: contraction (α_1); relaxation (β_2). Nonpregnant: relaxation (β_2)	Variable [10]
Sex Organs, Male	α_1	Ejaculation +++	Erection +++
Skin			
Pilomotor muscles	α_1	Contraction ++	—
Sweat glands	α_1	Localized secretion [11] +	Generalized secretion +++
Spleen Capsule	$\alpha_1; \beta_2$	Contraction +++; relaxation +	—

Table 5–1. RESPONSES OF EFFECTOR ORGANS TO AUTONOMIC NERVE IMPULSES (Continued)

EFFECTOR ORGANS	ADRENERGIC IMPULSES [1]		CHOLINERGIC IMPULSES [1]
	Receptor Type [2]	*Responses* [3]	*Responses* [3]
Adrenal Medulla		—	Secretion of epinephrine and norepinephrine (nicotinic effect)
Skeletal Muscle	β_2	Increased contractility; glycogenolysis; K^+ uptake	—
Liver	α; β_2	Glycogenolysis and gluconeogenesis [12] +++	—
Pancreas			
Acini	α	Decreased secretion +	Secretion ++
Islets (β cells)	α_2	Decreased secretion +++	—
	β_2	Increased secretion +	—
Fat Cells	α; β_1 (β_3)	Lipolysis [12] +++	—
Salivary Glands	α_1	Potassium and water secretion +	Potassium and water secretion +++
	β	Amylase secretion +	
Lacrimal Glands	α	Secretion +	Secretion +++
Nasopharyngeal Glands		—	Secretion ++
Pineal Gland	β	Melatonin synthesis	—
Posterior Pituitary	β_1	Antidiuretic hormone secretion	—

[1] The anatomical classes of adrenergic and cholinergic nerve fibers are described on page 86 and depicted in Figure 5–1 in red and blue, respectively. A dash signifies no known functional innervation. Subtypes of muscarinic cholinergic receptors are not indicated; most glands and smooth muscles appear to contain multiple subtypes, while the heart largely contains M_2 cholinergic receptors.

[2] Where a designation of subtype is not provided, the nature of the subtype has not been determined unequivocally.

[3] Responses are designated 1+ to 3+ to provide an approximate indication of the importance of adrenergic and cholinergic nerve activity in the control of the various organs and functions listed.

[4] Heart also contains α_1 and β_2 receptors, but they are less important for physiological responses.

[5] Dilatation predominates *in situ* due to metabolic autoregulatory phenomena.

[6] Cholinergic vasodilatation at these sites is of questionable physiological significance.

[7] Over the usual concentration range of physiologically released, circulating epinephrine, β-receptor response (vasodilatation) predominates in blood vessels of skeletal muscle and liver; α-receptor response (vasoconstriction), in blood vessels of other abdominal viscera. The renal and mesenteric vessels also contain specific dopaminergic receptors, activation of which causes dilatation (*see* review by Goldberg *et al.*, 1978).

[8] Sympathetic cholinergic system causes vasodilatation in skeletal muscle, but this is not involved in most physiological responses.

[9] It has been proposed that adrenergic fibers terminate at inhibitory β receptors on smooth muscle fibers, and at inhibitory α receptors on parasympathetic cholinergic (excitatory) ganglion cells of Auerbach's plexus.

[10] Depends on stage of menstrual cycle, amount of circulating estrogen and progesterone, and other factors.

[11] Palms of hands and some other sites ("adrenergic sweating").

[12] There is significant variation among species in the type of receptor that mediates certain metabolic responses; α and β responses have not been determined in man. A β_3 receptor has been cloned and may mediate responses in fat cells in some species.

The parasympathetic system is organized mainly for discrete and localized discharge and is concerned primarily with the functions of conservation of energy and maintenance of organ function during periods of minimal activity. It slows the heart rate, lowers the blood pressure, stimulates the gastrointestinal movements and secretions, aids absorption of nutrients, protects the retina from excessive light, and empties the urinary bladder and rectum. No useful purpose would be served in the body if the parasympathetic nerves all discharged at once.

NEUROHUMORAL TRANSMISSION

Nerve impulses elicit responses in smooth, cardiac, and skeletal muscles, exocrine glands, and postsynaptic neurons through liberation of specific chemical neurotransmitters. The steps involved and the evidence for them will be outlined in some detail because the concept of chemical mediation of nerve impulses profoundly affects our knowledge of the mechanism of action of drugs at these sites.

HISTORICAL ASPECTS

The earliest concrete proposal of a neurohumoral mechanism was made shortly after the turn of the present century. Lewandowsky (1898) and Langley (1901) noted independently the similarity between the effects of injection of extracts of the adrenal gland and stimulation of sympathetic nerves. A few years later, in 1905, T. R. Elliott, while a student with Langley at Cambridge, England, extended these observations and postulated that sympathetic nerve impulses release minute amounts of an epinephrine-like substance in immediate contact with effector cells. He considered this substance to be the chemical step in the process of transmission. He also noted that long after sympathetic nerves had degenerated, the effector organs still responded characteristically to the hormone of the adrenal medulla. In 1905, Langley suggested that effector cells have excitatory and inhibitory "receptive substances," and that the response to epinephrine depended on which type of substance was present. In 1907, Dixon was so impressed by the correspondence between the effects of the alkaloid muscarine and the responses to vagal stimulation that he advanced the important idea that the vagus nerve liberated a muscarine-like substance that acted as a chemical transmitter of its impulses. In the same year, Reid Hunt described the actions of acetylcholine (ACh) and other choline esters. In 1914, Dale thoroughly reinvestigated the pharmacological properties of ACh. He was so intrigued with the remarkable fidelity with which this drug reproduced the responses to stimulation of parasympathetic nerves that he introduced the term *parasympathomimetic* to characterize its effects. Dale also noted the brief duration of the action of this chemical and proposed that an esterase in the tissues rapidly splits ACh to acetic acid and choline, thereby terminating its action.

The brilliant researches of Otto Loewi, begun in 1921, provided the first proof of the chemical mediation of nerve impulses by the release of specific chemical agents. He stimulated the vagus nerve of a perfused (donor) frog heart and allowed the perfusion fluid to come in contact with a second (recipient) frog heart used as a test object. It was thus evident that a substance was liberated from the first organ that slowed the rate of the second. Loewi referred to this chemical substance as *Vagusstoff* ("vagus-substance"; parasympathin); subsequently, Loewi and Navratil (1926) presented evidence for its identification as ACh. Loewi also discovered that an accelerator substance similar to epinephrine was liberated into the perfusion fluid in summer, when the action of the sympathetic fibers in the frog's vagus, a mixed nerve, predominated over that of the inhibitory fibers. Loewi's discoveries were eventually confirmed and became universally accepted. Evidence that the cardiac vagus-substance is also ACh in mammals was obtained in 1933 by Feldberg and Krayer.

In addition to the role of ACh as the transmitter of all postganglionic parasympathetic fibers and of a few postganglionic sympathetic fibers, such as those to the sweat glands and the sympathetic vasodilator fibers, this substance has been shown to have transmitter function in three additional classes of nerves: preganglionic fibers of both the sympathetic and the parasympathetic systems, motor nerves to skeletal muscle, and certain neurons within the CNS.

Mention has already been made of Loewi's discovery of an accelerator substance released from frog hearts under certain conditions. In the same year, Cannon and Uridil (1921) reported that stimulation of the sympathetic hepatic nerves resulted in the release of an epinephrine-like substance that increased the blood pressure and the heart rate. Subsequent experiments, mainly by Cannon and coworkers, firmly established that this substance is the chemical mediator liberated by sympathetic nerve impulses at neuroeffector junctions. The mediator was originally called "sympathin" by Cannon.

In many of its pharmacological and chemical properties, Cannon's "sympathin" closely resembled epinephrine, but the two substances differed in certain important respects. When epinephrine is injected into the body, it elicits both excitatory and inhibitory effects. Thus, it accelerates the rate of the heart but simultaneously dilates certain vascular beds while constricting others. In contrast, the excitatory effects of "sympathin" could be elicited in the absence of dilatation of some vascular beds, with more marked increases in total peripheral resistance and diastolic blood pressure. As early as 1910, Barger and Dale noted that the effects of sympathetic nerve stimulation were more closely reproduced by the injection of sympathomimetic primary amines than by that of epinephrine or other secondary amines. The possibility that demethylated epinephrine (*norepinephrine*) might be "sympathin" had been repeatedly advanced by Z. M. Bacq and others, but definitive evidence for its role as the sympathetic nerve mediator was not obtained until specific assay methods were developed for the quantitative determination of small amounts of sympathomimetic amines in extracts of tissues and body fluids. von Euler in 1946 found that the sympathomimetic substance in highly purified extracts resembled norepinephrine by all criteria used. It is now known that norepinephrine is the predominant sympathomimetic substance in the postganglionic sympathetic nerves of mammals and is the adrenergic mediator liberated by their stimulation (*see* von Euler, 1972). Norepinephrine, its immediate precursor, dopamine, and epinephrine are also neurohumoral transmitters in the CNS (*see* Chapter 12).

EVIDENCE FOR NEUROHUMORAL TRANSMISSION

The concept of neurohumoral transmission was developed primarily to explain observations relating to the transmission of impulses from postganglionic autonomic fibers to effector cells. The general lines of evidence to support the concept have included (1) demonstration of the presence of a physiologically active compound and its biosynthetic enzymes at appropriate sites; (2) recovery of the compound from the perfusate of an innervated structure during periods of nerve stimulation, but not (or in greatly reduced amounts) in the absence of stimulation; (3) demonstration that the compound, when administered appropriately, is capable of producing responses identical to those to nerve stimulation; and (4) demonstration that the responses to nerve stimulation and to the administered compound are modified in the same manner by various drugs.

General acceptance of neurohumoral, rather than electrogenic, transmission at autonomic ganglia and the neuromuscular junction of skeletal muscle was withheld for a considerable period, chiefly for two reasons: (1) the extremely rapid time factors involved, in contrast to those seen at autonomic effector sites; and (2) discrepancies between the amount of the putative transmitter, ACh, recovered during nerve stimulation and that required to produce characteristic responses. Both objections have been answered by modern techniques of intracellular recording and microiontophoretic application of drugs.

Neurohumoral transmission in the peripheral and central nervous systems was once believed to conform to the hypothesis that each neuron contains only one transmitter substance. However, enkephalins, substance P, somatostatin, and other peptides have been found in nervous tissue, and these peptides can depolarize or hyperpolarize nerve terminals or postsynaptic cells (*see* Barker, 1983). Furthermore, histochemical, immunocytochemical, and autoradiographic studies have demonstrated that one or more of these peptides is present in the same neurons that contain one of the classical biogenic amine neurotransmitters (Bartfai *et al.*, 1988). For example, enkephalins are found in postganglionic sympathetic neurons and adrenal medullary chromaffin cells. VIP is apparently localized in peripheral cholinergic neurons that innervate exocrine glands. The VIP may be responsible for the vasodilatation that accompanies secretion following nerve stimulation. These observations suggest that in many instances synaptic transmission may be mediated by the release of more than one neurohumoral agent (*see* below).

STEPS INVOLVED IN NEUROHUMORAL TRANSMISSION

The sequence of events involved in neurohumoral transmission is of particular importance pharmacologically, since the actions of a great number of drugs are related directly to the individual steps. The term *conduction* is reserved for the passage of an impulse along an axon or muscle fiber; *transmission* refers to the passage of an impulse across a synaptic or neuroeffector junction. With the exception of the local anesthetics, very few drugs modify axonal conduction in the doses employed therapeutically. Hence, this process will be described only briefly.

Axonal Conduction. Current knowledge of axonal conduction stems largely from the investigative work of Hodgkin and Huxley (1952).

At rest, the interior of the typical mammalian axon is approximately 70 mV negative to the exterior. The resting potential is essentially a diffusion potential, based chiefly on the 40-fold higher concentration of K^+ in the axoplasm as compared with the extracellular fluid, and the relatively high permeability of the resting axonal membrane to this ion. Na^+ and Cl^- are present in higher concentrations in the extracellular fluid than in the axoplasm, but the axonal membrane at rest is considerably less permeable to these ions; hence their contribution to the resting potential is small. These ionic gradients are maintained by an energy-dependent active transport or pump mechanism, which involves an adenosine triphosphatase (ATPase) activated by Na^+ at the inner and by K^+ at the outer surface of the membrane (*see* Armstrong, 1974; Grundfest, 1975). In some excitable tissues an electrogenic Na^+ pump may also contribute to the net resting potential (Fleming, 1980).

In response to depolarization to a threshold level, an action potential (AP) or nerve impulse is initiated at a local region of the membrane. The action potential consists of two phases. The initial phase is caused by a rapid increase in the permeability of Na^+ through the voltage-sensitive Na^+ channel. The result is inward movement of Na^+ and a rapid depolarization from the resting potential, which continues to a positive overshoot. The second phase results from the rapid inactivation of the Na^+ channel and the delayed opening of a K^+ channel, which permits outward movement of K^+ to terminate the depolarization. Although not important in axonal conduction, Ca^{2+} channels in other tissues (*e.g.*, heart) contribute to the action potential by prolonging depolarization by an inward movement of Ca^{2+}. This influx of Ca^{2+} also serves as a stimulus to initiate intracellular events (Hille, 1984; *see also* Chapter 2).

The transmembrane ionic currents produce local circuit currents around the axon. As a result of such localized changes in membrane potential, adjacent inactive channels in the axon are activated, and excitation of the next excitable portion of the axonal membrane occurs. This brings about the propagation of the AP without decrement along the axon. The region that has undergone depolarization remains momentarily in a refractory state. In myelinated fibers, permeability changes occur only at the nodes of Ranvier, thus causing a rapidly progressing type of jumping, or saltatory, conduction. The puffer fish poison, tetrodotoxin, and a close congener found in some shellfish, saxitoxin, selectively block axonal conduction; they do so by preventing the increase in permeability to Na^+ associated with the rising phase of the AP. In contrast, batrachotoxin, an extremely potent steroidal alkaloid secreted by a South American frog, produces paralysis through a selective increase in Na^+ permeability, which induces a persistent depolarization. Scorpion toxins are peptides that also cause persistent depolarization, but they do this by inhibiting the inactivation process. The pharmacological aspects of axonal conduction have been reviewed by Strichartz and associates (1987) and by Wu and Narahashi (1988). Na^+ and Ca^{2+} channels are discussed in more detail in Chapters 15 and 32, respectively.

Junctional Transmission. The arrival of the action potential (AP) at the axonal terminals initiates a series of events that put into effect the neurohumoral transmission of an excitatory or inhibitory impulse across the synapse or neuroeffector junction (*see* reviews by Katz, 1966; Eccles, 1973). These events, diagrammed in Figure 5–2, are as follows:

1. *Release of the Transmitter.* The nonpeptide neurohumoral transmitters are largely synthesized in the region of the axonal terminals and stored there within synaptic vesicles. Peptide neurotransmitters (or precursor peptides) are transported down the axon from their site of synthesis in the cell body. During the resting state, there is a continual slow release of isolated quanta of the transmitter; this produces electrical responses at the postjunctional membrane (miniature end-plate potentials, mepps) that are associated with the maintenance of physiological responsiveness of the effector organ (*see* Katz, 1969). A low level of spontaneous activity within the motor units of skeletal muscle is particularly important, since skeletal muscle lacks inherent tone. The AP causes the synchronous release of several hundred quanta of neurotransmitter. The depolarization of the axonal terminal triggers this process; the critical step is the influx of Ca^{2+}, which enters the axonal cytoplasm and in some way promotes fusion between the axoplasmic membrane and those vesicles in close proximity to it. The contents of the vesicles are then discharged to the exterior by a process termed *exocytosis*. Other components of the vesicle, including enzymes and other proteins, are also released.

A variety of chemical substances can inhibit the neurally mediated release of either norepinephrine or ACh by interaction with receptors on the appropriate nerve terminals. Norepinephrine is able to interact with a presynaptic α_2-adrenergic receptor (termed an *autoreceptor*) and inhibit neurally mediated release of norepinephrine. Administration of α_2-adrenergic antagonists causes a marked increase in the release of norepinephrine per nerve impulse. In an analogous fashion, neurally mediated release of ACh from cholinergic neurons is inhibited by α_2-adrenergic agonists. Conversely, stimulation of presynaptic β_2-adrenergic receptors is associated with a modest enhancement of norepinephrine release. Adenosine, acetylcholine, dopamine, prostaglandins, and enkephalins all inhibit neurally mediated release of norepinephrine by means of interactions with specific presynaptic receptors (*see* Starke, 1987; Langer and Lehmann, 1988). These receptors probably exert their modulatory effects at least in part by inhibiting the function of prejunctional Ca^{2+} channels (Tsien *et al.*, 1988).

In cholinergic neurons, presynaptic muscarinic receptors have been detected at those synapses containing postjunctional muscarinic receptors. These receptors mediate inhibition of the evoked release of acetylcholine, and the output of acetylcholine is thus decreased with repetitive stimulation. The evoked release of ACh is also blocked by inhibitors of acetylcholinesterase (AChE), and it is enhanced by muscarinic antagonists (Kilbinger, 1984). Presynaptic muscarinic receptors also influence the release of norepinephrine from adrenergic neurons in the myocardium and vasculature, but they have not been detected in somatic motor nerves.

2. *Combination of the Transmitter with Postjunctional Receptors and Production of the Postjunctional Potential.* The transmitter diffuses across the synaptic or junctional cleft and combines with specialized receptors on the postjunctional membrane; this often results in a localized increase in the ionic permeability, or conductance, of the membrane. With certain exceptions, noted below, one of three types of permeability change can occur: (1) a generalized increase in the permeability to cations (no-

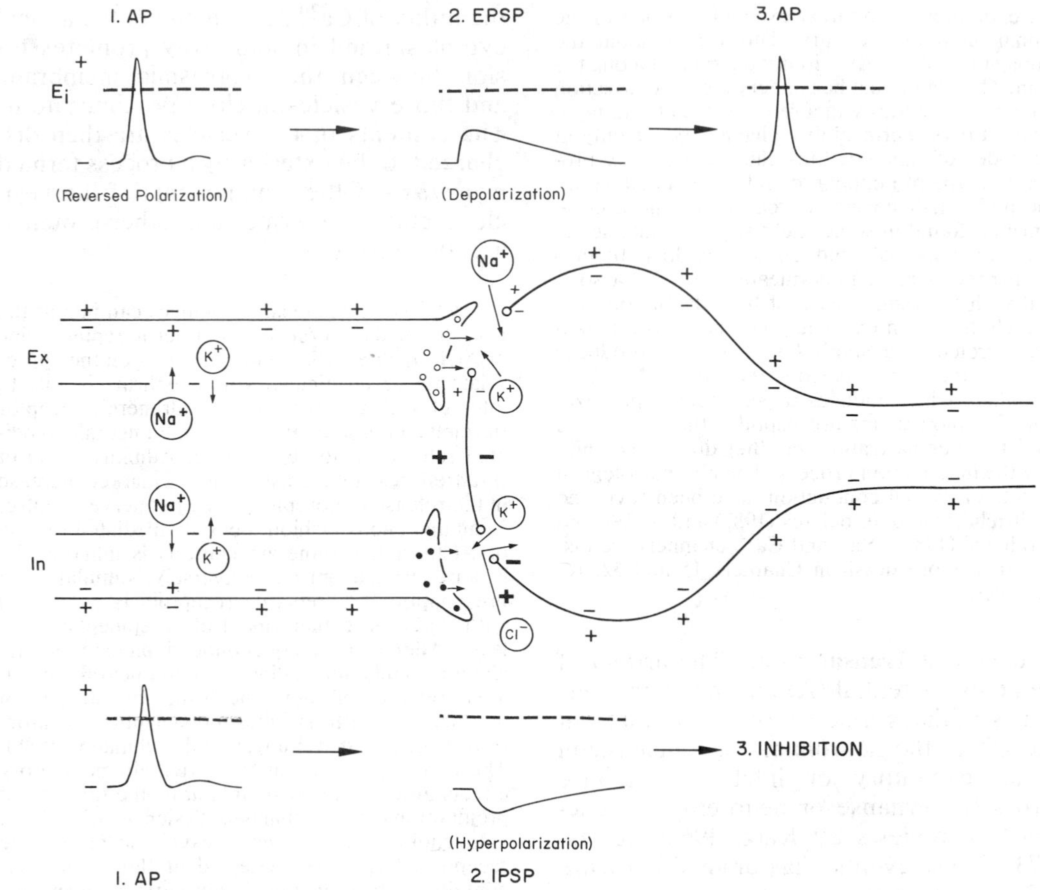

Figure 5–2. *Steps involved in excitatory* (Ex) *and inhibitory* (In) *neurohumoral transmission.*

1. The nerve action potential (AP), consisting in a self-propagated *reversal* of negativity (the internal potential, E_i, goes from a negative value, through zero potential, indicated by the broken line, to a positive value) of the axonal membrane, arrives at the presynaptic terminal and causes release of the excitatory (○) or inhibitory (●) transmitter.

2. Combination of the excitatory transmitter with postsynaptic receptors produces a localized depolarization, the excitatory postsynaptic potential (EPSP), through an increase in permeability to cations, most notably Na^+. The inhibitory transmitter causes a selective increase in permeability to K^+ or Cl^-, resulting in a localized hyperpolarization, the inhibitory postsynaptic potential (IPSP).

3. The EPSP initiates a conducted AP in the postsynaptic neuron; this can, however, be prevented by the hyperpolarization induced by a concurrent IPSP.

The transmitter is dissipated by enzymatic destruction, by reuptake into the presynaptic terminal or adjacent glial cells, or by diffusion. (Modified from Eccles, 1964, 1973; Katz, 1966; and others.)

tably Na^+, but occasionally Ca^{2+}), resulting in a localized depolarization of the membrane, that is, an *excitatory postsynaptic potential* (EPSP); (2) a selective increase in permeability to anions, resulting in stabilization or actual hyperpolarization of the membrane, which constitutes an *inhibitory postsynaptic potential* (IPSP); or (3) an increased permeability to K^+. Since K^+ can then exit the cell, hyperpolarization and stabilization of the membrane potential occur (an IPSP).

It should be emphasized that the potential changes associated with the EPSP and

IPSP at most sites are the results of passive fluxes of extracellular and intracellular ions down their concentration gradients. The changes in channel permeability that cause these potential changes are specifically regulated by the specialized postjunctional receptors for the neurotransmitter that initiates the response (*see* Chapter 2 and the remainder of this section). Under normal conditions, these receptors may be highly localized on the effector-cell surface, as seen at the neuromuscular junctions of skeletal muscle and other discrete synapses, or distributed in a more uniform fashion, as observed in smooth muscle.

By using microelectrodes that form high resistance seals on the surface of cells, it is possible to record electrical events associated with a single neurotransmitter-gated channel (*see* Hille, 1984). In the presence of an appropriate neurotransmitter, the channel opens rapidly to a high conductance state, remains open for about a millisecond, and then closes. A short square-wave pulse of current is observed as a result of the channel opening and closing. The summation of these microscopic events gives rise to the EPSP. The graded response to a neurotransmitter is usually related to the frequency of opening events rather than to the extent of opening or the duration of opening. High conductance ligand-gated ion channels usually permit passage of Na^+ or Cl^-; K^+ and Ca^{2+} are involved less frequently. These ligand-gated channels belong to a large family of proteins that includes the nicotinic cholinergic receptor, gamma-aminobutyric acid A receptors, glycine receptors, and receptors for the excitatory amino acid (*e.g.*, glutamate). Neurotransmitters can also modulate the function of channels for K^+ and Ca^{2+} indirectly. In these cases the receptor and channel are separate proteins and information is conveyed between them by a guanine nucleotide–binding regulatory protein (*see* Chapter 2). Other receptors for neurotransmitters act by influencing the synthesis of intracellular second messengers and do not necessarily cause a change in membrane potential. The most widely documented examples of receptor regulation of second messenger systems are the activation or inhibition of adenylyl cyclase and the increase in intracellular concentrations of Ca^{2+} that results from release of the ion from internal stores.

3. *Initiation of Postjunctional Activity*. If an EPSP exceeds a certain threshold value, it initiates a propagated AP in a postsynaptic neuron or a muscle AP in skeletal or cardiac muscle. In smooth muscle, in which propagated impulses are minimal, an EPSP may increase the rate of spontaneous depolarization and enhance muscle tone; in gland cells, it initiates secretion. An IPSP will tend to oppose excitatory potentials initiated by other neuronal sources at the same time and site. Whether a propagated impulse or other response ensues will depend on the algebraic sum of all these effects.

4. *Destruction or Dissipation of the Transmitter*. When impulses can be transmitted across junctions at frequencies up to several hundred per second, it is obvious that there should be an efficient means of disposing of the transmitter following each impulse. At most cholinergic junctions involved in rapid neurotransmission, high concentrations of acetylcholinesterase (AChE) are available for this purpose. Upon inhibition of AChE, removal of the transmitter is accomplished principally by diffusion. Under these circumstances, the effects of released ACh are potentiated and prolonged.

It is unlikely that enzymes are directly involved in rapidly terminating the action of the adrenergic transmitter at the immediate receptor site; this action is probably effected by a combination of simple diffusion and reuptake by the axonal terminals of most of the released norepinephrine (*see* Iversen, 1975). Termination of the action of amino acid transmitters results from their active transport into neurons and surrounding glia. Peptide neurotransmitters are hydrolyzed by various peptidases and dissipated by diffusion; specific uptake mechanisms have not been demonstrated for these substances.

5. *Nonelectrogenic Functions*. The continual quantal release of neurotransmitters in amounts not sufficient to elicit a postjunctional response is probably important in the transjunctional control of neurotransmitter action. The activity and turnover of enzymes involved in the synthesis and inactivation of neurotransmitters, the density of presynaptic and postsynaptic receptors, and other characteristics of synapses are probably controlled by trophic actions of neurotransmitters or other substances released by the neuron or the target cells (Thesleff, 1973; Fambrough, 1979; Richardson, 1988).

CHOLINERGIC TRANSMISSION

Two enzymes, choline acetyltransferase and acetylcholinesterase (AChE), are involved in the synthesis and degradation, respectively, of ACh.

Choline Acetyltransferase. Choline acetyltransferase catalyzes the final step in the synthesis of ACh—the acetylation of choline with acetyl coenzyme A (CoA) (*see* Tuček, 1988). The primary structure of choline acetyltransferase is known from molecular cloning (Berrard *et al.*, 1989), and immunocytochemical localization of the enzyme has proven useful for identification of cholinergic axons and nerve cell bodies.

Acetyl CoA for this reaction is derived from pyruvate via the multistep pyruvate dehydrogenase reaction or is synthesized by acetate thiokinase, which catalyzes the reaction of acetate with adenosine triphosphate (ATP) to form an enzyme-bound acyladenylate (acetyl AMP). In the presence of CoA, transacetylation and synthesis of acetyl CoA proceed.

Choline acetyltransferase, like other protein constituents of the neuron, is synthesized within the perikaryon and is then transported along the length of the axon to its terminal. The synaptic vesicles appear to be formed at the terminal, and the axonal terminals contain a large number of mitochondria, where acetyl CoA is synthesized. Choline is taken up from the extracellular fluid into the axoplasm by active transport. The final step in the synthesis occurs within the cytoplasm, following which most of the ACh is sequestered within the synaptic vesicles. Although moderately potent inhibitors of choline acetyltransferase exist (Cavallito *et al.*, 1969), they have no therapeutic utility, in part because they are relatively weak inhibitors of the enzyme *in vivo* and because the uptake of choline appears to be the rate-limiting step in the biosynthesis of ACh.

Transport of choline from the plasma into neurons is accomplished by distinct high- and low-affinity transport systems. The high-affinity system (K_m 1 to 5 μM) is unique to cholinergic neurons, is dependent on extracellular Na^+, and is inhibited by hemicholinium. This system is probably responsible for delivery of choline to the cholinergic nerve ending; much of this choline is recycled after hydrolysis of ACh by acetylcholinesterase. Plasma concentrations of choline approximate 10 μM; thus, the concentration of choline does not limit its availability to cholinergic neurons, at least in the periphery (where choline transport across the blood–brain barrier is not necessary) (*see* Jope, 1979; Ducis, 1988).

After synthesis, ACh is transported into and stored in synaptic vesicles. Vesamicol inhibits this transport system. The drug blocks evoked release of ACh without affecting influx of Ca^{2+} into the nerve ending, choline transport, or ACh synthesis (Parsons *et al.*, 1987).

Acetylcholinesterase. For ACh to serve as the neurohumoral agent in peripheral junctional transmission, the ester must be removed or inactivated within the time limits imposed by the response characteristics of visceral neuroeffector junctions, motor end-plates, and various types of neurons. At the neuromuscular junction, the mediator must be removed from the synapse almost immediately—with "flashlike suddenness," as Dale expressed it. Modern biophysical methods have revealed that the time required for hydrolysis of ACh is less than a millisecond. Choline has only 10^{-5} the vasodepressor potency of ACh.

Acetylcholinesterase (AChE; also known as specific or true ChE) is found in cholinergic neurons (dendrites, perikarya, and axons), in the vicinity of cholinergic synapses, and in other tissues. It is highly concentrated at the neuromuscular junction. Hydrolysis of ACh occurs in the immediate vicinity of the nerve ending. Butyrylcholinesterase (BuChE; also known as cholinesterase, ChE, serum esterase, or pseudo-ChE) is present in various types of glial or satellite cells but only to a limited extent in neuronal elements of the central and peripheral nervous systems. It is also present in the plasma, liver, and other organs; its physiological function is unknown. The ratios of AChE and BuChE change substantially during development of the nervous system. Although both types of enzyme can hydrolyze ACh and are inhibited by physostigmine, they can be distinguished by their rates of hydrolysis of butyrylcholine and by the use of selective inhibitors. Almost all the pharmacological effects of the anti-ChE agents (Chapter 7) are due to the inhibition of AChE, with the consequent accumulation of endogenous ACh.

AChE hydrolyzes ACh at a greater velocity than choline esters with acyl groups larger than acetate or propionate. The enzyme also hydrolyzes methacholine, and it is inhibited selectively by low concentrations of several *bis*-quaternary ammonium compounds and by other agents. BuChE, on the other hand, exhibits a maximal velocity of hydrolysis with butyrylcholine as a substrate; it does not hydrolyze methacholine; and it is more sensitive than AChE to inhibition by certain organophosphorus agents (*see* Chapter 7).

At the motor end-plates of skeletal muscle, most of the AChE is localized at the surface and infoldings of the postjunctional membrane. Accordingly, it is situated strategically for the rapid hydrolysis of ACh following the production of the end-plate potential (EPP). Several distinct molecular forms of the enzyme exist, and activity appears to be localized in both presynaptic and postsynaptic membranes and in the basal lamina in the neuromuscular junction. Both nerve and muscle have the capacity to synthesize AChE, and the enzyme present at the end-plate is derived from both tissues.

Storage and Release of Acetylcholine. Fatt and Katz (1952) recorded at the motor end-plate of skeletal muscle and observed the random occurrence of small (0.1 to 3.0 mV), spontaneous depolarizations at a frequency of approximately one per second. The magnitude of these miniature end-plate potentials (mepps) is considerably below the threshold required to fire a muscle AP; that they are due to the release of ACh is indicated by their enhancement by neostigmine (an anti-ChE agent) and their blockade by tubocurarine (an antagonist that acts at nicotinic receptors). This was the first evidence that ACh is released from motor-nerve endings in constant amounts, or *quanta*. The morphological counterpart of this phenomenon was discovered shortly thereafter in the form of synaptic vesicles (De Robertis and Bennett, 1955). The storage and release of ACh have been investigated most extensively at motor end-plates; nevertheless, most of the principles discovered at this locus probably apply to other sites of cholinergic transmission as well, and in many respects to noncholinergic transmission (*see* reviews by Hubbard, 1973; Krnjević, 1974; Reichardt and Kelly, 1983).

When an AP arrives at the motor-nerve terminal, there is an explosive release of 100 or more quanta (or vesicles) of ACh (Katz and Miledi, 1965). Depolarization of the terminal permits the influx of Ca^{2+} through a voltage-dependent channel. This influx of Ca^{2+} in some way facilitates the fusion of axonal and vesicular membranes at active zones, resulting in the extrusion of the contents of the vesicles. Ca^{2+} ionophores, which allow extracellular Ca^{2+} to permeate the nerve ending, also stimulate release of ACh. Release can be inhibited by excess Mg^{2+}.

Although there is general agreement regarding certain steps involved in the storage and release of ACh, many of the details are still unknown. Estimates of the ACh content of the synaptic vesicles range from 1000 to over 50,000 molecules per vesicle, and it has been calculated that a single motor-nerve terminal contains 300,000 or more vesicles. In addition, an uncertain but significant amount of ACh is present in the extravesicular cytoplasm. Recording the electrical events associated with the opening of single channels at the motor end-plate during continuous application of ACh has permitted estimation of the potential change induced by a single molecule of ACh (3×10^{-7} V); from such calculations, it is evident that even the lower estimate of the ACh content per vesicle (1000 molecules) is sufficient to account for the magnitude of the mepps (Katz and Miledi, 1972).

The release of ACh by exocytosis through the prejunctional membrane is inhibited by a toxin produced by *Clostridium botulinum;* it is one of the most potent toxins known. A small number of molecules of this toxin bind irreversibly to their sites of action, producing an essentially irreversible blockade of all cholinergic junctions (*see* Simpson, 1986). Death results from respiratory failure. Tetanus toxin has a similar mechanism of action. Black widow spider toxin has a site of action similar to that of botulinus toxin, but with the opposite effect. Clumping of vesicles at the prejunctional membrane is associated with the release of excessive amounts of ACh, followed by blockade of release.

Characteristics of Cholinergic Transmission at Various Sites. From the comparisons noted above, it is obvious that there are marked differences between various sites of cholinergic transmission with respect to general-architectural and fine-structural arrangements, the distributions of AChE, and the temporal factors involved in normal functioning. For example, in skeletal muscle the junctional sites occupy a small, discrete portion of the surface of the individual fibers and are relatively isolated from those of adjacent fibers; in the superior cervical ganglion, in contrast, approximately 100,000 ganglion cells are packed within a volume of a few cubic millimeters, and both the presynaptic and postsynaptic neuronal processes form complex networks. It is therefore to be expected that the specific features of cholinergic transmission will vary markedly at different sites.

Skeletal Muscle. Stimulation of a motor nerve results in the release of ACh from perfused muscle; close intraarterial injection of ACh produces muscular contraction similar to that elicited by stimulation of the motor nerve. The amount of ACh (10^{-17} mol) required to elicit an EPP following its microiontophoretic application to the motor end-plate of a rat diaphragm muscle fiber is equivalent to that recovered from each fiber following stimulation of the phrenic nerve (Krnjević and Mitchell, 1961).

The combination of ACh with the so-called nicotinic cholinergic receptors at the external surface of the postjunctional membrane induces an immediate, marked increase in permeability to cations. Upon activation of the receptor by ACh, its intrinsic channel opens for about 1 millisecond; during this interval about 50,000 sodium ions traverse the channel (Katz and Miledi, 1972). This process is the basis for the localized depolarizing EPP within the end-plate, which triggers the muscle AP. The latter in turn leads to contraction. Further details concerning these events and their modification by neuromuscular blocking agents are presented in Chapter 9.

Following section and degeneration of the motor nerve to skeletal muscle or of the postganglionic fibers to autonomic effectors, there is a marked reduction in the threshold doses of the transmitters and of certain other drugs required to elicit a response, that is, *denervation supersensitivity*. In skeletal muscle this change is accompanied by a spread of the cholinoceptive sites from the end-plate region to the adjacent portions of the sarcoplasmic membrane, which eventually involves the entire muscle surface. Embryonic muscle also exhibits this uniform sensitivity to ACh prior to innervation (Fambrough, 1979).

Autonomic Effectors. Stimulation or inhibition of autonomic effector cells occurs by activation of muscarinic cholinergic receptors (*see* below). In this case the effector is coupled to the receptor by a G protein (*see* Chapter 2). In contrast to skeletal muscle and neurons, smooth muscle and the cardiac conduction system (SA node, atrium, AV node, and the His–Purkinje system) normally exhibit intrinsic activity, both electrical and mechanical, that is modified but not initiated by nerve impulses. In the basal condition, smooth muscle exhibits waves of depolarization and/or spikes that are propagated from cell to cell at rates considerably slower than the AP of axons or skeletal muscle. The spikes are apparently initiated by rhythmic fluctuations in the membrane resting potential. In intestinal smooth muscle, the site of the pacemaker activity continually shifts, but in the heart spontaneous depolarizations normally arise from the SA node; however, under certain circumstances they can arise from any part of the conduction system (*see* Chapter 35).

The addition of ACh (0.1 to 1 μM) to isolated intestinal muscle causes a fall in the resting potential (*i.e.*, the membrane potential becomes less negative) and an increase in the frequency of spike production, accompanied by a rise in tension. A primary action of ACh in initiating these effects through muscarinic receptors is probably the partial depolarization of the cell membrane, brought about by an increase in Na^+ and, in some instances, Ca^{2+} conductances (Bolton, 1979; Hille, 1984). ACh can also produce contraction of some smooth muscles when the membrane has been completely depolarized by high concentrations of K^+, provided Ca^{2+} is present. Hence, ACh stimulates ion fluxes across membranes and/or mobilizes intracellular Ca^{2+} to cause contraction.

In the cardiac conduction system, particularly in the SA and the AV nodes, stimulation of the cholinergic innervation (of which the preganglionic fibers are in the vagus nerve) or the direct application of ACh causes inhibition, associated with hyperpolarization of the fiber membrane and a marked decrease in the rate of depolarization. These effects are due, at least in part, to a selective increase in permeability to K^+ (Trautwein *et al.*, 1956).

Autonomic Ganglia. The primary pathway of cholinergic transmission in autonomic ganglia is similar to that at the neuromuscular junction of skeletal muscle. Ganglion cells can be discharged by injecting very small amounts of ACh into the ganglion. The initial depolarization is the result of activation of nicotinic cholinergic receptors, which are ligand-gated cation channels.

Ganglionic transmission is a highly complex process, and several secondary transmitters or modulators are involved. These either enhance or diminish the sensitivity of the postganglionic cell to ACh. This sensitivity appears to be related to the membrane potential of the postsynaptic nerve cell body or its dendritic branches. Ganglionic transmission is discussed in more detail in Chapter 9.

Actions of Acetylcholine at Prejunctional Sites. Considerable attention has been focused on the possible involvement of prejunctional cholinoceptive sites in both cholinergic and noncholinergic transmission and in the actions of various drugs. The intraarterial injection of ACh or an anti-ChE agent (physostigmine or neostigmine) produces both fasciculations (synchronous contractions of the skeletal muscle fibers of entire motor units) and antidromic APs that are conducted from the terminals of the motor nerves to the ventral spinal roots. Both effects are blocked by curare. These and related observations suggest that the compounds can act at the prejunctional axonal terminals as well as at the postjunctional cholinoceptive sites (*see* Chapter 9).

Although cholinergic innervation of blood vessels is limited, prejunctional cholinergic muscarinic receptors appear to be present on sympathetic vasoconstrictor nerves (Steinsland *et al.*, 1973). The physiological role of these receptors is unclear, but their activation causes inhibition of neurally mediated release of norepinephrine (*see* Chapter 6). Because ACh is so rapidly hydrolyzed by local and circulating esterases, it is very unlikely that it plays a role as a circulating hormone analogous to that of epinephrine.

Dilatation of blood vessels in response to administered choline esters could involve several sites of action, including prejunctional inhibitory synapses on sympathetic fibers and inhibitory cholinergic receptors in the vasculature that are not innervated. The vasodilator effect of ACh on isolated blood vessels requires an intact endothelium. Activation of muscarinic receptors results in the liberation of a vasodilator substance (endothelium-derived relaxing factor) that diffuses to the smooth muscle and causes relaxation (*see* below; *see also* Furchgott, 1984).

Cholinergic Receptors and Signal Transduction. Sir Henry Dale noted that the various esters of choline elicited responses that were similar to those of either nicotine or muscarine, depending on the pharmacological preparation (Dale, 1914). A similarity in response was also noted between muscarine and nerve stimulation in those organs innervated by the craniosacral divisions of the autonomic nervous system. Thus, Dale suggested that acetylcholine was a neurotransmitter in the autonomic nervous system; he also stated that the compound had dual actions, which he termed a *nicotine action* (nicotinic) and a *muscarine action* (muscarinic).

The capacities of tubocurarine and atropine to block nicotinic and muscarinic effects of ACh, respectively, provided further support for the proposal of two distinct types of cholinergic receptors. Although Dale had access only to the plant alkaloids from *Amanita muscaria* and *Nicotiana tabacum* (and the chemical structures of the alkaloids were then unknown), this classification remains as the primary subdivision of cholinergic receptors. Its utility has survived the discovery of several distinct subtypes of nicotinic and muscarinic cholinergic receptors.

Although ACh and certain other compounds can stimulate both muscarinic and nicotinic receptors, a large number of other agonists and antagonists are very selective for one of the two major types of receptor, thus highlighting their very different properties. ACh itself is a flexible molecule, and indirect evidence suggests that the conformations of the neurotransmitter are distinct when it is bound to nicotinic or muscarinic receptors.

Nicotinic receptors are ligand-gated ion channels, and their activation always causes a rapid increase in cellular permeability to Na^+ and K^+, depolarization, and excitation. By contrast, muscarinic receptors belong to the class of so-called G protein–coupled receptors. Responses to muscarinic agonists are slower; they may be either excitatory or inhibitory, and they are not necessarily linked to changes in ion permeability.

The primary structures of various species of nicotinic receptors (Numa *et al.*, 1983) and muscarinic receptors (Kubo *et al.*, 1986) have been deduced by molecular cloning. That these two types of receptor belong to distinct families of proteins is not surprising, retrospectively, in view of their distinct differences in chemical specificity and function.

The nicotinic receptors are pentameric proteins that are composed of at least two distinct (but homologous) subunits. Each subunit contains multiple membrane-spanning regions (probably 4), and the individual subunits surround an internal channel. One of the subunits (designated α) is present in at least two copies and forms the ligand binding site on the receptor.

Muscarinic receptors are glycoproteins with molecular weights of approximately 80,000; as mentioned, they belong to the superfamily of receptor proteins whose functions are mediated by interaction with G proteins (*see* Chapter 2). As with other members of this receptor family, analysis of the hydrophobicity of their amino acid sequences predicts that they traverse the plasma membrane seven times.

Subtypes of Nicotinic Receptors. Based on the distinct actions of certain agonists and antagonists that interact with nicotinic receptors from skeletal muscle and ganglia, it has long been evident that all nicotinic receptors are not identical. Heterogeneity of this type of receptor was further revealed by molecular cloning. For example, the muscle receptor contains four distinct subunits in a pentameric complex ($\alpha_2\beta\delta\gamma$ or $\alpha_2\beta\delta\varepsilon$). Receptors in embryonic or denervated muscle contain a γ subunit, while an ε subunit replaces γ in adult innervated muscle. This gives rise to small differences in ligand selectivity, but the switch of subunits may be more important for dictating rates of turnover of the receptors or their tissue localization. Nicotinic receptors in the CNS also exist as pentamers, but they are composed of only two subunits, α and β. Further complexity arises because multiple forms of α and β have been detected (*see* Steinbach and Ifune, 1989). Each of the α and β subunits is found in discrete regions of the brain. It is not yet clear whether there are preferred matching pairs of α and β to form the pentamer or if all permutations of α and β are possible. The subtypes of nicotinic receptors are listed in Table 5–2; the structure and function of the nicotinic receptor are described in more detail in Chapter 9.

Subtypes of Muscarinic Receptors. Five subtypes of muscarinic cholinergic receptor have been detected by molecular cloning. Like the different forms of nicotinic receptors, these variants have distinct anatomical localizations and chemical specificities.

Table 5–2. CHARACTERISTICS OF SUBTYPES OF CHOLINERGIC RECEPTORS *

RECEPTOR	AGONISTS	ANTAGONISTS	TISSUE	RESPONSES	MOLECULAR MECHANISMS
Nicotinic					
Muscle (N_M)	Phenyltrimethyl-ammonium	Tubocurarine α-Bungarotoxin	Neuromuscular junction	End-plate depolarization, skeletal muscle contraction	Opening of cation channel in N_M receptor
Neuronal (N_N) [1]	Dimethylphenyl-piperazinium	Trimethaphan	Autonomic ganglia	Depolarization and firing of postganglionic neuron	Opening of cation channel in N_N receptor
			Adrenal medula	Secretion of catecholamines	
			CNS	Undefined	
Muscarinic					
M_1	Oxotremorine McN-A-343	Atropine Pirenzepine	Autonomic ganglia	Depolarization (late EPSP)	Stimulation of PLC with formation of IP_3 and DAG; increased cytosolic Ca^{2+}
			CNS [2]	Undefined	
M_2	—	Atropine AF-DX 115	Heart SA node	Slowed spontaneous depolarization; hyperpolarization	Activation of K^+ channels; inhibition of adenylyl cyclase
			Atrium	Shortened duration of action potential; decreased contractile force	
			AV node	Decreased conduction velocity	
			Ventricle	Slight decrease in contractile force	
M_3	—	Atropine Hexahydro-siladifenidol	Smooth muscle [3]	Contraction [4]	Stimulation of PLC with formation of IP_3 and DAG; increased cytosolic Ca^{2+}
			Secretory glands [3]	Increased secretion	

* This table provides examples of drugs that act on cholinergic receptors and of the location of subtypes of these receptors. Abbreviations are: excitatory postsynaptic potential (EPSP); phospholipase C (PLC); inositol-1,4,5-trisphosphate (IP_3); diacylglycerol (DAG).

[1] The nicotinic receptors of autonomic ganglia and the CNS contain a variety of different subunits; most of the subunits of receptors in the CNS are distinct from those in ganglia (*see* text).

[2] The CNS contains all known subtypes of muscarinic receptors.

[3] The subtypes in various smooth muscles or secretory glands have not been precisely determined, but are most likely to be mechanistically related to M_3 (or M_1) receptors.

[4] Relaxation occurs in sphincters in the urinary and gastrointestinal tracts, but this may result from the release of dilatory peptides from intrinsic ganglia or parasympathetic nerves; blood vessels relax as a consequence of release of factors from the endothelium (*see* text).

Unlike the nicotinic receptors, the muscarinic receptors act by two distinctly different mechanisms (*see* Table 5–2).

The diversity of muscarinic receptors was not suspected until the pharmacology of pirenzepine was examined in the late 1970s. Of the large number of muscarinic antagonists that had been studied over many decades, only pirenzepine showed the unique property of blocking gastric acid secretion at concentrations that did not affect several other responses to muscarinic agonists. These observations, subsequent study of other agonists and antagonists, and rapid advances in the cloning of complementary DNAs that encode muscarinic receptors have led to considerable inconsistency in nomenclature and difficulty in the unambiguous assignment of the pharmacological profile of a given response to a specific molecular entity (*i.e.*, receptor). By current convention, receptors that have been defined pharmacologically are designated as M_1, M_2, and M_3, while those that have been revealed by molecular cloning are termed m_1, m_2, m_3, m_4, and m_5 (Bonner, 1989). Fortunately, m_1, m_2, and m_3 appear to correspond to M_1, M_2, and M_3; there is less information about the nature and cellular location of the m_4 and m_5 receptors. Because of the correspondence of the first three subtypes of receptor and the unstable nature of such a dual system of classification, the distinction between "upper case" and "lower case" receptors will be ignored in this and subsequent chapters.

Information on the cellular locations of subtypes of muscarinic receptors is as yet somewhat fragmentary; however, a few generalizations can be made. M_1 receptors are found in ganglia and various secretory glands; M_2 receptors predominate in the myocardium and also appear to be found in smooth muscle; and M_3 receptors are located in smooth muscle and secretory glands. All five subtypes are found in the CNS. To confuse the issue further, most tissues contain several subtypes of muscarinic receptors, and the problem may be compounded by the presence of parasympathetic ganglia within the tissue.

The basic functions of muscarinic receptors are mediated by interactions with members of the family of G proteins and thus by G protein–induced changes in the functions of distinct membrane-bound effector molecules. Two pathways are currently appreciated. In one of these, muscarinic receptors (M_1, M_3, and M_5 subtypes) appear to activate an as yet unidentified G protein that is responsible for stimulation of phospholipase C activity; the immediate result is hydrolysis of phosphatidylinositol polyphosphates (which are components of the plasma membrane) to form inositol polyphosphates. Some of the inositol phosphate isomers (chiefly inositol-1,4,5-trisphosphate) cause release of intracellular Ca^{2+} from stores in the endoplasmic reticulum. Thus, these receptors mediate such Ca^{2+}-dependent phenomena as contraction of smooth muscle and secretion (*see* Chapter 2; *see also* Berridge, 1988). The second product of the phospholipase C reaction, diacylglycerol, activates protein kinase C (in conjunction with Ca^{2+}). This arm of the pathway plays a role in modulation of function or in the later phases of the functional response (Nishizuka, 1986).

A second pathway for mediation of responses to muscarinic agonists is evoked by activation of M_2 and M_4 receptors. These receptors interact with a distinct group of G proteins (in particular those termed G_i) with resultant inhibition of adenylyl cyclase, activation of K^+ channels (in the heart, for example), and modulation of the activity of Ca^{2+} channels in certain cell types (*see* Gilman, 1987; Brown and Birnbaumer, 1988; *see also* Chapter 2). The functional consequences of these effects are most clear in the myocardium, where inhibition of adenylyl cyclase and activation of K^+ conductances could account for both the negative chronotropic and inotropic effects of ACh.

Other cellular events such as the release of arachidonic acid and the activation of guanylyl cyclase can also result from activation of muscarinic receptors. However, these events may be secondary to changes in the concentrations of other intracellular mediators (*see* McKinney and Richelson, 1989).

ADRENERGIC TRANSMISSION

Under this general heading are included *norepinephrine*, the transmitter of most sympathetic postganglionic fibers and of certain tracts in the CNS, and *dopamine,* the predominant transmitter of the mammalian extrapyramidal system and of several mesocortical and mesolimbic neuronal pathways, as well as *epinephrine,* the major hormone of the adrenal medulla.

A tremendous amount of information about catecholamines and related compounds has accumulated in recent years, motivated in part by the importance of interactions between the endogenous catecholamines and many of the drugs used in the treatment of hypertension, mental disorders, and a variety of other conditions. The details of these interactions and of the pharmacology of the sympathomimetic amines themselves will be found in subsequent chapters. The basic physiological, biochemical, and pharmacological features are presented here.

Synthesis, Storage, and Release of Catecholamines. The synthesis of epinephrine from tyrosine, by the steps shown in Figure 5–3, was proposed by Blaschko in 1939. The enzymes involved have been identified and characterized. It is important to note that these enzymes exhibit broad substrate specificity; consequently, many other endogenous substances as well as certain drugs are similarly acted upon at the various steps. For example, 5-hydroxytryptamine (5-HT, serotonin) can be produced by L-aromatic amino acid decarboxylase (or dopa decarboxylase) from 5-hydroxy-L-tryptophan. Dopa decarboxylase can also convert the drug methyldopa to α-methyldopamine, which, in turn, is converted by dopamine β-hydroxylase to the "false transmitter," α-methylnorepinephrine.

The hydroxylation of tyrosine is generally regarded as the rate-limiting step in the biosynthesis of catecholamines (Weiner, 1979b), and tyrosine hydroxylase is activated following stimulation of adrenergic nerves or the adrenal medulla. The enzyme is a substrate for cyclic AMP–dependent and Ca^{2+}-calmodulin–sensitive protein kinases, and kinase-catalyzed phosphorylation is associated with increased hydroxylase activity (Yamauchi *et al.*, 1981; Weiner *et al.*, 1984). In addition, tyrosine hydroxylase is inhibited by catechol compounds in a

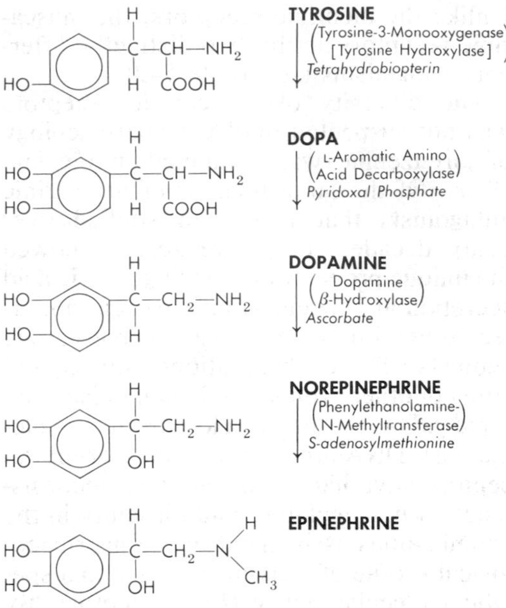

Figure 5–3. *Steps in the enzymatic synthesis of dopamine, norepinephrine, and epinephrine.*

The enzymes involved are shown in parentheses; essential cofactors, in italics. The final step occurs only in the adrenal medulla and in a few epinephrine-containing neuronal pathways in the brainstem.

manner that is competitive with its pterin cofactor, tetrahydrobiopterin. It is thus subject to end-product feedback inhibition (Weiner *et al.*, 1972).

Current knowledge concerning the cellular sites and mechanisms of synthesis, storage, and release of catecholamines has been derived from studies of both adrenergically innervated organs and adrenal medullary tissue. Nearly all the norepinephrine content of the former is confined to the postganglionic sympathetic fibers; it disappears within a few days after section of the nerves.

The main features of the mechanisms of synthesis, storage, and release of catecholamines and their modifications by drugs are summarized in Figure 5–4. The enzymes that participate in the formation of norepinephrine are synthesized in the cell bodies of the adrenergic neurons and are then transported along the axons to their terminals. Electron-dense vesicles, 0.05 to 0.2 μm in diameter, are found in the adrenergic nerve endings, and these vesicles or

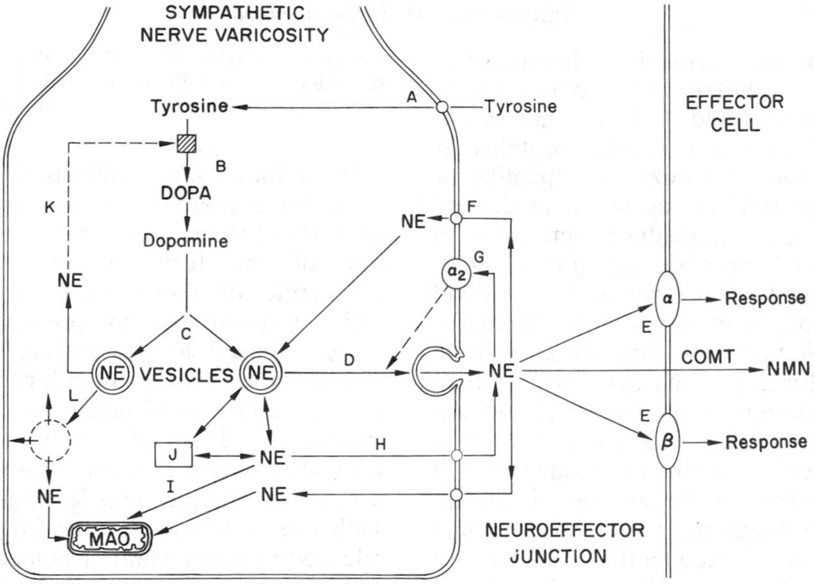

Figure 5–4. *Proposed sites of action of drugs on the synthesis, action, and fate of norepinephrine at sympathetic neuroeffector junctions.*

The events proposed to occur in this model of a sympathetic neuroeffector junction are as follows. Tyrosine is transported actively into the axoplasm (*A*) and is converted to dopa and then to dopamine by cytoplasmic enzymes (*B*). Dopamine is transported into the vesicles of the varicosity, where the synthesis and the storage of norepinephrine (NE) take place (*C*). An action potential causes an influx of Ca^{2+} into the nerve terminal (not shown), with subsequent fusion of the vesicle with the plasma membrane and exocytosis of NE (*D*). The transmitter then activates α and β receptors in the membrane of the postsynaptic cell (*E*). NE that penetrates into these cells (uptake-2) is probably rapidly inactivated by catechol-O-methyltransferase (COMT) to normetanephrine (NMN). The most important mechanism for termination of the action of NE in the junctional space is by active reuptake into the nerve (uptake-1) and the storage vesicles (*F*). Norepinephrine in the synaptic cleft can also activate presynaptic (α_2) receptors (*G*), the result of which is to inhibit further exocytotic release of norepinephrine (dashed line). Other potential neurotransmitters (*e.g.*, ATP and neuropeptide Y) may be stored in the same or a different population of vesicles.

NE can also be displaced from storage vesicles by sympathomimetic amines such as tyramine, which gain access to the nerve terminal by active uptake as in *F*. A portion of this NE is extruded by reversal of the uptake process (*H*) to interact with receptors. Another portion of the NE released in this manner, or by spontaneous diffusion, is deaminated by mitochondrial monoamine oxidase (MAO) (*I*). Observations suggest that only a fraction of the total NE content is available for release by either nerve stimulation or tyramine, and indicate that there may be functional pools of the transmitter that are held in reserve (*J*). These may be vesicles that reside deep within the nerve terminals.

The most important mechanism of regulation of NE synthesis involves the rate-limiting step, the hydroxylation of tyrosine. This regulation is complex but in part involves feedback inhibition by NE (*K*) and activation of the enzyme by cyclic AMP–dependent protein kinase and, perhaps, by Ca^{2+}-dependent protein kinases.

Sites of drug action in this scheme include:

1. Inhibition of MAO (*e.g.*, by pargyline) or COMT (no pharmacologically significant example of inhibitor).

2. Inhibition of plasma membrane uptake mechanism for NE (*F*) by tricyclic antidepressants or cocaine, making more NE available for binding to receptors.

3. Inhibition of vesicular storage of NE by reserpine and, in part, by guanethidine (*L*). The NE thereby released is normally inactivated by MAO. Guanethidine and bretylium also block coupling of the action potential to the release of NE.

4. Displacement of NE by indirectly acting sympathomimetic amines (*H*). Exocytosis of vesicular contents does not occur.

5. Direct interaction with adrenergic receptors by agonists and antagonists (*E, G*).

Anatomical elements are not drawn to scale. Mitochondria are about 0.25 μm in diameter and 0.75 μm long; vesicles, 0.05 μm; a nerve varicosity, 2 to 10 μm; the junctional space, 0.1 μm or more.

granules contain extremely high concentrations of catecholamines (approximately 21% dry weight) and ATP, in a molecular ratio of 4:1, as well as specific proteins, or *chromogranins,* the enzyme dopamine β-hydroxylase (DBH), ascorbic acid, and peptides (*e.g.,* enkephalin precursors). In the course of synthesis (*see* Figure 5–3), the hydroxylation of tyrosine to dopa and the decarboxylation of dopa to dopamine take place in the cytoplasm. About half the dopamine formed in the cytoplasm is then actively transported into the DBH-containing storage vesicles, where it is converted to norepinephrine; the remainder, which escaped capture by the vesicles, is deaminated to 3,4-dihydroxyphenylacetic acid (DOPAC) and subsequently O-methylated to homovanillic acid (HVA). The adrenal medulla has two distinct catecholamine-containing cell types: those with norepinephrine and those with primarily epinephrine. The latter cell population contains the enzyme phenylethanolamine-N-methyltransferase. In these cells, the norepinephrine formed in the granules leaves these structures, presumably by diffusion, and is methylated in the cytoplasm to epinephrine. Epinephrine then reenters the chromaffin granules, where it is stored until released. In the human adult, epinephrine accounts for approximately 80% of the catecholamines of the adrenal medulla, with norepinephrine making up most of the remainder. (*See* von Euler, 1972; Rubin, 1982.)

A major factor that controls the rate of synthesis of epinephrine, and hence the size of the store available for release from the adrenal medulla, is the level of glucocorticoids secreted by the adrenal cortex. The latter hormones are carried in high concentration, by the intraadrenal portal vascular system, directly to the adrenal medullary chromaffin cells, where they induce the synthesis of phenylethanolamine-N-methyltransferase (*see* Figure 5–3). The activities of both tyrosine hydroxylase and DBH are also increased in the adrenal medulla when the secretion of glucocorticoids is stimulated (Weiner, 1975). Thus, any stress that persists sufficiently to invoke an enhanced secretion of corticotropin mobilizes the appropriate hormones of both the adrenal cortex (predominantly cortisol) and medulla (epinephrine).

This remarkable relationship is present only in certain mammals, including man, where the adrenal chromaffin cells are enveloped entirely by steroid-secreting cortical cells. In the dogfish, for example, where the chromaffin cells and steroid-secreting cells are located in independent, noncontiguous glands, no epinephrine is formed.

In addition to its synthesis *de novo,* outlined above, there is a second major mechanism for replenishment of the norepinephrine of the terminal portions of the adrenergic fibers—namely, recapture by active transport of norepinephrine previously released to the extracellular fluid. This process is responsible for the termination of the effects of adrenergic impulses in most organs. In blood vessels and in tissues with wide synaptic gaps, recapture of released norepinephrine is less important. At such sites a relatively large fraction of the released neurotransmitter is inactivated by a combination of extraneuronal uptake (*see* below) and enzymatic breakdown and diffusion (Spector *et al.,* 1972). To effect the reuptake of norepinephrine into adrenergic nerve terminals and to maintain the concentration gradient of norepinephrine within the vesicles, at least two distinct carrier-mediated transport systems are involved: one across the axoplasmic membrane from the extracellular fluid to the cytoplasm; and the other from the cytoplasm into the storage vesicles.

Due to the relative ease of isolating pure preparations of granules, especially from the adrenal medulla, the transport system of the storage granule has been well characterized. It can concentrate catecholamines against a 200-fold gradient across the membrane of the chromaffin granule. This transport system requires ATP and Mg^{2+}, and it is blocked by low concentrations (40 nM) of reserpine. Uptake of catecholamine and ATP into isolated chromaffin granules appears to be driven by pH and potential gradients that are established by an ATP-dependent proton translocase (Winkler *et al.,* 1981).

The amine transport system across the axoplasmic membrane is Na^+ dependent and is blocked selectively by a number of drugs, including cocaine and the tricyclic antidepressants, such as imipramine. This transporter has a high affinity for norepinephrine and a somewhat lower affinity for epinephrine; the synthetic β-adrenergic agonist isoproterenol is not a substrate for this system. The neuronal uptake process has been termed *uptake-1* (Iversen, 1975). There is also an extraneuronal amine transport system, termed *uptake-2,* which exhibits a low affinity for norepinephrine, a somewhat higher affinity for epinephrine, and a still higher affinity for isoproterenol. This uptake process is quite ubiquitous and is present in glial, hepatic, myocardial, and other cells. Uptake-2 is not inhibited by imipramine or cocaine. It is probably of relatively little physiological importance unless the neuronal uptake mechanism is blocked (Iversen, 1975; Trendelenburg, 1980). It may be of greater importance in the disposition of circulating catecholamines than in the removal of amines that have been released from adrenergic nerve terminals.

Certain sympathomimetic drugs (*e.g.*, ephedrine, tyramine) produce most of their effects indirectly, chiefly by displacing norepinephrine from the nerve-ending binding sites to the extracellular fluid, where the released endogenous transmitter then acts at the receptor sites of the effector cells. The mechanisms by which indirectly acting sympathomimetic amines release norepinephrine from nerve endings are complex. All such agents are substrates for uptake-1. As a result of their transport across the neuronal membrane and release into the axoplasm, they make carrier available at the inner surface of the membrane for the outward transport of norepinephrine ("facilitated exchange diffusion"). In addition, these amines are able to mobilize norepinephrine stored in the vesicles by competing for the vesicular uptake process. Reserpine, which depletes vesicular stores of norepinephrine, also inhibits this uptake mechanism, but, in contrast with the indirectly acting sympathomimetic amines, it enters the adrenergic nerve ending by passive diffusion across the axonal membrane (Bönisch and Trendelenburg, 1988).

These actions of indirectly acting sympathomimetic amines are associated with the phenomenon of *tachyphylaxis*. For example, repeated administration of tyramine results in rapidly decreasing effectiveness, whereas the effect of repeated administration of norepinephrine is not reduced and, in fact, reverses the tachyphylaxis to tyramine. Although these phenomena have not been explained satisfactorily, several hypotheses have been proposed. One possible explanation of tachyphylaxis to tyramine and similarly acting sympathomimetic agents is that the pool of neurotransmitter available for displacement by these drugs is quite small relative to the total amount stored in the sympathetic nerve ending. This pool is presumed to reside in close proximity to the plasma membrane, and the norepinephrine of such vesicles may be replaced by the less potent amine following repeated administration of the latter substance. Alternatively, the repeated administration of an indirectly acting sympathomimetic amine may lead to its accumulation in the neuronal cytosol in sufficient concentration to inhibit competitively the transport of norepinephrine out of the nerve terminal. Administration of exogenous norepinephrine may then promote the egress of the amine by facilitated exchange diffusion, thereby restoring the original condition. In either event, neurotransmitter release by displacement is not associated with the release of DBH and does not require extracellular Ca^{2+}; thus, it is presumed not to involve exocytosis.

The full sequence of steps by which the nerve impulse effects the release of norepinephrine from adrenergic fibers is not known. In the adrenal medulla, the triggering event is the liberation of ACh by the preganglionic fibers and its interaction with nicotinic receptors on the chromaffin cells to produce a localized depolarization; a succeeding step is the entrance of Ca^{2+} into these cells, which results in the extrusion by exocytosis of the granular contents, including epinephrine, ATP, some neuroactive peptides or their precursors (Gilbert and Emson, 1983; Viveros and Wilson, 1983), chromogranins, and DBH (Weiner, 1979a; Winkler *et al.*, 1981). Ca^{2+} likewise plays an essential role in coupling the nerve impulse with the release of norepinephrine at adrenergic nerve terminals. Enhanced activity of the sympathetic nervous system is accompanied by an increased concentration of both DBH and chromogranins in the circulation, supporting the argument that the process of release following adrenergic nerve stimulation also involves exocytosis.

A group of homologous cytoplasmic proteins, the annexins, can promote the fusion of chromaffin granules *in vitro* in the presence of low concentrations of Ca^{2+} when certain unsaturated fatty acids (*e.g.*, arachidonic acid) are also present. The annexins interact specifically with acidic phospholipids that are enriched on the cytoplasmic faces of the plasma membrane and the membrane of chromaffin granules. One of the annexins, calpactin I, displays a sensitivity to Ca^{2+} that is sufficient to suggest that it may play an important role in the fusion of secretory granules with the plasma membrane, a process that precedes exocytosis (*see* Creutz *et al.*, 1990).

Adrenergic fibers can sustain the output of norepinephrine during prolonged periods of stimulation without exhausting their reserve supply, provided synthesis and uptake of the transmitter are unimpaired. To meet increased needs for norepinephrine, acute regulatory mechanisms come into play that involve activation of tyrosine hydroxylase (*see* above).

Termination of the Actions of Catecholamines. The actions of norepinephrine and epinephrine are terminated by (1) reuptake into nerve terminals; (2) dilution by diffusion out of the junctional cleft and uptake at extraneuronal sites; and (3) metabolic transformation. Two enzymes are important in the initial steps of metabolic transformation of catecholamines—monoamine oxidase (MAO) and catechol-O-methyltransferase (COMT) (*see* Axelrod, 1966; Kopin, 1972). However, it is evident that a powerful enzymatic mechanism, such as that provided by AChE, is absent from the adrenergic nervous system. The importance of neuronal reuptake of catecholamines is indicated by observations that inhibitors of this process (*e.g.*, cocaine, imipramine) potentiate the effects of the neurotransmitter; inhibitors of MAO and COMT have little effect. However, transmitter that is released *within* the nerve terminal is metabolized by MAO. COMT, particularly in the liver, plays a major role in the metabolism of endogenous circulating and administered catecholamines.

Both MAO and COMT are widely distributed throughout the body, including the brain; the highest concentrations of each are in the liver and the kidney. However, little or no COMT is found in adrenergic neurons. There are distinct differences in the cytological locations of the two enzymes; whereas MAO is associated chiefly with the outer surface of mitochondria, including those within the terminals of adrenergic fibers, COMT is located largely in the cytoplasm. These factors are of importance both in determining the primary metabolic pathways followed by catecholamines in various circumstances and in explaining the effects of certain drugs. Two different isozymes of MAO are found in widely varying proportions in different cells in the CNS and in peripheral tissues. Selective inhibitors of these two isozymes are available (*see* Chapters 18 and 20).

Most of the epinephrine and norepinephrine that enters the circulation, from the adrenal medulla or following administration, or that is released by exocytosis from adrenergic fibers is first methylated by COMT to metanephrine or normetanephrine, respectively (Figure 5–5). Norepinephrine that is released intraneuronally by drugs such as reserpine is initially deaminated by MAO to 3,4-dihydroxyphenylglycolaldehyde (DOPGAL) (*see* Figure 5–5). The aldehyde is reduced by aldehyde reductase to the glycol, 3,4-dihydroxyphenylethylene glycol (DOPEG) within the neuron. If the amine is deaminated at extraneuronal sites, such as the intestine or liver, the aldehyde is largely oxidized by aldehyde dehydrogenase to 3,4-dihydroxymandelic acid (DOMA). Most of the DOPEG formed in the neurons is converted to 3-methoxy-4-hydroxyphenylethylene glycol (MOPEG or MHPG) by O-methylation in the tissues before entering the plasma. The MOPEG that reaches the plasma is largely converted to 3-methoxy-4-hydroxymandelic acid (generally but incorrectly called vanillylmandelic acid [VMA]) or conjugated (mostly with sulfate and to a lesser extent with glucuronic acid) before excretion. These substances constitute the major metabolites of catecholamines excreted in the urine. The corresponding product of the metabolic degradation of dopamine, which contains no hydroxyl group in the side chain, is homovanillic acid (HVA). Other metabolic reactions are described in Figure 5–5. Measurement of the concentrations of catecholamines and their metabolites in blood and urine is useful in the diagnosis of pheochromocytoma—a catecholamine-secreting tumor of the adrenal medulla.

Inhibitors of MAO (*e.g.*, pargyline, nialamide) can cause an increase in the concentration of norepinephrine, dopamine, and 5-HT in the brain and other tissues accompanied by a variety of pharmacological effects. No striking pharmacological action can be attributed to the inhibition of COMT.

Classification of Adrenergic Receptors. Crucial to understanding the remarkably diverse effects of the catecholamines and related sympathomimetic agents is an understanding of the classification and properties of the different types of adrenergic

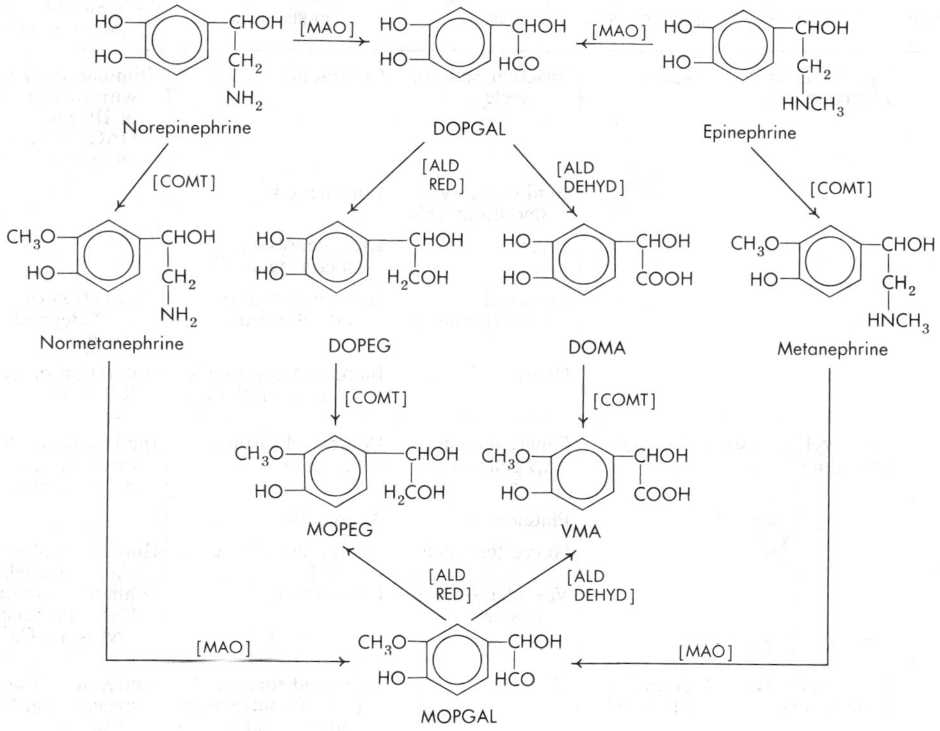

Figure 5–5. *Steps in the metabolic disposition of catecholamines.*

Both norepinephrine and epinephrine are first oxidatively deaminated by monoamine oxidase (MAO) to 3,4-dihydroxyphenylglycolaldehyde (DOPGAL) and then either reduced to 3,4-dihydroxyphenylethylene glycol (DOPEG) or oxidized to 3,4-dihydroxymandelic acid (DOMA). Alternatively, they can initially be methylated by catechol-O-methyltransferase (COMT) to normetanephrine and metanephrine, respectively. Most of the products of either type of reaction are then metabolized by the other enzyme to form the major excretory products, 3-methoxy-4-hydroxyphenylethylene glycol (MOPEG or MHPG) and 3-methoxy-4-hydroxymandelic acid (VMA). Free MOPEG is largely converted to VMA. The glycol and, to some extent, the O-methylated amines and the catecholamines may be conjugated to the corresponding sulfates or glucuronides. (MOPGAL = 3-methoxy-4-hydroxyphenylglycolaldehyde; ALD RED = aldehyde reductase; ALD DEHYD = aldehyde dehydrogenase.) (Modified from Axelrod, 1966; and others.)

receptors. Elucidation of the characteristics of these receptors and the biochemical and physiological pathways that they regulate has clarified and organized a wealth of information about the seemingly contradictory and variable effects of catecholamines on various organ systems. Although structurally related (*see* below), different adrenergic receptors regulate distinct physiological processes by controlling the synthesis or release of a variety of second messengers (*see* Table 5–3 and Figure 5–6).

Ahlquist (1948) first proposed that there was more than one adrenergic receptor; he based his hypothesis on a study of the abilities of epinephrine, norepinephrine, and other related agonists to regulate various physiological processes. It was known that these drugs can cause either contraction or relaxation of smooth muscle, depending on the site, the dose, and the agent chosen. For example, norepinephrine has potent excitatory effects on smooth muscle and correspondingly low activity as an inhibitor; isoproterenol displays the opposite pattern of activity. Epinephrine can both excite and inhibit smooth muscle. Thus, Ahlquist proposed the designations α and β for receptors on smooth muscle where catecholamines produce excitatory and inhibitory responses, respectively. (An exception is the gut, which is generally relaxed by ac-

Table 5–3. CHARACTERISTICS OF SUBTYPES OF ADRENERGIC RECEPTORS *

RECEPTOR	AGONISTS	ANTAGONISTS	TISSUE	RESPONSES	MOLECULAR MECHANISMS [1]
α_1 [2]	Epi $\geq$ NE $\gg$ Iso Phenylephrine	Prazosin	Vascular smooth muscle	Contraction	Stimulation of PLC with formation of IP_3 and DAG; increased cytosolic Ca^{2+}
			Genitourinary smooth muscle	Contraction	
			Liver [3]	Glycogenolysis; gluconeogenesis	
			Intestinal smooth muscle	Hyperpolarization and relaxation	(Activation of Ca^{2+}-dependent K^+ channels)
			Heart	Increased contractile force; arrhythmias	(Inhibition of transient K^+ current)
α_2 [2]	Epi $\geq$ NE $\gg$ Iso Clonidine	Yohimbine	Pancreatic islets (β cells)	Decreased insulin secretion	Inhibition of adenylyl cyclase; activation of K^+ channels
			Platelets	Aggregation	
			Nerve terminals	Decreased release of NE	(Inhibition of neuronal Ca^{2+} channels)
			Vascular smooth muscle	Contraction	(Enhanced influx of Ca^{2+}; increased cytosolic Ca^{2+})
β_1	Iso > Epi = NE Dobutamine	Metoprolol CGP 20712A	Heart	Increased force and rate of contraction and AV nodal conduction velocity	Activation of adenylyl cyclase and Ca^{2+} channels
			Juxtaglomerular cells	Increased renin secretion	
β_2	Iso > Epi $\gg$ NE Terbutaline	ICI 118551	Smooth muscle (vascular, bronchial, gastrointestinal, and genito-urinary)	Relaxation	Activation of adenylyl cyclase
			Skeletal muscle	Glycogenolysis; uptake of K^+	
			Liver [3]	Glycogenolysis; gluconeogenesis	
β_3 [4]	Iso = NE > Epi BRL 37344	ICI 118551 CGP 20712A	Adipose tissue	Lipolysis	Activation of adenylyl cyclase

* This table provides examples of drugs that act on adrenergic receptors and of the location of subtypes of adrenergic receptors. Abbreviations are: epinephrine (Epi); norepinephrine (NE); isoproterenol (Iso); phospholipase C (PLC); inositol-1,4,5-trisphosphate (IP_3); diacylglycerol (DAG).

[1] Entries in parentheses denote additional or alternative mechanisms that may be important in the responses of the tissue listed.

[2] At least two subtypes of α_1- and α_2-adrenergic receptors are known, but distinctions in their mechanism of action and tissue location have not been defined.

[3] In some species (*e.g.*, rat), metabolic responses in the liver are mediated by α_1 receptors, whereas in others (*e.g.*, dog) β_2 receptors are predominantly involved. Both types of receptors appear to contribute to responses in man.

[4] Metabolic responses in adipocytes and certain other tissues with atypical pharmacological characteristics may be mediated by this subtype of receptor. Most β-adrenergic antagonists (including propranolol) do not block these responses.

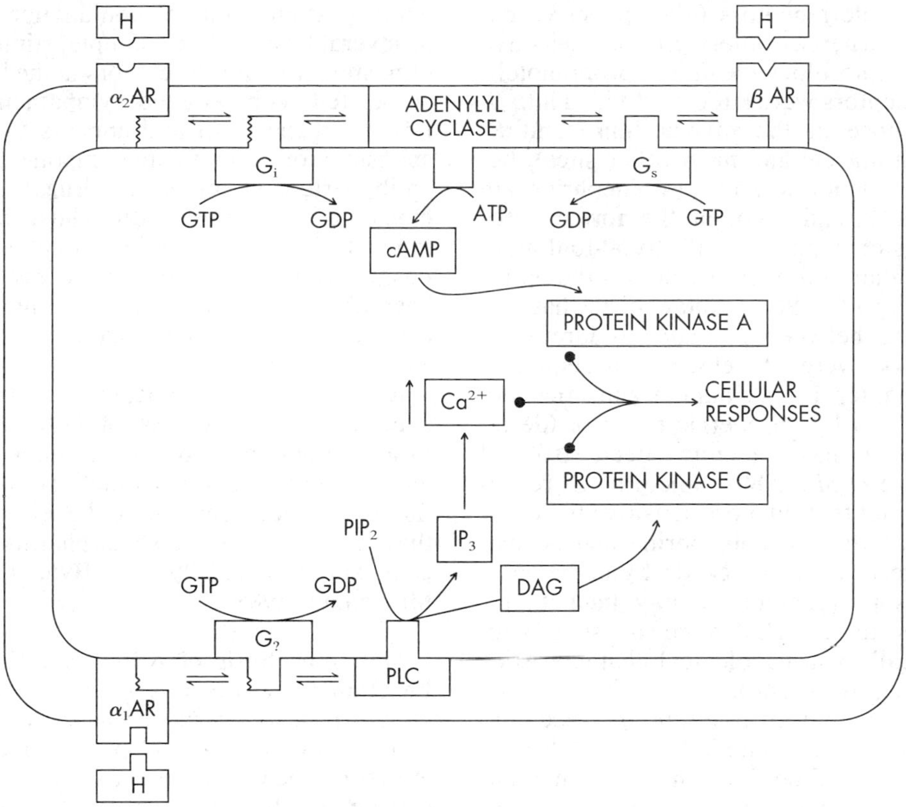

Figure 5–6. *Schematic representation of subtypes of α- and β-adrenergic receptors and their effector systems.*

Adenosine 3′,5′-monophosphate (cyclic AMP, *cAMP*) is synthesized by adenylyl cyclase at the cytoplasmic face of the plasma membrane consequent to activation of β-adrenergic receptors (*βAR*) by neurotransmitter or hormone (*H*). To accomplish the activation of adenylyl cyclase, the liganded receptor interacts with a stimulatory guanine nucleotide–binding regulatory protein (G_s) (*see* Chapter 2). A related regulatory protein (G_i) also binds GTP in response to interaction with α_2-adrenergic receptors (α_2AR) or other appropriate inhibitory receptors (*e.g.*, M_2-muscarinic receptors). The interaction of $G_i \cdot$ GTP with the components of the system causes inhibition of adenylyl cyclase. G_i can also modulate the function of certain ion channels and cause either activation (*e.g.*, K^+ channels) or inhibition (*e.g.*, voltage-gated Ca^{2+} channels) (not shown). The intracellular receptor for cyclic AMP is cyclic AMP–dependent protein kinase (*PROTEIN KINASE A*). When activated by cyclic AMP, the kinase phosphorylates a variety of cellular proteins and regulates their activities. The stimulation of α_1-adrenergic receptors (α_1AR) causes activation of a membrane-bound phospholipase C (*PLC*) by a process that is apparently mediated by an unidentified G protein ($G_?$). Phospholipase C hydrolyzes a membrane phospholipid, phosphatidylinositol-4,5-bisphosphate (PIP_2), resulting in the formation of diacylglycerol (*DAG*) and inositol-1,4,5-trisphosphate (IP_3). IP_3 causes the release of Ca^{2+} from intracellular stores, which then initiates a variety of cellular responses. Some of these responses result from activation of Ca^{2+}/calmodulin–dependent enzymes (*e.g.*, phosphorylase kinase, myosin light-chain kinase). DAG stimulates the activity of a Ca^{2+}-sensitive enzyme, protein kinase C, which phosphorylates a distinct set of substrates; some of these are also substrates for protein kinase A (*e.g.*, glycogen synthase).

tivation of either α or β receptors.) The rank order of potency of agonists is isoproterenol > epinephrine ≥ norepinephrine for β and epinephrine ≥ norepinephrine ≫ isoproterenol for α (*see* Table 5–3). This initial classification of adrenergic receptors was corroborated by the finding that certain antagonists produce selective blockade of the effects of adrenergic nerve impulses and sympathomimetic agents at α-adrenergic receptors (*e.g.*, phenoxybenzamine), whereas others produce selective β-adrenergic blockade (*e.g.*, propranolol).

β Receptors were later subdivided into β_1 (*e.g.*, those in the myocardium) and β_2 (smooth muscle and most other sites), because epinephrine and norepinephrine are essentially equipotent at the former sites whereas epinephrine is 10- to 50-fold more potent than norepinephrine at the latter (Lands *et al.*, 1967). Antagonists that discriminate between β_1- and β_2-adrenergic receptors were developed subsequently (*see* Chapter 11). A human gene that encodes a third β-adrenergic receptor (designated β_3) has recently been isolated (Emorine *et al.*, 1989). Since the β_3 receptor is about tenfold more sensitive to norepinephrine than to epinephrine and is relatively resistant to blockade by antagonists such as propranolol, it may mediate responses to catecholamine at sites with "atypical" pharmacological characteristics (*e.g.*, adipose tissue).

Heterogeneity of α-adrenergic receptors is also now appreciated. The initial distinction was based on functional and anatomical considerations when it was realized that norepinephrine and other α-adrenergic agonists could profoundly inhibit the release of norepinephrine from neurons (*see* Langer, 1980; Starke, 1987; *see also* Figure 5–4). Indeed, when sympathetic nerves are stimulated in the presence of certain α-adrenergic antagonists the amount of norepinephrine liberated by each nerve impulse increases markedly. This feedback inhibitory effect of norepinephrine on its release from nerve terminals is mediated by α receptors that are pharmacologically distinct from the classical postsynaptic α receptors. Accordingly, these presynaptic α receptors were designated α_2, whereas the postsynaptic "excitatory" α receptors were designated α_1 (*see* Langer and Lehmann, 1988). Compounds such as clonidine are more potent agonists at α_2 than at α_1 receptors; by contrast, phenylephrine and methoxamine selectively activate postsynaptic α_1 receptors. Although there is little evidence to suggest that α_1-adrenergic receptors function presynaptically in the autonomic nervous system, it is now clear that α_2-adrenergic receptors are also present at postjunctional or nonjunctional sites in several tissues. For example, stimulation of postjunctional α_2 receptors in the brain is associated with reduced sympathetic outflow from the CNS and appears to be responsible for a significant component of the antihypertensive effect of drugs such as clonidine (*see* Chapter 10). Thus, the anatomical concept of prejunctional α_2- and postjunctional α_1-adrenergic receptors has been abandoned in favor of pharmacological and functional classification (*see* Table 5–3).

Recent evidence indicates that there is additional heterogeneity of both α_1- and α_2-adrenergic receptors (α_{1A}, α_{1B}; α_{2A}, α_{2B}; *etc.*). Although distinct functional roles of these receptors remain to be elucidated, they can be distinguished pharmacologically and structurally (*see* Bylund, 1988; Minneman, 1988).

Molecular Basis of Adrenergic Receptor Function. The responses that follow activation of all types of adrenergic receptors appear to result from G protein–mediated effects on the generation of second messengers and on the activity of ion channels. As discussed in Chapter 2, these systems are thought to involve three interacting proteins—the receptor, the coupling G protein, and effector enzymes or ion channels. The pathways overlap broadly with those discussed for muscarinic receptors and are summarized in Table 5–3 and Figure 5–6.

Structure of Adrenergic Receptors. The adrenergic receptors constitute a family of closely related proteins. They are also related both structurally and functionally to receptors for a wide variety of other hormones and neurotransmitters that are coupled to G proteins. This wider family of receptors includes the muscarinic cholinergic receptors and even the visual "photon receptor," rhodopsin (Dohlman *et al.*, 1987; Lefkowitz and Caron, 1988). The adrenergic receptors are integral membrane glycoproteins; they have been purified and their genes have been cloned. A schematic diagram of this type of receptor is shown in Figure 2–1 (page 36). A major feature is their presumed topography, with seven transmembrane spanning domains, a series of interconnecting loops, glycosylated extracellular amino terminus, and a cytoplasmic carboxyl terminus. Examination of cloned receptors by site-directed labeling and mutagenesis has revealed that the conserved membrane spanning regions are crucially involved in the binding of ligands (Lefkowitz and Caron, 1988). These regions appear to create a ligand-binding pocket analogous to that formed by the membrane spanning regions of rhodopsin to accommodate the covalently attached chromophore, retinal (Applebury and Hargrave, 1986). The amino acid sequences within the third cytoplasmic loop appear to be particularly important for interaction between the receptor and the appropriate G protein. The consequences of this interaction are described in Chapter 2.

β-Adrenergic Receptors. All β-adrenergic receptors stimulate adenylyl cyclase; the interaction between the receptor and the enzyme is not direct but is mediated by a G protein that is called G_s (*see* Chapter 2; *see also* Gilman, 1987). Stimulation of the receptor leads to the accumulation of cyclic AMP, activation of the cyclic AMP–dependent protein kinase, and altered function of numerous cellular proteins as a result of their phosphorylation (*see* below). In addition, G_s can directly enhance the activation of voltage-sensitive Ca^{2+} channels in the plasma membrane of skeletal and cardiac muscle (Brown and Birnbaumer, 1988); this action may provide an additional means of regulating the function of these tissues.

Although the biochemical pathways have been delineated in detail in relatively few cases, the involvement of cyclic AMP–dependent protein kinase is well documented in the vast majority of responses that result from the stimulation of β-adrenergic receptors, and this enzyme is considered to be the intracellular receptor for cyclic AMP (Krebs and Beavo, 1979). It exists as a tetramer (R_2C_2), consisting of two regulatory (R) and two catalytic (C) subunits. Binding of cyclic AMP causes dissociation of the regulatory subunits with resultant activation of the catalytic subunits. Phosphorylation of various cellular proteins then causes responses that are characteristic of those produced by β-adrenergic agonists. When the stimulus is removed, dephosphorylation of the various protein substrates is catalyzed by phosphoprotein phosphatases.

A well-defined example of these mechanisms is the activation of hepatic glycogen phosphorylase, the enzyme that carries out the rate-limiting step in glycogenolysis, the conversion of glycogen to glucose 1-phosphate. This activation is itself the result of a cascade of phosphorylation reactions. Cyclic AMP–dependent protein kinase catalyzes the phosphorylation of phosphorylase kinase, thereby activating it; phosphorylase kinase then phosphorylates and activates phosphorylase. This sequence of successive phosphorylations permits considerable amplification of the initial signal. Thus, stimulation of only a few receptors is necessary to activate a large number of phosphorylase molecules in a very brief period of time.

Concurrent with the activation of hepatic glycogen phosphorylase, cyclic AMP-dependent protein kinase also catalyzes the phosphorylation and inactivation of another enzyme, glycogen synthase, that catalyzes the transfer of glycosyl units from UDP-glucose to glycogen. This effect decreases the net rate of synthesis of glycogen from glucose. The dual effect of cyclic AMP to enhance conversion of glycogen to glucose and to decrease the synthesis of glycogen from glucose summate to increase the output of glucose from the liver.

Similar types of reactions result in the activation of triglyceride lipase in adipose tissue, with resultant increased release of free fatty acids. The lipase is activated when it is phosphorylated by the cyclic AMP–dependent protein kinase. Catecholamines provide an increased supply of substrate for oxidative metabolism by this mechanism.

In the heart, stimulation of β-adrenergic receptors leads to positive inotropic and chronotropic responses. Increased intracellular concentrations of cyclic AMP and enhanced phosphorylation of proteins such as troponin and phospholamban are detected after β-adrenergic stimulation. Although these phosphorylation events appear to influence both the actions and the disposition of cellular Ca^{2+}, other events may also contribute to the inotropic response (England *et al.*, 1984).

Stimulation of β-adrenergic receptors also results in an increase in cyclic AMP concentrations and relaxation of smooth muscle; the membrane may become hyperpolarized and "spike" potentials caused by the activation of voltage-sensitive Ca^{2+} channels may disappear or become less frequent. Although cyclic AMP–dependent phosphorylation events that lead to a reduction of the cytosolic concentration of free Ca^{2+} are presumably involved, the precise mechanisms remain unknown (*see* Kamm and Stull, 1985).

α-Adrenergic Receptors. α_2-Adrenergic receptors inhibit adenylyl cyclase by interacting with G proteins termed G_i; intracellular concentrations of cyclic AMP are thus lowered and the state of activation of the cyclic AMP–dependent protein kinase is decreased. The G proteins that mediate inhibition of adenylyl cyclase can also activate K^+ conductances and inhibit voltage-sensitive Ca^{2+} channels (Limbird, 1988). Thus, α_2-adrenergic agonists cause hyperpolarization of cholinergic myenteric neurons by enhancing the activity of inwardly rectifying K^+ channels (Surprenant and North, 1988); this results in reduced release of ACh and is probably partly responsible for the inhibition of gastrointestinal motility that follows stimulation of the sympathetic nervous system. Similar actions may account for inhibition of the release of transmitter from noradrenergic nerve terminals (Zimanyi *et al.*, 1988), but inhibition of neuronal Ca^{2+} channels is also thought to be involved (*see* Tsien *et al.*, 1988).

Stimulation of α_1-adrenergic receptors increases intracellular concentrations of Ca^{2+} by several distinct mechanisms (*see* Minneman, 1988). The most firmly established pathway involves activation of a phospholipase C, apparently through an as yet unidentified G protein, and the hydrolysis of membrane-bound polyphosphoinositides; the result is generation of two second messengers—diacylglycerol and inositol-1,4,5-trisphosphate (IP_3) (*see* Chapter 2; *see also* Berridge, 1988). The latter compound stimulates the release of Ca^{2+} from intracellular stores. A major component of the responses that follow involves regulation of several protein kinases, including protein kinase C, which is activated by Ca^{2+} and diacylglycerol, as well as a group of Ca^{2+}- and calmodulin-sensitive protein kinases (Kakiuchi *et al.*, 1982; Nishizuka, 1986). For example, α_1-adrenergic receptors regulate hepatic glycogenolysis in some animal species; this effect results from the activation of phosphorylase kinase by the mobilized Ca^{2+} and is aided by the inhibition of glycogen synthase caused by protein kinase C–mediated phosphorylation (*see* Berridge, 1988). Protein kinase C phosphorylates many other cellular substrates, including membrane proteins such as channels, pumps, and ion-exchange proteins (including Ca^{2+}-transport ATPase). These effects presumably lead to regulation of various ion conductances.

Stimulation of α_1-adrenergic receptors also results in an influx of extracellular Ca^{2+} in many tissues, but the mechanisms are poorly understood. Activation of Ca^{2+} channels in the plasma membrane by IP_3 or one of its metabolites may be involved. In other circumstances, a distinct subtype of α_1 receptor may regulate Ca^{2+} channels more directly; α_2 receptors in vascular smooth muscle may exert a similar effect (*see* Minneman, 1988).

In most smooth muscles, the increased concentrations of intracellular Ca^{2+} ultimately cause contraction as a result of activation of Ca^{2+}-sensitive protein kinases such as the calmodulin-dependent myosin light chain kinase; phosphorylation of the light chain of myosin is associated with the development of tension (Murphy *et al.*, 1983; Kamm and Stull, 1985). By contrast, the increased concentrations of intracellular Ca^{2+} that result from stimulation of α_1-adrenergic receptors in gastrointestinal smooth muscle cause hyperpolarization and relaxation by activation of Ca^{2+}-dependent K^+ channels (*see* Bolton, 1979). Preferential availability of the Ca^{2+} to these channels is apparently involved (Nelemans and den Hertog, 1987), and α_1-adrenergic agonists cause contraction when K^+ channels are blocked (Maas and den Hertog, 1979).

Stimulation of α_1-adrenergic receptors in the heart and certain neurons causes inhibition of transient voltage-activated K^+ currents (Randle *et al.*, 1986; Fedida *et al.*, 1989). The mechanism is unknown, but involvement of IP_3 and/or diacylglycerol is suspected in cardiac tissues. This action may be partially responsible for the arrhythmogenic effects of sympathomimetic amines under some circumstances. Although similar actions may be involved in depolarizing responses to α_1-adrenergic agonists in certain smooth muscles (*e.g.*, vas deferens), direct evidence for this mechanism is lacking.

Localization of Adrenergic Receptors. Evidence suggests that α_1- and β_1-adrenergic receptors are located in the immediate vicinity of adrenergic nerve terminals in peripheral target organs, strategically placed to be activated during stimulation of these nerves. In addition to those located on nerve terminals, both α_2- and β_2-adrenergic receptors also appear to be situated in postjunctional regions that are relatively remote from sites of release of norepinephrine. The latter receptors may be stimulated preferentially by circulating catecholamines, particularly epinephrine. In some instances, the physiological role of these and other adrenergic receptors (*e.g.*, those on leukocytes and platelets) is not well understood.

Refractoriness to Catecholamines. Exposure of catecholamine-sensitive cells and tissues to adrenergic agonists causes a progressive diminution in their capacity to respond to such agents. This phenomenon is variously termed *refractoriness, desensitization,* or *tachyphylaxis,* and it significantly limits the therapeutic efficacy and duration of action of catecholamines and other agents (*see* Chapter 2). Although descriptions of such adaptive changes are common, mechanisms are incompletely understood. They have been studied extensively in cells that synthesize cyclic AMP in response to β-adrenergic agonists. Following the application of isoproterenol or similar drugs to such cells, their capacity to synthesize cyclic AMP may be markedly reduced within a few minutes.

There is evidence for multiple points of regulation of responsiveness, including the receptors, G proteins, adenylyl cyclase, cyclic nucleotide phosphodiesterase, and so on (Benovic *et al.*, 1988). The pattern of refractoriness varies according to the extent to which these different components are modified. In some cases, especially when the receptors themselves are altered, the desensitization may be limited to the actions of β-adrenergic agents. This is often termed *homologous desensitization*. In other cases, stimulation by a β-adrenergic agonist can cause diminished responsiveness to a wide variety of receptor-mediated stimulators of cyclic AMP synthesis. Although such *heterologous desensitization* may result from changes in receptors, it often involves perturbations of more distal elements in the signaling pathway as well.

Different types of receptor modifications occur upon stimulation by agonists, and these appear to contribute to decreased sensitivity to catecholamines. Receptors may be phosphorylated by several protein kinases; this leads to decreased efficiency of coupling of the receptor with G_s. One such kinase is the cyclic AMP–dependent protein kinase, which functions in what appears to be a feedback regulatory manner to dampen receptor function and thus decrease the stimulation of the kinase that is elicited by agonists. In addition, a special protein kinase, termed the β-adrenergic receptor kinase, phosphorylates the receptors only when they are occupied by an agonist (Benovic *et al.*, 1986).

Agonists also promote a rapid (minutes) and reversible sequestration (internalization) of their receptors and a slower (hours) "down regulation" of the receptors, in which the actual number of receptors in the cell declines. Both processes may contribute to desensitization, although the underlying mechanisms are poorly understood.

Responses to α_1-adrenergic agonists also display desensitization. Mechanisms include uncoupling of receptor and down regulation, as well as postreceptor alterations. Phosphorylation reactions may be mediated by protein kinase C (Sibley *et al.*, 1987).

Relationship Between the Nervous and the Endocrine Systems

The concept that "humors" are secreted at certain sites to act elsewhere in the body can be traced back to Aristotle. In modern terms, the theory of neurohumoral transmission by its very designation implies at least a superficial resemblance between the nervous and the endocrine systems. Yet it should now be clear that the similarities extend considerably deeper, particularly with respect to the autonomic nervous system. In the regulation of homeostasis, the autonomic nervous system is responsible for rapid adjustments to changes in the total environment, which it effects at both its ganglionic synapses and postganglionic terminals by the liberation of chemical agents that act transiently at their immediate sites of release. The endocrine system, in contrast, regulates slower, more generalized adaptations by releasing its hormonal agents into the systemic circulation to act at distant, widespread sites over periods of hours or days. Both systems have major central representations in the hypothalamus, where they are integrated with each other and with subcortical, cortical, and spinal influences. The neurohumoral theory may thus be said to provide a unitary concept of the functioning of the nervous and the endocrine systems, in which the differences are essentially only quantitative.

PHARMACOLOGICAL CONSIDERATIONS

The forcgoing sections contain numerous references to the actions of drugs considered primarily as tools for the dissection and elucidation of physiological mechanisms. Here will be presented a classification of drugs that act upon the peripheral nervous system and its effector organs at some stage of neurohumoral transmission. In the immediately succeeding chapters, as well as elsewhere in the text, the systematic pharmacology of the important members of each of these classes is described.

Each step involved in neurohumoral transmission (*see* Figure 5–2) represents a potential point of drug attack. This is depicted in the diagram of the adrenergic terminal and its postjunctional site, in Figure 5–4. Drugs that affect processes concerned in each step of transmission at both cholinergic and adrenergic junctions are summarized in Table 5–4, which lists representative agents that act by the mechanisms described below.

Interference with the Synthesis or Release of the Transmitter. *Cholinergic.* Hemicholinium (HC-3), a synthetic compound, blocks the transport system by which choline accumulates in the terminals of cholinergic fibers, thus limiting the synthesis of the ACh store available for release (Birks and MacIntosh, 1957). Vesamicol blocks

Table 5–4. TYPES OF ACTION OF REPRESENTATIVE AGENTS AT PERIPHERAL CHOLINERGIC AND ADRENERGIC SYNAPSES AND NEUROEFFECTOR JUNCTIONS

MECHANISM OF ACTION	SYSTEM	AGENTS	EFFECT
1. Interference with synthesis of transmitter	Cholinergic	Hemicholinium	Block of choline uptake with consequent depletion of ACh
	Adrenergic	α-Methyltyrosine	Depletion of norepinephrine
2. Metabolic transformation by same pathway as precursor of transmitter	Adrenergic	Methyldopa	Displacement of norepinephrine by false transmitter (α-methylnorepinephrine)
3. Blockade of transport system of membrane of nerve terminal	Adrenergic	Cocaine, imipramine	Accumulation of norepinephrine at receptors
4. Blockade of transport system of storage granule membrane	Adrenergic	Reserpine	Destruction of norepinephrine by mitochondrial MAO, and depletion from adrenergic terminals
5. Displacement of transmitter from axonal terminal	Cholinergic	Black widow spider venom	Cholinomimetic followed by anticholinergic
	Adrenergic	Amphetamine, tyramine	Sympathomimetic
6. Prevention of release of transmitter	Cholinergic	Botulinus toxin	Anticholinergic
	Adrenergic	Bretylium, guanethidine	Antiadrenergic
7. Mimicry of transmitter at postsynaptic receptor	Cholinergic		
	Muscarinic	Methacholine	Cholinomimetic
	Nicotinic	Nicotine	Cholinomimetic
	Adrenergic		
	$Alpha_1$	Phenylephrine	Sympathomimetic
	$Alpha_2$	Clonidine	Sympathomimetic (periphery) Reduced sympathetic outflow (CNS)
	$Beta_{1,2}$	Isoproterenol	Nonselective β-adrenomimetic
	$Beta_1$	Dobutamine	Selective cardiac stimulation
	$Beta_2$	Terbutaline	Selective inhibition of smooth muscle contraction
8. Blockade of endogenous transmitter at postsynaptic receptor	Cholinergic		
	Muscarinic	Atropine	Muscarinic blockade
	Nicotinic, N_M	Tubocurarine	Neuromuscular blockade
	Nicotinic, N_N	Trimethaphan	Ganglionic blockade
	Adrenergic		
	Alpha	Phenoxybenzamine	α-Adrenergic blockade
	$Beta_{1,2}$	Propranolol	β-Adrenergic blockade
	$Beta_1$	Metoprolol	Selective adrenergic blockade (cardiac)
9. Inhibition of enzymatic breakdown of transmitter	Cholinergic	Anti-ChE agents (physostigmine, di*iso*propyl phosphorofluoridate [DFP])	Cholinomimetic
	Adrenergic	MAO inhibitors (pargyline, nialamide, tranylcypromine)	Little direct effect on norepinephrine or sympathetic responses; potentiation of tyramine

the transport of ACh into its storage vesicles, thus preventing its release. Botulinus toxin prevents the release of ACh by all types of cholinergic fibers studied; death results from peripheral respiratory paralysis. Apparently, the toxin blocks release of vesicular ACh at the preterminal portion of the axon, but why this effect is confined to cholinergic fibers is not known (Simpson, 1986).

Adrenergic. α-Methyltyrosine (metyrosine) blocks the synthesis of norepinephrine by inhibiting tyrosine hydroxylase, the enzyme that catalyzes the rate-limiting step. On the other hand, methyldopa, an inhibitor of aromatic L-amino acid decarboxylase, is—like dopa itself—successively decarboxylated and hydroxylated in its side chain to form the putative "false neurotransmitter" α-methylnorepinephrine. Bretylium and guanethidine act by preventing the release of norepinephrine by the nerve impulse. However, both guanethidine and bretylium can transiently stimulate the release of norepinephrine, as a result of their ability to displace the amine from storage sites. Guanethidine can also partially deplete tissue stores of catecholamines by inhibition of the vesicular transport system for such amines.

Promotion of the Release of the Transmitter. *Cholinergic.* The ability of cholinergic agents to promote the release of ACh is limited, presumably because ACh and other cholinomimetic agents are quaternary ammonium compounds and do not readily cross the axonal membrane into the nerve ending. Black widow spider venom is known to cause a transient release of ACh before a permanent block is elicited (Simpson, 1986).

Adrenergic. Several drugs that promote the release of the adrenergic mediator have already been discussed. On the basis of the rate and the duration of the drug-induced release of norepinephrine from adrenergic terminals, one of two opposite effects can predominate. Thus, tyramine, ephedrine, amphetamine, and related drugs cause a relatively rapid, brief liberation of the transmitter and hence produce a sympathomimetic effect. On the other hand, reserpine, by blocking vesicular uptake of amines, produces a slow, prolonged release of the adrenergic transmitter within the nerve terminal, where it is largely metabolized by intraneuronal MAO. The resultant depletion of transmitter produces the equivalent of adrenergic blockade. Reserpine also causes the depletion of 5-HT, dopamine, and possibly other, unidentified, amines from central and peripheral sites, and many of its major effects may be consequent to the depletion of transmitters other than norepinephrine.

Combination with Postjunctional Receptor Sites. *Cholinergic.* The majority of therapeutically useful agents that affect the peripheral cholinergic systems are in this category, and much research on drug development in this area is directed to discovery of agents that interact with specific types of cholinergic receptors. Since ACh is the neurohumoral transmitter at various peripheral junctions, the postjunctional cholinergic receptors might be expected to share certain common features. However, it has long been known that individual drugs vary in potency, relative to ACh, at different cholinoceptive sites. Structural and functional differences between nicotinic and muscarinic cholinergic receptors are now well appreciated, and subtypes of these major categories have been defined more recently (*see* above).

The nicotinic receptors of autonomic ganglia and skeletal muscle are not identical; they respond differently to certain stimulating and blocking agents and they contain different polypeptide subunits (*see* Table 5–2). Dimethylphenylpiperazinium (DMPP) and phenyltrimethylammonium (PTMA) are selective stimulants of autonomic ganglion cells and end-plates of skeletal muscle, respectively. Tetraethylammonium, trimethaphan, and hexamethonium are selective ganglionic blocking agents. Although tubocurarine effectively blocks transmission at both motor end-plates and autonomic ganglia, its action at the former site predominates. Decamethonium, a depolarizing agent, produces selective neuromuscular blockade. The snake toxins, which cause neuromuscular paralysis, also exhibit selectivity for the nicotinic cholinergic receptor at the neuromuscular junction. Transmission at autonomic ganglia is further complicated by the presence of muscarinic receptors, in addition to the principal nicotinic receptors (*see* Chapter 9).

Muscarinic receptors, which mediate the effects of ACh at autonomic effector cells, can now be divided into five subclasses. Atropine blocks all the muscarinic responses to injected ACh and related cholinomimetic drugs, whether they are excitatory, as in the intestine, or inhibitory, as in the heart. Antagonists such as pirenzepine show selectivity for blocking particular muscarinic receptors. Such compounds yield additional therapeutic selectivity, and further developments can be anticipated in this area (*see* Chapter 8).

Adrenergic. A vast number of synthetic compounds that bear structural resemblance to the naturally occurring catecholamines can interact with α- or β-adrenergic receptors or both, and produce sympathomimetic effects (*see* Chapter 10). Phenylephrine acts selectively at α_1-receptor sites, while clonidine is a selective α_2 agonist. Isoproterenol exhibits agonist activity at both β_1- and β_2-adrenergic receptors. Preferential stimulation of cardiac β_1 receptors follows the administration of dobutamine. Terbutaline is an example of a drug with relatively selective action on β_2 receptors; that is, it produces effective bronchodilatation with minimal effects on the heart. The main features of adrenergic blockade, including the selectivity of various blocking agents for α and β receptors, have been mentioned (*see also* Chapter 11). Here too, partial dissociation of effects at β_1- and β_2-adrenergic receptors has been achieved, as exemplified by the β_1-blocking agent metoprolol, which blocks the cardiac actions of catecholamines without causing an equivalent degree of antagonism at bronchioles. Prazosin and yohimbine are representative of α_1- and α_2-adrenergic antagonists, respectively. Several important drugs that promote the release of norepinephrine or deplete the transmitter resemble, in their effects, activators or blockers of postjunctional receptors (*e.g.*, tyramine and reserpine, respectively).

Interference with the Destruction of the Transmitter. *Cholinergic.* The anti-ChE agents (Chapter 7) constitute a large group of compounds, the primary action of which is inhibition of AChE, with the consequent accumulation and action of endogenous ACh at sites of cholinergic transmission.

Adrenergic. The reuptake of norepinephrine by the adrenergic nerve terminals is probably the major mechanism for terminating its transmitter action. Interference with this process is the basis of the potentiating effect of cocaine on responses to adrenergic impulses and injected catecholamines. It has also been suggested that the antidepressant actions and some of the side effects of imipramine and related drugs are due to a similar action at adrenergic synapses in the CNS (*see* Chapter 18). Inhibitors of COMT, such as pyrogallol and tropolone, produce only slight enhancement of the actions of catecholamines, whereas MAO inhibitors, such as tranylcypromine, potentiate the effects of tyramine but not of catecholamines.

OTHER AUTONOMIC NEUROTRANSMITTERS

Evidence has accumulated in recent years that the vast majority of neurons in both the central and peripheral nervous systems contain more than one substance with potential or demonstrated activity at relevant postjunctional sites (*see* Bartfai *et al.*, 1988; Kow and Pfaff, 1988; *see also* Chapter 12). In some cases, especially in peripheral structures, it has been possible to demonstrate that two or more such substances are contained within individual nerve terminals and are released simultaneously upon nerve stimulation. Although the anatomical separation of the parasympathetic and sympathetic components of the autonomic nervous system and the actions of ACh and norepinephrine (their primary neurotransmitters) still provide the essential framework for studying autonomic function, a host of other chemical messengers such as purines, eicosanoids, and peptides modulate or mediate responses that follow stimulation of the preganglionic neurons of the autonomic nervous system. An expanded view of autonomic neurotransmission is thus evolving to include instances where substances other than ACh or norepinephrine are released and may function as cotransmitters, neuromodulators, or primary transmitters. Moreover, it is becoming evident that structures that are innervated by the autonomic nervous system frequently elaborate chemical messengers that may mediate all or a portion of the responses to stimulation of autonomic nerves. The origin of these active substances may be "local" neurons, such as enteric neurons in the gastrointestinal tract, or cells in close apposition to the target structures, such as those of the vascular endothelium.

The evidence for cotransmission, or for so-called nonadrenergic, noncholinergic transmission, in the autonomic nervous system usually includes many of the following items. (1) All or a portion of responses to stimulation of preganglionic or postganglionic nerves or to field stimulation of target structures persist in the presence of maximal concentrations of muscarinic antagonists and adrenergic blocking agents. (2) The candidate substance can be detected within nerve fibers that course through target tissues. (3) The substance can be recovered in the venous or perfusion effluent following electrical stimulation; such release should be blocked by tetrodotoxin. (4) Effects of electrical stimulation are mimicked by the application of the substance and are inhibited in the presence of specific antagonists (or antibodies). Because such antagonists are usually not available, reliance is often placed upon selective desensitization produced by prior exposure to the substance. A number of problems confound interpretation of such evidence. It is particularly difficult to eliminate the possibility that substances that fulfill all the criteria listed do not originate within the autonomic nervous system, at least as it is classically defined. In some instances, their origin can be traced to sensory fibers or to intrinsic neurons, even in blood vessels (Su *et al.*, 1987; Ando, 1988). Apparently negative items of evidence can also be misinterpreted; for example, there may be marked synergism between the candidate substance and either known or unknown transmitters (*see* Bartfai *et al.*, 1988; Kow and Pfaff, 1988).

It has long been known that ATP and ACh both exist in cholinergic vesicles (Dowdall *et al.*, 1974) and that ATP and catecholamines are both found within storage granules in nerves and the adrenal medulla (*see* above). ATP is released along with the transmitters, and either it or its metabolites may have a significant function in synaptic transmission in some circumstances (*see* below). In addition, ATP is thought to be a transmitter between nonadrenergic, noncholinergic nerve terminals and certain structures that are innervated by the autonomic nervous system, especially in the gastrointestinal and genitourinary tracts (Burnstock, 1969, 1986). More recently, attention has been focused on the rapidly growing list of peptides that are found in the adrenal medulla, nerve fibers or ganglia of the autonomic nervous system, or in the structures that are innervated by the autonomic nervous system. This list includes the enkephalins, substance P, somatostatin, gonadotropin-releasing hormone, cholecystokinin, calcitonin gene-related peptide, galanin, vasoactive intestinal peptide (VIP), and neuropeptide Y (NPY). The evidence for transmitter function in the autonomic nervous system is greatest for VIP and NPY, and further discussion is confined to these peptides and ATP.

Cotransmission in the Autonomic Nervous System. Both norepinephrine and ATP elicit excitation when released from certain adrenergic nerve terminals, such as those in the vas deferens and the vasculature. The response to ATP is rapid and that to norepinephrine is slower (Sneddon and Westfall, 1984). Sympathectomy and adrenergic neuron-depleting agents such as reserpine eliminate both phases of the response, consistent with storage of both substances in the same population of vesicles. In other cases, metabolism of ATP to adenosine in the extracellular space results in important modulatory effects. For example, blockade of adenosine receptors in afferent renal arterioles with theophylline causes vasodilatation and an increase in glomerular filtration rate (*see* Chapter 25); this results from the marked augmentation of norepinephrine-induced constriction produced by adenosine in these vessels. There is also evidence that adenosine exerts ongoing inhibitory effects on the release of transmitter, and the administration of antagonists such as theophylline results in increased concentrations of norepinephrine and dopamine-β-hydroxylase in the circulation.

The pioneering studies of Hökfelt and coworkers (Lundberg *et al.*, 1979), which demonstrated the existence of VIP and ACh in peripheral autonomic neurons, initiated interest in the possibility of peptidergic cotransmission in the autonomic nervous system. Subsequent work has confirmed the frequent association of these two substances in autonomic fibers, including parasympathetic fibers that innervate blood vessels in skeletal muscle and cholinergic sympathetic neurons that innervate sweat glands (Lindh *et al.*, 1989). The role of VIP in parasympathetic transmission has been most extensively studied in the regulation of salivary secretion. The evidence for cotransmission includes the release of VIP following stimulation of the chorda lingual nerve and the incomplete blockade by atropine of vasodilatation when the frequency of stimulation is raised (Fazekas *et al.*, 1987); the latter observation may indicate independent release of the two substances, which is consistent with histochemical evidence for storage of ACh and VIP in separate populations of vesicles. Synergism between ACh and VIP in stimulating vasodilatation and secretion has also been described.

NPY is widely distributed in the central and peripheral nervous systems, frequently in cells that also contain tyrosine hydroxylase (*see* McDonald, 1988; Wahlestedt *et al.*, 1989). Evidence for its corelease with catecholamines includes increases in plasma concentrations of NPY during stress-induced sympathoadrenal stimulation (Zukowska-Grojec and Vaz, 1988). Although direct evidence is limited, the distribution and actions of NPY suggest that it contributes to vasoconstriction produced by stimulation of the sympathetic nervous system. In other tissues such as the vas deferens, NPY may function only to modulate synaptic transmission by contributing to feedback inhibition of the release of norepinephrine (Donoso *et al.*, 1988).

Nonadrenergic, Noncholinergic Transmission. The smooth muscle of many structures that are innervated by the autonomic nervous system is relaxed following stimulation by field electrodes. Since such responses are frequently undiminished in the presence of adrenergic and muscarinic cholinergic antagonists, these observations have been taken as evidence for the existence of nonadrenergic, noncholinergic transmission in the autonomic nervous system.

Burnstock (1969, 1986) has compiled a great deal of evidence for the existence of so-called purinergic nerves in the gastrointestinal tract, genitourinary tract, and certain blood vessels; ATP has fulfilled all the criteria for a neurotransmitter listed above. However, in at least some circumstances, primary sensory axons may be an important source of ATP (*see* Burnstock, 1987). Although adenosine is generated from the released ATP, its function appears to be only modulatory by causing feedback inhibition of release of the transmitter.

In other tissues, such as the trachea, there is evidence that VIP mediates nonadrenergic, noncholinergic transmission (Venugopalan and O'Malley, 1988). The peptide may also be involved in a number of parasympathetic responses in the gastrointestinal tract, including the relaxation of sphincters in the stomach and intestine (*see* Fahrenkrug, 1989).

Modulation of Vascular Responses by Endothelium-Derived Factors. Furchgott and Zawadski demonstrated that an intact endothelium was necessary to achieve vascular relaxation in response to acetylcholine (*see* Furchgott, 1984). This inner layer of the blood vessel is now known to modulate autonomic and hormonal effects on the contractility of blood vessels. In response to a variety of vasoactive agents and even physical stimuli, the endothelial cells release short-lived vasodilator and, less commonly, vasoconstrictor substances called endothelium-derived relaxing factor (EDRF) and endothelium-derived contracting factor. Products of inflammation and platelet aggregation such as 5-hydroxytryptamine, histamine, bradykinin, purines, and thrombin exert all or part of their action by stimulating the release of EDRF. α_2-Adrenergic vasodilatation of coronary and splanchnic vessels is also due, in part, to EDRF (Vanhoutte, 1989). EDRF has chemical and pharmacological properties similar to those of nitric oxide (NO), and NO is generated by endothelial cells (Palmer *et al.*, 1987). However, other endothelium-derived factors may also be involved in vasodilatation and hyperpolarization of the smooth muscle cell. Full contractile responses of cerebral arteries also require an intact endothelium. Superoxide ($O_2 \cdot^-$) and a peptide termed *endothelin* appear to be involved in contraction mediated by the endothelium. The mechanisms of action of NO and superoxide remain open questions, although NO activates guanylyl cyclase (*see* Chapter 32) and superoxide may act by scavenging NO.

Ahlquist, R. P. A study of the adrenotropic receptors. *Am. J. Physiol.*, **1948**, *153*, 586–600.

Ando, K. Distribution and origin of vasoactive intestinal polypeptide (VIP)-immunoreactive, acetylcholinesterase-positive and adrenergic nerves of the cerebral arteries in the bent-winged bat (Mammalia: *Chiroptera*). *Cell Tissue Res.*, **1988**, *251*, 345–351.

Benovic, J. L.; Strasser, R. H.; Caron, M. G.; and Lefkowitz, R. J. Beta-adrenergic receptor kinase: identification of a novel protein kinase which phosphorylates the agonist-occupied form of the receptor. *Proc. Natl. Acad. Sci. U.S.A.*, **1986**, *83*, 2797–2801.

Berrard, S.; Bruce, A.; and Mallet, J. Molecular genetic approach to study the mammalian choline acetyltransferase. *Brain Res. Bull.*, **1989**, *22*, 147–153.

Bönisch, H., and Trendelenburg, U. The mechanism of action of indirectly acting sympathomimetic amines. In, *Catecholamines I*. (Trendelenburg, U., and Weiner, N., eds.) *Handbook of Experimental Pharmacology*, Vol. 90. Springer-Verlag, Berlin, **1988**, pp. 247–278.

Cannon, W. B., and Uridil, J. E. Studies on the conditions of activity in endocrine glands. VIII. Some effects on the denervated heart of stimulating the nerves of the liver. *Am. J. Physiol.*, **1921**, *58*, 353–354.

Cavallito, C. J.; Yun, H. S.; Smith, J. C.; and Foldes, F. F. Choline acetyltransferase inhibitors. Configurational and electronic features of styrylpyridine analogs. *J. Med. Chem.*, **1969**, *12*, 134–138.

Dale, H. H. The action of certain esters and ethers of choline, and their relation to muscarine. *J. Pharmacol. Exp. Ther.*, **1914**, *6*, 147–190.

De Robertis, E., and Bennett, H. S. Some features of the submicroscopic morphology of synapses in frog and earthworm. *J. Biophys. Biochem. Cytol.*, **1955**, *1*, 47–58.

Dohlman, H. G.; Bouvier, M.; Benovic, J. L.; Caron, M. G.; and Lefkowitz, R. J. The multiple membrane spanning topography of the β_2-adrenergic receptor. Localization of the sites of binding, glycosylation and regulatory phosphorylation by limited proteolysis. *J. Biol. Chem.*, **1987**, *262*, 14282–14288.

Donoso, V.; Silva, M.; St. Pierre, S.; and Huidobro-Toro, J. P. Neuropeptide Y (NPY), and endogenous presynaptic modulator of adrenergic neurotransmission in the rat *vas deferens:* structural and functional studies. *Peptides*, **1988**, *9*, 545–553.

Dowdall, M. J.; Boyne, A. F.; Whittaker, V. P. Adenosine triphosphate, a constituent of cholinergic synaptic vesicles. *Biochem. J.*, **1974**, *140*, 1–12.

Emorine, L. J.; Marullo, S.; Briend-Sutren, M.-M.; Patey, G.; Tate, K.; Delavier-Klutchko, C.; and Strosberg, D. Molecular characterization of the human β_3-adrenergic receptor. *Science*, **1989**, *245*, 1118–1121.

Fatt, P., and Katz, B. Spontaneous subthreshold activity at motor nerve endings. *J. Physiol. (Lond.)*, **1952**, *117*, 109–128.

Fazekas, A.; Gazelius, B.; Edwall, B.; Theodorsson-Norheim, E.; Blomquist, L.; and Lundberg, J. M. VIP and noncholinergic vasodilatation in rabbit submandibular gland. *Peptides*, **1987**, *8*, 13–20.

Fedida, D.; Shimoni, Y.; and Giles, W. R. A novel effect of norepinephrine on cardiac cells is mediated by alpha$_1$-adrenoceptors. *Am. J. Physiol.*, **1989**, *256*, H1500–H1504.

Hodgkin, A. L., and Huxley, A. F. A quantitative description of membrane current and its application to conduction and excitation in nerve. *J. Physiol. (Lond.)*, **1952**, *117*, 500–544.

Hökfelt, T., and others. Coexistence of peptides with classical neurotransmitters. *Experientia [Suppl.]*, **1989**, *56*, 154–179.

Katz, B., and Miledi, R. The measurement of synaptic delay, and the time course of acetylcholine release at the neuromuscular junction. *Proc. R. Soc. Lond. [Biol.]*, **1965**, *161*, 483–495.

———. The statistical nature of the acetylcholine potential and its molecular components. *J. Physiol. (Lond.)*, **1972**, *224*, 665–699.

Krnjević, K., and Mitchell, J. F. The release of acetylcholine in the isolated rat diaphragm. *J. Physiol. (Lond.)*, **1961**, *155*, 246–262.

Kubo, T., and others. Cloning sequencing and expression of the complementary DNA encoding the muscarinic acetylcholine receptor. *Nature*, **1986**, *323*, 411–416.

Lands, A. M.; Arnold, A.; McAuliff, J. P.; Luduena, F. P.; and Brown, R. G., Jr. Differentiation of receptor systems activated by sympathomimetic amines. *Nature*, **1967**, *214*, 597–598.

Langley, J. N. Observations on the physiological action of extracts of the supra-renal bodies. *Ibid.*, **1901**, *27*, 237–256.

Lewandowsky, M. Ueber eine Wirkung des Nebennieren-extractes auf das Auge. *Zentralbl. Physiol.*, **1898**, *12*, 599–600.

Lindh, B.; Lundberg, J. M.; and Hökfelt, T. NPY-, galanin-, VIP/PHI-, CGRP- and substance P-immunoreactive neuronal subpopulations in cat autonomic and sensory ganglia and their projections. *Cell Tissue Res.*, **1989**, *256*, 259–273.

Loewi, O., and Navratil, E. Über humorale Übertragbarkeit der Herznervenwirkung. X. Mitteilung. Über das Schicksal des Vagusstoff. *Pflügers Arch. Gesamte Physiol.*, **1926**, *214*, 678–688.

Lundberg, J. M.; Hökfelt, T.; Schultzberg, M.; Uvnäs-Wallensten, K.; Köhler, C.; and Said, S. I. Occurrence of vasoactive intestinal polypeptide (VIP)-like immunoreactivity in certain cholinergic neurons of the cat: evidence from combined immunohistochemistry and acetylcholinesterase staining. *Neuroscience*, **1979**, *4*, 1539–1559.

Maas, A. J., and den Hertog, A. The effect of apamin on the smooth muscle cells of the guinea-pig *taenia coli*. *Eur. J. Pharmacol.*, **1979**, *58*, 151–156.

Nelemans, A., and den Hertog, A. Calcium translocation during activation of α_1-adrenoceptor and voltage-operated channels in smooth muscle cells. *Eur. J. Pharmacol.*, **1987**, *140*, 39–46.

Palmer, R. M. J.; Ferrigo, A. G.; and Moncada, S. Nitric oxide release accounts for the biological activity of endothelium-derived relaxing factor. *Nature*, **1987**, *327*, 524–525.

Randle, J. C. R.; Bourque, C. W.; and Renaud, L. P. α_1-Adrenergic receptor activation depolarizes rat supraoptic neurosecretory neurons *in vitro*. *Am. J. Physiol.*, **1986**, *251*, R569–R574.

Sibley, D. R.; Daniel, K.; Strader, C. D.; and Lefkowitz, R. J. Phosphorylation of the beta-adrenergic receptor in intact cells: relationship to heterologous and homologous mechanisms of adenylate cyclase. *Arch. Biochem. Biophys.*, **1987**, *258*, 24–32.

Sneddon, P., and Westfall, D. P. Pharmacological evidence that adenosine trisphosphate and noradrenalin are cotransmitters in the guinea pig vas deferens. *J. Physiol. (Lond.)*, **1984**, *347*, 561–580.

Spector, S.; Tarver, J.; and Berkowitz, B. Effects of drugs and physiological factors in the disposition of catecholamines in blood vessels. *Pharmacol. Rev.*, **1972**, *24*, 191–202.

Steinsland, O. S.; Furchgott, R. F.; and Kirpekar, F. M. Inhibition of adrenergic neurotransmission by parasympathomimetics in the rabbit ear artery. *J. Pharmacol. Exp. Ther.*, **1973**, *184*, 346–356.

Su, H. C.; Bishop, A. E.; Power, R. F.; Hamada, Y.; and Polak, J. M. Dual intrinsic and extrinsic origins of CGRP- and NPY-immunoreactive nerves of rat gut and pancreas. *J. Neurosci.*, **1987**, *7*, 2674–2687.

Surprenant, A., and North, R. A. Mechanism of synaptic inhibition by noradrenaline acting at α_2-adrenoceptors. *Proc. R. Soc. Lond. [Biol.]*, **1988**, *234*, 85–114.

Trautwein, W.; Kuffler, S. W.; and Edwards, C. Changes in membrane characteristics of heart muscle during inhibition. *J. Gen. Physiol.*, **1956**, *40*, 135–145.

Venugopalan, C. S., and O'Malley, N. A. Cross-desensitization of VIP- and NANC-mediated inhibition of the guinea-pig tracheal pouch. *J. Auton. Pharmacol.*, **1988**, *8*, 53–61.

Viveros, O. H., and Wilson, S. P. The adrenal chromaffin cell as a model to study cosecretion of enkephalins and catecholamines. *J. Auton. Nerv. Syst.*, **1983**, *7*, 41–58.

Yamauchi, T.; Nakata, H.; and Fujisawa, H. A new activator protein that activates tryptophan-5-monooxygenase and tyrosine-3-monooxygenase in the presence of Ca^{++}-calmodulin dependent protein kinase. *J. Biol. Chem.*, **1981**, *256*, 5404–5409.

Zimanyi, I.; Folly, G.; and Vizi, E. S. Inhibition of K^+ permeability diminishes alpha$_2$-adrenoceptor mediated effects on norepinephrine release. *J. Neurosci. Res.*, **1988**, *20*, 102–108.

Zukowska-Grojec, Z., and Vaz, A. C. Role of neuropeptide Y (NPY) in cardiovascular responses to stress. *Synapse*, **1988**, *2*, 293–298.

Monographs and Reviews

Applebury, M. L., and Hargrave, P. A. Molecular biology of the visual pigments. *Vision Res.*, **1986**, *26*, 1881–1895.

Armstrong, C. M. Ionic pores, gates and gating currents. *Q. Rev. Biophys.*, **1974**, *7*, 179–209.

Axelrod, J. Methylation reactions in the formation and metabolism of catecholamines and other biogenic amines: the enzymatic conversion of norepinephrine (NE) to epinephrine (E). *Pharmacol. Rev.*, **1966**, *18*, 95–113.

Barker, J. L. Peptide effects on the excitability of single nerve cells. In, *Neuropeptides*. (Iversen, L. L.; Iversen, S. D.; and Snyder, S. H.; eds.) *Handbook of Psychopharmacology*, Vol. 16. Plenum Press, New York, **1983**, pp. 489–517.

Bartfai, T.; Iverfeldt, K.; Fisone, G.; and Serfözö, P. Regulation of the release of coexisting neurotransmitters. *Annu. Rev. Pharmacol. Toxicol.*, **1988**, *28*, 285–320.

Benovic, J. L.; Bouvier, M.; Caron, M. G.; and Lefkowitz, R. J. Regulation of adenylyl cyclase-coupled beta-adrenergic receptors. *Annu. Rev. Cell Biol.*, **1988**, *4*, 405–428.

Bernard, C. *Leçons sur les phénomènes de la vie communs aux animaux et aux végétaux*. Baillière, Paris, **1878–1879.** (Two volumes.)

Berridge, M. J. Inositol lipids and calcium signalling. *Proc. R. Soc. Lond. [Biol.]*, **1988**, *234*, 359–378.

Birks, R. I., and MacIntosh, F. C. Acetylcholine metabolism at nerve-endings. *Br. Med. Bull.*, **1957**, *13*, 157–161.

Bolton, T. B. Mechanisms of action of transmitters and other substances on smooth muscle. *Physiol. Rev.*, **1979**, *59*, 606–718.

Bonner, T. I. The molecular basis of muscarinic receptor diversity. *Trends Neurosci.*, **1989**, *12*, 148–151.

Brown, A. M., and Birnbaumer, L. Direct G protein gating of ion channels. *Am. J. Physiol.*, **1988**, *254*, H401–H410.

Burnstock, G. Evolution of the autonomic innervation of visceral and cardiovascular systems in vertebrates. *Pharmacol. Rev.*, **1969**, *21*, 247–324.

———. The changing face of autonomic neurotransmission. *Acta Physiol. Scand.*, **1986**, *126*, 67–91.

———. Mechanisms of interaction of peptide and nonpeptide vascular neurotransmitter systems. *J. Cardiovasc. Pharmacol.*, **1987**, *10*, Suppl. 12, S74–S81.

Bylund, D. B. Subtypes of alpha$_2$-adrenoceptors: pharmacological and molecular biological evidence converges. *Trends Pharmacol. Sci.*, **1988**, *9*, 356–361.

Cannon, W. B. Organization for physiological homeostasis. *Physiol. Rev.*, **1929**, *9*, 399–431.

———. *The Wisdom of the Body*. W. W. Norton & Co., Inc., New York, **1932**.

Creutz, C. E.; Drust, D. S.; Hamman, H. C.; Junker, M.; Kambouris, N. G.; Klein, J. R.; Nelson, M. R.; and Snyder, S. L. Calcium-dependent membrane-binding proteins as potential mediators of stimulus-secretion coupling. In, *Stimulus-Response Coupling: The Role of Intracellular Calcium*. (Dedman, J., and Smith, V., eds.) The Telford Press, West Caldwell, New Jersey, **1990**. In Press.

Dale, H. H. The beginnings and the prospects of neurohumoral transmission. *Pharmacol. Rev.*, **1954**, *6*, 7–13.

Ducis, I. The high-affinity choline uptake system. In, *The Cholinergic Synapse*. (Whittaker, V. P., ed.) *Handbook of Experimental Pharmacology*, Vol. 86. Springer-Verlag, Berlin, **1988**, pp. 409–446.

Duggan, A. W., and North, R. A. Electrophysiology of opioids. *Pharmacol. Rev.*, **1983**, *35*, 219–281.

Eccles, J. C. *The Physiology of Synapses*. Springer-Verlag, Berlin; Academic Press, Inc., New York, **1964**.

———. *The Understanding of the Brain*. McGraw-Hill Book Co., New York, **1973**.

England, P. J.; Pask, H. T.; and Mills, D. Cyclic AMP–dependent phosphorylation of cardiac contractile proteins. *Adv. Cyclic Nucleotide Protein Phosphorylation Res.*, **1984**, *17*, 383–390.

Fahrenkrug, J. VIP and autonomic neurotransmission. *Pharmacol. Ther.*, **1989**, *41*, 515–534.

Fambrough, D. M. Control of acetylcholine receptors in skeletal muscle. *Physiol. Rev.*, **1979**, *59*, 165–227.

Fleming, W. W. The electrogenic Na^+,K^+-pump in smooth muscle: physiologic and pharmacologic significance. *Annu. Rev. Pharmacol. Toxicol.*, **1980**, *20*, 129–149.

Furchgott, R. F. The role of endothelium in the responses of vascular smooth muscle to drugs. *Annu. Rev. Pharmacol. Toxicol.*, **1984**, *24*, 175–197.

Gabella, G. Structure of smooth muscles. In, *Smooth Muscle: An Assessment of Current Knowledge*. (Bülbring, E.; Brading, A. F.; Jones, A. W.; and Tomita, T.; eds.) University of Texas Press, Austin, **1981**, pp. 1–46.

Gilbert, R. F. T., and Emson, P. C. Neuronal coexistence of peptides with other putative transmitters. In, *Neuropeptides*. (Iversen, L. L.; Iversen, S. D.; and Snyder, S. H.; eds.) *Handbook of Psychopharmacology*, Vol. 16. Plenum Press, New York, **1983**, pp. 519–556.

Gilman, A. G. G proteins: transducers of receptor-generated signals. *Annu. Rev. Biochem.*, **1987**, *56*, 615–649.

Goldberg, L. I.; Volkman, P. H.; and Kohli, J. D. A comparison of the vascular dopamine receptor with other dopamine receptors. *Annu. Rev. Pharmacol. Toxicol.*, **1978**, *18*, 57–80.

Grundfest, H. Physiology of electrogenic excitable membranes. In, *The Nervous System*, Vol. 1. (Tower, D. B., ed.) Raven Press, New York, **1975**, pp. 153–164.

Hille, B. *Ion Channels of Excitability Membranes*. Sinauer Associates, Sunderland, Mass., **1984**.

Hubbard, J. I. Microphysiology of vertebrate neuromuscular transmission. *Physiol. Rev.*, **1973**, *53*, 674–723.

Iversen, L. L. Uptake processes for biogenic amines. In, *Handbook of Psychopharmacology*, Vol. 3. (Iversen, L. L.; Iversen, S. D.; and Snyder, S. H.; eds.) Plenum Press, New York, **1975**, pp. 381–442.

Jessell, T. M. Substance P in the nervous system. In, *Neuropeptides*. (Iversen, L. L.; Iversen, S. D.; and Snyder, S. H.; eds.) *Handbook of Psychopharmacology*, Vol. 16. Plenum Press, New York, **1983**, pp. 1–105.

Jope, R. S. High-affinity choline transport and acetyl CoA production in brain and their roles in the regulation of acetylcholine synthesis. *Brain Res. Rev.*, **1979**, *1*, 313–344.

Kakiuchi, S.; Hidaka, H.; and Means, A. R. (eds.). *Calmodulin and Intracellular Calcium Receptors*. Plenum Press, New York, **1982**.

Kamm, K. E., and Stull, J. T. Function of myosin and myosin light chain kinase in smooth muscle. *Annu. Rev. Pharmacol. Toxicol.*, **1985**, *25*, 593–620.

Katz, B. *Nerve, Muscle, and Synapse*. McGraw-Hill Book Co., New York, **1966**.

———. *The Release of Neural Transmitter Substances*. Charles C Thomas, Publisher, Springfield, Ill., **1969**.

Kilbinger, H. Presynaptic muscarine receptors modulating acetylcholine release. *Trends Pharmacol. Sci.*, **1984**, *5*, 103–105.

Kopin, I. J. Metabolic degradation of catecholamines. The relative importance of different pathways under physiological conditions and after administration of drugs. In, *Catecholamines*. (Blaschko, H., and Muscholl, E., eds.) *Handbuch der Experimentellen Pharmakologie*, Vol. 33. Springer-Verlag, Berlin, **1972**, pp. 271–282.

Kow, L.-M., and Pfaff, D. W. Neuromodulatory actions of peptides. *Annu. Rev. Pharmacol. Toxicol.*, **1988**, *28*, 163–188.

Krebs, E. G., and Beavo, J. A. Phosphorylation-dephosphorylation of enzymes. *Annu. Rev. Biochem.*, **1979**, *48*, 923–960.

Krnjević, K. Chemical nature of synaptic transmission in vertebrates. *Physiol. Rev.*, **1974**, *54*, 418–540.

Langer, S. Z. Presynaptic regulation of the release of catecholamines. *Pharmacol. Rev.*, **1980**, *32*, 337–362.

Langer, S. Z., and Lehmann, J. Presynaptic receptors on catecholamine neurons. In, *Catecholamines I*. (Trendelenberg, U., and Weiner, N., eds.) *Handbook of Experimental Pharmacology*, Vol. 90. Springer-Verlag, Berlin, **1988**, pp. 419–508.

Lefkowitz, R. J., and Caron, M. G. Adrenergic receptors: models for the study of receptors coupled to guanine nucleotide regulatory proteins. *J. Biol. Chem.*, **1988**, *263*, 4993–4996.

Limbird, L. E. Receptors linked to inhibition of adenylate cyclase: additional signaling mechanisms. *FASEB J.*, **1988**, *2*, 2686–2695.

McDonald, J. K. NPY and related substances. *Crit. Rev. Neurobiol.*, **1988**, *4*, 97–135.

McKinney, M., and Richelson, E. Muscarinic receptor regulation of cyclic GMP and eicosanoid production. In, *The Muscarinic Receptors*. (Brown, J. H., ed.) Humana Press, Clifton, N. J., **1989**, pp. 309–339.

Mancia, G., and Zanchetti, A. Hypothalamic control of autonomic function. In, *Handbook of the Hypothalamus*, Vol. 3, Pt. B. *Behavioral Studies of the Hypothalamus*. (Morgane, P. J., and Panksepp, J., eds.) Marcel Dekker, Inc., New York, **1981**, pp. 147–202.

Minneman, K. P. α_1-Adrenergic receptor subtypes, inositol phosphates, and sources of cell Ca^{2+}. *Pharmacol. Rev.*, **1988**, *40*, 87–119.

Morgane, P. J. Historical and modern concepts of hypothalamic organization and function. In, *Anatomy of the Hypothalamus*. (Morgane, P. J., and Panksepp, J., eds.) *Handbook of the Hypothalamus*, Vol. 1. Marcel Dekker, Inc., New York, **1981**, pp. 1–64.

Murphy, R. A.; Aksoy, M. O.; Dillon, P. F.; Gerthoffer, W. T.; and Kamm, K. E. The role of myosin light chain phosphorylation in regulation of the cross-bridge cycle. *Fed. Proc.*, **1983**, *42*, 51–56.

Nishizuka, Y. Studies and perspectives of protein kinase C. *Science*, **1986**, *233*, 305–312.

Numa, S.; Noda, M.; Takahashi, H.; Tanabe, T.; Toyosoto, M.; Furatani, Y.; and Kikyotani, S. Molecular structure of the acetylcholine receptor. *Cold Spring Harbor Symp. Quant. Biol.*, **1983**, *48*, 57–69.

Parsons, S. M.; Bahu, B. A.; Graez, M.; Kaufman, R.; and Korneich, W. D. Acetylcholine transport: fundamental properties and effects of pharmacological agents. *Ann. N.Y. Acad. Sci. U.S.A.*, **1987**, *493*, 220–233.

Pernow, B. Substance P. *Pharmacol. Rev.*, **1983**, *35*, 85–141.

Reichardt, L. F., and Kelly, R. B. A molecular description of nerve terminal function. *Annu. Rev. Biochem.*, **1983**, *52*, 871–926.

Richardson, G. P. Development of a cholinergic synapse: role of trophic factors. In, *The Cholinergic Synapse*. (Whittaker, V. P., ed.) *Handbook of Experimental Pharmacology*, Vol. 86. Springer-Verlag, Berlin, **1988**, pp. 81–102.

Rubin, R. P. *Calcium and Cellular Secretion*. Plenum Press, New York, **1982.**

Simpson, L. L. The molecular pharmacology of botulinium toxin and tetanus toxin. *Annu. Rev. Pharmacol. Toxicol.*, **1986**, *26*, 427–453.

Starke, K. Presynaptic α-autoreceptors. *Rev. Physiol. Biochem. Pharmacol.*, **1987**, *107*, 73–146.

Steinbach, J. H., and Ifune, C. How many kinds of nicotinic acetylcholine receptors are there? *Trends Neurosci.*, **1989**, *12*, 3–6.

Strichartz, G.; Rando, T.; and Wang, G. K. An integrated view of the molecular toxicology of sodium channel gating inexertable cells. *Annu. Rev. Neurosci.*, **1987**, *10*, 237–267.

Thesleff, S. Functional properties of receptors in striated muscle. In, *Drug Receptors*. (Rang, H. P., ed.) University Park Press, Baltimore, **1973**, pp. 121–133.

Trendelenburg, U. A kinetic analysis of the extraneuronal uptake and metabolism of catecholamines. *Rev. Physiol. Biochem. Pharmacol.*, **1980**, *87*, 33–115.

Tsien, R. W.; Lipscombe, D.; Madison, D. V.; Bleg, K. R.; and Fox, A. P. Multiple types of neuronal calcium channels and their selective modulation. *Trends Neurosci.*, **1988**, *11*, 431–438.

Tucek, S. Choline acetyltransferase and synthesis of acetylcholine. In, *The Cholinergic Synapse*. (Whittaker, V. P., ed.) *Handbook of Experimental Pharmacology*, Vol. 86. Springer-Verlag, Berlin, **1988**, pp. 125–166.

Vanhoutte, P. M. Endothelium and control of vascular function. *Hypertension*, **1989**, *13*, 658–667.

von Euler, U. S. Synthesis, uptake and storage of catecholamines in adrenergic nerves. The effects of drugs. In, *Catecholamines*. (Blaschko, H., and Muscholl, E., eds.) *Handbuch der Experimentellen Pharmakologie*, Vol. 33. Springer-Verlag, Berlin, **1972**, pp. 186–230.

———. Historical perspective: growth and impact of the concept of chemical neurotransmission. In, *Chemical Neurotransmission—75 Years*. (Stjärne, L.; Hedqvist, P.; Lagercrantz, H.; and Wennmalm, Å.; eds.) Academic Press, Ltd., London, **1981**, pp. 3–12.

Wahlestedt, C.; Ekman, R.; and Widerlov, E. Neuropeptide Y (NPY) and the central nervous system: distribution effects and possible relationship to neurological and psychiatric disorders. *Prog. Neuropsychopharmacol. Biol. Psychiatry*, **1989**, *13*, 31–54.

Weiner, N. Control of the biosynthesis of adrenal catecholamines by the adrenal medulla. In, *Adrenal Gland*, Vol. 6. Sect. 7, *Endocrinology. Handbook of Physiology*. (Blaschko, H.; Sayers, G.; and Smith, A. D.; eds.) American Physiological Society, Washington, D.C., **1975**, pp. 357–366.

———. Multiple factors regulating the release of norepinephrine consequent to nerve stimulation. *Fed. Proc.*, **1979a**, *38*, 2193–2202.

———. Tyrosine-3-monooxygenase (tyrosine hydroxylase). In, *Aromatic Amino Acid Hydroxylases: Biochemical and Physiological Aspects*. (Youdim, M. B. H., ed.) John Wiley & Sons, Inc., New York, **1979b**, pp. 141–190.

Weiner, N.; Cloutier, G.; Bjur, R.; and Pfeffer, R. I. Modification of norepinephrine synthesis in intact tissue by drugs and during short-term adrenergic nerve stimulation. *Pharmacol. Rev.*, **1972**, *24*, 203–232.

Weiner, N.; Yanagihara, N.; Tank, A. W.; Baizer, L.; and Langan, T. A. Studies of the mechanism of activation of tyrosine hydroxylase *in situ* in PC 12 cells. In, *Neurology and Neurobiology*. (Usdin, E.; Carlsson, A.; Dahlström, A.; and Engel, J.; eds.) *Catecholamines: Basic and Peripheral Mechanisms*, Vol. 8A. Alan R. Liss, Inc., New York, **1984**, pp. 173–181.

Winkler, H.; Fischer-Colbrie, F.; and Weber, A. Molecular organization of vesicles storing transmitter: chromaffin vesicles as a model. In, *Chemical Neurotransmission—75 Years*. (Stjärne, L.; Hedqvist, P.; Lagercrantz, H.; and Wennmalm, Å.; eds.) Academic Press, Ltd., London, **1981**, pp. 57–68.

Wu, C. H., and Narahashi, T. Mechanism of action of novel marine toxins on ion channels. *Annu. Rev. Pharmacol. Toxicol.*, **1988**, *28*, 141–162.

CHAPTER

6 CHOLINERGIC AGONISTS

Palmer Taylor

Cholinergic agonists have as their primary action the excitation or inhibition of autonomic effector cells that are innervated by postganglionic parasympathetic nerves. When acting in this capacity, they may be referred to as *parasympathomimetic agents*. Additional actions are exerted on ganglia, on the neuromuscular junction, on prejunctional sites in the autonomic nervous system, and on cells that do not receive extensive parasympathetic innervation but nevertheless possess cholinergic receptors. The drugs may be divided into two groups: (1) acetylcholine and several synthetic choline esters, and (2) the naturally occurring cholinomimetic alkaloids (particularly pilocarpine, muscarine, and arecoline) and their synthetic congeners. In addition, the anticholinesterase agents (Chapter 7) and the ganglionic stimulants (Chapter 9) have parasympathomimetic actions, but they also produce prominent effects at locations other than the postganglionic cholinergic effector site.

CHOLINE ESTERS

Acetylcholine (ACh) has virtually no therapeutic applications because of its diffuseness of action and its rapid hydrolysis by both acetylcholinesterase (AChE) and plasma butyrylcholinesterase. Consequently, numerous derivatives have been synthesized in attempts to obtain drugs with more selective and prolonged actions. Only the latter objective has met with much success.

History. ACh was first synthesized by Baeyer in 1867. Investigations culminating in its identification as a neurohumoral transmitter are described in Chapter 5.

Of the several hundred synthetic choline derivatives investigated, only methacholine, carbachol, and bethanechol have had clinical application. The structures of these compounds are shown in Table 6–1. Although methacholine, the β-methyl analog of ACh, was studied by Hunt and Taveau as early as 1911, it was not until the systematic investigations of this compound by Simonart (1932) and Starr and associates (1933) that the drug received adequate therapeutic trial. Carbachol, the carbamyl ester of choline, and bethanechol, its β-methyl analog, were synthesized in the early 1930s; their pharmacological actions were investigated by Molitor (1936) and others.

Mechanism of Action. The mechanisms of action of endogenous ACh at the postjunctional membranes of the effector cells and neurons that correspond to the four classes of cholinergic synapses are discussed in Chapter 5. By way of recapitulation, these synapses are (1) autonomic effector sites, innervated by postganglionic parasympathetic fibers; (2) sympathetic and parasympathetic ganglion cells and the adrenal medulla, innervated by preganglionic autonomic fibers; (3) motor end-plates on skeletal muscle, innervated by somatic motor nerves; and (4) certain synapses within the central nervous system (CNS). In addition, ACh acts on prejunctional re-

Table 6–1. STRUCTURAL FORMULAS OF CHOLINE, ACETYLCHOLINE, AND CHOLINE ESTERS EMPLOYED CLINICALLY

Choline chloride	$(CH_3)_3\overset{+}{N}CH_2CH_2OH$	Cl^-
Acetylcholine chloride	$(CH_3)_3\overset{+}{N}CH_2CH_2O\overset{\overset{O}{\|}}{C}CH_3$	Cl^-
Methacholine chloride	$(CH_3)_3\overset{+}{N}CH_2\underset{\underset{CH_3}{\vert}}{C}HO\overset{\overset{O}{\|}}{C}CH_3$	Cl^-
Carbachol chloride	$(CH_3)_3\overset{+}{N}CH_2CH_2O\overset{\overset{O}{\|}}{C}NH_2$	Cl^-
Bethanechol chloride	$(CH_3)_3\overset{+}{N}CH_2\underset{\underset{CH_3}{\vert}}{C}HO\overset{\overset{O}{\|}}{C}NH_2$	Cl^-

ceptors in the autonomic and central nervous systems. When ACh is administered systemically, it has the potential to act at all of these sites; however, as a quaternary ammonium compound its penetration into the CNS is limited, and butyrylcholinesterase in the plasma reduces the concentrations of ACh that reach areas in the periphery with low blood flow.

Since muscarine was characterized originally as acting relatively selectively at autonomic effector cells to produce qualitatively the same effects as ACh, actions of ACh and related drugs at these sites are referred to as *muscarinic*. Accordingly, the muscarinic, or parasympathomimetic, actions of the drugs considered in this chapter are practically equivalent to the effects of postganglionic parasympathetic nerve impulses listed in Table 5–1 (page 90); the differences between the actions of the classical muscarinic agonists are largely quantitative, with limited selectivity for one organ system or another. Muscarinic receptors are also present to a variable degree on autonomic ganglion cells and on certain cortical and subcortical neurons. These muscarinic receptors are often of the M_1 type and differ in chemical selectivity from those found predominantly on postganglionic effector sites in cardiac tissue and secretory organs. In addition, muscarinic agonists have secondary effects at ganglionic sites (*see* Chapter 9). All the actions of ACh and its congeners at muscarinic receptors can be blocked by atropine (*see* Chapter 8). The *nicotinic* actions of cholinergic agonists refer to their initial stimulation, and in high doses to subsequent blockade, of autonomic ganglion cells and the neuromuscular junction, actions comparable to those of nicotine.

Properties of Muscarinic Receptors. Muscarinic receptors were initially characterized in the periphery and the CNS by analysis of the responses of cells and tissues; this was followed by examination of the binding of various ligands to these receptors. The heterogeneity of muscarinic receptors was first revealed largely by the distinctive properties of McN-A-343 (an agonist) and pirenzepine (an antagonist); both of these compounds have greater affinity for receptors in the cerebral cortex and sympathetic ganglia (designated M_1) than they do for receptors in the heart or in various smooth muscles and glands (initially designated M_2). It is now clear that the muscarinic receptors in tissues innervated by postganglionic parasympathetic neurons are also heterogeneous, and antagonists have been developed that rather selectively block responses of the heart (M_2) and various glands (M_3) (*see* Chapters 5 and 8). The types of muscarinic receptors that mediate responses of smooth muscle appear to vary in different tissues, and their classification remains unclear.

Molecular cloning has recently revealed the existence of at least five structural variants of the muscarinic receptor (Bonner *et al.*, 1987; Symposium, 1988). Three of the products detected after expression of the individual genes appear to correspond to the pharmacologically defined receptors that are designated M_1, M_2, and M_3. All of the muscarinic receptors interact with members of a group of guanine nucleotide–binding regulatory proteins (G proteins) that regulate a variety of effector systems within cells (*see* Chapter 2). Thus, stimulation of M_1 or M_3 receptors causes hydrolysis of polyphosphoinositides and mobilization of intracellular Ca^{2+}, apparently as a consequence of a G protein–mediated activation of phospholipase C (*see* Chapter 5); this effect in turn results in a variety of Ca^{2+}-mediated events, either directly or as a consequence of the phosphorylation of certain proteins. M_2-muscarinic receptors regulate ion channels (*e.g.*, they enhance a K^+ conductance in cardiac atrial fibers) and inhibit adenylyl cyclase by interaction with a distinct G protein.

Structure–Activity Relationship. The structure–activity relationship of cholinergic agonists has been described in detail (Bebbington and Brimblecombe, 1965; Kosterlitz, 1967; Rand and Stafford, 1967). Attention is accorded here only to those drugs that are of therapeutic interest.

Acetyl-β-methylcholine (methacholine) differs from ACh chiefly in its greater duration and selectivity of action. Its action is more prolonged because it is hydrolyzed by AChE at a considerably slower rate than ACh and is almost totally resistant to hydrolysis by nonspecific cholinesterase or butyrylcholinesterase. Its selectivity is manifested by slight nicotinic and a predominance of muscarinic actions, the latter being most marked on the cardiovascular system (Table 6–2).

Carbachol and bethanechol, which are unsubstituted carbamoyl esters, are totally resistant to hydrolysis by either AChE or nonspecific cholinesterases; their half-lives are thus sufficiently long that they are distributed to areas of low blood flow. Bethanechol has mainly muscarinic actions, but both drugs act with some selectivity on the

Table 6–2. SOME PHARMACOLOGICAL PROPERTIES OF CHOLINE ESTERS

CHOLINE ESTER	SUSCEPTIBILITY TO CHOLINESTERASES	PHARMACOLOGICAL ACTIONS					
		Muscarinic					*Nicotinic*
		Cardiovascular	Gastrointestinal	Urinary Bladder	Eye (Topical)	Antagonism by Atropine	
Acetylcholine	+++	++	++	++	+	+++	++
Methacholine	+	+++	++	++	+	+++	+
Carbachol	−	+	+++	+++	++	+	+++
Bethanechol	−	±	+++	+++	++	+++	−

smooth muscle of the gastrointestinal tract and urinary bladder. Carbachol retains substantial nicotinic activity, particularly on autonomic ganglia. It is likely that both its peripheral and its ganglionic actions are due, in part, to the release of endogenous ACh from the terminals of cholinergic fibers.

PHARMACOLOGICAL PROPERTIES

Cardiovascular System. ACh has four primary effects on the cardiovascular system: vasodilatation, a decrease in cardiac rate (the negative chronotropic effect), a decrease in the rate of conduction in the specialized tissues of the sinoatrial (SA) and atrioventricular (AV) nodes (the negative dromotropic effect), and a decrease in the force of cardiac contraction (the negative inotropic effect). The last-named effect is of lesser significance in ventricular than in atrial muscle. Certain of the above effects can be obscured by the dampening of the direct effects of ACh by baroreceptor and other reflexes.

Although ACh is rarely given systemically as a drug, its cardiac actions are of importance because of the involvement of cholinergic vagal impulses in the actions of the cardiac glycosides, antiarrhythmic agents, and many other drugs. The intravenous injection of a small dose of ACh produces an evanescent fall in blood pressure owing to generalized vasodilatation, accompanied usually by reflex tachycardia. A considerably larger dose is required to elicit bradycardia or block of AV nodal conduction from a direct action of ACh on the heart. If large doses of ACh are injected after the administration of atropine, an increase in blood pressure is observed; the increase is caused by stimulation of release of catecholamines from the adrenal medulla and activation of sympathetic ganglia.

ACh produces dilatation of essentially all vascular beds, including the pulmonary and coronary vascular beds. Coronary vasodilatation may be elicited by cardiovascular reflexes or by direct electrical stimulation of the vagus (Feigl, 1975). However, neither parasympathetic vasodilator nor sympathetic vasoconstrictor tone plays a major role in the regulation of coronary blood flow, in comparison with the effects of local oxygen tension and autoregulatory metabolic factors such as adenosine (Berne and Rubio, 1979).

The dilatation of vascular beds by choline esters is due to the presence of muscarinic receptors, despite the lack of apparent cholinergic innervation of most blood vessels. The muscarinic receptors responsible for relaxation are located on the endothelial cells of the vasculature; when these receptors are stimulated, the endothelial cells release an unidentified mediator, endothelium-derived relaxing factor, that diffuses to adjacent smooth muscle cells and causes them to relax (Furchgott and Zawadzki, 1980; Vanhoutte, 1989). Vasodilatation may also arise secondarily from inhibition by ACh of norepinephrine release from adrenergic nerve endings. If the endothelium is damaged, ACh can stimulate receptors on vascular smooth muscle cells and cause vasoconstriction.

ACh has important actions on all types of specialized cardiac cells; the same is qualitatively true of vagal impulses, since cholinergic parasympathetic fibers are distributed extensively to the SA and AV nodes and the atrial muscle. Cholinergic innervation of the ventricular myocardium is sparse, and the parasympathetic fibers terminate predominantly on specialized conduction tissue such as the Purkinje fibers (Kent *et al.*, 1974; Priola *et al.*, 1977).

In the SA node, each normal cardiac impulse is initiated by the spontaneous depolarization of the pacemaker cells (*see* Chapter 35). At a critical level—the threshold potential—this depolarization initiates an action potential (AP). The AP is conducted over the course of the atrial muscle fibers to the AV node and thence through the Purkinje system to the ventricular muscle. ACh slows the heart rate by hyperpolarization and by decreasing the rate of spontaneous diastolic depolarization at the SA node; this action delays the attainment of the threshold potential and the succeeding events in the cardiac cycle.

In atrial muscle, ACh decreases the strength of contraction. It also shortens the durations of the AP and the effective refractory period. The rate of conduction in the normal atrium is usually unaffected; however, if disease produces partial depolarization or if certain arrhythmias are present, an increase in conduction velocity may be seen. The combination of these factors is the basis for the perpetuation or exacerbation by vagal impulses of atrial flutter or fibrillation arising at an ectopic focus. In contrast, primarily in the AV node and to a much lesser extent in the Purkinje conducting system, ACh slows conduction and increases the refractory period. The decrement in AV nodal conduction is usually responsible for the complete heart block that may be observed when large quantities of cholinergic agonists are administered systemically. With an increase in vagal tone, such as is produced by the digitalis glycosides, the increased refractory period can contribute to the reduction in the frequency with which aberrant atrial impulses are transmitted to the ventricle, and thus decrease the ventricular rate during atrial flutter or fibrillation.

In the ventricle, ACh, whether released by vagal stimulation or applied directly, also has a negative inotropic effect, although it is much smaller than that observed in the atrium. The effect is more obvious when contractility is enhanced by adrenergic stimulation (*see* Higgins *et al.*, 1973; Levy and Martin, 1979). Automaticity of Purkinje fibers is suppressed, and the threshold for ventricular fibrillation is increased (Kent *et al.*, 1974; Kent and Epstein, 1976). Sympathetic and vagal nerve terminals lie in close proximity, and muscarinic receptors are believed to exist at presynaptic as well as postsynaptic sites (*see* Watanabe, 1983). Inhibition of adrenergic stimulation of the heart arises from the capacity of ACh to modulate or depress the myocardium's response to catecholamines as well as from a capacity to inhibit the release of norepinephrine from sympathetic nerve endings. These effects can be explained in part by the inhibitory effect of muscarinic agonists on adenylyl cyclase activity.

The hypotension and bradycardia produced by constant intravenous infusion of high doses of methacholine are identical with those obtained with ACh, but the effective dose is only about 0.5% as large. After a subcutaneous dose of 20 mg, a transient fall in blood pressure and a compensatory tachycardia occur. The cardiovascular effects of carbachol and bethanechol ordinarily are less conspicuous following usual subcutaneous or oral doses that affect the gastrointestinal and urinary tracts; these generally consist only in a slight, transient fall in diastolic pressure accompanied by a mild reflex tachycardia.

Gastrointestinal System. All the compounds of this class are capable of producing increases in tone, amplitude of contractions, and peristaltic activity of the stomach and intestines, as well as enhanced secretory activity of the gastrointestinal tract. The enhanced motility may be accompanied by nausea, belching, vomiting, intestinal cramps, and defecation.

Urinary Tract. Carbachol and bethanechol, in contrast to ACh and methacholine, stimulate rather selectively the urinary tract as well as the gastrointestinal tract. The choline esters increase ureteral peristalsis, contract the detrusor muscle of the urinary bladder, increase the maximal voluntary voiding pressure, and decrease the capacity of the bladder. In addition, the trigone and external sphincter are relaxed. In animals with experimental lesions of the spinal cord or sacral roots, these drugs bring about satisfactory evacuation of the neurogenic bladder.

Miscellaneous Effects. ACh and its analogs stimulate secretion by all glands that receive parasympathetic innervation, including the lacrimal, tracheobronchial, salivary, digestive, and exocrine sweat glands. The effects on the respiratory system, in addition to increased tracheobronchial secretion, include bronchoconstriction and stimulation of the chemoreceptors of the carotid and aortic bodies. When instilled into the eye, they produce miosis.

The effects of ACh on autonomic ganglia and at the neuromuscular junction of skeletal muscle are described in Chapter 9. Muscarinic receptors are also found at presynaptic sites and, when stimulated, inhibit the release of norepinephrine or ACh (*see* Chapter 5).

Synergisms and Antagonisms. ACh and methacholine are hydrolyzed by AChE, and their effects are markedly enhanced by the prior administration of anticholinesterase (anti-ChE) agents. The latter drugs produce only additive effects with the stable analogs—carbachol and bethanechol.

The muscarinic actions of all the drugs of this class are blocked selectively by atropine, through competitive occupation of cholinergic receptor sites on the autonomic effector cells and on the muscarinic receptors of autonomic ganglion cells. The nicotinic actions of ACh and its derivatives at autonomic ganglia are blocked by hexamethonium and related drugs; their actions at the neuromuscular junction of skeletal muscle are antagonized by tubocurarine and other competitive blocking agents.

Preparations, Routes of Administration, and Dosage. *Acetylcholine chloride* is occasionally used as an intraocular solution (MIOCHOL). It is available in dual-chambered vials for the preparation of a 1% solution in 3% mannitol.

Methacholine chloride (acetyl-β-methylcholine chloride) (PROVOCHOLINE) is available as a powder for preparation of a solution that is used for diagnosis of bronchial hyperreactivity.

Bethanechol chloride (*carbamylmethylcholine chloride;* URECHOLINE, others) is available in tablets containing 5, 10, 25, or 50 mg and as an injection (5 mg/ml). It is used to stimulate contraction of the urinary bladder and gastrointestinal tract. The oral dose for adults varies from 10 to 50 mg, taken on an empty stomach to avoid nausea and vomiting; the subcutaneous dose is 2.5 to 5.0 mg. The single dose may be given two to four times daily. The drug should not be administered by the intramuscular or intravenous route.

Carbachol (*carbamylcholine chloride*) is used as an ophthalmic solution (ISOPTO CARBACHOL) in concentrations of 0.75, 1.5, 2.25, and 3.0%. It is also available as *carbachol intraocular solution* (MIOSTAT), a 0.01% solution that is used to produce miosis during ocular surgery. The solution (0.5 ml) is instilled into the anterior chamber.

Precautions, Toxicity, and Contraindications. Drugs of this class should be administered only by the oral or subcutaneous route for systemic effects; they are also used locally in the eye. If they are given intravenously or intramuscularly, their relative selectivity of action no longer holds, and the incidence and severity of toxic side effects is greatly increased. Should serious toxic reactions to these drugs arise, atropine sulfate (0.5 to 1.0 mg) should be given subcutaneously or intravenously. Epinephrine (0.3 to 1.0 mg, subcutaneously or intramuscularly) is also of value in overcoming severe cardiovascular or bronchoconstrictor responses.

Among the major contraindications to the use of the choline esters are asthma, hyperthyroidism, coronary insufficiency, and peptic ulcer. Their bronchoconstrictor action is liable to precipitate an asthmatic attack, and hyperthyroid patients may develop atrial fibrillation. Hypotension induced by these agents can severely reduce coronary blood flow, especially if it is already compromised. Bethanechol is less likely to cause untoward cardiovascular effects than are other choline esters. The gastric acid secretion produced by the choline esters can aggravate the symptoms of peptic ulcer. Other possible undesirable effects of the cholinergic agonists are flushing, sweating, abdominal cramps, belching, a sensation of tightness in the urinary bladder, difficulty in visual accommodation, headache, and salivation.

THERAPEUTIC USES

Bethanechol is used as a stimulant of the smooth muscle of the gastrointestinal tract and, particularly, the urinary bladder; carbachol is no longer available for these purposes because of its relatively larger component of nicotinic action at autonomic ganglia. The unpredictability of the intensity of response has virtually eliminated the use of methacholine as a vasodilator and cardiac vagomimetic agent.

Gastrointestinal Disorders. Bethanechol can be of value in certain cases of postoperative abdominal distention and gastric atony and retention or gastroparesis. The oral route is preferred; the usual dosage is 10 to 20 mg three or four times daily. Bethanechol is given by mouth before each main meal in cases without complete retention; when gastric retention is complete and nothing passes into the duodenum, the subcutaneous route is necessary because the drug is not adequately absorbed from the stomach. Bethanechol has likewise been used to advantage in certain patients with adynamic ileus secondary to toxic states. It may be necessary to insert a rectal tube to facilitate passage of flatus. The drug is also of value in selected cases of congenital megacolon. Bethanechol has been shown in some studies to be of benefit in the treatment of esophageal reflux (Saco *et al.*, 1982; Thanik *et al.*, 1982). Lower esophageal sphincter pressure and esophageal motility are increased, and acid reflux into the esophagus is decreased; however, symptomatic improvement does not necessarily correlate with these parameters.

Urinary Bladder Disorders. Bethanechol may be useful in combating urinary retention and inadequate emptying of the bladder when organic obstruction is absent, as in postoperative and postpartum urinary retention and in certain cases of chronic hypotonic, myogenic, or neurogenic bladder (Kaufman, 1986; Wein and Barrett, 1988). α-Adrenergic antagonists have been reported to be a useful adjunct in reducing outlet resistance of the internal sphincter. Bethanechol may enhance contractions of the detrusor muscle after spinal injury if the vesical reflex is intact, and some benefit has been noted in partial sensory or motor paralysis of the bladder. Catheterization can thus be avoided. For acute retention, 2.5 mg of the drug is injected subcutaneously; this dose can be repeated after 15 to 30 minutes if necessary. The stomach should be empty at the time the drug is injected. In chronic cases, 10 to 50 mg of the drug may be given orally two to four times daily until voluntary or automatic voiding begins; its administration is then slowly withdrawn. Too large a dose will result in detrusor–sphincter dyssynergia.

Ophthalmological Uses. Acetylcholine, 1%, or carbachol, 0.01%, is used in cataract extractions and certain other surgical procedures on the anterior segment when it is desired to produce miosis rapidly; the action of acetylcholine is brief. For the long-term therapy of noncongestive wide-angle glaucoma, carbachol (0.75 to 3.0%) has been employed. Carbachol will often reduce intraocular pressure in patients who have become resistant to pilocarpine or physostigmine. The fall in intraocular pressure may be preceded by a transient elevation, owing to an increase in the permeability of the blood–aqueous humor barrier and vasodilatation of small vessels.

CHOLINOMIMETIC NATURAL ALKALOIDS AND SYNTHETIC ANALOGS

The three major natural alkaloids in this group—pilocarpine, muscarine, and arecoline—have the same principal sites of action as the choline esters discussed above. Muscarine acts almost exclusively at muscarinic receptor sites, their classification as such being derived from this fact. Arecoline acts in addition at nicotinic receptors. Pilocarpine has a dominant muscarinic action, but it causes anomalous cardiovascular responses, and the sweat glands are particularly sensitive to the drug. Although these naturally occurring alkaloids are of great value as pharmacological tools, present clinical use is largely restricted to the employment of pilocarpine as a miotic agent. The recent elucidation of the existence and distinct tissue distribution of several subtypes of muscarinic receptors has renewed interest in synthetic analogs that enhance the tissue selectivity of muscarinic agonists.

History and Sources. Pilocarpine is the chief alkaloid obtained from the leaflets of South American shrubs of the genus *Pilocarpus*. Although it was long known by the natives that the chewing of leaves of *Pilocarpus* plants caused salivation, the first experiments were apparently performed in 1874 by a Brazilian physician named Coutinhou. The alkaloid was isolated in 1875, and shortly thereafter the actions of pilocarpine on the pupil and on the sweat and salivary glands were described by Weber.

The poisonous effects of certain species of mushrooms have been known since ancient times, but it was not until Schmiedeberg isolated the alkaloid muscarine from *Amanita muscaria* that the properties of the drug could be systematically investigated. Schmiedeberg and Koppe published the first careful pharmacological study of muscarine in 1869. The role played by muscarine in the development of the neurohumoral theory has been recounted in Chapter 5.

Arecoline is the chief alkaloid of areca or betel nuts, the seeds of *Areca catechu*. The betel nut has been consumed as a euphoretic by the natives of the East Indies from early times in a masticatory mixture known as betel and composed of the nut, shell lime, and leaves of *Piper betle*, a climbing species of pepper.

Structure–Activity Relationship. The muscarinic alkaloids show marked differences as well as interesting relationships in structure (Table 6–3). Arecoline and pilocarpine are tertiary amines. Muscarine, a quaternary ammonium compound, has three asymmetrical carbon atoms; all four pairs of enantiomorphs have been synthesized (Eugster *et al.*, 1958), including the naturally occurring L(+) form. Oxotremorine is a synthetic compound that is used as an investigative tool. In the periphery, it acts as a potent muscarinic agonist. Its parkinsonism-like central effects include tremor, ataxia, and spasticity, which result apparently from activation of muscarinic receptors in the basal ganglia and elsewhere (Cho *et al.*, 1962). The chemistry and pharmacology of many natural and synthetic muscarinic compounds have been reviewed by Bebbington and Brimblecombe (1965).

McN-A-343 (*see* Table 6–3) stimulates M_1 receptors with some selectivity. Upon systemic injection of McN-A-343, blood pressure and peripheral vascular resistance increase as a consequence of stimulation of sympathetic ganglia in the absence of stimulation of cardiac and vascular postganglionic muscarinic receptors (*see* Roszkowski, 1961). McN-A-343 also stimulates muscarinic receptors on inhibitory neurons in the myenteric plexus (Symposium, 1988).

PHARMACOLOGICAL PROPERTIES

Smooth Muscle. Pilocarpine, when applied locally to the eye, causes pupillary constriction, spasm of accommodation, and a transitory rise in intraocular pressure, followed by a more persistent fall. Miosis lasts from several hours to a day, but the effect on accommodation disappears in about 2 hours. The muscarinic alkaloids stimulate the smooth muscles of the intestinal tract, thereby increasing tone and motility; large doses cause marked spasm and tenesmus. The bronchial musculature is also stimulated; asthmatic patients uniformly respond to pilocarpine with a reduction in vital capacity, and a typical asthmatic attack may be precipitated. Pilocarpine and muscarine also enhance the tone and motility of the ureters, urinary bladder, gallbladder, and biliary ducts.

Exocrine Glands. Pilocarpine (10 to 15 mg, subcutaneously) causes marked diaphoresis in man; 2 to 3 liters of sweat may be secreted. Muscarine and arecoline are also potent diaphoretic agents. Accompanying side effects may include hiccough, salivation, nausea, vomiting, weakness, and occasionally collapse. These alkaloids also stimulate the salivary, lacrimal, gastric, pancreatic, and intestinal glands, and the mucous cells of the respiratory tract.

Cardiovascular System. The most prominent cardiovascular effects following the intravenous injection of extremely small doses (0.01 to

Table 6–3. STRUCTURAL FORMULAS OF CHOLINOMIMETIC NATURAL ALKALOIDS AND SYNTHETIC ANALOGS

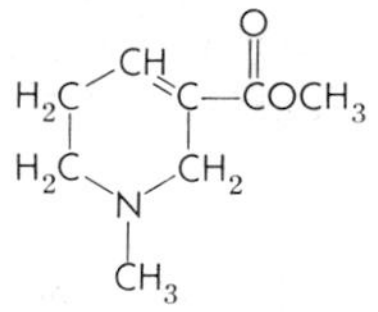

Arecoline

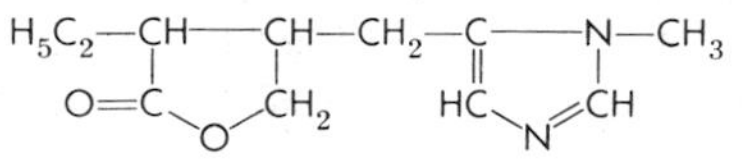

Pilocarpine

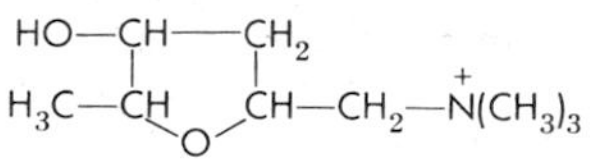

Muscarine

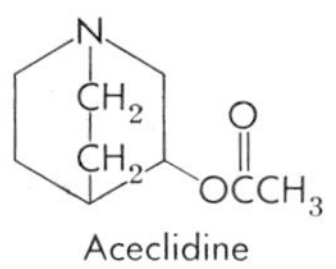

Aceclidine

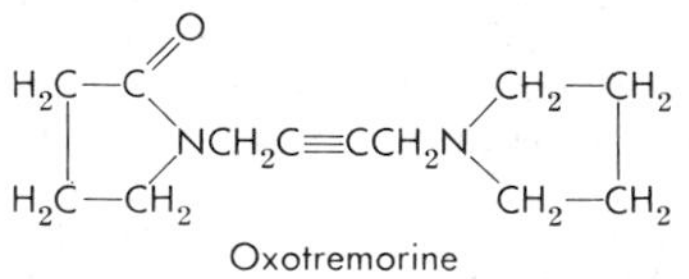

Oxotremorine

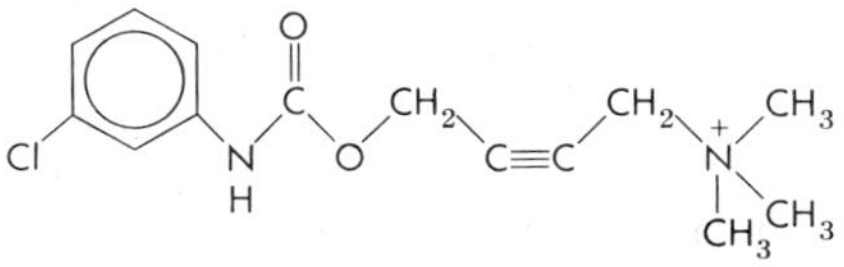

McN-A-343

0.03 μg/kg) of muscarine in various species are a marked fall in the blood pressure and a slowing or temporary cessation of the heart beat. The actions of pilocarpine on the cardiovascular system have not been explained satisfactorily. An intravenous injection of 0.1 mg/kg of pilocarpine produces a brief fall in blood pressure. However, if this is preceded by an appropriate dose of a nicotinic blocking agent, pilocarpine produces a marked rise in pressure. Both the vasodepressor and pressor responses are prevented by atropine; the latter effect is also abolished by α-adrenergic blocking agents (Levy and Ahlquist, 1962).

Central Nervous System. The intravenous injection of relatively small doses of pilocarpine, muscarine, and arecoline evokes a characteristic cortical arousal or activation response in cats, similar to that produced by the injection of ACh or anti-ChE agents or by electrical stimulation of the brainstem reticular formation. The arousal response to all these drugs is reduced or blocked by atropine and related agents (*see* Krnjević, 1974).

Toxicology. Poisoning from pilocarpine, muscarine, or arecoline is characterized chiefly by exaggeration of their various parasympathomimetic effects, and resembles that produced by consumption of mushrooms of the genus *Inocybe* (*see* below). Treatment consists of the parenteral administration of atropine and adequate measures to support the respiration and the circulation and to counteract pulmonary edema.

Preparations and Dosage. Preparations of pilocarpine include ophthalmic solutions of both *pilocarpine hydrochloride* and *pilocarpine nitrate*. Pilocarpine hydrochloride solutions usually include methylcellulose or a similar polymer and are available under a variety of trade names in concentrations ranging from 0.25 to 10%, while the concentrations of pilocarpine nitrate solutions range from 1 to 4%. Combinations of pilocarpine with epinephrine or physostigmine are also available.

A drug-delivery system (OCUSERT PILO-20 or -40) is available for achieving the sustained release of pilocarpine; it is placed in the cul-de-sac of the eyes. It is an elliptically shaped unit consisting of a pilocarpine-containing reservoir bounded by two layers of copolymer that control delivery of the drug. A relatively constant release of pilocarpine (20 or 40 μg per hour, corresponding to 1% and 2% pilocarpine solutions) is maintained for 7 days. However, variation in duration of action between individuals is substantial. Intraocular pressure may be effectively controlled without the stinging sensation and the myopia experienced immediately after the application of pilocarpine solution. Diurnal control of intraocular pressure may also be improved. Some patients find the foreign body uncomfortable and have difficulty inserting the device.

Aceclidine (GLAUCOSTAT, others) is a synthetic compound that resembles arecoline (*see* Table 6–3). In concentrations of 0.5 to 4.0%, it is approximately as effective as pilocarpine in reducing intraocular pressure in glaucoma (Romano, 1970). The drug is used in Europe but is not currently available in the United States.

THERAPEUTIC USES

Pilocarpine is used in the treatment of glaucoma, where it is generally administered as a 0.5 to 4.0% aqueous solution (*see* Chapter 7). It is usually better tolerated than are the anticholinesterases, and pilocarpine is the standard cholinergic agent for initial treatment of open-angle glaucoma. Reduction of intraocular pressure occurs within a few minutes and lasts 4 to 8 hours. The initial irritation and miosis can be bothersome, and care should be used when treating patients at risk for retinal detachment (Beasley and Fraunfelder, 1979). The miotic action of pilocarpine is useful in overcoming the mydriasis produced by atropine; alternated with mydriatics, pilocarpine is employed to break adhesions between the iris and the lens.

MUSHROOM POISONING (MYCETISM)

Mushroom poisoning has been known for centuries. The Greek poet Euripides (fifth century B.C.) is said to have lost his wife and three children from this cause. In recent years the number of cases of mushroom poisoning has been increasing as the result of the current popularity of the consumption of wild mushrooms (*see Medical Letter*, 1984). Various species of mushrooms contain many toxins, and species within the same genus may contain distinct toxins.

Although *Amanita muscaria* is the source from which muscarine was isolated, its content of the alkaloid is so low (approximately 0.003%) that muscarine cannot be responsible for the major toxic effects. Much higher concentrations of muscarine are present in various species of *Inocybe* and *Clitocybe*. The symptoms of intoxication attributable to muscarine develop within 30 to 60 minutes of ingestion; they include salivation, lacrimation, nausea, vomiting, headache, visual disturbances, abdominal colic, diarrhea, bronchospasm, bradycardia, hypotension, and shock. Treatment with atropine (1 to 2 mg intramuscularly every 30 minutes) effectively blocks these effects.

Intoxication produced by *A. muscaria* and related species arises from the anticholinergic and hallucinogenic properties of a variety of isoxazole derivatives. Symptoms include irritability, restlessness, ataxia, hallucinations, and delirium. Treatment is mainly supportive; atropine is contraindicated, and sedatives are of questionable value (Rumack and Salzman, 1978).

The most serious form of mycetism is produced by *Galerina* species and by *A. verna*, *A. virosa*, *A. ocreata*, and *A. phalloides*, which are fairly common in both North America and Europe (Ammirati *et al.*, 1985). These species account for over 90% of all fatal cases. The principal toxins are the amatoxins (α and β amanitin), a group of cyclic octapeptides that inhibit RNA polymerase II and hence block the synthesis of mRNA. This causes cell death, particularly in the gastrointestinal mucosa, liver, and kidneys. Initial symptoms, which are slow in onset, include diarrhea and abdominal cramps. Death occurs in 4 to 7 days from renal and hepatic failure (Rumack and Salzman, 1978). Treatment is largely supportive; thioctic acid may be an effective antidote in the treatment of this type of mushroom poisoning, but the evidence for this effect is based largely on anecdotal studies (Mitchel, 1980).

Beasley, H., and Fraunfelder, F. T. Retinal detachments and topical ocular miotics. *Ophthalmology (Rochester)*, **1979**, *85*, 95–98.

Bonner, T. L.; Buckley, N. J.; Young, A. C.; and Brann, M. R. Identification of a family of muscarinic receptor genes. *Science*, **1987**, *237*, 527–531.

Cho, A. K.; Haslett, W. L.; and Jenden, D. J. The peripheral actions of oxotremorine, a metabolite of tremorine. *J. Pharmacol. Exp. Ther.*, **1962**, *138*, 249–257.

Eugster, C. H.; Häfliger, F.; Denss, R.; and Girod, E. Die Spaltung von *d,l*-Muscarin in die optischen Antipoden. *Helv. Chim. Acta*, **1958**, *41*, 886–888.

Feigl, E. O. Reflex parasympathetic coronary vasodilatation elicited from cardiac receptors in the dog. *Circ. Res.*, **1975**, *37*, 175–182.

Furchgott, R. F., and Zawadzki, J. V. The obligatory role of endothelial cells in relaxation of arterial smooth muscle by acetylcholine. *Nature*, **1980**, *288*, 373–376.

Kent, K. M., and Epstein, S. E. Neural basis for the genesis and control of arrhythmias associated with myocardial infarction. *Cardiology*, **1976**, *61*, 61–74.

Kent, K. M.; Epstein, S. E.; Cooper, T.; and Jacobowitz, D. M. Cholinergic innervation of the canine and human ventricular conducting system. *Circulation*, **1974**, *50*, 948–955.

Levy, B., and Ahlquist, R. P. A study of sympathetic ganglionic stimulants. *J. Pharmacol. Exp. Ther.*, **1962**, *137*, 219–228.

Medical Letter. Mushroom poisoning. **1984**, *26*, 67–70.

Molitor, H. A comparative study of the effects of five choline compounds used in therapeutics: acetylcholine chloride, acetyl-beta-methycholine chloride, carbaminoyl choline, ethyl ether beta-methylcholine chloride, carbaminoyl beta-methylcholine chloride. *J. Pharmacol. Exp. Ther.*, **1936**, *58*, 337–360.

Priola, D. V.; Spurgeon, M. A.; and Geis, W. P. The intrinsic innervation of the canine heart: a functional study. *Circ. Res.*, **1977**, *40*, 50–56.

Romano, J. H. Double-blind cross-over comparison of aceclidine and pilocarpine in open-angle glaucoma. *Br. J. Ophthalmol.*, **1970**, *54*, 510–521.

Roszkowski, A. P. An unusual type of ganglionic stimulant. *J. Pharmacol. Exp. Ther.*, **1961**, *132*, 156–170.

Saco, L. S.; Orlando, R. C.; Levinson, S. L.; Buzymki, K. M.; Jones, J. D.; and Frakes, J. T. Double-blind controlled trial of bethanechol and antacid versus placebo and antacid in the treatment of erosive esophagitis. *Gastroenterology*, **1982**, *82*, 1369–1373.

Simonart, A. On the action of certain derivatives of choline. *J. Pharmacol. Exp. Ther.*, **1932**, *46*, 157–193.

Starr, I., Jr.; Elsom, K. A.; Reisinger, J. A.; and Richards, A. N. Acetyl-β-methylcholin: action on normal persons with note on action of ethyl ether of β-methylcholin. *Am. J. Med. Sci.*, **1933**, *186*, 313–323.

Thanik, K.; Chey, W. K.; Shak, A.; Hamilton, D.; and Nadelson, N. Bethanechol or cimetidine in the treatment of symptomatic reflex esophagitis. *Arch. Intern. Med.*, **1982**, *142*, 1479–1481.

Monographs and Reviews

Ammirati, J. F.; Traquair, J. A.; and Morgen, P. A. *Poisonous Mushrooms of the Northern United States and Canada*. Fitzhenry and Whiteside, Markham, Ontario, **1985**.

Bebbington, A., and Brimblecombe, R. W. Muscarinic receptors in the peripheral and central nervous systems. *Adv. Drug Res.*, **1965**, *2*, 143–172.

Berne, R. M., and Rubio, R. Coronary circulation. In, *The Cardiovascular System*, Vol. 1. (Berne, R. M., ed.) *Handbook of Physiology*, Sect. II. American Physiological Society, Bethesda, Md., **1979**, pp. 873–952.

Higgins, C. B.; Vatner, S. F.; and Braunwald, E. Parasympathetic control of the heart. *Pharmacol. Rev.*, **1973**, *25*, 119–155.

Kaufman, J. J. (ed.). *Current Urologic Therapy*. W. B. Saunders Co., Philadelphia, **1986**.

Kosterlitz, H. W. Effects of choline esters on smooth muscle and secretions. In, *Physiological Pharmacology*. Vol. 3, *The Nervous System—Part C: Autonomic Nervous System Drugs*. (Root, W. S., and Hofmann, F. G., eds.) Academic Press, Inc., New York, **1967**, pp. 97–161.

Krnjević, K. Chemical nature of synaptic transmission in vertebrates. *Physiol. Rev.*, **1974**, *54*, 418–540.

Levy, M. N., and Martin, P. J. Neural control of the heart. In, *The Cardiovascular System*, Vol. 1. (Berne, R. M., ed.) *Handbook of Physiology*, Sect. II. American Physiological Society, Bethesda, Md., **1979**, pp. 581–620.

Mitchel, D. H. *Amanita* mushroom poisoning. *Annu. Rev. Med.*, **1980**, *31*, 51–57.

Rand, M. J., and Stafford, A. Cardiovascular effects of choline esters. In, *Physiological Pharmacology*. Vol. 3, *The Nervous System—Part C: Autonomic Nervous System Drugs*. (Root, W. S., and Hofmann, F. G., eds.) Academic Press, Inc., New York, **1967**, pp. 1–95.

Rumack, B. H., and Salzman, E. *Mushroom Poisoning: Diagnosis and Treatment*. CRC Press, West Palm Beach, Fla., **1978**.

Symposium. (Various authors.) Subtypes of muscarinic receptors III. *Trends Pharmacol. Sci.*, **1988**, Suppl.

Vanhoutte, P. M. Endothelium and control of vascular function. *Hypertension*, **1989**, *13*, 658–667.

Watanabe, A. M. Cholinergic agonists and antagonists. In, *Cardiac Therapy*. (Rosen, M. R., and Hoffman, B. F., eds.) Martinus Nijhoff Publishing, Hingham, Mass., **1983**, pp. 95–144.

Wein, A. J., and Barrett, D. M. *Voiding Function and Dysfunction*. Yearbook Medical Publishers, Inc., Chicago, **1988**.

CHAPTER

7 ANTICHOLINESTERASE AGENTS

Palmer Taylor

The function of acetylcholinesterase (AChE) in terminating the action of acetylcholine (ACh) at the junctions of the various cholinergic nerve endings with their effector organs or postsynaptic sites is considered in Chapter 5. Drugs that inhibit AChE are called *anticholinesterase* (anti-ChE) agents. They cause ACh to accumulate at cholinergic receptor sites and thus are potentially capable of producing effects equivalent to excessive stimulation of cholinergic receptors throughout the central and peripheral nervous systems. In view of the widespread distribution of cholinergic neurons, it is not surprising that the anti-ChE agents as a group have received extensive application as toxic agents, in the form of agricultural insecticides and potential chemical-warfare "nerve gases." Nevertheless, several members of this class of compounds are used as therapeutic agents.

Prior to World War II, only the "reversible" anti-ChE agents were generally known, of which physostigmine is the outstanding example. Shortly before and during World War II, a comparatively new class of highly toxic chemicals, the organophosphates, was developed chiefly by Schrader, of I. G. Farbenindustrie, first as agricultural insecticides and later as potential chemical-warfare agents. The extreme toxicity of these compounds was found to be due to their "irreversible" inactivation of AChE, which resulted in long-lasting inhibitory activity. Since the pharmacological actions of both classes of anti-ChE agents are qualitatively similar, they will be discussed here as a group. Certain effects of anti-ChE agents and their interactions with other drugs at autonomic ganglia and the neuromuscular junction are described in Chapter 9.

History. Physostigmine, also called eserine, is an alkaloid obtained from the Calabar or ordeal bean, the dried ripe seed of *Physostigma venenosum* Balfour, a perennial plant found in tropical West Africa. The Calabar bean, also called Esére nut, chop nut, or bean of Etu Esére, was once used by native tribes of West Africa as an "ordeal poison" in trials for witchcraft.

The Calabar bean was brought to England in 1840 by Daniell, a British medical officer stationed in Calabar, and early investigations of its pharmacological properties were conducted by Christioson (1855), Fraser (1863), and Argyll-Robertson (1863). A pure alkaloid was isolated by Jobst and Hesse in 1864 and named *physostigmine*. The first therapeutic use of the drug was in 1877 by Laqueur, in the treatment of glaucoma, one of its clinical uses today. Interesting accounts of the history of physostigmine have been presented by Karczmar (1970) and Holmstedt (1972).

As a result of the basic research of Stedman (1929a, 1929b) and associates in elucidating the chemical basis of the activity of physostigmine, others began systematic investigations of a series of substituted phenyl esters of alkyl carbamic acids. Neostigmine, a most promising member of this series, was introduced into therapeutics in 1931 for its stimulant action on the intestinal tract. It was subsequently reported to be effective in the symptomatic treatment of myasthenia gravis.

It is remarkable that the first account of the synthesis of a highly potent compound of the organophosphorus anti-ChE series, tetraethyl pyrophosphate (TEPP), was published by Clermont in 1854, 10 years prior to the isolation of physostigmine. More remarkable still, as Holmstedt (1963) pointed out, is the fact that the investigator survived to report on the compound's taste; a few drops should have been lethal. Modern investigations of the organophosphorus compounds date from the 1932 publication of Lange and Krueger on the synthesis of dimethyl and diethyl phosphorofluoridates. The authors' statement that inhalation of these compounds caused a persistent choking sensation and blurred vision apparently was instrumental in leading Schrader to explore this class for insecticidal activity.

Upon synthesizing approximately 2000 compounds, Schrader (1952) defined the structural requirements for insecticidal (and, as learned subsequently, for anti-ChE) activity (*see* below). One compound in this early series, parathion, later became the most widely used insecticide of this class. Prior to and during World War II, the efforts of Schrader's group were directed toward the development of chemical-warfare agents. The synthesis of several compounds of much greater toxicity than parathion, such as sarin, soman, and tabun, was kept secret by the German government. Investigators in the Allied countries also followed Lange and

Krueger's lead in the search for potentially toxic compounds; di*iso*propyl phosphorofluoridate (DFP), synthesized by McCombie and Saunders (1946), was the organophosphorus compound studied most extensively by British and American scientists.

In the 1950s, a series of heterocyclic, aromatic, and naphthyl carbamates was synthesized and found to have a high degree of selective toxicity against insects and to be potent anti-ChE agents (Gysin, 1954). Among those currently employed as insecticides are 1-naphthyl N-methylcarbamate (carbaril or carbaryl; SEVIN) and 2-isopropoxyphenyl N-methylcarbamate (BAYGON) (*see* Hayes, 1982; Murphy, 1986; WHO, 1986a, 1986b).

Structure of Acetylcholinesterase. AChE exists in two classes of molecular forms: simple oligomers of homologous catalytic subunits (*i.e.*, monomers, dimers, and tetramers) and associations of heterologous subunits that form complex, elongated molecular structures (Massoulié and Toutant, 1988). The homologous oligomers often contain a glycophospholipid attached to the carboxyl terminus (Silman and Futerman, 1987) and are bound to the outer surface of the plasma membrane. The heterologous forms consist of tetramers of the catalytic subunit, but the tetramers in turn are linked by disulfide bonds to a collagen-containing filamentous structure (Lwebuga-Mukasa *et al.*, 1976; Rosenberry and Richardson, 1977). The molecular weights of these latter forms approach 10^6, and their structure is analogous to balloons attached to a branching stalk (Cartaud *et al.*, 1975). The composition of the elongated forms, their susceptibility to dissolution from the synapse by collagenases, and their retention in synaptic areas after degeneration of the nerve and muscle plasma membranes all indicate that these forms are localized in the outer basal lamina (basement membrane) of the synapse, rather than in the plasma membrane of the nerve ending or muscle end-plate. Deposition of the elongated forms occurs during synaptogenesis, and these forms are primarily found in junctional areas of skeletal muscle (Hall, 1973; Massoulié and Toutant, 1988).

Amino acid sequencing and molecular cloning reveal that a single gene encodes the catalytic subunits of the acetylcholinesterases. However, these proteins are heterogeneous, having distinctive carboxyl-termini ends; this heterogeneity arises as a result of alternative processing of mRNA (Schumacher *et al.*, 1986; Gibney *et al.*, 1988). Control of the expression of the particular catalytic subunit then dictates the posttranslational steps of subunit assembly and processing that yield the individual molecular species described above. A separate but structurally related gene encodes the butyrylcholinesterase found in plasma (Lockridge *et al.*, 1987). The cholinesterases are members of a superfamily of serine hydrolases, which includes several esterases not involved in nervous system function and, surprisingly, thyroglobulin (Schumacher *et al.*, 1986).

The active center of AChE consists of a negative subsite, which attracts the quaternary group of choline through both coulombic and hydrophobic forces, and an esteratic subsite, where nucleophilic attack occurs on the acyl carbon of the substrate (Figure 7–1, I–A). The catalytic mechanism resembles that of other serine esterases, where a serine hydroxyl group is rendered highly nucleophilic through a charge-relay system involving the close apposition of an imidazole group and, presumably, a carboxyl group on the enzyme. During enzymatic attack on the ester, a tetrahedral intermediate between enzyme and ester is formed (Figure 7–1, I–B) that collapses to an acetyl enzyme conjugate with the concomitant release of choline (Figure 7–1, I–C). The acetyl enzyme is labile to hydrolysis, which results in the formation of acetate and active enzyme (Figure 7–1, I–D) (*see* Froede and Wilson, 1971; Rosenberry, 1975). AChE is one of the most efficient enzymes known and has the capacity to hydrolyze 3×10^5 ACh molecules per molecule of enzyme per minute; this indicates a turnover time of 150 microseconds.

Mechanism of Action of AChE Inhibitors.

The mechanisms of action of compounds that typify the three classes of anti-ChE agents are also shown in Figure 7–1 (II, III, IV).

Quaternary compounds inhibit the enzyme reversibly by combining either at the active center or at a site spatially removed from the active center—the peripheral anionic site (Changeux, 1966; Taylor and Lappi, 1975). The potent reversible inhibitor edrophonium binds selectively to the active center. The complex is stabilized by interaction of the quaternary nitrogen at the anionic subsite and by hydrogen bonding (Wilson and Quan, 1958) (*see* Figure 7–1, II). Edrophonium has a brief duration of action owing to the reversibility of its binding to AChE and rapid renal elimination following systemic administration.

Drugs such as physostigmine and neostigmine that have a carbamyl ester linkage are hydrolyzed by AChE, but much more slowly than is ACh (Wilson *et al.*, 1960). Both the quaternary amine, neostigmine, and the tertiary amine, physostigmine, exist as cations at physiological pH. By serving as alternate substrates (*see* Figure 7–1, III–A, B), the alcohol moiety is cleaved, giving rise to the carbamoylated enzyme. In contrast to the acetyl enzyme, methylcarbamoyl AChE or dimethylcarbamoyl AChE is far more stable ($t_{1/2}$ for hydrolysis of the dimethylcarbamoyl enzyme is 15 to 30 minutes; *see* Figure 7–1, III–C) (Wilson and Harrison, 1961). Sequestration of the enzyme in its carbamoylated form thus precludes the enzyme-catalyzed hydrolysis of ACh for extended periods of time. *In vivo*, the duration of inhibition by the carbamoylating agents is 3 to 4 hours.

The organophosphorus inhibitors, such as DFP, serve as true hemisubstrates, since the resultant phosphorylated or phosphonylated enzyme is extremely stable (*see* Figure 7–1, IV–A, B). Reaction occurs at the esteratic subsite and is enhanced

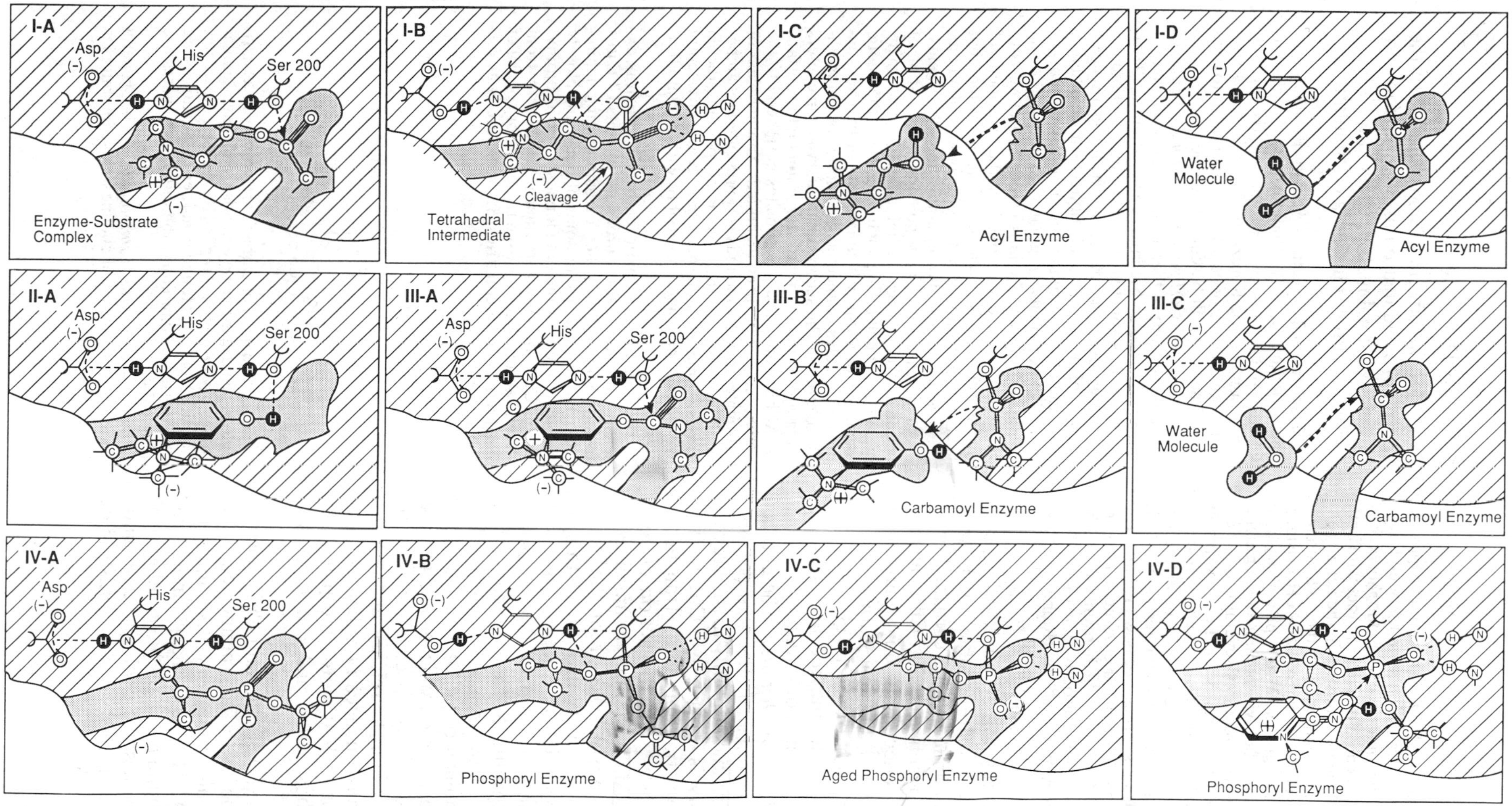

Figure 7–1. *Steps involved in the hydrolysis of acetylcholine by acetylcholinesterase and in the inhibition and reactivation of the enzyme.*

The processes are shown are follows: I–A, binding of substrate; I–B, attack of the serine hydroxyl with formation of the transient tetrahedral intermediate; I–C, loss of choline and formation of the acetyl enzyme; and I–D, deacylation of the enzyme by attack with H_2O. II–A, binding of the reversible inhibitor edrophonium to the active site. III–A, binding of neostigmine; III–B, formation of the carbamoylated enzyme; and III–C, hydrolysis of the carbamoylated enzyme. IV–A, binding of diisopropyl fluorophosphate; IV–B, formation of the phosphoryl enzyme; IV–C, formation of an aged form of the enzyme; and IV–D, attack by pralidoxime to regenerate active enzyme.

by the geometry of the tetrahedral phosphates, which resemble the transition state for acetyl ester hydrolysis. Certain quaternary organophosphorus compounds (*e.g.*, echothiophate) interact with both the esteratic and anionic subsites in the active center; this interaction contributes to the high potency and selectivity of these agents (*see* Holmstedt, 1963). If the alkyl groups in the phosphorylated enzyme are ethyl or methyl, spontaneous regeneration of active enzyme requires several hours. Secondary (as in DFP) or tertiary alkyl groups further enhance the stability of the phosphorylated enzyme, and significant regeneration of active enzyme is not observed. Hence, the return of AChE activity depends on synthesis of new enzyme. The stability of the phosphorylated enzyme is also enhanced through "aging," which results from the loss of one of the alkyl groups (*see* Figure 7–1, IV–C; *see also* Aldridge, 1976; Hobbiger, 1976).

From the foregoing account, it is apparent that the terms "reversible" and "irreversible," as applied to the carbamyl ester and organophosphorus anti-ChE agents, respectively, reflect only quantitative differences in rates of deacylation of the acylenzyme. Both chemical classes react covalently with the enzyme in essentially the same manner as does ACh.

Action at Effector Organs. The characteristic pharmacological effects of the anti-ChE agents are due primarily to the prevention of hydrolysis of ACh by AChE at sites of cholinergic transmission. Transmitter thus accumulates, and the action of ACh that is liberated by cholinergic impulses or that spontaneously leaks from the nerve ending is enhanced. With most of the organophosphorus agents, such as DFP, virtually all the acute effects of moderate doses are attributable to this action. For example, the characteristic miosis that follows local application of DFP to the eye is not observed after chronic postganglionic denervation of the eye because there is no source from which to release endogenous ACh. The consequences of enhanced concentrations of ACh at motor end-plates are unique to these sites and are discussed below.

Among the classical anti-ChE agents, physostigmine, a tertiary amine, can also block nicotinic receptors (Albuquerque *et al.*, 1987). The quaternary ammonium anti-ChE compounds all have additional direct actions at some cholinergic receptor sites, either as agonists or antagonists. For example, the effects of neostigmine on the spinal cord and neuromuscular junction are based on a combination of its anti-ChE activity and direct cholinergic stimulation.

Chemistry and Structure–Activity Relationships. The structure–activity relationships of anti-ChE drugs have been reviewed extensively (Holmstedt, 1963; Long, 1963; Karczmar, 1967; Usdin, 1970). Only those agents of general therapeutic or toxicological interest will be considered here.

"Reversible" Carbamate Inhibitors. Drugs of this class that are of therapeutic interest are shown in Table 7–1. From Stedman's early studies (1929a, 1929b), it was concluded that the essential moiety of the physostigmine molecule was the methyl carbamate of a basically substituted simple phenol. The quaternary ammonium derivative, neostigmine, is a compound of greater stability and equal or greater potency. Pyridostigmine is a close congener that is also employed in the treatment of myasthenia gravis. Analogs of neostigmine that lack the carbamoyl group, such as edrophonium, are less potent and shorter-acting anti-ChE agents.

An increase in anti-ChE potency and duration of action can result from the linking of two quaternary ammonium nuclei. One such example is the miotic agent demecarium, which consists of two neostigmine molecules connected by a series of ten methylene groups. The second quaternary group confers additional stability to the interaction on the surface of AChE, since negative subsites peripheral to the active center have been identified. Another class of *bis*-quaternary compounds is represented by ambenonium, used in the treatment of myasthenia gravis. Ambenonium does not react covalently with AChE but binds reversibly with a high affinity.

The insecticide carbaril (carbaryl), which is extensively used in garden products, inhibits ChE in a fashion identical to other carbamoylating inhibitors. The signs and symptoms of poisoning closely resemble those of the organophosphates (Murphy, 1986). Carbaril has a particularly low toxicity from dermal absorption. It is used topically for control of head lice in some countries. Its structure is as follows:

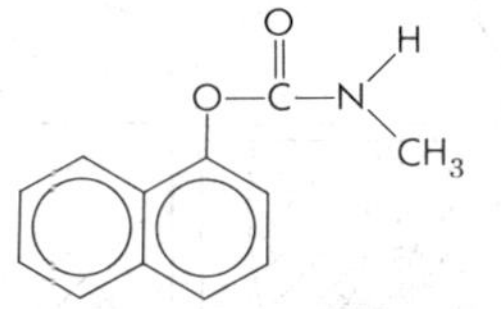

Carbaril

Several analogs of carbaril are employed as agricultural and garden insecticides and have similar inhibitory properties (*see* WHO, 1986b). However, not all carbamates found in garden formulations are cholinesterase inhibitors; the dithiocarbamates are fungicidal.

Organophosphorus Compounds. The general formula for this class of cholinesterase inhibitors is

Table 7–1. REPRESENTATIVE "REVERSIBLE" ANTICHOLINESTERASE AGENTS EMPLOYED CLINICALLY

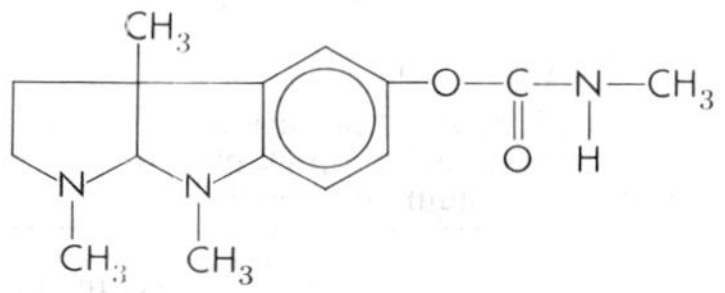

Physostigmine

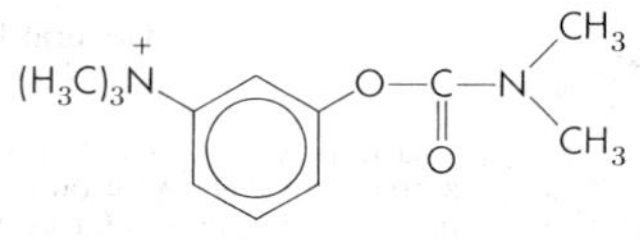

Neostigmine

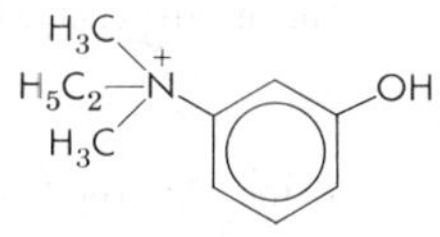

Edrophonium

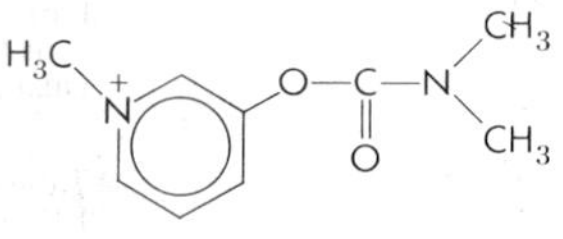

Pyridostigmine

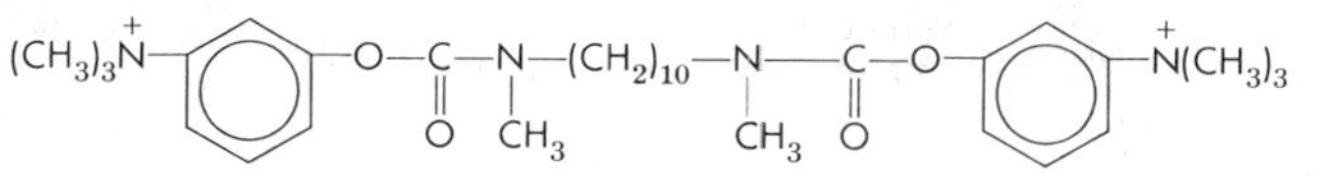

Demecarium

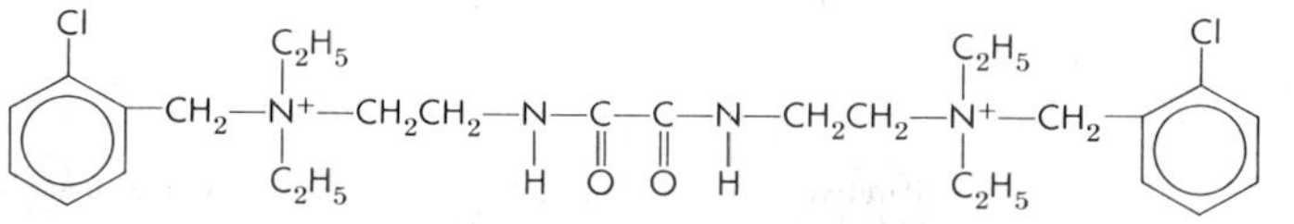

Ambenonium

presented in Table 7–2. A great variety of substituents is possible: R_1 and R_2 may be alkyl, alkoxy, aryloxy, amido, mercaptan, or other groups, and X, the leaving group, may represent a halide, cyanide, thiocyanate, phenoxy, thiophenoxy, phosphate, thiocholine, or carboxylate group (Holmstedt, 1963). For a compilation of the organophosphorus compounds and their toxicity, *see* Hayes (1982).

Di*iso*propyl phosphorofluoridate (DFP) is perhaps the most extensively studied compound of this general class as the result of its toxicological evaluation during World War II. It produces virtually irreversible inactivation of AChE and other esterases by alkylphosphorylation. Its high lipid solubility, low molecular weight, and volatility facilitate inhalation, transdermal absorption, and penetration into the central nervous system (CNS).

The "nerve gases"—tabun, sarin, and soman—are among the most potent synthetic toxic agents known; they are lethal to laboratory animals in submilligram doses.

Because of its low volatility and stability in aqueous solution, parathion (ETILON, FOLIDOL, NIRAN) became widely used as an insecticide. It continues to be used extensively in agriculture, but less hazardous compounds have become popular for home and garden use. Parathion itself is inactive in inhibiting AChE *in vitro;* paraoxon is the active metabolite. The sulfur-for-oxygen substitution is carried out predominantly in the liver by the mixed-function oxygenases. This reaction is also carried out less efficiently in the insect. Parathion has probably been responsible for more cases of accidental poisoning and death than any other organophosphorus compound. Other insecticides possessing the phosphorothiolate structure are widely employed for home, garden, and agricultural use. These include dimpylate (diazinon), fenthion, and chlorpyrifos.

Malathion (CHEMATHION, MALA-SPRAY) also requires replacement of a sulfur atom with oxygen *in vivo*. This insecticide can be detoxified by hydrolysis of the carboxyl ester linkage by plasma carboxylesterases. The detoxification reaction is much more rapid in mammals and birds than in insects, giving rise to an additional degree of selective toxicity (*see* Murphy, 1986; Costa *et al.*, 1987). In recent years, malathion has been employed in aerial spraying of relatively populous areas for control of Mediterranean fruit flies and mosquitoes. Little evidence for acute toxicity has been reported. The lethal dose in mammals is about 1 g/kg. Exposure to the skin results in a small fraction (< 10%) of systemic absorption.

Among the quaternary ammonium organophosphorus compounds (group E in Table 7–2), only echothiophate is useful clinically. Being positively charged, it is not volatile and does not readily penetrate the skin.

PHARMACOLOGICAL PROPERTIES

Generally, the pharmacological properties of anti-ChE agents can be predicted by knowing those loci where ACh is released

Table 7–2. CHEMICAL CLASSIFICATION OF REPRESENTATIVE ORGANOPHOSPHORUS COMPOUNDS OF PARTICULAR PHARMACOLOGICAL OR TOXICOLOGICAL INTEREST *

General formula (Schrader, 1952): 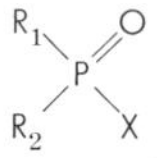

Group A, X = halogen, cyanide, or thiocyanate; group B, X = alkylthio, arylthio, alkoxy, or aryloxy; group C, thiol- or thionophosphorus compounds; group D, pyrophosphates and similar compounds; group E, quaternary ammonium compounds

GROUP	STRUCTURAL FORMULA	COMMON, CHEMICAL, AND OTHER NAMES	COMMENTS
A	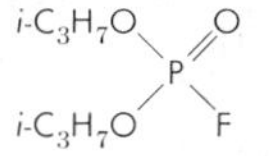	DFP; Isoflurophate (*see* trade names in text) Di*iso*propyl phosphorofluoridate	Potent, irreversible inactivator
	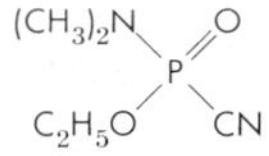	Tabun Ethyl N-dimethylphosphoramidocyanidate	Extremely toxic "nerve gas"
	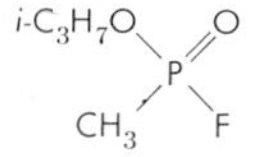	Sarin (GB) *Iso*propyl methylphosphonofluoridate	Extremely toxic "nerve gas"
	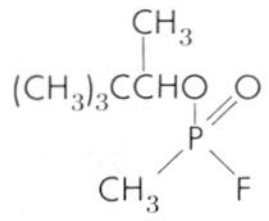	Soman Pinacolyl methylphosphonofluoridate	Extremely toxic "nerve gas"
B	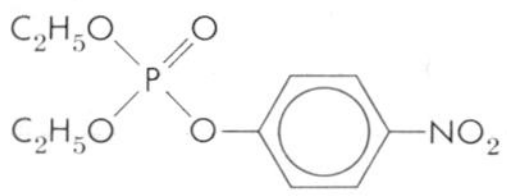	Paraoxon (MINTACOL), E 600 O,O-Diethyl O-(4-nitrophenyl)-phosphate	Active metabolite of parathion
C	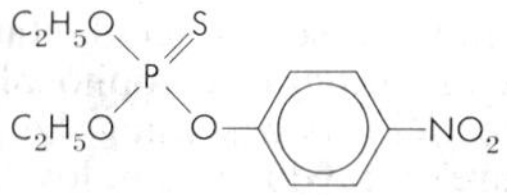	Parathion (*see* trade names in text) O,O-Diethyl O-(4-nitrophenyl)-phosphorothioate	Employed as agricultural insecticide, resulting in numerous cases of accidental poisoning
	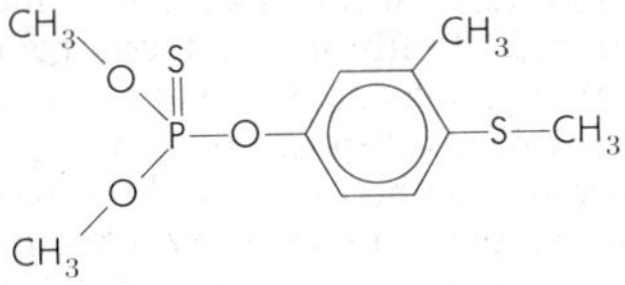	Fenthion O,O-Dimethyl O-4-methylthio-*m*-tolyl phosphorothioate	Insecticide with high lipid solubility; agricultural use
	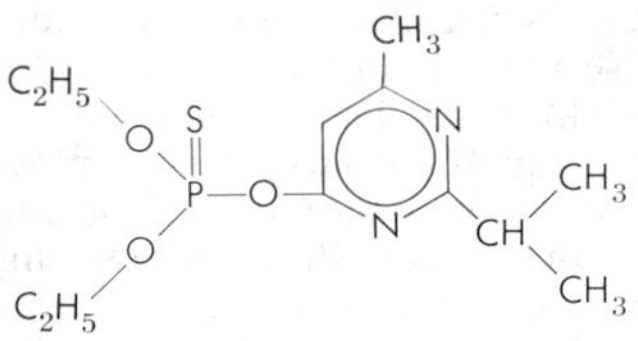	Dimpylate, Diazinon O,O-Diethyl 2-isopropyl-6-methyl-4-pyrimidinyl phosphorothioate	Insecticide in wide use for gardening and agriculture
	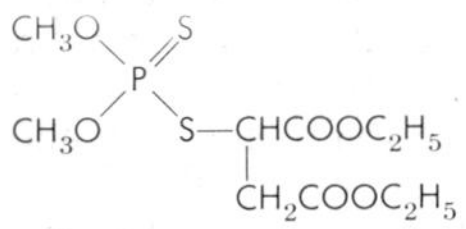	Malathion O,O-Dimethyl S-(1,2-dicarbethoxyethyl) phosphorodithioate	Widely employed insecticide of greater safety than parathion or other agents because of rapid detoxification by higher organisms
D	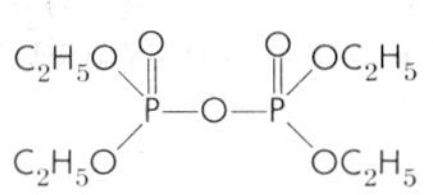	TEPP Tetraethyl pyrophosphate	Early insecticide
E	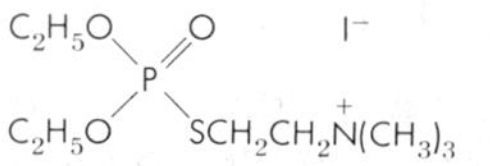	Echothiophate (PHOSPHOLINE IODIDE), MI-217 Diethoxyphosphinylthiocholine iodide	Extremely potent choline derivative; employed in treatment of glaucoma; relatively stable in aqueous solution

* After Holmstedt, 1963. *See also* Hobbiger, 1976; Hayes, 1982.

physiologically by nerve impulses, the degree of nerve impulse activity, and the responses of the corresponding effector organs to ACh (*see* Chapter 5). The anti-ChE agents can potentially produce all the following effects: (1) stimulation of muscarinic receptor responses at autonomic effector organs; (2) stimulation, followed by depression or paralysis, of all autonomic ganglia and skeletal muscle (nicotinic actions); and (3) stimulation, with occasional subsequent depression, of cholinergic receptor sites in the CNS. Following toxic or lethal doses of anti-ChE agents, most of these effects can be noted (*see* below). However, with smaller doses, particularly those used therapeutically, several modifying factors are significant. Compounds such as parathion become more toxic when distributed systemically, owing to conversion to the active form, paraoxon. In general, compounds containing a quaternary ammonium group do not penetrate cell membranes readily; hence, anti-ChE agents in this category are absorbed poorly from the gastrointestinal tract or across the skin and are excluded from the CNS by the blood–brain barrier after moderate doses. On the other hand, such compounds act relatively selectively at the neuromuscular junctions of skeletal muscle, exerting their action both as anti-ChE agents and as direct agonists. They have comparatively less effect at autonomic effector sites; their ganglionic actions are generally intermediate. In contrast, the more lipid-soluble agents are well absorbed after oral administration and have ubiquitous effects at both peripheral and central cholinergic receptor sites. The lipid-soluble organophosphates are also well absorbed through the skin, and the volatile agents are readily transferred across the alveolar membrane.

The actions of anti-ChE agents on autonomic effector cells and on cortical and subcortical sites in the CNS, where the receptors are largely of the muscarinic type, are blocked by atropine. Likewise, atropine blocks some of the excitatory actions of anti-ChE agents on autonomic ganglia, since stimulation of both nicotinic and muscarinic receptors is involved in ganglionic neurotransmission (*see* Chapter 9).

The main actions of anti-ChE agents that are of therapeutic importance are concerned with the eye, the intestine, and the skeletal neuromuscular junction; most of the other actions are of toxicological interest.

Eye. When applied locally to the conjunctiva, anti-ChE agents cause conjunctival hyperemia and constriction of the sphincter pupillae muscle around the pupillary margin of the iris (miosis) and the ciliary muscle (block of accommodation reflex with resultant focusing to near vision). Miosis is apparent in a few minutes, becomes maximal in 0.5 hour, and can last several hours to days. Although the pupil may be "pinpoint" in size, it generally contracts further when exposed to light. The block of accommodation is more transient and generally disappears before termination of the miosis. Intraocular pressure, when elevated, usually falls as the result of facilitation of outflow of the aqueous humor.

Gastrointestinal Tract. The actions of various anti-ChE agents on the gastrointestinal tract are nearly identical. In man, neostigmine enhances gastric contractions and increases the secretion of gastric acid. The drug tends to counteract the inhibition of gastric tone and motility induced by atropine, and enhances the stimulatory effect of morphine. After bilateral vagotomy, the effects of neostigmine on gastric motility are greatly reduced. The lower portion of the esophagus is stimulated by neostigmine; in patients with marked achalasia and dilatation of the esophagus, the drug can cause a salutary increase in tone and peristalsis.

Neostigmine augments the motor activity of the small and large bowel; the colon is particularly stimulated. Atony may be overcome or prevented, propulsive waves are increased in amplitude and frequency, and movement of intestinal contents is thus promoted. The total effect of anti-ChE agents on intestinal motility probably represents a combination of actions at the ganglion cells of Auerbach's plexus and at the smooth muscle fibers, as a result of the preservation of ACh released by the cholinergic preganglionic and postganglionic fibers, respectively.

Skeletal Neuromuscular Junction. Most of the effects of potent anti-ChE drugs on muscle fibers can be adequately explained on the basis of their inhibition of AChE at neuromuscular junctions. However, there is good evidence for an accessory direct action of neostigmine and other quaternary ammonium anti-ChE agents on skeletal muscle. For example, the intraarterial injection of neostigmine into chronically denervated muscle, or into normally innervated muscle in which essentially all the AChE has been inactivated by prior administration of DFP, evokes an immediate contraction, whereas physostigmine does not.

Normally, a single nerve impulse in a terminal motor-axon branch liberates enough ACh to produce a localized depolarization (end-plate potential) of sufficient magnitude to initiate a propagated muscle action potential. The ACh released is rapidly hydrolyzed by AChE, such that the lifetime of free ACh within the synapse (~200 microseconds) is shorter than the decay of the end-plate potential or the refractory period of the muscle (Colquhoun, 1979). Therefore, each nerve impulse gives rise to a single wave of depolarization. After inhibition of AChE the residence time of ACh in the synapse increases, allowing for rebinding of transmitter to multiple receptors. Successive stimulation at neighboring receptors results in a prolongation of the decay of the end-plate potential. Quanta released by individual nerve impulses are no longer isolated. This action destroys the synchrony between end-plate depolarizations and the development of the action potentials. Consequently, asynchronous excitation and fibrillation of muscle fibers are observed. With sufficient inhibition of AChE, depolarization of the end-plate predominates and blockade owing to depolarization ensues (*see* Chapter 9). When ACh persists in the synapse, it may also depolarize the axon terminal, resulting in antidromic firing of the motoneuron; this effect contributes to fasciculations, which involve the entire motor unit. The effect may result from a direct action on prejunctional sites or involve release of K^+ into the synapse.

The anti-ChE agents will reverse the antagonism caused by competitive neuromuscular blocking agents. Neostigmine is not usually effective against the skeletal muscle paralysis caused by succinylcholine, since this agent also produces neuromuscular blockade by depolarization. However, partial reversal can often be achieved if the duration of action of succinylcholine is prolonged and phase-II block is evident (Futter *et al.*, 1983; *see* Chapter 9).

Actions at Other Sites. Secretory glands that are innervated by postganglionic cholinergic fibers include the bronchial, lacrimal, sweat, salivary, gastric (antral G cells and parietal cells), intestinal, and acinar pancreatic glands. Low doses of anti-ChE agents cause, in general, augmentation of these glands' secretory responses to nerve stimulation, and higher doses actually produce an increase in the resting rate of secretion.

Anti-ChE agents cause contraction of smooth muscle fibers of the bronchioles and ureters, and the ureters may show increased peristaltic activity.

The cardiovascular actions of anti-ChE agents are complex, since they reflect both ganglionic and postganglionic effects of accumulated ACh on the heart and blood vessels. The predominant effect on the heart from the peripheral action of accumulated ACh is bradycardia, resulting in a fall in cardiac output. Higher doses usually cause a fall in blood pressure, often as a consequence of effects of anti-ChE agents on the medullary vasomotor centers of the CNS.

Anti-ChE agents shorten the effective refractory period of cardiac atrial muscle fibers, and increase the refractory period and conduction time of the SA and AV nodes. The blood vessels are in general dilated, although the coronary and pulmonary circulation may show the opposite response. At the ganglionic level, ACh first has an excitatory and at higher concentrations an inhibitory action. The excitatory action on the parasympathetic ganglion cells would tend to reinforce the diminished cardiac output, whereas the opposite sequence would result from the action of ACh on sympathetic ganglion cells. Excitation followed by inhibition is also produced by ACh at the medullary vasomotor and cardiac centers. All these effects are complicated further by the hypoxemia resulting from the bronchoconstrictor and secretory actions of increased ACh on the respiratory system; hypoxemia, in turn, would reinforce both sympathetic tone and ACh-induced discharge of epinephrine from the adrenal medulla. Hence, it is not surprising that a wide variety of hemodynamic effects has been reported following administration of anti-ChE agents.

At autonomic ganglia, as indicated above, low concentrations of ACh or of anti-ChE agents cause spontaneous firing of the ganglion cells in response to submaximal preganglionic stimulation. This effect results from the activation of both muscarinic and nicotinic receptors. The ganglionic blockade from higher concentrations of anti-ChE drugs results from persistent depolarization of the cell membrane induced at nicotinic receptors (*see* Chapter 9).

The effects of anti-ChE drugs on the CNS are likewise characterized by stimulation or facilitation at various sites, succeeded by inhibition or paralysis at higher concentrations. Hypoxemia is probably a major factor in CNS depression that appears after large doses of anti-ChE agents. The stimulant effects are antagonized by atropine, although not as completely as are the muscarinic effects at peripheral autonomic effector sites.

Absorption, Fate, and Excretion. Physostigmine is readily absorbed from the gastrointestinal tract, subcutaneous tissues, and mucous membranes. The conjunctival instillation of solutions of the drug may result in systemic effects if measures (*e.g.*, pressure on inner canthus) are not taken to prevent absorption from the nasal mucosa. The alkaloid is largely destroyed in the body, mainly by hydrolytic cleavage at the ester linkage by plasma esterases; renal excretion plays only a minor role in its disposal. In man, a 1-mg dose of physostigmine injected subcutaneously is largely destroyed in 2 hours.

Neostigmine and related quaternary ammonium drugs are absorbed poorly after oral administration, such that much larger doses are needed than by the parenteral route. Whereas the effective parenteral dose of neostigmine in man is 0.5 to 2.0 mg, the equivalent oral dose may be 15 to 30 mg or more. Large oral doses may prove toxic if intestinal absorption is enhanced for any reason. Neostigmine is destroyed by plasma esterases, and the quaternary alcohol and parent compound are excreted in the urine; the half-life of the drug is only 1 to 2 hours. Pyridostigmine and its quaternary alcohol are also the predominant entities found in urine after administration of this drug to man (Somani *et al.*, 1972; Cohan *et al.*, 1976; *see* Appendix II).

The commonly encountered organophosphorus anti-ChE agents are, with certain exceptions (*e.g.*, echothiophate), highly lipid-soluble liquids; many have high vapor pressures. The less volatile agents that are commonly used as agricultural insecticides (*e.g.*, parathion, malathion) are generally dispersed as aerosols or as dusts consisting of the organophosphorus compound adsorbed to an inert, finely particulate material. Consequently, the compounds are rapidly and effectively absorbed by practically all routes, including the gastrointestinal tract, as well as through the skin and mucous membranes following contact with moisture, and by the lungs after inhalation.

Following their absorption, most organophosphorus compounds are excreted almost entirely as hydrolysis products in the urine. Plasma and tissue enzymes are responsible for hydrolysis to the corresponding phosphoric and phosphonic acids. However, oxidative enzymes are also involved in the metabolism of some organophosphorus compounds.

The organophosphorus anti-ChE agents are hydrolyzed in the body by a group of enzymes known as A-esterases, or paroxonase, and by the cytochrome P_{450} system. Considerable variability exists in the human population for organophosphate metabolism by these routes (Omenn, 1987). The A-esterases are found in plasma and in the hepatic endoplasmic reticulum and can hydrolyze a large number of organophosphorus compounds (*e.g.*, DFP, tabun, sarin, paraoxon, TEPP) by splitting the anhydride, P—F, P—CN, or ester bond. The enzymes are not inhibited by organophosphorus compounds, presumably because the phosphorylated active-site serine residue reacts rapidly with water to regenerate the free form, in contrast to its high stability in the case of the cholinesterases. Acquired resistance of insects to certain insecticides of this class results from the adaptive elaboration of such enzymes. Malathion and other organophosphorus compounds containing carboxylesters undergo hydrolysis at these ester linkages. This reaction is catalyzed by plasma esterases that can be inhibited by organophosphorus compounds. Thus, the activity and toxicity from exposure to two organophosphorus insecticides may be supra-additive (Su *et al.*, 1971; Murphy, 1986).

TOXICOLOGY

The toxicological aspects of the anti-ChE agents are of practical importance to the physician. In addition to numerous cases of accidental intoxication from the use and manufacture of organophosphorus compounds as agricultural insecticides, these agents have been used frequently for homicidal and suicidal purposes, largely because of their accessibility. Occupational exposure occurs most commonly by the dermal and pulmonary routes, while oral ingestion is most common in cases of nonoccupational poisoning. In addition, chronic exposure to several organophosphorus compounds, in particular triarylphosphates, can produce a delayed neuropathy characterized by demyelination and axonal degeneration; these effects are apparently not due to inhibition of cholinesterases but rather to inhibition of a separate enzyme, termed the *neurotoxic esterase*. It is common practice to screen for this toxicity in the evaluation of the safety of new insecticides.

Acute Intoxication. The effects of acute intoxication by anti-ChE agents are manifested by muscarinic and nicotinic signs and symptoms and, except for compounds of extremely low lipid solubility, by signs referable to the CNS. Local effects are due to the action of vapors or aerosols at their site of contact with the eyes or respiratory tract, or to the local absorption after liquid contamination of the skin or mucous membranes, including those of the gastrointestinal tract. Systemic effects appear within minutes after inhalation of vapors or aerosols. In contrast, the onset of symptoms is delayed after gastrointestinal and percutaneous absorption. The duration of effects is determined largely by the properties of the compound: its lipid solubility, whether it must be activated, the stability of the organophosphorus–AChE bond, and whether "aging" of the phosphorylated enzyme has occurred.

After local exposure to vapors or aerosols or after their inhalation, ocular and respiratory effects generally appear first. Ocular effects include marked miosis, ocular pain, conjunctival congestion, diminished vision, ciliary spasm, and brow ache. With acute systemic absorption, miosis may not be evident due to sympathetic discharge in response to the hypotension. In addition to rhinorrhea and hyperemia of the upper respiratory tract, respiratory effects consist of "tightness" in the chest and wheezing respiration, caused by the combination of bronchoconstriction and increased bronchial secretion. Gastrointestinal symptoms occur earliest after ingestion, and include anorexia, nausea and vomiting, abdominal cramps, and diarrhea. With percutaneous absorption of liquid, localized sweating and muscular fasciculation in the immediate vicinity are generally the earliest manifestations. Additional muscarinic effects include those discussed under pharmacological properties; severe intoxication is manifested by extreme salivation, involuntary defecation and urination, sweating, lacrimation, penile erection, bradycardia, and hypotension.

Nicotinic actions at the neuromuscular junctions of skeletal muscle usually consist of fatigability and generalized weakness, involuntary twitchings, scattered fasciculations, and eventually severe weakness and paralysis; a central component of action may contribute to some of these effects. The most serious consequence of the neuromuscular actions is paralysis of the respiratory muscles.

The broad spectrum of effects on the CNS include confusion, ataxia, slurred speech, loss of reflexes, Cheyne–Stokes respiration, generalized convulsions, coma, and central respiratory paralysis. Actions on the vasomotor and other cardiovascular centers in the medulla oblongata lead to hypotension.

The time of death after a single acute exposure may range from less than 5 minutes to nearly 24 hours, depending upon the dose, route, agent, and other factors. The cause of death is primarily respiratory failure, usually accompanied by a secondary cardiovascular component. Muscarinic, nicotinic, and central actions all contribute to respiratory embarrassment; effects include laryngospasm, bronchoconstriction, increased tracheobronchial and salivary secretion, compromised voluntary control of the diaphragm and intercostal muscles, and central respiratory depression. Although the blood pressure may fall to alarmingly low levels and cardiac irregularities intervene, these effects probably result as much from hypoxemia as from the specific actions mentioned, since they are often reversed by the establishment of adequate pulmonary ventilation.

Diagnosis and Treatment. The diagnosis of severe, acute anti-ChE intoxication is readily made from the history of exposure and the characteristic signs and symptoms. In suspected cases of milder acute or chronic intoxication, determination of the ChE activities in erythrocytes and plasma will generally establish the diagnosis. Although these values vary considerably in the normal population, they will usually be depressed well below the normal range before any symptoms are evident.

Treatment is both specific and highly effective. Atropine in sufficient dosage (*see* below) effectively antagonizes the actions at muscarinic receptor sites, including increased tracheobronchial and salivary secretion, bronchoconstriction, bradycardia, and, to a moderate extent, peripheral ganglionic and central actions. Larger doses are required to get appreciable concentrations of atropine into the CNS. Atropine is virtually without effect against the peripheral neuromuscular activation and subsequent paralysis. The last-mentioned action of the anti-ChE agents as well as all other peripheral effects can be reversed by pralidoxime, a cholinesterase reactivator that is discussed in detail below.

In moderate or severe intoxication with an organophosphorus anti-ChE agent, the recommended adult dose of pralidoxime is 1 to 2 g, infused intravenously within not less than 5 minutes. If weakness is not relieved or if it recurs after 20 to 60 minutes, the dose may be repeated. Early treatment is very important to assure that the oxime reaches the phosphorylated AChE while the latter can still be reactivated. Many of the alkylphosphates are extremely lipid soluble, and, if extensive partitioning into body fat has occurred, the onset of toxicity may be delayed and symptoms may recur after initial treatment. In some cases it has been necessary to continue treatment with atropine and pralidoxime for several weeks.

In addition, certain general supportive measures are important. These include (1) termination of exposure, by removal of the patient or application of a gas mask if the atmosphere remains contaminated, removal and destruction of contaminated clothing, copious washing of contaminated skin or mucous membranes with water, or gastric lavage; (2) maintenance of a patent airway, including endobronchial aspiration; (3) artificial respiration, if required; (4) administration of oxygen; (5) alleviation of persistent convulsions with diazepam (5 to 10 mg, intravenously) or sodium thiopental (2.5% solution, intravenously); and (6) treatment of shock (*see* Wills, 1970).

Atropine should be given in adequate doses (usually very large). Following an initial injection of 2 to 4 mg, given intravenously if possible, otherwise intramuscularly, 2 mg should be given every 5 to 10 minutes until muscarinic symptoms disappear, if they reappear, or until signs of atropine toxicity appear. More than 200 mg may be required on the first day. A mild degree of atropine block should then be maintained for up to 48 hours or as long as symptoms are evident. Whereas the AChE reactivators can be of great benefit in the therapy of anti-ChE intoxication (*see* below), their use must be regarded as a supplement to the administration of atropine.

Cholinesterase Reactivators. Although the phosphorylated esteratic site of AChE undergoes hydrolytic regeneration at a slow or negligible rate, Wilson (1951) found that nucleophilic agents, such as hydroxylamine (NH_2OH), hydroxamic acids (RCONH-OH), and oximes (RCH=NOH), reactivate the enzyme more rapidly than does spontaneous hydrolysis. He reasoned that selective reactivation could be achieved by a site-directed nucleophile, wherein interaction of a quaternary nitrogen with the negative subsite of the active center would place the nucleophile in close apposition to the phosphorus. This goal was achieved to a remarkable degree by Wilson and Ginsburg (1955) with pyridine-2-aldoxime methyl chloride (2-PAM, pralidoxime; *see* Figure 7–1, IV–D, and below); reactivation with this compound occurs at a million times the rate of that with hydroxylamine. The oxime is oriented proximally to exert a nucleophilic attack on the phosphorus; the oxime-phosphonate is then split off, leaving the regenerated enzyme (Wilson, 1959).

A number of *bis*-quaternary oximes were subsequently shown to be even more potent as reactivators and as antidotes for nerve gas poisoning (*see* below; *see also* Ellin, 1982); an example is obidoxime chloride. The structures of pralidoxime and obidoxime are as follows:

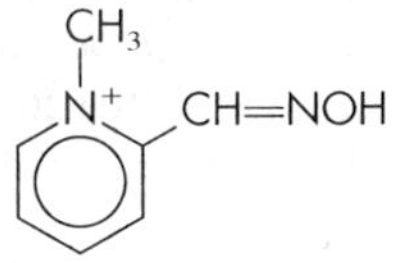

Pralidoxime

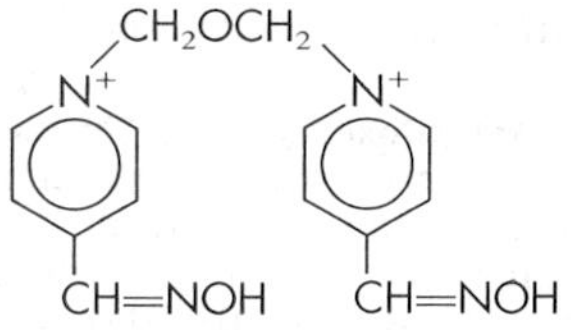

Obidoxime

The velocity of reactivation of phosphorylated AChE by pralidoxime varies with the nature of the phosphoryl group, and in general follows the same sequence as the order for spontaneous hydrolytic reactivation, that is, dimethylphosphoryl-AChE > diethylphosphoryl-AChE > di*iso*propylphosphoryl-AChE, and so forth. Furthermore, phosphorylated AChEs can undergo a fairly rapid process of "aging," so that within the course of minutes or hours they become completely resistant to the reactivators. The "aging" is probably due to the loss of one alkyl or alkoxy group, leaving a much more stable monoalkyl- or monoalkoxy-phosphoryl-AChE (Fleisher and Harris, 1965) (*see* Figure 7–1, III–C). Phosphonates containing tertiary alkoxy groups are more prone to "aging" than are the secondary or primary congeners (Aldridge, 1976). The oximes are not effective in antagonizing the toxicity of the more rapidly hydrolyzing carbamoyl ester inhibitors, and, since pralidoxime itself has weak anti-ChE activity, they are not recommended for the treatment of overdosage with neostigmine or physostigmine and are contraindicated in poisoning with carbaril (Hayes, 1982; Murphy, 1986).

Pharmacology, Toxicology, and Disposition. The reactivating action of oximes and hydroxamic acids *in vivo* is most marked at the skeletal neuromuscular junction. Following a dose of an organophosphorus compound that produces total blockade of transmission, the intravenous injection of an oxime can restore the response to stimulation of the motor nerve within a few minutes. Antidotal effects are less striking at autonomic effector sites and insignificant in the CNS.

High doses of pralidoxime and related compounds can in themselves cause neuromuscular blockade and other effects, including inhibition of AChE; such actions are minimal at the doses recommended for clinical use, 1 to 2 g intravenously. If pralidoxime is injected intravenously at a rate more rapid than 500 mg per minute, it can cause mild weakness, blurred vision, diplopia, dizziness, headache, nausea, and tachycardia.

The oximes as a group are largely metabolized by the liver, and the breakdown products are excreted by the kidney.

Chronic Neurotoxicity of Organophosphorus Compounds. Certain fluorine-containing alkylorganophosphorus anti-ChE agents (*e.g.*, DFP, mipafox) have in common with the triarylphosphates, of which triorthocresylphosphate (TOCP) is the classical example, the property of inducing delayed neurotoxicity. This syndrome first received widespread attention following the demonstration that TOCP, an adulterant of Jamaica ginger, was responsible for an outbreak of thousands of cases of paralysis that occurred in the United States during prohibition.

The clinical picture is that of a severe polyneuritis that begins several days after a single exposure to the toxic compound. It is manifested initially by mild sensory disturbances, ataxia, weakness, and ready fatigability of the legs, accompanied by reduced tendon reflexes and the presence of muscle twitching, fasciculation, and tenderness to palpation. In severe cases, the weakness may progress eventually to complete flaccid paralysis that, over the course of weeks or months, is often succeeded by a spastic paralysis with a concomitant exaggeration of reflexes. During these phases, the muscles show marked wasting. Recovery may require 2 or more years and may be incomplete.

Certain triarylphosphates and fluorine-containing alkylphosphates have the greatest propensity to produce the characteristic neurotoxic pattern, clinically and experimentally. Accordingly, it does not seem to be dependent upon inhibition of AChE or other cholinesterases. The pathological lesion, studied most thoroughly in the chicken, is characterized by axonal swelling, segmentation, and eventual breakdown into granular debris; the marked demyelination is probably secondary to the aforementioned axonal changes. Increasing evidence points to inhibition of a different esterase, termed a *neurotoxic esterase*, as being linked to the lesions (Abou-Donia, 1981; Johnson, 1982). Aging of the esterase–alkylphosphate conjugate in a manner similar to that described for AChE may be required for the genesis of the disease. No specific therapy is known. Experimental myopathies that result in generalized necrotic lesions and changes in end-plate cytostructure are also found after long-term treatment with organophosphates (Laskowski and Dettbarn, 1977).

PREPARATIONS

The compounds described here are those commonly used as anti-ChE drugs and cholinesterase reactivators in the United States. Conventional dosages and routes of administration are given in the discussion of therapeutic applications of these agents (*see* below).

Physostigmine salicylate (ANTILIRIUM) is available as a solution (1 mg/ml) for injection. *Physostigmine sulfate ophthalmic ointment* (0.25%) and *physostigmine salicylate ophthalmic solution* (0.25% and 0.5%) are also available.

Neostigmine bromide (PROSTIGMIN) is available for oral use in 15-mg tablets. *Neostigmine methylsulfate* (PROSTIGMIN) is marketed for parenteral injection in ampuls and vials containing 0.25, 0.5, or 1.0 mg/ml.

Ambenonium chloride (MYTELASE) is available for oral use in 10-mg tablets.

Pyridostigmine bromide (MESTINON, REGONOL) is available for oral use in 60-mg tablets, in 180-mg sustained-release tablets, and in a syrup that contains 12 mg/ml, as well as in an injectable form that contains 5 mg/ml.

Edrophonium chloride (TENSILON, others) is marketed for parenteral injection in ampuls and vials containing 10 mg/ml.

Demecarium bromide ophthalmic solution (HUMORSOL) is available in concentrations of 0.125 and 0.25%.

Echothiophate iodide for ophthalmic solution (PHOSPHOLINE IODIDE) is marketed as a powder in 1.5-, 3.0-, 6.25-, and 12.5-mg amounts. Solutions of appropriate strength must be freshly prepared in a diluent supplied by the manufacturer. Once prepared, the solution is stable for about 6 months if kept refrigerated.

Isoflurophate ophthalmic ointment (FLOROPRYL) contains 0.025% isoflurophate (di*iso*propyl phosphorofluoridate, DFP) in an anhydrous vehicle.

Pralidoxime chloride (PROTOPAM CHLORIDE) is the only AChE reactivator currently available for general use in the United States. It is dispensed in vials in 1-g amounts for solution in 20 ml of sterile water. It is also marketed in 500-mg tablets and in an auto-injector (600 mg/2 ml) for intramuscular administration.

Other reactivators of AChE not currently available in the United States include *obidoxime chloride* (TOXOGONIN), its analog *trimedoxime bromide* (TMB-4), and *diacetyl monoxime* (*see* Ellin, 1982). Obidoxime is more potent than pralidoxime; the recommended dose is 3 to 6 mg/kg, injected intramuscularly or intravenously over 5 to 10 minutes.

The dose of diacetyl monoxime is 1 g, injected intravenously at a rate of 200 mg per minute; unlike pralidoxime or obidoxime, it penetrates the blood–brain barrier and reactivates AChE in the CNS. Both drugs can be repeated in the same doses after 20 minutes.

THERAPEUTIC USES

Although anti-ChE agents have been recommended for the treatment of a wide variety of conditions, their widespread acceptability has been established mainly in four areas: atony of the smooth muscle of the intestinal tract and urinary bladder, glaucoma, myasthenia gravis, and termination of the effects of competitive neuromuscular blocking drugs (*see* Chapter 9). Physostigmine is also useful in the treatment of atropine intoxication (*see* below) and of poisoning with phenothiazines and tricyclic antidepressants (Chapter 18); it is also indicated for the treatment of Friedreich's or other inherited ataxias. Edrophonium can be used for terminating attacks of paroxysmal supraventricular tachycardia.

Paralytic Ileus and Atony of the Urinary Bladder. In the treatment of both these conditions, neostigmine is generally the most satisfactory of the anti-ChE agents. The direct parasympathomimetic agents, discussed in Chapter 6, are employed for the same purposes.

Neostigmine is used for the relief of abdominal distention from a variety of medical and surgical causes. The usual subcutaneous dose of neostigmine methylsulfate for postoperative paralytic ileus is 0.5 mg, given as needed. Peristaltic activity commences 10 to 30 minutes after parenteral administration, whereas 2 to 4 hours are required after oral administration of neostigmine bromide (15 to 30 mg). A rectal tube should be inserted to facilitate expulsion of gas, and it may be necessary to assist evacuation with a small low enema. The drug should not be used when the intestine or urinary bladder is obstructed, when peritonitis is present, when the viability of the bowel is doubtful, or when bowel dysfunction is a consequence of inflammatory disease. Other supportive measures include intubation and suction.

When neostigmine is used for the treatment of atony of the detrusor muscle of the urinary bladder, postoperative dysuria is relieved and the time interval between operation and spontaneous urination is shortened. The drug is used in the same dose and manner as in the management of paralytic ileus.

Glaucoma. Glaucoma is a disease complex characterized chiefly by an increase in intraocular pressure that, if sufficiently high and persistent, leads to damage to the optic disc at the juncture of the optic nerve and the retina; irreversible blindness can result. Of the three types of glaucoma—primary, secondary, and congenital—anti-ChE agents are of considerable value in the management of the primary as well as of certain categories of the secondary type (*e.g.*, aphakic glaucoma, following cataract extraction); the congenital type rarely responds to any therapy other than surgery. Primary glaucoma is subdivided into narrow-angle (acute congestive) and wide-angle (chronic simple) types, based on the configuration of the angle of the anterior chamber where reabsorption of the aqueous humor occurs. Anti-ChE agents produce a fall in intraocular pressure in both types of primary glaucoma, chiefly by lowering the resistance to outflow of the aqueous humor. Effects on the volumes of the various intraocular vascular beds (*e.g.*, those of the iris, ciliary body, *etc.*) and on the rate of secretion of the aqueous humor into the posterior chamber may contribute secondarily to the lowering of pressure, or conversely may produce a rise in pressure preceding the fall.

In narrow-angle glaucoma, the aqueous outflow is facilitated by the freeing of the entrance to the trabecular space at the canal of Schlemm from blockade by the iris, as the result of the drug-induced contraction of the sphincter muscle of the iris. In wide-angle glaucoma, there is no physical obstruction to the entry to the trabeculae; rather, the trabeculae, which are a meshwork of pores of small diameter, lose their patency. In this circumstance, contraction of the sphincter muscle of the iris and the ciliary muscle enhances tone and alignment of the trabecular network to improve resorption and outflow of aqueous humor through the network to the canal of Schlemm (*see* reviews by Schwartz, 1978; Kaufman *et al.*, 1984; Hoskins and Kass, 1989).

The foregoing distinctions are of great importance for therapy, since the roles of miotic drugs, including the anti-ChE agents, are quite different in the management of the two types of primary glaucoma. Narrow-angle glaucoma is nearly always a medical emergency in which the drugs are essential in controlling the acute attack, but the long-range management is often surgical (*e.g.*, peripheral or complete iridectomy). Wide-angle glaucoma, on the other hand, has a gradual, insidious onset and is not generally amenable to surgical improvement; in this type, control of intraocular pressure is usually dependent upon permanent drug therapy.

Narrow-angle glaucoma may be precipitated by the injudicious use of a mydriatic agent in patients over 40, or by a variety of factors that can cause pupillary dilatation or engorgement of intraocular vessels. The cardinal signs and symptoms include marked ocular inflammation, a semidilated pupil, severe pain, and nausea. Every effort must be made to reduce and then maintain intraocular pressure at the normal level. In general, an anti-ChE agent is not used in this condition. Therapy includes the intravenous administration of a carbonic anhydrase inhibitor, such as acetazolamide, to reduce the secretion of aqueous humor; in addition, an osmotic agent, such as mannitol (intravenously) or glycerin (orally) is administered to induce intraocular dehydration. Miosis is achieved by the application of pilocarpine. One or two drops of a 2 or 4% solution of pilocarpine nitrate is administered at 10- to 15-minute intervals for 1 hour; thereafter, the drug is given every 2 to 3 hours. Some ophthalmologists administer physostigmine salicylate in addition to pilocarpine.

Chronic wide-angle glaucoma and secondary glaucoma require careful consideration of the needs of the individual patient in selecting the drug or combination of drugs to be employed. The choices available include (1) parasympathomimetic agents (*e.g.*, pilocarpine nitrate, 1 to 4%; *see* Chapter 6); (2) anti-ChE agents that are short acting (*e.g.*, physostigmine salicylate, 0.25 and 0.5%) or long acting (demecarium bromide, 0.125 and 0.25%; echothiophate iodide, 0.03 to 0.25%; isoflurophate, 0.025%); (3) β-adrenergic antagonists such as timolol maleate (0.25 and 0.5%) or betaxolol (0.5%), an antagonist with β_1 selectivity; and paradoxically (4) adrenergic agonists (*e.g.*, epinephrine, 0.25 to 2%; phenylephrine, 10%; dipivefrin, 0.1%, a prodrug with improved penetration into the aqueous chambers that is converted to epinephrine by esterases; *see* Chapter 10). The β-adrenergic antagonists are administered at 12-hour intervals. They do not directly affect pupillary aperture but reduce production of aqueous humor (Boger *et al.*, 1978; Lotti *et al.*, 1984) and avoid the partial block of accommodation and the untoward effects of the long-acting anti-ChE agents. Adrenergic agonists are often most effective when used in combination with AChE inhibitors or cholinergic agonists. They reduce intraocular pressure by decreasing secretion of aqueous humor, and they prevent engorgement of small blood vessels. Combinations of β-adrenergic antagonists and cholinergic miotic agents are receiving increased attention. Potential systemic effects limit the use of adrenergic agonists and antagonists in certain respiratory and cardiovascular conditions (*see* Chapters 10 and 11).

Since the cholinergic agonists and cholinesterase inhibitors block accommodation, these agents produce transient blurring of far vision. The block of accommodation usually occurs after administration of relatively high doses and is of relatively short duration. With long-term administration of the cholinergic agonists and anti-ChE agents, this response diminishes.

Despite the convenience of less frequent administration and the high potency of long-acting anti-ChE agents, their use entails a greater risk of development of lenticular opacities and untoward autonomic effects (*see* below). Of the organophosphorus agents, DFP has the longest duration of action and is extremely potent when applied locally; solutions in peanut or sesame oil require instillation from once daily to once weekly, and may control intraocular pressure in severe cases that are resistant to other drugs. The oily vehicle is unpleasant to most patients. Consequently, DFP has largely been replaced by echothiophate.

Anti-ChE agents have been employed locally in the treatment of a variety of other ophthalmological conditions, including accommodative esotropia and myasthenia gravis confined to the extraocular and eyelid muscles. Adie (or tonic pupil) syndrome results from dysfunction of the ciliary body, perhaps because of local nerve degeneration. Low concentrations of physostigmine are reported to decrease the blurred vision and pain associated with this condition (Wirtschafter and Herman, 1980). In alternation with a mydriatic drug such as atropine, short-acting anti-ChE agents have proven useful for the breaking of adhesions between the iris and the lens or cornea. (For a complete account of the use of anti-ChE agents in ocular therapy, *see* Havener, 1983; Kaufman *et al.*, 1984; Hoskins and Kass, 1989.)

Untoward Effects. Treatment of glaucoma with potent, long-acting anti-ChE agents (including demecarium, echothiophate, and isoflurophate) for 6 months or longer carries a high risk of the development of a specific type of cataract, which begins as anterior subcapsular vacuoles (Shaffer and Hetherington, 1966). Although formation of spontaneous cataracts is quite common within comparable age groups, the incidence of lenticular opacities under such circumstances can be as high as 50%; the hazard is apparently increased in proportion to the strength of the solution, frequency of instillation, duration of therapy, and age of the patient. The underlying mechanism remains elusive (*see* Kaufman *et al.*, 1984).

Most of the studies that have implicated the long-acting anti-ChE agents in the formation of cataracts have been retrospective and uncontrolled. The reported incidence of cataracts attributable to such drugs may thus be distorted by selection of patients with more severe glaucoma; nevertheless, cataractogenesis should be considered when therapeutic decisions are made. Long-acting anti-ChE agents are, of course, not indicated when glaucoma can be controlled by β-adrenergic antagonists, parasympathomimetic drugs, physostigmine, or other agents. Since glaucoma leads to irreversible blindness if not adequately controlled, the long-acting cholinesterase inhibitors retain their therapeutic importance in situations where other agents are inadequate. At present, it seems clear that pilocarpine and other shorter-acting miotic drugs should be employed as long as they provide adequate control of intraocular tension. If they fail to do so, the hazards of cataract development must be balanced against those of increased intraocular pressure. When long-acting anti-ChE agents are used, patients should be examined for the appearance of lenticular opacities at intervals of 6 months or less.

Miscellaneous ocular side effects that may occur following local instillation of anti-ChE agents are headache, brow pain, blurred vision, pericorneal injection, congestive iritis, various allergic reactions, and, rarely, retinal detachment. When anti-ChE drugs are instilled intraconjunctivally at frequent intervals, sufficient absorption may occur to produce various systemic effects, which result from inhibition of AChE and butyryl-ChE. Hence, cholinergic autonomic function will be augmented, the duration of action of local anesthetics with an ester linkage will be prolonged (*see* Chapter 15), and the neuromuscular blockade produced by succinylcholine will be enhanced and prolonged (*see* Chapter 9). Individuals with vagotonia and allergies are at particular risk. Systemic absorption of the drug can be minimized by digital compression of the inner canthus of the eye during and for a short period following its instillation.

Myasthenia Gravis. Myasthenia gravis is a neuromuscular disease characterized by weakness and marked fatigability of skeletal muscle (*see* Drachman, 1987; DeBaets *et al.*, 1988); exacerbations and partial remissions occur frequently. Jolly (1895) noted the similarity between the symptoms of myasthenia gravis and curare poisoning in animals and suggested that physostigmine, an agent then known to antagonize curare, might be of therapeutic value. Forty years elapsed before his suggestion was given systematic trial (Walker, 1934).

The defect in myasthenia gravis is in synaptic transmission at the neuromuscular junction. When a motor nerve of a normal subject is stimulated at 25 Hz, electrical and mechanical responses are well sustained. A suitable margin of safety exists for maintenance of neuromuscular transmission. Initial responses in the myasthenic patient may be normal, but they diminish rapidly, which explains the difficulty in maintaining voluntary muscle activity for more than brief periods. When the patient is given an appropriate dose of neostigmine, the response to tetanic stimulation is improved, along with symptomatic improvement in muscle strength. The same dose of neostigmine in control subjects leads to a reduced response to tetanic stimulation, accompanied by fasciculations, local weakness, and repetitive action potentials in response to a single stimulus.

The relative importance of prejunctional and postjunctional defects in myasthenia gravis was a matter of considerable debate until Patrick and Lindstrom (1973) found that rabbits immunized with the nicotinic receptor purified from electric eels slowly developed muscular weakness and respiratory difficulties that resembled the symptoms of myasthenia gravis. The rabbits also exhibited decremental responses following repetitive nerve stimulation, enhanced sensitivity to curare, and symptomatic and electrophysiological improvement of neuromuscular transmission following administration of anti-ChE agents. Although this experimental allergic myasthenia gravis and the naturally occurring disease differ somewhat, this critical development of an animal model prompted intense investigation into whether the natural disease represented an autoimmune response directed toward the ACh receptor. Antireceptor antibody was soon identified in patients with myasthenia gravis (Almon *et al.*, 1974). Receptor-binding antibodies are now detectable in sera of 90% of patients with the disease, although the clinical status of the patient does not correlate precisely with the antibody titer (Lindstrom *et al.*, 1976; Drachman *et al.*, 1982). By use of the snake α-neurotoxins that bind with high affinity to the nicotinic receptor (*see* Chapter 9), Fambrough and associates (1973) were able to detect a 70 to 90% reduction in the number of receptors per end-plate in myasthenic patients. This finding provided crucial support for the hypothesis that a decrease in receptors in the postsynaptic membrane accounts for the defects of the disease.

The picture that emerges is that myasthenia gravis is caused by an autoimmune response primarily to the ACh receptor at the postjunctional end-plate. Antibodies, which are also present in plasma, reduce the number of receptors detectable either by toxin-binding assays or by electrophysiological measurements of ACh sensitivity (Drachman, 1987). The autoimmune reaction enhances receptor degradation (Drachman *et al.*, 1982). Immune complexes have been detected at the postsynaptic membrane, along with marked ultrastructural abnormalities in the synaptic cleft (Engel *et al.*, 1977). The latter appear to be a consequence of complement-mediated lysis of junctional folds in the end-plate. A related disease that also compromises neuromuscular transmission is Lambert–Eaton syndrome. Here, antibodies are directed against Ca^{2+} channels that are necessary for presynaptic release of ACh (Fukuoka *et al.*, 1987; Kim and Neher, 1988).

Diagnosis. Although the diagnosis can usually be made from the history, signs, and symptoms, its differentiation from certain neurasthenic, infectious, endocrine, neoplastic, and degenerative neuromuscular diseases may be difficult. However, myasthenia gravis is the only condition in which the aforementioned deficiencies can be improved dramatically by anti-ChE medication. The edrophonium test is performed by rapid intravenous injection of 2 mg of edrophonium chloride, followed 45 seconds later by an additional 8 mg if the first dose is without effect; a positive response consists of brief improvement in strength, unaccompanied by lingual fasciculation (which generally occurs in nonmyasthenic patients).

An excessive dose of an anti-ChE drug results in a cholinergic crisis. The condition is characterized by weakness resulting from generalized depolarization of the motor end-plate; other features result from overstimulation of muscarinic receptors. The weakness resulting from depolarization block may resemble myasthenic weakness, which is due to insufficient anti-ChE medication. The distinction is of obvious practical importance, since the former is treated by withholding, and the latter by administering, the anti-ChE agent. When the edrophonium test is performed cautiously, limiting the dose to 2 mg, and with facilities for respiratory resuscitation immediately available, a further decrease in strength indicates cholinergic crisis, while improvement signifies myasthenic weakness. Atropine sulfate, 0.4 to 0.6 mg or more intravenously, should be given immediately if a severe muscarinic reaction ensues (for complete details, *see* Osserman *et al.*, 1972).

Although a provocative test with 0.5 mg of tubocurarine to elicit muscular weakness has been used to confirm the diagnosis, the test is potentially hazardous. The quantitation of antireceptor antibodies in muscle biopsies or plasma is now widely employed.

Treatment. Neostigmine, pyridostigmine, and ambenonium are the standard anti-ChE drugs used in the symptomatic treatment of myasthenia gravis.

All can increase the response of myasthenic muscle to repetitive nerve impulses, primarily by the preservation of endogenous ACh; receptors over a greater cross-sectional area of the end-plate are then presumably exposed to concentrations of ACh that are sufficient for stimulation.

When the diagnosis of myasthenia gravis has been established, the optimal single oral dose of an anti-ChE agent can be determined empirically. Baseline recordings are made of grip strength, vital capacity, and a number of signs and symptoms that reflect the strength of various muscle groups. The patient is then given an oral dose of neostigmine (7.5 to 15 mg), pyridostigmine (30 to 60 mg), or ambenonium (2.5 to 5 mg). The improvement in muscle strength and changes in other signs and symptoms are noted at frequent intervals until there is a return to the basal state. After an hour or longer in the basal state, the drug is given again with the dose increased to one and one-half times the initial amount, and the same observations are repeated. This sequence is continued, with increasing increments of one half the initial dose, until the optimal response is obtained. The result can be confirmed by the edrophonium test. If the dose of the longer-acting anti-ChE agent was insufficient, a further improvement in muscle strength will result. If the dose was adequate or excessive, no further change or a reduction in muscle strength will be evident. The optimal single oral dose may range from the initial doses given above to more than five times these amounts.

The duration of action of these drugs is such that the interval between oral doses required to maintain a reasonably even level of strength is usually 2 to 4 hours for neostigmine, 3 to 6 hours for pyridostigmine, or 3 to 8 hours for ambenonium. However, the dose required may vary from day to day, and physical or emotional stress, intercurrent infections, and menstruation usually necessitate an increase in the frequency or size of the dose. In addition, unpredictable exacerbations and remissions of the myasthenic state may require adjustment of the dosage upward or downward. Although all patients with myasthenia gravis should be seen by a physician at regular intervals, most can be taught to modify their dosage regimens according to their changing requirements. Pyridostigmine is available in sustained-release tablets containing a total of 180 mg, of which 60 mg is released immediately and 120 mg over several hours; this preparation is of value in maintaining patients for 6- to 8-hour periods, but should be limited to use at bedtime. Muscarinic cardiovascular and gastrointestinal side effects of anti-ChE agents can generally be controlled by atropine or other anticholinergic drugs (Chapter 8). However, it should be recognized that anticholinergics mask the side effects of an excessive dose of an anticholinesterase. Many patients learn to titrate dosage by noting symptomatic improvement of muscle function and development of side effects. In most patients, tolerance develops eventually to the muscarinic effects, so that anticholinergic medication is not necessary. A number of drugs, including curariform agents and certain antibiotics and general anesthetics, interfere with neuromuscular transmission (*see* Chapter 9); their administration to patients with myasthenia gravis is hazardous without proper adjustment of anti-ChE dosage and other appropriate precautions.

In cases where administration of anti-ChE agents at optimal doses does not promote near-normal motor activity, other therapeutic measures should be considered. Controlled studies reveal that corticosteroids promote clinical improvement in a high percentage of patients (Engel, 1976). However, when treatment with steroids is continued over prolonged periods, a high incidence of side effects may result (*see* Chapter 60). Gradual lowering of maintenance doses and alternate-day regimens of short-acting steroids are used to minimize side effects. Initiation of steroid treatment augments muscle weakness; however, as the patient improves with continued administration of steroids, doses of anti-ChE drugs can be reduced (Drachman, 1987). Other immunosuppressive agents such as azathioprine and cyclosporine have also been beneficial in more advanced cases.

Thymectomy should be considered in myasthenia associated with a thymoma or when the disease is not adequately controlled by anti-ChE agents and steroids. The relative risks and benefits of the surgical procedure versus anti-ChE and corticosteroid treatment require careful assessment in each case (Rowland, 1980). Since the thymus contains myoid cells with nicotinic receptors (Schluep *et al.*, 1987) and a predominance of patients have thymic abnormalities, the thymus may be responsible for the initial pathogenesis. It is also the source of autoreactive T helper cells. However, the thymus is not required for perpetuation of the condition.

In keeping with the presumed autoimmune etiology of myasthenia gravis, plasmapheresis has been performed, with beneficial results, in patients who have remained disabled despite thymectomy and treatment with steroids and anti-ChE agents (Dau, 1981). Improvement in muscle strength correlates with the reduction of the titer of antibody directed against the cholinergic nicotinic receptor.

Intoxication by Anticholinergic Drugs. Many of the peripheral and central effects of poisoning by atropine and related antimuscarinic drugs (Chapter 8) can be reversed by intravenous injection of physostigmine. Many other drugs, such as the phenothiazines, antihistamines, and tricyclic antidepressants, have central, as well as peripheral, anticholinergic activity, and physostigmine salicylate may be useful in reversing the central anticholinergic syndrome produced by overdosage or an unusual reaction to these drugs (Aquilonius, 1977; Nilsson, 1982). The effectiveness of physostigmine as an antidote for the anticholinergic effects of these agents has been clearly documented. However, other toxic effects of the tricyclic antidepressants and phenothiazines, such as intraventricular conduction deficits and ventricular arrhythmias, are not reversed by physostigmine. In addition, the drug may precipitate seizures; hence, its usually small potential benefit must be weighed against this risk. The initial intravenous or intramuscular dose of physostigmine is 2 mg, with additional doses given as necessary. Physostigmine, a tertiary amine, crosses the blood–brain barrier, in contrast to the quaternary anti-AChE drugs. The use of anti-ChE agents to reverse the effects of competitive neuromuscular blocking agents is discussed in Chapter 9.

Alzheimer's Disease. A deficiency of functional cholinergic neurons, particularly those extending from the lateral basalis (Katzman and Thal, 1989), has been observed in patients with progressive dementia of the Alzheimer type. Physostigmine and a longer acting anti-ChE, tacrine (a tetrahydroacridine), have been used in the earlier stages of the disease to improve memory. Results have been variable, although some investigators have employed dosage schedules that appear to cause transient improvement (*see* Thal *et al.*, 1983). Long-term studies of several hundred patients are currently under way to evaluate the efficacy of anti-ChE agents (Giacobini and Becker, 1988).

Almon, R. R.; Andrew, C. G.; and Appel, S. H. Serum globulin in myasthenia gravis: inhibition of α-bungarotoxin binding to acetylcholine receptors. *Science,* **1974,** *186,* 55–57.

Argyll-Robertson, D. The Calabar bean as a new agent in ophthalmic practice. *Edinb. Med. J.,* **1863,** *8,* 815–820.

Boger, W.; Steinert, R.; Puliafito, C.; and Pavah-Langston, D. Clinical trial comparing timolol ophthalmic solution in patients with open angle glaucoma. *Am. J. Ophthalmol.,* **1978,** *86,* 8–18.

Cartaud, J.; Reiger, F.; Bon, S.; and Massoulié, J. Fine structure of electric eel acetylcholinesterase. *Brain Res.,* **1975,** *88,* 127–130.

Changeux, J. P. Responses of acetylcholinesterase from *Torpedo marmorata* to salts and curarizing drugs. *Mol. Pharmacol.,* **1966,** *2,* 369–392.

Christioson, R. On the properties of the ordeal bean of Old Calabar. *Mon. J. Med. (Lond.),* **1855,** *20,* 193–204.

Cohan, S. L.; Pohlmann, J. L. W.; Mikszewki, J.; and O'Doherty, D. S. The pharmacokinetics of pyridostigmine. *Neurology (Minneap.),* **1976,** *26,* 536–539.

Dau, P. C. Response to plasmapheresis and immunosuppressive drug therapy in sixty myasthenia gravis patients. *Ann. N.Y. Acad. Sci.,* **1981,** *377,* 700–708.

Drachman, D. B.; Adams, R. N.; Josifek, L. F.; and Self, S. G. Functional activities of autoantibodies to acetylcholine receptors and the clinical severity of myasthenia gravis. *N. Engl. J. Med.,* **1982,** *307,* 769–775.

Engel, A. G.; Lambert, E. H.; and Howard, F. M., Jr. Immune complexes (IgG and C3) at the motor endplate in myasthenia gravis. *Mayo Clin. Proc.,* **1977,** *52,* 267–280.

Engel, W. K. Myasthenia gravis: corticosteroids and anticholinesterases. *Ann. N.Y. Acad. Sci.,* **1976,** *274,* 623–630.

Fambrough, D. M.; Drachman, D. B.; and Satyamurti, S. Neuromuscular junction in myasthenia gravis: decreased acetylcholine receptors. *Science,* **1973,** *182,* 293–295.

Fleisher, J. H., and Harris, L. W. Dealkylation as a mechanism for aging of cholinesterase after poisoning with pinacolyl methylphosphonofluoridate. *Biochem. Pharmacol.,* **1965,** *14,* 641–650.

Fraser, T. R. On the characters, actions and therapeutical uses of the ordeal bean of Calabar (*Physostigma venenosum,* Balfour). *Edinb. Med. J.,* **1863,** *9,* 36–56, 123–132, 235–248.

Fukuoka, T.; Engel, A.; Lang, B.; Newson-Davis, J.; Prior, C.; and Wray, D. W. Lambert–Eaton myasthenic syndrome: I. Early morphological effects of IgG on the presynaptic membrane active zones. *Ann. Neurol.,* **1987,** *22,* 193–199.

Futter, M. E.; Donati, F.; Sodikor, A. S.; and Bevan, D. R. Neostigmine antagonism of succinylcholine phase II block: a comparison with pancuronium. *Can. Anaesth. Soc. J.,* **1983,** *30,* 575–580.

Gibney, G.; MacPhee-Quigley, K.; Thompson, B.; Vedvick, T.; Low, M. G.; Taylor, S. S.; and Taylor, P. Divergence in primary structures between the molecular forms of acetylcholinesterase. *J. Biol. Chem.,* **1988,** *263,* 1140–1145.

Gysin, H. Über einige neue Insektizide. *Chimia,* **1954,** *8,* 205–210, 221–228.

Hall, Z. W. Multiple forms of acetylcholinesterase and their distribution in endplate and non-endplate regions of rat diaphragm muscle. *J. Neurobiol.,* **1973,** *4,* 343–361.

Jolly, F. Pseudoparalysis myasthenica. *Neurol. Zentralbl.,* **1895,** *14,* 34.

Kim, Y. I., and Neher, E. IgG from patients with Lambert–Eaton syndrome blocks voltage-dependent calcium channels. *Science,* **1988,** *239,* 405–408.

Lindstrom, J. M.; Seybold, M. E.; Lennon, V. A.; Whittingham, S.; and Duane, D. D. Antibody to acetylcholine receptor in myasthenia gravis: prevalence, clinical correlates and diagnostic value. *Neurology (Minneap.),* **1976,** *26,* 1054–1059.

Lockridge, O.; Bartels, C. F.; Vaughan, T. A.; Wong, C. K.; Norton, S. E.; and Johnson, L. L. Complete amino acid sequence of human serum cholinesterase. *J. Biol. Chem.,* **1987,** *262,* 549–557.

Lwebuga-Mukasa, J. S.; Lappi, S.; and Taylor, P. Molecular forms of acetylcholinesterase from *Torpedo californica:* their relationship to synaptic membranes. *Biochemistry,* **1976,** *15,* 1425–1434.

McCombie, H., and Saunders, B. C. Alkyl fluorophosphonates: preparation and physiological properties. *Nature,* **1946,** *157,* 287–289.

Nilsson, E. Physostigmine treatment in various drug-induced intoxications. *Ann. Clin. Res.,* **1982,** *14,* 165–172.

Patrick, J. L., and Lindstrom, J. Autoimmune response to acetylcholine receptor. *Science,* **1973,** *180,* 871–872.

Rosenberry, T. L., and Richardson, J. M. Structure of 18S and 14S acetylcholinesterase. Identification of collagen-like subunits that are linked by disulfide bonds to catalytic subunits. *Biochemistry,* **1977,** *16,* 3550–3558.

Schluep, M.; Wilcox, N.; Vincent, A.; Prior, C.; Wray, D.; and Newson-Davis, J. Acetylcholine receptors in human thymic myoid cells in situ: an immunohistological study. *Ann. Neurol.,* **1987,** *22,* 212–222.

Schumacher, M.; Camp, S.; Maulet, Y.; Newton, M.; MacPhee-Quigley, K.; Friedmann, T.; Taylor, S. S.; and Taylor, P. Primary structure of *Torpedo californica* acetylcholinesterase deduced from its cDNA sequence. *Nature,* **1986,** *319,* 407–409.

Shaffer, R. N., and Hetherington, J., Jr. Anticholinesterase drugs and cataracts. *Am. J. Ophthalmol.,* **1966,** *62,* 613–618.

Silman, I., and Futerman, A. H. Modes of attachment of acetylcholinesterase to the surface membrane. *Eur. J. Biochem.,* **1987,** *170,* 11–22.

Somani, S. M.; Roberts, J. B.; and Wilson, A. Pyridostigmine metabolism in man. *Clin. Pharmacol. Ther.,* **1972,** *13,* 393–399.

Stedman, E. III. Studies on the relationship between chemical constitution and physiological action. Part II. The miotic activity of urethanes derived from the isomeric hydroxybenzyldimethylamines. *Biochem. J.,* **1929a,** *23,* 17–24.

———. Chemical constitution and miotic action. *Am. J. Physiol.*, **1929b**, *90*, 528–529.

Su, M.; Kinoshita, F. K.; Frawley, F. P.; and DuBois, K. P. Comparative inhibition of aliesterases and cholinesterases in rats fed eighteen organophosphorus insecticides. *Toxicol. Appl. Pharmacol.*, **1971**, *20*, 241–249.

Taylor, P., and Lappi, S. Interaction of fluorescent probes with acetylcholinesterase. The site and specificity of propidium binding. *Biochemistry*, **1975**, *14*, 1989–1997.

Thal, L. J.; Fuld, P. A.; Masur, D. M.; and Sharpless, N. S. Oral physostigmine and lecithin improve memory in Alzheimer's disease. *Ann. Neurol.*, **1983**, *13*, 491–496.

Walker, M. B. Treatment of myasthenia gravis with physostigmine. *Lancet*, **1934**, *1*, 1200–1201.

Wilson, I. B. Acetylcholinesterase. XI. Reversibility of tetraethyl pyrophosphate inhibition. *J. Biol. Chem.*, **1951**, *190*, 111–117.

Wilson, I. B., and Ginsburg, S. A powerful reactivator of alkyl phosphate–inhibited acetylcholinesterase. *Biochim. Biophys. Acta*, **1955**, *18*, 168–170.

Wilson, I. B., and Harrison, M. A. Turnover number of acetylcholinesterase. *J. Biol. Chem.*, **1961**, *236*, 2292–2295.

Wilson, I. B.; Hatch, M. A.; and Ginsburg, S. Carbamylation of acetylcholinesterase. *J. Biol. Chem.*, **1960**, *235*, 2312–2315.

Wilson, I. B., and Quan, C. Acetylcholinesterase: studies on molecular complementariness. *Arch. Biochem. Biophys.*, **1958**, *73*, 131–143.

Wirtschafter, J. D., and Herman, W. K. Low concentration eserine therapy for the tonic pupil (Adie) syndrome. *Ophthalmology (Rochester)*, **1980**, *87*, 1037–1043.

Monographs and Reviews

Abou-Donia, M. B. Organophosphorus ester-induced delayed neurotoxicity. *Annu. Rev. Pharmacol. Toxicol.*, **1981**, *21*, 511–548.

Albuquerque, E. X.; Aracava, Y.; Idriss, M.; Schönenberger, B.; Brassi, A.; and Deshpande, S. S. Activation and blockade of the nicotinic and glutaminergic synapses by reversible and irreversible cholinesterase inhibitors. In, *Neurobiology of Acetylcholine*. (Dun, N. J., and Perlman, R. L., eds.) Plenum Press, New York, **1987**, pp. 301–328.

Aldridge, W. N. Survey of major points of interest about reactions of cholinesterases. *Croat. Chem. Acta*, **1976**, *47*, 225–233.

Aquilonius, S.-M. Physostigmine in the treatment of drug overdose. In, *Cholinergic Mechanisms and Psychopharmacology*, Vol. 24. (Jenden, D. J., ed.) Plenum Press, New York, **1977**, pp. 817–825.

Colquhoun, D. The link between drug binding and response: theories and observations. In, *The Receptors: A Comprehensive Treatise*, Vol. I. (O'Brien, R. D., ed.) Plenum Press, New York, **1979**, pp. 93–142.

Costa, L. G.; Galli, C. L.; and Murphy, S. D. (eds.). *Toxicology of Pesticides: Experimental, Clinical, and Regulatory Perspectives. NATO Advanced Study Institute Series H*, Vol. 13. Springer-Verlag, Berlin, **1987**.

DeBaets, M. H.; Oosterhuis, H. J. G. H.; and Toyka, K. V. (eds.). *Myasthenia Gravis*, Vol. 25. *Monographs in Allergy*. S. Karger, Basel, **1988**.

Drachman, D. (ed.). Myasthenia gravis: biology and treatment. *Ann. N.Y. Acad. Sci.*, **1987**, *555*.

Ellin, R. I. Anomalies in theories and therapy of intoxication by potent organophosphorus anticholinesterase compounds. *Gen. Pharmacol.*, **1982**, *13*, 457–466.

Froede, H. C., and Wilson, I. B. Acetylcholinesterase. In, *The Enzymes*, Vol. 5. (Boyer, P. D., ed.) Academic Press, Inc., New York, **1971**, pp. 87–114.

Giacobini, E., and Becker, R. (eds.). *Current Research in Alzheimer Therapy*. Taylor and Francis, New York, **1988**.

Havener, W. H. *Ocular Pharmacology*, 5th ed. C. V. Mosby Co., St. Louis, **1983**.

Hayes, W. J., Jr. *Pesticide Studies in Man*, 2nd ed. The Williams & Wilkins Co., Baltimore, **1982**, pp. 284–435, 436–467.

Hobbiger, F. Pharmacology of anticholinesterase drugs. In, *Neuromuscular Junction*. (Zaimis, E., ed.) *Handbuch der Experimentellen Pharmakologie*, Vol. 42. Springer-Verlag, Berlin, **1976**, pp. 487–581.

Holmstedt, B. Structure–activity relationships of the organophosphorus anticholinesterase agents. In, *Cholinesterases and Anticholinesterase Agents*. (Koelle, G. B., ed.) *Handbuch der Experimentellen Pharmakologie*, Vol. 15. Springer-Verlag, Berlin, **1963**, pp. 428–485.

———. The ordeal bean of Old Calabar: the pageant of *Physostigma venenosum* in medicine. In, *Plants in the Development of Modern Medicine*. (Swain, T., ed.) Harvard University Press, Cambridge, Mass., **1972**, pp. 303–360.

Hoskins, H. D., Jr., and Kass, M. *Diagnosis and Therapy of the Glaucomas*, 6th ed. C. V. Mosby Co., St. Louis, **1989**, pp. 406–495.

Johnson, M. K. The target for initiation of delayed neurotoxicity by organophosphorus esters. In, *Reviews in Biochemical Toxicology*, Vol. 4. (Hodgson, E.; Band, E.; and Philpot, R. M.; eds.) Elsevier Publishing Co., New York, **1982**, pp. 141–272.

Karczmar, A. G. Pharmacologic, toxicologic, and therapeutic properties of anticholinesterase agents. In, *Physiological Pharmacology*. Vol. 3, *The Nervous System—Part C: Autonomic Nervous System Drugs*. (Root, W. S., and Hofmann, F. G., eds.) Academic Press, Inc., New York, **1967**, pp. 163–322.

———. History of the research with anticholinesterase agents. In, *Anticholinesterase Agents*, Vol. 1. *International Encyclopedia of Pharmacology and Therapeutics*, Sect. 13. (Karczmar, A. G., ed.) Pergamon Press, Ltd., Oxford, **1970**, pp. 1–44.

Katzman, R., and Thal, L. J. Neurochemistry of Alzheimer's disease. In, *Basic Neurochemistry: Molecular, Cellular, and Medical Aspects*, 4th ed. (Siegel, G. J.; Agranoff, B.; Albers, R. W.; and Molinoff, P.; eds.) Raven Press, New York, **1989**, pp. 827–838.

Kaufman, P. L.; Weidman, T.; and Robinson, J. R. Cholinergics. In, *Pharmacology of the Eye*. (Sears, M. L., ed.) *Handbook of Experimental Pharmacology*, Vol. 69. Springer-Verlag, Berlin, **1984**, pp. 149–192.

Laskowski, M. B., and Dettbarn, W. D. The pharmacology of experimental myopathies. *Annu. Rev. Pharmacol. Toxicol.*, **1977**, *17*, 387–409.

Long, J. P. Structure–activity relationships of the reversible anticholinesterase agents. In, *Cholinesterases and Anticholinesterase Agents*. (Koelle, G. B., ed.) *Handbuch der Experimentellen Pharmakologie*, Vol. 15. Springer-Verlag, Berlin, **1963**, pp. 374–427.

Lotti, V. J.; Le Douarec, S. C.; and Stone, C. A. Autonomic nervous system: adrenergic antagonists. In, *Pharmacology of the Eye*. (Sears, M. L., ed.) *Handbook of Experimental Pharmacology*, Vol. 69. Springer-Verlag, Berlin, **1984**, pp. 249–278.

Massoulié, J., and Toutant, J. P. Vertebrate cholinesterases: structure and types of interaction. In, *The Cholinergic Synapse*. (Whittaker, V. P., ed.) *Handbook of Experimental Pharmacology*, Vol. 86. Springer-Verlag, Berlin, **1988**, pp. 167–224.

Murphy, S. D. Pesticides. In, *Casarett and Doull's Toxicology: The Basic Science of Poisons*, 3rd ed. (Klaassen, C. D.; Amdur, M. O.; and Doull, J.; eds.) Macmillan Publishing Co., New York, **1986**, pp. 519–581.

Omenn, G. S. The role of genetic differences in human

susceptibility to pesticides. In, *Toxicology of Pesticides: Experimental, Clinical, and Regulatory Perspectives.* (Costa, L. G.; Galli, C. L.; and Murphy, S. D.; eds.) *NATO Advanced Study Institute Series H,* Vol. 13. Springer-Verlag, Berlin, **1987**, pp. 93–108.

Osserman, K. E.; Foldes, F. F.; and Genkins, G. Myasthenia gravis. In, *Neuromuscular Blocking and Stimulating Agents,* Vol. 11. *International Encyclopedia of Pharmacology and Therapeutics,* Sect. 14. (Cheymol, J., ed.) Pergamon Press, Ltd., Oxford, **1972,** pp. 561–618.

Rosenberry, T. L. Acetylcholinesterase. *Adv. Enzymol.,* **1975,** *43,* 103–213.

Rowland, L. P. Controversies about treatment of myasthenia gravis. *J. Neurol. Neurosurg. Psychiatry,* **1980,** *43,* 644–659.

Schrader, G. *Die Entwicklung neuer Insektizide auf Grundlage von Organischen Fluor- und Phosphorverbindungen.* Monographie No. 62, Verlag Chemie, Weinheim, **1952.**

Schwartz, B. The glaucomas. *N. Engl. J. Med.,* **1978,** *290,* 182–186.

Usdin, E. Reactions of cholinesterases with substrates inhibitors and reactivators. In, *Anticholinesterase Agents,* Vol. 1. *International Encyclopedia of Pharmacology and Therapeutics,* Sect. 13. (Karczmar, A. G., ed.) Pergamon Press, Ltd., Oxford, **1970,** pp. 47–354.

WHO. *Organophosphorus Insecticides: A General Introduction.* Environmental Health Criteria, No. 63. World Health Organization, Geneva, **1986a.**

———. *Carbamate Insecticides: A General Introduction.* Environmental Health Criteria, No. 64. World Health Organization, Geneva, **1986b.**

Wills, J. H. Toxicity of anticholinesterases and treatment of poisoning. In, *Anticholinesterase Agents,* Vol. 1. *International Encyclopedia of Pharmacology and Therapeutics,* Sect. 13. (Karczmar, A. G., ed.) Pergamon Press, Ltd., Oxford, **1970,** pp. 355–471.

Wilson, I. B. Molecular complementarity and antidotes for alkyl phosphate poisoning. *Fed. Proc.,* **1959,** *18,* 752–758.

CHAPTER

8 ATROPINE, SCOPOLAMINE, AND RELATED ANTIMUSCARINIC DRUGS

Joan Heller Brown

The drugs described in this chapter inhibit the actions of acetylcholine (ACh) on autonomic effectors innervated by postganglionic cholinergic nerves. They also inhibit the actions of ACh on neuronal and ganglionic muscarinic receptors and on smooth muscle cells that lack cholinergic innervation. Since they antagonize the muscarinic actions of ACh, they are known as *antimuscarinic* or *muscarinic cholinergic blocking agents*. Because the major effects of most members of this class of drugs are qualitatively similar to those of its best-known member, atropine, the term *atropine-like* is also used.

In general, antimuscarinic agents cause little blockade of the effects of ACh at nicotinic receptor sites. Thus, at autonomic ganglia, where transmission primarily involves an action of ACh on nicotinic receptors, atropine produces partial block only at relatively high doses. At the neuromuscular junction, where the receptors are principally or exclusively nicotinic, extremely high doses of atropine or related drugs are required to cause any degree of blockade. However, quaternary ammonium analogs of atropine and related drugs generally exhibit a greater degree of nicotinic blocking activity and, consequently, are likely to interfere with ganglionic or neuromuscular transmission in doses that more closely approximate those that produce muscarinic block. In the central nervous system (CNS), cholinergic transmission appears to be predominantly nicotinic in the spinal cord and both muscarinic and nicotinic at subcortical and cortical levels in the brain (*see* Chapter 12). Autoradiographic studies have revealed a widespread distribution of muscarinic receptors throughout the human brain (Palacios *et al.*, in Symposium, 1986a). Many or most of the CNS effects of therapeutic doses of atropine-like drugs are probably attributable to their central antimuscarinic actions. At high or toxic doses, the central effects of atropine and related drugs generally consist of stimulation followed by depression. Since quaternary compounds penetrate the blood–brain barrier poorly, antimuscarinic drugs of this type have little or no effect on the CNS.

Parasympathetic neuroeffector junctions in different organs are not equally sensitive to the antimuscarinic agents. However, the relative sensitivity of the parasympathetically innervated organs to blockade varies little among the antimuscarinic drugs currently available for clinical use. Small doses depress salivary and bronchial secretion and sweating. With larger doses, the pupil dilates, accommodation of the eye is inhibited, and vagal effects on the heart are blocked so that the heart rate is increased. Larger doses inhibit the parasympathetic control of the urinary bladder and gastrointestinal tract, thus inhibiting micturition and decreasing the tone and motility of the gut. Still larger doses are required to inhibit gastric secretion and motility. Thus, doses of atropine and most related antimuscarinic drugs that reduce gastrointestinal tone and depress gastric secretion also almost invariably affect salivary secretion, ocular accommodation, and micturition. This hierarchy of relative sensitivities is probably not a consequence of differences in the affinity of atropine for the muscarinic receptors at these sites, because this varies little among various cell types. More likely determinants include the degree to which the functions of various end organs are regulated by parasympathetic tone and the involvement of intramural neurons and reflexes.

The actions and effects of most clinically available antimuscarinic agents differ only quantitatively from those of atropine, which is considered in detail below as the prototype of the group. Recent evidence indicates, however, that subclasses of muscarinic receptors are present in both the CNS and peripheral organs (*see* Chapter 5; *see also* Hammer *et al.*, 1980; Symposium, 1984, 1986a, 1988). Following earlier pharmacological clues, direct support for this concept came from the discovery of pirenzepine, an antagonist with higher affinity for muscarinic receptors in autonomic and other peripheral ganglia than for those in cardiac or smooth muscle. Moreover, gastric acid secretion can be greatly reduced by doses of pirenzepine that have little or no effect on heart rate or salivary secretion (*see* Hirschowitz and Molina *and also* Stockbreugger *et al.*, in Symposium, 1984). Most recently, molecular cloning studies have demonstrated the existence of at least five human genes that encode structurally distinct muscarinic cholinergic receptors (Bonner *et al.*, 1987). These receptors differ not only in their ligand binding properties but also in their capacity to elicit particular functional responses. Thus, it is possible that the next decade may see the development of antimuscarinic drugs with far greater selectivity than those currently on the scene.

History. The naturally occurring antimuscarinic drugs are the alkaloids of the belladonna plants. The most important of these are atropine and scopolamine. Preparations of belladonna were known to the ancient Hindus and have been used by physicians for many centuries. During the time of the Roman Empire and in the Middle Ages the deadly nightshade plant was frequently used to produce obscure and often prolonged poisoning. This prompted Linné to name the shrub *Atropa belladonna,* after Atropos, the oldest of the Three Fates, who cuts the thread of life. Kahn-Jemshed (1984) has argued that Dr. Roger Chillingworth, the cuckolded husband of Hester Prynne in Hawthorne's *The Scarlet Letter,* took his revenge on the Reverend Arthur Dimmesdale, the adulterer, with an atropine-based concoction. The name *belladonna* derives from the alleged use of this preparation by Italian women to dilate their pupils; modern day fashion photographers are known to use this same device for visual appeal. In India the root and leaves of the Jimson weed plant were burned and the smoke inhaled to treat asthma. British colonists observed this ritual and introduced the belladonna alkaloids into Western medicine in the early 1800s.

Accurate study of the actions of belladonna dates from the isolation of atropine in pure form by Mein in 1831. In 1867, Bezold and Bloebaum showed that atropine blocked the cardiac effects of vagal stimulation, and 5 years later Heidenhain found that it prevented salivary secretion produced by stimulation of the chorda tympani. Many semisynthetic congeners of the belladonna alkaloids, usually quaternary ammonium derivatives, and a large number of synthetic antimuscarinic compounds have been prepared, primarily with the objective of depressing gastric secretion without undesired antimuscarinic effects on other organs. With the advent of pirenzepine and its congeners, this goal may yet be achieved.

ATROPINE, SCOPOLAMINE, AND RELATED BELLADONNA ALKALOIDS

Sources and Members. The belladonna drugs are widely distributed in nature, especially in the Solanaceae plants. *Atropa belladonna,* the deadly nightshade, yields mainly the alkaloid atropine (*dl*-hyoscyamine). The same alkaloid is found in *Datura stramonium,* known as Jamestown or Jimson weed, stinkweed, thorn-apple, and devil's apple. The alkaloid scopolamine (hyoscine) is found chiefly in the shrub *Hyoscyamus niger* (henbane) and *Scopolia carniolica.*

Chemistry. These alkaloids are organic esters formed by combination of an aromatic acid, tropic acid, and complex organic bases, either tropine (tropanol) or scopine. Scopine differs from tropine only in having an oxygen bridge between the carbon atoms designated as 6 and 7 in the structural formulas given in Table 8–1. Homatropine is a semisynthetic compound produced by combining the base tropine with mandelic acid. Methylatropine nitrate, methscopolamine bromide, and homatropine methylbromide are the corresponding quaternary ammonium derivatives, modified by the addition of a second methyl group to the nitrogen.

Structure–Activity Relationship. The intact ester of tropine and tropic acid is essential for the antimuscarinic action of atropine, since neither the free acid nor the base exhibits significant antimuscarinic activity. The presence of a free OH group in the acid portion of the ester is also important. Substitution of other aromatic acids for tropic acid modifies but does not necessarily abolish the antimuscarinic activity. When given parenterally, quaternary ammonium derivatives of atropine and scopolamine are, in general, more potent than their parent compounds in both antimuscarinic and ganglionic blocking activity, and lack CNS activity because of poor penetration into the brain. Given orally, they are poorly and unreliably absorbed, as are other quaternary ammonium compounds.

Both tropic and mandelic acids have an asymmetrical carbon atom (boldface **C** in the formulas in Table 8–1). Scopolamine is *l*-hyoscine and is much more active than *d*-hyoscine. Atropine is racemized during extraction and consists of a mixture of equal parts of *d*- and *l*-hyoscyamine, but the

Table 8–1. STRUCTURAL FORMULAS OF ATROPINE, SCOPOLAMINE, AND HOMATROPINE

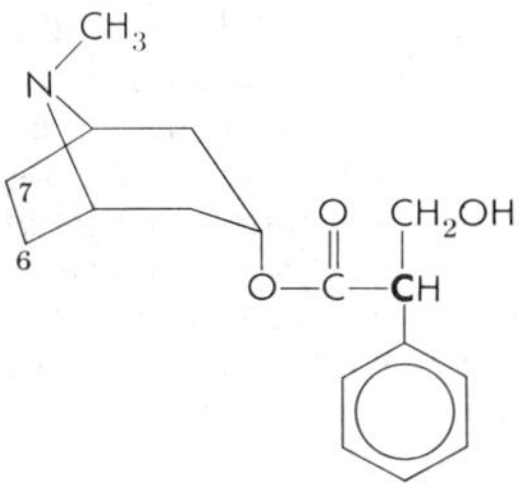

Atropine

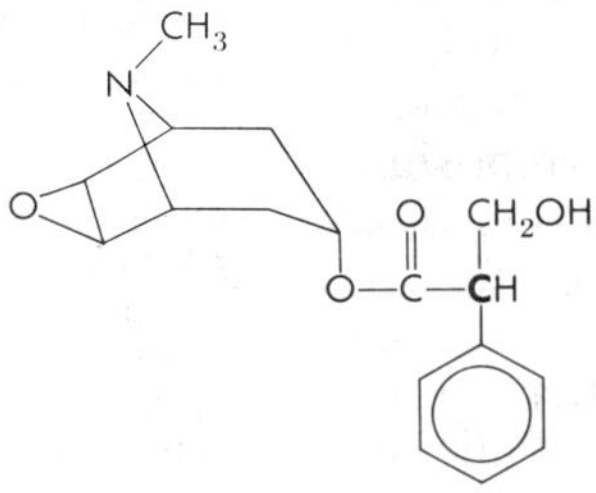

Scopolamine

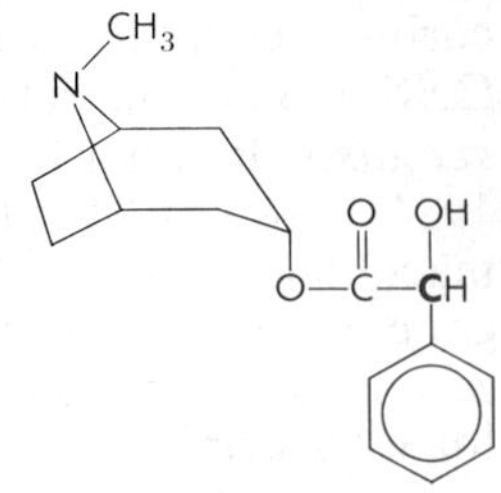

Homatropine

antimuscarinic activity is almost wholly due to the naturally occurring *l* form.

Mechanism of Action. Atropine and related compounds are competitive antagonists of the actions of ACh and other muscarinic agonists; they compete with such agonists for a common binding site on the muscarinic receptor (Yamamura and Snyder, 1974; Hulme *et al.*, 1978). The antagonism can therefore be overcome by increasing sufficiently the concentration of ACh at receptor sites of the effector organ. The receptors affected are those of peripheral structures that are either stimulated or inhibited by muscarine—that is, exocrine glands and smooth and cardiac muscle. Muscarinic receptors in ganglia and on intramural neurons are also affected. Antimuscarinic drugs inhibit responses to postganglionic cholinergic nerve stimulation less readily than they do responses to injected choline esters. The difference may be due to release of ACh by cholinergic nerve terminals so close to receptors that very high concentrations of the transmitter gain access to the receptors in the neuroeffector junction. In addition, diffusion and other factors may limit the concentration of antagonist that can be attained at these receptor sites.

Subtypes of Muscarinic Receptors. Studies of differential effects of muscarinic agonists (bethanechol and McN-A-343) on the tone of the lower esophageal sphincter led to the first discrimination between two different types of muscarinic receptors, which came to be designated M_1 (ganglionic) and M_2 (effector cell) (*see* Rattan and Goyal, in Symposium, 1984; *see also* Chapter 5). The use of ligand-binding techniques also revealed the existence of multiple muscarinic sites. Initially, only agonist ligands detected such heterogeneity; however, since the advent of pirenzepine, selective antagonists have been used to define at least three subtypes of muscarinic receptors. Pirenzepine binds with high affinity to sites in the cerebral cortex and sympathetic ganglia (M_1), but it has much lower affinity for those in cardiac muscle (M_2), as well as in smooth muscle and various glands (M_3) (*see* Watson *et al.*, in Symposium, 1984). Such data correlate well with the ability of pirenzepine to block agonist-induced responses that are mediated by muscarinic receptors in sympathetic and myenteric ganglia at concentrations considerably lower than those required to block responses that result from direct stimulation of receptors in various effector organs. Newer antagonists can further discriminate between muscarinic receptors in cardiac muscle and those in smooth muscle and various glands. For example, methoctramine displays selectivity for cardiac muscarinic receptors (*see* Melchiorre, 1988), while hexahydrosiladifenidol is relatively selective for glandular and smooth muscle receptors (*see* Ladinsky *et al.*, in Symposium, 1988).

The cloning of the cDNAs that encode muscarinic receptors has thus far detected five structural variants (*see* Chapter 5). When these receptors are expressed in cells, the properties of three of them (sometimes designated m_1, m_2, and m_3) correspond well with those defined pharmacologically (designated M_1, M_2, and M_3). Two additional structural variants have been cloned, but their relationship to pharmacologically defined receptors remains to be clarified.

The various muscarinic receptors regulate several effector systems within cells (*see* Chapters 2, 5, and 6). For example, stimulation of M_1 or M_3 receptors causes hydrolysis of polyphosphoinositides and the mobilization of intracellular Ca^{2+}, presumably as a result of a G protein–mediated activation of phospholipase C. M_2-muscarinic receptors regulate ion channels (*e.g.*, enhancement of a K^+ conductance in cardiac atrial fibers) and inhibit adenylyl cyclase by interaction with a G protein that is distinct from that utilized by M_1 and M_3 receptors.

PHARMACOLOGICAL PROPERTIES

Atropine and scopolamine differ quantitatively in antimuscarinic actions, particularly in their ability to affect the CNS. Atropine has almost no detectable effect on the CNS in doses that are used clinically. In contrast, scopolamine has prominent central effects at low therapeutic doses. The basis for this difference is probably the greater permeation of scopolamine through the blood–brain barrier. Because atropine has limited CNS effects it is given in preference to scopolamine for most purposes. When some central depressant effect is no disadvantage or is desired, as in preanesthetic medication, scopolamine is frequently administered.

Central Nervous System. Atropine in therapeutic doses (0.5 to 1.0 mg) causes only mild vagal excitation as a result of stimulation of the medulla and higher cerebral centers. The rate and occasionally the depth of breathing are increased, but this effect is probably the result of bronchiolar dilatation and the subsequent increase in physiological "dead space." With toxic doses of atropine, central excitation becomes more prominent, leading to restlessness, irritability, disorientation, hallucinations, or delirium (*see* discussion of atropine poisoning). With still larger doses, stimulation is followed by depression, leading to circulatory collapse and respiratory failure after a period of paralysis and coma.

Scopolamine in therapeutic doses normally causes CNS depression manifest as drowsiness, amnesia, fatigue, and dreamless sleep with a reduction in rapid-eye-movement (REM) sleep. It also causes euphoria and is therefore subject to some abuse. The depressant effects are sometimes sought when scopolamine is used as an adjunct to anesthetic agents or for preanesthetic medication. However, in the presence of severe pain, the same doses of scopolamine occasionally cause excitement, restlessness, hallucinations, or delirium. These excitatory effects, which resemble those of toxic doses of atropine, occur regularly after large doses of scopolamine.

Antitremor Activity. The belladonna alkaloids and related antimuscarinic agents have long been used in parkinsonism. These agents can be effective adjuncts to the recommended treatment with levodopa (*see* Chapter 20). Antimuscarinic drugs are also used to treat the extrapyramidal symptoms that commonly occur as side effects of antipsychotic drug therapy (*see* Chapter 18).

Vestibular Function. Scopolamine is effective in preventing motion sickness. This action is probably either on the cortex or more peripherally on the vestibular apparatus.

Other Effects. Atropine reduces the voltage and frequency of the alpha rhythm and consistently shifts the EEG rhythm to slow activity, an EEG pattern typical of drowsiness. Central cholinergic pathways are also believed to be important in the control of memory function. The memory loss that occurs in Alzheimer's disease is associated with degeneration of cholinergic neurons; however, these memory deficits are not accurately mimicked by treatment of human subjects with scopolamine (Beatty *et al.,* 1986).

Ganglia and Autonomic Nerves. Cholinergic neurotransmission in autonomic ganglia is mediated by activation of nicotinic cholinergic receptors, resulting in the generation of action potentials (*see* Chapters 5 and 9). In sympathetic ganglia, cholinergic agonists also cause the generation of slow excitatory postsynaptic potentials that are mediated by postganglionic muscarinic (M_1) cholinergic receptors. This response is particularly sensitive to pirenzepine (Brown *et al.,* 1980). A similar excitatory response is mediated by pirenzepine-sensitive muscarinic receptors on postganglionic neurons in the myenteric plexus (North *et al.,* 1985). The extent to which the slow excitatory response can alter impulse transmission through ganglia is not known, but the effects of pirenzepine on responses of end organs suggest a physiological modulatory function for the ganglionic M_1 receptor.

Pirenzepine inhibits gastric acid secretion at doses that have little effect on salivation or heart rate. Since the muscarinic receptors on the parietal cells do not appear to have a high affinity for pirenzepine, the M_1 receptor responsible for alterations in gastric acid secretion is postulated to be localized on postganglionic intramural neurons (*see* Goyal, 1988). Blockade of receptors on such neurons (rather than those at the neuroeffector junction) also appears to underlie the ability of pirenzepine to inhibit the relaxation of the lower esophageal sphincter. There is evidence that ganglia in the lung and in the heart may also be sites of action for certain muscarinic receptor antagonists (Barnes *et al.,* 1988; Wellstein and Pitschner, 1988).

Muscarinic receptors are present on presynaptic nerve terminals of autonomic neurons; their blockade augments transmitter release. These presynaptic receptors may be of either the M_1 or the M_2 subtype. Nonselective muscarinic blocking agents may therefore augment ACh release, partially counteracting the effects of postsynaptic receptor blockade.

The ultimate responses of end organs to blockade of muscarinic receptors on preganglionic or postganglionic neurons are difficult to predict. Inhibition of the slow excitatory potentials in ganglia may diminish the activity of postganglionic neurons that are cholinergic or adrenergic, or that contain other substances, as is the case for intramural neurons in the gut. Thus, while direct blockade at neuroeffector sites predictably reverses the usual effects of the parasympathetic nervous system, inhibition of ganglionic or neuronal sites may produce paradoxical responses.

Eye. The atropinic drugs block the responses of the sphincter muscle of the iris and the ciliary muscle of the lens to cholinergic stimulation (*see* Table 8–3, page 161). Thus, they dilate the pupil (mydriasis) and paralyze accommodation (cycloplegia). The wide pupillary dilatation results in photophobia; the lens is fixed for far vision, near objects are blurred, and micropsia sometimes occurs. The normal pupillary reflex constriction to light or upon convergence of the eyes is abolished. These effects can occur after either local or systemic administration of the alkaloids. However, conventional systemic doses of atropine (0.6 mg) have little ocular effect, in contrast to equal doses of scopolamine, which cause definite mydriasis and loss of accommodation. Locally applied atropine or scopolamine produces ocular effects of considerable duration; accommodation and pupillary reflexes may not fully recover for 7 to 12 days. The atropinic mydriatics differ from the sympathomimetic agents in that the latter cause pupillary dilatation without loss of accommodation. Pilocarpine, choline esters, physostigmine, and isoflurophate (DFP) in sufficient concentrations can reverse the ocular effects of atropinic drugs at least partially.

Atropine-like drugs administered systemically have little effect on intraocular pressure except in patients with narrow-angle glaucoma, where the pressure may occasionally rise dangerously. The rise in pressure occurs because the iris, crowded back into the angle of the anterior chamber of the eye, interferes with drainage of aqueous humor. The drugs may precipitate a first attack in unrecognized cases of this rare condition. In patients with open-angle glaucoma, a significant rise in pressure is unusual. Atropine-like drugs can generally be used safely in this latter condition, particularly if the patient is also adequately treated with an appropriate miotic agent.

Cardiovascular System. *Heart.* The main effect of atropine on the heart is to alter the rate. Although the dominant response is tachycardia, the heart rate often decreases transiently with average clinical doses (0.4 to 0.6 mg). The slowing is rarely marked, about 4 to 8 beats per minute, and is usually absent after rapid intravenous injection. There are no accompanying changes in blood pressure or cardiac output.

This paradoxical effect was once thought to be due to central vagal stimulation; however, such cardiac slowing is also seen with antimuscarinic drugs that do not readily enter the brain. Recent studies in man show that pirenzepine is equipotent with atropine in decreasing heart rate; its prior administration can prevent any further decrease by atropine. The data suggest that the decreased heart rate is produced through blockade of M_1 receptors on postganglionic parasympathetic neurons, thereby relieving the inhibitory effects of synaptic ACh on release of transmitter (Wellstein and Pitschner, 1988).

Larger doses of atropine cause progressively increasing tachycardia by blocking vagal effects on M_2 receptors on the SA nodal pacemaker. The resting heart rate is increased by about 35 to 40 beats per minute in young men given 2 mg of atropine intramuscularly; the maximal heart rate (*e.g.*, in response to exercise) is not altered by atropine. The influence of atropine is most noticeable in healthy young adults, in whom vagal tone is considerable. In infancy and old age, even large doses of atropine may fail to accelerate the heart. Atropine often produces cardiac arrhythmias, but without significant cardiovascular symptoms. Atrial arrhythmias and atrioventricular dissociation occur, the former most commonly in children given small doses that slow the heart, the latter usually in adults after small or large doses (Dauchot and Gravenstein, 1971; Hayes *et al.*, 1971).

With low doses of scopolamine (0.1 or 0.2 mg) the cardiac slowing is greater than with atropine. With higher doses, cardioacceleration occurs initially, but it is short lived and is followed within 30 minutes either by a return to the normal rate or by bradycardia. Thus, except for a short initial period, doses of scopolamine that produce ocular effects do not accelerate cardiac rate. With atropine, ocular effects are accompanied by tachycardia.

Adequate doses of atropine can abolish many types of reflex vagal cardiac slowing or asystole, for example, from inhalation of irritant vapors, stimulation of the carotid sinus, pressure on the eyeballs, peritoneal stimulation, or injection of contrast dye during cardiac catheterization. It also prevents or abruptly abolishes bradycardia or asystole caused by choline esters, anticholinesterase (anti-ChE) agents, or other parasympathomimetic drugs, as well as cardiac arrest from electrical stimulation of the vagus.

The removal of vagal influence on the heart by atropine may also cause changes in conduction. The velocity of AV conduction is increased; this effect can be shown to be independent of heart rate because the P–R interval is shortened even during atrial pacing. Atropine also shortens the functional refractory period of the AV node and can increase ventricular rate in patients who have atrial fibrillation or flutter. In certain cases of second-degree heart block (*e.g.*, Wenckebach AV block), in which vagal activity is an etiological factor (such as with digitalis toxicity), atropine may lessen the degree of block. In some patients with complete heart block, the idioventricular rate may be accelerated by atropine; in others it is stabilized. Atropine may improve the clinical condition of patients with early myocardial infarction by relieving severe sinus or nodal bradycardia or AV block (*see* Adgey *et al.*, 1968; and below).

Circulation. Atropine, in clinical doses, completely counteracts the peripheral vasodilatation and sharp fall in blood pressure caused by choline esters. In contrast, when given alone, its effect on blood vessels and blood pressure is neither striking nor constant. This result is expected, because most vascular beds probably lack significant cholinergic innervation and the cholinergic sympathetic vasodilator fibers to vessels supplying skeletal muscle do not appear to be involved to any important extent in the normal regulation of tone.

Toxic amounts of atropine usually, and therapeutic doses occasionally, dilate cutaneous blood vessels, especially those in the blush area (atropine flush). The mechanism of this anomalous vascular response is unknown. It may be a compensatory reaction permitting the radiation of heat to offset the atropine-induced rise in temperature that can accompany inhibition of sweating. On the other hand, it may represent a direct vasodilator action unrelated to cholinergic blockade.

Gastrointestinal Tract. Interest in the actions of antimuscarinic drugs on the stomach and intestine has led to their use as antispasmodic agents for gastrointestinal disorders and in the treatment of peptic ulcer. Although atropine can completely abolish the effects of ACh (and other parasympathomimetic drugs) on the gastrointestinal tract, it inhibits only incompletely the effects of vagal impulses. This difference is particularly striking in the effects of atropine on motility of the gut. Preganglionic vagal fibers innervating the gut synapse not only with postganglionic cholinergic fibers but also with a network of noncholinergic intramural neurons that form the enteric plexus. Since therapeutic doses of atropine do not block responses to gastrointestinal hormones or to noncholinergic neurohumoral transmitters, release of these substances from the intramural neurons can still effect changes in motility.

Secretion. Salivary secretion is particularly sensitive to inhibition by antimuscarinic agents, which can completely abolish the copious, watery, parasympathetically induced secretion. The mouth becomes dry, and swallowing and talking may become difficult.

Gastric secretion is reduced by antimuscarinic drugs. The doses that are necessary to decrease acid secretion also cause dry mouth, increase in heart rate, ocular disturbances, and other side effects. Secretion during the cephalic phase is markedly reduced by antimuscarinic drugs. The intestinal phase of gastric secretion is generally much less inhibited, whereas the basal (fasting) secretion of acid can be markedly reduced by atropine. The volume of secretion is usually reduced, but the concentration of acid is not necessarily lowered, possibly because secretion of HCO_3^- as well as of H^+ is blocked. The gastric cells that secrete mucin and proteolytic enzymes are more directly under vagal influence than are the acid-secreting cells, and atropine decreases the output of these organic constituents.

Motility. The belladonna alkaloids have marked effects on motility of the gastrointestinal tract. This reflects the predominantly parasympathetic motor control of the gut; sympathetic nerve impulses have a lesser role in the physiological regulation of tone and motility. The parasympathetic nerves enhance both tone and motility, and relax sphincters, thereby favoring the passage of chyme through the gut. However, the intestine has a complex system of intramural nerve plexuses that regulate motility independent of parasympathetic control; impulses from the CNS only modify the effects of the intrinsic reflexes. Some of the terminal neurons of the intramural plexuses are cholinergic, excitatory neurons; others are noncholinergic neurons that contain as yet unidentified neurotransmitters.

Both in normal subjects and in patients with gastrointestinal disease, full therapeutic doses of atropine produce definite and prolonged inhibitory effects on the motor activity of the stomach, duodenum, jejunum, ileum, and colon, characterized by a decrease in tone and in amplitude and frequency of peristaltic contractions. Relatively large doses are needed to produce such inhibition, possibly because concomitant blockade of muscarinic receptors in the myenteric plexus may have effects that are opposite to those produced by blockade of receptors on smooth muscle. Atropine can effectively block the excess motor activity of the gastrointestinal tract induced by parasympathomimetic drugs and anti-ChE agents.

Respiratory Tract. The parasympathetic nervous system plays a major role in regulating bronchomotor tone (Ziment and Au, 1986; Barnes *et al.*, 1988). A diverse set of stimuli cause reflex increases in parasympathetic activity that contribute to bronchoconstriction. Vagal fibers synapse in ganglia located in the airway wall; short postganglionic fibers end on muscarinic receptors that are concentrated in the larger airway smooth muscle. The submucosal glands are also innervated by parasympathetic neurons. Although anticholinergic agents were widely used as bronchodilators before the advent of epinephrine in the 1920s, they were supplanted thereafter by adrenergic agents and methylxanthines (*see* Chapter 25). Largely owing to the introduction of ipratropium, anticholinergic therapy of respiratory disease has been revived (*see* Symposium, 1987).

The belladonna alkaloids inhibit secretions of the nose, mouth, pharynx, and bronchi, and thus dry the mucous membranes of the respiratory tract. This action is especially marked if secretion is excessive, and is the basis for the use of atropine and scopolamine in preanesthetic medication. The ability of these agents to reduce the occurrence of laryngospasm during general anesthesia appears to be due to inhibition of respiratory tract secretions that can precipitate reflex laryngospasm. However, the depression of mucous secretion and the inhibition of mucociliary clearance are undesirable side effects of atropine in patients with airway disease. For unexplained reasons, ipratropium has little or no effect on the function of ciliated bronchial epithelium (*see* Gross, 1988).

The muscarinic antagonists are particularly effective against bronchoconstriction produced by parasympathomimetic drugs such as methacholine and anti-ChE agents. However, they only partially antagonize bronchoconstriction induced by histamine, bradykinin, or prostaglandin $F_{2\alpha}$, which presumably reflects the participation of parasympathetic efferents in the bronchial reflexes instigated by these agents. This action upon the indirect bronchoconstrictive effects of inflammatory mediators that are released during attacks of asthma forms the basis for the use of anticholinergic agents in the treatment of reversible airway disease (*see* Ziment and Au, 1986; Gross, 1988; *see also* Chapter 25).

Other Smooth Muscle. *Urinary Tract.* Intravenous urographic studies in man indicate that atropine (1.2 mg, intravenously) dilates the pelves, calyces, ureters, and bladder, and increases the visibility of the kidneys. Atropine decreases the normal tone and amplitude of contractions of the ureter and bladder, and often eliminates drug-induced enhancement of ureteral tone.

Biliary Tract. Atropine exerts a mild antispasmodic action on the gallbladder and bile ducts in man. However, this effect is not usually sufficient to overcome or prevent the marked spasm and increase in biliary duct pressure induced by opioids. The nitrites are more effective than atropine in this respect. Atropine has no consistent effect on the choledochal sphincter mechanism in man. Emptying of the human gallbladder in response to a fatty meal is delayed by prior administration of atropine. There is little basis for the use of atropine alone as a biliary antispasmodic.

Uterus. Uterine smooth muscle is innervated by parasympathetic fibers, but the effect of cholinergic impulses on uterine contractility is variable. Hence, atropine and scopolamine generally have negligible effects on the human uterus. Although the drugs cross the placental barrier, the fetus is apparently not adversely affected and the respiration of the newborn is not depressed.

Sweat Glands and Temperature. Small doses of atropine or scopolamine inhibit the activity of sweat glands, and the skin becomes hot and dry.

Sweating may be depressed enough to raise the body temperature, but only notably so after large doses or at high environmental temperatures. The anhidrotic action of atropine and stimulation of sweating by muscarinic agonists appeared for many years to be a pharmacological anomaly, as the sweat glands are supplied only by nerves that are anatomically sympathetic. However, these fibers are, in fact, mainly cholinergic.

In infants and small children moderate doses of belladonna alkaloids can induce "atropine fever." In atropine poisoning in infants, the temperature may reach 43° C or higher. Suppression of sweating is doubtless a considerable factor in the production of the fever, especially when the environmental temperature is high.

Absorption, Fate, and Excretion. The belladonna alkaloids are absorbed rapidly from the gastrointestinal tract. They also enter the circulation when applied locally to the mucosal surfaces of the body. Absorption from intact skin is limited. The quaternary ammonium derivatives of the belladonna alkaloids are poorly absorbed after an oral dose (Jonkman *et al.*, 1977); nevertheless, some of these compounds applied locally to the eye can cause mydriasis and cycloplegia. Atropine has a half-life of approximately 4 hours; hepatic metabolism accounts for the elimination of about half of a dose, and the remainder is excreted unchanged in the urine. Traces of atropine are found in various secretions, including breast milk.

Poisoning by Belladonna Alkaloids. The deliberate or accidental ingestion of belladonna alkaloids or other classes of drugs with atropinic properties is a major cause of poisonings. Many H_1-histaminergic blocking agents, phenothiazines, and tricyclic antidepressants have antimuscarinic activity and, in sufficient dosage, may produce syndromes that include features of atropine intoxication. Infants and young children are especially susceptible to the toxic effects of atropinic drugs (Rumack, 1973). Indeed, many cases of intoxication in children have resulted from conjunctival instillation of atropinic drugs for ophthalmic refraction and for other ocular effects (North and Kelly, 1987). Systemic absorption occurs either from the nasal mucosa after the drug has traversed the nasolacrimal duct or from the intestinal tract if it is swallowed. Delirium or toxic psychoses, without undue peripheral manifestations, have been reported in adults after instillation of atropine eyedrops. Transdermal preparations of scopolamine have been reported to cause toxic psychoses, especially in children and in the elderly (Wilkinson, 1987; Ziskind, 1988). Serious intoxication may occur in children who ingest berries or seeds containing belladonna alkaloids. Reports of stramonium poisoning due to tea made from Jimson weed seeds date as far back as 1676 in the United States and are described in *earlier editions* of this textbook.

El-Fakahany and Richelson (1983) have quantified the antimuscarinic activity of a series of antidepressants based on their ability to bind to muscarinic receptors in human brain. The range of antimuscarinic potencies is broad, but a number of these drugs show significant activity; protriptyline and amitriptyline are the most potent, with an affinity for the receptor that is approximately one tenth that reported for atropine. Since these drugs are administered in therapeutic doses considerably higher than the effective dose of atropine, antimuscarinic effects are often observed clinically (*see* Chapter 18). In addition, overdose with suicidal intent is a danger in the population using antidepressants. Treatment of intoxication by tricyclic antidepressants may require the administration of physostigmine (*see* below; *see also* Rumack, 1973; Aquilonius, 1978).

Fatalities from intoxication with atropine and scopolamine are rare, but they sometimes occur in children, in whom 10 mg or less may be lethal. Idiosyncratic reactions are more common with scopolamine than with atropine, and ordinary therapeutic doses sometimes cause alarming effects. Homatropine methylbromide is well tolerated in doses much larger than those used for therapy and is only about one fiftieth as toxic as atropine. Table 8–2 shows the doses of atropine giving undesirable responses or symptoms of overdosage. In cases of full-blown atropine poisoning, the syndrome may last 48 hours or longer. In addition to the effects described in Table 8–2, convulsions may occur. Depression and circulatory collapse are evident only in cases of severe intoxication; the blood pressure declines, respiration becomes inadequate, and death due to respiratory failure may follow after a period of paralysis and coma (*see* Shader and Greenblatt, 1972).

The diagnosis of atropine poisoning is suggested by the widespread paralysis of organs innervated by parasympathetic nerves. Intramuscular injection of 1 mg of the anti-ChE agent physostigmine may be used for confirmation. If the typical salivation, sweating, and intestinal hyperactivity do not occur, intoxication with atropine or a related agent is almost certain.

Measures to limit intestinal absorption should be initiated without delay if the poison has been taken

Table 8–2. EFFECTS OF ATROPINE IN RELATION TO DOSE

DOSE	EFFECTS
0.5 mg	Slight cardiac slowing; some dryness of mouth; inhibition of sweating
1.0 mg	Definite dryness of mouth; thirst; acceleration of heart, sometimes preceded by slowing; mild dilatation of pupil
2.0 mg	Rapid heart rate; palpitation; marked dryness of mouth; dilated pupils; some blurring of near vision
5.0 mg	All the above symptoms marked; speech disturbed; difficulty in swallowing; restlessness and fatigue; headache; dry, hot skin; difficulty in micturition; reduced intestinal peristalsis
10.0 mg and more	Above symptoms more marked; pulse rapid and weak; iris practically obliterated; vision very blurred; skin flushed, hot, dry, and scarlet; ataxia, restlessness, and excitement; hallucinations and delirium; coma

orally. For symptomatic treatment, physostigmine is the rational therapy. The slow intravenous injection of 1 to 4 mg of physostigmine (0.5 mg in children) rapidly abolishes the delirium and coma caused by large doses of atropine. Since physostigmine is metabolized rapidly, the patient may again lapse into coma within 1 to 2 hours, and repeated doses may be needed (*see* Ketchum *et al.*, 1973; Rumack, 1973). If marked excitement is present and more specific treatment is not available, diazepam is the most suitable agent for sedation and for control of convulsions. Large doses should be avoided because the central depressant action may coincide with the depression occurring late in atropinic poisoning. Phenothiazines should not be used because their antimuscarinic action is likely to intensify toxicity. Artificial respiration may be necessary. Ice bags and alcohol sponges help to reduce fever, especially in children.

Preparations, Dosage, and Routes of Administration. *Belladonna tincture* is a preparation that consists of an aqueous-alcoholic extract of belladonna leaf. The adult dose is 0.6 to 1.0 ml, which contains approximately 0.2 to 0.3 mg, respectively, of the alkaloids of the leaf (mainly atropine). *Belladonna extract* may be given in tablets; the dose is 15 mg, equivalent to slightly less than 0.2 mg of atropine. *Atropine* is the main alkaloid of belladonna as the free base. The readily soluble salt, *atropine sulfate,* is available in tablet form, as an injectable solution, as an ophthalmic solution and ointment, and as a solution to be given by nebulization. The average oral or parenteral dose of atropine sulfate for adults is 0.5 mg. *Scopolamine* (*l*-hyoscine) is marketed as the readily soluble salt, *scopolamine hydrobromide;* the adult parenteral dose is 0.3 to 0.6 mg. Scopolamine is also available in an ophthalmic solution and in transdermal patches (*see* below).

SYNTHETIC AND SEMISYNTHETIC SUBSTITUTES FOR BELLADONNA ALKALOIDS

The lack of selectivity of the belladonna alkaloids for those parasympathetic functions that might profitably be blocked in various diseases has led to intensive efforts to discover antimuscarinic drugs with more selective effects. Until recently, success has been limited, and the agents currently available are not wholly satisfactory.

The main differences in pharmacological properties are seen with compounds having a quaternary ammonium structure. These drugs are poorly and unreliably absorbed after oral administration, and valid comparisons of their potencies with those of the belladonna alkaloids can be made only after parenteral administration (Jonkman *et al.*, 1977). Penetration of the conjunctiva is also poor, so that most quaternary ammonium compounds are of little value in ophthalmology. Central effects are generally lacking, because these agents do not readily cross the blood–brain barrier. The quaternary ammonium compounds usually have a somewhat more prolonged action than the belladonna alkaloids; little is known of the fate and excretion of most of these agents. The most important pharmacodynamic difference is that the ratio of ganglionic blocking to antimuscarinic activity is greater for compounds with the quaternary ammonium structure than for tertiary amines because of their greater potency at nicotinic receptors; some of the side effects seen after high doses are due to ganglionic blockade. Thus, impotence and postural hypotension can occur in patients who are given these drugs. Poisoning with quaternary ammonium compounds may also cause a curariform neuromuscular block, leading to respiratory paralysis. Thus, toxic doses of these agents produce the usual manifestations of antimuscarinic poisoning with additional effects of ganglionic and, rarely, neuromuscular block, but usually without significant CNS involvement.

There is a clinical impression that the quaternary ammonium compounds have a relatively greater effect on gastrointestinal activity and that the doses necessary to treat gastrointestinal disorders are, consequently, somewhat more readily tolerated than are other agents of this type; this effect has been attributed to the additional element of ganglionic block. Nevertheless, most of these drugs, like atropine, generally control gastric secretion or gastrointestinal motility only at doses that also cause significant side effects due to muscarinic blockade at other sites. However, it has been suggested that propantheline, taken orally, can significantly reduce secretion of gastric acid stimulated by food to the same extent at low doses (15 mg per day) as when near-toxic doses are given (Feldman *et al.*, 1977).

QUATERNARY AMMONIUM ANTIMUSCARINIC COMPOUNDS

Methscopolamine. *Methscopolamine bromide* (PAMINE) is a quaternary ammonium derivative of scopolamine and therefore lacks the central actions of scopolamine. It is less potent than atropine and is poorly absorbed; however, its action is more prolonged, the usual oral dose (2.5 mg) acting for 6 to 8 hours. Its use has been limited chiefly to gastrointestinal diseases.

Homatropine. *Homatropine methylbromide* is less potent than atropine in antimuscarinic activity, but it is four times more potent as a ganglionic blocking agent. It is available in some combination products intended for relief of gastrointestinal spasm.

Methantheline. *Methantheline bromide* (BANTHINE) is a quaternary ammonium compound that differs from atropine in having a particularly high ratio of ganglionic blocking activity to antimuscarinic activity. Its structural formula is as follows:

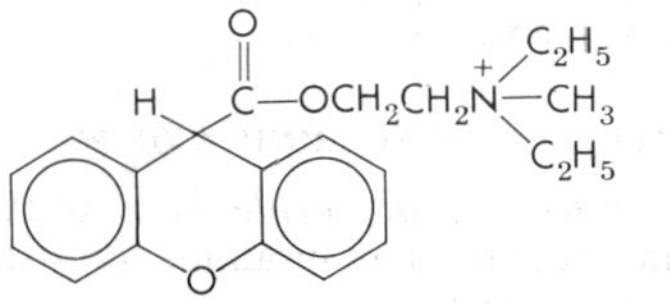

Methantheline

High doses may cause impotence, an effect rarely produced by purely antimuscarinic drugs and indicative of ganglionic block. Toxic doses may paralyze respiration by neuromuscular block. Restlessness, euphoria, fatigue, or, very rarely, acute psychotic episodes may be seen in occasional patients despite the relatively poor penetration of the drug into the CNS. Gastrointestinal effects of methantheline appear to be relatively greater than those of atropine, and many clinicians have the impression that the doses of methantheline used in the treatment of gastrointestinal disorders cause fewer antimuscarinic side effects than does atropine. The action is somewhat more prolonged than that of atropine, the effects of a therapeutic dose (50 to 100 mg) lasting 6 hours. An additional toxic manifestation unrelated to the blocking actions is the occasional appearance of skin rashes, including exfoliative dermatitis.

Propantheline. *Propantheline bromide* (PRO-BANTHINE) resembles methantheline chemically (isopropyl groups replace the ethyl substituents on the quaternary N atom). Its pharmacological properties are also similar to those of methantheline, but it is two to five times more potent. It is one of the more widely used of the synthetic antimuscarinic drugs. Very high doses block the skeletal neuromuscular junction. The usual clinical dose (15 mg) acts for about 6 hours.

Ipratropium. *Ipratropium bromide* is a quaternary ammonium compound formed by the introduction of an isopropyl group to the N atom of atropine. A somewhat less potent agent, *oxitropium bromide*, is currently under investigation in Europe; it is a quaternary ammonium derivative of scopolamine, formed by the introduction of an ethyl group. The structures of the parent alkaloids appear in Table 8–1.

Pharmacological Properties. Ipratropium bromide produces effects that are similar to those of atropine when each agent is administered parenterally (*see* Symposium, 1986b). These include bronchodilatation, tachycardia, and inhibition of salivary secretion. Although somewhat more potent than atropine in these actions, ipratropium lacks appreciable effect on the CNS and has greater inhibitory effects on ganglionic transmission, similar to other quaternary ammonium antimuscarinic agents. One unexpected and therapeutically important property of ipratropium is the relative lack of effect on the function of ciliated bronchial epithelium, compared with the marked inhibition of ciliary beating and mucociliary clearance produced by atropine; this difference is evident upon either local or parenteral administration and remains unexplained (*see* Wanner, in Symposium, 1986b). Hence, the use of ipratropium in patients with airway disease avoids the increased accumulation of lower airway secretions and the antagonism of β-adrenergic agonist–induced enhancement of mucociliary clearance encountered with atropine (*see* Foster and Bergofsky, in Symposium, 1986b).

When solutions are inhaled, the actions of ipratropium are confined almost exclusively to the mouth and airways. Even when administered in amounts many times the recommended dosage, little or no change occurs in heart rate, blood pressure, bladder function, intraocular pressure, or pupillary diameter. This selectivity results from the very inefficient absorption of the drug from the lungs or the gastrointestinal tract. The degree of bronchodilatation produced by ipratropium is thought to reflect the level of parasympathetic tone, supplemented by reflex activation of cholinergic pathways brought about by various stimuli. In normal subjects, the inhalation of ipratropium can provide virtually complete protection against the bronchoconstriction produced by the subsequent inhalation of such substances as sulfur dioxide, ozone, nebulized citric acid, or cigarette smoke. However, subjects with asthma or with demonstrable bronchial hyperresponsiveness are less well protected. Although ipratropium causes a marked reduction in sensitivity to methacholine in asthmatic subjects, only modest inhibition of responses to challenge with histamine, bradykinin, or prostaglandin $F_{1\alpha}$ is achieved, and little protection is provided against the bronchoconstriction induced by 5-hydroxytryptamine or the leukotrienes. Extensive reviews of the pharmacological properties of ipratropium bromide have appeared (*see* Massey and Gotz, 1985; Symposium, 1986b, 1987; Gross, 1988).

Absorption, Fate, and Excretion. Less than 1% of an inhaled dose of ipratropium bromide is absorbed systemically. As with most drugs administered by aerosol, about 90% of a dose is swallowed; most of the drug is not absorbed and appears in the feces. The small amount that is absorbed is eliminated from plasma with a half-time of about 3 hours. After inhalation, maximal responses usually develop over 30 to 90 minutes, and significant effects may persist for more than 4 hours. The pharmacokinetic properties of ipratropium bromide have been discussed in several reviews (*see* Pakes *et al.*, 1980; Massey and Gotz, 1985; Cugell, in Symposium, 1986b; Holgate, in Symposium, 1987; Gross, 1988).

Preparation and Dosage. Ipratropium bromide (ATROVENT) is available in the United States as a metered-dose inhaler that delivers 18 μg per spray. The recommended dosage is two inhalations four times daily, up to a maximum of 12 inhalations in 24 hours. The principal clinical use of ipratropium is in the treatment of chronic obstructive pulmonary disease; it is less effective in most asthmatic patients. The therapeutic use of ipratropium is discussed in Chapter 25.

Other Compounds. Other drugs in this category include *anisotropine methylbromide* (VALPIN), *clidinium bromide* (QUARZAN; also in combination with chlordiazepoxide as LIBRAX and others), *glycopyrrolate* (ROBINUL; also used parenterally in conjunction with anesthesia), *hexocyclium methylsulfate* (TRAL), *isopropamide iodide* (DARBID), *mepenzolate bromide* (CANTIL), and *tridihexethyl chloride* (PATHILON). Their structural formulas appear in *earlier editions* of this textbook. Many of these drugs, as well as the belladonna alkaloids, are found in a large number of combination products that include sedatives and, in some cases, other agents.

TERTIARY-AMINE ANTIMUSCARINIC COMPOUNDS

Certain of these agents are particularly useful in ophthalmology; included in this category are *homatropine hydrobromide* (ISOPTO HOMATROPINE) (a semisynthetic derivative of atropine; *see* Table 8–1), *cyclopentolate hydrochloride* (CYCLOGYL), and *tropicamide* (MYDRIACYL); the structural formulas of the latter two agents are as follows:

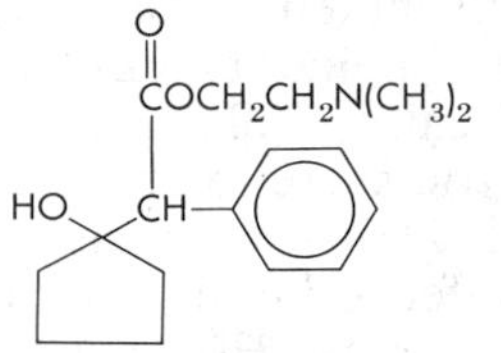

Cyclopentolate

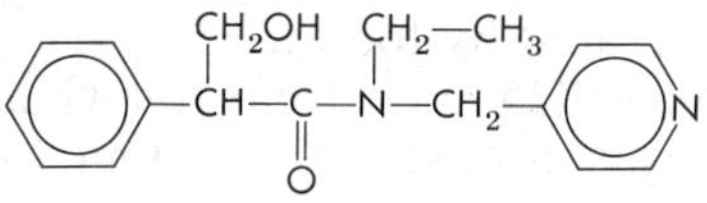

Tropicamide

These agents are preferred to atropine or scopolamine because of their shorter duration of action (Table 8–3). Additional information on the ophthalmological properties and preparations of these drugs is provided in Table 8–3.

The anticholinergic drugs used to treat parkinsonism and the extrapyramidal side effects of antipsychotic drugs are tertiary amines that can gain access to the CNS. Agents used primarily for these conditions include *benztropine mesylate* (COGENTIN) and *trihexyphenidyl hydrochloride* (ARTANE, others). These drugs are discussed in Chapter 20.

Tertiary amines used for their antispasmodic properties are *dicyclomine hydrochloride* (BENTYL, others), *oxyphencyclimine hydrochloride* (DARICON), *flavoxate hydrochloride* (URISPAS), and *oxybutynin chloride* (DITROPAN). The latter two are indicated specifically for urological disorders. These agents have weak anticholinergic properties but appear to exert a nonspecific direct relaxant effect on smooth muscle. In therapeutic doses they decrease spasm of the gastrointestinal tract, biliary tract, ureter, and uterus without producing characteristic atropine-like effects on the salivary, sweat, or gastrointestinal glands, the eye, or the cardiovascular system.

SELECTIVE ANTIMUSCARINIC COMPOUNDS

Pirenzepine hydrochloride is a tricyclic drug, similar in structure to imipramine; its structural formula is as follows:

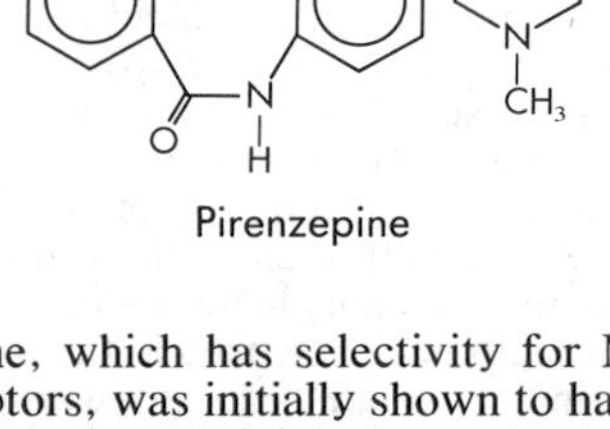

Pirenzepine

Pirenzepine, which has selectivity for M_1-muscarinic receptors, was initially shown to have greater gastrointestinal selectivity than other muscarinic

Table 8–3. MYDRIATIC AND CYCLOPLEGIC PROPERTIES OF ANTIMUSCARINIC AGENTS

DRUG	STRENGTH OF SOLUTION * (*percent*)	MYDRIASIS *Maximal* (*minutes*)	MYDRIASIS *Recovery* † (*days*)	PARALYSIS OF ACCOMMODATION *Maximal* (*minutes*)	PARALYSIS OF ACCOMMODATION *Recovery* ‡ (*days*)
Atropine sulfate	1.0	30–40	7–10	60–180	6–12
Scopolamine hydrobromide	0.5	20–30	3–7	30–60	3–7
Homatropine hydrobromide	1.0 §	40–60	1–3	30–60	1–3
Cyclopentolate hydrochloride	0.5–1.0	30–60	1	25–75	¼–1
Tropicamide	0.5–1.0 ‖	20–40	¼	30	<¼

* One instillation of 1 drop of solution. Preparations of ophthalmic solutions currently available in the United States include atropine sulfate, 0.5–3%; scopolamine hydrobromide, 0.25%; homatropine hydrobromide, 2 and 5%; cyclopentolate hydrochloride, 0.5–2%; and tropicamide, 0.5 and 1%.

† To within 1 mm of original pupillary diameter.

‡ To within 2 diopters of original accommodative power; ability to read fine print is possible by the third day after instillation of atropine or scopolamine and by 6 hours after homatropine.

§ Full mydriasis requires instillation of a 5% solution; cycloplegia may be incomplete.

‖ Adequate loss of accommodation lasting about 30 minutes requires instillation of a 1% solution.

antagonists (*see* Carmine and Brogden, 1985; Londong, 1986). The drug is used in the treatment of peptic ulcer in a number of countries, not currently including the United States. Therapeutic doses of 100 to 150 mg per day are required to achieve maximal rates of healing. At these doses the incidence of dry mouth and blurred vision is relatively low. Central effects are not seen because of the drug's low lipid solubility and limited penetration into the CNS.

Telenzepine is an analog of pirenzepine with a fourfold to tenfold greater potency for inhibition of gastric acid secretion; it has similar selectivity for M_1-muscarinic receptors (Londong, 1986). It also is not currently marketed in the United States.

AF-DX 116 is an analog of pirenzepine that differs markedly in its pharmacological properties. AF-DX 116 has its greatest affinity for cardiac (M_2) muscarinic receptors. It also displays cardioselectivity in human subjects (Pitschner *et al.*, 1989) and may be marketed for use in sinus bradycardia and AV block of vagal origin.

Other muscarinic antagonists under investigation include methoctramine and himbacine, which show selectivity for cardiac M_2 receptors, and hexahydrosiladifenidol, which shows selectivity for M_3 receptors in exocrine glands.

THERAPEUTIC USES OF ANTIMUSCARINIC DRUGS

Antimuscarinic drugs have been employed in a wide variety of clinical conditions, predominantly to inhibit effects of parasympathetic nervous system activity. The major limitation in the use of these drugs is often failure to obtain desired therapeutic responses without concomitant side effects. The latter usually are not serious but are sufficiently disturbing to decrease patient compliance, particularly during long-term administration.

Certain of the synthetic belladonna substitutes are used much more extensively than the natural alkaloids in a number of clinical conditions. In a few situations this preference is supported by evidence. With the discovery of subclasses of muscarinic receptors, more selective antimuscarinic agents may soon become available.

Gastrointestinal Tract. Antimuscarinic agents have been widely used in the management of peptic ulcer. Although these drugs can reduce gastric motility and the secretion of gastric acid, the doses required to produce these effects are usually associated with pronounced side effects, such as dryness of the mouth, loss of visual accommodation, photophobia, and difficulty in urination. As a consequence, patient compliance in the long-term management of symptoms of peptic ulcer with these drugs is poor. Although Feldman and coworkers (1977) reported that propantheline can inhibit the secretion of gastric acid (stimulated by food) in doses that produce minimal side effects, most investigators have concluded that the antimuscarinic agents that are currently available, even when administered in relatively high doses, are not unequivocally efficacious in the management of patients with peptic ulcer (Ivey, 1975).

The use of histamine H_2-receptor blocking agents has resulted in marked improvement in the treatment of peptic ulcer (*see* Chapters 23 and 37). These agents cause few side effects and have been generally considered to be the drugs of choice for inhibiting gastric acid secretion. Recently, pirenzepine has been developed for potential use in the treatment of ulcer. Because of its selectivity, pirenzepine clearly offers a marked improvement over atropine. In the current context, however, it is more useful to compare the efficacy and side effects of this agent with that of the H_2-blocking agents.

Most studies indicate that pirenzepine (100 to 150 mg per day) produces about the same rate of healing of duodenal ulcers as the H_2 blockers cimetidine or ranitidine; it may also be effective in preventing the recurrence of ulcers. Although less extensive data are available, similar results have been obtained in the treatment of gastric ulcers. Dry mouth has occurred in 14% and blurred vision in 2 to 5% of patients treated with pirenzepine, but these side effects necessitated withdrawal of the drug in fewer than 1% of the patients. There are indications that the concurrent administration of antimuscarinic drugs and H_2 blockers may produce synergistic effects, such that lower doses of each type of agent may be therapeutically effective. These studies in man have also provided support for the postulated localization of M_1 receptors at ganglionic sites, because pirenzepine has been found to be more potent in inhibiting gastric acid secretion produced as a result of neural stimuli than that induced by muscarinic agonists. The therapeutic efficacy and pharmacological properties of pirenzepine have been reviewed by Carmine and Brogden (1985); *see also* Londong (1986).

The belladonna alkaloids and their synthetic substitutes have also been used and recommended in a wide variety of conditions known or supposed to involve increased tone ("spasticity") or motility of the gastrointestinal tract. These agents can reduce tone and motility when administered in maximal tolerated doses, and they might be expected to have a real effect if the condition in question is in fact due to excessive smooth muscle contraction, a point that is often in doubt. Although antimuscarinic agents are commonly used in the management of irritable colon syndrome, there is no convincing evidence that these drugs are more effective than placebo in this condition.

The intestinal hypermotility and increased frequency of stools associated with administration of antihypertensive agents such as guanethidine are frequently well controlled by atropine-like drugs. Diarrhea sometimes associated with irritative conditions of the lower bowel, such as mild dysenteries and diverticulitis, may respond to such therapy. However, more severe conditions such as salmonella dysenteries, ulcerative colitis, and regional enteritis respond poorly.

The belladonna alkaloids and synthetic substitutes are very effective in reducing excessive salivation, such as that associated with heavy-metal poisoning or parkinsonism. They are also useful for blocking salivation in patients unable to swallow because of esophageal obstruction from tumors or stricture. The dosage must be adjusted carefully to avoid reducing secretion to the point where dry mouth is troublesome. Antimuscarinic agents can reduce the secretion of enzymes and HCO_3^- by the pancreas. Several agents, particularly methantheline and propantheline, have been tried in the treatment of acute pancreatitis; however, evidence for their efficacy in this condition remains entirely unconvincing.

Uses in Ophthalmology. Effects limited to the eye are obtained by local administration of an antimuscarinic drug to produce mydriasis and cycloplegia. Cycloplegia is not attainable without mydriasis and requires higher concentrations or more prolonged application of a given agent. Mydriasis is often necessary for thorough examination of the retina and optic disc and in the therapy of iridocyclitis and keratitis. The belladonna mydriatics may be alternated with miotics for breaking or preventing the development of adhesions between the iris and the lens. Complete cycloplegia may be necessary in the treatment of iridocyclitis and choroiditis and for accurate measurement of refractive errors. In instances where complete cycloplegia is required, agents such as atropine or scopolamine, which are more effective, are preferred to drugs such as cyclopentolate and tropicamide. Details of the drugs commonly used and the duration of action of the usual solutions are given in Table 8–3. Although the effect of a single drop of a solution of atropine on healthy eyes is very prolonged, in acute inflammation two or three instillations a day may be required to maintain a full effect. Atropine occasionally causes local irritation of the eye, and in susceptible persons it may produce swelling of the eyelids and conjunctivitis. With continued use, the conjunctivitis may become chronic. Therapy with topical antihistaminic agents may control the atropine conjunctivitis, or therapy may be continued with another agent (*e.g.,* scopolamine).

Shorter-acting substitutes for atropine or scopolamine are used when prolonged mydriasis and cycloplegia are not required or may pose a hazard to the patient. The standard agents for this purpose are homatropine, cyclopentolate, and tropicamide. Where mydriasis alone is desired, the weaker solutions of cyclopentolate or tropicamide may be used, if necessary in combination with a sympathomimetic drug such as phenylephrine.

It is of great importance to recognize patients who are predisposed to narrow-angle glaucoma. The ophthalmic use of any of the antimuscarinic drugs may increase intraocular pressure in eyes with a narrow angle between iris and cornea, precipitating an attack of acute glaucoma with the potential hazard of ensuing blindness. Systemic use of the antimuscarinic agents can also precipitate glaucoma in such predisposed patients. Although narrow-angle glaucoma is a rare condition, the use of drugs with antimuscarinic properties is not; careful ophthalmological evaluation, including examination with tonometer and gonioscope, should be undertaken to detect the possible presence of a narrow anterior chamber angle before starting therapy with these agents, particularly if therapy is to be intensive or prolonged. Mydriasis due to the shorter-acting agents may be counteracted by local application of pilocarpine (1 to 4%); mydriasis from atropine and scopolamine is usually only partly counteracted, even by physostigmine (0.25%) or isoflurophate (0.025%). In wide-angle glaucoma the drugs generally do not cause dangerous elevation of intraocular pressure, particularly if the patient is treated soon afterward with locally applied miotics.

The photophobia associated with mydriasis usually requires that the patient wear dark glasses. Although absorption into the bloodstream from the conjunctival sac is minimal, systemic toxicity can occur from an antimuscarinic agent that reaches more absorptive mucosal surfaces by way of the nasolacrimal duct. This danger should be minimized by exerting pressure on the inner canthus of the eye for a few minutes after each instillation. This precaution is particularly important in small children, who are highly susceptible to the toxic effects of belladonna alkaloids.

Respiratory Tract. Atropine and other belladonna alkaloids and substitutes reduce secretion in both the upper and lower respiratory tracts. This effect in the nasopharynx may provide some symptomatic relief of acute rhinitis associated with coryza or hay fever, but such therapy does not affect the natural course of the condition. It is probable that the contribution of antihistamines employed in "cold" mixtures is primarily due to their antimuscarinic properties, except in conditions with an allergic basis.

The belladonna alkaloids can induce bronchial dilatation and were formerly in common use as a remedy for bronchial asthma. They appear to have beneficial effects when obstruction of the airway is associated with chronic bronchitis or emphysema. However, when administered systemically, most antimuscarinic agents reduce the volume of bronchial secretion, which can result in decreased fluidity and subsequent inspissation of the residual secretion. This viscid material is difficult to remove from the respiratory tree, and its presence can dangerously obstruct airflow and predispose to infection.

Ipratropium bromide, a congener of methylatropine, has recently become available in the United States for use as a bronchodilator. As noted above, ipratropium does not produce adverse effects on mucociliary clearance, in contrast to atropine and other muscarinic antagonists. Thus, its anticholinergic properties can be safely exploited in the treatment of reversible airway disease. Moreover, the inhalation of solutions of the drug produces little or no systemic anticholinergic side effects. The therapeutic use of ipratropium bromide is discussed in Chapter 25.

Cardiovascular System. The cardiovascular effects of the antimuscarinic drugs are of limited clinical application. Generally, these agents are used in coronary care units for short-term interventions. Atropine is a specific antidote for the cardiovascular collapse that may result from the injudicious administration of a choline ester or an inhibitor of cholinesterase. It is also used to antagonize reflex vagal cardiac slowing.

Atropine may be of value in the initial treatment of patients with acute myocardial infarction in whom excessive vagal tone causes sinus or nodal bradycardia. Sinus bradycardia is the most common arrhythmia seen during acute myocardial infarction, especially of the inferior or posterior wall. Some experimental and clinical evidence suggests that bradycardia may be beneficial in limiting the size of the infarction and protecting the ischemic myocardium against ventricular arrhythmias (Myers *et al.,* 1974). On the other hand, bradycardia may be so severe as to lead to hypotension. In addition, the patient with very high vagal tone may develop AV block. Both of these events would lead to further clinical deterioration, and atropine may be beneficial in such cases (Watanabe, 1983). The therapeutic goals are to restore heart rate to a level sufficient to maintain adequate hemodynamic status and to eliminate AV nodal block. A total dose of 0.6 to 1 mg given intravenously is generally recommended. Dosing must be done judiciously; doses that are too low may cause a paradoxical bradycardia (*see* above), while excessive doses will cause tachycardia that may extend the infarct by increasing the demand for oxygen. Repeated doses of atropine should not be used because of the development of side effects such as CNS toxicity and urinary retention. Bradycardia, if persistent, should be controlled by the insertion of a pacemaker as soon as possible.

Atropine is occasionally useful in reducing the severe bradycardia and syncope associated with a hyperactive carotid sinus reflex. It has little effect on most ventricular rhythms. In some patients atropine may eliminate premature ventricular contractions associated with a very slow atrial rate. It may also reduce the degree of AV block when increased vagal tone is a major factor in the conduction defect, such as the second-degree AV block that can be produced by digitalis. Atropine is occasionally useful in the diagnosis of anomalous AV conduction (Wolff–Parkinson–White syndrome) by restoring the QRS complex to normal duration.

Central Nervous System. For many years the belladonna alkaloids and subsequently the tertiary-amine synthetic substitutes were the only agents helpful in the treatment of parkinsonism. Levodopa is now the treatment of choice, but alternative or concurrent therapy with antimuscarinic agents may be required in some patients (*see* Chapter 20). Synthetic agents such as benztropine have been shown to be efficacious in preventing dystonias or parkinsonian symptoms in patients treated with antipsychotic drugs (Arana *et al.,* 1988; *see also* Chapter 18).

The belladonna alkaloids were among the first drugs to be used in the prevention of motion sickness. Scopolamine is the most effective prophylactic agent for short (4- to 6-hour) exposures to severe motion, and probably for periods of up to several days. All agents used to combat motion sickness should be given prophylactically; they are much less effective after severe nausea or vomiting has developed. A preparation for the transdermal administration of scopolamine (TRANSDERM SCŌP) has been shown to be highly effective for the prevention of motion sickness (Price *et al.,* 1981). The drug is incorporated into a multilayered adhesive unit that is applied to the postauricular mastoid region. Absorption of the drug is especially efficient in this area. For optimal effects, the application should be made at least 4 hours before the antiemetic effect is required. The duration of action of the preparation is about 72 hours, during which time approximately 0.5 mg of scopolamine is delivered. Dry mouth is common, occurring in about two thirds of patients, and decreased production of saliva has been documented (Gordon *et al.*, 1985; Wilkinson, 1987). Drowsiness is not infrequent; blurred vision occurs in some individuals. Rare but severe psychotic episodes have also been reported (Wilkinson, 1987; Ziskind, 1988). (For further discussion of motion sickness, *see* Chapter 23.)

The sedation, tranquilization, and amnesia produced by scopolamine are useful in a variety of circumstances, including labor. In this situation it is almost always combined with agents that produce analgesia or sedation. Given alone in the presence of pain or severe anxiety, scopolamine may induce outbursts of uncontrolled behavior.

Uses in Anesthesia. The belladonna alkaloids were often used prior to the administration of a general anesthetic agent, mainly to inhibit excessive salivation and secretions of the respiratory tract; their concomitant bronchodilator action is also of value. The increasing use of relatively nonirritating anesthetics lessens the importance of antimuscarinic agents for this purpose. Scopolamine may contribute to tranquilization and amnesia (*see* Chapter 13). Atropine is commonly given with neostigmine to counteract its parasympathomimetic effects when the latter agent is used to end curarization after surgery. Serious cardiac arrhythmias have occasionally occurred, perhaps because of the initial cholinomimetic effects of atropine combined with those produced by neostigmine.

Genitourinary Tract. Atropine has often been given with an opioid in the treatment of renal colic in the hope that it will relax the ureteral smooth muscle; however, as in biliary colic, it probably does not make a major contribution to the relief of pain. The belladonna alkaloids and several synthetic substitutes can lower intravesicular pressure, increase capacity, and reduce the frequency of urinary bladder contractions by antagonizing the parasympathetic control of this organ. The block is less complete than in many other organs, but it has been taken as a basis for the use of such agents in enuresis in children, particularly when a progressive increase in bladder capacity is the objective; to reduce urinary frequency in spastic paraplegia; and to increase the capacity of the bladder in conditions in which irritation has led to hypertonicity. However, it has not been established that antimuscarinic drugs make a major contribution to the treatment of any of these conditions. Oxybutynin appears to be effective in the treatment of a range of unstable bladder conditions (Kirkali and Whitaker, 1987) but has significantly less anticholinergic and greater antispasmodic activity than atropine.

Anticholinesterase and Mushroom Poisoning. The use of atropine in large doses for the treatment of poisoning by anti-ChE organophosphorus insecticides is discussed in detail in Chapter 7. Atropine may also be used to antagonize the parasympathomimetic effects of neostigmine or other anti-ChE agents administered in the treatment of myasthenia gravis. It does not interfere with the salutary effects at the skeletal neuromuscular junction, and is particularly useful early in therapy, before tolerance to muscarinic side effects has developed.

Atropine is a specific antidote for the so-called rapid type of mushroom poisoning due to the cholinomimetic alkaloid muscarine, found in *Amanita muscaria* and a few other fungi. Atropine is of no value in the delayed type of mushroom poisoning due to the toxins of *A. phalloides* and certain other species of the same genus (*see* Chapter 6).

Adgey, A. A. J.; Geddes, J. S.; Mulholland, H. C.; Keegan, D. A. J.; and Pantridge, J. F. Incidence, significance, and management of early bradyarrhythmia complicating acute myocardial infarction. *Lancet*, **1968**, *2*, 1097–1101.

Aquilonius, S.-M. Physostigmine in the treatment of drug overdose. In, *Cholinergic Mechanisms and Psychopharmacology*, Vol. 24. (Jenden, D. J., ed.) Plenum Press, New York, **1978**, pp. 817–825.

Arana, G. W.; Goff, D. C.; Baldessarini, R. J.; and Keepers, G. A. Efficacy of anticholinergic prophylaxis for neuroleptic-induced acute dystonia. *Am. J. Psychiatry*, **1988**, *145*, 993–996.

Beatty, W. W.; Butters, N.; and Janowsky, D. S. Patterns of memory failure after scopolamine treatment: implications for cholinergic hypotheses of dementia. *Behav. Neural Biol.*, **1986**, *45*, 196–211.

Bonner, T. I.; Buckley, N. J.; Young, A. C.; and Brann, M. R. Identification of a family of muscarinic acetylcholine receptor genes. *Science*, **1987**, *237*, 527–532.

Brown, D. A.; Forward, A.; and Marsh, S. Antagonist discrimination between ganglionic and ileal muscarinic receptors. *Br. J. Pharmacol.*, **1980**, *71*, 362–364.

Dauchot, P., and Gravenstein, J. S. Effects of atropine on the electrocardiogram in different age groups. *Clin. Pharmacol. Ther.*, **1971**, *12*, 274–280.

El-Fakahany, E., and Richelson, E. Antagonism by antidepressants of muscarinic acetylcholine receptors of human brain. *Br. J. Pharmacol.*, **1983**, *78*, 97–102.

Feldman, M.; Richardson, C. T.; Peterson, W. L.; Walsh, J. H.; and Fordtran, J. S. Effect of low-dose propantheline on food-stimulated gastric acid secretion. *N. Engl. J. Med.*, **1977**, *297*, 1427–1430.

Gordon, C.; Ben-Aryeh, H.; Attias, J.; Szargel, R.; and Gutman, D. Effect of transdermal scopolamine on salivation. *J. Clin. Pharmacol.*, **1985**, *25*, 407–412.

Hammer, R.; Berrie, C. P.; Birdsall, N. J. M.; Burgen, A. S. V.; and Hulme, E. C. Pirenzepine distinguishes between different subclasses of muscarinic receptors. *Nature*, **1980**, *283*, 90–92.

Hayes, A. H., Jr.; Copelan, H. W.; and Ketchum, J. S. Effects of large intramuscular doses of atropine on cardiac rhythm. *Clin. Pharmacol. Ther.*, **1971**, *12*, 482–486.

Hulme, E. C.; Birdsall, N. J. M.; Burgen, A. S. V.; and Mehta, P. The binding of antagonists to brain muscarinic receptors. *Mol. Pharmacol.*, **1978**, *14*, 737–750.

Ivey, K. J. Anticholinergics: do they work in peptic ulcer? *Gastroenterology*, **1975**, *68*, 154–166.

Jonkman, J. H. G.; Van Bork, L. E.; Wijsbeek, J.; De Zeeuw, R. A.; and Orie, N. G. M. Variations in the bioavailability of thiazinamium methylsulfate. *Clin. Pharmacol. Ther.*, **1977**, *21*, 457–463.

Ketchum, J. S.; Sidell, F. R.; Crowell, E. B., Jr.; Aghajanian, G. K.; and Hayes, A. H., Jr. Atropine, scopolamine, and ditran: comparative pharmacology and antagonists in man. *Psychopharmacologia,* **1973,** *28,* 121–145.

Khan-Jemshed, A. Occasional notes: atropine poisoning in Hawthorne's *The Scarlet Letter. N. Engl. J. Med.,* **1984,** *311,* 414–416.

Kirkali, Z., and Whitaker, R. H. The use of oxybutynin in urological practice. *Int. Urol. Nephrol.,* **1987,** *19,* 385–391.

Myers, R. W.; Pearlman, A. S.; Hyman, R. M.; Goldstein, R. A.; Kent, K. M.; Goldstein, R. E.; and Epstein, S. E. Beneficial effects of vagal stimulation and bradycardia during experimental acute myocardial ischemia. *Circulation,* **1974,** *49,* 943–947.

North, R. A.; Slack, B. E.; and Surprenant, A. Muscarinic M_1 and M_2 receptors mediate depolarization and presynaptic inhibition in guinea-pig enteric nervous system. *J. Physiol.* [*Lond.*], **1985,** *368,* 435–452.

North, R. V., and Kelly, M. E. A review of the uses and adverse effects of topical administration of atropine. *Ophthalmic Physiol. Opt.,* **1987,** *7,* 109–114.

Pitschner, H. F.; Schulte, B.; Schlepper, M.; Palm, D.; and Wellstein, A. AF-DX 116 discriminates heart from gland M_2-cholinoceptors in man. *Life Sci.,* **1989,** *45,* 493–498.

Price, N. M.; Schmitt, L. G.; McGuire, J.; Shaw, J. E.; and Trobough, G. Transdermal scopolamine in the prevention of motion sickness at sea. *Clin. Pharmacol. Ther.,* **1981,** *29,* 414–419.

Rumack, B. H. Anticholinergic poisoning: treatment with physostigmine. *Pediatrics,* **1973,** *52,* 449–451.

Wellstein, A., and Pitschner, H. F. Complex dose–response curves of atropine in man explained by different functions of M1- and M2-cholinoceptors. *Naunyn Schmiedebergs Arch. Pharmacol.,* **1988,** *338,* 19–27.

Wilkinson, J. A. Side effects of transdermal scopolamine. *J. Emerg. Med.,* **1987,** *5,* 389–392.

Yamamura, H. I., and Snyder, S. H. Muscarinic cholinergic receptor binding in the longitudinal muscle of the guinea pig ileum with (^{3}H) quinuclidinyl benzilate. *Mol. Pharmacol.,* **1974,** *10,* 861–867.

Ziskind, A. A. Transdermal scopolamine-induced psychosis. *Postgrad. Med.,* **1988,** *84,* 73–76.

Monographs and Reviews

Barnes, P. J.; Minette, P.; and Maclagan, J. Muscarinic receptor subtypes in airways. *Trends Pharmacol. Sci.,* **1988,** *9,* 412–416.

Carmine, A. A., and Brogden, R. N. Pirenzepine: a review of its pharmacodynamic and pharmacokinetic properties and therapeutic efficacy in peptic ulcer disease and other allied diseases. *Drugs,* **1985,** *30,* 85–126.

Goyal, R. K. Identification, localization and classification of muscarinic receptor subtypes in the gut. *Life Sci.,* **1988,** *43,* 2209–2220.

Gross, N. J. Ipratropium bromide. *N. Engl. J. Med.,* **1988,** *319,* 486–494.

Londong, W. Present status and future perspectives of muscarinic receptor antagonists. *Scand. J. Gastroenterol.,* **1986,** *21,* 55–59.

Massey, K. L., and Gotz, V. P. Ipratropium bromide. *Drug Intell. Clin. Pharm.,* **1985,** *19,* 5–12.

Melchiorre, C. Polymethylene tetramines: a new generation of selective muscarinic antagonists. *Trends Pharmacol. Sci.,* **1988,** *9,* 216–220.

Pakes, G. E.; Brogden, R. N.; Heel, R. C.; Speight, T. M.; and Avery, G. S. Ipratropium bromide: a review of its pharmacological properties and therapeutic efficacy in asthma and chronic bronchitis. *Drugs,* **1980,** *20,* 237–266.

Shader, R. I., and Greenblatt, D. J. Belladonna alkaloids and synthetic anticholinergics: uses and toxicity. In, *Psychiatric Complications of Medical Drugs.* (Shader, R. I., ed.) Raven Press, New York, **1972,** pp. 103–147.

Symposium. (Various authors.) Subtypes of muscarinic receptors. (Hirschowitz, B. I.; Hammer, R.; Giachetti, A.; Keirns, J. J.; and Levine, R. R.; eds.) *Trends Pharmacol. Sci.,* **1984,** Suppl., 1–103.

Symposium. (Various authors.) Subtypes of muscarinic receptors II. (Levine, R. R.; Birdsall, N. J. M.; Giachetti, A.; Hammer, R.; Iversen, L. L.; Jenden, D. J.; and North, R. A.; eds.) *Trends Pharmacol. Sci.,* **1986a,** Suppl., 1–97.

Symposium. (Various authors.) Cholinergic pathway in obstructive airways disease. (Bergofsky, E. H., ed.) *Am. J. Med.,* **1986b,** *81,* 1–192.

Symposium. (Various authors.) Anticholinergic therapy—the state of the art. (Higenbottam, T. W.; Hoffbrand, B. I.; Howell, J. B. L.; and Morgan, S. A.; eds.) *Postgrad. Med. J.,* **1987,** *63,* Suppl. 1, 1–86.

Symposium. (Various authors.) Subtypes of muscarinic receptors III. (Levine, R. R.; Birdsall, N. J. M.; North, R. A.; Holman, M.; Watanabe, A.; and Iversen, L. L.; eds.) *Trends Pharmacol. Sci.,* **1988,** Suppl., 1–93.

Watanabe, A. M. Cholinergic agonists and antagonists. In, *Cardiac Therapy.* (Rosen, M. R., and Hoffman, B. F., eds.) Martinus Nijhoff, Boston, **1983,** pp. 95–144.

Ziment, I., and Au, J. P. Respiratory pharmacology: anticholinergic agents. *Clin. Chest Med.,* **1986,** *7,* 355–366.

CHAPTER

9 AGENTS ACTING AT THE NEUROMUSCULAR JUNCTION AND AUTONOMIC GANGLIA

Palmer Taylor

Several drugs employed clinically have as their major action the interruption or mimicry of transmission of the nerve impulse at the skeletal neuromuscular junction and/or autonomic ganglia. These agents can be classified together, since they interact with a common family of receptors; these receptors are called *nicotinic cholinergic,* since they are stimulated by both the natural transmitter acetylcholine and the alkaloid nicotine. Distinct subtypes of nicotinic receptors exist at the neuromuscular junction and the ganglia, and several pharmacological agents discriminate between them. Neuromuscular blocking agents are distinguished by whether or not they cause depolarization of the motor end plate and, for this reason, are classified either as *competitive* (*stabilizing*) agents, of which curare is the classical example, or as *depolarizing* agents, such as succinylcholine. Ganglionic agents usually act by stimulating or blocking nicotinic receptors on the postganglionic neuron.

The Nicotinic Cholinergic Receptor. The concept of the nicotinic cholinergic receptor, with which ACh combines to initiate the end-plate potential (EPP) in muscle or an excitatory postsynaptic potential (EPSP) in nerve, is introduced in Chapter 5. Classical studies of the actions of curare and nicotine made this the prototypical pharmacological receptor a century ago. By taking advantage of specialized evolutionary events related to cholinergic neurotransmission, it has been possible in recent years to isolate and characterize central and peripheral nicotinic receptors. These accomplishments represent landmarks in the development of molecular pharmacology.

The electric organs from the aquatic species of *Electrophorus* and, especially, *Torpedo* provide rich sources of receptor. The electric organ is derived embryologically from myoid tissue; however, in contrast to skeletal muscle, a significant fraction (30 to 40%) of the surface of the membrane is excitable and contains cholinergic receptors. In vertebrate skeletal muscle, motor end plates occupy 0.1% or less of the cell surface. The discovery of seemingly irreversible antagonism of neuromuscular transmission by an α toxin from venoms of the krait, *Bungarus multicinctus,* or varieties of the cobra, *Naja naja* (Chang and Lee, 1963), offered a suitable marker for identification of the receptor. The α toxins are peptides of about 8000 molecular weight that can be labeled with radioisotopes. The interaction of α toxins with the receptor was initially applied to an assay for identification of the isolated cholinergic receptor *in vitro* by Changeux and colleagues in 1970 (*see* Changeux *et al.,* 1984). The α toxins have extremely high affinities and slow rates of dissociation from the receptor, yet the interaction is noncovalent. *In situ* and *in vitro* their behavior resembles that expected for a high-affinity antagonist.

Purification of the receptor from *Torpedo* ultimately led to the isolation of complementary DNAs (cDNAs) that encode all of its subunits. These cDNAs, in turn, have permitted the cloning of genes for receptor subunits from mammalian neurons and muscle (Numa *et al.,* 1983). Comparative sequences and structures of the nicotinic receptor family have thus been analyzed, and several subtypes of receptor have been identified. By expressing these genes in cellular systems and recording the electrophysiological events that result from activation by agonists, researchers have been able to correlate the structural and functional properties of the molecule (Claudio *et al.,* 1987; Goldman *et al.,* 1988).

The nicotinic receptor in skeletal muscle and the electric organ is a pentamer composed of four distinct subunits in the stoichiometric ratio of $\alpha_2\beta\gamma\delta$. In muscle from adult animals the γ subunit is replaced by ε, and this gives rise to a receptor with slightly altered biophysical properties. The individual subunits are about 40% identical in their amino acid sequences, suggesting that they arose from a common primordial gene (Numa *et al.*, 1983). Only the α subunits carry the primary recognition sites for ACh, the reversible antagonists, and the snake α toxins. The binding of these ligands is mutually exclusive with each other. Each of the subunits has an extracellular and an intracellular exposure on the postsynaptic membrane. They are arranged in such a manner as to circumscribe an internally located channel in a fashion similar to petals on a lily (Changeux *et al.*, 1984; Unwin *et al.*, 1988; Figure 9–1). In each subunit are four short sequences of hydrophobic amino acid residues, which are the likely domains that span the membrane as α helices. The receptor is an asymmetrical molecule (14 nm × 8 nm) of 250,000 daltons, with the bulk of the nonmembrane spanning domain on the extracellular surface. The receptor in junctional areas (*i.e.*, the motor end plate in skeletal muscle and the central surface of the electric organ) is present in high densities (10,000/μm^2). This ordering of the receptors has allowed analysis of molecular structure at a resolution of about 10 Å (Unwin *et al.*, 1988; *see* Figure 9–1).

Measurements of membrane conductances demonstrate that rates of ion translocation are sufficiently rapid (5×10^7 ions per second) to require movement through an open channel, rather than by a rotating carrier of ions. Moreover, agonist-mediated changes in ion permeability (inward movement of Na^+ and outward movement of K^+) occur through a single class of channels (Dionne *et al.*, 1978). Thus, the agonist binding site is intimately coupled with an ion channel; binding of two agonist molecules results in a rapid conformational change that opens the channel, which is internal to the five subunits in the pentameric receptor molecule.

A plethora of cDNAs that encode nicotinic receptor subunits has been isolated from the central nervous system (CNS), ganglia, and tissues derived from the neural crest. In general, the neuronal nicotinic receptors exist as pentamers of only α and β subunits (presumably $\alpha_2\beta_3$). Genes for four distinct α subunits and two β subunits appear to be expressed in the CNS. Their sequences differ from those of their counterparts in muscle. When different combinations of α and β subunits are expressed, the resultant holoreceptors have different electrophysiological properties and pharmacological specificities. Messenger RNAs (mRNAs) for individual forms of each subunit are found in discrete regions of the brain; only one type of α and β subunit has been detected in ganglia (Goldman *et al.*, 1987). The neuronal nicotinic receptors are not blocked by the krait and cobra α toxins and they show enhanced sensitivity to nicotine and certain other agents.

NEUROMUSCULAR BLOCKING AGENTS

History, Sources, and Chemistry. *Curare* is a generic term for various South American arrow poisons. The drug has a long and romantic history. It has been used for centuries by the Indians along the Amazon and Orinoco Rivers and in other parts of that continent for killing wild animals used for food; death results from paralysis of skeletal muscles. The preparation of curare was long shrouded in mystery and was entrusted only to tribal witch doctors. Soon after the discovery of the American continent, Sir Walter Raleigh and other early explorers and botanists became interested in curare, and late in the sixteenth century samples of the native preparations were brought to Europe for examination and investigation. Following the pioneering work of the scientist-explorer von Humboldt, in 1805, the botanical sources of curare became the object of much field search. The curares from eastern Amazonia contain various species of *Strychnos* as their chief ingredient. It is noteworthy that most of the South American species of *Strychnos* examined contain chiefly quaternary, neuromuscular blocking alkaloids, whereas the Asiatic, African, and Australian species nearly all contain tertiary, strychnine-like alkaloids. Research on curare was greatly accelerated by the work of Gill (1940), who, after prolonged study of the native methods of preparing curare, brought to the United States a sufficient amount of the authentic drug to permit chemical and pharmacological investigations.

The modern clinical use of curare apparently dates from 1932, when West employed highly purified fractions in patients with tetanus and spastic disorders. The first trial of curare for promoting muscular relaxation in general anesthesia was reported by Griffith and Johnson (1942). The significant advantage of obtaining the desired degree of muscular relaxation without the use of dangerously high concentrations of anesthetic became recognized over the next decade.

The fascinating history of curare, the reports of early travelers, and the complex problems of botanical source, nomenclature, and chemical identification of the curare alkaloids have been presented in extensive reviews (*see* Bovet, 1972; McIntyre, 1972; Morowitz, 1986; and *previous editions* of this textbook).

The essential structure of tubocurarine was established by King in 1935. One of the nitrogen atoms was later found to be a tertiary amine (Table 9–1). A synthetic derivative, metocurine (formerly called dimethyl tubocurarine), contains three additional methyl groups, one of which quaternizes the nitrogen; the other two form methyl ethers at the phenolic hydroxyl groups. This compound possesses two to three times the potency of tubocurarine in man.

The most potent of all curare alkaloids are the toxiferines, obtained from *Strychnos toxifera*. A semisynthetic derivative, alcuronium chloride (*N,N'*-diallylnortoxiferinium dichloride) (*see* Table 9–1), is used clinically in Europe and elsewhere. The seeds of the trees and shrubs of the genus *Erythrina*, widely distributed in tropical and subtropical areas, contain substances with curare-like activity. A hydrogenated derivative, dihydro-β-erythroidine, of the parent alkaloid, erythroidine, has been subjected to clinical trial.

Gallamine (*see* Table 9–1) is one of a series of synthetic substitutes for curare described by Bovet

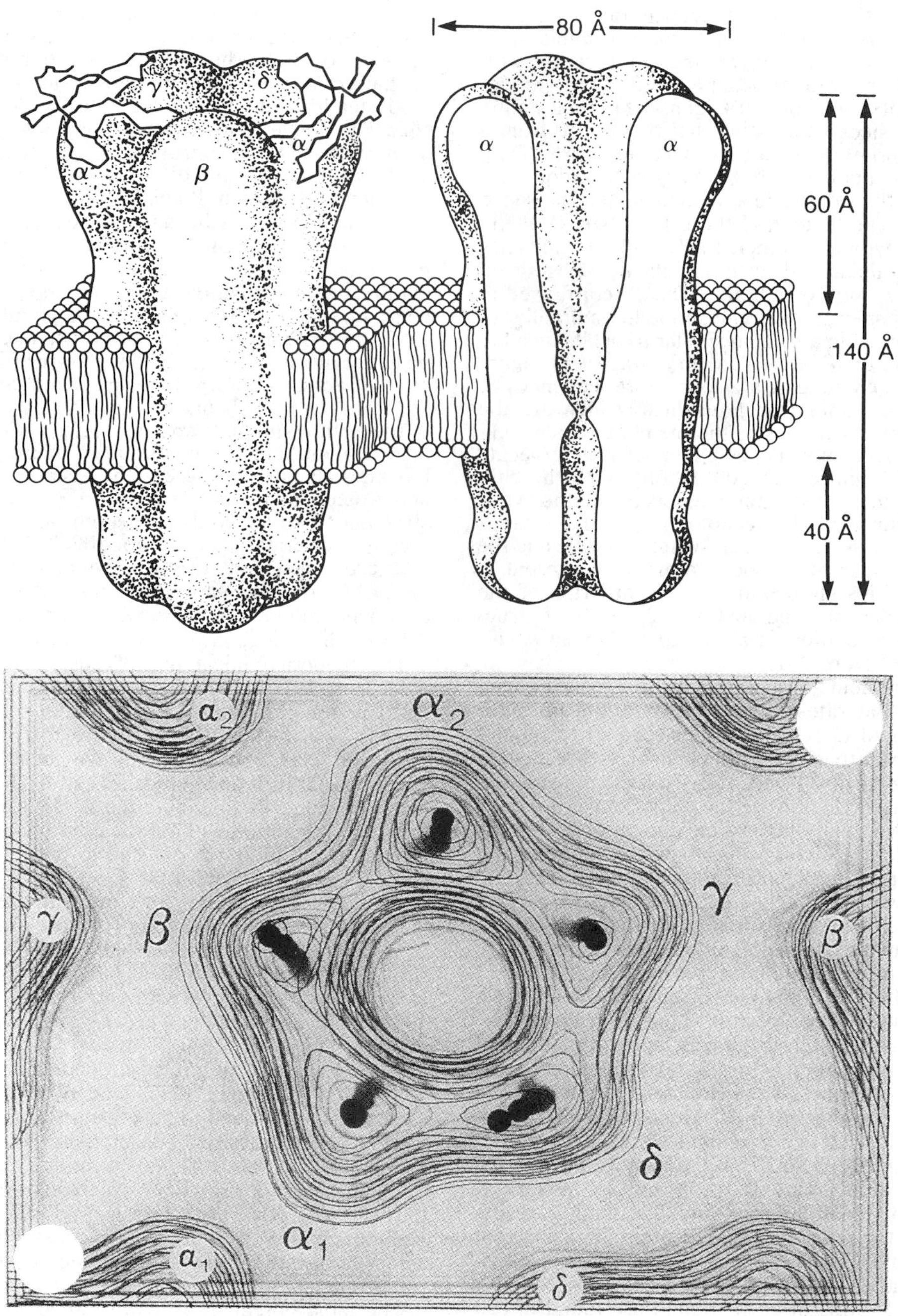

Figure 9–1. *Molecular structure of the nicotinic cholinergic receptor.*

The structure of the receptor is described in the text. A side view of a model of the receptor is shown at the top of the figure. The positions of the respective subunits (α, β, γ, and δ) in the pentamer are shown. The two leaf-like structures shown on the extracellular surface of the receptor are molecules of cobra α toxin that are bound primarily to the α subunits. The 40-Å extension into the cytoplasm is accentuated owing to the association of a protein (designated 43K) with the cytoplasmic surface of the receptor. A cross-sectional view of an electron-density map of the receptor is shown at the bottom of the figure. This view is taken 50 to 60 Å above the extracellular face of the membrane and clearly reveals the mouth of the channel. Densities from neighboring receptor molecules are also visible. (From Unwin *et al.*, 1988; Courtesy of *The Journal of Cell Biology*. © Rockefeller University Press.)

Table 9–1. STRUCTURAL FORMULAS OF MAJOR NEUROMUSCULAR BLOCKING AGENTS

COMPETITIVE AGENTS

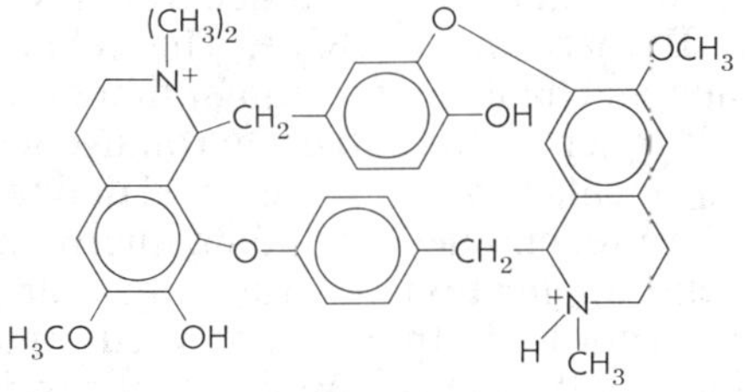

Tubocurarine

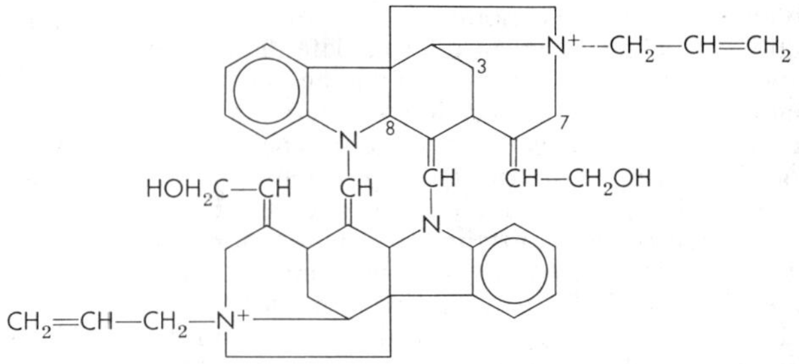

Alcuronium

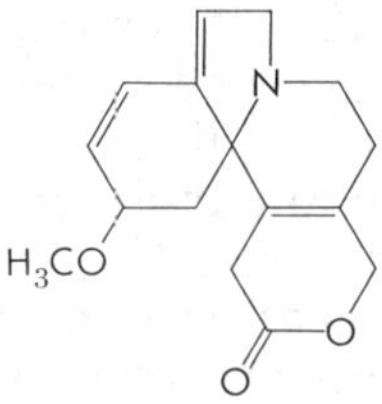

β-Erythroidine

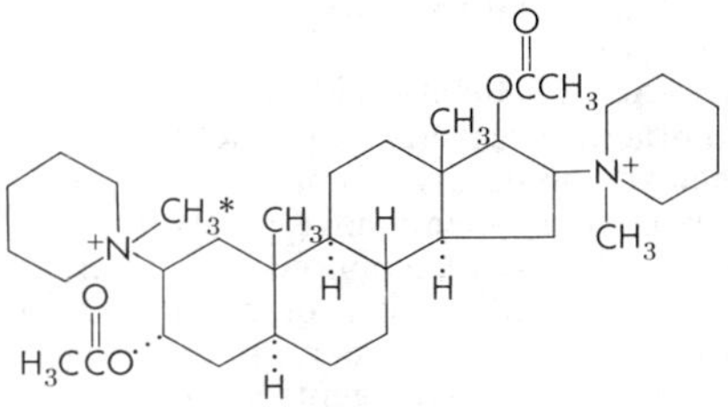

Pancuronium

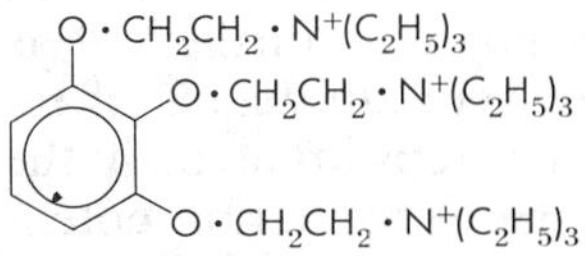

Gallamine

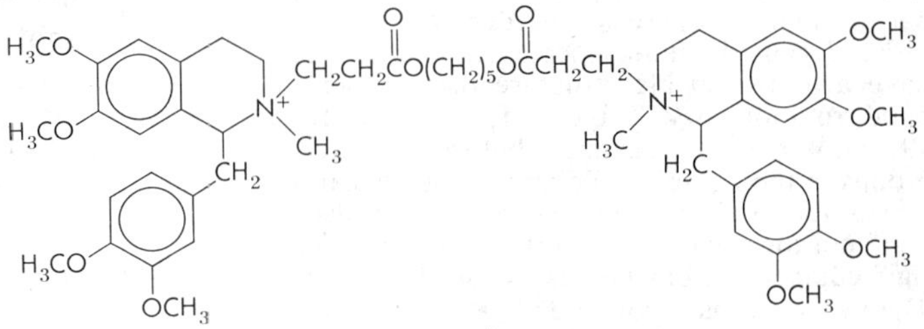

Atracurium

DEPOLARIZING AGENTS

$$(CH_3)_3\overset{+}{N}—(CH_2)_{10}—\overset{+}{N}(CH_3)_3$$

Decamethonium

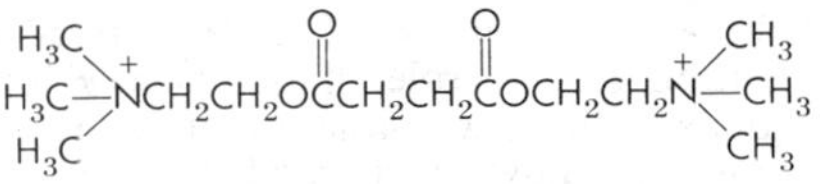

Succinylcholine

* The adjacent methyl group is absent in vecuronium.

and coworkers in 1949 (*see* review by Bovet, 1972). Exploration of the structure–activity relationships of the plant alkaloids led to the development of the polymethylene bis-trimethylammonium series (referred to herein by the generic term *methonium compounds*) (Barlow and Ing, 1948; Paton and Zaimis, 1949 *et seq*.). The most potent agent was found when the chain contained ten carbon atoms (decamethonium [C10], *see* Table 9–1). The member of the series containing six carbon atoms in the chain—hexamethonium (C6)—was found to be essentially devoid of neuromuscular blocking activity but is particularly effective as a ganglionic blocking agent (*see* below).

The use of curarized animals by Hunt and Taveau in 1906 in experiments on succinylcholine (*see* Table 9–1) prevented them from observing the neuromuscular blocking activity of the drug, and this property went unrecognized for more than 40 years. In 1949, the curariform action of the compound was described and its clinical application soon followed (*see* Dorkins, 1982).

Pancuronium is a member of a series of *bis*-quaternary ammonium steroids that were synthesized in 1964. Extensive pharmacological and clinical studies have shown that pancuronium is approximately five times as potent as tubocurarine as a competitive neuromuscular blocking agent, with minimal cardiovascular and little histamine-releasing or hormonal actions. Vecuronium is a congener of pancuronium in which the 2β-methyl group has been removed. This small modification has been shown to minimize cardiovascular effects. The potency of vecuronium is equivalent to or slightly greater than that of pancuronium (Agoston *et al.*, 1980). Atracurium, which is actually a mixture of about ten isomers, is another newer synthetic competitive blocking agent of intermediate duration of action. It undergoes both spontaneous and enzymatically catalyzed conversion to inactive metabolites and, hence, is less dependent on renal elimination for termination of its action (Hughes and Chapple, 1981). It is three to four times less potent than pancuronium. Fazadinium was developed in Great Britain as a competitive blocking agent. Its extensive metabolism by the liver (reduction of a diazo group) also makes it less dependent on renal elimination. Additional long-acting, competitive blocking agents, pipecuronium and doxacurium, are under clinical trial (Shanks, 1988).

Structure–Activity Relationships. For both theoretical and practical reasons, the structural features that distinguish competitive from depolarizing neuromuscular blocking agents have received particular attention. Although exceptions can be cited, a few useful generalizations can be made about the differences in structure between these two groups of agents. The competitive agents are for the most part relatively bulky, rigid molecules (*e.g.*, tubocurarine, the toxiferines, β-erythroidine, gallamine, pancuronium), whereas the depolarizing agents (*e.g.*, decamethonium, succinylcholine) generally have a more flexible structure that enables free bond rotation (*see* Table 9–1; *see also* Bovet, 1972). While the distance between quaternary groups in the flexible depolarizing agents can vary up to the limit of the maximal bond distance (1.45 nm for decamethonium), the distance for the rigid competitive blockers is usually 1.0 ± 0.1 nm. The *tris*-quaternary compound gallamine, the tertiary amine β-erythroidine, and fazadinium, in which the cationic charge is delocalized, represent exceptions to this generalization.

The functional relationship of curare to ACh focuses attention on the role of quaternary ammonium groups. Many well-known drugs (*e.g.*, atropine, quinine) show a marked increase in neuromuscular blocking potency when their nitrogen atom is quaternized. On the other hand, many nonquaternary ammonium compounds block the neuromuscular junction (*e.g.*, nicotine, β-erythroidine). The neuromuscular blocking activity of β-erythroidine is actually abolished by quaternization of the nitrogen atom. Other atoms can substitute for cationic quaternary nitrogen; thus, neuromuscular blocking activity has been reported for sulfonium, phosphonium, arsonium, stibonium, iodinium, platinum, and osmium compounds.

The *bis*-quaternary ammonium structure of most of the compounds pictured in Table 9–1 suggests that electrostatic or coulombic association occurs between the two cationic centers of the drug and certain anionic groups of the receptor site; for example, replacement of one quaternary moiety of decamethonium by a primary amine group results in a considerable loss of potency, which is likely a consequence of increased hydration of the cation.

PHARMACOLOGICAL PROPERTIES

Skeletal Muscle. The localization of the paralytic action of curare to the junction between nerve and muscle was first adequately described in the classical reports of Claude Bernard in the 1850s. The cellular locus and mechanism of action of tubocurarine and other competitive neuromuscular blocking agents have now been well defined by modern techniques, including microiontophoretic application of drugs and intracellular recording. In brief, tubocurarine combines with the nicotinic cholinergic receptor at the postjunctional membrane and thereby blocks competitively the transmitter action of ACh. When the drug is applied directly to the end plate of a single isolated muscle fiber, the muscle cell becomes insensitive to motor-nerve impulses and to directly applied ACh; however, the end-plate region and the remainder of the muscle fiber membrane retain their normal sensitivity to K^+, and the muscle fiber still responds to direct electrical stimulation.

To analyze the action of antagonists at the neuromuscular junction further, it is important to consider certain details of receptor activation. The steps involved in the release of ACh by the nerve action potential (AP), the development of miniature end-plate potentials (MEPPs; currents that arise from the spontaneous release of ACh), their summation to form a postjunctional end-plate potential (EPP), the triggering of the muscle AP, and contraction have been described in Chapter 5. In the past 20 years electrophysiological experimentation has revealed the electrical event associated with the opening and closing of the individual receptor channels associated with activation by agonist. The fundamental event elicited by agonist is an "all-or-none" opening and closing of channels, which gives rise to a square-wave pulse with an average open-channel conductance of 20 to 30 pS and a duration that is exponentially distributed around a time of about 1 msec. The duration of channel opening is far more dependent on the nature of the agonist than is the value of the open-channel conductance (Colquhoun, 1979).

The influence of increasing concentrations of the competitive antagonist tubocurarine is to diminish progressively the amplitude of the EPP. The amplitude of the EPP may fall to below 70% of its initial value before it is insufficient to initiate the propagated muscle AP; this provides a safety factor in neuromuscular transmission. Analysis of the antagonism of tubocurarine on single-channel events shows that it reduces the frequency of channel-opening events but does not affect the conductance or duration of opening for a single channel (Katz and Miledi, 1973). This behavior is precisely that expected for a competitive antagonist. At higher concentrations, curare and other competitive antagonists will block the channel directly in a fashion that is noncompetitive with agonists. The magnitude of this inhibition is dependent on membrane potential (Colquhoun *et al.*, 1979).

The duration of MEPPs parallels the lifetime of channel opening. Since the potentials are a consequence of the action of one or more quanta of ACh ($\sim 10^4$ molecules), individual molecules of ACh released into the synapse do not successively rebind to receptors to activate multiple channels before hydrolysis by acetylcholinesterase. The concentration of unbound ACh in the synapse diminishes more rapidly than does the decay of the end-plate current.

If anticholinesterase (anti-ChE) drugs are present, the EPP (or end-plate current) is prolonged, which is indicative of rebinding of transmitter to neighboring receptors before removal from the synapse. It is therefore not surprising that anti-ChE agents and tubocurarine are competitive, since increasing the duration of action of ACh in the synapse should favor occupation of the receptor by transmitter relative to tubocurarine. Tubocurarine also partially prevents the prolongation of the EPP by the anti-ChE compounds (Mageby and Terrar, 1975). This effect is, in part, a consequence of longer diffusion distances between unoccupied receptors and a diminished probability of agonist rebinding to neighboring receptors when antagonist is present.

At the level of the individual receptor molecules, simultaneous binding by two agonist molecules (one on each α subunit) is required for activation. Activation shows positive cooperativity, and thus occurs over a narrow range of concentrations (Dionne *et al.*, 1978; Taylor *et al.*, 1983). Although two competitive antagonist or snake α-toxin molecules can bind to each receptor molecule, also on the α subunits, the binding of one molecule of antagonist to each receptor is sufficient to render it nonfunctional (Sine and Taylor, 1981; Taylor *et al.*, 1983).

The depolarizing agents, such as succinylcholine and decamethonium, act by a different mechanism. Their initial action is to depolarize the membrane by opening channels in the same manner as ACh. However, since they persist at the neuromuscular junction, the depolarization is longer lasting, resulting in a brief period of repetitive excitation, which may be manifested by transient muscle fasciculations. This phase is followed by block of neuromuscular transmission and flaccid paralysis. The details of the sequence of excitation and depression vary with different species and muscles in the same species, so that the dominance of repetitive excitation, contracture, or block will differ. In man, the sequence of repetitive excitation (fasciculations) followed by block of transmission and neuromuscular paralysis is observed; however, even this sequence is influenced by such factors as the anesthetic agent used concurrently, the type of muscle, and the interval between doses of drug. Depolarization blockade exhibits several distinct differences from that produced by tubocurarine and related drugs; these differences are listed in Table 9–2.

A partial explanation of these distinctive features of neuromuscular blockade by the depolarizing agents was provided by the discovery by Burns and Paton (1951) that, in contrast to the stabilizing action of tubocurarine on the motor end plate, decamethonium produces an immediate and persistent depolarization of both the end plate and the immediately adjacent area of the sarcoplasmic membrane. Much the same result is obtained with high, paralyzing doses of ACh in the presence of an anti-ChE agent. Thus, it was assumed that neuromuscular blockade was due to the inability of the depolarized area within or just beyond the end plate to initiate propagated muscle APs in response to the continued depolarization of the end plate itself. However, this proposal did not fully explain several subsequent observations (*see* below).

Many of the characteristics listed in Table 9–2 of depolarizing blocking agents apply only to man and to the twitch ("white") muscles of the cat. In other muscles investigated in several species and in the slowly contracting soleus muscle of the cat, decamethonium and succinylcholine produce a blockade that combines certain features of both the depolarizing and the competitive agents described above and that has some characteristics not associated with either; Zaimis (1976) has termed this type of action a "dual" mechanism. In such cases, the depolarizing agents produce initially the characteristic fasciculations and potentiation of the maximal twitch, followed by the rapid onset of neuromuscular block; this block is potentiated by anti-ChE agents. However, following the onset of blockade,

Table 9–2. COMPARISON OF COMPETITIVE (TUBOCURARINE) AND DEPOLARIZING (DECAMETHONIUM) BLOCKING AGENTS *

	TUBOCURARINE	DECAMETHONIUM (C10)
Effect of tubocurarine chloride administered previously	Additive	Antagonistic
Effect of decamethonium administered previously	No effect, or antagonistic	Some tachyphylaxis; usually no cumulative effect
Effect on block of anticholinesterase agents	Reversal of block	No antagonism
Effect on motor end plate	Elevated threshold to acetylcholine; no depolarization	Partial, persisting depolarization
Initial excitatory effect on striated muscle	None	Transient fasciculations
Character of muscle response to indirect tetanic stimulation during *partial* block	Poorly sustained contraction	Well-sustained contraction
Effect on block of KCl or of a tetanus	Transient reversal of block	No antagonism
Effect of current applied to end-plate region:		
—cathodal	Lessens paralysis	Intensifies paralysis
—anodal	Intensifies paralysis	Lessens paralysis
Effect on block of lowering muscle temperature	Antagonism and shortening of block	Amplification and prolongation of block
Effect on denervated mammalian muscle	Transient fibrillation	Contracture

* Based on data in Paton and Zaimis, 1949, 1952; Zaimis, 1976; Zaimis and Head, 1976.

there is a poorly sustained response to tetanic stimulation of the motor nerve, intensification of the block by tubocurarine, and usual reversal by anti-ChE agents.

The dual action of the depolarizing blocking agents is also seen in intracellular recordings of membrane potential; when agonist is applied continuously, the initial depolarization is followed by a gradual repolarization (Elmqvist and Thesleff, 1962). The second phase, repolarization, resembles receptor desensitization (Katz and Thesleff, 1957).

In man, most of the early evidence indicated that decamethonium and succinylcholine produced a depolarization blockade, wherein anti-ChE drugs potentiate depolarization. However, behavior characteristic of a dual type of blockade has also been frequently reported under clinical circumstances. Here, with increasing concentrations of succinylcholine and in time, the block converts slowly from a depolarizing to a nondepolarizing type, termed *phase-I* and *phase-II* block (Durant and Katz, 1982). Zaimis (1976) has observed that the pattern of neuromuscular blockade produced by depolarizing drugs in anesthetized patients has changed. Prolonged apnea and slow recovery are now observed more frequently, and the characteristics of depolarization blockade are less evident following prolonged administration of succinylcholine or decamethonium. She suggested that the general anesthetic employed may be an important factor, with fluorinated hydrocarbons predisposing the system to nondepolarization blockade (*see also* Fogdall and Miller, 1975). Thus, the anesthetic may induce a change in the postsynaptic membrane such that certain features of neuromuscular blockade are accentuated.

During the initial phase of application, depolarizing agents produce channel opening, which can be measured by the statistical analysis of fluctuation of EPPs. The probability of channel opening associated with the binding of drug to the receptor is less with decamethonium than with ACh (Katz and Miledi, 1973). The diminished probability of channel opening would serve to classify decamethonium as a partial agonist at the end plate. Higher concentrations of decamethonium also block the channel directly and thereby interfere with ion permeability (Adams and Sakmann, 1978). In fact, this behavior can be seen at high concentrations of many nicotinic agonists and antagonists.

Although the observed fasciculations may also result from stimulation of the prejunctional motor-nerve terminal by the depolarizing agent, giving rise to stimulation of the motor unit in an antidromic fashion (Riker, 1975), the primary site of action of both competitive and depolarizing blocking agents is the postjunctional membrane (Katz and Miledi, 1965; Auerbach and Betz, 1971). Presynaptic actions of the competitive agents may become significant upon repetitive, high-frequency stimulation, since prejunctional nicotinic receptors may be involved in the mobilization of ACh for release from the nerve terminal (Bowman *et al.*, 1988).

Many ions, drugs, and toxins block neuromuscular transmission by other mechanisms, such as interference with the synthesis or release of ACh (*see* Chapter 5), but most of these agents are not employed clinically for this purpose. One exception is botulinus toxin, which has been administered locally into muscles of the orbit in the management of blepharospasm and strabismus (Elston *et al.*,

1985). This treatment produces a long-lasting interruption of neuromuscular transmission and reduction of spasmodic ocular movements. Another exception is dantrolene, which blocks release of Ca^{2+} from the sarcoplasmic reticulum and is used in the treatment of malignant hyperthermia (*see* below). The sites of action and interrelationship of several agents that serve as pharmacological tools are shown in Figure 9–2.

Sequence and Characteristics of Paralysis. When an appropriate dose of tubocurarine is injected intravenously in man, the onset of effects is rapid. Motor weakness gives way to a total flaccid paralysis. Small, rapidly moving muscles such as those of the fingers and eyes are involved before those of the limbs, neck, and trunk. Ultimately the intercostal muscles and finally the diaphragm are paralyzed, and respiration then ceases. Recovery of muscles usually occurs in the reverse order to that of their paralysis, and thus the diaphragm is ordinarily the first to regain function.

Prior to causing paralysis, depolarizing agents such as succinylcholine evoke transient muscular fasciculations, observed especially over the chest and abdomen; however, these are less common in the anesthetized patient. As the paralytic effect progresses, the neck, arm, and leg muscles are involved at a time when there is only slight weakness of facial, masticatory, lingual, pharyngeal, and laryngeal muscles; at this stage, respiratory muscular weakness is not pronounced and vital capacity is reduced only 25%.

After a single intravenous dose of 10 to 30 mg of succinylcholine, muscular fasciculation occurs briefly; then relaxation occurs

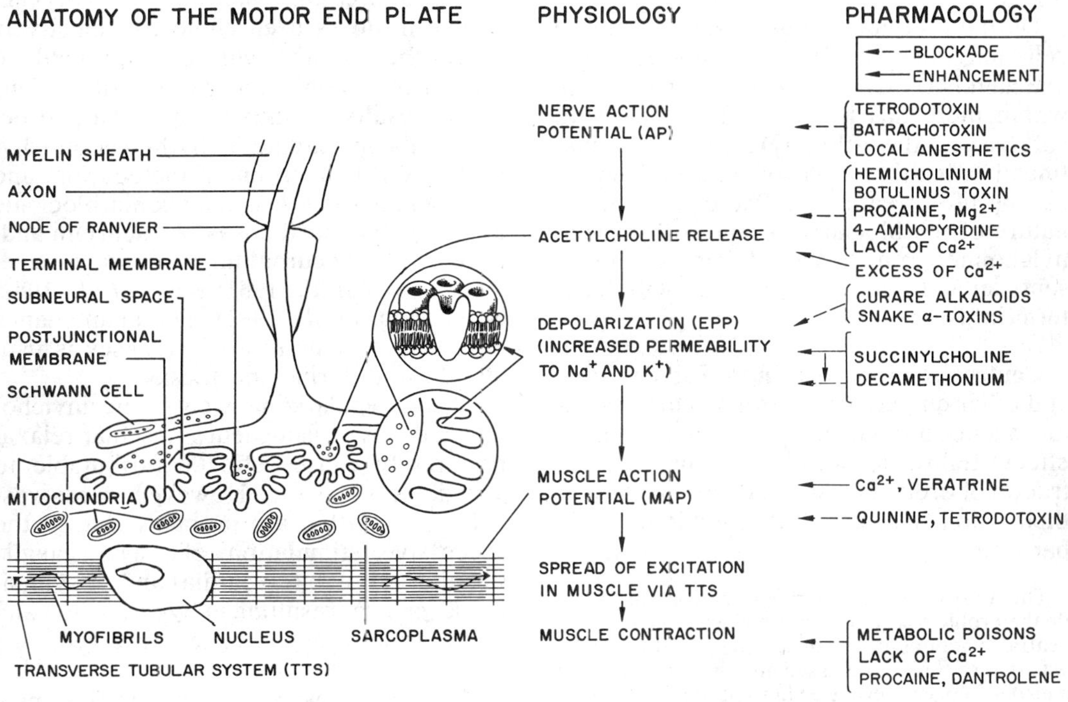

Figure 9–2. *Sites of action of agents at the neuromuscular junction and adjacent structures.*

The anatomy of the motor end plate, shown at the left, and the sequence of events from liberation of acetylcholine (ACh) by the nerve action potential (AP) to contraction of the muscle fiber, indicated in the middle column, are described in some detail in Chapter 5. The modification of these processes by various agents is shown on the right; the dashed arrows indicate inhibition or block; the solid arrows, enhancement or activation. The circled inserts are an enlargement of the indicated structures. The highest magnification depicts the receptor in the bilayer of the postsynaptic membrane. A more detailed view of the receptor is shown in Figure 9–1.

within 1 minute, becomes maximal within 2 minutes, and disappears as a rule within 5 minutes. Transient apnea usually occurs at the time of maximal effect. Muscular relaxation of longer duration can be achieved by repeated injections at appropriate intervals or by continuous intravenous infusion. Even after discontinuance of an infusion, the effects of the drug usually disappear rapidly because of its rapid hydrolysis by the butyrylcholinesterase of the plasma and liver. The degree of muscular relaxation can be altered within 30 to 60 seconds by a change in the rate of infusion. Muscle soreness may follow the administration of succinylcholine. Small doses of competitive blocking agents have been employed to minimize fasciculations and muscle pain caused by succinylcholine. However, this procedure is controversial, since it increases the requirement for the depolarizing drug.

During prolonged depolarization, muscle cells may lose significant quantities of K^+ and gain Na^+, Cl^-, and Ca^{2+}. In patients in whom there has been extensive injury to soft tissues, the efflux of K^+ following continued administration of succinylcholine can be life threatening. The change in the nature of the blockade produced by succinylcholine (from phase I to phase II) presents an additional complication with long-term infusion.

Central Nervous System. Tubocurarine and other quaternary neuromuscular blocking agents are virtually devoid of central effects following the intravenous administration of ordinary clinical doses because of their inability to penetrate the blood–brain barrier.

The most decisive experiment performed to settle the problem whether curare significantly affects central functions in the dose range used clinically was that of Smith and associates (1947). Smith (an anesthesiologist) permitted himself to receive intravenously two and one-half times the amount of tubocurarine necessary for paralysis of all skeletal muscles. Adequate respiratory exchange was maintained by artificial respiration. At no time was there any evidence of lapse of consciousness, clouding of sensorium, analgesia, or disturbance of special senses. Despite adequate artificially controlled respiration, "shortness of breath" was experienced, and the accumulation of unswallowed saliva in the pharynx caused the sensation of choking. The experience was decidedly unpleasant. It was concluded that tubocurarine given intravenously even in large doses has no significant central stimulant, depressant, or analgesic effect in man, and that its sole action in anesthesia is the peripheral paralytic effect on skeletal muscle.

Autonomic Ganglia. Neuromuscular blocking agents vary with respect to their relative potencies in producing ganglionic blockade. Just as at the motor end plate, ganglionic blockade by tubocurarine and other stabilizing drugs is antagonized effectively by anti-ChE agents; however, in ganglia, the antagonism is reinforced by the additional action of endogenous ACh at the muscarinic receptors of the ganglion cells (*see* below).

At the doses of tubocurarine used clinically, some degree of blockade is probably produced, both at autonomic ganglia and at the adrenal medulla, which results in a fall in blood pressure and tachycardia. Gallamine in doses used clinically selectively blocks the cardiac vagus nerve, probably at the postganglionic muscarinic sites. This action results in sinus tachycardia and occasionally in cardiac arrhythmias and hypertension. Pancuronium, metocurine, and alcuronium show less ganglionic blockade at common clinical doses. Atracurium and, particularly, vecuronium are even more selective (Son *et al.*, 1981; Basta *et al.*, 1982; Sutherland, *et al.*, 1983). The maintenance of cardiovascular reflex responses is usually desired during anesthesia.

Of the depolarizing agents, succinylcholine at doses causing neuromuscular relaxation rarely causes effects attributable to ganglionic blockade. However, cardiovascular effects that are probably due to the successive stimulation of vagal ganglia (manifested by bradycardia) and of sympathetic ganglia (resulting in hypertension and tachycardia) are sometimes observed.

Histamine Release. Tubocurarine produces typical histamine-like wheals when injected intracutaneously or intraarterially in man, and certain clinical responses to tubocurarine (bronchospasm, hypotension, excessive bronchial and salivary secretion) appear to be caused by the release of histamine. Metocurine, succinylcholine, and atracurium also cause histamine release, but to a lesser extent. Decamethonium, pancuronium, alcuronium, vecuronium, and gallamine have even less tendency to release histamine after intradermal or systemic injection (Bowman, 1982; Ertama, 1982).

Cardiovascular System. The rapid intravenous injection of large doses of tubocurarine in man may cause a rapid and severe fall in blood pressure. The major causes of the hypotension are peripheral vasodilatation from the release of histamine and sympathetic ganglionic blockade. Additional factors are diminished venous return owing to loss of skeletal muscle tone, diminished respiratory excursion, and the consequences of intermittent positive pressure in the airway for the purpose of restoring the adequacy of respiration. Pancuronium is unique in that rapid injection can increase blood pressure, possibly because of ganglionic stimulation. Little change in blood pressure or heart rate is noted upon injection of atracurium or vecuronium.

Miscellaneous Actions. Ganglionic blockade is chiefly responsible for the decreased tone and motility of the gastrointestinal tract. Succinylcholine may cause an increase in intraocular pressure. The depolarizing agents can release K^+ rapidly from intracellular sites; this may be a factor in production of the prolonged apnea that has been noted in patients who receive these drugs while in electrolyte imbalance (Dripps, 1976). Such alterations in the distribution of K^+ may be particularly important in patients with congestive heart failure who are receiving digitalis or diuretics. Caution should be used or depolarizing blocking agents should be avoided in patients with extensive soft-tissue trauma or burns. A higher dose of a competitive blocking agent is often indicated in these patients. Neonates may have an enhanced sensitivity to competitive neuromuscular blocking agents and some resistance to depolarizing drugs (Smith, 1976). Patients receiving long-term treatment with phenytoin show increased resistance to the competitive blocking agents (Ornstein *et al.*, 1987).

Synergisms and Antagonisms. The interactions between the competitive and depolarizing neuromuscular blocking agents have already been considered. From a clinical viewpoint, the most important pharmacological interactions of these drugs are with certain general anesthetics, certain antibiotics, Ca^{2+} channel blockers, and anti-ChE compounds.

Since the anti-ChE agents neostigmine, pyridostigmine, and edrophonium preserve endogenous ACh and also act directly on the neuromuscular junction, they can be used in the treatment of overdosage with tubocurarine or other competitive blocking agents. Similarly, upon completion of the surgical procedure many anesthesiologists employ neostigmine or edrophonium to reverse and decrease the duration of competitive neuromuscular blockade (Donati *et al.*, 1989). A muscarinic antagonist (atropine or glycopyrrolate) is used concomitantly to prevent stimulation of muscarinic receptors. The anti-ChE agents, however, are synergistic with the depolarizing blocking agents, particularly in their initial phase of action. Since they will not reverse neuromuscular blockade and, in fact, can enhance it, the distinction in the type of neuromuscular blocking agent must be clear.

Many inhalational anesthetics (*e.g.*, halothane, isoflurane, and enflurane) exert a stabilizing effect on the postjunctional membrane and therefore act synergistically with the competitive blocking agents. Consequently, when such blocking drugs are used for muscle relaxation as adjuncts to these anesthetics, their doses should be reduced (*see* Fogdall and Miller, 1975; Ali and Savarese, 1976).

Aminoglycoside antibiotics produce neuromuscular blockade by inhibiting ACh release from the preganglionic terminal (through competition with Ca^{2+}) and to a lesser extent by stabilizing the postjunctional membrane. The blockade is antagonized by calcium salts, but only inconsistently by anti-ChE agents (*see* Chapter 47). The tetracycline antibiotics can also produce neuromuscular blockade, possibly by chelation of Ca^{2+}. Additional antibiotics that have neuromuscular blocking action, through both presynaptic and postsynaptic actions, include polymyxin B, colistin, clindamycin, and lincomycin (*see* Sokoll and Gergis, 1981). When neuromuscular blocking agents are to be administered to patients who are receiving one of these antibiotics, special consideration should be given to the dose and to the judicious use of a calcium salt as an antagonist if recovery of spontaneous respiration is delayed. Ca^{2+}-channel blockers also enhance neuromuscular blockade produced by both competitive and depolarizing antagonists. It is not clear whether this is a result of a diminution of Ca^{2+}-dependent release of transmitter from the nerve ending or is a postsynaptic action (Durant *et al.*, 1984).

Miscellaneous drugs that may have significant interactions with either competitive or depolarizing neuromuscular blocking agents include trimethaphan, opioid analgesics, procaine, lidocaine, quinidine, phenelzine, phenytoin, propranolol, magnesium salts, corticosteroids, digitalis glycosides, chloroquine, catecholamines, and diuretics (*see* Zaimis, 1976; Argov and Mastaglia, 1979).

Toxicology. The important untoward responses of the neuromuscular blocking agents are prolonged apnea and cardiovascular collapse and those resulting from histamine release.

Failure of respiration to become adequate in the postoperative period may not always be due directly to the drug. An obstruction of the airway, decreased arterial carbon dioxide tension secondary to hyperventilation during the operative procedure, or the neuromuscular depressant effect of excessive amounts of neostigmine used to reverse the action of the competitive blocking drugs may also be implicated. Directly related factors may include alterations in body temperature (an increased temperature potentiating the competitive drugs, and a decreased temperature potentiating the depolarizing substances); electrolyte imbalance, particularly of K^+; decreased plasma cholinesterase, resulting in a reduction in the rate of destruction of succinylcholine; the presence of latent myasthenia gravis or of malignant disease such as oat-cell carcinoma of the bronchus (myasthenic syndrome); reduced blood flow to skeletal muscles causing delayed removal of the blocking drugs; and decreased elimination of the relaxants secondary to reduced renal function. Great care should be taken when administering muscle relaxants to dehydrated or severely ill patients.

A severe rapid rise in temperature occurs occasionally in patients receiving halothane and succinylcholine, and more rarely with other combinations of general anesthetics and neuromuscular blocking agents. This condition, known as *malignant hyperthermia,* has a familial tendency and an estimated incidence between 1 in 15,000 and 1 in 50,000. The inducing agent causes widespread muscular rigidity and enhanced heat production by muscle. The hyperthermia may be fatal, and steps must be taken to dissipate heat quickly. Subsequent muscle damage is usually evident. Malignant hyperthermia should be treated by rapid cooling, inhalation of 100% oxygen, and control of the acidosis that is generally present. Dantrolene is immediately administered intravenously. The drug blocks release of Ca^{2+} from the sarcoplasmic reticulum, which reduces muscle tone and heat production (Denborough, 1980; Rosenberg and Fletcher, 1987).

Treatment of respiratory paralysis should be by positive-pressure artificial respiration with oxygen and maintenance of a patent airway until the recovery of normal respiration is assured. With the competitive blocking agents, this may be hastened by the administration of neostigmine methylsulfate (0.5 to 2 mg, intravenously) or edrophonium (10 mg, intravenously, repeated as required).

Neostigmine antagonizes only the skeletal muscular blocking action of the competitive blocking agents effectively, and it may aggravate such side effects as hypotension or bronchospasm. In such circumstances, sympathomimetic amines may be given to support the blood pressure. Atropine or glycopyrrolate is administered to counteract muscarinic stimulation. The position of the patient should be such as to favor the return of venous blood from the flaccid musculature. Antihistamines are definitely beneficial to counteract the responses that follow the release of histamine, particularly if they are administered before the neuromuscular blocking agent.

Absorption, Fate, and Excretion. Quaternary ammonium neuromuscular blocking agents are very poorly and irregularly absorbed from the gastrointestinal tract. This fact was well known to the South American Indians, who ate with impunity the flesh of game killed with curare-poisoned arrows. Absorption is quite adequate from intramuscular sites.

When a single moderate dose of tubocurarine is injected intravenously, the action begins to wear off in about 20 minutes, yet some residual effect is still discernible after 2 to 4 hours or more. The brief duration of paralysis following the initial dose is due to redistribution of the drug; when repeated doses are administered, the tissues become saturated and factors of degradation and excretion then directly influence intensity and duration of action. In man, up to two thirds of an administered dose of tubocurarine is excreted in the urine over a period of several hours; smaller quantities appear in the bile, and a variable amount is metabolized (Gibaldi *et al.*, 1972; Crankshaw and Cohen, 1975). Insignificant amounts of tubocurarine cross the placenta.

Distribution and elimination of metocurine are similar to those of tubocurarine, as is its duration of action (Savarese *et al.*, 1977). Pancuronium is partially hydroxylated in the liver but also has a similar duration of action (Agoston *et al.*, 1977). Gallamine and decamethonium are almost entirely excreted by the kidney, with no apparent metabolic degradation. Atracurium is converted to less active metabolites by plasma esterases and by spontaneous nonenzymatic rearrangement (Hughes and Chapple, 1981; Basta *et al.*, 1982); this accounts for its briefer duration of action (about 30 minutes), which is about one half that of pancuronium. Vecuronium is metabolized to an appreciable extent, and its duration of action is also about one half that of pancuronium. The drug shows little cumulation with multiple doses (Agoston *et al.*, 1980; Fahey *et al.*, 1981).

The extremely brief duration of action of succinylcholine is due largely to its rapid hydrolysis by the butyrylcholinesterase of liver and plasma. The initial metabolite, succinylmonocholine, has a much weaker, predominantly competitive type of neuromuscular blocking action. Among the occasional patients who exhibit prolonged apnea following the administration of succinylcholine, a considerable number have an atypical plasma cholinesterase or a deficiency of the enzyme, due to allelic variations (McGuire *et al.*, 1989), hepatic disease, or a nutritional disturbance; however, in some the enzymatic activity in plasma is normal (Whittaker, 1986). A new short-acting depolarizing blocking agent, mivacurium, also owes its short duration of action to hydrolysis by cholinesterase (Shanks, 1988).

Preparations, Routes of Administration, and Dosages. Neuromuscular blocking agents are administered parenterally and nearly always intravenously. Detailed information on dosage can be found in anesthesiology textbooks (Kharkevich, 1986; Miller and Savarese, 1986; Azar, 1987). The neuromuscular blocking agents are potentially hazardous drugs. Consequently, they should be administered to patients only by anesthesiologists and other clinicians who have had extensive training in their use and in a setting where facilities for respiratory and cardiovascular resuscitation are immediately at hand.

Tubocurarine chloride is marketed as a solution containing 3 mg/ml. Because of its hypotensive effects, its use is declining. In light surgical anesthesia, 6 to 9 mg of the drug may be given as a single intravenous injection in adults. One half of this dose may be given after 3 to 5 minutes, if necessary, and small supplements given later, as required. With certain general anesthetics (halothane, isoflurane, and enflurane), lower doses should be used.

Metocurine iodide (METUBINE IODIDE) is available as a solution containing 2 mg/ml. Since this drug is about two times as potent as tubocurarine in man, the doses employed are only half those of the parent alkaloid.

Gallamine triethiodide (FLAXEDIL) is available as a solution containing 20 mg/ml. For muscular relaxation in conjunction with surgical anesthesia, gallamine triethiodide is usually injected intravenously in a dose of 1.0 mg/kg of body weight, and an additional 0.5 to 1.0 mg/kg may be given after 30 to 40 minutes, if necessary.

Pancuronium bromide (PAVULON) is available in solutions containing 1 or 2 mg/ml. The usual initial intravenous dose is 0.04 to 0.10 mg/kg.

Vecuronium bromide (NORCURON) is available in vials containing 10 mg. Usual initial doses are 0.08 to 0.1 mg/kg, administered intravenously. Additional doses of 0.01 to 0.015 mg/kg are given as necessary.

Atracurium besylate (TRACRIUM) is marketed as a solution (10 mg/ml); it should be administered intravenously at doses of 0.4 to 0.5 mg/kg initially. Maintenance doses are usually one fifth of the initial doses.

Succinylcholine chloride (ANECTINE, others) is marketed as a sterile powder and as a solution containing 20, 50, or 100 mg/ml. For brief surgical procedures in adults, the usual intravenous dose is 0.6 mg/kg, but the optimal dose varies considerably (0.3 to 1.1 mg/kg). For more prolonged procedures, the drug is given by intravenous drip infusion to obtain sustained muscular relaxation; the dose varies widely from patient to patient (0.5 to 5.0 mg or more per minute), and must be highly individualized. Moment-to-moment control of relaxation can be obtained by careful attention to the rate of infusion and the response of the patient.

Hexafluorenium bromide (MYLAXEN; hexamethylenebis [9-fluorenyldimethylammonium] dibromide) is a selective inhibitor of plasma cholinesterase with mild competitive neuromuscular blocking potency. It is given to prolong the blocking action of succinylcholine and to minimize the fasciculations that occur prior to neuromuscular block with this agent. The drug is available as a solution (20 mg/ml). Following an intravenous dose of hexafluorenium of 0.4 mg/kg (not to exceed a total dose of 36 mg), the initial dose of succinylcholine is 0.2 mg/kg, intravenously (not to exceed a total dose of 18 mg), which causes muscular relaxation for 20 to 30 minutes.

Alcuronium chloride (ALLOFERIN) is provided in ampuls containing 5 mg/ml; the recommended intravenous dose is 0.2 to 0.3 mg/kg initially. The drug is not marketed in the United States.

Fazadinium bromide is used in Europe as a rapidly acting competitive blocking agent. Its chief attributes lie in its rapid onset of action and metabolic degradation in patients with compromised renal function (Brittain and Tyers, 1973). The agent has yet to be marketed or tested extensively in the United States.

Decamethonium bromide is no longer marketed in the United States.

Measurement of Neuromuscular Blockade in Man. Assessment of neuromuscular block is usually performed by stimulation of the ulnar nerve. Responses are monitored from compound action potentials or muscle tension developed in the adductor pollicis muscle. Responses to repetitive or tetanic stimuli are most useful for evaluation of blockade of transmission since individual measurements of twitch tension must be related to control values obtained prior to the administration of drugs. Thus, stimulus schedules such as the "train of four" or responses to tetanic stimulation are preferred procedures (Waud and Waud, 1972; Ali and Savarese, 1976).

THERAPEUTIC USES

The main clinical use of the neuromuscular blocking agents is as an adjuvant in surgical anesthesia to obtain relaxation of skeletal muscle, particularly of the abdominal wall, so that operative manipulations are facilitated. With muscular relaxation no longer dependent upon the depth of general anesthesia, a much lighter level of anesthesia suffices. This situation is of obvious advantage since the risk of respiratory and cardiovascular depression is minimized. Moreover, the postanesthetic recovery period is shortened. Muscle relaxation is also of value in various orthopedic procedures, such as the correction of dislocations and the alignment of fractures. Neuromuscular blocking agents of short duration are often used to facilitate intubation with an endotracheal tube and have been used to facilitate laryngoscopy, bronchoscopy, and esophagoscopy in combination with a general anesthetic.

Use to Prevent Trauma During Electroshock Therapy. Electroconvulsive therapy of psychiatric disorders is occasionally complicated by trauma to the patient; the seizures induced may cause dislocations or fractures. Inasmuch as the muscular component of the convulsion is not essential for benefit from the procedure, neuromuscular blocking agents and thiopental are employed. The combination of the blocking drug, the anesthetic agent, and postictal depression usually results in respiratory depression or temporary apnea. An endotracheal tube and oxygen should always be available. An oropharyngeal airway should be inserted as soon as the jaw muscles relax (after the seizure) and provision made to prevent aspiration of mucus and saliva. Succinylcholine is most often used because of the brevity of its effect. A cuff may be applied to one extremity to prevent the effects of the drug in that limb; evidence of an effective electroshock is provided by contraction of the group of protected muscles.

Diagnostic Uses. Curare can be employed diagnostically for the detection of pain due to nerve-root compression masked by painful spasm of muscles involved in protective splinting. The use of tubocurarine to assist in the diagnosis of myasthenia gravis, and the potential hazards associated with this use, are presented in Chapter 7.

GANGLIONIC NEUROTRANSMISSION

Neurotransmission in autonomic ganglia has long been recognized to be a far more complex process than that described by a single neurotransmitter-receptor system, and intracellular recordings reveal at least four different changes in potential that can be elicited by stimulation of the preganglionic nerve (Eccles and Libet, 1961; Nishi and Koketsu, 1968; Weight *et al.*, 1979). The primary event involves the rapid depolarization of postsynaptic sites by ACh. The receptors are nicotinic, and the pathway is sensitive to classical nondepolarizing blocking agents such as hexamethonium. Activation of this primary pathway gives rise to an initial excitatory postsynaptic potential (EPSP). This rapid depolarization is primarily due to an inward Na^+ current through a neuronal type of nicotinic receptor channel (*see* above). The secondary pathways are thought to amplify or suppress this signal.

An action potential is generated in the postganglionic neuron when the initial EPSP attains a critical amplitude. In mammalian sympathetic ganglia *in vivo*, it may be necessary for multiple synapses to be activated before transmission is effective.

Iontophoretic application of ACh to the ganglion results in a depolarization with a latency of less than 1 msec; this decays over a period of 10 to 50 msec (Ascher *et al.*, 1979; MacDermott *et al.*, 1980). Measurements of single channel conductances indicate that the characteristics of nicotinic receptor channels of the ganglia and the neuromuscular junction are quite similar. In some ganglia, two types of fast channels have been detected (Gray and Rang, 1983).

The secondary events or pathways are insensitive to hexamethonium or other nicotinic antagonists. They include the slow EPSP, the late slow EPSP, and an inhibitory postsynaptic potential

(IPSP). The slow EPSP is generated by agonists acting on muscarinic receptors, and it is blocked by atropine or antagonists that are selective for M_1 muscarinic receptors (Libet, 1970; *see* Chapter 8). The slow EPSP has a longer latency and a duration of 30 to 60 seconds. In contrast, the late slow EPSP lasts for several minutes and is initiated by the action of peptides that are found in specific ganglia (*see* below). The peptides and ACh are released from the same nerve ending, but the enhanced stability of the peptide in the ganglion extends its sphere of influence to postsynaptic sites beyond those in immediate proximity to the nerve ending (Jan *et al.*, 1983). The slow EPSPs result from decreased K^+ conductance (Weight *et al.*, 1979). Depolarization activates a K^+ channel, and the muscarinic agonists or peptides suppress channel conductance. The K^+ conductance has been called an *M current,* and it regulates the sensitivity of the cell to repetitive fast-depolarizing events (Adams *et al.*, 1982).

Like the slow EPSP, the IPSP is unaffected by the classical ganglionic blocking agents but, in many systems, is sensitive to blockade by atropine. Substantial electrophysiological and morphological evidence has accumulated to suggest that catecholamines participate in the generation of the IPSP. Dopamine and norepinephrine cause hyperpolarization of ganglia, and both the IPSP and the catecholamine-induced hyperpolarization are blocked by α-adrenergic antagonists. Since the IPSP is sensitive in most systems to blockade by both atropine and α-adrenergic antagonists, ACh that is released at the preganglionic terminal may act on a catecholamine-containing interneuron to stimulate the release of dopamine or norepinephrine; the catecholamine, in turn, produces hyperpolarization (an IPSP) of the ganglion cell (Eccles and Libet, 1961; Libet, 1970). The muscarinic link in the IPSP is mediated through M_2 receptors (at least in some ganglia). Morphological studies indicate that catecholamine-containing cells are present in ganglia. These include the dopamine- or norepinephrine-containing small, intensely fluorescent (SIF) cells and adrenergic nerve terminals. The precise role played by the SIF cells and the electrogenic mechanism of the IPSP remain to be resolved (Eränkö *et al.*, 1980).

The relative importance of the secondary pathways and even the nature of the modulating transmitters appear to differ among individual ganglia and between parasympathetic and sympathetic ganglia. A variety of peptides, including luteinizing hormone–releasing hormone, substance P, angiotensin, vasoactive intestinal polypeptide, neuropeptide Y, and enkephalins, have been identified in ganglia by immunofluorescence, and they appear to be released upon preganglionic nerve stimulation (Sejnowski, 1982; Jan *et al.*, 1983). Precise details of their modulatory actions are not understood, but they appear to be most closely associated with the late slow EPSP and inhibition of the M current in various ganglia. Other neurotransmitter substances, such as 5-hydroxytryptamine (Wood and Mayer, 1979) and gamma-aminobutyric acid, are known to modify ganglionic transmission. It should be emphasized that the secondary synaptic events only modulate the initial EPSP. Conventional ganglionic blocking agents can inhibit ganglionic transmission completely; the same cannot be said for muscarinic antagonists or α-adrenergic agonists (*see* Weight *et al.*, 1979; Volle, 1980).

Drugs that stimulate cholinergic receptor sites on autonomic ganglia can be grouped into two major categories. The first group consists of drugs with nicotinic specificity, including nicotine itself. Their excitatory effects on ganglia are rapid in onset, are blocked by nondepolarizing ganglionic blocking agents, and mimic the initial EPSP. The second group is composed of agents such as muscarine, McN-A-343, and methacholine, and, in part, the anticholinesterase (anti-ChE) agents. Their excitatory effects on ganglia are delayed in onset, blocked by atropine-like drugs, and mimic the slow EPSP.

Ganglionic blocking agents impair transmission by actions at the primary nicotinic receptor and also may be classified into two groups. The first group includes those drugs that initially stimulate the ganglia by an ACh-like action and then block them because of a persistent depolarization (*e.g.*, nicotine); prolonged application of nicotine results in desensitization of the cholinergic receptor site and continued blockade. (*See* review by Volle, 1980.) The blockade of autonomic ganglia produced by the second group of blocking drugs, of which hexamethonium and trimethaphan can be regarded as prototypes, does not involve prior ganglionic stimulation or changes in the ganglionic potentials. These agents impair transmission either by competing with ACh for ganglionic cholinergic receptor sites or by blocking the channel when it is open. Trimethaphan acts by competition with ACh, analogous to the mechanism of action of curare at the neuromuscular junction. Hexamethonium appears to block the channel after it opens. This action shortens the duration of current flow, since the open channel either becomes occluded or closes (Rang, 1982; Gurney and Rang, 1984). Irrespective of the mechanism, the initial EPSP is blocked and ganglionic transmission is inhibited.

GANGLIONIC STIMULATING DRUGS

History. Two natural alkaloids, nicotine and lobeline, exhibit their primary actions by stimulating autonomic ganglia. Nicotine (Table 9–3) was first isolated from leaves of tobacco, *Nicotiana tabacum*, by Posselt and Reiman in 1828, and Orfila initiated the first pharmacological studies of the alkaloid in 1843. Langley and Dickinson (1889) painted the superior cervical ganglion of rabbits with nicotine and demonstrated that its site of action was the ganglion, rather than the preganglionic or postganglionic nerve fiber. Lobeline (α-lobeline) (*see* Table 9–3) was first obtained in crystalline form from *Lobelia inflata* (Indian tobacco) by Wieland in 1915. Lobeline has many of the same actions in the body as nicotine but is less potent.

A number of synthetic compounds also have prominent actions at ganglionic receptor sites. The actions of the onium compounds, of which tetramethylammonium (TMA) is the simplest prototype, were explored in considerable detail in the last half of the nineteenth century and in the early twentieth century. In 1951, Chen and coworkers described the ganglionic stimulating properties of 1,1-dimethyl-4-phenylpiperazinium (DMPP) iodide, a relatively specific ganglionic stimulant.

NICOTINE

Nicotine is of considerable medical significance because of its toxicity, presence in tobacco, and propensity for conferring a dependence on its users. The chronic effects of nicotine and the untoward effects of the chronic use of tobacco are considered in Chapter 22.

Table 9–3. GANGLIONIC STIMULANTS

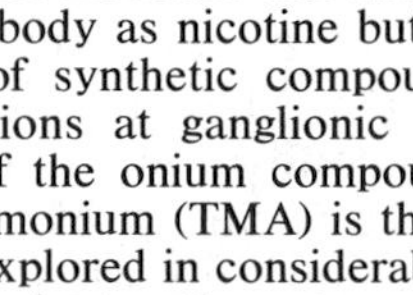

Nicotine

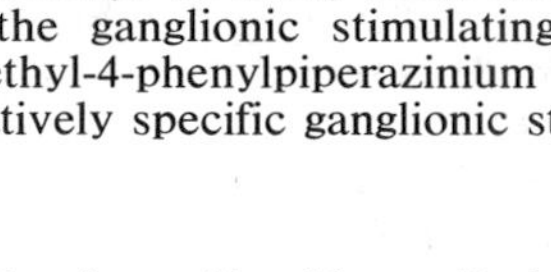

Lobeline

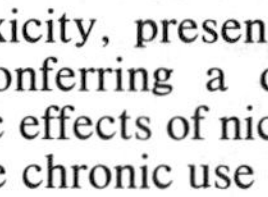

Tetramethylammonium (TMA)

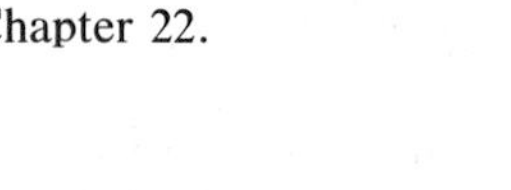

1,1-Dimethyl-4-phenylpiperazinium (DMPP)

Nicotine is one of the few natural liquid alkaloids. It is a colorless, volatile base ($pK_a = 8.5$) that turns brown and acquires the odor of tobacco on exposure to air.

Pharmacological Actions. The complex and often unpredictable changes that occur in the body after administration of nicotine are due not only to its actions on a variety of neuroeffector and chemosensitive sites but also to the fact that the alkaloid has both stimulant and depressant phases of action. The ultimate response of any one system represents the summation of the several different and opposing effects of nicotine. For example, the drug can increase the heart rate by excitation of sympathetic or paralysis of parasympathetic cardiac ganglia, and it can slow the heart rate by paralysis of sympathetic or stimulation of parasympathetic cardiac ganglia. In addition, the effects of the drug on the chemoreceptors of the carotid and aortic bodies and on medullary centers influence heart rate, as do also the cardiovascular compensatory reflexes resulting from changes in blood pressure caused by nicotine. Finally, nicotine causes a discharge of epinephrine from the adrenal medulla, and this hormone accelerates cardiac rate and raises blood pressure.

Peripheral Nervous System. The major action of nicotine consists initially in transient stimulation and subsequently in a more persistent depression of all autonomic ganglia. Small doses of nicotine stimulate the ganglion cells directly and facilitate the transmission of impulses. When larger doses of the drug are applied, the initial stimulation is followed very quickly by a blockade of transmission. Whereas stimulation of the ganglion cells coincides with their depolarization, depression of transmission by adequate doses of nicotine occurs both during the depolarization and after it has subsided. Nicotine also possesses a biphasic action on the adrenal medulla; small doses evoke the discharge of catecholamines, and larger doses prevent their release in response to splanchnic nerve stimulation.

Nicotine also causes the release of catecholamines in a number of isolated organs. This action results in a sympathomimetic response to nicotine that is blocked by drugs known to prevent the effects of catecholamines.

The effects of nicotine on the neuromuscular junction are similar to those on ganglia. However, with the exception of avian and denervated mammalian muscle, the stimulant phase is largely obscured by the rapidly developing paralysis. In the latter stage, nicotine also produces neuromuscular blockade by receptor desensitization.

Nicotine, like ACh, is known to stimulate a number of sensory receptors. These include mechanoreceptors that respond to stretch or pressure of the skin, mesentery, tongue, lung, and stomach; chemoreceptors of the carotid body; thermal receptors of the skin and tongue; and pain receptors. Prior administration of hexamethonium prevents the stimulation of the sensory receptors by nicotine, but has little, if any, effect on the activation of the sensory receptors by physiological stimuli.

Central Nervous System. Nicotine markedly stimulates the CNS. Appropriate doses produce tremors; with somewhat larger doses, the tremor is followed by convulsions. The excitation of respiration is a prominent action of nicotine; although large doses act directly on the medulla oblongata, smaller doses augment respiration reflexly by excitation of the chemoreceptors of the carotid and aortic bodies. Stimulation of the CNS is followed by depression, and death results from failure of respiration due to both central paralysis and peripheral blockade of muscles of respiration.

Nicotine and lobeline induce vomiting by both central and peripheral actions. The central component of the vomiting response is due to stimulation of the emetic chemoreceptor trigger zone in the area postrema of the medulla oblongata. In addition, nicotine activates vagal and spinal afferent nerves that form the sensory input of the reflex pathways involved in the act of vomiting.

Cardiovascular System. When administered intravenously to the dog, nicotine characteristically produces an increase in heart rate and blood pressure. The latter is usually a more sustained response. In general, the cardiovascular responses to nicotine are due to stimulation of sympathetic ganglia and the adrenal medulla, together with the discharge of catecholamines from sympathetic nerve endings. Also contributing to the sympathomimetic response to nicotine is the activation of chemoreceptors of the aortic and carotid bodies, which reflexly results in vasoconstriction, tachycardia, and elevated blood pressure.

Gastrointestinal Tract. The effects of the drug on the gastrointestinal tract are due largely to parasympathetic stimulation. The combined activation of parasympathetic ganglia and cholinergic nerve endings results in increased tone and motor activity of the bowel. Nausea, vomiting, and occasionally diarrhea are observed following systemic absorption of nicotine.

Exocrine Glands. Nicotine causes an initial stimulation of salivary and bronchial secretions that is followed by inhibition. Salivation caused by smoking is reflexly produced by the irritant smoke rather than by a systemic effect of nicotine.

Absorption, Fate, and Excretion. Nicotine is readily absorbed from the respiratory tract, buccal membranes, and skin (Benowitz, 1986). Severe poisoning has resulted from percutaneous absorption. Being a relatively strong base, its absorption from the stomach is limited unless intragastric pH is raised. Intestinal absorption is far more efficient. Nicotine in chewing tobacco, because it is more slowly absorbed than inhaled nicotine, has a longer duration of effect (Benowitz *et al.*, 1988).

Approximately 80 to 90% of nicotine is altered in the body, mainly in the liver but also in the kidney and lung. A significant fraction of inhaled nicotine is metabolized by the lung (Turner *et al.*, 1975). The major metabolites of nicotine are cotinine and nicotine-1′-N-oxide, which are formed respectively from oxidation of the α carbon and N-oxidation of the pyrrolidine ring. The half-life of nicotine following inhalation or parenteral administration is about 2 hours. Both nicotine and its metabolites are rapidly eliminated by the kidney (Russell and Feyerabend, 1978). The rate of urinary excretion of nicotine is dependent upon the pH of the urine; excretion diminishes when the urine is alkaline. Nicotine is also excreted in the milk of lactating women who smoke. The milk of heavy smokers may contain 0.5 mg per liter.

Acute Nicotine Poisoning. Poisoning from nicotine may occur from accidental ingestion of insecticide sprays in which nicotine is present as the effective agent or in children from ingestion of tobacco products. The acutely fatal dose of nicotine for an adult is probably about 60 mg of the base. Smoking tobacco usually contains 1 to 2% nicotine. Apparently the gastric absorption of nicotine from tobacco taken by mouth is delayed because of slowed gastric emptying, so that vomiting caused by the central effect of the initially absorbed fraction may remove much of the tobacco remaining in the gastrointestinal tract.

The onset of symptoms of acute, severe nicotine poisoning is rapid; they include nausea, salivation, abdominal pain, vomiting, diarrhea, cold sweat, headache, dizziness, disturbed hearing and vision, mental confusion, and marked weakness. Faintness and prostration ensue; the blood pressure falls; breathing is difficult; the pulse is weak, rapid, and irregular; and collapse may be followed by terminal convulsions. Death may result within a few minutes from respiratory failure.

Therapy. Vomiting should be induced with syrup of ipecac, or gastric lavage should be performed. Alkaline solutions should be avoided. A slurry of activated charcoal is then passed through the tube and left in the stomach. Respiratory assistance and treatment of shock may be necessary.

OTHER GANGLIONIC STIMULANTS

Stimulation of ganglia by TMA or DMPP differs from that produced by nicotine in that the initial stimulation is not followed by a dominant blocking action. Their stimulatory action results from an initial EPSP and is blocked by hexamethonium. DMPP is about three times more potent than nicotine. Parasympathomimetic drugs (muscarine, pilocarpine, and the synthetic choline esters) can also stimulate ganglia; however, their effects are usually obscured by stimulation of other neuroeffector sites. McN-A-343 represents an exception to this; in certain tissues its primary action appears to occur at muscarinic M_1 receptors in ganglia.

GANGLIONIC BLOCKING DRUGS

The chemical diversity of compounds that block autonomic ganglia without causing prior stimulation is shown in Table 9–4.

History and Structure–Activity Relationship. Although Marshall (1913) and Burn and Dale (1915) first described the "nicotine paralyzing" action of

Table 9–4. NONDEPOLARIZING GANGLIONIC BLOCKING AGENTS

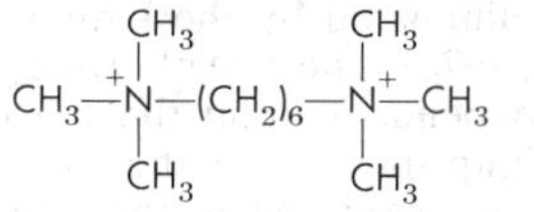
Hexamethonium (C6)

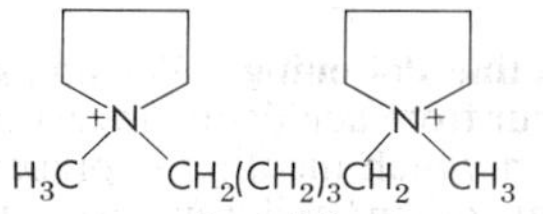
Pentolinium

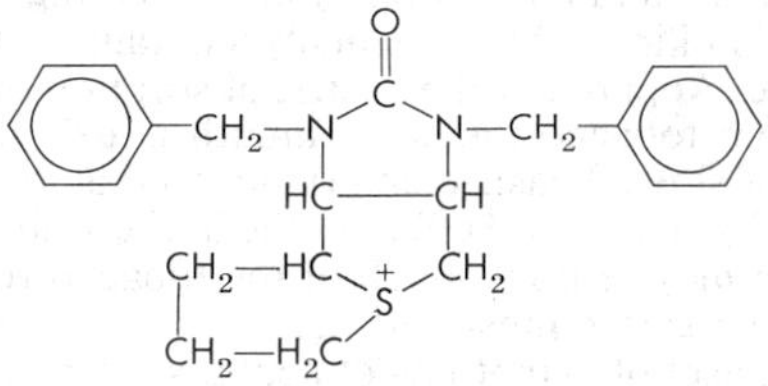
Trimethaphan

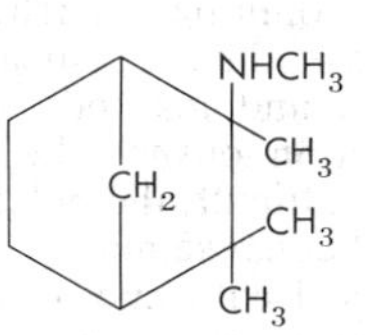
Mecamylamine

tetraethylammonium (TEA) on ganglia, TEA was largely overlooked until Acheson and Moe (1946) and Acheson and Pereira (1946) published their definitive analyses of the effects of the ion on the cardiovascular system and autonomic ganglia. They also proposed the use of TEA for the treatment of hypertension. The *bis*-quaternary ammonium salts were developed and studied independently by Barlow and Ing (1948) and Paton and Zaimis (1949, 1952). The prototypical ganglionic blocking drug in this series, hexamethonium (C6), has a bridge of six methylene groups between the two quaternary nitrogen atoms (*see* Table 9–4). C6 and its congener C5 have minimal neuromuscular and muscarinic blocking activity.

Subsequently, several series of *bis*-quaternary ammonium compounds were investigated for ganglionic blocking activity, and some drugs so discovered, such as pentolinium, have been employed clinically. Pentolinium has a longer duration of action than hexamethonium and was widely used to produce controlled hypotension in anesthesia after Enderby's favorable report in 1954. Triethylsulfoniums, like the quaternary and *bis*-quaternary ammonium ions, possess ganglionic blocking actions. This knowledge led to the development of sulfonium ganglionic blocking agents such as trimethaphan (*see* Table 9–4). The synthesis of secondary amines with ganglionic blocking activity represented a departure in the chemistry of these agents. The pharmacological properties of mecamylamine (*see* Table 9–4) were reported in the mid-1950s, and the drug was soon introduced into therapy. Pempidine, a tertiary amine with similar properties, was introduced shortly after mecamylamine.

Pharmacological Properties. Nearly all of the physiological alterations observed after the administration of ganglionic blocking agents can be attributed to the mechanisms already considered. These alterations can be anticipated with reasonable accuracy by a careful inspection of Figure 5–1 (facing page 86) and by knowing which division of the autonomic nervous system exercises dominant control of various organs (Table 9–5). For example, blockade of sympathetic ganglia interrupts adrenergic control of arterioles and results in vasodilatation, improved peripheral blood flow in some vascular beds, and a fall in blood pressure.

Generalized ganglionic blockade may result also in atony of the bladder and gastrointestinal tract, cycloplegia, xerostomia, diminished perspiration, and, by abolishing circulatory reflex pathways, postural hypotension. These changes represent the generally undesirable features of ganglionic blockade, which limit the therapeutic efficacy of ganglionic blocking agents.

Cardiovascular System. The importance of existing sympathetic tone in determining the degree to which blood pressure is lowered by ganglionic blockade is illustrated by the fact that blood pressure may be decreased only minimally in recumbent normotensive subjects but may fall markedly in sitting or standing subjects. Postural hypotension is a major problem in ambulatory patients receiving ganglionic blocking drugs; it is relieved to some extent by muscular activity and completely by recumbency. Sympathetically mediated vasomotor reflexes are inhibited, and the cold pressor response is reduced.

Changes in cardiac rate following ganglionic blockade depend largely on existing vagal tone. In man, mild tachycardia usually accompanies the hypotension, a sign that indicates fairly complete ganglionic blockade. However, a decrease may occur if the heart rate is initially high.

Cardiac output is often reduced by ganglionic blocking drugs in patients with normal cardiac function as a consequence of diminished venous return resulting from venous dilatation and peripheral pooling of blood. In patients with cardiac failure, ganglionic blockade frequently results in increased cardiac output due to a reduction in peripheral resistance. In hypertensive subjects, cardiac output, stroke volume, and left ventricular work are diminished.

Although total systemic vascular resistance is decreased in patients who receive ganglionic blocking agents, changes in blood flow and vascular resistance of individual vascular beds are variable. Skin temperature is elevated mostly in the hands and feet, and blood flow to the limbs may increase. Reduction of cerebral blood flow is small unless mean systemic blood pressure falls below 50 to

Table 9–5. USUAL PREDOMINANCE OF SYMPATHETIC (ADRENERGIC) OR PARASYMPATHETIC (CHOLINERGIC) TONE AT VARIOUS EFFECTOR SITES, WITH CONSEQUENT EFFECTS OF AUTONOMIC GANGLIONIC BLOCKADE

SITE	PREDOMINANT TONE	EFFECT OF GANGLIONIC BLOCKADE
Arterioles	Sympathetic (adrenergic)	Vasodilatation; increased peripheral blood flow; hypotension
Veins	Sympathetic (adrenergic)	Dilatation; peripheral pooling of blood; decreased venous return; decreased cardiac output
Heart	Parasympathetic (cholinergic)	Tachycardia
Iris	Parasympathetic (cholinergic)	Mydriasis
Ciliary muscle	Parasympathetic (cholinergic)	Cycloplegia
Gastrointestinal tract	Parasympathetic (cholinergic)	Reduced tone and motility; constipation
Urinary bladder	Parasympathetic (cholinergic)	Urinary retention
Salivary glands	Parasympathetic (cholinergic)	Xerostomia
Sweat glands	Sympathetic (cholinergic)	Anhidrosis

60 mm Hg. Skeletal muscle blood flow is unaltered, but splanchnic and renal blood flow decrease following the administration of a ganglionic blocking agent. Renal vascular resistance increases, and the rate of glomerular filtration falls. Trimethaphan appears to cause some vasodilatation by a direct mechanism.

Other Effects. Ganglionic blocking agents generally decrease gastrointestinal secretions and reduce the tone and motility of the gastrointestinal tract. Ganglionic blockade causes partial or total impairment of the voiding contractions of the urinary bladder, with a resultant increase in vesical capacity and incomplete voiding. This effect is due to blockade of parasympathetic ganglia along the efferent pathways of the spinal reflex concerned with micturition, so that bladder distention causes no urge to void. Penile erection and ejaculation are impaired. Ganglionic blockade causes incomplete mydriasis and partial loss of accommodation as a result of impaired transmission in the ciliary ganglion. Sweating is reduced.

Absorption, Fate, and Excretion. The absorption of quaternary ammonium and sulfonium compounds from the enteric tract is incomplete and unpredictable. This is due both to the limited ability of these ionized substances to penetrate cell membranes and to the depression of propulsive movements of the small intestine. Gastric emptying time may be so delayed that two or three doses may be retained in the stomach; the gastric contents may then suddenly enter the duodenum, and the absorption of the accumulated toxic amounts of drug can cause severe hypotension and collapse. Although the absorption of mecamylamine is less erratic, a danger exists of reduced bowel activity leading to frank paralytic ileus.

After absorption, the quaternary ammonium and sulfonium blocking agents are confined primarily to the extracellular space and are mostly excreted unchanged by the kidney. High concentrations of mecamylamine accumulate in the liver and kidney. Mecamylamine is excreted slowly by the kidney in unchanged form and has a relatively long duration of action.

Untoward Responses and Severe Reactions. Among the milder untoward responses observed are visual disturbances, dry mouth, conjunctival suffusion, urinary hesitancy, decreased potentia, subjective chilliness, moderate constipation, occasional diarrhea, abdominal discomfort, anorexia, heartburn, nausea, eructation and bitter taste, and the signs and symptoms of syncope caused by postural hypotension. These side effects tend to become less pronounced as administration of the drug is continued. More severe reactions include marked hypotension, constipation, syncope, paralytic ileus, urinary retention, and cycloplegia. Unlike the quaternary ganglionic blocking agents, which do not readily reach the CNS, large doses of mecamylamine can produce prominent central effects, resulting in tremors, mental confusion, seizures, mania, or depression.

Preparations, Routes of Administration, and Dosages. Of the ganglionic blocking agents that have appeared on the therapeutic scene, only mecamylamine and trimethaphan are currently utilized in the United States. Pempidine and pentolinium are still used to a limited extent in Europe.

Mecamylamine hydrochloride (INVERSINE) is available for oral administration in tablets containing 2.5 mg of the drug. The usual initial dose is 2.5 mg, given twice daily.

Trimethaphan camsylate (ARFONAD) is available as an injection (50 mg/ml). It possesses a short duration of action and is administered by intravenous drip. When administered in this manner, a 0.1% solution in 5% dextrose is employed.

Therapeutic Uses. Historically, the major therapeutic use of the ganglionic blocking agents was in the management of hypertensive cardiovascular disease. However, these drugs have been supplanted by superior agents for the treatment of chronic hypertension and hypertensive crisis (*see* Chapter 33). The only remaining use of ganglionic blockers in hypertension is for the initial control of blood pressure in patients with acute dissecting aortic aneurysm. Ganglionic blocking agents are ideal for this condition because they not only reduce blood pressure but also inhibit sympathetic reflexes and thereby reduce the rate of rise of pressure at the site of the tear. In such situations, trimethaphan is infused intravenously at a rate of 0.3 to 3 mg per minute with frequent monitoring of blood pressure. In the absence of symptoms or signs of renal, cerebral, or myocardial ischemia, the dose is increased until the pressure is in the low-normal range. Disappearance of pain is a sign that the dissection has stopped. A disadvantage of trimethaphan is the development of tolerance over the first 48 hours of therapy; this is in part related to fluid retention. Increased efficacy is obtained if the bed is tilted so that the legs are below the level of the heart. Since trimethaphan can stimulate the release of histamine, it should be used with caution in patients with a history of allergy.

An additional therapeutic use of the ganglionic blocking agents is in the production of controlled hypotension; a reduction in blood pressure during surgery may be sought deliberately to minimize hemorrhage in the operative field, to reduce blood loss in various orthopedic procedures, and to facilitate surgery on blood vessels (Leigh, 1975; Salem, 1978). Trimethaphan, as an infusion, may be used as an alternative to or in combination with sodium nitroprusside, since some patients are resistant to the latter drug. Trimethaphan blunts the sympathoadrenal stimulation caused by nitroprusside and reduces the required dosage (Fahmy, 1985).

Trimethaphan can be used in the management of autonomic hyperreflexia. This syndrome is typically seen in patients with injuries of the upper spinal cord and results from a massive sympathetic discharge. A common stimulus for such discharge is distention of the bladder; it is often associated with catheterization or irrigation of the bladder, cystoscopy, or transurethral resection. Since normal central inhibition of the reflex is lacking in such patients, the spinal reflex is dominant. It can be controlled successfully with ganglionic blocking agents (Basta *et al.*, 1977).

Acheson, G. H., and Moe, G. K. The action of tetraethylammonium ion on the mammalian circulation. *J. Pharmacol. Exp. Ther.*, **1946**, *87*, 220–236.

Acheson, G. H., and Pereira, S. A. The blocking effect of tetraethylammonium ion on the superior cervical ganglion of the cat. *J. Pharmacol. Exp. Ther.*, **1946**, *87*, 273–280.

Adams, P. R.; Brown, D. A.; and Constanti, A. Pharmacological inhibition of the M-current. *J. Physiol. (Lond.)*, **1982**, *332*, 223–262.

Adams, P. R., and Sakmann, B. Decamethonium both blocks and opens end plate channels. *Proc. Natl. Acad. Sci. U.S.A.*, **1978**, *75*, 2994–2998.

Agoston, S.; Crul, J. F.; Kersten, U. W.; and Scaf, A. H. J. Relationship of serum concentration of pancuronium to its neuromuscular activity in man. *Anesthesiology*, **1977**, *15*, 509–512.

Agoston, S.; Salt, P.; Newton, D.; Bencini, A.; Boomsma, P.; and Erdmann, W. The neuromuscular blocking action of Org NC 45, a new pancuronium derivative, in anaesthetized patients. *Br. J. Anaesth.*, **1980**, *52*, 53S–59S.

Ali, H. H., and Savarese, J. J. Monitoring of neuromuscular function. *Anesthesiology*, **1976**, *14*, 216–249.

Ascher, P.; Large, W. A.; and Rang, H. P. Studies on the mechanism of action of acetylcholine antagonists on rat parasympathetic ganglion cells. *J. Physiol. (Lond.)*, **1979**, *295*, 139–170.

Auerbach, A., and Betz, W. Does curare affect transmitter release? *J. Physiol. (Lond.)*, **1971**, *213*, 691–705.

Barlow, R. B., and Ing, H. R. Curare-like action of polymethylene *bis*-quaternary ammonium salts. *Br. J. Pharmacol. Chemother.*, **1948**, *3*, 298–304.

Basta, J. W.; Nlejadlik, K.; and Pallares, V. Autonomic hyperflexia: intraoperative control with pentolinium tartrate. *Br. J. Anaesth.*, **1977**, *49*, 1087–1090.

Basta, S. J.; Ali, H. H.; Savarese, J. J.; Sander, N.; Gionfriddo, M.; Clouter, G.; Lineberry, G.; and Cato, A. E. Clinical pharmacology of atracurium besylate: a new non-depolarizing muscle relaxant. *Anesth. Analg.*, **1982**, *61*, 723–729.

Benowitz, N. L. Clinical pharmacology of nicotine. *Annu. Rev. Med.*, **1986**, *37*, 21–32.

Benowitz, N. L.; Porchet, H.; Sheiner, L.; and Jacob, P., III. Nicotine absorption and cardiovascular effects with smokeless tobacco use: comparison with cigarettes and nicotine gum. *Clin. Pharmacol. Ther.*, **1988**, *44*, 23–28.

Brisson, A., and Unwin, P. N. T. Quaternary structure of the acetylcholine receptor. *Nature*, **1985**, *315*, 474–477.

Brittain, R. T., and Tyers, M. B. The pharmacology of AH 8165: a rapid-acting, short-lasting competitive neuromuscular blocking drug. *Br. J. Anaesth.*, **1973**, *45*, 837–843.

Burn, J. H., and Dale, H. H. The action of certain quaternary ammonium bases. *J. Pharmacol. Exp. Ther.*, **1915**, *6*, 417–438.

Burns, B. D., and Paton, W. D. M. Depolarization of the motor end-plate by decamethonium and acetylcholine. *J. Physiol. (Lond.)*, **1951**, *115*, 41–73.

Chang, C. C., and Lee, C. Y. Isolation of neurotoxins from the venom of *Bungarus multicinctus* and their modes of neuromuscular blocking action. *Arch. Int. Pharmacodyn. Ther.*, **1963**, *144*, 241–257.

Claudio, T.; Green, W. N.; Hartman, D. S.; Hayden, D.; Paulson, H. L.; Sigworth, F. J.; Sine, S.; and Swedlund, A. Genetic reconstitution of functional acetylcholine receptor channels in mouse fibroblasts. *Science*, **1987**, *238*, 1688–1697.

Colquhoun, D.; Dreyer, F.; and Sheridan, R. E. The actions of tubocurarine at the frog neuromuscular junction. *J. Physiol. (Lond.)*, **1979**, *293*, 247–284.

Dionne, V. E.; Steinbach, J. H.; and Stevens, C. F. An analysis of the dose-response relationship at voltage-clamped frog neuromuscular junctions. *J. Physiol. (Lond.)*, **1978**, *281*, 421–444.

Donati, F.; Smith, C. E.; and Bevan, D. R. Dose-response relationships for edrophonium and neostigmine as antagonists of moderate and profound atracurium blockade. *Anesth. Analg.*, **1989**, *68*, 13–19.

Durant, N. N.; Nguyen, N.; and Katz, R. L. Potentiation of neuromuscular blockade by verapamil. *Anesthesiology*, **1984**, *60*, 298–303.

Eccles, R. M., and Libet, B. Origin and blockade of the synaptic responses of curarized sympathetic ganglia. *J. Physiol. (Lond.)*, **1961**, *157*, 484–503.

Elston, J. S.; Lee, J. P.; Powell, C. M.; Hogg, C.; and Clark, P. Treatment of strabismus in adults with botulinum toxin A. *Br. J. Ophthalmol.*, **1985**, *69*, 718.

Ertama, P. M. Histamine liberation in surgical patients following administration of neuromuscular blocking drugs. *Ann. Clin. Res.*, **1982**, *14*, 27–31.

Fahey, M. R.; Morris, R. B.; Miller, R. D.; Sohn, Y. J.; Cronnelly, R.; and Gencarelli, P. Clinical pharmacology of ORG NC45. *Anesthesiology*, **1981**, *55*, 6–11.

Fahmy, N. R. Nitroprusside vs. a nitroprusside-trimethaphan mixture for induced hypotension, hemodynamic effects, and cyanide release. *Clin. Pharmacol. Ther.*, **1985**, *70*, 264–270.

Fogdall, R. P., and Miller, R. D. Neuromuscular effects of enflurane, alone and combined with *d*-tubocurarine, pancuronium and succinylcholine in man. *Anesthesiology*, **1975**, *42*, 173–178.

Gibaldi, M.; Levy, G.; and Hayton, W. L. Tubocurarine and renal failure. *Br. J. Anaesth.*, **1972**, *44*, 163–165.

Goldman, D.; Deneris, E.; Luyten, W.; Kochar, A.; Patrick, J.; and Heinemann, S. Members of a nicotinic acetylcholine receptor gene family are expressed in different regions of the mammalian central nervous system. *Cell*, **1987**, *48*, 965–973.

Gray, P. T. A., and Rang, H. P. Analysis of current noise evoked by nicotinic agonists in rat submandibular ganglion neurones. *Br. J. Pharmacol.*, **1983**, *80*, 235–240.

Griffith, H. R., and Johnson, G. E. The use of curare in general anesthesia. *Anesthesiology*, **1942**, *3*, 418–420.

Gurney, A. M., and Rang, H. P. The channel-blocking action of methonium compounds on rat submandibular ganglion cells. *Br. J. Pharmacol.*, **1984**, *82*, 623–642.

Hughes, R., and Chapple, D. J. The pharmacology of atracurium: a new competitive neuromuscular blocking agent. *Br. J. Anaesth.*, **1981**, *53*, 31–44.

Katz, B., and Miledi, R. Propagation of electric activity in motor nerve terminals. *Proc. R. Soc. Lond.* [*Biol.*], **1965**, *161*, 453–482.

———. The characteristics of "end plate noise" produced by different depolarizing drugs. *J. Physiol. (Lond.)*, **1973**, *231*, 549–574.

Katz, B., and Thesleff, S. A study of "desensitization" produced by acetylcholine at the motor end-plate. *J. Physiol. (Lond.)*, **1957**, *138*, 63–80.

Langley, J. N., and Dickinson, W. L. On the local paralysis of peripheral ganglia, and on the connexion of different classes of nerve fibers with them. *Proc. R. Soc. Lond.* [*Biol.*], **1889**, *46*, 423–431.

MacDermott, A. B.; Connor, E. A.; Dionne, V. E.; and Parsons, R. L. Voltage clamp study of fast excitatory synaptic currents in bullfrog sympathetic ganglion cells. *J. Gen. Physiol.*, **1980**, *75*, 39–60.

McGuire, M. C.; Nogueira, C. F.; Bartes, C. F.; Lightstone, H.; Majra, A.; Van der Spek, A. F. L.; Lockridge, O.; and LaDu, B. N. Identification of the structural mutation responsible for the dibucaine resistant variant form of human serum cholinesterase. *Proc. Natl. Acad. Sci. U.S.A.*, **1989**, *86*, 953–957.

Mageby, K., and Terrar, D. A. Factors affecting the time course of decay of end-plate currents: a possible cooperative action of acetylcholine on receptors at the frog neuromuscular junction. *J. Physiol. (Lond.)*, **1975**, *244*, 467–482.

Marshall, C. R. Studies on the pharmaceutical action of tetra-alkyl-ammonium compounds. *Trans. R. Soc. Edinb.*, **1913**, *1*, 17–40.

Nishi, S., and Koketsu, K. Early and late after-discharges of amphibian sympathetic ganglion cells. *J. Neurophysiol.*, **1968**, *31*, 109–121.

Ornstein, F.; Matteo, R. S.; Schwartz, A. E.; Silverberg, P. A.; Young, W. L.; and Diaz, J. The effect of phenytoin on the magnitude and duration of neuromuscular block following atracurium or vecuronium. *Anesthesiology*, **1987**, *67*, 191–196.

Paton, W. D. M., and Zaimis, E. J. The pharmacological actions of polymethylene bistrimethylammonium salts. *Br. J. Pharmacol. Chemother.*, **1949**, *4*, 381–400.

Rang, H. P. The action of ganglionic blocking drugs on the synaptic responses of submandibular ganglion cells. *Br. J. Pharmacol.*, **1982**, *75*, 151–168.

Savarese, J. J.; Ali, H. H.; and Antonio, R. P. The clinical pharmacology of metocurine. *Anesthesiology*, **1977**, *47*, 277–284.

Sine, S., and Taylor, P. Relationship between reversible antagonist occupancy and the functional capacity of the acetylcholine receptor. *J. Biol. Chem.*, **1981**, *256*, 6692–6698.

Smith, S. M.; Brown, H. O.; Toman, J. E. P.; and Goodman, L. S. The lack of cerebral effects of *d*-tubocurarine. *Anesthesiology*, **1947**, *8*, 1–14.

Son, S. L.; Waud, B. E.; and Waud, D. R. A comparison of the neuromuscular and vagolytic effects of ORG NC 45 and pancuronium. *Anesthesiology*, **1981**, *55*, 12–18.

Sutherland, G. A.; Squire, J. B.; Gibb, A. J.; and Marshall, I. G. Neuromuscular blocking and autonomic effects of vecuronium and atracurium in the anaesthetized cat. *Br. J. Anaesth.*, **1983**, *55*, 1119–1126.

Turner, D. M.; Armitage, A. K.; Briant, R. H.; and Dollery, C. T. Metabolism of nicotine by the isolated perfused dog lung. *Xenobiotica*, **1975**, *5*, 539–551.

Unwin, N.; Toyoshima, C.; and Kubalek, E. Arrangement of the acetylcholine receptor subunits in the resting and desensitized states determined by cryoelector microscopy of crystallized *Torpedo* postsynaptic membranes. *J. Cell Biol.*, **1988**, *107*, 1123–1138.

Waud, B. E., and Waud, D. R. The relation between the response to "train of four" stimulation and receptor occlusion during competitive neuromuscular block. *Anesthesiology*, **1972**, *37*, 413–416.

Wood, J. D., and Mayer, C. J. Serotonergic activation of tonic-type enteric neurons in guinea pig small bowel. *J. Neurophysiol.*, **1979**, *42*, 582–593.

Monographs and Reviews

Argov, Z., and Mastaglia, F. L. Disorders of neuromuscular transmission caused by drugs. *N. Engl. J. Med.*, **1979**, *301*, 409–413.

Azar, I. (ed.). *Muscle Relaxants: Side Effects and a Rational Approach to Selection*, Vol. 7. *Clinical Pharmacology Series*. Marcel Dekker, Inc., New York, **1987.**

Bovet, D. Synthetic inhibitors of neuromuscular transmission, chemical structures and structure activity relationships. In, *Neuromuscular Blocking and Stimulating Agents*, Vol. 1. *International Encyclopedia of Pharmacology and Therapeutics*, Sect. 14. (Cheymol, J., ed.) Pergamon Press, Ltd., Oxford, **1972**, pp. 243–294.

Bowman, W. C. Non-relaxant properties of neuromuscular blocking drugs. *Br. J. Anaesth.*, **1982**, *54*, 147–159.

Bowman, W. C.; Marshall, I. G.; Gibb, A. J.; and Harborne, A. J. Feedback control of neurotransmitter release at the neuromuscular junction. *Trends Pharmacol. Sci.*, **1988**, *9*, 14–20.

Changeux, J.-P.; Devilers-Thierry, A.; and Chemmuivilli, P. Acetylcholine receptor: an allosteric protein. *Science*, **1984**, *25*, 1335–1345.

Colquhoun, D. The link between drug binding and response: theories and observations. In, *The Receptors: A Comprehensive Treatise*. (O'Brien, R. D., ed.) Plenum Press, New York, **1979**, pp. 93–142.

Crankshaw, D. P., and Cohen, E. N. Uptake, distribution and elimination of skeletal muscle relaxants. In, *Muscle Relaxants*. (Katz, R., ed.) Excerpta Medica, Amsterdam, **1975**, pp. 125–141.

Denborough, M. The pathopharmacology of malignant hyperpyrexia. *Pharmacol. Ther.*, **1980**, *9*, 357–365.

Dorkins, H. R. Saxamethonium—the development of a modern drug from 1906 to the present day. *Med. Hist.*, **1982**, *26*, 145–168.

Dripps, R. D. The clinician looks at neuromuscular blocking drugs. In, *Neuromuscular Junction*. (Zaimis, E., ed.) Springer-Verlag, Berlin, **1976**, pp. 583–592.

Durant, N. N., and Katz, R. L. Saxamethonium. *Br. J. Anaesth.*, **1982**, *54*, 195–208.

Elmqvist, D., and Thesleff, S. Ideas regarding receptor desensitization at the motor end plate. *Rev. Can. Biol.*, **1962**, *21*, 220–234.

Eränkö, O.; Sonila, S.; and Päivärinta, H. *Histochemistry and Cell Biology of Autonomic Neurons, SIF Cells and Paraneurons*. Academic Press, Inc., New York, **1980.**

Gill, R. C. *White Waters and Black Magic*. Henry Holt & Co., New York, **1940.**

Jan, Y. N.; Bowers, C. W.; Branton, D.; Evans, L.; and Jan, L. Y. Peptides in neuronal function: studies using frog autonomic ganglia. *Cold Spring Harbor Symp. Quant. Biol.*, **1983**, *43*, 363–374.

Kharkevich, D. A. (ed.). *Neuromuscular Blocking Agents*, Vol. 79. *Handbook of Experimental Pharmacology*. Springer-Verlag, Berlin, **1986.**

Leigh, J. M. The history of controlled hypotension. *Br. J. Anaesth.*, **1975**, *47*, 745–749.

Libet, B. Generation of slow inhibitory and excitatory postsynaptic potentials. *Fed. Proc.*, **1970**, *29*, 1945–1956.

McIntyre, A. R. History of curare. In, *Neuromuscular Blocking and Stimulating Agents*, Vol. 1. *International Encyclopedia of Pharmacology and Therapeutics*, Sect. 14. (Cheymol, J., ed.) Pergamon Press, Ltd., Oxford, **1972**, pp. 187–203.

Miller, R. D., and Savarese, J. J. Pharmacology of muscle relaxants and their antagonists. In, *Anesthesia*, Vol. 2. (Miller, R. D., ed.) Churchill Livingstone, Inc., New York, **1986**, pp. 889–994.

Morowitz, H. J. Myasthenia gravis and arrows of fortune. *Hosp. Pract.* [*Off.*], **1986**, *21*, No. 3, 179–194.

Numa, S.; Noda, M.; Takahashi, H.; Tanabe, T.; Toyosato, M.; Furutani, Y.; and Kikyotani, S. Molecular structure of the nicotinic acetylcholine receptor. *Cold Spring Harbor Symp. Quant. Biol.*, **1983**, *48*, 57–70.

Paton, W. D. M., and Zaimis, E. J. The methonium compounds. *Pharmacol. Rev.*, **1952**, *4*, 219–253.

Riker, W. F. Prejunctional effects of neuromuscular blocking and facilitatory drugs. In, *Muscle Relaxants*. (Katz, R., ed.) Excerpta Medica, Amsterdam, **1975**, pp. 59–102.

Rosenberg, H., and Fletcher, J. E. Malignant hyperthermia. In, *Muscle Relaxants: Side Effects and a Rational Approach to Selection*, Vol. 7. (Azar, I., ed.) *Clinical Pharmacology Series*. Marcel Dekker, Inc., New York, **1987**, pp. 115–148.

Russell, M. A. H., and Feyerabend, C. Cigarette smoking: a dependence on high nicotine level boli. *Drug Metab. Rev.*, **1978**, *8*, 29–57.

Salem, M. R. Therapeutic uses of ganglionic blocking drugs. *Int. Anesthesiol. Clin.*, **1978**, *16*, 171–200.

Sejnowski, T. J. Peptidergic synaptic transmission in sympathetic ganglia. *Fed. Proc.*, **1982**, *41*, 2923–2928.

Shanks, C. A. What's new in skeletal muscle relaxants and their antagonists. In, *Anesthesiology Clinics of North America*, Vol. 6. (Fragen, R. J., ed.) W. B. Saunders Co., Philadelphia, **1988**, pp. 335–355.

Smith, S. C. Neuromuscular blocking drugs in man. In, *Neuromuscular Junction*. (Zaimis, E., ed.) Springer-Verlag, Berlin, **1976**, pp. 593–660.

Sokoll, M. D., and Gergis, S. D. Antibiotics and neuromuscular function. *Anesthesiology*, **1981**, *55*, 148–159.

Taylor, P.; Brown, R. D.; and Johnson, D. A. The linkage between ligand occupation and response of the nicotinic acetylcholine receptor. In, *Current Topics in Membranes and Transport*, Vol. 18. (Kleinzeller, A., and Martin, B. R., eds.) Academic Press, Inc., New York, **1983**, pp. 407–444.

Volle, R. L. Nicotinic ganglion-stimulating agents. In, *Pharmacology of Ganglionic Transmission*. (Kharkevich, D. A., ed.) Springer-Verlag, Berlin, **1980**, pp. 281–312.

Weight, F. F.; Schulman, J. A.; Smith, P. A.; and Busis, N. A. Long-lasting synaptic potentials and the modulation of synaptic transmission. *Fed. Proc.*, **1979**, *38*, 2084–2094.

Whittaker, S. M. Cholinesterase. In, *Monographs in Human Genetics*, Vol. 11. (Beckman, L., ed.) S. Karger, Basel, **1986**, p. 231.

Zaimis, E. The neuromuscular junction: area of uncertainty. In, *Neuromuscular Junction*. (Zaimis, E., ed.) Springer-Verlag, Berlin, **1976**, pp. 1–18.

Zaimis, E., and Head, S. Depolarizing neuromuscular blocking drugs. In, *Neuromuscular Junction*. (Zaimis, E., ed.) Springer-Verlag, Berlin, **1976**, pp. 365–420.

CHAPTER

10 CATECHOLAMINES AND SYMPATHOMIMETIC DRUGS

Brian B. Hoffman and Robert J. Lefkowitz

The sympathetic nervous system is vitally involved in the homeostatic regulation of a wide variety of functions, among which are heart rate, force of cardiac contraction, vasomotor tone, blood pressure, bronchial airway tone, and carbohydrate and fatty acid metabolism. Stimulation of the sympathetic nervous system normally occurs in response to physical activity, psychological stress, generalized allergic reactions, and other situations in which the organism is provoked. Because the functions that are mediated or modified by the sympathetic nervous system are diverse, agents that mimic or alter its activity are useful in the treatment of several clinical disorders, including hypertension, shock, cardiac failure and arrhythmias, asthma, allergy, and anaphylaxis.

The host of physiological and metabolic responses that follows stimulation of sympathetic nerves in mammals is usually mediated by the neurotransmitter norepinephrine. As part of the response to stress, the adrenal medulla is also stimulated, resulting in elevation of the concentrations of epinephrine and norepinephrine in the circulation. The actions of these two catecholamines are very similar at some sites but differ significantly at others. For example, both compounds stimulate the myocardium; however, epinephrine dilates blood vessels to skeletal muscle, whereas norepinephrine has a minimal constricting effect on them. Dopamine is a third, naturally occurring catecholamine. Although it is found predominantly in the basal ganglia of the central nervous system (CNS), dopaminergic nerve endings and specific receptors for this catecholamine have been identified elsewhere in the CNS and in the periphery. The role of the catecholamines in the CNS is detailed in Chapter 12 and elsewhere. As might be expected, sympathomimetic amines—naturally occurring catecholamines and drugs that mimic their actions—comprise one of the more extensively studied groups of pharmacological agents.

Most of the actions of such compounds can be classified into seven broad types: (1) a *peripheral excitatory action* on certain types of smooth muscle, such as those in blood vessels supplying skin and mucous membranes, and on gland cells, such as those in salivary and sweat glands; (2) a *peripheral inhibitory action* on certain other types of smooth muscle, such as those in the wall of the gut, in the bronchial tree, and in blood vessels supplying skeletal muscle; (3) a *cardiac excitatory action*, responsible for an increase in heart rate and force of contraction; (4) *metabolic actions*, such as an increase in rate of glycogenolysis in liver and muscle, and liberation of free fatty acids from adipose tissue; (5) *endocrine actions*, such as modulation of the secretion of insulin, renin, and pituitary hormones; (6) *CNS actions*, such as respiratory stimulation and, with some of the drugs, an increase in wakefulness, psychomotor activity, and a reduction in appetite; and (7) *presynaptic actions*, which result in either inhibition or facilitation of the release of neurotransmitters such as norepinephrine and acetylcholine. Physiologically, the inhibitory action is more important than the excitatory action. Many of these actions and the receptors that mediate them are summarized in Tables 5–1 (page 90) and 5–3 (page 108). All sympathomimetic drugs do not show each of the above types of action to the same degree. However, many of the differences in their effects are only quantitative, and description of the effects of each compound would be unnecessarily repetitive. Therefore, the pharmacological properties of these drugs as a class are described in detail for the prototypical agent, epinephrine.

Appreciation of the pharmacological properties of the drugs that are described in this chapter is critically dependent on understanding the classification, distribution, and mechanism of action of the various subtypes of adrenergic receptors (α_1, α_2, β_1, β_2). This information is presented in Chapter 5.

History. The pressor effect of suprarenal extracts was first shown by Oliver and Schäfer in 1895. The active principle was named *epinephrine* by Abel in 1899 and synthesized independently by Stolz and Dakin (*see* Hartung, 1931). The development of our knowledge of epinephrine and norepinephrine as neurohumoral transmitters is outlined in Chapter 5. Barger and Dale (1910) studied the pharmacological activity of a large series of synthetic amines related to epinephrine and termed their action *sympathomimetic*. This important study determined the basic structural requirements for activity. When it was later found that cocaine or chronic denervation of effector organs reduced the responses to ephedrine and tyramine but enhanced the effects of epinephrine, it became clear that the differences between sympathomimetic amines were not simply quantitative. It was suggested that epinephrine acted directly on the effector cell while ephedrine and tyramine had an indirect effect by acting on the nerve endings. The discovery that reserpine depletes tissues of norepinephrine (Bertler *et al.*, 1956) was followed by evidence that tyramine and certain other sympathomimetic amines do not act on tissues from animals that have been treated with reserpine; this too indicated that they act by releasing endogenous norepinephrine (Burn and Rand, 1958).

Chemistry and Structure–Activity Relationship of Sympathomimetic Amines. β-Phenylethylamine (Table 10–1) can be viewed as the parent compound of the sympathomimetic amines, consisting of a benzene ring and an ethylamine side chain. The structure permits substitutions to be made on the aromatic ring, the α- and β-carbon atoms, and the terminal amino group, to yield a great variety of compounds with sympathomimetic activity. Norepinephrine, epinephrine, dopamine, isoproterenol, and a few other agents have OH groups substituted in the 3 and 4 positions of the benzene ring. Since *o*-dihydroxybenzene is also known as *catechol,* sympathomimetic amines with these OH substitutions in the aromatic ring are termed *catecholamines*.

Many directly acting sympathomimetic drugs influence both α and β receptors, but the ratio of the α and β activity varies tremendously between drugs, in a continuous spectrum from an almost pure α activity (phenylephrine) to an almost pure β activity (isoproterenol). Despite the multiplicity of the sites of action of sympathomimetic amines, several generalizations can be made, as presented below.

Separation of Aromatic Ring and Amino Group. By far the greatest sympathomimetic activity occurs when two carbon atoms separate the ring from the amino group. This rule applies with few exceptions to all types of action.

Substitution on the Amino Group. The effects of amino substitution are most readily seen in the actions of catecholamines on α and β receptors. Increase in the size of the alkyl substituent increases β-receptor activity (*e.g.*, isoproterenol). Norepinephrine has, in general, rather feeble β_2 activity; this is greatly increased in epinephrine with the addition of a methyl group. A notable exception is phenylephrine, which has an N-methyl substituent but is almost a pure α agonist. Selective β_2-receptor stimulants require a large amino substituent, but depend on other substitutions for their selectivity for β_2 rather than for β_1 receptors. In general, the less the substitution on the amino group the greater is the selectivity for α activity, although N-methylation increases the potency of primary amines. Thus, α activity is maximal in epinephrine, less in norepinephrine, and almost absent in isoproterenol.

Substitution on the Aromatic Nucleus. Maximal α and β activity depends on the presence of OH groups in the 3 and 4 positions. When one or both of these groups are absent, without other aromatic substitution, the overall potency is reduced. Phenylephrine is thus less potent than epinephrine on both α and β receptors, with β activity almost completely absent. Recent studies of the β-adrenergic receptor reveal that the hydroxy groups on serine residues 204 and 207 likely form hydrogen bonds with the catechol hydroxy groups at positions 3 and 4, respectively (Strader *et al.*, 1989). It also appears that aspartate 113 is a point of electrostatic interaction with the amine group on the ligand. Since the serines are in the fifth membrane spanning region and the aspartate is in the third (*see* Chapter 5), it is likely that the catecholamines bind parallel to the plane of the membrane, forming a bridge between the two membrane spans.

Hydroxy groups in the 3 and 5 positions confer β_2-receptor selectivity on compounds with large amino substituents. Thus, metaproterenol, terbutaline, and other similar compounds relax the bronchial musculature in patients with asthma but cause less direct cardiac stimulation than do the nonselective drugs. The response to noncatecholamines is in part determined by their capacity to release norepinephrine from sites of storage. These agents thus cause effects that are mostly mediated by α and β_1 receptors, since norepinephrine is a weak β_2 agonist. Phenylethylamines that lack both hydroxy groups on the ring and the β-hydroxy group on the side chain act almost exclusively by causing the release of norepinephrine from adrenergic nerve terminals.

Since substitution of polar groups on the phenylethylamine structure makes the resultant compounds less lipophilic, unsubstituted or alkyl-substituted compounds cross the blood–brain barrier more readily and have more central activity. Thus, ephedrine, amphetamine, and methamphetamine exhibit considerable CNS activity. In addition, as mentioned, the absence of polar hydroxy groups results in a loss of direct peripheral sympathomimetic activity.

Table 10–1. CHEMICAL STRUCTURES AND MAIN CLINICAL USES OF IMPORTANT SYMPATHOMIMETIC DRUGS †

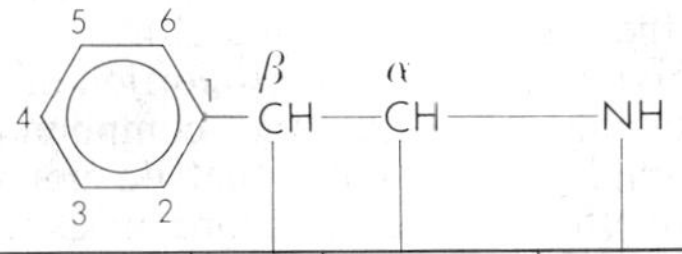

	Ring	β	α	NH	MAIN CLINICAL USES: *α Receptor* A N P V	*β Receptor* B C U	*CNS, 0*
Phenylethylamine		H	H	H			
Epinephrine	3-OH,4-OH	OH	H	CH_3	A, P,V	B,C	
Norepinephrine	3-OH,4-OH	OH	H	H	P		
Dopamine	3-OH,4-OH	H	H	H	P		
Dobutamine	3-OH,4-OH	H	H	1 *		C	
Colterol	3-OH,4-OH	OH	H	$C(CH_3)_3$		B	
Ethylnorepinephrine	3-OH,4-OH	OH	CH_2CH_3	H		B	
Isoproterenol	3-OH,4-OH	OH	H	$CH(CH_3)_2$		B,C	
Isoetharine	3-OH,4-OH	OH	CH_2CH_3	$CH(CH_3)_2$		B	
Metaproterenol	3-OH,5-OH	OH	H	$CH(CH_3)_2$		B	
Terbutaline	3-OH,5-OH	OH	H	$C(CH_3)_3$		B, U	
Metaraminol	3-OH	OH	CH_3	H	P		
Phenylephrine	3-OH	OH	H	CH_3	N,P		
Tyramine	4-OH	H	H	H			
Hydroxyamphetamine	4-OH	H	CH_3	H			
Ritodrine	4-OH	OH	CH_3	2 *		U	
Prenalterol	4-OH	OH ‡	H	$-CH(CH_3)_2$		C	
Methoxamine	$2-OCH_3,5-OCH_3$	OH	CH_3	H	P		
Albuterol	$3-CH_2OH,4-OH$	OH	H	$C(CH_3)_3$		B, U	
Amphetamine		H	CH_3	H			CNS, 0
Methamphetamine		H	CH_3	CH_3			CNS, 0
Benzphetamine		H	CH_3	3 *			0
Ephedrine		OH	CH_3	CH_3	N,P	B,C	
Phenylpropanolamine		OH	CH_3	H	N		0
Mephentermine		H	4 *	CH_3	N,P		
Phentermine		H	4 *	H			0
Fenfluramine	$3-CF_3$	H	CH_3	C_2H_5			0
Propylhexedrine	5 *	H	CH_3	CH_3	N		
Diethylpropion			6 *				0
Phenmetrazine			7 *				0
Phendimetrazine			8 *				0

1

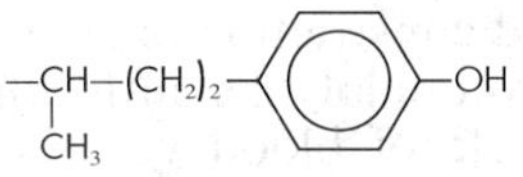

2

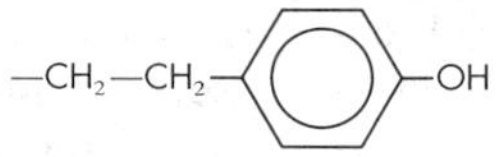

3

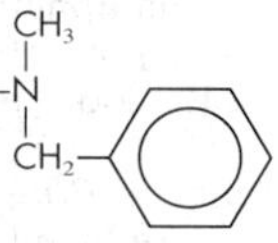

4

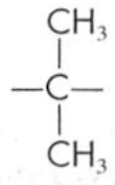

5

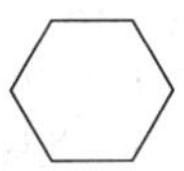

6

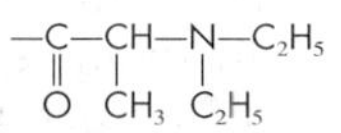

7

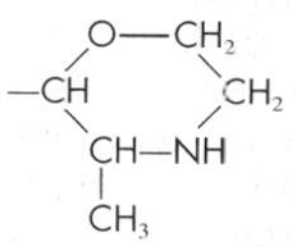

8

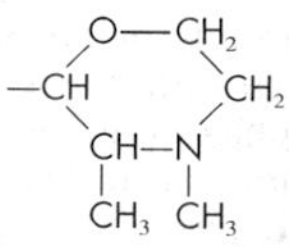

α Activity
A = Allergic reactions (includes β action)
N = Nasal decongestion
P = Pressor (may include β action)
V = Other local vasoconstriction (*e.g.*, in local anesthesia)

β Activity
B = Bronchodilator
C = Cardiac
U = Uterus

CNS = Central nervous system
0 = Anorectic

* Numbers bearing an asterisk refer to the substituents numbered in the bottom rows of the table; substituent 3 replaces the N atom, substituent 5 replaces the phenyl ring, and 6, 7, and 8 are attached directly to the phenyl ring, replacing the ethylamine side chain.

† The α and β in the prototypical formula refer to positions of the C atoms in the ethylamine side chain.

‡ Prenalterol has $—OCH_2—$ between the aromatic ring and the carbon atom designated as β in the prototypical formula.

Catecholamines have only a brief duration of action and are ineffective after oral administration because they are rapidly inactivated in the intestinal mucosa and in the liver before reaching the systemic circulation (*see* Chapter 5). Compounds without one or both OH substituents, particularly the 3-OH group, are not acted upon by catechol-O-methyltransferase (COMT), and their oral effectiveness and duration of action are enhanced.

Groups other than OH have been substituted on the aromatic ring. In general, potency on α receptors is reduced and β-receptor activity is minimal; the compounds may even block β receptors. For example, methoxamine, with methoxy substituents on positions 2 and 5, has highly selective α-stimulating activity and in large doses blocks β receptors. Albuterol, a selective β_2-receptor stimulant, has a CH_2OH substituent on position 3 and is an important exception to the general rule of low β activity.

Substitution on the α-Carbon Atom. This substitution blocks oxidation by monoamine oxidase (MAO), thus greatly prolonging the duration of action of noncatecholamines because their degradation depends largely on the action of MAO. The duration of action of drugs such as ephedrine or amphetamine is thus measured in hours rather than in minutes. Similarly, compounds with an α-methyl substituent persist in the nerve terminal and are more likely to release norepinephrine from sites of storage. Agents such as metaraminol thus exhibit a greater degree of indirect sympathomimetic activity.

Substitution on the β-Carbon Atom. Substitution of an OH group on the β carbon generally decreases actions within the CNS, largely because of the lower lipid solubility of such compounds. However, such substitution greatly enhances agonistic activity at both α and β receptors. Thus, ephedrine is less potent than methamphetamine as a central stimulant, but it is more powerful in dilating bronchioles and increasing blood pressure and heart rate.

Absence of the Benzene Ring. The capacity to stimulate the CNS is reduced without a corresponding decrease in α and β activity when the benzene ring is replaced by a saturated ring (*e.g.*, cyclopentamine, propylhexedrine), or by a different unsaturated ring (*e.g.*, naphazoline; Table 10–2). Naphazoline, in fact, is a powerful α-receptor stimulant, but it differs from most other sympathomimetic amines in that it depresses rather than stimulates the CNS, presumably because it, like clonidine and oxymetazoline, exhibits preferential effects on α_2 receptors (*see* below; *see also* Chapters 5 and 33).

The proportion of α to β receptor activity varies with the compound; however, in general the amines that do not possess a benzene ring have rather more marked α than β activity. Consequently, many of them are used primarily as nasal decongestants because of their vasoconstrictor properties.

Optical Isomerism. Substitution on either α or β carbon yields optical isomers. Levorotatory substitution on the β carbon confers the greater peripheral activity, so that the naturally occurring *l*-epinephrine and *l*-norepinephrine are at least ten times as potent as their unnatural *d* isomers. Dextrorotatory substitution on the α carbon generally provides a more potent compound than the *l* isomer in central stimulant activity. *d*-Amphetamine is more potent than *l*-amphetamine in central but not peripheral activity.

Physiological Basis of Adrenergic Receptor Function. An important factor in the response of any cell or organ to sympathomimetic amines is its density and proportion of α- and β-adrenergic receptors. For example, norepinephrine has relatively little capacity to increase bronchial air flow since the receptors in bronchial smooth muscle are largely of the β_2 type. In contrast, isoproterenol and epinephrine are potent bronchodilators. Cutaneous blood vessels possess α receptors almost exclusively; thus, norepinephrine and epinephrine cause marked constriction of such vessels, while isoproterenol has little effect. The smooth muscle of blood vessels that supply skeletal muscles has both β_2 and α receptors; activation of β_2 receptors causes vasodilatation, and stimulation of α receptors constricts these vessels. In such vessels the threshold concentration for activation of β_2 receptors by epinephrine is lower than that for α receptors, but when both

Table 10–2. CHEMICAL STRUCTURES OF IMIDAZOLINE DERIVATIVES

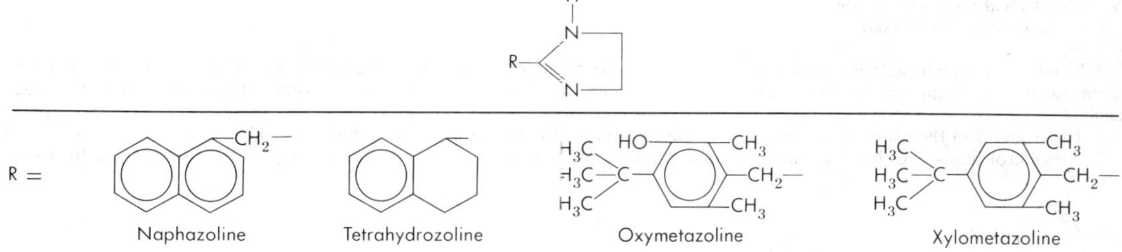

types of receptors are activated at high concentrations of epinephrine, the response to α receptors predominates.

The ultimate response of a target organ to sympathomimetic amines is dictated not only by the direct effects of the agents but also by the reflex homeostatic adjustments of the organism. One of the most striking effects of many sympathomimetic amines is a rise in arterial blood pressure caused by stimulation of vascular α receptors. This stimulation elicits compensatory reflexes that are mediated by the caroticoaortic baroreceptor system. As a result, sympathetic tone is diminished and vagal tone is enhanced; both responses result in bradycardia. This reflex effect is of special importance for drugs that have little capacity to activate β-adrenergic receptors directly.

Indirectly Acting Sympathomimetic Drugs. For many years it was presumed that all sympathomimetic amines produced their effects by acting directly on adrenergic receptors. However, this notion was dispelled by the finding that the effects of tyramine and many other noncatecholamines were reduced or abolished following chronic postganglionic adrenergic denervation or treatment with cocaine or reserpine. Under these circumstances, the effects of epinephrine and especially norepinephrine were often enhanced. These observations led to the proposal that tyramine and related amines acted indirectly, following uptake into the adrenergic nerve terminal, by stoichiometric displacement of norepinephrine from storage sites in the synaptic vesicles or from extravesicular binding sites (Burn and Rand, 1958). Norepinephrine could then exit from the adrenergic nerve terminal and interact with receptors to produce the sympathomimetic effects. The depletion of tissue stores of catecholamines that follows treatment with reserpine or degeneration of adrenergic nerve terminals would explain the lack of effect of tyramine under these conditions. In the presence of cocaine, the high-affinity neuronal transport system for catecholamines and certain congeners is inhibited, and tyramine and related amines are unable to enter the adrenergic nerve terminal. In this manner cocaine inhibits the actions of indirectly acting sympathomimetic amines, while potentiating the effects of directly acting agents that are normally removed from the synaptic cleft by this transport system (*see* Chapter 5).

In assessing the proportion of direct and indirect actions of a sympathomimetic amine, the most common experimental procedure is to compare the dose–response curve for the agent on a particular target tissue before and after treatment with reserpine (Trendelenburg, 1972). Those drugs whose actions are essentially unaltered after treatment with reserpine are classified as directly acting sympathomimetic amines (*e.g.*, norepinephrine, phenylephrine), while those whose actions are abolished are termed indirectly acting (*e.g.*, tyramine). Most agents exhibit some degree of residual sympathomimetic activity after the administration of reserpine, but higher doses of these amines are required to produce comparable effects. These are classified as mixed-acting sympathomimetic amines; that is, they have both direct and indirect actions. The proportion of direct and indirect actions can vary considerably between different tissues and species.

Since the actions of norepinephrine are more marked on α and β_1 receptors than on β_2 receptors, many noncatecholamines that release norepinephrine have predominantly α-receptor–mediated and cardiac effects. However, certain noncatecholamines with both direct and indirect effects on adrenergic receptors show significant β_2-agonistic activity and are used clinically for the effects that result. Thus, ephedrine, although dependent upon release of norepinephrine for some of its effects, relieves bronchospasm by its action on β_2 receptors in bronchial muscle, an effect virtually absent with norepinephrine. It must also be recalled that some noncatecholamines—phenylephrine, for example—act primarily and directly on effector cells. It is therefore impossible to predict precisely the characteristic effects of noncatecholamines simply on the basis that they all provoke the release of at least some norepinephrine.

False-Transmitter Concept. As indicated above, indirectly acting amines are taken up into adrenergic nerve terminals and storage vesicles, where they presumably replace norepinephrine in the storage complex. Phenylethylamines that lack a β-hydroxyl group are retained there poorly, but β-

hydroxylated phenylethylamines and compounds that subsequently become hydroxylated in the synaptic vesicle by dopamine β-hydroxylase are retained in the synaptic vesicle for relatively long periods of time (Musacchio *et al.*, 1965; Kopin, 1968). Such substances can produce a persistent diminution in the content of norepinephrine at functionally critical sites in the adrenergic nerve terminal. When the nerve is stimulated, the content of a relatively constant number of synaptic vesicles is presumably released by exocytosis. If these vesicles contain a considerable proportion of phenylethylamines that are much less potent than norepinephrine, activation of postsynaptic adrenergic receptors will be diminished.

This hypothesis, known as the *false-transmitter concept,* is a possible explanation for the hypotensive effect that results from the administration of inhibitors of MAO. Phenylethylamines are normally synthesized in the gastrointestinal tract as a result of the action of bacterial tyrosine decarboxylase. The tyramine that is formed in this fashion is usually oxidatively deaminated in the gastrointestinal tract and the liver, and the amine does not reach the systemic circulation in significant concentrations. However, when an MAO inhibitor is administered, tyramine may be absorbed systemically. It is transported into the adrenergic nerve terminal, where its catabolism is again prevented because of the inhibition of MAO at this site; it is then β-hydroxylated to octopamine and stored in the vesicles in this form. As a consequence, norepinephrine is gradually displaced, and stimulation of the nerve terminal results in the release of a relatively small amount of norepinephrine along with a fraction of octopamine. The latter amine has relatively little ability to activate either α- or β-adrenergic receptors. Thus, a functional impairment of sympathetic nerve transmission occurs with long-term administration of MAO inhibitors.

Despite such functional impairment, patients who have received MAO inhibitors may experience severe hypertensive crises if they ingest cheese, beer, or red wine. These and related foods, which are produced by a fermentation process, contain a large quantity of tyramine and, to a lesser degree, other phenylethylamines. When gastrointestinal and hepatic MAO is inhibited, the large quantity of tyramine that is ingested is absorbed rapidly and reaches the systemic circulation in high concentration. A massive and precipitous release of norepinephrine can result, with consequent hypertension that can be sufficiently severe to cause myocardial infarction or a cerebrovascular accident (*see* Chapter 18).

I. Endogenous Catecholamines

EPINEPHRINE

Epinephrine is a potent stimulator of both α- and β-adrenergic receptors, and its effects on target organs are thus complex. Most of the responses listed in Table 5–1 (page 90) are seen after injection of epinephrine, although the occurrence of sweating, piloerection, and mydriasis depends on the physiological state of the subject. Particularly prominent are the actions on the heart and the vascular and other smooth muscle.

Blood Pressure. Epinephrine is one of the most potent vasopressor drugs known. Given rapidly intravenously it evokes a characteristic effect on blood pressure, which rises rapidly to a peak that is proportional to the dose. The increase in systolic pressure is greater than the increase in diastolic pressure, so that the pulse pressure increases. As the response wanes, the mean pressure falls below normal before returning to the control level. Repeated doses of epinephrine continue to have the same pressor effect, in sharp contrast to amines that owe a major part of their effect to release of norepinephrine.

The mechanism of the rise in blood pressure due to epinephrine is threefold: a direct myocardial stimulation that increases the strength of ventricular contraction (positive inotropic action); an increased heart rate (positive chronotropic action); and, most important, vasoconstriction in many vascular beds, especially in the precapillary resistance vessels of skin, mucosa, and kidney, along with marked constriction of the veins. The pulse rate, at first accelerated, may be slowed markedly at the height of the rise of blood pressure by compensatory vagal discharge. Minute doses of epinephrine (0.1 μg/kg) may cause the blood pressure to fall. The depressor effect of small doses and the biphasic response to larger doses are due to greater sensitivity to epinephrine of vasodilator β_2 receptors than of constrictor α receptors.

The effects are somewhat different when the drug is given by slow intravenous infusion or by subcutaneous injection. Absorption of epinephrine after subcutaneous injection is slow owing to the drug's local vasoconstrictor action; the effects of doses as large as 0.5 to 1.5 mg can be duplicated by intravenous infusion at a rate of 10 to 30 μg per minute. There is a moderate increase in systolic pressure owing to increased cardiac contractile force and a rise in cardiac output (Figure 10–1). Peripheral resistance decreases, owing to the dominant action on β_2 receptors of vessels in skeletal muscle, where blood flow is enhanced; as a consequence, diastolic pressure usually falls. Since the mean blood pressure is not, as a rule, greatly elevated, compensatory baroreceptor reflexes do not appreciably antagonize the direct cardiac actions. Heart rate, cardiac output, stroke volume, and left ventricular work per beat are increased as a result of direct cardiac stimulation and increased venous return to the heart, which is reflected by an increase in right atrial pressure. At slightly higher rates of infusion, there may be no change or a slight rise in peripheral resistance and diastolic pressure, depending on the dose and the resultant ratio of α to β responses in the various vascular beds; compensatory reflexes may also come into play. The details of the effects of intravenous infusion of epinephrine, norepinephrine, and isoproterenol in man are compared in Table 10–3 and Figure 10–1.

Vascular Effects. The chief vascular action of epinephrine is exerted on the smaller arterioles and precapillary sphincters, although veins and large arteries also respond to the drug. Various vascular beds react differently, which results in a substantial redistribution of blood flow.

Injected epinephrine markedly reduces cutaneous blood flow, constricting precapillary vessels and subpapillary venules. Cutaneous vasoconstriction accounts for a marked decrease in blood flow in the hands and feet. The "aftercongestion" of mucosae following the vasoconstriction from locally applied epinephrine is probably due to changes in vascular reactivity as a result of

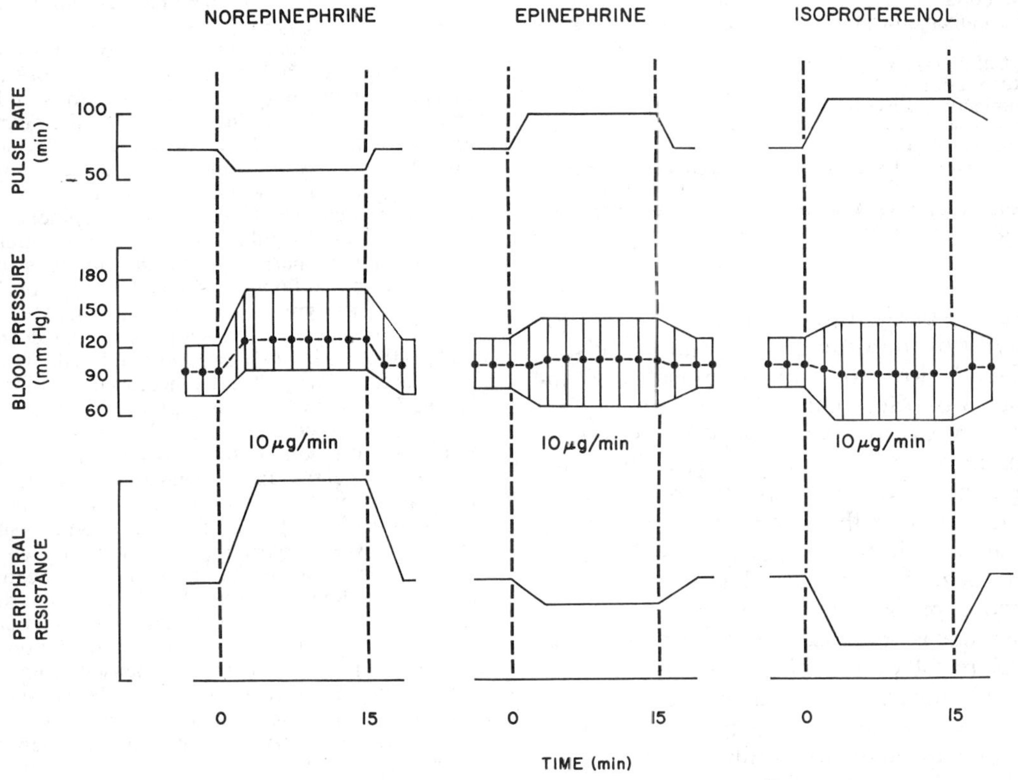

Figure 10–1. *The effects of intravenous infusion of norepinephrine, epinephrine, and isoproterenol in man.* (After Allwood, Cobbold, and Ginsburg, 1963. Courtesy of the *British Medical Bulletin.*)

Table 10–3. COMPARISON OF THE EFFECTS OF INTRAVENOUS INFUSION OF EPINEPHRINE AND NOREPINEPHRINE IN MAN *

	EPINEPHRINE	NOREPINEPHRINE
Cardiac		
Heart rate	+	− †
Stroke volume	++	++
Cardiac output	+++	0,−
Arrhythmias	++++	++++
Coronary blood flow	++	++
Blood Pressure		
Systolic arterial	+++	+++
Mean arterial	+	++
Diastolic arterial	+,0,−	++
Mean pulmonary	++	++
Peripheral Circulation		
Total peripheral resistance	−	++
Cerebral blood flow	+	0,−
Muscle blood flow	+++	0,−
Cutaneous blood flow	−−	−−
Renal blood flow	−	−
Splanchnic blood flow	+++	0,+
Metabolic Effects		
Oxygen consumption	++	0,+
Blood glucose	+++	0,+
Blood lactic acid	+++	0,+
Eosinopenic response	+	0
Central Nervous System		
Respiration	+	+
Subjective sensations	+	+

* 0.1 to 0.4 μg/kg/min

+ = increase; 0 = no change; − = decrease; † = after atropine, +

(After Goldenberg, Aranow, Smith, and Faber, 1950. Courtesy of *Archives of Internal Medicine*.)

tissue hypoxia rather than to β-receptor activity of the drug on mucosal vessels.

Blood flow to skeletal muscles is increased by therapeutic doses in man. This is due in part to a powerful β_2-receptor vasodilator action that is only partially counterbalanced by a vasoconstrictor action on the α receptors that are also present in the vascular bed. If an α-adrenergic blocking agent is given, the vasodilatation in muscle is more pronounced, the total peripheral resistance is decreased, and the mean blood pressure falls (epinephrine reversal). After the administration of a nonselective β-adrenergic antagonist, only vasoconstriction occurs, and the administration of epinephrine is associated with a considerable pressor effect. This marked rise in blood pressure is not elicited by epinephrine in the presence of a selective β_1 antagonist (Houben *et al.*, 1982).

The effect of epinephrine on cerebral circulation is related to systemic blood pressure. In usual therapeutic doses the drug has no significant constrictor action on cerebral arterioles; cerebral blood flow increases, and cerebrovascular resistance does not change. However, autoregulatory mechanisms tend to limit the increase in cerebral blood flow caused by increased blood pressure.

Intravenous infusion of 0.1 μg/kg per minute in man markedly increases hepatic blood flow and decreases splanchnic vascular resistance, concomitantly with a large increase in hepatic glucose output and in the consumption of oxygen as measured in the splanchnic vascular bed.

Doses of epinephrine that have little effect on mean arterial pressure consistently increase renal vascular resistance and reduce renal blood flow by as much as 40%. All segments of the renal vascular bed contribute to the increased resistance. Since the glomerular filtration rate is only slightly and variably altered, the filtration fraction is consistently increased. Excretion of Na^+, K^+, and Cl^- is decreased; urine volume may be increased, decreased, or unchanged. Maximal tubular reabsorptive and excretory capacities are unchanged. The secretion of renin is increased as a consequence of a direct action of epinephrine on β_1 receptors in the juxtaglomerular apparatus.

Arterial and venous pulmonary pressures are raised. Although direct pulmonary vasoconstriction can be shown under suitable conditions, redistribution of blood from the systemic to the pulmonary circulation, due to constriction of the more powerful musculature in the systemic great veins, doubtless plays an important part in the increase in pulmonary pressure. Overdosage of epinephrine may cause death by pulmonary edema precipitated by elevated pulmonary capillary filtration pressure.

Coronary blood flow is enhanced by epinephrine or by cardiac sympathetic stimulation. The increased flow occurs even with doses that do not increase the aortic blood pressure and is the result of two factors. The first is the increased duration of diastole (*see* below); this is partially offset by decreased blood flow during systole owing to more forceful contraction of the surrounding myocardium and an increase in mechanical compression of the coronary vessels. The increased flow during diastole is further enhanced if aortic blood pressure is elevated by epinephrine, and, as a consequence, total coronary flow may be increased. The second factor is a metabolic dilator effect that results from the increased strength of contraction and myocardial oxygen consumption. This vasodilatation is mediated in part by adenosine released from the cardiac myocytes (*see* Berne *et al.*, 1983), and it overrides a direct vasoconstrictor effect of epinephrine that results from activation of α receptors in coronary vessels.

Cardiac Effects. Epinephrine is a powerful cardiac stimulant. It acts directly on the predominant β_1 receptors of the myocardium and of the cells of the pacemaker and conducting tissues; β_2 and α receptors are also present in the heart. The heart rate increases and the rhythm is often altered. Cardiac systole is shorter and more powerful, cardiac output is enhanced, and the work of the heart and its oxygen consumption are markedly increased. Cardiac efficiency (work done relative to oxygen consumption) is lessened. Direct responses to epinephrine include increases in contractile force, accelerated rate of rise of isometric tension, enhanced rate of relaxation, decreased time to peak tension, increased excitability, acceleration of the rate of spontaneous beating, and induction of automaticity in specialized regions of the heart.

In accelerating the heart within the physiological range, epinephrine preferentially shortens systole so that the duration of diastole is usually not reduced. Epinephrine speeds the heart by accelerating the slow depolarization of SA nodal cells that takes place during diastole, that is, during phase 4 of the action potential. Thus, the transmembrane potential of the pacemaker cells falls more rapidly to the threshold level at which the action potential is initiated. The amplitude of the action potential and the maximal rate of depolarization (phase 0) are also increased. A shift in the location of the pacemaker within the SA node often occurs, indicating the activation of latent pacemaker cells. In Purkinje fibers, epinephrine also accelerates diastolic depolarization and may cause activation of latent pacemaker cells. These changes do not occur in atrial and ventricular muscle fibers, where epinephrine has little effect on the stable, phase-4 membrane potential after repolarization. If large doses of epinephrine are given, premature ventricular systoles occur and may herald more serious ventricular arrhythmias. This is rarely seen with conventional doses in man, but ventricular extrasystoles, tachycardia, or even fibrillation may be precipitated by release of endogenous epinephrine when the heart has been sensitized to this action of epinephrine by certain anesthetics or in cases of myocardial infarction. The mechanism of induction of these cardiac arrhythmias is not clear. However, α-adrenergic blocking agents protect against epinephrine-induced cardiac irregularities during anesthesia; protection is due in part to prevention of the rise in blood pressure (which sensitizes the myocardium to epinephrine-induced ectopic rhythms).

Some effects of epinephrine on cardiac tissues are largely secondary to the increase in heart rate, and are small or inconsistent in preparations where the heart rate is kept constant. For example, the effect of epinephrine on repolarization of atrium, Purkinje fibers, or ventricle is small if the heart rate is unchanged. When the heart rate is increased, the duration of the action potential is consistently shortened, and the refractory period is correspondingly decreased.

Conduction through the Purkinje system depends on the level of membrane potential at the time of excitation. Excessive reduction of this potential results in conduction disturbances, ranging from slowed conduction to complete block. Epinephrine often increases the membrane potential and improves conduction in Purkinje fibers that have been excessively depolarized.

Epinephrine normally shortens the refractory period of the human AV node, although doses that slow the heart through reflex vagal discharge may indirectly prolong it. Epinephrine also decreases the grade of AV block that occurs as a result of disease, drugs, or vagal stimulation. Supraventricular arrhythmias are apt to occur from the combination of epinephrine and cholinergic stimulation. Depression of sinus rate and AV conduction by vagal discharge probably plays a part in epinephrine-induced ventricular arrhythmias, since various drugs that block the vagal effect confer some protection. The action of epinephrine in enhancing cardiac automaticity and its action in causing arrhythmias are effectively antagonized by β-blocking agents such as propranolol. However, α_1 receptors exist in most regions of the heart, and their activation prolongs the refractory period and strengthens myocardial contractions (Schumann *et al.*, 1978; Benfey, 1982).

Cardiac arrhythmias have been recorded in man after inadvertent intravenous administration of conventional subcutaneous doses of epinephrine. Systolic and diastolic pressures rise alarmingly, resulting in cerebrovascular hemorrhage. Ventricular premature systoles can appear, which may be followed by multifocal ventricular tachycardia or ventricular fibrillation. Pulmonary edema may also occur.

Epinephrine decreases the amplitude of the T wave of the electrocardiogram (ECG) in normal persons. In animals given relatively larger doses, additional effects are seen on the T wave and S–T segment. After being decreased in amplitude, the T wave may become biphasic and the S–T segment deviates either above or below the isoelectric line. Such S–T segment changes are similar to those seen in patients with angina pectoris during spontaneous or epinephrine-induced attacks of pain. These electrical changes have therefore been attributed to myocardial ischemia.

Effects on Smooth Muscles. The effects of epinephrine on the smooth muscles of different organs and systems depend upon the type of adrenergic receptor in the muscle (Table 5–1, page 90). Gastrointestinal smooth muscle is, in general, relaxed by epinephrine. Intestinal tone and the frequency and amplitude of spontaneous contractions are reduced. The stomach is usually relaxed and the pyloric and ileocecal sphincters are contracted, but these effects depend upon the preexisting tone of the muscle. If tone is already high, epinephrine causes relaxation; if low, contraction.

The responses of uterine muscle to epinephrine vary with species, phase of the sexual cycle, state of gestation, and the dose given. Epinephrine contracts strips of pregnant or nonpregnant human uterus *in vitro* by interaction with α receptors. The effects of epinephrine on the human uterus *in situ,* however, differ. During the last month of pregnancy and at parturition, epinephrine inhibits uterine tone and contractions. More selective β_2-receptor stimulants, such as ritodrine or terbutaline, are used to delay premature labor (*see* Caritis, 1983; *see also* Chapter 39).

Epinephrine relaxes the detrusor muscle of the bladder as a result of activation of β receptors and contracts the trigone and sphincter muscles due to its α-agonistic activity. This can result in hesitancy in urination and may contribute to retention of urine in the bladder.

Respiratory Effects. Epinephrine affects respiration primarily by relaxing bronchial muscle. It has a powerful bronchodilator action, most evident when bronchial muscle is contracted because of disease, as in bronchial asthma, or in response to drugs or various autacoids. In such situations, epinephrine has a striking therapeutic effect as a physiological antagonist to substances that cause bronchoconstriction.

The beneficial effects of epinephrine in asthma may also arise from inhibition of antigen-induced release of inflammatory mediators from mast cells, and to a lesser extent from diminution of bronchial secretions and congestion within the mucosa. Inhibition of mast cell secretion is mediated by β_2-adrenergic receptors, while the effects on the mucosa are mediated by α receptors.

Effects on Central Nervous System. Because of the inability of this rather polar compound to enter the CNS, epinephrine in conventional therapeutic doses is not a powerful CNS stimulant. While the drug may cause restlessness, apprehension, headache, and tremor in many persons, these effects may in part be secondary to the effects of the catecholamine on the cardiovascular system, skeletal muscles, and intermediary metabolism.

Metabolic Effects. Epinephrine has a number of important influences on metabolic processes. Epinephrine elevates the concentrations of glucose and lactate in blood by mechanisms described in Chapter 5. Insulin secretion is inhibited via α_2 receptors and is enhanced by activation of β_2 receptors; the predominant effect seen with epinephrine is inhibition. Glucagon secretion is enhanced by an action on the β receptors of the α cells of pancreatic islets. Epinephrine also decreases the uptake of glucose by peripheral tissues, at least in part because of its effects on the secretion of insulin. Glycosuria rarely occurs. The effect of epinephrine to stimulate glycogenolysis in most tissues and in most species involves β receptors (*see* Chapter 5).

Epinephrine raises the concentration of free fatty acids in blood by stimulating β receptors in adipocytes. The result is activation of triglyceride lipase, which accelerates the breakdown of triglycerides to form free fatty acids and glycerol. The calorigenic action of epinephrine (increase in metabolism) is reflected in man by an increase of 20 to 30% in oxygen consumption after conventional doses. This effect is mainly due to enhanced breakdown of triglycerides in brown adipose tissue, providing an increase in oxidizable substrate. (*See* Himms-Hagen, 1972; Ellis, 1980; *see also* Chapter 5.)

Miscellaneous Effects. Epinephrine reduces circulating plasma volume by loss of protein-free fluid to the extracellular space, thereby increasing erythrocyte and plasma protein concentrations. However, conventional doses of epinephrine in man do not significantly alter plasma volume or packed red-cell volume under normal conditions, although such doses are reported to have variable effects in the presence of shock, hemorrhage, hypotension, and anesthesia. Epinephrine increases total leukocyte count but causes eosinopenia. Epinephrine has long been known to accelerate blood coagulation in animals and man, an effect probably due to increased activity of factor V.

The effects of epinephrine on secretory glands are not marked; in most glands secretion is usually inhibited, partly due to reduced blood flow caused by vasoconstriction. Epinephrine stimulates lacrimation and a scanty mucous secretion from salivary glands. Sweating and pilomotor activity are not seen after systemic administration of epinephrine, but occur after intradermal injection of very dilute solutions of either epinephrine or norepinephrine. Such effects are inhibited by α-blocking agents.

Mydriasis is readily seen during physiological sympathetic stimulation but not when epinephrine is instilled into the conjunctival sac of normal eyes. However, epinephrine usually lowers intraocular pressure from normal levels and in wide-angle glaucoma; the mechanism is not clear, but both reduced production of aqueous humor due to vasoconstriction and enhanced outflow probably occur (*see* Grant, 1969). Paradoxically, timolol and other β-receptor antagonists also reduce intraocular pressure and are useful in the treatment of glaucoma (*see* Chapter 7).

Although epinephrine does not directly excite skeletal muscle, it facilitates neuromuscular transmission, particularly that following prolonged rapid stimulation of the motor nerve. This effect appears to involve both α- and β-adrenergic receptors. Stimulation of the latter may increase cyclic AMP presynaptically, thereby facilitating the release of neurotransmitter (Weiner, 1980). In apparent contrast to the effects of α-receptor activation at presynaptic nerve terminals in the autonomic nervous system, stimulation of α-adrenergic receptors causes a more rapid increase in transmitter release from the somatic motoneuron, perhaps as a result of enhanced influx of Ca^{2+} (Bowman, 1981; Snider and Gerald, 1982). These actions may explain in part the ability of epinephrine (given intraarterially) to cause a brief increase in motor power of the injected limb of patients with myasthenia gravis. Given orally, ephedrine and amphetamine have this same effect; although these two drugs have been used clinically in this condition, the improvement in muscle strength does not approach that seen after neostigmine. Epinephrine also acts directly on white, fast-contracting muscle fibers to prolong the active state, thereby increasing peak tension. Of greater physiological and clinical importance is the capacity of epinephrine and selective β_2-adrenergic agonists to shorten the active state of red, slow-contracting mammalian muscle, apparently by accelerating the sequestration of cytosolic Ca^{2+}; this causes incomplete fusion of contractile events at physiological rates of nerve stimulation and a reduction in developed tension. These effects, together with a β-receptor–mediated enhancement of discharge of muscle spindles, are thought to be important in the production of the tremor that sometimes accompanies the use of adrenergic bronchodilators (*see* Bowman, 1981).

Epinephrine produces a transient rise in the concentration of K^+ in plasma, mainly due to release of the ion from the liver. This hyperkalemia is followed by a more prolonged fall in plasma K^+. During these changes hepatic K^+ rapidly enters the blood and is taken up by muscle. Subsequently, the pool of K^+ in muscle falls during the period of hypokalemia and is transferred to the liver. β_2-Adrenergic agonists, such as albuterol, have been used in the management of hyperkalemic familial periodic paralysis, which is characterized by episodic flaccid paralysis, hyperkalemia, and depolarization of skeletal muscle. Albuterol is apparently able to correct the impairment in the ability of the muscle to accumulate and retain K^+, presumably by stimulating the Na^+,K^+-ATPase (*see* Bowman, 1981).

Large or repeated doses of epinephrine or other sympathomimetic amines given to experimental animals lead to damage to arterial walls and myocardium, so severe as to cause the appearance of necrotic areas, indistinguishable in the heart from myocardial infarcts. The mechanism of this injury is not yet clear, but α and β receptor antagonists and Ca^{2+}-channel blockers may afford substantial protection against the damage. Similar lesions occur in many patients with pheochromocytoma or after prolonged infusions of norepinephrine.

Absorption, Fate, and Excretion. Epinephrine is not effective after oral administration because it is rapidly conjugated and oxidized in the gastrointestinal mucosa and liver. Absorption from subcutaneous tissues occurs slowly because of local vasoconstriction. Absorption is more rapid after intramuscular than after subcutaneous injection. When relatively concentrated solutions (1%) are nebulized and inhaled, the actions of the drug are largely restricted to the respiratory tract; however, systemic reactions such as arrhythmias may occur, particularly if larger amounts are used.

Epinephrine is rapidly inactivated in the body. The liver, which is rich in both of the enzymes responsible for destruction of circulating epinephrine (COMT and MAO), is particularly important in this regard (*see* Figure 5–5, page 107). Although only small amounts appear in the urine of normal persons, the urine of patients with pheochromocytoma contains relatively large amounts of epinephrine, norepinephrine, and their metabolites.

Preparations, Routes of Administration, and Dosage. *Epinephrine* is the *l* isomer of β-(3,4-dihydroxyphenyl)-α-methylaminoethanol (*see* Table 10–1). It is unstable in alkaline solution and on exposure to air or light, turning pink from oxidation to adrenochrome and then brown from formation of polymers. Epinephrine may be given by injection, usually subcutaneously, inhaled as an aerosol, or applied locally to mucous membranes or abraded surfaces as an aqueous solution.

Epinephrine injection is a 1:1000 or a 1:10,000 sterile solution of epinephrine hydrochloride in water. The usual adult dose given subcutaneously ranges from 0.3 to 0.5 mg. The intravenous route is used cautiously if an immediate and reliable effect is mandatory. If the solution is given by vein, it must be adequately diluted and injected *very slowly*. The dose is seldom as much as 0.25 mg, except for cardiac arrest, when 0.5 to 1.0 mg can be given every 5 minutes. Intracardiac injection is occasionally used for attempted resuscitation in emergencies (0.3 to 0.5 mg). An aqueous 1:200 suspension of crystalline epinephrine (SUS-PHRINE) has a prolonged duration of action because of its low solubility. Injected subcutaneously the usual adult dose is 0.1 to 0.3 ml, repeated no sooner than after 6 hours. *Epinephrine suspensions must never be injected intravenously.*

Epinephrine inhalation is a nonsterile 1% aqueous solution of epinephrine hydrochloride for oral (not nasal) inhalation, either from a nebulizer or from an intermittent positive-pressure breathing apparatus. It is used to relieve bronchial constriction. *Every precaution must be taken not to confuse this 1:100 solution with the 1:1000 solution designed for parenteral administration.* Injection of the 1:100 solution has caused death.

Epinephrine bitartrate is available as a 2% ophthalmic solution and as a pressurized aerosol (MEDIHALER-EPI, others) delivering measured doses of 0.3 mg (0.16 mg of epinephrine base) for oral inhalation.

Epinephrine hydrochloride (0.1 to 2%) and *epinephrine borate* (0.5 to 2%) are also available for topical ophthalmic use.

Toxicity, Side Effects, and Contraindications. Epinephrine may cause disturbing reactions, such as fear, anxiety, tenseness, restlessness, throbbing headache, tremor, weakness, dizziness, pallor, respiratory difficulty, and palpitation. The effects rapidly subside with rest, quiet, recumbency, and reassurance. Hyperthyroid and hypertensive individuals are particularly susceptible to the untoward and pressor responses to epinephrine. In psychoneurotic individuals, existing symptoms are often markedly aggravated by the administration of epinephrine.

More serious reactions include cerebral hemorrhage and cardiac arrhythmias. The use of large doses or the accidental rapid intravenous injection of epinephrine may result in cerebral hemorrhage from the sharp rise in blood pressure. Subarachnoid hemorrhage and hemiplegia have occurred even after a subcutaneous dose of 0.5 ml of the 1:1000 solution. Rapidly acting vasodilators such as the nitrites or sodium nitroprusside can counteract the marked pressor effects of large doses of epinephrine; α-adrenergic blocking agents may also be of use.

Ventricular arrhythmias may follow the administration of epinephrine. Fibrillation is particularly likely to occur if the drug is used unwisely during anesthesia, especially with halogenated hydrocarbon anesthetics, or in individuals with organic heart disease. Patients with long-standing bronchial asthma and a significant degree of emphysema, who have reached the age at which degenerative heart disease is prevalent, must be given epinephrine only with considerable caution. In patients suffering from shock, the drug may accentuate the underlying disorder. Anginal pain is readily induced by epinephrine in patients with angina pectoris.

The use of epinephrine is contraindicated in patients who are receiving nonselective β-adrenergic receptor blocking drugs, since its unopposed actions on vascular α_1-adrenergic receptors may lead to severe hypertension and cerebral hemorrhage.

Therapeutic Uses. Epinephrine has a variety of clinical uses. In general, these are based on the actions of the drug on blood vessels, heart, and bronchial muscle. The most common uses of epinephrine are to relieve respiratory distress due to bronchospasm, to provide rapid relief of hypersensitivity reactions to drugs and other allergens, and to prolong the action of local anesthetics. Its cardiac effects may be of use in restoring cardiac rhythm in patients with cardiac arrest due to various causes. It is also used as a topical hemostatic on bleeding surfaces. The therapeutic uses of epinephrine are discussed later in this chapter, in relation to other sympathomimetic drugs.

NOREPINEPHRINE (LEVARTERENOL)

Norepinephrine (levarterenol, *l*-noradrenaline, *l*-β-[3,4-dihydroxyphenyl]-α-aminoethanol) is the chemical mediator liberated by mammalian postganglionic adrenergic nerves. It differs from epinephrine only by lacking the methyl substitution in the amino group (*see* Table 10–1). Norepinephrine constitutes 10 to 20% of the catecholamine content of human adrenal medulla and as much as 97% in some pheochromocytomas. The history of its discovery and its role as a neurohumoral mediator are discussed in Chapter 5.

Pharmacological Properties. The pharmacological actions of norepinephrine and epinephrine have been extensively compared *in vivo* and *in vitro* (*see* Table 10–3). Both drugs are direct agonists on effector cells, and their actions differ mainly in the ratio of their effectiveness in stimulating α and β_2 receptors. Both are approximately equipotent in stimulating β_1 (cardiac) receptors. Norepinephrine is a potent agonist at α receptors and has little action on β_2 receptors; however, it is somewhat less potent than epinephrine on the α receptors of most organs.

Cardiovascular Effects. The cardiovascular effects of intravenous infusion of 10 μg of norepinephrine per minute in man are shown in Figure 10–1. Systolic and diastolic pressures and usually pulse pressure are increased. Cardiac output is unchanged or decreased, and the total peripheral resistance is raised. Compensatory vagal reflex activity slows the heart, overcoming the direct cardioaccelerator action, and thus increases the stroke volume. The peripheral vascular resistance increases in most vascular beds, and the blood flow is reduced through kidney, liver, and usually skeletal muscle. A marked venoconstriction contributes to the increased resistance. Glomerular filtration rate is maintained unless the decrease in renal blood flow is quite marked. Norepinephrine constricts mesenteric vessels and reduces splanchnic and hepatic blood flow in man. Coronary flow is substantially increased, probably due to both indirectly induced coronary dilatation, as with epinephrine, and elevated blood pressure. However, patients with Prinzmetal's variant angina may be supersensitive to the α-adrenergic vasoconstrictor effects of norepinephrine, epinephrine, and sympathetic nerve discharge. In such patients, endogenous or exogenous norepinephrine may reduce coronary blood flow. They can experience angina at rest even though their vascular bed may be relatively free of atherosclerotic lesions, and the decrease in coronary blood flow may be sufficiently great and prolonged to cause myocardial infarction (*see* Chapter 32).

Unlike epinephrine, small doses of norepinephrine do not cause vasodilatation or lower blood pressure, since the blood vessels of skeletal muscle constrict instead of dilate; α-blocking agents therefore abolish the pressor effects but do not cause significant reversal. The circulating blood volume is reduced by loss of protein-free fluid to the extracellular space, probably due to postcapillary venoconstriction. The usual ECG change is sinus bradycardia due to a reflex increase in vagal tone, with or without prolongation of the P–R interval. Nodal rhythm, AV dissociation, bigeminal rhythm, ventricular tachycardia, and fibrillation have also been observed.

Other Effects. Other responses to norepinephrine are not prominent in man. The drug causes hyperglycemia and other metabolic effects similar to those produced by epinephrine, but these are observed only when larger doses are given. Intradermal injection of suitable doses in man causes sweating that is not blocked by atropine. Increased frequency of contraction of the pregnant human uterus has been observed, but the effects on the other smooth muscles are slight.

Absorption, Fate, and Excretion. Norepinephrine, like epinephrine, is ineffective when given orally and is absorbed poorly from sites of subcutaneous injection. It is rapidly inactivated in the body by the same enzymes that methylate and oxidatively deaminate epinephrine (*see* above). Small amounts are normally found in the urine, but the excretion rate may be greatly increased in patients with pheochromocytoma.

Preparations, Route of Administration, and Dosage. *Norepinephrine bitartrate* (LEVOPHED BITARTRATE) is the water-soluble, crystalline monohydrate salt. Like epinephrine, it is readily oxidized. *Norepinephrine bitartrate injection* is usually given by intravenous infusion as a solution containing 4 μg/ml of norepinephrine base. The infusion is adjusted to obtain the desired pressor response. Normally the infusion of 2 to 4 μg of base per minute is adequate. The pressor response to the drug can be readily controlled since it disappears within 1 or 2 minutes after the infusion is stopped. In patients in whom intravenous infusion of large volumes of fluid is undesirable, less dilute solutions may be used cautiously.

Toxicity, Side Effects, and Precautions. The untoward effects of norepinephrine are similar to those of epinephrine, but they are usually less pronounced and less frequent. Anxiety, respiratory difficulty, awareness of the slow, forceful heart beat, and transient headache are the most common effects. Overdoses or conventional doses in hypersensitive persons (*e.g.*, hyperthyroid patients) cause severe hypertension with violent headache, photophobia, stabbing retrosternal pain, pallor, intense sweating, and vomiting. The risk of cardiac arrhythmias contraindicates the use of the drug during anesthesia with agents that sensitize the automatic tissue of the heart.

Care must be taken that necrosis and sloughing do not occur at the site of intravenous injection, due to extravasation of the drug. The infusion should be made high in the limb, preferably through a long plastic cannula extending centrally. Impaired circulation at injection sites, with or without extravasation of norepinephrine, may be relieved by infiltration of the area with phentolamine. Blood pressure must be determined frequently during the infusion and particularly during adjustment of the rate of the infusion. Blood pressure should not be raised to more than normotensive levels. Reduced blood flow to vital areas is a constant danger with the use of norepinephrine. The drug should not be used in pregnant women because of its contractile action on the pregnant uterus.

Therapeutic Uses and Status. Norepinephrine has only limited therapeutic value. The therapeutic use of norepinephrine and of other sympathomimetic amines in shock is discussed later in this chapter.

DOPAMINE

Dopamine (3,4-dihydroxyphenylethylamine) (*see* Table 10–1) is the immediate metabolic precursor of norepinephrine and epinephrine; it is a central neurotransmitter (Chapters 12, 18, and 20) and possesses important intrinsic pharmacological properties. Dopamine is a substrate for both MAO and COMT and thus is ineffective when administered orally.

Cardiovascular Effects. The cardiovascular effects of dopamine are mediated by several distinct types of receptors that vary in their affinity for the catecholamine (Goldberg and Rajfer, 1985). At low concentrations the primary interaction of dopamine is with vascular D_1-dopaminergic receptors, especially in the renal, mesenteric, and coronary beds. By activating adenylyl cyclase and raising intracellular concentrations of cyclic AMP (*see* Chapter 5), D_1-receptor stimulation leads to vasodilatation. Infusion of low doses of dopamine causes an increase in glomerular filtration rate, renal blood flow, and Na^+ excretion. As a consequence, dopamine is especially useful in the management of states of low cardiac output associated with compromised renal function, such as cardiogenic and hypovolemic shock.

At somewhat higher concentrations dopamine exerts a positive inotropic effect on the myocardium, acting via β_1-adrenergic receptors. Dopamine also causes the release of norepinephrine from nerve terminals, which contributes to its effects on the heart. Tachycardia is less prominent during infusion of dopamine than of isoproterenol (*see* below). Dopamine usually increases systolic and pulse pressure and either has no effect on diastolic blood pressure or increases it slightly. Total peripheral resistance is usually unchanged when low or intermediate doses of dopamine are given. This is probably due to the ability of dopamine to reduce regional arterial resistance in the mesentery and kidney while causing only minor increases in other vascular beds.

At high concentrations dopamine activates vascular α_1-adrenergic (and possibly tryptaminergic) receptors, leading to vasoconstriction. Accordingly, when dopamine is used in life-threatening states of shock, blood pressure and renal function must be monitored carefully (Higgins and Chernow, 1987).

Other Effects. Although there are specific dopaminergic receptors in the CNS, injected dopamine usually has no central effects because it does not readily cross the blood–brain barrier (*see* Chapters 12, 18, and 20).

Preparations, Route of Administration, and Dosage. *Dopamine hydrochloride* (INTROPIN) is marketed in solutions for injection that contain 40, 80, and 160 mg/ml. It is used only by the intravenous route. The drug is usually diluted to a concentration of 0.4 to 1.6 mg/ml and is administered at a rate of 2 to 5 μg/kg per minute initially; this rate may be increased gradually up to 20 to 50 μg/kg per minute or more as the clinical situation dictates. During the infusion, all patients require intermittent evaluation of blood volume and frequent assessment of myocardial function, perfusion of vital organs, and the production of urine. Most patients should receive intensive care, with monitoring of arterial and venous pressures and the ECG. Reduction in urine flow, tachycardia, and the development of arrhythmias may be indications to slow or terminate the infusion. The duration of action of dopamine is quite brief, and hence the rate of administration can be used to control the intensity of effect.

Precautions, Adverse Reactions, and Contraindications. Before dopamine is administered to patients in shock, hypovolemia should be corrected by transfusion of whole blood, plasma, or appropriate fluids. The patient must be monitored as indicated above. Untoward effects due to overdosage are generally attributable to excessive sympathomimetic activity (although this may also be the response to worsening shock).

Nausea, vomiting, tachycardia, anginal pain, arrhythmias, headache, hypertension, and vasoconstriction may be encountered during infusion of dopamine. Since the drug has an extremely short half-life in plasma, these effects usually disappear quickly if the infusion is slowed or interrupted. Rarely, the use of a short-acting α-blocking agent such as phentolamine may be required. Extravasation of large amounts of dopamine during infusion may cause ischemic necrosis and sloughing. Rarely, gangrene of the fingers or toes has followed the prolonged infusion of the drug. If this is threatened, local infiltration of the region with phentolamine should be instituted.

Dopamine should be avoided or used at a much reduced dosage (one tenth or less) if the patient has received an MAO inhibitor. Careful adjustment of dosage is also necessary for the patient who is taking tricyclic antidepressants.

Therapeutic Uses. Dopamine is useful in the treatment of some types of shock. It is particularly beneficial for patients with oliguria and with low or normal peripheral vascular resistance. The drug is also of value in the treatment of cardiogenic and septic shock, as well as profound hypotension following removal of pheochromocytoma. The management of shock is more fully discussed later in this chapter.

II. β-Adrenergic Agonists

β-Adrenergic agonists have been utilized in many clinical settings but now play major roles only in the treatment of bronchoconstriction in patients with asthma (reversible airway obstruction) or as cardiac stimulants. Epinephrine was first used as a bronchodilator at the beginning of this century, and ephedrine was introduced into Western medicine in 1924, although it had been used in China for thousands of years (Chen and Schmidt, 1930; Nelson, 1982; Seale, 1988). The next major advance was the development in the 1940s of isoproterenol, a pure β-adrenergic agonist; this provided a drug for asthma that lacked α-adrenergic activity. The more recent development of selective β_2 agonists has provided drugs with even more valuable characteristics—adequate oral bioavailability, lack of α-adrenergic activity, and diminished likelihood of adverse cardiovascular effects.

β-Adrenergic agonists that activate β receptors may be used to stimulate the rate and force of cardiac contraction. The chronotropic effect is useful in the emergency treatment of bradycardia or heart block, whereas the inotropic effect is useful when it is desirable to augment myocardial contractility. The various therapeutic uses of β-adrenergic agonists are discussed later in the chapter.

ISOPROTERENOL

Isoproterenol (isopropylarterenol, isopropylnorepinephrine, isoprenaline, isopropylnoradrenaline, *dl*-β-[3,4-dihydroxyphenyl]-α-isopropylaminoethanol) (*see* Table 10–1) is a potent nonselective β-adrenergic agonist with very low affinity for α-adrenergic receptors. Consequently, isoproterenol has powerful effects on all β receptors and almost no action at α receptors.

Pharmacological Actions. The major cardiovascular effects of isoproterenol (compared with epinephrine and norepinephrine) are illustrated in Figure 10–1. Intravenous infusion of isoproterenol in man lowers peripheral vascular resistance, primarily in skeletal muscle but also in renal and mesenteric vascular beds. Diastolic pressure falls. Renal blood flow is decreased in normotensive subjects but is increased markedly in shock. Systolic blood pressure may remain unchanged or rise, although mean arterial pressure typically falls. Cardiac output is increased because of the positive inotropic and chronotropic effects of the drug in the face of diminished peripheral vascular resistance. The cardiac effects of isoproterenol may lead to palpitations, sinus tachycardia, and more serious arrhythmias; large doses of isoproterenol may cause myocardial necrosis in animals.

Isoproterenol relaxes almost all varieties of smooth muscle when the tone is high, but this action is most pronounced on bronchial and gastrointestinal smooth muscle. It prevents or relieves bronchoconstriction, but tolerance to this effect develops with overuse of the drug. Its effect in asthma may be due in part to an additional action to inhibit antigen-induced release of histamine and other mediators of inflammation; this action is shared by selective β_2-receptor stimulants.

In man, isoproterenol causes less hyperglycemia than does epinephrine, in part because insulin secretion is stimulated by the strong β-adrenergic activation of pancreatic islet cells. Isoproterenol and epinephrine are equally effective in stimulating the release of free fatty acids and energy production.

Absorption, Fate, and Excretion. Isoproterenol is readily absorbed when given parenterally or as an aerosol. It is metabolized primarily in the liver and other tissues by COMT. Isoproterenol is a relatively poor substrate for MAO and is not taken up by sympathetic neurons to the same extent as are epinephrine and norepinephrine. The duration of action of isoproterenol may therefore be longer than that of epinephrine, but it is still brief.

Preparations, Routes of Administration, and Dosage. *Isoproterenol hydrochloride* (ISUPREL HCL) is a white, water-soluble powder; it is oxidized on exposure to air or alkali. *Isoproterenol hydrochloride inhalation* is available as a 0.25% aerosol (ISUPREL MISTOMETER, NORISODRINE AEROTROL) and as solutions (0.25 to 1%) for nebulization. For acute bronchial asthma, one or two inhalations are taken from a metered-dose inhaler four to six times daily. Alternatively, 5 to 15 deep inhalations of a 0.5% solution may be administered up to five times daily by nebulization. A usual dose to relieve bronchoconstriction in chronic obstructive pulmonary disease is 0.5 ml of the 0.5% solution. This is diluted to approximately 2.5 ml with water or isotonic saline solution and is given as a mist over 10 to 20 minutes up to five times a day. The drug is also available as *isoproterenol hydrochloride injection,* containing 200 μg/ml. In shock, 1 to 2 mg of the drug is diluted in 500 ml of 5% dextrose solution or normal saline and is infused at an initial rate of 0.5 to 5 mg/min in adults. *Isoproterenol sulfate* (MEDIHALER-ISO) is available as a suspension for use with an inhaler. Sublingual preparations of isoproterenol are unreliable, and their use is not recommended.

Toxicity and Side Effects. The acute toxicity of isoproterenol is much less than that of epinephrine. Palpitation, tachycardia, headache, and flushing of the skin are common; anginal pain, nausea, tremor, dizziness, weakness, and sweating are less frequent. Cardiac arrhythmias can occur readily, although they are not usually serious at moderate doses.

Therapeutic Uses. Isoproterenol may be used in emergencies to stimulate heart rate in patients with bradycardia or heart block, particularly in anticipation of inserting an artificial cardiac pacemaker. The use of isoproterenol in disorders such as asthma and shock has largely been replaced by other sympathomimetic drugs (*see* below).

DOBUTAMINE

Dobutamine resembles dopamine structurally but possesses a bulky aromatic substituent on the amino group (*see* Table 10–1). The pharmacological effects of dobutamine are due to direct interactions with both α- and β-adrenergic receptors; its actions do not appear to be a result of release of norepinephrine from sympathetic nerve endings, nor are they exerted via dopaminergic receptors (Leier, 1983). Although originally thought to be a relatively selective β_1-adrenergic agonist, it is now clear that the pharmacological effects of dobutamine are considerably more complex. Dobutamine possesses an asymmetric center; the two enantiomeric forms are present in the racemic mixture that is used clinically (Ruffolo *et al.,* 1981). The (−)-isomer of dobutamine is a potent agonist at α_1 receptors and is capable of causing marked pressor responses (Ruffolo and Yaden, 1983). By contrast, (+)-dobutamine is a potent α_1-receptor antagonist that can block the effects of (−)-dobutamine. The effects of these two isomers that are mediated via β-adrenergic receptors are more straightforward. The (+)-isomer is about ten times more potent as a β-receptor agonist than is the (−)-isomer; each isomer appears to be a full agonist. Dobutamine may have somewhat greater selectivity for β_1 than for β_2 receptors.

Cardiovascular Effects. The cardiovascular effects of racemic dobutamine represent a composite of the distinct pharmacological properties of the (−) and (+) stereoisomers. Dobutamine has relatively more prominent inotropic than chronotropic effects on the heart compared with isoproterenol. The explanation for this useful selectivity is not clear (Sonnenblick *et al.,* 1979). It may be due in part to the fact that peripheral resistance is relatively unchanged. Alternatively, cardiac α_1 receptors may contribute to the inotropic effect. At equivalent inotropic doses dobutamine enhances automaticity of the sinus node to a lesser extent than does isoproterenol; however, enhancement of atrioventricular and intraventricular conduction are similar for the two drugs (Sonnenblick *et al.*, 1979).

In animals, administration of dobutamine at a rate of 2.5 to 15 μg/kg per minute increases cardiac contractility and cardiac output. Total peripheral resistance is not much affected. The relative constancy of peripheral resistance presumably reflects counterbalancing of α_1 receptor-mediated vasoconstriction and β_2 receptor-mediated vasodilatation (Ruffolo, 1987). The heart rate increases only modestly when the rate of administration of dobutamine is maintained at less than 20 μg/kg per minute. After administration of β-blocking agents, infusion of dobutamine fails to increase cardiac output, but total peripheral resistance increases, confirming that dobutamine does have modest direct effects on α receptors in the vasculature.

Preparations, Route of Administration, and Dosage. *Dobutamine hydrochloride* (DOBUTREX) is supplied in 20-ml vials that contain the equivalent of 250 mg of dobutamine. The compound is dissolved in 10 ml of sterile water or 5% dextrose solution, and this solution is then further diluted to at least 50 ml for use by continuous intravenous infusion. The usual dose is 2.5 to 10 μg/kg per minute.

Adverse Effects. In some patients blood pressure and heart rate may increase significantly during administration of dobutamine; this may require reduction of the rate of infusion. Patients with a history of hypertension may be at greater risk of developing an exaggerated pressor response. Since dobutamine facilitates atrioventricular conduction, patients with atrial fibrillation are at risk of marked increases in ventricular response rates; digoxin or other measures may be required to prevent this problem. Some patients may develop ventricular ectopic activity. As with any inotropic agent, dobutamine may potentially increase the size of a myocardial infarction by increasing myocardial oxygen demand. This risk must be balanced against the patient's overall clinical status. The efficacy of dobutamine over a period of more than a few days is uncertain; there is evidence for the development of tolerance (Unverferth *et al.*, 1980). However, short-term infusions used intermittently over a period of months may improve exercise tolerance in some patients with congestive heart failure (Leier, 1983), although such treatment probably does not prolong survival (Krell *et al.*, 1986).

Therapeutic Uses. Dobutamine is indicated for the short-term treatment of cardiac decompensation that may occur after cardiac surgery or in patients with congestive heart failure or acute myocardial infarction. Dobutamine increases cardiac output and stroke volume in such patients, usually without a marked increase in heart rate. Alterations in blood pressure or peripheral resistance are usually minor, although some patients may have marked increases in blood pressure or heart rate.

Dobutamine has a half-life of about 2 minutes; the major metabolites are conjugates of dobutamine and 3-O-methyl dobutamine. The onset of effect is rapid. Consequently, a loading dose is not required and steady-state concentrations are generally achieved within 10 minutes of initiation of an infusion. The rate of infusion required to increase cardiac output typically is between 2.5 and 10 μg/kg per minute, although higher infusion rates are occasionally required. The rate and duration of the infusion are determined by the clinical and hemodynamic responses of the patient.

SELECTIVE β_2-ADRENERGIC AGONISTS

Some of the major adverse effects of β-adrenergic agonists in the treatment of asthma are caused by stimulation of β_1-adrenergic receptors in the heart. Accordingly, drugs with preferential affinity for β_2 receptors compared with β_1 receptors have been developed. However, this selectivity is not absolute, and it is lost at sufficiently high concentrations of these drugs.

A second strategy that has increased the usefulness of several β_2-selective agonists in the treatment of asthma has been structural modifications that result in lower rates of metabolism and enhanced oral bioavailability (compared with catecholamines). Modifications have included placing the hydroxy groups at the third and fifth positions of the phenyl ring or substituting another moiety for the hydroxy group at the third position. This has yielded drugs such as metaproterenol, terbutaline, and albuterol that are not substrates for COMT. Bulky substituents on the amino group of catecholamines contribute to β_2-adrenergic selectivity, decreased activity at α-adrenergic receptors, and decreased metabolism by MAO (Nelson, 1982).

A final strategy to enhance preferential activation of pulmonary β_2 receptors is the administration by inhalation of small doses of the drug in aerosol form. This approach typically leads to effective activation of β_2 receptors in the bronchi but very low systemic drug concentrations (Newhouse and Dolovich, 1986). Thus, there is less potential to activate cardiac β_1 receptors or to stimulate β_2 receptors in skeletal muscle that can cause tremor and thereby limit oral therapy.

Administration of β-adrenergic agonists by aerosol typically leads to a very rapid therapeutic response, generally within minutes. Although subcutaneous injection also causes prompt bronchodilatation, the peak effect of a drug given orally may be delayed for several hours (Dulfano and Glass, 1976). Aerosol therapy depends on the delivery of drug to the distal airways. This, in turn, depends on the size of the particles in the aerosol and respiratory parameters such as inspiratory flow rate, tidal volume, breath-holding time, and airway diameter (Newhouse and Dolovich, 1986). Only about 10% of an inhaled dose actually enters the lungs; much of the remainder is swallowed and may ultimately be absorbed. Successful aerosol therapy requires that each patient master the technique of drug administration. Many patients, particularly children and the elderly, do not use optimal techniques, often because of inadequate instructions (Kelly, 1985; Newhouse and Dolovich, 1986).

In the treatment of asthma, β-adrenergic agonists are used to activate pulmonary receptors that relax bronchial smooth muscle and decrease airway resistance. Although this action appears to be the major therapeutic effect of these drugs in patients with asthma, evidence suggests that β-adrenergic agonists may also suppress the release of leukotrienes and histamine from mast cells in lung tissue (Hughes *et al.*, 1983), enhance mucociliary function, decrease microvascular permeability, and possibly inhibit phospholipase A_2 (Seale, 1988). The relative importance of these actions in the treatment of human asthma remains to be determined.

A number of different β-adrenergic agonists are available for the treatment of airway obstruction. They vary in β_2 selectivity, ability to activate α-adrenergic receptors, potency, oral bioavailability, half-life of elimination, and availability of parenteral dosage formulations. Unfortunately, it remains difficult to rank the drugs in order of their β_2 selectivity in man. The adverse effects of these drugs are considered as a group after discussion of the individual agents. Their therapeutic uses are described at the end of the chapter.

METAPROTERENOL

Metaproterenol (orciprenaline), along with terbutaline and fenoterol, belong to the structural class of resorcinol bronchodilators that have hydroxy groups at the 3 and 5 positions of the phenyl ring (rather than the 3 and 4 positions as for catechols) (*see* Table 10–1). Consequently, metaproterenol is resistant to methylation by COMT and a substantial fraction (40%) is absorbed in active form after oral administration. It is excreted primarily as glucuronic acid conjugates. Metaproterenol is considered to be β_2 selective, although it is probably less selective than albuterol or terbutaline. Effects occur within minutes of inhalation and persist for several hours. After oral administration, onset of action is slower, but effects last 3 to 4 hours. Metaproterenol is used for the long-term treatment of obstructive airway diseases and to treat acute bronchospasm.

Preparations, Routes of Administration, and Dosage. *Metaproterenol sulfate* (ALUPENT, METAPREL) is available for oral inhalation as a micronized powder. The metered-dose inhaler contains 225 mg of the drug, and approximately 0.65 mg is nebulized per dose. Administration is generally performed by 2 or 3 deep inhalations, and this may be repeated at 3- to 4-hour intervals; the total daily dose should not exceed 12 inhalations. An oral inhalant solution can also be used. For oral administration, metaproterenol is supplied as 10- and 20-mg tablets. The usual adult dose is 20 mg, taken three or four times a day. A syrup (10 mg/5 ml) is suitable for use in children. The usual dose in children who are 6 to 9 years of age or who weigh less than 27 kg is 5 ml, given three or four times a day. Children over 9 years of age or who weigh more than 27 kg may receive 10 ml three or four times a day.

TERBUTALINE

Terbutaline is a β_2-selective bronchodilator. It contains a resorcinol ring and thus is not a substrate for methylation by COMT. It is effective when taken orally, subcutaneously, or by inhalation (Dulfano and Glass, 1976). Effects are observed rapidly after inhalation or parenteral administration; after inhalation this action may persist for 3 to 6 hours. With oral administration, the onset of effect may be delayed for 1 to 2 hours, although the duration of response is 4 to 8 hours. Terbutaline is used for the long-term treatment of obstructive airway diseases and to treat acute bronchospasm; furthermore, it is the only selective β_2 bronchodilator available for parenteral use for the emergency treatment of status asthmaticus.

Preparations, Routes of Administration, and Dosage. *Terbutaline sulfate* (BRETHAIRE, BRETHINE, BRICANYL) may be administered subcutaneously, orally, or by inhalation. Its use in children under 12 years of age is not recommended. The usual subcutaneous dose is 0.25 mg. If significant clinical improvement does not occur in 15 to 30 minutes, a second dose may be administered. A total dose of 0.5 mg should not be exceeded within a 4-hour period. The usual oral dose for adults is 5 mg, administered three times a day at intervals of approximately 6 hours. The inhalational dose is 2 sprays every 4 to 6 hours. Terbutaline is available in tablets containing either 2.5 or 5 mg of the drug, as an injection containing 1 mg/ml, and as an aerosol containing 0.2 mg per spray.

ALBUTEROL

Albuterol is a selective β_2-adrenergic agonist with pharmacological properties and therapeutic indications similar to those of terbutaline. It is administered either by inhalation or orally for the symptomatic relief of bronchospasm. When administered by inhalation, it produces significant bronchodilatation within 15 minutes and effects are demonstrable for 3 to 4 hours. The cardiovascular effects of albuterol are considerably less than those of isoproterenol when doses that produce comparable bronchodilatation are administered by inhalation (Ahrens and Smith, 1984).

Preparations, Routes of Administration, and Dosage. *Albuterol* (*salbutamol*) (PROVENTIL, VENTOLIN) is marketed in 2- and 4-mg tablets (as the sulfate) for oral administration, in 4-mg extended release tablets, and as an aerosol. Each inhalation delivers approximately 90 μg of the drug; no more than 2 inhalations every 4 to 6 hours is recommended. The initial oral dose is 2 to 4 mg, given three to four times daily; a total daily dose of 32 mg should not be exceeded. A syrup (2 mg/5 ml) is also available.

ISOETHARINE

Isoetharine was the first widely used drug with β_2 selectivity for the treatment of airway obstruction. However, its degree of selectivity for β_2-adrenergic receptors may not approach those of some of the other agents. Although resistant to metabolism by MAO, it is a catecholamine and thus is a good substrate for COMT (*see* Table 10–1). Consequently, it is used only by inhalation for the treatment of acute episodes of bronchoconstriction.

Isoetharine is available in solutions for nebulization (BRONKOSOL) or for pressurized inhalation (BRONKOMETER). Usually, treatment should not be repeated more often than every 4 hours, although in severe cases more frequent dosage may be necessary.

PIRBUTEROL

Pirbuterol is a relatively selective β_2 agonist. It is structurally identical to albuterol except for the substitution of a pyridine ring for the benzene ring (Richards and Brogden, 1985).

Pirbuterol acetate (MAXAIR) is available for inhalation therapy for adults and children 12 years of age and older. Two inhalations (total of 0.4 mg) may be repeated every 4 to 6 hours. One inhalation may be sufficient for some patients; the total daily dose should not exceed 12 inhalations.

BITOLTEROL

Bitolterol is a novel β_2 agonist in which the hydroxy groups in the catechol moiety are protected by esterification with 4-methylbenzoate. Esterases in the lung and other tissues hydrolyze this prodrug to the active form, colterol, or terbutylnorepinephrine (*see* Table 10–1). Animal studies have suggested that these esterases are present in higher concentration in lung than in tissues such as the heart (Nelson, 1986; Friedel and Brogden, 1988). The duration of effect of bitolterol after inhalation ranges from 3 to 6 hours.

Bitolterol mesylate (TORNALATE) is available for inhalation for adults and children over 12 years of age. The recommended dosage to relieve bronchospasm is two inhalations at an interval of at least 1 to 3 minutes, followed by a third inhalation if needed. Dosage should not exceed two inhalations every 4 hours or three inhalations every 6 hours. Each metered dose consists of 0.37 mg of the drug.

RITODRINE

Ritodrine is a selective β_2-adrenergic agonist that was developed specifically for use as a uterine relaxant. Nevertheless, its pharmacological properties closely resemble those of the other agents in this group. Ritodrine is the only β_2-adrenergic agonist that is currently approved in the United States for use to delay or prevent premature parturition; other drugs, such as terbutaline and fenoterol, have been used extensively for this purpose in Europe and elsewhere (*see* Caritis, 1983).

Ritodrine is rapidly but incompletely (30%) absorbed following oral administration, and 90% of the drug is excreted in the urine as inactive conjugates; about 50% of ritodrine is excreted unchanged after intravenous administration. The pharmacokinetic properties of ritodrine are complex and incompletely defined (*see* Caritis, 1983).

Therapeutic Uses. Ritodrine is administered intravenously to selected patients in order to arrest premature labor; if successful, oral therapy is then instituted. The preparations, dosage, indications, and contraindications for the use of ritodrine are presented in Chapter 39.

ADVERSE EFFECTS OF β_2 AGONISTS

The major adverse effects of β-adrenergic agonists occur as a result of excessive activation of β-adrenergic receptors. Patients with underlying cardiovascular disease are particularly at risk for significant reactions.

Skeletal muscle tremor is the most common adverse effect of the selective β_2-adrenergic agonists. This appears to be caused by an increase in the amplitude of movements within the frequency range of physiological tremors (Lulich *et al.*, 1986). Tolerance generally develops to this effect; it is not clear whether tolerance reflects desensitization of the β_2 receptors of skeletal muscle or adaptation within the CNS. This adverse effect can be minimized by starting oral therapy with a low dose of drug and progressively increasing the dose as tolerance to the tremor develops. Feelings of restlessness, apprehension, and anxiety may limit therapy with these drugs, particularly after oral or parenteral treatment.

Tachycardia is a common adverse effect of systemically administered β-adrenergic agonists. Stimulation of heart rate occurs primarily via β_1 receptors. It is uncertain to what extent the increase in heart rate is also due to activation of cardiac β_2 receptors or to reflex effects that stem from β_2 receptor-mediated peripheral vasodilatation. However, during a severe asthmatic attack heart rate may actually decrease during therapy with a β-adrenergic agonist, presumably because of improvement in pulmonary function with consequent reduction in endogenous sympathetic stimulation. In patients without cardiac disease, β agonists rarely cause significant arrhythmias or myocardial ischemia; however, patients with underlying coronary artery disease or preexisting arrhythmias are at much greater risk. The risk of adverse cardiovascular effects is also increased in patients who are receiving MAO inhibitors or tricyclic antidepressants.

Arterial oxygen tension may fall when treatment of patients with an acute exacerbation of asthma is begun; this may be due to drug-induced pulmonary vascular dilatation, which leads to increased mismatching of ventilation and perfusion. This effect is usually small and transient; supplemental oxygen should be given if necessary. Severe pulmonary edema has been reported in women receiving ritodrine or terbutaline for premature labor.

Large doses of β-adrenergic agonists may cause myocardial necrosis in laboratory animals. When given parenterally these drugs may also increase the concentrations of glucose, lactate, and free fatty acids in plasma and decrease the concentration of K^+. The fall in K^+ may be especially important in patients with cardiac disease, particularly those taking cardiac glycosides and diuretics. In some diabetic patients hyperglycemia may be worsened by these drugs, and higher doses of insulin may be required. All these adverse effects are far less likely with inhalation therapy than with parenteral or oral therapy.

Tolerance to β-adrenergic agonists has been studied extensively, both *in vitro* and *in vivo* (*see* Chapter 5). Long-term systemic administration of β-adrenergic agonists leads to "down-regulation" of β receptors in some tissues and decreased pharmacological responses. This has been demonstrated in patients with asthma. However, it appears likely that tolerance to the pulmonary effects of these drugs is not a major clinical problem in the majority of asthmatics who do not exceed recommended dosages of β-adrenergic agonists over prolonged periods (Jenne, 1982; Tattersfield, 1985).

III. α-Adrenergic Agonists

There are a number of drugs whose major clinical effects are due to activation of α-adrenergic receptors in vascular smooth muscle. As a result, peripheral vascular resistance is increased and blood pressure is maintained or elevated. Although the clinical utility of these drugs is limited, they may be useful in the treatment of some patients with hypotension or shock. Phenylephrine and methoxamine are directly acting vasoconstrictors and they are selective activators of α_1 receptors. Mephentermine and metaraminol act both directly and indirectly; that is, a portion of their effects is mediated by the release of endogenous norepinephrine.

METHOXAMINE

Methoxamine (*see* Table 10–1) is a relatively specific α_1-selective adrenergic agonist; as such, it causes a dose-related increase in peripheral vascular resistance. The drug may have different intrinsic activities at α_1 receptors in different tissues (Garcia-Sainz *et al.,* 1985). Methoxamine does not activate β-adrenergic receptors, nor does it cause stimulation of the CNS. However, at high concentrations methoxamine has some capacity to block β receptors. The major cardiovascular response to the drug is a rise in blood pressure, which is associated with sinus bradycardia because of activation of vagal reflexes; the slowing of the heart rate is largely blocked by atropine. Methoxamine may be used in the treatment of hypotensive states or to relieve attacks of paroxysmal atrial tachycardia, particularly those associated with hypotension. The vagal reflexes induced by the drug may terminate the arrhythmia successfully.

Preparations, Routes of Administration, and Dosage. *Methoxamine hydrochloride* (VASOXYL) is available as a solution (20 mg/ml). The drug is usually given intravenously. A dose of 3 to 5 mg is injected slowly to correct blood pressure; 10 mg may be given over 3 to 5 minutes for supraventricular tachycardias. To maintain control of blood pressure, methoxamine may be infused at a rate of 5 μg/min or a dose of 10 to 15 mg may be given intramuscularly. However, absorption from intramuscular sites of administration can be unreliable in hypotensive patients.

PHENYLEPHRINE

Phenylephrine is an α_1-selective agonist; it activates β-adrenergic receptors only at much higher concentrations. Chemically, phenylephrine differs from epinephrine only in lacking a hydroxy group in the 4 position on the benzene ring (*see* Table 10–1). The pharmacological effects of phenylephrine are similar to those of methoxamine. The drug causes marked arterial vasoconstriction during an intravenous infusion. Phenylephrine is also used as a nasal decongestant and as a mydriatic.

Preparations, Routes of Administration, and Dosage. *Phenylephrine hydrochloride* (NEO-SYNEPHRINE, others) is the *l* isomer. It is available as a solution (10 mg/ml) for parenteral use and in various nasal and ophthalmic solutions, as a nasal jelly, and as a viscous ophthalmic solution. Phenylephrine is also present in a large number of combination products, primarily for use as a decongestant. To prevent hypotension, particularly during spinal anesthesia, the usual dose is 2 to 3 mg, administered subcutaneously or intramuscularly. To treat hypotension in such situations, the drug is given intravenously and the dose is titrated according to the response; the usual dose is 0.2 to 0.5 mg. Intravenous doses of 0.5 to 1.0 mg are used to terminate paroxysmal supraventricular tachycardias.

MEPHENTERMINE

Mephentermine (*see* Table 10–1) is a sympathomimetic drug that acts both directly and indirectly; it has many similarities with ephedrine (*see* below). After an intramuscular injection, the onset of action is prompt (within 5 to 15 minutes), and effects may last for several hours. Since the drug releases norepinephrine, cardiac contraction is enhanced, and cardiac output and systolic and diastolic pressures are usually increased. The change in heart rate is variable, depending on the degree of vagal tone. Adverse effects are related to CNS stimulation, excessive rises in blood pressure, and arrhythmias. Mephentermine is used to prevent hypotension, which frequently accompanies spinal anesthesia.

Mephentermine sulfate (WYAMINE SULFATE) is available in solution for parenteral injection (15 and 30 mg/ml). Although the drug can be given intramuscularly, intravenous injection or infusion with titration of the dose according to the blood pressure response is generally preferable in the treatment of hypotension.

METARAMINOL

Metaraminol (*see* Table 10–1) is a sympathomimetic drug with prominent direct effects on vascular α-adrenergic receptors. Metaraminol is also an indirectly acting agent that stimulates the release of norepinephrine. The drug is used in the treatment of hypotensive states or to relieve attacks of paroxysmal atrial tachycardia, particularly those associated with hypotension.

Metaraminol bitartrate (ARAMINE) is available in solution (10 mg/ml) for parenteral administration. Absorption of the drug after subcutaneous or intramuscular injection is unreliable in hypotensive patients. Intravenous dosing should be titrated according to the change in blood pressure. A dose of 0.5 to 5 mg can be given initially, and blood pressure can then be maintained by infusion.

SELECTIVE α_2-ADRENERGIC AGONISTS

Selective α_2-adrenergic agonists are used primarily for the treatment of systemic hypertension. Their efficacy as antihypertensive agents is somewhat surprising, since many blood vessels contain postsynaptic α_2 receptors that promote vasoconstriction (*see* Chapter 5). Indeed, clonidine was initially developed as a vasoconstricting nasal decongestant. Its capacity to lower blood pressure results from activation of α_2-adrenergic receptors in the cardiovascular control centers of the CNS; such activation suppresses the outflow of sympathetic nervous system activity from the brain.

CLONIDINE

Clonidine, an imidazoline, was synthesized in the early 1960s and found to produce vasoconstriction that was mediated by α-adrenergic receptors. During clinical testing of the drug as a topical nasal decongestant, clonidine was found to cause hypotension, sedation, and bradycardia. The structural formula of clonidine is as follows:

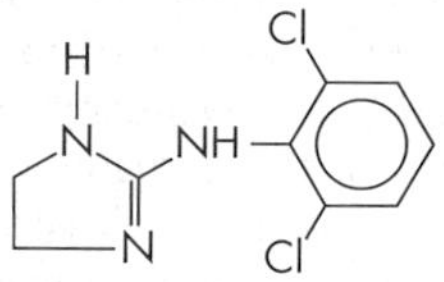

Clonidine

Pharmacological Effects. The major pharmacological effects of clonidine involve changes in blood pressure and heart rate, although the drug has a variety of other important actions. Intravenous infusion of clonidine causes an acute *rise* in blood pressure, apparently because of activation of postsynaptic α_2 receptors in vascular smooth muscle (Kobinger, 1978). The affinity of clonidine for these receptors is high, although the drug is a partial agonist with relatively low efficacy at these sites. The hypertensive response that follows parenteral administration of clonidine is not generally seen when the drug is given orally. However, even after intravenous administration, the transient vasoconstriction is followed by a more prolonged hypotensive response that results from decreased central outflow of impulses in the sympathetic nervous system. The exact mechanism by which clonidine lowers blood pressure is not completely understood. The effect appears to result from activation of α_2 receptors in the lower brainstem region, possibly in the nucleus tractus solitarius (Kobinger, 1978; Langer *et al.*, 1980). This central action has been demonstrated by infusing small amounts of the drug into the vertebral arteries or by injecting it directly into the cisterna magna.

Clonidine decreases discharges in sympathetic preganglionic fibers in the splanchnic nerve as well as in postganglionic fibers of cardiac nerves (Langer *et al.*, 1980). These effects are blocked by α_2-selective antagonists such as yohimbine. Clonidine also stimulates parasympathetic outflow, and this may contribute to the slowing of heart rate as a consequence of increased vagal tone. In addition, some of the antihypertensive effect of clonidine may be mediated by activation of presynaptic α_2 receptors that suppress the release of norepinephrine from peripheral nerve endings. Clonidine decreases the plasma concentration of norepinephrine and reduces its excretion in the urine.

Clonidine may also decrease the plasma concentrations of renin and aldosterone in some patients with hypertension (Lowenthal *et al.*, 1988).

Absorption, Fate, and Excretion. Clonidine is well absorbed after oral administration, and bioavailability is nearly 100%. The peak concentration in plasma and the maximal hypotensive effect are observed 1 to 3 hours after an oral dose. The elimination half-life of the drug ranges from 6 to 24 hours with a mean of about 12 hours (Lowenthal *et al.*, 1988). About half of an administered dose can be recovered unchanged in the urine, and the half-life of the drug may be increased with renal failure. The correlation is good between plasma concentrations of clonidine and its pharmacological effects. A transdermal delivery system permits continuous administration of clonidine as an alternative to oral therapy. The drug is released at an approximately constant rate for a week; 3 or 4 days are required to reach steady-state concentrations in plasma. When the patch is removed, plasma concentrations remain stable for about 8 hours and then decline gradually over a period of several days; this is associated with a rise in blood pressure (Langley and Heel, 1988; Lowenthal *et al.*, 1988).

Preparations, Routes of Administration, and Dosage. *Clonidine hydrochloride* (CATAPRES) is available in 0.1-, 0.2-, and 0.3-mg tablets. A transdermal delivery system (CATAPRES-TTS) is available that delivers clonidine into the circulation at rates of 0.1, 0.2, or 0.3 mg per day for 1 week. In the treatment of hypertension, therapy is usually started with oral doses of 0.1 mg twice daily or with the smallest transdermal patch. The dose is progressively elevated until the desired response is achieved. The maximum dose is 2.4 mg per day, although the usual range is 0.2 to 0.8 mg per day in divided doses. Some physicians use a more aggressive dosage regimen for the treatment of severe hypertension.

Adverse Effects. The major adverse effects of clonidine are dry mouth and sedation. These responses occur in at least 50% of patients and may require discontinuation of the drug. However, they may diminish in intensity after several weeks of therapy. Sexual dysfunction may also occur. Marked bradycardia is observed in some patients. These and some of the other adverse effects of clonidine are frequently related to dose, and their incidence may be lower with transdermal administration of clonidine, since antihypertensive efficacy may be achieved while avoiding the relatively high peak concentrations that occur after oral administration of the drug; however, this possibility requires further evaluation (Langley and Heel, 1988). About 15 to 20% of patients develop a contact dermatitis to the clonidine in the transdermal system. Withdrawal reactions follow abrupt discontinuation of long-term therapy with clonidine in some hypertensive patients (Parker and Atkinson, 1982; *see also* Chapter 33).

Therapeutic Uses. The major therapeutic use of clonidine is in the treatment of hypertension; this use is discussed in Chapter 33. Clonidine also has apparent efficacy in the treatment of a range of other disorders. Stimulation of the α_2-adrenergic receptors of cells in the gastrointestinal tract may increase absorption of sodium chloride and fluid and inhibit secretion of bicarbonate (Chang *et al.*, 1986). This finding may explain why clonidine has been found to improve diarrhea in some diabetic patients with autonomic neuropathy (Fedorak *et al.*, 1985). Clonidine is also useful in treating and preparing addicted subjects for withdrawal from narcotics (Gold *et al.*, 1978), alcohol (Bond, 1986), and tobacco (Glassman *et al.*, 1984, 1988) (*see* Chapter 22). Clonidine may help ameliorate some of the adverse sympathetic nervous activity associated with withdrawal from these agents, as well as decrease craving for the drug. The long-term benefits of clonidine in these settings and in neuropsychiatric disorders remains to be determined (Bond, 1986). Preliminary evidence suggests that clonidine may be useful in selected patients receiving anesthesia, because it may decrease the requirement for anesthetic and increase hemodynamic stability (Flacke *et al.*, 1987; Maze *et al.*, 1988; *see also* Chapter 14). Transdermal administration of clonidine may be useful in reducing the incidence of menopausal hot flashes (Nagamani *et al.*, 1987).

Acute administration of clonidine has been used in the differential diagnosis of patients with hypertension and suspected pheochromocytoma (*see* Chapter 33). In patients with primary hypertension, plasma concentrations of norepinephrine are markedly suppressed after a single dose of clonidine; this response is not observed in many patients with pheochromocytoma (Bravo *et al.*, 1981). The capacity of clonidine to activate postsynaptic α_2 receptors in vascular smooth muscle has been exploited in a limited number of patients whose autonomic failure is so severe that reflex sympathetic responses upon standing are absent; postural hypotension is thus marked. Since the central effect of clonidine is moot in these patients, the drug can elevate blood pressure and improve the symptoms of postural hypotension (Robertson *et al.*, 1983).

GUANFACINE

Guanfacine is a phenylacetyl-guanidine derivative. Its structural formula is as follows:

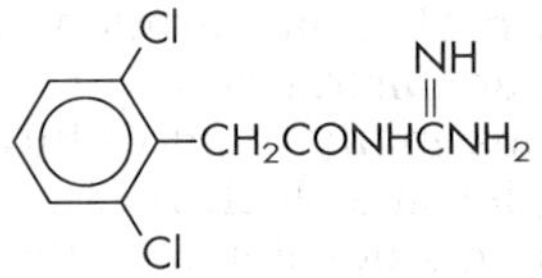

Guanfacine

Guanfacine is an α_2-adrenergic agonist that is more selective for α_2 receptors than is clonidine. Like clonidine, guanfacine lowers blood pressure by activation of central α_2 receptors with resultant suppression of sympathetic nervous system activity (Sorkin and Heel, 1986). The drug is well absorbed after oral administration and has a large volume of distribution (4 to 6 liters/kg). About 30% of guanfacine appears unchanged in the urine; the rest is metabolized. The half-time for elimination ranges from 12 to 24 hours. Guanfacine and clonidine appear to have similar efficacy for the treatment of hypertension. The pattern of adverse effects of the two drugs is also similar, although it has been suggested that some of these effects may be milder and occur less frequently with guanfacine (Sorkin and Heel, 1986). A withdrawal syndrome may occur after the abrupt discontinuation of guanfacine, but it appears to be less frequent and of milder intensity than the syndrome that follows withdrawal of clonidine. Part of this difference may relate to the longer half-life of guanfacine.

Guanfacine hydrochloride (TENEX) is available in 1-mg tablets. The initial dosage is usually 0.5 to 1 mg per day; this may be taken at bedtime to minimize problems with somnolence. If necessary, the dose may be increased in 1-mg increments at intervals of at least several weeks. Doses of 3 mg per day are generally adequate. If the therapeutic response is insufficient, a second drug such as a diuretic should be added.

GUANABENZ

Guanabenz and guanfacine are closely related chemically and pharmacologically. The structural formula of guanabenz is as follows:

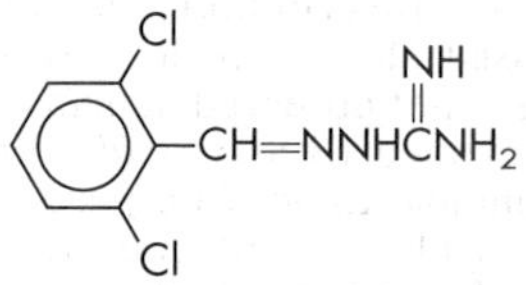

Guanabenz

Guanabenz is a centrally acting α_2 agonist that decreases blood pressure by a mechanism similar to those of clonidine and guanfacine (Holmes *et al.*, 1983). Guanabenz has a half-life of 4 to 6 hours and is extensively metabolized by the liver. Dosage adjustment may be necessary in patients with hepatic cirrhosis. The adverse effects caused by guanabenz (*e.g.*, dry mouth and sedation) are similar to those seen with clonidine.

Guanabenz acetate (WYTENSIN) is available in 4- and 8-mg tablets. For the treatment of hypertension, the initial dose is generally 4 mg twice daily. This may be increased by 4 to 8 mg per day every 1 to 2 weeks, depending on the therapeutic response. The maximum dose that has been studied is 32 mg taken twice daily.

METHYLDOPA

Methyldopa (α-methyl-3,4-dihydroxyphenylalanine) is a centrally acting antihypertensive agent. It is metabolized to α-methyl norepinephrine in the brain, and this compound is thought to activate central α_2-adrenergic receptors and lower blood pressure in a manner similar to that of clonidine. Methyldopa is described in detail in Chapter 33.

IV. Miscellaneous Adrenergic Agonists

AMPHETAMINE

Amphetamine, racemic β-phenylisopropylamine (*see* Table 10–1), has powerful CNS stimulant actions in addition to the peripheral α and β actions common to indirectly acting sympathomimetic drugs. Unlike epinephrine, it is effective after oral administration and its effects last for several hours.

Cardiovascular Responses. Amphetamine given orally raises both systolic and diastolic blood pressures. Heart rate is often reflexly slowed; with large doses, cardiac arrhythmias may occur. Cardiac output is not enhanced by therapeutic doses, and cerebral blood flow is little changed. The *l* isomer is slightly more potent than the *d* isomer in its cardiovascular actions.

Other Smooth Muscles. In general, smooth muscles respond to amphetamine as they do to other sympathomimetics. The contractile effect on the urinary bladder sphincter is particularly marked, and has been used in treating enuresis and incontinence. Pain and difficulty in micturition occasionally occur. The gastrointestinal effects of amphetamine are unpredictable. If enteric activity is pronounced, amphetamine may cause relaxation and delay the movement of intestinal contents; if the gut is already relaxed, the opposite effect may be seen. The response of the human uterus varies, but usually an increase in tone occurs.

Central Nervous System. Amphetamine is one of the most potent sympathomimetic amines in stimulating the CNS. It stimulates the medullary respiratory center, lessens the degree of central depression caused by various drugs, and produces other signs of stimulation of the CNS. These effects are thought to be due to cortical stimulation and possibly to stimulation of the reticular activating system. In contrast, the drug can obtund the maximal electroshock seizure discharge and prolong the ensuing period of depression. In elicitation of CNS excitatory effects, the *d* isomer (dextroamphetamine) is three to four times as potent as the *l* isomer.

In man, the psychic effects depend on the dose and the mental state and personality of the individual. The main results of an oral dose of 10 to 30 mg are as follows: wakefulness, alertness, and a decreased sense of fatigue; elevation of mood, with increased initiative, self-confidence, and ability to concentrate; often elation and euphoria; increase in motor and speech activity. Performance of only simple mental tasks is improved; and, although more work may be accomplished, the number of errors may increase. Physical performance—in athletes, for example—is improved, and the drug is often abused for this purpose. These effects are not invariable, and may be reversed by overdosage or repeated usage. Prolonged use or large doses are nearly always followed by mental depression and fatigue. Many individuals given amphetamine experience headache, palpitation, dizziness, vasomotor disturbances, agitation, confusion, dysphoria, apprehension, delirium, or fatigue. (*See* Chapter 22.)

Fatigue and Sleep. Prevention and reversal of fatigue by amphetamine have been studied extensively in the laboratory, in military field studies, and in athletics. In general, the duration of adequate performance is prolonged before fatigue appears and the effects of fatigue are at least partly reversed. The most striking improvement seen with amphetamine appears to occur when performance has been reduced by fatigue and lack of sleep. Such improvement may be partly due to alteration of unfavorable attitudes toward the task. However, amphetamine reduces the frequency of attention lapses that impair performance after prolonged sleep deprivation, and thus improves execution of tasks requiring sustained attention. The need for sleep may be postponed, but it obviously cannot be indefinitely avoided. When the drug is discontinued after long use, the pattern of sleep may take as long as 2 months to return to normal. (*See* reviews by Weiss and Laties, 1962; Oswald, 1968.)

Analgesia. Amphetamine and some other sympathomimetic amines have a small analgesic effect, but it is not sufficiently pronounced to be useful therapeutically. However, amphetamine can enhance the analgesia produced by morphine-like drugs (*see* Chapter 21).

Respiration. Amphetamine stimulates the respiratory center, increasing the rate and depth of respiration. In normal man, usual doses of the drug do not appreciably increase respiratory rate or minute volume. Nevertheless, when respiration is depressed by centrally acting drugs, amphetamine may stimulate respiration.

Depression of Appetite. Amphetamine and similar drugs have been widely used in the treatment of obesity, although the wisdom of this use is at best questionable. Weight loss in obese humans treated with amphetamine is almost entirely due to reduced food intake and only in small measure to increased metabolism. The site of action is probably in the lateral hypothalamic feeding center; injection of amphetamine into this area, but not into the ventromedial satiety center, suppresses food intake (*see* Blundell and Leshem, 1973). In man, tolerance to the appetite suppression develops rapidly. Hence, continuous weight reduction is not usually observed in obese individuals without dietary restrictions.

Mechanisms of Action in the CNS. Amphetamine appears to exert most or all of its effects in the CNS by releasing biogenic amines from their storage sites in the nerve terminals. The alerting effect of amphetamine, its anorectic effect, and at least a component of its locomotor-stimulating action are presumably mediated by release of norepinephrine from central noradrenergic neurons. These effects can be prevented by treatment of the animal with α-methyltyrosine, an inhibitor of tyrosine hydroxylase and, therefore, of catecholamine synthesis. Some aspects of locomotor activity and the stereotyped behavior induced by amphetamine are probably a consequence of the release of dopamine from dopaminergic nerve terminals, particularly in the neostriatum. Higher doses are required to produce these behavioral effects, and this correlates with the higher concentrations of amphetamine required to release dopamine from brain slices or synaptosomes *in vitro*. With still higher doses of amphetamine, disturbances of perception and overt psychotic behavior occur. These effects may be due to release of 5-hydroxytryptamine (5-HT) from tryptaminergic neurons and of dopamine in the mesolimbic system. In addition, amphetamine may exert direct agonistic effects on central receptors for 5-HT (*see* Weiner, 1972).

Preparations, Route of Administration, and Dosage. *Amphetamine sulfate* is available in 5- and 10-mg tablets. The *d* isomer is available as *dextroamphetamine sulfate* (DEXEDRINE, others) in 5- and 10-mg tablets, in an elixir (1 mg/ml), and in 5-, 10-, and 15-mg slow-release capsules. To treat exogenous obesity, doses of 5 to 10 mg of amphetamine are given 30 to 60 minutes before meals. For narcolepsy, the initial daily dose is 10 mg. The usual dosage range for attention-deficit hyperactivity disorder in children is 0.1 to 0.5 mg/kg. The amphetamines are schedule-II drugs under federal regulations (*see* Appendix I).

Toxicity and Side Effects. The acute toxic effects of amphetamine are usually extensions of its therapeutic actions and, as a rule, result from overdosage. The central effects commonly include restlessness, dizziness, tremor, hyperactive reflexes, talkativeness, tenseness, irritability, weakness, insomnia, fever, and sometimes euphoria. Confusion, assaultiveness, increased libido, anxiety, delirium, paranoid hallucinations, panic states, and suicidal or homicidal tendencies occur, especially in mentally ill patients. However, these psychotic effects can be elicited in any individual if sufficient quantities of amphetamine are ingested for a prolonged period. Fatigue and depression usually follow the central stimulation. Cardiovascular effects are common and include headache, chilliness, pallor or flushing, palpitation, cardiac arrhythmias, anginal pain, hypertension or hypotension, and circulatory collapse. Excessive sweating occurs. Symptoms referable to the gastrointestinal system include dry mouth, metallic taste, anorexia, nausea, vomiting, diarrhea, and abdominal cramps. Fatal poisoning usually terminates in convulsions and coma, and cerebral hemorrhages are the main pathological finding.

The toxic dose of amphetamine varies widely. Toxic manifestations occasionally occur as an idiosyncrasy after as little as 2 mg, but are rare with doses of less than 15 mg. Severe reactions have occurred with 30 mg, yet doses of 400 to 500 mg are not uniformly fatal. Larger doses can be tolerated after chronic use of the drug.

Treatment of acute amphetamine intoxication may include acidification of the urine by administration of ammonium chloride; this enhances the rate of elimination. Sedatives may be required for the CNS symptoms. Severe hypertension may require administration of sodium nitroprusside or an α-adrenergic antagonist.

Chronic intoxication with amphetamine causes symptoms similar to those of acute overdosage, but abnormal mental conditions are more common. Weight loss may be marked. A psychotic reaction with vivid hallucinations and paranoid delusions, often mistaken for schizophrenia, is the most common serious effect. Recovery is usually rapid after withdrawal of the drug, but occasionally the condition becomes chronic. In these persons amphetamine may act as a precipitating factor hastening the onset of an incipient schizophrenia (*see* Angrist and Gershon, 1972).

The abuse of amphetamine as a means of overcoming sleepiness and of increasing energy and alertness should be discouraged. The drug should be used only under medical supervision. The additional contraindications and precautions in the use of amphetamine are generally similar to those described above for epinephrine. Its use is inadvisable in patients with anorexia, insomnia, asthenia, psychopathic personality, or a history of homicidal or suicidal tendencies.

Dependence and Tolerance. Psychological dependence often occurs when amphetamine or dextroamphetamine is used chronically, as discussed in Chapter 22. Tolerance almost invariably develops to the anorexigenic effect of amphetamines, and is often seen also in the need for increasing doses to maintain improvement of mood in psychiatric patients. Tolerance is striking in individuals who are dependent on the drug, and a daily intake of 1700 mg without apparent ill effects has been reported. Development of tolerance is not invariable, and cases of narcolepsy have been treated for years without requiring an increase in the initially effective dose.

Therapeutic Uses. Amphetamine and dextroamphetamine are used chiefly for their CNS effects. Dextroamphetamine, with greater CNS action and less peripheral action, is generally preferred to amphetamine; it is used in obesity, narcolepsy, and attention-deficit hyperactivity disorder. These uses are discussed later in this chapter.

METHAMPHETAMINE

Methamphetamine is closely related chemically to amphetamine and ephedrine (*see* Table 10–1). Small doses have prominent central stimulant effects without significant peripheral actions; somewhat larger doses produce a sustained rise in systolic and diastolic blood pressures, due mainly to cardiac stimulation. Cardiac output is increased, although the heart rate may be reflexly slowed. Venous constriction causes peripheral venous pressure to increase. These factors tend to increase the venous return and, therefore, the cardiac output. Pulmonary arterial pressure is raised, probably secondary to increased cardiac output. Renal blood flow is also enhanced. Although moderate doses stimulate cardiac contraction, excessive doses depress the myocardium. (*See* Aviado, 1970.)

Methamphetamine hydrochloride (DESOXYN) is the *d* isomer. It is available in tablets containing 5 mg and in sustained-release tablets containing 5, 10, or 15 mg. The usual oral dose for central effects varies from 5 to 25 mg daily in single or divided doses, depending on the formulation used. Methamphetamine is a schedule-II drug under federal regulations (*see* Appendix I).

Methamphetamine is principally used for its central effects, which are more pronounced than those of amphetamine and are accompanied by less prominent peripheral actions. These uses are discussed below in the section of this chapter on therapeutic uses.

METHYLPHENIDATE

Methylphenidate is a piperidine derivative that is structurally related to amphetamine and has the following formula:

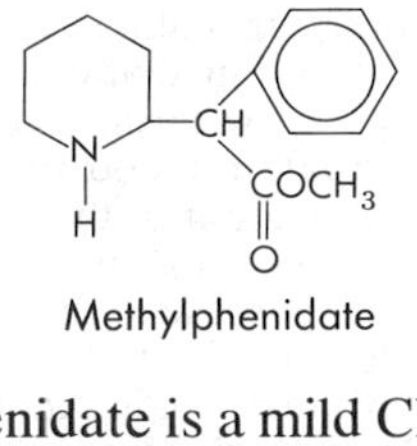

Methylphenidate

Methylphenidate is a mild CNS stimulant with more prominent effects on mental than on motor activities. However, large doses produce signs of generalized CNS stimulation that may lead to convulsions. Its pharmacological properties are essentially the same as those of the amphetamines. Methylphenidate also shares the abuse potential of the amphetamines.

Methylphenidate is readily absorbed after oral administration and reaches peak concentrations in plasma in about 2 hours. Its half-life in plasma is 1 to 2 hours, but concentrations in the brain exceed those in plasma. The main urinary metabolite is a deesterified product, ritalinic acid, which accounts for 80% of the dose.

Methylphenidate hydrochloride (RITALIN) is available as tablets that contain 5, 10, or 20 mg of drug. The usual adult dose is 10 mg, given two or three times daily. The initial dosage recommended for children with attention-deficit hyperactivity disorder is 5 mg taken twice daily. This may be increased gradually over a period of weeks to a maximum of 60 mg per day. The drug is given in equal portions before breakfast and lunch. Sustained-release tablets that contain 20 mg of the drug have a duration of action of approximately 8 hours and may be useful to reduce the frequency of dosage for some patients.

Methylphenidate is effective in the treatment of narcolepsy and the attention-deficit hyperactivity disorder, as described below.

PEMOLINE

Pemoline (CYLERT) is structurally dissimilar to methylphenidate but elicits similar changes in CNS function with minimal effects on the cardiovascular system. It is employed in treating the attention-deficit hyperactivity disorder and can be given once daily because of its long half-life. However, clinical improvement may be delayed by 3 to 4 weeks. The drug is available in tablets, and the usual daily dose is 56 to 75 mg.

EPHEDRINE

Ephedrine is both an α- and a β-adrenergic agonist; in addition, it enhances release of norepinephrine from sympathetic neurons. Ephedrine contains two asymmetrical carbon atoms (*see* Table 10–1); only *l*-ephedrine and racemic ephedrine are used clinically.

Pharmacological Actions. Ephedrine does not contain a catechol moiety, and it is effective after oral administration. The drug stimulates heart rate and cardiac output and variably increases peripheral resistance; as a result, ephedrine usually increases blood pressure. Stimulation of the α-adrenergic receptors of smooth muscle cells in the bladder base may increase the resistance to the outflow of urine. Activation of β-adrenergic receptors in the lungs promotes bronchodilatation. Ephedrine is a potent stimulator of the CNS, but less so than amphetamine. After oral administration, effects of the drug may persist for several hours. Ephedrine is eliminated in the urine largely as unchanged drug with a half-time of about 3 to 6 hours.

Preparations, Routes of Administration, and Dosage. *Ephedrine sulfate* is available in a parenteral formulation (25 or 50 mg/ml) for subcutaneous, intramuscular, or slow intravenous administration. The drug is also available for oral administration to patients with asthma or nasal congestion in capsules (25 or 50 mg) and syrups (11 or 20 mg per 5 ml). For the treatment of hypotension, the drug is administered parenterally and the dose is titrated according to the response. The usual oral dose is 25 to 50 mg repeated every 3 to 4 hours as required.

Therapeutic Uses and Toxicity. In the past, ephedrine was used to treat Stokes–Adams attacks with complete heart block and as a CNS stimulant in narcolepsy and depressive states. It has been replaced by alternative modes of treatment in each of these disorders. In addition, its use as a bronchodilator in patients with asthma has become much less extensive with the development of selective β_2 agonists. Ephedrine has been used to promote urinary continence, although its efficacy is not clear. Indeed, the drug may cause urinary retention, particularly in men with prostatic hypertrophy. Ephedrine has also been used to treat the hypotension that may occur with spinal anesthesia.

Untoward effects of ephedrine include the risk of hypertension and cardiac arrhythmias, particularly after parenteral administration. Insomnia is a common CNS side effect. Tachyphylaxis may occur with repetitive dosing.

ETHYLNOREPINEPHRINE

Ethylnorepinephrine hydrochloride (*see* Table 10–1) (BRONKEPHRINE) is primarily a β-adrenergic agonist. Its use is as a bronchodilator. The drug also has α-adrenergic agonist activity; this may cause local vasoconstriction and thereby reduce bronchial congestion. Ethylnorepinephrine is administered intramuscularly or subcutaneously. Bronchodilatation is achieved within 5 to 10 minutes and lasts about 1 to 2 hours. The drug is available in a solution for injection that contains 2 mg/ml, and the usual dose is 1 to 2 mg.

OTHER SYMPATHOMIMETIC AGENTS

Several sympathomimetic drugs are used primarily as vasoconstrictors for local application to the nasal mucous membrane or the eye. Their structures are depicted in Tables 10–1 and 10–2. Their nonproprietary and trade names as well as representative preparations are as follows: *propylhexedrine* (BENZEDREX), nasal inhaler (250 mg); *naphazoline hydrochloride,* 0.05% nasal spray or drops (PRIVINE) and 0.012 to 0.1% ophthalmic solution (NAPHCON, others); *tetrahydrozoline hydrochloride,* 0.05 and 0.1% nasal solutions (TYZINE) and 0.05% ophthalmic solution (VISINE, others); *oxymetazoline hydrochloride,* 0.025% ophthalmic solution (OCUCLEAR) and 0.025 and 0.05% nasal solution (spray or drops) (AFRIN, others); and *xylometazoline hydrochloride* (OTRIVIN), 0.05 and 0.1% nasal solutions (spray or drops).

Phenylephrine (*see* above), pseudoephedrine (a stereoisomer of ephedrine), and phenylpropanolamine are the sympathomimetic drugs most commonly used in oral preparations for the relief of nasal congestion. *Pseudoephedrine hydrochloride* (SUDAFED, others) is available in a variety of solid and liquid dosage forms. *Phenylpropanolamine hydrochloride* (PROPAGEST, others) shares the pharmacological properties of ephedrine and is approximately equal in potency except that it causes less CNS stimulation. The drug is available in tablets and capsules. In addition, numerous proprietary mixtures marketed for the oral treatment of nasal and sinus congestion contain one of these sympathomimetic amines, usually in combination with an H_1 antihistamine.

V. Therapeutic Uses of Sympathomimetic Drugs

The success that has attended efforts to develop therapeutic agents that can influence adrenergic receptors selectively and the variety of vital functions that are regulated by the sympathetic nervous system have resulted in a class of drugs with a large number of important therapeutic uses.

Shock. Shock is a clinical syndrome characterized by inadequate perfusion of tissues; it is usually associated with hypotension and ultimately with the failure of organ systems (Higgins and Chernow, 1987). Shock is an immediately life-threatening impairment of delivery of oxygen and nutrients to the organs of the body. Causes of shock include hypovolemia (due to dehydration or blood loss), cardiac failure (extensive myocardial infarction, severe arrhythmia, or cardiac mechanical defects such as ventricular septal defect), obstruction to cardiac output (due to pulmonary embolism, pericardial tamponade, or aortic dissection), and peripheral circulatory dysfunction (sepsis or anaphylaxis) (Balakumaran and Hugenholtz, 1986). The treatment of shock consists of specific efforts to reverse the underlying pathogenesis, as well as nonspecific measures aimed at correcting hemodynamic abnormalities. Regardless of the etiology, the accompanying fall in blood pressure generally leads to marked activation of the sympathetic nervous system. This in turn causes peripheral vasoconstriction and an increase in the rate and force of cardiac contraction. In the initial stages of shock these mechanisms may maintain blood pressure and cerebral blood flow, although there may be decreased blood flow to the kidneys, skin, and other organs leading to impaired production of urine and metabolic acidosis.

The initial therapy of shock involves basic measures to support life. It is essential to optimize blood volume, which often requires monitoring of hemodynamic parameters. Specific therapy (*e.g.*, antibiotics for patients in septic shock) should be initiated as soon as possible. If these measures do not lead to an adequate therapeutic response, it may be necessary to use vasoactive drugs in an effort to improve abnormalities in blood pressure and flow. Adrenergic agonists may be used in an attempt to increase myocardial contractility or modify peripheral vascular resistance. In general terms, β-adrenergic agonists increase heart rate and force of contraction, α-adrenergic agonists increase peripheral vascular resistance, and dopamine promotes dilatation of renal and splanchnic vascular beds, in addition to activating β- and α-adrenergic receptors.

Cardiogenic shock due to myocardial infarction has a poor prognosis; therapy is aimed at improving peripheral blood flow. In the setting of severely impaired cardiac output, falling blood pressure leads to intense sympathetic outflow and vasoconstriction. This may further decrease cardiac output as the damaged heart pumps against a higher peripheral resistance. Medical intervention is designed to optimize cardiac filling pressure (preload), myocardial contractility, and peripheral resistance (afterload). Preload may be increased by administration of intravenous fluids or reduced with drugs such as diuretics and nitrates. A number of sympathomimetic amines have been used to increase the force of contraction of the heart. Some of these drugs have disadvantages: isoproterenol is a powerful chronotropic agent and can greatly increase myocardial oxygen demands; norepinephrine intensifies peripheral vasoconstriction; and epinephrine increases heart rate and may predispose the heart to dangerous arrhythmias (Balakumaran and Hugenholtz, 1986). Dopamine is an effective inotropic agent that causes less increase in heart rate than does isoproterenol. Dopamine also promotes renal arterial dilatation; this may be useful in preserving renal function. At higher doses (greater than 10 to 20 μg/kg per minute) dopamine activates α-adrenergic receptors, causing peripheral and renal vasoconstriction. Dobutamine has complex pharmacological actions that are mediated by its stereoisomers; the clinical effects of the drug are to increase myocardial contractility with little increase in heart rate or peripheral resistance.

In some patients in shock, hypotension is so severe that vasoconstricting drugs are required to maintain a blood pressure that is adequate for perfusion of the CNS. α-Adrenergic agonists such as norepinephrine, phenylephrine, metaraminol, mephentermine, and methoxamine have been used for this purpose. This approach may be advantageous in patients with hypotension due to failure of the sympathetic nervous system (*e.g.*, after spinal anesthesia or injury). However, in patients with other forms of shock, such as cardiogenic shock, reflex vasoconstriction is generally intense, and α-adrenergic agonists may further compromise blood flow to organs such as the kidneys and gut as well as adversely increase the work of the heart. Indeed, vasodilating drugs such as nitroprusside are more likely to improve blood flow and decrease cardiac work in such patients by decreasing afterload if a minimally adequate blood pressure can be maintained.

The hemodynamic abnormalities in septic shock are complex and are not well understood. Most patients with septic shock initially have low or barely normal peripheral vascular resistance and normal or increased cardiac output. If the syndrome progresses, myocardial depression, increased peripheral resistance, and impaired tissue oxygenation occur (Higgins and Chernow, 1987). The primary treatment of septic shock is antibiotics; glucocorticoids have not been proven to be of benefit. Data on the comparative value of various adrenergic agents in the treatment of septic shock are limited (Chernow and Roth, 1986). Therapy with drugs such as dopamine or dobutamine is guided by hemodynamic monitoring with individualization of therapy depending on the patient's overall clinical condition.

Hypotension. Drugs with predominantly α-adrenergic activity can be used to raise blood pressure in patients with decreased peripheral resistance in conditions such as spinal anesthesia or intoxication with antihypertensive medications. However, hypotension *per se* is not an indication for treatment with these agents unless there is inadequate perfusion of organs such as the brain, heart, or kidneys. Furthermore, adequate replacement of fluid or blood may be more appropriate than drug therapy for many patients with hypotension. In patients with spinal anesthesia that interrupts sympathetic activation of the heart, injections of ephedrine increase heart rate as well as peripheral vascular resistance; tachyphylaxis may occur with repetitive injections, necessitating the use of a directly acting drug. Oral therapy with ephedrine or clonidine may be efficacious in selected patients with chronic postural hypotension due to autonomic nervous system dysfunction.

Hypertension. Centrally acting α_2-adrenergic agonists such as clonidine are useful in the treatment of hypertension. Drug therapy of hypertension is discussed in Chapter 33.

Cardiac Arrhythmias. Cardiopulmonary resuscitation in patients with cardiac arrest due to ventricular fibrillation, electromechanical dissociation, or asystole may be facilitated by drug treatment. Epinephrine is an important therapeutic agent in patients with cardiac arrest. The effectiveness of epinephrine compared with certain other catecholamines appears to be due to α-adrenergic receptor–mediated vasoconstriction; epinephrine and other α-adrenergic agonists increase diastolic pressure and improve coronary blood flow (Raehl, 1987). α-Adrenergic agonists also help to preserve cerebral blood flow during resuscitation. Cerebral blood vessels are relatively insensitive to the vasoconstricting effects of catecholamines and perfusion pressure is increased. Although it had been thought that the β-adrenergic effects of epinephrine on the heart made ventricular fibrillation more susceptible to conversion with electrical countershock, tests in animal models have not confirmed that view (Raehl, 1987). The optimal dose of epinephrine in patients with cardiac arrest is not known; however, the American Heart Association recommends 0.5 to 1.0 mg of epinephrine hydrochloride (for a 70-kg patient) intravenously at 5-minute intervals (Raehl,

1987). Once a cardiac rhythm has been restored, it may be necessary to treat arrhythmias, hypotension, or shock.

In patients with paroxysmal supraventricular tachycardias, particularly those associated with mild hypotension, careful infusion of an α-adrenergic agonist such as phenylephrine or methoxamine to raise blood pressure to about 160 mm of Hg may end the arrhythmia by reflexly increasing vagal tone. However, this method of treatment has largely been replaced by drugs such as Ca^{2+}-channel blockers and β-adrenergic antagonists and by electrical cardioversion (*see* Chapter 35). β-Adrenergic agonists such as isoproterenol may be used as adjunctive therapy with atropine in patients with marked bradycardia who are compromised hemodynamically; if long-term therapy is required, a cardiac pacemaker is usually the treatment of choice.

Congestive Heart Failure. Sympathetic stimulation of β-adrenergic receptors in the heart is a very important compensatory mechanism for maintenance of cardiac function in many patients with congestive heart failure (Francis and Cohn, 1986). Evidence indicates that responses mediated by β-adrenergic receptors are blunted in the failing human heart (Bristow *et al.*, 1985). Long-term therapy with β-adrenergic agonists as inotropic agents has met with only limited success in the treatment of congestive heart failure, possibly because the response to these drugs may be compromised by the condition and by the progressive development of desensitization during continuous therapy (*see* Chapter 5). The possibility that intermittent infusions of β agonists may lead to improved cardiac function requires further study. Paradoxically, interest has grown recently in the role of β-adrenergic antagonists and drugs such as clonidine that suppress sympathetic outflow in the treatment of selected patients with congestive heart failure. The rationale is to decrease β-adrenergic desensitization and to decrease the possibility that prolonged sympathetic stimulation of the heart may potentiate cardiac dysfunction. Assessment of the risks and benefits of this approach requires more extensive clinical testing.

Local Vascular Effects of α-Adrenergic Agonists. Epinephrine is used in many surgical procedures in the nose, throat, and larynx to shrink the mucosa and improve visualization by limiting hemorrhage. Simultaneous injection of epinephrine with local anesthetics retards the absorption of the anesthetic and increases the duration of anesthesia (*see* Chapter 15). Injection of α-adrenergic agonists into the penis may be useful in reversing priapism that may complicate the use of α-adrenergic antagonists in the treatment of impotence (*see* Chapter 11).

Nasal Decongestion. α-Adrenergic agonists are used extensively as nasal decongestants in patients with allergic or vasomotor rhinitis and in acute rhinitis in patients with upper respiratory infections (Empey and Medder, 1981). These drugs likely decrease resistance to airflow by decreasing the volume of the nasal mucosa; this may occur by activation of α-adrenergic receptors in venous capacitance vessels in nasal tissues that have erectile characteristics (Cole *et al.*, 1983). The receptors that mediate this effect appear to be α_1-adrenergic receptors. Interestingly, α_2 receptors may mediate contraction of arterioles that supply nutrition to the nasal mucosa (Andersson and Bende, 1984). Intense constriction of these vessels may cause structural damage of the mucosa (DeBernardis *et al.*, 1987). A major limitation of therapy with nasal decongestants is that loss in efficacy and "rebound" hyperemia and worsening of symptoms often occur with chronic use or when the drug is stopped. Although mechanisms are uncertain, possibilities include receptor desensitization and damage to the mucosa. Agonists that are selective for α_1 receptors may be less likely to induce mucosal damage (DeBernardis *et al.*, 1987).

For decongestion, α-adrenergic agonists may be administered either orally or topically. Oral ephedrine often causes CNS side effects. Pseudoephedrine is a stereoisomer of ephedrine that is less potent than ephedrine in producing tachycardia, increased blood pressure, or CNS stimulation (Empey and Medder, 1981). Phenylpropanolamine is similar to pseudoephedrine. Sympathomimetic decongestants should be used with great caution in patients with hypertension and in men with prostatic enlargement. These drugs are contraindicated in patients who are taking an MAO inhibitor. A variety of compounds (*see* above) are available for topical use in patients with rhinitis. Topical decongestants are particularly useful in acute rhinitis because of their more selective site of action, but they are prone to be used excessively by patients, leading to rebound congestion. Oral decongestants are much less likely to cause rebound congestion but carry a greater risk of inducing adverse systemic effects.

Asthma. A number of options are available for the treatment of patients with asthma: β-adrenergic agonists, methylxanthines, sodium cromoglycate, muscarinic cholinergic antagonists, and glucocorticoids. This subject is discussed in Chapter 25 (*see also* Chapters 8 and 60). β-Adrenergic agonists are the mainstay of treatment for most patients. Because of a lower incidence of adverse cardiovascular effects, selective β_2 agonists have largely replaced compounds such as isoproterenol. Administration of β_2 agonists by aerosol provides an effective form of prophylaxis against asthma induced by cold or exercise, as well as treatment for acute asthmatic attacks. However, education of the patient in the proper technique for administration of the drug is particularly important with aerosols. Although oral agents carry a greater risk of cardiovascular and CNS side effects, these may be more appropriate for patients who do not wish to use aerosols or who abuse them. Parenteral therapy with terbutaline is sometimes combined with aerosols or nebulized solutions in patients with severe refractory asthma who remain unresponsive to other treatments.

β-Adrenergic agonists are frequently given to

patients with chronic obstructive pulmonary disease who have a reversible bronchoconstrictive component to their disease. Some of these patients may have a more favorable response to other drugs, particularly the muscarinic cholinergic antagonists or methylxanthines. It is important to assess the symptomatic and objective effects of treatment with bronchodilators before proceeding indefinitely with drugs that may have no efficacy and that may cause adverse effects in this patient population.

Allergic Reactions. Epinephrine is the drug of choice to reverse the manifestations of serious, acute hypersensitivity reactions (*e.g.*, from a food, bee sting, or drug allergy). A subcutaneous injection of epinephrine rapidly relieves itching, hives, and swelling of lips, eyelids, and the tongue. This treatment may be lifesaving when edema of the glottis threatens patency of the airway or when there is hypotension or shock. In addition to its cardiovascular effects, epinephrine is thought to activate β-adrenergic receptors that suppress the release of mediators such as histamine or leukotrienes from mast cells. Although glucocorticoids and antihistamines are frequently administered to patients with severe hypersensitivity reactions, epinephrine remains the mainstay of treatment.

Ophthalmic Uses. Local application of various sympathomimetic amines (*e.g.*, phenylephrine or epinephrine) to the conjunctiva is used to dilate the pupil, usually to permit adequate examination of the fundus. This effect may last for several hours. These drugs do not cause cycloplegia; however, there is a small risk of inducing acute narrow-angle glaucoma in susceptible patients. Drugs in this category may be used to prevent the formation of synechiae in uveitis. Epinephrine and phenylephrine also decrease intraocular pressure in patients with wide-angle glaucoma. Interestingly, both β-adrenergic agonists and antagonists are capable of lowering intraocular pressure in patients with glaucoma (Potter, 1981).

Narcolepsy. Narcolepsy is characterized by hypersomnia, including attacks of sleep that may occur suddenly under conditions that are not normally conducive to sleepiness. Some patients respond to treatment with tricyclic antidepressants or MAO inhibitors (Zarcone, 1973). Alternatively, CNS stimulants such as amphetamine, dextroamphetamine, or methamphetamine may be useful. Therapy with amphetamines is complicated by the risk of abuse and the likelihood of the development of tolerance. Depression, irritability, and paranoia may also occur. Amphetamines may disturb nocturnal sleep, which increases the difficulty in avoiding day-time attacks of sleep in these patients (Zarcone, 1973). Pemoline is an alternative.

Weight Reduction. Obesity arises as a consequence of positive caloric balance. Optimally, weight loss is achieved by a gradual increase in energy expenditure from exercise combined with dieting to decrease the caloric intake. However, this obvious approach has a relatively low success rate. Consequently, alternative forms of treatment including surgery or medications have been developed in an effort to increase the likelihood of achieving and maintaining weight loss. Amphetamine was found to produce weight loss in early studies of patients with narcolepsy and was subsequently used in the treatment of obesity (Silverstone, 1986). The drug promotes weight loss by suppressing appetite, rather than by increasing energy expenditure. Other anorexiant drugs include methamphetamine, phentermine, benzphetamine, phendimetrazine, phenmetrazine, diethylpropion, mazindol, fenfluramine, and phenylpropanolamine. In short-term (up to 20 weeks), double-blind, controlled studies, amphetamine-like drugs have been shown to be more effective than placebo in promoting weight loss; the rate of weight loss is typically increased by about 0.5 pound per week with these drugs. There is little to choose between these drugs in terms of efficacy (Bray, 1976). However, long-term efficacy has not been demonstrated. In addition, other important issues have not yet been resolved; these include the selection of patients who might be benefited by these drugs, whether the drugs should be administered continuously or intermittently, and the duration of treatment (Silverstone, 1986). Adverse effects of treatment include the potential for drug abuse and habituation, serious worsening of hypertension (although in some patients blood pressure may actually fall, presumably as a consequence of weight loss), sleep disturbances, palpitations, dry mouth, and depression (particularly with fenfluramine). These agents may be effective as adjuncts in the treatment of obese patients. However, available evidence does not support the isolated use of these drugs in the absence of a more comprehensive program that stresses exercise and modification of diet.

Attention-Deficit Hyperactivity Disorder (ADHD). This syndrome, usually first evident in childhood, is characterized by excessive motor activity, difficulty in sustaining attention, and impulsiveness. Children with this disorder are frequently troubled by academic difficulties, impaired interpersonal relationships, and excitability. Academic underachievement is an additional important characteristic. A substantial number of children with this syndrome have characteristics that persist into adulthood, although in modified form (American Psychiatric Association, 1987). Behavioral therapy may be helpful in some patients.

There is evidence that catecholamines may be involved in the control of attention at the level of the cerebral cortex. A variety of stimulant drugs have been utilized in the treatment of ADHD, and they are particularly indicated in moderate-to-severe cases. Dextroamphetamine has been demonstrated to be more effective than placebo (Klein *et al.*, 1980); methylphenidate is also effective in children with ADHD, although information about the long-term efficacy of both drugs is limited. Treatment may start with a dose of 5 mg of methylphenidate in the morning and at lunch; the dose is gradually increased over a period of weeks depending on the response as judged by parents, teachers, and the physician. The total daily dose generally should not exceed 60 mg; because of its short duration of action, most children require two or three doses each day. The timing of doses is adjusted individually in accordance with rapidity of onset of effect and duration of action. Some children may not respond, and the drug should be discontinued after 1 month of dosage adjustment. Methylphenidate and dextroamphetamine probably have similar efficacy in ADHD. Pemoline appears to be less effective, although it may be used once daily in some children (Klein *et al.*, 1980). Potential adverse effects of these medications in children include insomnia, abdominal pain, anorexia, and weight loss that may be associated with suppression of growth. Minor symptoms may be transient or may respond to adjustment of dosage or administration of the drug with meals. Other drugs that have been utilized include tricyclic antidepressants, antipsychotic agents, and clonidine. There is evidence that stimulant medications are effective in adults with similar disorders (Chiarello and Cole, 1987).

Ahrens, R. C., and Smith, G. D. Albuterol: an adrenergic agent for use in the treatment of asthma. Pharmacology, pharmacokinetics and clinical use. *Pharmacotherapy,* **1984,** *4,* 105–120.

Andersson, K.-E., and Bende, M. Adrenoceptors in the control of human nasal mucosal blood flow. *Ann. Otol. Rhinol. Laryngol.,* **1984,** *93,* 179–182.

Barger, G., and Dale, H. H. Chemical structure and sympathomimetic action of amines. *J. Physiol. (Lond.),* **1910,** *41,* 19–59.

Benfey, B. G. Function of myocardial alpha-adrenoceptors. *Life Sci.,* **1982,** *31,* 101–112.

Bertler, A.; Carlsson, A.; and Rosengren, E. Release by reserpine of catecholamines from rabbit hearts. *Naturwissenschaften,* **1956,** *43,* 521.

Blundell, J. E., and Leshem, M. B. Dissociation of the anorexic effects of fenfluramine and amphetamine following intrahypothalamic injection. *Br. J. Pharmacol.,* **1973,** *47,* 183–185.

Bravo, E. L.; Tarazi, R. C.; Fouad, R. M.; Vidt, D. G.; and Gifford, R. W. The clonidine suppression test: a useful aid in the diagnosis of pheochromocytoma. *N. Engl. J. Med.,* **1981,** *305,* 623–626.

Burn, J. H., and Rand, M. J. The action of sympathomimetic amines in animals treated with reserpine. *J. Physiol. (Lond.),* **1958,** *144,* 314–336.

Chang, E. B.; Fedorak, R. N.; and Field, M. Experimental diabetic diarrhea in rats: intestinal mucosal denervation hypersensitivity and treatment with clonidine. *Gastroenterology,* **1986,** *91,* 564–569.

Cole, P.; Haight, J. S. J.; Cooper, P. W.; and Kassel, E. E. A computed tomographic study of nasal mucosa: effects of vasoactive substances. *J. Otolaryngol.,* **1983,** *12,* 58–60.

DeBernardis, J. F.; Winn, M.; Kerkman, D. J.; Kyncl, J. J.; Buckner, S.; and Horrom, B. A new nasal decongestant, A-57219: a comparison with oxymetazoline. *J. Pharm. Pharmacol.,* **1987,** *39,* 760–763.

Dulfano, M. J., and Glass, P. The bronchodilator effects of terbutaline: route of administration and patterns of response. *Ann. Allergy,* **1976,** *37,* 357–366.

Fedorak, R. N.; Field, M.; and Chang, E. B. Treatment of diabetic diarrhea with clonidine. *Ann. Intern. Med.,* **1985,** *102,* 197–199.

Flacke, J. W.; Bloor, B. C.; Flacke, W. E.; Wong, S.; Dazza, S.; Stead, S. W.; and Laks, H. Reduced narcotic requirements by clonidine with improved hemodynamic and adrenergic stability in patients undergoing coronary bypass surgery. *Anesthesia,* **1987,** *67,* 11–19.

Garcia-Sainz, J. A. G.; Molina, R. V.; Corvera, S.; Bahena, J. H.; Tsujimoto, G.; and Hoffman, B. B. Differential effects of adrenergic agonists and phorbol esters on the alpha-adrenoceptors of hepatocytes and aorta. *Eur. J. Pharmacol.,* **1985,** *112,* 393–397.

Glassman, A. H.; Jackson, W. K.; Walsh, B. T.; Roose, S. P.; and Rosenfeld, B. Cigarette craving, smoking withdrawal, and clonidine. *Science,* **1984,** *226,* 864–866.

Glassman, A. H.; Stetner, F.; Walsh, B. T.; Raizman, P. S.; Fleiss, J. L.; Cooper, T. B.; and Covey, L. S. Heavy smokers, smoking cessation, and clonidine. Results of a double-blind, randomized trial. *J.A.M.A.,* **1988,** *259,* 2863–2866.

Gold, M. S.; Redmond, D. E.; and Kleber, H. D. Clonidine blocks acute opiate withdrawal symptoms. *Lancet,* **1978,** *2,* 599–602.

Goldberg, L. I., and Rajfer, E. I. Dopamine receptors: applications in clinical cardiology. *Circulation,* **1985,** *72,* 245–248.

Goldenberg, M.; Aranow, H., Jr.; Smith, A. A.; and Faber, M. Pheochromocytoma and essential hypertensive vascular disease. *Arch. Intern. Med.,* **1950,** *86,* 823–836.

Hartung, W. H. Epinephrine and related compounds: influence of structure on physiologic activity. *Chem. Rev.,* **1931,** *9,* 389–465.

Holmes, B.; Brogden, R. N.; Heel, R. C.; Speight, T. M.; and Avery, G. S. Guanabenz. A review of its pharmacodynamic properties and therapeutic efficacy in hypertension. *Drugs,* **1983,** *26,* 212–229.

Houben, H.; Thien, T.; and van't Laar, A. Effect of low-dose epinephrine infusion on hemodynamics after selective and nonselective beta-blockade in hypertension. *Clin. Pharmacol. Ther.,* **1982,** *31,* 685–690.

Hughes, J. M.; Seale, J. P.; and Temple, D. M. Effect of fenoterol on immunological release of leukotrienes and histamine from human lung *in vitro*: selective antagonism by beta-adrenoceptor antagonists. *Eur. J. Pharmacol.,* **1983,** *95,* 239–245.

Kelly, H. W. New beta$_2$-adrenergic agonist aerosols. *Clin. Pharm.,* **1985,** *4,* 393–403.

Musacchio, J. M.; Kopin, I. J.; and Weise, V. K. Subcellular distribution of some sympathomimetic amines and their β-hydroxylated derivatives in the rat heart. *J. Pharmacol. Exp. Ther.,* **1965,** *148,* 22–28.

Nagamani, M.; Kelver, M. E.; and Smith, E. R. Treatment of menopausal hot flashes with transdermal administration of clonidine. *Am. J. Obstet. Gynecol.,* **1987,** *156,* 561–565.

Oliver, G., and Schäfer, E. A. The physiological effects of extracts from the suprarenal capsules. *J. Physiol. (Lond.),* **1895,** *18,* 230–276.

Robertson, D.; Goldberg, M. R.; Hollister, A. S.; Wade, D.; and Robertson, R. M. Clonidine raises blood pressure in severe idiopathic orthostatic hypotension. *Am J. Med.,* **1983,** *74,* 193–200.

Ruffolo, R. R., Jr.; Spradlin, T. A.; Pollock, G. D.; Waddell, J. E.; and Murphy, P. J. Alpha and beta adrenergic effects of the stereoisomers of dobutamine. *J. Pharmacol. Exp. Ther.,* **1981,** *219,* 447–452.

Ruffolo, R. R., Jr., and Yaden, E. M. Vascular effects of the stereoisomers of dobutamine. *J. Pharmacol. Exp. Ther.,* **1983,** *224,* 46–50.

Schumann, H. J.; Wagner, J.; Knorr, A.; Reidemeister, J. C.; Sadony, V.; and Schramm, G. Demonstration in human atrial preparations of alpha-adrenoceptors mediating positive inotropic effects. *Naunyn Schmiedebergs Arch. Pharmacol.,* **1978,** *302,* 333–336.

Snider, R. M., and Gerald, M. C. Studies on the mechanism of (+)-amphetamine enhancement of neuromuscu-

lar transmission: muscle contraction, electrophysiological and biochemical results. *J. Pharmacol. Exp. Ther.*, **1982**, *221*, 14–21.
Sonnenblick, E. H.; Frishman, W. H.; and LeJemtel, T. H. Dobutamine: a new synthetic cardioactive sympathetic amine. *N. Engl. J. Med.*, **1979**, *300*, 17–22.
Strader, C. D.; Candelore, M. R.; Hill, W. S.; Sigal, I. S.; and Dixon, R. A. F. Identification of two serine residues involved in agonist activation of the β-adrenergic receptor. *J. Biol. Chem.*, **1989**, *264*, 13572–13578.
Unverferth, D. V.; Blanford, M.; Dates, R. E.; and Leier, C. V. Tolerance to dobutamine after a 72 hour continuous infusion. *Am. J. Med.*, **1980**, *69*, 262–266.

Monographs and Reviews

Allwood, M. J.; Cobbold, A. F.; and Ginsburg, J. Peripheral vascular effects of noradrenaline, isopropylnoradrenaline and dopamine. *Br. Med. Bull.*, **1963**, *19*, 132–136.
American Psychiatric Association. Attention-deficit hyperactivity disorder. In, *Diagnostic and Statistical Manual of Mental Disorders*, 3rd ed., rev. American Psychiatric Association, Washington, D.C., **1987**, pp. 50–53.
Angrist, B. M., and Gershon, S. Psychiatric sequelae of amphetamine use. In, *Psychiatric Complications of Medical Drugs*. (Shader, R. I., ed.) Raven Press, New York, **1972**, pp. 175–199.
Aviado, D. M., Jr. *Sympathomimetic Drugs*. Charles C Thomas, Publisher, Springfield, Ill., **1970**.
Balakumaran, D., and Hugenholtz, P. G. Cardiogenic shock. Current concepts in management. *Drugs*, **1986**, *32*, 372–382.
Berne, R. M.; Winn, H. R.; Knabb, R. M.; Ely, S. W.; and Rubio, R. Blood flow regulation by adenosine in heart, brain, and skeletal muscle. In, *Regulatory Function of Adenosine*. (Berne, R. M.; Rall, T. W.; and Rubio, R.; eds.) Martinus Nijhoff, Boston, **1983**, pp. 293–317.
Bond, W. S. Psychiatric indications for clonidine: the neuropharmacologic and clinical basis. *J. Clin. Psychopharmacol.*, **1986**, *6*, 81–87.
Bowman, W. C. Effects of adrenergic activators and inhibitors on the skeletal muscles. In, *Adrenergic Activators and Inhibitors*. (Szekeres, L., ed.) *Handbook of Experimental Pharmacology*, Vol. 54, Pt. II. Springer-Verlag, Berlin, **1981**, pp. 47–128.
Bray, G. A. *The Obese Patient*, Vol. IX. *Major Problems in Internal Medicine*. (Smith, L. H., ed.) W. B. Saunders Co., Philadelphia, **1976**, pp. 353–410.
Bristow, M. R.; Kantrowitz, N. E.; Ginsburg, R.; and Fowler, M. B. Beta adrenergic functions in heart muscle disease and heart failure. *J. Mol. Cell Cardiol.*, **1985**, *17*, Suppl. 2, 41–52.
Caritis, S. N. Treatment of preterm labour. A review of therapeutic options. *Drugs*, **1983**, *26*, 243–261.
Chen, K. K., and Schmidt, C. F. Ephedrine and related substances. *Medicine (Baltimore)*, **1930**, *9*, 1–117.
Chernow, B., and Roth, B. L. Pharmacologic manipulation of the peripheral vasculature in shock: clinical and experimental approaches. *Circ. Shock*, **1986**, *18*, 141–155.
Chiarello, R. H., and Cole, J. O. The use of psychostimulants in general psychiatry. *Arch. Gen. Psychiatry*, **1987**, *44*, 286–295.
Ellis, S. Effects on the metabolism. In, *Adrenergic Activators and Inhibitors*. (Szekeres, L., ed.) *Handbook of Experimental Pharmacology*, Vol. 54, Pt. I. Springer-Verlag, Berlin, **1980**, pp. 319–349.
Empey, D. W., and Medder, K. T. Nasal decongestants. *Drugs*, **1981**, *21*, 438–443.
Francis, G. S., and Cohn, J. N. The autonomic nervous system in congestive heart failure. *Annu. Rev. Med.*, **1986**, *37*, 235–247.
Friedel, H. A., and Brogden, R. N. Bitolterol: a preliminary review of its pharmacological properties and therapeutic efficacy in reversible obstructive airways disease. *Drugs*, **1988**, *35*, 22–41.
Grant, W. M. Action of drugs on movement of ocular fluids. *Annu. Rev. Pharmacol.*, **1969**, *9*, 85–94.
Higgins, T. L., and Chernow, B. Pharmacotherapy of circulatory shock. *Dis. Mon.*, **1987**, *33*, 309–361.
Himms-Hagen, J. Effects of catecholamines on metabolism. In, *Catecholamines*. (Blaschko, H., and Muscholl, E., eds.) *Handbuch der Experimentellen Pharmakologie*, Vol. 33. Springer-Verlag, Berlin, **1972**, pp. 363–462.
Jenne, J. W. Whither beta-adrenergic tachyphylaxis? *J. Allergy Clin. Immunol.*, **1982**, *70*, 413–416.
Klein, D. F.; Gittleman, R.; Quitkin, F.; and Rifkin, A. Diagnosis and drug treatment of childhood disorders. In, *Diagnosis and Drug Treatment of Psychiatric Disorders: Adults and Children*, 2nd ed. The Williams & Wilkins Co., Baltimore, **1980**, pp. 590–775.
Kobinger, W. Central alpha-adrenergic systems as targets for hypotensive drugs. *Rev. Physiol. Biochem. Pharmacol.*, **1978**, *81*, 39–100.
Kopin, I. J. False adrenergic transmitters. *Annu. Rev. Pharmacol.*, **1968**, *8*, 377–394.
Krell, M. J.; Kline, E. M.; Bates, E. R.; Hodgson, J. M.; Dilworth, L. R.; Lanfer, N.; Vogel, R. A.; and Pitt, B. A. Intermittent ambulatory dobutamine infusions in patients with severe congestive heart failure. *Am. Heart J.*, **1986**, *112*, 787–791.
Langer, S. Z.; Cavero, I.; and Massingham, R. Recent developments in noradrenergic neurotransmission and its relevance to the mechanism of action of certain antihypertensive agents. *Hypertension*, **1980**, *2*, 372–382.
Langley, M. S., and Heel, R. C. Transdermal clonidine: a preliminary review of its pharmacodynamic properties and therapeutic efficacy. *Drugs*, **1988**, *35*, 123–142.
Leier, C. V. Dobutamine. *Ann. Intern. Med.*, **1983**, *99*, 490–496.
Lowenthal, D. T.; Matzek, K. M.; and MacGregor, T. R. Clinical pharmacokinetics of clonidine. *Clin. Pharmacokinet.* **1988**, *14*, 287–310.
Lulich, K. M.; Goldie, R. G.; Ryan, G.; and Paterson, J. W. Adverse reactions to beta$_2$-agonist bronchodilators. *Med. Toxicol.*, **1986**, *1*, 286–299.
Maze, M.; Segal, I. S.; and Bloor, B. C. Clonidine and other alpha$_2$ adrenergic agonists: strategies for the rational use of these novel anesthetic agents. *J. Clin. Anesth.*, **1988**, *1*, 146–157.
Nelson, H. S. Beta adrenergic agonists. *Chest*, **1982**, *82*, Suppl., 33S–38S.
———. Adrenergic therapy of bronchial asthma. *J. Allergy Clin. Immunol.*, **1986**, *77*, 771–785.
Newhouse, M. T., and Dolovich, M. B. Control of asthma by aerosols. *N. Engl. J. Med.*, **1986**, *315*, 870–874.
Oswald, I. Drugs and sleep. *Pharmacol. Rev.*, **1968**, *20*, 273–303.
Parker, M., and Atkinson, J. Withdrawal syndromes following cessation of treatment with antihypertensive drugs. *Gen. Pharmacol.*, **1982**, *13*, 79–85.
Potter, D. E. Adrenergic pharmacology of aqueous humor dynamics. *Pharmacol. Rev.*, **1981**, *33*, 133–153.
Raehl, C. L. Advances in drug therapy of cardiopulmonary arrest. *Clin. Pharm.*, **1987**, *6*, 118–139.
Richards, D. M., and Brogden, R. N. Pirbuterol: a preliminary review of its pharmacological properties and therapeutic efficacy in reversible bronchospastic disease. *Drugs* **1985**, *30*, 6–21.
Ruffolo, R. R. Review: the pharmacology of dobutamine. *Am. J. Med. Sci.*, **1987**, *294*, 244–248.
Seale, J. P. Whither beta-adrenoceptor agonists in the treatment of asthma? *Prog. Clin. Biol. Res.*, **1988**, *263*, 367–377.

Silverstone, T. Clinical use of appetite suppressants. *Drug Alcohol Depend.*, **1986,** *17,* 151–167.

Sorkin, E. M., and Heel, R. C. Guanfacine. A review of its pharmacodynamic and pharmacokinetic properties and therapeutic efficacy in the treatment of hypertension. *Drugs,* **1986,** *31,* 301–336.

Tattersfield, A. E. Tolerance to beta-agonists. *Bull. Eur. Physiopathol. Respir.*, **1985,** *21,* 1s–5s.

Trendelenburg, U. Factors infuencing the concentration of catecholamines at the receptors. In, *Catecholamines.* (Blaschko, H., and Muscholl, E., eds.) *Handbuch der Experimentellen Pharmakologie,* Vol. 33, Springer-Verlag, Berlin, **1972,** pp. 726–761.

Weiner, N. Pharmacology of central nervous system stimulants. In, *Drug Abuse: Proceedings of the International Conference.* (Zarafonetis, C. J. D., ed.) Lea & Febiger, Philadelphia, **1972,** pp. 243–251.

———. The role of cyclic nucleotides in the regulation of neurotransmitter release from adrenergic neurons by neuromodulators. In, *Essays in Neurochemistry and Neuropharmacology,* Vol. 4. (Youdim, M. B. H.; Lovenberg, W.; Sharman, D. F.; and Lagnado, J. R.; eds.) John Wiley & Sons, Inc., New York, **1980,** pp. 69–124.

Weiss, B., and Laties, V. G. Enhancement of human performance by caffeine and the amphetamines. *Pharmacol. Rev.*, **1962,** *14,* 1–36.

Zarcone, V. Narcolepsy. *N. Engl. J. Med.*, **1973,** *288,* 1156–1166.

CHAPTER

11 ADRENERGIC RECEPTOR ANTAGONISTS

Brian B. Hoffman and Robert J. Lefkowitz

There are many types of drugs that interfere with the function of the sympathetic nervous system and, thus, have profound effects on the physiology of sympathetically innervated organs. Several of these drugs are important in clinical medicine, particularly for the treatment of cardiovascular diseases. Drugs that decrease the amount of norepinephrine released as a consequence of sympathetic nerve stimulation are discussed in Chapter 33. Drugs that inhibit sympathetic nervous activity by suppressing sympathetic outflow from the brain are discussed in Chapters 10 and 33.

This chapter focuses on drugs termed adrenergic receptor antagonists, since they inhibit the interaction of norepinephrine, epinephrine, and other sympathomimetic drugs with adrenergic receptors. Almost all of the drugs considered herein are competitive antagonists in their interactions with either α- or β-adrenergic receptors; one exception is phenoxybenzamine, an irreversible antagonist that binds covalently to α-adrenergic receptors. There are important structural differences among the various types of adrenergic receptors (*see* Chapter 5). Since compounds have been developed that have different affinities for the various receptors, it is possible to interfere selectively with responses that result from stimulation of the sympathetic nervous system. For example, selective antagonists of β_1-adrenergic receptors block most actions of epinephrine and norepinephrine on the heart, while having less effect on β_2-adrenergic receptors in bronchial smooth muscle and no effect on vasoconstrictor responses mediated by α_1- or α_2-adrenergic receptors. A detailed knowledge of the autonomic nervous system and the sites of action of drugs that act on adrenergic receptors is essential for understanding the pharmacology and therapeutic uses of this important class of drugs. This background material is presented in Chapters 5 and 10. Because of their unique activity in the central nervous system (CNS), drugs that block dopaminergic receptors are considered in Chapter 18.

I. α-Adrenergic Receptor Antagonists

α-Adrenergic receptors mediate many of the important actions of endogenous catecholamines. Responses of particular relevance include α_1 receptor-mediated contraction of arterial and venous smooth muscle. α_2-Adrenergic receptors are involved in suppressing sympathetic output, increasing vagal tone, facilitating platelet aggregation, inhibiting the release of norepinephrine and acetylcholine from nerve endings, and regulating metabolic effects (such as suppression of insulin secretion and inhibition of lipolysis); α_2 receptors also mediate contraction of some arteries and veins.

α-Adrenergic antagonists have a wide spectrum of pharmacological specificities and are heterogeneous chemically. Some of these drugs have markedly different affinities for α_1 and α_2 receptors. For example, prazosin is much more potent in blocking α_1 than α_2 receptors (and is termed α_1 selective), whereas yohimbine is α_2 selective; phentolamine has similar affinity for both of these receptor subtypes. In addition, some of these drugs (*e.g.*, phenoxybenzamine) may have additional actions that are unrelated to adrenergic receptor blockade.

Chemistry. The structural formulas of a number of α-adrenergic antagonists are shown in Table 11–1. Although structurally diverse, these drugs can be divided into four groups: β-haloethylamine alkylating agents, imidazoline analogs, piperazinyl quinazolines, and indole derivatives.

Table 11–1. STRUCTURAL FORMULAS OF α-ADRENERGIC ANTAGONISTS

Alkylating agents

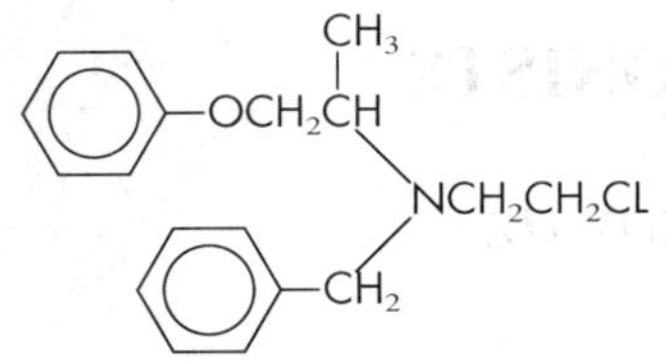

Phenoxybenzamine

Imidazolines

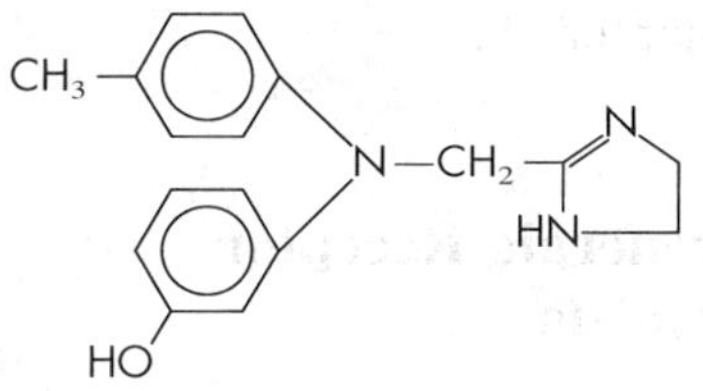

Phentolamine

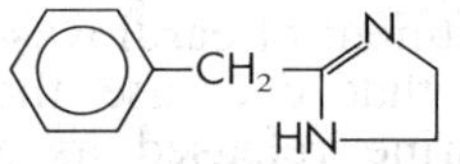

Tolazoline

Piperazinyl quinazolines

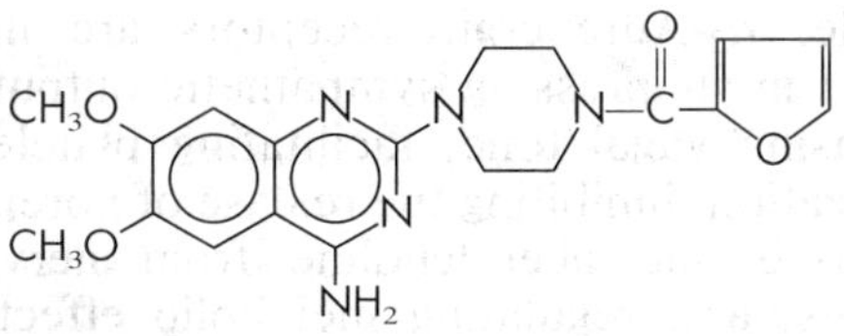

Prazosin

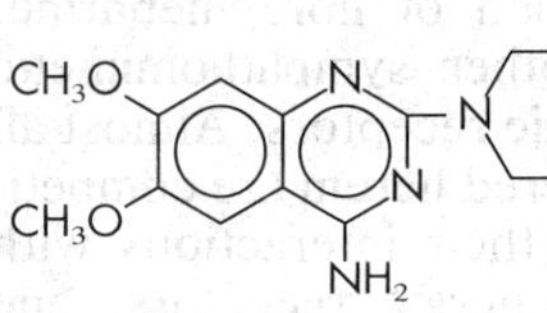

Terazosin

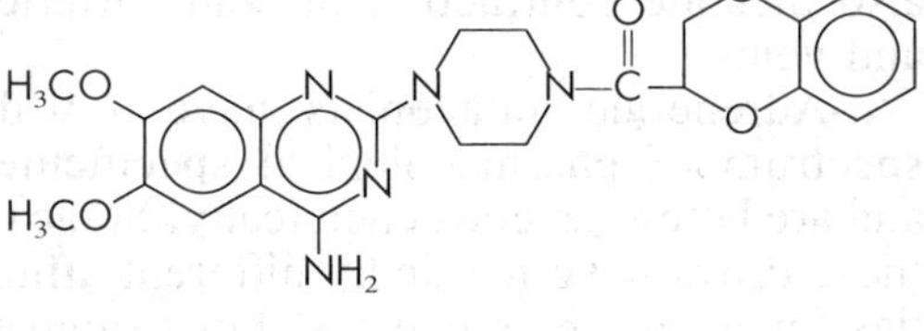

Doxazosin

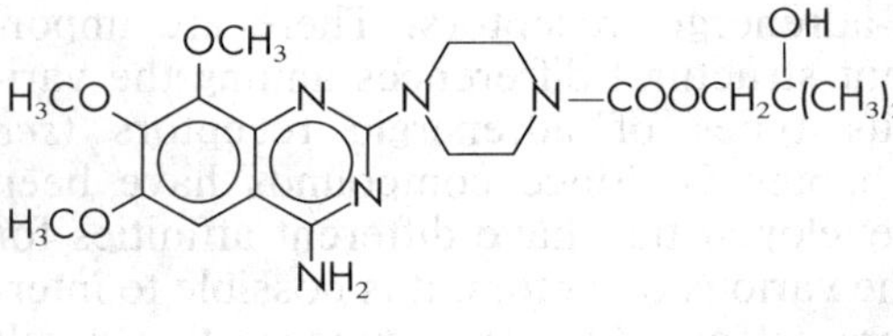

Trimazosin

Indoles

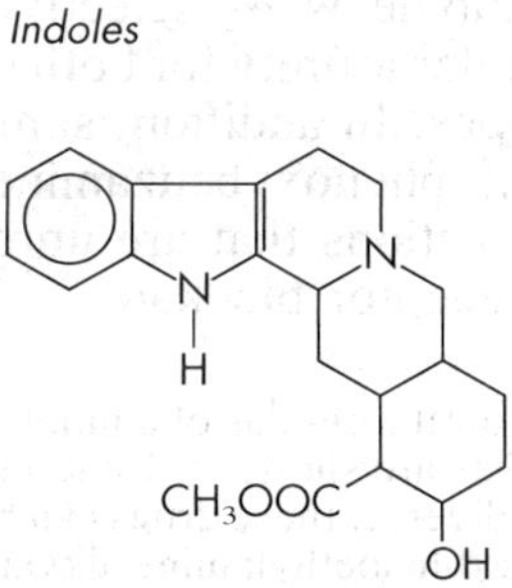

Yohimbine

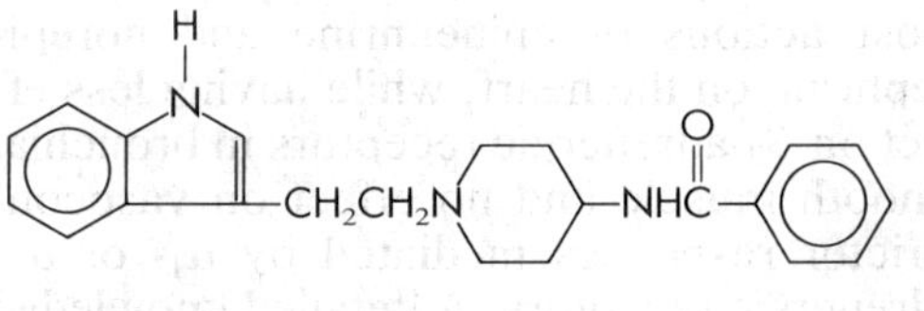

Indoramin

PHARMACOLOGICAL PROPERTIES

Cardiovascular System. The most important effects of α-adrenergic antagonists observed clinically are on the cardiovascular system. Actions in both the CNS and the periphery are involved, and the outcome depends on the cardiovascular status of the patient at the time of drug administration and the relative selectivity of the agent for α_1 or α_2 receptors.

α_1-Adrenergic Antagonists. Blockade of α_1-adrenergic receptors inhibits vasoconstriction induced by endogenous catecholamines; vasodilatation may occur in both arteriolar resistance vessels and veins. The result is a fall in blood pressure because of decreased peripheral vascular resistance. The magnitude of such effects depends on the activity of the sympathetic nervous system at the time the antagonist is administered and, thus, is less in supine than in upright subjects and is particularly marked if there is hypovolemia. For most α-adrenergic antagonists, the fall in blood pressure is opposed by baroreceptor reflexes that cause increases in heart rate and cardiac output, as well as fluid retention. These reflexes are exaggerated if the antagonist also blocks α_2 receptors on peripheral sympathetic nerve endings, leading to enhanced release of norepinephrine and increased stimulation of postsynaptic β_1 receptors in the heart and the juxtaglomerular cells (Langer, 1981; Starke, 1981; *see also* Chapter 5). Although stimulation of α_1-adrenergic receptors in the heart may cause an increased force of contraction, the importance of blockade at this site is uncertain.

Blockade of α_1-adrenergic receptors also inhibits vasoconstriction and the increase in blood pressure produced by the administration of a sympathomimetic amine. The pattern of effects depends upon the adrenergic agonist that is administered: pressor responses to phenylephrine can be completely suppressed; those to norepinephrine are only incompletely blocked because of residual stimulation of cardiac β_1 receptors; and pressor responses to epinephrine may be transformed to vasodepressor effects (epinephrine "reversal") because of residual stimulation of β_2 receptors in the vasculature with resultant vasodilatation.

α_2-Adrenergic Antagonists. α_2-Adrenergic receptors have an important role in regulation of the activity of the sympathetic nervous system, both peripherally and centrally. As mentioned above, activation of presynaptic α_2 receptors inhibits the release of norepinephrine from peripheral sympathetic nerve endings. Activation of α_2 receptors in the pontomedullary region of the CNS inhibits sympathetic nervous system activity and leads to a fall in blood pressure; these receptors are a site of action of drugs such as clonidine (*see* Chapter 10). Blockade of α_2-adrenergic receptors with selective antagonists such as yohimbine can thus increase sympathetic outflow and potentiate the release of norepinephrine from nerve endings, leading to activation of α_1 and β_1 receptors in the heart and peripheral vasculature with a consequent rise in blood pressure (Goldberg and Robertson, 1983). Antagonists that also block α_1 receptors give rise to similar effects on sympathetic outflow and release of norepinephrine, but the net increase in blood pressure is prevented by inhibition of vasoconstriction.

Although certain vascular beds contain α_2-adrenergic receptors that promote contraction of smooth muscle, it is thought that these receptors are preferentially stimulated by circulating catecholamines, whereas α_1 receptors are activated by norepinephrine released from sympathetic nerve fibers (Davey, 1987; van Zwieten, 1988). In other vascular beds, α_2 receptors promote vasodilatation by stimulating the release of endothelium-derived relaxing factor (Miller and Vanhoutte, 1985). However, the physiological role of vascular α_2-adrenergic receptors in the regulation of blood flow within various vascular beds is uncertain (Cubeddu, 1988), and the effects of α_2-adrenergic antagonists on the cardiovascular system are dominated by actions in the CNS and on sympathetic nerve endings.

Other Actions of α-Adrenergic Antagonists. α-Adrenergic antagonists can block α receptors that mediate contraction of nonvascular smooth muscle. For example, contraction of the trigone and sphincter muscles in the base of the urinary bladder may be inhibited, leading to decreased resistance to urinary outflow. Although α receptors may promote contraction of bronchial smooth muscle, the importance of this effect is minimal. Catecholamines increase the output of glucose from the liver; in man, this effect is mediated predominantly by β-adrenergic receptors, although α receptors may contribute (Rosen *et al.,* 1983). α_2-Adrenergic receptors facilitate platelet aggregation; the effect of blockade of these receptors *in vivo* is not clear. Activation of α_2 receptors in the pancreatic islets greatly suppresses insulin secretion; blockade of these receptors may facilitate insulin release (Kashiwagi *et al.,* 1986).

PHENOXYBENZAMINE AND RELATED HALOALKYLAMINES

Phenoxybenzamine and dibenamine are haloalkylamines that block α_1- and α_2-adrenergic receptors irreversibly. Although phenoxybenzamine may have slight selectivity for α_1 receptors, it is not clear if this has any significance in man.

Chemistry. Dibenamine is N,N-dibenzyl-β-chloroethylamine and differs from phenoxybenzamine only in the replacement of the phenoxyisopropyl moiety with a benzyl group. The haloalkylamine adrenergic blocking drugs are closely related chemically to the nitrogen mustards; like the latter, the tertiary amine cyclizes with the loss of chlorine to form a reactive ethyleniminium or aziridinium ion (*see* Chapter 52). The molecular configuration directly responsible for blockade is probably a highly reactive carbonium ion formed upon cleavage of the three-membered ring. It is presumed that the arylalkyl amine moiety of the molecule is responsible for the relative specificity of action of these agents, since the reactive intermediate can likely react with sulfhydryl, amino, and carboxyl groups in many proteins. Because of these chemical reactions, phenoxybenzamine is covalently conjugated with α-adrenergic receptors. Consequently, receptor blockade is uniquely irreversible, and restoration of cellular responsiveness to α-adrenergic agonists probably requires the synthesis of new receptors.

PHARMACOLOGICAL PROPERTIES

The major effects of phenoxybenzamine result from blockade of α-adrenergic receptors in smooth muscle. Phenoxybenzamine causes a progressive decrease in peripheral resistance and an increase in cardiac output that is due, in part, to reflex sympathetic nerve stimulation. Tachycardia may be accentuated by enhanced release of norepinephrine (because of α_2 blockade) and decreased inactivation of the amine because of inhibition of neuronal and extraneuronal uptake mechanisms (*see* below; *see also* Chapter 5). Pressor responses to exogenously administered catecholamines are impaired. Indeed, hypotensive responses to epinephrine occur because of unopposed β-adrenergic receptor-mediated vasodilatation. Although phenoxybenzamine has relatively little effect on supine blood pressure in normotensive subjects, there is a marked fall in blood pressure on standing because of antagonism of compensatory vasoconstriction. In addition, the ability to respond to hypovolemia and anesthetic-induced vasodilatation is impaired.

Phenoxybenzamine inhibits the uptake of catecholamines into both adrenergic nerve terminals and extraneuronal tissues (Cubeddu *et al.,* 1974). In addition to blockade of α-adrenergic receptors, substituted β-haloalkylamines irreversibly inhibit responses to 5-hydroxytryptamine (5-HT), histamine, and acetylcholine. However, somewhat higher doses of phenoxybenzamine are required to observe these effects as compared with those that produce blockade of α-adrenergic receptors. The general pharmacology of the haloalkylamines has been reviewed by Nickerson and Hollenberg (1967) and Furchgott (1972); a more detailed discussion can be found in *earlier editions* of this textbook.

The pharmacokinetic properties of phenoxybenzamine are not well understood. Absorption from the gastrointestinal tract is incomplete and variable, and only about 20 to 30% of the drug is absorbed in an active form after oral administration. The half-life of phenoxybenzamine is probably less than 24 hours. However, since the drug inactivates α-adrenergic receptors irreversibly, the duration of its effect is dependent not only on its presence but also on the rate of synthesis of α-adrenergic receptors. Many days may be required before the number of functional α-adrenergic receptors on the surface of target cells returns to normal (Hamilton *et al.,* 1982). However, blunted maximal responses to catecholamines may not be as persistent, since there are so-called "spare" α_1 receptors in vascular smooth muscle (Hamilton *et al.,* 1983).

Preparations, Routes of Administration, and Dosage. *Phenoxybenzamine hydrochloride* (DIBENZYLINE) is available in 10-mg capsules for oral use. The dosage for the treatment of pheochromocytoma is discussed below. For the treatment of urinary obstruction due to prostatic hypertrophy, the dose is usually 20 mg per day or less.

Therapeutic Uses. A major use of phenoxybenzamine is in the treatment of pheochromocytoma. Pheochromocytomas are tumors of the adrenal medulla and sympathetic neurons that secrete enormous quantities of catecholamines into the circulation. The usual result is hypertension, which may be episodic and severe. The vast majority of pheochromocytomas are treated surgically; however, phenoxybenzamine is frequently used to treat the patient in preparation for surgery. The drug controls episodes of severe hypertension and minimizes other adverse effects of catecholamines, such as contraction of plasma volume and injury of the myocardium. A conservative approach is to initiate treatment with phenoxybenzamine (at a dosage of 10 mg twice daily) 1 to 3 weeks before the operation. The dose is increased every other day until the desired effect on blood pressure is achieved. Therapy may be limited by postural hypotension; nasal stuffiness is another frequent side effect. The usual total daily dose of phenoxybenzamine in patients with pheochromocytoma is 40 to 120 mg given in two or three divided portions. Prolonged treatment with phenoxybenzamine may be necessary in patients with inoperable or malignant pheochromocytoma. In some patients, particularly those with malignant disease, administration of metyrosine may be a useful adjuvant (Brogden *et al.*, 1984). Metyrosine is a competitive inhibitor of tyrosine hydroxylase, the rate-limiting enzyme in the synthesis of catecholamines (*see* Chapters 5 and 33). β-Adrenergic antagonists are also used to treat pheochromocytoma, but only *after* the administration of an α blocker (*see* below).

Phenoxybenzamine is effective for the management of benign prostatic obstruction. Although surgery remains the definitive treatment, phenoxybenzamine may be useful in some patients who are not candidates for surgery, since blockade of α_1-adrenergic receptors in the prostate and bladder base may decrease both obstructive symptoms and the need to urinate at night (Caine *et al.*, 1981; Caine, 1985). The usual dosage is 10 or 20 mg per day, much lower than that required to treat pheochromocytoma. Phenoxybenzamine has been used to control the manifestations of autonomic hyperreflexia in patients with spinal cord transection (Sizemore and Winternitz, 1970).

Toxicity and Adverse Effects. The major adverse effect of phenoxybenzamine is postural hypotension. This is often accompanied by reflex tachycardia and other arrhythmias. Hypotension can be particularly severe in hypovolemic patients or under conditions that promote vasodilatation (administration of vasodilator drugs, exercise, ingestion of alcohol or large quantities of food). Reversible inhibition of ejaculation and aspermia after orgasm may occur because of impaired smooth muscle contraction in the vas deferens and ejaculatory ducts. Phenoxybenzamine has mutagenic activity in the Ames test, and repeated administration of phenoxybenzamine to experimental animals causes peritoneal sarcomas and lung tumors (IARC, 1980). The clinical significance of these findings is not known.

PHENTOLAMINE AND TOLAZOLINE

Phentolamine, an imidazoline, is a competitive α-adrenergic antagonist that has similar affinity for α_1 and α_2 receptors. As such, its effects on the cardiovascular system are very similar to those of phenoxybenzamine. Phentolamine can also block receptors for 5-HT, and it releases histamine from mast cells. Tolazoline is a related but somewhat less potent compound. Tolazoline and phentolamine stimulate gastrointestinal smooth muscle, an effect that is antagonized by atropine, and they also enhance gastric acid secretion. Tolazoline stimulates secretion by salivary, lacrimal, and sweat glands as well.

The pharmacokinetic properties of phentolamine are not known, although the drug is metabolized extensively. Tolazoline is well absorbed after oral administration and is excreted in the urine.

Preparations, Routes of Administration, and Dosage. *Phentolamine mesylate* (REGITINE) is available in 5-mg vials for intravenous or intramuscular administration. *Tolazoline hydrochloride* (PRISCOLINE) is available at a concentration of 25 mg/ml for intravenous injection.

Therapeutic Uses. Phentolamine is used in the short term to control hypertension in patients with pheochromocytoma. Rapid infusions of phentolamine may cause severe hypotension, and the drug should be administered cautiously; the usual dose is 5 mg. Phentolamine may also be useful to relieve pseudo-obstruction of the bowel in patients with pheochromocytoma; this condition may result from the inhibitory effects of catecholamines on intestinal smooth muscle. Phentolamine has been used locally to prevent dermal necrosis after the inadvertent extravasation of an α-adrenergic agonist. The drug may also be useful for the treatment of hypertensive crises that follow the abrupt withdrawal of clonidine or that may result from the ingestion of tyramine-containing foods during the use of nonselective inhibitors of monoamine oxidase (*see* Chapter 18). Although excessive activation of α-adrenergic receptors has an important role in the development of severe hypertension in these settings, there is little information comparing the safety and efficacy of phentolamine with that of other antihypertensive agents in the treatment of such patients. Direct, intracavernous injection of phentolamine (in combination with papaverine) has been proposed as a treatment for male sexual dysfunction (Sidi, 1988; Zentgraf *et al.*, 1988). The long-term efficacy of this treatment is not known. Intracavernous injection of phentolamine may cause orthostatic hypotension and priapism; pharmacological reversal of drug-induced erections can be achieved with an α-adrenergic agonist such as phenylephrine. Repetitive intrapenile injections may cause fibrotic reactions (Sidi, 1988). Tolazoline has been used in the treatment of persistent pulmonary hypertension of the newborn.

Toxicity and Adverse Effects. Hypotension is the major adverse effect of phentolamine. In addition, reflex cardiac stimulation may cause alarming tachycardia, cardiac arrhythmias, and ischemic cardiac events, including myocardial infarction. Gastrointestinal stimulation may result in abdominal pain, nausea, and exacerbation of peptic ulcer. Phentolamine should be used with particular caution in patients with coronary artery disease or a history of peptic ulcer.

PRAZOSIN AND RELATED DRUGS

Prazosin, the prototype of a family of agents that contain a piperazinyl quinazoline nucleus, is a very potent and selective α_1-adrenergic antagonist. Its affinity for α_1 receptors is about 1000-fold greater than that for α_2 receptors. Interestingly, the drug is also a relatively potent inhibitor of cyclic nucleotide phosphodiesterases, and it was originally synthesized for this purpose (Hess, 1975). The pharmacological properties of prazosin have been characterized extensively, and the drug is used frequently for the treatment of hypertension (*see* Chapter 33).

PHARMACOLOGICAL PROPERTIES.

Prazosin. The major effects of prazosin are a result of its blockade of α_1-adrenergic receptors in arterioles and veins. This leads to a fall in peripheral vascular resistance and in venous return to the heart. Administration of prazosin usually does not increase heart rate, a response that occurs frequently with other vasodilating drugs. Since prazosin has little or no α_2 blocking effects at concentrations achieved clinically, it probably does not promote the release of norepinephrine from sympathetic nerve endings in the heart. In addition, prazosin decreases cardiac preload and thus has little tendency to increase cardiac output and rate, in contrast to vasodilators such as hydralazine that have minimal dilatory effects on veins. Although the combination of reduced preload and selective α_1 receptor blockade might be sufficient to account for the relative absence of reflex tachycardia, prazosin may also have an action in the central nervous system (CNS) to suppress sympathetic outflow (*see* Cubeddu, 1988). Prazosin does appear to depress baroreflex function in hypertensive patients (Sasso and O'Connor, 1982; Elliott *et al.*, 1988).

Prazosin is well absorbed after oral administration, and bioavailability is about 70%. Peak concentrations of prazosin in plasma are generally reached 1 to 3 hours after an oral dose. The drug is tightly bound to plasma proteins (primarily α_1-acid-glycoprotein), and only 5% of the drug is free in the circulation; diseases that modify the concentration of this protein (*e.g.*, inflammatory processes) may change the free fraction (Rubin and Blaschke, 1980). Prazosin is extensively metabolized in the liver, and little unchanged drug is excreted by the kidneys. The plasma half-life is 3 hours, and the duration of action of the drug is 4 to 6 hours.

Terazosin. Terazosin is a close structural analog of prazosin. It is less potent than prazosin but retains high specificity for α_1 receptors. The major distinctions between the two drugs involve their pharmacokinetic properties. Terazosin is more soluble in water than is prazosin, and its bioavailability is high (> 90%) (Cubeddu, 1988; Frishman *et al.*, 1988); this may facilitate titration of dosage (Titmarsh and Monk, 1987). Furthermore, the half-time for elimination of terazosin is approximately 12 hours, and its duration of action may extend beyond 18 hours. Thus, the drug may be taken once daily to control hypertension in many patients. Only about 10% of terazosin is excreted unchanged in the urine.

Doxazosin. Doxazosin is another structural analog of prazosin. It too is a highly selective antagonist at α_1-adrenergic receptors, but it differs in its pharmacokinetic profile. The half-life of doxazosin is about 20 hours, and its duration of action may extend to 36 hours (Cubeddu, 1988; Young and Brogden, 1988). The bioavailability and extent of metabolism of doxazosin and prazosin are similar. The majority of the metabolites of doxazosin are eliminated in the feces. The hemodynamic effects of doxazosin appear to be similar to those of prazosin. For the treatment of hypertension, single daily doses range from 1 to 16 mg; average maintenance doses are 2 to 4 mg (Young and Brogden, 1988).

Trimazosin. The bioavailability, plasma half-life (3 hours), and extensive metabolism of trimazosin are reminiscent of prazosin. 1-Hydroxytrimazosin, a major metabolite in man, may have antihypertensive efficacy, and the delayed onset of the peak hypotensive effect of trimazosin may reflect the rate of appearance of this metabolite. Although therapeutic doses of trimazosin are 10- to 50-fold higher than those of prazosin, the drug is highly selective for α_1-adrenergic receptors. However, high doses of trimazosin may produce vasodilatation directly.

Preparations, Routes of Administration, and Dosage. *Prazosin hydrochloride* (MINIPRESS) is available in 1-, 2-, and 5-mg capsules. The initial dose should be 1 mg, usually given at bedtime so that the patient will remain recumbent for at least several hours; this reduces the risk of syncopal reactions that may follow the first dose of prazosin. Therapy is begun with 1 mg given two or three times daily, and the dose is titrated upward depending on the blood pressure. A maximal effect is generally observed with a total daily dose of 20 mg.

Terazosin hydrochloride (HYTRIN) is available in 1-, 2-, 5-, and 10-mg tablets. As with prazosin, it is essential that therapy be initiated with the 1-mg dose at bedtime. Terazosin is usually effective when given once or twice daily for hypertension. The dose of terazosin is titrated upward slowly, depending on the blood pressure, to a maximum of 20 mg per day.

Doxazosin and trimazosin are not available for general clinical use in the United States.

Adverse Effects. A major potential adverse effect of prazosin and its congeners is the so-called first-dose phenomenon; marked postural hypotension and syncope are sometimes seen 30 to 90 minutes after a patient takes an initial dose. Occasionally, syncopal episodes have also occurred with a rapid increase in dosage or with the addition of a second antihypertensive drug to the regimen of a patient who is already taking a large dose of prazosin. The mechanisms responsible for such exaggerated hypotensive responses or for the development of tolerance to these effects are not clear. The rapid development of both venous and arterial α_1-adrenergic receptor blockade without compensatory tachycardia may be crucial; an action in the CNS to reduce sympathetic outflow may also contribute (*see* above). The risk of the first-dose phenomenon is minimized by limiting the initial dose to 1 mg at bedtime, by increasing the dosage slowly, and by introducing additional antihypertensive drugs cautiously. Since postural hypotension may be a problem during long-term treatment with prazosin or its congeners, it is essential to check standing as well as recumbent blood pressure. Nonspecific adverse effects such as headache, dizziness, drowsiness, and nausea do not often limit treatment with prazosin. Although not as extensively documented, the adverse effects of the structural analogs of prazosin appear to be similar to those of the parent compound (Cubeddu, 1988).

Therapeutic Uses. Prazosin and its congeners have been used successfully in the treatment of primary systemic hypertension (*see* Chapter 33). The most important distinction among these drugs relates to their duration of action and thus the required dosing interval.

Congestive Heart Failure. α-Adrenergic antagonists have been used in the treatment of congestive heart failure, as have other vasodilating drugs. The short-term effects of prazosin in patients with congestive heart failure are due to dilatation of both arteries and veins, resulting in a reduction of preload and afterload (Colucci, 1982). This increases cardiac output and reduces pulmonary congestion. Although some studies have shown persistence of these therapeutic effects during continued administration of prazosin to patients with congestive heart failure, many appear to become tolerant to the drug during long-term therapy (*see* Colucci, 1982; Frishman and Charlap, 1988). It is uncertain if such tolerance results from regulatory mechanisms that promote retention of salt and water. In contrast to results obtained with inhibitors of angiotensin converting enzyme or a combination of hydralazine and an organic nitrate, prazosin has not been found to prolong life in patients with congestive heart failure (Cohn *et al.*, 1986).

Other Disorders. Although anecdotal evidence suggested that prazosin might be useful in the treatment of patients with variant angina (Prinzmetal's angina) due to coronary vasospasm, several small controlled trials have failed to demonstrate any clear benefit (Robertson *et al.*, 1983; Winniford *et al.*, 1983). Some studies have indicated that prazosin can decrease the incidence of digital vasospasm in patients with Raynaud's disease; however, its relative efficacy as compared with other vasodilators (*e.g.*, Ca^{2+}-channel blockers) is not known (Surwit *et al.*, 1984; Wollersheim *et al.*, 1986). Prazosin decreases ventricular arrhythmias induced by coronary artery ligation or reperfusion in laboratory animals (Sheridan *et al.*, 1980); the therapeutic potential for this use in man is not known (Davey, 1986). Prazosin might also be useful for the treatment of patients with mitral or aortic valvular insufficiency, presumably because of reduction of afterload; additional data are needed (Jebavy *et al.*, 1983; Stanaszek *et al.*, 1983).

α_1-Adrenergic receptors in the trigone muscle of the bladder and urethra contribute to the resistance to outflow of urine. Prazosin reduces such resistance in some patients with impaired bladder emptying caused by prostatic obstruction or parasympathetic decentralization from spinal injury (Kirby *et al.,* 1987; Andersson, 1988).

ERGOT ALKALOIDS

The ergot alkaloids were the first adrenergic blocking agents to be discovered, and most aspects of their general pharmacology were disclosed by the classical studies of Dale (1906). Ergot alkaloids exhibit a complex variety of pharmacological properties. To varying degrees, these agents act as partial agonists or antagonists at α-adrenergic, tryptaminergic, and dopaminergic receptors (Berde and Stürmer, 1978; *see* Table 39–2).

Chemistry. Details of the chemistry of the ergot alkaloids are presented in Chapter 39. In general, compounds of the ergonovine type, which lack a peptide side chain, have no adrenergic blocking activity. Of the natural ergot preparations, "ergotoxine" has the greatest α-adrenergic blocking potency. It is a mixture of three alkaloids—ergocornine, ergocristine, and ergocryptine; fortunately, these have very similar pharmacological properties. Dihydrogenation of the lysergic acid nucleus increases α-adrenergic blocking activity and decreases, but does not eliminate, the ability to stimulate smooth muscle by an action on tryptaminergic receptors.

PHARMACOLOGICAL PROPERTIES

Both the natural and the dihydrogenated peptide alkaloids produce α-adrenergic blockade. This is relatively persistent for a competitive antagonist, but it is of much shorter duration than that produced by phenoxybenzamine. These drugs also are effective antagonists of 5-HT. Although the hydrogenated ergot alkaloids are among the most potent α-adrenergic blocking agents known, a plethora of side effects prevent the administration of doses that could produce more than minimal blockade in man.

The most important effects of all the ergot alkaloids are due to actions on the CNS and direct stimulation of smooth muscle. The latter occurs in many different organs (*see* Chapter 39), and even dihydroergotoxine (ergoloid mesylates) has been observed to produce spastic contractions of the intestine in man.

The peptide ergot alkaloids can reverse the pressor response to epinephrine to a depressor action. However, all the natural ergot alkaloids cause a significant rise in blood pressure as a result of peripheral vasoconstriction, which is more pronounced in postcapillary than in precapillary vessels. Although hydrogenation reduces this action, dihydroergotamine is still an effective vasoconstrictor, and a residual constrictor action of dihydroergotoxine is also demonstrable. Ergotamine, ergonovine, and other ergot alkaloids can produce coronary vasoconstriction, often with associated ischemic changes and anginal pain in patients with coronary artery disease. The ergot alkaloids usually induce bradycardia even when the blood pressure is not increased. This is predominantly due to increased vagal activity, but a central reduction in sympathetic tone and direct myocardial depression may also be involved.

The pharmacology of the ergot alkaloids is discussed in more detail by Nickerson and Hollenberg (1967) and in a volume edited by Berde and Schild (1978).

Toxicity and Adverse Effects. The dose of dihydroergotoxine in man is strictly limited by the presence of nausea and vomiting. Prolonged or excessive administration of any of the natural peptide ergot alkaloids can cause vascular insufficiency and gangrene of the extremities. This is particularly likely to occur in the presence of preexisting vascular pathological processes or infection. In severe cases, prompt vasodilatation is essential. There have been no comparative studies on the treatment of this sporadic condition, but a direct-acting drug such as nitroprusside appears to be most effective (Carliner *et al.,* 1974). Toxic effects of the ergot alkaloids are described in more detail in Chapter 39.

Therapeutic Uses and Preparations. The primary uses of ergot alkaloids are to stimulate contraction of the uterus post partum and to relieve the pain of migraine. These and other applications are described in Chapter 39; the effect of bromocriptine on the secretion of prolactin is described in Chapter 56. The various preparations of ergot alkaloids are listed in Chapter 39.

MISCELLANEOUS α-ADRENERGIC ANTAGONISTS

Indoramin. Indoramin is a selective, competitive α_1 antagonist that has been used for the treatment of hypertension. Competitive antagonism of histamine H_1 and 5-HT receptors is also evident (Cubeddu, 1988). As a selective α_1 antagonist, indoramin lowers blood pressure without producing tachycardia. The drug also decreases the incidence of attacks of Raynaud's phenomenon (Holmes and Sorkin, 1986).

The bioavailability of indoramin is only about 30%; it probably undergoes extensive first-pass metabolism (Holmes and Sorkin, 1986). Little unchanged drug is excreted in the urine, and some of the metabolites may be biologically active. The elimination half-life is about 5 hours. Some of the adverse effects of indoramin include sedation, dry mouth, and failure of ejaculation. Although indoramin is an effective antihypertensive agent, it lacks a well-defined place in current therapy and is not available in the United States.

Labetalol. Labetalol, a potent β-adrenergic antagonist, competitively blocks α_1 receptors as well (*see* below).

Ketanserin. Although developed as a 5-HT antagonist, ketanserin also blocks α_1-adrenergic receptors. Ketanserin is discussed in Chapter 23.

Urapidil. Urapidil is a novel, selective α_1-adrenergic antagonist that has a chemical structure distinct from those of prazosin and related compounds. Blockade of peripheral α_1 receptors appears to be primarily responsible for the hypotension produced by urapidil, although it has actions in the CNS as well (Cubeddu, 1988; van Zwieten, 1988). After oral administration, the bioavailability of urapidil is about 80% (Kirsten *et al.*, 1988). The drug is extensively metabolized and has a half-life of 3 hours. The role of urapidil in the treatment of hypertension remains to be determined.

Yohimbine. Yohimbine is a competitive antagonist that is selective for α_2-adrenergic receptors. The compound is an indolealkylamine alkaloid, and is found in the bark of the *Pausinystalia yohimbe* tree and in *Rauwolfia* root; its structural resemblance to reserpine is apparent. Yohimbine readily enters the CNS, where it acts to increase blood pressure and heart rate; it also enhances motor activity and produces tremors. These actions are opposite to those of clonidine, an α_2 agonist (*see* Goldberg and Robertson, 1983). Yohimbine is also an antagonist of 5-HT. In the past, it has been used extensively to treat impotence. Although efficacy was never clearly demonstrated, there is renewed interest in the use of yohimbine in the treatment of male sexual dysfunction. The drug enhances sexual activity in male rats (Clark *et al.*, 1984), and it may benefit some patients with psychogenic impotence (Reid *et al.*, 1987). Several small studies suggest that yohimbine may also be useful for diabetic neuropathy and in the treatment of postural hypotension.

Neuroleptic Agents. Natural and synthetic compounds of several other chemical classes exhibit α-adrenergic blocking activity. Chlorpromazine, haloperidol, and other neuroleptic drugs of the phenothiazine and butyrophenone types produce significant α blockade in both laboratory animals and man. Chlorpromazine can also prolong and, under appropriate conditions, enhance the pressor response to norepinephrine, possibly as a result of the ability of this compound to block neuronal reuptake of the neurotransmitter. Haloperidol also inhibits dopamine-induced renal vasodilatation, which is not affected by the common α- or β-adrenergic blocking agents.

II. β-Adrenergic Receptor Antagonists

β-Adrenergic receptor antagonists have received enormous clinical attention because of their efficacy in the treatment of hypertension, ischemic heart disease, and certain arrhythmias. Ahlquist's hypothesis that the effects of catecholamines were mediated by activation of distinct α- and β-adrenergic receptors provided the initial impetus for the synthesis and pharmacological evaluation of β-adrenergic blocking agents (*see* Chapter 5). The first such selective agent was dichloroisoproterenol (Powell and Slater, 1958). However, this compound is a partial agonist, and this property was thought to preclude its safe clinical use. Sir James Black and his colleagues initiated a program in the late 1950s to develop additional agents of this type. Although the usefulness of their first antagonist, pronethalol, was limited by the production of thymic tumors in mice, propranolol soon followed (Black and Stephenson, 1962; Black and Prichard, 1973). Propranolol is a competitive β-adrenergic antagonist that is devoid of agonist activity, and it remains the prototype with which other β blockers are compared. Subsequent efforts to generate additional antagonists have resulted in compounds that can be distinguished by the following properties: relative affinity for β_1 and β_2 receptors, intrinsic sympathomimetic activity, blockade of α-adrenergic receptors, differences in lipid solubility, and general pharmacokinetic properties. Some of these distinguishing characteristics have clinical significance, and they help guide the appropriate choice of a β-adrenergic antagonist for individual patients.

Propranolol has equal affinity for β_1 and β_2 receptors; thus it is a nonselective β-adrenergic antagonist. Agents such as metoprolol and atenolol have somewhat greater affinity for β_1 than for β_2 receptors; these are examples of selective β_1 antagonists, even though the selectivity is not absolute. Propranolol is a pure antagonist, and it has no capacity to activate β-adrenergic receptors. Several β blockers (*e.g.*, pindolol and acebutolol) activate β receptors partially in the absence of catecholamines; however, the intrinsic activities of these drugs are far less than that of a full agonist such as isoproterenol. These partial agonists are said to have intrinsic sympathomimetic activity. Substantial sympathomimetic activity is obviously counterproductive to the response desired from a β-adrenergic antagonist; however, slight residual activity may, for example, prevent profound bradycardia or negative inotropy in a resting heart. Although most β antagonists do not block α-adrenergic receptors, labetalol is an example of an agent that blocks both α_1 and β receptors.

Chemistry. The structural formulas of some β-adrenergic antagonists in general use are shown in Table 11–2. The structural similarities between agonists and antagonists that act on β receptors are closer than those between α-receptor agonists and antagonists. Substitution of an isopropyl group or other bulky substituent on the amino nitrogen fa-

Table 11–2. STRUCTURAL FORMULAS OF β-ADRENERGIC ANTAGONISTS

Nonselective Antagonists

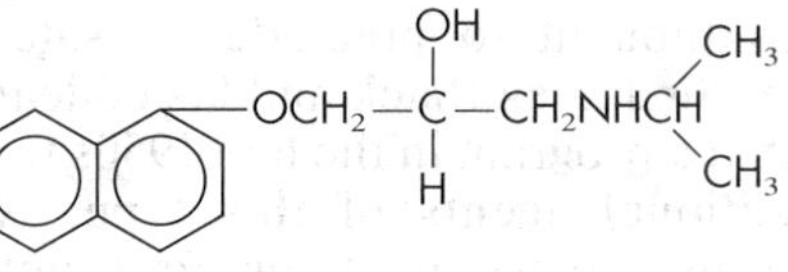

Propranolol

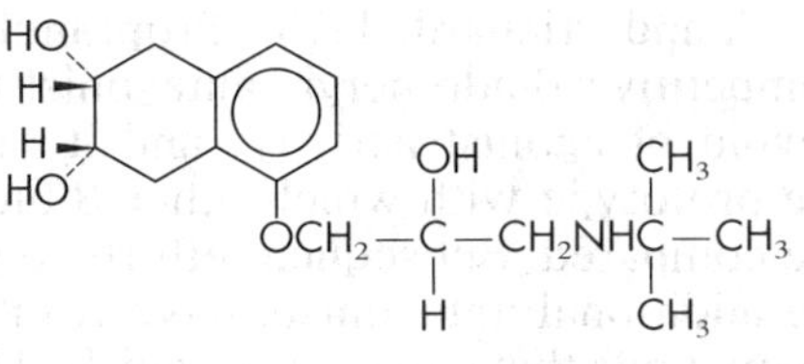

Nadolol

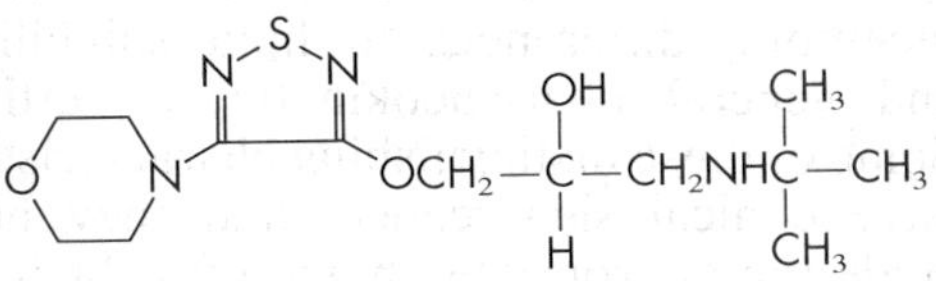

Timolol

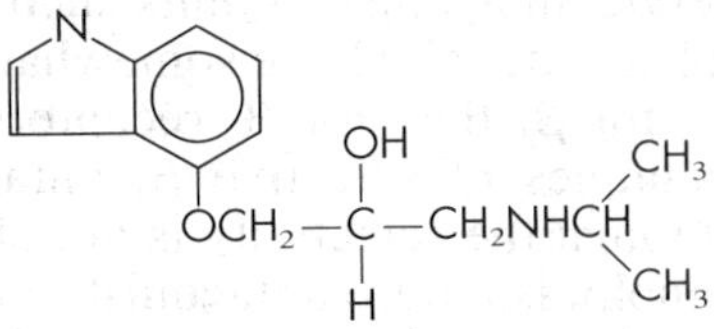

Pindolol

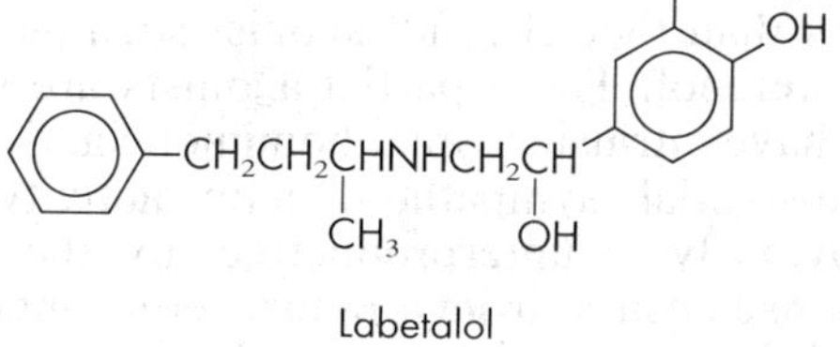

Labetalol

β_1–Selective Antagonists

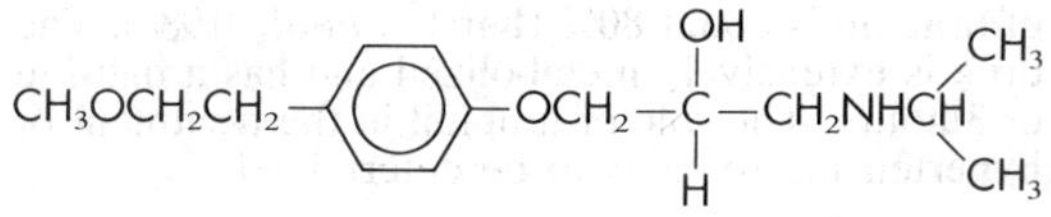

Metoprolol

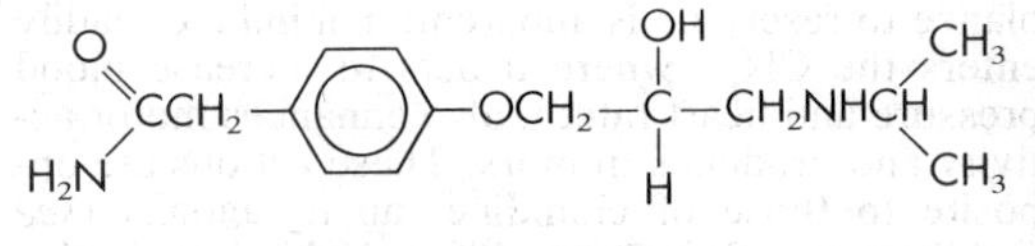

Atenolol

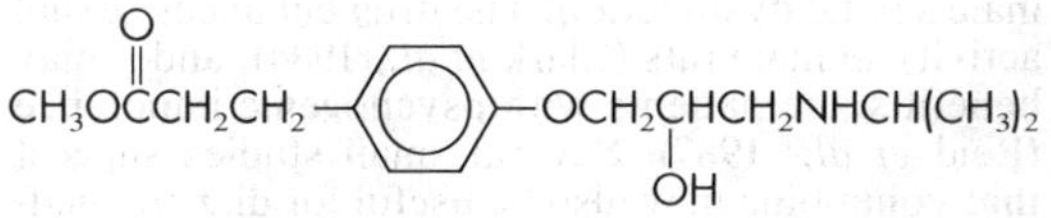

Esmolol

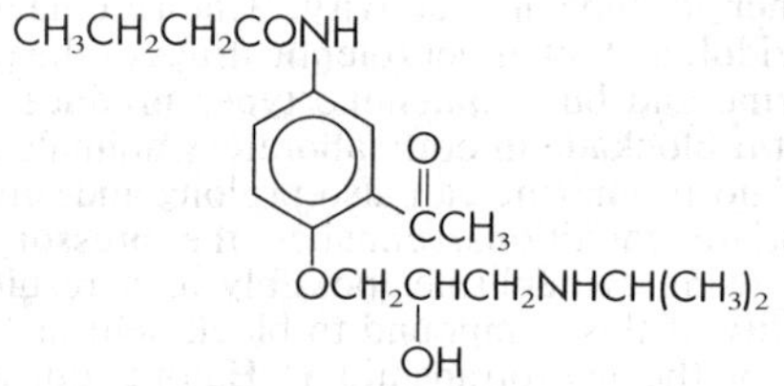

Acebutolol

vors interaction with β-adrenergic receptors. There is a rather wide tolerance for the nature of the aromatic moiety in the nonselective β antagonists; however, the structural tolerance for β_1-selective antagonists is far more constrained. The seven membrane-spanning regions of the β-adrenergic receptor appear to outline a cylindrical structure, and competitive antagonists bind to the receptor within the plane of the membrane, rather than on the extracellular surface (*see* Chapter 5). A reasonable proposal is that both agonists and antagonists bind within the cylinder and bridge two or more of the membrane-spanning regions.

PHARMACOLOGICAL PROPERTIES

As in the case of α-adrenergic blocking agents, the pharmacology of β-adrenergic blockade can be deduced from a knowledge of the responses elicited by the receptors in the various tissues and the activity of the sympathetic nerves that innervate these tissues (*see* Table 5–1). For example, β-receptor blockade has little effect on the normal heart of an individual at rest but has profound effects when sympathetic control of the heart is dominant, as during exercise or stress.

Cardiovascular System. The important therapeutic effects of β-adrenergic antagonists are on the cardiovascular system. It is important to distinguish these effects in normal subjects and in those with cardiovascular disease such as hypertension or myocardial ischemia.

Since catecholamines have positive chronotropic and inotropic actions, β-adrenergic antagonists slow the heart rate and decrease myocardial contractility. When stimulation of β receptors is low, this effect is correspondingly modest. However, when the sympathetic nervous system is activated, such as during exercise or stress, β-adrenergic antagonists attenuate the expected rise in heart rate. Short-term administration of β-adrenergic antagonists decreases cardiac output; peripheral resistance increases as a result of blockade of vascular β_2 receptors and compensatory sympathetic reflexes that activate vascular α-adrenergic receptors. Blood flow to most organs other than the brain is reduced (Nies *et al.*, 1973). Renal blood flow and glomerular filtration rate may decrease only modestly with nonselective β-receptor antagonists; these changes are generally unimportant in patients with normal renal function (Epstein and Oster, 1982). However, with long-term use of β-adrenergic antagonists, total peripheral resistance returns to initial values (Mimran and Ducailar, 1988). Drugs that have either intrinsic sympathomimetic activity or α blocking activity may lower peripheral vascular resistance in the short term (Frishman and Weksler, 1984).

β-Adrenergic antagonists have significant effects on cardiac rhythm and automaticity. Although it had been thought that these effects were due exclusively to blockade of β_1 receptors, β_2-adrenergic receptors may also be involved in regulating heart rate in man (Brodde, 1988). β-Adrenergic antagonists reduce sinus rate, decrease the spontaneous rate of depolarization of ectopic pacemakers, slow conduction in the atria and in the atrioventricular (AV) node, and increase the functional refractory period of the AV node.

Although high concentrations of many β blockers produce quinidine-like effects ("membrane-stabilizing activity"), it is doubtful that this is significant at usual doses of these agents. However, this effect may be important when there is overdosage. β-Adrenergic antagonists that lack membrane-stabilizing activity retain their antiarrhythmic efficacy (Shand, 1975).

The cardiovascular effects of β-adrenergic antagonists are most evident during dynamic exercise. In the presence of β-receptor blockade, the exercise-induced increases in heart rate and myocardial contractility are attenuated. However, the exercise-induced increase in cardiac output is less affected because of an increase in stroke volume (Shephard, 1982; Tesch, 1985; Van Baak, 1988). The effects of β-adrenergic antagonists on exercise are somewhat analogous to the changes that occur with normal aging. In the healthy elderly, catecholamine-induced increases in heart rate are attenuated as compared with younger individuals; however, the increase in cardiac output in older people may be preserved because of an increase in stroke volume during exercise. β Blockers tend to decrease work capacity, as assessed by their effects on intense short-term or more prolonged steady-state exertion (Kaiser *et al.*, 1986). Exercise performance may be impaired to a lesser extent by β_1-selective agents than by nonselective antagonists (Tesch, 1985). Blockade of β_2 receptors tends to blunt the increase in blood flow to active skeletal muscle during submaximal exercise (Van Baak, 1988). Blockade of β receptors may also attenuate catecholamine-induced activation of glucose metabolism and lipolysis.

Coronary arterial blood flow increases during exercise or stress to meet the metabolic demands of the heart. By increasing heart rate, contractility, and systolic pressure, catecholamines increase myocardial oxygen demand. However, in patients with coronary artery disease, fixed narrowing of these vessels attenuates the expected increase in flow, leading to myocardial ischemia. β-Adrenergic antagonists decrease the effects of catecholamines on the determinants of myocardial oxygen consumption. However, these agents may tend to increase the requirement for oxygen by increasing end-diastolic pressure and systolic ejection period. Usually the net effect is to improve the relationship between cardiac oxygen supply and demand; exercise tolerance is generally improved in patients with angina, whose capacity to exercise is limited by the development of chest pain.

Activity as Antihypertensive Agents. β-Adrenergic antagonists are not "hypotensive" agents in patients with normal blood pressure. However, these drugs do lower blood pressure in patients with hypertension. Despite their widespread use, the mechanisms responsible for this important clinical effect are not well understood. The release of renin from the juxtaglomerular apparatus is stimulated by the sympathetic nervous system, and this effect is blocked by β-adrenergic antagonists (*see* Chapter 31). However, the relationship between this phenomenon and the fall in blood pressure is not clear. Some investigators have found that the antihypertensive effect of propranolol is most marked in patients with elevated concentrations of plasma renin as compared with patients with low or normal concentrations of renin (Buhler *et al.*, 1972). However, pindolol is an effective antihypertensive agent that has little or no effect on plasma renin activity (Frishman, 1983).

Presynaptic β-adrenergic receptors potentiate the release of norepinephrine from sympathetic neurons; however, the importance of diminished release of norepinephrine to the antihypertensive effects of β-adrenergic antagonists is also uncertain. Although β blockers would not be expected to decrease the contractility of vascular smooth muscle, long-term administration of these drugs to hypertensive patients ultimately leads to a fall in peripheral vascular resistance (Man in't Veld *et al.*, 1988). The mechanism for this important effect is not known. However, this delayed fall in peripheral vascular resistance in the face of a persistent reduction of cardiac output appears to account for the bulk of the antihypertensive effects of these drugs. Although it has been hypothesized that central actions of β blockers may also contribute to their antihypertensive effects, there is relatively little evidence to support this theory.

Propranolol and other nonselective β-adrenergic antagonists inhibit the vasodilatation caused by isoproterenol and augment the pressor response to epinephrine. This is particularly significant in pheochromocytoma, for which β-adrenergic antagonists should be used only after adequate α-adrenergic blockade has been established. This avoids uncompensated α-receptor–mediated vasoconstriction caused by epinephrine secreted from the tumor. Pressor responses to nonselective β-adrenergic antagonists can also occur in other situations that involve increased sympathetic activity, such as hypoglycemic reactions in unstable diabetics and excessive use of tobacco (Cleophas and Kauw, 1988).

Pulmonary System. Nonselective β-adrenergic antagonists such as propranolol block β_2-adrenergic receptors in bronchial smooth muscle. This usually has little effect on pulmonary function in normal individuals. However, in patients with asthma or chronic obstructive pulmonary disease, such blockade can lead to life-threatening bronchoconstriction. Although β_1-selective antagonists or antagonists with intrinsic sympathomimetic activity may be less likely than propranolol to increase airway resistance in patients with asthma, these drugs should be used only with great caution, if at all, in patients with bronchospastic diseases.

Metabolic Effects. β-Adrenergic antagonists modify the metabolism of carbohydrates and lipids. Catecholamines promote glycogenolysis and mobilize glucose in response to hypoglycemia. Nonselective β blockers may adversely affect recovery from hypoglycemia in insulin-dependent diabetics. β-Adrenergic antagonists should be used with great caution in labile diabetics. A β_1-selective compound is preferable, since these drugs are less likely to delay recovery from hypoglycemia (Deacon and Barnett, 1976; Deacon *et al.*, 1977). All β blockers mask the tachycardia that is typically seen with hypoglycemia, denying the patient an important warning sign. Although insulin secretion is potentiated by β-adrenergic agonists, β blockade impairs insulin release only rarely.

β-Adrenergic receptors activate hormone-sensitive lipase in fat cells, leading to the release of free fatty acids into the circulation. This increased flux of fatty acids is an important energy source for exercising muscle. β-Adrenergic antagonists can attenuate the release of free fatty acids from adipose tissue. Nonetheless, nonselective β blockers modestly elevate plasma concentrations of triglycerides and decrease those of high-density lipoproteins in some patients. Concentrations of low-density lipoproteins do not usually change (Miller, 1987). Although the significance of these changes is not known, there is concern that they may be undesirable, particularly in patients with hypertension (Reaven and Hoffman, 1987). Selective β_1 antagonists and those with intrinsic sympathomimetic activity may cause these changes in lipid metabolism less frequently. The mechanism of these effects is not known.

β-Adrenergic agonists decrease the plasma concentration of K^+ by promoting the uptake of the ion, predominantly into skeletal muscle. At rest, an infusion of epinephrine causes a fall in the plasma concentration of K^+ (Brown *et al.*, 1983). The marked increase in the concentration of epinephrine that occurs with stress (such as myocardial infarction) may cause hypokalemia, which could predispose to cardiac arrhythmias (Struthers and Reid, 1984). The hypokalemic effect of epinephrine is blocked by an experimental antagonist, ICI 118551, that is selective for β_2- and β_3-adrenergic receptors (Brown *et al.*, 1983; Emorine *et al.*, 1989). Exercise causes an increase in the efflux of K^+ from skeletal muscle. Catecholamines tend to buffer the rise in K^+ by increasing its influx into muscle. β Blocking agents negate this buffering effect (Brown, 1985).

Other Effects. β-Adrenergic antagonists block catecholamine-induced tremor. They also block inhibition of mast-cell degranulation by catecholamines (*see* Chapter 25). β-Adrenergic antagonists may have effects on platelet function (*see* Frishman and Weksler, 1984).

NONSELECTIVE β-ADRENERGIC ANTAGONISTS

PROPRANOLOL

In view of the extensive experience with propranolol, it is a useful prototype (*see* Table 11–3). Propranolol interacts with β_1 and β_2 receptors with equal affinity, lacks intrinsic sympathomimetic activity, and does not block α-adrenergic receptors.

Absorption, Fate, and Excretion. Propranolol is highly lipophilic and is almost completely absorbed after oral administration. However, much of the drug is metabolized by the liver during its first passage through the portal circulation; on average, only about 25% reaches the systemic circulation. In addition, there is great interindividual variation in the presystemic clearance of propranolol by the liver; this contributes to enormous variability in plasma concentrations after oral administration of the drug (approximately 20-fold). The degree of hepatic extraction of propranolol declines as the dose is increased, and the bioavailability of propranolol may be increased by the ingestion of food and during long-term administration of the drug.

Propranolol has a large volume of distribution (4 liters/kg) and readily enters the CNS. Approximately 90% of the drug in the circulation is bound to plasma proteins. Propranolol is extensively metabolized, with most metabolites appearing in the urine. One product of hepatic metabolism is 4-hydroxypropranolol, which possesses some β-adrenergic antagonist activity (Shand, 1975; Oates *et al.*, 1977).

Analysis of the distribution of propranolol, its clearance by the liver, and its activity is complicated by the stereospecificity of these processes (Walle *et al.*, 1988). The (−)-enantiomers of propranolol and other β blockers are the active forms of the drug. This enantiomer of propranolol appears to

Table 11–3. PHARMACOLOGICAL CHARACTERISTICS OF β-ADRENERGIC ANTAGONISTS *

COMPOUND	INTRINSIC SYMPATHOMIMETIC ACTIVITY	MEMBRANE-STABILIZING ACTIVITY	LIPID SOLUBILITY (LOG KP †)	ORAL BIO-AVAILABILITY (%)	HALF-LIFE IN PLASMA (HOURS) ‡
I. Nonselective β- ($\beta_1 + \beta_2$) Adrenergic Antagonists					
Propranolol	0	++	3.65	~25	3–5
Nadolol	0	0	0.7	~35	10–20
Timolol	0	0	2.1	~50	3–5
Pindolol	++	±	1.75	~75	3–4
Labetalol §	— §	±	—	~20	4–6
II. Selective β_1-Adrenergic Antagonists					
Metoprolol	0	±	2.15	~40	3–4
Atenolol	0	0	0.23	~50	5–8
Esmolol	0	0	—	—	0.13
Acebutolol	+	+	1.9	~40	2–4

* Based on data in Drayer (1987), McDevitt (1987), and other references cited in the text.

† Kp refers to the octanol:water partition coefficient; propranolol and atenolol are at the lipophilic and hydrophilic extremes, respectively.

‡ The duration of effect, in general, is longer than might be expected from the plasma $t_{1/2}$.

§ Labetalol is also a potent α_1-adrenergic antagonist. *See* text for a description of the activities of the individual isomers of labetalol.

be cleared more slowly from the body than is the inactive enantiomer. The clearance of propranolol may vary with hepatic blood flow and liver disease, and it may also change during the administration of other drugs that affect hepatic metabolism. Monitoring of plasma concentrations of propranolol has found little application, since the clinical endpoints (reduction of blood pressure and heart rate) are readily determined. The relationships between the plasma concentrations of propranolol and its pharmacodynamic effects are complex; for example, despite its short half-life in plasma (about 4 hours), the antihypertensive effect of propranolol is sufficiently long-lived to permit administration once or twice daily. Some of the (−)-enantiomer of propranolol and other β blockers is taken up into sympathetic nerve endings and is released upon sympathetic nerve stimulation (Walle *et al.*, 1988).

A sustained-release formulation of propranolol has been developed to maintain therapeutic concentrations of propranolol in plasma throughout a 24-hour period (Nace and Wood, 1987). Suppression of exercise-induced tachycardia is maintained throughout the dosing interval, and patient compliance may be improved.

Preparations, Routes of Administration, and Dosage. *Propranolol hydrochloride* (INDERAL, IPRAN) is available in tablets that contain 10 to 90 mg of the drug for oral administration and at a concentration of 1 mg/ml for intravenous use. It is also available in sustained-release capsules (INDERAL LA) that contain 80, 120, or 160 mg.

For the treatment of hypertension and angina, the initial oral dose of propranolol is generally 40 to 80 mg per day. The dose may then be titrated upward until the optimal response is obtained. For the treatment of angina, the dose may be increased at intervals of less than 1 week, as indicated clinically. In hypertension, the full response of the blood pressure may not develop for several weeks. Typically, doses are less than 320 mg per day. If propranolol is taken twice daily for hypertension, blood pressure should be measured just prior to a dose to ensure that the duration of effect is sufficiently prolonged. Adequacy of β-adrenergic blockade can be assessed by measuring suppression of exercise-induced tachycardia. Propranolol may be administered intravenously for the management of life-threatening arrhythmias or to patients under anesthesia. Under these circumstances the usual dose is 1 to 3 mg, administered slowly (less than 1 mg per minute) with careful and frequent measurement of blood pressure, the electrocardiogram, and cardiac function. If an adequate response is not obtained, a second dose may be given after several minutes. If bradycardia is excessive, atropine should be administered to increase heart rate. Oral therapy should be initiated as soon as possible.

NADOLOL

Nadolol is a long-acting antagonist with equal affinity for β_1- and β_2-adrenergic receptors. It is devoid of both membrane-stabilizing and intrinsic sympathomimetic activity. A distinguishing characteristic of nadolol is its relatively long half-life.

Absorption, Fate, and Excretion. Nadolol is very soluble in water and is incompletely absorbed from the gut; its bioavailability is about 35% (Frishman, 1982). However, interindividual variability is less than with propranolol. The low solubility of nadolol in fat may result in lower concentrations of the drug in the brain as compared with more lipid-soluble β-adrenergic antagonists. Although it has frequently been suggested that the incidence of CNS side effects is lower with hydrophilic β-adrenergic antagonists, there are limited data from controlled trials to support this contention. Nadolol is not extensively metabolized and is largely excreted intact in the urine. The half-life of the drug in plasma is in the range of 12 to 20 hours; consequently, it generally is administered once daily. Nadolol may accumulate in patients with renal failure, and dosage should be reduced in such individuals.

Preparations, Routes of Administration, and Dosage. *Nadolol* (CORGARD) is available for oral administration in 20-, 40-, 80-, 120-, and 160-mg tablets. Therapy is usually begun with a daily dose of 40 mg. For angina, this may be increased every 3 to 7 days in 40- to 80-mg increments. The usual daily dose to treat angina or hypertension is 40 to 80 mg, but higher doses may be required. Dosage is titrated to clinical endpoints. In patients with renal dysfunction (creatinine clearance < 50 ml/min/1.73 m^2), dosage should be decreased or the dosing interval increased.

TIMOLOL

Timolol is a short-acting, potent, nonselective β-adrenergic antagonist. It has no intrinsic sympathomimetic activity and no membrane-stabilizing activity.

Absorption, Fate, and Excretion. Timolol is well absorbed from the gastrointestinal tract and is subject to moderate first-pass metabolism. It is metabolized extensively by the liver, and only a small amount of unchanged drug appears in the urine. The half-life in plasma is about 4 hours. Interestingly, the ocular formulation of timolol, used for the treatment of glaucoma, may be extensively absorbed systemically; adverse effects can occur in susceptible patients, such as those with asthma or congestive heart failure.

Preparations, Routes of Administration, and Dosage. *Timolol maleate* (BLOCADREN) is available in 5-, 10-, and 20-mg tablets. For the treatment of hypertension, the initial dosage is usually 10 mg taken twice daily. Maintenance doses should be titrated upward at weekly or greater intervals; generally, daily doses of 20 to 40 mg (maximum, 60 mg) are used. For long-term prophylactic use to prevent recurrence of myocardial infarction, timolol is administered in a dosage of 10 mg twice daily.

Timolol is also available as a 0.25% or 0.5% ophthalmic solution (TIMOPTIC) to lower intraocular pressure for the treatment of glaucoma. The initial dose is generally 1 drop of the 0.25% solution twice a day; if the response is not adequate, the dosage is increased to 1 drop of the 0.5% solution twice daily. If the response is adequate, the drug can then usually be administered once a day. Although mild ocular irritation is noted occasionally, major local adverse effects are unusual. However, as indicated above, plasma concentrations of timolol may become sufficiently high to block pulmonary and cardiac β-adrenergic receptors.

PINDOLOL

Pindolol is a nonselective β-adrenergic antagonist with prominent intrinsic sympathomimetic activity. It has low membrane-stabilizing activity and is moderately soluble in lipid.

Although limited data are available, β blockers with slight partial agonistic activity may produce smaller reductions in resting heart rate and blood pressure. Hence, such drugs may be preferred as antihypertensive agents in individuals with diminished cardiac reserve or a propensity for bradycardia. These agents still block exercise-induced increases in heart rate and cardiac output.

Absorption, Fate, and Excretion. Pindolol is almost completely absorbed after oral administration and has moderately high bioavailability. These properties tend to minimize interindividual variation in the plasma concentrations of the drug that are achieved after its oral administration. Approximately 50% of pindolol is ultimately metabolized in the liver. The principal metabolites are hydroxylated derivatives that are subsequently conjugated with either glucuronide or sulfate before renal excretion. The remainder of the drug is excreted unchanged in the urine. The plasma half-life of pindolol is about 4 hours; clearance is reduced in patients with renal failure.

Preparations, Routes of Administration, and Dosage. *Pindolol* (VISKEN) is available in 5- and 10-mg tablets. For hypertension, the usual initial dose is 5 mg twice daily. The maintenance dosage is typically a total of 15 to 40 mg per day, given in two or three divided doses; the maximum recommended daily dose is 60 mg per day. Doses are increased at intervals of several weeks in increments of 10 mg per day, depending on the response.

LABETALOL

Labetalol is representative of a relatively new class of drugs that act as competitive antagonists at both α_1- and β-adrenergic receptors. However, the compound has two optical centers, and the formulation used clinically contains equal amounts of its four diasteriomers (Gold *et al.*, 1982). The pharmacological properties of the drug are complex because each isomer displays different relative activities. The properties of the mixture include selective blockade of α_1- (as compared with α_2-) adrenergic receptors, blockade of β_1 and β_2 receptors, partial agonist activity at β_2 receptors, and inhibition of neuronal uptake of norepinephrine (cocaine-like effect; inhibitor of uptake$_1$). The potency of the mixture for β-adrenergic blockade is fivefold to tenfold that for α-adrenergic blockade (*see* Blakeley and Summers, 1977; Drew *et al.*, 1978; Gold *et al.*, 1982).

The pharmacological effects of labetalol have become clearer since the four isomers were separated and tested individually. The R,R isomer is about fourfold more potent as a β-adrenergic antagonist than is racemic labetalol, and it accounts for all of the β blockade produced by the mixture of isomers as an α_1 antagonist; this isomer is less than 20% as potent as the racemic mixture (Sybertz *et al.*, 1981; Gold *et al.*, 1982). The R,S isomer is almost devoid of either α- or β-adrenergic blocking effects. The S,R isomer has almost no β-adrenergic blocking activity yet is about fivefold more potent as an α_1 blocker than is racemic labetalol. The S,S isomer is devoid of β blocking activity and has a potency similar to racemic labetalol as an α_1-receptor antagonist (Gold *et al.*, 1982). The R,R isomer has some intrinsic sympathomimetic activity at β_2 receptors; this may contribute to vasodilatation (Baum *et al.*, 1981). Labetalol may also have some direct vasodilating capacity (Dage and Hsieh, 1980). The favorable spectrum of pharmacological properties of the R,R isomer of labetalol has prompted its clinical development. However, experience with this compound, *dilevalol* (UNICARD) is still limited.

The actions of labetalol on both α_1- and β-adrenergic receptors contribute to the fall in blood pressure observed in patients with hypertension. α_1-Receptor blockade leads to relaxation of arterial smooth muscle and vasodilatation, particularly in the upright position. The β_1 blockade also contributes to a fall in blood pressure, in part by blocking reflex sympathetic stimulation of the heart. In addition, the intrinsic sympathomimetic activity of labetalol at β_2 receptors may contribute to vasodilatation.

Absorption, Fate, and Excretion. Although labetalol is completely absorbed from the gut, there is extensive first-pass clearance; bioavailability is only about 20% and is quite variable (McNeil and Louis, 1984). Bioavailability may be increased by food intake. The drug is rapidly and extensively metabolized in the liver by oxidative biotransformation and glucuronidation; very little unchanged drug is found in the urine (Gal *et al.*, 1988). The rate of metabolism of labetalol is sensitive to changes in hepatic blood flow. The elimination half-life of the drug is 4 to 6 hours. There are no data on the pharmacokinetic properties of the individual isomers of labetalol.

Preparations, Routes of Administration, and Dosage. *Labetalol hydrochloride* (NORMODYNE, TRANDATE) is available in 100-, 200-, and 300-mg tablets. An intravenous formulation (5 mg/ml) is also available for the treatment of hypertensive emergencies. The initial oral dosage of labetalol is usually 100 mg twice daily. For the treatment of hypertension, the dose may be titrated upward every 2 to 3 days in increments of 100 mg twice daily. Both supine and standing blood pressure should be measured. The maintenance dose is generally in the range of 200 to 400 mg twice daily, although some patients may require 1200 to 2400 mg per day. In hypertensive emergencies, the response to intravenous injections of labetalol should be monitored closely. Initially, a dose of 20 mg (or 0.25 mg/kg) is given slowly over several minutes, and supine blood pressure is monitored. Additional injections of 40 or 80 mg can be given at 10-minute intervals until the desired blood pressure is achieved or a total of 300 mg has been administered. Alternatively, diluted solutions may be infused at a rate of 2 mg/min. Oral treatment should be initiated as soon as possible.

SELECTIVE β-ADRENERGIC ANTAGONISTS

METOPROLOL

Metoprolol is a selective β_1-adrenergic antagonist that is devoid of intrinsic sympathomimetic activity.

Absorption, Fate, and Excretion. Metoprolol is almost completely absorbed after oral administration, but bioavailability is relatively low (about 40%) because of first-pass metabolism. Plasma concentrations of the drug vary widely (up to 17 fold), perhaps because of genetically determined differences in the rate of metabolism (Benfield *et al.*, 1986). Metoprolol is extensively metabolized by the hepatic monooxygenase system, and only 10% of the administered drug is recovered unchanged in the urine. The half-life of metoprolol is 3 to 4 hours.

Preparations, Routes of Administration, and Dosage. *Metoprolol tartrate* (LOPRESSOR) is available for oral use in 50- and 100-mg tablets. For the treatment of hypertension, the usual initial dose is 100 mg per day. The drug is often effective when given once daily, although it is frequently used in two divided doses. Dosage may be increased at weekly intervals until optimal reduction of blood pressure is achieved. The usual maintenance dosage is 100 to 200 mg per day. If the drug is taken only once daily, it is important to confirm that blood pressure is controlled for the entire 24-hour period. Metoprolol is generally used in two divided doses for the treatment of stable angina. For the initial treatment of patients with acute myocardial infarction, an intravenous formulation of metoprolol tartrate is available at a concentration of 1 mg/ml. Three bolus injections of 5 mg each given at 2-minute intervals are recommended as soon as the patient's hemodynamic condition has stabilized. Blood pressure, heart rate, and the electrocardiogram should be monitored. If the patient tolerates the full intravenous dose, oral dosage (50 mg every 6 hours) is started 15 minutes later and is continued for 48 hours. Thereafter, a maintenance dosage of 100 mg twice daily is administered. In patients who do not tolerate the full intravenous dose, oral dosing is initiated with 25 or 50 mg every 6 hours as soon as the clinical situation permits. In patients with severe intolerance, treatment should be discontinued. Metoprolol is contraindicated for the treatment of acute myocardial infarction in patients with heart rates of less than 45 beats per minute, heart block greater than first degree (P–R interval greater than or equal to 0.24 second), systolic blood pressure less than 100 mm Hg, or moderate to severe heart failure.

ATENOLOL

Atenolol is a β_1-selective antagonist that is devoid of intrinsic sympathomimetic activity. Atenolol is very hydrophilic and appears to penetrate the brain to only a limited extent. Its half-life is somewhat longer than that of metoprolol.

Absorption, Fate, and Excretion. Atenolol is incompletely absorbed (about 50%), but most of the absorbed dose reaches the systemic circulation. There is relatively little variation in the plasma concentrations of atenolol as compared with most other β-adrenergic antagonists, and peak concentrations in different patients vary only over a fourfold range (Cruickshank, 1980). The drug is excreted largely unchanged in the urine, and the elimination half-life is about 5 to 8 hours. The drug accumulates in patients with renal failure, and dosage should be adjusted for patients whose creatinine clearance is less than 35 ml/min.

Preparations, Routes of Administration, and Dosage. *Atenolol* (TENORMIN) is available in 50- and 100-mg tablets for oral use. The initial dose of atenolol for the treatment of hypertension is usually 50 mg per day given once daily. If an adequate therapeutic response is not evident within several weeks, the daily dose may be increased to 100 mg; higher doses are unlikely to provide any greater antihypertensive effect.

ESMOLOL

Esmolol is a selective β_1 antagonist with a very short duration of action. It has little if any intrinsic sympathomimetic activity, and it lacks membrane-stabilizing actions. Esmolol is administered intravenously and is used when β blockade of short duration is desired or in critically ill patients in whom adverse effects of bradycardia, heart failure, or hypotension may necessitate rapid withdrawal of the drug.

Absorption, Fate, and Excretion. Esmolol has a half-life of about 8 minutes and an apparent volume of distribution of approximately 2 liters/kg (*see* Appendix II). The drug contains an ester linkage, and it is hydrolyzed rapidly by esterases in erythrocytes. The half-life of the carboxylic acid metabolite of esmolol is far longer (4 hours), and it accumulates during prolonged infusion of esmolol (*see* Benfield and Sorkin, 1987). However, this metabolite has very low potency as a β-adrenergic antagonist (1/500 of the potency of esmolol) (Reynolds *et al.*, 1986); it is excreted in the urine.

The onset and offset of β-adrenergic blockade with esmolol are rapid; peak hemodynamic effects occur within 6 to 10 minutes of administration of a loading dose, and there is substantial attenuation of β blockade within 20 minutes of stopping an infusion. Esmolol may have striking hypotensive effects in normal subjects, although the mechanism is uncertain (Reilly *et al.*, 1985).

Preparations, Routes of Administration, and Dosage. *Esmolol hydrochloride* (BREVIBLOC) is available in a concentrated solution (250 mg/ml) to be diluted prior to use, or in a solution (10 mg/ml) for intravenous administration. In the United States, esmolol is approved only for the treatment of supraventricular tachycardia. To initiate treatment, a loading dose of 500 μg/kg is infused over 1 minute; this is followed by infusion of 50 μg/kg per minute for 4 minutes. If an adequate therapeutic effect is not observed within 5 minutes, the same loading dose is repeated and the maintenance infusion is increased to 100 μg/kg per minute. The titration can be repeated with progressively greater 4-minute infusions (increments of 50 μg/kg per minute). As the desired endpoint (*e.g.*, lowered heart rate or blood pressure) is approached, the loading dose is omitted and the increment in the maintenance infusion is made more gradually (steps of 25 μg/kg per minute or less). Responses to esmolol usually occur with maintenance infusions of 50 to 200 μg/kg per minute; the safety of maintenance rates above 300 μg/kg per minute is not known. Infusions have been tolerated for up to 48 hours.

ACEBUTOLOL

Acebutolol is a selective β_1-adrenergic antagonist with some intrinsic sympathomimetic activity.

Absorption, Fate, and Excretion. Acebutolol is well absorbed, but it is extensively metabolized to an active metabolite, diacetolol, which accounts for most of the drug's activity (Singh *et al.*, 1985). The elimination half-life of acebutolol is typically about 3 hours, but the half-life of diacetolol is 8 to 12 hours; it is excreted in the urine.

Preparations, Routes of Administration, and Dosage. *Acebutolol hydrochloride* (SECTRAL) is available in 200- and 400-mg capsules. The initial dose in hypertension is usually 400 mg per day, which may be given in a single dose, but two divided doses may be required for adequate control of blood pressure. Optimal responses usually occur with doses of 400 to 800 mg per day (range 200 to 1200 mg). For treatment of ventricular arrhythmias, the drug should be given twice daily.

OTHER β-ADRENERGIC ANTAGONISTS

A plethora of other β-adrenergic antagonists have also been synthesized and evaluated to varying extents. Of those available in the United States, both *carteolol* (CARTROL) and *penbutolol* (LEVATOL) are nonselective β blockers; penbutolol has some intrinsic sympathomimetic activity. *Levobunolol* (BETAGAN LIQUIFILM), a nonselective antagonist, is available in a 0.5% ophthalmic solution for the treatment of glaucoma. *Betaxolol* (BETOPTIC) is a β_1-selective ophthalmic preparation. Betaxolol may be less likely to induce bronchospasm than are ophthalmic preparations of timolol or levobunolol. *Sotalol* is a nonselective antagonist that is devoid of membrane-stabilizing actions. However, it appears to have antiarrhythmic actions independent of its ability to block β-adrenergic receptors (*see* Singh *et al.*, 1987). Many other β blockers are marketed in countries other than the United States.

ADVERSE EFFECTS AND PRECAUTIONS

The most common adverse effects of β-adrenergic antagonists arise as pharmacological consequences of blockade of β receptors; serious adverse effects unrelated to β-receptor blockade are rare.

Cardiovascular System. β-Adrenergic antagonists may induce congestive heart failure in susceptible patients, since the sympathetic nervous system provides critical support for cardiac performance in many individuals with impaired myocardial function. Thus, β-adrenergic blockade may cause or exacerbate heart failure in patients with compensated heart failure, acute myocardial infarction, or cardiomegaly. It is not known if β-adrenergic antagonists that possess intrinsic sympathomimetic activity or peripheral vasodilating properties are safer in these settings.

Bradycardia is a normal response to β-adrenergic blockade; however, in patients with partial or complete atrioventricular conduction defects, β-adrenergic antagonists may cause life-threatening bradyarrhythmias. Particular caution is indicated in patients who are taking other drugs that may impair sinus-node function or atrioventricular conduction, such as verapamil or various antiarrhythmic agents.

Some patients complain of cold extremities while taking β-adrenergic antagonists. Symptoms of peripheral vascular disease may worsen, or Raynaud's phenomenon may develop. It is not known if selective β_1-adrenergic antagonists, drugs with intrinsic sympathomimetic activity at β_2 receptors, or drugs that possess α_1-blocking activity are less likely to exacerbate intermittent claudication.

Abrupt discontinuation of β-adrenergic antagonists after long-term treatment can exacerbate angina and may increase the risk of sudden death. The underlying mechanism is uncertain. However, it is well established that there is enhanced sensitivity to β-adrenergic agonists in patients who have undergone long-term treatment with certain β-adrenergic antagonists after the blocker is withdrawn abruptly. For example, chronotropic responses to isoproterenol are blunted in patients who are receiving β-adrenergic antagonists; however, abrupt discontinuation of propranolol leads to greater than normal sensitivity to isoproterenol. This increased sensitivity is evident several days after stopping propranolol and may persist for at least 1 week (Nattel *et al.*, 1979). Such enhanced sensitivity can be attenuated by tapering the dose of the β blocker for several weeks before discontinuation (Rangno *et al.*, 1982). Supersensitivity to isoproterenol has also been observed after abrupt discontinuation of metoprolol, but not of pindolol (Rangno and Langlois, 1982). The concentration of β-adrenergic receptors on circulating lymphocytes is increased in subjects who have received propranolol for long periods; pindolol has the opposite effect (Hedberg *et al.*, 1986). Optimal strategies for discontinuation of β blockers are not known, but it is prudent to decrease the dose gradually and to restrict exercise during this period.

Pulmonary Function. A major adverse effect of β-adrenergic antagonists is caused by blockade of β_2 receptors in bronchial smooth muscle. These receptors are particularly important for promoting bronchodilatation in patients with bronchospastic disease, and β blockers may cause a life-threatening increase in airway resistance in such patients. Drugs with selectivity for β_1 receptors or those with intrinsic sympathomimetic activity at β_2 receptors may be somewhat less likely to induce bronchospasm. However, the selectivity of current β blockers for β_1-adrenergic receptors is modest; consequently, these drugs should be avoided if at all possible in patients with asthma.

Central Nervous System. The side effects of β-adrenergic antagonists that are referable to the CNS include fatigue, sleep disturbances (including insomnia and nightmares), and depression. Interest has focused on the relationship between the incidence of these effects and the lipophilicity of the various β blockers. However, no clear correlation has emerged (Drayer, 1987; Gengo *et al.*, 1987).

Metabolism. As described above, β-adrenergic blockade may blunt recognition of hypoglycemia by patients; it may also delay recovery from insulin-induced hypoglycemia. β-Adrenergic antagonists should be used with great caution in diabetics who are prone to hypoglycemic reactions; β_1-selective agents may be preferable for these patients. β-Adrenergic antagonists cause an increased concentration of plasma triglycerides.

Miscellaneous. Nonspecific symptoms such as constipation, diarrhea, or indigestion are uncommon. The incidence of sexual dysfunction in men with hypertension who are treated with β-adrenergic antagonists is not clearly defined. Although experience with the use of β-adrenergic antagonists in pregnancy is increasing, information about the safety of these drugs during pregnancy is still limited (*see* Widerhorn *et al.*, 1987).

Overdosage. The manifestations of poisoning with β-adrenergic antagonists are dependent on the pharmacological properties of the ingested drug, particularly its β_1 selectivity, intrinsic sympathomimetic activity, and membrane-stabilizing properties (*see* Frishman *et al.*, 1984). Hypotension, bradycardia, prolonged AV conduction times, and widened QRS complexes are common manifestations of overdosage. Seizures and/or psychiatric depression may occur. Hypoglycemia is rare, and bronchospasm is uncommon in the absence of pulmonary disease. Therapy involves the usual supportive measures. Significant bradycardia should be treated initially with atropine, but a cardiac pacemaker is often required. Large doses of isoproterenol or an α-adrenergic agonist may be necessary to treat hypotension. Glucagon has positive chronotropic and inotropic effects on the heart that are independent of interactions with β-adrenergic receptors, and the drug has been useful in some patients.

Drug Interactions. Both pharmacokinetic and pharmacodynamic interactions have been noted between β-adrenergic blocking agents and other drugs. Aluminum salts, cholestyramine, and colestipol may decrease the absorption of β blockers. Drugs such as phenytoin, rifampin, and phenobarbital, as well as smoking, induce hepatic biotransformation enzymes and may decrease plasma concentrations of β-adrenergic antagonists that are metabolized extensively (*e.g.*, propranolol). Cimetidine and hydralazine may increase the bioavailability of agents such as propranolol and metoprolol by affecting hepatic blood flow. β-Adrenergic antagonists can impair the clearance of lidocaine.

Other drug interactions have pharmacodynamic explanations. For example, β-adrenergic antagonists and Ca^{2+}-channel blockers have additive effects on the cardiac conducting system. Additive effects on blood pressure between β blockers and other antihypertensive agents are often sought. However, the antihypertensive effects of β-adrenergic antagonists can be opposed by indomethacin and other nonsteroidal antiinflammatory drugs (*see* Chapter 26).

THERAPEUTIC USES

Cardiovascular Diseases. β-Adrenergic antagonists are used extensively in the treatment of hypertension (*see* Chapter 33) and angina (*see* Chapter 32). These drugs are also used frequently in the treatment of supraventricular and ventricular arrhythmias; this is discussed in Chapter 35.

A great deal of interest has focused on the use of β-adrenergic antagonists in the treatment of acute myocardial infarction and in the prevention of recurrences for those who have survived an initial attack. Several trials have shown that intravenous administration of β-adrenergic antagonists such as metoprolol or atenolol during the early phases of acute myocardial infarction may decrease mortality by about 10% (MIAMI Trial Research Group, 1985; ISIS-1 Group, 1986; Yusuf, 1987). The precise mechanism is not known, but the favorable effects of β-adrenergic antagonists may stem from decreased myocardial oxygen demand, redistribution of myocardial blood flow, reduction of the concentration of free fatty acids in plasma, and antiarrhythmic actions. For prevention of recurrences, propranolol, metoprolol, and timolol decrease the mortality rate when started within several weeks of a myocardial infarction (Olsson *et al.*, 1985; Furberg, 1987).

β-Adrenergic antagonists, particularly propranolol, are used in the treatment of hypertrophic obstructive cardiomyopathy. Propranolol is useful for relieving angina, palpitations, and syncope in patients with this disorder. Efficacy is probably related to partial relief of the pressure gradient along the outflow tract. Although β-adrenergic antagonists can precipitate congestive heart failure in susceptible patients, these drugs may be useful in the treatment of selected patients with dilated cardiomyopathy. One rationale for this use is that limited blockade of β_1 receptors could reduce the deleterious effects on myocardial function produced by the increased sympathetic stimulation that occurs in congestive heart failure. The results of this approach await the outcome of appropriate clinical trials. β-Adrenergic antagonists are used to treat arrhythmias in patients with mitral valve prolapse. These drugs may also have efficacy in some patients with postural hypotension, although the mechanism is not understood.

β-Blockers are used frequently in the medical management of acute dissecting aortic aneurysm; their usefulness comes from the reduction in the force of myocardial contraction and the rate of development of such force. Nitroprusside is an alternative, but when given in the absence of β-adrenergic blockade, it causes an undesirable tachycardia. β-Adrenergic antagonists are used to combat arrhythmias in patients with pheochromocytoma. However, it is very important to initiate treatment with an α-receptor blocker before a β antagonist is administered. Otherwise, hypertension may be exacerbated because of the loss of β_2-receptor mediated vasodilatation. β Blockers may also attenuate catecholamine-induced cardiomyopathy in this disease (Rosenbaum *et al.*, 1987).

Other Uses. Many of the signs and symptoms of hyperthyroidism are reminiscent of the manifestations of increased sympathetic nervous system activity. Indeed, there is some evidence that excess thyroid hormone increases the expression of β-adrenergic receptors in some types of cells. β-Adrenergic antagonists control many of the cardiovascular signs and symptoms of hyperthyroidism and are useful adjuvants to more definitive therapy (Feely and Peden, 1984). In addition, propranolol inhibits the peripheral conversion of thyroxine to triiodothyronine, an effect that may be independent of β blockade. However, caution is advised in patients with cardiac enlargement, since treatment with β-adrenergic blockers may cause congestive heart failure.

Propranolol, timolol, and metoprolol are effective for the prophylaxis of migraine (Tfelt-Hansen, 1986); the mechanism of this effect is not known, and these drugs are not useful for treatment of acute attacks of migraine (*see* Chapter 39).

Propranolol and other β blockers are effective in controlling acute panic symptoms in individuals who are required to perform in public or in other anxiety-provoking situations (Lader, 1988). Thus, public speakers may be calmed by the prophylactic administration of the drug and the performance of musicians may be improved (Brantigan *et al.*, 1982). Tachycardia, muscle tremors, and other evidence of increased sympathetic activity are reduced. Propranolol may also be useful in the treatment of essential tremor.

Timolol, betaxolol, and levobunolol are effective when used topically for the treatment of open-angle glaucoma. β-Adrenergic antagonists decrease intraocular pressure, probably by decreasing the rate of production of aqueous humor by the ciliary body (Lesar, 1987).

β Blockers may be of some value in the treatment of patients undergoing withdrawal from alcohol or those with akathisia. Although there have been suggestions that these drugs prevent variceal bleeding in patients with portal hypertension, additional information is required (Rector, 1986).

Selection of a β-Adrenergic Antagonist. The various β-adrenergic antagonists that are used for the treatment of hypertension and angina appear to have similar efficacy. Selection of the most appropriate drug for an individual patient should be based on pharmacokinetic and pharmacodynamic differences between the drugs, cost, and whether or not there are associated medical problems. For some diseases (*e.g.*, myocardial infarction, migraine), it should not be assumed that all members of this class of drugs are interchangeable; the appropriate drug should be selected from those that have documented efficacy for the disease. Selective β_1 antagonists are preferable in patients with bronchospasm, diabetes, peripheral vascular disease, or Raynaud's phenomenon. Although no clinical advantage of β-adrenergic antagonists with intrinsic sympathomimetic activity has been clearly established, such drugs might be preferable in patients with bradycardia. Selective β_1 antagonists or drugs with intrinsic sympathomimetic activity might also be preferable in patients with hyperlipidemia.

Baum, T.; Watkins, R. W.; Sybertz, E. J.; Vemulapalli, S.; Pula, K. K.; Eynon, E.; Nelson, S.; Vliet, G. V.; Glennon, J.; and Moran, R. M. Antihypertensive and hemodynamic actions of SCH 19927, the R,R-isomer and labetalol. *J. Pharmacol. Exp. Ther.*, **1981**, *218*, 444–452.

Black, J. W., and Stephenson, J. S. Pharmacology of a new *beta*-adrenergic receptor blocking compound. *Lancet*, **1962**, *2*, 311–314.

Blakeley, A. G., and Summers, R. J. The effects of labetalol (AH 5158) on adrenergic transmission in the cat spleen. *Br. J. Pharmacol.*, **1977**, *59*, 643–650.

Brantigan, C. O.; Brantigan, T. A.; and Joseph, N. Effect of beta blockade and beta stimulation on stage fright. *Am. J. Med.*, **1982**, *72*, 88–94.

Brown, M. J.; Brown, D. C.; and Murphy, M. B. Hypokalemia from beta$_2$-receptor stimulation by circulating epinephrine. *N. Engl. J. Med.*, **1983**, *309*, 1414–1419.

Buhler, F. R.; Laragh, J. H.; Baer, L.; Vaughn, D. E.; and Brunner, H. R. Propranolol inhibition of renin secretion. *N. Engl. J. Med.*, **1972**, *287*, 1209–1214.

Caine, M.; Perlberg, S.; and Shapiro, A. Phenoxybenzamine for benign prostatic obstruction: review of 200 cases. *Urology*, **1981**, *17*, 542–546.

Carliner, N. H.; Denune, D. P.; Finch, C. S., Jr.; and Goldberg, L. I. Sodium nitroprusside treatment of ergotamine-induced peripheral ischemia. *J.A.M.A.*, **1974**, *227*, 308–309.

Clark, J. T.; Smith, E. R.; and Davidson, J. M. Enhancement of sexual motivation in male rats by yohimbine. *Science*, **1984**, *225*, 847–849.

Cohn, J. N., and others. The effect of vasodilator therapy on mortality in chronic congestive heart failure: results of a Veterans Administration cooperative study. *N. Engl. J. Med.*, **1986**, *314*, 1547–1552.

Cubeddu, L. X.; Barnes, E.; Langer, S. Z.; and Weiner, N. Release of norepinephrine and dopamine-β-hydroxylase by nerve stimulation. I. Role of neuronal and extraneuronal uptake and of alpha presynaptic receptors. *J. Pharmacol. Exp. Ther.*, **1974**, *190*, 431–450.

Dage, R. C., and Hsieh, C. P. Direct vasodilatation by labetalol in anaesthetized dogs. *Br. J. Pharmacol.*, **1980**, *702*, 87–93.

Deacon, S. P., and Barnett, D. Comparison of atenolol and propranolol during insulin-induced hypoglycemia. *Br. Med. J.*, **1976**, *2*, 272–273.

Deacon, S. P.; Karunanuyake, A.; and Barnett, D. Acebutolol, atenolol and propranolol and metabolic responses to acute hypoglycemia in man. *Br. Med. J.*, **1977**, *2*, 1255–1257.

Drew, G. M.; Hilditch, A.; and Levy, G. P. Effect of labetalol on the uptake of [3H]-(−)-noradrenaline into the isolated vas deferens of the rat. *Br. J. Pharmacol.*, **1978**, *63*, 471–474.

Elliott, H. L.; Vincent, J.; Meredith, P. A.; and Reid, J. L. Relationship between plasma prazosin concentration and alpha-antagonism in humans: comparison of conventional and rate-controlled (Oros) formulations. *Clin. Pharmacol. Ther.*, **1988**, *43*, 582–587.

Emorine, L. J.; Marullo, S.; Briend-Sutren, M.-M.; Patey, G.; Tate, K.; Delavier-Klutchko, C.; and Strosberg, D. Molecular characterization of the human β_3-adrenergic receptor. *Science*, **1989**, *245*, 1118–1121.

Gal, J.; Zirrolli, J. A.; and Lichtenstein, P. S. Labetalol is metabolized oxidatively in humans. *Res. Commun. Chem. Pathol. Pharmacol.*, **1988**, *62*, 3–17.

Gengo, F. M.; Huntoon, L.; and McHugh, W. B. Lipid-soluble and water-soluble beta-blockers: comparison of the central nervous system depressant effect. *Arch. Intern. Med.*, **1987**, *147*, 39–43.

Gold, E. H.; Chang, W.; Cohen, M.; Baum, T.; Ehrreich, S.; Johnson, G.; Prioli, N.; and Sybertz, E. J. Synthesis and comparison of some cardiovascular properties of the stereoisomers of labetalol. *J. Med. Chem.*, **1982**, *25*, 1363–1370.

Hamilton, C.; Dalrymple, H.; and Reid, J. Recovery *in vivo* and *in vitro* of alpha-adrenoceptor responses and radioligand binding after phenoxybenzamine. *J. Cardiovasc. Pharmacol.*, **1982**, *4*, Suppl. 1, S125–S128.

Hamilton, C. A.; Reid, J. L.; and Sumner, D. J. Acute effects of phenoxybenzamine on alpha-adrenoceptor responses *in vivo* and *in vitro*: relation of *in vivo* pressor responses to the number of specific adrenoceptor binding sites. *J. Cardiovasc. Pharmacol.*, **1983**, *5*, 868–873.

Hedberg, A.; Gerber, J. G.; Nies, A. S.; Wolfe, B. B.; and Molinoff, P. B. Effects of pindolol and propranolol on beta adrenergic receptors on human lymphocytes. *J. Pharmacol. Exp. Ther.*, **1986**, *239*, 117–123.

ISIS-1 Group. Randomized trial of intravenous atenolol among 16027 cases of suspected myocardial infarction. *Lancet*, **1986**, *2*, 57–65.

Jebavy, P.; Koudelkova, E.; and Henzlova, M. Unloading effects of prazosin in patients with chronic aortic regurgitation. *Am. Heart J.*, **1983**, *105*, 567–574.

Kaiser, P.; Tesch, P. A.; Frisk-Holmberg, M.; Juhlin-Dannfelt, A.; and Kaiser, L. Effect of beta$_1$ and nonselective beta-blockade on work capacity and muscle metabolism. *Clin. Physiol.*, **1986**, *6*, 197–207.

Kashiwagi, A.; Harano, Y.; Suzuki, M.; Kojima, H.; Harada, M.; Nishio, Y.; and Shigeta, Y. New alpha$_2$ adrenergic blocker (DG-5128) improves insulin secretion and *in vivo* glucose disposal in NIDDM patients. *Diabetes*, **1986**, *35*, 1085–1089.

Kirby, R. S.; Coppinger, S. W.; Corcoran, M. O.; Chapple, C. R.; Flannigan, M.; and Milroy, E. J. Prazosin in the treatment of prostatic obstruction; a placebo-controlled study. *Br. J. Urol.*, **1987**, *60*, 136–142.

Kirsten, R.; Nelson, K.; Steinijans, V. W.; Zech, K.; and Haerlin, R. Clinical pharmacokinetics of urapidil. *Clin. Pharmacokinet.*, **1988**, *14*, 129–140.

MIAMI Trial Research Group. Metoprolol in acute myocardial infarction (MIAMI): a randomized placebo-controlled international study. *Eur. Heart J.*, **1985**, *6*, 199–226.

Miller, V. M., and Vanhoutte, P. M. Endothelial alpha$_2$-adrenoreceptors in canine pulmonary and systemic blood vessels. *Eur. J. Pharmacol.*, **1985**, *118*, 123–129.

Nattel, S.; Rangno, R. E.; and Van Loon, G. Mechanism of propranolol withdrawal phenomena. *Circulation*, **1979**, *59*, 1158–1164.

Nies, A. S.; Evans, G. H.; and Shand, D. G. Regional hemodynamic effects of beta-adrenergic blockade with propranolol in the unanesthetized primate. *Am. Heart J.*, **1973**, *85*, 97–102.

Olsson, G.; Rehnqvist, N.; Sjögren, A.; Erhardt, L.; and Lundman, T. Long-term treatment with metoprolol after myocardial infarction: effect on 3 year mortality and morbidity. *J. Am. Coll. Cardiol.*, **1985**, *5*, 1428–1437.

Powell, C. E., and Slater, I. H. Blocking of inhibitory adrenergic receptors by a dichloro analog of isoproterenol. *J. Pharmacol. Exp. Ther.*, **1958**, *122*, 480–488.

Rangno, R. E., and Langlois, S. Comparison of withdrawal phenomena after propranolol, metoprolol, and pindolol. *Am. Heart J.*, **1982**, *104*, 473–478.

Rangno, R. E.; Nattel, S.; and Lutterodt, A. Prevention of propranolol withdrawal mechanism by prolonged small dose propranolol schedule. *Am. J. Cardiol.*, **1982**, *49*, 828–833.

Reid, D.; Morales, A.; Harris, C.; Surridge, D. H. C.; Condra, M.; and Owen, J. Double-blind trial of yohimbine in treatment of psychogenic impotence. *Lancet*, **1987**, *2*, 421–423.

Reilly, C. S.; Wood, M.; Koshakji, R. P.; and Wood, A. J. J. Ultra-short-acting beta-blockade: a comparison with conventional beta-blockade. *Clin. Pharmacol. Ther.*, **1985**, *38*, 579–585.

Robertson, R. M.; Bernard, Y. D.; Carr, R. K.; and Robertson, D. Alpha-adrenergic blockade in vasotonic angina: lack of efficacy of specific $alpha_1$ receptor blockade with prazosin. *J. Am. Coll. Cardiol.*, **1983**, *2*, 1146–1150.

Rosen, S. G.; Clutter, W. E.; Shah, S. D.; Miller, J. P.; Bier, D. M.; and Cryer, P. E. Direct alpha-adrenergic stimulation of hepatic glucose production in human subjects. *Am. J. Physiol.*, **1983**, *245*, E616–E626.

Rosenbaum, J. S.; Ginsburg, R.; Billingham, M. E.; and Hoffman, B. B. Effects of adrenergic receptor antagonists on cardiac morphological and functional alterations in rats harboring pheochromocytoma. *J. Pharmacol. Exp. Ther.*, **1987**, *241*, 354–360.

Sasso, E. H., and O'Connor, D. T. Prazosin depression of baroreflex function in hypertensive man. *Eur. J. Clin. Pharmacol.*, **1982**, *22*, 7–14.

Sheridan, D. J.; Penkoske, P. A.; Sobel, B. E.; and Corr, P. B. Alpha adrenergic contributions to dysrhythmia during myocardial ischemia and reperfusion in cats. *J. Clin. Invest.*, **1980**, *65*, 161–171.

Sizemore, G. W., and Winternitz, W. W. Autonomic hyper-reflexia—suppression with alpha-adrenergic blocking agents. *N. Engl. J. Med.*, **1970**, *282*, 795.

Surwit, R. S.; Gilgor, R. S.; Allen, L. M.; and Duvic, M. A double-blind study of prazosin in the treatment of Raynaud's phenomenon in scleroderma. *Arch. Dermatol.*, **1984**, *120*, 329–331.

Sybertz, E. J.; Sabin, C. S.; Pula, K. K.; Vander Vliet, G.; Glennon, J.; Gold, E. H.; and Baum, T. Alpha and beta adrenoceptor blocking properties of labetalol and its R,R-isomer, SCH 19927. *J. Pharmacol. Exp. Ther.*, **1981**, *218*, 435–443.

Winniford, M. D.; Filipchuk, N.; and Hillis, L. D. Alpha-adrenergic blockade for variant angina: a long-term, double-blind, randomized trial. *Circulation*, **1983**, *67*, 1185–1188.

Wollersheim, H.; Thien, T.; Fennis, J.; van Elteren, P.; and van't Laar, A. Double-blind, placebo-controlled study of prazosin in Raynaud's phenomenon. *Clin. Pharmacol. Ther.*, **1986**, *40*, 219–225.

Monographs and Reviews

Andersson, K.-E. Current concepts in the treatment of disorders of micturition. *Drugs*, **1988**, *35*, 477–494.

Benfield, P.; Clissold, S. P.; and Brogden, R. N. Metoprolol. *Drugs*, **1986**, *31*, 376–429.

Benfield, P., and Sorkin, E. M. Esmolol: a preliminary review of its pharmacodynamic and pharmacokinetic properties, and therapeutic efficacy. *Drugs*, **1987**, *33*, 392–412.

Berde, B., and Schild, H. O. (eds.). *Ergot Alkaloids and Related Compounds. Handbuch der Experimentellen Pharmakologie*, Vol. 49. Springer-Verlag, Berlin, **1978.**

Berde, B., and Stürmer, E. Introduction to the pharmacology of ergot alkaloids and related compounds as a basis of their therapeutic application. In, *Ergot Alkaloids and Related Compounds*. (Berde, B., and Schild, H. O., eds.) *Handbuch der Experimentellen Pharmakologie*, Vol. 49. Springer-Verlag, Berlin, **1978**, pp. 1–28.

Black, J. W., and Prichard, B. N. C. Activation and blockade of β adrenoceptors in common cardiac disorders. *Br. Med. Bull.*, **1973**, *29*, 163–167.

Brodde, O. E. The functional importance of $beta_1$ and $beta_2$ adrenoceptors in the human heart. *Am. J. Cardiol.*, **1988**, *62*, 24C–29C.

Brogden, R. N.; Heel, R. C.; Speight, T. M.; and Avery, G. S. α-Methyl-*p*-tyrosine: a review of its pharmacology and clinical use. *Drugs*, **1984**, *21*, 81–89.

Brown, M. J. Hypokalemia from β_2-receptor stimulation by circulating epinephrine. *Am. J. Cardiol.*, **1985**, *56*, 3D–9D.

Caine, M. The place of pharmacologic treatment in benign prostatic hyperplasia. *Semin. Urol.*, **1985**, *3*, 311–316.

Cleophas, T. J., and Kauw, F. H. Pressor responses from noncardioselective beta-blockers. *Angiology*, **1988**, *39*, 587–596.

Colucci, W. S. Alpha-adrenergic receptor blockade with prazosin: consideration of hypertension, heart failure, and potential new applications. *Ann. Intern. Med.*, **1982**, *97*, 67–77.

Cruickshank, J. M. The clinical importance of cardioselectivity and lipophilicity in beta blockers. *Am. Heart J.*, **1980**, *100*, 160–178.

Cubeddu, L. X. New $alpha_1$-adrenergic receptor antagonists for the treatment of hypertension: role of vascular alpha receptors in the control of peripheral resistance. *Am. Heart J.*, **1988**, *116*, 133–162.

Dale, H. H. On some physiological actions of ergot. *J. Physiol. (Lond.)*, **1906**, *34*, 163–206.

Davey, M. Mechanism of alpha blockade for blood pressure control. *Am. J. Cardiol.*, **1987**, *59*, 18G–28G.

Davey, M. J. Alpha adrenoceptors—an overview. *J. Mol. Cell. Cardiol.*, **1986**, *18*, Suppl. 5, 1–15.

Drayer, D. E. Lipophilicity, hydrophilicity, and the central nervous system side effects of beta blockers. *Pharmacotherapy*, **1987**, *7*, 87–91.

Epstein, M., and Oster, J. R. Beta-blockers and the kidney. *Miner. Electrolyte Metab.*, **1982**, *8*, 237–254.

Feely, J., and Peden, N. Use of beta-adrenoceptor blocking drugs in hyperthyroidism. *Drugs*, **1984**, *27*, 425–446.

Frishman, W. H. Nadolol: a new beta-adrenoceptor antagonist. *N. Engl. J. Med.*, **1982**, *305*, 678–682.

———. Pindolol: a new beta-adrenoceptor antagonist with partial agonist activity. *Ibid.*, **1983**, *308*, 940–944.

Frishman, W. H., and Charlap, S. Alpha adrenergic blockers. *Med. Clin. North Am.*, **1988**, *72*, 427–440.

Frishman, W. H.; Eisen, G.; and Lapsker, J. Terazosin: a new long-acting $alpha_1$ adrenergic antagonist of hypertension. *Med. Clin. North Am.*, **1988**, *72*, 441–448.

Frishman, W. H.; Jacob, H.; Eisenberg, E.; and Spivack, C. R. Overdosage with beta-adrenoceptor blocking drugs: pharmacologic considerations and clinical management. In, *Clinical Pharmacology of the Beta Adrenoceptor Blocking Drugs*, 2nd ed. (Frishman, W. H., ed.) Appleton-Century-Crofts, Norwalk, Conn., **1984**, pp. 169–203.

Frishman, W. H., and Weksler, B. B. Effects of beta-adrenoceptor blocking agents on platelet function. In, *Clinical Pharmacology of the Beta Adrenoceptor Blocking Drugs*, 2nd ed. (Frishman, W. H., ed.) Appleton-Century-Crofts, Norwalk, Conn., **1984**, pp. 273–298.

Furberg, C. D. Secondary prevention trials after acute myocardial infarction. *Am. J. Cardiol.*, **1987**, *60*, 28A–32A.

Furchgott, R. F. The classification of adrenoceptors (adrenergic receptors). An evaluation from the standpoint of receptor theory. In, *Catecholamines*. (Blaschko, H., and Muscholl, E., eds.) *Handbuch der Experimentellen Pharmakologie*, Vol. 33. Springer-Verlag, Berlin, **1972**, pp. 283–335.

Goldberg, M. R., and Robertson, D. Yohimbine: a pharmacological probe of the $alpha_2$ adrenoreceptor. *Pharmacol. Rev.*, **1983**, *35*, 143–180.

Hess, H.-J. Prazosin: biochemistry and structure-activity studies. *Postgrad. Med.*, **1975**, *58*, 9–17.

Holmes, B., and Sorkin, E. M. Indoramin: a review of its pharmacodynamic and pharmacokinetic properties, and therapeutic efficacy in hypertension and related vascular, cardiovascular and airway diseases. *Drugs*, **1986**, *31*, 467–499.

IARC. Phenoxybenzamine and phenoxybenzamine hydrochloride. *IARC Monogr. Eval. Carcinog. Risk Chem. Hum.*, **1980**, *24*, 185–194.

Lader, M. Beta-adrenoceptor antagonists in neuropsychiatry: an update. *J. Clin. Psychiatry*, **1988**, *49*, 213–223.

Langer, S. Z. Presynaptic regulation of the release of catecholamines. *Pharmacol. Rev.*, **1981**, *32*, 337–362.

Lesar, T. S. Comparison of ophthalmic beta-blocking agents. *Clin. Pharm.*, **1987**, *6*, 451–463.

McDevitt, D. G. Comparison of pharmacokinetic properties of beta-adrenoceptor blocking drugs. *Eur. Heart J.*, **1987**, *8*, Suppl. M, 9–14.

McNeil, J. J., and Louis, W. J. Clinical pharmacokinetics of labetalol. *Clin. Pharmacokinet.*, **1984**, *9*, 157–167.

Man in't Veld, A. J.; Van den Meiracker, A. H.; and Schalekamp, M. A. Do beta-blockers really increase peripheral vascular resistance? Review of the literature and new observations under basal conditions. *Am. J. Hypertens.*, **1988**, *1*, 91–96.

Miller, N. E. Effects of adrenoceptor-blocking drugs on plasma lipoprotein concentrations. *Am. J. Cardiol.*, **1987**, *60*, 17E–23E.

Mimran, A., and Ducailar, G. Systemic and regional haemodynamic profile of diuretics and alpha- and beta-blockers. A review comparing acute and chronic effects. *Drugs*, **1988**, *35*, Suppl. 6, 60–69.

Nace, G. S., and Wood, A. J. Pharmacokinetics of long acting propranolol: implications for therapeutic use. *Clin. Pharmacokinet.*, **1987**, *13*, 51–64.

Nickerson, M., and Hollenberg, N. K. Blockade of α-adrenergic receptors. In, *Physiological Pharmacology*. Vol. 4, *The Nervous System—Part D: Autonomic Nervous System Drugs*. (Root, W. S., and Hofmann, F. G., eds.) Academic Press, New York, **1967**, pp. 243–305.

Oates, J. A.; Conolly, M. E.; Prichard, B. N. C.; Shand, D. G.; and Schapel, G. The clinical pharmacology of antihypertensive drugs. In, *Antihypertensive Agents*. (Gross, F., ed.) *Handbuch der Experimentellen Pharmakologie*, Vol. 39. Springer-Verlag, Berlin, **1977**, pp. 571–632.

Reaven, G. M., and Hoffman, B. B. A role for insulin in the aetiology and course of hypertension? *Lancet*, **1987**, *2*, 435–437.

Rector, W. G. Drug therapy for portal hypertension. *Ann. Intern. Med.*, **1986**, *105*, 96–107.

Reynolds, R. D.; Gorczynske, R. J.; and Quon, C. Y. Pharmacology and pharmacokinetics of esmolol. *J. Clin. Pharmacol.*, **1986**, *26*, Suppl. A, A3–A14.

Rubin, P., and Blaschke, T. Prazosin protein binding in health and disease. *Br. J. Clin. Pharmacol.*, **1980**, *9*, 177–182.

Shand, D. G. Propranolol. *N. Engl. J. Med.*, **1975**, *293*, 280–284.

Shephard, R. J. *Physiology and Biochemistry of Exercise*. Praeger, New York, **1982**, pp. 228–229.

Sidi, A. A. Vasoactive intracavernous pharmacotherapy. *Urol. Clin. North Am.*, **1988**, *15*, 95–101.

Singh, B. N.; Deedwania, P.; Nademanee, K.; Ward, A.; and Sorkin, E. M. Sotalol. *Drugs*, **1987**, *34*, 311–349.

Singh, B. N.; Thoden, W. R.; and Ward, A. Acebutolol. *Drugs*, **1985**, *29*, 531–569.

Stanaszek, W. F.; Kellerman, D.; Brogden, R. N.; and Romankiewicz, J. A. Prazosin update. A review of its pharmacological properties and therapeutic use in hypertension and congestive heart failure. *Drugs*, **1983**, *25*, 339–384.

Starke, D. Alpha-adrenoceptor subclassification. *Rev. Physiol. Biochem. Pharmacol.*, **1981**, *88*, 199–236.

Struthers, A. D., and Reid, J. L. The role of adrenal medullary catecholamines in potassium homeostasis. *Clin. Sci.*, **1984**, *66*, 377–382.

Tesch, P. A. Exercise performance and beta-blockade. *Sports Med.*, **1985**, *2*, 389–412.

Tfelt-Hansen, P. Efficacy of beta-blockers in migraine: a critical review. *Cephalalgia*, **1986**, *6*, Suppl. 5, 15–24.

Titmarsh, S., and Monk, S. P. Terazosin. A review of its pharmacodynamic and pharmacokinetic properties, and therapeutic efficacy in essential hypertension. *Drugs*, **1987**, *33*, 461–477.

Van Baak, M. A. Beta-adrenoceptor blockade and exercise: an update. *Sports Med.*, **1988**, *5*, 209–225.

van Zwieten, P. A. Antihypertensive drugs interacting with alpha- and beta-adrenoceptors: a review of basic pharmacology. *Drugs*, **1988**, *35*, Suppl. 6, 6–19.

Walle, T.; Webb, J. G.; Bagwell, E. E.; Walle, U. K.; Daniell, G. B.; and Gaffney, T. E. Stereoselective delivery and actions of beta receptor antagonists. *Biochem. Pharmacol.*, **1988**, *37*, 115–124.

Widerhorn, J.; Rubin, J. N.; Frishman, W. H.; and Elkayam, U. Cardiovascular drugs in pregnancy. *Cardiol. Clin.*, **1987**, *5*, 651–674.

Young, R. A., and Brogden, R. N. Doxazosin: a review of its pharmacodynamic and pharmacokinetic properties, and therapeutic efficacy in mild or moderate hypertension. *Drugs*, **1988**, *35*, 525–541.

Yusuf, S. Interventions that potentially limit myocardial infarct size: overview of clinical trials. *Am. J. Cardiol.*, **1987**, *60*, 11A–17A.

Zentgraf, M.; Baccouche, M.; and Junemann, K. P. Diagnosis and therapy of erectile dysfunction using papaverine and phentolamine. *Urol. Int.*, **1988**, *43*, 65–75.

SECTION

III

Drugs Acting on the Central Nervous System

CHAPTER

12 NEUROHUMORAL TRANSMISSION AND THE CENTRAL NERVOUS SYSTEM

Floyd E. Bloom

Drugs that act upon the central nervous system (CNS) influence the lives of everyone, everyday. These agents are invaluable therapeutically because they can produce specific physiological and psychological effects. Without general anesthetics, modern surgery would be impossible. Drugs that affect the CNS may selectively relieve pain or fever, suppress disorders of movement, or prevent seizures. They may induce sleep or arousal, reduce the desire to eat, or allay the tendency to vomit. They may be used to treat anxiety, mania, depression, or schizophrenia without altering consciousness. The brain may also be affected by drugs that are used to treat diseases of peripheral organs.

The nonmedical, self-use of CNS drugs is widely practiced. Socially acceptable stimulants and antianxiety agents produce stability, relief, and even pleasure for many. However, the excessive use of these and other drugs can adversely affect lives when their use leads to physical dependence on the drug or to toxic side effects, which may include lethal overdosage.

The unique quality of drugs that affect the nervous system and behavior places investigators who study the CNS in the midst of an extraordinary scientific challenge—the attempt to understand the cellular and molecular basis for the enormously complex and varied functions of the human brain. In this effort, pharmacologists have two major goals: to use drugs to dissect the mechanisms that operate in the normal CNS and to develop appropriate drugs to correct pathophysiological events in the abnormal CNS.

Approaches to the elucidation of the sites and mechanisms of action of CNS drugs demand an understanding of the cellular and molecular biology of the brain. Although knowledge of the anatomy, physiology, and chemistry of the nervous system is far from complete, the acceleration of interdisciplinary research on the CNS has led to remarkable progress. This chapter introduces guidelines and fundamental principles for the comprehensive analysis of drugs that affect the CNS. Specific therapeutic approaches to neurological and psychiatric disorders are discussed in the chapters that follow in this section.

ORGANIZATIONAL PRINCIPLES OF THE BRAIN

The brain is an assembly of interrelated neural systems that regulate their own and each other's activity in a dynamic, complex fashion. The large anatomical divisions provide a superficial classification of the distribution of brain functions.

MACROFUNCTIONS OF BRAIN REGIONS

Cerebral Cortex. The two cerebral hemispheres constitute the largest division of the brain. Regions of the cortex are classified in several ways: (1) by the modality of information processed (*e.g.*, sensory, including somatosensory, visual, auditory, and olfactory, as well as motor and associational); (2) by anatomical position (frontal, temporal, parietal, and occipital); and (3) by the geometrical relationship between cell types in the major cortical layers (so-called cytoarchitectonic classifications). The cerebral cortex exhibits a relatively uniform laminar appearance within any given local region. Columnar sets of approximately 100 vertically connected neurons are considered to form an elemental processing module. The specialized functions of a cortical region arise from the interplay upon this basic module of connections to and from both other regions of the cortex (corticocortical systems) and noncortical areas of the brain (subcortical systems). Varying numbers of adjacent columnar modules may be functionally, but transiently, linked into larger information-processing ensembles. The pathology of Alzheimer's disease, for example, destroys the integrity of the columnar modules and the corticocortical connections.

Mountcastle and Edelman (1978) view these columnar ensembles as "interconnected . . . nested distributed systems" and suggest that the associations are rapidly modifiable as information is processed. The 50 billion neurons of the human cortex provide an astronomical number of possibilities for such processing. Cortical areas termed *association areas* receive and somehow process information from primary cortical sensory regions to produce higher cortical functions such as abstract thought, memory, and consciousness (Rakic and Singer, 1988). The cerebral cortices also provide for supervisory integration of the autonomic nervous system, and they may integrate somatic and vegetative functions, including those of the cardiovascular and gastrointestinal systems.

Limbic System. This region, which consists of the *hippocampus, amygdaloid complex, septum, hypothalamus, olfactory* and *pyriform lobes, basal ganglia,* and parts of the *thalamus,* is sometimes called the visceral brain. These structures lie beneath the cortical mantle and act in a complex manner to integrate emotional state with motor and visceral activities.

Parts of the limbic system also participate individually in functions that are capable of more precise definition. Thus, the basal ganglia or neostriatum (the *caudate nucleus, putamen, globus pallidus,* and *lentiform nucleus*) form an essential segment of the *extrapyramidal motor system.* This system complements the function of the pyramidal (or voluntary) motor system; damage to the extrapyramidal system depresses the ability to initiate voluntary movements and causes disorders characterized by involuntary movements, such as the tremors and rigidity of Parkinson's disease or the uncontrollable limb movements of Huntington's chorea. Similarly, the hippocampus may be crucial to the formation of recent memory, since this function is lost in patients with extensive bilateral damage to the hippocampus or with Alzheimer's disease, which destroys the intrinsic structure of the hippocampus.

The *thalamus* lies in the center of the brain, beneath the cortex and basal ganglia and above the hypothalamus. The neurons of the thalamus are arranged into distinct clusters, or nuclei, which are either paired or midline structures. These nuclei act as relays between the incoming sensory pathways and the cortex, between the discrete regions of the thalamus and the hypothalamus, and between the basal ganglia and the association regions of the cerebral cortex. The thalamic nuclei and the basal ganglia also exert regulatory control over visceral functions; aphagia and adipsia, as well as general sensory neglect, follow damage to the corpus striatum.

The *hypothalamus* is the principal integrating region for the entire autonomic nervous system, and it regulates, among other functions, body temperature, water balance, intermediary metabolism, blood pressure, sexual and circadian cycles, secretion of the adenohypophysis, sleep, and emotion. Recent advances in the cytophysiological and chemical dissection of the hypothalamus have clarified the connections and possible functions of individual hypothalamic nuclei (Guillemin, 1978; Swanson, 1986).

Midbrain and Brainstem. The *mesencephalon, pons,* and *medulla oblongata* connect the cerebral hemispheres and thalamus-hypothalamus to the spinal cord. These "bridge portions" of the CNS contain most of the nuclei of the cranial nerves, as well as the major inflow and outflow tracts from the cortices and spinal cord. It is within these regions that the *reticular activating system* is found, which is an important but incompletely characterized region of gray matter linking peripheral sensory and motor events with higher levels of nervous integration. The major monoamine-containing neurons of the brain are found within this zone. These regions together represent the points of central integration for coordination of essential reflexive acts such as swallowing, vomiting, and those that involve the cardiovascular and respiratory systems; these areas also include the primary receptive regions for most visceral afferent sensory information. The reticular activating system is essential for the regulation of sleep, wakefulness, and level of arousal, as well as for coordination of eye movements. The fiber systems projecting from the reticular formation have been called "nonspecific" because the targets to which these fibers project are considerably more diffuse in distribution than are the connections from many other neurons (*e.g.*, specific thalamocortical projections). However, the reticular systems may innervate targets in a coherent, functional manner even though their targets are widely distributed (*see* Foote *et al.,* 1983; Aghajanian and Vandermaelen, 1986; Björklund and Lindvall, 1986).

Cerebellum. This small and highly organized cortical region arises from the posterior pons behind the cerebral hemispheres. Although it is also highly laminated and redundant in its detailed cytological organization, the lobules and folia of the cerebellum project onto specific deep cerebellar nuclei, which in turn make relatively selective projections to the motor cortex (by way of the thalamus) and to the brainstem nuclei concerned with vestibular (position-stabilization) function. The cerebellum is generally regarded as playing an important role in the maintenance of appropriate body posture in space. In addition to maintaining the proper tone of antigravity musculature and providing continuous feedback during volitional movements of the trunk and extremities, the cerebellum may also regulate heart rate, possibly to maintain blood flow despite changes in posture.

Spinal Cord. The spinal cord extends from the caudal end of the medulla oblongata to the lower lumbar vertebrae. Within this mass of nerve cells and tracts, the sensory information from skin, muscles, joints, and viscera is locally coordinated with motoneurons and with primary sensory relay cells that project to and receive signals from higher levels. The spinal cord is divided into anatomical segments (cervical, thoracic, lumbar, and sacral) that correspond to divisions of the peripheral nerves and spinal column. Ascending and descending tracts of the spinal cord are located within the white matter at the perimeter of the cord, while intersegmental connections and synaptic contacts are concentrated within the H-shaped internal mass of gray matter. Sensory information flows into the dorsal cord, and motor commands exit via the ventral portion. The preganglionic neurons of the autonomic nervous system are found in the intermediolateral columns of the gray matter. Autonomic reflexes (*e.g.*, changes in skin vasculature with alteration of temperature) can easily be elicited within local segments of the spinal cord, as shown by the maintenance of these reflexes after the cord is severed.

MICROANATOMY OF THE BRAIN

Cellular Organization of the Brain. Present understanding of the cellular organization of the CNS can be viewed simplistically according to three main patterns of neuronal connectivity (*see* Shepherd, 1988). In the first, *long-hierarchical* neuronal organizations are typically found in the primary sensory and motor pathways. Here the transmission of information is highly sequential, and interconnected neurons are related to each other in a hierarchical fashion. Primary receptors (in the retina, inner ear, olfactory epithelium, tongue, or skin) transmit first to primary relay cells, then to secondary relay cells, and finally to the primary sensory fields of the cerebral cortex. For motor output systems, the reverse sequence holds, descending from the motor cortex to the final common output of the spinal motoneuron. The essential feature of this hierarchical scheme of organization is that chains of neurons provide a precise flow of information, but such organization suffers the disadvantage that destruction of any link incapacitates the entire system. As yet, few specific neurotransmitters have been identified for any of the major links in the sensory or motor pathways. The final junction between motoneuron and muscle uses acetylcholine (ACh) as the transmitter. Substance P and other peptides may function in some sensory neurons (Nicoll *et al.*, 1980; Krieger *et al.*, 1983; Palkovits, 1988).

The second pattern of organization involves neurons whose connections are established mainly within the immediate vicinity of their location. Such local-circuit neurons are frequently small and may have very few processes. They are believed to regulate the flow of information through their small spatial domain, and they may do this *without* generating action potentials, which are essential for the long-distance transmission between hierarchically connected neurons. Local-circuit neurons appear to use many different transmitter substances, including the amino acids gamma-aminobutyrate (GABA), glycine, glutamate, and aspartate, as well as several families of peptides.

A third pattern of organization is utilized by certain neuronal systems of the hypothalamus, pons, and brainstem. These systems contain either a monoamine—norepinephrine (NE), dopamine (DA), or 5-hydroxytryptamine (5-HT)—or one of a number of peptides, including vasopressin, oxytocin, beta-endorphin, corticotropin-releasing hormone, or growth hormone-releasing hormone (*see* Swanson, 1986). From a single anatomical location, these neurons extend multiple-branched and divergent connections to many target cells, almost all of which lie outside of the brain region in which the neurons are located. In no case do these cells appear to be sequential elements within any known hierarchical system; rather, they appear to be special local-circuit neurons whose spatial domains are one to two orders of magnitude larger than the classical intraregional interneurons. For example, NE-containing neurons of the locus ceruleus project from the pons to the cerebellum, spinal cord, thalamus, and several cortical zones, but the function of these target regions is not obviously disrupted when the adrenergic fibers are destroyed experimentally, indicating their divergent but nonhierarchical structure. These systems could mediate linkages between regions that may require temporary integration. Many other long projecting systems that arise from the midbrain could also fit into this organizational scheme, which is neither hierarchical nor strictly local circuit. The neurotransmitters for most of these connections are not yet known.

Cell Biology of Neurons. Morphological properties of central neurons have been very useful for the description of their functional characteristics. Neurons are classified in many different ways, including designation according to function (sensory, motor, or interneuron), location, or identity of the transmitter they synthesize and release. Microscopic analysis focuses on their general shape, and, in particular, the number of extensions from the cell body. Most neurons have one axon, which carries signals from the cell of origin to other cells. Other processes extend from the nerve cell to receive synaptic contacts from other neurons; these processes, called dendrites, may branch in extremely complex patterns. Neurons exhibit the cytological characteristics of highly active secretory cells: large nuclei; large amounts of smooth and rough endoplasmic reticulum; and frequent clusters of specialized smooth endoplasmic reticulum (Golgi apparatus), where secretory products of the cell are packaged into membrane-bound organelles for transport out of the cell (Figure 12–1). The synaptic vesicles that are characteristic of distal axons are not easily observed within the neuronal cell body; larger vesicles seen in the Golgi zone may thus form the synaptic vesicles after transport to the nerve terminals. Neurons and their cellular extensions are rich in microtubules—elongated tubules approximately 24 nm in diameter. Their functions may be to support the elongated axons and dendrites and to assist in the reciprocal transport of essential macromolecules and organelles between the cell body and the distant axon or dendrites.

Synaptic Relationships. Synaptic arrangements in the CNS fall into a wide variety of morphological and functional forms that are specific for the cells involved. Specific synaptic connections that have one origin will tend to form contacts with particular surface zones of their target cells in a mosaic arrangement that may reflect the underlying distribution of chemical receptors. Electron microscopic observations of target neurons reveal two major structural details as characteristic of the site presumed to be the active zone of contact. The presynaptic structure is rich in small vesicles; their shape, size, and chemical properties vary with the identity of the neurotransmitter. Each vesicle probably contains several thousand molecules of transmitter, a number that approaches the lower estimate of transmitter molecules in a "quantum," the elemental package responsible for miniature postsynaptic potentials (*see* Chapter 5). In addition, the presynaptic and postsynaptic membranes exhibit a specialized attachment site, termed the *synaptolemma* by Bodian (1972).

Many spatial arrangements are possible within synaptic relationships (*see* Figure 12–1). The most common arrangement, typical of the hierarchical pathways, is the axodendritic or axosomatic arrangement in which the axons of the cell of origin make their functional contact with the dendrites or cell body of the target. In other cases, functional contacts may occur between the adjacent cell bodies (somasomatic) or between overlapping dendrites (dendrodendritic). Many local-circuit neurons do not possess distinct axons and yet enter into synaptic relationships through modified dendrites, sometimes termed *telodendrites;* these modified dendrites can be either the presynaptic or the postsynaptic element. Within the spinal cord, serial axoaxonic synapses are relatively frequent. Here, the axon of an interneuron ends upon the terminal of a long-distance neuron as that terminal contacts a dendrite in the dorsal horn. Many presynaptic axons contain local collections of typical synaptic vesicles with no opposed specialized synaptolemma. Release of transmitter may not occur at such sites.

The bioelectric properties of neurons and junctions in the CNS generally follow the outlines and details already described for the peripheral autonomic nervous system (*see* Chapter 5), except that a much more varied range of intracellular mechanisms has been discerned in the CNS (Bloom, 1988; Llinas, 1988; Nicoll, 1988).

There are many steps in the transmission of chemical messages from neurons to their target cells, and each step provides the potential for pharmacological intervention (*see* Chapter 5). Recent advances in our knowledge of the complexity of these mechanisms include (1) the identification of likely new neurotransmitters, especially small neuropeptides, and appreciation of their co-localization in individual nerve terminals with amino acid or aminergic transmitters (Rogawski and Barker, 1985; Hökfelt *et al.,* 1987; Blakely and Coyle, 1988; Ferrendelli *et al.,* 1988; Palkovits, 1988); (2) elucidation of mechanisms of regulation of neuronal excitability, including detailed aspects of the structure and function of transmitter- and voltage-regulated ion channels (Siggins and Gruol, 1986; Miller, 1987; Schofield *et al.,* 1987; Catterall, 1988); and (3) appreciation of mechanisms of regu-

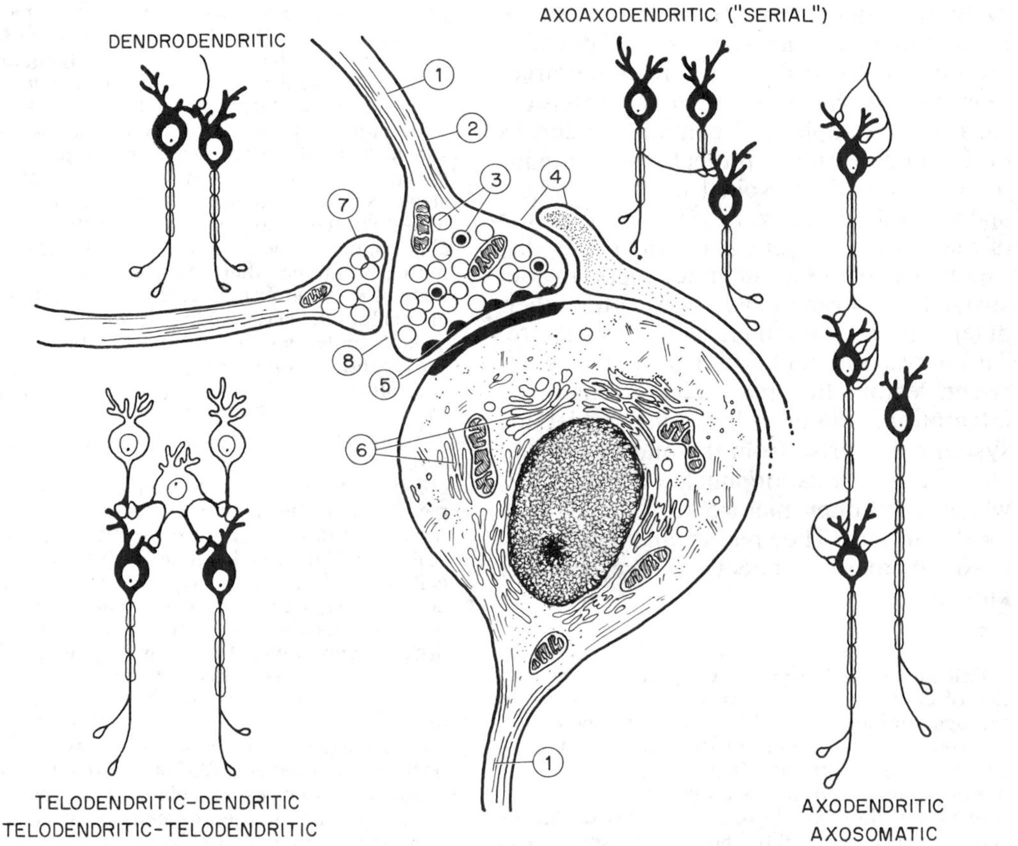

Figure 12–1. *Drug-sensitive sites in synaptic transmission.*

Schematic view of the drug-sensitive sites in some prototypical synaptic complexes. In the center, a postsynaptic neuron receives a somatic synapse (shown greatly oversized) from an axonic terminal; an axoaxonic terminal is shown in contact with this presynaptic nerve terminal. Drug-sensitive sites include: (*1*) microtubules responsible for orthograde and retrograde transport of macromolecules between the neuronal cell body and distal processes; (*2*) electrically conductive membranes; (*3*) sites for the synthesis and storage of transmitters; (*4*) sites for the active uptake of some transmitters into nerve terminals or glia; (*5*) sites for the release of transmitter and sites (receptors) to generate responses; (*6*) cytoplasmic organelles and postsynaptic membranes for maintenance of synaptic activity and for long-term mediation of altered physiological states; and (*7*) presynaptic receptors on adjacent presynaptic processes and (*8*) on nerve terminals (autoreceptors). Around the central neuron are schematic illustrations of the more common synaptic relationships in the CNS. (Modified from Bodian, 1972, and Cooper *et al.*, 1986.)

lation of second messenger synthesis and ion channel function by receptors that are linked to guanine nucleotide-binding regulatory proteins (G proteins), including characterization of the molecules that function in these complex pathways (Dohlman *et al.*, 1987; Gilman, 1987; Sigal *et al.*, 1988; Krupinski *et al.*, 1989).

In the simplest case, conceptually, the receptor is an oligomeric macromolecule whose subunits constitute the functional ion channel and also contain sites for regulation of the channel by the transmitter. Examples include receptors for GABA and glycine in the CNS (Greeningloh *et al.*, 1987; Akagi and Miledi, 1988) and the nicotinic cholinergic receptor (Conti-Tronconi *et al.*, 1985; Schmidt, 1988; *see* Chapter 9). Multiple forms of the mRNAs that encode one or more of the subunits of several ligand-regulated ion channels have been detected, and it is very likely that different forms of these receptors are expressed in various types of neurons (*see* Akagi and Miledi, 1988; Blair *et al.*, 1988).

The mechanism of action of many other receptors is clearly more complex and involves the concerted function of a series of interacting macromolecules. These include the plasma membrane-bound receptor itself, with its extracellularly oriented ligand-binding domain; membrane-associated G proteins, which act as transducers by coupling activation of the receptor to regulation of the activity of an effector; and the effector molecule of the pathway, which may be either a membrane-bound enzyme (*e.g.*, adenylyl cyclase) or an ion channel (*see* Chapters 2 and 5). There are many well-characterized examples of such complex arrangements, and complementary DNAs (cDNAs) that encode several receptors of this type have been cloned. These include muscarinic cholinergic receptors (Kubo *et al.*, 1986), both α- and β-adrenergic receptors (Dohlman *et al.*, 1987; Sigal *et al.*, 1988), certain types of tryptaminergic receptors (Julius *et al.*, 1988), and the receptor for neuropeptide K (Masu *et al.*, 1987). The receptors that have been characterized to date are constructed in a similar fashion, consisting of seven transmembrane spans, with intervening extracellular and cytoplasmic loops. The ligand-binding sites of these receptors are contributed by several amino acid residues that lie within the transmembrane-spanning segments. The cytoplasmic loops interact with the G protein. Depending on the receptor and the G protein involved, the ultimate result can be activation or inhibition of adenylyl cyclase, activation of one or more phospholipases, or regulation of the activity of a variety of ion channels (*e.g.*, for K^+ or Ca^{2+}).

IDENTIFICATION OF CENTRAL TRANSMITTERS

The rigorous scientific identification of the transmitter for a given central synaptic connection requires data to satisfy the same criteria that were utilized to demonstrate that ACh and NE were the predominant transmitters of the autonomic nervous system (*see* Chapter 5).

1. *The transmitter must be shown to be present in the presynaptic terminals of the synapse and in the neurons from which those presynaptic terminals arise.* Extensions of this criterion involve the demonstration that the presynaptic neuron synthesizes the transmitter substance, rather than simply storing it after accumulation from a nonneural source. Microscopic cytochemistry (*see* Cooper *et al.*, 1986) and subcellular fractionation and analysis of brain tissue are particularly useful to evaluate this criterion in the CNS. These techniques are often combined with the production in experimental animals of surgical or chemical lesions of presynaptic neurons or their tracts to demonstrate that the lesion causes the disappearance of the alleged transmitter from the target region.

2. *The transmitter must be released from the presynaptic nerve concomitantly with presynaptic nerve activity.* This criterion is generally evaluated by electrical stimulation of the nerve pathway *in vivo* and collection of the transmitter in an enriched extracellular fluid within the synaptic target area. However, devices for collection such as push-pull cannulas are still hundreds of times larger than individual synapses, and the sensitivity of the methods for detecting transmitters requires that collection extend for periods that are thousands of times longer than most known synaptic potentials. Thus, this "release" criterion has not yet been rigorously satisfied for single synapses in the CNS. However, methods have recently been developed that may provide sufficient sensitivity to permit collection of substances *in situ* within the spatial and temporal bounds of transmission at a single synapse (Lindefors *et al.*, 1987; Maysinger *et al.*, 1988). Release of transmitter can also be studied *in vitro* by ionic or electrical activation of thin brain slices or subcellular fractions that are enriched in nerve terminals. The release of all transmitter substances so far studied, including presumptive transmitter release from dendrites (Nedergaard *et al.*, 1988), is voltage-dependent and requires the influx of Ca^{2+} into the presynaptic terminal. However, transmitter release is relatively insensitive to extracellular Na^+ or to tetrodotoxin, which blocks transmembrane movement of Na^+.

3. *The effects of the alleged substance, when applied experimentally to the target cells, must be identical to the effects of stimulating the presynaptic pathway.* This criterion can be met loosely by qualitative comparisons (*e.g.*, both the substance and the pathway inhibit or excite the target cell). More convincing is the demonstration that the ionic conductances activated by the pathway are the same as those activated by the candidate transmitter. More specifically, the equilibrium value of the synaptic potential and the potential to which the cell is driven by the alleged transmitter should be identical (Werman, 1972). These tests require prolonged intracellular recording, which is difficult to achieve *in vivo*, especially for smaller or deeply placed target neurons. The use of preparations of brain slices *in vitro* may overcome such problems

(Lynch and Schubert, 1980; Siggins and Gruol, 1986; Llinas, 1988; Nicoll, 1988). Alternatively, the criterion can be satisfied less rigorously by demonstration of the pharmacological identity of receptors. In general, pharmacological antagonism of the pathway's actions and those of the candidate transmitter should be achieved by similar doses of the same drug. To be convincing, the antagonistic drug should not affect responses of the target neurons to other unrelated pathways or to chemically distinct transmitter candidates. Actions that are qualitatively identical to those that follow stimulation of the pathway should also be observed with synthetic agonists that mimic the transmitter. Pharmacological characterization of the actions of various agonists and antagonists will define various subsets of receptors for the presumed natural agonist (*e.g.*, muscarinic or nicotinic cholinergic receptors, β_1- or β_2-adrenergic receptors, *etc.*). At present, such definitions may be based on the functional response that is elicited or the relative potencies of agonists and antagonists, assessed either functionally or through ligand-binding assays.

Recent studies, especially those that have implicated peptides as transmitters in the central and peripheral nervous systems, suggest that many synapses may contain more than one transmitter substance (*see* Hökfelt *et al.*, 1987). Although rigorous proof is lacking, substances that coexist in a given synapse are presumed to be released together and to act jointly on the postsynaptic membrane. Clearly, if more than one substance transmits information, no single agonist or antagonist would necessarily provide faithful mimicry or total antagonism of activation of the presynaptic element.

Assessment of Receptor Properties. Central synaptic receptors may be characterized by examination of their ability to bind high-specific-activity radiolabeled agonists or antagonists or of the ability of other unlabeled compounds to compete for such binding sites (*see* Chapter 2). The specificity of such binding must be evaluated with care. Radioligand-binding assays can be used to quantify binding sites within a region, to follow their appearance throughout the phylogenetic scale and during brain development, and to determine how physiological or pharmacological manipulation regulates receptor number or affinity.

The properties of the cellular response to the transmitter can be studied electrophysiologically by the use of *microiontophoresis* (a combination of recordings from single cells and highly localized drug administration). The *patch clamp technique* can be used to study the electrical properties of single ionic channels and their regulation by neurotransmitters. These direct electrophysiological tests of neuronal responsiveness can provide qualitative and quantitative information on the effects of a putative transmitter substance (Siggins and Gruol, 1986; Nicoll, 1988). In some cases, receptor properties can also be studied biochemically when the activated receptor is coupled to an enzymatic reaction, such as the synthesis of a cyclic nucleotide.

With limitations, these biochemical and electrophysiological methods can provide quantitative information on the adaptive self-regulation of receptors for a neurotransmitter that follows pharmacological or pathological perturbations (*e.g.*, denervation supersensitivity, drug-induced subsensitivity, *etc.*). Drug-receptor interactions should be considered to be constantly modifiable relationships. Postsynaptic receptivity on CNS neurons is continuously regulated in terms of the number of receptive sites and the threshold required for generation of a response. Receptor number is often dependent upon the concentration of agonist to which the target cell is exposed. Thus, chronic excess of agonist can lead to a reduced number of receptors (desensitization or down-regulation) and consequently to subsensitivity or tolerance to the transmitter. A deficit of transmitter can lead to increased numbers of receptors and supersensitivity of the system (*see* Symposium, 1983). These adaptive processes become especially important when drugs are used to treat chronic illness of the CNS. *With prolonged periods of exposure to drug, the actual mechanisms underlying the therapeutic effect may differ strikingly from those that operate when the agent is first introduced into the system.* Similar adaptive modifications of neuronal systems can also occur at presynaptic sites, such as those concerned with transmitter synthesis, storage, reuptake, and release.

NEUROTRANSMITTERS, NEUROHORMONES, AND NEUROMODULATORS: CONTRASTING PRINCIPLES OF NEURONAL REGULATION

Neurotransmitters. The criteria for identification of synaptic transmitters rely heavily on the demonstrations that a substance contained in a neuron is secreted by that neuron to transmit information to its postsynaptic target. Given this level of functional description and a definite effect of neuron A on target cell B, a substance found in neuron A, secreted from neuron

A, and producing the effect of A on B would then operationally be the transmitter from A to B. Within this broad definition, substances may act to transmit their information in a variety of ways, many of which are only now beginning to be characterized as to mechanisms. In some cases, transmitters may produce minimal effects on bioelectric properties, yet activate or inactivate biochemical mechanisms necessary for responses to other circuits. Alternatively, the action of a transmitter may vary with the context of ongoing synaptic events—enhancing excitations or inhibitions, rather than operating to impose direct excitation or inhibition. Each chemical substance that fits within the broad definition of a transmitter may, therefore, require operational definition within the spatial and temporal domains in which a specific cell–cell circuit is defined. Those same properties may or may not be generalized to other cells that are contacted by the same presynaptic neurons, with the differences in operation related to differences in the postsynaptic receptor and the mechanisms by which the activated receptor produces its effect (Bloom, 1975).

Classically, electrophysiological signs of the action of a *bona fide* transmitter fall into two major categories: *excitation* (in which ion channels are opened to permit net influx of positively charged ions, leading to depolarization with a reduction in the electrical resistance of the membrane), and *inhibition* (in which selective ion movements lead to hyperpolarization, also with decreased membrane resistance). More recent work suggests there may be many "nonclassical" transmitter mechanisms operating in the CNS. In some cases, either depolarization or hyperpolarization is accompanied by a *decreased* ionic conductance (increased membrane resistance) as actions of the transmitter lead to the closure of ion channels (so-called leak channels) that are normally open in some resting neurons (Shepherd, 1988). For some transmitters, such as monoamines and some peptides, a "conditional" action may be involved. That is, a transmitter substance may enhance or suppress the response of the target neuron to classical excitatory or inhibitory transmitters while producing little or no change in membrane potential or ionic conductance when applied alone. Such conditional responses have been termed *modulatory*, and specific categories of modulation have been hypothesized (*see* Foote *et al.*, 1983; Aghajanian, 1985; North *et al.*, 1987; Bloom, 1988; Nicoll, 1988). Regardless of the mechanisms that underlie such synaptic operations, their temporal and biophysical characteristics differ substantially from the rapid onset-offset type of effect previously thought to describe all synaptic events. These differences have thus raised the issue of whether substances that produce slow synaptic effects should be described with the same term—*neurotransmitter*. Some of the alternate terms deserve brief survey with regard to mechanisms of drug action.

Neurohormones. Peptide-secreting cells of the hypothalamicohypophyseal circuits were originally described as neurosecretory cells, a form of neuron that was both fish and fowl, receiving synaptic information from other central neurons yet secreting their transmitter in a hormone-like fashion into the circulation (Scharrer, 1969; *see* Chapter 56). The transmitter of such neurons was termed a *neurohormone*—that is, a substance secreted into the blood by a neuron. However, this term has lost most of its original meaning because these hypothalamic neurons may also form traditional synapses with many central neurons (Krieger *et al.*, 1983; Swanson, 1986). Cytochemical evidence indicates that transmission at these sites is also mediated by the same substance that is secreted as a hormone from the posterior pituitary (oxytocin, antidiuretic hormone). Thus, the designation *hormone* relates to the site of release at the pituitary and does not necessarily describe all the actions of the peptide.

Neuromodulators. Florey (1967) employed the term *modulator* to describe substances that can influence neuronal activity differently than do neurotransmitters. In the context of this definition, the distinctive feature of a modulator is that it originates from cellular and nonsynaptic sites, yet influences the excitability of nerve cells. Florey specifically designated substances such as CO_2 and ammonia, arising from active neurons or glia, as potential modulators through nonsynaptic actions. Similarly, circulating steroid hormones as well as steroids produced in the nervous system (Coascogne *et al.,* 1987), locally released adenosine and other purines, and prostaglandins might all now be regarded as modulators.

Neuromediators. Substances that participate in the elicitation of the postsynaptic response to a transmitter fall under this heading. The clearest examples of such mediation are provided by the involvement of adenosine 3′,5′-monophosphate (cyclic AMP), and perhaps of guanosine 3′,5′-monophosphate (cyclic GMP), as second messengers at specific sites of synaptic transmission (Bloom, 1975; Greengard, 1978). However, it is technically difficult to demonstrate that a change in the concentration of cyclic nucleotides occurs prior to the generation of the synaptic potential and that this change in concentration is both necessary and sufficient for its generation. Possibly, the changes in the concentration of cyclic nucleotides that can be observed under certain conditions supplement and enhance the generation of the synaptic potentials. Activation of cyclic nucleotide–dependent protein phosphorylation reactions (*see* Chapters 2 and 5) can alter properties of membrane proteins that are known to be substrates in these reactions (Greengard, 1978; Nestler and Greengard, 1984). These possibilities are particularly pertinent to the action of the central catecholaminergic circuits described below.

ACTIONS OF DRUGS IN THE CNS

Specificity and Nonspecificity of CNS Drug Action. The effect of a drug is considered to be *specific* when it affects an identifiable molecular mechanism unique to target cells that bear receptors for that drug. Conversely, a drug is regarded as *nonspecific* when it produces effects on many different target cells and acts by diverse molecular mechanisms. This terminology thus distinguishes broad actions at many levels of the CNS through effects on specific molecular mechanisms (*e.g.,* atropine blockade of muscarinic receptors) from nonspecific actions. This separation is often a property of the dose–response relationship of the drug and the cell or mechanisms under scrutiny. Even a drug that is highly specific when tested at a low concentration may exhibit nonspecific actions at substantially higher doses. (For example, many specific antagonists of β-adrenergic receptors can also cause local anesthesia at high concentrations; similar nonspecific effects may be seen with tricyclic antidepressants at doses one to two orders of magnitude higher than those required to cause selective changes in rates of transmitter uptake or release.) Conversely, even generally acting drugs may not act equally on all levels of the CNS. For example, sedatives, hypnotics, and general anesthetics would have very limited utility if central neurons that control the respiratory and cardiovascular systems were not less sensitive to their actions. Drugs with specific actions may produce nonspecific effects when the dose and route of administration initially produce high tissue concentrations; their specificity of action becomes apparent only later, when the concentrations fall.

As the number of putative neurotransmitters has increased and as techniques have evolved for the analysis of the actions of drugs on specific target neurons, many drugs that have been regarded as having general actions have been found to exhibit actions that can be related to specific mechanisms. For example, the effects of the broadly acting stimulants strychnine and picrotoxin can now be attributed to interference with inhibitory actions that are mediated at receptors for glycine and GABA, respectively (Curtis *et al.,* 1971); similarly, barbiturates have been found to have relatively selective effects on synaptic mechanisms (Macdonald and McLean, 1982).

Drugs whose mechanisms currently appear to be primarily general or nonspecific are classed according to whether they produce behavioral depression or stimulation, while specifically acting CNS drugs can be classed more definitively according to their locus of action or specific therapeutic usefulness. It must be remembered that the absence of overt behavioral effects does not rule out the existence of important central actions for a given drug. For example, the impact of muscarinic cholinergic antagonists on the behavior of normal animals may be subtle, but these agents are used extensively in the treatment of movement disorders and motion sickness (*see* Chapters 8 and 20).

General (Nonspecific) CNS Depressants. This category includes the anesthetic gases and vapors, the aliphatic alcohols, and some hypnotic-sedative drugs. These agents share the ability to depress excitable tissue at all levels of the CNS by stabilizing neuronal membranes, leading to a decrease in the amount of transmitter released by the nerve impulse, as well as to general depression of postsynaptic responsiveness and ion movement. At subanesthetic concentrations, these agents (*e.g.*, ethanol) can exert rather specific effects on certain groups of neurons, which may account for differences in their behavioral effects, especially the propensity to produce dependence (*see* Koob and Bloom, 1988; *see also* Chapter 17).

General (Nonspecific) CNS Stimulants. The drugs that remain in this category are pentylenetetrazol and related agents that are capable of powerful excitation of the CNS and the methylxanthines, which have a much weaker stimulant action. Stimulation may be accomplished by one of two general mechanisms: by blockade of inhibition or by direct neuronal excitation (which may involve increased transmitter release, more prolonged transmitter action, labilization of the postsynaptic membrane, or decreased synaptic recovery time). A recently described class of drugs termed "nootropics" has been reputed to stimulate the brain in a more specific way such that learning is facilitated and the cognitive decline associated with aging or disease is overcome or retarded (*see* Heise, 1987). Although a general mechanism of action has yet to be elucidated, in experimental animals these drugs all prevent the disruption of memory consolidation that is produced by seizures or anoxia. The relationship of this action to their hypothesized therapeutic effect is unclear.

Drugs That Selectively Modify CNS Function. The agents in this group *may* cause either depression or excitation. In some instances, a drug may produce both effects simultaneously on different systems. Some agents in this category have little effect on the level of excitability in doses that are used therapeutically. The principal classes of these CNS drugs are the following: anticonvulsants, antiparkinsonism drugs, opioid and nonopioid analgesics, appetite suppressants, antiemetics, analgesic-antipyretics, certain stimulants, neuroleptics (antidepressants and antimanic and antipsychotic agents), tranquilizers, sedatives, and hypnotics.

Although selectivity of action may be remarkable, a drug usually affects several CNS functions to varying degrees. When only one constellation of effects is wanted in a therapeutic situation, the remaining effects of the drug are regarded as limitations in selectivity (*i.e.*, unwanted or side effects).

The specificity of a drug's action is frequently overestimated. This is partly due to the fact that the drug is identified with the effect that is implied by the class name. For example, levodopa, atropine and other muscarinic antagonists, and some antihistamines are all antiparkinsonism drugs, yet all have substantial additional effects that are therapeutically useful. However, since all centrally acting drugs are more or less selective, it will be profitable to consider some of the probable bases for their selectivity; such considerations are inseparable from discussion of the mechanisms of their action.

Blood–Brain Barrier. Apart from the exceptional instances in which drugs are introduced directly into the CNS, the concentration of the agent in the blood after oral or parenteral administration obviously has great bearing on the concentration in the CNS. However, this relationship is often not as simple as for peripheral structures.

Although not thoroughly defined anatomically, the *blood–brain barrier* represents an important boundary between the periphery and the CNS in the form of a permeability barrier to the passive diffusion of substances from the bloodstream into various regions of the CNS (*see* Pardridge, 1988). Evidence of the barrier is provided by the greatly diminished rate of access of chemicals from plasma to the brain (*see* Chapter 1). This phenomenon is much less prominent in the hypothalamus and in several small specialized organs lining the third and fourth ventricles of the brain: the median eminence, area postrema, pineal gland, subfornical organ, and subcommissural organ. In addition, there is little evidence of a barrier between the circulation and the peripheral nervous system (*e.g.,* sensory and autonomic nerves and ganglia). While severe limitations are imposed upon the diffusion of macromolecules, selective barriers to permeation also exist for small charged molecules such as neurotransmitters, their precursors and metabolites, and some drugs. These diffusional barriers are at present best conceived as a combination of the partition of solute across the vasculature (which governs passage by definable properties such as molecular weight, charge, and lipophilicity) and the presence or absence of energy-dependent transport systems. Active transport of certain agents may occur in either direction across the barrier. The diffusional barriers retard the movement of substances from brain to blood as well as from blood to brain, but the brain clears metabolites of transmitters into the cerebrospinal fluid by excretion through the acid transport system of the choroid plexus (*see* Wood, 1979). Substances that can rarely gain access to the brain from the bloodstream can often reach the brain after injection directly into the cerebrospinal fluid. Under certain conditions, it may be possible to open the blood–brain barrier, at least transiently, to permit the entry of chemotherapeutic agents (*see* Rapoport, 1988, for discussion).

General Characteristics of CNS Drugs. Combinations of centrally acting drugs are frequently administered to therapeutic advantage (*e.g.,* an anticholinergic drug and levodopa for Parkinson's disease). However, other combinations of drugs may be detrimental because of potentially dangerous additive or mutually antagonistic effects.

The effect of a CNS drug is additive with the physiological state and with the effects of other depressant and stimulant drugs. For example, anesthetics are less effective in a hyperexcitable subject than in a normal patient; the converse is true with respect to the effects of stimulants. In general, the depressant effects of drugs from all categories are additive (*e.g.,* the fatal combination of barbiturates or benzodiazepines with ethanol), as are the effects of stimulants. Therefore, respiration depressed by morphine is further impaired by depressant drugs, while stimulant drugs can augment the excitatory effects of morphine to produce vomiting and convulsions.

Antagonism between depressants and stimulants is variable. Some instances of true pharmacological antagonism among CNS drugs are known; for example, opioid antagonists are very selective in blocking the effects of opioid analgesics. However, the antagonism exhibited between two CNS drugs is usually physiological in nature. Thus, an individual who has received one drug cannot be returned entirely to normal by another.

The selective effects of drugs on specific neurotransmitter systems may be additive or competitive. This potential for drug interaction must be considered whenever such drugs are administered concurrently. To avoid such interactions, the prolonged duration of action of certain agents may necessitate a drug-free period before therapy with other drugs can be started. An excitatory effect on some functions is commonly observed with low concentrations of some depressant drugs owing either to depression of inhibitory systems or to a transient increase in the release of excitatory transmitters. Examples are the "stage of excitement" during induction of general anesthesia and the "stimulant" effects of alcohol. The excitatory phase occurs only with low concentrations of the depressant; uniform depression ensues with increasing drug concentration. The excitatory effects can be minimized, when appropriate, by pretreatment with a depressant drug that is devoid of such effects (*e.g.,* benzodiazepines in preanesthetic medication). Acute, excessive stimulation of the cerebrospinal axis is normally followed by depression (amphetamine, strychnine), which is in part the consequence of neuronal fatigue and exhaustion of stores of transmitters. This postictal depression is additive with the effects of depressant drugs. Acute, drug-induced depression is not, as a rule, followed by stimulation. However, chronic drug-induced sedation or depression is followed by prolonged hyperexcitability upon abrupt withdrawal of the medication (barbiturates, alcohol). This type of hyperexcitability can be effectively controlled by the same or another depressant drug (*see* Chapter 22).

Organization of CNS-Drug Interactions. The structural and functional properties of neurons provide a means to specify the possible sites at which drugs could interact specifically or generally in the CNS (*see* Figure 12–1). In this scheme, drugs that affect neuronal energy metabolism, membrane integrity, or transmembrane ionic equilibria would be generally acting compounds. Similarly general in action would be drugs that affect the two-way intracellular transport systems (*e.g.*, colchicine). These general effects can still exhibit different dose–response or time–response relationships among different neurons based, for example, on such neuronal properties as rate of firing, dependence of discharge on external stimuli or internal pacemakers, resting ionic fluxes, or axon length. In contrast, when drug actions can be related to specific aspects of the metabolism, release, or function of a neurotransmitter, the site, specificity, and mechanism of action of a drug can be defined by systematic studies of dose–response and time–response relationships. From such data the most sensitive, rapid, or persistent neuronal event can be identified.

Transmitter-dependent actions of drugs can be organized conveniently into *presynaptic* and *postsynaptic* categories. The presynaptic category includes all of the events in the perikaryon and nerve terminal that regulate transmitter synthesis (including the acquisition of adequate substrates and cofactors), storage, release, reuptake, and catabolism. Transmitter concentrations can be lowered by blockade of synthesis, storage, or both. The amount of transmitter released per impulse is generally stable but can also be regulated. For example, 5-HT produces a cyclic AMP-mediated phosphorylation of presynaptic membrane proteins in certain invertebrate neurons. This leads to increased influx of Ca^{2+} and release of transmitter at the affected synapse (Siegelbaum *et al.*, 1982). The effective concentration of transmitter may be increased by inhibition of reuptake or by blockade of catabolic enzymes. The transmitter that is released at a synapse can also exert actions upon the terminal from which it was released by interacting with receptors at these sites (termed *autoreceptors*). Activation of presynaptic autoreceptors can slow the rate of discharge of transmitter and thereby provide a feedback mechanism that controls the concentration of transmitter in the synaptic cleft (*see* Carlsson, 1975; *see also* Chapter 5).

The postsynaptic category includes all the events that follow release of the transmitter in the vicinity of the postsynaptic receptor—in particular, the molecular mechanisms by which occupation of the receptor by the transmitter produces changes in the properties of the membrane of the postsynaptic cell (shifts in membrane potential) as well as more enduring biochemical actions (changes in intracellular cyclic nucleotides, protein kinase activity, and related substrate proteins). Direct postsynaptic effects of drugs generally require relatively high affinity for the receptors or resistance to metabolic degradation. Each of these presynaptic or postsynaptic actions is potentially highly specific and can be envisioned as being restricted to a single, chemically defined subset of CNS cells.

CENTRAL NEUROTRANSMITTERS

In examining the effects of drugs on the CNS with reference to the neurotransmitters for specific circuits, attention should be devoted to the general organizational principles of neurons. The view that synapses represent drug-modifiable control points within neuronal networks thus requires the explicit delineation of the sites at which given neurotransmitters may operate and the degree of specificity or generality by which such sites may be affected. One principle that underlies the following summaries of individual transmitter substances is the chemical-specificity hypothesis of Dale (1935), which holds that a given neuron releases the same transmitter substance at every one of its synaptic terminals. In the face of growing indications that some neurons may contain more than one transmitter substance (Hökfelt *et al.,* 1980, 1987), Dale's hypothesis has been modified to indicate that a given neuron will secrete the same set of transmitters from all its terminals. However, even this view may require revision. For example, it is not clear whether a neuron that secretes a given peptide will process the precursor peptide to the same end product at all of its synaptic terminals. Table 12–1 provides an overview of the pharmacological properties of the amino acid and monoamine transmitters that have been most fully studied in the CNS.

Amino Acids. The CNS contains uniquely high concentrations of certain amino acids, notably glutamate and gamma-aminobutyrate (GABA); these amino acids are extremely potent in their ability to alter neuronal discharge. However, many physiologists were extremely reluctant to accept these simple substances as central neurotransmitters. This reluctance was based in part on conceptual problems of how to discriminate amino acids acting as transmitters from the same compounds acting as precursors for protein synthesis. The ubiquitous distribution of amino acids within the brain also posed problems in relating release to activity of a single neuronal circuit. Other important arguments against amino acids as transmitters were that they produced prompt, powerful, and readily reversible but redundant effects on every neuron tested; the dicarboxylic amino acids produced excitation, and the monocarboxylic ω-amino acids (*e.g.,* GABA, glycine, β-alanine, taurine) produced qualitatively similar inhibitions (Kelly and Beart, 1975). This redundancy of effect was taken as further support of a nonspecific action on neuronal discharge, and this view was seemingly supported by the early observations that iontophoretic application of amino acids produced excitations or inhibitions that differed from those produced by activation of relevant synapses. Research was also hampered by the facts that selective antagonists of the amino acids were not available and that no cytochemical methods were available that could visualize such junctions. In the past 20 years most of these conceptual arguments have proven to be unjustified, and the evidence is quite strong that certain amino acids, especially GABA, glycine, and glutamate, are central transmitters.

GABA was identified as a unique chemical constituent of brain in 1950, but its potency as a CNS depressant was not immediately recognized. In the crustacean stretch receptor, GABA mimicked the actions of stimulation of the inhibitory nerve, and picrotoxin antagonized both the effects of applied GABA and stimulation of the inhibitory nerve. Kravitz and coworkers (1963) demonstrated in the crustacean that GABA was the only inhibitory amino acid found exclusively in the inhibitory nerve and that the inhibitory potency of extracts of this nerve were accounted for by their content of GABA. Release of GABA was then correlated with the frequency of nerve stimulation. Intracellular recordings from the muscle indicated that the inhibitory nerve and GABA produced identical increases of Cl^- conductance in the muscle. These observations thus fully satisfy the criteria for identification of a transmitter (*see* Otsuka, 1973).

These same physiological and pharmacological properties were later found to be useful models in tests of a role for GABA in the CNS. Evidence strongly supports the idea that GABA mediates the inhibitory actions of local interneurons in the brain and that GABA may also mediate presynaptic inhibition within the spinal cord. Presumptive GABA-ergic inhibitory synapses have been demonstrated most clearly between cerebellar Purkinje neurons and their targets in Deiter's nucleus; between small interneurons and the major output cells of the cerebellar cortex, olfactory bulb, cuneate nucleus, hippocampus, and lateral septal nucleus; and between the vestibular nucleus and the trochlear motoneurons. GABA may also mediate the effects of inhibitory neurons within the cerebral cortex (*see* Kelly and Beart, 1975). The existence of a GABA-ergic pathway from caudate nucleus to substantia nigra is supported by neurochemical and cytochemical evidence (Kelly and Beart, 1975). Presumptive GABA-ergic neurons and nerve terminals have been localized with immunocytochemical methods that visualize glutamic acid decarboxylase. The reaction catalyzed by this pyridoxal phosphate–requiring enzyme provides the major source of GABA. The most useful drugs for confirmation of GABA-ergic mediation have been *bicuculline* and *picrotoxin;* however, many convulsants whose actions were previously unexplained (including penicillin and pentylenetetrazol) may also act as selective antagonists of GABA (Macdonald and McLean, 1982). Useful therapeutic effects have not yet been obtained by the use of agents that mimic GABA (such as muscimol), that inhibit the active reuptake of the transmitter (2,4-diaminobutyrate, nipecotic acid, and guvacine; *see* Johnston, 1978), or that alter the rate of synthesis or degradation of GABA (such as aminooxyacetic acid; *see* Iversen, 1978). Picrotoxin and bicuculline appear to antagonize the actions of GABA. However, while bicuculline competes with GABA for putative receptor binding sites, picrotoxin cannot (Iversen, 1978). Benzodiazepines can potentiate responses to GABA, apparently by interacting with a drug receptor located within the GABA-ergic receptor complex (Olsen, 1982). Two types of receptors for GABA have been proposed: GABA-A receptors, where muscimol is a potent agonist, bicuculline is a competitive antagonist, and binding of GABA may be enhanced by benzodiazepines, barbiturates, and certain steroids (*see* Chapter 17); and GABA-B sites, where baclofen is an agonist and GABA has a relatively low potency that is unaffected by benzodiazepines (Nicoll, 1988; Price and Bowery, 1988).

Glycine was found not to be a particularly potent agent when its inhibitory effects were first evaluated by the iontophoretic technique in spinal cord. However, Werman and associates (1968) assembled neurochemical and electrophysiological evidence that has established glycine as the inhibitory transmitter between spinal interneurons and motoneurons.

Glycine is the most abundant amino acid with inhibitory activity found in the ventral-quadrant gray matter of the spinal cord, and concentrations of glycine drop in proportion to the degeneration of ventral-quadrant interneurons following transient ischemia of the cord. Glycine has also been localized to spinal interneurons by electron-microscopic autoradiography. It is concentrated in nerve terminals that can be discriminated from those that accumulate GABA (Iversen, 1978). The hyperpolarization of motoneurons produced by iontophoretic application of glycine is relatively transient but approaches the equilibrium potential for the indirectly activated inhibitory postsynaptic potential; however, tests with GABA also indicate similar electrophysiological effects and a similar increase in Cl^- conductance. The major evidence that favors glycine as the mediator of intraspinal postsynaptic inhibition is the selective antagonism of its effects by strychnine. Strychnine does not usually antagonize responses to GABA (*see* Ryall, 1975), but it is able to inhibit the hyperpolarizing responses to β-alanine, another naturally occurring amino acid (*see* Zieglgänsberger, 1982). Glycine also appears to be the most likely inhibitory transmitter in the reticular formation (excluding the cuneate nucleus). Except for experiments with strychnine or strychnine-like antagonists, there has been little pharmacological manipulation of neurons that release glycine (*see* Gynther and Curtis, 1986).

Glutamate and *aspartate* are found in very high concentrations in brain, and both of these amino acids have extremely powerful excitatory effects on neurons in virtually every region of the CNS. However, the widespread distribution of these two dicarboxylic acids in the CNS and their roles in intermediary metabolism have tended to obscure the action that they might have as transmitters.

Although the existence of selective, high-affinity uptake systems for glutamate and aspartate is consistent with a transmitter role, efforts to establish either substance as an excitatory transmitter in the mammalian CNS have been hampered by the lack of convincingly selective receptor antagonists. However, over the past decade three subtypes of receptors for excitatory amino acids have been characterized pharmacologically, based on the relative potencies of synthetic agonists and the discovery of potent and selective antagonists. At present, these receptors are named for their respective prototypical agonists: kainate (blocked by lactonized kainate); quisqualate (blocked by 6-cyano-7-nitroquinoxaline-2,3-dione; CNXQ); and N-methyl-D-aspartate (NMDA) (blocked by 3-[2-carboxypiperazin-4-yl] propyl-1-phosphonic acid; CPP).

Although still somewhat circumstantial, both pharmacological and electrophysiological evidence has led to the widespread acceptance of the notion that either glutamate or aspartate (or, in some instances, perhaps both) functions as the principal transmitter for classical, fast synaptic excitation at various sites throughout the CNS (*see* Monaghan and Cotman, 1985; Lehmann *et al.*, 1987; Meldrum, 1987; Robinson and Coyle, 1987). There is also evidence that voltage-dependent cation channels that are regulated by NMDA receptors are major targets for certain drugs, including ketamine (a dissociative anesthetic) and its hallucinogenic analog, phencyclidine (PCP) (*see* Meldrum, 1987). These agents impede the flow of ions through such channels in a fashion analogous to the actions of local anesthetic agents on voltage-sensitive Na^+ channels. In experimental animals, local instillation of analogs of excitatory amino acids produces areas of neuronal death, while sparing nearby axons. These effects can be prevented by antagonists of NMDA receptors; it is possible that drugs with similar actions may prove therapeutically useful in salvaging neurons threatened by hypoxia following trauma or stroke (Gallo *et al.*, 1989).

Acetylcholine. After it was established that ACh is the transmitter at neuromuscular and parasympathetic neuroeffector junctions, as well as at the major synapse of autonomic ganglia (*see* Chapter 5), the amine began to receive considerable attention as a potential central neurotransmitter. Based on the finding of an irregular distribution within regions of the CNS and the observation that peripheral cholinergic drugs could produce marked behavioral effects after central administration, many were willing to consider that ACh might be "the" central neurotransmitter. In the late 1950s Eccles and colleagues demonstrated

Table 12–1. OVERVIEW OF THE PHARMACOLOGY OF AMINO ACID AND MONOAMINE TRANSMITTERS IN THE CENTRAL NERVOUS SYSTEM

TRANSMITTER	ANATOMY-CYTOLOGY	PRESYNAPTIC PHARMACOLOGY			POSTSYNAPTIC PHARMACOLOGY			
		Synthesis	*Storage*	*Reuptake*	*Receptor Subtypes and Agonists*	*Antagonists*	*Receptor Mechanisms* *	*Catabolism*
GABA	Supraspinal interneurons	—	—	2-Hydroxy-GABA, guvacine, and nipecotic acid inhibit	A: Muscimol	Bicuculline, picrotoxin	Increases chloride conductance; hyperpolarizes	Blocked with aminooxyacetic acid
					B: Baclofen	—	—	
Glycine	Spinal interneurons	—	—	—	Taurine (?), β-alanine (?)	Strychnine	Increases Cl^- conductance; hyperpolarizes	—
Glutamate; aspartate	Interneurons at all levels	—	—	—	Quisqualate, AMPA [a]	CNQX [b]	Increases cation conductance; depolarizes	—
					N-Me-D-aspartate	CPP [c]		
					Kainate	Lactonized kainate		
Acetylcholine	All levels; probable long and short connections	Hemicholinium blocks	—	Choline uptake can be enhanced with loading	M_1: Muscarine, McN-A-343 ‡	Quinuclidinyl benzoate, atropine, pirenzepine	Excitatory	Cholinesterase inhibitors block
					M_2: Bethanechol	Atropine	Inhibitory	
	Motoneuron–Renshaw cell				Nicotine	Dihydro-β-erythroidine	Excitatory	

Dopamine	All levels; short, medium, and long connections	α-Methyltyrosine inhibits; levodopa enhances	Tetrabenazine, reserpine, α-methyl-*m*-tyrosine inhibit; amphetamine releases; γ-hydroxybutyrate inhibits release	Benztropine, amitriptyline inhibit; 6-hydroxydopamine accumulates and is toxic	D_1: SKF 38393	SCH 23390	Activates adenylyl cyclase; inhibitory	Monoamine oxidase inhibitors block
					D_2: Apomorphine; quinpirole	Butyrophenones; s-sulpiride	Unlinked to or inhibits adenylyl cyclase; inhibitory	
Norepinephrine	All levels; long axons from pons and brainstem	Same as for dopamine; FLA-63 [d] and diethyldithiocarbamate inhibit dopamine β-hydroxylase	Reserpine, tetrabenazine, α-methyl-*m*-tyrosine inhibit; amphetamine releases	Desipramine inhibits; 6-hydroxydopamine accumulates and is toxic	α_1: Phenylephrine	Prazosin	—	Same as for dopamine
					α_2: Clonidine	Rauwolscine, yohimbine	Inhibitory	
					β_1: Dobutamine ‡	Metoprolol, practolol	Activates adenylyl cyclase; inhibitory and excitatory	
					β_2: Terbutaline ‡	Butoxamine ‡		
Epinephrine	Midbrain and brainstem to diencephalon	Same as for norepinephrine	Probably same as for norepinephrine	—	Probably same as for norepinephrine	Probably same as for norepinephrine	—	Probably same as for dopamine
5-Hydroxytryptamine	Midbrain and pons to all levels	*p*-Chlorophenylalanine blocks; tryptophan may increase	Reserpine, tetrabenazine inhibit	Clomipramine and fluoxetine inhibit; 5,7-dihydroxytryptamine accumulates and is toxic	$5\text{-}HT_{1A}$: LSD, 8-OH DPAT [e]	Metergoline	Inhibitory	Same as for dopamine
					$5\text{-}HT_2$: —	Spiperone methysergide	—	
					$5\text{-}HT_3$: —	MDL-7222	—	
Histamine	Posterior hypothalamus	—	Reserpine	—	H_1: Histamine	Mepyramine	—	—
					H_2: 2 Thiazolylethylamine	Cimetidine	Activates adenylyl cyclase	
					H_3: —	Thioperamide	—	

* Excitatory and inhibitory refer to the effects of agonists on the rates of firing of responsive neurons in the CNS.

‡ Predicted on the basis of peripheral actions.

[a] AMPA is DL-α-amino-3-hydroxy-5-methylisoxazole-4-propionate.

[b] CNQX is 6-cyano-7-nitroquinoxaline-2,3-dione.

[c] CPP is 3-(2-carboxypiperazin-4-yl)propyl-1-phosphonic acid.

[d] FLA-63 is *bis*-(1-methyl-4-homopiperazinyl-thiocarbonyl) disulfide.

[e] 8-OH DPAT is 8-hydroxy-2(di-*n*-propylamino)tetralin.

the recurrent excitation of spinal Renshaw neurons to be sensitive to nicotinic cholinergic antagonists; these cells were also found to be cholinoceptive. Such observations were consistent with the chemical and functional specificity of Dale's hypothesis that all branches of a neuron released the same transmitter substance and, in this case, produced similar types of postsynaptic action (*see* Eccles, 1964). Although the ability of ACh to elicit neuronal discharge has subsequently been replicated on scores of CNS cells (*see* Shepherd, 1988), the spinal Renshaw cell remains the best if not the sole example of a central nicotinic cholinergic junction (*see* McCormick and Prince, 1987; Madison *et al.*, 1987; Wada *et al.*, 1988).

In most regions of the CNS, the effects of ACh, assessed either by iontophoresis or by radioligand receptor-displacement assays (Kuhar, 1978), would appear to be generated by interaction with a mixture of nicotinic and muscarinic receptors. Several sets of presumptive cholinergic pathways have been proposed in addition to that of the motoneuron-Renshaw cell. These include the medial septal nucleus to dentate gyrus and subiculum of hippocampus habenula to interpeduncular nucleus; cortical interneurons to cortical pyramidal neurons; and thalamus, putamen, and caudate to neurons in the caudate. Cholinergic circuits are prominent in cerebral, limbic, and thalamic regions, and they include both long-divergent and local-circuit connections. Subsets of muscarinic cholinergic sites have also been described (Kerlavage *et al.*, 1987).

Thus, while ACh has long been the subject of intense investigation as a CNS transmitter, compelling evidence has been accumulated for only a few sites. The present data are fully in keeping with the possibility that both interregional and intraregional circuits may have ACh as their transmitter. When administered to man and animals, both cholinergic and anticholinergic drugs can cause marked behavioral effects (*see* Chapters 7 and 8; *see also* Iversen and Iversen, 1979).

Catecholamines. The brain contains separate neuronal systems that utilize three different catecholamines—*dopamine, norepinephrine,* and *epinephrine*. Each system is anatomically distinct and presumably serves separate functional roles. These systems have been extensively investigated with a variety of techniques, and a wealth of descriptive details is thus available for each (Björklund and Lindvall, 1986).

Dopamine. Although originally regarded only as a precursor of norepinephrine, assays of distinct regions of the CNS eventually revealed that the distributions of dopamine and norepinephrine are markedly different. In fact, more than half the CNS content of catecholamine is dopamine, and extremely high amounts are found in the basal ganglia (especially the caudate nucleus), the nucleus accumbens, the olfactory tubercle, the central nucleus of the amygdala, the median eminence, and restricted fields of the frontal cortex. Due to the availability of histochemical methods that can reveal all the catecholamines (formaldehyde- or glyoxylic acid-induced fluorescence; Dahlstrom and Fuxe, 1964) or immunohistochemical methods for enzymes that synthesize individual catecholamines (Hökfelt *et al.*, 1978), the anatomical connections of the dopamine-containing neurons are known with some precision, at least for the rodent brain. These studies indicate that dopaminergic neurons fall into three major morphological classes: (1) ultrashort neurons within the amacrine cells of the retina and periglomerular cells of the olfactory bulb; (2) intermediate-length neurons within the tuberobasal ventral hypothalamus that innervate the median eminence and intermediate lobe of the pituitary, incertohypothalamic neurons that connect the dorsal and posterior hypothalamus with the lateral septal nuclei, and small series of neurons within the perimeter of the dorsal motor nucleus of the vagus, the nucleus of the solitary tract, and the periaqueductal gray matter; and (3) long projections between the major dopamine-containing nuclei in the substantia nigra and ventral tegmentum and their targets in the striatum, in the limbic zones of the cerebral cortex, and in other major regions of the limbic system except the hippocampus (*see* Björklund and Lindvall, 1986). At the cellular level, the nature of the actions of dopamine remains somewhat controversial. While most iontophoretic studies indicate that inhibition is the predominant action, studies of the effects of electrical stimulation on transmembrane properties of the target neurons in the striatum suggest that there are depolarizing effects (Siggins and Gruol, 1986). Two subtypes of dopamine receptors have been characterized, and the complete amino acid sequence of one has been determined (Bunzow *et al.*, 1988); they continue to be the subject of intense study (*see* Seeman and Niznik, 1988). D_1 receptors activate, while D_2 receptors inhibit, adenylyl cyclase. Although the two forms of receptor are probably found mainly on different types of neurons, there is some evidence for their presence and interaction in individual cells. The D_1 receptor is approximately 15-fold more sensitive to dopamine than is the D_2 receptor. The clinical potency of antipsychotic agents appears to parallel their affinity for D_2 receptors (*see also* Chiodo and Bunney, 1987). Agents have been developed that are highly selective for D_1 and D_2 receptors. For example, SCH 23390 is a specific D_1 antagonist, and SKF 38393 is a potent and selective D_1 agonist.

Norepinephrine. There are relatively large amounts of norepinephrine within the hypothalamus and in certain zones of the limbic system, such as the central nucleus of the amygdala and the dentate gyrus of the hippocampus, but this catecholamine is also present in significant but lower amounts in most brain regions. Detailed mapping studies indicate that most noradrenergic neurons arise either in the locus ceruleus of the pons or in neurons of the lateral tegmental portion of the reticular formation. From these neurons, multiple branched axons innervate specific target cells in a large number of cortical, subcortical, and spinomedullary fields (Foote *et al.*, 1983).

Although norepinephrine has been firmly established as the transmitter at synapses between presumptive noradrenergic pathways and a wide variety of target neurons, a number of features to the mode of action of this biogenic amine have complicated the acquisition of convincing evidence. In large part, these problems reflect its "nonclassical" electrophysiological synaptic actions, which result in "state-dependent" or "enabling" effects. In some instances, the pharmacological properties of such synapses have been complex, with evidence for mediation by both α- and β-adrenergic receptors (*see* Siggins and Gruol, 1986; Bloom, 1988). For example, stimulation of the locus ceruleus depresses the spontaneous activity of target neurons in the cerebellum; this is associated with a slowly developing hyperpolarization and a decrease in membrane conductance. However, activation of the locus ceruleus affects the higher firing rates produced by stimulation of excitatory inputs to these neurons to a lesser degree, and excitatory postsynaptic potentials are enhanced. All consequences of activation of the locus ceruleus are emulated by the iontophoretic application of norepinephrine and are effectively blocked by β-adrenergic antagonists. Although the mechanisms underlying these effects are not at all clear, there is convincing evidence for intracellular mediation by cyclic AMP.

For the most part, the effects of activation of the locus ceruleus (or of application of norepinephrine) on target neurons in the cerebral cortex or hippocampus are similar to those observed in the cerebellum. However, several different features have been noted, especially in studies on hippocampal pyramidal cells. First, norepinephrine-induced inhibition of firing frequently appears to be mediated predominantly by α-adrenergic receptors (*see* Siggins and Gruol, 1986). Second, stimulation of β-adrenergic receptors can increase the firing rate of target neurons depolarized by stimulation of excitatory inputs (Madison and Nicoll, 1986). The latter effect results from the cyclic AMP-mediated inhibition of a Ca^{2+}-activated K^+ conductance and is associated with a reduction in the hyperpolarization that follows repetitive firing of action potentials. The mechanisms underlying the inhibitory effects mediated by α-adrenergic receptors are not understood. The involvement of cyclic AMP is considered to be one possibility because, in some circumstances, the stimulation of α-adrenergic receptors can promote accumulation of the cyclic nucleotide in the presence of heterologous agonists, such as adenosine (*see* Rall, 1972).

As in the periphery, four subtypes of adrenergic receptors have been described in the CNS (*i.e.*, α_1, α_2, β_1, and β_2). Even though the proportion varies from region to region, β_1-adrenergic receptors may be associated predominantly with neurons, while β_2-adrenergic receptors may be more characteristic of glial and vascular elements. Both α_1- and α_2-adrenergic receptors have been detected in regions of the CNS that are targets for noradrenergic neurons (*see* Bylund and U'Prichard, 1983; Ruffolo and Nichols, 1987). Clearly, further study is necessary to define the functions subserved by the various subtypes of adrenergic receptors.

Epinephrine. Neurons in the CNS that contain epinephrine were recognized relatively recently following the development of sensitive enzymatic assays for phenylethanolamine-N-methyltransferase (*see* Chapter 5) and immunocytochemical staining techniques for the enzyme (Hökfelt *et al.*, 1974). Epinephrine-containing neurons are found in the medullary reticular formation and make restricted connections to a few pontine and diencephalic nuclei, eventually coursing as far rostrally as the paraventricular nucleus of the dorsal midline thalamus. The physiological properties of these connections have not as yet been studied.

5-Hydroxytryptamine. Following the chemical determination that a biogenic substance found both in serum ("serotonin") and in gut ("enteramine") was 5-HT, assays for this substance revealed its presence in brain (Brodie and Shore, 1957). Since that time, studies of 5-HT have had a pivotal role in understanding the neuropharmacology of the CNS. Various cytochemical methods have been used to trace the central anatomy of 5-HT–containing neurons in several species (*see* Aghajanian and Vandermaelen, 1986). Tryptaminergic neurons are localized to some nine nuclei lying in or adjacent to the midline (raphe) regions of the pons and upper brainstem, corresponding to well-defined nuclear ensembles (Dahlstrom and Fuxe, 1964).

The more rostral raphe nuclei appear to innervate forebrain regions, while the more caudal raphe nuclei project within the brainstem and spinal cord. The median raphe nucleus contributes a major portion of the tryptaminergic innervation of the limbic system, and the dorsal raphe nucleus contributes a major portion of similar innervation of cortical regions and the neostriatum.

In the mammalian CNS, cells receiving cytochemically demonstrable tryptaminergic input, such as the suprachiasmatic nucleus, ventrolateral geniculate body, amygdala, and hippocampus, exhibit a uniform and dense investment of reactive terminals. Recordings obtained from such neurons show uniform inhibition after stimulation of the raphe neurons, and this effect is mimicked, at least qualitatively, by iontophoretic application of 5-HT.

At least in hippocampal pyramidal cells, such inhibition appears to result from membrane hyperpolarization caused by an *increase* in a K^+ conductance. On the other hand, stimulation of dorsal raphe neurons increases the firing of a variety of target cells, including those in the caudate-putamen and motor neurons in the facial nucleus and spinal cord. Although specific depletion of 5-HT reduces or eliminates such effects, the iontophoretic application of 5-HT produces excitatory actions that wax and wane more slowly than do those that follow stimulation of raphe neurons. This discrepancy may reflect the possible function of neuropeptides (*e.g.*, substance P) that frequently have been demonstrated within tryptaminergic neurons and nerve terminals. The excitation (or facilitation) induced by 5-HT appears to result from membrane depolarization associated with a *decrease* in a K^+ conductance. Within raphe nuclei, 5-HT exerts powerful inhibitory effects on tryptaminergic neurons by way of dendrodendritic synapses. Although apparently caused by an increase in a K^+ conductance, both the electrophysiological and pharmacological characteristics of these effects are clearly different from those associated with inhibition of hippocampal pyramidal cells (*see* Aghajanian and Vandermaelen, 1986).

Ligand-binding studies have defined a multitude of putative receptors for 5-HT. Depending on the species and region of the CNS examined, as many as six distinct subtypes have been detected (*see* Peroutka, 1988). The current nomenclature is confusing: four putative classes of 5-HT_1 sites (designated A through D); 5-HT_2; and 5-HT_3. The correlation between these data and the electrophysiological observations described above is still sketchy, but the site designated as 5-HT_{1A} appears to mediate the inhibitory effects on raphe neurons and hippocampal pyramidal cells because of the potent agonistic actions of such agents as 8-hydroxy-2(di-*n*-propylamino)tetralin (8-OH DPAT) (despite the different properties of the K^+ conductances influenced). Moreover, both stimulation and inhibition of adenylyl cyclase has been ascribed to 5-HT_{1A} receptors in different regions of the CNS. Those sites designated as 5-HT_2 may mediate excitatory effects, such as those described in the facial motor nucleus, because of the potent antagonistic actions of methysergide; these receptors appear to activate phospholipase C, with the resultant synthesis of inositol phosphates and diacylglycerol. Those sites designated as 5-HT_3 were first identified in peripheral structures, such as sympathetic ganglia and sensory nerves, where they mediate excitatory effects; although detected elsewhere in the CNS, their function is unknown (Kilpatrick *et al.*, 1987). Thus far, a cDNA that encodes the receptor designated as 5-HT_{1C} has been cloned and expressed in *Xenopus* oocytes and mouse fibroblasts (Lübbert *et al.*, 1987; Julius *et al.*, 1988). Although this receptor is especially concentrated in the choroid plexus, it is also expressed in neurons in many regions of the CNS; 5-HT_{1C} receptors also activate phospholipase C and thus increase intracellular concentrations of Ca^{2+}.

Many different classes of centrally active drugs can affect physiological or biochemical parameters of various tryptaminergic neuronal systems by influencing direct responses to 5-HT or its uptake, synthesis, storage, release, or catabolism. The list includes hallucinogens (such as lysergic acid diethylamide [LSD], N,N-dimethyltryptamine [DMT] and other tryptamine congeners, and mescaline), reserpine, chlorpromazine, tricyclic antidepressants, monoamine oxidase inhibitors, amphetamines (particularly the chloroamphetamines), Li^+, and morphine. These drugs have also been demonstrated to have effects on catecholamine-containing and other chemically defined neurons, making the functional importance of the effects on mechanisms that involve 5-HT difficult to interpret.

LSD is among the most interesting of the compounds that interact with 5-HT. In iontophoretic tests, LSD and 5-HT are both potent inhibitors of the firing of raphe (5-HT) neurons, but LSD and other hallucinogens are far less potent depressants than is 5-HT on neurons that receive innervation from the raphe. The inhibitory effect of LSD on raphe neurons offers a plausible explanation for the drug's hallucinogenic effects, namely, that they result from depression of activity in a system that tonically inhibits visual and other sensory inputs. However, typical LSD-induced behavior is still seen in animals with raphe nuclei destroyed or after blockade of the synthesis of 5-HT by *p*-chlorophenylalanine. Other evidence against this explanation of LSD-induced hallucinations is the potentiation of LSD by administration of the precursor of 5-HT, 5-hydroxytryptophan. More precise definition of the various functional roles of tryptaminergic pathways in the CNS awaits the results of studies utilizing more specific agents, whose number is steadily mounting.

Histamine. For many years, histamine and antihistamines that are active in the periphery have been known to produce significant effects on animal behavior. Only relatively recently, however, has evidence accumulated to suggest that histamine might be a central neurotransmitter. Biochemical detection of histamine synthesis by neurons, as well as direct cytochemical localization of these neurons, has established the validity of a histaminergic system in the CNS (*see* Schwartz *et al.*, 1986; Schwartz, 1988). Most of these neurons are located in the ventral posterior hypothalamus; they give rise to long ascending and descending tracts to the entire CNS that are typical of the patterns characteristic of other aminergic systems. Based on the presumptive central effects of histamine antagonists, the histaminergic system is thought to function in the regulation of arousal, body temperature, and vascular dynamics.

Three subtypes of histamine receptors have been described. H_1 receptors, the most prominent, may be located on glia and vessels as well as on neurons and may act to mobilize Ca^{2+} in receptive cells. H_2 receptors are directly linked to the activation of adenylyl cyclase, perhaps in concert with H_1 receptors in certain circumstances (Bertaccini and

Coruzzi, 1987). H_3 receptors, which have the greatest sensitivity to histamine, are localized much more selectively in basal ganglia and olfactory regions in the rat, but consequences of their activation remain unsettled (Schwartz, 1988). Unlike the monoamines and amino acid transmitters, there does not appear to be an active reuptake process for histamine after its release. In addition, no direct evidence has been obtained for histamine release *in vivo* or *in vitro* associated with neuronal activity.

Peptides. The continuing discovery of novel peptides in the CNS that are capable of regulating one or another aspect of neural function has produced considerable excitement, and an imposing catalog of previously unknown neuropeptides has accumulated (*see* Guillemin, 1978; Krieger, 1983; Krieger *et al.*, 1983; Hökfelt *et al.*, 1987). In addition, certain peptides previously thought to be restricted to the gut or to endocrine glands have also been found in the CNS. Relatively detailed maps are now available for neurons that show immunoreactivity to peptide-specific antisera. CNS peptides may function on their own or in concert with a coexisting transmitter. Some hypothalamic neurons may contain more than two possible transmitters (*see* Hökfelt *et al.*, 1983, 1987). At this time at least three schemes appear to have some utility in attempting to organize the peptidergic systems of neurons.

Organization by Peptide Families. Because of significant homology in amino acid sequences, families of related molecules can be defined (Blundell and Humbel, 1980; Niall, 1982). These families may be *ancestral* or *concurrent*. The ancestral relationship is illustrated by peptides such as the substance-P or the vasotocin family, in which species differences can be correlated with modest variations in peptide structure. The concurrent relationship is best exemplified by the endorphins and by the glucagon-secretin family. In the "superfamily" endorphin, three major systems of endorphin peptides (proopiomelanocortin, proenkephalin, and prodynorphin) exist in independent neuronal circuits (*see* Bloom, 1988). These arise from independent, but homologous, genes. The peptides all share some actions at receptors once classed generally as "opioid" and now undergoing progressive refinement (*see* Chapters 21 and 56). In the glucagon family, multiple and somewhat homologous peptides are found simultaneously in different cells of the same organism but in separate organ systems: glucagon and vasoactive intestinal polypeptide (VIP) in pancreatic islets; secretin in duodenal mucosa; VIP and related peptides in enteric, autonomic, and central neurons (*see* Blundell and Humbel, 1980; Iversen, 1983); and growth hormone–releasing factor in central neurons only (Guillemin *et al.*, 1982). The general metabolic effects produced by this family can be viewed as leading to increased blood glucose. To some degree, ancestral and concurrent relationships are not mutually exclusive, since multiple members of the substance-P family have now been reported (Nawa *et al.*, 1983); this may account for the apparent existence of subsets of receptors for substance P (Iversen *et al.*, 1982). The mammalian terminus of the vasotocin family shows two concurrent products as well, vasopressin and oxytocin, each having evolved to perform separate functions that were once executed by single vasotocin-related peptides in lower phyla.

Organization by Anatomic Pattern. Some peptide systems follow rather consistent anatomical organizations. Thus, the hypothalamic peptides oxytocin, vasopressin, proopiomelanocortin, luteinizing hormone–releasing hormone and growth hormone–releasing hormone all tend to be made by single large clusters of neurons that give off multibranched axons to several distant targets. Others, such as systems that contain somatostatin, cholecystokinin, and enkephalin, can have many forms, with patterns varying from moderately long, hierarchical connections to short-axon, local-circuit neurons that are widely distributed throughout the brain (*see* Krieger *et al.*, 1983).

Organization by Function. Since almost all peptides were identified initially on the basis of bioassays, their names reflect these functions (*e.g.*, thyrotropin-releasing hormone, vasoactive intestinal polypeptide, *etc.*). These names become trivial if more ubiquitous distributions and additional functions are discovered. Although some general integrative role might be hypothesized for widely separated neurons (and other cells) that make the same peptide, a more parsimonious view would be that each peptide has unique messenger roles at the cellular level and that these are used again and again in functionally similar pathways within large systems that differ in their overall functions (*see* Bloom, 1988).

Comparison with Other Transmitters. Peptides differ in several important respects from the monoamine and amino acid transmitters considered earlier. Synthesis of a peptide is performed in the rough endoplasmic reticulum, where mRNA for the propeptide can be translated into an amino acid sequence. The propeptide is then cleaved (processed) to the form that is secreted as the secretory vesicles are transported from the perinuclear cytoplasm to the nerve terminals. Further, no active reuptake mechanisms for peptides have been described; this increases the dependency of nerve terminals on distant sites of synthesis. Perhaps most importantly, linear chains of amino acids can assume many conformations at their receptors, making it difficult to detect the sequences and their steric relationships that are critical for activity.

The lack of predictive capability has severely limited the development of agonists or antagonists that will interact with specific receptors for peptides. Nature has also had limited success in this regard, since only one plant alkaloid, morphine, has been found to act selectively at peptidergic synapses. Fortunately for pharmacologists, morphine was discovered before the endorphins, or there might not yet be any example of a rigid molecule that is capable of acting at receptors for a peptide. The recent development of nonpeptide antagonists of cholecystokinin suggests that this also can be achieved by man (Chang and Lotti, 1986; Evans *et al.*, 1986).

PERSPECTIVES FOR FUTURE DEVELOPMENT

Concepts of the relationship between the actions of a drug and the functions of specific brain systems have progressed through three phases, particularly in the relatively brief history of psychopharmacology (Mandell, 1973). In the first phase, drug-induced changes in function were correlated directly with changes in the concentrations of neurotransmitters or their metabolites. An exemplary anomaly revealed at this stage was the relationship between the behavioral depression that follows administration of reserpine and the decreased storage of 5-HT (and also norepinephrine and dopamine) in the brain (Brodie and Shore, 1957). The time course of the change in behavior coincides initially with alterations in the content of biogenic amines; however, when the analysis is extended past the first 48 hours, it becomes clear that the concentrations of amines remain depressed while behavior returns toward normal.

A second phase of investigation began with demonstrations that many drugs with potent behavioral actions (*e.g.*, LSD, amphetamine, tricyclic antidepressants, antipsychotics) produced relatively minor changes in the concentrations of transmitters. Attempts were thus made to relate the effects of drugs to alterations in the dynamics of neuronal metabolism, from which it was hoped that information about changes in neuronal activity could be inferred. For example, estimates have been made of the turnover rates of neurotransmitters, and single-unit electrophysiological recordings have also been employed as indices of the effects of drugs on the functional activity of chemically characterized neuronal systems. This approach suffers from at least two problems that are also shared by experiments that rely on assessment of concentrations of transmitters. (1) Neurochemical experiments proceed on a time scale of minutes to hours, while neuronal events occur in milliseconds or seconds; changes that are measured may therefore be quite removed from those that occur at the primary site of action. (2) Neurotransmitters that have not yet been identified obviously cannot be measured. Because of these and other limitations, it is entirely possible for a drug treatment to induce changes that are correctly correlated, perhaps even selectively, with aspects of the metabolism or action of one or more transmitters, and yet the two effects—that on function and that on specific neuronal systems—may not be causally related.

Current efforts in CNS pharmacology are also in a third phase that focuses in part on the adaptive changes imposed on the nervous system by chronic treatment with drugs. It has become clear that the metabolic and functional changes observed initially do not persist and are replaced by changes that may in fact be opposite to those seen acutely. For example, tricyclic antidepressants, when given acutely, potentiate the cellular and behavioral effects of norepinephrine by inhibition of its reuptake. It has been inferred that depression results from a deficiency of catecholamine and that tricyclic antidepressants are effective by increasing the amounts of catecholamine at the postsynaptic receptor. However, in animals treated chronically with desmethylimipramine, sensitivity of β-adrenergic receptors is decreased, even though presynaptic reuptake of norepinephrine remains fully inhibited.

With the ability to clone, sequence, and express the genes that encode receptor molecules for neurotransmitters, a new era in drug development is approaching. Such studies have permitted the identification of novel receptor subtypes that were undetected by traditional pharmacological approaches; the pace of such discovery will accelerate. Receptor heterogeneity provides an opportunity for greater pharmacological selectivity. *In-situ* hybridization with appropriate probes facilitates unambiguous cellular localization of individual forms of a receptor, and expression of the receptor in cultured cell systems allows its characterization against a null background. In the future, molecular modeling based on the primary amino acid sequence of a receptor will make it possible to define the precise structure of the ligand-binding site and should permit synthesis of novel compounds tailored to these sites. Such data also make possible new methods to evaluate the regulation of receptor number and the precise nature of the protein–protein interactions by which ion-channel receptors and G protein–coupled receptors transduce their effects.

Future efforts to provide explanations for drug-induced neurological changes will undoubtedly continue to focus on synaptic transmitters and their mechanisms. If estimates of the complexity of brain-specific mRNA are any indication, many more transmitter peptides remain to be discovered (Milner and Sutcliffe, 1983). Use of recombinant DNA technology has already lengthened the list of putative transmitter peptides considerably (Tatemoto and Mutt, 1980; Tatemoto, 1982; Itoh *et al.*, 1983; Nawa *et al.*, 1983). As more transmitters are discovered and their neuronal systems are mapped, new target cells will become available for the study of unique or common mechanisms of action. In this regard it may be useful to consider three general properties by which neuronal circuits can be described and to employ them in efforts to correlate the molecular actions of drugs with their resulting neurological and behavioral effects. A *spatial domain* describes those areas of the brain or of peripheral receptive fields that feed signals to a given cell and those areas to which that cell sends its signals. A *temporal domain* describes the duration of the effects of a cell on its targets. A *functional domain* describes the molecular mechanisms by which the cell influences its targets. Within these three domains, neurons can be defined in terms of their transmitters, receptors, and functional location, as well as in the more classical categories of sensory, motor, or interneuronal. All these properties must be borne in mind simultaneously in the attempt to develop comprehensive explanations of the acute and chronic effects of drugs.

Aghajanian, G. K. Modulation of a transient outward current in serotonergic neurones by alpha 1-adrenoreceptors. *Nature,* **1985,** *315,* 501–503.

Akagi, H., and Miledi, R. Heterogeneity of glycine receptors and their messenger RNAs in rat brain and spinal cord. *Science,* **1988,** *242,* 270–273.

Blair, L. A. C.; Levitan, E. S.; Marshall, J.; Dionne, V. E.; and Barnard, E. A. Single subunits of the GABAa receptor form ion channels with properties of the native receptor. *Science,* **1988,** *242,* 577–579.

Brodie, B. B., and Shore, P. A. A concept for a role of serotonin and norepinephrine as chemical mediators in the brain. *Ann. N.Y. Acad. Sci.,* **1957,** *66,* 631–642.

Bunzow, J. R.; Van Tol, H. H. M.; Grandy, D. K.; Albert, P.; Salon, J.; Christi, M.; Machida, C. A.; Neve, K. A.; and Civelli, O. Cloning and expression of a rat D_2 dopamine receptor cDNA. *Nature,* **1988,** *336,* 783–787.

Chang, R. S. L., and Lotti, V. J. Biochemical and pharmacological characterization of an extremely potent and selective nonpeptide cholecystokinin antagonist. *Proc. Natl. Acad. Sci. U.S.A.,* **1986,** *83,* 4923–4926.

Chiodo, L. A., and Bunney, B. S. Population response of midbrain dopaminergic neurons to neuropeptides: further studies on time course and nondopaminergic neuronal influences. *J. Neurosci.,* **1987,** *7,* 629–633.

Coascogne, C. L.; Robel, P.; Gouezou, M.; Sananes, N.; Baulieu, E.-E.; and Waterman, M. Neurosteroids: cytochrome P-450_{scc} in rat brain. *Science,* **1987,** *237,* 1212–1215.

Conti-Tronconi, B. M.; Dunn, S. M. J.; Barnard, E. A.; Dolly, J. O.; Lai, F. A.; Ray, N.; and Raftery, M. A. Brain and muscle nicotinic acetylcholine receptors are different but homologous proteins. *Proc. Natl. Acad. Sci. U.S.A.,* **1985,** *82,* 5208–5212.

Curtis, D. R.; Duggan, A. W.; Felix, D.; Johnston, G. A. R.; and McLennan, H. Antagonism between bicuculline and GABA in the cat brain. *Brain Res.,* **1971,** *33,* 57–73.

Dahlstrom, A., and Fuxe, K. Evidence for the existence of monoamine-containing neurons in the central nervous system. I. Demonstration of monoamines in the cell bodies of brain stem neurons. *Acta Physiol. Scand.,* **1964,** *232,* Suppl. 62, 1–55.

Evans, B. E.; Bock, M. G.; Rittle, K. E.; DiPardo, R. M.; Whitter, W. L.; Veber, D. F.; Anderson, P. S.; and Freidinger, R. M. Design of potent, orally effective, nonpeptidal antagonists of the peptide hormone cholecystokinin. *Proc. Natl. Acad. Sci. U.S.A.,* **1986,** *83,* 4918–4922.

Gallo, V.; Giovannini, C.; and Levi, G. Quisqualic acid modulates kainate responses in cultured cerebellar granule cells. *J. Neurochem.,* **1989,** *52,* 10–16.

Greeningloh, G.; Rienitz, A.; Schmitt, B.; Methfessel, C.; Zensen, M.; Beyreuther, K.; Gundelfinger, E. D.; and Betz, H. The strychnine-binding subunit of the glycine receptor shows homology with nicotinic acetylcholine receptors. *Nature,* **1987,** *328,* 215–220.

Guillemin, R.; Brazeau, P.; Bohlen, P.; Esch, F.; Ling, N.; and Wehrenberg, W. B. Growth hormone-releasing factor from a human pancreatic tumor that caused acromegaly. *Science,* **1982,** *218,* 585–587.

Gynther, B. D., and Curtis, D. R. Pyridazinyl-GABA derivatives as GABA and glycine antagonists in the spinal cord of the cat. *Neurosci. Lett.,* **1986,** *68,* 211–215.

Hökfelt, T.; Fahrenkrug, J.; Tatemoto, K.; Mutt, V.; Werner, S.; Hulting, A. L.; Terenius, L.; and Chang, K. J. The PHI-27/corticotropin releasing factor/enkephalin immunoreactive hypothalamic neuron: possible morphological basis for integrated control of prolactin, corticotropin, and growth hormone secretion. *Proc. Natl. Acad. Sci. U.S.A.,* **1983,** *80,* 895–898.

Hökfelt, T.; Fuxe, K.; Goldstein, M.; and Johansson, O. Immunohistochemical evidence for the existence of adrenaline neurons in the rat brain. *Brain Res.,* **1974,** *66,* 235–251.

Itoh, N.; Obata, K. I.; Yanaihara, N.; and Okamoto, H. Human preprovasoactive intestinal polypeptide contains a novel PHI-27-like peptide, PHM-27. *Nature,* **1983,** *304,* 547–549.

Iversen, L. L.; Hanley, M. R.; Sandberg, B. E.; Lee, C. M.; Pinnock, R. D.; and Watson, S. P. Substance P receptors in the nervous system and possible receptor subtypes. *Ciba Found. Symp.,* **1982,** *91,* 186–205.

Julius, D.; MacDermott, A. B.; Axel, R.; and Jessell, T. M. Molecular characterization of a functional cDNA encoding the serotonin 1c receptor. *Science,* **1988,** *241,* 558–564.

Kilpatrick, G. J.; Jones, B. J.; and Tyers, M. B. Identification and distribution of 5-HT receptors in rat brain using radioligand binding. *Nature,* **1987,** *330,* 746–748.

Kravitz, E. A.; Kuffler, S. W.; and Potter, D. D. Gamma-aminobutyric acid and other blocking compounds in Crustacea. Their relative concentrations in separated motor and inhibitory axons. *J. Neurophysiol.,* **1963,** *26,* 739–751.

Krupinski, J.; Cousson, F.; Bakalyar, H. A.; Tang, W. J.; Feinstein, P. G.; Orth, K.; Slaughter, C.; Reed, R. R.; and Gilman, A. G. Adenylyl cyclase amino acid sequence: possible channel- or transporter-like structure. *Science,* **1989,** *244,* 1558–1564.

Kubo, T., and others. Cloning, sequencing and expression of complementary DNA encoding the muscarinic acetylcholine receptor. *Nature,* **1986,** *323,* 411–416.

Lehmann, J., and others. CPP, a selective n-methyl-d-aspartate (NMDA)-type receptor antagonist: characterization *in vitro* and *in vivo*. *J. Pharmacol. Exp. Ther.,* **1987,** *240,* 737–746.

Lindefors, N.; Brodin, E.; and Ungerstedt, U. Microdialysis combined with a sensitive radioimmunoassay. A technique for studying *in vivo* release of neuropeptides. *J. Pharmacol. Methods,* **1987,** *17,* 305–312.

Lübbert, H.; Hoffman, B. J.; Snutch, T. P.; van Dyke, T.; Levine, A. J.; Hartig, P. R.; Lester, H. A.; and Davidson, N. cDNA cloning of a serotonin 5-HT1C receptor by electrophysiological assays of mRNA-injected *Xenopus* oocytes. *Proc. Natl. Acad. Sci. U.S.A.,* **1987,** *84,* 4332–4336.

McCormick, D. A., and Prince, D. A. Acetylcholine causes rapid nicotinic excitation in the medial habenular nucleus of guinea pig, *in vitro*. *J. Neurosci.,* **1987,** *7,* 742–752.

Macdonald, R. L., and McLean, M. J. Cellular bases of barbiturate and phenytoin anticonvulsant drug action. *Epilepsia,* **1982,** *23,* Suppl. 1, S7–S18.

Madison, D. V.; Lancaster, B.; and Nicoll, R. A. Voltage clamp analysis of cholinergic action in the hippocampus. *J. Neurosci.,* **1987,** *7,* 733–741.

Madison, D. V., and Nicoll, R. A. Cyclic adenosine 3′-5′-monophosphate mediates receptor actions of noradrenaline in rat hippocampal pyramidal cells. *J. Physiol. (Lond.),* **1986,** *372,* 245–279.

Mandell, A. J. Redundant macromolecular mechanisms in central synaptic regulation. In, *New Concepts in Neurotransmitter Regulation.* (Mandell, A. J., ed.) Plenum Press, New York, **1973,** pp. 259–277.

Masu, Y.; Nakayama, K.; Tamaki, H.; Harada, Y.; Kuno, M.; and Nakanishi, S. cDNA cloning of bovine substance-K receptor through oocyte expression system. *Nature,* **1987,** *329,* 836–838.

Maysinger, D.; Herrera-Marschitz, M.; Carlsson, A.; Garofalo, L.; Cuello, A. C.; and Ungerstedt, U. Striatal and cortical acetylcholine release *in vivo* in rats with unilateral decortication: effects of treatment with monosialoganglioside GM1. *Brain Res.,* **1988,** *461,* 355–360.

Milner, R. J., and Sutcliffe, J. G. Gene expression in rat brain. *Nucleic Acids Res.,* **1983,** *11,* 5497–5520.

Monaghan, D. T., and Cotman, C. W. Distribution of N-methyl-D-aspartate-sensitive L-^{3}H-glutamate-binding sites in rat brain. *J. Neurosci.,* **1985,** *5,* 2909–2919.

Nawa, H.; Hirose, T.; Takashima, H.; Inayama, S.; and Nakanishi, S. Nucleotide sequences of cloned cDNAs for two types of bovine brain substance P precursor. *Nature,* **1983,** *306,* 32–36.

Nedergaard, S.; Bolam, J. P.; and Greenfield, S. A. Facilitation of a dendritic calcium conductance by 5-hydroxytryptamine in the substantia nigra. *Nature,* **1988,** *333,* 174–177.

North, R. A.; Williams, J. T.; Surprenant, A.; and Christie, M. J. Mu and delta receptors belong to a family of receptors that are coupled to potassium channels. *Proc. Natl. Acad. Sci. U.S.A.,* **1987,** *84,* 5487–5491.

Otsuka, M. Gamma aminobutyric acid and some other transmitter candidates in the nervous system. In, *Pharmacology and the Future of Man: Proceedings of the Fifth International Congress on Pharmacology,* Vol. 4. (Acheson, G. H., and Bloom, F. E., eds.) S. Karger, Basel, **1973,** pp. 186–201.

Rapoport, S. I. Osmotic opening of the blood-brain barrier. *Ann. Neurol.,* **1988,** *22,* 677–681.

Schofield, P. R., and others. Sequence and functional expression of the GABAa receptor shows a ligand-gated receptor super-family. *Nature,* **1987,** *328,* 221–227.

Siegelbaum, S. A.; Camardo, J. S.; and Kandel, E. R. Serotonin and cyclic AMP close single K+ channels in *Aplysia* sensory neurones. *Nature,* **1982,** *299,* 413.

Tatemoto, K. Neuropeptide Y: complete amino acid sequence of the brain peptide. *Proc. Natl. Acad. Sci. U.S.A.,* **1982,** *79,* 5485–5489.

Tatemoto, K., and Mutt, V. Isolation of two novel candidate hormones using a chemical method for finding naturally occurring polypeptides. *Nature,* **1980,** *285,* 417–418.

Wada, K.; Ballivet, M.; Boulter, J.; Connolly, J.; Wada, E.; Deneris, E. S.; Swanson, L. W.; Heinemann, S.; and Patrick, J. Functional expression of a new pharmacological subtype of brain nicotinic acetylcholine receptor. *Science,* **1988,** *240,* 330–332.

Werman, R.; Davidoff, R. A.; and Aprison, M. H. Inhibitory action of glycine on spinal neurons in the cat. *J. Neurophysiol.,* **1968,** *31,* 81–95.

Monographs and Reviews

Aghajanian, G. K., and Vandermaelen, C. P. Specific systems of the reticular core: serotonin. In, *Handbook of Physiology,* Vol. IV, Sect. 1. (Bloom, F. E., ed.) American Physiological Society, Bethesda, Md, **1986,** pp. 237–256.

Bertaccini, G., and Coruzzi, G. Histamine H2 receptor antagonists. In, *ISI Atlas of Science: Pharmacology,* Vol. 1. Institute for Scientific Information, Philadelphia, **1987,** pp. 181–186.

Björklund, A., and Lindvall, O. Catecholaminergic brain stem regulatory systems. In, *Handbook of Physiology,* Vol. IV, Sect. 1. (Bloom, F. E., ed.) American Physiological Society, Bethesda, Md, **1986,** pp. 155–236.

Blakely, R. D., and Coyle, J. T. The neurobiology of N-acetylaspartylglutamate. *Int. Rev. Neurobiol.,* **1988,** *30,* 39–100.

Bloom, F. E. The role of cyclic nucleotides in central synaptic function. *Rev. Physiol. Biochem. Pharmacol.,* **1975,** *74,* 1–103.

———. Neurotransmitters: past, present, and future directions. *FASEB J.,* **1988,** *2,* 32–41.

Blundell, T. L., and Humbel, R. E. Hormone families: pancreatic hormones and homologous growth factors. *Nature,* **1980,** *287,* 781–786.

Bodian, D. Neuron junctions: a revolutionary decade. *Anat. Rec.,* **1972,** *174,* 73–82.

Bylund, D. B., and U'Prichard, D. C. Characterization of α_1 and α_2 adrenergic receptors. *Int. Rev. Neurobiol.,* **1983,** *24,* 343–427.

Carlsson, A. Autoreceptors. In, *Pre- and Postsynaptic Receptors.* (Usdin, E., and Bunney, W. E., Jr., eds.) Marcel Dekker, Inc., New York, **1975,** pp. 49–65.

Catterall, W. A. Structure and function of voltage-sensitive ion channels. *Science*, **1988**, *242*, 50–61.

Cooper, J. R.; Bloom, F. E.; and Roth, R. H. *The Biochemical Basis of Neuropharmacology*, 5th ed. Oxford University Press, New York, **1986**.

Dale, H. H. Pharmacology and nerve endings. *Proc. R. Soc. Med.*, **1935**, *28*, 319–332.

Dohlman, H. G.; Caron, M. G.; and Lefkowitz, R. J. A family of receptors coupled to guanine nucleotide regulatory proteins. *Biochemistry*, **1987**, *26*, 2657–2664.

Eccles, J. C. *The Physiology of Synapses*. Academic Press, Inc., New York, **1964**.

Ferrendelli, J. A.; Collins, R. C.; and Johnson, E. M. (eds.). *Neurobiology of Amino Acids, Peptides, and Trophic Factors*. Kluwer Academic Publishers, Boston, **1988**.

Florey, E. Neurotransmitters and modulators in the animal kingdom. *Fed. Proc.*, **1967**, *26*, 1164–1176.

Foote, S. L.; Bloom, F. E.; and Aston-Jones, G. The nucleus locus coeruleus: new evidence of anatomical and physiological specificity. *Physiol. Rev.*, **1983**, *63*, 844–914.

Gilman, A. G. G proteins: transducers of receptor-generated signals. *Annu. Rev. Biochem.*, **1987**, *56*, 615–649.

Greengard, P. *Cyclic Nucleotides, Phosphorylated Proteins, and Neuronal Function: Distinguished Lecture Series of the Society of General Physiologists*, Vol. 1. Raven Press, New York, **1978**.

Guillemin, R. Peptides in the brain: the new endocrinology of the neuron. *Science*, **1978**, *202*, 390–402.

Heise, G. A. Facilitation of memory and cognition by drugs. *Trends Pharmacol. Sci.*, **1987**, *8*, 65–69.

Hökfelt, T.; Fuxe, K.; and Oernow, B. Coexistence of neuronal messengers: new principle in chemical transmission. *Prog. Brain Res.*, **1987**, *68*, 1–411.

Hökfelt, T.; Johansson, O.; Ljungdahl, A.; Lundberg, J. M.; and Schutzberg, M. Peptidergic neurons. *Nature*, **1980**, *284*, 515–521.

Hökfelt, T., and others. Aminergic and peptidergic pathways in the nervous system with special reference to the hypothalamus. In, *The Hypothalamus*. (Reichlin, S.; Baldessarini, R. J.; and Martin, J. B.; eds.) Raven Press, New York, **1978**, pp. 69–136.

Iversen, L. L. Biochemical psychopharmacology of GABA. In, *Psychopharmacology—A Generation of Progress*. (Lipton, M. A.; DiMascio, A.; and Killam, K. F.; eds.) Raven Press, New York, **1978**, pp. 25–38.

———. Nonopioid neuropeptides in mammalian CNS. *Annu. Rev. Pharmacol. Toxicol.*, **1983**, *23*, 1–27.

Iversen, S. D., and Iversen, L. L. *Behavioral Pharmacology*, 2nd ed. Oxford University Press, New York, **1979**.

Johnston, G. A. R. Neuropharmacology of amino acid inhibitory transmitters. *Annu. Rev. Pharmacol. Toxicol.*, **1978**, *18*, 269–289.

Kelly, J. S., and Beart, P. M. Amino acid receptors in CNS. II. GABA in supraspinal regions. In, *Handbook of Psychopharmacology*, Sect. I, Vol. 4. (Iversen, L. L.; Iversen, S. D.; and Snyder, S. H.; eds.) Plenum Press, New York, **1975**, pp. 129–209.

Kerlavage, A. R.; Frase, C. M.; and Venter, J. C. Muscarinic cholinergic receptor structure: molecular biological support for subtypes. *Trends Pharmacol. Sci.*, **1987**, *8*, 426–429.

Koob, G. F., and Bloom, F. E. Cellular and molecular mechanisms of drug dependence. *Science*, **1988**, *242*, 715–723.

Krieger, D. T. Brain peptides: what, where, and why? *Science*, **1983**, *222*, 975–985.

Krieger, D. T.; Brownstein, M. J.; and Martin, J. B. (eds.). *Brain Peptides*. John Wiley & Sons, Inc., New York, **1983**.

Kuhar, M. J. Central cholinergic pathways: physiologic and pharmacologic aspects. In, *Psychopharmacology—A Generation of Progress*. (Lipton, M. A.; DiMascio, A.; and Killam, K. F.; eds.) Raven Press, New York, **1978**, pp. 199–204.

Llinas, R.R. The intrinsic electrophysiological properties of mammalian neurons: insights into central nervous system function. *Science*, **1988**, *242*, 1654–1664.

Lynch, G., and Schubert, P. The use of *in vitro* brain slices for multidisciplinary studies of synaptic function. *Annu. Rev. Neurosci.*, **1980**, *3*, 1–22.

Meldrum, B. Excitatory amino acid receptors and selective antagonists. In, *ISI Atlas of Science: Pharmacology*, Vol. 1. Institute for Scientific Information, Philadelphia, **1987**, pp. 228–232.

Miller, R. J. Multiple Ca channels and neuronal function. *Science*, **1987**, *235*, 46–52.

Mountcastle, V. B., and Edelman, G. M. An organizing principle for cerebral function: the unit module and the distributed system. In, *The Mindful Brain*. (Edelman, G. M., and Mountcastle, V. B., eds.) The MIT Press, Cambridge, MA, **1978**, pp. 7–50.

Nestler, E. J., and Greengard, P. *Protein Phosphorylation in the Nervous System*. John Wiley & Sons, New York, **1984**.

Niall, H. D. The evolution of peptide hormones. *Annu. Rev. Physiol.*, **1982**, 44, 615–624.

Nicoll, R. A. The coupling of neurotransmitter receptors to ion channels in the brain. *Science*, **1988**, *241*, 545–551.

Nicoll, R. A.; Schenker, C.; and Leeman, S. E. Substance P as a transmitter candidate. *Annu. Rev. Neurosci.*, **1980**, *3*, 227–268.

Olsen, R. W. Drug interactions at the GABA receptor–ionophore complex. *Annu. Rev. Pharmacol. Toxicol.*, **1982**, *22*, 245–277.

Palkovits, M. Neuropeptides in the brain. In, *Frontiers in Neuroendocrinology*, Vol. 10. (Martini, L., and Ganong, W. F., eds.) Raven Press, New York, **1988**, pp. 1–44.

Pardridge, W. M. Recent advances in blood-brain barrier transport. *Annu. Rev. Pharmacol. Toxicol.*, **1988**, *28*, 25–39.

Peroutka, S. J. 5-Hydroxytryptamine receptor subtypes. *Annu. Rev. Neurosci.*, **1988**, *11*, 45–60.

Price, G. W., and Bowery, N. G. $GABA_a$ and $GABA_b$ receptor site distribution: an overview. In, *ISI Atlas of Science: Pharmacology*, Vol. 2. Institute for Scientific Information, Philadelphia, **1988**, pp. 136–140.

Rakic, P., and Singer, W. (eds.). *Neurobiology of Neocortex*. John Wiley & Sons, Inc., New York, **1988**.

Rall, T. W. Role of adenosine 3′-5′-monophosphate (cyclic AMP) in actions of catecholamines. *Pharmacol. Rev.*, **1972**, *24*, 399–409.

Robinson, M. B., and Coyle, J. T. Glutamate and related acidic excitatory neurotransmitters: from basic science to clinical application. *FASEB J.*, **1987**, *1*, 446–455.

Rogawski, M. A., and Barker, J. L. *Neurotransmitter Actions in the Vertebrate Nervous System*. Plenum Press, New York, **1985**.

Ruffolo, R. R., Jr., and Nichols, A. J. Drugs with combined α- and β-adrenoceptor blocking properties. In, *ISI Atlas of Science*, Vol. 1. Institute for Scientific Information, Philadelphia, **1987**, pp. 241–245.

Ryall, R. W. Amino acid receptors in CNS. I. GABA and glycine in spinal cord. In, *Handbook of Psychopharmacology*, Sect. I, Vol. 4. (Iversen, L. L.; Iversen, S. D.; and Snyder, S. H.; eds.) Plenum Press, New York, **1975**, pp. 83–128.

Scharrer, B. Neurohumors and neurohormones: definitions and terminology. *J. Neurovisc. Relat.*, **1969**, *9*, Suppl., 1–20.

Schmidt, J. Biochemistry of nicotinic acetylcholine receptors in the vertebrate brain. *Int. Rev. Neurobiol.*, **1988**, *30*, 1–38.

Schwartz, J.-C. Histamine receptors in brain. In, *ISI Atlas of Science: Pharmacology*, Vol. 1. Institute for Scientific Information, Philadelphia, **1988**, pp. 185–189.

Schwartz, J.-C.; Garbarg, M.; and Pollard, H. Histaminergic transmission in the brain. In, *Handbook of Physiology,* Vol. IV, Sect. 1 (Bloom, F. E., ed.) American Physiological Society, Bethesda, Md, **1986,** pp. 257–316.

Seeman, P., and Niznik, H. B. Dopamine D1 receptor pharmacology. In, *ISI Atlas of Science,* Vol. 2. Institute for Scientific Information, Philadelphia, **1988,** pp. 161–170.

Shepherd, G. M. *Neurobiology,* 2nd ed. Oxford University Press, New York, **1988.**

Sigal, I. S.; Dixon, R. A. F.; and Strader, C. D. Molecular biology of adrenergic receptors. In, *ISI Atlas of Science,* Vol. 2. Institute for Scientific Information, Philadelphia, **1988,** pp. 387–391.

Siggins, G. R., and Gruol, D. L. Mechanisms of transmitter action in the vertebrate central nervous system. In, *Handbook of Physiology,* Vol. IV, Sect. 1. (Bloom, F. E., ed.) American Physiological Society, Bethesda, Md, **1986,** pp. 1–114.

Swanson, L. W. Organization of mammalian neuroendocrine system. In, *Handbook of Physiology,* Vol. IV, Sect. 1. (Bloom, F. E., ed.) American Physiological Society, Bethesda, Md, **1986,** pp. 317–364.

Symposium. (Various authors.) Molecular mechanisms in the actions of drugs active in mania and depression. *Neuropharmacology,* **1983,** *22,* 359–446.

Werman, R. Amino acids as central transmitters. In, *Neurotransmitters: Proceedings of the Association for Research in Nervous and Mental Disease,* Vol. 50. (Kopin, I. J., ed.) The Williams & Wilkins Co., Baltimore, **1972,** pp. 147–180.

Wood, J. W. (ed.). *Neurobiology of the Cerebrospinal Fluid.* Plenum Press, New York, **1979.**

Zieglgänsberger, W. Actions of amino acids, amines and neuropeptides on target cells in the mammalian central nervous system. *Prog. Brain Res.,* **1982,** *55,* 297–320.

CHAPTER

13 HISTORY AND PRINCIPLES OF ANESTHESIOLOGY

Sean K. Kennedy and David E. Longnecker

I. History of Surgical Anesthesia

Anesthesia before 1846. Surgical procedures were uncommon before 1846. Understanding of the pathophysiology of disease and of the rationale for its treatment by surgery was rudimentary. Aseptic technique and the prevention of wound infection were almost unknown. In addition, the lack of satisfactory anesthesia was a major deterrent. Because of all these factors few operations were attempted and mortality was frequent. Typically, surgery was of an emergency nature—for example, amputation of a limb for open fracture or drainage of an abscess. Fine dissection and careful technique were not possible in patients for whom relief of pain was inadequate.

Some means of attempting to relieve surgical pain were available and, in fact, had been used since ancient times (Davison, 1965). Drugs like alcohol, hashish, and opium derivatives, taken by mouth, provided some consolation. Physical methods for the production of analgesia, such as packing a limb in ice or making it ischemic with a tourniquet, were occasionally used. Unconsciousness induced by a blow to the head or by strangulation did provide relief from pain, although at a high cost. However, the most common method used to achieve a relatively quiet surgical field was simple restraint of the patient by force. It is no wonder that surgery was looked upon as a last resort.

Although the analgesic properties of both nitrous oxide and diethyl ether had been known to a few for years, the agents were not used for medical purposes (Keys, 1963). Nitrous oxide was synthesized by Priestley in 1776, and both he and Humphry Davy some 20 years later commented upon its anesthetic properties (Faulconer and Keys, 1965). Davy in fact suggested that ". . . it may probably be used with advantage during surgical operations in which no great effusion of blood takes place." Another 20 years passed before Michael Faraday wrote that the inhalation of diethyl ether produced effects similar to those of nitrous oxide. However, except for their inhalation in carnival exhibitions or to produce "highs" at "ether frolics," these drugs were not used in man until the mid-nineteenth century.

Greene (1971) has presented an analysis of the reasons for the introduction of anesthesia in the 1840s. The time was then right, since concern for the well-being of one's fellows, a humanitarian attitude, was more prevalent than it had been in the previous century. "So long as witches were being burned in Salem, anesthesia could not be discovered 20 miles away in Boston." While humanitarian concern extended to the relief of pain, chemistry and medicine had simultaneously advanced to such an extent that a chemically pure drug could be prepared and then used with some degree of safety. There was, too, growth of the inquisitive spirit—a search for improvement of man's lot.

Public Demonstration of Ether Anesthesia. Dentists were instrumental in the introduction of both diethyl ether and nitrous oxide. They, even more than physicians, came into daily contact with persons complaining of pain; often, as a by-product of their work, they produced pain. It was at a stage show that Horace Wells, a dentist, noted that one of the participants, while under the influence of nitrous oxide, injured himself yet felt no pain. The next day Wells, while breathing nitrous oxide, had one of his own teeth extracted, painlessly, by a colleague. Shortly thereafter, in 1845, Wells attempted to demonstrate his discovery at the Massachusetts General Hospital in Boston. Unfortunately the patient cried out during the operation, and the demonstration was deemed a failure.

William T. G. Morton, a Boston dentist (and medical student), was familiar with the use of nitrous oxide from a previous association with Horace Wells. Morton learned of ether's anesthetic effects, thought it more promising, and practiced with it on animals and then on himself. Finally, he asked permission to demonstrate the drug's use, publicly, as a surgical anesthetic.

The story of this classical demonstration in 1846 has been retold countless times. The operating room ("ether dome") at the Massachusetts General Hospital remains as a memorial to the first public demonstration of surgical anesthesia. In the gallery of this room skeptical spectators gathered, for the news had spread that a second-year medical student had developed a method for abolishing surgical pain. The patient, Gilbert Abbott, was brought in and Dr. Warren, the surgeon, waited in formal morning clothes. Operating gowns, masks, gloves, surgical asepsis, and the bacterial origin of infection were entirely unknown at that time. Everyone was ready and waiting, including the strong men to hold down the struggling patient, but Morton did not appear. Fifteen minutes passed, and the surgeon, becoming impatient, took his scalpel and turning to the gallery said, "As Dr. Morton has not arrived, I presume he is otherwise engaged." While the audience smiled and the patient cringed, the surgeon turned to make his incision.

Just then Morton entered, his tardiness being due to the necessity for completing an apparatus with which to administer the ether. Warren stepped back, and pointing to the man strapped to the operating table said, "Well, sir, your patient is ready." Surrounded by a silent and unsympathetic audience, Morton went quietly to work. After a few minutes of ether inhalation, the patient was unconscious, whereupon Morton looked up and said, "Dr. Warren, *your* patient is ready." The operation was begun. The patient showed no sign of pain, yet he was alive and breathing. The strong men were not needed. When the operation was completed, Dr. Warren turned to the astonished audience and made the famous statement, "Gentlemen, this is no humbug." Dr. Henry J. Bigelow, an eminent surgeon attending the demonstration, remarked, "I have seen something today that will go around the world."

Following initial disbelief, news of the successful demonstration spread rapidly. Within a month, ether was in use in other cities of the United States and had been given in Great Britain as well. Its use was soon established as legitimate medical therapy.

The lives of those involved in the introduction of surgical anesthesia did not have so salubrious an outcome. Morton initially tried to patent the use of ether to produce anesthesia and, when this failed, patented instead his device for its administration. Considerable wrangling ensued as to who was the legitimate discoverer of anesthesia. Never receiving what he felt to be his due, Morton died an embittered man.

Charles Jackson, Morton's chemistry teacher at Harvard, also claimed priority in the discovery; it was he who had suggested that Morton use pure sulfuric ether. Jackson became insane, a fate that also befell Horace Wells, the man who had failed in the public demonstration of nitrous oxide anesthesia. Crawford Long, a physician in rural Georgia, had used ether anesthesia since 1842 but neglected to publish his experiences. He survived and prospered, but Morton rightfully receives credit for the introduction of surgical anesthesia. A monument erected by the citizens of Boston over the grave of Dr. Morton in Mt. Auburn Cemetery near Boston bears the following inscription, written by Dr. Jacob Bigelow:

WILLIAM T. G. MORTON
Inventor and Revealer of Anaesthetic Inhalation.
Before Whom, in All Time, Surgery Was Agony.
By Whom Pain in Surgery Was Averted and Annulled.
Since Whom Science Has Control of Pain.

Anesthesia after 1846. Although it is rarely used today, ether was the ideal "first" anesthetic. Chemically, it is readily made in pure form. It is relatively easy to administer, since it is a liquid at room temperature but is readily vaporized. Ether is potent, unlike nitrous oxide, and thus a few volumes percent can produce anesthesia without diluting the oxygen in room air to hypoxic levels. It supports both respiration and circulation, crucial properties at a time when human physiology was not understood well enough for assisted respiration and circulation to be possible. And ether is not toxic to vital organs.

The next anesthetic to receive wide use was chloroform. Introduced by the Scottish obstetrician James Simpson in 1847, it became quite popular, perhaps because of its more pleasant odor. Other than this and its nonflammability, there was little to recommend it (Sykes, 1960). The drug is a hepatotoxin and a severe cardiovascular depressant. Despite the relatively high incidence of intraoperative and postoperative death associated with the use of chloroform, it was championed, especially in Great Britain, for nearly 100 years (Duncum, 1947). Because of the danger and difficulty in administering chloroform, distinguished British physicians became interested in anesthetics and their administration, a trend that was not evident in the United States until 100 years later.

The course of anesthesiology in the United States, after the initial burst of enthusiasm, was one of slow change and limited progress (Vandam, 1973). Furthermore, despite the relative comfort that the surgical patient experienced, the amount and scope of surgery increased only slightly during the 1840s and 1850s (Greene, 1979). The incidence of mortality was little changed, for postoperative infection was still a serious problem. Only with the introduction of aseptic techniques 20 years after the discovery of anesthesia did surgery come into its own.

Other Anesthetic Agents. Nitrous oxide fell into disuse after the apparent failure in Boston in 1845. It was reintroduced in 1863 into American dental and surgical practice, largely through the efforts of a showman, entrepreneur, and partially trained physician, Gardner Q. Colton. In 1868, the administration of nitrous oxide with oxygen was described by Edmond Andrews, a Chicago surgeon, and soon thereafter the two gases became available in steel cylinders, greatly increasing their practicality (Thomas, 1975). Nitrous oxide is still widely used today.

The anesthetic properties of cyclopropane were accidentally discovered in 1929 when chemists were analyzing impurities in an isomer, propylene (Lucas, 1961). After extensive clinical trial at the University of Wisconsin, the drug was introduced into practice; cyclopropane was perhaps the most widely used general anesthetic for the next 30 years. However, with the increasing risk of explosion in the operating room brought about by the use of electronic equipment, the need for a safe, nonflammable anesthetic increased, and several groups pursued the search. Efforts by the British Research Council and by chemists at Imperial Chemical Industries were rewarded by the development of halothane, a nonflammable anesthetic that was introduced into clinical practice in 1956; it revolutionized inhalational anesthesia. Most of the newer agents, which are halogenated hydrocarbons and ethers, are modeled after halothane.

The skeletal muscle relaxants (neuromuscular blocking agents) were also discovered and their pharmacological properties demonstrated long before their introduction into clinical practice (McIntyre, 1959; Bennett, 1967). Curare, in crude form, had long been used by South American Indians as a poison on their arrow tips (*see* Chapter 9). Its first clinical use was in spastic disorders, where it could decrease muscle tone without compromising respiration excessively. It was then used to modify the violent muscle contractions associated with convulsive therapy of psychiatric disorders. Finally, in the 1940s, anesthesiologists used curare to provide the muscular relaxation that previously could be obtained only with deep levels of general anesthesia. Over the next half-dozen years several synthetic substitutes were used clinically. It is difficult to overemphasize the importance of muscle relaxants in anesthetic practice. Their use permits adequate conditions for surgery with light levels of general anesthesia; cardiovascular depression is thus minimized, and the patient awakens promptly when the anesthetic is discontinued.

Although the desirability of an intravenous anesthetic agent must have been apparent to physicians early in the twentieth century, the drugs at hand were few and unsatisfactory. The situation changed dramatically in 1935, when Lundy demonstrated the clinical usefulness of thiopental, a rapidly acting thiobarbiturate. It was originally considered useful as a sole anesthetic agent, but the doses required resulted in serious depression of the circulatory, respiratory, and nervous systems. Thiopental has, however, been enthusiastically accepted as an agent for the rapid induction of general anesthesia.

Various combinations of intravenous drugs from several classes have been used recently as anesthetic agents, usually together with nitrous oxide. The administration of short-acting opioids by constant intravenous infusion (with little or no potent inhalational agent) is an exciting current development in the practice of anesthesia.

II. Principles of the Administration of General Anesthetics

UPTAKE AND DISTRIBUTION OF INHALATIONAL ANESTHETICS

A firm understanding of general anesthesia requires appreciation of the pharmacokinetic properties of drugs that are inhaled. During general anesthesia produced with an inhalational agent, the depth of anesthesia varies directly with the tension of anesthetic agent in the brain, and the rates of induction and recovery depend upon the rate of change of tension in this tissue. The terms *tension* and *partial pressure* are used interchangeably. The tension of anesthetic agent in the brain is always approaching the tension in arterial blood. The factors that determine the tension of anesthetic gas in the arterial blood and in the brain can be considered under four headings: (1) concentration of the anesthetic agent in inspired gas, (2) pulmonary ventilation delivering the anesthetic to the lungs, (3) transfer of the gas from the alveoli to the blood flowing through the lungs, and (4) loss of the agent from the arterial blood to all the tissues of the body.

CONCENTRATION OF THE ANESTHETIC AGENT IN INSPIRED GAS

The tension of an individual gas in a mixture of gases is proportional to its concentration, and one often refers to them interchangeably when speaking of the inspired gases.

When a constant tension of anesthetic gas is inhaled, the tension in arterial blood approaches that of the agent in the inspired mixture, in the manner shown in Figure 13–1 for several different anesthetics. (The tension of the inspired vapor or gas is called the *inspired tension*.) For drugs such as nitrous oxide, the arterial tension reaches 90% of the inspired tension in about 20 minutes. When diethyl ether is administered, the approach to a steady state is much slower, and 90% of the inspired tension would be reached in arterial blood only after many hours. This difference is determined by the physical properties of the two agents (*see* below).

In practice, the inspired tension is rarely constant. An anesthetizing concentration of some agents may irritate the airway of an awake or lightly anesthetized patient, so that the inspired concentration must be increased slowly. In other cases, where the vapor is not irritating, the speed of induction may be increased by giving the inhalational anesthetic in concentrations greater than those ultimately desired. Anesthetic tensions are thus produced in blood and tissues sooner than would be possible if maintenance concentrations were used for induction. As anesthesia proceeds, the inspired concentration of anesthetic is reduced to a level suitable for the maintenance of anesthesia.

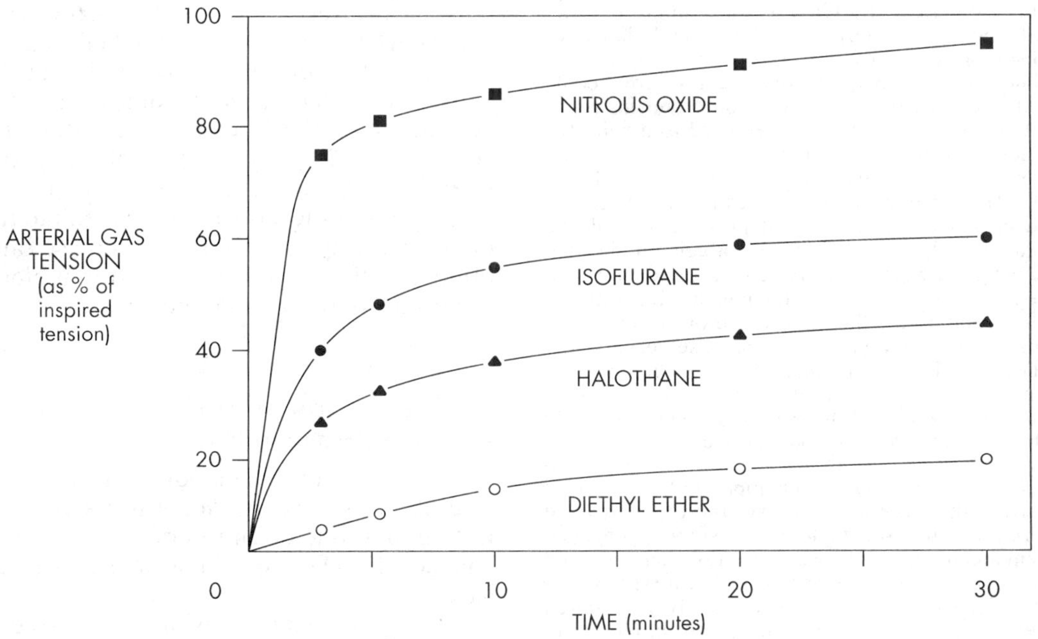

Figure 13–1. *The tensions of anesthetic gases in arterial blood.*

The curves demonstrate how arterial blood tension of the anesthetics increases toward the inspired tension. The increase in partial pressure is rapid for the relatively insoluble gases, and slower for those that are more soluble in blood. The course of events is illustrated here for an idealized situation, where the inhaled concentration remains constant, and pulmonary ventilation and cardiac output and its regional distribution remain constant at normal values. In fact, as anesthesia deepens, alveolar ventilation and cardiac output fall, and distribution of regional circulation and agent solubility are variably altered. These and other factors can result in up to an 11% difference between predicted and actual concentration (Cowles *et al.*, 1972). Alinear analyses have been proposed that take these factors into consideration (Smith *et al.*, 1972; Munson *et al.*, 1973). (From Dripps *et al.*, 1988; courtesy of W. B. Saunders Co.)

PULMONARY VENTILATION

Each inspiration delivers some anesthetic gas to the lung. If the respiratory minute ventilation is great, the tension of the anesthetic in alveoli increases quickly, as does its tension in arterial blood. Thus, the partial pressure of anesthetic gas in blood can be increased by overventilation during induction. Conversely, decreased ventilation (resulting, for instance, from respiratory depression caused by premedication or the anesthetic itself) can lead to a slower rate of change of alveolar and arterial gas tension.

The effects of the rate of respiration to slow or speed induction are transient for gases such as nitrous oxide that have low solubility in blood and tissues and thus equilibrate quickly. However, the volume of respiration exerts a more significant and prolonged effect on the rate of uptake of more soluble and slowly equilibrating drugs, such as diethyl ether. (For further discussion, *see* Eger, 1974.)

Although pulmonary ventilation influences the speed of induction of anesthesia, it does not alter the ultimate depth of anesthesia; this depends on the final tension of the anesthetic in brain, not on the rate of change of that tension.

TRANSFER OF ANESTHETIC GASES FROM ALVEOLI TO BLOOD

The normal alveolar membrane poses no barrier to the transfer of anesthetic gases in both directions. Although the diffusion of anesthetic gases may be normal, certain situations can occur during clinical anesthesia that impede the efficient transfer of gases into blood flowing through the lung. One of these is maldistribution of alveolar ventilation such as may occur in pulmonary emphysema. There is then a lower tension of anesthetic gas in the poorly ventilated alveoli, and thus a lower anesthetic tension in the blood leaving these alveoli. The contribution of this blood to the arterial pool results in slowing of the rate of change of tension of the anesthetic in arterial blood. Any mismatch of ventilation and perfusion in the lung that may occur as a result of a variety of pulmonary disorders produces a difference between alveolar and arterial tensions of anesthetic gases. This, too, results in slowing of the rate of induction of, or recovery from, anesthesia (*see* Eger, 1974).

In the absence of ventilation–perfusion disturbances, three factors determine how rapidly anesthetics pass from the inspired gases to blood. These are (1) the solubility of the agent in blood, (2) the rate of blood flow through the lung, and (3) the partial pressures of the agent in arterial and mixed venous blood.

Solubility of the Agent in Blood. This is usually expressed as the blood:gas partition coefficient, or λ, which represents the ratio of anesthetic concentration in blood to anesthetic concentration in a gas phase when the two are in equilibrium (*i.e.*, when the partial pressure is equal in both phases). The blood:gas partition coefficient is as high as 12 for very soluble agents such as methoxyflurane or diethyl ether, and as low as 0.47 for relatively insoluble anesthetics such as nitrous oxide. The more soluble an anesthetic is in blood, the more of it must be dissolved in blood to raise its partial pressure there appreciably. Therefore, the blood tension of soluble agents rises slowly. The potential reservoir for relatively insoluble gases is small and can be filled more quickly. Therefore, their tension in blood can increase more rapidly.

The blood:gas partition coefficients for the commonly used anesthetic agents are given in Table 14–1 (page 286). The feature of the curves in Figure 13–1 that is largely determined by the blood solubility of the agents is the height of the bend, or "knee," in the uptake curve. The more soluble the agent (*i.e.*, the higher the λ), the lower is the "knee" of the curve, and the slower is the approach of blood tension to that of the inhaled gases.

Rate of Pulmonary Blood Flow. The pulmonary blood flow (*i.e.*, the cardiac output) affects the rate at which anesthetics pass from the alveolar gases into the arterial blood. An increase in pulmonary blood flow slows the initial portion of the arterial tension curve; but the later part of the curve tends to catch up, with the overall result that there is little change in the total time required for complete equilibration. (For the reasons why this should be so, *see* Eger, 1974.)

Partial Pressures in Arterial and Mixed Venous Blood. After taking up anesthetic gas in the lung, the blood circulates to the tissues, and anesthetic gas is transferred from the blood to all tissues of the body. Blood cannot approach equilibrium with inhaled gas tension until this process, which tends to decrease the blood tension, is nearly complete. The mixed venous blood returning to the lungs has more anesthetic gas in it with each passage through the body. After a few minutes of anesthesia the difference between arterial (or alveolar) and mixed venous gas tension decreases continuously. Since the rate of diffusion across the pulmonary membrane is proportional to the difference between alveolar and mixed venous gas tensions, the volume of gas transferred to arterial blood during each minute decreases as time passes. Thus, arterial tension rises more slowly in the final portion of the curves in Figure 13–1.

LOSS OF ANESTHETIC GASES FROM ARTERIAL BLOOD TO TISSUES

When the inhalational agents are delivered by arterial blood to the tissues, the tension rises in tissues to approach that in arterial blood. The rate at which a gas passes into tissues depends on (1) the solubility of the gas in the tissues, (2) the rate at which the gas is delivered to the tissues (*i.e.*, the blood flow to the various areas of the body), and (3) the partial pressures of the gas in arterial blood and tissues. Note that these three factors affecting transfer of the gas from blood to tissue are similar to the three that affect transfer of the anesthetic from lung to blood (*see* above).

Solubility of Gas in Tissues. This is expressed as a tissue:blood partition coefficient, a concept analogous to the blood:gas partition coefficient previously discussed. With most anesthetic agents, the tissue:blood partition is near unity for many of the body's lean tissues; that is, these agents are equally soluble in lean tissue and blood. An anesthetic concentration in blood or tissue is the product of partial pressure and solubility. Thus, the concentration of most anesthetics in lean tissues, such as the gray matter of brain, approaches that in blood as tissue tension builds up toward arterial blood tension. On the other hand, the tissue:blood coefficient for all anesthetics is large for fatty tissues. The concentration of anesthetics in the fatty tissue is much greater than that in blood at the time of equilibrium (when tissue tension equals blood tension).

Tissue solubility is of importance in determining the slope of the final portion, or "tail," of the gas tension curves (*see* Figure 13–1). High tissue solubility, especially high fat solubility, tends to depress the rate of rise of the "tail" of the curve.

Tissue Blood Flow. The greater the blood flow to a tissue, the faster is the delivery of the anesthetic agent, and the more rapidly will its tension and concentration rise in that area. Thus, the concentration of an inert gas in brain approaches that in arterial blood more rapidly when cerebral blood flow is high, and more slowly when cerebral blood flow decreases.

Only tissues with high rates of blood flow will exhibit rapid rises in concentration of anesthetic, and only high-flow areas take up significant amounts of the agent during the early stages of anesthesia. Because blood flow to adipose tissue is very limited, anesthetic gases will be delivered to, and taken up by, fatty tissues so slowly that these tissues contain a significant amount of anesthetic agent only after a considerable time has elapsed.

Partial Pressures in Arterial Blood and Tissues. As the tissues take up anesthetic agent, the partial pressure of the gas in tissues increases toward that of the arterial blood. Since the rate at which gas diffuses from arterial blood to tissues varies with the partial-pressure difference between them, tissue concentration changes rapidly in the early minutes of anesthesia; however, as the tissue tension comes closer to the arterial tension, the tissue uptake of gas slows.

In summary, during the administration of an anesthetic, its tension in blood rises toward that in the inspired gas, at first rapidly, then more slowly. Tissue tensions increase concomitantly, approaching the arterial tension. The partial pressure increases most rapidly in tissues with high rates of blood flow, and lags considerably in areas where blood flow is lower.

ELIMINATION OF INHALATIONAL ANESTHETICS

The major factors that affect rate of elimination of the anesthetics are the same as those that are important in the uptake phase: pulmonary ventilation, blood flow, and solubility in blood and tissue. However, the administration of anesthesia is usually completed before arterial tension has reached inspired tension, and long before tissues of low blood flow or high gas solubility have reached inspired tension. As ventilation with anesthetic-free gas washes out the lungs, the arterial blood tension declines first, followed by that in the tissues. An example of tissue concentrations during 60 minutes of nitrous oxide inhalation and 45 minutes of washout is shown in Figure 13–2 (*see* Cowles *et al.*, 1968). Soon after elimination begins, the tension in lung and blood falls to very low (nonanesthetic) levels. Because of the high blood flow to brain, its tension of anesthetic gas decreases rapidly, accounting for the rapid awakening from anesthesia noted with relatively insoluble agents such as nitrous oxide. The agent persists for a longer time in tissues with lower blood flow such as muscle, and for even longer times in fat,

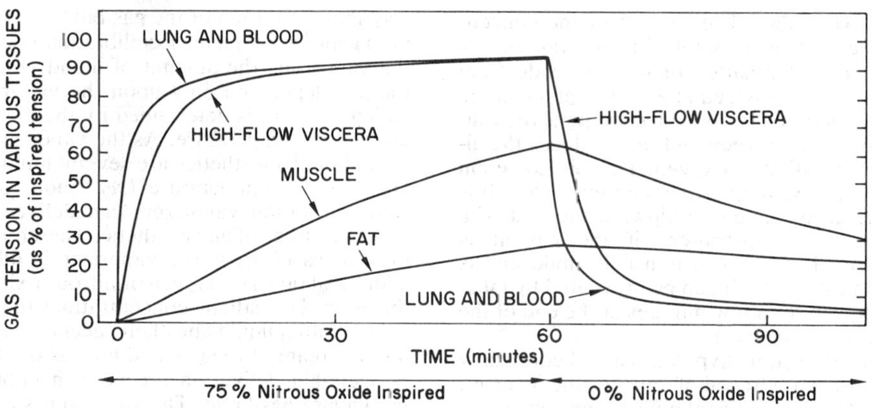

Figure 13–2. *Tissue tensions of an anesthetic gas during uptake and elimination.*

The curves demonstrate how tissue tensions of nitrous oxide approach the inspired tension during a 60-minute anesthetic uptake phase and a subsequent 45-minute elimination phase. The high-blood-flow viscera include brain, heart, and kidney. Liver and intestine have lower blood flows, and their tensions would lie between those of the high-blood-flow viscera and muscle. (Modified from Cowles *et al.*, 1968.)

where blood flow is very low, and from which the agent is therefore very slowly removed.

OTHER ROUTES OF ELIMINATION OF ANESTHETICS

The anesthetic gases are metabolized in the body to a variable extent. With most agents the amount metabolized is small. However, up to 15% of halothane and 70% of methoxyflurane are metabolized to various intermediate compounds, and in some cases to ionized halogens (*see* Chapter 14; *see also* Cohen, 1971). The bulk of metabolism of anesthetics occurs after clinical anesthesia has been discontinued, and is greatest for the more fat-soluble drugs (Berman *et al.*, 1973). The importance of the metabolism of anesthetic agents is not in the termination of their action; rather, metabolites of anesthetics may be responsible for certain of their toxic effects or aftereffects.

Additional small losses of anesthetic gases from the body occur by diffusion across skin and mucous membranes, and by means of urinary excretion of the agent or its breakdown products (Stoelting and Eger, 1969; Cohen, 1971).

MINOR EFFECTS

Minor pharmacokinetic effects distinguish the uptake, distribution, and elimination of gases such as nitrous oxide from those of relatively less solubility, such as nitrogen or helium.

Concentration Effect and Second-Gas Effect. The *concentration effect* may be defined as follows: when higher concentrations of an anesthetic gas are inhaled, arterial tension increases at a slightly greater rate than it would have if a lesser concentration of the anesthetic had been inhaled (*see* Eger, 1974). Consider a patient who is inhaling 75% nitrous oxide and 25% oxygen. Although nitrous oxide is relatively insoluble, when the inhaled concentration is high, the rate of uptake of the gas by blood and tissues may be as great as 1 liter per minute during the early minutes of anesthesia. As this volume of gas disappears from the lung, fresh gases are literally sucked into the lung from the breathing circuit to replace the volume taken up. The rate at which the inspired gas mixture is delivered to the lung is then 1 liter per minute greater than the minute ventilation would have provided without this effect. Therefore, the rate of rise of the arterial tension curve for nitrous oxide is increased during induction of anesthesia. However, if only 10% nitrous oxide is inhaled, the body's uptake of approximately 150 ml per minute results in no significant change in the rate of gas delivery to the lung, and there is little or no acceleration of the arterial tension.

The simultaneous presence of two anesthetic gases in the lung can introduce a closely related phenomenon known as the *second-gas effect*. An illustration may be taken in which 75% nitrous oxide and 1% enflurane are administered together with 24% oxygen. The same disappearance of 1 liter per minute of nitrous oxide from the lung into the body takes place, and the rate at which 1% enflurane is delivered to the alveoli becomes 1 liter per minute greater than the minute ventilation would otherwise have provided. As a result, the arterial tension of enflurane rises a little more rapidly in the presence of nitrous oxide.

Thus, the concentration effect results from the capacity of a rapidly absorbed gas to facilitate its own uptake. In the second-gas effect, a rapidly absorbed gas increases the rate of uptake of a second anesthetic gas (*see* Epstein *et al.*, 1964).

Diffusion Hypoxia. The reverse of the concentration effect can occur after nitrous oxide is discontinued. The elimination of nitrous oxide from blood to lung may proceed at a rate as great as the uptake. The additional gas added to the alveoli dilutes the available oxygen and thus reduces the alveolar concentration of oxygen. This phenomenon is known as *diffusion hypoxia* (*see* Fink, 1955). It is seen in the early minutes following the end of a nitrous oxide administration, if the patient is breathing air. The hypoxia is usually mild and is rarely a clinical threat. It can be prevented by inhalation of oxygen for a few minutes at the end of the anesthetic administration.

Although diffusion hypoxia can theoretically occur after the withdrawal of any anesthetic agent, its magnitude is insignificant unless high concentrations of a relatively soluble agent such as nitrous oxide have been inhaled for some time. Under these circumstances a considerable volume of inert gas has been dissolved in the body (up to 30 liters), and much of it is eliminated through the lungs in the first few minutes after its administration is discontinued. When lower concentrations of an agent (*e.g.*, 2% halothane) are inhaled, even after a long time only a few liters will have been taken up in the body. When administration is discontinued, the elimination of 100 ml per minute or less of halothane is not sufficient to dilute the alveolar oxygen to hypoxic levels.

Intertissue Diffusion. During the approach to equilibrium, the gas being inhaled may be present at different partial pressures in adjacent tissues, the partial pressure being higher in the areas with greater flow and in those where the gas is less soluble. The anesthetic will diffuse into the areas where its tension is lower. The rates of diffusion are such that gas tensions are not much affected in tissues with high blood flow and areas where the gas is relatively insoluble. However, tissue concentrations can be significantly changed by diffusion in areas where flow rates are low and gas solubility is high, as in adipose tissue (*see* Eger, 1973).

ADMINISTRATION OF INHALATIONAL ANESTHETICS

ANESTHETIC MACHINES

With these devices, the anesthesiologist is able to deliver measured quantities of anesthetic gases and oxygen through accurate flowmeters, and with the use of special vaporizers it is possible to add the vapor of volatile anesthetic liquids to the gas stream. The mixture of oxygen and anesthetic agents is then delivered to a breathing circuit for administration by inhalation.

Vaporizers. Liquid anesthetics may be vaporized by a gas stream that passes over the surface of the liquid or past a wick saturated with the liquid. A gas may also be passed through the liquid, as in "saturation-type" vaporizers. In these devices, gas bubbles pass through a liquid anesthetic in such a way that saturation of the gas bubbles with the liquid agent is complete. Equilibration occurs within the vaporizer, the amount of liquid volatilized by the gas depending only upon the vapor pressure, which, in turn, is determined by the particular liquid and its temperature. As the vapor pressures of many liquid anesthetics are several hundred mm of Hg at room temperature (*see* Table 14–1, page 286), saturation vaporizers can deliver excessive concentrations of an anesthetic. Therefore, the outflow of gases from the vaporizer is diluted with additional flows of oxygen or nitrous oxide to attain the desired anesthetic concentrations to be inhaled.

Most often liquid anesthetic agents are vaporized into a stream of oxygen and nitrous oxide by a vaporizer that delivers a precise concentration of a particular anesthetic. The vaporizer is constructed so that anesthetic concentration is accurately maintained over a range of gas flows and ambient temperatures.

Breathing Circuits. The gases and vapors are delivered into a system of wide-bore tubes with valves, a distensible bag that provides a reservoir for the gases, and a method for elimination of expired carbon dioxide. Gases are administered to the patient by means of a face mask or endotracheal tube. Two types of gas delivery systems are illustrated in Figure 13–3.

Low-Flow System (Circle System). Unidirectional valves near the connection of the circuit to the patient ensure that gases circulate in one direction around the circle. The exhaled carbon dioxide is absorbed chemically by a material such as soda lime. This system permits rebreathing of the exhaled gases, and only small amounts of fresh gas need be added through the flowmeters and vaporizer to replace the oxygen and the anesthetic gases taken up by the patient. If larger amounts of fresh gas are added, the excess is eliminated through the one-way pop-off valve. A distensible bag provides a reservoir of gas from which the patient can inhale. The bag partially empties during inhalation and refills during exhalation. The bag also provides a means for the assistance or control of respiration by the anesthesiologist, who can compress the bag and thus force gas into the patient's lungs. When pressure on the bag is released, the lungs empty and the bag refills.

Closed-Circuit Anesthesia. When the pop-off valve is closed and the gas flows are reduced to equal the amounts needed to replace uptake, the closed system is in steady state; the breathing bag empties and refills during the respiratory cycle, always to the same volumes. This technique is known as closed-circuit anesthesia, and is the most economical way to deliver inhalational agents. It minimizes losses of heat and water from the lungs; however, it requires careful attention to gas flows and the delivery of oxygen.

High-Flow System. The fresh gas inflow in this system moves to and fro as the patient inhales gases from the bag and exhales. Because the rate of gas inflow exceeds the amount of oxygen used and anesthetic taken up, the excess gas escapes

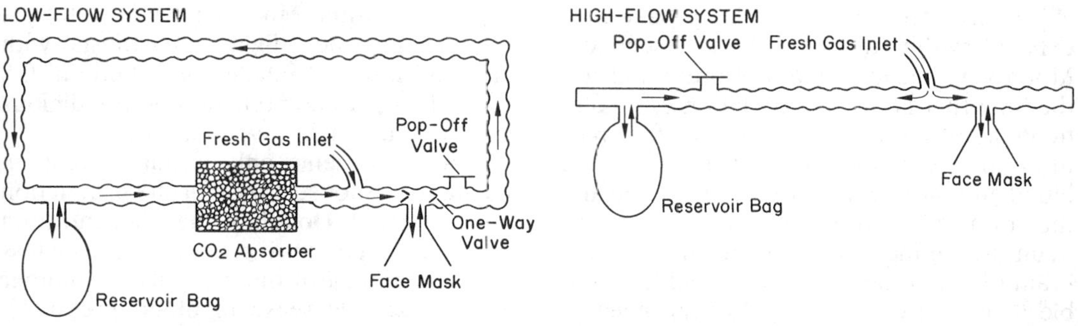

Figure 13–3. *Systems used for delivering inhalational anesthetics.*

Two breathing circuits are shown; they are made up of similar components arranged in slightly different ways. In the low-flow system, gas flow is unidirectional around the circle, and exhaled carbon dioxide is absorbed chemically. In the high-flow system, the movement of gases is bidirectional. As long as the inflow of fresh gas is approximately as great as the respiratory minute volume, carbon dioxide is diluted and washed out via the pop-off valve.

through the one-way pop-off valve, carrying the exhaled carbon dioxide with it.

Information on Exact Concentrations. With accurate flowmeters for gases and a dependable vaporizer for liquids, the anesthesiologist can determine the concentrations of anesthetics and oxygen delivered to the breathing circuit. However, rebreathing occurs in low-flow systems, and the gas mixture inhaled by the patient is not the same as that delivered to the breathing circuit. Elimination of nitrogen from the patient dilutes the gases in the system; humidification of the gases in the system lowers their concentrations somewhat; oxygen is lost from the system as the patient uses it for metabolic requirements; and anesthetic gases are taken up by the patient at a variable rate. Simultaneously, small amounts of oxygen and anesthetic must be added to the circuit. It is apparent that in a low-flow system, the inhaled gases are a mixture with a composition that is difficult to estimate. As the flow rates increase, the characteristics of the system change, and the inhaled gas concentrations approach the concentrations of fresh gases being delivered from the flowmeters and the vaporizer. Nitrous oxide is most frequently delivered in high-flow systems; the anesthesiologist is then assured of at least 20% inhaled oxygen and very nearly 80% inhaled concentration of this rather weak anesthetic gas.

Recently introduced techniques, such as mass spectroscopy, permit accurate and continuous measurement of the concentrations of inhaled and exhaled gases. This technique eliminates much of the uncertainty about delivery of anesthetics and allows accurate estimates of ventilation (P_{CO_2}) and depth of anesthesia from measurements of the composition of the exhaled gases.

Gas, Heat, and Water Exchange in Anesthesia Systems. Three liters of nitrogen may be eliminated from the lung and from tissues in the first hour of anesthesia if a nitrous oxide–oxygen mixture is inspired. This nitrogen must be exhausted from the breathing circuit if high concentrations of both oxygen and nitrous oxide are desired. Unlike carbon dioxide, nitrogen cannot be absorbed, but it can be eliminated by dilution and venting through a pop-off valve.

Water vapor and the heat to vaporize water are provided under normal conditions by the nasal turbinates. However, during anesthesia, the patient inspires dry gases through oropharyngeal or endotracheal tubes that bypass the nasal turbinates; cooling and drying of the tracheobronchial mucosa thus occur. Whereas the heat and water loss may be tolerable in a normal patient for a short operation, the small, the elderly, and those with large surfaces exposed by surgery benefit from the conservation of water and heat. This may be provided by the use of low-flow systems or by warming and humidifying inspired gases. Such measures are often undertaken in pediatric anesthesia.

DOSAGE AND POTENCY OF GENERAL ANESTHETICS

General anesthetics are among the most dangerous drugs approved for general use, in that the margin of safety in their use is small. Therapeutic indices range from about two to four. That is, the dose that produces circulatory failure may be only two to four times that which produces adequate anesthesia (Wolfson *et al.*, 1978). Thus, accurate methods are required for choosing the dose of an anesthetic and for evaluating the depth of anesthesia.

When a tablet is swallowed or a solution injected into a muscle, the dose is described in terms of the mass of drug that is administered. However, when a drug is inhaled as a gas or vapor, only a relatively small amount is actually absorbed; a very large fraction is exhaled within the next 1 or 2 seconds. Moreover, because it is the brain and not the lung that is the site of action of inhalational anesthetics, the agent must first partition between the alveolar gas and the blood and then again between the blood and the brain before exerting its action. It is difficult to define the concentration in the brain of experimental animals and impossible to measure it in man. Yet the need to specify a dose to permit the administration of general anesthesia is inescapable. Anesthesiologists have therefore accepted a measure of potency of inhalational agents known as MAC, which stands for *minimum alveolar concentration* of anesthetic at 1 atmosphere that produces immobility in 50% of patients or animals exposed to a noxious stimulus (Eger *et al.,* 1965). The rationale for using the alveolar concentration rather than that in the brain to measure a dose is based on the following considerations: concentration in the lung can be easily, frequently, and accurately measured; near equilibrium, the partial pressure of anesthetic in the lung and the partial pressure in the brain are almost equal; and relatively high blood flow to the brain results in rapid equilibration between blood and brain.

Among the characteristics of MAC that recommend it as a measure of anesthetic dose and potency are that MAC is invariant with a variety of noxious stimuli; that variability within individuals of a given species is small; that sex, height, weight, and duration of anesthesia do not alter MAC, although temperature and age do (Stevens *et al.,* 1975; Lerman *et al.,* 1983); and, finally, that doses of anesthetic agents appear to be additive (*i.e.,* one half of a MAC of one drug plus one half of a MAC of another drug will cause immobility following noxious stimulation in 50% of individuals tested) (Cullen *et al.,* 1969; Millar *et al.,* 1969).

The slopes of the dose–response curves for inhalational anesthetics are steep. Thus, although only 50% of individuals may fail to respond to stimulation at 1.0 MAC, 99% are unresponsive at a dose of 1.3 MAC (*see* de Jong and Eger, 1975). The latter concentration is, therefore, the surgically useful dose of each anesthetic if it is used without supplementation. Modern anesthesiologists tend to provide "light" anesthesia with concentrations of inhaled anesthetic of 0.8 to 1.2 MAC, in combination with judicious use of adjuvant intravenous drugs.

MAC represents only a single point on the dose–response curve for the production of anesthesia. Doubling the concentration of an anesthetic may produce more or less than a doubling of the intensity of another effect (*e.g.,* decrease in blood pressure), depending on the slope of the dose–response curve of that drug for that effect.

DEPTH OF ANESTHESIA

SIGNS AND STAGES OF ANESTHESIA

Between 1847 and 1858, John Snow described certain signs that helped him determine the depth of anesthesia in patients receiving chloroform or ether. These included the onset of rhythmic, automatic breathing and the loss of winking in response to touching the conjunctiva as surgical anesthesia was reached, and the gradual disappearance of intercostal muscle activity and cessation of eyeball movement as anesthesia was deepened. In 1920, Guedel, using these and other signs, outlined four stages of general anesthesia, dividing the third stage—surgical anesthesia—into four planes. Guedel's observations related primarily to ether, a substance with such great solubility in blood that the onset and progressive deepening of anesthesia were predictably slow. Opportunity was thus afforded the anesthesiologist to watch the unfolding of a series of changes involving respiration, muscle tone, and reflex activity. The somewhat arbitrary division is as follows: I—stage of analgesia; II—stage of delirium; III—stage of surgical anesthesia; IV—stage of medullary depression.

Although the classical signs and stages of anesthesia are partly recognizable during administration of many general anesthetics, they are often obscured by modern anesthetic techniques. Furthermore, Cullen and coworkers (1972) demonstrated that no single one of the major signs described by Guedel correlated satisfactorily with the measured alveolar concentrations of anesthetic during prolonged stable states. Thus, only the term "stage two" remains in common use today, signifying a state of delirium in the partially anesthetized patient.

A PRACTICAL APPROACH TO EVALUATING DEPTH OF ANESTHESIA

The following approach is useful for almost any general anesthetic. If the eyelids blink when the eyelashes are stroked, if the patient is swallowing, if respiration is irregular in rate and depth, and if one knows that not a great deal of anesthetic has been administered, surgical anesthesia is *not* present.

Loss of the eyelash reflex and the development of rhythmic respiration indicate the beginning of surgical anesthesia. If the skin incision is made at once, indications of "light" anesthesia may include an increase in respiratory rate or arterial blood pressure. Jaw muscles may become tight, and even if the mouth can be opened an attempt to insert an oral airway may stimulate gagging, coughing, vomiting, or laryngospasm.

As anesthesia deepens, these responses are reduced or abolished. With most of the general anesthetics, an increase in depth brings progressive reduction in respiratory tidal volume. Tracheal tug may become evident as accessory muscles of respiration come into play, diaphragmatic activity becomes jerky, and the lower chest is pulled in as the diaphragm descends. When the potent halogenated agents are used, arterial blood pressure tends to vary directly with the depth of anesthesia, and hypotension can be used as an imprecise index of dosage. Suggestions that anesthesia is becoming "lighter" include the formation of tears, apnea following peritoneal stimulation, increasing resistance to inflation of the lungs, and the return of the indices of light anesthesia listed above.

Severe respiratory depression, apnea, marked hypotension, or asystole must be regarded as evidence of deep anesthesia unless other causes—for example, the effect of muscle relaxants, blood loss, and hypoxia, or the influence of vagal reflexes—can explain these findings.

Thus, experience, combined with constant observation of the patient's responses to anesthetic drugs and to stimuli, permit estimation of depth of anesthesia. However, measurement of end-tidal concentrations of anesthetics is a more precise indicator of depth of anesthesia when inhalational agents are used.

The Electroencephalogram (EEG) as an Index of Depth of General Anesthesia. A number of workers have classified the EEG changes produced by the inhalational agents and barbiturates. However, use of the EEG as the sole index of anesthetic depth is unreliable, since many factors influence the activity of the central nervous system (CNS). Hypoxia, hypocarbia, hypoglycemia, hypothermia, and inadequate cerebral circulation can markedly alter the EEG at a time when anesthetic concentration remains constant. Furthermore, although EEG changes produced by a given agent may correlate with brain concentration, they also vary widely when different anesthetics are compared. (For a detailed examination of this subject, the reader should consult Clark and Rosner, 1973; Rosner and Clark, 1973; McDowall, 1976; Levy *et al.*, 1980.) Another approach is to use the evoked response to auditory, visual, or peripheral electrical stimulation. Averages of 100 or more such stimulations yield a relatively reproducible, multiphasic wave response; the characteristics of this response vary with depth of anesthesia (*see* Grundy, 1983; Thornton *et al.*, 1983).

PREANESTHETIC MEDICATION

Preanesthetic medication should decrease anxiety without producing excessive drowsiness, provide amnesia for the perioperative period while maintaining cooperation prior to loss of consciousness, and relieve preoperative pain if it is present. Secondary goals include reduction in the requirement for an inhalational anesthetic agent, minimization of undesirable side effects associated with some of these agents (notably salivation, bradycardia, coughing, and postanesthetic vomiting), and reduction of the volume and acidity of gastric contents. In addition, adequate premedication may help reduce stress responses in the perioperative period (Walsh *et al.*, 1987). The accomplishment of these multiple purposes usually requires the concomitant use of two or three drugs. The most commonly employed classes include sedative–hypnotics, antianxiety agents, opioids, antiemetics, histamine (H_2) antagonists, gastrokinetic agents, and anticholinergics. An informative, supportive preoperative visit by the anesthesiologist has long been known to be as effective as a traditional sedative–hypnotic drug (Egbert *et al.*, 1963). The wide variety of preanesthetic regimens in current use testifies to the lack of agreement on optimal combinations (*see* Moyers, 1989).

SEDATIVE–HYPNOTICS AND ANTIANXIETY AGENTS

Although drowsiness does not imply loss of all anxiety, most drugs in use for preanesthetic medication have some of both effects.

Benzodiazepines. These drugs have been used extensively for preanesthetic medication, and they have become even more useful since the development of agents with shorter durations of action and a greater propensity to cause amnesia. Despite the relative lack of respiratory and cardiac depression caused by benzodiazepines (*see* Chapter 17), there have been reports of respiratory arrest, particularly in the elderly. These drugs are not analgesics, and they rarely cause nausea or vomiting. Benzodiazepines can raise the threshold for CNS toxicity of local anesthetics (de Jong and Heavner, 1973). Diazepam has been most widely used in doses of 5 to 10 mg; it is active orally. However, diazepam is poorly soluble in water, and its absorption is unreliable after parenteral administration. Furthermore, the solvent used in parenteral preparations causes pain and phlebitis. The drug has little effect on respiration at usual doses, and it does not potentiate the respiratory depression produced by opioids (Aukburg *et al.,* 1976). Lorazepam may be given orally or parenterally, and it produces amnesia in most patients. The drug often causes prolonged sedation. The usual intramuscular dose is 0.05 mg/kg (to a maximum of 4 mg), given at least 2 hours prior to the operative procedure. Midazolam has become popular because of its combination of water solubility, rapid onset and short duration of action, and reliability. In usual doses for preanesthetic medication (0.07 mg/kg, given intramuscularly) it produces amnesia with few side effects (Fragen *et al.,* 1983). Mental function returns to normal within 4 hours (Reves *et al.,* 1985), making it a popular choice for ambulatory surgery and during regional anesthesia. Lorazepam and midazolam are less likely to produce cumulative effects than is diazepam.

Barbiturates. Pentobarbital and secobarbital are used occasionally to provide sedation and relieve apprehension before surgery. However, barbiturates may cause disorientation rather than sedation when the patient is in pain. Pentobarbital or secobarbital may be administered orally or intramuscularly to adults in doses of 100 to 200 mg, and to children in doses of 2 to 5 mg/kg (to a maximum of 100 mg). These drugs have a minimal depressant action on respiration and circulation and rarely produce nausea or vomiting. Tolerance to barbiturates is observed in patients who have been taking various classes of drugs, including other barbiturates and alcohol.

Antihistamines. Sedation is a variable side effect of these drugs. In the past, hydroxyzine, 25 to 100 mg intramuscularly, was widely used for preanesthetic medication; benzodiazepines are now used more commonly. Hydroxyzine produces minimal circulatory and respiratory depression and does not prolong anesthesia. Diphenhydramine (10 to 50 mg intravenously or intramuscularly) is a mild sedative as well as an H_1 blocker, and this combination of effects may be desirable in certain patients.

Phenothiazines. Phenothiazines have sedative, antiarrhythmic, antihistaminic, and antiemetic properties. They are occasionally combined in reduced dosage with a barbiturate or an opioid. Prolongation of postanesthetic sleep and greater respiratory depression are probable, and decrease in blood pressure is possible. The value of phenothiazines in premedication must be carefully weighed against their side effects. Phenothiazines used in premedication include promethazine and propiomazine, both in intramuscular doses of 20 to 40 mg.

Butyrophenones. The usual dose for premedication is 1.25 to 5 mg of droperidol. Antiemetic activity is present at low doses, and reasonable cardiovascular stability is maintained, despite slight α-adrenergic blocking activity. Both restlessness and extrapyramidal dyskinesia can occur, especially in children; these effects may be countered by the administration of atropine. When given alone, droperidol may produce dysphoria in an outwardly calm patient. Thus, it is generally given with a sedative or an opioid. Butyrophenones potentiate the actions of opioids.

OPIOIDS

Surgical pain is often severe, and even minor preoperative pain is deleterious to smooth induction of anesthesia. Opioids are thus frequently used for preanesthetic medication. The major difference among opioids that governs the choice for premedication is their duration of activity (*see* Chapter 21).

Morphine in doses of 8 to 12 mg intramuscularly is frequently used prior to operation, especially if pain is present. Its duration of action is such that it also minimizes the incidence of restlessness or excitation during emergence from general anesthesia. Preanesthetic medication with an opioid reduces by 10 to 20% the amount of general anesthetic required.

Unfortunately, morphine may have undesirable side effects. It often prolongs the awakening from general anesthesia, since its clinical effects persist for 4 to 6 hours. Its stimulant effect on smooth muscle may cause spasm of the bile duct or of the ureters. Wheezing may develop in patients with asthma. Constipation and urinary retention may be annoying. Nausea and vomiting are not uncommon. A vagotonic effect may be evidenced by bradycardia. Hypotension can occur after the use of morphine or other opioid analgesics. The respiratory depressant action of morphine may increase intracranial pressure as a result of retention of carbon dioxide and subsequent cerebral vasodilatation.

Meperidine is used occasionally in doses of 50 to 100 mg intramuscularly. It shares all the disadvantages of morphine, including depression of blood pressure and respiration.

Fentanyl is useful in some cases because of its short duration of action—1 to 2 hours. The usual dose is 0.05 to 0.10 mg intramuscularly.

ANTIEMETICS

The sequelae of the prophylactic administration of antiemetics (notably hypotension) are often as disturbing and frequent as emetic episodes. However, if a drug is otherwise useful in a given instance, its antiemetic effect is an additional welcome benefit. Droperidol and hydroxyzine are sometimes useful for their antiemetic effects. Benzquinamide is a mild vasopressor and hence does not share some of the drawbacks of other antiemetics.

ANTICHOLINERGIC DRUGS

The excessive respiratory tract secretions seen during administration of ether indicated the need for use of an anticholinergic drug prior to anesthesia. With the advent of less irritating anesthetic agents, secretions have become less of a problem. The emphasis has now shifted to the desire to counteract the vagal effects that may occur during anesthesia and surgery. If needed, vagal blockade is best accomplished immediately prior to the expected stimulus, thus sparing the patient a very dry mouth during the preoperative period.

Atropine produces oral dryness and blurred vision within 10 to 15 minutes after intramuscular injection of the standard 0.4- to 0.6-mg dose. The vagal blocking action of such an amount may not be sufficient to prevent parasympathetically induced cardiovascular effects such as hypotension and bradycardia that result from increase in ocular pressure, visceral traction, manipulation of the carotid sinus, or injection of multiple doses of succinylcholine. However, the intravenous injection of an additional dose of atropine often promptly restores the cardiac rate and the arterial pressure toward normal. Atropine is not contraindicated in patients with glaucoma. Increased intraocular pressure does not result from the doses recommended. Its use in febrile patients may be unwise because it depresses heat loss via sweating.

Scopolamine is usually given intramuscularly, in a dose of 0.4 to 0.6 mg. It is superior to atropine as an antisialogogue but is less effective in preventing reflex bradycardia during general anesthesia, particularly in children. The sedative effect of scopolamine is more marked than that of atropine; occasionally, however, patients become restless or disoriented after scopolamine, and the incidence of emergence excitement appears greater after its administration.

Glycopyrrolate, a longer-acting quaternary amine, produces less sedation than scopolamine and is a more effective antisialogogue than atropine. It is less likely to cause significant tachycardia than atropine, while it simultaneously blocks bradyarrhythmias more effectively (Odura, 1975; Myer and Tomeldan, 1979). Intraoperatively it is given intravenously in doses of 0.1 mg (for adults), which may be repeated at intervals of 2 to 3 minutes.

DRUGS THAT REDUCE THE ACIDITY AND VOLUME OF GASTRIC CONTENTS

The induction of general anesthesia eliminates the patient's ability to protect the airway should regurgitation of gastric contents occur. Decreasing the volume of gastric contents reduces the likelihood of regurgitation, and increasing their pH above 2.5 reduces damage to the lungs should aspiration occur.

H_2-Receptor Antagonists. Cimetidine and ranitidine selectively block H_2 receptors for histamine, decreasing gastric acid secretion, particularly when given in divided doses starting the night before surgery. There is no reliable effect on the volume of gastric fluid. Ranitidine causes fewer cardiovascular and CNS side effects than does cimetidine.

Antacids. Particulate antacids are generally more effective in raising gastric pH than soluble agents; however, they may cause more damage to the lungs should aspiration occur. Thus, nonparticulate antacids such as sodium citrate are generally preferred, even though they tend to increase the volume of gastric contents.

Gastrokinetic Agents. Metoclopramide is a dopaminergic antagonist that promotes gastrointestinal motility and pyloric relaxation, thus speeding gastric emptying (*see* Chapter 38). It does not affect acid secretion or gastric pH. Sodium citrate or anticholinergic agents may interfere with the action of metoclopramide. The combination of metoclopramide and an H_2-receptor antagonist appears to provide the best protection against pulmonary aspiration.

MOLECULAR MECHANISM OF ACTION OF GENERAL ANESTHETICS

A myriad of molecular species are capable of producing anesthesia, including inert gases (*e.g.*, xenon), simple inorganic and organic compounds (*e.g.*, nitrous oxide and chloroform), and more complex organic molecules (*e.g.*, halogenated alkanes and ethers). Yet there remains no satisfactory explanation as to how these drugs produce general anesthesia.

Most theories of anesthetic action are based on the physicochemical characteristics of the anesthetic drugs. These proposals relate closely to the correlation between the potency of an anesthetic agent and the solubility of the drug in oil, first demonstrated by Meyer (1899, 1901) and Overton (1901). The precise nature of this correlation is demonstrated in Figure 13–4, where the MAC value for a number of anesthetics is plotted versus the olive oil:gas partition coefficient at 37° C. Interpretation of this fundamental result is thought to be crucial to the understanding of the action of anesthetics.

The physical force that promotes the high relative solubility of molecules in oil compared with water is the so-called hydrophobic interaction. Molecules such as potent anesthetics that cannot form a significant number of hydrogen bonds and that are nonpolar distribute to sites in which they are removed from the aqueous environment. For this reason and because of the correlation of lipophilicity with anesthetic potency, it is believed that the major site of action of anesthetics is either the lipid matrix of the biological membrane or hydrophobic regions of specific membrane-bound proteins. Anesthetics can bind to proteins, presumably to hydrophobic sites.

Anesthesia in experimental animals can be reversed by the application of moderate pressure (~100 atmospheres) (Miller *et al.*, 1973). One interpretation of this observation is that a large change of volume may be crucially associated with the fundamental action of anesthetics. Phospholipids in artificial (model) membranes undergo a change of

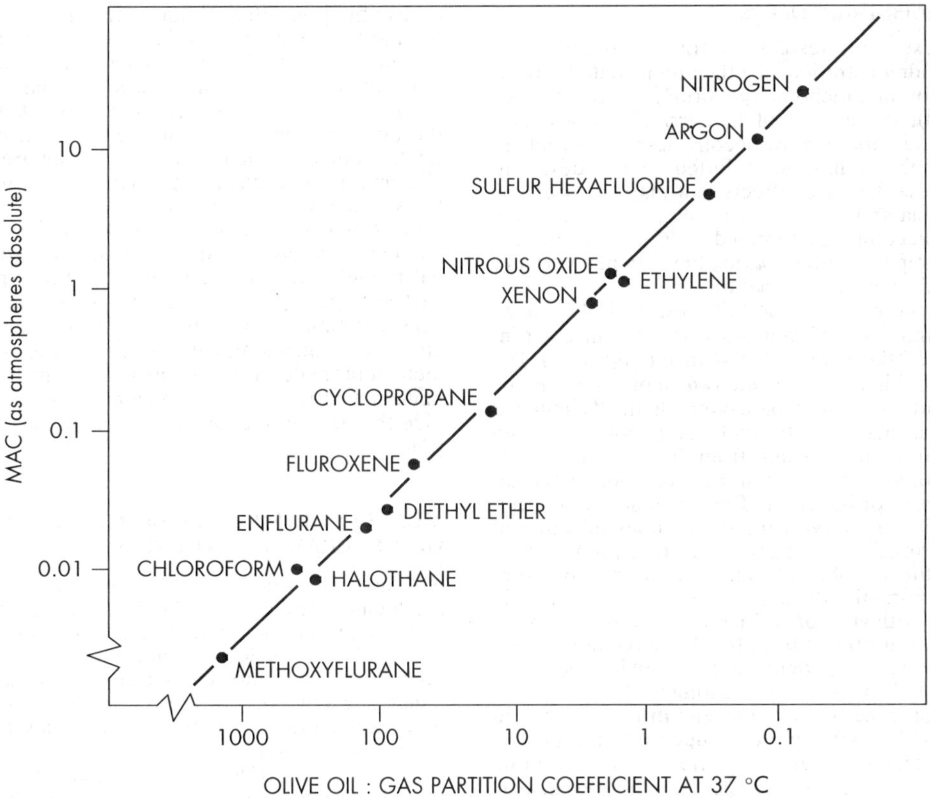

Figure 13–4. *The correlation of anesthetic potency with olive oil : gas partition coefficient.*

The correlation is shown for a number of general anesthetic agents and other inert gases not usually used for anesthesia. Note the log scales and the excellent correlation over a very wide range of fat solubilities and potencies (*see* Paton, 1974). (Modified from Eger *et al.*, 1969; Miller *et al.*, 1972.)

state as temperature is increased—the so-called gel–liquid crystalline transition of the phospholipid matrix. The temperature at which this reaction occurs is dependent on the identity of the phospholipid, and the change in state is associated with an increase in the molar volume of the lipid. If anesthetics are present, the transition from the gel to the liquid crystalline state of the phospholipids is more likely to happen; that is, it occurs at lower temperatures (Trudell *et al.*, 1973b). It is possible to rationalize the effect of pressure to reverse anesthesia based on such considerations. Furthermore, anesthetics broaden the melting curve for the gel–liquid crystalline transition (as if water melted between 0° and 5° C), indicative of a reduction in the number of phospholipid molecules that interact cooperatively at any time. The application of physical techniques, such as nuclear magnetic resonance and electron-spin resonance, indicates that anesthetics cause a local disordering of the lipid matrix (Trudell *et al.*, 1973a; Trudell and Hubbell, 1976). Because anesthetics appear to decrease the number of molecules of phospholipid that alternate simultaneously between the gel and liquid crystalline states, these drugs reduce the magnitude of fluctuations of volume that probably occur in dynamic biological membranes (Mountcastle *et al.*, 1978). It is hypothesized that such fluctuations are sufficiently large to be important in the regulation of the structural state of membrane-bound proteins (*e.g.*, their state of aggregation) and, therefore, of their functional properties (*see* Halsey, 1974; Halsey *et al.*, 1986). As inhibitors of such fluctuations, anesthetics could readily influence the fluxes of ions, which are crucial determinants of neuronal excitability, or other functions of membranes that are determined by the proteins that function in the milieu of a dynamic lipid matrix. (For a review of the mechanism of action of general anesthetics, *see* Richter, 1989.)

Aukburg, S. J.; Miller, J.; and Smith, T. C. Interaction between meperidine and diazepam on the ventilatory response to carbon dioxide. *Clin. Res.*, **1976**, *24*, 506a.

Bennett, A. E. How "Indian arrow poison" curare became a useful drug. *Anesthesiology*, **1967**, *28*, 446–451.

Berman, M. L.; Lowe, H. J.; Bochantin, J.; and Hagler, K. Uptake and elimination of methoxyflurane as influenced by enzyme induction in the rat. *Anesthesiology*, **1973**, *38*, 352–357.

Cowles, A. L.; Borgstedt, H. H.; and Gillies, A. J. Uptake and distribution of inhalation anesthetic agents in clinical practice. *Anesth. Analg.*, **1968**, *47*, 404–414.

———. The uptake and distribution of four inhalation anesthetics in dogs. *Anesthesiology*, **1972**, *36*, 558–570.

Cullen, D. J., and others. Clinical signs of anesthesia. *Anesthesiology*, **1972**, *36*, 21–36.

Cullen, S. C.; Eger, E. I., II; Cullen, B. F.; and Gregory, P. Observations on the anesthetic effect and the combination of xenon and halothane. *Anesthesiology*, **1969**, *31*, 305–309.

de Jong, R. H., and Eger, E. I., II. MAC expanded: AD_{50} and AD_{95} values of common inhalation anesthetics in man. *Anesthesiology*, **1975**, *42*, 384–389.

de Jong, R. H., and Heavner, J. E. Diazepam and lidocaine-induced cardiovascular changes. *Anesthesiology*, **1973**, *39*, 633–638.

Egbert, L. D.; Battit, G. E.; Turndorf, H.; and Becker, H. K. The value of a preoperative visit by an anesthetist. *J.A.M.A.*, **1963**, *185*, 533–555.

Eger, E. I., II. Intertissue diffusion of anesthetics. *Anesthesiology*, **1973**, *38*, 201.

———. (ed.). *Anesthetic Uptake and Action*. The Williams & Wilkins Co., Baltimore, **1974.**

Eger, E. I., II; Lundgren, C.; Miller, S. F.; and Stevens, W. C. Anesthetic potencies of sulfur hexafluoride, carbon tetrafluoride, chloroform and ETHRANE in dogs: correlation with the hydrate and lipid theories of anesthetic action. *Anesthesiology*, **1969**, *30*, 129–135.

Eger, E. I., II; Saidman, L. J.; and Brandstater, B. Minimum alveolar anesthetic concentration, a standard of anesthetic potency. *Anesthesiology*, **1965**, *26*, 756–763.

Epstein, R. M.; Rackow, H.; Salanitre, E.; and Wolf, G. Influence of the concentration effect on the uptake of anesthetic mixtures: the second gas effect. *Anesthesiology*, **1964**, *25*, 364–371.

Fink, B. R. Diffusion anoxia. *Anesthesiology*, **1955**, *16*, 511–519.

Fragen, R. J.; Funk, D. I.; Avram, M. J.; Costello, C.; and DeBruine, K. Midazolam versus hydroxyzine as intramuscular premedicant. *Can. Anaesth. Soc. J.*, **1983**, *30*, 136–141.

Greene, N. M. A consideration of factors in the discovery of anesthesia and their effects on its development. *Anesthesiology*, **1971**, *35*, 515–522.

———. Anesthesia and the development of surgery (1846–1896). *Anesth. Analg.*, **1979**, *58*, 5–12.

Halsey, M. J. Mechanisms of general anesthesia. In, *Anesthetic Uptake and Action*. (Eger, E. I., II, ed.) The Williams & Wilkins Co., Baltimore, **1974**, pp. 45–76.

Halsey, M. J.; Wardley-Smith, B.; and Wood, S. Pressure reversal of alphaxalone/alphadolone and methohexitone in tadpoles: evidence for different molecular sites for general anaesthesia. *Br. J. Pharmacol.*, **1986**, *89*, 299–305.

Lerman, J.; Robinson, S.; Willis, M. M.; and Gregory, G. A. Anesthetic requirements for halothane in young children 0–1 month and 1–8 months of age. *Anesthesiology*, **1983**, *59*, 421–424.

Lucas, G. H. The discovery of cyclopropane. *Anesth. Analg.*, **1961**, *40*, 15–27.

McDowall, D. G. Monitoring the brain. *Anesthesiology*, **1976**, *45*, 117–134.

McIntyre, A. R. Historical background, early use and development of muscle relaxants. *Anesthesiology*, **1959**, *20*, 409–415.

Meyer, H. H. Zur Theorie de Alkoholnarkose. I. Mitt. Welche Eigenschaft der Anästhetika bedingt ihre narkotische Wirkung? *Arch. Exp. Pathol. Pharmakol.*, **1899**, *42*, 109.

———. Zur Theorie der Alkoholnarkose. III. Mitt. Der Einfluss wechselnder Temperatur auf Wirkungsstärke und Teilungskoefficient der Narkotika. *Ibid.*, **1901**, *46*, 338.

Millar, R. D.; Wahrenbrock, E. A.; Schroeder, C. F.; Knipstein, T. W.; Eger, E. I., II; and Buechel, D. R. Ethylene-halothane anesthesia: addition or synergism? *Anesthesiology*, **1969**, *31*, 301–304.

Miller, K. W.; Paton, W. D. M.; Smith, E. B.; and Smith, R. A. Physicochemical approaches to the mode of action of general anesthetics. *Anesthesiology*, **1972**, *36*, 339–351.

Miller, K. W.; Paton, W. D. M.; Smith, R. A.; and Smith, E. B. The pressure reversal of general anesthesia and the critical volume hypothesis. *Mol. Pharmacol.*, **1973**, *9*, 131–143.

Mountcastle, D. B.; Biltonen, R. L.; and Halsey, M. J. Effect of anesthetics and pressure on the thermotropic behavior of multilamellar dipalmitoylphosphatidyl choline liposomes. *Proc. Natl. Acad. Sci. U.S.A.*, **1978**, *75*, 4906–4910.

Moyers, J. R. Preoperative medication. In, *Clinical Anesthesia*. (Barasch, P. G.; Cullen, B. F.; and Stoelting, R. K.; eds.) J. B. Lippincott Co., Philadelphia, **1989**, pp. 485–503.

Munson, E. S.; Eger, E. I., II; and Bowers, D. L. Effects of anesthetic-depressed ventilation and cardiac output on anesthetic uptake: a computer nonlinear simulation. *Anesthesiology*, **1973**, *38*, 251–259.

Myer, E. F., and Tomeldan, S. A. Glycopyrrolate compared with atropine in prevention of the oculocardiac reflex during eye-muscle surgery. *Anesthesiology*, **1979**, *51*, 350–352.

Odura, K. A. Glycopyrrolate methylbromide. Comparison with atropine sulfate. *Can. Anaesth. Soc. J.*, **1975**, *22*, 466–473.

Overton, E. *Studien über die Narkose zugleich ein Beitrag zur allgemeinen Pharmakologie*. G. Fischer, Jena, **1901.**

Reves, J. G.; Fragen, R. J.; Vinick, H. R.; and Greenblatt, D. J. Midazolam: pharmacology and uses. *Anesthesiology*, **1985**, *62*, 310–324.

Rosner, B. S., and Clark, D. L. Neurophysiologic effects of general anesthetics. II. Sequential regional actions in the brain. *Anesthesiology*, **1973**, *39*, 59–81.

Smith, N. T.; Zwart, A.; and Beneken, J. E. W. Interaction between the circulatory effects and the uptake and distribution of halothane: use of a multiple model. *Anesthesiology*, **1972**, *37*, 47–58.

Stevens, W. C.; Dolan, W. M.; Gibbons, R. T.; White, A.; Eger, E. I., II; Miller, R. D.; de Jong, R. H.; and Elashoff, R. M. Minimum alveolar concentrations (MAC) of isoflurane with and without nitrous oxide in patients of various ages. *Anesthesiology*, **1975**, *42*, 197–200.

Stoelting, R. K., and Eger, E. I., II. Percutaneous loss of nitrous oxide, cyclopropane, ether and halothane in man. *Anesthesiology*, **1969**, *30*, 278–289.

Thornton, C.; Catley, D. M.; Jordan, C.; Lehane, J. R.; Royston, D.; and Jones, J. G. Enflurane anaesthesia causes graded changes in the brainstem and early cortical auditory evoked response in man. *Br. J. Anaesth.*, **1983**, *55*, 479–486.

Trudell, J. R., and Hubbell, W. L. Localization of molecular halothane in phospholipid bilayer model nerve membranes. *Anesthesiology*, **1976**, *44*, 202.

Trudell, J. R.; Hubbell, W. L.; and Cohen, E. N. The effect of two inhalation anesthetics on the order of spin-labeled phospholipid vesicles. *Biochim. Biophys. Acta*, **1973a**, *291*, 321–327.

———. Pressure reversal of inhalation anesthetic-induced disorder in spin-labeled phospholipid vesicles. *Ibid.*, **1973b**, *291*, 328–334.

Vandam, L. D. Early American anesthetists—the origins of professionalism in anesthesia. *Anesthesiology*, **1973**, *38*, 264–274.

Walsh, J.; Puig, M. M.; Lovitz, M. A.; and Turndorf, H. Premedication abolishes the increase in plasma beta-endorphin observed in the immediate preoperative period. *Anesthesiology*, **1987**, *66*, 402–405.

Wolfson, B.; Hetrick, W. D.; Kake, C. L.; and Siker, E. S. Anesthetic indices—further data. *Anesthesiology,* **1978,** *48,* 187–190.

Monographs and Reviews

Clark, D. L., and Rosner, B. S. Neurophysiologic effects of general anesthetics. I. The electroencephalogram and sensory evoked responses in man. *Anesthesiology,* **1973,** *38,* 564–582.

Cohen, E. N. Metabolism of the volatile anesthetics. *Anesthesiology,* **1971,** *35,* 193–202.

Davison, M. H. A. *The Evolution of Anesthesia.* The Williams & Wilkins Co., Baltimore, **1965.**

Dripps, R. D.; Eckenhoff, J. E.; and Vandam, L. D. *Introduction to Anesthesia: The Principles of Safe Practice,* 7th ed. W. B. Saunders Co., Philadelphia, **1988,** p. 263.

Duncum, B. M. *The Development of Inhalation Anesthesia.* Oxford University Press, New York, **1947.**

Faulconer, A., and Keys, T. E. (eds.). *Foundations of Anesthesiology.* Charles C Thomas, Publisher, Springfield, Ill., **1965.**

Grundy, B. L. Intraoperative monitoring of sensory-evoked potentials. *Anesthesiology,* **1983,** *58,* 72–87.

Keys, T. E. *The History of Surgical Anesthesia.* Dover Publications, Inc., New York, **1963.**

Levy, W. J.; Shapiro, H. M.; Maruchak, G.; and Meathe, E. Automated EEG processing for intraoperative monitoring. *Anesthesiology,* **1980,** *53,* 223–236.

Paton, W. D. M. Unconventional anaesthetic molecules. In, *Molecular Mechanisms in General Anaesthesia.* (Halsey, M. J.; Millar, R. A.; and Sutton, J. A.; eds.) Churchill-Livingstone, Ltd., London, **1974,** pp. 48–64.

Richter, J. J. Mechanisms of general anesthesia. In, *Clinical Anesthesia.* (Barasch, P. G.; Cullen, B. F.; and Stoelting, R. K.; eds.) J. B. Lippincott Co., Philadelphia, **1989,** pp. 281–291.

Sykes, W. S. *Essays on the First Hundred Years of Anesthesia.* E. & S. Livingstone, Edinburgh, **1960.**

Thomas, K. B. *The Development of Anaesthetic Apparatus.* Blackwell Scientific Publications, Oxford, **1975.**

CHAPTER

14 GENERAL ANESTHETICS

Bryan E. Marshall and David E. Longnecker

The state of general anesthesia is a drug-induced absence of perception of all sensations. Depths of anesthesia appropriate for the conduct of surgical procedures can be achieved with a wide variety of drugs, either alone or, more often, in combinations. General anesthetics can be administered by a variety of routes, but intravenous or inhalational administration is preferred, because the effective dose and the time course of action are more predictable when these techniques are used. In this chapter the inhalational general anesthetic agents are described in some detail. The intravenous agents, including the barbiturates, benzodiazepines, opioids, and neuroleptics, are discussed in detail elsewhere (*see* Index) and, therefore, only their use for anesthesia will be presented here.

I. Inhalational Anesthetics

An ideal inhalational general anesthetic agent would be characterized by (1) rapid and pleasant induction of, and recovery from, anesthesia; (2) rapid changes in the depth of anesthesia; (3) adequate relaxation of skeletal muscles; (4) a wide margin of safety; and (5) the absence of toxic effects or other adverse properties in normal doses. However, the availability of ultra-short-acting intravenous agents, potent opioid analgesics with short durations of action, and specific muscle relaxants has reduced the necessity for the first three properties. The margin of safety of inhalational drugs has become less of an issue, since lower concentrations of the anesthetic can be administered in combination with useful intravenous supplements. The incidence of adverse effects is, therefore, the principal factor that now determines the acceptability of a general anesthetic agent.

The inhalational general anesthetic agents in wide use are nitrous oxide, halothane, enflurane, and isoflurane; methoxyflurane is usually employed only for analgesia during obstetrical procedures. The inorganic compound nitrous oxide (N_2O) is a gas at normal ambient temperature and pressure, whereas the other four agents are volatile organic liquids (Table 14–1). Certain generalizations are appropriate concerning the relative potency and the properties that result from their physical and chemical characteristics (*see also* Chapter 13).

Potency. A standard of comparison for potency of general anesthetic agents was elusive, but the introduction of the concept of *minimum alveolar concentration* (MAC; *see* Chapter 13; *see also* Eger, 1974) provided an important and practical definition. A dose of 1 MAC will prevent movement in response to surgical incision in 50% of subjects; doses that span the approximate range of 0.5 to 2 MAC are necessary for adequate anesthesia in individual patients. A dose of less than 1 MAC may also be effective when requirements are reduced by disease or the presence of other drugs. The values of MAC in Table 14–1 demonstrate both the wide range of relative potencies and the greater potencies of the volatile agents compared with nitrous oxide. Techniques for vaporization and administration of volatile anesthetic agents are described in Chapter 13. The saturated vapor pressures for the volatile anesthetics are shown in Table 14–1; also listed are the maximum concentrations of anesthetic vapor that can be delivered by an efficient vaporizer.

Induction of Anesthesia. None of the agents listed in Table 14–1 is irritating to breathe, and their odors are not unpleasant. The depth of anesthesia that can be achieved depends on the potency relative to the maximum amount of agent that can be vaporized. Table 14–1 illustrates the fact

Table 14–1. PROPERTIES OF INHALATIONAL ANESTHETIC AGENTS

ANESTHETIC	MAC * (%)	VAPOR PRESSURE (*mm Hg at 20°C*)	MAXIMUM VAPOR CONCENTRATION (*% at 20°C*)	BLOOD:GAS PARTITION COEFFICIENT (*at 37°C*)	OIL:GAS PARTITION COEFFICIENT (*at 37°C*)
Methoxyflurane	0.16	22.5	3	12.0	970
Halothane	0.75	243	32	2.3	224
Enflurane	1.68	175	23	1.9	98
Isoflurane	1.15	250	33	1.4	99
Nitrous oxide	105 †	Gas	—	0.47	1.4

* MAC = minimum alveolar concentration (*see* text for further definition).
† A value of MAC greater than 100% means that hyperbaric conditions would be required to reach 1 MAC.

that concentrations far higher than are usually necessary can be delivered when halothane, enflurane, and isoflurane are used. The speed with which induction of anesthesia can be accomplished is inversely related to the solubility of the agent in most body tissues (blood:gas partition coefficient), as described in Chapter 13. The greater the oil:gas partition coefficient (Table 14–1), the greater the capacity of fatty tissues to absorb the agent; this results in slower equilibration with fatty tissues and longer periods of elimination after discontinuation of the anesthetic following prolonged administration.

Most of what follows in this chapter concerns the pharmacological properties of anesthetic drugs. Their influences on the lungs, heart, and circulation, as well as the less apparent actions on other organ systems, are side effects that always accompany general anesthesia; accurate knowledge of these properties is required for safe management of the patient. Although inhalational anesthetics in current use are relatively inert and nontoxic, some are more prone than others to be metabolized. Certain metabolic products determine the long-term toxic effects that may follow the use of these drugs.

HALOTHANE

Chemistry and Physical Properties. *Halothane* (FLUOTHANE) is 2-bromo-2-chloro-1,1,1-trifluoroethane (Table 14–2). Mixtures of halothane with air or oxygen are not flammable or explosive. Partition coefficients and the MAC value for halothane are listed in Table 14–1.

With the exception of chromium, nickel, and titanium, most metals are tarnished or corroded by halothane. The compound interacts with rubber and some plastics, but not with polyethylene.

The solubility of halothane in rubber can theoretically slow the induction of and the emergence from anesthesia as a consequence of the uptake or release of the anesthetic from the rubber elements in the anesthesia circuit when low-flow techniques are used.

PHARMACOLOGICAL PROPERTIES

General Characteristics. The general and special properties of halothane are discussed in greater detail than are those of the other volatile agents because halothane represents the first of the series of drugs now in common use, and it is the standard to which others are compared. Halothane is a potent anesthetic agent with properties that allow a smooth and rather rapid loss of consciousness that progresses to anesthesia. However, the rapidity, convenience, and pleasantness associated with the intravenous administration of thiopental are usually preferred for induction of anesthe-

Table 14–2. STRUCTURES OF VOLATILE GENERAL ANESTHETIC AGENTS *

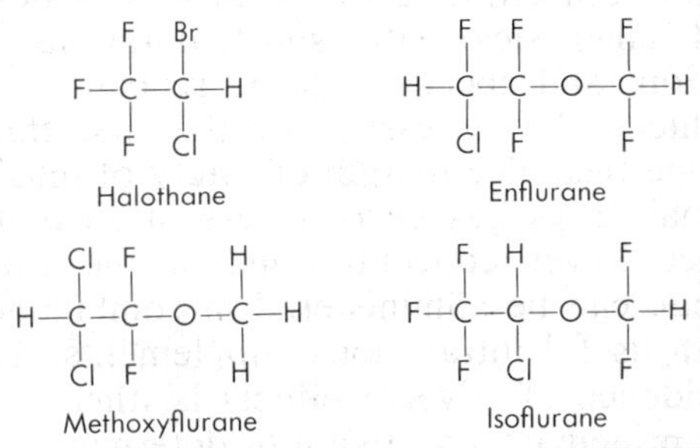

* Note the varying halogen substitutions and that all of the agents, except halothane, are ethers. While isoflurane and enflurane are isomers, there are some important differences in their pharmacological properties (*see* text).

sia; halothane is then introduced for maintenance of anesthesia during the surgical procedure. The circumstances and requirements of the surgical procedure determine whether the trachea is intubated; whether the patient is allowed to breathe spontaneously or is ventilated manually or mechanically; and whether additional drugs, such as muscle relaxants or analgesics, are administered.

Following its introduction in 1956, the clinical popularity of halothane was based primarily on its lack of flammability, the ease with which depth of anesthesia can be changed, the rapid awakening (less than 1 hour) when its administration is stopped, and the relatively low incidence of toxic effects associated with its use. However, the margin of safety of halothane is not wide; circulatory depression with profound reduction of arterial blood pressure is readily produced (Eger, 1974).

The signs of depth of anesthesia with halothane that are of most practical value are the blood pressure, which is progressively depressed, and the response to surgical stimulation (*e.g.*, pulse rate, blood pressure, movement, or even awakening). The concentration of anesthetic agent that is necessary in the inspired gas mixture for induction of anesthesia must be appropriately reduced as the alveolar concentration increases during maintenance if progressive increase in depth of anesthesia and decrease in blood pressure are to be avoided.

Circulation. Administration of halothane is characterized by a dose-dependent reduction of arterial blood pressure. Hypotension results from two main effects. First, the myocardium is depressed directly and cardiac output is decreased; second, the normal baroreceptor-mediated tachycardia in response to hypotension is obtunded. With halothane and the other commonly used volatile agents, anesthesia is not associated with increased sympathoadrenal activity; concentrations of catecholamines in blood do not increase (Perry *et al.*, 1974), and cardiovascular depression is evident. However, at clinical depths of anesthesia, sympathoadrenal response to stimulation is not abolished by halothane. An appropriate stimulus—for example, increased carbon dioxide tension or surgical stimulation—may cause an active sympathetic response with increases of blood pressure, heart rate, and concentrations of catecholamines in plasma.

Heart. When anesthesia is induced by inspiration of halothane at concentrations commonly necessary for surgical anesthesia (0.8 to 1.2%), cardiac output is reduced by 20 to 50% from the level characteristic of the awake state (Marshall *et al.*, 1969). Both increased concentration of halothane and reduced arterial carbon dioxide tension (hyperventilation) accentuate the reduction in cardiac output.

The contractility of preparations of heart muscle *in vitro* is depressed by halothane in a dose-dependent fashion. It is also generally agreed that myocardial contractility is reduced during halothane anesthesia in man (Sonntag *et al.*, 1978). However, after 2 to 5 hours of constant halothane anesthesia, all the cardiovascular changes (*i.e.*, hypotension, depressed cardiac output, and bradycardia) tend to return toward normal; this response has been attributed to sympathetic activation with time (Eger *et al.*, 1970). Animal studies have established that autoregulation of coronary flow remains intact and that any reduction of flow that is observed reflects the reduced oxygen consumption and work of the heart.

The negative inotropic effects of halothane appear to be due to a reduced concentration of intracellular Ca^{2+}, which is necessary to activate actomyosin. This reduction is attributable to actions of halothane on the sarcolemma that reduce the influx of Ca^{2+} through so-called slow channels. In addition, binding of Ca^{2+} by the plasma membrane is increased (Rusy and Komai, 1987), and the uptake and release of Ca^{2+} by the sarcoplasmic reticulum are impaired (Housmans and Murat, 1988).

Cardiac Rhythm. The heart rate is slowed during anesthesia with halothane. This is, in part, reversible by atropine and is due to reduction of cardiac sympathetic activity with consequent vagal predominance. However, direct, atropine-insensitive slowing of SA nodal discharge can be observed *in vitro;* both a reduced rate of phase-4 depolarization and an increased threshold for the generation of an action potential appear to be involved. During halothane anesthesia in man, vagal activity is further enhanced by manipulation of the airway. Sinus bradycardia, wandering pacemaker, or junctional rhythms are not uncommon at this time, but they are generally benign.

Tachyarrhythmias may also occur in the presence of halothane. Some of these may be of the reentrant type (*see* Chapter 35). Since halothane slows the conduction of impulses and also probably increases refractory periods in conducting tissue, it creates conditions conducive to reentry, a unidirectional block with slowed retrograde conduction (Atlee and Rusy, 1977).

Halothane may also increase the automaticity of the myocardium; this effect is exaggerated by adrenergic agonists and leads to propagated impulses from ectopic sites within the atria or ventricles. Increased secretion of endogenous epinephrine may result from stimulation during surgery, if anesthesia is insufficient, or from increased arterial tension of carbon dioxide, if ventilation is inadequate. Alternatively, exogenously administered epinephrine may initiate the arrhythmia. Tachyarrhythmias are unlikely if, in the presence of halothane anesthesia, ventilation is adequate and the use of epinephrine for hemostasis is limited to concentrations of 1:100,000 or less and the dose in adults does not exceed 0.1 mg in 10 minutes or 0.3 mg in 1 hour. Arrhythmias caused by halothane and epinephrine may be reduced by blockade of myocardial α_1-adrenergic receptors and increased by thiopental or ketamine (Maze *et al.,* 1985).

Although all the above-mentioned arrhythmias are generally benign in patients with a healthy myocardium, they may not be so in the presence of cardiac disease, hypoxia, acidosis, or electrolyte abnormalities.

Baroreceptor Control. Although early work demonstrated that halothane reduces afferent discharge by "resetting" the baroreceptors to respond around a lower "set point," depresses the vasomotor response of the brainstem, and reduces the sympathetic outflow that results, the observed changes are small. In addition, halothane has little effect on the response of preganglionic sympathetic neurons to stimulation of baroreceptors (Skovsted *et al.,* 1969). Thus, it is concluded that the predominant actions of halothane are at the effector sites in the heart that control cardiac rate and/or contractility.

Organ Blood Flow. Halothane influences the blood flow to every organ by both direct and indirect actions (Seyde and Longnecker, 1984). These include interference with the generation or action of factors derived from the endothelium that regulate the tone of vascular smooth muscle (Stone and Johns, 1989). In the skin and cerebral circulation, flow may increase as the vessels dilate. However, the cerebrovascular bed, as well as the renal and splanchnic circulations, loses some of its ability to autoregulate flow, and perfusion of these tissues decreases if blood pressure falls excessively. The coronary circulation remains responsive to myocardial needs for oxygen; vasodilatation occurs in poorly ventilated areas of the lung because of inhibition of pulmonary vasoconstriction that normally occurs in response to hypoxia.

In an individual patient, blood flow to each of these organs can be influenced by pH and carbon dioxide tension, posture, temperature, age, disease, and the administration of other drugs. It is, therefore, not surprising that conflicting results have been reported. However, it is agreed that, despite the differences from organ to organ, the total peripheral vascular resistance changes very little when hypotension occurs with halothane (Eger *et al.,* 1970; Sonntag *et al.,* 1978). Dilatation in one organ bed is offset by reduced flow in another, and, thus, generalized peripheral vasodilatation is not the primary cause of hypotension.

Respiration. If the patient anesthetized with halothane is allowed to breathe spontaneously, an increased partial pressure of carbon dioxide in the arterial blood is common and is indicative of ventilatory depression; there is also an increased difference between the partial pressure of oxygen in the alveolar gas and in the arterial blood, indicating less efficient exchange of gas. Halothane thus influences both ventilatory control and the efficiency of oxygen transfer. To compensate for these effects, ventilation is frequently assisted or controlled by manual or mechanical means, and the concentration of inspired oxygen is increased.

Ventilatory Control. Characteristically, respirations are rapid and shallow during halothane anesthesia. Minute volume is reduced, and arterial carbon dioxide tension is increased from 40 mm Hg to approximately 50 mm Hg. Halothane causes a dose-related reduction in the ventilatory response to carbon dioxide (Knill and Gelb, 1978). While the precise effects of the anesthetic on the function of central and peripheral chemoreceptors are uncertain, the changes in the ventilatory response to carbon dioxide and the altered pattern of breathing caused by halothane are probably predominantly mediated at central sites of action.

In the awake state, the total ventilatory response to carbon dioxide is altered little by denervation of peripheral chemoreceptors. Therefore, despite evidence that halothane depresses the activity of the carbon dioxide–stimulated carotid body, it seems unlikely that this effect can be responsible for the ventilatory depression that is observed.

The increased ventilation in response to arterial hypoxemia, which is mediated by the carotid bodies, is abolished by denervation and by halothane (Knill and Gelb, 1978). It follows that adequacy of oxygenation during anesthesia cannot be assessed by observing ventilatory exchange. However, halothane depresses responsiveness to carbon dioxide even when the blood is hyperoxic.

The above considerations lead to the conclusion that halothane-induced depression of respiratory sensitivity to carbon dioxide results from a central action on the respiratory centers themselves; inhibitory effects on inspiratory neurons of the tractus solitarius have been documented (Tabatabai *et al.*, 1987). However, the decreased overall sensitivity of the ventilatory response to carbon dioxide is greater than the depression of the neural drive (Pavlin and Hornbein, 1986).

Pulmonary Oxygen Transfer. Efficient transfer of oxygen from the alveolar gas to hemoglobin in the alveolar capillary red blood cell depends on a proper balance between alveolar ventilation and perfusion. This balance is importantly controlled by the effects of gravity and various structural mechanical factors, and fine adjustments are provided by changes in the tone of the smooth muscle of bronchial airways and pulmonary vessels. All these factors may be altered during halothane anesthesia. The influence of gravity obviously differs when the patient is in the horizontal position, particularly when ventilation is achieved by intermittent positive pressure. Halothane changes the movements of the thoracic cage (Tusiewicz *et al.*, 1977), depresses diaphragmatic function (Clergue *et al.*, 1986), alters lung volume (Laws, 1968), dilates constricted bronchial smooth muscle (a useful property in asthmatic patients) (Hirshman *et al.*, 1982), depresses mucociliary flow (Forbes, 1976), and inhibits pulmonary vascular constriction in the presence of hypoxia (Benumof and Wahrenbrock, 1975). The outcome is more or less impairment of oxygen exchange (Marshall and Marshall, 1985), with evidence of an increased fraction of blood to which no oxygen is added as it traverses the lungs (pulmonary shunt) and increased mismatching of ventilation and perfusion (Dueck *et al.*, 1980).

Nervous System. Electrical activity of the cerebral cortex recorded by a frontooccipital EEG shows progressive replacement of fast, low-voltage activity by slow waves of greater amplitude as halothane anesthesia is deepened. Surgical stimulation may reverse this pattern, and such arousal reactions may be associated with recall of intraoperative events by patients, as in a dream (Bimar and Bellville, 1977). This sequence resembles arousal of the brain by activation of the brainstem reticular formation, but reticular neuronal activity is depressed by halothane (Shimoji *et al.*, 1977).

Since cerebral blood flow generally increases during halothane anesthesia (*see* above), cerebrospinal fluid pressure increases (Lassen and Christensen, 1976). Halothane may thus aggravate conditions in which the intracranial pressure is elevated. The cerebral metabolic consumption of oxygen is reduced and the delivery of oxygen and substrates to the brain appears to be adequate, but there are marked regional differences (Eintrei *et al.*, 1985). After several hours of anesthesia with halothane the changes in cerebral blood flow and metabolism return toward normal (Warner *et al.*, 1985).

Recovery of mental function after even brief anesthesia with halothane is not complete for several hours, but this phenomenon probably contributes little to the more prolonged impairment of psychological performance that has been reported after major surgery. Shivering during recovery is common and probably represents both a response to heat loss and an ill-defined expression of neurological recovery.

Muscle. Relaxation of skeletal muscle is desirable or necessary for many surgical procedures. Anesthesia with halothane causes some relaxation by central depression; in addition, the duration and magnitude of the muscular relaxation induced by nondepolarizing skeletal muscle relaxants such as tubocurarine or pancuronium are increased. The mechanism of this effect is not known but appears to be based on increased sensitivity of the end-plate to the action of the competitive neuromuscular blocking agents (Waud, 1977).

Rarely, induction of anesthesia with halothane or any of the other halogenated inhalational anesthetics triggers an uncontrolled hypermetabolic reaction in the skeletal muscle of susceptible patients. The resultant syndrome of malignant hyperthermia is characterized by a rapid rise in body temperature and a massive increase in oxygen consumption and production of carbon dioxide; death may result unless the anesthetic is discontinued and treatment with dantrolene is begun promptly. This syndrome may be caused by a defect in the uptake of Ca^{2+} by the sarcoplasmic reticulum in genetically susceptible muscle (Gronert, 1980).

Uterine smooth muscle is relaxed by halothane. This effect is of sufficient magnitude to allow manipulation of the fetus (version) during the prenatal period. Inhibition of natural or induced uterine contractions by halothane during parturition may prolong the process of delivery, as well as increase blood loss. Thus, other agents or techniques may be preferred for the relief of obstetrical pain.

Kidney. Halothane causes dose-dependent reductions of renal blood flow and the rate of glomerular filtration; these parameters may be 40 to 50% of normal at 1 MAC (Mazze *et al.*, 1963). These effects can be attenuated by preoperative hydration and prevention of hypotension. Halothane does not interfere greatly with autoregulation of renal blood flow nor, in the normotensive state, with the distribution of flow between the renal cortex and medulla (Leighton and Bruce, 1975). Anesthesia is normally accompanied by the production of a small volume of concentrated urine. The changes in urine volume are probably secondary to circulatory responses and reduced glomerular filtration (Deutsch *et al.*, 1966). The renal effects of halothane anesthesia are rapidly reversed, and there is no evidence of postoperative renal impairment. In an occasional patient (usually elderly), retention of water postoperatively results in hyponatremia, reduced plasma osmolality, and mental confusion.

Liver and Gastrointestinal Tract. Compared with older agents (*e.g.*, ether and cyclopropane), the incidence and duration of postoperative nausea and vomiting are much reduced with the inhalational anesthetics in current use. Factors such as age, sex, site and duration of surgery, disease state, and other medications have a greater influence than does the specific inhalational agent selected. However, the injectable anesthetic agents generally result in an even lower incidence of nausea and vomiting.

Splanchnic and, therefore, hepatic blood flow is reduced by halothane as a passive consequence of reduced perfusion pressure, but there is no evidence of overt ischemia (Epstein *et al.*, 1966; Seyde and Longnecker, 1984). Hepatic cellular functions are, however, depressed, and halothane reduces the ability of the microsomal enzyme systems to metabolize drugs. The extent of this depression is similar to that produced by other inhalational anesthetics, and it is rapidly reversed when administration of halothane is stopped.

Hepatitis. Hepatitis that occurs in the postoperative period is most often due to transmission of hepatitis virus (*e.g.*, in transfused blood), involvement of the liver by disease processes, or damage by known hepatotoxic drugs. However, a retrospective analysis of the records of more than 850,000 administrations of anesthetics suggested a small incidence of hepatic necrosis in which the above etiological factors did not appear to be present (Summary of the National Halothane Study, 1966).

Typically, some 2 to 5 days after anesthesia and surgery, a fever develops, accompanied by anorexia, nausea, and vomiting. Occasionally, a rash occurs and analysis of blood reveals eosinophilia and biochemical abnormalities characteristic of hepatitis. There may be a progression to hepatic failure, and death occurs in about 50% of these patients. The incidence of the syndrome is low, approximately 1 in 10,000 anesthetic administrations in adults and much less in children. Since it is seen most often after repeated administrations of halothane over a short period of time, the term *halothane hepatitis* is used. The unpredictable occurrence of this syndrome is the principal reason that the use of halothane for anesthesia in adults has declined.

A possible basis for halothane hepatitis has been provided by the observation that halothane and all other general anesthetic agents are metabolized, at least to some extent (*see* below). Chemically reactive or immunogenic products may result. An excess of a toxic product or of a metabolite capable of inducing an immune response may be the primary factor that leads to hepatitis (Stock and Strunin, 1985).

Biotransformation. Approximately 60 to 80% of absorbed halothane is eliminated unchanged in the exhaled gas in the first 24 hours after its administration, and smaller amounts continue to be exhaled for several days or even weeks. Of the fraction not exhaled, as much as 50% undergoes biotransformation, and the rest is eliminated unchanged by other routes.

The mixed-function oxidase or cytochrome P_{450} system in the endoplasmic reticulum of the hepatocyte is responsible for this biotransformation. Chlorine and to a lesser extent bromine are removed from halothane; since the bond energy for C—F is nearly twice that for C—Br or C—Cl, little fluorine is removed. The urine contains organic fluorine-containing compounds, mostly trifluoroacetic acid (Sakai and Takaori, 1978). Induction of microsomal enzymes may follow repeated exposure to various drugs, including halothane, and metabolic breakdown may thereby be increased.

Several studies have suggested that occupational exposure to an environment containing halothane or other anesthetic agents for a prolonged period may result in an increased incidence of miscarriage of pregnancy (Vessey, 1978). While neither this nor suggestions of teratogenicity or carcinogenicity of halothane have been confirmed, effective steps to reduce environmental contamination are relatively simple and have been instituted in all areas where anesthesiology is practiced.

Evaluation. *Disadvantages and Limitations.* General anesthesia for surgery requires sleep, analgesia, suppression of visceral reflexes, and, to a variable extent, muscle relaxation; only the first is completely obtained with halothane. Analgesia must often be accomplished by the use of opioids or nitrous oxide, muscle relaxation is enhanced by specific relaxant drugs, and visceral reflexes are managed with other drugs as appropriate (*e.g.*, atropine for bradycardia or local anesthesia to obtund responses to visceral traction). Hypoxemia, hypotension, and transient arrhythmias may occur and sometimes require modification of the anesthetic technique; respiratory depression usually necessitates supplemental ventilation. Life-threatening hepatic necrosis occasionally follows exposure to halothane.

Advantages and Uses. Halothane is nonflammable and moderately potent; it has a relatively low blood:gas partition coefficient, and induction of and recovery from anesthesia are thus not prolonged. Induction is smooth because the larynx is not irritated and bronchospasm is uncommon. Nevertheless, thiopental is most commonly injected to induce sleep prior to the administration of halothane. Halothane is compatible with soda lime and may be used with oxygen to provide maximal oxygenation or combined with other gas mixtures such as nitrous oxide and oxygen. Its potential for inducing hypotension is sometimes utilized deliberately to reduce blood loss under carefully controlled conditions. Uterine relaxation can be valuable during version or extraction of a fetus.

Status. Halothane enjoyed wide popularity for over 25 years and was used for the entire range of surgical procedures. Its administration is associated with an excellent safety record (Summary of the National Halothane Study, 1966). Appropriate equipment is available for precise administration of this agent in all situations. However, the introduction of enflurane and isoflurane, together with the availability of a variety of intravenous agents, has dramatically reduced the use of halothane in more recent years.

ENFLURANE

Chemistry and Physical Properties. *Enflurane* (ETHRANE) is 2-chloro-1,1,2-trifluoroethyl difluoromethyl ether. It is a clear, colorless, nonflammable liquid with a mild, sweet odor. It is extremely stable chemically. It does not attack aluminum, tin, brass, iron, or copper. The partition coefficients and the MAC value for enflurane are listed in Table 14–1. Enflurane is soluble in rubber (partition coefficient = 74), and this property may prolong induction and recovery somewhat, as described for halothane.

PHARMACOLOGICAL PROPERTIES

General Characteristics. The physical properties of enflurane assure that induction of and emergence from anesthesia and adjustment of anesthetic depth during maintenance can be smooth and moderately rapid. Techniques of administration are very similar to those for halothane. Induction of anesthesia to depths appropriate for surgery may be achieved in less than 10 minutes when approximately 4% enflurane is inhaled. A short-acting barbiturate is usually infused intravenously to render the patient unconscious. As with any inhalational agent, the alveolar concentration approaches the inspired concentration with time, and the latter must be progressively reduced. Anesthesia is maintained with inspired concentrations of 1.5 to 3% enflurane.

There is mild stimulation of salivation and tracheobronchial secretions, but these effects are usually not troublesome. Laryngeal and pharyngeal reflexes are obtunded early, and excitement during induction is seldom observed.

The pupils remain small, and eye movements are not prominent; respiration is depressed, and ventilatory assistance is usually required; as with halothane, the most useful signs of depth of anesthesia are changes in arterial blood pressure, pulse rate, or movement in response to surgical stimulation.

Circulation. Arterial blood pressure decreases progressively as the depth of anesthesia increases with enflurane, to about the same degree as it does with halothane. Studies of the effects of the agent on the baroreceptor responses and preganglionic sympathetic activity are also similar (Skovsted and Price, 1972); adrenergic activity is reduced, and the concentration of circulating catecholamines is not increased (Göthert and Wendt, 1977).

In-vitro preparations of myocardium show dose-dependent, reversible depression of contractility (Shimosato *et al.*, 1969), similar to that caused by halothane at equivalent doses. In the intact animal, Merin and associates (1976) have demonstrated that depression of myocardial work is paralleled by diminished consumption of oxygen by the heart. There is no evidence of myocardial hypoxia.

The potent volatile anesthetic agents have a number of subtle differences with regard to their effects on blood flow to vital organs. Bradycardia does not usually occur during anesthesia with enflurane; the pulse rate remains constant. Cardiac output is not decreased as much as with halothane (Marshall *et al.*, 1971), at least at concentrations below 1.5 MAC, and the decreased blood pressure is due, in part, to greater peripheral vascular dilatation (Seyde and Longnecker, 1984). In response to surgical stimulation or hypercarbia, cardiovascular depression may be reversed and blood pressure and cardiac output return toward preanesthetic levels. Administration of a Ca^{2+}-channel blocker (Merin, 1987) or a β-adrenergic antagonist exaggerates enflurane-induced hypotension (Horan *et al.*, 1977); this effect is also observed with other anesthetic agents. Doses of general anesthetics are, therefore, often reduced in patients who are receiving such drugs.

Cardiac Rhythm. In addition to the absence of bradycardia with enflurane, the tendency to arrhythmias is also reduced.

Enflurane does not interfere with impulse conduction in the heart to the same extent as does halothane (Atlee and Rusy, 1977), and the heart is not as sensitized to catecholamines. Hypercarbia or the use of epinephrine for hemostasis or prolongation of the action of local anesthetic agents seldom promotes cardiac arrhythmias in patients receiving enflurane. Thus, somewhat more epinephrine can be used with enflurane than with halothane.

Respiration. Enflurane causes increasing respiratory depression as its concentration is increased. At the level of 1 MAC, the arterial tension of carbon dioxide is greater than with other anesthetics, and depression of the responses to both hypoxia and hypercarbia are greater than with halothane (Hirshman *et al.*, 1977). Curiously, and in contrast to halothane, tachypnea is less common. Assisted or controlled ventilation is usually employed; nevertheless, hyperventilation should be avoided to reduce the incidence of seizure activity (*see* below). As with all inhalational agents, pulmonary exchange of oxygen may become less efficient during anesthesia, and inspired oxygen concentrations of 35% or more are given to avoid hypoxemia, especially in the elderly. Enflurane causes bronchodilatation and usually inhibits bronchoconstriction.

Nervous System. The occurrence of tonic–clonic muscle activity in a small proportion of subjects was noted early in the clinical use of enflurane (Clark and Rosner, 1973). Subsequently it was demonstrated that a characteristic EEG pattern may emerge when higher concentrations of enflurane are used or when there is hypocarbia. A high-voltage, fast-frequency (14- to 18-Hz) pattern progresses to spike–dome complexes; these alternate with periods of electrical silence or frank seizure activity with motor movements. Jerking or twitching of the muscles of the jaw, face, neck, or limbs may be seen. The seizures are of short duration, are self-limited, and may be prevented by avoiding deep anesthesia and/or hyperventilation. This excitatory action of enflurane is not thought to be of special concern, and the drug does not appear to aggravate seizures in epileptic patients. Nevertheless, enflurane is best avoided in such patients.

The other effects of enflurane on the CNS are qualitatively similar to those of halothane. Cerebral oxygen consumption is reduced. Because of vasodilatation, cerebral blood flow is increased when perfusion pressure remains constant, and intracranial pressure is also increased. However, all these effects are less marked than with halothane (Eintrei *et al.*, 1985).

Muscle. Skeletal muscle relaxation increases with the depth of anesthesia and is greater than that produced by halothane (Rupp *et al.*, 1985). Relaxation may be sufficient for abdominal surgery. Competitive skeletal muscle relaxants are more effective in the presence of enflurane (Waud, 1977), and the administration of small doses of these agents allows the use of lighter stages of anesthesia. The muscle relaxant activity of enflurane is caused by actions in the CNS and at the postjunctional membrane of the neuromuscular junction; it is not reversed by neostigmine. Malignant hyperthermia can also occur when susceptible individuals are anesthetized with enflurane.

Uterine muscle is relaxed by enflurane, and increased blood loss may occur during parturition, cesarean section, or therapeutic abortion.

Kidney. Reductions of renal blood flow, glomerular filtration rate, and urine volume during anesthesia with enflurane are similar to those that occur with equivalent depths of anesthesia from halothane; the reductions are reversed rapidly when the anesthetic is discontinued.

Fluoride is a metabolite of enflurane (Mazze *et al.*, 1977; Sakai and Takaori, 1978); however, despite circulating concentrations (up to 20 μM) that far exceed those derived from halothane, concentrations of fluoride do not usually reach the threshold for renal toxicity ($> 40\ \mu$M). Even when there is renal failure in animals, plasma concentrations of fluoride decline rapidly after enflurane is discontinued, probably owing to entry of the anion into bone. It is probable that anesthesia with enflurane is safe in patients with renal disease as long as the depth and duration are not excessive.

Liver and Gastrointestinal Tract. No unusual effects on the gastrointestinal tract have been reported. Splanchnic blood flow is reduced in proportion to perfusion pressure, but delivery of oxygen is not compromised. Nausea and vomiting occur in the postoperative period in perhaps 3 to 15% of patients.

Evidence of hepatic impairment has been obtained during and after surgical anesthesia with enflurane. However, postanesthetic impairment is not apparent in volunteers and the hepatic effects of enflurane are rapidly reversed. Hepatic necrosis associated with repeated administration of enflurane has been reported, and another anesthetic agent should be selected if sensitivity is suspected from a previous administration of the drug (*see* above).

Biotransformation. About 80% of the enflurane that is administered can be recovered unchanged in the expired gas. Of the remainder, 2 to 10% is metabolized in the liver (Carpenter *et al.*, 1986). This quantity is small because the presence of fluorine and chlorine, the absence of bromine, and the incorporation of an ether bond in the molecule increase its stability. In addition, the oil:gas partition coefficient is less than that of other halogenated anesthetic agents. For this reason, enflurane leaves the fatty tissues more rapidly in the postoperative period and is available for degradation for a relatively brief time. Biotransformation may be increased if hepatic enzymes are induced. The metabolic products that have been identified include difluoromethoxydifluoroacetic acid and fluoride ion. The significance of circulating fluoride with regard to renal function is discussed above.

Evaluation. *Disadvantages and Limitations.* Deep anesthesia with enflurane is associated with respiratory and circulatory depression. Seizure activity may occur when concentrations of enflurane are relatively high, especially in the presence of hypocarbia. This agent should be avoided in patients who have preexisting abnormalities in the EEG or a history of a seizure disorder. Uterine relaxation caused by enflurane provides a relative contraindication to the use of deep levels of enflurane anesthesia during labor.

Advantages. Enflurane allows rapid, smooth adjustments of the depth of anesthesia with little change in pulse or respiratory rate. Although arrhythmias, postoperative shivering, nausea, and vomiting occur, they do so to a lesser extent than with halothane or methoxyflurane. Relaxation of skeletal muscle is often adequate for surgery, and interactions with competitive muscle relaxants allow smaller doses of enflurane or of relaxants to be used. If epinephrine is used parenterally with the same precautions as are described for halothane, arrhythmias are even less likely to occur than with the latter agent.

Status. Enflurane was introduced into general clinical use in 1973. It was utilized initially mainly as a substitute to avoid repeated administration of halothane, but it is now employed quite widely whenever an inhalational anesthetic agent is desired.

ISOFLURANE

Chemistry and Physical Properties. *Isoflurane* (FORANE) is 1-chloro-2,2,2-trifluoroethyl difluoromethyl ether. The chemical and physical properties of isoflurane are similar to those of its isomer enflurane (*see* Table 14–1). It is not flammable in air or oxygen. Its vapor pressure is high, and delivery of safe concentrations necessitates the use of a precision vaporizer.

PHARMACOLOGICAL PROPERTIES

General Characteristics. The properties of isoflurane are such that it allows a smooth and rapid induction of, and emergence from, general anesthesia. Isoflurane has a lower blood:gas solubility coefficient than enflurane; a smaller volume of anesthetic vapor must therefore be transferred to achieve the same tension in blood (or brain), and changes in anesthetic depth can thus be achieved more rapidly with isoflurane than with enflurane. Induction of anesthesia can be achieved in less than 10 minutes with an inhaled concentration of 3% isoflurane in oxygen, and this concentration is generally reduced to 1.5 to 2.5% for maintenance of anesthesia. Induction is usually assisted by the injection of a rapidly acting barbiturate. The use of other adjuvant drugs, such as opioids, nitrous oxide, and/or muscle relaxants, reduces the dose of volatile anesthetic that is required to achieve the conditions optimal for surgery.

The clinical signs by which depth of anesthesia is judged include progressive decreases in blood pressure and in respiratory volume and rate, as well as an increase in heart rate. When ventilation is controlled, changes in blood pressure and heart rate and responses to surgical stimulation are the most reliable indices. The pupils are small and responsive to light and are not a useful guide to depth of anesthesia with isoflurane. However, a variety of techniques based on analysis of the electrical activity of the brain have been introduced to assist with estimation of depth of anesthesia with isoflurane (Levy, 1987).

Circulation. Systemic arterial blood pressure decreases progressively with increasing depth during anesthesia with isoflurane, as it does with halothane and enflurane. However, in contrast to the latter agents, cardiac output is well maintained with isoflurane, and the hypotension is due to decreased vascular resistance (Seyde and Longnecker, 1984); vasodilatation occurs particularly in skin and muscle (Stevens *et al.*, 1971). Although negative inotropic effects are seen *in vitro,* they are less obvious with isoflurane than with halothane. Coronary vessels are dilated maximally at about 1.5 MAC of isoflurane. Coronary blood flow is maintained despite decreased myocardial oxygen consumption, suggesting that isoflurane may have a wider margin of cardiovascular safety than is provided by halothane or enflurane. However, in some patients with ischemic heart disease, regions of myocardium with narrowed vessels are dependent on blood supplied by collaterals, and dilatation of the normal coronary vessels by isoflurane may "steal" blood from the collateral vessels and exacerbate ischemia (Buffington *et al.*, 1988). Such changes are minimized by preventing hypotension and tachycardia.

Cardiac Rhythm. Isoflurane increases heart rate, but arrhythmias are not precipitated. Isoflurane does not interfere with atrioventricular conduction and does not sensitize the heart to catecholamines. When epinephrine is utilized for local hemostasis, three times the dose that induces arrhythmias in the presence of halothane is well tolerated with isoflurane.

Respiration. Isoflurane depresses respiration progressively as the concentration increases. With a concentration of 1 MAC, the arterial carbon dioxide tension is increased to about the same level as with halothane (~50 mm Hg), but the ventilatory responses to excess carbon dioxide or to hypoxia are depressed somewhat more than with the other volatile agents (Hirshman *et al.*, 1977). With spontaneous respiration, depression of ventilation is characterized by a reduction in tidal volume with little change in respiratory rate. Respiratory depression is exacerbated by premedication with opioids; assisted or controlled ventilation is generally employed to avoid excessive hypercarbia.

Reductions of pulmonary compliance and functional residual capacity, as well as inhibition of hypoxic pulmonary vasoconstriction, also contribute to the inefficiency of gas exchange that occurs with all the volatile agents (Carlsson *et al.*, 1987). Isoflurane reduces the tone of constricted bronchi in a manner similar to that of halothane (Hirshman *et al.*, 1982). Until adequate levels of anesthesia are attained, isoflurane may stimulate airway reflexes, resulting in increased secretions, coughing, and laryngospasm. The incidence of these effects is greatly reduced by the use of adequate preanesthetic medication and by induction of anesthesia with thiopental or another intravenous agent prior to the administration of isoflurane.

Nervous System. Cerebral blood flow is increased slightly during isoflurane anesthesia, while cerebral metabolism is reduced to an extent that is only slightly less than that with halothane. The cerebral circulation remains responsive to carbon dioxide, and cerebral blood flow, metabolism, and intracranial pressure are reduced by isoflurane and hypocarbia (McPherson *et al.*, 1989). For this reason, isoflurane is preferred during neurosurgery (Messick *et al.*, 1987); furthermore, the anesthetic may provide some protection from hypoxemic or ischemic injury of the brain (Newberg and Michenfelder, 1983). The EEG reveals progressive changes with increasing depth of anesthesia (Clark and Rosner, 1973). At 1 MAC, slow waves with increased voltage predominate; this pattern declines to burst suppression at 1.5 MAC and electrical silence at 2 MAC. Unlike its isomer, enflurane, convulsive activity is not observed with isoflurane.

Muscle. Isoflurane reduces the response of skeletal muscle to sustained nerve stimulation and enhances the neuromuscular blocking effects of both nondepolarizing and depolarizing muscle relaxants. It is more potent in this regard than halothane, and, for the same depth of anesthesia, only half as much tubocurarine may be required with isoflurane (or enflurane) to achieve satisfactory muscular relaxation. This effect is desirable, because it reduces the requirement for drugs and allows lighter levels of anesthesia. The muscle relaxant activity results from actions on the CNS and neuromuscular junction that are similar to those of enflurane; in addition, the increased muscle blood flow that accompanies anesthesia with isoflurane accelerates delivery and removal of neuromuscular blocking drugs. As with halothane and enflurane, malignant hyperthermia can occur during anesthesia with isoflurane. Uterine muscle is relaxed by isoflurane, as it is by the other agents, and it is not recommended for procedures that depend on adequate uterine contraction to limit blood loss.

Kidney. Depression of renal blood flow, the rate of glomerular filtration, and urinary flow accompanies anesthesia with isoflurane, as with all the volatile anesthetic agents. However, all changes in renal function observed during anesthesia are rapidly reversed during recovery. The quantity of fluoride released by metabolic degradation of isoflurane is small, and renal injury is not observed with single or repeated exposures. This agent is not contraindicated for patients with renal diseases.

Liver and Gastrointestinal Tract. The incidence of nausea and vomiting following isoflurane is similar to that for other halogenated anesthetics and is dependent on other factors, discussed above for halothane.

Blood flow to the liver and gastrointestinal tract is altered little by moderate levels of isoflurane anesthesia (Seyde and Longnecker, 1984); these flows decrease with increasing depth of anesthesia as the systemic arterial pressure declines. Tests of hepatic function show minimal changes, which are reversed with recovery from anesthesia. Hepatic failure has not been reported following the administration of isoflurane. Experience with this agent is still accumulating, but the limited extent to which isoflurane is metabolized encourages confidence that hepatotoxicity will occur less frequently than with halothane and enflurane.

Biotransformation. Only 0.2% of the isoflurane that enters the body is metabolized (Holaday *et al.*, 1975); this fraction is markedly less than the extent of metabolism of halothane or enflurane. The small quantities of fluoride and trifluoroacetic acid that are generated as degradation products of isoflurane are insufficient to cause cell damage, which accounts for the lack of renal or hepatic toxicity. Isoflurane does not appear to be a mutagen, teratogen, or carcinogen (Eger *et al.*, 1978).

Evaluation. *Disadvantages and Limitations.* Isoflurane has a more pungent odor than halothane; supplemental intravenous agents are used to overcome this drawback. Anesthesia with isoflurane is associated with progressive respiratory depression and hypotension. Uterine relaxation can be undesirable.

Advantages. The depth of anesthesia can be rapidly adjusted with isoflurane. Cardiac output is well sustained, and systemic (including coronary) vessels dilate. Arrhythmias are uncommon, and epinephrine can be used in greater amounts for hemostasis than with halothane. Isoflurane potentiates the action of muscle relaxants and reduces the dosage of such drugs that are required. Cerebral blood flow and intracranial pressure can be controlled during isoflurane anesthesia. Isoflurane is metabolized to only a minimal extent, and hepatic and renal toxicity have not been reported.

Status. Isoflurane was introduced in 1981, and it has become the most widely used inhalational anesthetic agent for the reasons detailed above.

METHOXYFLURANE

Chemistry and Physical Properties. *Methoxyflurane* (PENTHRANE) is 2,2-dichloro-1,1-difluoroethyl methyl ether (*see* Table 14–2). It is a clear, colorless liquid with a sweet, fruity odor. It is stable in the presence of soda lime and is nonflammable and nonexplosive in air or oxygen in anesthetic concentrations. Physical properties of methoxyflurane and its MAC value are listed in Table 14–1; it is very soluble in rubber (partition coefficient = 635).

PHARMACOLOGICAL PROPERTIES

General Characteristics. Methoxyflurane is the most potent of the inhalational agents. Because of its low vapor pressure at room temperature, the maximal inspired concentration that can be obtained is only 3%. Because of extreme solubility in rubber, as much as 30% of the administered drug may be absorbed by components of an anesthetic circuit, thus reducing the concentration available. Furthermore, the unusually large blood:gas partition coefficient reduces still further the alveolar and hence the arterial tension of the drug early in administration.

Methoxyflurane is metabolized extensively to fluoride and other nephrotoxic products (*see* below). For this reason its use is largely restricted to special situations.

Methoxyflurane does not relax the uterus and in normal doses has little effect on uterine contractions during labor. Thus, it is valuable for use in obstetrical practice, particularly for analgesia during the first stage of labor. Methoxyflurane may be self-administered by the patient by use of a special inhaler that limits the total dose to 15 ml of liquid methoxyflurane. The inhaled concentration is usually between 0.1% and 0.6%, and the patient learns to time the intermittent inhalations to anticipate the period when analgesia is desired. The technique has proven to be safe and practical.

Cardiovascular and respiratory depression with methoxyflurane are generally similar to those produced by halothane (Walker *et al.*, 1962). Systemic arterial blood pressure, pulse rate, and cardiac output are decreased progressively with increasing depth of anesthesia. Cardiac arrhythmias are not frequent, but sinus bradycardia may occur; it is responsive to atropine (Reynolds *et al.*, 1970).

During spontaneous respiration, changes in ventilatory minute volume are useful as a sign of depth of anesthesia. Methoxyflurane is not irritating to the respiratory tract. Secretions are not stimulated and bronchoconstriction does not occur.

Kidney. Renal blood flow, glomerular filtration rate, and urine flow are reduced, as they are with halothane. However, in the postoperative period, high-output renal failure may occur under certain circumstances. All patients who receive methoxyflurane have concentrations of circulating fluoride as a result of biotransformation of the anesthetic. When the administration of methoxyflurane exceeds the equivalent of a dose of 1 MAC for more than 2 hours, the concentration of fluoride in plasma may exceed 40 μM, and direct damage to the renal tubules occurs. The toxic syndrome is characterized by an inability to concentrate the urine, even in response to vasopressin (Cousins and Mazze, 1973). The resulting polyuria may result in dehydration, hypernatremia, and azotemia. In those who survive, recovery of renal function is usual, but it may take a year; mortality rates in such patients have been reported to be as high as 20%.

It is this complication that has curtailed the use of methoxyflurane. To avoid renal toxicity, the dose and duration must be limited. Justification of its use for analgesia in labor is based on intermittent administration of the agent immediately preceding each uterine contraction.

Biotransformation. Methoxyflurane is metabolized to a greater extent than any other inhalational agent (Sakai and Takaori, 1978). As much as 50 to 70% of the absorbed dose is metabolized in the liver to free fluoride, oxalic acid, difluoromethoxyacetic acid, and dichloroacetic acid. The first two substances, particularly fluoride, cause renal damage.

Two characteristics of methoxyflurane are responsible for this occurrence. The molecule, despite the ether bond, is more susceptible to metabolism than are the other halogenated methyl ethyl ethers. Probably of greater importance is the great propensity of methoxyflurane to diffuse into fatty tissues. The drug is released slowly from this reservoir and becomes available for biotransformation for many days. The peak concentration of free fluoride in the plasma is found on the second to fourth postanesthetic day. The concentration of fluoride that is achieved varies considerably. It is greater in obese subjects, in the elderly, and after induction of hepatic microsomal enzymes by drugs such as phenobarbital.

Evaluation. *Disadvantages and Limitations.* The potential renal toxicity of this agent dictates that it should not be used to achieve profound anesthesia nor for prolonged periods of time. Contraindications to its use include the presence of renal disease or the concomitant administration of drugs that induce hepatic enzymes or that are nephrotoxic. Respiratory and circulatory depression can be profound. Induction, maintenance, and adjustment of the depth of anesthesia are slow compared with halothane or enflurane.

Advantages and Uses. This agent was quite widely used for all types of anesthesia following its introduction into clinical practice in 1960. It is nonflammable, and it provides profound analgesia and good relaxation of skeletal muscles. Uterine contractions are not inhibited. Postoperative nausea and vomiting are not troublesome.

Status. As a result of its renal toxicity, the use of methoxyflurane as a general anesthetic is limited. It is valued mainly for its analgesic potency during labor, where intermittent administration of small doses does not result in sufficient accumulation of methoxyflurane or its metabolites to produce observable renal toxicity.

OTHER HALOGENATED ANESTHETICS

The search for improved general anesthetic agents has entailed the systematic synthesis and evaluation of a large number of halogenated compounds. Two such drugs that are presently undergoing clinical trials are worthy of mention.

Sevoflurane (fluoromethyl 2,2,2-trifluoro-1-[trifluoromethyl]ethyl ether) is a nonflammable, nonirritating agent with a MAC value of 1.7% and a blood:gas partition coefficient of 0.6 (Katoh and Ikeda, 1987). These properties result in a more rapid induction and termination of anesthesia with sevoflurane than are observed with the inhalational agents in current use. The circulatory and respiratory effects of sevoflurane resemble those of isoflurane. This agent is in clinical use in some countries, but evidence of instability in soda lime and of release of fluoride *in vivo* has delayed its approval in the United States.

Desflurane (I-653; difluoromethyl 1-fluoro 2,2,2-trifluoroethyl ether) is a nonflammable, nonirritating agent that is stable in soda lime; it has a MAC value of approximately 8 to 10% and a blood:gas partition coefficient of 0.42. Induction with this agent is smooth and rapid. The respiratory, hemodynamic, and electroencephalographic changes caused by desflurane are similar to those of isoflurane (Eger *et al.*, 1988; Weiskopf *et al.*, 1989).

NITROUS OXIDE

Chemistry and Physical Properties. *Nitrous oxide* (dinitrogen monoxide; N_2O) is a colorless gas without appreciable odor or taste. It is the only inorganic gas that is practical for clinical anesthesia. It is marketed in steel cylinders as a colorless liquid under pressure and in equilibrium with its gas phase. As it is released from the cylinder, some of the liquid nitrous oxide returns to the gaseous state; the pressure in the tank thus remains nearly constant until all the liquid has evaporated. The heat required for its vaporization is obtained from the walls of the cylinder and surrounding air, with the result that the tank becomes cold. Nitrous oxide is heavier than air. Although nitrous oxide is not flammable, it supports combustion as actively as does oxygen when it is present in proper concentration with a flammable anesthetic.

Nitrous oxide has relatively low solubility in blood, the blood:gas partition ratio at 37°C being 0.47. Other properties are listed in Table 14–1.

PHARMACOLOGICAL PROPERTIES

General Characteristics. Since Colton first administered nitrous oxide in 1844, it has passed through periods of greater or lesser popularity. It is currently used as an adjuvant during many procedures in which general anesthesia is employed.

Nitrous oxide can cause surgical anesthesia predictably only when administered under hyperbaric conditions. Paul Bert demonstrated this in 1879 by the use of 85% nitrous oxide in oxygen at 1.2 atmospheres in a pressure chamber. The MAC value is about 105%, but variability among individuals is considerable. Analgesia equivalent to that produced by morphine follows the inspiration of 20% nitrous oxide; some patients lose consciousness when breathing 30% nitrous oxide in oxygen, and most will become unconscious with 80%.

Nitrous oxide has been used as the sole anesthetic agent at inspired concentrations up to 80% and even beyond. In this situation the danger of hypoxia is obvious. The avoidance of hypoxic organ damage and the maintenance of satisfactory anesthesia for any but the briefest of procedures require maneuvering between very narrow limits, and this should no longer be attempted.

Another technique for the administration of nitrous oxide that has enjoyed considerable success includes induction of sleep by the intravenous administration of thiopental, accomplishment of skeletal muscle relaxation with neuromuscular blocking agents, and hyperventilation to reduce the arterial tension of carbon dioxide to approximately 25 mm Hg. It has been suggested that the total muscle paralysis and the absence of respiratory drive obtained with these maneuvers augment the analgesia provided by nitrous oxide. Conditions for surgery are excellent, organ functions are depressed minimally, and recovery is rapid. However, there have been several reports of recall by patients of events that occurred during this type of "anesthesia." The subjects are immobilized and unable to communicate and their unconsciousness cannot be assured without appropriate supplementation with potent inhalational agents or intravenous drugs such as opioids or benzodiazepines.

The value of nitrous oxide is as an adjuvant. In the presence of 70% nitrous oxide in oxygen, the concentration of potent inhalational agents can be reduced. Reductions of MAC values in these circumstances are from 0.75% to 0.29% for halothane, from 1.68% to 0.6% for enflurane, and from 1.15% to 0.5% for isoflurane. Smaller doses of the halogenated agents, combined with some nitrous oxide, result in less respiratory and circulatory depression and more rapid recovery.

The uptake and distribution of nitrous oxide are influenced in relatively unique ways by its physical properties (Eger, 1974). A normal adult breathing 70% nitrous oxide will achieve 90% equilibration in about 15 minutes. During this time, approximately 10 liters of nitrous oxide will have been absorbed from the alveolar gas into the body. This volume change is more than ten times that which occurs during the inhalation of 1% halothane. This large uptake of gas has two effects: the second-gas effect and the concentration effect (*see* Chapter 13). Clinically, the second-gas and concentration effects are useful during induction of anesthesia, since they increase the rapidity of uptake of a potent inhalational agent and also increase the alveolar concentration of oxygen, thus minimizing hypoxia. The reverse process occurs when the administration of nitrous oxide is discontinued (*see* Chapter 13). If air is abruptly substituted, the exchange of nitrous oxide from tissue and blood to alveolar gas results in a transient substantial decrease in the alveolar tension and, hence, the arterial tension of oxygen. This has been labeled *diffusional hypoxia* and can be a cause of postoperative hypoxemia, particularly when there also is respiratory depression following prolonged hyperventilation. Diffusional hypoxia has a limited time span, and adverse effects can be avoided by the administration of supplemental oxygen during the early recovery period.

Nitrous oxide exchanges with nitrogen whenever a nitrous oxide–containing mixture of gases is administered to a patient who had previously been breathing air. Since the blood : gas partition coefficient for nitrous oxide is 34 times that for nitrogen, a great deal more nitrous oxide is available for exchange. As a result, when nitrous oxide is administered, pockets of trapped gas in the body will expand as nitrogen leaves and is replaced by larger amounts of nitrous oxide. Such pockets may be found in an occluded middle ear, a pneumothorax, loops of intestine, lung, or renal cysts. Even air within the skull following a pneumoencephalogram is subject to expansion. This can result in large increases in pressure and volume, and nitrous oxide is thus best avoided in these circumstances.

Circulation. Nitrous oxide is generally employed as only one of several agents for general anesthesia. The potent inhalational agents have such marked effects on the cardiovascular system that the subtle influence of nitrous oxide may be easily overlooked.

When nitrous oxide is added to halothane in combined concentrations that do not alter the depth of anesthesia, the pupils dilate and the concentration of circulating norepinephrine increases. Under these conditions, arterial blood pressure, total peripheral vascular resistance, and cardiac output all rise (Hornbein *et al.*, 1969; Smith *et al.*, 1970). Increasing the depth of halothane anesthesia by the concurrent administration of nitrous oxide causes increased cerebral blood flow and decreased flow to the kidneys and splanchnic viscera without significant change in arterial pressure (Seyde *et al.*, 1986). Nitrous oxide depresses myocardial contractility *in vitro* but increases the responsiveness of vascular smooth muscle to epinephrine. The net effect of supplementation of halothane with nitrous oxide is a substantial reduction in the amount of halothane required to maintain anesthesia and, thus, less hypotension.

Supplementation of enflurane anesthesia with 70% nitrous oxide results in reduction of the concentration of enflurane that is required and in similar, but less marked, activation of the sympathetic nervous system (Smith *et al.*, 1978). Similarly, when nitrous oxide is administered with isoflurane, respiratory depression and systemic hypotension are less than with the same depth of anesthesia achieved with isoflurane alone. When combined with opioids, nitrous oxide causes only further circulatory depression.

Respiration. The effects of nitrous oxide on ventilatory drive are generally small. Slight or no depression of the response to carbon dioxide has been reported with 50% nitrous oxide; however, when nitrous oxide is added to other anesthetic agents, further depression is unequivocal (Hornbein *et al.*, 1969). The response to hypoxia is reduced when 50% nitrous oxide is given alone (Yacoub *et al.,* 1976).

The relatively nonspecific changes in respiratory function that may result in an increased difference between alveolar and arterial oxygen tension during general anesthesia reemphasize the importance of augmentation of the tension of inspired oxygen. However, continuous measurement of hemoglobin saturation with a pulse oximeter allows individual control of gas concentrations with safety.

Effects on Other Organs. Nitrous oxide does not exert adverse effects on the CNS. Cerebral blood flow remains responsive to carbon dioxide, and autoregulation continues as perfusion pressure changes in the presence of 70% nitrous oxide (Wollman *et al.,* 1965).

Skeletal muscle does not relax in the presence of 80% nitrous oxide, and blood flow to muscle does not change. Unlike the halogenated general anesthetics, nitrous oxide is most unlikely to trigger malignant hyperthermia.

The liver, kidneys, and gastrointestinal tract show no marked effects to nitrous oxide administration despite the changes in blood flow described previously, and there is no evidence of toxicity. Nausea or vomiting occurs postoperatively in approximately 15% of patients.

Methionine synthase, a vitamin B_{12}–dependent enzyme, is inactivated following very prolonged administration of nitrous oxide, and the subsequent interference with DNA synthesis prevents production of both leukocytes and red blood cells by bone marrow. These effects do not occur within the time frame of clinical surgery (Amess *et al.,* 1978). Oxidation of the cobalt atom in vitamin B_{12} by nitrous oxide can also cause megaloblastic changes in the bone marrow and a neuropathy in experimental animals (*see* Chapter 54). Although long-term inhalation of nitrous oxide has been used to treat pain, its value is limited by these side effects. Of more practical concern is the effect on operating-room personnel of long-term, low-dose exposure to the gas. As with halothane, there is little definitive evidence of adverse effects, although mild CNS depression is detectable at a concentration of 500 ppm. However, with simple procedures to prevent contamination, the atmosphere of an operating room should not contain more than 50 ppm of nitrous oxide. A neuropathy similar to that of vitamin B_{12} deficiency has been observed in dentists who use nitrous oxide as an anesthetic (Layzer, 1978).

Biotransformation. Nitrous oxide is rapidly and predominantly eliminated as such in the expired gas, and a little diffuses out through the skin. Sufficiently precise methods have not been found to determine to what extent biotransformation may occur.

Evaluation. *Disadvantages.* Nitrous oxide is a weak agent with no muscle relaxant activity, and attempts to provide adequate anesthesia may be accompanied by hypoxia if it is used alone. Transient postanesthetic hypoxia may also occur as large volumes of nitrous oxide are exhaled. Air pockets in closed spaces may expand in the abdomen, chest, and skull.

Advantages. Nitrous oxide is a nonflammable, nonirritating, and powerful analgesic agent; the onset of and recovery from its effects is very rapid, and it causes little or no toxicity during ordinary clinical use. Its principal application is as a supplement to other specific and/or potent agents, and this results in the use of smaller doses of the latter, shorter recovery time, and reduced likelihood of complications.

Status. As a sole agent, nitrous oxide is used intermittently to provide analgesia for dental procedures and during the first stage of parturition. In combination with other drugs, nitrous oxide is widely used for general anesthesia.

II. Intravenous Anesthetics

The requirements for general anesthesia and surgery may necessitate the administration of several intravenous drugs with different actions to ensure hypnosis, analgesia, relaxation, and control of visceral reflex responses. The use of intravenous drugs thus adds flexibility and permits the administration of lower doses of inhalational agents. Intravenous drugs are also frequently used to induce anesthesia rapidly.

In this section the special properties of barbiturates, benzodiazepines, opioids, and other agents that have utility in surgical procedures will be discussed. More detailed discussions of each class of drug and their uses in other circumstances are presented elsewhere (*see* Index).

BARBITURATES

A barbiturate with a duration of action appropriate to the requirements of surgery became available with the introduction of thiopental by Lundy in 1935. Its use during general anesthesia continues to exceed that of any other barbiturate.

Chemistry and Preparations. Thiopental is supplied for clinical use as the water-soluble sodium salt *thiopental sodium for injection* (PENTOTHAL). When thiopental sodium is diluted in sterile water, a 3.4% solution is isotonic; concentrations less than 2% may cause hemolysis. Other ultrashort-acting barbiturates include *methohexital sodium* (BREVITAL SODIUM) and *thiamylal sodium* (SURITAL).

PHARMACOLOGICAL PROPERTIES

Pharmacokinetics. Following a single intravenous anesthetic dose of thiopental sodium, unconsciousness occurs in 10 to 20 seconds (the time required for the drug to circulate from the arm to the brain). The depth of anesthesia may increase for up to 40 seconds and then decreases progressively until consciousness returns in 20 to 30 minutes. This sequence reflects the changes in concentration of thiopental at its sites of action in the brain and is a consequence of the initial distribution of the drug to the brain, followed by its subsequent redistribution to other tissues (plasma half-life is 3 minutes). This property is discussed fully in Chapters 1 and 17. At the time of awakening, the plasma concentration may be 10% of the peak value. When all tissues contain sufficient quantities of thiopental, redistribution does not result in such a precipitous drop of the concentrations in plasma, and the duration of action is prolonged. Thus, when too great a total quantity of thiopental is administered, recovery may require many hours (elimination half-time is 9 hours).

Thiopental is metabolized slowly in the liver, although this factor is not significant in limiting the duration of anesthesia except after excessive dosage. For methohexital, metabolic degradation may be of somewhat greater importance (Breimer, 1977). Other factors, such as the binding of thiopental by plasma proteins, change in the nonionized fraction of the drug following changes in blood pH, or changes in the distribution of blood flow, may also influence the depth of anesthesia, time of recovery, and duration of action.

General Anesthetic Action. The effects of barbiturates on the CNS are discussed in Chapter 17. The signs of anesthesia are not particularly characteristic; pupils are of small or normal size, eyeballs are fixed and usually central, eyelash and tendon reflexes are diminished, and respiration and circulation are somewhat depressed. However, thiopental and other barbiturates are poor analgesics and may even increase sensitivity to pain when administered in inadequate amounts. In these circumstances, evidence of sympathetic response becomes manifest with tachycardia, dilated pupils, tears, sweating, tachypnea, increased blood pressure, and movement or vocalization in response to surgery.

Respiration. Unlike some of the inhalational anesthetics, thiopental is not irritating to the respiratory tract, and yet coughing, laryngospasm, and even bronchospasm occur with some frequency. The basis of these reactions is unknown; they disappear as a deeper plane of anesthesia is established. The presence of saliva, the insertion of an airway, or partial obstruction by soft tissues may trigger one or all of these responses. Moderate doses of thiopental do not depress these airway reflexes.

Thiopental produces a dose-related depression of respiration that can be profound. Both the response to carbon dioxide and the response to hypoxia are reduced or even abolished (Hirshman *et al.,* 1975). Following a dose of thiopental sufficient to cause sleep, tidal volume is decreased, and, despite a small increase of respiratory rate, the minute volume is reduced; the functional residual capacity may be reduced, especially if coughing occurs (Bickler *et al.*, 1987); and the arterial tension of carbon dioxide rises slightly. Larger doses of thiopental cause more profound changes, and respiration is maintained only by movements of the diaphragm. Surgical manipulations provide a stimulus to respiration and, within limits, can offset the respiratory depression.

Circulation. In vivo, following the administration of an anesthetic dose of thiopental to a normal adult, the arterial blood pressure decreases only transiently and then returns essentially to normal. Cardiac output is usually decreased somewhat, but total peripheral vascular resistance is unchanged or increased. Blood flow to the skin and brain is decreased, but that to other organs remains essentially normal.

However, in the presence of hemorrhage or other form of hypovolemia, circulatory instability, sepsis, toxemia, or shock, the administration of a "normal" dose of thiopental may result in hypotension, circulatory collapse, and cardiac arrest. Thiopental or any other general anesthetic agent should be used very cautiously in patients with these conditions.

The baroreceptor system appears unaffected, but sympathetic nerve activity is reduced. Concentrations of catecholamines in plasma are not increased, and the heart is not sensitized to epinephrine. Arrhythmias are uncommon except in the presence of hypercarbia or arterial hypoxemia.

Cerebral blood flow and cerebral metabolic rate are reduced with thiopental and other barbiturates. Intracranial pressure is markedly reduced, and this effect is utilized clinically in anesthesia for neurosurgery or in other circumstances when elevated intracranial pressures are expected (Shapiro, 1975). Doses of thiopental sufficient to cause an isoelectric electroencephalogram protect the brain during ischemia (but not if cardiac arrest or head injury has already rendered the electroencephalogram isoelectric) (Michenfelder, 1986).

Other Organs. Relaxation of skeletal muscle is transient and occurs only at the onset of anesthesia. Thiopental has little effect on uterine contractions, but it does cross the placenta and depress the fetus. The functions of liver and kidney are depressed only with large doses, and then only transiently.

Clinical Use. Thiopental sodium is administered intravenously. It may be injected either as a single bolus, intermittently, or as a continuous infusion. The use of a continuous infusion increases the likelihood of overdosage, with a subsequent prolonged recovery period. For single or intermittent injections of thiopental sodium, the concentration employed should not exceed 2.5% in aqueous solution. Injections are most safely made into the side port of a flowing intravenous infusion of saline solution or 5% dextrose in water.

If concentrations greater than 2.5% are injected extravascularly, the pain may be severe and tissue necrosis can occur. Of even greater concern are the results of inadvertent intraarterial injection of concentrated solutions of thiopental. The arterial endothelium and deeper layers are immediately damaged and endarteritis follows, often with thrombosis exacerbated by subsequent arteriolar spasm. Vascular ischemia and even gangrene may result. Because damage to the arterial wall is instantaneous, the aim of treatment is to reduce the response and hence limit the lesion. If the infusion needle is still *in situ,* 5 to 10 ml of 1% procaine may serve to reduce the pain and the arteriospasm. Heparin may inhibit thrombosis, and a regional block of the sympathetic nerves may also induce arterial dilatation. Permanent and serious sequelae have not been reported to follow intraarterial injection of 2.5% solutions of thiopental and do not occur with 1% solutions of methohexital.

For induction of anesthesia in an adult patient, the usual procedure is to inject a 50-mg test dose moderately rapidly, observe the response, and then inject an additional 100 to 200 mg over 20 seconds. In a muscular, robust individual, as much as 500 mg may occasionally be necessary to induce general anesthesia. If the dose is injected too slowly, a stage of excitement may be encountered. Such excitatory movements are more common with methohexital. Conversely, if too much drug is injected too rapidly, profound anesthesia may supervene with apnea and hypotension. The usual response after a correctly chosen dose is for the patient to experience a faint taste of garlic, followed by a suppressed yawn and then the smooth, rapid appearance of sleep. There is an initial and transient period of relaxation, which may be appropriate for very short procedures such as correction of a dislocation, and the airway may become impaired by the infolding of soft tissues around the tongue and pharynx.

After this point the drugs to be used for maintenance of anesthesia can be administered. Most commonly, these will be an inhalational agent (with or without nitrous oxide), opioid analgesics, or muscle relaxants. For short procedures that are not especially painful, intermittent doses of thiopental combined with nitrous oxide are satisfactory, particularly if an analgesic was given preoperatively. A total dose of 1 g of thiopental should not generally be exceeded if prolonged recovery is to be avoided. The larger the initial dose of thiopental that is required, the larger the supplementary doses must be, even in patients of the same size. Patients who require a large initial dose of thiopental will awaken despite plasma concentrations that would normally cause sleep. Although the nature of this acute tolerance is obscure, it is important in its effects on total drug dosage.

Recovery following thiopental should be characterized by smooth, rapid awakening to consciousness. However, if there is postoperative pain, restlessness may become evident and analgesics should be given (an antianalgesic effect of thiopental at low circulating concentrations may be partially responsible). There is often shivering postoperatively as heat is generated to restore body temperature that has decreased during anesthesia and surgery. Postural hypotension may be encountered, and patients should not be moved too hurriedly.

Evaluation. *Disadvantages.* Most of the complications associated with the use of thiopental are minor and can be avoided or minimized by judicious use of the drug. Extravenous or intraarterial injection should be uncommon and, if concentrations no greater than 2.5% are used, are unlikely to cause serious damage. Cough, laryngospasm, and bronchospasm can be serious in certain patients, such as those with elevated intracranial pressure, penetrating injuries of the eye, pharyngeal infections, unstable aneurysms, or asthma. In each such case, adequate anesthesia should be ensured prior to stimulation of the airway.

Overdosage can occur if the specific requirements for each patient are not estimated correctly. There is no effective agent to antagonize the actions of the barbiturates. Hexobarbital and methohexital both cause a higher incidence of motor movements during induction of anesthesia.

The presence of variegate porphyria (South African) or acute intermittent porphyria constitutes an absolute contraindication to the use of barbiturates. In these two forms of porphyria, thiopental or other barbiturates may precipitate a widespread demyelination of peripheral and cranial nerves and disseminated lesions throughout the CNS, resulting in pain, weakness, and paralysis that may be life threatening. Other types of porphyria do not contraindicate the use of barbiturates; this has been a point of confusion.

Advantages. The outstanding advantages of thiopental are rapid, pleasant induction of anesthesia and fast recovery therefrom, with little postanesthetic excitement or vomiting. The use of methohexital is associated with even more rapid recovery of consciousness. These drugs may be given to induce anesthesia prior to administration of another agent, or they can be used alone to provide anesthesia for short procedures that are associated with little pain. They are useful to promote light sleep during regional local anesthesia and for quieting excitement or controlling convulsions.

Status. The ultrashort-acting barbiturates have an important place in the practice of anesthesiology. Thiopental sodium remains the standard for comparison. Thiamylal is very similar; methohexital is more potent and has a somewhat shorter duration of effect. General anesthesia is most often initiated by an injection of thiopental to induce sleep prior to administration of the agents that are necessary for the surgical procedure.

BENZODIAZEPINES

Benzodiazepines were first introduced for the treatment of anxiety, and a large number of these compounds with sedative, antianxiety, anticonvulsant, and muscle relaxant properties have now been synthesized (*see* Chapters 17, 18, 19, and 20). Hypnosis and unconsciousness may be produced with large doses of benzodiazepines, and diazepam, lorazepam, and midazolam have become widely used for preanesthetic medication and to supplement or to induce and maintain anesthesia.

Preparations. *Diazepam* (VALIUM) is insoluble in water and is supplied for injection in a solution of 5 mg of diazepam per milliliter of organic solvents; it should not be diluted. The solution is injected intravenously into the side port of a running intravenous infusion to minimize a burning sensation on injection and the possibility of venous thrombosis. *Lorazepam* (ATIVAN) is supplied at a concentration of 2 or 4 mg/ml of organic solvent for injection; this preparation should be diluted with an equal volume of a compatible solution immediately before intravenous administration. Lorazepam is somewhat less irritating than diazepam, but the same precautions should be observed during injection.

Midazolam (VERSED) is supplied as the hydrochloride at concentrations of 1 and 5 mg/ml. All three drugs can also be given intravenously. Midazolam and lorazepam are about three times more potent than diazepam. Otherwise, their pharmacological properties are similar.

PHARMACOLOGICAL PROPERTIES

Diazepam is discussed as the prototype, and the properties of lorazepam and midazolam are compared where appropriate.

Pharmacokinetics. Following an intravenous injection of 0.1 to 1 mg/kg of diazepam, the drug is rapidly distributed to the brain, but, unlike with thiopental, several minutes pass before the onset of drowsiness. The concentration in plasma declines rapidly owing to redistribution, with an initial half-time of 10 to 15 minutes; however, drowsiness often returns with an increased concentration of diazepam in plasma after 6 to 8 hours. This effect is probably due to absorption from the gastrointestinal tract after excretion in the bile. The onset of drowsiness is slightly less rapid after administration of lorazepam and is slightly more rapid with midazolam; the half-time of redistribution of lorazepam is more than twice that of diazepam. Midazolam and its active metabolite α-hydroxymidazolam are eliminated with half-lives of about 3 hours. Additional information is given in Chapter 17 and Appendix II.

General Anesthetic Action. *Central Nervous System.* The effects of the benzodiazepines on the CNS are described in detail in Chapters 17, 18, 19, and 20. In the doses used to supplement or induce anesthesia, these drugs cause sedation, reduction of anxiety, and amnesia in 50% or more of patients. The amnesia may last up to 6 hours and is characteristically antegrade, with little or no retrograde effect. CNS depression induced by benzodiazepines is partially antagonized by physostigmine (2 mg intravenously), probably owing to inhibition of acetylcholinesterase. If physostigmine is used for this purpose, atropine (1 mg intravenously) should be given to prevent excessive salivation, abdominal cramps, nausea, and vomiting. If the dose of diazepam is very large, the CNS depression may return as physostigmine is eliminated. The administration of aminophylline (1 to 2 mg/kg) can also antagonize CNS depression induced by benzodiazepines. However, both these approaches will probably become obsolete when the specific benzodiazepine antagonist flumazenil is released for general use (White *et al.,* 1989; *see also* Chapter 17).

Circulation and Respiration. By themselves, the benzodiazepines cause only moderate depression of the circulation and respiration. Large doses may cause a 15 to 20% decline in systemic blood pressure and vascular resistance. Changes in heart rate vary from a mild decrease to a moderate increase. If tachycardia occurs, it may compensate for a small decrease in stroke volume and thus limit the modest tendency toward reduction in cardiac output. Stability of the cardiovascular system has encouraged the use of these drugs for anesthesia in patients with cardiac impairment (particularly for diagnostic procedures) (Samuelson *et al.,* 1981). Benzodiazepines are not analgesics, nor can they produce a state of surgical anesthesia when used alone. It is thus necessary to combine several drugs to achieve surgical levels of anesthesia with a balance of sedation, analgesia, amnesia, relaxation, and freedom from reflex stimulation. When opioids are given concurrently with benzodiazepines, the combination may produce severe cardiovascular depression, probably as a result of a sympatholytic action. The same considerations apply to the respiratory effects of benzodiazepines, which are minimal by themselves but in combination with opioids may result in severe and prolonged depression of the respiratory response to hypoxia and to carbon dioxide (Forster *et al.,* 1980; Gross *et al.,* 1983). Transient apnea may follow the rapid injection of diazepam, and facilities for the support of respiration should always be available.

Other Organs. Diazepam neither causes emesis nor prevents it and has little effect on renal, hepatic, or reproductive functions. Although the drug induces relaxation of spastic muscle, which is centrally mediated, it has no effect on the neuromuscular junction and does not enhance or antagonize the actions of specific muscle relaxants. Diazepam crosses the placenta readily and can depress the fetus.

Use in Anesthesia. Diazepam (5 to 10 mg) may be administered orally, intramuscularly, or intravenously for preanesthetic medication about an hour before the patient is transported to the operating area. Benzodiazepines are useful as the sole agent for procedures that do not require analgesia, such as endoscopy, cardioversion, cardiac catheterization, and a spectrum of radiodiagnostic procedures. For induction of anesthesia, the benzodiazepines are given intravenously. However, it is important that the injection be given slowly and that the rate of administration not be so rapid that an excessive dose is given during the period of delayed onset of action. A total dose of 0.6 mg/kg of diazepam administered to an adult will usually result in a sequence of drowsiness, amnesia, and, finally, unconsciousness. Induction with midazolam or lorazepam is similar but requires approximately one third to one half the dose necessary for diazepam. A special application for the benzodiazepines is the control and prevention of seizures induced by local anesthetics during regional techniques. Benzodiazepines are also frequently employed as part of a technique of balanced anesthesia, combined with thiopental for rapid induction, muscle relaxants, analgesics, and, often, an inhalational anesthetic agent. Such a technique has the advantage of requiring a reduced dose of each drug while providing rapid and more precise control of side effects.

Status. The benzodiazepines are useful for their contribution to preanesthetic medication and to induction and maintenance of anesthesia. Midazolam is available as a water-soluble salt, and its injection is neither painful nor irritating. Furthermore, the onset of action of midazolam is shorter, its potency is greater, and its metabolic elimination is more rapid than that of diazepam; thus, it is preferred for induction and maintenance of anesthesia. Lorazepam is useful when antegrade amnesia is particularly desirable.

ETOMIDATE

Etomidate is a potent hypnotic agent without analgesic properties. It is supplied for injection in a solution containing 2 mg/ml (AMIDATE).

An intravenous injection of 0.3 mg/kg of etomidate to an adult patient will induce sleep that lasts for approximately 5 minutes. Cardiovascular and respiratory depression do not usually occur, although hypotension and carbon dioxide retention can happen occasionally. Involuntary muscle movements are a frequent occurrence and necessitate the administration of other drugs, such as diazepam. The induction of anesthesia with etomidate is usually followed by the administration of analgesic and muscle relaxant drugs and/or potent inhalational anesthetic agents. Nausea and vomiting are common during the recovery period, particularly when opioids have been used. Etomidate can inhibit adrenal steroidogenesis; concentrations of cortisol in plasma may be lowered even after a single injection of the drug, and increased mortality has been observed when etomidate was used for prolonged sedation of critically ill patients (Wagner *et al.*, 1984).

OPIOID ANALGESICS

The detailed pharmacology of the opioids is discussed in Chapter 21. Morphine, meperidine, fentanyl, sufentanil, alfentanil, or other analgesics are frequently employed as supplements during general anesthesia with inhalational or intravenous agents (Kitahata and Collins, 1982). For this purpose, intravenous doses of 1 to 2 mg of morphine, 10 to 25 mg of meperidine, 0.05 to 0.1 mg of fentanyl, 0.005 to 0.01 mg of sufentanil, and 0.15 to 0.3 mg of alfentanil are approximately equivalent and may provide analgesia for about 90, 45, 30, 15, and 20 minutes, respectively. Respiratory depression, mild decreases in blood pressure, some delay in awakening, and an appreciable incidence of postoperative nausea or vomiting accompany the use of these drugs.

In some situations, very large doses of opioids may be infused to obtain anesthesia. Morphine given slowly intravenously in doses of 1 to 3 mg/kg over 15 to 20 minutes induces analgesia and unconsciousness. Respiratory depression is severe, and ventilation must be mechanically controlled, often for extended periods of time. The addition of nitrous oxide adds further to the anesthesia, and administration of competitive skeletal muscle relaxants provides good conditions for surgery. It is perhaps unexpected that the cardiovascular system is not severely depressed with such large doses of morphine. Lowenstein and associates (1969) showed that patients with normal cardiac function experienced no significant changes, while an increase in cardiac output and stroke volume and a decrease in total peripheral resistance often occur in patients with cardiac disease. Blood flow to organs is maintained. For example, autoregulation of the cerebral circulation is unimpaired even at the higher dose range (3 mg/kg); similarly, renal function is well maintained.

The morphine–nitrous oxide technique has been used quite widely for cardiac surgery. Despite the large doses of morphine, some patients are evidently not sufficiently anesthetized and may become hypertensive during surgery; postoperative recall of events as a terrifying dream or psychosis may also occur.

When large doses of fentanyl (50 to 100 μg/kg) are administered slowly intravenously, profound analgesia and unconsciousness are induced. While this state is similar to that caused by morphine, the incidence of incomplete amnesia, hypotension, and hypertension is less than that associated with morphine; the duration of respiratory depression is also shorter. For these reasons, fentanyl and its newer congeners have largely replaced morphine for anesthesia; they are used particularly during cardiac surgery, usually combined with muscle relaxants and nitrous oxide or small doses of other inhalational anesthetics. Rigidity of respiratory muscles may be prominent during induction of anesthesia with large doses of opioids, and administration of a muscle relaxant may be necessary to permit artificial ventilation.

Following intravenous administration of fentanyl, the onset of action is within one circulation time. The drug is rapidly redistributed, and the duration of action is approximately 30 minutes. However, accumulation of fentanyl occurs with repeated administration or following injection of large doses, leading to a prolonged duration of sedation and respiratory depression. Fentanyl is metabolized by the liver and is eliminated with a half-life of 3.5 hours, but there is considerable variability and individual titration is essential to achieve the desired effect.

Alfentanil and sufentanil are newer and more potent opioid analgesics. *Alfentanil* (ALFENTA) has one third to one fourth the potency of fentanyl, and its duration of action is shorter by two thirds. *Sufentanil* (SUFENTA) has a potency about ten times that of fentanyl, and its duration of action is about one half as long, even after administration of large doses. These drugs can induce profound analgesia and, in sufficient doses, anesthesia; cardiovascular stability is impressive.

Status. Opioid analgesics are widely used to provide relief from pain during general anesthesia of all types. Judicious use of these agents intravenously can provide analgesia of rapid onset and appropriate duration; smaller doses of general anesthetics are then required. When large or repeated doses of opioids are administered for general anesthesia, sedation and respiratory depression can be prolonged and mechanical ventilation may be necessary. These effects can be reversed by the use of specific opioid antagonists (*see* Chapter 21). Small doses (increments of 0.05 to 0.2 mg) of naloxone may be repeated until the desired reversal is achieved; careful titration will prevent precipitous awakening and return of discomfort. The duration of action of naloxone is 60 to 90 minutes, and the patient must remain under close observation for recurrence of respiratory depression. Naltrexone and certain investigational opioid antagonists have a longer duration of action. Some practitioners prefer to employ the mixed opioid agonist–antagonists nalbuphine or butorphanol for anesthetic uses. Epidural and intrathecal opioid analgesia are discussed in Chapter 15.

NEUROLEPTIC–OPIOID COMBINATIONS

Neuroleptic compounds, such as the butyrophenone derivative *droperidol* (INAPSINE), produce a state of quiescence with reduced motor activity, reduced anxiety, and indifference to the surroundings. Sleep is not necessarily induced, and patients are responsive to commands. In addition to inducing neurolepsis, droperidol has adrenergic-blocking, antiemetic, antifibrillatory, and anticonvulsant actions, and it enhances the effects of other CNS depressants.

When a potent opioid analgesic such as fentanyl citrate is combined with droperidol, a state of neurolept analgesia is established, during which a variety of diagnostic or minor surgical procedures can be accomplished; these include endoscopy, radiological studies, burn dressings, and the like. Neurolept analgesia can be converted to neurolept anesthesia by the concurrent administration of 65% nitrous oxide in oxygen.

Clinical Use. Droperidol and fentanyl citrate may be used alone or together, the dose of each being adjusted individually, but most often a precompounded mixture (INNOVAR) is used. Each milliliter of this preparation contains 0.05 mg of fentanyl as the citrate salt and 2.5 mg of droperidol.

A useful technique for adults is to mix a dose of 0.1 ml/kg of INNOVAR in 250 ml of 5% dextrose in water and to infuse this solution intravenously over a period of 5 to 10 minutes. If the rate of infusion is too slow, delirium and excitement may occur, sometimes with laryngospasm. If the rate is too rapid, spasm of the chest wall may supervene, and respiratory exchange can become impossible, even by artificial means. This untoward response is easily managed by the intravenous administration of a rapidly acting neuromuscular blocking agent, such as succinylcholine. Normally, after approximately 3 to 4 minutes, the recipient appears to fall asleep and may cease to breathe, except on command. Should an endotracheal tube be required to ensure adequate ventilation, a smaller dose of the combination will suffice if the larynx and trachea are anesthetized by the topical application of a local anesthetic.

Circulatory effects of neurolept anesthesia are not generally marked. Droperidol has a slight α-adrenergic–blocking action that results in moderate hypotension. A parasympathomimetic effect of fentanyl accounts for bradycardia; administration of atropine will prevent this response. Cerebral blood flow and cerebral metabolism are not altered in human subjects, and elevated intracranial pressure may be reduced, provided that the arterial tension of carbon dioxide does not increase when respiration is depressed. Care should be taken to avoid abrupt changes in posture, since severe hypotension may be precipitated. Other than bradycardia, cardiac arrhythmias are rare, and the heart is not sensitized to the effects of epinephrine.

In contrast to the circulatory effects, respiratory depression is marked (Dunbar *et al.*, 1967). Assisted or controlled ventilation is necessary, and respiration of an oxygen-enriched gas mixture is desirable.

Droperidol has a prolonged duration of action (3 to 6 hours), whereas fentanyl exerts its analgesic effect for only about 30 minutes. Following induction of neurolept anesthesia, supplementary doses of fentanyl alone (1 μg/kg) are injected at intervals of approximately 20 minutes. Indications for additional doses include evidence of sympathetic activity with increasing pulse rate and blood pressure, sweating, and limb movements.

Recovery. Consciousness is recovered rapidly after the administration of nitrous oxide is stopped, but patients remain free from pain and drowsy, although arousable. Nausea or vomiting occurs in 5 to 10% of patients; confusion and a depressed mental state may become apparent.

Respiratory depression may persist into the postoperative period and can last 3 to 4 hours (Harper *et al.*, 1976). The opioid antagonist naloxone can reverse this respiratory depression (*see* above).

A side effect of droperidol is the occurrence of extrapyramidal muscle movements. Approximately 1% of patients receiving droperidol exhibit this side effect, which is sometimes delayed for 12 hours after the termination of anesthesia. The movements are self-limited and can be controlled with atropine or benztropine. Neurolept analgesia should not be used for patients with Parkinson's disease.

Status. Neurolept analgesia and neurolept anesthesia are safe and simple procedures, although induction of these states is slow. Circulatory changes are minimal unless the patient is hypovolemic or subjected to postural changes. Respiratory depression is severe but predictable. This is a useful technique in the elderly or the seriously ill or debilitated.

When neuromuscular blocking agents are also used, adequate conditions can be provided for all types of surgery, but the technique is generally not preferred over the use of potent inhalational agents for most types of major surgery. It has specialized uses for certain diagnostic procedures and for some types of peripheral operations.

DISSOCIATIVE ANESTHESIA

Some arylcycloalkylamines may induce a state of sedation, immobility, amnesia, and marked analgesia. The name *dissociative anesthesia* is derived from the strong feeling of dissociation from the environment that is experienced by the subject to whom such an agent is administered. This condition is similar to neurolept analgesia but results from the administration of a single drug (Winters *et al.*, 1972).

Phencyclidine was the first drug used for this purpose, but the frequent occurrence of unpleasant hallucinations and psychological problems soon led to its abandonment. These effects are much less frequent with *ketamine hydrochloride* (2-[*o*-chlorophenyl]-2-[methylamino] cyclohexanone hydrochloride; KETALAR).

Ketamine hydrochloride is supplied in solution for intravenous or intramuscular use in vials containing 10, 50, or 100 mg of ketamine base per milliliter.

Clinical Use. For the induction of dissociative anesthesia in an adult, ketamine hydrochloride is administered in a dose of 1 to 3 mg/kg over a period of about 1 minute. (A similar induction follows the intramuscular injection of 6.5 to 13 mg/kg.) A sensation of dissociation is noticed within 15 seconds, and unconsciousness becomes apparent within another 30 seconds. Intense analgesia and amnesia are established rapidly. Following a single dose, unconsciousness lasts 10 to 15 minutes and analgesia persists for some 40 minutes; amnesia may be evident for a period of 1 to 2 hours following the initial injection. If anesthesia of longer duration is necessary, supplementary doses of about one half of the initial amount may be administered.

Muscle tone may be increased, purposeless movements sometimes occur, and violent and irrational responses to stimuli are occasionally observed. A soothing and quiet environment is necessary for success with this technique.

Hypoxic or hypercarbic stimulation of respiration is not seriously affected following usual doses of ketamine (Hirshman *et al.*, 1975). Pharyngeal and laryngeal reflexes are retained, and, although the cough reflex is depressed, airway obstruction does not normally occur. Airway resistance is in fact decreased, and bronchospasm may be abolished (Bovill *et al.*, 1971). Pulmonary vascular resistance is not altered, and ketamine does not inhibit hypoxic pulmonary vasoconstriction. Arterial blood pressure increases by as much as 25%, and cardiac output and rate increase. When myocardial tissue is exposed to ketamine *in vitro*, depression of contractility occurs. The stimulation observed *in vivo* is attributed to increased sympathetic activity. When ketamine is used to induce anesthesia in hypovolemic patients, hypotension may occur, but the incidence is less than when inhalational agents are used. Cerebral blood flow, metabolic rate, and intracranial pressure are augmented (Lassen and Christensen, 1976). Intraocular pressure is unaltered.

Recovery. Unlike the barbiturates, ketamine does not act primarily on the reticular activating system in the brainstem; rather, it is believed to act on receptors in the cortex and the limbic system (Reich and Silvay, 1989). Perhaps this is why recovery after ketamine has some unusual features. Awakening often requires several hours and is not infrequently characterized by disagreeable dreams and even hallucinations. Sometimes these unpleasant occurrences may recur days or weeks later. Almost half of adults over the age of 30 years exhibit delirium or excitement, or experience visual disturbances. The incidence of such adverse psychological experiences is much lower in children and young adults and can be reduced by the prior administration of a benzodiazepine, particularly midazolam.

Status. Given in conjunction with diazepam, ketamine provides satisfactory anesthesia for a variety of special purposes. This regimen is particularly useful for trauma and emergency surgical procedures, repeated changes of dressings, radiological procedures in children, and even some cardiac surgical procedures.

PROPOFOL

Propofol (2,6-diisopropylphenol; DIPRIVAN) is chemically unrelated to the other intravenous anesthetic agents. The compound is an oil at room temperature and is supplied as a 1% emulsion.

General Anesthetic Action. An intravenous injection of propofol (2 mg/kg) induces anesthesia as rapidly as does thiopental (Cummings *et al.*, 1984). Some pain may occur at the site of injection, but it is rarely followed by phlebitis or thrombosis. Anesthesia may be maintained by continuous infusion of propofol combined with opioids, nitrous oxide, and/or other inhalational agents.

Propofol decreases systemic arterial pressure by approximately 30%, but this effect is due more to peripheral vasodilatation than to decreased cardiac output (Monk *et al.*, 1987). The systemic pressure returns to normal with intubation of the trachea. Propofol does not appear to cause arrhythmias or myocardial ischemia.

Following induction of anesthesia with propofol, respiration is so depressed that apnea may occur for 30 seconds; tidal volume, minute volume, and functional residual capacity are all subsequently reduced, as is the respiratory response to carbon dioxide. All these effects are augmented by premedication with opioids (Gold *et al.*, 1987).

Propofol does not impair hepatic or renal function. Cerebral blood flow, cerebral metabolic rate, and intracranial pressure appear to be reduced. There have been some reports of seizures or involuntary movements during induction or emergence from propofol-induced anesthesia. Interactions of propofol with neuromuscular blocking agents are not apparent.

The emergence from anesthesia with propofol is more rapid than that from thiopental and is characterized by minimal postoperative confusion. The incidences of nausea, vomiting, and headache are similar to those observed with thiopental (Grounds *et al.*, 1985).

Status. Propofol is a new agent, and it is not yet available in the United States. The rapid induction of anesthesia and recovery therefrom (even after prolonged infusion) suggest that it will be valuable for ambulatory patients who are undergoing brief procedures and for sedation in intensive care units.

α_2-ADRENERGIC AGONISTS

Clonidine, an antihypertensive agent with sedative properties, was noted to reduce the dose requirement for anesthetic and analgesic drugs (Kaukinen and Pyykko, 1979). These actions are due to stimulation of α_2-adrenergic receptors in the CNS.

An oral dose of clonidine (200 to 300 μg) administered 90 minutes before surgery results in sedation and reduction in anxiety. The required dose of anesthetic (either opioids or potent inhalational agents) is reduced, and cardiovascular stability is improved. Clonidine also has analgesic activity; this action is not accompanied by respiratory depression and is not reversed by naloxone (Flacke *et al.*, 1987).

A series of highly selective, centrally acting α_2-adrenergic agonists are currently being developed; compounds include azepexole and dexmedetomidine (Doze *et al.*, 1989). These drugs not only markedly reduce the dose requirements of anesthetic agents but may be capable of inducing anesthesia by themselves.

Amess, J. A. L.; Burman, J. F.; Rees, G. M.; Nancekievill, D. G.; and Mollin, D. L. Megaloblastic hemopoiesis in patients receiving nitrous oxide. *Lancet*, **1978**, *2*, 339–341.

Atlee, J. L., and Rusy, B. F. Atrioventricular conduction times and atrioventricular nodal conductivity during enflurane anesthesia in dogs. *Anesthesiology*, **1977**, *47*, 498–503.

Benumof, J., and Wahrenbrock, E. A. Local effects of anesthetic on regional hypoxic pulmonary vasoconstriction. *Anesthesiology*, **1975**, *43*, 525–532.

Bickler, P. E.; Dueck, R.; and Prutow, R. J. Effects of barbiturate anesthesia on functional residual capacity and ribcage/diaphragm contributions to ventilation. *Anesthesiology*, **1987**, *66*, 147–152.

Bimar, J., and Bellville, J. W. Arousal reaction during anesthesia in man. *Anesthesiology*, **1977**, *47*, 449–454.

Bovill, J. G.; Clarke, R. S. J.; Davis, E. A.; and Dundee, J. W. Some cardiovascular effects of ketamine in man. *Br. J. Pharmacol.*, **1971**, *41*, 411P–412P.

Breimer, D. D. Clinical pharmacokinetics of hypnotics. *Clin. Pharmacokinet.*, **1977**, *2*, 93–109.

Buffington, C. W.; Davis, K. B.; Gillispie, S.; and Pettinger, M. The prevalence of steal-prone coronary anatomy in patients with coronary artery disease: an analysis of the coronary artery surgery study registry. *Anesthesiology*, **1988**, *69*, 721–727.

Carlsson, A. J.; Bindslev, L.; and Hedenstierna, G. Hypoxia-induced pulmonary vasoconstriction in the human lung: the effect of isoflurane anesthesia. *Anesthesiology*, **1987**, *66*, 312–316.

Carpenter, R. L.; Eger, E. I., II; Johnson, B. H.; Unadkat, J. D.; and Sheiner, L. B. The extent of metabolism of inhaled anesthetics in humans. *Anesthesiology*, **1986**, *65*, 201–205.

Clark, D. L., and Rosner, B. D. Neurophysiologic effects of general anesthetics. 1. The electroencephalogram and sensory evoked responses in man. *Anesthesiology*, **1973**, *38*, 564–582.

Clergue, F.; Viires, N.; Lemesle, P.; Aubier, M.; Viars, P.; and Pariente, R. Effect of halothane on diaphragmatic muscle function in pentobarbital-anesthetized dogs. *Anesthesiology*, **1986**, *64*, 181–187.

Cousins, M. J., and Mazze, R. I. Methoxyflurane nephrotoxicity: a study of dose-response in man. *J.A.M.A.*, **1973**, *225*, 1611–1616.

Cummings, G. C.; Dixon, J.; Kay, N. H.; Windsor, J. P. W.; Major, E.; Morgan, M.; Sear, J. W.; Spence, A. A.; and Stephenson, D. K. Dose requirements of ICI 35, 868 (propofol, DIPRIVAN) in a new formulation for induction of anaesthesia. *Anaesthesia*, **1984**, *39*, 1168–1171.

Deutsch, S.; Goldberg, M.; Stephens, G. M.; and Wu, W. H. Effects of halothane anesthesia on renal function in normal man. *Anesthesiology*, **1966**, *27*, 793–804.

Doze, V. A.; Chen, B. X.; and Maze, M. Dexmedetomidine produces a hypnotic-anesthetic action in rats via activation of central alpha$_2$-adrenoceptors. *Anesthesiology*, **1989**, *71*, 75–79.

Dueck, R.; Young, I.; Clauson, J.; and Wagner, P. D. Altered distribution of pulmonary ventilation and blood flow following induction of inhalational anesthesia. *Anesthesiology*, **1980**, *52*, 113–125.

Dunbar, B. S.; Ovassapian, A.; Dripps, R. D.; and Smith, T. C. The respiratory response to carbon dioxide during INNOVAR–nitrous oxide anaesthesia in man. *Br. J. Anaesth.*, **1967**, *39*, 861–866.

Eger, E. I., II; Johnson, B. H.; Weiskopf, R. B.; Holmes, M. A.; Yasuda, N.; Targ, A.; and Rampil, I. J. Minimum alveolar concentration of I-653 and isoflurane in pigs: definition of a supramaximal stimulus. *Anesth. Analg.*, **1988**, *67*, 1174–1176.

Eger, E. I., II; Smith, N. T.; Stoelting, R. K.; Cullen, D. J.; Kadis, L. B.; and Whitcher, C. E. Cardiovascular effects of halothane in man. *Anesthesiology*, **1970**, *32*, 396–409.

Eger, E. I., II; White, A.; Brown, C.; Biava, C.; Corbett, T.; and Steven, W. A test of carcinogenicity of enflurane, isoflurane, halothane, methoxyflurane, and nitrous oxide in mice. *Anesth. Analg.*, **1978**, *57*, 678–694.

Eintrei, C.; Leszniewski, W.; and Carlsson, C. Local application of ^{133}Xenon for measurement of regional cerebral blood flow (rCBF) during halothane, enflurane, and isoflurane anesthesia in humans. *Anesthesiology*, **1985**, *63*, 391–394.

Epstein, R. M.; Deutsch, S.; Cooperman, L. H.; Clement, A. J.; and Price, H. L. Splanchnic circulation during halothane anesthesia and hypercapnia in normal man. *Anesthesiology*, **1966**, *27*, 654–661.

Flacke, J. W.; Bloor, B. C.; Flacke, W. E.; Wong, D.; Dazza, S.; Stead, S. W.; and Laks, H. Reduced narcotic requirement by clonidine with improved hemodynamic and adrenergic stability in patients undergoing coronary bypass surgery. *Anesthesiology*, **1987**, *67*, 11–19.

Forbes, A. R. Halothane depresses mucociliary flow in the trachea. *Anesthesiology*, **1976**, *45*, 59–63.

Forster, A.; Gardaz, J. P.; Suter, P. M.; and Gemperle, M. Respiratory depression by midazolam and diazepam. *Anesthesiology*, **1980**, *53*, 494–497.

Gold, M. I.; Abraham, E. C.; and Herrington, C. A controlled investigation of propofol, thiopentone and methohexitone. *Can. J. Anaesth.*, **1987**, *34*, 478–483.

Göthert, M., and Wendt, J. Inhibition of adrenal medullary catecholamine secretion by enflurane. I. Investigations *in vivo*. *Anesthesiology*, **1977**, *46*, 400–403.

Gronert, G. A. Malignant hyperthermia. *Anesthesiology*, **1980**, *53*, 395–423.

Gross, J. B.; Zebrowski, M. E.; Carel, W. D.; Gardner, S.; and Smith, T. C. Time course of ventilatory depression after thiopental and midazolam in normal subjects and in patients with chronic obstructive pulmonary disease. *Anesthesiology*, **1983**, *59*, 46–50.

Grounds, R. M.; Twigley, A. O.; Carli, F.; Whitwam, J. G.; and Morgan, M. The hemodynamic effects of intravenous induction. *Anaesthesia*, **1985**, *40*, 735–740.

Harper, M. H.; Hickey, R. F.; Cromwell, T. H.; and Linwood, S. The magnitude and duration of respiratory depression produced by fentanyl and fentanyl plus droperidol in man. *J. Pharmacol. Exp. Ther.*, **1976**, *199*, 464–468.

Hirshman, C. A.; Edelstein, G.; Peetz, S.; Wayne, R.; and Downes, H. Mechanism of action of inhalational anesthesia on airways. *Anesthesiology*, **1982**, *56*, 107–111.

Hirshman, C. A.; McCullough, R. E.; Cohen, P. J.; and Weil, J. V. Hypoxic ventilatory drive in dogs during thiopental, ketamine or pentobarbital anesthesia. *Anesthesiology*, **1975**, *43*, 628–634.

———. Depression of hypoxic ventilatory response by halothane, enflurane and isoflurane in dogs. *Br. J. Anaesth.*, **1977**, *49*, 957–963.

Holaday, D. A.; Fiseroua-Bergerova, V.; Latto, I. P.; and Zumbiel, M. A. Resistance of isoflurane to biotransformation in man. *Anesthesiology*, **1975**, *43*, 325–332.

Horan, B. F.; Prys-Roberts, C.; Hamilton, W. K.; and Roberts, J. G. Haemodynamic responses to enflurane anaesthesia and hypovolaemia in the dog and their modification by propranolol. *Br. J. Anaesth.*, **1977**, *49*, 1189–1197.

Hornbein, T. F.; Martin, W. E.; Bonica, J. J.; Freund, F. G.; and Parmentier, P. Nitrous oxide effects on the circulatory and ventilatory responses to halothane. *Anesthesiology*, **1969**, *31*, 250–260.

Housmans, P. R., and Murat, I. Comparative effects of halothane, enflurane and isoflurane at equipotent anesthetic concentrations on isolated ventricular myocardia of the ferret. *Anesthesiology*, **1988**, *69*, 451–463.

Katoh, T., and Ikeda, K. The minimum alveolar concentration (MAC) of sevoflurane in humans. *Anesthesiology*, **1987**, *66*, 301–303.

Kaukinen, S., and Pyykko, K. The potentiation of halothane anaesthesia by clonidine. *Acta Anaesthesiol. Scand.*, **1979**, *23*, 107–111.

Knill, R. L., and Gelb, A. W. Ventilatory responses to hypoxia and hypercapnia during halothane sedation and anesthesia in man. *Anesthesiology*, **1978**, *49*, 244–251.

Lassen, N. A., and Christensen, M. S. Physiology of cerebral blood flow. *Br. J. Anaesth.*, **1976**, *48*, 719–734.

Laws, A. K. Effects of induction of anaesthesia and muscle paralysis on functional residual capacity of the lungs. *Can. Anaesth. Soc. J.*, **1968**, *15*, 325–331.

Layzer, R. B. Myeloneuropathy after prolonged exposure to nitrous oxide. *Lancet*, **1978**, *2*, 1227–1230.

Leighton, K., and Bruce, C. Distribution of kidney blood flow: a comparison of methoxyflurane and halothane effects as measured by heated thermocouple. *Can. Anaesth. Soc. J.*, **1975**, *22*, 125–137.

Lowenstein, E.; Hallowell, P.; Levine, F. H.; Daggett, W. M.; Austen, W. G.; and Laver, M. B. Cardiovascular response to large doses of intravenous morphine in man. *N. Engl. J. Med.*, **1969**, *281*, 1389–1393.

McPherson, R. W.; Brian, J. E.; and Traystman, R. J. Cerebrovascular responsiveness to carbon dioxide in dogs with 1.4% and 2.87% isoflurane. *Anesthesiology*, **1989**, *70*, 843–850.

Marshall, B. E.; Cohen, P. J.; Klingenmaier, C. H.; and Aukburg, S. Pulmonary venous admixture before, during and after halothane:oxygen anesthesia in man. *J. Appl. Physiol.*, **1969**, *27*, 653–657.

Marshall, B. E.; Cohen, P. J.; Klingenmaier, C. H.; Neigh, J. L.; and Pender, J. W. Some pulmonary and cardiovascular effects of enflurane (ETHRANE) anaesthesia with varying $PaCO_2$ in man. *Br. J. Anaesth.*, **1971**, *43*, 996–1002.

Maze, M.; Hayward, E.; and Gaba, D. M. Alpha-adrenergic blockade raises epinephrine-arrhythmias threshold in halothane-anesthetized dogs in a dose-dependent fashion. *Anesthesiology*, **1985**, *63*, 611–615.

Mazze, R. I.; Calverley, R. K.; and Smith, N. T. Inorganic fluoride nephrotoxicity: prolonged enflurane and halothane anesthesia in volunteers. *Anesthesiology*, **1977**, *46*, 265–271.

Mazze, R. I.; Schwartz, F. D.; Slocum, H. C.; and Barry, K. G. Renal function during anesthesia and surgery. I. The effects of halothane anesthesia. *Anesthesiology*, **1963**, *24*, 279–284.

Merin, R. G. Calcium channel blocking drugs and anesthetics: is the drug interaction beneficial or detrimental? *Anesthesiology*, **1987**, *66*, 111–113.

Merin, R. G.; Kumazawa, T.; and Luka, N. L. Enflurane depresses myocardial function, perfusion and metabolism in the dog. *Anesthesiology*, **1976**, *45*, 501–507.

Messick, J. M., Jr.; Casement, B.; Sharbrough, F. W.; Milde, L. N.; Michenfelder, J. D.; and Sundt, J. M., Jr. Correlation of regional anesthesia for carotid endarterectomy: critical rCBF. *Anesthesiology*, **1987**, *66*, 344–349.

Michenfelder, J. D. A valid demonstration of barbiturate-induced brain protection in man—at last. *Anesthesiology*, **1986**, *64*, 140–142.

Monk, C. R.; Coates, D. P.; Prys-Roberts, C.; Turtle, M. J.; and Spelina, K. Haemodynamic effects of a prolonged infusion of propofol as a supplement to nitrous oxide anaesthesia. *Br. J. Anaesth.*, **1987**, *599*, 954–960.

Newberg, L. A., and Michenfelder, J. D. Cerebral protection by isoflurane during hypoxemia or ischemia. *Anesthesiology*, **1983**, *59*, 29–35.

Perry, L. B.; VanDyke, R. A.; and Theye, R. A. Sympathoadrenal and hemodynamic effects of isoflurane, halothane, and cyclopropane in dogs. *Anesthesiology*, **1974**, *40*, 465–470.

Reich, D. L., and Silvay, G. Ketamine: an update on the first twenty-five years of clinical experience. *Can. J. Anaesth.*, **1989**, *36*, 186–197.

Reynolds, A. K.; Chiz, J. F.; and Pasquet, A. F. Halothane and methoxyflurane. A comparison of their effects on cardiac pacemaker fibers. *Anesthesiology*, **1970**, *33*, 602–610.

Rupp, S. M.; McChristian, J. W.; and Miller, R. D. Neuromuscular effects of atracurium during halothane, nitrous oxide and enflurane, nitrous oxide anesthesia on humans. *Anesthesiology*, **1985**, *63*, 16–19.

Rusy, B. F., and Komai, H. Anesthetic depression of myocardial contractility: a review of possible mechanisms. *Anesthesiology*, **1987**, *67*, 745–766.

Sakai, T., and Takaori, M. Biodegradation of halothane, enflurane, and methoxyflurane. *Br. J. Anaesth.*, **1978**, *50*, 785–791.

Samuelson, P. M.; Reves, J. G.; Kouchoukos, N. T.; Smith, L. R.; and Dole, K. M. Hemodynamic responses to anesthetic induction with midazolam or diazepam in patients with ischemic heart disease. *Anesth. Analg.*, **1981**, *60*, 802–809.

Seyde, W. C.; Ellis, J. E.; and Longnecker, D. E. The addition of nitrous oxide to halothane decreases renal and splanchnic flow and increases cerebral blood flow in rats. *Br. J. Anaesth.*, **1986**, *58*, 63–68.

Seyde, W. C., and Longnecker, D. E. Anesthetic influences on regional hemodynamics in normal and hemorrhaged rats. *Anesthesiology*, **1984**, *61*, 686–698.

Shapiro, H. M. Intracranial hypertension: therapeutic and anesthetic considerations. *Anesthesiology*, **1975**, *43*, 445–471.

Shimoji, K.; Matsuki, M.; Shimizu, H.; Maruyama, Y.; and Aida, S. Dishabituation of mesencephalic reticular neurons by anesthetics. *Anesthesiology*, **1977**, *47*, 349–352.

Shimosato, S.; Sugai, N.; Iwatsuki, N.; and Etsten, B. E. The effect of ETHRANE on cardiac muscle mechanics. *Anesthesiology*, **1969**, *30*, 513–518.

Skovsted, P., and Price, H. L. The effects of ETHRANE on arterial pressure, preganglionic sympathetic activity and barostatic reflexes. *Anesthesiology*, **1972**, *36*, 257–262.

Skovsted, P.; Price, M. L.; and Price, H. L. The effects of halothane on arterial pressure, preganglionic sympathetic activity, and barostatic reflexes. *Anesthesiology*, **1969**, *31*, 507–514.

Smith, N. T.; Calverley, R. K.; Prys-Roberts, C.; Eger, E. I., II; and Jones, C. W. Impact of nitrous oxide on the circulation during enflurane anesthesia in man. *Anesthesiology*, **1978**, *48*, 345–349.

Smith, N. T.; Eger, E. I., II; Stoelting, R. K.; Whayne, T. F.; Cullen, D.; and Kadis, L. B. The cardiovascular and sympathomimetic responses to the addition of nitrous oxide to halothane in man. *Anesthesiology*, **1970**, *32*, 410–421.

Sonntag, H.; Donath, U.; Hillebrand, W.; Merin, R. G.; and Radke, J. Left ventricular function in conscious man and during halothane anesthesia. *Anesthesiology*, **1978**, *48*, 320–324.

Stevens, W. C.; Cromwell, T. H.; Halsey, M. J.; Eger, E. I., II; Shakespeare, T. F.; and Bahlman, S. H. The cardiovascular effects of a new inhalation anesthetic, FORANE, in human volunteers at constant arterial carbon dioxide tension. *Anesthesiology*, **1971**, *35*, 8–16.

Stock, J. G. L., and Strunin, L. Unexplained hepatitis following halothane. *Anesthesiology*, **1985**, *63*, 424–439.

Stone, D. J., and Johns, R. A. Endothelium-dependent effects of halothane, enflurane and isoflurane on isolated rat aortic vascular rings. *Anesthesiology*, **1989**, *71*, 126–132.

Summary of the National Halothane Study. *J.A.M.A.*, **1966**, *197*, 775–788.

Tabatabai, M.; Kitahata, L. M.; Yuge, O.; Matsumoto, M.; and Collins, J. G. Effect of halothane on medullary inspiratory neurons of the cat. *Anesthesiology*, **1987**, *66*, 176–180.

Tusiewicz, K.; Bryan, A. C.; and Froese, A. B. Contributions of changing rib cage–diaphragm interactions to the ventilatory depression of halothane anesthesia. *Anesthesiology*, **1977**, *47*, 327–337.

Vessey, M. P. Epidemiological studies of the occupational hazards of anaesthesia—a review. *Anaesthesia*, **1978**, *33*, 430–438.

Wagner, R. L.; White, P. F.; Kan, P. B.; Rosenthal, M. H.; and Feldman, D. Inhibition of adrenal steroidogenesis by the anesthetic etomidate. *N. Engl. J. Med.*, **1984**, *310*, 1415–1421.

Walker, J. A.; Eggers, G. W. N.; and Allen, C. R. Cardiovascular effects of methoxyflurane anesthesia in man. *Anesthesiology*, **1962**, *23*, 639–642.

Warner, D. S.; Boarin, D. J.; and Kassell, N. F. Cerebrovascular adaptation to prolonged halothane anesthesia is not related to cerebrospinal fluid pH. *Anesthesiology*, **1985**, *63*, 243–248.

Weiskopf, R. B.; Eger, E. I., II; Holmes, M. A.; Rampil, I. J.; Johnson, B.; Brown, J. G.; Yasuda, N.; and Targ, A. G. Epinephrine-induced premature ventricular contractions and changes in arterial blood pressure and heart rate during I-653, isoflurane and halothane. *Anesthesiology*, **1989**, *70*, 293–298.

White, P. F.; Shafer, A.; Boyle, W. A., III; Doze, V. A.; and Duncan, S. Benzodiazepine antagonism does not provoke a stress response. *Anesthesiology*, **1989**, *70*, 636–639.

Winters, W. D.; Ferrer-Allado, T.; and Guzman-Flores, C. The cataleptic state induced by ketamine: a review of the neuropharmacology of anesthesia. *Neuropharmacology*, **1972**, *11*, 303–315.

Wollman, H.; Alexander, S. C.; Cohen, P. J.; Smith, T. C.; Chase, P. E.; and van der Molen, R. A. Cerebral circulation during general anesthesia and hyperventilation in man. Thiopental induction to nitrous oxide and *d*-tubocurarine. *Anesthesiology*, **1965**, *26*, 329–334.

Yacoub, O.; Doell, D.; Kryger, M. H.; and Anthonisen, N. R. Depression of hypoxic ventilatory response by nitrous oxide. *Anesthesiology*, **1976**, *45*, 385–389.

Monographs and Reviews

Eger, E. I., II. *Anesthetic Uptake and Action*. The Williams & Wilkins Co., Baltimore, **1974.**

Kitahata, L. M., and Collins, J. G. *Narcotic Analgesics in Anesthesiology*. The Williams & Wilkins Co., Baltimore, **1982.**

Levy, W. J. Central nervous system monitoring. In, *Cardiac Anesthesia*, 2nd ed. (Kaplan, J. A., ed.) Grune and Stratton, Inc., New York, **1987**, pp. 319–338.

Marshall, B. E., and Marshall, C. Anesthesia and pulmonary circulation. In, *Effects of Anesthesia*. (Covino, B. G.; Fozzard, H. A.; Rehder, K.; and Strichartz, G. S.; eds.) American Physiological Society, Bethesda, Md., **1985**, pp. 121–136.

Pavlin, E. G., and Hornbein, T. F. Anesthesia and the control of ventilation. In, *The Respiratory System*, Vol. 2., Sect. 3, *Handbook of Physiology*. (Cherniak, N. S., and Widdicombe, J. G., eds.) American Physiological Society, Bethesda, Md., **1986**, pp. 793–813.

Waud, B. E. Neuromuscular blocking agents. In, *Current Problems in Anesthesia and Critical Care Medicine*, Vol. 4. (Brunner, E. A., ed.) Year Book Medical Publishers, Inc., Chicago, **1977**, pp. 5–47.

CHAPTER 15 LOCAL ANESTHETICS

J. Murdoch Ritchie and Nicholas M. Greene

GENERAL PHARMACOLOGY OF LOCAL ANESTHETICS

Local anesthetics are drugs that block nerve conduction when applied locally to nerve tissue in appropriate concentrations. They act on any part of the nervous system and on every type of nerve fiber. Thus, a local anesthetic in contact with a nerve trunk can cause both sensory and motor paralysis in the area innervated. The necessary practical advantage of the compounds that are termed local anesthetics is that their action is reversible; their use is followed by complete recovery in nerve function with no evidence of structural damage to nerve fibers or cells.

History. The first local anesthetic to be discovered was cocaine, an alkaloid contained in large amounts (0.6 to 1.8%) in the leaves of *Erythroxylon coca,* a shrub growing in the Andes Mountains 1000 to 3000 m above sea level. Vast quantities of these leaves are consumed annually by about 2 million inhabitants of the highlands of Peru, who chew or suck the leaves primed with plant ash for the sense of well-being it produces. The plant ash is alkaline and thereby releases the alkaloid in a form that can be absorbed across the mucous membranes of the mouth.

The pure alkaloid was first isolated in 1860 by Niemann, who noted that it had a bitter taste and produced a peculiar effect on the tongue, making it numb and almost devoid of sensation. Von Anrep in 1880 observed that the skin became insensitive to the prick of a pin when cocaine was infiltrated subcutaneously. He recommended that the alkaloid be used clinically as a local anesthetic. His suggestion, however, was not acted upon. The clinical use of cocaine was in fact initiated by two young Viennese physicians, Sigmund Freud and Karl Koller. In 1884, Freud made a general study of the physiological effects of cocaine (*see* Byck, 1987; Vandam, 1987). He was particularly impressed by the central actions of the drug and used it to wean one of his colleagues from morphine. He was successful in this attempt, but at the cost of producing one of the first-known cocaine addicts of modern times. Koller quickly appreciated that the anesthetizing properties of cocaine had great practical importance and soon introduced cocaine into ophthalmology as a local anesthetic. Within a short time, Hall in 1884 introduced local anesthesia into dentistry, and the next year Halsted, by demonstrating that cocaine could stop transmission in nerve trunks, laid the foundation for nerve block anesthesia in surgery. Corning in 1885 produced spinal anesthesia in dogs, but several years passed before his technique was employed in clinical surgery.

A chemical search for synthetic substitutes for cocaine started in 1892 with the work of Einhorn and his colleagues. This resulted in 1905 in the synthesis of procaine, which became the prototype for local anesthetic drugs for nearly half a century. The most widely used agents today are lidocaine, bupivacaine, and tetracaine.

Properties Desirable in Local Anesthetics. A good local anesthetic should combine several properties. It should not be irritating to the tissue to which it is applied, nor should it cause any permanent damage to nerve structure. Its systemic toxicity should be low because it is eventually absorbed from its site of application. The ideal local anesthetic must be effective regardless of whether it is injected into the tissue or applied locally to mucous membranes. It is usually important that the time required for the onset of anesthesia should be as short as possible. Furthermore, the action must last long enough to allow time for the contemplated surgery, yet not so long as to entail an extended period of recovery. Occasionally, a local anesthetic action lasting for days or even weeks or months is desirable, for example, in the control of chronic pain. Unfortunately, the available compounds employed for anesthesia of such long duration have high local toxicity. Neurolysis with slough and necrosis of surrounding tissues occur, and partial or complete transverse injury of the spinal cord with permanent paralysis may result if such a reaction occurs in the vicinity of the cord.

GENERAL PROPERTIES

The local anesthetics have many actions in common, and before discussing the pharmacology of the individual drugs these general properties will be considered. (For reviews, *see* Roth and Miller, 1986; Strichartz, 1987.)

Chemistry and Structure–Activity Relationship. Table 15–1 shows that the structure of typical anes-

Table 15–1. STRUCTURAL FORMULAS OF SELECTED LOCAL ANESTHETICS

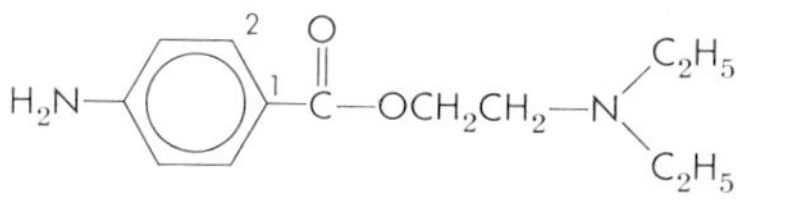

Procaine *

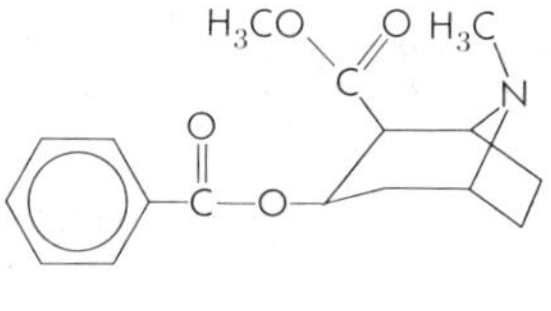

Cocaine

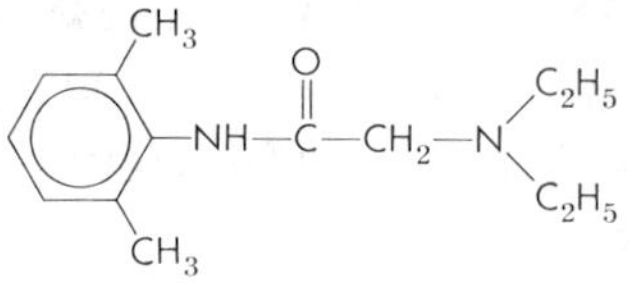

Lidocaine

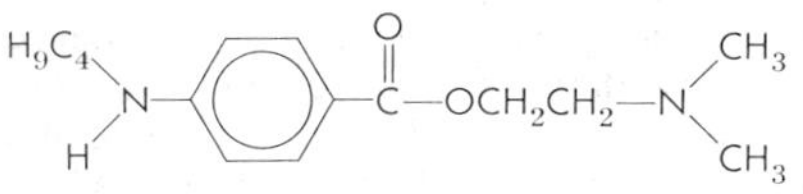

Tetracaine

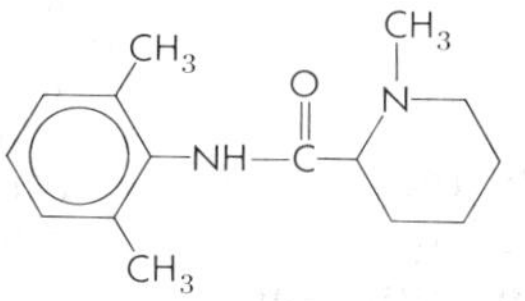

Mepivacaine †

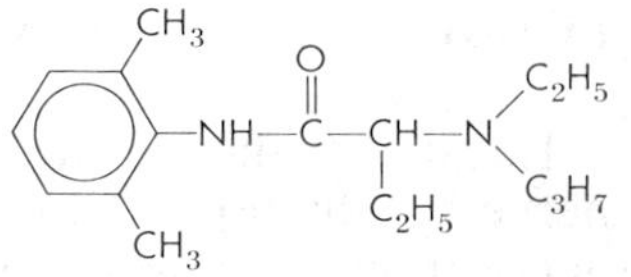

Etidocaine

* Chloroprocaine has a chlorine atom in position 2 of the aromatic moiety of procaine.
† Bupivacaine has a butyl group in place of the N-methyl substituent of mepivacaine.

thetics contains hydrophilic and hydrophobic domains that are separated by an intermediate alkyl chain. The hydrophilic group is usually a tertiary amine, but it may also be a secondary amine; the hydrophobic domain is an aromatic residue. Linkage to the aromatic group is of either the ester or amide type, and the nature of this bond determines certain of the pharmacological properties of these agents. The ester link is important because this bond is readily hydrolyzed during metabolic degradation and inactivation in the body. The structure–activity relationship and the physicochemical properties of local anesthetics have been reviewed by Courtney and Strichartz (1987). In brief, hydrophobicity increases both the potency and the duration of action of the local anesthetics. This arises because association of the drug at hydrophobic sites decreases the rate of hydrolysis by plasma esterases and enhances the partitioning of the drug to its sites of action. Hydrophobicity also increases potential toxicity, so little is gained in terms of therapeutic index if this parameter is increased.

Mechanism of Action. Local anesthetics prevent the generation and the conduction of the nerve impulse. Their main site of action is the cell membrane, since conduction block can be demonstrated in giant axons from which the axoplasm has been removed.

Local anesthetics block conduction by decreasing or preventing the large transient increase in the permeability of excitable membranes to Na^+ that is produced by a slight depolarization of the membrane (*see* Strichartz and Ritchie, 1987). This action of local anesthetics is due to their direct interaction with voltage-sensitive Na^+ channels. As the anesthetic action progressively develops in a nerve, the threshold for electrical excitability gradually increases, the rate of rise of the action potential declines, impulse conduction slows, and the safety factor for conduction decreases; these factors decrease the probability of propagation of the action potential, and nerve conduction fails.

Raising the concentration of Ca^{2+} in the medium bathing a nerve may relieve conduction block produced by local anesthetics. Relief occurs because Ca^{2+} alters the surface potential on the membrane, and hence the transmembrane electrical field. This, in turn, reduces the degree of inactivation of the Na^+ channels and the affinity of the latter for the local anesthetic molecules (*see* Hille, 1977).

In addition to Na^+ channels, local anesthetics can also bind to other membrane-bound proteins (*see* Butterworth and Strichartz, 1990). In particular, they can block K^+ channels as well (*see* Strichartz and Ritchie, 1987). However, since the interaction of local anesthetics with K^+ channels requires higher concentrations of drug, blockade of conduction is not accompanied by any large or consistent change in membrane potential.

Quaternary analogs of local anesthetics block conduction when applied internally to perfused giant axons of squid, but they are relatively ineffective when applied externally. These observations, together with others on the effects of varying pH on the potency of related tertiary amines, suggest that the site at which local anesthetics act, at least in their charged form, is accessible only from the inner surface of the membrane (Narahashi and Frazier, 1971; Strichartz and Ritchie, 1987). Local anesthetics applied externally must therefore first cross the membrane, in the uncharged form, before they can exert a blocking action.

Although a variety of physicochemical models have been proposed to explain how local anesthetics achieve conduction block (*see* Courtney and Strichartz, 1987), it is now generally accepted that the major mechanism of action of these drugs involves their interaction with a specific binding site within the Na^+ channel. However, whether or not all actions of local anesthetics are mediated by a common site remains unclear (Courtney and Strichartz, 1987; Strichartz and Ritchie, 1987).

Biochemical, biophysical, and molecular biological investigations during the past decade have led to a rapid expansion of knowledge about the Na^+ channel and other voltage-sensitive ion channels (*see* Catterall, 1988; Trimmer and Agnew, 1989). The Na^+ channel of the mammalian brain is a heterotrimeric complex of glycosylated proteins with an aggregate molecular size in excess of 300,000 daltons; the individual subunits are designed α (260 kilodaltons), β_1 (36 kilodaltons), and β_2 (33 kilodaltons). After incorporation of the purified polypeptides into phospholipid vesicles, Na^+ flux into the vesicles occurs in response to veratridine, a substance known to cause persistent activation of Na^+ channels. Only the α subunit is required to reconstitute channel function. Movement of Na^+ into the vesicles is blocked by the neurotoxins tetrodotoxin and saxitoxin (*see* below) and by local anesthetics (Tamkun *et al.*, 1984). The hydrophilic neurotoxins probably bind within the mouth of the channel, which is formed by the α subunit. By use of a nonpermeant quaternary analog of lidocaine, it is possible to show that local anesthetics and tetrodotoxin interact at opposite ends of the Na^+ channel (Rosenberg *et al.*, 1984). A simple model of the Na^+ channel in the plasma membrane is shown in Figure 15–1.

The large α subunit of the Na^+ channel contains four homologous domains, each of which appears to consist of six stretches of amino acid residues that are thought to criss-cross the plasma membrane (*see* Figure 15–1). The Na^+-selective transmembrane pore of the channel is presumed to reside in the center of a nearly symmetrical structure formed by the four homologous domains. The voltage-dependence of channel opening is hypothesized to reflect conformational changes that result from the movement of "gating charges" (voltage sensors) in response to changes in the transmembrane potential (Figure 15–2). Candidate voltage sensors are found in the so-called S4 transmembrane helix—one of the six transmembrane spans that is found in each of the four homologous domains of the channel. Although the S4 transmembrane helix is partly hydrophobic, it alone also contains positively charged amino acid residues at every third position that must move perpendicular to the plane of the membrane when the transmembrane potential is altered.

Radioactive neurotoxins and antibodies to the purified channel proteins have permitted visualization of Na^+ channels in plasma membranes of electrically excitable cells; their distribution is nonuniform. For example, the density of Na^+ channels in the internodal regions of myelinated axons is much lower than at the nodes of Ranvier. Thus, local anesthetics need have access only to the nodal regions in order to produce blockade of conduction.

Differential Sensitivity of Nerve Fibers to Local Anesthetics. As a general rule, small nerve fibers seem to be more susceptible to the action of local anesthetics than are large fibers. This was clearly established for the myelinated A fibers by Gasser and Erlanger (1929), who showed that when cocaine is applied to a cutaneous nerve the δ waves (from small cutaneous afferent fibers) are the first and the α waves (from large fibers) the last to disappear. The smallest mammalian nerve fibers are nonmyelinated and, on the whole, are blocked more readily than the myelinated fibers. However, the spectrum of sensitivity of the nonmyelinated fibers overlaps that of the myelinated fibers to some extent. Thus, some myelinated A δ fibers are blocked earlier, and with lower concentrations of anesthetic, than are most of the C fibers (Nathan and Sears, 1961). The sensitivity to local anesthetics is not determined by fiber size alone, therefore, but also by the anatomical fiber type. This finding is not surprising in view of the great difference between the physiological mode of conduction in the myelinated fibers, in which conduction is saltatory, and that of the nonmyelinated fibers, in which it is continuous. Still other factors may determine the susceptibility of a fiber to a local anesthetic. For example, in the rabbit vagus nerve the myelinated autonomic B fibers seem to have a greater safety factor for conduction than do the larger myelinated A fibers; this would account for their lower sensitivity to local anesthetics (*see* Raymond and Gissen, 1987).

Although there is general agreement on the differential rate of blockade produced by local anesthetics in fibers of different sizes and function, still in question is whether a similar differential effect obtains after sufficient time has been allowed for full equilibration of the local anesthetic with the tissue. Indeed, Franz and Perry (1974) found that *absolute* differential blockade occurred only when the length of nerve exposed to the anesthetic was limited to a few millimeters.

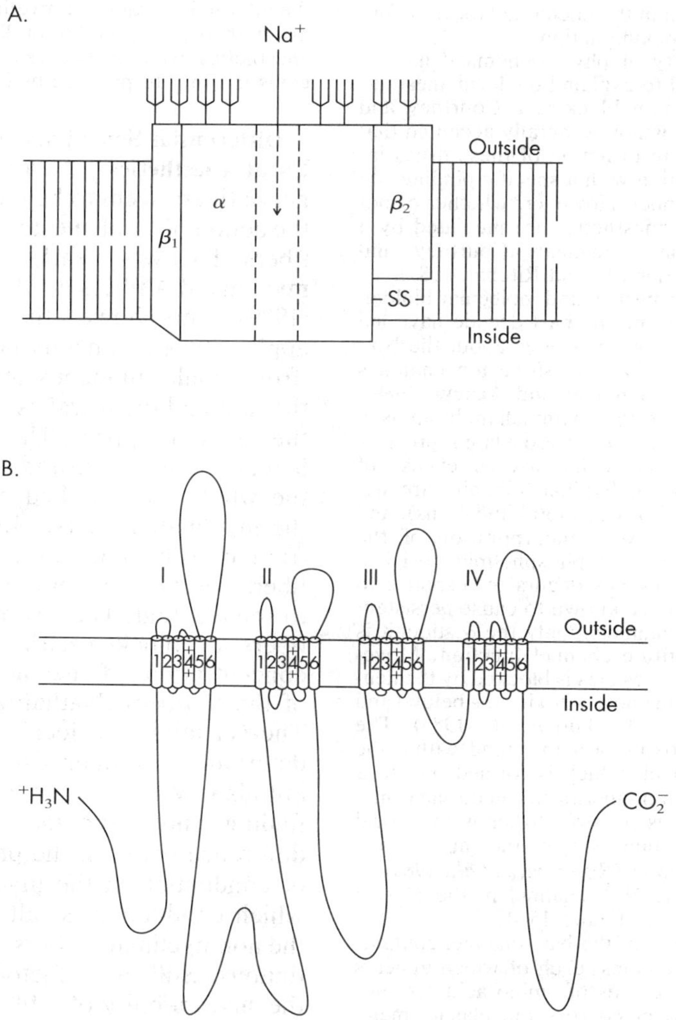

Figure 15–1. *Proteins of the voltage-sensitive Na^+ channel.*

(A) A model of the voltage-sensitive Na^+ channel from mammalian brain in the plasma membrane. The α and β_1 subunits interact noncovalently; the α and β_2 subunits are linked by disulfide bonds. The branched structures at the outer surface of the channel represent oligosaccharides. **(B)** Proposed transmembrane arrangement of the α subunit of the Na^+ channel. Four homologous domains (I–IV) each consist of six stretches of hydrophobic amino acid residues that are thought to cross the plasma membrane. The S4 segment contains positively charged residues (*see* Figure 15–2). (Modified from Catterall, 1988; copyright 1988 by the AAAS.)

The sensitivity of a fiber to local anesthetics does not seem to depend on whether it is sensory or motor. Although application of local anesthetic to a muscle-nerve trunk leads to blockade of contractions elicited reflexly before those elicited by electrical stimulation of the nerve, both muscle proprioceptive afferent and muscle efferent fibers are equally sensitive. These two types of fibers have the same diameter, which is larger than the γ motor fibers that supply the muscle spindles. It is the more rapid blockade of these smaller motor fibers, rather than the sensory fibers, that leads to the preferential loss of the muscle reflexes.

Computer simulation suggests that the safety factor for conduction in a homologous population of myelinated fibers (*e.g.*, in a somatic nerve) should be largely independent of fiber diameter except at very small diameters (Chiu and Ritchie, 1984). This independence agrees with the suggestion of Franz and Perry (1974) that differential block cannot result from differences in minimal concentrations necessary to block axons of different diameters. Rather, it results from differences in the critical lengths of axons that must be exposed to the anesthetic, smaller axons having shorter critical lengths because of their smaller internodal distances. In the

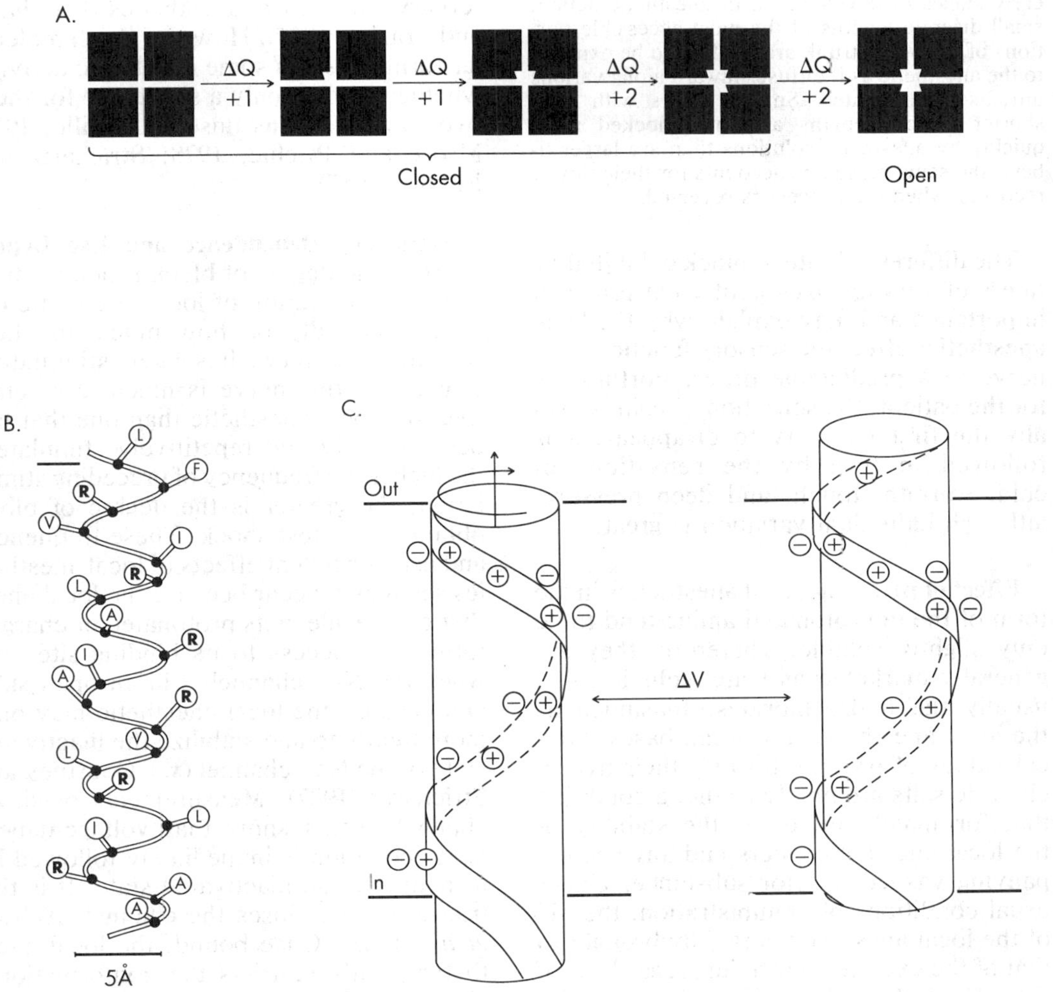

Figure 15–2. *Sliding helix model of voltage-dependent gating of the Na^+ channel.*

(A) The Na^+ channel α subunit is illustrated from a perspective perpendicular to the plane of the membrane as a square array of four homologous domains surrounding a central transmembrane pore. Depolarization causes a sequential series of voltage-driven conformational changes in the individual domains. After each domain has changed conformation, an open ion channel is formed. Each conformational change is associated with an outward transfer of protein-bound positive gating charge (ΔQ) across the membrane. **(B)** A ball-and-stick, three-dimensional representation of the S4 helix of domain IV of the Na^+ channel. Darkened circles represent the α carbon of each amino acid residue. Open circles show the direction of projection of the side chain of each residue away from the core of the helix. Nonpolar residues are illustrated by their single-letter code: F = Phe; A = Ala; I = Ile; L = Leu; V = Val; G = Gly; and T = Thr. Positively charged amino acids are illustrated in bold letters: R = Arg. **(C)** Movement of the S4 helix in response to membrane depolarization. The proposed transmembrane S4 helix is illustrated as a cylinder with a spiral ribbon of positive charge. At the resting membrane potential (left), all positively charged residues are paired with fixed negative charges on other transmembrane segments of the channel and the transmembrane segment is held in that position by the negative internal membrane potential. Depolarization reduces the force holding the positive charges in their inward position. The S4 helix is then proposed to undergo a spiral motion through a rotation of approximately 60° and an outward displacement of approximately 5 Å. This movement leaves an unpaired negative charge on the inward surface of the membrane and reveals an unpaired positive charge on the outward surface to give a net charge transfer (ΔQ) of +1. Note that all intramembranous positive charges are paired in both conformations. In domains III and IV, there are enough arginine residues to give a gating charge movement of +2. (From Catterall, 1988; copyright 1988 by the AAAS.)

early stages of development of anesthetic action, small discrete lengths of the most accessible portions of the nerve trunk are the first to be exposed to the anesthetic as it diffuses inward along various intrafascicular routes. Smaller fibers with their shorter critical lengths are thus blocked more quickly by anesthetic solutions than are larger fibers; the same reasoning accounts for their slower recovery when the process is reversed.

The differential rate of block exhibited by fibers of varying sizes is of great practical importance and may explain why the local anesthetics affect the sensory functions of a nerve in a predictable order. Fortunately for the patient, the sensation of pain is usually the first modality to disappear; it is followed in turn by the sensations of cold, warmth, touch, and deep pressure, although individual variation is great.

Effect of pH. The local anesthetics in the form of the unprotonated amine tend to be only slightly soluble. Therefore, they are generally marketed as water-soluble salts, usually the hydrochlorides. Inasmuch as the local anesthetics are weak bases (typical values of pK_a are 8 to 9), their hydrochloride salts are mildly acidic, a condition that fortunately increases the stability of the local anesthetic esters and any accompanying vasoconstrictor substance. Under usual conditions of administration, the pH of the local anesthetic is rapidly brought to that of the extracellular fluids, regardless of the pH of the solution in which it is injected.

Although the unprotonated species of the local anesthetic is necessary for diffusion through cellular membranes to reach its site of action, the cationic species apparently interacts preferentially with the Na^+ channels. This conclusion has been supported by the results of experiments on anesthetized mammalian nonmyelinated fibers (Ritchie and Greengard, 1966), in which conduction could be blocked or unblocked merely by setting the pH of the bathing medium at pH 7.2 or pH 9.6, respectively, without altering the amount of anesthetic present. The major role of the cation has also been clearly demonstrated by Narahashi and colleagues, who perfused the extracellular and axoplasmic surface of the giant squid axon with tertiary and quaternary amine local anesthetics (Narahashi and Frazier, 1971). However, both molecular forms possess some anesthetic activity; whether there is only a single site for these two forms remains unsettled (Hille, 1977; Mrose and Ritchie, 1978; Strichartz and Ritchie, 1987).

Frequency Dependence and Use Dependence. The degree of block produced by a given concentration of local anesthetic depends markedly on how much and how recently the nerve has been stimulated. Thus, a resting nerve is much less sensitive to a local anesthetic than one that has been recently and repetitively stimulated: the higher the frequency of preceding stimulation, the greater is the degree of block obtained to a test shock. These frequency- and use-dependent effects of local anesthetics seemingly occur because the local anesthetic molecule in its protonated or charged form gains access to its binding site only when the Na^+ channel is in an open state and because the local anesthetic may bind more tightly to and stabilize the inactivated state of the Na^+ channel (*see* Courtney and Strichartz, 1987). Measurements of single channel events show that voltage-dependent activation is immediately followed by formation of an inactivated state. It is this transition that closes the channel (Aldrich *et al.*, 1983). Once bound, the local anesthetic greatly restricts the conformational changes in the channel that underlie activation (Butterworth and Strichartz, 1990). Local anesthetics exhibit these properties to different extents, depending, for example, on their pK_a, lipid solubility, and molecular size.

Prolongation of Action by Vasoconstrictors. The duration of action of a local anesthetic is proportional to the time during which it is in contact with nerve. Consequently, procedures that keep the drug at the nerve prolong the period of anesthesia. Cocaine itself constricts blood vessels by potentiating the action of norepinephrine (*see* Chapters 5 and 10); therefore, it prevents its own absorption. In clinical practice the preparation of local anesthetic often contains a vasoconstrictor, usually epinephrine but occasionally phenylephrine. The vasoconstrictor performs a dual service. By decreasing the rate of absorption, it not only localizes the anesthetic at the desired site but also allows the rate at which it is destroyed in the body to keep pace with the rate at which it is absorbed into the circulation. This reduces its systemic toxicity.

Some of the vasoconstrictor agent may be absorbed systemically, occasionally to an extent sufficient to cause untoward reactions. There may also be a delay in wound healing, tissue edema, or necrosis after local anesthesia. These effects seem to occur in part because sympathomimetic amines increase the oxygen consumption of the tissue, and this, together with the vasoconstriction, leads to hypoxia and local tissue damage. This is particularly serious when local anesthetics are used in surgery on the digits, hands, or feet. Prolonged constriction of major arteries in the presence of limited collateral circulation can produce irreversible hypoxic damage, tissue necrosis, and gangrene. In addition, the local anesthetics themselves may interfere with the reparative processes of wound healing.

Pharmacological Actions. In addition to blocking conduction in nerve axons in the peripheral nervous system, local anesthetics interfere with the function of all organs in which conduction or transmission of impulses occurs. Thus, they have important effects on the central nervous system (CNS), the autonomic ganglia, the neuromuscular junction, and all forms of muscle (for reviews, *see* Covino, 1987; Garfield and Gugino, 1987; Gintant and Hoffman, 1987). The danger of such adverse reactions is proportional to the concentration of local anesthetic that is achieved in the circulation.

Central Nervous System. Following absorption, local anesthetics may cause stimulation of the CNS, producing restlessness and tremor that may proceed to clonic convulsions. In general, the more potent the anesthetic the more readily convulsions may be produced. Alterations of CNS activity are thus predictable from the local anesthetic agent in question and the blood concentration achieved. Unfortunately, electroencephalographic patterns give little or no consistent warning of impending convulsive activity (Covino, 1987). Central stimulation is followed by depression, and death is usually caused by respiratory failure.

The apparent stimulation and subsequent depression produced by applying local anesthetics to the CNS is presumably due solely to depression of neuronal activity; a selective depression of inhibitory neurons is thought to account for the excitatory phase *in vivo*. Rapid systemic administration of local anesthetics, or large doses of the more toxic agents administered locally, may produce death with only transient or no signs of CNS stimulation. Under these conditions the concentration of the drug probably rises so rapidly that all neurons are depressed simultaneously. The support of respiration is the essential feature of treatment in the late stage of intoxication. Diazepam administered intravenously is the drug of choice for both the prevention and the arrest of convulsions (*see* Chapter 19).

Although drowsiness is the most frequent complaint that emanates from the CNS actions of local anesthetics, lidocaine may produce dysphoria or euphoria and muscle twitching at a blood concentration of 5 μg/ml. However, both lidocaine and procaine may produce loss of consciousness that is preceded only by symptoms of sedation (*see* Covino, 1987). While shared to some extent by other local anesthetics, cocaine has a particularly prominent effect on mood and behavior (*see* Gawin and Ellingwood, 1988). These effects of cocaine and its potential for abuse are discussed in Chapter 22.

Neuromuscular Junction and Ganglionic Synapse. Local anesthetics also affect transmission at the neuromuscular junction. Procaine, for example, can block the response of skeletal muscle to maximal motor-nerve volleys and to acetylcholine at concentrations where the muscle responds normally to direct electrical stimulation. Similar effects occur at autonomic ganglia. Two modes of action can be discerned from biophysical analysis of the acetylcholine receptor channel. First, the local anesthetics break the square-wave conductance changes associated with individual channel openings and closings into a large number of very short opening and closing events (flickering). Second, they promote receptor desensitization. The particular mode of action depends on membrane voltage and the individual anesthetic (Neher and Steinbach, 1978; Koblin and Lester, 1979). Both of these events reduce the efficiency of neuromuscular transmission. The site on the nicotinic receptor to which local anesthetics bind is distinct from the agonist binding site, and it appears to be within the acetylcholine receptor channel.

Cardiovascular System. Following systemic absorption, local anesthetics act on the cardiovascular system (*see* Covino, 1987). The primary site of action is the myocardium, where decreases in electrical excitability, conduction rate, and force of contraction occur. In addition, most local anesthetics cause arteriolar dilatation. The cardiovascular effects are usually seen only after high systemic concentrations are attained and effects on the CNS are produced. However, on rare occasions small amounts of anesthetic employed for simple infiltration anesthesia will cause cardiovascular collapse and death. This probably results from cardiac arrest due to either an action on the pacemaker or the sudden onset of ventricular fibrillation. Such a reaction may follow inadvertent intravascular administration of the agent, particularly if epinephrine is present in the preparation. The effects of local anesthetics such as lidocaine and procainamide on the heart are presented in Chapter 35.

Smooth Muscle. The local anesthetics depress contractions in the intact bowel and in strips of isolated intestine (*see* Zipf and Dittmann, 1971). There is, however, little correlation between anesthetic potency and antispasmodic efficacy. They also relax vascular and bronchial smooth muscle, although low concentrations may initially produce contraction (*see* Covino, 1987).

Spinal and epidural anesthesia, as well as instillation of local anesthetics into the peritoneal cavity, cause sympathetic nervous system paralysis that can result in increased tone of gastrointestinal musculature. Most local anesthetics may increase the resting tone and decrease the contractions of isolated human uterine muscle; however, uterine contractions are seldom depressed during intrapartum regional anesthesia.

Hypersensitivity to Local Anesthetics. Rare individuals are hypersensitive to local anesthetics. The reaction may manifest itself as an allergic dermatitis or a typical asthmatic attack (*see* Covino, 1987). Hypersensitivity seems to occur most prominently with local anesthetics of the ester type and frequently extends to chemically related compounds. For example, individuals sensitive to procaine may also react to structurally similar compounds (*e.g.*, tetracaine). Although agents of the amide type are essentially free of this problem, solutions of such agents may contain preservatives that are not (Covino, 1987). Certain antihistamines are occasionally used as local anesthetics for individuals who have become hypersensitive to all the conventional agents. These antihistamines presumably do not share the specific antigenic determinants of the conventional local anesthetics.

Fate of Local Anesthetics. The metabolic fate of local anesthetics is of great practical importance because their toxicity depends largely on the balance between their rate of absorption and their rate of destruction. As noted above, the rate of absorption can be reduced considerably by the incorporation of a vasoconstrictor agent in the anesthetic solution. However, the rate of destruction of local anesthetics varies greatly, and this is a major factor in determining the safety of a particular agent. Binding of the anesthetic to tissues reduces the concentration of drug in the systemic circulation and, consequently, reduces toxicity. For example, in intravenous regional anesthesia of an extremity, about half of the original anesthetic dose is still tissue bound 30 minutes after release of the tourniquet; the lungs also bind large quantities of local anesthetic (Arthur, 1987).

Some of the common local anesthetics (*e.g.*, tetracaine) are esters, and their activity and toxicity are usually lost as the result of hydrolysis. This is accomplished primarily by a plasma esterase, probably plasma cholinesterase; the liver also participates. Since spinal fluid contains little or no esterase, anesthesia produced by the intrathecal injection of an anesthetic agent will persist until the local anesthetic agent has been absorbed into the blood.

The amide-linked local anesthetics are, in general, degraded by the hepatic endoplasmic reticulum, the initial reactions involving N-dealkylation and subsequent hydrolysis (Arthur, 1987). However, with prilocaine the initial step is hydrolytic, forming *o*-toluidine metabolites that can cause methemoglobinemia. Caution is indicated in the extensive use of amide-linked local anesthetics in patients with severe hepatic disease. The amide-linked local anesthetics are extensively (55 to 95%) bound to plasma proteins, particularly α_1-acid glycoprotein. Many factors increase (cancer, trauma, myocardial infarction, smoking, uremia) or decrease (oral contraceptive agents) the concentration of this protein in plasma. This results in changes in the amount of anesthetic delivered to the liver for metabolism, thus influencing systemic toxicity (*see* Arthur, 1987). Uptake by the lung may also play an important role in the distribution of amide-linked local anesthetics in the body (Arthur, 1987).

COCAINE

Source. Cocaine occurs in the leaves of *Erythroxylon coca* and other species of *Erythroxylon,* trees indigenous to Peru and Bolivia, where the leaves have been used for centuries by the natives to increase endurance and promote a sense of well-being.

Chemistry. Cocaine is benzoylmethylecgonine. Ecgonine is an amino alcohol base closely related to tropine, the amino alcohol in atropine. Cocaine is thus an ester of benzoic acid and a nitrogen-containing base. It has the fundamental structure previously described for the synthetic local anesthetics (*see* Table 15–1).

Pharmacological Actions. The most important action of cocaine clinically is its ability to block the initiation or conduction of the nerve impulse following local application. Its most striking systemic effect is stimulation of the CNS. In addition, cocaine has numerous important side actions (*see* Cregler and Mark, 1986).

Central Nervous System. Cocaine stimulates the CNS generally. In man, this is manifested first as a feeling of well-being and euphoria; sometimes dysphoria may result. These effects may be accompanied by garrulousness, restlessness, and excitement. After small amounts of cocaine, motor activity is well coordinated; however, as the dose is increased, tremors and eventually clonic-tonic convulsions result. The vasomotor and vomiting centers may also share in the stimulation, and emesis may result. Central stimulation is soon followed by depression. Eventually the vital medullary centers are depressed, and death results from respiratory failure. The cerebral actions of cocaine and the subject of cocaine abuse are discussed in Chapter 22.

Cardiovascular System. Small doses of cocaine given systemically may slow the heart as a result of central vagal stimulation, but after moderate doses the heart rate is increased. The increased cardiac rate probably results from increased central sympathetic stimulation as well as from the peripheral effects of cocaine on the sympathetic nervous system, as discussed below. Although the blood pressure may finally fall, there is at first a prominent rise in blood pressure owing to sympathetically mediated tachycardia and vasoconstriction. A large intravenous dose of cocaine may cause immediate death from arrhythmias, myocardial infarction, or cardiac failure caused by direct depression of heart muscle.

Body Temperature. Cocaine is markedly pyrogenic. The increased muscular activity attending stimulation by cocaine augments heat production; vasoconstriction decreases heat loss. Also, cocaine may have a direct action on the heat-regulating centers, for the onset of cocaine fever is often heralded by a chill, which indicates that the body is adjusting its temperature to a higher level. Cocaine pyrexia is often a striking feature of cocaine poisoning and can easily be elicited in animals by sublethal doses.

Sympathetic Nervous System. Cocaine potentiates the responses of sympathetically innervated organs to norepinephrine, sympathetic nerve stimulation, and, to a lesser degree, epinephrine. It is well established that cocaine blocks the uptake of catecholamines at adrenergic nerve endings; this uptake process is primarily responsible for terminating the actions of both adrenergic impulses and circulating catecholamines (*see* Chapter 5). Other local anesthetics do not share this capability to alter the uptake of norepinephrine, to produce sensitization to catecholamines, or to produce vasoconstriction and mydriasis. The peripheral component of the cardioacceleration produced by cocaine is probably of similar origin.

Local Anesthetic Actions. The most important local action of cocaine is its ability to block nerve conduction. Cocaine was once used extensively in ophthalmological procedures, but it causes sloughing of the corneal epithelium. Because of this, and because of its potential for abuse, cocaine is now restricted to topical use, especially in the upper respiratory passages. Even this use may be accompanied by severe toxicity.

Absorption, Fate, and Excretion. Cocaine is absorbed from all sites of application, including mucous membranes and the gastrointestinal mucosa (*see* Appendix II). Absorption is enhanced in the presence of inflammation, and systemic effects of the drug may thereby be markedly increased. For example, such may occur if cocaine is used in cystoscopy when the urinary bladder is inflamed.

After absorption, cocaine is degraded by plasma esterases and, at least in some animals, by hepatic enzymes. Small amounts are excreted unchanged in the urine. The half-life of cocaine in the plasma after oral or nasal administration is approximately 1 hour (*see* Fleming *et al.*, 1990).

Tolerance, Abuse, and Acute Poisoning. As noted, cocaine is often abused for its effects on the

CNS. The symptoms and treatment of poisoning and the misuse of cocaine are discussed in Chapter 22.

Preparations and Dosage. *Cocaine* and *cocaine hydrochloride* are the official preparations of the alkaloid. Cocaine is not prepared legitimately to be used internally or injected. Solutions used clinically for surface anesthesia usually vary from 1 to 4%, depending on the mucosa being anesthetized. Cocaine and epinephrine or other sympathomimetics should not be used concurrently.

Cocaine is included among the drugs controlled by the federal drug-abuse regulations (*see* Appendix I).

LIDOCAINE

Lidocaine, introduced in 1948, is now the most widely used local anesthetic. Its chemical structure is shown in Table 15–1.

Pharmacological Actions. The pharmacological actions that lidocaine shares with other local anesthetic drugs have been presented. Lidocaine produces more prompt, more intense, longer-lasting, and more extensive anesthesia than does an equal concentration of procaine. Unlike procaine it is an aminoethylamide. It is an agent of choice, therefore, in individuals sensitive to ester-type local anesthetics.

Absorption, Fate, and Excretion. Lidocaine is relatively quickly absorbed after parenteral administration and from the gastrointestinal tract. Although it is effective when used without any vasoconstrictor, in the presence of epinephrine the rate of absorption and the toxicity are decreased and the duration of action is prolonged. Lidocaine is dealkylated in the liver by mixed-function oxidases to monoethylglycine xylidide and glycine xylidide, which can be metabolized further to monoethylglycine and xylidide. Both monoethylglycine xylidide and glycine xylidide retain local anesthetic activity. In man about 75% of xylidide is excreted in the urine as the further metabolite 4-hydroxy-2,6-dimethylaniline (*see* Arthur, 1987).

Toxicity. Overdosage of lidocaine produces death from ventricular fibrillation or, if massive, cardiac arrest; procaine, on the other hand, tends to depress respiration rather than the circulation. Side effects of lidocaine are related to its CNS effects and include sleepiness, dizziness, paresthesias, altered mental status, coma, and seizures. The metabolites monoethylglycine xylidide and glycine xylidide may contribute to some of these side effects.

Preparations. *Lidocaine hydrochloride* (*lignocaine;* XYLOCAINE, others) is very soluble in water and alcohol. Preparations include injections, ointments, jelly, topical solutions, and topical aerosol for oral mucosa. Market preparations (0.5 to 20%), some with and without epinephrine (1:50,000 to 1:200,000), are suitable for infiltration (0.5 to 1%), block (1 to 2%), and topical mucosal anesthesia (1 to 5%).

Clinical Uses. Lidocaine has a variety of clinical uses as a local anesthetic. In addition, lidocaine is employed as an antiarrhythmic agent, as described in Chapter 35.

OTHER SYNTHETIC LOCAL ANESTHETICS

The number of synthetic local anesthetics is so large that it is impractical to consider all of them here.

Some local anesthetic agents are too toxic to be given by injection. Their use is restricted to topical application to the eye, the mucous membranes, or the skin. Many local anesthetics are suitable, however, for infiltration or injection to produce nerve block; some of them are also useful for topical application. The main categories of local anesthetics are given below; the agents are listed alphabetically.

LOCAL ANESTHETICS SUITABLE FOR INJECTION

Bupivacaine hydrochloride (MARCAINE, SENSORCAINE) is a widely used amide type of local anesthetic; its structure is identical to that of mepivacaine except that a butyl group replaces the methyl substituent on the amino nitrogen. It is a potent agent capable of producing prolonged anesthesia. Its mean duration of action is greater than that of tetracaine, while the toxicity of the two compounds is similar. As with other highly potent local anesthetics (such as tetracaine and etidocaine), bupivacaine can cause a variety of cardiac toxicities. In relatively low concentrations it slows conduction in various regions of the heart, and it may depress cardiac contractility (Covino, 1987). Recovery is relatively slow (*see* Courtney and Strichartz, 1987). Bupivacaine hydrochloride is available in solutions for injection (0.25, 0.5, and 0.75%) with or without epinephrine (1:200,000). The 0.75% solution should not be used for obstetrical anesthesia. A hyperbaric solution for spinal anesthesia is also available.

Chloroprocaine hydrochloride (NESACAINE) is a halogenated derivative of procaine, the pharmacological properties of which it shares almost completely. Its anesthetic potency is at least twice as great as that of procaine, and its toxicity is lower because of its more rapid metabolism. Questions have been raised about the possibility of neurological toxicity from the use of chloroprocaine in spinal anesthesia (*see* Covino, 1987). Some authors have attributed this toxicity to the presence of bisulfite as an antioxidant in the anesthetic solution (*see* Covino, 1987; however, *see also* Kalichman *et al.*, 1988). Chloroprocaine hydrochloride is available in solutions for injection (1.0, 2.0, and 3.0%).

Etidocaine hydrochloride (DURANEST) is a long-acting derivative of lidocaine. The time required for induction of anesthesia with etidocaine is about the same as that for lidocaine, but its analgesic action lasts two to three times longer. It is not employed for spinal anesthesia, but is useful for epidural and for all types of infiltration and regional anesthesia. Etidocaine hydrochloride is marketed in solutions for injection (1.0%) with or without epinephrine (1:200,000) and in a 1.5% solution with epinephrine (1:200,000).

Mepivacaine hydrochloride (CARBOCAINE, others) is a local anesthetic of the amide type (*see* Table 15–1). Its pharmacological properties are similar to those of lidocaine, which it resembles chemically. Its action is more rapid in onset and somewhat more prolonged than that of lidocaine. It has been employed for all types of infiltration and regional nerve block anesthesia. Mepivacaine hydrochloride is marketed in solutions for injection (1.0, 1.5, 2.0, and 3.0% without, and 2% with, levonordefrin as a vasoconstrictor).

Prilocaine hydrochloride (CITANEST) is a local anesthetic of the amide type. Its pharmacological properties resemble those of lidocaine. Its onset and duration of action are longer than those of lidocaine. Like lidocaine, it may produce sleepiness. A unique toxic aftereffect is methemoglobinemia, which is caused by its metabolites. Its use is now largely confined to dental procedures. Prilocaine hydrochloride is marketed in a solution for injection (4% with or without epinephrine).

Procaine hydrochloride (NOVOCAIN) was once used widely; it has largely been displaced by lidocaine and its congeners. Procaine (*see* Table 15–1) is hydrolyzed *in vivo* to produce paraaminobenzoic acid, which inhibits the action of sulfonamides. This fact is occasionally of practical significance. Procaine is rapidly absorbed following parenteral administration; vasoconstrictors may be added to procaine solutions to prolong its action. Solutions usually contain 0.25 to 0.5% procaine for infiltration anesthesia, 0.5 to 2% for peripheral nerve block, and 10% for spinal anesthesia. Procaine is largely ineffective when applied topically.

Tetracaine hydrochloride (PONTOCAINE) is a derivative of paraaminobenzoic acid (*see* Table 15–1). It is about ten times more toxic and more active than procaine after intravenous injection. For topical anesthesia of the eye, a 0.5% solution or ointment is used; for the mucous membranes of the nose and throat, a 2.0% solution. For spinal anesthesia, a total dose of 5 to 20 mg is adequate. The effects are longer lasting than those of procaine. Tetracaine hydrochloride for injection is available in solutions and in ampuls containing the dry salt. An ointment (0.5%) and cream (1%) for topical application to skin are also available.

LOCAL ANESTHETICS LARGELY RESTRICTED TO OPHTHALMOLOGICAL USE

While certain of the agents described above can be used in the eye, the following local anesthetic agents are largely restricted to the production of corneal anesthesia. Their main advantage over the prototype, cocaine, is that they produce little or no mydriasis or corneal injury.

Benoxinate hydrochloride is a benzoic acid ester related to procaine. A single instillation of 1 or 2 drops of a 0.4% solution produces within 60 seconds a sufficient degree of anesthesia to permit Schiötz tonometry. It is marketed as a 0.4% ophthalmic solution in combination with 0.25% fluorescein.

Proparacaine hydrochloride (ALCAINE, OPHTHAINE, others) is a benzoate ester, but it is chemically distinct from procaine, benoxinate, and tetracaine. This difference in chemical structure may explain the lack of cross-sensitization between proparacaine and other local anesthetic agents. It is about as potent as tetracaine. Unlike some topical anesthetics, proparacaine hydrochloride produces little or no initial irritation. It is available in a 0.5% ophthalmic solution for topical application.

LOCAL ANESTHETICS USED MAINLY TO ANESTHETIZE MUCOUS MEMBRANES AND SKIN

Some anesthetics are either too irritating or too ineffective to be applied to the eye. However, they are useful as topical anesthetic agents on the skin and/or mucous membranes. These preparations are effective in the symptomatic relief of anal and genital pruritus, poison ivy rashes, and numerous other acute and chronic dermatoses.

Dibucaine (*cinchocaine*, NUPERCAINAL) is a quinoline derivative. Its toxicity resulted in its removal from the United States market as an injectable preparation. It is currently available as a cream and an ointment for use on the skin.

Dyclonine hydrochloride (DYCLONE) has a rapid onset of action and a duration of effect comparable to that of procaine. It is absorbed through the skin and mucous membranes. The compound is used as a 0.5 or 1.0% solution for topical anesthesia in otolaryngology and for anogenital anesthesia.

Pramoxine hydrochloride (TRONOTHANE, others) is a surface anesthetic agent that is not of the benzoate ester type. Its distinct chemical structure is likely to minimize the danger of cross-sensitivity reactions in patients allergic to other local anesthetics. Pramoxine produces satisfactory surface anesthesia and is reasonably well tolerated on the skin and mucous membranes. It is too irritating to be used on the eye or in the nose. Preparations available for topical application include a 1% cream or lotion.

ANESTHETICS OF LOW SOLUBILITY

Some local anesthetics are poorly soluble in water and, consequently, too slowly absorbed to be toxic. They can be applied directly to wounds and ulcerated surfaces, where they remain localized for long periods of time to produce a sustained anesthetic action. Chemically, they are esters of paraaminobenzoic acid that lack the terminal amino group possessed by the previously described local anesthetics. The most important member of the series is *benzocaine* (*ethyl aminobenzoate;* AMERICAINE ANESTHETIC, others). Benzocaine is identical to procaine structurally, except that it lacks the terminal diethylamino group. It is incorporated into a large number of topical preparations.

Some salts of the tertiary amino group of local anesthetics are very insoluble. For example, the hydroiodide salt of tetracaine may produce anesthesia of 45 hours' duration when sprinkled in a surgical wound (Cherney, 1963).

Tetrodotoxin and Saxitoxin

These toxins are two of the most potent poisons known, the minimal lethal dose of each in the mouse being about 8 μg/kg. Both toxins are responsible for outbreaks of fatal poisoning in man. Tetrodotoxin is found in the gonads and other visceral tissues of some fish of the order Tetraodontiformes (to which the Japanese *fugu*, or puffer fish, belongs); it also occurs in the skin of some newts of the family Salamandridae and of the Costa Rican frog *Atelopus*. Saxitoxin, and possibly some related toxins, are elaborated by the dinoflagellates *Gonyaulax catanella* and *Gonyaulax tamerensis*, and are retained in the tissues of clams and other shellfish that eat these organisms. Given the right conditions of temperature and light the *Gonyaulax* may multiply so rapidly as to discolor the ocean—hence the term *red tide*. Shellfish feeding on *Gonyaulax* at this time become extremely toxic to man and are responsible for periodic outbreaks of paralytic shellfish poisoning (*see* Kao, 1972; Ritchie, 1980).

Although the toxins are chemically different from each other, their mechanism of action seems identical (*see* Ritchie, 1980). Both toxins, in nanomolar concentrations, specifically block the Na^+ channels in the membranes of excitable cells. As a result, the action potential is blocked. Not all Na^+ channels are equally sensitive to tetrodotoxin; the channels in cardiac and smooth muscle cells are largely resistant, and a tetrodotoxin-insensitive Na^+ channel is expressed when skeletal muscle is denervated. Blockade of vasomotor nerves, together with a relaxation of vascular smooth muscle, seems to be responsible for the hypotension that is characteristic of tetrodotoxin poisoning (Kao, 1972). Both toxins cause death by paralysis of the respiratory muscles. The treatment of severe cases of poisoning therefore requires artificial ventilation. Early gastric lavage and therapy to support the blood pressure are also indicated. If the patient survives paralytic shellfish poisoning for 24 hours, the prognosis is good (*see* Ogura, 1971; Schantz, 1971).

CLINICAL USES OF LOCAL ANESTHETICS

Local anesthesia is the loss of sensation without the loss of consciousness or the impairment of central control of vital functions. A major advantage, therefore, is that the physiological trespass associated with general anesthesia is avoided. Local anesthetics are not, however, devoid of the potential to produce deleterious side effects. The choice of a local anesthetic and the technique of its use are the determinants of such toxicity.

The following discussion concerns the pharmacological and physiological consequences of the use of local anesthetics, evaluated in terms of the potential advantages and disadvantages of local anesthetics under clinical conditions. Techniques for the administration of local anesthetics are described in detail elsewhere (Cousins and Bridenbaugh, 1988).

Surface Anesthesia

Anesthesia of mucous membranes of the nose, mouth, throat, tracheobronchial tree, esophagus, and genitourinary tract can be produced by direct application of aqueous solutions of salts of many local anesthetics. Tetracaine (2%), lidocaine (2 to 10%), and cocaine (1 to 4%) are most often used. Cocaine is used only in the nose, nasopharynx, mouth, throat, and ear. Procaine and other more polar local anesthetics are clinically unsatisfactory; they penetrate mucous membranes too poorly. Cocaine has the unique advantage of producing vasoconstriction as well as anesthesia. The shrinking of mucous membranes decreases operative bleeding while improving surgical visualization. Comparable vasoconstriction can be achieved with other local anesthetics by the addition of a low concentration of a vasoconstrictor such as phenylephrine (0.005%). Epinephrine, topically applied, has no significant local effect and does not prolong the duration of action of local anesthetics applied to mucous membranes because it penetrates mucous membranes too poorly. Maximal safe total dosages for topical anesthesia in a healthy 70-kg adult are 750 mg for lidocaine, 200 mg for cocaine, and 50 mg for tetracaine.

Peak anesthetic effect following topical application of cocaine or lidocaine occurs within 2 to 5 minutes (3 to 8 minutes with tetracaine), and anesthesia lasts for 30 to 45 minutes (30 to 60 minutes with tetracaine). Anesthesia is entirely superficial; it does not extend to submucosal structures. This technique does not alleviate joint pain or discomfort from subdermal inflammation or injury.

Local anesthetics are rapidly absorbed into the circulation following topical application to mucous membranes or denuded skin. Such topical anesthesia thus always carries the risk of systemic toxic reactions. Systemic toxicity has followed the use of local anesthetics to control discomfort associated with severe diaper rash in infants. Absorption is particularly rapid when local anesthetics are applied to the tracheobronchial tree. Concentrations in blood after instillation of local anesthetics into the airway are nearly the same as those that follow intravenous injection. Blood concentrations are lower and peak values are reached more slowly when a given amount of topical anesthetic is applied over a longer period of time. When topical anesthetics are applied to the mouth, nose, or throat, the patient should be cautioned to expectorate the excess solution of the anesthetic to avoid excessive absorption. Surface anesthetics for the skin and cornea have been described above.

INFILTRATION ANESTHESIA

Infiltration anesthesia consists in injection of a solution of local anesthetic directly into the tissue to be incised or mechanically stimulated. Infiltration anesthesia can be so superficial as to include only the skin. It can also include deeper structures, including intraabdominal organs when these, too, are infiltrated.

The duration of infiltration anesthesia can be approximately doubled by the addition of epinephrine (1:200,000; 5 μg/ml) to the solution; epinephrine also decreases peak concentrations of local anesthetics in blood. Epinephrine-containing solutions should not, however, be injected into tissues supplied by end arteries, for example, fingers and toes, ears, the nose, and the penis. To do so may result in gangrene. For the same reason, epinephrine should be avoided in solutions injected intracutaneously. Since epinephrine is also absorbed into the circulation, it should not be used in patients in whom adrenergic stimulation is undesirable.

The local anesthetics most frequently used for infiltration anesthesia are lidocaine (0.5 to 1.0%), procaine (0.5 to 1.0%), and bupivacaine (0.125 to 0.25%). When used without epinephrine, up to 4.5 mg/kg of lidocaine, 7 mg/kg of procaine, or 2.5 mg/kg of bupivacaine can be employed in adults. When epinephrine is added, these amounts can be increased by one third.

The advantage of infiltration anesthesia and other regional anesthetic techniques is that it is possible to provide good anesthesia without disruption of normal bodily functions. The chief disadvantage of infiltration anesthesia is that relatively large amounts of drug must be used to anesthetize relatively small areas. This is no problem with minor surgery. When major surgery is performed, however, the amount of local anesthetic that is required may make systemic toxic reactions likely. Whereas intraabdominal procedures are technically feasible under infiltration anesthesia, substantially better operating conditions are more readily and safely achieved either with lesser amounts of local anesthetic administered by other regional techniques or with general anesthesia.

FIELD BLOCK ANESTHESIA

Field block anesthesia is produced by subcutaneous injection of a solution of local anesthetic in such a manner as to interrupt nerve transmission proximal to the site to be anesthetized. For example, subcutaneous infiltration of the proximal portion of the volar surface of the forearm results in an extensive area of cutaneous anesthesia that starts 2 to 3 cm distal to the site of injection. The same principle can be applied with particular benefit to the scalp, the anterior abdominal wall, and the lower extremity.

The drugs used and the concentrations and doses recommended are the same as for infiltration anesthesia. The advantage of field block anesthesia is that less drug can be used to provide a greater area of anesthesia than when infiltration anesthesia is used. Knowledge of the relevant neuroanatomy is obviously essential for successful field block anesthesia.

NERVE BLOCK ANESTHESIA

Injection of a solution of a local anesthetic into or about individual peripheral nerves or nerve plexuses produces even greater areas of anesthesia with a smaller amount of drug than do the techniques described above. Blockade of mixed peripheral nerves and nerve plexuses also usually anesthetizes somatic motor nerves, a matter of importance in certain types of surgery. The areas of sensory and motor denervation usually start several centimeters distal to the site of injection. Particularly useful are blocks of the brachial plexus for procedures on the upper extremity distal to insertion of the deltoid, intercostal nerve blocks for anesthesia and relaxation of the anterior abdominal wall, cervical plexus block for surgery of the neck, sciatic and femoral nerve blocks for surgery distal to the knee, blocks of individual nerves at the wrist and at the ankle or blocks of individual nerves such as the median or ulnar at the elbow, and blocks of sensory cranial nerves.

The onset of sensory anesthesia following injection about a peripheral nerve depends on the pK_a of the anesthetic. The onset of action of lidocaine occurs in about 3 minutes; 35% of lidocaine is in the basic form at this pH. Onset of action of bupivacaine requires about 15 minutes; only 5 to 10% of bupivacaine is not protonated at pH 7.4. Latency is also determined by the need for diffusion of the agent from its site of injection to its site of action. Diffusion is more important in determining rapidity of onset when nerve plexuses are blocked than when single nerves are anesthetized. The latency of the anesthetic effect of lidocaine injected about the ulnar nerve is 3 minutes, but this value is nearly 15 minutes when the drug is injected about the brachial plexus. The latency of bupivacaine is over 20 minutes in brachial plexus block.

Duration of nerve block anesthesia depends on the physical characteristics of the local anesthetic used. Especially important are lipid solubility and protein binding. In general, local anesthetics can be divided into three categories: those with a short duration of action (20 to 45 minutes) following anesthetization of a mixed peripheral nerve, such as procaine; those with an intermediate duration of action (60 to 120 minutes), such as lidocaine and mepivacaine; and those with a long duration of action (400 to 450 minutes), such as tetracaine, bupivacaine, and etidocaine. Duration of nerve block anesthesia can be extended by increasing the amount of drug injected. However, this is of relatively limited value because the possibility of systemic toxic reactions is increased more than is the duration of action of the drug. Increasing the volume of anesthetic injected also increases the likelihood of spread of the solution to nearby structures that one may not wish to anesthetize. Duration of action can also be prolonged by the addition of epinephrine.

The types of nerve fibers that are blocked when a local anesthetic is injected about a mixed peripheral nerve depend on the concentration of drug used, nerve-fiber size, internodal distance, and frequency and pattern of nerve-impulse transmission (*see* above). Anatomical factors are similarly important. A mixed peripheral nerve or nerve trunk consists of individual nerves surrounded by an investing epineurium. The vascular supply is usually centrally located. When a local anesthetic is deposited about a peripheral nerve, it diffuses from the outer surface toward the core along a concentration gradient (Winnie *et al.*, 1977). Consequently, nerves located in the outer mantle of the mixed nerve are blocked first. These fibers are usually distributed to more proximal anatomical structures than are those situated near the core of the mixed nerve. If the volume and concentration of local anesthetic solution deposited about the nerve are adequate, the local anesthetic will eventually diffuse inwardly in amounts adequate to block even the most centrally located fibers. Lesser amounts of drug will block only nerves in the mantle and smaller and more sensitive central fibers. Furthermore, since uptake of local anesthetics usually occurs primarily in the core of a mixed nerve or nerve trunk where the vascular supply is located, the duration of blockade of centrally located nerves is shorter than that of more peripherally situated fibers.

Which local anesthetic is to be used for a nerve block, as well as the amount and concentration to be used, depends upon which nerves or plexuses are to be blocked, the types of fibers to be blocked, the duration of anesthesia required, and the size and physical status of the patient. Procaine (0.5 to 2.0% solution) and lidocaine (1.0 to 2.0% solution) can be used in the amounts recommended above under Infiltration Anesthesia. Mepivacaine (up to 7 mg/kg of a 1.0 to 3.0% solution) provides anesthesia that lasts about as long as that from lidocaine. Bupivacaine (0.25 to 0.75% solution) can be used when a long duration of action is required. Chloroprocaine (1 to 2% solution) is especially useful when a short duration of effect is desired; up to 11 mg/kg may be injected because chloroprocaine is so rapidly hydrolyzed by plasma cholinesterase. As with other regional anesthetic techniques, addition of 1:200,000 epinephrine prolongs duration and allows the use of greater amounts of local anesthetic.

Peak concentrations of local anesthetics in blood and the potential for systemic reactions depend on the amount injected, the physical characteristics of the local anesthetic, and whether epinephrine is used. They also are determined by the rate of blood flow to the site of injection. This is of particular importance in nerve block anesthesia. Peak concentrations of lidocaine in blood following injection of 400 mg for intercostal nerve blocks average 7 μg/ml; the same amount of lidocaine used for block of the brachial plexus results in peak concentrations in blood of approximately 3 μg/ml (Covino and Vassallo, 1976). For reference, the therapeutic range of concentrations for the antiarrhythmic effects of lidocaine is 1.5 to 6 μg/ml, and values in excess of 6 μg/ml are associated with CNS toxicity. The amounts of local anesthetic that can be safely injected as outlined in the preceding paragraph must, therefore, be adjusted according to the anatomical site of the nerve(s) to be blocked. Multiple nerve blocks (*e.g.*, intercostal block) require reduction in the amount of anesthetic that can be safely given because the surface area for absorption is increased. Nerve blocks in richly vascular areas must also be performed with less drug.

Successful nerve blocks depend upon thorough knowledge of neuroanatomy. Armed with such knowledge the expert anesthesiologist can predictably block any nerve by using one of two techniques. (1) The anesthesiologist can place the needle for injection in the same fascial compartment in which the nerve to be blocked lies and then inject a relatively large volume of anesthetic solution. Diffusion of the solution is restricted by anatomical boundaries, and an effective concentration can thus be delivered to the nerve. (2) The anesthesiologist can ensure that the tip of the needle lies immediately adjacent to the nerve to be blocked. Smaller amounts of local anesthetic need then be injected because of reliance on accurate placement of the drug. Assurance that the tip of the needle lies immediately adjacent to the nerve requires that a paresthesia be elicited; the most accurate placement is ensured when a paresthesia is produced by injection of the anesthetic solution.

Intravenous Regional Anesthesia

Intravenous regional anesthesia consists in the injection of local anesthetic solution into a vein of an extremity previously exsanguinated with an Esmarch bandage and kept exsanguinated by a pneumatic tourniquet placed on the upper part of the extremity and inflated above arterial pressure. Lidocaine (1.5 mg/kg of 0.5% solution) is frequently used for intravenous regional anesthesia of the upper extremity. Onset of anesthesia occurs in 2 to 3 minutes. When the tourniquet is released at the end of surgery, approximately 15 to 30% of the lidocaine injected into the isolated extremity enters the systemic circulation. Peak concentrations in blood, reached within 4 to 5 minutes, are less than those observed following brachial plexus or lumbar epidural block. Bupivacaine is not approved for use in intravenous regional anesthesia.

Intravenous regional anesthesia is not as effective in the lower as it is in the upper extremity. In the latter case it is used for operations at the level of or distal to the elbow. Intravenous regional anesthesia cannot be used when fractures or other tender lesions exist in the extremity because of pain produced by exsanguination with the Esmarch bandage. The safety of intravenous regional anesthesia depends upon maintenance of pressure in the tourniquet adequate to occlude arterial flow at all times.

Spinal Anesthesia

Spinal anesthesia is produced by injection of a local anesthetic into the lumbar subarachnoid space below the termination of the cord (second lumbar vertebra). Spread of the agent within the subarachnoid space and, thus, the level of anesthesia are controlled by the injection of solutions of greater or lesser specific gravity than cerebrospinal fluid; the patient is then placed in the head-up or head-down position. Addition of 10% glucose solution to that of the local anesthetic produces a solution of greater specific gravity than cerebrospinal fluid (hyperbaric spinal anesthesia). With the patient in the head-down position the glucose–local anesthetic solution then ascends into the subarachnoid space. The height that it achieves is determined by the volume of solution injected and the degree of tilt of the patient. Hyperbaric solutions remain in the distal subarachnoid space when injected with the patient sitting or in the head-up position. Hypobaric spinal anesthesia is produced by addition of sterile distilled water to the solution of local anesthetic. These mixtures are used less frequently than are hyperbaric solutions.

The concentration of local anesthetic in cerebrospinal fluid decreases rapidly after injection as the drug is bound to tissue and absorbed into the vascular system. Furthermore, within 10 to 15 minutes a hyperbaric solution becomes isobaric. At this point changes in position of the patient no longer affect distribution of the local anesthetic within the subarachnoid space. The level of anesthesia becomes "fixed."

Local anesthetics within the subarachnoid space act on superficial layers of the spinal cord, but their primary site of anesthetic action is on nerve fibers. Because the concentration of local anesthetic in spinal fluid decreases as a function of distance from the site of injection, zones of differential anesthesia develop. Since preganglionic sympathetic fibers are blocked by concentrations of local anesthetics that are inadequate to affect somatic sensory or motor fibers, the level of sympathetic denervation during hyperbaric spinal anesthesia extends an average of two spinal segments cephalad to the level that is unresponsive to painful stimuli. On the other hand, since somatic motor fibers are more resistant to the action of local anesthetics than are somatic sensory fibers, the level of motor blockade is an average of two spinal segments below the level made unresponsive to painful stimuli during hyperbaric spinal anesthesia.

The goal of spinal anesthesia is to block somatic sensory and motor fibers. The accompanying sympathetic denervation, however, alters physiological responses. Blood concentrations of local anesthetics during spinal anesthesia are relatively low and play no role in altering physiological responses. The amount of drug that is injected is too small, and the rate of absorption is too slow. The physiological effects of spinal anesthesia are largely those of sympathetic blockade, and the safe practice of spinal anesthesia requires comprehension of its consequences (Greene, 1981).

Cardiovascular Consequences of Sympathetic Blockade. The most cephalad preganglionic sympathetic fibers arise from the spinal cord at the level of the first thoracic segment. Because of the two-segment zone of differential sympathetic block, sympathetic denervation is complete when sensory anesthesia is obtained at the third thoracic segmental level. Since the physiological responses to spinal anesthesia depend upon the level of sympathetic denervation, the consequences of spinal anesthesia with sensory loss to midcervical levels are essentially the same as those associated with sensory effects that extend only to the third thoracic segmental level. Furthermore, sympathetic denervation by spinal anesthesia involves preganglionic fibers, and each preganglionic fiber ascends and descends in the paravertebral chain to synapse with up to 18 postganglionic fibers, which are then distributed peripherally in a nonsegmental manner (*see* Chapter 5). Thus, blockade of sympathetic fibers at, for example, the fourth thoracic segmental level is associated with diffuse peripheral responses that extend three or four segments above the peripheral sensory area that is innervated by fibers arising at the fourth thoracic segmental level.

Even low segmental levels of sensory spinal anesthesia are usually associated with some degree of sympathetic blockade. The most distal preganglionic sympathetic fibers arise from the spinal cord at the second lumbar segmental level. Spinal anesthetic solutions are usually injected between the third and fourth lumbar vertebrae. Turbulence associated with injection, together with subsequent diffusion of the local anesthetic in spinal fluid, almost invariably results in sympathetic blockade at the second lumbar segmental level, even when sensory denervation involves only low lumbar or sacral roots.

The most important consequence of the sympathetic blockade of spinal anesthesia is alteration of cardiovascular function. Arteries and arterioles dilate in sympathetically denervated areas; total peripheral vascular resistance and mean arterial blood pressure thus decrease. Reduction in blood pressure due to arterial and arteriolar vasodilatation during spinal anesthesia is, however, not proportional to the extent of the sympathetic block. Compensatory vasoconstriction occurs in areas where sympathetic innervation is intact. This increases regional vascular resistance and tends to restore blood pressure. Compensatory vasoconstriction occurs mainly in the upper extremities. However, even with total sympathetic blockade the decrease in total peripheral resistance averages no more than 12 to 14% in normal individuals. The change is relatively small because the smooth muscles of arteries and (especially) arterioles retain a certain degree of autonomous tone, and they do not dilate maximally. Because the decrease in total peripheral resistance is relatively minor in normal individuals, even with total sympathetic blockade during spinal anesthesia, severe arterial hypotension is not brought about by changes in the arterial side of the circulation.

The most important cardiovascular responses to spinal anesthesia are those that result from changes in the venous side of the circulation. Sympathetic tone to veins and venules is lost during spinal anesthesia to the same extent as is that to arteries and arterioles. Unlike arteries and arterioles, however, denervated veins and venules retain little autonomous tone. They can dilate maximally, and the extent to which they do is determined by intraluminal hydrostatic pressure. As they increase their capacity, they sequester within them a greater percentage of the blood volume, and venous return to the heart decreases. This can cause an appreciable fall in cardiac output and blood pressure.

The safety of spinal anesthesia thus depends upon maintenance of an adequate venous return to the heart. This is best accomplished by elevation of sympathetically blocked areas above the level of the right atrium. The slight (10° to 15°) head-down position is appropriate. In normal individuals in the slight head-down position, cardiac output remains normal even during total preganglionic sympathetic blockade. The head-up position, on the other hand, is associated with severe decreases in cardiac output and profound arterial hypotension. Cardiac arrest may occur. The head-up position should, of course, be used to restrict spread of hyperbaric anesthetic solutions in the subarachnoid space; however, if the level of anesthesia becomes unexpectedly high or if severe hypotension develops, the patient must unhesitatingly and immediately be placed in the head-down position. The resulting level of anesthesia may be embarrassingly high, but the patient will survive. Because adequate venous return is essential to the safe management of patients during spinal anesthesia, this form of anesthesia is contraindicated in the presence of hypovolemia from any cause.

Treatment of arterial hypotension during spinal anesthesia should, as a general rule, be initiated if systolic blood pressure falls by approximately 25% of normal *resting* levels. The patient is placed in the slight head-down position and oxygen is administered. Vasopressors are of some value but should not be relied upon exclusively. When used, vasopressors should be given intravenously in small doses. α-Adrenergic agonists, such as methoxamine and phenylephrine, are best avoided. The increase in peripheral vascular resistance produced by such agents may so increase afterload that the myocardium, already suffering from a decrease in preload, may fail acutely. Agents that increase blood pressure by increasing heart rate are also best avoided. Drugs that act solely by virtue of their positive inotropic effects are also of limited value in the absence of an adequate venous return. The most satisfactory vasopressors are those that decrease venous compliance. While no vasopressor acts solely on the venous circulation, agents such as mephentermine and ephedrine have desirable effects. They also have moderate positive inotropic effects, yet do not produce severe and undesirable increases in peripheral vascular resistance. Hypotension during spinal anesthesia may also be treated by the rapid intravenous infusion of balanced salt solutions, sometimes in amounts as great as 1.5 to 2 liters or more. However, while hypovolemia must be treated during spinal anesthesia (or any other type of anesthesia), the administration of large volumes of intravenous fluids to normovolemic patients rendered hypotensive by sympathetic blockade during spinal anesthesia may be questioned. Cardiac output is restored by rapid infusion of balanced salt solutions to the extent that venous return is increased, but the increase is accomplished by hemodilution, not by increasing the output of blood with a normal content of oxygen. Use of large volumes of intravenous fluids in this way also sharply increases the incidence of postoperative urinary retention and the need for catheterization.

Spinal anesthesia, in the absence of premedication with muscarinic blocking agents, is characterized by a decrease in pulse rate. The bradycardia is due to a combination of two factors: preganglionic blockade of cardiac accelerator fibers (first through fourth thoracic spinal segments), and responses of intrinsic stretch receptors in the right side of the heart that mediate chronotropic responses to changes in central venous and right atrial pressure. The role of intrinsic stretch receptors in regulation of heart rate during spinal anesthesia to midthoracic levels is illustrated by the effects of changes in posture on heart rate after the local anesthetic is fixed and changes in the level of anesthesia are no longer possible; lowering the patient's head increases pulse rate as venous return and right atrial pressure increase, while elevating the patient's head decreases pulse rate as venous return and right atrial pressure decrease.

Coronary blood flow decreases during spinal anesthesia in proportion to the decrease in mean aortic pressure. Myocardial work, however, also decreases. Myocardial oxygen requirements decrease because of the decrease in afterload, the decrease in preload, and the bradycardia. In normal individuals the decrease in the myocardial requirement for oxygen slightly exceeds the decrease in oxygen supply (coronary flow); the myocardium is thus relatively overperfused. It is not known whether the same relationship holds true in patients with coronary artery disease.

Cerebrovascular autoregulatory mechanisms maintain cerebral circulation at normal levels even though arterial hypotension may develop during spinal anesthesia. Only when mean aortic pressure decreases to the range of 55 to 60 mm Hg does cerebral blood flow begin to diminish. The level of blood pressure at which cerebrovascular autoregulation is no longer able to compensate for decreases in arterial perfusion pressure is greater in hypertensive than in normotensive patients. Thus, hypotension should be treated sooner in hypertensive patients than in normal subjects.

Renovascular autoregulation also compensates for changes in arterial blood pressure over a wide range. When arterial hypotension is severe enough to diminish renal blood flow, glomerular filtration and urinary output decrease, but circulation usually remains adequate to maintain the viability of glomerular and tubular cells. The oliguria is then transient and disappears as the effects of the spinal anesthetic wear off and blood pressure returns to normal.

Respiratory Complications. Pulmonary ventilation is little affected by spinal anesthesia. Even levels of sensory denervation high enough to include lower cervical dermatomes are associated with normal tensions of carbon dioxide and oxygen in arterial blood. The phrenic nerves remain unaffected during such high levels of anesthesia because of the existence of the two-segment zone of differential motor blockade mentioned above. The diaphragm compensates for intercostal paralysis, particularly since relaxation of the anterior abdominal wall associated with intercostal paralysis decreases resistance to descent of the diaphragm during inhalation. Diaphragmatic excursions during high spinal anesthesia may be impaired, however, in obese patients, in patients with ascites, in pregnant women at term, or in other situations in which intraabdominal pressure may be increased, including use of the extreme head-down or Trendelenburg position.

Although respiratory tidal volume and maximal inspiratory capacity are unaffected by high spinal anesthesia, forced expiration is impaired because of paralysis of the abdominal musculature. Patients with high spinal anesthesia are unable to cough normally. High spinal anesthesia may therefore be hazardous in patients with excessive tracheobronchial secretions.

Respiratory arrest, while rare, can occur during spinal anesthesia. Its most frequent cause is ischemic paralysis of the medullary respiratory centers associated with profound decreases in cardiac output and arterial blood pressure. Only a small percentage of such incidents is due to phrenic nerve paralysis during lumbar spinal anesthesia. Nor is apnea due to ascent of the local anesthetic in cerebrospinal fluid with direct depression of chemotactic respiratory neurons in the brainstem. Concentrations of local anesthetic in cisternal spinal fluid during high spinal anesthesia are inadequate to produce pharmacological effects; they are even lower in ventricular cerebrospinal fluid and have no effect on either vasomotor or respiratory nuclei in the medulla.

The fundamental importance of inadequate cerebral perfusion as the primary cause of apnea during spinal anesthesia is demonstrated by the observation that respiratory arrest almost always immediately precedes or follows cardiac arrest. Furthermore, prompt restoration of cardiac output by appropriate means will result in immediate restoration of ventilation. This would not occur if the apnea were due to phrenic nerve paralysis or to direct depression of the respiratory centers.

The incidence, magnitude, and type of postoperative respiratory complications are the same after spinal anesthesia (or other forms of regional anesthesia) as after general anesthesia for the same operative procedure. Postoperative respiratory complications are related to age, sex, smoking habits, use of narcotics, quality of intraoperative and postoperative ventilatory care, preexisting pulmonary disease, and, above all, the anatomical site and nature of the surgery. When these factors are taken into consideration, postoperative respiratory complications are not related to the type of anesthesia. Regional anesthesia, including spinal anesthesia, provides no advantage for the avoidance of pulmonary complications in the postoperative period.

Effects on Hepatic Function. Hepatic function is largely unaffected by spinal anesthesia, even in the presence of hypotension. Postoperative hepatic function is principally determined by the type and nature of the surgery performed. Spinal and other forms of regional anesthesia confer no special benefits in patients with liver disease.

Neurological Complications. Residual neurological deficits associated with spinal anesthesia are so rare in modern practice that, if they do occur, aggressive and complete diagnostic tests must be undertaken immediately to ensure that they are not due to other causes. When neurological deficits occur that are directly ascribable to spinal anesthesia, they may present themselves either immediately or they may develop days or a week or more after the procedure. Neurological complications with acute onset may be due to the injection of a local anesthetic with histotoxic properties or to the injection of an excessive concentration of a local anesthetic that normally does not cause histotoxicity. Tetracaine, procaine, and lidocaine are devoid of neurotoxicity. When neurological complications follow the use of these local anesthetics, they are, in the absence of chemical contamination of the solution, the result of injection in such a manner as to expose nerve roots and the spinal cord to excessive concentrations of the drug. They are not due to "allergic" responses to the agent.

Another cause of the immediate appearance of neurological deficits following spinal anesthesia is traumatic damage to a nerve root incurred during performance of the lumbar puncture. This characteristically involves a single nerve root. Nerve damage during lumbar puncture usually occurs when the needle is directed so far laterally that it impinges on a nerve root at its point of exit from the subarachnoid space through the dura—the point at which a nerve is sufficiently fixed to be susceptible to direct trauma. Such damage to a nerve root in the cauda equina is rare.

Neurological sequelae of spinal anesthesia that are delayed in onset are usually the result of chronic arachnoiditis; this is produced by the inadvertent injection of materials (lint, talc, *etc.*) or chemicals that initiate a chronic inflammatory response. Avoidance of this type of reaction depends upon meticulous attention to details of technique during administration of the drug and the use of equipment that is chemically uncontaminated as well as sterile.

Spinal anesthesia is commonly regarded as contraindicated in patients with preexisting disease of the spinal cord. No experimental evidence exists to support this hypothesis. It is, nonetheless, prudent to avoid spinal anesthesia in patients with progressive diseases of the spinal cord, since worsening of the disease may be blamed on the anesthetic agent or the procedure.

Headaches may follow any lumbar puncture, whether for diagnostic or anesthetic purpose. Characteristically postural in nature, these disappear when the patient is supine. The incidence of such headaches is related to the size of the needle used and to the age and sex of the patient. When 25-gauge needles are used, the incidence of headaches after spinal anesthesia is 1% or less (even in obstetrical patients, who constitute the most susceptible group). Spinal needles larger than 22-gauge should be avoided.

Dosage and Duration of Anesthesia. Dosages of local anesthetics used for spinal anesthesia vary according to the volume of the subarachnoid space (*i.e.*, the height of the patient), the segmental level of anesthesia desired, and the duration of anesthesia required. Although four local anesthetics (procaine, lidocaine, tetracaine and bupivacaine) are presently available for use in spinal anesthesia in the United States, only two—lidocaine and tetracaine—enjoy widespread clinical use. The concentration of tetracaine injected for spinal anesthesia should not exceed 0.5%; the injected concentration of lidocaine should not exceed 5%. When high thoracic levels of anesthesia are sought, 16 mg of tetracaine or 100 mg of lidocaine may be used.

The duration of spinal anesthesia is governed by the rate at which the local anesthetic is absorbed from the subarachnoid space, the spinal cord, and, after diffusion through the dura, the epidural space. Duration thus decreases with increases in the absorptive surface to which the drug is exposed as it spreads within the subarachnoid space. Duration also depends upon lipophilicity of the local anesthetic. Tetracaine, which is highly lipid soluble, provides 2 to 3 hours of anesthesia, while anesthesia with the less lipid-soluble lidocaine lasts about an hour. Epinephrine (0.2 to 0.5 mg) prolongs the duration of spinal anesthesia with tetracaine by about 30%. For reasons that remain to be clarified, epinephrine fails to produce significant prolongation of lidocaine-induced spinal anesthesia (Greene, 1983).

Evaluation of Spinal Anesthesia. Modern spinal anesthesia is a safe and effective technique. Its value is greatest during surgery involving the lower abdomen, the extremities, or the perineum. It is often combined with intravenous medication to provide sedation and amnesia. With low spinal anesthesia the potential for physiological trespass is less than that associated with general anesthesia. The same does not apply for high spinal anesthesia. The sympathetic blockade that accompanies levels of spinal anesthesia adequate for mid- or upper-abdominal surgery is so extensive that equally satisfactory and safer operating conditions are usually achieved by the administration of a general anesthetic and a neuromuscular blocking agent. Low spinal anesthesia and high spinal anesthesia are, in physiological terms, totally different techniques. One is frequently indicated, the other only rarely.

EPIDURAL ANESTHESIA

Injection of a solution of local anesthetic into the epidural space is a popular form of regional anesthesia. When injected into the lumbar, or less frequently, the thoracic area, the anesthetic acts in two places. It diffuses across the dura into the subarachnoid space, where it acts on nerve roots and the spinal cord much as it does when injected directly into the subarachnoid space during spinal anesthesia. The drug also diffuses into the paravertebral area through the intervertebral foramina, producing, in essence, multiple paravertebral nerve blocks. The former is the more important site of action. When local anesthetics are injected into the epidural space via the caudal canal (caudal anesthesia), the anesthetic acts less by diffusing across the dura and more by blocking nerves as they pass through the epidural space; diffusion through sacral foramina also plays an important role.

The choice of drugs to be used during epidural anesthesia is dictated primarily by the duration of anesthesia desired. Particularly popular are bupivacaine, when long duration is sought, and lidocaine, when intermediate duration is indicated. Chloroprocaine provides rapid onset and very short duration of action. However, its use in epidural anesthesia has been clouded by controversy regarding its potential to cause neurological complications if the drug is accidentally injected into the subarachnoid space. The duration of action of lidocaine is frequently prolonged (and its systemic toxicity decreased) by addition of epinephrine (1:200,000). Duration of anesthesia is also frequently extended by serial injections through a catheter placed in the epidural space.

The volumes of local anesthetic injected during epidural anesthesia are determined principally by the segmental level of anesthesia required. The larger the volume, the greater is the spread within the epidural space and the more extensive the area of anesthesia.

Concentrations of local anesthetic used are determined by the types of nerve fibers to be blocked. The highest concentrations are used when sympathetic, somatic sensory, and somatic motor blockade are required. Intermediate concentrations allow somatic sensory anesthesia without muscle relaxation. Low concentrations will block only preganglionic sympathetic fibers. The total amounts of drug that can be safely injected at one time are approximately the same as those mentioned above in the sections on Nerve Block Anesthesia and Infiltration Anesthesia. The technique of epidural anesthesia and the volumes, concentrations, and types of drugs used are described in detail by Cousins and Bridenbaugh (1988).

A significant difference between epidural and spinal anesthesia is that drugs used with the epidural technique are injected in amounts sufficient to produce high concentrations in blood following absorption. Peak concentrations of lidocaine in blood following injection of 400 mg (without epinephrine) into the lumbar epidural space average 3 to 4 μg/ml. The same amount of lidocaine injected into the caudal epidural space results in slightly higher values. Addition of epinephrine (1:200,000) to the lidocaine decreases peak concentrations in blood by about 25%. Peak concentrations of bupivacaine in blood average 1.0 μg/ml after the lumbar epidural injection of 150 mg. These concentrations are a function of the total dose of drug rather than the concentration or volume of solution following epidural or other forms of regional anesthesia, except for spinal anesthesia (Covino and Vassallo, 1976).

Another difference between epidural and spinal anesthesia is that there is no zone of differential sympathetic blockade with epidural anesthesia, and the level of sympathetic denervation is thus the same as the level of sensory denervation. On the other hand, the zone of differential motor blockade is four to five spinal segments with epidural anesthesia, whereas it is only two segments with spinal anesthesia.

Because epidural anesthesia is not associated with the zone of differential sympathetic blockade that is observed during spinal anesthesia, cardiovascular responses to epidural anesthesia would be expected to be less prominent. In practice, this is not the case; this potential advantage of epidural anesthesia is offset by the cardiovascular responses to the high concentration of anesthetic in blood that is achieved during epidural anesthesia. This is most apparent when, as is often the case, epinephrine is added to the epidural injection. The resulting concentration of epinephrine in blood is sufficient to produce significant β-adrenergic stimulation. As a consequence, peripheral vasodilatation is so pronounced that blood pressure decreases, even though cardiac output increases owing to the positive inotropic and chronotropic effects of epinephrine. The result is peripheral hyperperfusion and hypotension. Differences in cardiovascular responses to equal levels of spinal and epidural anesthesia are also observed when a local anesthetic such as lidocaine is used without epinephrine. The direct effects of the high concentration of lidocaine on peripheral smooth muscle and the effects of the agent on the heart may become significant. The magnitude of the differences in responses to equal sensory levels of spinal and epidural anesthesia varies, however, with the local anesthetic used for the epidural injection (assuming no epinephrine is used). Local anesthetics such as bupivacaine, which are highly lipid soluble, are distributed less into the circulation than are less lipid-soluble agents such as lidocaine.

High concentrations of local anesthetics in blood during epidural anesthesia are of special importance when this technique is used to control pain during labor and delivery. Local anesthetics cross the placenta, enter the fetal circulation, and may cause depression of the neonate (Scanlon *et al.*, 1974). The extent to which they do so is determined by dosage, the level of protein binding in both maternal and fetal blood (Tucker, *et al.*, 1970), placental blood flow, and solubility of the agent in fetal tissue. The persistence of abnormal neonatal neurobehavioral activity for 24 or even 48 hours after delivery may be related to placental transfer of local anesthetics during labor and delivery and to the relative inability of the neonate to metabolize the drugs, particularly those of the amide type. These potential hazards to the neonate can be offset to some extent by use of local anesthetics (*e.g.*, bupivacaine) that are less distributed into the circulation. On the other hand, should high plasma concentrations of bupivacaine be achieved, the resulting systemic toxicity may be less readily reversed.

The greater zone of differential motor blockade that results with epidural anesthesia means that this procedure has less effect on pulmonary ventilation than does an equal sensory level of spinal anesthesia. This potential benefit is offset, however, during abdominal operations, because higher sensory levels of epidural anesthesia must be achieved to obtain the same degree of surgical relaxation of abdominal muscles that is produced by spinal anesthesia.

Epidural and Intrathecal Opioid Analgesia. Small quantities of opioids injected intrathecally or epidurally produce analgesia in localized regions (Yaksh and Rudy, 1976). This observation led to the application of spinal analgesia during surgical procedures and for the relief of postoperative and chronic pain (Cousins and Mather, 1984). As with local anesthesia, analgesia is confined to sensory nerves that enter the spinal segments in the vicinity of the injection. Different subtypes of opioid receptors exist in the spinal cord. They have both a presynaptic location, where they inhibit the release of substance P from primary afferents, and a postsynaptic location, where they diminish activity of certain dorsal horn neurons in the spinothalamic tracts (Yaksh *et al.*, 1988; *see also* Chapters 5 and 21). Since conduction in autonomic, sensory, and motor nerves is not affected by the opioids, blood pressure, motor function, and nonnociceptive sensory perception are typically not influenced by such procedures. The volume-evoked micturition reflex is inhibited, which implicates opioid-containing neurons in this reflex pathway. Delayed respiratory depression is noted in a small number of patients who have received intrathecal injections. This appears to result from slow rostral movement of the opioid within the cerebrospinal fluid to the brainstem (Bromage *et al.*, 1982). The incidence of respiratory depression is likely to depend on body position and the specific gravity of the preparation that is administered intrathecally, and it is far lower or negligible with epidural injection of opioids.

Intrathecal or epidural use of opioids in gynecological, abdominal, and orthopedic surgery has increased substantially during the past decade. However, blockade of the nociceptive response is localized and is often not complete. These factors limit the use of spinal analgesia to certain procedures. The risk of circulatory depression is lessened when compared with the local anesthetics. The duration of analgesia with morphine is 12 to 14 hours, which provides coverage for the early postoperative period. Acceptance of spinal opioids for the control of postoperative pain is also increasing, and slow infusions of opioids are efficacious in the treatment of terminal cancer pain over periods of weeks. Tolerance develops over this period of time, but infusions in nontolerant individuals require doses of only about 5 mg of morphine per day. Such dosage reduces substantially the systemic complications of long-term administration of morphine, since higher brain centers are exposed to relatively small concentrations of the drug.

Aldrich, R. W.; Corey, D. P.; and Stevens, C. F. A reinterpretation of mammalian sodium channel gating based on single channel recording. *Nature,* **1983,** *306,* 436–441.

Bromage, P. R.; Camporesi, E. M.; Durant, P. A. C.; and Nielsen, C. H. Rostral spread of epidural morphine. *Anesthesiology,* **1982,** *56,* 431–436.

Cherney, L. S. Tetracaine hydroiodide: a long-lasting local anesthetic agent for the relief of pain. *Anesth. Analg.,* **1963,** *42,* 477–481.

Chiu, S. Y., and Ritchie, J. M. On the physiological role of potassium channels and the security of conduction in myelinated nerve fibres. *Proc. R. Soc. Lond.* [*Biol.*], **1984,** *220,* 415–422.

Cousins, M. J., and Mather, L. E. Intrathecal and epidural administration of opioids. *Anesthesiology,* **1984,** *61,* 276–310.

Franz, D. N., and Perry, R. S. Mechanisms for differential block among single myelinated and non-myelinated axons by procaine. *J. Physiol.* (*Lond.*), **1974,** *236,* 193–210.

Gasser, H. S., and Erlanger, J. The role of fiber size in the establishment of a nerve block by pressure or cocaine. *Am. J. Physiol.,* **1929,** *88,* 581–591.

Hille, B. Local anesthetics: hydrophilic and hydrophobic pathways for the drug-receptor reaction. *J. Gen. Physiol.,* **1977,** *69,* 497–515.

Kalichman, M. W.; Powell, H. C.; and Myers, R. R. Pathology of local anesthetic-induced nerve injury. *Acta Neuropathol.* (*Berl.*), **1988,** *75,* 583–589.

Koblin, D. D., and Lester, H. A. Voltage-dependent and voltage-independent blockade of acetylcholine receptors by local anesthetics in Electrophorus electroplaques. *Mol. Pharmacol.,* **1979,** *15,* 559–580.

Mrose, H., and Ritchie, J. M. Local anesthetics: do benzocaine and lidocaine act at the same site? *J. Gen. Physiol.,* **1978,** *71,* 223–225.

Nathan, P. W., and Sears, T. A. Some factors concerned in differential nerve block by local anaesthetics. *J. Physiol.* (*Lond.*), **1961,** *157,* 565–580.

Neher, E., and Steinbach, J. H. Local anesthetics transiently block currents through single acetylcholine receptor channels. *J. Physiol.* (*Lond.*), **1978,** *277,* 153–176.

Rosenberg, R. L.; Tomiko, S. A.; and Agnew, W. S. Reconstitution of neurotoxin-modulated ion transport by the voltage-regulated sodium channel isolated from the electroplax of *Electrophorus electricus. Proc. Natl. Acad. Sci. U.S.A.,* **1984,** *81,* 1239–1243.

Scanlon, J. W.; Brown, W. U., Jr.; Weiss, J. B.; and Alper, M. H. Neurobehavioral responses of newborn infants after maternal epidural anesthesia. *Anesthesiology,* **1974,** *40,* 121–128.

Tamkun, M. M.; Talvenheimo, J. A.; and Catterall, W. A. The sodium channel from rat brain: reconstitution of neurotoxin-activated ion flux and scorpion toxin binding from purified components. *J. Biol. Chem.,* **1984,** *259,* 1676–1688.

Tucker, G. T.; Boyes, R. N.; Bridenbaugh, P. O.; and Moore, D. C. Binding of anilide-type local anesthetics in human plasma. II. Implications *in vivo,* with special reference to transplacental distribution. *Anesthesiology,* **1970,** *35,* 304–314.

Winnie, A. P.; Tay, C. H.; Patel, K. P.; Ramanmurthy, S.; and Durrani, Z. Pharmacokinetics of local anesthetics during plexus blocks. *Anesth. Analg.,* **1977,** *56,* 852–861.

Yaksh, T. L., and Rudy, T. A. Analgesia mediated by a direct spinal action of narcotics. *Science,* **1976,** *192,* 1357–1358.

Monographs and Reviews

Arthur, G. R. Pharmacokinetics. In, *Local Anesthetics.* (Strichartz, G. R., ed.) *Handbook of Experimental Pharmacology,* Vol. 81. Springer-Verlag, Berlin, **1987,** pp. 165–186.

Butterworth, J. F., and Strichartz, G. R. Molecular mechanisms of local anesthesia: a review. *Anesthesiology,* **1990,** In Press.

Byck, R. Cocaine use and research: three histories. In, *Cocaine: Clinical and Behavioral Aspects.* (Fisher, S.; Raskin, A.; and Uhlenhutch, E. H.; eds.) Oxford University Press, New York, **1987,** pp. 3–20.

Catterall, W. A. Structure and function of voltage-sensitive ion channels. *Science,* **1988,** *242,* 50–61.

Courtney, K. R., and Strichartz, G. R. Structural elements which determine local anesthetic activity. In, *Local Anesthetics.* (Strichartz, G. R., ed.) *Handbook of Experimental Pharmacology,* Vol. 81. Springer-Verlag, Berlin, **1987,** pp. 53–94.

Cousins, M. J., and Bridenbaugh, P. O. (eds.). *Neural Blockade in Clinical Anesthesia and Management of Pain,* 2nd ed. J. B. Lippincott Co., Philadelphia, **1988.**

Covino, B. G. Toxicity and systemic effects of local anesthetic agents. In, *Local Anesthetics.* (Strichartz, G. R., ed.) *Handbook of Experimental Pharmacology,* Vol. 81. Springer-Verlag, Berlin, **1987,** pp. 187–212.

Covino, B. G., and Vassallo, H. G. *Local Anesthetics: Mechanisms of Action and Clinical Use.* Grune & Stratton, Inc., New York, **1976.**

Cregler, L. L., and Mark, H. Medical complications of cocaine abuse. *N. Engl. J. Med.,* **1986,** *315,* 1495–1499.

Fleming, J. A.; Byck, R.; and Barash, P. G. Pharmacology and therapeutic applications of cocaine. *Anesthesiology,* **1990,** In Press.

Garfield, J. M., and Gugino, L. Central effects of local anesthetics. In, *Local Anesthetics.* (Strichartz, G. R., ed.) *Handbook of Experimental Pharmacology,* Vol. 81. Springer-Verlag, Berlin, **1987,** pp. 253–284.

Gawin, F. H., and Ellingwood, E. H. Cocaine and other stimulants: actions, abuse, and treatment. *N. Engl. J. Med.,* **1988,** *318,* 1173–1182.

Gintant, G. A., and Hoffman, B. F. The role of local anesthetic effects in the actions of antiarrhythmic drugs. In, *Local Anesthetics.* (Strichartz, G. R., ed.) *Handbook of Experimental Pharmacology,* Vol. 81. Springer-Verlag, Berlin, **1987,** pp. 213–251.

Greene, N. M. *Physiology of Spinal Anesthesia,* 3rd ed. The Williams & Wilkins Co., Baltimore, **1981.**

———. Uptake and elimination of local anesthetics during spinal anesthesia. *Anesth. Analg.,* **1983,** *62,* 1013–1024.

Kao, C. Y. Pharmacology of tetrodotoxin and saxitoxin. *Fed. Proc.,* **1972,** *31,* 1117–1123.

Narahashi, T., and Frazier, D. T. Site of action and active form of local anesthetics. *Neurosci. Res.,* **1971,** *4,* 65–99.

Ogura, Y. Fugu (puffer-fish) poisoning and the pharmacology of crystalline tetrodotoxin poisoning. In, *Neuropoisons: Their Pathophysiological Actions.* Vol. 1, *Poisons of Animal Origin.* (Simpson, L. L., ed.) Plenum Press, New York, **1971,** pp. 139–156.

Raymond, S. A., and Gissen, A. J. Mechanism of differential nerve block. In, *Local Anesthetics.* (Strichartz, G. R., ed.) *Handbook of Experimental Pharmacology,* Vol. 81. Springer-Verlag, Berlin, **1987,** pp. 95–164.

Ritchie, J. M. Tetrodotoxin and saxitoxin and the sodium channels of excitable tissues. *Trends Pharmacol. Sci.,* **1980,** *1,* 275–279.

Ritchie, J. M., and Greengard, P. On the mode of action of local anesthetics. *Annu. Rev. Pharmacol.,* **1966,** *6,* 405–430.

Roth, S. H., and Miller, K. W. (eds.). *Molecular and Cellular Mechanisms of Anesthetics.* Plenum Press, New York, **1986.**

Schantz, E. J. Paralytic shellfish poisoning and saxitoxin. In, *Neuropoisons: Their Pathophysiological Actions.* Vol. 1, *Poisons of Animal Origin.* (Simpson, L. L., ed.) Plenum Press, New York, **1971,** pp. 159–168.

Strichartz, G. R. (ed.). *Local Anesthetics. Handbook of Experimental Pharmacology,* Vol. 81. Springer-Verlag, Berlin, **1987.**

Strichartz, G. R., and Ritchie, J. M. The action of local anesthetics on ion channels of excitable tissues. In, *Local Anesthetics.* (Strichartz, G. R., ed.) *Handbook of Experimental Pharmacology,* Vol. 81. Springer-Verlag, Berlin, **1987,** pp. 21–53.

Trimmer, J. S., and Agnew, W. S. Molecular diversity of voltage-sensitive Na channels. *Annu. Rev. Physiol.,* **1989,** *51,* 401–418.

Vandam, L. D. Some aspects of the history of local anesthesia. In, *Local Anesthetics.* (Strichartz, G. R., ed.) *Handbook of Experimental Pharmacology,* Vol. 81. Springer-Verlag, Berlin, **1987,** pp. 1–19.

Yaksh, T. L.; Al-Rodhan, N. R. F.; and Jensen, T. S. Sites of action of opiates in production of analgesia. In, *Progress in Brain Research,* Vol. 77. (Fields, H. L., and Besson, J. M., eds.) Elsevier, Amsterdam, **1988,** pp. 373–396.

Zipf, H. F., and Dittmann, E. C. General pharmacological effects of local anesthetics. In, *Local Anesthetics,* Vol. 1. *International Encyclopedia of Pharmacology and Therapeutics,* Sect. 8. (Lechat, P., ed.) Pergamon Press, Ltd., Oxford, **1971,** pp. 191–238.

CHAPTER

16 THE THERAPEUTIC GASES

Oxygen, Carbon Dioxide, Helium, and Water Vapor

Roderic G. Eckenhoff and David E. Longnecker

The therapeutic gases discussed in this chapter, most notably oxygen, are obviously not uniquely relevant to the central nervous system. They are placed in Section III primarily for proximity to the general anesthetic agents, many of which are also administered by inhalation.

OXYGEN

The importance of oxygen, water, and food to the animal organism is fundamental. Of these three basic essentials for the maintenance of life, the deprivation of oxygen leads to death most rapidly. Therapy with oxygen is useful or necessary for life in several diseases and intoxications that interfere with normal oxygenation of the blood or tissues. In addition, pure oxygen administered at ambient pressures greater than 1 atmosphere (100 kPa) has both unique applications as a therapeutic agent and multiple toxic effects.

History. Soon after Priestley's discovery of oxygen in 1772 and Lavoisier's elucidation of its role in respiration, oxygen therapy was introduced in England by Beddoes. His publication in 1794, entitled "Considerations on the Medicinal Use and Production of Factitious Airs," can be considered the beginning of inhalational therapy. Beddoes, overcome with enthusiasm for his project, treated all kinds of diseases with oxygen, including such diverse conditions as scrofula, leprosy, and paralysis. Such indiscriminate therapeutic applications naturally led to many failures, and Beddoes died a disconsolate man. It is interesting to note that Beddoes' collaborator was James Watt, engineer and inventor of the steam engine, and his assistant was Sir Humphry Davy. When Beddoes' experiments proved disappointing, Davy left the laboratory to pursue his own investigations on the properties of nitrous oxide. Davy's contribution to the history of anesthesia is mentioned in Chapter 13.

It was only following such pioneer investigations as those of Haldane, Hill, Barcroft, Krogh, L. J. Henderson, and Y. Henderson that oxygen therapy was placed on a sound physiological basis (*see* Sackner, 1974). Although Paul Bert had studied therapeutic aspects of hyperbaric oxygen in 1870, and identified oxygen toxicity (Bert, 1873), the extension of the "dose" of oxygen above 1 atmosphere for therapeutic purposes did not begin until the 1950s (*see* Lambertsen *et al.*, 1953; Boerema *et al.*, 1960).

Normal Oxygenation

Oxygen Cascade. Oxygen moves down a stepwise series of partial pressure gradients from the inspired air to the body's cells and their mitochondria. Air normally contains 20.9% oxygen, equivalent (at normal barometric pressure) to a partial pressure of 159 mm Hg (21 kPa). The partial pressure of oxygen decreases as the air is delivered to the distal airways and alveoli by inspiration—by dilution with carbon dioxide and water vapor and by uptake into the blood. If ventilation and perfusion are homogeneously distributed throughout the lung, the partial pressure of oxygen in the alveoli can be calculated to approximate 110 mm Hg (14.7 kPa). Diffusion of oxygen into the pulmonary capillary blood is driven by the gradient between the partial pressure of oxygen in mixed venous (pulmonary arterial) blood and that in the alveolar gas. Because of facilitated diffusion through an extremely thin barrier within the capillary (Hemmingsen and Scholander, 1960), the Po_2 of pulmonary end-capillary blood is normally within a few mm Hg of that in the alveolus. Regional inhomogeneity of ventilation and perfusion influences the size of this gradient, and thus the rate of equilibration and end-capillary Po_2.

The partial pressure of oxygen in systemic arterial blood (Pa_{O_2}) is slightly lower than that of mixed pulmonary capillary blood because of the addition of a small fraction of venous blood (shunt fraction). Together, the diffusional barrier, inhomogeneities of ventilation and perfusion, and the shunt fraction are the major causes of the alveolar-to-arterial oxygen gradient, which is normally 10 to 12 mm Hg when air is breathed and 30 to 50 mm Hg when 100% oxygen is inspired (Clark and Lambertsen, 1971a).

Oxygen is delivered to the tissue capillary beds by the circulation, and oxygen again follows a gradient out of the blood and into the cells and their mitochondria. As a result of this loss to the tissues, the Po_2 of venous blood is lower than that of arterial blood by about 55 mm Hg. However, the mean tissue Po_2 is much lower than the value in mixed venous blood because of the substantial diffusional barriers and ongoing utilization of oxygen in the tissues. Although the Po_2 at the site of oxygen utilization—the mitochondria—is not known, oxidative phosphorylation can continue at a Po_2 of only a few mm Hg (Robiolio *et al.*, 1989).

Blood Oxygen Content. Oxygen in blood is carried primarily in chemical combination with hemoglobin and to a small extent in physical solution in plasma. The quantity of oxygen combined with hemoglobin depends on the Po_2, as illustrated by the sigmoid-shaped oxyhemoglobin dissociation curve (Figure 16–1). When fully saturated, each gram of hemoglobin binds 1.31 ml of oxygen (Gregory, 1974). Hemoglobin is about 98% saturated when air is breathed under normal circumstances; thus, elevation of Po_2 by breathing mixtures enriched in oxygen can elevate the oxygen content of blood only by increasing the fraction dissolved in plasma. Because of the low solubility of oxygen in plasma (0.03 ml · liter^{-1} · mm Hg^{-1} at 37°C), breathing 100% oxygen can increase the amount of oxygen in blood by only 15 ml per liter; this is less than one third of normal metabolic demands. However, if the inspired Po_2 is increased to 3 atmospheres (304 kPa) in a hyperbaric chamber, the amount of oxygen dissolved in plasma is sufficient to meet metabolic demands in the absence of hemoglobin.

The oxygen content of mixed venous blood is lower than that of arterial blood by the amount utilized for metabolism—generally 50 to 60 ml per liter under normal conditions. When air is breathed, venous hemoglobin is about 70% saturated with oxygen; this value is increased to 100% when the inspired Po_2 is increased to 3 atmospheres (304 kPa). The lack of desaturation of hemoglobin under hyperbaric conditions has implications for the transport of carbon dioxide (*see* below).

OXYGEN DEPRIVATION

Knowledge of the causes and effects of oxygen deficiency is necessary for the intelligent therapeutic use of the gas. *Hypoxia* is a broad term used to denote insufficient oxygenation of the tissues. Since hypoxia can arise from a variety of causes, and because therapy is closely allied to etiology, a

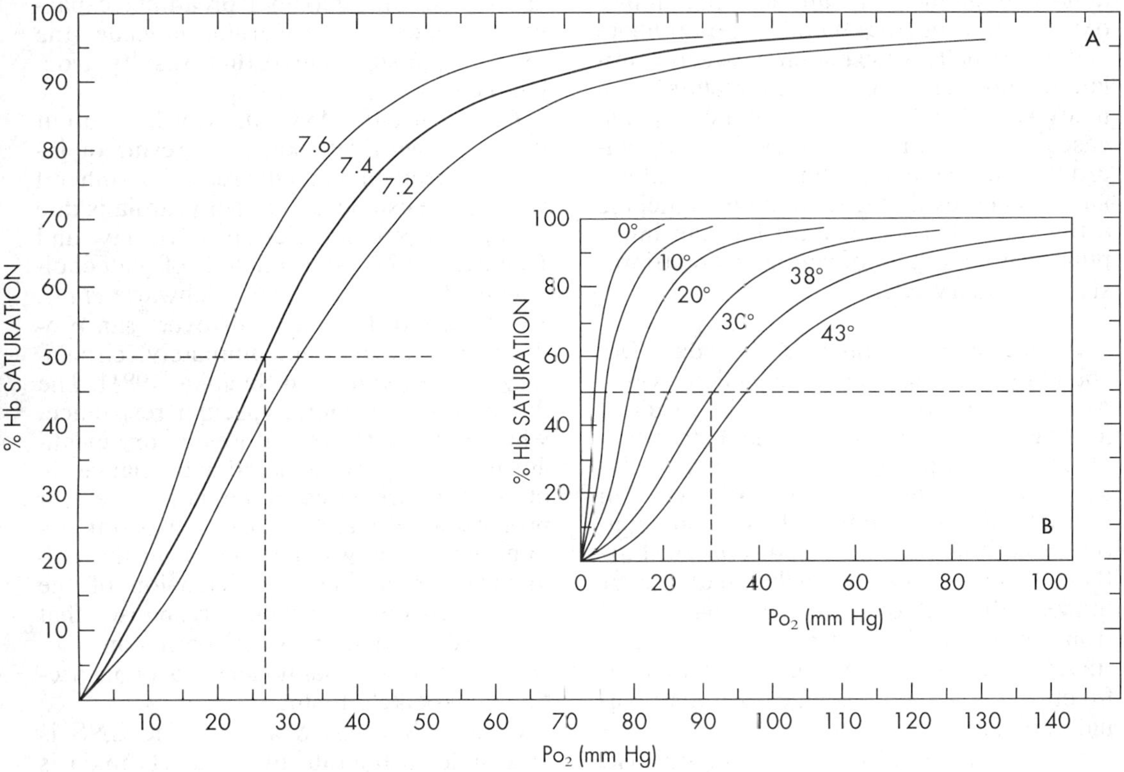

Figure 16–1. *Oxyhemoglobin dissociation curves for whole blood.*

The main diagram shows the effect of pH on the affinity of hemoglobin for oxygen. The inset shows the effect of temperature. An increase in temperature or a decrease in pH (as in a working muscle) aids in "unloading" oxygen from oxyhemoglobin. (Reproduced by permission from: Lambertsen, C. J. Transport of oxygen, carbon dioxide, and inert gases by the blood. (Mountcastle, ed.) *Med. Physiol.*, **1980,** *14,* 1725, Fig. 69–3. St. Louis, 1980, The C. V. Mosby Co.)

simple classification of causes of hypoxia is useful. Three categories can be delineated.

Prepulmonary Causes of Hypoxia. Hypoxia can be caused by inadequate delivery of oxygen to the lung. This may be the result of an inadequate partial pressure of inspired oxygen because of low barometric pressure (altitude) or low oxygen concentration (dilution). However, inadequate delivery of oxygen results more commonly from inadequate ventilation brought about by airway obstruction (laryngospasm, bronchospasm), muscular weakness (disease or neuromuscular blocking drugs), or impaired respiratory drive (central nervous system [CNS] disease, opioids, anesthetics).

Pulmonary Causes of Hypoxia. Despite normal delivery of oxygen to the lungs, abnormal pulmonary function can impair oxygenation of the blood. The ultimate cause is usually a mismatch between ventilation and perfusion, which results from many short- and long-term pulmonary diseases (*e.g.*, adult respiratory distress syndrome, asthma, emphysema). Other pulmonary processes that lead to hypoxia include a thickened barrier to diffusion and intrapulmonary shunting of venous blood (fibrosis, pulmonary edema).

Postpulmonary Causes of Hypoxia. Despite normal Pa_{O_2}, inadequate delivery of oxygen to the tissues may be the result of low cardiac output (shock), maldistribution of cardiac output (sepsis, vascular occlusion), or inadequate content of oxygen in arterial blood (anemia, hemoglobinopathies, carbon monoxide poisoning). Further, the tissues may be unable to extract or utilize sufficient oxygen. This may result from an unusually high metabolic demand (thyrotoxicosis, hyperpyrexia) or to malfunction of cellular enzyme systems (cyanide poisoning).

Several causes of hypoxia often coexist. For example, a victim of smoke inhalation may have inspired a low concentration of oxygen because of its consumption by the fire; airway obstruction may exist as a result of thermal injury and edema; and the content of oxygen in blood and its utilization by tissues may be reduced because of carbon monoxide poisoning. An organ with a marginal blood supply because of atherosclerosis may be seriously damaged if the Po_2 or oxygen content of its arterial supply is decreased only slightly.

Effects of Hypoxia. *Respiration.* Ventilatory rate and depth are both progressively increased during hypoxia as a result of stimulation of carotid and aortic chemoreceptors; minute ventilation almost doubles when normal individuals inspire gas with a Po_2 of 50 mm Hg. The hypocarbia that results from this hyperpnea attenuates the ventilatory response to hypoxia. Similarly, the ventilatory response to hypercarbia is enhanced in the presence of hypoxia (Lahiri *et al.,* 1981). Dyspnea is not always experienced with simple hypoxia; dyspnea occurs when the respiratory minute volume approaches the maximal breathing capacity. In general, little warning precedes the loss of consciousness that results from hypoxia.

Cardiovascular System. Cardiac output increases with hypoxia as a result of increased heart rate and decreased peripheral vascular resistance. The tachycardia is due to both CNS stimulation (Krasney and Koehler, 1977) and release of catecholamines (Cohen *et al.,* 1967; Schwartz *et al.,* 1981). Severe hypoxia, however, can produce bradycardia and, ultimately, circulatory failure (Kafer and Sugioka, 1981). The decrease in peripheral vascular resistance, which is mediated by autoregulatory mechanisms, is rarely associated with changes in blood pressure unless hypoxia is severe or prolonged. Hypoxia causes vasoconstriction and possibly hypertension in the pulmonary circulation—an extension of the normal regional vascular response that matches ventilation with perfusion (so-called "hypoxic pulmonary vasoconstriction") (Voelkel, 1986).

Central Nervous System. The CNS is least able to tolerate hypoxia. Hypoxia is accompanied initially by decreased intellectual capacity and impaired judgment and psychomotor ability; this state progresses to confusion and restlessness and ultimately to stupor, coma, and death as the Pa_{O_2} decreases below 30 to 40 mm Hg. As noted above, the victim is often unaware of this progression.

Cellular and Metabolic Effects. Delivery of oxygen to mitochondria slows as the partial pressure gradient from capillaries to tissues decreases. At a mitochondrial Po_2 of less than about 1 mm Hg (130 Pa), aerobic metabolism stops, and the less efficient anaerobic pathways of glycolysis become responsible for the production of cellular energy (Robiolio *et al.*, 1989). Ion gradients decrease because energy-dependent transport slows, and cellular functions (*e.g.*, action potentials, secretion) that rely upon the maintenance of ion gradients are impaired. The cellular concentrations of Na^+, Ca^{2+}, and H^+ increase, leading to cell death. Restoration of perfusion and oxygenation prior to hypoxic cell death can paradoxically result in an accelerated form of cell injury (the ischemia–reperfusion syndrome), thought to result from the generation of oxygen-free radicals (McCord, 1985). The ultimate mechanism of cell death and the point of irreversibility are not yet known.

Adaptation to Hypoxia. Long-term hypoxia results in adaptive physiological changes; these have been studied most thoroughly in persons exposed to high altitude. Persons living at high altitude have increased numbers of pulmonary alveoli, increased concentrations of hemoglobin in blood and myoglobin in muscle, and a decreased ventilatory response to hypoxia (Cruz *et al.*, 1980). Short-term exposure to altitude produces similar adaptive changes, although the precise mechanisms for the changes are not clear. In susceptible individuals, however, acute exposure to high altitude results in a syndrome characterized initially by headache, nausea, dyspnea, and impaired judgment, progressing to pulmonary and cerebral edema (Johnson and Rock, 1988). The mechanism for this acute mountain sickness may not be entirely related to hypoxia; a form of decompression sickness (*see* below under Hyperbaric Oxygen Therapy) may contribute to the pathophysiological process (Levine *et al.*, 1988). Mountain sickness is treated by inhalation of oxygen, descent to lower altitude, or a small increase in ambient pressure. Treatment with diuretics (carbonic anhydrase inhibitors) and steroids may also be helpful. The syndrome can be avoided by slow ascent to higher altitude, thereby permitting adaptation. A form of chronic mountain sickness has been described in which severe polycythemia results in altered blood rheology, which can lead ultimately to cardiac failure (Pugh, 1964).

EFFECTS OF OXYGEN INHALATION

The primary use for inhalation of oxygen is to reverse the effects of hypoxia; other consequences are usually minor. However, when breathed in excessive amounts, physiological adaptation to oxygen and toxic effects can both occur.

Respiration. Inhalation of oxygen at 1 atmosphere (100 kPa) or above causes a small and immediate respiratory depression in normal subjects, presumably owing to loss of tonic chemoreceptor activity. Minutes later, however, ventilation increases, owing to a paradoxical increase in the tension of carbon dioxide in tissues. This increase results from the increased concentration of oxyhemoglobin in venous blood, which causes less efficient removal of carbon dioxide from the tissues (Lambertsen *et al.*, 1953; Plewes and Farhi, 1983).

One of the ways in which carbon dioxide is carried by blood is in the form of bicarbonate. This mechanism of carbon dioxide transfer operates more readily when a hydrogen ion acceptor is made available, as occurs in the capillaries when oxyhemoglobin is converted to deoxyhemoglobin, a stronger base and therefore a better hydrogen ion acceptor. When large amounts of oxygen are carried in simple solution (*e.g.*, during hyperbaric oxygenation), the amount of physically dissolved oxygen may be sufficient to satisfy the requirements of tissue. Little or no oxygen is then extracted from oxyhemoglobin, and deoxyhemoglobin is not formed. Carbon dioxide is then carried away from tissues less efficiently, and the Pco_2 of the tissues rises by several mm Hg.

In patients whose CNS respiratory center is depressed by long-term retention of carbon dioxide, injury, or drugs, ventilation is maintained largely by stimulation of carotid and aortic chemoreceptors, commonly referred to as the *hypoxic drive* (Aubier *et al.*, 1980). Therefore, an acute rise in Pa_{O_2} as a result of inhalation of oxygen may further depress ventilation, resulting in pronounced respiratory acidosis. Careful titration of the concentration of inhaled oxygen, coupled with continuous ventilatory or oximetric monitoring (*see* below), often allows sufficient oxygenation without dangerous hypoventilation.

Expansion of poorly ventilated alveoli is maintained in part by the nitrogen content of alveolar gas. Inhalation of oxygen rapidly lowers the nitrogen content of alveoli and tissues, and if removal of oxygen from the alveoli exceeds delivery by ventilation, collapse may occur. This *absorption atelectasis* worsens oxygenation of blood by impairing the relationship between ventilation and perfusion; it can be prevented by the administration of as little as 5 to 10% nitrogen in the inspired gas (DuBois *et al.*, 1966).

Cardiovascular System. Aside from reversing the effects of hypoxia, the physiological effects of oxygen inhalation on the cardiovascular system are of little consequence. Heart rate and cardiac output are slightly reduced when 100% oxygen is breathed; blood pressure changes little. Pulmonary arterial pressure is decreased slightly because of removal of the vascular tone that is maintained by regional alveolar hypoxia (Voelkel, 1986).

Metabolism. Inhalation of 100% oxygen does not produce detectable changes in oxygen consumption, carbon dioxide production, respiratory quotient, or glucose utilization.

OXYGEN TOXICITY

During the course of evolution, the atmospheric concentration of oxygen increased as a result of the hydrolytic release of oxygen by newly evolved photosynthetic organisms. Mechanisms for production of energy by utilization of oxygen had to be coupled with mechanisms for defense against oxidative damage. These defense systems consist of enzymes (superoxide dismutase, glutathione peroxidase, catalase) and reducing agents (glutathione, ascorbate, iron). However, these mechanisms are inadequate when inspired concentrations of oxygen exceed normal for appreciable periods of time (Figure 16–2). Oxygen-induced toxicity probably results from increased production of reactive species such as superoxide anion, singlet oxygen, hydroxyl radical, and hydrogen peroxide (Turrens *et al.*, 1982). The oxidative damage that these substances initiate is propagated by lipid peroxidation and ulti-

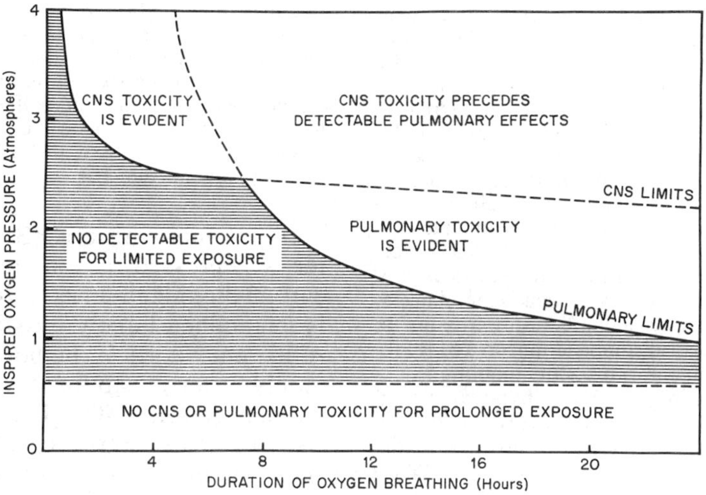

Figure 16–2. *Oxygen-toxicity limits in man.*

The two areas most affected are the CNS and the lungs. The occurrence of toxicity depends upon both the inspired oxygen pressure (Po_2) and the duration of exposure. The safe duration of exposure becomes shorter as the inspired Po_2 increases. Below ½ atmosphere of inspired oxygen, indefinite exposure appears to be safe; between ½ and approximately 2 atmospheres, pulmonary toxicity occurs after prolonged exposures but CNS effects are not detectable; above 2 atmospheres, CNS toxicity appears before pulmonary effects are detectable. (Adapted from Lambertsen, 1978.)

mately involves all components of the cell. Cell injury and death is presumed to result from loss of membrane integrity. Although high concentrations of oxygen affect all tissues adversely, differential sensitivity is observed because of both inherent tissue factors and the concentration of oxygen to which the tissue is continuously exposed.

Respiratory Tract. The pulmonary system is continuously exposed to the highest Po_2 of any organ system, and it is usually the first to be adversely affected by exposure to elevated concentrations of oxygen at ambient pressure. Inhalation of 100% oxygen for as little as 6 to 8 hours decreases the velocity of movement of tracheal mucous (Sackner *et al.*, 1975); symptoms of tracheobronchial irritation and "tightness" of the chest are observed in as little as 12 hours. Increased alveolar permeability and inflammation are apparent after 17 hours (Davis *et al.*, 1983), and decreased pulmonary function after 18 to 24 hours of continuous exposure (Clark, 1988). Although nausea, vomiting, and anorexia are prominent symptoms in human subjects exposed to 100% oxygen for more than 24 hours, survival time of otherwise normal primates is in excess of a week (Clark and Lambertsen, 1971b); death results from pulmonary edema and, ironically, hypoxia. Although the development and rate of progression of pulmonary oxygen toxicity are directly related to the partial pressure of oxygen in the inspired gas, the maximal "safe" partial pressure of oxygen is not entirely clear. However, prolonged exposure to 0.5 atmospheres (50 kPa) produces few symptoms in normal subjects and even allows recovery from acute pulmonary injury in animals (Cheney *et al.*, 1980) and man (Eckenhoff *et al.*, 1987). Absorption atelectasis (*see* above) is not an important contributor to pulmonary oxygen toxicity.

The precise pathophysiological mechanisms of pulmonary oxygen toxicity are not well understood. The pulmonary capillary endothelium is most sensitive (Crapo *et al.*, 1980), and endothelial injury results in progressive accumulation of interstitial and alveolar fluid and loss of capillary surface area, both of which impair gas transport. Granulocytes do not appear to have an important role in the pathophysiology of oxygen poisoning (Boyce *et al.*, 1989).

The treatment of oxygen toxicity relies on decreasing the inspired Po_2 and providing supportive measures; there are no specific pharmacological approaches. Some amelioration of toxicity in animals has been obtained by the parenteral administration of antioxidant enzymes in forms designed to gain access to the intracellular space (White *et al.*, 1989). Dramatic improvements in oxygen tolerance in animals have been produced by prior exposure to high concentrations of the gas (Kravetz *et al.*, 1980; Coursin *et al.*, 1987); paradoxically, prior hypoxia can also cause increased resistance to pulmonary oxygen toxicity (Frank, 1982). Similarly, oxygen tolerance by man can be increased by regular, brief interruptions of oxygen inhalation (Hendricks *et al.*, 1977; Clark, 1988). In animals, adaptation is associated with increased activities of cellular antioxidant enzymes, proliferation of alveolar type-II cells, and increased concentrations of alveolar surfactant (Crapo *et al.*, 1980; Holm *et al.*, 1988).

Central Nervous System. CNS oxygen toxicity is generally not seen when the partial pressure of inspired oxygen is less than 2 atmospheres (203 kPa); its occurrence is thus limited to a small number of hyperbaric applications. CNS toxicity usually occurs before pulmonary toxicity when oxygen is administered at partial pressures above 3 atmospheres (304 kPa) (*see* Figure 16–2); like pulmonary toxicity, susceptibility among individuals varies widely (Clark, 1982). The syndrome is characterized by convulsions, which may be preceded by visual symptoms or muscular twitching. Exercise and hypercarbia accelerate the appearance of symptoms. CNS toxicity is rapidly reversible when the partial pressure of inspired oxygen is reduced, and sequelae have not been described.

Retina. Exposure of neonates younger than 44 weeks' gestation to an increased Pa_{O_2} may be associated with the development of retrolental fibroplasia (Betts *et al.*, 1977); this effect is believed to be the result of aberrant angiogenesis in the developing eye (Kushner *et al.*, 1977; Ashton, 1979).

The changes may regress, or they may progress to blindness. The syndrome may be largely prevented by careful titration of oxygen concentrations to achieve a defined saturation of hemoglobin as detected by oximetry (*see* below). Oxygen-induced retinopathy in adults is rare, even after hyperbaric exposure.

PREPARATIONS

Oxygen is available as the compressed gas in steel cylinders, and a purity of 99% is referred to as "medical grade." Most hospitals have oxygen piped from insulated liquid oxygen containers to areas of frequent use. Oxygen cylinders and piping are color coded (green in the United States), and some form of mechanical indexing of valve connections is used to prevent the connection of other gases to oxygen systems.

METHODS OF ADMINISTRATION

Oxygen is administered by inhalation, except during extracorporeal circulation, when it is dissolved directly in the exteriorized blood. Devices for inhalation include nasal cannulae, masks, tents or hoods, and tracheal tubes.

Plastic or rubber tubing is used to deliver a low flow (2 to 5 l/min) of humidified oxygen into one or both nostrils. The nasopharynx acts as an oxygen reservoir, and this reservoir is diluted with room air during inhalation. The inspired oxygen concentration is variable, unpredictable, dependent on the patient's ventilatory pattern, and usually less than 35%.

A wide variety of masks that cover both the mouth and nose are available for administration of oxygen. Masks that lack sufficient flow rates to meet peak inspiratory demand will either entrain diluent room air through valves or draw on built-in reservoir bags that fill during exhalation. One-way valves in the bag and in the sides of the mask prevent rebreathing of expired gas. Such masks must be fit carefully to provide a tight seal around the face, and they must be monitored for proper operation of the valves and reservoir bag. The seal around the mask is critical for masks with a demand valve, since negative pressure must be generated to initiate the flow of oxygen. In practice, these demand (aviator) masks will deliver the highest concentration of oxygen, but they are probably the least comfortable for extended use. Seal and valving are less important with masks that deliver flows sufficient to meet peak inspiratory flow rates. However, since these masks produce high flow rates by dilution with room air, inspired oxygen concentrations are generally not higher than about 50%.

A known concentration of oxygen can be administered consistently by enlarging the inspiratory reservoir to encompass the entire head (with a hood) or a larger area (with a tent). These devices are comfortable and require little cooperation from the patient. Flow rates must be sufficient to prevent accumulation of carbon dioxide.

A tracheal tube that seals against the walls of the airway is the definitive means of delivering known concentrations of oxygen to the lungs. Ventilation is often accomplished mechanically. Such measures are used for those who are critically ill or who are undergoing procedures that may compromise ventilatory function.

MONITORING OF OXYGENATION

Monitoring and titration are required to meet the therapeutic goals of oxygen therapy and to avoid toxicity. Although cyanosis is a physical finding of substantial clinical importance, it is not a sensitive or reliable index for evaluation of oxygenation. Cyanosis appears when the concentration of deoxyhemoglobin in arterial blood is about 50 g per liter. Thus, as but one example, cyanosis may be absent when tissue hypoxia is due to anemia. Invasive approaches for evaluation of oxygenation include intermittent sampling of arterial or mixed venous blood for laboratory analysis of blood gases or placement of vascular cannulae that are capable of continuous measurements of oxygen tension. The latter method, which relies on fiberoptic oximetry, is most frequently used clinically for the continuous measurement of mixed venous hemoglobin saturation as an index of tissue requirements and extraction of oxygen, usually in critically ill patients.

Because of the inherent disadvantages of invasive techniques, noninvasive procedures for monitoring oxygen tensions have received much attention recently. Transcutaneous oximetry relies on diffusion of gases from cutaneous arteriovenous shunts (created by heating the skin) to a polarographic electrode applied to the skin. Transcutaneous oximetry has been used successfully to monitor oxygenation in children, but the physiology of cutaneous gas transport is complex and inadequately described; the technique is also subject to instability, and frequent calibration is necessary. A more popular continuous technique, pulse oximetry, relies on differential absorbance of light by oxyhemoglobin and deoxyhemoglobin in an accessible pulsatile tissue, such as a finger, nose, or ear. Application is simple and calibration is generally not required. Because pulse oximetry measures hemoglobin saturation and not Po_2, it is less useful when the Pao_2 exceeds that necessary for complete saturation of hemoglobin. However, it is very useful for monitoring the adequacy of oxygenation during procedures that require sedation or anesthesia or for titration of oxygen therapy in clinical situations where toxicity from oxygen is a concern.

THERAPEUTIC USES

Correction of Hypoxia. As stated above, the primary therapeutic use for oxygen is to correct hypoxia. However, hypoxia is most commonly a manifestation of an underlying disease, and administration of oxygen can thus be viewed as symptomatic or temporizing therapy. Only rarely is hypoxia due to a primary deficiency in the inspired gas. Because of the vast array of causes of hypoxia, it is reasonable that supplementation of the inspired gas alone will often not suffice to correct the problem. Efforts must be directed at correcting the cause of the hypoxia. For example, airway obstruction is unlikely to respond to an increase in inspired tension of oxygen without relief of the obstruction. The hypoxia of anemia will not respond to normobaric administration of oxygen without more fundamental efforts directed at increasing the concentration of hemoglobin. However, the hypoxia that results from most pulmonary diseases can be at least partially alleviated by administration of oxygen, hopefully allowing time for more definitive therapy to reverse the primary process. Thus, administration of oxygen is a basic and important treatment to be used in all forms of hypoxia, with the understanding that the response will vary in a way that is generally predictable from knowledge of the underlying pathophysiologic processes.

Reduction of the Partial Pressure of an Inert Gas. The predominant gas in most gas-filled spaces in the body (natural or acquired) is nitrogen. Since nitrogen is relatively insoluble, inhalation of high concentrations of oxygen (and thus low concentrations of nitrogen) rapidly lowers the total body partial pressure of nitrogen and provides a substantial gradient for removal of nitrogen from the gas spaces. Such spaces result from intestinal obstruction or ileus, pneumothorax, and air embolism. Administration of oxygen for air embolism is especially beneficial, since it also helps to relieve the localized hypoxia distal to the embolic (gas) vascular obstruction.

The acquired gas disease known as *decompression sickness* or *bends* represents another instance in which lowering of the tension of an inert gas in blood and tissues is a desired effect of inhalation of oxygen. In this case, lowering of the tissue tension of the inert gas prior to or during a barometric decompression (from hyperbaric conditions or to high altitude) reduces the degree of supersaturation that occurs after decompression to a degree where separation of a gas phase does not occur (*i.e.*, bubbles do not form). The time required to remove an inert gas depends on the nature of the gas, ventilation, cardiac output, tissue perfusion, and body composition. If a gas phase does form in either tissues or the vasculature, administration of oxygen is based on the same logic as described for gas embolism.

Oxygen as a Diluent. Oxygen is used as a diluent or carrier gas for the administration of other vapors and gases—primarily anesthetic agents. This utilization serves a dual purpose, since anesthetic agents commonly depress ventilation and circulation enough to require administration of supplemental oxygen to meet metabolic needs.

Hyperbaric Oxygen Therapy. The use of oxygen at increased pressure is close to a true pharmacological application of the gas. However, most of the indications for hyperbaric oxygen remain the relief of either generalized or localized hypoxia (*see* Davis, 1986; Thom, 1989a).

Hyperbaric oxygen is administered in a pressure chamber, of which there are two basic types—monoplace and multiplace. The modern monoplace chamber is made of transparent acrylic, accommodates a single patient, and is usually pressurized with oxygen; the patient does not wear a mask. The multiplace chamber is usually made of steel, accommodates more than two persons, and is usually pressurized with air while the patient breathes oxygen from a tight-fitting mask or circuit. The multiplace chamber is more suited for critically ill patients who require ventilation, monitoring, and constant attendance. The pressure achieved depends on the indication, and ranges from 2 to 6 atmospheres; however, the inhaled oxygen tension rarely exceeds 3 atmospheres.

Hyperbaric oxygen therapy has two important and not entirely separable components: increased hydrostatic pressure and increased oxygen tension. Both factors are necessary for the treatment of gas-lesion disease (decompression sickness, air embolism). Hydrostatic pressure reduces bubble volume, and oxygen increases the gradient for elimination of nitrogen and reduces hypoxia in downstream tissues. Increased oxygen tension is the primary therapeutic goal for most of the other indications for hyperbaric oxygen. For example, even a small increase in Po_2 in previously ischemic areas may enhance the bactericidal activity of leukocytes and angiogenesis. Thus, repetitive brief exposures to hyperbaric oxygen are a useful adjunct in the treatment of chronic refractory osteomyelitis, osteoradionecrosis, or crush injury or for the maintenance of compromised skin or tissue grafts or flaps. Furthermore, increased oxygen tension can itself be bacteriostatic; the spread of infection with *Clostridium perfringens* and production of toxin by the bacteria are slowed when oxygen tensions exceed 250 mm Hg (33 kPa), justifying the early use of hyperbaric oxygen in clostridial myonecrosis (gas gangrene).

Hyperbaric oxygen is also useful in selected instances of generalized hypoxia. In carbon monoxide poisoning, hemoglobin and myoglobin become unavailable for oxygen binding because of the high affinity of CO for these proteins. A high Po_2 facilitates competition of oxygen with CO for binding sites, permitting the resumption of normal delivery of oxygen to the tissues. Hyperbaric oxygen decreases the incidence of neurological sequelae after CO intoxication; this effect may be independent of the ability of hyperbaric oxygen to speed the elimination of CO (Thom, 1989b). The occasional use of hyperbaric oxygen in cyanide poisoning has a similar rationale. Hyperbaric oxygen may also be useful in severe, short-term anemia, since sufficient oxygen can be dissolved in the plasma at 3 atmospheres to meet metabolic needs. However, such treatment must be limited, since pulmonary and possibly CNS oxygen toxicity result from an increased Po_2 and not from an increased oxygen content in the blood.

Hyperbaric oxygen therapy has also been used in such diverse conditions as multiple sclerosis, traumatic spinal cord injury, cerebrovascular accidents, bone grafts and fractures, and leprosy. However, these uses are not justified by sufficient data from well-controlled clinical trials.

CARBON DIOXIDE

It was not until the end of the eighteenth century that Priestley discovered carbon dioxide and Lavoisier described its role in respiration. A century later Miesher demonstrated its effects on the respiration of man. The gas is of paramount importance in the regulation of many vital functions, and small changes in P_{CO_2} in the body have marked physiological effects.

Transfer and Elimination of Carbon Dioxide

Approximately 200 ml per minute of carbon dioxide are produced by the body's metabolism at rest, and up to ten times that much during heavy exercise. The gas diffuses readily from the cells that produce it into the bloodstream, where it is carried partly as bicarbonate ion, partly in chemical combination with hemoglobin and plasma proteins, and partly in solution at a partial pressure of about 46 mm Hg in mixed venous blood. It is transported to the lung, where it is normally exhaled at the same rate at which it is produced, leaving a partial pressure of about 40 mm Hg in the alveoli and in the arterial blood.

When carbon dioxide is inhaled, or when alveolar ventilation is decreased, the P_{CO_2} in arterial blood rises and its pH falls. This decrease in pH is referred to as *respiratory acidosis*. When overventilation lowers the P_{CO_2} of blood, the pH rises and *respiratory alkalosis* is present. As carbon dioxide can freely diffuse into and out of cells, the changes in blood P_{CO_2} and pH are soon reflected by intracellular changes of P_{CO_2} and pH (*see* Chapter 27).

Effects of Carbon Dioxide

Alterations of P_{CO_2} and pH have widespread effects in the body. Here a description will be given of the important effects of carbon dioxide on respiration, circulation, and the CNS. (For a more complete discussion of these and other effects, *see* Nunn, 1987.)

Respiration. Carbon dioxide is a potent stimulus to respiration. The inhalation of 2% carbon dioxide produces a measurable increase in both rate and depth of ventilation. Ten percent carbon dioxide can produce respiratory volumes of 75 l/min in normal individuals. Respiratory stimulation begins in seconds following the inhalation of even low concentrations of carbon dioxide, and maximal stimulation by the inhaled carbon dioxide is usually attained in less than 5 minutes (*see* Lourenco, 1976). The respiratory effects of carbon dioxide inhalation disappear within a few minutes after its withdrawal.

There are at least two sites where carbon dioxide acts to stimulate respiration. Respiratory integration areas in the brainstem are acted upon by impulses from medullary chemoreceptors and from peripheral arterial chemoreceptors. The mechanism by which carbon dioxide acts on these receptors involves the decrease in pH produced by the gas (*see* Neff and Talmage, 1978; Drysdale *et al.*, 1981). Elevated P_{CO_2} causes bronchodilatation, while hypocarbia causes constriction of airway smooth muscle; these responses may play a role in matching pulmonary ventilation and perfusion (Duane *et al.*, 1979).

Circulation. The circulatory effects of carbon dioxide are the result of its direct local effects and its centrally mediated effects on the autonomic nervous system. The direct effect of carbon dioxide on the heart results from pH changes and produces diminished contractility (van den Bos *et al.*, 1979). Cardiac rhythm is usually not affected. The direct effect on systemic blood vessels results in vasodilatation.

Carbon dioxide causes widespread activation of the sympathetic nervous system and an increase in the plasma concentrations of epinephrine, norepinephrine, angiotensin, and other vasoactive peptides (Staszewska-Barczak and Dusting, 1981). The response is mediated by various subcortical centers in the hypothalamus, brainstem reticular formation, and medulla. These areas can be excited locally by carbon dioxide, but they also receive afferents from the carotid and aortic chemoreceptors that are sensitive to changes in carbon dioxide in the blood. The results of sympathetic nervous system activation are, in general, opposite to the local effects of carbon dioxide. The sympathetic effects consist of an increase in cardiac contractility and heart rate and vasoconstriction.

The total circulatory response to carbon dioxide, therefore, is determined by the balance of the opposing effects on local tissues and the sympathetic nervous system effects. The overall effects of carbon dioxide inhalation in normal man are an increase in cardiac output and heart rate, an elevation of systolic and diastolic blood pressures, and an increase in pulse pressure (Rasmussen *et al.*, 1978; Lin *et al.*, 1983). In contrast to the effects of carbon dioxide on the heart, the local effects on blood vessels appear to exert more of an influence than do the sympathetically mediated vasoconstrictor effects, and total peripheral resistance decreases when carbon dioxide is breathed. The cerebral circulation, which does not have functionally important sympathetic innervation, undergoes significant dilatation when carbon dioxide is inhaled. Carbon dioxide is also a potent coronary vasodilator (Ely *et al.*, 1982).

In isolated cardiac preparations, carbon dioxide increases the threshold for catecholamine-induced arrhythmias (de Castuma *et al.*, 1977). In the intact organism, however, the amount of catecholamine released during hypercarbia may be sufficient to overwhelm this protective effect. Arrhythmias are especially likely to occur if the myocardium has been sensitized by inhalation of halogenated anesthetics.

The circulatory effects of hypocarbia consist of

decreased blood pressure, vascular dilatation in muscle, and vasoconstriction in skin, intestine, brain, kidney, and heart. If the hypocarbia results from voluntary hyperventilation, cardiac output and heart rate increase because of increased venous return and increased metabolic demands of the respiratory muscles. In contrast, mechanical hyperventilation reduces heart rate and cardiac output. This effect is probably related to the increased intrathoracic pressure caused by mechanical ventilation.

Central Nervous System. Hypercarbia depresses the excitability of the cerebral cortex and increases the threshold for the production of seizures by drugs or electroshock. It also increases the cutaneous pain threshold through a central action. This central depression is of importance in the therapeutic application of the gas, since carbon dioxide can accentuate preexisting CNS depression. However, when high concentrations of carbon dioxide (25 to 30%) are breathed, subcortical areas that have cortical projections are activated. This activation overcomes the depressant effect of carbon dioxide on the cortex and can result in convulsions. The inhalation of even higher concentrations of carbon dioxide (about 50%) produces marked cortical and subcortical depression of a type similar to that produced by anesthetic agents.

Chemistry, Preparations, and Methods of Administration

Carbon dioxide is marketed in metal cylinders as the pure gas or as carbon dioxide mixed with oxygen. It is usually administered by means of a face mask at a concentration of 5 to 10% in combination with oxygen. Another method for the temporary administration of carbon dioxide is by rebreathing—for example, from an anesthesia breathing circuit when the soda lime canister is bypassed or from something as simple as a paper bag.

Therapeutic Uses

Inhalation of carbon dioxide has been suggested as a means of therapy in many commonly encountered situations, but for most of these, other treatments are more effective and offer fewer disadvantages.

Uses in Anesthesia. Inhalation of carbon dioxide can increase the speed of induction and emergence from inhalational anesthesia by increasing minute ventilation and cerebral blood flow (*see* Chapter 13). However, some degree of respiratory acidosis is inevitable. Hypocarbia with its attendant respiratory alkalosis has some uses in anesthesia. It increases the apparent depth of anesthesia, and by constricting the cerebral vessels, it decreases brain size slightly and may facilitate the performance of neurosurgical operations.

Respiratory Depression. Although carbon dioxide stimulates respiration, it is not useful in situations where respiratory depression has resulted in hypercarbia or acidosis, since further depression of respiration can result.

Miscellaneous Uses. Inhalation of carbon dioxide is one of many suggested treatments for hiccoughs, and it has been successful in some cases. Sudden deafness has been treated successfully by inhalation of mixtures of carbon dioxide and oxygen, presumably because of increased cochlear circulation and delivery of oxygen (Fisch, 1983). Because it does not support combustion, carbon dioxide is often insufflated during endoscopic procedures when electrocauterization is used (Bigard *et al.*, 1979).

HELIUM

Helium is the most inert gas. Its low density, low solubility, and high thermal conductivity are the basis for the medical and diagnostic use of helium. The high velocity of sound transmission in helium causes voice distortion when subjects breath the gas.

History and Preparation. Helium was identified spectroscopically in the sun's atmosphere in 1868, as α radiation from uranium ore in 1895, and as a component in natural gas in 1905. The sole commercial source of helium is recovery after liquefaction of natural gas from fields in the western United States. It is marketed in compressed form in steel cylinders.

Methods of Administration. Helium is mixed with the desired concentration of oxygen and is administered by mask, mouthpiece, or tracheal tube. In certain hyperbaric applications, the entire surrounding atmosphere consists of a mixture of helium and oxygen.

Applications. The therapeutic and diagnostic uses of helium have been summarized by Mathewson (1982). It is used in pulmonary function testing, the treatment of respiratory obstruction, laser airway surgery, and selected hyperbaric applications.

Pulmonary Function Testing. Determination of residual lung volume, functional residual capacity, and related values requires a highly diffusible gas that is insoluble (and thus does not leave the lung), so that its dilution by gas in the lung can be measured. Of the inert gases, helium best meets these criteria. In practice, a single large breath of a known concentration of helium is administered, and the concentration of helium is then measured in the mixed expired gas; pulmonary volumes are derived by appropriate calculations.

Respiratory Obstruction. Under normal conditions, pulmonary gas flow is mostly laminar, especially in the distal airways. However, an increased flow rate or airway obstruction increases the component of flow that is turbulent. Helium has been used as a diluent for oxygen in cases of airway obstruction because flow rates under turbulent conditions are inversely related to the density of the gas, and the density of helium is substantially less than that of air (Chan-Yeung *et al.*, 1976). Indeed, measurable reductions in the work of breathing have been reported with inhalation of mixtures of helium and oxygen (DeWeese *et al.*, 1983). However, three factors reduce the effectiveness of this approach. First, oxygenation is usually the principal problem in airway obstruction, and the small increase in flow rate that is achieved with mixtures of helium and oxygen may not improve oxygenation beyond that achievable by breathing pure oxygen. Second, the necessary dilution of helium with oxygen increases the density of the mixture to become closer to that of air. Finally, the viscosity of helium exceeds that of air; high viscosity reduces gas flow in regions where laminar flow predominates.

Laser Airway Surgery. The high thermal conductivity of helium makes it useful during laser surgery on the airway. More rapid conduction of heat away from the point of contact of the laser beam with the airway reduces the spread of tissue damage and the likelihood that the ignition point of flammable materials in the airway will be reached. It also improves the flow rate of gas through the small endotracheal tubes that are commonly used for such operations.

It is a common misconception that the high thermal conductivity of helium increases respiratory heat loss, similar to the well-documented increase in conductive heat loss from the skin of divers who are surrounded by helium atmospheres (Flynn *et al.*, 1974). Because respiratory gas is always heated to body temperature, the heat *capacity*, and not the *conductivity*, of the mixture is the relevant index. The heat capacity of helium is less than that of air; thus, inhalation of helium–oxygen mixtures may actually reduce the respiratory component of overall heat loss.

Hyperbaric Applications. The depth and duration of diving activity are limited by oxygen toxicity, inert gas narcosis, and inert gas supersaturation on decompression (occasionally producing decompression sickness or "bends"). Oxygen toxicity becomes apparent with prolonged exposure to compressed air at 5 atmospheres or more (Eckenhoff *et al.*, 1987); this problem can be minimized by dilution of oxygen with an inert gas. Pure oxygen is used only rarely for diving. The use of helium as a diluent is based on its absolute lack of narcotic potential, even at exceedingly high pressures (Brauer and Way, 1970), and its relative insolubility in body tissues and fluids. The latter factor reduces the volume of dissolved helium after a hyperbaric exposure and thus reduces the time necessary for decompression and the likelihood of separation of a gas phase after decompression. The low density of helium also reduces the work of breathing in the otherwise dense hyperbaric atmosphere. In some undersea missions, subjects have lived in a helium–oxygen atmosphere. Problems encountered included distorted speech, increased loss of body heat, and gas emboli at the junction of skin and subcutaneous fat or of body fat and blood vessels. The latter is due to the phenomenon of isobaric counterdiffusion of nitrogen and helium (Lambertsen and Idicula, 1975).

WATER VAPOR

Because of extensive hydrogen bonding, water is a liquid with a large heat of vaporization, a high specific heat, and considerable ability to dissolve or disperse a wide variety of other compounds. Although inspired gas is normally humidified by the conducting airways, inhalation of supplemental amounts of water vapor can be an important therapeutic procedure.

Inspired air is warmed to body temperature and humidified to saturation by the time it reaches the larynx or upper trachea. While deep, rapid breathing may move the boundary of saturation into the lung, the air-conditioning function of the nasal turbinates and upper airway still provides the bulk of humidification. Normal man can tolerate a temporary shift in the site of humidification to the tracheobronchial tree during endotracheal anesthesia (Knudsen *et al.*, 1973) or the long-term shift that results from tracheostomy if no additional stress is placed on the airways. Since about 50 mg of water is needed for each liter of inspired dry gas to saturate it at body temperature, sedentary individuals require approximately 500 ml of water per day for this purpose.

Uses of Inspired Water. Water vapor is indicated for patients whose airways are chronically intubated; it decreases crusting of respiratory mucosa, liquefies thick secretions, promotes mucociliary clearance, limits the loss of body water, and tends to conserve body heat by limiting evaporation in the airway (Chalon *et al.*, 1979). In addition, inhalation of warmed humidified gases can help to warm hypothermic patients (Caldwell *et al.*, 1981).

Water aerosols may be used instead of water vapor. Either cool or warm aerosols may be soothing in laryngitis and croup. Aerosols also permit delivery to the respiratory tract of drugs such as bronchodilators, mucolytics, hydroscopics, steroids, and antibiotics (Pierce and Saltzman, 1974).

Methods of Administration. Inspired water may be provided as vapor from humidifiers or as vapor and particulate water from aerosol generators (nebulizers). Distilled water may be used; isotonic saline solutions are preferred for nebulizers (Shephard *et al.*, 1983).

Although the content of water vapor in inspired gas is limited to a maximum set by temperature, additional water may be administered with an aerosol generator. Control of the size of the aerosol particles permits some control over the site of deposition of the aerosol. Particles larger than 50 μm tend to settle rapidly or coalesce, and they are not inhaled. Particles of 10 to 20 μm tend to impact on the walls of the upper airway and trachea. Particles of 5 to 10 μm are deposited in medium-sized and small bronchi, while those of 1 to 5 μm may penetrate all the way to the alveolar ducts and alveoli. Most particles of less than 1 μm are exhaled in the subsequent breath. Aerosol deposition tends to be increased at points of increased airway resistance and collections of secretions (Kim *et al.*, 1983). Regardless of particle size, slow deep breaths favor more alveolar penetration of droplets, while fast short breaths favor upper airway deposition (Stahlhofen *et al.*, 1983).

Untoward Effects. Potential problems include thermal damage from overheated inspired gas, fluid overload from absorption of excess water, and coughing and bronchoconstriction from direct irritation of the bronchi by water droplets. Prior administration of lidocaine aerosol can inhibit coughing, and administration of bronchodilators or cromolyn sodium can inhibit bronchoconstriction (Shephard *et al.*, 1983). Thermal damage is due not only to the temperature of the gas but also to the heat of condensation of water (580 cal/g). Long-term inhalation of an aerosol mist can result in the net absorption of more than 500 ml of water a day by adult patients and disproportionately more (relative to weight) by children and infants. Humidification devices must be cleaned scrupulously to reduce the incidence of nosocomial infections (*see* Brain, 1980).

Ashton, N. The pathogenesis of retrolental fibroplasia. *Ophthalmology (Rochester)*, **1979**, *86*, 695–699.

Aubier, M.; Murciano, D.; Milic-Emili, J.; Touaty, E.; Daghfous, J.; Pariente, R.; and Derenne, J. P. Effects of the administration of O_2 on ventilation and blood gases in patients with chronic obstructive pulmonary disease during acute respiratory failure. *Am. Rev. Respir. Dis.*, **1980**, *122*, 747–754.

Bert, P. Experience sur l'empoisonment par l'oxygene. *Gaz. Méd. Paris*, **1873**, *28*, 387.

Betts, E. K.; Downes, J. J.; Schaffer, D. B.; and Johns, R. Retrolental fibroplasia and oxygen administration during general anesthesia. *Anesthesiology*, **1977**, *47*, 518–520.

Bigard, M.; Gaucher, P.; and Lassalle, C. Fatal colonic explosion during colonoscopic polypectomy. *Gastroenterology*, **1979**, *77*, 1307–1310.

Boerema, I.; Meyne, N. G.; Brummelkamp, W. K.; Bouma, S.; Mensch, M. H.; Kamermans, F.; Stern Hanf, M.; and Van Aalderen, W. Life without blood. *J. Cardiovasc. Surg. (Torino)*, **1960**, *1*, 133–146.

Boyce, N. W.; Campbell, D.; and Holdsworth, S. R. Granulocyte independence of pulmonary oxygen toxicity in the rat. *Exp. Lung Res.*, **1989**, *15*, 491–498.

Brauer, R. W., and Way, R. O. Relative narcotic potencies of hydrogen, helium, nitrogen and their mixtures. *J. Appl. Physiol.*, **1970**, *29*, 23–31.

Caldwell, C.; Crawford, R.; and Sinclair, I. Hypothermia after cardiopulmonary bypass in man. *Anesthesiology*, **1981**, *55*, 86–87.

Chalon, J.; Patel, C.; Ali, M.; Ramanathan, S.; Capan, L.; Tang, C. K.; and Turndorf, H. Humidity and the anesthetized patient. *Anesthesiology*, **1979**, *50*, 195–198.

Chan-Yeung, M.; Abboud, R.; Ming, S. T.; and MacLean, L. Effect of helium on maximum expiratory flow in patients with asthma before and during induced bronchoconstriction. *Am. Rev. Respir. Dis.*, **1976**, *113*, 434–443.

Cheney, F. W.; Huang, T. W.; and Gronka, R. The effects of 50% oxygen on the resolution of pulmonary injury. *Am. Rev. Respir. Dis.*, **1980**, *122*, 373–379.

Clark, J. M. Pulmonary limits of oxygen tolerance in man. *Exp. Lung Res.*, **1988**, *14*, 897–910.

Clark, J. M., and Lambertsen, C. J. Alveolar-arterial oxygen differences in man during exposure to inspired oxygen pressures of 0.2, 1.0, 2.0, and 3.5 ATA. *J. Appl. Physiol.*, **1971a**, *30*, 753–763.

———. Rate of development of pulmonary oxygen toxicity in man during oxygen breathing at 2.0 ATA. *Ibid.*, **1971b**, *30*, 739–752.

Cohen, P. J.; Alexander, S. C.; Smith, T. C.; Reivich, M.; and Wollman, H. Effects of hypoxia and normocarbia on cerebral blood flow and metabolism in conscious man. *J. Appl. Physiol.*, **1967**, *23*, 183–189.

Coursin, D. B.; Cihla, H. P.; Will, J. A.; and McCreary, J. L. Adaptation to chronic hyperoxia: biochemical effects and the response to subsequent lethal hyperoxia. *Am. Rev. Respir. Dis.*, **1987**, *135*, 1002–1006.

Crapo, J. D.; Barry, B. E.; Foscue, H. A.; and Shelburne, J. Structural and biochemical changes in rat lungs occurring during exposures to lethal and adaptive doses of oxygen. *Am. Rev. Respir. Dis.*, **1980**, *122*, 123–143.

Cruz, J. C.; Reeves, J. T.; Grover, R. F.; Maher, J. T.; McCullough, R. E.; Cymerman, A.; and Denniston, J. C. Ventilatory acclimatization to high altitude is prevented by CO_2 breathing. *Respiration*, **1980**, *39*, 121–130.

Davis, W. B.; Rennard, S. I.; Bitterman, P. B.; and Crystal, R. G. Pulmonary oxygen toxicity: early reversible changes in human alveolar structures induced by hyperoxia. *N. Engl. J. Med.*, **1983**, *309*, 878–883.

de Castuma, E. S.; Mattiazzi, A. R.; and Cingolani, H. E. Effect of hypercapnic acidosis on induction of arrhythmias by catecholamines in cat papillary muscles. *Arch. Int. Physiol. Biochim.*, **1977**, *85*, 509–518.

DeWeese, E. L.; Sullivan, T. Y.; and Yu, P. L. Ventilatory and occlusion pressure responses to helium breathing. *J. Appl. Physiol.*, **1983**, *54*, 1525–1531.

Drysdale, D. B.; Jensen, J. I.; and Cunningham, D. J. C. The short-latency respiratory response to sudden withdrawal of hypercapnia and hypoxia in man. *Q. J. Exp. Physiol.*, **1981**, *66*, 203–210.

Duane, S. F.; Weir, E. K.; Stewart, R. M.; and Niewoehner, D. E. Distal airway responses to changes in oxygen and carbon dioxide tensions. *Respir. Physiol.*, **1979**, *38*, 303–311.

DuBois, A. B.; Turaids, T.; Mammen, R. E.; and Nobrega, F. T. Pulmonary atelectasis in subjects breathing oxygen at sea level or at simulated altitude. *J. Appl. Physiol.*, **1966**, *21*, 828–836.

Eckenhoff, R. G.; Dougherty, J. H.; Messier, A. A.; Osborne, S. F.; and Parker, J. W. Progression of and recovery from pulmonary oxygen toxicity in humans exposed to 5 ATA air. *Aviat. Space Environ. Med.*, **1987**, *58*, 658–667.

Ely, S. W.; Sawyer, D. C.; and Scott, J. B. Local vasoactivity of oxygen and carbon dioxide in the right coronary circulation of the dog and pig. *J. Physiol. (Lond.)*, **1982**, *332*, 427–439.

Fisch, U. Management of sudden deafness. *Otolaryngol. Head Neck Surg.*, **1983**, *91*, 3–8.

Flynn, E. T.; Vorosmarti, J.; and Modell, H. I. Temperature requirements for the maintenance of thermal balance in high pressure helium–oxygen environments. U. S. Navy Experimental Diving Unit Report No. 21-73, Panama City, Fla., **1974**.

Frank, L. Protection from oxygen toxicity by pre-exposure to hypoxia: lung antioxidant enzyme role. *J. Appl. Physiol.*, **1982**, *53*, 475–482.

Gregory, I. C. The oxygen and carbon monoxide capacities of foetal and adult blood. *J. Physiol. (Lond.)*, **1974**, *236*, 625–634.

Hemmingsen, A., and Scholander, P. E. Specific transport of oxygen through hemoglobin solutions. *Science*, **1960**, *132*, 1379–1381.

Hendricks, P. L.; Hall, D. A.; Hunter, W. L.; and Haley, P. J. Extension of pulmonary oxygen tolerance in men at 2 ATA by intermittent oxygen exposure. *J. Appl. Physiol.*, **1977**, *42*, 593–599.

Holm, B. A.; Matalon, S.; Finkelstein, J. N.; and Notter,

R. H. Type II pneumocyte changes during hyperoxic lung injury and recovery. *J. Appl. Physiol.*, **1988**, *65*, 2672–2678.

Kim, C. S.; Brown, L. K.; Lewars, G. G.; and Sacknet, M. A. Depression of aerosol particles and flow resistance in mathematical and experimental airway models. *J. Appl. Physiol.*, **1983**, *55*, 154–163.

Knudsen, J.; Lomholt, N.; and Wisborg, K. Postoperative pulmonary complications using dry and humidified anesthetic gases. *Br. J. Anaesth.*, **1973**, *45*, 363–368.

Krasney, J. A., and Koehler, R. C. Influence of arterial hypoxia on cardiac and coronary dynamics in the conscious sinoaortic-denervated dog. *J. Appl. Physiol.*, **1977**, *43*, 1012–1018.

Kravetz, G.; Fisher, A. B.; and Forman, H. J. The oxygen-adapted rat model: tolerance to oxygen at 1.5 and 2 ATA. *Aviat. Space Environ. Med.*, **1980**, *51*, 775–777.

Kushner, B. J.; Essner, D.; Cohen, I. J.; and Flynn, J. T. Retrolental fibroplasia. II. Pathologic correlation. *Arch. Ophthalmol.*, **1977**, *95*, 29–38.

Lahiri, S.; Mokashi, A.; Mulligan, E.; and Nishino, T. Comparison of aortic and carotid chemoreceptor responses to hypercapnia and hypoxia. *J. Appl. Physiol.*, **1981**, *51*, 55–61.

Lambertsen, C. J., and Idicula, J. A. A new gas lesion syndrome in man induced by "isobaric gas counter diffusion." *J. Appl. Physiol.*, **1975**, *39*, 434–443.

Lambertsen, C. J.; Kough, R. H.; Cooper, D. Y.; Emmel, G. L.; Loeschcke, H. H.; and Schmidt, C. F. Oxygen toxicity. Effects in man of oxygen inhalation at 1 and 3.5 atmospheres upon blood gas transport, cerebral circulation and cerebral metabolism. *J. Appl. Physiol.*, **1953**, *5*, 471–486.

Levine, B. D.; Kubo, K.; Kobayashi, T.; Fukushima, M.; Shibamoto, T.; and Ueda, G. Role of barometric pressure in pulmonary fluid balance and oxygen transport. *J. Appl. Physiol.*, **1988**, *64*, 419–428.

Lin, Y. C.; Shida, K. K.; and Hong, S. K. Effects of hypercapnia, hypoxia, and rebreathing on circulatory response to apnea. *J. Appl. Physiol.*, **1983**, *54*, 172–177.

Lourenco, R. V. Clinical methods for the study of regulation of ventilation. *Chest*, **1976**, *70*, 109–195.

McCord, J. M. Oxygen-derived free radicals in postischemic tissue injury. *N. Engl. J. Med.*, **1985**, *312*, 159–163.

Mathewson, H. S. Helium—who needs it? *Respir. Care*, **1982**, *27*, 1400–1401.

Neff, T. A., and Talmage, P. Neuromuscular and chemical control of breathing. *Chest*, **1978**, *73*, 247–308.

Plewes, J. L., and Farhi, L. E. Peripheral circulatory responses to acute hyperoxia. *Undersea Biomed. Res.*, **1983**, *10*, 123–129.

Pugh, L. G. C. E. Cardiac output in muscular exercise at 5800 m (19,000 ft). *J. Appl. Physiol.*, **1964**, *19*, 441–447.

Rasmussen, J. P.; Dauchot, P. J.; DePalma, R. G.; Sorensen, B.; Regula, G.; Anton, A. H.; and Gravenstein, J. S. Cardiac function and hypercarbia. *Arch. Surg.*, **1978**, *113*, 1196–1200.

Robiolio, M.; Rumsey, W. L.; and Wilson, O. F. Oxygen diffusion and mitochondrial respiration in neuroblastoma cells. *Am. J. Physiol.*, **1989**, *256*, C1207–C1213.

Sackner, M. A. A history of oxygen usage in chronic obstructive pulmonary disease. *Am. Rev. Respir. Dis.*, **1974**, *110*, Suppl., 25–34.

Sackner, M. A.; Landa, J.; Hirsch, J.; and Zapata, A. Pulmonary effects of oxygen breathing. *Ann. Intern. Med.*, **1975**, *82*, 40–43.

Schwartz, S.; Frantz, R. A.; and Shoemaker, W. C. Sequential hemodynamic and oxygen transport responses in hypovolemia, anemia, and hypoxia. *Am. J. Physiol.*, **1981**, *241*, H864–H871.

Shephard, D.; Rizk, N. W.; Boushey, H. A.; and Bethel, R. A. Mechanism of cough and bronchoconstriction induced by distilled water aerosol. *Am. Rev. Respir. Dis.*, **1983**, *127*, 691–694.

Stahlhofen, W.; Gibhart, J.; Hayder, J.; and Scheuck, G. Disposition pattern of droplets from medical nebulizers in the human respiratory tract. *Bull. Eur. Physiopath. Respir.*, **1983**, *19*, 459–463.

Staszewska-Barczak, J., and Dusting, G. J. Importance of circulating angiotensin II for elevation of arterial pressure during acute hypercapnia in anaesthetized dogs. *Clin. Exp. Pharmacol. Physiol.*, **1981**, *8*, 189–201.

Turrens, J. F.; Freeman, B. A.; Levitt, J. G.; and Crapo, J. D. The effect of hyperoxia on superoxide production by lung submitochondrial particles. *Arch. Biochem. Biophys.*, **1982**, *217*, 401–410.

van den Bos, G. C.; Drake, A. J.; and Noble, M. I. M. The effect of carbon dioxide upon myocardial contractile performance, blood flow, and oxygen consumption. *J. Physiol. (Lond.)*, **1979**, *287*, 149–161.

Voelkel, N. F. Mechanisms of hypoxic pulmonary vasoconstriction. *Am. Rev. Respir. Dis.*, **1986**, *133*, 1186–1195.

White, C. W.; Jackson, J. H.; Abuchowski, A.; Kazo, G. M.; Mimmack, R. F.; Berger, E. M.; Freeman, B. A.; McCord, J. M.; and Repine, J. E. Polyethylene glycol-attached antioxidant enzymes decrease pulmonary oxygen toxicity in rats. *J. Appl. Physiol.*, **1989**, *66*, 584–590.

Monographs and Reviews

Brain, J. Aerosol and humidity therapy. *Am. Rev. Respir. Dis.*, **1980**, *122*, 17–21.

Clark, J. M. Oxygen toxicity. In, *The Physiology and Medicine of Diving*, 3rd ed. (Bennett, P. B., and Elliott, D. H., eds.) Best Publishing Co., San Pedro, Calif., **1982**, pp. 200–238.

Davis, J. C. *Hyperbaric Oxygen Therapy: A Committee Report*. Undersea Medical Society, Inc., Bethesda, Md., **1986.**

Johnson, T. S., and Rock, P. B. Acute mountain sickness. *N. Engl. J. Med.*, **1988**, *319*, 841–845.

Kafer, E. R., and Sugioka, K. Respiratory and cardiovascular responses to hypoxemia and the effects of anesthesia. *Int. Anesthesiol. Clin.*, **1981**, *19*, 85–122.

Lambertsen, C. J. Effects of hyperoxia on organs and their tissues. In, *Extrapulmonary Manifestations of Respiratory Disease*. (Robin, E. D., ed.) Vol. 8, *Lung Biology in Health and Disease*. (Lenfant, C., ed.) Marcel Dekker, Inc., New York, **1978**, pp. 239–303.

———. Transport of oxygen, carbon dioxide, and inert gases by the blood. In, *Medical Physiology*, 14th ed., Vol. 2. (Mountcastle, V. B., ed.) C. V. Mosby Co., St. Louis, **1980**, p. 1725.

Nunn, J. F. Carbon dioxide. In, *Applied Respiratory Physiology*, 3rd ed. Butterworths, London, **1987**, pp. 207–230.

Pierce, A. K., and Saltzman, H. A. The scientific basis of respiratory therapy (the Sugarloaf Conference). *Am. Rev. Respir. Dis.*, **1974**, *110*, Pt. 2, 1–204.

Thom, S. R. Hyperbaric oxygen therapy. *J. Intensive Care Med.*, **1989a**, *4*, 58–74.

———. Smoke inhalation. *Emerg. Med. Clin. North Am.*, **1989b**, *7*, 371–387.

CHAPTER

17 HYPNOTICS AND SEDATIVES; ETHANOL

Theodore W. Rall

Except for the benzodiazepines, the sedative-hypnotic drugs belong to a group of agents that depress the central nervous system (CNS) in a relatively nonselective, dose-dependent fashion, producing progressively calming or drowsiness (sedation), sleep (pharmacological hypnosis), unconsciousness, surgical anesthesia, coma, and fatal depression of respiration and cardiovascular regulation. They share these properties with a large number of chemicals, including the aliphatic alcohols, most notably ethanol. The CNS depressants also include the general anesthetics, and some sedative-hypnotic agents, notably certain barbiturates, are used at high doses to induce or maintain surgical anesthesia (*see* Chapter 14). Many sedative-hypnotic drugs have long been used at low doses to calm anxious patients; this role in "daytime sedation" is now largely restricted to the less dangerous benzodiazepines. The role of the benzodiazepines and other agents in the pharmacotherapy of anxiety will be discussed in Chapter 18. The present chapter emphasizes the hypnotic properties and uses of these drugs.

A *sedative* drug decreases activity, moderates excitement, and calms the recipient. A *hypnotic* drug produces drowsiness and facilitates the onset and maintenance of a state of sleep that resembles natural sleep in its electroencephalographic characteristics and from which the recipient may be easily aroused; the effect is sometimes called hypnosis, but the sleep induced by hypnotic drugs does not resemble the artificially induced passive state of suggestibility also called hypnosis. Sedation is a side effect of many drugs that are not general CNS depressants. Although such agents intensify the effects of CNS depressants, they cannot induce general anesthesia by themselves, and they usually produce more specific therapeutic effects at concentrations far lower than those causing substantial generalized depression of the CNS. By themselves, the benzodiazepines also cannot induce general anesthesia; although they produce coma at very high doses, they are virtually incapable of causing fatal respiratory depression or cardiovascular collapse. Moreover, certain congeners can specifically antagonize the actions of the benzodiazepines without eliciting significant effects in their absence. This constellation of properties sets the benzodiazepines apart from the other sedative-hypnotic drugs.

Some sedative-hypnotic drugs, particularly the benzodiazepines, are employed in other therapeutic settings. They are used as muscle relaxants (Chapter 20) and antiepileptic agents (Chapter 19) and to produce sedation and amnesia before or during operative procedures (Chapter 14). Although the benzodiazepines are used widely as antianxiety drugs, it is not certain whether their effects on wakefulness and anxiety are truly distinct, and separation of these topics in this textbook may represent an artificial division.

Ethanol shares many pharmacological properties with the nonbenzodiazepine sedative-hypnotic drugs. However, its usefulness in the treatment of sleep disorders is limited, and it may often be more disruptive than beneficial. Nevertheless, ethanol is consumed by a large number of persons for recreational purposes, and many ingest it chronically to the point of abuse. This chapter will emphasize those aspects of the actions of ethanol that allow comparison with the sedative-hypnotic agents. The abuse of ethanol and other CNS depressants is discussed in Chapter 22.

History. Since antiquity, potions have been used to induce sleep. History and folklore have provided accounts of both sinister and romantic uses of laudanum, alcoholic beverages, and various herbals to produce stupor, during which intrigue, adultery, or magical transformation could take place. Potions were also used for sedation and hypnosis, but they were too unpredictable to bequeath to modern medicine. The first agent to be specifically introduced as a sedative and soon thereafter as a hypnotic was bromide (1853, 1864). Only four more sedative-hypnotic drugs (chloral hydrate, paraldehyde, urethane, and sulfonal) were in use before 1900. Barbital was introduced in 1903 and phenobarbital in 1912. Their success spawned the synthesis and testing of over 2500 barbiturates, of which approximately 50 were distributed commercially. The barbiturates held the stage so dominantly that less than a dozen other sedative-hypnotics were successfully marketed before 1960, and several popular old drugs slipped into oblivion.

The partial separation of sedative-hypnotic-anesthetic from anticonvulsant properties, embodied in phenobarbital, led to searches for agents with more selective effects on the functions of the CNS. As a result, relatively nonsedative anticonvulsants, notably phenytoin and trimethadione, were developed in the late 1930s and early 1940s (*see* Chapter 19). The advent of chlorpromazine and meprobamate in the early 1950s, with their taming effects in animals, and the development of increasingly sophisticated methods for evaluating the behavioral effects of drugs set the stage in 1957 for the synthesis of chlordiazepoxide by Sternbach and the discovery of its unique pattern of actions by Randall (*see* Symposium, 1982). With its introduction into clinical medicine in 1961, chlordiazepoxide ushered in the era of benzodiazepines; more than 3000 have been synthesized, over 120 have been tested for biological activity, and about 35 are in clinical use in various parts of the world.

Most of the benzodiazepines that have reached the marketplace were selected for high anxiolytic potential relative to their potency to depress CNS function. Their extraordinary popularity in clinical medicine is due largely to their ability to relieve symptoms of anxiety with relatively little interference with cognitive function or wakefulness. Nevertheless, the benzodiazepines all possess sedative-hypnotic properties to varying degrees; these properties are extensively exploited clinically, especially to facilitate sleep. Mainly because of their remarkably low capacity to produce fatal CNS depression, the benzodiazepines have displaced the barbiturates as sedative-hypnotic agents.

BENZODIAZEPINES

Although the benzodiazepines in clinical use exert qualitatively similar effects, important quantitative differences in their pharmacodynamic spectra and pharmacokinetic properties have led to varying patterns of therapeutic application. There is reason to believe that a number of distinct mechanisms of action contribute in varying degrees to the sedative-hypnotic, muscle relaxant, anxiolytic, and anticonvulsant effects of the benzodiazepines. While only those benzodiazepines used primarily for hypnosis will be discussed in detail, this chapter will describe the general properties of the group and the important differences between individual agents (*see also* Chapters 18 and 19).

Chemistry. The structures of the benzodiazepines in use in the United States are shown in Table 17–1, as are those of a few related compounds to be discussed below.

The term *benzodiazepine* refers to the portion of the structure composed of a benzene ring (A) fused to a seven-membered diazepine ring (B). However, since all the important benzodiazepines contain a 5-aryl substituent (ring C) and a 1,4-diazepine ring, the term has come to mean the 5-aryl-1,4-benzodiazepines. Various modifications in the structure of the ring systems have yielded compounds with similar activities. These include 1,5-benzodiazepines (*e.g.*, clobazam) and the replacement of the fused benzene ring (A) with heteroaromatic systems such as thieno (*e.g.*, brotizolam) or pyrazolo (*see* Fryer, in Symposium, 1983a). The 5-aryl substituent greatly enhances potency but can be replaced by a five-membered ring fused to positions 3 and 4 to form an anthramycin.

The chemical nature of substituents at positions 1 to 3 can vary widely and can include triazolo or imidazo rings fused at positions 1 and 2. Electron-withdrawing groups at position 7 markedly enhance activity; electron-releasing or large groups at this position or substituents elsewhere in ring A reduce activity. Electron-withdrawing groups at the 2′ (or ortho) position in ring C enhance potency, while substituents elsewhere decrease activity (*see* Sternbach, in Symposium, 1973). Replacement of ring C with a keto function at position 5 and a methyl substituent at position 4 are important structural features of the benzodiazepine antagonist flumazenil (Ro 15–1788) (*see* Haefely *et al.*, in Symposium, 1983a).

PHARMACOLOGICAL PROPERTIES

The effects of the benzodiazepines virtually all result from actions of these drugs on the CNS. The most prominent of these effects are sedation, hypnosis, decreased anxiety, muscle relaxation, anterograde amnesia, and anticonvulsant activity. One benzodiazepine, alprazolam, appears to have antidepressant activity in certain clinical settings. Only two effects of these drugs appear to result from actions on peripheral tissues: coronary vasodilatation, seen after intravenous administration of therapeutic doses of certain benzodiazepines, and neu-

Table 17–1. BENZODIAZEPINES: NAMES AND STRUCTURES *

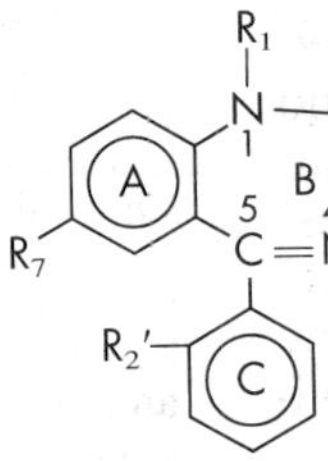

BENZODIAZEPINE	R_1	R_2	R_3	R_7	$R_{2'}$
Alprazolam	[Fused triazolo ring] [b]		—H	—Cl	—H
Brotizolam †	[Fused triazolo ring] [b]		—H	[Thieno ring A] [c]	—Cl
Chlordiazepoxide [a]	(—)	—NHCH$_3$	—H	—Cl	—H
Clobazam [a],†	—CH$_3$	=O	—H	—Cl	—H
Clonazepam	—H	=O	—H	—NO$_2$	—Cl
Clorazepate	—H	=O	—COO$^-$	—Cl	—H
Demoxepam [a],†,‡	—H	=O	—H	—Cl	—H
Diazepam	—CH$_3$	=O	—H	—Cl	—H
Flumazenil [a],†	[Fused imidazo ring] [d]		—H	—F	[=O at C$_5$] [e]
Flurazepam	—CH$_2$CH$_2$N(C$_2$H$_5$)$_2$	=O	—H	—Cl	—F
Halazepam	—CH$_2$CF$_3$	=O	—H	—Cl	—H
Lorazepam	—H	=O	—OH	—Cl	—Cl
Midazolam	[Fused imadazo ring] [f]		—H	—Cl	—F
Nitrazepam †	—H	=O	—H	—NO$_2$	—H
Nordazepam †,§	—H	=O	—H	—Cl	—H
Oxazepam	—H	=O	—OH	—Cl	—H
Prazepam	—CH$_2$—CH<(CH$_2$)$_2$ (cyclopropyl: CH$_2$, CH$_2$)	=O	—H	—Cl	—H
Quazepam†	—CH$_2$CF$_3$	=S	—H	—Cl	—F
Temazepam	—CH$_3$	=O	—OH	—Cl	—H
Triazolam	[Fused triazolo ring] [b]		—H	—Cl	—Cl

* Alphabetical footnotes refer to alterations of the general formula; symbolic footnotes are used for other comments.
† Not available for clinical use in the United States.
‡ Major metabolite of chlordiazepoxide.
§ Major metabolite of diazepam and others; also referred to as nordiazepam and desmethyldiazepam.
[a] No substituent at position 4, except for chlordiazepoxide and demoxepam, which are N-oxides; R_4 is —CH$_3$ in flumazenil, in which there is no double bond between positions 4 and 5; R_4 is =O in clobazam, in which position 4 is C and position 5 is N.

b 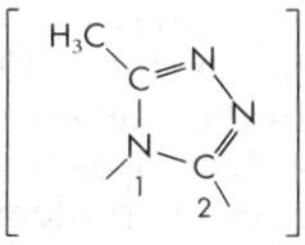

c 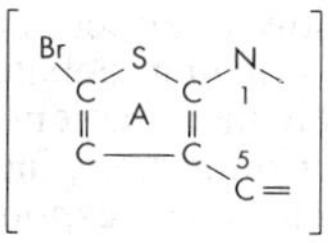

d 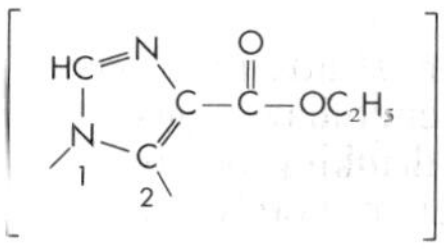

f 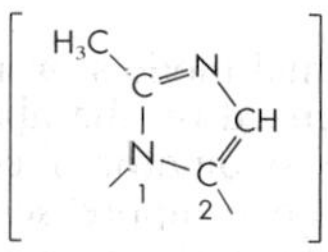

[e] No ring C.

romuscular blockade, seen only with very high doses.

Central Nervous System. While the benzodiazepines affect activity at all levels of the neuraxis, some structures are affected to a much greater extent than are others. In addition, some effects of the drugs are indirect. The benzodiazepines are not general neuronal depressants, as are the barbiturates. All the benzodiazepines have very similar pharmacological profiles. Nevertheless, the drugs differ in selectivity, and the clinical usefulness of individual benzodiazepines thus varies considerably.

As the dose of a benzodiazepine is increased, sedation progresses to hypnosis and then to stupor. The clinical literature often refers to the "anesthetic" effects and uses of certain benzodiazepines, but the drugs do not cause a true general anesthesia, since awareness usually persists and relaxation sufficient to allow surgery cannot be achieved. However, at "preanesthetic" doses, there is amnesia for events subsequent to the administration of the drug; this may create the illusion of previous anesthesia.

The question whether the so-called antianxiety effects of benzodiazepines are the same as or different from the sedative and hypnotic effects has not been resolved. Contributing to this uncertainty are the difficulty in defining and measuring sedation, the difficulty in assessing antianxiety effects in man (*see* Chapter 18), and the unproven validity of various models of anxiety in animals.

The pharmacological profile for a given benzodiazepine varies markedly from species to species. In some species, the subject may become alert before CNS depression is evident. For example, the 7-nitrobenzodiazepines induce hyperactivity in mice, rats, and monkeys, but not in most other species. Interestingly, muscle relaxation in cats and anticonvulsant activity against pentylenetetrazol in mice correlate better with the sedative, antianxiety, and hypnotic properties in man than do the actions to suppress motor activity, induce sleep, and release suppressed behavior in experimental animals.

In animal models of anxiety, most attention has been focused on the ability of benzodiazepines to increase locomotor, feeding, or drinking behavior that has been suppressed by novel or aversive stimuli. For example, animals have been tested in various ways in which behavior that had previously been rewarded by food or water is periodically punished by an electric shock. The time during which shocks are delivered is signaled by some auditory or visual cue, and untreated animals stop performing almost completely when the cue is perceived. The administration of a benzodiazepine can eliminate the difference in behavioral responses during the punished and unpunished periods, usually at doses that do not reduce the rate of unpunished responses or produce other signs of impaired motor function. Similarly, rats placed in an unfamiliar environment exhibit markedly reduced exploratory behavior ("neophobia"), while animals treated with benzodiazepines do not. Opioid analgesics and neuroleptic (antipsychotic) drugs do not increase suppressed behaviors, while phenobarbital and meprobamate usually do so only at doses that also reduce spontaneous or unpunished behaviors or produce ataxia. Descriptions of these and other experimental procedures, as well as discussions of their potential relationship to anxiety in man, can be found in the proceedings of several symposia (*see* Symposium, 1983a, 1983b, 1983c).

The ratio of the dose required to impair motor function to that necessary to increase punished behavior varies widely among the benzodiazepines and depends, not surprisingly, on the species and experimental protocol. While such data may have encouraged the marketing of some benzodiazepines (*e.g.*, flurazepam) only as sedative-hypnotic agents, they have not predicted with any accuracy the relative frequency or intensity of sedative effects among those benzodiazepines marketed as anxiolytic agents (*see* Linnoila, in Symposium, 1983a). To some degree, these discrepancies may have resulted from the fact that observations in animals were often made shortly after parenteral administration, and hence reflected principally the actions of the parent compound. By contrast, after oral administration, a number of benzodiazepines reach the systemic circulation to only a limited extent, if at all, and their effects result primarily from the actions of one or more metabolites (*see* below).

Studies on tolerance in animals are often cited to support the belief that disinhibitory effects of benzodiazepines are separate from their sedative-ataxic effects. For example, tolerance to the depressant effects on rewarded or neutral behavior occurs after several days of treatment with benzodiazepines; the disinhibitory effects of the drugs on punished behavior are augmented initially and decline after 3 to 4 weeks (*see* File, 1985). Although tolerance to the impairment of certain aspects of psychomotor performance (*e.g.*, visual tracking) in man is not usually observed (*see* Linnoila, in Symposium, 1983a), most patients who ingest benzodiazepines chronically report that drowsiness wanes over a few days (*see* Lader and Petursson, in Symposium, 1983c). The development of tolerance to the anxiolytic effects of benzodiazepines is a subject of ongoing debate (Lader and File, 1987). However, most patients maintain themselves on a fairly constant dose; increases or decreases in dosage appear to correspond to changes in problems or stresses. Nevertheless, some patients either do not reduce their dosage when stress is relieved or steadily escalate dosage without apparent reason (*see* Lader and Petursson, in Symposium, 1983c). Such behavior may be associated with the development of drug dependence (*see* Woods *et al.*, 1987).

Some benzodiazepines induce muscle hypotonia without interfering with normal locomotion. They also decrease decerebrate rigidity in cats and rigidity in patients with cerebral palsy. They increase the patellar reflex. In cats, muscle relaxation is effected in doses that are two (flurazepam) to four (clonazepam) orders of magnitude less than those that abolish the righting reflex. Diazepam is ten times more selective than meprobamate. However, this remarkable degree of selectivity is not seen in man; clonazepam in nonsedative doses does cause muscle relaxation in man, but diazepam and most other benzodiazepines do not. Tolerance occurs to both the muscle relaxant and ataxic effects of these drugs.

Experimentally, benzodiazepines inhibit seizure activity induced by either pentylenetetrazol or picrotoxin, but strychnine- and maximal electroshock-induced seizures are suppressed only with doses that also severely impair locomotor activity. Flunitrazepam, triazolam, clonazepam, bromazepam, nitrazepam, and nordazepam are more selective anticonvulsants than are other benzodiazepines. Benzodiazepines also suppress photic seizures in baboons and ethanol-withdrawal seizures in man. However, the development of tolerance to the anticonvulsant effects has limited the usefulness of benzodiazepines in the treatment of seizure disorders in man (*see* Chapter 19).

Although analgesic effects of benzodiazepines have been observed in experimental animals, only transient analgesia is apparent in human patients after intravenous administration. Such effects may actually involve the production of amnesia. However, it is clear that benzodiazepines do not cause hyperalgesia, unlike the barbiturates.

Effects on EEG and Sleep Stages. The effects of benzodiazepines on the waking EEG resemble those of other sedative-hypnotic drugs. Alpha activity is decreased, and there is an increase in low-voltage fast activity, especially beta activity. Tolerance occurs to these effects.

Benzodiazepine-induced alterations of the stages of sleep have been studied widely. An excellent compilation of findings and discussion of 66 studies may be found in the review by Kay and associates (1976) (*see also* Greenblatt and Shader, 1974; Mendelson *et al.*, 1977). With a few exceptions, the benzodiazepines are all rather similar in their effects on the important sleep parameters. It is difficult to assess the significance of these exceptions, and they will not be detailed here. Despite the fact that the exceptions are used for promotional purposes, variations in the pharmacokinetic properties of individual benzodiazepines are much more important determinants of the utility of these drugs for their effects on sleep than are differences in their pharmacodynamic properties.

Most benzodiazepines decrease sleep latency, especially when first used, and diminish the number of awakenings and the time spent in stage 0 (a stage of wakefulness). Time in stage 1 (descending drowsiness) is usually decreased, but this is variable. All benzodiazepines increase time spent in stage 2 (which is the major fraction of non–rapid-eye-movement [REM] sleep). Benzodiazepines prominently decrease the time spent in slow-wave sleep (SWS; stages 3 and 4); usually both stages 3 and 4 are shortened. The decrease in stage-4 sleep is accompanied by a reduction in night terrors and nightmares; however, if the decrease is marked, these phenomena may be shifted to the waking hours ("daymares").

Much attention has been paid to the effects on REM sleep. Most benzodiazepines increase REM latency (time from onset of spindle sleep to the first REM burst). The time spent in REM sleep is usually shortened; however, the number of cycles of REM sleep is usually increased, mostly late in the sleep time.

Benzodiazepines do not appear to lessen the relaxation of neck muscles that occurs at the onset of REM sleep. They diminish the frequency of eyeball movement and the magnitude of the bursts of tachycardia that occur during REM sleep and the fluctuations in skin resistance that occur in both stage-2 and REM sleep.

Despite the shortening of stage-4 and REM sleep, the net effect of administration of benzodiazepines is usually an increase in total sleep time. The effect is greatest in subjects with the shortest baseline total sleep time, for whom sleep time may triple. In addition, despite the increase in the number of REM cycles, the number of shifts to lighter sleep stages (1 and 0) and the amount of body movement are diminished. The nocturnal peaks in the concentration of growth hormone in plasma and the concentrations of prolactin and luteinizing hormone are not affected.

Use of benzodiazepines imparts a sense of deep or refreshing sleep, but it is uncertain to which effect on sleep parameters this feeling can be attributed. Some authors have ascribed it to the diminution in REM sleep, but this is not a consistent finding. Others attribute it to the suppression of SWS, but this, too, is inconsistent.

During chronic nocturnal use of benzodiazepines the effects on the various stages of sleep usually decline within a few nights but do not disappear. The number of dreams may double, although dreams usually are less bizarre. If after 3 to 4 weeks of nightly use of a benzodiazepine the drug is discontinued, there may be a considerable rebound in the amount and density of REM sleep. The number of dreams per night is about the same as before the drug was taken, but their bizarre character may increase. There is also usually a rebound in SWS, which may exceed the rebound in REM sleep.

Sites and Mechanisms of CNS Actions. The current predominant view is that most, if not all, of the actions of benzodiazepines are a result of potentiation of the neural inhibition that is mediated by gamma-aminobutyric acid (GABA). This idea is supported by behavioral and electrophysiological evidence that the effects of benzodiazepines are usually reduced or prevented by prior treatment with antagonists of GABA (*e.g.*, bicuculline) or inhibitors of the synthesis of the transmitter (*e.g.*, thiosemicarbazide). Although possible actions that lead to increased release of GABA cannot be excluded, most attention has been focused on the ability of benzodiazepines to potentiate the actions of GABA on neurons at all levels of the neuraxis. As a result of the detection and characterization of specific binding sites for benzodiazepines, a substantial body of biochemical evidence has accumulated that suggests a close molecular association between sites of action for GABA and the benzodiazepines. The various categories of evidence have been brought together by the discovery that certain congeners of the benzodiazepines are potent and selective inhibitors of both their biological effects and their binding to putative sites of action. One such antagonist (flumazenil) has been investigated extensively for potential clinical use in reversing the effects of high doses of benzodiazepines. Various aspects of the sites and mechanisms of action of the benzodiazepines have been reviewed (*see* Dubnick *et al.*, 1983; Barker *et al.*, 1986; Olsen *et al.*, 1986; Martin, 1987; Gardner, 1988; Polc, 1988) and have been the subject of several symposia (Symposium, 1983a, 1983b, 1983c, 1988a).

Although the GABA-potentiation hypothesis does not yet provide detailed explanations for the therapeutic actions of the benzodiazepines, it does supply a versatile framework with which to connect diverse observations. For example, the remarkable safety of the benzodiazepines can be accounted for by the self-limited nature of neuronal depression that requires the release of an endogenous inhibitory neurotransmitter to be expressed. While barbiturates have similar effects at low doses, they also can mimic the inhibitory actions of GABA at higher doses; thus, they can produce profound depression of the CNS (*see* below). Further, the ability of benzodiazepines to release suppressed behaviors as well as to produce sedation can be ascribed in part to potentiation of GABA-ergic pathways that serve to regulate the firing of neurons containing various monoamines (*see* Chapter 12); these neurons are known to promote behavioral arousal as well as to be important mediators of the inhibitory effects of fear and punishment on behavior. Finally, inhibitory effects on muscular hypertonia or the spread of seizure activity can be rationalized by potentiation of inhibitory GABA-ergic circuits at various levels of the neuraxis. However, a number of observations are not congruent with the exclusive nature of this view, especially those in which the effects of benzodiazepines are not sensitive to antagonists of GABA and/or do not appear to involve changes in chloride conductance (*see* Polc, 1988). Moreover, this hypothesis does not provide an explanation for the ability of relatively low concentrations of antagonists of adenosine receptors (*e.g.*, theophylline) to reverse the neuronal depressant or clinical effects of the benzodiazepines (*see* Phillis and O'Regan, 1988). Despite the impressive array of evidence supporting the GABA-potentiation theory, it does exclude the participation of other mechanisms of action.

In the vast majority of studies conducted *in vivo* or *in situ*, the local or systemic administration of benzodiazepines reduces the spontaneous or evoked electrical activity of major (large) neurons in all regions of the brain and spinal cord; significant effects can usually be detected at doses that are consistent with those used in man. The activity of these neurons is regulated in part by small inhibitory interneurons (predominantly GABA-ergic) arranged in both feedback and feedforward types of circuits (*see* Chapter 12). In the former, axonal branches activate the interneurons, which in turn inhibit the large neuron by way of axosomatic and, sometimes, axodendritic synapses. In feedforward circuits, some or all of the excitatory inputs to the large neuron send collateral axons to inhibitory interneurons that make synaptic contact with the large neuron and/or with excitatory nerve terminals; the latter arrangement is termed *presynaptic inhibition*. The magnitude of the effects produced by benzodiazepines can vary widely and depends upon such factors as the types of inhibitory circuits that are operating, the sources and intensity of ongoing excitatory input, and the manner in which experimental manipulations are performed and assessed. For example, the inhibitory synapses on the neuronal soma, especially those near the axon hillock, are the most powerful and are usually supplied predominantly by recurrent pathways. The synaptic or exogenous application of GABA to this region can prevent neuronal discharge. This involves a GABA-induced increase in the conductance of chloride, thereby shunting electrical currents that would otherwise depolarize the membrane of the initial segment. Accordingly, benzodiazepines markedly prolong the period that follows brief activation of recurrent GABA-ergic pathways, during which neither spontaneous nor applied excitatory stimuli can evoke neuronal discharge; this effect is reversed by bicuculline.

The effects of the benzodiazepines have also been studied extensively *in vitro*, using brain slices or cultured dissociated neurons. Until quite recently, the concentration of benzodiazepines required to produce GABA-potentiating effects *in vitro* was distressingly high (*e.g.*, 50 to 1000 nM). This can be compared with the concentration of unbound diazepam in the plasma and cerebrospinal fluid (CSF) of patients treated for anxiety (10 to 15 nM) or for status epilepticus (above 35 nM); the latter concentration is usually associated with marked sedation. For unexplained reasons, more recent studies have detected substantial enhancement of GABA-induced chloride currents in cultured neurons using either diazepam or clonazepam at 1 to 10 nM (*see* Macdonald and McLean, 1986). These effects appear to result from an increase in the frequency of bursts of openings of chloride channels induced by submaximal amounts of GABA (Twyman *et al.*, 1989). The benzodiazepines produced no effects on chloride conductances in the absence of GABA.

In other studies, however, these or lower concentrations of benzodiazepines have induced depressant effects on hippocampal pyramidal cells that were insensitive to either bicuculline or picrotoxin (*see* Polc, 1988). These effects have included selective inhibition of cholecystokinin-induced excitation and an enhancement of a Ca^{2+}-dependent K^+ conductance. In both instances, the effects were blocked by benzodiazepine antagonists. At higher concentrations (*e.g.*, 35 to 200 nM clonazepam or diazepam), GABA-independent inhibition of tetrodotoxin-sensitive Na^+ channels has been observed (*see* Macdonald and McLean, 1986). This frequency- and voltage-dependent effect results in reduction of sustained high-frequency, repetitive firing of action potentials, similar to the effects of several antiepileptic agents that are used in the treatment of tonic-clonic seizures (*e.g.*, phenytoin, carbamazepine; *see* Chapter 19). At still higher concentrations (above 1 μM), benzodiazepines can inhibit Ca^{2+} currents and Ca^{2+}-dependent release of neurotransmitters. It is not clear whether such effects involve direct actions of the benzodiazepines or reflect the participation of adenosine (*see* below). There have been no reports on the effect of flumazenil on benzodiazepine-induced inhibitions of Na^+ or Ca^{2+} currents.

Specific binding sites with high (nM) affinity for benzodiazepines have been detected in the CNS of various species, including man; the binding capacity is greatest in the cerebral cortex and least in the spinal cord. The affinity of these sites for benzodiazepines (but not for flumazenil) is enhanced by both GABA and chloride; conversely, benzodiazepines enhance the binding of GABA. The sedative barbiturates increase the binding of both GABA and the benzodiazepines in a chloride-dependent fashion, and these effects are blocked by certain convulsant agents, including picrotoxin (*see* below). These allosteric relationships are retained after solubilization of these receptors with detergent and purification to apparent homogeneity. The isolated macromolecular complex is an oligomer (possibly a tetramer) containing two closely related subunits; photoaffinity labelling experiments indicate that the binding sites for benzodiazepines and GABA-ergic agonists reside on the α and β subunits, respectively (*see* Barnard and Seeburg, in Symposium, 1988a). Recently, complementary DNAs that encode these subunits have been cloned, and RNA derived therefrom has been injected into *Xenopus* oocytes, yielding GABA-regulated chloride channels whose function was enhanced and inhibited by pentobarbital and picrotoxin, respectively. For reasons that have yet to be explained, these maneuvers did not result in the expression of channels that were sensitive to benzodiazepines (Levitan *et al.*, 1988). Thus, the intimate relationship between sites of action for the benzodiazepines and GABA-regulated chloride channels suggested by the biochemical experiments awaits further clarification.

Other evidence for the importance of the high-affinity binding sites in mediating the actions of the benzodiazepines includes a reasonably good correlation between relative binding affinities and relative potencies in producing various effects, especially the release of inhibited behaviors and antagonism of pentylenetetrazol-induced seizures, as long as appropriate adjustments are made for the formation of active metabolites. Most importantly, a number of compounds such as flumazenil compete with active benzodiazepines for such binding sites and antagonize their biological effects. While flumazenil itself is virtually devoid of biological activity, other antagonists display a limited range of benzodiazepine-like properties. The latter group is viewed as "partial agonists" in the classical sense. Still other compounds, many of which are β-carbolines, compete for binding but produce effects that are opposite to those of the benzodiazepines, including inhibition of GABA-induced chloride currents and promotion of seizures. Since their actions are also blocked by flumazenil and other antagonists and go beyond mere reversal of the actions of benzodiazepines, these agents have been called "inverse agonists" (*see* Gardner, 1988).

A number of issues remain unresolved, including an explanation for the different patterns of effects displayed by some of the benzodiazepines currently in clinical use. For example, clonazepam and clobazam produce less sedative-hypnotic effect for a given degree of protection against seizures than other members of the group. One view posits the existence of variant sites of action. Although different types of high-affinity binding sites for benzodiazepines have been detected in the brain, it has not been possible to assign any particular action to a given site. Nevertheless, there is evidence for several different forms of the α subunit of the GABA-regulated chloride channel, the presumed site of benzodiazepine action (Levitan *et al.*, 1988), and this possibility remains open. Another view ascribes differing patterns of pharmacological effects to the partial agonistic properties of a given agent (*see* Haefely, in Symposium, 1988a). In this view, sedative-hypnotic effects require a relatively high degree of occupancy of sites by a "full" agonist, and the relatively low sedative efficacy of some benzodiazepines (including clonazepam) is attributed to the fact that they are partial agonists. In support of this notion is the growing list of experimental compounds that have a limited ability to enhance the binding and electrophysiological actions of GABA as well as to produce sedation, and that also antagonize the sedative-hypnotic effects of presumed full-agonist benzodiazepines. Still other explanations invoke the participation of sites of action in addition to GABA-regulated chloride channels, especially for effects requiring higher concentrations of the benzodiazepines. As noted above, both Na^+ and Ca^{2+} channels become potential targets at concentrations greater than those associated with anxiolytic or antiepileptic effects. In addition, various benzodiazepines inhibit the uptake of adenosine and potentiate the actions of this endogenous neuronal depressant over this same range of concentrations (*see* Phillis and O'Regan, 1988).

The macromolecular complex containing GABA-regulated chloride channels also appears to be an important site of action of certain steroid anesthetic agents, including alfaxalone, which is in clinical use in Europe, and 3α-hydroxy,5α-dihydroprogesterone, a naturally occurring metabolite of progesterone (Gee *et al.*, 1987, 1988; Harrison *et al.*, 1987). These agents produce barbiturate-like effects, including enhancement of the binding of benzodiazepines and GABA-ergic agonists and promotion of GABA-induced chloride currents. At somewhat higher concentrations, the steroids activate chloride currents in the absence of GABA; this feature also resembles the effects of anesthetic barbiturates. Since glucocorticoids and certain of their metabolites can interact at these sites, it is possible that they may mediate some of the behavioral effects of various steroids.

Respiration. The benzodiazepines have only slight effects on respiration; hypnotic doses are without effect in normal subjects. Preanesthetic doses of diazepam and midazolam slightly depress alveolar ventilation and cause respiratory acidosis as the result of a decrease in hypoxic rather than hypercapnic drive. The rate of expiratory flow is depressed only under hypoxic conditions. In doses used for endoscopy, benzodiazepines decrease alveolar ventilation and P_{O_2}, increase P_{CO_2}, and may cause CO_2 narcosis in patients with chronic obstructive pulmonary disease (*see* Gross *et al.*, 1983; Dundee *et al.*, 1984). Furthermore, diazepam can cause apnea during anesthesia and also when given with opioids. Despite the occasional adverse interaction with opioids, the benzodiazepines do not alter the effect of meperidine on the response to CO_2 (*see* Greenblatt and Shader, 1974). It is noteworthy that in scores of cases of intoxication involving benzodiazepines the only patients who required respiratory assistance were those who had also taken another CNS-depressant drug, especially alcohol (Greenblatt *et al.*, 1977).

Cardiovascular System. The cardiovascular effects of benzodiazepines are minor, except in severe intoxication. In preanesthetic doses, all benzodiazepines decrease blood pressure and increase heart rate. With flunitrazepam and midazolam, the effects are secondary to a decrease in peripheral resistance (Seitz *et al.*, 1977), but with diazepam and lorazepam they are secondary to a decrease in left ventricular work and cardiac output (*see* Rao *et al.*, 1973; Al-Khudhairi *et al.*, 1982). Diazepam increases coronary flow in man (Ikram *et al.*, 1973), possibly by an action to increase interstitial concentrations of adenosine. In large doses, midazolam decreases considerably both cerebral blood flow and oxygen assimilation (Nugent *et al.*, 1982).

Gastrointestinal Tract. Benzodiazepines are thought by some gastroenterologists to improve a variety of "anxiety-related" gastrointestinal disorders. There is a paucity of evidence for direct actions. Benzodiazepines partially protect against stress ulcers in rats, and diazepam markedly decreases nocturnal gastric secretion in man.

Absorption, Fate, and Excretion. The physicochemical and pharmacokinetic properties of the benzodiazepines greatly affect their clinical utility. They all have high lipid:water distribution coefficients in the nonionized form; nevertheless, lipophilicity varies more than 50-fold according to the polarity and electronegativity of various substituents.

All of the benzodiazepines are essentially completely absorbed, with the exception of clorazepate; this drug is rapidly decarboxylated in gastric juice to N-desmethyldiazepam (nordazepam), which is subsequently absorbed completely. Some benzodiazepines (*e.g.*, prazepam and flurazepam) reach the systemic circulation only in the form of active metabolites. After oral administration the time to peak concentration in plasma ranges from 0.5 to 8 hours for the various benzodiazepines. Among those commonly used for their hypnotic effects, peak concentrations of triazolam occur in plasma within 1 hour, while the absorption of temazepam is somewhat slower and more variable. Peak concentrations of active metabolites of flurazepam are attained in 1 to 3 hours. With the exception of lorazepam and midazolam, the absorption of benzodiazepines tends to be erratic after intramuscular injection.

The benzodiazepines and their active metabolites bind to plasma proteins. The extent of binding correlates strongly with lipid solubility and ranges from about 70% for alprazolam to nearly 99% for diazepam. The concentration in the CSF is approximately equal to the concentration of free drug in plasma. While competition with other protein-bound drugs may occur, no clinically significant examples have been reported.

The plasma concentrations of most benzodiazepines exhibit patterns that are consistent with two-compartment models (*see* Chapter 1 and Appendix II), but three-compartment models appear to be more appropriate for the compounds with the highest lipid solubility. Accordingly, there is rapid uptake of benzodiazepines into the brain and other highly perfused organs after intravenous administration (or oral administration of a rapidly absorbed compound); rapid uptake is followed by a phase of redistribution into tissues that are less well perfused, especially muscle and fat. Redistribution is most rapid for drugs with the highest lipid solubility. In the regimens used for nighttime sedation, the rate of redistribution can sometimes have a greater influence than the rate of biotransformation on the duration of CNS effects (Dettli, in Symposium, 1986a). The kinetics of redistribution of diazepam and other lipophilic benzodiazepines is complicated by enterohepatic circulation. The volumes of distribution of the benzodiazepines are large (*see* Appendix II), and many are increased in elderly patients (Swift and Stevenson, in Symposium, 1983a). These drugs cross the placental barrier and are secreted into breast milk.

The benzodiazepines are metabolized extensively, particularly by several different microsomal enzyme systems in the liver. Because active metabolites are generated that are biotransformed more slowly than the parent compound, the duration of action of many benzodiazepines bears little relationship to the half-time of elimination of the drug that has been administered. For example, the half-life of flurazepam in plasma is 2 to 3 hours, but that of a major active metabolite (N-desalkylflurazepam) is 50 hours or more. Conversely, the rate of biotransformation of those agents that are inactivated by the initial reaction is an important determinant of their duration of action; these agents include oxazepam, lorazepam, temazepam, triazolam, and midazolam. Metabolism of the benzodiazepines occurs in three major stages. These and the relationships between the drugs and their metabolites are shown in Table 17–2.

For those benzodiazepines that bear a substituent at position 1 (or 2) of the diazepine ring, the initial and most rapid phase of metabolism involves modification and/or removal of the substituent. With the exception of triazolam, alprazolam, and midazolam, which contain either a fused triazolo or imidazo ring, the eventual products are N-desalkylated compounds; these are all biologically active. One such compound, nordazepam, is a major metabolite common to the biotransformation of diazepam, clorazepate, prazepam, and halazepam; it is also formed from demoxepam, an important metabolite of chlordiazepoxide. The second stage involves hydroxylation at position 3 and also usually yields an active derivative (*e.g.*, oxazepam from nordazepam). The rates of these reactions are usually very much slower than the first stage (half-times greater than 40 to 50 hours), such that appreciable accumulation of hydroxylated products with intact substituents at position 1 does not occur. The accumulation of small amounts of temazepam during the chronic administration of diazepam (not shown in Table 17–2) is an exception to this rule. The third major stage is the conjugation of the 3-hydroxyl compounds, principally with glucuronic acid; the half-times of these reactions are usually between 6 and 12 hours, and the products are invariably inactive. Conjugation is the only major route of metabolism available for oxazepam and lorazepam, and it is the preferred pathway for temazepam because of its slower conversion to oxazepam. Triazolam and alprazolam are metabolized principally by initial hydroxylation of the methyl group on the fused triazolo ring; the absence of a chlorine residue in ring C of alprazolam slows this reaction significantly. The products, sometimes referred to as α-hydroxylated compounds, are quite active but are metabolized very rapidly, primarily by conjugation with glucuronic acid, such that there is no appreciable accumulation of active metabolites. These drugs are also metabolized to a significant extent by hydroxylation at position 3 of the benzodiazepine ring; the rate of this reaction appears to be unusually swift compared with that for compounds without the triazolo ring. These metabolites are rapidly conjugated or oxidized further to benzophenone derivatives, and excreted. Midazolam is metabolized rapidly, primarily by hydroxylation of the methyl group on the fused imidazo ring; only small amounts of 3-hydroxyl compounds are formed (*see* Dundee *et al.*, 1984). The α-hydroxylated com-

Table 17–2. MAJOR METABOLIC RELATIONSHIPS BETWEEN SOME OF THE BENZODIAZEPINES *

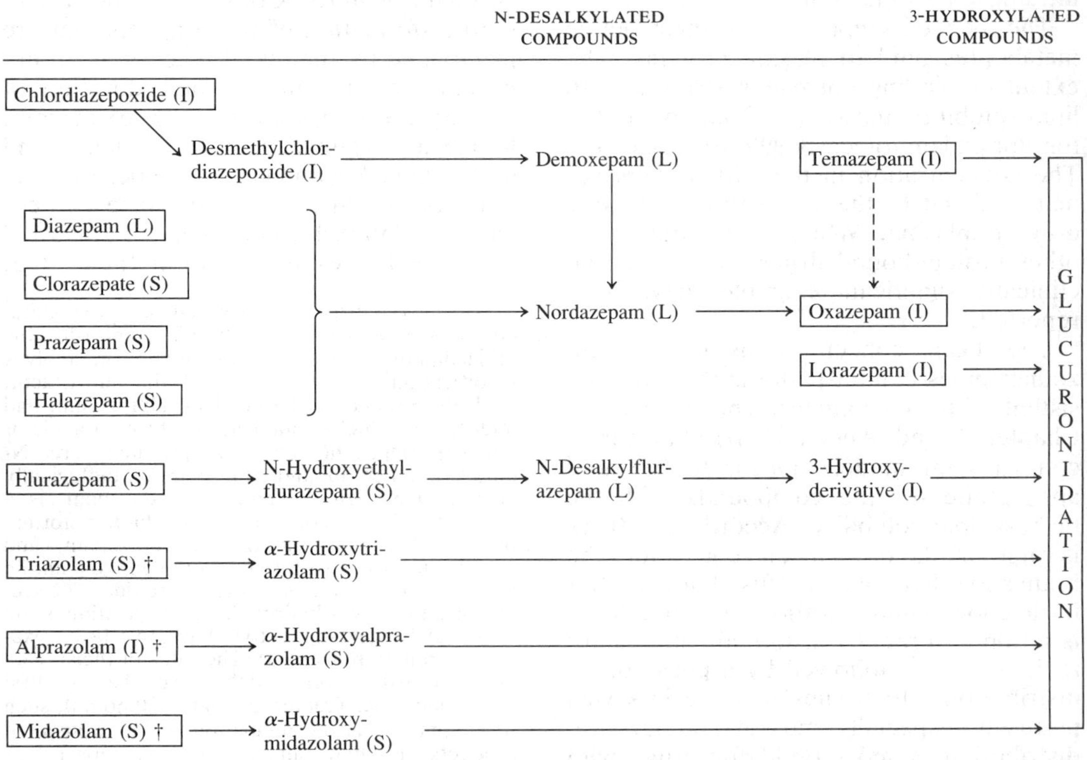

* Compounds enclosed in boxes are marketed in the United States. The approximate half-lives of the various compounds are denoted in parentheses: S = <6 hours; I = 6 to 20 hours; L = >20 hours. All compounds except clorazepate are biologically active; the activity of 3-hydroxydesalkylflurazepam has not been determined. Clonazepam (not shown) is an N-desalkyl compound, and it is metabolized primarily by reduction of the 7-NO_2 group to the corresponding amine (inactive), followed by acetylation; its half-life is 20 to 40 hours.

† *See* text for discussion of other pathways of metabolism.

pound, which has appreciable biological activity, is eliminated with a half-time of 1 hour after conjugation with glucuronic acid. Variable and sometimes substantial accumulation of this metabolite has been noted during intravenous infusions (Oldenhof *et al.,* 1988).

The aromatic rings (A and C) of the benzodiazepines are hydroxylated to only a small extent. The only important metabolism at these sites is the reduction of the 7-nitro substituents of clonazepam, nitrazepam, and flunitrazepam; the half-times of these reactions are usually 20 to 40 hours. The resulting amines are inactive and are acetylated to varying degrees before excretion.

Since the benzodiazepines apparently do not significantly induce the synthesis of hepatic microsomal enzymes, their chronic administration usually does not result in the accelerated metabolism of other substances or of the benzodiazepines. Cimetidine and oral contraceptives inhibit N-dealkylation and 3-hydroxylation of benzodiazepines. Ethanol, isoniazid, and phenytoin are less effective in this regard. These reactions are usually reduced to a greater extent in the aged and in patients with chronic liver disease than are those involving conjugation. However, the half-life of temazepam is markedly longer in elderly women compared with young adults or with men of the same age (Smith *et al.,* 1983).

Ideally, a useful hypnotic agent would have a rapid onset of action when taken at bedtime, a sufficiently sustained action to facilitate sleep throughout the night, and no residual action by the following morning. Among those benzodiazepines that are commonly used as hypnotic agents, triazolam theoretically fits this description most closely. Because of the slow rate of elimination of desalkylflurazepam, flurazepam might seem to be unsuitable for this purpose. However, in practice there appear to be some disadvantages to the use of agents that have a relatively rapid rate of disappearance; these disadvantages are not well defined at present but include the phenomena of "rebound" daytime anxiety and early-morning insomnia that are experienced by some patients. With careful selection of dosage, flurazepam and other benzodiazepines with slower rates of elimination than triazolam can be used effectively. The biotransformation and pharmacokinetic properties of the benzodiazepines have been reviewed by Breimer (1979), Bellantuono and associates (1980), Breimer and Jochemsen (in Symposium, 1981), Greenblatt and coworkers (1983a, 1983b, 1983c), and Schütz (1982), as well as in several symposia (Symposium, 1983a, 1983b).

Untoward Effects. At the time of peak concentration in plasma, hypnotic doses of benzodiazepines can be expected to cause varying degrees of lightheadedness, lassitude, increased reaction time, motor incoordination, ataxia, impairment of mental and psychomotor functions, disorganization of thought, confusion, dysarthria, anterograde amnesia, dry mouth, and a bitter taste. Cognition appears to be affected less than motor performance. All of these effects greatly impair driving and other psychomotor skills. When the drug is given at the intended time of sleep, they may not even be noticed, but the persistence of these effects during the waking hours is adverse. Interaction with ethanol may be especially serious. Significant residual effects have been observed after administration of hypnotic doses of a variety of benzodiazepines. For example, in one study the residual effects of two nightly 30-mg doses of flurazepam on driving performance were at least as great as those produced acutely by alcohol at a concentration of 100 mg/dl in blood, a level at which persons usually are considered to be legally intoxicated (*see* O'Hanlon and Volkerts, in Symposium, 1986a). Under the same conditions, significant effects of temazepam (20-mg doses) were not observed. These and other residual effects are clearly dose-related and can be insidious, since most subjects underestimate the degree of their impairment. The intensity and incidence of CNS toxicity generally increase with age; both pharmacokinetic and pharmacodynamic factors are involved (*see* Meyer, 1982; Swift *et al.*, in Symposium, 1983a). The effects of benzodiazepines on performance have been reviewed by Bond and Lader (in Symposium, 1981), by Linnoila (in Symposium, 1983a), and in recent Symposia (1986a, 1986b).

Other relatively common side effects of benzodiazepines are weakness, headache, blurred vision, vertigo, nausea and vomiting, epigastric distress, and diarrhea; joint pains, chest pains, and incontinence may occur in a few recipients. Anticonvulsant benzodiazepines sometimes actually increase the frequency of seizures in patients with epilepsy.

The possible adverse effects of alterations in the sleep pattern will be discussed at the end of this chapter.

Adverse Psychological Effects. Benzodiazepines may cause paradoxical effects. Nitrazepam frequently and flurazepam occasionally increase the incidence of nightmares, especially during the first week of use. Flurazepam occasionally causes garrulousness, anxiety, irritability, tachycardia, and sweating. Euphoria, restlessness, hallucinations, and hypomanic behavior have been reported to occur during use of various benzodiazepines. Antianxiety benzodiazepines have been reported to release bizarre uninhibited behavior in some users with low levels of anxiety; hostility and rage may occur in others. Paranoia, depression, and suicidal ideation occasionally also accompany the use of these agents. However, the incidence of such paradoxical reactions is extremely small (*see* Hall and Zisook, 1981).

Although benzodiazepines have a reputation for causing only a low incidence of abuse and dependence, the possibility of this adverse complication of chronic use must not be overlooked. Mild dependence may develop in many patients who have taken therapeutic doses of benzodiazepines on a regular basis for prolonged periods. Withdrawal symptoms may include temporary intensification of the problems that originally prompted their use (*e.g.*, insomnia, anxiety). Dysphoria, irritability, sweating, unpleasant dreams, tremors, anorexia, and faintness or dizziness may also occur. Hence, it is prudent to taper the dosage gradually when therapy is to be discontinued. During conventional treatment regimens, very few individuals increase their intake without instructions to do so, and very few manifest compulsive drug-seeking behavior upon discontinuation of a benzodiazepine. It is the patients who have histories of drug or alcohol abuse who are most apt to use these agents inappropriately, and abuse of benzodiazepines usually occurs as part of a pattern of abuse of multiple drugs. In such individuals, benzodiazepines are seldom preferred to barbiturates or even alcohol. The use of high doses of benzodiazepines over prolonged periods can lead to more severe symptoms after discontinuing the drug, including agitation, depression, panic, paranoia, myalgia, muscle twitches, and even convulsions. Dependence on benzodiazepines and their abuse have been reviewed by Marks (1978), Owen and Tyrer (1983), and Woods and colleagues (1987, 1988) as well as in several symposia (Symposium, 1983b, 1983c).

In spite of the adverse effects reviewed above, the benzodiazepines are relatively safe drugs. Even huge doses are rarely fatal unless other drugs are taken concomitantly. Ethanol is a common contributor to deaths involving benzodiazepines, and true coma is uncommon in the absence of another CNS depressant. Although overdosage with a benzodiazepine rarely causes severe cardiovascular or respiratory depression, therapeutic doses can further compromise respiration in patients with chronic obstructive pulmonary disease.

A wide variety of allergic, hepatotoxic, and hematologic reactions to the benzodiazepines may occur, but the incidence is quite low; these reactions have been associated with the use of flurazepam and triazolam, but not with temazepam. Large doses taken just prior to or during labor may cause hypothermia, hypotonia, and mild respiratory depression in the neonate. Abuse by the pregnant mother can result in a withdrawal syndrome in the newborn.

Except for additive effects with other sedative or hypnotic drugs, reports of clinically important, pharmacodynamic interactions between benzodiazepines and other drugs have been infrequent. Ethanol increases both the rate of absorption of benzodiazepines and the associated CNS depression. Valproate and benzodiazepines in combination may cause psychotic episodes. Pharmacokinetic interactions are mentioned above.

THERAPEUTIC USES

The use of the benzodiazepines as hypnotics and sedatives is discussed at the end of this chapter. (*See also* Mitler, 1981; McElnay *et al.*, 1982; Roth *et al.*, 1983.) Other uses of benzodiazepines are as antianxiety agents (Chapter 18), anticonvulsants (Chapter 19), muscle relaxants (Chapter 20), for preanesthetic medication (Chapter 13), and in anesthesia (Chapter 14).

Preparations and Dosage. The aqueous solubility of benzodiazepines ranges from less than 1/10,000 (chlordiazepoxide, lorazepam, oxazepam) to 1/2 (flurazepam hydrochloride). Solubilities in lipid are generally moderate; however, because of the generally low aqueous solubilities, lipid:water partition coefficients are usually high. The official names, trade names, preparations, and sedative and hypnotic doses of these agents are given in Table 17–3.

FLUMAZENIL

Flumazenil, an imidazobenzodiazepine (*see* Table 17–1), is the first specific benzodiazepine antagonist to undergo extensive clinical trial. As noted above, flumazenil binds with high affinity to specific sites, where it competitively antagonizes the binding and allosteric effects of benzodiazepines and other ligands. Both the electrophysiological and behavioral effects of agonist or inverse-agonist benzodiazepines or β-carbolines are also antagonized. In animal studies, the intrinsic pharmacological actions of flumazenil have been quite subtle; effects resembling those of inverse agonists have sometimes been detected at low doses, while slight benzodiazepine-like effects have often been evident at high doses. The underlying mechanisms for such effects are not at all clear; the various hypotheses range from antagonism of endogenous agonist and/or inverse-agonist substances to indirect actions, such as inhibition of adenosine uptake. The evidence for intrinsic activity in human subjects is even more vague, except for modest anticonvulsant effects at high doses.

Upon oral administration, flumazenil is subject to extensive first-pass hepatic metabolism, and less than 20% reaches the systemic circulation. Flumazenil rapidly enters the brain, reaching maximal concentrations within 5 to 10 minutes of injection. The half-time of elimination is somewhat less than 1 hour. Virtually no unchanged flumazenil is excreted in the urine, but little information is available on the nature or activity of metabolites. The brief duration of clinical effects suggests that active metabolites do not accumulate to an appreciable extent.

Flumazenil has been evaluated for its utility in reversing the sedation produced by benzodiazepines administered before or during anesthetic procedures. The intravenous administration of 0.3 to 1 mg of flumazenil is usually sufficient to abolish the effects of therapeutic doses of benzodiazepines within 1 to 2 minutes. There is some debate as to whether the improvement in respiration or consciousness is of significant value when the short-acting midazolam has been used, but its benefits are clear following the use of diazepam. Flumazenil will also awaken patients rendered comatose by the ingestion of excessive doses of benzodiazepines,

Table 17–3. **HALF-LIVES, DOSAGE FORMS, AND ORAL DOSAGES OF SEDATIVE-HYPNOTIC DRUGS**

DRUG CLASSES, NONPROPRIETARY NAMES, AND TRADE NAMES	HALF-LIFE (*hours*)	DOSAGE FORMS *	ADULT ORAL DOSAGE (*mg*)	
			Sedative †	*Hypnotic*
Benzodiazepines				
Chlordiazepoxide (LIBRIUM, others)	5–15	C,T,I	15–100, 1–3×d ‡	—
Clorazepate (dipotassium) (TRANXENE, others)	50–80 §	C,T	3.75–20, 2–4×d ‡	—
Diazepam (VALIUM, others)	30–60	T,ERC,I,L	5–10, 3–4×d ‡	—
Flurazepam HCl (DALMANE, others)	50–100 §	C	—	15–30
Lorazepam (ATIVAN, others)	10–20	T,I	—	2–4
Oxazepam (SERAX, others)	5–10	C,T	15–30, 3–4×d ‡	—
Temazepam (RESTORIL, others)	10–17	C	—	15–30
Triazolam (HALCION)	2–4	T	—	0.125–0.5
Barbiturates				
Amobarbital (sodium) (AMYTAL)	8–42	C,T,I,P	30–50, 2–3×d	65–200
Aprobarbital (ALURATE)	14–34	E	40, 3×d	40–160
Butabarbital (sodium) (BUTISOL SODIUM, others)	34–42	C,T,E	15–30, 3–4×d	50–100
Butalbital ‖	—	M ‖	—	—
Mephobarbital (MEBARAL)	11–67	T	32–100, 3–4×d	—
Pentobarbital (sodium) (NEMBUTAL)	15–48	C,E,I,S	20, 3–4×d	100
Phenobarbital (sodium) (LUMINAL SODIUM, others)	80–120	C,T,E,I	15–40, 2–3×d	100–320
Secobarbital (sodium) (SECONAL SODIUM)	15–40	C,T,I	30–50, 3–4×d	50–200
Talbutal (LOTUSATE)	—	T	15–40, 2–3×d	120
Miscellaneous				
Chloral hydrate (NOCTEC, others)	4–9.5 §	C,L,S	250, 3×d	500–1000
Ethchlorvynol (PLACIDYL)	10–25 ¶	C	100–200, 2–3×d	500–1000
Ethinamate (VALMID)	—	C	—	500–1000
Glutethimide (DORIDEN, other)	5–22	C,T	—	250–500
Meprobamate (MILTOWN, others)	6–17	ERC,T	400, 3–4×d	—
Methyprylon (NOLUDAR)	3–6	C,T	50–100, 3–4×d	200–400
Paraldehyde (PARAL)	4–10	L,I	2–5 ml, 2–4×d	10–30 ml

* C = capsule; E = elixir; ERC = extended-release capsule; I = injection; L = liquid; P = powder; S = suppository; T = tablet.

† Dose, number per day; dosages do not apply for extended-release forms.

‡ Approved as a sedative-hypnotic drug only for management of alcohol withdrawal; dose in a nontolerant individual would be smaller.

§ Half-life of the active metabolite, to which effects can be attributed.

‖ Marketed only in mixtures.

¶ For acute use, half-life of distribution phase (1–3 hours) may be more appropriate.

even when there is concurrent intoxication with other agents. In general, the administration of 1 to 10 mg of flumazenil intravenously results in a return to consciousness within 5 to 15 minutes, but additional doses may be required after 1 to 2 hours. Flumazenil is not effective in single-drug overdosages with either barbiturates or tricyclic antidepressants; variable or delayed effects have been reported in comatose patients intoxicated with alcohol. The properties and therapeutic uses of flumazenil have been reviewed by Brogden and Goa (1988).

Flumazenil has also been found to diminish the neurological deficits in patients with hepatic encephalopathy (*see* Basile and Gammal, 1988). Hepatic failure is thought to permit the assimilation of benzodiazepine-like substances contained in certain foods or produced by enteric bacteria, or to cause their accumulation in the CSF (Mullen *et al.*, 1988). Although flumazenil has no effect on the course of the underlying hepatic disease, it may prove useful in improving the mental status of patients with hepatic insufficiency.

BARBITURATES

The barbiturates once enjoyed a long period of extensive use as sedative-hypnotic drugs; however, except for a few specialized uses, they have been largely replaced by the much safer benzodiazepines. A more detailed description of the barbiturates can be found in the *fifth edition* of this textbook.

Chemistry. Barbituric acid is 2,4,6-trioxohexahydropyrimidine. The compound lacks central-depressant activity, but the presence of alkyl or aryl groups at position 5 confers sedative-hypnotic and sometimes other activities. The general structural formula for the barbiturates and the structures of those compounds available in the United States are shown in Table 17–4.

The carbonyl group at position 2 takes on acidic character because of lactam ("keto")–lactim ("enol") tautomerization favored by its location between the two electronegative amido nitrogens. The lactim form is favored in alkaline solution, and salts result.

Barbiturates in which the oxygen at C2 is replaced by sulfur are sometimes called thiobarbiturates. These compounds are more lipid-soluble than the corresponding oxybarbiturates. In general, structural changes that increase lipid solubility decrease duration of action, decrease latency to onset of activity, accelerate metabolic degradation, increase binding to albumin, and often increase hypnotic potency.

PHARMACOLOGICAL PROPERTIES

The barbiturates reversibly depress the activity of all excitable tissues. The CNS is exquisitely sensitive, and, even when barbiturates are given in anesthetic concentrations, direct effects on peripheral excitable tissues are weak. However, serious deficits in cardiovascular and other peripheral functions occur in acute barbiturate intoxication.

Table 17–4. BARBITURATES CURRENTLY AVAILABLE IN THE UNITED STATES: NAMES AND STRUCTURES

GENERAL FORMULA:

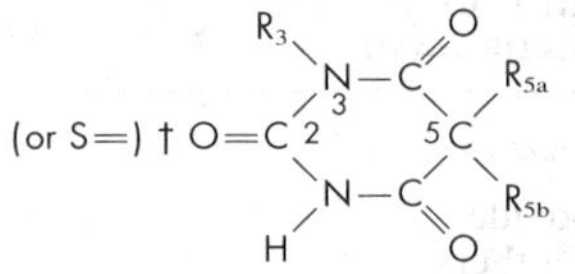

BARBITURATE	R_{5a}	R_{5b}
Amobarbital	ethyl	isopentyl
Aprobarbital	allyl	isopropyl
Butabarbital	ethyl	*sec*-butyl
Butalbital	allyl	isobutyl
Mephobarbital *	ethyl	phenyl
Metharbital *	ethyl	ethyl
Methohexital *	allyl	1-methyl-2-pentynyl
Pentobarbital	ethyl	1-methylbutyl
Phenobarbital	ethyl	phenyl
Secobarbital	allyl	1-methylbutyl
Talbutal	allyl	*sec*-butyl
Thiamylal †	allyl	1-methylbutyl
Thiopental †	ethyl	1-methylbutyl

* R_3 = H, except in mephobarbital, metharbital, and metho- hexital, where it is replaced by CH_3.

† O, except in thiamylal and thiopental, where it is replaced by S.

Central Nervous System. The barbiturates can produce all degrees of depression of the CNS, ranging from mild sedation to general anesthesia. The use of barbiturates for general anesthesia is discussed in Chapter 14. Certain barbiturates, particularly those containing a 5-phenyl substituent (phenobarbital, mephobarbital) have selective anticonvulsant activity (*see* Chapter 19). The antianxiety properties of the barbiturates are not equivalent to those exerted by the benzodiazepines, especially with respect to the degree of sedation that is produced. The barbiturates may have euphoriant effects, which, when maximal, are comparable to those of morphine.

Except for the anticonvulsant activities of phenobarbital and its congeners, the barbiturates possess a low degree of selectivity and therapeutic index. Thus, it is not possible to achieve a desired effect without evidence of general depression of the CNS. Pain perception and reaction are relatively unimpaired until the moment of unconsciousness, and in small doses the barbiturates increase the reaction to painful stimuli. Hence, they cannot be relied upon to produce sedation or sleep in the presence of even moderate pain.

In some individuals and in some circumstances, such as in the presence of pain, barbiturates cause overt excitement instead of sedation. The fact that such paradoxical excitement occurs with other CNS depressants suggests that it may result from depression of inhibitory centers. As with ethanol, the degree and quality of excitement are variable, depending on both personality and environment.

Effects on Stages of Sleep. Hypnotic doses of barbiturates alter the stages of sleep in a dose-dependent manner. They decrease sleep latency, decrease the number of stage shifts to stages 0 and 1 (number of awakenings), and decrease body movement. Stages 3 and 4 (slow-wave sleep, SWS) are generally shortened considerably. The latent period before REM sleep is prolonged, and total time spent in REM sleep, the number of REM cycles, and REM activity are diminished. With the short-acting barbiturates, these effects occur primarily during the first third of the night and are compensated for in the last third.

During repetitive nightly administration, some tolerance to the effects on sleep occurs within a few days, and the effect on total sleep time may be reduced by as much as 50% after 2 weeks of use. In all of nine studies reviewed by Kay and associates (1976), discontinuation led to rebound increases in all the parameters reported to be decreased by barbiturates. There may be an increase in REM sleep even if there was no reduction of this phenomenon during the time of drug administration. The effects of barbiturates on sleep have been reviewed by Kay and associates (1976) and Mendelson and coworkers (1977).

Tolerance. Both pharmacodynamic (functional) and pharmacokinetic tolerance to barbiturates can occur. The former contributes more to the decreased effect than does the latter. With chronic administration of gradually increasing doses, pharmacodynamic tolerance continues to develop over a period of weeks to months, depending upon the dosage schedule, whereas pharmacokinetic tolerance reaches its peak in a few days to a week. Tolerance to the effects on mood, sedation, and hypnosis occurs more readily and is greater than that to the anticonvulsant and lethal effects; thus, as tolerance increases, the therapeutic index decreases. When tolerance becomes maximal, the effective dose of a barbiturate may be increased by as much as six times; this is twofold to threefold greater than can be accounted for by enhanced metabolic disposition.

Although supervised chronic sedation for weeks to months with therapeutic doses of secobarbital or pentobarbital usually causes only a small degree of tolerance, decreased effects on sleep stages may occur. Moreover, the chronic disruption of the normal sleep pattern may in itself make sleep less satisfying. The result is that the dosage may be increased in an attempt to improve sleep and thereby enhance the probability or degree of tolerance.

Pharmacodynamic tolerance to barbiturates confers tolerance to all general CNS-depressant drugs, including ethanol. There may even be cross-tolerance to the pharmacodynamically dissimilar opioids and phencyclidine, only a part of which is due to induction of hepatic enzymes. There is some evidence of cross-tolerance to the antianxiety and hypnotic effects of benzodiazepines, but not to the muscle relaxant effects.

Abuse and Dependence. Like other CNS-depressant drugs, barbiturates are abused, and some individuals develop a dependence upon them. These topics are discussed in Chapter 22.

Sites and Mechanisms of Action on the CNS. Barbiturates act throughout the CNS, although not with equal potency in all regions. Nonanesthetic doses preferentially suppress polysynaptic responses. Facilitation is diminished, and inhibition is usually enhanced. The site of inhibition is either postsynaptic, as at cortical and cerebellar pyramidal cells and in the cuneate nucleus, substantia nigra, and thalamic relay neurons, or presynaptic, as in the spinal cord. Furthermore, inhibition occurs only at synapses where neurotransmission is mediated by GABA. The effect, however, may not be entirely mediated by GABA.

The barbiturates exert several distinct effects on excitatory and inhibitory synaptic transmission. For example, in cultures of spinal neurons, both hypnotic-anesthetic (*e.g.*, pentobarbital) and anticonvulsant barbiturates (*e.g.*, phenobarbital) potentiate GABA-induced increases in chloride conductance and reduce glutamate-induced depolarization at about the same concentrations (50 to 75 μM). At higher concentrations, the barbiturates depress Ca^{2+}-dependent action potentials, reduce the Ca^{2+}-dependent release of neurotransmitters, and enhance chloride conductance in the absence of GABA (so-called GABA-mimetic action). However, pentobarbital is much more potent than phenobarbital in producing these effects. Thus, the more selective anticonvulsant properties of phenobarbital and its higher therapeutic index might be explained by its lower capacity to produce profound depression of neuronal function as compared with the anesthetic barbiturates (*see* Macdonald and McLean, 1982).

The capacity of the barbiturates to facilitate GABA-ergic inhibition resembles some of the actions of the benzodiazepines, discussed above. However, promotion of GABA-induced chloride currents by barbiturates appears to result from prolongation of periods during which bursts of channel openings occur, rather than by increasing the frequency of bursts of channel openings (Twyman *et al.*, 1989). Moreover, barbiturates do not displace benzodiazepines from their binding sites. Instead, they enhance such binding; they also enhance the binding of GABA. These effects are almost completely dependent upon the presence of chloride or other anions that are known to permeate through chloride channels, and they are competitively antagonized by picrotoxin. These phenomena have been correlated with the ability of barbiturates to compete for specific binding sites for dihydropicrotoxinin and with the relative potency of barbiturates to cause general depression of the CNS. Of particular interest is the fact that phenobarbital is an impotent competitor for dihydropicrotoxinin binding sites and a weak enhancer of the binding of benzodiazepines and GABA. As noted above, these allosteric relationships are evident when mRNA that encodes the GABA-ergic receptor is expressed in *Xenopus* oocytes. Collectively, these observations indicate that a macromolecular complex composed of binding sites for GABA and a chloride channel is an important site of action for the depressant barbiturates. However, the relationship of these observations to the electrophysiological effects of the barbiturates is not at all clear, and they would appear to have little relevance to the anticonvulsant actions of phenobarbital.

Stereoisomers of barbiturates often display different anesthetic potencies (*see* Andrews and Mark, 1982). In some instances (*e.g.*, mephobarbital), one enantiomer has only excitant properties. The enantiomer with the lower CNS depressant activity has a lower capacity to enhance the binding of benzodiazepines and a greater potency as an antagonist at adenosine receptors (Lohse *et al.*, 1987). The significance of such correlations has yet to be established. At concentrations considerably above those at which effects on chloride and Ca^{2+} currents are observed, the barbiturates suppress high-frequency, repetitive firing of neurons. This appears to result from inhibition of voltage-dependent, tetrodotoxin-sensitive Na^+ channels. At still higher concentrations, voltage-dependent K^+ conductances are reduced.

The mechanisms of action of barbiturates have been reviewed by Ho and Harris (1981), Macdonald and McLean (1982, 1986), Richter and Holman (1982), and Olsen (1987).

Peripheral Nervous Structures. Barbiturates selectively depress transmission in autonomic ganglia and reduce nicotinic excitation by choline esters. This effect may account, at least in part, for the fall in blood pressure produced by intravenous oxybarbiturates and by severe barbiturate intoxication. At skeletal neuromuscular junctions, the blocking effects of both tubocurarine and decamethonium are enhanced during barbiturate anesthesia.

Respiration. Barbiturates depress both the respiratory drive and the mechanisms responsible for the rhythmic character of respiration. The neurogenic drive is diminished by hypnotic doses, but usually no more so than during natural sleep. *Neurogenic drive is essentially eliminated by a dose three times greater than that normally used to induce sleep.* Such doses also suppress the hypoxic drive and, to a lesser extent, the chemoreceptor drive. Thus, with increasing depth of depression of the CNS, the dominant respiratory drive shifts to the carotid and aortic bodies. At still higher doses, the powerful hypoxic drive also fails. However, the margin between the lighter planes of surgical anesthesia and dangerous respiratory depression is sufficient to permit the ultrashort-acting barbiturates to be used, with suitable precautions, as anesthetic agents.

The barbiturates only slightly depress protective reflexes until the degree of intoxication is sufficient to produce severe respiratory depression. Coughing, sneezing, hiccoughing, and laryngospasm may occur when barbiturates are employed as intravenous anesthetic agents. Indeed, laryngospasm is one of the chief complications of barbiturate anesthesia.

Cardiovascular System. When given orally in sedative or hypnotic doses, the barbiturates do not produce significant overt cardiovascular effects, except for a slight decrease in blood pressure and heart rate such as occurs in normal sleep. During thiopental anesthesia, there is usually either no change or a fall in mean arterial pressure. Hypotension is caused, in part, by partial inhibition of ganglionic transmission. In patients with congestive heart failure or hypovolemic shock whose reflexes are already operating maximally, barbiturates can cause an exaggerated fall in blood pressure. Because barbiturates impair reflex cardiovascular adjustments to inflation of the lung, positive-pressure respiration should be used cautiously and only when necessary to maintain adequate pulmonary ventilation in patients who are anesthetized or intoxicated with a barbiturate.

Apart from changes in blood pressure, the following cardiovascular changes have often been noted when thiopental and other intravenous thiobarbiturates are administered after conventional preanesthetic medication: a decrease in cardiac output and in renal plasma flow; an increase in total calculated peripheral resistance; an increase or no change in heart rate; and a decrease in cerebral blood flow, with a marked fall in CSF pressure. Cardiac arrhythmias are observed only rarely. In general, the effects of thiopental anesthesia on the cardiovascular system are benign in comparison with those of the volatile anesthetic agents. Direct depression of cardiac contractility occurs only when doses several times those required to cause anesthesia are administered, which probably contributes to the cardiovascular depression that accompanies acute barbiturate poisoning.

Gastrointestinal Tract. The oxybarbiturates tend to decrease the tonus of the gastrointestinal musculature and the amplitude of rhythmic contractions. The locus of action is partly peripheral and partly central, depending on the dose. A hypnotic dose does not significantly delay gastric emptying in man. The relief of various gastrointestinal symptoms by sedative doses is probably largely due to the central-depressant action.

Liver. The best-known effects of barbiturates on the liver are those on the microsomal drug-metabolizing system (*see* Chapter 1). Acutely, the barbiturates combine with cytochrome P_{450} and competitively interfere with the biotransformation of a number of other drugs as well as endogenous substrates, such as steroids. Thus, adverse drug interactions and potential endocrine imbalance can result. Other substrates may reciprocally inhibit barbiturate biotransformations. However, barbiturates do not inhibit the biotransformations of all drugs that are substrates of the microsomal enzyme system. The barbiturates need not be oxidized by the enzyme system in order to inhibit the biotransformation of other drugs.

The barbiturates cause a marked increase in the enzyme, protein, and lipid content of the hepatic smooth endoplasmic reticulum. This enzyme induction results in an increased rate of metabolism of a number of drugs and endogenous substances, including steroid hormones, cholesterol, bile salts, and vitamins K and D. Glucuronyl transferase activity is increased. Not all microsomal biotransformations of drugs and endogenous substrates are affected to the same degree, but a convenient rule of thumb is that, at maximal induction in man, the rates are approximately doubled. The inducing effect is not limited to the microsomal enzymes; for example, there is an increase in δ-aminolevulinic acid (ALA) synthetase, a mitochondrial enzyme, and aldehyde dehydrogenase, a cytoplasmic enzyme. The effect of barbiturates on ALA synthetase can cause dangerous exacerbations of disease in persons with intermittent porphyria.

The inducing effect of the barbiturates causes an increase in the rate of their own metabolism and accounts for part of the tolerance to the drugs. Many sedative-hypnotics, various anesthetics, and ethanol also are metabolized by and/or induce the microsomal enzymes, and cross-tolerance can occur on this basis. A number of other drugs and chlorinated hydrocarbon insecticides can also induce microsomal enzymes, but only under exceptional circumstances have they been shown to increase significantly the rate of elimination of barbiturates in man.

Choleresis results from treatment with phenobarbital but not other barbiturates. Both bile salt–dependent flow and bile salt–independent flow are increased by barbiturates in persons with cholestasis.

Kidney. Severe oliguria or anuria may occur in acute barbiturate poisoning, largely as a result of the marked hypotension.

Absorption, Fate, and Excretion. For sedative-hypnotic use, the barbiturates are usually administered orally. Such doses are rapidly and probably completely absorbed; sodium salts are absorbed more rapidly than the corresponding free acids, especially from liquid formulations. The onset of action varies from 10 to 60 minutes, depending upon the agent and the formulation, and is delayed by the presence of food in the stomach. When necessary, intramuscular injections of solutions of the sodium salts should be placed deep into large muscles in order to avoid the pain and possible necrosis that can result at more superficial sites. With some agents, special preparations are available for rectal administration. The intravenous route is usually reserved for the management of status epilepticus (phenobarbital sodium) or for the induction and/or maintenance of general anesthesia (*e.g.*, thiopental, methohexital).

Barbiturates are distributed widely and readily cross the placenta. Binding to plasma proteins is a function of lipid solubility and is greatest for thiopental, which is bound to the extent of 65% or more. The highly lipid-soluble barbiturates, led by those used to induce anesthesia, undergo redistribution after intravenous injection. Uptake into less vascular tissues, especially muscle and fat, leads to a decline in the concentration of barbiturate in the plasma and brain. With thiopental and methohexital, this results in the awakening of patients within 5 to 15 minutes of the injection of the usual anesthetic doses.

With the exception of the less lipid-soluble aprobarbital and phenobarbital, nearly complete metabolism and/or conjugation of barbiturates in the liver precedes their renal excretion. The oxidation of radicals at C5 is the most important biotransformation responsible for termination of biological activity. Oxidation results in the formation of alcohols, ketones, phenols, or carboxylic acids, which may appear in the urine as such or as glucuronic acid conjugates. In some instances (*e.g.*, phenobarbital), N-glucosylation is an important metabolic pathway. Other biotransformations include N-hydroxylation, desulfuration of thiobarbiturates to oxybarbiturates, opening of the barbituric acid ring, and N-dealkylation of N-alkylbarbiturates to active metabolites (*e.g.*, mephobarbital to phenobarbital). About 25% of phenobarbital and nearly all of aprobarbital are excreted unchanged in the urine. Their renal excretion can be greatly increased by osmotic diuresis and/or alkalinization of the urine.

The relationship between duration of action and half-time of elimination is complicated in part by the fact that enantiomers of optically active barbiturates often have both different biological potencies and rates of biotransformation; standard assays of the concentration of the agents in plasma do not distinguish between stereoisomers. Frequently, but not always, the more potent enantiomer is metabolized more rapidly (*see* Andrews and Mark, 1982). As with many other drugs, metabolic elimination is more rapid among young people than in the elderly and infants, and half-lives are increased during pregnancy, partly because of the expanded volume of distribution. Chronic liver disease, especially cirrhosis, often increases the half-life of the biotransformable barbiturates. Repeated administration, especially of phenobarbital, shortens the half-life of barbiturates that are metabolized as a result of the induction of microsomal enzymes (*see* above). The biotransformations and pharmacokinetics of the barbiturates have been reviewed by Freudenthal and Carroll (1973) and by Breimer (1977).

The data on half-lives given in Table 17–3 show that none of the barbiturates used for hypnosis in the United States appears to have an elimination half-life that is sufficiently short for virtually complete elimination to occur in 24 hours. Thus, all of these barbiturates will accumulate during repetitive administration unless appropriate adjustments in dosage are made. Furthermore, the persistence of the drug in plasma during the day favors the development of tolerance and abuse.

Untoward Effects. *Aftereffects.* Drowsiness may last for only a few hours after a hypnotic dose of barbiturate, but residual depression of the CNS (hangover) is sometimes frankly evident the following day. Even in the absence of overt evidence of residual depression, subtle distortions of mood and impairment of judgment and fine motor skills may be demonstrable. For example, a 200-mg dose of secobarbital has been shown to impair performance of driving or flying skills for 10 to 22 hours. Residual effects may also take the form of vertigo, nausea, vomiting, or diarrhea.

The aftereffects of barbiturates may sometimes be manifested as overt excitement. The user may awaken slightly intoxicated and feel euphoric and energetic; later, as the demands of daytime activities challenge possibly impaired faculties, the user may display irritability and temper. Aftereffects such as nightmares and night terrors may be caused by deprivation of REM and/or stage-4 sleep, especially after several nights of use.

Paradoxical Excitement. In some persons, barbiturates repeatedly produce excitement rather than depression, and the patient may appear to be inebriated. This type of idiosyncrasy is relatively common among geriatric and debilitated patients and occurs most frequently with phenobarbital and N-methylbarbiturates.

Pain. Rarely, the use of barbiturates results in localized or diffuse myalgic, neuralgic, or arthritic pain, especially in psychoneurotic patients with insomnia. Barbiturates may cause restlessness, excitement, and even delirium when given in the presence of pain.

Hypersensitivity. Allergic reactions occur especially in persons who tend to have asthma, urticaria, angioedema, and similar conditions. Hypersensitivity reactions in this category include localized swellings, particularly of the eyelids, cheeks, or lips, and erythematous dermatitis. Rarely, exfoliative dermatitis may be caused by phenobarbital and can prove fatal; the skin eruption may be associated with fever, delirium, and marked degenerative changes in the liver and other parenchymatous organs.

Drug Interactions. Barbiturates combine with other CNS depressants to cause severe depression; ethanol is the most frequent offender, and interactions with antihistamines are also common. Isoniazid, methylphenidate, and monoamine oxidase inhibitors also increase the CNS-depressant effects.

The greatest number of drug interactions results from induction of hepatic microsomal enzymes. As noted above, the disappearance of many drugs and endogenous substances is significantly accelerated. The metabolism of vitamin K is accelerated, which may be pertinent to reported instances of coagulation defects in neonates whose mothers were taking phenobarbital. Elderly patients may have low concentrations of Ca^{2+} in plasma as the probable result of accelerated elimination of vitamin D. Hepatic enzyme induction enhances metabolism of endogenous steroid hormones, which may cause endocrine disturbances. Barbiturates also induce the hepatic generation of toxic metabolites of chlorocarbon anesthetics and carbon tetrachloride and consequently promote lipid peroxidation, which facilitates the periportal necrosis of the liver caused by these agents.

Barbiturates competitively inhibit the metabolism of certain other drugs. The most important interaction of this type is with tricyclic antidepressants.

Although barbiturates compete with other weak acids for binding to plasma albumin, the only clinically important displacement is that of thyroxine. The absorptions of dicumarol and griseofulvin are decreased by barbiturates, especially phenobarbital.

Other Untoward Effects. Because barbiturates enhance porphyrin synthesis, they are absolutely contraindicated in patients with acute intermittent porphyria or porphyria variegata. In hypnotic doses, the effects of barbiturates on the control of respiration are minor; however, in the presence of pulmonary insufficiency, serious respiratory depression may occur and the drugs are thus contraindicated. Rapid intravenous injection of a barbiturate may cause cardiovascular collapse before anesthesia ensues, so that the CNS signs of depth of anesthesia may fail to give an adequate warning of impending toxicity. Blood pressure can fall to shock levels; even slow intravenous injection of barbiturates often produces apnea and occasionally laryngospasm, coughing, and other respiratory difficulties.

BARBITURATE POISONING

In part because of the ready availability of barbiturates, poisoning with these drugs is a major clinical problem; death occurs in a few percent of cases. Most of the cases are the result of deliberate attempts at suicide, but some are from accidental poisonings in children or in drug abusers. The lethal dose of barbiturate varies with many factors, but severe poisoning is likely to occur when more than ten times the full hypnotic dose has been ingested at once. The potentially fatal dose of phenobarbital is 6 to 10 g, whereas that of amobarbital, secobarbital, or pentobarbital is 2 to 3 g. The lowest concentration of drug in plasma associated with lethal overdosage has been 60 μg/ml for phenobarbital and barbital but only 10 μg/ml for shorter-acting agents such as amobarbital and pentobarbital; if alcohol or other depressant drugs are also present, the concentrations that can cause death are lower.

The signs and symptoms of barbiturate poisoning are referable especially to the CNS and the cardiovascular system. In severe intoxication, the patient is comatose; the deep reflexes may persist for some time despite coexistent coma. The Babinski sign is often positive. The pupils may be constricted and react to light, but late in the course of barbiturate poisoning hypoxic paralytic dilatation may appear. Respiration is affected early. Breathing may be either slow, or rapid and shallow; Cheyne-Stokes respiration may be present. Superficial observation of respiration may be misleading with regard to actual minute volume and to the degree of respiratory acidosis and cerebral hypoxia; arterial P_{CO_2} and P_{O_2} must be determined. Eventually, blood pressure falls owing to the direct effect of the drug and of hypoxia on medullary vasomotor centers; depression of cardiac contractility, sympathetic ganglia, and vascular smooth muscle also contribute. Hypothermia, sometimes with temperatures as low as 32° C, often occurs; during recovery, hyperthermia may occur. Pulmonary complications (atelectasis, edema, and bronchopneumonia) and renal failure are likely to be the fatal complications of severe barbiturate poisoning. Not uncommonly, patients suffering from acute barbiturate intoxication develop necrosis of sweat glands and bullous cutaneous lesions, which are not due to hypersensitivity or hypothermia but may be related to pressure necrosis from prolonged immobility. These lesions heal slowly, sometimes requiring many weeks.

The optimal treatment of acute barbiturate intoxication is based upon general supportive measures. Hemodialysis or hemoperfusion is only rarely necessary. A highly organized intensive care unit can reduce the mortality rate to less than 2%. Formerly, when CNS stimulants were used in attempts to antagonize barbiturates, mortality rates were as high as 40%. The present treatment is applicable in most respects for poisoning by any CNS depressant.

The depth of coma and adequacy of ventilation are first evaluated. If fewer than 24 hours have elapsed since ingestion, gastric lavage should be considered, since the barbiturate can reduce gastrointestinal motility. Lavage or emesis should be attempted only after precautions have been taken to avoid aspiration. After lavage, activated charcoal and a cathartic (usually sorbitol) should be administered. Repeated doses of charcoal (as long as bowel sounds are present) may shorten the half-life of phenobarbital but will do little for barbiturates that have a larger volume of distribution.

Constant attention must be given to the maintenance of a patent airway and to the prevention of pneumonia; oxygen should be administered. Measures to prevent or treat atelectasis should be taken. Blood P_{CO_2} and pH should be monitored, and mechanical ventilation should be initiated when indicated. Fever or radiological evidence of pneumonia calls for appropriate therapy. Measures should be taken to prevent further loss of body heat, but it is not universally agreed that it is necessary to restore the body temperature to normal.

In severe acute barbiturate intoxication, circulatory collapse is a major threat. Often the patient is admitted to the hospital with severe hypotension or shock, and dehydration is often severe. Hypovolemia must be corrected, and, if necessary, the blood pressure can be supported with dopamine.

Acute renal failure consequent to shock and hypoxia accounts for perhaps one sixth of the deaths. Anuria and uremia may ensue, even after the patient has recovered consciousness. In the event of renal failure, hemodialysis should be instituted. If renal and cardiac function are satisfactory and the patient is hydrated, forced diuresis and alkalinization of the urine will hasten the excretion of certain long-acting barbiturates, but this is rarely of sufficient clinical benefit to justify the risks. While such maneuvers can increase the renal clearance of pentobarbital by as much as 15 times, the total rate of detoxication is increased by only 15 to 25%, since little of this drug is usually excreted in the urine. Intoxication by barbiturates and its management have been reviewed by Gary and Tresnewsky (1983).

THERAPEUTIC USES

The use of barbiturates as sedative-hypnotic drugs has declined enormously because they lack specificity of effect in the CNS, they have a lower therapeutic index than do the benzodiazepines, tolerance occurs more frequently than with benzodiazepines, the liability for abuse is greater, and the number of drug interactions is considerable.

CNS Uses. The use of barbiturates as hypnotics is included in the general discussion on page 369.

Although barbiturates have largely been replaced by benzodiazepines and other compounds for daytime sedation, phenobarbital and butabarbital are still available as "sedatives" in a host of inefficacious combinations for the treatment of functional gastrointestinal disorders, urethral inflammation, hypertension, asthma, and coronary artery disease. They are also included in analgesic combinations, possibly counterproductively. Barbiturates, especially butabarbital and phenobarbital, are sometimes used to antagonize unwanted CNS-stimulant effects of various drugs, such as ephedrine, dextroamphetamine, and theophylline. While they may be superior to benzodiazepines in such cases, adjustment of dosage or substitution of alternative therapy is preferred.

Barbiturates are still employed in the emergency treatment of convulsions, such as occur in tetanus, eclampsia, status epilepticus, cerebral hemorrhage, and poisoning by convulsant drugs; however, benzodiazepines are generally superior in these uses. Phenobarbital sodium is most frequently used because of its anticonvulsant efficacy; however, even when administered intravenously, 15 minutes or more may be required for it to attain peak concentrations in the brain. If the patient has not been receiving barbiturates previously, a loading dose of phenobarbital of about 12 mg/kg given slowly and intravenously is usually required to achieve control of seizures. While the rapidity of onset of the ultrashort- and short-acting barbiturates would seem to have appeal, these drugs have a low ratio of anticonvulsant to hypnotic action. These drugs or inhalational agents are employed only when general anesthesia must be used to control seizures refractory to other measures. Diazepam is usually chosen for the emergency treatment of seizures. In addition, patients are often given a loading dose of phenytoin. The use of phenobarbital and mephobarbital in the symptomatic therapy of epilepsy is discussed in Chapter 19.

The ultrashort-acting agents continue to be employed as intravenous anesthetics (Chapter 14). Short- and ultrashort-acting barbiturates are occasionally used as adjuncts to other agents in the production of obstetrical anesthesia. Although several studies have failed to affirm gross depression of respiration in the neonate at birth, evaluation of the effects on the fetus and neonate is difficult; it is prudent to avoid the use of barbiturates in obstetrics.

The barbiturates are employed as diagnostic and therapeutic aids in psychiatry, in narcoanalysis and narcotherapy. They are used to activate latent abnormalities in the EEG. In low concentrations, amobarbital has been administered directly into the carotid artery prior to neurosurgery as a means of identifying the dominant cerebral hemisphere for speech.

Anesthetic doses of barbiturates attenuate cerebral edema resulting from surgery, head injury, or cerebral ischemia, and they may decrease infarct size and increase survival. General anesthetics do not provide protection. The procedure is not without serious danger, however, and the ultimate benefit to the patient has been questioned (*see* Marshall and Bowers, 1982; Michenfelder, 1982; Steer, 1982; Shapiro, 1985).

Hepatic Metabolic Uses. Because hepatic glucuronyl transferase and the bilirubin-binding Y protein are increased by the barbiturates, phenobarbital has been successfully used to treat hyperbilirubinemia and kernicterus in the neonate. The nondepressant barbiturate phetharbital (N-phenylbarbital) works equally well. Phenobarbital may improve the hepatic transport of bilirubin in patients with hemolytic jaundice. The effect of phenobarbital on bile salt metabolism and excretion has been employed in the treatment of selected cases of cholestasis.

Preparations and Dosage. Barbiturates are marketed in a vast array of preparations. In the United States, phenobarbital is an ingredient in more than 25 proprietary remedies, which are best ignored in favor of nonproprietary preparations. The hypnotic and sedative dosages of the barbiturates are listed in Table 17–3.

CHLORAL DERIVATIVES

The pharmacology and uses of the chloral derivatives are essentially the same, because they are all converted in the body to the same active intermediate. Only chloral hydrate remains available in the United States.

Chemistry. Chloral hydrate [$CCl_3CH(OH)_2$] is formed by adding one molecule of water to the carbonyl group of chloral (2,2,2-trichloroacetaldehyde). Its metabolite, trichloroethanol (CCl_3CH_2OH), is also an effective hypnotic.

Local Actions. Chloral hydrate is quite irritating to the skin and mucous membranes. Gastrointestinal side effects are particularly likely to occur if the drug is insufficiently diluted or if it is taken on an empty stomach.

Systemic Actions. Like the barbiturates, chloral hydrate has little analgesic activity, and excitement or delirium may be initiated by pain. The margin of safety is too narrow to permit the drug to be used as a general anesthetic agent.

During the first week of use of chloral hydrate, there is a decrease in the sleep latency and the number of awakenings, a variable change in total sleep time, and a slight decrease in SWS; REM sleep is rarely suppressed (*see* Kay *et al.*, 1976). There are claims that during repetitive nightly use, the effects on sleep disappear within 2 weeks; however, Hartmann (1976) reported that total sleep time and REM latency remain elevated, even though the number of awakenings is increased. After discontinuation of the drug, a significant rebound in REM sleep does not occur.

In therapeutic doses, chloral hydrate has little effect on respiration and blood pressure. Toxic doses produce severe respiratory depression and hypotension. In large doses, chloral hydrate depresses cardiac contractility and shortens the refractory period; untoward cardiac effects may occur when toxic doses are administered, especially to patients with heart disease.

The pharmacological properties of trichloroethanol closely resemble those of chloral hydrate. Chloral hydrate is rapidly reduced to trichloroethanol, with a half-time of a few minutes, and significant amounts of chloral hydrate have not been detected in the blood after its oral administration; therefore, its central-depressant effects are probably caused by trichloroethanol.

Distribution and Fate. Chloral hydrate and trichloroethanol are widely distributed throughout the body. Chloral hydrate is reduced to trichloroethanol, largely by alcohol dehydrogenase in the liver. Ethanol accelerates the reduction, because its own oxidation provides reduced nicotinamide adenine dinucleotide (NADH) to drive the reduction of chloral hydrate. A small but variable amount of chloral hydrate and a larger fraction of trichloroethanol are oxidized to trichloroacetic acid. Trichloroethanol is mainly conjugated with glucuronic acid, and the product (urochloralic acid) is excreted mostly into the urine and to a limited extent into the bile. The plasma half-life of trichloroethanol ranges from 4 to 12 hours. The pharmacokinetics of chloral hydrate and trichloroethanol have been reviewed by Breimer (1977).

Untoward Effects. The irritant actions of chloral hydrate give rise to an unpleasant taste, epigastric distress, nausea, occasional vomiting, and flatulence. Undesirable CNS effects include lightheadedness, malaise, ataxia, and nightmares. "Hangover" may also occur, although it is less common than with most barbiturates and some benzodiazepines. The tendency of hypnotics to cause persistent effects in the elderly is less pronounced with chloral hydrate than with agents that are metabolized by the hepatic microsomal enzyme system.

Rarely, patients exhibit idiosyncratic reactions to chloral hydrate and may be disoriented and incoherent and show paranoid behavior. Allergic reactions include erythema, scarlatiniform exanthems, urticaria, and eczematoid dermatitis. Eosinophilia and leukopenia may also occur. Chloral hydrate is contraindicated in patients with marked hepatic or renal impairment, and it should perhaps be avoided in patients with severe cardiac disease or gastritis.

There is a popular belief that chloral hydrate and ethanol in combination (the "Mickey Finn") are supra-additive. Its basis is presumed to be inhibition of the metabolism of ethanol by chloral and enhancement of the generation of trichloroethanol by ethanol, in addition to the combined depressant effect of the two drugs. Interactions of chloral hydrate with a number of acidic drugs have been noted; the most important of these is a transient enhancement of hypoprothrombinemia during the administration of oral anticoagulants.

Acute Intoxication. The toxic oral dose of chloral hydrate for adults is approximately 10 g. Poisoning by chloral hydrate resembles acute barbiturate intoxication, and the same supportive treatment is indicated. If the patient survives, icterus due to hepatic damage and albuminuria from renal irritation may appear.

Abuse and Dependence. The habitual use of chloral hydrate may result in the development of tolerance, physical dependence, and addiction, and sudden withdrawal may result in delirium and seizures with a high frequency of death, when untreated. The chloral habitué may suddenly exhibit acute intoxication and death may occur, either as a result of an overdose or a failure of the detoxification mechanism owing to hepatic damage. Parenchymatous renal injury may also occur.

Preparations and Dosage. The preparations and dosage of *chloral hydrate* are listed in Table 17–3. The often-recommended dose of 0.5 to 1 g has only a slight effect on sleep, and many individuals require as much as 2 g. To minimize irritation, solutions of the drug should be taken well diluted with water or fruit juice.

ETHCHLORVYNOL

Ethchlorvynol is a sedative-hypnotic drug with a rapid onset and short duration of action. It has the following structure:

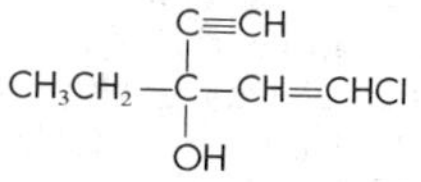

Ethchlorvynol

CNS Effects. Ethchlorvynol has anticonvulsant and muscle relaxant properties as well as sedative-hypnotic activity. Its effects on the CNS are very similar to those produced by barbiturates and other general CNS depressants. Ethchlorvynol causes changes in sleep latency and in the stages of sleep that are virtually identical to those produced by the shorter-acting barbiturates, both during administration and after withdrawal of the drug (*see* above).

Absorption and Fate. Oral ethchlorvynol acts within 15 to 30 minutes, and maximal concentrations in blood are attained in 1 to 1.5 hours. The apparent volume of distribution is about 4 liters per kilogram. The drug crosses the placental barrier. Two-compartment kinetics is manifested, with a distribution half-life of about 1 to 3 hours and an elimination half-life of 10 to 25 hours. After intoxicating doses, dose-dependent rates of elimination may be seen. Approximately 90% of the drug is destroyed in the liver.

Untoward Effects, Intoxication, and Abuse. The most common side effects caused by ethchlorvynol are mintlike aftertaste, dizziness, nausea, vomiting, hypotension, and facial numbness. Mild "hangover" is also relatively common. An occasional patient responds with profound hypnosis, muscular weakness, and syncope unrelated to marked hypotension. Idiosyncratic responses range from mild stimulation to marked excitement and hysteria. Ethchlorvynol should not be used with antidepressants, because delirium may result. Hypersensitivity reactions include urticaria, rare but sometimes fatal thrombocytopenia, and occasionally cholestatic jaundice. Because of a reported effect to suppress the anticipated response to dicumarol, the drug should be used cautiously in combination with drugs metabolized by the liver, and it is contraindicated in patients with intermittent porphyria.

The therapeutic index of ethchlorvynol is probably about the same as that of barbiturates with an intermediate duration of action. Acute intoxication resembles that produced by barbiturates, except for more severe respiratory depression and a relative bradycardia. The lethal dose usually ranges from 10 to 25 g, but death has followed a dose of 2.5 g in the presence of ethanol. Treatment is similar to that for acute barbiturate intoxication.

Chronic abuse of ethchlorvynol results in tolerance and physical dependence, and withdrawal symptoms may resemble delirium tremens and are sometimes suggestive of a schizophrenic reaction. They are especially severe in elderly patients.

Preparations and Dosage. These are listed in Table 17–3. A dose of 770 mg of ethchlorvynol is approximately equivalent to 100 mg of secobarbital.

GLUTETHIMIDE

Glutethimide is 3-ethyl-3-phenyl-2,6-piperidinedione and is similar to methyprylon (*see* below). Their structures are as follows:

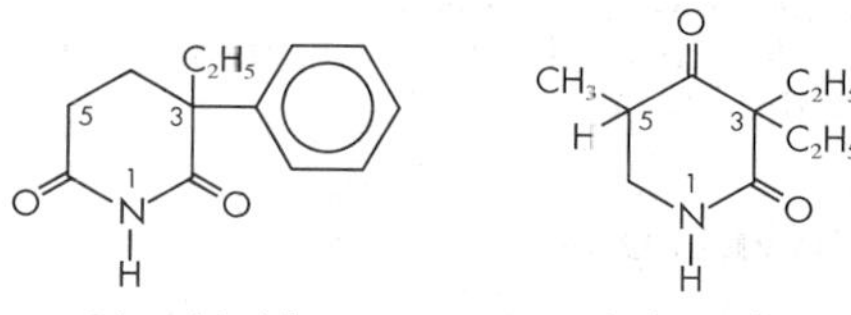

Glutethimide Methyprylon

Glutethimide has little to recommend its continued use as a sedative-hypnotic drug. Its addiction liability and the severity of withdrawal symptoms are equal to those of the barbiturates, and certain features of acute intoxication make its treatment more difficult.

Pharmacological Properties. The pharmacology of glutethimide is like that of barbiturates. The drug also exhibits pronounced anticholinergic activity.

Absorption and Fate. Glutethimide is quite erratically absorbed from the gastrointestinal tract. About 50% of the drug is bound to plasma proteins. More than 95% of glutethimide is metabolized in the liver; the half-life ranges from 5 to 22 hours. Active metabolites may accumulate after repetitive administration and during intoxication. Glutethimide induces hepatic microsomal enzymes.

Untoward Effects. With therapeutic doses, toxic side effects are rare and consist in "hangover," excitement, blurring of vision, gastric irritation, headache, and, infrequently, skin rashes, including exfoliative dermatitis. Thrombocytopenia, aplastic anemia, and leukopenia may also occur.

Acute Intoxication. The symptoms of acute intoxication are similar to those of barbiturate poisoning, with somewhat less severe respiratory depression. In addition, the antimuscarinic actions cause xerostomia, ileus, atony of the urinary bladder, and long-lasting mydriasis and hyperpyrexia, which may persist for hours after the patient regains consciousness. In some cases of glutethimide poisoning, occasional bouts of tonic muscular spasms, twitching, and even convulsions occur. A dose of 5 g is sufficient to produce severe intoxication, and the lethal dose is between 10 and 20 g. In acute intoxication, the plasma half-life may exceed 100 hours but averages about 40 hours. The management of intoxication is usually supportive, but hemodialysis may be useful to remove active metabolites and to shorten the coma.

Chronic Use and Abuse. Excessive use of glutethimide leads to tolerance and psychic and physical dependence. The abstinence syndrome includes tremulousness, nausea, tachycardia, fever, tonic muscle spasms, and generalized convulsions. The same symptoms occasionally occur in patients who have been taking glutethimide regularly in moderate doses (0.5 to 3 g daily) even when there is no evidence of abstention, and also in patients being treated for acute intoxication who have no previous history of drug abuse. In the latter case, tonic muscular spasms and, infrequently, generalized convulsions are seen.

Preparations and Dosage. These are listed in Table 17–3. It is difficult to justify the continued use of this agent.

METHYPRYLON

The structure of methyprylon is shown with that of glutethimide.

In a dose of 300 mg, the hypnotic effect of methyprylon is indistinguishable from that of 200 mg of secobarbital.

Approximately 97% of methyprylon appears to be metabolized. The metabolites are partly conjugated to glucuronides. The plasma half-life is 4 hours, but it is longer in acute intoxication. Methyprylon stimulates the hepatic microsomal enzyme system and δ-ALA synthetase; it should be avoided in patients with intermittent porphyria.

Untoward effects of methyprylon are not frequent, but include "hangover," nausea, vomiting, epigastric distress, diarrhea, esophagitis, headache, and rash. An idiosyncratic excitement occasionally occurs.

Acute intoxication resembles that caused by barbiturates, and the general principles of management are the same. Hypotension, shock, and pulmonary edema are more conspicuous features than is respiratory depression. Coma may last up to 5 days. Methyprylon is quite water-soluble, which facilitates dialysis. Death has occurred after ingestion of 6 g.

Habituation, tolerance, physical dependence, and addiction can occur. The abstinence syndrome is like that of the barbiturates.

The dosage and preparations are shown in Table 17–3.

MEPROBAMATE

Meprobamate is a *bis*-carbamate ester with the following structural formula:

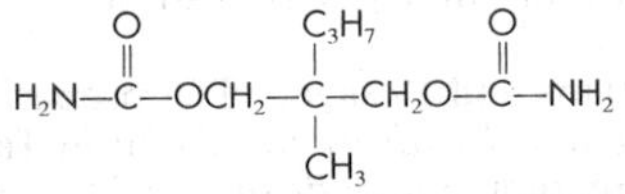

Meprobamate

Meprobamate was introduced as an antianxiety agent in 1955, and this remains its only approved use in the United States. However, it also became popular as a sedative-hypnotic drug, and it is discussed here mainly because of the continuing practice to use this drug for such purposes. The question of whether the sedative and antianxiety actions of meprobamate differ remains unanswered.

Pharmacological Properties. The properties of meprobamate resemble those of the benzodiazepines in a number of ways. Although it can cause widespread depression of the CNS, meprobamate does not produce anesthesia. In addition to taming aggressive animals, meprobamate can release suppressed behaviors at doses that cause little impairment of locomotor activity. Surprisingly, naloxone can block the latter effects. Despite these and a number of other experimental findings that are usually thought to correlate with antianxiety effects in man, clinical proof for the efficacy of meprobamate as a selective antianxiety agent is lacking.

As an anticonvulsant, meprobamate resembles ethosuximide more than the benzodiazepines, in that it antagonizes pentylenetetrazol and has little ability to modify seizures induced by maximal electrical shock in laboratory animals. In man, it suppresses absence seizures but may aggravate tonic-clonic epilepsy.

Meprobamate can depress polysynaptic reflexes in the spinal cord without affecting monosynaptic reflexes, and it is more selective than barbiturates in this respect. This effect is thought to contribute to its muscle relaxant properties. However, with clinical doses in man, the muscle relaxant effects are negligible; there may be some decrease in spasm as a result of a lessening of anxiety. Although meprobamate may sometimes produce modest hyperalgesia, it appears to have a mild analgesic effect in patients with musculoskeletal pain, and it enhances the analgesic effects of other drugs.

Absorption, Fate, and Excretion. Meprobamate is well absorbed when administered orally; peak concentrations in plasma are reached in 1 to 3 hours. There is little binding to plasma proteins. Most of the drug is metabolized in the liver, mainly to a side chain hydroxy derivative and a glucuronide; the remainder is excreted unchanged in the urine. The half-life of a single dose in plasma ranges from 6 to 17 hours, but it has been reported to be as long as 24 to 48 hours during chronic administration; the kinetics of elimination may be dependent on the dose. Meprobamate can induce some hepatic microsomal enzymes. It is not clear whether the drug induces the enzymes responsible for its own metabolism.

Untoward Effects and Intoxication. The major unwanted effects of sedative doses of meprobamate are drowsiness and ataxia. A single dose of 400 mg has little effect on the performance of psychometric tests; however, larger doses produce considerable impairment of learning and motor coordination and prolongation of reaction time. Meprobamate enhances the CNS depression produced by other drugs.

Hypotension may occur in response to meprobamate. Allergic reactions have been reported in a few percent of patients and appear most frequently in those with a history of dermatological or allergic conditions. Urticaria or an erythematous rash is the most common manifestation. Acute nonthrombocytopenic purpura has also been reported, and angioedema and bronchospasm have occurred occasionally.

Conflicting reports have appeared on the effects of exposure of the fetus to meprobamate; it is recommended that meprobamate not be taken during pregnancy, especially during the first trimester.

Induction of hepatic microsomal enzymes by meprobamate may result in exacerbation of intermittent porphyria and may also be the cause of various drug interactions. The elimination of warfarin, estrogens, and oral contraceptives is increased by large doses of meprobamate, but interactions appear to be slight when usual doses are taken.

The abuse of meprobamate has continued despite a substantial decrease in the clinical use of the drug. The drug is preferred to the benzodiazepines by subjects with a history of drug abuse (Roache and Griffiths, 1987). After long-term medication with doses usually in excess of 2.4 g a day for several weeks, abrupt discontinuation evokes a withdrawal syndrome usually characterized by anxiety, insomnia, tremors, gastrointestinal disturbances, and, frequently, hallucinations; generalized seizures occur in about 10% of cases. Mild symptoms sometimes occur after withdrawal from long-term use of doses as low as 1.6 g a day.

Moderate overdosage with meprobamate (blood concentrations of 30 to 100 μg/ml) may cause vertigo, ataxia, slurred speech, stupor, or light coma. Ingestions that result in concentrations of 100 to 200 μg/ml cause coma, hypotension, respiratory depression, shock, pulmonary edema, and heart failure. Lethal doses usually exceed 36 g and produce concentrations in blood above 200 μg/ml (Kintz *et al.*, 1988). The principles of the management of intoxication are those described for barbiturate intoxication (*see* above). Hemodialysis or hemoperfusion is indicated only if brainstem functions are inadequate. Hemoperfusion with charcoal is superior to hemodialysis and can rescue patients who present with plasma concentrations of meprobamate of nearly 200 μg/ml (Jacobsen *et al.*, 1987). An important aspect of intoxication with meprobamate is the formation of gastric bezoars, consisting of undissolved meprobamate tablets. As patients begin to awaken and intestinal motility improves, absorption of additional meprobamate can occur from the bezoar. This cycle can be broken by endoscopy, with mechanical removal of the bezoar.

Therapeutic Uses. Even though meprobamate is currently approved for use only as an antianxiety agent, it is also employed as a hypnotic agent in the treatment of insomnia. It has been advocated for hypnotic use in geriatric patients, for whom it has been reported to be as effective as flurazepam and flunitrazepam (Keston and Brocklehurst, 1974; Brocklehurst *et al.*, 1978), more predictable than chloral hydrate, and subject to fewer dosage problems than barbiturates and probably flurazepam. The sedative and hypnotic dosages are listed in Table 17–3.

PARALDEHYDE

Paraldehyde is a polymer of acetaldehyde, but it is perhaps best regarded as a polyether of cyclic structure, as follows:

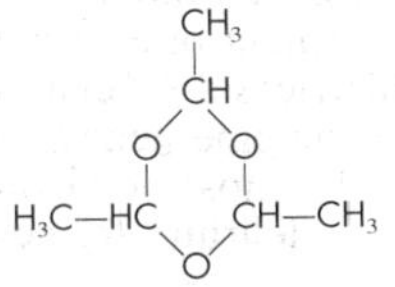

Paraldehyde

Because of some limited virtues and despite its disadvantages, paraldehyde has managed to survive a century of use; it deserves to be retired.

Pharmacological Properties. Paraldehyde is a rapidly acting hypnotic; after a therapeutic oral dose, sleep usually ensues in 10 to 15 minutes. The drug does not possess analgesic properties, and it may produce excitement or delirium in the presence of pain.

Paraldehyde has little effect on respiration and blood pressure in ordinary therapeutic doses. In large doses, it produces respiratory depression and hypotension.

Pharmacokinetics. Oral paraldehyde is rapidly absorbed and widely distributed; the drug readily crosses the placental barrier. With hypnotic doses, 70 to 80% is metabolized in the liver, most of the remainder is exhaled, and a small amount is excreted in urine. Its half-time of elimination is 4 to 10 hours. In hepatic insufficiency, the rate of elimination is slowed, and the proportion excreted in the expired air is increased. It is believed that paraldehyde is depolymerized to acetaldehyde in the liver and then oxidized by aldehyde dehydrogenase to acetic acid, which is ultimately metabolized to carbon dioxide and water.

Untoward Effects and Poisoning. Paraldehyde has a strong aromatic odor and a disagreeable taste. Orally, it is irritating to the throat and stomach, and it is rarely administered parenterally because of its injurious effects on tissues.

Intoxication with paraldehyde is uncommon only because its use has been essentially restricted to hospitalized or institutionalized patients. The lethal dose has ranged from 25 g to 150 g.

Patients poisoned by paraldehyde commonly exhibit very rapid, labored respiratory movements. Acidosis, bleeding gastritis, muscular irritability, azotemia, oliguria, albuminuria, leukocytosis, fatty changes in the liver and kidney with toxic hepatitis and nephrosis, pulmonary hemorrhages and edema, and dilatation of the right ventricle have all been observed in cases of severe acute or chronic paraldehyde poisoning.

Chronic paraldehyde intoxication results in tolerance and dependence. The paraldehyde addict may become acquainted with the drug when it is used in the treatment of alcoholism and then, surprisingly in view of its disagreeable taste and odor, prefer it to alcohol. Paraldehyde addiction resembles alcoholism, and sudden withdrawal may result in delirium tremens and vivid hallucinations.

Therapeutic Uses. Paraldehyde has been used chiefly for the treatment of abstinence phenomena and other psychiatric states characterized by excitement, and for the emergency treatment of convulsive episodes. Its most persisting use has been in the treatment of delirium tremens.

Preparations and Dosage. The hypnotic dose is shown in Table 17–3. When given rectally as a retention enema, the drug is usually added to 1 or 2 volumes of olive oil.

MISCELLANEOUS SEDATIVE-HYPNOTIC DRUGS

Ethinamate. Ethinamate is a urethane with the following structure:

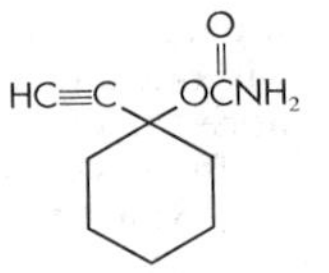

Ethinamate

It has a rapid onset and a short duration of action. Ethinamate is inactivated at least partly by the liver, by hydroxylation of the cyclohexyl ring; the product is conjugated and excreted as the glucuronide. Side effects of ethinamate include nausea, occasional vomiting, and, infrequently, rash. Idiosyncratic excitement may be noted, especially in children. Fever and thrombocytopenia occur rarely. The lethal dose is unknown; death has resulted from the ingestion of 15 g. Long-term use of larger-than-recommended doses may lead to psychic and physical dependence. The abstinence syndrome is similar to that for the barbiturates. It is stated that 500 mg of ethinamate is equivalent to 100 mg of secobarbital, but some studies have found this dose to be little better than a placebo.

Others. Etomidate (AMIDATE) is used in the United States and other countries as an intravenous anesthetic, often in combination with fentanyl. It is advantageous because it lacks pulmonary- and vascular-depressant activity, although it has a negative inotropic effect on the heart. Its pharmacology and anesthetic uses are described in Chapter 14. It is also used abroad as a sedative-hypnotic drug in intensive care units, during intermittent positive-pressure breathing, in epidural anesthesia, and in other situations. Because it is administered only intravenously, its use is limited to hospital settings. The myoclonus seen after anesthetic doses is not seen after sedative-hypnotic doses.

Clomethiazole has sedative, muscle relaxant, and anticonvulsant properties. It is used outside the United States for hypnosis in elderly and institutionalized patients, for preanesthetic sedation, and, especially, in the management of withdrawal from ethanol (*see* Symposium, 1986b). Given alone, its effects on respiration are slight, and the therapeutic index is high. However, deaths from adverse interactions with ethanol are relatively frequent.

Nonprescription Hypnotic Drugs. An advisory review panel of the United States Food and Drug Administration has recommended that, except for certain antihistamines (doxylamine, diphenhydramine, and pyrilamine), all putative active ingredients be eliminated from nonprescription sleep aids. Despite the prominent sedative side effects encountered during their use in the treatment of allergic diseases (*see* Chapter 23), these antihistamines are not consistently effective in the treatment of sleep disorders. Contributory factors may include the rapid development of tolerance and the inadequacy of the doses that are currently approved. Nevertheless, these doses sometimes produce prominent residual daytime CNS depression. For example, the elimination half-life of doxylamine is about 9 hours. Diphenhydramine, with a half-life of about 4 hours, might have an advantage with regard to residual effects.

MANAGEMENT OF INSOMNIA

Few clinical disorders have been more casually and carelessly treated than insomnia. Insomnia has many causes, and an accurate differential diagnosis is required before treatment should be considered. Prescription of a hypnotic without regard to the underlying disturbance subjects the patient to the risk of abuse, may mask the signs and symptoms of a pernicious disease, and may dangerously exacerbate an unrecognized sleep apnea. Furthermore, behavioral therapy, psychotherapy, or nonhypnotic drugs may be superior to hypnotic drugs when the insomnia has a specific cause. For example, dextroamphetamine or similar drugs may improve sleep in some hyperkinetic patients and those with Parkinson's disease; other examples include antidepressants for those with endogenous depression, phenothiazines or haloperidol for psychotics, phenytoin when there are paroxysmal nightmares, analgesics when sleep is impaired by (even subliminal) pain, and so forth.

Even when no specific pathological etiology can be identified, insomnia may nevertheless relate to identifiable causes, such as ingestion of food or coffee near bedtime, various drugs, or a host of other factors. Only when specific causes cannot be eliminated or compensated for should a nonspecific, hypnotic drug be considered.

Nature does not compel man to sleep 8 hours a day, and many persons function well on much less sleep. Sometimes simple assurance of this fact is sufficient to improve sleep or at least to decrease the concern about nocturnal sleeplessness. A relaxing activity before bedtime is often efficacious.

When insomnia is expected to be transient, as in minor situational stress or jet lag, the use of hypnotic drugs may be justifiable, depending upon assessment of the situation and of personality factors. Unless there is a need for concurrent daytime sedation, a drug with a short half-life is indicated. In this setting, treatment should be limited to one to three nights.

In short-term insomnia, as when there is grief, short-term illness, a change in occupational status, or temporary family or occupational stress, a drug can be prescribed and the patient should be counseled. The antianxiety action of the benzodiazepines assists in such situations. Treatment should begin with a small dose, to be increased gradually if necessary. The drug should be discontinued for at least one or two nights after one or two nights of acceptable sleep have been obtained. Treatment should not exceed 3 weeks. Discontinuation should be accomplished gradually. Whether a hypnotic drug with a short half-life or an antianxiety drug with a longer half-life is prescribed depends upon the perceived contribution of anxiety to the insomnia and the acceptability of diminished daytime alertness. During the course of treatment, the patient should be monitored to assess problems resulting from accumulation of drug, alterations in sleep pattern, and tolerance.

The use of sedative-hypnotic drugs in the treatment of long-term insomnia is controversial, not only because of the likelihood of tolerance and potential drug abuse but also because this condition is often secondary to disorders that are manageable by psychotherapy, physical therapy, chronotherapy, or nonhypnotic drugs. When there is no specific identifiable cause for the insomnia, psychosocial-behavioral therapies are indicated; hypnotic drugs may be used in the early stages in conjunction with such treatment. A hypnotic drug should be administered no more frequently than every third night in order to avoid adverse alterations in sleep pattern, drug accumulation, and tolerance. The drug should be discontinued gradually after 3 to 6 months, or even earlier. Upon discontinuation, drugs that have relatively slow rates of elimination produce a lower incidence or intensity of withdrawal symptoms, including rebound insomnia. However, such drugs may also produce more residual daytime effects than do those with shorter half-lives of elimination. The latter drugs may thus offer advantages if used on an intermittent schedule or in elderly patients, in whom residual cognitive impairment is especially frequent. However, the incidence and severity of residual daytime sequelae do not always correlate with the half-life of the hypnotic drug or its active metabolites. The responses in patients with severe, chronic insomnia are often quite erratic (*see* Nicholson, 1981; Linnoila *et al.*, 1982).

Much has been made of the importance of prescribing a short-acting hypnotic drug for patients who have prolonged sleep latency but who sleep well once sleep ensues, and a drug with a longer duration of action for those who awaken early and have difficulty in returning to sleep. For the former, triazolam has both a short onset and duration of action. For the latter, temazepam has acceptable properties, although flurazepam also suffices. However, for the elderly early waker, sleep counseling may often be sufficient. For those who awaken early with feelings of panic, psychotherapy and/ or antidepressant drugs are probably more appropriate. The actual prolongation of total sleep time by shortening latency or decreasing the number of "mini-awakenings" often does not amount to more than 20 to 40 minutes; this is not an appreciable amount of sleep. Consequently, the most important role of the physician may be to convince the patient that a short period of wakefulness is less serious than are the potential complications of dependence on hypnotics.

There has been an emphasis on the effects of drugs on the stages of sleep and especially on reductions in REM sleep. However, except for the number of "mini-awakenings," the sleep pattern often fails to relate to the sense of refreshing sleep. Thus, the emphasis has shifted to the patient's subjective evaluation of sleep and of the impact of the drug on daytime performance.

There are situations in which alterations in sleep pattern during and after use of hypnotic drugs may have special relevance. Since night terrors and somnambulism most frequently occur during stage 4 of sleep, drugs that shorten or lighten this stage may be indicated. However, caution is in order, since, with some hypnotics, rebound effects on stage 4 may be quite severe or protracted. Furthermore, strong suppression of stage 4 may cause the emergence of day terrors or of suicidal ideation. Similarly, nightmares that normally occur during REM sleep may transfer to stage 2. Nocturnal enuresis may be prevented by drugs that suppress REM sleep. Suppression of REM sleep may also improve endogenous depression.

Except when specific drug therapy or nonpharmacological interventions are indicated, benzodiazepines should be considered to be the hypnotic drugs of choice, since they have better therapeutic indices, fewer drug interactions, less effect on respiration, and lower abuse liability than do the barbiturates and the other prescription hypnotic drugs available in the United States. The treatment of insomnia and related sleep disorders has been reviewed by Mendelson (1980), Borkovec (1982), Kales and coworkers (1982), Seidel and Dement (1982), Wincor (1982), and Kales and Kales (1983).

ETHANOL

Alcoholic beverages have been used since the dawn of history, beginning with fermented beverages of relatively low alcohol content. When the Arabs introduced the then recent technique of distilling into Europe in the Middle Ages, the alchemists believed that alcohol was the long-sought elixir of life. Alcohol was therefore held to be a remedy for practically all diseases, as indicated by the term *whisky* (Gaelic: *usquebaugh,* meaning "water of life"). It is now recognized that the therapeutic value of ethanol is extremely limited and that chronic ingestion of excessive amounts is a major social and medical problem.

PHARMACOLOGICAL PROPERTIES

Central Nervous System. Although laymen may view alcoholic drinks as stimulating, ethanol is a primary and continuous depressant of the CNS. As with other CNS depressants, the apparent stimulation results from depression of inhibitory control mechanisms in the brain. The first mental processes to be affected are those that depend on training and previous experience and that usually make for sobriety and self-restraint. Memory, concentration, and insight are dulled and then lost. Confidence abounds, the personality becomes expansive and vivacious, and uncontrolled mood swings and emotional outbursts may be evident. These psychic changes are accompanied by sensory and motor disturbances. As intoxication becomes more advanced, a general impairment of nervous function occurs and a condition of general anesthesia ultimately prevails. However, there is little margin between the full surgical anesthetic dose and that which is dangerous to respiration.

In general, the effects of ethanol on the CNS are proportional to its concentration in the blood. However, the effects are more marked when the concentration is rising than when it is falling. The neurological and physiological effects of ethanol have been reviewed by Wallgren and Barry (1970), Kissin and Begleiter (1974), and Gross (1977); in a report by the U.S. Department of Health, Education, and Welfare (1978); and by Majchrowicz and Noble (1979).

Chronic excessive ingestion of ethanol is directly associated with serious neurological and mental disorders (*e.g.*, brain damage, memory loss, sleep disturbances, and psychoses). Individuals who regularly ingest ethanol also have an increased risk of experiencing unprovoked seizures; the risk appears to be dose-related (Ng *et al.*, 1988). Since the first seizure can occur during periods in which consumption is escalating, this phenomenon appears to be distinct from seizures induced by withdrawal from ethanol. In addition, nutritional and vitamin deficiencies, incident to the poor food intake or the faulty gastrointestinal and hepatic function of the alcoholic (*see* Hillman, 1974), seem to cause many neuropsychiatric syndromes that are common in alcoholics, such as Wernicke's encephalopathy, Korsakoff's psychosis, polyneuritis, and nicotinic acid deficiency encephalopathy (*see* Turner *et al.*, 1977; *see also* Chapter 63).

Respiration. Moderate amounts of ethanol in man may stimulate or depress respiration; the ventilatory response to carbon dioxide is, however, always depressed. Large amounts (sufficient to produce a blood concentration of 400 mg/dl or more) produce dangerous or lethal depression of respiration.

Sleep. Acute and chronic administration of ethanol produces a variety of effects on sleep (*see* Mendelson, 1979; Roth *et al.*, 1985). In normal persons, the acute use of ethanol at bedtime reduces initial latency to sleep and REM sleep and increases deep non-REM sleep. However, wake time during the latter part of the sleep period is increased, and the reduction in sleep latency and other measures dissipates with three or more nightly ingestions, followed by a rebound increase in wake time upon discontinuation. A survey revealed that a surprising number of men believed that nighttime ingestion of ethanol reduced the quality of their sleep (Urponen *et al.*, 1988). In patients with mild or severe obstructive sleep apnea, ingestion of ethanol before bedtime consistently increases the frequency and severity of apneic episodes and the associated hypoxia (*see* Roth *et al.*, 1985). In chronic alcoholics, marked fragmentation of sleep occurs, with sleep interrupted by frequent awakenings.

Cardiovascular System. The immediate effects of ethanol on the circulation are relatively minor (Wallgren and Barry, 1970). The blood pressure, cardiac output, and force of myocardial contraction do not change greatly after a moderate amount of ethanol. The pulse rate may increase, but this is usually due to muscular activity or reflex stimulation. The cardiovascular depression that is observed in acute severe alcoholic intoxication is due mainly to central vasomotor factors and to the respiratory depression. However, long-term excessive use of ethanol has largely irreversible deleterious effects on the heart (Urbano-Marquez *et al.*, 1989), and may be the major cause of cardiomyopathy in the Western world (*see* Rubin, 1979; Altura, 1982).

Ethanol in moderate doses causes vasodilatation, especially of the cutaneous vessels, and produces warm, flushed skin. The vasodilatation results partly from central vasomotor depression and partly from a direct vasodilating action of ethanol on blood vessels (Altura and Altura, 1982). No beneficial increase in coronary blood flow occurs in man. Indeed, in individuals with classical stable angina and proven coronary artery disease, ethanol decreases the duration of exercise required to precipitate angina and to produce changes in the ECG that are characteristic of myocardial ischemia (Regan, 1982).

Ethanol administered to human subjects in doses sufficient to produce facial vasodilatation and mild inebriation causes no change in cerebral blood flow or cerebral vascular resistance. However, a plasma concentration associated with severe alcoholic intoxication (300 mg/dl) does indeed markedly increase mean cerebral blood flow and diminish cerebrovascular resistance, despite reduced cerebral oxygen uptake. This pattern of effects of ethanol appears to arise in part because of regional differences in the properties of blood vessels as well as variable indirect effects. The latter include the release of catecholamines from the adrenal medulla and the ability of low concentrations of ethanol to potentiate the vasoconstriction induced by various agents (*see* Pohorecky and Brick, 1988). Although intoxicating doses can produce widespread vasodilatation, moderate doses of ethanol can cause appreciable vasoconstriction in such vital areas as the heart and the brain. Hence, there is no rational basis for the use of ethanol as a vasodilator in patients with cerebrovascular disease. Furthermore, several studies indicate that regular use of large amounts of ethanol is a risk factor for development of hypertension and stroke (*see* Klatsky *et al.*, 1981; Kannel, in Symposium, 1988c).

Plasma Lipoproteins. In contrast to the potential deleterious effects of ethanol on the cardiovascular system described above, several studies show a clear negative correlation between chronic ingestion of *small* amounts of ethanol and the incidence of coronary heart disease. This protective effect seems to occur because ethanol increases the concentration of high-density lipoproteins and decreases that of low-density lipoproteins in plasma (*see* Symposium, 1988c). The lower the concentration of high-density lipoprotein in blood, the greater is the risk of coronary heart disease (*see* Chapter 36).

Skeletal Muscle. Although small doses of ethanol may lessen the appreciation of fatigue and increase muscular work, large doses cause CNS depression and thereby decrease the amount of muscular work accomplished. Such doses also cause reversible damage to muscle, signified by a marked increase in the activity of creatine phosphokinase in plasma. Most patients with chronic alcoholism show electromyographical changes, and many show evidence of a skeletal myopathy similar to the alcoholic cardiomyopathy (Rubin, 1979; Urbano-Marquez *et al.*, 1989).

Body Temperature. Ingestion of ethanol causes a feeling of warmth because alcohol enhances cutaneous and gastric blood flow. Increased sweating may also occur. Heat is therefore lost more rapidly, and the internal temperature consequently falls. With large amounts of ethanol, the central temperature-regulating mechanism itself becomes depressed and the fall in body temperature may become pronounced (*see* Pohorecky and Brick, 1988). The action of alcohol in lowering body temperature is naturally greater and more dangerous when the environmental temperature is low.

Gastrointestinal Tract. Gastric secretions, like salivary secretions, are usually stimulated psychically by ethanol, especially if the individual likes it. The gastric juice produced in this way is rich in acid and normal in pepsin content. Ethanol may also reflexly stimulate the secretion of salivary and gastric juice by exciting sensory endings in the buccal and gastric mucosae. Finally, ethanol may evoke gastric secretion through a more direct action on the stomach, possibly involving the release of gastrin. The release of histamine has also been implicated. The various physiological mechanisms involved have been reviewed by Glass and colleagues (1979). Alcohol is a very effective stimulus for gastric acid secretion, and, clearly, the drinking of alcoholic beverages is inadvisable in patients with peptic ulcer.

The presence in the stomach of ethanol in concentrations of about 10% results in a gastric secretion rich in acid, but it is poor in pepsin unless psychic secretion is also elicited. At concentrations above 20%, gastric secretion tends to be inhibited and peptic activity is depressed. Strong alcoholic drinks, of 40% concentration and over, are quite irritating to the mucosa and cause congestive hyperemia and inflammation, with an accompanying loss of plasma protein into the gastrointestinal lumen. In such high concentrations ethanol produces an erosive gastritis (*see* Lorber *et al.*, 1974; Glass *et al.*, 1979). The gastric damage produced by aspirin is much enhanced by ethanol.

The habitual use of immoderate amounts of ethanol may lead to constipation or diarrhea, depending on the composition of the diet or the irritant action of certain flavoring oils. Alcohol taken in moderate amounts does not significantly influence the motor activity of the colon, but taken to the point of intoxication it results in virtual cessation of gastrointestinal secretory and motor functions. Absorption is delayed, and pylorospasm and vomiting may occur independently of any reflex due to local irritation.

Ethanol contributes to the production of lesions of the esophagus and duodenum and is also an etiological factor in acute and chronic pancreatitis (Pirola and Lieber, 1974; Turner *et al.*, 1977). The pancreatitis appears to occur because ethanol produces not only increased secretion but also an obstruction of the pancreatic duct (*see* Wallgren and Barry, 1970), perhaps as a result of increased plasma concentrations of secretin that have been observed to follow the ingestion of ethanol by normal human subjects (Straus *et al.*, 1975).

Liver. The acute ingestion of ethanol, even in intoxicating doses, probably produces little lasting change in hepatic function. However, consumed on a regular basis, ethanol produces a constellation of dose-related deleterious effects that appear to result principally from its metabolism (*see* Lieber, 1988a, 1988b). Although malnutrition can intensify hepatic damage, an excellent nutritional status does not prevent the development of alcoholic hepatitis or its progression to cirrhosis.

The accumulation of fat in the liver is an early event and can occur in normal individuals after the ingestion of relatively small amounts of ethanol. This results from inhibition of both the tricarboxylic acid cycle and the oxidation of fat, in part due to the generation of excess NADH produced by the action of alcohol dehydrogenase. A portion of the ingested ethanol is metabolized by microsomal mixed-function oxidases that are subject to induction by ethanol and other agents. The product of all these reactions, acetaldehyde, is a reactive and toxic substance that can form adducts with proteins and other compounds, leading to inhibition of a wide variety of enzymes and generation of immunogenic derivatives.

The regular ingestion of more than moderate amounts of alcohol leads to increased accumulation of acetaldehyde, in part due to reduced activity of acetaldehyde dehydrogenase. The acetaldehyde is thought to cause a host of deleterious effects, including enhanced lipid peroxidation and damage to mitochondrial and other cellular membranes; depletion of glutathione; depletion of vitamins and trace metals, especially pyridoxine, vitamin A, zinc, and selenium; and decreased transport and secretion of proteins through inhibition of the polymerization of tubulin. This view can account for the engorging of hepatocytes with protein, fat, and water that progresses to the necrosis and fibrosis found in cirrhotic livers, as well as the various metabolic disturbances observed in alcoholic individuals. Moreover, the association of the chronic ingestion of ethanol with an increased incidence of cancer and the enhanced toxicity of certain drugs (*e.g.*, acetaminophen) can be explained by induction of microsomal oxidases coupled with depletion of glutathione, leading to increased accumulation of activated carcinogens or toxic metabolites.

Teratogenic Effects. Although suspected for centuries, the fetal alcohol syndrome has only been fully described relatively recently (*see* Beattie, in Symposium, 1988c; Warren and Bast, 1988). The abnormality consists in CNS dysfunction (such as low IQ and microcephaly), slowness in growth, a characteristic cluster of facial abnormalities (such as short palpebral fissures, hypoplastic upper lip, and short nose), and a variable set of major and minor malformations. These features may be due, at least in part, to a direct action of ethanol (or of acetaldehyde) to inhibit embryonic cellular proliferation early in gestation (Brown *et al.*, 1979). There may also be selective fetal malnutrition through injury to the placenta (*see* Fisher and Karl, 1988). In addition to their characteristic morphological and neurological abnormalities, children with the fetal alcohol syndrome have a greatly increased susceptibility to both life-threatening and minor infectious diseases. Such children have extensive impairment of their immune system, which might well explain this susceptibility (Johnson *et al.*, 1981).

Ethanol seems to be the most frequent cause of teratogenically induced mental deficiency that is known in the Western world; even moderate drinking of alcohol is clearly contraindicated during pregnancy. Depending on the population studied, the incidence of the full-blown fetal alcohol syndrome ranges from 1 in 300 to 1 in 2000 live births; it is 1 in 3 in infants of alcoholic mothers (Council Report, 1983). The smallest quantity of ethanol ingestion reported to be associated with the fetal alcohol syndrome is about 75 ml (2.5 oz) daily (*see* Council Report, 1983). Although it is not clear whether there is any safe lower limit, there is no evidence for any adverse effects associated with very modest consumption of alcohol (*e.g.*, a single daily glass of wine; 15 ml [0.5 oz] of alcohol). Reduction of the mother's drinking early in pregnancy seems to reduce the severity of the syndrome (Rossett *et al.*, 1981).

Other effects on the fetus occur with excessive drinking (Council Report, 1983). For example, stillbirths and spontaneous abortions are two to three times as frequent in women who have three or more drinks daily as in those who have less than one drink a day. The pattern of wakefulness and sleep in the newborn may also be disturbed. There may be a decrease in birth weight, and various minor physical abnormalities are found (Tennes and Blackard, 1980).

Sexual Functions. It is a popular notion that ethanol is an aphrodisiac; indeed, aggressive sexual behavior is often seen after alcohol ingestion, usually as a result of a loss of inhibition and restraint. Shakespeare, however, realized that inebriation interferes with coitus. In *Macbeth*, for example, the following conversation occurs (act 2, scene 3):

MACDUFF: What three things does drink especially provoke?

PORTER: Marry, sir, nose-painting, sleep, and urine. Lechery, sir, it provokes, and unprovokes; it provokes the desire, but it takes away the performance. . . .

The experiments of Gantt (1952) on the effects of ethanol on the sexual reflexes of normal dogs support the observations of Shakespeare; in neurotic dogs, ethanol has some therapeutic value. Objective measurements in human beings of penile tumescence and vaginal pressure show that ethanol significantly decreases sexual responsiveness in both men and women (Wilson, 1977).

In men, chronic ingestion of ethanol may lead to impotence, sterility, testicular atrophy, and gynecomastia. This feminization in alcoholic men has a dual origin. First, alcohol-induced hepatic injury leads to a hyperestrogenization and a reduced rate of production of testosterone; second, by increasing the activity of the enzymes of the hepatic endoplasmic reticulum, ethanol markedly increases the rate of metabolic inactivation of testosterone (Van Thiel and Lester, 1976; Turner *et al.*, 1977). This ethanol-induced dysfunction is reversible in some abstinent alcoholics, but only if there has been no gonadal atrophy (Van Thiel *et al.*, 1983).

Kidney. That ethanol exerts a diuretic effect has been established by a number of investigators and by most consumers. Although the large amount of fluid ordinarily ingested with alcoholic beverages undoubtedly contributes, ethanol in itself produces a marked diuretic response in man by virtue of inhibition of ADH secretion and resultant decrease in renal tubular reabsorption of water. The diuretic effect is roughly proportional to the blood alcohol concentration and occurs when the concentration is rising but not when it is stationary or falling (*see* Wallgren and Barry, 1970). Indeed, ethanol in repeated doses may have an antidiuretic effect. (*See* Beard and Sargent, 1979, for a review.)

Biogenic Amines. Concentrations of catecholamines in blood are elevated by ethanol, largely owing to their release from the adrenal medulla. The increased concentration of circulating catecholamines may be partly responsible for the transient hyperglycemia, the pupillary dilatation, and the slight rise in blood pressure that often occur during the early stages of intoxication. Experiments in animals have shown a wide variety of effects of ethanol on biogenic amines in the CNS; the most consistent of these is the increased turnover of norepinephrine while the concentration of ethanol is rising following its acute administration, or during its long-term administration (*see* Pohorecky and Brick, 1988). The fact that naloxone can prevent or reverse such effects, as well as many of the manifestations of alcohol intoxication, has invited numerous speculations on possible relationships between the actions of opioids and ethanol.

Blood. Alcohol produces a number of hematological effects (*see* Lindenbaum, 1974). Some, such as sideroblastic and megaloblastic anemias, occur because alcohol interferes with several aspects of folate metabolism and transport, as well as with its normal pattern of storage and release from the liver (*see* Hillman and Steinberg, 1982). These effects are rapidly reversible with the onset of abstinence. Other effects, such as thrombocytopenia and vacuolization of the precursors of red and white cells, occur even when the diet is adequate and seem to result from a direct depressant action of ethanol on the bone marrow. There is also a depression of leukocyte migration into inflamed areas, which may partly account for the poor resistance of alcoholics to infection.

Mechanism of Action. For many years it has been thought that ethanol and other aliphatic alcohols, as well as the barbiturates and the volatile anesthetic agents, exerted their depressant effects on the CNS by dissolving in lipid membranes, thereby perturbing the function of ion channels and other proteins embedded therein. The most compelling evidence was the excellent correlation between lipid solubility and anesthetic potency (*see* Chapter 13). This hypothesis has been refined by the application of various physical techniques that showed that anesthetics caused a local disordering in the lipid matrix, also referred to as membrane fluidization. Since Chin and Goldstein (1981) reported the membrane-fluidizing effects of ethanol, a number of investigators have shown a correlation between the degree of intoxication and the extent of ethanol-induced disordering of membranes (*see* Wood and Schroeder, 1988). Included was the demonstration that synaptosomal membranes from an alcohol-resistant strain of mice are less strongly disordered by ethanol *in vitro* than are those from a related strain of alcohol-sensitive mice.

Further refinements in this hypothesis have resulted in the view that the interactions of ethanol and related compounds are not uniform throughout the lipid bilayer (Wood and Schroeder, 1988). Rather, there are differential effects in regions or domains, reflecting the nonuniform distribution of various phospholipids and cholesterol within the membrane. Moreover, the hydrophobic domains of membrane-bound proteins (or perhaps water-soluble proteins) represent additional targets for anesthetic agents. Although effects at anesthetic or higher concentrations may well reflect the consequences of the fluidization of the bulk membrane and be closely related to the total number of molecules dissolved therein, actions at subanesthetic concentrations may also depend upon the three-dimensional structure of the molecules in question. In this way, such phenomena as the differing potencies of enantiomers of barbiturates (*see* above) or the convulsant properties of close relatives of halogenated anesthetic agents, notably flurothyl, may be explained.

Attention has also been focused on the capacity of ethanol to augment GABA-mediated synaptic inhibition as well as fluxes of chloride (*see* Ticku and Kulkarni, 1988). Such effects, as well as the sedative-ataxic actions of ethanol, are inhibited by bicuculline, a specific antagonist at GABA-ergic receptors. The binding of certain convulsant agents is also inhibited allosterically by ethanol, and higher concentrations of ethanol increase chloride permeability in the absence of GABA. All of these properties closely resemble those of the anesthetic barbiturates, and they are shared by other aliphatic alcohols and a variety of anesthetic agents at their respective anesthetic concentrations (Mehta and Ticku, 1988; Moody *et al.*, 1988). Such actions are not well correlated with fluidizing effects on the bulk membrane (Huidobro-Toro *et al.*, 1988). The actions of ethanol on these parameters *in vitro* were exaggerated in preparations from an alcohol-sensitive strain of mice (long-sleep) compared with their more resistant (short-sleep) counterparts (McIntyre *et al.*, 1988). It is interesting that long-sleep mice are also more sensitive to the sedative effects of adenosine analogs and to the excitant effects of theophylline (Proctor and Dunwiddie, 1984), and that selection for sensitivity to diazepam-induced ataxia produced a strain of mice that was also more sensitive to ethanol (Allan *et al.*, 1988).

The apparent relationship of an important target for the action of ethanol to sites of action for the barbiturates and benzodiazepines prompted examination of the impact of benzodiazepine antagonists on ethanol-induced intoxication. One such agent (Ro 15–4513), closely related structurally to flumazenil (*see* above), has been reported to antagonize the effects of ethanol on motor coordination and on the release of punished behavior, as well as on chloride permeability *in vitro* (Suzdak *et al.*, 1986). The effects of pentobarbital on chloride permeability and on punished behavior were not affected. However, the specificity of this agent has been questioned because of its proconvulsant actions and its ability to exert at least some electrophysiological effects that are not antagonized by flumazenil (*see* Lister and Nutt, 1987, 1988). The potential therapeutic utility of such an agent has also been questioned because it might encourage the use of excessive amounts of alcohol. It would also thoroughly confuse the medicolegal relationship between concentrations of ethanol in the blood and degree of impaired driving performance.

Absorption, Fate, and Excretion. Ethanol is rapidly absorbed from the stomach, small intestine, and colon. The time from the last drink to maximal concentrations in blood usually ranges from 30 to 90 minutes. Vaporized ethanol can be absorbed through the lungs, and fatal intoxication has occurred as a result of its inhalation.

Many factors modify the absorption of ethanol from the stomach. At first absorption is rapid, but then it decreases to a very slow rate although the gastric concentration is still high. If the emptying of the stomach is delayed, for example, by the presence of food, the subsequent absorption of ethanol from the intestine will also be delayed. Absorption from the small intestine is extremely rapid and complete, and it is largely independent of the presence of food in the stomach or intestine. Indeed, the time of gastric emptying and, consequently, of the onset of the phase of extremely rapid intestinal absorption may well be the prime factor that determines the wide variety of rates of absorption of ingested ethanol that is seen in different individuals and under different conditions.

After absorption, ethanol is fairly uniformly distributed throughout all tissues and all fluids of the body. The placenta is permeable to ethanol; thus, alcohol gains free access to the fetal circulation.

Between 90 and 98% of the ethanol that enters the body is completely oxidized. The metabolism of ethanol differs from that of most substances in that the rate of oxidation is relatively constant with time, and it is little increased by raising the concentration in the blood (zero-order kinetics). The amount of ethanol oxidized per unit of time is roughly proportional to body weight and probably to liver weight. In the adult, the average rate at which ethanol can be metabolized is 120 mg/kg per hour, or about 30 ml (1 oz) in 3 hours. The oxidation of ethanol occurs chiefly in the liver, initiated principally by alcohol dehydrogenase, which is a zinc-containing enzyme that utilizes NAD as the hydrogen acceptor (*see* Sytkowski and Vallee, 1979). The product, acetaldehyde, is converted to acetyl CoA, which is then oxidized through the citric acid cycle or utilized in the various anabolic reactions involved in the synthesis of cholesterol, fatty acids, and other tissue constituents.

As noted above, ethanol can also be metabolized to acetaldehyde by the microsomal mixed-function oxidases that occur in the smooth endoplasmic reticulum of the liver. The extent to which this system metabolizes ethanol in man is probably very small, but its contribution increases as the concentration of ethanol rises, especially in individuals who consume alcohol regularly. It also provides one basis for the known interactions between ethanol and the host of other drugs also metabolized by this system (*see* Teschke *et al.*, 1977; Pirola, 1978).

There is genetic polymorphism of both alcohol dehydrogenase and aldehyde dehydrogenase; the variants have different catalytic properties and are found with different frequencies in various racial populations (*see* Bosron *et al.*, 1988). This may account in part for variations in the rate of metabolism of ethanol observed among different individuals. Moreover, deficiency in one variant of aldehyde dehydrogenase is associated with increased accumulation of acetaldehyde and more intense adverse symptoms after the acute ingestion of ethanol; this deficiency may also cause a greater frequency of long-term effects.

Ethanol can be a ready, albeit expensive, source of energy that is utilized more rapidly than most foods because it is quickly absorbed from the gastrointestinal tract and requires no preliminary digestion. The energy released per gram of ethanol is approximately 7 kcal. However, the ingestion of alcohol in addition to a diet that is otherwise adequate in essential nutrients and calories often results in weight loss (*see* Lieber, 1988a, 1988b). It is thought that this is principally a consequence of toxic effects of ethanol and/or acetaldehyde on mitochondria, with a reduction in the efficiency of oxidative phosphorylation. The dietary deficiencies that often accompany alcoholism exaggerate such effects.

Normally, about 2% of ingested ethanol escapes oxidation; under special circumstances, such as when large doses have been consumed, this value may be as high as 10%. Although small amounts of ethanol can be detected in various secretions, most of the ethanol that escapes oxidation is excreted through the kidneys and lungs. At most, the concentration in the urine is slightly greater than, and the concentration in the alveolar air only 0.05%, that of the blood.

Interactions with Other Drugs. The effects of ethanol are augmented by other agents that depress the function of the CNS and may be very much enhanced in a person who has also taken sedatives, hypnotics, anticonvulsants, antidepressants, antianxiety drugs, or analgesic agents such as propoxyphene or opioids. Psychopharmacological agents are now so widely used that it is important for the physician to warn patients given such medication of the enhanced effects of alcohol and of the consequent increased danger of driving an automobile after drinking alcohol.

Ethanol can interfere with the therapeutic actions of a wide variety of drugs by altering their metabolism. For example, acute ingestion of ethanol reduces the clearance of phenytoin because both drugs compete for the same hepatic microsomal oxidase system (*see* above; *see also* Sandor *et al.,* 1981). However, in the chronic drinker, there is enzyme induction by alcohol, and a period of abstinence leads to an enhanced rate of clearance of phenytoin (*see* Kissin, 1974; Hoyumpa and Schenker, 1982). In such individuals, the half-life of tolbutamide and perhaps that of similar agents is decreased. In part, this may explain the unpredictable fluctuations of plasma glucose that can result from the combination of ethanol and an oral hypoglycemic agent. An additional hypoglycemic action of ethanol may also be involved, in that ethanol sometimes markedly increases the effects of insulin. As noted above, the hepatic toxicity of acetaminophen is enhanced in individuals who consume ethanol regularly, presumably because of the increased formation of toxic intermediates and the depletion of hepatic glutathione.

Unusual side effects may occur when ethanol is taken in association with other drugs. For example, patients treated with metronidazole, cephalosporins, or oral hypoglycemic agents may experience unpleasant symptoms similar to those experienced by patients who ingest alcohol while taking disulfiram. This presumably results from inhibition of acetaldehyde dehydrogenase (*see* below).

Tolerance and Addiction to Alcohol. The repeated use of alcohol results in the development of tolerance, so that larger doses must be taken to produce characteristic effects. However, the degree of tolerance is not as marked as for morphine and nicotine. Tolerance and addiction to alcohol are discussed in Chapter 22.

Acute Alcohol Intoxication. The characteristic signs and symptoms of alcohol intoxication are well known. Nevertheless, the erroneous diagnosis of drunkenness is often made in patients who appear inebriated, but who have not ingested ethanol. Diabetic coma, for example, may be mistaken for severe alcoholic intoxication. Drug intoxications, cardiovascular accidents, and fractured skulls seem to be common causes for the diagnostic errors (*see* Morgan and Cagan, 1974). The odor of the breath, which is not due to any ethanol vapor but to impurities in the alcoholic beverages or to other causes, is a notoriously unreliable guide and may often be seriously misleading. For medicolegal purposes, the concentration of ethanol in the blood, exhaled air, or urine should be determined.

Treatment. In general, the therapy of acute alcohol intoxication where the patient is somnolent or comatose does not differ significantly from that of acute central depression caused by conventional general anesthetics or hypnotics (*see* above). The stomach may be lavaged, but care must be taken to prevent pulmonary aspiration of the return flow. Since ethanol is freely miscible with water, it lends itself ideally to removal by hemodialysis (*see* Morgan and Cagan, 1974). Increased intracranial pressure owing to cerebral edema is treated by the usual medical measures, such as hypertonic solutions given intravenously.

Acute alcohol intoxication is not always associated with coma, and therapy is not usually required. It is sufficient to wait while the patient's tissues metabolize the ingested ethanol until sobriety ensues. However, some individuals may display extremely violent behavior. Sedatives and antipsychotic agents have been employed to quiet such patients. Great care must be taken, however, when sedatives are used to treat a patient who has ingested an excessive amount of a CNS depressant. The subject of acute alcohol intoxication has been extensively reviewed by various authors (*e.g.*, Morgan and Cagan, 1974).

Concentration of Ethanol in Body Fluids in Relation to Alcohol Intoxication. It is generally agreed that threshold effects (such as an increased reaction time, diminished fine motor control, and an impaired critical faculty) appear when the concentration of ethanol in the blood is 20 to 30 mg/dl; more than 50% of persons are grossly intoxicated when the concentration is 150 mg/dl. The average concentration in fatal cases is about 400 mg/dl (Committee on Medicolegal Problems, 1968).

The determination of ethanol in body fluids is often important for medicolegal purposes, to establish how much was ingested. The concentration of ethanol in the blood may be determined directly. Alternatively, it can be estimated from the concentration either in expired air, which is about 0.05% that in the blood or, less frequently, in the urine, which is about 130% that in the blood.

Diagnosis of Intoxication. All but a few states have passed laws embodying the recommendations of the National Safety Council and the American Medical Association concerning the driving of motor vehicles by persons who are drunk. If the defendant's blood has a concentration of ethanol of 100 mg/dl or over, he should be considered as being under the influence of intoxicating beverages; if 50 mg/dl or under, not under the influence; if between 50 and 100 mg/dl, this fact must be considered only with other competent positive evidence with regard to the guilt or innocence of the defendant. The importance of such legislation is emphasized by the fact that the average person with a blood ethanol concentration of 100 or 150 mg/dl is 7 or 25 times, respectively, more likely to have a fatal accident than the driver with no ethanol in his blood (*see* reports by U.S. Department of Health, Education, and Welfare, 1974, 1978).

Many factors, such as weight and the rate of absorption from the gastrointestinal tract, determine the concentration of ethanol in the blood produced by the ingestion of a given amount of ethanol. On the average, ingestion of 44 g of ethanol taken as whisky (4 oz) on an empty stomach results in a maximal blood concentration of 67 to 92 mg/dl; after a mixed meal, 30 to 53 mg/dl. Ingestion of the same amount of ethanol taken as conventional-strength beer (1.2 liters) on an empty stomach results in a maximal blood concentration of 41 to 49 mg/dl; after a mixed meal, 23 to 29 mg/dl. For individuals with normal hepatic function, ethanol is metabolized at a rate of about 120 mg/kg per hour (*see* Appendix II). One rule of thumb advocated by some is to wait 1 hour for every one or two drinks consumed before attempting to drive an automobile.

Contraindications. Contraindications to the use of alcohol largely follow from toxicological considerations. Patients with hepatic disease or gastrointestinal ulcers should not use alcohol. Alcohol should be avoided by patients with alcoholic skeletal or cardiac myopathy. Clearly, it should be taken only in great moderation, or not at all, by pregnant women, and alcohol should usually be forbidden to patients who were once addicted to it (*see* Chapter 22). In general, the use of alcohol in the presence of any particular disease is a matter that the physician and patient must decide in each individual case.

Therapeutic Uses. Ethanol and alcoholic beverages are widely used by the laity for numerous ailments; their legitimate uses in medicine are few.

External. Ethanol is an excellent solvent for many drugs and is frequently employed as a vehicle for medicinal mixtures. Ethanol is a solvent for the toxicodendrol causing ivy poisoning; early and thorough washing of the affected parts with alcohol may abort or lessen the severity of the dermatitis. Ethanol cools the skin when it is allowed to evaporate, and ethanol sponges are therefore used to treat fever. It is also rubefacient and is included in liniments. Ethanol (50 to 70% by volume) is employed as a rubbing agent on the skin of bedridden patients to prevent decubitus ulcers. It is also used to decrease sweating, and is an ingredient of many anhidrotic and astringent lotions. Ethanol still remains the most popular skin disinfectant.

Injection for Relief of Pain. Dehydrated alcohol may be injected in the close proximity of nerves or sympathetic ganglia for the relief of the long-lasting pain that occurs in trigeminal neuralgia, inoperable carcinoma, and other conditions. Epidural, subarachnoid, and lumbar paravertebral injections of ethanol have also been employed in appropriate circumstances. For example, lumbar paravertebral injections of ethanol may destroy sympathetic ganglia and thereby produce vasodilatation, relieve pain, and promote healing of lesions in patients with vascular disease of the lower extremities.

Systemic Uses. With the possible exception of its use as an emergency tocolytic agent (*see* Chapter 39), the therapeutic utility of systemically administered ethanol is confined to the treatment of poisoning by methyl alcohol and ethylene glycol (*see* Chapter 67). This use is based on the fact that the metabolism of methanol and ethylene glycol to toxic metabolites is initiated predominantly by alcohol dehydrogenase, albeit at a slower rate than that for ethanol.

Alcohol is widely employed for its hypnotic and antipyretic effects. However, alcohol taken at bedtime can have a disruptive effect on sleep and reduce the desired sense of refreshment (*see* above). In addition, alcoholic beverages have been used for generations to check impending "head colds." Perhaps the greatest therapeutic advantage of such therapy is to make the patient drowsy and sleepy and thus stay in bed. Hamburger (1936) humorously advised the following therapy, culled from an old English book, to be instituted at the first inkling of a cold, namely, to hang one's hat on the bedpost, drink from a bottle of good whisky until two hats appear, and then get into bed and stay there.

DISULFIRAM

History. Tetraethylthiuram disulfide (*disulfiram*) was used in the rubber industry as an antioxidant. Workers exposed to disulfiram developed a hypersensitivity to ethanol. Two Danish physicians, who had taken disulfiram in the course of an investigation of its potential anthelmintic usefulness and who became ill at a cocktail party, were quick to realize that the compound had altered their response to alcohol. They then initiated a series of pharmacological and clinical studies that provided the basis for the use of disulfiram as an adjunct in the treatment of chronic alcoholism. Similar sensitization is produced by various congeners of disulfiram, cyanamide, the fungus *Coprinus atramentarius,* the hypoglycemic sulfonylureas, metronidazole, certain cephalosporins, and the ingestion of animal charcoal (*see* Kitson, 1977; Eneanya *et al.,* 1981).

Mechanism of Action. Disulfiram, given by itself, is a relatively nontoxic substance. However, disulfiram markedly alters the intermediary metabolism of alcohol. When ethanol is given to an individual previously treated with disulfiram, the blood acetaldehyde concentration rises five to ten times higher than in an untreated individual. This effect is accompanied by marked signs and symptoms, known as the *acetaldehyde syndrome.* Within about 5 to 10 minutes the face feels hot, and soon afterwards it is flushed and scarlet in appearance. As the vasodilatation spreads over the whole body, intense throbbing is felt in the head and neck, and a pulsating headache may develop. Respiratory difficulties, nausea, copious vomiting, sweating, thirst, chest pain, considerable hypotension, orthostatic syncope, marked uneasiness, weakness, vertigo, blurred vision, and confusion are observed. The facial flush is replaced by pallor, and the blood pressure may fall to shock level. As little as 7 ml of alcohol will cause mild symptoms in sensitive persons, and the effect, once elicited, lasts between 30 minutes and several hours. After the symptoms wear off, the patient is exhausted and may sleep for several hours.

Most of the signs and symptoms observed after the ingestion of disulfiram plus alcohol are attributable to the resulting increase in the concentration of acetaldehyde in the body. They can, in fact, be produced in normal humans by the intravenous injection of acetaldehyde. Acetaldehyde is produced as a result of the initial oxidation of ethanol by the alcohol dehydrogenase of the liver. It does not accumulate in the tissues because it is further oxidized almost as soon as it is formed, primarily by the enzyme aldehyde dehydrogenase. In the presence of disulfiram, however, the concentration of acetaldehyde rises because disulfiram appears to react with crucial sulfhydryl groups in both the cytosolic and the mitochondrial forms of this enzyme, thereby producing irreversible inactivation (Sanny and Weiner, 1987). Recovery of activity is not achieved by removal of the drug and must await synthesis of new molecules of enzyme (*see* Kitson, 1977). It is not clear whether diethyldithiocarbamate, the major metabolite of disulfiram, is involved in this action to any extent, even though it combines extensively with proteins in blood and tissues. Diethyldithiocarbamate is an avid chelator of copper and other metals and thereby inhibits the activity of several metalloenzymes, including dopamine β-hydroxylase and alcohol dehydrogenase. The latter action would account for the increased concentration of ethanol in blood sometimes reported during treatment with disulfiram. Inhibition of dopamine β-hydroxylase, with a consequent reduction of norepinephrine synthesis in sympathetic nerve terminals, may provide an explanation for the hypotension that is characteristic of the disulfiram–ethanol reaction.

Disulfiram can inhibit most enzymes with crucial sulfhydryl groups, and it thus has a wide spectrum of biological effects. It inhibits hepatic microsomal drug-metabolizing enzymes and thereby interferes with the metabolism of phenytoin, chlordiazepoxide, barbiturates, and other drugs (Eneanya *et al.,* 1981).

Absorption, Fate, and Excretion. About 80% of an oral dose of disulfiram is absorbed rapidly from the gastrointestinal tract. However, only small amounts of disulfiram appear in blood because of its rapid reduction to diethyldithiocarbamate, principally by the glutathione reductase system in erythrocytes. Nonenzymatic reduction through interaction with the sulfhydryl groups of albumin may also be important (Agarwal *et al.,* 1986). Diethyldithiocarbamate is metabolized further in the liver, primarily by conjugation with glucuronic acid (*see* Eneanya *et al.,* 1981).

Toxic Reactions and Contraindications. Disulfiram by itself is largely, but not completely, innocuous. It may cause acneform eruptions, allergic dermatitis, urticaria, lassitude, fatigue, tremor, restlessness, reduced sexual potency, headache, dizziness, a garlic-like or metallic taste, and mild gastrointestinal disturbances. Hepatotoxicity, peripheral neuropathies, psychosis, and acetonemia have also been reported (*see* Eneanya *et al.,* 1981). The hepatic toxicity of disulfiram may be enhanced by the ingestion of ethanol (Iber *et al.,* 1987). The concentrations of nickel in blood rise progressively during treatment with disulfiram and may increase 10- to 20-fold within 4 months (Hopfer *et al.,* 1987). Evidently, diethyldithiocarbamate forms a complex with the metal and promotes its absorption. Similarly, disulfiram enhances the absorption and toxicity of lead in rats (Oskarsson *et al.,* 1986). Since the accumulation of these metals in the brain is also promoted, it would seem prudent to avoid the use of disulfiram in patients who are apt to encounter them in their environment. Disulfiram may be teratogenic and should not be used during pregnancy. Alarming reactions may result from the ingestion of even small amounts of alcohol in persons being treated with disulfiram, and sudden and unexplained fatalities have occurred. Obviously the use of disulfiram as a therapeutic agent is not without danger, and it should be attempted only under careful medical and nursing supervision. Patients must be warned that, as long as they are taking disulfiram, the ingestion of alcohol in any form will make them sick and may endanger their life. Patients must learn to avoid disguised forms of alcohol, such as sauces, fermented vinegar, cough syrups, and even aftershave lotions and backrubs.

Chemistry, Preparations, and Dosage. The chemical structure of disulfiram is as follows:

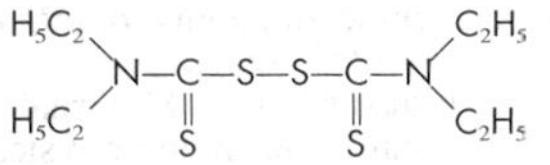

Disulfiram

Disulfiram (ANTABUSE) is available in the form of oral tablets that contain 250 or 500 mg of the drug. Disulfiram should be administered only by a physician, and therapy is usually commenced in the hospital. The drug should never be administered until the patient has abstained from alcohol for at least 12 hours. In the initial phase of treatment, a maximal daily dose of 500 mg is given for 1 to 2 weeks. Maintenance dosage then ranges from 125 to 500 mg daily, depending on tolerance to side effects. Unless sedation is prominent, the daily dose should be taken in the morning, the time when the resolve not to drink may be strongest. Sensitization to alcohol may last as long as 14 days after the last ingestion of disulfiram because of the slow rate of restoration of aldehyde dehydrogenase.

Therapeutic Use. The only therapeutic use of disulfiram is in the treatment of chronic alcoholism. Disulfiram is not a cure for alcoholism; it merely affords the volunteer a crutch by which the sincere desire to stop drinking can be fortified. The rationale for its use is that the patients know that if they are to avoid the devastating experience of the "acetaldehyde syndrome" they cannot drink for at least 3 or 4 days after taking disulfiram. *Calcium carbimide* (*citrated calcium cyanamide;* TEMPOSIL) has similar but briefer effects. It is not available in the United States. This subject is further discussed in Chapter 22, which deals with the therapy of drug abuse.

Agarwal, R. P.; Phillips, M.; McPherson, R. A.; and Hensley, P. Serum albumin and the metabolism of disulfiram. *Biochem. Pharmacol.*, **1986**, *35*, 3341–3347.

Al-Khudhairi, D.; Whitwam, J. G.; Chakrabarti, M. K.; Askitopoulou, H.; Grundy, E. M.; and Powrie, S. Haemodynamic effects of midazolam and thiopentone during induction of anaesthesia for coronary artery surgery. *Br. J. Anaesth.*, **1982**, *54*, 831–835.

Allan, A. M.; Gallaher, E. J.; Gionet, S. E.; and Harris, R. A. Genetic selection for benzodiazepine ataxia produces functional changes in the γ-aminobutyric acid receptor chloride channel complex. *Brain Res.*, **1988**, *452*, 118–126.

Altura, B. M., and Altura, B. T. Microvascular and vascular smooth muscle actions of ethanol, acetaldehyde, and acetate. *Fed. Proc.*, **1982**, *41*, 2447–2451.

Brocklehurst J. C.; Carty, M. H.; and Skorecki, J. The use of a kymograph in a comparative trial of flunitrazepam and meprobamate in elderly patients. *Curr. Med. Res. Opin.*, **1978**, *5*, 663–668.

Brown, N. A.; Goulding, E. H.; and Fabro, S. Ethanol embryotoxicity: direct effects on mammalian embryos *in vitro*. *Science*, **1979**, *206*, 573–575.

Chin, J. H., and Goldstein, D. B. Membrane-disordering action of ethanol. *Mol. Pharmacol.*, **1981**, *19*, 425–431.

Gantt, W. H. Effect of alcohol on the sexual reflexes of normal and neurotic male dogs. *Psychosom. Med.*, **1952**, *14*, 174–181.

Gee, K. W.; Bolger, M. B.; Brinton, R. E.; Coirini, H.; and McEwen, B. S. Steroid modulation of the chloride ionophore in rat brain: structure-activity requirements, regional dependence and mechanism of action. *J. Pharmacol. Exp. Ther.*, **1988**, *246*, 803–812.

Gee, K. W.; Chang, W.-C.; Brinton, R. E.; and McEwen, B. S. GABA-dependent modulation of the Cl^- ionophore by steroids in rat brain. *Eur. J. Pharmacol.*, **1987**, *136*, 419–423.

Greenblatt, D. J.; Allen, M. D.; Noel, B. J.; and Shader, R. I. Acute overdosage with benzodiazepine derivatives. *Clin. Pharmacol. Ther.*, **1977**, *4*, 497–514.

Gross, J. B.; Zebrowski, M. E.; Carel, W. D.; Gardner, S.; and Smith, T. C. Time course of ventilatory depression after thiopental and midazolam in normal subjects and in patients with chronic obstructive pulmonary disease. *Anesthesiology*, **1983**, *58*, 540–544.

Hall, R. C., and Zisook, S. Paradoxical reactions to benzodiazepines. *Br. J. Clin. Pharmacol.*, **1981**, *11*, Suppl. 1, 99S–104S.

Hamburger, L. P. Some minor ailments: their importance in the medical curriculum. *Yale J. Biol. Med.*, **1936**, *8*, 365–386.

Harrison, N. L.; Majewska, M. D.; Harrington, J. W.; and Barker, J. L. Structure-activity relationships for steroid interaction with the γ-aminobutyric acid A receptor complex. *J. Pharmacol. Exp. Ther.*, **1987**, *241*, 346–353.

Hartmann, E. Long-term administration of psychotropic drugs: effects on human sleep. In, *Pharmacology of Sleep*. (Williams, R. L., and Karacan, I., eds.) John Wiley & Sons, Inc., New York, **1976**, pp. 211–223.

Hopfer, S. M.; Linden, J. V.; Rezuke, W. N.; O'Brien, J. E.; Smith, L.; Watters, F.; and Sunderman, F. W., Jr. Increased nickel concentrations in body fluids of patients with chronic alcoholism during disulfiram therapy. *Res. Commun. Chem. Pathol. Pharmacol.*, **1987**, *55*, 101–109.

Huidobro-Toro, J. P.; Bleck, V.; Allan, A. M.; and Harris, R. A. Neurochemical actions of anesthetic drugs on the γ-aminobutyric acid receptor-chloride channel complex. *J. Pharmacol. Exp. Ther.*, **1988**, *242*, 963–969.

Iber, F. L.; Lee, K.; Lacoursier, R.; and Fuller, R. Liver toxicity encountered in the Veterans Administration trial of disulfiram in alcoholics. *Alcoholism (NY)*, **1987**, *11*, 301–304.

Ikram, H.; Rubin, A. P.; and Jewkes, R. F. Effect of diazepam on myocardial blood flow of patients with and without coronary artery disease. *Br. Heart J.*, **1973**, *35*, 626–630.

Jacobsen, D.; Wiik-Larsen, E.; Saltvedt, E.; and Bredesen, J. E. Meprobamate kinetics during and after terminated hemoperfusion in acute intoxications. *J. Toxicol. Clin. Toxicol.*, **1987**, *25*, 317–331.

Johnson, S.; Knight, R.; Marmar, D. J.; and Steele, R. W. Immune deficiency in fetal alcohol syndrome. *Pediatr. Res.*, **1981**, *15*, 908–911.

Keston, M., and Brocklehurst, J. C. Flurazepam and meprobamate: a clinical trial. *Age Ageing*, **1974**, *3*, 54–58.

Kintz, P.; Tracqui, A.; Mangin, P.; and Lugnier, A. A. Fatal meprobamate self-poisoning. *Am. J. Forensic Med. Pathol.*, **1988**, *9*, 139–140.

Lader, M., and File, S. The biological basis of benzodiazepine dependence. *Psychol. Med.*, **1987**, *17*, 539–547.

Levitan, E. S., and others. Structural and functional basis for $GABA_A$ receptor heterogeneity. *Nature*, **1988**, *335*, 76–79.

Linnoila, M.; Ervin, C. W.; and Brendle, A. Efficacy and side-effects of flunitrazepam and pentobarbital in severely insomniac patients. *J. Clin. Pharmacol.*, **1982**, *22*, 14–19.

Lister, R. G., and Nutt, D. J. Is Ro 15-4513 a specific alcohol antagonist? *Trends Neurosci.*, **1987**, *10*, 223–225.

Lohse, M. J.; Böser, S.; Klotz, K.-N.; and Schwabe, U. Affinities of barbiturates for the GABA-receptor complex and A_1 adenosine receptors: a possible explanation of their excitatory effects. *Naunyn Schmiedebergs Arch. Pharmacol.*, **1987**, *336*, 211–217.

McIntyre, T. D.; Trullas, R.; and Skolnick, P. Differences in the biophysical properties of the benzodiazepine/γ-aminobutyric acid receptor chloride channel complex in the long-sleep and short-sleep mouse lines. *J. Neurochem.*, **1988**, *51*, 642–647.

Mehta, A. K., and Ticku, M. K. Ethanol potentiation of GABAergic transmission in cultured spinal cord neurons involves γ-aminobutyric $acid_A$-gated chloride channels. *J. Pharmacol. Exp. Ther.*, **1988**, *246*, 558–564.

Michenfelder, J. D. Barbiturates for brain resuscitation: yes and no. *Anesthesiology*, **1982**, *57*, 74–75.

Moody, E. J.; Suzdak, P. D.; Paul, S. M.; and Skolnick, P. Modulation of the benzodiazepine/γ-aminobutyric acid receptor chloride channel complex by inhalation anesthetics. *J. Neurochem.*, **1988**, *51*, 1386–1393.

Mullen, K. D.; Martin, J. V.; Mendelson, W. B.; Bassett, M. L.; and Jones, E. A. Could an endogenous benzodiazepine ligand contribute to hepatic encephalopathy? *Lancet*, **1988**, *1*, 457–459.

Ng, S. K. C.; Hauser, W. A.; Brust, J. C. M.; and Susser, M. Alcohol consumption and withdrawal in new-onset seizures. *N. Engl. J. Med.*, **1988**, *319*, 666–673.

Nugent, M.; Artru, A. A.; and Michenfelder, J. D. Cerebral metabolic, vascular and protective effects of midazolam maleate. Comparison to diazepam. *Anesthesiology*, **1982**, *56*, 172–176.

Oldenhof, H.; de Jong, M.; Steenhoek, A.; and Janknegt, R. Clinical pharmacokinetics of midazolam in intensive care patients, a wide interpatient variability? *Clin. Pharmacol. Ther.*, **1988**, *43*, 263–269.

Oskarsson, A.; Olson, L.; Palmer, M. R.; Lind, B.; Bjorklund, H.; and Hoffer, B. Increased lead concentration in brain and potentiation of lead-induced neuronal depression in rats after combined treatment with lead and disulfiram. *Environ. Res.*, **1986**, *41*, 623–632.

Proctor, W. R., and Dunwiddie, T. V. Behavioral sensitivity to purinergic drugs parallels ethanol sensitivity in selectively bred mice. *Science*, **1984**, *224*, 519–521.

Rao, S.; Sherbaniuk, R. W.; Prasad, K.; Lee, S. J. K.; and Sproule, B. J. Cardiopulmonary effects of diazepam. *Clin. Pharmacol. Ther.*, **1973**, *14*, 182–189.

Regan, T. J. Regional circulatory responses to alcohol and its congeners. *Fed. Proc.*, **1982**, *41*, 2438–2442.

Roache, J. D., and Griffiths, R. R. Lorazepam and meprobamate dose effects in humans: behavioral effects and abuse liability. *J. Pharmacol. Exp. Ther.*, **1987**, *243*, 978–988.

Rossett, H. L.; Weiner, L.; and Edelin, K. C. Strategy for prevention of fetal alcohol effects. *Obstet. Gynecol.*, **1981**, *57*, 1–7.

Rubin, E. Alcoholic myopathy in heart and skeletal muscles. *N. Engl. J. Med.*, **1979**, *301*, 28–33.

Sandor, P.; Sellers, E. M.; Dumbrell, M.; and Khouw, V. Effect of short- and long-term alcohol abuse on phenytoin kinetics in chronic alcoholics. *Clin. Pharmacol. Ther.*, **1981**, *30*, 390–397.

Sanny, C. G., and Weiner, H. Inactivation of horse liver mitochondrial aldehyde dehydrogenase by disulfiram: evidence that disulfiram is not an active-site-directed reagent. *Biochem. J.*, **1987**, *242*, 499–503.

Seitz, W.; Hempelman, G.; and Piepenbrock, S. Zur kardiovaskulären Wirkung von Flunitrazepam (ROHYPNOL, Ro-5-4200). *Anaesthesist*, **1977**, *26*, 249–256.

Smith, R. B.; Divoll, M.; Gillespie, W. R.; and Greenblatt, D. J. Effect of subject age and gender on the pharmacokinetics of oral triazolam and temazepam. *J. Clin. Psychopharmacol.*, **1983**, *3*, 172–176.

Straus, E.; Urbach, H.-J.; and Yalow, R. S. Alcohol-stimulated secretion of immunoreactive secretin. *N. Engl. J. Med.*, **1975**, *293*, 1031–1032.

Suzdak, P. D.; Glowa, J. R.; Crawley, J. N.; Schwartz, R. D.; Skolnick, P.; and Paul, S. M. A selective imidazobenzodiazepine antagonist of ethanol in the rat. *Science*, **1986**, *234*, 1243–1247.

Tennes, K., and Blackard, C. Maternal alcohol consumption, birthweight, and minor physical abnormalities. *Am. J. Obstet. Gynecol.*, **1980**, *138*, 774–780.

Teschke, R.; Matsuzaki, S.; Ohnishi, K.; Hasumura, Y.; and Lieber, C. S. Metabolism of alcohol at high concentrations: role and biochemical nature of the hepatic microsomal oxidizing system. *Adv. Exp. Med. Biol.*, **1977**, *85A*, 257–280.

Twyman, R. E.; Rogers, C. J.; and Macdonald, R. L. Differential regulation of γ-aminobutyric acid receptor channels by diazepam and phenobarbital. *Ann. Neurol.*, **1989**, *25*, 213–220.

Urbano-Marquez, A.; Estruch, R.; Navarro-Lopez, F.; Grau, J. M.; Mont, L.; and Rubin, E. The effects of alcoholism on skeletal and cardiac muscle. *N. Engl. J. Med.*, **1989**, *320*, 409–415.

Urponen, H.; Vuori, I.; Hasan, J.; and Partinen, M. Self-evaluations of factors promoting and disturbing sleep: an epidemiological survey in Finland. *Soc. Sci. Med.*, **1988**, *26*, 443–450.

Van Thiel, D. H.; Gavaler, J. S.; and Sanghvi, A. Recovery of sexual function in abstinent alcoholic men. *Gastroenterology*, **1983**, *84*, 677–682.

Van Thiel, D. H., and Lester, R. Sex and alcohol: a second peek. *N. Engl. J. Med.*, **1976**, *295*, 835–836.

Wilson, G. T. Alcohol and human sexual behavior. *Behav. Res. Ther.*, **1977**, *15*, 239–252.

Woods, J. H.; Katz, J. L.; and Winger, G. W. Use and abuse of benzodiazepines. *J.A.M.A.*, **1988**, *260*, 3476–3480.

Monographs and Reviews

Altura, B. T. Cardiovascular effects of alcohol and alcoholism. *Fed. Proc.*, **1982**, *41*, 2437–2477.

Andrews, P. R., and Mark, L. C. Structural specificity of barbiturates and related drugs. *Anesthesiology*, **1982**, *57*, 314–320.

Barker, J. L.; Harrison, N. L.; and Mariani, A. P. Benzodiazepine pharmacology of cultured mammalian CNS neurons. *Life Sci.*, **1986**, *39*, 1959–1968.

Basile, A. S., and Gammal, S. H. Evidence for the involvement of the benzodiazepine receptor complex in hepatic encephalopathy. *Clin. Neuropharmacol.*, **1988**, *11*, 401–422.

Beard, J. D., and Sargent, W. Q. Water and electrolyte metabolism following ethanol intake and during acute withdrawal from ethanol. In, *Biochemistry and Pharmacology of Ethanol*, Vol. 2. (Majchrowicz, E., and Noble, E. P., eds.) Plenum Press, New York, **1979**, pp. 3–16.

Bellantuono, C.; Reggi, V.; Tognoni, G.; and Garattini, S. Benzodiazepines: clinical pharmacology and therapeutic use. *Drugs*, **1980**, *19*, 195–219.

Borkovec, T. D. Insomnia. *J. Consult. Clin. Psychol.*, **1982**, *50*, 880–895.

Bosron, W. F.; Lumeng, L.; and Li, T. K. Genetic polymorphism of enzymes of alcohol metabolism and susceptibility to alcoholic liver disease. *Mol. Aspects Med.*, **1988**, *10*, 147–158.

Breimer, D. D. Clinical pharmacokinetics of hypnotics. *Clin. Pharmacokinet.*, **1977**, *2*, 93–109.

———. Pharmacokinetics and metabolism of various benzodiazepines used as hypnotics. *Br. J. Clin. Pharmacol.*, **1979**, *8*, Suppl. 1, 7S–13S.

Brogden, R. N., and Goa, K. L. Flumazenil: a preliminary review of its benzodiazepine antagonist properties, intrinsic activity and therapeutic use. *Drugs*, **1988**, *35*, 448–467.

Committee on Medicolegal Problems. *Alcohol and the Impaired Driver: A Manual on the Medicolegal Aspects of Chemical Tests for Intoxication*. American Medical Association, Chicago, **1968**.

Council Report. Fetal effects of maternal alcohol use. *J.A.M.A.*, **1983**, *249*, 2517–2521.

Dubnick, B.; Lippa, A. S.; Klepner, C. A.; Coupet, J.; Greenblatt, E. N.; and Beer, B. The separation of 3H-benzodiazepine binding sites in brain and of benzodiazepine pharmacological properties. *Pharmacol. Biochem. Behav.*, **1983**, *18*, 311–318.

Dundee, J. W.; Halliday, N. J.; Harper, K. W.; and Brogden, R. N. Midazolam: a review of its pharmacological properties and therapeutic use. *Drugs*, **1984**, *28*, 519–543.

Eneanya, D. L.; Bianchine, J. R.; Duran, D. O.; and Andresen, B. D. The actions and metabolic fate of disulfiram. *Annu. Rev. Pharmacol. Toxicol.*, **1981**, *21*, 575–596.

File, S. E. Tolerance to the behavioral actions of benzodiazepines. *Neurosci. Behav. Rev.*, **1985**, *9*, 113–121.

Fisher, S. E., and Karl, P. I. Maternal ethanol use and selective fetal malnutrition. *Recent Dev. Alcohol.*, **1988**, *6*, 277–289.

Freudenthal, R. I., and Carroll, F. I. Metabolism of certain commonly used barbiturates. *Drug Metab. Rev.*, **1973**, *2*, 265–278.

Gardner, C. R. Functional *in vivo* correlates of the benzodiazepine agonist-inverse agonist continuum. *Prog. Neurobiol.*, **1988**, *31*, 425–476.

Gary, N. E., and Tresnewsky, O. Clinical aspects of drug intoxication: barbiturates and a potpourri of other sedatives, hypnotics, and tranquilizers. *Heart Lung*, **1983**, *12*, 122–127.

Glass, G. B. J.; Slomiany, B. L.; and Slomiany, A. Biochemical and pathological derangements of the gastrointestinal tract following acute and chronic digestion of ethanol. In, *Biochemistry and Pharmacology of Ethanol*, Vol. 1. (Majchrowicz, E., and Noble, E. P., eds.) Plenum Press, New York, **1979**, pp. 551–586.

Greenblatt, D. J.; Divoll, M.; Abernethy, D. R.; Ochs, H. R.; and Shader, R. I. Benzodiazepine kinetics: implications for therapeutics and pharmacogeriatrics. *Drug Metab. Rev.*, **1983a**, *14*, 251–292.

———. Clinical pharmacokinetics of the newer benzodiazepines. *Clin. Pharmacokinet.*, **1983b**, *8*, 233–252.

Greenblatt, D. J., and Shader, R. I. *Benzodiazepines in Clinical Practice*. Raven Press, New York, **1974**.

Greenblatt, D. J.; Shader, R. I.; and Abernethy, D. R. Current status of benzodiazepines. *N. Engl. J. Med.*, **1983c**, *309*, 354–358, 410–416.

Gross, M. M. (ed.). *Alcohol Intoxication and Withdrawal*. Vols. A and B, *Advances in Experimental Medicine and Biology*. Plenum Press, New York, **1977**.

Hillman, R. S., and Steinberg, S. E. The effects of alcohol on folate metabolism. *Annu. Rev. Med.*, **1982**, *33*, 345–354.

Hillman, R. W. Alcoholism and malnutrition. In, *The Biology of Alcoholism*. Vol. 3, *Clinical Pathology*. (Kissin, B., and Begleiter, H., eds.) Plenum Press, New York, **1974**, pp. 513–586.

Ho, I. K., and Harris, R. A. Mechanism of action of barbiturates. *Annu. Rev. Pharmacol. Toxicol.*, **1981**, *21*, 83–111.

Hoyumpa, A. M., and Schenker, S. Major drug interactions: effect of liver disease, alcohol and malnutrition. *Annu. Rev. Med.*, **1982**, *33*, 113–149.

Kales, A., and Kales, J. Sleep laboratory studies of hypnotic drugs: efficacy and withdrawal effects. *J. Clin. Psychopharmacol.*, **1983**, *3*, 140–150.

Kales, A.; Kales, J.; and Soldatos, C. R. Insomnia and other sleep disorders. *Med. Clin. North Am.*, **1982**, *66*, 971–991.

Kay, D. C.; Blackburn, A. B.; Buckingham, J. A.; and Karacan, I. Human pharmacology of sleep. In, *Pharmacology of Sleep*. (Williams, R. L., and Karacan, I., eds.) John Wiley & Sons, Inc., New York, **1976**, pp. 83–210.

Kissin, B. Interactions of ethyl alcohol and other drugs. In, *The Biology of Alcoholism*. Vol. 3, *Clinical Pathology*. (Kissin, B., and Begleiter, H., eds.) Plenum Press, New York, **1974**, pp. 109–161.

Kissin, B., and Begleiter, H. (eds.). *The Biology of Alcoholism*. Vol. 3, *Clinical Pathology*. Plenum Press, New York, **1974**.

Kitson, T. M. The disulfiram–ethanol reaction. *J. Stud. Alcohol*, **1977**, *38*, 96–113.

Klatsky, A. L.; Friedman, G. D.; and Siegelaub, A. B. Alcohol and mortality. A ten-year Kaiser-Permanente experience. *Ann. Intern. Med.*, **1981**, *95*, 139–145.

Lieber, C. S. The influence of alcohol on nutritional status. *Nutr. Rev.*, **1988a**, *46*, 241–254.

———. Biochemical and molecular basis of alcohol-induced injury to liver and other tissues. *N. Engl. J. Med.*, **1988b**, *319*, 1639–1650.

Lindenbaum, J. Hematologic effects of alcohol. In, *The Biology of Alcoholism*. Vol. 3, *Clinical Pathology*. (Kissin, B., and Begleiter, H., eds.) Plenum Press, New York, **1974**, pp. 461–480.

Lister, R. G., and Nutt, D. J. Ro 15-4513 and its interaction with ethanol. *Adv. Alcohol Subst. Abuse*, **1988**, *7*, 119–123.

Lorber, S. H.; Dinoso, V. P., Jr.; and Chey, W. Y. Diseases of the gastrointestinal tract. In, *The Biology of Alcoholism*. Vol. 3, *Clinical Pathology*. (Kissin, B., and Begleiter, H., eds.) Plenum Press, New York, **1974**, pp. 339–357.

McElnay, J. C.; Jones, M. E.; and Alexander, B. Temazepam (RESTORIL, Sandoz Pharmaceuticals). *Drug Intell. Clin. Pharm.*, **1982**, *16*, 650–656.

Macdonald, R. L., and McLean, M. J. Cellular bases of barbiturate and phenytoin anticonvulsant drug action. *Epilepsia*, **1982**, *23*, Suppl. 1, S7–S18.

———. Anticonvulsant drugs: mechanisms of action. *Adv. Neurol.*, **1986**, *44*, 713–735.

Majchrowicz, E., and Noble, E. P. (eds.). *Biochemistry and Pharmacology of Ethanol*, Vols. 1–3. Plenum Press, New York, **1979**.

Marks, J. *The Benzodiazepines: Use, Overuse, Misuse, Abuse*. MTP Press, Ltd., Lancaster, **1978**, pp. 1–111.

Marshall, L. F., and Bowers, S. A. Medical management of head injury. *Clin. Neurosurg.*, **1982**, *29*, 312–325.

Martin, I. L. The benzodiazepines and their receptors: 25 years of progress. *Neuropharmacology*, **1987**, *26*, 957–970.

Mendelson, W. B. Pharmacologic and electrophysiologic effects of ethanol in relation to sleep. In, *Biochemistry and Pharmacology of Ethanol*, Vol. 2. (Majchrowicz, E., and Noble, E. P., eds.) Plenum Press, New York, **1979**, pp. 467–484.

———. *The Use and Misuse of Sleeping Pills: A Clinical Guide*. Plenum Medical Book Co., New York, **1980**.

Mendelson, W. B.; Gillin, J. C.; and Wyatt, R. J. *Human Sleep and Its Disorders*. Plenum Press, New York, **1977**.

Meyer, B. R. Benzodiazepines in the elderly. *Med. Clin. North Am.*, **1982**, *66*, 1017–1035.
Mitler, M. M. Evaluation of temazepam as a hypnotic. *Pharmacotherapy*, **1981**, *1*, 3–13.
Morgan, R., and Cagan, E. J. Acute alcohol intoxication, the disulfiram reaction, and methyl alcohol intoxication. In, *The Biology of Alcoholism*. Vol. 3, *Clinical Pathology*. (Kissin, B., and Begleiter, H., eds.) Plenum Press, New York, **1974**, pp. 163–189.
Nicholson, A. N. The use of short- and long-acting hypnotics in clinical medicine. *Br. J. Clin. Pharmacol.*, **1981**, *11*, 615–695.
Olsen, R. W. GABA-drug interactions. *Prog. Drug Res.*, **1987**, *31*, 224–238.
Olsen, R. W.; Yang, J.; King, R. G.; Dilber, A.; Stauber, G. B.; and Ransom, R. W. Barbiturate and benzodiazepine modulation of GABA receptor binding and function. *Life Sci.*, **1986**, *39*, 1969–1976.
Owen, R. T., and Tyrer, P. Benzodiazepine dependence. *Drugs*, **1983**, *25*, 385–398.
Phillis, J. W., and O'Regan, M. H. The role of adenosine in the central actions of the benzodiazepines. *Prog. Neuropsychopharmacol. Biol. Psychiatry*, **1988**, *12*, 389–404.
Pirola, R. C. *Drug Metabolism and Alcohol*. University Park Press, Baltimore, **1978**.
Pirola, R. C., and Lieber, C. S. Acute and chronic pancreatitis. In, *The Biology of Alcoholism*. Vol. 3, *Clinical Pathology*. (Kissin, B., and Begleiter, H., eds.) Plenum Press, New York, **1974**, pp. 359–402.
Pohorecky, L. A., and Brick, J. Pharmacology of ethanol. *Pharmacol. Ther.*, **1988**, *36*, 335–427.
Polc, P. Electrophysiology of benzodiazepine receptor ligands: multiple mechanisms and sites of action. *Prog. Neurobiol.*, **1988**, *31*, 349–423.
Richter, J. A., and Holman, J. R. Barbiturates: their *in-vivo* effects and potential biochemical mechanisms. *Prog. Neurobiol.*, **1982**, *18*, 275–319.
Roth, T.; Roehrs, T. A.; and Zorick, F. J. Pharmacology and hypnotic efficacy of triazolam. *Pharmacotherapy*, **1983**, *3*, 137–148.
Roth, T.; Roehrs, T.; Zorick, F.; and Conway, W. Pharmacological effects of sedative-hypnotics, narcotic analgesics, and alcohol during sleep. *Med. Clin. North Am.*, **1985**, *69*, 1281–1288.
Schütz, H. *Benzodiazepines—A Handbook: Basic Data, Pharmacokinetics, and Comprehensive Literature*. Springer-Verlag, Berlin, **1982**.
Seidel, W. F., and Dement, W. C. Sleepiness in insomnia: evaluation and treatment. *Sleep*, **1982**, *5*, Suppl. 2, S182–S190.
Shapiro, H. M. Barbiturates in brain ischaemia. *Br. J. Anaesth.*, **1985**, *57*, 82–95.
Steer, C. R. Barbiturate therapy in the management of cerebral ischemia. *Dev. Med. Child Neurol.*, **1982**, *24*, 219–231.
Symposium. (Various authors.) *The Benzodiazepines*. (Garattini, S.; Mussini, E.; and Randall, L. O.; eds.) Raven Press, New York, **1973**.
Symposium. (Various authors.) *Psychopharmacology of Sleep*. (Wheatly, D., ed.) Raven Press, New York, **1981**.
Symposium. (Various authors.) *Pharmacology of Benzodiazepines*. (Usdin, E.; Skolnick, P.; Tallman, J. F.; Greenblatt, D.; and Paul, S. M.; eds.) Macmillan Press, Ltd., London, **1982**.
Symposium. (Various authors.) *The Benzodiazepines: From Molecular Biology to Clinical Practice*. (Costa, E., ed.) Raven Press, New York, **1983a**.
Symposium. (Various authors.) *Benzodiazepines Divided: A Multidisciplinary Review*. (Trimble, M. R., ed.) John Wiley & Sons, Ltd., Chichester, **1983b**.
Symposium. (Various authors.) *Anxiolytes: Neurochemical, Behavioral and Clinical Perspectives*. (Malick, J. B.; Enna, S. J.; and Yamamura, H. I.; eds.) Raven Press, New York, **1983c**.
Symposium. (Various authors.) Modern hypnotics and performance. (Nicholson, A.; Hippius, H.; Rüther, E.; and Dunbar, G.; eds.) *Acta Psychiatr. Scand.*, **1986a**, *74*, Suppl. 332, 3–174.
Symposium. (Various authors.) Chlormethiazole 25 years: recent developments and historical perspectives. (Evans, J. G.; Feuerlein, W.; Glatt, M. M.; Kanowski, S.; and Scott, D. B.; eds.) *Acta Psychiatr. Scand.*, **1986b**, *73*, Suppl. 329, 5–198.
Symposium. (Various authors.) Chloride channels and their modulation by neurotransmitters and drugs. (Biggio, G., and Costa, E., eds.) *Adv. Biochem. Psychopharmacol.*, **1988a**, *45*, 1–375.
Symposium. (Various authors.) Benzodiazepine receptor ligands, memory and information processing. (Hindmarch, I., and Ott, H., eds.) *Psychopharmacol. Ser.*, **1988b**, *6*, 3–303.
Symposium. (Various authors.) Nutrition and alcohol. (Mathers, J. C.; Quarterman, J.; and Gurr, M. I.; eds.) *Proc. Nutr. Soc.*, **1988c**, *47*, 79–133.
Sytkowski, A. J., and Vallee, B. L. Metalloenzymes and ethanol metabolism. In, *Biochemistry and Pharmacology of Ethanol*, Vol. 1. (Majchrowicz, E., and Noble, E. P., eds.) Plenum Press, New York, **1979**, pp. 43–63.
Ticku, M. K., and Kulkarni, S. K. Molecular interactions of ethanol with GABAergic system and potential of Ro 15-4513 as an ethanol antagonist. *Pharmacol. Biochem. Behav.*, **1988**, *30*, 501–510.
Turner, T. B.; Mezey, E.; and Kimball, A. W. Measurement of alcohol-related effects in man: chronic effects in relation to levels of alcohol consumption. *Johns Hopkins Med. J.*, **1977**, *5*, 235–248, 273–286.
U.S. Department of Health, Education, and Welfare. *Alcohol and Health*. (Second and Third Special Reports to the Congress from the Secretary of Health, Education, and Welfare.) The Department, Washington, D. C., **1974, 1978**.
Wallgren, H., and Barry, H., III. *Actions of Alcohol*, Vols. I and II. American Elsevier Publishing Co., Inc., New York, **1970**.
Warren, K. R., and Bast, R. J. Alcohol-related birth defects: an update. *Public Health Rep.*, **1988**, *103*, 638–642.
Wincor, M. Z. Insomnia and the new benzodiazepines. *Clin. Pharm.*, **1982**, *1*, 425–432.
Wood, W. G., and Schroeder, F. Membrane effects of ethanol: bulk lipid versus lipid domains. *Life Sci.*, **1988**, *43*, 467–475.
Woods, J. H.; Katz, J. L.; and Winger, G. Abuse liability of benzodiazepines. *Pharmacol. Rev.*, **1987**, *39*, 254–390.

CHAPTER

18 DRUGS AND THE TREATMENT OF PSYCHIATRIC DISORDERS

Ross J. Baldessarini

The use of drugs with well-demonstrated efficacy in psychiatric disorders has become widespread since the mid-1950s. Today, about 10 to 20% of prescriptions written in the United States are for medications intended to affect mental processes, namely, to sedate, stimulate, or otherwise change mood, thinking, or behavior. This practice reflects both the high frequency of primary emotional disorders and the nearly inevitable emotional, psychological, and social reactions of persons with medical illnesses. In addition, many drugs used for other purposes also modify emotions and cognition either as part of their usual actions or as toxic effects of overdosage (*see* especially Chapter 22). This chapter discusses agents used primarily for the treatment of psychiatric disorders.

Although alternative schemes exist, the agents described herein are placed into three major categories. *Antipsychotic* or *neuroleptic drugs* are those used to treat very severe psychiatric illnesses, the psychoses; they have beneficial effects on mood and thought but carry the risk of producing characteristic side effects that mimic neurological diseases. *Mood-stabilizing drugs* (notably, lithium salts and certain anticonvulsants) and *antidepressants* (mood-elevating agents) are those used to treat affective disorders and related conditions. *Antianxiety-sedative agents,* particularly the benzodiazepines, are those used for the drug therapy of anxiety states.

The use of drugs in the treatment of psychiatric disorders is complicated by diagnostic uncertainties characteristic of clinical psychiatry. However, psychiatric diagnosis continues to gain objectivity, coherence, and reliability. The association between specific clinical syndromes and predictable responses to psychotropic drugs has supported the impressive recent progress in this area. Testable hypotheses about possible biological bases of severe psychiatric illnesses have been stimulated by knowledge of the mechanisms of action of psychotropic agents, assisted by the emergence of a medical discipline commonly known as *biological psychiatry*. The diagnostic terminology and criteria currently employed in the United States are well described in the *Diagnostic and Statistical Manual of Mental Disorders* of the American Psychiatric Association (1987).

History. Modification of behavior, mood, and emotion by drugs has always been a favorite indulgence of mankind. The use of psychoactive drugs evolved along two related paths. The first was in the use of drugs to modify normal behavior and to produce altered states of feeling for religious, ceremonial, or recreational purposes. The second was to alleviate mental ailments. A fascinating account of the early history and characteristics of many psychoactive compounds is presented by Lewin (1924). More modern reviews are those of Efron and associates (1967), Caldwell (1978), and Schultes (1978). In 1845, Moreau proposed that hashish intoxication provided a model psychosis useful in the study of insanity. Three decades later, Freud presented his study of cocaine and suggested its potential uses in pharmacotherapy. Soon thereafter, Kraepelin founded the first laboratory of clinical psychopharmacology in Germany and evaluated psychological effects of drugs in man. In 1931, Sen and Bose published the first report of the use of *Rauwolfia serpentina* in the treatment of insanity (*see* Shore and Giachetti, 1978). Insulin shock, pentylenetetrazol-induced convulsions, and electroconvulsive therapy followed in 1933, 1934, and 1937, respectively. Treatment of both major depression and schizophrenia thus became available. Amphetamine was the first synthetic drug to provide a model psychosis. In 1943, Hofmann ingested a minute amount of lysergic acid diethylamide (LSD; lysergide) and experienced its psychic effects. His report of the high potency of LSD made more popular the concept that a toxic metabolic product might be a cause of mental illness. Accounts of this and other early experiments in psychopharmacology have been presented by the original participants (*see* Ayd and Blackwell, 1970).

The first modern report on the treatment of psychotic excitement or mania with lithium salts was that of Cade (1949). This discovery was slow in gaining general acceptance by the medical community. In 1950, chlorpromazine was synthesized in France. The recognition of the unique effects of chlorpromazine by Laborit and colleagues (1952) and its use in psychiatric patients by Delay and Deniker (1952) marked the beginnings of modern psychopharmacology. The history of this revolutionary era in psychiatric therapy is recounted by Ayd and Blackwell (1970), Swazey (1974), and Caldwell (1978). The term *tranquilizer* was introduced in the early 1950s by Yonkman to characterize the psychic effect of reserpine. Despite its popularity, this ambiguous and misleading term is not used in this chapter.

A report on meprobamate by Berger (1954) marked the beginning of investigations of modern sedatives with useful antianxiety properties. An antitubercular drug, iproniazid, was introduced in the early 1950s and was soon recognized as a monoamine oxidase inhibitor and antidepressant (Kline, 1958; Crane, 1959); in 1958, Kuhn recognized the antidepressant effect of imipramine. The first of the antianxiety benzodiazepines, chlordiazepoxide, was developed by Sternbach in 1957. In the following year Janssen discovered the antipsychotic properties of haloperidol, a butyrophenone (*see* Janssen, 1974), and thus still another class of antipsychotic agents became available. During the 1960s the expansion of psychopharmacological research was rapid, and many new theories of psychoactive drug effects were introduced. The clinical efficacy of many of these agents was firmly established during that decade.

In recent years, emphasis has centered on biogenic amines and their receptors in the CNS, their probable mediation of many effects of psychotropic drugs, and their possible causal involvement in mental illness. In addition, much attention is being paid to the liabilities of treatment with psychotherapeutic drugs, especially their limited efficacy in severe or chronic mental illnesses, their risk of sometimes serious toxic effects, and the limitations of screening and testing methods used to develop new agents, most of which offer few advantages over drugs available for four decades. A balanced view of their advantages and disadvantages is emerging. While not nearly the curative "wonder drugs" they promised to be initially, antipsychotic, mood-stabilizing, and antidepressant agents used to treat the most severe mental illnesses have had a remarkable impact on psychiatric practice and theory—an impact that can legitimately be called revolutionary.

Nosology. The several classes of therapeutic psychotropic agents are fairly selective in their ability to modify the symptoms of mental illnesses. The optimal use of such drugs thus requires experience in the differential diagnosis of psychiatric conditions (*see* Kaplan and Sadock, 1985; American Psychiatric Association, 1987). A few salient aspects of psychiatric nosology are summarized briefly here, and additional information is provided in the discussion of the specific classes of drugs.

A most important distinction is made between the *psychoses* and the less severe conditions commonly called the *neuroses* (or psychoneuroses). The psychoses are among the most severe psychiatric disorders, in which there is not only a marked impairment of behavior but also a serious inability to think coherently, to comprehend reality, or to gain insight into these abnormalities; the psychoses often include delusions and hallucinations. The psychotic disorders include organic conditions (notably, delirium and dementia), which typically are associated with definable toxic, metabolic, or neuropathologic changes and are characterized by confusion, disorientation, and memory disturbances as well as behavioral disorganization. Other psychotic conditions are designated as idiopathic (or "functional") disorders, for which underlying causes remain obscure. The latter are characterized by the retention of orientation and memory in the presence of severely disordered thought or reasoning, emotion, and behavior. Those primary disorders characterized by abnormal emotion or mood (depression, dysphoria, irritability, lability of emotion, elation, or mania) are called *major affective* or *manic-depressive disorders* (Pope and Lipinski, 1978; Baldessarini, 1983). These may ("bipolar" illnesses) or may not ("nonbipolar" illnesses) include periods of elation, irritability, or excitement alternating with severe depression and autonomic changes, notably insomnia or hypersomnia, anorexia, and altered daily rhythms of mood, activity, temperature, or neuroendocrine function. In addition, depression can occur as a milder disorder or as a symptom of other psychiatric or medical illnesses. The idiopathic psychoses characterized mainly by chronically disordered thinking and emotional withdrawal and often associated with paranoid delusions and auditory hallucinations are called *schizophrenia*. Acute or recurrent idiopathic psychoses also occur that bear an uncertain relationship to schizophrenia or the major affective disorders. In addition, there are disorders marked by more or less isolated delusions; these may represent a separate category of illness called *delusional disorder* or *paranoia*.

Antipsychotic drugs exert beneficial effects in virtually all classes of psychotic illness, and, contrary to a common misconception, are *not* selective for schizophrenia. Moreover, antidepressant drugs that are especially beneficial in severe depression can also exert useful effects on less severe depressive syndromes and on conditions that are not obviously depressive in nature (*e.g.*, panic attacks, bulimia nervosa, chronic pain, obsessive-compulsive disorder, and attention deficit–hyperactivity disorders). Thus, in general, psychotropic drugs are not disease-specific; they provide clinical benefit for specific syndromes or complexes of symptoms.

The less pervasive psychiatric disorders include notably the neuroses. While the ability to comprehend reality is retained, suffering and disability are sometimes very severe. Neuroses may be acute and transient or, more commonly, persistent or recurrent. Their symptoms may include mood changes (anxiety, panic, dysphoria) or limited abnormalities of thought (obsessions, irrational fears) or of behavior (rituals or compulsions, pseudoneurological or "hysterical" conversion signs). In such disorders, drugs may have some beneficial effects, particularly by modifying associated anxiety and depression.

Some so-called personality disorders may or may not respond to medical intervention; these conditions include characteristic personality styles (*e.g.*, avoidant, paranoid, withdrawn, dependent). Other disorders involve patterns of behavior (*e.g.*, abuse of alcohol or other substances, deviant eating patterns, hypochondriasis, antisocial or perverse behavior) that may run counter to societal expectations. Typically, drugs are not effective in such chronic conditions except when episodes of panic, anxiety, or depression occur; they may also be effective in some cases of bulimia or obsessive-compulsive disorder or in cases of withdrawal from addicting substances (*see* Chapter 22).

Biological Hypotheses in Mental Illness. The introduction in the 1950s of relatively effective and selective drugs for the management of schizophrenic and manic-depressive patients encouraged formulation of biological concepts of the pathogenesis of these major mental illnesses. In addition, other agents were discovered that mimic some of the symptoms of severe mental illnesses. These include LSD, which induces hallucinations and altered emotional states, and antihypertensive agents such as reserpine, which can cause depression. A leading hypothesis to arise from such considerations was based on data that indicated that antidepressants enhance the biological activity of monoamine neurotransmitters in the CNS and that antiadrenergic compounds may induce depression. These observations led to speculation that a deficiency of amine neurotransmission in the CNS might be causative of depression or that an excess could result in mania. Further, since antipsychotic agents antagonize the actions of dopamine as a neurotransmitter in the forebrain, it was proposed that there may be a state of functional overactivity of dopamine in the limbic system or cerebral cortex in schizophrenia or mania. Alternatively, an endogenous psychotomimetic compound might be produced either uniquely or in excessive quantities in psychotic patients.

This "pharmacocentric" approach to the construction of hypotheses is appealing and has gained support from studies of the actions of antipsychotic and antidepressant drugs over the past 4 decades. In turn, the plausibility of such biological hypotheses has encouraged interest in genetic studies, as well as in clinical biochemical studies. Despite extensive efforts, the attempts to document metabolic changes in human subjects predicted by these hypotheses have not, on balance, provided consistent or compelling corroboration (Baldessarini, 1983; Losonczy *et al.*, 1987; Meltzer and Lowy, 1987; Siever, 1987). Moreover, genetic studies have provided evidence that inheritance can account for only a portion of the causation of mental illnesses, leaving room for environmental and psychological hypotheses. Thus, the hopes of the 1950s and 1960s for the discovery of clearly defined, genetically determined inborn errors of metabolism to explain psychiatric disease have not yet been realized.

The antipsychotic, antimanic, and antidepressant drugs have effects on cortical, limbic, hypothalamic, and brainstem mechanisms that are of fundamental importance in the regulation of arousal, consciousness, affect, and autonomic functions. It is entirely possible that physiological and pharmacological modification of these brain regions has important behavioral consequences and useful clinical effects regardless of the fundamental nature or cause of the mental disorder in question.

Even if the most generous interpretations of the actions of psychotropic drugs could be taken to provide insights into the clinical pathophysiology or the etiology of mental illnesses, many other serious problems remain. They include biological heterogeneity, even within groups of the most carefully diagnosed patients. In addition, the lack of disease specificity of psychotropic drugs tends to minimize the chances of finding a discrete metabolic correlate for a specific disease. Finally, the technical problems associated with attempts to study changes in the metabolism or the postmortem chemistry of the human CNS are formidable. Among these are artifacts introduced by drug treatment itself.

In summary, the available information does not permit a conclusion as to whether crucial, discrete biological lesions are the basis of the most severe mental illnesses (other than the deliria and dementias). Moreover, it is not necessary to presume that such a basis is operative in order to provide effective medical treatment for psychiatric patients. Furthermore, it would be clinical folly to underestimate the importance of psychological and social factors in the manifestations of mental illnesses or to overlook psychological aspects of the conduct of biological therapies (Baldessarini, 1985).

Evaluation of Psychotropic Drugs. Although evaluating the efficacy of any drug is problematic, the difficulties in evaluating psychoactive drugs are particularly severe. The essential characteristics of human mental disorders cannot be reproduced in animals. Cognition, communication, and social relationships in animals are difficult to compare with human achievements in these areas. Thus, screening procedures in animals are of limited utility for the discovery of unique therapeutic agents. In addition, clinical evaluation of new drugs is hampered by inhomogeneity of diagnostic groups and difficulty in application of valid, sensitive measurements of the effects of therapy. As a consequence, the results of clinical trials of psychotropic agents are sometimes equivocal or inconsistent. Reviews of the principles and problems in establishing the efficacy and safety of psychotropic drugs are available (Hardesty and Burdock, 1978; Baldessarini, 1983, 1985).

I. Drugs Used in the Treatment of Psychoses

Several classes of drugs are effective in the symptomatic treatment of psychoses. They are most appropriately used in the therapy of schizophrenia, organic psychoses, the manic phase of manic-depressive illness, and other acute idiopathic psychotic illnesses. Their occasional use may be indicated in severe depression with psychotic features and in the management of patients with organic psychotic disorders. Effective antipsychotic compounds include the *phenothiazines,* structurally similar *thioxanthenes,* and *dibenzodiazepines* and *dibenzoxazepines;* the *butyrophenones* (phenylbutylpiperidines) and *diphenylbutylpiperidines;* the *indolones* and other heterocyclic compounds; and the less effective *rauwolfia alkaloids* and related amine-depleting agents. Since these chemically dissimilar drugs share many properties, information about their pharmacology and clinical uses is presented for the group as a whole. Particular attention is paid to chlorpromazine, the oldest representative of the phenothiazine-thioxanthene group of antipsychotic agents, and haloperidol, the original butyrophenone and representative of several related classes of aromatic butylpiperidine derivatives.

The use of antipsychotic (neuroleptic) agents is widespread, as is evident from the fact that hundreds of millions of patients have been treated with them since their introduction in the 1950s. Although the antipsychotic drugs have had a revolutionary, beneficial impact on medical and psychiatric practice, their liabilities, especially their almost relentless association with extrapyramidal neurological effects, must also be emphasized (*see* Baldessarini, 1984b, 1985; Tarsy and Baldessarini, 1986).

PHENOTHIAZINES AND OTHER ANTIPSYCHOTIC AGENTS

Antipsychotic agents are primarily used in the management of patients with psychotic or other serious psychiatric illnesses. However, these drugs have other clinically useful properties, including antiemetic, antinausea, and antihistaminic effects and the ability to potentiate analgesics, sedatives, and general anesthetics; many of these actions are discussed elsewhere in this text (*see* Index). At the present time, more than three dozen neuroleptic drugs are used in psychiatric conditions; still others are marketed primarily for other uses.

History. The history of the antipsychotic agents is especially well summarized by Swazey (1974) and Caldwell (1978). In the early 1950s, some antipsychotic effects were obtained with natural extracts of the *Rauwolfia* plant and then with large doses of pure reserpine, which was isolated, characterized, and synthesized by Woodward. Although reserpine and related compounds that share its ability to deplete monoamines from their vesicular storage sites in neurons exert antipsychotic effects, these are relatively weak and are typically associated with severe side effects, including hypotension and psychotic depression. Thus, the clinical utility of reserpine has primarily been as an antihypertensive agent (*see* Chapter 33).

Phenothiazine compounds were synthesized in Europe in the late nineteenth century as part of the development of aniline dyes such as methylene blue. In the late 1930s a phenothiazine derivative, promethazine, was found to have antihistaminic and strong sedative effects. Attempts to treat agitation in psychiatric patients with promethazine and other antihistamines followed in the 1940s, but with little success.

Meanwhile, the ability of promethazine to prolong barbiturate sleeping time in rodents was discovered, and the drug was introduced into clinical anesthesia as a potentiating agent (Laborit *et al.,* 1952). This work prompted a search for other phenothiazine derivatives with anesthesia-potentiating actions, and in 1949–1950 Charpentier synthesized chlorpromazine. Soon thereafter, Laborit and colleagues described the ability of this compound to potentiate anesthetics and produce "artificial hibernation." Chlorpromazine by itself did not cause a loss of consciousness but produced only diminished arousal and a tendency to sleep. These central actions became known as *ataractic* or *neuroleptic.*

The first attempts to treat mental illness with chlorpromazine alone were made in Paris in 1951 and early 1952 by Paraire and Sigwald. In 1952, Delay and Deniker began their important early work with chlorpromazine. They were convinced that chlorpromazine achieved more than symptomatic relief of agitation or anxiety and that it had an ameliorative effect upon psychotic processes with diverse symptomatology. In 1954, Lehmann and Hanrahan reported the initial use of chlorpromazine in North America for the treatment of psychomotor excitement and manic states. Clinical studies soon revealed that the most important use of chlorpromazine was in the treatment of psychotic states.

Chemistry and Structure–Activity Relationship. This topic has been reviewed by Biel and coworkers (1978). Phenothiazine has a three-ring structure in which two benzene rings are linked by a sulfur and a nitrogen atom (*see* Table 18–1, page 396). If the nitrogen at position 10 is replaced by a carbon atom with a double bond to the side chain, the compound becomes a thioxanthene.

Substitution of an electron-withdrawing group at position 2 increases the efficacy of phenothiazines and other tricyclic congeners. The nature of the substituent at position 10 also influences pharmacological activity. As can be seen in Table 18–1, the phenothiazines and thioxanthenes can be divided into three groups on the basis of substitution at this site. The group with an *aliphatic* side chain includes chlorpromazine and triflupromazine among the phenothiazines; these compounds are relatively low in potency (but not in clinical efficacy). Those with a *piperidine* moiety in the side chain include thioridazine and mesoridazine. There appears to be a lower incidence of extrapyramidal side effects with this substitution, at least in the case of thioridazine, possibly due to increased antimuscarinic activity. The most potent phenothiazine antipsychotic compounds have a *piperazine* (or piperazinyl) group; fluphenazine and trifluoperazine are examples. Use of these potent compounds entails a greater risk of inducing acute extrapyramidal effects but less tendency to produce sedation or autonomic side effects such as hypotension, unless unusually large doses are employed. Several piperazine phenothiazines have been esterified with long-chain fatty acids to produce slowly absorbed and hydrolyzed, long-acting, lipophilic prodrugs. Fluphenazine enanthate and decanoate are the only such derivatives currently available in the United States; the decanoate of haloperidol is also available.

The thioxanthenes are also available with aliphatic and piperazine substituents. The analog of chlorpromazine among the thioxanthenes is chlorprothixene. The piperazine-substituted thioxanthenes include clopenthixol, flupentixol, piflutixol, and thiothixene; they are all potent and effective antipsychotic agents, although only thiothixene is currently available in the United States. Since thioxanthenes have an olefinic double bond between the central-ring carbon atom at position 10 and the side chain, geometric isomers exist; the *cis* (or α) isomers are the more active.

The phenothiazines and thioxanthenes used in psychiatry have three carbon atoms interposed between position 10 of the central ring and the first amino nitrogen atom of the side chain at this position; in addition, the amine is always tertiary. This structure of neuroleptic compounds contrasts with that of antihistaminic phenothiazines (*e.g.*, promethazine) or strongly anticholinergic phenothiazines (*e.g.*, ethopropazine, diethazine), which have only two carbon atoms separating the amino group from position 10 of the central ring; addition of a fourth carbon atom also results in a loss of neuroleptic activity. When one or two of the methyl or other substituents of the tertiary amino group of the side chain are removed (as can occur in the natural metabolism of chlorpromazine), there is a progressive loss of activity; increasing the size of amino N-alkyl substituents also leads to a reduction of activity.

The structure–activity relationship has also been studied in detail for butyrophenones and their congeners. The largest group of butyrophenones includes substituted piperidine compounds that are analogs of haloperidol. Among these is spiperone, one of the most potent neuroleptics yet discovered. In addition, there are several investigational piperazine-substituted butyrophenones and a short-acting tetrahydropyridine derivative, droperidol, which is used almost exclusively in anesthesia because of its marked sedative properties.

A closely related family of drugs are the diphenylbutylpiperidines. These compounds include pimozide, fluspirilene, and penfluridol; pimozide is available in the United States, primarily for the treatment of Tourette's syndrome. These agents are both very potent and long-acting (several days to a week or more) even after oral administration, unlike most other neuroleptic agents.

Several other classes of heterocyclic compounds have neuroleptic or antipsychotic effects, but too few are available or sufficiently well characterized to permit conclusions regarding structure–activity relationships (*see* Neumeyer, 1989). These include a small number of indole compounds (notably, molindone and oxypertine) and several piperazine-substituted tricyclic compounds with various seven-membered central rings. These latter agents bear some resemblance to the imipramine-like antidepressant drugs and include dibenzoxazepines (notably, loxapine, a typical neuroleptic) and dibenzodiazepines (notably, clozapine, a so-called "atypical" antipsychotic agent that seems to have minimal central antidopaminergic activity). Other congeners, such as fluperlapine, remain experimental.

Other heterocyclic compounds include butaclamol, a pentacyclic compound with active (dextrorotatory) and inactive enantiomeric forms that have been useful in characterization of the stereochemistry of the sites of action of neuroleptic agents. Sulpiride is one of a series of substituted benzamides (which includes metoclopramide) with some neuroleptic activity. However, their hydrophilic properties may account for their limited penetration into the CNS and their low potency. Newer experimental benzamides (*e.g.*, raclopride) are in clinical trials. The availability of drugs such as clozapine, sulpiride, and, to some extent, thioridazine is encouraging, since they represent at least partial exceptions to the association of neurological side effects with antipsychotic actions.

PHARMACOLOGICAL PROPERTIES

The antipsychotic drugs share many pharmacological effects and therapeutic applications. Chlorpromazine and haloperidol are commonly taken as prototypes for the group. Many antipsychotic drugs, and especially chlorpromazine and other agents of low potency, have sedative effects. These are especially conspicuous early in treatment, although tolerance to this effect is typical; sedation may not be noticeable when very agitated psychotic patients are treated. Antipsychotic drugs also have antianxiety effects. However, this class of agents is not generally used for such a purpose, largely because of their autonomic and neurological side effects, which paradoxically can include severe anxiety and restlessness (akathisia).

The term *neuroleptic,* which was introduced to denote the effects of chlorpromazine and reserpine on psychiatric patients, was intended to contrast the effects of these agents with those of classical CNS depressants. The neuroleptic syndrome consists in suppression of spontaneous movements and complex behavior, while spinal reflexes and unconditioned nociceptive-avoidance behaviors remain intact. In man, the neuroleptic drugs reduce initiative and interest in the environment, and they reduce displays of emotion or affect. Initially, there may be some slowness in response to external stimuli and drowsiness. However, subjects are easily aroused, capable of giving appropriate answers to direct questions, and seem to have intact intellectual functions; ataxia, incoordination, or dysarthria do not occur at ordinary doses. Typically, psychotic patients soon become less agitated and restless, and withdrawn or autistic patients sometimes become more responsive and communicative. Aggressive and impulsive behavior diminishes. Gradually (usually over a period of days), psychotic symptoms of hallucinations, delusions, and disorganized or incoherent thinking tend to disappear. Early clinical reports of the effects of chlorpromazine also described neurological effects, including bradykinesia, mild rigidity, some tremor, and occasional subjective restlessness (akathisia), that resemble those of Parkinson's disease.

Although the original use of the term *neuroleptic* appears to have encompassed the whole unique syndrome just described and is widely used as a synonym for *antipsychotic*, there is now a tendency to use the term *neuroleptic* to emphasize the more neurological aspects of the syndrome (*i.e.*, the parkinsonian and other extrapyramidal effects). The description of drugs such as clozapine that are clearly antipsychotic and have little extrapyramidal action has reinforced this trend. At the present time, virtually all antipsychotic drugs available in the United States also have effects on movement and posture and can thus be called neuroleptic. However, the more general and hopeful term *antipsychotic* is commonly used and may be preferable.

General Psychophysiological and Behavioral Effects. In animals and in man, the most prominent observable effects of typical neuroleptic agents are strikingly similar. In low doses, operant behavior is reduced but spinal reflexes are unchanged. Exploratory behavior is diminished, and responses to a variety of stimuli are fewer, slower, and smaller, although the ability to discriminate stimuli is retained. Conditioned avoidance behaviors are selectively inhibited, while unconditioned escape or avoidance responses are not. Highly reinforcing self-stimulation of the animal brain (typically with electrodes placed in the monoamine-rich medial forebrain bundle) is blocked, although the capacity to press the stimulation-inducing lever is not lost. Behavioral activation, stimulated environmentally or pharmacologically, is blocked. Feeding is inhibited. Most neuroleptics block the emesis, hyperactivity, and aggression induced by apomorphine and other dopaminergic agonists. In high doses, most neuroleptic agents induce characteristic cataleptic immobility that allows the animal to be placed in abnormal postures that persist. Muscle tone is increased, and ptosis is typical. The animal appears to be indifferent to most stimuli, although it continues to withdraw from those that are noxious or painful. Many learned tasks can still be performed if sufficient stimulation and motivation are provided. Even very high doses of most neuroleptics do not induce coma, and the lethal dose is extraordinarily high. Many of these effects are well summarized by Fielding and Lal (1978).

Effects on Motor Activity. Nearly all of the neuroleptic agents used in psychiatry can diminish spontaneous motor activity in every species of animal studied, including man. However, one of the more disturbing side effects of these agents in man, akathisia, is manifested by an increase in restless activity. The cataleptic immobility of animals treated with neuroleptics, described above, resembles the catatonia seen in some psychotic patients and in a variety of metabolic and neurological disorders affecting the CNS. In man, catatonic signs, along with other features of schizophrenia, are sometimes relieved by antipsychotic agents. However, rigidity and bradykinesia, which can mimic catatonia, can be induced in patients, especially by large doses of the more potent neuroleptic agents, and reversed by removal of the drug or the addition of an antiparkinsonian agent (*see* Fielding and Lal, 1978; Janssen and Van Bever, 1978).

Phenothiazines and other antipsychotic drugs characteristically produce parkinsonism and other extrapyramidal effects. Theories concerning the mechanisms underlying these extrapyramidal reactions, as well as descriptions of their clinical presentations and management, are given below.

Chlorpromazine causes skeletal muscular relaxation in some types of spastic conditions. Since it has little effect at spinal levels, actions on motor activity must be mediated at a higher level, perhaps in the basal ganglia. The drug does not produce blockade of the neuromuscular junction.

Effects on Sleep. The effect of antipsychotic drugs on sleep patterns is not consistent, but they tend to normalize sleep disturbances characteristic of many psychoses. The ability to prolong and enhance the effect of opioid and hypnotic drugs appears to parallel the sedative rather than the neuroleptic potency of the particular agent. Thus, the more potent neuroleptic agents that do not cause drowsiness also do not enhance hypnosis produced by other drugs.

Effects on Conditioned Responses. Chlorpromazine and other neuroleptics impair the ability of animals to make a conditioned avoidance response to a learned sensory cue that signals the onset of punishing shock avoidable by moving to a safe place in an experimental chamber. Under the influence of small doses of these drugs, animals ignore the warning signal but still attempt to escape once the shock is applied. General CNS depressants affect both avoidance (the conditioned response) and escape (the unconditioned response) to approximately the same extent, and only in doses that produce ataxia or hypnosis. Passive avoidance behavior, requiring immobility, is also suppressed by neuroleptic drugs, in contrast to what might be expected in the case of drugs that suppress locomotion nonspecifically.

Since correlations between antipsychotic effectiveness and conditioned avoidance tests are quite good for many types of neuroleptic agents, they have become an important basis for screening procedures in pharmaceutical psychopharmacology laboratories. Despite their empirical utility and quantitative characteristics, effects on conditioned avoidance have not provided important insights into the basis of antipsychotic effects in man. For example, the effects of neuroleptic drugs on conditioned avoidance are subject to tolerance and are blocked by anticholinergic agents, while their clinical antipsychotic actions are not. Moreover, the extraordinarily close correlation between the potencies of drugs in conditioned avoidance tests and their ability to block the behavioral effects of dopaminergic agonists such as amphetamine or apomorphine suggests that such avoidance tests may be specifically selective for drugs with extrapyramidal and other neurological effects. The limited ability of the atypical and perhaps more selective antipsychotic drugs, such as clozapine and sulpiride, to antagonize dopamine agonists or to block conditioned avoidance responses in animal behavioral tests also supports this interpretation. (*See* Barchas *et al.*, 1978; Fielding and Lal, 1978; Janssen and Van Bever, 1978.)

Effects on Complex Behavior. Antipsychotic drugs impair vigilance in human subjects performing a variety of tasks, such as continuous rotor-pursuit and tapping-speed tests. The drugs produce relatively little impairment of digit-symbol substitution, a test of intellectual functioning. On the other hand, secobarbital causes greater impairment in performance in digit-symbol substitution than in continuous performance and other vigilance tests.

Effects on Specific Areas of the Nervous System. The effects of antipsychotic drugs are apparent at all levels in the nervous system. Although the actions underlying the antipsychotic and many of the neurological effects of antipsychotic drugs remain uncertain, theories based on their ability to antagonize the actions of dopamine as a neurotransmitter in the basal ganglia and limbic portions of the forebrain have become most prominent and are supported by a large body of data.

Cortex. Since psychosis involves a disorder of higher functions and thought processes, cortical effects of antipsychotic drugs are of great interest. Much attention has been drawn to the effects of neuroleptics on dopaminergic projections to the prefrontal and deep-temporal (limbic) regions of the cerebral cortex and to the relative sparing of these areas from adaptive changes in dopamine metabolism that are suggestive of tolerance to actions of neuroleptics. However, little information is available about specific effects on the cortex that sheds light on the mechanisms of action of antipsychotic drugs.

Seizure Threshold. Many neuroleptic drugs can lower the seizure threshold and induce discharge patterns in the EEG that are associated with epileptic seizure disorders. Aliphatic phenothiazines with low potency (such as chlorpromazine) seem particularly able to do this, while the more potent piperazine phenothiazines and thioxanthenes (notably, fluphenazine and thiothixene) seem least likely to have this effect (Itil, 1978). The butyrophenones have variable and unpredictable effects on seizure activity; molindone may have the least activity of this type. Overt seizures associated with the administration of antipsychotic drugs are more likely to be seen in patients who have either a history of epilepsy or a condition that predisposes to seizures. Neuroleptic agents, especially low-potency phenothiazines and thioxanthenes, should be used with *extreme caution,* if at all, in untreated epileptic patients and in patients undergoing withdrawal from central depressants such as alcohol or barbiturates. Antipsychotic drugs, especially the piperazines, can be used safely in epileptics if moderate doses are attained gradually and if concomitant anticonvulsant drug therapy is maintained (*see* Chapter 19).

Basal Ganglia. Because the extrapyramidal effects of nearly all of the clinically used antipsychotic drugs are prominent, a great deal of interest has centered on the actions of these drugs in the basal ganglia, notably the caudate nucleus, putamen, globus pallidus, and allied nuclei, which play a crucial role in the control of posture and the involuntary (extrapyramidal) aspects of movement. Current understanding of the role of a deficiency of dopamine in this region in the pathogenesis of Parkinson's disease, the demonstration that neuroleptic agents act as antagonists of dopaminergic receptors, and the striking resemblance between the clinical manifestations of Parkinson's disease and the neurological effects of neuroleptic drugs, all have focused attention on the role of a deficiency of dopamine activity in some of the neuroleptic-induced extrapyramidal effects.

The hypothesis that interference with the transmitter function of dopamine in the mammalian forebrain might contribute to the neurological and possibly also the antipsychotic effects of the neuroleptic drugs arose from the observation that neuroleptic drugs consistently increased the concentrations of the metabolites of dopamine but had variable effects on the metabolism of other neurotransmitters. The importance of dopamine was also supported by histochemical studies, which indicated a preferential distribution of dopamine-containing fibers between midbrain and the basal ganglia (notably, the nigroneostriatal tract), and within the hypothalamus (*see* Chapter 12). Other dopamine-containing neurons project from midbrain tegmental nuclei to forebrain regions associated with the limbic system, as well as to temporal and prefrontal cerebral cortical areas closely related to the limbic system. A somewhat simplistic, but attractive, concept arose: many extrapyramidal neurological effects of the antipsychotic drugs might be mediated by antidopaminergic effects in the basal ganglia. Their antipsychotic effects might be mediated by antagonism of dopaminergic neurotransmission in the limbic, mesocortical, and hypothalamic systems.

Antagonism of dopamine-mediated synaptic neurotransmission is an important action of neuroleptic drugs (Carlsson, 1978; Creese *et al.,* 1978; Baldessarini and Tarsy, 1979). Thus, drugs with neuroleptic actions, but not their inactive congeners, increase the rate of production of dopamine metabolites, the rate of conversion of the precursor amino acid tyrosine to dopamine and its metabolites, and the rate of firing of putative dopamine-containing cells in the midbrain. These effects have usually been interpreted to represent adaptive responses of neuronal systems that tend to reduce the impact of the presumed interruption of synaptic transmission at dopaminergic terminals in the forebrain. Supporting evidence for such an interpretation includes the observation that small doses of neuroleptic drugs block behavioral or neuroendocrine effects of dopaminergic agonists. An example is stereotypical gnawing behavior in the rat induced by apomorphine. Neuroleptic drugs also block the effects of agonists on a dopamine-sensitive adenylyl cyclase system in caudate and limbic tissue. Notably, atypical antipsychotic drugs such as clozapine are characterized by their relative lack of action in such tests.

Radioligand-binding assays for dopaminergic receptors have been used to define more precisely the mechanism of action of neuroleptic agents. These assays use membrane fractions, typically from mammalian caudate tissue, as a source of receptors and radiolabeled neuroleptic drugs or dopaminergic agonists as ligands (*see* Creese *et al.*, 1978; Snyder *et al.*, 1978; Seeman, 1980; Faedda *et al.*, 1989). Estimates of the clinical potency of most types of antipsychotic drugs correlate best with their relative potency *in vitro* to inhibit binding of these ligands to putative D_2-dopaminergic sites (*see* Chapter 12). This correlation is obscured to some extent by the additional correlation between clinical potency and the relative ease with which compounds reach the CNS (Sunderland and Cohen, 1987). Nevertheless, almost all of the clinically effective antipsychotic agents have characteristically high affinity for D_2 sites. Although some neuroleptics (especially the thioxanthenes and some phenothiazines) bind avidly to D_1 sites, those with relatively high affinity for D_1 receptors also bind to and block D_2 receptors (Peroutka and Snyder, 1980b; Faedda *et al.*, 1989). The butyrophenones (*e.g.*, haloperidol) are relatively selective, and the benzamides (*e.g.*, sulpiride) have very high selectivity for D_2 receptors (Seeman, 1980). Atypical antipsychotic agents such as clozapine have weak antidopaminergic activity and little propensity to produce extrapyramidal side effects; they are, however, potent α_1-adrenergic antagonists, as are many other antipsychotic agents (Peroutka and Snyder, 1980b; Cohen and Lipinski, 1986a). Agents with selective antiadrenergic actions in the CNS have not been evaluated for potential antipsychotic efficacy.

Thus, many antipsychotic drugs interfere with the actions of dopamine as a neurotransmitter. Although their antidopaminergic effects may well account for the diverse extrapyramidal effects of the neuroleptic drugs, the properties of agents such as clozapine cast some doubt on the necessity for dopaminergic antagonism in order to produce antipsychotic actions.

Limbic System. Dopaminergic projections from the midbrain terminate on septal nuclei, the olfactory tubercle, the amygdala, and other structures within the temporal and prefrontal lobes of the cerebrum. Because of the dopamine hypothesis just reviewed, much attention has also been given to the mesolimbic and mesocortical systems as possible sites of mediation of some of the antipsychotic effects of these agents. Speculations about the pathophysiology of the idiopathic psychoses such as schizophrenia have for many years centered around the limbic area. Such speculation has been given indirect encouragement by repeated "natural experiments" that have associated psychotic mental phenomena with lesions of the temporal lobe and other portions of the limbic system (*see* Losonczy *et al.*, 1987).

Many of the behavioral, neurophysiological, biochemical, and pharmacological findings about the dopaminergic system of the basal ganglia have been extended to mesolimbic and mesocortical tissue. Certain important effects of antipsychotic drugs are similar in extrapyramidal and limbic regions, including those on ligand-binding assays for dopaminergic receptors (Creese *et al.*, 1978). However, the extrapyramidal and antipsychotic actions of the neuroleptic drugs differ in a number of ways. For example, while several of the acute extrapyramidal effects of neuroleptic drugs tend to diminish or to disappear with time or when anticholinergic drugs are administered concurrently, this is not characteristic of the antipsychotic effects. However, it must be recalled that different dopaminergic systems are not identical, either functionally or in the physiological regulation of their responses to drugs (*see* Bunney and Aghajanian, 1978; Moore and Kelly, 1978; Sulser and Robinson, 1978; Wolf and Roth, 1987). For example, while anticholinergic agents block the increase in turnover of dopamine in the basal ganglia induced by neuroleptic agents, they seem not to do so in limbic areas containing dopaminergic terminals. Further, the development of tolerance to the effect of antipsychotic drugs to enhance the turnover of dopamine is not as prominent in limbic as in extrapyramidal areas. For further discussions of this topic, *see* Carlsson (1978).

Hypothalamus. In addition to neurological and antipsychotic effects that appear to be mediated in part by antidopaminergic actions of the neuroleptic drugs, endocrine changes occur, owing to effects of these agents on the hypothalamus or pituitary, that may also involve dopamine. Prominent among these is the ability of most neuroleptic drugs to increase the secretion of prolactin in man.

The effect of neuroleptic agents on prolactin secretion is probably due to a blockade of the tuberoinfundibular dopaminergic system that projects from the arcuate nucleus of the hypothalamus to the median eminence by a direct antagonistic action at dopaminergic receptors localized on cells of the anterior pituitary. The existence of D_2-dopaminergic receptors in the pituitary itself, as well as morphological evidence of an intimate relationship between dopamine-containing neurosecretory terminals in the median eminence and the small blood vessels of the hypophyseal portal system, supports the hypothesis that dopamine is the prolactin release-inhibiting hormone known to exist in the hypothalamus (*see* Reichlin and Boyd, 1978; *see also* Chapter 56).

Correlations between the potencies of neuroleptic drugs to stimulate prolactin secretion and to cause behavioral effects are excellent, and they prevail for many classes of drugs (Meltzer *et al.*, 1978; Sachar, 1978). There are, however, a few discrepancies. The effects of neuroleptic drugs on prolactin secretion tend to occur at lower doses than do their antipsychotic effects; this may reflect their action outside the blood–brain barrier in the inferior hypothalamus or in the pituitary gland. Little or no tolerance develops to the effect of antipsychotic drugs on prolactin, even after years of treatment. However, the effect is rapidly reversible when the drugs are discontinued (Overall, 1978). This effect of antipsychotic agents is presumed to be responsible for the breast engorgement and galactorrhea that is sometimes associated with their use, even in male patients.

The effects of neuroleptics on other hypothalamic neuroendocrine functions are much less well characterized, although it is known that they inhibit the release of growth hormone and chlorpromazine may reduce the secretion of corticotropin-regulatory hormone in response to stress. In addition to neuroendocrine effects, it is likely that the other autonomic effects of some antipsychotic drugs may be mediated by the hypothalamus. An important example is the poikilothermic effect of chlorpromazine, which impairs the ability to regulate body temperature such that hypo- or hyperthermia may result, depending on the ambient temperature.

Brainstem. Clinical doses of the neuroleptics usually have little effect on respiration. However, vasomotor reflexes mediated by either the hypothalamus or the brainstem are depressed by relatively low doses of chlorpromazine. This effect might occur at many points in the reflex pathway, and the net result is a centrally mediated fall in blood pressure. Even in cases of acute overdosage with suicidal intent, the phenothiazines usually do not cause life-threatening coma or suppression of vital functions; this contributes importantly to their safety.

Chemoreceptor Trigger Zone (CTZ). Most neuroleptic agents have a marked protective action against the nausea- and emesis-inducing effects of apomorphine and certain ergot alkaloids, all of which can interact with central dopaminergic receptors in the CTZ of the medulla. The antiemetic effect of most neuroleptics occurs with very low doses. However, thioridazine, uniquely, has no clinical efficacy as an antiemetic in man. Drugs or other stimuli that cause emesis by an action on the nodose ganglion or locally on the gastrointestinal tract are not antagonized by antipsychotic drugs, but potent piperazines and butyrophenones are sometimes effective against nausea caused by vestibular stimulation. Several antipsychotic agents have become especially popular for the treatment of nausea and vomiting (*see* Chapter 38).

Autonomic Nervous System. Since various antipsychotic agents have peripheral cholinergic blocking activity, α-adrenergic blocking actions, and adrenergic activity (secondary to the block of neuronal reuptake of amines), their effects on the autonomic nervous system are complex and unpredictable. Antihistaminic and antitryptaminergic effects of these agents further complicate the picture.

Chlorpromazine has significant α-adrenergic antagonistic activity and can block the pressor effects of norepinephrine. The relative potencies of several antipsychotic drugs as α-adrenergic antagonists can be ranked as follows: relatively strong (piperacetazine > droperidol > triflupromazine > chlorpromazine); moderate (thioridazine > fluphenazine > haloperidol); relatively weak (trifluoperazine > clozapine > pimozide). Since piperazines and haloperidol are used in low doses to produce antipsychotic effects, it follows that they should show little antiadrenergic activity in patients; indeed, this seems to be true (*see* Creese *et al.*, 1978; Janssen and Van Bever, 1978; Snyder *et al.*, 1978).

The cholinergic blocking effects of antipsychotic drugs are relatively weak, but the blurring of vision commonly experienced with chlorpromazine may be due to an anticholinergic action on the ciliary muscle. Chlorpromazine regularly produces miosis in man, which can be due to α-adrenergic blockade. Other phenothiazines can cause mydriasis; this is especially likely to occur with thioridazine, which is the most potent muscarinic antagonist of the group. Chlorpromazine has intermediate antimuscarinic potency and can cause constipation and decreased gastric secretion and motility. Decreased sweating and salivation are probably additional manifestations of the anticholinergic effects of the phenothiazines. Urinary retention is rare, but can occur in males with prostatism. Anticholinergic effects are least frequently caused by piperazines and other potent neuroleptics, including haloperidol (*see* Snyder *et al.*, 1978). The anticholinergic status of clozapine remains controversial; it is very potent in several tests *in vitro* but does not seem to be active *in vivo*.

The phenothiazines inhibit ejaculation without interfering with erection. Thioridazine produces this effect with some regularity, sometimes limiting its acceptance by male patients. Attribution of this effect to adrenergic blockade is logical but unsubstantiated inasmuch as thioridazine is less potent than chlorpromazine in its antiadrenergic effects.

For further discussion of the autonomic pharmacology of the phenothiazines, *see* Gordon (1974) and Klein and colleagues (1980).

Endocrine System. The effects of neuroleptic drugs on hypothalamic regulatory hormones result in profound changes in the endocrine system, as mentioned above with respect to increased secretion of prolactin. As a result of the latter derangement, galactorrhea and gynecomastia can occur. Chlorpromazine can also reduce urinary concentrations of gonadotropins, as well as those of estrogens and progestins. This action may contribute to the amenorrhea that is sometimes seen in women treated with chlorpromazine.

Since antipsychotic drugs are used chronically and thus cause prolonged elevations of concentrations of prolactin, concern has arisen over a possible increased risk of carcinoma of the breast. To date, there is no evidence that the use of antipsychotic agents entails this risk (Overall, 1978; Schyve *et al.*, 1978). Nevertheless, neuroleptic and other agents that stimulate the secretion of prolactin should be avoided in patients with established carcinoma of the breast.

Nonreproductive endocrinological functions are also affected. Chlorpromazine may cause a decrease in the secretion of adrenocorticosteroids as a result of diminished release of corticotropin. It interferes with the secretion of pituitary growth hormone, but neuroleptics are poor therapy for acromegaly. There is no evidence that neuroleptics retard growth or development of children. In addition, chlorpromazine can decrease the secretion of neurohypophyseal hormones. Weight gain and an increase in appetite occur with all phenothiazines but perhaps less with haloperidol and molindone. Chlorpromazine may also impair glucose tolerance and insulin release to a clinically appreciable degree in some "prediabetic" patients (Erle *et al.*, 1977); however, this effect is not known to occur with other neuroleptic agents. Peripheral edema occurs in 1 to 3% of patients and may be of endocrine origin.

Kidney. Chlorpromazine may have weak diuretic effects in animals and man, owing either to a depressant action on the secretion of antidiuretic hormone (ADH), to inhibition of reabsorption of water and electrolytes by a direct action on the renal tubule, or to both. The slight fall in blood pressure that occurs with chlorpromazine is not associated with a significant change in glomerular filtration rate; indeed, renal blood flow tends to increase.

Cardiovascular System. The actions of chlorpromazine on the cardiovascular system are complex because the drug produces direct effects on the heart and blood vessels, and also indirect ones through actions on CNS and autonomic reflexes. In normal man, the intravenous administration of chlorpromazine causes orthostatic hypotension, due to a combination of central actions and peripheral α-adrenergic blockade, and reflex tachycardia. Oral therapy causes mild hypotension, systolic blood pressure being affected more than diastolic. Tolerance develops to the hypotensive effect, so that after several weeks of administration the pressures return toward normal. However, some degree of orthostatic hypotension may persist indefinitely, especially in elderly patients (*see* Ray *et al.*, 1987). Orthostatic hypotension occurs more frequently with chlorpromazine and thioridazine, and less so with piperazine derivatives, haloperidol, loxapine, or molindone. Because of its vasodilating action due both to its effects on the autonomic nervous system and to a direct action on blood vessels, chlorpromazine may increase coronary blood flow.

Chlorpromazine has a direct negative inotropic action and a quinidine-like antiarrhythmic effect on the heart. ECG changes include prolongation of the Q–T and P–R intervals, blunting of T waves, and depression of the S–T segment. Thioridazine, in particular, causes a high incidence of Q–T and T wave changes and can produce ventricular arrhythmias and sudden death. These effects are uncommon when potent antipsychotic agents are administered.

Liver. Aside from the hypersensitivity reactions occasionally seen after administration of the antipsychotic drugs, such as an obstructive form of jaundice (*see* below), these agents have no characteristic hepatic effects. The drugs may be used in patients with hepatic disease, but caution is advisable. Since their metabolism may be delayed or modified, they may compromise an already diseased liver.

Miscellaneous Pharmacological Effects. There are reports of interactions of antipsychotic drugs with central neurohumors other than dopamine that may contribute to their antipsychotic effects or other actions (*see* Carlsson, 1978). For example, many neuroleptics enhance the turnover of acetylcholine, especially in the basal ganglia, perhaps secondary to the blockade of dopamine receptors on cholinergic neurons. In addition, as discussed above, there is an inverse relationship between antimuscarinic potency of antipsychotic drugs in the brain and the likelihood of extrapyramidal effects (Snyder *et al.*, 1978). Although chlorpromazine and a few other low-potency phenothiazines have mild antagonistic actions at receptors for histamine, this effect is not shared by all antipsychotic drugs. Antagonistic interactions are also known to occur at receptors for 5-hydroxytryptamine (5-HT), including those designated as 5-HT_2 in the forebrain. The significance of this effect is not certain, but several experimental agents have been developed with relatively potent and selective 5-HT_2 antagonistic activity (*e.g.*, ketanserin); their status as antipsychotic agents is unproven.

Absorption, Distribution, Fate, and Excretion. The study of the pharmacokinetics and metabolism of the antipsychotic drugs has been an active aspect of their evaluation. A few generalizations with clinical relevance can be drawn. Some antipsychotic drugs tend to have erratic and unpredictable patterns of absorption, particularly after oral administration and even when liquid preparations are used. Parenteral (intramuscular) administration can increase the bioavailability of active drug by four to ten times. The drugs are highly lipophilic, highly membrane- or protein-bound, and accumulate in the brain, lung, and other tissues with a high blood supply; they also enter the fetal circulation quite easily. It is virtually impossible (and usually not necessary) to remove these agents by dialysis.

The pharmacokinetics of antipsychotic drugs follows a multiphasic pattern. The usually stated elimination half-lives with respect to total concentrations in plasma are typically 20 to 40 hours, but complex patterns of elimination may occur with some agents. The biological effects of single doses of most neuroleptics usually persist for at least 24 hours; this encourages the common practice of giving the entire daily dose at one time, once the patient has accommodated to the initial side effects of the drug. Elimination from the plasma may be more rapid than from sites of high lipid content and binding, notably in the CNS, but direct pharmacokinetic studies on this issue are few and inconclusive. Metabolites of some agents have been detected in the urine for as long as several months after the drug has been discontinued. Slow removal of drug may contribute to the typically slow rate of exacerbation of psychosis after stopping drug treatment. Repository preparations of esters of neuroleptic drugs are absorbed and eliminated much more slowly than are oral preparations. For example, whereas half of an oral dose of fluphenazine hydrochloride is eliminated in about 20 hours, the elimination half-time for a depot of the enanthate or the decanoate ester is 2 to 3 or 7 to 10 days, respectively.

The main routes of metabolism of the antipsychotic drugs are by oxidative processes mediated largely by hepatic microsomal and other drug-metabolizing enzymes. Conjugation with glucuronic acid is a prominent route of metabolism. Hydrophilic metabolites of these drugs are excreted in the urine and, to some extent, in the bile. Most oxidized metabolites of antipsychotic drugs are biologically inactive, but a few are not (notably, 7-hydroxychlorpromazine, mesoridazine, and several N-demethylated metabolites) and may contribute to the biological activity of the parent substance, as well as complicate the problem of correlating assays of drug in blood with clinical effects. The less potent antipsychotic drugs may induce their own hepatic metabolism, since concentrations of chlorpromazine and other phenothiazines in blood are lower after several weeks of treatment with the same dosage; it is also possible that alterations of gastrointestinal motility are partially responsible. The fetus, the infant, and the elderly have diminished capacity to metabolize and eliminate antipsychotic agents; children tend to metabolize these drugs more rapidly than do adults (Morselli, 1977; Popper, 1987).

The pharmacokinetics of antipsychotic drugs has been reviewed by Cooper and associates (1976), Morselli (1977), Baldessarini (1984b), and Baldessarini and colleagues (1988).

Detailed comments on the pharmacokinetics can be offered for only a few agents, such as chlorpromazine and haloperidol, that have been well studied. However, the complex metabolism of chlorpromazine limits its usefulness as a model agent. The absorption of tablets of chlorpromazine is erratic, although the bioavailability seems to be increased somewhat by the use of liquid concentrates, as is true for many of the antipsychotic agents. Peak concentrations in plasma are attained in about 2 to 4 hours. Intramuscular administration of the drug avoids much of the first-pass metabolism in the liver (and possibly also the gut) and provides measurable concentrations in plasma within 15 to 30 minutes; bioavailability may be increased up to tenfold, but the clinical dose usually is decreased by three- to fourfold. The gastrointestinal absorption of chlorpromazine is modified unpredictably by food and is probably decreased by antacids. There is controversy as to whether the concurrent administration of anticholinergic antiparkinsonian agents diminishes the intestinal absorption of some neuroleptic agents (Simpson *et al.*, 1980). Chlorpromazine and other antipsychotic agents bind significantly to membranes and to plasma proteins. Typically, over 85% of the drug in plasma is bound to albumin. Concentrations of some neuroleptics (*e.g.*, haloperidol) in brain can be more than ten times those in the blood (Sunderland and Cohen, 1987), and their apparent volume of distribution may be as high as 20 liters per kilogram. Disappearance of chlorpromazine from plasma includes a rapid distribution phase ($t_{1/2}$ about 2 hours) and a slower early elimination phase ($t_{1/2}$ about 30 hours), but markedly variable values have been reported; the half-life of elimination from human brain is unknown. The elimination of haloperidol from human plasma is also not a log-linear function, such that the apparent half-life increases with time; very slow terminal-elimination rates ($t_{1/2} > 1$ week) may ultimately be attained.

Attempts to correlate plasma concentrations of chlorpromazine or its metabolites with clinical responses have not been especially successful (*see* Cooper *et al.*, 1976; Baldessarini *et al.*, 1988). Studies have revealed that wide variations (at least tenfold) in plasma concentrations occur among individuals. Although it appears that plasma concentrations of chlorpromazine below 30 ng/ml are not likely to produce an adequate antipsychotic response and that levels above 750 ng/ml are likely to be associated with unacceptable toxicity (*see* Rivera-Calimlin and Hershey, 1984), it is not yet possible to state the concentrations in plasma that are likely to be associated with optimal clinical responses.

As many as 10 or 12 metabolites of chlorpromazine occur in man in appreciable quantities (Morselli, 1977). Quantitatively, the most important of these are nor$_2$-chlorpromazine (doubly demethylated), chlorophenothiazine (removal of entire side chain), methoxy and hydroxy products, and glucuronide conjugates of the hydroxylated compounds. In the urine, 7-hydroxylated and dealkylated (nor_2) metabolites and their conjugates predominate.

There is less information about other phenothiazines. Thioridazine has been studied relatively well (Gottschalk *et al.*, 1975). Its pharmacokinetics and metabolism are similar to those of chlorpromazine, but the strong anticholinergic action of thioridazine on the gut may modify its own absorption. Major metabolites include sulfoxy products at ring-position 5 (inactive) or at the substituent at position 2 (including the active metabolite, mesoridazine). Demethylation of the piperidine ring is very rapid, but the activity of this metabolite is unknown. It is known that concentrations of thioridazine in plasma are relatively high (hundreds of nanograms per milliliter), possibly owing to its relative hydrophilicity, and it is suspected that mesoridazine is an important contributor to neuroleptic activity.

The biotransformation of the thioxanthenes is similar to that of chlorpromazine, except that metabolism to sulfoxides is common and ring-hydroxylated products are uncommon. Piperazine derivatives of the phenothiazines and thioxanthenes are also handled much like chlorpromazine, although metabolism of the piperidine ring itself occurs. Haloperidol and other butyrophenones are metabolized primarily by an N-dealkylation reaction; the resultant fragments can be conjugated with glucuronic acid, and it is believed that all of the metabolites of haloperidol are inactive (Forsman and Öhman, 1974), with the possible exception of a hydroxylated product formed by reduction of the keto moiety that may be re-oxidized to haloperidol (Korpi *et al.*, 1983). Typical plasma concentrations of haloperidol encountered clinically are about 10 to 30 ng/ml (Baldessarini *et al.*, 1988).

Tolerance and Physical Dependence. The antipsychotic drugs are not addicting, as the term is defined in Chapter 22. However, some degree of physical dependence may occur. Some authors have reported the occurrence of muscular discomfort and difficulty in sleeping that develop several days after abrupt discontinuation.

Tolerance develops to the sedative effects of chlorpromazine and other phenothiazines over a period of days or weeks. Tolerance to antipsychotic drugs and cross-tolerance among the agents are also demonstrable in behavioral and biochemical experiments in animals, particularly those directed toward evaluation of the blockade of dopaminergic receptors in the basal ganglia (*see* Baldessarini and Tarsy, 1979). This form of tolerance may be less prominent in limbic and cortical areas of the forebrain. One correlate of tolerance in forebrain dopaminergic systems is the development of disuse supersensitivity of those systems, possibly mediated by changes in the receptors for the neurotransmitter. This mechanism may underlie the clinical phenomenon of withdrawal-emergent dyskinesias (choreoathetosis on abrupt discontinuation of antipsychotic agents, especially following prolonged use of high doses of potent agents) (Baldessarini *et al.*, 1980). Although cross-tolerance for some effects may occur among neuroleptic drugs, clinical problems occur in making rapid changes from high doses of one type of agent to another; sedation, hypotension, and other autonomic effects or acute extrapyramidal reactions can result.

Preparations and Dosage. Since the number of agents with known neuroleptic or antipsychotic effects is large, Table 18–1 summarizes only those that are currently marketed in the United States. A few available agents are excluded that are now known to have inferior antipsychotic effects or that are no longer commonly used in psychiatric patients. These include promazine hydrochloride (SPARINE) and reserpine and other rauwolfia alkaloids. Prochlorperazine (COMPAZINE) has questionable utility as an antipsychotic agent and frequently produces acute extrapyramidal reactions; it is thus not commonly employed in psychiatry, although it is used as an antiemetic. Thiethylperazine (TORECAN), which is currently marketed only as an antiemetic, is a potent dopaminergic antagonist with many neuroleptic-like properties; at high doses it may be an efficacious antipsychotic agent (Rotrosen *et al.*, 1978). The United States has been slow to accept many psychotropic agents that are in common use in other countries; thus, many more thioxanthenes, butyrophenones, diphenylbutylpiperidines, benzamides, and long-acting repository preparations of neuroleptic agents are available in other countries.

Toxic Reactions and Side Effects. The antipsychotic drugs have a high therapeutic index and are remarkably safe agents. Furthermore, most phenothiazines have a relatively flat dose–response curve and can be used over a wide range of dosages. Although occasional deaths from overdosage have been reported, it is rare if the patient is given medical care and if an overdosage is not complicated by the concurrent ingestion of alcohol or other drugs. Based on animal data, the therapeutic index is lowest for thioridazine (20) and chlorpromazine (200) and is in excess of 1000 for the more potent agents (Janssen and Van Bever, 1978). Adult patients have survived doses of chlorpromazine up to 10 g, and deaths from an overdose of haloperidol appear to be unknown.

Side effects are often extensions of the many pharmacological actions of the drugs, which have already been discussed. The most important are those on the CNS, cardiovascular system, autonomic nervous system, and endocrine functions. The extrapyramidal effects, which are of great importance, are discussed in detail below.

Table 18–1. SELECTED ANTIPSYCHOTIC DRUGS: CHEMICAL STRUCTURES, DOSES, DOSAGE FORMS, AND SIDE EFFECTS *

NONPROPRIETARY NAME / TRADE NAME		DOSE AND DOSAGE FORMS †				SIDE EFFECTS		
Phenothiazines 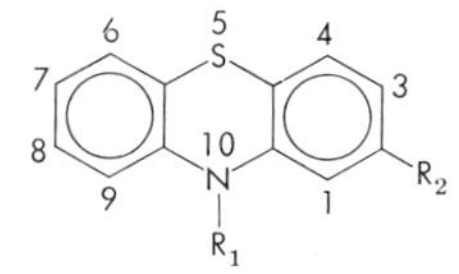		*Adult Antipsychotic Oral Dose Range—Daily Dosage*			*Single Intramuscular Dose ‡*	*Sedative Effects*	*Extra-pyramidal Effects*	*Hypotensive Effects*
R_1	R_2	Usual (mg)	Extreme § (mg)	Dosage forms	Usual (mg)			
Chlorpromazine hydrochloride $-(CH_2)_3-N(CH_3)_2$ THORAZINE, others	—Cl	200–800	30–2000	O,SR,L,I,S	25–50	+++	++	I.M. +++ Oral ++
Trifluprormazine hydrochloride $-(CH_2)_3-N(CH_3)_2$ VESPRIN	$-CF_3$			I	20–60	++	+++	++
Mesoridazine besylate 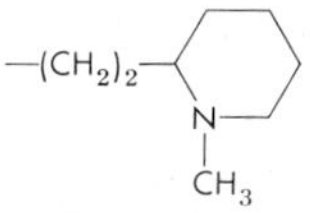 SERENTIL	$-S(=O)CH_3$	75–300	30–400	O,L,I	25	+++	+	++
Thioridazine hydrochloride 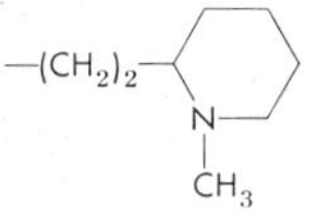 MELLARIL, MILLAZINE	$-SCH_3$	150–600	20–800	O,L		+++	+	++
Acetophenazine maleate 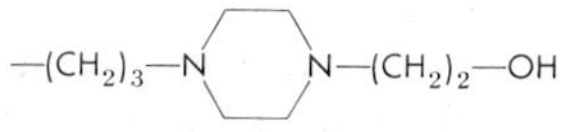 TINDAL	$-COCH_3$	40–120	40–600	O		++	++	+
Fluphenazine hydrochloride Fluphenazine enanthate Fluphenazine decanoate 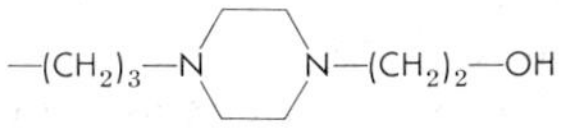 PERMITIL and PROLIXIN (HYDROCHLORIDES) (PROLIXIN ENANTHATE) and DECANOATE)	$-CF_3$	2–20	0.5–30	O,L,I	1.25–2.5 (decanoate or enanthate: 12.5–50 every 1–4 weeks)	+	+++	+
Perphenazine 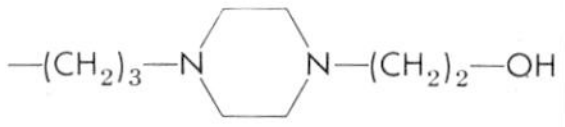 TRILAFON	—Cl	8–32	4–64	O,L,I	5–10	++	++	+
Trifluoperazine hydrochloride 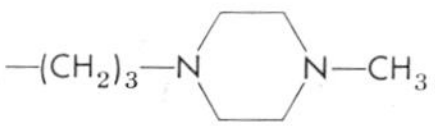 STELAZINE, SUPRAZINE	$-CF_3$	5–20	2–30	O,L,I	1–2	+	+++	+

Table 18–1. SELECTED ANTIPSYCHOTIC DRUGS: CHEMICAL STRUCTURES, DOSES, DOSAGE FORMS, AND SIDE EFFECTS * (Continued)

NONPROPRIETARY NAME / TRADE NAME		DOSE AND DOSAGE FORMS †			SIDE EFFECTS		
Thioxanthenes ‖		*Adult Antipsychotic Oral Dose Range—Daily Dosage*		*Single Intramuscular Dose* ‡	*Sedative Effects*	*Extra-pyramidal Effects*	*Hypotensive Effects*
R_1	R_2	Usual (mg)	Extreme § (mg)	Usual (mg)			
Chlorprothixene ‖ CH—$(CH_2)_2$—$N(CH_3)_2$ TARACTAN	—Cl	50–400	30–600	25–50	+++	++	++
		O,L,I					
Thiothixene hydrochloride 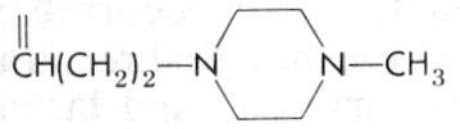 NAVANE	—SO_2 $N(CH_3)_2$	5–30	2–30	2–4	+ to ++	++	++
		O,L,I					
Other Heterocyclic Compounds							
Haloperidol and haloperidol decanoate 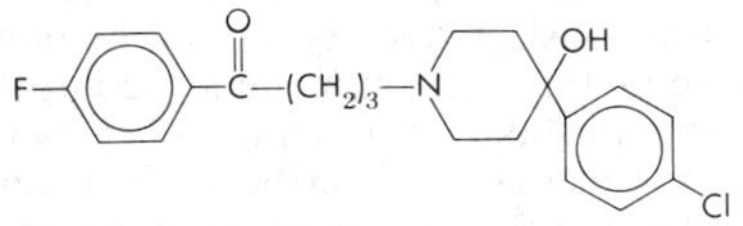 HALDOL, HALPERON		2–20	1–30	2–5 (haloperidol decanoate: 25–250 every 2–4 weeks)	+	+++	+
		O,L,I					
Loxapine succinate 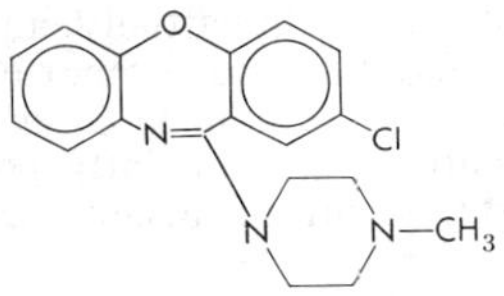 LOXITANE		60–100	20–250	12.5–50	+	++	+
		O,L,I					
Molindone hydrochloride 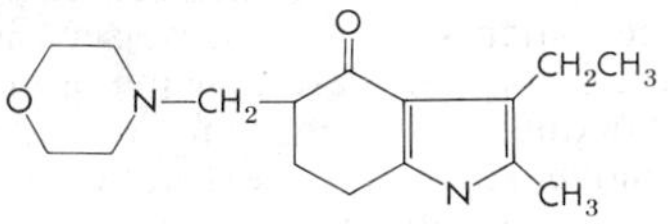 MOBAN		50–225	15–400		++	+	0
		O,L					
Pimozide 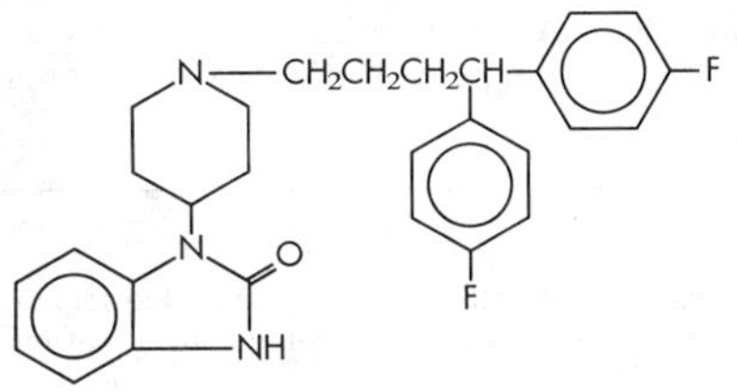 ORAP		2–6	1–10		+	+++	+
		O					

Footnotes for Table 18–1 will be found on page 398.

Other dangerous effects are agranulocytosis and pigmentary degeneration of the retina, both of which are rare (*see* below).

Therapeutic doses of phenothiazines may cause faintness, palpitation, and anticholinergic effects including nasal stuffiness, dry mouth, blurred vision, constipation, and, in males with prostatism, urinary retention. The patient may complain of being cold, drowsy, or weak. The most troublesome cardiovascular side effect is orthostatic hypotension, which may result in syncope. A fall in blood pressure is most likely to occur from administration of the phenothiazines with aliphatic side chains. Congeners of the piperazine type, as well as other potent neuroleptic agents, produce less hypotension.

Neurological Side Effects. A variety of neurological syndromes, involving particularly the extrapyramidal system, occur following the use of almost all antipsychotic drugs. These reactions are particularly prominent during treatment with the high-potency neuroleptic agents (tricyclic piperazines and butyrophenones). There is less likelihood of acute extrapyramidal side effects with thioridazine as well as with clozapine or other experimental atypical antipsychotic agents. The neurological effects associated with antipsychotic drugs have been reviewed in detail (Baldessarini *et al.*, 1980; Baldessarini, 1984b; Tarsy and Baldessarini, 1986).

Six varieties of neurological syndromes are characteristic of antipsychotic drugs. Four of these (acute dystonia, akathisia, parkinsonism, and the rare neuroleptic malignant syndrome) usually appear concomitantly with the administration of the drug, and two (the rare perioral tremor and tardive dyskinesia) are late-appearing syndromes that occur following prolonged treatment for many months or years. The clinical features of these syndromes and guidelines for their management are summarized in Table 18–2.

Acute dystonic reactions are occasionally seen with the initiation of antipsychotic drug therapy. Facial grimacing and torticollis can occur and may be associated with oculogyric crisis. These syndromes may be mistaken for hysterical reaction or seizures, but they respond dramatically to parenteral administration of anticholinergic antiparkinsonian drugs. Oral administration of anticholinergic agents can also prevent dystonia, particularly in young male patients who have been given high-potency neuroleptic drugs (Arana *et al.*, 1988). Although treated readily, acute dystonic reactions are terrifying to patients; sudden death has occurred in rare instances, perhaps due to the impaired respiration caused by dystonia of pharyngeal and laryngeal muscles.

Akathisia refers to strong subjective feelings of distress or discomfort, often referred to the legs, as well as to a compelling need to be in constant movement rather than to follow any specific movement pattern. The patient feels that he must get up and walk or continuously move about, and he may be unable to keep this tendency under control. Akathisia can be mistaken for agitation in psychotic patients; the distinction is critical, since agitation might be treated with an increase in dosage. Because the response of akathisia to antiparkinsonian drugs is frequently unsatisfactory, treatment typically requires reduction of antipsychotic drug dosage. Antianxiety agents may help partially, and moderate doses of propranolol have been reported to be beneficial in many cases (Lipinski *et al.*, 1984). This common syndrome is frequently not diagnosed and often interferes with the acceptance of neuroleptic treatment.

A *parkinsonian syndrome* that may be indistinguishable from idiopathic parkinsonism may develop during administration of antipsychotic drugs. Its incidence varies with different agents (*see* Table 18–1), and in some patients it may not be seen at all. Clinically, there is a generalized slowing of volitional movement (akinesia) with mask facies and a reduction in arm movements. The most noticeable signs are rigidity and tremor at rest, especially involving the upper extremities. "Pill-rolling" movements may be seen, although this is not as prominent in neuroleptic-induced as in idiopathic parkinsonism. Parkinsonian side effects may be mistaken for depression since the flat facial expres-

---

Footnotes for Table 18–1

* Antipsychotic agents for use in children under age 12 years include chlorpromazine, chlorprothixene (>6 years), thioridazine, and triflupromazine (among agents of low potency); and prochlorperazine and trifluoperazine (>6 years) (among agents of high potency). Haloperidol (orally) has also been used extensively in children. *See* page 404.

† Dosage forms are indicated as follows: I = injection; L = oral liquid; O = oral solid; S = suppository; SR = oral, sustained release.

‡ Except for the enanthate and decanoate forms of fluphenazine and haloperidol decanoate, dosage can be given intramuscularly up to every 6 hours for agitated patients. Haloperidol lactate has been given intravenously; this is experimental.

§ Extreme dosage ranges are occasionally exceeded cautiously and only when other appropriate measures have failed.

|| Carbon replaces nitrogen in position 10 of the general formula for the phenothiazines.

Table 18–2. NEUROLOGICAL SIDE EFFECTS OF NEUROLEPTIC DRUGS

REACTION	FEATURES	TIME OF MAXIMAL RISK	PROPOSED MECHANISM	TREATMENT
Acute dystonia	Spasm of muscles of tongue, face, neck, back; may mimic seizures; *not* hysteria	1 to 5 days	Unknown	Many treatments can alter, but effects of antiparkinsonian agents are diagnostic and curative *
Akathisia	Motor restlessness; *not* anxiety or "agitation"	5 to 60 days	Unknown	Reduce dose or change drug; antiparkinsonian agents †, benzodiazepines, or propranolol ‡ may help
Parkinsonism	Bradykinesia, rigidity, variable tremor, mask facies, shuffling gait	5 to 30 days	Antagonism of dopamine	Antiparkinsonian agents helpful †
Malignant syndrome	Catatonia, stupor, fever, unstable blood pressure, myoglobinemia; can be fatal	Weeks; can persist for days after stopping neuroleptic	Antagonism of dopamine may contribute	Stop neuroleptic immediately; dantrolene or bromocriptine may help §; antiparkinsonian agents not effective
Perioral tremor ("rabbit" syndrome)	Perioral tremor (may be a late variant of parkinsonism)	After months or years of treatment	Unknown	Antiparkinsonian agents often help †
Tardive dyskinesia	Oral-facial dyskinesia; widespread choreoathetosis or dystonia	After months or years of treatment (worse on withdrawal)	Excess function of dopamine hypothesized	Prevention crucial; treatment unsatisfactory

* Many drugs have been claimed to be helpful for acute dystonia. Among the most commonly employed treatments are diphenhydramine hydrochloride, 25 or 50 mg intramuscularly, or benztropine mesylate, 1 or 2 mg intramuscularly or slowly intravenously, followed by oral medication with the same agent for a period of days to perhaps several weeks thereafter.

† For details regarding the use of oral antiparkinsonian agents, *see* the text and Chapter 20.

‡ Propranolol is often effective in relatively low doses (20–80 mg per day). Selective β_1-adrenergic antagonists are less effective.

§ Despite the response to dantrolene, there is no evidence of an abnormality of Ca^{2+} transport in skeletal muscle; with lingering neuroleptic effects, bromocriptine may be tolerated in large doses (10–40 mg per day).

sion and retarded movements resemble signs of depression. This reaction is usually managed by use of either antiparkinsonian agents with anticholinergic properties or amantadine; the use of levodopa or bromocriptine incurs the risk of inducing agitation and worsening the psychotic illness (*see* Chapter 20).

A rarer disorder, *neuroleptic malignant syndrome*, resembles a very severe form of parkinsonism with catatonia, fluctuations in the intensity of tremor, signs of autonomic instability (labile pulse and blood pressure, hyperthermia), stupor, elevation of creatine kinase in plasma, and sometimes myoglobinemia. In its most severe form, this syndrome may persist for more than a week after stopping the offending agent. Since mortality is high (over 10%), immediate medical attention is required. This reaction has been associated with various types of neuroleptics, but its prevalence may be greater when relatively high doses of the more potent agents are used, especially when they are administered parenterally. Aside from immediate cessation of neuroleptic treatment and provision of supportive care, specific treatment is unsatisfactory; administration of dantrolene or the dopaminergic agonist bromocriptine may be helpful (Caroff *et al.*, 1983; Levenson, 1985). Although dantrolene is also used to manage the syndrome of malignant hyperthermia induced by general anesthetics, the neuroleptic-induced form of catatonia and hyperthermia is probably not associated with a defect in Ca^{2+} metabolism in skeletal muscle (Caroff *et al.*, 1983; Levenson, 1985; *see also* Chapter 14).

A rare movement disorder that can appear late in the treatment of chronically ill patients with antipsychotic agents is *perioral tremor*, sometimes referred to as the "rabbit syndrome" (Jus *et al.*, 1974) because of the peculiar movements that characterize this condition. While sometimes categorized with other tardive (late or slowly evolving) dyskinesias, the latter term is usually reserved for choreoathetotic reactions. The "rabbit syndrome," in fact, shares many features with parkinsonism, since the tremor has a frequency of about 5 to 7 Hz and there is a favorable response to anticholinergic agents and to the removal of the offending agent.

Tardive dyskinesia is a late-appearing neurological syndrome associated with antipsychotic drug use. It occurs more frequently in older patients, and the prevalence averages about 15 to 20% in chronically institutionalized patients; however, because of spontaneous remissions, from 2 to 5% of patients will be experiencing this syndrome at any given time. It has been associated with every class of neuroleptic agent in common clinical use. The incidence appears to be very low with the atypical antipsychotic agent clozapine. Tardive dyskinesia is characterized by stereotypical, repetitive, involuntary movements consisting in sucking and smacking of the lips, lateral jaw movements, and pushing or twisting of the tongue. There may be choreiform or purposeless, quick movements of the extremities. Slower, more dystonic, athetoid movements and postures of the extremities, trunk, and neck may also be seen, especially in younger males. All of these movements disappear during sleep, as they do in parkinsonism. Although the tardive dyskinesias may be partially suppressed by the administration of antipsychotic drugs, this form of treatment is employed only in very compelling circumstances, such as severely incapacitating dyskinesia, particularly with continuing psychosis. Symptoms sometimes persist indefinitely after discontinuation of the medication, although they often diminish or disappear with time (weeks or as long as 1 to 3 years), especially in younger patients (Glazer *et al.*, 1984). Antiparkinsonian drugs typically exacerbate tardive dyskinesias and other forms of choreoathetosis, such as in Huntington's disease, and no adequate therapy has as yet been devised (Jeste and Wyatt, 1982); the best approach is preventive (*see* below).

There is no established neuropathology in tardive dyskinesia, and its pathophysiology remains obscure. It has been hypothesized that compensatory increases in the function of dopamine as a neurotransmitter in the basal ganglia may be involved. This idea is supported by the dissimilarities of therapeutic responses in patients with Parkinson's disease and those with tardive dyskinesia, and by the similarities in responses of patients with other choreoathetotic dyskinesias such as Huntington's disease. Thus, antidopaminergic drugs tend to suppress the manifestations of tardive dyskinesia or Huntington's disease, while dopaminergic agonists worsen these conditions; in contrast to parkinsonism, antimuscarinic agents tend to worsen tardive dyskinesia, but cholinergic agents usually are ineffective. In addition, abundant data now support the concept of disuse supersensitivity of dopaminergic systems in the animal brain. Since supersensitivity to dopaminergic agonists tends not to persist for more than a few weeks after exposure to antagonists of the transmitter, this phenomenon is most likely to play a role in those variants of tardive dyskinesia that resolve rapidly; these are usually referred to as *withdrawal-emergent dyskinesias*. The theoretical and clinical aspects of this problem have been reviewed in detail elsewhere (Baldessarini and Tarsy, 1979; Baldessarini *et al.*, 1980; Jeste and Wyatt, 1982; Tarsy and Baldessarini, 1986).

It is important to prevent the neurological syndromes that complicate the use of antipsychotic drugs. Certain therapeutic guidelines should be followed. Routine use of antiparkinsonian agents in an attempt to avoid early extrapyramidal reactions is usually unnecessary and adds complexity, side effects, and expense to the treatment regimen. Antiparkinsonian agents are best reserved for cases of *overt* extrapyramidal reactions that respond favorably to such intervention. The need for such agents for the treatment of acute dystonic reactions ordinarily diminishes with time, but parkinsonism and akathisia tend to persist. The thoughtful and conservative use of antipsychotic drugs in patients with chronic or frequently recurrent psychotic disorders almost certainly can reduce the risk of tardive dyskinesia. Although reduction of the dose of an antipsychotic agent is the best way to minimize its neurological side effects, this may not be practical in a patient with uncontrollable psychotic illness. The best preventive practice is to use the minimum effective dose of an antipsychotic drug for long-term therapy and to discontinue treatment as soon as it seems reasonable to do so or if a satisfactory response cannot be obtained.

Jaundice. Jaundice was observed in patients shortly after the introduction of chlorpromazine; the incidence was low and has decreased further since the 1960s. This change may be due to improved quality of the products or to the increased use of more potent agents, which tend to have less systemic toxicity than do the low-potency phenothiazines. Commonly occurring during the second to fourth week of therapy, the jaundice is generally mild, and pruritus is rare. The reaction is probably a manifestation of hypersensitivity, since eosinophilic infiltration of the liver as well as eosinophilia occur; there is no correlation with dose. Desensitization to chlorpromazine may occur with repeated administration, and jaundice may or may not recur if the same neuroleptic agent is given again. When the psychiatric disorder calls for uninterrupted drug therapy for a patient with neuroleptic-induced jaundice, it is probably safest to use low doses of a potent, dissimilar agent.

Blood Dyscrasias. Mild leukocytosis, leukopenia, and eosinophilia occasionally occur with phenothiazine medication. It is difficult to determine whether a leukopenia occurring during the administration of a phenothiazine is a forewarning of impending agranulocytosis. This serious but rare complication occurs in not more than 1 in 10,000 patients receiving chlorpromazine or other low-potency agents, particularly in high doses; it usually appears within the first 8 to 12 weeks of treatment (DuComb and Baldessarini, 1977). Suppression of the bone marrow or, less commonly, agranulocytosis has particularly been associated with use of clozapine; the incidence approaches 1% and close monitoring of the patient is recommended. Since the onset of blood dyscrasia may be sudden, the appearance of an apparent upper respiratory infection in a patient being treated with an antipsychotic drug should be followed immediately by a complete blood count.

Skin Reactions. Dermatological reactions to the phenothiazines are common. Urticaria or dermatitis occurs in about 5% of patients receiving chlorpromazine. Several types of skin disorders may occur. The first is a hypersensitivity reaction that may be urticarial, maculopapular, petechial, or edematous. It usually occurs between the first and eighth week of treatment. The skin clears following discontinuation of the drug and may remain so even if drug therapy is reinstituted. Secondly, contact dermatitis may occur in personnel who handle chlorpromazine, and there may be a certain degree of cross-sensitivity to the other phenothiazines. Thirdly, photosensitivity occurs; the reaction resembles that seen with severe sunburn. An effective sunscreen preparation should be prescribed for outpatients during the summer. Abnormal gray-blue pigmentation induced by long-term administration of low-potency phenothiazines in high doses can occur but is rare with current practices.

Epithelial keratopathy is often observed in patients on long-term therapy with chlorpromazine, and opacities in the cornea and in the lens of the eye have also been noted. In extreme cases the deposits in the lens may result in impairment of vision. Active treatment of this condition (*e.g.*, with penicillamine) has not been especially helpful, and the deposits tend to disappear spontaneously, although slowly, following discontinuation of the low-potency drug usually implicated. Pigmentary retinopathy has been reported, particularly following doses of thioridazine in excess of 1000 mg per day; a maximal daily dose of 800 mg is currently recommended.

Interactions with Other Drugs. The phenothiazines and thioxanthenes, especially those of low potency, affect the actions of a number of other drugs, sometimes with important clinical consequences (*see* Kaufman, 1976). Chlorpromazine was originally introduced to potentiate central depressants in anesthesiology. Such drugs can strongly potentiate sedatives and analgesics prescribed for medical purposes, as well as alcohol, nonprescription sedatives and hypnotics, antihistamines, and cold remedies. Chlorpromazine increases the miotic and sedative effects of morphine and may increase its analgesic actions. Furthermore, the drug markedly increases the respiratory depression produced by meperidine and can be expected to have similar effects when administered concurrently with other opioids. Obviously, neuroleptic drugs will inhibit the actions of direct dopaminergic agonists and of levodopa.

Other interactive effects can be manifest on the cardiovascular system. Chlorpromazine and some other antipsychotic drugs, as well as their N-demethylated metabolites, may block the antihypertensive effects of guanethidine, probably by blocking its uptake into sympathetic nerves. The more potent antipsychotic agents as well as molindone are less likely to cause this effect. Low-potency phenothiazines can promote postural hypotension, possibly due to their α-adrenergic blocking properties. Thus, the interaction between phenothiazines and antihypertensive agents can be unpredictable.

Thioridazine may partially nullify the inotropic effect of digitalis by its quinidine-like action, which can cause myocardial depression, decreased efficiency of repolarization, and increased risk of tachyarrhythmias. The antimuscarinic action of thioridazine can cause tachycardia and enhance the peripheral and central effects (confusion, delirium) of other anticholinergic agents, such as the tricyclic antidepressants and antiparkinsonian agents.

Sedatives or anticonvulsants (*e.g.*, phenytoin, phenobarbital, carbamazepine) that induce microsomal drug-metabolizing enzymes can enhance the metabolism of antipsychotic agents, sometimes with significant clinical consequences (Loga *et al.*, 1975) .

DRUG TREATMENT OF PSYCHOSES

The antipsychotic drugs are not specific for the diagnostic type of psychosis to be treated. They are clearly effective in acute psychoses of unknown etiology, including mania, acute idiopathic psychoses, and acute exacerbations of schizophrenia; the greatest amount of controlled clinical data exists for the acute and chronic phases of schizophrenia. In addition, antipsychotic drugs are used empirically in many other disorders, whether idiopathic or organic, in which psychotic symptoms and severe agitation are prominent.

The fact that phenothiazines and other neuroleptic agents are indeed antipsychotic was slow to gain acceptance. However, many clinical trials and 4 decades of clinical experience have established that these agents are effective and that they are superior to agents such as the benzodiazepines or to alternatives such as electroconvulsive shock or other medical or psychological therapies (*see* Donaldson *et al.*, 1986). The "target" symptoms for which the neuroleptic agents seem to be especially effective include tension, hyperactivity, combativeness, hostility, hallucinations, acute delusions, insomnia, anorexia, poor self-care, negativism, and sometimes withdrawal and seclusiveness; less likely is improvement in insight, judgment, memory, and orientation. The most favorable prognosis is for patients with acute illnesses of brief duration who had relatively healthy personalities prior to the illness.

Despite the great success of the antipsychotic drugs, their use alone does not constitute optimal care of psychotic patients. The acute care, protection, and support of acutely psychotic patients, as well as mastery of techniques employed in their long-term care and rehabilitation, are important medical skills. Many detailed reviews of the clinical use of antipsychotic drugs are available (Klein *et al.*, 1980; Bassuk *et al.*, 1983; Baldessarini, 1984b, 1985).

No one drug or combination of drugs has a selective effect on a particular symptom complex in groups of psychotic patients; although individual patients appear to do better with one agent than another, this can only be determined by trial and error. It is important to simplify the treatment regimen and to ensure that the patient is receiving the drug. In cases of severe and dangerous noncompliance, the patient can be treated with injections of fluphenazine decanoate, haloperidol decanoate, or other long-acting preparations. Since delusional paranoid patients frequently believe that the medicine is "poison," they are often given long-acting injectable preparations.

Since the choice of a drug cannot be made on the basis of anticipated therapeutic effect, the selection of a particular medication for treatment often depends on side effects. If a patient has responded well to a drug in the past, it probably should be used again. If the patient has a history of cardiovascular disease or stroke and the threat from hypotension is serious, a potent neuroleptic should be used in the smallest dose that is effective (*see* Table 18–1). If it seems important to minimize the risk of acute extrapyramidal symptoms, thioridazine should be considered. If the patient would be seriously discomforted by interference with ejaculation or if there are serious risks of cardiovascular or other autonomic toxicity, thioridazine should be avoided. If sedative effects are undesirable, a potent agent is preferable. Small doses of antipsychotic drugs of high or moderate potency may be safest in the elderly. If the patient has compromised hepatic function or if there is a potential threat of jaundice, low doses of a high-potency agent may be used. The physician's experience with a particular drug may outweigh all other considerations. Skill in the use of antipsychotic drugs depends on selection of an adequate but not excessive dose, knowledge of what to expect, and judgment as to when to stop therapy or change drugs.

Some patients do not respond satisfactorily to antipsychotic drug treatment, and many chronically disorganized schizophrenic patients, while helped during periods of acute exacerbation of their disease, may show unsatisfactory responses between the more acute phases of illness. The individual nonresponder cannot be identified beforehand with certainty, and a small subgroup of patients does poorly or sometimes even becomes worse on medication. If a patient does not improve after a course of adequate treatment and fails to respond to another drug given in adequate dosage, therapy should be discontinued and the diagnosis reevaluated.

Usually 2 to 3 weeks or more are required to demonstrate obvious positive effects in hospitalized schizophrenics. Maximum benefit may require 6 weeks to 6 months in chronically psychotic patients. In contrast, improvement of some acutely psychotic patients can be seen within 24 to 48 hours. Aggressive parenteral administration of an antipsychotic drug at the start of an acute psychosis has not been found to increase the rate of appearance of therapeutic responses (Baldessarini *et al.*, 1988). Sedative or anxiolytic agents, such as the benzodiazepines, can be used for brief periods during the initiation of therapy with neuroleptic drugs; they are not effective in the long-term treatment of chronically psychotic and, especially, schizophrenic patients. After the initial response, drugs are usually used in conjunction with psychological, supportive, and rehabilitative treatments.

There is no convincing evidence that combinations of antipsychotic drugs offer any advantage. A combination of an antipsychotic drug and an antidepressant may be useful in some cases, especially in depressed psychotic patients or in cases of agitated major depression with psychotic features. However, the suggestion that a tricyclic antidepressant or a stimulant can reduce apathy and withdrawal in schizophrenia is not proven, and the hypothesis that diphenylbutylpiperidines, benzamides, or atypical agents are especially valuable against such "negative" symptoms of schizophrenia requires further study.

Optimal dosage of antipsychotic drugs is difficult to determine because of the ill-defined dose–response relationships for both the antipsychotic and neurotoxic effects and the difficulties in defining an end point of therapeutic response. The typical effective dose of chlorpromazine is approximately 300 to 500 mg daily; 5 to 15 mg of haloperidol daily usually produces clearly apparent antipsychotic effects. Doses of as little as 50 to

200 mg of chlorpromazine (or 2 to 6 mg of haloperidol or fluphenazine) daily may be effective and better tolerated by some patients, especially after the initial improvement of acute symptoms (Davis and Garver, 1978; Cole, 1982; Baldessarini *et al.*, 1988). Careful observation of the patient's changing response is the best guide to dosage.

In the treatment of acute psychoses, the dose of antipsychotic drug is increased during the first few days to achieve control of symptoms. The dose is then adjusted during the next several weeks as the patient's condition warrants. Parenteral medication sometimes is indicated for acutely agitated patients; 5 mg of haloperidol or fluphenazine or comparable doses of another agent are given intramuscularly (and almost never by other routes). The desired response can usually be obtained by additional doses at intervals of 4 to 8 hours for the first 24 to 72 hours because the appearance of effects may be delayed for several hours. Rarely is it necessary to administer more than 20 to 30 mg of fluphenazine or haloperidol (or an equivalent amount of another agent) per 24 hours. Severe and otherwise poorly controlled agitation can usually be managed safely by use of adjunctive sedation (*e.g.*, with a benzodiazepine such as lorazepam) and close supervision in a secure setting. One must remain alert for acute dystonic reactions, which are especially likely early in the aggressive use of potent neuroleptics. Hypotension is most likely to occur if an agent of low potency, such as chlorpromazine, is given by injection. Some antipsychotic drugs, including fluphenazine, other piperazines, and haloperidol, have been given in doses of several hundred milligrams a day without disaster, although such high doses of potent agents do not yield significantly superior results in the treatment of acute or chronic psychosis, and may yield inferior antipsychotic effects as well as increased risks of neurological and other side effects (Aubree and Lader, 1980; Cole, 1982; Baldessarini *et al.*, 1988). After an initial period of stabilization, regimens based on a single daily dose (typically about 5 to 15 mg per day of haloperidol, fluphenazine, or their equivalent) are effective and safe; they may also allow some degree of selection of the time at which unwanted effects occur so as to minimize the patient's discomfort.

Table 18–1 (page 396) gives usual and extreme ranges of dosage for antipsychotic drugs used in the United States. These ranges are only guidelines, and they have been established, for the most part, in the treatment of schizophrenic or manic patients. Higher doses have been used, but are considered experimental. While acutely disturbed inpatients may require higher doses of an antipsychotic drug than do more stable outpatients, the concept that a low or flexible maintenance dose will suffice during follow-up care of a partially recovered or chronic psychotic patient is supported by several appropriately controlled trials (Kane *et al.*, 1983; Carpenter *et al.*, 1987; Baldessarini *et al.*, 1988).

The duration of treatment has received a great deal of attention. In a review of nearly 30 controlled prospective studies involving close to 3500 schizophrenic patients, the mean overall relapse rate was 58% for those patients who were withdrawn from antipsychotic drugs and given a placebo, compared with only 16% of those who continued on drug therapy (Davis, 1975; Baldessarini, 1984b, 1985; Baldessarini *et al.*, 1988). Dosage in chronic cases can often be lowered to 50 to 200 mg of chlorpromazine (or its equivalent) per day without signs of relapse (Baldessarini *et al.*, 1988). Flexible therapy in which dosage is adjusted to changing current requirements can be useful and can reduce the incidence of side effects. Effective maintenance with injections of the decanoate ester of fluphenazine or haloperidol every 2 to 4 weeks is well established and commonly practiced (Kane *et al.*, 1983).

The treatment of organic mental syndromes (*i.e.*, delirium or dementia) is another accepted use of the antipsychotic drugs. They may be administered temporarily, while a specific and correctable structural, infectious, metabolic, or toxic cause is vigorously sought. They are sometimes used for prolonged periods when no correctable cause can be found. Once again, there are no drugs of choice or clearly established dosage guidelines (*see* Prien, 1973). In patients with acute "brain syndromes" without likelihood of seizures, frequent small doses (*e.g.*, 2 to 6 mg) of haloperidol or a piperazine may be effective in controlling agitation. Agents with low potency should be avoided because of their greater tendency to produce sedation, hypotension, and seizures. The potent antipsychotic drugs are much less likely to cause additional confusion, as is common when sedatives are given to delirious or demented patients. The intravenous administration of extraordinarily high doses of haloperidol (*e.g.*, more than 500 mg in 24 hours) has been used experimentally in postoperative or intensive care settings to manage extreme agitation in critically ill patients for whom ordinary sedation is considered excessively risky (Tesar *et al.*, 1985).

The use of antipsychotic drugs in mania and depression has met with some success. Haloperidol and chlorpromazine are both effective in the treatment of mania and are often used concomitantly with the institution of lithium therapy (*see* below). In fact, it is often impractical to attempt to manage a manic patient with lithium alone during the first week of illness, when the antipsychotic drugs are usually required; sedative doses of anxiolytic agents may also be used. No adequately controlled studies of possible long-term preventive effects of antipsychotic drugs in manic-depressive illness have been conducted. The treatment of depression with neuroleptics is more controversial. Controlled studies have demonstrated the efficacy of several antipsychotic drugs in some depressed patients, especially those with striking agitation or psychotic delusions (*see* Chan *et al.*, 1987).

Anxiety has been considered a possible indication for the use of antipsychotic drugs, especially in small doses. In view of the wide range of disturbing and serious side effects, the routine use of these drugs for such a purpose is inappropriate. However, for patients who have crippling anxiety that does not respond to sedative-antianxiety drugs or to treatment with antidepressant agents, a brief trial of an antipsychotic agent might be warranted.

The status of the drug treatment of childhood psychosis and other behavioral disorders of children is confused by diagnostic inconsistencies and a paucity of controlled studies. Neuroleptics can benefit children with disorders characterized by features that occur in adult psychoses. Low doses of the more potent agents are usually preferred in an attempt to avoid interference with daytime activities or performance in school (Biederman and Jellinek, 1984). Attention disorder with hyperactivity responds poorly to antipsychotic agents but uniquely well to certain stimulant drugs, especially dextroamphetamine and methylphenidate (Zametkin and Rapoport, 1987), and possibly also to some tricyclic antidepressants (*see* Biederman *et al.*, 1986). Information on dosages of antipsychotic drugs for children is limited, as is the number of drugs currently approved in the United States for use in preadolescents. The recommended doses of antipsychotic agents for school-aged children with moderate degrees of agitation are lower than those for acutely psychotic children, who may require doses similar to those used in adults (total milligrams per day) (*see* Anders and Ciaranello, 1977; Werry, 1978; Biederman and Jellinek, 1984; Baldessarini, 1985; Popper, 1987; *see also* Table 18–1). Most relevant experience is with chlorpromazine, for which the recommended single dose is approximately 0.5 mg/kg of body weight, given at intervals of 4 to 6 hours orally or 6 to 8 hours intramuscularly. Suggested dosage limits are 200 mg per day (orally) for preadolescents, 75 mg per day (intramuscularly) for children age 5 to 12 years or weighing 23 to 45 kg, and 40 mg per day (intramuscularly) for children under 5 years of age or 23 kg of body weight. Usual single doses for other agents of relatively low potency are triflupromazine, 0.25 mg/kg; thioridazine, 0.25 to 0.5 mg/kg; and chlorprothixene, 0.5 to 1.0 mg/kg, to a total of 100 mg/day (over the age of 6). For neuroleptics of high potency, daily doses are trifluoperazine, 1 to 15 mg (6 to 12 years of age) and 1 to 30 mg (over 12 years of age); fluphenazine, 0.05 to 0.10 mg/kg, up to 10 mg (over 5 years of age); and perphenazine, 0.05 to 0.10 mg/kg, up to 6 mg (over 1 year of age). Haloperidol has been used in children, especially for Gilles de la Tourette's syndrome, and is recommended for use in a dosage of 2 to 16 mg per day in children over 12 years of age.

Poor tolerance of the side effects of the antipsychotic drugs often limits the dosage that can be given to elderly patients. One should proceed cautiously, using small, divided doses of agents with moderate or high potency, with the expectation that the very elderly will require doses that are one half or less of those needed for young adults (*see* Prien and Cole, 1978; Raskin *et al.*, 1981).

MISCELLANEOUS MEDICAL USES FOR NEUROLEPTIC DRUGS

Neuroleptic drugs have a variety of uses in addition to the treatment of psychiatric patients. Predominant among these are the treatment of nausea and vomiting, alcoholic hallucinosis, certain neuropsychiatric diseases marked by movement disorders (notably, Gilles de la Tourette's syndrome and Huntington's disease), and, occasionally, pruritus (for which trimeprazine is recommended) and intractable hiccough.

Nausea and Vomiting. Chlorpromazine and certain other antipsychotic agents can prevent vomiting of specific etiologies when given in relatively low, nonsedative doses. This use is discussed in Chapter 38.

Other Neuropsychiatric Disorders. Antipsychotic drugs are useful in the management of several syndromes with psychiatric features that are also characterized by movement disorders. These include, in particular, *Gilles de la Tourette's syndrome* (marked by tics, other involuntary movements, grunts, and vocalizations that are frequently obscene) (*see* Shapiro *et al.*, 1973; Van Woert *et al.*, 1976) and *Huntington's disease* (marked by severe and progressive choreoathetosis, psychiatric symptoms and dementia, with a clear genetic basis) (*see* Chase, 1976). Haloperidol is currently regarded as the drug of choice for these conditions, although it is probably not unique in its antidyskinetic actions. Pimozide, a diphenylbutylpiperidine, is also available for the treatment of Gilles de la Tourette's syndrome (typically in daily doses of 2 to 10 mg), although it has been used as an antipsychotic agent in Europe. Since pimozide carries some risk of impairing cardiac repolarization, it should be discontinued if the Q–T interval exceeds 470 msec, especially in a child. Clonidine may also be effective in Tourette's syndrome (Cohen *et al.*, 1980).

Hiccough. An interesting use of chlorpromazine is in the control of intractable hiccough. The mechanism of action in this disorder is unknown.

Withdrawal Syndromes. Antipsychotic drugs are *not* useful in the management of withdrawal from opioids, and their use in the management of withdrawal from barbiturates and other sedatives is contraindicated, owing to the high risk of seizures. This risk also precludes the use of neuroleptics during withdrawal from alcohol. However, they can be used safely and effectively in certain psychoses associated with chronic alcoholism—especially the syndrome known as *alcoholic hallucinosis* (*see* Kaplan and Sadock, 1985).

II. Drugs Used in the Treatment of Disorders of Mood

Affective disorders—*major depression* and *mania* (or *bipolar manic-depressive illness*)—are characterized by changes in mood as the primary clinical manifestation. Either extreme of mood may be associated with psychosis, manifested as disordered or delusional thinking and perceptions, often congruent with the predominant mood. Conversely, psychotic disorders may have associated or secondary changes in mood; the same is true of many medical illnesses. This overlap of disorders may lead to errors in diagnosis and clinical management (American Psychiatric Association, 1987). With a lifetime morbid risk of between 5 and 10% in the general population, major depression is one of the most common of the major mental illnesses; it should be distinguished from normal grief, sadness and disappointment, and the dysphoria or demoralization often associated with medical illness. The condition is underdiagnosed and frequently undertreated (Keller *et al.*, 1986). Major depression is characterized by feelings of intense sadness and despair, mental slowing and loss of concentration, pessimistic worry, agitation, and self-deprecation. Physical changes also occur, particularly in severe or "melancholic" depression; these include insomnia or hypersomnia, anorexia and weight loss (or sometimes overeating), decreased energy and libido, and disruption of the normal circadian rhythms of activity, body temperature, and many endocrine functions. Perhaps 10 to 15% of individuals with this disorder display suicidal behavior during their lifetime. The condition responds well to tricyclic or other antidepressant drugs, monoamine oxidase inhibitors, or, in severe or treatment-resistant cases, electroconvulsive treatment (ECT). The decision to treat with an antidepressant drug is guided by the presenting clinical syndrome and its severity, and by the patient's personal and family history. Most of the antidepressant agents exert important actions on the metabolism of monoamine neurotransmitters and their receptors. Their therapeutic effectiveness and actions, together with strong evidence for genetic predisposition, have led to speculation that the biological basis of major mood disorders may include abnormal function of monoamine neurotransmission. However, the direct evidence for this view is limited and inconsistent (*see* Murphy *et al.*, 1978; Praag, 1978; Baldessarini, 1983).

Mania and the alternation of mania and depression (bipolar affective disorder) are less common than nonbipolar major depression. Mania and its milder form (hypomania) are treated with antipsychotic drugs or lithium salts in the short term and lithium salts or certain anticonvulsants for longer-term prevention of recurrences. Mania is characterized by excessive elation, typically tinged with dysphoria or marked by irritability, severe insomnia, hyperactivity, uncontrollable speech and activity, and impaired judgment. The selection and management of appropriate treatment for depression and mania are discussed below.

TRICYCLIC ANTIDEPRESSANTS

Imipramine, amitriptyline, their N-demethyl derivatives, and other closely related compounds are the drugs currently most widely used for the treatment of major depression. Because of their structure (*see* below), they are often referred to as the "tricyclic" antidepressants. Their efficacy in alleviating major depression is well established, and support for their use in other psychiatric disorders is growing.

History. Häfliger and Schindler in the late 1940s synthesized a series of more than 40 derivatives of iminodibenzyl for possible use as antihistamines, sedatives, analgesics, and antiparkinsonian drugs. One of these was *imipramine,* a dibenzazepine compound, which differs from the phenothiazines only by replacement of the sulfur with an ethylene bridge to produce a seven-membered central ring. Following screening in animals, a few compounds, including imipramine, were selected on the basis of sedative or hypnotic properties for therapeutic trial.

During clinical investigation of these phenothiazine analogs, Kuhn (1958) found fortuitously that, unlike the phenothiazines, imipramine was relatively ineffective in quieting agitated psychotic patients. Instead, it apparently bestowed remarkable benefit upon certain depressed patients. Since then, indisputable evidence for the effectiveness of this compound has accumulated (*see* Hollister, 1978; Klein *et al.*, 1980; Herrington and Lader, 1981).

Chemistry and Structure–Activity Relationship. The search for compounds related chemically to imipramine has yielded, to date, nine analogs that are in common clinical use in the United States. In addition to the dibenzazepines, imipramine and its secondary-amine congener (and major metabolite) *desipramine,* there are *amitriptyline* and its N-demethylated metabolite *nortriptyline* (dibenzocycloheptadienes), as well as *doxepin* (a dibenzoxepine) and *protriptyline* (a dibenzocycloheptatriene). Additional structurally related agents approved for general use in the United States are *trimipramine* (a dibenzazepine); maprotiline (containing an additional ethylene bridge across the central six-carbon ring); and *amoxapine* (a dibenzoxazepine with mixed antidepressant and neuroleptic properties) (Cohen *et al.*, 1982). Since these agents all have a three-ring molecular core and produce therapeutic responses in most patients with major depression, the trivial name *tricyclic antidepressants* is used for this group. To varying degrees, these agents also share the capability of inhibiting the neuronal uptake of norepinephrine.

Some of the newer antidepressant agents that are in clinical use in Europe and elsewhere have a variety of chemical structures and pharmacological properties that differ from the tricyclic antidepressants. These are sometimes referred to as "atypical antidepressants" to distinguish them from both the monoamine oxidase inhibitors and the tricyclic antidepressants. Atypical antidepressants that are currently marketed in the United States include *trazodone*, a complex heterocyclic compound that is thought to potentiate the actions of 5-HT, and *fluoxetine*, a phenyltolylpropylamine that is a potent and selective inhibitor of the neuronal uptake of 5-HT. *Clomipramine* (3-chloroimipramine), which inhibits the neuronal uptake of both 5-HT and norepinephrine, has been in use for many years in Canada and Europe. Although still investigational in the United States, clomipramine is being evaluated for possible use in the treatment of obsessive-compulsive disorder. Under development are other drugs that potentiate the action of 5-HT; these include some analogs of fluoxetine (*e.g.*, *fluvoxamine*), as well as compounds with novel structures (*e.g.*, *citalopram*). A number of other agents have been marketed for brief periods before withdrawal because of the detection of various unacceptable or dangerous side effects. These include *zimeldine*, a selective inhibitor of 5-HT uptake, and two atypical antidepressants with stimulant properties (*bupropion* and *nomifensine*); the latter is an inhibitor of the neuronal uptake of both norepinephrine and dopamine.

Two anticonvulsant agents are undergoing evaluation for the treatment of mania and for stabilization of mood in manic-depressive patients, especially those who can not be controlled adequately with lithium salts: *carbamazepine*, a derivative of iminostilbene with a carbamyl group at the 5 position, and *valproic acid* (dipropylacetic acid), a branched chain carboxylic acid (*see* Post *et al.*, 1983; McElroy and Pope, 1988; *see also* Chapter 19).

The structures of the available tricyclic and atypical antidepressant compounds are given in Table 18–3. Although dibenzazepines seem to be similar to the phenothiazines chemically, the ethylene group of imipramine's middle ring imparts dissimilar stereochemical properties and prevents conjugation among the rings, as occurs with the phenothiazines. The demethylated congener of imipramine—desipramine—resembles imipramine as an antidepressant, although there are some dissimilarities as discussed below. While it had been suggested that desipramine might be the agent responsible for therapeutic responses to imipramine, desipramine is no more effective or rapidly acting than imipramine. The same generalizations can be made from the comparison between amitriptyline and nortriptyline. The latter pair are the structural homologs of the thioxanthenes among the antipsychotic drugs (*cf.* Tables 18–3 and 18–1). The chemistry and structure–activity relationship of a variety of antidepressant agents are discussed by Maxwell and White (1978), Usdin (1978), and Nieforth and Cohen (1989).

PHARMACOLOGICAL PROPERTIES

Our understanding of the pharmacological properties of this class of agents is quite incomplete. Since it is the oldest and best studied, imipramine will be discussed as a prototype.

Central Nervous System. One might expect an effective antidepressant drug to have a stimulating or mood-elevating effect when given to a normal subject. Although this may occur with the monoamine oxidase (MAO) inhibitors and some atypical, stimulant-like antidepressants, it is not true of the tricyclic antidepressants.

The administration of therapeutic doses of imipramine to normal subjects produces sleepiness, lightheadedness, a slight fall in blood pressure, and certain anticholinergic effects (*e.g.*, dry mouth, blurred vision). Gait may become unsteady; subjects feel tired and clumsy and have difficulty in concentrating and thinking. These effects are perceived as unpleasant and cause dysphoria.

In contrast, if the drug is given over a period of time to depressed patients, an elevation of mood occurs. *About 2 to 3 weeks must pass before the therapeutic effects of the drug are evident.* For this reason, the tricyclic antidepressants cannot be prescribed on an "as-needed" basis. The explanation of the slow onset of effects remains a matter of conjecture. No agent of the tricyclic antidepressant group acts more rapidly on the core symptoms of major depression than does imipramine. With some antidepressants, sedative or antianxiety effects (or the stimulant-like effects of others) may appear within a few days of treatment.

Table 18–3. TRICYCLIC AND ATYPICAL ANTIDEPRESSANTS

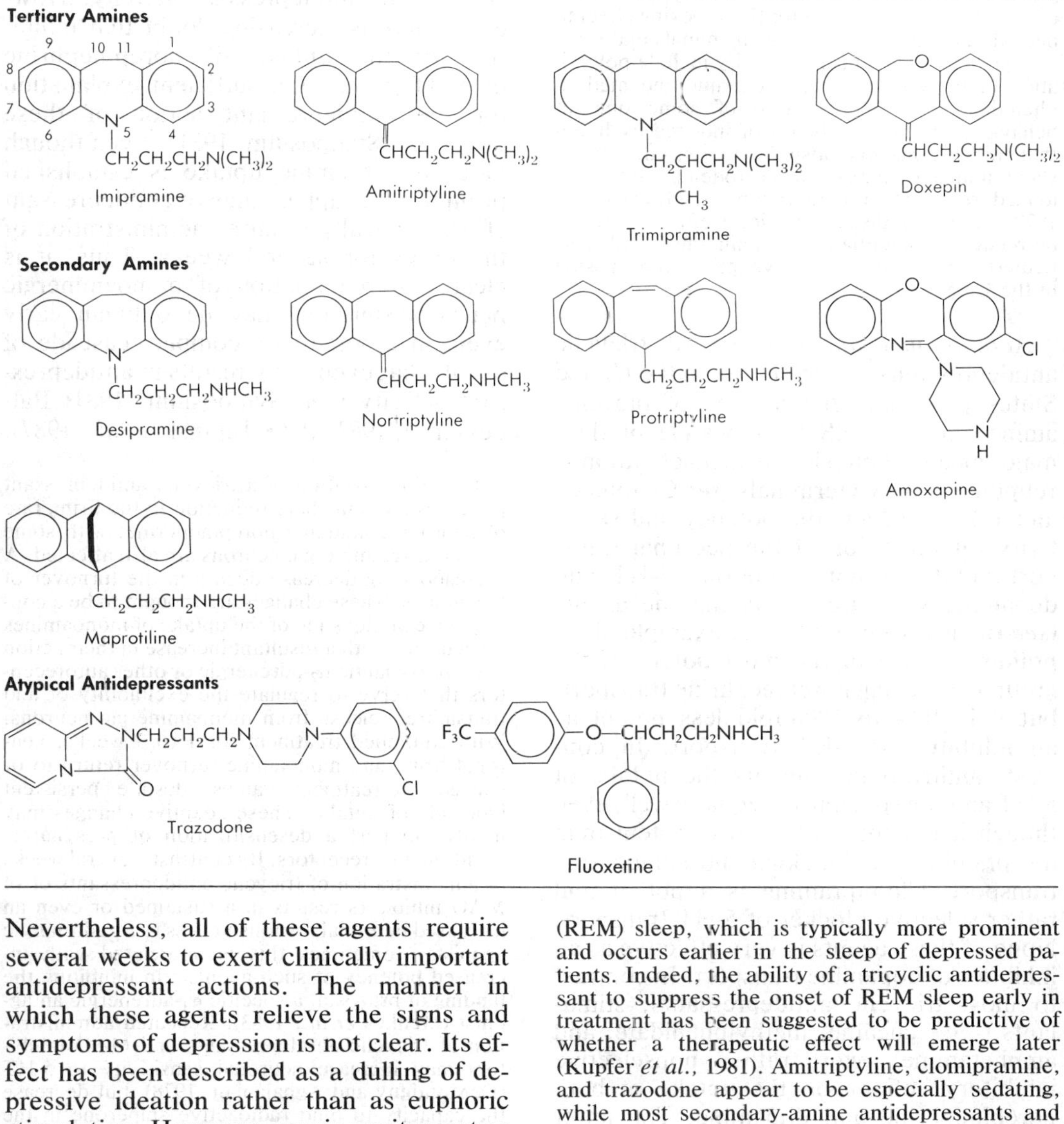

Nevertheless, all of these agents require several weeks to exert clinically important antidepressant actions. The manner in which these agents relieve the signs and symptoms of depression is not clear. Its effect has been described as a dulling of depressive ideation rather than as euphoric stimulation. However, manic excitement as well as euphoria and insomnia can be induced in susceptible patients, which contributes to the conclusion that antidepressant agents have clinically important mood-elevating actions.

Effects on Sleep. The tricyclic antidepressants occasionally have been used as hypnotics because of their sedative property; this effect may be useful in the initial therapy of a depressed patient who is not sleeping well. The imipramine-like drugs decrease the number of awakenings, increase stage-4 sleep, and markedly increase the latency and decrease the total time spent in rapid-eye-movement (REM) sleep, which is typically more prominent and occurs earlier in the sleep of depressed patients. Indeed, the ability of a tricyclic antidepressant to suppress the onset of REM sleep early in treatment has been suggested to be predictive of whether a therapeutic effect will emerge later (Kupfer *et al.,* 1981). Amitriptyline, clomipramine, and trazodone appear to be especially sedating, while most secondary-amine antidepressants and fluoxetine are less so.

Effects on Animal Behavior. Despite its clinical antidepressant effects, imipramine produces depression of spontaneous motor activity in laboratory animals. It impairs both acquisition and performance of conditioned avoidance responses. In all these tests, it is less potent than chlorpromazine, although it bears some similarities to diazepam. Effects on hexobarbital- or alcohol-induced sedation are unpredictable; ataxia and mild hypothermia are usual.

Although imipramine decreases spontaneous motor activity in animals, it is also capable of stimulating a variety of behavior patterns. Blockade of the reserpine-induced sedative or "depressive" patterns in animals is a characteristic of all the tricyclic antidepressants. The latter drugs must be given before reserpine because an intact CNS store of amines must be present for this blocking effect to become evident. Other effects in animals that seem to represent stimulant-like activity include potentiation of the effects of amphetamine and methylphenidate and augmentation of some operant behaviors. Aggressive behavior induced by hypothalamic lesions can also be increased, as can shock-induced aggression in rodents after prolonged treatment with imipramine (*see* Lowe *et al.*, 1978). Many of these behavioral effects seem to be related to potentiation of amine-mediated (particularly noradrenergic) synaptic transmission in the CNS.

Actions on Brain Amines. All tricyclic antidepressants in current use in the United States potentiate the actions of biogenic amines in the CNS by blockade of their major means of physiological inactivation—reuptake at nerve terminals (*see* Chapters 5 and 12). However, the potency and selectivity for inhibition of the neuronal transport (uptake) of norepinephrine, 5-HT, and dopamine vary greatly among the agents (*see* Baldessarini, 1985). For example, desipramine is one of the most potent of the group in blocking norepinephrine transport, but it is 100- to 1000-fold less potent as an inhibitor of 5-HT transport. In contrast, amitriptyline inhibits the uptake of 5-HT and norepinephrine equally well, even though it is about 20-fold less potent than desipramine in blocking norepinephrine transport. Clomipramine is a potent and rather selective blocker of 5-HT transport. None of these agents is very effective as an inhibitor of dopamine transport. In contrast to most tricyclic antidepressants, stimulants (*e.g.*, cocaine, methylphenidate, and amphetamine) exert rather nonselective inhibitory actions on the uptake of both norepinephrine and dopamine. The latter drugs are poor antidepressants in severe, melancholic depression, despite the fact that they have stimulant and even euphoriant effects in some people.

A few tentative generalizations may be made from these observations, together with the clinical and behavioral effects of antidepressant drugs. First, blockade of dopamine transport seems to be associated with stimulant rather than antidepressant activity. Second, inhibition of 5-HT uptake may well contribute to antidepressant activity. Finally, inhibitory actions on the uptake of norepinephrine seem to correspond with antidepressant activity. However, there is increasing doubt that inhibition of the uptake of norepinephrine or 5-HT *per se* is a sufficient explanation for the antidepressant action of these drugs (*see* Symposium, 1981). Even though blockade of amine uptake is established promptly, the appearance of antidepressant effects typically requires administration of the drugs for several weeks. Thus, it is clear that potentiation of monoaminergic neurotransmission may be only an early event in a potentially complex cascade of events that eventually results in antidepressant activity (*see* Symposium, 1981; Baldessarini, 1983, 1985; Lipinski *et al.*, 1987).

The administration of a tricyclic antidepressant produces an immediate reduction in the firing rate of neurons containing norepinephrine; with some agents, tryptaminergic neurons are also affected. A corresponding decrease occurs in the turnover of the amines. These changes are thought to be a consequence of blockade of the uptake of monoamines by neurons, with a resultant increase in their action upon presynaptic α_2-adrenergic or other autoreceptors that serve to regulate the excitability of and transmitter release from monoaminergic neurons. With continued treatment for 1 to 3 weeks, neuronal firing and monoamine turnover return to or exceed pretreatment values, despite persistent blockade of uptake. These adaptive changes may involve in part a desensitization of presynaptic α_2-adrenergic receptors. By contrast, several weeks of administration of tricyclic antidepressants or of MAO inhibitors results in a sustained or even an increased neuronal responsiveness to α_1-adrenergic agonists; sometimes this is associated with increased potency of such agonists in inhibiting the binding of prazosin, a specific α_1-adrenergic antagonist (Menkes *et al.*, 1983). Repeated administration of tricyclic antidepressants and MAO inhibitors may increase neuronal sensitivity to 5-HT (DeMontigny and Aghajanian, 1978), but decrease the capacity to bind radioactive spiperone in the cerebral cortex, suggesting a reduced number of 5-HT_2 receptors (Peroutka and Snyder, 1980a). Finally, prolonged administration of tricyclic antidepressants, atypical antidepressants, MAO inhibitors, or electroconvulsive shock *reduces* the number of β-adrenergic binding sites and the responsiveness of brain tissue to β-adrenergic agonists (*see* Sulser and Mobley, 1980). The relationship of these adaptive changes to the emergence of therapeutic responses is not known, but it seems clear that the various modalities useful in the treatment of major depression can produce similar alterations in the function of monoaminergic systems by a variety of pharmacological mechanisms.

Hypothetically, the acute reduction in turnover and release of norepinephrine, coupled with a sustained or an increased sensitivity to α_1-adrenergic agonists during antidepressant treatment, may lead to an eventual increase in the efficacy of transmission through postsynaptic α_1 receptors. This latter effect might be a consequence of the modest α_1-adrenergic antagonistic properties of most antidepressant agents (*see* below), while their low affinity for other adrenergic sites would permit the increased intrasynaptic concentrations of norepinephrine to produce desensitization or down-regulation of α_2- and β-adrenergic receptors. In addition, this moderate affinity for α_1-adrenergic receptors may represent an important distinction between true antidepressants and stimulants, which lack affinity for adrenergic or dopaminergic receptors and tend to develop rapid loss of efficacy on repeated administration (*see* Baldessarini, 1983, 1985; Lipinski *et al.,* 1987).

Tricyclic antidepressants also act as antagonists at receptors for various neurohormones; these include moderate to high affinity at muscarinic cholinergic (Snyder and Yamamura, 1977), α_1-adrenergic (U'Prichard *et al.,* 1978), and both H_1- and H_2-histaminergic receptors (Richelson, 1979). Both the pattern and potency of these effects differ widely among the various agents. For example, amitriptyline is one of the most potent of the group in blocking muscarinic cholinergic, H_1-histaminergic, and α_1-adrenergic receptors, while desipramine is 10- to 100-fold less potent than amitriptyline. These actions do not correlate with antidepressant potency, but they are probably related to various untoward effects, such as confusion, sedation, and postural hypotension.

Autonomic Nervous System. The principal effects of the tricyclic antidepressants on the function of the autonomic nervous system are believed to result from inhibition of norepinephrine transport into adrenergic nerve terminals and from antagonism of muscarinic cholinergic and α_1-adrenergic responses to the autonomic neurotransmitters. For example, the blurred vision, dry mouth, constipation, and urinary retention produced by therapeutic doses of tricyclic antidepressants are manifestations of anticholinergic actions. Amitriptyline causes a high incidence of these effects, while desipramine is less prone to do so (Blackwell *et al.,* 1978); trazodone and other atypical antidepressants have very weak anticholinergic properties (*see* Baldessarini, 1983, 1985). Since the autonomic changes that accompany depression may include some of these symptoms, the distinction between symptoms of disease and side effects of drugs may be difficult.

Cardiovascular System. In therapeutic doses, the tricyclic antidepressants have significant effects on the cardiovascular system; with overdose these effects may be life-threatening (*see* Burrows *et al.,* 1976; Cassem, 1982). In man, the most common manifestation of such effects is postural hypotension, arising in part from peripheral α-adrenergic blockade. Mild sinus tachycardia is also frequently observed, probably as a consequence of both inhibition of norepinephrine uptake and blockade of muscarinic receptors. The most prominent ECG changes found during the use of imipramine and its congeners include inversion or flattening of the T waves and evidence of prolonged conduction times at all levels of the intracardiac conduction system. Direct depression of the myocardium can also be prominent. While these actions resemble those of quinidine and can produce antiarrhythmic effects, potentially dangerous interactions may occur in the presence of preexisting conduction defects (Glassman and Bigger, 1981). Ventricular arrhythmias can be precipitated, particularly when bundle-branch block is present. In addition, tricyclic antidepressants enhance the effects of other cardiac depressant drugs. Acute studies in animals suggest that the newer antidepressants (trazodone and fluoxetine, in particular) have less intense depressant effects on cardiac conduction. Moreover, clinical studies indicate that trazodone has minimal effects on cardiac conduction and usually produces a slight sinus bradycardia instead of tachycardia (*see* Van De Merwe *et al.,* 1984). However, the relative safety of trazodone, fluoxetine, and similar atypical antidepressant agents during chronic administration to patients with cardiac disease requires further evaluation.

Since the tricyclic antidepressants can cause orthostatic hypotension, produce arrhythmias, and interact in deleterious ways with other drugs (*see* below), great caution must be observed in their use in patients with cardiac disease. Unfortunately, since many depressed patients are in an age group in which cardiac problems are common and coexistence of depressive illness and cardiovascular disease is frequent, the physician is faced with a dilemma. Milder cases may be self-limited, or treatment for anxiety and insomnia may suffice. However, antidepressants can be used in severely depressed patients; moderate, divided doses of the secondary amines (desipramine, nortriptyline) are currently preferred, and newer atypical antidepressants such as fluoxetine may also prove useful. For some severely depressed cardiac patients, ECT may be an option.

Absorption, Distribution, Fate, and Excretion. Imipramine and other tricyclic antidepressants are fairly well absorbed after oral administration. Although they are usually used initially in divided doses, their relatively long half-lives and rather wide range of tolerated concentrations permit a gradual transition toward a single daily dose given at bedtime. This is most safely done for doses up to the equivalent of 150 mg of imipramine. High doses of these strongly anticholinergic agents can slow gastrointestinal activity and gastric emptying time, resulting in slower or erratic absorption of these and other drugs taken concomitantly; this can complicate the management of acute overdosage. Concentrations in plasma typically peak within 2 to 8 hours, but this can be delayed for over 12 hours. Intramuscular administration of some tricyclic antidepressants (including clomipramine) can be performed under unusual circumstances, particularly with severely depressed, anorexic patients who may refuse oral medication.

Once absorbed, these lipophilic drugs are widely distributed; their pharmacokinetic properties are similar to those of the phenothiazines. They are strongly bound to plasma protein and to constituents of tissues. The latter fact accounts for their large volumes of apparent distribution, which are typically 10 to 50 liters per kilogram. The concentrations of these drugs in plasma that have been suggested to correlate best with satisfactory antidepressant responses range between 50 and 300 ng/ml. Toxic effects of these drugs can be expected when their concentrations in plasma rise above 1 μg/ml and can occur at even half this value (*see* Glassman and Perel, 1978; Amsterdam *et al.*, 1980; Baldessarini, 1983, 1985). However, the measurement of concentrations of antidepressants in blood has not been shown to be a useful guide for treatment or in predicting the outcome of an overdose.

The tricyclic antidepressants are oxidized by hepatic microsomal enzymes, followed by conjugation with glucuronic acid. The major route of metabolism of imipramine is to the active product desipramine; biotransformation of either compound occurs largely by oxidation to 2-hydroxy metabolites, which retain some ability to block the uptake of amines and may have particularly prominent cardiac depressant actions (*see* Kutcher *et al.*, 1986). In contrast, amitriptyline (while mainly demethylated to nortriptyline) and nortriptyline undergo preferential oxidation at the 10 position; the 10-hydroxy metabolites may have some biological activity. The conjugation of hydroxylated metabolites with glucuronic acid extinguishes any remaining biological activity. Although the demethylated metabolites of imipramine and amitriptyline possess antidepressant activity, it is not known to what extent they account for the activity of the parent drugs. These demethylated products can accumulate in concentrations approaching, or even exceeding, those of their precursors. Doxepin also appears to be converted to an active metabolite, nordoxepin, by N-demethylation (Ziegler *et al.*, 1978). Relatively little information has been published on the metabolism of the newer antidepressants in man. Amoxapine is primarily converted to the active 8-hydroxy metabolite. Fluoxetine is known to be N-demethylated to norfluoxetine, which has very long-lasting biological activity.

The inactivation and elimination of tricyclic antidepressants occur over a period of several days, and half-lives range from about 20 hours for amitriptyline to an extreme of about 80 hours for protriptyline or over 160 hours for norfluoxetine; other agents have intermediate values (*see* Appendix II). Half-lives of the N-demethylated tricyclic antidepressants typically are at least twice those of the corresponding tertiary amines. It follows that most tricyclic antidepressants should be inactivated and excreted within a week after termination of treatment, with notable exceptions being ordinary doses of protriptyline or fluoxetine and overdosage with the other agents. As with many other drugs, antidepressants are metabolized more rapidly by children and more slowly by patients over 60 years of age compared with young adults (*see* Nies *et al.*, 1977; Geller *et al.*, 1987; Popper, 1987); dosages should be adjusted accordingly.

The pharmacokinetic properties of these agents are discussed by Morselli (1977) and

Amsterdam and associates (1980); *see also* Appendix II.

Tolerance and Physical Dependence. Some tolerance to the anticholinergic effects tends to develop with continued use of imipramine. Occasional patients show physical dependence on the tricyclic antidepressants. A withdrawal syndrome consisting in malaise, chills, coryza, and muscle aching has been reported to follow abrupt discontinuation of high doses of imipramine (Shatan, 1966). Thus it is wise to discontinue a tricyclic antidepressant gradually over a week or longer. Despite these occasional problems, it is important to emphasize that tricyclic antidepressants frequently have been used for prolonged periods (years) by patients with severe recurring depression with only occasional reports of tolerance to their desirable effects (*see* Davis, 1976; Cohen and Baldessarini, 1985).

Preparations, Routes of Administration, and Dosage. These are presented in Table 18–4. A further consideration of dosage and the use of antidepressant drugs appears below.

Toxic Reactions and Side Effects. Significant side effects of tricyclic antidepressant drugs are relatively common, and estimates of prevalence have run as high as 5% (Bryant *et al.,* 1987; Pollack and Rosenbaum, 1987). Most of these reactions involve antimuscarinic effects of the drugs and cerebral intoxication, but cardiac toxicity and orthostatic hypotension also represent serious problems. Clinical consequences of the antimuscarinic effects include dry mouth and a sour or metallic taste, epigastric distress, constipation, dizziness, tachycardia, palpitations, blurred vision, and urinary retention. Special precautions should be taken in men with prostatic hypertrophy. Paradoxically, excessive sweating is a fairly common complaint; the mechanism of this response is not known. Weakness and fatigue are attributable to central effects of the drugs. Older patients suffer more from dizziness, postural hypotension, constipation, delayed micturition, edema, and muscle tremors. Very rarely, amitriptyline may cause inappropriate secretion of ADH. Trazodone, but not the other antidepressant agents, can cause priapism and permanent impotence (Lansky and Selzer, 1984).

Another undesirable effect of antidepressant drugs (and apparently of all effective forms of medical treatment of depression) is a transition in certain patients from depression to hypomanic or manic excitement. This striking feature of bipolar manic-depressive illness is sometimes re-

Table 18–4. ANTIDEPRESSANT DRUGS: DOSAGE FORMS AND DOSES

NONPROPRIETARY NAME	TRADE NAMES	DOSAGE FORMS *	USUAL DAILY DOSE (*mg*) †	EXTREME DAILY DOSE (*mg*) †,‡
Tricyclics				
Amitriptyline HCl	ELAVIL, others	O,I	50–150	40–300
Amoxapine	ASENDIN	O	200–300	50–600
Desipramine HCl	NORPRAMIN, PERTOFRANE	O	75–200	25–300
Doxepin HCl	ADAPIN, SINEQUAN	O,L	75–150	25–300
Imipramine HCl	JANIMINE, TOFRANIL, others	O,I	50–200	30–300
Maprotiline HCl	LUDIOMIL	O	75–150	25–200
Nortriptyline HCl	PAMELOR	O,L	75–100	20–150
Protriptyline HCl	VIVACTIL	O	15–40	15–60
Trimipramine maleate	SURMONTIL	O	50–150	50–300
Atypical				
Fluoxetine HCl	PROZAC	O	40–60	20–80
Trazodone HCl	DESYREL	O	150–200	50–600
Monoamine Oxidase Inhibitors				
Isocarboxazid	MARPLAN	O	10–30	10–30
Phenelzine sulfate	NARDIL	O	15–30	15–90
Tranylcypromine sulfate	PARNATE	O	20–30	10–40

* Dosage forms: O = oral solid; I = injection; L = oral liquid.

† Oral doses.

‡ Extreme doses are for very young and very elderly patients at the low end and for hospital use in severe or treatment-resistant depression at the high end. In addition, owing to the long biological half-life of MAO inhibition, small doses of MAO inhibitors are used after several days to weeks of treatment.

ferred to as the "switch process" (Goodwin, 1983). In addition to manic reactions to tricyclic antidepressants, confusion or delirium is common. These may be seen in approximately 10% of treated patients (and in over 30% of patients over age 50). These drug-related problems are frequently overlooked or misinterpreted as being part of the primary illness, particularly in the elderly. These symptoms may be secondary to central anticholinergic activity, and small doses of physostigmine may aid in the diagnosis in some cases (*see* Granacher and Baldessarini, 1975). Among the CNS problems associated with tricyclic antidepressants, extrapyramidal reactions are rare, although tremor is not unusual. A fine tremor occurs in perhaps 10% of patients receiving a tricyclic agent; the prevalence of this effect is much higher in elderly patients, particularly when high doses of drug are administered. Tremor may respond to small doses of propranolol. In the therapy of CNS-based toxic or psychiatric reactions to tricyclic antidepressants, antipsychotic drugs are to be avoided, except for the management of manic reactions or severe agitation. They may exacerbate toxic confusional states, rather than help them. In any of these reactions, whether manic or toxic-organic, the best first step is to stop the antidepressant. Physostigmine may be effective in some cases, and, if sedation is urgently required, small doses of a benzodiazepine may be considered. Another toxic effect of tricyclic antidepressants is an increased risk of tonic-clonic seizures. This risk appears to be especially great with maprotiline in doses above 250 mg per day (Rotblatt, 1982). Desipramine may have relatively less effect on seizure thresholds. In cases of overdosage, the incidence of seizures with amoxapine is especially high (Litovitz and Troutman, 1983).

Although loss of accommodation is a common ophthalmological side effect of any strongly anticholinergic agent, including most typical tricyclic antidepressants, the precipitation of glaucoma, while potentially a risk, is a rare event. The risk is probably highest in elderly patients with the narrow-angle type of glaucoma. Tricyclic antidepressants can be used in patients with glaucoma, provided that pilocarpine eyedrops or an equivalent medication is continued. The most rational choice of an antidepressant in such a case would be trazodone, desipramine, or fluoxetine.

Various types of cardiovascular difficulties have already been discussed. In the absence of cardiac disease, the principal problem associated with imipramine-like agents is postural hypotension, which can be severe (*see* Ray *et al.*, 1987; Roose *et al.*, 1987). It is often helpful to change medication to an agent (such as nortriptyline or desipramine) with less α-adrenergic blocking activity, to reduce or divide doses, and to instruct patients in the need to rise slowly from a recumbent position. Tricyclic antidepressants, especially the tertiary amines and protriptyline, are to be avoided in the period following an acute myocardial infarction, in the presence of defects in bundle-branch conduction, or when other cardiac depressants are being administered. Mild congestive heart failure and the presence of many cardiac arrhythmias are not necessarily contraindications to the use of an antidepressant when depression and its associated medical risks are severe and appropriate medical care is provided. In fact, the antiarrhythmic effects of some of the tricyclic antidepressants may actually be advantageous in some cardiac patients (*see* Glassman and Bigger, 1981; Cassem, 1982; Veith *et al.*, 1982; McGrath *et al.*, 1987; Roose *et al.*, 1987).

Children seem to be especially vulnerable to cardiotoxic and seizure-inducing effects of high doses of tricyclic compounds (Morselli, 1977; Popper, 1987). Deaths have occurred in children after accidental or deliberate overdosage with only a few hundred milligrams of drug.

Miscellaneous toxic effects of tricyclic antidepressants include jaundice, agranulocytosis, and rashes, but these are very infrequent. Weight gain is a common side effect of most antidepressants except fluoxetine (Berken *et al.*, 1984); increased appetite is usually implicated. Delay of orgasm and orgasmic impotence have been described in men and women. The safety of antidepressants during pregnancy and lactation or in the treatment of young children is not well established. Epidemiological evidence concerning the possibility of teratogenic effects of the tricyclic agents is unconvincing (*see* Goldberg and DiMascio, 1978). For severe depression during pregnancy and lactation, ECT may be a relatively safe and effective alternative.

Acute poisoning with tricyclic antidepressants is common and potentially life-threatening. Unfortunately, most of the drugs used in the treatment of severe disorders of mood are potentially lethal in doses commonly available to patients with an increased risk of suicide. Deaths have been reported with doses of approximately 2000 mg of imipramine (or the equivalent of another drug), and severe intoxication can be expected at doses above 1000 mg. As a general rule, *it is unwise to dispense more than a week's supply of an antidepressant to an acutely depressed patient.*

The presentation of symptoms and the course of events in acute poisoning with a tricyclic antidepressant is often complex (Nicotra *et al.*, 1981; Boehnert and Lovejoy, 1985). A typical pattern is a brief phase of excitement and restlessness, sometimes with myoclonus, tonic-clonic seizures, or dystonia, followed by rapid development of coma, often with depressed respiration, hypoxia, depressed reflexes, hypothermia, and hypotension. Especially with antidepressants that have relatively strong antimuscarinic potency, anticholinergic effects are striking, with mydriasis, flushed dry skin and dry mucosae, absent bowel sounds, urinary retention, and tachycardia or other cardiac arrhythmias. At this crucial stage the patient must be treated in an intensive care unit. Gastric lavage sometimes is used early in treatment. Although dialysis and diuresis are useless in such cases, administration of activated charcoal to adsorb the drug in the gut has some demonstrated utility (Crome *et al.*, 1977). The comatose phase disappears gradually, usually over 1 to 3 days, depending on the severity of the poisoning. A period of excitement and delirium is then typical, again with prominent anticholinergic signs. Even when this phase of delirious intoxication has passed, the risk of life-threatening cardiac arrhythmias continues for at least several days, requiring close medical supervision (*see* Boehnert and Lovejoy, 1985).

The efficacy and safety of various pharmacological interventions to counter tricyclic poisoning remain unsettled. Although physostigmine salicylate can sometimes produce dramatic effects to alleviate many of the antimuscarinic, cardiotoxic, and neurotoxic features of this syndrome, its safety and efficacy seem to be greater in cases of mild intoxication, characterized by confusion and delirium but with stable vital functions and the absence of coma, seizures, or life-threatening cardiac arrhythmias (Granacher and Baldessarini, 1975). In any event, physostigmine should not substitute for the aggressive use of other life-support measures (Krenzelok *et al.*, 1981).

Cardiac toxicity and hypotension in such poisonings can be especially difficult to manage. The heart is usually hyperactive, with supraventricular tachycardia and a high cardiac output. The effects of the drugs on the His-Purkinje conduction system are manifest by a prolonged duration of the QRS complex. Cardiac glycosides and antiarrhythmic drugs such as quinidine or procainamide are contraindicated, but phenytoin has been given safely and may simultaneously be useful to suppress the convulsive seizures that are often present. In addition, β-adrenergic antagonists and lidocaine have been recommended. Diazepam has been used to control seizures and myoclonic and dystonic features of tricyclic antidepressant poisoning. Aside from the problems of management created by the specific effects of tricyclic antidepressants, hypoxia, hypertension or hypotension, and metabolic acidosis may have to be treated. In the presence of high concentrations of tricyclic antidepressants, the effects of α-adrenergic agonists, used as pressor agents, may be unpredictable, and maintenance of intravascular volume may be difficult to achieve.

Interactions with Other Drugs. The tricyclic antidepressants are involved in several clinically important drug interactions (*see* Baldessarini, 1985; Hansten, 1985). The binding of tricyclic antidepressants to plasma albumin can be reduced by competition with phenytoin, phenylbutazone, aspirin, aminopyrine, scopolamine, and phenothiazines. Other interactions that may also potentiate the effects of tricyclic antidepressants can result from interference with their metabolism in the liver. This effect has been associated with neuroleptic drugs, methylphenidate, and certain steroids, including oral contraceptives. In the opposite direction, barbiturates and certain other sedatives, as well as cigarette smoking, can increase the hepatic metabolism of the antidepressants by inducing microsomal enzyme systems; benzodiazepines do not seem to have this effect.

Antidepressants potentiate the effects of alcohol and probably other sedatives. The anticholinergic activity of tricyclic antidepressants makes it important to monitor the results if the drugs must be used simultaneously with antiparkinsonian agents, antipsychotic drugs of low potency (especially thioridazine), or other compounds with antimuscarinic activity. The tricyclic antidepressants have prominent and potentially dangerous potentiative interactions with biogenic amines, such as norepinephrine, which normally are removed from their site of action by neuronal uptake. However, they block the effects of indirectly acting amines, such as tyramine, which must be taken up by sympathetic neurons to cause the release of norepinephrine. Presumably by a similar mechanism, tricyclic antidepressants prevent the action of adrenergic neuron blocking agents such as guanethidine. This effect may be less noticeable with trimipramine, trazodone, and perhaps fluoxetine, which are less potent blockers of reuptake of norepinephrine by sympathetic neurons. While its peripheral effects are blocked, the CNS stimulation produced by amphetamine may be potentiated by tricyclic antidepressants. This results from the inability of these drugs to interfere with amphetamine-induced release of dopamine from CNS neurons, combined with inhibition of the hepatic metabolism of amphetamine by tricyclic antidepressants (*see* Iversen *et al.*, 1978).

Tricyclic agents and trazodone can block the centrally mediated antihypertensive action of clonidine. A particularly severe, but rare, interaction has been noted following the concurrent administration of an MAO inhibitor and a tricyclic antidepressant. The resultant syndrome can include severe CNS toxicity, marked by hyperpyrexia, convulsions, and coma. Although this reaction is rare and the two classes of antidepressant agents have been combined safely (*see* White and Simpson, 1981), this use should be regarded as unusual and controversial, since the interaction has a potentially catastrophic outcome. There is insufficient evidence that treatment with tricyclic agents plus MAO inhibitors is more efficacious than aggressive use of either type of antidepressant alone. Tricyclic antidepressants can be used safely during a course of ECT, but the dose prior to each treatment is usually omitted.

Therapeutic Uses. The use of tricyclic antidepressants in depressed patients is discussed below (*see* page 422).

Several other possible indications for these drugs have been suggested (Klein *et al.*, 1980; Baldessarini, 1985). *Enuresis* in children over 6 years of age has been accepted as a possible use for imipramine (in doses up to 2.5 mg/kg, or 50 mg total, daily). This effect is temporary but it occurs without delay; it may also be obtained with incontinent elderly patients. Since recognition of major depression in children is increasing and since the syndrome of attention disorder with hyperactivity may also respond to these agents, the use of imipramine and other antidepressants in this age group is becoming more accepted (Biederman and Jellinek, 1984; Puig-Antich, 1987). Because of the more efficient clearance of tricyclic antidepressants in children, effective doses may be up to twice the adult doses on a mg/kg basis (*see* Biederman *et al.*, 1986; Popper, 1987).

Other areas of suggested use that remain investigational include certain syndromes that may mimic depression, overlap diagnostically with depression, or be accompanied by or complicated by secondary depression. These include *alcoholism, bulimia* (*see* Pope and Hudson, 1986), *severe anxiety syndromes* that are characterized by panic reactions (Klein *et al.*, 1980), and some cases of *obsessive-compulsive disorder*. The latter disorder seems to be most likely to respond to agents that potentiate 5-HT; clomipramine is the most extensively evaluated, and fluoxetine is being studied (Insel and Zohar, 1987). Some cases of *chronic pain, neuralgias, migraine, sleep apnea, fibromyalgia,* and *irritable bowel syndrome* may also respond to an antidepressant agent (Ries *et al.*, 1984; Greenbaum *et al.*, 1987; Mendelson, 1987; France and Krishnan, 1988; Goldenberg, 1989). Also, evidence suggests that some antidepressants, notably doxepin, may be of benefit in the treatment of patients with *peptic ulcer*. It is not certain whether the blockade of muscarinic and H_2-histaminergic receptors by these agents can account completely for these effects.

MONOAMINE OXIDASE (MAO) INHIBITORS

The MAO inhibitors comprise a chemically heterogeneous group of drugs that have in common the ability to block oxidative deamination of naturally occurring monoamines. Although MAO inhibitors are probably as effective as tricyclic antidepressants in the treatment of major depression, the complex, sometimes severe, and often unpredictable interactions between MAO inhibitors and many drugs and food-derived amines make their medical use difficult and potentially hazardous. Thus, the use of MAO inhibitors in psychiatry has become limited as the tricyclic and newer atypical antidepressants have come to dominate the treatment of depression and allied conditions. MAO inhibitors are used most often when tricyclic antidepressants give an unsatisfactory result and when ECT is inappropriate or refused. In addition, certain neurotic illnesses with depressive features, and also with anxiety and phobias, may respond especially favorably to these drugs. (*See* Robinson *et al.*, 1978; Klein *et al.*, 1980; Baldessarini, 1984a, 1985.)

History. In 1951, *isoniazid* and its isopropyl derivative, *iproniazid,* were developed for the treatment of tuberculosis. It was soon found that iproniazid had mood-elevating effects in tuberculous patients. In 1952, Zeller and coworkers found that iproniazid, in contrast to isoniazid, was capable of inhibiting the enzyme MAO. Following investigations by Kline and colleagues and by Crane it was applied in psychiatry for the treatment of depressed patients. MAO inhibitors had an important impact on the development of modern biological psychiatry. (For reviews of this topic, *see* Weil-Malherbe, 1967; Ayd and Blackwell, 1970; Baldessarini, 1983.)

Chemistry and Structure–Activity Relationship. The first MAO inhibitors to be used in the treatment of depression were derivatives of hydrazine, a highly hepatotoxic substance. *Phenelzine* is the hydrazine analog of phenethylamine, a substrate for MAO; *isocarboxazid* is a hydrazide derivative that probably must be converted to the corresponding hydrazine to produce long-lasting inhibition of MAO. Subsequently, compounds unrelated to hydrazine were found to be potent MAO inhibitors. Several of these agents were structurally related to amphetamine and were synthesized in an attempt to enhance central stimulant properties. Cyclization of the side chain of amphetamine resulted in the MAO inhibitor *tranylcypromine*. Experimental MAO inhibitors include a series of propargylamines that contain an acetylenic bond. Details of the structure–activity relationship and the chemistry of these agents can be found elsewhere (*see* Biel *et al.*, 1978; Maxwell and White, 1978). Structures of the MAO inhibitors currently available in the United States are as follows:

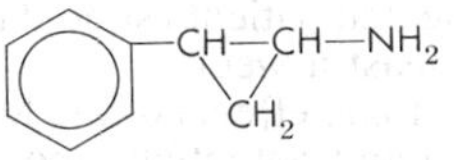

Tranylcypromine

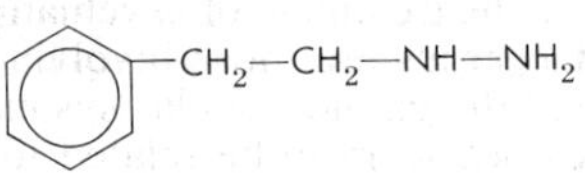

Phenelzine

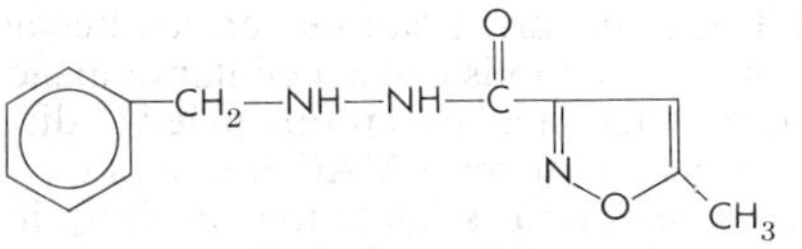

Isocarboxazid

PHARMACOLOGICAL PROPERTIES

MAO inhibitors exert their effects mainly on organ systems influenced by sympathomimetic amines and 5-HT. These agents inhibit not only MAO but other enzymes as well, and they interfere with the hepatic metabolism of many drugs. In addition, they are believed to exert effects not directly related to enzyme inhibition. MAO is a flavin-containing enzyme that is localized in mitochondrial membranes, whether in nerve terminals, the liver, or other organs. It is biochemically dissimilar to other nonspecific amine oxidases found, for example, in plasma. It is closely linked functionally with an aldehyde reductase in all tissues, but the products of these reactions can be carboxylic acids *or* alcohols, depending on the substrate and the tissue. MAO is important in regulating the metabolic degradation of catecholamines and 5-HT in neural or target tissues, and hepatic MAO has a crucial defensive role in inactivating circulating monoamines or those, such as tyramine, that originate in the gut and are absorbed into the portal circulation.

There are at least two types of MAO, which display dissimilar preferences for substrates and differential sensitivities to selective inhibitors; these were originally defined by sensitivity to clorgiline and preference for 5-HT (MAO-A) and by sensitivity to selegiline (deprenyl) and preference for phenylethylamine (MAO-B). (These selective inhibitors are examples of propargylamines, mentioned above.) The two types of MAO appear to be distinct molecular entities that exist in various proportions in different tissues. For example, human placenta and intestinal mucosa contain only MAO-A, and this type appears to be predominant in the peripheral noradrenergic nerve terminals of the rat. In contrast, human platelets contain only MAO-B, while about equal amounts of both types are found in the liver and brain of most species. The MAO inhibitors currently in therapeutic use are relatively nonselective, but selective inhibitors may offer advantages in certain clinical settings. Only selective inhibitors of MAO-A (*e.g.*, clorgiline) appear to have efficacy in the treatment of major depression; all of these agents remain experimental. Recently, a series of selective inhibitors of MAO-A have been developed whose actions are rapidly reversible (*e.g.*, *brofaromine, cimoxatone, moclobemide*). These agents appear to be clinically effective and to have much less ability to potentiate the pressor actions of tyramine than do the nonselective MAO inhibitors (*see* Delini-Stula *et al.*, 1988). Extensive discussions of these and other aspects of MAO and its inhibitors are available (*see* Symposium, 1979; Baldessarini, 1984a). (*See also* Chapters 5 and 20.)

The MAO inhibitors in clinical use are site-directed, irreversible ("suicide") inhibitors (*see* Singer, in Symposium, 1979). The hydrazines (phenelzine and the putative active metabolite of isocarboxazid) and the acetylenic agents (pargyline, clorgiline, and selegiline) attack and inactivate the flavin prosthetic group following their oxidation to reactive intermediates by MAO. The chemistry of inhibition by cyclopropylamines (tranylcypromine) is less certain, but appears to involve the reaction of a sulfhydryl group in the active center of the enzyme following the formation of an imine by the action of MAO. In the clinical setting, maximal inhibition is usually achieved within a few days, although the antidepressant effect of these drugs may be delayed for 2 or 3 weeks. Up to 2 weeks may be required to restore amine metabolism to normal following withdrawal of the drugs, presumably because of the necessity for synthesis of the enzyme; reversal following tranylcypromine is only slightly more rapid, possibly reflecting slow, spontaneous decomposition of the enzyme-inhibitor adduct. Behavioral effects of tranylcypromine are also produced more rapidly, perhaps owing to acute amphetamine-like stimulant actions.

Evaluation of MAO activity in human subjects taking these drugs has led to the impression that favorable clinical responses are likely to occur when platelet MAO is inhibited by at least 85% (Robinson *et al.*, 1978). This relationship is best established for phenelzine, but it has encouraged more aggressive dosing with MAO inhibitors to seek their maximal therapeutic potential.

The capacity of MAO inhibitors to act as antidepressants has most often been assumed to reflect the increased availability of one or more monoamines in the CNS or sympathetic nervous system, although this assumption has been difficult to prove. One problem is that the acute biochemical and pharmacological actions of MAO inhibitors precede their palliative effects in psychiatric illnesses by as long as 2 or more weeks. Reasons for this delay of therapeutic effects remain unexplained, but they are reminiscent of the delayed effect of the tricyclic antidepressants.

Effects on Sleep. MAO inhibitors are highly effective suppressors of REM sleep. This effect has been used therapeutically in the treatment of narcolepsy. Moreover, when they are effective in the treatment of depression, MAO inhibitors correct the accompanying disorder of sleep, whether it is an increase or decrease of sleep time.

Animal Behavior. The administration of single doses of an MAO inhibitor produces either minor changes in the behavior of animals or none at all, even when concentrations of dopamine, norepinephrine, and 5-HT in the CNS are significantly elevated. However, when these drugs are combined with other agents, marked effects may be seen. Thus, in animals pretreated with MAO inhibitors, reserpine and tetrabenazine produce excitement rather than sedation (probably because of protection of monoamines released from intracellular storage); by contrast, hexobarbital-induced sleeping time is prolonged, and the actions of many other CNS depressants and stimulants may be augmented.

Cardiovascular System. The predominant cardiovascular effect associated with the use of MAO inhibitors is orthostatic hypotension, usually with only minor elevations of basal diastolic or systolic pressure; occasionally, a significant elevation in blood pressure may be seen that is apparently unrelated to exposure to exogenous pressor substances (*see* Keck *et al.*, 1989). In hypertensive patients, MAO inhibitors lower blood pressure and provide symptomatic relief in angina pectoris. Although pargyline is available for this indication, its use as an antihypertensive agent is essentially extinct (*see previous editions* of this textbook).

Absorption, Fate, and Excretion. The MAO inhibitors are absorbed readily when given by mouth; they are not given parenterally. These drugs produce maximal inhibition of MAO within 5 to 10 days. Little information is available on their pharmacokinetics. Although their biological activity is prolonged owing to the characteristics of their interaction with the enzyme, their clinical efficacy appears to be reduced when the drug is given less frequently than once daily.

The hydrazide MAO inhibitors are thought to be cleaved, with resultant liberation of active products (*e.g.*, hydrazines). They are inactivated primarily by acetylation. About one half the population in the United States and Europe (and more in certain Orientals) are "slow acetylators" of hydrazine-type drugs, including phenelzine, and this may contribute to the exaggerated effects observed in some patients given conventional doses of phenelzine.

Preparations and Dosage. These are presented in Table 18–4. A further consideration of dosage and the clinical use of these agents appears below.

Toxic Reactions and Side Effects. Toxic reactions from overdosage may occur in a matter of hours despite the long delay in onset of a therapeutic response. Effects of overdosage include agitation, hallucinations, hyperreflexia, hyperpyrexia, and convulsions. Both hypotension and hypertension also occur. Treatment of such intoxication presents a problem. Conservative treatment aimed at maintaining normal temperature, respiration, blood pressure, and proper fluid and electrolyte balance is often successful. Since the inhibition of MAO is irreversible, late toxic effects may appear. Severely intoxicated patients should be observed in hospital for at least a week.

The potential toxic effects of the MAO inhibitors are more varied and potentially more serious than are those of most other groups of therapeutic agents used in the treatment of psychiatric patients. The most dangerous are those involving the liver, the brain, and the cardiovascular system. Hepatotoxicity does not seem to be related to dosage or duration of therapy, and the incidence with currently used MAO inhibitors is low. Nevertheless, when it does occur, it can be serious because the hydrazine compounds cause cellular damage to the hepatic parenchyma. This problem led to discontinuation of use of several MAO inhibitors.

Excessive central stimulation resulting in tremors, insomnia, and hyperhidrosis may occur and might be considered extensions of the pharmacological effects. Agitation and hypomanic behavior may also occur, and on rare occasions hallucinations and confusion are observed, as are convulsions. Peripheral neuropathy following the use of hydrazines may be related to a pyridoxine deficiency.

Orthostatic hypotension occurs with use of all the MAO inhibitors currently employed. The immediate condition readily yields to recumbency, but the dose may have to be reduced or the medication withdrawn.

A variety of other less serious side effects have been reported, including dizziness and vertigo (perhaps related to orthostatic hypotension), headache, inhibition of ejaculation, difficulty in urination, weakness, fatigue, dry mouth, blurred vision, and skin rashes. Constipation is common, but the cause is not known. Phenelzine seems especially likely to exert such effects, even though significant antimuscarinic activity has not been detected *in vitro*.

Interactions with Other Drugs. The paucity of grossly observable signs following the administration of MAO inhibitors is deceptive, for major changes have occurred in the body's capacity to handle endogenous or exogenous biogenic amines and to respond normally to a wide spectrum of pharmacological agents (Baldessarini, 1985; Hansten, 1985). Administration of precursors of biogenic amines may cause marked effects when administered following MAO inhibitors. Thus, the concurrent administration of levodopa and an MAO inhibitor produces agitation and hypertension. The actions of sympathomimetic amines are similarly potentiated. The effect is greater with indirectly acting amines (*e.g.*, amphetamine and tyramine) than with directly acting amines, which are potentiated in man to a greater degree by the tricyclic antidepressants. Since administered catecholamines are inactivated largely by catechol-O-methyltransferase and by neuronal uptake, the MAO inhibitors have less effect in prolonging and intensifying their action. On the other hand, inasmuch as certain sympathomimetic amines such as amphetamine and tyramine act peripherally, primarily by releasing the stores of catecholamines in nerve endings, and since the concentration of amines is raised by MAO inhibitors, profound potentiation of effects such as pressor responses may be expected (*see* below).

MAO inhibitors also interfere with detoxification mechanisms for certain other drugs. They prolong and intensify the effects of central-depressant agents, such as general anesthetics, sedatives, antihistamines, alcohol, and potent analgesics; of anticholinergic agents, particularly those used in the treatment of parkinsonism; and of antidepressant agents, especially imipramine and amitriptyline. A serious hyperpyrexic reaction occurs after the concomitant use of meperidine or perhaps other phenylpiperidine analgesics. This reaction may be mediated by the release of 5-HT (*see* Kaufman, 1976).

Hypertensive crisis is a most serious toxic effect of MAO inhibitors related to drug interaction. Hypertensive crises were noted to be associated with the ingestion of cheese in patients receiving MAO inhibitors. Acting on the suggestion of an alert pharmacist, Blackwell suggested that certain cheeses might contain a pressor amine or substance capable of liberating stored catecholamines (*see* Ayd and Blackwell, 1970). Tyramine was soon implicated as the culpable substance. The average meal of natural or aged cheeses contains enough tyramine to provoke a marked rise in blood pressure and other cardiovascular changes. As a result of inhibition of MAO, tyramine and other monoamines in food or produced by bacteria in the gut escape oxidative deamination in the liver and other organs and release catecholamines that are present in supranormal amounts in nerve endings and the adrenal medulla. Other foods implicated in this syndrome include beer, wine, pickled herring, snails, chicken liver, yeast, large quantities of coffee, citrus fruits, canned figs, broad beans (which contain dopa), and chocolate and cream or their products. Since more than 10 mg of tyramine seems to be required to produce significant hypertension, the most dangerous foods are aged cheeses and yeast products used as food supplements (*see* Folks, 1983). Patients being treated with an MAO inhibitor and their families should be given a list of foods to be avoided and a general warning about the use of *any* medication by the patient without permission. Care must be exercised even here, since certain depressed patients have used such a list as a compilation of potential suicidal agents.

In certain instances, intracranial bleeding has occurred, and death has sometimes followed. Headache is a common symptom, and fever frequently accompanies the hypertensive episode. Opioids should never be used for such headaches, and blood pressure should be evaluated immediately when a patient taking an MAO inhibitor reports a severe throbbing headache. The hypertensive syndrome is clinically similar to that seen in pheochromocytoma. Such episodes may also be encountered when MAO inhibitors are used with sympathomimetic amines, methyldopa, or dopamine. Acute increases in blood pressure also can follow the initial doses of reserpine and adrenergic neuron blocking agents such as guanethidine, when these are given concurrently with an MAO inhibitor. It should be noted that tranylcypromine can cause a reaction if administered when the effect of phenelzine is still present. Switching a patient from one MAO inhibitor to another or to a tricyclic antidepressant requires that a rest period of 2 weeks intervenes. A short-acting α-adrenergic blocking agent (*e.g.*, phentolamine, 2 to 5 mg, intravenously) is recommended for treatment of the hypertensive crisis; intravenous nitroprusside can also be used.

The actual incidence of serious side effects is difficult to determine. It has been estimated that 3.5 million patients had used tranylcypromine by 1970 and, of these, perhaps 50 persons sustained cerebrovascular accidents and 15 died. There is no evidence that the relative incidence of hypertensive crises is any greater with tranylcypromine than with the other agents in this class. However, tranylcypromine is not recommended for use in patients over 60 years of age, or in those with cardiac disease or hypertension or at risk of stroke; it is questionable whether *any* irreversible MAO inhibitor should be used by patients in these categories.

It is important to distinguish between the hypertensive interaction of MAO inhibitors and pressor amines and the potentially catastrophic interaction between MAO inhibitors and tricyclic antidepressants. The latter reaction is characterized by high fever and cerebral excitation, with variable degrees of hypertension; its mechanism is obscure. Tricyclic antidepressants may protect against the pressor effects of indirectly acting sympathomimetic amines such as tyramine, which must be transported into sympathetic nerve terminals to exert their action.

Therapeutic Uses. The MAO inhibitors have been used primarily in the treatment of *depression* and certain *phobic-anxiety* states. They may also be of value in the treatment of *bulimia, posttraumatic reactions,* and other *obsessive-compulsive,* ruminative disorders. Their possible use in *narcolepsy* is mentioned above. MAO inhibitors have been reserved mainly for patients refractory to other treatments. The use of MAO inhibitors in psychiatry is discussed below, with other drug treatments for disorders of mood (page 422).

LITHIUM SALTS

Lithium salts were introduced into psychiatry in 1949 for the treatment of mania. However, they were not accepted in the United States for this use until 1970, in part due to reluctance of American physicians to accept the safety of this treatment. This resistance was the result of reports of severe intoxication with lithium chloride from its uncontrolled use as a substitute for sodium chloride in patients with cardiac disease. Evidence for both the safety and the efficacy of lithium salts in the treatment of mania and the prevention of recurrent attacks of manic-depressive illness is now highly impressive. Many details of the pharmacology and uses of lithium salts in psychiatry and medicine are reviewed elsewhere (Johnson, 1980; Herrington and Lader, 1981; Jefferson *et al.*, 1983).

History. Lithium urate is quite soluble, and, accordingly, lithium salts were used in the nineteenth century as a treatment of gout. Lithium bromide was employed in that era as a sedative (including its use in manic patients) and anticonvulsant as well. Thereafter, lithium salts were little used until the late 1940s, when lithium chloride was employed as a salt substitute for cardiac and other chronically ill patients. This ill-advised usage led to several reports of severe intoxication and death and to considerable notoriety concerning lithium salts within the medical profession. Cade in Australia, while looking for toxic nitrogenous substances in the urine of mental patients for testing in guinea pigs, administered lithium salts to the animals in an attempt to increase the solubility of urates. Lithium carbonate made the animals lethargic, and, in an inductive leap, Cade gave lithium carbonate to several agitated or manic psychiatric patients. In 1949, he reported that this treatment seemed to have a specific effect in mania. For a more detailed account of the early development of lithium salts in psychiatric therapeutics, *see* Schou (1968) and Ayd and Blackwell (1970).

Chemistry. Lithium is the lightest of the alkali metals (group Ia); the salts of this monovalent cation share some characteristics with those of Na^+ and K^+, but not others. Li^+ is readily assayed in biological fluids by flame-photometric and atomic-absorption spectrophotometric methods. Traces of the ion occur in animal tissues, but it has no known physiological role. It is abundant in some alkaline mineral-spring waters. Both lithium carbonate and lithium citrate are currently in therapeutic use in the United States.

PHARMACOLOGICAL PROPERTIES

Therapeutic concentrations of Li^+ have almost no discernible psychotropic effects in normal man. It is not a sedative, depressant, or euphoriant, and this characteristic differentiates Li^+ from other psychotropic agents. The general biology and pharmacology of Li^+ have been reviewed in detail by Schou (1969). The mechanism of action of Li^+ as a mood-stabilizing agent remains unknown, although effects on biological membranes and synaptic neurotransmission are suspected.

An important characteristic of Li^+ is that it has a relatively small gradient of distribution across biological membranes, unlike Na^+ and K^+; although it can replace Na^+ in supporting a single action potential in a nerve cell, it is not an adequate "substrate" for the Na^+ pump and it cannot, therefore, maintain membrane potentials. It is uncertain whether important interactions occur between Li^+ (at therapeutic concentrations of about 1 mEq per liter) and the transport of other monovalent or divalent cations by nerve cells.

Central Nervous System. In addition to speculations about altered distribution of ions in the CNS, much attention has centered on the effects of low concentrations of Li^+ on the metabolism of the biogenic monoamines that have been implicated in the pathophysiology of mood disorders.

In animal brain tissue, Li^+ at concentrations of 1 to 10 mEq per liter inhibits the depolarization-provoked and Ca^{2+}-dependent release of norepinephrine and dopamine, but *not* 5-HT, from nerve terminals (Baldessarini and Vogt, 1988). Li^+ may even enhance the release of 5-HT, especially in the hippocampus (Treiser *et al.*, 1981). It may also slightly alter the reuptake and presynaptic storage of catecholamines in directions consistent with increased inactivation of the amines. The ion has little effect on catecholamine-sensitive adenylyl cyclase activity or on the binding of ligands to putative adrenergic receptors in brain tissue, although there is some inconsistent evidence that Li^+ can inhibit the effects of receptor blocking agents to cause supersensitivity in such systems (Pert *et al.*, 1978; Bloom *et al.*, 1983). Li^+ has been noted to modify hormonal responses mediated by adenylyl cyclase in other tissues (*see* below). The effects of Li^+ on the distribution of Na^+, Ca^{2+}, and Mg^{2+} and on glucose metabolism have all been suggested to contribute to the antimanic or mood-stabilizing effects of the ion, but none of these hypotheses has been substantiated.

In recent years, evidence has accumulated for an important second-messenger role for inositol trisphosphate and diacylglycerides (*see* Chapter 2). These compounds are released by hydrolysis of membrane phosphatidylinositides as a result of activation of receptors for numerous neurohormones. Lithium ion (at a concentration of 1 mM) inhibits the hydrolysis of inositol-l-phosphate in brain and other tissues. As a result, Li^+ can decrease the content of phosphatidylinositides of cells that are stimulated intensely and that are insulated from exogenous sources of inositol (*e.g.*, neurons in the CNS). Depletion of phosphatidylinositides may reduce the responsiveness of neurons to muscarinic cholinergic, α-adrenergic, or other stimuli. Hypothetically, treatment with Li^+ could selectively modulate the function of hyperactive neurons that contribute to the manic state (*see* Berridge *et al.*, 1982; Berridge, 1984; Worley *et al.*, 1988; Casebolt and Jope, 1989).

Absorption, Distribution, and Excretion. Lithium ions are absorbed readily and almost completely from the gastrointestinal tract. Complete absorption occurs in about 8 hours, with peak concentrations in plasma occurring 2 to 4 hours after an oral dose. Slow-release preparations of lithium carbonate provide a slower rate of absorption and thereby minimize early peaks in plasma concentrations of the ion. However, absorption can be more variable and the incidence of lower intestinal tract symptoms may be increased. Li^+ is initially distributed in the extracellular fluid and then gradually accumulated in various tissues to different degrees. The concentration gradients across cellular membranes are much smaller than those for Na^+ and K^+. The final volume of distribution (0.7 to 0.9 liter per kilogram) is slightly higher than that of total body water. Passage through the blood–brain barrier is slow, and when a steady state is achieved the concentration of Li^+ in the cerebrospinal fluid is about 40 to 50% of the concentration in plasma. There is no evidence of the ion binding to plasma proteins.

Approximately 95% of a single dose of Li^+ is eliminated in the urine. About one third to two thirds of an acute dose is excreted during a 6- to 12-hour initial phase of excretion, followed by a slow excretion over the next 10 to 14 days. The elimination half-life averages 20 to 24 hours. With repeated administration, Li^+ excretion increases during the first 5 to 6 days until steady state is reached between ingestion and excretion. When therapy with Li^+ is stopped, there is a rapid phase of renal excretion followed by a slow 10- to 14-day phase. Since 80% of the filtered Li^+ is reabsorbed by the proximal renal tubules, clearance of Li^+ by the kidney is about 20% of that for creatinine, ranging between 15 and 30 ml per minute. This is somewhat lower in elderly patients (10 to 15 ml per minute) and higher in young persons. Loading with Na^+ produces a small enhancement of Li^+ excretion, but Na^+ depletion promotes a clinically important degree of retention of Li^+.

Because of the low therapeutic index for Li^+ (as low as 2 or 3), concentrations in plasma or serum must be determined to facilitate the safe use of the drug. This is usually done daily in the treatment of acutely manic patients. Indeed, the risks of such early treatment are sufficiently great that one can postpone treatment with Li^+ until some degree of behavioral control and metabolic stability have been attained with antipsychotic drugs or sedatives. Although the concentration of Li^+ in blood is usually measured at a trough of the oscillations that result from repetitive administration, the peaks can be two or three times higher than the steady-state concentration. When the peaks are reached, intoxication may result. (This can occur even when concentrations in morning samples of plasma are in the acceptable range of around 1 mEq per liter.) Evidence suggests that single daily doses, with relatively large oscillations of the plasma concentration of Li^+, may reduce the polyuria sometimes associated with this treatment (Plenge *et al.*, 1982). Nevertheless, because of the very low margin of safety of Li^+ and because of its short half-life during initial distribution, divided daily doses are used and even slow-release formulations typically are given two or three times daily.

Although the pharmacokinetics of Li^+ varies considerably between subjects, it is relatively stable in an individual patient. However, well-established regimens can be complicated by occasional periods of Na^+ loss, as may occur with an intercurrent medical illness, or with losses or restrictions of fluids and electrolytes; heavy sweating may be an exception due to a preferential secretion of Li^+ over Na^+ in sweat (*see* Jefferson *et al.*, 1982). Hence, all patients should have plasma concentrations checked at least occasionally. The relatively stable and characteristic pharmacokinetics of Li^+ in each patient makes it possible to predict dosage requirements of an individual based on the results of administration of a small test dose of lithium carbonate, followed by a single plasma assay 24 hours later (Cooper and Simpson, 1978).

Most of the renal tubular reabsorption of Li^+ seems to occur in the proximal tubule. Nevertheless, its retention can be increased by any diuretic that leads to depletion of Na^+ (*e.g.*, amiloride, ethacrynic acid, furosemide, and thiazides) (Himmelhoch *et al.*, 1977; DePaulo *et al.*, 1981). Renal excretion can be increased somewhat by the administration of osmotic diuretics, acetazolamide, or aminophylline, although this is of little help in the management of Li^+-induced toxicity. Triamterene may increase excretion of Li^+, suggesting that some reabsorption of the ion may occur in the distal nephron; however, spironolactone does not increase the excretion of Li^+. Some nonsteroidal antiinflammatory agents (*e.g.*, indomethacin and phenylbutazone) can facilitate renal proximal tubular resorption of Li^+ and thereby increase concentrations in plasma (*see* DePaulo *et al.*, 1981).

Less than 1% of ingested Li^+ leaves the human body in the feces, and 4 to 5% is excreted in the sweat. Li^+ is secreted in saliva in concentrations about twice those in plasma, while its concentration in tears is about equal to that in plasma. It is feasible to analyze these fluids instead of plasma to monitor concentrations of Li^+ (Brenner *et al.*, 1982; Selinger *et al.*, 1982). Since the ion is also secreted in human milk, women receiving Li^+ should not breast-feed infants.

Preparations and Dosage. Preparations currently used in the United States are 150-, 300-, and 600-mg tablets or capsules of Li_2CO_3. Slow-release preparations of lithium carbonate are also available, as are liquid preparations of lithium citrate. In Europe and elsewhere, salts other than the carbonate have been used. The carbonate salt is favored for tablets and capsules because it is relatively less hygroscopic and less irritating to the gut than other salts, especially the chloride salt.

Li^+ is not prescribed merely by dose; instead, owing to the very low therapeutic index, determination of the concentration of the ion in blood is crucial. Li^+ cannot be used with adequate safety in patients who cannot be tested regularly. The concentration that is currently considered to be effective and acceptably safe is between 0.75 and 1.25 mEq per liter; the range of 1.0 to 1.25 mEq per liter is favored for treatment of manic or hypomanic patients. Somewhat lower values (0.75 to 1.0 mEq per liter) are considered adequate and safer for long-term use for prevention of recurrent manic-depressive illness; some patients may not relapse at concentrations as low as 0.5 to 0.75 mEq per liter (Maj *et al.*, 1986). These concentrations refer to serum or plasma samples obtained at 10 ± 2 hours after the last oral dose of the day. The recommended concentration is often attained by doses of 900 to 1500 mg of lithium carbonate per day in outpatients and 1200 to 2400 mg per day in hospitalized manic patients; the optimal dose tends to be larger in younger and heavier individuals.

Toxic Reactions and Side Effects. The occurrence of toxicity is related to the plasma concentration of Li^+ and its rate of rise following administration. Acute intoxication is characterized by vomiting, profuse diarrhea, coarse tremor, ataxia, coma, and convulsions. Symptoms of milder toxicity are most likely to occur at the absorptive peak of Li^+ and include nausea, vomiting, abdominal pain, diarrhea, sedation, and fine tremor. The more serious effects involve the nervous system and consist in mental confusion, hyperreflexia, gross tremor, dysarthria, seizures, and cranial-nerve and focal neurological signs, progressing to coma and death (Saron and Gaind, 1973). Other toxic effects are cardiac arrhythmias, hypotension, and albuminuria.

Therapy with Li^+ is associated initially with a transient increase in the excretion of 17-hydroxycorticosteroids, Na^+, K^+, and water. This effect is usually not sustained beyond 24 hours. In the subsequent 4 to 5 days, the excretion of K^+ becomes normal, Na^+ is retained, and, in some cases, pretibial edema forms. Na^+ retention has been associated with increased aldosterone secretion and responds to administration of spironolactone; however, this maneuver incurs the risk of promoting the retention of Li^+ and increasing its concentration in plasma. Edema and Na^+ retention frequently disappear spontaneously after several days.

A small number of patients treated with Li^+ develop a benign, diffuse, nontender thyroid enlargement, suggestive of compromised thyroid function. In patients treated with Li^+ thyroid ^{131}I uptake is increased, plasma protein-bound iodine and free thyroxine tend to be slightly low, and thyroid-stimulating hormone (TSH) secretion may be moderately elevated. These effects appear to result from interference with the iodination of tyrosine and, therefore, the synthesis of thyroxine. However, patients usually remain euthyroid and obvious hypothyroidism is rare. In patients who do develop goiter, discontinuation of Li^+ or treatment with thyroid hormone results in shrinkage of the gland. In rats, the ion inhibits thyrotropin activation of thyroid adenylyl cyclase; inhibitory effects of Li^+ have been noted on the synthesis of cyclic AMP in several other situations (Forrest, 1975).

Treatment with Li^+ has also been associated occasionally with changes in Ca^{2+} metabolism that resemble those of hyperparathyroidism (Franks *et al.*, 1982).

Polydipsia and polyuria occur in patients treated with Li^+, occasionally to a disturbing degree. Cases of acquired nephrogenic diabetes insipidus have been reported in patients maintained at therapeutic plasma concentrations of the ion. Typically, mild polyuria appears early in treatment and then disappears. Late-developing polyuria is an indication to evaluate renal function, lower the dose of Li^+, or consider addition of a thiazide diuretic or a K^+-sparing agent such as amiloride to counteract the polyuria (*see* DePaulo *et al.*, 1981; Battle *et al.*, 1985). The polyuria disappears with termination of Li^+ therapy. The mechanism of this effect may involve inhibition of the action of antidiuretic hormone (ADH) on renal adenylyl cyclase, resulting in decreased ADH stimulation of renal reabsorption of water. However, there is also evidence that Li^+ may exert an action at steps beyond cyclic AMP synthesis to alter renal function. The effect of Li^+ on water metabolism is not sufficiently predictable to be therapeutically useful in treatment of the syndrome of inappropriate secretion of ADH. Evidence of chronic inflammatory changes in biopsied renal tissue has been found in a minority of patients given Li^+ for prolonged periods. Since there is little indication of progressive, clinically significant impairment of renal function, these are considered incidental findings by most experts; nevertheless, plasma creatinine and urine volume should be monitored during long-term use of Li^+ (*see* DePaulo *et al.*, 1981).

Li^+ also has a weak action on carbohydrate metabolism that resembles somewhat that of insulin. In rats, Li^+ causes an increase in skeletal muscle glycogen accompanied by severe depletion of glycogen from the liver.

The prolonged use of Li^+ causes a benign and reversible depression of the T wave of the ECG, an effect not related to depletion of Na^+ or K^+.

Li^+ causes EEG changes characterized by diffuse slowing, widened frequency spectrum, and potentiation with disorganization of background rhythm. There are conflicting reports with regard to Li^+ and convulsive disorders. Seizures have been reported in nonepileptic patients with plasma concentrations of Li^+ in the therapeutic range. Myesthenia gravis may worsen during treatment with Li^+ (Neil *et al.*, 1976).

A benign, sustained increase in circulating polymorphonuclear leukocytes occurs during the chronic use of Li^+ and is reversed within a week after termination of treatment.

Allergic reactions such as dermatitis and vasculitis can occur with Li^+ administration.

In pregnancy, concomitant use of natriuretics and low-Na^+ diets can contribute to maternal and neonatal Li^+ intoxication, and during postpartum diuresis one can anticipate potentially toxic retention of Li^+ by the mother. The use of Li^+ in pregnancy has been associated with neonatal goiter, CNS depression, hypotonia, and cardiac murmur. All these conditions reverse with time. More ominously, epidemiological data suggest that the use of Li^+ in early pregnancy may be associated with a severalfold increase in the incidence of cardiovascular anomalies of the newborn (especially Ebstein's malformation) (Goldberg and DiMascio, 1978; Källén and Tandberg, 1983). For these reasons, the safety of lithium salts in pregnancy is at least uncertain, and such use is not recommended.

Treatment of Lithium Intoxication. There is no specific antidote for Li^+ intoxication, and treatment is supportive. Care must be taken to assure that the patient is not Na^+- and water-depleted. If renal function is adequate, excretion can be accelerated slightly with osmotic diuresis and intravenous sodium bicarbonate solution. Dialysis is the most effective means of removing the ion from the body and should be considered in severe poisonings. When the concentration of Li^+ in plasma is lowered by dialysis or other means, recovery is still slow, suggesting that the intracellular concentration of Li^+ may be the prime determinant of the appearance of clinical toxicity.

Interactions with Other Drugs. Interactions between Li^+ and diuretics have been discussed above. Thiazide diuretics as well as amiloride may correct the nephrogenic diabetes insipidus caused by Li^+. Li^+ is often used in conjunction with antipsychotic, sedative, and antidepressant drugs. A few case reports have suggested a risk of increased CNS toxicity of Li^+ when it is combined with haloperidol; however, this finding is at variance with more than a decade of experience with this combination (*see* Tupin and Schuller, 1978). The antipsychotic drugs may prevent nausea, which can be a sign of Li^+ toxicity. Urinary retention owing to the anticholinergic effects of the tricyclic antidepressants can become particularly uncomfortable in the presence of Li^+-induced diuresis. There is, however, no absolute contraindication to the concurrent use of Li^- and other psychotropic drugs.

Therapeutic Uses. The use of Li^+ in *manic-depressive illness* is discussed below. Treatment with Li^+ is ideally conducted only in patients with normal Na^+ intake and with normal cardiac and renal function. Very occasionally, patients with severe systemic illnesses can be treated with Li^+, provided the indications are sufficiently compelling. Its use in otherwise-healthy adults or adolescents for acute mania or the prevention of recurrences of bipolar manic-depressive illness are the only indications currently approved in the United States. In addition, based on compelling evidence of efficacy, it is also sometimes used as an alternative to tricyclic antidepressants in severe recurrent depression (nonbipolar manic-depressive illness) and as a supplement to antidepressant treatment in acute, major depression (*see* DeMontigny *et al.*, 1981; Ramsey and Mendels, 1981; Baldessarini and Tohen, 1988). These beneficial effects may be associated with the presence of clinical features also found in bipolar affective disorder (*see* Baldessarini, 1983, 1985). Growing clinical experience also suggests the utility of Li^+ in the management of childhood disorders that are marked by episodic changes in mood and behavior and that bear an uncertain relationship to bipolar disorder in adults (*see* DeLong and Nieman, 1983).

DRUG TREATMENT OF DISORDERS OF MOOD

Disorders of mood (*affective disorders*) are extremely common in general medical practice, as well as in psychiatry. The severity of these conditions covers an extraordinarily broad range, from normal grief reactions to severe, incapacitating, and sometimes fatal psychosis. The lifetime risk of suicide in major affective disorders is about 10 to 15%, but this statistic does not begin to represent the morbidity and cost of this group of underdiagnosed illnesses. Clearly, not all of human grief, misery, and disappointments are indications for medical treatment, and even severe affective disorders have a high rate of spontaneous remission, provided that sufficient time (often a matter of months) passes. The antidepressant agents or lithium salts are thus generally reserved for the more severe and otherwise incapacitating disorders of mood, and the most satisfactory results tend to occur in patients who have severe illnesses with "endogenous" or "melancholic" characteristics (*see* Baldessarini, 1983, 1985; American Psychiatric Association, 1987). The data from clinical research in support of the efficacy of antidepressant agents and of lithium salts are totally convincing (*see* Klein *et al.*, 1980; Herrington and Lader, 1981; Baldessarini, 1983, 1985; Baldessarini and Tohen, 1988). Nevertheless, many shortcomings and problems continue to be associated with all drugs used to treat affective disorders. In addition to less-than-dramatic efficacy in some cases, virtually all the drugs used to treat disorders of mood are potentially lethal when acute overdosage occurs and can cause appreciable morbidity even with careful clinical use.

The tricyclic agents are the most widely used antidepressants. They are all apparently similar in efficacy for depression, provided that adequate doses are used for a sufficient period of time. Effective doses, calculated in terms of imipramine or its equivalent of a similar drug, are currently estimated to exceed 125 mg per day; doses above 250 mg per day are best reserved for severely ill inpatients (Simpson *et al.*, 1976; Stewart *et al.*, 1980; Keller *et al.*, 1986). Since the onset of action of all antidepressant drugs is delayed for up to 2 or 3 weeks, a trial of treatment with an adequate dose cannot be judged a failure for at least 4 to 6 weeks.

Secondary considerations govern the selection of a specific antidepressant. If some sedation seems desirable early in treatment, amitriptyline, doxepin, or trazodone may be selected. If anticholinergic side effects are to be avoided, desipramine, fluoxetine, or trazodone may be a rational choice. Prior success with a specific agent is an additional consideration. The tertiary-amine tricyclic antidepressants are highly effective and commonly used; however, if they fail to produce satisfactory results, it is probably best to increase the dose before changing to other agents, such as the secondary-amine tricyclic antidepressants. This advice is based on research that suggests a complex biphasic relationship between the concentration of drug in blood and the clinical response for nortriptyline; this relationship may or may not exist for other agents (*see* Baldessarini, 1983, 1985).

Disappointing responses to antidepressant therapy usually result from the use of inadequate doses or too short a therapeutic trial. Unless a patient is very debilitated or unusually sensitive to the side effects of a tricyclic antidepressant, it is best to begin treatment with the equivalent of about 50 mg of imipramine per day and to increase the dose rapidly to 150 mg or more per day. For severely ill hospitalized patients, the dose can be raised to 300 mg per day, although little added benefit and much more toxicity are likely to result. It is also wise to avoid single doses above 150 mg in outpatients. Because of the high rate of relapse within the first year following recovery from an acute, severe depressive illness, treatment usually is continued for at least several months (Prien and Kupfer, 1986). In this phase of treatment, doses below 100 mg per day of imipramine or its equivalent are less likely to be effective, and, as an approximate guideline, 100 to 150 mg per day for at least 3 to 6 months can be tried. Some physicians have attempted to discontinue treatment gradually over several months, in accordance with the clinical response observed. Increasing evidence suggests that the prolonged use of a tricyclic antidepressant agent alone or combined with a lithium salt can have important ameliorative or preventive effects on recurrent, nonbipolar depression (*see* Klein *et al.*, 1980; Bialos *et al.*, 1982; Baldessarini and Tohen, 1988). While formal, controlled studies of long-term use of antidepressants have rarely exceeded 1 year, clinical experience indicates that many patients continue to obtain clinical benefit, safely, with imipramine-like agents for several years. The literature contains a few case reports of possible "tolerance" to the therapeutic effects of antidepressants after prolonged use. Sometimes this loss of benefit may be overcome by increasing the dose of antidepressant, by temporary addition of Li^+ or a small dose of a neuroleptic agent, or by changing to a dissimilar antidepressant (Cohen and Baldessarini, 1985).

Although acute mania is a primary indication for the use of lithium carbonate, it is, in practice, an inferior agent for the management of severe manic attacks. These episodes represent a serious medical problem and require hospitalization for the protection and careful medical management of the patient. While a few mildly hypomanic patients can be managed successfully as outpatients with Li^+ alone, it is more common to begin treatment of severely manic patients with antipsychotic doses of a neuroleptic drug (the type selected makes little difference). A benzodiazepine can also be used temporarily for sedation. As the intake of food and fluids becomes stable and the patient becomes more cooperative over several days, Li^+ can then be introduced gradually and with greater safety. While long-term benefits of antipsychotic drugs in bipolar disorders of mood have yet to be proven, the *preventive* effects of lithium carbonate have become its most compelling clinical indication. This is most clear with bipolar affective disorders, but Li^+ is probably also efficacious in the prevention of the emergence of recurrent depression. Tricyclic antidepressants, given alone, are usually contraindicated in bipolar illness, except to treat acute depressive phases, because of their tendency to destabilize mood and provoke a "switch" to mania or hypomania. Even in acute depressive phases, bipolar patients are probably best managed with an antidepressant plus a lithium salt. In view of the very low therapeutic index for Li^+, it is important to be circumspect when recommending a prolonged regimen involving Li^+. Factors that enter into this decision include the severity of the illness, the frequency of recurrence, and the probable reliability of the patient.

The use of Li^+ in mania, and especially in the long-term prevention of manic-depressive illness, is sometimes only partially effective. Alternative or supplementary treatments currently under clinical investigation include the use of certain agents developed as anticonvulsants, especially those that are effective in temporal lobe epilepsy. Most experience has been accumulated with carbamazepine, but encouraging results also have been reported with valproate. There is no evidence that these agents are efficacious in depression. They are used in doses that are recommended for the treatment of epilepsy; close monitoring is required to avoid side effects on bone marrow or the liver (*see* Post *et al.*, 1983; McElroy and Pope, 1988; *see also* Chapter 19). Benzodiazepines such as clonazepam or lorazepam are sometimes used as sedatives early in acute mania, but they do not have demonstrated efficacy in long-term prevention of manic-depressive recurrences (Cohen and Lipinski, 1986b; Rosenbaum, 1987). Other experimental agents that have had limited assessment in the treatment of mania include various antihypertensive agents, including clonidine and Ca^{2+}-channel blockers such as verapamil; their effects appear to be weak, inconsistent, or temporary (Cohen and Lipinski, 1986b).

Other forms of treatment of depression have not been well established or are no longer regularly employed, with the important exception of ECT. This remains the most rapid and effective treatment for severe acute depression and is sometimes lifesaving for acutely suicidal patients (*see* Avery and Winokur, 1977; Freeman *et al.*, 1978). The MAO inhibitors are generally considered drugs of second choice for the treatment of severe depression, even though the evidence for efficacy of adequate doses of tranylcypromine or phenelzine is convincing. The efficacy of isocarboxazid is less certain, and use of this agent is rare. Despite the favorable results obtained with tranylcypromine and with doses of phenelzine above 45 mg per day, the potential for unwanted reactions has limited their acceptance by many clinicians and patients. Nevertheless, MAO inhibitors sometimes are tried when a vigorous trial of a tricyclic antidepressant has been unsatisfactory and when ECT is refused. In addition, MAO inhibitors may have selective benefits for conditions other than depression, including neurotic illnesses marked by phobias and anxiety or panic as well as dysphoria. Similar benefits may, however, be found with imipramine-like agents; thus, indications for the MAO inhibitors are limited and must be weighed against their potential toxicity and their complex interactions with many other drugs. Stimulants, with or without added sedatives, are an outmoded and ineffective treatment for severe depression. However, some clinicians continue to find utility and safety in the short-term treatment of selected patients with a stimulant such as methylphenidate or amphetamine. These include patients with mild dysphoria or lack of energy associated with medical illnesses, as well as some geriatric patients; however, none of these possible indications has been investigated systematically (Chiarello and Cole, 1987).

III. Drugs Used in the Treatment of Anxiety

Sedatives with useful antianxiety effects are consistently among the most commonly prescribed drugs. The appropriate generic term for this group of agents remains uncertain, and terms such as *antianxiety agents*, *anxiolytics,* and *tranquilizers* represent to some extent wishful thinking and the impact of advertising. Drugs used to treat anxiety are sedatives or at least have many properties in common with traditional sedatives, such as the barbiturates. Even the benzodiazepines have sedative properties, particularly when relatively high doses are given. The wide diversity of compounds used to treat anxiety greatly complicates attempts to make generalizations about them. Many of these drugs are discussed in other chapters of this text (*see* Chapters 17, 19, and 22). This section covers only a limited group of agents that are commonly used to treat anxiety and mild dysphoria, and only this use is emphasized. Since the benzodiazepines dominate this field, they are given the most attention. Several reviews of the pharmacology of these drugs, particularly the benzodiazepines, are available (*see* Hollister *et al.,* 1980; Rosenbaum, 1982, 1987; Symposium, 1982; Greenblatt *et al.,* 1983; Lader, 1984; *see also* Chapter 17).

History. Man has sought chemical agents to modify the effects of stress and the feelings of discomfort, tension, anxiety, and dysphoria throughout recorded history. Many of these efforts have led to the development of agents that are often classed as sedatives, and the single most widely used of these is one of the oldest—ethanol. In the last century, bromide salts and compounds similar in effect to alcohol, including paraldehyde and chloral hydrate, were introduced into medical practice as sedatives; these were followed in the early 1900s by the introduction of the barbiturates. The barbiturates were the dominant antianxiety agents throughout the first half of this century; however, by the 1950s concern had arisen about their propensity to induce tolerance, physical dependence, and potentially lethal reactions during withdrawal, and this encouraged the search for safer agents. Compounds such as meprobamate were the initial result. Despite the popularity of some of these compounds for daytime sedation or for hypnotic effects, an awareness developed that they shared many of the undesirable properties of barbiturates. These properties included an unclear separation between their useful antianxiety effects and excessive sedation as well as an impressive propensity to cause physical dependence and severe acute intoxication on overdosage. This set the scene for the discovery of chlordiazepoxide in the late 1950s and the introduction of more than a dozen benzodiazepine congeners since that time. This class of sedatives has come to dominate the market and medical practice; in recent years, diazepam, alprazolam, lorazepam, and their congeners have been among the front-runners in terms of numbers of prescriptions written for all drugs used in medical practice.

BENZODIAZEPINES

Nine benzodiazepine derivatives are presently recommended for the treatment of anxiety. In their order of introduction, they are *chlordiazepoxide, diazepam, oxazepam, clorazepate, lorazepam, prazepam, alprazolam,* and *halazepam;* in addition *clonazepam* (noted more for its potent anticonvulsant properties) is sometimes used in the treatment of panic disorder (*see* Rosenbaum, 1987). Although commonly used for treating anxiety, these drugs share other therapeutic indications—notably sedation and induction of sleep. While other benzodiazepines are advertised with an emphasis on sedative or hypnotic effects, the differences between them and the nine recommended for anxiety are subtle and possibly insignificant in some cases (*see* Greenblatt *et al.,* 1983). These other indications are discussed elsewhere (*see* Index).

History. The first successful benzodiazepine, *chlordiazepoxide,* was developed by Sternbach's group at the Roche Laboratories in the late 1950s. Tests in animals indicated that chlordiazepoxide had interesting muscle-relaxant and spinal reflex–blocking properties. It also produced "taming" of a number of species of animals in doses much lower than those producing ataxia or measurable hypnosis. These findings led to the clinical trial of the drug in man for the determination of antianxiety effects (*see* Symposium, 1982.)

Chemistry. Over 2000 benzodiazepines have been synthesized. The structure–activity relationship of this group has been reviewed by Sternbach (in Symposium, 1982). Structures of benzodiazepines commonly recommended for treatment of anxiety are shown in Chapter 17 (Table 17–1, page 347) (*see also* Neumeyer, 1989).

PHARMACOLOGICAL PROPERTIES

Chlordiazepoxide and diazepam can be considered prototypical drugs for their class. They have achieved wide use as antianxiety agents.

Central Nervous System. *Behavioral and Neurophysiological Effects.* The effects of the benzodiazepines in the relief of anxiety can readily be demonstrated in experimental animals. In conflict punishment procedures, benzodiazepines greatly reduce the suppressive effects of punishment. Positive effects in this experimental model are not seen with antidepressants and antipsychotics.

Difficulties in evaluating the therapeutic efficacy of psychotropic drugs in man are particularly great in the case of the antianxiety drugs, owing largely to the contribution of nonpharmacological factors to the treatment of anxiety; disparate results have thus been obtained. Many studies have shown that benzodiazepines are more effective than a placebo in the treatment of varied groups of anxious neurotic patients. However, negative results have also been reported (*see* Klein *et al.*, 1980; Rosenbaum, 1982). The clinical popularity of these drugs apparently is the result of a combination of their pharmacological actions, their relative safety, and an extraordinary demand for agents of this type by both doctors and patients.

In common with barbiturates, chlordiazepoxide blocks EEG arousal from stimulation of the brainstem reticular formation. Central-depressant actions of diazepam and other benzodiazepines on spinal reflexes occur and are in part mediated by the brainstem reticular system. Like meprobamate and the barbiturates, chlordiazepoxide depresses the duration of electrical afterdischarge in the limbic system, including the septal region, the amygdala, the hippocampus, and the hypothalamus. Virtually all benzodiazepines increase seizure threshold and are anticonvulsant. Clonazepam, diazepam, and clorazepate are used clinically for this purpose (*see* Chapter 19).

There is also much interest in the effects of benzodiazepines on neurotransmission in the CNS that is mediated by gamma-aminobutyric acid (GABA). This research has been stimulated by electrophysiological observations of the benzodiazepines' potentiation of the inhibitory effects of GABA, as well as by the discovery of specific binding sites for benzodiazepines in various brain regions. These sites are believed to occur in a macromolecular complex that includes GABA receptors and a chloride channel. The binding of benzodiazepines can be modulated by both GABA and chloride even after solubilization and extensive purification of the binding sites. Imidazodiazepine and β-carboline compounds have been found that can competitively inhibit the binding and the biological actions of the benzodiazepines. At concentrations in the therapeutic range, benzodiazepines also can reduce the excitability of some neurons by actions that involve neither GABA nor alterations in membrane permeability to chloride. Thus, cellular mechanisms in addition to the facilitation of GABA-mediated chloride conductance may contribute to the behavioral effects of benzodiazepines. (*See* Skolnick and Paul, 1982; Study and Barker, 1982; Symposium, 1982, 1983, 1988; Polc, 1988; *see also* Chapters 17 and 19.)

Effects on Sleep. Benzodiazepines can be used effectively as hypnotics in conjunction with their use as antianxiety drugs (Chapter 17). They seem to have only mild capacity to suppress REM sleep, but they do have a tendency to suppress the deeper phases of sleep, especially stage 4 (while *increasing* total sleep time). The significance of this finding is not known, but diazepam has been used in the treatment of "night terrors" that arise out of stage-4 sleep.

Cardiovascular and Respiratory Systems. The cardiovascular effects of the benzodiazepines are mild, and this encourages their frequent use in cardiac patients. Diazepam, in an intravenous dose of 5 to 10 mg, causes a slight decrease in respiration, blood pressure, and left ventricular stroke work. Increase in heart rate and decrease in cardiac output can also occur. The effects are minimal, and it is unlikely that benzodiazepines given in usual therapeutic doses by the oral route significantly depress cardiovascular function.

Skeletal Muscle. Diazepam and other benzodiazepines are widely used as muscle relaxants, although controlled studies have been inconsistent in showing an advantage of benzodiazepines over either placebo or aspirin. Some muscle relaxation occurs after administration of any of the CNS depressants, and the advantages of the benzodiazepines appear to be small when given orally (*see* Chapter 20).

Absorption, Distribution, Fate, and Excretion. Prazepam, clonazepam, and oxazepam are absorbed relatively slowly following oral administration, and peak concentrations in plasma may not be attained for hours. In contrast, diazepam is absorbed rapidly, reaching peak concentrations in about an hour in adults, and as quickly as 15 to 30 minutes in children.

Alprazolam, chlordiazepoxide, halazepam, and lorazepam have intermediate rates of absorption. Clorazepate and prazepam do not appear as such in the blood. Clorazepate is quickly decarboxylated in the gastrointestinal tract, and the product, N-desmethyldiazepam (*nordazepam*), is rapidly absorbed; prazepam is absorbed slowly and is transformed primarily to nordazepam by the liver before reaching the systemic circulation (*see* Greenblatt *et al.*, 1981). With the exception of lorazepam, the benzodiazepines are unpredictably absorbed following intramuscular injection (*see* Greenblatt *et al.*, 1983). Most of the benzodiazepines are bound to plasma protein to a great extent (85 to 95%)—a factor that limits the efficacy of dialysis in the treatment of acute poisonings. The apparent volumes of distribution for most benzodiazepines are about 1 to 3 liters per kilogram. Secondary peaks in the plasma concentration have been described for several benzodiazepines, for example, at 6 to 12 hours after an oral dose of diazepam. These are most likely due to enterohepatic recirculation.

The pharmacokinetic parameters that have been reported for these agents can often be misleading because active metabolites with long half-lives can markedly alter the duration of effects. For example, the formation of nordazepam from diazepam can extend the duration of effect by twofold or threefold. Even more striking is the fact that halazepam (half-life in plasma of 2 to 4 hours) is metabolized principally to nordazepam, which has a half-life of up to 100 hours. Nordazepam is subsequently hydroxylated to another active compound, oxazepam, before inactivation by conjugation with glucuronic acid is finally achieved. The metabolism of the benzodiazepines is described further in Chapter 17 and summarized in Table 17–2 (page 354).

The usually stated half-life for the elimination phase of the more lipophilic benzodiazepines does not adequately depict the kinetics of the early distributive phase, which can be important clinically. For example, the distributive (alpha) half-life of diazepam is about 1 hour, while the elimination (beta) half-life is about 1.5 days initially and even longer after prolonged treatment. Diazepam is rapidly absorbed and delivered to highly perfused tissues, including the brain, where the effect is produced. The drug is then redistributed to less well perfused tissues. Thus, diazepam has a rapid onset and a relatively brief duration of action after a single dose due to redistribution out of the brain, even though the elimination half-life is long. Moreover, while correlations between plasma concentrations of benzodiazepines and clinical effects are imperfect (*see* Greenblatt and Shader, 1987), concentrations in plasma only twice those usually considered to be effective are associated with undesirable degrees of sedation. For this reason, the benzodiazepines are *not* effectively or safely given once a day, despite their relatively long elimination half-lives; doses should be divided into two to four portions for the treatment of daytime anxiety.

The benzodiazepines as a class tend to have minimal pharmacokinetic interactions with other drugs, although their oxidative metabolism may be inhibited by cimetidine, disulfiram, isoniazid, and oral contraceptives, while it appears to be increased by rifampin. The premature neonate and the elderly may have half-lives for diazepam that are three or four times longer than those of young adults, children, or even full-term neonates. In addition, severe hepatic disease can increase the half-life of diazepam by a factor of two to five. Since formation of glucuronides is not restricted to hepatic endoplasmic reticulum, oxazepam, lorazepam, and possibly alprazolam may be safer agents for patients with severely impaired hepatic function, if they are given in small divided doses. Oxazepam may be safer for elderly patients because of its relatively short duration of action. Most of the benzodiazepines are excreted almost entirely in the urine and in the form of oxidized and glucuronide-conjugated metabolites (*see* Chapter 17).

Information on the pharmacokinetic properties and metabolism of the benzodiazepines is described by Morselli (1977) and Greenblatt and Shader (1987). (*See also* Symposium, 1982, and Appendix II.)

Tolerance and Physical Dependence. High doses of benzodiazepines must be given for long periods of time and then abruptly withdrawn before marked withdrawal symptoms, occasionally including seizures, appear (*see* Allquander, 1978). Because of the long half-lives and conversion to active metabolites with long durations of action, withdrawal or abstinence symptoms after prolonged use may not appear for a week or more after abrupt discontinuation of the drug and are likely to be mild (Lader and Olajide, 1987; Rickels *et al.*, 1988). In most instances after tapered withdrawal of usual doses of long-acting agents, no abstinence syndrome occurs. However, some observations suggest that those benzodiazepines with relatively short durations of action may be associated with the emergence of symptoms of anxiety between doses; difficulty in discontinuing treatment or a tendency to increase doses has also been noted. It is not clear to what extent these phenomena represent tolerance or mild withdrawal reactions, in contrast to the re-emergence of primary symptoms for which the treatment was originally given. Alprazolam and lorazepam appear to be most often associated with such reactions. Some clinicians have found that substitution of a longer-acting benzodiazepine (*e.g.*, 1 mg of clonazepam for each mg of alprazolam or lorazepam) can provide more sustained anxiolytic effects and facilitate gradual withdrawal (*see* Rosenbaum, 1987).

Toxic Reactions and Side Effects. The expected side effects of CNS depressants of drowsiness and ataxia are extensions of the pharmacological actions of these drugs.

With diazepam, antianxiety effects can be expected at blood concentrations of 300 to 400 ng/ml, while some sedative effects and psychomotor impairment begin at similar concentrations and gross CNS intoxication can be expected at concentrations over 900 to 1000 ng/ml (*see* Morselli, 1977). Therapeutic concentrations of chlordiazepoxide are approximately 700 to 1000 ng/ml.

An increase in hostility and irritability, and vivid or disturbing dreams, are sometimes associated with the benzodiazepines. In addition, one of the most common causes of reversible confusional states in the elderly is the overuse of sedatives of all kinds, including what would ordinarily be referred to as "small" doses of benzodiazepines.

In general, the clinical toxicity of the benzodiazepines is low. Weight gain, which may be the result of renewed appetite, occurs in some patients. Among the other toxic reactions seen with chlordiazepoxide are skin rash, nausea, headache, impairment of sexual function, vertigo, and lightheadedness. Agranulocytosis and hepatic reactions have been reported very rarely. Menstrual irregularities have been noted, and women may fail to ovulate while taking benzodiazepines.

Overdosage with the benzodiazepines is frequent, but serious sequelae are rare unless other drugs or ethanol are also taken. A few deaths have been reported at doses greater than 700 mg of diazepam or chlordiazepoxide. The striking advantage of this group of drugs is the remarkable margin of safety. Treatment for overdosage is purely supportive of respiratory and cardiovascular function. The discovery that certain imidazobenzodiazepines have selective, antagonistic effects against the benzodiazepines might herald the development of clinically useful antidotes for states of intoxication (*see* Hunkeler *et al.*, 1981; *see also* Chapter 17).

The question of teratogenic effects of benzodiazepines or other toxic effects on the fetus is controversial (*see* Safra and Oakley, 1975; Morselli, 1977; Goldberg and DiMascio, 1978). The most persistent, but still unproven, suggestion has been that there may be a small increase in the risk of midline cleft deformities of the lip or palate, although these remain well below the overall risk of birth defects (about 2 to 5% in the general population) and are correctable by surgery. Benzodiazepines depress CNS function in the neonate, and especially in the premature newborn. Concentrations of these drugs in umbilical cord blood may exceed those in the maternal circulation; as mentioned, the fetus and newborn are much less able to metabolize benzodiazepines than are adults.

Interactions with Other Drugs. These are infrequent with the benzodiazepines, and, except for an additive effect with other CNS depressants, they are usually not significant. Minor pharmacokinetic interactions have been mentioned above. Heavy cigarette smoking may decrease the effectiveness of usual doses of these drugs.

Preparations, Routes of Administration, and Dosage. These are presented in Table 18–5.

Therapeutic Uses. The benzodiazepines are used primarily in the treatment of *anxiety* (*see* below). Other uses of these drugs are described elsewhere in the text (*see* Index).

OTHER SEDATIVES USED FOR ANXIETY

Many other classes of drugs that act on the CNS have been used for daytime sedation and the treatment of anxiety. Many of these uses are now virtually obsolete. Such drugs include the propanediol carbamates (notably, *meprobamate*), the barbiturates (*see* Chapter 17), and many other pharmacologically similar nonbarbiturates (*e.g.*, *chlormezanone*). The dosage forms and the usual sedative-hypnotic doses of many of these drugs are provided in Table 17–3 (page 357). The demise of these agents in modern psychiatric practice is due primarily to their tendency to cause unwanted degrees of sedation or frank intoxication at the dosage required to alleviate anxiety; meprobamate and the barbiturates present additional problems, particularly their liability to produce tolerance, physical dependence, severe withdrawal reactions, and life-threatening toxicity with overdosage.

Table 18–5. COMPOUNDS USED FOR ANXIETY: DOSAGE FORMS AND DOSES

NONPROPRIETARY NAME	TRADE NAME	DOSAGE FORMS *	USUAL DAILY DOSE (*mg*) †	EXTREME DAILY DOSE (*mg*)
Benzodiazepines				
Alprazolam	XANAX	O	0.75–1.5	0.5–4
Chlordiazepoxide	LIBRIUM, others	O,I	15–40	10–100
			25–100 (parenteral; may repeat in 2–4 hr)	25–300 (parenteral)
Clonazepam ‡	KLONOPIN	O	1.5–10	0.5–20
Clorazepate	TRANXENE	O §	15–60	7.5–90
Diazepam	VALIUM, others	O §,I,L	4–40	2–40
			2–20 (parenteral; may repeat in 3–4 hr)	
Halazepam	PAXIPAM	O	60–160	20–160
Lorazepam	ATIVAN, others	O,I	2–6	1–10
			2–4 (parenteral)	
Oxazepam	SERAX, ZAXOPAM	O	30–60	30–120
Prazepam	CENTRAX	O	20–40	10–60
Atypical Agent				
Buspirone	BUSPAR	O	20–30	15–60

* Dosage forms: O = oral solid; I = injection; L = oral liquid.

† The daily doses are given as total milligrams per day, assuming doses are divided into two or four portions per day. Single parenteral doses are given for chlordiazepoxide and diazepam. All doses are for adults or adolescents. For children 6 to 12 years of age, chlordiazepoxide may be given orally in divided daily doses of 10 to 30 mg. Diazepam may be given in divided daily doses of 3 to 10 mg to children over 6 months of age. For younger children, consult the manufacturer's instructions. Clorazepate is not recommended for children less than 9 years of age.

‡ Clonazepam is used primarily as an anticonvulsant, but has been used in panic disorder, as an adjunctive treatment of acute mania, and to facilitate withdrawal from other benzodiazepines that have a shorter duration of action.

§ Clorazepate is also available as slow-release tablets (TRANXENE-SD) to be taken once daily. Diazepam is also available in slow-release capsules (VALRELEASE).

Other drugs that have been used in the treatment of anxiety include certain anticholinergic agents and antihistamines. Among these is *hydroxyzine*, an antihistamine that is widely prescribed for the treatment of anxiety. The popularity of hydroxyzine is surprising in view of studies that suggest that it is not an effective antianxiety agent unless given in doses (400 mg per day) that produce marked sedation (*see* Rickels, 1977; Goldberg, 1984). Hydroxyzine is also used intramuscularly as a preanesthetic medication for its sedative, anticholinergic, and antiemetic effects (*see* Chapter 13). *Propranolol* and other β-adrenergic antagonists can reduce the autonomic symptoms associated with specific situational phobias.

An entirely new class of drugs with potential utility in the treatment of anxiety is the azaspirodecanediones, currently represented by *buspirone* (*see* Table 18–5). Originally developed as a potential antipsychotic agent, buspirone has a pattern of pharmacological properties that is distinct from that of the benzodiazepines, including an inability to influence the binding of either the benzodiazepines or GABA, a lack of anticonvulsant activity, and minimal interaction with CNS depressants (*see* Eison, 1984). Buspirone behaves as a selective antagonist at 5-HT_{1A} receptors (*see* Chapter 12); its potency as a dopaminergic antagonist is relatively low, and thus the risk of inducing extrapyramidal side effects at the doses used to treat anxiety is small. Clinical studies indicate that buspirone is an effective antianxiety agent that produces relatively little sedation; there also appears to be little risk of producing tolerance or dependence (Rickels *et al.*, 1988). It is not effective in panic disorder (*see* Goldberg, 1984; Taylor, 1988). Its use during or following withdrawal from a benzodiazepine is complicated by the lack of cross-tolerance between the two classes of agents, and buspirone fails to protect against symptoms of withdrawal from a benzodiazepine. Analogs of buspirone (*e.g., tiaspirone, gepirone*) are being evaluated as possible antianxiety, antidepressant, or antipsychotic agents.

DRUG TREATMENT OF ANXIETY

Anxiety is not only a cardinal symptom of many psychiatric disorders but also an almost-inevitable component of many medical and surgical conditions. Indeed, it is a universal human emotion, closely allied with appropriate fear, and often serving psychobiologically adaptive purposes. A most important clinical generalization is that anxiety is rather infrequently a "disease" in itself. The anxiety that is typically associated with the "psychoneurotic" disorders cannot be readily explained in biological or psychological terms; one hypothesis suggests an overactivity of adrenergic systems in the CNS (*see* Hoehn-Saric, 1982; Gorman *et al.*, 1987). In addition, symptoms of anxiety commonly are associated with depression and especially with dysthymic disorder ("neurotic" depression), panic disorder, agoraphobia and other specific phobias, obsessive-compulsive disorder, and many personality disorders. Sometimes, despite a thoughtful evaluation of a patient, no treatable primary illness is found, or, if one is found and treated, it may be desirable to deal directly with the anxiety at the same time. In such situations, antianxiety medications are frequently and appropriately used (*see* Hollister *et al.*, 1980; Rosenbaum, 1982; Bassuk *et al.*, 1983; Greenblatt *et al.*, 1983; Lader, 1984).

Currently, the most useful antianxiety drugs are the benzodiazepines. The specific drug chosen seems to make little difference. In patients with impaired hepatic function or in the elderly, oxazepam is currently favored; since lorazepam and alprazolam have similar characteristics, they may be suitable alternatives if administered in small, divided doses. Chlordiazepoxide and diazepam have been used extensively in children.

Clinical experience strongly indicates that the most favorable responses to the benzodiazepines are obtained in situations that involve relatively acute anxiety reactions in medical or psychiatric patients who have either modifiable primary illnesses or primary anxiety disorders. However, this group of anxious patients also has a high response rate to placebo and is likely to undergo spontaneous improvement. Antianxiety drugs are also used in the management of more persistent or recurrent anxiety associated with the neuroses; guidelines for their appropriate use are less clear in these situations. Although there has been concern about the potential for habituation and abuse of sedatives, recent studies suggest that physicians tend to be conservative and may even undertreat patients with anxiety. They may either withhold drug unless symptoms or dysfunction are severe or interrupt treatment within a few weeks, causing a high proportion of relapses. However, patients with very long-lasting or persistent patterns of dissatisfaction or insecurity or those who have diagnosable personality disorders (*see* American Psychiatric Association, 1987) may be particularly difficult to treat successfully with antianxiety agents. They may be at higher risk of a gradual escalation of dose, physical dependence, or impulsive overdosing. Nevertheless, data suggest that such abuses are relatively infrequent or, when one considers the millions of patients using such drugs, even rare (*see* Greenblatt *et al.*, 1983). Moreover, sustained benefits of benzodiazepine treatment can be demonstrated for at least several months (*see* Fabre *et al.*, 1981; Hollister *et al.*, 1981).

An important recent advance is the separation of various types of anxiety disorders, including those characterized by panic and phobias as well as other, more generalized, anxiety disorders. Among features that help to make such distinctions are apparently preferential responses of panic disorder and some phobias to tricyclic antidepressants or to MAO inhibitors (*see* Sheehan *et al.*, 1980; Pohl *et al.*, 1982; Shader *et al.*, 1982; Charney *et al.*, 1986). Certain benzodiazepines, notably lorazepam, clonazepam, and alprazolam, may have useful effects in panic disorder, and they are commonly tried before treating this disorder with an antidepressant or MAO inhibitor. Use of these or other benzodiazepines to sedate acutely psychotic or manic patients as a temporary adjunct to the use of an antipsychotic agent or Li^+ was discussed above. Although commonly used in the clinical management of mild depressive syndromes marked by anxiety and insomnia, evidence for true mood-elevating effects of benzodiazepines is generally lacking; there are suggestions that alprazolam might have such an effect, at least in relatively mild cases of depression. (*See* Sheehan, 1980; Chouinard *et al.*, 1982; Fawcett *et al.*, 1987.)

Other agents have been tried experimentally in anxiety. β-Adrenergic antagonists have been used to block the peripheral autonomic manifestations of anxiety, but controlled trials generally do not show better results than those obtained with the benzodiazepines, with the exception of specific, situational phobias (performance anxiety, "stage fright") (*see* Kathol *et al.*, 1980). Other methods of treatment, including psychotherapy and behavioral techniques, are discussed by Lader (1984). There are important, nonpharmacological factors that bear on the use and effects of antianxiety drugs. Discussions of the nonspecific and placebo aspects of such treatment, as well as the general topic of the evaluation and treatment of anxiety, are provided by Rosenbaum (1982), Greenblatt and colleagues (1983), and Lader (1984). Aspects of the abuse of sedatives are reviewed by Cole and colleagues (1981) and Woods and colleagues (1987). The current status of some of the effective sedative-antianxiety agents as federally controlled substances is reviewed in Appendix I.

Amsterdam, J.; Brunswick, D.; and Mendels, J. The clinical application of tricyclic antidepressant pharmacokinetics and plasma levels. *Am. J. Psychiatry*, **1980**, *137*, 653–662.

Arana, G. W.; Goff, D.; and Baldessarini, R. J. Efficacy of anticholinergic prophylaxis of neuroleptic-induced acute dystonia. *Am. J. Psychiatry*, **1988**, *145*, 993–996.

Aubree, J. C., and Lader, M. H. High and very high dosage antipsychotics: a critical review. *J. Clin. Psychiatry*, **1980**, *41*, 341–350.

Avery, D., and Winokur, G. The efficacy of electroconvulsive therapy and antidepressants in depression. *Biol. Psychiatry*, **1977**, *12*, 507–523.

Baldessarini, R. J. Treatment of depression by altering monoamine metabolism: precursors and metabolic inhibitors. *Psychopharmacol. Bull.*, **1984a**, *20*, 224–239.

Baldessarini, R. J.; Cohen, B. M.; and Teicher, M. H. Significance of neuroleptic dose and plasma level in the pharmacologic treatment of psychoses. *Arch. Gen. Psychiatry*, **1988**, *45*, 79–91.

Baldessarini, R. J., and Tohen, M. Is there a long-term protective effect of mood-altering drugs in unipolar depressive disorder? In, *Psychopharmacology: Current Trends*. (Casey, D. E., and Christensen, A. V., eds.) Springer-Verlag, Berlin, **1988**, pp. 130–139.

Baldessarini, R. J., and Vogt, M. Release of ^{3}H-dopamine and analogous monoamines from rat striatal tissue. *Cell. Mol. Neurobiol.*, **1988**, *8*, 205–216.

Battle, D. C.; Von Riotte, A. B.; Gaviria, M.; and Grupp, M. Amelioration of polyuria by amiloride in patients receiving long-term lithium therapy. *N. Engl. J. Med.*, **1985**, *312*, 408–414.

Berger, F. M. The pharmacological properties of 2-methyl-2-*n*-propyl-1,3 propanediol dicarbamate (MILTOWN), a new interneuronal blocking agent. *J. Pharmacol. Exp. Ther.*, **1954**, *112*, 413–423.

Berken, G. H.; Weinstein, D. O.; and Stern, W. C. Weight gain: a side-effect of tricyclic antidepressants. *J. Affective Disord.*, **1984**, *7*, 133–138.

Berridge, M. J. Inositol trisphosphate and diacylglycerol as second messengers. *Biochem. J.*, **1984**, *220*, 345–360.

Berridge, M. J.; Downes, C. P.; and Hanley, M. R. Lithium amplifies agonist-dependent phosphatidylinositol responses in brain and salivary glands. *Biochem. J.*, **1982**, *206*, 587–595.

Bialos, D.; Giller, E.; and Jatlow, P. Recurrence of depression after the discontinuation of long-term amitriptyline treatment. *Am. J. Psychiatry*, **1982**, *139*, 325–329.

Biederman, J.; Gastfriend, D. R.; and Jellinek, M. S. Desipramine in the treatment of children with attention deficit disorder. *J. Clin. Psychopharmacol.*, **1986**, *6*, 359–363.

Biederman, J., and Jellinek, M. A. Psychopharmacology in children. *N. Engl. J. Med.*, **1984**, *310*, 968–972.

Blackwell, B.; Stefopoulos, A.; and Enders, P. Anticholinergic activity of two tricyclic antidepressants. *Am. J. Psychiatry*, **1978**, *135*, 722–724.

Bloom, F. E.; Baetge, G.; Deyo, S.; Ettenberg, A.; Koda, L.; Magisretti, P. J.; Shoemaker, W. J.; and Staunton, D. A. Chemical and physiological aspects of the actions of lithium and antidepressant drugs. *Neuropharmacology*, **1983**, *22*, 359–365.

Boehnert, M. T., and Lovejoy, F. J., Jr. Value of the QRS duration vs. the serum drug level in predicting seizures and ventricular arrhythmias after an acute overdose of tricyclic antidepressants. *N. Engl. J. Med.*, **1985**, *313*, 474–479.

Brenner, R.; Cooper, T. B.; Yablonski, M. E.; Lieberman, J. A.; Lesser, M.; Siris, S. G.; and Rifkin, A. E. Measurement of lithium concentrations in human tears. *Am. J. Psychiatry*, **1982**, *139*, 678–679.

Bryant, S. G.; Fisher, S.; and Kluge, R. M. Long-term vs. short-term amitriptyline side effects as measured by a postmarketing surveillance system. *J. Clin. Psychopharmacol.*, **1987**, *7*, 78–82.

Bunney, B. S., and Aghajanian, G. K. Mesolimbic and mesocortical dopaminergic systems: physiology and pharmacology. In, *Psychopharmacology: A Generation of Progress*. (Lipton, M. A.; DiMascio, A.; and Killam, K. F.; eds.) Raven Press, New York, **1978**, pp. 159–169.

Burrows, G. D.; Vohra, J.; Hunt, D.; Sloman, J. G.; Soggins, B. A.; and Davies, B. Cardiac effects of different tricyclic antidepressant drugs. *Br. J. Psychiatry*, **1976**, *129*, 335–341.

Cade, J. F. J. Lithium salts in the treatment of psychotic excitement. *Med. J. Aust.*, **1949**, *2*, 349–352.

Carlsson, A. Mechanism of action of neuroleptic drugs. In, *Psychopharmacology: A Generation of Progress*. (Lipton, M. A.; DiMascio, A.; and Killam, K. F.; eds.) Raven Press, New York, **1978**, pp. 1057–1070.

Caroff, S.; Rosenberg, H.; and Gerber, J. C. Neuroleptic malignant syndrome and malignant hyperthermia. *J. Clin. Psychopharmacol.*, **1983**, *3*, 120–121.

Carpenter, W. T., Jr.; Heinrichs, D. W.; and Hanlon, T. E. A comparative trial of pharmacologic strategies in schizophrenia. *Am. J. Psychiatry*, **1987**, *144*, 1466–1470.

Casebolt, T. L., and Jope, R. S. Long-term lithium treatment selectively reduces receptor-coupled inositol phospholipid hydrolysis in rat brain. *Biol. Psychiatry*, **1989**, *25*, 329–340.

Cassem, N. Cardiovascular effects of antidepressants. *J. Clin. Psychiatry*, **1982**, *43*, 22–28.

Chan, C. H.; Janicak, P. G.; Davis, J. M.; Altman, E.; Andriukaitis, S.; and Hedeker, D. Response of psychotic and nonpsychotic depressed patients to tricyclic antidepressants. *J. Clin. Psychiatry*, **1987**, *48*, 197–200.

Charney, D. S.; Woods, S. W.; Goodman, W. K.; Rifkin, B.; Kirch, M.; Aiken, B.; Quadrino, L. M.; and Heninger, G. R. Drug treatment of panic disorder: the comparative efficacy of imipramine, alprazolam, and trazodone. *J. Clin. Psychiatry*, **1986**, *47*, 580–586.

Chiarello, R. J., and Cole, J. O. The use of psychostimulants in general psychiatry: a reconsideration. *Arch. Gen. Psychiatry*, **1987**, *44*, 286–295.

Chouinard, G.; Annable, L.; Fontaine, R.; and Solyom, L. Alprazolam in the treatment of generalized anxiety and panic disorders. *Psychopharmacology (Berlin)*, **1982**, *77*, 229–233.

Cohen, B. J.; Harris, P. Q.; Altesman, R. I.; and Cole, J. O. Amoxapine: a neuroleptic as well as an antidepressant? *Am. J. Psychiatry*, **1982**, *139*, 1165–1167.

Cohen, B. M., and Baldessarini, R. J. Tolerance to the therapeutic effects of antidepressant agents. *Am. J. Psychiatry*, **1985**, *182*, 489–490.

Cohen, B. M., and Lipinski, J. F. *In vivo* potencies of antipsychotic drugs in blocking alpha-1 and dopamine D-2 receptors: implications for drug mechanisms of action. *Life Sci.*, **1986a**, *39*, 2571–2580.

———. Treatment of acute psychosis with non-neuroleptic agents. *Psychosomatics*, **1986b**, *27*, Suppl., 7–16.

Cohen, D. J.; Detlor, J.; and Young, J. G. Clonidine ameliorates Gilles de la Tourette syndrome. *Arch. Gen. Psychiatry*, **1980**, *37*, 1350–1357.

Cole, J. O. Antipsychotic drugs: is more better? *McLean Hosp. J.*, **1982**, *7*, 61–87.

Cole, J. O.; Haskell, D. S.; and Orzack, M. H. Problems with the benzodiazepines: an assessment of the available evidence. *McLean Hosp. J.*, **1981**, *6*, 46–74.

Cooper, T. B., and Simpson, G. M. Kinetics of lithium and clinical response. In, *Psychopharmacology: A Generation of Progress*. (Lipton, M. A.; DiMascio, A.; and Killam, K. F.; eds.) Raven Press, New York, **1978**, pp. 923–931.

Crane, G. E. Iproniazid (MARSILID) phosphate, a therapeutic agent for mental disorders and debilitating disease. *Psychiatr. Res. Rep.*, **1959**, *8*, 142–152.

Creese, I.; Burt, D.; and Snyder, S. H. Biochemical actions of neuroleptic drugs: focus on dopamine receptor. In, *Handbook of Psychopharmacology*, Vol. 10. (Iversen, L. L.; Iversen, S. D.; and Snyder, S. H.; eds.) Plenum Press, New York, **1978**, pp. 37–89.

Crome, P.; Dawling, S.; and Braithwaite, R. A. Effect of activated charcoal on absorption of nortriptyline. *Lancet*, **1977**, *2*, 1203–1205.

Delay, J., and Deniker, P. Trente-huit cas de psychoses traitées par la cure prolongée et continue de 4560 RP. Le Congrès des Al. et Neurol. de Langue Fr. In, *Compte rendu du Congrès*. Masson et Cie, Paris, **1952.**

Delini-Stula, A.; Radeke, E.; and Waldmeier, P. S. Basic and clinical aspects of the new monoamine oxidase inhibitors. In, *Psychopharmacology: Current Trends.* (Casey, D. E., and Christensen, A. V., eds.) Springer-Verlag, Berlin, **1988**, pp. 147–158.

DeLong, G. R., and Nieman, G. W. Lithium-induced behavior changes in children with symptoms suggesting manic-depressive illness. *Psychopharmacol. Bull.*, **1983**, *19*, 258–265.

DeMontigny, C., and Aghajanian, G. K. Tricyclic antidepressants: long-term treatment increases responsivity of rat forebrain neurons to serotonin. *Science,* **1978**, *202*, 1303–1305.

DeMontigny, C.; Grunberg, F.; Mayer, A.; and Deschenes, J.-P. Lithium induces rapid relief of depression in tricyclic antidepressant non-responders. *Br. J. Psychiatry*, **1981**, *138*, 252–256.

DePaulo, J. R., Jr.; Correa, E. I.; and Sapir, D. G. Renal toxicity of lithium and its implications. *Johns Hopkins Med. J.*, **1981**, *149*, 15–21.

Donaldson, S.; Gelenberg, A. J.; and Baldessarini, R. J. Alternative treatments for schizophrenic psychoses. In, *American Handbook of Psychiatry*, Vol. 8. (Berger, P., and Brodie, H. K. H., eds.) Academic Press, Inc., New York, **1986**, pp. 513–535.

DuComb, L., and Baldessarini, R. J. Timing and risk of bone marrow depression by psychotropic drugs. *Am. J. Psychiatry*, **1977**, *134*, 1294–1295.

Erle, G.; Basso, M.; Federspil, G.; Sicolo, N.; and Scandellari, C. Effect of chlorpromazine on blood glucose and plasma insulin in man. *Eur. J. Clin. Pharmacol.*, **1977**, *11*, 15–18.

Fabre, L. F.; McLendon, D. M.; and Stephens, A. G. Comparison of the therapeutic effect, tolerance and safety of benzodiazepines administered for six months to out-patients with chronic anxiety neurosis. *J. Int. Med. Res.*, **1981**, *246*, 1568–1570.

Faedda, G.; Kula, N. S.; and Baldessarini, R. J. Pharmacology of binding of ^{3}H-SCH-23390 to D-1 dopaminergic receptor sites in rat striatal tissue. *Biochem. Pharmacol.*, **1989**, *38*, 473–480.

Fawcett, J.; Edwards, J. H.; Kravitz, H. M.; and Jeffriess, H. Alprazolam: an antidepressant? Alprazolam, desipramine, and an alprazolam-desipramine combination in the treatment of adult depressed outpatients. *J. Clin. Psychopharmacol.*, **1987**, *7*, 295–310.

Folks, D. G. Monoamine oxidase inhibitors: reappraisal of dietary considerations. *J. Clin. Psychopharmacol.*, **1983**, *3*, 249–252.

Forrest, J. J., Jr. Lithium inhibition of cAMP-mediated hormones: a caution. *N. Engl. J. Med.*, **1975**, *292*, 423–424.

Forsman, A., and Öhman, R. On the pharmacokinetics of haloperidol. *Nord. Psykiatr. Tidskr.*, **1974**, *28*, 441–448.

France, R. D., and Krishnan, K. R. R. Psychotropic drugs in chronic pain. In, *Chronic Pain.* (France, R. D., and Krishnan, K. R. R., eds.) American Psychiatric Press, Washington, DC, **1988**, pp. 322–374.

Franks, R. D.; Dabovsky, S. L.; Lifshitz, M.; Coen, P.; Subryan, V.; and Walter, S. H. Long-term lithium therapy causes hyperparathyroidism. *Arch. Gen. Psychiatry*, **1982**, *39*, 1074–1077.

Freeman, C. P.; Basson, J. V.; and Crighton, A. Double-blind controlled trial of electroconvulsive therapy (ECT) and simulated ECT in depressive illness. *Lancet*, **1978**, *1*, 738–740.

Geller, B.; Cooper, T. B.; Schluchter, M. D.; Warham, J. E.; and Carr, L. G. Child and adolescent nortriptyline single dose pharmacokinetic parameters: final report. *J. Clin. Psychopharmacol.*, **1987**, *7*, 321–323.

Glassman, A. H., and Bigger, J. T., Jr. Cardiovascular effects of therapeutic doses of tricyclic antidepressants. *Arch. Gen. Psychiatry*, **1981**, *38*, 815–820.

Glazer, W. M.; Moore, D. C.; Schooler, N. R.; Brenner, L. M.; and Morgenstern, H. Tardive dyskinesia: a discontinuation study. *Arch. Gen. Psychiatry*, **1984**, *41*, 623–627.

Goldberg, H. L., and DiMascio, A. Psychotropic drugs in pregnancy. In, *Psychopharmacology: A Generation of Progress.* (Lipton, M. A.; DiMascio, A.; and Killam, K. F.; eds.) Raven Press, New York, **1978**, pp. 1047–1055.

Goldenberg, D. L. Treatment of fibromyalgia syndrome. *Rheum. Dis. Clin. North Am.*, **1989**, *15*, 61–71.

Goodwin, F. K. The impact of tricyclic antidepressants and lithium on the course of recurrent affective disorders. *McLean Hosp. J.*, **1983**, *8*, 1–16.

Gorman, J. M.; Fyer, M. R.; Liebowitz, M. R.; and Klein, D. F. Pharmacologic provocation of panic attacks. In, *Psychopharmacology: The Third Generation of Progress.* (Meltzer, H. Y., ed.) Raven Press, New York, **1987**, pp. 985–993.

Gottschalk, L. A.; Biener, R.; Noble, E.; Birch, H.; Wilbert, D.; and Heizer, J. Thioridazine plasma levels and clinical response. *Compr. Psychiatry*, **1975**, *16*, 323–337.

Granacher, R. P., and Baldessarini, R. J. Physostigmine in the acute anticholinergic syndrome associated with antidepressant and antiparkinson drugs. *Arch. Gen. Psychiatry*, **1975**, *32*, 375–380.

Greenbaum, D. S., and others. Effects of desipramine on irritable bowel syndrome compared with atropine and placebo. *Dig. Dis. Sci.*, **1987**, *32*, 257–266.

Greenblatt, D. J., and Shader, R. I. Pharmacokinetics of antianxiety drugs. In, *Psychopharmacology: The Third Generation of Progress.* (Meltzer, H. Y., ed.) Raven Press, New York, **1987**, pp. 1377–1386.

Greenblatt, D. J.; Shader, R. I.; and Abernethy, D. R. Current status of benzodiazepines. *N. Engl. J. Med.*, **1983**, *309*, 354–358, 410–416.

Greenblatt, D. J.; Shader, R. I.; Divoll, M.; and Harmatz, J. S. Benzodiazepines: a summary of pharmacokinetic properties. *Br. J. Clin. Pharmacol.*, **1981**, *11*, 11S–16S.

Hardesty, A. S., and Burdock, E. I. Quantitative clinical evaluation in psychopharmacology. In, *Psychopharmacology: A Generation of Progress.* (Lipton, M. A.; DiMascio, A.; and Killam, K. F.; eds.) Raven Press, New York, **1978**, pp. 871–878.

Himmelhoch, J. M.; Poust, R. I.; and Mallinger, A. G. Adjustment of lithium dose during lithium-chlorothiazide therapy. *Clin. Pharmacol. Ther.*, **1977**, *22*, 225–227.

Hoehn-Saric, R. Neurotransmitters in anxiety. *Arch. Gen. Psychiatry*, **1982**, *39*, 735–742.

Hollister, L. E. Tricyclic antidepressants. *N. Engl. J. Med.*, **1978**, *299*, 1106–1109, 1168–1172.

Hollister, L. E.; Conley, F. K.; Britt, R. H.; and Shuer, L. Long-term use of diazepam. *J.A.M.A.*, **1981**, *246*, 1568–1570.

Hollister, L. E.; Greenblatt, D. J.; Rickels, K.; Ayd, F. J.; and Greiner, G. E. Benzodiazepines: current update. *Psychosomatics*, **1980**, *21*, Suppl., 1–32.

Hunkeler, W.; Möhler, H.; Pieri, L.; Polc, P.; Bonetti, E. P.; Cumin, R.; Schaffner, R.; and Haefely, W. Selective antagonists of benzodiazepines. *Nature*, **1981**, *290*, 514–516.

Insel, T. R., and Zohar, J. Psychopharmacologic approaches to obsessive-compulsive disorder. In, *Psychopharmacology: The Third Generation of Progress.* (Meltzer, H. Y., ed.) Raven Press, New York, **1987**, pp. 1205–1210.

Jefferson, J. W.; Greist, J. H.; Clagnaz, P. J.; Eischens, R. R.; Marten, W. C.; and Eversen, M. A. Effect of strenuous exercise on serum lithium level in man. *Am. J. Psychiatry*, **1982**, *139*, 1593–1595.

Jus, K.; Jus, A.; Gautier, J.; Villeneuve, A.; Pires, P.; Pineau, R.; and Villeneuve, R. Studies of the actions of certain pharmacological agents on tardive dyskinesia and on the rabbit syndrome. *Int. J. Clin. Pharmacol.*, **1974**, *9*, 138–145.

Källén, B., and Tandberg, A. Lithium and pregnancy: a cohort study on manic-depressive women. *Acta Psychiatr. Scand.*, **1983**, *68*, 134–139.

Kane, J. M.; Rifkin, A.; Woerner, M.; Reardon, G.; Sarantoakos, S.; Schiebel, D.; and Ramos-Lorenzi, J. Low-dose neuroleptic treatment of outpatient schizophrenics. *Arch. Gen. Psychiatry*, **1983**, *40*, 893–896.

Kathol, R. G.; Noyes, R., Jr.; Sylmen, D. J.; Crowe, R. R.; Clancy, J.; and Kerber, R. E. Propranolol in chronic anxiety disorders. *Arch. Gen. Psychiatry*, **1980**, *37*, 1361–1365.

Keck, P. E., Jr.; Vuckovic, A.; Pope, H. G., Jr.; Nierenberg, A. A.; Gribble, G. W.; and White, K. Acute cardiovascular response to monoamine oxidase inhibitors: a prospective assessment. *J. Clin. Psychopharmacol.*, **1989**, *9*, 203–206.

Keller, M. B.; Lavori, P. W.; Klerman, G. L.; Andreasen, N. C.; Endicott, J.; Coryell, W.; Fawcett, J.; Rice, J. P.; and Hirschfeld, R. M. Low levels and lack of predictors of somatotherapy and psychotherapy received by depressed patients. *Arch. Gen. Psychiatry*, **1986**, *43*, 458–466.

Kline, N. S. Clinical experience with iproniazid (MARSILID). *J. Clin. Exp. Psychopathol.*, **1958**, *19*, Suppl., 72–78.

Korpi, E. R.; Phelps, B. H.; Granger, H.; Chang, W.-H.; Linnoila, M.; Meek, J. L.; and Wyatt, R. J. Simultaneous determination of haloperidol and its reduced metabolite in serum and plasma by isocratic liquid chromatography with electrochemical detection. *Clin. Chem.*, **1983**, *29*, 626–628.

Krenzelok, E. P.; North, D. S.; and Elkins, B. R. Physostigmine's use questioned for amoxapine overdose. *Am. J. Hosp. Pharm.*, **1981**, *38*, 1882–1889.

Kuhn, R. The treatment of depressive states with G22355 (imipramine hydrochloride). *Am. J. Psychiatry*, **1958**, *115*, 459–464.

Kupfer, D. J.; Spiker, D. G.; Coble, P. A.; Neil, J. F.; Ulrich, R.; and Shaw, D. H. Sleep and treatment prediction in endogenous depression. *Am. J. Psychiatry*, **1981**, *138*, 429–434.

Kutcher, S. P.; Reid, K.; Dubben, J. D.; and Shulman, K. I. Electrocardiographic changes and therapeutic desipramine and 2-hydroxy-desipramine concentrations in elderly depressives. *Br. J. Psychiatry*, **1986**, *148*, 676–679.

Laborit, H.; Huguenard, P.; and Alluaume, R. Un nouveau stabilisateur vegetatif, le 4560 RP. *Presse Méd.*, **1952**, *60*, 206–208.

Lader, M., and Olajide, D. A comparison of buspirone and placebo in relieving benzodiazepine withdrawal symptoms. *J. Clin. Psychopharmacol.*, **1987**, *7*, 11–15.

Lansky, M. R., and Selzer, J. Priapism associated with trazodone therapy: case report. *J. Clin. Psychiatry*, **1984**, *45*, 232–233.

Levenson, J. L. Neuroleptic malignant syndrome. *Am. J. Psychiatry*, **1985**, *142*, 1137–1145.

Lipinski, J. F.; Cohen, B. M.; Zubenko, G. S.; and Waternaux, C. Adrenoreceptors and the pharmacology of affective illness: a unifying hypothesis. *Life Sci.*, **1987**, *40*, 1947–1963.

Lipinski, J. F.; Zubenko, G.; Cohen, B. M.; and Barreira, P. Propranolol in the treatment of neuroleptic-induced akathisia. *Am. J. Psychiatry*, **1984**, *141*, 412–415.

Litovitz, T. L., and Troutman, W. G. Amoxapine overdose: seizures and fatalities. *J.A.M.A.*, **1983**, *250*, 1069–1071.

Loga, S.; Curry, S.; and Lader, M. Interactions of orphenadrine and phenobarbitone with chlorpromazine: plasma concentrations and effects in man. *Br. J. Clin. Pharmacol.*, **1975**, *2*, 197–208.

Losonczy, M. F.; Davidson, M.; and Davis, K. L. The dopamine hypothesis of schizophrenia. In, *Psychopharmacology: The Third Generation of Progress.* (Meltzer, H. Y., ed.) Raven Press, New York, **1987**, pp. 715–726.

McGrath, P. J.; Blood, D. K.; Stewart, J. W.; Harrison, W.; Quitkin, F. M.; Tricamo, E.; and Markowitz, J. A comparative study of the electrocardiographic effects of phenelzine, tricyclic antidepressants, mianserin, and placebo. *J. Clin. Psychopharmacol.*, **1987**, *7*, 335–339.

Maj, M.; Arena, F.; Lovero, N.; Pirozzi, R.; and Kemali, D. Factors associated with responses to lithium prophylaxis in DSMIII major depression and bipolar disorder. *Pharmacopsychiatry*, **1986**, *19*, 420–423.

Maxwell, R. A., and White, H. L. Tricyclic and monoamine oxidase inhibitor antidepressants: structure-activity relationships. In, *Handbook of Psychopharmacology*, Vol. 14. (Iversen, L. L.; Iversen, S. D.; and Snyder, S. H.; eds.) Plenum Press, New York, **1978**, pp. 83–155.

Meltzer, H. Y.; Goode, D. J.; and Fang, V. S. The effect of psychotropic drugs on endocrine function. In, *Psychopharmacology: A Generation of Progress.* (Lipton, M. A.; DiMascio, A.; and Killam, K. F.; eds.) Raven Press, New York, **1978**, pp. 509–529.

Meltzer, H. Y., and Lowy, M. T. The serotonin hypothesis of depression. In, *Psychopharmacology: The Third Generation of Progress.* (Meltzer, H. Y., ed.) Raven Press, New York, **1987**, pp. 513–526.

Menkes, D. B.; Aghajanian, G. K.; and Gallager, D. W. Chronic antidepressant treatment enhances agonist affinity of brain α_1-adrenoreceptors. *Eur. J. Pharmacol.*, **1983**, *87*, 35–41.

Moore, K. E., and Kelly, P. H. Biochemical pharmacology of mesolimbic and mesocortical dopaminergic neurons. In, *Psychopharmacology: A Generation of Progress.* (Lipton, M. A.; DiMascio, A.; and Killam, K. F.; eds.) Raven Press, New York, **1978**, pp. 221–234.

Morselli, P. L. Psychotropic drugs. In, *Drug Disposition during Development.* (Morselli, P. L., ed.) Spectrum Publications, Inc., New York, **1977**, pp. 431–474.

Neil, J. F.; Himmelhoch, J. M.; and Licata, S. M. Emergence of myasthenia gravis during treatment with lithium carbonate. *Arch. Gen. Psychiatry*, **1976**, *33*, 1090–1092.

Neumeyer, J. L. Neuroleptics and anxiolytic agents. In, *Principles of Medicinal Chemistry*, 3rd ed. (Foye, W. E., ed.) Lea & Febiger, Philadelphia, **1989**, pp. 189–221.

Nicotra, M. B.; Rivera, M.; Pool, J. L.; and Noall, M. W. Tricyclic antidepressant overdose: clinical and pharmacological observations. *Clin. Toxicol.*, **1981**, *18*, 599–613.

Nieforth, K. A., and Cohen, M. L. Central nervous system stimulants. In, *Principles of Medicinal Chemistry*, 3rd ed. (Foye, W. E., ed.) Lea & Febiger, Philadelphia, **1989**, pp. 277–309.

Nies, A.; Robinson, D. S.; Friedman, M. J.; Green, R.; Cooper, T. B.; Ravaris, C. L.; and Ives, J. O. Relationship between age and tricyclic antidepressant plasma levels. *Am. J. Psychiatry*, **1977**, *134*, 790–793.

Overall, J. E. Prior psychiatric treatment and the development of breast cancer. *Arch. Gen. Psychiatry*, **1978**, *35*, 898–899.

Peroutka, S. J., and Snyder, S. H. Long-term antidepressant treatment decreases spiroperidol-labeled serotonin receptor binding. *Science*, **1980a**, *210*, 88–90.

———. Relationship of neuroleptic drug effects at brain dopamine, serotonin, α-adrenergic, and histamine receptors to clinical potency. *Am. J. Psychiatry*, **1980b**, *137*, 1518–1522.

Pert, A.; Rosenblatt, J. E.; Sivit, C.; Pert, C. B.; and Bunney, W. E., Jr. Long-term treatment with lithium prevents the development of dopamine receptor supersensitivity. *Science*, **1978**, *201*, 171–173.

Plenge, P.; Mellerup, E. T.; Bolwig, T. G.; Brun, C.; Hetmar, O.; Ladefoged, J.; Larsen, S.; and Rafaelsen, O. J.

Lithium treatment: does the kidney prefer one daily dose instead of two? *Acta Psychiatr. Scand.*, **1982**, *66*, 121–128.

Pohl, R.; Berchou, R.; and Rainey, J. M. Tricyclic antidepressants and monoamine oxidase inhibitors in the treatment of agoraphobia. *J. Clin. Psychopharmacol.*, **1982**, *2*, 399–407.

Pollack, M. H., and Rosenbaum, J. F. Management of antidepressant-induced side effects: a practical guide for the clinician. *J. Clin. Psychiatry*, **1987**, *48*, 3–8.

Pope, H. G., Jr., and Hudson, J. I. Antidepressant drug therapy for bulimia: current studies. *J. Clin. Psychiatry*, **1986**, *47*, 339–345.

Prien, R. F., and Kupfer, D. J. Continuation drug therapy for major depressive episodes: how long should it be maintained? *Am. J. Psychiatry*, **1986**, *143*, 18–23.

Puig-Antich, J. Affective disorders in children and adolescents: diagnostic validity and psychobiology. In, *Psychopharmacology: The Third Generation of Progress*. (Meltzer, H. Y., ed.) Raven Press, New York, **1987**, pp. 843–859.

Ray, W. A.; Griffin, M. R.; Schaffner, W.; Baugh, D. K.; and Milton, L. J., III. Psychotropic drug use and the risk of hip fracture. *N. Engl. J. Med.*, **1987**, *316*, 363–369.

Richelson, E. Tricyclic antidepressants and H_1 receptors. *Mayo Clin. Proc.*, **1979**, *54*, 669–674.

Rickels, K.; Schweizer, E.; Csanalosi, I.; Case, G.; and Chung, H. Long-term treatment of anxiety and risk of withdrawal: prospective comparison of chlorazepate and buspirone. *Arch. Gen. Psychiatry*, **1988**, *45*, 444–450.

Ries, R. K.; Gilbert, D. A.; and Katon, W. Tricyclic antidepressant therapy for peptic ulcer disease. *Arch. Intern. Med.*, **1984**, *144*, 566–569.

Robinson, D. S.; Nies, A.; Ravaris, C. L.; Ives, J. O.; and Bartlett, D. Clinical pharmacology of phenelzine. *Arch. Gen. Psychiatry*, **1978**, *35*, 629–635.

Roose, S. P.; Glassman, A. H.; Giardina, E. G.; Walsh, B. T.; Woodring, S.; and Bigger, J. T. Tricyclic antidepressants in depressed patients with cardiac conduction disease. *Arch. Gen. Psychiatry*, **1987**, *44*, 273–275.

Rosenbaum, J. F. The drug treatment of anxiety. *N. Engl. J. Med.*, **1982**, *306*, 401–404.

———. (ed.). New uses for clonazepam in psychiatry. *J. Clin. Psychiatry*, **1987**, *48*, Suppl. 3, 1–56.

Rotblatt, M. D. Antidepressants and seizures. *Drug Intell. Clin. Pharm.*, **1982**, *16*, 749–750.

Rotrosen, J.; Angrist, B. M.; Gershon, S.; Aronson, M.; Gruen, P.; Sachar, E.; Denning, R. K.; Matthysse, S.; Stanley, M.; and Wilk, S. Thiethylperazine. *Arch. Gen. Psychiatry*, **1978**, *35*, 1112–1118.

Sachar, E. J. Neuroendocrine responses to psychotropic drugs. In, *Psychopharmacology: A Generation of Progress*. (Lipton, M. A.; DiMascio, A.; and Killam, K. F.; eds.) Raven Press, New York, **1978**, pp. 499–507.

Safra, M. J., and Oakley, G. P., Jr. Association between cleft lip with or without cleft palate and prenatal exposure to diazepam. *Lancet*, **1975**, *2*, 478–480.

Saron, B. M., and Gaind, R. Lithium. *Clin. Toxicol.*, **1973**, *6*, 257–269.

Schou, M. Lithium in psychiatric therapy and prophylaxis. *J. Psychiatr. Res.*, **1968**, *6*, 67–95.

Schyve, P. M.; Smithline, F.; and Meltzer, H. Y. Neuroleptic-induced prolactin level elevation and breast cancer: an emerging issue. *Arch. Gen. Psychiatry*, **1978**, *35*, 1291–1301.

Seeman, P. Brain dopamine receptors. *Pharmacol. Rev.*, **1980**, *32*, 229–313.

Selinger, D.; Simmons, S.; Hailer, A. W.; Nurnberger, J. I., Jr.; and Gershon, E. S. An effective method for measuring salivary lithium in patients on anticholinergic drugs. *Biol. Psychiatry*, **1982**, *17*, 1145–1155.

Shader, R. I.; Goodman, M.; and Gever, J. Panic disorders: current perspectives. *J. Clin. Psychopharmacol.*, **1982**, *2*, Suppl., 2–10.

Shapiro, A. K.; Shapiro, E.; and Wayne, H. L. Treatment of Tourette's syndrome with haloperidol. Review of 34 cases. *Arch. Gen. Psychiatry*, **1973**, *28*, 92–97.

Shatan, C. Withdrawal symptoms after abrupt termination of imipramine. *Can. Psychiatr. Assoc. J.*, **1966**, *2*, 150–157.

Sheehan, D. V. Panic attacks and phobias. *N. Engl. J. Med.*, **1980**, *307*, 156–158.

Sheehan, D. V.; Ballenger, J.; and Jacobson, G. Treatment of endogenous anxiety with phobic, hysterical, and hypochondriacal symptoms. *Arch. Gen. Psychiatry*, **1980**, *37*, 51–59.

Siever, L. J. Role of noradrenergic mechanisms in the etiology of the affective disorders. In, *Psychopharmacology: The Third Generation of Progress*. (Meltzer, H. Y., ed.) Raven Press, New York, **1987**, pp. 493–504.

Simpson, G. M.; Cooper, T. B.; Bark, N.; Sud, I.; and Lee, H. J. Effect of antiparkinsonian medication on plasma levels of chlorpromazine. *Arch. Gen. Psychiatry*, **1980**, *37*, 205–208.

Simpson, G. M.; Lee, J. H.; Cuculic, Z.; and Kellner, R. Two dosages of imipramine in hospitalized endogenous and neurotic depressives. *Arch. Gen. Psychiatry*, **1976**, *33*, 1093–1102.

Skolnick, P., and Paul, S. M. Benzodiazepine receptors in the central nervous system. *Int. Rev. Neurobiol.*, **1982**, *23*, 103–140.

Snyder, S. H.; U'Prichard, D.; and Greenberg, D. A. Neurotransmitter receptor binding in the brain. In, *Psychopharmacology: A Generation of Progress*. (Lipton, M. A.; DiMascio, A.; and Killam, K. F.; eds.) Raven Press, New York, **1978**, pp. 361–370.

Snyder, S. H., and Yamamura, H. Antidepressants and the muscarinic acetylcholine receptor. *Arch. Gen. Psychiatry*, **1977**, *34*, 236–239.

Stewart, J. H.; Quitkin, F.; Fyer, A.; Rifkin, A.; McGrath, T.; Liebowitz, M.; Rosnick, L.; and Klein, D. F. Efficacy of desipramine in endogenomorphically depressed patients. *J. Affective Disord.*, **1980**, *2*, 165–176.

Study, R. E., and Barker, J. L. Cellular mechanisms of benzodiazepine action. *J.A.M.A.*, **1982**, *247*, 2147–2151.

Sulser, F., and Robinson, S. E. Clinical implications of pharmacological differences among antipsychotic drugs. In, *Psychopharmacology: A Generation of Progress*. (Lipton, M. A.; DiMascio, A.; and Killam, K. F.; eds.) Raven Press, New York, **1978**, pp. 943–954.

Sunderland, T., and Cohen, B. M. Blood to brain distribution of neuroleptics. *Psychiatry Res.*, **1987**, *20*, 299–305.

Tarsy, D., and Baldessarini, R. J. Clinical and pathophysiologic features of movement disorders induced by psychotherapeutic agents. In, *Movement Disorders*. (Shah, N., and Donald, A., eds.) Plenum Press, New York, **1986**, pp. 365–389.

Taylor, D. P. Buspirone, a new approach to the treatment of anxiety. *FASEB J.*, **1988**, *2*, 2445–2452.

Tesar, G. E.; Murray, G. B.; and Cassem, E. H. Use of high-dose intravenous haloperidol in the treatment of agitated cardiac patients. *J. Clin. Psychopharmacol.*, **1985**, *5*, 344–347.

Treiser, S. L.; Cascio, C. S.; O'Donohue, T. L.; Thoa, N. B.; Jacobowitz, D. M.; and Kellar, K. J. Lithium increases serotonin release and decreases serotonin receptors in the hippocampus. *Science*, **1981**, *213*, 1529–1531.

Tupin, J. P., and Schuller, A. B. Lithium and haloperidol incompatibility reviewed. *Psychiatr. J. Univ. Ottawa*, **1978**, *3*, 245–251.

U'Prichard, D. C.; Greenberg, D. A.; Sheehan, P. P.; and Snyder, S. H. Tricyclic antidepressants: therapeutic properties and affinity for alpha-noradrenergic receptor binding sites in the brain. *Science*, **1978**, *199*, 197–198.

Van De Merwe, T. J.; Silverstone, T.; Ankier, S. I.; Warrington, S. J.; and Turner, P. A double-blind non-crossover placebo-controlled study between group comparison of trazodone and amitriptyline on cardiovascular function in major depressive disorder. *Psychopathology,* **1984,** *17,* Suppl. 2, 64–76.

Veith, R. C.; Raskind, M. A.; and Caldwell, J. H. Cardiovascular effects of tricyclic antidepressants in depressed patients with chronic heart disease. *N. Engl. J. Med.,* **1982,** *306,* 954–959.

White, K., and Simpson, G. Combined MAOI–tricyclic antidepressant treatment: a reevaluation. *J. Clin. Psychopharmacol.,* **1981,** *1,* 264–282.

Wolf, M., and Roth, R. Dopamine autoreceptors. In, *Structure and Function of Dopamine Receptors: Receptor Biochemistry and Methodology,* Vol. 8. (Creese, I., and Fraser, C. M., eds.) Alan R. Liss, Inc., New York, **1987,** pp. 45–96.

Worley, P. F.; Heller, W. A.; Snyder, S. H.; and Baraban, J. M. Lithium blocks a phosphoinositide-mediated cholinergic response in hippocampal slices. *Science,* **1988,** *239,* 1428–1429.

Zametkin, A. J., and Rapoport, J. L. Noradrenergic hypothesis of attention deficit disorder with hyperactivity: a critical review. In, *Psychopharmacology: The Third Generation of Progress.* (Meltzer, H. Y., ed.) Raven Press, New York, **1987,** pp. 837–842.

Ziegler, V. E.; Biggs, J. T.; and Wylie, L. T. Doxepin kinetics. *Clin. Pharmacol. Ther.,* **1978,** *23,* 573–579.

Monographs and Reviews

Allquander, C. Dependence on sedative and hypnotic drugs. *Acta Psychiatr. Scand.* [*Suppl.*], **1978,** *270,* 1–120.

American Psychiatric Association. *Diagnostic and Statistical Manual of Mental Disorders,* 3rd ed., Revised. APA Press, Inc., Washington, D.C., **1987.**

Anders, T. F., and Ciaranello, R. Psychopharmacology of childhood disorders. In, *Psychopharmacology: From Theory to Practice.* (Barchas, J. D.; Berger, P. A.; Ciaranello, R.; and Elliott, G. R.; eds.) Oxford University Press, New York, **1977,** pp. 407–447.

Ayd, F. J., Jr., and Blackwell, B. (eds.). *Discoveries in Biological Psychiatry.* J. B. Lippincott Co., Philadelphia, **1970.**

Baldessarini, R. J. *Biomedical Aspects of Depression.* American Psychiatric Press, Inc., Washington, D.C., **1983.**

———. Antipsychotic agents. In, *The Psychiatric Therapies.* (Karasu, B., ed.) American Psychiatric Association, Washington, DC, **1984b,** pp. 119–170.

———. *Chemotherapy in Psychiatry: Principles and Practice,* 2nd ed. Harvard University Press, Cambridge, MA, **1985.**

Baldessarini, R. J.; Cole, J. O.; Davis, J. M.; Gardos, G.; Simpson, G.; and Tarsy, D. *Tardive Dyskinesia.* Task Force Report No. 18, American Psychiatric Association, Washington, D.C., **1980.**

Baldessarini, R. J., and Tarsy, D. Relationship of the actions of neuroleptic drugs to the pathophysiology of tardive dyskinesia. *Int. Rev. Neurobiol.,* **1979,** *21,* 1–45.

Barchas, J. D.; Berger, P. A.; Matthysse, S.; and Wyatt, R. J. The biochemistry of affective disorders and schizophrenia. In, *Principles of Psychopharmacology,* 2nd ed. (Clark, W. G., and del Guidice, J., eds.) Academic Press, Inc., New York, **1978,** pp. 105–132.

Bassuk, E. L.; Schoonover, S. C.; and Gelenberg, A. J. *The Practitioner's Guide to Psychoactive Drugs,* 2nd ed. Plenum Medical Book Publishing Co., New York, **1983.**

Biel, J. H.; Bopp, B.; and Mitchell, B. D. Chemistry and structure-activity relationships of psychotropic drugs. In, *Principles of Psychopharmacology,* 2nd ed. (Clark, W. G., and del Guidice, J., eds.) Academic Press, Inc., New York, **1978,** pp. 140–168.

Caldwell, A. E. History of psychopharmacology. In, *Principles of Psychopharmacology,* 2nd ed. (Clark, W. G., and del Guidice, J., eds.) Academic Press, Inc., New York, **1978,** pp. 9–40.

Chase, T. N. Rational approaches to the pharmacotherapy of chorea. In, *The Basal Ganglia.* Association for Research in Nervous and Mental Disease Publications, Vol. 55. (Yahr, M. D., ed.) Raven Press, New York, **1976,** pp. 337–350.

Cooper, T. B.; Simpson, G. M.; and Lee, H. J. Thymoleptic and neuroleptic drug plasma levels in psychiatry: current status. *Int. Rev. Neurobiol.,* **1976,** *19,* 269–309.

Davis, J. M. Overview: maintenance therapy in psychiatry. I. Schizophrenia. *Am. J. Psychiatry,* **1975,** *132,* 1237–1245.

———. Overview: maintenance therapy in psychiatry. II. Affective disorders. *Ibid.,* **1976,** *133,* 1–13.

Davis, J. M., and Garver, D. L. Neuroleptics: clinical use in psychiatry. In, *Handbook of Psychopharmacology,* Vol. 10. (Iversen, L. L.; Iversen, S. D.; and Snyder, S. H.; eds.) Plenum Press, New York, **1978,** pp. 129–164.

Efron, D. H.; Holmstedt, B.; and Kline, N. S. (eds.). *Ethnopharmacologic Search for Psychoactive Drugs.* Public Health Service Publication No. 67–1645, U.S. Government Printing Office, Washington, D.C., **1967.**

Eison, M. S. Use of animal models: toward anxioselective drugs. *Psychopathology,* **1984,** *17,* Suppl. 1, 37–44.

Fielding, S., and Lal, H. Behavioral actions of neuroleptics. In, *Handbook of Psychopharmacology,* Vol. 10. (Iversen, L. L.; Iversen, S. D.; and Snyder, S. H.; eds.) Plenum Press, New York, **1978,** pp. 91–128.

Glassman, A. H., and Perel, J. M. Tricyclic blood levels and clinical outcome: a review of the art. In, *Psychopharmacology: A Generation of Progress.* (Lipton, M. A.; DiMascio, A.; and Killam, K. F.; eds.) Raven Press, New York, **1978,** pp. 917–921.

Goldberg, H. L. Benzodiazepine and nonbenzodiazepine anxiolytics. *Psychopathology,* **1984,** *17,* Suppl. 1, 45–55.

Gordon, M. *Psychopharmacological Agents,* Vols. II and III. Academic Press, Inc., New York, **1967** and **1974.**

Hansten, P. D. *Drug Interactions,* 5th ed. Lea & Febiger, Philadelphia, **1985.**

Herrington, R. N., and Lader, M. H. Chap. 1, Antidepressant drugs. Chap. 2, Lithium. In, *Handbook of Biological Psychiatry.* Pt. V, *Drug Treatment in Psychiatry—Psychotropic Drugs.* (Praag, H. M. van, ed.) Marcel Dekker, Inc., New York, **1981,** pp. 1–72.

Itil, T. M. Effects of psychotropic drugs on qualitatively and quantitatively analyzed human EEG. In, *Principles of Psychopharmacology,* 2nd ed. (Clark, W. G., and del Guidice, J., eds.) Academic Press, Inc., New York, **1978,** pp. 261–277.

Iversen, L. L.; Iversen, S. D.; and Snyder, S. H. (eds.). *Affective Disorders: Drug Actions in Animals and Man. Handbook of Psychopharmacology,* Vol. 14. Plenum Press, New York, **1978.**

Janssen, P. A. Butyrophenones and diphenylbutylpiperidines. In, *Psychopharmacological Agents,* Vol. 3. (Gordon, M., ed.) Academic Press, Inc., New York, **1974,** pp. 128–158.

Janssen, P. A., and Van Bever, W. F. Preclinical psychopharmacology of neuroleptics. In, *Principles of Psychopharmacology,* 2nd ed. (Clark, W. G., and del Guidice, J., eds.) Academic Press, Inc., New York, **1978,** pp. 279–295.

Jefferson, J. W.; Greist, J. H.; and Ackerman, D. L. *Lithium Encyclopedia for Clinical Practice.* Lithium

Information Center, Department of Psychiatry, University of Wisconsin, Madison, **1983.**

Jeste, D. V., and Wyatt, R. J. *Understanding and Treating Tardive Dyskinesia*. The Guilford Press, New York, **1982.**

Johnson, F. N. (ed.). *Handbook of Lithium Therapy*. University Park Press, Baltimore, **1980.**

Kaplan, H. I., and Sadock, B. J. (eds.). *Comprehensive Textbook of Psychiatry*, 4th ed. The Williams & Wilkins Co., Baltimore, **1985.**

Kaufman, J. S. Drug interactions involving psychotherapeutic agents. In, *Drug Treatment of Mental Disorders*. (Simpson, L. L., ed.) Raven Press, New York, **1976,** pp. 289–309.

Klein, D. F.; Gittelman, R.; Quitkin, F.; and Rifkin, A. *Diagnosis and Drug Treatment of Psychiatric Disorders: Adults and Children*, 2nd ed. The Williams & Wilkins Co., Baltimore, **1980.**

Lader, M. Antianxiety drugs in the psychiatric therapies. In, *The Psychiatric Therapies*. (Karasu, B., ed.) American Psychiatric Association, Washington, D.C., **1984,** pp. 53–84.

Lewin, L. *Phantastica, Narcotic and Stimulating Drugs; Their Use and Abuse*. Berlin, **1924;** English translation, London, **1931;** E. P. Dutton & Co., New York, **1931.**

Lowe, M. C.; Horita, A.; Gelenberg, A. J.; and Klerman, G. L. Preclinical pharmacology of antidepressants. In, *Principles of Psychopharmacology*, 2nd ed. (Clark, W. G., and del Guidice, J., eds.) Academic Press, Inc., New York, **1978,** pp. 311–323.

McElroy, S. M., and Pope, H. G., Jr. *Use of Anticonvulsants in Psychiatry: Recent Advances*. Oxford Health Care, Clifton, NJ, **1988.**

Mendelson, W. B. *Human Sleep: Research and Clinical Care*. Plenum Press, New York, **1987.**

Murphy, D. L.; Campbell, I.; and Costa, J. L. Current status of the indoleamine hypothesis of the affective disorders. In, *Psychopharmacology: A Generation of Progress*. (Lipton, M. A.; DiMascio, A.; and Killam, K. F.; eds.) Raven Press, New York, **1978,** pp. 1235–1248.

Polc, P. Electrophysiology of benzodiazepine receptor ligands: multiple mechanisms and sites of action. *Prog. Neurobiol.*, **1988,** *31*, 349–423.

Pope, H. G., and Lipinski, J. F. Diagnosis in schizophrenia and manic-depressive illness. *Arch. Gen. Psychiatry*, **1978,** *35*, 811–828.

Popper, C. (ed.). *Psychiatric Pharmacosciences of Children and Adolescents*. American Psychiatric Press, Washington, DC, **1987.**

Post, R. M.; Uhde, T. W.; Rubinow, D. R.; Ballenger, J. C.; and Gold, P. W. Biochemical effects of carbamazepine: relationship to its mechanisms of action in affective illness. *Prog. Neuropsychopharmacol. Biol. Psychiatry*, **1983,** *7*, 263–271.

Praag, H. M. van. Amine hypotheses of affective disorders. In, *Handbook of Psychopharmacology*, Vol. 13. (Iversen, L. L.; Iversen, S. D.; and Snyder, S. H.; eds.) Plenum Press, New York, **1978,** pp. 187–297.

Prien, R. F. Chemotherapy in chronic organic brain syndrome—a review of the literature. *Psychopharmacol. Bull.*, **1973,** *9*, 5–20.

Prien, R. F., and Cole, J. O. The use of psychopharmacological drugs in the aged. In, *Principles of Psychopharmacology*, 2nd ed. (Clark, W. G., and del Guidice, J., eds.) Academic Press, Inc., New York, **1978,** pp. 593–605.

Ramsey, T. A., and Mendels, J. Lithium as an antidepressant. In, *Antidepressants: Neurochemical, Behavioral and Clinical Perspectives*. (Enna, S. J.; Malick, J. B.; and Richelson, E.; eds.) Raven Press, New York, **1981,** pp. 175–182.

Raskin, A.; Robinson, D. S.; and Levine, J. *Age and the Pharmacology of Psychoactive Drugs*. Elsevier-North Holland, Inc., New York, **1981.**

Reichlin, S., and Boyd, A. E., III. Neural control of prolactin secretion in man. *Psychoneuroendocrinology*, **1978,** *3*, 113–130.

Rickels, K. Drug treatment of anxiety. In, *Psychopharmacology in the Practice of Medicine*. (Jarvik, M. E., ed.) Appleton-Century-Crofts, New York, **1977,** pp. 309–324.

Rivera-Calimlin, L., and Hershey, L. Neuroleptic concentrations and clinical response. *Annu. Rev. Pharmacol. Toxicol.*, **1984,** *24*, 361–386.

Schou, M. The biology and pharmacology of lithium: a bibliography. *Psychopharmacol. Bull.*, **1969,** *5*, 33–62.

Schultes, R. E. Ethnopharmacological significance of psychotropic drugs of vegetal origin. In, *Principles of Psychopharmacology*, 2nd ed. (Clark, W. G., and del Guidice, J., eds.) Academic Press, Inc., New York, **1978,** pp. 41–70.

Shore, P. A., and Giachetti, A. Reserpine: basic and clinical pharmacology. In, *Handbook of Psychopharmacology*, Vol. 10. (Iversen, L. L.; Iversen, S. D.; and Snyder, S. H.; eds.) Plenum Press, New York, **1978,** pp. 197–219.

Sulser, F., and Mobley, P. L. Biochemical effects of antidepressants in animals. In, *Psychotropic Agents: Antipsychotics and Antidepressants*. Vol. 55, Pt. I, *Handbook of Experimental Pharmacology*. (Hoffmeister, F., and Stille, G., eds.) Springer-Verlag, Berlin, **1980,** pp. 471–490.

Swazey, J. P. *Chlorpromazine in Psychiatry: A Study in Therapeutic Innovation*. M.I.T. Press, Cambridge, MA, **1974.**

Symposium. (Various authors.) *Monoamine Oxidase: Structure, Function and Altered Functions*. (Singer, T. P.; Von Korff, D. W.; and Murphy, D. L.; eds.) Academic Press, Inc., New York, **1979.**

Symposium. (Various authors.) *Antidepressants: Neurochemical, Behavioral, and Clinical Perspectives*. (Enna, S. J.; Malick, J. B.; and Richelson, E.; eds.) Raven Press, New York, **1981.**

Symposium. (Various authors.) *Pharmacology of Benzodiazepines*. (Usdin, E.; Skolnick, P.; Tallman, J. F., Jr.; Greenblatt, D.; and Paul, S. M.; eds.) Macmillan Press Ltd., London, **1982.**

Symposium. (Various authors.) *Anxiolytes: Neurochemical, Behavioral and Clinical Perspectives*. (Malick, J. B.; Enna, S. J.; and Yamamura, H. I.; eds.) Raven Press, New York, **1983.**

Symposium. (Various authors.) Chloride channels and their modulation by neurotransmitters and drugs. (Biggio, G., and Costa, E., eds.) *Adv. Biochem. Psychopharmacol.*, **1988,** *45*.

Usdin, E. Classification of psychotropic drugs. In, *Principles of Psychopharmacology*, 2nd ed. (Clark, W. G., and del Guidice, J., eds.) Academic Press, Inc., New York, **1978,** pp. 193–246.

Van Woert, M. H.; Jutkowitz, R.; Rosenbaum, D.; and Bowers, M. B., Jr. Gilles de la Tourette's syndrome: biochemical approaches. In, *The Basal Ganglia*. Association for Research in Nervous and Mental Disease Publications, Vol. 55. (Yahr, M. D., ed.) Raven Press, New York, **1976,** pp. 459–465.

Weil-Malherbe, H. The biochemistry of the functional psychoses. *Adv. Enzymol.*, **1967,** *29*, 479–553.

Werry, J. S. (ed.). *Pediatric Psychopharmacology: The Use of Behavior Modifying Drugs in Children*. Brunner/Mazel, Inc., New York, **1978.**

Woods, J. H.; Katz, J. L.; and Winger, G. Abuse liability of benzodiazepines. *Pharmacol. Rev.*, **1987,** *39*, 254–390.

CHAPTER

19 DRUGS EFFECTIVE IN THE THERAPY OF THE EPILEPSIES

Theodore W. Rall and Leonard S. Schleifer

GENERAL CONSIDERATIONS

Classification of Epileptic Seizures. The term *epilepsies* is a collective designation for a group of central nervous system (CNS) disorders having in common the repeated occurrence of sudden and transitory episodes (seizures) of abnormal phenomena of motor (convulsion), sensory, autonomic, or psychic origin. The seizures are nearly always correlated with abnormal and excessive discharges in the brain, which can be recorded on an electroencephalogram (EEG).

Epilepsy afflicts at least 1 to 2 million people in the United States and about 20 to 40 million people worldwide (*see* Delgado-Escueta *et al.*, in Symposium, 1986a). The disease is more common in children than in adults, with a prevalence of about 8 per 1000 children below the age of 7 years (*see* Nelson and Ellenberg, in Symposium, 1987a). The term *primary,* or *idiopathic, epilepsy* denotes those cases where no cause for the seizures can be identified. *Secondary,* or *symptomatic, epilepsy* designates the disorder when it is associated with such factors as trauma, neoplasm, infection, developmental abnormalities, or cerebrovascular disease. Although certain metabolic disorders or metabolic diseases of neurons may underlie symptomatic epilepsy (*see* Tharp, in Symposium, 1987a), the convulsions that may accompany severe systemic metabolic disturbances (such as hypoglycemia) should not be classified as epilepsy. The detection of factors that contribute to secondary epilepsy has been facilitated by the advent of improved diagnostic procedures, such as computerized axial tomography and nuclear magnetic resonance scanning of the brain.

For purposes of drug treatment, it is more useful to classify patients according to the type of seizure they experience. A simplified form of the proposal from the Commission on Classification and Terminology of the International League Against Epilepsy (1981), based on the clinical manifestations of the attacks and the pattern of the EEG, is presented in Table 19–1. A more complete description of the various types of seizures has been provided by Browne (Symposium, 1983a) and by Delgado-Escueta and coworkers (1983). The most recent proposal from the Commission on Classification (1985) subdivides each category of epileptic seizures according to etiology, either idiopathic or symptomatic. To date, this refinement has had more impact on the overall therapeutic strategy than on the choice of antiepileptic agent.

Nature and Mechanisms of Seizures. Almost a century ago John Hughlings Jackson, the father of modern concepts of epilepsy, proposed that seizures were caused by "occasional, sudden, excessive, rapid and local discharges of gray matter," and that a generalized convulsion resulted when normal brain tissue was invaded by the seizure activity initiated in the abnormal focus. In the intervening years little has been added to Jackson's concepts except for the electrical proof of their correctness. The EEG amply demonstrates that seizures are associated with abnormal and sometimes massive electrical discharges in the brain and serves as the basic method of differential diagnosis of the epilepsies.

The pathophysiology of epilepsy is poorly understood. In no instance has the abnormal function of neurons or of aggregates of neurons that is responsible for the genesis of seizures been unambiguously identified (*see* Symposium 1986a, 1987a). Undoubtedly, epileptogenesis involves the complex interaction of multiple causative factors. Macroscopic lesions of the brain can produce epilepsy.

Table 19–1. CLASSIFICATION OF EPILEPTIC SEIZURES *

SEIZURE TYPE †		CHARACTERISTICS
I. *Partial Seizures* (Focal, Local Seizures)	A. Simple partial seizures	Various manifestations, without impairment of consciousness, including convulsions confined to a single limb or muscle group (*Jacksonian motor epilepsy*), specific and localized sensory disturbances (*Jacksonian sensory epilepsy*), and other limited signs and symptoms depending upon the particular cortical area producing the abnormal discharge
	B. Complex partial seizures	Attacks of confused behavior, with impairment of consciousness, with a wide variety of clinical manifestations, associated with bizarre generalized EEG activity during the seizure but with evidence of anterior temporal lobe focal abnormalities even in the interseizure period in many cases
	C. Partial seizures secondarily generalized	
II. *Generalized Seizures* (Convulsive or Nonconvulsive)	A.1. Absence seizures	Brief and abrupt loss of consciousness associated with high-voltage, bilaterally synchronous, 3-per-second spike-and-wave pattern in the EEG, usually with some symmetrical clonic motor activity varying from eyelid blinking to jerking of the entire body, sometimes with no motor activity
	A.2. Atypical absence seizures	Attacks with slower onset and cessation than is usual for absence seizures, associated with a more heterogeneous EEG
	B. Myoclonic seizures	Isolated clonic jerks associated with brief bursts of multiple spikes in the EEG
	C. Clonic seizures	Rhythmic clonic contractions of all muscles, loss of consciousness, and marked autonomic manifestations
	D. Tonic seizures	Opisthotonus, loss of consciousness, and marked autonomic manifestations
	E. Tonic-clonic (*grand mal*) seizures	Major convulsions, usually a sequence of maximal tonic spasm of all body musculature followed by synchronous clonic jerking and a prolonged depression of all central functions
	F. Atonic seizures	Loss of postural tone, with sagging of the head or falling

* Modified from the proposal from the Commission on Classification and Terminology of the International League Against Epilepsy (1981).

† Additional seizure types are presently unclassified owing to incomplete data.

Certain types of lesions (*e.g.*, traumatic hemorrhage) are more likely to lead to secondary epilepsy than are others (*e.g.*, ischemic stroke). At the microscopic level, glial proliferation and loss of neurons in brain tissue from epileptic patients have been reported repeatedly, together with evidence for loss of inhibitory synaptic elements containing gamma-aminobutyric acid (GABA) (*see* Ribak, in Symposium, 1986a). However, it is not clear whether such changes preceded the development of epileptic foci or whether they might represent the consequences of seizures and simply contribute to the spread of seizure discharges. By definition, gross or microscopic pathology is absent in patients with idiopathic epilepsy, probably including some with inherited disorders. The complexity of epileptogenesis is also indicated by the existence of over 100 human Mendelian traits that are associated with increased risk of seizures. Moreover, apparently identical seizure disorders can occur both in the presence and absence of a particular inherited metabolic defect (*see* Anderson *et al.,* in Symposium, 1986a; Tharp, in Symposium, 1987a).

Investigation of various animal models has also provided ample evidence for heterogeneity in the mechanisms of epileptogenesis (*see* Symposium, 1972; 1986a). Two well-studied examples are particularly instructive. One involves the application of alumina cream to the motor cortex of the monkey or other species (*see* Wilder, in Symposium, 1972; Delgado-Escueta *et al.*, in Symposium, 1986a). Spontaneous convulsive seizures eventually emerge that generalize from a focal onset. Groups of neurons that discharge synchronously at high frequency can be found near the original site of application. The number of terminals and small neurons that contain glutamate decarboxylase are reduced within this focus and in adjacent tissue (*see* Ribak, in Symposium, 1986a). Such evidence for reduced function of inhibitory pathways that utilize GABA is congruent with the production of epileptiform discharges in groups of neurons exposed to drugs that are known to interfere with the function of GABA, including penicillin, picrotoxin, pentylenetetrazol, and bicuculline.

The second example is provided by an inbred strain of Mongolian gerbil, in which myoclonic or tonic-clonic seizures gradually develop about 50 days after birth (*see* Paul and Scheibel, in Symposium, 1986a). One interesting microscopic finding is that the number of neurons and terminals that contain GABA is *increased* in the hippocampus of these animals (*see* Ribak, in Symposium, 1986a). These terminals appear to be located on inhibitory basket cells, giving rise to the notion of epileptogenesis by "disinhibition."

A similar, apparently paradoxical arrangement has been found in the *tottering* mutant mouse. Animals with this single-gene recessive mutation display a stereotyped triad of ataxia, intermittent focal myoclonic seizures, and generalized seizures that appears in the third postnatal week (*see* Noebels, in Symposium, 1986a). The only apparent cellular pathology is a selective overgrowth of axons from neurons in the locus ceruleus, leading to elevated concentrations of norepinephrine in terminal projection fields, including the neocortex, hippocampus, cerebellum, and thalamus. Treatment of neonatal animals with the selective neurotoxin 6-hydroxydopamine prevents the later appearance of seizures in adult animals; instillation of this agent into the locus ceruleus of adults produces a temporary but rapidly appearing reduction in seizure discharges. This is in marked contrast to the ability of 6-hydroxydopamine and other maneuvers that reduce noradrenergic transmission in the CNS to *enhance* the production of seizures in a wide variety of other animal models (*see* Chauvel and Trottier, in Symposium, 1986a).

Although it appears that the establishment of a chronic epileptic focus is apt to be associated with local structural or neurochemical abnormalities in small aggregates of neurons, it is unlikely that the progressive entrainment of adjacent tissue (*ictal initiation*) and the emergence of electrical or behavioral seizures (*ictal propagation*) involve similar detectable pathology. The strongest evidence for this notion comes from the investigation of kindling, which involves the delivery of brief, initially subliminal electrical or chemical stimuli to various areas of the brain, usually the amygdala (*see* Wasterlain *et al.,* and McNamara, in Symposium, 1986a). After 10 to 15 days of once-daily stimulation, the duration and intensity of after-discharges reach a stable maximum, and a characteristic behavioral seizure is produced. Subsequent stimulations, even at intervals of several months, regularly elicit seizures. Microscopic evidence for significant structural damage is lacking. It would appear that the synaptic delivery of electrical discharges of sufficient intensity or frequency can produce adaptive changes in groups of neurons such that there is progressive recruitment of neuronal circuits; these changes can be detected only by electrophysiological techniques. The adaptive changes may involve processes similar to those responsible for long-term potentiation, a phenomenon that is produced by high-frequency stimulation of inputs to the hippocampus and leads to an enhancement of excitatory synaptic potentials (*see* McIntyre and Racine, 1986).

Mechanisms of Action of Antiepileptic Agents. There are two general ways in which drugs might abolish or attenuate seizures: through effects on pathologically altered neurons of seizure foci to prevent or reduce their excessive discharge, and through effects that would reduce the spread of excitation from seizure foci and prevent detonation and disruption of function of normal aggregates of neurons. Most, if not all, antiepileptic agents that are presently available act at least in part by the second mechanism, since all modify the ability of the brain to respond to various seizure-evoking stimuli. Although a variety of neurophysiological effects of such drugs have been noted, especially effects on inhibitory systems that involve GABA, investigators frequently fail to define those effects that might be prominent at therapeutic concentrations of free drug in plasma or those that are not characteristic of local anesthetics or sedatives. Thus, it must be admitted that mechanisms of action of antiepileptic agents are only poorly understood.

Chemical Structure and Antiepileptic Selectivity. The useful antiepileptic agents belong to several chemical classes. Most of the drugs introduced before 1965 are closely related in structure to phenobarbital, the oldest member of this therapeutic class. These include the hydantoins, the deoxybarbiturates, the oxazolidinediones, and the succinimides. The agents introduced after 1965 include benzodiazepines (clonazepam and clorazepate), an iminostilbene (carbamazepine), and a branched-chain carboxylic acid (valproic acid). The structure–activity relationships of these and other classes of compounds have been summarized (*see* Symposium, 1977). Many thousands of compounds have been screened in industrial laboratories and by the Antiepileptic Drug Development Program of the National Institute of Neurological and Communicative Disorders and Stroke (*see* Gladding *et al.*, 1985); a number of active compounds with novel structures have been identified and are undergoing clinical trial (*see* Schäfer, 1985). These screening tests have relied heavily on the capacity of the drugs to modify the effects of maximal electric shock (inhibition of tonic hindlimb extension) and to elevate the dose of pentylenetetrazol required to precipitate tonic-clonic convulsions. Although the former test usually predicts activity against generalized tonic-clonic and cortical focal convulsions and the latter against absence seizures, there are a number of important exceptions to this generalization. Continued development of model systems for the detection and evaluation of potential therapeutic agents is needed, and the use of genetically based or kindling models is currently being emphasized.

Therapeutic Aspects. The ideal antiepileptic drug would obviously suppress all seizures without causing any unwanted effects. Unfortunately, the drugs used currently not only fail to control seizure activity in some patients, but they frequently cause side effects that range in severity from minimal impairment of the CNS to death from aplastic anemia or hepatic failure. The physician who treats patients with epilepsy is thus faced with the task of selecting the appropriate drug or combination of drugs that best controls seizures in an individual patient at an acceptable level of untoward effects. It is generally held that complete control of seizures can be achieved in up to 50% of patients and that possibly another 25% can be improved significantly. The degree of success is greater in newly diagnosed patients and is dependent on such factors as the type of seizure, the family history, and the extent of associated neurological abnormalities (Elwes *et al.*, 1984).

For the purposes of drug therapy the classification of seizures given above may be further condensed. *Absence seizures* respond well to one group of drugs, and *generalized tonic-clonic convulsions* are usually adequately controlled by a second. *Complex partial seizures* tend to be refractory to therapy but may respond to agents in the second group. *Infantile spasms* and *akinetic, atonic,* and *myoclonic seizures* are a group for which therapy is generally unsatisfactory. In order to minimize toxicity, treatment with a single drug is usually sought (*see* Wilder, in Symposium, 1987c). If seizures are not controlled at adequate plasma concentrations of the initial agent, substitution of a second drug is generally preferred to the concurrent administration of another agent. However, multiple-drug therapy may be required, especially when two or more types of seizure occur in the same patient.

The general principles of the drug therapy of the epilepsies are summarized below, following discussion of the individual agents. Details of diagnosis and therapy can be found in the monographs and reviews listed at the end of the chapter.

Plasma Concentrations of Antiepileptic Drugs. Measurement of drug concentrations in plasma greatly facilitates antiepileptic medication, especially when therapy is initiated, after dosage adjustments, in the event of therapeutic failure, when toxic effects appear, or when multiple-drug therapy is instituted (*see* Hvidberg, 1985). However, for some drugs clinical effects do not correlate well with concentrations in plasma, and recommended concentrations are only guidelines for therapy. The ultimate therapeutic regimen must be determined by clinical assessment of effect and toxicity.

HYDANTOINS

PHENYTOIN

Phenytoin is a primary drug for all types of epilepsy except absence seizures. It has been more thoroughly studied in the laboratory and clinic than any other antiepileptic agent.

History. Phenytoin was first synthesized in 1908 by Biltz, but its anticonvulsant activity was not discovered until 1938 (Merritt and Putnam, 1938a). In contrast to the earlier accidental discovery of the anticonvulsant properties of bromide and phenobarbital, phenytoin was the product of a search among nonsedative structural relatives of phenobarbital for agents capable of suppressing electroshock convulsions in laboratory animals. It was introduced for the symptomatic treatment of epilepsy in the same year (Merritt and Putnam, 1938b). The discovery of phenytoin was a signal advance. Since this agent is not a sedative in ordinary doses, it established that antiepileptics need not impair consciousness and encouraged the search for drugs with selective anticonvulsant action.

Structure–Activity Relationship. Phenytoin has the following structural formula:

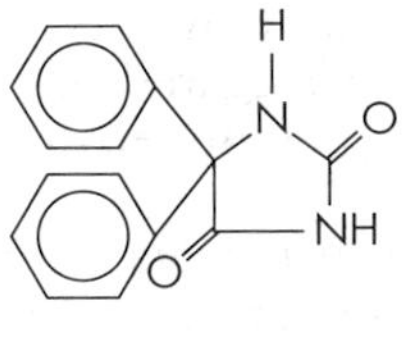

Phenytoin

A 5-phenyl or other aromatic substituent appears essential for activity against generalized tonic-clonic seizures. Alkyl substituents in position 5 contribute to sedation, a property absent in phenytoin. The 5 carbon permits asymmetry, as in mephenytoin, but there appears to be little difference in activity between isomers. (*See* Vida and Gerry, in Symposium, 1977.)

Pharmacological Effects. *Central Nervous System.* Phenytoin exerts antiepileptic activity without causing general depression of the CNS. In toxic doses it may produce excitatory signs and at lethal levels a type of decerebrate rigidity. The most easily demonstrated properties of phenytoin are its ability to limit the development of maximal seizure activity and to reduce the spread of the seizure process from an active focus. Both features are undoubtedly related to its clinical usefulness. Phenytoin can induce complete remission of generalized tonic-clonic and certain partial seizures but does not completely eliminate the sensory aura or other prodromal signs.

The anticonvulsant properties of phenytoin have been reviewed by Jones and Wimbish (1985). Unlike phenobarbital, phenytoin does not elevate the threshold for seizures induced by injection of such convulsant drugs as strychnine, picrotoxin, or pentylenetetrazol. It also has only limited ability to elevate the threshold for electroshock seizures. Phenytoin does, however, restore abnormally increased excitability toward normal.

Probably the most significant effect of phenytoin is its ability to modify the pattern of maximal electroshock seizures. The characteristic tonic phase can be abolished completely, but the residual clonic seizure may be exaggerated and prolonged. The drug produces similar alterations in the convulsions of psychiatric patients undergoing electroconvulsive therapy and in maximal seizures induced in animals by picrotoxin and pentylenetetrazol. This seizure-modifying action is also observed with other antiepileptics that are effective against generalized tonic-clonic seizures.

As noted, the ability of phenytoin to reduce the duration of afterdischarge and to limit the spread of seizure activity is more prominent than its effect on threshold for stimulation. It is thus surprising that phenytoin does not consistently retard the process of kindling in various animal species; this is in contrast to results with phenobarbital, carbamazepine, valproate, and certain benzodiazepines (*see* Wada, 1977). The prophylactic effect of phenytoin in human posttraumatic epilepsy has also been variable and difficult to evaluate (*see* Mutani, in Symposium, 1983b).

Mechanism of Action. Phenytoin exerts a stabilizing effect on excitable membranes of a variety of cells, including neurons and cardiac myocytes. It can decrease resting fluxes of Na^+ as well as Na^+ currents that flow during action potentials or chemically induced depolarizations (*see* Jones and Wimbish, 1985). The latter effects probably result from inhibition of voltage-sensitive Na^+ channels (Willow and Catterall, 1982). Phenytoin-induced inhibition of Na^+ currents is dependent on both voltage and frequency (Willow *et al.*, 1985) and thus resembles the action of local anesthetics (*see* Chapter 15). As a result, phenytoin suppresses episodes of repetitive neuronal firing that are induced by passage of intracellular current (*see* Macdonald and McLean, in Symposium, 1986a). Such effects can be achieved at therapeutically relevant concentrations of the drug (below 10 μM).

At concentrations in excess of 10 μM, phenytoin delays the activation of outward K^+ currents during action potentials in nerves, leading to an increased refractory period (*see* Yaari *et al.*, 1986). Phenytoin can also reduce the size and duration of

Ca^{2+}-dependent action potentials in cultured neurons at about 20 μM (McLean and Macdonald, 1983). Moreover, Narahashi (1988) observed that phenytoin affects a rapidly inactivating type of Ca^{2+} channel in neurons and that its inhibitory effects are intensified by membrane depolarization. Since dose–response relationships were not studied, it is not clear whether therapeutic concentrations of phenytoin can influence Ca^{2+} currents in neurons under certain circumstances, such as during high-frequency discharge.

Pharmacokinetic Properties. The pharmacokinetic characteristics of phenytoin are markedly influenced by its limited aqueous solubility and by dose-dependent elimination. Its inactivation by the hepatic microsomal enzyme system is susceptible to alteration by other drugs.

Phenytoin is a weak acid with a pK_a of about 8.3; its aqueous solubility is limited, even in the intestine. Upon intramuscular injection, the drug precipitates at the injection site and is absorbed slowly and unpredictably.

Absorption of phenytoin after oral ingestion is slow, sometimes variable, and occasionally incomplete. Significant differences in bioavailability of oral pharmaceutical preparations have been detected. Peak concentration in plasma may occur as early as 3 hours after a single dose or as late as 12 hours. Slow absorption during chronic medication blunts the fluctuations of drug concentration between doses. After absorption, phenytoin is rapidly distributed into all tissues.

Phenytoin is extensively (about 90%) bound to plasma proteins, mainly albumin. A greater fraction remains unbound in the neonate, in patients with hypoalbuminemia, and in uremic patients (*see* Appendix II). Fractional binding in tissues, including brain, is about the same as in plasma. Thus, the apparent volume of distribution of phenytoin is about 0.6 liter per kilogram but is about ten times larger when calculated on the basis of unbound drug. The concentration in the cerebrospinal fluid (CSF) is equal to the unbound fraction in plasma.

Less than 5% of phenytoin is excreted unchanged in the urine. The remainder is metabolized primarily in the hepatic endoplasmic reticulum. The major metabolite, the parahydroxyphenyl derivative, is inactive. It accounts for 60 to 70% of a single dose of the drug and a somewhat smaller fraction during chronic medication. It is excreted initially in the bile and subsequently in the urine, in large part as the glucuronide. Other apparently inactive metabolites include the dihydroxy catechol and its 3-methoxy derivative, and the dihydrodiol. At plasma concentrations below 10 μg/ml, elimination is exponential (first order); plasma half-life ranges between 6 and 24 hours. At higher concentrations, dose-dependent elimination is apparent; plasma half-life increases with concentration (dose), perhaps because the hydroxylation reaction approaches saturation or is inhibited by the metabolites. Values of 20 to 60 hours are often found at therapeutic concentrations. A genetically determined limitation in ability to metabolize phenytoin has been detected. The pharmacokinetic properties of phenytoin have been reviewed by Perucca and Richens (1985a) and by Jones and Wimbish (1985).

Toxicity. The toxic effects of phenytoin depend upon the route of administration, the duration of exposure, and the dosage. When it is administered intravenously at an excessive rate in the emergency treatment of cardiac arrhythmias or status epilepticus, the most notable toxic signs are cardiac arrhythmias, with or without hypotension, and/or CNS depression. Although cardiac toxicity occurs more frequently in older patients and in those with known cardiac disease, it can also develop in young, healthy patients (Earnest *et al.*, 1983). These complications can be minimized by slow administration of dilute solutions of the drug. Acute oral overdosage features primarily signs referable to the cerebellum and vestibular system; high doses can produce marked cerebellar atrophy (Masur *et al.*, 1989). Toxic effects associated with chronic medication are also primarily dose-related cerebellar-vestibular effects but include other CNS effects, behavioral changes, increased frequency of seizures, gastrointestinal symptoms, gingival hyperplasia, osteomalacia, and megaloblastic anemia. Hirsutism is an annoying untoward effect in young females. Usually, these phenomena can be made bearable by proper adjustment of dosage. Serious adverse effects, including those on the skin, bone marrow, and liver, are probably manifestations of drug allergy. Although rare, they necessitate withdrawal of the drug. Moderate elevation of the concentrations in plasma of enzymes that are used to assess hepatic function are sometimes observed; since these changes are transient and may result in part from induced synthesis of the enzymes, they do not necessitate withdrawal of the drug (Aiges *et al.*, 1980). The toxicity of phenytoin has been extensively reviewed in a Symposium (1982a).

Central and peripheral nervous system toxicity is the most consistent effect of phenytoin overdosage. Nystagmus, ataxia, diplopia, and vertigo and other cerebellar-vestibular effects are common. Blurred vision, mydriasis, ophthalmoplegia, and hyperactive tendon reflexes also occur. Behavioral effects include hyperactivity, silliness, confusion, dullness, drowsiness, and hallucinations. An increased frequency of seizures may occur in epileptic patients who have received excessive amounts of phenytoin, but the incidence may be lower than previously thought (Osorio *et al.*, 1989). Although phenytoin has been implicated in the irreversible cerebellar damage noted in some epileptic patients, similar findings were described before the introduction of this agent. This condition may thus be a consequence of repeated seizures (*see* Dam, in Symposium, 1982a). Electrophysiological evidence of peripheral neuropathy can occur in up to 30% of patients receiving phenytoin, but this phenomenon is rarely of clinical significance.

Gingival hyperplasia occurs in about 20% of all patients during chronic therapy and is probably the most common manifestation of phenytoin toxicity in children and young adolescents. It may be more frequent in those individuals who also develop coarsened facial features. The overgrowth of tissue appears to involve altered collagen metabolism (Hassell and Gilbert, 1983). Toothless portions of the gums are not affected. The condition does not necessarily require withdrawal of medication, and it can be minimized by good oral hygiene.

Gastrointestinal disturbances, including nausea, vomiting, epigastric pain, and anorexia, can be reduced by taking the drug with meals or in more frequent divided doses.

A variety of endocrine effects have been reported. Inhibition of release of antidiuretic hormone (ADH) has been observed in patients with inappropriate ADH secretion. Hyperglycemia and glycosuria appear to be due to inhibition of insulin secretion. Osteomalacia, with hypocalcemia and elevated alkaline phosphatase activity, has been attributed to both altered metabolism of vitamin D and inhibition of intestinal absorption of Ca^{2+}. Phenytoin also increases the metabolism of vitamin K and reduces the concentration of vitamin K–dependent proteins that are important for normal Ca^{2+} metabolism in bone (Keith *et al.*, 1983). This may explain why the osteomalacia is not always ameliorated by the administration of vitamin D.

Hypersensitivity reactions include morbilliform rash in 2 to 5% of patients and occasionally more serious skin reactions, including Stevens–Johnson syndrome. Systemic lupus erythematosus and potentially fatal hepatic necrosis have been reported rarely. Hematological reactions include neutropenia and leukopenia. A few instances of red-cell aplasia, agranulocytosis, and mild thrombocytopenia have also been reported. Aplastic anemia has been associated with hydantoins other than phenytoin (*see* Pisciotta, in Symposium, 1982a). Megaloblastic anemia has been attributed to altered folate absorption but probably also involves altered folate metabolism. It is rare and responds to administration of folic acid. Similar effects have been reported during medication with phenobarbital, primidone, and mephenytoin. Lymphadenopathy, resembling Hodgkin's disease and malignant lymphoma, is associated with reduced immunoglobulin A (IgA) production. Hypoprothrombinemia and hemorrhage have occurred in the newborn of mothers who received phenytoin during pregnancy; vitamin K is effective treatment or prophylaxis.

Preparations, Routes of Administration, and Dosages. *Phenytoin sodium* (*diphenylhydantoin sodium;* DILANTIN, DIPHENYLAN) is available as 30- and 100-mg capsules with both slow and rapid rates of dissolution for oral use, and as a solution (50 mg/ml) in a special solvent for parenteral use. Preparations of phenytoin include 50-mg tablets and oral suspensions. Various preparations of phenytoin differ significantly in both bioavailability and rate of absorption, and patients should thus be treated with the drug product of a single manufacturer.

Choice and adjustment of the dosage of phenytoin and interpretation of measured concentrations of the drug in plasma must be dominated by recognition of the dose-dependent kinetics of elimination of the drug. As dosage is increased, plasma half-life and the time required to attain the plateau state increase. *Plasma drug concentration increases disproportionately as dosage is increased.* The concentration of phenytoin can increase from subtherapeutic to toxic levels with small (*e.g.*, 50 mg per day) increments of dosage.

Initial daily dosage for adults is 3 to 5 mg/kg (300 mg daily). Dosage is subsequently adjusted, preferably with monitoring of plasma concentration, as needed for control of seizures or as limited by toxicity. Increments in dosage may be made at 1-week intervals at low dosage but at 2-week intervals when dosage exceeds 300 mg daily. Doses greater than 600 mg daily are rarely tolerated if taken regularly, although they may be necessary in occasional patients. Because of its relatively long half-life and slow absorption, a single daily dose is often satisfactory for adults, but gastric intolerance or the use of rapidly absorbed formulations often dictates divided dosage. Divided dosage is recommended for children (4 to 8 mg/kg per day). If a loading dose is deemed necessary, 600 to 1000 mg, in divided portions over 8 to 12 hours, will provide effective plasma concentrations within 24 hours in most patients.

Intravenous administration of phenytoin should not exceed 50 mg per minute for adults and should be followed by the injection of saline to reduce the local venous irritation that results from the alkalinity of solutions of the drug. A slower rate is preferred, especially in elderly patients, but a continuous infusion is usually not recommended. Intramuscular administration is not appropriate because of erratic absorption and tissue damage at the site of injection.

Plasma Drug Concentrations. A good correlation is usually observed between the total concentration of phenytoin in plasma and the clinical effect. Thus, control of seizures is generally obtained with concentrations above 10 μg/ml, while toxic effects such as nystagmus develop at concentrations around 20 μg/ml. Ataxia is apparent at 30 μg/ml and lethargy at about 40 μg/ml.

The degree of protein binding of phenytoin and, therefore, the concentration of free drug in plasma at any given total concentration may vary from patient to patient. Such factors can confuse interpretation of measured concentrations of the drug. Since both efficacy and toxicity are dependent on the concentration of unbound drug, some patients will achieve adequate control of seizures without evidence of toxicity only when the total concentration of phenytoin is above the usual therapeutic range. More commonly, patients will experience toxicity when the total concentration of phenytoin in plasma is within the accepted therapeutic range because binding to plasma proteins is reduced (*e.g.*, by uremia, hypoalbuminemia, or other drugs). In such cases the concentration of free phenytoin should be measured as the basis for adjustment of dosage.

Drug Interactions. Concurrent administration of chloramphenicol, dicumarol, disulfiram, isoniazid, cimetidine, or certain sulfonamides can increase the concentration of phenytoin in plasma by decreasing its rate of metabolism. Inhibition of inactivation of phenytoin should be suspected for other agents that are also hydroxylated by the microsomal enzyme system. Various agents, including sulfisoxazole, salicylates, and tolbutamide can compete for binding sites on plasma proteins. Since this can increase the metabolic clearance and lower the total concentration of phenytoin, there may be little effect on the concentration of free drug in plasma at steady state. By contrast, valproate and phenylbutazone reduce both the rate of metabolism of phenytoin and its binding to plasma proteins. Although this may have little effect on the total plasma concentration, the fraction of free drug may increase substantially (*see* Perucca and Richens, 1985b).

Carbamazepine, which may enhance the metabolism of phenytoin, causes a well-documented *decrease* in phenytoin concentration. Conversely, phenytoin reduces the concentration of carbamazepine. Phenytoin increases the rate of clearance of theophylline, and plasma concentrations of phenytoin are also reduced when the two drugs are given concurrently. The latter effect may be due to enhanced metabolism and/or decreased absorption of phenytoin.

Interaction between phenytoin and phenobarbital is variable. Phenobarbital may increase the biotransformation of phenytoin by induction of the hepatic microsomal enzyme system, but may also decrease its inactivation, apparently by competitive inhibition. In addition, phenobarbital may reduce the oral absorption of phenytoin. Conversely, the phenobarbital concentration is sometimes increased by phenytoin. Ethanol has similar opposing effects on the inactivation of phenytoin.

Phenytoin has been demonstrated to enhance the metabolism of corticosteroids and may decrease the effectiveness of oral contraceptives. The suggested mechanism for this effect is an induction of metabolizing enzymes, although phenytoin is only a weak inducer of the hepatic microsomal enzyme system in man.

Therapeutic Uses. *Epilepsy.* Phenytoin is one of the more widely used antiepileptic agents, and it is effective in most forms of epilepsy except absence seizures. The use of phenytoin and other agents in the therapy of epilepsies is discussed further at the end of this chapter.

Other Uses. Some cases of trigeminal and related neuralgias respond well to phenytoin, but carbamazepine is the preferred agent. The use of phenytoin in the treatment of cardiac arrhythmias is discussed in Chapter 35.

OTHER HYDANTOINS

Mephenytoin. *Mephenytoin* (MESANTOIN), 3-methyl-5,5-phenylethylhydantoin, is N-demethylated to 5,5-phenylethylhydantoin. During chronic administration of mephenytoin, this active metabolite constitutes most of the total hydantoins in plasma and probably accounts, at least in part, for the therapeutic benefit and toxicity of chronic medication with mephenytoin (*see* Jones and Wimbish, 1985).

Pharmacological Effects and Metabolism. Mephenytoin is active in most anticonvulsant tests in animals. Unlike phenytoin, it antagonizes the effects of pentylenetetrazol, elevates seizure threshold, and is a sedative. Also unlike phenytoin, mephenytoin is rapidly absorbed after oral administration. Both mephenytoin and its N-demethylated metabolite are converted to inactive hydroxylated products in a stereospecific fashion by hepatic microsomal enzymes. As a result of the hydroxylation, conjugation, and excretion of the S-enantiomer, the active R-enantiomer—5,5-phenylethylhydantoin—accumulates in plasma. It is possible that the serious toxicity associated with mephenytoin results from the formation of arene oxide intermediates during the hydroxylation reaction.

Therapeutic Uses and Toxicity. Mephenytoin was introduced in 1945 for the treatment of epilepsy. Its antiepileptic spectrum is similar to that of phenytoin, and it may exacerbate absence seizures. The half-life of the active metabolite is about 95 hours in patients previously exposed to various other anticonvulsants. Although mephenytoin causes less ataxia, gingival hyperplasia, gastric distress, and hirsutism than does phenytoin and less sedation than does phenobarbital, serious toxicity is common. These adverse effects include morbilliform rash (in 10% of patients), fever, lymphadenopathy, aplastic anemia, leukopenia, pancytopenia, agranulocytosis, hepatotoxicity, periarteritis nodosa, and lupus erythematosus. Consequently, mephenytoin is generally used only in patients who fail to respond to or do not tolerate safer agents.

Preparations and Dosages. Typical daily dosage is 200 to 600 mg in adults and 100 to 400 mg in children. The drug is available in 100-mg tablets.

Ethotoin. *Ethotoin* (PEGANONE) is 3-ethyl-5-phenylhydantoin. Introduced in 1957, it appeared to be of some value in the treatment of complex partial as well as generalized tonic-clonic seizures and to be relatively free of the typical adverse effects of phenytoin (*see* Kupferberg, in Symposium, 1982a). However, because of its low efficacy, it is used only occasionally, mostly as an adjunct to other agents, in the therapy of generalized tonic-clonic seizures. The usual daily dose for adults is 2 to 3 g. Ethotoin is available in 250- and 500-mg tablets.

Skin rash, gastrointestinal distress, and drowsiness are the common adverse effects of ethotoin. Lymphadenopathy has also been reported. Metabolites, produced by the hepatic microsomal enzymes, include the N-dealkyl and parahydroxyphenyl derivatives and 5-hydroxy-5-phenylhydantoin (*see* Jones and Wimbish, 1985). The half-life in plasma is about 5 hours and does not appear to change with increasing dosage.

ANTICONVULSANT BARBITURATES

The pharmacology of the barbiturates as a class is considered in Chapter 17; discussion in this chapter is limited to the two barbiturates used for therapy of the epilepsies. Although still marketed, a third barbiturate (metharbital) has virtually disappeared from the therapeutic scene.

PHENOBARBITAL

Phenobarbital was the first effective organic antiepileptic agent (Hauptmann, 1912). It has relatively low toxicity, is inexpensive, and is still one of the more effective and widely used drugs for this purpose.

Structure–Activity Relationship. The structural formula of phenobarbital (5-phenyl-5-ethylbarbituric acid) is shown in Table 17–4 (page 358). The structure–activity relationship of the barbiturates has been studied extensively and summarized by Vida and Gerry (in Symposium, 1977). Maximal anticonvulsant activity is obtained when one substituent at position 5 is a phenyl group. The 5,5-diphenyl derivative has less anticonvulsant potency than phenobarbital but is virtually devoid of hypnotic activity. By contrast, 5,5-dibenzyl barbituric acid causes convulsions.

Anticonvulsant Properties. Most barbiturates have anticonvulsant properties. However, the capacity of some of these agents, such as phenobarbital, to exert maximal anticonvulsant action at doses below those required for hypnosis determines their clinical utility as antiepileptics. Phenobarbital is active in most anticonvulsant tests in animals but is relatively nonselective. It limits the spread of seizure activity and also elevates seizure threshold.

The ability of some barbiturates to be selective anticonvulsants suggests that different mechanisms of action are involved in the anticonvulsant and hypnotic effects. Based on the electrophysiological effects of various barbiturates in dissociated cell cultures of mammalian spinal cord neurons, Macdonald and McLean (Symposium, 1986a) have proposed that the low potency of phenobarbital (relative to that of pentobarbital) both in producing GABA-like increases in the conductance of chloride and in reducing Ca^{2+}-dependent release of neurotransmitters may account for the relatively selective effects of anticonvulsant barbiturates. Further, the ability of phenobarbital at therapeutic concentrations to reduce the excitatory effects of glutamate and to augment the inhibitory effects of GABA may be important to its anticonvulsant activity. Other distinctions between hypnotic and anticonvulsant barbiturates have been noted with respect to effects on the ability of brain membranes to bind certain drugs. Phenobarbital is much less potent than pentobarbital in displacing dihydropicrotoxinin and in enhancing the binding of GABA and various benzodiazepines (*see* Olsen, 1987). The relationship of these observations to the electrophysiological effects of barbiturates is not clearly understood.

Pharmacokinetic Properties. Oral absorption of phenobarbital is complete but somewhat slow; peak concentrations in plasma occur several hours after a single dose. It is 40 to 60% bound to plasma proteins and bound to a similar extent in tissues, including brain. The volume of distribution is approximately 0.5 liter per kilogram. The pK_a of phenobarbital is 7.3, and up to 25% of a dose is eliminated by pH-dependent renal excretion of the unchanged drug; the remainder is inactivated by hepatic microsomal enzymes. One major metabolite, the parahydroxyphenyl derivative, is inactive and is excreted in the urine partly as the glucuronide conjugate. Another major metabolite is the N-glucoside derivative. The plasma half-life of phenobarbital is about 100 hours in adults; it is somewhat longer in neonates, while it is shorter and more variable in children.

Toxicity. The adverse effects of phenobarbital have been reviewed by Mattson and Cramer (Symposium, 1982a). Sedation, the most frequent undesired effect of phenobarbital, is apparent to some extent in all patients upon initiation of therapy, but tolerance develops during chronic medication. Nystagmus and ataxia occur at excessive dosage. Phenobarbital sometimes produces irritability and hyperactivity in children, and agitation and confusion in the elderly.

Scarlatiniform or morbilliform rash, possibly with other manifestations of drug allergy, occurs in 1 to 2% of patients. Exfoliative dermatitis is rare. Hypoprothrombinemia with hemorrhage has been observed in the newborn of mothers who have received phenobarbital during pregnancy; vitamin K is effective for treatment or prophylaxis. Megaloblastic anemia that responds to folate and osteomalacia that responds to high doses of vitamin D occur during chronic phenobarbital therapy of epilepsy, as they do during phenytoin medication. Other adverse effects of phenobarbital are discussed in Chapter 17.

Preparations, Routes of Administration, and Dosages. *Phenobarbital* and *phenobarbital sodium* (LUMINAL SODIUM, others) are available in a variety of dosage forms for oral and parenteral use. The usual oral daily dose for adults is 1 to 5 mg/kg (60 to 250 mg). Since plasma half-life averages 100 hours, weeks are required to attain the plateau state. Double dosage for the initial 4 days provides an effective plasma drug concentration more promptly, but sedation will be prominent. The usual initial daily dose for children is 3 to 6 mg/kg, in two divided portions. Dosage is subsequently increased or adjusted, as required for control of seizures or as limited by toxicity.

Plasma Drug Concentrations. During long-term therapy in adults, the plasma concentration of phenobarbital averages 10 μg/ml per daily dose of 1 mg/kg; in children, the value is 5 to 7 μg/ml per 1 mg/kg. Although a precise relationship between therapeutic results and concentration of drug in plasma does not exist, plasma concentrations of 10 to 35 μg/ml are usually recommended for control of epilepsy; 15 μg/ml is the minimum for prophylaxis against febrile convulsions.

The relationship between plasma concentration of phenobarbital and adverse effects varies with the development of tolerance. Sedation, nystagmus, and ataxia are usually absent at concentrations below 30 μg/ml during long-term therapy, but adverse effects may be apparent for several days at lower concentrations when therapy is initiated or whenever the dosage is increased. Concentrations greater than 60 μg/ml may be associated with marked intoxication in the nontolerant individual.

Since significant behavioral toxicity may be present despite the absence of overt signs of toxicity, the tendency to maintain patients, particularly children, on excessively high doses of phenobarbital should be resisted. Plasma phenobarbital concentration should be increased above 30 to 40 μg/ml only if the increment is adequately tolerated and only if it contributes significantly to control of seizures. (*See* Booker, in Symposium, 1982a.)

Drug Interactions. Interactions between phenobarbital and other drugs usually involve induction of the hepatic microsomal enzyme system by phenobarbital (*see* Chapters 1 and 17). The variable interaction with phenytoin has been discussed above. Concentrations of phenobarbital in plasma may be elevated by as much as 40% during concurrent administration of valproic acid (*see* below).

Therapeutic Uses. Phenobarbital is an effective agent for generalized tonic-clonic and partial seizures. Its efficacy, low toxicity, and low cost make it an important agent for these types of epilepsy. However, its sedative effects and its tendency to disturb behavior in children have reduced its use as a primary agent. The use of phenobarbital in the therapy of the epilepsies is discussed further at the end of this chapter.

OTHER BARBITURATES

Mephobarbital. *Mephobarbital* (MEBARAL) is N-methylphenobarbital. It is N-demethylated in the hepatic endoplasmic reticulum, and most of its activity during long-term therapy can be attributed to the accumulation of phenobarbital. Consequently, the pharmacological properties, toxicity, and clinical uses of mephobarbital are the same as those for phenobarbital. However, oral absorption of mephobarbital is usually incomplete, and its dose is approximately twice that of phenobarbital. The plasma concentration of phenobarbital provides a guide to adjustment of mephobarbital dosage. (*See* Eadie, in Symposium, 1982a.)

DEOXYBARBITURATES

PRIMIDONE

Primidone is an effective agent for treatment of all types of epilepsy except absence seizures.

Chemistry. Primidone may be viewed as a congener of phenobarbital in which the carbonyl oxygen of the urea moiety is replaced by two hydrogen atoms:

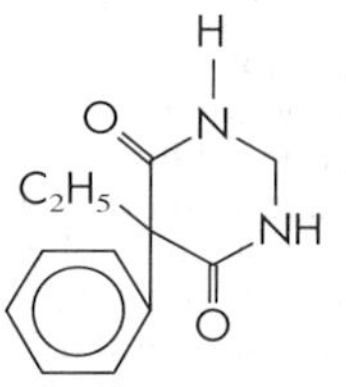

Primidone

Anticonvulsant Properties. Primidone resembles phenobarbital in many laboratory anticonvulsant effects, but it is much less potent than phenobarbital in antagonizing seizures induced by pentylenetetrazol (*see* Woodbury and Pippenger, in Symposium, 1982a). The anticonvulsant effects of primidone are attributed to both the drug and its active metabolites, principally phenobarbital (*see* Frey, 1985).

Pharmacokinetic Properties. Primidone is rapidly and almost completely absorbed after oral administration, although individual variability can be great. Peak concentrations in plasma are usually observed approximately 3 hours after ingestion. The plasma half-life of primidone is variable; mean values ranging from 5 to 15 hours have been reported (*see* Schottelius, in Symposium, 1982a; Frey, 1985).

Primidone is converted to two active metabolites, phenobarbital and phenylethylmalonamide (PEMA). Primidone and PEMA are bound to plasma proteins to only a small extent, whereas about half of phenobarbital is so bound. The half-life of PEMA in plasma is 16 hours; both it and phenobarbital accumulate during long-term therapy. The appearance of phenobarbital in plasma may be delayed several days upon initiation of therapy with primidone. Approximately 40% of the drug is excreted unchanged in the urine; unconjugated PEMA and, to a lesser extent, phenobarbital and its metabolites constitute the remainder.

Toxicity. The toxicity of primidone has been reviewed by Leppik and Cloyd (Symposium, 1982a). The more common complaints are sedation, vertigo, dizziness, nausea, vomiting, ataxia, diplopia, and nystagmus. Patients may also experience an acute feeling of intoxication immediately following administration of primidone. This occurs before there is any significant metabolism of the drug. The relationship of adverse effects to dosage is complex, since they result from both the parent drug and its two active metabolites and since tolerance develops during long-term therapy. Side effects are occasionally quite severe when therapy is initiated.

Serious adverse effects are relatively uncommon, but maculopapular and morbilliform rash, leukopenia, thrombocytopenia, systemic lupus erythematosus, and lymphadenopathy have been reported. Acute psychotic reactions, usually in patients with complex partial seizures, have also occurred. Hemorrhagic disease in the neonate, megaloblastic anemia, and osteomalacia similar to those discussed previously in connection with phenytoin and phenobarbital have also been described.

Preparations and Dosages. *Primidone* (MYSOLINE) is available as 50- and 250-mg tablets and as an oral suspension (250 mg/5 ml). The usual daily dose for adults is 750 to 1500 mg, given in divided doses; for children under age 8, 10 to 25 mg/kg. Therapy should be initiated at a lower dosage (*e.g.*, 100 to 125 mg per day for adults) and increased gradually. Lower dosages may be possible or necessary when the drug is used concurrently with phenytoin.

Plasma Drug Concentrations. The relationship between the dose of primidone and the concentration of the drug and its active metabolites in plasma shows marked individual variability. During long-term therapy, the plasma concentrations of primidone and phenobarbital average 1 μg/ml and 2 μg/ml, respectively, per daily dose of 1 mg/kg of primidone. The plasma concentration of PEMA is usually intermediate between those of primidone and phenobarbital. There is no clear relationship between the concentrations of primidone or its metabolites in plasma and therapeutic effect. As an initial guide, the dosage of primidone may be adjusted primarily with reference to the concentration of phenobarbital, as outlined previously for administered phenobarbital, and secondarily with reference to the concentration of the parent drug. Concentrations of primidone greater than 10 μg/ml are usually associated with significant toxic side effects. A disproportionately high primidone:phenobarbital concentration ratio during long-term therapy usually implies that medication has not been taken sufficiently regularly for phenobarbital to accumulate. (*See* Fincham and Schottelius, in Symposium, 1982a.)

Drug Interactions. Phenytoin has been reported to increase the conversion of primidone to phenobarbital. Other drug interactions to be anticipated are those for phenobarbital.

Therapeutic Uses. Primidone is useful against generalized tonic-clonic and both simple and complex partial seizures. While it may be effective alone in patients who are refractory to other medications, primidone is generally used concurrently with phenytoin or carbamazepine. Its use in combination with phenobarbital is illogical. Primidone is ineffective against absence seizures but is sometimes useful against myoclonic seizures in young children. The therapeutic use of primidone and other antiepileptic agents is discussed further at the end of this chapter.

IMINOSTILBENES

CARBAMAZEPINE

Carbamazepine was approved in the United States for use as an antiepileptic agent in 1974. It has been employed since the 1960s for the treatment of trigeminal neuralgia. It is now considered to be a primary drug for the treatment of all types of epilepsy except absence seizures.

Chemistry. Carbamazepine is related chemically to the tricyclic antidepressants. It is a derivative of iminostilbene with a carbamyl group at the 5 position; this moiety is essential for potent antiepileptic activity. The structural formula of carbamazepine is as follows:

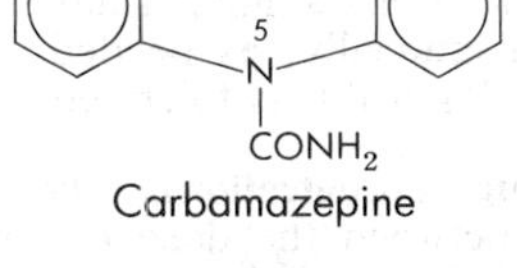

Carbamazepine

Pharmacological Effects. Although the effects of carbamazepine in animals and man resemble those of phenytoin in many ways, the two drugs differ in a number of potentially important ways (*see* Julien, in Symposium, 1982a). For example, carbamazepine is more effective than phenytoin in reducing stimulus-induced discharges in the amygdala of kindled rats (Albright, 1983) and in blocking pentylenetetrazol-induced seizures (*see* Schmutz, 1985). Further, it can produce therapeutic responses in manic-depressive patients, including some in whom lithium carbonate is not effective (*see* Symposium, 1988a). Finally, carbamazepine has antidiuretic effects that are sometimes associated with reduced concentrations of ADH in plasma (*see* Masland, in Symposium, 1982a). The mechanisms responsible for these effects of carbamazepine are not clearly understood.

Carbamazepine and phenytoin have virtually identical actions on Na^+ channels (Willow and Catterall, 1982; Willow *et al.*, 1985); both are thought to produce differential inhibition of high-frequency discharges in and around epileptic foci with minimal disruption of normal neuronal traffic (*see* Macdonald and McLean, in Symposium, 1986a; Macdonald, 1988).

Therapeutic doses of carbamazepine increase the rate of firing of noradrenergic neurons in the locus ceruleus of the rat (Olpe and Jones, 1983). Since phenytoin does not have similar effects, the relationship of this observation to the therapeutic effects of carbamazepine is not clear. However, both clonidine (which inhibits discharge of noradrenergic neurons) and selective depletion of norepinephrine in the brain antagonize the anticonvulsant effects of carbamazepine. Thus, the capacity to increase discharge of noradrenergic neurons may contribute to the antiepileptic actions of the drug.

Carbamazepine competes with specific ligands for several binding sites of neurochemical interest (*see* Post, in Symposium, 1988a). The drug acts as an antagonist at adenosine receptors, an effect that may be more relevant to antidepressant rather than to anticonvulsant actions. Carbamazepine also appears to interact with the so-called "peripheral type" of binding site for benzodiazepines that is thought to be involved in the regulation of Ca^{2+} channels. Although one specific ligand for this site (Ro 5–4864) can reverse the anticonvulsant effects of carbamazepine, the importance of this interaction in therapeutic situations is not yet established.

Pharmacokinetic Properties. The pharmacokinetic characteristics of carbamazepine are complex. They are influenced by its limited aqueous solubility and by the ability of many antiepileptic drugs, including carbamazepine itself, to increase its conversion to an active metabolite by hepatic oxidative enzymes.

Carbamazepine is absorbed slowly and erratically after oral administration. Peak concentrations in plasma are usually observed 4 to 8 hours after oral ingestion but may be delayed by as much as 24 hours, especially following the administration of a large dose (*see* Morselli and Bossi, in Symposium, 1982a). The drug distributes rapidly into all tissues. Binding to plasma proteins occurs to the extent of about 75%, and concentrations in the CSF appear to correspond to the concentration of free drug in plasma.

The predominant pathway of metabolism in man involves conversion to the 10,11-epoxide (*see* Faigle and Feldman, in Symposium, 1982a). This metabolite is as active as the parent compound in various animals, and its concentrations in plasma and brain may reach 50% of those of carbamazepine, especially during the concurrent administration of phenytoin or phenobarbital. The 10,11-epoxide is metabolized further to inactive compounds, which are excreted in the urine principally as glucuronides. Carbamazepine is also inactivated by conjugation and hydroxylation. Less than 3% of the drug is recovered in the urine as the parent compound or the epoxide. During long-term therapy, the half-life of carbamazepine in plasma averages between 10 and 20 hours. Because of induction of drug-metabolizing enzymes, the half-life is much longer in individuals who have received only a single dose. In patients who are receiving phenobarbital or phenytoin, the average half-life is reduced to 9 to 10 hours. The half-life of the 10,11-epoxide is somewhat shorter than that of the parent compound.

Toxicity. Acute intoxication with carbamazepine can result in stupor or coma, hyperirritability, convulsions, and respiratory depression (*see* Masland, in Symposium, 1982a). During long-term therapy, the more frequent untoward effects of the drug include drowsiness, vertigo, ataxia, diplopia, and blurred vision. The frequency of seizures may increase, especially with overdosage. Other adverse effects include nausea, vomiting, serious hematological toxicity (aplastic anemia, agranulocytosis), and hypersensitivity reactions (dermatitis, eosinophilia, lymphadenopathy, splenomegaly). A late complication of therapy with carbamazepine is retention of water, with decreased osmolality and concentration of Na^+ in plasma, especially in elderly patients with cardiac disease.

Some tolerance develops to the neurotoxic effects of carbamazepine, and they can be minimized by gradual increase in dosage or adjustment of maintenance dosage. Various hepatic or pancreatic abnormalities have been reported during therapy with carbamazepine, most commonly a transient elevation of hepatic enzymes in plasma in 5 to 10% of patients. A transient mild leukopenia occurs in about 10% of patients during initiation of therapy and usually resolves within the first 4 months of continued treatment; transient thrombocytopenia has also been noted. In about 2% of patients, a persistent leukopenia may develop that requires withdrawal of the drug. The initial concern that aplastic anemia might be a frequent complication of long-term therapy with carbamazepine has not materialized. The total number of cases reported through 1986 is 25, with 9 fatalities (*see* Pellock, in Symposium, 1987b). In the majority of cases, the administration of multiple drugs or the presence of another underlying disease has made it difficult to establish a causal relationship. In any event, the prevalence of aplastic anemia appears to be about 1 in 200,000 patients who are treated with the drug. It is not clear whether monitoring of hematological function can avert the development of irreversible aplastic anemia (*see* Hart and Easton, 1982; Pisciotta, in Symposium, 1982a). Although carbamazepine is carcinogenic in rats, it remains to be determined whether it is carcinogenic in man. The induction of fetal malformations during the treatment of pregnant women is discussed below.

Preparations and Dosages. *Carbamazepine* (TEGRETOL) is available in 100- and 200-mg tablets and as a suspension (20 mg/ml) for oral administration. Therapy for epilepsy is usually started at a dosage of 200 mg, taken twice daily to minimize side effects. Dosage is then increased gradually to 600 to 1200 mg per day for adults and 20 to 30 mg/kg for children. Division of the daily intake into three or four doses is usually recommended to minimize fluctuations in plasma concentrations.

Therapy for trigeminal neuralgia is generally started at a dose of 200 mg per day; the dose may be increased gradually, as needed, to a level of 1200 mg per day if this is tolerated.

Plasma Drug Concentrations. There is no simple relationship between the dose of carbamazepine and concentrations of the drug in plasma (*see* Cereghino, in Symposium, 1982a). Therapeutic concentrations are reported to be 6 to 12 μg/ml, although considerable variation occurs. Side effects referable to the CNS are frequent at concentrations above 9 μg/ml.

Drug Interactions. Phenobarbital, phenytoin, and valproate may increase the metabolism of carbamazepine (Theodore *et al.*, 1989); carbamazepine may enhance the biotransformation of phenytoin as well as the conversion of primidone to phenobarbital. Administration of carbamazepine may lower concentrations of valproate given concurrently. Carbamazepine reduces both the plasma concentration and therapeutic effect of haloperidol (*see* Levy and Kerr, in Symposium, 1988a). The metabolism of carbamazepine may be inhibited by propoxyphene and erythromycin (*see* Levy and Patlick, in Symposium, 1982a).

Therapeutic Uses. Carbamazepine is useful in patients with generalized tonic-clonic and both simple and complex partial seizures. When it is used, renal and hepatic function and hematological parameters should be monitored. The therapeutic use of carbamazepine is discussed further at the end of this chapter.

Carbamazepine was introduced by Blom in the early 1960s and is now the primary agent for treatment of trigeminal and glossopharyngeal neuralgias. It is also effective for lightning tabetic pain. Most patients with neuralgia are benefited initially, but only 70% obtain continuing relief. Adverse effects have required discontinuation of medication in 5 to 20% of patients. The therapeutic range of plasma concentrations for antiepileptic therapy serves as a guideline for its use in neuralgia. Concurrent medication with phenytoin may be useful when carbamazepine alone is not satisfactory. Carbamazepine has also found use in the treatment of bipolar affective disorders (*see* Symposium, 1988a), a use that is discussed further in Chapter 18.

SUCCINIMIDES

ETHOSUXIMIDE

The succinimides evolved from a systematic search for effective agents less toxic than the oxazolidinediones for the treatment of absence seizures. Ethosuximide is a primary agent for this type of epilepsy.

Structure–Activity Relationship. Ethosuximide has the following structural formula:

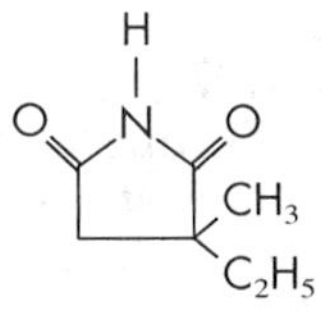

Ethosuximide

The structure–activity relationship of the succinimides is in accord with that for other anticonvulsant classes. Methsuximide and phensuximide have phenyl substituents and are more active against maximal electroshock seizures. Ethosuximide, with alkyl substituents, is the most active of the succinimides against seizures induced by pentylenetetrazol and is the most selective for clinical absence seizures.

Pharmacological Effects. The anticonvulsant spectrum of ethosuximide in animals resembles that of trimethadione. The most prominent characteristic of both drugs is protection against the convulsant action of pentylenetetrazol. Ethosuximide also elevates threshold for electroshock seizures, but it abolishes the tonic extensor component of maximal electroshock seizures only in anesthetic doses (*see* Ferrendelli and Klunk, in Symposium, 1982a; Teschendorf and Kretzschmar, 1985). There is little information about the mechanism of action of ethosuximide. Unlike phenytoin and carbamazepine, it does not inhibit voltage-gated Na^+ channels; unlike phenobarbital and clonazepam, it does not enhance the postsynaptic actions of GABA (*see* De Deyn and Macdonald, 1989).

Pharmacokinetic Properties. Absorption of ethosuximide appears to be complete, and peak concentrations occur in plasma within about 3 hours after a single oral dose. Ethosuximide is not significantly bound to plasma proteins; during long-term therapy, the concentration in the CSF is similar to that in plasma. The apparent volume of distribution averages 0.7 liter per kilogram (*see* Glazko and Chang, in Symposium, 1982a).

In man, 25% of the drug is excreted unchanged in the urine. The remainder is metabolized by hepatic microsomal enzymes. The major metabolite, the hydroxyethyl derivative, accounts for about 40% of administered drug, is inactive, and is excreted as such and as the glucuronide in the urine. Other metabolites include other hydroxylated products. The plasma half-life of ethosuximide averages between 40 and 50 hours in adults and approximately 30 hours in children.

Toxicity. The toxicity of ethosuximide has been reviewed by Dreifuss (Symposium, 1982a). The most common dose-related side effects are gastrointestinal complaints (nausea, vomiting, and anorexia) and CNS effects (drowsiness, lethargy, euphoria, dizziness, headache, and hiccough). Some tolerance to these effects develops. Parkinson-like symptoms and photophobia have also been reported. Restlessness, agitation, anxiety, aggressiveness, inability to concentrate, and other behavioral effects have occurred primarily in patients with a prior history of psychiatric disturbance.

Urticaria and other skin reactions, including Stevens–Johnson syndrome, as well as systemic lupus erythematosus, eosinophilia, leukopenia, thrombocytopenia, pancytopenia, and aplastic anemia have also been attributed to the drug. The leukopenia may be transient, despite continuation of the drug, but several deaths have resulted from bone-marrow depression. Renal or hepatic toxicity has not been reported.

Preparations and Dosages. *Ethosuximide* (ZARONTIN) is available for oral administration as 250-mg capsules and as a syrup (250 mg/5 ml). An initial daily dose of 250 mg in children (3 to 6 years old) and 500 mg in older children and adults is increased by 250-mg increments at weekly intervals until seizures are adequately controlled or toxicity intervenes. Divided dosage is occasionally required to prevent nausea or drowsiness associated with single daily dosage. The usual maintenance dose is 20 mg/kg. Increased caution is required if the daily dose exceeds 1500 mg in adults or 750 to 1000 mg in children.

Plasma Drug Concentrations. During long-term therapy, the plasma concentration of ethosuximide averages about 2 μg/ml per daily dose of 1 mg/kg. However, because of variation, concentrations in plasma cannot be predicted accurately. The plateau state is attained in 4 to 6 days in children; longer times are required in adults. A plasma concentration of 40 to 100 μg/ml is required for satisfactory control of absence seizures in most patients (*see* Sherwin, in Symposium, 1982a). A relationship between plasma concentration and adverse effects has not been established. Concentrations as high as 160 μg/ml have been tolerated without excessive toxicity.

Therapeutic Uses. Ethosuximide is more effective than trimethadione against absence seizures and has a lower risk of serious adverse effects; it is an important therapeutic agent for this type of epilepsy. The use of ethosuximide and the other antiepileptic agents is discussed further at the end of the chapter.

OTHER SUCCINIMIDES

Methsuximide. Methsuximide, N,2-dimethyl-2-phenylsuccinimide, was introduced in 1956 for the therapy of absence seizures (*see* Porter and Kupferberg, in Symposium, 1982a). Ethosuximide subsequently proved more effective. Methsuximide, particularly when given concurrently with other drugs, may also be useful in the treatment of complex partial seizures. Adverse gastrointestinal and central effects are similar in pattern to those of ethosuximide. Severe depression, skin rash, fever, periorbital edema, leukopenia, aplastic anemia, nephropathy, and hepatotoxicity have also been reported.

Methsuximide (CELONTIN) is available as 150- and 300-mg capsules. Medication is initiated with 300 mg daily. The usual daily dose for adults is 600 to 1200 mg. Patients receiving higher doses, especially in multiple-drug therapy, should be carefully monitored.

Methsuximide is rapidly absorbed and metabolized by hepatic microsomal enzymes to the N-demethyl and various parahydroxyphenyl derivatives. The half-life of methsuximide in plasma is less than 2 hours, while that of the active N-demethyl metabolite is about 40 hours. During long-term administration of methsuximide, therapeutic responses are associated with plasma concentrations of 20 to 40 μg/ml of the metabolite or 0.04 to 0.08 μg/ml of the parent drug.

Phensuximide. The first succinimide introduced for the therapy of absence seizures was phensuximide (N-methyl-2-phenylsuccinimide). Low efficacy has relegated it to secondary status. Adverse gastrointestinal and central effects are similar to those for ethosuximide. A dreamlike state, skin rash, fever, granulocytopenia, leukopenia, and reversible nephropathy have also been reported.

Phensuximide (MILONTIN) is available as 500-mg capsules. The usual daily dose is 1 to 3 g, regardless of age. Phensuximide is rapidly absorbed and converted to the N-demethyl and various hydroxylated metabolites. The N-demethyl derivative, which is suspected of being an active species, has a half-life in plasma similar to that of the parent drug (about 8 hours) and is metabolized to 2-phenylsuccinamic acid. At steady state, the plasma concentration of the N-demethyl derivative is about 30% that of phensuximide (*see* Porter and Kupferberg, in Symposium, 1982a).

VALPROIC ACID

Valproic acid was approved for use in the United States in 1978 after more than a decade of use in Europe. The antiepileptic properties of valproate were discovered serendipitously when it was employed as a vehicle for other compounds that were being screened for antiepileptic activity (*see* Symposium, 1982a).

Chemistry. Valproic acid (*n*-dipropylacetic acid) is a simple branched-chain carboxylic acid; its structural formula is as follows:

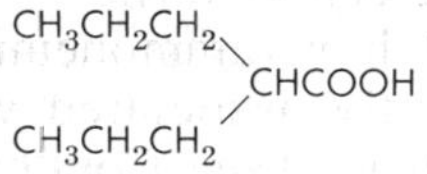

Valproic Acid

Certain other branched-chain carboxylic acids have potencies similar to that of valproic acid in antagonizing pentylenetetrazol-induced convulsions. However, increasing the number of carbon atoms to nine introduces marked sedative properties. Straight-chain acids have little or no activity. The primary amide of valproic acid is about twice as potent as the parent compound (*see* Murray and Kier, in Symposium, 1977; Keane *et al.*, 1983).

Pharmacological Effects. Valproic acid has antiepileptic activity against a variety of types of seizures while causing only minimal sedation and other CNS side effects. Valproate prevents pentylenetetrazol-induced seizures in mice with a potency somewhat greater than that of ethosuximide, but it also eliminates hindlimb extension in mice subjected to maximal electroshock at only slightly higher doses (*see* Löscher, 1985). Since its potency in the latter test is considerably less than that of phenytoin, valproate was initially used in the treatment of absence seizures. However, the use of valproate is currently being expanded to include the treatment of generalized tonic-clonic seizures (*see* Symposium, 1987c, 1988b).

Valproate is effective in a wide variety of model systems (*see* Löscher, 1985). For example, it can prevent seizures induced by the administration of GABA antagonists (*e.g.*, picrotoxin) or of inhibitors of GABA synthesis (*e.g.*, isoniazid), as well as those induced by sensory stimuli in seizure-prone strains of animals or by electrical stimuli in kindled animals. In cats, valproate inhibits the spread of seizure discharges from cortical lesions produced by implantation of alumina cream or cobalt, and can prevent establishment of the kindling phenomenon at relatively low doses. Although many of these results are predictive of utility in the treatment of absence seizures, no other antiepileptic agent displays such a broad pattern of activity.

Current hypotheses on the mechanism of action of valproate have centered on potential interactions with voltage-sensitive Na^+ channels (*see* Macdonald, 1988) and on the possible enhancement of GABA accumulation (*see* Löscher, 1985). Valproate markedly inhibits repetitive firing of cultured neurons at therapeutically relevant concentrations (2 to 10 μg/ml). These effects resemble those produced by phenytoin and carbamazepine, including their dependency on frequency and voltage. Although valproate has no effect on responses to GABA, it does increase the amount of GABA that can be recovered from brain after the drug is administered to animals.

In vitro, valproate can stimulate the activity of glutamic acid decarboxylase and inhibit GABA transaminase, but the concentrations required are greater than those that occur during therapy. However, the metabolism of valproate (*see* below) generates several active compounds, one of which (2-propyl-2-pentenoic acid, or 2-en-valproic acid) accumulates in brain during long-term administration of the drug. Moreover, an anticonvulsant effect outlasts the sojourn of valproate in plasma and brain following its chronic administration and withdrawal. Although 2-en-valproic acid has no effect on repetitive firing, it can cause accumulation of GABA *in vivo* at anticonvulsant doses. Hence, it is possible that this or another metabolite plays a role in the actions of valproate.

Pharmacokinetic Properties. Valproic acid is rapidly and completely absorbed after oral administration. Peak concentration in plasma is observed in 1 to 4 hours, although it can be delayed for several hours if the drug is administered in enteric-coated tablets or is ingested with meals. The apparent volume of distribution for valproate is about 0.2 liter per kilogram. Its extent of binding to plasma proteins is usually about 90%, but the fraction bound is reduced as the total concentration of valproate is increased through the therapeutic range. Although concentrations of valproate in CSF suggest equilibration with free drug in the blood, there is evidence for carrier-mediated transport of valproate both into and out of the CSF (*see* Löscher, 1985).

Almost no valproate is excreted unchanged in the urine or feces. When given in therapeutic doses, the majority of the drug is converted to the conjugate ester of glucuronic acid, while mitochondrial metabolism (both β-oxidation and ω-oxidation) accounts for the remainder. Some of these metabolites, notably 2-propyl-2-pentenoic acid and 2-propyl-4-pentenoic acid, are nearly as potent anticonvulsant agents as the parent compound; however, only the former (2-en-valproic acid) accumulates in plasma and brain to a potentially significant extent (*see* above). The half-life of valproate is approximately 15 hours but is reduced in patients taking other antiepileptic drugs (*see* Chapman *et al.*, 1982; *see also* Appendix II).

Toxicity. The toxicity of valproic acid has been reviewed by Dreifuss (Symposium, 1983c) and by Löscher (1985). The most common side effects are transient gastrointestinal symptoms, including anorexia, nausea, and vomiting in about 16% of patients. Effects on the CNS include sedation, ataxia, and tremor; these symptoms occur infrequently and usually respond to a decrease in dosage. Rash, alopecia, and stimulation of appetite have been observed occasionally. Valproic acid has several effects on hepatic function. Elevation of hepatic enzymes in plasma is observed in up to 40% of patients and often occurs asymptomatically during the first several months of therapy. A rare complication is a fulminant hepatitis that is frequently fatal (*see* Dreifuss and Langer, in Symposium, 1987c). Pathological examination reveals a microvesicular steatosis without evidence of inflammation or hypersensitivity reaction. Through 1984, the overall incidence of hepatic failure was about 1 in 10,000 patients using the drug. However, the cases were very unevenly distributed among the patient population. Children below 2 years of age with other medical conditions who were given multiple antiepileptic agents were especially likely to suffer fatal hepatic injury. At the other extreme, there were no deaths reported for patients over the age of 10 years who received only valproate. More recent data have confirmed this pattern (Dreifuss *et al.*, 1989). Despite increased usage, the overall incidence of hepatic fatalities has declined to about 1 in 50,000 patients, apparently due in part to the increased use of valproate as the sole antiepileptic agent. Other antiepileptic drugs, administered concurrently, may enhance the formation of toxic intermediates of valproate metabolism and/or exert independent hepatotoxic effects. This type of interaction may also occur with other potentially hepatotoxic agents, such as the salicylates. The occurrence of fulminant hepatitis is not consistently preceded by abnormal tests of hepatic function, making advanced detection difficult. Acute pancreatitis and hyperammonemia have also been frequently associated with the use of valproic acid. (*See* Coulter and Allen, 1981; Mattson and Cramer, in Symposium, 1983a.)

Preparations and Dosages. *Valproic acid* (DEPAKENE, others) is available in 250-mg capsules and in a syrup containing the sodium salt (equivalent to 250 mg of valproic acid per 5 ml). The initial daily dose is usually 15 mg/kg, and this is increased at weekly intervals by 5 to 10 mg/kg per day to a maximum daily dose of 60 mg/kg. Divided doses should be given when the total daily dose exceeds 250 mg.

Divalproex sodium (DEPAKOTE) is a stable coordination compound containing equal molar proportions of valproic acid and sodium valproate. It reportedly causes a lower incidence of gastrointestinal side effects. Divalproex sodium is available in 125-, 250- and 500-mg tablets.

Plasma Drug Concentrations. The concentration of valproate in plasma that appears to be associated with therapeutic effects is approximately 30 to 100 μg/ml (Appendix II). However, the correlation between this concentration and efficacy is poor. There appears to be a threshold at about 30 to 50 μg/ml; this is the concentration at which binding sites on plasma albumin begin to become saturated (*see* Chapman *et al.*, 1982).

Drug Interactions. The interaction between valproate and phenobarbital is well-documented. Concentrations of phenobarbital in plasma rise by as much as 40% when valproate is given concurrently. The underlying mechanism probably involves inhibition of phenobarbital metabolism; its half-life is prolonged and urinary excretion of unchanged drug is increased. Valproate may also inhibit the metabolism of phenytoin, but a change in its total concentration in plasma may not occur because of the simultaneous displacement of phenytoin from protein binding sites. Nevertheless, an increase in the concentration of free drug is possible (*see* Perucca and Richens, 1985b). The concurrent administration of valproate and clonazepam has been associated with the development of absence status epilepticus; however, this complication appears to be rare (Browne, 1980).

Therapeutic Uses. The therapeutic uses of valproic acid in epilepsy have been reviewed by Dreifuss (*see* Symposium, 1983c) and in two recent symposia (1987c, 1988b). Although there has been more experience with its use in the treatment of absence seizures, valproate has been shown to be effective in a wide variety of partial and generalized seizures. The therapeutic uses of valproate in epilepsy are discussed further at the end of this chapter.

OXAZOLIDINEDIONES

TRIMETHADIONE

Although no longer the clinical agent of choice, trimethadione has been extensively studied in the laboratory and clinic, and, in this regard, it may still be considered a prototype for agents useful against absence seizures.

History. The demonstration by Perlstein and the confirmation by many others of the selectivity of trimethadione in the treatment of absence seizures was an important advance in the therapy of the epilepsies (*see* Withrow, in Symposium, 1980). It provided the first clear indication that drugs could be selective for the various types of epilepsy and spurred research on the basic physiological mechanism of absence seizures, which previously had been refractory to therapy.

Structure–Activity Relationship. Trimethadione has the following structural formula:

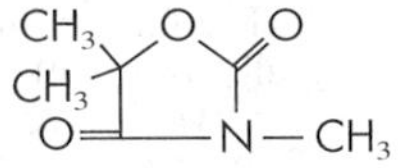

Trimethadione

The alkyl substituents on the carbon in position 5 appear important for the selectivity of the oxazolidinediones both as antagonists of pentylenetetrazol in animals and as clinically useful agents in the therapy of absence seizures. The same is true for the succinimides. The structure–activity relationship for these compounds has been reviewed by Close and Spielman (1961).

Pharmacological Effects. The outstanding anticonvulsant property of trimethadione in laboratory animals is its protective effect against pentylenetetrazol seizures, in which property it differs markedly from phenytoin (Toman and Goodman, 1948). Conversely, it is far inferior to phenytoin in its ability to modify the maximal electroshock seizure pattern. Dimethadione, the N-demethyl metabolite of trimethadione, is active and resembles the parent drug in most respects.

As is the case for ethosuximide, investigation of the mechanism of action of trimethadione has revealed little beyond demonstration of its selective effects in clinical and experimental seizures and of the differences between its electrophysiological effects and those of phenytoin.

Pharmacokinetic Properties. Trimethadione is rapidly absorbed from the gastrointestinal tract; the peak plasma concentration after a single dose occurs in 0.5 to 2 hours. It is not bound significantly to plasma proteins and is uniformly distributed in tissues. Trimethadione is largely demethylated by the hepatic microsomal enzymes to the active metabolite dimethadione. Dimethadione is not further metabolized but is excreted unchanged in the urine with a half-life of 6 to 13 days. During long-term therapy, the metabolite accumulates and is largely responsible for the anticonvulsant effects (*see* Symposium, 1982a).

Toxicity. The most common undesired effects of trimethadione are sedation and hemeralopia (blurring of vision in bright light, or glare effect). Hemeralopia does not usually require discontinuation of medication and can be overcome by the use of tinted glasses. Children are not as susceptible as adults. Drowsiness tends to diminish with continued medication.

Less common but more serious untoward effects include exfoliative dermatitis and other skin rashes, blood dyscrasias, hepatitis, and nephrosis. Fatalities have been reported. Moderate neutropenia is not uncommon (incidence as high as 20%); fulminating pancytopenia and aplastic anemia have occurred. Lupus erythematosus and lymphadenopathy have been observed. A myasthenic syndrome has also been reported (*see* Booker, in Symposium, 1982a).

Preparations and Dosages. *Trimethadione* (TRIDIONE) is available for oral use as 300-mg capsules, 150-mg chewable tablets, and a flavored solution (40 mg/ml). The usual daily dose is 900 to 2400 mg for adults and 20 to 60 mg/kg (300 to 900 mg) for children. However, larger doses are sometimes necessary.

Plasma Drug Concentrations. During chronic medication, the plasma concentration of trimethadione averages 0.6 μg/ml per daily dose of 1 mg/kg. Plasma concentrations of the active metabolite, dimethadione, are 20 times higher (12 μg/ml per 1 mg/kg) and provide the guide for adjustment of dosage. Several weeks are required to attain the plateau state both when therapy is initiated and when the dosage is changed. A disproportionately high trimethadione:dimethadione concentration ratio usually implies that the patient has not been taking medication regularly. The plasma concentration of dimethadione must usually be maintained above 700 μg/ml for control of seizures. The relationship between plasma concentration and adverse effects has not been established (*see* Booker, in Symposium, 1982a).

Therapeutic Uses. Trimethadione is used only in the treatment of absence seizures, and usually only in patients who are inadequately controlled by or do not tolerate other agents. Because of its potential for serious toxicity, treatment with trimethadione necessitates close medical supervision of the patient, especially during the initial year of therapy. The therapeutic use of trimethadione and other agents in the treatment of absence seizures is discussed further at the end of the chapter.

PARAMETHADIONE

Paramethadione differs from trimethadione only in the replacement by an ethyl substituent of one of the methyl groups on the carbon in the 5 position. Its pharmacological properties, therapeutic uses, dosage, and toxicity are similar to those of trimethadione.

Paramethadione (PARADIONE) is available in 150- and 300-mg capsules and in a solution (300 mg/ml).

Although the undesired effects of paramethadione and trimethadione are similar, the reported incidence of serious adverse effects may be less for paramethadione (*see* Symposium, 1982a). More importantly, perhaps, individuals who do not tolerate one of the oxazolidinediones may tolerate the other.

Paramethadione is N-demethylated in the hepatic endoplasmic reticulum to an active metabolite that is slowly excreted in the urine. The metabolite accumulates during long-term therapy and is probably responsible for most of the anticonvulsant activity of the parent drug.

BENZODIAZEPINES

The benzodiazepines are employed clinically primarily as sedative-antianxiety drugs; their pharmacology is presented in detail in Chapters 17 and 18. Discussion in this chapter is limited to consideration of their usefulness in the therapy of the epilepsies. A large number of benzodiazepines have broad antiepileptic properties, but only clonazepam and clorazepate have been approved in the United States for the long-term treatment of certain types of seizures; clobazam is being examined as an alternative that may cause less sedation. Nitrazepam is being evaluated for the treatment of infantile spasms. Diazepam has a well-defined role in the management of status epilepticus, while the utility of lorazepam and clonazepam is under investigation.

Chemistry. The structures of the benzodiazepines are presented in Table 17–1 (page 347). The structure–activity relationship for the anticonvulsant effect of the benzodiazepines has been summarized by Popp (Symposium, 1977).

Anticonvulsant Properties. In animals, prevention of pentylenetetrazol-induced seizures by the benzodiazepines is much more prominent than their modification of the maximal electroshock seizure pattern. Clonazepam is unusually potent in antagonizing the effects of pentylenetetrazol, but it is almost without action on seizures induced by maximal electroshock (Swinyard and Castellion, 1966). Nevertheless, in experimental models of epilepsy, benzodiazepines, including clonazepam, suppress the spread of seizure activity produced by epileptogenic foci in the cortex, thalamus, and limbic structures but do not abolish the abnormal discharge of the focus. Further, both diazepam and clonazepam suppress stimulus-induced generalized convulsions in kindled rats, but they produce little or no reduction in stimulus-induced afterdischarges (Albright and Burnham, 1980). In agreement with these observations in animals, clonazepam has anticonvulsant activity in patients with a wide variety of seizure disorders, with the notable exception of generalized tonic-clonic seizures (*see* Browne, in Symposium, 1983a).

The current view is that the anticonvulsant actions of the benzodiazepines, as well as other effects that occur at nonsedating doses, result in large part from their ability to enhance GABA-induced increases in the conductance of chloride (*see* Symposium, 1982b; Meldrum and Chapman, in Symposium, 1986b; Mennini *et al.*, 1987; Olsen, 1987). At therapeutically relevant concentrations, diazepam and other active benzodiazepines augment the inhibitory effects produced by stimulating various GABAergic pathways and enlarge GABA-induced changes in membrane potential. The latter effect is associated with an increased frequency of bursts of openings of chloride channels (Twyman *et al.*, 1989). Extensive biochemical evidence suggests a close molecular association between specific binding sites for benzodiazepines and GABA-regulated chloride channels (*see* Chapter 17). Nevertheless, there may be other mechanisms by which benzodiazepines reduce the excitability of neurons. These include enhancement of Ca^{2+}-dependent K^+ conductances and of adenosine accumulation, neither of which requires GABA (*see* Chapter 17).

At higher concentrations, diazepam and many other benzodiazepines can reduce sustained high-frequency firing of neurons, similar to the effects of phenytoin, carbamazepine, and valproate (*see* Macdonald and McLean, in Symposium, 1986a). Although these concentrations correspond to those achieved in patients during treatment of status epilepticus with diazepam, they are considerably higher than those associated with anticonvulsant or anxiolytic effects in ambulatory patients.

Pharmacokinetic Properties. Benzodiazepines are well absorbed after oral administration, and concentrations in plasma are usually maximal within 1 to 4 hours (*see* Symposium, 1982a; Browne, in Symposium, 1983a). After intravenous administration, they are redistributed in a manner typical of that for highly lipid-soluble agents (*see* Chapter 1). Central effects develop promptly but wane rapidly as the drugs move to other tissues. Diazepam is redistributed especially rapidly, with a half-time of about 1 hour. The extent of binding of benzodiazepines to plasma proteins correlates with lipid solubility, ranging from approximately 99% for diazepam to about 85% for clonazepam (*see* Appendix II).

The major metabolite of diazepam, N-desmethyldiazepam, is somewhat less active than the parent drug and may behave as a partial agonist (*see* Mennini *et al.*, 1987). This metabolite is also produced by the rapid decarboxylation of clorazepate following its ingestion. Both diazepam and N-desmethyldiazepam are slowly hydroxylated to other active metabolites, such as oxazepam. The half-life of diazepam in plasma averages between 1 and 2 days, while that of N-desmethyldiazepam is about 60 hours. The metabolism of clobazam, a 1,5-benzodiazepine, proceeds through a similar sequence and at about the same rate as that of diazepam. Both clonazepam and nitrazepam are metabolized principally by reduction of the nitro group to produce inactive 7-amino derivatives. Less than 1% of each drug is recovered unchanged in the urine. The half-lives of clonazepam and nitrazepam in plasma average about 1 day. Lorazepam is metabolized chiefly by conjugation with glucuronic acid; its half-life in plasma is about 14 hours.

Toxicity. The acute toxicity of benzodiazepines is low relative to usual clinical dosage. For example, oral ingestion of as much as 60 mg (small child) or 100 mg (adult) of clonazepam has occurred without permanent sequelae (*see* Pinder *et al.*, 1976); therapy consisted of gastric lavage and supportive measures. Cardiovascular and respiratory depression may occur after the intravenous administration of diazepam, clonazepam, or lorazepam, particularly if other anticonvulsants or central depressants have been administered previously (*see* Symposium, 1983d).

The principal side effects of long-term oral therapy with clonazepam are drowsiness and lethargy. These occur in about 50% of patients initially but tend to subside with continued administration. Muscular incoordination and ataxia are less frequent. Although these symptoms can usually be kept to tolerable levels by reducing the dosage or the rate at which it is increased, they sometimes force discontinuation of the drug. Other side effects include hypotonia, dysarthria, and dizziness. Behavioral disturbances, especially in children, can be very troublesome; these include aggression, hyperactivity, irritability, and difficulty in concentration. Both anorexia and hyperphagia have been reported. Increased salivary and bronchial secretions may cause difficulties in children. Seizures are sometimes exacerbated (*see* Browne, in Symposium, 1983a), and status epilepticus may be precipitated if the drug is discontinued abruptly. Sedation, hypotonia, and behavioral disturbances may be less frequent and less severe during treatment with clobazam than with clonazepam (*see* Farrell, in Symposium, 1986b). Other aspects of the toxicity of the benzodiazepines are discussed in Chapters 17 and 18.

Preparations, Routes of Administration, and Dosages. *Clonazepam* (KLONOPIN) is available as 0.5-, 1-, and 2-mg tablets. The initial dose for adults should not exceed 1.5 mg per day, and for children it is 0.01 to 0.03 mg/kg per day. The dose-dependent side effects are reduced if two or three divided doses are given each day. The dose may be increased every 3 days by up to 0.25 to 0.5 mg per day in children and 0.5 to 1 mg per day in adults. The maximal recommended dose is 20 mg per day for adults and 0.2 mg/kg per day for children. In children, each 0.05 mg/kg per day produces an increase in the concentration of clonazepam in plasma of about 25 ng/ml.

Clorazepate dipotassium (TRANXENE) is available in a variety of tablets and capsules. The maximal initial dose is 22.5 mg per day in three portions for adults and 15 mg per day in two doses for children. Daily doses should be increased by no more than 7.5 mg in any given week. The maximal recommended dose is 90 mg per day for adults and 60 mg per day for children. Clorazepate is not recommended for children under the age of 9.

Diazepam (VALIUM, others) is available as 2-, 5-, and 10-mg tablets, as 15-mg sustained-release capsules, and in solutions for oral administration or injection. For status epilepticus, diazepam is administered intravenously and at a rate of no more than 5 mg per minute. The usual dose for adults is 5 to 10 mg, as required; this may be repeated at intervals of 10 to 15 minutes, up to a maximal dose of 30 mg. If necessary, this regimen can be repeated in 2 to 4 hours, but no more than 100 mg should be administered in a 24-hour period. An alternate regimen has also been recommended (*see* Symposium, 1983d); initial therapy includes the infusion of 20 mg of diazepam over a period of 10 minutes or until seizures stop.

Plasma Drug Concentrations. Effective concentrations of clonazepam in plasma range from 5 to 70 ng/ml. The values for N-desmethyldiazepam formed by the decarboxylation of clorazepate range from 0.5 to 1.9 μg/ml. However, similar ranges of concentrations are observed in patients who have poor therapeutic responses or various side effects (*see* Browne, in Symposium, 1983a). Thus, neither clear-cut minimal therapeutic concentrations nor usually toxic concentrations can be stated.

Therapeutic Uses. Clonazepam is useful in the therapy of absence seizures as well as myoclonic seizures in children. However, tolerance to its antiepileptic effects usually develops after 1 to 6 months of administration, after which some patients will no longer respond to clonazepam at any dosage. While diazepam is currently the agent of choice for the treatment of status epilepticus, its relatively short duration of action is a disadvantage. Although diazepam is not useful as an oral agent for the treatment of seizure disorders, clorazepate is effective in combination with certain other drugs in the treatment of partial seizures. These applications are discussed further at the end of the chapter. Other uses of the benzodiazepines are described primarily in Chapters 17 and 18.

OTHER ANTIEPILEPTIC AGENTS

Phenacemide. Introduced in 1949, phenacemide (phenylacetylurea) is the straight-chain analog of 5-phenylhydantoin. Even if its efficacy remained unchallenged, its clinical value would be severely limited by its potential for serious toxicity. Adverse reactions include behavioral effects, gastrointestinal symptoms, rash, hepatitis, aplastic anemia, and nephritis. Phenacemide can be used as adjunctive therapy in the treatment of complex partial seizures refractory to other agents. Periodic assessment of hepatic, renal, and bone marrow function is mandatory.

Phenacemide (PHENURONE) is available as 500-mg tablets. The usual daily dose in adults varies from 1.5 to 5 g. Phenacemide is almost completely absorbed from the gastrointestinal tract. Biotransformation by hepatic microsomal enzymes includes inactivation by *p*-hydroxylation of the phenyl substituent. Unchanged drug is not excreted in the urine (*see* Browne, in Symposium, 1983a).

Acetazolamide. Acetazolamide, the prototype for the carbonic anhydrase inhibitors, is discussed in Chapter 28. Its anticonvulsant actions have been discussed in *previous editions* of this textbook and have been reviewed by Woodbury and Kemp (Symposium, 1982a). Although it is sometimes effective against absence seizures, its usefulness is limited by the rapid development of tolerance. Adverse effects are minimal when it is used in moderate dosage for limited periods.

Progabide. Progabide (4-[(4-chlorophenyl)(5-fluoro-2-hydroxyphenyl)-methylene] aminobutanamide) is an analog of the amide derivative of GABA. This compound behaves as an agonist at receptors for GABA, and it was developed as a result of hypotheses concerning the role of GABA in epileptogenesis and in the anticonvulsant actions of a number of antiepileptic drugs (*see* Bergmann, 1985). Progabide and its principal metabolite, the deamidated derivative, display anticonvulsant activity in a wide variety of animal models, including antagonism of pentylenetetrazol and modification of seizures induced by maximal electroshock. However, the therapeutic status of progabide remains uncertain. Despite early enthusiasm, controlled clinical evaluation has produced mixed results (*see* Leppik *et al.,* 1987).

GENERAL PRINCIPLES AND CHOICE OF DRUGS FOR THE THERAPY OF THE EPILEPSIES

Early diagnosis and treatment of seizure disorders with a single appropriate agent offers the best prospect of achieving prolonged seizure-free periods with the lowest risk of toxicity (*see* Smith *et al.,* in Symposium, 1987b; Reynolds, 1988). Although this dictum represents an extrapolation from studies on adult patients with partial or generalized tonic-clonic seizures, it is reinforced by classical ideas about the progressive, "autocatalytic" nature of epilepsy and by observations on the kindling phenomenon in animals. Hence, there is an increasing tendency to institute treatment after the first seizure. This places even more emphasis on accurate diagnosis and the exclusion of patients who have experienced other neurological events that might be mistaken for a seizure (*e.g.,* fainting) or those who have experienced a single seizure precipitated by a reversible abnormality (*e.g.,* hypoglycemia). Furthermore, an attempt should be made to ascertain the cause of the epilepsy with the hope of discovering a correctable lesion, either structural or metabolic. This is more likely in the very young patient or in the patient whose first seizure appears during adulthood. Once the decision has been made to use drugs to control the seizures, and this is often the case even if a specific etiology is found, the goal of therapy is to keep the patient free of seizures without interfering with normal function.

In most instances, *medication should be initiated with a single drug*. Initial dosage is usually that expected to provide a plasma drug concentration during the plateau state at least in the lower portion of the range associated with clinical efficacy. However, to minimize dose-related adverse effects, therapy with some drugs is initiated at reduced dosage. Loading dosage is employed only if the urgency for control of seizures exceeds the risk of adverse effects during the initial therapy. Initial results should be assessed with appropriate regard for the time required to attain the plateau state, the usual variability of incidence of seizures, and the anticipation that some tolerance usually develops to the sedative and other minor adverse effects of these drugs. Dosage is increased at appropriate intervals, as required for control of seizures or as limited by toxicity, and such adjustment is preferably assisted by monitoring of drug concentrations in plasma.

If a single drug fails to provide adequate control of seizures in maximal tolerated dosage and if compliance has been confirmed, *another drug should be substituted.* Unless serious adverse effects of the drug dictate otherwise, dosage should always be reduced gradually when a drug is being discontinued, to minimize the risk of precipitating status epilepticus. No drug should be discarded as useless unless toxicity prevents increased dosage. In the event that therapy with a second drug is also inadequate, many physicians substitute still another drug before instituting a combined-drug regimen (if a suitable alternative is available). The frequency and severity of toxicity are reduced by avoiding regimens with two or more drugs (*see* Bourgeois, 1988). Moreover, the efficacy of two drugs in combination for a given type of seizure appears to be additive at best. Nevertheless, some patients (particularly those with more than one type of seizure) will not be controlled adequately without the use of two or more antiepileptic agents simultaneously. This should be recognized as a more difficult and risky therapeutic situation by both the physician and the patient.

Essential to optimal management of epilepsy is the filling-out of a seizure chart by the patient or a relative; frequent visits to the physician or seizure clinic, particularly in the early period of treatment, since hematological and other possible side effects require consideration of a change in medication; and long-term follow-up, including repetition of EEG and neurological examination. Most crucial for successful management is regularity of medication, since faulty compliance is the most frequent cause for failure of therapy with antiepileptic drugs.

Measurement of plasma drug concentration at appropriate intervals greatly facilitates the initial adjustment of dosage for individual differences in drug elimination and the subsequent adjustment of dosage to minimize dose-related adverse effects without sacrifice of seizure control. Periodic monitoring during maintenance therapy can detect failure of the patient to take the medication as prescribed; for the patient with infrequent seizures and apparent control, periodic monitoring can provide assurance that seizure control is, in fact, being maintained. Knowledge of plasma drug concentration can be especially helpful during multiple-drug therapy. If toxicity occurs, monitoring helps to identify the particular drug responsible, and, if pharmacokinetic drug interaction occurs, it can guide readjustment of dosage.

Duration of Therapy. In an attempt to provide guidelines for withdrawal of anticonvulsant drugs, Thurston and coworkers (1982) studied the effects of withdrawing treatment from 148 children who had been free of seizures for 4 years; 28% of the children had a recurrence of seizures during the next 15 to 23 years. Most of these were children who had focal seizures. The recurrence rates were lowest in children who had only tonic-clonic (14%) or absence (12%) seizures. Neurological dysfunction was associated with a high rate of recurrence (46%).

In a prospective study, the treatment of patients with generalized or partial seizures was stopped after 2 seizure-free years; only patients who had been treated with a single drug (phenytoin, carbamazepine, or valproate) were included (Callaghan *et al.*, 1988). The overall rate of relapse (within 3 years) was 34% in both children and adults. Although only 92 patients were studied, the risk of relapse was apparently greatest for patients with complex partial seizures or those who had a persistently abnormal EEG. The risk of relapse was also apparently greatest in those patients who had been treated with valproate, and it was lower in those who had received carbamazepine. Although these and other results are encouraging, it is not yet possible to provide clear guidelines for the selection of patients for withdrawal from therapy (*see* Pedley, 1988). Such decisions must be made on an individual basis, weighing both the medical and psychosocial consequences of recurrence of seizures against the potential toxicity associated with prolonged therapy.

If a decision to withdraw antiepileptic drugs is made, such withdrawal should be done gradually over a period of months. The risk of status epilepticus is great with abrupt cessation of therapy.

Generalized Tonic-Clonic and Simple Partial Seizures. Carbamazepine and phenytoin are the principal agents used to treat generalized tonic-clonic seizures and simple partial seizures. In a large multicenter trial, phenobarbital and primidone were less likely to provide complete control of seizures when used alone as initial treatment (Mattson *et al.,* 1985); they are considered to be alternatives when therapy with carbamazepine or phenytoin is unsuccessful (*see Medical Letter,* 1989). Although valproate has not yet been approved for use in the United States for the treatment of partial or generalized tonic-clonic seizures, several studies indicate that its efficacy in these conditions is equal to that of either carbamazepine or phenytoin when used in single-drug regimens (Callaghan *et al.,* 1985; *see also* Symposium, 1987c, 1988b). The combination of carbamazepine and phenytoin is most apt to be utilized if single-drug therapy is unsuccessful, but there have been no controlled trials to substantiate this choice. Combinations of primidone and phenobarbital are obviously not rational, since phenobarbital is a major metabolite of primidone.

Absence Seizures. The best current data indicate that ethosuximide and valproate are equally effective in the treatment of absence seizures (*see* Mikati and Browne, 1988). Between 50 and 75% of newly diagnosed patients can be rendered free of seizures. In the event that tonic-clonic seizures are present or emerge during therapy, valproate is the agent of first choice; a combination of ethosuximide and phenobarbital might be preferred in children below the age of 3 years because of the higher incidence of fatal valproate-induced hepatic injury in this age group.

Clonazepam is also effective in the treatment of absence seizures, particularly those with a myoclonic component. However, because tolerance may develop to the antiepileptic effects, other agents are generally preferred.

Complex Partial Seizures. The treatment of complex partial seizures is generally less effective than is that of generalized or absence seizures. Drugs used for generalized tonic-clonic seizures are employed; carbamazepine, phenytoin, and valproate appear to be equally effective. Essential to appropriate therapy is differentiation between absence seizures and complex partial seizures. The latter are characterized by an aura, a duration of 1 to 2 minutes, and postictal confusion. Absence seizures are characterized by an abrupt onset of loss of consciousness, a duration of 5 to 20 seconds, and a characteristic 3-per-second spike-and-wave activity in the EEG (*see* Solomon *et al.,* 1983). The agents used to treat absence seizures are generally ineffective for complex partial seizures.

Febrile Convulsions. Two to four percent of children experience a convulsion associated with a febrile illness. About 33% of these children will have another febrile convulsion, and 2 to 3% become epileptic in later years. This is a sixfold increase in risk compared with the general population.

The treatment, if any, of febrile seizures is controversial (*see* Fishman, 1979). Several alternatives have been proposed, including no treatment, regular treatment with phenobarbital, or initiation of phenobarbital at the onset of a febrile illness. The latter course of action is doomed to failure because of the pharmacokinetic properties of phenobarbital. It takes several days to reach effective concentrations in blood, and the use of a sufficient loading dose results in toxic effects.

One approach to the problem of febrile seizures is to institute long-term therapy in those children who are at greatest risk for a recurrence of seizures. This includes children who have their first seizure before 18 months of age, those who have significant neurological abnormalities, and those in whom the seizures last more than 15 minutes or are complex in nature. The presence of two of these risk factors increases to 13% the likelihood of developing epilepsy. However, there is no evidence that prophylactic treatment reduces this risk. When a decision to treat is made, phenobarbital is the drug of choice. Although valproate is equally effective, it is associated with an increased incidence of hepatic injury in young children. Moreover, some authors have expressed concern that valproate might interact with certain viral infections in a fashion similar to that of salicylates. Continuous prophylaxis with carbamazepine or phenytoin is not effective in preventing febrile seizures. If the child has experienced no seizures for 30 months and is otherwise normal, therapy is usually discontinued (*see* Fishman, 1979; Freeman, 1980; Mikati and Browne, 1988).

Seizures in Infants and Young Children. Infantile myoclonic spasms with hypsarhythmia are refractory to the usual antiepileptic agents; corticotropin or the adrenocorticosteroids are the agents of choice. Valproic acid has been used successfully in some patients. Clonazepam may be a useful adjunct, but tolerance often develops.

Valproate may be effective against myoclonic, akinetic, and atonic seizures in young children and is considered by some experts to be the agent of choice. Clonazepam is also useful in such cases. Phenytoin is relatively ineffective and may produce restlessness and hyperactivity when given to young children.

Posttraumatic Epilepsy. Head injuries can predispose to the development of epilepsy; with penetrating wounds the risk may be as high as 30 to 40%. Some evidence suggests that prophylactic therapy may be effective in preventing the development of a seizure disorder in such cases. The agents effective for treatment of focal seizures and generalized tonic-clonic convulsions are employed.

Status Epilepticus and Other Convulsive Emergencies. Status epilepticus is a neurological emergency; left untreated, it may be fatal. In addition to specific drug therapy, supportive care is essential. Attention must be paid to electrolyte abnormalities, cardiac arrhythmias, dehydration, hypoglycemia, and the possibility of hypotensive shock. Diazepam, administered intravenously, is the agent of choice for control of status epilepticus; the dosage is discussed above. It is effective in 80 to 90% of cases, largely independent of seizure type or etiology, but is least likely to work when the seizures are symptomatic of acute brain lesions. The use of either lorazepam or clonazepam as alternatives to diazepam is being evaluated. Lorazepam appears to offer the advantage of persistence of effective concentrations in plasma and brain for several hours, without appreciable delay in onset of action. Phenytoin, administered intravenously at a maximal rate of 50 mg per minute, may also be employed and is preferred by some physicians; a loading dose of 500 to 1000 mg is needed to achieve effective concentrations in plasma so that a therapeutic response usually occurs only after 15 to 20 minutes. For this reason, some investigators have advocated the simultaneous intravenous administration of both diazepam and phenytoin (*see* Symposium, 1983d). Therapy may also be initiated by the rapid intravenous infusion of phenobarbital (10 to 20 mg/kg) at the rate of 60 mg per minute. Whatever agent is employed, equipment for maintenance of an airway and for mechanical support of ventilation must be immediately available. If seizures continue despite treatment, general anesthesia may be required. Paralysis of the skeletal musculature with a neuromuscular blocking agent does not affect seizure activity in the CNS but can sometimes be helpful to limit acidosis and rhabdomyolysis. After seizures are controlled, appropriate long-term antiepileptic therapy should be initiated.

Convulsive emergencies associated with drug poisoning and drug-induced seizures in previously nonepileptic patients during medication with agents such as the local anesthetics may also be controlled by diazepam and phenobarbital or another barbiturate. The control of drug-withdrawal seizures associated with abuse of alcohol, barbiturates, or related sedative-hypnotics is discussed in Chapter 22.

Antiepileptic Therapy and Pregnancy. Rates of stillbirth and infant mortality are higher for epileptic mothers, and children of epileptic mothers who received anticonvulsant medication during the early months of pregnancy have an increased incidence of a variety of birth defects. The risk is approximately 7%, compared to 2 to 3% for the general population. It is difficult to differentiate the effects of repeated seizures, teratogenic effects of anticonvulsants, and genetic factors. However, the evidence that indicts antiepileptic drugs includes (1) higher concentrations of antiepileptic drugs in the plasma of mothers with malformed children than in mothers with healthy children; (2) lower rates of malformation in children of untreated epileptic mothers compared with mothers who received antiepileptic therapy; and (3) higher rates of malformation in offspring exposed *in utero* to combinations of agents than in those exposed to a single drug (*see* Yerby, in Symposium, 1987b). Evidence for a teratogenic effect is greatest for trimethadione (Zackai *et al.*, 1975). Spina bifida has been associated with maternal use of valproate, and the risk of a neural tube defect in offspring may be increased 20-fold. The formation of epoxide intermediates during the metabolism of carbamazepine and phenytoin has also been implicated in the induction of fetal malformations (Lindhout *et al.*, 1984; Jones *et al.*, 1989). The accumulation of such epoxides increases progressively as other agents are added to therapeutic regimens; the incidence of malformations is the greatest with the combination of carbamazepine, valproate, and either phenytoin or phenobarbital.

Malformations associated with the use of carbamazepine during pregnancy include craniofacial defects, fingernail hypoplasia, and delay of development. Although a "fetal hydantoin syndrome" has been described (Hanson and Smith, 1975), its existence as a direct consequence of exposure to phenytoin is controversial (*see* Janz, in Symposium, 1982c).

Abrupt discontinuation of antiepileptic medication incurs a definite risk of status epilepticus and its hazards for the fetus and mother. For these reasons, antiepileptic medication should *not* be discontinued in pregnant epileptic women for whom the medication is necessary for the prevention of major seizures. However, depending upon the frequency and severity of seizures in the individual patient, cautious reduction of dosage to a minimum may be feasible and advisable, particularly in the first trimester. Therapeutic abortion should be considered when trimethadione has been used during pregnancy. Folic acid deficiency, if present, should be corrected. Monitoring of anticonvulsant drug concentrations should be performed to detect alterations of drug metabolism during pregnancy, especially during the last trimester when increased drug clearance may require adjustment of dosage. The therapy of seizure disorders during pregnancy has been reviewed by Dalessio (1985) and by Yerby (Symposium, 1987b).

The newborn of mothers who received phenobarbital, primidone, or phenytoin during pregnancy may also develop a deficiency of vitamin K–dependent clotting factors, and serious hemorrhage may occur during the first 24 hours of life. Bleeding can be prevented by administration of vitamin K.

Aiges, H. W.; Daum, F.; Olson, M.; Kahn, E.; and Teichberg, S. The effects of phenobarbital and diphenylhydantoin on liver function and morphology. *J. Pediatr.*, **1980**, *97*, 22–26.

Albright, P. S. Effects of carbamazepine, clonazepam, and phenytoin on seizure threshold in amygdala and cortex. *Exp. Neurol.*, **1983**, *79*, 11–17.

Albright, P. S., and Burnham, W. M. Development of a new pharmacological seizure model: effects of anticonvulsants on cortical- and amygdala-kindled seizures in the rat. *Epilepsia*, **1980**, *21*, 681–689.

Bergmann, K. J. Progabide: a new GABA-mimetic agent in clinical use. *Clin. Neuropharmacol.*, **1985**, *8*, 13–26.

Browne, T. R. Valproic acid. *N. Engl. J. Med.*, **1980**, *302*, 661–666.

Callaghan, N.; Garrett, A.; and Goggin, T. Withdrawal of anticonvulsant drugs in patients free of seizures for two years. *N. Engl. J. Med.*, **1988**, *318*, 942–946.

Callaghan, N.; Kenny, R. A.; O'Neill, B.; Crowley, M.; and Goggin, T. A prospective study between carbamazepine, phenytoin and sodium valproate as monotherapy in previously untreated and recently diagnosed patients with epilepsy. *J. Neurol. Neurosurg. Psychiatry*, **1985**, *48*, 639–644.

Commission on Classification and Terminology of the International League Against Epilepsy. Proposal for revised clinical and electroencephalographic classification of epileptic seizures. *Epilepsia*, **1981**, *22*, 489–501.

———. Proposal for a classification of epilepsies and epileptic syndromes. *Ibid.*, **1985**, *26*, 268–278.

Coulter, D. L., and Allen, R. J. Hyperammonemia with valproic acid therapy. *J. Pediatr.*, **1981**, *99*, 317–319.

De Deyn, P. P., and Macdonald, R. L. Effects of antiepileptic drugs on GABA responses and on reduction of GABA responses by PTZ and DMCM on mouse neurons in cell culture. *Epilepsia*, **1989**, *30*, 17–25.

Dreifuss, F. E.; Langer, D. H.; Moline, K. A.; and Maxwell, J. E. Valproic acid hepatic fatalities. *Neurology*, **1989**, *39*, 201–207.

Earnest, M. P.; Marx, J. A.; and Drury, L. R. Complications of intravenous phenytoin for acute treatment of seizures. *J.A.M.A.*, **1983**, *249*, 762–765.

Elwes, R. D. C.; Johnson, A. L.; Shorvon, S. D.; and Reynolds, E. H. The prognosis for seizure control in newly diagnosed epilepsy. *N. Engl. J. Med.*, **1984**, *311*, 944–947.

Fishman, M. A. Febrile seizures: the treatment controversy. *J. Pediatr.*, **1979**, *94*, 174–184.

Freeman, J. M. Febrile seizures: a consensus of their significance, evaluation, and treatment. *Pediatrics*, **1980**, *66*, 1009–1012.

Hanson, J. W., and Smith, D. W. The fetal hydantoin syndrome. *J. Pediatr.*, **1975**, *87*, 285–290.

Hart, R. G., and Easton, J. D. Carbamazepine and hematological monitoring. *Ann. Neurol.*, **1982**, *11*, 309–312.

Hassell, T. M., and Gilbert, G. H. Phenytoin sensitivity of fibroblasts as the basis for susceptibility to gingival enlargement. *Am. J. Pathol.*, **1983**, *112*, 218–223.

Hauptmann, A. LUMINAL bei Epilepsie. *Munch. Med. Wochenschr.*, **1912**, *59*, 1907–1909.

Jones, K. L.; Lacro, R. V.; Johnson, K. A.; and Adams, J. Pattern of malformations in the children of women treated with carbamazepine during pregnancy. *N. Engl. J. Med.*, **1989**, *320*, 1661–1666.

Keane, P. E.; Simiand, J.; Mendes, E.; Santucci, V.; and Morre, M. The effects of analogues of valproic acid on seizures induced by pentylenetetrazol and GABA content in brain of mice. *Neuropharmacology*, **1983**, *22*, 875–879.

Keith, D. A.; Gundberg, C. M.; Japour, A.; Aronoff, J.; Alvarez, N.; and Gallop, P. M. Vitamin K–dependent proteins and anticonvulsant medication. *Clin. Pharmacol. Ther.*, **1983**, *34*, 529–532.

Leppik, I. E., and others. A controlled study of progabide in partial seizures: methodology and results. *Neurology*, **1987**, *37*, 963–968.

Lindhout, D.; Höppener, R.; and Meinardi, H. Teratogenicity of antiepileptic drug combinations with special emphasis on epoxidation (of carbamazepine). *Epilepsia*, **1984**, *25*, 77–83.

McIntyre, D. C., and Racine, R. J. Kindling mechanisms: current progress on an experimental epilepsy model. *Prog. Neurobiol.*, **1986**, *27*, 1–12.

McLean, M. J., and Macdonald, R. L. Multiple actions of phenytoin on mouse spinal cord neurons in cell culture. *J. Pharmacol. Exp. Ther.*, **1983**, *227*, 779–789.

Macdonald, R. L. Anticonvulsant drug actions on neurons in cell culture. *J. Neural Transm.*, **1988**, *72*, 173–183.

Masur, H.; Elger, C. E.; Ludolph, A. C.; and Galanski, M. Cerebellar atrophy following acute intoxication with phenytoin. *Neurology*, **1989**, *39*, 432–433.

Mattson, R. H., and others. Comparison of carbamazepine, phenobarbital, phenytoin, and primidone in partial and secondarily generalized tonic-clonic seizures. *N. Engl. J. Med.*, **1985**, *313*, 145–151.

Medical Letter. Drugs for epilepsy. **1989**, *31*, 1–4.

Mennini, R.; Caccia, S.; and Garattini, S. Mechanism of action of anxiolytic drugs. *Prog. Drug Res.*, **1987**, *31*, 315–347.

Merritt, H. H., and Putnam, T. J. A new series of anticonvulsant drugs tested by experiments on animals. *Arch. Neurol. Psychiatry*, **1938a**, *39*, 1003–1015.

———. Sodium diphenyl hydantoinate in treatment of convulsive disorders. *J.A.M.A.*, **1938b**, *111*, 1068–1073.

Olpe, H. R., and Jones, R. S. G. The action of anticonvulsant drugs on the firing of locus coeruleus neurons: selective, activating effect of carbamazepine. *Eur. J. Pharmacol.*, **1983**, *91*, 107–110.

Osorio, I.; Burnstine, T. H.; Remler, B.; Manon-Espaillat, R.; and Reed, R. C. Phenytoin-induced seizures: a paradoxical effect at toxic concentrations in epileptic patients. *Epilepsia*, **1989**, *30*, 230–234.

Pedley, T. A. Discontinuing antiepileptic drugs. *N. Engl. J. Med.*, **1988**, *318*, 982–984.

Swinyard, E. A., and Castellion, A. W. Anticonvulsant properties of some benzodiazepines. *J. Pharmacol. Exp. Ther.*, **1966**, *151*, 369–375.
Theodore, W. H.; Narang, P. K.; Holmes, M. D.; Reeves, P.; and Nice, F. J. Carbamazepine and its epoxide: relation of plasma levels to toxicity and seizure control. *Ann. Neurol.*, **1989**, *25*, 194–196.
Thurston, J. H.; Thurston, L. D.; Hixon, B. B.; and Keller, A. J. Prognosis in childhood epilepsy. Additional follow-up of 148 children 15 to 23 years after withdrawal of anticonvulsant therapy. *N. Engl. J. Med.*, **1982**, *306*, 831–836.
Twyman, R. E.; Rogers, C. J.; and Macdonald, R. L. Differential regulation of γ-aminobutyric acid receptor channels by diazepam and phenobarbital. *Ann. Neurol.*, **1989**, *25*, 213–220.
Willow, M., and Catterall, W. A. Inhibition of binding of [^{3}H] batrachotoxinin a 20-α-benzoate to sodium channels by the anticonvulsant drugs diphenylhydantoin and carbamazepine. *Mol. Pharmacol.*, **1982**, *22*, 627–635.
Willow, M.; Gonoi, R.; and Catterall, W. A. Voltage clamp analysis of the inhibitory actions of diphenylhydantoin and carbamazepine on voltage-sensitive sodium channels in neuroblastoma cells. *Mol. Pharmacol.*, **1985**, *27*, 549–558.
Yaari, Y.; Selzer, M. E.; and Pincus, J. H. Phenytoin: mechanisms of its anticonvulsant action. *Ann. Neurol.*, **1986**, *20*, 171–184.
Zackai, E. H.; Mellman, W. J.; Neiderer, B.; and Hanson, J. W. The fetal trimethadione syndrome. *J. Pediatr.*, **1975**, *87*, 280–284.

Monographs and Reviews

Bourgeois, B. F. D. Problems of combination drug therapy in children. *Epilepsia*, **1988**, *29*, Suppl. 3, S20–S24.
Chapman, A.; Keane, P. E.; Meldrum, B. S.; Simiand, J.; and Vernieres, J. C. Mechanism of anticonvulsant action of valproate. *Prog. Neurobiol.*, **1982**, *19*, 315–359.
Close, W. J., and Spielman, M. A. Anticonvulsant drugs. In, *Medicinal Chemistry*, Vol. 5. (Hartung, W. H., ed.) John Wiley & Sons, Inc., New York, **1961**.
Dalessio, D. J. Current concepts: seizure disorders and pregnancy. *N. Engl. J Med.*, **1985**, *312*, 559–563.
Delgado-Escueta, A. V.; Treiman, D. M.; and Walsh, G. O. The treatable epilepsies. *N. Engl. J. Med.*, **1983**, *308*, 1508–1514, 1576–1584.
Frey, H.-H. Primidone. In, *Antiepileptic Drugs*. (Frey, H.-H., and Janz, D., eds.) *Handbook of Experimental Pharmacology*, Vol. 74. Springer-Verlag, Berlin, **1985**, pp. 283–289.
Gladding, G. D.; Kupferberg, H. J.; and Swinyard, E. A. Antiepileptic drug development program. In, *Antiepileptic Drugs*. (Frey, H.-H., and Janz, D., eds.) *Handbook of Experimental Pharmacology*, Vol. 74. Springer-Verlag, Berlin, **1985**, pp. 342–347.
Hvidberg, E. F. Monitoring antiepileptic drug levels. In, *Antiepileptic Drugs*. (Frey, H.-H., and Janz, D., eds.) *Handbook of Experimental Pharmacology*, Vol. 74. Springer-Verlag, Berlin, **1985**, pp. 725–765.
Jones, G. L., and Wimbish, G. H. Hydantoins. In, *Antiepileptic Drugs*. (Frey, H.-H., and Janz, D., eds.) *Handbook of Experimental Pharmacology*, Vol. 74. Springer-Verlag, Berlin, **1985**, pp. 351–419.
Löscher, W. Valproic acid. In, *Antiepileptic Drugs*. (Frey, H.-H., and Janz, D., eds.) *Handbook of Experimental Pharmacology*, Vol. 74. Springer-Verlag, Berlin, **1985**, pp. 507–537.
Mikati, M. A., and Browne, T. R. Comparative efficacy of antiepileptic drugs. *Clin. Neuropharmacol.*, **1988**, *11*, 130–140.
Narahashi, T. Drugs acting on calcium channels. In, *Calcium Drugs in Action*. (Baker, P. F., ed.) *Handbook of Experimental Pharmacology*, Vol. 83. Springer-Verlag, Berlin, **1988**, pp. 255–274.
Olsen, R. W. GABA-drug interactions. *Prog. Drug Res.*, **1987**, *31*, 224–238.
Perucca, E., and Richens, A. Clinical pharmacokinetics of antiepileptic drugs. In, *Antiepileptic Drugs*. (Frey, H.-H., and Janz, D., eds.) *Handbook of Experimental Pharmacology*, Vol. 74. Springer-Verlag, Berlin, **1985a**, pp. 661–723.
———. Antiepileptic drug interactions. In, *Antiepileptic Drugs*. (Frey, H.-H., and Janz, D., eds.) *Handbook of Experimental Pharmacology*, Vol. 74. Springer-Verlag, Berlin, **1985b**, pp. 831–855.
Pinder, R. M.; Brogden, R. N.; Speight, T. M.; and Avery, G. S. Clonazepam: a review of its pharmacological properties and therapeutic efficacy in epilepsy. *Drugs*, **1976**, *12*, 321–361.
Reynolds, E. H. The prevention of chronic epilepsy. *Epilepsia*, **1988**, *29*, Suppl. 1, S25–S28.
Schäfer, H. Chemical constitution and pharmacological effect. In, *Antiepileptic Drugs*. (Frey, H.-H., and Janz, D., eds.) *Handbook of Experimental Pharmacology*, Vol. 74. Springer-Verlag, Berlin, **1985**, pp. 199–245.
Schmutz, M. Carbamazepine. In, *Antiepileptic Drugs*. (Frey, H.-H., and Janz, D., eds.) *Handbook of Experimental Pharmacology*, Vol. 74. Springer-Verlag, Berlin, **1985**, pp. 479–506.
Solomon, G. E.; Kutt, H.; and Plum, F. *Clinical Management of Seizures: A Guide for the Physician*, 2nd ed. W. B. Saunders Co., Philadelphia, **1983**.
Symposium. (Various authors.) *Experimental Models of Epilepsy: A Manual for the Laboratory Worker*. (Purpura, D. P.; Penry, J. K.; Tower, D.; Woodbury, D. M.; and Walter, R.; eds.) Raven Press, New York, **1972**.
Symposium. (Various authors.) *Anticonvulsants*. (Vida, J. A., ed.) Academic Press, Inc., New York, **1977**.
Symposium. (Various authors.) *Antiepileptic Drugs: Mechanisms of Action. Advances in Neurology*, Vol. 27. (Glaser, G. H.; Penry, J. K.; and Woodbury, D. M.; eds.) Raven Press, New York, **1980**.
Symposium. (Various authors.) *Antiepileptic Drugs*, 2nd ed. (Woodbury, D. M.; Penry, J. K.; and Pippenger, C. E.; eds.) Raven Press, New York, **1982a**.
Symposium. (Various authors.) *Pharmacology of Benzodiazepines*. (Usdin, E.; Skolnick, P.; Tallman, J. F., Jr.; Greenblatt, D.; and Paul, S. M.; eds.) Macmillan Press, Ltd., London, **1982b**.
Symposium. (Various authors.) *Epilepsy, Pregnancy, and the Child*. (Janz, D.; Dam, M.; Richens, A.; Bossi, L.; Helgo, H.; and Schmidt, D.; eds.) Raven Press, New York, **1982c**.
Symposium. (Various authors.) *Epilepsy: Diagnosis and Management*. (Browne, T. R., and Feldman, R. G., eds.) Little, Brown & Co., Boston, **1983a**.
Symposium. (Various authors.) *Epilepsy: An Update on Research and Therapy. Progress in Clinical and Biological Research* Vol. 124. (Nistico, G.; Perri, R. D.; and Meinardi, H. eds.) Alan R. Liss, Inc., New York, **1983b**.
Symposium. (Various authors.) *Recent Advances in Epilepsy. I*. (Pedley, T. A., and Meldrum, B. S., eds.) Churchill Livingstone, Inc., New York, **1983c**.
Symposium. (Various authors.) *Status Epilepticus: Mechanisms of Brain Damage and Treatment. Advances in Neurology*, Vol. 34. (Delgado-Escueta, A. V.; Wasterlain, C. G.; Treiman, D. M.; and Porter, R. J.; eds.) Raven Press, New York, **1983d**.
Symposium. (Various authors.) Basic mechanisms of the epilepsies: molecular and cellular approaches. (Delgado-Escueta, A. V.; Ward, A. A., Jr.; Woodbury, D. M.; and Porter, R. J.; eds.) *Adv. Neurol.*, **1986a**, *44*, 1–120.
Symposium. (Various authors.) Recent contributions of

benzodiazepines to the management of epilepsy. (Trimble, M. R., ed.) *Epilepsia,* **1986b,** *27,* Suppl. 1, S1–S52.

Symposium. (Various authors.) Pediatric aspects of epilepsy. (Pedley, T. A., ed.) *Epilepsia,* **1987a,** *28,* Suppl. 1, S1–S109.

Symposium. (Various authors.) Carbamazepine's place in antiepileptic drug therapy. (Dodson, W. E., and Trimble, M. R., eds.) *Epilepsia,* **1987b,** *28,* Suppl. 3, S1–S87.

Symposium. (Various authors.) Divalproex/valproate monotherapy: an international perspective. (Ferrendelli, J. A., ed.) *Epilepsia,* **1987c,** *28,* Suppl. 2, S1–S29.

Symposium. (Various authors.) *J. Clin. Psychiatry,* **1988a,** *49,* Suppl., 4–62.

Symposium. (Various authors.) Valproate monotherapy in the treatment of epilepsy. (Penry, J. K., ed.) *Am. J. Med.,* **1988b,** *84,* 1–41.

Teschendorf, H. J., and Kretzschmar, R. Succinimides. In, *Antiepileptic Drugs.* (Frey, H.-H., and Janz, D., eds.) *Handbook of Experimental Pharmacology,* Vol. 74. Springer-Verlag, Berlin, **1985,** pp. 557–575.

Toman, J. E. P., and Goodman, L. S. Anticonvulsants. *Physiol. Rev.,* **1948,** *28,* 409–432.

Wada, J. A. Pharmacological prophylaxis in the kindling model of epilepsy. *Arch. Neurol.,* **1977,** *34,* 389–395.

CHAPTER

20 DRUGS FOR PARKINSON'S DISEASE, SPASTICITY, AND ACUTE MUSCLE SPASMS

Jesse M. Cedarbaum and Leonard S. Schleifer

Most of the drugs described in this chapter have in common the ability to improve skeletal muscle function primarily by actions on the central nervous system (CNS). These drugs fall into two distinct categories on the basis of their pharmacological properties and their therapeutic uses. The first group acts particularly on the basal ganglia; its members exert either dopaminergic or anticholinergic effects, and are useful for the treatment of Parkinson's disease and related disorders. Levodopa is the prototype of centrally acting dopaminergic drugs, while trihexyphenidyl is the prototypical centrally acting anticholinergic agent. Most members of the second group of drugs—those used to treat spasticity and acute muscle spasms—depress with varying degrees of selectivity certain neuronal systems that control muscle tone. Dantrolene, however, acts directly on skeletal muscle.

I. Drugs for Parkinson's Disease

Parkinsonism: Clinical Overview. Parkinsonism is a clinical syndrome comprised of four cardinal features: bradykinesia (slowness and poverty of movement), muscular rigidity (perceived by the examiner as an increase in the resistance of the muscles to passive movement), resting tremor (which usually abates during voluntary movement), and abnormalities of posture and gait. Idiopathic Parkinson's disease, which was first described by James Parkinson in 1817 as *paralysis agitans*, or the "shaking palsy," is a common neurodegenerative disease and is the most common cause of the parkinsonian syndrome. The incidence of Parkinson's disease increases with age: it afflicts approximately 1% of all adults over the age of 65 worldwide, and usually becomes manifest after the age of 55 (Martilla, 1983). The primary neurological features of Parkinson's disease give rise to a number of functional disabilities, including inability to walk, a mask-like facial expression, and impairment of speech and skilled acts such as writing and even eating. Without treatment, the end stage of the illness is a rigid, akinetic state in which patients are incapable of caring for themselves, and in which death is usually due to complications of immobility, such as pulmonary embolism or aspiration or hypostatic pneumonias. Major advances in the pharmacotherapy of parkinsonism over the past 25 years have markedly reduced morbidity from the disease and represent a triumph of rational pharmacology.

Despite advances in the understanding of the pathophysiology and the treatment of parkinsonism, its cause remains unknown. Genetic factors do not appear to play an important role in most cases of Parkinson's disease, although familial cases have been documented (Ward *et al.*, 1983). The lack of evidence that Parkinson's disease is a genetically determined loss of neuronal function has prompted vigorous searches for environmental causes (*e.g.*, infections and toxins).

Although no etiological factor has been documented for the vast majority of cases, a toxin has recently been shown to be responsible for the appearance of Parkinson's disease in exposed individuals. MPTP (N-methyl-4-phenyl-1,2,3,6-tetrahydropyridine), a commercial compound used in organic synthesis, causes a syndrome that resembles Parkinson's disease when administered to primates (Burns *et al.*, 1983). Development of this animal model of the disease followed observation of the occurrence of irreversible parkinsonism in a number of drug addicts and a chemist; they were exposed to the compound because of its presence (as a side product) in a preparation of a meperidine analog that was used illegally in California (Langston *et al.*, 1983). MPTP-induced parkinsonism is pathologically and biochemically similar to the idiopathic disease, and it responds favorably to the administration of antiparkinsonian drugs. It has been speculated that substances like MPTP may be widespread in the environment, and there is concern that repeated exposure to small quantities of such chemicals, combined with the effects of aging, may be an etiological factor in the development of parkinsonism (Blume, 1983).

A parkinsonism-like syndrome may also arise as an untoward effect of certain drugs. Agents that produce such a syndrome have in common the capacity to prevent the action of the neurotransmitter dopamine in the basal ganglia of the brain. For example, antipsychotic drugs such as the phenothiazines and butyrophenones block postsynaptic receptors for dopamine and cause extrapyramidal symptoms that resemble parkinsonism, especially in older patients (*see* Chapter 18). In contrast, reserpine produces a parkinsonism-like syndrome by depleting dopamine available for release by the presynaptic neuron.

Progressive supranuclear palsy, olivopontocerebellar degeneration, Shy-Drager syndrome, carbon monoxide poisoning, manganese poisoning, and Wilson's disease commonly are associated with certain symptoms that are characteristic of Parkinson's disease. However, in these rare disorders, parkinsonism is only one aspect of a more widespread cerebral disorder. With the exception of manganese poisoning, standard antiparkinsonian drugs produce little improvement in these conditions.

Parkinsonism: A Striatal Dopamine–Deficiency Syndrome. Now-classical investigations performed in the 1950s and 1960s clearly established the basal ganglia of the brain and specifically the nigrostriatal dopaminergic system as the site of the fundamental lesion in Parkinson's disease; there is a marked deficiency in the dopaminergic innervation of the basal ganglia owing to degeneration of neurons in the substantia nigra (Ehringer and Hornykiewicz, 1960). The pigmented neurons of the substantia nigra normally utilize dopamine as their neurotransmitter (*see* Chapter 12). The loss of this catecholamine from the basal ganglia has been shown to underlie all of the major motor manifestations of parkinsonism, although symptoms emerge only when such depletion exceeds 80 or 90%. Restoration of dopaminergic transmission by a variety of substances to be discussed below restores motor function in parkinsonism and forms the central strategy in virtually all current drug regimens for treatment of the disease.

Among the panoply of other neurotransmitters contained in the basal ganglia, only acetylcholine is currently known to be of significance in the pharmacotherapy of parkinsonism. A simplistic, but useful, neurochemical model of the function of the basal ganglia suggests that the neostriatum (caudate nucleus and putamen) normally contains balanced inhibitory dopaminergic and excitatory cholinergic components (Duvoisin, 1967). Although cholinergic neurons are not damaged in Parkinson's disease, the decrease in dopaminergic activity results in a relative excess of cholinergic influence. Consequently, a second (although historically older) strategy for the treatment of parkinsonism is to block cholinergic activity in an attempt to restore the balance of dopaminergic and cholinergic tone in the striatum. Furthermore, dopaminergic agonists and cholinergic (muscarinic) antagonists are often combined effectively.

The circuitry of the basal ganglia (extrapyramidal system) forms a loop superimposed upon the output of the motor cortex; this loop apparently monitors ongoing movement in order to prepare the motor system for the next movement in a sequence. This system has no direct influence on the final common pathway of motor function at the level of the spinal cord. The circuitry of the system is constituted such that information from the motor, sensory, and association cortices is conveyed to the neostriatum (caudate nucleus and putamen) and then to the other elements of the basal ganglia (globus pallidus, subthalamic nucleus, and substantia nigra) by both direct and indirect pathways (*see* Figure 20–1). The return limb of the loop emanates principally from the pars reticulata of the substantia nigra to a nucleus in the thalamus; from there, information is relayed first to the premotor

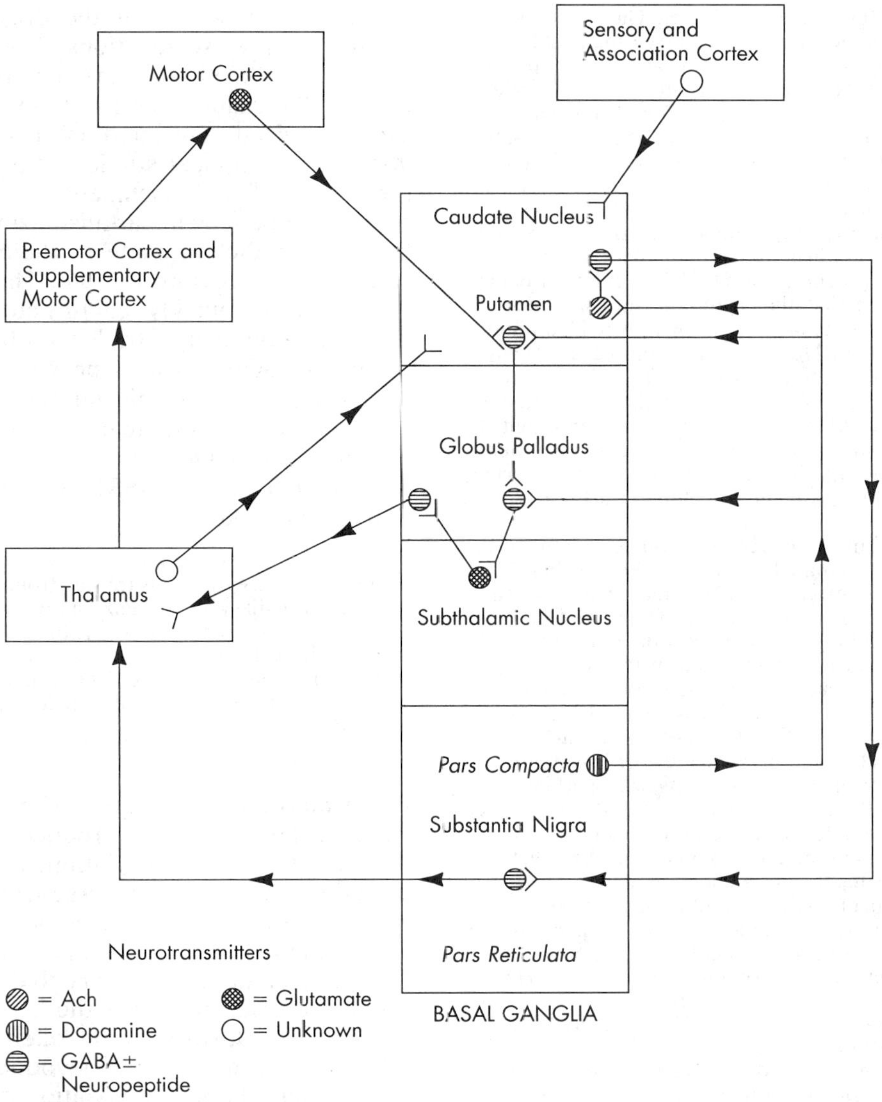

Figure 20–1. *Simplified diagram of the neuronal circuits and neurotransmitters of the basal ganglia.* (*See* text for explanation.)

and supplementary motor cortices and then back to the motor cortex itself.

There are numerous interconnections among the various elements of the basal ganglia, some of which are shown in Figure 20–1. However, the most important pathways in the pathogenesis and treatment of Parkinson's disease appear to be those that connect the caudate nucleus-putamen with the substantia nigra. Dopamine-containing afferents arise from the pars compacta of the substantia nigra; it is these cells that degenerate in Parkinson's disease. These dopaminergic neurons terminate on all neuronal cell types in the caudate-putamen, including large aspiny cholinergic interneurons and medium spiny and aspiny neurons that contain gamma-aminobutyric acid (GABA). The GABA-ergic neurons are the principal source of projections to other structures, especially the pars reticulata of the substantia nigra. The GABA-ergic neurons also contain one of a number of peptides, such as substance P, somatostatin, an enkephalin, or a dynorphin. Thus, it appears the role of dopaminergic projections to the striatum is to modify the effects of other inputs to interneurons and output neurons within this structure.

The understanding that parkinsonism is a syndrome of dopamine deficiency and the discovery of levodopa as an important drug for the treatment of the disease were the logical culmination of a series of related basic and clinical observations (*see* review by Hornykiewicz, 1973b). The first may have been the clinical finding that reserpine could induce a parkinsonism-like syndrome as a dose-dependent side effect. Reserpine was later shown to release and thereby deplete stores of 5-hydroxytryptamine (5-HT) and catecholamines in the brain. Subsequently, Carlsson and coworkers (1957) found that the akinesia and sedation produced by reserpine in mice could be reversed by the administration of 3,4-dihydroxyphenylalanine (dopa; the metabolic precursor of dopamine) but not of 5-hydroxytryptophan, the precursor of 5-HT. The relevant clinical observation that the phenothiazines also may induce symptoms of parkinsonism provided another clue that helped focus attention on the basal ganglia as a site of action for this important class of drugs. The presence of dopamine in the brain, first reported by Montagu (1957), was confirmed by Carlsson and coworkers, who also showed depletion of the putative neurotransmitter by reserpine and its replenishment by dopa (Carlsson *et al.*, 1957).

Measurements of regional concentrations of dopamine in human brains provided the basic link between laboratory studies and clinical applications. Bertler and Rosengren (1959) and Carlsson (1959) found that about 80% of the dopamine in the human brain is concentrated in the basal ganglia, mostly in the caudate nucleus and putamen (corpus striatum). The pivotal discovery by Ehringer and Hornykiewicz (1960) that there is a marked deficiency of striatal dopamine (10% or less of normal) in the basal ganglia of patients with parkinsonism furnished the crucial evidence. The degree of deficiency correlated with the loss of melanin-containing neurons in the pars compacta of the substantia nigra, the most consistent pathological finding of parkinsonism. Recent studies have also demonstrated a moderate deficiency of dopamine as well as reductions in the concentrations of other neurotransmitters (*e.g.*, norepinephrine and 5-HT) in several regions of the cerebral cortex of such patients (Hornykiewicz and Kish, in Symposium, 1984). Parkinson's disease may be caused by an aggravation of the normal aging process, to which dopamine-containing neurons are especially sensitive (Rinne, 1982; Mann and Yates, 1983; Calne, 1984).

LEVODOPA

Since dopamine does not cross the blood–brain barrier when administered systemically, it has no therapeutic effect in parkinsonism. However, levodopa (L-3,4-dihydroxyphenylalanine), the immediate metabolic precursor of dopamine, is transported into the brain by the large, neutral amino acid transporter and permeates into striatal tissue, where it is decarboxylated to dopamine. Initial clinical trials with small intravenous doses of D,L-dopa provided encouraging results, but the drug caused prominent adverse reactions. Cotzias and associates (1967) first clearly demonstrated that small, gradual increments in oral dosage minimized unwanted effects of D,L-dopa. These clinical studies demonstrated the value of replenishment of depleted stores of dopamine in parkinsonism and fulfilled the prediction made by the basic scientists in the previous decade. The clinical findings were quickly confirmed and extended in a number of trials with the active isomer, levodopa, which proved more effective than the racemic mixture. Several extensive reviews on the use of levodopa in parkinsonism have been published (*see* Nutt and Fellman, 1984; Quinn, 1984; Cedarbaum, 1987).

Chemistry. Levodopa is formed from L-tyrosine as an intermediary in the enzymatic synthesis of catecholamines. Dopamine is synthesized directly from levodopa by a cytoplasmic enzyme, aromatic L-amino acid decarboxylase. The structures of levodopa and dopamine are shown in Figure 20–2 (page 469).

Pharmacological Effects. The main effects of levodopa are produced by the product of its decarboxylation, dopamine; levodopa, as such, is practically inert pharmacologically. Since about 95% of orally administered levodopa is rapidly decarboxylated in the periphery to dopamine, which does not penetrate the blood–brain barrier, large doses must be taken to allow sufficient accumulation of levodopa in the brain, where its decarboxylation raises the central dopamine concentration. The concurrent administration of peripherally acting inhibitors of dopa decarboxylase can reduce the required dose of levodopa (*see* below).

Approximately 75% of patients with parkinsonism respond well to levodopa, enjoying more than a 50% reduction in the severity of their symptoms. Therapeutic response in some patients is seemingly "miraculous," especially at the outset. Essentially all signs and symptoms of parkinsonism except dementia and postural instability can respond to the administration of this agent (Cedarbaum and McDowell, 1986).

Central Nervous System. The pharmacological effects of levodopa on muscle tone and movement are not seen in normal individuals. However, in the patient with parkinsonism, continued therapy often results in significant reductions in bradykinesia, rigidity, and tremor. Amelioration of the cardinal symptoms of parkinsonism is accompanied by similar improvements in overall functional ability. Secondary motor manifestations such as disturbances in facial expression, speech, handwriting, swallowing, and respiration are proportionately improved.

Psychic Effects. In many patients, levodopa at least partially relieves the changes in mood that are characteristic of Parkinson's disease. Early in therapy, feelings of apathy are generally replaced by increased vigor and a sense of well-being. The result is described as a general alerting response characterized by apparent improvement in mental function and an increased interest in self, surroundings, and family. However, a significant number of patients develop serious behavioral side effects, which are discussed below. Dementia, which is present in a significant number of patients with parkinsonism, predisposes to the development of such behavioral side effects.

Cardiovascular System. Peripheral decarboxylation of levodopa markedly increases the concentration of dopamine in blood. Dopamine is a pharmacologically active catecholamine with effects on α- and β-adrenergic receptors, although its potency is much less than that of epinephrine, norepinephrine, or isoproterenol (*see* Chapter 10). Dopamine also activates vascular dopaminergic receptors and can release norepinephrine from adrenergic neurons. The reluctance of early investigators to test the effects of high doses of levodopa for parkinsonism rested largely on the expectation of potentially toxic cardiovascular effects, particularly hypertension and cardiac arrhythmias. Contrary to such expectation, therapeutic doses of levodopa frequently cause only modest and asymptomatic orthostatic hypotension; tolerance to this effect develops within a few weeks of chronic treatment. The mechanism by which levodopa produces hypotension is not fully understood, but both central and peripheral actions may be involved.

Therapeutic doses of levodopa produce cardiac stimulation by an action of dopamine on β_1-adrenergic receptors. Transient tachycardia and other cardiac arrhythmias may occur in some patients, and myocardial contractility may be increased for several hours after a large dose of levodopa, especially early in therapy. Tolerance to these effects also develops after several weeks of chronic treatment. The cardiac effects of levodopa are usually blocked by β-adrenergic antagonists such as propranolol.

Oral administration of levodopa to patients with severe congestive heart failure can produce a diuresis and sustained improvement in cardiac function (Rajfer *et al.*, 1984). Peak hemodynamic responses occur 1 hour after ingestion of the drug; these include an increase in cardiac index and a decrease in systemic vascular resistance. The effects may be due to the activation of both β_1-adrenergic and dopaminergic receptors.

Metabolic and Endocrine Effects. The tuberoinfundibular neurons of the hypothalamus comprise a major central dopaminergic system. These neurons play an important and as yet incompletely defined role in the modulation of hypothalamic-pituitary function (*see* Chapter 56). Dopamine inhibits the secretion of prolactin in man, at least in part by a direct action on the relevant cells of the adenohypophysis. Thus, levodopa and other dopaminergic agonists decrease the secretion of prolactin, while dopaminergic antagonists have the opposite effect. However, studies suggest that hypothalamic regulation of the adenohypophysis may be abnormal in Parkinson's disease (Langston and Forno, 1978). Consequently, the release of growth hormone that is noted in response to the administration of levodopa in normal subjects (*see* Chapter 56) is minimal or absent when levodopa is administered to patients with Parkinson's disease (Eddy *et al.*, 1971). A hypothalamic defect in the regulation of growth hormone might explain why earlier predictions of the production of acromegaly (or diabetes mellitus) in patients receiving levodopa have proven to be false. Inhibition of prolactin secretion by analogs of dopamine is useful in a variety of clinical situations.

Mechanism of Action. Since abundant evidence suggests that parkinsonism is a syndrome of deficiency of striatal dopamine, it follows that levodopa would act by replenishing these depleted stores. Evidence in favor of this mechanism includes a positive correlation between the symptoms of Parkinson's disease and loss of nigrostriatal neurons. Conversion of levodopa to dopamine has been demonstrated in human brain (Lloyd *et al.*, 1973). Furthermore, the brains of patients with Parkinson's disease who had received high doses of levodopa until death contain concentrations of dopamine in the striatum that are five to eight times higher than those in untreated patients (Davidson *et al.*, 1971). These findings indicate that the capacity of the nigrostriatal system to synthesize and store dopamine is not completely lost in patients with parkinsonism. The striatal concentration of aromatic L-amino acid decarboxylase, the enzyme that converts levodopa to dopamine, is markedly reduced in parkinsonism, but sufficient enzymatic activity apparently remains to account for the partial replenishment of dopamine following the administration of levodopa (*see* Hornykiewicz, 1973a). The exact cellular locus of this decarboxylase activity is unknown. Possibilities include residual dopaminergic nerve terminals, nondopaminergic neurons and their terminals, and glial elements (Duvoisin and Mytilineau, 1978; Hefti *et al.*, 1981).

The actions of dopamine have been studied at the molecular level, and receptors for dopamine have been identified and studied with ligand-binding techniques. The general conclusion is that there are at least two types of receptors for dopamine, designated D_1 and D_2 (*see* Table 12–1, page 258; *see also* Seeman and Grigoriadis, 1987). D_1 receptors can be preferentially labeled with thioxanthenes or certain phenothiazines and appear to stimulate adenylyl cyclase activity; D_2 receptors are preferentially labeled with butyrophenones and are thought to inhibit adenylyl cyclase in some cases or to be unlinked to the enzyme in others. Dopamine binds with approximately equal affinity to both receptor subtypes. D_1 receptors appear to be predominantly located on cell bodies and presynaptic terminals of intrinsic striatal neurons. D_2 receptors are located on neuronal cell bodies in the striatum and on the presynaptic terminals of dopaminergic nigrostriatal axons (Boyson *et al.*, 1986). Despite the fact that dopamine clearly *stimulates* adenylyl cyclase activity in homogenates of the basal ganglia, most investigators believe that the beneficial effects of levodopa (and other dopaminergic agonists; *see* below) in parkinsonism are mediated via D_2 receptors. Furthermore, the capacity of certain antipsychotic drugs to induce parkinsonism is also thought to be mediated predominantly by blockade of D_2 receptors. However, D_1 and D_2 agonists selectively stimulate different components of behavior, and maximal dopaminergic stimulation is achieved in experimental animals only when both populations of dopamine receptors are activated (Barone *et al.*, 1986; Koller and Herbster, 1988). Because both D_1 and D_2 receptors are present at both presynaptic and postsynaptic sites in the striatum, it has been difficult to draw a clear picture of dopaminergic function at the receptor level. Incongruities in data exist, including the fact that D_1 receptors appear to be inhibitory and D_2 excitatory in electrophysiological experiments (Ohno *et al.*, 1987), yet the overall effect of dopamine itself appears to be inhibitory to neuronal firing in the striatum (*see* review by Schmidt, 1982).

Absorption, Distribution, Fate, and Excretion. Levodopa is rapidly absorbed from the small bowel by an active transport system for aromatic amino acids. Concentrations of the drug in plasma usually peak between 0.5 and 2 hours after an oral dose. The half-life in plasma is short—only 1 to 3 hours. The rate of absorption of levodopa is greatly dependent upon the rate of gastric emptying, the pH of gastric juice, and the length of time the drug is exposed to the degradative enzymes of the gastric and intestinal mucosae. For example, sluggish gastric emptying (caused either by intrinsic factors, meals, or anticholinergic drugs), hyperacidity of gastric juice, and competition for absorption sites in the small bowel by amino acids each may interfere with the bioavailability of levodopa (Bianchine and Shaw, 1976). Thus, Nutt and associates (1984) found that administration of levodopa with meals delayed absorption of the drug and reduced peak concentrations in plasma by 30%.

More than 95% of levodopa is decarboxylated in the periphery by the widely distributed aromatic L-amino acid decarboxylase (when an inhibitor of this enzyme is not given concurrently). The drug is extensively decarboxylated in the mucosa of the gastrointestinal tract, which is rich in decarboxylase, so that relatively little unchanged drug reaches the cerebral circulation and probably less than 1% penetrates into the CNS. Inhibition of peripheral decarboxylase markedly increases the fraction of administered levodopa that remains unmetabolized and available to cross the blood–brain barrier.

The principal metabolic pathways for levodopa are depicted in Figure 20–2. A

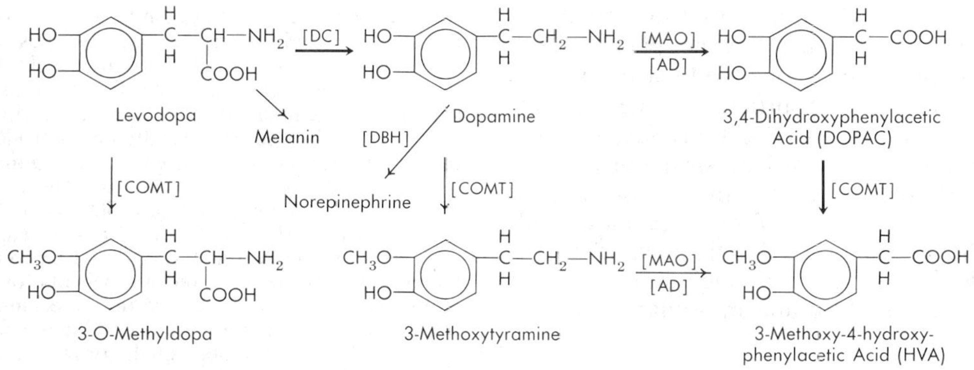

Figure 20–2. *Important catabolic pathways of levodopa* (L-*dopa*).

Major pathways are shown by heavy arrows; minor pathways, by light arrows. *AD* = aldehyde dehydrogenase; *COMT* = catechol-O-methyltransferase; *DBH* = dopamine β-hydroxylase; *DC* = aromatic L-amino acid decarboxylase; *MAO* = monoamine oxidase. (For biosynthetic pathway, *see* Figure 5–3, p. 102.)

small amount is methylated to 3-O-methyldopa, which accumulates in the CNS and periphery because of its long half-life. Most administered levodopa is converted to dopamine, small amounts of which are in turn metabolized to norepinephrine and epinephrine. Biotransformation of dopamine proceeds rapidly to yield the principal excretion products, 3,4-dihydroxyphenylacetic acid (DOPAC) and 3-methoxy-4-hydroxyphenylacetic acid (homovanillic acid; HVA). At least 30 metabolites of levodopa have been identified. Some evidence indicates that the metabolism of levodopa may be accelerated during prolonged therapy, possibly because of enzyme induction.

Metabolites of dopamine are rapidly excreted in the urine; about 80% of a radioactively labeled dose is recovered within 24 hours. DOPAC and HVA account for up to 50% of the administered dose. These metabolites, as well as small amounts of levodopa and dopamine, also appear in the cerebrospinal fluid. Negligible amounts are found in the feces. After prolonged therapy with levodopa, the ratio of DOPAC to HVA excreted may increase, probably reflecting a depletion of methyl donors necessary for metabolism by catechol-O-methyl transferase; it is estimated that about three fourths of dietary methionine is utilized for the metabolism of large therapeutic doses of levodopa. The pharmacokinetic properties of levodopa have been reviewed by Nutt and Fellman (1984) and by Cedarbaum (1987).

Side Effects and Toxicity. Careful and judicious administration of levodopa to an informed and cooperative patient is essential to optimize the ratio of benefit to toxicity. The majority of patients with Parkinson's disease who are treated with levodopa experience side effects. Their intensity and type vary greatly at different stages of therapy. Although many are relatively innocuous, others are troublesome and necessitate reduction in dosage or complete withdrawal of the drug. Side effects are generally dose dependent and reversible. Elderly patients are especially intolerant of large doses. The concurrent administration of levodopa and a peripheral inhibitor of dopa decarboxylase is the most effective means of decreasing the extracerebral side effects of levodopa (*see* below).

The most common side effects *early* in therapy with levodopa are nausea and vomiting. Cardiac arrhythmias occur in some patients, especially those with preexisting disturbances in cardiac conduction. The majority of patients on *long-term* therapy develop abnormal involuntary movements, which vary considerably in pattern and severity and often limit the tolerated dosage of levodopa. Levodopa produces psychiatric disturbances in a significant proportion of patients; these frequently limit the dose that can be tolerated. All side effects are reversible and can generally be controlled by a reduction in dosage.

Because of these potential side effects, it is important to exercise very special care in the administration of levodopa to patients with coronary insufficiency, cardiac arrhythmias, occlusive cerebrovascular disease, affective disorders, or major psychoses. Furthermore, abrupt withdrawal or reduction in dosage of levodopa may result in the appearance of a malignant neuroleptic-like syndrome, including elevated body temperature and muscular rigidity.

Gastrointestinal. About 80% of patients experience anorexia, nausea, vomiting, and/or epigastric distress early in the course of treatment with levodopa. These effects are caused partially by stimulation of the medullary emetic center and are more likely to occur if dosage is increased too rapidly, if individual doses are too large, or if the drug is taken without food. Anorexia may result in transient weight loss in some patients. These symptoms are controlled by concurrent administration of food, lowering of dosage, or concurrent administration of a "peripheral" inhibitor of dopa decarboxylase, which can dramatically reduce the incidence of gastrointestinal side effects of levodopa (*see* below). Although certain phenothiazines are highly effective antiemetic drugs, they should not be used for the control of nausea in this situation, since they interfere with the action of dopamine at striatal receptor sites. Gastrointestinal side effects tend to disappear with continuing therapy as tolerance develops. Supplementation of the regimen with an additional quantity of decarboxylase inhibitor or administration of domperidone (MOTILIUM, others), an antiemetic dopamine antagonist that does not cross the blood–brain barrier, may be effective if nausea persists. (Domperidone is not generally available in the United States.) Bleeding and perforation of peptic ulcers have been reported in a few patients.

Hypotension. About 30% of patients develop orthostatic hypotension early in therapy. It is usually asymptomatic, but some patients experience dizziness and, rarely, syncope. Careful regulation of dosage is necessary in such individuals, and the usual measures for controlling orthostatic hypotension should be employed. Despite continuation of therapy, blood pressure tends to return to values that obtained prior to treatment. The mechanism that underlies this effect remains unclear.

Cardiac Irregularities. Cardiac arrhythmias are not uncommon in the older-age group of patients with Parkinson's disease; consequently, a direct association between the development of an arrhythmia and therapy with levodopa is difficult to establish. However, the β-adrenergic action of dopamine on the heart, as well as direct β-adrenergic receptor stimulation by other catecholamine metabolites of the drug, presents a potentially serious side effect of levodopa. Fortunately, the incidence of arrhythmias is low, particularly in patients who are treated concurrently with a peripheral dopa decarboxylase inhibitor. Sinus tachycardia, atrial and ventricular extrasystoles, atrial flutter and fibrillation, and ventricular tachycardia have been reported. These cardiac arrhythmias, which are more likely to occur in patients with coronary artery disease, can usually be controlled by the administration of a β-adrenergic antagonist.

Abnormal Involuntary Movements. These movements appear in approximately 50% of patients within 2 to 4 months after the initiation of treatment with levodopa. Unfortunately, they often coincide temporally with what would otherwise be optimal improvement. They appear with increasing frequency as drug administration continues and are directly related to the dose of the drug and to the degree of clinical improvement. About 80% of patients on full therapeutic doses for a year or longer will develop some abnormal movements.

The abnormal involuntary movements are presumed to be due to "supersensitivity" of postsynaptic dopaminergic receptors (Lee *et al.*, 1978) and are variable in type. Buccolingual movements, grimacing, head bobbing, and various choreiform or dystonic movements of the arms, legs, or trunk can occur alone or in varying combinations. Rarely, exaggerated respiratory movements can produce an irregular gasping pattern or hyperventilation. Tolerance does not develop to this side effect; in fact, the symptoms tend to increase in severity if the dosage is not reduced. Although such movements are abolished by a decrease in the dose of levodopa, it is unfortunate that this maneuver reduces the therapeutic efficacy of levodopa as well (*see* below). Therefore, the physician must carefully titrate the dose and time of administration of levodopa to maximize the therapeutic benefit while minimizing side effects. These abnormal involuntary movements are the most important dose-limiting side effect of levodopa. No satisfactory means, pharmacological or otherwise, has been found to antagonize this side effect selectively.

Behavioral Disturbances. Levodopa can cause hallucinations, paranoia, mania, insomnia, anxiety, nightmares, and emotional depression, particularly in elderly patients. The actions of levodopa on the hypothalamus may cause renewed sexual interest, and this can cause additional behavioral changes.

Serious behavioral disturbances occur in about 15% of patients who receive levodopa and usually require reduction of dosage or, for some, complete withdrawal of the drug. One of the more common disturbances resembles an organic brain syndrome and is characterized by confusion, sometimes progressing to frank delirium. Although the mental depression of many patients is often improved by levodopa, some appear to develop a more severe depression, which in a few cases has led to suicidal gestures. Tricyclic antidepressant drugs have been helpful in some cases. Fully developed psychotic reactions with paranoid delusions or hallucinations are most likely to occur in patients with a history of mental disorder, organic brain syndrome including dementia, or postencephalitic parkinsonism. A few patients develop classical symptoms of hypomania, one manifestation of which may be inappropriate or excessive sexual behavior.

Inhibitors of Aromatic L-Amino Acid Decarboxylase. Concurrent administration of levodopa with an inhibitor of aromatic L-amino acid (dopa) decarboxylase that is unable to penetrate into the CNS greatly diminishes the decarboxylation of levodopa in peripheral tissues. Such reduction allows a greater proportion of levodopa to reach the desired receptor sites in the neostriatum. Concentrations of levodopa in plasma are higher and the half-life is longer after concurrent administration of a decarboxylase inhibitor and levodopa than when levodopa is given alone (Bianchine and Shaw, 1976; Nutt *et al.,* 1985). *Carbidopa* is the only such inhibitor that is clinically available in the United States, and it is supplied in combination with levodopa. *Benserazide* has similar properties and is marketed in Canada and elsewhere (Palfreyman *et al.,* 1978). Carbidopa has the following structure:

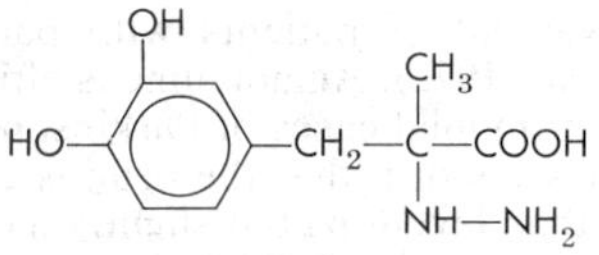

Carbidopa

Several clinical studies have clearly demonstrated distinct advantages of combined therapy with a decarboxylase inhibitor and levodopa. These may be summarized as follows: (1) The optimally effective dose of levodopa can be reduced by about 75%. (2) Nausea and vomiting from stimulation of dopaminergic receptors in the medullary emetic center are largely eliminated. Likewise, the cardiac side effects are diminished or prevented. (3) Effective dosage of levodopa can be achieved much more quickly during initial therapy since the necessity to develop tolerance to the peripheral effects of dopamine is minimized. (4) Antagonism of the therapeutic efficacy of levodopa by pyridoxine is avoided (*see* below). (5) The percentage of patients who are improved and the degree of improvement appear to be somewhat greater than with levodopa alone (Yahr, 1978; Calne, 1984).

However, problems of therapy arising from the CNS actions of levodopa are not resolved by the concomitant use of peripheral decarboxylase inhibitors. Abnormal involuntary movements not only occur with the same frequency but also tend to develop earlier in therapy and may be more severe. Adverse mental effects also occur with about the same frequency but appear earlier in the course of therapy.

Untoward Effects. In recommended doses the peripheral decarboxylase inhibitors that are currently employed are essentially devoid of obvious pharmacological activity when administered alone, and toxic effects have not been observed (Chase and Watanabe, 1972; Papavasiliou *et al.,* 1972). However, when administered in combination with levodopa, these drugs enhance, quantitatively, both the beneficial and the adverse effects of levodopa that are referable to the CNS.

Interactions of Levodopa and Levodopa–Decarboxylase Inhibitor Combinations with Other Drugs. Decarboxylation of levodopa to dopamine is catalyzed by the pyridoxine-dependent enzyme L-amino acid decarboxylase, and doses of pyridoxine that are only modestly in excess of the recommended dietary allowance enhance the extracerebral metabolism of levodopa. Consequently, when administered with levodopa, pyridoxine may completely reverse its therapeutic effect or promptly reduce its toxic side effects, depending on the clinical circumstances. Patients should be aware that pyridoxine is present in many multivitamin preparations in amounts in excess of 5 mg. A multivitamin preparation that does not contain pyridoxine is available. It is important to note that, when levodopa is coadministered with an inhibitor of L-amino acid decarboxylase, the interactive antagonistic effect of pyridoxine is lost (Yahr, 1975), since the inhibitor binds to the pyridoxal binding site on the enzyme.

Antipsychotic drugs, such as phenothiazines, butyrophenones, and reserpine, can produce a parkinsonism-like syndrome. Reserpine acts by depleting stores of central dopamine, while the other agents block receptors for dopamine. Since these drugs nullify the therapeutic effects of levodopa, they are contraindicated. This possible etiological drug factor should be considered in every newly diagnosed case of parkinsonism. If the exposure to these antipsychotic drugs was short, it is likely that their prompt withdrawal alone will cause disappearance of symptoms of parkinsonism. As previously mentioned, the phenothiazines should not be used to combat the emetic or behavioral side effects of levodopa.

Nonspecific monoamine oxidase inhibitors, such as phenelzine and isocarboxazid, interfere with inactivation of dopamine, norepinephrine, and other catecholamines. Hence, they exaggerate, unpredictably, the central effects of levodopa and its catecholamine metabolites; hypertensive crisis and hyperpyrexia are very real and dangerous sequelae of their administration with levodopa. An MAO inhibitor should be withdrawn at least 14 days prior to the administration of levodopa. It is interesting to note that selegiline (deprenyl), a selective inhibitor of monoamine oxidase B, has recently been released for use in the treatment of Parkinson's disease (*see* below).

Anticholinergic drugs, such as trihexyphenidyl, benztropine, procyclidine, and others, act synergistically with levodopa to improve certain symptoms of parkinsonism, especially tremor. However, large doses of anticholinergic drugs can slow gastric emptying sufficiently to cause a delay in the absorption of levodopa by the small bowel (Algeri *et al.,* 1976). This effect can be so pronounced as to detract from the therapeutic benefit of levodopa.

Preparations and Dosage. *Levodopa* (DOPAR, LARODOPA) is available for oral use as tablets or capsules containing 100, 250, or 500 mg of the drug. Fixed-dose combinations of levodopa and carbidopa are available in scored tablets that contain 10 or 25 mg of carbidopa in combination with 100 mg of levodopa (SINEMET 10/100 or 25/100) or that contain 25 mg of carbidopa and 250 mg of levodopa (SINEMET 25/250). SINEMET CR contains 200 mg of levodopa and 50 mg of carbidopa in a controlled-release matrix. Physicians can obtain carbidopa as a single agent (LODOSYN) upon request of the manufacturer for use in special patients who require a different ratio of carbidopa to levodopa than those available in these fixed-dose combinations.

In current practice, levodopa is almost always administered in combination with a peripheral inhibitor of dopa decarboxylase. However, in certain situations, levodopa is still administered alone, for example to patients who are extremely sensitive to the production of involuntary movements by even the smallest dose of a combined preparation. Levodopa may also be added to a regimen to titrate the dosage for patients who require slight modifications of therapy. Generally, treatment is initiated with three or four tablets (100 mg of levodopa, 25 mg of carbidopa) daily in divided doses. This provides an amount of carbidopa sufficient to inhibit peripheral dopa decarboxylase activity maximally in most patients. If a greater therapeutic effect is needed, the dose can be increased progressively to a daily maximum of about 2000 mg of levodopa and 200 mg of carbidopa. The optimal maintenance dosage is determined by careful titration in each patient. The controlled-release preparation is indicated for patients with advanced disease who experience fluctuations in therapeutic response and a short duration of effect from individual doses of the standard preparations (Cedarbaum, 1989). For patients treated previously with levodopa alone, dosage with levodopa must be withheld overnight (at least 8 hours) before starting the combination of levodopa and carbidopa. As a first approximation, the total daily dosage of levodopa must be reduced by approximately 75%.

AMANTADINE

Amantadine, introduced as an antiviral agent for the prophylaxis of A_2 influenza (*see* Chapter 51), was unexpectedly found to cause symptomatic improvement of patients with parkinsonism (Schwab *et al.,* 1972). Amantadine is efficacious as a single agent in mild cases of Parkinson's disease. Many studies confirm that the drug is clearly less efficacious than levodopa but slightly more so than the anticholinergic drugs (Mawdsley *et al.,* 1972). Amantadine acts maximally within a few days but often appears to lose a portion of its efficacy within 6 to 8 months of continuous treatment. Many patients who are obtaining near-maximal or waning benefits from levodopa generally experience some additional improvement from amantadine because of synergistic actions of the two drugs.

Amantadine is readily absorbed from the gastrointestinal tract and has a relatively long duration of action. It is excreted unchanged in the urine and, therefore, can accumulate in the body when renal function is inadequate.

Mechanism of Action. The precise mechanism of action of amantadine remains to be elucidated. The drug releases dopamine from peripheral neuronal storage sites of animals who have received infusions of the transmitters; this peripheral effect suggests that amantadine might exert a similar action on the residual, intact dopaminergic terminals in the striatum of parkinsonian patients. Amantadine causes release of dopamine from central neurons and facilitates its release by nerve impulses. Amantadine has also been shown to delay the reuptake of dopamine by neural cells, and it may have anticholinergic effects as well (*see* Lang, in Symposium, 1984).

Untoward Effects. Compared with levodopa or anticholinergic agents, amantadine is relatively free of side effects. When unwanted effects do occur, they are generally mild, often transient, and always reversible. Their incidence and severity increase markedly when the daily dose exceeds 200 mg. Hallucinations, confusion, and nightmares are more common when the drug is administered concurrently with anticholinergic agents or when the patient has an underlying cognitive impairment. Insomnia, dizziness, lethargy, drowsiness, and slurred speech have also been reported. Nausea, vomiting, anorexia, and constipation occur infrequently.

Long-term use of amantadine may result in the appearance of livedo reticularis in the lower extremities. Although this complication is often cosmetically unacceptable, it merely reflects the local release of catecholamines with resultant vasoconstriction.

Preparations and Dosage. *Amantadine hydrochloride* (SYMMETREL, SYMADINE) is available as 100-mg capsules and in a syrup containing 50 mg/5 ml. The usual dose is 100 mg, given twice daily.

DOPAMINERGIC AGONISTS

The efficacy of levodopa wanes over time in many patients with Parkinson's disease. Since the drug must be converted to dopamine in regions of a brain where the basic pathology involves loss of the capacity to perform that function, interest has turned to the development of directly acting dopaminergic agonists. Some of these compounds and their structural similarity to dopamine are illustrated in Figure 20–3. The first family of compounds to be investigated were the aporphines (apomorphine and N-propylnoraporphine). Interest was subsequently focused on a series of ergot derivatives—bromocriptine, lisuride, and pergolide. Most recently, a number of nonergot compounds that are highly selective for either D_1 or D_2 receptors have been investigated. The efficacy, if any, of these latter compounds in the management of Parkinson's disease remains to be determined.

APORPHINES

Apomorphine, commonly used as an emetic in

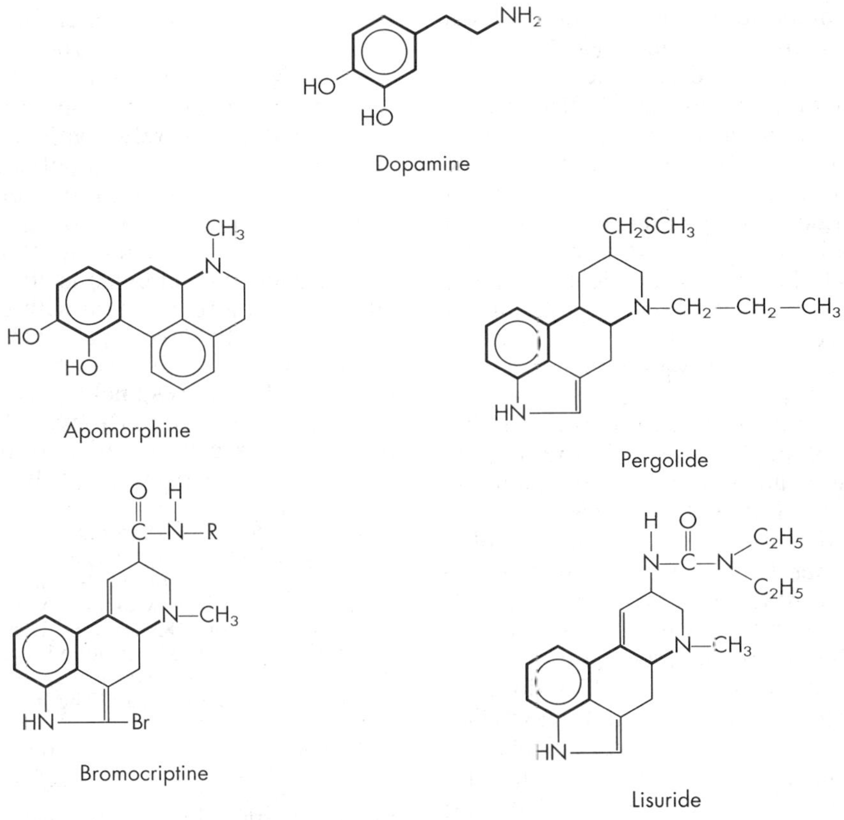

Figure 20–3. *Structural similarities (heavy lines) between dopamine, apomorphine, and selected ergolines.*

the management of oral ingestion of certain poisons or oral drug overdosage, was the first dopaminergic agonist reported to have beneficial effects in Parkinson's disease. Because of renal damage associated with the chronic administration of large doses of apomorphine, Cotzias and associates (1976) shifted their investigations to N-propylnoraporphine, an analog of apomorphine. Although this drug is clearly efficacious in the treatment of parkinsonism, nausea and vomiting are major impediments to its widespread use.

ERGOLINES

Several ergot derivatives demonstrate dopaminergic activity in animal models of parkinsonism and mimic the neuroendocrinological effects of dopamine on the secretion of prolactin and growth hormone. These derivatives include bromocriptine, lisuride, and pergolide. Despite the fact that the three drugs differ in their pharmacokinetic properties and their spectra of activities at the different populations of dopamine receptors, they appear to be very similar in clinical efficacy (LeWitt *et al.*, 1983). Bromocriptine has been studied most thoroughly and hence logically serves as a prototype for the ergolines. Its structure is shown in Figure 20–3. Bromocriptine is a derivative of lysergic acid (*see* Table 39–1, page 941). The addition of the bromine atom renders this alkaloid a potent dopaminergic agonist at D_2 receptors and an antagonist at D_1 sites (Markstein, 1981). Virtually all the pharmacological actions of bromocriptine result from stimulation of dopamine receptors in the CNS, cardiovascular system, pituitary-hypothalamic axis (Chapter 56), and gastrointestinal tract.

Bromocriptine has several roles in the treatment of parkinsonism. Currently, its main use is as an adjunct to levodopa in the management of patients with parkinsonism who experience excessive "on-off" phenomenon (*see* below) or who are not reasonably controlled with levodopa (LeWitt and Calne, 1981). In patients who are unable to tolerate levodopa because of excessive involuntary movements, high doses of bromocriptine (50 to 100 mg) may elicit therapeutic responses that are equivalent to those obtained with levodopa. Optimal clinical results, with a lessened tendency to produce involuntary movements, may be achieved by a combination of submaximal doses of bromocriptine and levodopa (Lieberman *et al.*, 1979). Poor control of symptoms toward the end of a dosage interval may also be minimized.

Bromocriptine is rapidly but only partially (about 30%) absorbed from the gastrointestinal tract (Burns and Calne, 1983). First-pass metabolism is extensive, such that systemic bioavailability is only a small fraction of the administered dose. Peak concentrations in plasma are found 1.5 to 3 hours after oral administration, and the half-life in plasma is about 3 hours. Many of the metabolites of bromocriptine have not been identified, but they do not appear to be active; most are excreted in the bile.

Adverse effects of bromocriptine are generally related to its activity as a dopaminergic agonist. Initial side effects include nausea, vomiting, and postural hypotension. Unlike the case with levodopa, bromocriptine may cause a "first-dose phenomenon," manifested by sudden cardiovascular collapse (Linch *et al.*, 1978); caution should also be exercised with patients who are taking antihypertensive medications. Visual and auditory hallucinations are more frequent with bromocriptine than with levodopa. Rarely, patients may develop inflammatory pleuropulmonary reactions or, even more rarely, erythromelalgia—a peculiar red, weepy skin eruption on the lower extremities. Symptomatic hypotension and cutaneous livedo reticularis are far more common with bromocriptine than with levodopa. Bromocriptine does, however, cause less dyskinesia than does levodopa, presumably because of its ability to stimulate D_2 receptors while blocking D_1 receptors. Alcohol intolerance and digital vasospasm may also be noted.

Bromocriptine mesylate (PARLODEL) is available in 2.5-mg tablets and 5-mg capsules. It is used as an adjunct to levodopa for the treatment of Parkinson's disease (with or without a peripheral decarboxylase inhibitor) (Keller and Daprada, 1979). The initial dose of bromocriptine is 1.25 mg, given twice daily with meals. This is increased every 2 to 4 weeks by 2.5 mg per day. The maximal dose is 100 mg per day.

Bromocriptine is also indicated for the therapy of hyperprolactinemia in a variety of clinical situations, including lactation, infertility, and amenorrhea-galactorrhea. In addition, it has been used as an adjunctive agent in the treatment of pituitary tumors associated with hyperprolactinemia or acromegaly (*see* Chapter 56). The initial dose of bromocriptine in the therapy of hyperprolactinemia is 1.25 to 2.5 mg, and most patients respond to a total daily dose of 5 to 7.5 mg. The uses of bromocriptine has been reviewed by Vance and associates (1984).

In contrast to bromocriptine, pergolide (*see* Figure 20–3) stimulates both D_2 and, to a lesser extent, D_1 receptors; it is among the most potent dopaminergic agonists (Goldstein *et al.*, 1980). Pergolide is as effective as bromocriptine in relieving parkinsonian signs and symptoms, but in a dose range of 0.1 to 7 mg per day (LeWitt *et al.*, 1983). Although a single dose of pergolide depresses prolactin secretion for over 36 hours, the duration of its antiparkinsonian action is much shorter, and most patients require two or three daily doses. Pergolide has less tendency to cause nausea and orthostatic hypotension than does bromocriptine. Pergolide may be efficacious in patients who have lost responsiveness to bromocriptine and vice versa.

Pergolide mesylate (PERMAX) is available as scored tablets that contain 0.25, 0.5, or 1.0 mg. Dosing is initiated with one half of a 0.25-mg tablet twice daily. As with bromocriptine, slow upward titration of the dose of pergolide with concomitant downward adjustment of the dose of levodopa is required.

Lisuride (*see* Figure 20–3), like bromocriptine, is a D_2 agonist and a D_1 antagonist. In addition, lisuride stimulates receptors for 5-HT, which may account for its increased capacity to cause hallucinations and other mental side effects. Because of its water solubility, lisuride may find a role in the management of patients with parkinsonism who are unable to take oral medications (*e.g.*, following major surgery); it may also be given as a chronic infusion (*see* Parkes *et al.*, 1981; Obeso *et al.*, 1986). Neither pergolide nor lisuride is generally available in the United States.

SELEGILINE

There are two isoenzymes that oxidize monoamines. While both isoenzymes (monoamine oxidase [MAO] A and B) are present in the periphery and inactivate monoamines of intestinal origin, the isoenzyme MAO-B predominates in certain regions of the CNS (*see* Chapter 18). Selegiline (deprenyl; phenylisopropyl-N-methylpropynylamine) is a highly selective inhibitor of MAO-B (Knoll, 1983; Riederer *et al.*, 1983). In striking contrast to the known nonspecific MAO inhibitors (*e.g.*, phenelzine and isocarboxazid), selegiline (at a dose of 5 to 10 mg per day) does not cause profound and potentially lethal potentiation of the effects of catecholamines when administered concurrently with an indirectly acting sympathomimetic amine. For example, a patient receiving selegiline may eat cheeses that contain tyramine or take levodopa without danger. However, administration of selegiline does inhibit the intracerebral metabolic degradation of dopamine. The resultant preservation of dopamine in the basal ganglia appears to enhance the therapeutic efficacy of levodopa. Consequently, when selegiline is added to the therapeutic regimen, the dose of levodopa can be reduced and the interval between doses lengthened without loss of therapeutic benefit. Although clinical trials with this compound indicate beneficial effects, the improvement may be poorly sustained (Yahr *et al.*, 1983; Golbe *et al.*, 1988). The drug is of limited value in patients with advanced disease.

Selegiline can prevent the appearance of MPTP-induced parkinsonism in experimental animals (*see* above); this effect results from inhibition of the conversion of MPTP to the putative toxic metabolite (1-methyl-4-phenylpyridinium ion) by MAO-B. These observations have led to speculation that selegiline might alter the progression of idiopathic Parkinson's disease by reducing the generation of potentially neurotoxic substances from either endogenous or exogenous compounds. In a recent study that involved a relatively small number of patients with early, previously untreated Parkinson's disease, the administration of selegiline postponed the need to initiate therapy with levodopa by about 8 months (Tetrud and Langston, 1989). Although encouraging, it is not clear whether these results reflect slowing of the degeneration of nigral dopaminergic neurons or represent only symptomatic treatment of early stages of the disease.

Selegiline hydrochloride (ELDEPRYL) is available in 5-mg tablets. The recommended dosage is 5 mg taken twice daily; daily doses of more than 10 mg usually do not provide additional benefit and substantially increase the risk of interaction with sympathomimetic amines or dietary tyramine. After 2 to 3 days, the dosage of levodopa/carbidopa (if given concurrently) can be gradually reduced, generally by 10 to 30%; further reduction is indicated if dopaminergic side effects appear or intensify (*e.g.*, dyskinesias, hallucinations).

ANTICHOLINERGIC DRUGS

Anticholinergic agents were the most effective drugs for treatment of Parkinson's disease for more than a century. However, the introduction of levodopa and decarboxylase inhibitors has relegated anticholinergics to a supportive role in the treatment of the disorder. Nonetheless, the anticholinergic drugs are still useful for patients with minimal symptoms, for those unable to tolerate levodopa because of side effects or contraindications, and for those who are not benefited by levodopa. Furthermore, more than half the patients who derive therapeutic benefit from levodopa experience further amelioration of symptoms after supplemental treatment with an anticholinergic drug. These drugs are also useful to alleviate the parkinsonian syndrome induced by antipsychotic drugs.

The deficiency of dopamine in the striatum of patients with parkinsonism intensifies the excitatory effects of the cholinergic system within the striatum. Anticholinergics aid such patients by blunting this component of the nigrostriatal pathway (Calne, 1978).

Pharmacological Effects. Trihexyphenidyl, the prototype of this group of drugs, is a muscarinic antagonist that qualitatively resembles the belladonna alkaloids in its pharmacological actions and side effects (*see* Chapter 8). Although it is widely believed that trihexyphenidyl and other antimuscarinic agents most favorably influence parkinsonian tremor and are less effective in improving rigidity and bradykinesia, all symptoms are relieved to a comparable extent. However, trihexyphenidyl is much less effective than levodopa. Among the secondary symptoms of parkinsonism, the anticholinergic agents improve excessive sialorrhea by inhibiting salivary secretion. Although the peripheral anticholinergic actions of the synthetic compounds selected for use in Parkinson's disease are less prominent than are those of the natural antimuscarinic alkaloids such as atropine, side effects of cycloplegia, constipation, and urinary retention may become troublesome, especially for the aged patient. Mental confusion, delirium, somnolence, and hallucinations also may limit the utility of these drugs. Although there are essentially no pharmacological differences among the anticholinergic agents commonly used in parkinsonism, certain patients clearly appear to tolerate one preparation better than another.

The anticholinergic drugs used for the treatment of Parkinson's disease are listed in Table 20–1, as is the antihistamine diphenhydramine; the latter drug possesses some central anticholinergic properties, which are probably the basis of its salutary effect in parkinsonism. Diphenhydramine is well tolerated, especially by elderly patients, but it is not as efficacious as are the anticholinergic agents. Its sedative effect may be helpful in certain patients.

Pharmacokinetic Properties of Anticholinergic Antiparkinsonian Drugs. There is surprisingly little information on the pharmacokinetic properties of these anticholinergic drugs. For trihexyphenidyl, procyclidine, and biperiden, peak concentrations in plasma are reached between 1 and 2 hours after an oral dose, and terminal elimination half-lives are between 10 and 12 hours (*see* Cedarbaum, 1987). Comparable data are not available for benztropine and ethopropazine. For those drugs for which information is available, it appears that twice-daily dosing should be appropriate for most patients, although in clinical practice more frequent dosing is often employed. Little is known of the pathways for metabolism and elimination of these drugs.

Preparations and Dosage. Patients should be started at the lower end of the range of daily doses listed in Table 20–1; this amount should be divided into two to four equal portions. Dosage should then be gradually increased until maximal improvement is seen or, more likely, until the onset of intolerable side effects. It is especially important to tailor the medication to achieve the optimal balance between control of the disabling symptoms and the adverse reactions to the drugs. The optimal dose of a given drug for a particular individual cannot be stated. In general, elderly patients are less able to tolerate large doses of the drugs than are young patients. The drugs with prominent peripheral anticholinergic effects must be used with great caution in individuals suffering from narrow-angle glaucoma or urinary retention secondary to disorders of the prostate.

THERAPEUTIC USES OF DRUGS FOR PARKINSON'S DISEASE

Many aspects of the clinical use of levodopa, the combination of levodopa and carbidopa, and other dopaminergic drugs have been described in the preceding pages. The combination of levodopa with a decarboxylase inhibitor is now the most effective preparation available for treatment of Parkinson's disease (Calne, 1984). A major controversy in the treatment of Parkinson's disease centers around the timing of initiation of treatment with levodopa. Some favor delaying such therapy, since there is evidence that relates drug-induced dyskinesias and fluctuations of response ("on-off" phenomenon) to the duration of therapy with levodopa (Lesser *et al.*, 1979; Fahn and Bressman, 1984). However, a number of investigators have concluded that drug-induced dyskinesias and fluctuations of response are a manifestation of the progression of the underlying disease rather than of the duration of levodopa therapy (Blin *et al.*, 1988). Recent evidence also suggests that there is less excess mortality and a slower progression of the severity of

Table 20–1. MISCELLANEOUS DRUGS FOR PARKINSONISM

DRUG CLASS, NONPROPRIETARY NAME, AND TRADE NAME	CHEMICAL STRUCTURE	DOSAGE FORMS *	RANGE OF AVERAGE DAILY DOSE
Anticholinergic Agents			
Benztropine mesylate (COGENTIN)	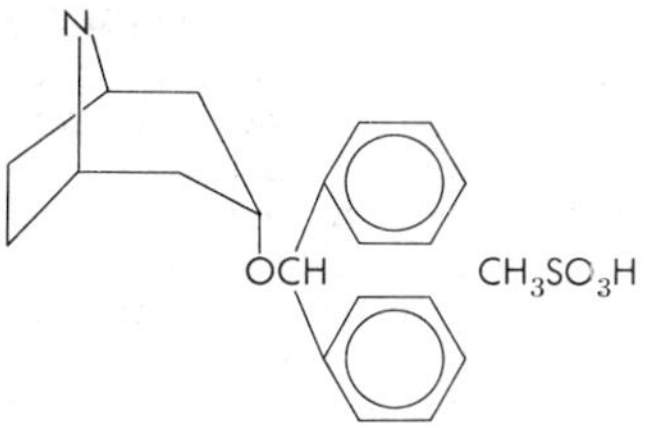	T, I	0.5–6 mg
Trihexyphenidyl hydrochloride (ARTANE, others)	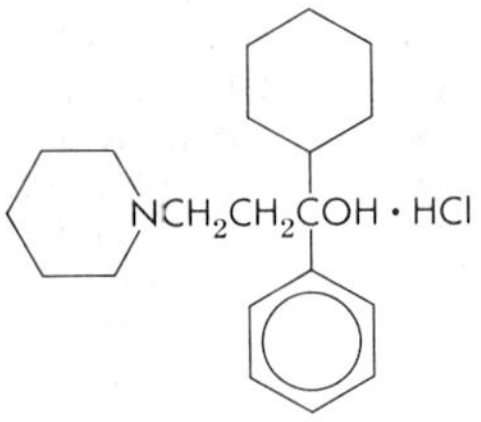	T, C(S), E	1–15 mg
Procyclidine hydrochloride (KEMADRIN)	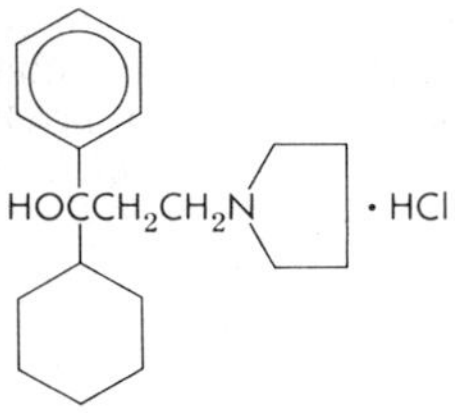	T	7.5–20 mg
Biperiden hydrochloride (AKINETON)	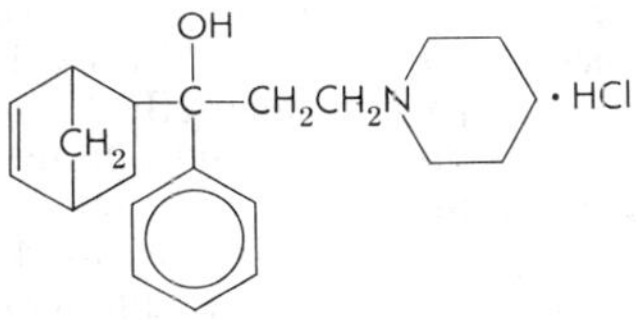	T, I †	2–8 mg
Ethopropazine hydrochloride ‡ (PARSIDOL)	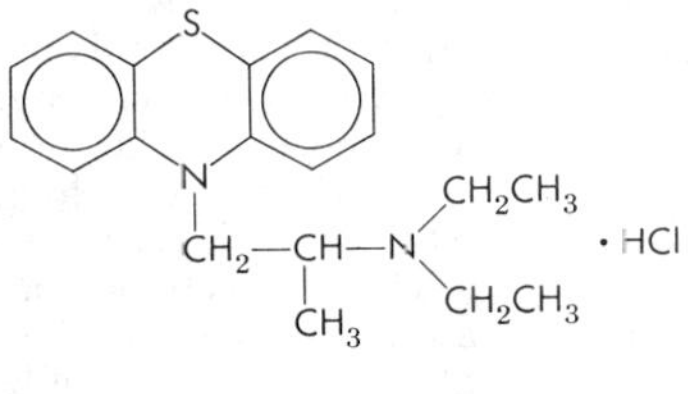	T	50–600 mg
Antihistamine			
Diphenhydramine hydrochloride (BENADRYL, others)	*See* Chapter 23	C, T, E, S, I	75–400 mg

* T = tablet; I = injection; C(S) = sustained-release capsule; E = elixir; C = capsule; S = syrup.
† As biperiden lactate.
‡ Ethopropazine is a phenothiazine with significant anticholinergic activity.

symptoms when treatment with levodopa is initiated relatively soon after Parkinson's disease is diagnosed (Hoehn, 1983; Diamond *et al.*, 1987). This obviously supports the view that treatment with levodopa should be initiated early in the course of the illness (Markham and Diamond, 1981; Muenter, 1984).

Yahr (1978) distinguished two phases of treatment with levodopa. First is an initial induction phase that lasts several weeks, followed by a long-term maintenance phase. During the induction phase, the daily dosage of levodopa is increased slowly to minimize the likelihood of side effects such as insomnia, nausea, and anorexia. *One critical factor in successful therapy during this phase is the careful and slow titration of dosage for each patient.* Too rapid an increase in dosage may result in a therapeutic failure because of side effects and toxicity. The full benefits of treatment with levodopa become apparent during the maintenance phase, where smooth, day-long control of parkinsonism is often achieved with three or four daily doses of levodopa plus carbidopa. However, some time between 2 and 5 years after the initiation of therapy, a variety of problems begin to emerge. First are often dyskinesias, or abnormal involuntary movements and fluctuation in motor performance (Fahn, 1981; Marsden *et al*, 1981).

Dyskinesias, which may be choreic, athetoid, or dystonic in form, are thought to be due to "supersensitivity" of striatal dopamine receptors, which, in turn, may be due to denervation (loss of normal dopaminergic input) (Lee *et al.*, 1978). At about this time, the patient may become aware of the presence of parkinsonian symptoms upon arising in the morning that are relieved within 30 to 60 minutes of taking the first dose of the day of levodopa. Attempts to eliminate dyskinesias by reducing the dosage of levodopa result in a briefer therapeutic response per dose—the so-called "short-duration response." The dyskinesias superimpose themselves upon the waxing and waning of the response cycle, usually occurring at the peak of the therapeutic effect ("peak-dose" dyskinesia). However, as time goes on patients may become unable to achieve any degree of mobility without experiencing some degree of involuntary movement. Ten to fifteen percent of patients, rather than having peak-dose dyskinesia, will experience a burst of involuntary (usually dystonic) movement at the beginning and end of each dose cycle, with a period of relatively good motor function in between (the diphasic dyskinesia or dystonia-improvement-dystonia syndrome) (Muenter *et al.*, 1977). Dietary factors and erratic gastric emptying may further complicate the picture, making the response to levodopa seem random and totally unrelated temporally to ingestion of the drug (the "random on-off" or "yo-yo" phenomenon). Often at this stage the patient may switch within seconds from a state of relatively good mobility to one of severe parkinsonism, giving rise to the term "on-off" phenomenon. Such fluctuations in therapeutic response afflict more than 50% of parkinsonian patients treated for 5 years or more with levodopa or levodopa/decarboxylase inhibitor combinations. With increasing duration of treatment (and of the underlying disease), the figure may approach 90% (Cedarbaum and McDowell, 1986).

Fluctuating motor performance in levodopa-treated parkinsonian patients can, to at least a certain extent, be explained by the pharmacokinetics of levodopa itself (*see* reviews by Nutt and Fellman, 1984, and by Cedarbaum, 1987). Most patients have a threshold concentration of levodopa in plasma above which antiparkinsonian effects are apparent (Marion *et al.*, 1986); this presumably reflects the provision of adequate amounts of dopamine in the brain. In patients with early and mild disease, there is apparently a sufficient reserve of dopamine synthetic and storage capacity to maintain adequate concentrations of the neurotransmitter despite relatively infrequent dosing with levodopa. Thus, plasma concentrations of levodopa may fall to below threshold levels without adverse consequences. However, as degeneration of the nigrostriatal tract progresses, the capacity of the system to synthesize and, particularly, to store dopamine becomes progressively compromised. At a certain point, the brain becomes dependent on a moment-to-moment basis upon levodopa in the plasma to provide a substrate for dopamine synthesis, and fluctuations in motor performance appear (Spencer and Wooten, 1984). Thus, Chase and coworkers elegantly demonstrated that the duration of the beneficial effects of levodopa shortens progressively with increasing severity of motor fluctuations, despite the fact that the elimination half-life of levodopa is relatively uniform among parkinsonian patients (Fabbrini *et al.*, 1987). The same investigators have also demonstrated that continuous intravenous infusion of levodopa increases the threshold concentration of levodopa in plasma for the production of dyskinesias relative to the threshold for producing antiparkinsonian effects (Mouradian *et al.*, 1988). This finding suggests that fluctuations in the concentrations of dopamine may facilitate the development of the receptor supersensitivity that is presumed to underlie the generation of levodopa-induced involuntary movements.

In studying the pharmacodynamics of levodopa, Nutt and Woodward (1986) observed that the antiparkinsonian effect appeared to be all-or-nothing; that is, beyond a certain concentration of levodopa in plasma, only the duration, but not the magnitude, of the antiparkinsonian effect increased. However, the severity of dyskinesias does increase with increasing concentrations of levodopa. In practical terms, this means that reducing the dose of levodopa to avoid dyskinesia will invariably lead to a shortened duration of antiparkinsonian effect and perhaps, in the long run, to increased susceptibility to dyskinesias themselves.

The management of motor fluctuations centers around maneuvers designed to prolong the action of individual doses of levodopa. Controlled-release preparations represent attempts to prolong the absorptive phase of drug administration, thereby smoothing the concentration–time curve. The rationale for the concurrent administration of levodopa and selegiline is to achieve the same effect by inhibiting degradation of dopamine in the brain. The dopaminergic agonists bromocriptine and pergolide have longer elimination half-lives than does levodopa; replacing a portion of a patient's requirement for levodopa with one of these drugs may "fill in the gap" in the levodopa dose cycle.

Sweet and McDowell (1975) and Cedarbaum and McDowell (1986) reviewed the outcome of 100 patients 5 and 16 years after starting levodopa. The adjusted death rate among patients receiving levodopa was less at 5 years but by 16 years again approached that of the prelevodopa era. The average "functional" status of the patients approached pretreatment levels after 5 years, and by 16 years all surviving patients were functioning less well than they did at the time of initiation of therapy. Thus, while levodopa does not cure Parkinson's disease, it does provide symptomatic relief for a long time and remains the most effective treatment available for this illness. It makes possible a more self-sufficient existence for a longer time than was possible before the drug became available.

Drug-Induced Parkinsonism. Parkinsonism, acute dyskinesia, and dystonias that are induced by the phenothiazines and other antipsychotic agents usually respond readily to low doses of anticholinergic drugs. There is some controversy over whether anticholinergic agents should be administered routinely upon the initiation of long-term treatment with antipsychotic drugs in an attempt to prevent or delay the appearance of these symptoms of parkinsonism (*see* Chapter 18).

Miscellaneous Uses of Drugs for Parkinson's Disease. The efficacy of levodopa in Parkinson's disease has prompted clinical trials of the drug for a number of other neurological conditions characterized by disordered extrapyramidal function, such as torsion dystonia, cerebral palsy, and progressive supranuclear palsy. The results have been unimpressive. Levodopa has not been found to be useful for the treatment of any psychiatric disorder; in fact, the drug tends to exacerbate latent or active psychotic states, both organic and functional. In addition, dopaminergic agents are not useful in controlling or reversing the extrapyramidal side effects induced by antipsychotic drugs such as the phenothiazines and butyrophenones, since the latter agents presumably block the activation of dopaminergic receptors.

II. Drug Therapy of Spasticity and Acute Muscle Spasms

Spasticity. Spasticity is not a single disorder. The term is applied relatively globally to abnormalities of regulation of skeletal muscle tone that result from lesions of the descending motor pathways at various levels in the CNS. A predominant component of such conditions is hyperexcitability of tonic stretch reflexes. Tendon jerks are exaggerated, painful flexor spasms may occur, and muscle weakness and a loss of dexterity almost always occur.

The pathophysiology of spasticity is poorly understood but usually appears to include dysfunction of descending pathways (*e.g.*, corticospinal, vestibulospinal, reticulospinal) that exert control over the motoneurons. Disease is rarely limited to the primary corticospinal (pyramidal) tract. The peripheral reflex arcs, although hyperactive because of abnormal control from higher centers, do not appear to be primarily involved in the pathological process. Nevertheless, sites in these arcs, which include afferent fibers from the skin and muscle spindles, interneurons within the spinal cord, and efferent fibers to intrafusal and extrafusal muscle fibers, may be targets for pharmacological intervention to control spasticity. The most effective agents for control of spasticity include two that act predominantly within the CNS, baclofen and diazepam, and one, dantrolene, that acts directly on skeletal muscle. An excellent review of the drug therapy of spasticity has been written by Young and Delwaide (1981).

BACLOFEN

Baclofen is a derivative of the inhibitory neurotransmitter gamma-aminobutyric acid (GABA), and experimentation on its mechanism of action has been guided by this fact. Its structural formula is as follows:

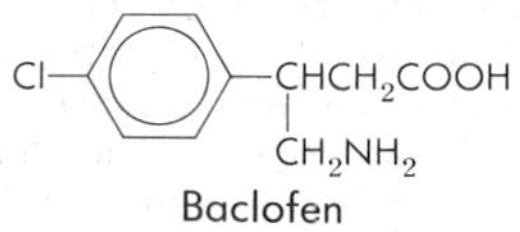

Baclofen

Baclofen is particularly useful in reducing the frequency and severity of flexor or extensor spasms and reducing increased flexor tone. Since it is effective in patients with complete spinal transections, its primary site of action appears to be in the spinal cord.

Baclofen is believed to exert its antispastic effects by depressing monosynaptic and polysynaptic transmission in the spinal cord. The drug reduces excitatory postsynaptic potentials in motoneurons in the ventral horn without affecting their membrane potential or input resistance (Fukuda *et al.*, 1977). These effects superficially resemble those of GABA, which is released by interneurons in the spinal cord and depolarizes the axonal terminals of primary afferent fibers; this results in presynaptic inhibition of motoneurons. While bicuculline blocks these actions of GABA, the effects of baclofen are not so antagonized.

Baclofen does not cause depolarization of primary afferent nerve terminals, but it does appear to cause a decrease in the release of excitatory transmitters onto motor neurons by increasing the threshold for excitation of primary afferent terminals in the spinal cord (Yu *et al.*, 1987). While the underlying mechanisms are not clearly understood, observations of neurons in various regions of the CNS suggest that baclofen can hyperpolarize some cells by increasing K^+ conductance (Newberry and Nicoll, 1984) and can inhibit the function of Ca^{2+} channels in others (Dolphin and Scott, 1986). One or both of these actions could contribute to decreased release of excitatory transmitters from primary afferent terminals. For example, baclofen blocks a voltage-dependent inward Ca^{2+} current in cultured sensory neurons from dorsal root ganglia of the rat. At higher concentrations, it augments a slow, Ca^{2+}-dependent outward K^+ current (Dolphin and Scott, 1986); this results in a shortening of Ca^{2+}-mediated spikes in axon terminals and a reduction of release of the putative excitatory transmitters glutamate and aspartate. There is no evidence that baclofen can increase chloride conductance, the most prominent action of GABA. Since both GABA and baclofen can produce similar bicuculline-insensitive effects under some circumstances, two classes of receptors for GABA (GABA-A and GABA-B) have been proposed. This hypothesis is supported by the demonstration of stereospecific binding sites for *l*-baclofen; such binding is inhibited by GABA but not by bicuculline or many GABA-mimetic compounds (Bowery *et al.*, 1980). Thus, baclofen may act as an agonist at GABA-B (bicuculline-insensitive) receptors. Presynaptic GABA-B receptors, capable of inhibiting release of a variety of neurotransmitters, have been found in many areas of the CNS. In the spinal cord they appear to be concentrated in laminae I to IV of the dorsal horn, the region of major termination of afferent sensory fibers (Price *et al.*, 1984).

Baclofen is absorbed rapidly after oral administration, and it has a half-life in plasma of about 3 to 4 hours. It is largely excreted unchanged by the kidney. The use of baclofen may be limited by its adverse effects, which include drowsiness, insomnia, dizziness, weakness, ataxia, and mental confusion. The drug is poorly tolerated by elderly individuals. Sudden withdrawal of baclofen after long-term administration may cause auditory and visual hallucinations, anxiety, and tachycardia. Coma, respiratory depression, and seizures have been reported following significant overdosage. The threshold for initiation of seizures may be lower in patients with epilepsy.

Preparations and Dosage. *Baclofen* (LIORESAL) is available in 10- and 20-mg tablets. Determination of optimal dosage in individual patients requires careful titration. Treatment is initiated with an oral dosage of 5 mg twice daily; the dosage is escalated as required at 3-day intervals until the maximal dosage (20 mg four times daily) is reached. Occasionally, total doses of 100 to 150 mg per day may be beneficial. Abrupt withdrawal of the drug should be avoided. Baclofen should be administered cautiously and in decreased dosage to patients with impaired renal function.

Intrathecal infusion of baclofen is currently under investigation for the long-term treatment of patients whose spasticity is not adequately controlled by oral administration of the drug. In one preliminary study of severely affected patients with either spinal cord injuries or multiple sclerosis, delivery of baclofen into the lumbar subarachnoid space was achieved with a surgically implanted pump (Penn *et al.*, 1989). Marked improvement of symptoms was maintained over a period of 1 to 3 years by the administration of doses of baclofen that averaged 340 μg per day; drowsiness and confusion were not evident.

Therapeutic Uses. Baclofen is most effective in the treatment of spasticity caused by multiple sclerosis or other diseases of the spinal cord, particularly traumatic lesions. Baclofen is also occasionally useful in patients with focal dystonic movements, including torticollis (wry neck) and Miege's syndrome (blepharospasm/oromandibular dystonia). Similar to other muscle relaxants, it may impair the patient's ability to walk or stand. It is not recommended for the management of the spasticity that occurs following stroke or other cerebral lesions (Young and Delwaide, 1981).

DIAZEPAM

Diazepam and the other benzodiazepines are discussed in detail in Chapters 17 and 18. The presumed mechanism of action of the benzodiazepines is to enhance the efficiency of GABA-ergic transmission, as discussed in Chapter 17. At the level of the spinal cord, this action may be manifest by enhancement of presynaptic inhibition of afferent neuronal terminals in the primary reflex arc. Diazepam is particularly useful for treatment of patients with spinal cord lesions, although it is probably not as effective as baclofen in relieving intermittent flexor spasms (Young and Delwaide, 1981). The drug may occasionally be useful in patients with cerebral palsy. Sedation can limit the efficacy of diazepam as a muscle relaxant, although its sedative and anxiolytic properties may be of value in certain patients (Lossius *et al.*, 1980). The dose of diazepam should be titrated upward gradually to minimize unwanted effects, particularly sedation.

DANTROLENE

Dantrolene is unique in comparison with baclofen and diazepam in that it exerts its effects by direct actions on skeletal muscle (Van Winkle, 1976; Davidoff, 1978). Dantrolene has the following chemical structure:

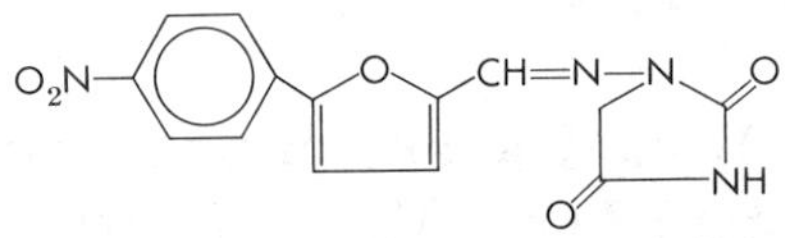

Dantrolene

Pharmacological Properties. Dantrolene reduces contraction of skeletal muscle by a direct action on excitation-contraction coupling, apparently by decreasing the amount of Ca^{2+} released from the sarcoplasmic reticulum (Van Winkle, 1976). Although the drug does depress the CNS, it does not appear to produce antispastic effects by actions on neurons. Dantrolene diminishes the force of electrically induced twitches in man without altering muscle action potentials, and it reduces reflex more than voluntary contraction (Herman *et al.*, 1972). The latter effect appears to be due to preferential actions on "fast" as compared with "slow" skeletal muscle fibers. Dantrolene does not affect neuromuscular transmission, nor does it change the electrical properties of skeletal muscle membranes (Davidoff, 1978).

In patients with upper motoneuron lesions, spasticity is generally diminished by treatment with dantrolene, and functional capacity is often improved. Unfortunately, the drug also tends to cause a generalized muscle weakness that negates functional improvement.

Absorption of dantrolene from the gastrointestinal tract is slow and incomplete but sufficiently consistent to provide dose-related concentrations in plasma. The mean half-life of the drug in adults is about 9 hours after a 100-mg dose. It is slowly metabolized by the liver, and the 5-hydroxy and acetamido metabolites are excreted with unchanged drug in the urine.

Untoward Effects and Precautions. Dantrolene has a serious potential to cause hepatotoxicity. Fatal hepatitis has been reported in approximately 0.1 to 0.2% of patients treated with the drug for 60 days or longer. Symptomatic hepatitis may occur in 0.5% of patients treated with dantrolene for more than 60 days, while chemical abnormalities of hepatic function are noted in up to 1%. In view of this potential for hepatic injury, long-term administration of dantrolene should be halted if clear benefits are not evident within 45 days, and hepatic function should be monitored. The most common major side effect of dantrolene is weakness, an extension of its effect on skeletal muscle. Although weakness may be transient or mild, its persistence in some ambulatory patients may compromise therapeutic benefit. Euphoria, lightheadedness, dizziness, drowsiness, and fatigue often occur early in treatment, but these side effects are generally transient; nevertheless, patients should be cautioned against driving or participating in hazardous activities. Although the diarrhea that occurs in some patients can usually be controlled by a more gradual increase in dosage, it may necessitate withdrawal of the drug.

Preparations and Dosage. *Dantrolene sodium* (DANTRIUM) is available for oral use in capsules containing 25, 50, or 100 mg of the drug. The starting dose of 25 mg once a day is gradually increased in increments of 25 mg every 4 to 7 days to a maximal dose of 400 mg daily, given in four divided doses. For children, the recommended starting dose of 0.5 mg/kg twice a day is gradually increased to a maximum of 3 mg/kg four times a day, but not to exceed 400 mg daily. Dantrolene is also available for intravenous administration.

Therapeutic Uses. Dantrolene can relieve spasticity, but the weakness it produces may handicap the patient more than the spasticity it relieves. In view of its mechanism of action, it would appear to make little difference as to the cause of the spasticity. Dantrolene provides significant and sustained reduction of spasticity and improves functional capacity for many paraplegic and hemiplegic patients; it reduces clonus, mass-reflex movements, and abnormal resistance to passive stretch. About one half of patients with athetoid cerebral palsy and a smaller fraction of those with multiple sclerosis are also sufficiently improved to warrant continued treatment. Because of the muscle weakness caused by dantrolene, its major utility is in nonambulatory patients whose nursing care is made difficult by muscle contraction and for whom relief of spasticity warrants the risk of hepatotoxicity (Pinder *et al.*, 1977; Davidoff, 1978; Young and Delwaide, 1981).

Dantrolene plays a unique role in the management of the malignant hyperthermia syndrome. This rare, dominantly inherited syndrome is usually precipitated by the administration of neuromuscular blocking agents or inhalational anesthetics during surgery (*see* Chapter 9). Vigorous contraction of skeletal muscle apparently occurs as a result of excessive release of Ca^{2+} from the sarcoplasmic reticulum, leading to a rapid and dangerous rise in body temperature, rhabdomyolysis, and renal failure. Dantrolene should be administered intravenously as soon as the syndrome of malignant hyperthermia is recognized; the initial dose is 1 mg/kg, repeated as necessary to a total of 10 mg/kg. Supportive measures are also important. These include discontinuation of anesthetics, administration of oxygen, management of acidosis and fever, and attention to urine output and water and electrolyte balance. Oral administration of dantrolene (1 to 2 mg/kg four times a day) may be necessary for 1 to 3 days to prevent recurrence of the condition. Dantrolene may be given prophylactically (prior to surgery) to patients who are judged to be susceptible to this syndrome. Dantrolene has also been used for the treatment of neuroleptic malignant syndrome.

THERAPEUTIC STATUS

No completely satisfactory form of therapy is available for alleviation of skeletal muscle spasticity (Davidoff, 1978; Young and Delwaide, 1981). Although drugs such as baclofen, diazepam, and dantrolene are capable of providing variable relief of spasticity in given circumstances, troublesome muscle weakness, adverse effects on gait, and a variety of other side effects minimize their overall usefulness. These drugs may temporarily abate some of the symptoms of cerebral palsy, but they have a minor role in the overall management of this disorder. Muscle relaxants are of little value in Parkinson's disease or in other dysfunctions resulting from diseases of the brain.

DRUG THERAPY OF ACUTE MUSCLE SPASMS

A variety of conditions (*e.g.*, trauma, inflammation, anxiety, and pain) can be associated with acute muscle spasms. Several drugs have been employed in attempts to alleviate such spasms, including *carisoprodol* (SOMA, others), *metaxalone* (SKELAXIN), and *cyclobenzaprine hydrochloride* (FLEXERIL). The efficacy of these compounds is difficult to assess because of the lack of well-controlled clinical studies. It is not clear that these agents offer any advantage over diazepam, sedatives, or analgesics. While some of these drugs have been vaguely characterized as interneuronal blocking agents, their limited efficacy may be due solely to general depression of the CNS. The pharmacological properties of these drugs are described in *earlier editions* of this textbook (*see also* Elenbaas, 1980). Such agents are not useful in the treatment of spasticity associated with chronic neurological disease.

Algeri, S.; Cerletti, C.; Curclo, M.; Morselli, P. L.; Bonollo, L.; Buniva, G.; Minazzi, M.; and Minoli, G. Effect of anticholinergic drugs on gastro-intestinal absorption of L-dopa in rats and in man. *Eur. J. Pharmacol.*, **1976**, *35*, 293–299.

Barone, P.; Davis, T. A.; Braun, A. R.; and Chase, T. N. Dopaminergic mechanisms and motor function: characterization of D-1 and D-2 dopamine receptor interactions. *Eur. J. Pharmacol.*, **1986**, *123*, 109–114.

Bertler, A., and Rosengren, E. Occurrence and distribution of dopamine in brain and other tissues. *Experientia*, **1959**, *15*, 10–11.

Blin, J.; Bonnet, A.-M.; and Agid, Y. Does levodopa aggravate Parkinson's disease? *Neurology*, **1988**, *38*, 1410–1416.

Blume, E. Street drugs yield Parkinson's model. *J.A.M.A.*, **1983**, *250*, 13–14.

Bowery, N. G.; Hill, D. R.; Hudson, A. I.; Doble, A.; Middlemiss, D. N.; Shaw, J.; and Turnbull, M. (−)Baclofen decreases neurotransmitter release in mammalian CNS by an action at a novel GABA receptor. *Nature*, **1980**, *283*, 92–94.

Boyson, S. J.; McGonigle, P.; and Molinoff, P. B. Quantitative autoradiographic localization of the D1 and D2 subtypes of dopamine receptors in brain. *J. Neurosci.*, **1986**, *6*, 3177–3188.

Burns, R. S., and Calne, D. B. Disposition of dopaminergic ergot compounds following oral administration. In, *Lisuride and Other Dopaminomimetics*. (Calne, D. B.; Horowski, D. B.; McDonald, R. J.; and Wuttke, W.; eds.) Raven Press, New York, **1983**, pp. 153–159.

Burns, R. S.; Chiueh, C. C.; Markey, S. P.; Ebert, M. H.; Jacobwitz, D. M.; and Kopin, I. J. A primate model of parkinsonism: selective destruction of dopaminergic neurons in the pars compacta of the substantia nigra by *N*-methyl-4-phenyl-1,2,3,6-tetrahydropyridine. *Proc. Natl. Acad. Sci. U.S.A.*, **1983**, *80*, 4546–4550.

Calne, D. B. Parkinsonism, clinical and neuropharmacologic aspects. *Postgrad. Med.*, **1978**, *64*, 82–88.

———. Progress in Parkinson's disease. *N. Engl. J. Med.*, **1984**, *310*, 523–524.

Carlsson, A. The occurrence, distribution, and physiological role of catecholamines in the nervous system. *Pharmacol. Rev.*, **1959**, *11*, 490–493.

Carlsson, A.; Lindqvist, M.; and Magnusson, T. 3,4-Dihydroxyphenylalanine and 5-hydroxytryptophan as reserpine antagonists. *Nature*, **1957**, *180*, 1200.

Cedarbaum, J. M. The promise and limitations of oral controlled-release levodopa administration. *Clin. Neuropharmacol.*, **1989**, *12*, 147–169.

Cedarbaum, J. M., and McDowell, F. H. Sixteen-year follow-up of 100 patients begun on levodopa in 1968: emerging problems. In, *Advances in Neurology*, Vol. 45. (Yahr, M. D., and Bergmann, K. J., eds.) Raven Press, New York, **1986**, pp. 469–472.

Chase, T. N., and Watanabe, A. M. Methyldopahydrazine as an adjunct to L-dopa therapy in parkinsonism. *Neurology*, **1972**, *22*, 384–392.

Cotzias, G. C.; Papavasiliou, P. S.; Tolosa, E. S.; Mendez, J. S.; and Bell-Midura, M. Treatment of parkinsonism with aporphines: possible role of growth hormone. *N. Engl. J. Med.*, **1976**, *294*, 567–572.

Cotzias, G. C.; Van Woert, M. H.; and Schiffer, L. M. Aromatic amino acids and modification of parkinsonism. *N. Engl. J. Med.*, **1967**, *276*, 374–379.

Davidson, L.; Lloyd, K.; and Hornykiewicz, O. L-DOPA treatment in Parkinson's disease: effect on dopamine and related substances in discrete brain regions. *Experientia*, **1971**, *27*, 1048–1049.

Diamond, S. G.; Markham, C. H.; Hoehn, M. M.; McDowell, F. H.; and Muenter, M. D. Multi-center study of Parkinson mortality with early versus later dopa treatment. *Ann. Neurol.*, **1987**, *22*, 8–12.

Dolphin, A. C., and Scott, R. Y. Inhibition of calcium currents in cultured rat dorsal root ganglion neurons by baclofen. *Br. J. Pharmacol.*, **1986**, *88*, 213–220.

Duvoisin, R. C. Cholinergic-anticholinergic antagonism in parkinsonism. *Arch. Neurol.*, **1967**, *17*, 124–136.

Duvoisin, R. C., and Mytilineau, C. Where is L-DOPA decarboxylated in the striatum after 6-hydroxydopamine nigrotomy? *Brain Res.*, **1978**, *152*, 369–373.

Eddy, R. L.; Jones, A. L.; Chakmakjian, Z. H.; and Silverthorne, M. C. Effect of levodopa (L-dopa) on human hypophyseal trophic hormone release. *J. Clin. Endocrinol. Metab.*, **1971**, *33*, 709–712.

Ehringer, H., and Hornykiewicz, O. Verteilung von Noradrenalin und Dopamin (3-hydroxytyramin) im Gehirn des Menschen und ihr Verhalten bei Erkrankungen des extrapyramidalen Systems. *Klin. Wochenschr.*, **1960**, *38*, 1236–1239.

Fabbrini, G.; Juncos, J.; Mouradian, M. M.; Cerrati, C.; and Chase, T. N. Levodopa pharmacokinetic mechanisms and motor fluctuations in Parkinson's disease. *Ann. Neurol.*, **1987**, *21*, 370–376.

Fahn, S., and Bressman, S. Should levodopa therapy for parkinsonism be started early or late? Evidence against early treatment. *Can. J. Neurol. Sci.*, **1984**, *11*, 200–206.

Fukuda, T.; Kudo, Y.; and Ono, H. Effects of β-(*p*-chlorophenyl)-GABA (baclofen) on spinal synaptic activity. *Eur. J. Pharmacol.*, **1977**, *44*, 17–24.

Golbe, L. I.; Lieberman, A. N.; Muenter, M. D.; Ahlskog, J. E.; Gopinathan, G.; Neophytides, A. N.; Foo, S.-H.; and Duvoisin, R. C. Deprenyl in the treatment of symptom fluctuations in advanced Parkinson's disease. *Clin. Neuropharmacol.*, **1988**, *11*, 45–55.

Goldstein, M.; Lieberman, A.; Lew, J. S.; Asano, T.; Rosenfeld, M. R.; and Makman, M. H. Interaction of pergolide with central dopamine receptors. *Proc. Natl. Acad. Sci. U.S.A.*, **1980**, *77*, 3725–3728.

Hefti, F.; Melamed, E.; and Wurtman, R. J. The site of dopamine formation in rat striatum after L-DOPA administration. *J. Pharmacol. Exp. Ther.*, **1981**, *217*, 189–197.

Herman, R.; Mayer, N.; and Mecomber, S. A. Clinical pharmaco-physiology of dantrolene sodium. *Am. J. Phys. Med.*, **1972**, *51*, 296–311.

Hoehn, M. M. M. Parkinsonism treated with levodopa: progression and mortality. *J. Neural Transm.*, **1983**, Suppl. 19, 253–264.

Hornykiewicz, O. Dopamine in the basal ganglia. *Br. Med. Bull.*, **1973a**, *29*, 172–178.

Keller, H. H., and Daprada, M. Central dopamine agonistic activity and microsomal biotransformation of lisuride, lergotrile and bromocriptine. *Life Sci.*, **1979**, *24*, 1211–1222.

Knoll, J. Deprenyl (selegiline): the history of its development and pharmacological action. *Acta Neurol. Scand.*, **1983**, Suppl. 95, 57–80.

Koller, W. C., and Herbster, L. D1 and D2 dopamine receptor mechanisms in dopaminergic behaviors. *Clin. Neuropharmacol.*, **1988**, *11*, 221–231.

Langston, J. W.; Ballard, P.; Tetrud, J. W.; and Irwin, I. Chronic parkinsonism in humans due to a product of meperidine-analog synthesis. *Science*, **1983**, *219*, 979–980.

Langston, J. W., and Forno, L. S. The hypothalamus in Parkinson's disease. *Ann. Neurol.*, **1978**, *3*, 129–133.

Lee, T.; Seeman, P.; Rajput, A.; Farlay, I. J.; and Hornykiewicz, O. Receptor basis for dopaminergic supersensitivity in Parkinson's disease. *Nature*, **1978**, *273*, 59–61.

Lesser, R. P.; Fahn, S.; Snider, S. R.; Cote, L. J.; Isgreen, W. P.; and Barrett, R. E. Analysis of the clinical problems in parkinsonism and the complications of long-term levodopa therapy. *Neurology*, **1979**, *29*, 1253–1260.

LeWitt, P. A., and Calne, D. B. Recent advances in the treatment of Parkinson's disease. The role of bromocriptine. *J. Neural Transm.*, **1981**, *51*, 175–184.

LeWitt, P. A.; Ward, C. D.; Larsen, T. A.; and Calne, D. B. Comparison of pergolide and bromocriptine therapy in parkinsonism. *Neurology*, **1983**, *33*, 1009–1014.

Lieberman, A. N.; Kupersmith, M.; Gopinathan, G.; Estey, E.; Goodgold, A.; and Goldstein, M. Bromocriptine in Parkinson's disease: further studies. *Neurology*, **1979**, *29*, 363–369.

Linch, D. C.; Shaw, K. M.; Muhlemann, M. F.; and Ross, E. J. Bromocriptine-induced postural hypotension in acromegaly. *Lancet*, **1978**, *1*, 320.

Lloyd, K. G.; Davidson, L.; and Hornykiewicz, O. Metabolism of levodopa in the human brain. *Adv. Neurol.*, **1973**, *3*, 173–188.

Lossius, R.; Dietrichson, P.; and Lunde, P. K. M. Effect of diazepam and desmethyl-diazepam in spasticity and rigidity: a quantitative study of reflexes and plasma concentrations. *Acta Neurol. Scand.*, **1980**, *61*, 378–383.

Mann, D. M. A., and Yates, P. O. Possible role of neuromelanin in the pathogenesis of Parkinson's disease. *Mech. Ageing Dev.*, **1983**, *21*, 193–203.

Marion, M. H.; Stocci, F.; Quinn, N. P.; Jenner, P.; and Marsden, C. D. Repeated levodopa infusions in fluctuating Parkinson's disease: clinical and pharmacological data. *Clin. Neuropharmacol.*, **1986**, *9*, 165–181.

Markham, C. H., and Diamond, S. G. Evidence to support early levodopa therapy in Parkinson's disease. *Neurology*, **1981**, *31*, 125–131.

Markstein, R. Neurochemical effects of some ergot derivatives: a basis for their antiparkinson actions. *J. Neural Transm.*, **1981**, *51*, 49–59.

Martilla, R. J. Diagnosis and epidemiology of Parkinson's disease. *Acta Neurol. Scand.*, **1983**, Suppl. 95, 9–17.

Mawdsley, C.; Williams, I. R.; Pullar, I. A.; Davidson, D. L.; and Kinloch, N. E. Treatment of parkinsonism by amantadine and levodopa. *Clin. Pharmacol. Ther.*, **1972**, *13*, 575–583.

Montagu, K. A. Catechol compounds in rat tissues and in brains of different animals. *Nature*, **1957**, *180*, 244–245.

Mouradian, M. M.; Heuser, I. J. E.; Baronti, F.; and Chase, T. N. Modifications of central pharmacodynamics of levodopa by its constant infusion. *Neurology*, **1988**, *38*, Suppl. 1, 178.

Muenter, M. D. Should levodopa therapy be started early or late? *Can. J. Neurol. Sci.*, **1984**, *11*, 195–199.

Muenter, M. D.; Sharples, N. S.; Tyce, G. M.; and Darey, F. L. Patterns of dystonia ("I-D-I" and "D-I-D") in response to L-dopa therapy for Parkinson's disease. *Mayo Clin. Proc.*, **1977**, *52*, 163–164.

Newberry, N. R., and Nicoll, R. A. Direct hyperpolarizing action of baclofen on hippocampal pyramidal cells. *Nature*, **1984**, *308*, 450–452.

Nutt, J. G., and Woodward, W. R. Levodopa pharmacokinetics and pharmacodynamics in fluctuating parkinsonian patients. *Neurology*, **1986**, *36*, 739–744.

Nutt, J. G.; Woodward, W. R.; and Anderson, J. L. The effect of carbidopa on the pharmacokinetics of intravenously administered levodopa: the mechanism of action in the treatment of parkinsonism. *Ann. Neurol.*, **1985**, *18*, 537–543.

Nutt, J. G.; Woodward, W. R.; Hammerstad, J. P.; Carter, J. H.; and Anderson, J. L. The "on-off" phenomenon in Parkinson's disease. *N. Engl. J. Med.*, **1984**, *310*, 483–488.

Obeso, J. A.; Luquin, M. R.; and Martinez-Lage, J. M. Intravenous lisuride corrects oscillations in motor performance in Parkinson's disease. *Ann. Neurol.*, **1986**, *19*, 31–35.

Ohno, Y.; Sasa, M.; and Takaori, S. Coexistence of inhibitory dopamine D-1 and excitatory D-2 receptors on the same caudate nucleus neurons. *Life Sci.*, **1987**, *40*, 1937–1945.

Palfreyman, M. G.; Danzin, C.; Bey, P.; Jung, M. J.; Riberbeau-Gayon, G.; Aubry, M.; Vevert, J. P.; and Sjoerdsma, A. Difluoromethyl dopa, a new enzyme-activated irreversible inhibitor of aromatic L-amino acid decarboxylase. *J. Neurochem.*, **1978**, *31*, 927–932.

Papavasiliou, P. S.; Cotzias, G. C.; Duby, S. E.; Steck, A. J.; Fehling, C.; and Bell, M. A. Levodopa in parkinsonism: potentiation of central effects with a peripheral inhibitor. *N. Engl. J. Med.*, **1972**, *285*, 8–14.

Parkes, J. D.; Schacter, M.; Marsden, C. D.; Smith, B.; and Wilson, A. Lisuride in parkinsonism. *Ann. Neurol.*, **1981**, *9*, 48–52.

Penn, R. D.; Savoy, S. M.; Corcos, D.; Latash, M.; Gottlieb, G.; Parke, B.; and Kroin, J. S. Intrathecal baclofen for severe spinal spasticity. *N. Engl. J. Med.*, **1989**, *320*, 1517–1521.

Price, G. W.; Wilkin, G. P.; Turnbull, M. J.; and Bowery, N. G. Are baclofen-sensitive $GABA_B$ receptors present on primary afferent terminals of the spinal cord? *Nature*, **1984**, *307*, 71–74.

Rajfer, S. I.; Anton, A. H.; Rossen, J. D.; and Goldberg, L. I. Beneficial hemodynamic effects of oral levodopa in heart failure. *N. Engl. J. Med.*, **1984**, *310*, 1357–1362.

Riederer, P.; Jellinger, K.; Danielczyk, W.; Seemann, D.; Ulm, G.; Reynolds, G. P.; Birkmayer, W.; and Koppel, H. Combination treatment with selective monoamine oxidase inhibitors and dopaminergic agonists in Parkinson's disease: biochemical and clinical observations. In, *Experimental Therapeutics of Movement Disorders*. (Fahn, S.; Calne, D. B.; and Shoulson, I.; eds.) Vol. 37, *Advances in Neurology*. Raven Press, New York, **1983**, pp. 159–176.

Schwab, R. S.; Poskanzer, D. C.; England, A. C.; and Young, R. R. Amantadine in Parkinson's disease. Review of more than two years' experience. *J.A.M.A.*, **1972**, *222*, 792–795.

Spencer, S. E., and Wooten, G. F. Altered pharmacokinetics of L-dopa metabolism in rat striatum deprived of dopaminergic innervation. *Neurology*, **1984**, *34*, 1609–1611.

Tetrud, J. W., and Langston, J. W. The effect of deprenyl (selegiline) on the natural history of Parkinson's disease. *Science*, **1989**, *245*, 519–522.

Van Winkle, W. B. Calcium release from skeletal muscle sarcoplasmic reticulum: site of action of dantrolene sodium? *Science*, **1976**, *193*, 1130–1131.

Ward, C. D.; Duvoisin, R. C.; Ince, S. E.; Nutt, J. G.; Eldridge, R.; and Calne, D. B. Parkinson's disease in 65 pairs of twins and in a set of quadruplets. *Neurology*, **1983**, *33*, 815–824.

Yahr, M. D.; Mendoza, M. R.; Moros, D.; and Bergmann, K. J. Treatment of Parkinson's disease in early and late phases. Use of pharmacological agents with special reference to deprenyl (SELEGILINE). *Acta Neurol. Scand.*, **1983**, Suppl. 95, 95–102.

Yu, Y. B.; Duchen, M. R.; and Biscoe, J. T. Primary afferent terminal excitability in the normal and spastic mutant mouse spinal cord. *Eur. J. Pharmacol.*, **1987**, *141*, 371–382.

Monographs and Reviews

Bianchine, J. R., and Shaw, G. M. Clinical pharmacokinetics of levodopa in Parkinson's disease. *Clin. Pharmacokinet.*, **1976,** *1,* 313–358.

Cedarbaum, J. M. Clinical pharmacokinetics of antiparkinsonian drugs. *Clin. Pharmacokinet.*, **1987,** *13,* 141–178.

Davidoff, R. A. Pharmacology of spasticity. *Neurology*, **1978,** *28,* 46–51.

Elenbaas, J. K. Centrally acting oral skeletal muscle relaxants. *Am. J. Hosp. Pharm.*, **1980,** *37,* 1313–1323.

Fahn, S. Fluctuations in disability in Parkinson's disease: pathophysiological aspects. In, *Movement Disorders.* (Marsden, C. D., and Fahn, S., eds.) Butterworth Scientific, Boston, **1981,** pp. 123–145.

Hornykiewicz, O. Parkinson's disease: from brain homogenate to treatment. *Fed. Proc.*, **1973b,** *32,* 183–190.

Marsden, C. D.; Parkes, J. D.; and Quinn, N. Fluctuations in disability in Parkinson's disease: clinical aspects. In, *Movement Disorders.* (Marsden, C. D., and Fahn, S., eds.) Butterworth Scientific, Boston, **1981,** pp. 96–122.

Nutt, J. G., and Fellman, J. H. Pharmacokinetics of levodopa. *Clin. Neuropharmacol.*, **1984,** *7,* 35–49.

Pinder, R. M.; Brogden, R. N.; Speight, T. M.; and Avery, G. S. Dantrolene sodium: a review of its pharmacological properties and therapeutic efficacy in spasticity. *Drugs,* **1977,** *3,* 3–23.

Quinn, N. P. Anti-parkinsonian drugs today. *Drugs,* **1984,** *28,* 236–262.

Rinne, U. K. Parkinson's disease as a model for changes in dopamine receptor dynamics with aging. *Gerontology,* **1982,** *28,* Suppl. 1, 35–52.

Schmidt, W. Depletion of dopamine in the striatum as an experimental model of parkinsonism: direct effects and adaptive mechanisms. *Prog. Neurobiol.*, **1982,** *18,* 121–166.

Seeman, P., and Grigoriadis, D. Dopamine receptors in brain and periphery. *Neurochem. Int.*, **1987,** *10,* 1–25.

Sweet, R. D., and McDowell, F. H. Five years' treatment of Parkinson's disease with levodopa: therapeutic results and survival of 100 patients. *Ann. Intern. Med.*, **1975,** *83,* 456–463.

Symposium. (Various authors.) Current concepts and controversies in Parkinson's disease. *Can. J. Neurol. Sci.*, **1984,** *11,* Suppl. 1, 89–240.

Vance, M. L.; Evans, W. S.; and Thorner, M. O. Bromocriptine. *Ann. Intern. Med.*, **1984,** *100,* 78–91.

Yahr, M. D. Levodopa. *Ann. Intern. Med.*, **1975,** *83,* 677–682.

———. Overview of present day treatment of Parkinson's disease. *J. Neural Transm.*, **1978,** *43,* 227–238.

Young, R. R., and Delwaide, P. J. Drug therapy: spasticity. *N. Engl. J. Med.*, **1981,** *304,* 28–33, 96–99.

CHAPTER

21 OPIOID ANALGESICS AND ANTAGONISTS

Jerome H. Jaffe and William R. Martin

This chapter presents the pharmacological properties of the opioids (opioid agonists) and the opioid antagonists. The term *opioid* is used here to designate a group of drugs that are, to varying degrees, opium- or morphine-like in their properties. The opioids are employed primarily as analgesics, but they have many other pharmacological effects as well. Opioids interact with several closely related groups of receptors, and they share some of the properties of three families of neuropeptides, the *enkephalins,* the *endorphins,* and the *dynorphins.*

History. Although the psychological effects of opium may have been known to the ancient Sumerians, the first undisputed reference to poppy juice is found in the writings of Theophrastus in the third century B.C. The word *opium* itself is derived from the Greek name for juice, the drug being obtained from the juice of the poppy, *Papaver somniferum.* Arabian physicians were well versed in the uses of opium; Arabian traders introduced the drug to the Orient, where it was employed mainly for the control of dysenteries. Paracelsus (1493–1541) is credited with repopularizing the use of opium in Europe; it had fallen into disfavor because of its toxicity. By the middle of the sixteenth century, the uses of opium that are still valid were fairly well understood, and, in 1680, Sydenham wrote, "Among the remedies which it has pleased Almighty God to give to man to relieve his sufferings, none is so universal and so efficacious as opium."

In the eighteenth century opium smoking became popular in the Orient. In Europe, the ready availability of opium led to some degree of overuse, but the problem of opium eating never became as prevalent or as socially destructive as the abuse of alcohol.

Opium contains more than 20 distinct alkaloids. In 1806, Sertürner reported the isolation of a pure substance in opium that he named morphine, after Morpheus, the Greek god of dreams. The discovery of other alkaloids in opium quickly followed that of morphine (codeine by Robiquet in 1832, papaverine by Merck in 1848). By the middle of the nineteenth century the use of pure alkaloids rather than crude opium preparations began to spread throughout the medical world.

In the United States, opioid abuse was accentuated by the unrestricted availability of opium that prevailed until the early years of this century and by the influx of opium-smoking immigrants from the Orient. In addition, the invention of the hypodermic needle led to the parenteral use of morphine and to a more severe variety of compulsive drug abuse.

The problem of addiction to opioids stimulated a search for potent analgesics that would be free of the potential to produce addiction. Just prior to and following World War II, synthetic compounds such as meperidine and methadone were introduced into clinical medicine, but proved to have typical morphine-like actions. However, nalorphine, a derivative of morphine, was found to antagonize the effects of morphine and was used as an antidote for morphine poisoning in the early 1950s. In 1954, Lasagna and Beecher reported that nalorphine had analgesic actions in postoperative patients despite its antagonistic actions. Although nalorphine frequently produced anxiety and dysphoria and, hence, was not clinically useful as an analgesic, the discovery of its analgesic effects stimulated research that led to the development of new drugs, such as the relatively pure antagonist naloxone and compounds with mixed actions (*e.g.,* pentazocine, butorphanol, and buprenorphine). Such agents not only enlarged the range of available therapeutic entities but also, in conjunction with the subsequent discovery of receptors for opioids and endogenous peptides that bind to these receptors, helped to change our views about the actions of the opioids.

By 1967, Martin and coworkers had concluded that the complex interactions among morphine-like drugs, antagonists, and mixed agonist-antagonists could best be explained by the existence of more than one type of receptor for the opioids and related drugs. In 1973, following a methodological approach developed by Goldstein and coworkers, three groups of investigators independently described stereospecific binding sites for opioid drugs in the mammalian nervous system. This discovery was soon followed by the isolation of two morphine-like pentapeptides from pig brain by Hughes, Kosterlitz, and their coworkers. Within months, Goldstein and colleagues reported the presence of peptide-like substances in the pituitary gland with opioid activity. Over a remarkably brief period, subsequent research revealed that there are three distinct families of opioid peptides and multiple categories of opioid receptors. These developments have been reviewed by Bloom (1983), Akil and colleagues (1984), and Goldstein (1984).

Terminology. The term *opiate* was once used to designate drugs derived from opium—morphine, codeine, and the many semisynthetic congeners of morphine. Soon after the development of totally synthetic entities with morphine-like actions, the word *opioid* was coined to refer in a generic sense to all drugs, natural and synthetic, with morphine-like actions. With time, *opioid* has also been used to refer to antagonists of morphine-like drugs as well as to receptors that combine with such agents.

The term *narcotic* was obsolete long before the discovery of endogenous opioid-like ligands and receptors for these substances. Derived from the Greek word for stupor and at one time applied to any drug that induced sleep, it was, for a number of years, used to refer to morphine-like strong analgesics. With the development of mixed agonist-antagonists, some of which do not suppress morphine-like physical dependence, and with the increasing use of the term in a legal context to refer to any substance that can cause dependence, the term *narcotic* is no longer useful in a pharmacological context. However, it is not likely to disappear soon.

Endogenous Opioid Peptides. Three distinct families of peptides have been identified thus far: the *enkephalins,* the *endorphins,* and the *dynorphins*. Each family is derived from a distinct precursor polypeptide and has a characteristic anatomical distribution. These precursors are now designated as proenkephalin (also proenkephalin A), pro-opiomelanocortin (POMC), and prodynorphin (also proenkephalin B). Figure 21–1 depicts some of the biologically active peptides, both opioid and nonopioid, that are derived from these precursors. For example, POMC contains the amino acid sequence for melanocyte-stimulating hormone (γ-MSH), adrenocorticotropin (ACTH), and β-lipotropin (β-LPH); within the 91 amino acid sequence of β-LPH are found β-endorphin and β-MSH. Although β-endorphin contains the sequence for met-enkephalin at its amino terminus, it is not converted to this peptide; instead, met-enkephalin is derived from the processing of proenkephalin. Prodynorphin yields more than seven peptides that contain leu-enkephalin, including dynorphin A(1–17), which can be cleaved further to dynorphin A(1–8), dynorphin B(1–13), and α- and β-neoendorphin, which differ from each other by only one amino acid. A more detailed description of the peptides derived from these precursors is provided by Höllt (1986).

The precursor molecules and the peptides derived therefrom are not confined to the central nervous system (CNS), and they are distributed in a specific fashion (*see* Chapter 12). The distribution of peptides from POMC is relatively limited. Their location within the CNS includes the arcuate nucleus, which projects its fibers widely to limbic and brainstem areas; some POMC-containing fibers descend to the spinal cord (*see* Lewis *et al.*, 1987). In the human brain the distribution of POMC corresponds to areas where electrical stimulation can produce pain relief (Pilcher *et al.*, 1988). Peptides from POMC occur in both the pars intermedia and the pars distalis of the pituitary. They are also contained in pancreatic islet cells.

The peptides from prodynorphin and proenkephalin are distributed widely throughout the CNS, where they are frequently found together in the same region; although each family of peptides usually occurs in different groups of neurons, in a few instances more than one family is expressed within the same neuron (Weihe *et al.*, 1988). Of particular note, proenkephalin peptides are present in areas of the CNS that are presumed to be related to the perception of pain (*e.g.*, laminae I and II of the spinal cord, the spinal trigeminal nucleus, and the periaqueductal gray), to the modulation of affective behavior (*e.g.*, amygdala, hippocampus, locus ceruleus, and the cerebral cortex), and to the regulation of the autonomic nervous system (medulla oblongata) and neuroendocrinological functions (median eminence). Although there are a few long enkephalinergic fiber tracts, these peptides are contained primarily in interneurons with short axons. The peptides from proenkephalin are also found in the adrenal medulla and in nerve plexuses and exocrine glands of the stomach and intestine.

Not all cells that make a given precursor polypeptide store and release the same mixture of active opioid peptides. These differences are thought to arise from variations in the cellular complement of peptidases that produce and degrade the active opioid fragments. Although the endogenous opioid peptides appear to function as neurotransmitters, modulators of neurotransmission, or neurohormones, their role in physiological processes is not completely understood. The elucidation of the physiological role of the opioid peptides has been made more difficult by their frequent coexistence with other putative neurotransmitters (peptides or biogenic amines) within a given neuron.

Other Endogenous Opioids. In addition to peptides, it now appears that morphine, codeine, and related morphinans occur naturally in mammalian tissues; they are usually found in a conjugated form or bound to proteins. Hepatic metabolic pathways that might accomplish the synthesis of morphine have been described in the rat (Donnerer *et al.*, 1987; Weitz *et al.*, 1987).

Multiple Opioid Receptors. Studies of the binding of various ligands in brain and

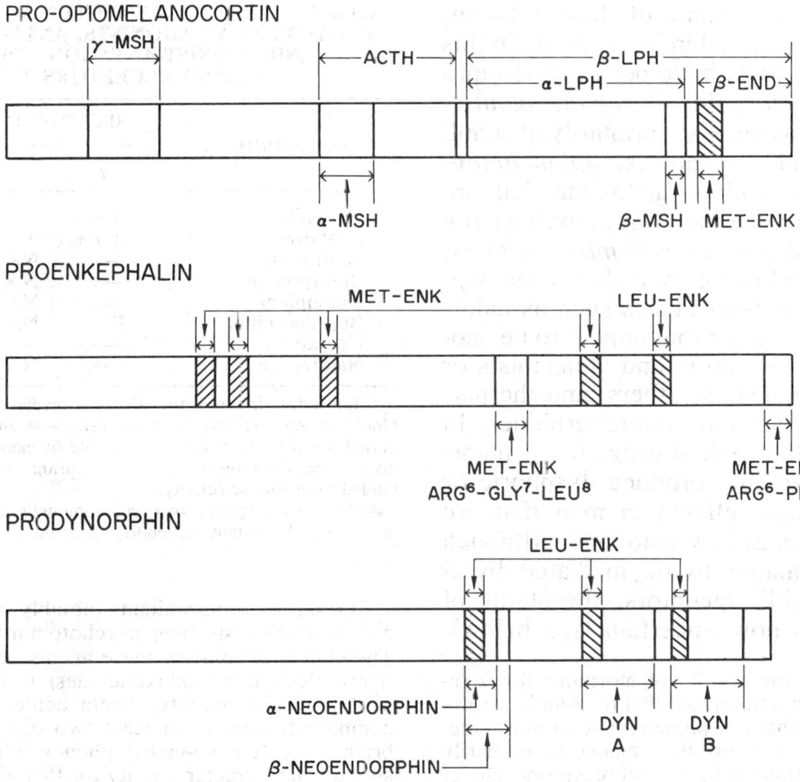

Figure 21–1. *Schematic representation of the structures of the protein precursors of the three families of opioid peptides.*

Abbreviations: ENK = enkephalin; DYN = dynorphin; END = endorphin. Other abbreviations are defined in the text. The sequence of met-enkephalin is Tyr-Gly-Gly-Phe-Met, while that of leu-enkephalin is Tyr-Gly-Gly-Phe-Leu. (Modified from Akil *et al.*, 1984.)

other organs suggest the existence of a multitude of distinct types of receptors that can interact with opioid drugs or endogenous peptides. There is reasonably firm evidence for three major categories of opioid receptors in the CNS, designated μ (mu), κ (kappa), and δ (delta); in addition, two subtypes of each category have been identified tentatively. Molecular cloning and expression of individual receptors will greatly facilitate the unraveling of this complex issue in the near future. The antagonist naloxone binds with high but variable affinity to all of these receptors, and "naloxone-sensitive" is often (but perhaps incorrectly) used synonymously with "opioid" in describing the actions of a given drug.

Inferences have been drawn from these data that attempt to relate pharmacological effects of opioid drugs to interactions with a particular constellation of receptors. For example, analgesia is thought to involve activation of μ receptors (largely at supraspinal sites) and κ receptors (principally within the spinal cord); δ receptors may also be involved, but the relative contribution of spinal and supraspinal sites is controversial (*see* below). Moreover, a given opioid drug may interact to a variable extent with all three types of receptors and act as an agonist, a partial agonist, or an antagonist at each (*see* Martin, 1983). It should be clear that our understanding of the detailed pharmacodynamic properties of opioid agonists and antagonists is in its infancy.

The profile of receptor interactions of opioid drugs in man is inferred both from clinical observations and from guarded extrapolation of their pharmacological properties in animals. Some of these relationships are summarized in Table 21–1. In this chapter the opioids have been divided into three groups: *morphine-like opioid agonists* (those acting as agonists primarily at μ and perhaps at κ and δ receptors); *opioid antagonists* (agents such as naloxone that are essentially devoid of agonist activity at any receptor); and *opioids with mixed actions*. The last-named category includes the agonist-antagonists (substances such as nalorphine or pentazocine that appear to be agonists at some receptors and antagonists or very weak agonists at others) and the partial agonists (such as buprenorphine). In addition, certain opioid drugs (*e.g.*, nalorphine, pentazocine) produce dysphoric or psychotomimetic effects in man that are poorly antagonized by naloxone. Although initially postulated to be mediated by σ (sigma)-"opioid" receptors, the status of these sites is now uncertain (*see* below).

Even though the affinity of morphine for μ receptors is only about tenfold that for δ and κ receptors, it is likely that morphine and other morphine-like opioid agonists produce analgesia primarily through interaction with μ-opioid receptors. This is best judged from the properties of sufentanil, a potent analgesic that binds about 200-fold more tightly to μ than to κ or δ receptors and exhibits a high degree of cross-tolerance with morphine-like agonists. Other consequences of μ-receptor activation include respiratory depression, miosis, reduced gastrointestinal motility, and feelings of well-being (euphoria). Two apparently distinct types of μ receptors have been detected based on their relative affinities for agonists: μ_1 (higher affinity), postulated to mediate supraspinal analgesic actions; and μ_2 (lower affinity), postulated to mediate respiratory depression and gastrointestinal actions, among others (*see* Pasternak, 1988).

Certain benzomorphan relatives of pentazocine interact quite selectively with κ receptors. These agonists produce analgesia that is undiminished in animals made tolerant to μ agonists and that results from actions primarily in the spinal cord; they cause less intense miosis and respiratory depression than do μ agonists. Instead of euphoria, κ agonists produce dysphoric, psychotomimetic effects (disoriented and/or depersonalized feelings) (Pfeiffer *et al.*, 1986).

The consequences of stimulating δ opioid receptors in man are uncertain because of the lack of selective agonists that can traverse the blood–brain barrier. In animals, relatively specific δ agonists (such as D-pen^2-D-pen^5-enkephalin; DPDPE [pen = penicillamine]) produce analgesia and positive reinforcing effects at supraspinal sites and antinociception for thermal stimuli at spinal sites (*see* Millan, 1986; Heyman *et al.*, 1988).

Table 21–1. SUMMARY OF THE ACTIONS OF PROTOTYPICAL AGONISTS, ANTAGONISTS, AND AGONIST-ANTAGONISTS AT OPIOID RECEPTORS *

COMPOUND	RECEPTOR TYPES		
	μ	δ	κ
Morphine	++	+	+
Fentanyl	+++	+	+
Pentazocine	—	NA	++
Butorphanol	—	NA	++
Nalbuphine	—	NA	++
Buprenorphine	P	NA	—
Naloxone	—	—	—
Nalorphine †	—	NA	+

* For a description of the effects of receptor activation or blockade, *see* the text. + = agonist; — = antagonist; P = partial agonist; NA = data unavailable or inadequate. For a given drug, the ratio of symbols at various receptors is intended to denote selectivity.

† Produces dysphoric or psychotomimetic effects at relatively high doses that are poorly antagonized by naloxone.

Certain benzomorphinans (notably pentazocine) can produce disturbing psychotomimetic effects. The effects of some of these agents are not effectively blocked by naloxone, despite their prominent κ-agonist activity. Pentazocine and related compounds bind to at least two distinct sites in brain. One (the so-called phencyclidine or PCP site) displays greater affinity for PCP than for benzomorphinans and appears to participate in inhibitory regulation of glutamate (and N-methyl-D-aspartate-) gated cation channels (*see* Chapters 12 and 22). The other (σ site) binds PCP less tightly than benzomorphinans. The σ site also binds numerous compounds that contain phenylpiperidine or piperazine moieties, and many of these drugs also interact with D_2-dopaminergic receptors (*see* Largent *et al.*, 1987). The function of the σ site is of considerable interest, including its potential role in mediating the naloxone-insensitive psychotomimetic effects of certain opioids.

Not surprisingly, the endogenous opioid peptides have a range of affinities for different types of receptors. For example, met-enkephalin–arg^6–gly^7–leu^8 has equal affinity for μ and δ binding sites, but other peptides derived from proenkephalin show a marked preference for δ sites. All the peptides from prodynorphin bind predominantly to κ sites. In the CNS and peripheral tissues, β-endorphin binds to both μ and δ receptors (*see* Akil *et al.*, 1984).

Opioid Receptor Mechanisms. Although biochemical and pharmacological evidence indicates that μ, δ, and κ receptors are distinct molecular entities, all three classes of opioid receptors share a number of characteristics. First, they all appear to function primarily by exerting inhibitory modulation of synaptic transmission in both the CNS and the myenteric plexus. Although their location varies, they are often found on presynaptic nerve terminals, where their action results in decreased release of excitatory neurotransmitters. Second, they all appear to be coupled to guanine nucleotide–

binding regulatory proteins (G proteins). Thus, it can be anticipated that opioids regulate the transmembrane signaling systems that are characteristically initiated by this type of receptor (*e.g.*, regulation of adenylyl cyclase, various ion channels, phospholipases, *etc.; see* Chapter 2). A few general patterns have emerged thus far. The consequences of the activation of μ and δ receptors are usually very similar or identical and are distinctly different from those resulting from activation of κ receptors. For example, stimulation of either μ (locus ceruleus neurons) or δ (enteric neurons) receptors can produce activation of inwardly rectifying K^+ channels and membrane hyperpolarization. Both μ and δ agonists can also inhibit adenylyl cyclase in many regions of the brain. By contrast, κ agonists have been found to influence Ca^{2+} channels; inhibition of voltage-dependent, dihydropyridine-insensitive (N-type) channels is produced in myenteric and dorsal root ganglion neurons. It is not yet clear whether these effects are a direct result of G protein–channel interactions or whether they involve the hydrolysis of phosphoinositides.

There are a few interesting exceptions to this general pattern. For example, δ agonists can prolong the duration of action potentials in cultured sensory neurons, apparently by reducing a voltage-sensitive K^+ conductance; evidence suggests that opioid receptor-induced *stimulation* of adenylyl cyclase may be involved in this response (Chen *et al.*, 1988). Opioid receptor function has been reviewed by McFadzean (1988) and by Simonds (1988).

MORPHINE AND RELATED OPIOIDS

There are now many compounds that produce analgesia and other effects similar to those produced by morphine. Some of these may have some special properties, but none has proven to be clinically superior in relieving pain. Morphine remains the standard against which new analgesics are measured. Because the laboratory synthesis of morphine is difficult, the drug is still obtained from opium or extracted from poppy straw.

Source and Composition of Opium. Opium is obtained from the unripe seed capsules of the poppy plant, *Papaver somniferum*. The milky juice derived therefrom is dried and powdered to make powdered opium, which contains a number of alkaloids. Only a few—morphine, codeine, and papaverine—have clinical usefulness. These alkaloids can be divided into two distinct chemical classes, *phenanthrenes* and *benzylisoquinolines*. The principal phenanthrenes are morphine (10% of opium), codeine (0.5%), and thebaine (0.2%). The principal benzylisoquinolines are papaverine (1.0%), which is a smooth muscle relaxant (*see* Chapter 32), and noscapine (6.0%).

Chemistry of Morphine and Related Opioids. The structure of morphine is as follows:

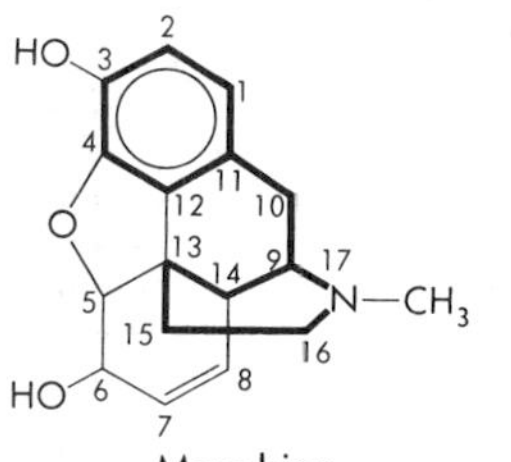

Morphine

Many semisynthetic derivatives are made by relatively simple modifications of the morphine or thebaine molecule. Codeine is methylmorphine, the methyl substitution being on the phenolic OH. Thebaine differs from morphine only in that both OH groups are methylated and that the ring has two double bonds ($\Delta^{6,7}$, $\Delta^{8,14}$). It has little analgesic action, but thebaine is a precursor of several important 14-OH compounds, such as oxycodone and naloxone. Certain derivatives of thebaine are more than 1000 times as potent as morphine (*e.g.*, etorphine). Diacetylmorphine, or heroin, is made from morphine by acetylation at the 3 and 6 positions. Apomorphine, which can also be prepared from morphine, is a potent emetic and dopaminergic agonist (*see* Chapter 20). Hydromorphone, oxymorphone, hydrocodone, and oxycodone are also made by modifying the morphine molecule. The structural relationship between morphine and some of its surrogates and antagonists is shown in Table 21–2.

Structure–Activity Relationship of the Morphine-Like Opioids. In addition to morphine, codeine, and the semisynthetic derivatives of the natural opium alkaloids, a number of other structurally distinct chemical classes of drugs have pharmacological actions similar to those of morphine. Clinically useful compounds include the morphinans, benzomorphans, methadones, phenylpiperidines, and propionanilides. Although the two-dimensional representations of these chemically diverse compounds appear to be quite different, molecular models show certain common characteristics; these are indicated by the heavy lines in the structure of morphine shown above. Among the important properties of the opioids that can be altered by structural modification are their affinity for various species of opioid receptors, agonistic versus antagonistic activity, lipid solubility, and resistance to metabolic breakdown. For example, blockade of the phenolic hydroxyl at position 3, as in codeine and heroin, drastically reduces binding to μ receptors; these compounds are converted to the potent analgesics, morphine and 6-acetyl morphine, respectively, *in vivo*.

The discovery of endogenous peptides with preferential affinities for various types of opioid receptors has added new dimensions to the study of structure–activity relationships. Scores of peptide congeners have been synthesized, and a certain number of selective agonists and antagonists have

Table 21–2. STRUCTURES OF OPIOIDS AND OPIOID ANTAGONISTS CHEMICALLY RELATED TO MORPHINE

NONPROPRIETARY NAME	CHEMICAL RADICALS AND POSITIONS *			OTHER CHANGES †
	3	*6*	*17*	
Morphine	—OH	—OH	$—CH_3$	—
Heroin	$—OCOCH_3$	$—OCOCH_3$	$—CH_3$	—
Hydromorphone	—OH	=O	$—CH_3$	(1)
Oxymorphone	—OH	=O	$—CH_3$	(1), (2)
Levorphanol	—OH	—H	$—CH_3$	(1), (3)
Levallorphan	—OH	—H	$—CH_2CH{=}CH_2$	(1), (3)
Codeine	$—OCH_3$	—OH	$—CH_3$	—
Hydrocodone	$—OCH_3$	=O	$—CH_3$	(1)
Oxycodone	$—OCH_3$	=O	$—CH_3$	(1), (2)
Nalmefene	—OH	$=CH_2$	$—CH_2$— 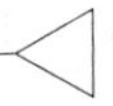	(1), (2)
Nalorphine	—OH	—OH	$—CH_2CH{=}CH_2$	—
Naloxone	—OH	=O	$—CH_2CH{=}CH_2$	(1), (2)
Naltrexone	—OH	=O	$—CH_2$— 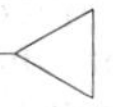	(1), (2)
Buprenorphine	—OH	$—OCH_3$	$—CH_2$— 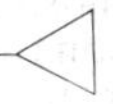	(1), (2), (4)
Butorphanol	—OH	—H	$—CH_2$— 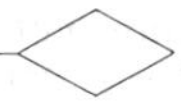	(2), (3)
Nalbuphine	—OH	—OH	$—CH_2$— 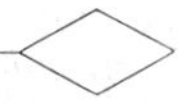	(1), (2)

* The numbers 3, 6, and 17 refer to positions in the morphine molecule, as shown above.
† Other changes in the morphine molecule are as follows:
(1) Single instead of double bond between C7 and C8.
(2) OH added to C14.
(3) No oxygen between C4 and C5.
(4) *Endo*etheno bridge between C6 and C14; 1-hydroxy-1,2,2-trimethylpropyl substitution on C7.

been characterized (*see* Heyman *et al.,* 1988; Kramer *et al.,* 1989).

PHARMACOLOGICAL PROPERTIES

Morphine and related μ-agonist opioids produce their major effects on the CNS and the bowel by acting as agonists, particularly at μ receptors. However, they also have appreciable affinity for δ and κ receptors. The effects are remarkably diverse and include analgesia, drowsiness, changes in mood, respiratory depression, decreased gastrointestinal motility, nausea, vomiting, and alterations of the endocrine and autonomic nervous systems. For reviews, *see* Martin and Sloan (1977), Duggan and North (1983), and Martin (1983).

Central Nervous System. In man, morphine-like drugs produce analgesia, drowsiness, changes in mood, and mental clouding. A significant feature of the analgesia is that it occurs without loss of consciousness. When therapeutic doses of morphine are given to patients with pain, they report that the pain is less intense, less discomforting, or entirely gone; drowsiness commonly occurs. In addition to relief of distress, some patients experience euphoria.

When morphine in the same dose is given to a presumably normal, pain-free individual, the experience is not always pleasant. Nausea is common, and vomiting may also occur. There may be feelings of drowsiness, difficulty in mentation, apathy, and lessened physical activity. As the dose is increased, the subjective, analgesic, and toxic effects, including respiratory depression, become more pronounced. Even large doses of morphine are not anticonvulsant and usually do not cause slurred speech, emotional lability, or significant motor incoordination.

Analgesia. The relief of pain by morphine-like opioids is relatively selective, in that other sensory modalities are not obtunded. Patients frequently report that the pain is still present but that they feel more comfortable (*see* below). Continuous dull pain is relieved more effectively than sharp intermittent pain, but with sufficient amounts of morphine it is possible to relieve even the severe pain associated with renal or biliary colic.

Any meaningful discussion of the action of analgesic agents must include some distinction between *pain as a specific sensation,* subserved by distinct neurophysiological structures, and *pain as suffering* (the original sensation plus the reactions evoked by the sensation). It is generally agreed that all types of painful experiences, whether produced experimentally or occurring clinically as a result of pathology, include both the original sensation and the reaction to that sensation. It is also important to distinguish between pain caused by stimulation of nociceptive receptors and transmitted over intact neural pathways (nociceptive pain) and pain that is caused by damage to neural structures, often involving neural supersensitivity (neuropathic pain). Although nociceptive pain is usually responsive to opioid analgesics, neuropathic pain typically responds poorly (McQuay, 1988).

In clinical situations, pain cannot be terminated at will, and the meaning of the sensation and the distress it engenders are markedly affected by the individual's previous experiences and current expectations. In experimentally produced pain, measurements of the effects of morphine on pain threshold have not always been consistent; some workers find that opioids reliably elevate the threshold, while many others do not obtain consistent changes. By contrast, moderate doses of morphine-like analgesics are quite effective in relieving clinical pain and increasing the capacity to tolerate experimentally induced pain. Opioids obtund the response to painful stimuli at several loci in the CNS. Not only is the sensation of pain altered by opioid analgesics, but the affective response is changed as well. This latter effect is best assessed by asking patients with clinical pain about the degree of relief produced by the drug administered. When pain does not evoke its usual responses (anxiety, fear, panic, and suffering), a patient's ability to tolerate the pain may be markedly increased even when the capacity to perceive the sensation is relatively unaltered. It is clear, however, that alteration of the emotional reaction to painful stimuli is not the sole mechanism of analgesia. Intrathecal administration of opioids can produce profound segmental analgesia without causing significant alteration of motor or sensory functions or subjective effects (*see* Yaksh and Noueihed, 1985; Yaksh, 1988).

Mechanisms and Sites of Opioid-Induced Analgesia. Opioid-induced analgesia is due to actions at several sites within the CNS; both spinal and multiple supraspinal sites have been identified. Morphine and other μ-opioid agonists selectively inhibit various nociceptive reflexes and induce profound analgesia when administered intrathecally or instilled locally into the dorsal horn of the spinal cord; other sensory modalities (*e.g.*, touch) are usually unaffected. At least three mechanisms appear to be involved. Opioid receptors on the terminals of primary afferent nerves mediate inhibition of the release of neurotransmitters, including substance P. Morphine also antagonizes the effects of exogenously administered substance P by exerting postsynaptic inhibitory actions on interneurons and on the output neurons of the spinothalamic tract that conveys nociceptive information to higher centers in the brain. Both δ and κ agonists appear to act similarly; however, κ agonists suppress noxious thermal stimuli only slightly, and their maximal effects on visceral pain are distinctly lower (*see* Lewis *et al.*, 1987).

Profound analgesia can also be produced by the instillation of morphine into the third ventricle or in various sites in the midbrain and medulla, most notably the periaqueductal gray matter and the nucleus raphe magnus. Either electrical or chemical stimulation at these sites also induces analgesia that is antagonized by naloxone, suggesting mediation by endogenous opioid peptides. Although the circuitry has not been clearly defined, all of these maneuvers result in enhanced activity in descending aminergic bulbospinal pathways that exert inhibitory effects on the processing of nociceptive information in the spinal cord. The instillation of δ agonists appears to be equally effective, even after blockade of μ receptors. Despite the fact that the periaqueductal gray matter is richly endowed with κ receptors and dynorphin peptides, the administration of selective κ agonists by this route is without appreciable effect.

The total amount of morphine required to produce equivalent analgesia is reduced up to tenfold by its simultaneous administration at both spinal and supraspinal sites (*see* Advokat, 1988). Hence, the effects are apparently synergistic. Similar mechanisms may also be involved in the enhancement of opioid-induced analgesia by agonists that act at receptors for various biogenic amines. The sites and mechanisms of opioid-induced analgesia have been reviewed in a recent symposium (1988a).

Mechanism of Other CNS Effects. High doses of opioids can produce muscular rigidity in man. Chest wall rigidity severe enough to compromise respiration is not uncommon during anesthesia with fentanyl, alfentanil, and sufentanil (*see* Monk, 1988). Opioids and endogenous peptides cause catalepsy, circling, and stereotypical behavior in rats and other animals. These effects are probably related to actions at opioid receptors in the substantia nigra and striatum, and involve interactions with both dopaminergic and GABA-ergic neurons.

The mechanism by which opioids produce euphoria, tranquility, and other alterations of mood is also not entirely clear. Microinjection of μ opioids into the ventral tegmentum activates dopaminergic neurons that project to the nucleus accumbens; this pathway is postulated to be a critical element in the reinforcing effects of opioids and, by inference, opioid-induced euphoria. Animals will work to receive such injections or injections into the nucleus accumbens itself or its projection areas. The administration of dopaminergic antagonists does not consistently prevent the reinforcing effects of opioids, suggesting that some nondopaminergic mechanisms may also play a role. The neural systems that mediate opioid reinforcement in the ventral tegmentum appear to be distinct from those involved in the classical manifestations of physical dependence and analgesia (Wise and Bozarth, 1987; Koob and Bloom, 1988). The activation of δ receptors may also produce reinforcing effects. In contrast to μ agonists, κ agonists inhibit the firing of dopamine-containing cells in the substantia nigra and inhibit dopamine release from cortical and striatal neurons (Walker *et al.*, 1987; Werling *et al.*, 1988); as mentioned above, they produce dysphoric effects rather than euphoria.

The locus ceruleus contains both noradrenergic neurons and high concentrations of opioid receptors and is postulated to play a critical role in feelings of alarm, panic, fear, and anxiety. Activity in the locus ceruleus is inhibited by both exogenous opioids and endogenous opioid-like peptides. The role of the locus ceruleus in opioid withdrawal is discussed in Chapter 22.

Effects on the Hypothalamus. Opioids alter the equilibrium point of the hypothalamic heat-regulatory mechanisms, such that body temperature usually falls slightly. However, chronic high dosage may increase body temperature (*see* Martin, 1983).

Neuroendocrine Effects. Morphine acts in the hypothalamus to inhibit the release of gonadotropin-releasing hormone (GnRH) and corticotropin-releasing factor (CRF), thus decreasing circulating concentrations of luteinizing hormone (LH), follicle-stimulating hormone (FSH), ACTH, and β-endorphin; the last two peptides are usually released simultaneously from corticotrophs in the pituitary. As a result of the decreased concentrations of pituitary trophic hormones, the concentrations of testosterone and cortisol in plasma decline. Secretion of thyrotropin is relatively unaffected.

The administration of μ opioids increases the concentration of prolactin (PRL) in plasma, probably by reducing the dopaminergic inhibition of its secretion. Although some opioids enhance the secretion of growth hormone, the administration of morphine or β-endorphin has little effect on the concentration of the hormone in plasma. With chronic administration, tolerance develops to the effects of morphine on hypothalamic releasing factors. Observations in patients maintained on methadone reflect this phenomenon: in women, menstrual cycles that had been disrupted by intermittent use of heroin return to normal; in men, circulating concentrations of LH and testosterone are usually within the normal range.

Although κ agonists inhibit the release of antidiuretic hormone (ADH) and cause diuresis, the administration of μ-opioid agonists tends to have antidiuretic effects in man. The effects of opioids on neuroendocrine function have been reviewed by Howlett and Rees (1986) and by Grossman (1988).

Pupil. Morphine and most μ and κ opioid agonists cause constriction of the pupil (in man). Miosis is due to an excitatory action on the autonomic segment of the nucleus of the oculomotor nerve. Following toxic doses of μ agonist opioids, *the miosis is marked and pinpoint pupils are pathognomonic;* however, marked mydriasis occurs when asphyxia intervenes. Some tolerance to the miotic effect develops, but addicts with high circulating concentrations of opioids continue to have constricted pupils. Therapeutic doses of morphine increase accommodative power and lower intraocular tension in both normal and glaucomatous eyes.

Excitatory Effects. In animals, high doses of morphine and related opioids produce convulsions. Several mechanisms appear to be involved, and different types of opioids produce seizures with different characteristics. Morphine-like drugs excite certain groups of neurons, especially hippocampal pyramidal cells; these excitatory effects probably result from inhibition of the release of GABA by interneurons (*see* Symposium, 1988b). Selective δ agonists produce similar effects. These actions may contribute to the seizures that are produced by some agents at doses only moderately higher than those required for analgesia, especially in children. However, with most opioids, convulsions occur only at doses far in excess of those required to produce profound analgesia, and seizures are not seen when potent μ agonists are used to produce anesthesia.

Naloxone is more potent in antagonizing convulsions produced by some opioids (*e.g.*, morphine, methadone, and *d*-propoxyphene) than those produced by others (*e.g.*, meperidine). The production of convulsant metabolites of the latter agent may be partially responsible (*see* below). Anticonvulsant agents may not always be effective in suppressing opioid-induced seizures.

Respiration. Morphine-like opioids depress respiration, at least in part by virtue of a direct effect on the brainstem respiratory centers. The respiratory depression is discernible even with doses too small to disturb consciousness, and increases progressively as the dose is increased. In man, death from morphine poisoning is nearly always due to respiratory arrest. Therapeutic doses of morphine in man depress all phases of respiratory activity (rate, minute volume, and tidal exchange) and may also produce irregular and periodic breathing. The diminished respiratory volume is due primarily to a slower rate of breathing, and with toxic amounts the rate may fall to 3 or 4 per minute.

Maximal respiratory depression occurs within 5 to 10 minutes after intravenous administration of morphine or within 30 or 90 minutes following intramuscular or subcutaneous administration, respectively. Maximal depressant effects occur more rapidly with more lipid-soluble agents. Following therapeutic doses, respiratory minute volume may be reduced for as long as 4 to 5 hours.

The primary mechanism of respiratory depression by opioids involves a reduction in the responsiveness of the brainstem respiratory centers to carbon dioxide. They also depress the pontine and medullary centers involved in regulating respiratory rhythmicity and the responsiveness of medullary respiratory centers to electrical stimulation (*see* Martin, 1983).

Hypoxic stimulation of the chemoreceptors may still be effective when opioids have decreased the responsiveness to CO_2, and the inhalation of high tensions of O_2 may thus produce apnea. After large doses of morphine or other μ agonists, patients will breathe if instructed to do so, but without such instruction they may remain relatively apneic.

Because of the accumulation of CO_2, respiratory rate and sometimes even minute volume can be unreliable indicators of the degree of respiratory depression that has been produced by morphine. Natural sleep also produces a decrease in the sensitivity of the medullary center to CO_2, and the effects of morphine and sleep are additive.

Numerous studies have compared morphine and morphine-like opioids with respect to their ratios of analgesic to respiratory-depressant activities. Most studies have found that, when equianalgesic doses are used, the degree of respiratory depression observed with morphine-like opioids is not significantly different from that seen with morphine. However, the partial agonist and agonist-antagonist opioids are less likely to cause severe respiratory depression and are far less commonly associated with death caused by overdosage (*see* below).

High concentrations of opioid receptors, as well as endogenous peptides, are found in the medullary areas believed to be important in ventilatory control. As mentioned previously, respiratory depression may be mediated by a subpopulation of μ receptors (μ_2), distinct from those that are involved in the production of analgesia (μ_1); there is also evidence that κ and δ receptors play some part in the respiratory-depressant effects of morphine. However, severe respiratory depression is less likely after the administration of large doses of selective κ agonists.

Cough. Morphine and related opioids also depress the cough reflex, at least in part by a direct effect on a cough center in the medulla. There is, however, no obligatory relationship between depression of respiration and depression of coughing, and effective antitussive agents are available that do not depress respiration (*see* below). Suppression of cough by such agents appears to involve receptors in the medulla that are less sensitive to naloxone than are those responsible for analgesia.

Nauseant and Emetic Effects. Nausea and vomiting produced by morphine-like drugs are unpleasant side effects caused by direct stimulation of the chemoreceptor trigger zone (CTZ) for emesis, in the area postrema of the medulla. Certain individuals never vomit after morphine, whereas others do so each time the drug is administered.

Nausea and vomiting are relatively uncommon in recumbent patients given therapeutic doses of morphine, but nausea occurs in approximately 40% and vomiting in 15% of ambulatory patients given 15 mg of the drug subcutaneously. This suggests that a vestibular component is also operative. Indeed, it has been shown that the nauseant and emetic effects of morphine in man are markedly enhanced by vestibular stimulation, and that morphine and related synthetic analgesics produce an increase in vestibular sensitivity. All clinically useful μ-agonist opioids produce some degree of nausea and vomiting. Careful, controlled clinical studies usually demonstrate that in equianalgesic dosage the incidence of such side effects is not significantly lower than that seen with morphine. Drugs that are useful in motion sickness are sometimes helpful in reducing opioid-induced nausea in ambulatory patients; phenothiazines are also useful (*see* Chapter 38).

Cardiovascular System. In the supine patient, therapeutic doses of morphine-like opioids have no major effect on blood pressure or cardiac rate and rhythm. Such doses do produce peripheral vasodilatation, reduced peripheral resistance, and an inhibition of baroreceptor reflexes. Therefore, when supine patients assume the head-up position, orthostatic hypotension and fainting may occur. The peripheral arteriolar and venous dilatation produced by morphine involves several mechanisms. Morphine and some other opioids provoke the release of histamine, which sometimes plays a large role in the hypotension. However, vasodilatation is usually only partially blocked by H_1 antagonists, but it is effectively reversed by naloxone. Morphine also blunts the reflex vasoconstriction caused by increased P_{CO_2}.

Effects on the myocardium are not significant in normal man. In patients with coronary artery disease but no acute medical problems, 8 to 15 mg of morphine intravenously produces a decrease in oxygen consumption, left ventricular end-diastolic pressure, and cardiac work; effects on cardiac index are usually slight (Sethna *et al.*, 1982). In patients with acute myocardial infarction, the cardiovascular responses to morphine may be more variable than in normal subjects, and the magnitude of changes (*e.g.*, the decrease in blood pressure) may be more pronounced (*see* Roth *et al.*, 1988).

Very large doses of morphine can be used to produce anesthesia; however, decreased peripheral resistance and blood pressure are troublesome. Fentanyl and sufentanil, which are potent and selective μ agonists, are less likely to cause hemodynamic instability during surgery, in part because they do not cause the release of histamine (*see* Monk, 1988).

Morphine-like opioids should be used with caution in patients who have a decreased blood volume, since these agents can aggravate hypovolemic shock. Morphine should be used with great care in patients with cor pulmonale, since deaths following ordinary therapeutic doses have been reported. The concurrent use of certain phenothiazines may increase the risk of morphine-induced hypotension.

Cerebral circulation is not directly affected by therapeutic doses of morphine. However, opioid-induced respiratory depression and CO_2 retention can result in cerebral vasodilatation and an increase in cerebrospinal fluid pressure; the pressure increase does not occur when P_{CO_2} is maintained at normal levels by artificial ventilation.

Gastrointestinal Tract. *Stomach.* Morphine and other μ agonists usually decrease the secretion of hydrochloric acid, although stimulation is sometimes evident. Activation of opioid receptors on parietal cells enhances secretion, but indirect effects, including increased secretion of somatostatin from the pancreas and reduced release of acetylcholine, appear to be dominant in most circumstances (*see* Kromer, 1988). Relatively low doses of morphine decrease gastric motility, thereby prolonging gastric emptying time; this can increase the likelihood of esophageal reflux (*see* Duthie and Nimmo, 1987). The tone of the antral portion of the stomach and of the first part of the duodenum is increased, which often makes therapeutic intubation of the duodenum more difficult. Passage of the gastric contents through the duodenum may be delayed by as much as 12 hours, and the absorption of orally administered drugs is retarded.

Small Intestine. Morphine diminishes biliary, pancreatic, and intestinal secretions (Dooley *et al.*, 1988) and delays digestion of food in the small intestine. Resting tone is increased, and periodic spasms are observed. The amplitude of the nonpropulsive type of rhythmic, segmental contractions is usually enhanced, but propulsive contractions are markedly decreased. The upper part of the small intestine, particularly the duodenum, is affected more than the ileum. A period of relative atony may follow the hypertonicity. Water is absorbed more completely because of the delayed passage of the bowel contents and intestinal secretion is decreased; this increases the viscosity of the bowel contents.

In the presence of intestinal hypersecretion that may be associated with diarrhea, morphine-like drugs inhibit the transfer of fluid and electrolytes into the lumen by naloxone-sensitive actions on the intestinal mucosa and within the CNS. Enterocytes may possess opioid receptors, but this hypothesis is controversial. However, it is clear that opioids exert important effects on the submucosal plexus that lead to a decrease in the basal secretion by enterocytes and inhibition of the stimulatory effects of acetylcholine, prostaglandin E_2, and vasoactive intestinal peptide. The effects of opioids initiated either in the CNS or the submucosal plexus may be mediated in large part by the release of norepinephrine and stimulation of α_2-adrenergic receptors on enterocytes (*see* Coupar, 1987). The actions of opioids on intestinal secretion have been reviewed by Awouters and colleagues (1983), Manara and Bianchetti (1985), and Kromer (1988).

Large Intestine. Propulsive peristaltic waves in the colon are diminished or abolished after morphine administration, and tone is increased to the point of spasm. The resulting delay in the passage of the contents causes considerable desiccation of the feces, which, in turn, retards its advance through the colon. The amplitude of the nonpropulsive type of rhythmic contractions of the colon is usually enhanced. The tone of the anal sphincter is greatly augmented, and the reflex relaxation response to rectal distention is reduced. These actions, combined with inattention to the normal sensory stimuli for the defecation reflex owing to the central actions of the drug, contribute to morphine-induced constipation.

Mechanism of Action on the Bowel. The usual gastrointestinal effects of morphine are primarily mediated by μ- and δ-opioid receptors in the bowel. However, injection of opioids into the cerebral ventricles or in the vicinity of the spinal cord can inhibit gastrointestinal propulsive activity as long as the extrinsic innervation to the bowel is intact. The relatively poor penetration of morphine into the CNS may explain how preparations such as paregoric can produce constipation at less than analgesic doses and may account for troublesome gastrointestinal side effects during the use of oral morphine for the treatment of cancer pain (*see* Manara and Bianchetti, 1985). Although some tolerance develops to the effects of opioids on gastrointestinal motility, patients who take opioids chronically remain constipated.

Biliary Tract. After the subcutaneous injection of 10 mg of morphine sulfate the sphincter of Oddi constricts and the pressure in the common bile duct may rise more than tenfold within 15 minutes; this effect may persist for 2 hours or more. Fluid pressure may also increase in the gallbladder and produce symptoms that may vary from epigastric distress to typical biliary colic.

Some patients with biliary colic may experience exacerbation rather than relief of pain when given these drugs. Spasm of the sphincter of Oddi is probably responsible for the elevations of plasma amylase and lipase that are sometimes found after patients are given morphine. Atropine only partially prevents morphine-induced biliary spasm, but opioid antagonists prevent or relieve it. Nitroglycerin (0.6 to 1.2 mg) administered sublingually also decreases the elevated intrabiliary pressure (*see* Staritz, 1988). Opioids such as meperidine, fentanyl, and some of the agonist-antagonists (*e.g.*, butorphanol and nalbuphine) seem to produce less pronounced increases in biliary pressure.

Other Smooth Muscle. *Ureter and Urinary Bladder.* Therapeutic doses of morphine may increase the tone and amplitude of contractions of the ureter, although the response is quite variable. When the antidiuretic effects of the drug are prominent and urine flow decreases, the ureter may become quiescent.

Morphine inhibits the urinary voiding reflex, and both the tone of the external sphincter and the volume of the bladder are increased; catheterization is sometimes required following therapeutic doses of morphine. Stimulation of either μ or δ receptors in the brain or in the spinal cord exerts similar actions on bladder motility (*see* Yaksh and Noueihed, 1985; Dray and Nunan, 1987). Tolerance develops to these effects of opioids on the bladder.

Uterus. Therapeutic doses of morphine may prolong labor. If the uterus has been made hyperactive by oxytocics, morphine tends to restore tone, frequency, and amplitude of contractions to normal. In addition, the central effects of morphine may affect the degree to which the parturient is able to cooperate in the delivery. Neonatal mortality may thus be increased by the injudicious use of morphine-like opioids during labor as a result of these factors and the high sensitivity of the neonate to the respiratory-depressant effect of these drugs.

Skin. Therapeutic doses of morphine cause dilatation of cutaneous blood vessels. The skin of the face, neck, and upper thorax frequently becomes flushed. These changes may, in part, be due to the release of histamine and may be responsible for the sweating and some of the pruritus that occasionally follow the systemic administration of morphine. Histamine release probably accounts for the urticaria commonly seen at the site of injection; this is not mediated by opioid receptors and is not blocked by naloxone. It is seen with morphine and meperidine, but not with oxymorphone, methadone, fentanyl, or sufentanil (*see* Duthie and Nimmo, 1987). Pruritus may, in part, involve effects of opioids on neurons, since it is provoked by opioids that do not release histamine and is quickly abolished by small doses of naloxone (*see* Ballantyne *et al.*, 1988).

Immune System. Although some opioid peptides can produce a number of naloxone-sensitive effects on the function of macrophages and leukocytes, morphine itself is active in relatively few instances. The most firmly established effect of morphine is its ability to inhibit the formation of rosettes by human lymphocytes. The administration of morphine to animals causes suppression of the cytotoxic activity of natural killer cells and enhances the growth of implanted tumors. Of interest, these effects are mediated by actions within the CNS. By contrast, β-endorphin enhances the cytotoxic activity of human monocytes *in vitro* and increases the recruitment of precursor cells into the killer cell population; this peptide can also exert a potent chemotactic effect on these cells. A novel type of receptor (designated ε) may be involved. These effects, combined with the synthesis of POMC and preproenkephalin by various cells of the immune system, have stimulated study of the potential role of opioids in the regulation of immune function (*see* Sibinga and Goldstein, 1988).

Tolerance, Physical Dependence, and Liability for Abuse. The development of tolerance and physical dependence with repeated use is a characteristic feature of all the opioid drugs, and the possibility of developing drug dependence is one of the major limitations of their clinical use. It is important to emphasize that the overall liability for abuse of an agent is not established by any one single factor; rather, it is a composite based on a number of factors. These include (1) the capacity of the drug to produce the kind of physical dependence in which drug withdrawal causes sufficient distress to bring about drug-seeking behavior; (2) its ability to suppress withdrawal symptoms caused by withdrawal of other agents; (3) the degree to which it induces reinforcing subjective effects, including euphoria, similar to those produced by morphine and other μ agonists; (4) the patterns of toxicity that occur when the dose is increased beyond the usual therapeutic range; and (5) physical characteristics of the drug, such as water solubility, that may determine whether it is likely to be abused by the parenteral route. There is considerable evidence that the overall abuse liability of some of the agonist-antagonist opioids is lower than that of μ-agonist opioids. Although selective κ agonists can produce a type of physical dependence, they are not reinforcing in animals (Gmerek *et al.*, 1987) and produce little euphoria in humans. The implications of the differences in abuse potential for the choice of agents in therapy are discussed below, and the characteristics of the morphine withdrawal syndrome and the subject of compulsive drug use are elaborated in detail in Chapter 22.

Absorption, Distribution, Fate, and Excretion. *Absorption.* In general, the opioids are readily absorbed from the gastrointestinal tract; absorption through the rectal mucosa is adequate and a few agents (*e.g.*, morphine, hydromorphone) are available in suppositories. The more lipophilic opioids are readily absorbed through the nasal or buccal mucosa, and the latter route of administration is under investigation (Weinberg *et al.*, 1988); those with the greatest lipid solubility can also be absorbed transdermally. Opioids are readily absorbed after subcutaneous or intramuscular injection and can adequately penetrate the spinal cord following epidural or intrathecal administration.

With most opioids, including morphine, the effect of a given dose is less after oral than after parenteral administration, due to variable but significant first-pass metabolism in the liver. For example, the bioavailability of oral preparations of morphine is only about 25%. The shape of the time–effect curve also varies with the route of administration, so that the duration of action is often somewhat longer with the oral route. If adjustment is made for variability of first-pass metabolism and clearance, it is possible to achieve adequate relief of pain by the oral administration of morphine. Satisfactory analgesia in cancer patients has been associated with a very broad range of steady-state concentrations of morphine in plasma (16 to 364 ng/ml) (Neumann *et al.*, 1982).

When morphine and most opioids are given intravenously, they act promptly. However, the more lipid-soluble compounds act more rapidly than morphine after subcutaneous administration because of differences in the rates of absorption and entry into the CNS. When opioids such as morphine are given initially, their durations of analgesic action show relatively little variation (*see* Table 21–3). Other effects may persist longer than analgesia, and some drugs may accumulate with repeated administration.

Distribution and Fate. When therapeutic concentrations of morphine are present in plasma, about one third of the drug is protein bound. Morphine itself does not persist in tissues, and 24 hours after the last dose tissue concentrations are quite low.

Although the primary site of action of morphine is in the CNS, in the adult only small quantities pass the blood–brain barrier. Compared with other more lipid-soluble opioids such as codeine, heroin, and methadone, morphine crosses the blood–brain barrier at a considerably lower rate.

Small amounts of morphine introduced epidurally or directly into the spinal canal can produce profound analgesia that may last 12 to 24 hours (*see* Yaksh and Noueihed, 1985). However, there is rostral spread of the drug in spinal fluid, and prominent untoward effects, especially respiratory depression, can emerge later at a time when analgesia may no longer be present. With highly lipophilic agents such as hydromorphone or fentanyl, rapid absorption by neural tissues produces very localized effects and segmental analgesia. The duration of action is shorter because of distribution of the drug in the systemic circulation, and the severity of respiratory depression is largely proportional to its concentration in plasma (*see* Gustafsson and Wiesenfeld-Hallin, 1988).

Table 21–3. A COMPARISON OF OPIOID ANALGESICS WITH RESPECT TO DOSAGE, DURATION OF ACTION, AND SOME DISTINGUISHING FEATURES [a]

NONPROPRIETARY NAME	TRADE NAME	ROUTE [b]	DOSE [c] (*mg*)	DURATION OF ACTION [d] (*hrs*)	PLASMA HALF-LIFE [e] (*hrs*)	DISTINGUISHING FEATURES [f]
Morphine		IM, SC	10	4–5	2	*see* text
		O	60	4–7		
Heroin		IM, SC	5	4–5	0.5	1
(diacetylmorphine)		O	60	4–5		
Hydromorphone	DILAUDID	IM, SC	1.3	4–5	2–3	
(dihydromorphenone)		O	7.5	4–6		
Oxymorphone	NUMORPHAN	IM, SC	1	4–6	2–3	9
(dihydrohydroxy-morphinone)		R	5	4–6		
Levorphanol	LEVO-DROMORAN	IM, SC	2	4–5	12–16	8
		O	4	4–7		
Methadone	DOLOPHINE	IM	10	4–5	15–40	8
		O	20	4–6		
Meperidine	DEMEROL,	IM, SC	75	3–5	3–4	
(pethidine)	PETHADOL	O	300	4–6		
Fentanyl	SUBLIMAZE	IM	0.1	1–2	3–4	9
Codeine		IM	130	4–6	2–4	5, 7
		O	200	4–6		
		O	10–20 [g]			
Hydrocodone	HYCODAN,	O	5–10 [h]	4–5	4	5, 6, 7
(dihydrocodeinone)	others	O	5–10 [g]			
Drocode	SYNALGOS-DC,	O	32 [h]	4–5	4	5, 6, 7
(dihydrocodeine)	COMPAL					
Oxycodone (dihydro-hydroxycodeinone)	ROXICODONE	O	5–10 [h]	4–5	—	5
Propoxyphene	DARVON, others	O	65 [h]	4–6	6–12	2, 7
Buprenorphine	BUPRENEX	IM	0.4	4–5	5	3, 9, 11
		SL	0.8	5–6		
Pentazocine	TALWIN	IM, SC	30–60	4–6	4–5	2, 10, 11, 12
		O	180	4–7		
Nalbuphine	NUBAIN	IM	10	4–6	2–3	4, 9, 11
Butorphanol	STADOL	IM	2	4–6	2.5–3.5	4, 9, 11

a. Except where noted, these opioids are all marketed in the United States and are listed in Schedule II of the United States Controlled Substances Act (*see* Appendix I). The doses and durations of action in this table are based in part on Foley (1985).

b. IM = intramuscular; SC = subcutaneous; O = oral; SL = sublingual; R = rectal.

c. Except where noted, dose is the amount that produces approximately the same analgesic effect as 10 mg of morphine administered intramuscularly or subcutaneously.

d. Average duration of action for the first single dose.

e. Average terminal half-life of parent molecule; some drugs have active metabolites with different half-lives.

f. 1 = Schedule I (manufacture or importation into the United States illegal); 2 = Schedule IV; 3 = Schedule V; 4 = not scheduled; 5 = some combination analgesic or antitussive preparations are listed in Schedules III or V, depending on their content of opioid; 6 = marketed in the United States only in combination with additional ingredients; 7 = traditionally used orally primarily for treatment of moderate pain; 8 = may exhibit cumulative effects with repeated administration; 9 = oral forms not available; 10 = marked irritation occurs at injection sites; 11 = may produce withdrawal symptoms in individuals who are physically dependent on μ agonists; 12 = may produce psychotomimetic effects at higher doses.

g. Oral antitussive dose.

h. Doses for moderate pain that are not necessarily equivalent to 10 mg of subcutaneous morphine.

The major pathway for the metabolism of morphine is conjugation with glucuronic acid to form both active and inactive products; morphine-6-glucuronide is more potent than morphine (Paul *et al.*, 1989). In young adults, the half-life of morphine is about 2 hours; the half-life of morphine-6-glucuronide is somewhat longer. Children achieve adult values by 6 months of age. In older patients, the volume of distribution is considerably smaller and initial concentrations of morphine are correspondingly higher (Owen *et al.*, 1983).

Excretion. Little morphine is excreted unchanged. It is eliminated by glomerular filtration, mainly as morphine-3-glucuronide; 90% of total excretion takes place during the first day. Enterohepatic circulation of morphine and its glucuronides occurs, which accounts for small amounts of morphine in the feces and in the urine for several days after the last dose.

Codeine, in contrast to morphine, is approximately 60% as effective orally as parenterally, both as an analgesic and as a respiratory depressant. Very few opioids have so high an oral–parenteral potency ratio; levorphanol, oxycodone, and methadone also share this attribute. The greater oral efficacy of these drugs is due to less first-pass metabolism in the liver. Once absorbed, codeine is metabolized by the liver and excreted chiefly in the urine, largely in inactive forms. A small fraction (approximately 10%) of administered codeine is demethylated to form morphine, and both free and conjugated morphine can be found in the urine after therapeutic doses of codeine. Codeine has an exceptionally low affinity for opioid receptors, and the analgesic effect of codeine is due to its conversion to morphine. However, its antitussive actions probably involve distinct receptors that bind codeine itself. The half-life of codeine in plasma is 2 to 4 hours.

Heroin (diacetylmorphine) is rapidly hydrolyzed to 6-monoacetylmorphine (6-MAM), which, in turn, is hydrolyzed to morphine. Both heroin and 6-MAM are more lipid soluble than morphine and enter the brain more readily. Current evidence suggests that morphine and 6-MAM are responsible for the pharmacological actions of heroin. Heroin is mainly excreted in the urine, largely as free and conjugated morphine.

The absorption, fate, and distribution of morphine-like drugs have been reviewed by Misra (1978) and by Chan and Matzke (1987).

Untoward Effects and Precautions. Morphine and related opioids produce a wide spectrum of unwanted effects, including respiratory depression, nausea, vomiting, dizziness, mental clouding, dysphoria, pruritus, constipation, increased pressure in the biliary tract, urinary retention, and hypotension. The bases of these effects have been described above. Rarely, a patient may develop a delirium. Increased sensitivity to pain after the analgesia has worn off may also occur.

A number of factors may alter a patient's sensitivity to opioid analgesics, including the integrity of the blood–brain barrier. For example, when morphine is administered to the mother prior to delivery, the newborn infant may exhibit respiratory depression even though the drug produced no significant depression in the mother. More lipophilic opioids such as meperidine cause relatively less respiratory depression in the newborn in doses that produce analgesia in the mother. In adults, the duration of the analgesia produced by morphine increases progressively with age; however, the degree of analgesia that is obtained with a given dose changes little (*see* Kaiko, 1980). Changes in pharmacokinetic parameters can only partially explain these observations. The patient with severe pain may tolerate larger doses of morphine (three to four therapeutic doses over a period of a few hours) but may exhibit subjective symptoms and respiratory depression should the pain suddenly subside.

All the opioid analgesics are metabolized by the liver, and the drugs should be used with caution in patients with hepatic disease, since increased bioavailability after oral administration or cumulative effects may occur (*see* Säwe *et al.*, 1981). Renal disease also significantly alters the pharmacokinetics of morphine, codeine, drocode (dihydrocodeine), meperidine, and propoxyphene. Although single doses of morphine are well tolerated, the active metabolite, morphine-6-glucuronide, may accumulate and symptoms of opioid overdose may result (*see* Chan and Matzke, 1987). This metabolite may also accumulate during repeated administration of codeine to patients with impaired renal function. When meperidine is given to such patients, the accumulation of normeperidine may cause tremor and seizures (Kaiko *et al.*, 1983); the repeated administration of propoxyphene may lead to naloxone-insensitive cardiac toxicity caused by the accumulation of norpropoxyphene (*see* Chan and Matzke, 1987).

Morphine and related opioids must be used with great caution in any situation in which respiratory reserve is decreased, such as emphysema, kyphoscoliosis, or even severe obesity. In patients with chronic cor pulmonale, death has occurred following therapeutic doses of morphine. Although many patients with such conditions seem to be functioning within normal limits, they are already utilizing compensatory mechanisms, such as increased respiratory rate. Many have chronically elevated levels of plasma CO_2, and may be less sensitive to the stimulating actions of CO_2. The further imposition of the depressant effects of opioids can be disastrous.

The respiratory-depressant effects of morphine and the related capacity to elevate intracranial pressure may be markedly exaggerated in the presence of head injury or of an already elevated cerebrospinal fluid pressure produced by trauma. Therefore, while head injury *per se* does not constitute an absolute contraindication to the use of opioids, the possibility of exaggerated depression of respiration must be considered. In addition, opioids may aggravate the effects of cerebral and spinal ischemia (*see* below). Finally, since opioids produce mental clouding and side effects such as miosis and vomiting, which are important signs in following the clinical course of patients with head injuries, the advisability of their use must be carefully weighed.

Opioids can precipitate attacks of asthma in anesthetized patients, but the risk does not seem to be high. During an asthmatic attack morphine and related drugs should be avoided, since they depress the cough reflex and respiration and tend to dry secretions. Some opioids also release histamine, which can produce additional bronchoconstriction.

Patients with reduced blood volume are considerably more susceptible to the hypotensive effects of morphine and related drugs, and these agents must be used cautiously in patients with hypotension from any cause. The basis for this susceptibility and the uses of opioid antagonists in shock are discussed below.

Allergic phenomena occur with opioid analgesics, but they are not common. They are usually manifested as urticaria and other types of skin rashes such as fixed eruptions; contact dermatitis in nurses and pharmaceutical workers also occurs. Wheals at the site of injection of morphine, codeine, and related drugs are probably caused by the release of histamine. Anaphylactoid reactions have been reported after intravenous administration of codeine and morphine, but such reactions are quite rare; however, it has been suggested, but not proven, that such reactions are responsible for some of the sudden deaths, episodes of pulmonary edema, and other complications that occur among addicts who use heroin intravenously (*see* Chapter 22).

Interactions with Other Drugs. The depressant effects of some opioids may be exaggerated and prolonged by phenothiazines, monoamine oxidase inhibitors, and tricyclic antidepressants; the mechanisms of these supra-additive effects are not fully understood, but may involve alterations in the rate of metabolic transformation of the opioid or alterations in neurotransmitters involved in the actions of opioids. Some, but not all, phenothiazines reduce the amount of opioid required to produce a given level of analgesia. However, depending on the specific agent, the respiratory-depressant effects also seem to be enhanced, the degree of sedation is increased, and the hypotensive effects of phenothiazines become an additional complication. Some phenothiazine derivatives enhance the sedative effects, but at the same time seem to be antianalgesic and increase the amount of opioid required to produce satisfactory relief from pain. Small doses of amphetamine substantially increase the analgesic and euphoriant effects of morphine and may decrease its sedative side effects. A number of antihistamines exhibit modest analgesic actions; some (*e.g.*, hydroxyzine) enhance the analgesic effects of low doses of opioids (*see* Rumore and Schlichting, 1986). Tricyclic antidepressants such as desipramine and amitriptyline are used in the treatment of chronic neuropathic pain but do not appear to have intrinsic analgesic actions in acute pain; however, desipramine may enhance morphine analgesia postoperatively (Levine *et al.*, 1986). The analgesic synergism between opioids and aspirin-like drugs is discussed below and in Chapter 26.

Preparations, Routes of Administration, and Dosage. Opium tincture, purified opium alkaloids, and paregoric (camphorated opium tincture) remain available for clinical use but are not recommended.

Morphine. Solutions of *morphine sulfate* (ROXANOL) are available for oral use (from 2 to 20 mg/ml) and for injection (from 2 to 15 mg/ml); tablets, controlled-release tablets, and rectal suppositories are also available. Preservative-free solutions (0.5 and 1 mg/ml) are intended for intravenous, epidural, or intrathecal injection.

Subcutaneously or intramuscularly, 10 mg/70 kg of body weight is generally considered to be an optimal initial dose of morphine and provides satisfactory analgesia in approximately 70% of patients with moderate-to-severe pain (*e.g.*, postoperative pain) with only a moderate incidence of side effects. Subsequent doses may be higher or lower, depending on the analgesic response and the side effects produced. The usual oral adult dose of morphine is 10 to 30 mg. However, controlled studies have shown that, on average, oral administration is only about one sixth as effective as parenteral administration. There is wide variability in first-pass metabolism, and the dose should be titrated to the patient's needs (*see* below).

Morphine may be given intravenously for the control of severe postoperative pain and restlessness, for preoperative medication, for minor surgical procedures when general anesthesia is not indicated, for severe cardiac pain, and for renal colic; it is also used for pulmonary edema. The usual dose is 2.5 to 10 mg. Maximal respiratory depression is manifest within 10 minutes. Opioids can also be given epidurally and intrathecally for postoperative analgesia and when more traditional routes no longer afford adequate pain control. Special isobaric solutions without preservatives are used for this purpose.

The dose of morphine for infants and children is 0.1 to 0.2 mg/kg (maximum 15 mg), injected subcutaneously or intramuscularly.

Codeine. Codeine is available as *codeine sulfate* and *codeine phosphate;* both salts are supplied as tablets (15 to 60 mg). Codeine phosphate is available for injection. It is contained in numerous analgesic combinations (liquids, tablets, and capsules) and in various antitussive combinations (liquids and capsules).

Although a dose of 120 mg of codeine, administered subcutaneously, produces analgesia equivalent to that resulting from 10 mg of morphine, codeine has no advantage over morphine when used parenterally. However, it has a high oral–parenteral potency ratio; in terms of total analgesia, codeine is about 60% as potent when given orally as when injected intramuscularly. In this respect it has definite advantages over morphine. Orally, a dose of 30 mg of codeine is approximately equianalgesic with 325 to 600 mg of aspirin. While the analgesic effects of opioids and aspirin-like drugs are usually additive, the analgesia produced by a combination of these two drugs at this dosage level sometimes exceeds that of 60 mg of codeine (*see* Beaver, 1988). Codeine (15 to 20 mg orally) reduces the frequency of pathological cough, and progressively greater cough suppression is seen as the dose is increased up to 60 mg (Matthys *et al.*, 1983). The abuse liability of codeine is lower than that of morphine, as discussed more fully in Chapter 22.

Other Semisynthetic Morphine and Codeine Derivatives. There are many drugs that can substitute for morphine and codeine. Their names, doses, and special characteristics are shown in Table 21–3.

Hydromorphone hydrochloride (DILAUDID) is available in tablets (1 to 4 mg) and in rectal suppositories. Solutions for injection (from 1 to 10 mg/ml) are also available. Plasma concentrations of hydromorphone above 4 ng/ml are usually required for adequate relief of pain (Reidenberg *et al.*, 1988). *Oxycodone hydrochloride* (ROXICODONE) is about as potent as morphine and is nearly ten times more potent than codeine. Like codeine, it is about one half as potent orally as parenterally. It is available in 5-mg tablets, as a solution, and in combination with other analgesics. *Oxymorphone hydrochloride* (NUMORPHAN) is available as a solution for injection and in rectal suppositories. *Hydrocodone bitartrate* is used in combination with other ingredients in proprietary antitussive and analgesic-antipyretic mixtures.

Diacetylmorphine (heroin) is not available for therapeutic use in the United States. Given intramuscularly to cancer patients with postoperative pain, it is about twice as potent as morphine. While peak analgesic effects occur a few minutes earlier than with morphine, its duration of action is not significantly different. Heroin does not appear to have any unique therapeutic advantages over the available opioids (*see* Kaiko *et al.*, 1981; Sawynok, 1986).

ACUTE OPIOID TOXICITY

Acute opioid toxicity may result from clinical overdosage, accidental overdosage in addicts, or attempts at suicide. Occasionally, a delayed type of toxicity may occur from the injection of an opioid into chilled skin areas or in patients with low blood pressure and shock. The drug is not fully absorbed, and, therefore, a subsequent dose may be given. When normal circulation is established, an excessive amount may suddenly be absorbed. It is difficult to state the exact amount of any opioid that is toxic or lethal to man. Recent experiences with methadone indicate that in nontolerant individuals serious toxicity may follow the oral ingestion of 40 to 60 mg. Older literature suggests that, in the case of morphine, a normal, pain-free adult is not likely to die after oral doses of less than 120 mg, or to have serious toxicity with less than 30 mg parenterally.

Symptoms and Diagnosis. The patient who has taken an overdose of an opioid is usually stuporous or, if a large overdose has been taken, in a profound coma. The respiratory rate is quite low (sometimes only 2 to 4 per minute), and cyanosis may be present. As respiratory exchange becomes poorer, blood pressure, at first maintained near normal, falls progressively. If adequate oxygenation is restored early, the blood pressure will improve; if hypoxia persists untreated, however, there may be capillary damage, and measures to combat shock may then be required. The pupils are symmetrical and pinpoint in size; however, if hypoxia is severe, they may be dilated. Urine formation is depressed. Body temperature falls, and the skin becomes cold and clammy. The skeletal muscles are flaccid, the jaw is relaxed, and the tongue may fall back and block the airway. Frank convulsions may occasionally be noted in infants and children. When death occurs, it is nearly always due to respiratory failure. Even if respiration is restored, death may still occur as a result of complications, such as pneumonia or shock, that develop during the period of coma. Noncardiogenic pulmonary edema is commonly seen with opioid poisoning. It is probably not due to contaminants or to anaphylactoid reactions, and has been observed following toxic doses of morphine, methadone, propoxyphene, and uncontaminated heroin.

The triad of coma, pinpoint pupils, and depressed respiration strongly suggests opioid poisoning. The finding of needle marks suggestive of addiction further supports the diagnosis. Mixed poisonings, however, are not uncommon. Examination of the urine and gastric contents for various drugs may aid in diagnosis, but the results usually become available too late to influence treatment.

Treatment. The first step is to establish a patent airway and ventilate the patient. Opioid antagonists such as naloxone can produce dramatic reversal of the severe respiratory depression (*see* below), and the use of naloxone is the treatment of choice. The safest approach is the administration of small intravenous doses (*e.g.*, 0.4 to 2 mg of naloxone); this dose should be repeated after 2 to 3 minutes if no effect is seen. For children, the initial dose is 0.01 mg/kg. If no effect is seen after a total dose of 10 mg, one can reasonably question the accuracy of the diagnosis. Pulmonary edema sometimes associated with opioid overdosage may be countered by positive-pressure respiration. Tonic-clonic seizures, occasionally seen as part of the toxic syndrome with meperidine and propoxyphene, are ameliorated by treatment with naloxone.

The presence of general CNS depressants does not prevent the salutary effect of naloxone, and in cases of mixed intoxications the situation will be improved largely due to antagonism of the respiratory-depressant effects of the opioid. However, some evidence indicates that naloxone and naltrexone may also antagonize some of the depressant actions of sedative-hypnotics (*see* below). One need not attempt to restore the patient to full consciousness. The duration of action of the available antagonists is shorter than that of many opioids; hence, patients must be carefully watched, lest they slip back into coma. This is particularly important when the overdosage is due to methadone or *l*-acetylmethadol. The depressant effects of these drugs may persist for 24 to 72 hours, and fatalities have occurred as a result of premature discontinuation of naloxone.

The use of excessive doses of an opioid antagonist to treat acute poisoning in an addict may precipitate a severe withdrawal syndrome that cannot be readily suppressed during the period of action of the antagonist. Treatment with naloxone may also result in a rebound increase in activity of the sympathetic nervous system, which may occasionally cause cardiac arrhythmias and pulmonary edema (*see* Duthie and Nimmo, 1987).

Toxicity owing to overdose of pentazocine and other opioids with mixed actions may require higher doses of naloxone. The pharmacological actions of opioid antagonists are discussed in more detail below.

THERAPEUTIC USES

Sir William Osler referred to morphine as "God's own medicine." Morphine-like drugs are still important in the treatment of severe pain and the pain of terminal illness, but physicians now have other options for many conditions that involve moderate pain.

General Principles. Opioid analgesics provide symptomatic relief of pain, cough, or diarrhea, but generally the underlying disease remains. The physician must weigh the benefits of this relief against its risk to the patient, which may be quite different in an acute compared with a chronic disease.

In acute problems, opioids may obscure the progress of the disease or the location or intensity of pain. However, relief of pain can also facilitate history taking, examination, and the patient's ability to tolerate diagnostic procedures. Patients should not be inadequately evaluated because of the physician's unwillingness to prescribe analgesics.

The problems that arise in the relief of pain associated with chronic conditions involve more complex considerations. Repeated daily administration will eventually produce some tolerance to the therapeutic effects of the drug, and some degree of physical dependence as well. The degree will depend on the particular drug, the frequency of administration, and the quantity administered. Because the risk of developing drug dependence is always present, a decision to control any chronic symptom, especially pain, by the repeated administration of an opioid must be made carefully. When pain is due to chronic nonmalignant disease, measures other than opioid drugs should be employed to relieve chronic pain if they are effective and available. Such measures include the use of aspirin-like drugs, local nerve block, antidepressant drugs, electrical stimulation, acupuncture, hypnosis, or behavioral modification (*see* Foley, 1985). Even when pain is due to cancer, the generally accepted procedure is to use aspirin-like drugs until they no longer adequately control the pain.

In the usual doses, morphine-like drugs relieve suffering by altering the emotional component of the painful experience as well as by producing analgesia. Control of pain, especially chronic pain, must include attention to both psychological factors and the social impact of the illness that sometimes play a dominant role in determining the suffering experienced by the patient. In addition to emotional support, the physician must also consider the substantial variability in both the patient's capacity to tolerate pain and the response to opioids. These factors may depend in part on the ability of the patient to mobilize endogenous opioids and other antinociceptive systems (*see* Millan, 1986). As a result, some patients may require considerably more than the average dose of a drug to experience any relief from pain; others, perhaps because of more rapid metabolic disposition, may require a drug at shorter intervals. Some clinicians, out of an exaggerated concern for the possibility of inducing addiction, tend to prescribe initial doses of opioids that are too low or too infrequent to alleviate pain, and then respond to the patient's continued complaints with an even more exaggerated concern about drug dependence, despite the high probability that the request for more drug is only the expected consequence of the inadequate dosage initially prescribed (*see* Sriwatanakul *et al.*, 1983). Infants and children are probably more apt to receive inadequate treatment for pain than are adults; if an illness or procedure causes pain for an adult, there is no reason to assume that it will produce less pain for a child (*see* Yaster and Deshpande, 1988). It is useful to remember that the typical initial dose of morphine (10 mg/70 kg) relieves postoperative pain satisfactorily in only two thirds of patients.

Pain. *Selection of a Drug.* In equianalgesic doses, morphine and most of its μ-agonist surrogates produce approximately the same incidence and degree of unwanted side effects (*see* Table 21–3). Nevertheless, some patients may have side effects with one agent and not with another. Some drugs have shorter durations of action, others are particularly efficacious when given by mouth, and a few are considered to have a lower risk for producing opioid dependence. Still others (*e.g.*, hydromorphone) are more soluble or more potent, which may allow the injection of adequate doses in a reasonable volume, or are available as rectal suppositories, which can be a useful alternative to injection when nausea precludes oral administration. The availability of a wide range of agents provides a therapeutic flexibility that is too often underutilized (*see* Foley, 1985; Bovill, 1987).

For many types of pain, aspirin or any of a number of aspirin-like antiinflammatory drugs provide relief equivalent to 60 mg of oral codeine; in some instances, their effects are equivalent to 8 mg or more of parenteral morphine. These drugs may have special advantages in the management of pain from bone metastases (*see* Foley, 1985). If relief of pain is insufficient, these drugs can then be combined with orally effective morphine-like agents, such as codeine, or with agonist-antagonist opioids. Because they exert their effects by different mechanisms, combinations of these two classes of drugs can usually achieve an analgesic effect that would otherwise require a higher dose of opioid, but with fewer side effects. In treating chronic pain not associated with terminal illness, the amount of the agonist-antagonist opioid component in such combinations should be increased until adverse side effects appear before changing to a μ-agonist opioid such as morphine.

It may also be helpful to employ other agents (adjuvants) that enhance opioid analgesia and that may add beneficial effects of their own. For example, the combination of an opioid with a small dose of amphetamine may augment analgesia while reducing the sedative effects. Certain antidepressants, such as amitriptyline and desipramine, may also enhance opioid analgesia, and they may have analgesic actions in some types of neuropathic (deafferentation) pain for which opioids are often ineffective (*see* McQuay, 1988). Other potentially useful adjuvants include certain antihistamines, anticonvulsants such as carbamazepine and phenytoin, and glucocorticoids.

When the pain is associated with biliary spasm, meperidine or one of the agonist-antagonist opioids may produce less increase in the spasm than will an equianalgesic dose of morphine or a similar agent. When the pain is likely to be of short duration (*e.g.*, diagnostic procedures, cystoscopy, orthopedic manipulation, *etc.*), a drug with a shorter duration of action, such as alfentanil, might be preferable to morphine or oxycodone.

Pain of Terminal Illness and Cancer Pain. Although they are not requisite or even desirable in all cases of terminal illness, the analgesia, tranquility, and even the euphoria afforded by the use of opioids can make the final days far less distressing for the patient and family. Some degree of physical dependence and tolerance develops whenever an opioid is given in therapeutic dosage several times a day over a prolonged period. In patients with painful terminal illnesses such considerations should not in any way prevent physicians from fulfilling their primary obligation to ease the patient's discomfort. The physician should not wait until the pain becomes agonizing; *no patient should ever wish for death because of a physician's reluctance to use adequate amounts of effective opioids.* Indeed, it is not acceptable to wait until the final days or weeks, and the physician must utilize those measures that will allow the patient to be as free of pain and as functional as possible. This may sometimes entail the regular use of opioid analgesics in substantial doses (*see* below). Such patients, while they may be physically dependent, are not considered "addicts" even though they may need large doses on a regular basis. Newer definitions of drug dependence (addiction) that have been developed by national and international groups emphasize the distinction between physical dependence and addiction. Physical dependence alone does not fulfill the criteria for drug addiction (*see* Chapter 22).

Most clinicians who are experienced in the management of chronic pain associated with malignant disease or terminal illness recommend that opioids be administered at sufficiently short, fixed intervals so that pain is continually under control and patients do not dread its return. Less drug is needed to prevent the recurrence of pain than to relieve it. Morphine remains the opioid of choice in most of these situations, and the route and dose should be adjusted to the needs of the individual patient. Many clinicians find that oral morphine is adequate in most situations. Sustained-release preparations of oral morphine are now available that can be administered at 8- to 12-hour intervals. Superior control of pain can often be achieved with fewer side effects using the same daily dose (Meed *et al.*, 1987); a decrease in the fluctuation of plasma concentrations of morphine may be partially responsible.

Constipation is an exceedingly common problem when opioids are used, and the use of stool softeners and laxatives should be initiated early. Amphetamines have demonstrable mood-elevating and analgesic effects and enhance opioid-induced analgesia. However, not all terminal patients require the euphoriant effects of amphetamine and some experience side effects. Controlled studies demonstrate no superiority of oral heroin over oral morphine. Similarly, after adjustment is made for potency, parenteral heroin is not superior to morphine in terms of analgesia, effects on mood, or side effects (*see* Sawynok, 1986). Although tolerance does develop to oral opioids, many patients obtain relief from the same dosage for weeks or months.

When opioids and other analgesics are no longer satisfactory, nerve block, chordotomy, or other types of neurosurgical intervention such as neurostimulation may be required if the nature of the lesion permits. Epidural or intrathecal administration of opioids may be useful when administration of opioids by usual routes no longer yields adequate relief of pain (*see* Chapter 15). While tolerance may develop, the technique can be used with ambulatory patients over periods of weeks or months (*see* Gustafsson and Wiesenfeld-Hallin, 1988). Moreover, portable devices have been developed that permit the patient to control the parenteral administration of an opioid while remaining ambulatory (Kerr *et al.*, 1988). These devices use a pump that infuses the drug from a reservoir at a rate that can be tailored to the needs of the patient, and they include mechanisms to limit dosage and/or allow the patient to self-administer an additional "rescue" dose if there is a transient change in the intensity of pain. Administration by the intravenous, intramuscular, subcutaneous, or intraspinal route can be employed.

Postoperative Pain. When pain is not too severe, oral codeine or oxycodone combined with aspirin-like drugs often provides adequate analgesia without the side effects associated with the use of usual doses of morphine. When pain is more severe, opioid analgesics are used in the immediate postoperative period. However, if used excessively, they may prevent the early recognition of complications, decrease the effectiveness of coughing, decrease respiratory ventilation, predispose to pneumonitis, reduce bowel motility, and cause urinary retention. Used properly, however, the reduction of pain may increase the patient's ability to breathe deeply, cooperate with respiratory therapy procedures, cough voluntarily, and ambulate. The use of fixed doses given "as needed" without consideration of individual requirements often leads to unnecessary suffering. Moreover, delays in administration of doses often lead to subtherapeutic plasma concentrations of drug. As a result, an increasing number of hospitals employ patient-controlled analgesia (PCA), utilizing the devices described above. With short-acting opioids such as morphine, serious toxicity or excessive use by the patient rarely occurs. The concern that self-administration of opioids intravenously would increase the likelihood of drug addiction has not materialized. Both adult and pediatric patients generally prefer PCA to traditional intramuscular injections for control of postoperative pain (Rodgers *et al.*, 1988).

Headache. Headache is often a recurrent problem, sometimes reflecting emotional disturbances, and opioid analgesics, with the possible exception of codeine, should not be employed unless all other measures have failed. Even then, considerable care should be employed to minimize the development of drug dependence.

Obstetrical Analgesia. The use of morphine-like drugs in obstetrical analgesia is a highly specialized field requiring experience and sound judgment to ensure effective analgesia, safety for the fetus, and minimal interference with the progress of labor. All the available morphine-like opioids are powerful respiratory depressants, and the fetus seems more susceptible to their respiratory-depressant effects than does the mother. In equianalgesic doses, morphine and methadone appear somewhat more depressant to the fetus than are meperidine and closely related drugs. The pharmacological basis for this difference has been discussed above. The differences are sufficient to justify the selection of meperidine-like drugs in preference to morphine for obstetrical use (*see* below).

Cough. The antitussive effect of opioid drugs can be demonstrated experimentally against the coughing induced by electrical stimulation of the medulla or by chemical or mechanical irritation of the respiratory tract. With several opioids, the dose required to suppress cough induced by these techniques is lower than that required for analgesia; this finding is consistent with other evidence that suggests that distinct receptors mediate the antitussive actions of opioids. A 10- or 20-mg oral dose of codeine, although ineffective for analgesia, produces a demonstrable antitussive effect, and higher doses of codeine produce even more suppression of chronic cough. A number of effective nonopioid, nonaddictive antitussives are now available for clinical use (*see* below).

Dyspnea. Morphine is used to alleviate the dyspnea of acute left ventricular failure and pulmonary edema, in which the response to intravenous morphine may be dramatic. The mechanism underlying this relief is still not clear. It may involve an alteration of the patient's reaction to impaired respiratory function and an indirect reduction of the work of the heart due to reduced fear and apprehension. However, it is more probable that the major benefit is due to cardiovascular effects, such as decreased peripheral resistance and an increased capacity of the peripheral and splanchnic vascular compartments (*see* Vismara *et al.,* 1976). Nitroglycerine, which also causes vasodilatation, may be superior to morphine in this condition (Hoffman and Reynolds, 1987). In patients with normal blood gases but severe breathlessness due to chronic obstruction of airflow ("pink puffers"), drocode (dihydrocodeine), 15 mg orally before exercise, reduces the feeling of breathlessness and increases exercise tolerance (Johnson *et al.,* 1983). Opioids are contraindicated in pulmonary edema due to respiratory irritants unless severe pain is also present; contraindications to their use in asthma have already been discussed.

Constipating Effects. The morphine-like opioids are effective agents for causing constipation or treating diarrhea. Mild constipation and a drier stool are often desirable after ileostomy or colostomy, and the constipating action is especially valuable in treating exhausting diarrhea and dysenteries due to a number of causes. As in the case for cough, it requires considerably less morphine to affect the gut than to produce analgesia. Traditionally, opium preparations rather than the pure alkaloids have been used. Synthetic opioids also produce a decrease in bowel motility as well as counteract the excessive secretion that accompanies some forms of diarrhea; several of these, such as diphenoxylate, loperamide, and difenoxin, are used exclusively for this purpose (*see* below).

Special Anesthesia. High doses of morphine or other opioids have been used as the primary anesthetic agents in certain surgical procedures. Although respiration is so depressed that physical assistance is required, patients can retain consciousness (*see* Chapter 14). Opioids can also be injected intrathecally or epidurally to relieve postoperative and chronic pain (*see* Chapter 15).

LEVORPHANOL AND CONGENERS

Levorphanol is the only commercially available opioid agonist of the morphinan series. The *d* isomer (dextrorphan) is relatively devoid of analgesic action. The structure of levorphanol is indicated in Table 21–2.

The pharmacological effects of levorphanol closely parallel those of morphine. However, clinical reports suggest that it produces less nausea and vomiting. The nonanalgesic isomer dextrorphan possesses considerable antitussive activity (*see* below). Although levorphanol is less effective when given orally, its oral–parenteral potency ratio is comparable to that of codeine and oxycodone. The average adult dose (2 mg subcutaneously) produces analgesia for a period of time somewhat longer than that for morphine (*see* Table 21–3). Levorphanol is metabolized less rapidly and has a half-life of about 12 to 16 hours; repeated administration at short intervals may thus lead to accumulation of the drug in plasma (*see* Foley, 1985). The drug is available as *levorphanol tartrate* (LEVO-DROMORAN) in 2-mg tablets and as a solution (2 mg/ml) for injection.

MEPERIDINE AND CONGENERS

Chemistry. The structural formulas of meperidine, a phenylpiperidine, and some of its congeners are shown in Table 21–4.

PHARMACOLOGICAL PROPERTIES

Meperidine is predominantly a μ agonist, and it exerts its chief pharmacological actions on the CNS and the neural elements in the bowel.

Central Nervous System. Meperidine produces a pattern of effects similar but not identical to that described for morphine.

Analgesia. The analgesic effects of meperidine are detectable about 15 minutes after oral administration, reach a peak in about 2 hours, and subside gradually over several hours. The onset of analgesic effect is faster (within 10 minutes) after subcutaneous or intramuscular administration and reaches a peak in about 1 hour that corresponds closely to peak concentrations in plasma. In clinical use, the duration of effective analgesia is approximately 3 to 5 hours.

In general, 75 to 100 mg of meperidine given parenterally is approximately equivalent to 10 mg of morphine, and, in equianalgesic doses, meperidine produces as much sedation, respiratory depression, and euphoria as does morphine. In terms of total analgesic effect, meperidine is less than one half as effective when given by mouth as

Table 21–4. CHEMICAL STRUCTURES OF PIPERIDINE AND PHENYLPIPERIDINE ANALGESICS

COMPOUND	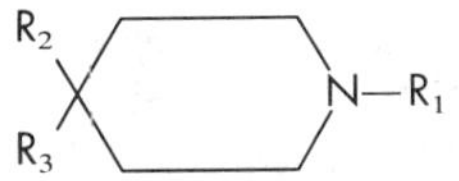		
	R_1	R_2	R_3
Meperidine	$-CH_3$	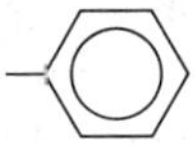	$-\underset{\substack{\| \\ O}}{C}OCH_2CH_3$
Diphenoxylate	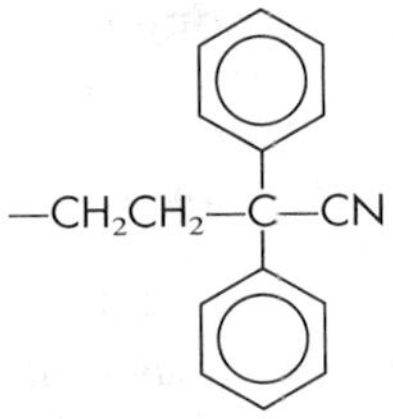	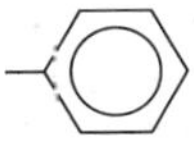	$-\underset{\substack{\| \\ O}}{C}OCH_2CH_3$
Loperamide	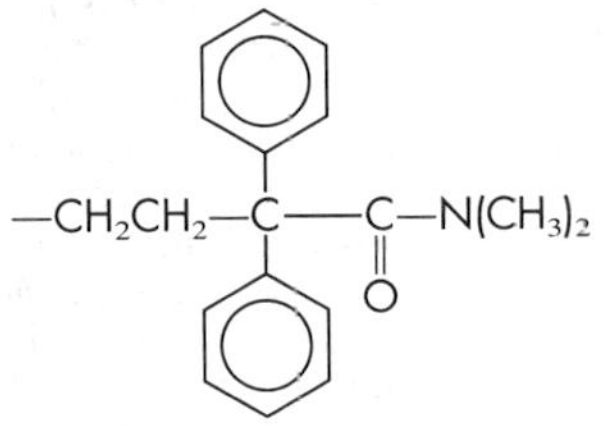	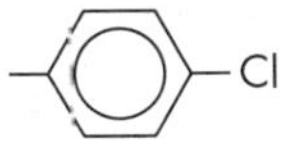	—OH
Fentanyl	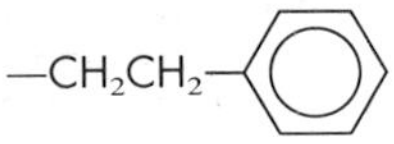	—H	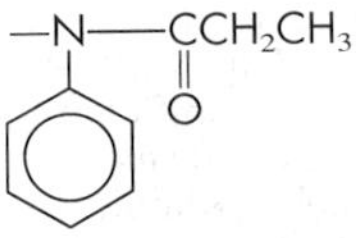
Sufentanil	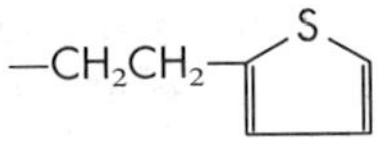	$-CH_2OCH_3$	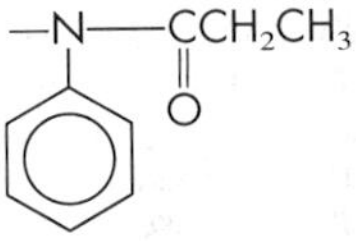
Alfentanil	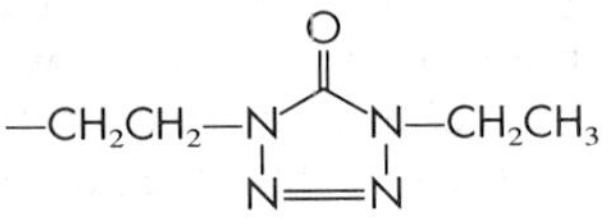	$-CH_2OCH_3$	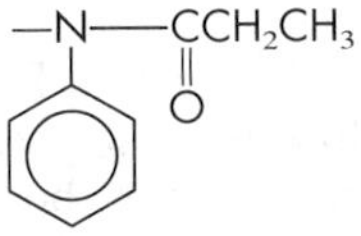

when administered parenterally; this is consistent with observations that its oral bioavailability is 40 to 60%. A few patients may experience dysphoria.

Other CNS Actions. Peak respiratory depression is observed within 1 hour after intramuscular administration, and there is a return toward normal starting at about 2 hours, although minute volume is usually measurably depressed for as long as 4 hours (*see* Edwards *et al.*, 1982). Like other opioids, meperidine causes pupillary constriction, increases the sensitivity of the labyrinthine apparatus, and has effects on the secretion of pituitary hormones similar to those of morphine. Meperidine differs from morphine in that toxic doses sometimes cause CNS excitation, characterized by tremors, muscle twitches, and seizures; these effects are due largely to a metabolite, normeperidine (*see* below).

Cardiovascular System. The effects of meperidine on the cardiovascular system generally resemble those of morphine, including the ability to release histamine upon parenteral administration (Lee *et al.,* 1976). Intramuscular administration of meperidine does not significantly affect heart rate, but intravenous administration frequently produces an increased rate that is sometimes alarming. As with morphine, respiratory depression is responsible for an accumulation of CO_2, which, in turn, produces cerebrovascular dilatation, increase in cerebral blood flow, and elevation of cerebrospinal fluid pressure.

Smooth Muscle. Meperidine has effects on certain smooth muscles qualitatively similar to those observed with other opioids but less intense relative to its analgesic actions.

Meperidine does not cause as much constipation when given over prolonged periods of time; this may be related to its greater facility to enter the CNS, thereby producing analgesia at lower concentrations in the periphery. After equianalgesic doses, the rise in pressure in the common bile duct induced by meperidine is less than that caused by morphine but greater than that by codeine. Nevertheless, clinical doses of meperidine slow gastric emptying sufficiently to delay absorption of other drugs significantly.

The uterus of nonpregnant women is usually mildly stimulated by meperidine. Administered prior to an oxytocic, meperidine does not exert any antagonistic effect. Therapeutic doses given during active labor do not delay the birth process; in fact, the frequency, duration, and amplitude of uterine contractions may sometimes be increased (Fishburne, 1982; Zimmer *et al.,* 1988). The drug does not interfere with normal postpartum contraction or involution of the uterus, and it does not increase the incidence of postpartum hemorrhage.

Absorption, Fate, and Excretion. Meperidine is absorbed by all routes of administration, but the rate of absorption may be erratic after intramuscular injection. The peak plasma concentration usually occurs at about 45 minutes, but the range is wide. After oral administration, only about 50% of the drug escapes first-pass metabolism to enter the circulation, and peak concentrations in plasma are usually observed in 1 to 2 hours (Herman *et al.,* 1985).

Meperidine is metabolized chiefly in the liver, with a half-time of about 3 hours. In patients with cirrhosis, the bioavailability of meperidine is increased to as much as 80% and the half-lives of both meperidine and normeperidine are prolonged. Approximately 60% of meperidine in plasma is protein bound.

In man, meperidine is hydrolyzed to meperidinic acid, which, in turn, is partially conjugated. Meperidine is also N-demethylated to normeperidine, which may then be hydrolyzed to normeperidinic acid and subsequently conjugated. The clinical significance of the formation of normeperidine is discussed further under toxicity. Only a small amount of meperidine is excreted unchanged.

Preparations, Routes of Administration, and Dosage. *Meperidine hydrochloride* (*pethidine,* DEMEROL, PETHADOL) is available for oral use in tablets (50 and 100 mg) and as a syrup, and in solutions for parenteral use. Subcutaneous or intramuscular administration causes local irritation and tissue induration, and frequent repetition may lead to severe fibrosis of muscle tissue. The dose varies with the clinical situation. Most patients with moderate-to-severe pain are relieved by 100 mg parenterally. The effectiveness of the drug by the oral route is not reduced to the same degree as is that of morphine, but its oral–parenteral potency ratio is lower than that of codeine. Doses for infants and children average 1 to 1.8 mg/kg.

Untoward Effects, Precautions, and Contraindications. The pattern and overall incidence of untoward effects that follow the use of meperidine are similar to those observed after equianalgesic doses of morphine, except that constipation and urinary retention are less common. Patients who experience nausea and vomiting with morphine may not do so with meperidine; the converse may also be true. As with other opioids, tolerance develops to some of these effects. The contraindications are generally the same as for other opioids. In patients or addicts who are tolerant to the depressant effects of meperidine, large doses repeated at short intervals produce tremors, muscle twitches, dilated pupils, hyperactive reflexes, and convulsions. These excitatory symptoms are due to the accumulation of normeperidine, which has a half-life of 15 to 20 hours compared with 3 hours for meperidine. Since normeperidine is eliminated by both the kidney and the liver, decreased renal or hepatic function increases the likelihood of such toxicity (Kaiko *et al.*, 1983). Opioid antagonists can block the convulsant effect of normeperidine in the mouse.

Interaction with Other Drugs. Severe reactions may follow the administration of meperidine to patients being treated with monoamine oxidase (MAO) inhibitors. Two types of syndromes may be seen: severe respiratory depression or excitation, delirium, hyperpyrexia, and convulsions. Similar interactions with MAO inhibitors have not been observed with other opioids.

Chlorpromazine increases the respiratory-depressant effects of meperidine, as do tricyclic antidepressants; this is not true of diazepam. Concurrent administration of drugs such as promethazine or chlorpromazine may also greatly enhance meperidine-induced sedation without slowing clearance of the drug. Treatment with phenobarbital or phenytoin increases systemic clearance and decreases oral bioavailability of meperidine; this is associated with an elevation of the concentration of normeperidine in plasma (*see* Edwards *et al.*, 1982). As with morphine, concomitant administration of amphetamine has been reported to enhance the analgesic effects of meperidine and its congeners.

Tolerance, Physical Dependence, and Liability for Abuse. As with other μ agonists, repeated administration of therapeutic doses at short intervals can produce tolerance; however, tolerance to meperidine develops slowly if the interval is greater than 3 to 4 hours. Even when tolerance develops to the respiratory-depressant effects, high doses given at frequent intervals may produce an excitatory syndrome, including hallucinations and seizures, probably as a result of the accumulation of normeperidine (*see* above; *see also* Chapter 22).

The pattern of withdrawal symptoms after abrupt discontinuation of meperidine differs from that after morphine in that the autonomic effects are fewer and the symptoms develop more rapidly and are of shorter duration. The abuse potential of the clinically available meperidine congeners is similar to that of meperidine.

THERAPEUTIC USES

The major use of meperidine is for analgesia. Unlike morphine and its congeners, meperidine is not useful for the treatment of cough or diarrhea.

Analgesia. Meperidine can be used in any situation where an opioid analgesic is required. However, in a number of clinical conditions its lesser spasmogenic effects or its better oral efficacy make meperidine preferable to morphine.

The concentrations of meperidine in plasma required to produce satisfactory analgesia range from 100 to 800 ng/ml (average, 500 ng/ml); in any given patient, the analgesic concentration appears to remain relatively constant over time (Glynn and Mather, 1982). In some circumstances, a decrease in concentration of as little as 10% can result in a marked reduction in analgesia. As a result, some clinicians now recommend continuous intravenous infusion or parenteral administration "on demand" to reduce fluctuations in analgesic effects. The administration of about 25 mg of meperidine per hour will usually yield concentrations of 500 ng/ml in plasma (Edwards *et al.*, 1982).

Meperidine crosses the placental barrier and even in reasonable analgesic doses causes a significant increase in the percentage of babies who show delayed respiration, decreased respiratory minute volume, or decreased oxygen saturation, or who require resuscitation. Both fetal and maternal respiratory depression induced by meperidine can be treated with naloxone. The fraction of drug that is bound to protein is lower in the fetus; concentrations of free drug may thus be considerably higher than in the mother. Nevertheless, meperidine produces less respiratory depression in the newborn than does an equianalgesic dose of morphine or methadone (*see* Fishburne, 1982).

CONGENERS OF MEPERIDINE

Diphenoxylate. Diphenoxylate is a meperidine congener that has a definite constipating effect in man. Its only recognized use is in the treatment of diarrhea. Although single doses in the therapeutic range (*see* below) produce little or no morphine-like subjective effects, at high doses (40 to 60 mg) the drug shows typical opioid activity, including euphoria, suppression of morphine abstinence, and a morphine-like physical dependence after chronic administration. Diphenoxylate is unusual in that even its salts are virtually insoluble in aqueous solution, thus obviating the possibility of abuse by the parenteral route. *Diphenoxylate hydrochloride* is available only in combination with atropine sulfate (LOMOTIL, others), in tablets and as a liquid. Each tablet or 5 ml contains 2.5 mg of diphenoxylate and 25 μg of atropine sulfate. The recommended daily dosage of diphenoxylate for treatment of diarrhea in adults is 20 mg, in divided doses. *Difenoxin* (difenoxylic acid) is one of the metabolites of diphenoxylate; it has actions similar to those of the parent compound.

Loperamide. Loperamide, like diphenoxylate, is a piperidine derivative (*see* Table 21–4). It slows gastrointestinal motility by effects on the circular and longitudinal muscles of the intestine, presumably as a result of its interactions with opioid receptors in the intestine. Some part of its antidiarrheal effect may be due to a reduction of gastrointestinal secretion (*see* above; *see also* Manara and Bianchetti, 1985; Coupar, 1987; Kromer, 1988).

In controlling chronic diarrhea, loperamide is as effective as diphenoxylate. In clinical studies, the most common side effect is abdominal cramps. Little tolerance develops to its constipating effect.

In human volunteers taking large doses, concentrations of loperamide in plasma peak about 4 hours after ingestion; this long latency may be due to inhibition of gastrointestinal motility and to enterohepatic circulation of the drug. The apparent elimination half-time is 7 to 14 hours. Loperamide is not well absorbed after oral administration and, in addition, apparently does not penetrate well into the brain; these properties contribute to the selectivity of its action. A large proportion of the drug is excreted in the feces.

The drug is unlikely to be abused parenterally because of its low solubility; large doses of loperamide given to human volunteers do not elicit pleasurable effects typical of opioids. Its overall potential for abuse is probably lower than that of diphenoxylate (*see* Awouters *et al.*, 1983). The drug is available as *loperamide hydrochloride* (IMODIUM) in 2-mg capsules and as a liquid (1 mg/5 ml). The usual dosage is 4 to 8 mg per day; the daily dose should not exceed 16 mg.

FENTANYL

Fentanyl is a synthetic opioid related to the phenylpiperidines (*see* Table 21–4). It is primarily a μ agonist and is estimated to be 80 times as potent as morphine as an analgesic. The respiratory-depressant effect of fentanyl is of shorter duration than that of meperidine; its analgesic and euphoric effects are antagonized by opioid antagonists, but are not significantly prolonged or intensified by droperidol, a neuroleptic agent with which it is usually combined for use as an intravenous anesthetic (*see* Chapter 14). The subjective effects of the combination depend on the relative proportions of the two agents. High doses of fentanyl produce marked muscular rigidity, possibly as a result of the effects of opioids on dopaminergic transmission in the striatum; this effect can be antagonized by naloxone. Fentanyl is usually used for anesthesia, but it can also be used for postoperative analgesia. *Fentanyl citrate* (SUBLIMAZE) is available as a solution for injection. It is also supplied as a fixed-dose combination with droperidol (INNOVAR). Congeners of fentanyl, such as *sufentanil citrate* (SUFENTA) and *alfentanil hydrochloride* (ALFENTA) are also very potent and relatively selective μ agonists. They are approved for use in general anesthesia (*see* Chapter 14), but have also been used intrathecally, epidurally, and for postoperative analgesia. Their structures are shown in Table 21–4.

METHADONE AND CONGENERS

Methadone is primarily a μ agonist with pharmacological properties qualitatively similar to those of morphine.

Chemistry. Methadone has the following structural formula:

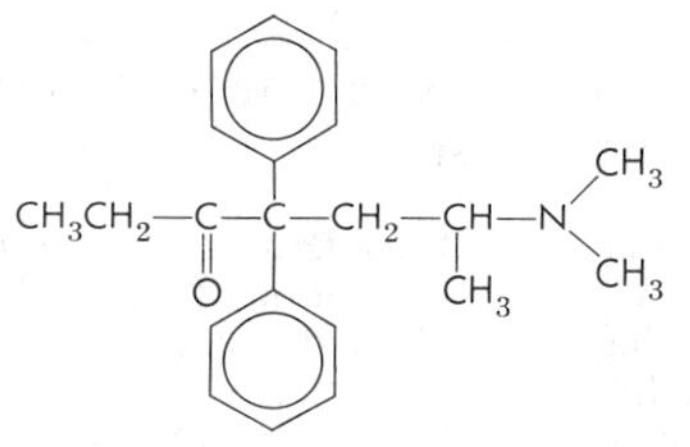

Methadone

The analgesic activity of the racemate is almost entirely the result of its content of *l*-methadone, which is 8 to 50 times more potent than the *d* isomer; *d*-methadone also lacks significant respiratory-depressant action and addiction liability, but it does possess antitussive activity.

Several structurally related congeners of methadone are in clinical use; as analgesics, these drugs have no demonstrable superiority over the parent compound. The dose, durations of action, and other effects of the congeners are compared with those of other opioid analgesics in Table 21–3.

Pharmacological Actions. The outstanding properties of methadone are its effective analgesic activity, its efficacy by the oral route, its extended duration of action in suppressing withdrawal symptoms in physically dependent individuals, and its tendency to show persistent effects with repeated administration. Miotic and respiratory-depressant effects can be detected for more than 24 hours after a single dose and, upon repeated administration, marked sedation is seen in some patients. Effects on cough, bowel motility, biliary tone, and the secretion of pituitary hormones are qualitatively similar to those of morphine.

Absorption, Fate, and Excretion. Methadone is well absorbed from the gastrointestinal tract and can be detected in plasma within 30 minutes after oral ingestion; it reaches peak concentrations at about 4 hours. After therapeutic doses, about 90% of methadone is bound to plasma proteins. Peak concentrations occur in the brain within 1 or 2 hours after subcutaneous or intramuscular administration, and this correlates well with the intensity and duration of analgesia. Methadone can also be absorbed from the buccal mucosa (Weinberg *et al.*, 1988).

Methadone undergoes extensive biotransformation in the liver. The major metabolites, the results of N-demethylation and cyclization to form pyrrolidines and pyrroline, are excreted in the urine and the bile along with small amounts of unchanged drug. The amount of methadone excreted in the urine is increased when the urine is acidified. The half-life of methadone is about 1 to 1.5 days (*see* Appendix II).

Methadone appears to be firmly bound to protein in various tissues, including brain. After repeated administration there is gradual accumulation in tissues. When administration is discontinued, low concentrations are maintained in plasma by slow release from extravascular binding sites (*see* Kreek, 1979); this process probably accounts for the relatively mild but protracted withdrawal syndrome.

The use of methadone in the treatment of compulsive heroin users has revived interest in other methadone congeners, such as *α-dl-* and *l*-acetylmethadol (methadyl acetate). In subjects physically dependent on *α-dl*-acetylmethadol, opioid withdrawal symptoms are not perceived for 72 to 96 hours after the last oral dose, and most subjects are entirely comfortable when given a single dose of the drug as infrequently as every 72 hours (*see* Ling *et al.*, 1978). The relatively slow onset and protracted duration of action of this drug, which is probably inactive, are thought to be due in part to its conversion to active metabolites (noracetylmethadol, dinoracetylmethadol, and normethadol) that are slowly further metabolized or excreted.

Preparations, Routes of Administration, and Dosage. *Methadone hydrochloride* (DOLOPHINE HCL) is available in tablets (5 and 10 mg) and in solutions for oral use, and as a solution for parenteral administration. The oral analgesic dose for adults is 2.5 to 15 mg, depending upon the severity of the pain and the response of the patient; the initial parenteral dose is usually 2.5 to 10 mg. The average minimal effective analgesic concentration in blood is about 30 ng/ml (Gourlay *et al.*, 1986).

In the United States, special controls on methadone have been enacted in an effort to prevent its unregulated large-scale use in the treatment of opioid addiction. Specialized dosage forms used in opioid addiction include tablets containing 40 mg of the drug.

Side Effects, Toxicity, Drug Interactions, and Precautions. Side effects, toxicity, and conditions that alter sensitivity, as well as the treatment of acute intoxication, are similar to those described for morphine. During long-term administration there may be excessive sweating, lymphocytosis, and increased concentrations of prolactin, albumin, and globulins in the plasma. Rifampin and phenytoin accelerate the metabolism of methadone and can precipitate withdrawal symptoms (*see* Kreek, 1979).

Tolerance, Physical Dependence, and Liability for Abuse. Volunteer postaddicts who received subcutaneous or oral methadone daily developed partial tolerance to the nauseant, anorectic, miotic, sedative, respiratory-depressant, and cardiovascular effects of methadone. Tolerance develops more slowly to methadone than to morphine in some patients, especially with respect to the depressant effects. However, this may be related in part to cumulative effects of the drug or its metabolites. Tolerance to the constipating effect of methadone does not develop as fully as does tolerance to other effects. The behavior of the addicts who use methadone parenterally is strikingly similar to that of the morphine addict, but many former heroin users treated with oral methadone show virtually no overt behavioral effects (*see* Chapter 22).

Development of physical dependence during the long-term administration of methadone can be demonstrated by drug withdrawal or by administration of an opioid antagonist. Subcutaneous administration of 10 to 20 mg of methadone to former opioid addicts produces definite euphoria, equal in duration to that caused by morphine, and its overall abuse potential is comparable to that of morphine.

Therapeutic Uses. The primary uses of methadone are relief of pain, treatment of opioid abstinence syndromes, and treatment of heroin users. It is not widely used as an antiperistaltic agent. It should be used with extreme caution, if at all, in labor.

Analgesia. The onset of analgesia occurs 10 to 20 minutes following parenteral administration and 30 to 60 minutes after oral medication. Despite its longer plasma half-life, the duration of the analgesic action of single doses is essentially the same as that of morphine. With repeated usage, cumulative effects are seen, so that either lower dosage or longer intervals between doses become possible. In contrast to morphine, methadone and many of its congeners retain a considerable degree of their effectiveness when given orally. In terms of total analgesic effects, methadone given orally is about 50% as effective as the same dose administered intramuscularly; however, the oral–parenteral potency ratio is considerably lower when peak analgesic effect is considered. In equianalgesic doses, the pattern and incidence of untoward effects caused by methadone and morphine are similar.

PROPOXYPHENE

Of the four stereoisomers, only the alpha racemate, known as propoxyphene, has analgesic activity. Its analgesic effect resides in the dextrorotatory isomer, *d*-propoxyphene (dextropropoxyphene). However, levopropoxyphene seems to have some antitussive activity. As can be seen from the following formula, propoxyphene is related structurally to methadone.

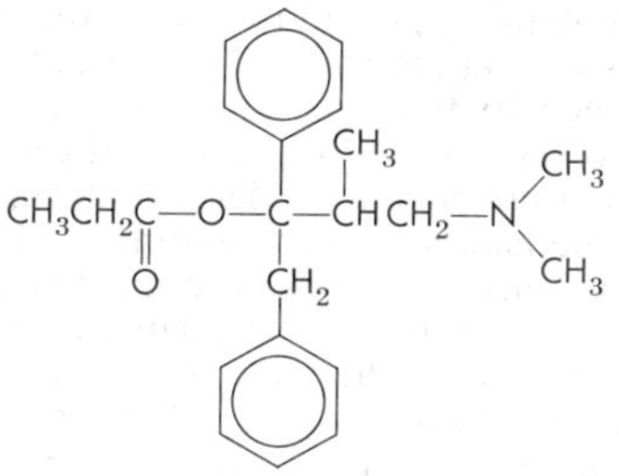

Propoxyphene

Pharmacological Actions. Although slightly less selective than morphine, propoxyphene binds primarily to μ-opioid receptors and produces analgesia and other CNS effects that are similar to those seen with morphine-like opioids. It is likely that at equianalgesic doses the incidence of side effects such as nausea, anorexia, constipation, abdominal pain, and drowsiness would be similar to those of codeine.

As an analgesic, propoxyphene is about one half to two thirds as potent as codeine given orally. Ninety to 120 mg of propoxyphene hydrochloride administered orally would equal the analgesic effects of 60 mg of codeine, a dose that usually produces about as much analgesia as 600 mg of aspirin. Combinations of propoxyphene and aspirin (like combinations of codeine and aspirin) afford a higher level of analgesia than does either agent given alone (Beaver, 1988).

Absorption, Fate, and Excretion. Following oral administration, concentrations of propoxyphene in plasma reach their highest values at 1 to 2 hours. There is great variability between subjects in the rate of clearance and the plasma concentrations that are achieved. The average half-life of propoxyphene in plasma after a single dose is from 6 to 12 hours, which is longer than that of codeine. In man, the major route of metabolism is N-demethylation to yield norpropoxyphene. The half-life of norpropoxyphene is about 30 hours, and its accumulation with repeated doses may be responsible for some of the observed toxicity (*see* Chan and Matzke, 1987).

Toxicity. Given orally, propoxyphene is approximately one third as potent as orally administered codeine in depressing respiration. Moderately toxic doses usually produce CNS and respiratory depression, but with still-larger doses the clinical picture may be complicated by convulsions in addition to respiratory depression. Delusions, hallucinations, confusion, cardiotoxicity, and pulmonary edema have also been noted. Respiratory-depressant effects are significantly enhanced when ethanol or sedative-hypnotic agents are ingested concurrently. Naloxone antagonizes the respiratory-depressant, convulsant, and some of the cardiotoxic effects of propoxyphene.

Liability for Abuse. Very large doses (800 mg of the hydrochloride or 1200 mg of the napsylate per day) reduce the intensity of the morphine withdrawal syndrome somewhat less effectively than do 1500-mg doses of codeine. Maximal tolerated doses are equivalent to daily doses of 20 to 25 mg of morphine, given subcutaneously. Use of higher doses of propoxyphene is prevented by untoward side effects and the occurrence of toxic psychoses. Very large doses produce some respiratory depression in morphine-tolerant addicts, suggesting that cross-tolerance between propoxyphene and morphine is incomplete. Abrupt discontinuation of chronically administered propoxyphene hydrochloride (up to 800 mg per day, given for almost 2 months) results in mild abstinence phenomena, and large oral doses (300 to 600 mg) produce subjective effects that are considered pleasurable by post-addicts. The drug is quite irritating when administered either intravenously or subcutaneously, so that abuse by these routes results in severe damage to veins and soft tissues. The incidence of abuse (corrected for the number of equianalgesic doses) has been approximately the same as with codeine.

Preparations, Route of Administration, Dosage, and Therapeutic Uses. The only recognized use of propoxyphene is for the treatment of mild-to-moderate pain that is not adequately relieved by aspirin. Given acutely, the commonly prescribed combination of 32 mg of propoxyphene with aspirin may not produce more analgesia than aspirin alone. The wide popularity of propoxyphene in clinical situations in which codeine was once used is largely a result of unrealistic overconcern about the addictive potential of codeine.

Propoxyphene hydrochloride (DARVON, DOLENE, others) is available in 32- and 65-mg capsules; *propoxyphene napsylate* (DARVON-N) is available in 100-mg tablets or as a suspension. Combinations of propoxyphene with aspirin or acetaminophen are also marketed in tablets and capsules.

OPIOIDS WITH MIXED ACTIONS: AGONIST-ANTAGONISTS AND PARTIAL AGONISTS

Most of the drugs to be discussed in this section presumably bind to the μ receptor and can therefore compete with other substances for these sites, but either they exert no actions (*i.e.*, they are *competitive antagonists* at the μ receptor) or they exert only limited actions (*i.e.*, they are *partial agonists* at the μ receptor). Drugs such as nalorphine, cyclazocine, and nalbuphine are competitive antagonists at the μ receptor (and block the effects of morphine-like drugs), yet they appear to exert partial agonistic actions at other receptors, including the δ and κ receptors. Pentazocine qualitatively resembles these three agents, but it appears to be either a weaker antagonist or a partial agonist at μ receptors and to have more powerful agonistic actions at κ receptors; buprenorphine behaves as a partial μ agonist (*see* Table 21–1).

PENTAZOCINE

Pentazocine was synthesized as part of a deliberate effort to develop an effective analgesic with little or no abuse potential. It has both agonistic actions and weak opioid antagonistic activity. The pharmacology of pentazocine has been reviewed by Brogden and associates (1973).

Chemistry. Pentazocine is a benzomorphan derivative with the following structural formula:

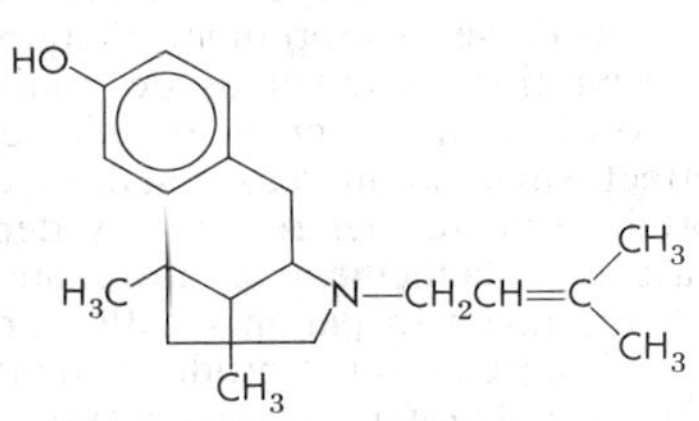

Pentazocine

The compound has a large substituent on the nitrogen atom that is analogous to position 17 of morphine. This structural feature is common to a number of opioids with antagonist or agonist-antagonist activity. The analgesic and respiratory-depressant activity of the racemate is due mainly to the *l* isomer.

Pharmacological Actions. The pattern of CNS effects produced by pentazocine is generally similar to that of the morphine-like opioids, including analgesia, sedation, and respiratory depression. It is probable that some of the analgesic effects of pentazocine are due to agonistic actions at κ opioid receptors. A dose of approximately 20 mg, administered parenterally, produces the same degree of respiratory depression as does a 10-mg dose of morphine. Increasing the dose of pentazocine beyond 30 mg does not ordinarily produce proportionate increases in respiratory depression. However, at doses of 60 to 90 mg, nalorphine-like dysphoric and psychotomimetic effects may occur that can be antagonized by naloxone; these effects are probably due to actions at κ-opioid receptors.

The effects of low doses of pentazocine on the gastrointestinal tract are qualitatively similar to those of the μ-agonist opioids. Doses of 30 to 45 mg increase the transit time through the intestinal tract. The drug produces less elevation of biliary pressure than does an equianalgesic dose of morphine; however, its effects are somewhat greater than those of buprenorphine (Staritz, 1988).

The cardiovascular responses to pentazocine differ from those seen with typical μ agonists, in that high doses cause an increase in blood pressure and heart rate. In patients with coronary artery disease, pentazocine (intravenously) elevates mean aortic pressure, left ventricular end-diastolic pressure, and mean pulmonary artery pressure, and causes an increase in cardiac work (Alderman *et al.*, 1972; Lee *et al.*, 1976). A rise in the concentrations of catecholamines in plasma may account for its effects on blood pressure.

Pentazocine acts as a weak antagonist or a partial agonist at μ-opioid receptors. It does not antagonize the respiratory depression produced by morphine; however, when given to patients who have been receiving μ-agonist opioids on a regular basis, it may precipitate withdrawal symptoms. In patients tolerant to morphine-like opioids, pentazocine reduces the analgesia produced by their administration, even when clear-cut withdrawal symptoms are not precipitated.

Absorption, Fate, and Excretion. Pentazocine is well absorbed from the gastrointestinal tract and from subcutaneous and intramuscular sites. Concentrations in plasma coincide closely with the onset, duration, and intensity of analgesia; peak values occur 15 minutes to 1 hour after intramuscular administration and 1 to 3 hours after oral administration. The half-life in plasma is about 4 hours. First-pass metabolism in the liver is extensive, and only about one half of pentazocine enters the systemic circulation.

The action of the drug is terminated largely by biotransformation in the liver; the metabolites, products of the oxidation of the terminal methyl groups and glucuronide conjugates, are excreted by the kidney. There is considerable variability between individuals in terms of rate of pentazocine metabolism, and this may account for the variability of analgesic response. Pentazocine passes the placental barrier but to a lesser extent than does meperidine.

Preparations, Routes of Administration, and Dosage. *Pentazocine lactate* (TALWIN) is available as a solution for injection. In an effort to reduce the use of tablets as a source of injectable pentazocine, tablets for oral use now contain *pentazocine hydrochloride* (equivalent to 50 mg of the base) and *naloxone hydrochloride* (equivalent to 0.5 mg of the base) (TALWIN NX). After oral ingestion, naloxone is destroyed rapidly by the liver; however, if the material is dissolved and injected, the naloxone produces aversive effects in subjects dependent on opioids. Tablets containing mixtures of pentazocine with aspirin or acetaminophen are also available. In terms of analgesic effect, 30 to 60 mg of pentazocine given parenterally is approximately equivalent to 10 mg of morphine. An oral dose of about 50 mg of pentazocine results in analgesia equivalent to that produced by 60 mg of codeine orally.

Side Effects, Toxicity, and Precautions. The most commonly reported untoward effects are sedation, sweating, and dizziness or lightheadedness; nausea also occurs, but vomiting is less common than with morphine. Nalorphine-like psychotomimetic effects such as uncontrollable or weird thoughts, anxiety, nightmares, and hallucinations are seen with increasing frequency with parenteral doses above 60 mg. Epidemiological data suggest that overdose with pentazocine alone rarely causes death. High doses produce marked respiratory depression associated with increased blood pressure and tachycardia. The respiratory depression is antagonized by naloxone. Pentazocine is irritating when administered subcutaneously or intramuscularly. Repeated injections over long periods may cause extensive fibrosis of subcutaneous and muscular tissue. Patients who have been receiving opioids on a regular basis may experience abstinence signs and symptoms when given pentazocine. After an opioid-free interval of 1 to 2 days, it is usually possible to administer pentazocine without producing such withdrawal effects.

Tolerance, Physical Dependence, and Liability for Abuse. With frequent and repeated use, tolerance develops to the analgesic and subjective effects of pentazocine. Given intravenously or subcutaneously to postaddicts, pentazocine (40 mg) produces essentially morphine-like effects; when the dose is increased to 60 mg, the effects begin to resemble the nervousness and loss of energy produced by nalorphine. However, pentazocine does not prevent or ameliorate the morphine withdrawal syndrome. Instead, when high doses of pentazocine are given to subjects dependent on morphine, it precipitates withdrawal symptoms because of its antagonistic actions at the μ receptor.

After long-term administration (60 to 90 mg every 4 hours), postaddicts develop physical dependence that can be demonstrated by abrupt withdrawal or by the administration of naloxone. The withdrawal syndrome after chronic doses of more than 500 mg per day includes abdominal cramps, anxiety, chills, elevated temperature, vomiting, lacrimation, and sweating. Although milder in intensity than withdrawal from morphine, the syndrome is associated with drug-seeking behavior.

Pentazocine was subject to no special controls when it was initially released for general use. However, it is now included under schedule IV of the Federal Controlled Substances Act because the combination of pentazocine and the antihistamine tripelennamine, used intravenously, became popular in the addict subculture of several large urban areas. Administered intravenously to former addicts, tripelennamine produces euphoric effects that are additive to those of pentazocine. Pentazocine withdrawal symptoms can be managed by gradual reduction of pentazocine itself or by substitution of μ agonists, such as morphine or methadone. A syndrome of withdrawal from pentazocine has also been observed in neonates.

Therapeutic Uses. Pentazocine is used as an analgesic, often in individuals who have chronic severe pain or in those who have drug-abuse problems. Although the risk of drug dependence definitely exists, it is lower than that associated with the use of morphine-like drugs in similar circumstances. Because abuse patterns appear to be less likely to develop with oral administration, this route should be used whenever possible.

NALBUPHINE

Nalbuphine is structurally related to both naloxone and oxymorphone (*see* Table 21–2). It is an agonist-antagonist opioid with a spectrum of effects that qualitatively resembles those of pentazocine; however, nalbuphine is a more potent antagonist at μ receptors and is less likely to produce dysphoric side effects than is pentazocine.

Pharmacological Actions and Side Effects. An intramuscular dose of 10 mg of nalbuphine causes analgesia equivalent to that which follows the administration of 10 mg of morphine; the onset and duration of both analgesic and subjective effects are similar to those of morphine. Nalbuphine depresses respiration as much as do equianalgesic doses of morphine; however, nalbuphine exhibits a ceiling effect, such that increases in dosage beyond 30 mg produce no further respiratory depression. In contrast to pentazocine and butorphanol, 10 mg of nalbuphine given to patients with stable coronary artery disease does not produce an increase in cardiac index, pulmonary arterial pressure, or cardiac work, and systemic blood pressure is not significantly altered; these indices are also relatively stable when nalbuphine is given to patients with acute myocardial infarction (*see* Roth *et al.*, 1988). Its gastrointestinal effects are probably similar to those of pentazocine. Nalbuphine produces few side effects at doses of 10 mg or less; sedation, sweating, and headache are the most common. At much higher doses (70 mg) side effects resemble those of nalorphine (dysphoria, racing thoughts, and distortions of body image). Nalbuphine is metabolized in the liver and has a half-life in plasma of 2 to 3 hours. Given orally, nalbuphine is 20 to 25% as potent as when given intramuscularly.

Tolerance, Physical Dependence, and Liability for Abuse. Postaddicts "like" the effects of single (8-mg) doses of nalbuphine as much as they do those of low doses of morphine. When the dose of nalbuphine is increased to 72 mg, the degree of "liking" and euphoria is increased only slightly, and sedative as well as nalorphine-like side effects begin to occur.

In subjects dependent on low doses of morphine (60 mg per day), nalbuphine precipitates an abstinence syndrome. During the first week of administration, experimental subjects usually identify nalbuphine as morphine-like. After 7 days (daily dose of 142 mg), subjects begin to complain of headache, difficulty in concentration, strange thoughts and dreams, irritability, and depression. The administration of 4 mg of naloxone produces an abstinence syndrome and subjects demand drugs for relief. The withdrawal syndrome is similar in intensity to that seen with pentazocine. The potential for abuse of parenteral nalbuphine in subjects not dependent on μ agonists is probably similar to that of parenteral pentazocine. Since its release for use in 1979, few cases of abuse of nalbuphine have been reported, and it has not been listed in any schedule of the Federal Controlled Substances Act.

Therapeutic Uses, Routes of Administration, Dosage, and Preparations. Nalbuphine is used to produce analgesia. Because it is an agonist-antagonist, administration to patients who have been receiving morphine-like opioids may create difficulties unless a brief drug-free interval is interposed. *Nalbuphine hydrochloride* (NUBAIN) is supplied as an injectable solution (10 or 20 mg/ml) for intramuscular, subcutaneous, or intravenous use. The usual adult dose is 10 mg every 3 to 6 hours; this may be increased to 20 mg in nontolerant individuals.

BUTORPHANOL

Butorphanol is a morphinan congener with a profile of actions similar to those of pentazocine. The structural formula of butorphanol is shown in Table 21–1.

Pharmacological Actions and Side Effects. In postoperative patients, a parenteral dose of 2 to 3 mg of butorphanol produces analgesia and respiratory depression approximately equal to that produced by 10 mg of morphine or 80 mg of meperidine; the onset, peak, and duration of action are similar to those that follow the administration of morphine. The plasma half-life of butorphanol is about 3 hours; higher values are observed in the elderly. Like pentazocine and other drugs whose actions are hypothesized to be exerted primarily on κ receptors, the increase in respiratory depression is much less pronounced as the dose is increased than it is with morphine and other μ-receptor agonists. Like pentazocine, analgesic doses of butorphanol produce an increase in pulmonary arterial pressure and in the work of the heart; systemic arterial pressure is slightly decreased (Popio *et al.*, 1978).

The major side effects of butorphanol are drowsiness, weakness, sweating, feelings of floating, and nausea. While the incidence of psychotomimetic side effects is lower than that with equianalgesic doses of pentazocine, they are qualitatively similar.

Tolerance, Physical Dependence, and Liability for Abuse. Single doses of butorphanol cause subjective effects that resemble those produced by cyclazocine, pentazocine, and nalorphine, rather than those produced by morphine. In subjects who are dependent on 60 mg of morphine per day, butorphanol neither suppresses nor precipitates a withdrawal syndrome. However, it does precipitate a withdrawal syndrome in patients maintained on methadone, suggesting that butorphanol has weak antagonistic actions at μ-opioid receptors (*see* Table 21–1). Postaddicts stabilized on 12 mg of butorphanol four times a day complain of drowsiness, constipation, difficulty in urinating, and inability to sleep. The drug is identified much more frequently as a barbiturate than as an opioid, and postaddicts express indifference or mild dislike for it. After long-term administration of butorphanol, the administration of 4 mg of naloxone or abrupt withdrawal of the drug produces a withdrawal syndrome characterized by discomfort and requests for medicine for relief. The syndrome resembles that which follows the use of cyclazocine and is largely over by the eighth day. Butorphanol is not included in any schedule of the Federal Controlled Substances Act, and few cases of abuse have been reported since its introduction in 1978.

Therapeutic Uses, Routes of Administration, Dosage, and Preparations. *Butorphanol tartrate* (STADOL) is available only in solutions for parenteral use. It is better suited for the relief of acute rather than chronic pain. Because of its side effects on the heart, it is less useful than morphine or meperidine in patients with congestive heart failure or myocardial infarction. The usual dose is between 1 and 4 mg of the tartrate given intramuscularly or 0.5 to 2 mg given intravenously; this may be repeated every 3 to 4 hours.

BUPRENORPHINE

Buprenorphine is a semisynthetic, highly lipophilic opioid derived from thebaine (*see* Table 21–2). It is 25 to 50 times more potent than morphine.

Pharmacological Actions and Side Effects. Buprenorphine produces analgesia and other CNS effects that are qualitatively similar to those of morphine. About 0.4 mg of buprenorphine is equianalgesic with 10 mg of morphine given intramuscularly (Wallenstein *et al.*, 1986). Although variable, the duration of analgesia is usually longer than that of morphine. Some of the subjective and respiratory-depressant effects are unequivocally slower in onset and longer lasting than those of morphine. For example, peak miosis occurs about 6 hours after intramuscular injection, while maximal respiratory depression is observed at about 3 hours.

Buprenorphine appears to be a partial μ agonist. Depending on the dose, buprenorphine may cause symptoms of abstinence in patients who have been receiving μ-receptor agonists (morphine-like drugs) for several weeks. It antagonizes the respiratory depression produced by anesthetic doses of fentanyl about as well as naloxone, without completely preventing opioid pain relief (Boysen *et al.*, 1988). In outpatients dependent on 30 mg of oral methadone, 2 mg of buprenorphine sublingually neither precipitates abstinence nor produces opioid effects, although such doses may suppress opioid withdrawal symptoms (*see* Bickel *et al.*, 1988). Although respiratory depression has not been a major problem in clinical trials, it is not clear whether there is a ceiling for this effect (as is seen with nalbuphine and pentazocine). The respiratory depression and other effects of buprenorphine can be prevented by prior administration of naloxone, but they are not readily reversed by high doses of naloxone once the effects have been produced.

This suggests that buprenorphine dissociates very slowly from opioid receptors. Cardiovascular and other side effects (sedation, nausea, vomiting, dizziness, sweating, and headache) appear to be similar to those of morphine-like opioids. In several species, buprenorphine appears to exert antagonist actions at κ receptors. The clinical significance of this property is not yet apparent.

Buprenorphine is relatively well absorbed by most routes, including the sublingual; 0.4 to 0.8 mg of the drug administered sublingually produces satisfactory analgesia in postoperative patients. Concentrations in blood peak within 5 minutes after intramuscular injection and within 2 hours after oral or sublingual administration. While the half-life in plasma has been reported to be about 3 hours, this value bears little relationship to the rate of disappearance of effects. Both N-dealkylated and conjugated metabolites are detected in the urine, but most of the drug is excreted unchanged in the feces. About 96% of the circulating drug is bound to protein.

Tolerance, Physical Dependence, and Liability for Abuse. In postaddicts, subcutaneous doses of buprenorphine ranging from 0.2 to 2 mg produce typical morphine-like effects, including euphoria and pupillary constriction. Miosis is detectable for 72 hours. During long-term administration of buprenorphine (8 mg subcutaneously or 8 to 16 mg sublingually per day), subjects identify the drug as morphine-like, and the subjective and physiological effects of parenteral morphine (in doses of up to 120 mg) are prevented or markedly attenuated. This attenuation or "blockade" persists for more than 30 hours after the last dose of buprenorphine. When buprenorphine is discontinued, a withdrawal syndrome develops that is delayed in onset for 2 days to 2 weeks; this consists in typical, but generally not very severe, morphine-like withdrawal signs and symptoms, and it persists for about 1 to 2 weeks. Some individuals demand drugs for relief (Jasinski *et al.*, 1978; Bickel *et al.*, 1988; Fudala *et al.*, 1989). Primarily because of the less intense withdrawal syndrome, the potential for abuse of buprenorphine is probably less than that of morphine.

Therapeutic Uses, Route of Administration, and Dosage. *Buprenorphine* may be used as an analgesic; it also appears to be useful as a maintenance drug for opioid-dependent subjects but is not yet approved for this purpose. The usual intramuscular or intravenous dose for analgesia is 0.3 mg, given every 6 hours. Sublingual doses of 0.4 to 0.8 mg produce effective analgesia, and doses of 6 to 8 mg appear to be about equal to 60 mg of methadone as a maintenance agent. Currently, only a parenteral preparation (BUPRENEX) is available, containing 0.3 mg of buprenorphine in 1 ml.

OTHER AGONIST-ANTAGONISTS

Meptazinol is an agonist-antagonist opioid that is about one tenth as potent as morphine in producing analgesia. Its duration of action is somewhat shorter than that of morphine. Meptazinol also has cholinergic actions that may contribute to its analgesic effects (*see* Holmes and Ward, 1985). Nevertheless, its analgesic actions are antagonized by naloxone, and it can precipitate withdrawal in animals dependent on μ agonists. The potential for abuse of meptazinol is less than that of morphine because dysphoric side effects appear when the dose is increased.

Dezocine, an aminotetralin, is another agonist-antagonist; its potency and duration of analgesic effect are similar to those of morphine. Increasing the dose above 30 mg/70 kg does not produce progressively more severe respiratory depression. In postaddicts, its subjective effects are similar to those of μ-agonist opioids (Jasinski and Preston, 1985).

OPIOID ANTAGONISTS

Under ordinary circumstances, the drugs to be discussed in this section produce few effects unless opioids with agonistic actions have been administered previously. However, when the endogenous opioid systems are activated, as in shock or certain forms of stress, the administration of an opioid antagonist alone has visible consequences. These agents have obvious therapeutic utility in the treatment of overdosage with opioids. As the understanding of the role of endogenous opioid systems in pathophysiological states increases, additional therapeutic indications for these antagonists may develop.

Chemistry. Relatively minor changes in the structure of an opioid can convert a drug that is primarily an agonist into one with antagonistic actions at one or more types of opioid receptors. The most common such substitution is that of a larger moiety (*e.g.*, an allyl or methylcyclopropyl group) for the N-methyl group that is typical of the μ-opioid agonists. Such substitutions transform morphine to nalorphine, levorphanol to levallorphan, and oxymorphone to naloxone or naltrexone (*see* Table 21–2). In some cases, congeners are produced that are competitive antagonists at μ receptors but that also have agonistic actions at κ receptors. Nalorphine and levallorphan have such properties. Other congeners, especially naloxone and naltrexone, appear to be devoid of agonistic actions and probably interact with all types of opioid receptors, albeit with widely different affinities (*see* Martin, 1983).

Nalmefene is a relatively pure μ antagonist that is more potent than naloxone (Dixon *et al.*, 1986); it is currently undergoing clinical trials. A number of other nonpeptide antagonists have recently been developed that are relatively selective for individual types of opioid receptors. These include cypridime (μ), naltrindole (δ), and nor-binaltorphimine (κ) (*see* Haynes, 1988; Portoghese, 1989). Their actions in man have not been studied.

PHARMACOLOGICAL PROPERTIES

If endogenous opioid systems have not been activated, the pharmacological actions of opioid antagonists depend upon whether an opioid agonist has been administered previously, the pharmacological profile of that opioid, and the degree to which physical dependence on an opioid has developed.

Effects in the Absence of Opioid Drugs. In man, subcutaneous doses of naloxone (up to 12 mg) produce no discernible subjective effects, and 24 mg causes only slight drowsiness. Naltrexone also appears to be a relatively pure antagonist, but with higher oral efficacy and a longer duration of action. At high doses, both naloxone and naltrexone may have some special agonistic effects. However, these are of little clinical significance. At doses in excess of 0.3 mg/kg of naloxone, normal subjects show increased systolic blood pressure and decreased performance on tests of memory. High doses of naltrexone appeared to cause mild dysphoria in one study but almost no subjective effects in several others (*see* Gonzalez and Brogden, 1988).

The subjective effects of nalorphine and levallorphan in man depend largely upon the dose, the subject, and the situation. For example, in patients with postoperative pain, a dose of 10 to 15 mg of nalorphine is about as effective as 10 mg of morphine in producing analgesia. This appears to be a result of agonistic actions at κ-opioid receptors. At such doses, a significant percentage of patients experience unpleasant reactions that range from anxiety and vivid, disturbing "unreal" daydreams to frank hallucinations. These dysphoric and psychotomimetic effects may also reflect agonistic actions at κ-opioid receptors; however, actions at PCP or σ sites may be involved as well (*see* above).

Nalorphine and levallorphan produce some degree of respiratory depression, presumably due to actions at κ receptors. However, the ceiling on the maximal respiratory depression that is produced appears to be relatively low.

Although high doses of antagonists might be expected to alter the actions of endogenous opioid peptides, the detectable effects are usually both subtle and limited. There appear to be several explanations for this apparent paradox. Endogenous opioids both enhance and inhibit the perception of pain. If antagonists interfere with both of these processes to the same degree, there may be little net change. However, when endogenous opioid systems are activated by pain, stress, or exercise, the effects of opioid antagonists on endogenous peptides become detectable. Thus, although naloxone does not consistently alter tolerance of experimentally induced pain in human subjects, it does decrease tolerance in those who normally have high pain thresholds. Naloxone also antagonizes the analgesic effects of placebo medication and increases the pain that patients may be experiencing. The analgesia that is produced by low-frequency stimulation of acupuncture needles is antagonized by opioid antagonists; such analgesia may involve activation of opioid peptidergic systems to some extent (*see* Pomeranz and Bibic, 1988). In both man and animals, various forms of acute and chronic stress induce some degree of analgesia. The physiological systems that mediate this analgesia vary with the nature and duration of the stress; both opioid and nonopioid systems are involved. Some forms of stress-induced analgesia are antagonized by naloxone (*see* Akil *et al.*, 1984; Cannon and Liebeskind, 1987).

In animals, the administration of naloxone will reverse or attenuate the hypotension associated with shock of diverse origins, including that caused by anaphylaxis, endotoxin, hypovolemia, and injury to the spinal cord; opioid agonists aggravate these conditions (*see* McNicholas and Martin, 1984; Amir, 1988). Naloxone apparently acts to antagonize the actions of endogenous opioids that are mobilized by pain or stress and that are involved in the regulation of blood pressure by the CNS. Although neural damage that follows trauma to the spinal cord or cerebral ischemia also appears to involve endogenous opioids, it is not certain whether opioid antagonists can prevent damage to these or other organs and/or increase rates of survival. Nevertheless, opioid antagonists can reduce the extent of injury in some animal models (Faden, 1988); in these instances the stimulation of κ receptors by dynorphins appears to be involved. Moreover, a few reports suggest that naloxone may have beneficial effects in patients with septic shock or with cerebral ischemia of diverse origins (Czlonkowska and Cyrta, 1988; Roberts *et al.*, 1988). However, the therapeutic utility of opioid antagonists in these conditions remains to be clarified.

As noted above, endogenous opioid peptides participate in the regulation of pituitary secretion, apparently by exerting tonic inhibitory effects on the release of certain hypothalamic hormones (*see* Chapter 56). Thus, the administration of naloxone or naltrexone increases the secretion of gonadotropin-releasing hormone and corticotropin-releasing factor and elevates the plasma concentrations of LH, FSH, and ACTH, as well as the hormones produced by their target organs. Antagonists do not consistently alter basal or stress-induced concentrations of prolactin in plasma in men; paradoxically, naloxone *stimulates* the release of prolactin in women. Opioid antagonists augment the increases in plasma concentrations of cortisol and catecholamines that normally accompany stress or exercise. However, exercise-induced elevation of mood is not significantly altered by opioid antagonists. The neuroendocrine effects of opioid antagonists have been reviewed by Howlett and Rees (1986) and by Staessen and coworkers (1988).

Endogenous opioid peptides probably have some role in the regulation of feeding or energy metabolism, because opioid antagonists increase energy expenditure and interrupt hibernation in appropriate species and induce weight loss in genetically obese rats. The antagonists also prevent stress-induced overeating and obesity in rats. These observations have led to the experimental use of opioid antagonists in the treatment of human obesity, especially that associated with stress-induced eating disorders. However, naltrexone does not accelerate weight loss in very obese subjects, even though short-term administration of opioid antagonists reduces food intake in both lean and obese individuals (Atkinson, 1987).

Antagonistic Actions. Small doses (0.4 to 0.8 mg) of naloxone given intramuscularly or intravenously in man prevent or promptly reverse the effects of μ-opioid agonists. In patients with respiratory depression, an increase in respiratory rate is seen within 1 or 2 minutes. Sedative effects are reversed, and blood pressure, if depressed, returns to normal. Higher doses of naloxone are required to antagonize the respiratory depressant effects of buprenorphine; 1 mg of naloxone intravenously completely blocks the effects of 25 mg of heroin. Naloxone reverses the psychotomimetic and dysphoric effects of agonist-antagonists such as pentazocine, but much higher doses (10 to 15 mg) are required. The duration of antagonistic effects depends on the dose but is usually 1 to 4 hours. Antagonism of opioid effects by naloxone is often accompanied by "overshoot" phenomena; for example, respiratory rate depressed by opioids transiently becomes higher than that prior to the period of depression. This "overshoot" is probably related to the "unmasking" of acute physical dependence. Rebound release of catecholamines may cause cardiac arrhythmias (*see* below).

Effects in Physical Dependence. In subjects who are dependent on morphine-like opioids, small subcutaneous doses of naloxone (0.5 mg) precipitate a moderate-to-severe withdrawal syndrome that is very similar to that seen after abrupt withdrawal of opioids, except that the syndrome appears within minutes after administration and subsides in about 2 hours. The severity and duration of the syndrome are related to the dose of the antagonist and the degree and type of dependence. Higher doses of naloxone will precipitate a withdrawal syndrome in patients dependent on pentazocine, butorphanol, or nalbuphine. Naloxone produces "overshoot" phenomena suggestive of early acute physical dependence 6 to 24 hours after a single dose of a μ agonist (*see* Heishman *et al.*, 1989).

Tolerance, Physical Dependence, and Liability for Abuse. Even after prolonged administration of high doses, discontinuation of naloxone is not followed by any recognizable withdrawal syndrome, and the withdrawal of naltrexone, another relatively pure antagonist, produces very few signs and symptoms. However, long-term administration of antagonists increases the density of opioid receptors in brain and causes a temporary exaggeration of responses to the subsequent administration of opioid agonists (Yoburn *et al.*, 1988). Naltrexone and naloxone have little or no potential for abuse.

Absorption, Fate, and Excretion. Although absorbed readily from the gastrointestinal tract, naloxone is almost completely metabolized by the liver before reaching the systemic circulation and thus must be administered parenterally. The drug is absorbed rapidly from parenteral sites of injection and is metabolized in the liver, primarily by conjugation with glucuronic acid; other metabolites are produced in small amounts. The duration of action of naloxone is about 1 to 4 hours; its half-life in plasma is about 1 hour.

Compared with naloxone, naltrexone retains much more of its efficacy by the oral route, and its duration of action approaches 24 hours after moderate oral doses. Peak concentrations in plasma are reached within 1 to 2 hours and then decline with an apparent half-life of about 3 hours; this value does not change with long-term use. Naltrexone is metabolized to 6-naltrexol, which is a weaker antagonist but has a longer half-life. The drug is much more potent than naloxone, and 100-mg oral doses given to patients addicted to opioids produce concentrations in tissues sufficient to block for 48 hours the euphorigenic effects of 25-mg intravenous doses of heroin (*see* Gonzalez and Brogden, 1988).

Preparations and Routes of Administration. *Naloxone hydrochloride* (NARCAN) is available in solutions for injection. It is the drug of choice in most situations where an opioid antagonistic effect is required. An injectable preparation is also available for use in neonates. *Naltrexone hydrochloride* (TREXAN) is available in 50-mg tablets for the maintenance of the opioid-free state in former addicts. *Levallorphan* and *nalorphine* are no longer available in the United States.

THERAPEUTIC USES

Opioid antagonists have established uses in the treatment of opioid-induced toxicity, especially respiratory depression; in the diagnosis of physical dependence on opioids; and as therapeutic agents in the treatment of compulsive users of opioids, as discussed in Chapter 22. Their potential utility in the treatment of shock, stroke, spinal cord and brain trauma, and other disorders that may involve mobilization of endogenous opioid peptides remains to be established.

Treatment of Opioid Overdosage. The dramatic effects of opioid antagonists in reversing opioid-induced respiratory depression in the adult have already been discussed. Opioid antagonists have also been effectively employed to decrease neonatal respiratory depression secondary to the administration of opioids to the mother. In the neonate, the initial dose is 10 μg/kg, given intravenously, intramuscularly, or subcutaneously. All known opioids, even in reasonable therapeutic doses, produce a significant increase in the incidence of depression of respiration in the neonate compared with deliveries in which no general anesthetic or opioid is used (Fishburne, 1982). However, naloxone has no benefit in neonatal asphyxia unrelated to exogenous opioids.

CENTRALLY ACTIVE ANTITUSSIVE AGENTS

Cough is a useful physiological mechanism serving to clear the respiratory passages of foreign material and excess secretions. It should not be suppressed indiscriminately. There are, however, many situations in which cough does not serve any useful purpose but may, instead, only annoy the patient or prevent rest and sleep. In such situations the physician should use a drug that will reduce the frequency or intensity of the coughing. The cough reflex is complex, involving the central and peripheral nervous systems as well as the smooth muscle of the bronchial tree. It has been suggested that irritation of the bronchial mucosa causes bronchoconstriction, which, in turn, stimulates cough receptors (which probably represent a specialized type of stretch receptor) located in tracheobronchial passages. Afferent conduction from these receptors is via fibers in the vagus nerve; central components of the reflex probably involve several mechanisms or centers that are distinct from the mechanisms involved in the regulation of respiration.

The drugs that can affect this complex mechanism directly or indirectly are quite diverse. For example, cough may be the first or only symptom in bronchial asthma or allergy, and in such cases bronchodilators (*e.g.*, β_2-adrenergic agonists) have been shown to reduce cough without having any significant central effects; other drugs might act primarily on the central or the peripheral nervous system components of the cough reflex. The early literature on antitussives has been reviewed by Eddy and associates (1969). This section describes a few of the many drugs that have been in clinical use and that are believed to act on the nervous system in modifying cough.

A number of drugs are known to reduce cough as a result of their central actions, although the exact mechanisms are still not entirely clear. Included among them are the opioid analgesics discussed above (codeine, hydrocodone, and hydromorphone are the opioids most commonly used to prevent cough), as well as a number of nonopioid agents.

In selecting a specific centrally active agent for a particular patient, the significant considerations are its antitussive efficacy against pathological cough and the incidence and type of side effects to be expected. In the overwhelming majority of situations requiring a cough suppressant, liability for abuse need not be a major consideration. Most of the nonopioid agents now offered as antitussives are effective against cough induced by a variety of experimental techniques. However, the ability of these tests to predict clinical efficacy is limited.

Dextromethorphan. *Dextromethorphan* (*d*-3-methoxy-N-methylmorphinan) is the *d* isomer of the codeine analog of levorphanol; however, unlike the *l* isomer, it has no analgesic or addictive properties. The drug acts centrally to elevate the threshold for coughing. Its effectiveness in patients with pathological cough has been demonstrated in controlled studies; its potency is nearly equal to that of codeine. Compared with codeine, dextromethorphan produces fewer subjective and gastrointestinal side effects (Matthys *et al.*, 1983). In therapeutic dosage the drug does not inhibit ciliary activity, and its antitussive effects persist for 5 to 6 hours. Its toxicity is quite low, but extremely high doses may produce CNS depression.

Sites that bind dextromethorphan with high affinity have been identified in membranes from various regions of the brain (Craviso and Musacchio, 1983). Two other known antitussives, carbetapentane and caramiphen, also bind avidly to this site, but codeine, levopropoxyphene, and other antitussive opioids (as well as naloxone) are not bound. Although noscapine (*see* below) enhances the affinity of dextromethorphan, it appears to interact with distinct binding sites (Karlsson and Dahlström, 1988). The relationship of these binding sites to antitussive actions is not known; however, these observations, coupled with the ability of naloxone to antagonize the antitussive effects of codeine but not those of dextromethorphan, indicate that cough suppression can be achieved by a number of different mechanisms.

The average adult dosage of *dextromethorphan hydrobromide* is 10 to 30 mg three to six times daily; however, as is the case with codeine, higher doses are often required. The drug is generally marketed for "over-the-counter" sale in syrups and lozenges, or in combinations with antihistamines and other agents.

Other Drugs. *Levopropoxyphene napsylate,* in doses of 50 to 100 mg orally, appears to suppress cough to about the same degree as does 30 mg of dextromethorphan. Unlike dextropropoxyphene, levopropoxyphene has little or no analgesic activity.

Noscapine is a naturally occurring opium alkaloid of the benzylisoquinoline group; except for its antitussive effect, it has no significant actions on the CNS in doses within the therapeutic range. The drug is a potent releaser of histamine, and large doses cause bronchoconstriction and transient hypotension.

Other drugs that have been used as centrally acting antitussives include *carbetapentane, caramiphen, chlophedianol, diphenhydramine,* and *glaucine.* Each is a member of a distinct pharmacological class unrelated to the opioids. The mechanism of action of diphenhydramine, an antihistamine, is unclear. Although sedative effects are common, paradoxical excitement may be seen in infants; dryness of mucous membranes caused by anticholinergic effects and thickening of mucus may be a disadvantage. In general, the toxicity of these agents is low, but controlled clinical studies are still insufficient to determine whether they merit consideration as alternatives to more thoroughly studied agents.

Pholcodine (3-O-[2-morpholinoethyl]morphine) is used clinically in many countries outside the United States. Although structurally related to the opioids, it has no opioid-like actions because the substitution at the 3-position is not removed by metabolism. Pholcodine is at least as effective as codeine; it has a long half-life and can be given once or twice daily (*see* Findlay, 1988).

Benzonatate (TESSALON) is a long-chain polyglycol derivative chemically related to procaine and believed to exert its antitussive action on stretch or cough receptors in the lung, as well as by a central mechanism. It has been administered by all routes; the oral dosage is 100 mg three times daily, but higher doses have been used.

Alderman, E. L.; Barry, W. H.; Graham, A. F.; and Harrison, D. C. Hemodynamic effects of morphine and pentazocine differ in cardiac patients. *N. Engl. J. Med.*, **1972**, *287*, 623–627.

Atkinson, R. L. Opioid regulation of food intake and body weight in humans. *Fed. Proc.*, **1987**, *46*, 178–182.

Beaver, W. T. Impact of non-narcotic oral analgesics on pain management. *Am. J. Med.*, **1988**, *84*, Suppl. 5A, 3–15.

Bickel, W. K.; Stitzer, M. L.; Bigelow, G. E.; Liebson, I. A.; Jasinski, D. R.; and Johnson, R. E. Buprenorphine: dose-related blockade of opioid challenge effects in opioid dependent subjects. *J. Pharmacol. Exp. Ther.*, **1988**, *247*, 47–53.

Boysen, K.; Hertel, S.; Chraemmer-Jorgensen, B.; Risbo, A.; and Poulsen, N. J. Buprenorphine antagonism of ventilatory depression following fentanyl anesthesia. *Acta Anaesthesiol. Scand.*, **1988**, *32*, 490–492.

Chen, G. G.; Chalazonitis, A.; Shen, K. F.; and Crain, S. M. Inhibitor of cyclic AMP-dependent protein kinase blocks opioid-induced prolongation of the action potential of mouse sensory ganglion neurons in dissociated cell cultures. *Brain Res.*, **1988**, *462*, 372–377.

Craviso, G. L., and Musacchio, J. M. High-affinity dextromethorphan binding sites in guinea pig brain. *Mol. Pharmacol.*, **1983**, *23*, 629–640.

Czlonkowska, A., and Cyrta, B. Effect of naloxone on acute stroke. *Pharmacopsychiatry*, **1988**, *21*, 98–100.

Dixon, R.; Howes, J.; Gentile, J.; Hsu, H.-B.; Hsiao, J.; Garg, D.; Weidler, D.; Meyer, M.; and Tuttle, R. Nalmefene: intravenous safety and kinetics of a new opioid antagonist. *Clin. Pharmacol. Ther.*, **1986**, *39*, 49–53.

Donnerer, J.; Cardinale, G.; Coffey, J.; Lisek, C. A.; Jardine, I.; and Spector, S. Chemical characterization and regulation of endogenous morphine and codeine in the rat. *J. Pharmacol. Exp. Ther.*, **1987**, *242*, 583–587.

Dooley, C. P.; Saad, C.; and Valenzuela, J. E. Studies of the role of opioids in control of human pancreatic secretion. *Dig. Dis. Sci.*, **1988**, *33*, 598–604.

Dray, A., and Nunan, L. Supraspinal and spinal mechanisms in morphine-induced inhibition of reflex urinary bladder contractions in the rat. *Neuroscience*, **1987**, *22*, 281–287.

Edwards, D. J.; Svensson, C. K.; Visco, J. P.; and Lalka, D. Clinical pharmacokinetics of pethidine: 1982. *Clin. Pharmacokinet.*, **1982**, *7*, 421–433.

Fudala, P. J.; Johnson, R. E.; and Bunker, E. Abrupt withdrawal of buprenorphine following chronic administration. *Clin. Pharmacol. Ther.*, **1989**, *45*, 186.

Glynn, C. J., and Mather, L. E. Clinical pharmacokinetics applied to patients with intractable pain; studies with pethidine. *Pain*, **1982**, *13*, 237–246.

Gmerek, D. E.; Dykstra, L. A.; and Woods, J. H. Kappa opioids in rhesus monkeys. III. Dependence associated with chronic administration. *J. Pharmacol. Exp. Ther.*, **1987**, *242*, 428–436.

Gourlay, G. K.; Cherry, D. A.; and Cousins, M. J. A comparative study of the efficacy and pharmacokinetics of oral methadone and morphine in the treatment of severe pain in patients with cancer. *Pain*, **1986**, *25*, 297–312.

Heishman, S. J.; Stitzer, M. L.; Bigelow, G. E.; and Liebson, I. A. Acute opioid physical dependence in postaddict humans: naloxone dose effects after brief morphine exposure. *J. Pharmacol. Exp. Ther.*, **1989**, *248*, 127–134.

Herman, R. J.; McAllister, C. B.; Branch, R. A.; and Wilkinson, G. R. Effects of age on meperidine disposition. *Clin. Pharmacol. Ther.*, **1985**, *37*, 19–24.

Heyman, J. S.; Vaught, J. L.; Raffa, R. B.; and Porreca, F. Can supraspinal delta-opioid receptors mediate antinociception? *Trends Pharmacol. Sci.*, **1988**, *9*, 134–138.

Hoffman, J. R., and Reynolds, S. Comparison of nitroglycerin, morphine, and furosemide in treatment of presumed pre-hospital pulmonary edema. *Chest*, **1987**, *92*, 586–593.

Jasinski, D. R.; Pevnick, J. S.; and Griffith, J. D. Human pharmacology and abuse potential of the analgesic buprenorphine. *Arch. Gen. Psychiatry*, **1978**, *35*, 501–516.

Jasinski, D. R., and Preston, K. L. Assessment of dezocine for morphine-like subjective effects and miosis. *Clin. Pharmacol. Ther.*, **1985**, *38*, 544–548.

Johnson, M. A.; Woodcock, A. A.; and Geddes, D. M. Dihydrocodeine for breathlessness in "pink puffers." *Br. Med. J.*, *[Clin. Res.]* **1983**, *286*, 675–677.

Kaiko, R. F. Age and morphine analgesia in cancer patients with postoperative pain. *Clin. Pharmacol. Ther.*, **1980**, *28*, 823–826.

Kaiko, R. F.; Foley, K. M.; Grabinski, P. Y.; Heidrich, G.; Rogers, A. G.; Inturrisi, C. E.; and Reidenberg, M. M. Central nervous system excitatory effects of meperidine in cancer patients. *Ann. Neurol.*, **1983**, *13*, 180–185.

Kaiko, R. F.; Wallenstein, S. L.; Rogers, A. G.; Grabinski, P. Y.; and Houde, R. W. Analgesic and mood effects of heroin and morphine in cancer patients with postoperative pain. *N. Engl. J. Med.*, **1981**, *304*, 1501–1505.

Karlsson, M. D., and Dahlström, N. A. Characterization of high-affinity binding for the antitussive [3H]noscapine in guinea pig brain tissue. *Eur. J. Pharmacol.*, **1988**, *12*, 195–203.

Kerr, I. G.; Sone, M.; Deangelis, C.; Iscoe, N.; MacKenzie, R.; and Schueller, T. Continuous narcotic infusion with patient-controlled analgesia for chronic cancer pain in outpatients. *Ann. Intern. Med.*, **1988**, *108*, 554–557.

Kramer, T. H.; Shook, J. E.; Kazmierski, W.; Ayres, E. A.; Wire, W. S.; Hruby, V. J.; and Burks, T. F. Novel peptidic Mu opioid antagonists: pharmacologic characterization *in vitro* and *in vivo*. *J. Pharmacol. Exp. Ther.*, **1989**, *249*, 544–551.

Kreek, M. J. Methadone in treatment: physiological and pharmacological issues. In, *Handbook on Drug Abuse*. (Dupont, R. I.; Goldstein, A.; and O'Donnell, J.; eds.) U.S. Government Printing Office, Washington, D. C., **1979**, pp. 57–86.

Largent, B. L.; Wikström, H.; Gundlach, A. L.; and Snyder, S. H. Structural determinants of σ receptor affinity. *Mol. Pharmacol.*, **1987**, *32*, 772–784.

Lee, G.; DeMaria, A.; Amsterdam, E. A.; Realyvasquez, E.; Angel, J.; Morrison, S.; and Mason, D. T. Comparative effects of morphine, meperidine and pentazocine on cardiocirculatory dynamics in patients with acute myocardial infarction. *Am. J. Med.*, **1976**, *60*, 949–955.

Levine, J. D.; Gordon, N. C.; Smith, R.; and McBryde, R. Desipramine enhances opiate postoperative analgesia. *Pain*, **1986**, *27*, 45–49.

Ling, W.; Klett, C. J.; and Gillis, R. D. A cooperative clinical study of methadyl acetate. *Arch. Gen. Psychiatry*, **1978**, *35*, 345–353.

Matthys, H.; Bleicher, B.; and Bleicher, U. Dextromethorphan and codeine: objective assessment of antitussive activity in patients with chronic cough. *J. Int. Med. Res.*, **1983**, *11*, 92–100.

Meed, S. D.; Kleinman, P. M.; Kantor, T. G.; Blum, R. H.; and Savarese, J. J. Management of cancer pain with oral controlled-release morphine sulfate. *J. Clin. Pharmacol.*, **1987**, *27*, 155–161.

Neumann, P. B.; Henriksen, H.; Grosman, N.; and Christensen, C. B. Plasma morphine concentrations during chronic oral administration in patients with cancer pain. *Pain*, **1982**, *13*, 247–252.

Owen, J. A.; Sitar, D. S.; Berger, L.; Brownell, L.; Duke, P. C.; and Mitenko, P. A. Age-related morphine kinetics. *Clin. Pharmacol. Ther.*, **1983**, *34*, 364–368.

Paul, D.; Standifer, K. M.; Inturrisi, C. E.; and Pasternak, G. W. Pharmacological characterization of morphine-6β-glucuronide, a very potent morphine metabolite. *J. Pharmacol. Exp. Ther.*, **1989**, *251*, 477–483.

Pfeiffer, A.; Brantl, V.; Herz, A.; and Emrich, H. M. Psychotomimesis mediated by κ opiate receptors. *Science*, **1986**, *233*, 774–776.

Pilcher, W. H.; Joseph, S. A.; and McDonald, J. V. Immunocytochemical localization of pro-opiomelanocortin neurons in human brain areas subserving stimulation analgesia. *J. Neurosurg.*, **1988**, *68*, 621–629.

Pomeranz, B., and Bibic, L. Electroacupuncture suppresses a nociceptive reflex: naltrexone prevents but does not reverse this effect. *Brain Res.*, **1988**, *452*, 227–231.

Popio, K. A.; Jackson, D. H.; Ross, A. M.; Schreiner, B. F.; and Yu, P. N. Hemodynamic and respiratory depressant effects of morphine and butorphanol. *Clin. Pharmacol. Ther.*, **1978**, *23*, 281–287.

Reidenberg, M. M.; Goodman, H.; Erle, H.; Gray, G.; Lorenzo, B.; Leipzig, R. M.; Meyer, B. R.; and Drayer, D. W. Hydromorphone levels and pain control in patients with severe chronic pain. *Clin. Pharmacol. Ther.*, **1988**, *44*, 376–382.

Roberts, D. E.; Dobson, K. E.; Hall, K. W.; and Light, R. B. Effects of prolonged naloxone infusion in septic shock. *Lancet*, **1988**, *2*, 699–702.

Rodgers, B. M.; Webb, C. J.; Stergios, D.; and Newman, B. M. Patient-controlled analgesia in pediatric surgery. *J. Pediatr. Surg.*, **1988**, *23*, 259–262.

Roth, A.; Keren, G.; Gluck, A.; Braun, S.; and Lanaido, S. Comparison of nalbuphine hydrochloride versus morphine sulfate for acute myocardial infarction with elevated pulmonary artery wedge pressure. *Am. J. Cardiol.*, **1988**, *62*, 551–555.

Säwe, J.; Dahlström, B.; Paalzow, L.; and Rane, A. Morphine kinetics in cancer patients. *Clin. Pharmacol. Ther.*, **1981**, *30*, 629–635.

Sethna, D. H.; Moffitt, E. A.; Gray, R. J.; Bussell, J.; Raymond, M.; Conklin, C.; Shell, W. E.; and Matloff, J. M. Cardiovascular effects of morphine in patients with coronary arterial disease. *Anesth. Analg.*, **1982**, *61*, 109–114.

Sriwatanakul, K.; Weis, O. F.; Alloza, J. L.; Kelvie, W.; Weintraub, M.; and Lasagna, L. Analysis of narcotic analgesic usage in the treatment of postoperative pain. *J.A.M.A.*, **1983**, *250*, 926–929.

Staessen, J.; Fiocchi, R.; Bouillon, R.; Fagard, R.; Hespel, P.; Lignen, P.; Moerman, E.; and Amery, A. Effects of opioid antagonism of the haemodynamic and hormonal responses to exercise. *Clin. Sci.*, **1988**, *75*, 293–300.

Vismara, L. A.; Leamon, D. M.; and Zelis, R. The effects of morphine on venous tone in patients with acute pulmonary edema. *Circulation*, **1976**, *54*, 335–337.

Walker, J. M.; Thompson, L. A.; Frascella, J.; and Friederich, M. W. Opposite effects of μ and κ opiates on the firing-rate of dopamine cells in the substantia nigra of the rat. *Eur. J. Pharmacol.*, **1987**, *28*, 53–59.

Wallenstein, S. L.; Kaiko, R. F.; Rogers, A. G.; and Houde, R. W. Crossover trials in clinical analgesic assays: studies of buprenorphine and morphine. *Pharmacotherapy*, **1986**, *6*, 228–235.

Weihe, E.; Millan, M. J.; Leibold, A.; Nohr, D.; and Herz, A. Co-localization of proenkephalin- and prodynorphin-derived opioid peptides in laminae IV/V spinal neurons revealed in arthritic rats. *Neurosci. Lett.*, **1988**, *29*, 187–192.

Weinberg, D. S.; Inturrisi, C. E.; Reidenberg, B.; Moulin, D. W.; Nip, T. J.; Wallenstein, S.; Houde, R. W.; and Foley, K. M. Sublingual absorption of selected opioid analgesics. *Clin. Pharmacol. Ther.*, **1988**, *44*, 335–342.

Weitz, C. J.; Faull, K. F.; and Goldstein, A. Synthesis of the skeleton of the morphine molecule by mammalian liver. *Nature*, **1987**, *330*, 674–677.

Werling, L. L.; Frattali, A.; Portoghese, P. S.; Takemori, A. E.; and Cox, B. M. Kappa receptor regulation of dopamine release from striatum and cortex of rats and guinea pigs. *J. Pharmacol. Exp. Ther.*, **1988**, *246*, 282–286.

Yoburn, B. C.; Luke, M. C.; Pasternak, G. W.; and Inturrisi, C. E. Upregulation of opioid receptor subtypes correlates with potency changes of morphine and DADLE. *Life Sci.*, **1988**, *43*, 1319–1324.

Zimmer, E. Z.; Divon, M. Y.; and Vadosz, A. Influence of meperidine on fetal movements and heart rate beat to beat variability in the active phase of labor. *Am. J. Perinatol.*, **1988**, *5*, 197–200.

Monographs and Reviews

Advokat, C. The role of descending inhibition in morphine-induced analgesia. *Trends Pharmacol. Sci.*, **1988**, *9*, 330–334.

Akil, H.; Watson, S. J.; Young, E.; Lewis, M. E.; Khachaturian, H.; and Walker, J. M. Endogenous opioids: biology and function. *Annu. Rev. Neurosci.*, **1984**, *7*, 223–255.

Amir, S. Anaphylactic shock: catecholamine actions in the responses to opioid antagonists. *Prog. Clin. Biol. Res.*, **1988**, *264*, 265–274.

Awouters, F.; Niemegeers, C. J. E.; and Janssen, P. A. J. Pharmacology of antidiarrheal drugs. *Annu. Rev. Pharmacol. Toxicol.*, **1983**, *23*, 279–301.

Ballantyne, J. C.; Loach, A. B.; and Carr, D. B. Itching after epidural and spinal opiates. *Pain*, **1988**, *33*, 149–160.

Bloom, F. E. The endorphins: a growing family of pharmacologically pertinent peptides. *Annu. Rev. Pharmacol. Toxicol.*, **1983**, *23*, 151–170.

Bovill, J. G. Which potent opioid? Important criteria for selection. *Drugs*, **1987**, *33*, 520–530.

Brogden, R. N.; Speight, T. M.; and Avery, G. S. Pentazocine: a review of its pharmacological properties, therapeutic efficacy and dependence liability. *Drugs*, **1973**, *5*, 6–91.

Cannon, J. T., and Liebeskind, J. C. Analgesic effects of electrical brain stimulation and stress. In, *Pain and Headache*, Vol. 9. *Neurotransmitters and Pain Control.* (Akil, H., and Lewis, J. W., eds.) S. Karger, Basel, **1987**, pp. 283–294.

Chan, G. L. C., and Matzke, G. R. Effects of renal insufficiency on the pharmacokinetics and pharmacodynamics of opioid analgesics. *Drug Intell. Clin. Pharm.*, **1987**, *21*, 773–783.

Coupar, I. M. Opioid action on the intestine: the importance of the intestinal mucosa. *Life Sci.*, **1987**, *41*, 917–925.

Duggan, A. W., and North, R. A. Electrophysiology of opioids. *Pharmacol. Rev.*, **1983**, *35*, 219–282.

Duthie, D. J. R., and Nimmo, W. S. Adverse effects of opioid analgesic drugs. *Br. J. Anaesth.*, **1987**, *59*, 61–77.

Eddy, N. B.; Friebel, H.; Hohn, K.; and Halbach, H. Codeine and its alternates for pain and cough relief. *Bull. WHO*, **1969**, *40*, 639–719.

Faden, A. I. Role of thyrotropin-releasing hormone and opiate receptor antagonists in limiting central nervous system injury. *Adv. Neurol.*, **1988**, *47*, 531–546.

Findlay, J. W. Pholcodine. *J. Clin. Pharmacol. Ther.*, **1988**, *13*, 5–17.

Fishburne, J. I. Systemic analgesia during labor. *Clin. Perinatol.*, **1982**, *9*, 29–53.

Foley, K. M. The treatment of cancer pain. *N. Engl. J. Med.*, **1985**, *313*, 84–95.

Goldstein, A. Opioid peptides: function and significance. In, *Opioids: Past, Present and Future.* (Collier, H. O. J.; Hughes, J.; Rance, M. J.; and Tyers, M. B.; eds.) Tayler & Frances Ltd., London, **1984**, pp. 127–143.

Gonzalez, J. P., and Brogden, R. N. Naltrexone: a review of its pharmacodynamic and pharmacokinetic properties and therapeutic efficacy in the management of opioid dependence. *Drugs*, **1988**, *35*, 192–213.

Grossman, A. Opioids and stress in man. *J. Endocrinol.*, **1988**, *119*, 377–381.

Gustafsson, L. L., and Wiesenfeld-Hallin, Z. Spinal opioid analgesia. A critical update. *Drugs*, **1988**, *35*, 597–603.

Haynes, L. Opioid receptors and signal transduction. *Trends Pharmacol. Sci.*, **1988**, *9*, 309–311.

Höllt, V. Opioid peptide processing and receptor selectivity. *Annu. Rev. Pharmacol. Toxicol.*, **1986**, *26*, 59–77.

Holmes, B., and Ward, A. Meptazinol. A review of its pharmacodynamic and pharmacokinetic properties and therapeutic efficacy. *Drugs*, **1985**, *30*, 285–312.

Howlett, T. A., and Rees, L. H. Endogenous opioid peptides and hypothalamo-pituitary function. *Annu. Rev. Physiol.*, **1986**, *48*, 527–537.

Koob, G. F., and Bloom, F. E. Cellular and molecular mechanisms of drug dependence. *Science*, **1988**, *242*, 715–723.

Kromer, W. Endogenous and exogenous opioids in the control of gastrointestinal motility and secretion. *Pharmacol. Rev.*, **1988**, *40*, 121–162.

Lewis, J.; Mansour, A.; Khachaturian, H.; Watson, S. J.; and Akil, H. Opioids and pain regulation. In, *Pain and Headache*, Vol. 9. *Neurotransmitters and Pain Con-*

trol. (Akil, H., and Lewis, J. W., eds.) S. Karger, Basel, **1987**, pp. 129–159.

McFadzean, I. The ionic mechanisms underlying opioid actions. *Neuropeptides*, **1988**, *11*, 173–180.

McNicholas, L. F., and Martin, W. R. New and experimental therapeutic roles for naloxone and related opioid antagonists. *Drugs*, **1984**, *27*, 81–93.

McQuay, H. J. Pharmacological treatment of neuralgic and neuropathic pain. *Cancer Surv.*, **1988**, *7*, 141–159.

Manara, L., and Bianchetti, A. The central and peripheral influences of opioids on gastrointestinal propulsion. *Annu. Rev. Pharmacol. Toxicol.*, **1985**, *25*, 249–273.

Martin, W. R. Pharmacology of opioids. *Pharmacol. Rev.*, **1983**, *35*, 283–323.

Martin, W. R., and Sloan, J. W. Neuropharmacology and neurochemistry of subjective effects, analgesia, tolerance, and dependence produced by narcotic analgesics. In, *Handbook of Experimental Pharmacology*. Vol. 45/I, *Drug Addiction I: Morphine, Sedative/Hypnotic and Alcohol Dependence*. (Martin, W. R., ed.) Springer-Verlag, Berlin, **1977**, pp. 43–158.

Millan, M. J. Multiple opioid systems and pain. *Pain*, **1986**, *27*, 303–347.

Misra, A. L. Metabolism of opiates. In, *Factors Affecting the Action of Narcotics*. (Adler, M. L.; Manara, L.; and Samanin, R.; eds.) Raven Press, New York, **1978**, pp. 297–343.

Monk, J. Sufentanil: a review. *Drugs*, **1988**, *36*, 249–381.

Pasternak, G. W. Multiple morphine and enkephalin receptors and the relief of pain. *J.A.M.A.*, **1988**, *259*, 1362–1367.

Portoghese, P. S. Bivalent ligands and the message-address concept in the design of selective opioid receptor antagonists. *Trends Pharmacol. Sci.*, **1989**, *10*, 230–235.

Rumore, M. M., and Schlichting, D. A. Clinical efficacy of antihistaminics as analgesics. *Pain*, **1986**, *25*, 7–22.

Sawynok, J. The therapeutic use of heroin: a review of the pharmacological literature. *Can. J. Physiol. Pharmacol.*, **1986**, *64*, 1–6.

Sibinga, N. E. S., and Goldstein, A. Opioid peptides and opioid receptors in cells of the immune system. *Annu. Rev. Immunol.*, **1988**, *6*, 219–249.

Simonds, W. F. The molecular basis of opioid receptor function. *Endocr. Rev.*, **1988**, *9*, 200–212.

Staritz, M. Pharmacology of the sphincter of Oddi. *Endoscopy*, **1988**, *20*, Suppl. 1, 171–174.

Symposium. (Various authors.) Pain modulation. (Fields, H. L., and Besson, J.-M., eds.) *Prog. Brain Res.*, **1988a**, *77*, 1–454.

Symposium. (Various authors.) Opioids in the hippocampus. (McGinty, J. F., and Friedman, D. P., eds.) *Natl. Inst. Drug Abuse Res. Mongr. Ser.*, **1988b**, *82*, 1–145.

Wise, R. A., and Bozarth, M. A. A psychomotor stimulant theory of addiction. *Psychol. Rev.*, **1987**, *94*, 469–492.

Yaksh, T. L. CNS mechanisms of pain and analgesia. *Cancer Surv.*, **1988**, *7*, 55–67.

Yaksh, T. L., and Noueihed, R. The physiology and pharmacology of spinal opiates. *Annu. Rev. Pharmacol. Toxicol.*, **1985**, *25*, 433–462.

Yaster, M., and Deshpande, J. K. Management of pediatric pain with opioid analgesics. *J. Pediatr.*, **1988**, *113*, 421–429.

CHAPTER

22 DRUG ADDICTION AND DRUG ABUSE

Jerome H. Jaffe

As far back as recorded history, every society has used drugs that produce effects on mood, thought, and feeling. Moreover, there were always a few individuals who digressed from custom with respect to the time, the amount, and the situation in which these drugs were to be used. Thus, both the nonmedical use of drugs and the problem of drug abuse are as old as civilization itself.

Problems of Terminology. *Drug abuse* refers to the use, usually by self-administration, of any drug in a manner that deviates from the approved medical or social patterns within a given culture. The term conveys the notion of social disapproval, and it is not necessarily descriptive of any particular pattern of drug use or its potential adverse consequences.

Since this definition is largely a social one, it is not surprising that for any particular drug there is a great variation in what is considered abuse, not only from culture to culture but also from time to time and from one situation to another within the same culture. For example, in Western society, chronic intoxication with alcohol is considered drug abuse, yet on certain occasions gross intoxication with alcohol is not. The use of medically prescribed opioid analgesics for the relief of pain is quite proper; however, the self-administration of the same drugs, in the same dosages, for relief of depression or tension or to induce euphoria is considered flagrant abuse.

Government agencies refer to any use of an illicit substance as drug abuse, regardless of the consequences or ubiquity of such use. In this context, even the occasional use of opioids or marihuana is considered drug abuse, but that of alcohol or tobacco is not. In contrast, the occasional use of illicit drugs does not constitute evidence of a psychiatric disorder unless it leads to adverse effects for the individual (*see* American Psychiatric Association, 1987). In this context, patterns of drug use that do lead to adverse effects may be referred to as drug abuse, even though they do not meet established criteria for drug dependence (*see* below).

Nonmedical drug use is a term that encompasses behaviors ranging from the occasional use of alcohol to compulsive use of opioids, and includes behaviors that may or may not be associated with adverse effects. Nonmedical drug use may consist in experimental use of a drug on one or a few occasions, because of curiosity about its effects or to conform to the expectations of peer groups. It may also involve casual or "recreational" use of modest amounts of a drug for its pleasurable effects, or circumstantial use, in which certain drug effects are sought because they are helpful in particular circumstances, as when students or truck drivers take amphetamines to alleviate fatigue. These various forms of nonmedical use may then lead to more intensive patterns of use in terms of frequency or amount and, in some cases, to patterns of dependence or compulsive drug use.

Drug Dependence. One of the hazards in the use of drugs to alter mood and feeling is that some individuals eventually develop a dependence on the drug. They continue to take it in the absence of medical indications, often despite adverse social and medical consequences, and they behave as if the effects of the drugs are needed for continued well-being. The intensity of this "need" or dependence may vary from a mild desire to a "craving" or "compulsion" to use the drug, and, when the availability of the drug is uncertain, individuals may exhibit a preoccupation with its procurement.

Drug dependence can be defined as a syndrome in which the use of a drug is given a much higher priority than other behaviors that once had higher value. The dependence syndrome is not absolute, but exists in degrees, and its intensity is gauged by the behaviors that are associated with the use of the drug. No sharp line separates drug dependence from nondependent but recurrent drug use. In its extreme form, drug dependence is associated with compulsive drug-using behavior, and it exhibits the characteristics of a chronic relapsing disorder (*see* Edwards *et al.*, 1981).

Dependence on a drug *per se* is not necessarily cause for concern. If the substance used has low toxicity and is relatively inexpensive (*e.g.*, caffeine), a drug-using behavior may meet the criteria for dependence but may not constitute a significant medical or social problem. More commonly, however, drug dependence is detrimental both to the user and to society. However, in weighing detrimental effects, one must consider both the pattern of use by a given individual and the available alternatives. For example, many would take the view that some individuals should be permitted to take opioids under appropriate supervision if the alternative is severe psychiatric impairment or uncontrolled use of opioids or other destructive psychoactive agents.

Drug dependence is commonly, but not necessarily, associated with the development of tolerance and physical dependence. *Tolerance* has developed when, after repeated administration, a given dose of a drug produces a decreased effect or when increasingly larger doses must be taken to obtain the effects observed with the original dose. *Physical dependence* refers to an altered physiological state (neuroadaptation) produced by the repeated administration of a drug, which necessitates the continued administration of the drug to prevent the appearance of a withdrawal or abstinence syndrome that is characteristic for the particular drug. The theoretical bases for the phenomena of tolerance and physical dependence are discussed below. The existence of drug dependence has recently been defined based on the presence of three or more of the following criteria (*see* American Psychiatric Association, 1987): (1) taking the substance more often or in larger amounts than intended; (2) unsuccessful efforts to terminate or reduce drug use; (3) large amounts of time spent acquiring or using the drug or recovering from its effects; (4) frequent intoxication or withdrawal symptoms; (5) abandonment of social or occupational activities because of drug use; (6) continued use despite adverse psychological or physical effects; (7) marked tolerance; and (8) frequent use of the drug to relieve withdrawal symptoms.

Addiction. The term *addiction,* like the term *abuse,* has been used in so many ways that it can no longer be employed without further qualification or elaboration. However, it is not likely that the term will be dropped from the language. In this chapter, the term *addiction* is used to connote a severe degree of drug dependence that is an extreme on a continuum of involvement with drug use. The term conveys a quantitative rather than a qualitative sense of the degree to which drug use pervades the total life activity of the user and of the range of circumstances in which drug use controls the user's behavior. Anyone who is addicted would be considered drug dependent by the criteria described above. However, the term *addiction* cannot be used interchangeably with *physical dependence* as that term is used here. It is possible to be physically dependent on drugs without being addicted and, in some special circumstances, to be addicted without being physically dependent (*see* below).

The use of the terms *drug dependence,* to denote a behavioral syndrome, and *physical dependence,* to refer to biological changes that underlie withdrawal syndromes, causes confusion. To reduce some of this confusion, the term *neuroadaptation* has been proposed as a substitute for *physical dependence* (*see* Edwards *et al.*, 1981).

GENESIS OF DRUG USE AND DEPENDENCE

Whether the use of a drug is socially acceptable or subject to extreme disapproval, many factors determine who will experiment with the drug and experience its effects; other factors influence who will continue to use it casually and who will progress from casual to intensive or compulsive use.

Experimentation is largely a matter of availability, curiosity, the attitude and drug-using behavior of one's friends, the social acceptability of a given form of drug use, the risks believed to be associated with experimental use, and the tendency of the individual to seek out novel situations and respect social norms. The emphasis here will be on the interactions of man and drug, and on those aspects of the interaction that are relevant to clinical situations and to the development of dependence.

Drugs as Reinforcers. Man's tendency to take drugs is shared with other mammals. Laboratory animals can learn to self-administer most of the drugs commonly used for nonmedical purposes, including opioids, barbiturates, ethanol, anesthetic gases, local anesthetics, volatile solvents, central nervous system (CNS) stimulants, phencyclidine, nicotine, and caffeine. Whether an animal will self-administer a drug depends on a number of factors, including the properties of the drug itself, the route of administration, the size of the individual dose, the amount of work required to obtain a dose and the time between the work and the drug administration (schedule of reinforcement), the presence of other drugs, and the kinds of drugs the animal has been given previously (*see* Johanson and Schuster, 1981). With certain notable exceptions, animals given continuous access show patterns of self-administration that are often strikingly similar to those exhibited by human users of the same drug. Such observations suggest that preexisting psychopathology is not a requisite for initial or even continued drug taking, and that drugs themselves are powerful reinforcers, even in the absence of physical dependence.

Drugs are not equally powerful as reinforcers in animals. Nicotine is self-administered under a narrower range of conditions than are opioids or cocaine; caffeine is a relatively weak reinforcer, and it is often quite difficult to train animals to self-administer ethanol. To date, there is no reliable animal model for the self-administration of cannabinoids. Some drugs (*e.g.*, chlorpromazine) are never self-administered; they appear instead to have aversive properties, and animals learn to avoid behaviors that result in small injections of such agents. On the other hand, animals will press a lever more than four thousand times to get a single injection of cocaine, and when given free access, they generally self-administer high daily doses that may produce severe toxic effects and induce self-mutilating behavior. With stimulants such as amphetamine and cocaine, periods of self-imposed abstinence alternate with periods of drug administration; generally the animals die of toxic effects and inanition after a period of several weeks of continuous use. If saline solution is substituted for cocaine or amphetamine, there is a burst of rapid lever pressing for several hours, then abruptly all responding ceases and is not resumed. However, a small "priming" dose of a reinforcing drug reinitiates the drug-taking behavior. Animals self-administering morphine gradually raise the daily dose over a period of weeks, then self-administer the drug at a steady rate that avoids both gross toxicity and withdrawal symptoms. When saline solution is substituted for morphine, however, the animal continues to press the lever (except during the peak of withdrawal) and does so at a slow but steady rate over a period of weeks (*see* Johanson and Schuster, 1981).

Drug-using behavior and reinforcement can become linked with environmental signals (*e.g.*, a light or tone), such that the signals function as secondary reinforcers. Drug-seeking behavior may then persist for long periods with only occasional reinforcement by the drug itself (*see* Young and Herling, 1986).

Mechanisms of Primary Reinforcement. The reinforcing effects of a number of psychoactive drugs involve dopaminergic systems that originate in the ventral tegmental area (VTA) of the brain and make connections with the nucleus accumbens and either directly or indirectly with the limbic cortex, ventral pallidum, and frontal cortex. Activation of this mesocorticolimbic system by electrical stimulation, a variety of drugs, or natural reinforcers (*e.g.*, food) results in release of dopamine in the nucleus accumbens. This release is associated with rewarding or reinforcing events (Hernandez and Hoebel, 1988; Koob and Bloom, 1988; Wise, 1988).

No category of drugs acts exclusively on the mesocorticolimbic system, and different classes of pharmacological agents activate the dopaminergic system by different mechanisms. For example, μ- and δ-agonist opioids inhibit neurons that tonically inhibit dopaminergic neurons in the VTA, while cocaine causes an increase in the synaptic concentration of dopamine by inhibition of its reuptake. Amphetamine has similar effects on reuptake of dopamine, and it also releases the neurotransmitter from intracellular stores. Drugs that are reinforcing also decrease the intensity of electrical stimulation in the VTA or medial forebrain bundle needed to produce reinforcing effects. Dopaminergic antagonists such as pimozide or opioid antagonists raise the threshold for electrical self-stimulation.

Tolerance and Physical Dependence. In addition to the primary reinforcing effects, other factors come into play during long-term drug use that profoundly affect the pattern of use and the likelihood that the drug use will be continued. Among these factors are the capacities of some substances to produce tolerance and/or physical dependence. These phenomena, as previously defined, are often assumed to be inextricably linked to each other and to the problem of compulsive drug use. Neither of these assumptions is valid. Tolerance and physical dependence develop not only with opioids, ethanol, and hypnotics but also after long-term administration of a wide variety of drugs that are not self-administered by animals or used compulsively by man. Such drugs include anticholinergics, dopaminergic antagonists, and imipramine. Rebound withdrawal effects may also be seen after abrupt discontinuation of β-adrenergic antagonists, Ca^{2+}-channel blockers, or α_2-adrenergic agonists (*see* Raftery, 1984). Nor does physical dependence invariably occur in every situation where tolerance develops. Tolerance is a general phenomenon observed with a host of substances, and many independent mechanisms are involved (*see* Chapters 1 and 2).

It is possible to distinguish two varieties of acquired pharmacological tolerance: dispositional and pharmacodynamic. Dispositional tolerance results from changes in the pharmacokinetic properties of the agent in the organism, such that reduced concentrations are present at the sites of drug action. The most common mechanism is an increased rate of metabolism. Dispositional tolerance has relatively little effect on the peak intensity of action and does not usually result in more than a threefold decrease in sensitivity. Pharmacodynamic tolerance results from adaptive changes within affected systems, such that the response is reduced in the presence of a given concentration of the drug. When behavioral phenomena are evaluated, tolerance usually develops more rapidly and to a greater degree when the effect of the drug has a behavioral "cost" to the organism (*i.e.*, when the capacity to earn a reward or avoid punishment is impaired) than when it does not. Thus, rats tested daily on a moving belt develop more tolerance to the ataxic effects of ethanol when it is administered before the test than afterward; the slowest development of tolerance occurs when daily testing is omitted. Similar relationships between behavioral conditions and the development of tolerance have been observed with opioids, marihuana, and amphetamines. (*See* Goudie and Demellweek, 1986; Tabakoff and Hoffman, 1987.)

Tolerance to Opioids. Tolerance does not develop uniformly to all the actions of opioid drugs. There may be complete tolerance to some actions, while responses to others are relatively unaltered. Tolerance to opioids is characterized by a shortened duration and decreased intensity of the analgesic, euphorigenic, sedative, and other CNS-depressant effects as well as by a marked elevation in the average lethal dose. Although animals that are tolerant to opioids may metabolize them somewhat more rapidly, most of the tolerance is due to adaptation of cells in the nervous system to the drug's action.

Although tolerance itself does not necessarily affect the likelihood of continued use, it can affect patterns of use by increasing the amount of drug that must be taken to produce a given effect (*e.g.*, euphoria). The use of increased amounts may in turn enhance the risk of toxic effects or produce other problems if the drug is expensive or obtained illicitly.

Tolerance to opioid drugs can develop with remarkable rapidity. Former morphine addicts can attain a dosage of 500 mg of morphine per day within 10 days. However, even with prolonged administration of opioids to experimental animals, there appears to be little tolerance to the facilitatory effect of such drugs on electrical self-stimulation of the brain or to their capacity to serve as discriminative stimuli (*see* Kornetsky *et al.*, 1979).

At some doses, the degree of tolerance to opioids depends on the environmental conditions under which they are given (*see* Goudie and Demellweek, 1986). Certain forms of long-lasting residual tolerance are also apparent; animals and human subjects previously dependent on opioids become physically dependent more rapidly on reexposure.

Tolerance to Ethanol, Barbiturates, and Related Hypnotics. Animals made tolerant to barbiturates or ethanol show significantly less sedation and ataxia than do nontolerant animals at the same blood concentrations. However, as the blood concentrations are increased, there is progressively less difference between tolerant and nontolerant animals in the degree of CNS depression. In contrast to the tolerance seen with opioids, animals tolerant to ethanol or barbiturates show only modest elevation of the lethal blood concentration. If the use of the CNS depressant has produced only ataxia and has been insufficient to depress respiration to some degree, there is little or no tolerance to the respiratory-depressant and lethal effects of the drug. It appears that only those systems that have been challenged or altered by the agent display tolerance to its effects (Okamoto *et al.*, 1978).

In the case of barbiturates such as pentobarbital, ethanol, and a number of nonbarbiturate hypnotics (glutethimide, meprobamate, *etc.*), a more rapid enzymatic degradation of the drug can also be demonstrated in tolerant animals. Thus, in the same animal, both pharmacodynamic and dispositional tolerance contribute to the decreased duration and intensity of the response to a given dose of drug.

With these groups of drugs, as with the opioids, tolerance does not directly increase the probability of continued or compulsive use. However, tolerance to toxic effects may not develop in parallel with tolerance to CNS depression and, in the case of ethanol particularly, the consumption of more drug in order to obtain CNS effects may increase the likelihood of direct damage to organs such as the brain and liver. Furthermore, the shortened duration of action may increase the frequency of drug taking, thereby increasing the number of times that drug-taking behavior will be reinforced.

Some aspects of tolerance to general CNS depressants develop with surprising rapidity. Thus, in man, when the blood concentration is falling after administration of a large dose of ethanol, the signs and symptoms of intoxication disappear at a concentration that was associated with gross intoxication when the blood level was rising. The degree of such acute CNS tolerance (as measured by the blood concentration of the drug when signs of ataxia disappear) seems directly related to the depth of the CNS depression that was produced by the drug. Acute tolerance also appears to develop with some benzodiazepines (Rosenberg and Chiu, 1985). It is not clear whether the mechanisms underlying acute tolerance are related to those involved in the tolerance that develops over longer periods. Tolerance to ethanol and related general CNS depressants has been reviewed by Smith (1977) and Tabakoff and Hoffman (1987). Tolerance to CNS sympathomimetics, nicotine, cannabinoids, and psychedelics is also discussed under clinical characteristics of their abuse.

Physical Dependence. Physical dependence has been studied after long-term administration of opioids, CNS depressants (ethanol, barbiturates, related hypnotics, and benzodiazepines), amphetamines, cocaine, cannabinoids, phencyclidine, and nicotine. The withdrawal symptoms associated with many of these classes of agents are generally characterized by rebound effects in those physiological systems that were initially modified by the drug. For example, CNS depressants elevate the seizure threshold, but spontaneous seizures may be seen during their withdrawal. Amphetamines and cocaine alleviate fatigue, suppress appetite, and elevate mood; withdrawal from these drugs is characterized by lack of energy, hyperphagia, and depression. However, it is not certain whether all the complex patterns of signs and symptoms seen during withdrawal from μ-agonist opioids or general depressants should be considered rebound effects, nor whether such a generalization is applicable to the syndromes observed after abrupt withdrawal of drugs such as nicotine, caffeine, clonidine, or opioids that do not act at μ receptors.

The time required to produce physical dependence on any drug depends on a number of factors, but the most important for many drugs seem to be the degree to which the drug alters CNS function and the continuity of this alteration. However, whether a withdrawal syndrome is clinically observable depends on the criteria for withdrawal symptoms, the sensitivity of methods used to detect withdrawal, and the rate at which the drug is removed from its site of action.

Patients who have received therapeutic doses of morphine several times a day for 1 to 2 weeks will have only mild symptoms that may not be recognized as withdrawal symptomatology when the drug is stopped; symptoms are even less pronounced when the opioid is one that is slowly eliminated (such as levorphanol or methadone). However, if the drug is not simply discontinued but an opioid antagonist (naloxone) is used to induce withdrawal, it is possible to demonstrate withdrawal symptoms in man 6 to 8 hours after a single therapeutic dose of morphine, indicating the presence of an otherwise-subclinical level of physical dependence (Bickel *et al.,* 1988; Heishman *et al.,* 1989). In short, the phenomenon of physical dependence on opioids is initiated by the first dose, and this rapid development has important clinical implications (*see* below).

The time required to produce physical dependence with general CNS depressants or benzodiazepines is likewise short; when rapidly metabolized drugs are used, the earliest signs of rebound excitability can be detected after surprisingly brief periods of CNS depression. A single large dose of ethanol produces an elevation of the threshold for chemically induced seizures that is followed by a period of subnormal threshold. After 3 days of continuous exposure to ethanol, mice develop marked physical dependence, with spontaneous seizures upon abrupt withdrawal. In cats, a withdrawal syndrome can be precipitated with a specific benzodiazepine antagonist 24 hours after administration of flurazepam (Rosenberg and Chiu, 1985). In man, it may require weeks of mild intoxication with short-acting barbiturates to produce clinically significant physical dependence, but some patients who are kept deeply intoxicated (semicomatose) for 16 to 20 hours per day, for 10 to 12 days, become so physically dependent that they develop seizures and delirium on abrupt withdrawal. If rebound changes in the EEG or insomnia are used as criteria, only 1 or 2 weeks of ordinary dosage at night is enough to induce low levels of physical dependence on CNS depressants and benzodiazepines (*see* Woods *et al.*, 1987).

The early onset of the adaptational processes that eventually produce grossly observable withdrawal symptoms has obvious implications not only for the problem of deciding just when physical dependence is present but also for the problem of determining the causes of drug dependence or compulsive drug use. It is quite conceivable that individuals who use short-acting drugs to induce euphoria or reduce tensions can perceive a relative dysphoria or an exacerbation of these same tensions (rebound effects) as the drug effects wane. Such increases in unpleasant feelings might then contribute to the motivation to repeat the use of the drug, and the alleviation of withdrawal phenomena might increase the effectiveness of the drug as a reinforcer of drug-using behavior. Similar subtle post-drug-use effects are also seen with amphetamines, cocaine, short-acting benzodiazepines, and possibly with nicotine.

The relationship of tolerance and physical dependence to drug-seeking behavior and compulsive drug use is complex and differs with drug categories. For example, it is difficult to show in animal models that physical dependence on ethanol increases ethanol intake (*see* Cappell and LeBlanc, 1981; Winger, 1988). The notion that physical dependence increases drug-seeking behavior and the reinforcing effects of the drug is best established for the opioids, but even with this group of drugs other factors appear to be more potent determinants of behavior. For example, although some degree of physical dependence develops in medical patients who receive opioids regularly for more than a few days, the overwhelming majority of such patients do not exhibit drug-seeking behavior and do not become compulsive users. Even those who administer such drugs to themselves for brief periods discontinue the drug when the medical condition is relieved. A large proportion of the young men who served in the United States Army in Vietnam used heroin, and about half of this group became physically dependent. Nevertheless, a substantial percentage simply stopped their use of heroin before their return to the United States, and many did so without benefit of any special treatment (*see* Robins, 1974). Similarly, many patients who develop some degree of physical dependence in the course of treatment with benzodiazepines are able to tolerate low-level withdrawal symptoms upon discontinuation, while others seem less able to do so. Wide individual differences in the capacity to tolerate withdrawal symptoms are also seen among cigarette smokers. The basis for this variability is still not clear. Thus, although some compulsive users attribute their drug problems entirely to "getting hooked" (either iatrogenically or in the course of using drugs illicitly), physical dependence is currently viewed not so much as a direct cause of drug dependence but as one of several factors that contribute to its development and to the tendency to relapse after withdrawal (*see* below).

Degree of Physical Dependence and Locus of Changes. Although it is possible to demonstrate changes in the biochemical and physiological properties of tissues (*e.g.*, brain, intestine) in dependent animals (*see* Redmond and Krystal, 1984; Tabakoff and Hoffman, 1987), the degree of physical dependence in the whole organism is still measured by the severity of the withdrawal syndrome produced either by abrupt withdrawal or by use of drug antagonists.

It is now quite clear that changes occur throughout the entire neuraxis during the development of physical dependence on CNS depressants, benzodiazepines, and, probably, ethanol (*see* Smith, 1977; Rosenberg and Okamoto, 1978). In view of the distribution and widespread effects of endogenous opioid-like peptides (*see* Chapters 12 and 21), it is not surprising that adaptive changes to the administration of exogenous opioids and withdrawal phenomena can be demonstrated throughout the autonomic and central nervous systems. Withdrawal hyperexcitability is observed in decerebrate animals, in the spinal cord of man, and in animals after cord transection. With local administration, the spinal cord or other structures can be made physically dependent on opioids with minimal involvement of the rest of the CNS (*see* Yaksh and Noueihed, 1985). Neural structures that subserve the expression of the classical manifestations of physical dependence on opioids appear to be distinct from those that are critical for the reinforcing effects of these agents (*see* Koob and Bloom, 1988; Wise, 1988).

Cross-Dependence. The ability of one drug to suppress the manifestations of physical dependence produced by another and to maintain the physically dependent state is referred to as *cross-dependence*. Cross-dependence may be partial or complete, symmetrical or asymmetrical.

Most sedative–hypnotics show a reasonable degree of cross-dependence with each other and with ethanol and the benzodiazepines. There is also some cross-dependence between barbiturates and volatile anesthetics. Although the mechanism of action of these agents differs, it is thought that they all share some capacity to influence the Cl^- channel that is regulated by gamma-aminobutyric acid (*see* Nutt *et al.*, 1989; *see also* Chapter 17).

Cross-tolerance and cross-dependence

among opioids develop only between those agents that act at the same type of opioid receptor (*see* Chapter 21). Thus, physical dependence induced by a specific δ agonist may be adequately suppressed by a less specific agent such as morphine that acts at both μ and δ receptors, but that induced by morphine is only partially suppressed by a specific δ agonist. This is an example of asymmetrical cross-dependence.

If a long-acting drug such as methadone is substituted over several days for morphine, abrupt discontinuation produces a withdrawal syndrome characteristic of the long-acting drug rather than that of morphine. This aspect of cross-dependence has important clinical implications, since the withdrawal symptoms that occur with drugs with longer half-lives (methadone, phenobarbital, diazepam) are generally less severe but more protracted. This phenomenon is the basis for the substitution treatment of physical dependence for both opioids and CNS depressants.

Mechanisms of Physical Dependence. Most theories postulate some form of CNS counteradaptation to the agonistic actions of the drugs. In view of knowledge of negative-feedback control of the activities of neurons by recurrent neural pathways and of the activities of regulatory molecules (such as receptors) and important metabolic pathways, it would be amazing if such counteradaptation did not occur. In the case of opioids and CNS depressants, long-term administration produces a "latent counteradaptation" in neural systems affected by the drugs that becomes manifest in the form of rebound or overshoot phenomena when the drugs are stopped or when an antagonist is administered. The underactivity of neural systems that often follows discontinuation of cocaine or amphetamine can also be viewed as a manifestation of latent counteradaptation. A number of mechanisms have been proposed to explain these changes, some of which help to account for the observation that physical dependence is generally accompanied by tolerance, and that the two phenomena develop and decay at about the same rate. However, there is growing evidence that for some drugs, notably ethanol, it is possible to distinguish the mechanisms responsible for tolerance from those responsible for physical dependence (*see* below). For any given drug, it is likely that a complete explanation of physical dependence will require a description of the adaptive changes induced in cells that express specific receptors for the drug and thus are directly affected (within-system adaptation), as well as those induced in other neural systems that are indirectly affected by the drug (between-system adaptation) (*see* Koob and Bloom, 1988).

The mechanisms responsible for opioid-induced physical dependence are among the most thoroughly studied. Although an increase in the number of opioid receptors follows the long-term administration of antagonists, the continuous administration of opioid agonists does not change the number or affinity of such receptors in the CNS (*see* Akil *et al.*, 1984; Morris *et al.*, 1988). However, adaptive changes in the second messenger systems that are altered by stimulation of opioid receptors can be detected. For example, in some brain regions (such as the locus ceruleus) the effects of μ and δ opioids include inhibition of adenylyl cyclase, an action mediated by the inhibitory guanine nucleotide–binding regulatory protein, G_i; this effect is shared with α_2-adrenergic agonists. The long-term administration of morphine causes a compensatory increase in adenylyl cyclase activity, and excessive production of cyclic AMP may be partially responsible for the rebound excitability of neurons in the locus ceruleus that typically occurs during opioid withdrawal. Moreover, the common intracellular mechanism helps to explain the utility of clonidine and other α_2-adrenergic agonists in suppressing some elements of the opioid withdrawal syndrome (*see* below). However, changes in the activity of adenylyl cyclase in the locus ceruleus do not develop as rapidly as do some manifestations of physical dependence, and failure to find similar changes in other regions of the CNS indicates that other mechanisms must also be operative (*see* Duman *et al.*, 1988). These mechanisms may involve changes in the linkage of opioid receptors to other effector systems, including K^+ channels (Aghajanian and Wang, 1987; Christie *et al.*, 1987). In addition, long-term administration of morphine decreases the synthesis of proenkephalin in the striatum, and some aspects of opioid withdrawal may reflect a lag in the return of enkephalin concentrations to normal (Uhl *et al.*, 1988). Additional discussion of the mechanisms involved in the development of dependence, tolerance, and withdrawal syndromes can be found in Redmond and Krystal (1984), Tabakoff and Hoffman (1987), Koob and Bloom (1988), and Nutt and colleagues (1989).

Learning, Conditioning, and Relapse. Within the framework of learning theory, drug use, whether casual or compulsive, can be viewed as behavior that is maintained by its consequences; consequences that strengthen a behavior pattern are reinforcers. Drugs may reinforce the antecedent drug-taking behavior by inducing pleasurable effects (positive reinforcement) or by terminating some aversive or unpleasant situation (negative reinforcement), as when a drug alleviates pain or anxiety. Some aspects of reinforcement that are linked to more remote consequences are not easily categorized. This is the case when control of weight is a stated motive for continued use of nicotine or other drugs. Secondary or social reinforcement entirely independent of pharmacological effects may also play a role, as is the case when drug use results in special status, membership in a desired group, or the approval of friends. Sometimes social reinforcement maintains initial drug-using behavior until the individual comes to appreciate the primary drug effect or becomes tolerant to some initial aversive effects of the particular drug. This seems to be the case with many young people who do not like the initial effects of tobacco or who perceive nothing pleasurable about the initial effects of smoking marihuana. Although it is not as widely appreciated, many naive individuals find the effects of an initial dose of heroin, with its associated nausea and vomiting, somewhat unpleasant; however, social reinforcement may maintain the behavior until tolerance develops to these effects.

The development of physical dependence opens possibilities for another variety of reinforcement; each time drug use alleviates withdrawal distress the antecedent drug-using behavior is further reinforced. Even when tolerance attenuates the initial reinforcing effects, drugs that induce certain varieties of physical dependence produce a regularly recurring sense of dysphoria or distress that is immediately eliminated by another dose of the drug. Dysphoria need not be severe for its regular alleviation to reinforce behavior. During the withdrawal state, drug use can simultaneously alleviate distress and in some cases produce euphoria, a particularly powerful reinforcement (*see* Wikler, 1980).

The correlation is not always high between the degree to which withdrawal from a given class of drugs threatens physical well-being and the degree to which withdrawal generates aversive states and increases the reinforcing effects of the drug. Withdrawal from nicotine never threatens physical well-being, but it regularly motivates continued smoking. By contrast, some users of ethanol or hypnotics elect to stop such use abruptly, even though doing so may cause delirium and life-threatening seizures.

It is uncertain to what extent the positive reinforcing (euphorigenic) effects of drugs continue to contribute to their reinforcing effects once tolerance develops. After as little as 5 days of self-administration of ethanol or heroin in a laboratory setting, alcoholics or heroin addicts show more depression, dysphoria, and anxiety than a sense of well-being. In the case of opioids, however, there is a brief period immediately after each dose when mood is elevated (Meyer and Mirin, 1979). Patients tolerant to most of the effects of large doses of methadone still experience some positive effects on mood at about the time the concentration of methadone reaches peak values in plasma after each daily dose.

The significance of such positive reinforcing effects also varies with the class of drug. For example, many people who become dependent on benzodiazepines continue to take them, not for their positive reinforcing effects, but to avoid emergence of antecedent anxiety or of withdrawal symptoms (Busto *et al.*, 1986; Woods *et al.*, 1987). Both actions are properly considered examples of negative reinforcement.

A protracted period of physiological and psychological abnormalities commonly follows the acute syndrome caused by withdrawal of opioids, and this condition can persist for weeks. Since the subjective sense of not being quite normal is immediately relieved by very small doses of opioid drugs, the protracted abstinence syndrome may predispose to relapse by creating a prolonged period of increased vulnerability, during which the effects of opioids are especially reinforcing (*see* Cushman and Dole, 1973; Martin *et al.*, 1973). Such a protracted state may also exist following withdrawal of other drugs that cause dependence. After withdrawal of ethanol, other CNS depressants, or benzodiazepines, sleep and mood may be disturbed for many weeks. It is not clear how long the anhedonia associated with withdrawal of cocaine or amphetamine persists (*see* below).

In both animals and man, drug effects, withdrawal phenomena, and relief of withdrawal symptoms by drugs can be conditioned to environmental stimuli. Such conditioning helps to explain how the rituals and circumstances surrounding drug use can act as secondary reinforcers, and how the mere taking of an inert pill or the use of a needle and syringe containing no drug can evoke the feelings (including euphoria or relief of withdrawal symptoms) previously produced when the pill or syringe contained an active substance. The observation that withdrawal distress can become conditioned to the environment in which it occurs may underlie reports that former opioid addicts may experience sensations very similar to withdrawal symptoms, including an intensified craving for drugs, when they return to an environment where drugs are available. Alcoholics may have similar experiences, particularly when they are exposed to the sight and smell of alcohol. The conditions that elicit the most severe withdrawal and the most intense "craving" are those associated with the availability and use of the drug, rather than those associated with withdrawal (*e.g.*, being offered some heroin or cocaine by a friend or watching someone else use the drug). These are also the circumstances that increase craving in recently abstinent alcoholics and cigarette smokers. Moreover, such stimuli can elicit craving and the memory of drug-induced euphoria without other elements of drug withdrawal (Childress *et al.,* 1986; O'Brien *et al.,* 1988). Positive reinforcing effects and memories of these effects evoked by a variety of stimuli may be sufficient in some individuals to account for the initial development of drug taking, escalation to compulsive drug use, and relapse after successful detoxification (*see* Wise, 1988). Nevertheless, evidence is good that continuation of use is primarily motivated by avoidance of withdrawal (*see* below).

Vulnerability. In man, drugs may produce effects experienced as pleasurable, novel, or tension-reducing, but these effects are not such powerful reinforcers that repetitive drug use is inevitable. Much research has centered on why some individuals stop after experimentation, others continue drug use but do not become dependent, and still others become compulsive drug users.

Individuals who later become regular users of socially disapproved drugs or abusers of ethanol tend to be more impulsive, more interested in new experiences, more rebellious with respect to social norms, less tolerant of frustration, and less concerned with avoiding self-harm. Early childhood aggression is also a predictor of later problems with drug use. Certain psychiatric diagnostic categories are regularly overrepresented among those who seek treatment for alcoholism and drug dependency. These include depressive disorders, anxiety disorders, and antisocial personality (Rounsaville *et al.,* 1982; Hesselbrock *et al.,* 1985). Despite these findings, no single recognized addictive personality or constellation of traits has been identified that is equally applicable to all varieties of drug-dependent individuals. Indeed, given the different pharmacological effects of various drugs, it would be surprising if all dependent drug users were similar.

There are many factors that could contribute to increased vulnerability to continued or compulsive drug use. Some individuals may experience a more intense response to the initial reinforcing properties of the drugs, such as a more intense euphoria or a more profound reduction of unpleasant feelings of anger, depression, or anxiety. Such intense reactions, in turn, could be due to differences in sensitivity to drug effects or to initially higher levels of distress. Thus, for some, drug use may be viewed as self-treatment for internal distress. Although the agent selected or the pattern of use may sometimes run counter to social norms, for some individuals the alternative may be a state of tension, anger, or depression that may be felt to be intolerable. On the other hand, the contributory factors may be entirely social, as in the case of young people who continue to smoke cigarettes more to conform to the pressures from friends than because of an especially intense need for the pharmacological effects of nicotine. Still other possibilities include differences in intensity of adverse effects of the drugs or in the intensity of withdrawal phenomena as experienced by different users (*see* above). For any given pattern of continued drug use the outcome is the result of an interaction between social, biological, and environmental factors.

Genetic Factors. Evidence for a genetic predisposition to alcoholism is growing. For example, rats bred to prefer ethanol over water spontaneously drink enough to become physically dependent, recover from acute intoxication at higher blood alcohol concentrations, and retain tolerance longer (Li, 1988). In man, two types of alcoholics have been described, each with distinct personality profiles and different patterns of inheritance, onset of problem drinking, and subjective responses to alcohol (*see* Cloninger *et al.,* 1989). Although no clear genetic basis for vulnerability to other forms of drug abuse has yet been demonstrated, there is some evidence for a genetic contribution to antisocial personality, which is a risk factor for both alcoholism and most other drug dependence.

Sociological Factors. Social factors have a major influence on which individuals have access to various drugs, and social attitudes, as well as the laws of any given country, determine which drugs are acceptable for casual or "recreational" use and which are prohibited. In addition, the nature of a society often determines the kinds of unpleasant feelings induced in its members, as well as the kinds of behaviors that are viewed as socially acceptable. In general, when the use of a drug is widely accepted, the number of users tends to be large and their personal characteristics quite diverse. When a particular form of drug use meets with severe disapproval, those who use it despite such sanctions tend to be very different from the average person in society in terms of attitudes and emotional adjustment even before use. Consequently, a high proportion may become compulsive users, sometimes leading to the conclusion that the particular drug is "more addicting" than those drugs used by larger and more diverse populations. Drugs may indeed differ in the degree to which they induce dependence, but the ratio of experimenters to addicts is not always a valid measure of the liability of a drug to cause dependence.

Those who use any legal or illegal drug are likely to use more than one drug. Furthermore, the use of more socially acceptable drugs, such as ethanol or tobacco, and the use of marihuana (sometimes known as "gateway drugs") precede the use of more disapproved drugs in a predictable pattern. In the United States, the earlier the experimentation with marijuana occurs, the greater the likelihood of later use of heroin or cocaine (*see* Kandel *et al.*, 1986).

Long-term drug use may establish a complex equilibrium among family members, and abstinence on the part of the user, with its attendant changes in behavior and role, can induce tension in other members of the family. Relapse to drugs or alcohol sometimes restores the previous pathological equilibrium. Cultural attitudes toward addicts and alcoholics and the legal or medical complications of drug use further increase the drug user's difficulties in obtaining realistic gratifications (alternative reinforcers) and simultaneously foster return to an environment (the local bar or group of drug users) where the drug is available, and where its use has been repeatedly reinforced.

CLINICAL CHARACTERISTICS

Most of the pharmacological agents commonly used for subjective purposes (excluding caffeine) can be placed into eight major classes, as follows: (1) opioids, (2) CNS depressants, (3) psychostimulants such as cocaine or amphetamine, (4) nicotine and tobacco, (5) cannabinoids, (6) psychedelics (hallucinogens, psychotomimetics, psychotogens), (7) arylcyclohexylamines (*e.g.*, phencyclidine), and (8) inhalants (*e.g.*, nitrous oxide, ethyl ether, volatile solvents). Although the agents within each class have many actions in common, differences also exist, and the classification is offered merely for its didactic convenience.

The following discussion is a condensed description of the actions and patterns of abuse of each of these drug categories. However, these drugs are rarely used singly. For example, opioid abusers commonly smoke cigarettes and use and abuse alcohol, cannabis, sedatives, stimulants, and cocaine. Similarly, alcoholics smoke heavily and typically use and abuse anxiolytics. Although in many instances there is dependence on only a single category of drugs, abuse of multiple drugs is common, particularly among individuals who use illicit drugs.

OPIOIDS

Extent and Patterns of Use. In the late 1960s the use of heroin increased considerably, in both the United States and Great Britain. Some of the reasons for the increase included changes in social attitudes toward drug use and toward established social norms in general, increased availability of drugs, and the substantial increase in the adolescent population (a result of the sharp increase in births following World War II), with its associated social changes. In 1988, less than 0.5% of young adults (age 18 to 25) reported having tried heroin at some time in their lives, although fewer had used it recently or had used it on a daily basis.

In the United States there are three basic patterns of opioid use and dependence. One involves individuals whose drug use begins in the context of medical treatment and who obtain their initial supplies through medical channels. This group constitutes a very small percentage of the addicted population. Another pattern begins with experimental or "recreational" drug use and progresses to more intensive use; this pattern involves primarily adolescents and young adults, with males outnumbering females. Most of these individuals are introduced to the drug by other users. Thus, drug use spreads from one friend to another in epidemic fashion. A third pattern involves users who begin in one or another of the preceding ways but later switch to oral opioids (methadone) obtained from organized treatment programs.

A user's first experience with opioids is often unpleasant, with nausea and vomiting as the outstanding features. Some may not try again for days or weeks; others, however, discover a new world of inner satisfaction with the first dose and make a conscious decision to continue to use the drug as frequently as their finances will permit. The most common pattern may be to try the drug once or twice and then, with awareness of the dangers, to avoid it thereafter. Despite the medical and legal risks, where group values support opioid use and relatively pure drugs are easily available, a very high percentage of users may become physically dependent. In 1971, about 42% of United States Army enlisted men in Vietnam used opioids at least once, and about half of these individuals reported that at some time during their year in Vietnam they were physically dependent (*see* Robins, 1974).

The incidence of opioid addiction among physicians, nurses, and those in the related health professions is many times higher than in any group with comparable educational background. Over the past decade, nonmedical drug use has increased among medical students, as it has in the general population (McAuliffe *et al.*, 1986). Many physician-addicts have stated that they first took opioids to overcome fatigue or depression or to alleviate some bodily ailment. However, the original motive is not necessarily the major determinant of the consequences of the addiction that later develops. Considering the frequency with which opioid analgesics are used in clinical medicine, addiction as a complication of medical treatment is quite uncommon. When it does occur, the pattern it follows depends on both the emotional adjustment of the patient prior to involvement with opioids and the source of the drug. Those individuals who are not seriously disturbed emotionally and who continue to obtain it from physicians or treatment programs may avoid many of the problems associated with illicit drugs.

Rapid intravenous injection of an opioid produces a warm flushing of the skin and sensations in the lower abdomen described by addicts as similar in intensity and quality to sexual orgasm; this feeling lasts for about 45 seconds and is known as a "rush," "kick," or "thrill." It is uncertain how much tolerance develops to this effect. Although heroin is the most commonly used illicit opioid, it has few special pharmacological properties that account for its popularity. Given subcutaneously, even experienced users cannot reliably distinguish heroin from morphine—understandably so, since heroin is rapidly converted into morphine in the body. However, heroin is more lipid soluble than morphine and, when the two drugs are given intravenously, heroin crosses the blood–brain barrier more rapidly. In the brain, heroin is rapidly deacetylated to 6-monoacetyl morphine, which is pharmacologically active, and then to morphine.

Symptoms and Effects of Compulsive Use. The behavior, social adjustment, and medical problems observed among opioid users and addicts are surprisingly varied. Experience with thousands of patients maintained on high daily doses of methadone for periods of up to 15 years has shown no direct injurious effects (Kreek, 1983). Good health and productive work are thus not incompatible with regular use of opioids. However, it is now clear that the behavior of the individual prior to opioid use and the purposes and patterns of use play a large role in determining the social and physiological consequences.

When chronic opioid users in England were able to obtain pure heroin from legitimate medical sources at no cost, the patterns of social adjustment were extremely varied and were similar to those observed in the United States. Four major patterns were noted: (1) "stables"—patients who were legitimately employed, did not engage in criminal activity, did not associate with other addicts, and did not buy extra heroin illicitly; (2) "junkies"—patients who were the opposite of the stable patients in these respects; (3) "loners"—patients who were on welfare rather than engaging in crime, did not associate with other addicts, but did use a wide variety of drugs not prescribed by treatment clinics; and (4) "two-worlders"—patients who were employed but associated with other addicts, bought extra drugs, and engaged in criminal activities. The disorganized behavior and criminality of the "junkies" and the organized behavior of the "stables" antedated the addiction. Despite the legal source of drugs, those receiving heroin at London clinics had a high incidence of infections (due to neglect of hygienic procedures or to shared needles) and a surprisingly high mortality rate, ranging from 2 to 6% per year. A follow-up study of young heroin addicts treated at London clinics revealed that 7 years later only 48% were still using opioids (43% obtained drugs from the clinics); 32% were abstinent and not abusing other drugs, and 12% were dead (*see* Stimson and Oppenheimer, 1982).

The health and social adjustment of patients maintained on oral methadone in the United States are equally varied. Many such patients hold jobs, raise children, commit no crimes, and use no socially disapproved drugs. Yet other patients continue to commit crimes, do not obtain employment, and use other drugs or excessive amounts of alcohol. A substantial number experience significant depression (*see* Rounsaville *et al.,* 1982). The mortality rate among patients in maintenance programs is higher than that among others of comparable age and socioeconomic status, but the general consensus is that the high rate is not related to the effects of oral methadone *per se,* but directly or indirectly to problems that antedated methadone use, to the excessive use of alcohol and other drugs, or to infection with human immunodeficiency virus (HIV).

Similar variations in patterns of behavior, social adjustment, and impaired health have been noted among heroin addicts in the United States who utilize exclusively illegal sources for their drugs. Undoubtedly, the high cost and impurities of illicit drugs in the United States exact their toll. Many women earn their drug money through prostitution, and the incidence of venereal disease is high. The average annual death rate among young-adult heroin addicts is several times higher than that for nonaddicts of similar age and ethnic backgrounds. In the younger group, much of this increase is due to fatal opioid overdosage that may be an accidental outcome of the dangerous fluctuations in the purity of illicit heroin or to combinations of opioids with ethanol or other CNS depressants. Considering the high prevalence of depression among opioid addicts, some apparent overdoses may be deliberate. Another frequent cause of sudden death has been termed an "anaphylactoid reaction," which probably results from the intravenous injection of a drug containing certain impurities. The suicide rate among addicts is considerably higher than that of the general population, and a surprisingly high percentage die violent deaths at the hands of others. The medical complications common among drug users include infections (*e.g.*, septicemia, endocarditis, hepatitis, acquired immune deficiency syndrome, tetanus, tuberculosis, and pulmonary, cerebral, and subcutaneous abscesses) due to shared needles and unhygienic procedures, foreign-body emboli, granulomata due to injection of contaminants, and a variety of neurological, musculoskeletal, and other lesions that may be due to hypersensitivity reactions or to toxic impurities in drugs produced in illicit laboratories.

Opioids reduce pain, aggression, and sexual drives, and their use, therefore, is unlikely to induce crime. However, many individuals committed crimes prior to the use of opioids, and they do not necessarily stop when opioid use begins. In addition, many individuals who did not engage in crime previously may begin to do so in order to obtain money to buy opioids, since the cost is usually beyond the amount they can obtain legitimately. In general, the number of crimes goes up while addicts are using illicit opioids and other drugs, such as cocaine, and goes down when they are abstinent or enter treatment (*see* Anglin *et al.*, 1981; Nurco *et al.*, 1988).

Tolerance, Physical Dependence, and Withdrawal Symptoms. A remarkable degree of tolerance develops to the respiratory-depressant, analgesic, sedative, emetic, and euphorigenic effects of μ-agonist opioids; however, the rate at which this tolerance develops, in either the addict or the medical patient, depends in part on the pattern of use. With intermittent use, it is possible to obtain for an indefinite period desired analgesic and sedative effects from doses in the therapeutic range. It is only when drug action is more or less continuous that significant tolerance develops. Thus, if the drug is used frequently, the addict who is primarily seeking to get a "rush" or to maintain a state of dreamy indifference (a "high") must constantly increase the dose. In this way, some addicts can build up to phenomenally large doses (*e.g.*, 2 g of morphine intravenously over a period of 2.5 hours without significant change in blood pressure, pulse rate, or respiration). Although the lethal dose is greatly altered in tolerant individuals, a dose always exists that is capable of producing death from respiratory depression. Moreover, tolerance to opioids largely disappears when withdrawal has been completed, and many addicts have taken fatal overdoses by returning to their previous dosage immediately after undergoing withdrawal.

Tolerance does not develop equally or at the same rate to all the effects of opioids, and even users highly tolerant to respiratory-depressant effects continue to exhibit some degree of miosis and to complain of constipation. Subjects who are maintained on daily oral doses of 100 mg of methadone for more than 8 weeks still seem sedated and apathetic and have constricted pupils and decreased respiratory rates (Martin *et al.*, 1973). However, experience with thousands of patients maintained on methadone for periods of several years suggests that, while constipation is a continuing problem, substantial sedation and apathy are easily managed by reductions in dosage.

Even after several years of constant dosage of methadone, there is less than complete tolerance to several effects of the drug. In addition to constipation, insomnia and decreased sexual function persist in 10 to 20% of patients, and about 50% complain of excessive sweating. Sensitivity of the CNS respiratory center to stimulation by CO_2 is diminished. Altered hypothalamic–pituitary function may also persist, although most patients on high doses of methadone have normal concentrations of testosterone, follicle-stimulating hormone (FSH), and luteinizing hormone (LH). However, plasma concentrations of prolactin peak each day at about the same time as does the concentration of methadone, about 4 hours after an oral dose (*see* Kreek, 1983).

Meperidine addicts may use large daily doses (3 to 4 g per day), but significant tolerance does not develop to the drug's excitant and atropine-like actions, which are due largely to a metabolite, normeperidine. When very high doses of meperidine are used, even the tolerant addict may show dilated pupils, increased muscular activity, twitching, tremors, mental confusion, and, occasionally, tonic–clonic seizures.

In general, there is a high degree of cross-tolerance and cross-dependence among opioids with actions at the same receptor type, but little or no cross-tolerance between opioids that act selectively at different receptors. Since most available opioids are not completely selective and have some affinity for each of the various receptors, the extent of cross-tolerance between different opioids is variable (*see* Chapter 21).

The character and the severity of the withdrawal symptoms that appear when an opioid is discontinued depend upon many factors, including the particular drug, the total daily dose used, the duration of use, and the health and personality of the addict.

It is helpful to view the total clinical picture of the abstinence syndrome as made up of purposive behavior, which is highly dependent on the observer and the environment and directed at getting more drug, and nonpurposive behavior, which is not goal oriented and which is relatively independent of the observer and the environment. The purposive phenomena, including complaints, pleas, demands, manipulations, and simulations, are as varied as the imagination of the drug-using population. In the hospital setting, they are considerably less pronounced when patients are certain that their behavior does not affect the decision to give them a drug.

In the case of morphine, heroin, or μ agonists with similar durations of action, nonpurposive symptoms, such as lacrimation, rhinorrhea, yawning, and sweating, appear about 8 to 12 hours after the last dose. About 12 to 14 hours after the last dose, the addict may fall into a tossing, restless sleep that may last several hours but from which he awakens more restless and more miserable than before. As the syndrome progresses, additional signs and symptoms appear, consisting of dilated pupils, anorexia, gooseflesh, restlessness, irritability, and tremor. With morphine and heroin, nonpurposive symptoms reach their peak at 48 to 72 hours. As the syndrome approaches peak intensity, the patient exhibits increasing irritability, insomnia, marked anorexia, violent yawning, severe sneezing, lacrimation, and coryza. Weakness and depression are pronounced. Nausea and vomiting are common, as are intestinal spasm and diarrhea. Heart rate and blood pressure are elevated. Marked chilliness, alternating with flushing and excessive sweating, is characteristic. Pilomotor activity resulting in waves of gooseflesh is prominent, and the skin resembles that of a plucked turkey. This feature is the basis of the expression "cold turkey" to signify abrupt withdrawal without treatment. Abdominal cramps and pains in the bones and muscles of the back and extremities are also characteristic, as are the muscle spasms and kicking movements that may be the basis for the expression "kicking the habit." The respiratory response to CO_2, which is decreased during opioid administration, is exaggerated during withdrawal. Rebound phenomena are also observed in the endocrine system. Leukocytosis is common, and white-cell counts above 14,000/mm^3 are often seen.

The failure to take food and fluids, combined with vomiting, sweating, and diarrhea, results in marked weight loss, dehydration, ketosis, and disturbance in acid–base balance. Occasionally there is cardiovascular collapse. However, seizures do not occur and the withdrawal syndrome is rarely life-threatening. At any point in the course of withdrawal, the administration of a suitable opioid will completely and dramatically suppress the symptoms of withdrawal. Without treatment, the acute phase of the morphine withdrawal syndrome runs its course; most of the grossly observable symptoms disappear in 7 to 10 days, but it is not certain how long it takes to restore physiological equilibrium completely.

The early opioid abstinence syndrome characterized by the signs and symptoms described above may be followed by a protracted abstinence syndrome, during which a number of physiological variables attain subnormal values. For example, a period of hyposensitivity to the respiratory-stimulant effects of CO_2 persists for many weeks after the exaggerated sensitivity of the early abstinence period subsides. In addition, there seem to be subtle behavioral manifestations that include an incapacity to tolerate stress, a poor self-image, and overconcern about discomfort. It is not unreasonable to postulate that these altered states contribute to the tendency of compulsive opioid users to relapse after withdrawal.

The abrupt withdrawal of methadone produces a syndrome that is qualitatively similar to that of morphine, but it develops more slowly and is more prolonged, although usually less intense. The addict has few or no symptoms until 24 to 48 hours after the last dose, and then complains of weakness, anxiety, anorexia, insomnia, abdominal discomfort, headache, sweating, pain in muscles and bones, and hot and cold flashes. As with morphine withdrawal, there is nausea, vomiting, and an increase in body temperature, blood pressure, pulse, respiratory rate, and pupillary size. In general, after abrupt withdrawal, the primary or early abstinence syndrome reaches its maximal intensity by about the third day and may not begin to decrease until the third week; apparent recovery may not occur until the sixth or seventh week. The early abstinence syndrome is followed by a secondary or protracted abstinence syndrome in which a number of previously elevated physiological parameters attain and remain at subnormal values through the twenty-fourth postwithdrawal week and concomitant psychological disturbances occur, such as tiredness, weakness, hypochondriasis, and feelings of lessened efficiency (Martin *et al.*, 1973). Even with very slow reduction in dosage, patients who have been maintained on high doses of methadone or methadyl acetate experience qualitatively similar withdrawal symptoms during and following the period of dosage reduction (Senay *et al.*, 1977; Judson *et al.*, 1983).

The meperidine abstinence syndrome usually develops within 3 hours after the last dose, reaches its peak within 8 to 12 hours, and then declines, so that few symptoms are apparent after 4 to 5 days. Craving may be intense, but the nonpurposive autonomic signs, while present, are not as prominent; the pupils may not be widely dilated, and there is usually little nausea, vomiting, or diarrhea. However, at peak intensity the muscle twitching, restlessness, and nervousness may be worse than during morphine withdrawal.

Withdrawal symptoms after other opioids that act at μ receptors are qualitatively similar to those after morphine, and they seem to follow the general rule that drugs with shorter durations of action tend to produce shorter, more intense abstinence syndromes while drugs that are slowly eliminated produce withdrawal syndromes that are prolonged but mild. Some differences between the syndrome seen upon withdrawal of μ agonists and that seen with partial agonists and with agonist–antagonists are described in Chapter 21.

Withdrawal in the Newborn. Babies born to mothers who have been regularly taking opioid agonists or agonist–antagonists prior to delivery will be physically dependent. The signs of withdrawal include irritability and excessive and high-pitched crying, tremors, frantic sucking of fists, hyperactive reflexes, increased respiratory rate, increased stools, sneezing, yawning, vomiting, and fever. With heroin, signs most commonly appear within the first day of life; they may not appear for several days with methadone. The intensity of the syndrome does not always correlate with the duration of maternal opioid use or dose. The use of paregoric (0.2 ml orally every 3 to 4 hours, increased as needed until symptoms are controlled) seems to be a rational and effective approach to management of such withdrawal when there is no question of simultaneous dependence on alcohol or other sedatives. Although withdrawal symptoms are generally more severe in babies born to mothers who have been maintained on methadone, compared with those who have been using heroin, the greater opportunity to provide prenatal care to the mother maintained on methadone results in a significant decrease in overall fetal distress and mortality.

When the mother is maintained on methadone any reduction of dosage must be gradual and the fetus must be monitored carefully because withdrawal of an opioid is potentially lethal for the fetus (*see* Finnegan, 1988).

Opioid Antagonists. The abstinence syndromes described above are those seen when opioids are abruptly withdrawn. If, however, an antagonist such as naloxone is given, a withdrawal syndrome develops within a few minutes after parenteral administration and reaches its peak intensity within 30 minutes. Until some of the antagonist is eliminated, even large doses of previously used opioid cannot always suppress the syndrome; partial suppression is possible by using large doses of opioid, but this may then produce respiratory depression as the action of the antagonist wanes. Depending on the dose of the antagonist, precipitated withdrawal is usually more severe than that seen after abrupt withdrawal of the drug, especially with an opioid that has a long duration of action.

GENERAL CNS DEPRESSANTS: BARBITURATES AND RELATED SEDATIVE–HYPNOTIC DRUGS

In general, the subjective effects of barbiturates and related sedatives and antianxiety agents are similar but not identical to those of ethanol, and the effects vary considerably with the dose, the situation, and the personality of the user.

Prevalence, Agents Employed, and Patterns of Use. The incidence and prevalence of nonmedical use of barbiturates, benzodiazepines, and related drugs exceeds that of the opioids. Although nonmedical use has declined over the past decade, in 1988 6% of young adults reported nonmedical use of sedatives, with 1% describing some use in the preceding month. About 8% indicated some experience with nonmedical use of tranquilizers.

Opioid users frequently take barbiturates, benzodiazepines, or other sedatives to augment the effects of weak illicit heroin or to produce psychological effects when they have become tolerant to prescribed opioids. Many heroin users and patients maintained on methadone are physically dependent on both opioids and sedatives. Some alcoholics use sedatives to relieve the ethanol withdrawal syndrome or to produce a state of intoxication devoid of the odor of alcohol. The short-acting barbiturates such as pentobarbital (''yellow jackets'') or secobarbital (''red devils'') are preferred to long-acting agents such as phenobarbital. Nonbarbiturates such as meprobamate, glutethimide, methyprylon, methaqualone, and some of the shorter-acting benzodiazepines are also abused. Paraldehyde and chloral hydrate, subject to considerable abuse in the past, have now been largely replaced by the other agents mentioned.

Chlordiazepoxide and certain other benzodiazepines that have minimal euphoriant actions and relatively slow onset of effects are uncommon as drugs of abuse. Normal subjects do not find benzodiazepines to be particularly reinforcing. However, for some individuals, including alcoholics and sedative abusers, certain benzodiazepines are reinforcing. More lipid-soluble agents, such as diazepam, alprazolam, and lorazepam, have a more prompt onset of action and appear to be more likely to be used for nonmedical purposes; some sedative abusers prefer them over short-acting barbiturates (*see* Woods *et al.*, 1987; Ciraulo *et al.*, 1988).

The patterns of nonmedical use of sedative–hypnotics are exceedingly varied. They range from infrequent sprees of gross intoxication, lasting a few days, to the prolonged, compulsive, daily use of huge quantities and a preoccupation with securing and maintaining adequate supplies. Some users may never exhibit gross intoxication but may, nevertheless, take drugs several times a day. The original contact with the drug may have been through a physician's prescription or through illicit drug trade. In the medical patient, the development of the problem may be a gradual one, beginning with prolonged use for insomnia or anxiety and progressing through increased dosage at night to a few capsules for sedation in the morning. Eventually, the drug is a major part of the user's life. Neither the patient taking benzodiazepines for anxiety or insomnia over a period of months nor the prescribing physician may recognize the existence of dependence. Both may assume that the anxiety, tremulousness, and insomnia that emerge when the drug is discontinued is a return of the original anxiety or insomnia. In some situations, no sharp line can be drawn between appropriate use and drug dependence. Most users take the drugs orally, but a few individuals inject barbiturates intravenously or intramuscularly. Such users can be recognized by the large abscesses that cover the accessible areas of their bodies.

The combination of amphetamines and barbiturates produces more elevation of mood than either drug alone. The mechanisms of this supra-additive effect are not clear, but competition for the same microsomal enzyme system and hence production of higher blood concentrations of the drugs may be partially responsible.

The amount of hypnotic that may be taken varies considerably, but an average daily dose of 1.5 g of short-acting barbiturate is not uncommon, and some individuals have consumed as much as 2.5 g daily over many months. Similar multiples of the usual daily therapeutic doses are taken by the compulsive users of meprobamate, glutethimide, and methyprylon. Abusers of benzodiazepines may ingest several hundred milligrams of diazepam or its equivalent every day. For references, *see* reviews by Smith (1977) and Woods and colleagues (1987).

Signs and Symptoms. Because tolerance develops to most of the actions of this group of drugs, there may be no apparent signs of long-term use. For the patient taking regular doses of barbiturates or benzodiazepines for sleep, the only manifestation may be a rebound insomnia and some anxiety when the drug is stopped. Some users, however, attempt to maintain a state of intoxication. In these individuals, the acute and the chronic effects of mild intoxication with CNS depressants resemble those of intoxication with alcohol. The individual who is intoxicated with a barbiturate shows a general sluggishness, difficulty in thinking, slowness and slurring of speech, poor comprehension and memory, faulty judgment, narrowed range of attention, emotional lability, and exaggeration of basic personality traits. Irritability, quarrelsomeness, and moroseness are common. There may be laughing or crying without provocation, untidiness in personal habits, hostile and paranoid ideas, and suicidal tendencies (*see* Smith, 1977). Similar patterns of increasing irritability may be seen when sedative abusers are given high doses of diazepam chronically. Interestingly, such subjects seem less aware of their mood changes and behavioral impairments when taking diazepam than when ingesting high doses of barbiturates (Griffiths *et al.*, 1983). Long-term intoxication with all pharmacologically similar agents has not been studied in as controlled a manner, but the clinical descriptions of isolated cases of abuse of high doses of meprobamate, glutethimide, and methaqualone are quite similar to the picture of chronic barbiturate intoxication. Neurological effects described here are those for barbiturates. These effects include thick, slurred speech, nystagmus, diplopia, strabismus, difficulty in visual accommodation, vertigo, ataxic gait, positive Romberg's sign, hypotonia, dysmetria, and decreased superficial reflexes; deep reflexes, pupillary responses, and sensation are usually unaltered.

Tolerance, Physical Dependence, and Withdrawal Symptoms. Long-term intoxication with short-acting barbiturates and related hypnotics results in both drug-disposition and pharmacodynamic tolerance. Pharmacodynamic tolerance also develops to most of the actions of benzodiazepines, but drug-disposition tolerance is less marked. Indeed, the slow accumulation of active metabolites of certain benzodiazepines tends to obscure the development of adaptive changes in the CNS. It is characteristic of adaptation to this class of agents that, while there may be considerable tolerance to the sedative and intoxicating effects, the lethal dose is not much greater in addicts than in normal individuals. Consequently, acute barbiturate or meprobamate poisoning may be accidentally or willfully superimposed on chronic intoxication at any time. Cross-tolerance between various agents in this group is common, but not all combinations have been studied. Benzodiazepines appear to be considerably safer than barbiturates and related sedatives, since acute overdosage is much less likely to produce fatal respiratory depression.

There are marked similarities between the withdrawal syndromes seen with all the sedative–hypnotic drugs. Although these syndromes are not identical (*see* Woods *et al.,* 1987), it still seems justified to use the term *general depressant withdrawal syndrome* to refer to the manifestations of withdrawal from any of these agents. In its mildest form, this syndrome may consist only of paroxysmal EEG abnormalities, rebound increases in rapid-eye-movement (REM) sleep, insomnia, or anxiety. Somewhat greater degrees of physical dependence result in tremulousness and weakness, in addition to anxiety and insomnia. When the syndrome is severe, there may be, in addition, tonic–clonic seizures and delirium. In contrast to opioid withdrawal, the withdrawal syndrome with these drugs can be a life-threatening medical emergency.

Former addicts can ingest 0.2 g of pentobarbital per day over many months without the development of any obvious manifestations of physical dependence on abrupt withdrawal. However, after 0.6 g per day for 1 to 2 months, 50% of subjects show withdrawal symptoms such as insomnia, anorexia, tremor, and EEG changes, and 10% may have a single seizure. When subjects are continuously intoxicated (0.9 to 2.2 g per day) for several months, 75% may have seizures and 66% delirium, and all experience insomnia, tremor, and anorexia on abrupt withdrawal.

Subjects given hypnotic drugs in ordinary doses for several weeks show tolerance to the hypnotic effects. Rebound increases in percentage of REM sleep and insomnia are often seen when such drugs are discontinued.

The typical course of withdrawal from large amounts of short-acting barbiturates is as follows: over the first 12 to 16 hours, as the concentration of the drug in blood declines and the intoxication clears, the patient seems to improve but then becomes increasingly restless, anxious, tremulous, and weak, and may complain of abdominal cramps and nausea. Vomiting, orthostatic hypotension, coarse tremors, and increased deep tendon reflexes may also be present. With the short-acting barbiturates and meprobamate, the symptoms usually reach their peak during the second and third days of abstinence; convulsions, when they occur, are usually seen within this period. The number of seizures varies from a single one to status epilepticus.

With the longer-acting barbiturates, symptoms may not begin until the second or third day and reach their peak more slowly. Seizures may not occur at all or may happen as late as the seventh to eighth day. When the rate of elimination of the barbiturate is slower than 20% per day, EEG changes and withdrawal symptoms may not be seen. Thus, clinical studies are consistent with laboratory studies that show that the onset and intensity of withdrawal are related to the rate at which active drug leaves the CNS. However, this self-tapering effect does not assure that only trivial symptoms will follow the abrupt discontinuation of long-acting drugs.

Patients who have seizures as a result of withdrawal of a barbiturate may begin to show improvement after the third day, but more than half go on to develop delirium. Anxiety mounts with time, and frightening dreams may be succeeded by a refractory insomnia. Visual hallucinations, usually of a persecutory nature, may occur, generally at the same time that sensorial clouding begins. Disorientation for time and place completes the picture of a full-blown delirium. Once the delirium develops, even the administration of large doses of barbiturate may not suppress it immediately. This is true also of the delirium that develops during the withdrawal of ethanol. The reason for this relative irreversibility is not clear. During the delirium, which usually occurs between the fourth and seventh day, agitation and hyperthermia can lead to exhaustion, cardiovascular collapse, and death. However, the withdrawal syndrome, even if untreated, usually clears by about the eighth day.

Some patients who have been taking benzodiazepines experience withdrawal phenomena even when the dose is tapered slowly, and there are reports of withdrawal syndromes occurring when patients are switched from a long-acting benzodiazepine to a shorter-acting congener. The benzodiazepine withdrawal syndrome commonly includes insomnia, restlessness, dizziness, nausea, abdominal pain, paresthesias, increased sensitivity to light and sound, tinnitus, headache, inability to concentrate, sweating, fatigue, and muscle twitching. Seizures may occur but are uncommon. The syndrome may persist for 10 days to several weeks. Withdrawal symptoms may occur after stopping ordinary therapeutic doses of benzodiazepines (*e.g.,* 5 to 40 mg of diazepam) that have been taken for several months. Although generally mild even with abrupt withdrawal, the symptoms cause sufficient distress to motivate continued drug taking (Busto *et al.*, 1986).

Babies born to mothers physically dependent on general CNS depressants or benzodiazepines will manifest withdrawal syndromes of varying severity. The signs are similar to those seen in the opioid withdrawal syndrome of the newborn; treatment involves the use of a general CNS depressant or a benzodiazepine, rather than an opioid or a phenothiazine.

ALCOHOL

Extent of Use. In the United States, two thirds of all adults use alcohol occasionally, and at least 12% of the users can be considered "heavy" drinkers. The lifetime risk of alcohol dependence or abuse is estimated at about 13%, with the risk for men far higher than for women (*see* Cloninger *et al.*, 1989).

Mechanisms of Reinforcing Actions. Despite the enthusiasm of some researchers for linking the reinforcing effects of all psychoactive drugs to dopaminergic systems (*see* above), others have concluded that no consistent relationship has been established between the reinforcing effects of ethanol and any single neurotransmitter system (*see* Tabakoff and Hoffman, 1987; Bloom, 1989). For example, rats bred to self-administer ethanol have reduced concentrations of 5-hydroxytryptamine (5-HT) in the brain. Moreover, inhibitors of 5-HT uptake into neurons decrease self-administration of alcohol by animals and by human subjects who were heavy drinkers (*see* Tabakoff and Hoffman, 1987).

People seem to use alcohol for a number of reasons. Cloninger and coworkers (1989) have proposed that type-II alcoholics (characterized by high novelty-seeking and low harm-avoidance behavior) drink to experience euphoric effects, while type-I alcoholics (with low novelty-seeking and high harm-avoidance behavior) drink to alleviate anxiety. However, other modes of reinforcement must come into play with long-term use since, after the first few days of drinking, alcoholics in laboratory settings often become more anxious and more depressed as drinking continues (*see* Mendelson and Mello, 1979).

Tolerance, Physical Dependence, and Special Complications. Long-term use of ethanol results in an increased capacity to metabolize ethanol, which declines after several weeks of abstinence, so that abstinent alcoholics and normal individuals metabolize ethanol at about the same rate. Chronic use of alcohol also produces pharmacodynamic tolerance, so that a higher blood concentration is necessary to produce intoxication in tolerant than in normal individuals. Some alcoholics can perform well on difficult tasks when their blood alcohol concentrations are above 200 mg/dl, twice the value that in most states is legally defined as significant intoxication. However, as is the case with barbiturates, there is no marked elevation of the lethal dose, and severe acute intoxication with respiratory depression may be superimposed on chronic alcoholic intoxication at any time (*see* Mendelson and Mello, 1979).

Cross-tolerance between ethanol and other drugs may be due to pharmacodynamic tolerance in the CNS or to more rapid metabolism, since the use of alcohol increases hepatic microsomal enzyme activity. Individuals tolerant to ethanol usually show cross-tolerance to general anesthetics; this cross-tolerance is probably a result of pharmacodynamic tolerance. There is also cross-tolerance to a variety of other sedative–hypnotics, including the benzodiazepines, which results from both pharmacodynamic (CNS) tolerance and from more rapid metabolism. However, cross-tolerance is seen only in the relatively sober alcoholic. When concentrations of ethanol in blood are high, the effects of other drugs are additive to those of ethanol. In addition, there is some mutual inhibition of metabolism as a result of competition for shared enzymatic systems (*see* Smith, 1977; Sellers and Busto, 1982). There is no obvious cross-tolerance between ethanol and opioids.

Long-term maintenance of high concentrations of ethanol in blood produces a state of physical dependence. The signs and symptoms of the alcohol withdrawal syndrome are similar but not entirely identical to those described above for barbiturate and benzodiazepine withdrawal. The intensity of the alcohol withdrawal syndrome correlates only partially with the amount of ethanol consumed and the duration of use. The low correlation is probably due to the way in which ethanol is metabolized. The body is able to metabolize the alcoholic content of about 30 ml (1 oz) of whisky in an hour (*see* Chapter 17). If the intake is sufficiently spread out over the day, each dose of ethanol may be metabolized without any substantial increase in blood concentration. On the other hand, the ingestion of only modestly larger amounts, but spaced so that the body's metabolic capacity is exceeded (*e.g.*, 120 ml [4 oz] of whisky every 3 hours), can produce much higher blood concentrations, which can induce clinically significant physical dependence in a matter of a few days (*see* above). Withdrawal phenomena most commonly appear within 12 to 72 hours after total cessation of drinking. However, even a relative decline in blood concentration (*e.g.*, from 300 to 100 mg/dl) may precipitate the syndrome, and such declines may occur with changes in the pattern of drinking, as well as with decreases in the total daily intake (*see* Mendelson and Mello, 1979).

With minimal levels of dependence, the entire syndrome may consist of disturbed sleep, nausea, weakness, anxiety, and mild tremors that last for less than a day. When dependence is severe, these symptoms are only prodromal, and the withdrawal phenomena may take the form of one or more of three overlapping syndromes—the tremulous syndrome, alcohol-related seizure disorders, and delirium tremens. As is the case with sedative–hypnotics, the alcohol withdrawal syndrome can be life-threatening.

The tremors, which appear within a few hours after the last drink, may be mild or so marked that the patient may be unable to lift a glass. They are often accompanied by nausea, anxiety, and sweating. There may be cramps, vomiting, hyperreflexia, and elevated blood pressure. Nightmares, disturbed sleep, and orthostatic hypotension are also part of the syndrome. The REM phase of sleep, which is depressed by alcohol, shows a rebound increase during alcohol withdrawal. The patient may begin to "see things," at first only when the eyes are closed, but later even when the eyes are open. Insight is at first retained, and the patient remains oriented. The hallucinations may be transient and the syndrome at this point is still referred to as *uncomplicated alcohol withdrawal*. Should hallucinations persist, the syndrome is designated *alcoholic hallucinosis*. Tonic–clonic seizures are most likely to occur within the first 24 hours after withdrawal. If the syndrome progresses further, insight is lost; the patient becomes weaker, more confused, disoriented, and agitated, and may be terrified by persecutory hallucinations. These are often so vivid that, even after recovery, patients sometimes doubt their unreality. Hyperthermia is common, and exhaustion and cardiovascular collapse may occur. At this stage, which appears around the third day of withdrawal, the picture is that of the *tremulous delirium*, first described by Thomas Sutton in 1813, and now called *alcohol withdrawal delirium* or *delirium tremens*.

The acute alcohol abstinence syndrome is self-limited. If the patient does not die, recovery usually occurs within 5 to 7 days, without treatment. However, even with continued abstinence, disturbed brain function, as measured by neuropsychological testing or the EEG, may persist for many months (*see* Grant, 1987). In rats, both aging and repeated episodes of alcohol withdrawal result in more severe syndromes in later cycles. Clinicians believe this is also true for alcoholics.

Babies born to mothers who drink heavily during pregnancy not only experience alcohol withdrawal after delivery but may also be mentally retarded and have other developmental abnormalities (*see* Chapter 17).

A number of special problems are seen in chronic alcoholics that are not apparent with some other types of drug abuse. Many of these are thought to be related to nutritional deficiencies that result from the capacity of alcohol to supply calories and depress appetite without supplying vitamins and essential amino acids. Problems include peripheral polyneuropathies, glossitis, stomatitis, pellagra, nutritional amblyopia, anemia, Wernicke's encephalopathy, and some components of Korsakoff's psychosis, which is characterized by profound impairment of recent memory. However, other disorders, such as acute gastritis, pancreatitis, fatty liver, cirrhosis of the liver, and damage to cardiac and skeletal muscle, once thought to be related to nutritional abnormalities, are due directly or indirectly to toxic effects of ethanol itself. Use of ethanol is also implicated in adult-onset seizures unrelated to withdrawal. Some additional problems, such as malabsorption, disturbances in regulation of glucose metabolism, and altered gonadal function, may be related to impairment of pancreatic or hepatic function. Moderate-to-high levels of alcohol use are associated with a number of types of cancer, including breast cancer in women (*see* Korsten and Lieber, 1985; Lieber, 1988; Ng *et al.*, 1988). Recently detoxified alcoholics frequently exhibit depressive symptoms and subtle cognitive deficits, especially in short-term memory. These symptoms are believed to result from direct toxic effects of alcohol on the brain and usually improve over weeks to months without treatment (*see* Grant, 1987).

COCAINE, AMPHETAMINE, AND RELATED PSYCHOSTIMULANTS

Extent of Use. It has been estimated that more than 20 million people in the United States have used cocaine. In 1988, 5% of young adults (18 to 25 years old) reported using cocaine and 2% reported using a stimulant other than cocaine during the 30 days prior to the survey. In recent years, increased use of cocaine by injection of its salts and by inhalation of the free alkaloid base ("crack") has been responsible for many serious toxic reactions and escalating crime rates.

Actions and Patterns of Use. The subjective effects of the psychostimulants, like those of all centrally active drugs, are dependent on the user, the environment, the dose of the drug, and the route of administration. For example, moderate doses of amphetamine given orally to normal subjects commonly produce an elevation of mood, a sense of increased energy and alertness, and decreased appetite; task performance that has been impaired by fatigue or boredom is improved. Some individuals may become anxious, irritable, or loquacious, and insomnia is common. As the dose is increased toward toxic levels, the effects of individual experiences and of environment become less significant. The general pharmacology of these agents is described in Chapter 10.

When equated for differences in potency, a number of other psychostimulants can produce subjective effects that resemble those of amphetamine. These drugs include dextroamphetamine, methamphetamine, phenmetrazine, methylphenidate, and diethylpropion. Another distinct member of this group is (−)-cathinone, the active ingredient in freshly gathered leaves of the Khat shrub (*Catha edulis*); its actions are quite similar to those of amphetamine (*see* below).

Some congeners of amphetamine with substitutions in the aromatic ring (*e.g.*, fenfluramine) do not produce amphetamine-like subjective effects and have little or no potential for reinforcement (*see* Griffiths *et al.*, 1978). Phenylpropanolamine suppresses appetite but is not self-administered by animals or recognized as amphetamine-like by human subjects, even at doses several times higher than those needed to produce anorexia. Mazindol also appears to be less reinforcing in man than amphetamine.

Cocaine users describe the euphoric effects of cocaine in terms that are almost indistinguishable from those used by amphetamine users. In the laboratory, subjects familiar with cocaine cannot distinguish between the subjective effects of 16 mg of cocaine and those of 10 mg of dextroamphetamine when both are given intravenously (Fischman and Schuster, 1982). However, the duration of cocaine's effects is relatively brief; it has a half-life of only 50 minutes, while the half-life of amphetamine is about 10 hours, and that of methamphetamine is about 5 hours. Like amphetamine, cocaine reduces the sense of fatigue and the decrement in performance caused by sleep deprivation. The toxic syndrome seen with cocaine seems clinically indistinguishable from that produced by amphetamines. In addition, animals exhibit similar patterns of self-administration of cocaine and amphetamine (*see* Fischman, 1988; Gawin and Ellinwood, 1988). Because of its recent widespread use, cocaine will be discussed as the prototype of this group of drugs.

Patterns of cocaine use show considerable variability. In the United States, cocaine hydrochloride (also called "coke," "snow," "gold dust," and "lady") is sold as a water-soluble powder that varies greatly in purity; it is often diluted with procaine. The powder is usually taken intranasally ("snorted"), but is also administered intravenously. Use of cocaine usually begins with intermittent experimentation. It is estimated that about 20% of those who experiment with the drug intranasally go on to become regular users, and about 25% of these progress to dependency. Heavy intranasal users may take the drug in bouts or binges, often using it until their supply is exhausted. Intravenous (or inhaled) cocaine may be taken as frequently as every 10 to 15 minutes. A cocaine binge usually lasts about 12 hours, but it may go on for several days. Among those who seek treatment, a substantial proportion use large amounts of the drug daily. However, because a typical pattern of dependent use consists of binges that are punctuated by brief periods of abstinence, individuals who do not use cocaine and amphetamine on a daily basis may still be severely dependent and out of control.

Cocaine and amphetamine-like psychostimulants produce an elevation of mood (euphoria) and a sense of increased self-esteem, well-being, and mental and physical capacity. Appetite and need for sleep are decreased. In the early stages of use, the increased energy and sociability may elicit positive responses from friends and associates. These positive experiences tend to lead to frequent use of the drug in increasing doses. Eventually, the socially reinforcing experiences are supplanted by a focus on drug-induced euphoria (*see* Gawin and Ellinwood, 1988).

Use of cocaine may be associated with heightened sexual interest. This, combined with disinhibition, grandiosity, and impaired judgment, often leads to promiscuous or atypical sexual acts under circumstances that foster transmission of venereal diseases, including infection with HIV. Many users claim that orgasm is delayed, permitting extended periods of sexual activity that culminate in seemingly more intense orgasms. Nevertheless, sexual dysfunction is a common complaint among those who seek treatment.

Unlike the user of morphine, whose drives are usually decreased, the user of cocaine-like psychostimulants may be excited, disinhibited, and hyperactive. With the development of toxic CNS symptoms, which are common among heavy users, anxiety, hypervigilance, suspiciousness, and persecutory fears occur. Insight is at first retained, but reality testing is eventually lost, and the user may act aggressively or even homicidally against those imagined to be persecutors.

In the 1980s, smoking of cocaine as the free base ("crack") became popular. Cocaine base is prepared from the hydrochloride salt by alkalinization and extraction with organic solvents. Cocaine base begins to vaporize at about 90°C; higher temperatures cause decomposition. At the temperature of burning tobacco, 400° to 600°C, only about 6% of the drug survives pyrolysis. Even in the glass pipes favored by cocaine users, more than half of the drug is destroyed (Perez-Reyes *et al.*, 1982; Jeffcoat *et al.*, 1989). Heating cocaine base produces an aerosol of particles about 2 to 3 microns in diameter and a small amount of vaporized drug (Snyder *et al.*, 1988). When smoked, cocaine base is rapidly and efficiently absorbed from the lungs; within a few minutes 50 mg can produce peak concentrations in plasma that are nearly as great as maximal values achieved about 40 minutes after nasal insufflation of 106 mg of crystalline cocaine hydrochloride (Jeffcoat *et al.*, 1989).

Immediately following inhalation or intravenous administration of cocaine, the user may experience an intense sensation (usually referred to as a "rush" or "flash") that lasts only a few minutes and is generally described as extremely pleasurable. Intranasal use of cocaine hydrochloride or oral use of amphetamines produces euphoria (a "high"), but not the sensation of a "rush." Cocaine penetrates the brain rapidly. After intravenous administration (and presumably inhalation), concentrations of cocaine in brain far exceed those in plasma; penetration into the brain is followed by redistribution to other tissues. It is thought that the sharp contrast between these high but brief concentrations in brain and the subsequent rapid decline generates the intense drive to use more drug within a very brief period. Crack users may progress from experimentation to dependence in a matter of weeks. With intranasal use, the experience is less intense and the decline in brain concentrations is modified by the slower absorption from the constricted mucous membranes. The urge to repeat the drug experience correlates better with the distribution half-life than with the terminal half-life of cocaine in plasma. The latter is nearly 1 hour, but crack users may have a craving to repeat the drug 10 to 30 minutes after use. Those who use cocaine intranasally may take the drug every 40 to 60 minutes if it is available. After long-term high-dose use, there is apparently some sequestration of unmetabolized cocaine in peripheral tissues; the drug can be detected in plasma for 5 to 10 days after intake is stopped (Cone and Weddington, 1989).

During early phases of intravenous use of amphetamine or methamphetamine, three or four doses of 20 to 40 mg are usually considered sufficient to obtain pleasurable effects. Those who inject these psychostimulants intravenously may dissolve oral tablets or use crystalline methamphetamine ("crystal") manufactured in illegal laboratories. As with cocaine, there may be a sensation of a "flash" or "rush" after intravenous use that does not occur after oral or intranasal use.

Some individuals apparently can use psychostimulants for months or years without developing a toxic paranoid syndrome; nevertheless, such symptoms can develop in the course of a single "run." The user may continue to inject the drug every 2 to 3 hours around the clock for periods of several days, going without food or sleep. Methamphetamine users have been reported to inject as much as 1 g intravenously every few hours during a "run." Such an episode commonly ends when the user is out of drug or is too disorganized to continue. Stopping use is followed within a few hours by a deep sleep ("crashing") that lasts 12 to 18 hours or longer, depending on the duration of the "run." Except for some differences in time course, the cocaine and amphetamine withdrawal syndromes are quite similar (*see* below).

A small percentage of people who take psychostimulants that have been prescribed for control of obesity become dependent on the drug. Although some seem able to restrict drug intake and function productively, others who become dependent escalate their drug use and exhibit progressive social and occupational deterioration, punctuated by periods of hospitalization for somatic and psychotoxic complications. A similar variability in risk of progression characterizes the use of cocaine.

Important factors in vulnerability to dependence include the dose and route of administration of the drug. For example, natives living high in the Andes chew the leaves of the coca bush (*Erythroxylon coca*) to produce a sense of decreased hunger and fatigue and of increased well being. Andean natives appear to have little difficulty discontinuing use of coca when they move to lower altitudes. In contrast, the smoking of coca paste (60 to 80% cocaine sulfate) by people living in urban areas of Peru is associated with a variety of psychopathological states, toxic effects, and severe dependence.

However, the risk of developing dependence is not limited to persons who use drugs intravenously or smoke cocaine as the base. Severe dependence with psychological, physical, and vocational impairment is also seen among those who use cocaine intranasally. Other vulnerability factors may include associated affective and personality disorders, such as antisocial personality. When dependence is extreme, all other interests—food, family, safety, reputation, and even survival—become secondary to acquiring and using the drug. It is not clear whether the dependence syndrome caused by amphetamine or cocaine are as persistent as that produced by the opioids. In the United States, the waves of amphetamine use did not leave large numbers of chronic users in their wake. However, many intravenous amphetamine users eventually became heroin users. Little is known of the natural history of cocaine dependence, but recovery from intranasal use of cocaine without a shift to other drugs is often possible.

Mechanisms of Reinforcing Action. Because of their similarities, the psychological and toxic effects of cocaine and amphetamine-like drugs will be discussed together. However, there are several important distinctions among the mechanisms by which cocaine and amphetamines produce their reinforcing actions and toxic effects that have implications for the treatment of dependence and toxicity.

The reinforcing effects of cocaine are thought to result from its capacity to increase synaptic concentrations of dopamine by inhibition of its uptake into neurons, primarily those originating in the ventral tegmental area of the brain and projecting to structures such as the nucleus accumbens, ventral pallidum, and frontal cortex (*see* Ritz *et al.*, 1987; Koob and Bloom, 1988; Wise, 1988). However, not every drug that inhibits dopamine uptake produces euphoria or is self-administered.

Amphetamine and related phenylethylamines also interact with transporters responsible for the uptake of dopamine, norepinephrine, and 5-HT, as well as with α_2-adrenergic receptors. However, the reinforcing effects of these agents are not well correlated with actions at any of these sites; in fact, there is an inverse correlation with affinity at sites for uptake of 5-HT (Ritz and Kuhar, 1989). The latter fact may account for the capacity of inhibitors of 5-HT uptake to reduce the self-administration of amphetamine, although these agents do not appear to inhibit self-administration of cocaine. Thus, it seems likely that the major mechanism by which amphetamine-like drugs produce their reinforcing effects is their well-known capacity to release newly synthesized dopamine from intraneuronal stores. The release of other neurotransmitters along with inhibition of their reuptake may account for other aspects of the actions of these drugs, including their toxic effects (*see* below). Cathinone also appears to release intraneuronal stores of dopamine. Its psychological, behavioral, cardiovascular, and toxic effects in animals and man are quite similar to those of amphetamine (*see* Kalix, 1986).

Toxicity. Cocaine can produce severe toxicity, sometimes unexpectedly, even under conditions of careful clinical use. The recent epidemic of cocaine abuse has reemphasized its toxic potential. In addition to psychiatric disorders (*see* below), the more common serious toxic effects induced by cocaine include cardiac arrhythmias, myocardial ischemia or infarction, myocarditis, high-output congestive heart failure, dilated cardiomyopathy, cerebrovascular spasm with transient neural ischemia or infarct of brain or spinal cord, intracerebral hemorrhage, aortic dissection, rhabdomyolysis with acute renal and hepatic failure, disseminated intravascular coagulation, convulsions, hyperpyrexia, and respiratory depression. While individuals with preexisting coronary disease or a history of convulsions are at higher risk of cardiac and CNS toxicity, cocaine has induced fatal cardiovascular and CNS events in young individuals with normal coronary and cerebral arteries and no history of seizures. Although complications are more common after large doses of cocaine are taken intravenously or by inhalation, they may also be seen after modest doses or intranasal use. (For references, *see* Isner *et al.*, 1986; Gawin and Ellinwood, 1988; Mody *et al.*, 1988; Roth *et al.*, 1988; Cregler, 1989.)

The correlation between sensitivity to cocaine's effects on the cardiovascular system and sensitivity to its euphorigenic effects is not high. Consequently, the cocaine abuser who uses subjective effects to regulate dosage can easily reach levels that have toxic effects on other systems. Dopamine, which has a central role in the reinforcing effects of cocaine, has little role in its cardiovascular toxicity; the latter is probably related primarily to blockade of reuptake of norepinephrine and to release of adrenal catecholamines. Coronary vasoconstriction and myocardial sensitization are probably the main factors responsible for ischemia, infarcts, and arrhythmias; ischemia of skeletal muscle or a direct toxic action may account for the rhabdomyolysis. Endothelial injury induced by vasoconstriction leads to formation of thrombi and may cause some delayed adverse cardiovascular effects. Long-term use of cocaine may induce a myocarditis or dilated cardiomyopathy even when there is no acute event (*see* Karch and Billingham, 1988). The contribution of cocaine's local anesthetic actions to cardiac complications is not certain.

Cocaine lowers the seizure threshold, and seizures are the most common neurological complication of cocaine use. This toxicity probably results from the local anesthetic actions of cocaine that become manifest at high concentrations. However, seizures and loss of consciousness may also be secondary to cardiac events.

Amphetamine-like drugs, which both release catecholamines from interneuronal stores and prevent their subsequent reuptake, produce many of the same cardiovascular effects seen with cocaine; however, some of the CNS toxicity differs. In animals, high doses of amphetamine-like drugs produce permanent degeneration of dopaminergic neurons, apparently because of the formation of 6-hydroxydopamine, a selective neurotoxin. In high doses, many amphetamine-like drugs can inhibit monoamine oxidase and the neurotoxin may arise from autooxidation of dopamine that escapes enzymatic degradation (*see* Gawin and Ellinwood, 1988). Although there is some controversy, cocaine does not appear to produce similar neuronal damage. Since cocaine neither releases dopamine nor inhibits its metabolic degradation, this difference in neurotoxicity is not entirely surprising. Prolonged anhedonia, occasionally seen following use of high doses of amphetamine, may be caused by drug-induced damage to dopaminergic elements in the reward system. The incidence and permanence of amphetamine-induced anhedonia is not certain (*see* Gawin and Ellinwood, 1988). There is little evidence for similar cocaine-induced syndromes in man.

Acute intoxication from amphetamine-like drugs is more likely to occur in the neophyte user. The acute toxic syndrome includes dizziness, tremor, irritability, confusion, hallucinations, chest pain, palpitations, hypertension, sweating, and cardiac arrhythmias. Death is usually preceded by hyperpyrexia, convulsions, and shock.

Women who use cocaine during pregnancy are more likely to have spontaneous abortions in the first trimester and to experience placental abruption or infarction and fetal death late in pregnancy. Ingestion of cocaine can induce the sudden onset of uterine contractions, fetal tachycardia, and excessive fetal activity. The likelihood of precipitous labor and maternal hemorrhage is also increased. Most of the toxicity is probably due to the vasoconstrictive effects of the drug. In addition, the appetite-suppressing effects of all the psychostimulants contribute to the vitamin deficiencies that are common among users and, together with maternal neglect of prenatal care, further complicate pregnancy and fetal development. It is not certain whether cocaine is teratogenic; there appears to be an increased incidence of sudden infant death among babies born to cocaine-dependent mothers (*see* Ryan *et al.*, 1987; Chasnoff *et al.*, 1989).

Treatment of acute cocaine-induced cardiovascular toxicity is aimed at reducing excessive effects of catecholamines and dealing with complications (*e.g.*, arrhythmias, infarcts). Although nonselective β-adrenergic blocking agents have been used, unopposed vascular α-adrenergic stimulation may continue to cause hypertension. Drugs such as labetalol, which block both α- and β-adrenergic receptors, seem better suited to the situation. Similar considerations argue for the use of labetalol to treat amphetamine toxicity. In addition, Ca^{2+}-channel blockers such as nifedipine or nitrendipine may be useful. The latter drug can reduce the acute toxic effects of cocaine in animal models (*see* Lathers *et al.*, 1988). Nifedipine appears to attenuate some of the subjective effects of cocaine as well. The intravenous administration of diazepam has been used to control seizures induced by either cocaine or amphetamine. Physical means to prevent hyperthermia and support respiration may be required. Acidification of the urine to accelerate the excretion of amphetamine is also indicated. Chlorpromazine antagonizes many effects of amphetamine, including the elevated blood pressure. However, in rodent models of cocaine toxicity, only selective antagonists of D_1-dopaminergic receptors were effective in preventing death.

Tolerance. Tolerance develops to some of the central effects of cocaine. However, there is sensitization rather than tolerance for other effects (*see* below). Some tolerance develops to the brief, euphoric "rush" after a single intravenous dose; within an hour or so the dose must be escalated in order to experience effects of equal intensity. Some small degree of tolerance to effects on heart rate and blood pressure develops during the infusion of cocaine over the course of 4 hours (Ambre *et al.*, 1988); however, it is unlikely that significant tolerance to its cardiovascular actions is usually achieved, since even long-term users can experience major toxic effects. In surveys, a substantial percentage of heavy users of cocaine report that they require more cocaine to produce the same subjective effects (*e.g.*, elevation of mood) experienced earlier in the course of use.

Amphetamine users also develop tolerance to some of its central effects (*e.g.*, euphorigenic, anorectic, hyperthermic, and lethal actions), and the long-term user often increases the dose to continue to obtain the desired effect. Some amphetamine users are able to take several hundred milligrams per day over prolonged periods. By suppressing appetite, high doses of amphetamine may foster ketosis; since amphetamine is excreted much more rapidly in acidic urine, some of the apparent tolerance may be due to more rapid elimination of the drug. As with cocaine, sensitivity to other effects on the CNS is increased (*see* below). Cross-tolerance among the amphetamine-like sympathomimetic agents has been observed clinically, and cross-tolerance between the anorectic effect of cocaine and amphetamine has been demonstrated in rats (Woolverton *et al.*, 1978). By contrast, tolerance does not develop to the psychotoxic effects of either cocaine or amphetamine-like drugs, and a toxic psychosis may occur after periods of weeks or months of continued use.

Psychotoxicity. Cocaine users may report increased anxiety within hours after use begins, even as aspects of the euphoria are declining. Similarly, suspiciousness and paranoia can develop within a few hours after initiating the use of high doses of cocaine (Sherer *et al.*, 1988), and fully developed paranoid ideation with visual hallucinations may develop within the course of a 24-hour bout of use. Among heavy users, perceptual changes and pseudohallucinations often occur. The most common of these are tactile ("cocaine bugs" in the skin) and visual ("snow lights").

Similar toxic signs and symptoms appear as higher and more frequent doses of amphetamine-like drugs are used; these include bruxism, touching and picking of the face and extremities, suspiciousness, and a feeling of being watched. In addition, the user seems preoccupied with his or her own thinking processes and with "meanings" and "essences." Stereotypical, repetitious behavior is common. Many users who later show a full-blown toxic psychosis exhibit a compulsion to take apart mechanical objects. They also have a compulsion to put them together, but are usually too disorganized to do so.

Both cocaine and amphetamine users commonly attempt to antagonize various toxic symptoms with other drugs. The mixture of an opioid and either cocaine or amphetamine is known as a "speedball." Many cocaine and amphetamine users simultaneously consume large amounts of barbiturates or alcohol.

The fully developed toxic syndrome from the use of psychostimulants is characterized by vivid visual, auditory, and sometimes tactile hallucinations. The paranoid ideation, loosening of associations, and changes in affect occur in association with a clear sensorium. In chronic amphetamine users, there may be a striking paucity of sympathomimetic effects, and the blood pressure is not unduly elevated. It is often extremely difficult to differentiate this syndrome from a schizophrenic reaction. The syndrome may be seen as early as 36 to 48 hours after the ingestion of a single large dose of amphetamine; in apparently sensitive individuals, psychosis may be produced by 55 to 75 mg of dextroamphetamine. With high enough doses, psychosis can probably be induced in anyone. Unless the individual continues to use the drug, the amphetamine psychosis usually clears within a week, the hallucinations being the first symptoms to disappear; the cocaine-induced psychosis clears somewhat more rapidly. Paranoid delusions and excitement due to amphetamine and cocaine are suppressed by dopaminergic antagonists, such as haloperidol (*see* Gawin and Ellinwood, 1988). Acidification of the urine, which facilitates excretion of amphetamine, also shortens the duration of the psychosis. Persons who develop a toxic psychosis may have a lowered threshold for such toxicity during subsequent episodes of use.

Sensitization. Coincident with the tolerance described above, cocaine and amphetamine-like drugs also produce sensitization, which is sometimes called "reverse tolerance." For example, in rodents or primates, single daily doses of cocaine or amphetamine that do not initially produce hyperactivity and stereotyped behavior gradually begin to induce such behaviors when repeated over a period of several weeks. The drugs need not be given daily, and, although reversible, the effects are still detectable weeks after the last dose. There is cross-sensitization between cocaine and amphetamine. This type of sensitization is believed to be mediated by release of dopamine in the striatum, and it can be induced by injections of amphetamine into areas of the midbrain that contain dopaminergic cell bodies (Kalivas and Weber, 1988; Kalivas *et al.*, 1988). It is postulated that such sensitization is the basis for the stereotyped behavior observed in individuals who use large amounts of amphetamine and cocaine on a long-term basis. Another form of sensitization associated with use of cocaine appears to be analogous to chemical kindling (*see* Chapter 19); repeated administration of subconvulsant doses of cocaine (or lidocaine) eventually produces seizures, and spontaneous seizures may also develop (Weiss *et al.*, 1989). In contrast to cocaine, amphetamine-like drugs have an anticonvulsant effect. It has been suggested that an analogous process may be involved in the panic attacks reported by a significant proportion of cocaine users (Louie *et al.*, 1989).

Physical Dependence and Withdrawal Symptoms. After long-term use of either cocaine or amphetamine, or even after a binge of a few days, abrupt cessation is commonly followed by depression, anxiety, and craving for the drug that is soon followed by general fatigue and a need for sleep ("crash"). Upon initial awakening, there is hyperphagia, continued sleepiness, depression, and anhedonia. Mood returns to normal over a period of days, although in some cases dysphoria and anhedonia may persist for weeks. Craving for the drug may wax and wane over the subsequent several weeks in response to emotions and cocaine-related stimuli (*see* Gawin and Ellinwood, 1988). Although these signs and symptoms meet the criteria for a withdrawal syndrome (*see* American Psychiatric Association, 1987), there are no grossly observable physiological disruptions that necessitate gradual withdrawal of the drug.

The role of withdrawal-induced dysphoria, hyperphagia, lethargy, anhedonia, and depression in perpetuating the use of these drugs is not clear. Although some users report that persistent anhedonia is a factor in relapse, they are more likely to report that relapse was associated with a wide variety of stimuli that evoked memories of the euphorigenic effects (*see* Gawin and Ellinwood, 1988).

NICOTINE AND TOBACCO

The chemistry and the acute pharmacological effects of nicotine are considered in Chapter 9. In this section, the discussion centers on the use and effects of tobacco products.

History. Crewmen who accompanied Columbus to the New World were the first Europeans to observe the smoking of tobacco. In the following century the smoking of tobacco spread throughout the world, despite vigorous official opposition and, in some cases, draconian penalties. The tobacco plant was named *Nicotiana tabacum* in honor of Jean Nicot, who promoted its importation and cultivation in the belief that it had medicinal value. Nicotine was first isolated from the leaves by Posselt and Reiman in 1828. In the mid-nineteenth century, new varieties of tobacco, changes in the technology of curing the leaf, and machinery for mass production facilitated the spread of a new product—the cigarette—cheaper and neater than cigars and yielding a smoke so mild that it could be inhaled. In the United States, per-capita consumption of cigarettes has been declining since 1973. In 1988, 27% of adults were still smokers, but only 19% of high school seniors were regular smokers. Smokeless tobacco (snuff and chewing tobacco) is now used by 8% of young men. The rationale for considering use of tobacco as a form of drug dependence is presented by Jaffe (1990) and in the report of the Surgeon General (1988).

Chemical Composition of Tobacco. About 4000 compounds are generated by the burning of tobacco; the smoke can be separated into gaseous and particulate phases. The composition of the actual smoke delivered to the smoker depends not only on the composition of the tobacco but also on how densely it is packed, the length of the column of tobacco, the characteristics of the filter and the paper, and the temperature at which the tobacco is burned. Rapid drawing of the smoke raises the temperature of the burning tip and changes the size of the particles and the composition of both the gaseous and particulate phases. These changes may in turn alter what is trapped in the filter. It is possible to specify the amounts of nicotine, "tar," and carbon monoxide delivered by a given cigarette when it is smoked by a machine under constant conditions, as is now done by governmental agencies in many countries. However, smokers do not usually conform to the smoking style of the machine.

Among the components of the gaseous phase that produce undesirable effects are carbon monoxide, carbon dioxide, nitrogen oxides, ammonia, volatile nitrosamines, hydrogen cyanide, volatile sulfur-containing compounds, nitriles and other nitrogen-containing compounds, volatile hydrocarbons, alcohols, and aldehydes and ketones (*e.g.*, acetaldehyde, formaldehyde, and acrolein). Some of the last-named substances are potent inhibitors of ciliary movement. The particulate phase contains nicotine, water, and "tar"; "tar" is what remains after the moisture and nicotine are subtracted and consists primarily of polycyclic aromatic hydrocarbons, some of which are documented carcinogens. Among these are nonvolatile nitrosamines and aromatic amines, which are believed to play a causative role in bladder cancer, and polycyclic hydrocarbons such as benzo[a]pyrene, an exceedingly potent carcinogen. The "tar" also contains numerous other compounds, including metallic ions and several radioactive compounds (*e.g.*, polonium 210). The components most likely to contribute to the health hazards of smoking are carbon monoxide, nicotine, and "tar"; probable contributors to the health hazards of smoking are acrolein, hydrocyanic acid, nitric oxide, nitrogen dioxide, cresols, and amphenols; suspected hazards include a host of other chemicals (*see* Surgeon General, 1979).

When a cigarette is smoked on a standard machine, the delivery of "tar" varies from 0.5 to 35 mg and that of nicotine from 0.05 to 2.0 mg (1985 average, 1.0 mg). The actual content of nicotine in tobacco can vary from 0.2 to 5%, but is generally between 1 and 2% for smoking tobaccos. It is present in the protonated form in almost all cigarette tobaccos. Because of a more alkaline pH, it is present in the more readily absorbed, unprotonated form in cigars, pipe tobaccos, and smokeless tobaccos (*see* Surgeon General, 1979).

Effects on the CNS. Nicotine is self-administered by animals, but it is less powerful as a reinforcer than is amphetamine or cocaine. Nicotine appears to have very specific properties as a stimulus; its effects are not confused with those of other drugs. These properties appear to involve both stereospecific receptors for nicotine and dopaminergic pathways. They can be blocked with mecamylamine, but not with muscarinic cholinergic or adrenergic blocking agents (*see* Benowitz, 1988; Surgeon General, 1988). Nicotine, as absorbed by the typical smoker, causes an increase in hand tremor and an alerting pattern in the EEG (low-voltage, fast activity); however, at the same time, there is decreased tone in some skeletal muscles (*e.g.,* the quadriceps), decreased amplitude in the electromyogram, and a decrease in deep-tendon reflexes. These effects may involve stimulation of the Renshaw cells in the spinal cord. The smoking of one or two cigarettes after a few hours of abstinence produces a significant rise in the concentrations of several hormones and neurotransmitters in plasma. Nicotine causes nausea and vomiting, in part by stimulating the chemoreceptor trigger zone of the medulla oblongata and by activating the vagal reflexes involved in the act of vomiting (*see* Chapter 38).

Nicotine facilitates memory, reduces aggression, and decreases weight gain. Smokers weigh an average of 5 to 10 pounds less than nonsmokers. The nicotine in tobacco appears to suppress appetite for sweeter tasting food and to increase energy expenditure both at rest and during exercise (Perkins *et al.,* 1989).

Many of nicotine's effects could, in theory, be reinforcing. These include the alerting and facilitation of memory or attention, the decrease in irritability and the capacity to alter appetite and suppress weight gain. However, in man these effects may be incidental to some primary reinforcing action. When smokers are given nicotine intravenously in doses of about 1.5 mg, they report that the effects are pleasant and they show increased scores on scales devised to measure the euphorigenic effects of morphine and amphetamine (Henningfield *et al.,* 1983). It is postulated that some of the reinforcing effects involve increased activity in mesolimbic dopaminergic neurons.

Absorption and Elimination. The nicotine in cigarette smoke, suspended on minute particles of "tar," is quickly absorbed from the lung, almost with the efficiency of intravenous administration. The compound reaches the brain within 8 seconds after inhalation. Nicotine in cigarette smoke, which is somewhat acidic, is not well absorbed from the mouth; pipe and cigar smoke, which is more alkaline (pH 8.5), is probably better absorbed, but the concentration of nicotine in the plasma of those who do not inhale cigars is low compared with those who do inhale cigarettes. Peak concentrations of nicotine in plasma after a cigarette is smoked are typically 25 to 50 ng/ml (Benowitz, 1988). Typical time courses for the appearance of nicotine in plasma after the use of nicotine gum and several forms of tobacco are shown in Figure 22–1.

The time course for elimination of nicotine is multiexponential. Following a single cigarette, concentrations decline rapidly (over 5 to 10 minutes), primarily reflecting distribution. After long-term smoking, the elimination half-life of nicotine is approximately 2 hours. For the average smoker, concentrations of nicotine in plasma are somewhat higher at the end of the day. Nicotine is oxidized to its major metabolite, cotinine, which causes few or no cardiovascular or subjective effects. Since cotinine is cleared more slowly (half-life of about 19 hours), it is a better measure of overall intake than nicotine itself (*see* Benowitz, 1988).

Chronic Toxicity of Tobacco. Chronic use of tobacco is causally linked to a variety of serious diseases, ranging from coronary artery disease to lung cancer. The likelihood of developing any one of these disorders increases with the degree of exposure (measured in cigarettes per day, or "pack years"). For example, for all male smokers, the overall mortality ratio is about 1.7 compared with nonsmokers. The ratio is 2.0 for those who smoke two packs daily, and it is higher among inhalers than noninhalers. For women, smoking a little over a pack a day is associated with a fivefold increase in fatal coronary heart disease (Willett *et al.,* 1987). Cigar smoking increases mortality in proportion to the number

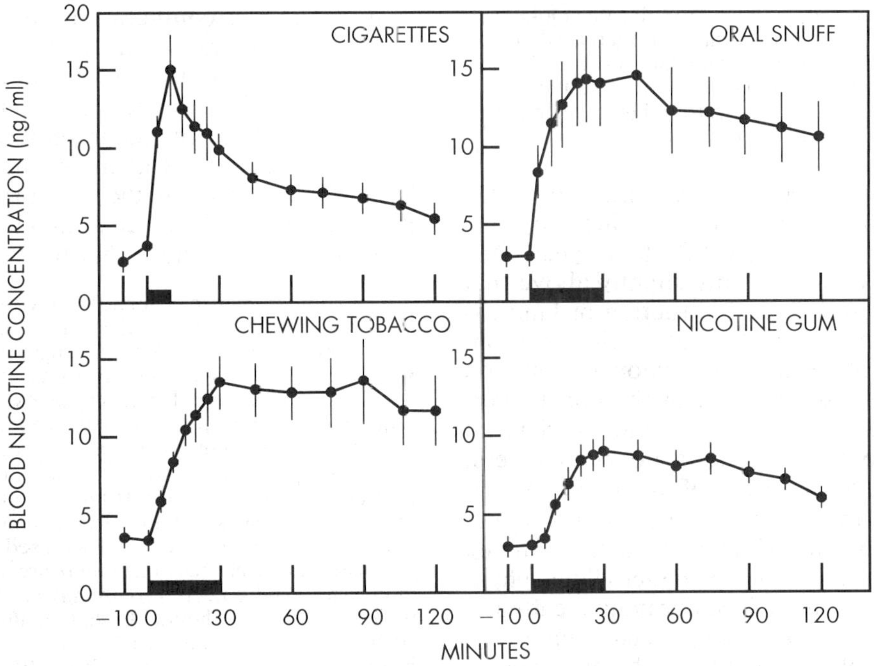

Figure 22–1. *Blood concentrations of nicotine during and after cigarette smoking, oral snuff, chewing tobacco, and nicotine gum.*

Data represent average values for 10 subjects; vertical bars indicate the standard error. Shaded bars above time axis indicate period of exposure to tobacco or nicotine gum. (Reproduced by permission from: Benowitz *et al.* Nicotine absorption and cardiovascular effects with smokeless tobacco use: comparison with cigarettes and nicotine gum. *Clin. Pharmacol. Ther.*, **1988**, *44*, 23–28. St. Louis, 1988, The C. V. Mosby Co.)

smoked, but not as sharply as for cigarettes. The differences between cigarette, pipe, and cigar smokers is probably related to the lesser inhalation among the latter two groups, which leads to lower exposure to all constituents of smoke. The smoking of tobacco continues to be described as the largest preventable cause of death in the United States.

Evidence indicates that the different diseases that are related to the use of tobacco may be caused, at least in part, by different constituents of tobacco or tobacco smoke. The catalog of tobacco-related diseases is extensive, and only the more important in terms of prevalence and seriousness can be mentioned here. Cardiovascular diseases related to tobacco include coronary artery disease, cerebrovascular disease, and peripheral vascular disease. Carbon monoxide (and related hypoxia) and the effects of nicotine on cardiac rhythm, free fatty acids in plasma, lipoproteins, and the coagulability of blood may play a role in the acceleration of atherosclerosis and in sudden cardiac death. Smokers have a threefold increase in frequency and a twelvefold increase in duration of silent ischemic episodes (Barry *et al.,* 1989). Smoking elevates concentrations of low-density and very-low-density lipoproteins and shortens the survival time of arterial grafts and arteriovenous fistulas used to facilitate dialysis. Neoplastic diseases (cancer of the lung, larynx, oral cavity, esophagus, bladder, and pancreas) are probably due to one or more of the known carcinogens in the smoke, rather than to nicotine or carbon monoxide. Chronic obstructive lung disease is probably caused by effects on proteolytic enzymes, interference with immune mechanisms, and inhibition of clearance mechanisms. Impairment of respiratory function can be detected in young adults after only a few years of smoking (*see* Surgeon General, 1979). The ciliotoxic actions of tobacco smoke and its ability to inhibit pulmonary clearance mechanisms probably account for the remarkable synergism between tobacco smoke and such environmental carcinogens as asbestos in increasing mortality from lung cancer. The mechanisms by which smoking reduces fertility and increases the incidence of spontaneous abortion, abruptio placenta, and premature rupture of the membranes are unclear. Smoking also significantly reduces the birth weight of children born to women who smoke during pregnancy, and increases the likelihood of perinatal mortality and of sudden death of infants. Smokers have more sleep difficulties than do nonsmokers and tend to exhibit more depression, irritability, and anxiety. Nonsmokers who are passively exposed to tobacco smoke over prolonged periods may have an increased risk of pulmonary dysfunction and lung cancer. Passive inhalation of smoke may also increase the risk of acute and chronic respiratory illness in children (*see* Fielding and Phenow, 1988).

The likelihood of development of a disorder related to smoking is reduced by cessation. Over a period of 5 to 10 years, the risk falls to a level only slightly above that of the nonsmoker. Destruction of lung tissue is not reversible, but, with cessation, the rate of decline in pulmonary function begins to resemble that of the nonsmoker.

Smokers metabolize a wide variety of drugs more rapidly than do nonsmokers, probably as a result of induction of enzymes in the intestinal mucosa or the liver by components of tobacco smoke. Among the drugs affected are theophylline, phenacetin, propranolol, imipramine, caffeine, oxazepam, and nordazepam (*see* Benowitz, 1988). Smokers may require higher doses of opioids to obtain relief from pain, may be less sedated by benzodiazepines, and may obtain less antianginal effect from nifedipine, atenolol, or propranolol. Not all differences arise from altered rates of drug metabolism. Enzymatic activities begin to return toward baseline within a few days of cessation of smoking. Changes in drug metabolism may become more problematic as more hospitals adopt no-smoking policies.

Tolerance, Dependence, and Relapse. Tolerance develops to some of the effects of nicotine. Following one or two cigarettes, even the chronic smoker still exhibits an increase in blood pressure, pulse rate, and hand tremor; decreased skin temperature; and increases in the plasma concentrations of certain hormones. However, the dizziness, nausea, and vomiting experienced by nontolerant individuals do not occur unless the smoker's customary intake is exceeded substantially. Furthermore, although regular smokers report that injections of nicotine are pleasant, nonsmokers describe unpleasant reactions (*see* Henningfield *et al.*, 1983). Smokers appear to metabolize nicotine more rapidly than do nonsmokers, but it is likely that tolerance is due primarily to pharmacodynamic changes rather than to alterations in drug disposition. There are conflicting reports on the duration of tolerance. In some studies of animals it appeared to disappear within 24 to 48 hours of abstinence; in others it persisted for months. In human smokers, some aspects of tolerance wax and wane rapidly. The first cigarette of the day produces a much greater cardiovascular and subjective response than do those that follow.

Cessation of the use of tobacco may be followed by a withdrawal syndrome that varies in intensity from person to person. There is uncertainty about what factors are responsible for its variability and little information on what levels of exposure are required to induce physical dependence in man. The most consistent symptoms (in addition to "craving" for tobacco, which subsides over a period of days to weeks) are irritability, impatience, anxiety, restlessness, and difficulty in concentrating. Drowsiness, headaches, increased appetite, and sleep disturbances (insomnia) are also common. The syndrome is prompt in onset, usually within the first 24 hours. Cognitive impairment, such as decreased short-term memory, can be objectively demonstrated for at least 10 days, but some smokers complain that certain problems, such as increased appetite and inability to concentrate, persist for weeks or months. In some cases it is uncertain whether the specific problem represents an effect of withdrawal or a return to the status quo that existed before the individual started smoking. Among the objective findings that quickly follow cessation of smoking are changes in the EEG, with a decrease in high-frequency activity characteristic of arousal and an increase in low-frequency activity characteristic of drowsiness and hypoarousal. Decreases in performance on tests of vigilance and psychomotor performance and increases in hostility are detectable within hours. There is a decrease in heart rate, blood pressure, and plasma epinephrine, while skin temperature and peripheral blood flow increase. Weight gain is a common finding. Cough and other respiratory difficulties show improvement, and, over a period of weeks to months, smoking-induced acceleration in degradation of other drugs approaches the norm for nonsmokers. Some evidence indicates that a higher intake of nicotine is associated with more severe withdrawal and more difficulty in giving up cigarettes, but other factors are probably just as important. Previously depressed smokers may experience an exacerbation of depression that is alleviated by return to smoking. Craving for cigarettes seems to exhibit a diurnal variation and is low on arising and rises to a peak in the evening. The syndrome of withdrawal from tobacco can be suppressed to some degree by nicotine. Use of buffered nicotine chewing gum reduces the irritability, anxiety, difficulty in concentrating, and somatic complaints that are associated with withdrawal, but it is less reliable or relatively ineffective in controlling insomnia and craving for tobacco (Hughes *et al.*, 1984). Nicotine gum may prevent the weight gain associated with cessation of tobacco use. To what degree the craving (either caused directly by withdrawal or elicited by environmental stimuli that have become conditioned to the use of tobacco) contributes to relapse among smokers is uncertain. In women, particularly, other motives, such as the weight-suppressing actions of nicotine, appear to play some role. Of those who seek some sort of formal help with their problem, about two thirds actually stop for at least a few days; but of these, only 20 to 40% are still abstinent 12 months later. The cessation rate is not much higher even for those who try to stop smoking after a myocardial infarction.

In the context of a formal cessation program, the use of nicotine gum, now available in a number of countries including the United States, significantly increases the number of smokers who remain abstinent for 1 year and is of greater help to those smokers who have the highest degree of dependence on nicotine. More heavily dependent smokers are helped even more by gum that contains 4 mg of nicotine, a dosage form not yet available in the United States (*see* Surgeon General, 1988; Tønnesen *et al.*, 1988). The effectiveness of nicotine gum is dependent on the manner in which it is prescribed and the extra effort that is made in helping the patient to stop smoking. When nicotine gum is prescribed as an adjunct to a doctor's unsolicited advice to stop smoking, it adds only slightly to the small impact of the admonition. Transdermal patches and a nasal spray containing nicotine have also been developed; both seem to be useful in increasing the probability of successful cessation. Use of the nasal spray results in plasma concentrations of nicotine that approach those achieved by smoking.

Gum containing nicotine (NICORETTE) is available in boxes of 96 pieces, each of which contains 2 mg of nicotine bound to an ion-exchange resin. The nicotine is released during chewing and is absorbed through the buccal mucosa. The patient must be instructed to chew slowly, to avoid swallowing, and to avoid the simultaneous use of liquids like coffee or carbonated beverages that lower buccal pH. Chewed at a rate of one piece per hour, cardiovascular effects are minimal; however, the concentration of nicotine in blood does not reach the trough level obtained by smoking one cigarette per hour (*see* Figure 22–1). At higher rates of chewing, the gum causes release of catecholamines and the expected cardiovascular effects. The drug is contraindicated or must be used with caution in patients with recent myocardial infarction, serious arrhythmias, or vasospastic disease. Gum containing a larger amount of nicotine (4 mg) increases the contractility of the normal myocardium but decreases contractility in regions of ischemia. On balance, however, the risk incurred by using gum may be less than the risks from nicotine and carbon monoxide if the patient does not stop smoking. The most common side effects of nicotine gum are hiccoughs, nausea, and vomiting. Withdrawal symptoms may be experienced when nicotine gum is discontinued. Clonidine has been reported to reduce craving for cigarettes associated with attempts at abstinence.

Titration. Most heavy smokers behave as if they are attempting to adjust their concentration of nicotine within relatively narrow limits. When given cigarettes with a high content of nicotine, they reduce the number smoked and alter their puffing patterns, and thereby achieve concentrations of nicotine in plasma only slightly greater than those to which they are accustomed. When given cigarettes with exceedingly low nicotine content, they change patterns of puffing or increase the number of cigarettes smoked in order to avoid declines in plasma nicotine concentrations, but the regulation is less precise. Titration is of considerable clinical significance, since smokers who switch to "low tar and nicotine" cigarettes generally alter their puffing patterns in a manner that minimizes the potential benefit. Most "switchers" take in as much or more carbon monoxide than previously. Plasma concentrations of nicotine and cotinine may be somewhat lower, reflecting a slightly reduced intake of particulates, but there is little evidence of any benefit to health (*see* Benowitz, 1988).

CANNABINOIDS (MARIHUANA)

Extent of Use. Marihuana, also known as "grass," "weed," "pot," and "reefer," is still by far the most commonly used illicit drug in the United States; about 55% of young adults report some lifetime experience with the drug. There is, however, a downward trend. Among high-school seniors, the use of marihuana in the month before survey has declined steadily from 37% in 1978 to 18% in 1988. The incidence of daily use among high school seniors is currently reported to be 2.7%.

History and Source. *Cannabis,* obtained from the flowering tops of hemp plants, is a very ancient drug. Other names for cannabis or its products include hashish, charas, bhang, ganja, dagga, and marihuana. The common hemp is an herbaceous annual, of which *Cannabis sativa* is the sole species and *Cannabis sativa* var. *indica* and var. *americana* are two varieties. While all parts of both the male and the female plant contain psychoactive substances (cannabinoids), the highest cannabinoid concentrations are found in the flowering tops. In the Middle East and North Africa the dried resinous exudate of the tops is called hashish; in the Far East it is called charas. The dried leaves and flowering shoots of the plant, containing smaller amounts of the active substance, are called bhang, and the resinous mass from the small leaves and brackets of inflorescence is called ganja. In the United States, the term *marihuana* is used to refer to any part of the plant or extract therefrom that induces somatic and psychic changes in man. Most commonly, the plant is cut, dried, chopped, and incorporated into cigarettes. Marihuana is sometimes contaminated with herbicides, with *Salmo-*

nella and *Aspergillus*, and, depending on the region in which it is grown, with mercury.

Chemistry. The hemp plant synthesizes at least 400 chemicals, of which more than 60 are cannabinoids. The three most abundant include cannabinol (CBN), cannabidiol (CBD), and several isomers of tetrahydrocannabinol. The isomer responsible for most of the characteristic psychological effects of marihuana is *l*-Δ^9-tetrahydrocannabinol (Δ^9-THC), also referred to as *l*-Δ^1-THC. The effects of *l*-Δ^8-THC, which occurs in minute amounts in marihuana, are similar to those of *l*-Δ^9-THC.

Δ^9-THC has the following structure:

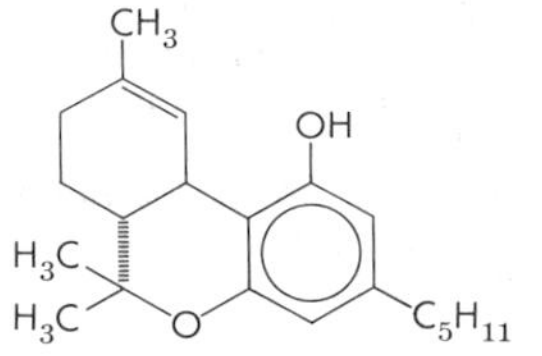

Tetrahydrocannabinol (Δ^9-THC)

Most other cannabinoids are not psychoactive, but they may interact with Δ^9-THC and either increase or decrease its potency. Many derivatives of tetrahydrocannabinol have been synthesized and studied; some of these are more potent than the natural plant products and may have potential therapeutic uses (*see* Dewey, 1986; Razdan, 1986). Hundreds of additional compounds are produced by pyrolysis when cannabis products are smoked. Several of these are also found in tobacco smoke, and they may be important in the long-term toxicity from use of cannabis.

Pharmacological Effects in Animals. In monkeys, both Δ^9-THC and Δ^8-THC produce sedation, decrease in aggressive behavior, loss of ability or motivation to perform complex tasks, and apparent hallucinations. Chronic high dosage produces a dose-related depression of ovarian function, decreases in concentrations of LH and FSH, and anovulatory menstrual cycles; tolerance may develop to these effects. Decreased spermatogenesis has also been reported. Δ^9-THC and several of its synthetic congeners have a number of actions not unlike those of the barbiturates. They exhibit anticonvulsant activity, raise the threshold for EEG and behavioral arousal, and depress polysynaptic reflexes (*see* Maykut, 1985; Dewey, 1986).

Mechanism of Action. Cannabinoids have multiple actions, and not all cannabinoids produce the same pattern of actions. The mechanism of action is poorly understood, but it is highly unlikely that any single receptor site or mechanism will account for the multiple effects. Although high-affinity binding sites have been identified in liver and brain, their characteristics cannot be correlated with any particular action of the cannabinoids. Proposed mechanisms include interactions with lipids in cell membranes to increase fluidity; Δ^9-THC and its active 11-hydroxy metabolite (but not the inactive CBD and CBN) increase membrane fluidity. Alteration of the synthesis of prostaglandins has also been suggested as a mechanism for some actions of cannabinoids. However, whether synthesis is increased or decreased seems to depend on the tissue studied, and some metabolites of Δ^9-THC have actions opposite to those of the parent compound (Martin, 1986; Reichman *et al.*, 1988).

Pharmacological Effects in Man. Δ^9-THC exerts its most prominent effects on the CNS and cardiovascular system. Behavioral responses vary as a function of dose, route of administration, setting, the experience and expectations of subjects, and individual vulnerability to certain psychotoxic effects.

In the United States, the Δ^9-THC content of marihuana ranges broadly from 0.5 to 11%. Furthermore, as with tobacco, the amount of active material that reaches the bloodstream is highly dependent on the smoking technique and the amount altered by pyrolysis.

CNS Effects. An oral dose of 20 mg of Δ^9-THC or the smoking of a cigarette containing 2% Δ^9-THC produces effects on mood, memory, motor coordination, cognitive ability, sensorium, time sense, and self-perception. Most commonly there is an increased sense of well-being or euphoria, accompanied by feelings of relaxation and sleepiness when subjects are alone; where users can interact, sleepiness is less pronounced and there is often spontaneous laughter (for references, *see* Maykut, 1985; Hollister, 1986, 1988). The sleepiness contrasts with the effects of LSD and related hallucinogens, which induce a state of arousal. Short-term memory is impaired, and the capacity to carry out tasks requiring multiple mental steps deteriorates. This effect on memory-dependent, goal-directed behavior has been called "temporal disintegration," and is correlated with a tendency to confuse past, present, and future, and with depersonalization—a sense of strangeness and unreality about the self.

Balance and stability of stance are affected even at low doses, effects that are more apparent when the eyes are closed. Decreases in muscle strength and hand steadiness can be demonstrated. Performance of relatively simple motor tasks and simple reaction times are relatively unimpaired until higher doses are reached. More complex processes, including perception, attention, and information processing, which are involved in driving and flying, are impaired by doses equivalent to one or two cigarettes; the impairment persists for 4 to 8 hours, well beyond the time that the user perceives the subjective effects of the drug. The impairment is apparent to trained observers: 94% of subjects failed a roadside sobriety test 90 minutes after smoking marihuana; 60% still failed after 150 minutes (*see* Hollister, 1986, 1988). The impairment produced by alcohol is additive to that induced by marihuana.

Marihuana smokers frequently report increased hunger, dry mouth and throat, more vivid visual imagery, and a keener sense of hearing. Subtle visual and auditory stimuli previously ignored may take on a novel quality, and the nondominant senses of touch, taste, and smell seem to be enhanced. Yet, in usual social doses, marihuana decreases empathy and the perception of emotions in others; clarity of sequential dialogue is impaired, and irrelevant ideas and words intrude into the stream of communication. Altered perception of time is a consistent effect of cannabinoids. Time seems to pass more slowly—minutes may seem like hours.

The effects of a single dose of marihuana on the surface EEG are not prominent; an increased abundance of alpha waves is the effect reported most commonly. REM sleep is reduced. Some tolerance develops to these effects.

Psychotoxic Effects. Higher doses of Δ^9-THC can induce frank hallucinations, delusions, and paranoid feelings. Thinking becomes confused and disorganized; depersonalization and altered time sense are accentuated. Anxiety reaching panic proportions may replace euphoria, often as a result of the feeling that the drug-induced state will never end. With high enough doses, the clinical picture is that of a toxic psychosis with hallucinations, depersonalization, and loss of insight; this reaction can occur acutely or only after months of use. Most users are able to regulate their intake in order to avoid the excessive dosage that produces these unpleasant effects. However, peak subjective effects of smoked cannabis occur 20 to 30 minutes after inhalation, and they lag somewhat behind concentrations of Δ^9-THC in plasma. Regulation of effect is thus imprecise. Because of the high prevalence of marihuana use, dysphoric reactions and psychiatric emergencies as a result of smoking marihuana are no longer uncommon. Use of marihuana can also cause an acute exacerbation of symptomatology in stabilized schizophrenics, and is an independent risk factor for the development of schizophrenia (Andreasson *et al.*, 1987). It is one of the common precipitants of "flashbacks" in former users of LSD (*see* Hollister, 1986). Although there are similarities between the subjective effects of Δ^9-THC at high doses and those of LSD, cannabinoids are a separate and distinct pharmacological class.

Chronic marihuana users may exhibit apathy; dullness; impairment of judgment, concentration, and memory; and loss of interest in personal appearance and pursuit of conventional goals. This has been called the "amotivational syndrome." It is clear that this syndrome may be due in part to factors other than the use of cannabis, and it is difficult to know the contribution of drug use in any given case. Cessation may lead to gradual improvement over a period of several weeks. At present there is no evidence to suggest that any personality changes are due to irreversible organic brain damage. However, the possibility of an adverse effect of frequent or chronic low levels of intoxication on developing personality cannot be dismissed, especially in view of the long-lasting structural and functional changes in hippocampal neurons that can be produced by the long-term administration of Δ^9-THC to animals.

Because marihuana use, especially at an early age, is highly correlated with use of other illicit drugs, it is often difficult to disentangle the effects of marihuana from those of other drugs. Heavy use of marihuana in adolescence strongly predicts continued use in young adulthood. Use of marihuana and illicit drugs in adolescence also predicts increased delinquency, unemployment, divorce, abortions, and health problems, even when an effort is made to control for individual differences (Kandel *et al.*, 1986). Persons who use only moderate amounts of marihuana, especially females, are likely to discontinue use when they assume family responsibilities (Kandel and Raveis, 1989).

Cardiovascular Effects. The most consistent effects on the cardiovascular system are an increase in heart rate, an increase in systolic blood pressure while supine, decreased blood pressure while standing, and a marked reddening of the conjunctivae. Propranolol, a β-adrenergic blocking agent, and clonidine, an α_2-adrenergic agonist, prevent or diminish the tachycardia produced by Δ^9-THC, but they do not interfere with the subjective and behavioral effects. The increase in heart rate is dose related, and its onset and duration correlate well with concentrations of Δ^9-THC in blood. Increases of 20 to 50 beats per minute are usual, but a tachycardia of 140 beats per minute is not uncommon. Myocardial oxygen demand is increased. In patients with angina, exercise time to angina is decreased by nearly 50% by one marihuana cigarette (*see* Hollister, 1988). Long-term use of cannabis causes an as-yet-unexplained increase in plasma volume.

Immune System. Cannabinoids suppress cellular and humoral immune responses in animals and *in vitro*. Juvenile animals appear to be more affected than are adults. The extent of the immunosuppressive effect varies with the tissue examined. Cannabinoids can also impair synthesis of nucleic acids and proteins. The practical significance of these findings remains unclear. Mice treated with Δ^9-THC show enhanced susceptibility to gram-negative bacteria. However, clinical experience has not yet shown that cannabis users are more susceptible to infection. There is little correlation between the potency of cannabinoids in producing psychic effects and their capacity to suppress immune response or inhibit protein synthesis. Although cannabis is teratogenic in high doses in some species, no such effects have been definitively linked to the use of cannabinoids by man.

Endocrine Effects. Conflicting data have been reported on the effects of chronic high doses of marihuana on human sexual function. In men, lowered concentrations of testosterone and reversible inhibition of spermatogenesis have been reported. Women may be more sensitive. A single marihuana cigarette can suppress plasma LH during the luteal phase of the menstrual cycle (Mendelson *et al.*, 1986); this property may account for the observation that anovulatory cycles are frequently associated with smoking marihuana. When the mother is exposed to cannabis during pregnancy, the offspring tend to have lower birth weight, shorter gestation periods, and more malformations. There is also more frequent meconium staining and longer labor. Offspring may exhibit persistent effects on behavior, which are most evident in terms of learning and responses to stimuli (*see* Hollister, 1986, 1988).

Respiratory Effects. Although no consistent changes occur in respiratory rate, long-term smoking of marihuana and hashish has long been associated with bronchitis and asthma; such smoking adversely affects pulmonary function and the bronchial epithelium, even in young people. However, the acute response to Δ^9-THC (given orally, intravenously, or by aerosol) is a significant and relatively long-lasting bronchodilatation to which little tolerance develops. This effect is seen in both normal subjects and asthmatics. The "tar" produced by pyrolysis of marihuana is more carcinogenic to animals than is that derived from tobacco. Because the smoke is inhaled more deeply and held longer in the lungs, smoking marihuana introduces four times more particulates (tar) into the lung than does smoking a tobacco cigarette (Wu *et al.*, 1988). It is likely, therefore, that even one or two such cigarettes per day will increase the risk of lung cancer.

Other Effects. Pupillary size is not significantly altered by marihuana, but intraocular pressure is decreased because of effects on the ocular vasculature. Δ^9-THC and selected synthetic congeners have antiemetic effects that are equal to those of metoclopramide in reducing nausea caused by cancer chemotherapy (*see* Vincent *et al.*, 1983; Hollister, 1988; *see also* Chapter 38).

Absorption, Fate, and Excretion. The systemic availability of Δ^9-THC from smoking a marihuana cigarette varies from 2% to 50%, depending on the technique used by the smoker (*see* Hollister, 1988). Thus, a 1-g cigarette that contains 2% Δ^9-THC could deliver from 0.4 to 10 mg of the drug to the circulation. The bioavailability of oral Δ^9-THC ranges from 4 to 12%, depending on the vehicle.

Pharmacological effects occur within minutes after smoking begins; plasma concentrations reach their peak within 7 to 10 minutes; physiological and subjective effects are not maximal for 20 to 30 minutes. The subjective effects of a cigarette seldom last longer than 2 or 3 hours. After oral administration, the onset of effects usually occurs at about 30 to 60 minutes; peak effects may not occur until the second or third hour and correlate well with plasma concentrations of drug.

Δ^9-THC is rapidly converted into an active metabolite, 11-hydroxy-Δ^9-THC, which produces effects identical to those of the parent compound. 11-Hydroxy-Δ^9-THC is, in turn, converted into more polar, inactive metabolites, which are then excreted in the urine and feces. One of the more common metabolites is 11-nor-Δ^9-THC-9-carboxylic acid, but approximately 80 compounds have now been identified. Metabolites excreted in the bile may be reabsorbed. Very little unmetabolized Δ^9-THC is found in the urine. After reaching their peaks, plasma concentrations of Δ^9-THC and 11-hydroxy-Δ^9-THC fall rapidly at first (half-time of minutes), reflecting the redistribution of these lipophilic compounds to lipid-rich tissues. This first phase of rapid decline is followed by a much slower terminal phase; the half-time for elimination is about 30 hours. This is consistent with the fact that traces of Δ^9-THC and its metabolites persist in the plasma of man for several days or even weeks and can also be detected in urine (*see* Maykut, 1985; Hollister, 1988; Johansson *et al.*, 1988). Under some circumstances, passive inhalation of smoke can result in sufficient absorption of cannabinoids to produce positive responses on sensitive tests for urinary metabolites. Consumption of repeated oral doses of Δ^9-THC for several days or its daily smoking for several weeks does not seem to produce clinically detectable evidence of accumulation, although accumulation of inactive metabolites is likely. Long-term marihuana smokers metabolize Δ^9-THC more rapidly than do nonsmokers. Marihuana also alters the metabolism of barbiturates and ethanol.

Tolerance and Physical Dependence. In animals, tolerance develops to the lethal, hypothermic, and some of the behavioral effects of cannabinoids. Although in certain species the degree of tolerance is remarkable, it may not develop to all the effects of the drug. Most of the tolerance is due to functional or pharmacodynamic adaptations of the CNS, rather than to a more rapid metabolic disposition (*see* Maykut, 1985; Dewey, 1986).

Reports from many countries indicate that a number of regular users of hashish consume amounts of Δ^9-THC that would produce toxic effects in most Western users. When volunteers are given Δ^9-THC orally every 4 hours (maximal dose of 210 mg per day), tolerance develops to drug-induced changes of mood, tachycardia, decrease in skin temperature, increase in body temperature, decrease in intraocular pressure, changes in the EEG, and impairment of performance on psychomotor tests. Tolerance to the cardiac effects develops within a few days and decays relatively quickly (48 hours) (*see* Jones *et al.*, 1976). If, however, the total dosage used is low, subjects continue to experience a "high" after the first cigarette of the day. Experienced users may actually report more subjective effects from smoking marihuana than naive subjects. However, they generally show less impairment of perceptual and motor functions, as well as smaller increases in heart rate.

Some degree of cross-tolerance between alcohol or opioids and Δ^9-THC has been observed in animals (*see* Dewey, 1986). However, there is no cross-tolerance between cannabinoids and the psychedelics (hallucinogens).

A withdrawal syndrome has been observed under laboratory conditions when volunteers have taken high doses of Δ^9-THC every few hours for several weeks. Signs and symptoms included irritability, restlessness, nervousness, decreased appetite, weight loss, insomnia, rebound increase in REM sleep, tremor, chills, and increased body temperature. Overall, the syndrome is relatively mild, begins within a few hours after cessation of drug administration, and lasts 4 to 5 days. The relationship between this relatively mild syndrome and cannabis-seeking behavior, if any, is unclear (Jones *et al.*, 1976).

Therapeutic Uses. Marihuana, Δ^9-THC, and certain synthetic analogs have one established and several potential therapeutic applications. Some synthetic cannabinoids may find use as analgesics or anticonvulsants. The capacity of some natural and synthetic cannabinoids to lower intraocular pressure has had little clinical utility to date. Δ^9-THC and a synthetic cannabinoid, nabilone, are now available for oral use as antiemetics (*see* Chapter 38). They are indicated for control of nausea associated with chemotherapy when patients do not respond adequately to other regimens. Because it produces subjective effects similar to those of Δ^9-THC, nabilone is included in Schedule II of the Controlled Substance Act.

The most serious side effects of nabilone are depersonalization and dysphoria, which, while uncommon, may be especially disturbing for older patients. More common side effects include vertigo, dizziness, drowsiness, dry mouth, and difficulty in concentrating. Nabilone (and, by inference, Δ^9-THC) increases the psychomotor impairment produced by diazepam, alcohol, and codeine.

PSYCHEDELICS (HALLUCINOGENS, PSYCHOTOMIMETICS, PSYCHOTOGENS)

Under certain conditions, or at toxic dosage, several classes of drugs (anticholinergics, bromides, antimalarials, opioid antagonists, cocaine, amphetamines, and corticosteroids) can induce illusions, hallucinations, delusions, paranoid ideations, and other alterations of mood and thinking that are observed in spontaneously occurring psychotic states. However, despite the legal terminology that defines lysergic acid diethylamide (LSD) and related drugs as hallucinogens, the production of hallucinations is not the most useful way to describe the very interesting pharmacological effects of this group of drugs.

The psychedelic drugs to be discussed here can, indeed, produce such pathological effects as the terms *hallucinogenic, psychotomimetic,* and *psychotogenic* imply, but the feature that distinguishes the psychedelic agents from other classes of drugs is their capacity reliably to induce states of altered perception, thought, and feeling that are not experienced otherwise except in dreams or at times of religious exaltation.

Most descriptions of the "psychedelic state" include several major effects. There is heightened awareness of sensory input, often accompanied by an enhanced sense of clarity, but a diminished control over what is experienced. Frequently there is a feeling that one part of the self seems to be a passive observer (a "spectator ego") rather than an active organizing and directing force, while another part of the self participates and receives the vivid and unusual sensory experiences. The attention of the user is turned inward, preempted by the seeming clarity and portentous quality of his or her own thinking processes. In this state the slightest sensation may take on profound meaning. Commonly, there is a diminished capacity to differentiate the boundaries of one object from another and of the self from the environment. Associated with the loss of boundaries there may be a sense of union with "mankind" or the "cosmos" (Freedman, 1968).

Despite increased understanding of the mechanism of action of these drugs (*see* below), the choice of which agents to include or exclude remains somewhat arbitrary. A number of them produce many, but not all, of the pharmacological effects of prototypical psychedelic drugs such as LSD and mescaline; others may produce a variety of additional effects distinct from those of the prototypical agents or they may produce LSD-like effects at one dose level and amphetamine-like effects as the dose is increased. Most of the drugs that are generally included among the psychedelics are related either to the indolealkylamines, such as LSD, psilocybin, psilocin, dimethyltryptamine (DMT), and diethyltryptamine (DET), or to the phenylethylamines (mescaline) or phenylisopropylamines, such as 2,5-dimethoxy-4-methylamphetamine (DOM, "STP"). At low dosage, dimethoxyamphetamine (DMA) has primarily LSD-like effects, but it is more like amphetamine as the dose is raised. Martin and Sloan (1977) have proposed three criteria for categorizing LSD-like drugs: (1) subjective effects and neurophysiological actions; (2) cross-tolerance between compounds; and (3) response to selective antagonists. By application of these criteria they classified a variety of compounds that produce changes in perception and mood into five categories: (I) LSD-like: LSD, mescaline, psilocybin, psilocin; (II) probably LSD-like: DMA, DOM, tryptamine, DMT, numerous congeners of lysergic acid; (III) probably LSD-like but with other properties: 3,4-methylenedioxyamphetamine (MDA), 5-methoxy-3,4-methylenedioxyamphetamine (MMDA); (IV) probably not LSD-like: D-2-bromlysergic acid diethylamide (BOL), 5-hydroxytryptophan; and (V) not LSD-like: amphetamine, β-phenethylamine (PEA), 2,5-dimethoxy-4-ethylamphetamine (DOET), bufotenine, L-LSD, scopolamine, Δ^9-THC. Since that time, additional LSD-like drugs and drugs with mixed actions such as 3,4-methylenedioxymethamphetamine (MDMA, "ecstasy") have been studied; ligand-binding techniques have been refined and more selective antagonists have been developed. However, the basic concept of a spectrum of drugs ranging from those that are like LSD to those that are not has not changed.

A number of compounds produce alterations of mood and perception that are so obviously distinct as to merit separate discussion. Included among these are phencyclidine, certain opioid agonist–antagonists (considered in Chapter 21), and inhalants such as nitrous oxide and certain volatile solvents.

LSD and Related Compounds. *History and Patterns of Use.* Drugs that induce psychedelic effects have been used for centuries. The peyote cactus (containing mescaline) and mushrooms (containing psilocin) were being used by the natives of Mexico and the Southwestern United States at the time of the Spanish conquest. There was a brief period of scientific interest in mescaline at the beginning of this century and again in the 1930s. However, Hoffman's discovery in 1943 of the psychedelic effects of LSD and its remarkable potency stimulated interest among scientists who felt its study might help facilitate understanding of mental illness. In the 1950s hundreds of scientific papers were written on the effects of LSD on biological systems *in vitro,* animal behavior, patients with a wide range of physical and mental illnesses, and normal human volunteers. The effects of LSD then caught the attention of students, writers, and others more interested in its possibilities for self-exploration than for scientific investigation. Within a matter of a few years its use had spread among young people. By 1970, LSD was included in the same regulatory category as heroin. The drug, which is relatively easy to manufacture, remains available and is still used. However, the frequency of use has been declining. By 1988, only 14% of young adults had ever used such drugs, and less than 2% had used them within the 30 days prior to the survey.

Chemistry. The structures of LSD, mescaline, psilocin, and several related compounds are shown in Table 22–1. The diversity of compounds included here precludes a consideration of structure–activity relationships.

Mechanism of Action. LSD and related psychedelic drugs have actions at multiple sites in the CNS, from the cortex to the spinal cord. Some of the best studied of these involve agonistic actions at presynaptic receptors for 5-HT in the midbrain, where the firing rate of neurons in the dorsal raphe nuclei is sharply reduced after small doses of LSD are administered systemically. 5-HT itself is inhibitory when applied iontophoretically to 5-HT–containing neurons in the dorsal raphe nuclei or to those neurons of the forebrain to which the dorsal raphe neurons project.

There appear to be at least five subtypes of 5-HT receptors (*see* Chapter 23). As selective agonists and antagonists for these receptor subtypes have been developed, evidence has mounted that LSD and related agents act relatively selectively at the 5-HT_2 receptor. However, whether LSD acts as an agonist or partial agonist and whether it acts exclusively at 5-HT_2 receptors is not yet settled (*see* Pierce and Peroutka, 1988; Sanders-Bush *et al.,* 1988; McKenna *et al.,* 1989). The actions of LSD and mescaline on the locus ceruleus (decreased spontaneous activity, but enhancement of activation by peripheral stimuli) are blocked by ritanserin, a selective 5-HT_2 antagonist (Rasmussen and Aghajanian, 1986). Although LSD is more potent than 5-HT in stimulating phosphoinositide hydrolysis mediated by 5-HT_2 receptors, the maximum response to LSD is only 25% of that to 5-HT, suggesting that it is a partial agonist. The administration of LSD causes a decreased capacity to bind 5-HT_2 antagonists such as ketanserin in brain, an effect that can be detected within a few hours after single high doses (Buckholtz *et al.,* 1988). Thus, down regulation of receptors may account in part for the rapid development of tolerance to LSD and related agents.

Pharmacological Effects. In man, oral doses of LSD as low as 20 to 25 μg produce CNS effects in susceptible individuals. At such doses detectable effects on other organ systems are few.

Some of the features that distinguish the psychedelic state from other effects produced by drugs have already been described. In addition, LSD produces somatic effects that are largely sympathomimetic in nature, such as pupillary dilatation, increase in blood pressure, tachycardia, hyperreflexia, tremor, nausea, piloerection, muscular weakness, and increased body temperature.

Following oral doses of 0.5 to 2 μg/kg, the somatic symptoms are usually perceived within a few minutes. These include dizziness, weakness, drowsiness, nausea, and paresthesias. They may be followed by a feeling of inner tension relieved by laughing or crying. Several feelings may seem to coexist at the same time, although euphoric effects

Table 22–1. STRUCTURAL FORMULAS AND CLASSIFICATION OF SELECTED PSYCHEDELIC DRUGS *

LSD-LIKE

Indoleamines

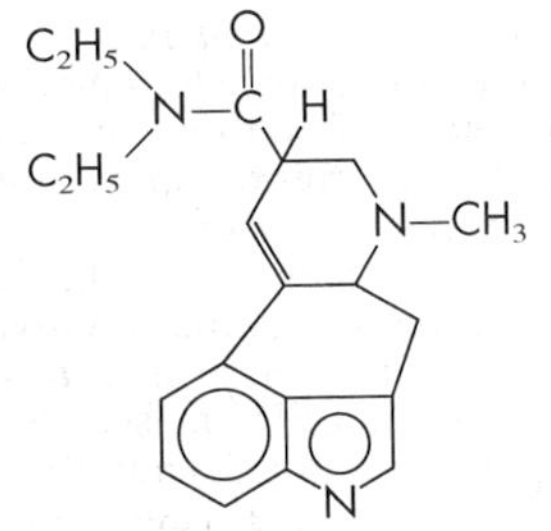

LSD

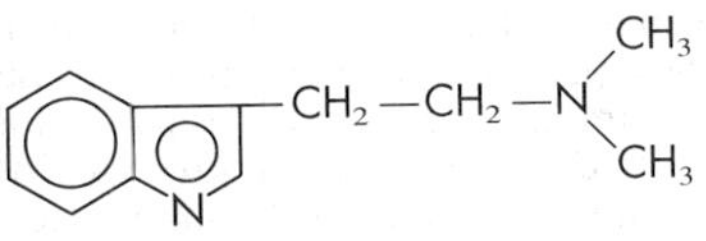

DMT

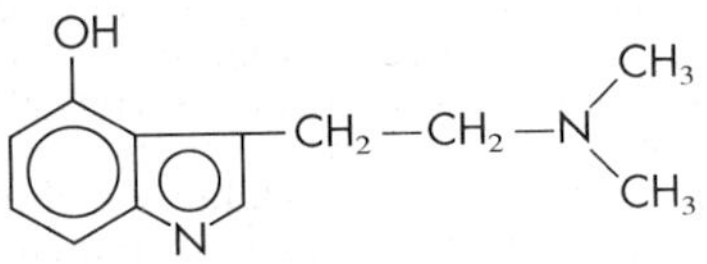

Psilocin

β-Phenethylamines

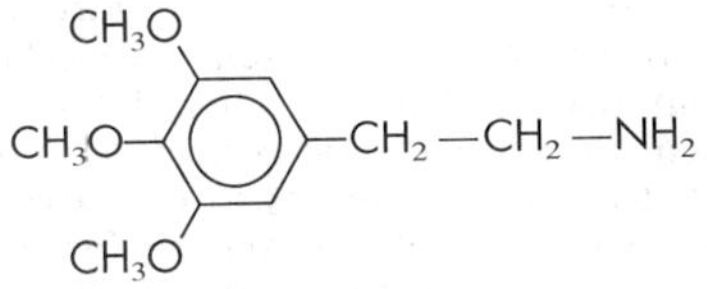

Mescaline

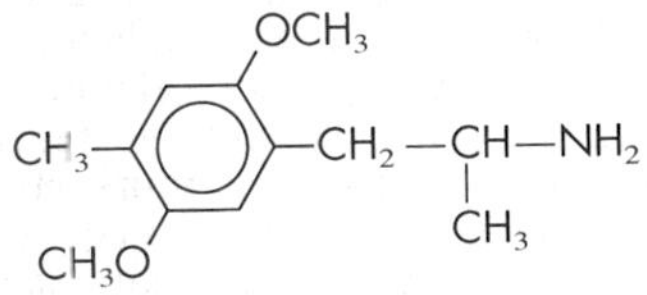

DOM

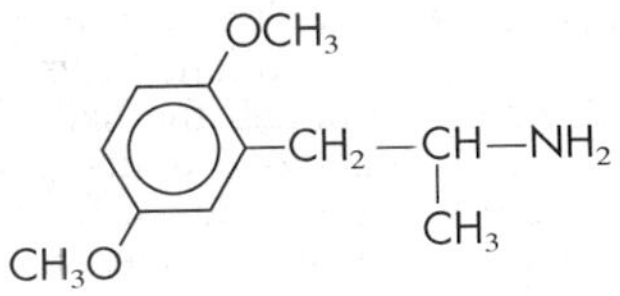

DMA

MIXED

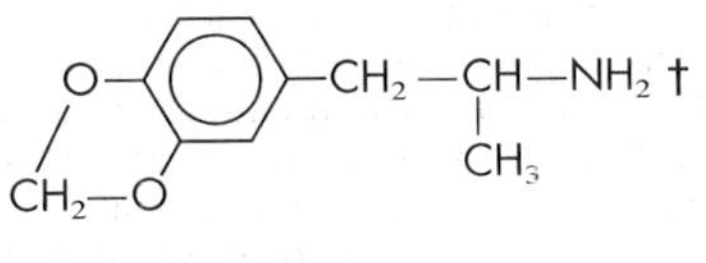

MDA

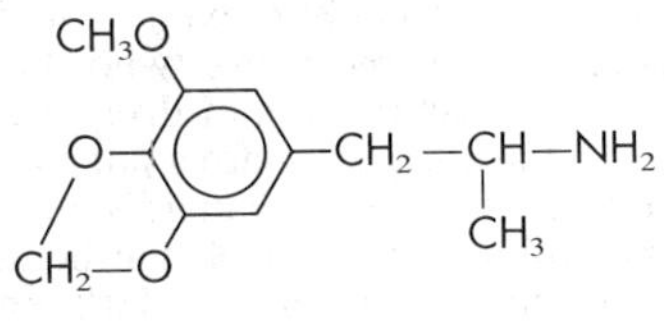

MMDA

AMPHETAMINE-LIKE

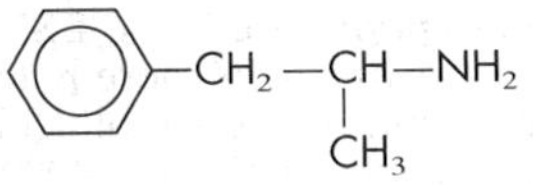

Amphetamine

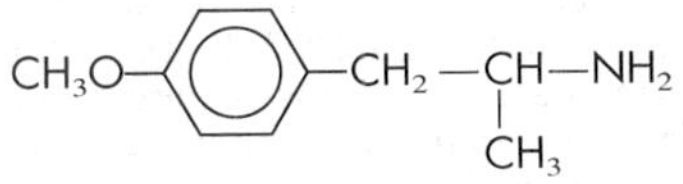

p-Methoxyamphetamine

* Based on classification of Martin and associates, 1978.
† MDMA differs from MDA only by the presence of —CH_3 on the nitrogen.

tend to predominate. In the second or third hour, visual illusions, wavelike recurrences of perceptual changes (*e.g.*, micropsia, macropsia), and affective symptoms may occur. Afterimages are prolonged, and the overlapping of present and preceding perceptions occurs. Some subjects recognize these confluences, whereas others elaborate them into hallucinations. In contrast to naturally occurring psychoses, auditory hallucinations are rare. Synesthesias, the overflow from one sensory modality to another, may occur. Colors are heard and sounds may be seen. Subjective time is also seriously altered, so that clock time seems to pass extremely slowly. The loss of boundaries and the fear of fragmentation create a need for a structuring or supporting environment and experienced companions. During the "trip," thoughts and memories can vividly emerge under self-guidance or unexpectedly, to the user's distress. Mood may be labile, shifting from depression to gaiety, from elation to fear. Tension and anxiety may mount and reach panic proportions. After about 4 to 5 hours, if a major panic episode does not occur, there may be a sense of detachment and the conviction that one is magically in control.

Between the dose ranges of 1 to 16 μg/kg, the intensity of the psychophysiological effects of LSD is proportional to the dose. The entire syndrome, including the pupillary dilatation, begins to clear after about 12 hours, although the half-life of the drug in man is approximately 3 hours (*see* Freedman, 1969). There is little evidence for long-term changes in personality, beliefs, values, or behavior produced by the drug.

Although the patterns of psychological and biochemical effects seen with other agents are quite similar to those with LSD, there are significant differences in potency, absorption, metabolism, duration of action, the slope of dose–response curves, and in potential neurotoxicity. DMT, for example, is inactive by mouth and must be injected, sniffed, or smoked to produce effects. LSD is longer acting and more than 100 times more potent than psilocybin and psilocin, the active alkaloids in the Mexican "magic mushroom"; it is 4000 times more potent than mescaline in producing altered states of consciousness. There may also be some differences in the frequency of somatic effects, such as more vomiting with mescaline. The effects of an oral dose of mescaline (about 5 mg/kg) persist for about 12 hours. DOM and DOET are particularly interesting in that at low doses they produce mild euphoria and enhanced self-awareness without perceptual distortion or hallucinogenic effects. At higher doses DOM has typical psychedelic activity. Most of the pharmacological actions of LSD, and, presumably, drugs with similar profiles can be blocked by 5-HT antagonists such as ketanserin and cyproheptadine, as well as by chlorpromazine and haloperidol, which also have considerable affinity for 5-HT_2 receptors (Rasmussen and Aghajanian, 1988).

In the mid-1980s, MDMA ("ecstasy") gained popularity, especially among college students, as a "recreational" drug. Because it was not initially listed in the Controlled Substances Act, its synthesis and sale were legal for a brief period, and it was used by some psychiatrists to facilitate psychotherapy. Like its close analog, MDA, to which it is metabolized in man, it has both psychedelic and amphetamine-like properties (Peroutka *et al.*, 1988; Verebey *et al.*, 1988). Unlike LSD, it is self-administered by laboratory animals (Lamb and Griffiths, 1987).

Tolerance, Toxicity, and Physical Dependence. A high degree of tolerance to the behavioral effects of LSD develops after three or four daily doses; sensitivity returns after a comparable drug-free interval. Down regulation of receptors may be one mechanism responsible for behavioral tolerance (*see* above). Tolerance to the cardiovascular effects is less pronounced. There is considerable cross-tolerance between LSD, mescaline, and psilocybin, but none between LSD and the amphetamines or between LSD-like drugs and scopolamine or Δ^9-THC. Curiously, DMT induces little cross-tolerance to LSD, perhaps because of the short duration of action of DMT.

In general, these drugs do not give rise to patterns of repetitive use over prolonged periods. The most common psychedelic-use pattern is the occasional "trip," separated by intervals of weeks or months during which marihuana is used with variable frequency. Withdrawal phenomena are not seen after abrupt discontinuation of LSD-like drugs. In man, deaths attributable to direct effects of LSD are unknown, although fatal accidents and suicides have occurred during states of LSD intoxication. The incidence of spontaneous abortion and fetal abnormalities appears to be higher among women who use illicit LSD, but the effects of pure LSD on pregnancy and the fetus remain uncertain. There appears to be no striking increase in genetic abnormalities or congenital malformations among American Indian tribes that have used mescaline for several generations.

The evidence for significant psychological hazards in the use of psychedelic agents is unambiguous. The most common adverse effect is a temporary (24-hour) episode of panic—a "bad trip." This can be treated by reassurance in a supportive and familiar environment ("talking down"), antianxiety agents, or induction of sleep with barbiturates. Although phenothiazines antagonize the effects of LSD, they are usually not needed. Such "bad trips" cannot be reliably prevented and have been experienced even by users who had previous "good trips." Recurrences of drug effects without the drug—"flashbacks"—are a puzzling phenomenon; they occur in more than 15% of users. Commonly precipitated by use of marihuana, anxiety, fatigue, or movement into a dark environment, "flashbacks" may persist intermittently for several years after the last exposure to LSD. They are exacerbated by the use of phenothiazines. In some individuals the use of psychedelics can precipitate serious depressions, paranoid behavior, or prolonged psychotic episodes. Whether such episodes would have occurred without the drug is not clear. Prolonged psychotic episodes following repeated use of LSD tend to resemble naturally occurring schizophreniform psychotic states, and the prognosis appears to be similar (*see* Vardy and Kay, 1983). It is possible that repeated use of LSD can induce subtle deficits in the capacity for abstract thinking.

MDMA and MDA produce a relatively selective destruction of tryptaminergic nerve terminals, especially in the hypothalamus and cerebral cortex of rats and nonhuman primates; catecholaminergic neurons are largely spared. Although some recovery occurs over a period of several months, it is incomplete. Since the dose required to produce this toxicity is only two to four times the acute hallucinogenic dose in man, the possibility of long-term neurotoxicity from the use of these agents must be considered (Battaglia *et al.*, 1987).

Therapeutic Uses. LSD was once proposed as an aid in psychotherapy and as an adjunct to the treatment of alcoholism and opioid addiction. In each situation, the use has been abandoned either because controlled studies have failed to demonstrate the value of LSD or because the elaborate precautions required to minimize adverse psychological reactions dampened enthusiasm and rendered its therapeutic use impractical. More recently, MDMA has been advocated as an adjunct to psychotherapy. No controlled studies have been published, and serious concerns have been raised about the potential for neurotoxicity (*see* above).

ARYLCYCLOHEXYLAMINES

Phencyclidine and Related Compounds. *History, Source, and Patterns of Use.* Phencyclidine, developed in the 1950s, was first used as an anesthetic for animals and, for a short time, as a general anesthetic in man. It fell into disuse quickly because patients experienced delirium when they emerged from anesthesia. Phencyclidine gained popularity in the early 1970s, when it became available as a drug to be smoked or "snorted." Use then declined sharply, so that by 1988, only 3% of high school seniors reported any experience with it, compared with about 13% in 1979. The compound is relatively easy to synthesize, and it is known among drug abusers by a number of street names, among which are "angel dust," "crystal," and "PCP." It is no longer used as a veterinary anesthetic, and the drug that is used illicitly is produced in clandestine laboratories and varies widely in purity. Phencyclidine is sometimes misrepresented as LSD, mescaline, or Δ^9-THC; thus the true extent of exposure may be underestimated. Many congeners with similar profiles of effects are now known, and some have been produced illicitly.

Chemistry. Phencyclidine is one of a group of arylcyclohexylamines. A related compound, ketamine, is still used as an anesthetic in man. The structural formula of phencyclidine is as follows:

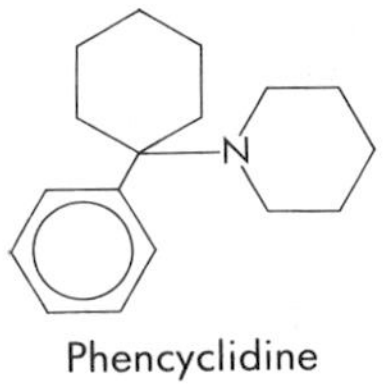

Phencyclidine

Pharmacological Actions. Phencyclidine and related arylcyclohexylamines have CNS-stimulant, CNS-depressant, hallucinogenic, and analgesic actions. The term *dissociative anesthetic* has been used to describe these drugs; they appear to represent a distinct category of agents in terms of their actions, as well as in terms of their properties in animal models.

In man, small doses of phencyclidine produce a subjective sense of intoxication, with staggering gait, slurred speech, nystagmus, and numbness of the extremities. Depending on the dose, users may exhibit sweating, catatonic muscular rigidity, and a blank stare; they may also experience changes in body image and disorganized thought, drowsiness, and apathy. There may be hostile and bizarre behavior. Amnesia for the episode may occur. With increasing dosage analgesia is more marked, and anesthesia, stupor, or coma may occur, although the eyes may remain open. Sensory impulses reach the cortex, but the individual experiences them in a distorted form. Heart rate and blood pressure are elevated; there is hypersalivation, sweating, fever, repetitive movements, and muscle rigidity on stimulation. At even higher doses prolonged coma, muscle rigidity, and convulsions may occur (*see* Aniline and Pitts, 1982).

At the height of its popularity, use of the drug once a week was typical. Some users engaged in 2- to 3-day binges or "runs" that were followed by prolonged sleep, from which the user awoke depressed and disoriented. Chronic users may ingest up to 1 g in 24 hours.

Monkeys with implanted catheters do not administer LSD to themselves, but they do self-administer phencyclidine. Few drugs seem to induce so wide a range of subjective effects. Among those effects that users seem to like are increased sensitivity to external stimuli, stimulation, mood elevation, and a sense of intoxication. Other effects, some of which appear to occur with every use, are described as unwanted; these include perceptual disturbances, restlessness, disorientation, and anxiety. The typical "high" from a single dose lasts 4 to 6 hours and is followed by an extended "coming-down" period.

Mechanism of Action. Phencyclidine and its congeners bind with high affinity to several distinct sites in the CNS, but it is not certain whether these represent important sites of its action. One such site, which is also characterized by high affinity for opioids such as *n*-allylnormetazocine and for certain butyrophenones (*e.g.*, haloperidol), has been designated the σ site. Although formerly thought to mediate the dysphoric effects of certain opioids, the function of σ sites is currently unknown (*see* Chapter 21). At present, most attention is focused on the capacity of phencyclidine, ketamine, and certain related compounds to block the cation channel that is regulated by one type of receptor for excitatory amino acids, the N-methyl-D-aspartate (NMDA) receptor (*see* Monaghan *et al.*, 1989; Wroblewski and Danysz, 1989; *see also* Chapter 12). Phencyclidine inhibits the flux of cations (principally Ca^{2+}) that is initiated by glutamate and/or aspartate, and it can prevent the production of long-term potentiation in the hippocampus that results from high-frequency stimulation of certain neural pathways. In addition, phencyclidine and related compounds can reduce the neuronal death caused by prolonged ischemia or the local application of excitatory neurotoxins. Although of potential clinical utility in the treatment of stroke, agents with the latter actions have not yet been found that are devoid of unacceptable psychotoxicity.

Phencyclidine can inhibit the uptake of dopamine and norepinephrine, and its administration results in increased concentrations of dopamine in the nucleus accumbens of free-moving animals (Dunwiddie and Alford, 1987; Hernandez *et al.,* 1988). The relationship of these actions to those at the NMDA receptor or to its behavioral effects have not been defined.

Absorption, Fate, and Excretion. Phencyclidine is well absorbed following all routes of administration. The parent compound may be hydroxylated, and these metabolites are conjugated with glucuronic acid. While some of the metabolites are active, most of the pharmacological effects are due to phencyclidine itself. Only a small fraction of the drug is excreted unchanged. Phencyclidine is a weak base, and lowering urinary pH (to below 5.0) with ammonium chloride markedly accelerates its excretion. There is considerable gastroenteric recirculation, and continuous gastric suction can be of value in the treatment of overdosage. In cases of overdose, the half-life of phencyclidine appears to be about 3 days, but this value can be shortened to about 1 day by continuous gastric suction and acidification of the urine (Aniline and Pitts, 1982).

Tolerance and Physical Dependence. In animals, tolerance develops to some of the behavioral and toxic effects of phencyclidine, but the extent varies with the species and with the neurotransmitter systems affected (Leccese *et al.,* 1986; Nabeshima *et al.,* 1987). Abrupt withdrawal after long-term use is followed by fearfulness, tremors, and facial twitches (*see* Balster and Wessinger, 1983). Clinical observations suggest that tolerance also develops in man; in addition, some chronic users make vague complaints about craving after stopping. Chronic users of large doses report persistent difficulties with recent memory, speech, and thinking that last from 6 months to 1 year after stopping. Personality changes ranging from social withdrawal and isolation to states of anxiety, nervousness, and severe depression have also been reported.

Toxicity and Treatment of Overdose. The frequency of adverse effects is uncertain, but deaths due to direct toxicity, violent behavior, and accidents have been reported. Phencyclidine can cause acute behavioral toxicity (intoxication, aggression, brief confusional states), coma or convulsions (from severe overdosage), and psychotic states. The last-named condition may be long lasting. People with schizophrenia may be particularly vulnerable to the psychotogenic actions of phencyclidine.

Treatment of overdosage is symptomatic and is directed at protecting the patient and others from the effects of impaired behavior and judgment and at supporting vital functions. Hastening excretion by continuous gastric suction and acidification of the urine can substantially shorten the half-life of the drug but can also increase the risk of renal failure if significant rhabdomyolysis and myoglobinuria are present. Hypersalivation may require suction, respiratory depression may require artificial ventilation, and fever may require external cooling. Convulsions have been treated with diazepam and hypertension with hydralazine. Clinicians advise isolation of patients from external stimuli to the degree compatible with support of vital functions and control of violent or self-destructive behavior. Excessive muscle contractions may aggravate rhabdomyolysis. Coma may be preceded or followed by delirium, paranoia, and assaultive behavior, and arrangements must take this into consideration. Haloperidol appears to be effective in treating phencyclidine psychosis (Giannini *et al.,* 1987). A psychotic phase may last several weeks after a single dose of phencyclidine (*see* Aniline and Pitts, 1982).

MISCELLANEOUS SUBSTANCES USED FOR SUBJECTIVE EFFECTS

The catalog of agents that have been used to produce subjective changes is impressive, and each generation not only adds a few new substances but seems impelled to reevaluate the old.

Inhalants: Anesthetic Gases and Solvents. The intoxicating and euphorigenic effects of both nitrous oxide and ethyl ether were recognized before their potential as anesthetics was appreciated. In the nineteenth century, efforts to reduce alcoholism in Ireland by means of ether were markedly successful, but the use of ether became so widespread that it was necessary to take steps to reeducate the public to the use of alcohol. When access to alcohol or other intoxicants is restricted by finances, laws, or incarceration, substances with marked toxicity such as antifreeze, paint thinner, and other industrial solvents may be used. Since adolescents are usually prohibited from using alcoholic beverages, "glue sniffing" may fall into this category. However, prohibition of alcohol cannot fully explain such behavior. Physicians, dentists, and nurses with access to a wide variety of drugs have been known to inhale anesthetic gases, sometimes with catastrophic outcomes for themselves and their patients. The alkyl nitrites (butyl, isobutyl, and amyl), used medically as vasodilators, became popular as aphrodisiacs in the 1980s. Inhalation of these agents is said to intensify and prolong orgasm. In 1988, about 12% of young adults (aged 18 to 25) indicated some experience with inhalants. Relatively infrequent inhalation of amyl nitrite can induce a significant suppression of immune function (*see* Dax *et al.,* 1988).

Animals will administer nitrous oxide, chloroform, and solvents (*e.g.,* toluene) to themselves; however, only a few of the many compounds have been systematically studied. Mice made tolerant to nitrous oxide are not cross-tolerant to barbiturates, although cross-tolerance and cross-dependence between barbiturates and chloroform have been reported. Although high doses of these substances produce depression of the CNS, low doses of most of these "anesthetics" and solvents produce increased activity that is usually thought to be due to disinhibition.

Because toxicity varies greatly with the specific substance, it can be discussed only in general terms. The causes of fatalities are not clear; most appear to involve cardiac arrhythmias. Inhalation of volatile material from a plastic bag (a common practice) may result in hypoxia as well as an extremely high concentration of vapor. Aerosol propellants containing fluorinated hydrocarbons produce cardiac arrhythmias, and ischemia increases sensitivity to fluorocarbon-induced arrhythmias. Chlorinated solvents (*e.g.*, trichloroethylene) depress myocardial contractility, and sympathetic activity is thereby increased reflexly. Ketones can produce pulmonary hypertension. Neurological impairment may occur with a variety of solvents. Peripheral neuropathies and progressive, fatal neurological deterioration have followed the "huffing" of lacquer thinner. Although the specific causative agents are not known with certainty because of the complexity of the mixtures, animal studies suggest that n-hexane is more likely to produce peripheral neuropathy, and toluene has been associated with diffuse CNS atrophy and renal damage (*see* Rosenberg *et al.*, 1988).

Other Agents. In large amounts, the common household spice nutmeg produces marked subjective changes. It is commonly used for this purpose by the inmates of prisons. The oral ingestion of the equivalent of two grated nutmegs produces, after a latency of several hours, leaden feelings in the extremities and a mental state that may include feelings of depersonalization and unreality. Agitation and apprehension are also common. Dry mouth, thirst, rapid heart rate, and red, flushed face are common and may mimic atropine poisoning.

The medically inappropriate, excessive use of nonopioid analgesic mixtures has been reported (*see* Chapter 26). Such use, however, is not characterized by extreme psychological dependence. Conceivably, excessive use of such drugs may be related to the mood-elevating effects of the caffeine contained in some preparations, or to certain misconceptions about the capacity of such mixtures to relieve tension and increase the user's ability to concentrate on tedious tasks.

Approximately 80% of the world's population consumes caffeine. Per capita consumption among adults in the United States is about 200 mg per day (*see* Chapter 25). Caffeine is a weak reinforcer in laboratory animals and man. In contrast to cocaine and amphetamine, it does not induce intense feelings of euphoria, but it does produce some modest increase in the sense of well being. Although tolerance and physical dependence are not necessary for these pleasurable and reinforcing effects, caffeine is more likely to induce dysphoria and anxiety in those who do not use it regularly. Some degree of physical dependence commonly develops after the daily ingestion of more than 400 to 600 mg of caffeine for 1 to 2 weeks.

The most characteristic symptom of caffeine withdrawal is headache. Fatigue, lethargy, and some anxiety are also common. These symptoms appear within 12 to 24 hours after use of caffeine is stopped, and they last 2 to 7 days (*see* Griffiths and Woodson, 1988). Although some subjects may experience severe symptoms, the degree of impairment and the long-term consequences of its use are judged to be too low for dependence on caffeine to be considered a psychiatric disorder (*see* American Psychiatric Association, 1987). Nevertheless, the long-term intake of more than 250 mg of caffeine per day may be associated with restlessness, nervousness, excitement, insomnia, muscle twitching, rambling flow of thought, and psychomotor agitation, in addition to cardiac and gastrointestinal disturbances. There may also be aggravation of panic disorder or depression (Greden, 1981).

For untold generations, peyote, ololiuqui (from the seeds of the morning glory, *Rivea corymbosa*), and "magic mushrooms" have been used by the Indians of the North American continent to produce altered states of consciousness. Throughout the world, many other substances are used for similar mind- and mood-changing effects. These include the use of kava in the South Pacific, indole-containing snuff among the Amazonian Indians in Brazil, and fly agaric among the Uralic-speaking tribes of Siberia. A discussion of the pharmacology and the patterns of use of these substances is beyond the scope of this chapter. The interested reader should consult Efron and associates (1967).

Designer Drugs. During the 1970s and 1980s clandestine laboratories began to synthesize drugs of several types that were potent reinforcers; however, because these compounds were not specifically listed in the Controlled Substances Act, their manufacture and sale were not at first subject to criminal penalties. These so-called "designer drugs" included several opioids. Certain derivatives of fentanyl (α-methyl fentanyl and 3-methyl fentanyl; both called "China white") are particularly potent and caused sporadic outbreaks of death from overdosage. A congener of meperidine was contaminated with N-methyl-4-phenyl-1,2,3,6-tetrahydropyridine (MPTP), a neurotoxin that causes irreversible Parkinsonism (*see* Chapter 20). Although originally synthesized for legitimate research purposes, several substituted derivatives of amphetamine with euphorigenic and mild hallucinogenic effects also came to be called "designer drugs" when their "recreational" use came to public attention; an example is MDMA ("ecstacy"; *see* above).

TREATMENT

The indications for treatment vary with the drugs being used as well as with the social and cultural factors determining the particular pattern of drug use. Some patterns of drug use, such as weekly use of marihuana, do not require treatment any more than does the occasional smoking of tobacco or the social use of alcohol. Such casual use is not without hazard, and it may jeopardize vocational status, especially as programs for testing the presence of drugs in body fluids expand. However, such patterns of use do not necessarily constitute a treatable disorder. It is likely that changing views about drug use will continue to create gray areas where the indications for treatment are unclear. However, there is general agreement that treatment is appropriate for the adverse consequences of drug use and for the compulsive drug user who voluntarily seeks help.

The management of withdrawal syndromes can usually be achieved with minimal risk and a high probability of success using available pharmacological agents. The more difficult task is helping the patient avoid relapse following withdrawal. This section provides a summary of withdrawal techniques and a brief survey of some common approaches to rehabilitation and prevention of relapse, with emphasis on those approaches that utilize pharmacological agents.

WITHDRAWAL TECHNIQUES

Successful withdrawal from any of the drugs discussed in this chapter can be accomplished on an ambulatory basis. However, withdrawal is usually more easily and more rapidly accomplished in an inpatient or residential setting where stimuli associated with drug use and access to drugs can be minimized, and the withdrawal syndrome can be observed and appropriately treated. Such treatment is obviously more costly than ambulatory care, and the additional cost is not always justified by better outcome or greater safety (*see* below).

Certain general principles apply irrespective of the particular drug or drugs the patient has been using. The degree of physical dependence, if any, that may have developed to each drug the patient has been using should be estimated. A medical history should be taken and a physical examination carried out, to determine whether there are any indications that the usual withdrawal techniques should be modified. For example, a more gradual reduction of opioids would be appropriate in patients with angina pectoris, ulcerative colitis, pulmonary insufficiency, or other debilitating illness. Needless to say, patients who are experiencing severe pain from obvious causes are not appropriate candidates for withdrawal of opioid analgesics until some alternative method of managing the pain is available. Clonidine, which has some analgesic properties, is sometimes particularly useful in this situation. The major decisions that must then be made are what setting is most appropriate for treatment and whether use of pharmacological agents will reduce risk and discomfort and increase chances of successful withdrawal.

Estimating the degree of physical dependence on opioids or on general CNS depressants from the history alone is difficult, since patients may not know the purity of the drugs they have been using and often distort their history of drug use. They may exaggerate their usage considerably and may also claim to be using large quantities of barbiturates or other sedatives in the hope that they will be given more generous amounts of opioids or hypnotics. Conversely, some may completely deny the intake of barbiturates, even when they have been using a sufficient quantity to produce a dangerous degree of physical dependence. Others, who have used paregoric or cough medicines in an alcoholic vehicle, are often unaware of the large amounts of alcohol they consume. The possibility of physical dependence on general CNS depressants should always be considered when a patient who has had sufficient opioids to suppress withdrawal symptoms remains sleepless and jittery. Physicians and nurses may attempt to minimize the extent of their use. The difficulty in getting an accurate history necessitates greater reliance on observation of the patient.

Withdrawal syndromes are observed after abrupt cessation of other types of drugs (CNS stimulants, tobacco, arylcyclohexylamines, and cannabis). There is no consensus on how the syndromes are best managed. Nicotine gum can reduce elements of tobacco withdrawal (*see* above), and a number of agents have been studied for control of symptoms of withdrawal from cocaine.

Withdrawal of Opioids. Even with very gradual reduction in dosage, most patients will perceive some withdrawal symptoms. It may be possible, of course, to gradually reduce the drug the patient was using (heroin, morphine, meperidine, *etc.*) over a period of several days. However, for reasons already discussed, methadone is quite suitable for suppressing withdrawal symptoms and can be substituted for any of the natural or synthetic μ-agonist opioid analgesics currently in use. With methadone substitution (in an inpatient or residential setting) now considered the standard technique, the opioid withdrawal symptoms are rarely worse than those of a moderate "influenza-like" syndrome. However, newer methods that use other drugs, settings, and time frames may have advantages (*see* below).

The dose of methadone will vary with the degree of physical dependence and the medical condition of the patient. The patient is observed and, if significant withdrawal symptoms appear, an initial dose of methadone that rarely needs to exceed 15 to 20 mg is given orally. Additional methadone can be given if the symptoms are not suppressed or each time withdrawal symptoms reappear. It is rarely necessary to give more than 80 mg of methadone over the first 24 hours. Compared with its analgesic effects, methadone is more potent and acts longer to suppress withdrawal symptoms. Usually 1 mg of methadone orally can substitute for the parenteral administration of 4 mg of morphine, 2 mg of heroin, or 20 mg of meperidine. Reduction can be started as soon as the dose for stabilization has been determined. It need not be given more frequently than twice a day. In hospitalized patients, reduction each day of 20% of the total daily dose is well tolerated and causes little discomfort. The majority of inpatients can be completely withdrawn from opioids in less than 10 days, although mild abstinence symptoms may persist for a number of days after the last dose of methadone. The protracted abstinence syndrome has been described above.

Discontinuation of methadone after a period of social stabilization (usually 6 to 18 months) can produce a protracted period of withdrawal. Nevertheless, former heroin addicts maintained on methadone have been gradually withdrawn from methadone entirely on an ambulatory basis. Even though the dosage is reduced very slowly (*e.g.*, by less than 10% of the stabilization dose per week or by as little as 3 mg per week), many of these patients experience opioid withdrawal symptoms when the daily dose of methadone is reduced to about 10 to 30 mg. Exceedingly gradual reduction of dosage is more likely to be successful for ambulatory patients (Senay *et al.*, 1977). Among the symptoms experienced over a period lasting up to several months after withdrawal are insomnia, irritability, restlessness, malaise, pain, fatigue, premature ejaculation, and gastrointestinal hyperactivity (Cushman and Dole, 1973).

Clonidine, a centrally acting α_2-adrenergic agonist, can suppress some components of the opioid withdrawal syndrome and has been used to facilitate ambulatory withdrawal, to shorten the time required to complete inpatient withdrawal, or to begin treatment with naltrexone. With ambulatory patients maintained on 20 to 30 mg of methadone per day, the opioid can be abruptly discontinued, and clonidine given for 7 to 10 days (10 to 17 μg/kg per day in divided doses) to suppress symptoms; clonidine is then withdrawn over 3 to 4 days. A similar procedure can be used for withdrawal of other opioids. Somewhat higher doses of clonidine (*e.g.*, 25 μg/kg per day) can be used for inpatients. In an experimental procedure used by Charney and associates (1986), patients who had been stabilized on methadone (mean dose, 32 mg per day) were given clonidine and naltrexone orally, initially at doses of 5 μg/kg and 1 mg, respectively, at the time that methadone was discontinued. The doses of clonidine and naltrexone were increased every four hours, and the dose of clonidine was adjusted on the basis of the intensity of withdrawal symptoms. The patients were discharged after 6 days and were maintained thereafter on naltrexone.

The primary side effects of clonidine are dry mouth, sedation, and orthostatic hypotension. Clonidine is more effective in suppressing the autonomic signs and symptoms of withdrawal (*e.g.*, nausea, vomiting, diarrhea) than the subjective discomfort or craving. Anxiety, restlessness, insomnia, and muscular aching are suppressed only minimally. Other α_2-adrenergic agonists (*e.g.*, guanabenz) are also useful in ameliorating some aspects of the opioid withdrawal syndrome. Except for α_2-adrenergic agonists, no nonopioid is of proven value in the treatment of opioid withdrawal, including the phenothiazines. Nighttime sedation with a barbiturate or a related sedative–hypnotic may be helpful, but complete suppression of opioid withdrawal symptoms with such agents cannot be achieved. Ca^{2+}-channel blockers decrease the severity of opioid withdrawal in rats (Pellegrini-Giampietro *et al.*, 1988).

Withdrawal of General CNS Depressants (Barbiturates and Related Drugs). Abrupt withdrawal of general CNS depressants that have been used in high doses over prolonged periods can be fatal. Therefore, abrupt withdrawal is not considered a safe technique, and the administration of a suitable general CNS depressant is usually started before major withdrawal symptoms develop. Pentobarbital (orally) can be substituted for any barbiturate the patient has been using. It is probably also a suitable substitute for glutethimide, paraldehyde, chloral hydrate, and meprobamate and for the suppression of the alcohol withdrawal syndrome. Sufficient pentobarbital should be given to produce mild intoxication, that is, slight ataxia, nystagmus, and slurred speech. Most patients require from 0.2 to 0.4 g every 6 hours, but some may need up to 2.5 g over a 24-hour period. The daily dose can be estimated from the response to a 200-mg pentobarbital test dose. Once a level of mild intoxication has been achieved, the dosage of pentobarbital should be maintained for at least 24 to 36 hours. At this level, the patient should be free of tremulousness, irritability, and insomnia. The amount of barbiturate required for this initial period becomes the stabilization level.

Once the stabilization level has been established and the patient observed for 1 to 2 days, gradual withdrawal can be started. Most patients can tolerate reductions of 0.1 g of pentobarbital per day without significant discomfort. Patients who are taking large amounts of lesser-known sedatives should probably be gradually withdrawn from the original drug of abuse without substitution therapy.

Many clinicians prefer phenobarbital for managing withdrawal from any sedative–hypnotic agent. The advantages of phenobarbital over pentobarbital are its long half-life, its superior anticonvulsant properties (which are associated with well-defined concentrations of the drug in blood), and a lower potential for abuse. Phenobarbital is administered at a dose of 90 to 120 mg per hour until the patient becomes drowsy or intoxicated. The phenobarbital is then discontinued, and the clinical signs and the concentration of phenobarbital in plasma are monitored. Because of its long half-life (about 90 hours in such patients), additional doses of phenobarbital are rarely necessary (except in those patients in whom the half-life is less than 40 hours). Fluctuations in requirements for short-acting barbiturates and drug-seeking behavior by patients are thereby minimized (Robinson *et al.*, 1981).

Withdrawal of Alcohol. Certain distinctions between the overall effects of long-term abuse of alcohol and those of other general CNS depressants necessitate differences in the therapeutic approach. Chronic ingestion of large amounts of alcohol is very frequently associated with various degrees of malnutrition and avitaminosis, especially vitamin B deficiencies. Some alcoholics may be dehydrated because of vomiting caused by alcoholic gastritis or withdrawal. Vitamins and attention to fluid balance are a necessary part of treatment, but these are obviously not substitutes for measures to control the general-depressant withdrawal syndrome.

As is the case with mild degrees of physical dependence of any type, in the milder forms of alcohol withdrawal a wide variety of drugs (phenothiazines, sedatives, antianxiety agents, β-adrenergic blockers) or simply nutritional supplements and good nursing care will provide some symptomatic relief. Indeed, although screening is a problem and the procedure involves risk for patients with medical problems or significant physical dependence, many alcoholics are now routinely withdrawn on an outpatient or day-hospital basis without the use of pharmacological agents other than vitamins (*see* Jaffe and Ciraulo, 1984; Kranzler and Orrok, 1989).

When there is a significant degree of physical dependence, drugs that show cross-dependence with alcohol are demonstrably superior in reducing mortality and morbidity to those that do not show such cross-dependence. Unfortunately, the tremulousness, anxiety, and insomnia, which in mildly dependent patients may be the most severe withdrawal symptoms, may in others be the prodrome of more severe epileptiform and delirious states. It is not possible to know in advance which patients are only mildly physically dependent and which patients will develop delirium tremens. Since delirium tremens always carries with it a certain risk of a fatal outcome, it seems appropriate to treat all but the mildest cases of alcohol withdrawal with agents that show cross-dependence with alcohol. Patients with histories of delirium tremens or seizures should be assumed to be at higher risk for severe withdrawal symptoms.

Its short duration of action and narrow range of safety make alcohol a poor therapeutic agent. In practice, it is abruptly stopped and longer-acting agents are substituted. If given in adequate quantities, pentobarbital, phenobarbital, chloral hydrate, paraldehyde, several benzodiazepines, clomethiazole, valproic acid, and carbamazepine have all been shown to be effective in preventing the development of withdrawal symptoms or suppressing the syndrome once it develops (*see* Kranzler and Orrok, 1989). The general technique is similar to that used in the management of physical dependence on barbiturates, in that the patient is brought to a level of stabilization in which he or she exhibits either no withdrawal symptoms or only mild intoxication and the drug is then gradually withdrawn. In the United States, the benzodiazepines are most commonly used for alcohol withdrawal. Chlordiazepoxide and diazepam are popular because the slow elimination of their active metabolites results in a smooth and gradual withdrawal. However, there is no evidence that any one long-acting benzodiazepine is superior to another in suppressing withdrawal (Kranzler and Orrok, 1989; Nutt *et al.*, 1989). Clomethiazole is commonly used in Europe and Australia. The long duration of action and slow elimination of most benzodiazepines make their use in the treatment of physical dependence on alcohol analogous to the use of methadone in the treatment of physical dependence on opioids. The rate at which the dosage of the benzodiazepine should subsequently be reduced has not been carefully studied; the clinician's adjustment of doses should be guided by the degree of intoxication and the appearance of tremulousness and insomnia. Some researchers have given diazepam at 2-hour intervals until all signs of withdrawal are suppressed. No further drug is given because nordazepam, the principal active metabolite, has a very long half-life (*see* Chapter 17; *see also* Sellers *et al.*, 1983). If seizures occur, diazepam should probably be given. Valproic acid and clomethiazole are also effective. Some clinicians use phenytoin in alcohol withdrawal, but the value of this procedure in patients without a history of seizures unrelated to the use of alcohol is questionable. Dopaminergic antagonists, such as haloperidol, are still utilized to control hallucinations once the period of risk for seizures has passed (generally the first 48 hours of withdrawal). For references, *see* Gessner (1979) and Kranzler and Orrok (1989).

Withdrawal of Benzodiazepines. After long-term use of benzodiazepines, withdrawal syndromes may be seen even in patients who do not exceed therapeutic doses (Busto *et al.*, 1986; Woods *et al.*, 1987). The syndromes seen with the shorter-acting drugs, such as triazolam or temazepam, are more rapid in onset, and they tend to be more intense and of shorter duration than those seen with longer-acting agents, such as flurazepam or diazepam; the latter should be self-tapering.

In practice, however, it is often necessary to reduce dosage of even the longer-acting agents gradually over several weeks to prevent emergence of anxiety, tremulousness, headache, tinnitus, perceptual changes, or severe insomnia. Withdrawal of shorter-acting agents is best accomplished by switching to a longer-acting benzodiazepine, followed by tapering of that dosage over a period of several days or weeks. However, long-term abstinence is enhanced when cognitive techniques are used to help patients learn to cope with anxiety (Sanchez-Craig *et al.*, 1987).

Withdrawal of Stimulants, Nicotine, and Other Drugs. Although the abrupt withdrawal of psychedelics, cocaine or amphetamine-like drugs, or tobacco does not cause syndromes that require medical treatment, these syndromes do cause aversive physiological and psychological disturbances that may contribute to relapse. Administration of dopaminergic agonists (*e.g.*, bromocriptine) or tricyclic antidepressants has been suggested for the treatment of the fatigue, irritability, depression, and hypersomnolence that may develop after withdrawal of amphetamines or cocaine, and these agents are also used as adjuncts to long-term therapy. Nicotine, administered in chewing gum, transdermal patches, or nasal sprays, ameliorates the tobacco withdrawal syndrome and, like tricyclic antidepressants, may be used over a more protracted period as an adjunct to a more comprehensive effort to alter drug-taking behavior (*see* below).

Withdrawal Techniques in Mixed Patterns of Abuse. It is not uncommon to encounter individuals who are simultaneously physically dependent on opioids and general CNS depressants or on opioids and cocaine. The therapeutic regimen in such situations combines the procedures described above. General CNS depressants are given in sufficient quantity to produce mild intoxication, and a stabilization dose is determined. At the same time the patient is observed for the autonomic signs of opioid withdrawal, and sufficient methadone or another suitable opioid is given to suppress such symptoms. While the dose of the CNS depressant is held constant, the opioid is reduced as previously described. When withdrawal from opioids is complete, the dose of the CNS depressant is then reduced gradually. Simultaneous withdrawal of both classes of drugs at appropriate rates is not contraindicated, but this procedure requires considerable experience, since insomnia, weakness, and restlessness occur in both syndromes.

Modification of Behavior Following Withdrawal

A number of very different approaches are currently used for modifying drug-taking behavior and helping patients avoid relapse. Some place emphasis on emotional problems that are believed to increase vulnerability to compulsive drug use; others aim at providing alternative gratifications or modifying life styles; still others use various forms of external pressure and threats of adverse consequences to change drug-use patterns; some employ pharmacological agents to modify the response to the drugs themselves. More recently, there has been a greater emphasis on combining self-help groups with cognitive techniques designed to teach participants how to deal with stress and to avoid situations that increase craving for drugs (McAuliffe and Ch'ien, 1986). In practice, several of these procedures may be combined in any one treatment program. Although similar themes appear in programs designed to modify compulsive use of different drugs, the great differences in pharmacological effects and social attitudes and legal consequences associated with use of different drugs make it appropriate to discuss treatment approaches to each drug separately.

The nonpharmacological methods can be only briefly summarized here.

In evaluating any treatment it is essential to recognize that recovery, or at least periods of substantial improvement, commonly occurs for all forms of drug dependence even with little or no formal intervention. For example, among United States Army personnel who began to use heroin in Vietnam, major changes in associates and environment led to rapid abandonment of illicit use of opioids (Robins, 1974). Since drug abusers typically use a number of different drugs and may be dependent on more than one simultaneously, cessation of opioid use does not necessarily mean total abstinence from all substances among those who seek treatment for opioid dependence. Some patients continue to abuse cocaine or alcohol, and most continue to smoke cigarettes. Some alcoholics can drink ethanol after detoxification without immediately relapsing to pathological use. However, in general, such controlled use is observed only in those who have not been severely dependent. For the heavily dependent cigarette smoker, opioid or cocaine addict, or alcoholic, any use regularly and quickly leads to compulsive use once again.

Hospitalization and Psychotherapy. For patients with mild-to-moderate physical dependence on alcohol, there may be little difference between treatment in an inpatient unit and that on an ambulatory basis using daily visits, vitamins, and benzodiazepines (at least when outcome is measured after 6 months) (*see* Hayashida *et al.,* 1989). On the other hand, opioid addicts seem far more likely to achieve complete withdrawal as inpatients than as outpatients (Gossop *et al.,* 1986). However, the relapse rate for such patients after short- or long-term hospitalization is consistently high.

There is little evidence that traditional individual psychotherapy alone is of value in the treatment of the compulsive drug user, although experienced clinicians report that it is useful for selected patients. However, cognitive or expressive psychotherapy has improved the outcome of patients with a poor prognosis in methadone programs, and specialized forms of group psychotherapy and cognitive self-help groups are demonstrably useful in preventing relapse. There is no way of predicting the type of drug user who will be helped by one or another of the many techniques now in use. However, those who have severe psychiatric difficulties tend to do poorly in almost every program, while those with the fewest problems and most skills and social assets do well in almost any program (McLellan *et al.,* 1983; Rounsaville *et al.,* 1987).

Voluntary Groups and Self-Regulatory Communities. Alcoholics Anonymous, Narcotics Anonymous, Phoenix House, Daytop Village, and similar groups have been helpful in the rehabilitation of certain types of compulsive drug users. Their efficacy may be due to a number of factors, including a reduction in the sense of isolation and a gratification of the need to belong. Equally important is the absence of a hard line between "patient" and "staff." The organizations are usually operated by former drug users, and the new member is immediately confronted by individuals who at once convey understanding and concern and provide role models for responsible behavior. Also important is the participation itself, which keeps the individual away from the environment in which drug use occurred and in the company of people who share concerns about drug use in a way that amounts to a ritualization of sobriety. Although a substantial proportion of treated alcoholics make contact with Alcoholics Anonymous at some point, it is not clear what proportion derive benefit. A more recent development is self-help groups that use cognitive approaches to prevention of relapse. Only a small percentage of compulsive opioid users seem motivated to seek admission to self-regulating residential centers; fewer still actually enter after learning what is expected of members, and many leave within weeks after joining. Those who remain in residential programs do well while they are members, and many continue to do well after they leave, provided they have stayed for more than a few months.

Supervisory–Deterrent Approaches. Some approaches that emphasize the maintenance of abstinence involve a period in a hospital, prison, or special facility followed by careful supervision of the individual in the community. If the chemical analysis of urine specimens or other body fluids or tissues indicates return to drug use, the supervisee, who has usually been paroled or civilly committed to the program, is reinstitutionalized. This appears to reduce the frequency of return to drug use among those who have been arrested or convicted of crimes. Similar to this approach are programs for professionals and employees who sign a binding contract that specifies that continued licensure or employment is contingent on abstinence as measured by urine or breath tests. In both of these situations, the deterrent effect of adverse consequences should drug use be detected is thought to be the critical element. Such an arrangement is believed to be an important factor in rehabilitating physicians who are impaired by use of drugs (Shore, 1987). In theory, this approach can be used with all types of drug abuse and dependence. Urine testing for drugs of abuse has become a highly sophisticated procedure with elaborate systems for tracking specimens and minimizing false positives. Although not fully standardized, analysis of hair samples can sometimes detect drugs for as long as several months after use (*see* Arnold, 1987).

Role of Pharmacological Agents Following Withdrawal. With every form of drug dependence, other drugs have been tried as therapeutic agents on a variety of theoretical grounds. Sometimes the therapeutic agents are directed at some postulated underlying psychological difficulty (*e.g.,* anxiety or depression) that is believed to contribute to the motivation to use the drug of dependence. Sometimes the therapeutic agent is intended to be a less toxic substitute, in whole or in part, for the effects of the drug being used, or at least to suppress any subclinical withdrawal phenomena (*e.g.*, oral or transdermal nicotine for inhaled tobacco; oral methadone, buprenorphine, or methadyl acetate for injected heroin). Some agents may be directed at drug-induced changes that contribute to craving following withdrawal. Other agents are intended to interfere in a variety of ways with the reinforcing or satisfying properties of the dependence-producing drug (*e.g.*, opioid antagonists), or to create situations where their use becomes unpleasant (*e.g.*, disulfiram).

Opioid Maintenance. Methadone maintenance was originally based on the hypothesis that, as a result of repeated use of opioids, the addict has sustained a metabolic alteration such that opioids produce a euphoria not experienced by nonaddicts, and that for months or years after withdrawal the addict experiences a feeling of abnormality (opioid hunger) relieved only by opioids. Since the original pilot studies of Dole and Nyswander, the use of this approach has been greatly expanded and the procedures and dosages have been substantially modified. Most commonly the procedure consists of the daily administration of 40 to 100 mg of methadone, orally in a flavored vehicle, combined with efforts at social rehabilitation. At the stabilization level (achieved by gradually increasing the dose over a period of several weeks), there is a high degree of cross-tolerance to all opioids so that the euphoric effects of even high doses of intravenous opioid are sharply diminished. While many patients report little or no craving for illicit opioids, in most treatment programs and under experimental conditions there are usually some patients who continue to seek out and use intravenous opioids despite the attenuated effects. Methadone does not prevent patients from experiencing the effects of alcohol, cocaine, or other nonopioids. Abuse of such drugs is a problem for some patients. Methadone maintenance explicitly emphasizes law-abiding behavior and abstinence from illicit opioids, rather than abstinence *per se*, and its relative efficacy in reaching its goals is well documented (*see* Simpson *et al.*, 1982). The methadone-maintenance approach is subject to special regulations. Despite its effectiveness in suppressing intravenous use of opioids, thereby substantially reducing the prevalence of HIV infection among those who stay in treatment (Ball *et al.*, 1988), it is still criticized by some as substituting one drug for another.

The duration of action of methadone is such that it need be given only once a day. Although the concentrations of methadone in plasma do change over the course of 24 hours (*see* Chapter 21), the decline is usually not sufficient to produce perceptible withdrawal phenomena in most patients. Therefore, the ingestion of all medication can be supervised by scheduled visits to the clinic. However, patients who take drugs that cause increased rates of methadone metabolism (*e.g.*, rifampin, phenobarbital, phenytoin) may have trough concentrations well below 100 ng/ml, even when they are maintained on doses of more than 100 mg of methadone per day. These patients may be unable to tolerate once-a-day dosing (Bell *et al.*, 1988). Patients who are employed, socially stable, and who require no support services have derived considerable benefit from experimental arrangements that permit them to obtain monthly supplies of methadone from private physicians (Novick *et al.*, 1988). How best to balance concern about the possibility of illicit diversion of methadone against the great burden of frequent visits to clinic remains controversial.

In one study of British addicts, new patients were randomly assigned to treatment with either intravenous heroin or oral methadone. After 1 year, those who had been given intravenous heroin were more likely to be in treatment at the clinic using prescribed intravenous drugs. Those originally assigned to oral methadone were more likely to have dropped out of treatment. Some of these dropouts stopped using opioids entirely, but a significant percentage was found to be using intravenous opioids obtained from the illicit drug traffic (Hartnoll *et al.*, 1980).

Concern about illicit diversion of methadone has led to efforts to develop longer-acting opioids for clinical use. One such drug is methadyl acetate (acetylmethadol), which suppresses opioid withdrawal for up to 72 hours after a single dose and, theoretically, all doses can be ingested under direct supervision when patients come to the clinic three times per week. In clinical trials it appears to be similar to methadone in its overall effects. Methadyl acetate is still an investigational drug.

Buprenorphine, a partial μ-opioid agonist (*see* Chapter 21), may be a useful alternative to methadone or methadyl acetate for maintenance purposes. It markedly attenuates the subjective effects of large doses of morphine; in laboratory settings, addicts given buprenorphine sharply decrease self-administration of intravenous heroin (Mello and Mendelson, 1980). Although buprenorphine produces morphine-like subjective effects and respiratory depression at low doses, higher doses do not cause correspondingly more intense respiratory depression (Jasinski *et al.*, 1978). After several weeks of sublingual administration of 4 to 8 mg per day, abrupt discontinuation of buprenorphine produces withdrawal symptoms that are gradual in onset and not very severe. For some patients, it may be possible to administer buprenorphine every 48 hours. Because it is a partial agonist, it is possible to substitute buprenorphine for low doses of methadone or heroin without precipitating severe withdrawal symptoms.

Opioid Antagonists. When the opioid receptors in the CNS are continuously occupied by antagonists, the effects of ordinary doses of opioids are attenuated or entirely blocked, and even the repeated administration of opioids for several weeks does not induce a significant degree of physical dependence.

Theoretically, the use of sufficiently high doses of opioid antagonists might help prevent reinforcement of drug taking and reinitiation of physical dependence. Prevention of the development of physical dependence in ambulatory patients may be of considerable value in that it may stop occasional illicit use from progressing quickly into regular and compulsive use. The patient who takes an antagonist behaves as if opioids are, for practical purposes, unavailable. This serves to decrease craving (Meyer and Mirin, 1979). Patients must first be withdrawn from opioids, since antagonists precipitate severe abstinence symptoms in individuals who are physically dependent.

Naltrexone is orally effective, seems relatively free of side effects, and, depending on the dose, can produce receptor blockade for more than 24 hours. Given orally at doses of 50 mg per day, it provides almost continuous blockade of the subjective effects of exogenous opioids. However, few patients continue to take naltrexone for more than 30 to 60 days. A few investigators have noted that the large doses commonly used produce subtle aversive side effects (*e.g.*, loss of energy) that could contribute to patients' reluctance to continue taking the drug. Experienced clinicians believe that naltrexone is useful for selected patients during the immediate period after withdrawal (*see* Gonzales and Brogden, 1988). Techniques for rapid initiation of treatment with naltrexone are discussed above.

Cocaine and Amphetamine Dependence. Several pharmacological agents have been tried as adjuncts for the treatment of cocaine dependence. For example, on the assumption that the anhedonia and craving are related to depletion of dopamine or desensitization of dopaminergic reward systems, there have been clinical trials of levodopa, dopaminergic agonists such as bromocriptine, and amantadine. Although there have been reports of a decrease in craving during acute phases of withdrawal, the effects have been neither robust nor reliably replicated.

Currently, the pharmacological approach that produces the most consistent effect is the use of tricyclic antidepressants such as desipramine. After a lag time of 1 to 2 weeks, desipramine (in doses that approach those used for the treatment of depression) appears to reduce craving for cocaine and to increase the number of ambulatory patients who can abstain from cocaine for several weeks. However, the drop-out rate is high, and little information is available on the drug-using behavior of the subjects after completion of treatment. The mechanism of this salutary effect is uncertain. It is postulated that antidepressants increase functional activity in reward systems by altering cocaine-induced supersensitivity at dopaminergic autoreceptors. Low doses of flupentixol are also postulated to reduce craving for cocaine by blocking these autoreceptors (Gawin and Ellinwood, 1988; Gawin *et al.*, 1989a, 1989b).

Pharmacotherapy for amphetamine dependence has received less systematic attention, although some clinical trials suggest that tricyclic antidepressants alleviate craving and anhedonia. However, the dopaminergic neurotoxicity that can result from abuse of high doses of amphetamine may compromise therapy.

Other Pharmacological Procedures. Maintenance approaches for compulsive users of ethanol, other general CNS depressants, and benzodiazepines do not appear to hold great promise. With the exception of those few patients who function well while taking small doses of such drugs and do poorly when withdrawn, most practitioners strive for total withdrawal. For the very heavy smoker, nicotine in the form of chewing gum appears to have value in alleviating withdrawal and reducing the probability of relapse to smoking (Surgeon General, 1988; Tønnesen *et al.*, 1988). In some cases, former smokers use the gum over many months as a less toxic substitute for nicotine inhaled in tobacco smoke (*see* above). Nicotine-containing nasal sprays and transdermal patches are under investigation. Clonidine has been reported to reduce craving for tobacco in some smokers (Glassman *et al.*, 1988).

Disulfiram and related agents have been used in the treatment of alcoholism for a number of years. When an individual who has been taking disulfiram ingests alcohol, a syndrome characterized by nausea, vomiting, flushing and hypotension, anxiety, and palpitations develops within minutes. The details of the administration and the potential hazards of disulfiram and related agents are discussed in Chapter 17. Disulfiram can be administered only with the patient's cooperation and, therefore, is useful only for selected patients. Other factors being equal, patients who take disulfiram relapse less rapidly than those who do not. The major factor associated with total abstinence appears to be compliance or the willingness to ingest the disulfiram, rather than its capacity to produce an aversive reaction (Fuller *et al.*, 1986). Although depot forms of disulfiram have been employed, there is little evidence that they yield effective plasma concentrations of the drug (*see* Kranzler and Orrok, 1989).

Conditioned aversion techniques have been tried in alcoholism, smoking, and other forms of drug abuse. This technique usually involves the administration of an emetic agent (apomorphine or ipecac), followed shortly thereafter by a dose of the drug (*e.g.*, a small amount of whisky or other agent) so that nausea and vomiting occur soon after the drug is ingested. In this way, the taking of alcohol or the drug of abuse becomes a conditioned stimulus that produces a sensation of nausea. Enthusiasm for the aversion techniques in the treatment of alcoholism has declined as their limitations have become clearer. However, there is a renewed interest in the use of apomorphine in subemetic doses as a dopaminergic agonist that reduces anxiety and craving for alcohol, and several optimistic clinical reports have been published (*see* Kranzler and Orrok,

1989). When smokers are encouraged to inhale more smoke than they are accustomed to, the smoke becomes aversive. This technique has been used in treatment with some reported success.

Drug Treatment of Postwithdrawal Mental Disturbances. As noted previously, the majority of alcoholics and opioid-dependent patients have diagnosable disorders in addition to drug dependence. The most common are various forms of depression, antisocial personality, anxiety disorders, alcoholism in opioid addicts, and drug dependence (usually involving sedatives, stimulants, or opioids) in alcoholics (Rounsaville *et al.*, 1982; Hesselbrock *et al.*, 1985). Depressive states, unstable mood, and insomnia are common during the months immediately following withdrawal of either alcohol or opioids. Some smokers with histories of depression may experience an increase in depressive symptoms when they try to quit. Because of the risk of dependence, most practitioners avoid the use of benzodiazepines or other sedatives in the management of alcoholism or other types of drug dependence. In alcoholics who experience anxiety following withdrawal, buspirone and β-adrenergic blockers are reported to reduce both anxiety and termination of treatment (*see* Kranzler and Orrok, 1989). Although patients who abstain from the use of illicit drugs commonly experience some spontaneous improvement in mood, a significant percentage report persistent depression. Tricyclic antidepressants are frequently prescribed, but evidence for their efficacy is scant (*see* Jaffe and Ciraulo, 1984; Kranzler and Orrok, 1989). Lithium has been reported to increase the likelihood of abstinence and reduce the incidence of relapse in some alcoholics, but it is uncertain which alcoholics are most likely to benefit; the effect does not appear to be related to the antidepressant actions of lithium. As with disulfiram, compliance with treatment is the best predictor of abstinence (Clark and Fawcett, 1989).

Role of the Medical Profession in Prevention

Since there is a relationship between the availability of certain drugs and the prevalence of their self-administration, all modern nations regulate the manufacture, prescription, and dispensing of those drugs considered to have a liability for abuse. The development of reasonable regulations requires efforts in several areas, including (1) methods for assessing the likelihood that a particular drug will be self-administered; (2) guidelines for classifying drugs in order to provide for different degrees of control at the levels of manufacturing, prescribing, and dispensing; and (3) general guidelines for medical practitioners who must prescribe these drugs for patients. The use of drugs with potential for abuse in the treatment of compulsive drug users creates special problems because of the belief that such individuals are particularly likely to sell or give some of their prescribed medication to others. There is also a belief that prescribing such drugs for drug abusers may aggravate and prolong the dependence syndrome.

Addicting and Nonaddicting Drugs: Assessing Liability for Abuse. Evaluation of the likelihood that a given drug will produce effects that might lead to its abuse is accomplished by determining whether animals will administer the new drug to themselves and how many properties it shares in animals and drug-experienced volunteers with prototypical drugs known to be abused. Both of these approaches have limitations. For example, animals do not self-administer psychedelics or Δ^9-THC, but they will self-administer caffeine, procaine, and clonidine.

With the availability of opioids that do not act principally at μ receptors, the assessment of abuse liability has become more complex. In general, a drug is considered to be nonopioid with respect to liability for abuse if (1) it does not suppress the μ-agonist opioid withdrawal syndrome when tested in subjects physically dependent on morphine, (2) it does not produce morphine-like physical dependence when given chronically, and (3) postaddicts neither consistently identify it as "dope" (morphine-like) nor repeatedly request it when offered the opportunity to do so. If a compound is found to share all these key characteristics with morphine, it is considered to have a high liability for abuse and is recommended for controls comparable to those applied to morphine-like drugs. However, some drugs share a few characteristics but not others. For example, drugs such as nalbuphine, butorphanol, buprenorphine, and loperamide may be somewhat morphine-like with respect to one or two characteristics; however, because of differences in solubility or toxicity or because they appear to exhibit a ceiling effect in inducing euphoria, they are considered to present a lower order of risk. Such agents may be recommended for less stringent controls than those applied to the prototypical morphine-like opioids. New drugs that have pharmacological actions similar to those of amphetamines, benzodiazepines, general CNS depressants, or cannabinoids are now required to be evaluated for potential for abuse prior to marketing for general use. The procedures for assessing potential for abuse have been summarized by Brady and Lukas (1984).

Treating the Compulsive Drug User. In the United States, the effort to control drug availability previously included severe restrictions on the use of opioids and certain other controlled drugs in the treatment of compulsive drug users. Musto (1988) has documented the history of the interactions between the medical profession and regulatory authorities. This situation has changed substantially since 1970, and opioids are now used both for easing withdrawal and for maintenance. However, it is likely that changes will continue to be made in laws and rules as practitioners and regulators strive for a balance between flexibility for treatment and control of illicit diversion. At present, continued administration of opioids to patients with chronic, incurable, and painful conditions is not considered "maintenance of an addiction" and, although the practice varies from state to state, such individuals are not generally reported to health authorities as opioid addicts.

The treatment of compulsive opioid users who do not have an obvious medical problem is more complicated. Methadone and similar drugs for both the ambulatory withdrawal and maintenance treatment of heroin addiction are now used in the treatment of more than 80,000 individuals at several hundred separate centers throughout the United States, as well as in several European countries. Federal and some state governments have promulgated regulations that legitimize the use of methadone, but at the same time attempt to minimize the amount of take-home medication permitted in such programs and to reduce the likelihood that patients will obtain methadone from more than one source. It is still medically appropriate to administer an opioid to relieve acute withdrawal symptoms. However, it is expected that, where there are nearby specialized detoxification or maintenance programs, the patient will be referred to these specialized facilities. The use of opioid maintenance is restricted to specially licensed centers and to clinicians affiliated with them. Interested clinicians should contact the appropriate state and federal agencies for current regulations.

Thus far no specific regulations or constraints at the federal level prohibit the use of CNS stimulants or depressants in the treatment of compulsive users of nonopioid drugs. However, with a few exceptions, long-term maintenance on these drugs is of little benefit to the patient, and a number of state medical boards have taken disciplinary actions against physicians who were too casual in prescribing CNS depressants and stimulants for purposes other than the traditional. Similar sanctions have not been applied to those who prescribe benzodiazepines for patients who became physically dependent during the course of treatment for anxiety.

In practice, the physician must often administer opioids or sedatives even to persons who seem predisposed to develop dependence on such drugs. There are a few general rules applicable to opioids that, if followed in all cases, will reduce, but obviously not eliminate, the probability of such a complication. The patient should not be given an opioid when another drug of lower potential for abuse will suffice. The use of agonist–antagonists may be less risky when problems are anticipated. The patient who is not terminally ill should not be permitted to self-administer such drugs parenterally as an outpatient. Only a few days' supply should be dispensed at any given time, and a return to nonopioids should be undertaken as soon as the situation permits. If the drug has been administered repeatedly for more than a few weeks, a change to a long-acting drug a few days prior to discontinuation will minimize withdrawal symptomatology. On the other hand, the tendency to avoid the use of opioid analgesics should not be carried to unwarranted extremes; the patient who needs a potent analgesic should not be left in pain because of the physician's fear of causing addiction.

Drugs given for the relief of fluctuating levels of pain, anxiety, or feelings of depression can be taken in several ways. They can be requested or taken by the patient each time the distress becomes too intense to tolerate—that is, for relief of distress, or they can be taken in anticipation of the recurrence of distress—that is, to avoid distress. With respect to inducing drug dependence, both ways carry risks. When used for relief, minimal amounts of drug will be used, since the time of drug action will correspond to the time when its action is required. In theory, however, each time relief is promptly obtained, the act of self-administration of the drug will be reinforced. Prescribing drugs with slower onset and longer duration of action may minimize this reinforcement process, but the likelihood of physical dependence is not reduced. Self-administration to avoid distress may be less reinforcing of each drug-taking act, but the patient never waits long enough to find out whether the drug is needed at all. Even the idea of discontinuing may cause anticipation of the return of distress. From a pharmacological viewpoint, the avoidance schedule leads to the regular and frequent use of unnecessary amounts of drug. Although there are no easy solutions to this therapeutic dilemma, the physician should be aware of the factors that may be operative. In both postoperative and terminally ill patients who do not have histories of drug abuse, self-administration of opioids for relief of pain does not appear to be associated with a higher incidence of drug dependence. The low incidence of problems may reflect either patient selection or some difference between relief of pain and relief of other aversive affects as reinforcers. In the case of patients who are terminally ill, opioid drugs should be given to prevent the recurrence of pain, rather than "as needed" (*see* Chapter 21). Less drug is needed when it is given before pain becomes intense. Concerns about physical dependence in such cases should be secondary.

A final caveat is in order. Physicians and other health care professionals with easy access to potent drugs are at relatively high risk for developing drug dependence (Murray, 1978; McAuliffe *et al.*, 1986). Health care professionals would do well to remember this, not only when treating patients but also whenever they consider treating themselves.

Aghajanian, G. K., and Wang, Y. Y. Common α_2- and opiate-effector mechanisms in the locus coeruleus: intracellular studies in brain slices. *Neuropharmacology*, **1987**, *26*, 793–799.

Ambre, J. J.; Belknap, S. M.; Nelson, J.; Ruo, T. I.; Shin, S.-G.; and Atkinson, A. J., Jr. Acute tolerance to cocaine in humans. *Clin. Pharmacol. Ther.*, **1988**, *44*, 1–8.

Andreasson, S.; Allebeck, P.; Engstrom, A.; and Rydberg, U. Cannabis and schizophrenia: a longitudinal study of Swedish conscripts. *Lancet*, **1987**, *2*, 1483–1486.

Anglin, M. D.; McGlothlin, W. H.; and Speckart, G. The effect of parole on methadone patient behavior. *Am. J. Drug Alcohol Abuse*, **1981**, *8*, 153–170.

Arnold, W. Radioimmunological hair analysis for narcotics and substitutes. *J. Clin. Chem. Clin. Biochem.*, **1987**, *25*, 753–757.

Ball, J. C.; Lange, W. R.; Myers, C. P.; and Friedman, S. R. Reducing the risk of AIDS through methadone maintenance treatment. *J. Health Soc. Behav.*, **1988**, *29*, 214–226.

Barry, J.; Mead, K.; Nabel, E. G.; Rocco, M. B.; Campbell, S.; Fenton, T.; Mudge, G. H., Jr.; and Selwyn, A. Effect of smoking on the activity of ischemic heart disease. *J.A.M.A.*, **1989**, *3*, 398–401.

Battaglia, G.; Yeh, S. Y.; O'Hearn, E.; Molliver, M. E.; Kuhar, M. J.; and De Souza, E. B. 3,4-Methylenedioxymethamphetamine and 3,4-methylenedioxyamphetamine destroy serotonin terminals in rat brain: quantification of neurodegeneration by measurement of [^{3}H]paroxetine-labeled serotonin uptake sites. *J. Pharmacol. Exp. Ther.*, **1987**, *242*, 911–916.

Bell, J.; Seres, V.; Bowron, P.; Lewis, J.; and Batey, R. The use of serum methadone levels in patients receiving methadone maintenance. *Clin. Pharmacol. Ther.*, **1988**, *43*, 623–629.

Benowitz, N. L.; Porchet, H.; Sheiner, L.; and Jacob, P., III. Nicotine absorption and cardiovascular effects with smokeless tobacco use: comparison with cigarettes and nicotine gum. *Clin. Pharmacol. Ther.*, **1988**, *44*, 23–28.

Bickel, W. K.; Stitzer, M. L.; Bigelow, G. E.; Liebson, I. A.; Jasinski, D. R.; and Johnson, R. E. Buprenorphine: dose-related blockade of opioid challenge effects in opioid dependent subjects. *J. Pharmacol. Exp. Ther.*, **1988**, *247*, 47–53.

Buckholtz, N. L.; Zhou, D. F.; and Freedman, D. X. Serotonin$_2$ agonist administration down-regulates rat brain serotonin$_2$ receptors. *Life Sci.*, **1988**, *42*, 2439–2445.

Busto, U.; Sellers, E. M.; Naranjo, C. A.; Cappell, H.; Sanchez-Craig, M.; and Sykora, K. Withdrawal reaction after long-term therapeutic use of benzodiazepines. *N. Engl. J. Med.*, **1986**, *313*, 854–859.

Charney, D. S.; Heninger, G. R.; and Kelber, H. D. The combined use of clonidine and naltrexone as a rapid, safe, and effective treatment of abrupt withdrawal from methadone. *Am. J. Psychiatry*, **1986**, *143*, 831–837.

Chasnoff, I. J.; Hunt, C. E.; and Kaplan, D. Prenatal cocaine exposure is associated with respiratory pattern abnormalities. *Am. J. Dis. Child.*, **1989**, *143*, 583–587.

Childress, A. R.; McLellan, A. T.; and O'Brien, C. P. Abstinent opiate abusers exhibit conditioned craving, conditioned withdrawal, and reductions in both through extinction. *Br. J. Addict.*, **1986**, *81*, 701–706.

Christie, M. J.; Williams, J. T.; and North, R. A. Cellular mechanisms of opioid tolerance: studies in single brain neurons. *Mol. Pharmacol.*, **1987**, *32*, 633–638.

Ciraulo, D. A.; Barnhill, J. G.; Greenblatt, D. J.; Shader, R. I.; Ciraulo, A. M.; Tarmey, M. F.; Molloy, M. A.; and Foti, M. E. Abuse liability and clinical pharmacokinetics of alprazolam in alcoholic men. *J. Clin. Psychiatry*, **1988**, *49*, 333–337.

Cone, E. J., and Weddington, W. W., Jr. Prolonged occurrence of cocaine in human saliva and urine after chronic use. *J. Anal. Toxicol.*, **1989**, *13*, 65–68.

Cushman, P., and Dole, V. P. Detoxification of rehabilitated methadone-maintained patients. *J.A.M.A.*, **1973**, *226*, 747–752.

Dax, E. M.; Nagel, J. E.; Lange, W. R.; Adler, W. H.; and Jaffe, J. H. Effects of nitrites on the immune system of humans. *Natl. Inst. Drug Abuse Res. Monogr. Ser.*, **1988**, *83*, 75–80.

Duman, R. S.; Tallman, J. F.; and Nestler, E. J. Acute and chronic opiate-regulation of adenylate cyclase in brain: specific effects in locus coeruleus. *J. Pharmacol. Exp. Ther.*, **1988**, *246*, 1033–1039.

Dunwiddie, T. V., and Alford, C. Electrophysiological actions of phencyclidine in hippocampal slices from the rat. *Neuropharmacology*, **1987**, *26*, 1267–1273.

Fielding, J. E., and Phenow, K. J. Health effects of involuntary smoking. *N. Engl. J. Med.*, **1988**, *319*, 1452–1460.

Fischman, M. W., and Schuster, C. R. Cocaine self-administration in humans. *Fed. Proc.*, **1982**, *41*, 241–246.

Freedman, D. X. The use and abuse of LSD. *Arch. Gen. Psychiatry*, **1968**, *18*, 300–347.

Fuller, R. K., and others. Disulfiram treatment of alcoholism. A Veterans Administration cooperative study. *J.A.M.A.*, **1986**, *256*, 1449–1455.

Gawin, F. H.; Allen, D.; and Humblestone, B. Outpatient treatment of "crack" cocaine smoking with flupenthixol decanoate: a preliminary report. *Arch. Gen. Psychiatry*, **1989a**, *46*, 322–325.

Gawin, F. H.; Kleber, H. D.; Byck, R.; Rounsaville, B. J.; Kosten, T. R.; Jatlow, P. I.; and Morgan, C. Desipramine facilitation of initial cocaine abstinence. *Arch. Gen. Psychiatry*, **1989b**, *46*, 117–121.

Giannini, A. J.; Loiselle, R. H.; DiMarzio, L. E.; and Giannini, M. C. Augmentation of haloperidol by ascorbic acid in phencyclidine intoxication. *Am. J. Psychiatry*, **1987**, *144*, 1207–1209.

Glassman, A. H.; Stetner, F.; Walsh, B. T.; Raizman, P. S.; Fleiss, J. L.; Cooper, T. B.; and Covey, L. S. Heavy smokers, smoking cessation, and clonidine. Results of a double-blind, randomized trial. *J.A.M.A.*, **1988**, *259*, 2863–2866.

Gossop, M.; Johns, A.; and Green, L. Opiate withdrawal: inpatient versus outpatient programmes and preferred versus random assignment to treatment. *Br. Med. J.*, **1986**, *293*, 103–104.

Griffiths, R. R.; Bigelow, G. E.; and Liebson, E. Differential effects of diazepam and pentobarbital on mood and behavior. *Arch. Gen. Psychiatry*, **1983**, *40*, 865–873.

Griffiths, R. R.; Brady, J. V.; and Snell, J. D. Progressive-ratio performance maintained by drug infusions: comparison of cocaine, diethylpropion, chlorphentermine, and fenfluramine. *Psychopharmacology*, **1978**, *56*, 5–13.

Hartnoll, R. L.; Mitcheson, M. C.; Battersby, A.; Brown, G.; Ellis, M.; Fleming, P.; and Hedley, N. Evaluation of heroin maintenance in controlled trial. *Arch. Gen. Psychiatry*, **1980**, *37*, 877–884.

Hayashida, M.; Alterman, A. I.; McLellan, T. A.; O'Brien, C. P.; Purtill, J. J.; Volpicelli, J. R.; Raphaelson, A. H.; and Hall, C. P. Comparative effectiveness and costs of inpatient and outpatient detoxification of patients with mild-to-moderate alcohol withdrawal syndrome. *N. Engl. J. Med.*, **1989**, *320*, 358–366.

Heishman, S. J.; Stitzer, M. L.; Bigelow, G. E.; and Liebson, I. A. Acute opioid physical dependence in postaddict humans: naloxone dose effects after brief morphine exposure. *J. Pharmacol. Exp. Ther.*, **1989**, *248*, 127–134.

Henningfield, J. E.; Miyasato, K.; and Jasinski, D. R. Cigarette smokers self-administer intravenous nicotine. *Pharmacol. Biochem. Behav.*, **1983**, *19*, 887–890.

Hernandez, L.; Auerbach, S.; and Hoebel, B. G. Phencyclidine (PCP) injected in the nucleus accumbens increases extracellular dopamine and serotonin as measured by microdialysis. *Life Sci.*, **1988**, *42*, 1713–1723.

Hernandez, L., and Hoebel, B. G. Food reward and cocaine increase extracellular dopamine in the nucleus accumbens as measured by microdialysis. *Life Sci.*, **1988**, *42*, 1705–1712.

Hesselbrock, M.; Meyer, R.; and Keener, J. Psychopathology in hospitalized alcoholics. *Arch. Gen. Psychiatry,* **1985,** *42,* 1050–1055.

Hughes, J. R.; Hatsukami, D. K.; Pickens, R. W.; Krahn, D.; Malin, S.; and Luknic, A. Effect of nicotine on the tobacco withdrawal syndrome. *Psychopharmacology,* **1984,** *83,* 82–87.

Isner, J. M.; Estes, N. A. M., III; Thompson, P. D.; Costanzo-Nordin, M. R.; Subramanian, R.; Miller, G.; Katsas, G.; Sweeney, K.; and Sturner, W. Q. Acute cardiac events temporally related to cocaine abuse. *N. Engl. J. Med.,* **1986,** *315,* 1438–1443.

Jasinski, D. R.; Pevnick, J. S.; and Griffith, J. D. Human pharmacology and abuse potential of the analgesic buprenorphine. *Arch. Gen. Psychiatry,* **1978,** *35,* 501–516.

Jeffcoat, A. R.; Perez-Reyes, M.; Hill, J. M.; Sadler, B. M.; and Cook, C. E. Cocaine disposition in humans after intravenous injection, nasal insufflation (snorting), or smoking. *Drug Metab. Dispos.,* **1989,** *17,* 153–159.

Johansson, E.; Agurell, S.; Hollister, L. E.; and Halldin, M. M. Prolonged apparent half-life of Δ1-tetrahydrocannabinol in plasma of chronic marijuana users. *J. Pharm. Pharmacol.,* **1988,** *40,* 374–375.

Jones, R. T.; Benowitz, N.; and Bachman, J. Clinical studies of cannabis tolerance and dependence. *Ann. N.Y. Acad. Sci.,* **1976,** *282,* 221–239.

Judson, B. A.; Goldstein, A.; and Inturrisi, C. E. Methadyl acetate (LAAM) in the treatment of heroin addicts. *Arch. Gen. Psychiatry,* **1983,** *40,* 834–840.

Kalivas, P. W.; Duffy, P.; DuMars, L. A.; and Skinner, C. Behavioral and neurochemical effects of acute and daily cocaine administration in rats. *J. Pharmacol. Exp. Ther.,* **1988,** *245,* 485–492.

Kalivas, P. W., and Weber, B. Amphetamine injection into the ventral mesencephalon sensitizes rats to peripheral amphetamine and cocaine. *J. Pharmacol. Exp. Ther.,* **1988,** *245,* 1095–1102.

Kalix, P. The releasing effect of the isomers of the alkaloid cathinone at central and peripheral catecholamine storage sites. *Neuropharmacology,* **1986,** *25,* 499–501.

Kandel, D. B.; Davies, M.; Karus, D.; and Yamaguchi, K. The consequences in young adulthood of adolescent drug involvement. *Arch. Gen. Psychiatry,* **1986,** *43,* 746–754.

Kandel, D. B., and Raveis, V. H. Cessation of illicit drug use in young adulthood. *Arch. Gen. Psychiatry,* **1989,** *46,* 109–116.

Kornetsky, C.; Esposito, R. U.; McLean, S.; and Jacobson, J. O. Intracranial self-stimulation thresholds. *Arch. Gen. Psychiatry,* **1979,** *36,* 289–292.

Lamb, R. J., and Griffiths, R. R. Self-injection of d, 1-3, 4-methylenedioxymethamphetamine (MDMA) in the baboon. *Psychopharmacology (Berlin),* **1987,** *91,* 268–272.

Lathers, C. M.; Tyau, L. S. Y.; Spino, M. M.; and Agarwal, I. Cocaine-induced seizures, arrhythmias and sudden death. *J. Clin. Pharmacol.,* **1988,** *28,* 584–593.

Leccese, A. P.; Marquis, K. L.; Mattia, A.; and Moreton, J. E. The anticonvulsant and behavioral effects of phencyclidine and ketamine following chronic treatment in rats. *Behav. Brain Res.,* **1986,** *22,* 257–264.

Li, T. K. Studies of mechanisms of aberrant alcohol-seeking behavior in an animal model. In, *Alcoholism: Origins and Outcome.* (Rose, R. M., and Barrett, J., eds.) Raven Press, New York, **1988,** pp. 209–218.

Louie, A. K.; Lannon, R. A.; and Ketter, T. A. Treatment of cocaine-induced panic disorder. *Am. J. Psychiatry,* **1989,** *146,* 40–44.

McAuliffe, W. E., and Ch'ien, J. M. N. Recovery training and self help: a relapse-prevention program for treated opiate addicts. *J. Subst. Abuse Treat.,* **1986,** *3,* 9–20.

McAuliffe, W. E.; Rohman, M.; Santangelo, S.; Feldman, B.; Magnuson, E.; Sobol, A.; and Weissman, J. Psychoactive drug use among practicing physicians and medical students. *N. Engl. J. Med.,* **1986,** *315,* 805–810.

McKenna, D. J.; Nazarali, A. J.; Hoffman, A. J.; Nichols, D. E.; Mathis, C. A.; and Saavedra, J. M. Common receptors for hallucinogens in rat brain: a comparative autoradiographic study using [^{125}I]LSD and [^{125}I]DOI, a new psychotomimetic radioligand. *Brain Res.,* **1989,** *476,* 45–56.

McLellan, A. T.; Luborsky, L.; Woody, G. E.; O'Brien, C. P.; and Druley, K. E. Predicting response to alcohol and drug abuse treatments. *Arch. Gen. Psychiatry,* **1983,** *40,* 620–625.

Martin, W. R.; Jasinski, D. R.; Haertzen, C. A.; Kay, D. C.; Jones, B. E.; Mansky, P. A.; and Carpenter, R. W. Methadone—a reevaluation. *Arch. Gen. Psychiatry,* **1973,** *28,* 286–295.

Martin, W. R.; Vaupel, D. B.; Nozaki, M.; and Bright, L. D. The identification of LSD-like hallucinogens using the chronic spinal dog. *Drug Alcohol Depend.,* **1978,** *3,* 113–123.

Mello, N. K., and Mendelson, J. H. Buprenorphine suppresses heroin use by heroin addicts. *Science,* **1980,** *207,* 657–659.

Mendelson, J. H.; Mello, N. K.; Ellingboe, J.; Skupny, A. S. T.; Lex, B. W.; and Griffin, M. Marihuana smoking suppresses luteinizing hormone in women. *J. Pharmacol. Exp. Ther.,* **1986,** *237,* 862–866.

Mody, C. K.; Miller, B. L.; McIntyre, H. B.; Cobb, S. K.; and Goldberg, M. A. Neurologic complications of cocaine abuse. *Neurology,* **1988,** *38,* 1189–1193.

Morris, B. J.; Millan, M. J.; and Herz, A. Antagonist-induced opioid receptor up-regulation. II. Regionally specific modulation of mu, delta and kappa binding sites in rat brain revealed by quantitative autoradiography. *J. Pharmacol. Exp. Ther.,* **1988,** *247,* 729–736.

Murray, R. M. The health of doctors: a review. *J. R. Coll. Physicians Lond.,* **1978,** *12,* 403–415.

Nabeshima, T.; Fukaya, H.; Yamaguchi, K.; Ishikawa, K.; Furukawa, H.; and Kameyama, T. Development of tolerance and supersensitivity to phencyclidine in rats after repeated administration of phencyclidine. *Eur. J. Pharmacol.,* **1987,** *135,* 23–33.

Ng, S. K. C.; Hauser, W. A.; Brust, J. C. M.; and Susser, M. Alcohol consumption and withdrawal in new-onset seizures. *N. Engl. J. Med.,* **1988,** *319,* 666–673.

Novick, D.; Joseph, H.; Richman, B.; Salsitz, E.; Pascarelli, E.; Des Jarlais, D.; Dole, V.; and Nyswander, M. Medical maintenance: a new model for continuing treatment of socially rehabilitated methadone maintenance patients. *J.A.M.A.,* **1988,** *259,* 3299–3302.

Nurco, D. N.; Kinlock, T. W.; Hanlon, T. E.; and Ball, J. C. Non-narcotic drug use over an addiction career—a study of heroin addicts in Baltimore and New York City. *Compr. Psychiatry,* **1988,** *29,* 450–459.

O'Brien, C. P.; Childress, A. R.; Arndt, I. O.; McLellan, T.; Woody, G. E.; and Maany, I. Pharmacological and behavioral treatment of cocaine dependence: controlled studies. *J. Clin. Psychiatry,* **1988,** *49,* 17–22.

Okamoto, M.; Boisse, N. R.; Rosenberg, H. C.; and Rosen, R. Characteristics of functional tolerance during barbiturate physical dependency production. *J. Pharmacol. Exp. Ther.,* **1978,** *207,* 906–915.

Pellegrini-Giampietro, D. E.; Bacciottini, L.; Carla, V.; and Moroni, F. Morphine withdrawal in cortical slices: suppression by $Ca2^{+}$-channel inhibitors of abstinence-induced [^{3}H]-noradrenaline release. *Br. J. Pharmacol.,* **1988,** *93,* 535–540.

Perez-Reyes, M.; Di Guiseppi, S.; Ondrusek, G.; Jeffcoat, A. R.; and Cook, C. E. Free-base cocaine smoking. *Clin. Pharmacol. Ther.,* **1982,** *32,* 459–465.

Perkins, K. A.; Epstein, L. H.; Marks, B. L.; Stiller, R. L.; and Jacob, R. G. The effect of nicotine on energy expenditure during light physical activity. *N. Engl. J. Med.*, **1989**, *320*, 898–903.

Peroutka, S. J.; Newman, H.; and Harris, H. Subjective effects of 3,4-methylenedioxymethamphetamine in recreational users. *Neuropsychopharmacology*, **1988**, *1*, 273–278.

Pierce, P. A., and Peroutka, S. J. Antagonism of 5-hydroxytryptamine$_2$ receptor-mediated phosphatidylinositol turnover by *d*-lysergic acid diethylamide. *J. Pharmacol. Exp. Ther.*, **1988**, *247*, 918–925.

Raftery, E. B. Cardiovascular drug withdrawal syndromes. A potential problem with calcium antagonists? *Drugs*, **1984**, *28*, 371–374.

Rasmussen, K., and Aghajanian, G. K. Effect of hallucinogens on spontaneous and sensory-evoked locus coeruleus unit activity in the rat: reversal by selective 5-HT$_2$ antagonists. *Brain Res.*, **1986**, *385*, 395–400.

———. Potency of antipsychotics in reversing the effects of a hallucinogenic drug on locus coeruleus neurons correlates with 5-HT$_2$ binding affinity. *Neuropsychopharmacology*, **1988**, *1*, 101–107.

Reichman, M.; Nen, W.; and Hokin, L. E. Δ^9-Tetrahydrocannabinol increases arachidonic acid levels in guinea pig cerebral cortex slices. *Mol. Pharmacol.*, **1988**, *34*, 823–828.

Ritz, M. C., and Kuhar, M. J. Relationship between self-administration of amphetamine and monoamine receptors in brain; comparison with cocaine. *J. Pharmacol. Exp. Ther.*, **1989**, *248*, 1010–1017.

Ritz, M. C.; Lamb, R. J.; Goldberg, S. R.; and Kuhar, M. J. Cocaine receptors on dopamine transporters are related to self administration of cocaine. *Science*, **1987**, *237*, 1219–1223.

Robinson, G. M.; Sellers, E. M.; and Janecek, E. Barbiturate and hypnosedative withdrawal by a multiple oral phenobarbital loading dose technique. *Clin. Pharmacol. Ther.*, **1981**, *30*, 71–76.

Rosenberg, H. C., and Okamoto, M. Loss of inhibition in the spinal cord during barbiturate withdrawal. *J. Pharmacol. Exp. Ther.*, **1978**, *205*, 563–568.

Rosenberg, N. L.; Kleinschmidt-DeMasters, B. K.; Davis, K. A.; Dreisbach, J. N.; Hormes, J. T.; and Filley, C. M. Toluene abuse causes diffuse central nervous system white matter changes. *Ann. Neurol.*, **1988**, *23*, 611–614.

Roth, D.; Alarcon, F. J.; Fernandez, J. A.; Preston, R. A.; and Bourgoignie, J. J. Acute rhabdomyolysis associated with cocaine intoxication. *N. Engl. J. Med.*, **1988**, *319*, 673–677.

Rounsaville, B. J.; Dolinsky, Z. S.; Babor, T. F.; and Meyer, R. E. Psychopathology as a predictor of treatment outcome in alcoholics. *Arch. Gen. Psychiatry*, **1987**, *44*, 505–513.

Rounsaville, B. J.; Weissman, M. M.; Kleber, H.; and Wilber, C. Heterogeneity of psychiatric diagnosis in treated opiate addicts. *Arch. Gen. Psychiatry*, **1982**, *39*, 161–166.

Sanchez-Craig, M.; Cappell, H.; Busto, U.; and Kay, G. Cognitive-behavioural treatment for benzodiazepine dependence: a comparison of gradual versus abrupt cessation of drug intake. *Br. J. Addict.*, **1987**, *82*, 1317–1327.

Sanders-Bush, E.; Burris, K. D.; and Knoth, K. Lysergic acid diethylamide and 2,5-dimethoxy-4-methylamphetamine are partial agonists at serotonin receptors linked to phosphoinositide hydrolysis. *J. Pharmacol. Exp. Ther.*, **1988**, *246*, 924–928.

Sellers, E. M., and Busto, U. Benzodiazepines and ethanol: assessment of the effects and consequences of psychotropic drug interactions. *J. Clin. Psychopharmacol.*, **1982**, *2*, 249–262.

Sellers, E. M.; Naranjo, C. A.; Harrison, M.; Devenyi, P.; Roach, C.; and Sykora, K. Diazepam loading: simplified treatment of alcohol withdrawal. *Clin. Pharmacol. Ther.*, **1983**, *34*, 822–826.

Senay, E. C.; Dorus, W.; Goldberg, F.; and Thornton, W. Withdrawal from methadone maintenance: rate of withdrawal and expectation. *Arch. Gen. Psychiatry*, **1977**, *34*, 361–367.

Sherer, M. A.; Kumor, K. M.; Cone, E. J.; and Jaffe, J. H. Suspiciousness induced by four-hour intravenous infusions of cocaine—preliminary findings. *Arch. Gen. Psychiatry*, **1988**, *45*, 673–677.

Shore, J. H. The Oregon experience with impaired physicians on probation. An eight-year follow-up. *J.A.M.A.*, **1987**, *257*, 2931–2934.

Simpson, D. D.; Joe, G. W.; and Bracy, S. A. Six-year follow-up of opioid addicts after admission to treatment. *Arch. Gen. Psychiatry*, **1982**, *39*, 1318–1326.

Snyder, C. A.; Wood, R. W.; Graefe, J. F.; Bowers, A.; and Magar, K. "Crack smoke" is a respirable aerosol of cocaine base. *Pharmacol. Biochem. Behav.*, **1988**, *29*, 93–95.

Tønnesen, P.; Fryd, V.; Hansen, M.; Helsted, J.; Gunnersen, A. B.; Forchammer, H.; and Stockner, M. Effects of nicotine chewing gum in combination with group counseling on the cessation of smoking. *N. Engl. J. Med.*, **1988**, *318*, 15–18.

Uhl, G. R.; Ryan, J. P.; and Schwartz, J. P. Morphine alters preproenkephalin gene expression. *Brain Res.*, **1988**, *459*, 391–397.

Vardy, M. M., and Kay, S. R. LSD psychosis or LSD-induced schizophrenia? *Arch. Gen. Psychiatry*, **1983**, *40*, 877–883.

Verebey, K.; Alrazi, J.; and Jaffe, J. H. Complications of "ecstasy" (MDMA). *J.A.M.A.*, **1988**, *259*, 1649–1650.

Weiss, S. R. B.; Post, R. M.; Szele, F.; Woodward, R.; and Nierenberg, J. Chronic carbamazepine inhibits the development of local anesthetic seizures kindled by cocaine and lidocaine. *Brain Res.*, **1989**, *497*, 72–79.

Willett, W. C.; Green, A.; Stampfer, M. J.; Speizer, F. E.; Colditz, G. A.; Rosner, B.; Monson, R. R.; Stason, W.; and Hennekens, C. H. Relative and absolute excess risks of coronary heart disease among women who smoke cigarettes. *N. Engl. J. Med.*, **1987**, *317*, 1303–1310.

Winger, G. Effects of ethanol withdrawal on ethanol-reinforced responding in rhesus monkeys. *Drug Alcohol Depend.*, **1988**, *22*, 235–240.

Woolverton, W. L.; Kandel, D.; and Schuster, C. R. Tolerance and cross-tolerance to cocaine and *d*-amphetamine. *J. Pharmacol. Exp. Ther.*, **1978**, *205*, 525–535.

Wu, T.-C.; Tashkin, D. P.; Djahed, B.; and Rose, J. E. Pulmonary hazards of smoking marijuana as compared with tobacco. *N. Engl. J. Med.*, **1988**, *318*, 347–351.

Monographs and Reviews

Akil, H.; Watson, S. J.; Young, E.; Lewis, M. E.; Khachaturian, H.; and Walker, J. M. Endogenous opioids: biology and function. *Annu. Rev. Neurosci.*, **1984**, *7*, 223–255.

American Psychiatric Association. *Diagnostic and Statistical Manual of Mental Disorders*, 3rd ed. revised. The American Psychiatric Association, Washington, D. C., **1987**.

Aniline, O., and Pitts, F. N., Jr. Phencyclidine (PCP): a review and perspectives. *CRC Crit. Rev. Toxicol.*, **1982**, *10*, 145–177.

Balster, R. L., and Wessinger, W. D. Central nervous system depressant effects of phencyclidine. In, *Phencyclidine and Related Arylcyclohexylamines: Present and Future Applications*. (Kamenka, J.-M.; Domino, E. F.; and Geneste, P.; eds.) NPP Books, Ann Arbor, Mich., **1983**, pp. 291–309.

Benowitz, N. L. Pharmacologic aspects of cigarette

smoking and nicotine addiction. *N. Engl. J. Med.*, **1988**, *319*, 1318–1330.

Bloom, F. E. Neurobiology of alcohol action and alcoholism. *Annu. Rev. Psychiatry*, **1989**, *8*, 347–360.

Brady, J. V., and Lukas, S. E. (eds.). *Testing Drugs for Physical Dependence Potential and Abuse Liability*. National Institute on Drug Abuse Research Monograph Series, Department of Health and Human Services Publication No. (ADM) 84-1332, U.S. Government Printing Office, Washington, D. C., **1984.**

Cappell, H., and LeBlanc, A. E. Tolerance and physical dependence: do they play a role in alcohol and drug self-administration? In, *Research Advances in Alcohol and Drug Problems*, Vol. 6. (Israel, Y.; Glaser, F. B.; Kalant, H.; Popham, R. E.; Schmidt, W.; and Smart, R. G.; eds.) Plenum Press, New York, **1981**, pp. 159–196.

Clark, D. C., and Fawcett, J. Does lithium carbonate therapy for alcoholism deter relapse drinking? *Recent Dev. Alcohol.*, **1989**, *7*, 315–328.

Cloninger, C. R.; Dinwiddie, S. H.; and Reich, T. Epidemiology and genetics of alcoholism. *Annu. Rev. Psychiatry*, **1989**, *8*, 331–346.

Cregler, L. L. Adverse consequences of cocaine abuse. *J. Natl. Med. Assoc.*, **1989**, *81*, 27–38.

Dewey, W. L. Cannabinoid pharmacology. *Pharmacol. Rev.*, **1986**, *38*, 151–178.

Edwards, G.; Arif, A.; and Hodgson, R. Nomenclature and classification of drug- and alcohol-related problems: a WHO memorandum. *Bull. WHO*, **1981**, *59*, 225–242.

Efron, D. H.; Holmstedt, B.; and Kline, N. S. (eds.). *Ethnopharmacologic Search for Psychoactive Drugs*. Public Health Service Publication No. 1645, U.S. Government Printing Office, Washington, D. C., **1967.**

Finnegan, L. P. Influence of maternal drug dependence on the newborn. In, *Toxicologic and Pharmacologic Principles in Pediatrics*. (Kacew, S., and Lock, S., eds.) Hemisphere Publishing Corp., New York, **1988**, pp. 183–198.

Fischman, M. W. Behavioral pharmacology of cocaine. *J. Clin. Psychiatry*, **1988**, *49*, 7–10.

Freedman, D. X. The psychopharmacology of hallucinogenic agents. *Annu. Rev. Med.*, **1969**, *20*, 409–418.

Gawin, F. H., and Ellinwood, E. H., Jr. Cocaine and other stimulants: actions, abuse, and treatment. *N. Engl. J. Med.*, **1988**, *318*, 1173–1182.

Gessner, P. K. Drug therapy of the alcohol withdrawal syndrome. In, *The Biochemistry and Pharmacology of Ethanol*. (Majchrowicz, E., and Noble, E., eds.) Plenum Press, New York, **1979**, pp. 375–435.

Gonzales, J. P., and Brogden, R. N. Naltrexone: a review. *Drugs*, **1988**, *35*, 192–213.

Goudie, A. J., and Demellweek, C. Conditioning factors in drug tolerance. In, *Behavioral Analysis of Drug Dependence*. (Goldberg, S. R., and Stolerman, I. P., eds.) Academic Press, Inc., New York, **1986**, pp. 225–285.

Grant, I. Alcohol and the brain: neuropsychological correlates. *J. Consult. Clin. Psychol.*, **1987**, *55*, 310–324.

Greden, J. F. Caffeinism and caffeine withdrawal. In, *Substance Abuse: Clinical Problems and Perspectives*. (Lowinson, J. H., and Ruiz, P., eds.) The Williams & Wilkins Co., Baltimore, **1981**, pp. 274–286.

Griffiths, R. R., and Woodson, P. P. Caffeine physical dependence: a review of human and laboratory animal studies. *Psychopharmacology (Berlin)*, **1988**, *94*, 437–451.

Hollister, L. E. Health aspects of cannabis. *Pharmacol. Rev.*, **1986**, *38*, 1–20.

———. Cannabis—1988. *Acta Psychiatr. Scand. [Suppl. 345]*, **1988**, *78*, 108–118.

Jaffe, J. H. Tobacco smoking and nicotine dependence. In, *Nicotine Psychopharmacology: Molecular, Cellular and Behavioural Aspects*. (Wonnacott, S.; Russell, M. A. H.; and Stolerman, I. P.; eds.) Oxford University Press, Oxford, **1990**, pp. 1–37.

Jaffe, J. H., and Ciraulo, D. A. Drugs used in the treatment of alcoholism. In, *The Diagnosis and Treatment of Alcoholism*. (Mendelson, J. H., and Mello, N. K., eds.) McGraw-Hill Book Co., New York, **1984**, pp. 355–389.

Johanson, C. E., and Schuster, C. R. Animal models of drug self-administration. In, *Advances in Substance Abuse; Behavioral and Biological Research*, Vol. II. (Mello, N. K., ed.) JAI Press, Inc., Greenwich, Conn., **1981**, pp. 219–297.

Karch, S. B., and Billingham, M. E. The pathology and etiology of cocaine-induced heart disease. *Arch. Pathol. Lab. Med.*, **1988**, *112*, 225–230.

Koob, G. F., and Bloom, F. E. Cellular and molecular mechanisms of drug dependence. *Science*, **1988**, *242*, 715–723.

Korsten, M. A., and Lieber, C. S. Medical complications of alcoholism. In, *The Diagnosis and Treatment of Alcoholism*. (Mendelson, J. H., and Mello, N. K., eds.) McGraw-Hill Book Company, New York, **1985**, pp. 21–64.

Kranzler, H. R., and Orrok, B. The pharmacotherapy of alcoholism. *Annu. Rev. Psychiatry*, **1989**, *8*, 397–417.

Kreek, M. J. Health consequences associated with the use of methadone. *N.I.D.A. Treatment Res. Monogr. Ser.*, **1983**, (ADM)83–1281, 456–482.

Lieber, C. S. Biochemical and molecular basis of alcohol-induced injury to liver and other tissues. *N. Engl. J. Med.*, **1988**, *319*, 1639–1650.

Martin, B. R. Cellular effects of cannabinoids. *Pharmacol. Rev.*, **1986**, *38*, 45–74.

Martin, W. R., and Sloan, J. W. Pharmacology and classification of LSD-like hallucinogens. In, *Drug Addiction II: Amphetamine, Psychotogen, and Marihuana Dependence*. (Martin, W. R., ed.) *Handbuch der Experimentellen Pharmakologie*, Vol. 45, Pt. 2. Springer-Verlag, Berlin, **1977**, pp. 305–368.

Maykut, M. O. Health consequences of acute and chronic marihuana use. *Prog. Neuropsychopharmacol. Biol. Psychiatry*, **1985**, *9*, 209–238.

Mendelson, J. H., and Mello, N. K. Biologic concomitants of alcoholism. *N. Engl. J. Med.*, **1979**, *301*, 912–921.

Meyer, R. E., and Mirin, S. M. *The Heroin Stimulus: Implication for a Theory of Addiction*. Plenum Press, New York, **1979.**

Monaghan, D. T.; Bridges, R. J.; and Cotman, C. W. The excitatory amino acid receptors: their classes, pharmacology, and distinct properties in the function of the central nervous system. *Annu. Rev. Pharmacol. Toxicol.*, **1989**, *29*, 365–402.

Musto, D. F. *The American Disease: Origins of Narcotic Control*. Oxford University Press, New York, **1988.**

Nutt, D.; Adinoff, B.; and Linnoila, M. Benzodiazepines in the treatment of alcoholism. *Recent Dev. Alcohol.*, **1989**, *7*, 283–313.

Razdan, R. K. Structure–activity relationships in cannabinoids. *Pharmacol. Rev.*, **1986**, *38*, 75–150.

Redmond, D. E., Jr., and Krystal, J. H. Multiple mechanisms of withdrawal from opioid drugs. *Annu. Rev. Neurosci.*, **1984**, *7*, 443–478.

Robins, L. *The Vietnam Drug User Returns: Final Report, Sept. 1973*. Special Action Office Monograph, Ser. A, No. 2, U.S. Government Printing Office, Washington, D. C., **1974.**

Rosenberg, H. C., and Chiu, T. H. Time course for development of benzodiazepine tolerance and physical dependence. *Neurosci. Biobehav. Rev.*, **1985**, *9*, 123–131.

Ryan, L.; Ehrlich, S.; and Finnegan, L. P. Cocaine abuse in pregnancy: effects on the fetus and newborn. *Natl. Inst. Drug Abuse Res. Monogr. Ser.*, **1987**, *76*, 280.

Smith, C. M. The pharmacology of sedative/hypnotics, alcohol, and anesthetics: sites and mechanisms of action. In, *Drug Addiction I: Morphine, Sedative/Hypnotic and Alcohol Dependence*. (Martin, W. R., ed.) *Handbuch der Experimentellen Pharmakologie*, Vol. 45, Pt. 1. Springer-Verlag, Berlin, **1977**, pp. 413–587.

Stimson, G. V., and Oppenheimer, E. *Heroin Addiction: Treatment and Control in Britain*. Tavistock Publications, London, **1982.**

Surgeon General. *Smoking and Health*. (Office of Smoking and Health, eds.) Department of Health, Education, and Welfare Publication No. (PHS) 79–50066, U.S. Government Printing Office, Washington, D. C., **1979.**

———. *The Health Consequences of Smoking. Nicotine Addiction*. (Office of Smoking and Health, eds.) Department of Health and Human Services Publication No. (CDC) 88-8406. U.S. Government Printing Office, Washington, D. C., **1988.**

Tabakoff, B., and Hoffman, P. L. Biochemical pharmacology of alcohol. In, *Psychopharmacology: The Third Generation of Progress*. (Meltzer, H. Y., ed.) Raven Press, New York, **1987**, pp. 1521–1526.

Vincent, B. J.; McQuiston, D. J.; Einhorn, L. H.; Nagy, C. M.; and Brames, M. J. Review of cannabinoids and their antiemetic effectiveness. *Drugs*, **1983**, *25*, 52–62.

Wikler, A. *Opioid Dependence: Mechanisms and Treatment*. Plenum Press, New York, **1980.**

Wise, R. The neurobiology of craving: implications for the understanding and treatment of addiction. *J. Abnorm. Psychol.*, **1988**, *97*, 118–132.

Woods, J. H.; Katz, J. L.; and Winger, G. Abuse liability of benzodiazepines. *Pharmacol. Rev.*, **1987**, *39*, 251–419.

Wroblewski, J. T., and Danysz, W. Modulation of glutamate receptors: molecular mechanisms and functional implications. *Annu. Rev. Pharmacol. Toxicol.*, **1989**, *29*, 441–474.

Yaksh, T. L., and Noueihed, R. The physiology and pharmacology of spinal opiates. *Annu. Rev. Pharmacol. Toxicol.*, **1985**, *25*, 433–462.

Young, A., and Herling, S. Drugs as reinforcers: studies in laboratory animals. In, *Behavioral Analysis of Drug Dependence*. (Goldberg, S. R., and Stolerman, I. P., eds.) Academic Press, Inc., New York, **1986**, pp. 9–67.

SECTION

IV

Autacoids; Drug Therapy of Inflammation

INTRODUCTION

James C. Garrison and Theodore W. Rall

The substances that are considered in this section have diverse physiological and pharmacological activities. They are grouped together in large part because they participate, at least in some settings, in physiological or pathophysiological responses to injury. At the same time, the opportunity is taken to discuss drugs that antagonize their actions or inhibit their elaboration, wherever such drugs are available. Included in Chapter 23 are discussions of histamine, bradykinin, and 5-hydroxytryptamine (5-HT) and their respective antagonists. Chapter 24 is devoted to lipid substances that are generated by biotransformation of the products of the selective hydrolysis of membrane phospholipids—the eicosanoids (prostaglandins, thromboxanes, and leukotrienes) and platelet-activating factor. Chapter 25 addresses the methylxanthines, which have as one of their major actions the capacity to block receptors for adenosine. Also discussed are a number of other drugs that are useful for the treatment of asthma. Chapter 26 deals with aspirin and aspirin-like drugs (nonsteroidal antiinflammatory agents), which owe their therapeutic utility in large part to their capacity to inhibit the synthesis of prostaglandins and thromboxanes.

This section thus includes discussion of an array of substances that are normally present in the body or may be formed there; although these substances function in humoral regulation, they cannot conveniently be classed with other members of this broad group, such as the hormones and neurotransmitters. Because these substances usually have a brief lifetime and act near their sites of synthesis, they have often been described as local hormones. However, unlike true hormones, which reach their sites of action via the bloodstream, these substances often conduct their affairs closeted from the circulation, such as in the confines of an inflammatory lesion. Hence, the term *autacoid,* from the Greek *autos* ("self") and *akos* ("medicinal agent" or "remedy"), seems more appropriate and will be used in this section. This term was once a rival of hormone and was revived for use in this setting by William W. Douglas in *earlier editions* of this textbook.

In many ways, the grouping of these substances under the rubric of "autacoids" is arbitrary. Not included here are an array of peptides that are elaborated by specialized cells within certain endocrine glands and in glands of the digestive system, whose actions are often exerted primarily on neighboring cells; these are usually described as *paracrine* hormones and include compounds such as somatostatin and gastrin. Indeed, histamine has important paracrine functions in the regulation of gastric acid secretion; these will be considered in Chapter 37. Since many of these substances are also distributed by the circulation for additional actions at more distant locations, they may well deserve to be called hormones. A more significant omission is the burgeoning array of cytokines or lymphokines that mediate the complex interactions involved in humoral and cellular immune responses.

In part, these substances share with autacoids their participation in inflammation and local regulatory function. Moreover, their actions often include the generation of autacoids; a notable example is the pyrogenic action of interleukin-1, which is mediated by the formation of prostaglandins. As a result, certain aspects of the functions of lymphokines are discussed in Chapter 26. Immunosuppressive agents appear to exert their effects by inhibiting the elaboration and/or action of lymphokines; an important example is the capacity of cyclosporine to suppress the synthesis of interleukin-2. Immunosuppressants are emerging as potentially important therapeutic agents in combating the destructive effects of synovial inflammation in patients with aggressive forms of rheumatoid arthritis, and their interference with the functions of lymphokines is considered in Chapter 53. Finally, in addition to their capacity to suppress the formation of eicosanoids, the glucocorticoids produce their antiinflammatory and immunosuppressant effects by inhibiting the synthesis and action of several cytokines; this role is discussed in Chapter 60. However they are defined, autacoids and related locally acting substances are clearly part and parcel of the physiological and pathological phenomena that provide the rationale for drug therapy; their existence provides numerous possibilities for therapeutic intervention by the use of drugs that mimic or antagonize their actions or interfere with their synthesis or metabolism.

CHAPTER 23 HISTAMINE, BRADYKININ, 5-HYDROXYTRYPTAMINE, AND THEIR ANTAGONISTS

James C. Garrison

HISTAMINE

History. The history of β-aminoethylimidazole, or histamine, parallels that of acetylcholine (ACh). Both compounds were synthesized as chemical curiosities before their biological significance was recognized; both were first detected as uterine stimulants in extracts of ergot, from which they were subsequently isolated; and both proved to be contaminants of ergot that resulted from bacterial action.

When Dale and Laidlaw (1910, 1911) subjected histamine to intensive pharmacological study, they discovered that it stimulated a host of smooth muscles and had an intense vasodepressor action. Remarkably, they pointed out that the immediate signs displayed by a sensitized animal when injected with a normally inert protein closely resemble those of poisoning by histamine. These comments anticipated by many years the discovery of the presence of histamine in the body and its release during immediate hypersensitivity reactions and upon cellular injury. It was not until 1927 that Best, Dale, Dudley, and Thorpe isolated histamine from impeccably fresh samples of liver and lung, thereby establishing that this amine is a natural constituent of the body. Demonstrations of its presence in a variety of other tissues soon followed—hence the name *histamine* after the Greek word for tissue, *histos*.

Meanwhile, Lewis and his colleagues had amassed evidence that a substance with the properties of histamine ("H-substance") was liberated from the cells of the skin by injurious stimuli, including the reaction of antigen with antibody (Lewis, 1927). Given the chemical evidence of histamine's presence in the body, there remained little impediment to supposing that Lewis' "H-substance" was histamine itself. Now, more than 60 years later, it is evident that endogenous histamine plays a role in the immediate allergic response and is an important regulator of gastric acid secretion; its role as a neurotransmitter in the central nervous system (CNS) is also being defined.

Early suspicions that histamine acts through more than one receptor have been borne out, and it is clear that there are at least three distinct classes of receptors for histamine, designated H_1 (Ash and Schild, 1966), H_2 (Black *et al.*, 1972), and H_3 (Arrang *et al.*, 1987). H_1 receptors are blocked selectively by the classical "antihistamines" (such as pyrilamine) developed around 1940, while H_2-

blocking drugs were introduced in the early 1970s. The discovery of H_2 antagonists has contributed greatly to the resurgence of interest in histamine in biology and clinical medicine. The H_3 receptor has been characterized by yet another distinct set of agonists and antagonists that were developed in the mid 1980s.

Chemistry. Histamine is a hydrophilic molecule comprised of an imidazole ring and an amino group connected by two methylene groups. The pharmacologically active form at all histamine receptors is the monocationic $N\gamma$—H tautomer—that is, the charged form of the species depicted in Table 23–1, although different chemical properties of this monocation may be involved in interactions with the H_1 and H_2 receptors (Ganellin, in Ganellin and Parsons, 1982). The three classes of histamine receptors can be activated differentially by analogs of histamine (*see* Table 23–1). Thus, 2-methylhistamine preferentially elicits responses mediated by H_1 receptors, whereas 4(5)-methylhistamine has a preferential effect on H_2 receptors (Black *et al.*, 1972). A chiral analog of histamine with restricted conformational freedom, (R) α-methylhistamine, is the preferred agonist at H_3-receptor sites (Arrang *et al.*, 1987).

DISTRIBUTION AND BIOSYNTHESIS OF HISTAMINE

Distribution. Histamine is widely, if unevenly, distributed throughout the animal kingdom and is present in many venoms, bacteria, and plants (Reite, 1972). Almost all mammalian tissues contain histamine in amounts ranging from less than 1 to more than 100 μg/g. Concentrations in plasma and other body fluids are generally very low, but human cerebrospinal fluid contains significant amounts (Khandelwal *et al.*, 1982). The mast cell is the predominant storage site for histamine in most tissues (*see* below). Thus the concentration of histamine is particularly high in tissues that contain large numbers of mast cells, such as skin, the mucosa of the bronchial tree, and the intestinal mucosa. However, some tissues synthesize and turn over histamine at a remarkably fast rate, even though their content of the amine may be modest.

Synthesis, Storage, and Degradation. Histamine that is ingested or formed by bacteria in the gastrointestinal tract is rapidly metabolized and eliminated in the urine (*see* below). Every mammalian tissue that contains histamine is capable of synthesizing it from histidine by virtue of its content of L-histidine decarboxylase. The chief site of histamine storage in most tissues is the mast cell; in the blood, it is the basophil. These cells synthesize histamine and store it in secretory granules along with heparin, eosinophil chemotactic factor (ECF-A), neutrophil chemotactic factor (NCF-A), and certain enzymes (*see* Plaut and Lichtenstein, in Ganellin and Parsons, 1982). The turnover rate of histamine in secretory granules is slow, and when tissues rich in mast cells are depleted of their stores of histamine, it may take weeks before concentrations of the autacoid return to normal. Non–mast-cell sites of histamine formation or storage include cells of the epidermis, cells in the gastric mucosa, neurons within the CNS, and cells in regenerating or rapidly growing tissues. Turnover is rapid at these sites, since the histamine is continuously released rather than stored. This factor contributes significantly to the daily excretion of histamine and its metabolites in the urine. Since L-histidine decarboxylase is an inducible enzyme, the histamine-forming capacity at such non–mast-cell sites is subject to regulation by various physiological and other factors.

There are two major paths of histamine metabolism in man. The more important of these involves ring methylation and is catalyzed by the enzyme histamine-N-methyltransferase, which is widely distributed. Most of the product, N-methylhistamine, is converted by monoamine oxidase (MAO) to N-methyl imidazole acetic acid. Alternatively, histamine undergoes oxidative deamination catalyzed mainly by the nonspecific enzyme diamine oxidase (DAO). The products are imidazole acetic acid and, eventually, its riboside. The metabolites have little or no activity and are excreted in the urine. The relative roles of these enzymes in the metabolism of endogenous histamine have not yet been established. Some inhibitors of histamine synthesis and degradation are known, but these are of little clinical interest (*see* Wetterquist, 1978).

FUNCTIONS OF ENDOGENOUS HISTAMINE

Histamine has important, but limited, physiological roles. Because histamine is one of the preformed mediators stored in the mast cell, its release as a result of the interaction of antigen with IgE antibodies on the surface of the mast cell plays a central role in immediate hypersensitivity and allergic responses. The actions of histamine on bronchial smooth muscle and blood vessels account in part for the symptoms of the allergic response. In addition, certain clinically useful drugs can act directly on mast cells to release histamine, thereby explaining some of their untoward effects. Histamine has a major role in the regulation of gastric acid secretion, and its function as a neurotransmitter in the CNS has recently come into focus.

Role in Allergic Responses. The principal target cells of immediate hypersensitivity reactions are mast cells and basophils. Histamine is stored within the secretory granules of these cells along with a heparin–protein complex to which it is bound loosely. Other pharmacologically active substances are also present; these include eosinophil chemotactic factor of anaphylaxis (ECF-A), neutrophil chemotactic factor, and enzymes such as β-glucuronidase, neutral proteases, superoxide dismutase, and peroxidase. As part of the allergic

Table 23–1. STRUCTURE OF HISTAMINE AND SOME H_1, H_2, AND H_3 AGONISTS

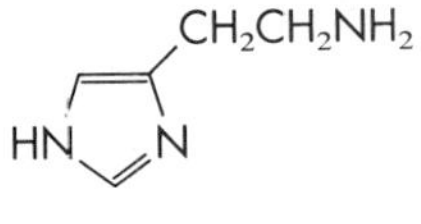

Histamine

H_1-Receptor Agonists

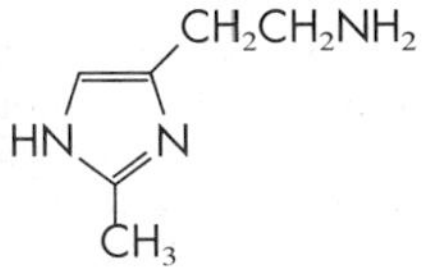

2-Methylhistamine (8:1) *

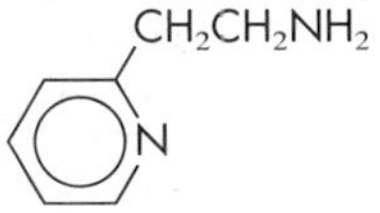

2-Pyridylethylamine (30:1)

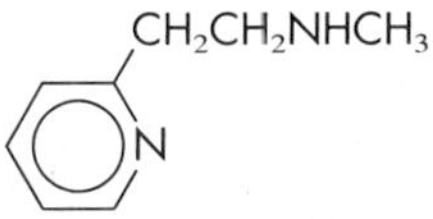

Betahistine (40:1)

2-Thiazolylethylamine (90:1)

H_2-Receptor Agonists

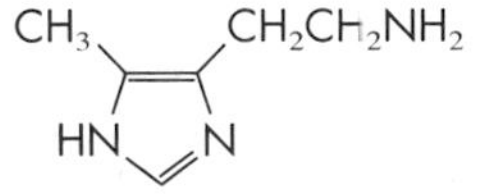

4(5)-Methylhistamine (170:1)

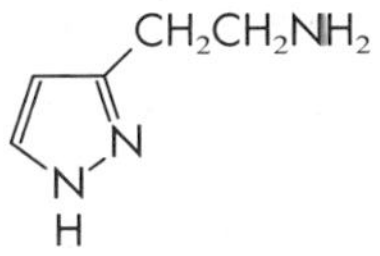

Betazole (10:1)

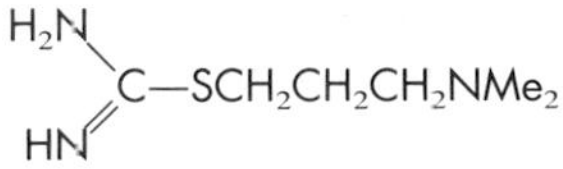

Dimaprit (2000:1)

Impromidine (10,000:1)

H_3-Receptor Agonist

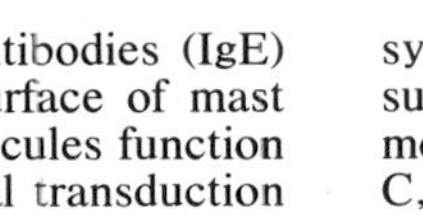

(R) α-Methylhistamine (15:1)

* The ratios in parentheses indicate approximate relative activities of the various compounds at the three receptor types (H_1:H_2 for the H_1 agonists; H_2:H_1 for the H_2 agonists; and H_3:H_1 for (R) α-methylhistamine). For further details, *see* Ganellin, in Ganellin and Parsons (1982); Arrang *et al.* (1987).

response to an antigen, reaginic antibodies (IgE) are generated and bound to the surface of mast cells and basophils. These IgE molecules function as receptors and interact with signal transduction systems in the membranes of sensitized cells. Upon subsequent exposure, the antigen bridges the IgE molecules and causes activation of phospholipase C, leading to the generation of inositol-1,4,5-trisphosphate and diacylglycerols and an elevation of intracellular Ca^{2+} (*see* Cunha-Melo *et al.*, 1987; *see also* Chapter 2). These events trigger the extrusion of the contents of secretory granules by exocytosis. The secretory behavior of mast cells and basophils is identical to that of various endocrine and exocrine glands and conforms to a general pattern of stimulus-secretion coupling in which a secretagogue-induced rise in the intracellular concentration of Ca^{2+} serves to initiate exocytosis (Douglas, 1968, 1978). The mechanism by which the rise in Ca^{2+} leads to fusion of the secretory granule with the plasma membrane is not fully elucidated, but it is likely to involve activation of Ca^{2+}/calmodulin–dependent protein kinases and protein kinase C (*see* Chapter 2).

Release of Other Autacoids. The classical histamine hypothesis provides only a partial explanation for the spectrum of effects that results from immediate hypersensitivity reactions. In addition to activation of phospholipase C and the hydrolysis of inositol phospholipids, stimulation of IgE receptors also activates phospholipase A_2, leading to the production of a host of mediators, including platelet-activating factor (PAF) and metabolites of arachidonic acid. Leukotriene D_4, which is generated in this way, stimulates contraction of the smooth muscle of the bronchial tree and may be a dominant factor in allergic conditions such as asthma (*see* Mathews, 1982; Dahlén *et al.*, 1983; *see also* Chapters 24 and 25). Kinins are also generated during some allergic responses (*see* below). Thus, the mast cell secretes a variety of inflammatory compounds in addition to histamine, and each contributes to varying extents to the major symptoms of the allergic response: constriction of the bronchi, decrease in blood pressure, increased capillary permeability, and edema formation (*see* below).

Regulation of Mediator Release. The wide variety of mediators released during the allergic response explains the ineffectiveness of drug therapy focused on a single mediator. Thus, considerable emphasis has been placed on the regulation of mediator release from mast cells and basophils, and these cells do contain receptors linked to signalling systems that can enhance or block the IgE-induced release of mediators.

Agents that act at muscarinic or α-adrenergic receptors enhance the release of mediators, although this effect is of little clinical significance (*see* Beaven, 1976). Significant inhibition of the secretory response can be achieved with epinephrine and related drugs that act through β-adrenergic receptors. The effect is the result of accumulation of adenosine 3′,5′-monophosphate (cyclic AMP). However, the beneficial effects of β-adrenergic agonists in allergic states such as asthma are due mainly to their relaxant effect on bronchial smooth muscle. Histamine itself, acting through H_2 receptors on mast cells and basophils, can reduce the secretory response. Histamine can also inhibit the secretion of lysosomal enzymes from neutrophils and of antibodies and lymphokines from lymphocytes. For the most part, these diverse "antiinflammatory" effects, which are mediated by H_2 receptors, are of modest intensity and have limited clinical significance (*see* Symposium, 1981, 1982; Lagunoff *et al.*, 1983; Larsen and Henson, 1983; Ishizaka, 1984). In contrast, cromolyn sodium owes its clinical utility to its capacity to inhibit the release of mediators from mast and other cells in the lung (*see* Chapter 25).

Histamine Release by Drugs, Peptides, Venoms, and Other Agents. Many compounds, including a large number of therapeutic agents, stimulate release of histamine from mast cells directly and without prior sensitization. Responses of this sort are most likely to occur following intravenous injections of certain categories of substances, particularly those that are organic bases. Among these bases are amides, amidines, quaternary ammonium compounds, pyridinium compounds, piperidines, alkaloids, and antibiotic bases. Tubocurarine, succinylcholine, morphine, radiocontrast media, and certain carbohydrate plasma expanders may also elicit the response. The phenomenon is one of clinical concern, for it accounts for many unexpected anaphylactoid reactions (*see* Lorenz *et al.*, 1981; Symposium, 1982; Weck and Bundgaard, 1983).

In addition to therapeutic agents, certain experimental compounds stimulate the release of histamine as their dominant pharmacological characteristic. The archetype is the polybasic substance known as compound 48/80. This is a mixture of low-molecular-weight polymers of *p*-methoxy-N-methylphenethylamine, of which the hexamer is most active (*see* Lagunoff *et al.*, 1983).

Basic polypeptides are often effective histamine releasers, and their potency generally increases with the number of basic groups over a limited range. Polymyxin B is very active; others include bradykinin and substance P. Since basic polypeptides are released upon tissue injury or are present in venoms, they constitute pathophysiological stimuli to secretion for mast cells and basophils. Anaphylotoxins (C3a and C5a), which are low-molecular-weight peptides that are cleaved from the complement system, may act similarly.

Within seconds of the intravenous injection of a histamine liberator, human subjects experience a burning, itching sensation. This effect, most marked in the palms of the hand and in the face, scalp, and ears, is soon followed by a feeling of intense warmth. The skin reddens, and the color rapidly spreads over the trunk. Blood pressure falls, the heart rate accelerates, and the subject complains of headache. After a few minutes, blood pressure recovers, and edema and crops of giant hives on the skin appear. There is colic, nausea, hypersecretion of acid, and moderate bronchospasm. The effect becomes less intense with successive injections as the mast-cell stores of histamine are depleted. Histamine liberators do not deplete tissues of non–mast-cell histamine.

Mechanism. All of the above-mentioned histamine-releasing substances can activate the secretory response of mast cells or basophils by causing a rise in intracellular Ca^{2+}. Some are ionophores and transport Ca^{2+} into the cell; others, such as the anaphylotoxins, appear to act like specific antigens to increase membrane permeability to Ca^{2+}. Still others, such as mastoparan (a peptide from wasp venom), may bypass cell-surface receptors and directly stimulate guanine nucleotide–binding regulatory proteins (G proteins), which then activate phospholipase C (Higashijima *et al.*, 1988). Basic histamine releasers, such as compound 48/80 and polymyxin B, act principally by mobilizing Ca^{2+} from cellular stores (*see* Metcalfe *et al.*, 1981; Lagunoff *et al.*, 1983).

Histamine Release by Other Means. Clinical conditions in which release of histamine occurs in response to other stimuli include cold urticaria, cholinergic urticaria, and solar urticaria. Some of these involve specific secretory responses of the mast cells and, indeed, cell-fixed IgE (*see* Salvaggio, 1982). However, histamine release also occurs whenever there is nonspecific cell damage from any cause. The redness and urticaria that follow scratching of the skin is a familiar example.

Growths of Mast Cells and Basophils. In urticaria pigmentosa (mastocytosis), mast cells aggregate in the upper corium and give rise to pigmented cutaneous lesions that urticate when stroked. In systemic mastocytosis, similar aggregates are also found in other organs. Patients with these syndromes suffer a constellation of signs and symptoms attributable to excessive histamine release, including urticaria, dermographism, pruritus, headache, weakness, hypotension, flushing of the face, and a variety of gastrointestinal effects such as peptic ulceration. The signs and symptoms are precipitated or exacerbated by a variety of stimuli—the friction of toweling the skin or exposure to drugs that release histamine directly or to which patients are allergic. In myelogenous leukemia, excessive numbers of basophils are present in the blood and raise its histamine content to high levels. Gastric carcinoid tumors secrete histamine, and this action apparently contributes to the patchy "geographical" flush.

Gastric Acid Secretion. Histamine is a powerful gastric secretagogue and evokes a copious secretion of acid from parietal cells by acting on H_2 receptors. The output of pepsin and intrinsic factor is also increased. However, the secretion of acid is also evoked by stimulation of the vagus nerve and by the enteric hormone gastrin. In addition, there appear to be cells in the gastric mucosa that contain somatostatin, which can inhibit secretion of acid by parietal cells; the release of somatostatin is inhibited by acetylcholine. The interplay among these endogenous regulators has not been precisely defined. However, it is clear that histamine is the dominant physiological mediator of acid secretion because blockade of H_2 receptors can not only eradicate acid secretion in response to histamine, but also cause nearly complete inhibition of responses to gastrin or vagal stimulation. This area is discussed in more detail in Chapter 37.

Central Nervous System. There is substantial evidence that histamine functions as a neurotransmitter in the CNS. Histamine, histidine decarboxylase, and enzymes that catalyze the degradation of histamine are distributed nonuniformly in the CNS and are concentrated in synaptosomal fractions of brain homogenates. High concentrations of H_1 receptors are found in the thalamus, hypothalamus, and certain regions of the cerebellum and forebrain (*see* Bouthenet *et al.*, 1988). Histamine-containing neurons may participate in the regulation of drinking, body temperature, and the secretion of antidiuretic hormone, as well as in the control of blood pressure and the perception of pain. Both H_1 and H_2 receptors seem to be involved in these responses (*see* Hough, 1988). In addition, H_3 receptors appear to be present on histaminergic nerve terminals, where they may regulate the synthesis and release of histamine. These receptors would be analogous to other presynaptic receptors that exert feedback regulation of neurotransmitter release (*see* Arrang *et al.*, 1987).

PHARMACOLOGICAL EFFECTS: H_1 AND H_2 RECEPTORS

Once released, histamine can exert local or widespread effects on smooth muscles and glands. The autacoid contracts many smooth muscles, such as those of the bronchi and gut, but powerfully relaxes others, including those of small blood vessels. It is also a potent stimulus to gastric acid secretion. Effects attributable to these actions dominate the overall response to histamine; however, there are other effects, such as formation of edema and stimulation of sensory nerve endings. Many of these effects, such as bronchoconstriction and contraction of the gut, are mediated by H_1 receptors (Ash and Schild, 1966), which are readily blocked by pyrilamine and other classical antihistamines (now more properly described as H_1 antagonists). Other effects, most notably gastric secretion, are the results of activation of H_2 receptors and, accordingly, can be inhibited by H_2 antagonists (Black *et al.*, 1972). Some responses, such as the hypotension that results from vascular dilatation, are mediated by both H_1 and H_2 receptors. (The H_3 receptor appears to exist only in the CNS.)

Cardiovascular System. Histamine characteristically causes dilatation of the finer blood vessels, resulting in flushing, lowered total peripheral resistance, and a fall in systemic blood pressure. In addition, histamine tends to increase capillary permeability. Its effects on the heart are generally less important. (*See* Rocha e Silva, 1978; Levi *et al.*, in Ganellin and Parsons, 1982.)

Vasodilatation. Loosely referred to as "capillary dilatation," this is the characteristic action of histamine on the vascular tree, and it is by far the most important in man. It involves both H_1 and H_2 receptors distributed throughout the resistance vessels in most vascular beds; however, quantitative differences are apparent in the degree of dilatation that occurs in various beds. Activation of either type of receptor can elicit maximal vasodilatation, but the responses differ in their sensitivity to histamine, in the duration of the effect, and in the mechanism of their production. H_1 receptors have the higher affinity for histamine and mediate a dilator response that is relatively rapid in onset and short lived. By contrast, activation of H_2 receptors causes dilatation that develops more slowly and is more sustained. As a result, H_1 antagonists effectively counter small dilator responses to low concentrations of histamine but only blunt the initial phase of larger responses to higher concentrations of the amine. H_2 receptors are located on vascular smooth muscle cells, and the vasodilator effects produced by their stimulation are mediated by cyclic AMP; H_1 receptors reside on endothelial cells, and their stimulation leads to the formation of local vasodilator substances (*see* below).

Increased "Capillary" Permeability. This classical effect of histamine on the fine vessels results in outward passage of plasma protein and fluid into the extracellular spaces, an increase in the flow of lymph and its protein content, and formation of edema. H_1 receptors are clearly important for this response; whether H_2 receptors also participate is uncertain.

Increased permeability results mainly from actions of histamine on postcapillary venules, where histamine causes the endothelial cells to contract and separate at their boundaries and thus to expose the basement membrane, which is freely permeable to plasma protein and fluid. The gaps between endothelial cells may also permit passage of particles such as platelets that become trapped between the cells and the basement membrane. The active separation of the endothelial cells is favored by the dilatation of the small venules. An additional factor favoring increased transcapillary movement of fluid and macromolecules may be increased transcapillary vesicular transport (*see* Altura and Halevy, 1978).

Triple Response. If histamine is injected intradermally, it elicits a characteristic phenomenon known as the "triple response" (Lewis, 1927). This is comprised of (1) a localized red spot, extending for a few millimeters around the site of injection, that appears within a few seconds and reaches a maximum in about a minute; (2) a brighter red flush, or "flare," extending about 1 cm or so beyond the original red spot and developing more slowly; and (3) a wheal that is discernible in 1 to 2 minutes and occupies the same area as the original small red spot at the injection site. The red spot results from the direct vasodilatory effect of histamine, the flush is due to histamine-induced stimulation of axon reflexes that cause vasodilatation indirectly, and the wheal reflects histamine's capacity to cause edema.

Constriction of Larger Vessels. Histamine tends to constrict larger blood vessels, in some species more than in others. In rodents the effect extends to the level of the arterioles and may overshadow dilatation of the finer blood vessels. A net increase in total peripheral resistance and an elevation of blood pressure can be observed.

Heart. Histamine has direct actions on the heart that affect both contractility and electrical events. It increases the force of contraction of both atrial and ventricular muscle by promoting the influx of Ca^{2+}, and it speeds heart rate by hastening diastolic depolarization in the SA node. It also acts directly to slow AV conduction, to increase automaticity, and, in high doses especially, to elicit arrhythmias. With the exception of slowed AV conduction, which involves mainly H_1 receptors, all these effects are largely attributable to H_2 receptors. If histamine is given intravenously, direct cardiac effects of histamine are not prominent and are overshadowed by baroreceptor reflexes elicited by the reduced blood pressure.

Histamine Shock. Histamine given in large doses or released during systemic anaphylaxis causes a profound and progressive fall in blood pressure. As the small blood vessels dilate, they trap large amounts of blood, and as their permeability increases, plasma escapes from the circulation. These effects diminish effective blood volume, reduce venous return, and greatly lower cardiac output. The condition resembles surgical or traumatic shock (*see* Symposium, 1982).

Extravascular Smooth Muscle. Histamine stimulates, or more rarely relaxes, various smooth muscles. Contraction is due to activation of H_1 receptors and relaxation (for the most part) to activation of H_2 receptors. Responses vary widely, even in individuals (*see* Parsons, in Ganellin and

Parsons, 1982). Bronchial muscle of guinea pigs is exquisitely sensitive, and bronchoconstriction leads to death. Minute doses of histamine will also evoke intense bronchoconstriction in patients with bronchial asthma and certain other pulmonary diseases; in normal man the effect is much less pronounced. Although the spasmogenic influence of H_1 receptors is dominant in human bronchial muscle, H_2 receptors with dilator function are also present. Thus, histamine-induced bronchospasm *in vitro* is potentiated slightly by H_2 blockade. In asthmatic subjects in particular, histamine-induced bronchospasm may involve an additional, reflex component that arises from irritation of afferent vagal nerve endings (*see* Eyre and Chand, in Ganellin and Parsons, 1982; Nadel and Barnes, 1984).

The uterus of some species contracts to histamine; in the human uterus, gravid or not, the response is negligible. Responses of intestinal muscle also vary with species and region, but the classical effect is contraction. Bladder, ureter, gallbladder, iris, and many other smooth muscle preparations are affected little or inconsistently by histamine.

Exocrine Glands. As mentioned above, histamine is an important physiological regulator of gastric acid secretion. This effect is mediated by H_2 receptors (*see* Chapter 37).

Nerve Endings: Pain, Itch, and Indirect Effects. Histamine stimulates various nerve endings. Thus, when released in the epidermis, it causes itch; in the dermis, it evokes pain, sometimes accompanied by itching. Stimulant actions on one or another type of nerve ending, including autonomic afferents and efferents, have been mentioned above as factors that contribute to the "flare" component of the triple response and to indirect effects of histamine on the bronchi and other organs. In the periphery, neuronal receptors for histamine are generally of the H_1 type (*see* Rocha e Silva, 1978; Ganellin and Parsons, 1982).

Mechanism of Action. Based on pharmacological criteria, there are at least three types of membrane-bound receptor for histamine; although structural information is not yet available, they will almost certainly resemble other receptors that interact with signal-transducing G proteins in the plasma membrane (*see* Chapter 2; *see also* Ganellin, in Ganellin and Parsons, 1982; Arrang *et al.*, 1987). H_1 receptors are coupled to phospholipase C, and their activation leads to synthesis of inositol-1,4,5-trisphosphate (IP_3) and diacylglycerols from phospholipids in the cell membrane; IP_3 causes a rapid release of Ca^{2+} from the endoplasmic reticulum. Diacylglycerols (and Ca^{2+}) activate protein kinase C, while Ca^{2+} activates Ca^{2+}/calmodulin–dependent protein kinases and phospholipase A_2 in the target cell to generate the characteristic response (*see* Chapter 2). H_2 receptors are linked to the stimulation of adenylyl cyclase and thus to the activation of cyclic AMP–dependent protein kinase in the target cell. The signaling mechanism used by H_3 receptors is not known; inhibitory coupling to adenylyl cyclase has been proposed (Arrang *et al.*, 1987).

In the smooth muscle of large blood vessels, bronchi, and intestine, the stimulation of H_1 receptors and the resultant IP_3-mediated release of intracellular Ca^{2+} leads to activation of the Ca^{2+}/calmodulin–dependent myosin light chain kinase. This enzyme phosphorylates the 20,000-dalton myosin light chain, with resultant enhancement of cross-bridge cycling and contraction (*see* Kamm and Stull, 1985; Somlyo *et al.*, 1988; Griendling and Alexander, 1990). The effects of histamine on sensory nerves are also mediated by H_1 receptors, but the sequence of events has not been defined.

As mentioned above, the vasodilator effects of histamine are mediated by both H_1 and H_2 receptors that are located on different cell types in the vascular bed: H_1 receptors on the vascular endothelial cells and H_2 receptors on smooth muscle cells. Activation of H_1 receptors leads to increased intracellular Ca^{2+}, activation of phospholipase A_2, and the local production of endothelium-derived relaxing factor (EDRF). EDRF diffuses to the smooth muscle cell, where it activates a soluble guanylyl cyclase and causes the accumulation of guanosine 3′,5′-monophosphate (cyclic GMP). Stimulation of a cyclic GMP–dependent protein kinase and a decrease in intracellular Ca^{2+} are thought to be involved in the relaxation caused by this cyclic nucleotide. The activation of phospholipase A_2 in endothelial cells also leads to the formation of prostaglandins, predominantly prostacyclin (PGI_2); this vasodilator makes an important contribution to endothelium-mediated vasodilatation in some vascular beds.

The mechanism of cyclic AMP–mediated relaxation of smooth muscle is not entirely clear, but it is presumed to involve a decrease in intracellular Ca^{2+} (*see* Kamm and Stull, 1985; Taylor *et al.*, 1989). Cyclic AMP–mediated actions in the heart, mast cells, basophils, and other tissues are also incompletely understood, but the effects of histamine that are mediated by H_2 receptors would obviously be produced in the same fashion as those resulting from stimulation of β-adrenergic receptors (*see* Chapter 5) or other receptors that are linked to the activation of adenylyl cyclase.

CLINICAL USES

The practical applications of histamine and its congeners are limited to minor uses as diagnostic agents. The ability of intradermal histamine to cause itching, wheal, and "flare" is commonly used in clinical trials to assess the efficacy of H_1 antagonists (*see* below). The fact that the "flare" is mediated by axon reflexes allows a test of the integrity of sensory nerves in certain neurological conditions. Because of its distressing side effects, histamine has been replaced by pentagastrin in tests of gastric acid secretion (*see* Chapter 37). Histamine (administered by inhalation) is still used to assess bronchial reactivity.

Drugs with histamine-like activity that act preferentially or selectively on H_1 or H_2 receptors offer some advantage over histamine, but their uses are also very modest. A moderately selective H_1 agonist, betahistine, has had limited clinical use as a vasodilator and is available for investigational use (*see* Ganellin and Parsons, 1982).

H_2 agonists have been used in tests of gastric secretory function. Betazole (3-pyrazolylethylamine; *see* Table 23–1) has only 2% of the potency of histamine at H_2 receptors, but its potency at H_1 receptors is still less (about 0.2%). Nevertheless, the residual H_1 activity causes adverse effects. Although the H_2 agonist impromidine (*see* Table 23–1) has a 10,000-fold selectivity for H_2 receptors, it produces cardiovascular side effects (*see* Porro *et al.*, 1982). The possible utility of impromidine for stimulation of the myocardium is being explored (*see* Baumann *et al.*, 1984).

Preparations. *Histamine phosphate* is available for injection in preparations containing 0.275, 0.55, and 2.75 mg/ml. It is readily absorbed after parenteral administration and acts rapidly and evanescently.

HISTAMINE ANTAGONISTS: H_1 ANTAGONISTS

Although antagonists that act selectively at the three types of histaminergic receptors have been developed, this discussion is confined to the properties and clinical uses of H_1 antagonists. Specific H_2 antagonists (*e.g.*, cimetidine, ranitidine) are used extensively in the treatment of peptic ulcers; these are discussed in Chapter 37. Antagonists that act at H_3 receptors are also known (*e.g.*, thioperamide), but the potential utility of such agents has yet to be defined.

History. Histamine-blocking activity was first detected in 1937 by Bovet and Staub in one of a series of amines with a phenolic ether function. The substance, 2-isopropyl-5-methylphenoxyethyldiethylamine, protected guinea pigs against several lethal doses of histamine, antagonized histamine-induced spasm of various smooth muscles, and lessened the symptoms of anaphylactic shock. This drug was too toxic for clinical use, but by 1944, Bovet and his colleagues had described pyrilamine maleate, which is still one of the most specific and effective histamine antagonists of this category. The discovery of the highly effective histamine antagonists diphenhydramine and tripelennamine soon followed (*see* Bovet, 1950; Ganellin, in Ganellin and Parsons, 1982).

By the early 1950s many compounds with histamine-blocking activity were available to physicians, but they uniformly failed to inhibit certain responses to histamine, most conspicuously gastric acid secretion. The discovery by Black and colleagues of a new class of drugs that blocked histamine-induced gastric acid secretion provided new pharmacological tools with which to explore the functions of endogenous histamine, and it ushered in a major new class of therapeutic agents (*see* Chapter 37).

Structure–Activity Relationship. All of the available antagonists are reversible, competitive inhibitors of the interaction of histamine with H_1 receptors. Like histamine, many H_1 antagonists contain a substituted ethylamine moiety, 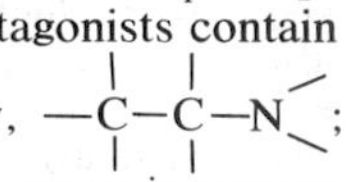; unlike histamine, which has a primary amino group and a single aromatic ring, most H_1 antagonists have a tertiary amino group linked by a two- or three-atom chain to two aromatic substituents and conform to the general formula:

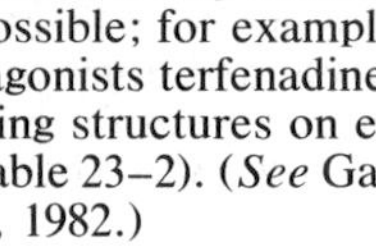

where Ar is aryl and X is a nitrogen or carbon atom or a —C—O— ether linkage to the β-aminoethyl side chain. Sometimes the two aromatic rings are bridged, as in the tricyclic derivatives, or the ethylamine may be part of a ring structure. Other variations are also possible; for example, the newer piperidine H_1 antagonists terfenadine and astemizole have aromatic ring structures on either side of the carbon chain (Table 23–2). (*See* Ganellin, in Ganellin and Parsons, 1982.)

PHARMACOLOGICAL PROPERTIES

Most H_1 antagonists have similar pharmacological actions and therapeutic applications and conveniently can be discussed together. Their effects are largely predictable from knowledge of the responses to histamine that involve interaction with H_1 receptors.

Smooth Muscle. H_1 antagonists inhibit most responses of smooth muscle to histamine. Antagonism of the constrictor action

Table 23–2. REPRESENTATIVE H_1 ANTAGONISTS

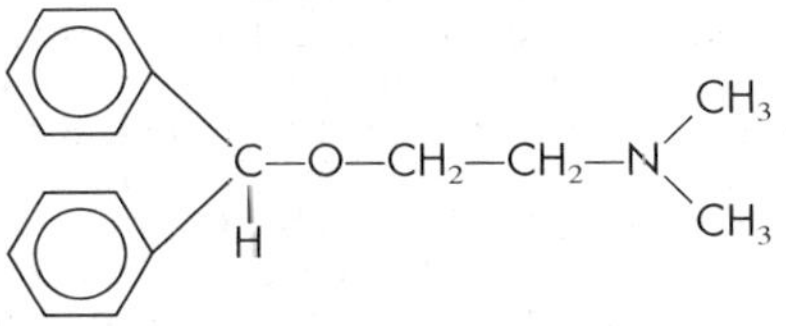

Diphenhydramine * (an ethanolamine)

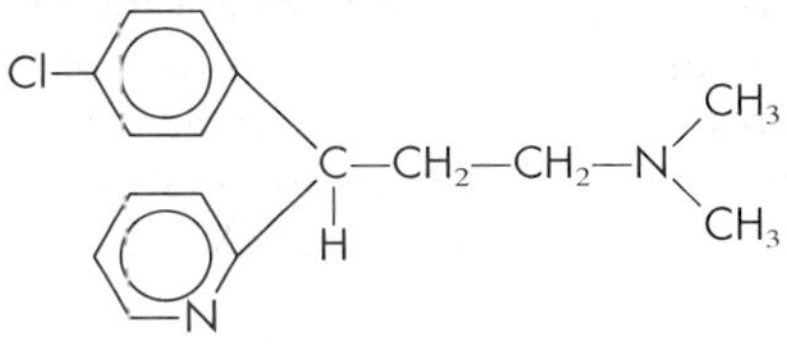

Chlorpheniramine † (an alkylamine)

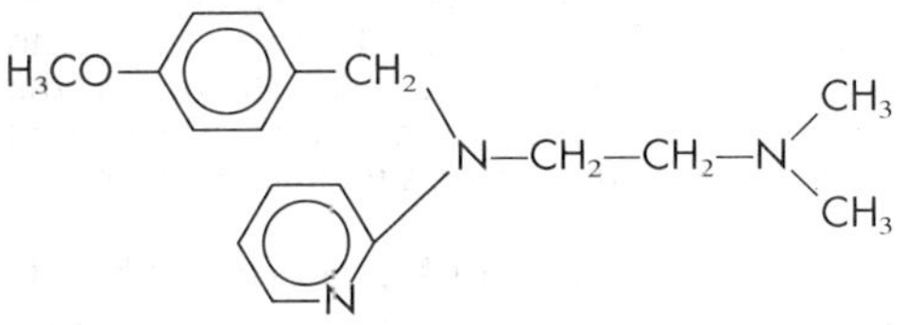

Pyrilamine ‡ (an ethylenediamine)

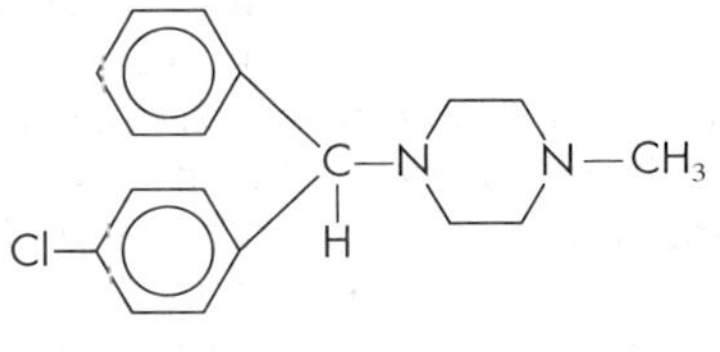

Chlorcyclizine § (a piperazine)

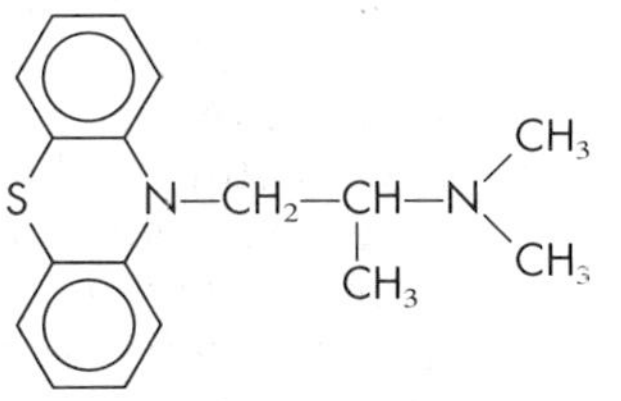

Promethazine (a phenothiazine)

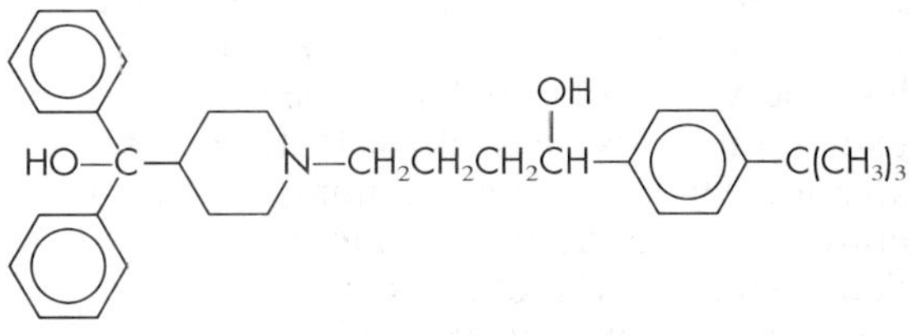

Terfenadine (a piperidine)

* Dimenhydrinate is a combination of diphenhydramine and 8-chlorotheophylline in equal molecular proportions.
† Pheniramine is the same less Cl.
‡ Tripelennamine is the same less H_3CO.
§ Cyclizine is the same less Cl.

of histamine on respiratory smooth muscle is easily shown *in vivo* or *in vitro*. In guinea pigs, for example, death by asphyxia follows quite small doses of histamine, yet the animal may survive a hundred lethal doses of histamine if given an H_1 antagonist. In the same species, striking protection is also afforded against anaphylactic bronchospasm. This is not so in man, because allergic bronchoconstriction is caused primarily by mediators such as leukotrienes and platelet-activating factor (*see* Chapter 24).

Within the vascular tree, the H_1 antagonists inhibit both the vasoconstrictor effects of histamine and, to a degree, the more rapid vasodilator effects that are mediated by H_1 receptors on endothelial cells. Residual vasodilatation reflects the involvement of H_2 receptors on smooth muscle and can be suppressed only by the concurrent administration of an H_2 antagonist. Effects of the histamine antagonists on histamine-induced changes in systemic blood pressure parallel these vascular effects.

Capillary Permeability. H_1 antagonists strongly block the action of histamine that results in increased capillary permeability and formation of edema and wheal.

"Flare" and Itch. The "flare" component of the triple response and the itching caused by intradermal injection of histamine are two different manifestations of the action of histamine on nerve endings. H_1 antagonists suppress both.

Exocrine Glands. Gastric secretion is not inhibited at all by H_1 antagonists, and they inconstantly suppress histamine-evoked salivary, lacrimal, and other exocrine secretions. The atropine-like properties of many of these agents may, however, contribute to lessened secretion in cholinergically innervated glands and reduce ongoing secretion in, for example, the respiratory tree.

Immediate Hypersensitivity Reactions: Anaphylaxis and Allergy. During hypersensitivity reactions, histamine is one of many potent autacoids released (*see* above), and its relative contribution to the ensuing symptoms varies widely with species and tissue. The protection afforded by histamine antagonists obviously varies accordingly. In man, some phenomena, including edema formation and itch, are fairly well controlled; others, such as hypotension, are less so. Bronchoconstriction is reduced little, if at all (*see* Dahlén *et al.*, 1983).

Central Nervous System. All H_1 antagonists studied to date can bind to H_1 receptors in the CNS (*see* Sorkin and Heel, 1985; Hough, 1988). However, a newer group of agents (*e.g.*, terfenadine, astemizole) are largely excluded from the brain when given in therapeutic doses (Sorkin and Heel, 1985; Krstenansky and Cluxton, 1987). The older H_1 antagonists can both stimulate and depress the CNS. Stimulation is occasionally encountered in patients given conventional doses, who become restless, nervous, and unable to sleep. Central excitation is also a striking feature of poisoning, which not uncommonly results in convulsions, particularly in infants. Central depression, on the other hand, is the usual accompaniment of therapeutic doses of the older H_1 antagonists. Diminished alertness, slowed reaction times, and somnolence are common manifestations. Some of the H_1 antagonists are more likely to depress the CNS than others, and patients vary in their susceptibility and responses to individual drugs. The ethanolamines (*e.g.*, diphenhydramine; *see* Table 23–2) are particularly prone to cause sedation. An antitussive effect reflects another and, perhaps, unrelated central action. The underlying mechanisms of these CNS actions are unknown.

An interesting and useful property of certain H_1 antagonists is the capacity to counter motion sickness. This effect was first observed with dimenhydrinate and subsequently with diphenhydramine (the active moiety of dimenhydrinate), various piperazine derivatives, and promethazine. The latter drug has perhaps the strongest muscarinic blocking activity among these agents and is among the most effective of the H_1 antagonists in combating motion sickness (*see* below). Since scopolamine is the most potent drug for the prevention of motion sickness (*see* Chapter 8), it is possible that the anticholinergic properties of certain H_1 antagonists are largely responsible for this effect.

Anticholinergic Effects. Many of the H_1 antagonists tend to inhibit responses to acetylcholine that are mediated by muscarinic receptors. These atropine-like actions are sufficiently prominent in some of the drugs to be manifest during clinical usage (*see* below). Among the older H_1 antagonists, pyrilamine is one of the least liable to produce this effect. The newer agents, terfenadine and astemizole, have no effect on muscarinic receptors (*see* Sorkin and Heel, 1985).

Local Anesthetic Effect. Some H_1 antagonists possess local anesthetic activity, and a few are more potent than procaine. Promethazine and pyrilamine are especially active. However, the concentrations required for this effect are several orders higher than those that antagonize histamine.

Absorption, Fate, and Excretion. The H_1 antagonists are well absorbed from the gastrointestinal tract. Following oral administration, peak plasma concentrations are achieved in 2 to 3 hours and effects usually last 4 to 6 hours; however, some of the drugs are much longer acting (Table 23–3).

Extensive studies of the metabolic fate of the older H_1 antagonists are limited. Diphenhydramine, given orally, reaches a maximal concentration in the blood in about 2 hours, remains at about this level for another 2 hours, and then falls exponentially with a plasma elimination half-time of about 8 hours. The drug is widely distributed throughout the body, including the CNS. Little, if any, is excreted unchanged in the urine; most appears there as metabolites. Other H_1 antagonists appear to be eliminated in much the same way (*see* reviews by Witiak and Lewis, 1978; Paton and Webster, 1985).

Information on the concentrations of these drugs achieved in the skin and mucous membranes is lacking. However, significant inhibition of "wheal-and-flare" responses to the intradermal injection of histamine or allergen may persist for 36 hours or more after treatment with some longer-acting H_1 antagonists, even when concentrations of the drugs in plasma are very low. Such results emphasize the need for flexibility in the interpretation of the recommended dosage schedules (*see* Table 23–3); less frequent dosage may suffice. Like many other drugs that are metabolized extensively, H_1 antagonists are eliminated more rapidly by children than by adults and more slowly in those with severe liver disease. H_1 blockers are among the many

Table 23–3. PREPARATIONS AND DOSAGE OF REPRESENTATIVE H_1-BLOCKING AGENTS *

CLASS AND NONPROPRIETARY NAME	TRADE NAME	DURATION OF ACTION (HOURS)	PREPARATIONS †	SINGLE DOSE (ADULT)
Ethanolamines				
Diphenhydramine hydrochloride	BENADRYL; others	4–6	O, L, I, T	25–50 mg
Dimenhydrinate	DRAMAMINE; others	4–6	O, L, I	50–100 mg
Carbinoxamine maleate	CLISTIN	3–4	O	4–8 mg
Ethylenediamines				
Pyrilamine maleate		4–6	O	25–50 mg
Tripelennamine hydrochloride	PBZ	4–6	O	25–50 mg; 100 mg (sustained release)
Tripelennamine citrate	PBZ		L	37.5–75 mg
Alkylamines				
Chlorpheniramine maleate	CHLOR-TRIMETON; others	4–6	O, L, I	4 mg 8–12 mg (sustained release) 5–20 mg (injection)
Brompheniramine maleate	DIMETANE; others	4–6	O, L, I	4 mg 8–12 mg (sustained release) 5–20 mg (injection)
Piperazines				
Hydroxyzine hydrochloride	ATARAX; others	6–24	O, L, I	25 mg
Hydroxyzine pamoate	VISTARIL	6–24	O, L	25 mg
Cyclizine hydrochloride	MAREZINE	4–6	O	50 mg
Cyclizine lactate	MAREZINE	4–6	I	50 mg
Meclizine hydrochloride	ANTIVERT; others	12–24	O	25–50 mg
Phenothiazines				
Promethazine hydrochloride	PHENERGAN; others	4–6	O, L, I, S	25 mg
Piperidines				
Terfenadine	SELDANE	12–24	O	60 mg
Astemizole	HISMANAL	< 24	O	10 mg (maintenance)

* For a discussion of phenothiazines, *see* Chapter 18.

† Preparations are designated as follows: O = oral solids; L = oral liquids; I = injection; S = suppository; T = topical. Many H_1-blocking agents are also available in preparations that contain multiple drugs.

drugs that induce hepatic microsomal enzymes, and they may facilitate their own metabolism (*see* Paton and Webster, 1985; Simons and Simons, 1988).

The newer H_1 antagonists terfenadine and astemizole do not penetrate the CNS and are metabolized to compounds that are active H_1 antagonists. Peak plasma concentrations of terfenadine occur 1 to 2 hours after oral administration. Although its plasma half-life is 4 to 5 hours, the drug is able to suppress the wheal and flare response to histamine or allergen for more than 12 hours, suggesting that the active metabolite is in part responsible for the effects of the compound. After oral administration of astemizole, maximal concentrations are achieved in 2 to 4 hours. The drug is extensively bound to plasma proteins and disappears from plasma with a half-life of about 20 hours. Astemizole is metabolized in the liver, principally to desmethylastemizole, which is also an active H_1 antagonist. Since the latter compound has a half-life of about 12 days, several weeks are required to reach steady-state concentrations of active compounds (astemizole plus metabolites) (*see* Paton and Webster, 1985; Sorkin and Heel, 1985; Krstenansky and Cluxton, 1987).

Side Effects. Although the side effects of the H_1 antagonists are rarely serious and often disappear with continued therapy, they are sometimes so troublesome that the drug must be withdrawn.

The side effect with the highest incidence, and the one common to all H_1 antagonists other than terfenadine or astemizole, is sedation (*see* Carruthers *et al.,* 1978). Although this may be a desirable adjunct in the treatment of some patients, it may interfere with the patient's daytime activities. Concurrent ingestion of alcohol or other CNS depressants produces an additive effect that impairs motor skills. Other untoward reactions referable to central actions include dizziness, tinnitus, lassitude, incoordination, fatigue, blurred vision, diplopia, euphoria, nervousness, insomnia, and tremors.

The next most frequent side effects involve the digestive tract and include loss of appetite, nausea, vomiting, epigastric distress, and constipation or diarrhea. Their incidence may be reduced by giving the drug with meals. Astemizole appears to increase appetite and cause weight gain. Other side effects that are apparently caused by the antimuscarinic actions of some of the older agents include dryness of the mouth and respiratory passages, sometimes inducing cough, urinary retention or frequency, and dysuria. These effects are not observed with terfenadine or astemizole. Palpitation, hypotension, headache, tightness of the chest, and tingling and weakness of the hands may also occur with the older agents.

Drug allergy may develop when H_1 antagonists are given orally, but more commonly it results from topical application. Allergic dermatitis is not uncommon; other hypersensitivity reactions include drug fever and photosensitization. Hematological complications such as leukopenia, agranulocytosis, and hemolytic anemia are very rare. Teratogenic effects have been noted in response to piperazine compounds, but extensive clinical studies have not demonstrated any association between the use of such H_1 antagonists and fetal anomalies in man. Since H_1 antagonists interfere with skin tests for allergy, they must be withdrawn well before such tests are performed.

In acute poisoning with H_1 antagonists, their central excitatory effects constitute the greatest danger. The syndrome includes hallucinations, excitement, ataxia, incoordination, athetosis, and convulsions. Fixed, dilated pupils with a flushed face, together with sinus tachycardia, urinary retention, dry mouth, and fever, lend the syndrome a remarkable similarity to that of atropine poisoning. Terminally, there is deepening coma with cardiorespiratory collapse and death, usually within 2 to 18 hours. Treatment is along general symptomatic and supportive lines.

Preparations. A needlessly large number of H_1 antagonists are available. The nonsedating H_1 antagonists terfenadine and astemizole offer advantages over the older agents for symptoms of allergy but are more costly. The brief discussion that follows is intended to provide an indication of the different classes of these drugs and their properties. Representative preparations are listed in Table 23–3.

Ethanolamines (Prototype: Diphenhydramine). The drugs in this group possess significant antimuscarinic activity and have a pronounced tendency to induce sedation. With conventional doses, about half of those who are treated with these drugs experience somnolence. The incidence of gastrointestinal side effects, however, is low with this group.

Ethylenediamines (Prototype: Pyrilamine). These include some of the most specific H_1 antagonists. Although their central effects are relatively feeble, somnolence occurs in a fair proportion of patients. Gastrointestinal side effects are quite common.

Alkylamines (Prototype: Chlorpheniramine). These are among the most potent H_1 antagonists. The drugs are not so prone as some H_1 antagonists to produce drowsiness and are among the more suitable agents for daytime use; but again, a significant proportion of patients do experience sedation. Side effects involving CNS stimulation are more common in this than in other groups.

Piperazines (Prototype: Chlorcyclizine). The oldest member of this group, chlorcyclizine, has a more prolonged action and produces a comparatively low incidence of drowsiness. Hydroxyzine is a long-acting compound that is widely used for skin allergies; its considerable central-depressant activity may contribute to its prominent antipruritic action. Cyclizine and meclizine have been used primarily to counter motion sickness, although promethazine and diphenhydramine (dimenhydrinate) are more effective (as is scopolamine; *see* below).

Phenothiazines (Prototype: Promethazine). Most drugs of this class are H_1 antagonists and also possess considerable anticholinergic activity. Promethazine, which has prominent sedative effects, and its many congeners are now used primarily for their antiemetic effects (*see* Chapter 38).

Piperidines (Prototype: Terfenadine). H_1 antagonists of this class include terfenadine and astemizole. These agents are highly selective for H_1 receptors and are devoid of significant anticholinergic actions. Together with these drugs' poor penetration into the CNS, these properties appear to account for the low incidence of side effects. Other nonsedating H_1 antagonists under study include loratadine (a piperidine), mequitazine (a phenothiazine), and cetirizine (a piperazine).

Therapeutic Uses. H_1 antagonists have an established and valued place in the symptomatic treatment of various immediate hypersensitivity reactions. In addition, the central properties of some of the series are of therapeutic value for suppressing motion sickness or for sedation.

Diseases of Allergy. H_1 antagonists are most useful in acute exudative types of allergy that present with symptoms of rhinitis, urticaria, and conjunctivitis. Their effect, however, is purely palliative and confined to the suppression of symptoms attributable to the histamine released by the antigen–antibody reaction. The drugs do not diminish the intensity of this reaction, which is the cause of the various hypersensitivity diseases. In bronchial asthma, histamine antagonists are singularly ineffectual. Similarly, in the treatment of systemic anaphylaxis, in which autacoids other than histamine play major roles, the mainstay of therapy is epinephrine, with histamine antagonists having only a subordinate and adjuvant role. The same is true for severe angioedema, in which laryngeal swelling constitutes a threat to life.

Other allergies of the respiratory tract are more amenable to therapy with H_1 antagonists. The best results are obtained in seasonal rhinitis and conjunctivitis (hay fever, pollinosis), in which these drugs relieve the sneezing, rhinorrhea, and itching of eyes, nose, and throat. A gratifying response is obtained in most patients, especially at the beginning of the season when pollen counts are low; however, the drugs are less effective when the allergens are in abundance, when exposure to them is prolonged, and when nasal congestion has become prominent. In contrast to the older agents, astemizole has been shown to be effective in suppressing symptoms of perennial vasomotor rhinitis (*see* Wihl *et al.*, 1985).

Certain of the allergic dermatoses respond favorably to H_1 antagonists. Benefit is most striking in acute urticaria, although the itching in this condition is perhaps better controlled than are the edema and the erythema. Chronic urticaria is less responsive, but some benefit may occur in a fair proportion of patients. Furthermore, the combined use of H_1 and H_2 antagonists is effective for some individuals if therapy with an H_1 antagonist has failed (*see* Chapter 37). Angioedema is also responsive to treatment with H_1 antagonists, but the paramount importance of epinephrine in the severe attack must be reemphasized, especially in the life-threatening involvement of the larynx. Here, however, it may be appropriate to administer additionally an H_1 antagonist by the intravenous route. H_1 antagonists also have a place in the treatment of itching pruritides. Some relief may be obtained in many patients suffering from atopic dermatitis and contact dermatitis (although topical corticosteroids are more valuable) and in such diverse conditions as insect bites and ivy poisoning. Various other pruritides without an allergic basis sometimes respond to antihistamine therapy, usually when the drugs are applied topically but sometimes when they are given orally. However, the possibility of producing allergic dermatitis with local application of H_1 antagonists must be recognized. Since these drugs inhibit allergic dermatoses, they should be withdrawn well before skin testing for allergies.

The urticarial and edematous lesions of serum sickness respond to H_1 antagonists, but fever and arthralgia often do not. Gastrointestinal allergies are seldom benefited significantly by these drugs.

Many drug reactions attributable to allergic phenomena respond to therapy with H_1 antagonists, particularly those characterized by itch, urticaria, and angioedema; reactions of the serum-sickness type also respond to intensive treatment. However, explosive release of histamine generally calls for treatment with epinephrine, with H_1 antagonists being accorded a subsidiary role. Nevertheless, prophylactic treatment with an H_1 antagonist may suffice to reduce symptoms to a tolerable level when a drug known to be a histamine liberator is to be given. Extensive discussion of the effects of H_1 antagonists in allergic and related conditions may be found in the articles by Beaven (1978), Hahn (1978), Burland and Mills (in Ganellin and Parsons, 1982), Salvaggio (1982), and Symposium (1982).

Common Cold. Despite persistent popular belief, H_1 antagonists are without value in combating the common cold. The weak anticholinergic effects of the older agents may tend to lessen rhinorrhea, but this drying effect may do more harm than good, as may also their tendency to induce somnolence (*see* West *et al.*, 1975).

Motion Sickness, Vertigo, and Sedation. Although scopolamine, given orally, parenterally, or transdermally, is the most effective of all drugs for the prophylaxis and treatment of motion sickness, some H_1 antagonists are useful in a broad range of milder conditions and offer the advantage of fewer adverse effects. These include dimenhydrinate and the piperazines (cyclizine, meclizine, and others). Promethazine is more potent and more effective and its additional antiemetic properties may be of value in reducing vomiting, but its pronounced sedative action is usually disadvantageous (*see* Graybiel *et al.*, 1975; Wood, 1979). Whenever possible, the various drugs should be administered an hour or so before the anticipated motion.

Some H_1 antagonists, notably dimenhydrinate and meclizine, are often of benefit in vestibular disturbances, such as Ménière's disease, and in other types of true vertigo (*see* Cohen and deJong, 1972). The same drugs and promethazine have some lesser usefulness in treating the nausea and vomiting subsequent to chemotherapy or radiation therapy for malignancies; however, more effective antiemetic drugs are available (*see* Chapter 38).

Diphenhydramine can be used to reverse the extrapyramidal side effects caused by phenothiazines. The anticholinergic actions of this agent can also be utilized in the early stages of treatment of patients with Parkinson's disease (*see* Chapter 20).

The tendency of certain of the H_1 blockers to produce somnolence has led to their use as hypnotics. H_1 antagonists, principally diphenhydramine, are often present in various proprietary remedies for insomnia that are sold "over the counter." While these remedies are generally ineffective in the recommended doses, some sensitive individuals may derive benefit (*see* Faingold, 1978). The sedative and mild antianxiety activities of hydroxyzine and diphenhydramine have contributed to their use as weak anxiolytics.

BRADYKININ AND KALLIDIN AND THEIR ANTAGONISTS

A variety of factors including tissue damage, allergic reactions, viral infections, and other inflammatory events activate a series of proteolytic reactions that generate bradykinin and kallidin in the plasma. These peptides are autacoids that act locally to produce pain, vasodilatation, increased vascular permeability, and the synthesis of prostaglandins. Thus, they comprise a subset of the large number of mediators that contribute to the inflammatory response.

History. The old observation that urine, injected intravenously, lowers blood pressure led to the discovery of the kinins. In the 1920s and 1930s, Frey and his associates Kraut and Werle characterized the hypotensive substance and showed that similar material could be obtained from saliva, plasma, and a variety of tissues. Since the pancreas was a rich source, they named this material kallikrein after an old Greek synonym for that organ, *kallikréas*. By 1937, Werle, Götze, and Keppler had established that kallikreins generate a pharmacologically active substance from some inactive precursor present in plasma. In 1948, Werle and Berek named the active substance *kallidin* and showed it to be a polypeptide cleaved from a plasma globulin that they termed *kallidinogen* (*see* Werle, 1970).

Interest in the field intensified when Rocha e Silva and associates (1949) reported that trypsin and certain snake venoms acted on plasma globulin to produce a substance that lowered blood pressure and caused a slowly developing contraction of the gut. Because of this slow response, they named this substance *bradykinin,* a term derived from the Greek words *bradys,* meaning "slow," and *kinein,* meaning "to move." In 1960, the nonapeptide bradykinin was isolated by Elliott and coworkers and synthesized by Boissonnas and associates. Shortly thereafter, kallidin was found to be a decapeptide—bradykinin with an additional lysine residue at the amino terminus. These substances are members of a group of polypeptides with related chemical structures and pharmacological properties that are widely distributed in nature. For the whole group the generic term *kinins* has been adopted, and kallidin and bradykinin are referred to as plasma kinins (*see* Bertaccini, 1976; Erdös, 1979; Fritz *et al.*, 1983). In the mid 1980s, peptide antagonists of bradykinin were developed, providing new tools with which to explore the functions of kinins (*see* Vavrek and Stewart, 1985).

THE ENDOGENOUS KALLIKREIN–KININOGEN–KININ SYSTEM

Synthesis and Metabolism of Kinins. Bradykinin is a nonapeptide with the following amino acid sequence: Arg-Pro-Pro-Gly-Phe-Ser-Pro-Phe-Arg. Kallidin has an additional lysine residue at the amino-terminal position and is sometimes referred to as lysyl-bradykinin. The two peptides are cleaved from α_2 globulins that are synthesized by the liver and circulate in the plasma. These precursors are termed *kininogens*. There are two kininogens, high-molecular-weight (HMW) and low-molecular-weight (LMW) kininogen. A number of serine proteases will generate kinins, but the highly specific proteases that release bradykinin and kallidin from the kininogens are termed *kallikreins* (*see* Figure 23–1 and below).

Kallikreins. The kallikreins circulate in plasma in an inactive state and must be activated by other proteases. Two kallikreins act on the kininogens: plasma kallikrein and tissue kallikrein. These are distinct enzymes, and they are activated by different mechanisms. Plasma prekallikrein is an inactive protein of about 88,000 daltons that is bound in a 1:1 complex with its substrate, HMW kininogen. The cascade is restrained by the protease inhibitors present in plasma. Among the most important are the inhibitor of the activated first component of complement ($C\bar{1}$ INH) and α_2-macroglobulin. Plasma prekallikrein is cleaved and activated by Hageman factor (HF; factor XII; a protease that is common to both the kinin and the intrinsic coagulation cascades) to the active 36,000-dalton moiety, kallikrein. Hageman factor itself is activated by contact with negatively charged surfaces such as collagen. Importantly, as indicated by the dotted lines in Figure 23–1, kallikrein further activates Hageman factor, thereby exerting a positive feedback on the system (*see* Proud and Kaplan, 1988).

Glandular or tissue kallikrein is a smaller protein

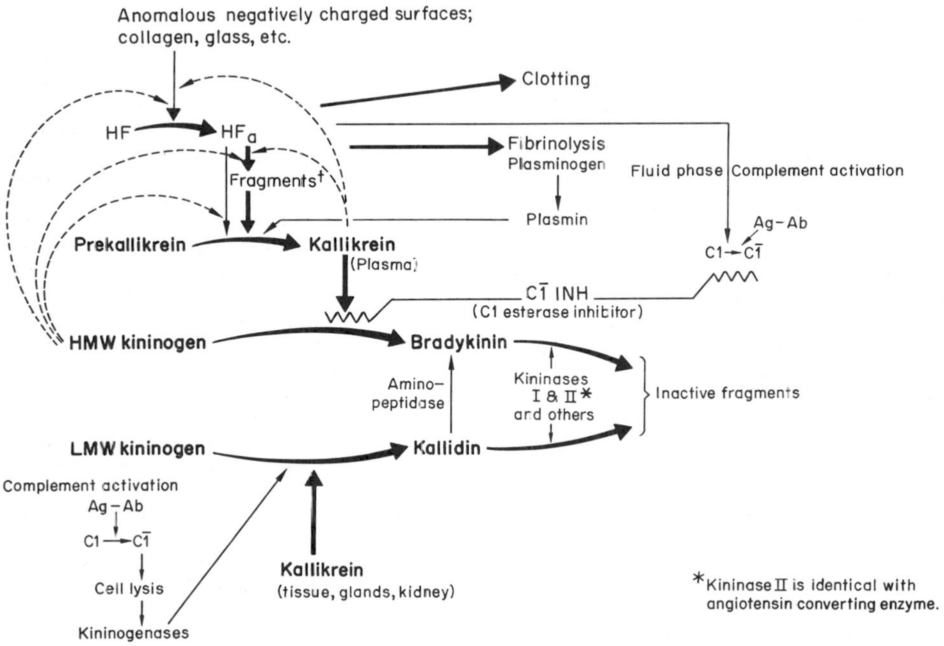

Figure 23–1. *Formation and destruction of the kinins.*

Bradykinin and kallidin are formed, respectively, by plasma and tissue kallikreins. Note the relationship of the plasma kinin–forming system to other Hageman factor (HF)–dependent processes, notably blood clotting and fibrinolysis. Two components of the kinin cascade—prekallikrein and high-molecular-weight (HMW) kininogen—are essential for HF activation and function and hence are also clotting factors (*see* Chapter 55). Their points of interaction are indicated by the dashed arrows; note especially the strong positive feedback provided by kallikrein, which is a major HF activator in the fluid phase and mainly responsible for the formation of the HF fragments (†) that are potent kallikrein activators. The kallikrein-inhibiting effect of complement C1 esterase inhibitor (C1̄ INH) is indicated; this agent is the primary inhibitor of plasma kallikrein. Other plasma protease inhibitors, α_2-macroglobulin and α_1-antitrypsin, act at the same site. The latter seems to be of more importance, however, with regard to inhibition of tissue kallikrein. The activation of complement by antigen–antibody complexes (Ag–Ab), leading to cell lysis liberating kininogenases, is indicated, along with fluid-phase activation of complement by HF_a. Negative-feedback, restraining mechanisms and other complexities are omitted. Note that kininase II is the same enzyme (dipeptidyl carboxypeptidase) as angiotensin converting enzyme (*see* Chapter 31).

(molecular weight of 29,000) that is synthesized in a number of tissues; it acts locally near its site of origin (Fukushima *et al.*, 1985; Evans *et al.*, 1988). A fragment of 24 amino acids is removed from this protein to form the active enzyme, but the endogenous protease responsible for this reaction has not been identified. The synthesis of tissue prekallikrein is regulated by a number of factors, including aldosterone in the kidney and salivary gland and androgens in certain other glands. The secretion of the tissue prekallikrein may also be regulated; for example, its secretion from the pancreas is enhanced by stimulation of the vagus nerve (*see* Proud and Kaplan, 1988; Margolius, 1989).

Kininogens. The two substrates for the kallikreins, HMW and LMW kininogen, are products of a single gene that arise by alternative processing of mRNA. The HMW kininogen contains 626 amino acid residues; the internal bradykinin sequence of 9 amino acid residues connects an amino-terminal "heavy chain" sequence (362 amino acids) and a carboxyl-terminal "light chain" sequence (255 amino acids). LMW kininogen is identical to the larger form of the protein from the amino terminus through the bradykinin sequence; its short "light chain" differs (Takagaki *et al.*, 1985). HMW kininogen is cleaved by plasma and tissue kallikrein to yield bradykinin and kallidin, respectively. LMW kininogen is a substrate only for the tissue kallikrein and the product is kallidin (*see* Nakanishi, 1987).

Metabolism. The decapeptide kallidin is about as active as the nonapeptide bradykinin and need not be converted to the latter to exert its characteristic effects. Some conversion of kallidin to bradykinin occurs as the amino-terminal lysine residue is removed by a plasma aminopeptidase. However, this reaction is slow relative to the rate of inactivation by hydrolysis at the carboxyl terminus. The minimal effective structure required to elicit the classical responses is that of the nonapeptide.

The kinins have an evanescent existence—their half-life in plasma is only about 15 seconds. Moreover, in a single passage through the pulmonary vascular bed some 80 to 90% of the kinins may be destroyed (*see* Ryan, 1982). The principal catabolizing enzyme in the lung and in other vascular beds is a dipeptidyl carboxypeptidase, known in this context as kininase II and in another as angiotensin converting enzyme (*see* Chapter 31). Removal of the carboxyl-terminal dipeptide abolishes kinin-like activity. A slower-acting enzyme, arginine carboxypeptidase (carboxypeptidase-N; kininase I), removes the carboxyl-terminal arginine residue (*see* Erdös, 1979; Fritz *et al.,* 1983). This too usually abolishes kinin-like activity; however, the des-Arg kinins that are formed may be active in some damaged tissues, where a different type of receptor for the kinins is apparently induced (*see* Marceau *et al.,* 1983; Regoli, 1987).

FUNCTIONS OF ENDOGENOUS KALLIKREINS AND KININS

Although the mechanisms for synthesis and degradation of the kinins are now understood in detail, the physiological roles of the peptides are being uncovered at a much slower rate. However, the discovery of effective bradykinin antagonists (*see* below) has helped to establish a role for the peptides in mediating nociception; other potential functions include participation in the regulation of blood pressure and the maintenance of fluid and electrolyte balance by the kidney. However, the most important function of the kinins appears to be their substantial role in the inflammatory response.

Pain. The algesic properties of bradykinin are well appreciated (Clark, 1979). Bradykinin receptors in the nervous system are localized to sites that are involved in nociception, including the superficial layers of the spinal cord, thin unmyelinated fibers, and cells in sensory ganglia. When applied to these sites, bradykinin elicits pain (Steranka *et al.,* 1988). In addition, bradykinin antagonists block the pain that is produced when bradykinin is applied to the exposed base of a blister on human skin as well as the generation of pain in several animal models (Steranka *et al.,* 1989).

Effects on Renal Function and Blood Pressure. Kinins affect the composition and volume of urine. They enhance the electrogenic transport of chloride in the collecting duct by stimulating receptors on the basolateral surface of the tubule cell. This effect, combined with the fact that tissue concentrations of renal kallikrein are increased by aldosterone, has suggested that kinins may be involved in the local regulation of renal function (Margolius, 1989). Although speculation about a role for the kinins in the regulation of blood pressure has been spurred by the knowledge that kininase II is identical with angiotensin converting enzyme, most studies using bradykinin antagonists have provided little support for this notion. However, the kinin system may be activated to blunt the effects of pressor agents (*see* Gavras and Gavras, 1988; Steranka *et al.,* 1989; Burch *et al.,* 1990).

Inflammation. Kinins mimic the manifestations of inflammation (*see* below), and measurement of the components of the kinin cascade and the effects of bradykinin antagonists indicate that kinins participate in a variety of inflammatory disorders. These include rhinitis caused by the inhalation of antigen, as well as that associated with rhinoviral infection (Proud and Kaplan, 1988; Burch *et al.,* 1990). Kinins are also involved in the manifestations of disorders such as hereditary angioedema. This disease, which results from defects in the complement inhibitor, $C\bar{1}$ INH (*see* above), is characterized by episodic swelling, laryngeal edema, and abdominal pain. Bradykinin is formed during such episodes, and there is depletion of the components of the kinin cascade (Proud and Kaplan, 1988). Kinins may also participate in inflammatory responses to urate deposits in gout, as well as those associated with endotoxic shock and disseminated intravascular coagulation (Proud and Kaplan, 1988; Burch *et al.,* 1990).

PHARMACOLOGICAL PROPERTIES

The plasma kinins are potent vasodilators. They increase capillary permeability and produce edema; they evoke pain and reflexes by acting on nerve endings; and they contract various smooth muscles. In all these respects bradykinin and kallidin behave very similarly (*see* Erdös, 1979; Regoli and Barabé, 1980; Marceau *et al.,* 1983). Furthermore, the responses to bradykinin are similar to those produced by stimulation of H_1 receptors (Table 23–4).

Cardiovascular System. *Blood Vessels.* On a molar basis, kinins are about ten times more potent than histamine in causing vasodilatation. If injected intravenously in man they cause flushing in the blush area and conjunctival injection. Blood vessels in muscle, kidney, viscera, and various glands are also dilated, as are coronary and cerebral vessels; throbbing headache may occur. Certain of these direct effects may be complemented by the ability of kinins to stimulate the release of histamine from mast cells. Dilatation of systemic arterioles causes a sharp fall in systolic and diastolic blood pressures. The dilatation is mediated by endothelial cells (*see* below). In contrast, large arteries and most veins, large and small, tend to be contracted by the kinins. Kinins promote dilatation of the fetal pulmonary artery, closure of the ductus arteriosus, and constriction of the umbilical vessels, all of which occur in the adjustment from fetal to neonatal circulation.

Heart. Cardiac muscle is not directly affected by bradykinin, but the fall in total peripheral resistance and systemic blood pressure owing to vasodilatation, combined with contraction of the large veins and increased venous return, causes a reflex increase in heart rate and increased cardiac output.

Table 23–4. COMPARISON OF SELECTED RESPONSES TO HISTAMINE, BRADYKININ, AND 5-HT

TISSUE OR CELL TYPE	HISTAMINE *Receptor*	HISTAMINE *Response*	BRADYKININ *Receptor*	BRADYKININ *Response*	5-HT *Receptor*	5-HT *Response*
Arteries	H_1	Contraction	B_1 *	Contraction	5-HT_2	Contraction
Arterioles	H_1	Relaxation (via EDRF) †	B_2	Relaxation (via EDRF)	5-HT_1	Relaxation (via EDRF)
	H_2	Relaxation	—	—	5-HT_1	Relaxation
Venules	H_1	Contraction	B_2	Relaxation (via EDRF)	5-HT_2	Contraction
	H_2	Relaxation	—	—	—	—
Veins	H_1	Contraction	B_1 *	Contraction	5-HT_2	Contraction
	—	—	—	—	5-HT_1	Relaxation
Endothelial cells						
Release of mediators	H_1	Release of EDRF	B_2	Release of EDRF	5-HT_1	Release of EDRF
Contraction	H_1	Increased permeability	B_2	Increased permeability	— ‡	—
Autonomic nerves	—	—	—	—	5-HT_1	Decreased release of NE †
Sensory nerves	H_1	Depolarization (itch, pain)	B_2	Depolarization (pain)	5-HT_3	Depolarization (itch, pain)
Mast cells	H_2	Decreased release of mediators	?	Histamine release	—	—
Platelets	—	—	—	—	5-HT_2	Stimulate aggregation

* Synthesis of B_1 receptors is induced by tissue damage. The normal response is dilatation via B_2 receptors.
† EDRF = endothelium-derived relaxing factor; NE = norepinephrine.
‡ 5-HT does not markedly increase vascular permeability in man.

Vascular Permeability and Edema Formation. The plasma kinins increase permeability in the microcirculation. The effect, like that of histamine (and 5-HT in some species), is exerted on the small venules and involves separation of the junctions between endothelial cells. This, together with an increased hydrostatic pressure gradient, causes edema. Such edema, coupled with stimulation of nerve endings (*see* below), results in a "wheal-and-flare" response to intradermal injections in man.

Extravascular Smooth Muscle. Various smooth muscle preparations contract in response to the kinins. The rat uterus is especially sensitive. It was the characteristic, slowly developing contraction of the isolated guinea pig ileum that prompted the name *bradykinin*. Tracheobronchial constriction is prominent in guinea pigs, but dilatation as well as constriction may occur in other species. In man, bronchial smooth muscle is contracted. Respiratory distress can be provoked by inhalation of kinins by asthmatics.

Stimulation of Nerve Endings and Production of Pain. The plasma kinins are powerful algesic agents (*see* above). For example, they cause an intense, burning pain when applied to the exposed base of a blister and a throbbing, burning pain in the hand when injected into the brachial artery.

Mechanism of Action. Evidence suggests the existence of three types of receptors for kinins. Those designated B_1 are most sensitive to the carboxyl-terminal des-Arg metabolites of bradykinin and kallidin and mediate contraction of vascular smooth muscle. The synthesis of B_1 receptors appears to be induced by trauma or pathological insults (Regoli, 1987). Selective B_1-receptor antagonists have been synthesized (*see* below). In contrast, B_2 receptors are most sensitive to the intact peptides. They appear to mediate the majority of the effects of bradykinin, including vasodilatation, increased vascular permeability, smooth muscle contraction, and pain (Regoli, 1987; Steranka *et al.*, 1989). Current B_2 antagonists do not discriminate between B_1 and B_2 receptors (*see* below). The possibility of a B_3 receptor is based on the observation that bradykinin-induced contraction in guinea pig tracheal smooth muscle is not blocked by known B_1 or B_2 antagonists (Farmer *et al.*, 1989).

Stimulation of B_2 receptors causes activation of phospholipase C and increased concentrations of cytosolic Ca^{2+}, as described above for the H_1 receptor. Stimulation of B_2 receptors also activates phospholipase A_2 (perhaps via increased Ca^{2+}), resulting in the synthesis of various eicosanoids. Increased intracellular Ca^{2+} causes contraction of smooth muscle, and stimulation of pain fibers may be mediated similarly (Fasolato *et al.*, 1988). Bradykinin-induced vasodilatation is mediated by the production of EDRF and prostaglandins by vascular endothelial cells (*see* above and Peach *et al.*, 1985; Jacob *et al.*, 1988; Furchgott and Vanhoutte, 1989).

Inhibitors of Kallikreins and Kinins. Although peptide inhibitors of kallikrein are available, progress has been more substantial in the development of selective antagonists of the kinins.

Receptor Antagonists. The first competitive bradykinin antagonist, [D-Phe[7]]bradykinin, was described by Vavrek and Stewart (1985). Two types of antagonists have been developed subsequently—those that block both B_1 and B_2 receptors and those that are selective for the B_1 receptor. The most selective and potent B_1 antagonists are des-$Arg^9[Leu^8]$bradykinin and des-$Arg^{10}[Leu^9]$kallidin (Burch *et al.*, 1990). An example of an antagonist that acts on both B_1 and B_2 receptors is D-Arg[4-hydroxy-Pro^3-D-Phe^7]bradykinin. Analogs of this type block the majority of the biological effects of kinins that are mediated by B_2 receptors (*see* above and Burch *et al.*, 1990). Unfortunately, the compounds that are currently available have very short half-lives *in vivo*.

Kallikrein Inhibitors. Inhibitors of kallikreins such as *aprotinin* (TRASYLOL, others) have been used in the past in attempts to treat acute pancreatitis and carcinoid syndrome (*see* Fritz *et al.*, 1983). Newer compounds are based on the structure of the Arg-Ser cleavage site in bovine kininogen (Okunishi *et al.*, 1985, 1987).

Therapeutic Uses. In initial trials, the nonselective bradykinin antagonist D-Arg[4-hydroxy-Pro^3-D-Phe^7]bradykinin has produced encouraging results in the relief of cold symptoms caused by the rhinovirus, in the suppression of pain from burns, and in the treatment of allergic asthma (Steranka *et al.*, 1989; Burch *et al.*, 1990).

5-HYDROXYTRYPTAMINE AND ITS ANTAGONISTS

5-Hydroxytryptamine (5-HT) is found in high concentrations in platelets, the enterochromaffin cells located throughout the gastrointestinal tract, and in certain regions of the brain. The physiological role of 5-HT as a neurotransmitter in the CNS is clearly established (*see* Chapter 12). 5-HT released from platelets appears to participate in hemostasis. It may play a role in certain vasospastic diseases and produce some of the manifestations of carcinoid, a syndrome caused by tumors of the enterochromaffin cell.

History. A vasoconstrictor material appears in serum when blood is allowed to clot. In the late 1940s, the substance appeared in another context during a search for humoral pressor agents such as angiotensin that might explain arterial hypertension. In this work the vasoconstrictor was a "pest," to be eliminated before the other enquiry could proceed. In 1948, investigators at the Cleveland Clinic crystallized the substance and named it serotonin (Rapport *et al.*, 1948); shortly thereafter, Rapport deduced that the active moiety was 5-HT.

Independently, in the 1930s Erspamer and colleagues began to characterize the substance that imparts peculiar histochemical properties to enterochromaffin cells of the gastrointestinal mucosa. Their experiments led them to discover, first in the mucosa and later in other tissues, a gut-stimulating factor, which they termed *enteramine*. By the late 1940s, Erspamer had shown that it was present in many tissues of vertebrates and invertebrates and had suggested that it was an indole alkylamine. In 1952, Erspamer and Asero identified enteramine as 5-HT (*see* Erspamer, 1966a).

Thus, by the time 5-HT had been identified chemically, a mass of evidence indicated that it was widely distributed and possessed a variety of pharmacological actions. Interest was heightened greatly by the discovery of 5-HT in the brain, the observations that lysergic acid diethylamide (LSD) and other potent hallucinogens were structurally similar to 5-HT and inhibited smooth muscle responses to 5-HT (Gaddum, 1953; Woolley and Shaw, 1954), and the finding that reserpine lowered the concentration of 5-HT in the brain (*see* Brodie and Shore, 1957).

Source and Chemistry. 5-HT is 3-(β-aminoethyl)-5-hydroxyindole. Like histamine, it is widely distributed in the animal and plant kingdoms. It occurs in vertebrates; in tunicates, mollusks, arthropods, and coelenterates; and in fruits and nuts. It is also present in numerous venoms, including those of the common stinging nettle, wasps, and scorpions.

Numerous synthetic or naturally occurring congeners of 5-HT have varying degrees of peripheral and central pharmacological activity. Particularly noteworthy are the "tryptamines" of plant origin with potent effects on brain function. For example, N,N-dimethyltryptamine (DMT) and its 5-hydroxy derivative (bufotenine) are active principles of the cahobe bean found along the shores of the Caribbean and used in aboriginal rites to induce mental changes. Both of these compounds can be formed in the mammal by N-methylation of tryptamine and 5-HT, respectively. In addition to the recognizable 4-substituted tryptamine moiety in LSD, the active ingredients of various hallucinogenic mushrooms are also 4-substituted tryptamine derivatives (*e.g.*, psilocine is 4-hydroxy-N,N-dimethyltryptamine). (*See* Weil-Malherbe, 1978; Ho *et al.*, 1982; *see also* Chapters 12 and 22.)

ENDOGENOUS 5-HYDROXYTRYPTAMINE: DISTRIBUTION, BIOSYNTHESIS, AND METABOLISM

Distribution. About 90% of the 5-HT present in the adult human body (about 10 mg) is located in the enterochromaffin cells of the gastrointestinal tract; most of the remainder is present in platelets and the CNS. Although mast cells of some species contain 5-HT, human mast cells do not (*see* Erspamer, 1966a, 1966b; Essman, 1978b).

Synthesis, Uptake, and Storage. The 5-HT found in enterochromaffin cells and neurons is synthesized *in situ* from tryptophan; platelets acquire 5-HT from their environment (*see* below). Tryptophan is first hydroxylated to 5-hydroxytryptophan (5-HTP) by the enzyme tryptophan-5-hydroxylase (the activity of which is rate-limiting), and is then decarboxylated to 5-HT by the nonspecific aromatic L-amino acid decarboxylase. 5-HT is then taken up into secretory granules and stored. The mechanisms for sequestration of 5-HT in storage granules are similar to those for catecholamines. Thus, drugs such as reserpine that disrupt the storage of catecholamines also impair the storage of 5-HT. Platelets actively accumulate 5-HT during their passage through the intestinal blood vessels, where they encounter relatively high concentrations of 5-HT that result from its secretion by enterochromaffin cells. The transport systems for 5-HT that are found in platelets and tryptaminergic neurons resemble those for neuronal reuptake of catecholamines and are influenced by many of the tricyclic antidepressant drugs. An amount of 5-HT roughly equal to that present in the body is synthesized each day. Turnover times of 5-HT in brain and gastrointestinal tract have been estimated at about 1 and 17 hours, respectively. (*See* Bosin, 1978; De Clerck and Vanhoutte, 1982; and Ho *et al.*, 1982.)

Absorption, Metabolism, and Excretion. Most 5-HT, endogenous or ingested, undergoes oxidative deamination by MAO to form 5-hydroxyindoleacetaldehyde. This is promptly degraded, mainly by further oxidation, to 5-hydroxyindoleacetic acid (5-HIAA) by aldehyde dehydrogenase; 5-hydroxyindoleacetaldehyde is also reduced (by alcohol dehydrogenase) to 5-hydroxytryptophol (5-HTOL). The three enzymes are present in liver and in various tissues that contain 5-HT, including the brain. The principal metabolite, 5-HIAA, is excreted in the urine, along with much smaller amounts of 5-HTOL, mainly as the glucuronide or sulfate. About 2 to 10 mg of 5-HIAA is excreted daily by the normal adult as a result of metabolism of endogenous 5-HT. Larger amounts are excreted by patients with malignant carcinoid, providing a reliable diagnostic test for the disease (*see* Feldman and O'Dorisio, 1986). Ingestion of ethyl alcohol diverts 5-hydroxyindoleacetaldehyde from the oxidative route to the reductive pathway because of the elevated concentration of NADH. This greatly increases excretion of 5-HTOL and correspondingly reduces that of 5-HIAA (*see* Bosin, 1978; Youdim and Ashkenazi, in Ho *et al.*, 1982).

ENDOGENOUS 5-HYDROXYTRYPTAMINE: FUNCTIONS

A major function of 5-HT is to serve as the chemical transmitter for tryptaminergic neurons within the brain. In addition, 5-HT serves as a precursor for the pineal hormone melatonin. In the periphery, 5-HT may play a role in regulating gastrointestinal motility; it is secreted by carcinoid tumors. 5-HT released from platelets appears to participate in hemostasis and may account for the vasospasm that accompanies certain vascular diseases. The peripheral effects of 5-HT are discussed below; its role in the CNS is described in Chapter 12.

Enterochromaffin System. The physiological function of enterochromaffin cells is still uncertain. In addition to 5-HT, they may contain the peptides substance P and motilin, which are potent autacoids in their own right (*see* Polak *et al.*, in De Clerck and Vanhoutte, 1982). However, intestinal enterochromaffin cells show a basal secretion of 5-HT that is augmented by mechanical stimulation, hypertonicity, norepinephrine, and vagal stimulation (*see* Ahlman and Dahlström, in De Clerck and Vanhoutte, 1982). In addition, 5-HT appears to be involved in the neural network that regulates intestinal motility (*see* Wood, 1987).

Tumors of 5-HT–Forming Cells: Malignant Carcinoid. Tumors of enterochromaffin or related cells (carcinoid tumors) may synthesize and release large amounts of 5-HT along with other autacoids. The 5-HT contributes to the symptoms of diarrhea, bronchoconstriction, and edema; vasodilatation and flushing may be primarily due to the release of substance P and the formation of kinins (*see* Creutzfeldt and Stöckmann, 1987). With massive tumors, so much tryptophan may be diverted to 5-HT synthesis that niacin synthesis suffers and pellagra results.

Platelets. During aggregation at sites of vascular injury, platelets release 5-HT along with ADP, metabolites of arachidonate (*e.g.*, thromboxane A_2), and other mediators. The platelet membrane contains 5-HT receptors (designated 5-HT_2) that enhance aggregation when stimulated. Activation of this receptor normally produces a weak response; however, in the presence of low concentrations of other agonists such as collagen, 5-HT can produce maximal activation of platelets. Thus, during the adhesion–aggregation reaction, 5-HT (acting in concert with thromboxane A_2) can amplify the platelet aggregation reaction and speed clot formation. Since the vascular endothelial cells may be damaged at the site of injury, 5-HT can also act directly on the smooth muscle of the vessel wall, thereby causing contraction and aiding hemostasis (*see* De Clerck *et al.*, 1984; Houston and Vanhoutte, 1986; Hollenberg, 1988).

Vascular Disease. Based on the effects of ketanserin, a selective 5-HT_2 antagonist (*see* below), there is some evidence that 5-HT released from platelets may play a role in causing the vasoconstriction that is apparent in certain vascular diseases (*e.g.*, atherosclerosis, Raynaud's phenomenon, spasm of newly formed collateral arteries, and certain types of essential hypertension) (*see* Houston and Vanhoutte, 1986; Hollenberg, 1988).

PHARMACOLOGICAL ACTIONS

5-HT both stimulates and inhibits nerves and smooth muscles in the cardiovascular, respiratory, and gastrointestinal systems. The receptors for

5-HT are divided into three major types, designated 5-HT_1, 5-HT_2, and 5-HT_3; these exist on a number of different cells (*see* below; *see also* Bradley *et al.*, 1986). Thus, administration of 5-HT to an intact animal or isolated preparation produces a wide spectrum of responses that are complicated by the species, the physiological state, or the integrity of the preparation. However, 5-HT rarely circulates in the plasma, and the physiologically relevant responses appear to be those produced locally in the vascular system by release of 5-HT from platelets (*see* Houston and Vanhoutte, 1986; Hollenberg, 1988). Detailed accounts of the responses of the intact organism to administration of 5-HT can be found in *previous editions* of this textbook. (*See also* Erspamer, 1966b; Essman, 1978a; De Clerck and Vanhoutte, 1982; Ho *et al.*, 1982.)

Cardiovascular System. Acting via 5-HT_1 and 5-HT_2 receptors (*see* below), 5-HT can directly stimulate or relax smooth muscle, influence the release of norepinephrine from adrenergic nerves, and stimulate endothelial cells to release EDRF and prostaglandins. The integrated response of a given blood vessel depends on the intensity of these different stimuli. However, the general response is similar to that produced by histamine or bradykinin (*see* Table 23–4).

Vasoconstriction. Stimulation of 5-HT_2 receptors in smooth muscle cells produces contraction of most vessels, including most arteries, veins, and venules. However, in some cases, such as the basilar artery in man, 5-HT–induced contraction is apparently mediated by 5-HT_1 receptors. This vasoconstriction is the classical response to 5-HT and is responsible for the terms vasotonin and serotonin. The splanchnic, renal, pulmonary, and cerebral beds are particularly affected. In addition to its direct effects on vascular smooth muscle, 5-HT amplifies the effects of other contractile agonists, such as norepinephrine, histamine, or angiotensin II. All of these effects are thought to aid in the hemostatic actions of platelets, especially in damaged vessels where the ability of endothelial cells to mediate vasodilatation is compromised (De Clerck *et al.*, 1984; Houston and Vanhoutte, 1986).

Vasodilatation. 5-HT can cause vasodilatation via its actions on several cell types in the vasculature. 5-HT_1 receptors on endothelial cells mediate the release of EDRF and prostaglandins, which act locally on smooth muscle cells to cause relaxation (Peach *et al.*, 1985). These effects are most prominent in small vessels, such as arterioles in skeletal muscle (De Clerck *et al.*, 1984). Stimulation of 5-HT_1 receptors on sympathetic nerve terminals causes inhibition of the release of norepinephrine, an effect that also promotes a reduction in vascular tone. Stimulation of 5-HT_1 receptors in the smooth muscle of some vessels may also cause vasodilatation (Bradley *et al.*, 1986). 5-HT does not alter capillary permeability to any appreciable extent.

Blood Pressure. 5-HT does not appear to regulate blood pressure in the normal animal. However, when platelets become activated in certain disease states, 5-HT may increase blood pressure (*see* above).

Heart. 5-HT produces positive inotropic and chronotropic effects that are mediated by 5-HT_1 receptors (*see* Bradley *et al.*, 1986). These effects may be blunted by stimulation of 5-HT_3 receptors on afferent nerves of baroreceptors and chemoreceptors. 5-HT_3 receptors are also present on vagal nerve endings in the coronary bed, and their stimulation initiates the coronary chemoreflex (Bezold–Jarisch reflex), characterized by inhibition of sympathetic outflow and increased activity of the cardiac (efferent) vagus, leading to profound bradycardia and hypotension.

Smooth Muscle. *Alimentary Tract.* 5-HT increases the motility of the small intestine; the motility of the stomach and large intestine may also be enhanced, but the usual response is inhibition. These inhibitory responses are mediated by 5-HT receptors located on both neural and muscle cells (*see* Wood, 1987). For example, in the isolated human colon, ganglion cells in both circular and longitudinal muscle layers participate; in addition, both muscle layers are relaxed directly.

Other Smooth Muscle. 5-HT can directly stimulate the smooth muscle of the uterus and bronchi to contract (Bradley *et al.*, 1986). Afferent nerves to the bronchi may also be stimulated by 5-HT, causing an increase in respiratory rate. The effects on the bronchi are exacerbated in asthmatic individuals and can also become apparent in patients with carcinoid, many of whom exhibit symptoms of asthma (Creutzfeldt and Stöckman, 1987).

Nerve Endings. 5-HT can stimulate or inhibit nerves, depending on the site and the type of receptor involved. As noted above, activation of 5-HT_1 receptors on adrenergic nerve terminals inhibits the release of the norepinephrine elicited by stimulation of the sympathetic nervous system. 5-HT_3 receptors located on various sensory neurons mediate a depolarizing response, which may account for the ability of 5-HT to cause pain and itching, as well as respiratory stimulation and cardiovascular reflexes (Bradley *et al.*, 1986).

Mechanism of Action. *5-HT Receptors.* In addition to the three "major" classes of receptors for 5-HT (1 through 3), 5-HT_1 receptors have been further subdivided (A through D) (*see* Bradley *et al.*, 1986; Peroutka, 1988). This complex nomenclature has evolved principally from the pharmacological characterization of responses and ligand-binding sites in various tissues; however, all observations do not fit into this scheme consistently (*see* Chapter 12). Relatively few agonists or antagonists have been developed that interact selectively with only one type of 5-HT receptor; ketanserin, a 5-HT_2 antagonist, is one of a few notable examples (*see* below).

The primary structures of the receptors designated 5-HT_{1A}, 5-HT_{1C}, and 5-HT_2 have been deduced from the sequences of their cloned complementary DNAs (Lübbert *et al.*, 1987; Fargin *et al.*, 1988; Pritchett *et al.*, 1988). These proteins resemble other G protein–linked membrane-bound receptors (*see* Chapter 2).

5-HT Effector Systems. Although there are many gaps, the effects of 5-HT in the periphery can be understood in terms of the effector systems that are activated by individual receptors (*see* Table 23–4). Thus, cardiac inotropic or direct vasodilatory effects produced by activation of 5-HT_1 receptors may reflect mediation by 5-HT_{1A} receptors, which are known to stimulate adenylyl cyclase. Indirect vasodilatory responses mediated by EDRF may result from the stimulation of endothelial 5-HT_{1C} receptors, since this receptor is known to activate phospholipase C (*see* Peroutka, 1988). 5-HT_2 receptors are also coupled to phospholipase C (de Chaffoy de Courcelles *et al.*, 1985), and their stimulation in vascular and other smooth muscles causes an increase in intracellular Ca^{2+}. 5-HT_{1B} and 5-HT_{1D} receptors appear to inhibit adenylyl cyclase (*see* Peroutka, 1988). One or both of these receptors may mediate inhibition of norepinephrine release from sympathetic nerve endings. By analogy with cardiac muscarinic receptors (*see* Chapter 5), these 5-HT receptors may also activate a K^+ channel, an action that could contribute to this effect. The 5-HT_3–mediated depolarization of sensory nerves may result from the activation of an as yet undefined cation channel (Derkach *et al.*, 1989).

5-HT ANTAGONISTS

Ergot alkaloids and related compounds are antagonists at receptors for 5-HT, particularly on smooth muscle (*see* Chapter 39); in this group the lysergic acid derivatives such as the diethylamide (LSD), 2-bromo-LSD, and 1-methyl-*d*-lysergic acid butanolamide (methysergide, *see* below) are especially potent. Many indole compounds are also 5-HT antagonists. However, progress in understanding the complex responses to 5-HT has been hampered by the lack of potent and selective antagonists for the various types of 5-HT receptors. For example, the two drugs that are usually classified as 5-HT antagonists—methysergide and cyproheptadine—have other prominent pharmacological activities; thus, the latter has been used as a potent H_1 antagonist. The utility of a selective antagonist is exemplified by ketanserin. Although it has some α_1-adrenergic blocking and other activities, it is highly selective for 5-HT_2 receptors (*see* Bradley *et al.*, 1986).

Ketanserin. This agent is the prototype of a novel series of 5-HT antagonists (*see* Van Nueten *et al.*, 1981; Janssen, 1983). It has the following structure:

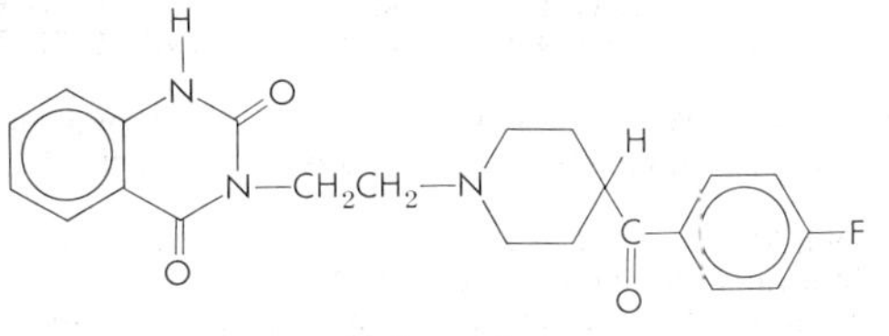

Ketanserin

As mentioned, ketanserin blocks 5-HT_2 receptors and has no significant effect on 5-HT_3 or the various subtypes of 5-HT_1 receptors. It is important to note, however, that ketanserin does have affinity for α_1-adrenergic receptors, histamine H_1 receptors, and dopamine receptors (*see* Janssen, 1983).

Ketanserin blocks the receptor responsible for 5-HT–induced contraction of most vascular smooth muscle and enhancement of platelet aggregation. Thus, it is being investigated for use in diseases where excess vascular tone may be caused by release of 5-HT from platelets; these include certain forms of hypertension, intermittent claudication, and Raynaud's phenomenon. However, because of its ability to block α_1-adrenergic receptors, the mechanism of ketanserin's antihypertensive effect is not clear. It has been proposed that actions at both types of receptor may be necessary (Vanhoutte *et al.*, 1988).

Ketanserin lowers blood pressure in man. The drug appears to reduce the tone of both capacitance and resistance vessels. The degree of reduction of blood pressure is similar to that seen with β-adrenergic antagonists or diuretics. Severe side effects have not been documented; minor reactions include sedation, dry mouth, dizziness, and nausea. The drug does not appear to affect the renin–angiotensin system, the secretion of pituitary hormones, renal blood flow, or glomerular filtration rate. Although ketanserin inhibits 5-HT–induced aggregation of platelets, it does not greatly reduce the ability of other agonists to cause aggregation.

The oral bioavailability of ketanserin is about 50%. The compound has a half-life of 12 to 25 hours in plasma, and it is eliminated primarily by hepatic metabolism (Vanhoutte *et al.*, 1988). Ketanserin is currently undergoing clinical trials in the United States. It is available elsewhere in 20- and 40-mg tablets (SUFREXAL) for oral administration. The usual dosage for the treatment of hypertension or vasospastic diseases is 40 to 80 mg per day in two divided doses.

Methysergide. This drug (1-methyl-*d*-lysergic acid butanolamide) is a congener of methylergonovine and of LSD. Its structure is shown in Table 39–1. It inhibits the vasoconstrictor and pressor effects of 5-HT as well as the action of the amine on a variety of extravascular smooth muscles and other cells. Although methysergide is an ergot derivative, it has only feeble vasoconstrictor and oxytocic activity.

Methysergide has been used for the prophylactic treatment of migraine and other vascular headaches, including Horton's syndrome. The protective effect of methysergide takes 1 to 2 days to develop and as long to wane when treatment is terminated. Rebound headaches may occur when the drug is withdrawn. Methysergide is without benefit when given during an acute attack. Since the mechanism of migraine and vascular headaches is unknown, it is not clear why methysergide or any of the other effective agents should be of value (*see* Chapter 39).

Methysergide can also be used to combat diarrhea and malabsorption in patients with carcinoid and may be beneficial in the postgastrectomy dumping syndrome. Both of these conditions have a 5-HT–mediated component. However, the drug is not effective against other substances (*e.g.*, kinins) that are released by carcinoid tumors (*see* above). For this reason, the preferred agent is a somatostatin analog, octreotide acetate, which inhibits the secretion of all of the mediators that are secreted by these tumors (*see* Chapter 56).

Untoward Effects. These are usually mild and transient, but may be severe enough to require withdrawal of the drug. The most common are gastrointestinal and include heartburn, diarrhea, cramps, nausea, and vomiting. Effects attributable to central actions include unsteadiness, drowsiness, weakness, lightheadedness, nervousness, insomnia, confusion, excitement, euphoria, hallucinations, and even frank psychotic episodes. There may be either loss of appetite or weight gain. Reactions suggestive of vascular insufficiency have been observed in a few patients, and exacerbation of angina pectoris has been noted. One infrequent but potentially serious complication of prolonged treatment is inflammatory fibrosis. Depending on the site, this condition gives rise to various syndromes, including retroperitoneal fibrosis, pleuropulmonary fibrosis, and coronary and endocardial fibrosis. Usually the fibrosis regresses after withdrawal of the drug, but it may not, and persistent cardiac valvular damage has been reported. Because of this danger, treatment should be interrupted for 3 weeks or more every 6 months, and other prophylactic drugs for migraine are preferred.

Preparation and Dosage. Methysergide maleate (SANSERT) is available in 2-mg tablets. The adult dose is 4 to 8 mg daily, in divided doses taken with food.

Cyproheptadine. This compound has the following structural formula:

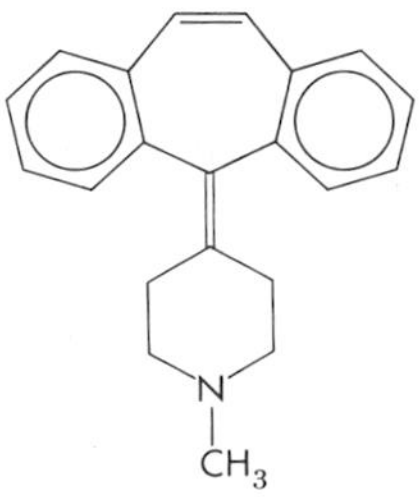

Cyproheptadine

Its structure resembles that of the phenothiazine H_1 antagonists, and, indeed, it is an effective H_1 blocker. It is discussed here because it also has prominent 5-HT–blocking activity on various smooth muscles. In addition, it has weak anticholinergic activity and possesses mild central-depressant properties.

Uses and Side Effects. Cyproheptadine shares the properties and uses of other H_1 blockers (*see* above). It appears to be about as effective as hydroxyzine in controlling skin allergies, particularly the accompanying pruritus. It also appears to be useful in cold urticaria (*see* Salvaggio, 1982). In allergic conditions its actions as a 5-HT antagonist are irrelevant, since 5-HT is not involved in human allergic responses. The 5-HT–antagonizing properties of cyproheptadine have been used in the postgastrectomy dumping syndrome, intestinal hypermotility of carcinoid, and some other conditions that do involve the release of 5-HT. However, octreotide acetate is now preferred for suppressing the symptoms of carcinoid (*see* above).

Side effects of cyproheptadine include drowsiness, dry mouth, and many other effects common to H_1 antagonists (*see* above). Weight gain and increased growth in children have been observed. The mechanism may involve interference with regulation of the secretion of growth hormone (*see* Fernstrom, in Ho *et al.*, 1982).

Preparations. Cyproheptadine hydrochloride (PERIACTIN) is available as tablets (4 mg) and as a syrup (2 mg/5 ml). The usual dosage for adults is 4 mg three or four times per day. The total daily dose should not exceed 0.5 mg/kg.

Arrang, J.-M.; Garbarg, M.; Lancelot, J.-C.; Lecomte, J.-M.; Pollard, H.; Robba, M.; Schunack, W.; and Schwartz, J.-C. Highly potent and selective ligands for histamine H_3-receptors. *Nature,* **1987,** *327,* 117–123.

Ash, A. S. F., and Schild, H. O. Receptors mediating some actions of histamine. *Br. J. Pharmacol.,* **1966,** *27,* 427–439.

Baumann, G.; Felix, S. B.; Heidecke, C. D.; Riess, F.; Loher, U.; Ludwig, L.; and Blomer, H. Apparent superiority of H_2-receptor stimulation and simultaneous β-blockade over conventional treatment of β-sympathomimetic drugs in post-acute myocardial infarction: cardiac effects of impromidine—a new specific H_2-receptor agonist—in the surviving catecholamine-insensitive myocardium. *Agents Actions,* **1984,** *15,* 216–228.

Black, J. W.; Duncan, W. A. M.; Durant, C. J.; Ganellin, C. R.; and Parsons, E. M. Definition and antagonism of histamine H_2-receptors. *Nature,* **1972,** *236,* 385–390.

Bouthenet, M. L.; Ruat, M.; Sales, N.; Garbarg, M.; and Schwartz, J. C. A detailed mapping of histamine H_1-receptors in guinea-pig central nervous system established by autoradiography with [^{125}I]iodobolpyramine. *Neuroscience,* **1988,** *26,* 553–600.

Bradley, P. B.; Engel, G.; Feniuk, W.; Fozard, J. R.; Humphrey, P. A.; Middlemiss, D. N.; Mylecharane, E. J.; Richardson, B. P.; and Saxena, P. R. Proposals for the classification and nomenclature of functional receptors for 5-hydroxytryptamine. *Neuropharmacology,* **1986,** *25,* 563–576.

Brodie, B. B., and Shore, P. A. A concept for a role of serotonin and norepinephrine as chemical mediators in the brain. *Ann. N.Y. Acad. Sci.,* **1957,** *66,* 631–642.

Carruthers, S. G.; Shoeman, D. W.; Hignite, C. E.; and Azarnoff, D. L. Correlation between plasma diphenhydramine level and sedative and antihistamine effects. *Clin. Pharmacol. Ther.,* **1978,** *23,* 375–382.

Cohen, B., and deJong, J. M. B. V. Meclizine and placebo in treating vertigo of vestibular origin. Relative efficacy in a double-blind study. *Arch. Neurol.,* **1972,** *27,* 129–135.

Creutzfeldt, W., and Stöckman, F. Carcinoids and carcinoid syndrome. *Am. J. Med.,* **1987,** *82,* Suppl. 5B, 4–16.

Cunha-Melo, J. R.; Dean, N. M.; Moyer, J. D.; Maeyama, K.; and Beaven, M. A. The kinetics of phosphoinositide hydrolysis in rat basophilic leukemia (RBL-2H3) cells varies with the type of IgE receptor cross-linking agent used. *J. Biol. Chem.,* **1987,** *262,* 11455–11463.

Dahlén, S. E.; Hansson, G.; Hedquist, P.; Bjorck, T.;

Granstrom, E.; and Dahlen, B. Allergen challenge of lung tissue from asthmatics elicits bronchial contraction that correlates with the release of leukotrienes C_4, D_4 and E_4. *Proc. Natl. Acad. Sci. U.S.A.*, **1983**, *80*, 1712–1716.

Dale, H. H., and Laidlaw, P. P. The physiological action of β-imidazolylethylamine. *J. Physiol. (Lond.)*, **1910**, *41*, 318–344.

———. Further observations on the action of β-imidazolylethylamine. *Ibid.*, **1911**, *43*, 182–195.

de Chaffoy de Courcelles, D.; Leysen, J. E.; De Clerck, F.; Van Belle, H.; and Janssen, P. A. J. Evidence that phospholipid turnover is the signal transducing system coupled to serotonin-S_2 receptor sites. *J. Biol. Chem.*, **1985**, *260*, 7603–7608.

Derkach, V.; Surprenant, A.; and North, R. A. 5-HT_3 receptors are membrane ion channels. *Nature*, **1989**, *339*, 706–709.

Douglas, W. W. Stimulus-secretion coupling: the concept and clues from chromaffin and other cells. The First Gaddum Memorial Lecture. *Br. J. Pharmacol.*, **1968**, *34*, 451–474.

———. Stimulus-secretion coupling: variations on the theme of calcium activated exocytosis involving cellular and extracellular sources of calcium. In, *Respiratory Tract Mucus*. Ciba Foundation Symposium, Vol. 54. Elsevier/Excerpta Medica/North Holland, Amsterdam, **1978**, pp. 61–90.

Evans, B. A., and others. Structure and chromosomal localization of the renal kallikrein gene. *Biochemistry*, **1988**, *27*, 3124–3129.

Fargin, A.; Raymond, J. R.; Lohse, M. J.; Kobilka, B. K.; Caron, M. G.; and Lefkowitz, R. J. The genomic clone G-21, which resembles a β-adrenergic receptor sequence encodes the 5-HT_{1a} receptor. *Nature*, **1988**, *335*, 358–360.

Farmer, S. G.; Burch, R. M.; Meeker, S. A.; and Wilkins, D. E. Evidence for a pulmonary B_3 bradykinin receptor. *Mol. Pharmacol.*, **1989**, *36*, 1–8.

Fasolato, C.; Pandiella, A.; Meldolesi, J.; and Pozzan, T. Generation of inositol phosphates, cytosolic Ca^{2+}, and ionic fluxes in Pc12 cells treated with bradykinin. *J. Biol. Chem.*, **1988**, *263*, 17350–17359.

Feldman, J. M., and O'Dorisio, T. M. Role of neuropeptides and serotonin in the diagnosis of carcinoid tumors. *Am. J. Med.*, **1986**, *81*, Suppl. 6B, 41–48.

Fukushima, D.; Kitamura, N.; and Nakanishi, S. Nucleotide sequence of cloned cDNA for human pancreatic kallikrein. *Biochemistry*, **1985**, *24*, 8037–8043.

Gaddum, J. H. Antagonism between LSD and 5-hydroxytryptamine. *J. Physiol. (Lond.)*, **1953**, *121*, 15P.

Graybiel, A.; Wood, C. D.; Knepton, J.; Hoche, J. P.; and Perkins, G. F. Human assay of antimotion sickness drugs. *Aviat. Space Environ. Med.*, **1975**, *46*, 1107–1118.

Higashijima, T.; Uzu, S.; Nakamjima, T.; and Ross, E. M. Mastoparan, a peptide toxin from wasp venom, mimics receptors by activating GTP-binding regulatory proteins (G proteins). *J. Biol. Chem.*, **1988**, *263*, 6491–6494.

Jacob, R.; Merritt, J. E.; Hallam, T. J.; and Rink, T. J. Repetitive spikes in cytoplasmic calcium evoked by histamine in human endothelial cells. *Nature*, **1988**, *335*, 40–45.

Janssen, P. A. J. 5-HT_2 receptor blockade to study serotonin-induced pathology. *Trends Pharmacol. Sci.*, **1983**, *5*, 198–206.

Khandelwal, J. K.; Hough, L. B.; and Green, J. P. Histamine and some of its metabolites in human body fluids. *Klin. Wochenschr.*, **1982**, *60*, 914–918.

Lübbert, H.; Hoffman, B. J.; Snutch, T. P.; Van Dyke, T.; Levine, A. J.; Hartig, P. R.; Lester, H. A.; and Davidson, N. cDNA cloning of a serotonin 5-HT_{1c} receptor by electrophysiological assays of mRNA-injected *Xenopus* oocytes. *Proc. Natl. Acad. Sci. U.S.A.*, **1987**, *84*, 4332–4336.

Okunishi, H.; Burton, J.; and Spragg, J. Specificity of substrate analogue inhibitors of human urinary kallikrein. *Hypertension*, **1985**, *7*, Suppl. I, I72–I75.

Okunishi, H.; Spragg, J.; and Burton, J. *In vivo* assay of specific kallikrein inhibitors. *Vasodepressor Hormones*, **1987**, *22*, 381–390.

Porro, G. B.; Grossi, E.; Petrillo, M.; and Sangaletti, O. A comparison of pentagastrin and impromidine as gastric secretagogues in duodenal ulcer patients. *Curr. Ther. Res.*, **1982**, *31*, 1–6.

Pritchett, D. B.; Bach, A. W. J.; Wozny, M.; Taleb, O.; Dal Toso, R.; Shih, J. C.; and Seeburg, P. H. Structure and functional expression of cloned rat serotonin 5HT-2 receptor. *EMBO J.*, **1988**, *7*, 4135–4140.

Rapport, M. M.; Green, A. A.; and Page, I. H. Serum vasoconstrictor (serotonin). IV. Isolation and characterization. *J. Biol. Chem.*, **1948**, *176*, 1243–1251.

Rocha e Silva, M.; Beraldo, W. T.; and Rosenfeld, G. Bradykinin, a hypotensive and smooth muscle stimulating factor released from plasma globulin by snake venoms and by trypsin. *Am. J. Physiol.*, **1949**, *156*, 261–273.

Simons, F. E. R., and Simons, K. J. H_1 receptor antagonist treatment of chronic rhinitis. *J. Allergy Clin. Immunol.*, **1988**, *81*, 975–980.

Somlyo, A. P.; Walker, J. W.; Goldman, Y. E.; Trentham, D. R.; Kobayashi, F. R. S. S.; Kitazawa, T.; and Somlyo, A. V. Inositol trisphosphate, calcium and muscle contraction. *Philos. Trans. R. Soc. Lond.* [*Biol.*], **1988**, *320*, 399–414.

Steranka, L. R.; Manning, D. C.; DeHaas, C. J.; Ferkany, J. W.; Borosky, S. A.; Connor, J. R.; Vavrek, R. J.; Stewart, J. M.; and Snyder, S. H. Bradykinin as a pain mediator: receptors are localized to sensory neurons, and antagonists have analgesic actions. *Proc. Natl. Acad. Sci. U.S.A.*, **1988**, *85*, 3245–3249.

Takagaki, Y.; Kitamura, N.; and Nakanishi, S. Cloning and sequence analysis of cDNAs for human high molecular weight prekininogens. *J. Biol. Chem.*, **1985**, *260*, 8601–8609.

Taylor, D. A.; Bowman, B. F.; and Stull, J. T. Cytoplasmic Ca^{2+} is a primary determinant for myosin phosphorylation in smooth muscle cells. *J. Biol. Chem.*, **1989**, *264*, 6207–6213.

Van Nueten, J. M.; Janssen, P. A. J.; Van Beek, J.; Xhonneux, R.; Verbeuren, T. J.; and Vanhoutte, P. M. Vascular effects of ketanserin (R 41 468), a novel antagonist of 5-HT_2 serotonergic receptors. *J. Pharmacol. Exp. Ther.*, **1981**, *218*, 217–230.

Vavrek, R. J., and Stewart, J. M. Competitive antagonists of bradykinin. *Peptides*, **1985**, *6*, 161–164.

West, S.; Brandon, B.; Stolley, P.; and Rumrill, R. A review of antihistamines and the common cold. *Pediatrics*, **1975**, *56*, 100–107.

Wihl, J.-A.; Petersen, B. N.; Petersen, L. N.; Gundersen, G.; Bresson, K.; and Mygind, N. Effect of the nonsedative H_1-receptor antagonist astemisole in perennial allergic and nonallergic rhinitis. *J. Allergy Clin. Immunol.*, **1985**, *75*, 720–727.

Woolley, D. W., and Shaw, E. A biochemical and pharmacological suggestion about certain mental disorders. *Science*, **1954**, *119*, 587–588.

Monographs and Reviews

Altura, B. M., and Halevy, S. Cardiovascular actions of histamine. In, *Histamine II and Anti-Histaminics: Chemistry, Metabolism and Physiological and Pharmacological Actions.* (Rocha e Silva, M., ed.) *Handbuch der Experimentellen Pharmakologie*, Vol. 18, Pt. 2. Springer-Verlag, Berlin, **1978**, pp. 1–39.

Beaven, M. A. Histamine. *N. Engl. J. Med.*, **1976**, *294*, 30–36.

———. *Histamine: Its Role in Physiological and Pathological Processes.* S. Karger, Basel, **1978**.

Bertaccini, G. Active polypeptides of nonmammalian origin. *Pharmacol. Rev.*, **1976**, *28*, 127–177.

Bosin, T. R. Serotonin metabolism. In, *Availability, Localization and Disposition*. Vol. 1, *Serotonin in Health and Disease*. (Essman, W. B., ed.) Spectrum Publications, Inc., New York, **1978**, pp. 181–300.

Bovet, D. Introduction to antihistamine agents and antergan derivatives. *Ann. N.Y. Acad. Sci.*, **1950**, *50*, 1089–1126.

Burch, R. M.; Farmer, S. G.; and Steranka, L. R. Bradykinin receptor antagonists. *Med. Res. Rev.*, **1990**, *10*, 143–175.

Clark, W. G. Kinins and the peripheral and central nervous systems. In, *Bradykinin, Kallidin and Kallikrein*. (Erdös, E. G., ed.) *Handbuch der Experimentellen Pharmakologie*, Vol. 25. Springer-Verlag, Berlin, **1979**, pp. 312–346.

De Clerck, F. F., and Vanhoutte, M. (eds.). *5-Hydroxytryptamine in Peripheral Reactions*. Raven Press, New York, **1982.**

De Clerck, F.; Van Neuten, J. M.; and Reneman, R. S. Platelet-vessel wall interactions implication of 5-hydroxytryptamine. *Agents Actions*, **1984**, *15*, 612–626.

Erdös, E. G. (ed.). *Bradykinin, Kallidin and Kallikrein. Handbuch der Experimentellen Pharmakologie*, Vol. 25, Suppl. Springer-Verlag, Berlin, **1979.**

Erspamer, V. Occurrence of indolealkylamines in nature. In, *5-Hydroxytryptamine and Related Indolealkylamines*. (Erspamer, V., ed.) *Handbuch der Experimentellen Pharmakologie*, Vol. 19. Springer-Verlag, Berlin, **1966a**, pp. 132–181.

——— (ed.). *5-Hydroxytryptamine and Related Indolealkylamines. Handbuch der Experimentellen Pharmakologie*, Vol. 19. Springer-Verlag, Berlin, **1966b.**

Essman, W. B. (ed.). *Serotonin in Health and Disease*, Vol. 1. *Availability, Localization and Disposition*. Spectrum Publications, Inc., New York, **1978a.**

———. Serotonin distribution in tissues and fluids. In, *Availability, Localization and Disposition*. Vol. 1, *Serotonin in Health and Disease*. (Essman, W. B., ed.) Spectrum Publications, Inc., New York, **1978b**, pp. 15–179.

Faingold, C. L. Antihistamines as central nervous system depressants. In, *Histamine II and Anti-Histaminics: Chemistry, Metabolism and Physiological and Pharmacological Actions*. (Rocha e Silva, M., ed.) *Handbuch der Experimentellen Pharmakologie*, Vol. 18, Pt. 2. Springer-Verlag, Berlin, **1978**, pp. 561–573.

Fritz, H.; Back, N.; Dietze, G.; and Haberland, G. L. (eds.). Kinins-III. *Adv. Exp. Med. Biol.*, **1983**, *156A*, 1–701; *156B*, 705–1222.

Furchgott, R. F., and Vanhoutte, P. M. Endothelium-derived relaxing and contracting factors. *FASEB J.*, **1989**, *3*, 2007–2018.

Ganellin, C. R., and Parsons, M. E. (eds.). *Pharmacology of Histamine Receptors*. Wright/PSG, Bristol, Mass., **1982.**

Gavras, I., and Gavras, H. Anti-hormones and blood pressure: bradykinin antagonists in blood pressure regulation. *Kidney Int.*, **1988**, *34*, Suppl. 26, S60–S62.

Griendling, K. K., and Alexander, R. W. Angiotensin, other pressors, and the transduction of vascular smooth muscle contraction. In, *Hypertension: Pathophysiology, Diagnosis and Management*, Vol. 1. (Laragh, J. H., and Brenner, B. M., eds.) Raven Press, Ltd., New York, **1990**, pp. 583–600.

Hahn, F. Antianaphylactic and antiallergic effects. In, *Histamine II and Anti-Histaminics: Chemistry, Metabolism and Physiological and Pharmacological Actions*. (Rocha e Silva, M., ed.) *Handbuch der Experimentellen Pharmakologie*, Vol. 18, Pt. 2. Springer-Verlag, Berlin, **1978**, pp. 439–504.

Ho, B. T.; Schoolar, J. C.; and Usdin, E. (eds.). Serotonin in biological psychiatry. *Adv. Biochem. Psychopharmacol.*, **1982**, *34*, 1–338.

Hollenberg, N. K. Serotonin and vascular responses. *Annu. Rev. Pharmacol. Toxicol.*, **1988**, *28*, 41–59.

Hough, L. B. Cellular localization and possible functions for brain histamine: recent progress. *Prob. Neurobiol.*, **1988**, *30*, 469–505.

Houston, D. S., and Vanhoutte, P. M. Serotonin and the vascular system: role in health and disease, and implications for therapy. *Drugs*, **1986**, *31*, 149–163.

Ishizaka, K. (ed.). Mast cell activation and mediator release. *Prog. Allergy*, **1984**, *34*, 1–338.

Kamm, K. E., and Stull, J. T. The function of myosin and myosin light chain kinase phosphorylation in smooth muscle. *Annu. Rev. Pharmacol. Toxicol.*, **1985**, *25*, 593–620.

Krstenansky, P. M., and Cluxton, R. J., Jr. Astemizole: a long-acting, nonsedating antihistamine. *Drug Intell. Clin. Pharm.*, **1987**, *21*, 947–953.

Lagunoff, D.; Martin, T. W.; and Read, G. Agents that release histamine from mast cells. *Annu. Rev. Pharmacol. Toxicol.*, **1983**, *23*, 331–351.

Larsen, G. L., and Henson, P. M. Mediators of inflammation. *Annu. Rev. Immunol.*, **1983**, *1*, 335–359.

Lewis, T. *The Blood Vessels of the Human Skin and Their Responses*. Shaw & Sons, Ltd., London, **1927.**

Lorenz, W.; Doenicke, A.; Schoning, B.; and Neugebauer, E. The role of histamine in adverse reactions to intravenous agents. In, *Adverse Reactions to Anaesthetic Drugs*. (Thornton, J. A., ed.) Elsevier/North Holland, Amsterdam, **1981**, pp. 169–238.

Marceau, F.; Lussier, A.; Regoli, D.; and Giroud, J. P. Pharmacology of kinins: their relevance to tissue injury and inflammation. *Gen. Pharmacol.*, **1983**, *14*, 209–229.

Margolius, H. S. Tissue kallikreins and kinins: regulation and roles in hypertensive and diabetic diseases. *Annu. Rev. Pharmacol. Toxicol.*, **1989**, *29*, 343–364.

Mathews, K. P. Respiratory atopic disease. *J.A.M.A.*, **1982**, *248*, 2587–2610.

Metcalfe, D. D.; Kaliner, M.; and Donlon, M. A. The mast cell. *CRC Crit. Rev. Immunol.*, **1981**, *3*, 23–74.

Nadel, J. A., and Barnes, P. J. Autonomic regulation of the airways. *Annu. Rev. Med.*, **1984**, *35*, 451–467.

Nakanishi, S. Substance P precursor and kininogen: their structures, gene organizations, and regulation. *Physiol. Rev.*, **1987**, *67*, 1117–1142.

Paton, D. M., and Webster, D. R. Clinical pharmacokinetics of H_1-receptor antagonists (the antihistamines). *Clin. Pharmacokinet.*, **1985**, *10*, 477–497.

Peach, M. J.; Loeb, A. L.; Singer, H. A.; and Saye, J. Endothelium-derived vascular relaxing factor. *Hypertension*, **1985**, *7*, Suppl. I, I94–I100.

Peroutka, S. J. 5-Hydroxytryptamine receptor subtypes. *Annu. Rev. Neurosci.*, **1988**, *11*, 45–60.

Proud, D., and Kaplan, A. P. Kinin formation: mechanisms and role in inflammatory disorders. *Annu. Rev. Immunol.*, **1988**, *6*, 49–83.

Regoli, D. Kinins. *Br. Med. Bull.*, **1987**, *43*, 270–284.

Regoli, D., and Barabé, J. Pharmacology of bradykinin and related kinins. *Pharmacol. Rev.*, **1980**, *32*, 1–47.

Reite, O. B. Comparative physiology of histamine. *Physiol. Rev.*, **1972**, *52*, 778–819.

Rocha e Silva, M. (ed.). *Histamine II and Anti-Histaminics: Chemistry, Metabolism and Physiological and Pharmacological Actions. Handbuch der Experimentellen Pharmakologie*, Vol. 18, Pt. 2. Springer-Verlag, Berlin, **1978.**

Ryan, J. W. Processing of the endogenous polypeptides by the lungs. *Annu. Rev. Physiol.*, **1982**, *44*, 241–255.

Salvaggio, J. E. (ed.). Primer on allergic and immunologic diseases. *J.A.M.A.*, **1982**, *248*, 2579–2772.

Sorkin, E. M., and Heel, R. C. Terfenadine: a review of its pharmacodynamic properties and therapeutic efficacy. *Drugs*, **1985**, *29*, 34–56.

Steranka, L. R.; Farmer, S. G.; and Burch, R. M. Antagonists of B_2 bradykinin receptors. *FASEB J.*, **1989**, *3*, 2019–2025.

Symposium. (Various authors.) *Biochemistry of the Acute Allergic Reaction*. Fourth International Symposium. (Becker, E. L.; Simon, A. S.; and Austen, K. F.; eds.) Alan R Liss, Inc., New York, **1981.**

Symposium. (Various authors.) *Histamine and Antihistamines in Anaesthesia and Surgery*. (Ahnefeld, F. W.; Doenicke, A.; and Lorenz, W.; eds.) *Klin. Wochenschr.*, **1982**, *60*, 871–1062.

Vanhoutte, P., and others. Serotoninergic mechanisms in hypertension: focus on the effects of ketanserin. *Hypertension*, **1988**, *11*, 111–133.

Weck, A. L. D., and Bundgaard, H. (eds.). *Allergic Reactions to Drugs. Handbook of Experimental Pharmacology*, Vol. 63. Springer-Verlag, Berlin, **1983.**

Weil-Malherbe, H. Serotonin and schizophrenia. In, *The Central Nervous System*. Vol. 3, *Serotonin in Health and Disease*. (Essman, W. B., ed.) Spectrum Publications, Inc., New York, **1978**, pp. 231–291.

Werle, E. Discovery of the most important kallikreins and kallikrein inhibitors. In, *Bradykinin, Kallidin and Kallikrein*. (Erdös, E. G., ed.) *Handbuch der Experimentellen Pharmakologie*, Vol. 25. Springer-Verlag, Berlin, **1970**, pp. 1–6.

Wetterquist, H. Histamine metabolism and excretion. In, *Histamine II and Anti-Histaminics: Chemistry, Metabolism and Physiological and Pharmacological Actions*. (Rocha e Silva, M., ed.) *Handbuch der Experimentellen Pharmakologie*, Vol. 18, Pt. 2. Springer-Verlag, Berlin, **1978**, pp. 131–150.

Witiak, D. T., and Lewis, N. J. Absorption, distribution, metabolism, and elimination of antihistamines. In, *Histamine II and Anti-Histaminics: Chemistry, Metabolism and Physiological and Pharmacological Actions*. (Rocha e Silva, M., ed.) *Handbuch der Experimentellen Pharmakologie*, Vol. 18, Pt. 2. Springer-Verlag, Berlin, **1978**, 513–560.

Wood, C. D. Antimotion sickness and antiemetic drugs. *Drugs*, **1979**, *17*, 471–479.

Wood, J. D. Physiology of the enteric nervous system. In, *Physiology of the Gastrointestinal Tract*. (Johnson, L. R., ed.) Raven Press, New York, **1987**, pp. 67–109.

CHAPTER 24 LIPID-DERIVED AUTACOIDS: EICOSANOIDS AND PLATELET-ACTIVATING FACTOR

William B. Campbell

Two distinct families of autacoids that are derived from membrane phospholipids have been identified: the eicosanoids, which are formed from certain polyunsaturated fatty acids (principally, arachidonic acid), include the prostaglandins, prostacyclin, thromboxane A_2, and the leukotrienes; and modified phospholipids, currently represented by platelet-activating factor (PAF). The eicosanoids are extremely prevalent and have been detected in almost every tissue and body fluid. Their production increases in response to diverse stimuli, and they produce a broad spectrum of biological effects. Although its precursors are widely distributed, PAF is formed by a smaller number of cell types, principally circulating leukocytes and platelets and endothelial cells. However, because of the wide distribution of these cells, the actions of PAF can be manifest in virtually every organ and tissue of the body.

EICOSANOIDS

History. In 1930 two American gynecologists, Kurzrok and Lieb, observed that strips of human uterus relax or contract when exposed to human semen. A few years later, Goldblatt in England and Euler in Sweden independently reported smooth muscle–contracting and vasodepressor activity in seminal fluid and accessory reproductive glands, and Euler identified the active material as a lipid-soluble acid, which he named "prostaglandin" (*see* Euler, 1973). More than 20 years passed before the demonstration that prostaglandin was in fact a family of unique compounds; the structure of two of these, prostaglandin E_1 (PGE_1) and $PGF_{1\alpha}$, were elucidated in 1962 (*see* Bergström and Samuelsson, 1968). More prostaglandins were soon characterized and these, like the others, proved to be 20-carbon unsaturated carboxylic acids with a cyclopentane ring. When the general structure of the prostaglandins became apparent, their kinship with essential fatty acids was recognized, and in 1964 Bergström and coworkers and van Dorp and associates independently achieved the biosynthesis of PGE_2 from arachidonic acid using homogenates of sheep seminal vesicle (*see* Samuelsson, 1972).

The past 25 years have witnessed a number of exceedingly important discoveries in this area. Realization that the "classically known" prostaglandins constitute only a fraction of the physiologically active products of arachidonate metabolism resulted from discovery of thromboxane A_2 (TXA_2) (Hamberg *et al.,* 1975), prostacyclin (PGI_2) (Moncada *et al.,* 1976), and the leukotrienes (Samuelsson, 1983). The discovery by Vane, Smith, and Willis in 1971 that aspirin and related drugs inhibit prostaglandin biosynthesis provided insight into the mechanism of action of these drugs, as well as an important tool for investigation of the role of these autacoids.

Chemistry and Biosynthesis. The families of prostaglandins, leukotrienes, and related compounds are called eicosanoids because they are derived from 20-carbon essential fatty acids that contain three, four, or five double bonds: 8,11,14-eicosatrienoic acid (dihomo-γ-linolenic acid), 5,8,11,14-eicosatetraenoic acid (arachidonic acid) (*see* Figure 24–1), and 5,8,11,14,17-eicosapentaenoic acid. In man, arachidonate is the most abundant precursor, and it is either derived from dietary linoleic acid (9,12-octadecadienoic acid) or is ingested as a dietary constituent. Arachidonate is then esterified to the phospholipids of cell membranes or other complex lipids. Since the concentration of free arachidonate in the cell is very low, the biosynthesis of eicosanoids depends primarily upon its availability to the eicosanoid-synthesizing enzymes; this results from its release from cellular stores of lipid by acyl hydrolases. The enhanced biosynthesis of the eicosanoids is closely regulated and occurs in response to widely divergent physical, chemical, and hormonal stimuli.

Hormones, autacoids, and other substances augment the biosynthesis of eicosanoids by interacting with plasma membrane–bound receptors that are coupled to guanine nucleotide–binding regulatory proteins (G proteins; *see* Chapter 2). This results in either the direct activation of phospholipases (C and/or A_2) or in elevated cytosolic concentrations of Ca^{2+}, which can also activate these enzymes (Okajima and Ui, 1984; Burch and Axelrod, 1987). Physical stimuli are believed to cause an influx of Ca^{2+} by perturbing the cell membrane, thereby activating phospholipase A_2. Phospholipase A_2 hydrolyzes the *sn*-2 ester bond of membrane phospholipids (particularly phosphatidylcholine and phosphatidylethanolamine) with the release of arachidonate. In contrast, phospholipase C cleaves the phosphodiester bond, resulting in the formation of a 1,2-diglyceride. Arachidonate is then released from the diglyceride by the sequential actions of diglyceride lipase and monoglyceride lipase (Okazaki *et al.*, 1981). Once released, a portion of the arachidonate is rapidly metabolized to oxygenated products by several distinct enzyme systems, including *cyclooxygenase* or one of several *lipoxygenases*.

Products of Cyclooxygenase. The prostaglandins can be considered analogs of an unnatural compound with the trivial name *prostanoic acid,* the structure of which is as follows:

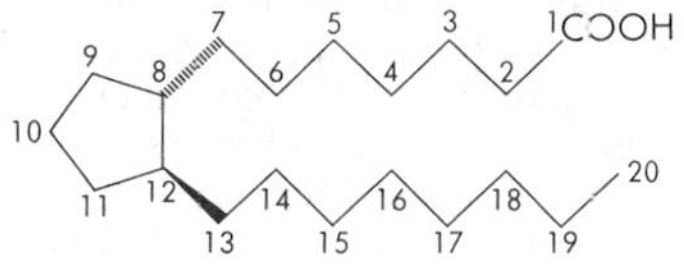

They fall into several main classes, designated by letters and distinguished by substitutions on the cyclopentane ring.

Prostaglandins of the E and D series are hydroxy ketones, while the F_α prostaglandins are 1,3-diols (*see* Figure 24–1). They are products of the metabolism of prostaglandins G (PGG) and H (PGH). PGA, PGB, and PGC are unsaturated ketones that arise nonenzymatically from PGE during extraction procedures; it is unlikely that they occur biologically. Prostacyclin (PGI_2) has a double-ring structure; in addition to a cyclopentane ring, a second ring is formed by an oxygen bridge between carbons 6 and 9. Thromboxanes (TX) contain a six-member oxane ring instead of the cyclopentane ring of the prostaglandins. Both PGI_2 and the thromboxanes also result from the metabolism of prostaglandins G and H (*see* Figure 24–1). The main classes are further subdivided in accord with the number of double bonds in the side chains. This is indicated by subscript 1, 2, or 3, and reflects the fatty acid precursor in most instances. Prostaglandins derived from arachidonate carry the subscript 2 and are the major prostaglandins in mammals. There is little evidence that prostaglandins of the 1 or 3 series are important under normal circumstances.

Synthesis of prostaglandins is accomplished in a stepwise manner by a ubiquitous complex of microsomal enzymes. The first enzyme in this synthetic pathway is prostaglandin endoperoxide synthase, also called *fatty acid cyclooxygenase*. The enzyme has two distinct activities: an endoperoxide synthase activity that oxygenates and cyclizes the unesterified precursor fatty acid to form the cyclic endoperoxide PGG, and a peroxidase activity that converts PGG to PGH (*see* Hamberg *et al.*, 1974). The endoperoxides are chemically unstable, but they can be transformed enzymatically into a variety of products, including PGI, TXA, PGE, PGF, or PGD (*see* Figure 24–1; Samuelsson *et al.*, 1975; Needleman *et al.*, 1986). Isomerases for the synthesis of PGE_2 and PGD_2 have been identified. A 9-keto reductase catalyzes the interconversion of PGE_2 and $PGF_{2\alpha}$ in some tissues.

The endoperoxide PGH_2 is also metabolized into two unstable and highly active compounds (Figure 24–1). Thromboxane A_2 (TXA_2) is formed by *thromboxane synthase*; TXA_2 breaks down nonenzymatically ($t_{1/2}$ = 3 minutes) into the stable thromboxane B_2 (TXB_2). PGI_2 is formed from PGH_2 by *prostacyclin synthase;* it is hydrolyzed nonenzymatically ($t_{1/2}$ = 3 minutes) to 6-keto-$PGF_{1\alpha}$.

Although most tissues are able to synthesize the prostaglandin endoperoxide intermediates from free arachidonate, their fate varies in each tissue and depends on the complement of enzymes (synthases or isomerases) that are present and on their relative abundance. For example, lung and spleen are able to synthesize the whole range of products. In contrast, platelets contain thromboxane synthase as the principal enzyme that metabolizes the endoperoxide, while endothelial cells contain primarily prostacyclin synthase.

Products of Lipoxygenases. Lipoxygenases are a family of cytosolic enzymes that catalyze the oxygenation of polyenic fatty acids to corresponding lipid hydroperoxides (*see* Samuelsson, 1983; Needleman *et al.*, 1986; Yamamoto, 1989). The enzymes require a fatty acid substrate with two *cis* double bonds separated by a methylene group. Arachidonate, which contains several double bonds in this configuration, is metabolized to a number of products with the hydroperoxy group in different positions. For arachidonate, these metabolites are called hydroperoxyeicosatetraenoic acids (*HPETEs*). Lipoxygenases differ in their specificity for placing the hydroperoxy group, and tissues differ in the lipoxygenase(s) that they contain. For example, platelets have only 12-lipoxygenase and synthesize 12-HPETE, whereas leukocytes contain both 5-lipoxygenase and 12-lipoxygenase and produce both 5-HPETE and 12-HPETE (*see* Figure 24–2).

The HPETEs are unstable intermediates, analogous to PGG or PGH, and are further metabolized by a variety of enzymes. All HPETEs may be converted to their corresponding hydroxy fatty acid (HETE) either by a peroxidase or nonenzymatically. 12-HPETE can also undergo a catalyzed molecular rearrangement to epoxy-hydroxyeicosatrienoic acids called *hepoxilins*. Similarly, leukocytes convert 15-HPETE to trihydroxylated metabolites called *lipoxins*.

The 5-lipoxygenase is perhaps the most important of these enzymes, since it leads to the synthesis of the *leukotrienes* (LTs) (Figure 24–2; *see* Samuelsson, 1983; Samuelsson *et al.*, 1987). Leukotriene A (LTA) synthase is associated with 5-lipoxygenase and promotes the rearrangement of 5-HPETE to an unstable 5,6-epoxide, known as leukotriene A_4 (LTA_4) (Borgeat and Samuelsson, 1979); LTA_4 may be transformed by LTA hydrolase to a 5,12-dihydroxyeicosatetraenoic acid known as leukotriene B_4 (LTB_4); alternatively, it may be conjugated with glutathione to form LTC_4 (Murphy *et al.*, 1979). Leukotriene D_4 (LTD_4) is produced by the removal of glutamic acid from LTC_4, and LTE_4 results from the subsequent cleavage of glycine; the reincorporation of glutamic acid yields a γ-glutamylcysteinyl derivative called LTF_4 (*see* Samuelsson, 1983; Piper, 1984; Samuelsson *et al.*, 1987). It is now generally accepted that a mixture of LTC_4 and LTD_4 makes up the material originally known as the "slow-reacting substance of anaphylaxis" (SRS-A), first described by Feldberg and Kellaway (1938).

Products of Cytochrome P_{450}. Arachidonate is metabolized by enzymes that contain cytochrome P_{450} to a variety of metabolites including HETEs, epoxyeicosatrienoic acids, and 19- or 20-hydroxy arachidonate (*see* Fitzpatrick and Murphy, 1989). The physiological importance of this pathway remains to be clarified.

Inhibitors of Eicosanoid Biosynthesis. Many of the biosynthetic steps described above can be inhibited by drugs. Inhibition of phospholipase A_2 decreases the release of the precursor fatty acid and thus the synthesis of all metabolites derived therefrom. Since phospholipase A_2 is activated by Ca^{2+} and calmodulin, it may be inhibited by drugs that reduce the availability of Ca^{2+}. Glucocorticoids also inhibit phospholipase A_2, but they do so indirectly by inducing the synthesis of a protein (*lipocortin*) that inhibits the enzyme (Flower and Blackwell, 1979). Other cellular proteins such as the *calpactins* may also regulate the phospholipases by binding the phospholipid substrate in a complex with Ca^{2+} and actin. The calpactins appear to be distinct from lipocortin, and their synthesis is not induced by glucocorticoids.

Aspirin and related anti-inflammatory drugs were originally found to interfere with the liberation of prostaglandins from spleen and platelets and to prevent the synthesis of prostaglandins from arachidonate in tissue homogenates (Vane, 1971). It is now known that these drugs inhibit the cyclooxygenase enzyme and, as a result, inhibit the synthesis of PGG_2, PGH_2, and all that flows therefrom. However, these drugs do not inhibit the metabolism of arachidonate by lipoxygenases. In fact, inhibition of cyclooxygenase can lead to increased formation of leukotrienes, perhaps by increasing the amount of arachidonate that is available to the lipoxygenases (*see* Piper, 1984). Inhibition of cyclooxygenase provides an important basis for understanding many of the therapeutic and other effects of these agents (*see* Chapter 26).

Since different metabolites of the prostaglandin endoperoxides sometimes produce opposite biological effects (*see* below), there should be advantages in the development of compounds that preferentially inhibit one or another of the enzymes that isomerize the endoperoxides (*see* Moncada and Vane, 1979). For example, there is current interest in drugs such as *dazoxiben* that inhibit thromboxane synthase preferentially (Patrignani *et al.*, 1984). These compounds have antithrombotic effects *in vivo* by selectively reducing the formation of TXA_2 (which promotes platelet aggregation and vasoconstriction) without interfering with the production of PGI_2 (which inhibits aggregation and produces vasodilatation).

Analogs of the natural fatty acid precursors can serve as competitive inhibitors of the formation of both prostaglandins and the products of lipoxygenases. One such inhibitor is the acetylenic analog of arachidonic acid, 5,8,11,14-eicosatetraynoic acid (*see* Figure 24–1). Since leukotrienes may function as inflammatory mediators, an intense effort is underway to discover selective inhibitors of lipoxygenases, particularly 5-lipoxygenase.

Catabolism. Efficient mechanisms exist for the catabolism and inactivation of most eicosanoids. For example, about 95% of infused PGE_2 is inactivated during one passage through the pulmonary circulation. Because of the unique position of the lungs between the venous and arterial circulation, the pulmonary vascular bed constitutes an important filter for many substances (including some prostaglandins) that act locally prior to their release into the venous circulation.

Broadly speaking, the enzymatic catabolic reactions are of two types: an initial (relatively rapid) step, catalyzed by widely distributed prostaglandin-specific enzymes, wherein prostaglandins lose most of their biological activity, and a second (relatively slow) step in which these metabolites are oxidized by enzymes probably identical to those responsible for the β and ω oxidation of most

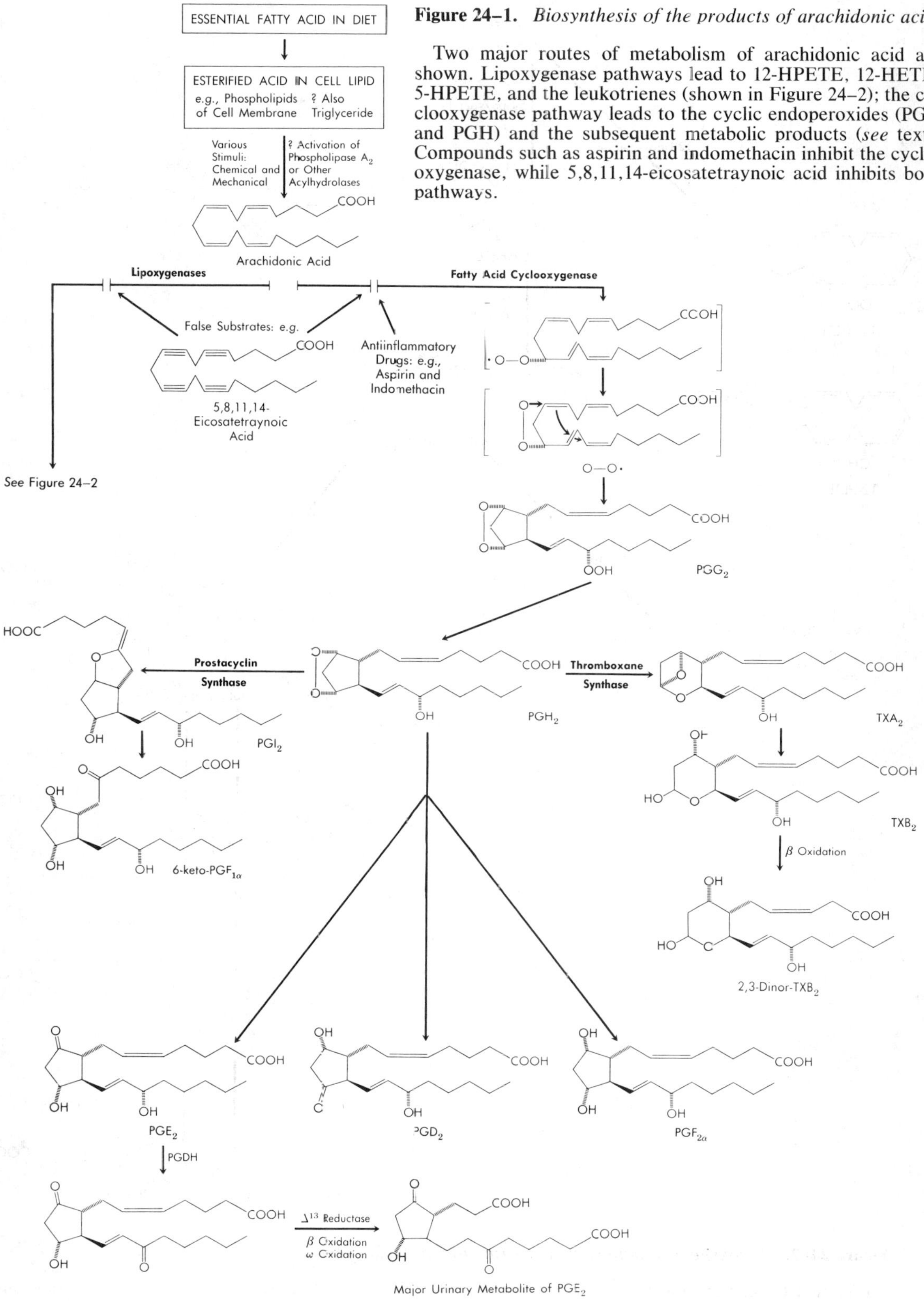

Figure 24–1. *Biosynthesis of the products of arachidonic acid.*

Two major routes of metabolism of arachidonic acid are shown. Lipoxygenase pathways lead to 12-HPETE, 12-HETE, 5-HPETE, and the leukotrienes (shown in Figure 24–2); the cyclooxygenase pathway leads to the cyclic endoperoxides (PGG and PGH) and the subsequent metabolic products (*see* text). Compounds such as aspirin and indomethacin inhibit the cyclooxygenase, while 5,8,11,14-eicosatetraynoic acid inhibits both pathways.

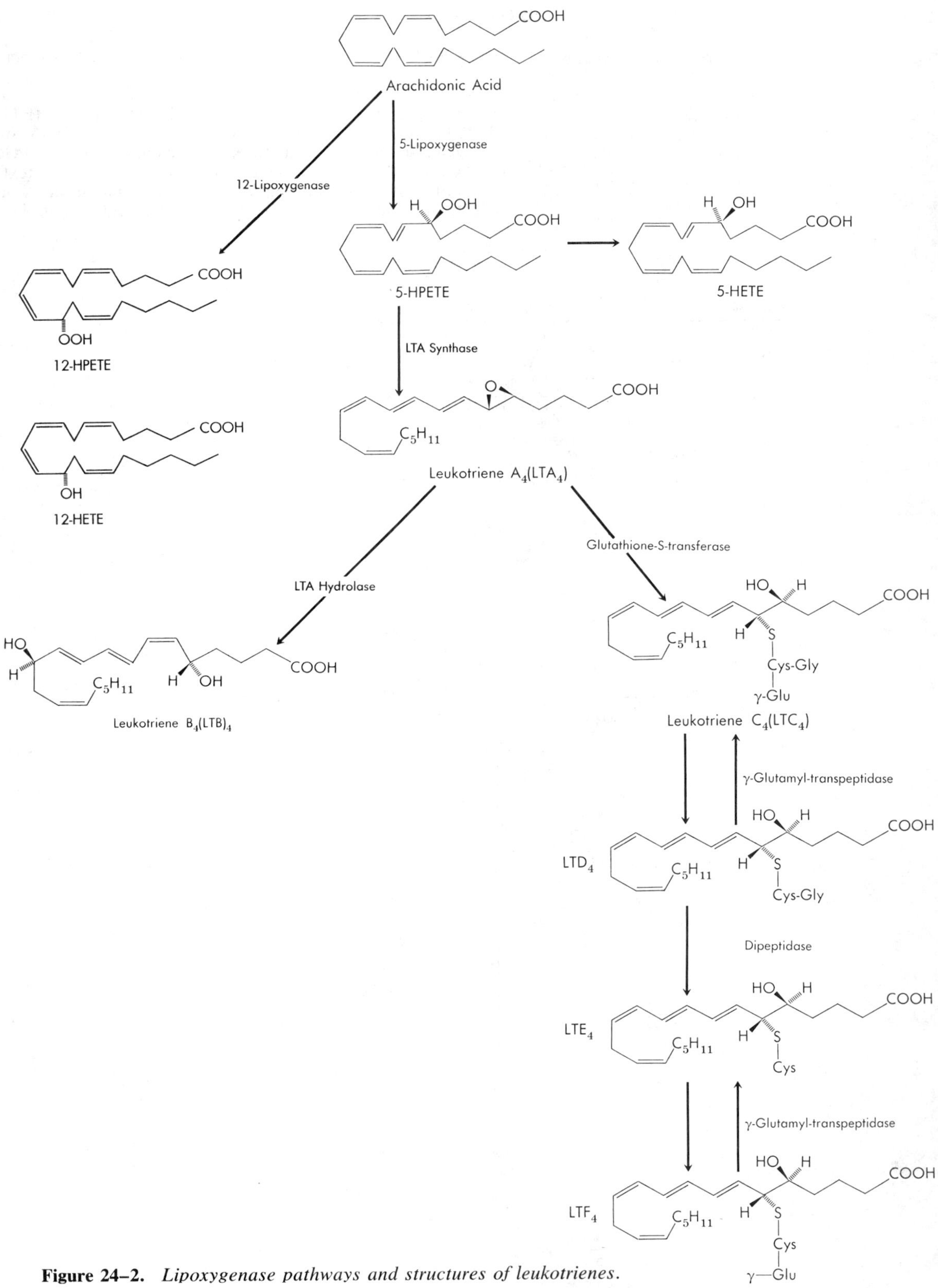

Figure 24–2. *Lipoxygenase pathways and structures of leukotrienes.* (*See* text for explanation.)

fatty acids. The initial step is the oxidation of the 15-OH group to the corresponding ketone by prostaglandin 15-OH dehydrogenase (PGDH). The 15-keto compound is then reduced to the 13,14-dihydro derivative, a reaction catalyzed by prostaglandin Δ^{13}-reductase. Subsequent steps consist of β and ω oxidation of the side chains of the prostaglandins, giving rise to a polar dicarboxylic acid, which is excreted in the urine as the major metabolite of both PGE_1 and PGE_2 (*see* Figure 24–1); these reactions take place particularly in the liver.

The metabolism of TXA_2 in man has been inferred from investigation of the fate of TXB_2 (Roberts *et al.*, 1981). Although up to 20 metabolites have been identified in urine, by far the most abundant is 2,3-dinor-TXB_2 (*see* Figure 24–1).

The degradation of PGI_2 apparently begins with its spontaneous hydrolysis in blood to 6-keto-$PGF_{1\alpha}$. The metabolism of this compound in man involves the same steps as those for PGE_2 and $PGF_{2\alpha}$ (Rosenkranz *et al.*, 1980).

The degradation of LTC_4 occurs in the lungs, kidney, and liver (Denzlinger *et al.*, 1986). The initial steps involve its conversion to LTE_4 and this results in a loss in biological activity. Leukotriene C_4 may also be inactivated by oxidation to a sulfoxide. The principal route of inactivation of LTB_4 is by ω oxidation.

Pharmacological Properties

No other autacoids show more numerous and diverse effects than do prostaglandins and other metabolites of arachidonate. Not only is the spectrum of actions broad, but also different compounds show different activities, both qualitatively and quantitatively. It would be overly confusing to present the myriad of pharmacological effects that have been ascribed to these substances and even more so to delve into the activities of their synthetic analogs. This discussion is limited to activities that are thought to be the most important.

Cardiovascular System. In most species (including man) and in most vascular beds, the PGEs are potent vasodilators. The dilatation appears to involve arterioles, precapillaries, sphincters, and postcapillary venules; large veins are not affected by PGEs. However, PGEs are not universally vasodilatory; constrictor effects have been noted at selected sites (*see* Bergström *et al.*, 1968).

Similarly, PGD_2 causes both vasodilation and vasoconstriction; however, in most vascular beds, including the mesenteric, coronary, and renal, vasodilatation occurs at lower concentrations than does vasoconstriction. An exception is the pulmonary circulation in which PGD_2 causes only vasoconstriction. Responses to $PGF_{2\alpha}$ vary with species and vascular bed. It is a potent constrictor of both pulmonary arteries and veins in man (Spannhake *et al.*, 1981; Giles and Leff, 1988). Superficial veins of the hand in man and large-capacitance veins in various animals are contracted by $PGF_{2\alpha}$ (*see* Nakano, 1973).

Systemic blood pressure generally falls in response to PGEs, and blood flow to most organs, including the heart, mesentery, and kidney, is increased. These effects are particularly striking in some hypertensive patients (*see* Lee, 1974). Blood pressure is increased by $PGF_{2\alpha}$ in some experimental animals due to venoconstriction; however, in man, $PGF_{2\alpha}$ does not alter blood pressure.

Cardiac output is generally increased by PGs E and F. Weak, direct inotropic effects have been noted in various isolated preparations. In the intact animal, however, increased force of contraction as well as increased heart rate is in large measure a reflex consequence of fall in total peripheral resistance.

Prostaglandin endoperoxides have variable effects in vascular beds. Their major effects are a result of intrinsic vasoconstrictor activity coupled with vasodilatation due to rapid conversion to a prostaglandin that is a vasodilator (probably PGI_2). They are rapidly converted into PGI_2 during passage through the lungs.

Thromboxane A_2 is intrinsically a potent vasoconstrictor. It contracts vascular smooth muscle *in vitro* (Bhagwat *et al.*, 1985), and it is a powerful vasoconstrictor in the whole animal and in isolated vascular beds (Bunting *et al.*, 1987).

The intravenous administration of PGI_2 causes prominent hypotension; it is about five times more potent than PGE_2 in producing this effect. The reduction in blood pressure is accompanied by a reflex increase in heart rate (*see* Hirsh *et al.*, 1981). The compound relaxes essentially all isolated preparations of vascular smooth muscle that have been tested. PGI_2 is not inactivated during passage through the lungs, and it is thought to be a physiological modulator of vascular tone that functions to oppose the actions of vasoconstrictors.

In man, LTC_4 and LTD_4 cause hypotension (*see* Feuerstein, 1984; Piper, 1984). This may result in part from a decrease in intravascular volume and in cardiac contractility that is secondary to a marked, leukotriene-induced reduction in coronary blood flow. Although LTC_4 and LTD_4 have little effect on most large arteries or veins, coronary arteries and distal segments of the pulmonary artery are contracted by nanomolar concentrations of these agents (Berkowitz *et al.*, 1984). The renal vasculature is resistant to this constrictor action, but the mesenteric vasculature is not.

The leukotrienes have prominent effects on the microvasculature. LTC_4 and LTD_4 appear to act on the endothelial lining of postcapillary venules to cause exudation of plasma; they are more than 1000-fold more potent than histamine in this regard (*see* Feuerstein, 1984; Piper, 1984). In higher concentrations, LTC_4 and LTD_4 constrict arterioles and reduce exudation of plasma.

Blood. Eicosanoids modify the function of the formed elements of the blood; in some instances, these actions reflect their physiological role. The prostaglandins and related products exert powerful actions on platelets. PGI_2 inhibits the aggregation of human platelets *in vitro* at concentrations between 1 and 10 nM. This fact and the observation that PGI_2 is synthesized by the vascular endothelium have led to the suggestion that the substance controls the aggregation of platelets *in vivo* and contributes to the nonthrombogenic properties of the vascular wall (*see* Moncada and Vane, 1979).

TXA_2 is a major product of arachidonate metabolism in platelets (Hamberg *et al.*, 1975). It is a very powerful inducer of platelet aggregation and the platelet release reaction and is thought to be a physiological mediator of platelet aggregation. Pathways of platelet aggregation that are dependent on the generation of TXA_2 are sensitive to the inhibitory action of aspirin (*see* Chapter 26; Moncada and Vane, 1979).

LTB_4 is a potent chemotactic agent for polymorphonuclear leukocytes, eosinophils, and monocytes; other leukotrienes do not share this action (*see* Piper, 1984). Its potency is comparable to that of various chemotactic peptides and PAF. In higher concentrations, LTB_4 stimulates the aggregation of polymorphonuclear leukocytes and promotes degranulation and the generation of superoxide. LTB_4 promotes adhesion of neutrophils to vascular endothelial cells and their transendothelial migration (Bray *et al.*, 1981); application of LTB_4 to the skin promotes the local accumulation of neutrophils (*see* Davies *et al.*, 1984).

Prostaglandins inhibit lymphocyte function and proliferation and suppress the immunological response. PGE_2 inhibits the differentiation of B lymphocytes into antibody-secreting plasma cells to depress the humoral antibody response. It also inhibits mitogen-stimulated proliferation of T lymphocytes and the release of lymphokines by sensitized T lymphocytes. Exogenously administered prostaglandins have been reported to prolong skin allograft survival (*see* Goodwin and Webb, 1980; Goldyne and Stobo, 1981; Davies *et al.*, 1984).

Smooth Muscle. Prostaglandins contract or relax many smooth muscles beside those of the vasculature. The leukotrienes (*e.g.*, LTD_4) contract most smooth muscles.

Bronchial and Tracheal Muscle. In general, PGFs and PGD_2 contract and PGEs relax bronchial and tracheal muscle. Asthmatic individuals are particularly sensitive to $PGF_{2\alpha}$, which causes intense bronchospasm. Although both PGE_1 and PGE_2 can produce bronchodilatation when given to such patients by aerosol, bronchoconstriction is sometimes observed (*see* Mathe *et al.*, 1977; Spannhake *et al.*, 1981). Prostaglandin endoperoxides and TXA_2 constrict human bronchial smooth muscle *in vitro*. PGI_2 causes bronchodilatation in most species; human bronchial tissue is particularly sensitive, and PGIs antagonize bronchoconstriction that is induced by other agents. However, as with PGEs, variable effects are produced in asthmatic patients.

LTC_4 and LTD_4 are powerful bronchoconstrictors in many species, including man (*see* Piper, 1984; Drazen and Austen, 1987). They act principally on smooth muscle in peripheral airways and are 1000 times more potent than histamine both *in vitro* and *in vivo*.

Uterus. Strips of nonpregnant human uterus are contracted by PGFs but relaxed by PGEs. The contractile response is most prominent before menstruation, whereas relaxation is greatest at mid-cycle (*see* Bergström *et al.*, 1968). Uterine strips from pregnant women are uniformly contracted by PGFs *and* by low concentrations of PGE_2; PGI_2 and high concentrations of

PGE_2 produce relaxation. The intravenous infusion of PGE_2 or $PGF_{2\alpha}$ to pregnant women produces a dose-dependent increase in uterine tone as well as the frequency and intensity of rhythmic uterine contraction. Uterine responsiveness to prostaglandins increases as pregnancy progresses; however, the increase is far less than that to oxytocin (*see* Chapter 39; Behrman and Anderson, 1974).

Gastrointestinal Muscle. In the main, longitudinal muscle from stomach to colon is contracted by both PGEs and PGFs, while circular muscle generally relaxes in response to PGEs and contracts in response to PGFs. Prostaglandin endoperoxides, TXA_2, and PGI_2 produce contraction but are less active than the PGEs or PGFs on gastrointestinal smooth muscle. The leukotrienes have potent contractile effects. Prostaglandins reduce transit times in the small intestine and colon. Diarrhea, cramps, and reflux of bile have been noted in response to oral PGE; these are common side effects (along with nausea and vomiting) in patients given prostaglandins for abortion (Bennett, 1977; Wilson and Kaymakcalan, 1981).

Gastric and Intestinal Secretions. PGEs and PGI_2 inhibit gastric acid secretion stimulated by feeding, histamine, or gastrin. Volume of secretion, acidity, and content of pepsin are all reduced, probably by an action exerted directly on the secretory cells. In addition, these prostaglandins are vasodilators in the gastric mucosa, and PGI_2 may be involved in the local regulation of blood flow. Mucus secretion in the stomach and small intestine is increased by prostaglandins. These effects help to maintain the integrity of the gastric mucosa. Furthermore, PGEs and their analogs inhibit gastric damage caused by a variety of ulcerogenic agents in experimental animals and promote healing of duodenal and gastric ulcers in man. PGEs and PGFs stimulate the movement of water and electrolytes into the intestinal lumen. Such effects may underlie the watery diarrhea that follows the oral or parenteral administration of prostaglandins. By contrast, PGI_2 does not induce diarrhea; indeed, it prevents that provoked by other prostaglandins (*see* Wilson and Kaymakcalan, 1981; Sontag, 1986).

Kidney and Urine Formation. Prostaglandins influence renal salt and water excretion by alterations in renal blood flow and by direct effects on renal tubules. PGE_2 and PGI_2 infused directly into the renal arteries of dogs increase renal blood flow and provoke diuresis, natriuresis, and kaliuresis; there is little change in the rate of glomerular filtration (Dunn and Hood, 1977). TXA_2 decreases renal blood flow and the rate of glomerular filtration. PGEs inhibit water reabsorption induced by antidiuretic hormone (ADH) (*see* Dunn and Hood, 1977). PGE_2 also inhibits chloride reabsorption in the thick ascending limb of the loop of Henle in the rabbit (Stokes, 1979). In addition, PGI_2, PGE_2, and PGD_2 cause the secretion of renin from the renal cortex, apparently through a direct effect on the granular juxtaglomerular cells (Keeton and Campbell, 1980).

Central Nervous System. Although a large number of observations have been made on the effects of prostaglandins in the central nervous system (CNS), evidence for a particular physiological role has yet to emerge. Both stimulant and depressant effects of prostaglandins on the CNS have been reported following their injection into the cerebral ventricles, and the firing rates of individual brain cells may be increased or decreased after iontophoretic application of these agents. The release of PGE_2 in the hypothalamus has been proposed to explain the genesis of pyrogen-induced fever. However, there is evidence that contradicts this hypothesis (*see* Wolfe, 1982; Davies *et al.*, 1984).

Afferent Nerves and Pain. PGEs cause pain when injected intradermally; these effects are generally not as immediate or intense as those caused by bradykinin or histamine, but they outlast those caused by the other autacoids. PGEs and PGI_2 sensitize the afferent nerve endings to the effects of chemical or mechanical stimuli by lowering the threshold of the nociceptors. Hyperalgesia is also produced by LTB_4. The release of these prostaglandins and of LTB_4 during the inflammatory process thus serves as an amplification system for the pain mechanism (*see* Moncada *et al.*, 1978; Davies *et al.*, 1984). The role of PGE_2 and PGI_2 in inflammation is discussed in Chapter 26.

Endocrine System. A variety of endocrine tissues respond to prostaglandins. In a number of species, the systemic administration of PGE_2 increases circulating concentrations of ACTH, growth hormone, prolactin, and the gonadotropins; the last-named effect appears to involve a hypothalamic site of action (*see* Behrman, 1979). Other effects include stimulation of steroid production by the adrenals, stimulation of insulin release, thyrotropin-like effects on the thyroid, and LH-like effects on isolated ovarian tissue, causing increased progesterone secretion from the corpus luteum. This last effect, observed *in vitro*, contrasts with the luteolytic effects of prostaglandins *in vivo* in many species, but not in pregnant women. This property is possessed especially but not uniquely by $PGF_{2\alpha}$ (*see* Behrman and Anderson, 1974; Goldberg and Ramwell, 1975; Horton and Poyser, 1976).

Metabolic Effects. PGEs inhibit the basal rate of lipolysis from adipose tissue *in vitro* and also lipolysis stimulated by exposure to catecholamines or other lipolytic hormones. Such effects have also been noted *in vivo* in various species, including man, but are more capricious. PGEs also have some insulin-like effects on carbohydrate metabolism and exert parathyroid hormone–like effects that result in mobilization of Ca^{2+} from bone in tissue culture.

Mechanism of Action. The diversity of the effects of prostanoids is explained by the existence of a number of distinct receptors that mediate their actions. One scheme for classifying these receptors in platelets and smooth muscle is based primarily on the pattern of effects and the relative potencies of natural and synthetic agonists (Kennedy *et al.*, 1982; Coleman *et al.*, 1984); this scheme has been largely substantiated by ligand-binding studies and by the discovery of relatively selective antagonists (*see* Halushka *et al.*, 1989) and is summarized in Table 24–1. The receptors have been named for the natural prostaglandin for which they have the greatest apparent affinity and have been divided into five main types, designated DP (PGD), FP (PGF), IP (PGI_2), TP (TXA_2), and EP (PGE). The last two named types have been further subdivided into EP_1 (smooth muscle contraction), EP_2 (smooth muscle relaxation), TP_τ (smooth muscle contraction), and TP_α (platelet aggregation). Table 24–1 also indicates the effects of the natural prostaglandins on smooth muscle tone and platelet aggregation when each receptor is stimulated.

As with many other receptors, the prostanoid receptors are coupled to effector mechanisms through G proteins (*see* Halushka *et al.*, 1989). To date, two second messenger systems have been associated with the action of prostanoids in platelets and smooth muscle; namely, stimulation of adenylyl cyclase (enhanced accumulation of cyclic AMP) and stimulation of phospholipase C (enhanced formation of inositol-1,4,5-trisphosphate leading to an increase in cytosolic Ca^{2+}, and diacylglycerols) (*see* Table 24–1). PGE antagonizes the lipolytic actions of epinephrine (rat adipocytes) and the effects of antidiuretic hormone (toad bladder) at least in part by inhibition of adenylyl cyclase.

The actions of prostanoids have been most thoroughly studied in platelets. The prostaglandin endoperoxides and TXA_2 stimulate the TP_α receptor and thereby cause platelet clumping and facilitation of aggregation. These effects are associated with activation of phospholipase C and subsequent release of intracellular Ca^{2+} (Owen and Le Breton, 1981). Ca^{2+} promotes aggregation and production of additional TXA_2. PGI_2 binds to IP receptors and activates adenylyl cyclase; inhibition of platelet aggregation by cyclic AMP is associated with a decrease in intracellular Ca^{2+} (Owen and Le Breton, 1981). PGD_2 interacts with a distinct receptor (DP) that also stimulates adenylyl cyclase. PGE_1 appears to act through IP receptors; PGE_2 may act on both IP and DP receptors.

Three distinct receptors for leukotrienes (LTB_4, LTC_4, and LTD_4/LTE_4) have also been identified pharmacologically and by ligand-binding techniques (*see* Halushka *et al.*, 1989). All of these appear to activate phospholipase C.

Other metabolites of the lipoxygenase and epoxygenase pathways (*e.g.*, HETEs, lipoxins, hepoxilins) possess biological activities; at present, however, there is no evidence for the existence of conventional receptors. It is possible that lipoxygenase metabolites function as intracellular second messengers. For example, some neurotransmitters stimulate the synthesis in neural tissue of an unidentified product of the 12-lipoxygenase pathway that appears to regulate the opening of a K^+ channel (Piomelli *et al.*, 1987). An analogous situation may also exist in myocardial cells.

Table 24–1. CLASSIFICATION OF PROSTAGLANDIN RECEPTORS *

PG RECEPTOR SUBTYPE	PLATELET AGGREGATION	SMOOTH MUSCLE TONE	NATURAL AGONIST	SECOND MESSENGER
DP	−		PGD_2	cAMP
EP_1		+	PGE, $PGF_{2\alpha}$	$IP_3/DAG/Ca^{2+}$
EP_2		−	PGE	cAMP
FP		+	$PGF_{2\alpha}$	$IP_3/DAG/Ca^{2+}$
IP	−	−	PGI_2 (PGE)	cAMP
TP_τ		+	TXA_2, PGH_2, (PGD_2, $PGF_{2\alpha}$)	$IP_3/DAG/Ca^{2+}$
TP_α	+		TXA_2, PGH_2	$IP_3/DAG/Ca^{2+}$

* This table lists the seven prostanoid receptors proposed to date, the responses mediated by the receptors on platelet aggregation and smooth muscle activity, and the proposed intracellular second messengers mediating the responses. Stimulation of aggregation is indicated by a +, while inhibition is indicated by a −. cAMP = adenosine 3′,5′-monophosphate; IP_3 = inositol-1,4,5-trisphosphate; DAG = diacylglycerol.

Receptor Antagonists. There are as yet no potent antagonists of the prostaglandins. However, some compounds are effective in selected tests *in vitro*, and a few of these may be of practical value *in vivo*.

Several compounds have been described that selectively antagonize responses to TXA_2 and the endoperoxides (*e.g.*, PGH_2). Certain of these are prostanoids with a bicycloheptane ring (Ogletree *et al.*, 1985); another is 13-azaprostanoic acid (Le Breton *et al.*, 1979). These drugs inhibit platelet aggregation stimulated by collagen, arachidonate, and PGH_2 (but not that induced by ADP) both *in vitro* and *in vivo*. They also block the bronchoconstriction and vasoconstriction that is induced by arachidonate and analogs that mimic TXA_2. These compounds reduce the formation of arterial and venous thrombi and the size of myocardial infarcts in experimental animals. Nonprostanoid antagonists of TXA_2 have also been developed (Hall *et al.*, 1987). One of these compounds, sulotroban, is an orally effective sulfonamide derivative that inhibits platelet aggregation and prolongs bleeding time when administered to normal subjects or patients with atherosclerotic disease. The clinical utility of agents with this pharmacological spectrum remains to be determined.

Orally active antagonists of leukotrienes are also being characterized (Fleisch *et al.*, 1985; Jones *et al.*, 1989). These agents inhibit the bronchoconstriction, wheal formation, and vascular leakage caused by LTD_4. They also reduce antigen-induced bronchoconstriction (*see* Snyder and Fleisch, 1989).

ENDOGENOUS PROSTAGLANDINS AND LEUKOTRIENES: POSSIBLE FUNCTIONS IN PHYSIOLOGICAL AND PATHOLOGICAL PROCESSES

Because eicosanoids can be formed by virtually every cell, it is not unreasonable to suspect that each pharmacological effect may reflect a physiological or pathophysiological function. Such suspicions have been nurtured and presented in countless hypotheses bearing on just about every bodily function.

Platelets. An area in which there has been considerable interest is the elucidation of the role played by prostaglandin endoperoxides and TXA_2 in platelet aggregation and by PGI_2 in the prevention of such aggregation. It is generally accepted that stimulation of platelets to aggregate leads to activation of membrane phospholipases with the consequent release of arachidonate and its transformation into prostaglandin endoperoxides and TXA_2. These substances induce platelet aggregation. However, this pathway is not the only mechanism for the induction of platelet aggregation, since, for example, thrombin aggregates platelets without the release of arachidonate. However, the importance of the thromboxane pathway is implied by the fact that aspirin and antagonists of TP receptors inhibit the second phase of platelet aggregation and induce a mild hemostatic defect in man (Hamberg *et al.*, 1974; Le Breton *et al.*, 1979).

PGI_2 that is generated in the vessel wall may be the physiological antagonist of this system; it inhibits platelet aggregation and contributes to the nonthrombogenic properties of the endothelium. According to this concept, PGI_2 and TXA_2 represent biologically opposite poles of a mechanism for regulating platelet–vessel wall interaction and the formation of hemostatic plugs and intra-arterial thrombi (*see* Moncada and Vane, 1979).

Reproduction and Parturition. Much interest is attached to the possible involvement of prostaglandins in reproductive physiology. Their very high concentrations in human semen, coupled with the substantial absorption of prostaglandins by the vagina, have encouraged speculation that prostaglandins deposited during coitus may facilitate conception by actions on the cervix, uterine body, fallopian tubes, and transport of semen. Although there is some correlation between lowered concentrations of prostaglandins in semen and certain cases of male infertility, the role of the eicosanoids in semen remains obscure.

During pregnancy in the human female, the capacity of the fetal membranes to elaborate prostaglandins rises progressively. Concentrations of prostaglandins in blood and amniotic fluid are elevated during labor, but it is not certain whether this is a major determinant of the onset of labor or only serves to sustain uterine contractions that have been initiated by oxytocin. In any event, inhibitors of cyclooxygenase increase the length of gestation, prolong the duration of spontaneous labor, and interrupt premature labor. The last-named effect has prompted clinical investigation of these agents for the prevention of premature delivery. Although effective, their potential impact on fetal development (*e.g.*, premature closure of the ductus arteriosus), together with the availability of other tocolytic agents, has limited the use of cyclooxygenase inhibitors for this purpose (*see* Chapter 39).

$PGF_{2\alpha}$ produced in the uterus is a luteolytic hormone in some subprimate species. This knowledge has led to the development of prostaglandin analogs for veterinary use in synchronizing estrus in farm animals in order to simplify breeding procedures; they are also used to provide safe, early abortions before the animals are sent to market. The possible roles of prostaglandins in reproductive processes have been reviewed by Goldberg and Ramwell (1975) and by Horton and Poyser (1976).

Vascular and Pulmonary Smooth Muscle. Local generation of PGE_2 and PGI_2 modulate vascular tone. They appear to function to counteract the effects of circulating vasoconstrictor autacoids and to maintain blood flow to vital organs (Aiken and Vane, 1973). These prostaglandins have also been implicated in the maintenance of patency of the ductus arteriosus. This hypothesis has been strengthened by the fact that aspirin-like drugs induce closure of a patent ductus in neonates (*see* Chapter 26; Coceani *et al.*, 1980). Prostaglandins might also play a role in the maintenance of placental blood flow.

A complex mixture of autacoids is released when sensitized lung tissue is challenged by the appropriate antigen. Various prostaglandins and leukotrienes are prominent components of this mixture. While both bronchodilator (PGE_2) and bronchoconstrictor (*e.g.*, $PGF_{2\alpha}$, TXA_2, LTC_4) substances are released, responses to the peptidoleukotrienes probably dominate during allergic constriction of the airway (*see* Piper, 1984). Included in the evidence for this conclusion is the ineffectiveness of inhibitors of cyclooxygenase and of histaminergic antagonists in the treatment of human asthma and the protection afforded by leukotriene antagonists in antigen-induced bronchoconstriction. Moreover, the relatively slow metabolism of the leukotrienes in lung tissue contributes to the long-lasting bronchoconstriction that follows challenge with antigen and may be a factor in the high bronchial tone that is observed in asthmatics in periods between acute attacks.

Kidney. Prostaglandins probably modulate renal blood flow and may serve to regulate urine formation by both renovascular and tubular effects. Additional roles in the regulation of the secretion of renin are also likely. The elaboration of PGE_2 and PGI_2 is increased by factors that reduce renal blood flow (*e.g.*, stimulation of sympathetic nerves and angiotensin). Under these circumstances, inhibitors of cyclooxygenase augment the renovasoconstriction that is produced by such stimuli (Aiken and Vane, 1973). In addition, the effects of ADH on the reabsorption of water may be restrained by the concomitant production and action of PGE_2.

Increased biosynthesis of prostaglandins has been associated with Bartter's syndrome. This is a rare disease characterized by low-to-normal blood pressure, decreased sensitivity to angiotensin, hyperreninemia, hyperaldosteronism, and excessive loss of K^+. There is also an increased granulation of renal medullary interstitial cells and an increased excretion of prostaglandins in the urine. After long-term administration of inhibitors of cyclooxygenase, sensitivity to angiotensin, plasma renin values, and the concentration of aldosterone in plasma return to normal. Although plasma K^+ rises, it remains low, and urinary wasting of K^+ persists. Whether an increase in prostaglandin biosynthesis is the cause of Bartter's syndrome or a reflection of a more basic physiological defect is not known (*see* Ferris, 1978).

Inflammatory and Immune Responses. Prostaglandins and leukotrienes are released by a host of mechanical, thermal, chemical, bacterial, and other insults, and they contribute importantly to the genesis of the signs and symptoms of inflammation (*see* Moncada *et al.*, 1978; Samuelsson, 1983; Davies *et al.*, 1984). The peptidoleukotrienes have powerful effects on vascular permeability, while LTB_4 is a potent chemoattractant for polymorphonuclear leukocytes and can promote exudation of plasma by mobilizing this source of additional inflammatory mediators. Although prostaglandins do not appear to have direct effects on vascular permeability, both PGE_2 and PGI_2 markedly enhance edema formation and leukocyte infiltration by promoting blood flow in the inflamed region. Moreover, they potentiate the pain-producing activity of bradykinin and other autacoids (*see* Chapter 23). However, PGEs inhibit the participation of lymphocytes in delayed hypersensitivity reactions. Moreover, they inhibit the release of hydrolases and lysosomal enzymes from human neutrophils as well as from mouse peritoneal macrophages.

Some experimental tumors in animals and certain spontaneous human tumors (medullary carcinoma of the thyroid, renal-cell adenocarcinoma, carcinoma of the breast) are accompanied by increased concentrations of local or circulating prostaglandins, bone metastasis, and hypercalcemia. Since the PGEs have potent osteolytic activity, it has been suggested that they are implicated in some cases of hypercalcemia. Some studies have implicated platelet aggregation and the effects of prostaglandins thereon in the hematogenous metastasis of tumors. Pretreatment of animals with inhibitors of thromboxane synthase reduces the formation of tumor colonies, although the administration of such agents after the injection of tumor cells is without effect. The infusion of PGI_2 either before or after the injection of cells markedly inhibits the establishment of tumor colonies. These effects have been attributed to inhibition of platelet aggregation, rather than to vasodilatation (*see* Honn *et al.*, 1983).

THERAPEUTIC USES

As described above, there has been intense interest in the effects of the prostaglandins on the female reproductive system. Their action as *abortifacients* when given early in pregnancy is clearly established. However, initial hopes that they might provide a simple, convenient means of postimplantation "contraception," perhaps given as a vaginal suppository, have not been fulfilled. Moreover, the abortifacient action of prostaglandins may be inconstant and often incomplete, and may be accompanied by side effects (Behrman and Anderson, 1974). Nevertheless, prostaglandins appear to be of value in missed abortion and molar gestation, and they have been widely used for the induction of midtrimester abortion. While PGE_2 or $PGF_{2\alpha}$ can induce labor at term, they may have more value when used to facilitate labor by promoting ripening and dilatation of the cervix. These actions of prostaglandins are considered more fully in Chapter 39.

The capacity of several prostaglandin analogs to suppress gastric ulceration is a property of therapeutic importance. Analogs of PGE_1 (*rioprostil* and *misoprostol*) and of PGE_2 (*enprostil, arbaprostil,* and *trimoprostil*) have been tested clinically. Misoprostol has recently been released for general use; its structure is as follows:

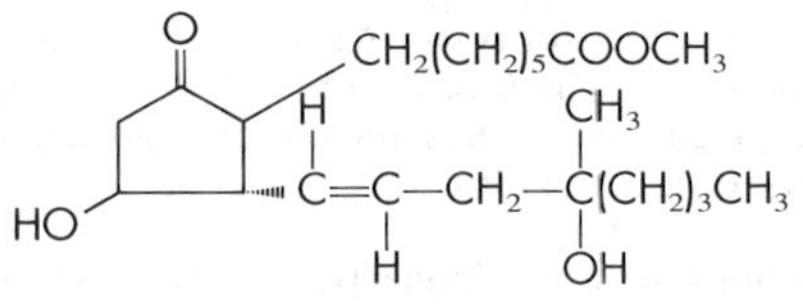

Misoprostol

When given in doses that suppress gastric acid secretion, these drugs appear to heal gastric ulcers about as effectively as the H_2 antagonists (*see* Chapter 37); however, relief of ulcerogenic pain and healing of duodenal ulcers has not been achieved consistently with misoprostol. The drug is currently used primarily for the prevention of ulcers that often occur during long-term treatment with aspirin-like drugs. Although diarrhea is frequently observed, it is mild and usually does not force discontinuation of therapy. *Misoprostol* (CYTOTEC) is rapidly absorbed and is converted to the equally active misoprostol acid with a half-time of 30 to 60 minutes; little information is available on the pharmacokinetic properties of this active metabolite (*see* Sontag, 1986; Monk and Clissold, 1987). Misoprostol is available in 200-μg tablets for the prevention of gastric ulcers in patients who are at risk for development of such ulcers during long-term therapy with aspirin-like drugs. The recommended dosage is 200 μg four times daily. The drug should not be administered to pregnant women because of its uterotonic activity.

PGE_1 or PGI_2 has been administered by intra-arterial or intravenous infusion to patients with severe peripheral vascular disease. In the absence of complete arterial occlusion, dramatic and long-lasting improvement has been observed after a brief infusion (Clifford *et al.*, 1980; Pardy *et al.*, 1980; Belch *et al.*, 1983).

Although the use of drugs that inhibit platelet aggregation in the treatment of acute myocardial infarction is controversial, there is evidence that PGI_2 and its analogs (*carbacyclin* and *iloprost*) reduce ischemic damage in experimental models. However, beneficial effects have not been demonstrated in man. PGI_2 and iloprost decrease arterial pressure, inhibit platelet aggregation, and reduce pulmonary resistance in normal subjects and patients with angina pectoris (Firth *et al.*, 1983; Bugiardini *et al.*, 1985). Unfortunately, chest pain typical of angina pectoris and evidence of myocardial ischemia is noted with these agents in some patients with severe coronary artery disease. These ischemic episodes apparently result from drug-induced dilatation of small coronary vessels, which diverts blood flow *away* from the ischemic zone. This effect apparently overrides the benefit of inhibition of platelet aggregation and limits the usefulness of these prostanoids in some patients with ischemic heart disease (*see* Hirsh *et al.*, 1981).

Both PGE_1 and PGI_2 are valuable for improving the harvest and storage of blood platelets for therapeutic transfusion. Clinical experience with cardiopulmonary bypass, charcoal hemoperfusion, and renal dialysis indicates that PGI_2 is also useful in the prevention of platelet aggregation in extracorporeal circulation systems. In addition, PGI_2 may be used in place of heparin during dialysis in patients with renal disease, and it may have advantages for those in whom the use of heparin is contraindicated (Zusman *et al.*, 1981).

PGE_1 may be used in the treatment of impotence. Intracavernous injection of PGE_1 causes complete or partial erection in impotent patients who do not have disorders of the vascular system or cavernous body damage (Ishii *et al.*, 1989). The erection lasts for one to three hours and is sufficient for sexual intercourse. PGE_1 is as effective as papaverine, but it does not cause prolonged erection and priapism.

The pulmonary blood vessels, particularly the ductus arteriosus in neonates, are sensitive to the vasodilatory effect of PGE_1 and PGI_2. These prostaglandins are used to increase pulmonary blood flow and oxygenation of blood in infants with congenital heart defects that restrict pulmonary or systemic blood flow. Under such circumstances, dilatation of the ductus arteriosus improves blood flow and tissue oxygenation. At present, only PGE_1 (*alprostadil*) is available for this purpose in the United States; PGI_2 (*epoprostenol*) is available in Europe. Alprostadil (PROSTIN VR PEDIATRIC) is usually infused intravenously at an initial rate of 0.05 to 0.1 μg/kg per minute, with subsequent reductions to the lowest dosage that maintains the response. Apnea is observed in about 10% of neonates so treated, particularly in those who weigh less than 2 kg at birth. The treatment is considered palliative until corrective surgery can be performed.

PLATELET-ACTIVATING FACTOR

History. In 1971, Henson demonstrated that a soluble factor was released from leukocytes and caused platelets to aggregate. Benveniste and his coworkers confirmed these observations and named the substance *platelet-activating factor* (PAF); their research indicated that the compound was a polar lipid. During this period, Muirhead described an antihypertensive polar renal lipid (APRL) produced by interstitial cells of the renal medulla. Sufficient evidence had accumulated by 1979 to conclude that PAF and APRL were identical. Hanahan and coworkers then synthesized acetylglyceryletherphosphorylcholine (AGEPC) and determined that this phospholipid had chemical and biological properties identical to those of PAF (Demopoulos *et al.*, 1979). Subsequently, the structures of PAF and APRL were determined independently and were found to be identical to that of AGEPC (Blank *et al.*, 1979; Hanahan *et al.*, 1980; Polonsky *et al.*, 1980). Of the names for the compound, platelet-activating factor has gained the greatest acceptance, despite the fact that the lipid has many biological actions in addition to those on platelets (*see* Hanahan, 1986; Braquet *et al.*, 1987; Snyder, 1989).

Chemistry and Biosynthesis. PAF is 1-O-alkyl-2-acetyl-*sn*-glycero-3-phosphocholine. Its structure is as follows:

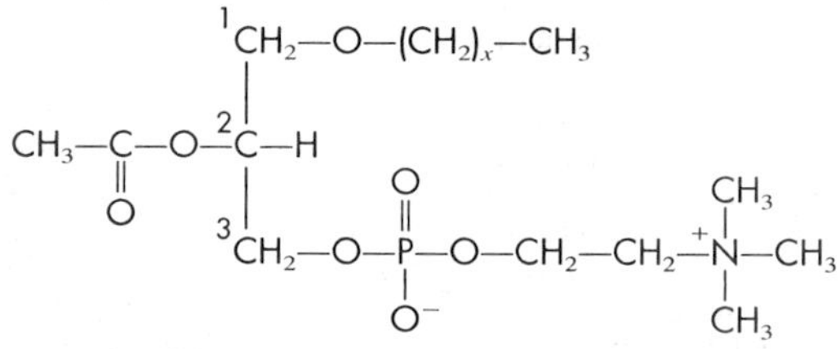

Platelet-Activating Factor (x = 11 to 17)

In contrast to the two long-chain acyl groups that are present in phosphatidylcholine, PAF contains a long-chain alkyl group joined to the glycerol backbone in an ether linkage at position 1 and an acetyl group at position 2. PAF actually represents a family of phospholipids, because the alkyl group at position 1 can vary in length from 12 to 18 carbon atoms. In human neutrophils, PAF consists predominantly of a mixture of the 16- and 18-carbon ethers, but its composition may change when cells are stimulated.

Like the eicosanoids, PAF is not stored in cells but is synthesized in response to stimulation. The precursor of PAF is 1-O-alkyl-2-acyl-glycerophosphocholine—a lipid found in high concentrations in the membranes of many types of cells. The 2-acyl substituents include an abundance of arachidonate. PAF is synthesized from this substrate in two steps (*see* Figure 24–3). The first involves the action of phospholipase A_2, with the formation of 1-O-alkyl-2-lyso-glycerophosphocholine (lyso-PAF) and a free fatty acid (usually arachidonate) (Chilton *et al.*, 1984). In some cells (*e.g.*, neutrophils) this reaction represents a major source of the arachidonate that is metabolized to prostaglandins and leukotrienes. In the second step, lyso-PAF is acetylated by acetyl coenzyme A in a reaction catalyzed by lyso-PAF acetyltransferase. This represents the rate-limiting step. The synthesis of PAF may be stimulated during antigen–antibody reactions or by a variety of agents, including chemotactic peptides, thrombin, collagen, and other autacoids; PAF can also stimulate its own formation. Both the phospholipase and acetyltransferase are Ca^{2+}-dependent enzymes, and PAF synthesis is regulated by the availability of Ca^{2+} (*see* Hanahan, 1986; Snyder, 1989).

The inactivation of PAF also occurs in two steps (*see* Figure 24–3) (Chilton *et al.*, 1983). Initially, the acetyl group of PAF is removed by PAF acetylhydrolase to form lyso-PAF; this enzyme is present in both cells and plasma. Lyso-PAF is then converted to a 1-O-alkyl-2-acyl-glycerophosphocholine by an acyltransferase. This latter step is inhibited by Ca^{2+}.

PAF is synthesized by platelets, neutrophils, monocytes, mast cells, eosinophils, renal mesangial cells, renal medullary cells, and vascular endothelial cells (*see* Braquet *et al.*, 1987). In most instances, stimulation of PAF synthesis results in the release of PAF and lyso-PAF from the cell. However, in some cells (*e.g.*, endothelial cells) PAF is not released and exerts its effects intracellularly (McIntyre *et al.*, 1986).

Pharmacological Properties. *Cardiovascular System.* PAF is a potent vasodilator, and it lowers peripheral vascular resistance and systemic blood pressure when injected intravenously (Blank *et al.*, 1979). PAF-induced vasodilatation is independent of effects on the sympathetic innervation or arachidonate metabolism (Sybertz *et al.*, 1985). However, the effects of PAF on the coronary circulation are a mixture of direct and indirect actions. The intracoronary administration of small amounts of PAF increases coronary blood flow by a mechanism that involves the release of a platelet-derived vasodilator (Jackson *et al.*, 1986). At higher doses, coronary blood flow is decreased by the formation of intravascular aggregates of platelets and/or the formation of TXA_2 (Sybertz *et al.*, 1985). The pulmonary vasculature is also constricted by PAF, and a similar mechanism is thought to be involved. Intradermal injection of PAF causes an initial vasoconstriction followed by a typical wheal and flare.

PAF increases vascular permeability and promotes the movement of fluid out of the vasculature (McManus *et al.*, 1981). As with substances such as histamine and bradykinin, the increase in permeability is due to contraction of venular endothelial cells, but PAF is 1000-fold more potent (Humphrey *et al.*, 1984).

Platelets. PAF is a potent stimulator of platelet aggregation *in vitro* (Demopoulos *et al.*, 1979). Aggregation is accompanied by the release of TXA_2 and the granular contents of the platelet; however, PAF does not require the presence of TXA_2 or other aggregating agents to produce this effect. The intravenous injection of PAF causes formation of intravascular platelet aggregates and thrombocytopenia (McManus *et al.*, 1981).

Leukocytes. PAF stimulates polymorphonuclear leukocytes to aggregate, to release leukotrienes and lysosomal enzymes, and to generate superoxide. Since LTB_4 is more potent, it is thought to mediate the effects of PAF (Lin *et al.*, 1982). Similarly, PAF promotes aggregation of monocytes and degranulation of eosinophils.

PAF is a chemotactic factor for eosinophils, neutrophils, and monocytes (Goetzl *et al.*, 1980). It also promotes the adherence of neutrophils to endothelial cells and their diapedesis. When given systemically, PAF causes leukocytopenia, with neutrophils showing the greatest decline (McManus *et al.*, 1981). Intradermal injection causes the accumulation of neutrophils and mononuclear cells at the site of injection, and inhaled PAF increases the infiltration of eosinophils into the airways.

Smooth Muscle. PAF generally contracts gastrointestinal, uterine, and pulmonary smooth muscle, apparently by both direct and indirect mechanisms. PAF enhances the amplitude of spontaneous uterine contractions; quiescent muscle contracts rapidly in a phasic fashion. These contractions are inhibited by inhibitors of prostaglandin synthesis.

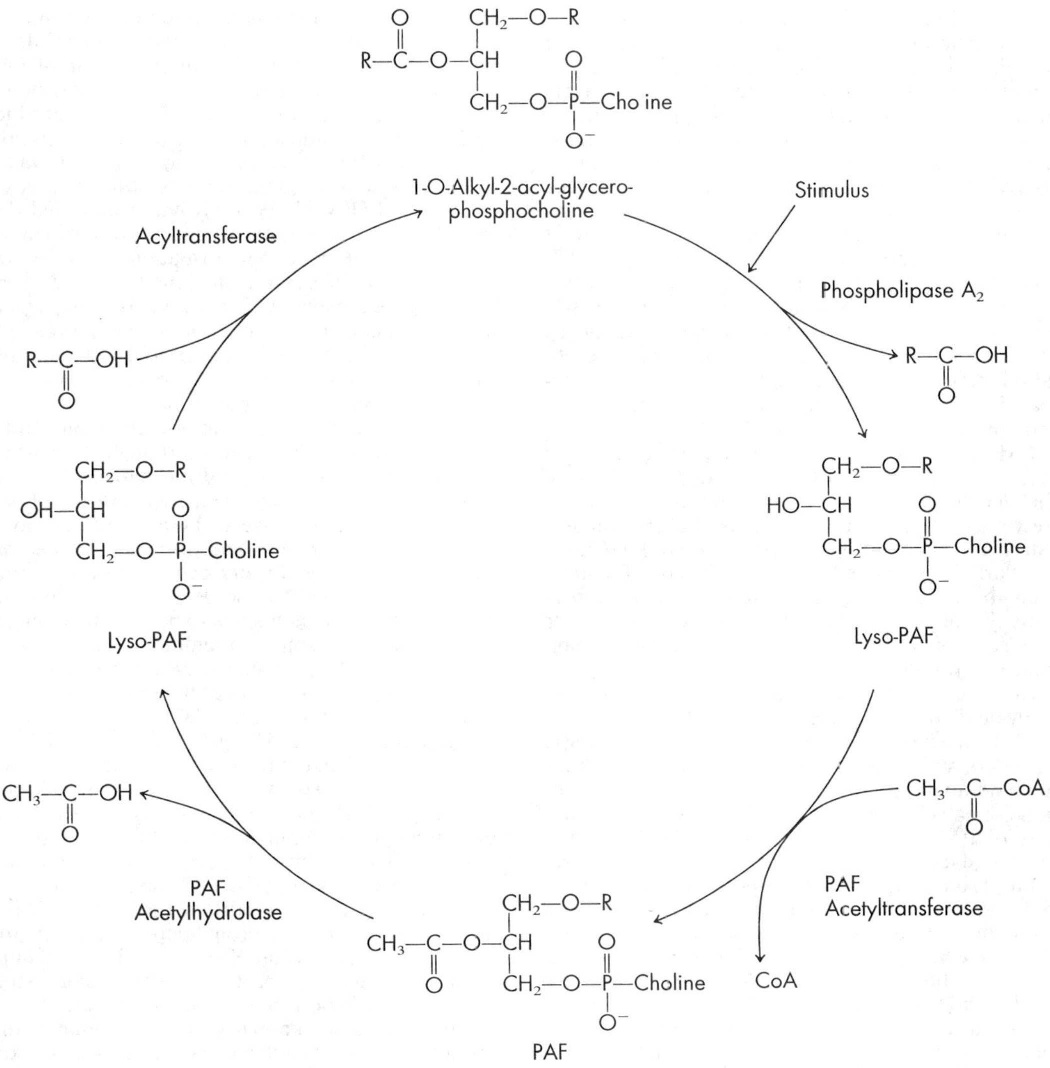

Figure 24–3. *Synthesis and degradation of platelet-activating factor* (PAF).

RCOOH is a mixture of fatty acids but is enriched in arachidonic acid; it may be metabolized to eicosanoids. CoA represents coenzyme A.

PAF does not affect tracheal smooth muscle but contracts the smooth muscle of peripheral airways (Stimler and O'Flaherty, 1983). Although controversial, most evidence suggests that another autacoid (*e.g.*, LTC_4 or TXA_2) mediates this effect. When given by aerosol, PAF increases airway resistance and increases the responsiveness to other bronchoconstrictors (Cuss *et al.*, 1986). This bronchial hyperresponsiveness occurs after a delay of up to 3 days in man and may persist for 1 to 4 weeks. PAF also increases mucus secretion and the permeability of pulmonary microvessels; this results in fluid accumulation in the mucosal and submucosal regions of the trachea and bronchi.

Stomach. In addition to contracting the fundus of the stomach, PAF is the most potent known ulcerogen. When given intravenously, it causes hemorrhagic erosions of the gastric mucosa that extend into the submucosa.

Kidney. When infused intrarenally in animals, PAF decreases renal blood flow, glomerular filtration rate, urine volume, and excretion of Na^+ (Schlondorff and Neuwirth, 1986). These effects are not due to the formation of platelet aggregates but are the result of a direct action on the renal circulation. PAF also stimulates the release of vasodilator prostaglandins, which tends to counteract the renal vasoconstriction.

Mechanism of Action. In most circumstances, PAF appears to exert its actions by stimulating G protein–linked, cell-surface receptors; high-affinity binding sites have been detected in the plasma membranes of a number of cell types (Braquet *et al.,* 1987; Hwang, 1988). Lyso-PAF is inactive, and biological activity is markedly reduced by relatively small changes in structure. In many cases stimulation of these receptors causes activation of phospholipases C and A_2, with resultant formation of inositol phosphates, diacylglycerol, and arachidonate (Kawaguchi and Yasuda, 1986; Schwertschlag and Whorton, 1988). Thus, prostaglandins, TXA_2, or leukotrienes may function as extracellular mediators of the effects of PAF. In addition, the binding of PAF to its receptor unmasks cell-surface binding sites for fibrinogen that promote platelet aggregation directly.

PAF may also exert actions without exiting the cell. The clearest example is provided by the endothelial cell. Synthesis of PAF is stimulated by a variety of factors, but it is not released extracellularly (McIntyre *et al.,* 1986). Accumulation of PAF intracellularly is associated with the adhesion of neutrophils to the surface of the endothelial cells, apparently because PAF promotes the expression or exposure of surface proteins that recognize and bind neutrophils.

Receptor Antagonists. Many compounds have been described that selectively inhibit the actions of PAF *in vivo* and *in vitro* (Braquet *et al.,* 1987; Saunders and Handley, 1987). These drugs inhibit the binding of PAF to its receptor and block its actions selectively. Among these antagonists are analogs of PAF with modifications in the 3-position of the glycerol backbone, a number of natural plant products, and, surprisingly, triazolobenzodiazepines such as alprazolam and triazolam. Of the natural products, a series of terpenes isolated from the Chinese tree *Ginkgo biloba* are potent and selective; the most active is *ginkgolide B* (Braquet *et al.,* 1987). The development of PAF antagonists is still in its early stages, and their clinical utility has not been established. However, the involvement of PAF in inflammation, asthma, and reproduction suggests that such antagonists may have therapeutic application.

Physiological and Pathological Functions of PAF. Unlike the eicosanoids, PAF is synthesized by a select assortment of cells; this is presumed to limit its participation in various physiological and pathological processes.

Platelets. Since PAF is synthesized by platelets and promotes aggregation, it was proposed to be the mediator of thrombin-induced aggregation (so-called alternate pathway). However, PAF antagonists fail to block thrombin-induced aggregation, even though they prolong bleeding time and prevent thrombus formation in some experimental models. Thus, PAF does not function as an independent mediator of aggregation but contributes to thrombus formation in a manner analogous to TXA_2 and ADP.

Reproduction and Parturition. PAF may be involved in ovulation, implantation, and parturition. Rupture of the follicle is inhibited in experimental animals by the PAF antagonist, ginkgolide B (Abisogun *et al.,* 1989); the administration of PAF restores ovulation. Following ovulation and subsequent fertilization, the embryo begins to produce PAF, which promotes platelet aggregation and the release of platelet factors that appear to stimulate activation and implantation of the blastocyst (Spinks and O'Neill, 1987). It has been noted that not all human embryos produced by fertilization *in vitro* generate PAF, and formation of PAF is correlated with successful implantation and pregnancy. The capacity to form PAF is being evaluated as a means for selecting human embryos with the greatest potential for successful implantation. These findings also suggest the potential utility of PAF antagonists in contraception.

PAF is found in the amniotic fluid only after labor commences. This PAF is thought to contribute to parturition by several mechanisms. It may cause contraction of the myometrium directly, or it may promote the release of PGE_2 (and additional PAF) from amnion cells and promote uterine contractions indirectly. In any event, the importance of PAF is indicated by the delay in parturition induced by PAF antagonists in experimental animals. Interestingly, the source of amnionic PAF appears to be the fetal lung, which may provide a link between fetal development and the initiation of parturition (*see* Johnston *et al.,* 1987).

Inflammatory and Allergic Responses. PAF is elaborated by leukocytes and mast cells and exerts proinflammatory effects. For example, intradermal injection of PAF duplicates many of the signs and symptoms of inflammation, including increased vascular permeability, hyperalgesia, edema, and infiltration of neutrophils. PAF also produces effects that suggest its importance in asthma. When inhaled, it is a potent bronchoconstrictor, it promotes the accumulation of eosinophils in the lung, it causes tracheal and bronchial edema, and it stimulates the secretion of mucus. Moreover, PAF is the only autacoid known to produce long-lasting bronchial hyperresponsiveness. The plasma concentration of PAF is increased in experimental anaphylactic shock, and the administration of PAF reproduces many of its signs and symptoms, suggesting a role for the autacoid in this condition. Despite the broad implications of these observations, the effects of PAF antagonists have been rather limited. Although they reverse the bronchoconstriction of anaphylactic shock and improve survival, the impact of PAF antagonists on animal models of asthma and inflammation has been disappointing. These results may reflect the complexity of these pathological conditions and the inherent limitations of the animal models (*see* Braquet *et al.,*1987; Saunders and Handley, 1987). Nevertheless, the potential role of PAF in these conditions may eventually warrant the evaluation of PAF antagonists in patients.

Abisogun, A. O.; Braquet, P.; and Tsafriri, A. The involvement of platelet activating factor in ovulation. *Science,* **1989,** *243,* 381–383.

Aiken, J. W., and Vane, J. R. Intrarenal prostaglandin

release attenuates the renal vasoconstrictor activity of angiotensin. *J. Pharmacol. Exp. Ther.*, **1973**, *184*, 678–687.

Belch, J. J. F.; McArdle, B.; Pollock, J. G.; Forbes, C. D.; McKay, A.; Leiberman, P.; Lowe, G. D. O.; and Prentice, C. R. M. Epoprostenol (prostacyclin) and severe arterial disease. A double-blind trial. *Lancet*, **1983**, *1*, 315–317.

Berkowitz, B. A.; Zabko-Potapovich, B.; Valocik, R.; and Gleason, J. G. Effects of the leukotrienes on the vasculature and blood pressure of different species. *J. Pharmacol. Exp. Ther.*, **1984**, *229*, 105–112.

Bhagwat, S. S.; Hamann, P. R.; Still, W. C.; Bunting, S.; and Fitzpatrick, F. A. Synthesis and structure of the platelet aggregation factor thromboxane A_2. *Nature*, **1985**, *315*, 511–513.

Blank, M. L.; Snyder, F.; Byers, L. W.; Brooks, B.; and Muirhead, E. E. Antihypertensive activity of an alkyl ether analog of phosphatidylcholine. *Biochem. Biophys. Res. Commun.*, **1979**, *90*, 1194–1200.

Borgeat, P., and Samuelsson, B. Arachidonic acid metabolism in polymorphonuclear leukocytes: unstable intermediate in formation of dihydroxy acids. *Proc. Natl. Acad. Sci. U.S.A.*, **1979**, *76*, 3213–3217.

Bray, M. A.; Ford-Hutchinson, A. W.; and Smith, M. J. H. Leukotriene B_4: an inflammatory mediator *in vivo*. *Prostaglandins*, **1981**, *22*, 213–222.

Bugiardini, R.; Galvani, M.; Ferrini, D.; Gridelli, C.; Tollemeto, D.; Mari, L.; Puddu, P.; and Lenzi, S. Myocardial ischemia induced by prostacyclin and iloprost. *Clin. Pharmacol. Ther.*, **1985**, *38*, 101–108.

Bunting, S.; Buchanan, L. V.; Holzgrefe, H. H.; and Fitzpatrick, F. A. Pharmacology of synthetic thromboxane A_2. In, *Advances in Prostaglandin, Thromboxane, and Leukotriene Research*. (Samuelsson, B.; Paoletti, R.; and Ramwell, P. W.; eds.) Raven Press, New York, **1987**, pp. 192–198.

Burch, R. M., and Axelrod, J. Dissociation of bradykinin-induced prostaglandin formation from phosphatidylinositol turnover in Swiss 3T3 fibroblasts: evidence for G protein regulation of phospholipase A_2. *Proc. Natl. Acad. Sci. U.S.A.*, **1987**, *84*, 6374–6378.

Chilton, F. H.; Ellis, J. M.; Olson, S. C.; and Wykle, R. L. 1-O-alkyl-2-arachidonoyl-*sn*-glycero-3-phosphocholine. *J. Biol. Chem.*, **1984**, *259*, 12014–12019.

Chilton, F. H.; O'Flaherty, J. T.; Ellis, J. M.; Swendsen, C. L.; and Wykle, R. L. Metabolic fate of platelet-activating factor in neutrophils. *J. Biol. Chem.*, **1983**, *258*, 6357–6361.

Clifford, P. C.; Martin, M. F. R.; Sheddon, E. J.; Kirby, J. D.; Baird, R. N.; and Dieppe, P. A. Treatment of vasospastic disease with prostaglandin E_1. *Br. Med. J.* [*Clin. Res.*], **1980**, *281*, 1031–1039.

Cuss, F. M.; Dixon, C. M. S.; and Barnes, P. J. Effects of inhaled platelet activating factor on pulmonary function and bronchial responsiveness in man. *Lancet*, **1986**, *1*, 189–192.

Demopoulos, C. A.; Pinckard, R. N.; and Hanahan, D. J. Evidence for 1-O-alkyl-2-acetyl-*sn*-glyceryl-3-phosphorylcholine as the active component (a new class of lipid chemical mediators). *J. Biol. Chem.*, **1979**, *254*, 9355–9358.

Denzlinger, C.; Guhlmann, A.; Scheuber, P. H.; Wilker, D.; Hammer, D. K.; and Keppler, D. Metabolism and analysis of cysteinyl leukotrienes in the monkey. *J. Biol. Chem.*, **1986**, *261*, 15601–15606.

Feldberg, W., and Kellaway, C. H. Liberation of histamine and formation of lysocithin-like substances by cobra venom. *J. Physiol.* (*Lond.*), **1938**, *94*, 187–226.

Firth, B. G.; Winniford, M. D.; Campbell, W. B.; and Hillis, L. D. Hemodynamic effects of intravenous prostacyclin in stable angina pectoris. *Am. J. Cardiol.*, **1983**, *52*, 439–443.

Fleisch, J. H.; Rinkema, L. E.; Haisch, K. D.; Swanson-Bean, D.; Goodson, T.; Ho, P. P. K.; and Marshall, W. S. LY171883, 1- < 2-hydroxy-3-propyl-4- < -(1H-tetrazol-5-yl) butoxy > phenyl > ethanone, an orally active leukotriene D_4 antagonist. *J. Pharmacol. Exp. Ther.*, **1985**, *233*, 148–157.

Flower, R. J., and Blackwell, G. J. Anti-inflammatory steroids induce biosynthesis of a phospholipase A_2 inhibitor which prevents prostaglandin generation. *Nature*, **1979**, *278*, 456–459.

Goetzl, E. J.; Derian, C. K.; Tauber, A. I.; and Valone, F. H. Novel effects of 1-O-hexadecyl-2-acyl-*sn*-glycero-3-phosphorylcholine mediators on human leukocyte function: delineation of the specific roles of the acyl substituents. *Biochem. Biophys. Res. Commun.*, **1980**, *94*, 881–888.

Hall, R. A., and others. Pharmacology of L-655,240 3([1-(4-chlorobenzyl)-5-fluoro-3-methyl-indol-2-yl],2,-2-dimethylpropanoic acid): a potent, selective thromboxane/prostaglandin endoperoxide antagonist. *Eur. J. Pharmacol.*, **1987**, *135*, 193–201.

Hamberg, M.; Svensson, J.; and Samuelsson, B. Thromboxane: a new group of biologically active compounds derived from prostaglandin endoperoxides. *Proc. Natl. Acad. Sci. U.S.A.*, **1975**, *72*, 2994–2998.

Hamberg, M.; Svensson, J.; Wakabayashi, T.; and Samuelsson, B. Isolation and structure of two prostaglandin endoperoxides that cause platelet aggregation. *Proc. Natl. Acad. Sci. U.S.A.*, **1974**, *71*, 345–349.

Hanahan, D. J.; Demopoulos, C. A.; Liehr, J.; and Pinckard, R. N. Identification of platelet activating factor isolated from rabbit basophils as acetyl glyceryl ether phosphorylcholine. *J. Biol. Chem.*, **1980**, *255*, 5514–5516.

Humphrey, D. M.; McManus, L. M.; Hanahan, D. J.; and Pinckard, R. N. Morphologic basis of increased vascular permeability induced by acetyl glyceryl ether phosphorylcholine. *Lab. Invest.*, **1984**, *50*, 16–25.

Hwang, S.-B. Identification of a second putative receptor of platelet-activating factor from human polymorphonuclear leukocytes. *J. Biol. Chem.*, **1988**, *263*, 3225–3233.

Ishii, N.; Watanabe, H.; Irisawa, C.; Kikuchi, Y.; Kubota, Y.; Kawamura, S.; Suzuki, K.; Chiba, R.; Tokiwa, M.; and Shirai, M. Intracavernous injection of prostaglandin E_1 for the treatment of erectile impotence. *J. Urol.*, **1989**, *141*, 323–325.

Jackson, C. V.; Schumacher, W. A.; Kunkel, S. L.; Driscoll, E. M.; and Lucchesi, B. R. Platelet-activating factor and the release of a platelet-derived coronary artery vasodilator substance in the canine. *Circ. Res.*, **1986**, *58*, 218–229.

Jones, T. R., and others. Pharmacology of L-660,711 (MK-571): a novel potent and selective leukotriene D_4 receptor antagonist. *Can. J. Physiol. Pharmacol.*, **1989**, *67*, 17–28.

Kawaguchi, H., and Yasuda, H. Effect of platelet-activating factor on arachidonic acid metabolism in renal epithelial cells. *Biochim. Biophys. Acta*, **1986**, *875*, 525–534.

Kennedy, I.; Coleman, R. A.; Humphrey, P. P. A.; Levy, G. P.; and Lumley, P. Studies on the characterization of prostanoid receptors: a proposed classification. *Prostaglandins*, **1982**, *24*, 667–689.

Le Breton, G. C.; Venton, D. L.; Enke, S. E.; and Halushka, P. V. 13-Azaprostanoic acid: a specific antagonist of the human blood platelet thromboxane/endoperoxide receptor. *Proc. Natl. Acad. Sci. U.S.A.*, **1979**, *76*, 4097–4101.

Lin, A. H.; Morton, D. R.; and Gorman, R. R. Acetyl glyceryl ether phosphorylcholine stimulates leukotriene B_4 synthesis in human polymorphonuclear leukocytes. *J. Clin. Invest.*, **1982**, *70*, 1058–1065.

McIntyre, T. M.; Zimmerman, G. A.; and Prescott, S. M. Leukotrienes C_4 and D_4 stimulate human endothelial cells to synthesize platelet-activating factor and bind neutrophils. *Proc. Natl. Acad. Sci. U.S.A.*, **1986**, *83*, 2204–2208.

McManus, L. M.; Pinckard, R. N.; Fitzpatrick, F. A.; O'Rourke, R. A.; Crawford, M. H.; and Hanahan, D. J. Acetyl glyceryl ether phosphorylcholine: intravascular alterations following intravenous infusion into the baboon. *Lab. Invest.*, **1981**, *45*, 303–307.

Moncada, S.; Gryglewski, R.; Bunting, S.; and Vane, J. R. An enzyme isolated from arteries transforms prostaglandin endoperoxides to an unstable substance that inhibits platelet aggregation. *Nature*, **1976**, *263*, 663–665.

Murphy, R. C.; Hammarstrom, S.; and Samuelsson, B. Leukotriene C: a slow-reacting substance from murine mastocytoma cells. *Proc. Natl. Acad. Sci. U.S.A.*, **1979**, *76*, 4275–4279.

Ogletree, M. L.; Harris, D. N.; Greenberg, R.; Haslanger, M. F.; and Nakane, M. Pharmacological actions of SQ 29,548, a novel selective thromboxane antagonist. *J. Pharmacol. Exp. Ther.*, **1985**, *234*, 435–441.

Okajima, F., and Ui, M. ADP-ribosylation of the specific membrane protein by islet-activating protein, pertussis toxin, associated with inhibition of a chemotactic peptide-induced arachidonate release in neutrophils. *J. Biol. Chem.*, **1984**, *259*, 13863–13871.

Okazaki, T.; Sagawa, N.; Okita, J. R.; Bleasdale, J. E.; MacDonald, P. C.; and Johnston, J. M. Diacylglycerol metabolism and arachidonic acid release in human fetal membranes and decidua vera. *J. Biol. Chem.*, **1981**, *256*, 7316–7321.

Owen, N. E., and Le Breton, G. C. Ca^{2+} mobilization in blood platelets as visualized by chlortetracycline fluorescence. *Am. J. Physiol.*, **1981**, *241*, 613–619.

Pardy, B. J.; Lewis, J. D.; and Eastcott, H. H. G. Preliminary experience with prostaglandins E_1 and I_2 in peripheral vascular disease. *Surgery*, **1980**, *88*, 826–832.

Patrignani, P.; Filabozzi, P.; Catella, F.; Pugliese, F.; and Patrono, C. Differential effects of dazoxiben, a selective thromboxane-synthase inhibitor, on platelet and renal prostaglandin-endoperoxide metabolism. *J. Pharmacol. Exp. Ther.*, **1984**, *228*, 472–477.

Piomelli, D.; Volterra, A.; Dale, N.; Siegelbaum, S. A.; Kandel, E. R.; Schwartz, J. H.; and Belardetti, F. Lipoxygenase metabolites of arachidonic acid as second messengers for presynaptic inhibition of *Aplysia* sensory cells. *Nature*, **1987**, *238*, 38–43.

Polonsky, J.; Tence, M.; Varenne, P.; Das, B. C.; Lunel, J.; and Benveniste, J. Release of 1-O-alkylglyceryl 3-phosphorylcholine, O-deacetyl platelet-activating factor, from leukocytes: chemical ionization mass spectrometry of phospholipids. *Proc. Natl. Acad. Sci. U.S.A.*, **1980**, *77*, 7019–7023.

Roberts, L. J.; Sweetman, B. J.; and Oates, J. A. Metabolism of thromboxane B_2 in man. Identification of twenty urinary metabolites. *J. Biol. Chem.*, **1981**, *256*, 8384–8393.

Rosenkranz, B.; Fischer, C.; Weimer, K. E.; and Frolich, J. C. Metabolism of prostacyclin and 6-keto-prostaglandin $F_{1\alpha}$ in man. *J. Biol. Chem.*, **1980**, *255*, 10194–10198.

Schwertschlag, U. S., and Whorton, A. R. Platelet-activating factor-induced homologous and heterologous desensitization in cultured vascular smooth muscle cells. *J. Biol. Chem.*, **1988**, *263*, 13791–13796.

Spinks, N. R., and O'Neill, C. Embryo-derived platelet-activating factor is essential for establishment of pregnancy in the mouse. *Lancet*, **1987**, *1*, 106–107.

Stimler, N. P., and O'Flaherty, J. T. Spasmogenic properties of platelet-activating factor: evidence for a direct mechanism in the contractile response of pulmonary tissues. *Am. J. Pathol.*, **1983**, *113*, 75–84.

Stokes, J. B. Effect of prostaglandin E_2 on chloride transport across the rabbit thick ascending limb of Henle: selective inhibition of the medullary portion. *J. Clin. Invest.*, **1979**, *64*, 495–502.

Sybertz, E. J.; Watkins, R. W.; Baum, T.; Pula, K.; and Rivelli, M. Cardiac, coronary and peripheral vascular effects of acetyl glyceryl ether phosphorylcholine in the anesthetized dog. *J. Pharmacol. Exp. Ther.*, **1985**, *232*, 156–162.

Vane, J. R. Inhibition of prostaglandin synthesis as a mechanism of action for aspirin-like drugs. *Nature* [*New Biol.*], **1971**, *231*, 232–235.

Zusman, R. M.; Rubin, R. H.; Cato, A. E.; Cocchetto, D. M.; Crow, J. W.; and Tolkoff-Rubin, N. Hemodialysis using prostacyclin instead of heparin as the sole antithrombotic agent. *N. Engl. J. Med.*, **1981**, *304*, 934–939.

Monographs and Reviews

Behrman, H. R. Prostaglandins in hypothalamo-pituitary and ovarian function. *Annu. Rev. Physiol.*, **1979**, *41*, 685–700.

Behrman, H. R., and Anderson, G. G. Prostaglandins in reproduction. *Arch. Intern. Med.*, **1974**, *133*, 77–84.

Bennett, A. The role of prostaglandins in gastrointestinal tone and motility. In, *Prostaglandins and Thromboxanes*. (Berti, F.; Samuelsson, B.; and Velo, G. P.; eds.) Plenum Press, New York, **1977**, pp. 275–285.

Bergström, S.; Carlson, L. A.; and Weeks, J. R. The prostaglandins: a family of biologically active lipids. *Pharmacol. Rev.*, **1968**, *20*, 1–48.

Bergström, S., and Samuelsson, B. The prostaglandins. *Endeavour*, **1968**, *27*, 109–113.

Braquet, R.; Touqui, L.; Shen, T. Y.; and Vargartif, B. B. Perspectives in platelet-activating factor research. *Pharmacol. Rev.*, **1987**, *39*, 97–145.

Coceani, F.; Olley, P. M.; and Lock, J. E. Prostaglandins, ductus arteriosus, pulmonary circulation: current concepts and clinical potential. *Eur. J. Clin. Pharmacol.*, **1980**, *18*, 75–81.

Coleman, R. A.; Humphrey, P. P. A.; Kennedy, I.; and Lumley, P. Prostanoid receptors—the development of a working classification. *Trends Pharmacol. Sci.*, **1984**, *5*, 303–306.

Davies, P.; Bailey, P. J.; and Goldenberg, M. M. The role of arachidonic acid oxygenation products in pain and inflammation. *Annu. Rev. Immunol.*, **1984**, *2*, 335–357.

Drazen, J. M., and Austen, K. F. Leukotrienes and airway responses. *Am. Rev. Respir. Dis.*, **1987**, *136*, 985–998.

Dunn, M. J., and Hood, V. L. Prostaglandins in the kidney. *Am. J. Physiol.*, **1977**, *233*, F169–F184.

Euler, U. S. von. Some aspects of the actions of prostaglandins. The First Heymans Memorial Lecture. *Arch. Int. Pharmacodyn. Ther.*, **1973**, *202*, Suppl., 295–307.

Ferris, T. F. Prostaglandins, potassium and Bartter's syndrome. *J. Lab. Clin. Med.*, **1978**, *92*, 663–668.

Feuerstein, G. Leukotrienes and the cardiovascular system. *Prostaglandins*, **1984**, *27*, 781–802.

Fitzpatrick, F. A., and Murphy, R. C. Cytochrome P-450 metabolism of arachidonic acid: formation and biological actions of "epoxygenase"-derived eicosanoids. *Pharmacol. Rev.*, **1989**, *40*, 229–241.

Giles, H., and Leff, P. The biology and pharmacology of PGD_2. *Prostaglandins*, **1988**, *35*, 277–300.

Goldberg, V. J., and Ramwell, P. W. Role of prostaglandins in reproduction. *Physiol. Rev.*, **1975**, *55*, 325–351.

Goldyne, M. E., and Stobo, J. D. Immunoregulatory role of prostaglandins and related lipids. *CRC Crit. Rev. Immunol.*, **1981**, *1*, 189–223.

Goodwin, J. S., and Webb, D. R. Regulation of the immune response by prostaglandins. *Clin. Immunol. Immunopathol.*, **1980**, *15*, 106–122.

Halushka, P. V.; Mais, D. E.; Mayeux, P. R.; and Morinelli, T. A. Thromboxane, prostaglandin and leukotriene receptors. *Annu. Rev. Pharmacol. Toxicol.*, **1989**, *29*, 213–219.

Hanahan, D. J. Platelet activating factor: a biologically active phosphoglyceride. *Annu. Rev. Biochem.*, **1986**, *55*, 483–509.

Hirsh, P. D.; Campbell, W. B.; Willerson, J. T.; and Hillis, L. D. Prostaglandins and ischemic heart disease. *Am. J. Med.*, **1981**, *71*, 1009–1026.

Honn, K. V.; Busse, W. D.; and Sloane, B. F. Prostacyclin and thromboxanes: implications for their role in tumor cell metastasis. *Biochem. Pharmacol.*, **1983**, *32*, 1–11.

Horton, E. W., and Poyser, N. L. Uterine luteolytic hormone. A physiological role for prostaglandin $F_{2\alpha}$. *Physiol. Rev.*, **1976**, *56*, 595–651.

Johnston, J. M.; Bleasdale, J. E.; and Hoffman, D. R. Functions of PAF in reproduction and development: involvement of PAF in fetal lung maturation and parturition. In, *Platelet-Activating Factor and Related Lipid Mediators*. (Snyder, F., ed.) Plenum Publishing Corporation, New York, **1987**, pp. 375–401.

Keeton, T. K., and Campbell, W. B. The pharmacologic alteration of renin release. *Pharmacol. Rev.*, **1980**, *32*, 81–227.

Lee, J. B. Cardiovascular renal effects of prostaglandins. *Arch. Intern. Med.*, **1974**, *133*, 56–76.

Mathe, A. A.; Hedqvist, P.; Strandberg, K.; and Leslie, C. A. Aspects of prostaglandin function in the lung. *N. Engl. J. Med.*, **1977**, *296*, 850–855, 910–914.

Moncada, S.; Ferreira, S. H.; and Vane, J. R. Pain and inflammatory mediators. In, *Inflammation. Handbook of Experimental Pharmacology*, Vol. 50. (Ferreira, S. H., and Vane, J. R., eds.) Springer-Verlag, Berlin, **1978**, pp. 588–616.

Moncada, S., and Vane, J. R. Pharmacology and endogenous roles of prostaglandin endoperoxides, thromboxane A_2 and prostacyclin. *Pharmacol. Rev.*, **1979**, *30*, 293–331.

Monk, J. P., and Clissold, S. P. Misoprostol: a preliminary review of its pharmacodynamic and pharmacokinetic properties, and therapeutic efficacy in the treatment of peptic ulcer disease. *Drugs*, **1987**, *33*, 1–30.

Nakano, J. General pharmacology of prostaglandins. In, *The Prostaglandins: Pharmacological and Therapeutic Advances*. (Cuthbert, M. F., ed.) J. B. Lippincott Co., Philadelphia, **1973**, pp. 23–124.

Needleman, P.; Turk, J.; Jakschik, B. A.; Morrison, A. R.; and Lefkowith, J. B. Arachidonic acid metabolism. *Annu. Rev. Biochem.*, **1986**, *55*, 69–102.

Piper, P. J. Formation and actions of leukotrienes. *Physiol. Rev.*, **1984**, *64*, 744–761.

Samuelsson, B. Biosynthesis of prostaglandins. *Fed. Proc.*, **1972**, *31*, 1442–1460.

———. Leukotrienes: mediators of immediate hypersensitivity reactions and inflammation. *Science*, **1983**, *220*, 568–575.

Samuelsson, B.; Dahlen, S-E.; Lindgren, J. A.; Rouzer, C. A.; and Serhan, C. N. Leukotrienes and lipoxins: structures, biosynthesis, and biological effects. *Science*, **1987**, *237*, 1085–1272.

Samuelsson, B.; Granstrom, E.; Green, K.; Hamberg, M.; and Hammarstrom, S. Prostaglandins. *Annu. Rev. Biochem.*, **1975**, *44*, 669–694.

Saunders, R. N., and Handley, D. A. Platelet-activating factor antagonists. *Annu. Rev. Pharmacol. Toxicol.*, **1987**, *27*, 237–255.

Schlondorff, D., and Neuwirth, R. Platelet-activating factor and the kidney. *Am. J. Physiol.*, **1986**, *251*, F1–F11.

Snyder, D. W., and Fleisch, J. H. Leukotriene receptor antagonists as potential therapeutic agents. *Annu. Rev. Pharmacol. Toxicol.*, **1989**, *29*, 123–143.

Snyder, F. Biochemistry of platelet-activating factor: a unique class of biologically active phospholipids. *Proc. Soc. Exp. Biol. Med.*, **1989**, *190*, 125–135.

Sontag, S. J. Prostaglandins in peptic ulcer disease: an overview of current status and future directions. *Drugs*, **1986**, *32*, 445–457.

Spannhake, E. W.; Hyman, A. L.; and Kadowitz, P. J. Bronchoactive metabolites of arachidonic acid and their role in airway function. *Prostaglandins*, **1981**, *22*, 1013–1026.

Wilson, D. E., and Kaymakcalan, H. Prostaglandins: gastrointestinal effects and peptic ulcer disease. *Med. Clin. North Am.*, **1981**, *65*, 773–787.

Wolfe, L. S. Eicosanoids: prostaglandins, thromboxanes, leukotrienes, and other derivatives of carbon-20 unsaturated fatty acids. *J. Neurochem.*, **1982**, *38*, 1–14.

Yamamoto, S. Mammalian lipoxygenases: molecular and catalytic properties. *Prostaglandins Leukotrienes Essent. Fatty Acids*, **1989**, *35*, 219–229.

CHAPTER

25 DRUGS USED IN THE TREATMENT OF ASTHMA

The Methylxanthines, Cromolyn Sodium, and Other Agents

Theodore W. Rall

Reversible airway obstruction—asthma—is the most common of the breathing disorders; perhaps 10% of all children may be afflicted sufficiently to require treatment (Weinberger, 1987). In adults, chronic obstructive pulmonary disease (COPD), may include a component of ongoing or antecedent bronchospasm, and therapeutic strategies for the treatment of COPD often resemble those for asthma.

Methylxanthines, initially in the form of strong coffee, have been employed to treat asthma for over a century (Salter, 1859), and theophylline is often incorporated into current therapeutic regimens. This chapter will present the pharmacological properties and therapeutic uses of the methylxanthines and of *cromolyn sodium*, another useful agent in the treatment of asthma. The *β_2-adrenergic agonists* are the mainstay of such regimens, and discussion of their role in treatment will be included here; their pharmacological properties are presented in Chapter 10. The use of *adrenocortical steroids* and *muscarinic cholinergic antagonists* (primarily *ipratropium bromide*) will also be discussed; their general properties are presented in Chapters 60 and 8, respectively.

More recently, the methylxanthines have been found to be of value in the treatment of apnea in preterm infants, an extension of an earlier, but largely extinct use as a general stimulant of respiration. The use of *doxapram*, another centrally acting stimulant, will also be mentioned as it has recently been revived for the treatment of methylxanthine-resistant apnea.

Pathophysiology of Asthma. It is generally agreed that asthma constitutes an inflammatory state in which the airways are narrowed chronically by edema and episodically by a variety of spasmogens that are released from resident and infiltrating cells. Asthmatic individuals display hyperresponsiveness to both chemical and physical stimuli, which not only precipitate immediate bronchoconstriction but may also cause an episode several hours later. This "late response" apparently involves recruitment of circulating cells that are called forth by chemotactic factors, and they may serve to maintain or intensify the inflammatory state. Although individual attacks are often provoked by nonallergic stimuli, it is believed that environmental allergens are responsible for maintenance of the underlying hyperresponsiveness in the vast majority of patients.

The sequence of events involved in immediate and late responses, as well as the role of various tissue elements and chemical mediators, have not been clearly defined. Investigation of these issues is complicated by important species-dependent factors in animal models of asthma and by tissue-specific properties of inflammatory cells. The classical example is that of histamine, which plays a prominent role in the bronchoconstriction induced by antigen in sensitized guinea pigs. By contrast, histamine receptor antagonists have only a modest effect in human asthma. Moreover, while mast cells in the lung undoubtedly play an important pathophysiological role and are among the targets for therapeutic agents, it has been difficult to document the mechanism of action of certain drugs, especially cromolyn sodium, because the properties of mast cells *in vitro* appear to depend upon the tissue and species from which they are obtained. The list of known or suspected mediators that are either released or generated as a result of contact with allergens has mounted steadily, and currently includes histamine, prostanoids (*e.g.*, thromboxane), leukotrienes (*e.g.*, leukotriene D_4 and leukotriene B_4), and, most recently, platelet-activating factor (PAF). The release of acetylcholine and neuropeptides such as substance P from parasympathetic nerves has also been implicated. The list of potential cellular participants has grown too, and now includes mast cells, autonomic and sensory nerves, and infiltrating inflammatory elements (eosinophils, basophils, neutrophils, platelets, and monocytes). Moreover, inflammation-induced damage to the bronchial epithelium is thought to be important; in addition to a reduction in its functions as a barrier, metabolic derangements occur, including loss of a postulated epithelium-derived relaxing factor with properties similar to those of the endothelium-derived relaxing factor in blood vessels (*see* Chapter 5).

As appreciation of the complexity of the pathophysiology of asthma has increased, certainty as to the mechanism of action and cellular targets of therapeutic agents has decreased. For example, there is controversy as to whether theophylline produces bronchodilatation primarily by causing direct relaxation of bronchial smooth muscle or whether indirect effects, such as reduction of the release and action of spasmogens, are more important. Moreover, the ability of the methylxanthines to block adenosine receptors has focused attention on the potential role of adenosine in asthma. On the positive side, these uncertainties have unleashed a host of investigations into the nature and role of various chemical mediators, and they have encouraged the development of specific inhibitors of the formation and action of thromboxane and the leukotrienes, as well as antagonists for PAF and adenosine. These and related issues have been reviewed in several recent symposia (Symposium, 1986a, 1987a, 1988a, 1988b, 1988c).

THE METHYLXANTHINES

Source and History. Theophylline, caffeine, and theobromine are three closely related alkaloids that occur in plants widely distributed geographically. It is believed that paleolithic man discovered the principal caffeine-containing plants throughout the world and made beverages from them. At least half the population of the world consumes tea (containing caffeine and small amounts of theophylline and theobromine), prepared from the leaves of *Thea sinensis,* a bush native to southern China and now extensively cultivated in other countries. Cocoa and chocolate, from the seeds of *Theobroma cacao,* contain theobromine and some caffeine. Coffee, the most important source of caffeine in the American diet, is extracted from the fruit of *Coffea arabica* and related species. Cola-flavored drinks usually contain considerable amounts of caffeine, in part because of their content of extracts of the nuts of *Cola acuminata* (the guru nuts chewed by the natives of the Sudan) and in part because of the addition of caffeine as such in their production (*see* Graham, 1978).

The basis for the popularity of all the caffeine-containing beverages has been the ancient belief that these beverages had stimulant and antisoporific actions that elevated mood, decreased fatigue, and increased capacity for work. For example, legend credits the discovery of coffee to a prior of an Arabian convent. Shepherds reported that goats that had eaten the berries of the coffee plant gamboled and frisked about all through the night instead of sleeping. The prior, mindful of the long nights of prayer that he had to endure, instructed the shepherds to pick the berries so that he might make a beverage from them.

Classical pharmacological studies, principally of caffeine, during the first half of this century confirmed these experiences and revealed that methylxanthines possess other important pharmacological properties as well. These properties were exploited for a number of years in a variety of therapeutic applications; many of these have now been replaced by more effective agents. However, in recent years there has been a resurgence of interest in the therapeutic use of the natural methylxanthines and synthetic derivatives thereof, principally as a result of increased knowledge of their cellular basis of action and their pharmacokinetic properties.

Chemistry. Caffeine, theophylline, and theobromine are methylated xanthines. Xanthine itself is dioxypurine and is structurally related to uric acid. Caffeine is 1,3,7-trimethylxanthine; theophylline, 1,3-dimethylxanthine; and theobromine, 3,7-dimethylxanthine. The structural formulas of xanthine and the three naturally occurring xanthine derivatives are as follows:

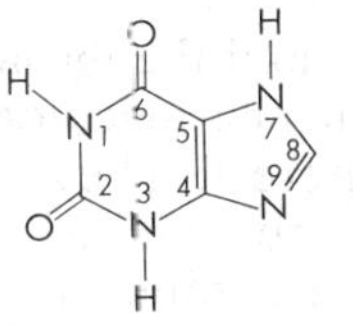

Xanthine

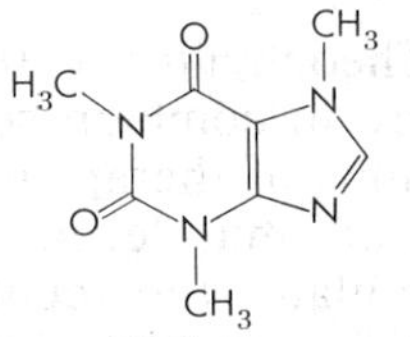

Caffeine

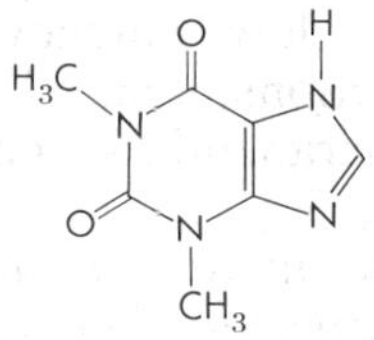

Theophylline

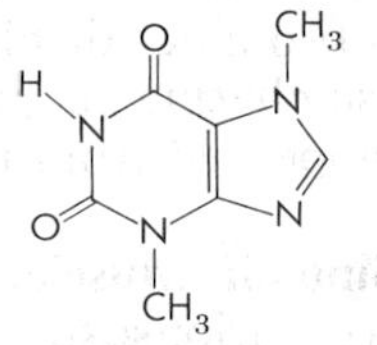

Theobromine

The solubility of the methylxanthines is low and is much enhanced by the formation of complexes (usually 1:1) with a wide variety of compounds. The most notable of such complexes is that between theophylline and ethylenediamine (to form *aminophylline*). The formation of complex double salts (*e.g.*, caffeine and sodium benzoate) or true salts (*e.g.*, *choline theophyllinate [oxtriphylline]*) also enhances aqueous solubility. These salts or complexes dissociate to yield the parent methylxanthines when dissolved in aqueous solution and should not be confused with covalently modified derivatives such as *dyphylline* (1,3-dimethyl-7-(2,3-dihydroxypropyl)-xanthine).

A large number of derivatives of the methylxanthines have been prepared and examined for their ability to inhibit cyclic nucleotide phosphodiesterases and to antagonize receptor-mediated actions of adenosine (the two best-characterized cellular actions of the methylxanthines). In general, both activities are reduced in derivatives that lack substituents at position 1 or contain substituents at position 7, as compared with the corresponding dialkylxanthine (*see* Persson, in Symposium, 1985). For example, the order of potency for the naturally occurring methylxanthines is theophylline > caffeine > theobromine. Congeners of theophylline with larger nonpolar substituents at positions 1 and 3 usually display enhancement of both activities (Choi *et al.*, 1988). Addition of aromatic, cyclohexyl, or cyclopentyl groups at position 8 usually increases affinity for adenosine receptors markedly but reduces inhibition of cyclic nucleotide phosphodiesterases (Martinson *et al.*, 1987). Although neither caffeine nor theophylline discriminates between the subtypes of adenosine receptors (*see* below), certain derivatives of 1,3-dipropyl-8-phenylxanthine display marked selectivity for A_1 receptors, while some analogs of caffeine display appreciable selectivity for A_2 receptors (*see* Daly *et al.*, and Bruns *et al.*, in Symposium, 1987b). In addition, certain nonxanthine compounds, notably the triazoloquinazolines, are potent antagonists at adenosine receptors (*see* Williams and Jarvis, in Symposium, 1988d).

PHARMACOLOGICAL PROPERTIES

Theophylline, caffeine, and theobromine share in common several pharmacological actions of therapeutic interest. They relax smooth muscle, notably bronchial muscle, stimulate the central nervous system (CNS), stimulate cardiac muscle, and act on the kidney to produce diuresis. Since theobromine displays a low potency in these pharmacological actions, it has all but disappeared from the therapeutic scene.

Smooth Muscle. The methylxanthines relax various smooth muscles. The most important action in this respect is their ability to relax the smooth muscles of the bronchi, especially if the bronchi have been constricted either experimentally by a spasmogen or clinically in asthma. Theophylline is the most effective of the xanthines and produces a definite increase in vital capacity. It is, therefore, of value in the treatment of bronchial asthma.

The mechanisms underlying theophylline-induced bronchodilatation *in vitro*, much less those operating *in vivo*, are not at all clear. In general, the concentrations of methylxanthines that produce bronchodilatation *in vivo* are considerably lower than those required to relax various preparations of airway muscle studied *in vitro*. For example, concentrations of theophylline greater than 50 μM are required to relax bronchiolar segments from human lung previously contracted by carbachol (Finney *et al.*, 1985); this corresponds to the concentration of free drug attained at the top of the therapeutic range (20 μg/ml). One prominent explanation of the effect *in vitro* is based on the ability of methylxanthines to inhibit cyclic nucleotide phosphodiesterases and on the association between increased accumulation of adenosine 3′,5′-monophosphate (cyclic AMP) or of guanosine 3′,5′-monophosphate (cyclic GMP) and the relaxation of smooth muscle. Supporting evidence for this idea includes the correlation between the potency of various xanthine derivatives to induce relaxation and to inhibit the hydrolysis of cyclic AMP, as well as their ability to potentiate relaxation induced by β_2-adrenergic agonists, which is thought to be mediated by cyclic AMP (*see* Symposium, 1985). However, such correlations are not evident *in vivo*, and numerous investigations in man have failed to indicate that combinations of theophylline and β_2-adrenergic agonists produce synergistic therapeutic responses (*see* Handslip *et al.*, 1981). Although there is evidence that release of catecholamines participates in theophylline-induced bronchodilatation in short-term animal studies, it is unlikely that such a mechanism operates during the long-term treatment of human asthma (*see* Persson, in Symposium, 1985). The potential role of blockade of adenosine receptors in theophylline-induced bronchodilatation *in vivo* will be discussed in a later section.

Central Nervous System. Theophylline and caffeine are potent stimulants of the CNS; theobromine is virtually inactive in this respect. Traditionally, caffeine has been considered the most potent of the methylxanthines; however, theophylline produces more profound and potentially more dangerous CNS stimulation than does caffeine.

Persons ingesting caffeine or caffeine-containing beverages usually experience less drowsiness, less fatigue, and a more rapid and clearer flow of thought. Comparable salutary effects of low doses of theophylline have not been investigated. As the dose of caffeine or theophylline is increased, signs of progressive CNS stimulation are produced, including nervousness or anxiety, restlessness, insomnia, tremors, and hyperesthesia. At still higher doses, focal and generalized convulsions are produced; theophylline is clearly more potent than caffeine in this regard. Such seizures, occasionally refractory to anticonvulsant agents, have sometimes occurred in patients when the blood concentration of theophylline was only about 50% above the top of the accepted therapeutic range.

Methylxanthines also stimulate the medullary respiratory centers. This action is particularly prominent in pathophysiological states such as Cheyne–Stokes respiration, apnea of preterm infants, and when respiration is depressed by drugs such as opioids. The methylxanthines appear to increase the sensitivity of medullary centers to the stimulatory actions of CO_2, and respiratory minute volume is increased at any given value of alveolar P_{CO_2}. Both methylxanthines may produce nausea and vomiting; this probably involves CNS actions, at least in part. Theophylline-induced emesis is common when concentrations in plasma exceed 15 μg/ml, which includes the upper part of the recommended range of therapeutic concentrations.

The ingestion of 85 to 250 mg of caffeine, the amount contained in 1 to 3 cups of coffee, produces an increased capacity for sustained intellectual effort and decreases reaction time; however, tasks involving delicate muscular coordination and accurate timing or arithmetic skills may be adversely affected (*see* Curatolo and Robertson, 1983; Arnaud, 1987). Similarly, the ability of asthmatic children to perform repetitive tasks requiring concentration declines during periods of medication with theophylline (Furukawa *et al.*, 1988). Patients with panic disorders may be particularly sensitive to the effects of the methylxanthines. In one study, the majority of such individuals given doses of caffeine that resulted in plasma concentrations of about 8 μg/ml experienced anxiety, fear, and other symptoms characteristic of their panic attacks (Charney *et al.*, 1985). Since the long-term ingestion of caffeine (and presumably theophylline) can produce tolerance and evidence of physical dependence (*see* Griffiths and Woodson, 1988), history of exposure to methylxanthines will influence the effects of a given dose. Hence, enhanced alertness, energy, and ability to concentrate could reflect alleviation of withdrawal symptoms in some instances.

Stimulatory effects of low doses of methylxanthines are evident in individuals whose CNS function has been depressed by certain agents. For example, aminophylline (2 mg/kg) can rapidly reverse the narcosis induced by as much as 100 mg of morphine given intravenously to produce anesthesia (Stirt, 1983), and there is evidence that methylxanthines can specifically antagonize a number of the actions of opioids, including analgesia. For example, intrathecal injection of either caffeine or theophylline in amounts that do not produce hyperalgesia elevates the analgetic ED_{50} for morphine in mice (DeLander and Hopkins, 1986). This apparently reflects the participation of adenosine in the actions of opioids (*see* Fredholm *et al.*, in Symposium, 1987b). By contrast, there is little evidence to support the popular belief that caffeine can improve mental function during intoxication with ethanol (*see* Curatolo and Robertson, 1983).

Cardiovascular System. Caffeine and theophylline, especially the latter, have prominent actions on the circulatory system. The capacity of theophylline to produce modest decreases in peripheral vascular resistance, sometimes powerful cardiac stimulation, increased perfusion of most organs, and diuresis was exploited in the past for the emergency treatment of congestive heart failure. However, the use of more effective vasodilators, specific inotropic agents, and diuretics is now preferred.

The actions of the methylxanthines on the circulatory system are complex and sometimes antagonistic, and the resultant effects largely depend upon the conditions prevailing at the time of their administration, the dose used, and the history of exposure to methylxanthines. In addition to effects on the vagal and vasomotor centers in the brain stem, there is an array of more or less direct actions on vascular and cardiac tissues in combination with indirect peripheral actions that are mediated by catecholamines and possibly by the renin–angiotensin system. Therefore, the observation of a single function, for example, the blood pressure, is deceiving because the drugs may act on a variety of circulatory factors in such a way that the blood pressure may remain essentially unchanged.

Heart. The administration of 250 to 350 mg of caffeine to methylxanthine-naive individuals may produce small decreases in heart rate and modest increases in both systolic and diastolic blood pressure, but such doses are usually without effect on these parameters in those who consume caffeine regularly. There is controversy as to whether circulating catecholamines or plasma renin activity is increased significantly in caffeine-naive subjects; however, it is generally agreed that little change occurs in chronic users. These issues have been reviewed by Myers (1988a).

Infusions of theophylline that lead to plasma concentrations of 10 to 20 μg/ml produce modest increases in heart rate and changes in cardiac parameters consistent with an increase in contractile force and decreased preload (Ogilvie *et al.*, 1977). In normal individuals, any rise in cardiac output may be brief and may be followed by a fall below the initial level. In patients with heart failure, however, the venous pressure is initially rather high;

consequently, the cardiac stimulation and decreased venous pressure produced by theophylline leads to a marked increase in cardiac output that persists for 30 minutes or more. Similar plasma concentrations of theophylline in methylxanthine-naive subjects also produce substantial increases in circulating epinephrine (Vestal *et al.*, 1983). Parallel observations on hemodynamic responses or on changes in plasma catecholamine concentrations have not been reported for patients receiving long-term therapeutic doses of theophylline. In view of the effects of caffeine (*see* above), it is unlikely that any hemodynamic effects of theophylline in such patients are caused by catecholamines (*see* Ogilvie, in Symposium, 1985).

At higher concentrations, both caffeine and theophylline produce definite tachycardia; sensitive individuals may experience other arrhythmias, such as premature ventricular contractions. Arrhythmias may also be encountered in persons who use caffeine-containing beverages to excess. However, it appears that the risk of inducing cardiac arrhythmias in normal subjects is quite low and that patients with ischemic heart disease or pre-existing ventricular ectopy can usually tolerate moderate amounts of caffeine without provoking an appreciable increase in the frequency of arrhythmias (Myers, 1988b).

Blood Vessels. The effects of therapeutic doses of caffeine or theophylline on peripheral blood flow or vascular resistance in man are variable. The conflicting patterns of hemodynamic effects that have been observed suggest that the methylxanthines have little direct action on the major resistance vessels. It is more likely that any change in peripheral vascular resistance results from primary actions on the brain stem (caffeine) or the heart (theophylline), with modification or reinforcement by autonomic reflexes and changes in the concentrations of circulating catecholamines (*see* above).

Most effects of methylxanthines on regional blood flow or vascular resistance in human subjects are also variable. However, it has been repeatedly demonstrated that methylxanthines cause a marked increase in cerebrovascular resistance with an accompanying decrease in cerebral blood flow and oxygen tension (Wechsler *et al.*, 1950; Moyer *et al.*, 1952). This apparently reflects the ability of the xanthines to block adenosine-induced vasodilatation and the prominent role of adenosine in cerebrovascular autoregulation (Morii *et al.*, 1987; Bowton *et al.*, 1988).

The xanthines can increase coronary blood flow in man. They also increase the work of the heart. The outstanding question is whether the blood supply to the myocardium increases to a greater extent than does the oxygen demand. Theophylline enhances the production of endogenous adenosine in the heart as well as antagonizes the capacity of this autacoid to dilate coronary arteries (*see* Berne *et al.*, in Symposium, 1987b).

In vitro, it has generally been found that methylxanthines (about 0.2 mM or above) cause relaxation of vascular smooth muscle in the presence of various stimulators of contraction (*e.g.*, norepinephrine, angiotensin, K^+). While relaxation probably results from a reduction of the cytosolic concentration of Ca^{2+}, it is not clear to what extent the methylxanthines alter Ca^{2+} binding and transport directly or influence these functions indirectly by means of changes in cyclic nucleotide metabolism. However, at concentrations close to those in the therapeutic range, the effects of methylxanthines are variable and depend upon the locale of the vascular bed and the experimental conditions employed.

Skeletal Muscle. It has long been known that caffeine increases the capacity for muscular work in man. For example, the ingestion of caffeine (6 mg/kg) improves the racing performance of cross-country skiers, particularly at high altitudes (Berglund and Hemmingsson, 1982). However, it is not clear to what extent this effect involves direct actions of caffeine on neuromuscular transmission or whether usual doses of theophylline produce similar effects. At therapeutic concentrations, both caffeine and theophylline can improve diaphragmatic contractility and reduce diaphragmatic fatigue in normal human subjects and in patients with COPD (*see* Aubier, in Symposium, 1985). Although these effects are not accompanied by increased discharge of the phrenic nerve, it is not clear whether improved neuromuscular transmission or increased muscular contractility is of greater relative importance. In any event, these effects may contribute to the improvement of ventilatory function and to the decreased sensation of dyspnea produced by theophylline in many patients with COPD. At much higher concentrations (0.5 to 1 mM), caffeine and, to a lesser extent, theophylline clearly augment the contractility of striated muscle. The possible role of the mobilization of intracellular Ca^{2+} in such circumstances is discussed in *earlier editions* of this textbook.

Diuretic Actions. Methylxanthines, especially theophylline, increase the production of urine, and the patterns of enhanced excretion of water and electrolytes are very similar to those produced by the thiazides (Maren, 1961). The underlying mechanisms remain a subject of continuing controversy, particularly with regard to the relative contribution of hemodynamic and intra-renal actions (*see* Spielman *et al.*, in Symposium, 1987b). In most animal studies, theophylline has been found to increase the glomerular filtration rate (GFR) and renal blood flow, especially in the medulla (*see* Osswald, in Symposium, 1985). However, the infusion of aminophylline (3.5 mg/kg) into normal human subjects appears to inhibit solute reabsorption in both the proximal nephron and the diluting segment without changing appreciably either GFR or total renal blood flow; no additional effects are produced by theophylline in the presence of furosemide (Brater *et al.*, 1983). By contrast, the administration of aminophylline (400 mg) does produce additional excretion of Na^+, Cl^-, and K^+ in patients with congestive heart failure during treatment with high-ceiling diuretics (Sigurd and Olesen, 1978).

Secretion. Methylxanthines augment release of the secretory products of a number of endocrine and exocrine tissues. One exception to this general statement is the ability of methylxanthines to inhibit secretion by mast cells and possibly other sources of mediators of inflammation. A number of the therapeutic and toxic properties of methylxanthines probably involve actions on secretory processes. However, the quantitative contribution of such actions has not often been delineated.

Gastric Secretion. Man is relatively sensitive to the effects of methylxanthines on gastric secretion, and moderate oral or parenteral doses of caffeine cause secretion of both acid and pepsin (*see* Debas *et al.*, 1971). Although never directly compared, theophylline would appear to be at least as potent as caffeine in this regard. Both direct actions on parietal cells and indirect effects resulting from actions within the CNS may be involved (Glavin *et al.*, 1987). The observation that adenosine is a potent inhibitor of histamine-induced acid secretion by the parietal cell suggests one mechanism for this effect (Gerber *et al.*, 1985). While atropine may partially inhibit caffeine-induced secretion of acid, the prior administration of cimetidine, an H_2-receptor antagonist, completely prevents the response to even relatively high doses of caffeine (Cano *et al.*, 1976).

It has been long known (and perhaps forgotten) that beverages made from roasted grain containing no caffeine stimulate acid secretion in man as much as does coffee (Öhnell and Berg, 1931). Decaffeinated coffee is only slightly less potent than the natural product in enhancing the secretion of gastrin and acid, and both are about twice as effective as is an equivalent amount of caffeine (Cohen and Booth, 1975; Acquaviva *et al.*, 1986).

Secretion of Other Substances. Therapeutic concentrations of caffeine or theophylline can increase the concentration of circulating catecholamines and can augment renin activity in the plasma of human subjects who have previously abstained from ingestion of methylxanthines. Since propranolol does not prevent the increase in plasma renin activity, catecholamines are probably not involved in this response (Zehner *et al.*, 1975). Administration of theophylline results in increases in the plasma concentrations of gastrin (Feurle *et al.*, 1976) and parathyroid hormone (Bowser *et al.*, 1975). Epinephrine can also produce the latter effect, and thus it is not clear whether this represents a direct action of the methylxanthine. While high concentrations of theophylline cause significant increases in circulating insulin, therapeutic concentrations are usually without effect (Vestal *et al.*, 1983). Theophylline can also potentiate the insulinemic responses to infusions of secretin and cholecystokinin–pancreozymin (Serrano-Ríos *et al.*, 1974).

The release of histamine from rat peritoneal mast cells produced by a variety of stimuli can usually be inhibited only by relatively high concentrations of theophylline (0.2 to 2.5 mM). However, much lower concentrations (below 0.1 mM) are effective in antagonizing the augmentation of histamine release produced by adenosine acting in concert with antigen or a calcium ionophore (Marquardt *et al.*, 1978; Sydbom and Fredholm, 1982). By contrast, theophylline can promote the release of myeloperoxidase from stimulated human neutrophils by antagonizing adenosine-induced inhibition of such secretion (*see* Iannone *et al.*, in Symposium, 1987b). Despite these apparently contradictory observations, theophylline is thought to exert some anti-inflammatory actions as part of its therapeutic effects in human asthma (*see* Symposium, 1985), and caffeine displays definite anti-inflammatory activity in various model systems, including the ability to enhance the effects of aspirin-like drugs (Vinegar *et al.*, 1976).

Metabolic Responses. The administration of caffeine (4 to 8 mg/kg) to normal or obese human subjects elevates the concentration of free fatty acids in plasma and increases the basal metabolic rate (Acheson *et al.*, 1980); therapeutic concentrations of theophylline produce similar effects on free fatty acids (Vestal *et al.*, 1983). It is not clear if the release and action of catecholamines are essential for the production of these metabolic responses.

Cellular Basis for the Action of Methylxanthines. Three basic cellular actions of the methylxanthines have received major attention in studies to explain their diverse effects. Listed in order of their increasing sensitivity to methylxanthines, they are (1) those associated with translocations of intracellular calcium, (2) those mediated by increasing accumulation of cyclic nucleotides, and (3) those mediated by blockade of receptors for adenosine. Of particular importance is the question of what types of actions contribute appreciably to the effects of methylxanthines in the therapeutic dose range. The concentration of free theophylline in plasma rarely exceeds 50 μM during therapy. At the present state of knowledge, this fact alone appears to eliminate the participation of the first category of actions to the therapeutic effects of theophylline. Except for the possible contribution of effects on the accumulation of cyclic GMP, the second category can also be excluded. This would leave the anti-adenosine action as the leading candidate (*see* Rall, 1982). There are also several other types of actions that have received relatively little attention to date but that might prove to be very important in certain effects of the methylxanthines. These include their potentiation of inhibitors of prostaglandin synthesis (*see* Vinegar *et al.*, 1976), and the possibility that methylxanthines reduce the uptake and/or metabolism of catecholamines in nonneural tissues (*see* Kalsner, 1971; Kalsner *et al.*, 1975). Further investigation will be required to establish the contribution of these actions to both the immediate effect of the methylxanthines and those involving the release of catecholamines.

At high concentrations (0.5 to 1 mM) caffeine interferes with the uptake and storage of Ca^{2+} by the sarcoplasmic reticulum in striated muscle. This action can account for observations that such concentrations of caffeine increase the strength and duration of contractions in both skeletal and cardiac muscle. Theophylline is less potent in this regard. Although similar actions could contribute to the ability of methylxanthines to enhance secretion in certain tissues, it is unlikely that they have an important role at therapeutic concentrations of theophylline. This topic is discussed in greater detail in *earlier editions* of this textbook.

The ability of methylxanthines to inhibit cyclic nucleotide phosphodiesterases is often cited to explain their therapeutic effects; however, there is little compelling evidence for such a view. Concentrations of theophylline of about 0.5 mM are required to increase the concentration of cyclic nucleotides in cells, usually only when their synthesis has been increased by hormonal or other stimuli. Potentiation of the responses to stimuli that are known or suspected to be mediated by cyclic AMP requires concentrations of at least 0.1 to 0.2 mM. However, at therapeutic concentrations (20 to 50 μM), theophylline produces minimal inhibition of the hydrolysis of cyclic AMP and potentiates hormone-induced responses known to be mediated by this nucleotide only in systems in which adenosine inhibits such effects (*see* Rall, 1982; Symposium, 1985). Although enhancement of the accumulation of cyclic GMP might participate in theophylline-induced relaxation of smooth muscle (*see* Murad, in Symposium, 1985), the release of inflammatory mediators from mast cells is promoted by stimuli that increase the concentration of cyclic GMP. In addition, with our present knowledge, effects on the metabolism of cyclic GMP would not provide explanations for the actions of the methylxanthines in the heart and the CNS.

By contrast, methylxanthines act as competitive antagonists at adenosine receptors at concentrations well within the therapeutic range. The effects of exogenous adenosine are very often opposite to those of the methylxanthines (*see* below), and the removal of ambient adenosine in some experimental settings (by the addition of adenosine deaminase) will reproduce and obtund the actions of the methylxanthines.

Adenosine as an Autacoid. Over the past 20 years, evidence has accumulated that adenosine functions as an autacoid and that its actions are mediated by specific receptors that reside in the plasma membranes of virtually every cell (*see* Symposium, 1983; 1987b). Increased concentrations of adenosine appear in the extracellular space when the delivery of oxygen is reduced or when the utilization of adenosine triphosphate (ATP) in tissues is raised (*e.g.*, during muscular contraction, secretion, or active transport of ions). The pattern of its actions suggests that one major function of adenosine is to assist in maintaining a balance between the availability and the utilization of oxygen in a given region. For example, adenosine dilates cerebral and coronary blood vessels and slows the rate of discharge of neurons in the CNS and of cardiac pacemaker cells. Acting in concert with norepinephrine or angiotensin, adenosine constricts the afferent arterioles in the kidney, thereby decreasing the GFR and the absorptive work of renal tubules, and it can reduce the deleterious effects of renal hypoxemia. There is considerable controversy, however, as to the relative importance of adenosine in the production of functional or post-occlusion hyperemia in skeletal muscle.

Adenosine also appears to participate in numerous local regulatory mechanisms, especially at synapses in the CNS and at neuroeffector junctions in the periphery. For example, adenosine inhibits the release of neurotransmitters from presynaptic structures; in this case, the nucleoside may be derived in part from ATP that is released together with the primary neurotransmitter from synaptic vesicles. In addition, adenosine sometimes modifies the response to neurotransmitters postjunctionally. For example, the presence of adenosine will cause α-adrenergic agonists to produce an increased accumulation of cyclic AMP in brain tissue. The interaction of adenosine and angiotensin at afferent arterioles in renal glomeruli is another example. Individually, adenosine produces modest vasodilatation, while angiotensin has little effect; when the two agents are combined, marked vasoconstriction results.

Adenosine Receptors. Receptors for adenosine are sometimes referred to as P_1 purinergic receptors; they should not be confused with those that mediate the actions of ATP in such tissues as the gastrointestinal tract and vascular endothelium (P_2 receptors; *see* Chapter 5). P_2 receptors have a far greater sensitivity to ATP than to adenosine and are not subject to blockade by methylxanthines. Two general categories of receptors for adenosine (P_1 receptors) have been identified, initially on the basis of whether they activate (A_2) or inhibit (A_1) adenylyl cyclase and subsequently by their relative sensitivity to various analogs of adenosine. Evidence for two subtypes of A_2 receptors in brain tissue has also appeared, based on relatively high (A_{2a}) and low (A_{2b}) affinity for adenosine and certain of its analogs. Although theophylline is more potent than caffeine, they display nearly identical affinity for all types of adenosine receptors. However, antagonists with relative specificity for either A_1 or A_2 receptors have been developed (*see* page

620). Compounds such as *enprofylline* (3-propylxanthine) that lack substituents at position 1 have relatively poor affinity for most adenosine receptors but may be more effective antagonists than theophylline at A_{2b} receptors.

It is now recognized that adenosine receptors are linked through appropriate guanine nucleotide-binding regulatory proteins (G proteins) not only to adenylyl cyclase but also to other effector systems. For example, the conductance of one type of K^+ channel in cardiac atrial tissue is increased by the stimulation of A_1 receptors. This action is probably mediated by a direct action of a G protein on the channel and does not involve the reduced synthesis of cyclic AMP. Long-term administration of methylxanthines produces an increase in both the number of A_1 binding sites and the concentration of pertussis toxin–sensitive G proteins in brain (Ramkumar *et al.*, 1988). Such effects may be involved in the generation of tolerance to some of the neural actions of the methylxanthines (*see* above).

Adenosine in Asthma. Although actions of adenosine that might be relevant to the pathophysiology of human asthma have not yet been firmly established, the therapeutic efficacy of the methylxanthines suggests that a significant role exists. Moreover, the inhalation of adenosine can precipitate marked bronchoconstriction in asthmatic patients but is without appreciable effect in normal subjects (*see* Holgate *et al.*, in Symposium, 1985; 1987b). The fact that enprofylline appears to be about fivefold more potent than theophylline as a bronchodilator in asthmatic patients but is relatively ineffective as an adenosine antagonist in most tissues has been cited as evidence against an important role both for adenosine in asthma and for antagonism of adenosine in the therapeutic effects of theophylline in asthma (*see* Symposium, 1985). However, the ability of enprofylline to block A_{2b} receptors in the CNS leaves open the possibility that similar receptors function in asthma and that both theophylline and enprofylline have similar mechanisms of action.

Toxicology. Fatal poisoning in man by the ingestion of caffeine is rare (*see* Curatolo and Robertson, 1983). Although the short-term lethal dose of caffeine in adults appears to be about 5 to 10 g, untoward reactions may be observed following the ingestion of 1 g (15 mg/kg; plasma concentrations above 30 μg/ml). These are mainly referable to the central nervous and circulatory systems. Insomnia, restlessness, and excitement are the early symptoms, which may progress to mild delirium; emesis and convulsions are also prominent. The muscles become tense and tremulous. Tachycardia and extrasystoles are frequent, and respiration is quickened.

Fatal intoxications with theophylline have been much more frequent than with caffeine. Rapid intravenous administration of therapeutic doses of *aminophylline* (500 mg) sometimes results in sudden death that is probably due to cardiac arrhythmias, and the drug should be injected slowly over 20 to 40 minutes to avoid severe toxic symptoms. These include headache, palpitation, dizziness, nausea, hypotension, and precordial pain. Additional symptoms of toxicity are tachycardia, severe restlessness, agitation, and emesis; these effects are associated with plasma concentrations of more than 20 μg/ml. Focal and generalized seizures can also occur, sometimes without prior signs of toxicity.

Most toxicity is the result of repeated administration of theophylline by either oral or parenteral routes. Although convulsions and death have occurred at plasma concentrations as low as 25 μg/ml, seizures are relatively rare at concentrations below 40 μg/ml (*see* Goldberg *et al.*, in Symposium, 1986a). Patients with long-term theophylline intoxication appear to be much more prone to seizures than those who experience short-term overdoses. Such a dependence upon the history of exposure to theophylline may contribute to the difficulty in establishing a relationship between the severity of toxic symptoms and the concentration of the drug in plasma (Aitken and Martin, 1987; Bertino and Walker, 1987), and greater caution is advised in treating intoxicated patients who have been ingesting theophylline regularly (*see* Paloucek and Rodvold, 1988). Treatment may include prophylactic administration of diazepam, perhaps together with phenytoin or phenobarbital; phenytoin may also be a useful alternative to lidocaine in the treatment of serious ventricular arrhythmias. Once seizures appear, they may be refractory to anticonvulsant therapy, and it may be necessary to resort to general anesthesia and other measures used in the treatment of status epilepticus (*see* Goldberg *et al.*, in Symposium, 1986a).

The widespread use of sustained-release preparations of theophylline has renewed emphasis on measures to prevent continued absorption, particularly the use of oral activated charcoal and of sorbitol as a cathartic (Goldberg *et al.*, 1987); multiple doses of oral charcoal will also accelerate clearance of theophylline. However, when plasma concentrations exceed 100 μg/ml, invasive measures are usually required, especially hemoperfusion through charcoal cartridges (*see* Paloucek and Rodvold, 1988).

Mutagenic and Carcinogenic Effects. Caffeine induces chromosomal abnormalities both in plant cells and in mammalian cells in culture and has potent mutagenic effects on microorganisms either alone or in combination with other mutagens (*see* Timson, 1977). These effects seem to be associated with inhibition of DNA-repair processes. They are observed only with concentrations of caffeine that are much in excess of those that follow the ingestion of beverages and medications. Furthermore, available evidence suggests that caffeine is neither mutagenic by itself nor in combination with known mutagens in mammals. At very high doses, caffeine appears to have some teratogenic activity in mammals, and in 1980 the United States Food and Drug Administration issued a warning advising pregnant women to limit their exposure to caffeine largely on this basis. However, subsequent studies have found no association between maternal consumption of caffeine and the incidence of malformations or of low birth weight in offspring (*see* Curatolo and Robertson, 1983; Leviton, 1988). At moderate doses, caffeine would seem to pose little risk of developmental toxicity for the human fetus.

Epidemiological studies have suggested that consumption of coffee is associated with cancer of the pancreas, kidney, and lower urinary tract. However, these studies contain serious flaws, such as the selection of inappropriate groups of patients for controls and the failure to exclude smoking as a confounding variable (*see* Curatolo and Robertson, 1983). There is no clear evidence that the consumption of caffeine is causally related to the development of cancer in these organs. Similarly, the postulated association of benign fibrocystic disease or of cancer of the breast with the consumption of methylxanthines has not been validated by recent investigations (*see* Phelps and Phelps, 1988).

Relation to Myocardial Infarction. There has been controversy over a possible deleterious effect of caffeine in the etiology of acute myocardial infarction. However, the results of a number of studies indicate that coffee drinking is associated with little, if any, increased incidence of coronary heart disease (*see* Curatolo and Robertson, 1983).

Behavioral Toxicity. As noted above, moderate doses of caffeine can provoke intense feelings of anxiety, fear, or panic in some individuals. Even subjects with a history of light-to-moderate use of caffeine experience tension, anxiety, and dysphoria after ingesting 400 mg or more of the drug (*see* Griffiths and Woodson, in Symposium, 1988d). In infants who have received treatment for apnea of prematurity, theophylline may produce persistent changes in sleep–wake patterns (Thoman *et al.*, 1985), but long-term effects on behavior or on cognitive development have yet to be identified (*see* Aranda *et al.*, in Symposium, 1986a). There has been mounting concern that the treatment of asthmatic children with theophylline might produce depression, hyperactivity, or other behavioral toxicity. Even though it is difficult to factor out specific effects of theophylline from those caused by the illness or by other features of the treatment regimen, many investigators believe that most children will benefit from the use of alternative means of controlling their symptoms.

Absorption, Fate, and Excretion. The methylxanthines are readily absorbed after oral, rectal, or parenteral administration. Theophylline administered in liquids or uncoated tablets is rapidly and completely absorbed. Absorption is also complete from some, but not all, sustained-release formulations (*see* Hendeles and Weinberger, 1982). In the absence of food, solutions or uncoated tablets of theophylline produce maximal concentrations in plasma within 2 hours; caffeine is more rapidly absorbed, and maximal plasma concentrations are achieved within 1 hour. Numerous sustained-release preparations of theophylline have appeared in recent years, designed for dosing intervals of 8, 12, or 24 hours. These preparations cause marked interpatient variability with regard to the rate and extent of absorption and especially the effect of food and time of administration on these parameters (*see* Symposium, 1986a). Thus, it has become necessary to calibrate a given preparation in a given patient and to avoid substitution of one apparently similar product for another.

Food ordinarily slows the rate of absorption of theophylline but does not limit its extent. With sustained-release preparations, food may decrease the bioavailability of theophylline in some products but may increase it in others. Recumbency or sleep may also reduce the rate or extent of absorption to an important degree. These factors make it difficult to maintain relatively constant concentrations of theophylline in plasma throughout the day. Fortunately, it has also become apparent that the concentrations required to alleviate asthmatic symptoms do not remain constant, and the emphasis has shifted toward designing dosing regimens that ensure peak concentrations in the early morning hours when symptoms frequently worsen (*see* Symposium, 1988e).

Theophylline is completely and very rapidly absorbed when small volumes of solutions of aminophylline are administered as an enema (Bolme *et al.*, 1979). Use of rectal suppositories results in slow and erratic absorption. Intramuscular injection of soluble preparations of theophylline (*e.g.*, aminophylline) produces long-lasting local pain; this route of administration should not be used. Parenteral or rectal administration does not obviate production of gastrointestinal distress, nausea, and vomiting. These symptoms are clearly a function of the concentration of theophylline in plasma.

Methylxanthines are distributed into all body compartments; they cross the placenta and pass into breast milk. The apparent volume of distribution is similar for both caffeine and theophylline and usually is between 0.4 and 0.6 liter/kg. These values are considerably higher in premature infants. Theophylline is bound to plasma proteins to a greater extent than is caffeine, and the fraction bound declines as the concentration of methylxanthine increases. At therapeutic concentrations, the protein binding of theophylline averages about 60%, but it is decreased to about 40% in newborn infants and in adults with hepatic cirrhosis (*see* Hendeles and Weinberger, 1982).

Methylxanthines are eliminated primarily by metabolism in the liver. Less than 20% and 5% of administered theophylline and caffeine, respectively, are recovered in the urine unchanged. Caffeine has a half-life in plasma of 3 to 7 hours; this increases by about twofold in women during the later stages of pregnancy or with long-term use of oral contraceptive steroids. In premature infants, the rate of elimination of both methylxanthines is quite slow. The average half-life for caffeine is more than 50 hours, while the mean values for theophylline obtained in various studies range between 20 and 36 hours. However, the latter values include the extensive conversion of theophylline to caffeine in these infants (*see* Symposium, 1981; Roberts, 1984).

There is marked interindividual variation in the rate of elimination of theophylline due to both genetic and environmental factors, and fourfold differences are not uncommon (*see* Lesko, in Symposium, 1986a). The half-life averages about 3.5 hours in young children, while values of 8 or 9 hours are more typical of adults. In most patients the drug obeys first-order elimination kinetics within the therapeutic range. However, at higher concentrations zero-order kinetics becomes evident because of saturation of metabolic enzymes. This prolongs the decline of theophylline concentrations to nontoxic levels.

The disposition of methylxanthines is also influenced by the presence of other agents or of disease (*see* Jonkman, in Symposium, 1986a). For example, the clearance of theophylline is increased nearly twofold during the administration of phenytoin or barbiturates; cigarette smoking, rifampin, or oral contraceptives produce smaller but appreciable increases in theophylline clearance. By contrast, the administration of cimetidine or of certain macrolide antibiotics (*e.g.*, erythromycin) reduces the clearance of theophylline. Although there have been reports to the contrary, neither glucocorticoids nor immunization with purified subvirion influenza vaccine appear to have a significant effect, although acute viral infections and interferon can reduce theophylline clearance. The half-life of theophylline can be quite prolonged in patients with hepatic cirrhosis, congestive heart failure, or acute pulmonary congestion, and values of more than 60 hours have been observed.

Caffeine is metabolized by demethylation and by oxidation at position 8 (*see* Arnaud, 1987). The major pathway in man proceeds through the formation of paraxanthine (1,7-dimethylxanthine), leading to the principal urinary metabolites, 1-methylxanthine, 1-methyluric acid, and an acetylated uracil derivative. Minor pathways involve the formation and metabolism of theophylline and theobromine. The major pathway of theophylline metabolism involves 8-hydroxylation, resulting in the formation and excretion of 1,3-dimethyluric acid (*see* Rowe *et al.*, 1988). Considerable demethylation also occurs, leading to the formation of 1-methylxanthine, which is nearly completely converted to 1-methyluric acid by xanthine oxidase before excretion, and of 3-methylxanthine, which accumulates in plasma and is excreted as such. There is no evidence that the methylxanthines are converted to uric acid or that their ingestion exacerbates gout.

Although scarcely detectable in adults, the conversion of theophylline to caffeine is an important metabolic pathway in preterm infants (*see* Symposium, 1981; Roberts, 1984). Caffeine accumulates in plasma to a concentration that approximates 25% of that of theophylline and is one of the urinary products. About 50% of the theophylline administered to such infants appears in the urine unchanged; the excretion of 1,3-dimethyluric acid, 1-methyluric acid, and caffeine accounts for nearly all of the remainder.

Other Xanthine Derivatives. *Dyphylline.* Dyphylline is 7-(2,3-dihydroxypropyl) theophylline. This substance is a chemical entity distinct from theophylline, and no evidence exists for its transformation to theophylline to any degree after administration. Since its introduction in 1946, dyphylline has been extensively used in the treatment of asthma; however, investigation of its efficacy and pharmacokinetic properties has been limited. Oral formulations are incompletely absorbed, and the half-time of elimination is about 2 hours. Since dyphylline appears to be only about one fifth as potent as theophylline as a bronchodilator in patients, both the doses recommended and the claims made for this compound seem unjustified. Nevertheless, dyphylline is marketed extensively.

Enprofylline. Enprofylline (3-propylxanthine) has been extensively investigated in Europe for use in the treatment of asthma (*see* Symposium, 1985). This agent is more potent than theophylline as a bronchodilator in asthmatic patients without producing obvious effects on the CNS, renal function, or cerebrovascular resistance. Although it has little effect on gastric secretion, the incidence of gastrointestinal disturbances is at least as great as with theophylline, and tachycardia is more prominent.

As noted above, enprofylline is a poor antagonist of adenosine at most, but not all types, of adenosine receptors. At least 90% of enprofylline is excreted unchanged in the urine; tubular secretion plays a substantial role. The half-time of elimination is less than 2 hours and is prolonged in individuals with reduced creatinine clearance. The drug is well absorbed after oral administration, and sustained-release preparations are under development. Enprofylline is not yet available in the United States.

Pentoxifylline. Pentoxifylline (1-[5-oxohexyl]-3,7-dimethylxanthine) is considered to be a derivative of theobromine. Although it is without demonstrated utility as a bronchodilator, pentoxifylline has been approved in the United States for use in the treatment of patients with intermittent claudication due to chronic occlusive arterial disease. Clinical studies indicate that pentoxifylline can lengthen the distance walked before the onset of claudication; there is also more direct evidence for increased blood flow in the ischemic limbs of such patients, as well as decreased paresthesias, cramps, and pain at rest (*see* Ward and Clissold, 1987). Not all investigators are enthusiastic, however, and some report that only 20 to 30% of patients may experience significant long-lasting benefit (*see* Green and McNamara, 1988). Pentoxifylline may also be of value in the treatment of cerebrovascular disease, and it is under investigation for possible use in other vascular disorders, including those associated with diabetes; its use in the treatment of the crises of sickle cell disease is also being evaluated. Except for the latter, in which clinical responses may occur within 24 to 48 hours, 2 to 6 weeks usually must elapse before beneficial effects are evident. Pentoxifylline does not appear to act as a vasodilator, and therapeutic doses are not associated with significant changes in heart rate, cardiac output, or peripheral vascular resistance. Clinical responses to long-term oral administration of pentoxifylline are thought to result primarily from improved flexibility of erythrocytes and reduced blood viscosity; a decreased concentration of fibrinogen may contribute to the latter. Reduced function of platelets and of granulocytes may also be involved (Hammerschmidt *et al.,* 1988; Rossignol *et al.,* 1988). However, the mechanism of action of pentoxifylline is poorly defined at present. Pentoxifylline (TRENTAL) is available in 400-mg controlled-release tablets. The usual dose is 400 mg, taken three times a day with meals.

Preparations and Routes of Administration. The xanthines are weakly basic alkaloids. For oral administration either the free base or one of the salts may be used; for parenteral administration, however, it is necessary to employ one of the salts.

Caffeine is available in tablets (100, 150, and 200 mg) and in capsules containing pellets for timed release (200 and 250 mg). *Citrated caffeine* is a mixture of equal parts of caffeine and citric acid and is available in 65-mg tablets. *Caffeine and sodium benzoate injection* is a mixture of approximately equal parts of caffeine and sodium benzoate. It is available for intramuscular injection. *Theophylline* is available in a wide range of dosages (50 to 500 mg) in tablets, tablets designed for timed release, capsules, and capsules containing coated pellets for timed release. The bioavailability of some timed-release preparations has not been documented. Oral liquid and intravenous preparations are also available. Theophylline is a component in dozens of proprietary mixtures that usually also contain a nonselective adrenergic agonist, most frequently ephedrine. Self-medication with one of these mixtures can increase the hazards of therapy with theophylline because patients are frequently unaware of their content of theophylline.

Aminophylline (theophylline ethylenediamine) is the most widely used of the soluble theophylline salts. It contains 86% anhydrous theophylline. It is available as solutions for intravenous injection or infusion, tablets, sustained-release tablets, solutions for both oral and rectal administration, and rectal suppositories.

Oxtriphylline, also called *choline theophyllinate,* contains 64% anhydrous theophylline. Tablets (partially enteric coated) and an elixir are available, as are sustained-release tablets and a syrup.

Theophylline sodium glycinate contains 46% anhydrous theophylline and is freely soluble in water. It is available as an elixir for oral administration.

THERAPEUTIC USES

The diverse pharmacological actions of the methylxanthines have found many therapeutic applications. Those currently in vogue include the extensive use of theophylline. Preparations are employed extensively to relax bronchial smooth muscle in the treatment of asthma and to relieve dyspnea in the treatment of chronic obstructive pulmonary disease. These applications will be discussed at the end of this chapter. At higher doses, caffeine can also be used in the treatment of asthma (Becker *et al.,* 1984). However, its use offers no advantages over that of theophylline. The stimulatory effects of the methylxanthines on the CNS are widely exploited to increase alertness and to allay drowsiness or fatigue, largely through the ingestion of caffeine-containing beverages or tablets. More importantly, both caffeine and theophylline have found application in the treatment of the prolonged apnea that is sometimes observed in preterm infants. Caffeine, in probably subtherapeutic amounts, is incorporated into a number of "over-the-counter" preparations used for analgesia or to produce diuresis.

Apnea of Preterm Infants. Episodes of prolonged apnea, lasting more than 15 seconds and accompanied by bradycardia, are not infrequent occurrences in premature infants. They pose the threat of recurrent hypoxemia and neurological damage. While they are often associated with serious systemic illness, no specific cause is found in many instances. Beginning with the work of Kuzemko and Paala (1973), methylxanthines have undergone numerous clinical trials for the treatment of apnea of undetermined origin. The oral or intravenous administration of methylxanthines can eliminate episodes of apnea that last more than 20 seconds and markedly reduces the number of episodes of shorter duration (*see* Symposium, 1981; Roberts, 1984; Aranda *et al.*, in Symposium, 1986a). Satisfactory responses may occur with concentrations of theophylline in plasma of 4 to 8 μg/ml, but concentrations of nearly 13 μg/ml are more frequently required (Muttitt *et al.*, 1988). Still higher concentrations may produce a more regular pattern of respiration without further reduction in the frequency of episodes of apnea and bradycardia, and these are usually associated with a definite tachycardia. Therapeutic concentrations are achieved with loading doses of about 5 mg/kg of theophylline (calculated as the free base) and can be maintained with 2 mg/kg given every 12 or 24 hours (*see* Roberts, 1984). Although caffeine was initially used less frequently than theophylline, some physicians now prefer it because the dosing regimens are simpler and more predictable. Moreover, the administration of theophylline leads to the accumulation of substantial amounts of caffeine in these infants (*see* above). Somewhat higher concentrations are required, but the available data indicate that caffeine is equally effective. The recommended loading dose is 10 mg/kg of caffeine, with maintenance doses of 2.5 mg/kg per day (*see* Roberts, 1984).

Although effects on growth or development of infants following treatment with methylxanthines have not been detected, the evidence is far from definitive. Therapy is thus continued for as brief a period as possible, usually only a few weeks.

Approximately 20% of infants may not respond adequately at theophylline concentrations of 15 μg/ml or when caffeine concentrations reach 25 μg/ml. Recent studies indicate that about 80% of such "refractory" infants can be treated successfully by the cautious addition of *doxapram hydrochloride* (DOPRAM) to the regimen (Barrington *et al.*, 1987).

Doxapram is not a xanthine but is one of a very few stimulants of central respiratory centers that remain in clinical use. At sufficient dosage, doxapram can stimulate the cerebrospinal axis at all levels; it appears to act by enhancing excitation rather than by blocking central inhibition. Although doxapram can produce tonic–clonic convulsions similar to those that follow the administration of pentylenetetrazol, it does not share this agent's ability to promote seizure activity in certain animal models of epilepsy (Albertson *et al.*, 1983). Doxapram administered intravenously in low doses selectively stimulates respiration in normal human subjects; both tidal volume and respiratory frequency are increased (Calverley *et al.*, 1983; Burki, 1984). However, doxapram increases ventilation without significant change in respiratory frequency in human neonates (Barrington *et al.*, 1986).

Therapeutic responses of infants to doxapram have been associated with concentrations in plasma ranging from 1.5 to 6 μg/ml (Barrington *et al.*, 1987; Beaudry *et al.*, 1988). In such infants, the apparent volume of distribution is quite large (about 4 liters/kg), and the half-life of the drug ranges from below 6 to above 10 hours. It must be remembered that the preceding observations in neonates have all been made in the presence of "therapeutic" concentrations of theophylline (10 to 20 μg/ml). Treatment is initiated by the continuous infusion of 0.5 mg/kg of doxapram hydrochloride per hour, and the dose is increased at intervals of 24 to 48 hours until it reaches 2.0 mg/kg per hour or until the frequency of apneic episodes is reduced to two per 6 hours or less. Although higher doses will stimulate ventilation, no further reduction in the frequency of apnea is apparent, and a marked increase in blood pressure is produced. Preparations of doxapram that contain benzyl alcohol should not be used in the treatment of immature infants. It is not known if the methylxanthine can be withdrawn during treatment with doxapram. Thus far, the use of combinations of a methylxanthine and doxapram within these limits has not been associated with the production of seizures or other signs of acute toxicity. The use of doxapram in the treatment of neonatal apnea is investigational in the United States.

Miscellaneous Uses. Caffeine is rarely used in treating cases of poisoning by central depressants. The drug is given by intramuscular injection, usually as caffeine and sodium benzoate (0.5 g). Other approaches are preferred (*see* Chapter 17). Low doses of the methylxanthines specifically antagonize opioid-induced respiratory depression (*see* above). However, it is not clear whether they are less apt to reduce analgesia or to precipitate withdrawal symptoms in physically dependent individuals than is naloxone, and their use in the treatment of opioid overdosage has not been extensive (*see* Bowdle, 1988).

Caffeine in combination with an analgesic, such as aspirin, is widely employed in the treatment of ordinary types of headache. There are few data to substantiate its efficacy for this purpose. Caffeine is also used in combination with an ergot alkaloid in the treatment of migraine (*see* Chapter 39).

XANTHINE BEVERAGES

It has been estimated that the per-capita intake of caffeine in the United States averages between 170 and 200 mg per day (*see* Graham, 1978; Clementz and Dailey, 1988). About 90% of this amount results from drinking coffee. Depending upon the alkaloid content of the coffee bean and the method of brewing, 1 cup of coffee contains about 85 mg of caffeine, while 1 cup of tea contains about 50 mg of caffeine and 1 mg of theophylline; cocoa contains about 250 mg of theobromine and 5 mg of caffeine per cup. A 12-oz (360-ml) bottle of a cola drink contains 40 to 50 mg of caffeine, half of which is added by the manufacturer as the alkaloid.

The xanthine beverages present a medical problem in that a large fraction of the population consumes enough caffeine to produce substantial effects on a number of organ systems. Hence, the physician should give due consideration to the possible contribution of caffeine to the presenting signs and symptoms of patients, as well as to its potential interaction with any contemplated therapeutic regimen. Patients with active peptic ulcer should restrict their intake of both caffeine-containing and roasted-grain beverages.

Overindulgence in xanthine beverages may lead to a condition that might be considered one of long-term poisoning. There are also rare persons who are so sensitive to caffeine that even a single cup of coffee will cause a response bordering on the toxic. Central nervous system stimulation results in restlessness and disturbed sleep; myocardial stimulation is reflected in premature systoles and tachycardia. The essential oils of coffee may cause some gastrointestinal irritation, and diarrhea is a common symptom. The high tannin content of tea, on the other hand, is apt to cause constipation.

There is no doubt that a certain degree of tolerance and of psychic dependence (*i.e.*, habituation) develops to the xanthine beverages (*see* Clementz and Dailey, 1988; Griffiths and Woodson, in Symposium, 1988d). This is probably true even in individuals who do not partake to excess. However, the morning cup of coffee is so much a part of American and European dietary habit that one seldom looks upon its consumption as a drug habit. The feeling of well-being and the increased performance it affords, although possibly obtained at the expense of decreased efficiency later in the day, are experiences that few individuals care to give up.

CROMOLYN SODIUM

History and Chemistry. Cromolyn was synthesized in 1965 as part of an attempt to improve upon the bronchodilator activity of *khellin*, a chromone (benzopyrone) derived from the plant *Ammi visnaga*, which had been used by the ancient Egyptians for its spasmolytic properties (*see* Shapiro and König, 1985). Although devoid of the bronchodilating capability of the parent compound, cromolyn was found to inhibit antigen-induced bronchospasm as well as the release of histamine and other autacoids from sensitized mast cells. Cromolyn has been used in the United States for the treatment of asthma since 1973. The initial clinical results were disappointing, in retrospect largely due to a misplaced emphasis on the hope that it would reduce or eliminate the need for systemic glucocorticoids in the treatment of patients with relatively severe asthma. However, its therapeutic role has been reevaluated in recent years, and cromolyn has emerged as a first-line agent in the treatment of mild-to-moderate asthma. *Nedocromil,* a compound with similar chemical and biological properties, is currently under investigation in asthmatic patients (*see* Gonzalez and Brogden, 1987). Cromolyn sodium (disodium cromoglycate) and nedocromil sodium have the following structures:

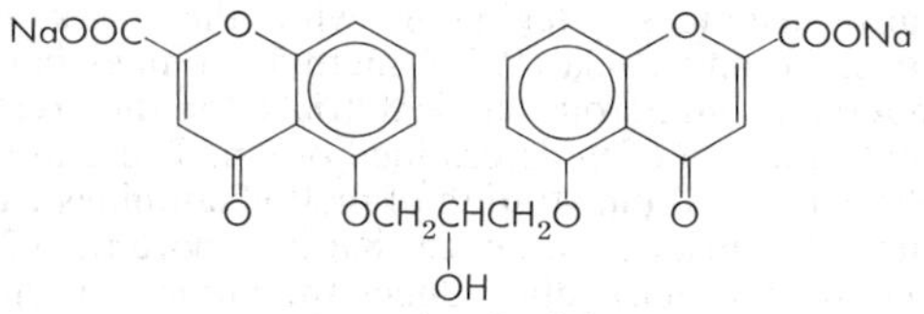

Cromolyn Sodium

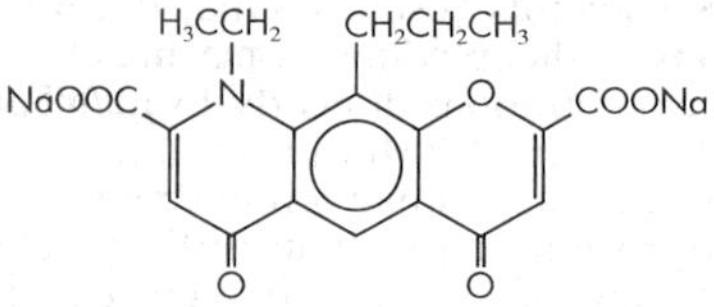

Nedocromil Sodium

Pharmacological Effects. One important action of cromolyn is believed to involve inhibition of the degranulation of pulmonary mast cells by a variety of stimuli, including the interaction between cell-bound IgE and specific antigen (*see* Shapiro and König, 1985; Murphy and Kelly, 1987). The release of histamine and other granular contents, as well as the production of leukotrienes, can be shown to be markedly reduced *in vitro* by cromolyn. However, its efficacy and potency are highly dependent upon the source of the mast cells. For example, human mast cells obtained by bronchoalveolar lavage are quite sensitive to cromolyn, while those prepared from lung fragments require high concentrations of the drug for inhibition of IgE-dependent release of mediators. More recently, attention has been focused on the ability of cromolyn to reverse various functional changes in leukocytes, such as increased expression of membrane-bound receptors, in white cells obtained from the blood of asthmatic subjects undergoing allergen challenge. Moreover, low concentrations (100 nM) of cromolyn can suppress completely the activating effects of chemoattractant peptides on human neutrophils, eosinophils, or monocytes (Kay *et al.*, 1987). Nedocromil produces similar effects at somewhat lower concentrations (Moqbel *et al.*, 1988).

Cromolyn does not relax bronchial or

other smooth muscles *in vitro*. Nor does it reduce responses of these muscles to a variety of pharmacological spasmogens, either *in vitro* or in the short term *in vivo*. However, during long-term administration of cromolyn, the bronchoconstriction induced by challenge of asthmatic patients with allergen, histamine, or exercise is usually reduced to an important degree. Hence, the therapeutic effects of cromolyn are primarily prophylactic and appear to result from the inhibition of release of inflammatory mediators from several cell types, as well as from a reduction in the burden of infiltrating cells.

The mechanism of action of cromolyn remains relatively poorly defined. Most attention has been focused on the ability of cromolyn to reduce the accumulation of intracellular Ca^{2+} induced by antigen in sensitized mast cells (White *et al.*, 1984). One biochemical correlate of the reduction of histamine release from mast cells by cromolyn is the enhanced phosphorylation of a 78,000-dalton protein (Wells and Mann, 1983). Unfortunately, these observations have been made using rather high concentrations of cromolyn (50 to 200 μM), and their relationship to therapeutic responses has yet to be established.

Absorption, Fate, and Excretion. Only about 1% of an oral dose of cromolyn is absorbed, and its therapeutic effects are achieved by local administration. For asthma, cromolyn is given by inhalation, using either solutions (delivered by aerosol spray or power-operated nebulizer) or powdered drug (mixed with lactose and delivered by a special turbo inhaler). The distribution of drug in the lung and the extent of systemic absorption depend upon the inhalation technique. For example, the delivery of powdered drug is markedly influenced by the rate of inspiratory flow and the duration of breath-holding after inhalation, and adequate dosing may require prior inhalation of a β-adrenergic bronchodilator. The bronchodilator also minimizes bronchospasm induced by the powder or spray. Under the best of circumstances, 10% or less of an inhaled dose of cromolyn is absorbed systemically. Once absorbed, the drug is excreted unchanged in the urine and the bile in about equal proportions. Peak concentrations in plasma occur within 15 minutes of inhalation, and excretion begins after some delay, such that the biological half-life ranges from 45 to 100 minutes. The terminal half-time of elimination following intravenous administration is about 20 minutes. The pharmacokinetic properties of cromolyn have been reviewed by Shapiro and König (1985) and by Murphy and Kelly (1987).

Toxicity. Cromolyn is generally well tolerated by patients. Adverse reactions are infrequent and minor; these include bronchospasm, cough or wheezing, laryngeal edema, joint swelling and pain, angioedema, headache, rash, and nausea. Such reactions have been reported at a frequency of less than 1 in 10,000 patients (*see* Murphy and Kelly, 1987). Very rare instances of anaphylaxis have also been documented.

Preparations and Dosage. *Cromolyn sodium for inhalation* (INTAL) is available in capsules that contain 20 mg of the finely powdered drug mixed with lactose. The contents of the capsule are inhaled by means of a special turbo inhaler, usually four times daily at regular intervals. Alternatively, a solution containing 10 mg/ml of the drug can be used with a power-operated nebulizer; this solution is compatible for mixing with a number of β-adrenergic bronchodilators and acetylcysteine. The dose for asthma is two sprays (800 μg per spray), four times daily. For prevention of exercise-induced bronchospasm, two sprays are administered 10 to 15 minutes before exercise. A 4% liquid nasal spray (NASALCROM) is available in a pump that delivers a metered spray containing 5.2 mg with each compression. The recommended dose is one spray in each nostril three to six times a day. A 4% ophthalmic solution (OPTICROM) is also available; 1 to 2 drops are used in each eye four to six times daily.

Clinical Use. The main use of cromolyn is in the prophylactic treatment of bronchial asthma. When inhaled several times daily, cromolyn will inhibit both the immediate and the late asthmatic responses to antigenic challenge or to exercise. With regular use for more than 2 to 3 months, there is evidence of reduced bronchial hyperreactivity, as measured by response to challenge with histamine or methacholine (*see* Murphy and Kelly, 1987). The role of cromolyn in the treatment of asthma is discussed further at the end of this chapter.

Cromolyn, in the form of a nasal spray, has beneficial effects in the prophylactic treatment of allergic rhinitis (*see* Shapiro and König, 1985). Treatment of seasonal rhinitis should commence with the appearance of symptoms. While the frequency of administration constitutes a disadvantage, the use of cromolyn avoids the complications of long-term therapy with topical decongestants, as well as the adverse effects of systemic decongestants or of antihistamines. Topical application of solutions of cromolyn has been shown to be of value in the treatment of allergic or vernal conjunctivitis, as well as of giant papillary conjunctivitis, and has often allowed reduction in the use of topical corticosteroids.

THERAPY OF ASTHMA AND CHRONIC OBSTRUCTIVE PULMONARY DISEASE

Asthma and chronic obstructive pulmonary disease are a heterogeneous group of conditions that share the common characteristic of impeded airflow in the lung sufficient to cause such symptoms as wheezing, labored breathing, or dyspnea. Individuals so afflicted may be subject to life-threatening episodes of acute respiratory distress precipitated by upper respiratory infections, exposure to environmental pollutants, or other stimuli. Asthma, sometimes referred to as reversible airway disease, is usually thought of as a disease of the young, since it is encountered in more than 10% of children (Weinberger, 1987). Although long-term remissions are frequent, asthma may recur in adult life as such or as a component of other pulmonary disease. When asthma, defined in terms of airway hyperresponsiveness, is encountered in adults over the age of about 40, it is usually included in the general category of chronic obstructive pulmonary disease (COPD), which also includes chronic bronchitis and emphysema. The compromised pulmonary function in these conditions has a major anatomical and largely irreversible basis, including hypertrophied bronchial lumens, destroyed or dilated alveolar air spaces, and decreased supportive connective tissue. In recent years, the prevalence of COPD has increased sharply in the United States, such that by 1981 it afflicted about 17 million patients and was the fifth leading cause of death; this upward trend is expected to continue through the end of the decade (*see* Boyars, 1988). Prevention, early diagnosis, and treatment of COPD are thus major health issues.

In addition to age, cigarette smoking and prior episodes of asthma are risk factors in the progression of COPD, and treatment includes cessation of smoking and avoidance of other pollutants. Because viral infection can trigger airway disease, yearly vaccinations against influenza and prophylaxis with amantadine are frequently recommended, as is early intervention with antibiotics to treat exacerbations of bronchitis (*see* Boyars, 1988). Similarly, immunotherapy and identification and avoidance of allergens may be valuable in the treatment of some young asthmatic patients (*see* Weinberger, 1987; Stafford, 1988; Chapman *et al.*, in Symposium, 1988a); avoidance of foods containing certain additives, such as sulfites, may also be helpful (*see* Adelman and Spector, 1988). While all important, these aspects of the treatment of asthma and COPD are beyond the scope of this discussion.

Asthma. The frequency and intensity of symptoms experienced by a patient will obviously dictate the therapeutic approach, as well as the adjustments to changes in the status of a given patient. Mild, periodic episodes of bronchoconstriction can often be managed simply by the inhalation of β_2-adrenergic agonists at the onset of symptoms or immediately before a provoking stimulus, such as exercise. At the other extreme, severe chronic asthma may require the use of several agents, including adrenocortical steroids administered systemically on a regular basis. The vast majority of patients fall somewhere in between; these individuals can be managed with regimens in which some degree of bronchodilatation is maintained by the systemic administration of an agent such as theophylline or in which the degree of bronchial hyperresponsiveness is controlled or reduced by the regular inhalation of adrenocortical steroids or cromolyn sodium. One or more of these strategies is supplemented by the periodic inhalation of a bronchodilator, most frequently a β_2-adrenergic agonist.

β-Adrenergic Agonists. Inhalation of a selective β_2-adrenergic agonist is the preferred form of bronchodilator therapy. Metered-dose aerosol formulations offer the greatest convenience and portability, although some patients have difficulty mastering the proper delivery technique without the aid of a "spacer." Nebulizer solutions may be more useful for more intensive therapy in the home or hospital. There seems to be little basis for choice among the newer, more selective agents, such as *albuterol, terbutaline, pirbuterol,* or *bitolterol.* The latter drug may produce a longer period of useful bronchodilatation than the 2 to 3 hours provided by the others, perhaps because it must be converted to *colterol* (the active compound) in the lung before further metabolism commences (*see* Friedel and Brogden, 1988); however, its disagreeable taste has discouraged widespread use. *Metaproterenol* and *isoetharine* are somewhat shorter-acting and less selective for β_2-adrenergic receptors, while *isoproterenol* activates both β_1- and β_2-adrenergic receptors equally and has a still shorter duration of action. Formerly a mainstay of therapy, *epinephrine* finds its greatest use in low-strength nonprescription inhalers appropriate only for patients with very mild intermittent symptoms.

Inhalation of a selective β_2-adrenergic agonist usually produces excellent bronchodilatation or short-term protection against a challenge without appreciable cardiac or other systemic effects, especially in the younger asthmatic population. Exceeding the recommended dosage will intensify such side effects, but a far greater danger in the use of these agents results from the tendency of patients to continue self-medication during periods when their symptoms are escalating. Patients should be encouraged to seek medical attention as soon as possible after they detect a marked decline in the efficacy of their usual therapeutic regimen in order to avoid a serious medical emergency. The use of orally administered adrenergic agonists for bronchodilatation has not gained wide acceptance, largely because of the greater risk of producing side effects, especially cardiac and metabolic disturbances. Even though stimulation of β-adrenergic receptors has been shown to inhibit the release of inflammatory mediators from mast cells, long-term administration of β_2-adrenergic agonists, either orally or by inhalation, does not reduce bronchial hyperresponsiveness. Thus, other approaches for the treatment of chronic symptoms are preferred. For additional information on adrenergic agonists, *see* Chapter 10.

Ipratropium bromide. The inhalation of anticholinergic alkaloids (including atropine) was at one time the mainstay of the treatment of asthma. With the introduction of adrenergic bronchodilators, anticholinergic therapy of airway disease became nearly extinct because of the undesirable systemic side effects (*see* Chapter 8). Moreover, atropine causes thickening of bronchial secretions and inhibits the beating of epithelial cilia, which combine to reduce mucociliary clearance in patients with inflamed airways. However, ipratropium (and perhaps other quaternary anticholinergic agents) does not inhibit mucociliary clearance for as yet unexplained reasons, and its actions are confined almost exclusively to the mouth and airways when solutions are inhaled.

In asthmatic subjects, the inhalation of ipratropium affords marked protection against the bronchoconstriction produced by the subsequent inhalation of such substances as sulfur dioxide, ozone, or methacholine; responses to histamine or bradykinin are only modestly inhibited, and there is little protection against leukotriene-induced bronchoconstriction. The degree of protection against challenge with allergens, exercise, or breathing cold dry air varies among asthmatic subjects. This presumably reflects differences in the amount of ongoing parasympathetic tone and in the degree to which reflex activation of cholinergic pathways participates in the generation of symptoms in individual patients. Hence, the therapeutic utility of ipratropium must be assessed on an individual basis.

The bronchodilatation produced by ipratropium in asthmatic subjects develops more slowly and is usually less intense than that produced by adrenergic agonists. By contrast, patients with COPD are often less responsive to adrenergic agonists, and ipratropium is frequently equally effective (*see* below). Nevertheless, some asthmatic patients may experience a useful and long-lasting response. Clinical trials suggest that the sequential inhalation of a β-adrenergic agonist followed by ipratropium may produce bronchodilatation that is sustained for 4 to 6 hours, and an aerosol formulation (DUOVENT) of a combination of ipratropium bromide with *fenoterol* is being evaluated in Europe. The pharmacological properties and therapeutic uses of ipratropium have been reviewed by Gross (1988). (*See also* Symposium, 1986b, 1987d, and Chapter 8.)

Theophylline. The oral administration of theophylline-containing preparations has been used to produce bronchodilatation for over 50 years. The efficacy of theophylline is unquestioned, and, with supplemental inhalation of β_2-adrenergic agonists, successful treatment of most patients with moderately severe chronic asthma has been a reality for nearly 20 years. However, the margin of safety is relatively narrow; the minimum therapeutic concentration in plasma is 6 to 10 μg/ml, and unacceptable symptoms of toxicity usually appear at or above 20 μg/ml. Still higher concentrations can lead to serious CNS toxicity, which includes seizures; long-term ingestion of theophylline is a predisposing factor in such toxicity (*see* above). Moreover, the clearance of theophylline is influenced by genetic, developmental, and environmental factors to an important degree. Thus, it is necessary to titrate the dosage cautiously against clinical observations of beneficial or toxic effects, with periodic determination of the concentration of the drug in plasma.

Therapy is usually initiated by the administration of 16 mg/kg per day of theophylline (calculated as the free base) up to a maximum of 400 mg per day for at least 3 days (*see* Weinberger, 1987). This minimizes the early side effects of nausea, vomiting, nervousness, and insomnia, which often subside with continued therapy, and virtually eliminates the possibility of exceeding concentrations of 20 μg/ml in the plasma of patients over the age of 1 year who do not have compromised hepatic or cardiac function. Thereafter, the dosage is increased in two successive stages to between 18 and 22 mg/kg per day (up to a maximum of 800 mg per day), depending upon the age and clinical response of the patient, allowing at least 3 days between adjustments. The plasma concentration of theophylline is determined before a further adjustment in dosage is made. Fortunately, such determinations can now be made rapidly from small volumes of blood. Although extended-release preparations of theophylline usually allow twice-daily dosing, variations in the rate and extent of absorption of such preparations require individualized calibration of dosing regimens for each patient and preparation.

Unlike the oral administration of β-adrenergic agonists, long-term therapy with theophylline permits undiminished responses to inhaled β_2-adrenergic agonists, and the availability of extended-release preparations of theophylline offers the opportunity to design regimens that can minimize the emergence of nocturnal symptoms (*see* Symposium, 1988e). Although theophylline can reduce or block the secondary or "late" responses to challenge with exercise or allergen that are experienced by some patients, there is little evidence that long-term therapy has substantial effects on the underlying bronchial hyperresponsiveness in such patients (Dutoit *et al.*, 1987). This, coupled with the inherent difficulty in designing safe therapeutic regimens and the growing concern over the potential for behavioral toxicity in children, has led some investigators to advocate the use of cromolyn sodium or inhaled adrenocortical steroids instead of theophylline (*see* Furukawa, 1988). Hence, the once-dominant status of theophylline in the treatment of asthma is currently undergoing reevaluation.

Cromolyn Sodium. With the growing appreciation of the role of inflammatory processes in the initiation, maintenance, and exacerbation of bronchial hyperresponsiveness, increased attention has been focused on the utility of cromolyn in the treatment of asthma that is not adequately controlled by the inhalation of β-adrenergic agonists (*see* Cockcroft, 1987; O'Byrne *et al.*, 1987; McFadden, in Symposium, 1988a). The inhalation of cromolyn sodium four times daily can reduce chronic and exercise-induced symptoms to the point that they can be controlled by periodic inhalation of a β_2-adrenergic agonist. However, not all patients will respond adequately, and cromolyn appears to be of greatest value in patients whose asthma is thought to be due to current exposure to allergens. With long-term use, evidence of reduced bronchial hyperresponsiveness can usually be obtained, and reduction in the frequency of administration may be possible after several months. It must be remembered that cromolyn is not a bronchodilator and cannot be used to treat an acute episode. Moreover, the proper administration of cromolyn may be impossible in the presence of bronchoconstriction, and prior inhalation of a bronchodilator may be necessary. Cromolyn can also be used prophylactically shortly before exercise or exposure to a known allergen. In this case, both the short-term obstructive response and the subsequent increase in bronchial reactivity can be prevented.

Adrenocortical Steroids. Although the systemic administration of adrenocortical steroids, chiefly *prednisone*, has long been employed in the treatment of patients with severe chronic asthma or those who are experiencing acute exacerbations of their symptoms, the more recent development of aerosol formulations has prompted a reevaluation of the therapeutic role of these agents (*see* Johnson, 1987; König, 1988). The most frequently used inhalational agents are *beclomethasone dipropionate, triamcinolone acetonide,* and *flunisolide*. Less information is available about the use of *dexamethasone sodium phosphate*. Another promising agent, *budesonide,* is available in Europe and elsewhere. Patients who respond inadequately to a trial with cromolyn are now viewed as candidates for the use of inhaled adrenocortical steroids, initially at the recommended maintenance dosage (two inhalations 3 to 4 times daily for adults; flunisolide is used twice daily). If symptoms are not controlled adequately, some investigators advocate a temporary increase in dosage by about fourfold (perhaps with the addition of theophylline) before resorting to the systemic administration of adrenocortical steroids. This approach can often restore the effectiveness of inhaled β-adrenergic agonists and reduce bronchial hyperresponsiveness. In contrast to cromolyn, a dose of steroid inhaled shortly before a challenge with allergen has relatively little effect on the initial obstructive response, even though the late response will be suppressed.

The systemic side effects of inhaled adrenocortical steroids are relatively minor. Even at the maximal recommended doses (*e.g.*, 840 μg per day of beclomethasone dipropionate), appreciable suppression of the hypothalamic–pituitary–adrenal axis is difficult to document. Oropharyngeal candidiasis and, more frequently, dysphonia are encountered; however, their incidence can be reduced substantially by rinsing the mouth and throat with water after each use and by employing spacer or reservoir devices attached to the dispenser to decrease the deposition of drug in the oral cavity (*see* Johnson, 1987). The adverse effects of the systemic administration of adrenocortical steroids are well known (*see* Chapter 60), but treatment for brief periods (5 to 10 days) causes relatively little dose-related toxicity. Hence, substantial doses of adrenocortical steroids (*e.g.*, 30 mg of prednisone twice daily for 5 days for children over 3 years of age) are often used to treat acute exacerbations of asthma (Weinberger, 1988). Although an additional week of therapy at somewhat reduced dosage may be required, the steroids can be withdrawn abruptly once control of the symptoms by other medications has been restored; any suppression of adrenal function appears to dissipate within 1 to 2 weeks. More protracted bouts of severe asthma may require long-term, alternate-day therapy, with the usual precautions upon cessation (*see* Bartoszek and Szefler, 1987).

Status Asthmaticus. Severe exacerbations of asthma require emergency treatment. For many years, the standard therapy included the administration of *epinephrine* subcutaneously and *aminophylline* intravenously. However, current approaches emphasize the use of inhaled β_2-adrenergic agonists to achieve bronchodilatation (*see* Dean and Brown, 1988). The injection of a β-adrenergic agonist (*e.g., terbutaline sulfate*) is of value if a patient cannot cooperate with the administration of inhaled medication. After determination of its concentration in plasma, the cautious infusion of *aminophylline* (up to 6 mg/kg) may provide additional benefit in this circumstance. The inhalation of the β_2-adrenergic agonist should be supervised and can be accomplished with either nebulizers or metered-dose inhalers; the treatment can be repeated every 30 minutes until maximal bronchodilatation or significant tachycardia occurs. Although adrenocortical steroids do not produce any immediate improvement in respiratory function, their administration early in the course of treatment is recommended (*see* Dean and Brown, 1988). Some advocate the intravenous administration of very high doses initially (*e.g.*, 60 to 125 mg of *methylprednisolone sodium succinate* every 6 hours), with gradual reduction in dosage once the patient has responded. With such high doses, it is prudent to institute appropriate prophylactic treatment to avoid gastric ulceration.

Chronic Obstructive Pulmonary Disease. The pharmacological treatment of COPD resembles that of asthma largely because it is the asthmatic component of a patient's disease that is most amenable to therapy. At present, the use of inhaled β_2-adrenergic agonists combined with oral theophylline is emphasized (*see* Symposium, 1987c; Boyars, 1988). In some patients, the presence of theophylline appears to enhance the efficacy of the inhaled agents; in others who have a more profound response to β-adrenergic agonists, theophylline fails to produce additional bronchodilatation beyond that achieved by maximal doses of the inhaled drug. Both classes of agents increase mucociliary clearance, which is of value in the treatment of chronic bronchitis. Although there is some controversy, theophylline appears to have beneficial effects on fatigued respiratory muscles, leading to enhanced respiration and a decreased sensation of dyspnea. Ipratropium bromide has only recently been approved for use in the treatment of patients with COPD, and its ultimate utility as a bronchodilator is yet to be determined. In contrast to its relatively small effects in asthmatic patients, this agent usually produces about the same degree of bronchodilatation in patients with COPD as do maximal doses of β-adrenergic agonists. The main drawback to the incorporation of ipratropium into therapeutic regimens is the added complexity of manipulating another inhaled medication by patients who often have difficulty using metered-dose inhalers. It remains to be seen if mixtures of ipratropium and β_2-adrenergic agonists can be formulated into aerosols with ratios of ingredients appropriate for the treatment of a variety of patients. Except for the treatment of acute bronchospastic episodes, the role of adrenocortical steroids in the therapy of COPD is uncertain.

Acheson, J. J.; Zahorska-Markiewiez, B.; Pittet, P.; Anantharaman, K.; and Jéquier, E. Caffeine and coffee: their influence on metabolic rate and substrate utilization in normal weight and obese individuals. *Am. J. Clin. Nutr.*, **1980**, *33*, 989–997.

Acquaviva, F.; DeFrancesco, A.; Andriulli, A.; Piantino, P.; Arrigoni, A.; Massarenti, P.; and Balzola, F. Effect of regular and decaffeinated coffee on serum gastrin levels. *J. Clin. Gastroenterol.*, **1986**, *8*, 150–153.

Aitken, M. L., and Martin, E. R. Life-threatening theophylline toxicity is not predictable by serum levels. *Chest*, **1987**, *91*, 10–14.

Albertson, T. E.; Stark, L. G.; and Joy, R. M. The effects of doxapram, diazepam, phenobarbital and pentylenetetrazol on suprathreshold and threshold stimulations in amygdaloid kindled rats. *Neuropharmacology*, **1983**, *22*, 245–248.

Barrington, K. J.; Finer, N. N.; Peters, K. L.; and Barton, J. Physiologic effects of doxapram in idiopathic apnea of prematurity. *J. Pediatr.*, **1986**, *108*, 124–129.

Barrington, K. J.; Finer, N. N.; Torok-Both, G.; Jamali, F.; and Coutts, R. T. Dose-response relationship of doxapram in the therapy for refractory idiopathic apnea of prematurity. *Pediatrics*, **1987**, *80*, 22–27.

Beaudry, M. A.; Bradley, J. M.; Gramlich, L. M.; and LeGatt, D. Pharmacokinetics of doxapram in idiopathic apnea of prematurity. *Dev. Pharmacol. Ther.*, **1988**, *11*, 65–72.

Becker, A. B.; Simons, K. J.; Gillespei, R. N.; and Simons, F. E. R. The bronchodilator effects and pharmacokinetics of caffeine in asthma. *N. Engl. J. Med.*, **1984**, *310*, 743–746.

Berglund, B., and Hemmingsson, P. Effects of caffeine ingestion on exercise performance at low and high altitudes in cross-country skiers. *Int. J. Sports Med.*, **1982**, *3*, 234–236.

Bertino, J. S., Jr., and Walker, J. W. Reassessment of theophylline toxicity. Serum concentrations, clinical course, and treatment. *Arch. Intern. Med.*, **1987**, *147*, 757–760.

Bolme, P.; Edlund, P.-O.; Eriksson, M.; Paalzow, L.; and Winbladh, B. Pharmacokinetics of theophylline in young children with asthma: a comparison of rectal enema and suppositories. *Eur. J. Clin. Pharmacol.*, **1979**, *16*, 133–139.

Bowdle, T. A. Clinical pharmacology of antagonists of narcotic-induced respiratory depression. *Acute Care*, **1988**, *12*, Suppl. 1, 70–76.

Bowser, E. W.; Hargis, G. K.; Henderson, W. J.; and Williams, G. A. Parathyroid hormone secretion in the rat: effect of aminophylline. *Proc. Soc. Exp. Biol. Med.*, **1975**, *148*, 344–346.

Bowton, D. L.; Haddon, W. S.; Prough, D. S.; Adair, N.; Alford, P. T.; and Stump, D. A. Theophylline effect on the cerebral blood flow response to hypoxemia. *Chest*, **1988**, *94*, 371–375.

Brater, D. C.; Kaojaren, S.; and Chennavasin, P. Pharmacodynamics of the diuretic effects of aminophylline and acetazolamide alone and combined with furosemide in normal subjects. *J. Pharmacol. Exp. Ther.*, **1983**, *227*, 92–97.

Burki, N. K. Ventilatory effects of doxapram in conscious human subjects. *Chest*, **1984**, *85*, 600–604.

Calverley, P. M.; Robson, R. H.; Wraith, P. K.; Prescott, L. F.; and Flenley, D. C. The ventilatory effects of doxapram in normal man. *Clin. Sci.*, **1983**, *65*, 65–69.

Cano, R.; Isenberg, J. I.; and Grossman, M. I. Cimetidine inhibits caffeine-stimulated gastric acid secretion in man. *Gastroenterology*, **1976**, *70*, 1055–1057.

Charney, D. S.; Heniger, G. R.; and Jatlow, P. I. Increased anxiogenic effects of caffeine in panic disorders. *Arch. Gen. Psychiatry*, **1985**, *42*, 233–243.

Choi, O. H.; Shamim, M. T.; Padgett, W. L.; and Daly, J. W. Caffeine and theophylline analogues: correlation of behavioral effects with activity as adenosine receptor antagonists and as phosphodiesterase inhibitors. *Life Sci.*, **1988**, *43*, 387–398.

Clementz, G. L., and Dailey, J. W. Psychotropic effects of caffeine. *Am. Fam. Physician*, **1988**, *37*, 167–172.

Cohen, S., and Booth, G. H. Gastric acid secretion and lower-esophageal-sphincter pressure in response to coffee and caffeine. *N. Engl. J. Med.*, **1975**, *293*, 897–899.

Debas, H. T.; Cohen, M. M.; Holubitsky, I. B.; and Harrison, R. C. Caffeine-stimulated gastric acid and pepsin secretion: dose-response studies. *Scand. J. Gastroenterol.*, **1971**, *6*, 453–457.

DeLander, G. E., and Hopkins, C. J. Spinal adenosine modulates descending antinociceptive pathways stimulated by morphine. *J. Pharmacol. Exp. Ther.*, **1986**, *239*, 88–93.

Dutoit, J. I.; Salome, C. M.; and Woolcock, A. J. Inhaled corticosteroids reduce the severity of bronchial hyperresponsiveness in asthma but oral theophylline does not. *Am. Rev. Respir. Dis.*, **1987**, *136*, 1174–1178.

Feurle, G.; Arnold, R.; Helmstädter, V.; and Creutzfeldt, W. The effect of intravenous theophylline ethylenediamine on serum gastrin concentration in control subjects and patients with duodenal ulcers and Zollinger–Ellison syndrome. *Digestion*, **1976**, *14*, 227–231.

Finney, M. J.; Karlsson, J. A.; and Persson, C. G. Effects of bronchoconstrictors and bronchodilators on a novel human small airway preparation. *Br. J. Pharmacol.*, **1985**, *85*, 29–36.

Furukawa, C. T.; DuHamel, T. R.; Weimer, L.; Shapiro, G. G.; Pierson, W. E.; and Bierman, C. W. Cognitive and behavioral findings in children taking theophylline. *J. Allergy Clin. Immunol.*, **1988**, *81*, 83–88.

Gerber, J. G.; Nies, A. S.; and Payne, N. A. Adenosine receptors on canine parietal cells modulate gastric acid secretion to histamine. *J. Pharmacol. Exp. Ther.*, **1985**, *233*, 623–627.

Glavin, G. B.; Westerberg, V. S.; and Geiger, J. D. Modulation of gastric acid secretion by adenosine in conscious rats. *Can. J. Physiol. Pharmacol.*, **1987**, *65*, 1182–1185.

Goldberg, M. J.; Spector, R.; Park, G. D.; Johnson, G. F.; and Roberts, P. The effect of sorbitol and activated charcoal on serum theophylline concentrations after slow-release theophylline. *Clin. Pharmacol. Ther.*, **1987**, *41*, 108–111.

Green, R. M., and McNamara, J. The effects of pentoxifylline on patients with intermittent claudication. *J. Vasc. Surg.*, **1988**, *7*, 356–362.

Hammerschmidt, D. E.; Kotasek, D.; McCarthy, T.; Huh, P. W.; Freyburger, G.; and Vercellotti, G. M. Pentoxifylline inhibits granulocyte and platelet function, including granulocyte priming by platelet activating factor. *J. Lab. Clin. Med.*, **1988**, *112*, 254–263.

Handslip, P. D. J.; Dart, A. M.; and Davies, B. H. Intravenous salbutamol and aminophylline in asthma: a search for synergy. *Thorax*, **1981**, *36*, 741–744.

Kalsner, S. Mechanism of potentiation of contractor responses to catecholamines by methylxanthines in aortic strips. *Br. J. Pharmacol.*, **1971**, *43*, 379–388.

Kalsner, S.; Frew, R. D.; and Smith, G. M. Mechanism of methylxanthine sensitization of norepinephrine responses in a coronary artery. *Am. J. Physiol.*, **1975**, *228*, 1702–1707.

Kay, A. B.; Walsh, G. M.; Moqbel, R.; MacDonald, A. J.; Nagakura, T.; Carroll, M. P.; and Richerson, H. B. Disodium cromoglycate inhibits activation of human inflammatory cells *in vitro*. *J. Allergy Clin. Immunol.*, **1987**, *80*, 1–8.

Kuzemko, J. A., and Paala, J. Apnoeic attacks in the newborn treated with aminophylline. *Arch. Dis. Child.*, **1973**, *48*, 404–406.

Leviton, A. Caffeine consumption and the risk of reproductive hazards. *J. Reprod. Med.*, **1988**, *88*, 175–178.

Maren, T. H. The additive renal effect of oral aminophylline and trichlormethiazide in man. *Clin. Res.*, **1961**, *9*, 57.

Marquardt, D. L.; Parker, C. W.; and Sullivan, T. J. Potentiation of mast cell mediator release by adenosine. *J. Immunol.*, **1978**, *120*, 871–878.

Martinson, E. A.; Johnson, R. A.; and Wells, J. N. Potent adenosine receptor antagonists that are selective for the A_1 receptor subtype. *Mol. Pharmacol.*, **1987**, *31*, 247–252.

Moqbel, R.; Cromwell, O.; Walsh, G. M.; Wardlaw, A. J.; Kurlak, L.; and Kay, A. B. Effects of nedocromil sodium (TILADE) on the activation of human eosinophils and neutrophils and the release of histamine from mast cells. *Allergy*, **1988**, *43*, 268–276.

Morii, S.; Ngai, A. C.; Ko, K. R.; and Winn, H. R. Role of adenosine in regulation of cerebral blood flow: effects of theophylline during normoxia and hypoxia. *Am. J. Physiol.*, **1987**, *253*, H165–H175.

Moyer, J. H.; Tashnek, A. B.; Miller, S. I.; Snyder, H.; and Bowman, R. O. The effect of theophylline with ethylenediamine (aminophylline) and caffeine on cerebral hemodynamics and cerebrospinal fluid pressure in patients with hypertension headaches. *Am. J. Med. Sci.*, **1952**, *224*, 377–385.

Muttitt, S. C.; Tierney, A. J.; and Finer, N. N. The dose response of theophylline in the treatment of apnea of prematurity. *J. Pediatr.*, **1988**, *112*, 115–121.

Myers, M. G. Effects of caffeine on blood pressure. *Arch. Intern. Med.*, **1988a**, *148*, 1189–1193.

———. Caffeine and cardiac arrhythmias. *Chest*, **1988b**, *94*, 4.

Ogilvie, R. I.; Fernandez, P. G.; and Winsberg, F. Cardiovascular response to increasing theophylline concentrations. *Eur. J. Clin. Pharmacol.*, **1977**, *12*, 409–414.

Öhnell, H., and Berg, H. Zur Frage über die Ventrikelfunktion nach verabreichung verschiedener Arten von Kaffee. *Acta Med. Scand.*, **1931**, *76*, 491–520.

Paloucek, F. P., and Rodvold, K. A. Evaluation of theophylline overdoses and toxicities. *Ann. Emerg. Med.*, **1988**, *17*, 135–144.

Phelps, H. M., and Phelps, C. E. Caffeine ingestion and breast cancer. *Cancer*, **1988**, *61*, 1051–1054.

Ramkumar, V.; Bumgarner, J. R.; Jacobson, K. A.; and Stiles, G. L. Multiple components of the A_1 adenosine receptor–adenylate cyclase system are regulated in rat cerebral cortex by chronic caffeine ingestion. *J. Clin. Invest.*, **1988**, *82*, 242–247.

Rossignol, L.; Plantavid, M.; Chap, H.; and Douste-Blazy, L. Effects of two methylxanthines, pentoxifylline and propentofylline, on arachidonic acid metabolism in platelets stimulated by thrombin. *Biochem. Pharmacol.*, **1988**, *37*, 3229–3236.

Rowe, D. J. F.; Watson, I. D.; Williams, J.; and Berry, D. J. The clinical use and measurement of theophylline. *Ann. Clin. Biochem.*, **1988**, *25*, 4–23.

Salter, H. On some points in the treatment and clinical history of asthma. *Edinburgh Med. J.*, **1859**, *4*, 1109–1115.

Serrano-Ríos, M.; Hawkins, F. G.; Esobar-Jiménez, F.; and Rodriguez-Miñón, J. L. The effect of aminophylline on insulin release induced by secretin and cholecystokinin–pancreozymin in normal humans. *J. Clin. Endocrinol. Metab.*, **1974**, *38*, 194–199.

Sigurd, B., and Olesen, K. H. Comparative natriuretic and diuretic efficacy of theophylline ethylenediamine and of bendroflumethiazide during long-term treatment with the potent diuretic bumetanide. *Acta Med. Scand.*, **1978**, *203*, 113–119.

Stirt, J. A. Aminophylline may act as a morphine antagonist. *Anaesthesia*, **1983**, *38*, 275–278.

Sydbom, A., and Fredholm, B. B. On the mechanism by which theophylline inhibits histamine release from rat mast cells. *Acta Physiol. Scand.*, **1982**, *114*, 243–251.

Thoman, E. B.; Davis, D. H.; Raye, J. R.; Philipps, A. F.; Rowe, J. C.; and Denenberg, V. H. Theophylline affects sleep-wake state development in premature infants. *Neuropediatrics*, **1985**, *16*, 13–18.

Vestal, R. E.; Eriksson, C. E.; Musser, B.; Ozaki, L. K.; and Halter, J. B. Effect of intravenous aminophylline on plasma levels of catecholamines and related cardiovascular and metabolic responses in man. *Circulation*, **1983**, *67*, 162–171.

Vinegar, R.; Truax, J. F.; Selph, J. L.; Welch, R. M.; and White, H. L. Potentiation of the anti-inflammatory and analgesic activity of aspirin by caffeine in the rat. *Proc. Soc. Exp. Biol. Med.*, **1976**, *151*, 556–560.

Wechsler, R. L.; Kleiss, L. M.; and Kety, S. S. The effects of intravenously administered aminophylline on cerebral circulation and metabolism in man. *J. Clin. Invest.*, **1950**, *29*, 28–30.

Weinberger, M. Corticosteroids for exacerbations of asthma: current status of the controversy. *Pediatrics*, **1988**, *81*, 726–729.

Wells, E., and Mann, J. Phosphorylation of a mast cell protein in response to treatment with anti-allergic compounds. Implications for the mode of action of sodium cromoglycate. *Biochem. Pharmacol.*, **1983**, *32*, 837–842.

White, J. R.; Ishizaka, T.; Ishizaka, K.; and Sha'afi, R. I. Direct demonstration of increased intracellular concentration of free calcium as measured by quin-2 in stimulated rat peritoneal mast cell. *Proc. Natl. Acad. Sci. U.S.A.*, **1984**, *81*, 3978–3982.

Zehner, J.; Klaus, D.; Klumpp, F.; and Lemke, R. The influence of propranolol, practolol, and theophylline on the plasma renin activity. *Res. Exp. Med. (Berl.)*, **1975**, *166*, 275–282.

Monographs and Reviews

Adelman, D. C., and Spector, S. L. Update on asthma therapy. *Compr. Ther.*, **1988**, *14*, 67–74.

Arnaud, M. J. The pharmacology of caffeine. *Prog. Drug Res.*, **1987**, *31*, 273–313.
Bartoszek, M., and Szefler, S. J. Corticosteroid therapy in adolescent patients. *J. Adolesc. Health Care*, **1987**, *8*, 84–91.
Boyars, M. C. COPD in the ambulatory elderly: management update. *Geriatrics*, **1988**, *43*, 29–40.
Cockcroft, D. W. Airway hyperresponsiveness: therapeutic implications. *Ann. Allergy*, **1987**, *59*, 405–414.
Curatolo, P. W., and Robertson, D. The health consequences of caffeine. *Ann. Intern. Med.*, **1983**, *98*, 641–653.
Dean, N. C., and Brown, J. K. Status asthmaticus: early institution of treatment. *Postgrad. Med.*, **1988**, *84*, 103–114.
Friedel, H. A., and Brogden, R. N. Bitolterol: a preliminary review of its pharmacological properties and therapeutic efficacy in reversible obstructive airways disease. *Drugs*, **1988**, *35*, 22–41.
Furukawa, C. T. Comparative trials including a $beta_2$ adrenergic agonist, a methylxanthine, and a mast cell stabilizer. *Ann. Allergy*, **1988**, *60*, 472–476.
Gonzalez, J. P., and Brogden, R. N. Nedocromil sodium. A preliminary review of its pharmacodynamic and pharmacokinetic properties, and therapeutic efficacy in the treatment of reversible obstructive airways disease. *Drugs*, **1987**, *34*, 560–577.
Graham, D. M. Caffeine—its identity, dietary sources, intake and biological effects. *Nutr. Rev.*, **1978**, *36*, 97–102.
Griffiths, R. R., and Woodson, P. P. Caffeine physical dependence: a review of human and laboratory animal studies. *Psychopharmacology (Berlin)*, **1988**, *94*, 437–451.
Gross, N. J. Ipratropium bromide. *N. Engl. J. Med.*, **1988**, *319*, 486–494.
Hendeles, L., and Weinberger, M. Improved efficacy and safety of theophylline in the control of airway hyperreactivity. *Pharmacol. Ther.*, **1982**, *18*, 91–105.
Johnson, C. E. Aerosol corticosteroids for the treatment of asthma. *Drug Intell. Clin. Pharm.*, **1987**, *21*, 784–790.
König, P. Inhaled corticosteroids—their present and future role in the management of asthma. *J. Allergy Clin. Immunol.*, **1988**, *82*, 297–306.
Murphy, S., and Kelly, H. W. Cromolyn sodium: a review of mechanisms and clinical use in asthma. *Drug Intell. Clin. Pharm.*, **1987**, *21*, 22–35.
O'Byrne, P. M.; Dolovich, J.; and Hargreave, F. E. Late asthmatic responses. *Am. Rev. Respir. Dis.*, **1987**, *136*, 740–751.
Rall, T. W. Evolution of the mechanism of action of methylxanthines: from calcium mobilizers to antagonists of adenosine receptors. *Pharmacologist*, **1982**, *24*, 277–287.
Roberts, R. J. *Drug Therapy in Infants: Pharmacologic Principles and Clinical Experience*. W. B. Saunders Co., Philadelphia, **1984**.
Shapiro, G. G., and König, P. Cromolyn sodium: a review. *Pharmacotherapy*, **1985**, *5*, 156–170.
Stafford, C. T. New concepts in chronic asthma: what is the impact on therapy? *Postgrad. Med.*, **1988**, *84*, 86–98.
Symposium. (Various authors.) Developmental pharmacology of the methylxanthines. (Soyka, L. F., ed.) *Semin. Perinatol.*, **1981**, *5*, 303–408.
Symposium. (Various authors.) *Regulatory Function of Adenosine*. (Berne, R. M.; Rall, T. W.; and Rubio, R.; eds.) Martinus Nijhoff, Boston, **1983**.
Symposium. (Various authors.) *Anti-asthma Xanthines and Adenosine*. (Andersson, K.-E., and Persson, C. G. A., eds.) Excerpta Medica, Amsterdam, **1985**.
Symposium. (Various authors.) Update on theophylline. (Grant, J. A., and Ellis, E. F., eds.) *J. Allergy Clin. Immunol.*, **1986a**, *78*, 669–824.
Symposium. (Various authors.) Cholinergic pathway in obstructive airways disease. (Bergofsky, E. H., ed.) *Am. J. Med.*, **1986b**, *81*, 1–192.
Symposium. (Various authors.) Airway smooth muscle and disease workshop. *Am. Rev. Respir. Dis.*, **1987a**, *136*, S1–S73.
Symposium. (Various authors.) *Proceedings of the Third International Symposium on Adenosine. Topics and Perspectives in Adenosine Research*. (Gerlach, E., and Becker, B. F., eds.) Springer-Verlag, Berlin, **1987b**.
Symposium. (Various authors.) Rationale for the use of theophylline in COPD. *Chest*, **1987c**, *92*, 1S–51S.
Symposium. (Various authors.) Anticholinergic therapy—the state of the art. *Postgrad. Med. J.*, **1987d**, *63*, Suppl., 1–86.
Symposium. (Various authors.) Basic mechanisms of asthma: role of inflammation. *Chest*, **1988a**, *94*, 175–190.
Symposium. (Various authors.) Mechanisms in asthma: pharmacology, physiology, and management. (Armour, C. L., and Black, J. L., eds.) *Prog. Clin. Biol. Res.*, **1988b**, *263*, 1–436.
Symposium. (Various authors.) Bronchial hyperreactivity: mediators and mechanisms. *J. Allergy Clin. Immunol.*, **1988c**, *81*, 111–162.
Symposium. (Various authors.) Progress in understanding the relationship between the adenosine receptor system and actions of methylxanthines. (Carney, J. M., and Katz, J. L., eds.) *Pharmacol. Biochem. Behav.*, **1988d**, *29*, 407–441.
Symposium. (Various authors.) Asthma: a nocturnal disease. (McFadden, E. R., Jr., ed.) *Am. J. Med.*, **1988e**, *85*, 1–70.
Timson, J. Caffeine. *Mutat. Res.*, **1977**, *47*, 1–52.
Ward, A., and Clissold, S. P. Pentoxifylline: a review of its pharmacodynamic and pharmacokinetic properties, and its therapeutic efficacy. *Drugs*, **1987**, *34*, 50–97.
Weinberger, M. Pharmacologic management of asthma. *J. Adolesc. Health Care*, **1987**, *8*, 74–83.

CHAPTER

26 ANALGESIC–ANTIPYRETICS AND ANTIINFLAMMATORY AGENTS; DRUGS EMPLOYED IN THE TREATMENT OF RHEUMATOID ARTHRITIS AND GOUT

Paul A. Insel

In this chapter drugs that are antiinflammatory, analgesic, and antipyretic will be considered; their mechanisms of action differ from those of the antiinflammatory steroids and the opioid analgesics. Also discussed are certain drugs (*e.g.*, gold compounds and others) that may modify the progression of rheumatoid arthritis, although they are not antiinflammatory in the classical sense. Finally, drugs used in the treatment of gout, such as colchicine and allopurinol, are discussed. Several other agents are employed to suppress the manifestations of inflammation but are described in other sections of the textbook. These include the adrenocorticosteroids, antagonists of histamine and 5-hydroxytryptamine, and immunosuppressive agents.

The antiinflammatory, analgesic, and antipyretic drugs are a heterogeneous group of compounds, often chemically unrelated (although most of them are organic acids), which nevertheless share certain therapeutic actions and side effects. The prototype is aspirin; hence these compounds are often referred to as *aspirin-like drugs;* they are also frequently designated as *nonsteroidal antiinflammatory drugs* (NSAIDs).

There has been substantial progress in elucidating the mechanism of action of aspirin-like drugs, although a precise understanding of their therapeutic activities and side effects is still lacking. Inhibition of cyclooxygenase, the enzyme responsible for the biosynthesis of the prostaglandins and certain related autacoids, is generally thought to be a major facet of the mechanism of action of aspirin-like drugs. Some of their shared properties will first be considered; then the more important drugs will be discussed in some detail.

History. The medicinal effect of the bark of willow and certain other plants has been known to several cultures for centuries. In England in the mid-eighteenth century, Reverend Edmund Stone described in a letter to the president of the Royal Society "an account of the success of the bark of the willow in the cure of agues" (fever). Since the willow grew in damp or wet areas "where agues chiefly abound," Stone reasoned that it would probably possess curative properties appropriate to that condition.

The active ingredient in the willow bark was a bitter glycoside called *salicin,* first isolated in a pure form in 1829 by Leroux, who also demonstrated its antipyretic effect. On hydrolysis, salicin yields glucose and salicylic alcohol. The latter can be converted into salicylic acid, either *in vivo* or by chemical manipulation. Sodium salicylate was first used for the treatment of rheumatic fever and as an antipyretic in 1875, and the discovery of its uricosuric effects and of its usefulness in the treatment of gout soon followed. The enormous success of this drug prompted Hoffman, a chemist employed by Bayer, to prepare acetylsalicylic acid based on the earlier, but forgotten, work of Gerhardt in 1853. After demonstration of its antiinflammatory effects, this compound was introduced into medicine in 1899 by Dreser under the name of *aspirin.* The name is said to have been derived from *Spiraea,* the plant species from which salicylic acid was once prepared.

The synthetic salicylates soon displaced the more expensive compounds obtained from natural sources. By the early years of this century the chief therapeutic actions of aspirin were known. Toward the end of the nineteenth century, other drugs were discovered that shared some or all of these actions; among these, only derivatives of para-aminophenol (*e.g.*, acetaminophen) are used today. Beginning with indomethacin, a host of new agents has been introduced into medicine in various countries during the past 20 years.

MECHANISM OF ACTION OF NONSTEROIDAL ANTIINFLAMMATORY DRUGS

Although this class of drugs had been known to inhibit a wide variety of reactions *in vitro,* no convincing relationship could be established with their known antiinflammatory, antipyretic, and analgesic effects. In 1971, Vane and associates and Smith and Willis demonstrated that low concentrations of aspirin and indomethacin inhibited the enzymatic production of prostaglandins (*see* Chapter 24). There was, at that time, some evidence that prostaglandins participated in the pathogenesis of inflammation and fever, and this reinforced the hypothesis that inhibition of the biosynthesis of these autacoids could explain a number of the clinical actions of the drugs (*see* Higgs *et al.,* in Symposium, 1983a). Numerous subsequent observations have solidified this point of view, including the discoveries that prostaglandins are released whenever cells are damaged, they appear in inflammatory exudates, and nonsteroidal antiinflammatory drugs inhibit the biosynthesis and release of prostaglandins in all cells tested. However, the nonsteroidal antiinflammatory drugs do not generally inhibit the formation of eicosanoids such as the leukotrienes, which also contribute to inflammation, nor do they affect the synthesis of numerous other inflammatory mediators. Furthermore, these drugs may have other actions that contribute to their therapeutic effects in the treatment of rheumatoid arthritis (*see* below).

Inflammation. The inflammatory process involves a series of events that can be elicited by numerous stimuli (*e.g.,* infectious agents, ischemia, antigen–antibody interactions, and thermal or other physical injury). Each type of stimulus provokes a characteristic pattern of response that represents a relatively minor variation on a theme. At a macroscopic level, the response is usually accompanied by the familiar clinical signs of erythema, edema, tenderness (hyperalgesia), and pain. Inflammatory responses occur in three distinct phases, each apparently mediated by different mechanisms: (1) an acute transient phase, characterized by local vasodilatation and increased capillary permeability; (2) a delayed, subacute phase, most prominently characterized by infiltration of leukocytes and phagocytic cells; and (3) a chronic proliferative phase, in which tissue degeneration and fibrosis occur.

Many mediators of the inflammatory process have been identified. Histamine was one of the earliest candidates, and several H_1 antagonists have long been available; however, they are useful only for the treatment of vascular events in the early transient phase of inflammation (*see* Chapter 23). Bradykinin and 5-hydroxytryptamine (5-HT) may also have a role, but their antagonists also ameliorate only certain types of inflammatory responses (*see* Chapter 23). There has been a considerable effort to develop effective inhibitors of the formation or action of the leukotrienes, but their clinical usefulness has yet to be determined. Another lipid autacoid, platelet-activating factor (PAF), has recently been indicted as an important mediator of inflammation, and inhibitors of its synthesis and action are under study (*see* Chapter 24).

The effects produced by intradermal, intravenous, or intraarterial injections of small amounts of prostaglandins are strongly reminiscent of inflammation. Prostaglandin E_2 (PGE_2) and prostacyclin (PGI_2) cause erythema and an increase in local blood flow. With PGE_2, such effects may persist for up to 10 hours, and they include the capacity to counteract the vasoconstrictor effects of substances such as norepinephrine and angiotensin. These properties are not generally shared by other inflammatory mediators. In contrast to their long-lasting effects on cutaneous vessels and superficial veins, prostaglandin-induced vasodilatation in other vascular beds vanishes within a few minutes.

Although PGE_1 and PGE_2 (but not $PGF_{2\alpha}$) cause edema when injected into the hind paw of rats, it is not clear if they can increase vascular permeability (leakage) in the postcapillary and collecting venules without the participation of other inflammatory mediators (*e.g.,* bradykinin, histamine, leukotriene C_4). In addition, there is a clear synergism between PGE_1 and bradykinin when these two compounds are given together. Prostaglandins are also unlikely to be directly involved in chemotactic responses, even though they may promote the migration of leukocytes into an inflamed area by increasing blood flow. One potent chemotactic substance, leukotriene B_4, is a product of the lipoxygenase pathway of arachidonate metabolism (*see* Chapter 24; Larsen and Henson, 1983). Although high concentrations of aspirin-like drugs can inhibit cell migration, inhibition of lipoxygenase does not appear to be involved.

Rheumatoid Arthritis. Although the pathogenesis of rheumatoid arthritis is largely unknown, it is generally agreed that it represents an autoimmune disease that involves both the humoral and cellular arms of the immune response (*see* Zvaifler, 1988; Cooke and Scudamore, 1989). A complex interaction of genetic, immunological, and local factors has been invoked to account for the differing patterns of joint involvement and progression of disease among patients with rheumatoid arthritis; viral or other infections may also be involved in the initiation and/or exacerbations of the disease. The process is thought to be initiated by a hypothetical joint-seeking ("arthrotropic") antigen that is processed and presented by macrophages to T lymphocytes in conjunction with a major histocompatibility antigen in the synovial membrane. The interaction of this complex with T-cell receptors, together with the actions of macrophage-derived cytokines, results in the activation, differentiation, and clonal expansion of T cells. These elements of the cellular immune response are accompanied by microvascular injury and an inflammatory reaction that includes development of an exudative synovial fluid that contains many neutrophils. Although activation of B lymphocytes and the humoral immune response is also clearly evident, most of the antibodies that are generated are IgGs of unknown specificity that apparently arise from polyclonal activation of B cells, rather than from a response to a specific antigen. Some of the antibodies are IgMs that are directed against determinants in the Fc fragment of IgG (rheumatoid factors); their concentration in the systemic circulation often parallels the intensity of articular disease.

Although this scenario does not adequately explain the persistence of rheumatoid arthritis and the fluctuations in its intensity that are observed in many patients, the notion that activated T cells "drive" the process is consistent with a number of observations (*see* Lipsky *et al.*, 1989). These include the presence of large numbers of activated memory ($CD4^+$) T cells and of T cell–derived cytokines in synovial tissue or fluid, improvement of patients after thoracic duct drainage or total lymphoid irradiation, and the therapeutic effects of cyclosporine and the cytotoxic agents (*e.g.*, methotrexate, cyclophosphamide). However, other cells and their products are likely to be involved in the perpetuation of disease and may also exert inhibitory or immunosuppressive effects that may be partially responsible for fluctuations in its intensity. Nevertheless, the reasons for persistence and fluctuation of rheumatoid inflammation are poorly understood. Competing ideas include persistent antigenic stimulation with cycles of positive and negative responses; alternatively, there may be repeated introduction of antigens into the synovium, each followed by the evolution and resolution of an immune reaction.

Many cytokines have been found in the rheumatoid synovium (*see* Lipsky *et al.*, 1989); one of the most prominent of these is interleukin-1 (IL-1). Increased concentrations of IL-1 are present in the plasma of patients with active rheumatoid arthritis and may be partially responsible for some of the systemic manifestations of the disease. IL-1 is released from many cells (most notably mononuclear phagocytes) in response to physical or chemical activation of the inflammatory process and appears to have a central role in both humoral and cellular immune reactions (*see* Dinarello, 1988).

Although some of the effects of IL-1 may be regarded as antiinflammatory (*e.g.*, increased production of gamma-interferon), other actions promote inflammation; these include mobilization of polymorphonuclear leukocytes from bone marrow and stimulation of their function, stimulation of the production of lymphokines by T lymphocytes, and promotion of adherence of leukocytes to endothelial cells. Other actions of IL-1 contribute to the fibrosis and tissue degeneration of the chronic proliferative phase of inflammation; these include stimulation of fibroblast proliferation, induction of collagenase by chondrocytes and synovial cells, and activation of osteoblasts/osteoclasts.

Of the available antiinflammatory drugs, only the adrenocorticosteroids are known to interfere with the synthesis and/or actions of cytokines such as IL-1 or tumor necrosis factor (*see* Chapter 60). Although some of the actions of these cytokines are accompanied by the release of prostaglandins and/or thromboxane A_2, only their pyrogenic effects are blocked by inhibitors of cyclooxygenase (*see* below). In addition, many of the actions of the prostaglandins are inhibitory to the immune response, including suppression of the function of helper T cells and B cells and inhibition of the production of IL-1. Thus, it is difficult to ascribe the antirheumatoid effects of aspirin-like drugs solely to inhibition of prostaglandin synthesis. It has been proposed that salicylate and certain other aspirin-like drugs can directly inhibit the activation and function of neutrophils, even though prostaglandins exert similar inhibitory activity (*see* Weissmann, in Symposium, 1987a). However, high concentrations of the drugs are required for such effects to be manifest *in vitro*, and the relationship of these observations to therapeutic responses to the drugs remains controversial.

Pain. The aspirin-like drugs are usually classified as mild analgesics, but this classification is not altogether correct. A consideration of the type of pain as well as its intensity is important in the assessment of analgesic efficacy. In some forms of postoperative pain, for example, the aspirin-like drugs can be superior to the opioid analgesics. Moreover they are particularly effective in settings in which inflammation has caused sensitization of pain receptors to normally painless mechanical or chemical stimuli.

Prostaglandins are associated particularly with the development of pain that accompanies injury or inflammation. Large doses of PGE_2 or $PGF_{2\alpha}$, given to women by intramuscular or subcutaneous injection to induce abortion, cause intense local pain. Prostaglandins can also cause headache and vascular pain when infused intravenously. Although the doses of prostaglandins required to elicit pain are high in comparison with the concentrations expected *in vivo,* sensitization to painful stimuli (hyperalgesia) occurs when even minute amounts of PGE_1 are given intradermally. Moreover, subdermal infusion of mixtures of PGE_1 with small, subthreshold amounts of either bradykinin or histamine causes marked pain.

The capacity of prostaglandins to sensitize pain receptors to mechanical and chemical stimulation has been confirmed by electrophysiological measurements and appears to result from a lowering of the threshold of the polymodal nociceptors of C fibers (Perl, 1976). In general, the aspirin-like drugs do not affect the hyperalgesia or the pain caused by direct action of prostaglandins, consistent with the notion that it is their synthesis that is inhibited.

Fever. Regulation of body temperature requires a delicate balance between the production and loss of heat, and the hypothalamus regulates the set point at which body temperature is maintained. In fever, this set point is elevated, and aspirin-like drugs promote its return to normal. These drugs do not influence body temperature when it is elevated by such factors as exercise or increases in the ambient temperature.

Fever may be a result of infection or one of the sequelae of tissue damage, inflammation, graft rejection, malignancy, or other disease states. A common feature of these conditions is the enhanced formation of cytokines such as IL-1 or tumor necrosis factor by neutrophils and other cells; this induces the synthesis of PGE_2 in vascular organs in the preoptic hypothalamic area. The prostaglandin acts within the hypothalamus to produce the resultant elevation of body temperature by processes that appear to be mediated by cyclic AMP. Aspirin-like drugs suppress this response by inhibiting the synthesis of PGE_2 (Dascombe, 1985; Stitt and Nadel, 1986). The evidence for this scenario includes the ability of prostaglandins, especially PGE_2, to produce fever when infused into the cerebral ventricles or when injected into the hypothalamus. In addition, fever is a frequent side effect of prostaglandins when they are administered to women as abortifacients. The fever produced by the administration of agents that enhance the synthesis of IL-1 and other cytokines, but not that caused by prostaglandins, is reduced by aspirin-like drugs (*see* Milton, 1982).

Inhibition of Prostaglandin Biosynthesis by Aspirin-like Drugs. Inhibition of prostaglandin biosynthesis by aspirin, indomethacin, or similar compounds has been demonstrated in many systems both *in vitro* and *in vivo*. This effect is dependent only on the drug reaching the cyclooxygenase enzyme. The distribution and pharmacokinetic properties of each agent thus have an important bearing on the drug's activity.

Aspirin-like drugs inhibit or interfere with a variety of other enzymes and cellular systems; however, few such actions occur at concentrations that inhibit the cyclooxygenase. It is more likely that inhibition of other enzymes may contribute to the toxic effects of these drugs, particularly with overdosage.

There is good evidence that therapeutic doses of aspirin-like compounds reduce prostaglandin biosynthesis in man. Such doses inhibit the production of prostaglandins by human platelets and reduce the prostaglandin content of human semen, urine, and the synovial fluid of arthritic knee joints. There is also a reasonably good rank–order correlation between the potency of these drugs as inhibitors of cyclooxygenase and their antiinflammatory activity (Vane and Botting, 1987). The only outstanding exception is indomethacin, which is apparently more potent in antiinflammatory tests than in the enzyme inhibition assay. In addition, there is a high degree of stereospecificity for antiinflammatory activity and inhibition of cyclooxygenase among several pairs of enantiomers of α-methyl arylacetic acids; in each instance the *d* isomer is more potent. Another example of this type of selectivity is provided by the drug sulindac; it is a prodrug that is only weakly active and is converted *in vivo* to a highly active antiinflammatory metabolite. Likewise, the drug itself has little ability to inhibit prostaglandin biosynthesis, but the sulfide metabolite is a potent inhibitor. Nevertheless, actions in addition to inhibition of cyclooxygenase may be involved in the therapeutic effects of aspirin-like drugs in the treatment of rheumatoid arthritis (*see* above). Furthermore, the degree to which microsomal preparations of cyclooxygenase from different tissues are inhibited by aspirin-like drugs varies considerably. This variability may result because there are multiple forms of the enzyme, and thus it may be possible to design drugs with greater tissue specificity.

Mode of Inhibitory Action. Aspirin-like drugs inhibit the conversion of arachidonic acid to the unstable endoperoxide intermediate, PGG_2, a reaction that is catalyzed by the cyclooxygenase (*see* Chapter 24). Individual agents have differing mechanisms for inhibition of cyclooxygenase; some are competitive inhibitors, but many exert effects that disappear only slowly. Others, most notably acetaminophen, can block the enzyme only in an environment that is low in peroxides (*e.g.*, the hypothalamus) (Marshall *et al.*, 1987). This may explain the poor antiinflammatory activity of acetaminophen, since sites of inflammation usually contain high concentrations of peroxides that are generated by leukocytes. Aspirin acetylates a serine at or near the active site of cyclooxygenase (Roth and Siok, 1978). Platelets are especially susceptible to this action because they have little or no capacity for protein biosynthesis and thus cannot regenerate the enzyme. In practical terms this means that a single dose of aspirin will inhibit the platelet cyclooxygenase for the life of the platelet (8 to 11 days); in man, a daily dose as small as 40 mg is sufficient to produce this effect. In contrast to aspirin, salicylic acid has no acetylating capacity. Nevertheless, it is as active as aspirin in reducing the synthesis of prostaglandins *in vivo*.

SHARED THERAPEUTIC ACTIVITIES AND SIDE EFFECTS OF ASPIRIN-LIKE DRUGS

All aspirin-like drugs are antipyretic, analgesic, and antiinflammatory, but there are important differences in their activities. For example, acetaminophen is antipyretic and analgesic but is only weakly antiinflammatory. The reasons for such differences are not fully understood, but differential sensitivity of enzymes in the target tissues may be important (*see* above).

When employed as analgesics, these drugs are usually effective only against pain of low-to-moderate intensity. Although their maximal effects are much lower, they lack the unwanted effects of the opioids on the central nervous system (CNS), including respiratory depression and the development of physical dependence. Aspirin-like drugs do not change the perception of sensory modalities other than pain. Chronic postoperative pain or pain arising from inflammation is particularly well controlled by aspirin-like drugs, whereas pain arising from the hollow viscera is usually not relieved.

As antipyretics, aspirin-like drugs reduce the body temperature in febrile states. Although all such drugs are antipyretics and analgesics, some are not suitable for either routine or prolonged use because of toxicity; phenylbutazone is an example.

These drugs find their chief clinical application as antiinflammatory agents in the treatment of musculoskeletal disorders, such as rheumatoid arthritis, osteoarthritis, and ankylosing spondylitis. In general, aspirin-like drugs provide only symptomatic relief from the pain and inflammation associated with the disease and do not arrest the progression of pathological injury to tissue during severe episodes.

In addition to sharing many therapeutic activities, aspirin-like drugs share several unwanted effects. The most common is a propensity to induce gastric or intestinal ulceration that can sometimes be accompanied by anemia from the resultant blood loss. Aspirin-like drugs vary considerably in their tendency to cause such erosions and ulcers (*see* individual sections). Gastric damage by these agents can be brought about by at least two distinct mechanisms. Although local irritation by orally administered drugs allows back diffusion of acid into the gastric mucosa and induces tissue damage, parenteral administration can also cause damage and bleeding. This appears to be correlated with inhibition of the biosynthesis of gastric prostaglandins, especially PGI_2 and PGE_2 (Isselbacher, in Symposium, 1987a, 1988a). These eicosanoids inhibit acid secretion by the stomach and promote the secretion of cytoprotective mucus in the intestine; inhibition of their synthesis may render the stomach more susceptible to damage.

Other side effects of these drugs that probably depend upon blockade of the synthesis of endogenous prostaglandins include disturbances in platelet function, the prolongation of gestation or spontaneous labor, and changes in renal function. Platelet function appears to be disturbed because aspirin-like drugs prevent the formation by the platelets of thromboxane A_2 (TXA_2), a potent aggregating agent. This accounts for the tendency of these drugs to increase the bleeding time. As mentioned, aspirin is a particularly effective inhibitor of platelet function; this ''side effect'' has been exploited in the prophylactic treatment of thromboembolic disorders. Prolongation of gestation by aspirin-like drugs has been demonstrated in both experimental animals and women. Prostaglandins of the E and F series are potent uterotropic agents, and their biosynthesis by the uterus increases dramatically in the hours before parturition. It is thus hypothesized that prostaglandins have a major role in the initiation and progression of labor and delivery (*see* Chapter 39).

Aspirin-like drugs have little effect on renal function in normal human subjects, presumably because the production of vasodilatory prostaglandins has only a minor role in Na^+-replete individuals. However, these drugs decrease renal blood flow and the rate of glomerular filtration in patients with congestive heart failure, hepatic cirrhosis with ascites, or chronic renal disease or in those who are hypovolemic for any reason (*see* Clive and Stoff, 1984; Pirson and van Ypersele de Strihou, 1986; Patrono and Dunn, 1987; Oates *et al.*, 1988); acute renal failure may be precipitated under these circumstances. In all of these settings renal perfusion is more dependent upon prostaglandins that cause vasodilatation and that can oppose the vasoconstrictive influences of norepinephrine and angiotensin II that result from the activation of pressor reflexes.

In addition to their hemodynamic effects in the kidney, aspirin-like drugs promote the retention of salt and water by reducing the prostaglandin-induced inhibition of both the reabsorption of chloride and the action of antidiuretic hormone. This may cause edema in some patients who are treated with an aspirin-like drug; it may also reduce the effectiveness of antihypertensive regimens (*see* Patrono and Dunn, 1987; Oates *et al.*, 1988). These drugs promote hyperkalemia by several mechanisms, including enhanced reabsorption of K^+ as a result of decreased availability of Na^+ at distal tubular sites and suppression of the prostaglandin-induced secretion of renin. The latter effect may account in part for the usefulness of aspirin-like drugs in the treatment of Bartter's syndrome, which is characterized by hypokalemia, hyperreninemia, hyperaldosteronism, juxtaglomerular hyperplasia, normotension, and resistance to the pressor effect of angiotensin II. Excessive production of renal prostaglandins may play an important part in the pathogenesis of this syndrome.

Although nephropathy is uncommonly associated with the long-term use of individual aspirin-like drugs, the abuse of analgesic mixtures has been linked to the development of renal injury, including papillary necrosis and chronic interstitial nephritis (*see* Kincaid-Smith, 1986). The injury is often insidious in onset, is usually manifest initially as reduced tubular function and concentrating ability, and may progress to irreversible renal insufficiency if misuse of analgesics continues. Females are involved more frequently than are males, and there is often a history of recurring urinary tract infection. Emotional disturbances are common, and other drugs may be abused concurrently. Despite numerous clinical observations and experimental studies in animals and man, crucial details of the problem remain unclear. Phenacetin was suggested to be the nephrotoxic component of analgesic mixtures and, therefore, was removed from these products. Although the incidence of analgesic nephropathy in some countries has subsequently declined, this has not been a universal result, especially in Australia. It is thus possible that chronic abuse of any aspirin-like drug or analgesic mixture may cause renal injury in the susceptible individual (*see* Maher, 1984). An acute interstitial nephritis can also occur as a rare complication of the use of aspirin-like drugs (Pirson and van Ypersele de Strihou, 1986).

Two other uses of aspirin-like drugs that depend upon their capacity to block prostaglandin biosynthesis also deserve mention. Prostaglandins have been implicated in the maintenance of patency of the ductus arteriosus, and indomethacin and related agents have been used in neonates to close the ductus when it has remained patent. The release of prostaglandins by the endometrium during menstruation may be a cause of severe cramps and other symptoms of primary dysmenorrhea; treatment of this condition with aspirin-like drugs has met with considerable success (*see* Shapiro, 1988).

Certain individuals display intolerance to aspirin and most aspirin-like drugs; this is manifest by symptoms that range from vasomotor rhinitis with profuse watery secretions, angioneurotic edema, generalized urticaria, and bronchial asthma to laryngeal edema and bronchoconstriction, hypotension, and shock. Although rare in children, this syndrome may occur in 20 to 25% of middle-aged patients with asthma, nasal polyps, or chronic urticaria (*see* Szczeklik, 1986; Oates *et al.*, 1988). Despite the resemblance to anaphylaxis, this reaction does not appear to be immunological in nature. Moreover, an individual who is intolerant to one aspirin-like drug may react when exposed to any of a variety of such agents, despite their chemical diversity. The underlying mechanism is unknown, but a common factor appears to be the ability of the drugs to inhibit cyclooxygenase. This has prompted the hypothesis that the reaction reflects the diversion of arachidonic acid metabolism toward the formation of increased amounts of leukotrienes and other products of lipoxygenase pathways (*see* Szczeklik, 1986; Stevenson and Lewis, 1987; Oates *et al.*, 1988). However, this view is as yet unproven and it does not explain why only a minority of patients with asthma or other predisposing conditions display the reaction.

Choice of Drug to Be Prescribed. The choice of an agent as an antipyretic or analgesic is seldom a problem. It is in the field of rheumatology that the decision becomes complex (*see* Hess and Tangnijkul, 1986). The choice among aspirin-like agents for the treatment of arthritides is largely empirical. A drug may be chosen and given for a week or more; if the therapeutic effect is adequate, treatment should be continued unless toxicity occurs. Large variations are possible in the response of individuals to different aspirin-like drugs, even when they are closely allied members of the same chemical family. Thus, a patient may do well on one propionic acid derivative (such as ibuprofen) but not on another. This may indicate that these drugs share (unequally) different types of therapeutic actions. Discussion of principles of the use of aspirin-like drugs is provided in several symposia and a monograph (Symposium, 1983a, 1983b, 1984; Lewis and Furst, 1987).

All the drugs in this chapter, with the exception of the *p*-aminophenol derivatives, have a tendency to cause gastrointestinal side effects, which may range from mild dyspepsia and heartburn to ulceration of the stomach or duodenum, sometimes with fatal results. Hypersensitivity to aspirin is a contraindication to therapy with any of the drugs discussed in this chapter; administration of any one of these could provoke a life-threatening reaction reminiscent of anaphylactic shock (*see* above).

When dealing with a child, the choice of drugs is considerably restricted, and only drugs that have been extensively tested in children should be used. This commonly means that only aspirin, naproxen, or tolmetin should be prescribed. However, the association of Reye's syndrome in children with the administration of aspirin for the treatment of febrile viral illnesses precludes its use in this setting. The use of any of the aspirin-like drugs in pregnant women is generally not recommended. If such a drug must be given to a pregnant woman, low doses of aspirin are probably the safest. Although toxic doses of salicylates cause teratogenic effects in animals, there is no evidence to suggest that salicylates in moderate doses have teratogenic effects on the human fetus. In any case, aspirin should be discontinued prior to the anticipated time of parturition in order to avoid complications such as prolongation of labor, increased risk of postpartum hemorrhage, and intrauterine closure of the ductus arteriosus.

Many aspirin-like drugs bind firmly to plasma proteins and thus may displace certain other drugs from the binding sites. Such interactions can occur in patients given salicylates or phenylbutazone together with warfarin, a sulfonylurea hypoglycemic agent, or methotrexate; the dosage of such agents may require adjustment, or concurrent administration should be avoided. The problem with warfarin is accentuated because almost all of the aspirin-like drugs disturb normal platelet function.

Initially, fairly low doses of the agent chosen should be prescribed to determine the patient's reaction. When the patient has problems with sleeping because of pain or morning stiffness, a larger single dose of the drug may be given at night; as an alternative, single doses of another drug (*e.g.*, 50 to 100 mg of indomethacin) may be given to supplement existing medication without much danger of serious side effects. A week is generally long enough to determine the effect of a given drug. If the drug is effective, treatment should be continued, reducing the dose if possible and stopping it altogether if it is no longer necessary. Side effects usually appear in the first weeks of therapy. If the patient does not respond, another compound should be tried, since there is a marked variation in the response of individuals to different but closely related drugs.

For mild arthropathies, the scheme outlined above, together with rest and physical therapy, will probably be effective. However, patients with a more debilitating disease may not respond adequately. In such cases, more aggressive therapy should be initiated with aspirin or another agent. It is best to avoid continuous combination therapy with more than one aspirin-like drug; there is little evidence of extra benefit to the patient, and the incidence of side effects is generally additive.

For the seriously debilitated patient who cannot tolerate these drugs or in whom they are not adequately effective, other forms of therapy should be considered. Gold, hydroxychloroquine, and penicillamine are discussed in a separate section of this chapter. Other relevant drugs include immunosuppressive agents (Chapter 53) and glucocorticoids (Chapter 60).

A final important consideration is the cost of therapy, particularly since these agents are frequently used on a long-term basis. Generally speaking, aspirin is very inexpensive, ibuprofen has become less costly than phenylbutazone and indomethacin, and the cost of the newer drugs can be very high.

THE SALICYLATES

Despite the introduction of many new drugs, aspirin (acetylsalicylic acid) is still the most widely prescribed analgesic–antipyretic and antiinflammatory agent, and it is the standard for the comparison and evaluation of the others. Prodigious amounts of the drug are consumed in the United States; some estimates place the quantity as high as 10 to 20 thousand tons annually. The layman relies upon it as the common household analgesic; yet, because the drug is so generally available, its usefulness is often underrated. Despite the efficacy and safety of aspirin as an analgesic and antirheumatic agent, it is necessary to be aware of its role in Reye's syndrome and as a common cause of lethal drug poisoning in young children, as well as its potential for serious toxicity if used improperly.

The older literature on salicylates has been summarized by Hanzlik (1927). More recent reviews of some of the clinical pharmacology appear in several symposia (1983a, 1983c) and in a monograph (Rainsford, 1985a).

Chemistry. Salicylic acid (orthohydroxybenzoic acid) is so irritating that it can only be used externally; therefore, various derivatives of this acid have been synthesized for systemic use. These comprise two large classes, namely, esters of salicylic acid obtained by substitution in the carboxyl group and salicylate esters of organic acids in which the carboxyl group of salicylic acid is retained and substitution is made in the OH group. For example, aspirin is an ester of acetic acid. In addition, there are salts of salicylic acid. The chemical relationships can be seen from the structural formulas shown in Table 26–1.

Structure–Activity Relationship. Salicylates generally act by virtue of their content of salicylic acid, although some of the unique effects of aspirin are due to its capacity to acetylate proteins (*see* below). Substitutions on the carboxyl or hydroxyl groups change the potency or toxicity of the compound. The *ortho* position of the OH group is an important feature for the action of salicylate. Benzoic acid, C_6H_5COOH, shares many of the actions of salicylic acid but is much weaker. The effects of simple substitutions on the benzene ring have been extensively studied, and new salicylate derivatives are still being synthesized. A difluorophenyl derivative, diflunisal, is also available for clinical use.

PHARMACOLOGICAL PROPERTIES

Analgesia. As noted above, the types of pain usually relieved by salicylates are those of low intensity that arise from integumental structures rather than from viscera, especially headache, myalgia, and arthralgia. The salicylates are more widely used for pain relief than is any other class of drugs. Long-term use does not lead to tolerance or addiction, and toxicity is lower than that of opioid analgesics. The salicylates alleviate pain by virtue of a peripheral action (*see* above); direct effects on the CNS may also be involved.

Antipyresis. As discussed above, salicylates usually lower elevated body temperatures rapidly and effectively. However, moderate doses that produce this effect also increase oxygen consumption and metabolic rate. In toxic doses, these compounds have a pyretic effect that results in sweating; this enhances the dehydration that occurs in salicylate intoxication (*see* below).

Table 26–1. STRUCTURAL FORMULAS OF THE SALICYLATES

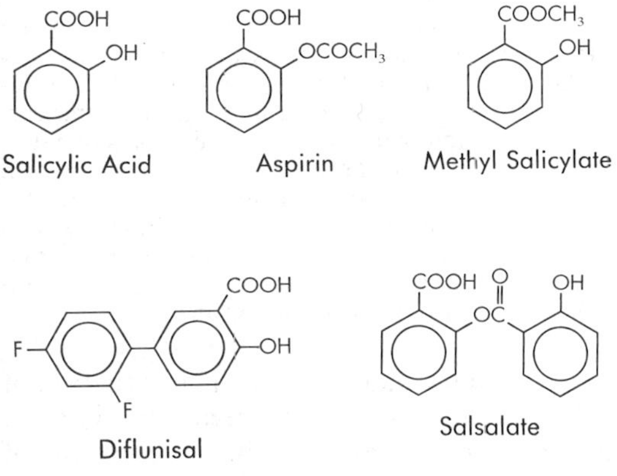

Miscellaneous Neurological Effects. In high doses, salicylates have toxic effects on the CNS, consisting of stimulation (including convulsions) followed by depression. Confusion, dizziness, tinnitus, high-tone deafness, delirium, psychosis, stupor, and coma may occur. The tinnitus and hearing loss caused by salicylate poisoning are due to increased labyrinthine pressure or an effect on the hair cells of the cochlea. Tinnitus is typically observed at salicylate concentrations of 200 to 450 μg/ml, and there is a close relation between the extent of hearing loss and the concentration of salicylate in plasma. The symptoms are completely reversible within 2 or 3 days after withdrawal of the drug.

Salicylates induce nausea and vomiting, which result from stimulation of sites that are accessible from the cerebrospinal fluid (CSF), probably in the medullary chemoreceptor trigger zone (CTZ). In man, centrally induced nausea and vomiting generally appear at plasma salicylate concentrations of about 270 μg/ml, but these same effects may occur at much lower plasma values as a result of local gastric irritation.

Respiration. The effects of salicylate on respiration are important because they contribute to the serious acid–base balance disturbances that characterize poisoning by this class of compounds. Salicylates stimulate respiration directly and indirectly. Full therapeutic doses of salicylates increase oxygen consumption and CO_2 production (especially in skeletal muscle); these effects are a result of salicylate-induced uncoupling of oxidative phosphorylation (*see* below). The increased production of CO_2 stimulates respiration. The increased alveolar ventilation balances the increased CO_2 production, and thus plasma CO_2 tension (P_{CO_2}) does not change. The initial increase in alveolar ventilation is characterized mainly by an increase in depth of respiration and only a slight increase in rate. If the respiratory response to CO_2 has been depressed by the administration of a barbiturate or an opioid, salicylates will cause a marked increase in plasma P_{CO_2} and respiratory acidosis.

Salicylate directly stimulates the respiratory center in the medulla. This results in marked hyperventilation, characterized by an increase in depth and a pronounced increase in rate. Patients with salicylate poisoning may have prominent increases in respiratory minute volume, and respiratory alkalosis ensues. Plasma salicylate concentrations of 350 μg/ml are nearly always associated with hyperventilation in man, and marked hyperpnea occurs when the level approaches 500 μg/ml.

A depressant effect of salicylate on the medulla appears after high doses or after prolonged exposure. Toxic doses of salicylates cause central respiratory paralysis as well as circulatory collapse secondary to vasomotor depression. Since enhanced CO_2 production continues, respiratory acidosis ensues (*see* below).

Acid–Base Balance and Electrolyte Pattern. Therapeutic doses of salicylate produce definite changes in the acid–base balance and electrolyte pattern. The initial event, as discussed above, is respiratory alkalosis. Compensation for the respiratory alkalosis is achieved by increased renal excretion of bicarbonate, which is accompanied by Na^+ and K^+; plasma bicarbonate is thus lowered, and blood pH returns toward normal. This is the stage of compensated respiratory alkalosis. This stage is most often seen in adults given intensive salicylate therapy and seldom proceeds further.

Subsequent changes in acid–base status generally occur only when toxic doses of salicylates are ingested by infants and children and occasionally after large doses in adults. In infants and children, the phase of respiratory alkalosis may not be observed, since the child with salicylate intoxication is rarely seen early enough. The stage generally present is characterized by a decrease in blood pH, a low plasma bicarbonate concentration, and a normal or nearly normal plasma P_{CO_2}; except for the P_{CO_2}, these changes resemble those of metabolic acidosis. However, in reality there is a combination of respiratory acidosis and metabolic acidosis produced as follows. The enhanced production of CO_2 outstrips its alveolar excretion because of direct salicylate-induced depression of respiration; consequently, plasma P_{CO_2} increases and blood pH decreases. Since the concentration of bicarbonate in plasma is already low because of increased renal bicarbonate excretion, the acid–base status at this stage is essentially an uncompensated respiratory acidosis. Superimposed, however, is a true metabolic acidosis caused by accumulation of acids as a result of three processes. First, toxic concentrations of salicylates displace about 2 to 3 mEq per liter of plasma bicarbonate. Second, vasomotor depression caused by toxic doses of salicylate impairs renal function with consequent accumulation of strong acids of metabolic origin, namely, sulfuric and phosphoric acids. Third, organic acids accumulate secondary to salicylate-induced derangement of carbohydrate metabolism, especially pyruvic, lactic, and acetoacetic acids.

The series of events that produce acid–base disturbances in salicylate intoxication also cause alterations of water and electrolyte balance. The low plasma P_{CO_2} leads to decreased renal tubular reabsorption of bicarbonate and increased renal excretion of Na^+, K^+, and water (*see* introduction to Section VI). In addition, water is lost by salicylate-induced sweating and by insensible water loss through the lungs during hyperventilation, and dehydration rapidly occurs. Since more water than electrolyte is lost through the lungs and by sweating, the dehydration is associated with hypernatremia. Prolonged exposure to high doses of salicylate also causes depletion of K^+ due to both renal and extrarenal factors.

Cardiovascular Effects. Ordinary therapeutic doses of salicylates have no important direct cardiovascular actions. The peripheral vessels tend to dilate after large doses because of a direct effect on their smooth muscle. Toxic amounts depress the circulation directly and by central vasomotor paralysis.

In patients given large doses of sodium salicylate or aspirin, such as the doses used in acute rheumatic fever, the circulating plasma volume increases (about 20%), the hematocrit falls, and cardiac output and work are increased. Consequently, in patients with clear evidence of carditis, such alterations can cause congestive failure and pulmonary edema. High doses of salicylates can also produce noncardiogenic pulmonary edema, particularly in older patients who are ingesting salicylates regularly over a long term.

Gastrointestinal Effects. The ingestion of salicylate may result in epigastric distress, nausea, and vomiting. The mechanism of the emetic effect is discussed above. Salicylate may also cause gastric ulceration; exacerbation of peptic ulcer symptoms (heartburn, dyspepsia), gastrointestinal hemorrhage, and erosive gastritis have all been reported in patients on high-dose therapy, but may occur rarely with low doses as a hypersensitivity response. Salicylate-induced gastric bleeding is painless and may lead to an iron-deficiency anemia.

The daily ingestion of 4 or 5 g of aspirin, a dose that produces plasma salicylate concentrations in the usual range for antiinflammatory therapy (120 to 350 μg/ml), results in an average fecal blood loss of about 3 to 8 ml per day as compared with approximately 0.6 ml per day in untreated subjects (Leonards and Levy, 1973). Gastroscopic or direct examination in salicylate-treated subjects reveals discrete ulcerative and hemorrhagic lesions of the gastric mucosa; in many cases, multiple hemorrhagic lesions with sharply demarcated areas of focal necrosis are observed. The incidence of bleeding is highest with salicylates that dissolve slowly and deposit as particles in the gastric mucosal folds.

As discussed above, the mechanisms by which salicylates injure gastric mucosal cells are complex (*see* Ivey, in Symposium, 1988a). Deleterious effects result from local actions (*e.g.*, "back diffusion" of acid), which cause injury to mucosal cells and the submucosal capillaries with subsequent necrosis and bleeding, and from effects secondary to inhibition of prostaglandin synthesis (*e.g.*, increased acid secretion and decreased mucus production). There may also be an increased tendency to bleed because of impaired platelet aggregation.

Hepatic and Renal Effects. Salicylates can produce at least two forms of hepatic injury. In one form, hepatotoxicity is dose dependent and is usually associated with plasma concentrations that are maintained above 150 μg/ml. The vast majority of cases occur in patients with connective tissue disorders. There are usually no symptoms, and elevated enzyme (transaminase) activities in plasma are the principal indications of hepatic damage. About 5% of the patients also have hepatomegaly, anorexia, and nausea, and jaundice may be present; in these instances, salicylates should be discontinued because of the potential hazard of fatal hepatic necrosis. For these and other reasons, restriction of salicylates has been advised in patients with chronic liver disease.

Considerable evidence implicates the use of salicylates as an important factor in the severe hepatic injury and encephalopathy observed in Reye's syndrome (*see* Heubi *et al.*, 1987; Hurwitz *et al.*, 1987; Pinsky *et al.*, 1988). This syndrome is a rare but often fatal consequence of infection with varicella and various other viruses, especially the influenza virus. Although a causal relationship between salicylates and Reye's syndrome has not been established, there is a strong epidemiological association. It has been proposed that aspirin and the viral illness may act to damage mitochondria, perhaps preferentially in genetically predisposed individuals (Heubi *et al.*, 1987; Pinsky *et al.*, 1988). The use of salicylates in children or adolescents with chickenpox or influenza is contraindicated.

As discussed above, salicylates can cause retention of salt and water as well as acute reduction of renal function in patients with congestive heart failure or hypovolemia. Although long-term use of salicylates alone is rarely associated with nephrotoxicity, the prolonged and excessive ingestion of analgesic mixtures containing salicylates in combination with acetaminophen or salicylamide can produce papillary necrosis and interstitial nephritis (Clive and Stoff, 1984).

Uricosuric Effects. The effects of salicylates on uric acid excretion are markedly dependent on dose. Low doses (1 or 2 g per day) may decrease urate excretion and elevate plasma urate concentrations; intermediate doses (2 or 3 g per day) usually do not alter urate excretion; large doses (over 5 g per day) induce uricosuria and lower plasma urate levels. Such large doses are poorly tolerated. Even small doses of salicylate can block the effects of probenecid and other uricosuric agents that decrease tubular reabsorption of uric acid (*see* Chapter 30).

Effects on the Blood. Ingestion of aspirin by normal individuals causes a definite prolongation of the bleeding time. For example, a single dose of 0.65 g of aspirin approximately doubles the mean bleeding time of normal persons for a period of 4 to 7 days. This effect is probably due to acetylation of platelet cyclooxygenase and the consequent reduced formation of TXA_2.

Patients with severe hepatic damage, hypoprothrombinemia, vitamin K deficiency, or hemophilia should avoid aspirin because the inhibition of platelet hemostasis can result in hemorrhage. If conditions permit, aspirin therapy should be stopped at least 1 week prior to surgery; care should also be exercised in the use of aspirin during long-term treatment with oral anticoagulant agents because of the possible danger of blood loss from the gastric mucosa. However, the intentional use of aspirin is being investigated for the prophylaxis of thromboembolic disease, especially in the coronary and cerebral circulation (*see* Reilly and Fitzgerald, 1988; *see also* Chapter 55).

Salicylates do not ordinarily alter the leukocyte, platelet, or erythrocyte count, the hematocrit, or the hemoglobin content. In acute rheumatic fever, salicylate therapy can reduce leukocytosis and the elevated erythrocyte sedimentation rate. The plasma iron concentration is markedly decreased and erythrocyte survival time is shortened by doses of 3 to 4 g per day. Aspirin is included among the drugs that can cause a mild degree of hemolysis in individuals with a deficiency of glucose-6-phosphate dehydrogenase.

Effects on Rheumatic, Inflammatory, and Immunological Processes, and on Connective Tissue Metabolism. For almost 100 years the salicylates have retained their preeminent position in the treatment of the rheumatic diseases. Although they suppress the clinical signs and even improve the histological picture in acute rheumatic fever, subsequent tissue damage such as cardiac lesions and other visceral involvement is unaffected. In addition to their action on prostaglandin biosynthesis, the mechanism of action of the salicylates in rheumatic disease may also involve effects on other cellular and immunological processes in mesenchymal and connective tissues.

Because of the known relationship between rheumatic fever and immunological processes, attention has been directed to the capacity of salicylates to suppress a variety of antigen–antibody reactions. These include the inhibition of antibody production, of antigen–antibody aggregation, and of antigen-induced release of histamine. Salicylates also induce a nonspecific stabilization of capillary permeability during immunological insults. The concentrations of salicylates needed to produce these effects are high, and the relationship of these effects to the antirheumatic efficacy of salicylates is yet to be determined.

Salicylates can also influence the metabolism of connective tissue, and these effects may be involved in their antiinflammatory action. For example, salicylates can affect the composition, biosynthesis, or metabolism of connective tissue mucopolysaccharides in the ground substance that provides barriers to spread of infection and inflammation.

Metabolic Effects. The salicylates have multiple effects on metabolic processes, some of which have already been discussed. Only a few pertinent aspects will be presented here.

Oxidative Phosphorylation. The uncoupling of oxidative phosphorylation by salicylate is similar to that induced by 2,4-dinitrophenol. The effect may occur with doses of salicylate used in the treatment of rheumatoid arthritis and can result in the inhibition of a number of adenosine triphosphate (ATP)–dependent reactions. Other consequences include the salicylate-induced increase in oxygen uptake and carbon dioxide production described above, the depletion of hepatic glycogen, and the pyretic effect of toxic doses of salicylate. Salicylate in toxic doses may decrease aerobic metabolism as a result of inhibition of various dehydrogenases, by competing with the pyridine nucleotide coenzymes, and inhibition of some oxidases that require nucleotides as coenzymes, such as xanthine oxidase.

Carbohydrate Metabolism. Large doses of salicylates may cause hyperglycemia and glycosuria and deplete liver and muscle glycogen; these effects are partly explained by the release of epinephrine. Such doses also reduce aerobic metabolism of glucose, increase glucose-6-phosphatase activity, and promote the secretion of glucocorticoids.

Nitrogen Metabolism. Salicylate in toxic doses causes a significant negative nitrogen balance, characterized by an aminoaciduria. Although adrenocortical activation may contribute to the negative nitrogen balance by enhancing protein catabolism, the mechanism of the aminoaciduria produced by salicylates is poorly understood.

Fat Metabolism. Salicylates reduce lipogenesis by partially blocking incorporation of acetate into fatty acids; they also inhibit epinephrine-stimulated lipolysis in fat cells and displace long-chain fatty acids from binding sites on human plasma proteins. The combination of these effects leads to increased entry and enhanced oxidation of fatty acids in muscle, liver, and other tissues, and to decreased plasma concentrations of free fatty acids, phospholipid, and cholesterol; the oxidation of ketone bodies is also increased.

Endocrine Effects. *Adrenal Cortex.* Very large doses of salicylate stimulate steroid secretion by the adrenal cortex through an effect on the hypothalamus and transiently increase plasma concentrations of free adrenocorticosteroids by displacement from plasma proteins. However, it is clear that the antiinflammatory effects of salicylate are independent of these effects on adrenocorticosteroids.

Thyroid Gland. Long-term administration of salicylate decreases thyroidal uptake and clearance of iodine, but increases oxygen consumption and rate of disappearance of thyroxine and triiodothyronine from the circulation. These effects are probably due to the competitive displacement by salicylate of thyroxine and triiodothyronine from transthyretin and the thyroxine-binding globulin in plasma.

Salicylates and Pregnancy. There is no evidence that moderate therapeutic doses of salicylates cause fetal damage in human beings; however, babies born to women who ingest salicylates for long periods may have significantly reduced weights at birth. In addition, there is an increase in perinatal mortality, anemia, antepartum and postpartum hemorrhage, prolonged gestation, and complicated deliveries (*see* above).

Local Irritant Effects. Salicylic acid is quite irritating to skin and mucosa and destroys epithelial cells. The keratolytic action of the free acid is employed for the local treatment of warts, corns, fungal infections, and certain types of eczematous dermatitis. The tissue cells swell, soften, and desquamate. The salts of salicylic acid are innocuous to the unbroken skin; however, if the free acid is released in the stomach, the gastric mucosa may be irritated. Methyl salicylate (oil of wintergreen) is irritating to both skin and gastric mucosa and is only used externally.

Pharmacokinetics and Metabolism. These important aspects of the salicylates have been reviewed by Davison (1971).

Absorption. Orally ingested salicylates are absorbed rapidly, partly from the stomach but mostly from the upper small intestine. Appreciable concentrations are found in plasma in less than 30 minutes; after a single dose, a peak value is reached in about 2 hours and then gradually declines. Rate of absorption is determined by many factors, particularly the disintegration and dissolution rates if tablets are given, the pH at the mucosal surfaces, and gastric emptying time.

Salicylate absorption occurs by passive diffusion primarily of nondissociated salicylic acid or acetylsalicylic acid across gastrointestinal membranes and hence is influenced by gastric pH. Even though salicylate is more ionized as the pH is increased, a rise in pH also increases the solubility of salicylate, and the overall effect is to enhance absorption. As a result, there is little meaningful difference between the rates of absorption of sodium salicylate, aspirin, and the numerous buffered preparations of salicylates. The presence of food delays absorption of salicylates.

Rectal absorption of salicylate is usually slower, incomplete, and unreliable; rectal administration is therefore not advisable when high plasma concentrations of the drug are required. Salicylic acid is rapidly absorbed from the intact skin, especially when applied in oily liniments or ointments, and systemic poisoning has occurred from its application to large areas of skin. Methyl salicylate is likewise speedily absorbed when applied cutaneously; its gastrointestinal absorption may be delayed many hours, and, therefore, gastric lavage should be performed even in cases of poisoning that are seen late.

When nonionized salicylic acid in the gastric lumen enters mucosal cells, large amounts of salicylate can accumulate because of dissociation to the ionized species at the intracellular pH. As a result, gastric mucosal damage may occur.

Distribution. After absorption, salicylate is distributed throughout most body tissues and most transcellular fluids, primarily by pH-dependent passive processes. Salicylate is actively transported by a low-capacity, saturable system out of the CSF across the choroid plexus. The drug readily crosses the placental barrier.

The volumes of distribution of usual doses of aspirin and sodium salicylate in normal subjects average about 170 ml/kg of body weight; at high therapeutic doses, this volume increases to about 500 ml/kg because of saturation of binding sites on plasma proteins. Ingested aspirin is mainly absorbed as such, but some enters the systemic circulation as salicylic acid, because of hydrolysis by esterases in the gastrointestinal mucosa and the liver. Aspirin can be detected in the plasma only for a short time as a result of hydrolysis in plasma, liver, and erythrocytes; for example, 30 minutes after a dose of 0.65 g, only 27% of the total plasma salicylate is in the acetylated form. As a result, plasma concentrations of aspirin are always low and rarely exceed 20 μg/ml at ordinary therapeutic doses. Methyl salicylate is also rapidly hydrolyzed to salicylic acid, mainly in the liver.

At concentrations encountered clinically, from 80 to 90% of the salicylate is bound to plasma proteins, especially albumin; this fraction declines as plasma concentrations are increased. In addition, hypoalbuminemia, as may occur in rheumatoid arthritis, is associated with a proportionately higher level of free salicylate in the plasma. Salicylate competes with a variety of compounds for plasma protein binding sites; these include thyroxine, triiodothyronine, penicillin, phenytoin, sulfinpyrazone, bilirubin, uric acid, and naproxen. Aspirin is bound to a more limited extent; however, it acetylates human plasma albumin *in vivo* by reaction with the ε-amino group of lysine; this acetylation may change the binding of drugs to albumin. Hormones, DNA, platelets, and hemoglobin and other proteins are also acetylated.

Biotransformation and Excretion. The biotransformation of salicylate takes place in many tissues, but particularly in the hepatic endoplasmic reticulum and mitochondria. The three chief metabolic products are salicyluric acid (the glycine conjugate), the ether or phenolic glucuronide, and the ester or acyl glucuronide. In addition, a small fraction is oxidized to gentisic acid (2,5-dihydroxybenzoic acid) and to 2,3-dihydroxybenzoic and 2,3,5-trihydroxybenzoic acids; gentisuric acid, the glycine conjugate of gentisic acid, is also formed.

Salicylates are excreted in the urine as free salicylic acid (10%), salicyluric acid (75%), salicylic phenolic (10%) and acyl (5%) glucuronides, and gentisic acid (<1%). However, excretion of free salicylate is extremely variable and depends upon both the dose and the urinary pH. In alkaline urine, more than 30% of the ingested drug may be eliminated as free salicylate, whereas in acidic urine this may be as low as 2%.

The plasma half-life for aspirin is approximately 15 minutes; that for salicylate is 2 to 3 hours in low doses and about 12 hours at usual antiinflammatory doses. The half-life of salicylate may be as long as 15 to 30 hours at high therapeutic doses or when there is intoxication. This dose-dependent elimination is the result of the limited ability of the liver to form salicyluric acid and the phenolic glucuronide, and a larger proportion of unchanged drug is excreted in the urine at higher doses.

The plasma concentration of salicylate is increased by conditions that decrease glomerular filtration rate or reduce its secretion by the proximal tubule, such as renal disease or the presence of inhibitors that compete for the transport system (*e.g.*, probenecid). Changes in urinary pH also have significant effects on salicylate excretion; for example, the clearance of salicylate is about four times as great at pH 8.0 as at pH 6.0, and it is well above the glomerular filtration rate at pH 8.0. High rates of urine flow decrease tubular reabsorption, whereas the opposite is true in oliguria. The conjugates of salicylic acid with glycine and glucuronic acid do not readily back diffuse across the renal tubular cells. Their excretion, therefore, is both by glomerular filtration and proximal tubular secretion and is not pH dependent.

Preparations, Routes of Administration, and Dosage. The two most commonly used preparations of salicylate for systemic effects are sodium salicylate and aspirin (acetylsalicylic acid).

Sodium salicylate is available in regular or enteric-coated tablets that contain 325 or 650 mg of drug and in an injectable solution for parenteral use. *Aspirin* is available in regular or enteric-coated tablets ranging from 65 to 975 mg and in suppositories; timed-release tablets are also marketed.

The dose of salicylate depends on the condition being treated. The usual single dose of aspirin in adults is 300 mg to 1.0 g. This may be repeated every 4 hours. More intensive dosage regimens are employed in acute rheumatic fever and rheumatoid arthritis (*see* below).

The route of administration is nearly always oral. Parenteral administration is rarely necessary. The rectal administration of aspirin suppositories may be necessary in infants or when oral medication is not retained. Salicylates are conveniently taken in tablets or capsules with a full glass of water to minimize gastric irritation. Aspirin is poorly soluble, has many chemical incompatibilities, and should be dispensed only in solid dry form. Timed-release preparations are of limited value, since the half-time for elimination of salicylate is so long, particularly during high-dose therapy. Absorption from enteric-coated tablets is sometimes incomplete, but these formulations may produce less gastrointestinal irritation. Preparations of aspirin containing alkali or buffer are sometimes better tolerated, but alkalinization of the urine, which may occur, can shorten the plasma half-life of salicylates considerably (*see* above).

Other salicylates that are available for systemic use include *salsalate* (salicylsalicylic acid; DICALCID); it is hydrolyzed to salicylic acid during and after absorption. The drug is available in 500- and 750-mg tablets and 500-mg capsules; the maximal daily dose is 3 g given in 2 to 4 divided doses. *Salicylamide,* which is not metabolized to salicylate *in vivo,* has antipyretic, analgesic, and antiinflammatory effects similar to those of salicylate. It remains available only in certain combination preparations. Sodium thiosalicylate (injection), choline salicylate (oral liquid), and magnesium salicylate (tablets) are also available. A combination of choline and magnesium salicylates (TRILISATE) is formulated to contain 500 mg of salicylate per 5 ml (oral liquid) or 500 to 1000 mg per tablet; 1 to 3 doses per day may be given. The nonacetylated salicylates appear to produce a lower incidence of gastrointestinal ulceration and have less effect on platelet aggregation than does aspirin. Diflunisal is discussed below.

Mesalamine (5-aminosalicylic acid) is a salicylate that is used for its local effects in the treatment of inflammatory bowel disease. The drug is not effective orally because it is poorly absorbed and is inactivated before reaching the lower intestine. It is currently available as a rectal suspension enema (ROWASA) for treatment of mild-to-moderate proctosigmoiditis; formulations that deliver the intact drug to the lower intestine are under investigation (Schroeder *et al.,* 1987). *Sulfasalazine* (salicylazosulfapyridine; AZULFIDINE, AZALINE) contains mesalamine linked covalently to sulfapyridine (*see* Chapter 45); it is poorly absorbed after oral administration, but it is cleaved to its active components by bacteria in the colon. The drug is of benefit in the treatment of inflammatory bowel disease, principally because of the local actions of mesalamine. Sulfasalazine has also been used in the treatment of rheumatoid arthritis and ankylosing spondylitis (*see* Symposium, 1986a, 1988b); sulfapyridine, which is absorbed systemically, appears to be the most important therapeutic component in these conditions.

Methyl salicylate (*sweet birch oil, wintergreen oil, gaultheria oil, betula oil*) is employed only for cutaneous counterirritation and is distributed in the form of salves, liniments, and other preparations. *Salicylic acid* is primarily used for local application as a keratolytic agent in plasters, liquids, creams, ointments, and other topical preparations. However, a transdermal patch containing 15% salicylic acid has recently been marketed for systemic therapy.

TOXIC EFFECTS

As a result of their wide use and ready availability, salicylates are frequently the cause of intoxication. Poisoning or serious intoxication often occurs in children and is sometimes fatal. The drug should not be viewed as a harmless household remedy.

Hypersensitivity is also a cause of untoward responses to salicylate. Furthermore, renal or hepatic insufficiency or hypoprothrombinemia or other bleeding disorders enhance the possibility of salicylate toxicity. Children with fever and dehydration are particularly prone to intoxication from relatively small doses of salicylate. In addition, the use of aspirin is contraindicated in children and adolescents with febrile viral illnesses because of the risk of Reye's syndrome. Many of the unwanted effects that are common to the aspirin-like drugs are discussed above.

Salicylate Intoxication. The fatal dose varies with the preparation of salicylate. From 10 to 30 g of sodium salicylate or aspirin has caused death in adults, but much larger amounts (130 g of aspirin, in one case) have been ingested without fatal outcome. The lethal dose of methyl salicylate is considerably less than that of sodium salicylate. As little as 4 ml (4.7 g) of methyl salicylate may be fatal in children.

Symptoms and Signs. Mild chronic salicylate intoxication is termed salicylism. When fully developed, the syndrome includes headache, dizziness, ringing in the ears, difficulty in hearing, dimness of vision, mental confusion, lassitude, drowsiness, sweating, thirst, hyperventilation, nausea, vomiting, and occasionally diarrhea. A more severe degree of salicylate intoxication is characterized by more pronounced CNS disturbances (including generalized convulsions and coma), skin eruptions, and marked alterations in acid–base balance. Fever is usually prominent, especially in children. Dehydration often occurs as a result of hyperpyrexia, sweating, vomiting, and the loss of water vapor during hyperventilation. Gastrointestinal symptoms are often present; about 50% of individuals with plasma salicylate concentrations of more than 300 μg/ml experience nausea.

A prominent feature of salicylate intoxication is the disturbance in acid–base balance and electrolyte composition of the plasma described above. The most severe metabolic disturbances occur in infants and very young children who become intoxicated as the result of therapeutic overdosage; most of the acidotic patients seen with salicylate intoxication are in this group.

Hemorrhagic phenomena are occasionally seen during salicylate poisoning, the mechanism and significance of which have been discussed. Petechial hemorrhages are a prominent postmortem feature. Thrombocytopenic purpura is a rare complication. While hyperglycemia may occur during salicylate intoxication, hypoglycemia may be a serious consequence of toxicity in young children. It should be seriously considered in any young child with coma, convulsions, or cardiovascular collapse.

Severe toxic encephalopathy may be a prominent feature of salicylate poisoning and may be difficult to differentiate from rheumatic encephalopathy. As poisoning progresses, central stimulation is replaced by increasing depression, stupor, and coma. Cardiovascular collapse and respiratory insufficiency ensue, and terminal asphyxial convulsions and pulmonary edema sometimes appear. Death usually results from respiratory failure after a period of unconsciousness.

Salicylate toxicity in adults may not be readily diagnosed because such patients usually become intoxicated from their therapeutic regimen; there is no history of acute overdosage. Prominent features of toxicity in this group are noncardiogenic pulmonary edema, nonfocal neurological abnormalities, and laboratory findings that include acid–base abnormalities, unexplained ketosis, and a prolonged prothrombin time (Anderson *et al.,* 1976).

Symptoms of poisoning by methyl salicylate differ little from those described for aspirin. Central excitation, intense hyperpnea, and hyperpyrexia are prominent features. The odor of the drug can easily be detected on the breath and in the urine and vomitus. Poisoning by salicylic acid differs only in the increased prominence of gastrointestinal symptoms due to the marked local irritation.

Treatment. Salicylate poisoning represents an acute medical emergency, and death may result despite all recommended procedures. The treatment is largely symptomatic. Salicylate medication is withdrawn as soon as intoxication is suspected. The patient should be hospitalized, particularly in cases of poisoning with methyl salicylate. Blood should be obtained for plasma salicylate determinations and acid–base and electrolyte studies. The salicylate concentration is reasonably well correlated with clinical severity, when corrected for the duration of the intoxication, and is of value in assessing the type of therapy to be instituted. Since absorption of salicylate from the gastrointestinal tract may be delayed for many hours after an overdose, measures to reduce such absorption should always be employed. These include induction of emesis, gastric lavage, administration of activated charcoal, or a combination of these.

Hyperthermia and dehydration are the immediate threats to life, and the initial therapy must be directed to their correction and to the maintenance of adequate renal function. External sponging with tepid water or alcohol should be provided quickly to any child with very high fever. Adequate amounts of intravenous fluids must be given promptly. The type and amount of solutions to be employed depend upon the interpretation of the laboratory data on acid–base balance. If the patient presents with an acidosis, correction of the low blood pH is essential, especially since acidosis results in a shift of salicylate from plasma into brain and other tissues. Bicarbonate solution should be infused intravenously, if possible, in sufficient quantity to maintain alkaline diuresis. Correction of ketosis and hypoglycemia by administration of glucose is also essential for complete control of the metabolic acidosis; however, the ketosis clears only slowly. If K^+ deficiency occurs during salicylate intoxication, it should be treated by adding the cation to the intravenous fluids once it has been determined that urine formation is adequate. Plasma transfusion may be beneficial, especially if the shock syndrome intervenes. Hemorrhagic phenomena may necessitate whole-blood transfusion and vitamin K (phytonadione).

Measures to rid the body of salicylate rapidly should be undertaken immediately. Forced diuresis with alkalinizing solution appears to be better than alkali alone; however, this may be dangerous in adults who are prone to develop pulmonary edema. In severe intoxication, hemodialysis is the most effective measure available for the removal of salicylate and for the correction of the electrolyte and acid–base disturbances. Hemodialysis should be considered in patients with salicylate concentrations above 1000 μg/ml, in those with severe acid–base disturbances whose clinical condition is deteriorating despite otherwise-appropriate therapy, and in those who have associated serious disease, particularly cardiac, pulmonary, or renal disease. (*See* Brenner and Simon, 1982; Meredith and Vale, 1986.)

Aspirin Hypersensitivity. Aspirin hypersensitivity or intolerance is discussed above. It is important to recognize this syndrome even though it is rather uncommon, since the administration of aspirin and many other aspirin-like drugs may result in severe and possibly fatal reactions. The nonacetylated salicylates appear to be considerably less apt to produce these reactions as compared with aspirin and other agents. Treatment of such responses does not differ from that ordinarily employed in acute anaphylactic reactions. Epinephrine is the drug of choice and usually controls angioedema and urticaria without difficulty.

THERAPEUTIC USES

There are many systemic and a few local uses of the salicylates. Several are based on tradition and empirical results rather than on a clear understanding of the mechanism of therapeutic benefit.

Systemic Uses. *Antipyresis.* Antipyretic therapy is reserved for patients in whom fever in itself may be deleterious, and for those who experience considerable relief when a fever is lowered. Little is known about the relationship between fever and the acceleration of inflammatory or immune processes; it may at times be a protective physiological mechanism. The course of the patient's illness may be obscured by the relief of symptoms and the reduction of fever from the use of antipyretic drugs. The antipyretic dose of salicylate for adults is 325 to 650 mg orally every 4 hours; for children, 50 to 75 mg/kg per day is given in four to six divided doses, not to exceed a total daily dose of 3.6 g.

Analgesia. Salicylate is valuable for the nonspecific relief of certain types of pain, for example, headache, arthritis, dysmenorrhea, neuralgia, and myalgia. For this purpose, it is prescribed in the same doses and manner as for antipyresis.

Acute Rheumatic Fever. In this disease, the salicylates suppress the acute exudative inflammatory process but do not affect the duration or progression of the disease or the later phases of granulomatous inflammation or scar formation. Nevertheless, if a patient has severe carditis and heart failure, the nonspecific antiinflammatory effect of salicylates and particularly of adrenocorticosteroids may be invaluable in reducing the burden upon the heart.

For maximal suppression of rheumatic inflammation, doses that provide a plasma salicylate concentration of 150 to 300 μg/ml should be maintained, but polyarthritis and fever usually respond to smaller amounts. For adults, a total daily dosage of 5 to 8 g, given at intervals in 1-g amounts, usually suffices. Children are given 100 mg/kg per day, in divided portions every 4 to 6 hours, for up to 1 week; the dose is then reduced in stepwise fashion at weekly intervals to 60 to 75 mg/kg per day and maintained as long as necessary. Anorexia, tinnitus, nausea, and vomiting are common during the first 3 or 4 days of therapy, but tend to subside despite continuation of medication. Ordinarily, full doses are continued until at least 2 weeks after the patient is asymptomatic and all evidence of active inflammation has disappeared. The drug is then gradually discontinued over a period of 7 to 10 days. If symptoms and signs of the disease reappear, salicylate therapy is reinstituted. Therapy with glucocorticoids does not yield overall results superior to those obtained with the salicylates; salicylate and glucocorticoids are additive in their effects. If carditis is not evident, salicylates and not steroids should be used. However, if acute severe carditis is present, most investigators believe adrenocorticosteroids should be given instead of salicylates, at least initially.

Rheumatoid Arthritis. Despite the development of the newer antiinflammatory agents, salicylates are still regarded as the standard with which other drugs should be compared for the treatment of rheumatoid arthritis. In addition to the analgesia that allows more effective therapeutic exercises, there is improvement in appetite and a feeling of well-being. Salicylates also reduce the inflammation in joint tissues and surrounding structures. Damage to joints is the most difficult aspect of rheumatoid arthritis to manage, and any agent that reduces the inflammation is important in lessening or delaying the development of crippling. Salicylates can be shown to produce objectively measurable antiinflammatory changes when given in large doses for long periods to patients with active rheumatoid disease. Large doses of salicylates, such as those used for rheumatic fever (4 to 6 g daily), are advised, but some patients respond well to less.

The majority of patients with rheumatoid arthritis can be controlled with salicylates alone or with other aspirin-like antiinflammatory agents. Some require therapy with more toxic drugs, such as gold salts, hydroxychloroquine, penicillamine, adrenocorticosteroids, or immunosuppressive agents.

Other Uses. Because of the potent and long-lasting effect of low doses of aspirin on platelet function, this drug is used in the treatment or prophylaxis of diseases associated with platelet hyperaggregability, such as coronary artery disease and postoperative deep-vein thrombosis (*see* Chapter 55). The effectiveness of such therapy appears to depend upon blockade of TXA_2 synthesis by platelets without preventing production of PGI_2 by endothelial cells (*see* Chapters 24 and 55). Although the optimal dosage has not been established, the frequency of beneficial effects appear to be greater when the dose of aspirin is 325 mg per day or lower. In the largest study to date, the ingestion of 325 mg of aspirin every other day reduced the incidence of myocardial infarction in male physicians by more than 40%; no effect was detected on the incidence of stroke (Steering Committee of the Physicians' Health Study Research Group, 1989).

A relative excess of TXA_2 over PGI_2 has been implicated in the genesis of preeclampsia and hypertension induced by pregnancy (*see* Lubbe, 1987). The administration of 60 or 100 mg of aspirin per day to pregnant women who have a high risk of developing hypertension reduces the formation of thromboxane A_2 without changing the production of PGI_2 and may lower the incidence of preeclampsia (Benigni *et al.*, 1989; Schiff *et al.*, 1989).

Relationship of Plasma Salicylate Concentration to Therapeutic Effect and Toxicity. For optimal antiinflammatory effect for patients with rheumatic diseases, plasma salicylate concentrations of 150 to 300 μg/ml are required. In this range, the clearance of the drug is nearly constant (despite the fact that saturation of metabolic capacity is approached) because the fraction of drug that is free and thus available for metabolism or excretion increases as binding sites on plasma proteins are saturated. The total concentration of salicylate in plasma is thus a relatively linear function of dose. It is important to individualize the total dose of aspirin, especially because the range of plasma salicylate concentrations needed for optimal antiinflammatory effects may overlap that at which tinnitus is noted. Tinnitus may be a reliable index of therapeutic plasma concentration in patients with normal hearing, but obviously not in those with a preexisting hearing loss. Hyperventilation generally occurs at concentrations greater than 350 μg/ml, and other signs of intoxication, such as acidosis, at concentrations greater than 460 μg/ml. Single analgesic–antipyretic doses of salicylate usually yield plasma concentrations below 60 μg/ml.

The plasma concentration of salicylate is generally little affected by other drugs, but concurrent administration of aspirin lowers the concentrations of indomethacin, naproxen, and fenoprofen, at least in part by displacement from plasma proteins. Important adverse interactions of aspirin with warfarin and methotrexate are mentioned above. Other interactions of aspirin include the antagonism of spironolactone-induced natriuresis and the blockade of the active transport of penicillin from CSF to blood.

Local Uses. Salicylic acid is applied topically as a keratolytic agent. In combination with benzoic acid, it is often prescribed for epidermophytosis. Salicylic acid is also employed as a wart and corn remover (10 to 20% in collodion).

Methyl salicylate is reserved for external use as a counterirritant. It is employed for painful muscles or joints and distributed in an ointment, liniment, or other preparation. Absorption of methyl salicylate can occur through the skin, and death has resulted from systemic poisoning from the local misapplication of the drug. It is a common pediatric poison, and its use should be strongly discouraged. It is also used as a flavoring agent.

DIFLUNISAL

Diflunisal is a difluorophenyl derivative of salicylic acid (*see* Table 26–1); it is not converted to salicylic acid *in vivo*. Diflunisal is more potent than aspirin in antiinflammatory tests in animals and appears to be a competitive inhibitor of cyclooxygenase. However, it is largely devoid of antipyretic effects, perhaps because of poor penetration into the CNS. The drug has been used primarily as an analgesic in the treatment of osteoarthritis and musculoskeletal strains or sprains; in these circumstances it is about three to four times more potent than aspirin. Diflunisal does not produce auditory side effects and appears to cause fewer and less intense gastrointestinal and antiplatelet effects than does aspirin.

Diflunisal is almost completely absorbed after oral administration, and peak concentrations occur in plasma within 2 to 3 hours. It is extensively bound to plasma albumin (99%). Diflunisal appears in the milk of lactating women; its penetration into the CNS is uncertain. About 90% of the drug is excreted as glucuronides, and its rate of elimination is dependent upon dosage. At the usual analgesic dose (500 to 750 mg per day) the plasma half-life ranges between 8 and 12 hours. (For reviews, *see* Brogden *et al.*, 1980; Davies, 1983; van Winzum *et al.*, in Symposium, 1983a.)

Diflunisal (DOLOBID) is marketed in 250- and 500-mg tablets. For mild-to-moderate pain, the usual initial dose is 500 to 1000 mg, followed by 250 to 500 mg every 8 to 12 hours. For rheumatoid arthritis or osteoarthritis, 250 to 500 mg is administered twice daily; maintenance dosage should not exceed 1.5 g per day.

PYRAZOLON DERIVATIVES

This group of drugs includes phenylbutazone, oxyphenbutazone, antipyrine, aminopyrine, dipyrone, and a more recent addition, apazone (azapropazone). With the exception of apazone, these drugs have been in clinical use for many years; although not a first-line drug, phenylbutazone is the most important from the therapeutic viewpoint, while antipyrine, dipyrone, and aminopyrine are seldom used today. Apazone is not yet available in the United States.

PHENYLBUTAZONE

Phenylbutazone was introduced in 1949 for the treatment of rheumatoid arthritis and allied disorders. Although it is an effective antiinflammatory agent, serious toxicity limits its use in long-term therapy. Its structural formula is as follows:

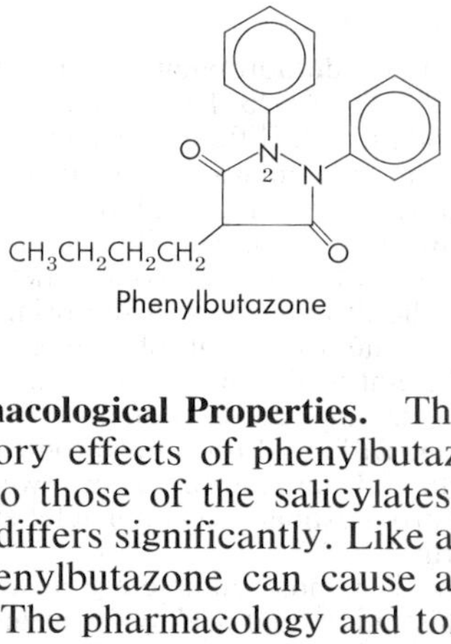

Phenylbutazone

Pharmacological Properties. The antiinflammatory effects of phenylbutazone are similar to those of the salicylates, but its toxicity differs significantly. Like aminopyrine, phenylbutazone can cause agranulocytosis. The pharmacology and toxicology of phenylbutazone and its metabolites and congeners have been reviewed in a symposium (Symposium, 1983a) and by Schuster and associates (Rainsford, 1985a).

Antiinflammatory Effects. Phenylbutazone has prominent antiinflammatory effects, and its frequent use to enhance the performance of race horses is well known. Somewhat similar effects are demonstrable in patients with rheumatoid arthritis and related disorders.

Antipyretic and Analgesic Effects. The antipyretic effect of phenylbutazone has been little studied in man. For pain of nonrheumatic origin, its analgesic efficacy is inferior to that of salicylates. Because of its toxicity, phenylbutazone should not be used routinely as an analgesic or antipyretic.

Uricosuric Effect. In doses of about 600 mg per day, phenylbutazone has a mild uricosuric effect, probably attributable to one of its metabolites that decreases tubular reabsorption of uric acid. Low concentrations of the drug inhibit tubular secretion of uric acid and cause retention of urate. A congener, sulfinpyrazone, is a much more effective uricosuric agent and is useful for the treatment of chronic gout (*see* below and Chapter 30).

Effects on Water and Electrolytes. Phenylbutazone causes significant retention of Na^+ and chloride, accompanied by a reduction in urine volume; edema may result. The excretion of K^+ is not changed. Plasma volume frequently increases by as much as 50%, and, as a result, cardiac decompensation and acute pulmonary edema have occurred in patients given the drug.

Other Effects. Phenylbutazone reduces the uptake of iodine by the thyroid gland, apparently secondary to inhibition of biosynthesis of organic iodine compounds. Goiter and myxedema may occasionally result from this effect.

Pharmacokinetics and Metabolism. Phenylbutazone is rapidly and completely absorbed from the gastrointestinal tract or the rectum, and the peak concentration in plasma is reached in 2 hours. After therapeutic doses, more than 98% of phenylbutazone is bound to plasma proteins. The half-life of phenylbutazone in plasma is very long—50 to 65 hours. The drug penetrates into the synovial spaces and reaches a concentration about one half of that in the plasma; significant concentrations may persist in the joints for up to 3 weeks after treatment is discontinued.

Phenylbutazone undergoes extensive metabolic transformation in man. The most significant primary reactions involve glucuronidation and hydroxylation of the phenyl rings or the butyl side chain. The conjugates are excreted in the urine and represent the bulk of the excreted drug. Oxyphenbutazone, a metabolite of phenylbutazone, has antirheumatic and Na^+-retaining activities similar to those of the parent drug. Oxyphenbutazone is also extensively bound to plasma proteins and has a half-life in plasma of several days. It accumulates significantly during long-term administration of phenylbutazone and contributes to the pharmacological and toxic effects of the parent drug. Only a trace of unchanged phenylbutazone is excreted in the urine. Oxyphenbutazone is excreted mainly as the O-glucuronide.

Drug Interactions. Other antiinflammatory agents, oral anticoagulant drugs, oral hypoglycemics, sulfonamides, and other drugs may be displaced from binding to plasma proteins by phenylbutazone. The net result depends upon the drug and its disposition after being displaced. The well-documented increased risk of bleeding associated with concurrent phenylbutazone–warfarin medication in part involves such displacement; more importantly, phenylbutazone also reduces the clearance of the more active stereoisomer of warfarin. Displacement of plasma protein–bound thyroid hormone complicates the interpretation of thyroid function tests.

Phenylbutazone may cause induction of hepatic microsomal enzymes, and it may also inhibit inactivation of other drugs that are hydroxylated by the microsomal system. It has been said to increase the effect of insulin.

Toxic Effects. Phenylbutazone is poorly tolerated by many patients. Some type of side effect is noted in 10 to 45% of patients, and medication may have to be discontinued in 10 to 15%. Nausea, vomiting, epigastric discomfort, and skin rashes are the most frequently reported untoward effects. Diarrhea, vertigo, insomnia, euphoria, nervousness, hematuria, and blurred vision have also been observed. In addition, water and electrolyte retention and edema formation occur.

More serious forms of adverse effects include peptic ulcer (or its reactivation) with hemorrhage or perforation, hypersensitivity reactions of the serum-sickness type, ulcerative stomatitis, hepatitis, nephritis, aplastic anemia, leukopenia, agranulocytosis, and thrombocytopenia. A number of deaths have occurred, especially from aplastic anemia and agranulocytosis.

When phenylbutazone is given, the patient should be closely supervised and his blood should be examined frequently; weight should also be checked to warn of undue retention of Na^+. The drug should be given only for short periods (not more than 1 week). Even then, the incidence of disturbing side effects is about 10%. The patient must be told to discontinue the drug and promptly report to the physician if he develops fever, sore throat or other oral lesions, skin rash, pruritus, jaundice, weight gain, or tarry stools. The drug is contraindicated in patients with hypertension; cardiac, renal, or hepatic dysfunction; or a history of peptic ulcer, blood dyscrasia, or hypersensitivity to the drug. The toxic effects of the drug are more severe in elderly persons, and its use in this group is inadvisable; its use in children under the age of 14 is also not recommended.

Preparations, Route of Administration, and Dosage. *Phenylbutazone* (BUTAZOLIDIN) is available in 100-mg coated tablets and capsules for oral administration. Daily doses of 300 to 600 mg for brief periods provide maximal therapeutic effects (higher doses only increase toxicity), but the disease may subsequently be adequately controlled by doses as low as 100 to 200 mg per day. The drug should be taken with meals to lessen gastric irritation.

Therapeutic Uses. At the present time, phenylbutazone is not considered to be the drug of choice for any condition, although it is still occasionally used for the treatment of acute gout and for rheumatoid arthritis and allied disorders. Phenylbutazone should be employed only after other drugs have failed and then only after careful consideration of the risks involved as compared with the advantage to the patient. Moreover, phenylbutazone should only be used for acute exacerbations of gout or rheumatoid arthritis and not for long-term treatment. Indiscriminate use of phenylbutazone in the therapy of trivial acute or chronic musculoskeletal disorders can only be condemned.

Phenylbutazone is an alternative to colchicine in acute gout; however, other antiinflammatory agents that have a lower incidence of side effects are generally preferred. Dosage recommendations have varied, but most often an initial dose of 400 mg is given, followed by 100 mg every 4 hours for no more than 1 week, or less if articular inflammation subsides. The drug should not be used prophylactically nor as a uricosuric agent.

Phenylbutazone has a limited role for relief of acute exacerbations of rheumatoid arthritis that are not relieved by any other measures. Synovitis is often reduced by a brief regimen (300 to 600 mg on the first day, followed by no more than 400 mg daily for 3 to 7 days). Because of the high incidence of adverse effects, long-term therapy is not recommended. Brief courses of the drug, if justified, may be of similar benefit for acute exacerbations of ankylosing spondylitis and osteoarthritis.

OXYPHENBUTAZONE

Oxyphenbutazone is a *p*-hydroxy analog of phenylbutazone (on the N-1 phenyl group) and one of the active metabolites of the parent drug. Various aspects of its pharmacology and metabolism are discussed above, in comparison with phenylbutazone. Oxyphenbutazone has the same spectrum of activity, therapeutic uses, interactions, and toxicity as the parent compound, and it shares the same indications, dangers, and contraindications for clinical use. Oxyphenbutazone is said to cause somewhat less gastric irritation.

Oxyphenbutazone is marketed in 100-mg tablets. It should be taken in three or four divided portions with meals to lessen gastric irritation. Dosage of oxyphenbutazone is the same as that of phenylbutazone.

ANTIPYRINE AND AMINOPYRINE

Antipyrine (phenazone) and aminopyrine (amidopyrine) were introduced into medicine in the late nineteenth century as antipyretics and subsequently were also widely used as analgesics and antiinflammatory agents. However, clinical use of aminopyrine was sharply curtailed after its potentially fatal bone-marrow toxicity, agranulocytosis, was recognized, and antipyrine has also lost favor. Both drugs have disappeared from the therapeutic scene in the United States, but antipyrine is still employed in some countries, usually in analgesic mixtures. A variety of related pyrazolon derivatives has also enjoyed sporadic popularity, for example, dipyrone. It, too, can cause agranulocytosis. A full description of the pharmacological properties of these drugs may be found in *earlier editions* of this textbook.

APAZONE (AZAPROPAZONE)

Apazone is a pyrazolon, aspirin-like agent with a spectrum of activity very similar to that of phenylbutazone, although it is much less toxic. Thus, it is antiinflammatory, analgesic, and antipyretic. In addition, apazone is a potent uricosuric agent and is particularly useful for the treatment of acute gout. The drug is not currently available in the United States. The structural formula of apazone is as follows:

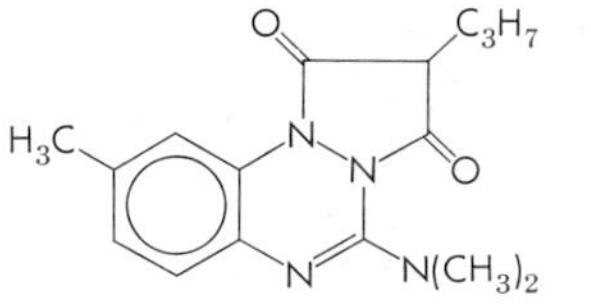

Apazone

Apazone is rapidly and probably almost completely absorbed from the gastrointestinal tract after oral administration to man; peak concentrations in plasma are achieved 4 hours later. The compound is extensively bound to plasma proteins (>95%), and the biological half-life is about 20 to 24 hours. The drug penetrates slowly into the synovial fluid. Most of the drug (about 65%) is excreted in the urine unchanged; approximately 20% is present as the 6-hydroxy derivative. There may be significant enterohepatic cycling.

Clinical experience to date suggests that apazone is generally well tolerated. Mild gastrointestinal side effects (nausea, epigastric pain, dyspepsia) occur in about 3% of patients. Skin rashes are also observed in 3% of patients, while CNS effects (headache, vertigo) are reported less frequently. The overall incidence of untoward reactions is probably 6 to 10%.

Because apazone is an inhibitor of cyclooxygenase, all precautions discussed above for the group are applicable. It should not be given to patients who have experienced aspirin-induced bronchospasm. Since the drug binds extensively to albumin, its adverse interactions with other agents may resemble those of phenylbutazone. There is no evidence that apazone causes agranulocytosis.

Apazone has been advocated for the treatment of rheumatoid arthritis, osteoarthritis, and gout. The usual dose is 1200 mg per day (in divided doses), but this may be reduced to 900 mg for maintenance therapy; elderly patients should receive lower doses. For the treatment of acute gout, an initial dose of 2400 mg (in four portions) is given on the first day, followed by daily doses of 1800 mg until the acute attack has subsided; daily maintenance doses of 1200 mg are then administered until symptoms disappear. (For a review, *see* Walker, in Rainsford, 1985b.)

PARA-AMINOPHENOL DERIVATIVES

The so-called coal tar analgesics, phenacetin and its active metabolite acetaminophen, are effective alternatives to aspirin as analgesic–antipyretic agents; however, unlike aspirin, their antiinflammatory activity is weak and seldom clinically useful. Acetaminophen has less overall toxicity and is thus preferred to phenacetin.

Because acetaminophen is well tolerated, lacks many of the side effects of aspirin, and is available without prescription, it has earned a prominent place as a common household analgesic. However, acute overdosage causes fatal hepatic damage, and the number of self-poisonings and suicides with acetaminophen has grown alarmingly in recent years. In addition, many individuals, physicians included, seem unaware of the poor antiinflammatory activity of acetaminophen.

History. Acetanilide is the parent member of this group of drugs. It was introduced into medicine in 1886 under the name of antifebrin by Cahn and Hepp, who had accidentally discovered its antipyretic action. However, acetanilide proved to be excessively toxic. In the search for less toxic compounds, para-aminophenol was tried in the belief that the body oxidized acetanilide to this compound. Toxicity was not lessened, however, and a number of chemical derivatives of para-aminophenol were then tested. One of the more satisfactory of these was phenacetin (acetophenetidin). It was introduced into therapy in 1887 and was extensively employed in analgesic mixtures until it was implicated in analgesic-abuse nephropathy (*see* above).

Acetaminophen (paracetamol; N-acetyl-*p*-aminophenol) was first used in medicine by von Mering in 1893. However, it has gained popularity only since 1949, after it was recognized as the major active metabolite of both acetanilide and phenacetin.

Chemistry. The relationship between the drugs of this group and their metabolites is shown in Table 26–2. The antipyretic activity of the compounds resides in the aminobenzene structure. Introduction of other radicals into the hydroxyl group of para-aminophenol and into the free amino group of aniline reduces toxicity without loss of antipyretic action. Best results are obtained with phenolic alkyl ethers (*e.g.*, phenacetin) and with the amides (*e.g.*, acetaminophen, phenacetin).

Pharmacological Properties. Acetaminophen and phenacetin have analgesic and antipyretic effects that do not differ significantly from those of aspirin. However, as mentioned, they have only weak antiinflammatory effects. Minor metabolites contribute significantly to the toxic effects

Table 26–2. STRUCTURAL FORMULAS OF MAJOR PARA-AMINOPHENOL DERIVATIVES, AND THEIR INTERRELATIONS

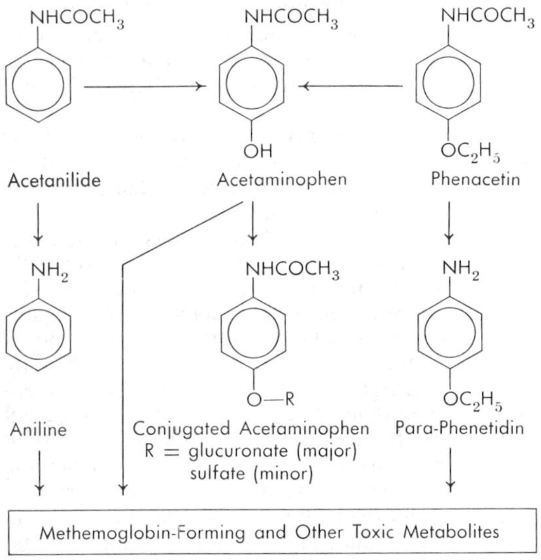

of both drugs. The pharmacological properties of acetaminophen have been reviewed by Clissold (1986).

Exactly why acetaminophen is an effective analgesic–antipyretic but only a weak antiinflammatory agent has not been satisfactorily explained. An antiinflammatory effect can be demonstrated in animal models, but only at doses considerably in excess of those required for analgesia. Acetaminophen is only a weak inhibitor of prostaglandin biosynthesis, although there is some evidence to suggest that it may be more effective against enzymes in the CNS than those in the periphery, perhaps because of the high concentrations of peroxides that are found in inflammatory lesions (Marshall *et al.*, 1987).

Subjective Effects and Liability for Abuse. Phenacetin has been said to cause relaxation, drowsiness, euphoria, stimulation, and increased efficiency; such effects have been thought to contribute to its liability for abuse. In patients, minor subjective effects may well occur secondary to relief of pain or fever. Restlessness and excitement may occur for 3 or 4 days after discontinuation of long-term administration of phenacetin.

Other Effects. Single or repeated therapeutic doses of phenacetin or acetaminophen have no effect on the cardiovascular and respiratory systems. Acid–base changes do not occur. Neither drug produces the gastric irritation, erosion, or bleeding that may occur after administration of salicylates. They have no effects on platelets, bleeding time, or the excretion of uric acid.

Pharmacokinetics and Metabolism. Acetaminophen and phenacetin are metabolized primarily by the hepatic microsomal enzymes. The metabolic pathways for the two drugs are rather different, except, of course, that a considerable proportion of phenacetin is dealkylated to acetaminophen.

Acetaminophen is rapidly and almost completely absorbed from the gastrointestinal tract. The concentration in plasma reaches a peak in 30 to 60 minutes, and the half-life in plasma is about 2 hours after therapeutic doses. Acetaminophen is relatively uniformly distributed throughout most body fluids. Binding of the drug to plasma proteins is variable; only 20 to 50% may be bound at the concentrations encountered during acute intoxication. After therapeutic doses, 90 to 100% of the drug may be recovered in the urine within the first day, primarily after hepatic conjugation with glucuronic acid (about 60%), sulfuric acid (about 35%), or cysteine (about 3%); small amounts of hydroxylated and deacetylated metabolites have also been detected. Children have less capacity for glucuronidation of the drug than do adults. A small proportion of acetaminophen undergoes cytochrome P_{450}-mediated N-hydroxylation to form N-acetyl-benzoquinoneimine, a highly reactive intermediate (*see* Figure 1–4, page 19). This metabolite normally reacts with sulfhydryl groups in glutathione. However, after large doses of acetaminophen the metabolite is formed in amounts sufficient to deplete hepatic glutathione; under these circumstances, reaction with sulfhydryl groups in hepatic proteins is increased and hepatic necrosis can result.

In the normal individual, 75 to 80% of phenacetin is rapidly metabolized to acetaminophen (*see* Table 26–2). The peak concentration of phenacetin in plasma usually occurs in about 1 hour and that of acetaminophen derived therefrom in 1 to 2 hours. Phenacetin is converted to at least a dozen other metabolites, by N-deacetylation to para-phenetidin and by hydroxylation and further metabolism of phenacetin and para-phenetidin. An unknown metabolite, but an oxidizing agent, is responsible for formation of methemoglobin and hemolysis of red blood cells. Individuals with a genetically determined limitation in their ability to metabolize phenacetin to acetaminophen convert a greater fraction of phenacetin to toxic metabolites, possibly with propensity for serious methemoglobin formation and hemolysis. Less than 1% of phenacetin is excreted unchanged in the urine.

Toxic Effects. In recommended therapeutic dosage, acetaminophen and phenacetin are usually well tolerated. Skin rash and other allergic reactions occur occasionally. The rash is usually erythematous or urticarial, but sometimes it is more serious and may be accompanied by drug fever and mucosal lesions. Patients who show hypersensitivity reactions to the salicylates only rarely exhibit sensitivity to acetaminophen and related drugs (Szczeklik, 1986; Stevenson and Lewis, 1987). In a few isolated cases, the use of acetaminophen has been associated with neutropenia, thrombocytopenia, and pancytopenia.

Despite the fact that acetaminophen is a metabolite of phenacetin, the signs and symptoms of acute intoxication with the two compounds are markedly different. The most serious adverse effect of acute overdosage of acetaminophen is a dose-dependent, potentially fatal hepatic necrosis. Renal tubular necrosis (also seen with phenacetin) and hypoglycemic coma may also occur. Phenacetin may cause methemoglobinemia and hemolytic anemia as a form of acute toxicity, but more commonly as a consequence of chronic overdosage. Lethal doses of phenacetin are not associated with hepatic damage, but with cyanosis, respiratory depression, and cardiac arrest. Acetaminophen is much less likely to cause the formation of methemoglobin and has not been incriminated in the hemolytic reactions. The nephrotoxicity associated with chronic abuse of acetaminophen, phenacetin, and other analgesics has been discussed above.

Hepatotoxicity. In adults, hepatotoxicity may occur after ingestion of a single dose of 10 to 15 g (150 to 250 mg/kg) of acetaminophen; doses of 20 to 25 g or more are potentially fatal. The mechanism of this effect is discussed above (*see also* Chapter 1). Symptoms during the first 2 days of acute poisoning by acetaminophen may not reflect the potential seriousness of the intoxication. Nausea, vomiting, anorexia, and abdominal pain occur during the initial 24 hours and may persist for a week or more. Clinical indications of hepatic damage become manifest within 2 to 4 days of ingestion of toxic doses. Initially, plasma transaminases are elevated (sometimes markedly so), and the concentration of bilirubin in plasma may be increased; in addition, the prothrombin time is prolonged. Perhaps 10% of poisoned patients who do not receive specific treatment develop severe liver damage; of these, 10 to 20% eventually die of hepatic failure. Acute renal failure also occurs in some patients. Biopsy of the liver reveals centrilobular necrosis with sparing of the periportal area. In nonfatal cases, the hepatic lesions are reversible over a period of weeks or months.

Severe liver damage (with levels of aspartate aminotransferase activity in excess of 1000 I.U. per liter of plasma) occurs in 90% of patients with plasma concentrations of acetaminophen greater than 300 μg/ml at 4 hours or 45 μg/ml at 15 hours after the ingestion of the drug. Minimal hepatic damage can be anticipated when the drug concentration is less than 120 μg/ml at 4 hours or 30 μg/ml at 12 hours after ingestion. The potential severity of hepatic necrosis can also be predicted from the half-life of acetaminophen observed in the patient; values greater than 4 hours imply that necrosis will occur, while values greater than 12 hours suggest that hepatic coma is likely.

Treatment. Early diagnosis is vital in the treatment of overdosage with acetaminophen, and methods are available for the rapid determination of concentrations of the drug in plasma. However, therapy should not be delayed while awaiting laboratory results if the history suggests a significant overdosage. Vigorous supportive therapy is essential when intoxication is severe. Gastric lavage should be performed in all cases, preferably within 4 hours of the ingestion. Activated charcoal is usually *not* administered because it can absorb the antidote, N-acetylcysteine, and reduce its efficacy (*see* below).

The principal antidotal treatment is the administration of sulfhydryl compounds, which probably act, in part, by replenishing hepatic stores of glutathione. N-acetylcysteine is particularly effective when given orally. The drug is recommended if less than 24 hours has elapsed since ingestion of acetaminophen, although treatment with N-acetylcysteine is more effective when given less than 10 hours after ingestion (Smilkstein *et al.*, 1988). An oral loading dose of 140 mg/kg is given, followed by the administration of 70 mg/kg every 4 hours for 17 doses. Treatment should begin immediately upon suspecting a significant acetaminophen overdosage, and it is terminated if assays of acetaminophen in plasma indicate that the risk of hepatotoxicity is low. *Acetylcysteine* (MUCOMYST, MUCOSOL) is available as a sterile 10 or 20% solution in vials containing 4, 10, and 30 ml. The solution is diluted with soft drinks or water to achieve a 5% solution and should be consumed within 1 hour of preparation. An intravenous form of acetylcysteine is available in Europe, where it is considered the treatment of choice. Consultation may be obtained from the Rocky Mountain Poison Center, Denver,

Colorado (Tel.: 800–525–6115). (*See* Prescott and Critchley, 1983; Smilkstein *et al.*, 1988.)

Other Toxic Effects. Phenacetin-induced hemolytic anemia and the methemoglobinemia that follows poisoning with acetanilide or phenacetin are discussed in *earlier editions* of this textbook.

Preparations, Routes of Administration, and Dosage. *Acetaminophen* (*paracetamol;* N-acetyl-*p*-aminophenol) is marketed under many trade names (*e.g.*, TEMPRA, TYLENOL). Preparations include tablets (160, 325, 500, 650 mg), capsules (325 and 500 mg), suppositories, chewable tablets, wafers, elixirs, and solutions. The conventional oral dose of acetaminophen is 325 to 1000 mg (650 mg rectally); the total daily dose should not exceed 4000 mg. For children, the single dose is 40 to 480 mg, depending upon age and weight; no more than five doses should be administered in 24 hours. A dose of 10 mg/kg may also be used. Acetaminophen should not be administered for more than 10 days or to young children except upon advice of a physician.

Phenacetin has been employed only in analgesic mixtures. In recent years it has been removed from almost all such mixtures. In some instances acetaminophen has been included to replace it.

Therapeutic Uses. Acetaminophen is a suitable substitute for aspirin for its analgesic or antipyretic uses; it is particularly valuable for patients in whom aspirin is contraindicated (*e.g.*, those with peptic ulcer) or when the prolongation of bleeding time caused by aspirin would be a disadvantage.

INDOMETHACIN AND SULINDAC

Indomethacin was the product of a laboratory search for drugs with antiinflammatory properties. It was introduced in 1963 for the treatment of rheumatoid arthritis and related disorders. Although indomethacin is widely used and is effective, toxicity often limits its use. Sulindac was developed in an attempt to find a less toxic but effective congener of indomethacin. The development, chemistry, and pharmacology of both drugs have been reviewed by Rhymer and Gengos (Symposium, 1983a) and by Shen (Rainsford, 1985a).

INDOMETHACIN

Chemistry. The structural formula of indomethacin, a methylated indole derivative, is as follows:

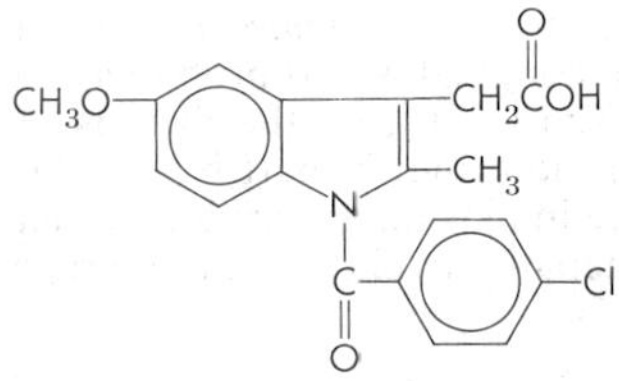

Indomethacin

Pharmacological Properties. Indomethacin has prominent antiinflammatory and analgesic–antipyretic properties similar to those of the salicylates.

The antiinflammatory effects of indomethacin are evident in patients with rheumatoid and other types of arthritis, including acute gout. Although indomethacin is more potent than aspirin, doses that are tolerated by patients with rheumatoid arthritis usually do not produce effects that are superior to those of salicylate. Indomethacin has analgesic properties distinct from its antiinflammatory effects, and there is evidence for both a central and a peripheral action; it is also an antipyretic.

Indomethacin is a potent inhibitor of the prostaglandin-forming cyclooxygenase; it also inhibits the motility of polymorphonuclear leukocytes. Like many other aspirin-like drugs, indomethacin uncouples oxidative phosphorylation in supratherapeutic concentrations and depresses the biosynthesis of mucopolysaccharides.

Pharmacokinetics and Metabolism. Indomethacin is rapidly and almost completely absorbed from the gastrointestinal tract after oral ingestion. The peak concentration in plasma is attained within 2 hours in the fasting subject but may be somewhat delayed when the drug is taken after meals. The concentrations in plasma required for an antiinflammatory effect have not been definitely determined but are probably less than 1 μg/ml. Steady-state concentrations in plasma after long-term administration are approximately 0.5 μg/ml. Indomethacin is 90% bound to plasma proteins and also extensively bound to tissues. The concentration of the drug in the CSF is low, but its concentration in synovial fluid is equal to that in plasma within 5 hours of administration.

Indomethacin is largely converted to inactive metabolites, including those formed by O-demethylation (about 50%), conjugation with glucuronic acid (about 10%), and N-deacylation. Some of these metabolites are detectable in plasma, and free and conjugated metabolites are eliminated in the urine, bile, and feces. There is enterohepatic cycling of the conjugates and probably of indomethacin itself. Ten to 20% of the drug is excreted unchanged in the urine, in part by tubular secretion. The half-life in plasma is variable, perhaps because of enterohepatic cycling, but averages about 3 hours.

Drug Interactions. The total plasma concentration of indomethacin plus its inactive metabolites is increased by concurrent administration of probenecid, possibly because of reduced tubular secretion of the former. However, it has not been determined whether the dosage of indomethacin must be adjusted when the two drugs are employed together. Indomethacin does not interfere with the uricosuric effect of probenecid. Indomethacin is said not to modify the effect of the oral anticoagulant agents. However, concurrent administration could be hazardous because of the increased risk of gastrointestinal bleeding. Indomethacin antagonizes the natriuretic and antihypertensive effects of furosemide; the antihypertensive effects of thiazide diuretics, β-adrenergic blocking agents, or inhibitors of angiotensin converting enzyme may also be reduced. Acute renal failure associated with the concomitant administration of indomethacin and triamterene has been reported (*see* Clive and Stoff, 1984).

Toxic Effects. A very high percentage (35 to 50%) of patients receiving usual therapeutic doses of indomethacin experience untoward symptoms, and about 20% must discontinue its use. Most adverse effects are dose related.

Gastrointestinal complaints and complications consist of anorexia, nausea, and abdominal pain. Single ulcers or multiple ulceration of the entire upper gastrointestinal tract, sometimes with perforations and hemorrhage, has been reported. Occult blood loss may lead to anemia in the absence of ulceration. Acute pancreatitis has also been reported. Diarrhea may occur and is sometimes associated with ulcerative lesions of the bowel. Hepatic involvement is rare, although some fatal cases of hepatitis and jaundice have been reported. The most frequent CNS effect (indeed, the most common side effect) is severe frontal headache, occurring in 25 to 50% of patients who take the drug for long periods. Dizziness, vertigo, light-headedness, and mental confusion are also frequent. Severe depression, psychosis, hallucinations, and suicide have occurred.

Hematopoietic reactions include neutropenia, thrombocytopenia, and, rarely, aplastic anemia. Platelet function is impaired by indomethacin. Hypersensitivity reactions are manifested as rashes, itching, urticaria, and, more seriously, acute attacks of asthma. Patients sensitive to aspirin may exhibit cross-reactivity to indomethacin. Indomethacin should not be used in pregnant women, nursing mothers, persons operating machinery, or patients with psychiatric disorders, epilepsy, or parkinsonism. It is also contraindicated in individuals with renal disease or ulcerative lesions of the stomach or intestines.

Preparations, Routes of Administration, and Dosage. *Indomethacin* (INDOCIN, others) is available for oral use in capsules containing 25, 50, or 75 mg of the drug, and in sustained-release capsules (75 mg); it is also supplied in 50-mg suppositories and as an oral suspension (25 mg/5 ml).

The initial dose is 25 mg, two or three times daily, and this can be increased in 25- or 50-mg increments at weekly intervals until the total daily dose is 150 to 200 mg. Few patients tolerate more than 150 mg per day without severe side effects. Most patients respond within 4 to 6 days, but some require substantially longer treatment. The drug should be taken in divided portions with food or antacids or immediately after meals to lessen gastric distress. A dose of indomethacin taken with milk at bedtime is said to reduce the incidence of morning headache.

Indomethacin is also available for intravenous injection as the sodium trihydrate (INDOCIN I.V.) to induce closure of a patent ductus arteriosus in neonates.

Therapeutic Uses. Because of the high incidence and severity of side effects associated with long-term administration, indomethacin must not be routinely used as an analgesic or antipyretic. However, it has proven useful as an antipyretic in certain settings (*e.g.*, Hodgkin's disease) when the fever has been refractory to other agents. Indomethacin has become an accepted part of the rheumatologist's armamentarium and a standard (together with aspirin) against which to measure the activity of other, newer drugs.

Clinical trials of indomethacin as an antiinflammatory agent have been reviewed by Rhymer and Gengos (in Symposium, 1983a). The majority of these trials have demonstrated that indomethacin relieves pain, reduces swelling and tenderness of the joints, increases grip strength, and decreases the duration of morning stiffness. In these actions the drug is superior to placebo and equivalent to phenylbutazone; estimates of its potency relative to salicylates vary between 10 and 40 times higher. Overall, about two thirds of patients benefit from treatment with indomethacin; however, if 75 to 100 mg of the drug fails to provide benefit within 2 to 4 weeks, alternative therapy must be considered. The incidence and severity of side effects with indomethacin are particularly annoying, but a useful way of employing the undoubted potency of the drug, perhaps in combination with other and better-tolerated daytime therapy, is to give a large single dose (up to 100 mg) at bedtime. This enables the patient to obtain a better-quality sleep, reduces the severity and length of morning stiffness, and provides good analgesia until midmorning. The side effects of indomethacin are apparently better tolerated when it is given at night.

Indomethacin is often more effective than aspirin in the treatment of ankylosing spondylitis and osteoarthrosis. It is also very effective in the treatment of acute gout, although it is not uricosuric.

Patients with Bartter's syndrome have been successfully treated with indomethacin, as well as with other inhibitors of prostaglandin synthetase (*see* Clive and Stoff, 1984). The results are frequently dramatic; however, the condition of the patients may deteriorate rapidly when therapy is discontinued, and the long-term therapy necessary to control the disease requires administration of a drug that is better tolerated.

Cardiac failure in neonates caused by a patent ductus arteriosus may be controlled by the administration of indomethacin. A typical regimen involves the intravenous administration of 0.1 to 0.2 mg/kg every 12 hours for three doses. Successful closure can be expected in more than 70% of neonates who are treated with the drug. Such therapy is indicated primarily in premature infants who weigh between 500 and 1750 g, who have a hemodynamically significant patent ductus arteriosus, and in whom other supportive maneuvers have been attempted. The principal limitation of this approach is renal toxicity, and therapy is stopped if the output of urine falls below 0.6 ml/kg per hour. Renal failure, enterocolitis, thrombocytopenia, or hyperbilirubinemia contraindicates the use of indomethacin.

SULINDAC

Chemistry. Sulindac is closely related to indomethacin; its structural formula is as follows:

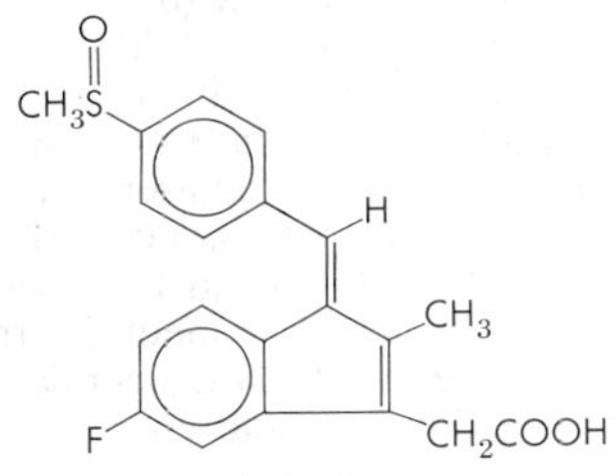

Sulindac

It is unlikely that sulindac itself has much therapeutic efficacy; most of its pharmacological activity resides in its sulfide metabolite.

Pharmacological Properties. In laboratory studies, sulindac exhibits the classical activities of aspirin-like drugs. In all tests, sulindac is less than half as potent as indomethacin.

Because sulindac is a prodrug, it appears to be either inactive or relatively weak in many tests, whereas its sulfide metabolite may be very active. This especially applies to tests where little or no metabolism can occur. The sulfide metabolite is more than 500 times more potent than sulindac as an inhibitor of cyclooxygenase. These observations may help to explain the somewhat lower incidence of gastrointestinal toxicity of sulindac as compared with indomethacin, since the gastric or intestinal mucosa is not exposed to high concentrations of an active drug during oral administration. Nevertheless, gastrointestinal toxicity is more common with sulindac than with many other aspirin-like drugs. Sulindac may also be unusual in that some clinical studies indicate that it does not alter the urinary excretion of prostaglandins or alter renal function (*see* Patrono and Dunn, 1987). However, if a "renal-sparing" effect exists, it is only relative, and the drug must be used with caution in patients who are dependent upon the synthesis of prostaglandins in the kidney for maintenance of renal function (*see* above).

Pharmacokinetics and Metabolism. The metabolism and pharmacokinetics of sulindac are complex and vary enormously among species. After oral administration in man, about 90% of the drug is absorbed. Peak concentrations of sulindac in plasma are attained within 1 hour, while those of the sulfide metabolite occur about 2 hours after the oral administration of sulindac.

Sulindac undergoes two major biotransformations in addition to conjugation reactions. It is oxidized to the sulfone and then reversibly reduced to the sulfide. It is this latter metabolite that is the active moiety, although all three compounds are found in comparable concentrations in human plasma. The half-life of sulindac itself is about 7 hours, but the active sulfide has a half-life as long as 18 hours. Sulindac and its metabolites undergo extensive enterohepatic circulation. There seems to be little or no placental transfer of the drug, but it is present in breast milk. Sulindac and the sulfone and sulfide metabolites are all extensively bound to plasma protein.

Little of the sulfide or its conjugates is found in urine. The principal components that are excreted in urine are the sulfone and its conjugate, which account for nearly 30% of an administered dose; sulindac and its conjugates account for about 20%. Up to 25% of an oral dose may appear as metabolites in the feces.

Preparations, Route of Administration, and Dosage. *Sulindac* (CLINORIL) is available as 150- and 200-mg tablets. The most common dosage for adults is 150 to 200 mg twice a day, although dosage should be optimized for each individual. The maximal daily dose is 400 mg. The drug is usually given with food to reduce gastric discomfort, although this may delay absorption and reduce the concentration in plasma.

Toxic Effects. Although the incidence of toxicity is lower than with indomethacin, untoward reactions to sulindac are common.

Gastrointestinal side effects are seen in nearly 20% of patients, although these are generally mild. Abdominal pain and nausea are the most frequent complaints. CNS side effects are seen in up to 10% of patients, with drowsiness, dizziness, headache, and nervousness being those most frequently reported. Skin rash and pruritus occur in 5% of patients. Transient elevations of hepatic enzymes in plasma are less common. Sulindac can precipitate a severe reaction in patients who are sensitive to aspirin; platelet function may also be impaired and bleeding time prolonged.

Therapeutic Uses. Sulindac has been used mainly for the treatment of rheumatoid arthritis, osteoarthrosis, and ankylosing spondylitis. The drug has also been used with success in the treatment of acute gout. The analgesic and antiinflammatory effects exerted by sulindac (400 mg per day) are comparable to those achieved with aspirin (4 g per day), ibuprofen (1200 mg per day), indomethacin (125 mg per day), and phenylbutazone (400 to 600 mg per day) (*see* Rhymer, in Symposium, 1983a).

THE FENAMATES

The fenamates are a family of aspirin-like drugs that are derivatives of N-phenylanthranilic acid. They include mefenamic, meclofenamic, flufenamic, tolfenamic, and etofenamic acids.

Although the biological activity of this group of drugs was discovered in the 1950s, the fenamates have not gained widespread clinical acceptance. They frequently cause side effects; diarrhea, in particular, may be very severe. Therapeutically, they also have no clear advantages over several other aspirin-like drugs.

Mefenamic acid and meclofenamate are the only members of the series available in the United States. The use of mefenamic acid is indicated only for analgesia and for relief of the symptoms of primary dysmenorrhea. While meclofenamate is employed in the treatment of rheumatoid arthritis and osteoarthritis, it is not recommended as initial therapy. Flufenamic acid is used in many other countries, as is mefenamic acid, for its antiinflammatory effects. Other members of the series will not be discussed further.

Chemistry. Mefenamic acid and meclofenamate are both N-substituted phenylanthranilic acids. Their structures are as follows:

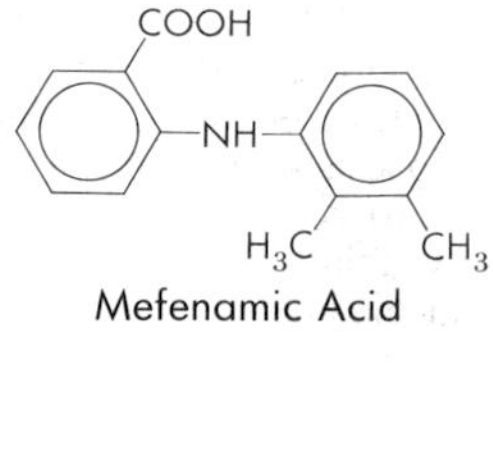

Mefenamic Acid

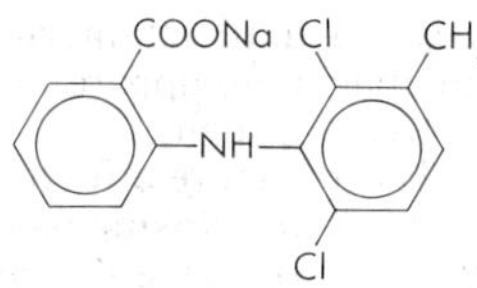

Meclofenamate Sodium

Pharmacological Properties. In tests of antiinflammatory activity, mefenamic acid is about half as potent and flufenamic acid about 1.5 times as potent as phenylbutazone. Both drugs also have antipyretic and analgesic properties. In tests of analgesia, mefenamic acid was the only fenamate to display a central as well as a peripheral action.

The fenamates appear to owe these properties to their capacity to inhibit cyclooxygenase. Unlike the other aspirin-like drugs, certain of the fenamates (especially meclofenamic acid) also appear to antagonize certain effects of prostaglandins.

Pharmacokinetic Properties. Peak concentrations in plasma are reached in 0.5 to 2 hours after a single oral dose of meclofenamate and in 2 to 4 hours for mefenamic acid. The two agents have similar half-lives in plasma (2 to 4 hours). In man, approximately 50% of a dose of mefenamic acid is excreted in the urine, primarily as the conjugated 3-hydroxymethyl metabolite and the 3-carboxyl metabolite and its conjugates. Twenty percent of the drug is recovered in the feces, mainly as the unconjugated 3-carboxyl metabolite.

Preparations, Route of Administration, and Dosage. *Mefenamic acid* (PONSTEL) is available in 250-mg capsules for oral administration. For acute pain, the initial dose is 500 mg; thereafter, 250 mg may be given every 6 hours with food. The drug is not recommended for use in children or pregnant women, and it should not be given for longer than 7 days. *Meclofenamate sodium* (MECLOMEN) is available in capsules or tablets containing the equivalent of 50 or 100 mg of meclofenamic acid. The usual daily dose is 200 to 400 mg in three or four portions. Dosage requires adjustment for the individual but should not exceed 400 mg per day. The drug is not recommended for children.

Toxic Effects and Precautions. The most common side effects (occurring in approximately 25% of all patients) involve the gastrointestinal system. Usually these take the form of dyspepsia or upper gastrointestinal discomfort, although diarrhea, which may be severe and associated with steatorrhea and inflammation of the bowel, is also relatively common.

Other reactions that have been noted less frequently include transient abnormalities of hepatic and renal function, CNS effects, and skin rashes. A potentially serious side effect seen in isolated cases is a hemolytic anemia, which may be of an autoimmune type.

The fenamates are contraindicated in patients with a history of gastrointestinal disease. If diarrhea or skin rash appears, the drug should be stopped at once. The physician and patient should watch for signs of hemolytic anemia. The fenamates can cause bronchoconstriction in patients who are sensitive to aspirin and can affect platelet function.

Therapeutic Uses. As an analgesic agent, mefenamic acid has been used to relieve pain arising from rheumatic conditions, soft-tissue injuries, other painful musculoskeletal conditions, and dysmenorrhea. Toxicity limits its usefulness and it appears to offer no advantage over other analgesic agents. As antiinflammatory agents, mefenamic acid and meclofenamate have been mainly tested in short-term trials in the treatment of osteoarthritis and rheumatoid arthritis and appear to offer no advantage over other aspirin-like drugs.

TOLMETIN

Tolmetin is an antiinflammatory, analgesic, and antipyretic agent that was introduced into clinical practice in the United States in 1976. Tolmetin, in recommended doses, appears to be approximately equivalent in efficacy to moderate doses of aspirin; it is usually better tolerated. The structural formula of tolmetin is as follows:

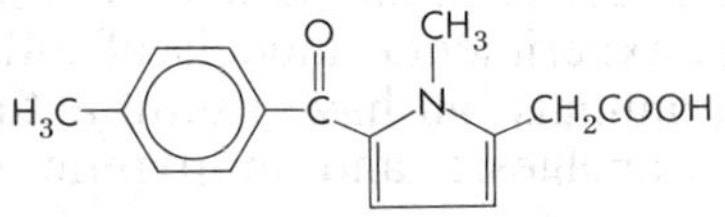

Tolmetin

Pharmacological Properties. Tolmetin is an effective antiinflammatory agent that also exerts antipyretic and analgesic effects. Like most of the other drugs considered in this chapter, tolmetin causes gastric erosions and prolongs bleeding time. The pharmacology of tolmetin has been reviewed by Ehrlich (in Symposium, 1983a) and by Wong (Rainsford, 1985b).

Pharmacokinetics and Metabolism. Tolmetin is rapidly and completely absorbed after oral administration in man; the concentrations achieved in plasma are not reduced by the concomitant administration of antacids. Peak concentrations are achieved 20 to 60 minutes after oral administration, and the half-life in plasma is about 5 hours. Accumulation of the drug in synovial fluid begins within 2 hours and persists for up to 8 hours after a single oral dose.

After absorption, tolmetin is extensively (99%) bound to plasma proteins. Virtually all of the drug can be recovered in the urine after 24 hours; some is unchanged but most is conjugated or otherwise metabolized. The major metabolic transformation involves oxidation of the para-methyl group to a carboxylic acid.

Preparations, Route of Administration, and Dosage. *Tolmetin sodium* (TOLECTIN) is supplied as 200-mg tablets and 400-mg capsules for oral use. The recommended initial dose is 400 mg three times daily, and it is suggested that one of these doses be taken at bedtime and another on awakening. The response to the drug is usually seen within a week, and the dose can then be adjusted; the usual range is 600 to 1800 mg per day in divided doses. The maximal recommended dose is 2 g per day. The drug may be given with meals, milk, or antacids other than sodium bicarbonate to lessen abdominal discomfort; however, peak plasma concentrations and bioavailability are significantly reduced when taken with food. The recommended initial daily dose for children (2 years and older) is 20 mg/kg per day in three or four divided doses. Maintenance dosage ranges from 15 to 30 mg/kg per day.

Toxic Effects. Side effects occur in 25 to 40% of patients who take tolmetin, and 5 to 10% discontinue use of the drug. Gastrointestinal side effects are the most common, with epigastric pain (15% incidence), dyspepsia, nausea, and vomiting being the chief manifestations. Gastric and duodenal ulceration has also been observed. CNS side effects, including nervousness, anxiety, insomnia, drowsiness, and visual disturbance, are less common and are said to be neither as frequent nor as severe as those caused by indomethacin. Similarly, the incidence of tinnitus, deafness, and vertigo is less than occurs with aspirin. It should be assumed that tolmetin will probably precipitate bronchoconstriction in patients who are hypersensitive to aspirin. In addition, there have been several reports of severe anaphylactoid reactions to tolmetin in patients who are not sensitive to aspirin and other aspirin-like drugs.

Drug Interactions. Despite its extensive binding to albumin, tolmetin does not interfere with concurrent treatment with warfarin or oral hypoglycemic agents.

Therapeutic Uses. Tolmetin is approved in the United States for the treatment of osteoarthritis, rheumatoid arthritis, and the juvenile form of the disease; it has also been used in the treatment of ankylosing spondylitis. In rheumatoid arthritis, many investigators have compared tolmetin (0.8 to 1.6 g per day) with aspirin (4 to 4.5 g per day) or indomethacin (100 to 150 mg per day). In general, there has been little difference in therapeutic efficacy. Tolmetin may be tolerated somewhat better than aspirin in equally effective doses. Similar results have been obtained with related arthritides and with soft-tissue injuries (*see* Ehrlich, in Symposium, 1983a).

PROPIONIC ACID DERIVATIVES

These drugs represent a group of effective, useful aspirin-like agents. They may offer significant advantages over aspirin, indomethacin, and the pyrazolon derivatives for many patients, since they are usually better tolerated. Nevertheless, propionic acid derivatives share all of the detrimental features of the entire class of drugs. Furthermore, their rapid proliferation in number and heavy promotion of these drugs make it difficult for the physician to choose rationally between members of the group and between propionic acid derivatives and the more established agents. The similarities between drugs in this class (and certain of the others discussed above) are far more striking than are the differences.

Ibuprofen, naproxen, flurbiprofen, fenoprofen, and ketoprofen are described individually below. These drugs are currently available in the United States, but several additional agents in this class are in use or under study in other countries. These include fenbufen, pirprofen, oxaprozin, indoprofen, and tiaprofenic acid. Ibuprofen was the first member of this class to come into general use, so experience with this drug is greater. It is available for sale without a prescription in the United States. The most distinctive feature among the others may probably be claimed by naproxen; its longer half-life makes twice-daily administration feasible. The structural formulas of these drugs are shown in Table 26–3.

Pharmacological Properties. The pharmacodynamic properties of the propionic acid derivatives do not differ significantly. While the compounds do vary in potency, this is not of obvious clinical significance. All are effective antiinflammatory agents in various experimental models of inflammation in animals; all have useful antiinflammatory, analgesic, and antipyretic activity in man.

All of these compounds can cause gastrointestinal erosions (gastric, duodenal, and intestinal) in experimental animals. All pro-

Table 26–3. STRUCTURAL FORMULAS OF ANTIINFLAMMATORY PROPIONIC ACID DERIVATIVES

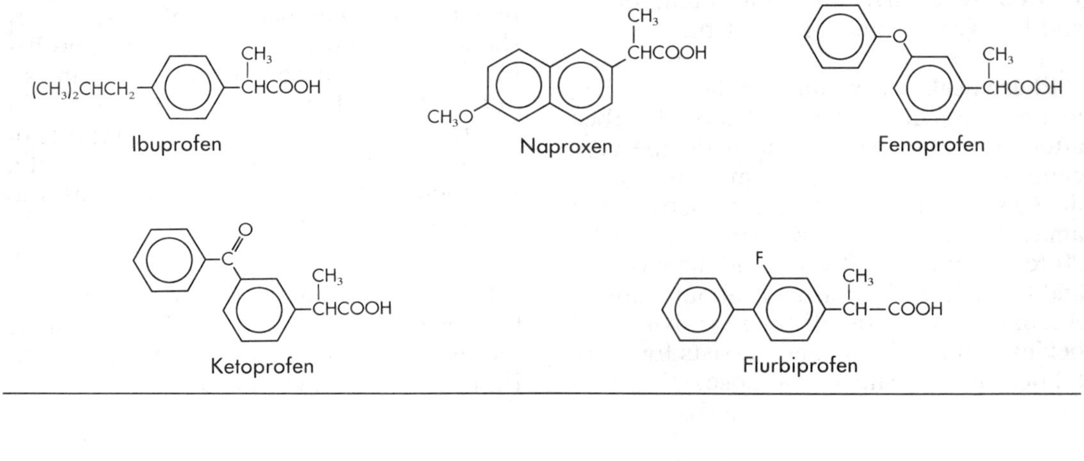

duce gastrointestinal side effects in man, although these are usually less severe than with aspirin. Certain propionic acid derivatives (*e.g.*, penoxaprofen) have produced a high incidence of hepatotoxicity, which has led to their removal from the market. The possibility that this may occur with other drugs in this class must be considered.

The propionic acid derivatives are effective inhibitors of the cyclooxygenase responsible for the biosynthesis of prostaglandins, although there is considerable variation in their potency. For example, naproxen is approximately 20 times more potent than aspirin, while ibuprofen, fenoprofen, and aspirin are roughly equipotent in this action. All of these agents alter platelet function and prolong bleeding time, and it should be assumed that any patient who is intolerant of aspirin may also suffer a severe reaction after administration of one of these drugs. Some of the propionic acid derivatives have prominent inhibitory effects on the migration and other functions of leukocytes. Naproxen is particularly potent in this regard.

Drug Interactions. The potential adverse drug interactions of particular concern with this group derive from their high degree of binding to albumin in plasma. However, the propionic acid derivatives do not alter the effects of the oral hypoglycemic drugs or warfarin. Nevertheless, the physician should be prepared to adjust the dosage of warfarin because these drugs impair platelet function and may cause gastrointestinal lesions.

As discussed above, the propionic acid derivatives can be expected to reduce the diuretic and natriuretic effects of furosemide as well as the antihypertensive effects of such agents as the thiazide diuretics, β-adrenergic antagonists, and inhibitors of angiotensin converting enzyme (*see* Clive and Stoff, 1984; Oates *et al.*, 1988). These effects probably result from the inhibition of the synthesis of renal or vascular prostaglandins (*see* above).

IBUPROFEN

Ibuprofen has been discussed in detail by Kantor (1979) and by Adams and Buckler (in Symposium, 1983a).

Pharmacokinetics and Metabolism. Ibuprofen is rapidly absorbed after oral administration in man, and peak concentrations in plasma are observed after 1 to 2 hours. The half-life in plasma is about 2 hours. Absorption is also efficient, although slower, from suppositories.

Ibuprofen is extensively (99%) bound to plasma proteins, but the drug occupies only a fraction of the total drug-binding sites at usual concentrations. Ibuprofen passes slowly into the synovial spaces and may remain there in higher concentration as the concentrations in plasma decline. In experimental animals, ibuprofen and its metabolites pass easily across the placenta.

The excretion of ibuprofen is rapid and complete. More than 90% of an ingested dose is excreted in the urine as metabolites or their conjugates, and no ibuprofen *per se* is found in the urine. The major metabolites are a hydroxylated and a carboxylated compound.

Preparations, Route of Administration, and Dosage. *Ibuprofen* (MOTRIN, RUFEN) is supplied as tablets containing 200 to 800 mg; only the 200-mg tablets (ADVIL, NUPRIN, others) are available without a prescription.

For rheumatoid arthritis and osteoarthritis, daily doses of up to 3200 mg in divided portions may be given, although the usual total dose is 1200 to 1800 mg. It may also be possible to reduce the dosage for maintenance purposes. For mild-to-moderate pain, especially that of primary dysmenorrhea, the usual dosage is 400 mg every 4 to 6 hours as needed. The drug may be given with milk or food to minimize gastrointestinal side effects. The safety and efficacy of ibuprofen in children have not been established.

Toxic Effects. Ibuprofen has been used in patients with known peptic ulceration or a history of gastric intolerance to other aspirin-like agents. Nevertheless, therapy must usually be discontinued in 10 to 15% of patients because of intolerance to the drug.

Gastrointestinal side effects are experienced by 5 to 15% of patients taking ibuprofen; epigastric pain, nausea, heartburn, and sensations of "fullness" in the gastrointestinal tract are the usual difficulties. However, the incidence of these side effects is less with ibuprofen than with aspirin or indomethacin. Occult blood loss is uncommon.

Other side effects of ibuprofen have been reported less frequently. They include thrombocytopenia, skin rashes, headache, dizziness and blurred vision, and, in a few cases, toxic amblyopia, fluid retention, and edema. Patients who develop ocular disturbances should discontinue the use of ibuprofen.

Ibuprofen is not recommended for use by pregnant women, or by those who are breast-feeding their infants.

NAPROXEN

The pharmacological properties and therapeutic uses of naproxen have been reviewed by Segre (in Symposium, 1983a) and by Allison and colleagues (Rainsford, 1985b).

Pharmacokinetics and Metabolism. Naproxen is fully absorbed when administered orally. The rapidity, but not the extent, of absorption is influenced by the presence of food in the stomach. Peak concentrations in plasma occur within 2 to 4 hours and may be achieved more rapidly after the administration of naproxen sodium. Absorption may be accelerated by the concurrent administration of sodium bicarbonate or reduced by magnesium oxide or aluminum hydroxide. Naproxen is also absorbed rectally, but peak concentrations in plasma are achieved more slowly. The half-life of naproxen in plasma is about 14 hours; this value is increased about twofold in elderly subjects and may necessitate adjustment of dosage.

Metabolites of naproxen are almost entirely excreted in the urine. About 30% of the drug undergoes 6-demethylation, and most of this metabolite, as well as naproxen itself, is excreted as the glucuronide or other conjugates.

Naproxen is almost completely (99%) bound to plasma protein following normal therapeutic doses. Naproxen crosses the placenta and appears in the milk of lactating women at approximately 1% of the maternal plasma concentration.

Preparations, Route of Administration, and Dosage. *Naproxen* (NAPROSYN) is available in 250-, 375-, and 500-mg tablets and a suspension (125 mg/5 ml) for oral administration. *Naproxen sodium* (ANAPROX) is marketed in tablets containing 275 or 550 mg of the salt (equivalent to 250 or 500 mg of naproxen). For rheumatoid arthritis, osteoarthritis, and ankylosing spondylitis, the usual dosage of naproxen is 250 to 500 mg, given twice daily; this is adjusted depending on the clinical response. For juvenile arthritis in children over 2 years of age, approximately 10 mg/kg per day is given in two divided doses. For acute gout, the usual initial dose of naproxen is 750 mg, followed by 250 mg every 8 hours until the attack has subsided. For mild-to-moderate pain, especially that associated with primary dysmenorrhea, bursitis, and acute tendinitis, the initial dose is 500 mg, followed by 250 mg every 6 to 8 hours. The drug may be given with meals if gastric discomfort is experienced.

Toxic Effects. Although the incidence of gastrointestinal and CNS side effects is about equal to that caused by indomethacin, naproxen is better tolerated in both regards. Gastrointestinal complications have ranged from relatively mild dyspepsia, gastric discomfort, and heartburn to nausea, vomiting, and gastric bleeding. CNS side effects range from drowsiness, headache, dizziness, and sweating to fatigue, depression, and ototoxicity. Less common reactions include pruritus and a variety of dermatological problems. A few instances of jaundice, impairment of renal function, angioneurotic edema, thrombocytopenia, and agranulocytosis have been reported.

FENOPROFEN

The pharmacological properties and therapeutic uses of fenoprofen have been reviewed by Burt and coworkers (Symposium, 1983a).

Pharmacokinetics and Metabolism. Oral doses of fenoprofen are readily, if incompletely (85%), absorbed. The presence of food in the stomach retards absorption and lowers peak concentrations in plasma, which are usually achieved within 2 hours. The concomitant administration of antacids does not seem to alter the concentrations that are achieved.

After absorption, fenoprofen is almost completely (99%) bound to plasma albumin. The drug is extensively (>90%) metabolized and excreted almost entirely in the urine. Fenoprofen undergoes metabolic transformation to the 4-hydroxy analog. The glucuronic acid conjugate of fenoprofen itself and 4-hydroxy fenoprofen are formed in almost equal amounts and together account for 90% of the excreted drug. The half-life of fenoprofen in plasma is about 3 hours.

Preparations, Route of Administration, and Dosage. *Fenoprofen calcium* (NALFON) is available in capsules and tablets containing 200 to 600 mg of the active drug for oral administration. The recommended dosage to treat rheumatoid arthritis or osteoarthritis is 300 to 600 mg, given three to four times a day, but this may be increased to a maximum of 3.2 g per day. For mild-to-moderate pain, the usual dosage is 200 mg every 4 to 6 hours. Fenoprofen may be administered with meals. The drug is not currently recommended for children.

Toxic Effects. The most frequently reported side effects have been gastrointestinal ones; abdominal discomfort and dyspepsia occur in about 15% of patients. Constipation and nausea have also been reported. These side effects are almost always less intense than with equipotent doses of aspirin and force discontinuation of therapy in a small percentage of patients. Nevertheless, care should be exercised when giving the drug to patients with a history of gastrointestinal ulceration or other pathology. Other side effects include skin rash and, less frequently, CNS effects such as tinnitus, dizziness, lassitude, confusion, and anorexia.

KETOPROFEN

Ketoprofen shares the pharmacological properties of other propionic acid derivatives; these have been reviewed by Harris and Vávra (Rainsford, 1985b) and Vávra (Lewis and Furst, 1987). Although it is a cyclooxygenase inhibitor, ketoprofen is said to stabilize lysosomal membranes and it may antagonize the actions of bradykinin.

Pharmacokinetics and Metabolism. Ketoprofen is rapidly absorbed after oral administration and maximal concentrations in plasma are achieved within 1 to 2 hours; food reduces the rate but not the extent of absorption. The drug is extensively bound to plasma proteins (99%), and it has a half-life in plasma of about 2 hours; slightly longer half-lives are observed in elderly subjects. Ketoprofen is conjugated with glucuronic acid in the liver, and the conjugate is excreted in the urine. Patients with impaired renal function eliminate the drug more slowly.

Preparations, Route of Administration, and Dosage. *Ketoprofen* (ORUDIS) is available as 25-, 50-, and 75-mg capsules. The recommended daily dosage to treat arthritic conditions is 150 to 300 mg, given in three or four divided doses; the lowest effective dose should be used. For nonarthritic pain, 25 to 50 mg given every 6 to 8 hours may be sufficient.

Toxic Effects. Dyspepsia and other gastrointestinal side effects have been observed in about 30% of patients, but these side effects are generally mild and are less frequent than those in patients treated with aspirin; untoward effects are reduced when the drug is taken with food, milk, or antacids. Ketoprofen can cause fluid retention and increased plasma concentrations of creatinine. These effects are generally transient and occur in the absence of symptoms, but they are more common in patients who are receiving diuretics or in those over the age of 60. Renal function should be monitored in such patients.

FLURBIPROFEN

Flurbiprofen has been available for over a decade in various combination preparations, and the drug has recently been marketed as a single entity in the United States.

The pharmacological properties, therapeutic indications, and adverse effects of flurbiprofen are similar to those of other antiinflammatory derivatives of propionic acid (*see* Smith *et al.*, in Rainsford, 1985b). The drug is well absorbed orally, and peak plasma concentrations occur within 1 to 2 hours. Flurbiprofen is extensively metabolized by hydroxylation and conjugation in the liver; its half-life in plasma is about 6 hours.

Flurbiprofen (ANSAID) is available in 50- and 100-mg tablets. The recommended daily dosage for rheumatoid arthritis and osteoarthritis is 200 to 300 mg in two to four divided doses.

THERAPEUTIC USES

The approved indications for the use of one or another of the propionic acid derivatives include the symptomatic treatment of rheumatoid arthritis, osteoarthritis, ankylosing spondylitis, and acute gouty arthritis; they are also used as analgesics, for acute tendinitis and bursitis, and for primary dysmenorrhea.

Clinical studies indicate that the propionic acid derivatives are comparable to aspirin for the control of the signs and symptoms of rheumatoid arthritis and osteoarthritis. In patients with rheumatoid arthritis there is a reduction in joint swelling, pain, and duration of morning stiffness. By objective measurements, strength, mobility, and stamina are improved. In general, the intensity of untoward effects is less than that associated with the ingestion of indomethacin or high doses of aspirin. However, aspirin is considerably less expensive for those who can tolerate it.

Although all of these agents may be of benefit in the treatment of ankylosing spondylitis, only naproxen has received approval for this use in the United States. As mentioned previously, naproxen appears to exert a prominent inhibitory effect on the migration of leukocytes; this may contribute to its efficacy in the treatment of acute attacks of gout. Clinical studies have indicated that the propionic acid derivatives may be as effective as aspirin in the treatment of juvenile arthritis. However, except for naproxen, the data are as yet insufficient to establish their safety for long-term use in children.

These agents are also effective for symptomatic relief from pain associated with injuries to soft tissues, and they have been used to relieve pain post partum and after oral, ophthalmic, and other types of surgery. Both ibuprofen and naproxen are more effective than aspirin for relief of pain from dysmenorrhea. Indeed, the effectiveness of ibuprofen in this condition was one important reason for its release in 1984 for over-the-counter use.

It is difficult to find data on which to base a rational choice between the members of this group of drugs, if in fact one can be made. However, in studies that compared the activity of several members of this group, patients preferred naproxen in terms of analgesia and relief of morning stiffness (*see* Huskisson, in Symposium, 1983a; Hart and Huskisson, 1984). With regard to side effects, naproxen was the best tolerated, followed by ibuprofen and fenoprofen. There was considerable interpatient variation in the preference for a single drug and also between the designation of the best and the worst drug. Unfortunately, it is probably impossible to predict *a priori* which drug will be most suitable for any given individual. Nevertheless, more than 50% of patients with rheumatoid arthritis will probably achieve adequate symptomatic relief by the use of one or another of the propionic acid derivatives, and many clinicians favor their use instead of aspirin in such patients.

PIROXICAM

Piroxicam is one of the oxicam derivatives, a class of enolic acids that possesses antiinflammatory, analgesic, and antipyretic activity. Other oxicams have been developed and are under study (*e.g.*, tenoxicam). Piroxicam is the only drug in this class that is currently available in the United States. In recommended doses, piroxicam appears to be the equivalent of aspirin, indomethacin, or naproxen for the long-term treatment of rheumatoid arthritis or osteoarthritis. It may be tolerated better than aspirin or indomethacin. The principal advantage of piroxicam is its long half-life, which permits the administration of a single daily dose. The pharmacological properties and therapeutic uses of piroxicam have been reviewed in a symposium (Symposium, 1982), by Wiseman (Rainsford, 1985b), and by Lombardino and Wiseman (in Lewis and Furst, 1987). The structural formula of piroxicam is as follows:

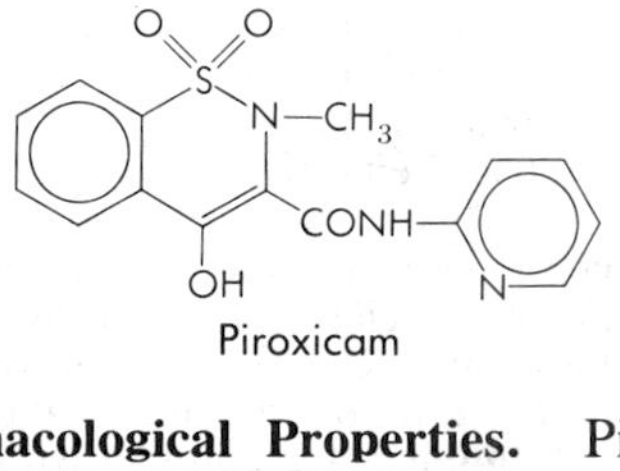

Piroxicam

Pharmacological Properties. Piroxicam is an effective antiinflammatory agent; it is about equal in potency to indomethacin as an inhibitor of prostaglandin biosynthesis *in vitro*. Piroxicam can also inhibit activation of neutrophils even when products of cyclooxygenase are present; hence, additional modes of antiinflammatory action have been proposed (Abramson *et al.*, 1985; Lombardino and Wiseman, in Lewis and Furst, 1987). Piroxicam exerts antipyretic and analgesic effects in experimental animals and man. As with other aspirin-like drugs, piroxicam can cause gastric erosions and it prolongs bleeding time.

Pharmacokinetics and Metabolism. Piroxicam is completely absorbed after oral administration; peak concentrations in plasma occur within 2 to 4 hours. Neither food nor antacids alter the rate or extent of absorption. There is enterohepatic cycling of piroxicam, and estimates of the half-life in plasma have been variable; a mean value appears to be about 50 hours.

After absorption, piroxicam is extensively (99%) bound to plasma proteins. At steady state (*e.g.*, after 7 to 12 days), concentrations of piroxicam in plasma and synovial fluid are approximately equal. Less than 5% of the drug is excreted in the urine unchanged. The major metabolic transformation in man is hydroxylation of the pyridyl ring, and this inactive metabolite and its glucuronide conjugate account for about 60% of the drug excreted in the urine and feces.

Preparations, Route of Administration, and Dosage. *Piroxicam* (FELDENE) is available in 10- and 20-mg capsules for oral administration. The usual daily dose for the relief of signs and symptoms of rheumatoid arthritis or osteoarthritis is 20 mg; if desired, this may be given in two portions. Since steady-state concentrations in plasma are not reached for 7 to 12 days, maximal therapeutic responses should not be expected for 2 weeks, even though they may be evident earlier. It has been suggested that satisfactory responses are associated with concentrations in plasma of greater than 5 to 6 μg/ml.

Toxic Effects. The reported incidence of adverse effects in patients who take piroxicam is about 20%; approximately 5% of patients stop using the drug because of side effects. Gastrointestinal reactions are the most common; the incidence of peptic ulcer is less than 1%. As with other aspirin-like drugs, piroxicam alters the function of platelets, and it should be assumed that piroxicam will precipitate bronchoconstriction in patients who are hypersensitive to aspirin.

Therapeutic Uses. Piroxicam is approved in the United States for the treatment of rheumatoid arthritis and osteoarthritis. It has also been used in the treatment of ankylosing spondylitis, acute musculoskeletal disorders, dysmenorrhea, postoperative pain, and acute gout.

DICLOFENAC

Diclofenac is the first of a series of phenylacetic acid derivatives that have been developed as antiinflammatory agents. Details of its pharmacology are discussed in a symposium (Symposium, 1986b) and a review by Liauw and associates (in Lewis and Furst, 1987). The structure of diclofenac is as follows:

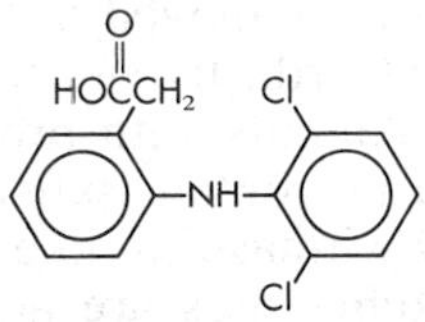

Diclofenac

Pharmacological Properties. Diclofenac possesses analgesic, antipyretic, and antiinflammatory activities; it is an inhibitor of cyclooxygenase, and its potency is substantially greater than that of indomethacin, naproxen, or several other agents. In addition, diclofenac appears to reduce intracellular concentrations of free arachidonate in leukocytes, perhaps by altering the release or uptake of the fatty acid.

Pharmacokinetics and Metabolism. Diclofenac is rapidly and completely absorbed after oral administration; peak concentrations in plasma are reached within 2 to 3 hours. Administration with food slows the rate but does not alter the extent of absorption. There is a substantial first-pass effect, such that only about 50% of diclofenac is available systemically. The drug is extensively bound to plasma proteins (99%), and its half-life in plasma is 1 to 2 hours. Diclofenac accumulates in synovial fluid after oral administration, which may explain the duration of therapeutic effect that is considerably longer than the plasma half-life. Diclofenac is metabolized in the liver to 4-hydroxydiclofenac, the principal metabolite, and other hydroxylated forms; after glucuronidation and sulfation, the metabolites are excreted in the urine (65%) and bile (35%).

Preparations, Route of Administration, and Dosage. *Diclofenac sodium* (VOLTAREN) is available as 25-, 50-, and 75-mg enteric-coated tablets. For the symptomatic relief of rheumatoid arthritis, the usual daily dosage is 150 to 200 mg given in two to four divided portions; for osteoarthritis, 100 to 150 mg is given daily in two or three divided doses; for ankylosing spondylitis, 100 to 125 mg is given daily in four or five divided doses.

Toxic Effects. Diclofenac produces side effects in about 20% of patients, and approximately 2% of patients discontinue therapy as a result. Gastrointestinal effects are the most common, and bleeding and ulceration or perforation of the intestinal wall have been observed. Elevation of hepatic transaminase activities in plasma occurs in about 15% of patients. Although usually moderate, these values may increase more than threefold in a small percentage of patients—often those who are being treated for osteoarthritis. The elevations in transaminases are usually reversible and are only rarely associated with clinical evidence of hepatic disease. Transaminase activities should be evaluated during the first 8 weeks of therapy, and the drug should be discontinued if abnormal values persist or if other signs or symptoms develop. Other untoward responses to diclofenac include CNS effects, skin rashes, allergic reactions, fluid retention and edema, and rarely, impairment of renal function. The drug is not recommended for children, nursing mothers, or pregnant women.

Therapeutic Uses. Diclofenac is approved in the United States for the long-term symptomatic treatment of rheumatoid arthritis, osteoarthritis, and ankylosing spondylitis. It may also be useful for short-term treatment of acute musculoskeletal injury, acute painful shoulder (bicipital tendinitis and subdeltoid bursitis), postoperative pain, and dysmenorrhea.

OTHER NONSTEROIDAL ANTIINFLAMMATORY DRUGS

A large number of antiinflammatory agents are under development or are under clinical study in the United States and elsewhere (*see* Rainsford, 1985b; Lewis and Furst, 1987). Although some are members of classes of drugs discussed above, others have novel structures and apparently different mechanisms of action. Two of the most important of these agents are etodolac and nabumetone; their structures are as follows:

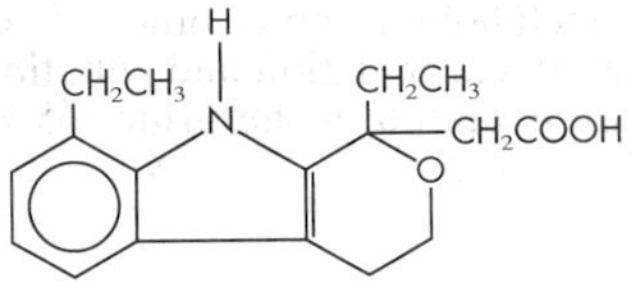

Etodolac

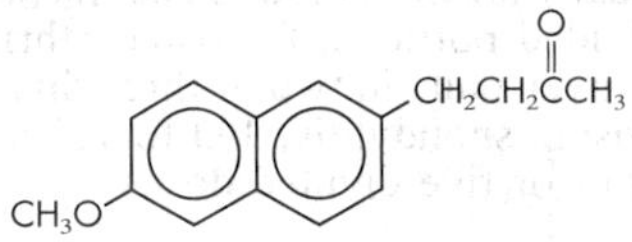

Nabumetone

Etodolac. This compound is an inhibitor of cyclooxygenase, and it possesses antiinflammatory activity. However, there is an unusually large difference between doses that produce antiinflammatory effects and those that cause gastric irritation in experimental animals. This may result from a relatively limited effect on the production of PGE_2 in the gastric mucosa.

Etodolac is rapidly and well absorbed orally, and it is about 99% bound to plasma proteins. It is actively metabolized by the liver to various metabolites that are largely excreted in the urine. The drug may undergo enterohepatic circulation in man; its half-life in plasma is about 7 hours.

A single oral dose of etodolac provides postoperative analgesia that typically lasts for 6 to 8 hours. Etodolac also appears to be effective in the treatment of osteoarthritis and rheumatoid arthritis. Although gastrointestinal irritation and ulceration are the most common manifestations of toxicity, these side effects appear to occur less frequently with etodolac than with certain other aspirin-like drugs. About 5% of patients who have taken the drug for up to 1 year discontinue treatment because of side effects, which also include skin rashes and CNS effects. (For further discussion of etodolac, *see* Lynch and Brogden, 1986, and Lewis and Furst, 1987.)

Nabumetone. Nabumetone is a weak inhibitor of cyclooxygenase *in vitro*, but it is an active antiinflammatory drug in various experimental models; it also possesses antipyretic and analgesic activities. In experimental animals, nabumetone appears to cause less gastric damage than do other antiinflammatory agents.

Nabumetone is absorbed rapidly and is converted in the liver to one or more active metabolites, principally 6-methoxy-2-naphthylacetic acid, a potent inhibitor of cyclooxygenase. This metabolite is inactivated by O-demethylation in the liver and is then conjugated before excretion.

Clinical trials with nabumetone have indicated substantial efficacy in the treatment of rheumatoid arthritis and osteoarthritis, with a relatively low incidence of side effects. However, only small numbers of patients have received the drug for more than 1 year. The drug also appears to be effective in the short-term treatment of soft-tissue injuries.

Side effects of treatment with nabumetone include lower bowel complaints, skin rash, headache, dizziness, heartburn, tinnitus, and pruritus. Thus far, the incidence of gastric ulceration has been much lower with nabumetone than with other aspirin-like drugs. This may result from the fact that an active compound is generated only after absorption of the administered drug. (For further discussion of nabumetone, *see* Symposium, 1987b, and Friedel and Todd, 1988.)

GOLD

Gold, in elemental form, has been employed for centuries as an antipruritic to relieve the itching palm. In more modern times, the observation by Robert Koch in 1890 that gold inhibited *Mycobacterium tuberculosis in vitro* led to trials in arthritis and lupus erythematosus, thought by some to be tuberculous manifestations. The favorable observations of Forestier (1929) were largely responsible for stimulating interest in gold therapy (chrysotherapy). At present, gold is employed in the treatment of rheumatoid arthritis; its use is usually reserved for patients with progressive disease who do not obtain satisfactory relief from therapy with aspirin-like drugs. However, gold compounds are among a small number of agents that are capable of arresting the progress of the disease and inducing apparent remissions in some patients; these are sometimes called disease-modifying drugs. Since degenerative lesions do not regress once formed, there is an increasing tendency to attempt to induce remission early in the course of the disease. Such therapy is most often initiated with gold.

Chemistry. The significant preparations of gold are all compounds in which the gold is attached to sulfur. The more water-soluble compounds employed in therapy contain hydrophilic groups in addition to the aurothio group. The structural formulas of aurothioglucose, gold sodium thiomalate, and auranofin are as follows:

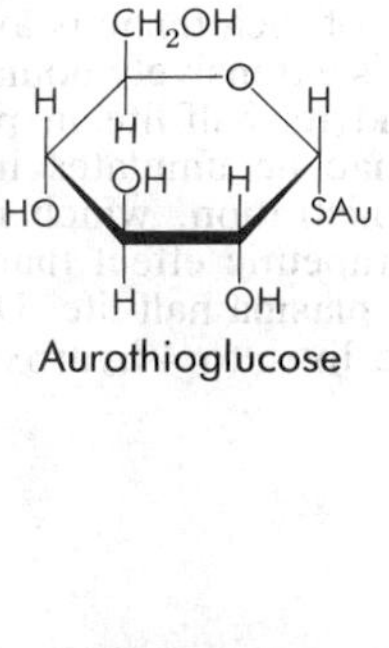

Aurothioglucose

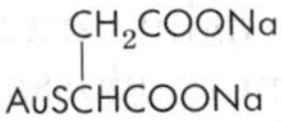

Gold Sodium Thiomalate

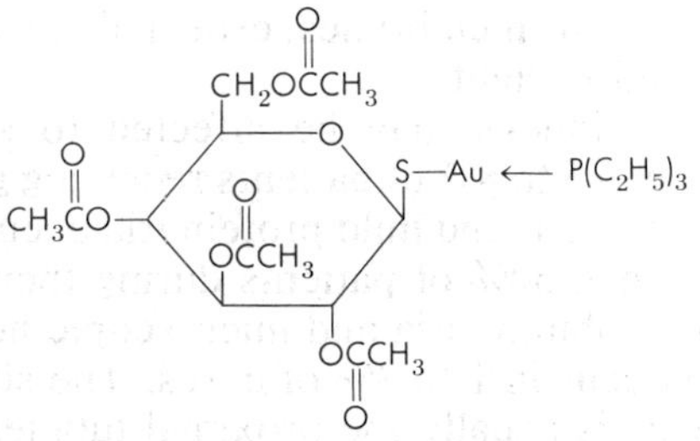

Auranofin

Monovalent gold has a relatively strong affinity for sulfur, weak affinities for carbon and nitrogen, and almost no affinity for oxygen, except in chelates. The high affinity for sulfur and the inhibitory effect of gold salts on various enzymes have suggested that the therapeutic effects of gold salts might derive from inhibition of sulfhydryl systems. However, other sulfhydryl inhibitors do not appear to have therapeutic actions in common with gold.

Pharmacological Properties. Gold compounds can suppress or prevent, but not cure, experimental arthritis and synovitis due to a number of infectious and chemical agents. Gold compounds have minimal antiinflammatory effects in other circumstances and cause only a gradual reduction of the signs and symptoms of inflammation associated with rheumatoid arthritis. Although many effects of these drugs have been observed, which, if any, are related to the therapeutic effects of gold in rheumatoid arthritis is unknown. Perhaps the best hypotheses relate to the capacity of gold compounds to inhibit the maturation and function of mononuclear phagocytes, thereby suppressing immune responsiveness (*see* Tsokos, 1987). Decreased concentrations of rheumatoid factor and immunoglobulins are often observed in patients who are treated with gold.

In experimental animals, gold is sequestered in organs that are rich in mononuclear phagocytes, and it selectively accumulates in the lysosomes of type-A synovial cells and other macrophages within the inflamed synovium of patients who are treated with gold compounds. Moreover, the administration of gold thiomalate to animals depresses the migration and phagocytic activity of macrophages in inflammatory exudates, and chrysotherapy reduces the augmented phagocytic capacity of blood monocytes from patients with rheumatoid arthritis. Other mechanisms of action of gold compounds have been suggested, but none is generally accepted. These include inhibition of prostaglandin synthesis, interference with complement activation, cross-linking of collagen, and inhibition of the activity of lysosomal and other enzymes.

Absorption, Distribution, and Excretion. *Aurothioglucose and Gold Sodium Thiomalate.* These more water-soluble gold compounds are rapidly absorbed after intramuscular injection, and peak concentrations in blood are reached in 2 to 6 hours, unless the drug is suspended in oil. These agents are erratically absorbed when administered orally. Tissue distribution depends not only on the type of compound administered but also on the time after administration and probably on the duration of treatment. Early in the course of therapy, several percent of the total body content of gold is in the blood, where it is first bound (about 95%) to albumin, and the concentration in synovial fluid eventually reaches about half that in plasma. With continued therapy, the concentration of gold in the synovium of affected joints is about ten times that of skeletal muscle, bone, or fat. Gold deposits are also found in macrophages of many tissues, as well as in proximal tubular epithelium, seminiferous tubules, hepatocytes, and adrenocortical cells.

The pharmacokinetic properties of gold in these compounds are complex and vary with the dose and the duration of treatment. The plasma half-life is about 7 days for a 50-mg dose. With successive doses the half-life lengthens, and values of weeks or months may be observed after prolonged therapy, reflecting the avid binding of gold in tissues. After a cumulative dose of 1 g of gold, about 60% of the amount administered is retained in the body. After termination of treatment, urinary excretion of gold can be detected for as long as a year, even though concentrations in blood fall to the normal trace amounts in about 40 to 80 days. Substantial quantities of gold have been found in the liver and skin of patients many years after the cessation of therapy. The excretion of gold is 60 to 90% renal and 10 to 40% fecal, the latter probably mostly by biliary secretion. Sulfhydryl agents, such as dimercaprol, penicillamine, and N-acetylcysteine, increase the excretion of gold. The pharmacokinetics of gold has been reviewed by Blocka and coworkers (1986).

Auranofin. Auranofin is a more hydrophobic gold-containing compound that is more readily absorbed after oral administration (to the extent of about 25%). Steady-state concentrations of gold in plasma are proportional to the doses and are reached after 8 to 12 weeks of treatment. Therapeutic doses of auranofin (6 mg per day) lead to concentrations of gold in plasma that are generally lower than those achieved with conventional parenteral therapy, and the accumulation of gold during a 6-month course of treatment with auranofin is only about 20% of that found with injectable gold compounds. Studies in animals suggest that auranofin binds to tissues to a lesser extent than does gold sodium thiomalate. After cessation of treatment, the half-life of gold in the body is about 80 days (*see* Chaffman *et al.*, 1984). Auranofin is predominantly excreted in the feces.

Preparations, Routes of Administration, and Dosage. *Aurothioglucose* (SOLGANAL) contains approximately 50% gold. Although it is water soluble, it is employed as a sterile suspension in a suitable fixed oil. The commercial preparation contains 50 mg/ml. *Gold sodium thiomalate* (MYOCHRYSINE) also contains approximately 50% gold and is very soluble in water. It is available as a sterile aqueous solution for injection. Both compounds should be administered intramuscularly.

The optimal intramuscular dosage schedule for the treatment of rheumatoid arthritis is still debated. Moreover, some rheumatologists use the same dosage regimen for either compound while others do not. The usual dose is 10 mg of either gold compound in the first week as a test dose, followed by 25 mg in the second and third weeks. Thereafter, either 25 to 50 mg (gold sodium thiomalate) or 50 mg (aurothioglucose) is administered at weekly intervals until the cumulative dose reaches 1 g. A favorable response may not be evident for a few months. If a remission occurs, treatment is continued but the dose is reduced or the dosage interval is increased. For example, 25 to 50 mg may be administered every 2 weeks for up to 20 weeks, followed by a dose every 3 weeks for an additional 18 weeks; thereafter a monthly-interval schedule may be followed for an indefinite period. If neither significant toxicity nor clinical response is apparent after the administration of 1 g of gold sodium thiomalate, a gradual increase in dosage may be considered; the weekly dose of this compound should not exceed 100 mg.

Auranofin (RIDAURA) contains about 29% gold and is available in 3-mg capsules for oral administration. For active rheumatoid arthritis, the daily dosage is 6 mg, which is given in one or two portions; some patients may require 9 mg daily in three divided doses. This higher dosage should not be instituted until the lower dosage has been given for 6 months, and therapy should be discontinued after 3 additional months if the response is still inadequate. Although patients have been maintained successfully on auranofin for several years, the optimal duration of therapy has not been determined.

Toxic Effects. The most common toxic effects that are associated with the therapeutic use of gold are those that involve the skin and the mucous membranes, usually of the mouth. These occur in about 15% of all patients. While clearly dose related, these effects do not correlate well with the concentration of gold in plasma (*see* Rothermich, in Symposium, 1983a). Cutaneous reactions may vary in severity from simple erythema to severe exfoliative dermatitis. Lesions of the mucous membranes include stomatitis, pharyngitis, tracheitis, gastritis, colitis, and vaginitis; glossitis is fairly common. As with silver, a gray-to-blue pigmentation (chrysiasis) may occur in the skin and mucous membranes, especially in areas exposed to light.

The kidneys may be affected to some degree in 5 to 8% of patients receiving gold, and transient and mild proteinuria occurs in more than 50% of patients during therapy. Heavy albuminuria and microscopic hematuria occur in 1 to 3% of cases. The site of damage is usually the proximal tubules. In addition, a gold-induced nephrosis can occur; the predominant lesion is membranous glomerulonephritis that is usually reversible.

Severe blood dyscrasias may also occur. Thrombocytopenia is observed in about 1% of patients. Most often this appears to be an immunological disturbance that results in an accelerated degradation of platelets. Occasionally the thrombocytopenia is a consequence of effects upon the bone marrow. In either case, withdrawal of the drug usually leads to recovery, but fatalities have occurred. Leukopenia, agranulocytosis, and aplastic anemia may also occur; aplastic anemia is rare but often fatal. When panmyelopathy results from aurotherapy, the concentrations of coproporphyrin and δ-aminolevulinic acid (δ-ALA) in urine may increase, as in lead poisoning. Eosinophilia is common, and many rheumatologists temporarily discontinue gold therapy when it occurs.

Gold may cause a variety of other severe toxic reactions, including encephalitis, peripheral neuritis, hepatitis, pulmonary infiltrates, and nitritoid (vasomotor) crisis. Fortunately, the incidence of serious reactions is low, and they generally are the result of failure to discontinue therapy when earlier, less serious symptoms occur.

Auranofin appears to be better tolerated than are the injectable gold compounds, and the incidence and severity of mucocutaneous and hematological side effects are less. However, auranofin produces a high incidence of gastrointestinal disturbances, which are sometimes troublesome and lead to discontinuation of therapy by about 5% of patients receiving the drug. About half of patients have a change in bowel habits (more frequent or loose stools often associated with abdominal cramping). Proteinuria is much less common with auranofin than with parenteral preparations, and the incidence of nephrotoxicity may also be less.

Avoidance and Treatment. Regular examination of the skin, buccal mucosa, urine, and blood, including cell and platelet counts, should be made. It is the practice in many arthritis clinics to initiate therapy with small doses of gold and to increase the dose gradually. Although untoward effects are not eliminated by this procedure, the severity of the reactions that occur early is somewhat reduced. If an untoward response occurs, therapy should be withheld until it subsides completely. If the reaction is a rash or stomatitis, antihistamines and glucocorticoids may be administered, the latter systemically and/or topically. Glucocorticoids are also indicated in gold-induced nephrosis.

If the reaction to gold therapy is not serious, injections of parenteral gold preparations may be cautiously resumed 2 or 3 weeks after the toxic reaction has subsided. Maintenance dosage should be two thirds to three fourths that previously planned. However, many experts decline to use the drug again, once toxicity has occurred. For auranofin, a decrease in dosage can also be attempted, but therapeutic responses may not be obtained.

If a severe reaction to gold occurs or if the above-mentioned steps fail to control the toxic effects, treatment with dimercaprol or penicillamine should be instituted. The administration of dimercaprol may shorten a therapeutic remission induced by gold.

Therapeutic Uses. Gold compounds find their chief therapeutic application in rheumatoid arthritis. Although these compounds can cause serious toxicity, they are among the most effective agents available for the treatment of rapidly progressive forms of the disease. Since other effective drugs (*e.g.*, penicillamine, methotrexate) can produce significantly more toxicity during long-term therapy, gold compounds are usually chosen to initiate therapy of rheumatoid arthritis when the goal is to attempt to halt its progression (*see* Rothermich, in Symposium, 1983a; Symposium, 1986c; Tsokos, 1987).

At present, gold is used in early, active arthritis that progresses despite an adequate regimen of aspirin-like drugs, rest, and physical therapy. Both subjective and objective manifestations of rheumatoid arthritis are improved. Gold compounds often arrest the progression of the disease in involved joints, at least temporarily; prevent involvement of unaffected joints; improve grip strength and morning stiffness; and decrease the erythrocyte sedimentation rate and abnormal plasma glycoprotein and fibrinogen levels. Gold should not be used if the disease is mild and is usually of little benefit when the disease is advanced. It has been estimated that chrysotherapy will induce a protracted remission in about 15% of patients, improve symptoms in 60 to 70% of patients, and must be discontinued in 15 to 20% of patients because of toxicity; about 10 to 15% of patients do not respond. The duration of the remission after discontinuation of treatment with gold is extremely variable (from 1 to 18 months). Although the recurrence is usually not as severe as the original disease and the majority of patients respond favorably to a second course of gold therapy, many rheumatologists prefer to continue treatment indefinitely without waiting for a relapse to occur. After 3 to 6 years of either continuous or discontinuous therapy, more than 50% of patients who had responded initially have terminated their treatment because of relapse or delayed toxicity (*see* Pinals, in Symposium, 1983d).

Therapy with gold is sometimes beneficial in juvenile rheumatoid arthritis, palindromic rheumatism, psoriatic arthritis, Sjögren's syndrome, nondisseminated lupus erythematosus, and pemphigus. Except for injectable preparations in the treatment of juvenile forms of arthritis, the use of gold in these conditions has not been approved in the United States.

Contraindications. Gold therapy is contraindicated in patients with renal disease, hepatic dysfunction or a history of infectious hepatitis, or hematological disorders. Gold should not be readministered to patients who have developed severe hematological or renal toxicity during a course of chrysotherapy; auranofin should not be administered after the occurrence of several additional gold-induced disorders, including pulmonary fibrosis, necrotizing enterocolitis, and exfoliative dermatitis. Gold is contraindicated during pregnancy or breast feeding. Patients who have recently had radiation should not receive gold because of its depressant action on hematopoietic tissue. Concomitant use of antimalarials, immunosuppressants, phenylbutazone, or oxyphenbutazone is contraindicated because of the potential of these drugs to cause blood dyscrasias. Urticaria, eczema, and colitis are also considered to be contraindications to the use of the metal. Finally, gold is poorly tolerated by elderly individuals.

OTHER DRUGS FOR RHEUMATOID ARTHRITIS

In addition to nonsteroidal antiinflammatory agents and gold, other drugs are also used for the treatment of rheumatoid arthritis. These include immunosuppressive agents, glucocorticoids, penicillamine, and hydroxychloroquine. With the exception of glucocorticoids, these drugs resemble gold salts in that they do not possess antiinflammatory or analgesic properties and their therapeutic effects become evident only after several weeks or months of treatment. They are generally reserved for patients who are refractory to therapeutic regimens that include rest, physiotherapy, and aspirin-like drugs, and in many instances, for those who do not tolerate or respond to treatment with gold. Although they are often grouped with gold as so-called disease-modifying antiarthritic drugs, these compounds are unlikely to induce remissions and are less apt to retard synovial erosion than is gold in patients with severe active rheumatoid arthritis (*see* Ward, 1988).

Although glucocorticoids can often produce dramatic symptomatic improvement, they do not arrest the progress of rheumatoid arthritis and are used only as adjuvants to other treatment because of their long-term toxicity (*see* Chapter 60). Immunosuppressants sometimes relieve joint inflammation when chrysotherapy has failed, but each of these drugs has its unique and significant toxicities (*see* Chapter 53). Of the cytotoxic immunosuppressants, only azathioprine and low oral doses of methotrexate have been approved for the treatment of rheumatoid arthritis; the use of cyclosporine, a novel immunosuppressant, is under investigation.

Even though their mechanisms of action are not understood, hydroxychloroquine and penicillamine are useful, orally effective alternatives to gold in the treatment of patients with early, mild, and nonerosive disease (*see* Ward, 1988). The latter drug is more apt to produce serious toxicity, including various cutaneous lesions, blood dyscrasias, and a number of autoimmune syndromes (*see* Chapter 66). Therapy with penicillamine is initiated with single daily doses of 125 to 250 mg; the dosage is gradually increased at 1- to 3-month intervals to a maximum of 1 to 1.5 g per day. Many patients will respond to less than 500 to 750 mg per day.

Hydroxychloroquine shares the toxicity of other 4-aminoquinoline antimalarials (*see* Chapter 41). Of greatest concern during the long-term treatment of rheumatoid arthritis is the danger of producing irreversible retinal damage. The risk of corneal deposits and ocular toxicity appears to be less for hydroxychloroquine than for chloroquine at the usual antirheumatic doses (*see* Easterbrook, 1988; Rynes, 1988). Therapy is initiated with 400 to 600 mg of hydroxychloroquine sulfate per day, taken with food or milk. After a satisfactory response is obtained (usually within 1 to 3 months), the daily dose is reduced to 200 to 400 mg. Ophthalmological examinations should be performed before treatment is begun and every 3 months thereafter.

DRUGS EMPLOYED IN THE TREATMENT OF GOUT

An acute attack of gout occurs as a result of an inflammatory reaction to crystals of sodium urate (the end product of purine metabolism in man) that are deposited in the joint tissue. The inflammatory response involves local infiltration of granulocytes, which phagocytize the urate crystals. Lactate production is high in synovial tissues and in the leukocytes associated with the inflammatory process, and this favors a local decrease in pH that fosters further deposition of uric acid.

Several therapeutic strategies can be used to counter attacks of gout. Uricosuric drugs increase the excretion of uric acid, thus reducing concentrations in plasma. Colchicine is specifically efficacious in gout, probably secondary to an effect on the mobility of granulocytes. Allopurinol is a selective inhibitor of the terminal steps of the biosynthesis of uric acid. Although prostaglandins may be implicated in the pain and inflammation, there is no evidence that they contribute to the pathogenesis of gout; nevertheless, aspirin-like drugs usually afford symptomatic relief, and some of them are uricosuric as well (*see* Gibson, in Lewis and Furst, 1987).

The pharmacology of aspirin-like drugs is described in the previous section. Discussion in this section is limited to colchicine, allopurinol, and the clinical use of the uricosuric agents. The basic pharmacology of uricosuric drugs is presented in Chapter 30. A useful volume on uric acid that contains major sections on the pathogenesis and therapy of gout is that edited by Kelley and Weiner (1978).

COLCHICINE

Colchicine is a unique antiinflammatory agent in that it is largely effective only against gouty arthritis. It provides dramatic relief of acute attacks of gout and is an effective prophylactic agent against such attacks.

History. Colchicine is an alkaloid of *Colchicum autumnale* (autumn crocus, meadow saffron). Although the poisonous action of colchicum was known to Dioscorides, preparations of the plant were not recommended for pain of articular origin until the sixth century A.D. Colchicum was introduced for the therapy of acute gout by von Störck in 1763, and its specificity for this syndrome soon resulted in its incorporation in a number of "gout mixtures" popularized by charlatans. Benjamin Franklin, himself a sufferer from gout, is reputed to have introduced colchicum therapy in the United States. The alkaloid colchicine was isolated from colchicum in 1820 by Pelletier and Caventou.

Chemistry. The structural formula of colchicine is as follows:

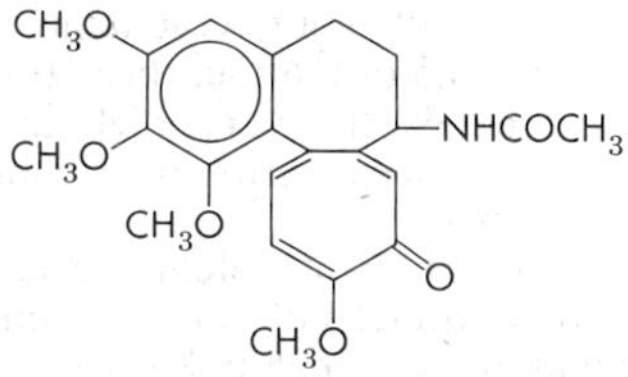

Colchicine

The structure–activity relationship of colchicine and related agents has been discussed by Wallace (1961).

Pharmacological Properties. The antiinflammatory effect of colchicine in acute gouty arthritis is relatively selective for this disorder. Colchicine is only occasionally effective in other types of arthritis; it is not an analgesic and does not provide relief of other types of pain.

Colchicine is an antimitotic agent and is widely employed as an experimental tool in the study of cell division and function.

Effect in Gout. Colchicine does not influence the renal excretion of uric acid or its concentration in blood. By virtue of its ability to bind to microtubular protein (tubulin), colchicine interferes with the function of the mitotic spindles and causes depolymerization and disappearance of the fibrillar microtubules in granulocytes and other motile cells. This action is apparently the basis for the beneficial effect of colchicine, namely, the inhibition of the migration of granulocytes into the inflamed area. This reduces the release of lactic acid and proinflammatory enzymes that occurs during phagocytosis and breaks the cycle that leads to the inflammatory response. However, there are a number of apparently contradictory observations that cannot be accommodated by this simple hypothesis (*see* Wallace and Ertel, 1978).

Neutrophils exposed to urate crystals ingest them and produce a glycoprotein, which may be the causative agent of acute gouty arthritis. Injected into joints, this substance produces a profound arthritis that is histologically indistinguishable from that caused by direct injection of urate crystals. Although it does not prevent phagocytosis of urate crystals, colchicine appears to prevent the elaboration by leukocytes of the glycoprotein that causes the joint pain and inflammation.

Effect on Cell Division. Colchicine can arrest plant and animal cell division *in vitro* and *in vivo*. Mitosis is arrested in metaphase, due to failure of spindle formation. Cells with the highest rates of division are affected earliest. High concentrations may completely prevent cells from entering mitosis, and they often die. The action is also characteristic of the vinca alkaloids (vincristine and vinblastine), podophyllotoxin, and griseofulvin.

Other Effects. Colchicine inhibits the release of histamine-containing granules from mast cells, the secretion of insulin from beta cells of pancreatic islets, and the movement of melanin granules in melanophores; all of these processes may involve the translocation of granules by the microtubular system.

Colchicine also exhibits a variety of other pharmacological effects. It lowers body temperature, increases the sensitivity to central depressants, depresses the respiratory center, enhances the response to sympathomimetic agents, constricts blood vessels, and induces hypertension by central vasomotor stimulation. It enhances gastrointestinal activity by neurogenic stimulation but depresses it by a direct effect, and alters neuromuscular function.

Pharmacokinetics and Metabolism. Colchicine is rapidly absorbed after oral administration, and peak concentrations occur in plasma by 0.5 to 2 hours. Large amounts of the drug and metabolites enter the intestinal tract in the bile and intestinal secretions, and this fact, plus the rapid turnover of intestinal epithelium, probably explains the prominence of intestinal manifestations in colchicine poisoning. The kidney, liver, and spleen also contain high concentrations of colchicine, but it is apparently largely excluded from heart, skeletal muscle, and brain. The drug can be detected in leukocytes and in the urine for at least 9 days after a single intravenous dose.

Colchicine is metabolized to a mixture of compounds *in vitro*. Most of the drug is excreted in the feces; however, in normal individuals, 10 to 20% of the drug is excreted in the urine. In patients with liver disease, hepatic uptake and elimination are reduced and a greater fraction of the drug is excreted in the urine.

Toxic Effects. Colchicine is well tolerated in moderate dosage. The most common side effects reflect the action of the drug on the rapidly proliferating epithelial cells in the gastrointestinal tract, especially in the jejunum. Nausea, vomiting, diarrhea, and abdominal pain are the most common and earliest untoward effects of colchicine overdosage. To avoid more serious toxicity, administration of the drug is discontinued as soon as these symptoms occur. There is a latent period of several hours or more between the administration of the drug and the onset of symptoms. This interval is not altered by dosage or route of administration. For this reason, and because of individual variation, adverse effects may be unavoidable during an initial course of medication with colchicine. However, the patient often remains relatively consistent in his response to the drug, and therefore toxicity can be minimized or avoided during subsequent courses of therapy. The drug is equally effective when given intravenously; the onset of the therapeutic effect may be faster, and the gastrointestinal side effects may be almost completely avoided.

In acute poisoning with colchicine, there is hemorrhagic gastroenteritis, extensive vascular damage, nephrotoxicity, muscular depression, and an ascending paralysis of the CNS.

Colchicine produces a temporary leukopenia that is soon replaced by a leukocytosis, sometimes due to a striking increase in the number of basophilic granulocytes. The site of action is apparently directly on the bone marrow. Myopathy and neuropathy have also been noted with colchicine treatment, especially in patients with decreased renal function (Kuncl *et al.,* 1987). Long-term administration of colchicine entails some risk of agranulocytosis, aplastic anemia, myopathy, and alopecia; azoospermia has also been described.

Preparations. *Colchicine* is available as 0.5- and 0.6-mg tablets; they should be stored in tight, light-resistant containers. A sterile solution (0.5 mg/ml) is also available for injection.

Therapeutic Uses. Colchicine provides dramatic relief from acute attacks of gout. The effect is sufficiently selective that the drug has been used for diagnostic purposes, but the test is not infallible. Colchicine also has an established role to prevent and to abort acute attacks of gout (*see* Rodnan, 1982; Talbott, in Symposium, 1983a). However, its toxicity and the availability of alternative agents that may be less toxic have lessened its usefulness (*see* Roberts *et al.,* 1987).

Acute Attacks. When colchicine is given promptly within the first few hours of an attack, less than 5% of patients fail to obtain relief. Pain, swelling, and redness abate within 12 hours and are completely gone in 48 to 72 hours. The usual doses are 0.5 to 1.2 mg, taken at intervals of 1 to 2 hours until either the pain disappears or gastrointestinal symptoms develop. The total dose usually required to alleviate an attack is 4 to 10 mg, and the latter amount should not be exceeded. Opioids or other drugs may be required for the diarrhea. In subsequent attacks, the patient may be able to stop medication short of the amount that causes toxic reactions. Colchicine can be administered intravenously, and there may be distinct advantages to this route for some patients (*see* Roberts *et al.,* 1987; Wallace and Singer, 1988). Although a number of regimens have been used, a single dose of 2 mg, diluted in 10 to 20 ml of 0.9% sodium chloride solution, is usually adequate; a total dose of 4 mg should not be exceeded. To avoid cumulative toxicity, treatment with colchicine should not be repeated within 3 (oral) or 7 (intravenous) days.

Great care should be exercised in prescribing colchicine for elderly patients, and for those with cardiac, renal, hepatic, or gastrointestinal disease. In these patients and in those who do not tolerate or respond to colchicine, indomethacin or another aspirin-like drug is preferred.

Prophylactic Uses. For patients with chronic gout, colchicine has established value as a prophylactic agent, especially when there is frequent recurrence of attacks. Prophylactic medication is also indicated upon initiation of long-term medication with allopurinol or the uricosuric agents, since acute attacks often increase in frequency during the early months of such therapy.

The prophylactic dose of colchicine depends upon the frequency and severity of prior attacks. As little as 0.5 mg two to four times a week may suffice; as much as 1.8 mg per day may be required by some patients. Colchicine should be taken in larger abortive doses immediately upon the first twinge of articular pain or the appearance of any prodrome of an acute attack. Before and after surgery in patients with gout, colchicine should be given for 3 days (0.5 or 0.6 mg, three times a day); this greatly reduces the very high incidence of acute attacks of gouty arthritis precipitated by operative procedures.

Daily administration of colchicine is useful for the prevention of attacks of familial Mediterranean fever (familial paroxysmal polyserositis) and for prevention and treatment of amyloidosis in such patients (Zemer *et al.,* 1986). Colchicine appears to benefit patients with primary biliary cirrhosis, although the underlying disease may not be altered (Bodenheimer *et al.,* 1988). Colchicine has been approved as an orphan drug to arrest the progression of neurological disability caused by multiple sclerosis. It has also been employed to treat a variety of skin disorders, including psoriasis and Behçet's syndrome (*see* Aram, 1983).

ALLOPURINOL

Allopurinol is effective for the treatment of both the primary hyperuricemia of gout and that secondary to hematological disorders or antineoplastic therapy. In contrast to the uricosuric agents that increase the renal excretion of urate, allopurinol inhibits the terminal steps in uric acid biosynthesis. Since overproduction of uric acid is a contributing factor in most patients with gout and a characteristic of most types of secondary hyperuricemia, allopurinol represents a rational approach to therapy.

History. The introduction of allopurinol by Hitchings, Elion, and associates provides an elegant example of the development of a drug on a rational biochemical basis. Originally synthesized as a candidate for an antineoplastic agent, allopurinol was found to lack antimetabolite activity but it proved to be a substrate for and an inhibitor of xanthine oxidase. Allopurinol delays inactivation of mercaptopurine by xanthine oxidase and reduces the plasma concentration and renal excretion of uric acid. Subsequent clinical study for treatment of gout by Rundles and coworkers was successful and quickly confirmed (*see* Elion, 1978).

Chemistry and Pharmacological Properties. Allopurinol, an analog of hypoxanthine, has the following structural formula:

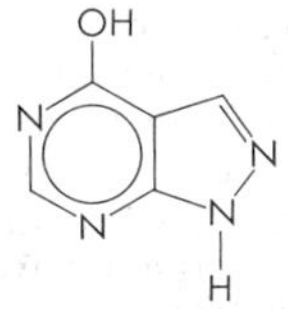

Allopurinol

Both allopurinol and its primary metabolite, alloxanthine (oxypurinol), are inhibitors of xanthine oxidase. Inhibition of this enzyme accounts for the major pharmacological effects of allopurinol (*see* Elion, 1978).

In man, uric acid is formed primarily by the xanthine oxidase–catalyzed oxidation of hypoxanthine and xanthine. At low concentrations, allopurinol is a substrate for and competitive inhibitor of the enzyme; at high concentrations, it is a noncompetitive inhibitor. Alloxanthine, the metabolite of allopurinol formed by the action of xanthine oxidase, is a noncompetitive inhibitor of the enzyme; the formation of this compound, together with its long persistence in tissues, is undoubtedly responsible for much of the pharmacological activity of allopurinol. Inhibition of uric acid biosynthesis reduces its plasma concentration and urinary excretion and increases the plasma concentrations and renal excretion of the more soluble oxypurine precursors.

In the absence of allopurinol, the urinary content of purines is almost solely uric acid. During treatment with allopurinol, the urinary purines are divided among hypoxanthine, xanthine, and uric acid. Since each has its independent solubility, the concentration of uric acid in plasma is reduced without exposing the urinary tract to an excessive load of uric acid and the likelihood of calculus formation. By lowering the uric acid concentration in plasma below its limit of solubility, allopurinol facilitates the dissolution of tophi and prevents the development or progression of chronic gouty arthritis. The formation of uric acid stones virtually disappears with therapy, and this prevents the development of nephropathy. The incidence of acute attacks of arthritis may increase during the early months of therapy but is subsequently reduced.

Tissue deposition of xanthine and hypoxanthine usually does not occur during allopurinol therapy because the renal clearance of the oxypurines is rapid; their plasma concentrations are only slightly increased and do not exceed their solubility. Although xanthine constitutes about 50% of total oxypurine excreted in the urine and is relatively insoluble, xanthine stone formation during allopurinol therapy has occurred only occasionally in patients with very high uric acid production prior to treatment. The risk can be minimized by alkalinization of the urine and by increasing the daily fluid intake during the administration of allopurinol. In some patients, the allopurinol-induced increase in excretion of oxypurines is less than the reduction in uric acid excretion; this disparity is primarily a result of reutilization of oxypurines and feedback inhibition of *de-novo* purine biosynthesis.

Pharmacokinetics and Metabolism. Allopurinol is absorbed relatively rapidly after oral ingestion, and peak plasma concentration is reached within 30 to 60 minutes. About 20% is excreted in the feces in 48 to 72 hours, presumably as unabsorbed drug. Allopurinol is rapidly cleared from plasma with a half-time of 2 to 3 hours, primarily by conversion to alloxanthine. Less than 10% of a single dose or about 30% of the drug ingested during long-term medication is excreted unchanged in the urine. Self-inhibition of the metabolism of allopurinol to alloxanthine explains this dose-dependent elimination. Alloxanthine is slowly excreted in the urine by the net balance of glomerular filtration and probenecid-sensitive tubular reabsorption. The plasma half-life of alloxanthine is 18 to 30 hours in patients with normal renal function and increases in proportion to the reduction of glomerular filtration in patients with renal impairment.

Allopurinol and its metabolite alloxanthine are distributed in total tissue water, with the exception of brain, in which their concentration is about one third that in other tissues. Neither compound is bound to plasma proteins. The plasma concentrations of the two compounds do not correlate well with therapeutic or toxic effects.

Drug Interactions. Interactions between allopurinol and probenecid and other uricosuric agents and those between allopurinol and mercaptopurine (and its derivative azathioprine) have been alluded to above. Allopurinol may also interfere with the hepatic inactivation of other drugs, including the oral anticoagulant agents. Although the effect is variable and of clinical significance only in some patients, increased monitoring of prothrombin activity is recommended in patients receiving both medications.

Whether the increased incidence of skin rash in patients receiving concurrent allopurinol–ampicillin medication, compared with that observed when these agents are administered individually, should be ascribed to allopurinol or to hyperuricemia remains to be established. Hypersensitivity reactions have been reported in patients with compromised renal function who are receiving a combination of allopurinol and a thiazide diuretic. The concomitant administration of allopurinol and theophylline leads to increased accumulation of an active metabolite of theophylline, 1-methylxanthine; the concentration of theophylline in plasma may also be increased.

Toxic Effects. Allopurinol is well tolerated by most patients. The most common adverse effects are hypersensitivity reactions. They may occur even after months or years of medication. The effects usually subside within a few days after medication is discontinued. Serious reactions preclude further use of the drug.

Attacks of acute gout may occur more frequently during the initial months of allopurinol medication and may require concurrent prophylactic therapy with colchicine (*see* above).

The cutaneous reaction caused by allopurinol is predominantly a pruritic, erythematous, or maculopapular eruption, but occasionally the lesion is exfoliative, urticarial, or purpuric. Fever, malaise, and muscle aching may also occur. Such effects are noted in about 3% of patients with normal renal function but more frequently in those with renal impairment.

Transient leukopenia or leukocytosis and eosinophilia are rare reactions but may require cessation of therapy. Hepatomegaly and elevated levels of transaminase activities in plasma may also occur. There have been isolated reports of peripheral neuritis, bone-marrow depression, and cataracts. Eosinophilia with epidermal necrolysis has resulted in renal failure.

Undesirable side effects such as headache, drowsiness, nausea, vomiting, vertigo, diarrhea, and gastric irritation occur occasionally but usually do not require that therapy be stopped.

Preparations, Route of Administration, and Dosage. *Allopurinol* (ZYLOPRIM, others) is available as 100- and 300-mg tablets for oral use.

For control of hyperuricemia in gout, the aim of therapy is to reduce the plasma uric acid concentration below 6 mg/dl (360 μM). Medication must not be initiated during an acute attack of gouty arthritis, and it is started at low doses to minimize the risk of precipitating such attacks. Concurrent prophylactic administration of colchicine is also recommended during and sometimes beyond the initial months of therapy. Fluid intake should be sufficient to maintain daily urinary volume above 2 liters; slightly alkaline urine is preferred. An initial daily dose of 100 mg is increased by 100-mg increments at weekly intervals to a maximum of 800 mg per day. The usual daily maintenance dose for adults is 200 to 300 mg for those with mild gout and 400 to 600 mg for patients with moderately severe tophaceous gout. Daily doses in excess of 300 mg should be given in divided portions. Dosage must be reduced in patients with renal impairment in proportion to the reduction in glomerular filtration (Hande *et al.*, 1984); for example, no more than 200 mg per day should be used in patients whose creatinine clearance is 10 to 20 ml/min.

In the treatment of secondary hyperuricemias, as for the prevention of uric acid nephropathy during vigorous treatment of certain neoplastic diseases, a dose of 600 to 800 mg daily for 2 to 3 days is advisable, together with a high fluid intake. In children with secondary hyperuricemias associated with malignancies, the usual daily dose is 150 to 300 mg, depending upon age.

Therapeutic Uses. Allopurinol provides effective therapy for both the primary hyperuricemia of gout and that secondary to polycythemia vera, myeloid metaplasia, or other blood dyscrasias.

Allopurinol is contraindicated in patients who have exhibited serious adverse effects from the medication, nursing mothers, and children, except those with malignancy or certain inborn errors of purine metabolism.

In gout, allopurinol is generally used in the severe chronic forms characterized by one or more of the following conditions: gouty nephropathy, tophaceous deposits, renal urate stones, impaired renal function, or hyperuricemia not readily controlled by the uricosuric drugs.

When given in effective doses and over prolonged periods, allopurinol fosters resorption of tophi and improvement of joint function in patients with tophaceous gout. By decreasing the amount of uric acid excreted and thereby preventing the development of nephrolithiasis, allopurinol eliminates the major cause of renal injury in patients with gout. It also appears likely that gouty nephropathy can be reversed by the drug if therapy is begun at a reasonably early stage, before renal function is severely compromised; however, there is little evidence of improvement in advanced renal disease.

Since attacks of acute gout occur in patients taking allopurinol, particularly during the initial stage of treatment, colchicine is used prophylactically when therapy is begun and continued if necessary to prevent such attacks. Concurrent allopurinol and uricosuric therapy is also employed occasionally, especially in patients with large tophaceous deposits in whom it is desirable both to reduce production and to increase elimination of uric acid. Such combined medication is valid, but interaction between these drugs is sometimes complex. The uricosuric agents increase the renal excretion of alloxanthine and thus cause a reduction in allopurinol effect. Conversely, allopurinol may delay elimination of probenecid and increase its concentration in plasma.

Allopurinol is also administered prophylactically to reduce the hyperuricemia and to prevent urate deposition or renal calculi in patients with leukemias, lymphomas, or other malignancies, particularly when antineoplastic or radiation therapy is initiated. Allopurinol inhibits the enzymatic inactivation of mercaptopurine by xanthine oxidase. Thus, when allopurinol is used concomitantly with oral mercaptopurine or azathioprine, dosage of the antineoplastic agent must be reduced to one fourth to one third of the usual dose. The risk of bone-marrow suppression is also increased when allopurinol is administered with cytotoxic agents that are not metabolized by xanthine oxidase, particularly cyclophosphamide.

The iatrogenic hyperuricemia sometimes induced by the thiazides and other drugs can be prevented or reversed by concurrent allopurinol medication, although this is rarely necessary. Allopurinol is also useful in lowering the high plasma concentrations of uric acid in patients with Lesch–Nyhan syndrome and thereby prevents the complications resulting from hyperuricemia; there is no evidence that it alters the progressive neurological and behavioral abnormalities characteristic of the disease.

CLINICAL USE OF URICOSURIC AGENTS

As described in Chapter 30, the uricosuric agents act directly on the renal tubule to increase the rate of excretion of uric acid. Although many agents share this property, only a few, primarily probenecid and sulfinpyrazone, are used clinically as uricosuric agents. Benzbromarone is not available for general use in the United States but is used elsewhere, especially in patients with renal insufficiency. In the clinical use of uricosuric drugs, it must be kept in mind that they can alter the plasma binding, distribution, and renal excretion of other organic acids, whether these are naturally occurring substances or drugs and drug metabolites.

Gout. The use of probenecid and sulfinpyrazone for the mobilization of uric acid in chronic gout is well established. In about two thirds of patients, these agents cause uric acid to be excreted at a rate sufficient to exceed that of formation and thereby promptly lower the plasma uric acid concentration. Although the intravenous administration of large doses of these drugs can cause a fivefold to sevenfold increase in the renal clearance of urate, continuous oral administration to patients with tophaceous gout approximately doubles the daily excretion of urates. In such patients, continued administration prevents the formation of new tophi and causes gradual shrinkage, or even disappearance, of old tophi. In gouty arthritis, there is a reduction in the swelling of chronically enlarged joints and a dramatic degree of rehabilitation may be achieved in patients who suffer severe pain and limitation of joint movement. In patients who do not respond well to uricosuric agents because of impaired renal function, allopurinol is especially useful, as described above. In patients with gouty nephropathy, allopurinol offers additional advantage over the uricosuric agents in that the daily excretion of uric acid is reduced rather than increased. Its administration is compatible with the simultaneous use of the uricosuric agents if necessary.

Neither the uricosuric agents nor allopurinol alters the course of acute attacks of gout or supplants the use of colchicine and antiinflammatory agents in their management. Indeed, the acute attacks may increase in frequency or severity during the early months of therapy when urate is being mobilized from affected joints. Therefore, therapy with uricosuric agents should not be initiated during an acute attack but may be continued if already begun. Colchicine in small doses (0.5 to 1.8 mg per day) may be administered at this period (or at any time) to reduce the frequency of attacks. When an acute attack occurs, it is treated with full doses of colchicine or an antiinflammatory drug such as indomethacin or naproxen. The use of salicylates is contraindicated because they antagonize the action of probenecid and sulfinpyrazone.

In the treatment of gout, the uricosuric drugs are given continually in the lowest dose that will maintain satisfactory plasma uric acid concentrations. Since the pK_a of uric acid is 5.6 and the solubility of the undissociated form is very low, maintaining the output of a large volume of alkaline urine minimizes its intrarenal deposition. This precaution is essential during the early weeks of therapy when uric acid excretion is large, especially in patients with a history of renal disease associated with the passage of urate stones or gravel. Eventual improvement in renal function in patients with gouty nephropathy has been reported, but it is uncommon. The use of allopurinol permits a more favorable prognosis in such patients. (For detailed evaluations of uricosuric agents, *see* Boss and Seegmiller, 1979; Rodnan, 1982.)

Other Hyperuricemic States. Uricosuric agents are useful for the control of the hyperuricemia resulting from the use of the cytotoxic antineoplastic agents or from diseases that involve accelerated formation and destruction of blood cells. Uricosuric agents are also rarely required to manage hyperuricemia in other settings, such as therapy with diuretics, levodopa, and ethambutol, and in certain disease states, including toxemia of pregnancy, diabetic ketosis, and uremia. The hyperuricemia usually remains asymptomatic, but attacks of gout or renal precipitation of urate may occur.

Selection of Agents for the Treatment of Gout and Hyperuricemia. Acute attacks of gout are effectively treated with colchicine or an aspirin-like drug, as discussed above. After the acute arthritis has responded to therapy, the patient should be evaluated in order to select a rational regimen for long-term management. Elevated concentrations of uric acid in plasma and the observation of crystals of urate in the aspirated fluid from an affected joint establish the diagnosis of hyperuricemia and symptomatic gout. When evaluated on a diet that is low in purines, patients with hyperuricemia can be categorized with regard to quantities of uric acid excreted in the urine. About 80 to 90% of such individuals excrete less than 600 mg of uric acid daily; the remainder excrete more than this amount due to excessive synthesis of urate. The former group can be managed effectively with uricosuric agents; the latter, however, is logically treated with allopurinol. If deposits of urate are evident as tophi, renal stones, or renal insufficiency, allopurinol is generally the preferred drug. During the first several months of treatment with allopurinol, colchicine may be given simultaneously to prevent acute attacks of gout. Patients with mild-to-moderate hyperuricemia (7 to 9 mg/dl) (420 to 530 μM) who do not have arthritis should be advised to drink large amounts of fluids and follow a diet low in purines. Drug-induced hyperuricemia is most commonly caused by diuretics (*see* Chapter 28); acute attacks of gout are only rarely caused by such agents. However, hyperuricemia that accompanies chemotherapy or radiotherapy for various neoplasms may be considerably more severe and is usually treated prophylactically with allopurinol and hydration.

Abramson, S.; Korchak, H.; Ludewig, R.; Edelson, H.; Haines, K.; Levin, R. I.; Herman, R.; Rider, L.; Kimmel, S.; and Weissmann, G. Modes of action of aspirin-like drugs. *Proc. Natl. Acad. Sci. U.S.A.*, **1985**, *82*, 7227–7231.

Anderson, R. J.; Potts, D. E.; Gabow, P. A.; Rumack, B. H.; and Schrier, R. W. Unrecognized adult salicylate intoxication. *Ann. Intern. Med.*, **1976**, *85*, 745–748.

Benigni, A., and others. Effect of low-dose aspirin on fetal and maternal generation of thromboxane by platelets in women at risk for pregnancy-induced hypertension. *N. Engl. J. Med.*, **1989**, *321*, 357–362.

Bodenheimer, H.; Schaffner, F.; and Pezzullo, J. Evaluation of colchicine therapy in primary biliary cirrhosis. *Gastroenterology*, **1988**, *95*, 124–129.

Forestier, J. L'aurothérapie dans les rhumatismes chronique. *Bull. Mém. Soc. Méd. Hôp. Paris*, **1929**, *53*, 323–327.

Hande, K. R.; Noone, R. M.; and Stone, W. J. Severe allopurinol toxicity. Description and guidelines for prevention in patients with renal insufficiency. *Am. J. Med.*, **1984**, *76*, 47–56.

Hurwitz, E. S., and others. Public Health Service study of Reye's syndrome and medications: report of the main study. *J.A.M.A.*, **1987**, *257*, 1905–1911.

Kantor, T. G. Ibuprofen. *Ann. Intern. Med.*, **1979**, *91*, 877–882.

Kuncl, R. W.; Duncan, G.; Watson, D.; Alderson, K.; Rogawski, M. A.; and Peper, M. Colchicine myopathy and neuropathy. *N. Engl. J. Med.*, **1987**, *316*, 1562–1568.

Leonards, J. R., and Levy, G. Gastrointestinal blood loss during prolonged aspirin administration. *N. Engl. J. Med.*, **1973**, *289*, 1020–1022.

Maher, J. F. Analgesic nephropathy. *Am. J. Med.*, **1984**, *76*, 345–348.

Marshall, P. J.; Kulmacz, R. J.; and Lands, W. E. M. Constraints on prostaglandin biosynthesis in tissues. *J. Biol. Chem.*, **1987**, *262*, 3510–3517.

Perl, E. R. Sensitization of nociceptors and its relation to sensation. *Advances in Pain Research and Therapy*, Vol. I. (Bonica, J. J., and Albe-Fersard, D., eds.) Raven Press, New York, **1976**, pp. 17–34.

Pinsky, P.; Hurwitz, E. S.; Schonberger, L. B.; and Gunn, W. J. Reye's syndrome and aspirin. Evidence for a dose–response effect. *J.A.M.A.*, **1988**, *260*, 657–661.

Roth, G. R., and Siok, C. J. Acetylation of the NH_2-terminal serine of prostaglandin synthetase by aspirin. *J. Biol. Chem.*, **1978**, *253*, 3782–3784.

Schiff, E., and others. The use of aspirin to prevent pregnancy-induced hypertension and lower the ratio of thromboxane A_2 to prostacyclin in relatively high risk pregnancies. *N. Engl. J. Med.*, **1989**, *321*, 351–356.

Schroeder, K. W.; Tremaine, W. J.; and Ilstrup, D. M. Coated oral 5-aminosalicylic acid therapy for mildly to moderately active ulcerative colitis. *N. Engl. J. Med.*, **1987**, *317*, 1625–1629.

Smilkstein, M. J.; Knapp, G. L.; Kulig, K. W.; and Rumack, B. H. Efficacy of oral N-acetylcysteine in the treatment of acetaminophen overdose. *N. Engl. J. Med.*, **1988**, *319*, 1557–1562.

Steering Committee of the Physicians' Health Study Research Group. Final report on the aspirin component of the ongoing Physicians' Health Study. *N. Engl. J. Med.*, **1989**, *321*, 129–135.

Vane, J. R. and Botting, R. Inflammation and the mechanism of action of antiinflammatory drugs. *FASEB J.*, **1987**, *1*, 89–96.

Wallace, S. L. Colchicine: clinical pharmacology in acute gouty arthritis. *Am. J. Med.*, **1961**, *30*, 439–448.

Zemer, D.; Pras, M.; Sohar, E.; Modon, M.; Cabili, S.; and Gafni, J. Colchicine in the prevention and treatment of amyloidosis of familial Mediterranean fever. *N. Engl. J. Med.*, **1986**, *314*, 1001–1005.

Monographs and Reviews

Aram, H. Colchicine in dermatologic therapy. *Int. J. Dermatol.*, **1983**, *22*, 566–569.

Blocka, K. L. N.; Paulus, H. E.; and Furst, D. E. Clinical pharmacokinetics of oral and injectable gold compounds. *Clin. Pharmacokinet.*, **1986**, *11*, 133–143.

Boss, G. R., and Seegmiller, J. E. Hyperuricemia and gout: classification, complications, and management. *N. Engl. J. Med.*, **1979**, *300*, 1459–1468.

Brenner, B. E., and Simon, R. R. Management of salicylate intoxication. *Drugs*, **1982**, *24*, 335–340.

Brogden, R. N.; Heel, R. C.; Pakes, G. E.; Speight, T. M.; and Avery, G. S. Diflunisal: a review of its pharmacological properties and therapeutic use in pain and musculoskeletal strains and sprains and pain in osteoarthritis. *Drugs*, **1980**, *19*, 84–106.

Chaffman, M.; Brogden, R. N.; Heel, R. C.; Speight, T. M.; and Avery, G. S. Auranofin: a preliminary review of its pharmacological properties and therapeutic use in rheumatoid arthritis. *Drugs*, **1984**, *27*, 378–424.

Clissold, S. P. Paracetamol and phenacetin. *Drugs*, **1986**, *32*, Suppl. 4, 46–59.

Clive, D. M., and Stoff, J. S. Renal syndromes associated with nonsteroidal antiinflammatory drugs. *N. Engl. J. Med.*, **1984**, *310*, 563–572.

Cooke, T. D. V., and Scudamore, R. A. Studies in the pathogenesis of rheumatoid arthritis. *Br. J. Rheumatol.*, **1989**, *28*, 243–250; 330–340.

Dascombe, M. J. The pharmacology of fever. *Prog. Neurobiol.*, **1985**, *25*, 327–373.

Davies, R. O. Review of the animal and clinical pharmacology of diflunisal. *Pharmacotherapy*, **1983**, *3*, 9S–22S.

Davison, C. Salicylate metabolism in man. *Ann. N.Y. Acad. Sci.*, **1971**, *179*, 249–268.

Dinarello, C. A. Biology of interleukin 1. *FASEB J.*, **1988**, *2*, 108–115.

Easterbrook, M. Ocular effects and safety of antimalarial agents. *Am. J. Med.*, **1988**, *86*, 23–29.

Elion, G. B. Allopurinol and other inhibitors of urate synthesis. In, *Uric Acid. Handbuch der Experimentellen Pharmakologie*, Vol. 51. (Kelley, W. N., and Weiner, I. M., eds.) Springer-Verlag, Berlin, **1978**, pp. 485–514.

Friedel, H. A., and Todd, P. A. Nabumetone: a preliminary review of its pharmacodynamics and pharmacokinetic properties and therapeutic efficacy in rheumatic diseases. *Drugs*, **1988**, *35*, 504–524.

Hanzlik, P. J. *Actions and Uses of the Salicylates and Cinchophen in Medicine*. Williams & Wilkins, Baltimore, **1927**.

Hart, F. D., and Huskisson, E. C. Non-steroidal antiinflammatory drugs. Current status and rational therapeutic use. *Drugs*, **1984**, *27*, 232–255.

Hess, E. V., and Tangnijkul, Y. A rational approach to NSAID therapy. *Ration. Drug Ther.*, **1986**, *20*, 1–6.

Heubi, J. E.; Partin, J. C.; Partin, J. S.; and Schubert, W. K. Reye's syndrome: current concepts. *Hepatology*, **1987**, *7*, 155–164.

Kelley, W. N., and Weiner, I. M. (eds.). *Uric Acid. Handbuch der Experimentellen Pharmakologie*, Vol. 51. Springer-Verlag, Berlin, **1978**.

Kincaid-Smith, P. Effects of non-narcotic analgesics on the kidney. *Drugs*, **1986**, *32*, Suppl. 4, 109–128.

Larsen, G. L., and Henson, P. M. Mediators of inflammation. *Annu. Rev. Immunol.*, **1983**, *1*, 335–359.

Lewis, A. J., and Furst, D. W. (eds.). *Nonsteroidal Anti-Inflammatory Drugs. Mechanisms and Clinical Use*. Marcel Dekker, New York, **1987**.

Lipsky, P. E.; Davis, L. S.; Cush, J. J.; and Oppenheimer-Marks, N. The role of cytokines in the pathogenesis of rheumatoid arthritis. *Springer Semin. Immunopathol.*, **1989**, *11*, 123–162.

Lubbe, W. F. Low dose aspirin in prevention of toxemia of pregnancy. Does it have a place? *Drugs*, **1987**, *34*, 515–518.

Lynch, S., and Brogden, R. N. Etodolac: a preliminary review of its pharmacodynamic activity and therapeutic use. *Drugs*, **1986**, *31*, 288–300.

Meredith, T. J., and Vale, J. A. Non-narcotic analgesics. Problems of overdosage. *Drugs*, **1986**, *32*, Suppl. 4, 177–205.

Milton, A. S. Prostaglandins in fever and the mode of action of antipyretic drugs. In, *Pyretics and Antipyretics. Handbook of Experimental Pharmacology*, Vol. 60. (Milton, A. S., ed.) Springer-Verlag, Berlin, **1982**, pp. 257–303.

Oates, J. A.; Fitzgerald, G. A.; Branch, R. A.; Jackson, E. K.; Knapp, H. R.; and Roberts, L. J. Clinical implications of prostaglandin and thromboxane formation. *N. Engl. J. Med.*, **1988**, *319*, 689–698, 757–767.

Patrono, C., and Dunn, M. J. The clinical significance of inhibition of renal prostaglandin synthesis. *Kidney Int.*, **1987**, *32*, 1–12.

Pirson, Y., and van Ypersele de Strihou, C. Renal side effects of nonsteroidal anti-inflammatory drugs: clinical relevance. *Am. J. Kidney Dis.*, **1986**, *8*, 337–344.

Prescott, L. F., and Critchley, J. A. J. H. The treatment of acetaminophen poisoning. *Annu. Rev. Pharmacol. Toxicol.*, **1983**, *23*, 87–101.

Rainsford, K. O. (ed.). *Inflammation Mechanisms and Actions of Traditional Drugs*, Vol. I. *Anti-Inflammatory and Anti-Rheumatic Drugs*. CRC Press, Boca Raton, Fla., **1985a**.

———. *Newer Anti-Inflammatory Drugs*, Vol. II. *Anti-Inflammatory and Anti-Rheumatic Drugs*. CRC Press, Boca Raton, Fla., **1985b**.

Reilly, I. A. G., and Fitzgerald, G. A. Aspirin in cardiovascular disease. *Drugs*, **1988**, *35*, 154–176.

Roberts, W. N.; Liang, M. H.; and Stern, S. H. Colchicine in acute gout. *J.A.M.A.*, **1987**, *257*, 1920–1922.

Rodnan, G. P. Treatment of the gout and other forms of crystal-induced arthritis. *Bull. Rheum. Dis.*, **1982**, *32*, 43–53.

Rynes, R. I. Hydroxychloroquine treatment of rheumatoid arthritis. *Am. J. Med.*, **1988**, *85*, 18–22.

Shapiro, S. S. Treatment of dysmenorrhea and premenstrual syndrome with nonsteroidal anti-inflammatory drugs. *Drugs*, **1988**, *36*, 475–490.

Stevenson, D. D., and Lewis, R. A. Proposed mechanisms of aspirin sensitivity reaction. *J. Allergy Clin. Immunol.*, **1987**, *80*, 788–790.

Stitt, J. Y., and Nadel, E. R. (eds.). An international symposium to debate current issues in thermal physiology. Part I. *Yale J. Biol. Med.*, **1986**, *59*, 89–178.

Symposium. (Various authors.) Pharmacology, efficacy, and safety of a new class of anti-inflammatory agents: a review of piroxicam. *Am. J. Med.*, **1982**, *72*, No. 2A, 1–90.

Symposium. (Various authors.) *Anti-Rheumatic Drugs*. (Huskisson, E. C., ed.) Praeger Publishers, New York, **1983a**.

Symposium. (Various authors.) Antipyretic analgesic therapy. Current world wide status. *Am. J. Med.*, **1983b**, *75*, No. 5A, 1–140.

Symposium. (Various authors.) New perspectives on aspirin therapy. *Am. J. Med.*, **1983c**, *74*, No. 6A, 1–109.

Symposium. (Various authors.) Management of rheumatoid arthritis and osteoarthritis. *Am. J. Med.*, **1983d**, *75*, No. 4B, 1–91.

Symposium. (Various authors.) Symposium for rational pharmacotherapy: the nonsteroidal antiinflammatory drugs (NSAIDs). *Drug Intell. Clin. Pharm.*, **1984**, *18*, 34–58.

Symposium. (Various authors.) Enteric coated sulphasalazine in rheumatoid arthritis. *Drugs*, **1986a**, *32*, Suppl. 1, 1–80.

Symposium. (Various authors.) Inflammatory disease and the role of VOLTAREN (diclofenac sodium). *Am. J. Med.*, **1986b**, *80*, Suppl. 4B, 1–87.

Symposium. (Various authors.) RIDAURA (auranofin). *Scand. J. Rheumatol.*, **1986c**, Suppl. 6, 1–95.

Symposium. (Various authors.) Arachidonic acid metabolism and inflammation. Therapeutic implications. *Drugs*, **1987a**, *33*, Suppl. 1, 1–66.

Symposium. (Various authors.) Nabumetone: a new nonsteroidal anti-inflammatory drug. Criteria for therapeutic selection. *Am. J. Med.*, **1987b**, *83*, Suppl. 4B, 1–22.

Symposium. (Various authors.) Nonsteroidal anti-inflammatory drug-induced gastrointestinal damage. *Am. J. Med.*, **1988a**, *84*, Suppl. 2A, 1–52.

Symposium. (Various authors.) Sulfasalazine in rheumatic diseases. *J. Rheumatol.*, **1988b**, *15*, Suppl. 16, 1–42.

Szczeklik, A. Analgesics, allergy and asthma. *Drugs*, **1986**, *32*, Suppl. 4, 148–163.

Tsokos, G. C. Immunomodulatory treatment in patients with rheumatic diseases: mechanisms of action. *Semin. Arthritis Rheum.*, **1987**, *17*, 24–38.

Wallace, S. L., and Ertel, N. H. Pharmacology of drugs used in the treatment of acute gout. In, *Uric Acid. Handbuch der Experimentellen Pharmakologie*, Vol. 51. (Kelley, W. N., and Weiner, I. M., eds.) Springer-Verlag, Berlin, **1978**, pp. 525–555.

Wallace, S. L., and Singer, J. Z. Review: systemic toxicity associated with intravenous administration of colchicine—guidelines for use. *J. Rheumatol.*, **1988**, *15*, 495–499.

Ward, J. R. Role of disease-modifying antirheumatic drugs versus cytotoxic agents in the therapy of rheumatoid arthritis. *Am. J. Med.*, **1988**, *85*, 39–44.

Zvaifler, N. J. New perspectives on the pathogenesis of rheumatoid arthritis. *Am. J. Med.*, **1988**, *85*, 12–17.

SECTION

V

Water, Salts, and Ions

Normal inorganic constituents of the body may be considered as pharmacological agents when they are administered to repair either acute or chronic states of deficiency. These compounds fall into several groups. Those that contribute to the osmolality, the pH, or the volume of the body fluids are considered in this section, while those that have a more unique relationship to the function of specific organs are discussed elsewhere. Thus, Ca^{2+} and phosphate are considered together with the agents that are primarily responsible for their regulation—vitamin D, parathyroid hormone, and calcitonin (Chapter 62); iodide is presented with other agents that are relevant to the function of the thyroid gland (Chapter 57), and the salts of iron are discussed in the context of hematopoiesis (Chapter 54). Drugs that are inorganic ions, such as Li^+ (Chapter 18), are described in chapters most appropriate to their therapeutic utility, while metallic ions that are primarily of toxicological importance are grouped in Chapter 66. It is not within the scope of this textbook to consider the role of trace elements in nutrition.

CHAPTER

27 AGENTS AFFECTING VOLUME AND COMPOSITION OF BODY FLUIDS

Gilbert H. Mudge and Irwin M. Weiner

The volume and composition of the body fluids vary tremendously from one compartment to another and from one cell type to another, and are maintained remarkably constant despite the vicissitudes of daily life and the stresses imposed by disease. The regulatory mechanisms reside in the central nervous system (CNS), the heart, the lungs, the gastrointestinal tract, and the kidneys.

Disturbances in fluid and electrolyte metabolism involve four major properties of the body fluids—volume, osmolality, hydrogen ion concentration (pH), and the concentrations of other specific ions. In some diseases an abnormality in one property may dominate the picture. However, severely ill patients often have multiple disturbances that coexist and interact.

Throughout this chapter, guidelines for therapy are suggested. The reader should be aware that these represent an approach that is an approximation for an average patient. The physician must examine the details of management as carefully as in any other therapeutic regimen in clinical medicine.

DISTURBANCES OF VOLUME AND OSMOLALITY

The Distribution and Composition of Body Fluids

Distribution of Body Fluids. It is convenient to consider total body water as divided into three "compartments": (1) the intracellular compartment; (2) the extracellular compartment, which consists of the plasma and the interstitial fluids; and (3) the transcellular compartment, which includes the fluids within the tracheobronchial tree, the gastrointestinal tract, the excretory systems of the kidneys and glands, and the humors of the eyes. The transcellular compartment is relatively small and is generally not considered in calculations of quantities of fluid necessary to repair abnormalities.

In the lean individual, the volume of total body water is equivalent to approximately 70% of body weight. This figure can be much lower in an obese individual, about 50% of body weight, since adipose tissue contains little water. The relative distribution of total body water between the two main compartments is approximately the same in lean and obese individuals, and only the former will be considered in the following discussion.

Water is distributed between the intracellular and extracellular compartments in the ratio of 5:2. Thus, when total body water is equivalent to 70% of body weight, intracellular water accounts for 50% and extracellular water for 20% of body weight.

Composition of Body Fluids. The two major compartments differ greatly in their composition (*see* Table 27–1). Moreover, neither compartment is completely homogeneous, and the compositions of various cell types differ. Skeletal muscle is used as an example because it represents the largest volume of cells in the body.

Table 27–1. CONCENTRATION OF MAJOR ELECTROLYTES IN PLASMA AND SKELETAL MUSCLE WATER *

ELECTROLYTE	PLASMA	MUSCLE
	mEq/l	
Cations		
Sodium	140	10
Potassium	4	150
Calcium	5	—
Magnesium	2	40
Anions		
Chloride	102	—
Bicarbonate	26	10
Phosphate + sulfate	3	150
Organic anions	5	—
Protein	15	40

* The variations in values among healthy individuals are not indicated in the table. Clinical laboratories indicate their normal ranges in their reports.

Plasma is the most accessible component of the extracellular fluid, and it differs from interstitial fluid in several respects. The protein concentration of plasma is higher because capillaries exhibit only limited permeability to macromolecules. The concentration of Ca^{2+} is higher because it is bound, in part, to protein. Plasma and interstitial fluid also differ in their concentrations of the monovalent anions and cations. These differences are the result of two factors: (1) the water content of plasma is lower since it contains more protein; (2) the presence of impermeable but charged proteins (Donnan effect) influences the distribution of ions. These differences are relatively small and need not be considered in most therapeutic interventions.

The vast difference in composition between the intracellular and extracellular compartments is, of course, the result of permeability barriers and of the transport mechanisms, both active and passive, that exist in the plasma membranes of cells. Among the most prominent of these mechanisms is the adenosine triphosphatase that is activated by Na^+ and K^+ (Na^+,K^+-ATPase). A detailed analysis of these phenomena is beyond the scope of this chapter.

Osmotic Pressure. Virtually all cell membranes are freely permeable to water. The chief determinant of the movement of water from one major compartment to another is a difference in effective osmolality. Those solutes that can permeate the plasma membrane freely influence the total osmolality of both compartments, but they do not lead to net movement of water. Conversely, nonpermeant solutes do contribute to effective osmolality.

At steady state the total osmolalities of the two major compartments are the same. For example, if a man drinks water faster than he can excrete it, he develops a positive water balance. This water gains access initially to the extracellular space, where it expands the volume and dilutes the solutes (hyponatremia). The decrease in effective osmolality (increase in the activity of water) is accompanied by a net movement of water molecules from the extracellular space to the intracellular fluid. Obviously, this will cease when the two fluids are once again of equal osmolality, albeit lower than initially. The result is the distribution of the increment of water through the volume of total body water.

Interstitial and Plasma Volumes. The same basic principles apply to the steady-state distribution of volume between these two components of the extracellular space. The vascular endothelium is permeable to water and to most of the solutes. However, as indicated earlier, it is relatively impermeable to the larger molecular species such as proteins. The segregation of these molecules within the vascular component enhances osmolality, and if there were no counteracting force all the extracellular fluid would move into the plasma. In the regulation of fluid distribution between the vascular and interstitial fluids, the counteracting force is the hydrostatic pressure within the vascular system. The balance of these forces—the Starling forces—is the determinant of the steady-state distribution of volume between the two compartments. These forces are usually so adjusted that about one fourth of the extracellular fluid is within the confines of the vascular system and the remainder is in the interstitial space.

Net shifts between the compartments do occur when these Starling forces are dislocated. An increase in the hydrostatic pressure may permit a greater rate of transudation than reabsorption. The same effect may be noted when there is hypoproteinemia and the colloidal oncotic pressure is thereby diminished. In both circumstances, there is a net movement of volume to the interstitial fluid compartment. The overall effect may be mitigated partially by another system of vessels, namely, the lymphatic system.

One of the important therapeutic implications is that the plasma volume cannot specifically be increased unless the administered fluid contains a colloidal agent. The administration of saline solution to a subject who has lost blood will reexpand the extracellular fluid volume, but most of the expansion will occur in the interstitial compartment.

EXTERNAL EXCHANGES OF WATER AND SOLUTE

The Balance Principle. With the exceptions that are noted below, one may consider that water and the major solutes do not undergo metabolic alteration. Hence, concentrations within the body fluids represent the balance between intake and output, both for water and the solute in question. By general usage, if a patient gains (or loses) something, he or she is in positive (or negative) balance. If no significant changes occur, the balance is neutral. The latter is often referred to as "being in balance," and this is the condition of the normal subject who is neither gaining nor losing weight (Table 27–2).

The proper management of many patients includes an accurate record of intake and output and daily weights. This is particularly true of severely ill patients with complex disturbances. Intake includes oral intake, infusions, transfusions, and so forth. Output includes urine, vomitus, and fecal and other intestinal losses. Except for research purposes, insensible losses through the lungs and skin are not measured; average values are used.

The initial state may have two connotations. It may refer to the value presumed to have been present in the state of health (*e.g.*, body water estimated from a patient's normal weight), or it may refer to any state during an illness prior to the initiation of a specific treatment.

From an accurate knowledge of the external balance, or even from a thoughtful guess as to its probable value, it is possible to deduce many pathophysiological mechanisms. Changes in the balance of water and solute may occur simultaneously, but their independent contributions should be evaluated separately.

It should be emphasized that the effect of a change in external balance on the composition of the body fluids is independent of the discrete physiological mechanism that is involved. For example, the loss of 10 liters of water has essentially the same effect on the residual body fluids, whether due to excessive losses through the skin or to the passage of very dilute urine in uncontrolled diabetes insipidus.

Table 27–2. REPRESENTATIVE "NORMAL" VALUES OF FLUID AND ELECTROLYTE INTAKE AND OUTPUT *

	INTAKE		OUTPUT		
	Oral	*Metabolism*	*Urine*	*Feces*	*Insensible*
Water as fluid, ml	1200	0	1500	100	900
Water in food, ml	1000	300			
Nitrogen, g	13	0	12	1.0	0
Sodium, mmol	75	0	74	0.5	0.5
Potassium, mmol	50	0	45	5.0	0
Chloride, mmol	75	0	74	0.5	0.5
Nonvolatile acid, mEq	0	70	70	0	0
Volatile acid, mEq	0	14,000	0	0	14,000

* A single value is selected for each entry to facilitate comparison of intake and output, and all are adjusted to depict a zero net external balance. Nonvolatile acids are largely phosphoric and sulfuric acid residues of metabolism. Volatile acid is exclusively carbon dioxide. All values refer to the amount per 24 hours.

Fixed and Labile Ions and Solutes. It is useful to bear in mind the distinction between fixed and labile solutes. In the case of charged particles, a fixed ion is one that exists in the ionic form under all physiological circumstances. This holds true for Na^+, K^+, and chloride. Through metabolic alterations, labile ions may either be generated from nonionic precursors or converted to nonionic end products. Thus, labile ions may be added to or removed from the body fluids in a form other than that of the charged ion. For example, the ammonium cation (NH_4^+) can be converted to urea in the liver, and also synthesized from amino acids in the kidney. Bicarbonate (HCO_3^-) is labile since at the proper pH it can be converted to H_2CO_3, and thence to its volatile form, CO_2. Another example is the formation of lactate from glucose. In addition, the ion of a weak acid or base may be buffered so as to change its ionic equivalence (*e.g.*, monobasic and dibasic phosphate). This is not metabolic alteration in the usual sense, but it does denote a degree of lability.

Consideration of Basal Requirements. A summary of average values for the intake and output of water and the major electrolytes is given in Table 27–2. These values presuppose average diet and physical activity, a normal state of metabolism, and no abnormal losses. There is considerable variation from one individual to another and moderate variation from day to day. The composition of important fluids that may be lost from the body is given in Table 27–3.

Table 27–3. PRODUCTION RATES AND COMPOSITION OF VARIOUS BODY FLUIDS *

	VOLUME	COMPOSITION			
		Na^+	*K^+*	*Cl^-*	*HCO_3^-*
	ml/24 hr	*mM*			
Cutaneous sweat	100–200	50–80	5	40–85	—
Gastrointestinal					
Saliva	1500	10	30	10	10–20
Gastric fluid	2500	10–115	1–35	90–150	0–15
Bile	500	130–160	3–12	90–120	40–50
Pancreatic fluid	700	115–150	3–8	55–95	60–120
Intestinal fluids	3000				
Jejunum	—	85–150	2–10	45–125	—
Ileum	—	85–120	3–10	60–130	—
Ileostomy (old)	—	40–50	3–5	20–30	—
Cecostomy	—	45–135	5–45	20–90	—
Feces					
Normal	100	5	50	5	—
Diarrhea (cholera)	—	130	20	100	50

* Data are summarized from the literature for both average values and their ranges, and refer to an adult in a temperate climate engaging in mild physical activity.

CLINICAL DISTURBANCES OF VOLUME AND OSMOLALITY

Table 27–4 contains idealized descriptions of acute disturbances in salt and water balance. With more chronic disturbances, compensatory physiological adjustments make the classification less accurate. Some of the conditions are usually accompanied by changes in acid–base balance; these changes are not mentioned in the table. For purposes of these descriptions it is assumed that the number of erythrocytes and the total mass of protein in the circulation have not changed.

The classification is based on changes in both volume and osmolality of the extracellular fluid. Changes in intracellular volume may be in the same or the opposite direction, depending on the condition. Examination of the table reveals the inadequacy of the terms *dehydration* and *overhydration*.

Na^+ Concentration as an Index of Plasma Osmolality. Since Na^+ is the major extracellular solute, its concentration may be used as an index of osmolality, directly for the extracellular fluid and indirectly for the intracellular fluid. As a first approximation, osmolality is twice the Na^+ concentration. This estimate is not valid in two instances.

Pseudohyponatremia. This is a condition in which the concentration of Na^+ in the plasma is abnormally low when analyzed by conventional methods (which depend on aliquots measured volumetrically), but in which the concentration would be normal if referred to plasma water. The discrepancy occurs when the concentration of macromolecules is abnormally high and hence the percentage of plasma water is abnormally low, a condition found most commonly with hyperlipemia or marked hyperproteinemia.

Na^+ as a False Index. This occurs, even with corrections for plasma water, in the presence of an abnormally high concentration of other solutes that are effective extracellular osmotic particles. It may be seen with severe hyperglycemia in diabetes mellitus or following the infusion of large amounts of glucose and after the administration of a nonmetabolizable extracellular solute such as mannitol. Glucose slowly gains access to the intracellular space by carrier-mediated transport. Thus, if the concentration in plasma rises abruptly, glucose acts at least transiently as if it were confined to the extracellular space. This may lead to hyperosmolality without hypernatremia and, indeed, because of shifts of water from the intracellular to the extracellular space, may be associated with hyponatremia. The simplest method of evaluation is to determine the concentrations of Na^+ and glucose separately, convert these to osmolar terms, and add them together.

Isotonic Contraction. This occurs when extracellular electrolytes and water are lost in isotonic proportions. The most common example is the loss of isotonic fluid from the gastrointestinal tract; cholera is the classical disease. This type of disturbance may be complicated by acid–base changes. Loss of strongly acidic fluid from the stom-

Table 27–4. TYPES OF ACUTE CHANGES IN VOLUME AND OSMOLALITY *

ACUTE EXTRACELLULAR CHANGE	CLINICAL EXAMPLE †	Δ VOLUME		Δ CONC. PLASMA SODIUM	Δ HEMATOCRIT	Δ CONC. PLASMA PROTEIN
		Δ *ECW*	Δ *ICW*			
Isotonic contraction	Cholera	↓	0	0	↑	↑
Hypertonic contraction	Excess sweating	↓	↓	↑	0	↑
Hypotonic contraction	Adrenal insufficiency	↓	↑	↓	↑	↑
Isotonic expansion	Isotonic saline	↑	0	0	↓	↓
Hypertonic expansion	Hypertonic saline	↑	↓	↑	↓	↓
Hypotonic expansion	Water intoxication	↑	↑	↓	0	↓

* For discussion of hematocrit, *see* text. Direction of change is shown by arrows. Δ=change; 0 = no change; ECW = extracellular water; ICW = intracellular water.

† Isotonic and hypertonic saline refer to infusions.

ach leads to metabolic alkalosis; loss of alkaline bile and pancreatic fluid, or the less alkaline fluid of severe diarrhea, leads to metabolic acidosis. In each instance the concentration of Na^+ in plasma remains normal. The repair of the condition requires an expansion of the extracellular fluid volume with a solution whose main cation is Na^+. In severe conditions, specific expansion of plasma volume with colloidal solutions may be required initially to maintain arterial pressure.

Hypertonic Contraction. This type of dehydration is observed in any circumstance in which water is lost in excess of Na^+. The classical example is exposure on a life raft to the unremitting impact of the tropical sun. In more common clinical conditions it occurs when a patient is unable to drink water owing to a clouded sensorium and too little water is provided parenterally. Other circumstances include diabetes insipidus, excessive sweating (of a hypotonic fluid), and osmotic diuresis. In uncontrolled diabetes mellitus, the high concentration of glucose (a labile solute) is additive to the negative external balance of water in causing extracellular hypertonicity. The external loss of Na^+ and water decreases extracellular fluid volume, but there is partial compensation for this reduction because the simultaneous extracellular hypertonicity results in redistribution of water from the intracellular to the extracellular compartment. On theoretical grounds there should be no change in hematocrit if there were a pure loss of water, since this would occur proportionately from the plasma and the erythrocytes. In most clinical examples, there is also a negative balance of Na^+ and a rise in the hematocrit.

Hypotonic Contraction. This occurs when Na^+ is lost in excess of water. Chief among these conditions are chronic renal insufficiency and adrenocortical insufficiency. It also occurs commonly when isotonic fluid losses are treated with water (isotonic glucose solution) and too little or no salt. Essentially the same mechanism is involved when physical exercise in a hot, dry climate is associated with the drinking of water but without the ingestion of salt tablets to replace the loss of salt through perspiration. In this condition the concentration of Na^+ in the plasma is reduced, and water moves from extracellular fluid into the cells. Thus, the extracellular fluid is reduced by loss to both the external environment and the cells.

Isotonic Expansion. This is the proportional retention of Na^+ and water and is the basis of generalized edema resulting from cardiac, hepatic, or renal disease. The extracellular compartment may also be expanded by the injudicious use of isotonic saline solution in the overzealous treatment of contraction. When renal function is normal, even major fluctuations in dietary salt intake rarely give rise to isotonic expansion, at least in the adult. With generalized edema, the concentration of Na^+ in the plasma is often normal, although a slight degree of hyponatremia is not uncommon because of retention of some excess water as well.

Hypertonic Expansion. This occurs when Na^+ is retained in excess of water. In its simplest form it results from the rapid and excessive infusion of hypertonic saline. The most common clinical example probably occurs in infants improperly treated for diarrhea when the concentration of administered salt is erroneously high. Salt poisoning has also been reported in infants following the accidental addition of sodium chloride instead of sugar to the formula. In these instances, hypertonicity may be extreme. Fatality from severe hypernatremia is due primarily to damage to the CNS.

Hypotonic Expansion. This occurs with retention of water in excess of Na^+. The simplest example is water intoxication owing to the excessive ingestion of water. The concentrations of Na^+ and protein in the plasma fall by dilution. Since water distributes itself throughout the body fluids, both the extracellular and the intracellular volumes are increased. Excessive ingestion of water is sometimes encountered in emotionally disturbed patients. The dominant symptoms are weakness and confusion, and this may progress to coma and generalized seizures.

Another more complicated example of hypotonic expansion is seen in some patients with edema. In rare instances, during its spontaneous development, edema is associated with a significantly greater retention of water than of salt, often referred to as dilutional hyponatremia. Far more frequently this results from the excessive use of diuretics, which may produce an imbalance between the losses of salt and water. The syndrome of the inappropriate secretion of antidiuretic hormone also produces hypotonic expansion.

TREATMENT OF FLUID AND ELECTROLYTE DEFICITS

The basic objective of therapy is to restore the volume and composition of the body fluids to normal. However, this requires extensive qualification insofar as priorities are concerned. The present discussion is limited to water and salt balance. The more complex derangements involving blood loss and protein depletion will be considered separately.

Volume Contraction. This is a life-threatening condition because it impairs the circulation. Blood volume decreases, cardiac output falls, and the integrity of the microcirculation is compromised. This occurs whether volume contraction is isotonic, hypertonic, or hypotonic, even though, as outlined above, there are important differences between them. Given volume depletion of sufficient magnitude to threaten life, the prompt infusion of isotonic sodium chloride solution is indicated; indeed, it is difficult to contrive a contraindication.

The volume of fluid that needs to be replaced varies enormously. As an extreme example, intravenous therapy at the rate of 100 ml per minute for the first 1000 ml has been considered necessary for the successful treatment of cholera. Most conditions require far less dramatic treatment. Attention should also be directed to the speed with which the volume depletion developed. For example, a 4-kg weight loss due to the loss of gastrointestinal fluids is far more debilitating if it occurs over 2 to 3 hours than over a period of days or weeks. A general rule is to replace one half of the estimated volume loss in the first 12 to 24 hours of treatment.

Disorders of Osmolality. Even with moderately severe hyponatremia or hypernatremia, the disorder frequently may be corrected with isotonic saline solution, provided renal function is normal. Given an adequate supply of raw materials the kidney is a remarkably effective regulator of the osmolality of the body. This is accomplished by the excretion of urine at a concentration appropriate for the correction of the underlying disturbance.

However, if the disturbance in osmolality is severe, it is proper to treat this directly. Clinical judgment should be based on the actual physiological consequences of the disorder, and not on blood chemistry values considered in isolation. As is the case with disturbances of volume, the effect of change in osmolality varies in importance depending on the speed of its development. For example, extreme hyponatremia may be asymptomatic if it develops slowly over months but not if it occurs in a few hours.

In addition to the diffusion of water, intracellular osmolality within the CNS is regulated by mechanisms specific for brain tissue. These mechanisms involve both the gain and loss of ions and the formation and degradation of "idiogenic osmoles" (*see* Arieff and DeFronzo, 1985). Since both of these processes are slow relative to the diffusion of water, it is not advisable to correct osmolality immediately and completely in either hypoosmotic or hyperosmotic states. A reasonable goal is to restore the extracellular osmolality one third to one half of the way toward normal within 1 day and to change plasma Na^+ by no more than 1 mM per hour. Except in extreme circumstances, this regimen leads to major symptomatic and physiological improvement (Sterns *et al.*, 1989). In some cases of dilutional hyponatremia, it is often debatable whether specific therapy is justified, either because of the absence of any detectable harm or because of the ineffectiveness of such measures (*see* Chapter 28).

Requirements to Correct Disturbances in Osmolality. As an example, how much salt would be required to elevate to 130 mM a plasma Na^+ concentration of 120 mM? For a 70-kg subject without gross volume deficits or excesses, one may assume a total body water volume of 50 liters. Although the administered Na^+ will be distributed in the volume of the extracellular fluid, it will exert an osmotic effect to move fluid into that compartment from the intracellular space. This will diminish the increment in extracellular osmolality and will increase intracellular osmolality. The concentration of Na^+ in the plasma will not rise by the desired increment of 10 mM until the osmolality of both the intracellular and extracellular compartments has been raised to a similar extent. Thus, 50 liters × 10 mM equals 500 mmol of Na^+. In this example the volume that is added with the hypertonic saline solution is ignored. A calculation based exclusively on the extracellular volume would be in error. Using TBW for total body water, [Na] for Na^+ concentration in plasma, and subscripts 1 and 2 for the initial and final states, if TBW is kept constant and one solves for electrolyte balance, then:

$$(TBW_1 \times [Na]_1) + \text{Na Balance} = TBW_2 \times [Na]_2$$
$$50 \times 120 \quad + 500 \quad = 50 \quad \times 130$$

The same principle applies to the calculation of water requirements for the treatment of hypernatremia. Thus, for the same subject, if the initial concentration of Na^+ in the plasma was 175 mM, diluting it to 160 mM would require a positive water balance of 4.7 liters; with the same equation, now keeping electrolyte content constant, and solving for the change in fluid balance, then:

$$TBW_1 \times [Na]_1 = TBW_2 \times [Na]_2$$
$$50 \times 175 \quad = 54.7 \quad \times 160$$

Simple modifications of these equations may be used to estimate requirements involving changes in both volume and osmolality.

Techniques of Administration of Fluid. While fluids can be administered by mouth, gavage, hypodermoclysis, or vein, acute emergencies dictate that fluid replacement be initiated intravenously. With intravenous administration, due consideration must be given to the status of the cardiovascular system. If cardiac function is impaired and large volumes of fluid are thought to be indicated, either the central venous or pulmonary venous pressure should be monitored. If the venous pressure rises substantially, the rate of infusion should be decreased or the infusion should be terminated.

Oral intake and administration by gavage should obviously be avoided in the presence of nausea or vomiting or when the patient is unconscious and likely to aspirate. Until recently the oral route was ineffective when large volumes of fluid had to be given. However, modern techniques of oral rehydration therapy have had a dramatic impact, especially in areas where diarrhea from cholera and other causes is a major public health problem. The new techniques are based on the fact that the addition of glucose to electrolyte solutions greatly increases the intestinal absorption of electrolyte and water. In cases of cholera, once initial dehydration has been corrected intravenously, it is possible to provide further replacement orally. This fact has major implications with regard to cost and other practical matters related to the preparation of sterile intravenous solutions under less-than-optimal conditions. Enhancement of Na^+ absorption by glucose probably involves both the provision of an energy source for active transport as well as the cotransport of sugar and electrolyte in a manner analogous to that of the renal tubule (*see* Introduction to Section VI). Carbohydrates other than glucose may also be effective but have been used less widely (*see* McQuestion, 1983). The solution recommended by the World Health Organization contains 2% dextrose, 0.35% NaCl, 0.25% $NaHCO_3$, and 0.15% KCl.

Fluids Available for the Repair of Contraction. Many commercially prepared solutions are available for replacement of fluid deficits. Some that are in frequent use include (1) 0.45%, 0.9%, 3%, and 5% NaCl in water; (2) 2.5%, 5%, and 10% dextrose in water; (3) mixtures of dextrose and NaCl in varying concentrations; (4) 5% $NaHCO_3$ in water; (5) mixtures of KCl (0.075 to 0.3%) with NaCl and dextrose; and (6) Ringer's injection with or without lactate or lactate plus dextrose. Several points warrant emphasis: (1) These solutions consist of simple compounds that are chemically compatible in virtually all proportions, with the exception of calcium salts, which have limited solubility. (2) The pH range may extend from 3.5 to 8. However, the solutions are not buffered and, therefore, the pH in this range has no effect on systemic acid–base balance, except when bicarbonate or its precursors are included or when enormous volumes of fluid are given. The pH of the solution may affect the stability and possible compatibility of other drugs that are added to it. (3) Of prime pharmacological importance is the actual composition of the infused fluid, expressed either as millimoles (mmol), milliequivalents (mEq), or milliosmoles (mOsmol) per liter. However, for pharmaceutical formulation, gravimetric terminology is essential. (4) Unfortunately, by common usage a trivial and inconsistent nomenclature has become widespread. The original term *normal physiological saline* has evolved to *normal saline,* which is 154 mM. (This usage of *normal* is different from that used in chemistry.) (5) Repair solutions consist of both fixed and labile solutes. The latter are of two types. For example, in the metabolism of precursors of bicarbonate (*e.g.*, lactate), one anion is replaced by another and osmolality does not change. However, in the metabolism of glucose to CO_2 and water, the osmolality attributable to glucose disappears. In these situations the CO_2 and water, which are end-products of metabolism, are inconsequential with regard to effective osmolality.

Due to the flexibility and effectiveness of physiological homeostatic mechanisms, the repair solution utilized need not be identical to the calculated deficit if the disturbance is minor or short-lived. However, for major disturbances, especially those in which large volumes of intake and output may be anticipated, the composition of the repair solution should resemble that of the calculated imbalance quite closely. The incorporation of glucose into intravenous solutions has become increasingly popular. This is a useful source of calories. Nevertheless, when there is a high turnover of fluid, the total amount of glucose infused must be monitored. As an approximation for adults, if the amount infused exceeds 500 g per day, persistent hyperglycemia, glycosuria, and polyuria may result.

Solutions of less than 110 mOsmol per liter should not be infused into peripheral veins, since they may cause hemolysis. (Solutions of 0.9% NaCl or 5% dextrose in water are isosmotic with plasma.) Very hypertonic infusions are best given into large central veins, where they are rapidly diluted.

CORRECTION OF PLASMA AND BLOOD VOLUME

When the plasma volume is contracted as the result of simple loss of fluid and electrolyte, as in cholera, the defect may be corrected in many patients by the simple replacement of saline. When the initial losses are of a more complex nature, as in hemorrhagic shock, these same solutions also have the capacity to improve cardiovascular function transiently. In such a setting, the volume of saline (or equivalent) that is required is far greater than the initial loss of whole blood. Nevertheless, saline should be employed as an initial emergency measure. The best substitute for the loss of whole blood is obviously suitable and adequately cross-matched whole blood. However, when plasma volume is critically jeopardized, the use of colloid-containing solutions is another interim measure that is more efficacious than saline.

Natural Products. There are several types of solutions that contain natural colloids. Products of human origin carry the risk of transmitting hepatitis (hepatitis virus B or virus C) or the virus responsible for acquired immunodeficiency syndrome (AIDS). For units of plasma derived from a single donor, this risk is no greater than for a single transfusion of whole blood. Preparations of pooled plasma are heated during manufacture to minimize this risk. Some commercial preparations of plasma proteins contain low concentrations of prekallikrein activators (Hageman-factor fragments). These have a hypotensive action, which may worsen the condition for which plasma proteins are prescribed (Colman, 1978). Human albumin, produced in bacteria by recombinant DNA techniques, would be a valuable preparation.

Synthetic Products. The search for synthetic compounds has been stimulated by the limited availability of natural products. Substances that are specifically designed to restore plasma volume must have oncotic properties comparable to plasma. Replacements for whole blood must in addition have adequate capacity to carry oxygen. These products also have various applications in the preparation of organs for transplantation and in the operation of various bypass machines required in cardiovascular surgery.

In addition to the properties just mentioned, desirable characteristics of a plasma expander include (1) adequate time in the circulation; (2) absence of other pharmacological actions; (3) absence of antigenic, allergenic, or pyrogenic effects; (4) absence of interference with typing or cross-matching of blood; (5) stability during long periods of storage and under wide variations of environmental temperature; (6) ease of sterilization; and (7) viscosity characteristics suitable for infusion. A number of substances have been studied in the past. Those of current interest are briefly described below.

Dextran. This compound is formed by the action of a bacterium, *Leuconostoc mesenteroides*. It has suitable oncotic properties but no oxygen-carrying capacity.

Chemistry and Pharmacodynamic Properties. In its original form, dextran is a branched polysaccharide of about 200,000 glucose units, with a molecular weight of approximately 40 million. The glucose units in the main chain are bound together through 1:6 glucosidic linkages; those in the shorter branches through 1:4 linkages. By partial hydrolysis and fractionation, dextran can be converted to polysaccharides of any desired molecular weight.

Two forms of dextran are currently available. One has an average molecular weight of either 70,000 or 75,000 (depending on the pharmaceutical preparation), and the other has an average molecular weight of 40,000. Both agents expand plasma volume. The lower-molecular-weight dextran may well have advantages; its administration not only corrects hypovolemia but also appears to improve the microcirculation independently of simple volume expansion. It minimizes the sludging of blood that may accompany shock. In an individual who has sustained a loss of whole blood or plasma, a single infusion of dextran increases the circulating blood volume and improves the hemodynamic status for 24 hours or longer.

Distribution, Metabolic Fate, and Excretion. Following the infusion of dextran, the molecules of smaller molecular weight are excreted by the kidney. However, the remainder traverses the capillary wall very slowly and is slowly oxidized over a period of a few weeks. The persistence of dextran and its ultimate metabolic disposal are desirable features.

Untoward Reactions. Dextran appears to have no significant deleterious effects on renal, hepatic, or other vital functions. However, when glomerular filtration rate is reduced, the excessive tubular reabsorption of water may increase the concentration of dextran in the tubular fluid, such that viscosity impedes the flow of fluid through the tubule; this may cause acute renal failure.

Dextran is a potent antigen. This is true of both the native polysaccharide and the hydrolysis products. Furthermore, dextran occurs in commercial sugar, and dextran-producing organisms can be found in the human gastrointestinal tract. Therefore, a small percentage of individuals who have never received dextran have antibodies to the polysaccharide in the circulation.

The incidence of sensitivity reactions is extremely variable, depending upon the preparation employed. As the technique of manufacture has improved, the number of untoward responses has diminished. Untoward reactions consist of itching, urticaria, joint pains, and other side effects, and are relatively mild in character. Their incidence in normal individuals is less than 10%.

The antigenic activity of dextran would seem to preclude its repeated use. However, when given in the massive doses that are employed for infusion, antibody production does not occur, owing presumably to the phenomenon of "immunological paralysis." Indeed, the incidence of anaphylactoid reactions to colloidal volume expanders such as plasma protein solutions, dextran, and hetastarch is remarkably low and is significantly less than that for transfusions or for many drugs.

Dextran may interfere with typing, cross-matching, or Rh determinations, but this effect is unpredictable. It may produce a hemostatic defect described as an acquired form of von Willebrand's disease. The uses of dextran for its antiplatelet and antithrombotic effects are discussed in Chapter 55.

Clinical Status. Dextran possesses most of the attributes of an ideal plasma expander, its chief defect being antigenicity. It has been successfully used in the treatment of the circulatory inadequacies associated with the hypovolemia attending the loss of both whole blood and plasma.

Hetastarch. This synthetic polymer, also known as hydroxyethyl starch, is prepared from amylopectin by the introduction of hydroxyethyl ether groups into its glucose residues. The purpose of the modification is to retard the degradation of the polymer. This preparation bears many similarities to dextran. Hetastarch has an average molecular weight of 450,000, with a range from 10,000 to 1,000,000. Molecules with the lower molecular weights are readily excreted in the urine, and, with the usual preparation, about 40% of the dose is excreted within 24 hours. The molecules of higher molecular weight are metabolized slowly; only about 1% of a dose persists after 2 weeks.

Like dextran, hetastarch is used for its oncotic properties; it has no oxygen-carrying capacity. In the management of shock and in postoperative cardiac patients, hetastarch has the same efficacy as albumin as far as major hemodynamic effects are concerned (Puri *et al.*, 1983). Hetastarch is said to have fewer antigenic properties than dextran.

Hemoglobin Solutions. Stroma-free solutions of hemoglobin are well tolerated, and they can expand plasma volume and increase oxygen-carrying capacity in experimental animals. A major problem with their use is the short period of intravascular retention of hemoglobin due to renal excretion. Another problem involves hemoglobin's excessively high affinity for oxygen when it is free in solution. Elimination of these undesired effects is being approached by chemical modification and polymerization of the protein (Symposium, 1982).

Perfluorochemicals. These compounds dissolve oxygen rather than binding it as a chelate. Emulsions of two perfluorochemicals together with hetastarch (FLUOSOL-DA) act as oncotic agents with oxygen-carrying capacity. In a clinical trial of severely anemic patients, untoward reactions were minimal and as much as 24% of the oxygen consumed was furnished by the preparation. These agents are still in an experimental stage (Tremper *et al.*, 1982).

Preparations. *Plasma protein fraction* (PLASMANATE, PLASMA-PLEX, others) is a sterile aqueous solution containing 5% human plasma proteins in sodium chloride solution, of which not less than 83% is albumin and the remainder is α- and β-globulins; it is osmotically equivalent to plasma. Manufacturers minimize the risk of transmitting hepatitis B virus by heating the solution at 60° C for 10 hours. The initial dose may be 250 or 500 ml for treatment of shock.

Albumin human (ALBUMINAR, ALBUTEIN, others) is a sterile preparation of 5 or 25% serum albumin obtained by fractionating blood from human donors. The 5% solution is osmotically equivalent to plasma. Risk of hepatitis B virus is minimized by heating in the same manner as described above. These preparations have 130 to 160 mEq of sodium chloride per liter.

Dextran. Two forms of dextran, which differ in molecular size, are available for use as plasma expanders. *Dextran 70 injection* (GENTRAN 70, MACRODEX) contains 6% dextran (average molecular weight 70,000) in 0.9% sodium chloride solution or 5% dextrose in water. *Dextran 75 injection* (GENTRAN 75) is virtually identical but with an average molecular weight of 75,000. *Dextran 40 injection* (GENTRAN 40, 10% LMD, RHEOMACRODEX) contains 10% dextran 40 (average molecular weight 40,000) in 0.9% sodium chloride solution or 5% dextrose in water. The molecular weight of the former preparation approximates that of human plasma albumin; the smaller molecular size of the latter preparation is said to have the advantage of retarding rouleau formation and sludging of red blood cells. Both preparations are available in units of 500 ml.

Hetastarch injection (HESPAN) is prepared as a 6% solution in 0.9% sodium chloride in units of 500 ml.

PROBLEMS OF CARBOHYDRATES, FATS, AND PROTEINS

In the absence of the normal dietary intake of foodstuffs, intravenous glucose protects against the development of ketosis and minimizes protein wasting. On a short-term basis, one should administer approximately 100 g of glucose per day to an adult.

Parenteral Nutrition. This technique is important in the management of patients with severe intestinal dysfunction, trauma, or various surgical complications. A positive nitrogen balance can be achieved and maintained for at least several months, and some patients are maintained on parenteral nutrition for years.

The basic nutrient solution consists of hypertonic dextrose (20 to 25% or more) and amino acids in addition to electrolytes, vitamins, and trace elements. The need for hypertonic solutions is dictated by the limits of water intake. The infusion is given through a percutaneous catheter inserted into a large branch of the superior vena cava. This placement permits prompt adjustment of osmolality by dilution. Rigid sterile surgical technique is essential. A peristaltic pump should be used to drive the infusion. The use of in-line filters greatly reduces the incidence of infection. Ancillary medications should be given by another route. Pharmaceutical incompatibilities, including incompatibilities with electrolytes such as Ca^{2+}, bicarbonate, phosphate, and sulfate, must be avoided.

The regimen should be initiated gradually, then kept constant from day to day and carefully monitored. Mild glycosuria is common but may subside after stimulation of endogenous insulin production. However, severe glycosuria may lead to excessive water loss and hypertonic contraction of body fluids. With adequate amounts of Na^+, K^+, Mg^{2+}, chloride, and bicarbonate, electrolyte imbalance may be avoided. Prolonged hypophosphatemia may lead to serious neurological and hematological complications, and phosphate is a requirement. Hyperammonemia may occur, particularly in infants, and can be prevented by reducing the nitrogenous content of the infusion. Parenteral administration of fat is required to provide essential components for the synthesis of cellular membranes; it also helps to meet caloric requirements. Most formulations provide more-than-adequate quantities of trace elements and vitamins. However, unexpected instances of deficiencies have been reported.

Preparations. In addition to the previously mentioned solutions of electrolytes and simple sugars, the following solutions are used in parenteral alimentation.

Amino Acids. *Amino acid injection* (AMINOSYN, TRAVASOL, others) consists of approximately 15 amino acids (both essential and nonessential), with total amino acid content varying from 3 to 15%. Formulations vary as to total osmolality and are available with or without added electrolytes. The proportion of amino acids also varies slightly between preparations. A solution of 3.5% amino acids is only slightly hypertonic and may be administered by peripheral vein; more concentrated solutions are intended for infusion by central vein and are usually mixed with hypertonic glucose solution to provide additional caloric intake. Other preparations of amino acids (*e.g.*, NEPHRAMINE, which contains primarily essential amino acids) are designed for patients with renal failure. Additional formulations are available for use in hepatic failure (HEPATAMINE) or high metabolic stress (FREAMINE HBC, others).

Fat Emulsion. Emulsions of 10 and 20% fat (INTRALIPID, others) are prepared from refined soybean or safflower oil, egg-yolk phospholipids, and glycerin. The major fatty acids are linoleic, oleic, palmitic, stearic, and linolenic. The preparation is isotonic and may be administered into a peripheral vein. It should not be mixed with other solutions employed in parenteral alimentation.

ACID–BASE DISTURBANCES

Abnormalities of the pH of body fluids are frequently encountered and are of major clinical importance.

An *acid* may be defined as a substance that can provide a hydrogen ion (proton donor), and a *base* is a substance that can accept a hydrogen ion, as follows:

$$\text{Acid} \rightleftharpoons \text{Base} + H^+$$

The negative logarithm of the equilibrium constant for this reversible reaction is termed the pK_a. pK_a is a measure of the intrinsic tendency of the proton donor to dissociate and to form the acceptor. Proton donors with low values of pK_a have the greatest tendency to dissociate and are commonly referred to as strong acids. The Henderson–Hasselbalch equation expresses the pH of a solution as a function of the concentrations of the acid–base pair and the value of pK_a:

$$\text{pH} = pK_a + \log \frac{[\text{Base}]}{[\text{Acid}]}$$

This equation makes clear the fact that the pH is determined by the pK_a and the ratio of the concentrations of the acid–base pair.

Since many different substances may coexist in solution, and since a solution can have only a single hydrogen ion concentration or pH, it follows that the ratios of each buffer pair must vary in order to satisfy the general equation:

$$pH = pK_{a_I} + \log \frac{[Base]_I}{[Acid]_I} = pK_{a_{II}} + \log \frac{[Base]_{II}}{[Acid]_{II}}$$

in which I and II refer to different chemical entities.

Acidemia and *alkalemia* refer, respectively, to an abnormal decrease or increase in the pH of the blood. *Acidosis* and *alkalosis* refer, respectively, to clinical states that can lead to either acidemia or alkalemia. However, in each condition the extent to which there is an actual change in pH depends in part on the degree of compensation, which varies in most clinical disturbances.

For reasons that will be amplified, it is most convenient to evaluate clinical disturbances of pH by reference to the $HCO_3^-:H_2CO_3$ system rather than to other proton acceptors or donors. It is also conventional to refer to the partial pressure of carbon dioxide (P_{CO_2}) rather than to the concentration of H_2CO_3.

There are four primary types of alteration of the ratio of HCO_3^- to P_{CO_2} (Table 27–5). They involve respiratory disorders in which the initial disturbance is either a decrease in P_{CO_2} (respiratory alkalosis) or an increase in P_{CO_2} (respiratory acidosis), and metabolic disorders in which the initial disturbance is either a decrease in HCO_3^- (metabolic acidosis) or an increase in HCO_3^- (metabolic alkalosis). Complex disorders with more than a single initiating factor may occur. These are discussed by Narins and Emmett (1980).

Mechanisms of Compensation. The responses that tend to minimize any deviation in pH are both chemical and physiological in nature.

Buffers. For significant buffering to occur in biological fluids, the pK_a of the compound in question must be within the pH range of those fluids. Buffering is maximally efficient when the ratio of proton acceptor to donor is unity, *i.e.*, when pH = pK_a. Total buffering capacity also depends on the concentration of the buffer itself.

The Bicarbonate–Carbonic Acid System. This system has unique importance when compared with other buffers, particularly because it is the major buffer system in the body that is subject to physiological regulation. Carbonic acid is the principal acidic end-product of metabolism (*see* Table 27–2). Unlike other proton donors, H_2CO_3 is converted to a volatile form (CO_2) that is exhaled through the lungs; unlike the macromolecular buffers, HCO_3^- and H_2CO_3 can be excreted by the kidney and their ratio in the urine can be regulated physiologically. In addition, the buffer pair can be administered separately as "drugs": the proton acceptor, HCO_3^-, as a simple salt, usually Na^+, and the proton donor as CO_2 gas by inhalation. With a change in the ratio between proton donor and acceptor in this

Table 27–5. PLASMA VALUES IN ACID–BASE DISORDERS: SUMMARY OF PROMPT AND DELAYED CHANGES

CONDITION	INITIAL ABNORMALITY	DIRECTION OF CHANGE IN PLASMA COMPOSITION					
		Prompt				*Delayed* *	
		P_{CO_2}	HCO_3^-	pH	Cl^-	HCO_3^-	Cl^-
Respiratory alkalosis	↓ P_{CO_2}	↓	↓ †	↑	0	↓	↑
Acute respiratory acidosis	↑ P_{CO_2}	↑	↑ †	↓	0	—	—
Chronic respiratory acidosis	↑ P_{CO_2}	↑	↑ †	↓	↓	↑	↓
Metabolic acidosis	↓ HCO_3^-	↓ ‡	↓	↓	0, ↑	↑	± or ↑
Metabolic alkalosis	↑ HCO_3^-	↑ ‡	↑	↑	↓	↓	↑

* The delayed changes are the result of renal compensatory mechanisms that alter the rate of excretion of bicarbonate, titratable acid, ammonium, or chloride. Renal compensation is usually maximally effective after several days but varies with the nature of the abnormality. In metabolic alkalosis, the delayed change also includes the development of organic acidemia. In metabolic acidosis, the plasma chloride concentration varies depending on the cause of the acidosis, *i.e.*, a gain of HCl or of other acids.

† Chemical effect of P_{CO_2} on nonbicarbonate buffers (*see* text).

‡ Physiological effect of change in ventilation.

system, other buffers in the same fluid must also change. The nonbicarbonate buffers include principally hemoglobin, other proteins, and phosphate. The pK_a of carbonic acid is 6.1. Thus, the ratio of the bicarbonate–carbonic acid system at a pH of 7.4 is 20:1. Although a buffer pair is more efficient when the ratio is close to 1, the unique physiological control of this system makes it highly effective even at a ratio of 20:1.

Ion Exchange. Cations such as Na^+ and K^+, and perhaps Mg^{2+} and Ca^{2+}, from muscle, bone, and other tissues can exchange for H^+ in the extracellular fluid, and this factor plays a significant role in the moderation of alterations in acid–base equilibrium. The exchange of anions probably plays a much less important role, except for the shift of chloride and bicarbonate that occurs across the red-cell membrane.

Respiratory Regulation. In terms of quantity alone, the lungs play the major role in the daily excretion of acid. Approximately 10 mmol of CO_2 are generated and expired each minute. The CNS is responsive to Pco_2 and pH and regulates the rate and depth of respiratory activity. A depression in pH promptly increases alveolar ventilation, which, in turn, serves to eliminate more acid as CO_2.

Renal Regulation. In terms of combating an acidosis, one can view the major role of the kidney as reabsorbing all the filtered bicarbonate and, in addition, generating new bicarbonate that is formed by the excretion of H^+ as either NH_4^+ or titratable acid. Since the usual diet gives rise to nonvolatile acids that must be eliminated by the kidney, this mechanism is normally in operation. In the renal compensation for alkalosis, particularly metabolic alkalosis produced by the excessive intake of $NaHCO_3$, the amount of filtered bicarbonate is increased and is only partially reabsorbed. Thus, bicarbonate is excreted in the urine, mainly as the Na^+ salt.

Laboratory Diagnosis of Acid–Base Disturbances. The most common laboratory measurements are the pH and Pco_2 of the blood, and the total CO_2 content of the serum. Determination of the pH of freshly voided urine specimens is useful and simple. The calculation of the anion gap is also exceedingly helpful and may provide important insight into etiology. In normal plasma (with all values in mM) the difference between the concentration of Na^+ (140) and the sum of the concentrations of bicarbonate (25) and chloride (105) is 10. A normal range is 8 to 12. Since the anion gap represents the difference between two relatively large numbers, it is subject to cumulative analytical error. An abnormally high concentration of an anion other than chloride or bicarbonate, or accumulation of an abnormal anion, may be detected by the anion gap. Major endogenous anions that are involved include β-hydroxybutyrate, acetoacetate, lactate, phosphate, and sulfate.

MAJOR ACID–BASE DISORDERS

Respiratory Alkalosis. This condition is caused by primary hyperventilation, which increases the elimination of CO_2 by the lungs and thus lowers the Pco_2 and raises the pH of the blood. Mild respiratory alkalosis is encountered in a number of different situations, including mechanical hyperventilation, hypoxia, pulmonary embolism, sepsis, hepatic failure, pulmonary disease, and drug administration (particularly salicylates). More severe alkalosis with tetany, paresthesias, or confusion may be seen with hysterical overbreathing or lesions of the CNS.

Mild asymptomatic alkalosis requires no specific treatment. With hysterical hyperventilation, symptoms may be alleviated by rebreathing into a paper bag. Sedation may also be employed in combination with breathing a gas mixture containing CO_2 (usually 5%).

Respiratory Acidosis. The primary disorder is the retention of carbon dioxide because of impaired ventilation. The increase in Pco_2 lowers the ratio of $HCO_3^-:Pco_2$ and hence decreases pH. The acidosis is partially buffered by the tissues. The kidney responds slowly by increasing the reabsorption of bicarbonate at the expense of chloride.

Retention of carbon dioxide results from two main causes: depression of the respiratory center in the medulla and pathological changes in the alveoli or airways. In both instances respiratory minute volume may decline progressively due to diminishing responsiveness of the medulla to changes in Pco_2 and pH. Respiratory drive may become inadequate and totally dependent on impulses arising from the hypoxic carotid body. The administration of oxygen may result in apnea (*see* Chapter 16). This does not mean that patients with respiratory acidosis should not receive oxygen, but that mechanical respiration is essential in treatment.

Obviously, the most important aspects of therapy relate to an improvement in the basic cause underlying the hypoventilation. However, in severe respiratory acidosis, particularly in asthmatic patients, it may be essential to correct the derangement of pH directly by the infusion of sodium bicarbonate solution. At a more normal pH the bronchodilator drugs become more effective and the basic pulmonary disorder may be alleviated (Menitove and Goldring, 1983).

Metabolic Acidosis. This disturbance commonly results from a loss of proton acceptors (such as bicarbonate during severe diarrhea) or from the accession of proton donors (such as keto acids, lactic acid) that either appear during metabolic or circulatory disorders or arise from the administration of an acidifying salt (such as ammonium chloride) or as an acidic metabolite of a poison such as methanol (formic acid) (*see* Chapter 67). Insight into the etiology may be gained from the anion gap; this is increased by the keto acids and lactic acid or by other organic acids. In renal insufficiency the abnormally large anion gap is attributable to phosphate and sulfate. If acidosis is the result of the administration of ammonium chloride, the anion gap is normal since the increased chloride is accounted for in the measurement. Respiratory compensation involves hyperventilation, which occurs promptly. Renal compensation involves the increased excretion of H^+ in the form of titratable acidity and NH_4^+.

No effort is made herein to detail the specific therapy for the many types of acidosis. However, the role of adequate renal function should be emphasized. Since metabolic acidosis is often accompanied by volume depletion, renal blood flow may be compromised and the kidneys may be unable to excrete appropriate amounts of titratable acid and NH_4^+. This problem may be corrected by the administration of isotonic sodium chloride solution.

When metabolic acidosis is acute and severe, cautious treatment with sodium bicarbonate may be warranted. However, this therapy is controversial, particularly when the acidosis is caused by the accumulation of lactate or keto acids (Narins and Cohen, 1987). With proper therapy of the underlying condition (*e.g.*, diabetes), the organ anions will be metabolized to generate bicarbonate, and the acidosis will resolve without the use of exogenous bicarbonate. If bicarbonate is used in the management of acidosis, the goal of therapy is to restore the plasma concentration of bicarbonate approximately halfway to normal. Because of the persistently high rate of lactic acid production in lactic acidosis, undertreatment is more likely to occur in this condition than in other forms of metabolic acidosis. Overtreatment is to be avoided, since the rapid conversion from acidosis to alkalosis may be harmful. Even a partial correction of the plasma bicarbonate may produce a disequilibrium between the pH of the plasma and that of the intracellular and cerebrospinal fluids. This results from the slow rate at which bicarbonate crosses cell membranes and the blood–brain barrier. As a consequence, the fluids that influence the respiratory center directly remain more acidic than normal and hyperventilation is maintained. The resultant hypocapnia, combined with the partially corrected bicarbonate concentration in the peripheral blood, may lead to alkalosis. In some cases of acidosis with impaired CNS function, the stimulus to respiration comes from chemoreceptors in the carotid body that are sensitive to the low extracellular pH. Treatment of acidosis with bicarbonate in this situation will reduce the respiratory drive and increase arterial P_{CO_2}; this may lead to a decrease in pH within cells and the cerebrospinal fluid, despite the elevation of extracellular pH.

The dose of bicarbonate is usually calculated on the empirical assumption that the ion is distributed in a volume equivalent to 50% of body weight. This is an approximation that includes diverse buffer reactions in both extracellular and intracellular fluids. In more chronic diseases, such as chronic renal insufficiency, the metabolic acidosis can be ameliorated with the use of sodium bicarbonate or preparations of sodium citrate.

Metabolic Alkalosis. This disorder is characterized by an increase in the concentration of bicarbonate in the extracellular fluid. Metabolic alkalosis can be induced by the loss of H^+, as in vomiting acidic gastric secretions, or by the administration of alkalinizing salts, such as sodium bicarbonate. Respiratory compensation consists of hypoventilation. Despite considerable variation between patients, the degree of hypoventilation is approximately proportional to the initial increment in plasma bicarbonate. The respiratory response significantly blunts the increase in pH but may also produce mild hypoxia. The latter is usually not sufficient to counteract the hypoventilation. Renal compensation involves the urinary excretion of sodium bicarbonate, a response that is well documented when alkalosis is produced by the administration of sodium bicarbonate and is associated with expansion of extracellular fluid volume. However, when metabolic alkalosis is accompanied by volume depletion, little or no sodium bicarbonate may be excreted by the kidney and the pH of the urine may remain low. The renal excretion of bicarbonate requires the obligatory excretion of an accompanying fixed cation, principally Na^+. When volume is reduced or Na^+ is depleted, mechanisms to promote the retention of Na^+ are implemented. Bicarbonate is retained simultaneously despite persistent alkalosis. It should be emphasized that Na^+ depletion during metabolic alkalosis is the most frequent cause of paradoxical aciduria. This situation should be monitored by the frequent determination of urinary pH. A third compensatory mechanism in metabolic alkalosis involves the accumulation of organic acids in the plasma. These may be estimated by the anion gap. Such acids significantly lower the concentration of bicarbonate in plasma (*see* Madias *et al.*, 1979).

In most cases acute metabolic alkalosis may be corrected by the administration of adequate amounts of sodium chloride solution. The ability of a neutral salt to correct an acid–base disturbance is based on physiological rather than chemical mechanisms. In the case of alkalosis due to vomiting, the body is depleted of water, H^+, chloride, and, to a lesser extent, Na^+. Once an adequate extracellular volume is reestablished, normal renal mechanisms become effective and Na^+, along with bicarbonate, is excreted in the urine. The complex relationship of K^+ to alkalosis is considered in a separate section below.

Severe metabolic alkalosis may be life threatening. In rare instances, the severity of symptoms requires direct correction of the abnormal pH itself. This can be accomplished with an acidifying salt such as ammonium chloride since, in the presence of normal hepatic function, the alkalosis can be corrected without waiting for renal mechanisms to come into play. Hepatic failure is a contraindication to the administration of ammonium chloride, as it may precipitate encephalopathy. The administration of 0.1 N hydrochloric acid by catheter into a large central vein may be employed in instances in which it is desired to lower the systemic pH promptly and directly without reliance on either renal or hepatic mechanisms. The infused acid is immediately buffered by the circulating blood, although mild hemolysis may occur; if administered into a peripheral vein, severe thrombophlebitis can result. This procedure should be considered as a heroic measure that is to be used only when more conventional therapy has failed (Arieff and DeFronzo, 1985).

Alkalinization or Acidification of the Urine. In some situations the primary purpose of therapy is to change the pH of the urine. When renal function is normal, this is readily accomplished by the administration of either alkalinizing or acidifying salts. Such a maneuver produces only a modest distortion in systemic acid–base balance. However, in edema-forming states, when the renal reabsorption of Na^+ is inappropriately high, alkalinizing salts are poorly excreted. Furthermore, in the presence of renal insufficiency, the capacity of the kidney to compensate for acidosis is diminished, and acidifying salts may have harmful systemic effects.

One goal of alkalinization of the urine (to a pH greater than 7.4) is to increase the solubility of certain weak acids that are more soluble as salts than as undissociated acids. This is indicated when the concentration of the acid in the urine is excessively high. Examples include cystine, in cystinuria; uric acid, in spontaneous hyperuricemia or following the administration of oncolytic or uricosuric agents; methotrexate, in high-dosage therapy; and the administration of certain sulfonamides. A second goal is to increase the excretory rate of lipid-soluble organic acids whose reabsorption is accomplished by diffusion of the nonionized species. Examples include the treatment of overdosage of salicylate or phenobarbital.

An alternate approach to the administration of an alkalinizing salt is to utilize an inhibitor of carbonic anhydrase such as acetazolamide (*see* Chapter 28). When sodium bicarbonate is administered, large doses (10 to 15 g per day) are required to keep the urine persistently alkaline throughout the 24-hour period. When acetazolamide increases bicarbonate excretion, it depletes the body stores of the anion, which tends to reduce the efficacy of the drug. It thus may be logical to prescribe both acetazolamide and sodium bicarbonate. Their actions on the pH of the urine are complementary. However, it should be kept in mind that acetazolamide may competitively inhibit the tubular secretion of other organic acids.

The urine is purposely rendered more acidic than normal either to increase the renal excretion of lipid-soluble organic bases or to provide conditions appropriate for a specific pharmacological effect (for example, the activity of some urinary tract antiseptics).

Preparations for the Treatment of Acid–Base Disturbances. *Sodium bicarbonate* has been discussed above. Precursors of bicarbonate include *lactate* and *acetate*.

Citrate and citric acid oral solutions are a palatable form in which to prescribe an alkalinizing agent. A typical formulation (BICITRA) contains 500 mg of sodium citrate and 334 mg of citric acid per 5 ml (1 mmol/ml of Na^+).

Tromethamine (THAM) is a synthetic buffer (*tris*-[hydroxymethyl]aminomethane); it is available as a 0.3 M solution adjusted to pH 8.6 with acetic acid. It is also supplied as a powder (THAM-E) to be dissolved in 1 liter of sterile water. Each liter contains 300 mmol (36 g) of tromethamine, 30 mmol of sodium chloride, and 5 mmol of potassium chloride. The use of tromethamine is contraindicated in pregnant women or patients with uremia or chronic respiratory acidosis. It should not be given for longer than 1 day except in life-threatening situations.

AMMONIUM AND ACID-FORMING SALTS

The ammonium ion is toxic in high concentrations, but it serves a major role in the maintenance of acid–base balance. It is a proton donor that dissociates to H^+ and NH_3, and the dissociation constant (pK_a 9.3) is such that, in the pH range of blood, NH_4^+ constitutes about 99% of the total ammonia ($NH_3 + NH_4^+$).

Endogenous Metabolism. Normally about 20% of the urea produced in the body diffuses into the gut, where it is converted by bacteria to ammonia and carbon dioxide. Intestinal bacteria also produce ammonia from dietary proteins. The ammonia is absorbed and converted back to urea in the liver by way of the ornithine (urea) cycle.

Renal Excretion. The ammonia that is formed by the kidney is excreted when the urine is acidic, but is largely returned to the systemic circulation if the urine is alkaline. In an acidic urine, NH_3 accepts a proton and exists almost entirely as NH_4^+. Under normal states of metabolism, about 70 mEq of nonvolatile acid is generated per day (*see* Table 27–2); about one half of this is excreted as ammonium salts; the remainder is excreted as titratable acid. Renal production of ammonia is stimulated by acidosis; ammonia buffers urinary acid and allows further secretion of protons into the tubular fluid.

Toxicity. Patients with severe hepatic disease and portal hypertension often develop hepatic encephalopathy. This is manifested by disturbance of consciousness, asterixis, and EEG abnormalities. Since the syndrome is most often associated with elevated concentrations of ammonia in blood, and since it can be provoked by feeding of protein as well as by ingestion of ammonium salts, it is thought to represent, in part, ammonia toxicity to the brain. The occurrence of hyperammonemia in children and infants can be the result of various defects in the enzymes of the urea cycle.

Pharmacological Actions. Ammonium chloride is useful for correction of metabolic acidosis when sodium chloride is contraindicated in the edematous patient. The acidifying action depends on the conversion by the liver of ammonium ions to urea with the generation of protons. Ammonium salts are thus contraindicated in hepatic insufficiency. Ammonium chloride, which has a fixed anion, is an acidifying salt; ammonium carbonate and ammonium bicarbonate, which have a labile anion, are not acidifying.

Solutions of ammonium hydroxide are local irritants. When applied to the skin in low concentration, they have a rubefacient action, and in high concentrations they are vesicant. Ammonium salts are sometimes employed as expectorants; their use as diuretics is now obsolete.

Preparations. *Ammonium chloride* is available as an injection or tablets. *Aromatic ammonia spirit* is a solution of ammonia, ammonium carbonate, and various essential oils in 70% alcohol; it has been used as a reflex stimulant.

Reversal of Intoxication with Ammonia. Several measures have been advocated for the management of encephalopathy associated with hepatic failure. Dietary intake of protein should be curtailed. Neomycin may be used to reduce the number of ammonia-producing microorganisms in the intestine. Lactulose is a disaccharide that is metabolized by intestinal bacteria to organic acids in the lower intestinal tract. The acidification of the intestinal contents retards the nonionic diffusion of ammonia and amines from the colon to the blood. Therapy with arginine has been advocated because it acts as a precursor of ornithine in the urea cycle in the liver; glutamate has been advocated because it reacts with ammonia in the enzymatic synthesis of glutamine (Flannery *et al.*, 1982).

POTASSIUM

K^+ is the predominant intracellular cation. It plays a vital role in the maintenance of electrical excitability of nerve and muscle. K^+ also plays an important role in the genesis and correction of imbalances of acid–base metabolism. Potassium salts are thus important therapeutic agents, but they are extremely dangerous if used improperly.

PHYSIOLOGICAL REGULATION

Absorption and Distribution. Active ion transport systems maintain a high gradient of K^+ across cell membranes; while the plasma concentration is 4 to 5 mM, the intracellular concentration is approximately 150 mM, with modest variation from one cell type to another. Almost all the dietary K^+ is absorbed from the gastrointestinal tract, and in the steady state the amount of K^+ excreted in the urine is thus essentially equal to that in the diet. In the fluids within the intestinal tract the K^+ concentration is two to three times greater than that in the plasma (*see* Table 27–3). In the adult, the daily intake varies with dietary habits and is usually in the range of 50 to 100 mmol.

Excretion. Renal mechanisms are of paramount importance in maintaining both the total body K^+ and its concentration in the plasma within narrow limits. K^+ is freely filtered at the glomerulus and is almost completely reabsorbed in the proximal tubule. The amount excreted in the urine, which is normally equivalent to 10% of the amount filtered, gains access to the tubular fluid by tubular secretion. This occurs in the late distal convoluted tubule and in the collecting duct.

Enhanced delivery of Na^+ to the late distal tubule tends to increase K^+ secretion by two mechanisms. Enhanced delivery of Na^+ is accompanied by enhanced reabsorption of the ion. The major mechanism for Na^+ reabsorption in this part of the nephron is electrogenic, *i.e.*, the more Na^+ that is reabsorbed, the more the tubular lumen becomes electronegative. The electronegativity of the lumen provides a driving force for the secretion of K^+. Second, enhanced delivery of Na^+ to this region of the nephron is associated with an enhanced delivery of fluid. The latter increases K^+ secretion in most circumstances. This increase in K^+ secretion is critically dependent on the presence of the antidiuretic hormone (ADH). When the hormone is absent (hypothalamic diabetes insipidus), ineffective (nephrogenic diabetes insipidus), or its secretion is suppressed (water diuresis), the increased flow to the distal tubule does not result in increased secretion of K^+. At the usual concentrations of ADH in the circulation, an acute increase in the excretion of Na^+ is usually accompanied by increased excretion of K^+, while a decrease in Na^+ excretion is usually accompanied by a decrease in K^+ excretion.

Aldosterone stimulates distal Na^+ reabsorption and K^+ secretion. Clinical conditions that enhance the secretion of aldosterone are characterized by K^+ loss.

Adaptation to K^+ Loads. When the intake of K^+ is increased, the resultant degree of hyperkalemia depends on the prior intake of K^+. Hyperkalemia is greater if prior intake has been low and smaller if prior intake has been higher. Since ingested K^+ is virtually completely absorbed in the upper intestinal tract, it is apparent that this adaptation involves mechanisms of excretion and redistribution.

The increased rate of urinary excretion is achieved by increased tubular secretion of K^+. Hyperkalemia stimulates the secretion of aldosterone by the adrenal cortex; it also directly enhances the Na^+,K^+-ATPase activity in the kidney, an enzyme critically involved in the adaptive response (Hayslett and Binder, 1982). When other physiological variables are kept constant, K^+ loading normally produces an enormous increase in K^+ excretion at the expense of only slight hyperkalemia (Young, 1982).

The major extrarenal adaptation involves the uptake of K^+ by tissues, principally muscle and liver. Hyperkalemia stimulates the release of insulin, which in turn facilitates the cellular uptake of K^+ in muscle independently of any action of the hormone on carbohydrate metabolism. Hyperkalemia also stimulates the secretion of glucagon. Although this hormone increases plasma K^+ by an action on the liver, it also has a hypokalemic action that results from its stimulation of the renal excretion of K^+. Thus, both the adrenals and the pancreas play a role in the adaptation to K^+ loads. When the function of both glands is compromised, subjects may be predisposed to hyperkalemia. This may occur when K^+ loads are given to patients with diabetes mellitus who, at the same time, are subject to either spontaneous hypoaldosteronism or its iatrogenic equivalent in the form of K^+-sparing diuretics. Conversely, when high K^+ intake is suddenly terminated, adrenocortical hyperfunction may persist, leading to hypokalemia that can cause paralysis (Duggin and Price, 1974).

The sympathetic nervous system is also involved in the regulation of cellular and plasma concentrations of K^+. With the increasing use of specific sympathetic blocking agents, these relationships are assuming greater clinical importance. Epinephrine causes an initial rise in plasma K^+ due to the release of the ion from liver, followed by a decrease due to uptake of K^+ by both liver and skeletal muscle. The rise in plasma K^+ is mediated by α receptors, the fall by β receptors. These adrenergic effects do not depend on insulin. When the plasma K^+ is slightly elevated by other factors, it is possible that the effects of β-adrenergic receptor blockade may be additive and lead to hyperkalemia of a dangerous degree (Arieff and DeFronzo, 1985).

During excessive intake of K^+ the amount of the ion secreted into the colon increases; it is excreted in the feces. As in the distal tubule of the kidney, Na^+,K^+-ATPase is involved. The intestinal excretion of K^+ is far less important in the normal subject than in the patient with chronic renal insufficiency, in whom a major fraction of dietary K^+ may be eliminated by this route.

K^+ Metabolism and Acid–Base Balance. This subject involves both ion-exchange mechanisms across the membranes of many types of cells as well as the excretory function of the kidney. In addition, the physiological disposition of H^+ and K^+ may be influenced, at least in part independently of each other, by the balance of other cations and anions.

Cellular Equilibria. The intracellular concentrations of both K^+ and H^+ are higher than those of the extracellular fluid. When the extracellular concentration of H^+ is increased, as in acidosis, there is a shift of K^+ from cells to extracellular fluid. When the extracellular concentration of H^+ is decreased, K^+ moves into cells. Thus, extracellular acidosis produces hyperkalemia, and extracellular alkalosis produces hypokalemia. A change of 0.1 unit in plasma pH can be accompanied by a change of opposite sign of 0.6 mM in the plasma concentration of K^+.

When a change in the concentration of K^+ is the initiating event, the distribution of H^+ may also be affected. In severe K^+ depletion, when the ion leaves the cell it exchanges with extracellular Na^+ and H^+ to preserve electroneutrality. This redistribution of H^+ results in extracellular alkalosis and intracellular acidosis. The opposite tends to occur in hyperkalemia (Adler and Fraley, 1977).

Renal Mechanisms. Deprivation of dietary K^+ initially increases urinary pH slightly and also stimulates the renal synthesis of ammonia (Tannen, 1977). Since urinary pH controls the excretion of both titratable acid and ammonia, the immediate overall effect is to diminish net acid excretion. If the concomitant loss of K^+ is mild, the decreased elimination of acid results in metabolic acidosis. However, if K^+ depletion becomes more extensive, systemic metabolic alkalosis and intracellular acidosis develop.

Considered together, the data suggest that near the normal range of K^+ balance, the ion has a regulatory role in the determination of urinary pH and ammonia synthesis, but that with severe K^+ depletion, additional mechanisms supervene.

Direct micropuncture studies of distal tubule function have revealed a complex relationship between H^+ and K^+. The salient features are as follows: (1) Alkalemia stimulates and acidemia inhibits the tubular secretion of K^+. (2) Inhibition of fluid reabsorption in the proximal tubule during acidosis enhances delivery of fluid to the distal segment and thus increases K^+ secretion. This counteracts the direct inhibitory effect of low plasma pH. (3) K^+ secretion appears not to be influenced by the pH of the tubular fluid itself. (4) The augmentation of K^+ secretion in alkalosis may involve two additional factors: the increased delivery of Na^+ and water to the distal segment and the inhibition of distal K^+ reabsorption as the result of a low tubular fluid concentration of chloride (Stanton and Giebisch, 1982).

PATHOLOGICAL CONDITIONS

The metabolism of K^+ may be considered pathological when its concentration in either the extracellular or intracellular fluid is above or below normal. The concentration in both compartments must be appraised for a complete understanding of K^+ imbalance.

Measurement of Extracellular K^+. The concentration of K^+ in the plasma can be directly measured. Pseudohypokalemia may be encountered in the same conditions that produce pseudohyponatremia, that is, those in which the plasma water content is abnormally low. Pseudohyperkalemia occurs with marked thrombocytosis or leukocytosis. K^+ leaks from the cells during the clotting process; true values are obtained with plasma from blood that is harvested with anticoagulants. Falsely high values are also obtained in the absence of hemolysis with samples of venous blood from patients with sickle-cell anemia. Hemolysis in shed blood also produces falsely high estimates of the plasma concentration. However, an elevated K^+ concentration in serum or plasma from patients with intravascular hemolysis may be a true representation of the concentration *in vivo*.

Since both hypokalemia and hyperkalemia directly influence the electrical activity of the heart, the ECG may be employed as a guide. This is particularly useful when there is a diagnostic emergency and when the concentration must be monitored sequentially during K^+ replacement therapy.

Measurement of Intracellular K^+. Measurement of the intracellular concentration of K^+ is virtually synonymous with measurement of total body K^+. Skeletal muscle accounts for the bulk of the total intracellular store.

Attempts to obtain accurate measurements of intracellular stores have been frustrating. The concentration of K^+ in the plasma is of only limited value. In those conditions in which extracellular and intracellular concentrations change in the same direction—that is, in otherwise uncomplicated K^+ depletion—there may be only a slight fall in the plasma concentration while the intracellular concentration may vary from almost normal to clearly low values. Other conditions in which the extracellular and intracellular concentrations diverge because of the movement of K^+ from one compartment to the other include acute alkalosis or acidosis and hypokalemic periodic paralysis. Since the erythrocyte and leukocyte may be readily sampled, their content of K^+ may be measured directly. However, these data correlate poorly with total body stores.

In the usual clinical situation, an evaluation of total body K^+ must depend on other sources of information. A careful analysis of the patient's history is probably the single most important step. Particular attention must be given to the quantitative aspects of dietary intake and abnormal fluid losses, especially from the gastrointestinal tract.

Hyperkalemia. *Causes.* Hyperkalemia results from a variety of causes: a sudden increase in K^+ intake, either by mouth or by vein; severe tissue trauma; acute rhabdomyolysis; acute or sometimes chronic acidosis; untreated Addison's disease; the rare metabolic disorder hyperkalemic periodic paralysis; an acute increase in osmolality, as may occur after the infusion of hypertonic mannitol or, in a more special case, with the induction of hyperglycemia in diabetic patients who are also deficient in aldosterone; the action of glucagon; the acute stimulation of α-adrenergic receptors; β-adrenergic receptor blockade; and the improper use of K^+-sparing diuretics (Knochel, 1977). Hyperkalemia is not observed during chronic renal failure except as an almost terminal event (due to the effectiveness of both the renal and intestinal adaptive mechanisms). However, in each of the above-listed conditions the degree of hyperkalemia will be accentuated by renal insufficiency.

Consequences. Deleterious effects on the electrical activity of the heart are by far the most important consequences of hyperkalemia. At modest levels of elevation (plasma K^+ of 5 to 7 mM), the T waves become increased in height, or "tented"; the P–R interval lengthens; and the P wave ultimately disappears. At higher concentrations of K^+ (8 to 9 mM) there is a profound depression in impulse generation and conduction in all cardiac tissues, widening of the QRS complex, and eventual asystole, sometimes preceded by ventricular tachycardia or fibrillation. The absolute concentration of K^+ in plasma at which these changes occur varies.

Increase in Total Body K^+. As indicated above in the discussion of adaptation to high-potassium intake, it is difficult to increase total body K^+ significantly above normal.

Hypokalemia. *Causes.* The most common cause of hypokalemia is depletion of total body K^+. However, the plasma concentration may also fall without any change in external balance, and hence without depletion, as a result of acute alkalosis, treatment with insulin, hypokalemic periodic paralysis, and stimulation of β-adrenergic receptors.

Consequences. Since hypokalemia and depletion of K^+ often coexist, it is difficult to attribute the sequelae specifically to one condition or the other. It is probable that the abnormalities associated with neuromuscular dysfunction are primarily correlated with the degree of hypokalemia. These include impaired neuromuscular function, which may vary from minimal weakness to frank paralysis; intestinal dilatation and ileus; and abnormalities of myocardial function with disturbed ECG patterns such as prolongation of the Q–T interval, a broad and flat T wave, appearance of a U wave, depression of the S–T segment, and defects in conduction.

Decrease in Total Body K^+. *Types of K^+ Depletion.* Three subgroups have important implications for guidelines to therapy. First, simple depletion occurs when extracellular and intracellular concentrations are reduced by approximately the same amount. Transmembrane potentials are unchanged, and conduction abnormalities are not observed. Second, the intracellular stores may be excessively lowered relative to extracellular concentrations when membrane function is disturbed. Third, a diminished capacity for K^+, or pseudodepletion, may occur when the total cellular mass is reduced with little or no change in the composition of the residual cells (Patrick, 1977).

This classification is admittedly an oversimplification, but it provides a useful framework. For example, mild starvation may lead to pseudodepletion, but severe starvation causes all three types. The inability of cell membranes to maintain normal gradients is seen in uremia, thyrotoxicosis, severe and prolonged hypoxia, and simultaneous deficiencies in pancreatic and adrenocortical function. Cardiac glycosides also produce this type of defect. As a more complex example, depletion of K^+ may produce rhabdomyolysis. If the depletion is sufficiently severe (approximately 25 to 30% of normal body stores), the integrity of the muscle cell membrane becomes secondarily impaired, leading to a further loss of intracellular K^+ (Knochel, 1978).

Causes of K^+ Depletion. The most common causes of K^+ depletion are associated with an increased rate of excretion by either the kidneys or the gastrointestinal tract. Increased renal excretion occurs in the following conditions: therapy with diuretics; the administration of large doses of anionic drugs that achieve high concentrations in the urine (*e.g.*, aminosalicylic acid and penicillin G and related antibiotics); primary disorders of renal function, such as renal tubular acidosis; secondary disorders of tubular function induced by amphotericin B or by deficiency of Mg^{2+}; primary hyperaldosteronism; and excessive ingestion of licorice or other compounds with mineralocorticoid activity. Secondary hyperaldosteronism markedly enhances the K^+ loss, particularly with the use of diuretics. The administration of sodium bicarbonate acutely increases K^+ excretion, but the effect may be short-lived since both hypokalemia and expansion of extracellular volume suppress production of aldosterone (Sanderson, 1954).

Increased elimination of K^+ via the gastrointestinal tract occurs with the loss of any gastrointestinal fluid (vomitus, diarrhea, or surgical drainage), chronic abuse of laxatives, the malabsorption syndromes, and mucus-secreting villous adenomas of the small intestine. Malabsorption syndromes frequently cause hypocalcemia, which tends to counterbalance the effect of hypokalemia on neuromuscular function.

Although the concentration of K^+ in perspiration is only about 10 mM, cutaneous losses from excessive exercise in a hot environment can result in significant depletion (Knochel, 1978).

Relationship to Metabolic Alkalosis. The popular term *hypokalemic hypochloremic metabolic alkalosis* is an unfortunate collection of redundancies that no longer denotes what was originally intended. First, except in the most contrived experimental situation, all instances of metabolic alkalosis are hypochloremic. And second, due to shifts of K^+ from extracellular to intracellular space, all instances of alkalosis are hypokalemic. The phrase was originally used to describe cases of metabolic alkalosis in which the acid–base imbalance could be corrected only after repair of the simultaneous depletion of both K^+ and chloride. As an example, consider the metabolic alkalosis that results from the loss of chloride and H^+ in the vomitus. There may also be a substantial loss of K^+ in the urine and gastric juice with the production of hypokalemia. Even with K^+ deficits as high as 500 mmol (in adults), the underlying acid–base deficit may be corrected by administration of sodium chloride without repair of the K^+ deficit (Kassirer and Schwartz, 1966). However, when K^+ depletion is more severe, potassium salts are required to correct the alkalosis; administration of sodium chloride will only repair depletion of extracellular fluid volume without correcting the alkalosis.

Metabolic alkalosis has been divided into two categories—sodium chloride–responsive and sodium chloride–resistant. Two separate but related factors are involved: the renal conservation of chloride during alkalosis and the requirement for sodium chloride compared with potassium chloride for repair. In sodium chloride–responsive alkalosis, the kidney effectively conserves chloride by reducing the urinary concentration to 10 mM or less. Acid–base balance can be corrected with sodium chloride. To minimize concomitant hypokalemia, the administration of small amounts of potassium chloride may or may not be considered desirable. In sodium chloride–resistant alkalosis, the kidney fails to conserve chloride effectively and, despite the often severe hypochloremia, the concentration of chloride in the urine is greater than 10 mM. When sodium chloride is administered, extracellular fluid volume may be repaired temporarily, but the sodium and chloride are promptly jettisoned in the urine. Chloride-wasting nephropathy is an appropriate descriptive term (Garella *et al.*, 1970). The disorder is corrected by the administration of K^+. Prior to treatment, both types of alkalosis are characterized by hypochloremia, hypokalemia, and paradoxical aciduria. The single test that best distinguishes between the two categories is determination of the concentration of chloride in urine (in the absence of diuretic drugs). In general, the degree of K^+ depletion is greater in sodium chloride–resistant alkalosis.

Paradoxical aciduria is the excretion of an acidic urine in the presence of metabolic alkalosis. Its relationship to contraction of extracellular volume and Na^+ depletion has been discussed previously. With alkalosis induced by the high-ceiling diuretics, the urine is acidic during the diuretic phase, when Na^+ and chloride are excreted, as well as in the postdiuretic phase, when Na^+ is conserved. Thus, severe K^+ depletion is only one of the conditions that produce paradoxical aciduria.

Effect of Diuretics. As described in Chapter 28, several classes of diuretics increase the excretion of K^+. This is regularly observed acutely, but the consequences of chronic therapy with diuretics are more controversial. In patients with uncomplicated hypertension, the daily administration of diuretics produces a slight reduction in plasma K^+ concentration and either little or no change in total body K^+. In edematous patients the results are more variable. One might anticipate that to the extent that these patients have secondary hyperaldosteronism, they would also be more prone to diuretic-induced losses of K^+. The validity of this concept is amply supported by the high incidence of severe K^+ deficiency in a series of patients treated simultaneously with diuretics and carbenoxolone, an agent with mineralocorticoid activity (Knochel, 1978).

The problem is further complicated by the effects of diuretics on acid–base balance. When edema fluid is rapidly mobilized by high-ceiling diuretics, the resulting alkalosis is largely of the subtraction type. When the same diuretics are used chronically to maintain the patient free of edema, persistence of the alkalosis must involve the negative chloride balance itself, as well as the associated response of the renal acidification mechanisms. With chronic diuretic therapy, despite the association of alkalosis and hypokalemia, there is no evidence in the vast majority of patients that K^+ depletion itself is a cause of the alkalosis.

Consequences of K^+ Depletion. The effects of hypokalemia, listed above, are also seen when intracellular K^+ is depleted. In addition, tolerance to carbohydrate is reduced. Polyuria that is resistant to ADH is a prominent symptom. A deficit of K^+ appears to increase the renal synthesis of prostaglandins, which in turn decrease the effect of ADH on permeability of the distal nephron to water. The disorder is responsive to indomethacin, an inhibitor of prostaglandin synthesis.

PHARMACOLOGICAL CONSIDERATIONS

Transient Volume of Distribution. When K^+ is administered as a drug, the factors that govern its distribution are of major importance. It is not possible to increase the total body content of K^+ significantly above normal. However, it is very easy to raise the extracellular concentration excessively. For example, if mild hypokalemia is treated injudiciously, one may suddenly find that the plasma concentration of K^+ has risen alarmingly (*e.g.*, from 3 to 9 mM). This does not represent a significant increment in total body K^+, of which only about 2% is located extracellularly. However, it is the concentration in the extracellular fluid that determines life-threatening toxicity. Therefore, even though the administered K^+ is eventually destined either to be excreted or taken up by cells, knowledge of the transient concentration achieved in the plasma must govern the use of K^+ as a therapeutic agent.

Indications and Rationale for Treatment with K^+. As a practical matter one should distinguish between prophylaxis and replacement and, in states of K^+ depletion, between acute and chronic conditions. In addition, it is essential to consider as a separate group those patients who are receiving cardiac glycosides.

Indications. The unequivocal indication for the therapeutic administration of K^+ is profound muscular weakness associated with hypokalemia, with or without corresponding abnormalities in cardiac conduction. One should include hypokalemia of all origins, including the specific disease entity of hypokalemic periodic paralysis. Also to be considered are those conditions, particularly diabetic ketoacidosis, in which standard treatment may be *anticipated* to produce acute and severe hypokalemia.

Replacement of K^+ is also indicated in those cases of metabolic alkalosis with K^+ depletion that are resistant to sodium chloride.

In either acute or chronic disorders of acid–base or fluid balance, K^+ may be indicated either to correct or prevent the disturbances attributable to hypokalemia. The goal of therapy is to elevate the plasma concentration of the ion to the low-normal range. K^+ supplementation should be considered if (1) the concentration of K^+ in plasma is less than 2.5 mM on repeated occasions, even if the patient is asymptomatic; (2) the concentration of K^+ is between 2.5 and 3.0 mM with symptoms or electrocardiographic findings suggestive of hypokalemia; or (3) the plasma K^+ concentration is consistently between 3.0 and 3.5 mM and there are clear-cut symptoms or electrocardiographic signs of hypokalemia.

Since digitalis and K^+ have competitive affinities for myocardial Na^+,K^+-ATPase, the actions of digitalis are accentuated by hypokalemia. Therefore, the criteria for supplementation with K^+ are altered for patients who are receiving a digitalis glycoside. In such individuals it is advisable to maintain the plasma K^+ concentration at 3.2 mM or higher. Although digitalis-related arrhythmias are accentuated by hypokalemia, there is no evidence that they are influenced by the absolute concentration of K^+ within the normal range for plasma (*i.e.*, from 3.5 to 5.0 mM). The role of K^+ in the treatment of digitalis intoxication is considered in Chapter 34.

The prophylactic administration of K^+ cannot be justified when the plasma concentration is normal, except for patients with hypokalemic periodic paralysis. In this disorder the concentration of K^+ is often normal during asymptomatic periods, but the frequency of attacks may be diminished by high K^+ intake.

Contraindications. Supplementation with K^+ is contraindicated when K^+-sparing diuretics are prescribed, with the possible exception of patients with Bartter's syndrome. Chronic renal insufficiency is a contraindication, probably for two reasons. First, the urinary excretion of K^+ normally provides a fortunate safety mechanism in the event of transient hyperkalemia. Second, cellular uptake of K^+ may be defective during chronic renal insufficiency. In acute renal failure, K^+ intake should be reduced to the lowest possible level. Tubular secretion of K^+ may be defective in patients with sickle-cell anemia, and supplementation can induce dangerous hyperkalemia (DeFronzo *et al.*, 1979).

Potassium salts have a somewhat unpleasant taste, and they can be irritating to the gastrointestinal tract; many patients do not take the prescribed dose. Many salt substitutes contain K^+ as the cation and can produce severe hyperkalemia if used inappropriately.

In the common situation in which diuretics are chronically prescribed, patients may also receive digitalis for underlying heart failure. As indicated above, alkalosis and hypokalemia may result. Supplementation with potassium chloride is warranted to control the plasma concentration of K^+ and to replenish chloride without Na^+. In the vast majority of such patients, K^+ is not necessary for the correction of alkalosis. However, in rare instances an exceptional degree of alkalosis, hyponatremia, and K^+ depletion were acutely induced by thiazides (Fichman *et al.*, 1971).

Oral Administration of K^+. Potassium chloride is the preferred salt for most situations because of the frequency with which deficits of K^+ and chloride coexist. This salt has a moderately unpleasant taste. For the prophylaxis of hypokalemia during chronic diuretic therapy, a total oral dose of K^+ of 20 to 50 mmol per day in divided portions is effective for most patients. This is given in addition to dietary intake, which may be quite variable.

Intravenous Administration of K^+. In acute illness when the oral administration of K^+ is not possible, it may be administered intravenously. A number of factors must be considered. The following doses are for adults.

Since the normal K^+ intake is 50 to 100 mmol per day, it is rare that a larger amount is warranted. In patients with K^+ depletion this amount slowly but adequately corrects the deficit. With extreme depletion or with high rates of ongoing loss, larger doses may be required. The recommended maximal rate of administration varies from 10 to 30 mmol per hour. If an infusion rate of greater than 30 mmol per hour is considered to be essential, the ECG should be monitored continuously so that the earliest indication of hyperkalemia may be detected. When infused into a peripheral vein, concentrations of potassium chloride up to 40 mM are usually tolerated and do not produce localized pain. If higher concentrations are required because of the concomitant need to minimize fluid intake, a central vein should be employed. When high concentrations are used, even brief errors in the rate of administration can cause cardiotoxicity. It is therefore recommended that the total amount of ion in the infusion system should not exceed 10 mmol when the K^+ concentration in the infusion is 80 mM or higher. In this case a fluid volume up to 100 ml can be conveniently administered by SOLUSET or similar device with a very low rate of infusion of fluid. The available dose of K^+ may be renewed as indicated by the clinical situation.

Toxicity of Potassium Salts. The cardiac toxicity of hyperkalemia is one of the leading causes of iatrogenic morbidity and mortality. Enteric-coated tablets of potassium chloride and other slow-release formulations can be irritating to the gastrointestinal tract and cause ulceration. The rather bad-tasting solutions of potassium chloride may limit the patient's compliance.

Treatment of Hyperkalemia. The acute management of this problem includes, first and foremost, the termination of the administration of K^+, if this is the cause. Additional treatment includes the intravenous administration of a calcium salt, glucose, insulin, and sodium bicarbonate. Ion-exchange resins such as sodium polystyrene sulfonate, administered by mouth or by rectum, are also useful. If the above measures fail, either peritoneal or extracorporeal dialysis may be lifesaving.

Preparations to Repair K^+ Depletion and to Control Hyperkalemia. Preparations of potassium chloride for oral administration are supplied in a vast array of formulations (liquids, powders, and effervescent tablets) and flavors, a reflection of their lack of palatability. Liquids contain from 10 to 40 mmol per 15 ml. Enteric-coated tablets, controlled-release tablets that contain a wax matrix, and controlled-release capsules are also available. *Potassium chloride injection* is a sterile solution of potassium chloride in water. It is usually marketed as a 15% (2 mmol/ml) solution. This solution should never be administered as such but must be suitably diluted. Various other potassium salts are also available.

Cation-Exchange Resins. Exchange resins are useful to lower the concentrations of K^+ in plasma and other body fluids. One of the most efficient is *sodium polystyrene sulfonate* (KAYEXALATE, SPS), which exchanges Na^+ for K^+. It may be given by mouth, through a nasogastric tube, instilled as an enema, or inserted in the rectum in a dialysis bag to facilitate recovery. The resin should be retained in the rectum for at least 30 to 60 minutes. When administered orally, a laxative such as sorbitol may be given concurrently to avoid fecal impaction. The use of resins by mouth is often avoided because of the presence of nausea and vomiting. The usual oral dose is 15 g of the resin one to four times daily. It should be suspended in a palatable vehicle.

When used as an enema, 30 to 50 g of the resin in 100 ml of a suitable vehicle is inserted through a large Foley catheter with the 30-ml Foley bag inflated. The rectal tube is clamped and the material left in the rectum for the period indicated above. The clamp is then released and the material expelled by the patient. Such enemas are given at 6-hour intervals until the plasma K^+ concentration is within a safe range.

Calcium Gluconate. Calcium gluconate may be a very useful agent in combating the deleterious effects of hyperkalemia on the heart. It may be administered directly intravenously as a 10% solution while the ECG is monitored. The usual dose is 5 to 30 ml, but as much as 50 ml of a 10% solution can be administered safely if given slowly. Following this, another 50 ml of the calcium gluconate (10%) can be placed in a larger volume of fluid (dextrose injection, *etc.*) and administered more slowly. Available preparations are described in Chapter 62.

MAGNESIUM

Mg^{2+} is the second most plentiful cation of the intracellular fluids. It is essential for the activity of many enzymes and plays an important role in neurochemical transmission and muscular excitability. Deficits are accompanied by a variety of structural and functional disturbances (*see* Mordes and Wacker, 1978; Rude and Singer, 1981).

The average 70-kg adult has about 1000 mmol (2000 mEq) of Mg^{2+} in his body. About 50% of this is in bone, 45% exists as an intracellular cation, and 5% is in the extracellular fluid. Intracellular concentrations of Mg^{2+} range from 2.5 to 15 mmol/kg. The concentration in plasma is 0.75 to 1.1 mM (1.5 to 2.2 mEq per liter), with about two thirds as free cation and one third bound to plasma proteins. Intracellular and extracellular concentrations of Mg^{2+} can vary independently, and a deficit in one compartment may not be accompanied by a significant change in the other. About 30% of the Mg^{2+} in the skeleton represents an exchangeable pool. Mobilization of the cation from this pool in bone is fairly rapid in children but not in adults.

Absorption and Excretion. The average adult in the United States ingests about 10 to 20 mmol of Mg^{2+} a day, and of this approximately one third is absorbed from the gastrointestinal tract. Absorption occurs largely in the upper small bowel.

Mg^{2+} is excreted principally by the kidney, and, under normal conditions, 3 to 5% of the filtered ion is excreted in the urine. Most of the reabsorption of Mg^{2+} occurs in the proximal tubule (Massry, 1977). Renal excretion of Mg^{2+} is increased by many diuretic agents, and hypomagnesemia can occur as a complication of diuretic therapy. Small amounts of Mg^{2+} are excreted in milk and saliva.

PHYSIOLOGICAL AND PHARMACOLOGICAL ACTIONS

Enzyme Systems. Mg^{2+} is a cofactor of all enzymes involved in phosphate transfer reactions that utilize adenosine triphosphate (ATP) and other nucleotide triphosphates as substrates. Many other enzymes are also influenced by this ion.

Mg^{2+} plays a vital role in the reversible association of intracellular particles and in the binding of macromolecules to subcellular organelles. For example, the binding of mRNA to ribosomes is Mg^{2+}-dependent, as is the functional integrity of ribosomal subunits.

Central Nervous System. Certain of the effects of Mg^{2+} on the nervous system are similar to those of Ca^{2+}. Hypomagnesemia causes increased irritability, disorientation, convulsions, and psychotic behavior.

The flaccid, anesthesia-like state that is produced by the intravenous administration of high doses of magnesium sulfate is probably due to peripheral neuromuscular blockade. In a carefully monitored study of two subjects in whom the plasma concentration of Mg^{2+} was raised to 7.5 mM, the ensuing profound muscular paralysis was unaccompanied by any significant loss of sensation or consciousness (Somjen *et al.*, 1966).

Neuromuscular System. Mg^{2+} has a direct depressant effect on skeletal muscle. In addition, excess Mg^{2+} decreases acetylcholine release by motor-nerve impulses, reduces the sensitivity of the motor end-plate to applied acetylcholine, and decreases the amplitude of the motor end-plate potential. The most critical of these effects is inhibition of acetylcholine release. The actions of increased Mg^{2+} on neuromuscular function are antagonized by Ca^{2+}. The administration of magnesium sulfate in preeclampsia and eclampsia potentiates neuromuscular blockade produced by tubocurarine, vecuronium, and succinylcholine (Ghoneim and Long, 1970). Abnormally low concentrations of Mg^{2+} in the extracellular fluid result in increased acetylcholine release and increased muscle excitability that can produce tetany.

Cardiovascular System. Certain of the cardiac effects of excess Mg^{2+} are similar to those of K^+. High concentrations of Mg^{2+} (5 to 7.5 mM) cause increased conduction time with lengthened P–R and QRS intervals of the ECG. Mg^{2+} slows the rate of S–A nodal impulse formation. Higher concentrations of Mg^{2+} produce cardiac arrest in diastole.

ABNORMALITIES OF Mg^{2+} METABOLISM

Hypomagnesemia. In the course of several months on a Mg^{2+}-deficient regimen, volunteer subjects have developed hypomagnesemia, with inconsistent occurrence of hypokalemia and hypocalcemia. They sometimes exhibited neuromuscular disorders akin to those seen in hypocalcemia.

Mg^{2+} deficiency can occur in diarrhea and steatorrhea; in chronic alcoholism; with prolonged intravenous feeding with Mg^{2+}-free solutions; during hemodialysis; and in diabetes mellitus, pancreatitis, postdiuretic electrolyte imbalance, renal tubular damage, and primary aldosteronism. Mg^{2+} deficiency is therefore often associated with hypokalemia and hypocalcemia.

Hypomagnesemia, as well as a decrease in total body stores of Mg^{2+}, frequently occurs in chronic alcoholic patients. The factors responsible probably include increased renal excretion of Mg^{2+}, decreased dietary intake of Mg^{2+}, vomiting and diarrhea, and hyperaldosteronism in the presence of hepatic cirrhosis. This observation and the similarity between the signs and symptoms of experimental Mg^{2+} deficiency in experimental animals and those of delirium tremens have led to the hypothesis that hypomagnesemia is a causative factor in the latter condition. However, convincing evidence of this is lacking. As part of the total treatment program for chronic alcoholism, the plasma concentrations of Mg^{2+} and of Ca^{2+}, which is also frequently decreased, should be determined and corrected if found to be low (*see* Rude and Singer, 1981).

When deficits of Mg^{2+} and K^+ coexist, correction of the Mg^{2+} deficit may be necessary in order to correct that of K^+. This interaction of the two ions is thought to be mediated by the effect of adrenal steroids on renal excretion (Güllner *et al.*, 1981).

During rapid growth periods in newborns and children, hypomagnesemia has been associated with poor intake or excessive losses. A low concentration of Mg^{2+} in plasma in newborns who are fed cow's milk or artificial formulas is apparently related to a high phosphate:Mg^{2+} ratio in these diets. In infancy the symptoms reliably associated with hypomagnesemia are seizures, hyperirritability, exaggerated tendon reflexes, and increased muscle tone. There is frequently a concomitant hypocalcemia that is resistant to therapy with Ca^{2+} and vitamin D. Symptoms may be corrected by the replacement of Mg^{2+} (Cockburn *et al.*, 1973). Mg^{2+} therapy also appears to be important in correcting hypocalcemia in infants. Oral administration of Ca^{2+} for treatment of hypocalcemia without regard to decreased Mg^{2+} may only exacerbate a Mg^{2+} deficiency by reducing intestinal absorption of the cation.

Hypomagnesemia in protein-calorie malnutrition is well documented. Conflicting reports exist on the significance of Mg^{2+} therapy in reducing the mortality rate in such patients (Rosen *et al.*, 1970).

Mg^{2+} deficiency, particularly if severe, can lead to a form of hypocalcemia that persists despite increased Ca^{2+} intake until the deficit of Mg^{2+} is repaired. Several factors may be involved, including parathyroid dysfunction and an altered equilibrium between Ca^{2+} in bone and extracellular fluid (Massry, 1977). If tetany is present, it is reversed by the administration of Mg^{2+} but not of Ca^{2+}. Other interrelationships between Mg^{2+}, Ca^{2+}, and the parathyroid glands are discussed in Chapter 62.

Hypermagnesemia. An elevated Mg^{2+} concentration in plasma is usually due to renal insufficiency. The use of magnesium sulfate as a cathartic in patients with impaired renal function can lead to severe toxicity, as can chronic ingestion of Mg^{2+}-containing antacids by such individuals. Mg^{2+} cathartics may undergo excessively rapid absorption in patients with large gastrojejunal stomas. As plasma concentrations of Mg^{2+} begin to exceed 2 mM, the deep-tendon reflexes are decreased and may be absent at levels approaching 5 mM. At 6 to 7.5 mM respiratory paralysis is a potential hazard; the respiratory effects can be antagonized to some extent by the intravenous administration of calcium salts. The concentration of Mg^{2+} in the plasma at which complete heart block occurs may be quite variable (*see* Mordes and Wacker, 1978).

Plasma concentrations of Mg^{2+} increase in the fetus and approach the maternal blood values after magnesium sulfate administration in eclampsia and preeclampsia. The neonate may be drowsy and exhibit respiratory difficulties and diminished muscle tone. However, Stone and Pritchard (1970) found no relationship between the plasma Mg^{2+} concentration of blood collected from the umbilical cord and the Apgar score. In infants who suffer hypoxia during delivery, hypermagnesemia can result, and the plasma Mg^{2+} concentration is inversely correlated with the Apgar score (Engel and Elin, 1970).

Preparations. *Magnesium citrate, sulfate,* and *hydroxide* are the preparations usually employed for their action on the gastrointestinal tract. There are many Mg^{2+} preparations used as antacids. For parenteral medication, magnesium sulfate is usually employed. The dosage is expressed in terms of the hydrated salt, $MgSO_4 \cdot 7H_2O$. One gram of this salt is equivalent to 4.06 mmol (8.12 mEq) of Mg^{2+}. *Magnesium sulfate injection* is available in concentrations ranging from 10 to 50%.

Therapeutic Uses. *Gastrointestinal Uses.* The uses of magnesium salts as cathartics (Chapter 38) and as antacids (Chapter 37) are discussed elsewhere.

Local Use. Skin burns from hydrofluoric acid are a serious industrial hazard. Infiltration of the contaminated area with magnesium salts has been recommended on the basis of animal experiments (Harris and Rumack, 1981).

Central Depression. Magnesium sulfate is used in the treatment of seizures associated with acute nephritis and with eclampsia of pregnancy. The dose for children is 0.1 to 0.2 ml/kg of body weight (0.08 to 0.16 mmol/kg) of a 20% solution administered intramuscularly. In the treatment of patients with toxemia of pregnancy, Rogers and associates (1969) have developed a system of initial and sustaining dosage, based on body weight. It is possible to attain unduly high plasma concentrations, and the patient must be carefully monitored both clinically and chemically. If Mg^{2+} therapy of this sort is to be used, a preparation of a calcium salt should be readily available for intravenous injection to counteract the potential serious hazard of Mg^{2+} intoxication. A clinical sign of significance is the presence of deep-tendon reflexes. As long as these are active, it is probable that the patient will not develop respiratory paralysis. The use of magnesium salts for tocolysis is discussed in Chapter 39.

Hypomagnesemia. The treatment for severe Mg^{2+} deficiency is intravenous administration of magnesium sulfate; it should be injected extremely slowly with observance of the same precautions as described above. Two to four g may be given daily in divided doses (8 to 16 mmol).

Adler, S., and Fraley, D. S. Potassium and intracellular pH. *Kidney Int.*, **1977**, *11*, 433–442.

Cockburn, F.; Brown, J. K.; Belton, N. R.; and Forfar, J. O. Neonatal convulsions associated with primary disturbances of calcium, potassium, and magnesium metabolism. *Arch. Dis. Child.*, **1973**, *48*, 99–108.

Colman, R. W. Paradoxical hypotension after volume expansion with plasma protein fraction. *N. Engl. J. Med.*, **1978**, *299*, 97–98.

DeFronzo, R. A.; Taufield, P. A.; Black, H.; McPhedran, P.; and Cooke, C. R. Impaired renal tubular potassium secretion in sickle cell disease. *Ann. Intern. Med.*, **1979**, *90*, 310–316.

Duggin, G. G., and Price, M. A. Hypokalemic muscular paresis in migratory Papua/New Guineans. *Lancet*, **1974**, *1*, 649–651.

Engel, R. R., and Elin, R. J. Hypermagnesemia from birth asphyxia. *J. Pediatr.*, **1970**, *77*, 631–637.

Fichman, M. P.; Vorherr, H.; Kleeman, C. R.; and Telfer, N. Diuretic-induced hyponatremia. *Ann. Intern. Med.*, **1971**, *75*, 853–863.

Garella, S.; Chazan, J. A.; and Cohen, J. J. Saline-resistant metabolic alkalosis or "chloride-wasting nephropathy." *Ann. Intern. Med.*, **1970**, *73*, 31–38.

Ghoneim, M. M., and Long, J. P. The interaction between magnesium and other neuromuscular blocking agents. *Anesthesiology*, **1970**, *32*, 23–27.

Güllner, H.-G.; Gill, J. R., Jr.; and Bartter, F. C. Correction of hypokalemia by magnesium repletion in familial hypokalemic alkalosis with tubulopathy. *Am. J. Med.*, **1981**, *71*, 578–582.

Harris, J. C., and Rumack, B. H. Comparative efficacy of injectable calcium and magnesium salts in the therapy of hydrofluoric acid burns. *Clin. Toxicol.*, **1981**, *18*, 1027–1032.

Kassirer, J. P., and Schwartz, W. B. Correction of metabolic alkalosis in man without repair of potassium deficiency. *Am. J. Med.*, **1966**, *40*, 19–26.

Knochel, J. P. Role of glucoregulatory hormones in potassium homeostasis. *Kidney Int.*, **1977**, *11*, 443–452.

———. Rhabdomyolysis and effects of potassium deficiency on muscle structure and function. *Cardiovasc. Med.*, **1978**, *3*, 247–261.

Madias, N. E.; Ayus, J. C.; and Adrogué, H. J. Increased anion gap in metabolic alkalosis: the role of plasma-protein equivalency. *N. Engl. J. Med.*, **1979**, *300*, 1421–1423.

Menitove, S. M., and Goldring, R. M. Combined ventricular and bicarbonate strategy in the management of status asthmaticus. *Am. J. Med.*, **1983**, *74*, 898–901.

Patrick, J. Assessment of body potassium stores. *Kidney Int.*, **1977**, *11*, 476–490.

Puri, V. K.; Howard, M.; Paidipaty, B. B.; and Singh, S. Resuscitation in hypovolemia and shock: a prospective study of hydroxyethyl starch and albumin. *Crit. Care Med.*, **1983**, *11*, 518–523.

Rogers, S. F.; Flowers, C. E., Jr.; and Alexander, J. A. Aggressive toxemia management. *Obstet. Gynecol.*, **1969**, *33*, 724–728.

Rosen, E. U.; Campbell, P. G.; and Moosa, G. M. Hypomagnesemia and magnesium therapy in protein-calorie malnutrition. *J. Pediatr.*, **1970**, *77*, 709–714.

Sanderson, P. H. Renal response to massive alkali loading in the human subject. In, *Ciba Foundation Symposium on the Kidney*. (Lewis, A. A. G., and Wolstenholme, G. E. W., eds.) Little, Brown & Co., Boston, **1954**, pp. 165–174.

Somjen, G.; Hilmy, M.; and Stephen, C. R. Failure to anesthetize human subjects by intravenous administration of magnesium sulfate. *J. Pharmacol. Exp. Ther.*, **1966**, *154*, 652–659.

Sterns, R. H.; Thomas, D. J.; and Herndon, R. M. Brain dehydration and neurologic deterioration after rapid correction of hyponatremia. *Kidney Int.*, **1989**, *35*, 69–75.

Stone, S. R., and Pritchard, J. A. Effects of maternally administered magnesium sulfate on the neonate. *Obstet. Gynecol.*, **1970**, *35*, 574–577.

Tannen, R. L. Relationship of renal ammonia production and potassium homeostasis. *Kidney Int.*, **1977**, *11*, 453–465.

Tremper, K. K.; Freidman, A. E.; Levine, E. M.; Lapin, R.; and Camarillo, D. The preoperative treatment of severely anemic patients with a perfluorochemical oxygen-transport fluid, fluosol-DA. *N. Engl. J. Med.*, **1982**, *307*, 277–283.

Young, D. B. Relationship between plasma potassium concentration and renal potassium excretion. *Am. J. Physiol.*, **1982**, *242*, F599–F603.

Monographs and Reviews

Arieff, A. I., and DeFronzo, R. A. *Fluid, Electrolyte and Acid-Base Disorders*. Churchill Livingstone, Inc., New York, **1985.**

Flannery, D. B.; Hsia, Y. E.; and Wolf, B. Current status of hyperammonemic syndromes. *Hepatology*, **1982**, *2*, 495–506.

Hayslett, J. P., and Binder, H. J. Mechanism of potassium adaptation. *Am. J. Physiol.*, **1982**, *243*, F103–F112.

McQuestion, M. J. (ed.). *Oral Rehydration Therapy: An Annotated Bibliography*. Pan American Health Organization, Washington, D. C., **1983.**

Massry, S. G. Pharmacology of magnesium. *Annu. Rev. Pharmacol. Toxicol.*, **1977**, *17*, 67–82.

Mordes, J. P., and Wacker, W. E. C. Excess magnesium. *Pharmacol. Rev.*, **1978**, *29*, 273–300.

Narins, R. G., and Cohen, J. J. Bicarbonate therapy for organic acidosis: the case for its continued use. *Ann. Intern. Med.*, **1987**, *106*, 615–618.

Narins, R. G., and Emmett, M. Simple and mixed acid-base disorders: a practical approach. *Medicine (Baltimore)*, **1980**, *59*, 161–187.

Rude, R. K., and Singer, F. R. Magnesium deficiency and excess. *Annu. Rev. Med.*, **1981**, *32*, 245–259.

Stanton, B. A., and Giebisch, G. H. Regulation of potassium homeostasis. In, *Functional Regulation at the Cellular and Molecular Levels*. (Corradino, R. A., ed.) Elsevier North Holland, Inc., New York, **1982**, pp. 259–283.

Symposium. (Various authors.) Acellular oxygen-delivery resuscitation fluids. (DeVenuto, F., ed.) *Crit. Care Med.*, **1982**, *10*, 237–293.

SECTION

VI

Drugs Affecting Renal Function and Electrolyte Metabolism

INTRODUCTION

Irwin M. Weiner

The important homeostatic role of the kidney in maintaining the volume and the composition of the body fluids has already been stressed in the preceding chapter. It is not surprising, therefore, that drugs that alter renal function comprise an indispensable group of therapeutic agents. The most widely used drugs in this group are the diuretics, which may be classified chemically or, preferably, according to the physiological functions that they affect. Some of the diuretics have therapeutic applications in addition to those that result from alterations of excretory function. It should also be noted that the kidney is the major excretory organ for many therapeutic agents and their metabolites. Consequently, renal malfunction may markedly affect the rate of excretion and hence the duration of drug action or the extent of drug toxicity.

PHYSIOLOGICAL CONSIDERATIONS

The majority of excretory products appear in the glomerular filtrate and are incompletely reabsorbed by the renal tubules. Some substances can also be secreted by the renal tubular cells into the tubular urine and thus be eliminated from the body. Certain substances, moreover, undergo both reabsorption and secretion. As used here, the terms *reabsorption* and *secretion* refer to the direction of transport without implication as to underlying cellular mechanisms. Therefore, the factors that are important in the determination of volume and composition of urine are (1) glomerular filtration, (2) tubular reabsorption, and (3) tubular secretion.

Glomerular Filtration. Filtration in the glomerulus is subject to the same physical laws that govern the transport of fluid and solutes across any capillary membrane. The filtering force is the hydrostatic pressure of the blood derived from the work of the heart. The plasma proteins and substances bound to them do not penetrate the normal glomerular membrane to an appreciable extent. All other constituents of plasma are filtered.

Although the rate of glomerular filtration is a very important aspect of renal function, drugs that affect the rate of filtration will not be discussed in this section. A common cause of reduction in the filtration rate is disease that alters the permeability or surface area of the glomerular capillary bed. There is no drug available to correct this abnormality. Another common cause of reduction in filtration rate is reduced renal blood flow secondary to heart failure. For its correction, attention is directed to the heart rather than to the kidney. Many drugs used in the treatment of hypertension reduce renal blood flow and filtration rate, but these represent undesirable side effects. Drugs with marked hemodynamic action, such as epinephrine, alter filtration rate and urine flow by affecting arterial pressure and afferent and efferent renal arteriolar resistance, but no therapeutic application is made of these actions. Finally, there are a few agents, such as dopamine, that significantly increase renal blood flow and filtration rate. Experience has demonstrated that one can alter the rate of excretion of many substances much more effectively by drugs that alter tubular function than by those that change filtration rate.

Tubular Transport of Inorganic Compounds. The importance of the reabsorptive function of the renal tubules to the body economy cannot be overemphasized and can best be illustrated by a few numerical considerations. The rate of glomerular filtration in the average adult is approximately 125 ml per minute. In such an individual, the total extracellular fluid volume is approximately 12.5 liters. Thus, a volume equivalent to that of the extracellular fluid is filtered across the glomerular capillary bed within a period of 100 minutes. During this time approximately 100 ml of urine reaches the bladder. Therefore, the tubules normally reabsorb over 99% of the glomerular filtrate. Obviously, the composition of the tubular reabsorbate must closely approximate that of the extracellular fluid; otherwise, extreme distortions in the composition of the extracellular fluid would soon result. Reabsorption is largely achieved by active transport of electrolyte and other solutes from tubular fluid to tubular cell and thence to the extracellular fluid. This involves the expenditure of energy derived from metabolic activity.

Tubular Reabsorption of Sodium Ions. It is convenient to consider the overall relationship between the reabsorption of solute and of water in terms of the sodium ion (*see* Figure VI–1). Sodium salts constitute by far the largest fraction of the filtered solutes and are reabsorbed in almost all segments of the nephron. The movement of Na^+ across the tubular epithelium occurs in large part through the epithelial cells, the transcellular route. In addition, a portion of Na^+ reabsorption occurs in the spaces between cells, the paracellular pathway. Transcellular transport may be divided into two processes: (1) the movement of Na^+ from the tubular fluid into the tubular cells and (2) the extrusion of Na^+ from the cells into the peritubular or extracellular fluid. The latter process involves the active transport of Na^+ against an electrochemical gradient. This gradient is the result of the negative intracellular potential and the relatively low concentration of Na^+ in the intracellular fluid. The major basolateral transport mechanism is essentially similar in all segments of the nephron (Figure VI–1, *G*). The energy for active extrusion is derived from the hydrolysis of adenosine triphosphate (ATP), and the pump is a Na^+,K^+–ATPase. This enzyme is often referred to as the "sodium pump." The cardiac glycosides are potent inhibitors of Na^+,K^+–ATPase and, under experimental conditions, can inhibit active reabsorption of Na^+ in all segments of the nephron. A second mechanism for extrusion of Na^+ from tubular cells will be discussed below in the section on bicarbonate reabsorption; although it plays a minor quantitative role, it is important physiologically.

A number of separate mechanisms are involved in the movement of Na^+ across the luminal membrane from the tubular fluid into the tubular cells. These mechanisms differ with respect to location in the nephron, sensitivity to drugs, and biophysical and biochemical aspects of the transport process. Thus far, five major types of mechanism for entry of Na^+ have been identified (*see* Figure VI–1). *A*, The direct entry of Na^+ *per se* along a favorable electrochemical gradient; *B*, the entry of Na^+, coupled to the entry of an organic solute or phosphate; *C*, the entry of Na^+ in exchange for a proton moving in the opposite direction; *D*, the entry of sodium ions each coupled to the simultaneous entry of one potassium and two chloride ions; and *E*, the entry of sodium ions each coupled to the entry of a single chloride ion. In *B*, the entry of Na^+ may be coupled to that of a nonelectrolyte (*e.g.*, glucose) or to an ion, such as phosphate, an amino acid, lactate, or other organic anion. The macromolecules that are responsible for the entry of Na^+ into the tubular cells are, in some instances, the receptors for important classes of diuretics.

These mechanisms for entry of Na^+ differ in the extent to which they are electrogenic (*i.e.*, capable of generating a current). For example, the movement of Na^+ *per se* (*A*) is

MECHANISMS OF SODIUM TRANSPORT ACROSS TUBULAR EPITHELIUM

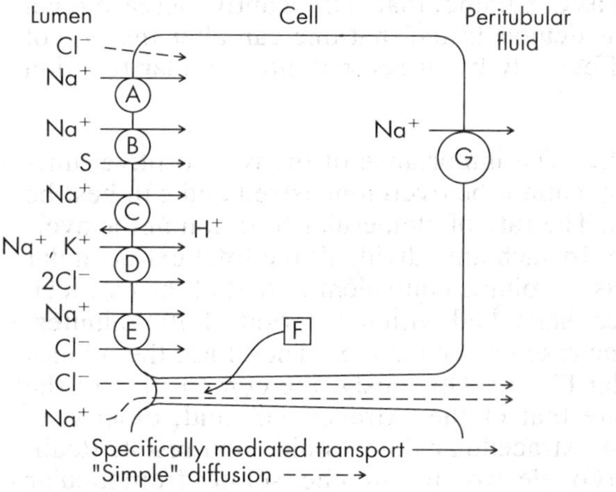

A Na^+ entry *per se*
B Na^+ cotransport with glucose, organic acids, or phosphate
C Na^+–H^+ exchange
D Na^+–K^+–$2Cl^-$ cotransport
E Na^+–Cl^- cotransport
F Cl^- diffusion, Na^+ following
G Active Na^+ extrusion (Na^+,K^+–ATPase)

FUNCTIONAL ORGANIZATION OF THE NEPHRON

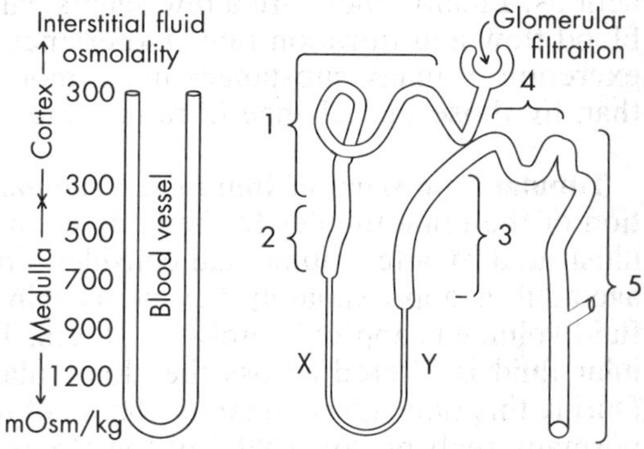

NUMBER	NAME	TYPE OF Na^+ ENTRY
1	Proximal convoluted tubule	A, B, C
2	Late proximal tubule	A, F
3	Thick ascending limb of Henle's loop	D
4	Distal convolution	E
5	Late distal tubule and collecting system	A, C

Figure VI–1. *Schematic summary of the major mechanisms for the renal tubular reabsorption of sodium and the relationship of these to the functional organization of the kidney.*

In the left panel the mechanisms of Na^+ uptake and extrusion are shown in simplified fashion as if all the mechanisms existed in a single hypothetical cell. In the right panel the regions of the nephron are shown (denoted numerically), as are the sites at which the various transport processes are localized. The right panel also shows the *countercurrent system*. The vertical axis depicts the isosmotic cortex and the hyperosmotic medulla. Region 3 is the site of the Na^+–K^+–$2Cl^-$ cotransport mechanism, but it is impermeable to water. This generates interstitial hyperosmolarity. The osmolarity of this space is also influenced by passive processes in the thin descending limb (X) and thin ascending limb (Y) of the loop of Henle, as well as by active and passive processes in the collecting duct (lower part of region 5).

The active ATP-dependent extrusion of Na^+ is localized to the basolateral membrane. To avoid confusion, this diagram excludes the buffer reactions consequent to Na^+–H^+ exchange, the movements of K^+, and the movements of anions at the basolateral membrane. Quantitatively, reabsorption of Na^+ in each region is approximately in the rank order $1 > 2 = 3 > 4 > 5$. It is unknown exactly to what extent this order fluctuates in disease states.

The principal natriuretic actions of the major classes of diuretics can be summarized according to the segmental site (numerical) and to the susceptible cellular mechanism (alphabetical): osmotic diuretics, 1-A, 2-A, 2-F, and indirectly 3-D; inhibitors of carbonic anhydrase, 1-C; thiazides, 4-E; high-ceiling diuretics, 3-D; potassium-sparing diuretics, 5-A.

electrogenic, as is the cotransport of Na^+ with glucose (*B*). However, the cotransport of Na^+ with a monovalent anion such as lactate (another example of a type-*B* mechanism) and mechanisms *C, D,* and *E* are not electrogenic. The electrogenic inward movement of Na^+ *per se* results in only a very small degree of charge separation, and this process causes the secondary or compensatory flow of other ions to maintain macroscopic electroneutrality. This is primarily accomplished by the separate entry of chloride into the cell. In this instance, Na^+ and Cl^- move in the same direction but by different mechanisms. This is to be distinguished from the cotransport of Na^+ and Cl^- (*E*), for which a single mechanism is involved.

A striking characteristic of the proximal tubule is the isosmotic nature of reabsorption. As much as 80% of the filtered solute is reabsorbed in this segment, and the permeability to water is so high that osmotically proportional amounts of water are reabsorbed at the same time.

As will be explained later, most of the filtered bicarbonate is reabsorbed by Na^+–H^+ exchange very early in the proximal tubule (Figure VI–1, *1–C*). The cotransport of Na^+ with anions other than chloride also occurs in the same segment (*1–B*). As a result of these two processes and because of the nature of isosmotic proximal tubular reabsorption, there is a marked increase in the concentration of chloride in the tubular fluid, while the concentration of Na^+ does not change. This results in an electrochemical gradient that is favorable for the passive reabsorption of chloride. Na^+ is available to move secondarily in order to preserve electroneutrality. These ion movements, the paracellular pathway (*F*), occur in the late proximal tubule through the intercellular spaces. In this instance Na^+ transport does not require the activity of the Na^+,K^+–ATPase. Although the immediate steps in reabsorption by this mechanism are passive in nature, it should be appreciated that the favorable gradient for diffusion of chloride is generated by active transcellular transport of Na^+ at upstream sites in the early proximal segment. Osmotic diuretics such as mannitol dilute the concentrations of Na^+ and Cl^- in the tubular fluid, and some of their natriuretic action may be attributed to interference with such "passive" reabsorption.

In the thick ascending limb (region 3) the tubule is relatively impermeable to water, despite the active reabsorption of solute. This has two consequences. First, there is a fall in the concentration of Na^+ and Cl^- in the tubular fluid, reaching a minimal value usually in the first portion of the distal convolution; second, the concentrations of Na^+ and Cl^- become elevated in the interstitial fluid. A concentration gradient across the tubular epithelium is thus established by active transport at the site of low water permeability. This gradient then becomes multiplied in a longitudinal direction by the countercurrent mechanism, such that within the interstitial fluid a large osmotic gradient becomes established between the isosmotic renal cortex and the hyperosmotic medulla and papilla. The osmotic gradients are partly maintained by the relatively meager blood flow to the medullary region. The contribution of Na^+ reabsorption in the segments indicated as region 5 in Figure VI–1 is uniquely important because it occurs in the portion of the nephron susceptible to the action of antidiuretic hormone (ADH). In the presence of ADH, there is a high permeability to water in this segment. As a result, the tubular fluid, particularly within the collecting ducts, equilibrates with the hyperosmotic interstitium and is then discharged at the end of the collecting duct as a hypertonic or concentrated solution. In the absence of ADH, this portion of the nephron is relatively impermeable to water, and the reabsorption of sodium chloride in regions 3, 4, and 5 progressively lowers the osmolality of the tubular fluid; as a result, the voided urine is characteristically hypoosmotic, or dilute.

The absolute amount of Na^+ reabsorbed in the distal nephron is determined not only by the amount filtered but also by the proportion of the filtrate that has already undergone reabsorption at more proximal sites. This fraction may vary over a wide range, particularly in pathological conditions associated with edema formation or oliguria.

Hydrogen Ion Secretion. It has long been known that the kidney has an important role in maintaining acid–base balance. This applies to normal conditions but increases in importance as a homeostatic compensation to metabolic acidosis. The renal response to this condition can be described as follows: (1) the complete reabsorption of filtered sodium bicarbonate, (2) the acidification of the urinary buffers (*i.e.*, the production of titratable acid), (3) the excretion of fixed anions in combination with NH_4^+ rather than Na^+, and (4) the adjustment of urinary pH. All of these factors are manifestations of a single underlying mechanism, H^+ secretion.

In normal circumstances most of the filtered bicarbonate disappears from the lumen early in the proximal tubule; the process is mediated largely if not entirely by the Na^+–H^+ exchange mechanism. It is important to recognize that the disappearance of bicarbonate from the lumen does not represent reabsorption of the ion in the conventional sense. It represents the destruction of bicarbonate in the lumen and, simultaneously, the synthesis of bicarbonate in the tubular cell; the ion is then extruded from the cell across the basolateral membrane. The equations for the lumenal destructive reaction are as follows. Step 1: $HCO_3^- \rightleftharpoons CO_2 + OH^-$; Step 2: $OH^- + H^+ \rightleftharpoons H_2O$; Sum: $HCO_3^- + H^+ \rightleftharpoons CO_2 + H_2O$. The reaction is driven to the right by the introduction of protons into the lumen via the exchange mechanism and by the removal of CO_2, which is readily diffusible. Step 1 is catalyzed by a membrane-bound isozyme of carbonic anhydrase.

The equation for the intracellular synthetic reaction is $OH^- + CO_2 \rightleftharpoons HCO_3^-$. This reaction is driven to the right by a steady source of intracellular hydroxyl ions, engendered by the loss of H^+ into the lumen, and by the removal of HCO_3^- across the basolateral membrane. The reaction is catalyzed by a soluble, intracellular form of carbonic anhydrase. The extrusion of bicarbonate is effected by a Na^+-HCO_3^- cotransporter that carries these ions in a ratio of 1:3 and that derives its force from the relatively negative intracellular electrical potential.

The cells of the tubules can synthesize more bicarbonate than is destroyed in the tubular lumen. It is this property that allows the kidney to correct a metabolic acidosis. This "extra" bicarbonate is produced by the same synthetic reaction mentioned above; it requires a steady supply of OH^-, which is provided by the secretion of H^+ into the lumen in exchange for Na^+. However, the tubules have a limited ability to sustain a pH gradient. For example, the most acidic urine achievable in man has a pH of about 4.4. Thus, for Na^+–H^+ exchange (or any other urine-acidifying mechanism) to progress it is necessary that there be sinks for protons in the tubular lumen. One major sink is provided by the buffers, mainly phosphate, in the glomerular filtrate. The other major sink is ammonia, which is synthesized in the kidney. The conversion of NH_3 to NH_4^+ in the lumen effectively traps a proton.

Potassium Ion Reabsorption and Secretion. K^+ is an unusual fixed cation in that it undergoes both tubular reabsorption and secretion. Reabsorption occurs largely in the proximal tubule and the thick ascending limb, secretion in the distal tubule. Since the major fraction of the filtered K^+ is reabsorbed and since this process is relatively inflexible, it follows, therefore, that physiological variations in the amount of K^+ actually excreted may be attributed to the distal secretory mechanism (region 5 of Figure VI–1). As judged by the action of many diuretic agents, the volume of unreabsorbed glomerular filtrate that flows through the distal tubule is one of the determinants of the rate of secretion of K^+. Thus, some drugs have the dual effect of increasing the urinary excretion of both Na^+ and K^+, the former by inhibition of reabsorption and the latter by augmentation of secretion.

Reabsorption of Calcium Ions. In general, the reabsorption of Ca^{2+} resembles that of Na^+ in the various segments of the nephron. Indeed, in short-term experiments in which Na^+ excretion is manipulated, Ca^{2+} excretion follows in a closely parallel manner. However, reabsorption of Ca^{2+} and Na^+ can be dissociated to meet the separate needs to regulate the concentration of each ion. For example, parathyroid hormone enhances Ca^{2+} reabsorption relative to that of Na^+. This enhancement occurs in the distal tubule and the immediately succeeding segment. The thiazide diuretics decrease Na^+ reabsorption in the distal tubule (region 4) while they simultaneously increase Ca^{2+} reabsorption. This action is independent of parathyroid hormone.

Tubular Transport of Organic Compounds. In the preceding discussion the number of different chemical compounds (*i.e.*, inorganic electrolytes) that were considered is small as compared with the total number of organic compounds that are present in the plasma and thus are candidates for renal tubular transport.

In general, endogenous substances such as glucose, amino acids, and other essentials are filtered and then reabsorbed. They do not appear in the voided urine unless presented to the tubules in unusually large amounts, so that transport capacity is exceeded. Although reabsorption of such compounds occurs by highly specific mechanisms that can be inhibited experimentally by a variety of agents, these inhibitors have no application in therapeutics. Indeed, drug-induced glucosuria or aminoaciduria is a manifestation of nephrotoxicity.

Two major mechanisms for secretion of organic compounds have been identified—one for organic acids, the other for organic bases; both are localized in the proximal tubule. In general, substances that affect one system do not affect the other. Whereas the processes of filtration and secretion increase the amount of a substance present in the tubular fluid, the amount ultimately excreted depends on the degree of reabsorption. This may occur both in the proximal tubule and in more distal segments.

In order to encompass all the foreign organic compounds that have been studied, it is essential to consider two separate mechanisms for their reabsorption. The first, diffusion, proceeds at a rate that is primarily dependent on the lipid solubility of the compound in question. If the molecule is an acid or a base, the pK_a of the compound and the pH of the tubular fluid are also important, since the nonionized form may be far better able to permeate the tubular epithelium. The rate of formation of urine (time available for reabsorption) is another important variable. These factors are discussed in Chapter 1. A carrier-mediated mechanism of reabsorption has been clearly shown for a number of foreign compounds; this is often difficult to demonstrate because of the quantitatively more important role of diffusion. In fact, little distinction need be made between endogenous and exogenous organic solutes with respect to carrier-mediated reabsorption and secretion. For example, uric acid, an endogenous product of metabolism, is reabsorbed by the same carrier-mediated mechanisms as are many organic acids. The complications that arise from the effects of a drug on one or both components of a bidirectional transport system are discussed in Chapter 30.

CHAPTER 28 DIURETICS AND OTHER AGENTS EMPLOYED IN THE MOBILIZATION OF EDEMA FLUID

Irwin M. Weiner

Diuretics are agents that increase the rate of urine formation. By common usage the term *diuresis* has two separate connotations: one refers to the increase in urine volume *per se,* the other to the net loss of solute and water. Under some conditions, the maintenance of an adequate urine volume in itself justifies the use of diuretic agents. However, by far the most important indication is the mobilization of edema fluid, that is, the production of a negative fluid balance such that extracellular volume is returned toward normal. The use of some of these agents in the therapy of hypertension is discussed in Chapter 33.

General Considerations. Except for the osmotic diuretics, the drugs that are considered in this chapter act directly on the tubular epithelia. For the most part, these direct actions are site specific, *i.e.,* a drug will act on one or another tubular segment, but not on all of them. However, sites that are not attacked directly may well be affected indirectly. First, consider the fact that the various segments of the nephron are arranged in series; a change in the behavior of one segment will alter conditions for the downstream segments. Second, the organism reacts to the diuretic-induced diminution of the extracellular fluid volume with hemodynamic, neural, and endocrine mechanisms that tend to conserve water and solutes. This is seen clearly in the normal subject given a diuretic on each of several consecutive days. An appreciable diuresis occurs on the first day, a lesser diuresis on the second, and no diuresis on the third (*see* Breslau *et al.,* 1976). Conservative mechanisms may result in increased reabsorption of salt and water at sites upstream to the site of action of a diuretic as well as downstream.

It should also be recognized that all drugs in this class have a tendency to distort the composition of the body fluids. Several factors contribute to these phenomena. First, the direct action of the drug may cause the selective excretion of a single type of ion. For example, inhibitors of carbonic anhydrase specifically deplete the body of bicarbonate. Second, the distortion in the pattern of axial flow in the nephron results in abnormal function; for example, increased flow in the distal tubule enhances excretion of K^+. Third, the conservative mechanisms that come into play as a result of volume depletion are capable of causing selective abnormalities in the concentrations of individual ions.

Extrarenal Sites of Drug Action. Many of the newer diuretics have proven to be useful in the investigation of electrolyte transport in organs other than the kidney. Not surprisingly, these studies have revealed fundamental mechanisms common to many tissues. However, these are not reviewed systematically in this chapter unless the action at the extrarenal site occurs with reasonable dosages and is of sufficient magnitude to be clinically important.

OSMOTIC DIURETICS

The term *osmotic diuretic* is used for certain solutes that have the following attributes in common: (1) they are freely filterable at the glomerulus; (2) they undergo limited reabsorption by the renal tubule; and (3) they are relatively inert by conventional pharmacological criteria. These agents are administered in sufficiently large quantities to contribute significantly to the osmolality of the plasma, the glomerular filtrate, and the tubular fluid. Mannitol is the most frequently used of the osmotic diuretics. Other agents include urea, glycerin, and isosorbide.

Mechanism of Diuretic Action. Sodium salts are the major solutes in proximal tubular fluid. Since the epithelium of this segment cannot maintain a substantial osmotic gradient, Na^+ and water are normally reabsorbed from the tubular fluid in the same ratio as exists in the glomerular filtrate. Thus, the concentration of Na^+ in the lumen remains essentially constant (*see* Introduction to Section VI). However, a nonreabsorbable solute in the proximal tubular lumen becomes progressively concentrated as fluid is reabsorbed, and this produces a counterforce to the normal reabsorption of water. Consequently, relatively more Na^+ than water is reabsorbed and the luminal concentration of Na^+ begins to fall.

The net reabsorption of Na^+ diminishes because of three factors: (1) the concentration of Na^+ in the tubular fluid becomes abnormally low, such that the driving force for its entry into the tubular cell diminishes; (2) there is an increased flux of Na^+ from the peritubular fluid back into the lumen as a result of the abnormal concentration gradient that becomes established in that direction; and (3) mannitol causes an increase in renal medullary blood flow through a prostaglandin-mediated mechanism. This results in a partial washout of the normal medullary hypertonicity, with a consequent decrease in net reabsorption of Na^+ in the thin ascending limb of Henle's loop (Lang, 1987). The overall result is an enhanced rate of urine flow associated with a relatively smaller increment in the excretion of salts. It is the increase in urine flow that is the primary basis of therapeutic efficacy.

Osmotic diuresis is sometimes an incidental phenomenon. In severe hyperglycemia the mechanism for reabsorption of glucose becomes saturated and the unreabsorbed portion acts as an osmotic diuretic. Urographic and angiographic radiocontrast agents have all the attributes of osmotic diuretics described above. The renal tubule is impermeable to the iodinated organic moiety that provides radioopacity. With most radiological procedures, the induced diuresis is short lived and has relatively little impact on fluid and electrolyte balance.

Therapeutic Uses. Mannitol is the agent most frequently employed in the prophylaxis and early treatment of acute renal failure in conditions as diverse as cardiovascular operations, severe traumatic injury, operations in the presence of severe jaundice, and management of hemolytic transfusion reactions. In each of these conditions, a precipitous fall in the flow of urine may be anticipated either as the result of an acutely reduced filtration rate or from acute changes in tubular permeability. The latter may be the consequence of the presence of a noxious agent within the tubular fluid in excessively high concentrations. In these situations, mannitol exerts an osmotic effect within the tubular fluid, inhibits water reabsorption, and maintains the rate of urine flow. As a consequence, the concentration of the toxic agent within the tubular fluid does not reach the excessively high levels that otherwise would have been achieved by the more complete reabsorption of water. The early use of osmotic diuretics seems to protect the kidney against damage. The maintenance of an adequate flow of relatively dilute urine is probably the single most important factor.

In the oliguric state that attends an acute reduction in the rate of glomerular filtration, the reabsorption of endogenous solutes is nearly complete. In this setting drugs that selectively inhibit solute reabsorption in one or another tubular segment may fail to enhance urine flow; other segments of the nephron may still complete the reabsorption. However, under these conditions the osmotic diuretics usually retain their efficacy. Even though the filtration rate is reduced, mannitol is still filtered at the glomerulus. Tubular impermeability to mannitol is not altered by acute renal ischemia of short duration. Hence, the mannitol that is filtered is also excreted in the voided urine. Unreabsorbed solute limits the back diffusion of water. As a consequence, urine volume can be maintained even in the presence of decreased glomerular function. Nephrotoxic agents and prolonged, severe renal ischemia may damage the tubular epithelium and produce acute tubular necrosis with oliguria. The tubule is then no longer selectively impermeable, and osmotic diuretics become ineffective.

Mannitol is also used for the reduction of the pressure and volume of the cerebrospinal fluid. By elevating the osmolality of the plasma, the diffusion of water back into the plasma is enhanced. However, the degree of success is quite variable (*see* Prockop, 1976). Mannitol, glycerin, and isosorbide are also used for the short-term reduction of intraocular pressure, particularly preoperatively and postoperatively in patients who require ocular surgery. They are also useful in certain other ophthalmological conditions.

Toxicity. Mannitol is distributed in the extracellular fluid, and consequently, the short-term administration of hypertonic solutions in amounts sufficient to make a significant contribution to extracellular osmolarity will inevitably be accompanied by an acute expansion of extracellular fluid volume. In the patient with cardiac decompensation, this represents an undesirable hazard. A variety of signs and symptoms suggestive of hypersensitivity reactions has occurred in occasional patients. Urea is more irritating to tissues and may cause thrombosis or pain if extravasation occurs. Glycerin is metabolized and can cause hyperglycemia and glycosuria. Headache, nausea, and vomiting are relatively common sequelae of the administration of any osmotic diuretic.

Preparations and Dosage. *Mannitol* (OSMITROL) is available for intravenous infusion in concentrations of 5 to 25% in volumes ranging from 50 to 1000 ml of water. The compound is not absorbed from the gastrointestinal tract. The adult dose for promotion of diuresis ranges from 50 to 200 g over a 24-hour period of infusion; the rate is generally adjusted to maintain a urinary output of at least 30 to 50 ml per hour. It should be preceded by a test dose in patients with marked oliguria or questionable adequacy of renal function. Plasma volume should also be assessed by determination of central venous or pulmonary arterial pressure, since correction of plasma volume should precede or accompany the use of these agents for oliguria. The recommended test dose is 200 mg/kg, infused over 3 to 5 minutes; if the first or a second test dose fails to promote a urinary flow greater than 30 ml per hour for 2 to 3 hours, the patient's status should be reevaluated before continuing therapy. The dose for the reduction of intracranial pressure and brain mass before or after neurosurgery, or for the reduction of intraocular tension during an acute attack of congestive glaucoma or for ophthalmic surgery, is 1.5 to 2 g/kg, given as a 15 to 25% solution over a period of 30 to 60 minutes. Contraindications to the administration of mannitol include renal disease of sufficient severity to produce anuria, marked pulmonary congestion or edema, marked dehydration, and intracranial hemorrhage, unless craniotomy is to be performed. The infusion of mannitol should be terminated if the patient shows signs of progressive renal dysfunction, heart failure, or pulmonary congestion.

A sterile preparation of *urea* (UREAPHIL) is available that may be reconstituted for intravenous use. When administered in this manner, the solution contains 30% urea and either 5 or 10% dextrose or invert sugar (equal parts of dextrose and fructose), the latter substances being necessary to prevent the hemolysis produced by pure solutions of urea. Intravenous doses of 1 to 1.5 g of urea per kilogram of body weight are optimal in preparation for neurosurgical procedures or for reduction of intraocular pressure. On a molar basis urea is less effective as a diuretic than is mannitol, since approximately 50% of the compound is reabsorbed from the tubular fluid.

Glycerin (OSMOGLYN) is given orally, particularly for use prior to ophthalmological procedures. Since the agent is rapidly metabolized, it produces relatively little diuresis. The dose for adults is 1 to 1.5 g/kg, and it is given as a 50% solution. The total daily dose should not exceed 120 g. Maximal reduction of intraocular pressure occurs 1 hour after its administration, and the effect disappears after 5 hours.

Isosorbide (ISMOTIC) is also used orally for ophthalmological purposes. The effects observed are generally similar to those of glycerin, although diuresis is greater and hyperglycemia does not occur. Dosage may range from 1 to 3 g/kg and may be given two to four times daily.

INHIBITORS OF CARBONIC ANHYDRASE

Acetazolamide is the prototype of a class of agents that have had limited usefulness as diuretics but have had a major role in the development of fundamental renal physiology and pharmacology. These drugs are used frequently in the treatment of glaucoma and for the prevention of acute mountain sickness.

History. In the early 1930s, Roughton discovered the enzyme carbonic anhydrase in erythrocytes. The enzyme has subsequently been found in many tissues, including the renal cortex, gastric mucosa, pancreas, eye, and central nervous system (CNS). When sulfanilamide was introduced as a chemotherapeutic agent, metabolic acidosis was recognized as a side effect. The drug was found to inhibit carbonic anhydrase *in vitro* and to inhibit the normal acidification of the urine *in vivo*. Subsequent studies with more potent inhibitors established the role of carbonic anhydrase in renal transport (Maren, 1967).

Chemistry. Among the enormous number of sulfonamides that have been synthesized and tested, acetazolamide has been studied the most extensively as an inhibitor of carbonic anhydrase. The other drugs of this class that are available in the United States are dichlorphenamide and methazolamide. Their structural formulas are as follows:

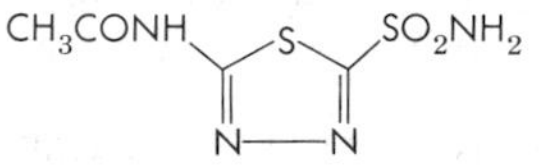

Acetazolamide

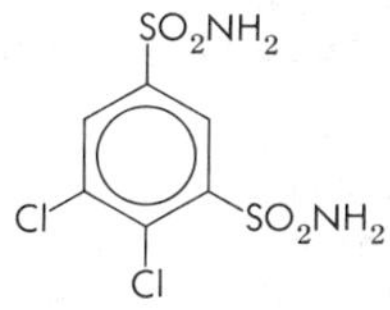

Dichlorphenamide

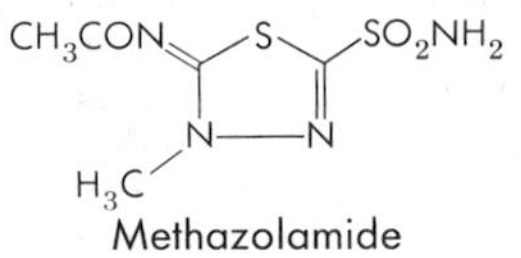

Methazolamide

Carbonic anhydrase inhibitory activity is abolished by N-sulfamyl substitutions (Maren, 1976).

Mechanism of Action. Acetazolamide is a potent, reversible inhibitor of carbonic anhydrase. The concentration of the drug required for 50% inhibition of the enzyme from the renal cortex is about 10 nM. The reaction catalyzed by the enzyme ($CO_2 + OH^- \rightleftharpoons HCO_3^-$) is discussed in the Introduction to Section VI. This reaction can occur in the absence of the enzyme, but the rate is too slow to allow normal physiological function. In general, the enzyme is normally present in tissues in huge excess. More than 99% of enzyme activity in the kidney must be inhibited before physiological effects become apparent. The enzyme itself is the dominant tissue component to which the inhibitors become bound.

Action on the Kidney. Following the administration of acetazolamide, the urine volume promptly increases. The normally acidic pH becomes alkaline. The urinary concentration of bicarbonate increases and is matched by Na^+ and substantial amounts of K^+ (Table 28–1). The urinary concentration of chloride falls. The increased alkalinity of the urine is necessarily accompanied by a decrease in the excretion of titratable acid and of ammonia.

The above sequence of events may be attributed to the inhibition of H^+ secretion by the renal tubule. This inhibition is indirect and, in the proximal tubule, is the consequence of inhibition of cytoplasmic carbonic anhydrase, which decreases the availability of protons for Na^+–H^+ exchange. In addition, carbonic anhydrase bound to the brush-border membrane is also inhibited. This slows the destruction of bicarbonate in the lumen and, thereby, the diffusion of CO_2 into the tubular cell. The overall effect is that bicarbonate reabsorption in the proximal tubule is reduced by some 80%. More than half of this rejected bicarbonate is reabsorbed in later segments of the nephron by mechanisms that do not involve carbonic anhydrase and that are not yet fully characterized. Acetazolamide also inhibits H^+ secretion by some segments of the distal nephron (Preisig *et al.*, 1987).

Effect on Plasma Composition. Acetazolamide increases the urinary excretion of bicarbonate and fixed cation, mostly Na^+. As a result, the concentration of bicarbonate in the extracellular fluid decreases and metabolic acidosis results. In metabolic acidosis, the renal response to acetazolamide is greatly reduced; conversely, it is enhanced with metabolic alkalosis. Factors in addition to the amount of filtered bicarbonate must be determinants of drug action since the extracellular alkalosis resulting from depletion of K^+ (with presumed intracellular acidosis) decreases the diuretic response.

Acetazolamide produces a marked increase in K^+ excretion, attributable to enhanced secretion in the distal nephron. The effects on K^+ are most prominent on short-term administration.

Eye. Carbonic anhydrase is present in a number of intraocular structures, including the ciliary processes, which produce the high concentration of bicarbonate in the aqueous humor. Acetazolamide reduces the rate of aqueous humor formation; intraocular pressure in patients with glaucoma is correspondingly reduced. This action of the drug appears to be independent of systemic acid–base balance (*see* Maren, 1967).

Gastrointestinal Tract. Under appropriate experimental conditions, it is possible to implicate carbonic anhydrase in the formation of gastric and pancreatic juice and to block secretion by enzyme

Table 28–1. URINARY ELECTROLYTE COMPOSITION DURING DIURESIS *

	VOLUME (*ml/min*)	pH	Na^+	K^+	Cl^-	HCO_3^-
			(*mM*)			
Control	1	6	50	15	60	1
Mannitol	10	6.5	90	15	110	4
Acetazolamide	3	8.2	70	60	15	120
Benzothiadiazides (thiazides)	3	7.4	150	25	150	25
High-ceiling diuretics	8	6	140	10	155	1
Potassium-sparing diuretics	2	7.2	130	5	110	15
Aminophylline	3	6	150	15	160	1

* Data are representative of results that would be observed in man or dog during normal hydration and acid–base balance. Such findings are readily reproducible during the peak of diuresis and following a single maximally effective dose. However, a significant range of urinary values may be anticipated: *a single value is given here solely to facilitate comparison of one drug with another.* Excretion rates are obtainable as the product of urinary volume and composition.

inhibition. These processes are relatively insensitive to ordinary doses of carbonic anhydrase inhibitors, and these pharmacological effects have no therapeutic applications.

Central Nervous System. An action of acetazolamide on the CNS was first suggested by the frequency of paresthesias and somnolence as side effects. Subsequently, the drug was found to inhibit epileptic seizures and to decrease the rate of formation of spinal fluid. Metabolic acidosis from ketogenic diets diminishes epileptic seizures, and acetazolamide, by virtue of its action on the kidney, leads to the production of a systemic acidosis. However, there is undoubtedly a more direct action on CNS function. An increase in local CO_2 tension may result from inhibition of the enzyme in the brain, the choroid plexus, or the erythrocytes of the cerebral blood. The exact role of carbonic anhydrase in brain function remains unknown. Acetazolamide may reduce the rate of cerebrospinal fluid formation by the choroid plexus, but it may also transiently elevate cerebrospinal fluid pressure as a result of an increase in intracranial blood flow (Laux and Raichle, 1978).

Respiration. The transport of CO_2 in the blood is related to the carbonic anhydrase activity of the circulating erythrocytes. Acetazolamide creates a disequilibrium in the CO_2 transport system, giving rise to increased CO_2 tensions in the tissues and a relatively decreased tension in the expired gas.

Absorption, Fate, and Excretion. Acetazolamide is readily absorbed from the gastrointestinal tract. Peak concentrations in plasma occur within 2 hours. The drug is excreted by the kidney; both active tubular secretion and passive reabsorption are involved. Excretion is complete within 24 hours. Acetazolamide is tightly bound to carbonic anhydrase and, consequently, is present in greater amounts in those tissues in which the enzyme is present in high concentration, particularly the erythrocytes and the renal cortex. Some carbonic anhydrase inhibitors do not penetrate the erythrocyte. Thus, renal and systemic drug actions may be dissociated on the basis of drug distribution (*see* Maren, 1967). Acetazolamide is not metabolized.

Preparations and Dosage. *Acetazolamide* (DIAMOX, others) is available as 125- or 250-mg tablets and as sustained-release capsules containing 500 mg. An effective single oral dose is 250 to 500 mg. Vials of *acetazolamide sodium* are available for parenteral administration. When used as a diuretic, it should be given once daily or every other day. To achieve a sustained metabolic acidosis, the drug should be given at intervals of 8 hours. Doses of 250 to 1000 mg per day (divided for amounts over 250 mg) are used for treatment of chronic simple glaucoma. *Dichlorphenamide* (DARANIDE) is available as 50-mg tablets. Optimal effects have been achieved with initial doses of 200 mg per day. *Methazolamide* (NEPTAZANE) is available as 25- and 50-mg tablets; the usual dose is 100 to 300 mg per day.

Clinical Toxicity. Serious toxic reactions are infrequent. With large doses, many patients exhibit drowsiness and paresthesias. In hepatic cirrhosis, episodes of disorientation may be induced; it has been postulated that urinary alkalinization diverts ammonia of renal origin from the urine into the systemic circulation. Hypersensitivity reactions are relatively rare. They consist of fever, skin reactions, bone-marrow depression, and sulfonamide-like renal lesions. Calculus formation and ureteral colic have been attributed to the marked reduction in urinary citrate produced by acetazolamide associated with either no change or even a rise in urinary Ca^{2+}. Acetazolamide depresses the uptake of iodide by the thyroid gland. However, drugs of this class are not therapeutically useful as antithyroid agents. Teratogenic effects have been demonstrated in animals, and it is recommended that these drugs not be administered during pregnancy. Since carbonic anhydrase inhibitors alkalinize the urine, they interfere with the action of methenamine as a urinary tract antiseptic. Drug-induced osteomalacia has been reported with the simultaneous use of phenytoin.

Therapeutic Uses. The most common application of carbonic anhydrase inhibitors is to reduce intraocular pressure (in the treatment of glaucoma). Their value in the management of absence seizures is limited by the rapid development of tolerance. Acetazolamide is rarely administered as a diuretic but may be useful for alkalinization of the urine. The clinical situations in which such alkalinization is appropriate are discussed in Chapter 27. Acetazolamide appears to have a beneficial effect in the management of periodic paralysis even when associated with hypokalemia (Griggs *et al.,* 1970). It has been postulated that the induced acidosis raises the extracellular concentration of K^+ locally in the microcirculation of muscle. Acetazolamide is also effective in ameliorating the symptoms of acute mountain sickness (Larson *et al.,* 1982).

BENZOTHIADIAZIDES AND RELATED AGENTS

History. This class of diuretics provides an instructive example of the manner in which newly synthesized agents may be endowed with unanticipated efficacious properties. They were synthesized in an attempt to enhance the potency of inhibitors of carbonic anhydrase. An unanticipated chemical reaction produced substances with new pharmacological properties. The voided urine contained increased amounts of chloride, a response significantly different from that evoked by the parent compounds (*see* Beyer, 1958). Subsequent studies indicated that the effect of the benzothiadiazides is independent of any action on carbonic anhydrase.

Chlorothiazide provided the first serious challenge to the mercurial diuretics, an obsolete class of organometallic compounds that dominated therapy in this area for over 30 years.

Chemistry and Structure–Activity Relationship. Most compounds of this group are analogs of 1,2,4-benzothiadiazine-1,1-dioxide (*see* Table 28–2 for the parent structural formula and the substituents of the analogs that have received the most intensive study). As a group they can be designated as the "benzothiadiazide," or "thiazide," diuretics. Some compounds have hyperglycemic activity, for which the structural requirements differ from those for diuresis (Wales *et al.,* 1968).

It should be emphasized that all thiazides thus far carefully examined have parallel dose–response curves and comparable maximal chloruretic effects. This implies that they have a common mechanism of action. The various analogs differ primarily in the dose required to produce a given effect and not in their optimal therapeutic response.

There are some other sulfonamide diuretics that differ chemically from the thiazides by the nature of the heterocyclic ring. However, their pharmacological action is indistinguishable from that of the thiazides. They have the following structures:

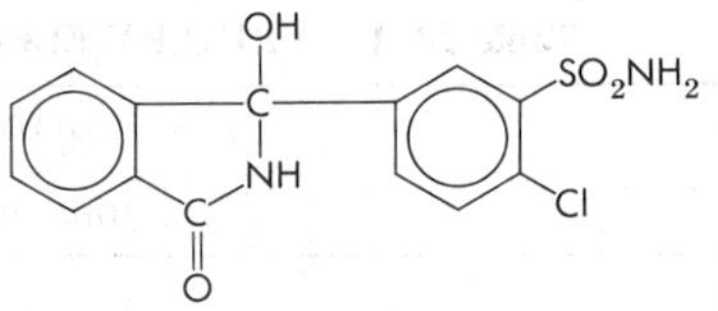

Chlorthalidone

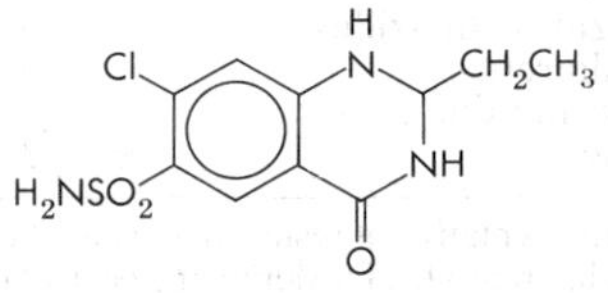

Quinethazone

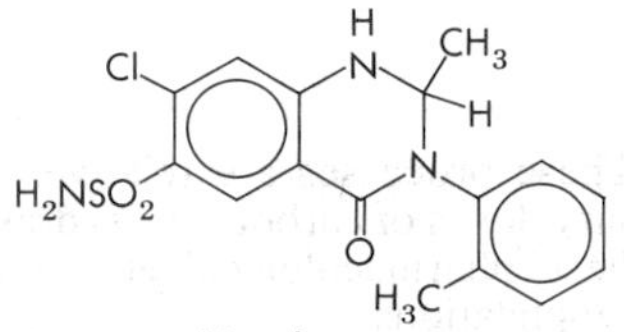

Metolazone

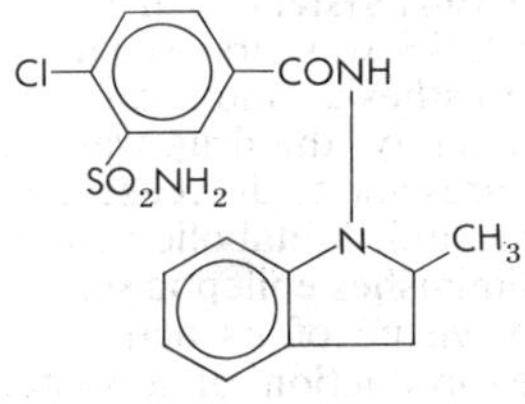

Indapamide

Mechanism of Renal Action. Thiazides act directly on the kidney to increase the excretion of sodium chloride and water; they also increase excretion of K^+. The thiazides vary widely in their potency as carbonic anhydrase inhibitors. Those that are active in this respect may, at sufficient dosage, have the same effect on bicarbonate excretion as does acetazolamide. However, this phenomenon is seldom encountered clinically. The use of thiazides as antihypertensive agents is considered in Chapter 33. In patients with diabetes insipidus, the thiazides actually *decrease* urinary volume (*see* Chapter 29).

Like many other organic acids, the thiazides are actively secreted in the proximal tubule. This secretion may be curtailed by competitors such as probenecid (*see* Chapter 30). In some circumstances, probenecid can inhibit the diuretic response to a thiazide, suggesting that the diuretic must be in the tubular fluid in order to exert its effect. The major, if not exclusive, site of action of thiazides is the early distal tubule. In distal tubular microperfusion studies, reabsorption of Na^+ was inhibited when chlorothiazide was added only to the fluid perfusing the lumen, a result consistent with the effects of probenecid. The action of thiazides is attributable to blockade of electroneutral Na^+–Cl^- cotransport (mechanism *E* in Figure VI–1, page 710; *see* Velázquez, 1987). The maximal rate of Na^+ excretion induced by thiazides is modest relative to that achievable with some other types of diuretics. This results from the fact that about 90% of filtered Na^+ is reabsorbed before the tubular fluid reaches the site of action of the thiazides.

Thiazide-induced increases in excretion of K^+ are most readily seen in short-term studies; they may be small during long-term administration (*see* Table 28–1). The nephron segments responsible for secretion of K^+ are distal to the site of action of thiazides, and the drug-induced enhancement of flow through these distal segments is a stimulant to K^+ secretion. Another factor that determines K^+ secretion, the transepithelial electrical potential, is not influenced by thiazides. Although minor differences in the kaliuresis caused by different thiazides have been observed in special circumstances, these have no practical consequences.

The glomerular filtration rate may be reduced by the thiazides, particularly with intravenous administration. This is presumably the result of a direct action on the renal vasculature. It has little significance in the interpretation of primary drug action but may be of clinical importance, particularly in patients with diminished renal reserve.

Thiazides may increase the concentration of urate in plasma. Two factors are involved. The first is an enhanced reabsorption of urate in the proximal tubule; this is secondary to enhanced reabsorption of fluid caused by a diuretic-induced contraction of extracellular fluid volume. Second, thiazides may inhibit the tubular excretion of urate (*see* Chapter 30). The increase in uric acid concentration may have little significance, since the incidence of acute attacks of gout is primarily related to the concentration of uric acid in plasma before treatment with a thiazide.

Unlike some other natriuretic agents, the thiazides decrease the renal excretion of Ca^{2+}. This is a result of a direct action on the early distal tubule (Stier and Itskovitz, 1986). The excretion of Mg^{2+} is enhanced by the thiazides, leading to hypomagnesemia.

Iodide and bromide are excreted by renal mechanisms qualitatively similar to those for chloride. Thus, all chloruretic agents may be useful in the management of bromide intoxication. In addition, increased excretion of iodide, particularly with prolonged diuretic therapy, may produce slight iodine depletion.

Effect on Composition of Extracellular Fluid. The thiazides tend to produce less distortion of the composition of the extracellular fluid than do other diuretic agents. This is in part the result of the relatively modest intensity of diuresis produced by these drugs.

Absorption, Fate, and Distribution. Chlorothiazide is poorly absorbed from the gastrointestinal tract, to the extent of about 10%. The other drugs in this class that have been studied have much greater bioavailability (*see* Appendix II). Bile acid–binding resins (colestipol and cholestyramine) may impair absorption of the thiazides. Most thiazides cause a demonstrable diuretic effect within an hour after oral administration. However, the persistence of the drugs in the body varies greatly; for example, the half-life of chlorothiazide in plasma is 1.5 hours, while that for chlorthalidone is 44 hours. The durations of diuretic action of the thiazides and related agents are summarized in Table 28–2. Differences are due to variation in rates of renal tubular secretion and clearance, metabolism, and enterohepatic circulation. The range of volumes of distribution is also great. Several of the drugs in this class are known to be highly concentrated in erythrocytes, probably as a result of binding to carbonic anhydrase. Binding to plasma proteins varies considerably among these agents; there is no correlation of this factor with half-life.

Table 28–2. SUMMARY OF CHEMICAL STRUCTURES AND DIURETIC PROPERTIES OF THE BENZOTHIADIAZIDES AND RELATED AGENTS *

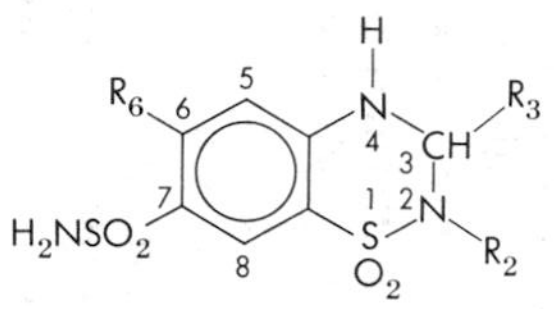

Agent †	R_2	R_3	R_6	RANGE OF OPTIMALLY EFFECTIVE ORAL DIURETIC DOSE IN MAN	RELATIVE ORAL NATRIURETIC MAXIMAL RESPONSE IN MAN	EQUIEFFECTIVE CHLORURETIC I.V. DOSE IN THE DOG	CARBONIC ANHYDRASE 50% INHIBITION IN VITRO	DURATION OF ACTION
				mg/day		*mg/kg*	*M*	*Hours*
Chlorothiazide ‡	H	H	Cl	500–2000	1	1.25	2×10^{-6}	6–12
Hydrochlorothiazide	H	H	Cl	25–100	1.8	0.05	2×10^{-5}	6–12
Hydroflumethiazide	H	H	CF_3	25–200	1.6	0.25	2×10^{-4}	6–12
Bendroflumethiazide	H	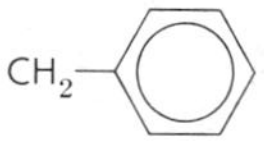	CF_3	2.5–15	2.3	0.01	3×10^{-4}	6–12
Benzthiazide ‡	H	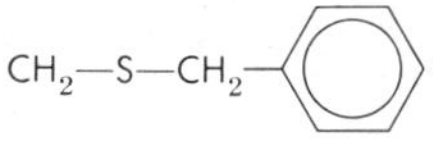	Cl	50–150	1.6	0.01–0.05	*ca.* 10^{-7}	6–12
Trichlormethiazide	H	$CHCl_2$	Cl	1–4	2.1	0.01	6×10^{-5}	24
Methyclothiazide	CH_3	CH_2Cl	Cl	2.5–10	2.3	——	——	24
Polythiazide	CH_3	$CH_2SCH_2CF_3$	Cl	1–4	2.5	0.01–0.03	5×10^{-7}	24–48
Cyclothiazide	H	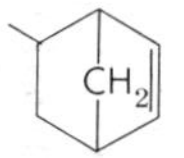	Cl	1–2	——	——	——	18–24
Chlorthalidone	——	——	——	25–100	2.3	0.25	3×10^{-7}	24–72
Quinethazone	——	——	——	50–100	1	——	——	18–24
Metolazone	——	——	——	2.5–20	1	0.1	5×10^{-5}	12–24
Acetazolamide	——	——	——	250–375	0.3	——	7×10^{-8}	——
Indapamide	——	——	——	2.5–5	1	0.3	——	24–36

* Note the general agreement between the optimal oral dosage for man relative to the equieffective dosage by intravenous administration in the dog. The relative oral natriuretic response in man is based on the method of Ford (1961), who used careful metabolic regimens and doses in the general range indicated. The numerical values refer to potency ratios, with the natriuretic response to a standard dose of chlorothiazide being given the value of 1. Despite the extremely wide range of effective oral dosage, the usual natriuretic response by this assay varies less than threefold.

† The above-listed agents are available under the following nonproprietary and selected trade names: Chlorothiazide: DIURIL. Hydrochlorothiazide: HYDRODIURIL. Hydroflumethiazide: SALURON. Bendroflumethiazide: NATURETIN. Benzthiazide: EXNA. Trichlormethiazide: METAHYDRIN. Methyclothiazide: ENDURON. Polythiazide: RENESE. Cyclothiazide: ANHYDRON. Chlorthalidone: HYGROTON. Quinethazone: HYDROMOX. Metolazone: DIULO. Acetazolamide: DIAMOX. Indapamide: LOZOL.

‡ Unsaturated between C 3 and N 4.

Clinical Toxicity. In animals the demonstrable toxic dose of all the thiazides is many times that required for their pharmacological action. For example, large short-term doses can depress CNS function. Clinical toxicity is relatively rare and usually results from unexpected hypersensitivity. Cases of purpura, dermatitis with photosensitivity, depression of the formed elements of the blood, acute pancreatitis, and necrotizing vasculitis have been reported.

Diuretic-induced hypokalemia is discussed in Chapter 27 along with the indications for K^+ supplementation. Alternatively, the thiazides have been prescribed in combination with a K^+-sparing diuretic (*see* below) in order to obtain an additive diuretic effect with maintenance of K^+ balance. The plasma uric acid is frequently elevated. For reasons that are unexplained, prolonged therapy with thiazides on rare occasions gives rise to hypercalcemia and hypophosphatemia that simulate hyperparathyroidism.

Borderline renal and/or hepatic insufficiency may be unpredictably aggravated by the thiazides. In patients, particularly those with hypertensive disease and decreased renal reserve, the manifestations of renal insufficiency may be aggravated after intensive or prolonged courses of thiazides that lead to excessive depletion of fluid and electrolytes. In patients with cirrhosis of the liver, deterioration of mental function, including the onset of coma, has been attributed to thiazide therapy. Many observers have noted a correlation with hypokalemia and alkalosis. Increased concentrations of ammonia in the blood have been reported. Cholestatic hepatitis has also been observed.

The thiazides may induce hyperglycemia and aggravate preexisting diabetes mellitus; the pharmacological effect of the oral hypoglycemic agents may also be reduced. Three apparently relevant factors have been identified in the rat: diminished insulin secretion in response to elevation of plasma glucose, enhanced glycogenolysis, and diminished glycogenesis (Hoskins and Jackson, 1978). Clinical studies indicate that depletion of K^+ has a role in glucose intolerance, probably by inhibition of insulin secretion (Tannen, 1985). Thiazides cause increases in the concentrations of cholesterol and triglycerides in plasma by unknown mechanisms. It is not known if this effect enhances the risk of atherosclerosis (Ames, 1986).

Preparations and Dosage. The thiazides are available as tablets for oral administration. The wide range of dosage is indicated in Table 28–2. A preparation of the sodium salt of chlorothiazide is available for intravenous administration when that route is required.

The shorter-acting thiazides are often given in divided daily doses. The longer-acting compounds have a duration of action of 24 hours or more and need be given only once daily (*see* Table 28–2). A single daily dose is often preferable to improve patient compliance with a regimen of antihypertensive therapy. Fixed-dose preparations of a thiazide with an aldosterone antagonist or other K^+-sparing diuretic are available and can be employed to advantage when the maintenance of K^+ balance presents a problem (*see* below).

Therapeutic Uses. The thiazides are the diuretics of choice in the management of edema due to mild-to-moderate congestive heart failure. Edema due to chronic hepatic or renal disease may also respond favorably. The use of the thiazides to treat hypertensive disease is discussed in Chapter 33. Less common usage includes the treatment of diabetes insipidus (*see* Chapter 29) and the management of hypercalciuria in patients who have recurrent urinary calculi composed of calcium salts (Sutton, 1985; Stier and Itskovitz, 1986).

HIGH-CEILING DIURETICS

The term *high-ceiling* has been used to denote a group of diuretics that have a distinctive action on renal tubular function. The peak diuresis is far greater than that observed with other agents. The main site of action is the thick ascending limb of the loop of Henle. The agents are thus often called *loop diuretics*. Three drugs of this class are in clinical use in the United States: ethacrynic acid, furosemide, and bumetanide. There are a number of other such compounds, some of which are in clinical use in other countries (Greger and Wangemann, 1987).

Chemistry and Structure–Activity Relationship. The agents available in the United States have the following structures:

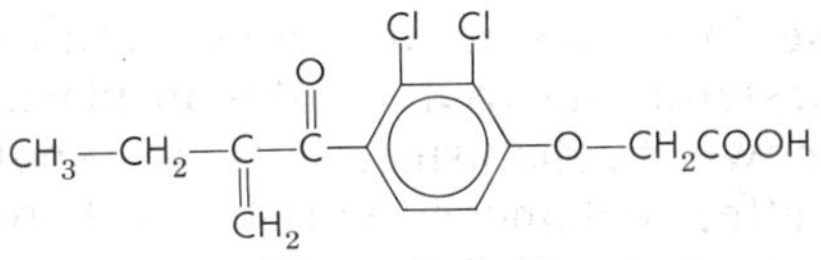

Ethacrynic Acid

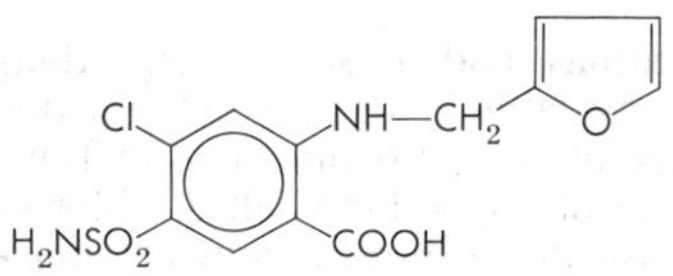

Furosemide

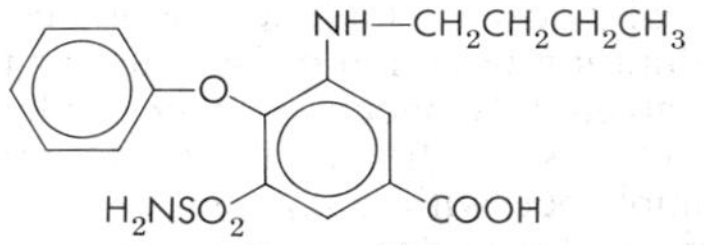

Bumetanide

These drugs share few structural features, and they constitute a pharmacological rather than a chemical class. Ethacrynic acid contains an α,β-unsaturated ketone moiety, which confers on it a high degree of reactivity toward sulfhydryl groups. It was synthesized in an attempt to mimic the sulfhydryl reactivity of the mercurial diuretics. It is clear from the other structures shown above that this is not a prerequisite for diuretic activity. However, it remains unsettled whether such reactivity is crucial for the action of ethacrynic acid. Furosemide is a derivative of anthranilic acid. Bumetanide is a 3-aminobenzoic acid derivative. It has a higher milligram potency than furosemide, but in other respects the compounds are similar.

Mechanism of Diuretic Action. In general, the time of onset and the duration of diuresis achieved with the agents in this class are shorter than those with the thiazides. The brevity of action is determined in large part by pharmacokinetic factors; the intensity of diuresis also calls compensatory mechanisms into play.

The high-ceiling diuretics act primarily to inhibit electrolyte reabsorption in the thick ascending limb of the loop of Henle. There are two major lines of evidence for this contention. First, micropuncture experiments demonstrate a greatly enhanced delivery of Na^+ and Cl^- to the beginning of the distal tubule. Second, in microperfusion experiments *in vitro* there is complete inhibition of sodium chloride transport in the thick ascending limb at luminal concentrations of drug in the range expected to occur *in vivo*. The drugs act at the luminal face of the epithelial cells to inhibit the Na^+–K^+–$2Cl^-$ cotransport mechanism (*see* Figure VI–1; Greger and Wangemann, 1987).

These agents tend to increase renal blood flow without increasing filtration rate, especially after intravenous injection. Such a change in renal hemodynamics reduces fluid and electrolyte reabsorption in the proximal tubule and may augment the initial diuretic response (*see* below). The increase in renal blood flow is relatively short lived. With the reduction of extracellular fluid volume that is induced by diuresis, there is a tendency for renal blood flow to decrease; this sets the stage for increased reabsorption from the proximal tubule. The latter phenomenon may be thought of as a compensatory mechanism that limits delivery of solute to the thick ascending limb, thereby diminishing the diuresis. The question of a minor direct action of high-ceiling diuretics on the proximal tubule remains controversial. Both furosemide and bumetanide are inhibitors of carbonic anhydrase (both are sulfonamides), but these activities are too weak to contribute to a proximal diuresis except when massive doses are employed. Ethacrynic acid is not a carbonic anhydrase inhibitor. Actions of high-ceiling diuretics in segments distal to the thick ascending limb have not been firmly established. However, the magnitude of the diuresis engendered by these drugs suggests that there may be multiple secondary sites of action (*see* Table 28–1).

The increase in K^+ excretion and the elevation in the concentration of uric acid in plasma are reminiscent of similar phenomena encountered with the thiazide diuretics; they probably result from the same mechanisms as those discussed for the thiazides.

Diuretics of this class enhance the excretion of both Ca^{2+} and Mg^{2+} to an extent approximately proportional to the increase in Na^+ excretion. Unlike the thiazides, high-ceiling diuretics do not increase Ca^{2+} reabsorption in the distal tubule. The calciuric action of these agents is the basis for their use in symptomatic hypercalcemia (Sutton, 1985).

High-ceiling diuretics increase the excretion of titratable acid and ammonia. This phenomenon, which is thought to be due to effects on the distal nephron, is one of the factors in the genesis and maintenance of diuretic-induced metabolic alkalosis (Bosch *et al.,* 1977).

Hemodynamic Actions. The ability of high-ceiling diuretics to enhance renal blood flow has already been mentioned. However, this effect is not always obtained. Depending on the experimental conditions, including the dose and rate of administration of the diuretic, either an increase or decrease in renal blood flow may occur. These changes are of interest, since they indicate that the renal actions are more complicated than simply an increase in the excretion of solute. When furosemide increases renal blood flow, there is a redistribution of flow from medulla to cortex and within the cortex. Acute diuresis increases intraluminal pressure and transiently reduces the filtration rate (Mudge *et al.,* 1975). This raises the possibility that diuretic-induced redistribution of blood flow might be directly mediated by changes in pressure. However, many studies have indicated a more complicated mechanism that involves both prostaglandins and renin. The renal secretion of these substances is increased by the high-ceiling diuretics. Stimulation of renin release results from both the effect of vascular dilatation on the juxtaglomerular apparatus and that of reduced reabsorption of sodium chloride in the region of the macula densa. Indomethacin, in doses adequate to inhibit the synthesis of prostaglandins, blocks the increase in renal blood flow and the increased secretion of prostaglandins and renin produced by furosemide. Although the effect is relatively small, it is clear that treatment with indomethacin blunts the natriuretic response to furosemide and that this is not mediated by a pharmacokinetic interaction (Brater, 1985).

In patients with pulmonary edema high-ceiling diuretics increase systemic venous capacitance, thereby decreasing left ventricular filling pressure. This is a short-term action, and it can be of benefit before the onset of diuresis (Dikshit *et al.,* 1973). This effect is inhibited by indomethacin.

Extrarenal Sites of Action. In isolated systems and with high doses, these agents act on electrolyte transport in a variety of tissues. Most of these actions have no known clinical implications. An exception is the action on the inner ear, consisting of a depression of the cochlear microphonic and neural potentials, and a transient increase in the Na^+ and K^+ concentrations in the endolymph. This may result from a direct toxic action on the hair cells (Rybak, 1982, 1988).

Effect on Composition of Extracellular Fluid. Metabolic alkalosis may result from the use of the high-ceiling diuretics. When the mobilization of edema fluid is rapid, the alkalosis largely results from a contraction of extracellular fluid volume. With long-term therapy, the dietary intake of salt and the urinary excretion of H^+ and K^+ become important factors. This is discussed in Chapter 27. Alkalosis is frequently accompanied by hyponatremia, but each is produced by a separate mechanism.

Absorption, Distribution, and Excretion. The high-ceiling diuretics are readily absorbed from the gastrointestinal tract, although to variable degrees. For example, the bioavailability of furosemide is about 60%, while that of bumetanide is nearly 100%. Ethacrynic acid, furosemide, and bumetanide are extensively bound to plasma proteins, but they are rapidly secreted by the organic acid transport system of the proximal tubule. In this manner they gain access to the tubular fluid and eventually to their site of action more distally. Furosemide has been particularly well studied in this context. Probenecid inhibits the secretion of furosemide into the tubular urine, and the dose–response curve for furosemide is shifted to the right when expressed in terms of the concentration of the diuretic in plasma (Figure 28–1). When the response is plotted as a function of the rate of excretion of furosemide, it is unchanged. Thus, the interaction between these two compounds occurs at the level of tubular secretion and not at the site of action of the diuretic. There is a complex interplay of several factors, including duration of action, that determines the extent to which inhibition of secretion influences the overall diuretic response (Brater, 1983).

About two thirds of an intravenous dose of ethacrynic acid is excreted by the kidneys, the remainder by the liver. The major urinary products are the unchanged drug and conjugates with sulfhydryl compounds, mainly cysteine and N-acetylcysteine. A large fraction of furosemide is excreted as such and a lesser fraction as a glucuronide. About half of bumetanide is excreted unchanged in the urine; metabolites are also observed. The half-lives of all of these diuretics are short (1 to 2 hours); each has a duration of action in the range of 3 to 6 hours.

Clinical Toxicity. Two generalizations may be made from extensive experience with ethacrynic acid and furosemide: ab-

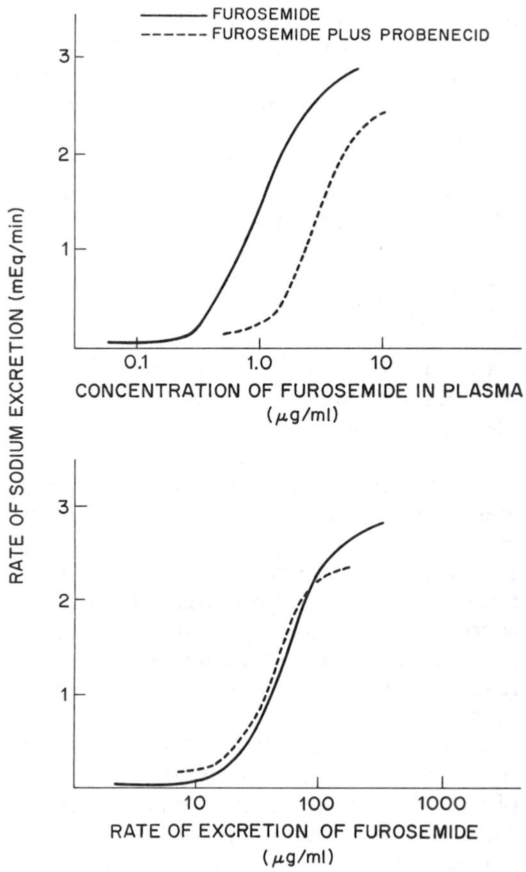

Figure 28–1. *The effect of probenecid on diuretic response curves for furosemide in human subjects.*

The upper panel depicts response as a function of the concentration of furosemide in plasma, while the lower panel is expressed as a function of the rate of excretion of furosemide. Probenecid inhibits the secretion of furosemide, such that at any concentration of furosemide in plasma the quantity of furosemide delivered to its site of action is diminished. This phenomenon accounts for the shift in the concentration-response curve (upper panel). On the other hand, probenecid does not directly interfere with the action of furosemide. Consequently, the curves in the lower panel are virtually superimposable. (Modified from Brater, 1983.)

normalities of fluid and electrolyte imbalance are the most common forms of clinical toxicity (*see* discussion at end of this chapter), and side effects unrelated to the primary action of these drugs are quite rare. Hyperuricemia is relatively common, but in most patients it represents little more than a chemical abnormality. Other reactions include gastrointestinal disturbances (with or without bleeding), depression of formed elements in the blood, skin rashes, paresthesias, and hepatic dysfunction. Cross-sensitivity may occur between furosemide and other sulfonamides. Gastrointestinal side effects are much more frequent with ethacrynic acid than furosemide. Furosemide and the thiazides have been implicated as causes of allergic interstitial nephritis, leading to reversible renal failure. A decrease in tolerance to carbohydrate may occur, but to a lesser extent than with the thiazides. Acute hypoglycemia of unexplained origin has been reported as a manifestation of overdosage. Because of their effect on offspring in experimental animals, the high-ceiling diuretics should not be prescribed during pregnancy unless absolutely necessary.

The development of deafness, either transient or permanent, is a serious and rare complication of treatment with ethacrynic acid. Transient deafness has also been reported with furosemide. Drug-induced changes in the electrolyte composition of the endolymph represent a possible mechanism (Rybak, 1982). From available data, it appears that ototoxicity from diuretics is unique to this class of drugs. If another potentially ototoxic drug, such as an aminoglycoside antibiotic, is being administered and concurrent diuretic therapy is indicated, it is advisable to use a diuretic agent from another class, for example, a thiazide.

The high-ceiling diuretics may interact adversely with other drugs. Ethacrynic acid and furosemide are significantly bound to plasma albumin and may compete for sites on the protein with drugs such as warfarin and clofibrate. The renal clearance of Li^+ is decreased during long-term therapy with diuretics (when there is depletion of Na^+), and concurrent use should be avoided unless concentrations of Li^+ in plasma can be monitored very carefully. The nephrotoxicity produced by cephaloridine is increased by furosemide, and one should be judicious in the use of any cephalosporin in conjunction with furosemide or ethacrynic acid.

Preparations. *Ethacrynic acid* (EDECRIN) is available for oral use as 25- and 50-mg tablets. The usual dose for adults is from 50 to 200 mg per day. The optimal dose should be determined for each patient, starting with minimal amounts. The sodium salt of ethacrynic acid is available for intravenous use; the usual dose is 50 mg or 0.5 to 1 mg/kg.

Furosemide (LASIX, others) is available as 20-, 40-, and 80-mg tablets and in oral solutions. In adults, the usual initial dosage ranges from 20 to 80 mg daily. If the initial dose is ineffective, it may be increased at 6-hour intervals until a response is obtained. The effective dose is then administered one to three times daily, depending on the desired response. Most patients will require less than 600 mg of furosemide per day. The usual pediatric dose is 2 mg/kg, which may be titrated up to 6 mg/kg. A preparation is also available for parenteral administration, either intravenously or intramuscularly. The recommended adult dose by this route is 20 or 40 mg. If the response is inadequate, the dose can be increased after not less than 2 hours. Once the desired effect is obtained, the dose should be given once or twice daily to control edema. The usual pediatric dose is 1 mg/kg, which may be titrated to a maximum of 6 mg/kg.

Bumetanide (BUMEX) is available for oral use as 0.5-, 1.0-, and 2.0-mg tablets. The usual dose for adults ranges from 0.5 to 2.0 mg, generally given once daily. A second or third dose may be given at 4- to 5-hour intervals up to a maximum of 10 mg daily. Alternate-day therapy or intermittent dosing for 3 to 4 days followed by 1- to 2-day rest periods may be the safest and most effective method for continued control of edema. In patients with hepatic failure, the dosage should be kept to a minimum and adjusted very carefully. Bumetanide is also available for parenteral administration. The usual initial dose is 0.5 to 1.0 mg, intravenously or intramuscularly. A second or third dose may be given at 2- to 3-hour intervals, up to a maximum of 10 mg daily.

Therapeutic Uses. Due to the lower incidence of gastrointestinal reactions and a less precipitous dose–response curve, furosemide and bumetanide are prescribed much more frequently than is ethacrynic acid. The high-ceiling diuretics are effective for the treatment of edema of cardiac, hepatic, or renal origin. The oral route should be used unless impractical or the clinical situation demands a very prompt diuresis, in which case intravenous or intramuscular administration may be employed. This applies particularly to the management of acute pulmonary edema. In this condition the favorable hemodynamic changes and the rapid reduction of the volume of extracellular fluid are of sufficient magnitude to reduce venous return and pulmonary congestion. In the management of refractory edema, the high-ceiling agents may be used in conjunction with other types of diuretics, such as a thiazide or a K^+-sparing drug, but there is no rationale for administering two high-ceiling agents concomitantly.

In the presence of nephrosis or chronic renal failure, doses of furosemide far higher than usual may be required. The reason for this is not well established. It has been suggested that the high protein content in the tubular fluid of patients with the nephrotic syndrome inhibits diuresis by binding the diuretic. In addition, patients with uremia have a decreased rate of tubular secretion of furosemide (Brater, 1985). Furosemide is metabolized to a reactive intermediate that produces hepatic necrosis in experimental animals. At the usual clinical dose hepatic toxicity is not observed, but the possible occurrence of this undesirable effect should be kept in mind when the massive doses sometimes employed in renal failure must be given. The high-ceiling diuretics have also been used in patients with early acute renal failure, but results are inconclusive. The drugs are contraindicated once anuric renal failure is unequivocally established. In symptomatic hypercalcemia, the high-ceiling diuretics may lower the concentration of Ca^{2+} in plasma by increasing its urinary excretion. When employed for this purpose, the replacement of urinary losses of Na^+ and Cl^- is required (Sutton, 1985).

ALDOSTERONE ANTAGONISTS

The role of adrenocorticosteroids in the regulation of electrolyte and water balance is discussed in Chapter 60. With insight into the chemistry of the steroids and with more complete knowledge of their physiological function, it has been possible to synthesize competitive antagonists that are useful as diuretics.

SPIRONOLACTONE

Chemistry. A number of 17-spirolactone steroids have been employed, of which spironolactone appears to have the greatest selectivity and efficacy. Its structural formula is as follows:

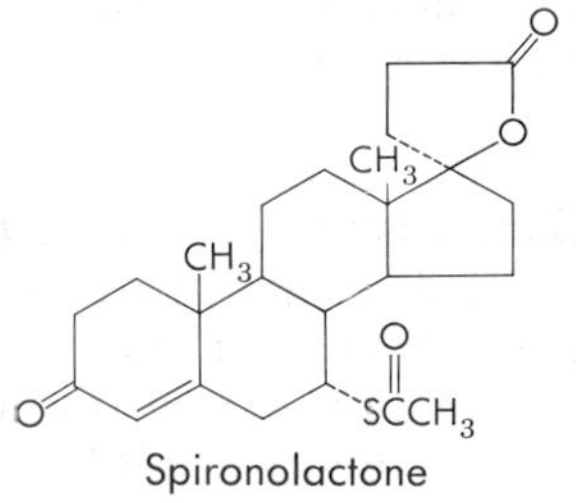

Spironolactone

Mechanism of Diuretic Action. Compounds of this type are competitive antagonists of the actions of mineralocorticoids, of which aldosterone is the most potent naturally occurring compound. The mineralocorticoid receptor is a soluble, cytoplasmic protein that is presumed to exist in active and inactive allosteric conformations (*see* Chapter 60). Spironolactone binds to the receptor and is thought to prevent it from assuming the active conformation. As a consequence, the entire chain of biochemical events that leads to the synthesis of physiologically active transport proteins is aborted (Horisberger and Giebisch, 1987).

Aldosterone receptors are present in several tissues, including the salivary glands, colon, and several segments of the nephron. In the present context, the most important target cells are those of the late distal tubule and collecting system. The overall action of aldosterone is to enhance reabsorption of Na^+ and secretion of K^+. Implicit in the foregoing description of mechanism are two phenomena that are amply supported by experimental evidence: first, spironolactone is effective only in the presence of either endogenous or exogenous aldosterone; second, the action of the antagonist may be overcome by increasing the concentration of aldosterone (Horisberger and Giebisch, 1987).

Under controlled conditions the urinary $Na^+:K^+$ ratio serves as an indirect index of aldosterone activity. The ratio can be greatly increased in response to the administration of spironolactone. Spironolactone also increases Ca^{2+} excretion through a direct effect on tubular transport (Stier and Itskovitz, 1986).

At relatively high concentrations, spironolactone can inhibit the biosynthesis of aldosterone. Theoretically, such an action could result in diuretic activity. However, it is unlikely that this action occurs at therapeutic concentrations.

Absorption, Distribution, and Excretion. About 70% of an oral dose of spironolactone is absorbed. The compound is metabolized to a significant extent during its first passage through the liver, and there is considerable enterohepatic circulation. Binding to plasma proteins is extensive. Virtually no unmetabolized drug appears in the urine.

Canrenone is a major metabolite of spironolactone, and it can be interconverted enzymatically with its hydrolytic product, canrenoate. Their structures are as follows:

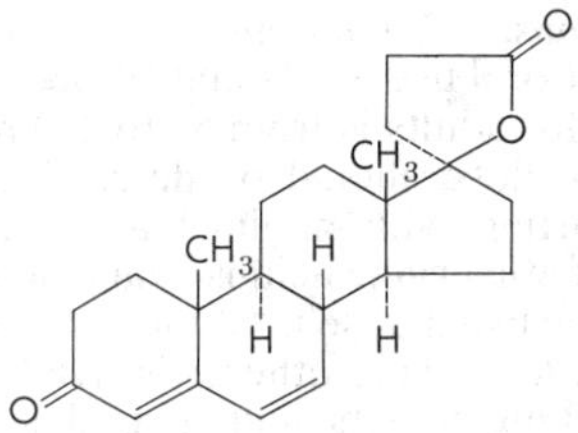

Canrenone

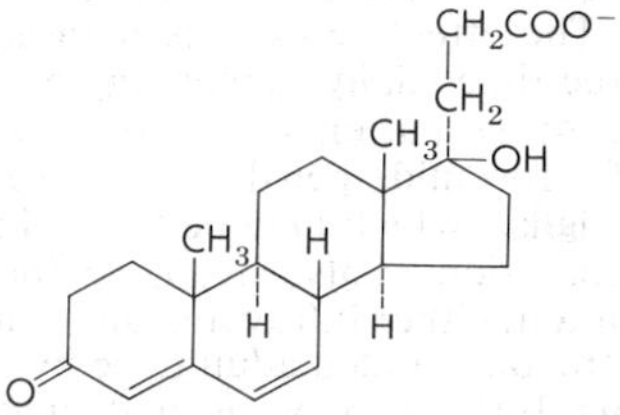

Canrenoate

Canrenone is an active aldosterone antagonist, and its formation contributes to, but does not account fully for, the biological activity of spironolactone. Canrenoate has no intrinsic activity, but it can exert biological effects by virtue of its interconversion with canrenone. Salicylates may interfere with the tubular secretion of canrenone and thereby decrease the effectiveness of spironolactone. The potassium salt of canrenoate is a water-soluble substance that can be administered parenterally. Both canrenone and potassium canrenoate are used clinically in some countries, but they are not available in the United States (Corvol *et al.*, 1981).

Clinical Toxicity. The most serious toxic effects of spironolactone result from hyperkalemia. Although hyperkalemia is almost certain to occur when the drug is injudiciously administered in conjunction with a high intake of K^+, it may also happen even when ordinary doses are given simultaneously with a thiazide to patients with severe renal insufficiency. A number of minor reactions have also been reported that are usually reversible when the drug is discontinued. Of these, the most common are gynecomastia, androgen-like side effects, and minor gastrointestinal symptoms. Spironolactone has been shown to be tumorigenic when administered for long periods to rats in high doses.

Preparations and Dosage. *Spironolactone* (ALDACTONE) is available in 25-, 50-, and 100-mg oral tablets. It is effective in an initial daily dose of 100 mg, given in single or divided doses. The dose may range from 25 to 200 mg daily in adults. Dosage in children should be initiated at 3.3 mg/kg per day. Spironolactone may also be given in doses of 400 mg per day as a diagnostic test for primary hyperaldosteronism and in doses of 100 to 400 mg daily in preparation for surgery after such a diagnosis. A fixed-dose combination of either 25 or 50 mg of both hydrochlorothiazide and spironolactone is also available (ALDACTAZIDE, others). Dosage should be determined by titration of the individual agents.

Therapeutic Uses. The aldosterone antagonists are widely used in the treatment of hypertension and in the management of refractory edema. Frequently, they are employed in conjunction with other diuretic agents to prevent excessive loss of K^+. The efficacy of such combinations has been substantiated by clinical experience in the treatment of congestive heart failure, cirrhosis of the liver, and the nephrotic syndrome. However, the quantitative effects are not exactly predictable, due to the complex interactions of the primary disease, the degree of secondary hyperaldosteronism, and the actions of the diuretics given concomitantly.

Competitive aldosterone antagonists, as well as other K^+-retaining agents, are also useful in both the diagnosis and the management of those rare metabolic and renal diseases associated with hypokalemia and K^+ depletion (*see* Liddle, 1966).

OTHER POTASSIUM-SPARING DIURETICS

The two drugs of this class that are in clinical use are triamterene and amiloride. Their actions are independent of those of the mineralocorticoids. Both drugs possess moderate natriuretic activity, sufficient for the maintenance of some patients. However, they are used most frequently for their effects on K^+ excretion.

Chemistry. Both triamterene and amiloride are organic bases. They have the following structures:

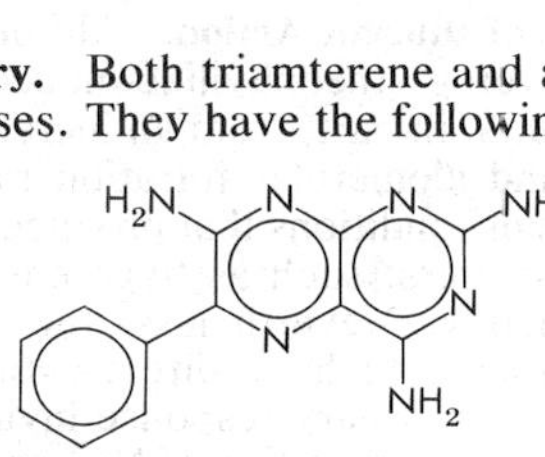

Triamterene

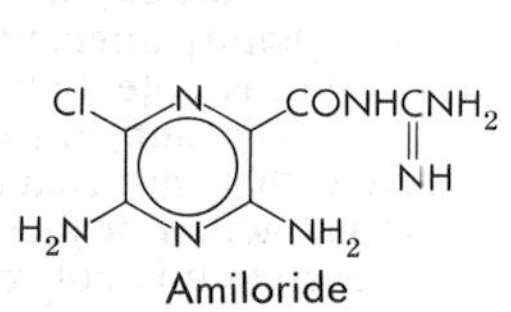

Amiloride

Triamterene is a pteridine with structural resemblance to folic acid and some of the inhibitors of dihydrofolate reductase. It is a weak inhibitor of the enzyme *in vivo*. Amiloride is a pyrazinoylguanidine.

Mechanism of Diuretic Action. Although triamterene is the older of the two drugs in this therapeutic class, amiloride has been studied more thoroughly. This is in large part attributable to the fact that amiloride is much more soluble in aqueous solution. To the extent that comparable studies are available, the drugs seem to have identical actions.

These agents interfere with transport in the late segments of the nephron. They induce a modest increase in the excretion of Na^+, mostly accompanied by chloride as the anion (*see* Table 28–1). Under ordinary circumstances there is little change in the excretion of K^+, although sometimes there is a slight increase. However, when excretion of K^+ is high because of increased intake, administration of another diuretic, or an excess of mineralocorticoid, these drugs cause a sharp decrease in its excretion. In many respects these effects resemble those of spironolactone, but it is quite clear that these drugs are not aldosterone antagonists. Their primary action is to inhibit the electrogenic entry of sodium (*see* Figure VI–1, *5–A*). This mechanism for permeation of Na^+ is quite widespread, and amiloride has been particularly useful in studies of Na^+ transport in a wide variety of systems (Benos, 1982). In some of these, amiloride acts as a competitive inhibitor of Na^+ transport; in others, the inhibition does not conform to competitive kinetics. This issue is not settled for the mammalian nephron.

Because of the interruption of electrogenic Na^+ transport by these agents, the electrical potential across the tubular epithelium falls. The reduction or elimination of this potential, which is one of the driving forces for secretion of K^+, is probably the basis of the K^+-sparing effect (Horisberger and Giebisch, 1987). The K^+-sparing diuretics may also cause slight alkalinization of the urine, which is attributable to inhibition of proton secretion in the distal nephron. These compounds are not inhibitors of carbonic anhydrase. Amiloride is an inhibitor of the Na^+–H^+ exchange mechanism of the proximal tubule and of the Na^+,K^+–ATPase. These latter actions require much higher concentrations of the drug than can be achieved *in vivo*. Amiloride decreases excretion of Ca^{2+}, an action that is additive to that of chlorothiazide (Sutton, 1985; Stier and Itskovitz, 1986).

Absorption, Distribution, and Excretion. Amiloride and triamterene are available only for oral use. About 50% of an oral dose of each agent is absorbed. Triamterene is about 60% bound to plasma proteins; amiloride is bound to a lesser extent. Both drugs have apparent volumes of distribution that are greater than body water (*see* Appendix II). Amiloride is not metabolized. The metabolism of triamterene is very extensive, and some of the metabolites have diuretic activity. Both drugs are secreted in the proximal tubule, presumably by the organic cation secretory mechanism.

Clinical Toxicity. The most serious toxic effect is hyperkalemia, which is a direct consequence of the major action of the drugs. Triamterene produces relatively few other side effects. The most common are nausea, vomiting, leg cramps, and dizziness. Slight-to-moderate azotemia is relatively common. This does not appear to be directly related to electrolyte and water imbalance and is reversible. Megaloblastic anemia has been reported in patients with alcoholic cirrhosis, presumably due to inhibition of dihydrofolate reductase in patients with reduced stores and intake of folic acid. Some patients receiving triamterene (about 1 in 1500) have developed nephrolithiasis, with high concentrations of triamterene and its metabolites in the stone.

The most common side effects of amiloride, aside from hyperkalemia, are nausea, vomiting, diarrhea, and headache.

Preparations. *Triamterene* (DYRENIUM) is administered only by the oral route. It is marketed in capsules containing 50 or 100 mg. The usual initial dose is 100 mg, given twice daily. The maximal daily dose is 300 mg. The maintenance dose should be determined for the individual patient and may be as low as 100 mg every other day. The fixed-dose combination of triamterene (50 mg) and hydrochlorothiazide (25 mg) (DYAZIDE) is available in capsules, one or two given twice daily. Other dosage forms of this combination are also available (MAXZIDE).

Amiloride hydrochloride (MIDAMOR) is available for oral use as 5-mg tablets. The usual dose is 5 to 10 mg per day. The maintenance dose should be determined for each patient individually. The fixed-dose combination of amiloride hydrochloride (5 mg) and hydrochlorothiazide (50 mg) (MODURETIC) is available in tablets. The usual dose is one or two tablets per day.

Therapeutic Uses. Some patients with *edema* have a satisfactory diuretic response to a K^+-sparing diuretic alone. However, the available clinical data suggest that the greatest usefulness of these drugs may be in conjunction with other diuretic agents. In general, the administration of a K^+-sparing diuretic with another natriuretic compound augments natriuresis and reduces loss of K^+. With concurrent drug therapy, it is this latter effect that is more consistently observed. Therefore, the rationale of concomitant drug therapy is primarily in relation to K^+ metabolism. Hansen and Bender (1967) summarized the experience obtained from several hundred patients maintained on long-term regimens with triamterene alone, hydrochlorothiazide alone, and both drugs together, and showed that both drugs together provided the highest incidence of normal values of K^+ in plasma. Because of the real possibility of inducing serious hyperkalemia, patients treated with a K^+-sparing diuretic should not receive supplements of K^+. Caution is also advised when these drugs are used concurrently with an inhibitor of angiotensin converting enzyme, since the latter drugs reduce the secretion of aldosterone. Similarly, triamterene or amiloride should not be prescribed with spironolactone; an unexpectedly high degree of hyperkalemia has occurred when this was done.

METHYLXANTHINES

The methylxanthines have long been known for their diuretic action. Their additional pharmacological properties are discussed in Chapter 25. Of the methylxanthines, theophylline has the greatest action on the kidney.

Mechanism of Diuretic Action. Although there is some controversy, theophylline-induced diuresis probably results, in part, from an increase in renal blood flow and glomerular filtration rate. This is most obvious in conditions that produce reductions in these parameters, such as hypotension or cardiac insufficiency. Nevertheless, the methylxanthines also appear to have direct actions on the renal tubule. The urinary response involves an increase in the rate of excretion of Na^+ and Cl^-, with no significant effect on urinary acidification. Diuretic action is only slightly affected by changes in acid–base balance but is potentiated by the coadministration of carbonic anhydrase inhibitors. It has been postulated that intracellular pH directly affects the intrarenal action of these agents. Augmentation of K^+ excretion is not remarkable. The renal actions of the methylxanthines appear to result, in part, from blockade of receptors for adenosine and reflect the participation of this autacoid in the regulation of renal function (Fredholm, 1984).

Clinical Application. The methylxanthines are rarely employed as primary diuretics. However, when used for other purposes, particularly as bronchodilators, the coexistence of their diuretic action should be kept in mind.

THE CLINICAL USE OF DIURETICS

Pathological Physiology of Edema Formation. In a healthy subject, changes in dietary intake or variations in the extrarenal loss of fluid and electrolytes are accompanied by fine adjustments in the rate of renal excretion. Edema can obviously result either from an abnormally high intake of water and electrolytes or from abnormally low rates of their excretion. When fluids are administered parenterally with excessive vigor, edema can certainly be produced. However, when cardiac and renal function are normal, the condition is short lived. In the usual edematous states, the underlying abnormality evokes a decreased rate of Na^+ excretion. The retention of this cation is accompanied by retention of extracellular anion and a proportional amount of water and, as a result, the increased volume of extracellular fluid is usually of normal composition and osmolality.

In many edematous states, increased rates of aldosterone secretion have been correlated with increased tubular reabsorption of Na^+. In addition, particularly in cardiac decompensation, the glomerular filtration rate may be reduced. However, quantitative studies, both in disease and under experimental conditions, have failed to provide a predictable relationship between the rate of Na^+ excretion and either the amount of Na^+ filtered or the concentration of aldosterone. For this reason, additional factors must be considered.

The atriopeptins or atrial natriuretic peptides are secreted by mammalian atria in response to stretch, as occurs when the extracellular fluid volume is increased. These peptides are derived from a precursor, atriopeptigen. The atriopeptins increase the excretion of Na^+ and water; they also relax vascular and intestinal smooth muscle (for review, *see* Cody *et al.*, 1987). The circulating concentrations of atriopeptins are elevated in patients with congestive heart failure, but their actions are overridden by factors that cause retention of Na^+.

There is some evidence for the existence of an endogenous substance (endoxin) that enhances the excretion of Na^+ by inhibiting the Na^+,K^+–ATPase. The nature of this material and its physiological importance are still obscure (Kelly, 1987).

Indications for the Use of Diuretics. When edema accumulates, three therapeutic approaches are available to mobilize the fluid and thereafter maintain the constancy of the extracellular fluid volume. The first is to correct the primary disease. This is, of course, the most desirable goal. The second is to suppress renal tubular reabsorptive capacity by the use of diuretics. The third is to reduce the intake of sodium salts.

Diuretics are usually the first drugs to be used in the management of congestive heart failure. Although they do not influence cardiac function directly, the diuretics reduce cardiac preload, pulmonary congestion, and edema. It may be possible to manage the mildest forms of cardiac failure with diuretics alone; however, most patients will ultimately require additional therapy with digitalis and/or vasodilators (*see* Chapters 31, 32, and 34).

The diuretics are extensively employed in the management of ascites, especially when associated with cirrhosis of the liver. Periodic administration either eliminates the necessity for or reduces the interval between paracenteses. Not only does a diuretic regimen contribute to the comfort of the patient, but also his meager protein reserves are spared inasmuch as significant amounts of protein are lost when ascitic fluid is mechanically withdrawn. With mild, asymptomatic, or residual ascites, no useful purpose is served in attempting to make the patient completely free of edema if this involves the persistent administration of diuretics and the production of hypovolemia or electrolyte imbalances.

As a general rule, chronic renal disease that causes edema may be treated in the same manner as other edematous states, with the recognition that these patients are more subject to electrolyte imbalance. In the presence of primary renal disease there is often a lesser effect of the diuretic on tubular function. In the case of the high-ceiling diuretics, particularly furosemide, an increased dose is required (Brater, 1985). The thiazides are relatively less effective and in high doses may decrease the glomerular filtration rate.

In the nephrotic syndrome, the response to diuretic agents is often disappointing. Although hypoproteinemia is a major pathogenic factor, the administration of albumin produces a minimal and unpredictable diuretic response. The important role of the corticosteroids in the management of the nephrotic syndrome is discussed in Chapter 60.

In incipient acute renal failure, diuretics have been used in the hope of diminishing further renal damage. Protection has been obtained in experimental models, and several intrarenal mechanisms may be involved. Unfortunately, such administration of diuretics has been of limited clinical utility (Tiller and Mudge, 1980).

Complications of Diuretic Therapy. With the availability of powerful diuretics, there has been an increased incidence of complications that may be directly attributed to the diuresis itself. It should be remembered that the goal of diuretic therapy is the mobilization of edema fluid in such a manner that the volume and composition of the extracellular fluid is restored toward normal. The excessively rapid mobilization of edema may lead to malaise and asthenia. Rapid changes in the pressure–flow relationships in the cardiovascular system may, even in the presence of an expanded extracellular fluid volume, give rise to symptoms usually associated with hypovolemia. In intensive long-term therapy, the diuretic-induced renal loss of sodium chloride may lead to extracellular fluid depletion, with or without hyponatremia. The condition usually responds to discontinuation of the diuretic agent and the liberalization of sodium chloride intake in the diet. Both these conditions are relatively rare.

A far more common condition, particularly in congestive heart failure and hepatic cirrhosis, is chronic dilutional hyponatremia. This is associated with persistent edema and expanded extracellular volume. It may occur solely as a result of the underlying disease, but is most often seen as a consequence of diuretic therapy, especially in patients who drink more than the usual quantities of fluids. The physiological defect is the inability to excrete an adequately dilute urine. This is attributed to an inadequate Na^+ load to the diluting segments of the nephron. Water restriction is the most direct therapeutic approach, but it may be complicated by uncontrollable thirst.

Severe hyponatremia with plasma Na^+ concentrations below 120 mM is a rare, life-threatening complication of diuretic therapy. Thus far it has been described only in patients receiving thiazides. The condition comes on rapidly, 2 to 12 days after therapy is initiated. Most patients afflicted by this complication are small, aged women. Excessive intake of water is believed to have a prominent role in the pathogenesis. It is not known if the excessive intake of water is spontaneous or an effect provoked by the drug (Friedman *et al.*, 1989).

The problems of diuretic-induced alkalosis and depletion of K^+ are discussed above and in Chapter 27. In addition, hyperkalemia may result if K^+-sparing diuretics are used injudiciously or if K^+ supplements are administered simultaneously.

Both extracellular and intracellular Mg^{2+} depletion may result from the use of diuretics. Since Mg^{2+} and K^+ deficits may interact, the problem is complex and warrants extensive evaluation (*see* Chapter 27). Depending on the type of diuretic employed, concentrations of Ca^{2+} in plasma may increase or decrease, as discussed above.

Refractory Edema. The increasing attention being given to so-called refractory edema is, in fact, partly attributable to the high degree of success in the management of the less severely ill patient. This has enabled many patients with cardiac decompensation to survive longer in an edema-free state. With the progression of the underlying disease, these patients consequently tend to become edematous at a time when their cardiac reserve is significantly more impaired than in the earlier years of their illness. With many drugs, diuretic efficacy is decreased by hyponatremia. Additional factors in drug refractoriness are the reduction in glomerular filtration rate and increased reabsorption of Na^+ in the proximal tubule, with consequent reduction of delivery of Na^+ to the portions of the nephron that are influenced by the diuretic.

When a patient becomes refractory to a diuretic, the entire regimen should be reevaluated. In some instances, adjustments of dosage may suffice. Bed rest itself may restore drug responsiveness, due to improvement in the renal circulation. Abnormalities of extracellular fluid composition should be sought and corrected. The administration of additional diuretics may be appropriate. As a general rule, patients who are refractory to a diuretic of moderate efficacy, such as the thiazides, will show a more satisfactory response to high-ceiling diuretics.

Use of Multiple Diuretics and Adjuvant Agents. The availability of many different types of diuretics and many different compounds of the same type has provided the temptation to alter the diuretic regimen at frequent intervals. In the initial management of the edematous subject, when mobilization of edema fluid is the primary goal of therapy, the changing status of the patient warrants appropriate adjustments in dosage schedules and also in the agents selected for use. However, in long-term management of edema, the best therapeutic results are often obtained with a purposefully constant therapeutic regimen.

Despite the widespread use of high-ceiling diuretics for the treatment of chronic edema, especially of cardiac origin, one may properly raise the question of their overuse in situations in which other diuretics, although less effective by conventional standards, might equally well achieve the desired therapeutic goal with less risk of overtreatment.

In the severely edematous patient, it is becoming

apparent that, if a single diuretic agent proves ineffective, it is proper to use more than one type of diuretic agent. Of course, nothing is to be gained by the administration of two drugs of the same type, such as two different thiazides. Specific examples of rational concurrent therapy with diuretics include the combination of a K^+-sparing diuretic with a thiazide or a high-ceiling agent or the combination of a high-ceiling diuretic with a thiazide-like drug (*see* Wollam *et al.*, 1982).

Beyer, K. H. The mechanism of action of chlorothiazide. *Ann. N.Y. Acad. Sci.*, **1958**, *71*, 363–379.

Bosch, J. P.; Goldstein, M. H.; Levitt, M. F.; and Kahn, T. Effect of chronic furosemide administration on hydrogen and sodium excretion in the dog. *Am. J. Physiol.*, **1977**, *232*, F397–F404.

Breslau, N.; Moses, A. M.; and Weiner, I. M. The role of volume contraction in the hypocalciuric action of chlorothiazide. *Kidney Int.*, **1976**, *10*, 164–170.

Dikshit, K.; Vyden, J. K.; Forrester, J. S.; Chatterjee, K.; Prakash, R.; and Swan, H. J. C. Renal and extrarenal hemodynamic effects of furosemide in congestive heart failure after acute myocardial infarction. *N. Engl. J. Med.*, **1973**, *288*, 1087–1090.

Friedman, E.; Shadel, M.; Halkin, H.; and Farfel, Z. Thiazide-induced hyponatremia. Reproducibility by single dose rechallenge and an analysis of pathogenesis. *Ann. Intern. Med.*, **1989**, *110*, 24–30.

Griggs, R. C.; Engel, W. K.; and Resnick, J. S. Acetazolamide treatment of hypokalemic periodic paralysis. Prevention of attacks and improvement of persistent weakness. *Ann. Intern. Med.*, **1970**, *73*, 39–48.

Hansen, K. B., and Bender, A. D. Changes in serum potassium levels occurring in patients treated with triamterene and triamterene-hydrochlorothiazide combination. *Clin. Pharmacol. Ther.*, **1967**, *8*, 392–399.

Hoskins, B., and Jackson, C. M., III. The mechanism of chlorothiazide-induced carbohydrate intolerance. *J. Pharmacol. Exp. Ther.*, **1978**, *206*, 423–430.

Larson, E. B.; Roach, R. C.; Schoene, R. B.; and Hornbein, T. F. Acute mountain sickness and acetazolamide. *J.A.M.A.*, **1982**, *248*, 328–332.

Laux, B. E., and Raichle, M. E. The effect of acetazolamide on cerebral blood flow and oxygen utilization in the rhesus monkey. *J. Clin. Invest.*, **1978**, *62*, 585–592.

Maren, T. H. Relations between structure and biological activity of sulfonamides. *Annu. Rev. Pharmacol. Toxicol.*, **1976**, *16*, 309–327.

Mudge, G. H.; Cooke, W. J.; and Berndt, W. P. Electrolyte excretion and free-water production during onset of acute diuresis. *Am. J. Physiol.*, **1975**, *228*, 1304–1312.

Prockop, L. D. The pharmacology of increased intracranial pressure. In, *Clinical Neuropharmacology.* (Klawans, H. L., ed.) Raven Press, New York, **1976**, pp. 147–171.

Rybak, L. P. Ototoxicity of ethacrynic acid (a persistent clinical problem). *J. Laringol. Otol.*, **1988**, *102*, 518–520.

Tannen, R. L. Diuretic-induced hypokalemia. *Kidney Int.*, **1985**, *28*, 988–1000.

Wales, J. K.; Krees, S. V.; Grant, A. M.; Viktora, J. K.; and Wolff, F. W. Structure–activity relationships of benzothiadiazine compounds as hyperglycemic agents. *J. Pharmacol. Exp. Ther.*, **1968**, *164*, 421–432.

Wollam, G. L.; Tarazi, R. C.; Bravo, E. L.; and Dustan, H. P. Diuretic potency of combined hydrochlorothiazide and furosemide therapy in patients with azotemia. *Am. J. Med.*, **1982**, *72*, 929–938.

Monographs and Reviews

Ames, R. P. The effects of antihypertensive drugs on serum lipids and lipoproteins. I. Diuretics. *Drugs*, **1986**, *32*, 260–278.

Benos, D. J. Amiloride: a molecular probe of sodium transport in tissues and cells. *Am. J. Physiol.*, **1982**, *242*, C131–C145.

Brater, D. C. Pharmacodynamic considerations in the use of diuretics. *Annu. Rev. Pharmacol. Toxicol.*, **1983**, *23*, 45–62.

———. Resistance to loop diuretics. Why it happens and what to do about it. *Drugs*, **1985**, *30*, 427–443.

Cody, R. J.; Atlas, S. A.; and Laragh, J. H. Physiologic and pharmacologic studies of atrial natriuretic factor: a natriuretic and vasoactive peptide. *J. Clin. Pharmacol.*, **1987**, *27*, 927–936.

Corvol, P.; Claire, M.; Oblin, M. E.; Geering, K.; and Rossier, B. Mechanism of the antimineralocorticoid effects of spirolactones. *Kidney Int.*, **1981**, *20*, 1–6.

Fredholm, B. B. Cardiovascular and renal actions of methylxanthines. In, *The Methylxanthine Beverages and Foods: Chemistry, Consumption and Health Effects.* (Spiller, G. A., ed.) Alan R. Liss, Inc., New York, **1984**, pp. 303–330.

Greger, R., and Wangemann, P. Loop diuretics. *Renal Physiol.*, **1987**, *10*, 174–183.

Horisberger, J.-D., and Giebisch, G. Potassium-sparing diuretics. *Renal Physiol.*, **1987**, *10*, 198–220.

Kelly, R. A. Endogenous cardiac glycosidelike compounds. *Hypertension*, **1987**, *10*, 187–192.

Lang, F. Osmotic diuresis. *Renal Physiol.*, **1987**, *10*, 160–173.

Liddle, G. W. Aldosterone antagonists and triamterene. *Ann. N.Y. Acad. Sci.*, **1966**, *139*, 466–470.

Maren, T. H. Carbonic anhydrase: chemistry, physiology, and inhibition. *Physiol. Rev.*, **1967**, *47*, 595–781.

Preisig, P. A.; Toto, R. D.; and Alpern, R. J. Carbonic anhydrase inhibitors. *Renal Physiol.*, **1987**, *10*, 136–159.

Rybak, L. P. Pathophysiology of furosemide ototoxicity. *J. Otolaryngol.*, **1982**, *11*, 127–133.

Stier, C. T., Jr., and Itskovitz, H. D. Renal calcium metabolism. *Annu. Rev. Pharmacol. Toxicol.*, **1986**, *26*, 101–116.

Sutton, R. A. L. Diuretics and calcium metabolism. *Am. J. Kidney Dis.*, **1985**, *5*, 4–9.

Tiller, D. J., and Mudge, G. H. Pharmacologic agents used in the management of acute renal failure. *Kidney Int.*, **1980**, *18*, 700–711.

Velázquez, H. Thiazide diuretics. *Renal Physiol.*, **1987**, *10*, 184–197.

CHAPTER

29 AGENTS AFFECTING THE RENAL CONSERVATION OF WATER

Richard M. Hays

ANTIDIURETIC HORMONE

Evolutionary precursors of antidiuretic hormone (ADH) were present in the central nervous systems of early aquatic species, and they have a water-conserving function in fish. However, with the emergence of life on land ADH became the mediator of a remarkable regulatory system for the conservation of water. The hormone is released by the posterior pituitary under conditions of water deprivation (when plasma osmolality is elevated) or when extracellular volume is depleted (irrespective of the level of plasma osmolality). In amphibia, the target organs for ADH are skin and the urinary bladder; in other vertebrates, including man, the site of action is the renal collecting duct. In each of these target tissues, ADH acts by increasing the permeability of the cell membrane to water, thus permitting water to move passively down an osmotic gradient across skin, bladder, or collecting duct into the extracellular compartment.

In view of the long evolutionary history of the hormone, it is not surprising that ADH acts at sites in the nephron other than the collecting duct and on tissues other than the kidney. It is a potent vasopressor; indeed, the name *vasopressin* was originally chosen on the basis of its vasoconstrictor action. It is a neurotransmitter, and, among its actions in the central nervous system (CNS), it appears to have a role in the secretion of adrenocorticotropic hormone (ACTH) and in the regulation of circulation, temperature, and other visceral functions. ADH also promotes the release of coagulation factors by the vascular endothelium. These renal and nonrenal actions of ADH will be discussed in this chapter.

Chemistry. duVigneaud and coworkers (1954) determined the structures of ADH and oxytocin and accomplished the complete synthesis of each. This was an unprecedented achievement at a time when the synthesis of even small peptides required years of effort; duVigneaud was awarded the Nobel Prize in 1955. Studies in his laboratory established principles of the structure–activity relationship that underlie much of the current effort to design peptides for therapeutic purposes. The structures of 8-arginine vasopressin (the neurohypophyseal peptide found in all mammals except swine), 8-lysine vasopressin (*lypressin,* the swine peptide), and oxytocin (the oxytocic and milk-ejecting peptide, *see* Chapter 39) are shown in Table 29–1. All are nonapeptides with two cysteine residues forming a bridge between positions 1 and 6. Integrity of the disulfide bond is essential for biological activity, and amino acid substitutions dictate specific physiological actions. Thus, a basic amino acid residue in position 8 confers antidiuretic activity, while isoleucine in position 3 promotes oxytocic activity.

The development of techniques for solid-phase peptide synthesis made it possible to synthesize and screen great numbers of analogs of ADH, and, in 1967, Zaoral and coworkers announced the synthesis of 1-deamino-8-D-arginine vasopressin (dDAVP, *desmopressin*; Table 29–1), now the preferred drug for the treatment of ADH-sensitive diabetes insipidus (Zaoral *et al.*, 1967). Deamination at position 1 renders the molecule less subject to the action of peptidases. It is this resistance to degradation that is the most important factor in the superior antidiuretic activity of desmopressin, since the natural hormone is hydrolyzed rapidly *in vivo* by a variety of enzymes in kidney, liver, brain, and elsewhere. The substitution of D- for L-arginine in position 8 sharply decreases pressor activity and thus greatly increases the ratio of antidiuretic to pressor effects. Synthetic peptides that have selective pressor activity have also been designed; one example, 2-phenylalanine-8-lysine vasopressin (*felypressin*), is in use in Europe as a vasoconstrictor.

Recently, a series of potent and specific antagonists of the antidiuretic action of ADH has been synthesized (Manning *et al.*, 1987). Two examples (analogs 1 and 2) are shown in Table 29–1. The antagonists inhibit binding of ADH to its receptor and activation of adenylyl cyclase by ADH in membrane preparations from a number of species. However, one potential antagonist proved to be antidiu-

Table 29–1. CHEMICAL STRUCTURES AND ACTIVITIES OF NATIVE AND SYNTHETIC ANTIDIURETIC PEPTIDES

	ACTIVITY * (Relative to Arginine Vasopressin) *Antidiuretic*	*Pressor*
Native Peptides		
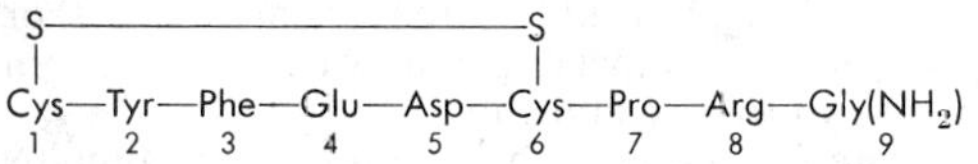 8-Arginine Vasopressin (ADH, AVP; mammals)	100	100
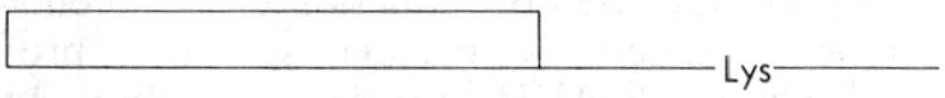 8-Lysine Vasopressin (lypressin, LVP; swine)	80	60
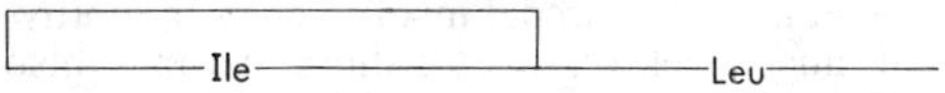 Oxytocin	1	1
Synthetic Antidiuretic Peptide		
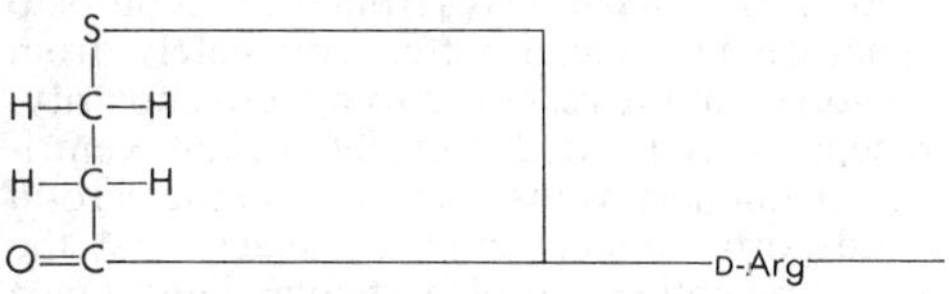 1-Deamino-8-D-Arginine Vasopressin (desmopressin, dDAVP)	1200	0.39
Synthetic ADH Antagonists		
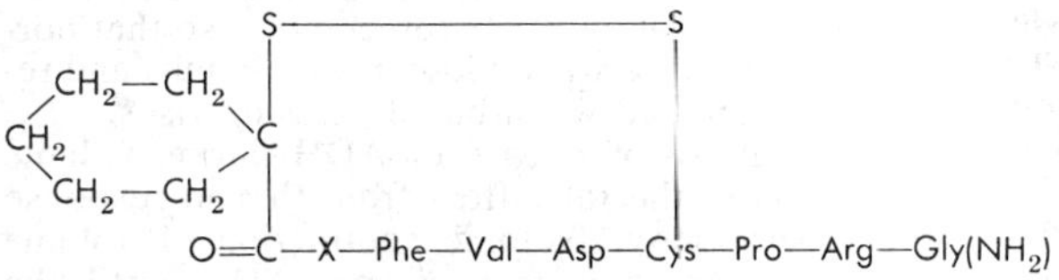		

Analogs

1. X † = D-Tyr
2. X = O-Ethyl-tyr
3. X = D-Phe
4. X = D-Ile

* Assayed in the rat.
† X refers to substituent shown in position 2 of structure to the left.

retic rather than water diuretic when tested in human subjects (Allison *et al.*, 1988), and clinically effective antagonists of ADH are still not available.

PHYSIOLOGICAL AND PATHOPHYSIOLOGICAL CONSIDERATIONS

Antidiuresis in the mammal involves a hypothalamiconeurohypophyseal system for the synthesis, storage, and release of ADH and a renal system for hormonally regulated concentration of the urine. At almost every point, pharmacological agents, as well as disease, can modify the normal chain of events.

Anatomy. The hypothalamiconeurohypophyseal tract is an extended neurosecretory system; the perikarya are located in specific hypothalamic nuclei, and their long axons traverse the supraopticohypophyseal tract to terminate in the median eminence and pars nervosa of the posterior pituitary. Interruption of the tract at any level produces retrograde degeneration of the cell bodies and axons. However, interruption below the level of the median eminence does not result in clinical diabetes insipidus, since axons terminating in the median eminence are spared and secrete adequate amounts of ADH. Lesions above the level of the median eminence generally result in diabetes insipidus.

Synthesis. In man, ADH and oxytocin are synthesized primarily at two hypothalamic sites: the supraoptic and paraventricular nuclei. There is good evidence that ADH and oxytocin are synthesized predominantly in separate neurons. A relatively large and biologically inactive precursor (prohormone) containing ADH, a neurophysin (proteins that bind ADH and oxytocin), and a glycopeptide is synthesized on ribosomes; incorporated into large (0.1 to 0.3 μm), membrane-enclosed granules; and then split into several moieties (ADH-neurophysin, intact and truncated glycopeptides) during the movement of the granules from the perikaryon down the axon to their storage position in the terminal bulbs of the axons (*see* North, 1987). *Dynorphin* is also incorporated into ADH-containing granules; when released, it appears to inhibit the secretion of oxytocin (Bondy *et al.*, 1988).

Transport and Storage. The process of axonal transport of the granules is relatively rapid; newly synthesized neurohypophyseal hormones arrive at the posterior lobe within 30 minutes of a stimulus such as hemorrhage. The axons involved in transport of granules have two destinations, carrying ADH and neurophysins not only to the classical storage sites in the neurohypophysis but also to the external zone of the median eminence, where they enter the adenohypophyseal portal circulation and play a role as corticotropin-releasing factors.

Secretion. Much of our current understanding of the secretion of ADH comes from the morphological studies of Douglas and associates (Douglas, 1973) and from techniques for the study of the hypothalamiconeurohypophyseal system in organ culture (*see* Sladek and Armstrong, 1987). Briefly, the neurosecretory system functions as a conventional neuron. Incoming impulses from osmoreceptors, higher cerebral centers, vascular baroreceptors, and other sites converge on the nerve bodies in the supraventricular or paraventricular nuclei. Stimulation leads to depolarization of the nerve membrane, which is propagated to the terminal bulb. The resultant influx of Ca^{2+} promotes fusion of granules with the membrane of the bulb and exocytosis of the granular contents. Neurophysins, as well as ADH, oxytocin, and dynorphin are released.

Physiological Stimuli for the Secretion of ADH. The two principal physiological stimuli for the secretion of ADH are an increase in plasma osmolality and a decrease in extracellular volume. Other stimuli include pain, nausea, and hypoxia.

Hyperosmolality. An increase of less than 2% in the osmolality of blood perfusing the hypothalamus produces a sharp antidiuresis. Antidiuresis is stimulated by hypertonic saline or sucrose solution, but not by hypertonic urea, suggesting that actual osmotic shrinkage of some receptor cell is necessary. The osmoreceptors are thought to function as a complex network of cells, which are located in the organum vasculosum laminae terminalis of the third ventricle, the lateral hypothalamus, the preoptic area, and the supraoptic nucleus itself. All respond to changes in osmolality and contribute to the final signal for secretion of ADH.

The pattern of secretion of ADH in response to hyperosmolality is shown in Figure 29–1, *A*. The threshold for secretion is approximately 280 mOsm/kg; below this level, ADH is barely detectable in plasma. Above threshold, the concentration of ADH in plasma rises rapidly as osmolality increases. Patients with fully developed ADH-sensitive diabetes insipidus are unable to increase the rate of secretion of ADH, while patients with partial disease show a range of concentrations in plasma. Subjects with nephrogenic diabetes insipidus (failure of the kidney to respond to ADH) or psychogenic polydipsia secrete ADH normally in response to hyperosmolality.

Volume Depletion. The second major stimulus for the secretion of ADH is depletion of extracellular fluid volume. Hemorrhage, depletion of Na^+, or other short-term causes of reduction of extracellular volume, irrespective of plasma osmolality, produce a discharge of ADH into the circulation. In addition to these short-term stimuli, more long-term conditions (*e.g.*, cardiac failure, hepatic cirrhosis with ascites, adrenal insufficiency, hypothyroidism, and excessive use of diuretics) may also be associated with abnormally high concentrations of ADH in plasma.

The baroreceptors that mediate this type of release and the neural pathways from the receptors to the hypothalamic nuclei differ completely from those involved in the response to hyperosmolarity. Baroreceptors are located in the left atrium, ventricles, and pulmonary veins, as well as in the carotid sinus and aorta. Recent studies suggest that the ventricular receptors are of particular importance (Wang *et al.*, 1988). Impulses from these receptors are relayed to the hypothalamus via afferent pathways in the vagus and the glossopharyngeal nerves. Secretion of ADH is believed to be under tonic inhibitory control by the baroreceptors, so that hormone is released when blood pressure falls and release is inhibited when blood pressure rises.

The pattern of release of ADH during volume depletion in the rat differs from that in response to hypertonicity. Isotonic contraction of volume causes little change in plasma ADH until the loss approaches 10%, after which concentrations of ADH increase exponentially. This response eventually exceeds that of hypertonicity (Figure 29–1, *B*).

Other Mediators of ADH Secretion. There is a large and often contradictory literature on mediators of ADH secretion in the CNS (*see* Sladek and Armstrong, 1987). Agents for which there is good evidence for a stimulatory action include angiotensin II, prostaglandins, acetylcholine, substance P, and vasoactive intestinal polypeptide; inhibitors include opioids, gamma-aminobutyric acid, and atrial natriuretic peptide (Schwartz *et al.*, 1986). Of the agents listed, a few deserve comment.

Angiotensin II is a potent dipsogen, and there is evidence that it has a role in both the stimulation of thirst and the secretion of ADH in response to volume depletion. Circulating angiotensin II binds to receptors in the organum vasculosum and the subfornical organ of the anterior wall of the third ventricle. These sites lack a blood–brain barrier, and it is from them and their neural projections that stimulation of ADH secretion appears to be initiated

(McKinley *et al.*, 1988). Angiotensin II synthesized within the brain may also stimulate thirst and ADH secretion, acting at sites such as the median preoptic nucleus (McKinley *et al.*, 1988).

In general, the endogenous opioid peptides (β-endorphin, enkephalin, and dynorphin) appear to inhibit ADH secretion (*see* Sladek and Armstrong, 1987). Atrial natriuretic peptide, whose peripheral actions in the kidney include natriuresis, inhibits the secretion of ADH. This may be an action of the circulating hormone or it may be an action of the peptide produced centrally (Sladek and Armstrong, 1987). This effect of atrial natriuretic peptide could be of importance in conditions of volume overload, when high concentrations of the peptide would limit fluid retention (Ramsay *et al.*, 1988). Prostaglandins may have a role in both the osmotic and the nonosmotic secretion of ADH.

Pharmacological Agents and the Secretion of ADH. A number of pharmacological agents alter the osmolality of urine, and, in many cases, it has been hypothesized that their action involves stimulation or inhibition of the secretion of ADH. Direct renal effects, as well as effects on blood pressure, may also be present; this complicates interpretation of mechanism of action (*see* Robertson and Berl, 1986).

Stimulators. These include vinca alkaloids, cyclophosphamide, clofibrate, tricyclic antidepressants, nicotine, isoproterenol, carbamazepine, insulin, morphine, and colchicine. Li^+, which inhibits the effect of ADH on the kidney, also enhances secretion of the hormone (Robertson and Berl, 1986).

Inhibitors. Ethanol and phenytoin inhibit the secretion of ADH. Both mineralocorticoids and glucocorticoids exert an inhibitory role, but for different reasons. Mineralocorticoids are essential for the maintenance of normal extracellular volume; their absence results in volume depletion and baroreceptor-mediated secretion of ADH. Glucocorticoids may inhibit secretion of ADH by a central action, but they may also reduce cardiac stroke volume, triggering secretion of ADH mediated by baroreceptors (*see* Schrier and Bichet, 1981).

Pathophysiology. *ADH-Sensitive Diabetes Insipidus.* ADH-sensitive diabetes insipidus, also referred to as central or neurogenic diabetes insipidus, results from the failure to secrete adequate quantities of ADH. The result is polyuria and the excretion of a dilute urine (specific gravity, 1.001 to 1.005). Trauma or surgery in the region of the pituitary and hypothalamus, malignancy, and infiltrative lesions are well-recognized causes of this condition; there are also familial and idiopathic varieties of the disease. Acute, postoperative diabetes insipidus may be transient in nature. Diabetes insipidus may also occur during pregnancy or in the postpartum period. A rare form, unresponsive to arginine vasopressin but responsive to desmopressin (dDAVP), has been described by Durr and coworkers (1987); this was attributed to abnormally high activities of plasma "vasopressinase," which rapidly inactivates vasopressin but not desmopressin.

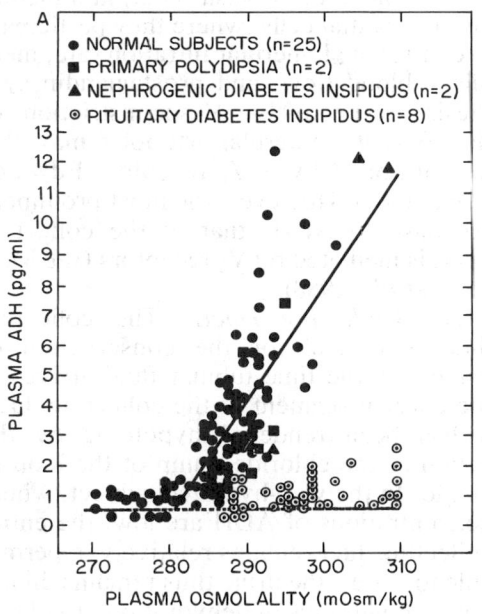

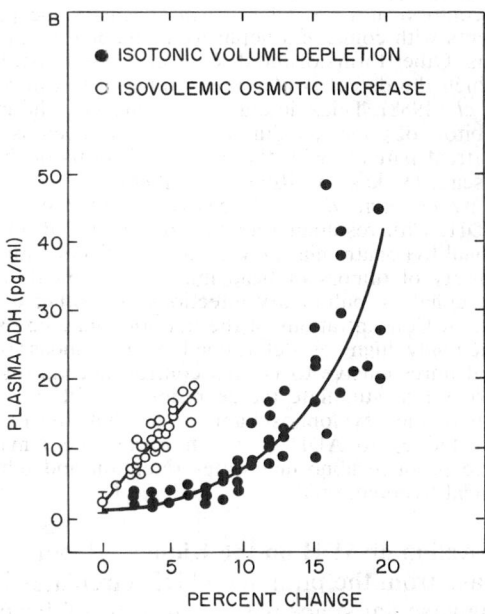

Figure 29–1. *Patterns of secretion of ADH.*

A. Effect of osmolality on the concentration of ADH in plasma. (After Robertson, Mahr, Athar, and Sinha, 1973. Courtesy of *Journal of Clinical Investigation.*)

B. Comparison of the effects of an increase in osmolality and a decrease in extracellular volume (both expressed as percent change) on the concentration of ADH in plasma. (After Dunn, Brennan, Nelson, and Robertson, 1973. Courtesy of *Journal of Clinical Investigation.*)

The appropriate diagnosis of ADH-sensitive diabetes insipidus requires differentiation from other causes of polyuria (*e.g.*, diabetes mellitus, various natriuretic syndromes, primary polydipsia, *etc.*). The diagnosis of diabetes insipidus is confirmed by showing that the patient is unable to reduce urine volume and increase urine osmolality after a period of carefully observed fluid deprivation. Finally, it is necessary to distinguish the ADH-sensitive condition from nephrogenic diabetes insipidus (failure of the kidney to respond to ADH) by administration of the hormone. Patients with ADH-sensitive diabetes insipidus show a prompt increase in urine osmolality (to levels significantly above that of plasma) if given vasopressin intravenously (1 ml per minute of a solution containing 5 units per liter of aqueous vasopressin) or desmopressin subcutaneously (1 μg). Patients with nephrogenic diabetes insipidus show little or no response. For a more complete discussion of diagnostic procedures, *see* Vokes and Robertson (1988).

Nephrogenic Diabetes Insipidus. Nephrogenic diabetes insipidus, a failure of the renal tubule to respond to ADH, has many causes. Drugs that interfere with the ability to respond to ADH are discussed below. Renal disease may cause hyposthenuria and polyuria, especially when the structure or function of the distal tubule and collecting duct are disproportionately affected. Hypercalcemia and hypokalemia can also interfere with the action of ADH.

Congenital forms of nephrogenic diabetes insipidus are well known, although rare. Recent studies by Bichet and colleagues (1988) suggest that a specific subtype of receptors for ADH (so-called V_2 receptors) may be defective in at least some patients with congenital nephrogenic diabetes insipidus. Other forms of the disease may also exist, in which the defect is at a postreceptor site (Moses *et al.*, 1988). Thiazide diuretics, amiloride, and inhibitors of prostaglandin synthesis have been used to treat patients with the congenital forms of this disease (Vokes and Robertson, 1988).

Water Retention. Excessive production of ADH, with resultant retention of water and dilutional hyponatremia, may occur in patients with a variety of tumors or head injuries, meningitis or encephalitis, pulmonary infections, and other diseases. Concentrations of the hormone may be exceedingly high, as determined by immunoassay, and unresponsive to normal control mechanisms. Drugs that stimulate the secretion of ADH (*e.g.*, vincristine, cyclophosphamide) or that sensitize the kidney to ADH (*e.g.*, chlorpropamide) may also produce abnormal water retention and dilutional hyponatremia.

Action of ADH on the Kidney. Upon release from the pituitary, ADH circulates in the vascular space with a half-time of disappearance of 17 to 35 minutes in the human adult. Several factors are responsible for removal of the hormone from the circulation. As mentioned above, enzymatic cleavage by peptidases is the most important.

The cellular actions of ADH are mediated by interactions of the hormone with at least two types of receptors, termed V_1 and V_2. V_1 receptors are located on vascular smooth muscle cells, hepatocytes, platelets, and some cells in the kidney (Michell *et al.*, 1979). These receptors are coupled to the phospholipase C that is responsible for hydrolysis of phosphatidylinositol-4,5-bisphosphate and the resultant generation of inositol-1,4,5-trisphosphate and diacylglycerol. Thus, many of the cellular effects of ADH at these sites are mediated by Ca^{2+} (*see* Chapter 2). A variant V_1 receptor (termed V_{1b}) has been described in the adenohypophysis (Jard *et al.*, 1986). V_2 receptors, which have a much greater affinity for ADH than do the V_1 subtype, stimulate adenylyl cyclase activity; these receptors are located on the cells of the renal collecting duct and the thick ascending limb of Henle's loop (*see* Figure VI–1, page 710).

There are several sites of action of ADH in the kidney, and both V_1 and V_2 receptors participate in renal responses to the hormone. V_1 receptors are found on glomerular mesangial cells, vasa recta, and medullary interstitial cells, where they participate in control of glomerular filtration rate, medullary blood flow, and prostaglandin synthesis, respectively. Vasoconstriction of the efferent glomerular arteriolae may also be controlled by a V_1 receptor (Edwards *et al.*, 1989). However, the most prominent response to ADH, that of the collecting duct, is mediated by V_2 receptors (*see* Margolis *et al.*, 1988).

The Collecting Duct. The collecting duct is critical for the conservation of water. By the time tubular fluid arrives at the cortical segment of the collecting duct, it has been rendered hypotonic by the action of the chloride pump of the loop of Henle. In the well-hydrated subject, where concentrations of ADH are low, the entire collecting duct remains relatively impermeable to water; the urine thus remains dilute. Under conditions of dehydration or volume depletion, on the other hand, concentrations of ADH are significantly elevated, and the cortical and medullary segments of the collecting duct become permeable to water. There is an osmotic gradient between the dilute tubular urine and the peritubular interstitial fluid, which becomes more pronounced in the medullary and papillary segments. Water moves passively down this concentration gradient and is reabsorbed from the tubule; the final osmolality of the urine may be as high as 1200 mOsm/kg in man. A significant saving of water is thus possible.

The binding of ADH to V_2 receptors on the basolateral (nutrient) surface of the principal (and possibly the intercalated) cells of the collecting duct initiates a sequence of steps that eventually increases the permeability of the opposite (luminal) cell surface to water. The sequence of steps is one of many examples in which cyclic AMP appears to serve as the intracellular mediator of the actions of a hormone on its target cell. The agonist-bound V_2 receptor activates the adenylyl cyclase system at the basolateral membrane, with resultant accumulation of cyclic AMP intracellularly. Cyclic AMP, in turn, initiates a series of events that ultimately increases the permeability of the luminal membrane. The exact nature of these events and their relationship to one another are not completely understood, but they include the activation of cyclic AMP–dependent protein kinase and changes in cytoskeletal structure. Channel-containing cytoplasmic vesicles fuse with the luminal membrane, and incorporation of these channels into the membrane appears to be responsible for increasing the permeability to water (Chevalier *et al.*, 1974; Brown, 1989; Hays, 1990). V_1 receptors are also present on the principal cells of the collecting duct (Burnatowska-Hledin and Spielman, 1989). Their activation is presumed to modulate the response that is initiated by the V_2 system.

Endogenous Modulators of the Renal Response. Prostaglandins are generated by medullary interstitial cells, and ADH stimulates prostaglandin biosynthesis through V_1 receptors. Prostaglandins of the E series inhibit ADH-stimulated water flow (Sonnenberg and Smith, 1988). The activation of protein kinase C, which also results from stimulation of V_1 receptors, produces an additional inhibition of ADH-stimulated water flow (Schlondorff and Levine, 1985). Atrial natriuretic peptide attenuates ADH-stimulated water flow in both the cortical and inner medullary collecting ducts, probably via cyclic GMP (Nonoguchi *et al.*, 1988).

Pharmacological Agents That Modify the Renal Response to ADH. Chlorpropamide, acetaminophen, and indomethacin enhance the action of ADH. This may be explained in part by inhibition of renal prostaglandin synthesis. Thus, these agents "sensitize" the kidney to concentrations of ADH that ordinarily would be too low to stimulate reabsorption of water.

A number of pharmacological agents inhibit the antidiuretic action of the hormone to the point of producing ADH-resistant polyuria (nephrogenic diabetes insipidus). Li^+ is of particular importance because of its wide use in the treatment of manic–depressive disorders (*see* Chapter 18). The polyuria is usually reversible upon discontinuation of the drug (Ramsay and Cox, 1982). Li^+ inhibits vasopressin-sensitive adenylyl cyclase, perhaps by an action at the level of the stimulatory guanine nucleotide–binding regulatory (G) protein (Goldberg *et al.*, 1988). Patients receiving Li^+ who develop nephrogenic diabetes insipidus may be helped by the administration of amiloride, which blocks the entry of Li^+ from tubular urine into renal epithelial cells (Batlle *et al.*, 1985). Indomethacin may also reduce the polyuria (Grindlinger and Boylan, 1987). The antibiotic demeclocycline causes defects in the ability of the kidney to produce a concentrated urine in a high percentage of patients and can produce symptomatic polyuria and polydipsia. The ability of demeclocycline to antagonize the action of ADH has been used successfully to promote diuresis in patients with water intoxication due to inappropriate secretion of ADH (Forrest *et al.*, 1978).

Nonrenal Actions of ADH. As mentioned, ADH and related peptides are old hormones in evolutionary terms, and they are found in species that have no mechanisms for the concentration of urine. It is thus not surprising that there are actions of ADH in mammals in addition to those on the kidney.

Cardiovascular System. The pressor effect of ADH occurs only at concentrations that are significantly higher than those required for maximal antidiuresis. Vasoconstriction is general, and smooth muscle of most parts of the vasculature can be affected. Circulation in the skin and the gastrointestinal tract is markedly reduced, the coronary vessels are not exempt, and pulmonary arterial pressure also rises. Given the vasoconstrictor effects of ADH, it is not surprising that there have been numerous studies of its role in the maintenance of vascular tone and in human hypertension. ADH may indeed be important in the maintenance of vascular tone. Dogs with diabetes insipidus, for example, have an impaired ability to maintain blood pressure following blood loss. In patients with congestive heart failure, ADH may contribute to systemic vascular resistance; injection of V_1 antagonists has been reported to improve hemodynamic function in such patients (Thibonnier, 1988). Thus far, there has been no convincing evidence for a role of ADH in the cause of human hypertension (*see* Thibonnier, 1988).

A vasodilatory action of ADH can be elicited when the hormone is given in the presence of a V_1 antagonist (Liard, 1988). Cardiac output increases and total peripheral resistance falls. The same response is seen when specific antidiuretic (V_2) agonists such as desmopressin are given, suggesting that vasodilatation is mediated by V_2 receptors in the vasculature.

The effects of ADH on the heart are largely indirect and are the result of coronary vasoconstriction, decreased coronary blood flow, and reflexly induced alterations in vagal and sympathetic tone. In man, the effects of ADH on coronary blood flow can be demonstrated readily, especially if large doses are employed. The cardiac actions of the hormone are of more than academic interest. Some patients with coronary insufficiency experience anginal pain even in response to the relatively small amounts of ADH required to control diabetes insipidus. ADH-induced myocardial ischemia has led to severe reactions and even death. This is an important consideration in relation to the use of ADH in the control of gastrointestinal hemorrhage (*see* below). If coronary blood flow is maintained at normal levels, one can demonstrate a modest, V_1 receptor–mediated positive inotropic effect of ADH on the isolated rat heart (Walker *et al.*, 1988).

Other Smooth Muscle. The stimulatory effects of ADH on smooth muscle also occur in the gastrointestinal tract. The response is elicited only by large doses. The smooth muscle of the uterus is stimulated by large doses of ADH at all stages of the menstrual cycle and during gestation.

Blood Coagulation. Desmopressin (dDAVP) and ADH raise the circulating levels of coagulation factor VIII and von Willebrand factor when given to healthy subjects, patients with mild-to-moderate hemophilia, and patients with type-I von Willebrand's disease (Mannucci, 1988). Although the mechanism of this effect is somewhat obscure, it is presumed to involve the secretion of von Willebrand factor from vascular endothelial cells and of factor VIII from hepatocytes. Desmopressin has thus become a valuable nontransfusional form of prophylaxis prior to surgery or treatment during bleeding episodes in patients with these disorders. However, not all patients with von Willebrand's disease respond to treatment (*see* Mannucci, 1988). Desmopressin can cause thrombocytopenia in patients with type-IIB von Willebrand's disease, and cryoprecipitate is the treatment of choice in this condition. Desmopressin is also effective in shortening the bleeding time in many patients with uremia, cirrhosis, and congenital platelet dysfunctions (Mannucci, 1988). The use of desmopressin in major surgical procedures is currently being evaluated.

Central Nervous System. There is growing recognition of the role of ADH as a neurotransmitter (*see* Gash *et al.*, 1987; Jolles, 1987). Autonomic effects that may result from the actions of ADH in the CNS include bradycardia, increase in respiratory rate, suppression of fever, and modulation of sleep patterns. Pathways to the brain stem and spinal cord may be involved in the central autonomic regulation of the circulation (Schmid *et al.*, 1984). Learned behavior may be influenced by ADH (deWied, 1980), although recent studies have suggested that visceral autonomic effects of ADH, rather than direct modulation of memory processes, may be involved (Gash *et al.*, 1987). Secretion of ACTH is enhanced by ADH that arrives at the anterior pituitary via a pathway that secretes the peptide into the hypophyseal portal blood. However, ADH is not the principal corticotropin-releasing factor.

Absorption, Fate, and Excretion. When ADH, lypressin, and their congeners are given orally, they are quickly inactivated by trypsin, which cleaves the 8–9 peptide link. ADH in aqueous solution may be given by the intravenous, intramuscular, or subcutaneous route and by the nasal insufflation of powders or sprays. Due to rapid inactivation by a number of enzymes that cleave the peptide at several sites, the effects are brief after intravenous administration unless the hormone is given by continuous infusion. An exception is desmopressin, which is found in the circulation for a prolonged period when absorbed from the nasal mucous membranes. Repository forms, such as *vasopressin tannate in oil,* are effective for 48 to 96 hours after intramuscular injection.

The half-life of ADH in the circulation is 17 to 35 minutes, due particularly to inactivation by peptidases in various tissues. The kidney and the liver are of major importance in the removal of ADH from the circulation, although urinary clearance is only a small fraction of the total in man (Moses and Steciak, 1986).

Preparations, Bioassay, and Unitage. ADH is available in two types of preparations. One is an extract in which no separation of the antidiuretic and oxytocic principles has been made. It is assayed for its oxytocic activity, which parallels antidiuretic activity. Activity is expressed in terms of USP *posterior pituitary units. Posterior pituitary injection* [PITUITRIN (S)] is a sterile aqueous extract of the gland that contains the equivalent of 20 USP posterior pituitary units per milliliter.

Vasopressin injection (PITRESSIN) is prepared synthetically. It is assayed for pressor activity rather than antidiuretic activity, but these are identical, unit for unit. The test method is the blood pressure of the rat. Activity is designated as *pressor units* and is determined by comparison with a USP standard.

Desmopressin acetate (dDAVP) is marketed as an aqueous solution containing 0.1 mg/ml of the synthetic peptide. The preparation is available in a screw-top vial containing 2.5 ml; it includes an applicator tube for intranasal administration. A solution for injection is also marketed.

Lypressin (DIAPID) is available as a nasal spray containing 0.185 mg/ml of synthetic 8-L-lysine vasopressin equivalent to 50 USP posterior pituitary (pressor) units per milliliter. One spray into a nostril provides approximately 2 pressor units.

Vasopressin tannate (PITRESSIN TANNATE IN OIL) is a water-insoluble tannate of the antidiuretic principle. It is marketed suspended in peanut oil. Each milliliter contains 5 pressor units.

THERAPEUTIC USES

The actions of ADH on the kidney and the circulation provide the basis for therapeutic applications of the hormone. ADH is also used in the control of certain bleeding disorders.

Antidiuretic Action. Once the diagnosis of ADH-sensitive diabetes insipidus has been made, the administration of vasopressin provides effective and immediate therapy, with reduction of urine volume to normal. With the exception of patients who experience transient diabetes insipidus as a result of head injury or surgery in the area of the pituitary, therapy is lifelong. Desmopressin, administered intranasally, is the drug of choice for most patients.

Numerous clinical trials (*see* Cobb *et al.,* 1978) have demonstrated that desmopressin is an effective agent in both adults and children and has few side effects. The duration of effect from a single intranasal dose is from 6 to 20 hours, and twice-daily administration has proven to be effective in the majority of patients. There is considerable variability in the dose of desmopressin required to maintain normal urine volume (2.5 to 20 μg twice daily), and the dosage must be tailored to the needs of the individual patient. In view of the high cost of the drug and the importance of avoiding water intoxication, it has been suggested that the schedule of administration be adjusted to determine the minimal amount required (Cobb *et al.,* 1978). An initial dose of 2.5 μg can be used, and therapy should first be directed toward the control of nocturia. An equivalent or higher morning dose controls daytime polyuria in most patients, although a third dose may occasionally be needed in the afternoon. Resistance to desmopressin may develop (Cobb *et al.,* 1978). Administration of more than 40 to 50 μg may cause headache.

Recent clinical trials in Europe indicate that desmopressin administered orally to children in tablet form controls polyuria effectively; as much as 20 times the intranasal dose is required (Fjellestad-Paulsen *et al.,* 1987a). The oral form of desmopressin is not presently available in the United States.

There has been a limited, but encouraging experience with desmopressin for the treatment of children with nocturnal enuresis; many children were cured or showed improvement (Fjellestad-Paulsen *et al.,* 1987b). Patients with autonomic failure appear to have less nocturnal polyuria and postural hypotension following treatment with desmopressin (Mathias *et al.,* 1986).

Vasopressin tannate in oil suspension was the standard therapy for vasopressin-sensitive diabetes insipidus, and this preparation can be used for the treatment of patients who are refractory to desmopressin or who experience significant side effects. Given as an intramuscular injection (2 to 5 units every 2 or 3 days), it produces a satisfactory antidiuresis in virtually all patients. Care must be used in preparing the ampul for use; it should be warmed in the hand and mixed until the hormone is distributed in the suspension. In view of the inconvenience of intramuscular injection and its side effects (*see* below), vasopressin tannate is less desirable than desmopressin, especially in children.

Vasopressin injection, the aqueous form of ADH, has no place in the long-term therapy of diabetes insipidus. Given intravenously, it has two uses: as an alternative to desmopressin in the initial diagnostic evaluation of patients with suspected diabetes insipidus and to control polyuria in the patient with diabetes insipidus who has recently undergone surgery (*e.g.*, hypophysectomy) or experienced head trauma. Under these circumstances polyuria may be transient, and long-acting agents may produce water intoxication.

Lypressin, synthetic lysine vasopressin administered as a nasal spray, produces antidiuresis if administered approximately every 4 to 6 hours. Its short duration of action limits its effectiveness, especially in cases of severe diabetes insipidus.

Pressor Action. Despite its name, vasopressin should not be employed as a pressor agent. If it is desired to produce systemic peripheral vasoconstriction, preference should be given to appropriate sympathomimetic amines that can increase peripheral resistance without reducing coronary blood flow. However, an exception has been made for the use of vasopressin as an adjunct in the control of bleeding esophageal varices, acute hemorrhagic gastritis, and during abdominal surgery in patients with portal hypertension. When large doses (10 to 20 units in 15 minutes) are infused in normal subjects or in patients with cirrhosis and portal hypertension, there is a marked decrease in portal blood flow and pressure lasting approximately 30 minutes. Only a moderate rise in arterial pressure occurs. This effect on portal circulation is attributable to marked splanchnic vasoconstriction. Infusion of vasopressin directly into the superior mesenteric artery has not proven superior to systemic infusion in the case of bleeding esophageal varices. Infusion of vasopressin into the left gastric artery of patients with acute hemorrhagic gastritis has, however, been effective (Peterson, 1989). Simultaneous administration of nitroglycerin has been reported to reverse the cardiotoxic effects of vasopressin while enhancing the beneficial splanchnic effects of the drug (Gimson *et al.*, 1986).

Bleeding Disorders. Reference has been made above to the action of desmopressin in von Willebrand's disease and moderately severe hemophilia. Mannucci (1988) has suggested that the response of any given patient to desmopressin be determined at the time of diagnosis or 1 to 2 weeks before elective surgery to assess the extent of the increase in factor VIII or von Willebrand factor. Desmopressin, given intravenously at a dose of 0.3 μg/kg, increases factor VIII and von Willebrand factor for more than 6 hours. Desmopressin can be given at intervals of 12 to 24 hours, depending on the clinical response and the severity of the bleeding. Subcutaneous administration of the same dose of desmopressin is also effective, especially when self-administration is involved. Progressive unresponsiveness to desmopressin may occur over 4 to 5 days in some hemophiliacs treated with the drug at closely spaced intervals.

Untoward Reactions and Contraindications. After the injection of large doses of vasopressin, marked facial pallor as a result of cutaneous vasoconstriction is commonly observed. Increased intestinal activity is likely to cause nausea, belching, cramps, and an urge to defecate. Women are apt to experience uterine cramps of a menstrual character. Most serious, however, is the effect on the coronary circulation. Individuals suffering from vascular disease, especially disease of the coronary arteries, should never receive vasopressin, except in the small doses needed for the treatment of diabetes insipidus. Sometimes even these small doses may cause myocardial ischemia. Other cardiac complications include arrhythmias and decreased cardiac output. Peripheral vasoconstriction and gangrene have been encountered in patients receiving large doses of vasopressin. Allergic reactions, ranging from urticaria to anaphylaxis, may also occur.

Complications of the administration of vasopressin tannate include sterile abscesses and abdominal pain. As mentioned, there is a possibility of water intoxication with the use of any of these antidiuretic agents.

BENZOTHIADIAZIDES

Chlorothiazide and other benzothiadiazide (thiazide) diuretics paradoxically cause a reduction in the polyuria of patients with diabetes insipidus. Other potent natriuretic agents, such as ethacrynic acid, have also been successfully employed.

Since effective agents are available for the treatment of ADH-sensitive diabetes insipidus, the principal use of the thiazide diuretics is in the treatment of the ADH-resistant (nephrogenic) disease. In infants with diabetes insipidus resistant to ADH, the antidiuretic effect may be of crucial importance, since the uncontrolled polyuria may exceed the child's capacity to imbibe and absorb fluids.

The mechanism of the antidiuretic effect is not yet completely understood. Most investigators agree that the natriuretic action of the thiazides has an important role and that depletion of salt is essential for antidiuresis. Under these conditions, there is excessive reabsorption of sodium chloride in the proximal tubule, with resultant reduction of volume delivered to the distal tubule. Consequently, less free water can be formed, and the polyuria is diminished.

Therapeutic Use. Chlorothiazide and its congeners are less effective than vasopressin in the treatment of pituitary diabetes insipidus but are useful for patients who experience undesirable side effects or allergic reactions after vasopressin and invaluable for those who have nephrogenic diabetes insipidus. Since their antidiuretic effects appear to parallel their ability to cause natriuresis, they are given in doses similar to those used for the mobilization of edema fluid. Chlorothiazide, 1.0 to 1.5 g, or hydrochlorothiazide, 50 to 150 mg, in daily divided doses, have been most frequently employed. Reduction of urine volume to 50% or less of pretreatment volumes is considered to be a good response. Moderate restriction of sodium chloride intake has been shown to enhance the antidiuretic effect.

Among the most common of the side effects encountered is depletion of K^+. Other untoward effects of the thiazides are described in Chapter 28, as are the chemistry, pharmacology, and preparations of these agents.

INHIBITORS OF PROSTAGLANDIN SYNTHESIS

There are a number of case reports describing the effectiveness of indomethacin in the treatment of hereditary nephrogenic diabetes insipidus (*see* Libber *et al.*, 1986). Other inhibitors of prostaglandin synthesis (e.g., ibuprofen) appear to be less effective. Doses of 2 mg/kg per day of indomethacin reduce urine volume significantly. The mechanism of action is unclear, but it may involve a decrease in glomerular filtration rate, an increase in medullary solute concentration, or an enhanced proximal reabsorption of fluid. In view of the reduction in glomerular filtration noted in some series, creatinine clearance should be determined at regular intervals.

A single case report describes amelioration of Li^+-induced polyuria by indomethacin (Grindlinger and Boylan, 1987). Such treatment might be useful during the acute phase of polyuria in patients who are receiving Li^+.

Batlle, D. C.; von Riotte, A. B.; Gaviria, M.; and Grupp, M. Amelioration of polyuria by amiloride in patients receiving long-term lithium therapy. *N. Engl. J. Med.*, **1985**, *312*, 408–414.

Bichet, D. G.; Razi, M.; Lonergan, M.; Arthus, M. F.; Papukna, V.; Kortas, C.; and Barjon, J. N. Hemodynamic and coagulation responses to 1-desamino [8-D-arginine] vasopressin in patients with congenital nephrogenic diabetes insipidus. *N. Engl. J. Med.*, **1988**, *318*, 881–887.

Bondy, C. A.; Gainer, H.; and Russel, J. T. Dynorphin A inhibits and naloxone increases the electrically stimulated release of oxytocin but not vasopressin from the terminals of the neural lobe. *Endocrinology*, **1988**, *122*, 1321–1327.

Burnatowska-Hledin, M. A., and Spielman, W. S. Vasopressin V_1 receptors on the principal cells of the rabbit cortical collecting tubule: stimulation of cytosolic free calcium and inositol phosphate production via coupling to a pertussis toxin substrate. *J. Clin. Invest.*, **1989**, *83*, 84–89.

Chevalier, J.; Bourguet, J.; and Hugon, J. S. Membrane associated particles: distribution in frog urinary bladder epithelium at rest and after oxytocin treatment. *Cell Tissue Res.*, **1974**, *152*, 129–140.

Cobb, W. E.; Spare, S.; and Reichlin, S. Neurogenic diabetes insipidus: management with dDAVP (1-desamino-8-D-arginine vasopressin). *Ann. Intern. Med.*, **1978**, *88*, 183–188.

Dunn, F. L.; Brennan, T. J.; Nelson, A. E.; and Robertson, G. L. The role of blood osmolality and volume in regulating vasopressin secretion in the rat. *J. Clin. Invest.*, **1973**, *52*, 3212–3219.

Durr, J. A.; Hoggard, J. G.; Hunt, J. M.; and Schrier, R. W. Diabetes insipidus in pregnancy associated with abnormally high circulating vasopressinase activity. *N. Engl. J. Med.*, **1987**, *316*, 1070–1074.

duVigneaud, V.; Gish, D. T.; and Katsoyannis, P. G. A synthetic preparation possessing biological properties associated with arginine vasopressin. *J. Am. Chem. Soc.*, **1954**, *76*, 4751–4752.

Edwards, R. M.; Trizna, W.; and Kinter, L. B. Renal microvascular effects of vasopressin and vasopressin antagonists. *Am. J. Physiol.*, **1989**, *256*, F274–F278.

Fjellestad-Paulsen, A.; Tubiana-Rufi, N.; Harris, A.; and Czernichow, P. Central diabetes insipidus in children: antidiuretic effect and pharmacokinetics of intranasal and peroral 1-deamino-8-D-arginine vasopressin. *Acta Endocrinol. (Copenh.)*, **1987a**, *115*, 307–312.

Fjellestad-Paulsen, A.; Wille, S.; and Harris, A. S. Comparison of intranasal and oral desmopressin for nocturnal enuresis. *Arch. Dis. Child.*, **1987b**, *62*, 674–677.

Forrest, J. N., Jr.; Cox, M.; Hong, C.; Morrison, G.; Bia, M.; and Singer, I. Superiority of demeclocycline over lithium in the treatment of chronic syndrome of inappropriate antidiuretic hormone. *N. Engl. J. Med.*, **1978**, *298*, 173–177.

Gimson, A. E. S.; Westaby, D.; Hegarty, J.; Watson, A.; and Williams, R. A randomized trial of vasopressin and vasopressin plus nitroglycerin in the control of acute variceal hemorrhage. *Hepatology*, **1986**, *6*, 410–413.

Goldberg, H.; Clayman, P.; and Skorecki, K. Mechanism of Li inhibition of vasopressin-sensitive adenylate cyclase in cultured renal epithelial cells. *Am. J. Physiol.*, **1988**, *255*, F995–F1002.

Grindlinger, G. A., and Boylan, M. J. Amelioration by indomethacin of lithium-induced polyuria. *Crit. Care Med.*, **1987**, *15*, 538–539.

Jard, S.; Gaillard, R. C.; Guillon, G.; Marie, J.; Schoenenberg, P.; Muller, A. F.; Manning, M.; and Sawyer, W. H. Vasopressin antagonists allow demonstration of a novel type of vasopressin receptor in the rat adenohypophysis. *Mol. Pharmacol.*, **1986**, *30*, 171–177.

Libber, S.; Harrison, H.; and Spector, D. Treatment of nephrogenic diabetes insipidus with prostaglandin synthesis inhibitors. *J. Pediatr.*, **1986**, *108*, 305–311.

Mathias, C. J.; Fosbraey, P.; daCosta, D. F.; Thornley, A.; and Bannister, R. The effect of desmopressin on nocturnal polyuria, overnight weight loss, and morning postural hypotension in patients with autonomic failure. *Br. Med. J.*, **1986**, *293*, 353–354.

Michell, R. H.; Kirk, C. J.; and Billah, M. M. Hormonal stimulation of phosphatidylinositol breakdown with particular reference to the hepatic effects of vasopressin. *Biochem. Soc. Trans.*, **1979**, *7*, 861–865.

Moses, A. M.; Miller, J. L.; and Levine, M. A. Two distinct pathophysiological mechanisms in congenital nephrogenic diabetes insipidus. *J. Clin. Endocrinol. Metab.*, **1988**, *66*, 1259–1264.

Moses, A. M., and Steciak, E. Urinary and metabolic clearances of arginine vasopressin in normal subjects. *Am. J. Physiol.*, **1986**, *252*, R365–R370.

Nonoguchi, H.; Sands, J. M.; and Knepper, M. A. Atrial natriuretic factor inhibits vasopressin-stimulated osmotic water permeability in rat inner medullary collecting duct. *J. Clin. Invest.*, **1988**, *82*, 1383–1390.

Robertson, G. L.; Mahr, E. A.; Athar, S.; and Sinha, T.

Development and clinical application of a new method for the radioimmunoassay of arginine vasopressin in human plasma. *J. Clin. Invest.*, **1973**, *52*, 2340–2352.

Schlondorff, D., and Levine, S. D. Inhibition of vasopressin-stimulated water flow in toad bladder by phorbol myristate acetate, dioctanoylglycerol and RHC-80267. *J. Clin. Invest.*, **1985**, *76*, 1071–1078.

Schmid, P. G.; Sharabi, F. M.; Guo, G. B.; Ahbound, F. M.; and Thames, M. D. Vasopressin and oxytocin in the neural control of the circulation. *Fed. Proc.*, **1984**, *43*, 97–102.

Sonnenberg, W. K., and Smith, W. L. Regulation of cyclic AMP metabolism in rabbit cortical collecting tubule cells by prostaglandins. *J. Biol. Chem.*, **1988**, *263*, 6155–6160.

Walker, B. R.; Childs, M. E.; and Adams, E. M. Direct cardiac effects of vasopressin: role of V_1- and V_2-vasopressinergic receptors. *Am. J. Physiol.*, **1988**, *255*, H261–H265.

Wang, B. C.; Flora-Ginter, G.; Leadley, R. J., Jr.; and Goetz, K. L. Ventricular receptors stimulate vasopressin release during hemorrhage. *Am. J. Physiol.*, **1988**, *254*, R204–R211.

Zaoral, M.; Kole, J.; and Sorm, F. Amino acids and peptides. LXXI. Synthesis of 1-deamino-8-D-aminobutyrine-vasopressin, 1-deamino-8-D-lysine vasopressin, and 1-deamino-8-D-arginine vasopressin. *Coll. Czech. Chem. Commun.*, **1967**, *32*, 1250–1257.

Monographs and Reviews

Allison, N. L.; Albrightson-Winslow, C. R.; Brooks, D. P.; Stassen, F. L.; Huffman, W. F.; Stote, R. M.; and Kinter, L. B. Species heterogeneity and antidiuretic hormone antagonists: what are the predictors? In, *Vasopressin: Cellular and Integrative Functions*. (Cowley, A. W., Jr.; Liard, J.-F.; and Ausiello, D. A.; eds.) Raven Press, New York, **1988**, pp. 207–214.

Brown, D. Membrane recycling and epithelial cell function. *Am. J. Physiol.*, **1989**, *256*, F1–F12.

deWied, D. Behavioral actions of neurohypophysial peptides. *Proc. R. Soc. Lond.* [*Biol.*], **1980**, *210*, 183–195.

Douglas, W. W. How do neurons secrete peptides? Exocytosis and its consequences, including "synaptic vesicle" formation in the hypothalamoneurohypophyseal system. *Prog. Brain Res.*, **1973**, *39*, 21–39.

Gash, D. M.; Herman, J. P.; and Thomas, G. J. Vasopressin and animal behavior. In, *Vasopressin: Principles and Properties*. (Gash, D. M., and Boer, G. J., eds.) Plenum Press, New York, **1987**, pp. 517–547.

Hays, R. M. Water transport in epithelia. In, *Comparative Physiology: Basic Principles in Transport*, Vol. II. (Kinne, R., ed.) A. G. Karger, Basel, **1990**, pp. 1–30.

Jolles, J. Vasopressin and human behavior. In, *Vasopressin: Principles and Properties*. (Gash, D. M., and Boer, G. J., eds.) Plenum Press, New York, **1987**, pp. 549–578.

Liard, J.-F. Acute hemodynamic effects of antidiuretic agonists. In, *Vasopressin: Cellular and Integrative Functions*. (Cowley, A. E., Jr.; Liard, J.-F.; and Ausiello, D. A.; eds.) Raven Press, New York, **1988**, pp. 461–466.

McKinley, M. J.; Allen, A.; Congiu, M.; Denton, D. A.; Mendelsohn, F. A. O.; Oldfield, B. J.; and Wessinger, R. S. Central integration of osmoregulatory vasopressin secretion, thirst, and sodium excretion. In, *Vasopressin: Cellular and Integrative Functions*. (Cowley, A. W., Jr.; Liard, J.-F.; and Ausiello, D. A.; eds.) Raven Press, New York, **1988**, pp. 185–191.

Manning, M.; Bankowski, K.; and Sawyer, W. H. Selective agonists and antagonists of vasopressin. In, *Vasopressin: Principles and Properties*. (Gash, D. M., and Boer, G. J., eds.) Plenum Press, New York, **1987**, pp. 335–368.

Mannucci, P. M. Desmopressin: a nontransfusional form of treatment for congenital and acquired bleeding disorders. *Blood*, **1988**, *72*, 1449–1455.

Margolis, B.; Angel, J.; Kremer, S.; and Skorecki, K. Vasopressin action in the kidney—overview and glomerular actions. In, *Vasopressin: Cellular and Integrative Functions*. (Cowley, A. W., Jr.; Liard, J.-F.; and Ausiello, D. A.; eds.) Raven Press, New York, **1988**, pp. 97–106.

North, W. G. Biosynthesis of vasopressin and neurophysins. In, *Vasopressin: Principles and Properties*. (Gash, D. M., and Boer, G. J., eds.) Plenum Press, New York, **1987**, pp. 175–209.

Peterson, W. L. Gastrointestinal bleeding. In, *Gastrointestinal Disease*. (Sleisenger, M. H., and Fordtran, J. S., eds.) W. B. Saunders Co., Philadelphia, **1989**, pp. 406–407.

Ramsay, D. J.; Thrasher, T. N.; and Keil, L. C. Neurohumoral influences on vasopressin. In, *Vasopressin: Cellular and Integrative Functions*. (Cowley, A. W., Jr.; Liard, J.-F.; and Ausiello, D. A.; eds.) Raven Press, New York, **1988**, pp. 169–176.

Ramsay, T. A., and Cox, M. Lithium and the kidney: a review. *Am. J. Psychiatry*, **1982**, *139*, 443–449.

Robertson, G. L., and Berl, T. Water metabolism. In, *The Kidney*, 3rd ed. (Brenner, B. M., and Rector, F. C., Jr., eds.) W. B. Saunders Co., Philadelphia, **1986**, pp. 385–482.

Schrier, R. W., and Bichet, D. G. Osmotic and nonosmotic control of vasopressin release and the pathogenesis of impaired water excretion in adrenal, thyroid, and edematous disorders. *J. Lab. Clin. Med.*, **1981**, *98*, 1–15.

Schwartz, D.; Katsube, N. C.; and Needleman, P. Atriopeptins in fluid and electrolyte homeostasis. *Fed. Proc.*, **1986**, *45*, 2361–2365.

Sladek, C. D., and Armstrong, W. E. Effect of neurotransmitters and neuropeptides on vasopressin release. In, *Vasopressin: Principles and Properties*. (Gash, D. M., and Boer, G. J., eds.) Plenum Press, New York, **1987**, pp. 275–333.

Thibonnier, M. Vasopressin and blood pressure. *Kidney Int.*, **1988**, *34*, Suppl. 25, S52–S56.

Vokes, T. J., and Robertson, G. L. Disorders of antidiuretic hormone. *Endocrinol. Metab. Clin. North Am.*, **1988**, *17*, 281–299.

CHAPTER

30 INHIBITORS OF TUBULAR TRANSPORT OF ORGANIC COMPOUNDS

Irwin M. Weiner

The physiological factors that influence the renal excretion of organic compounds have been considered in Chapter 1 and in the Introduction to Section VI. Pharmacological agents can change the rate of excretion of other drugs and endogenous chemicals by affecting (1) the glomerular filtration rate, (2) the extent of binding to plasma proteins, (3) the rate of urine flow, (4) the pH of urine, or (5) the activity of tubular transport mechanisms. This chapter describes a class of agents that act on the tubular transport of certain drugs and of urate, all of which are organic anions. Although certain cationic drugs may interfere with the tubular secretion of organic bases, there are no therapeutic agents specifically designed to inhibit the renal transport of organic cations (Rennick, 1981).

The renal transport mechanisms for organic anions have been identified only in the proximal tubule. The most thoroughly studied is that for the secretion of para-aminohippurate (PAH) and a great variety of other organic anions (Møller and Sheikh, 1982). The overall process of secretion requires, first, the uptake of PAH from interstitial fluid across the basolateral membrane into the cell and, second, the subsequent movement of PAH from the cell across the brush-border membrane into the tubular fluid. The first step involves concentration; PAH in intracellular fluid is driven to levels much higher than that in the interstitial fluid. This process is mediated by a *transporter*—an integral constituent of the basolateral membrane that can be saturated and inhibited competitively. This transporter operates as an anion exchanger—exchanging a molecule of PAH for a molecule of a normal anionic metabolite, such as α-ketoglutarate. The anionic metabolite may be synthesized in the tubular cell or enter the cell by a Na^+-dependent mechanism of the type described in the Introduction to Section VI (Pritchard, 1987; Shimada *et al.*, 1987). In the second step of PAH secretion, PAH moves from a high intracellular concentration to a lower concentration in the tubular fluid. In some species this is specifically mediated by a transporter in the brush-border membrane that is also saturable and subject to competitive inhibition (Guggino *et al.*, 1983).

Many anionic drugs and metabolites of drugs are secreted by this two-step mechanism, and such compounds, when present simultaneously, may interfere with the secretion of one another. The competition for secretion observed *in vivo* is a reflection of events at the basolateral membrane. The transporter in this membrane has a smaller capacity and a higher affinity for its substrates than does that in the brush-border membrane (Ross and Holohan, 1983). Although competition for secretion occurs frequently, it is not always apparent *in vivo*. To illustrate this point, consider the action of probenecid, the prototypical inhibitor of secretion, on the renal excretion of two organic anions—penicillin and salicylate. Probenecid itself is a highly lipid-soluble carboxylic acid. It is completely reabsorbed in an acidic urine, while net tubular secretion is apparent in an alkaline urine. Penicillin is also secreted by the tubule, but it is a much more polar compound and, therefore, is not extensively reabsorbed. The effect of probenecid is to decrease the excretion of penicillin by inhibition of its secretion, regardless of whether the urine is acidic or alkaline. In contrast, the action of probenecid on the excretion of salicylate is apparent only when the urine is alkaline. When the urine is acidic, the passive reabsorption of both salicylate and probenecid is virtually complete and thus any interaction between the two at the secretory level is not reflected in the voided urine. It is possible to take advantage of competition for secretion in order to prolong the action of a therapeutic agent (*see* below). In other instances it is a potentially dangerous situation to have retention of one drug induced by another (Nierenberg, 1983).

Action of Uricosuric Agents. A uricosuric agent is a drug that increases the rate of excretion of uric acid. There is perhaps no other class of therapeutic agents for which the observations in their entirety appear so inconsistent and at times contradictory. This results from the complexity of the transport mechanisms, as well as the marked species variation of individual mechanisms and their sensitivity to drug action. Birds, reptiles, and some mammals demonstrate net secretion of urate; in some mammalian species both net secretion and net reabsorption can be observed; and in others, including man, net reabsorption is found almost invariably. In animals that demonstrate net secretion, the mechanism is analogous, and in some instances identical, to the mechanism for the secretion of PAH. In man and other species that demonstrate net reabsorption, the reabsorptive process is mediated by a specific transporter and it is inhibitable. Finally, in all species that have been studied thoroughly, the major transport mechanism, either secretion or reabsorption, is opposed by a smaller flux operating in the opposite direction; that is, there is bidirectional transport. In most instances the smaller flux is specifically mediated (Roch-Ramel and Weiner, 1980). As a consequence of all these factors, a drug that is uricosuric in one species may produce urate retention in another; within one species a drug may cause either urate retention or uricosuria, depending on the dose; and one uricosuric drug may either add to or inhibit the action of another.

In man, uric acid is largely reabsorbed; the amount excreted is usually about 10% of that filtered. Studies with brush-border membranes from other animals that also demonstrate net reabsorption of urate indicate that the first step in reabsorption is the uptake of urate from tubular fluid by the same transporter that allows PAH to move from cell to lumen. This transporter can act as an anion exchanger. Thus, urate in the tubular fluid can be exchanged for either an organic or an inorganic anion moving in the opposite direction. It has been suggested that the anionic compositions of luminal and intracellular fluids are such that reabsorption of urate is favored. In the case of PAH, the high intracellular concentration produced by the transporter in the basolateral membrane is sufficient to overcome the reabsorptive tendency of the brush-border transporter (Guggino *et al.*, 1983). The exit step for urate at the basolateral membrane is also mediated by an anion exchanger. This exchanger has no affinity for PAH (Kahn and Weinman, 1985). Probenecid and other uricosuric drugs, when present in the lumen, compete with urate for the brush-border transporter, thereby inhibiting its reabsorption. Thus, the same drug, probenecid, inhibits the secretion of one anion (*e.g.*, PAH) by an action at the basolateral membrane and inhibits the reabsorption of another anion (*e.g.*, urate) by an action at the luminal membrane.

The *paradoxical effect of uricosuric agents* refers to the fact that, depending on dosage, a drug may either decrease or increase the excretion of uric acid. Decreased excretion usually occurs at a low dosage, while increased excretion is observed at a higher dosage. Not all agents show this phenomenon. With some drugs, such as salicylate, the biphasic effect may be seen within the normal dosage range; with pyrazinamide, reduction of the excretion of uric acid is the dominant action except at extremely high (experimental) doses (Fanelli and Weiner, 1973). Two mechanisms for a drug-induced decrease in excretion of urate have been advanced; they are not mutually exclusive. The first presumes that the small secretory movement of urate is mediated by a mechanism separate from that for the secretion of PAH. This secretory mechanism is thought to be extremely sensitive to low concentrations of compounds such as salicylate and pyrazinamide (Fanelli and Weiner, 1973). Higher concentrations of these substances may inhibit urate reabsorption in the usual manner. The second proposal suggests that the urate-retaining anionic drug gains access to the intracellular fluid by an independent mechanism and promotes reabsorption of urate across the brush border by anion exchange (Guggino *et al.*, 1983).

There are two mechanisms by which one drug may nullify the uricosuric action of another. First, the drug may inhibit the secretion of the uricosuric agent, thereby denying it access to its site of action, the luminal aspect of the brush border. Second, the inhibition of urate secretion by one drug may counterbalance the inhibition of urate reabsorption by the other (Fanelli and Weiner, 1979). There are situations in which two uricosuric agents administered together almost completely nullify each other's actions (*see*, for example, Yü *et al.*, 1963). In such an instance one of the drugs (A) must have a strong paradoxical action. Drug B inhibits the secretion of A, thereby preventing its uricosuric action but not its urate-retaining action. The latter effect balances the uricosuric action of drug B.

There are a great many compounds that have uricosuric activity, but only a few are prescribed for this purpose. Some have other primary pharmacological actions, and their ability to increase urate excretion is either incidental or unexpected. In all instances the active compound is probably either an anionic drug or an anionic metabolite. On the other hand, there are a number of drugs and toxins that cause retention of urate. Both classes of compounds have been reviewed by Emmerson (1978).

PROBENECID

History. Probenecid was developed as a result of a planned approach to achieve a specific objective. When penicillin was first introduced, it was in critically short supply and the rapid renal excretion of the antibiotic was thus of practical significance. For this reason, Beyer and associates began a study to find an organic acid that would depress the tubular secretion of penicillin in the manner described above. The first compound to be evaluated clinically was CARINAMIDE. It proved to be effective, but the drug was secreted by the renal tubules fairly rapidly and it was necessary to give frequent doses. This problem was overcome with the discovery of probenecid (Beyer *et al.*, 1951).

Chemistry. Probenecid is a highly lipid-soluble benzoic acid derivative (pK_a 3.4) with the following structural formula:

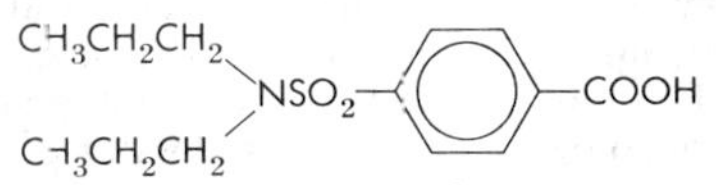

Probenecid

Various congeners of probenecid have been studied. Increasing the size of the N-alkyl substitution results in more efficient compounds. Optimal activity appears in probenecid, the N-dipropyl derivative. Gutman (1966) has reviewed the structure–activity relationship of probenecid congeners and that of other uricosuric drugs.

Pharmacological Actions. The actions of probenecid are largely confined to inhibition of the transport of organic acids across epithelial barriers. This is most important for the renal tubule, in which tubular secretion of many drugs and drug metabolites is inhibited (Weiner *et al.*, 1964; Diamond, 1978). The renal action of probenecid reduces the concentrations of certain compounds in urine and raises them in plasma. This is a desirable therapeutic effect in the case of penicillin and related antibiotics that have a beneficial systemic action, but it may be undesirable with an agent such as nitrofurantoin when it is employed as a urinary antiseptic. When tubular secretion of a substance is inhibited, its final concentration in the urine is determined by the degree of filtration, which in turn is a function of binding to plasma protein, and by the degree of reabsorption. The significance of each of these factors varies widely with different compounds.

Uric Acid. Uric acid is the only important endogenous compound whose excretion is known to be increased by probenecid. This results from inhibition of its reabsorption (*see* above). The uricosuric action of probenecid is blunted by the administration of salicylates.

Miscellaneous Substances. Probenecid inhibits the tubular secretion of a number of drugs, such as indomethacin, methotrexate, dyphylline, and the active metabolite of clofibrate, but there is no clinical indication for the coadministration of probenecid in most instances. In the case of a number of endogenous or exogenous organic acids whose rate of excretion is determined for diagnostic purposes, misleading values may be obtained if the patient is receiving probenecid.

Cerebrospinal Fluid. Probenecid inhibits the transport of 5-hydroxyindoleacetic acid (5-HIAA) and other acidic metabolites of cerebral monoamines from the subarachnoid space to the plasma. This has been the subject of interest in psychopharmacology (*see* Van der Poel *et al.,* 1977). The transport of drugs such as penicillin G may also be affected (Spector and Lorenzo, 1974).

Biliary Excretion. Since probenecid and some of its metabolites may be secreted into the bile, it is not surprising that probenecid depresses the biliary secretion of other compounds, including the diagnostic agents indocyanine green and sulfobromophthalein (BSP). The inhibition of biliary secretion also has implications in the use of rifampin for the treatment of tuberculosis. Higher concentrations of the antibiotic are achieved in plasma if probenecid is administered concurrently (Guarino and Schanker, 1968; Kenwright and Levi, 1973).

Absorption, Fate, and Excretion. Probenecid is completely absorbed after oral administration. Peak concentrations in plasma are reached in 2 to 4 hours. The half-life of the drug in plasma is dose dependent and varies from less than 5 hours to more than 8 hours over the therapeutic range (*see* Appendix II). Between 85 and 95% of the drug is bound to plasma albumin. The small unbound portion gains access to the glomerular filtrate; a much larger portion is actively secreted by the proximal tubule. The high lipid solubility of the undissociated form results in virtually complete absorption by back diffusion unless the urine is markedly alkaline. A small amount of probenecid glucuronide appears in the urine. It is also hydroxylated to metabolites that retain their carboxyl function and have uricosuric activity (Israeli *et al.,* 1972).

Preparation and Dosage. *Probenecid* (BENEMID, PROBALAN) is marketed as oral tablets (500 mg). The dose schedule depends upon the objectives of therapy. To block the renal excretion of penicillin effectively, a total daily dose of 2 g is employed in adults. This is administered in four divided doses. For children weighing less than 50 kg, an initial dose of 25 mg/kg is followed by maintenance doses of 10 mg/kg given four times daily. In the treatment of chronic gout, 250 mg is given twice daily for 1 week, following which 500 mg is administered twice daily. In some patients it may be necessary to increase the daily dosage gradually to a maximum of 2 g, given in four divided portions. Liberal fluid intake should be maintained throughout therapy.

Adjunct in Penicillin Therapy. The oral administration of probenecid in conjunction with penicillin G results in higher and more prolonged concentrations of the antibiotic in plasma than when penicillin is given alone. The elevation in the plasma level is at least twofold and sometimes much greater. Although the reduction of a daily dose of penicillin G from 1 million to 500,000 units has very little significance, a reduction by 50% or more may be of importance for convenience in the treatment of resistant infections that may require the administration of penicillin G in very large doses. This combined regimen may also be useful to minimize the amount of K^+ that is administered to some patients who receive very large doses of penicillin.

Probenecid is also included in certain regimens that can be completed during one visit to the physician for the treatment and prophylaxis of gonococcal infections (*see* Chapter 46).

Untoward Reactions and Precautions. Probenecid is well tolerated by most patients. Some degree of gastrointestinal irritation is experienced by at least 2% of patients; the incidence is considerably higher after large doses. Caution is advised in administering probenecid to patients with a history of peptic ulcer. Most reports place the incidence of hypersensitivity reactions, usually mild skin rashes, between 2 and 4%. More serious hypersensitivity reactions occur, but they are rare. The nephrotic syndrome has been reported as a toxic reaction. The appearance of a rash during the concurrent administration of probenecid and penicillin G or a congener presents the physician with an awkward diagnostic dilemma. The compound also increases to some degree the concentration of sulfonamide in the blood. Huge overdosage of probenecid results in stimulation of the central nervous system, convulsions, and death from respiratory failure.

SULFINPYRAZONE

History. Despite its therapeutic efficacy as an anti-inflammatory and uricosuric agent, phenylbutazone (*see* Chapter 26) has undesirable side effects severe enough to preclude its continuous use. For this reason, a number of congeners were evaluated for uricosuric and anti-inflammatory activity. One of these, in which a phenylthioethyl configuration replaces the butyl side chain of the parent compound, displayed promising activity. When the metabolites of the new compound were studied, it was found that side chain oxidation *in vivo* led to the formation of the sulfoxide, sulfinpyrazone, which was a potent uricosuric agent (Gutman *et al.,* 1960).

Chemistry. The chemical structure of sulfinpyrazone is as follows:

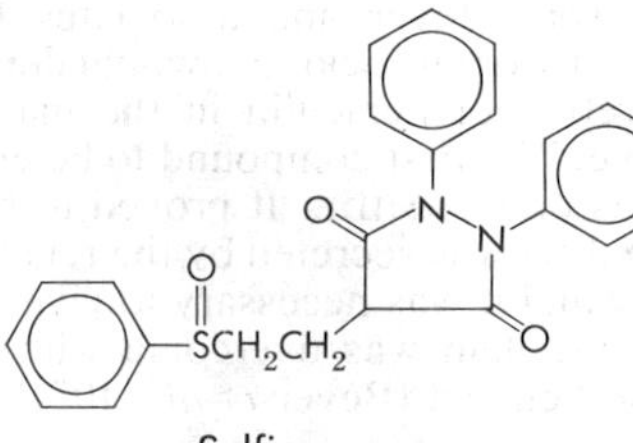

Sulfinpyrazone

It is a strong organic acid (pK_a 2.8) that readily forms soluble salts. Burns and coworkers (1958) studied a number of congeners; they found that a low pK_a and polar side chain substitutions favor uricosuric activity (*see also* Gutman, 1966).

Pharmacological Actions. Sulfinpyrazone in sufficient dosage is a potent inhibitor of the renal tubular reabsorption of uric acid. As with other uricosuric agents, small doses may reduce the excretion of uric acid. Like probenecid, sulfinpyrazone reduces the renal tubular secretion of many other organic anions. The drug may induce hypoglycemia by inhibiting the metabolism of the sulfonylurea oral hypoglycemic agents; hepatic metabolism of warfarin is also impaired. The uricosuric action of sulfinpyrazone is additive to that of probenecid and phenylbutazone but is mutually antagonistic to that of salicylates (Yü *et al.*, 1963).

Sulfinpyrazone lacks the anti-inflammatory and analgesic properties of its congener, phenylbutazone.

Platelet Aggregation. The inhibitory effect of sulfinpyrazone on platelet function is discussed in Chapter 55.

Absorption, Fate, and Excretion. Sulfinpyrazone is well absorbed after oral administration. It is strongly bound to plasma albumin (98 to 99%), and displaces other anionic drugs that have their highest affinity for the same binding site (site I) (Sudlow *et al.*, 1975). The half-life of the drug in plasma after its intravenous injection is about 4 hours. After oral administration, however, its uricosuric effect may persist for as long as 10 hours. Although little sulfinpyrazone is available for filtration at the glomerulus, it is secreted by the proximal tubule and undergoes little passive back diffusion. Approximately half of the orally administered dose appears in the urine within 24 hours. Most of the drug (90%) in the urine is unchanged; the remainder is eliminated as the N^1-*p*-hydroxyphenyl metabolite, which also is a potent uricosuric substance (*see* Gutman *et al.*, 1960; Dayton *et al.*, 1961).

Preparations and Dosage. *Sulfinpyrazone* (ANTURANE, APRAZONE) is available as 100-mg tablets and 200-mg capsules. For the treatment of chronic gout, the initial dosage is 100 to 200 mg given twice daily. After the first week, the dosage may be gradually increased until a satisfactory lowering of plasma uric acid is achieved and maintained. This may require from 200 to 800 mg per day, divided in two to four doses and preferably given with meals or milk; a liberal fluid intake should be maintained. Larger doses are poorly tolerated and unlikely to produce a further uricosuric effect in the resistant patient.

Untoward Reactions and Precautions. Gastrointestinal irritation occurs in 10 to 15% of all patients receiving sulfinpyrazone, and occasionally a patient may require discontinuance of its use. Gastric distress is lessened when the drug is taken in divided doses with meals. Sulfinpyrazone should be given to patients with a history of peptic ulcer only with the greatest caution. Hypersensitivity reactions, usually a rash with fever, do occur, but less frequently than with probenecid. The severe blood dyscrasias and salt and water retention, hazards of phenylbutazone therapy (*see* Chapter 26), have not been observed during sulfinpyrazone therapy. However, depression of hematopoiesis has been demonstrated experimentally, and periodic blood-cell counts are therefore advised during prolonged therapy.

BENZBROMARONE

This is a potent uricosuric agent that is used in Europe. It has the following structural formula:

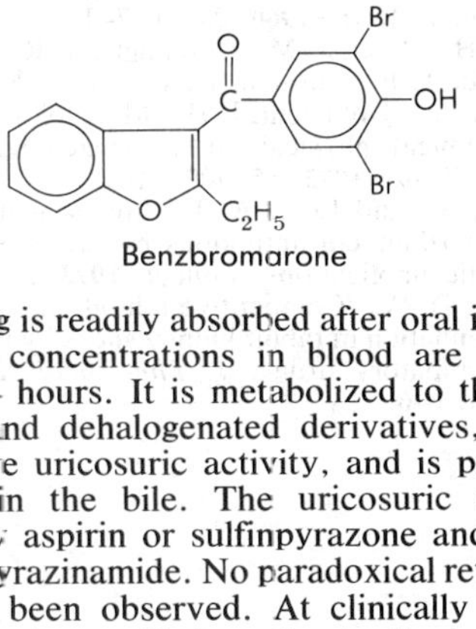

Benzbromarone

The drug is readily absorbed after oral ingestion, and peak concentrations in blood are achieved in about 4 hours. It is metabolized to the monobromine and dehalogenated derivatives, both of which have uricosuric activity, and is principally excreted in the bile. The uricosuric action is blunted by aspirin or sulfinpyrazone and is abolished by pyrazinamide. No paradoxical retention of urate has been observed. At clinically effective doses there is no effect on the synthesis of urate. Therefore, benzbromarone probably reduces the concentration of urate in plasma solely by inhibiting its tubular reabsorption. Its action on the tubular transport of other organic acids has not been systematically examined.

Benzbromarone is of interest as a member of a newer chemical class of uricosuric agents. As the micronized powder it is effective in a single daily dose of 40 to 80 mg, which makes it significantly more potent than other uricosuric drugs. It may be useful clinically in patients who are either allergic or refractory to other drugs used for the treatment of gout (Diamond, 1978).

THE CLINICAL USE OF URICOSURIC AGENTS

This subject is described in Chapter 26 in conjunction with the discussion of other types of drugs that are also used for the treatment of gout and other syndromes characterized by hyperuricemia.

Beyer, K. H.; Russo, H. F.; Tillson, E. K.; Miller, A. K.; Verwey, W. F.; and Gass, S. R. BENEMID, *p*-(di-*n*-propylsulfamyl)-benzoic acid: its renal affinity and its elimination. *Am. J. Physiol.*, **1951**, *166*, 625–640.

Burns, J. J.; Yü, T.-F.; Dayton, P. G.; Berger, L.; Gutman, A. B.; and Brodie, B. B. Relationship between pK_a and uricosuric activity in phenylbutazone analogues. *Nature*, **1958**, *182*, 1162–1163.

Dayton, P. G.; Sicam, L. E.; Landrau, M.; and Burns, J. J. Metabolism of sulfinpyrazone and other thio analogues of phenylbutazone in man. *J. Pharmacol. Exp. Ther.*, **1961**, *132*, 287–390.

Fanelli, G. M., Jr., and Weiner, I. M. Pyrazinoate excretion in the chimpanzee: relation to urate disposition and the actions of uricosuric drugs. *J. Clin. Invest.*, **1973**, *52*, 1946–1957.

———. Urate excretion: drug interactions. *J. Pharmacol. Exp. Ther.*, **1979**, *210*, 186–195.

Guarino, A. M., and Schanker, L. S. Biliary excretion of probenecid and its glucuronide. *J. Pharmacol. Exp. Ther.*, **1968**, *164*, 387–395.

Guggino, S. E.; Martin, G. J.; and Aronson, P. S. Specificity and modes of the anion exchanger in dog renal microvillus membranes. *Am. J. Physiol.*, **1983**, *244*, F612–F621.

Gutman, A. B.; Dayton, P. G.; Yü, T.-F.; Berger, L.; Chen, W.; Sicam, L. E.; and Burns, J. J. A study of the inverse relationship between pK_a and rate of renal excretion of phenylbutazone analogues in man and dogs. *Am. J. Med.*, **1960**, *29*, 1017–1033.

Israeli, Z. H.; Perel, J. M.; Cunningham, R. F.; Dayton, P. G.; Yü, T.-F.; Gutman, A. B.; Long, K. R.; Long, R. C., Jr.; and Goldstein, J. H. Metabolites of probenecid. Chemical, physical, and pharmacological studies. *J. Med. Chem.*, **1972**, *15*, 709–716.

Kenwright, S., and Levi, A. J. Impairment of hepatic uptake of rifamycin antibiotics by probenecid and its therapeutic implications. *Lancet*, **1973**, *2*, 1401–1405.

Nierenberg, D. W. Competitive inhibition of methotrexate accumulation in rabbit kidney slices by nonsteroidal anti-inflammatory drugs. *J. Pharmacol. Exp. Ther.*, **1983**, *226*, 1–6.

Pritchard, J. B. Luminal and peritubular steps in renal transport of p-aminohippurate. *Biochim. Biophys. Acta*, **1987**, *906*, 295–308.

Shimada, H.; Moewes, B.; and Burckhardt, G. Indirect coupling to Na^+ of p-aminohippuric acid uptake into rat renal basolateral membrane vesicles. *Am. J. Physiol.*, **1987**, *253*, F795–F801.

Spector, R., and Lorenzo, A. V. The effects of salicylate and probenecid on the cerebrospinal fluid transport of penicillin, aminosalicylic acid and iodide. *J. Pharmacol. Exp. Ther.*, **1974**, *188*, 55–65.

Sudlow, G.; Birkett, D. J.; and Wade, D. N. The characterization of two specific drug binding sites on human serum albumin. *Mol. Pharmacol.*, **1975**, *11*, 824–832.

Monographs and Reviews

Diamond, H. S. Uricosuric drugs. In, *Uric Acid.* (Kelley, W. N., and Weiner, I. M., eds.) Springer-Verlag, Berlin, **1978**, pp. 459–484.

Emmerson, B. T. Abnormal urate excretion associated with renal and systemic disorders, drugs, and toxins. In, *Uric Acid.* (Kelley, W. N., and Weiner, I. M., eds.) Springer-Verlag, Berlin, **1978**, pp. 287–324.

Gutman, A. B. Uricosuric drugs, with special reference to probenecid and sulfinpyrazone. *Adv. Pharmacol.*, **1966**, *4*, 91–142.

Kahn, A. M., and Weinman, E. J. Urate transport in the proximal tubule: *in vivo* and vesicle studies. *Am. J. Physiol.*, **1985**, *249*, F789–F798.

Møller, J. V., and Sheikh, M. I. The renal organic anion transport system: pharmacological, physiological, and biochemical aspects. *Pharmacol. Rev.*, **1982**, *34*, 315–358.

Rennick, B. R. Renal tubule transport of organic cations. *Am. J. Physiol.*, **1981**, *240*, F83–F89.

Roch-Ramel, F., and Weiner, I. M. Renal excretion of urate: factors determining the actions of drugs. *Kidney Int.*, **1980**, *18*, 665–676.

Ross, C. R., and Holohan, P. D. Transport of organic anions and cations in isolated renal plasma membranes. *Annu. Rev. Pharmacol. Toxicol.*, **1983**, *23*, 65–85.

Van der Poel, F. W.; Van Praag, H. M.; and Korf, J. Evidence for a probenecid-sensitive transport system of acid monoamine metabolites from the spinal subarachnoid space. *Psychopharmacology*, **1977**, *52*, 35–40.

Weiner, I. M.; Blanchard, K. C.; and Mudge, G. H. Factors influencing renal excretion of foreign organic acids. *Am. J. Physiol.*, **1964**, *207*, 953–963.

Yü, T.-F.; Dayton, P. G.; and Gutman, A. B. Mutual suppression of the uricosuric effects of sulfinpyrazone and salicylate: a study in interactions between drugs. *J. Clin. Invest.*, **1963**, *42*, 1330–1339.

SECTION

VII Cardiovascular Drugs

A major pharmacological action of a number of drugs is their ability to alter cardiovascular function; these agents will be considered in this section. Many additional drugs, however, also have a marked influence on the heart and blood vessels; they are described elsewhere in connection with their other important pharmacodynamic properties.

CHAPTER

31 RENIN AND ANGIOTENSIN

James C. Garrison and Michael J. Peach

THE RENIN–ANGIOTENSIN SYSTEM

History. In 1898, Tiegerstedt and Bergman found that crude saline extracts of the kidney contained a pressor principle, which they named *renin*. Their discovery had an obvious bearing on the problem of arterial hypertension and its relation to kidney disease that had been posed by Richard Bright's work some 60 years earlier. However, relatively little interest was generated until 1934, when Goldblatt and his colleagues showed convincingly that it was possible to produce persistent hypertension in dogs by constricting the renal arteries. In 1940, Braun-Menéndez and his colleagues in Argentina and Page and Helmer at the Cleveland Clinic reported that renin was an enzyme that acted on a plasma protein substrate to catalyze the formation of the actual pressor material, a peptide, which was named *hypertensin* by the former group and *angiotonin* by the latter. These two terms persisted for nearly 20 years, until it was agreed to rename the pressor substance *angiotensin* and to call the plasma substrate *angiotensinogen*. In the mid-1950s, two forms of angiotensin were recognized, the first a decapeptide (angiotensin I) and the second an octapeptide (angiotensin II) formed from angiotensin I by enzymatic cleavage by another enzyme, termed *angiotensin converting enzyme*. The octapeptide was shown to be the more active form, and its synthesis in 1957 by Schwyzer and by Bumpus made the material available for intensive study (*see* Page and Bumpus, 1974; Skeggs, 1984).

Further progress came in 1958, when Gross suggested that the renin–angiotensin system was involved in the regulation of aldosterone secretion. It was soon shown that the kidneys are important for such regulation and that synthetic angiotensin, in minute amounts, stimulates the production of aldosterone in man. Moreover, elevated rates of renin secretion were noted upon experimental reduction of Na^+ concentration in plasma (*see* Gross, 1968). Thus, the renin–angiotensin system came to be recognized as a mechanism to stimulate aldosterone synthesis and secretion and an important physiological mechanism in the homeostatic regulation of blood volume and pressure and of the electrolyte composition of body fluids.

In the 1970s, pharmacological agents were introduced that either inhibited the formation of angiotensins or blocked their actions at receptors. These inhibitors have illuminated the homeostatic functions of the renin–angiotensin system and have revealed its important role in the maintenance of elevated blood pressure in hypertensive states of diverse etiology. These findings led to the development of a new and broadly efficacious class of antihypertensive drugs, the inhibitors of angiotensin converting enzyme.

COMPONENTS OF THE RENIN–ANGIOTENSIN SYSTEM

The renin–angiotensin system is an important element of the interrelated mechanisms that regulate hemodynamics and water and electrolyte balance. Factors that lower blood volume, renal perfusion pressure, or the concentration of Na^+ in plasma tend to activate the system, while factors that increase these parameters tend to suppress its function (Figure 31–1).

An overview of the pathways for synthesis and degradation of the angiotensins *in vivo* is shown in Figure 31–2. The process is initiated when the enzyme renin acts on angiotensinogen (renin substrate), an α_2-globulin, to release the decapeptide angiotensin I (angiotensin-[1-10]). This decapeptide is cleaved by angiotensin converting enzyme (ACE) to yield the active angiotensin II (angiotensin-[1-8]octapeptide). This, in turn, undergoes hydrolysis by an aminopeptidase to yield the heptapeptide angiotensin III (angiotensin-[2-8]heptapeptide), which is also active. Further cleavage yields peptides with little activity. In an alternative (minor) path, converting enzyme and aminopeptidase act in the opposite sequence such that the decapeptide, angiotensin I, is hydrolyzed first to [des-Asp^1] angiotensin I, which, like the parent compound, has limited activity. It is then cleaved by converting enzyme to form angiotensin III (*see* Skeggs, 1984).

Renin. The rate-limiting factor in the production of the dominant hormone of the system, angiotensin II, is the amount of renin in the plasma. The main source of renin is the kidney. It is synthesized, stored, and secreted into the renal arterial circulation by the granular juxtaglomerular cells that lie in the walls of the afferent arterioles as they enter the glomeruli. Renin and the other components of the renin–angiotensin system are also found in the central nervous system (CNS) (*see* below).

Human renin is an aspartyl protease that attacks only a restricted number of substrates. Its principal natural substrate is a circulating α_2-globulin, angiotensinogen (*see* below). Renin cleaves the bond between residues 10 and 11 at the amino terminus of this protein to generate angiotensin I (*see* Figure 31–2). The active form of renin is a glycoprotein that contains 340 amino acids. It is synthesized as a preproenzyme of 406 amino acid residues that is processed to prorenin, a mature but inactive form of the protein. Prorenin is finally activated by an as yet uncharacterized protease that removes 46 amino acid residues from its amino terminus. A gene that encodes renin has been cloned, and the recombinant human enzyme has been crystallized and studied by X-ray diffraction. It is similar to other aspartyl proteases, in that it has a bilobal structure with a cleft that forms the active site (*see* Imai *et al.*, 1983; Inagami, 1989; Sielecki *et al.*, 1989). Knowledge of the properties of the protein is being exploited for the development of novel renin inhibitors (*see* below).

Renin and prorenin are both stored in the juxtaglomerular cells and circulate in the blood; the concentration of prorenin in the circulation is about tenfold greater than that of the active enzyme. The half-life of circulating renin is about 15 minutes. The physiological status of circulating prorenin is uncertain. Closely related forms of renin (isorenin) are synthesized in some other tissues. The mouse submaxillary gland is extraordinarily rich in renin and prorenin, and study of this tissue has provided critical information about their structures and processing (*see* Corvol *et al.*, 1983).

Control of Renin Secretion. The secretion of renin from juxtaglomerular cells is

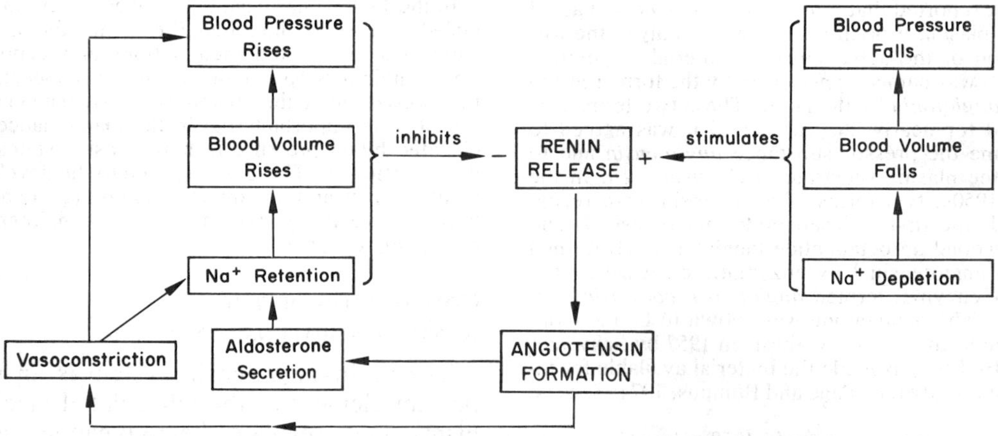

Figure 31–1. *A schematic portrayal of the homeostatic roles of the renin–angiotensin system.*

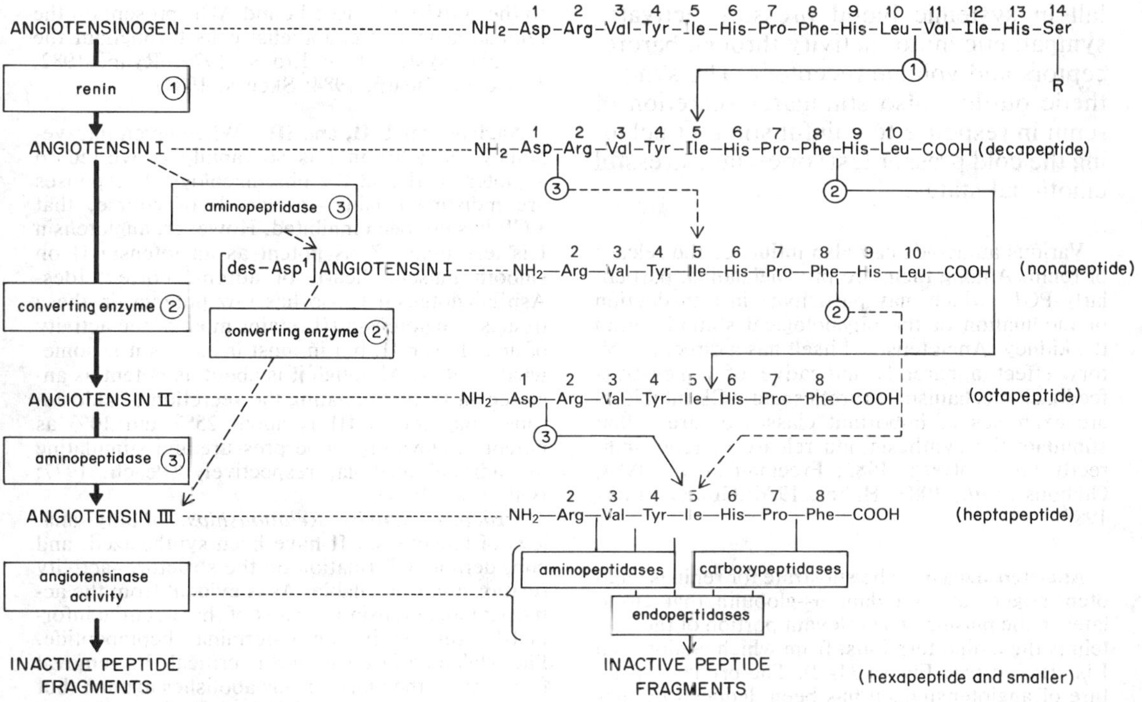

Figure 31–2. *Formation and destruction of angiotensin.*

The left-hand scheme is complemented by the diagram on the right of structures and sites of enzymatic cleavage (the numbers within circles correspond to those assigned to the enzymes within the boxes). The solid arrows show the classic paths, while the dashed arrows indicate an alternative (minor) path. The structures of the angiotensins shown are those found in man, horse, rat, and pig; the bovine form has valine in the 5 position. The sequence of human angiotensinogen is depicted (Tewksbury *et al.*, 1981; Imai *et al.*, 1983).

controlled by three mechanisms—two acting locally within the kidney and the third acting through the CNS and mediated by norepinephrine released from sympathetic nerves (*see* Figure 31–1).

The first intrarenal mechanism is mechanical; factors that tend to lower renal perfusion pressure increase the secretion of renin. These include a fall in systemic blood pressure from any cause, such as diminished cardiac output, lowered total peripheral resistance, or reduction in blood volume through hemorrhage or a deficiency of Na^+; local vascular effects, such as renal arterial or aortic stenosis, can also augment secretion. The immediate stimulus to secretion is believed to be reduction in the tension within the wall of the glomerular afferent arterial vessel.

The second intrarenal mechanism is ionic; reduction of Na^+ concentration in the early distal tubule stimulates the secretion of renin. This effect is not exerted directly on the juxtaglomerular cells but is apparently mediated by events in the renal tubule of the same glomerulus, particularly the macula densa region located at the site where the distal tubule descends past the afferent and efferent arterioles. It is believed that the macula densa monitors the ionic environment of the tubular fluid and relays to the juxtaglomerular cells the stimulus for secretion. The macula densa cells abut the juxtaglomerular cells and constitute with the latter (and some other specialized cells) the juxtaglomerular apparatus.

The third mechanism is mediated by the release of norepinephrine from postganglionic sympathetic nerve terminals; activation of β_1-adrenergic receptors on juxtaglomerular cells enhances renin secretion. The sympathetic innervation conveys the neural influences on renin secretion that are determined by reflex and other factors. Thus, a fall in systemic blood pressure activates sympathetic motor activity through baroreceptors and volume receptors. The sympathetic outflow also stimulates secretion of renin in response to painful stimuli (including the cold pressor test) or certain stressful emotional states.

Various autacoids can also influence the release of renin. Among them are prostaglandins, particularly PGI_2, which may participate in transduction or modulation of the physiological stimuli within the kidney. Angiotensin II itself has a direct inhibitory effect apparently indicative of a negative-feedback mechanism. Diuretics and ACE inhibitors are examples of important classes of drugs that stimulate the synthesis and release of renin indirectly (*see* Torretti, 1982; Freeman *et al.*, 1984; Gibbons *et al.*, 1984; Haber, 1986; Gomez *et al.*, 1988).

Angiotensinogen. The substrate for renin is angiotensinogen, an abundant α_2-globulin that circulates in the plasma. The relevant portion of the protein is the amino terminus, from which angiotensin I is cleaved (*see* Figure 31–2). The primary structure of angiotensinogen has been deduced by molecular cloning (Kageyama *et al.*, 1984). Angiotensinogen is synthesized primarily in the liver, although messenger RNA that encodes the protein is also abundant in fat, certain regions of the CNS, and kidney (*see* Campbell and Habener, 1986; Cassis *et al.*, 1988). Angiotensinogen is continuously synthesized and secreted by the liver, and its synthesis is stimulated by a number of hormones, including glucocorticoids, thyroid hormone, and angiotensin II itself (*see* Dzau and Herrmann, 1982; Ben-Ari and Garrison, 1988). Nevertheless, the concentration of angiotensinogen in plasma does not limit the rate of synthesis of angiotensin II.

Angiotensin Converting Enzyme (ACE; Kininase II; Dipeptidyl Carboxypeptidase). This enzyme was discovered serendipitously, in plasma, as the factor responsible for conversion of angiotensin I into angiotensin II (*see* Skeggs, 1984). Human ACE is a large protein, containing 1278 amino acid residues. It appears to have two homologous domains, each with a catalytic site and a region for binding Zn^{2+} (Soubrier *et al.*, 1988; Bernstein *et al.*, 1989). The enzyme is rather nonspecific and cleaves dipeptide units from substrates with diverse amino acid sequences. Preferred substrates have only one free carboxyl group in the carboxyl-terminal amino acid, and proline must not be the penultimate amino acid; thus the enzyme does not degrade angiotensin II. Bradykinin is one of the many natural substrates for ACE, and the enzyme is the same as that designated kininase II, which inactivates bradykinin and other potent vasodilator peptides (*see* Chapter 23). Although slow conversion of angiotensin I to angiotensin II occurs in plasma, the very rapid metabolism that occurs *in vivo* is due largely to the activity of tissue-bound ACE present on the luminal aspect of endothelial cells throughout the vascular system (*see* Erdös, 1979; Ryan, 1982; Doyle and Bearn, 1984; Skeggs, 1984).

Angiotensins I, II, and III. When given intravenously, angiotensin I is so rapidly converted to angiotensin II that the pharmacological responses are indistinguishable—provided, of course, that ACE has not been inhibited. However, angiotensin I is less than 1% as potent as angiotensin II on smooth muscle, heart, or adrenal cortex; [des-Asp^1]angiotensin I also has low potency in these tissues. Angiotensin III retains most of the activity of angiotensin II, but in most instances it is somewhat weaker. Although it is about as potent as angiotensin II in stimulating the secretion of aldosterone, angiotensin III is about 25% and 10% as potent in elevating blood pressure and stimulating the adrenal medulla, respectively (Peach, 1977; Bell *et al.*, 1984).

Structure–Activity Relationships. Many analogs of angiotensin II have been synthesized, and considerable information on the structure–activity relationship is available. As is evident from the activity of angiotensin III, most of the essential information resides in the C-terminal heptapeptide. Phenylalanine in position 8 is critical. Its removal from any of the angiotensins abolishes agonist (but not necessarily antagonist) activity in peripheral tissues. Des-phe^8-angiotensin II is active in the CNS, however, where it is as potent as angiotensin in stimulating the secretion of antidiuretic hormone (ADH), but it has no pressor or dipsogenic actions (Schiavone *et al.*, 1988). The other aromatic residues in positions 4 and 6, the guanido group in position 2, and the C-terminal carboxyl are thought to be involved in binding to the receptor site. Position 1 is not critical (thus the efficacy of angiotensin III), but replacement of aspartic acid in position 1 with sarcosine (N-methylglycine) enhances binding and slows hydrolysis by rendering the peptide refractory to an important subgroup of aminopeptidases that are specific for aspartic or glutamic acid ("Asp-aminopeptidase"; "angiotensinase A"). Such a substitution, combined with that of alanine or isoleucine in place of phenylalanine in position 8, yields potent angiotensin II antagonists; saralasin (Sar^1-Ala^8-angiotensin II) is an example (*see* below). (*See* Page and Bumpus, 1974; Regoli *et al.*, 1974; Bumpus, 1977.)

Angiotensinases. This term is applied to various peptidases that are involved in the degradation and inactivation of angiotensin II; none is specific. Among them are aminopeptidases, the activity of which may also contribute to the formation of active angiotensins. One aminopeptidase—Asp-aminopeptidase, or angiotensinase A—is specific for aspartic (or glutamic) acid, and its action terminates with the formation of the [des-Asp^1] compounds. In some tissues a considerable portion of angiotensin I is converted to [des-Asp^1]angiotensin I; in the adrenal gland the fraction is as large as one half. These and other reactions are shown in Figure 31–2.

FUNCTIONS OF THE RENIN–ANGIOTENSIN SYSTEM

The renin–angiotensin system plays a major role in the regulation of fluid and electrolyte balance, blood pressure, and blood volume via its circulating hormone, angiotensin II. The primary effects of angiotensin II are to stimulate the synthesis and secretion of aldosterone by the adrenal cortex and to raise blood pressure via direct constriction of the smooth muscle of the arterioles. However, the hormone has numerous other effects, including stimulation of the heart and the sympathetic nervous system; these effects complement the direct vascular effects and contribute to the increase in blood pressure caused by angiotensin. Effects in the CNS, such as stimulation of water consumption and increased secretion of ADH, complement the actions of aldosterone and contribute to positive fluid balance.

Adrenal Cortex. The renin–angiotensin–aldosterone axis is an important element in the regulation of Na^+ balance. Angiotensin stimulates the zona glomerulosa of the adrenal cortex to increase the synthesis and secretion of aldosterone, and it exerts trophic and permissive influences that augment other stimuli (*e.g.*, hormonal or ionic). Increased output of aldosterone is elicited by very low concentrations of angiotensin that have little or no effect on blood pressure. Aldosterone, in turn, acts on the distal tubule and collecting duct in the kidney to cause retention of Na^+ and excretion of K^+ and H^+. The stimulant effect of angiotensin on the synthesis and release of aldosterone is enhanced under conditions of hyponatremia or hyperkalemia and is reduced when concentrations of these cations in plasma are altered in the opposite direction. Such changes in sensitivity are believed to be due to alterations of the number of receptors for angiotensin on the zona glomerulosa cells as well as to adrenocortical hyperplasia in the Na^+-depleted state (*see* Davis and Freeman, 1976; Bell *et al.*, 1984).

Kidney. Angiotensin II has three effects on renal function other than its indirect effects mediated by aldosterone. Angiotensin influences urine formation by (1) constricting the arterioles surrounding the glomerulus; (2) decreasing the permeability of the filtration apparatus; and (3) stimulating Na^+/H^+ exchange in the proximal tubule. Both the rise in systemic blood pressure, which increases renal perfusion pressure, and the vasoconstrictor effect on efferent glomerular arterioles tend to enhance glomerular filtration. Vasoconstriction of the afferent arterioles has the opposite effect, as does the action of angiotensin on the glomerular capillaries, where a contractile response of mesangial cells (and possibly endothelial cells) shrinks the structure and reduces the surface area available for filtration, thus lowering the permeability coefficient. The outcome of these opposing effects depends on the concentration of angiotensin and the status of the circulatory and renal systems. In healthy man, the typical response to an elevation in the concentration of angiotensin is antidiuresis and antinatriuresis, accompanied by reduced rates of effective renal plasma flow and glomerular filtration. However, certain hypertensive individuals and patients with hepatic cirrhosis and ascites or other cardiovascular–renal deficiencies (where the renin–angiotensin system is already activated) respond to a further increase in angiotensin with diuresis and natriuresis (*see* Symposium, 1983a, 1984; Ménard *et al.*, 1984). Angiotensin can also enhance bicarbonate reabsorption in the early proximal tubule of the rat. Approximately 20 to 30% of the bicarbonate handled by the nephron may be affected by this mechanism (Liu and Cogan, 1987).

Peripheral Autonomic Nervous System. In addition to central enhancement of sympathetic outflow, angiotensin facilitates peripheral sympathetic transmission, both by augmenting the output of norepinephrine from the nerve terminals and by amplifying the responses of effector cells to the neurotransmitter (*see* Peach, 1986, 1988). High concentrations of the peptide stimulate ganglion cells directly.

Adrenal Medulla. Angiotensin stimulates the release of catecholamines from the adrenal medulla by depolarizing the chromaffin cells. Although this response is of little importance physiologically, intense and dangerous responses have followed the administration of angiotensin to individuals with pheochromocytoma.

Cardiovascular System. Stimulation of the cardiovascular system by angiotensin involves a constellation of effects, among which are direct stimulation of vascular and cardiac muscle, facilitation of sympathetic transmission in the periphery, and stimulation of central sympathetic outflow. Moreover, reflex responses, especially those involving baroreceptors, may obtund or mask the primary ability of angiotensin to generate a strong pressor response.

Blood Vessels. Angiotensin constricts precapillary arterioles and, to a lesser but significant extent, postcapillary venules. The peptide has a direct action on vascular smooth muscle; this is augmented by facilitation of the activity of the sympathetic nervous system. In man, the direct action seems to account for most of the increase in total peripheral resistance; however, in certain vascular beds, such as those of the hand and the foot, vasoconstriction has a large sympathetic component, since it is much reduced by α-adrenergic antagonists.

The vasoconstrictor effect of angiotensin is strongest in the vessels of the skin, splanchnic region, and kidney; blood flow in these regions falls sharply following an increase in the plasma concentration of angiotensin. The effect is less in the vessels of the brain and still weaker in the lung and skeletal muscle. In these regions blood flow may actually increase, especially following small changes in the concentration of the peptide, because the relatively weak vasoconstrictor response is opposed by the elevated systemic blood pressure. Nevertheless, with high circulating concentrations of angiotensin cerebral blood flow tends to fall and coronary insufficiency may occur.

Heart. Angiotensin increases the entry of Ca^{2+} via voltage-sensitive channels during the plateau phase of the action potential in atrial and ventricular myocytes. This action prolongs the plateau phase and increases the force of contraction. Angiotensin has no direct effect on heart rate; however, by increasing systemic blood pressure and baroreceptor discharge, it may initiate reflex vagal activity sufficient to slow the heart and raise end-diastolic pressure. The decrease in heart rate and cardiac output may be less than expected from the increase in blood pressure because the peptide tends to increase heart rate and force of contraction by its facilitatory actions on sympathetic outflow. The rise in central venous pressure is generally modest, since angiotensin has a comparatively feeble constrictor effect on the larger veins and hence reduces venous capacity much less than does, for example, norepinephrine. As a result of these various factors cardiac output generally falls. Despite this, the work of the heart often increases as a result of the elevated systemic blood pressure and increased mechanical load, and this may contribute to coronary insufficiency.

Blood Pressure. Modest changes in plasma concentrations of angiotensin increase blood pressure as a result of the direct cardiovascular actions of the peptide; these actions may account, at least in part, for the role of the renin–angiotensin system in hypertension (*see* below). On a molar basis, angiotensin II is about 40 times more potent than norepinephrine. When a single moderate dose is injected intravenously, systemic blood pressure begins to rise within about 10 seconds, rapidly reaches maximum, and returns to normal within a few minutes. When the drug is infused continuously, blood pressure is maintained at an elevated level for hours or days. Indeed, with such infusion the effectiveness of angiotensin may even increase with time; infusions that are initially without observable effect may cause hypertension if continued for days. Angiotensin commonly causes a moderate rise in pulmonary arterial pressure that is due less, perhaps, to its feeble pulmonary vasoconstrictor action than to an increase of pressure in the pulmonary vein as end-diastolic pressure rises.

Involvement in Regulation of Blood Pressure. As indicated in Figure 31–1, factors that lower blood pressure or volume tend to stimulate renin secretion, while factors that raise blood pressure or volume have the opposite effect. The renin–angiotensin system is thus one of the many layers of physiological controls of systemic blood pressure. Blockade of the system has minor effects on the blood pressure of normal, Na^+-replete individuals. However, normotensive subjects who have been depleted of Na^+ by diet or diuretics experience a consistent decrease in blood pressure when treated with an inhibitor of renin or ACE or an antagonist of angiotensin II. Physiological stimuli may act through the baroreceptor reflex mechanism to stimulate secretion of renin. Stronger pathophysiological stimuli, such as hemorrhage, recruit additional local renal mechanisms for stimulation of renin secretion. The combination of sympathetically mediated stimuli and intrarenal mechanisms produces a synergistic effect.

The renin–angiotensin system contributes to hypertension of diverse etiologies. The role of angiotensin II in supporting blood pressure is most clearly understood in patients with malignant hypertension or with hypertension resulting from stenosis of the renal artery, where plasma renin activity (PRA) is usually elevated (*see* Symposium, 1983a; Laragh, 1984). Inhibitors of the renin–angiotensin system (receptor antagonists or ACE inhibitors) commonly cause a marked fall in blood pressure in such individuals (*see* below). However, there is no simple relationship between excess secretion of renin (as reflected by PRA) and blood pressure in the large population of individuals with essential hypertension. Indeed, most patients with hypertension do not have high PRA; PRA and plasma concentrations of angiotensin II are distributed through the same broad range of values that are found in normotensive individuals, and about 25% of hypertensive patients have a value for PRA below that expected from their daily intake of Na^+ (*see* Laragh, 1984). Although this finding might suggest that the renin–angiotensin system plays only a limited role in the etiology of hypertension, the fact that ACE inhibitors lower blood pressure in a large fraction of hypertensive patients with normal PRA indicates that the renin–angiotensin system is supporting the blood pressure in these individuals. Although the mechanisms underlying these findings have yet to be clarified, these observations tend to dispel the notion that the renin–angiotensin system is involved in elevating blood pressure only in those with frank renal disease. Thus, inhibitors of ACE are an important and useful class of antihypertensive agents (*see* below).

Extravascular Smooth Muscle. Effects of angiotensin on smooth muscle other than that in blood vessels are generally weak, but contractions are readily elicited in preparations such as guinea pig ileum and rat uterus *in vitro*. Besides direct stimulation of the smooth muscle cells, angiotensin can elicit indirect effects—contraction or relaxation—by exciting cholinergic or adrenergic ganglion cells or nerve endings.

Central Nervous System. The brain contains all the components of a renin–angiotensin system wholly independent of the peripheral system. Moreover, histochemical methods have revealed angiotensin-like immunoreactivity at many sites within the CNS. This suggests the possibility that angiotensin II serves as a neurotransmitter or modulator. In addition, angiotensin II formed in the vascular system gains access to those specialized periventricular regions of the brain that lack the blood–brain barrier and elicits a variety of responses (*see* Fitzsimons, 1980; Ferrario, 1983; Ganong, 1984).

Central Sympathetic Stimulation. Small amounts of angiotensin infused into the vertebral arteries cause a sustained rise in systemic blood pressure. This effect is mediated by increased sympathetic outflow and is due to effects of the hormone in the area postrema.

Drinking and Hydration. Angiotensin has a centrally mediated dipsogenic effect that can be observed following intravenous injection as well as after injection of the peptide into the third ventricle or surrounding areas. The concentrations of angiotensin II that elicit this effect are within the range observed during mild depletion of Na^+. The preoptic region and subfornical organ are particularly sensitive. Hunger for food is suppressed in favor of drinking (*see* Fitzsimons, 1980; Elfont and Fitzsimons, 1983).

Secretion of ADH. Angiotensin increases activity in supraoptic neurons when injected into the brain or third ventricle and induces secretion of ADH. It also enhances release of ADH from the neurohypophysis *in vitro*. Increased secretion of ADH has been noted less consistently after intravenous injections (*see* Ganong, 1984).

Mechanism of Angiotensin Action. The effects of angiotensin are exerted through specific receptors on cell surfaces, which can be blocked selectively by peptide and nonpeptide antagonists (*see* below). Angiotensin II receptors are coupled to effector systems via guanine nucleotide–binding regulatory proteins (G proteins) (*see* Guillemette *et al.*, 1986; Peach, 1986). Depending on the tissue, the effector systems include adenylyl cyclase (which is inhibited) or a phospholipase C (which is stimulated). Clear evidence for distinct types of receptors that are coupled to different effector systems is lacking but would hardly be surprising. In most cells, stimulation of angiotensin II receptors leads to the hydrolysis of phosphatidylinositol 4,5-bisphosphate, with generation of inositol-1,4,5-trisphosphate and diacylglycerol as second messengers (*see* Chapter 2). The resulting increase in the intracellular concentration of Ca^{2+} and activation of Ca^{2+}/calmodulin-dependent myosin light-chain kinase appear to account for the capacity of angiotensin II to contract smooth muscle (*see* Kamm and Stull, 1985; Griendling and Alexander, 1990). In the adrenal cortex, where angiotensin II stimulates the synthesis of aldosterone, the exact role of Ca^{2+}-dependent protein kinases is unclear (*see* Quinn and Williams, 1988; Barrett *et al.*, 1989).

Angiotensin II activates phospholipases other than phospholipase C. Stimulation of phospholipase A_2 leads to increased synthesis of eicosanoids, which may mediate some of the effects of angiotensin II in the kidney. In the adrenal, liver, and kidney, the peptide inhibits adenylyl cyclase, especially if the enzyme is activated by other hormones or neurotransmitters (*see* Peach, 1986). Angiotensin II also depolarizes cells in the adrenal medulla and sympathetic ganglia. In cardiac cells, angiotensin II prolongs the plateau phase of the action potential that is caused by opening of voltage-sensitive Ca^{2+} channels. In these cases depolarization leads to an increased influx of Ca^{2+}, which presumably augments the release of catecholamines from the adrenal medulla and neurotransmitters from ganglion cells; it may also account for some of the peptide's positive inotropic effect in cardiac tissue (*see* Peach, 1988).

CLINICAL CONSIDERATIONS

Angiotensin itself is of limited therapeutic utility, and most clinical interest focuses on inhibitors of renin and ACE. Nevertheless, the peptide has occasionally been used as an alternative to sympathomimetic amines, where its unique properties offer some advantage—for example, in hypotensive crises encountered during the administration of halogenated anesthetics, where catecholamine-induced cardiac arrhythmias are a potential hazard. With the advent of drugs that inhibit endogenous formation of angiotensin II and precipitate grave hypotension in some patients, the use of angiotensin as an antidote may increase.

The pressor effects of angiotensin are well sustained and are unlikely to be accompanied by disturbing cardiac arrhythmias or to be followed by hypotension. Moreover, the peptide does not cause spasm of the vein into which it is infused. However, neither does it significantly constrict the capacitance vessels, increase venous return, or stimulate cardiac output. Too-rapid infusion of angiotensin may raise systemic blood pressure to dangerous heights. Profound reflex bradycardia and, occasionally, ventricular escape rhythms may occur.

Preparation. *Angiotensin amide* (HYPERTENSIN), the amide of angiotensin II (1-L-asparaginyl-5-L-valyl angiotensin octapeptide), is the preparation that has been used clinically. It is not available commercially in the United States. The drug is given slowly by intravenous infusion at a rate of about 0.01 to 0.2 μg/kg per minute. Blood pressure must be monitored closely.

INHIBITORS OF THE RENIN–ANGIOTENSIN SYSTEM

Two classes of effective inhibitors of the renin–angiotensin system have been identified: angiotensin II antagonists, which block receptors for the peptide, and angiotensin converting enzyme inhibitors, which slow the rate of formation of angiotensin II. Drugs of the latter type, exemplified by captopril, have proven to be effective in a surprisingly broad range of patients with essential hypertension, as well as in those with renovascular hypertension. This finding, in turn, has heightened interest in alternative approaches to inhibition of the renin–angiotensin system. Some recent experimental results with inhibitors of renin appear promising (*see* below). Moreover, inhibition of the secretion of renin from the juxtaglomerular cells contributes to the antihypertensive effects of β-adrenergic antagonists and other inhibitors of sympathetic function (*see* Chapters 11 and 33).

ANTAGONISTS OF ANGIOTENSIN II

Most antagonists of angiotensin II are slightly modified congeners in which agonist activity is profoundly attenuated by replacement of phenylalanine in position 8 with some other amino acid; in addition, stability is enhanced by substitutions that slow degradation and thus prolong the life of a given compound in the circulation. The best studied of these molecules combines alanine in position 8 with sarcosine (N-methylglycine) in position 1; the "blocked" amino acid sarcosine not only slows degradation of the peptide but also increases its affinity for the receptor. This substance—[Sar^1, Val^5, Ala^8]angiotensin-(1-8)octapeptide, or saralasin—was introduced by Pals and associates in 1971, who showed that it effectively antagonized the pressor effects of angiotensin II in rats and lowered blood pressure in renin-dependent hypertensive animals. The possible clinical utility of saralasin and other inhibitors of the renin–angiotensin system became apparent when saralasin was shown not only to block pressor responses to injected angiotensin but also to lower blood pressure in certain renin-dependent hypertensive patients and even in normal subjects who were depleted of Na^+ (*see* Atlas *et al.*, 1983; Laragh, 1984).

A series of carboxybenzyl–chloroimidazole compounds have recently been described that are also competitive antagonists of angiotensin II (*see* Wong *et al.*, 1989). The most potent compound, EXP 6803, has high affinity and selectivity for angiotensin II receptors and decreases blood pressure in models of renovascular hypertension. This group of compounds offers hope for the development of orally effective compounds that block the actions of angiotensin.

Pharmacological Properties. Saralasin and related analogs with aliphatic carboxyl-terminal substitutions compete with angiotensin II for its receptors. In the absence of angiotensin II, these analogs are weak partial agonists (*see* Bumpus, 1977; Peach, 1986). When given by intravenous infusion to healthy individuals or to patients with hypertension, saralasin commonly causes a transient rise in blood pressure that lasts for 1 to 2 minutes; its action then evolves in different ways, depending largely on the concentration of endogenous angiotensin II. In the normal, Na^+-replete individual, the pressor response tends to be relatively well sustained. In the Na^+-depleted individual, the increase in blood pressure is transient and there may be a depressor phase. In individuals with hypertension, there is a correspondence between the dependency of the condition on renin and the response. Thus, saralasin commonly causes a fall in systemic blood pressure in patients with renovascular hypertension, whereas sharp, sustained pressor responses may be encountered in patients with so-called low-renin essential hypertension and hyperaldosteronism. In the past, saralasin was used as an aid in the differential diagnosis of hypertension and in the assessment of renovascular hypertension that might be corrected by surgery. However, because the blood pressure responses were complicated by the residual agonist activity of the compound and were subject to Na^+ balance and other variables, false-positive and false-negative results were so common that the drug is no longer used clinically. A better index of the participation of renin in hypertensive states is provided by inhibitors of converting enzyme (*see* Laragh, 1984).

INHIBITORS OF ANGIOTENSIN CONVERTING ENZYME

History. In the 1960s, Ferreira and colleagues found that the venoms of pit vipers contain factors that intensify responses to bradykinin. These bradykinin potentiating factors (BPFs) proved to be a family of peptides of 5 to 13 amino acid residues that were shown to inhibit an enzyme that catalyzes the degradation and inactivation of bradykinin (now known as kininase II). Erdös and associates established that angiotensin converting enzyme and kininase II are one and the same enzyme: a peptidyl dipeptidase (or dipeptidyl carboxypeptidase). Thus, a single enzyme catalyzes both the synthesis of angiotensin II, a potent pressor substance, and the destruction of bradykinin, a potent vasodilator.

Following the discovery of the BPFs, the nonapeptide $BPF_{9\alpha}$ (teprotide) was synthesized and tested in man. It was found to lower blood pressure in many patients with essential hypertension more consistently than did the angiotensin II antagonists. Teprotide also exerted beneficial effects in patients with heart failure. These important observations encouraged the search for compounds that, in contrast to peptides, would be effective orally.

The orally effective converting enzyme inhibitor captopril (Cushman *et al.*, 1977) was developed by a rational approach that involved analysis of the inhibitory action of teprotide; inferences about the action of converting enzyme on its substrates; and analogy with carboxypeptidase A, which was known to be inhibited by D-benzylsuccinic acid. Ondetti and Cushman and their colleagues argued that inhibition of converting enzyme might be produced by succinyl amino acids that corresponded in length to the dipeptide cleaved by converting enzyme. This hypothesis proved to be true and led ultimately to the synthesis of a series of carboxy alkanoyl or mercapto alkanoyl derivatives that acted as potent competitive inhibitors of the enzyme (*see* Petrillo and Ondetti, 1982). Most active (with a K_i of 1.7 nM) was D-3-mercapto-methylpropanoyl-L-proline or captopril (*see* below).

Pharmacological Effects of ACE Inhibition. The essential effect of these agents on the renin–angiotensin system is to inhibit conversion of the relatively inactive angiotensin I to the active angiotensin II (or the conversion of [des-Asp[1]]angiotensin I to angiotensin III). In this way they attenuate or abolish responses to angiotensin I, but not to angiotensin II.

The converting enzyme inhibitors are highly specific drugs. They do not interact, directly, with other components of the renin–angiotensin system. Although they inhibit the degradation of bradykinin and potentiate its hypotensive action, the principal pharmacological and clinical effects of ACE inhibitors seem to arise from suppression of synthesis of angiotensin II. Nevertheless, it must be remembered that these inhibitors, albeit quite specific at the level of the enzyme, act on an enzyme with many substrates. In addition, recent evidence suggests that ACE inhibitors may also affect other enzymes, including those involved in the generation of prostaglandins (*see* Zusman, 1987). (*See* Antonaccio, 1982; Romankiewicz *et al.*, 1983; Doyle and Bearn, 1984; Symposium, 1984; Frohlich, 1989.)

Cardiovascular System. In healthy, Na^+-replete animals and man, a single oral dose of an ACE inhibitor has little or no effect on supine or erect systemic blood pressure (Atlas *et al.*, 1983). Repeated doses over a period of several days, however, cause a small, consistent reduction in blood pressure and a subtle blunting of compensatory postural reflexes. By contrast, even a single dose of these inhibitors lowers blood pressure substantially in normal subjects when they have been depleted of Na^+. This effect is accompanied by a clear fall in total peripheral resistance and reflects the activation of the renin–

angiotensin system by restriction of dietary Na^+.

Effects in Hypertension. Inhibition of ACE lowers systemic arteriolar resistance and mean, diastolic, and systolic blood pressures in various hypertensive states. The effects are readily observed in animal models of renal or genetic hypertension. In human subjects with hypertension (with the exception of that due to primary aldosteronism), ACE inhibitors commonly lower blood pressure. The initial change in blood pressure tends to be positively correlated with PRA and angiotensin II concentrations prior to treatment. However, as treatment is continued, a greater number of patients show a sizable reduction in blood pressure, and the antihypertensive effect then correlates poorly or not at all with pretreatment values of PRA. This result, which is as yet little understood, presents a challenge to current understanding of the mechanisms of hypertension. At the same time it confers on drugs of this class a welcome breadth of clinical utility as antihypertensive agents.

The fall in systemic blood pressure observed in hypertensive individuals treated with ACE inhibitors results from a reduction of total peripheral resistance in which there seems to be a somewhat variable participation by different vascular beds. The kidney is a notable exception to this variability, in that there is a prominent vasodilator effect and increased blood flow is a relatively constant finding (*see* Symposium, 1984). This is perhaps not surprising, since the renal vessels are exceptionally sensitive to the vasoconstrictor actions of angiotensin II. Increased renal flow occurs without an increase in glomerular filtration rate; in fact, the filtration fraction is reduced. Both the afferent and efferent arterioles are dilated, and the hydrostatic pressure in the glomerulus does not change (Frohlich, 1989). Blood flow in cerebral and coronary beds, where autoregulatory phenomena are prominent, is generally well maintained.

Besides causing systemic arteriolar dilatation, ACE inhibitors increase the compliance of large arteries, which contributes to a reduction of systolic pressure. Cardiac function in patients with uncomplicated hypertension is generally little changed, although stroke volume and cardiac output may increase slightly with sustained treatment. Baroreceptor function and cardiovascular reflexes are not compromised, and responses to postural changes and exercise are little impaired. Yet surprisingly, even when a substantial lowering of blood pressure is achieved, heart rate and concentrations of catecholamines in plasma generally increase only slightly, if at all. This perhaps reflects an alteration of baroreceptor function with increased arterial compliance and the loss of the normal tonic influence of angiotensin II on the sympathetic nervous system.

Secretion of aldosterone in the general population of hypertensive individuals is reduced, but not seriously impaired, by inhibition of converting enzyme. The stimulation that results from postural changes, in which angiotensin plays a prominent role, is attenuated. However, aldosterone output is maintained at adequate levels by other stimuli of steroidogenesis, such as adrenocorticotropic hormone (ACTH) and K^+. The activity of these secretagogues on the zona glomerulosa of the adrenal cortex requires, at most, only very small trophic or permissive amounts of angiotensin II, which are always present because inhibition of converting enzyme is never complete. Excessive retention of K^+ is encountered only in patients taking supplemental K^+ or a K^+-sparing diuretic.

Effects in Chronic Congestive Heart Failure. This condition presents a complex pathophysiological profile (*see* Chapter 34). Inhibition of converting enzyme commonly reduces afterload, and both cardiac output and cardiac index increase, as do indices of stroke work and stroke volume. Heart rate generally is reduced. Systemic blood pressure falls, sometimes steeply at the outset, but tends to return toward initial levels. Renovascular resistance falls sharply, and renal blood flow increases. Natriuresis occurs as a result of the improved renal hemodynamics and the reduced stimulus to secretion of aldosterone by angiotensin II. The excess volume of body fluids contracts, which reduces venous return to the right heart. A further reduction results from venodilatation and an increased capacity of the venous bed.

Venodilatation is another somewhat unexpected effect of inhibition of converting enzyme, for angiotensin II has little acute venoconstrictor activity. Nevertheless, long-term infusion of angiotensin II has been reported to increase venous tone *in vivo,* perhaps by some central or peripheral interaction with the sympathetic nervous system (*see* Schwartz and Chatterjee, 1983; Johns and Ayers, 1984). The response to the converting enzyme inhibitor also involves reductions of pulmonary arterial pressure, pulmonary capillary wedge pressure, and left atrial and left ventricular filling pressures (preload). The better hemodynamic performance results in increased tolerance of exercise. Cerebral and coronary blood flows usually are well maintained, even when systemic blood pressure is very substantially reduced (*see* Symposium, 1982, 1983b, 1984; Romankiewicz *et al.,* 1983; Schwartz and Chatterjee, 1983).

In addition to the beneficial hemodynamic effects in heart failure, ACE inhibitors decrease the mass and wall thickness of the left ventricle in patients with hypertension. Such changes, which can be detected after therapy with ACE inhibitors for as short a period as 3 months, resemble those that are seen with inhibitors of the sympathetic nervous system, β-adrenergic antagonists, and Ca^{2+}-channel blockers. Resting cardiac performance is improved following regression of left ventricular hypertrophy, even if blood pressure is allowed to return to the hypertensive range (Schmieder *et al.,* 1989). In rats, ACE inhibitors also protect against the congestive failure that follows myocardial infarction; studies are now in progress in patients who have had an infarct (*see* Frohlich, 1989). In one small study captopril attenuated the progressive ventricular enlargement and improved exercise capacity in patients who had suffered an anterior myocardial infarction (Pfeffer *et al.,* 1988).

Precautions and Adverse Reactions to ACE Inhibitors. Untoward reactions occasionally appear to be a specific result of inhibition of converting enzyme. A steep fall in blood pressure may occur, for example, following the first dose of an ACE inhibitor in patients with severe hypertension who have been treated with multidrug regimens that include diuretics. A similar reaction may occur in patients with congestive heart failure, especially when they have been vigorously treated with diuretics. Care should be exercised in patients who are likely to be depleted of salt and water. Treatment should be initiated with very small doses of the inhibitor and preferably at an interval after withdrawal of the diuretic. The latter can be given again subsequently, if necessary. Inhibition of converting enzyme can also induce renal insufficiency in patients with bilateral renal stenosis or with stenosis of the artery to a single remaining kidney. This effect is apparently caused by reduction of the concentration of angiotensin II, which is needed in such conditions to constrict the efferent glomerular arterioles and maintain adequate glomerular filtration. Adaptive renal autoregulatory mechanisms are absent in these patients and renal failure or paradoxical malignant hypertension may occur. Angioedema also has been reported. Despite some reduction in the concentration of aldosterone, significant retention of K^+ is rarely encountered.

Less severe side effects include skin rash and loss of sense of taste. Both effects disappear with discontinuation of the agents and may not reappear if therapy is reinstated. Although these side effects were initially attributed to the presence of the sulfhydryl group in captopril, they also occur with other ACE inhibitors. A disturbing cough may occur during long-term treatment with an ACE inhibitor; this too disappears when the drug is discontinued.

Two rare but major side effects of ACE inhibitor are proteinuria and neutropenia. Proteinuria (more than 1 g per day) occurs particularly in patients with renal parenchymal disease. Although the frequency of neutropenia is low, it occurs predominantly in patients with hypertension that complicates collagen–vascular or renal parenchymal disease.

Metabolic side effects are not encountered during long-term therapy with ACE inhibitors. The drugs do not alter carbohydrate metabolism or plasma concentrations of uric acid, lipoproteins, and cholesterol (*see* Frohlich, 1989). However, there is usually a striking compensatory increase in renin secretion, leading to high concentrations of renin and angiotensin I.

Captopril. Captopril is D-3-mercapto-methyl-propionyl-L-proline; its structure is as follows:

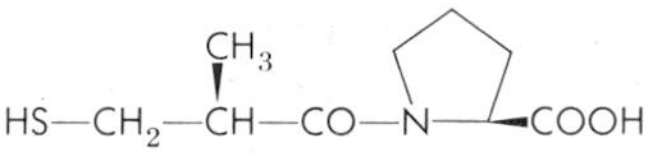

Captopril

Absorption, Fate, and Excretion. Captopril is rapidly absorbed when given orally. Bioavailability averages about 65% and is reduced significantly by food; the drug is thus generally given 1 hour before meals. Peak concentrations in plasma occur within an hour, and the drug is cleared rapidly (half-life of approximately 2 hours). However, a single, small oral dose (20 mg) of captopril abolishes the pressor effect of angiotensin I for more than 2 hours, and about 4 hours are needed for 50% recovery of the original response (*see* Symposium, 1982). Nearly all of the drug is eliminated in the urine, about 40% as captopril itself and the rest as metabolites (disulfide dimer and mixed disulfides). Excretion is slowed in patients with impaired renal function.

Captopril is generally well tolerated. In one large series of patients who received about 350 mg of captopril daily, the estimated 4-year cumulative frequency of discontinuation of the drug because of side effects was less than 12%. This compares favorably with the value for other standard antihypertensive agents (*e.g.,* the corresponding value is 15% for propranolol) (*see* Symposium, 1989). Subsequent studies with smaller doses of captopril (<150 mg per day) indicate a lower incidence of side effects.

Preparation and Dosage. Captopril (CAPOTEN) is available in tablets containing 12.5, 25, 50, or 100 mg. The drug should be taken 1 hour before meals. The recommended initial dosage for adults is 25 mg two or three times a day. This is increased, as necessary, after 2 weeks to 50 mg three times daily. However, recent experience indicates that twice-daily dosing commonly suffices and most patients should not receive daily doses in excess of 150 mg. A much smaller dosage, 6.25 mg or less three times daily, is appropriate for initiation of therapy in patients with heart failure or in others who have received intensive therapy with diuretics. Reduced dosage is also indicated for patients with impaired renal function.

Enalapril. This newer inhibitor of converting enzyme has a mechanism of action and spectrum of pharmacological effects and therapeutic applications that are characteristic of those described for captopril. The structure of enalapril is as follows:

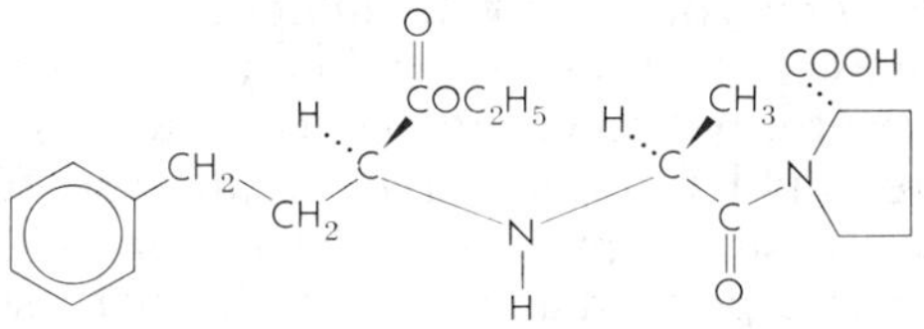

Enalapril

Enalapril is a prodrug that is not itself highly active—it must be hydrolyzed to the active parent dicarboxylic acid, enalaprilate. This conversion is accomplished by a serum esterase. Enalaprilate is a potent inhibitor of ACE with a K_i of about 0.2 nM. Although it also contains a "proline surrogate," enalaprilate differs from captopril in that it is an analog of a tripeptide rather than of a dipeptide.

Enalapril (but not enalaprilate) is rapidly absorbed when given orally, and bioavailability is little affected by food. Plasma concentrations of enalaprilate reach a maximum only after 3 to 4 hours. The onset of action after oral administration is thus slower than with captopril, and peak reduction in blood pressure occurs some 4 to 6 hours after ingestion. By contrast, responses to enalaprilate given intravenously are apparent in 15 minutes (*see* Symposium, 1983b; Doyle and Bearn, 1984; Joint National Committee, 1984).

Enalapril is efficacious in the same broad range of hypertensive conditions as captopril, although the main focus has been on essential hypertension (usually mild to moderate) and on chronic congestive heart failure. However, enalapril has several distinctive features. While of minor significance, it is considerably more potent than captopril. Of greater interest is the prolonged duration of action of enalapril; enalaprilate binds more tightly to converting enzyme and persists longer in the plasma (*see* Appendix II). This property often allows effective treatment with a single daily dose, although twice-daily dosage may sometimes be more appropriate. Furthermore, the incidences of rash and disturbance of taste appear to be lower; however, both neutropenia and proteinuria, although rare, have been encountered. Hemodynamic side effects, cough, and angioedema occur with similar frequency.

Preparations and Dosage. *Enalapril maleate* (VASOTEC) is available for oral use as tablets containing 2.5, 5, 10, or 20 mg. Daily dose ranges from a total of 10 mg to 40 mg (occasionally 80 mg), given once or in two divided doses. *Enalaprilat injection* (enalaprilate) is provided in a solution for injection that contains 1.25 mg/ml.

Lisinopril. This compound is the lysine analog of enalaprilate. Its structure is as follows:

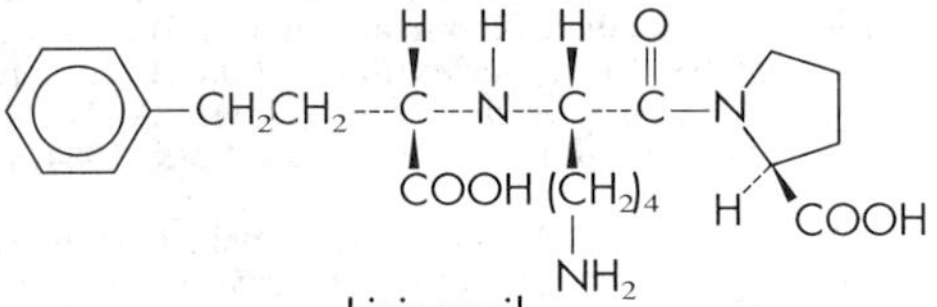

Lisinopril

Unlike enalapril, lisinopril itself is active. In addition, it has a long duration of action, with near maximal effects still evident 24 hours after a single dose. Lisinopril is slowly and incompletely (30%) absorbed after oral administration; peak concentrations in plasma are achieved within 6 to 8 hours. It is cleared as the intact compound by the kidney, and its half-life in plasma is about 12 hours (*see* Armayor and Lopez, 1988; Lancaster and Todd, 1988). Although the pharmacodynamic effects of lisinopril are comparable to those of other ACE inhibitors, it is noteworthy that short-term treatment (10 to 12 weeks) with the drug causes a significant decrease in cardiac output. Lisinopril causes a decrease in venous return, and intravascular volume is redistributed from the pulmonary bed to the periphery. It may also cause a negative inotropic effect (*see* Garavaglia *et al.*, 1988).

Preparation and Dosage. *Lisinopril* (PRINIVIL, ZESTRIL) is available for oral use as tablets containing 5, 10, 20, and 40 mg. The initial dose is 10 mg per day; this can be increased to 20 to 40 mg to be taken once daily, often in the evening.

Therapeutic Uses of ACE Inhibitors. *Hypertension.* Converting enzyme inhibitors have a broad range of usefulness. Although a maximal lowering of blood pressure may take some weeks to develop, a significant reduction in blood pressure may be achieved in many hypertensive patients with relatively few adverse reactions; this is especially true when an ACE inhibitor is used concurrently with a diuretic. When used as the sole antihypertensive agent, ACE inhibitors are roughly comparable in their activity to a thiazide diuretic or a β-adrenergic antagonist, and they lower blood pressure significantly in about half of patients with moderate essential hypertension. When used with a thiazide diuretic, this fraction rises to more than 80%. The concurrent administration of a β-adrenergic blocking agent also enhances the response, but to a lesser extent. This is perhaps because the β-adrenergic blockers owe their efficacy, in part, to inhibition of renin release (*see* Chapter 33).

It is apparent that drugs of this class offer several advantages. Since they have no direct sympatholytic activity, cardiovascular reflexes are retained, responses to exercise and posture are not disrupted, and postural hypotension is rare. Unlike β-adrenergic antagonists, they are not contraindicated in patients with bronchial asthma or diabetes (*see* Chapter 11). In contrast to the thiazide diuretics, they do not cause hypokalemia, hyperuricemia, hyperglycemia, or hyperlipidemia. Indeed, they oppose the secondary hyperaldosteronism produced by the diuretics and ameliorate or prevent the hypokalemia. Furthermore, they are well tolerated and have relatively little tendency to cause side effects such as lethargy, weakness, and sexual dysfunction that not uncommonly diminish the quality of life and undermine compliance of patients on multidrug antihypertensive therapy. Indeed, patients formerly treated with such regimens have reported an improved sense of well-being during treatment with a converting enzyme inhibitor. (*See* Symposium, 1982, 1983b, 1984, 1989; Johnston *et al.*, 1984.)

Some less common hypertensive conditions in which converting enzyme inhibitors appear to be particularly useful include malignant hypertension, renovascular hypertension, hypertensive crisis of scleroderma, and dialysis-resistant hypertension in end-stage renal failure (*see* reviews just cited; *see also* Chapter 33).

Chronic Congestive Heart Failure. Vasodilators have a valued place in the management of acute heart failure, but their utility in chronic congestive failure has been more limited (*see* Smith and Braunwald, 1984; *see also* Chapter 32). Converting enzyme inhibitors not only induce systemic arteriolar dilatation, and thereby reduce afterload, but they also cause venodilatation, lessen fluid retention, and thus reduce preload. These and other beneficial effects described above lead to increased cardiac output, amelioration of signs and symptoms of congestion, increased exercise tolerance, improved clinical status, and prolongation of life for patients in end-stage congestive heart failure. Although initially indicated for patients inadequately controlled by digitalis and diuretics, converting enzyme inhibitors are now being used at earlier stages of cardiac decompensation. (*See* Romankiewicz *et al.*, 1983; Schwartz and Chatterjee, 1983; Symposium, 1982, 1983b, 1984, 1989.)

RENIN INHIBITORS

Inhibitors of renin are attracting increasing interest both as analytical tools and as possible therapeutic agents (*see* Haber, 1984, 1986; Inagami, 1989). Various highly active inhibitors have been described, and some have potent hypotensive activity in man when given intravenously. Inhibitors containing as few as three amino acid residues have been described. Several analogs of these peptides block renin activity after oral administration (*see* Pals *et al.*, 1986; DeForrest *et al.*, 1989). Unfortunately, these agents are poorly absorbed from the gastrointestinal tract and are rapidly eliminated from the blood. Nevertheless, progress has been significant and it seems possible that clinically useful compounds of this type may become available.

Bell, J. B. G.; Chu, F. W.; Tait, J. F.; Tait, S. A. S.; and Khosla, M. The use of the superfusion approach with rat adrenal capsular cells to compare the steroidogenic potencies of angiotensin analogues, without the effects of peptide degradation. *Proc. R. Soc. Lond.* [*Biol.*], **1984,** *221,* 21–30.

Ben-Ari, E. T., and Garrison, J. C. Regulation of angiotensinogen mRNA accumulation in rat hepatocytes. *Am. J. Physiol.,* **1988,** *255,* E70–E79.

Bernstein, K. E.; Martin, B. M.; Edwards, A. S.; and Bernstein, E. A. Mouse angiotensin-converting enzyme is a protein composed of two homologous domains. *J. Biol. Chem.,* **1989,** *264,* 11945–11951.

Campbell, D. J., and Habener, J. F. Angiotensinogen gene is expressed and differentially regulated in multiple tissues of the rat. *J. Clin. Invest.,* **1986,** *78,* 31–39.

Cassis, L. C.; Saye, J.; and Peach, M. J. Location and regulation of rat angiotensinogen messenger RNA. *Hypertension,* **1988,** *11,* 591–596.

Corvol, P.; Panthier, J. J.; Foote, S.; and Rougeon, F. Structure of the mouse submaxillary gland renin precursor and a model for renin processing. *Hypertension,* **1983,** *5,* Suppl. 1, I3–I9.

Cushman, D. W.; Cheung, H. S.; Sabo, E. F.; and Ondetti, M. A. Design of potent competitive inhibitors of angiotensin-converting enzyme. Carboxyalkanoyl and mercaptoalkanoyl amino acids. *Biochemistry,* **1977,** *16,* 5484–5491.

DeForrest, J. M.; Waldron, T. L.; Oehl, R. S.; Scalese, R. J.; Free, C. A.; Weller, H. N.; and Ryono, D. E. Pharmacology of novel imidazole alcohol inhibitors of primate renin. *J. Hypertens.,* **1989,** *7,* Suppl. 2, S15–S19.

Dzau, V. J., and Herrmann, H. C. Hormonal control of angiotensinogen production. *Life Sci.,* **1982,** *30,* 577–584.

Elfont, R. M., and Fitzsimons, J. T. Renin dependence of captopril-induced drinking after ureteric ligation in the rat. *J. Physiol.* (*Lond.*), **1983,** *343,* 17–30.

Garavaglia, G. E.; Messerli, F. H.; Nunez, B. D.; Schmieder, R. E.; and Frohlich, E. D. Immediate and short-term cardiovascular effects of a new converting enzyme inhibitor (lisinopril) in essential hypertension. *Am. J. Cardiol.,* **1988,** *62,* 912–916.

Gomez, R. A.; Lynch, K. R.; Chevalier, R. L.; Everett, A. D.; Johns, D. W.; Wilfong, N.; Peach, M. J.; and Carey, R. M. Renin and angiotensinogen gene expression and intrarenal renin distribution during ACE inhibition. *Am. J. Physiol.,* **1988,** *254,* F900–F906.

Guillemette, G.; Guillon, G.; Marie, J.; Balestre, M.-N.; Escher, E.; and Jard, S. High yield photoaffinity labeling of angiotensin II receptors. *Mol. Pharmacol.,* **1986,** *30,* 544–551.

Haber, E. Control of renin action: inhibitors and antibodies. In, *Hypertension and the Angiotensin System: Therapeutic Approaches.* (Doyle, A. E., and Bearn, A. G., eds.) Raven Press, New York, **1984,** pp. 138–148.

Imai, T.; Miyazaki, H.; Hirose, S.; Hori, H.; Hayashi, T.; Kageyama, R.; Ohkubo, H.; Nakanishi, S.; and Murakami, K. Cloning and sequence analysis of cDNA for human renin precursor. *Proc. Natl. Acad. Sci. U.S.A.,* **1983,** *80,* 7405–7409.

Inagami, T. Structure and function of renin. *J. Hypertens.,* **1989,** *7,* Suppl. 2, S3–S8.

Johns, D. W., and Ayers, C. R. Dilation of forearm blood vessels after angiotensin converting-enzyme inhibition by captopril in hypertensive patients. *Hypertension,* **1984,** *6,* 545–550.

Kageyama, R.; Ohkubo, H.; and Nakanishi, S. Primary structure of human preangiotensinogen deduced from the cloned cDNA sequence. *Biochemistry,* **1984,** *23,* 3603–3609.

Laragh, J. H. Conceptual diagnostic and therapeutic dimensions of renin-system profiling of hypertensive disorders and of congestive heart failure: four new research frontiers. In, *Hypertension and the Angiotensin System: Therapeutic Approaches.* (Doyle, A. E., and Bearn, A. G., eds.) Raven Press, New York, **1984,** pp. 47–72.

Liu, F.-Y., and Cogan, M. G. Angiotensin II: a potent regulator of acidification in the rat early proximal convoluted tubule. *J. Clin. Invest.,* **1987,** *80,* 272–275.

Ménard, J.; Alhenc-Gelas, F.; Gardes, J.; Misumi, J.; and Corvol, P. Intrarenal formation of and role of angiotensins: practical implications. In, *Hypertension and the Angiotensin System: Therapeutic Approaches.* (Doyle, A. E., and Bearn, A. G., eds.) Raven Press, New York, **1984,** pp. 109–121.

Pals, D. T.; Thaisrivongs, S.; Lawson, J. A.; Kati, W. M.; Turner, S. R.; DeGraaf, G. L.; Harris, D. W.; and Johnson, G. A. An orally active inhibitor of renin. *Hypertension,* **1986,** *8,* 1105–1112.

Pfeffer, M. A.; Lamas, G. A.; Vaughan, D. E.; Parisi, A. F.; and Braunwald, E. Effect of captopril on progressive ventricular dilatation after myocardial infarction. *N. Engl. J. Med.,* **1988,** *319,* 80–86.

Schiavone, M. T.; Santos, R. A. S.; Brosnihan, K. B.; Khosla, M. C.; and Ferrario, C. M. Release of vasopressin from the rat hypothalamo-neurohypophysial system by angiotensin-(1-7) heptapeptide. *Proc. Natl. Acad. Sci. U.S.A.,* **1988,** *85,* 4095–4098.

Sielecki, A. R.; Hayakawa, K.; Fujinaga, M.; Murphy, M. E. P.; Fraser, M.; Muir, A. K.; Carilli, C. T.; Lewicki, J. A.; Baxter, J. D.; and James, M. N. G. Structure of recombinant human renin, a target for cardiovascular-active drugs, at 2.5 A resolution. *Science,* **1989,** *243,* 1346–1351.

Skeggs, L. T., Jr. Historical overview of the renin–angiotensin system. In, *Hypertension and the Angiotensin System: Therapeutic Approaches.* (Doyle, A. E., and Bearn, A. G., eds.) Raven Press, New York, **1984,** pp. 31–45.

Soubrier, F.; Alhenc-Gelas, F.; Hubert, C.; Allegrini, J.; John, M.; Tregear, G.; and Corvol, P. Two putative active centers in human angiotensin I-converting enzyme revealed by molecular cloning. *Proc. Natl. Acad. Sci. U.S.A.,* **1988,** *85,* 9386–9390.

Tewksbury, D. A.; Dart, R. A.; and Travis, J. The amino terminal amino acid sequence of human angiotensinogen. *Biochem. Biophys. Res. Commun.*, **1981**, *99*, 1311–1315.

Wong, P. C.; Price, W. A., Jr.; Chiu, A. T.; Thoolen, M. J. M. C.; Duncia, J. V.; Johnson, A. L.; and Timmermans, P. B. M. W. M. Nonpeptide angiotensin II receptor antagonists. IV. EXP6155 and EXP6803. *Hypertension*, **1989**, *13*, 489–497.

Zusman, R. M. Effects of converting-enzyme inhibitors on the renin–angiotensin–aldosterone, bradykinin, and arachidonic acid–prostaglandin systems: correlation of chemical structure and biologic activity. *Am. J. Kidney Dis.*, **1987**, *X*, Suppl. 1, 13–23.

Monographs and Reviews

Antonaccio, M. J. Angiotensin converting enzyme (ACE) inhibitors. *Annu. Rev. Pharmacol. Toxicol.*, **1982**, *22*, 57–87.

Armayor, G. M., and Lopez, L. M. Lisinopril: a new angiotensin-converting enzyme inhibitor. *Drug Intell. Clin. Pharm.*, **1988**, *22*, 365–372.

Atlas, S. A.; Niarchos, A. P.; and Case, D. B. Inhibitors of the renin–angiotensin system. Effects on blood pressure, aldosterone secretion and renal function. *Am. J. Nephrol.*, **1983**, *3*, 118–127.

Barrett, P. Q.; Bollag, W. B.; Isales, C. M.; McCarthy, R. T.; and Rassmussen, H. The role of Ca^{2+} in the regulation of aldosterone secretion. *Endocr. Rev.*, *10*, **1989**, pp. 496–518.

Bumpus, F. M. Mechanisms and sites of action of newer angiotensin agonists and antagonists in terms of activity and receptor. *Fed. Proc.*, **1977**, *36*, 2128–2132.

Davis, J. O., and Freeman, R. H. Mechanisms regulating renin release. *Physiol. Rev.*, **1976**, *56*, 1–56.

Doyle, A. E., and Bearn, A. G. (eds.). *Hypertension and the Angiotensin System: Therapeutic Approaches.* Raven Press, New York, **1984**.

Erdös, E. G. (ed.). *Bradykinin, Kallidin and Kallikrein. Handbuch der Experimentellen Pharmakologie,* Vol. 25, Suppl., Springer-Verlag, Berlin, **1979**.

Ferrario, C. M. Neurogenic actions of angiotensin II. *Hypertension*, **1983**, *5*, Suppl. V, V73–V79.

Fitzsimons, J. T. Angiotensin stimulation of the central nervous system. *Rev. Physiol. Biochem. Pharmacol.*, **1980**, *87*, 117–167.

Freeman, R. H.; Davis, J. O.; and Villareal, D. Role of renal prostaglandins in the control of renin release. *Circ. Res.*, **1984**, *54*, 1–9.

Frohlich, E. D. Angiotensin converting enzyme inhibitors: present and future. *Hypertension*, **1989**, *13*, Suppl. 1, I125–I130.

Ganong, W. F. The brain renin–angiotensin system. *Annu. Rev. Physiol.*, **1984**, *46*, 17–31.

Gibbons, G. H.; Dzau, V. J.; Farhi, E. R.; and Barger, A. C. Interaction of signals influencing renin release. *Annu. Rev. Physiol.*, **1984**, *46*, 291–308.

Griendling, K. K., and Alexander, R. W. Angiotensin, other pressors, and the transduction of vascular smooth muscle contraction. In, *Hypertension: Pathophysiology, Diagnosis, and Management,* Vol. 1. (Laragh, J. H., and Brenner, B. M., eds.) Raven Press, New York, **1990**, pp. 583–600.

Gross, F. The regulation of aldosterone secretion by the renin–angiotensin system under various conditions. *Acta Endocrinol. (Kbh.)*, **1968**, Suppl. 124, 41–64.

Haber, E. Agents which inhibit the renin-angiotensin system. In, *Kidney Hormones,* Vol. 3. (Fisher, J. W., ed.) Academic Press, Inc., London, **1986**, pp. 309–331.

Johnston, C. I.; Arnolda, L.; and Hiwatari, M. Angiotensin-converting enzyme inhibitors in the treatment of hypertension. *Drugs,* **1984**, *27*, 271–277.

Joint National Committee. The 1984 Report of the Joint National Committee on Detection, Evaluation, and Treatment of High Blood Pressure. *Arch. Intern. Med.*, **1984**, *144*, 1045–1057.

Kamm, K. E., and Stull, J. T. The function of myosin and myosin light chain kinase phosphorylation in smooth muscle. *Annu. Rev. Pharmacol. Toxicol.*, **1985**, *25*, 593–620.

Lancaster, S. G., and Todd, P. A. Lisinopril. A preliminary review of its pharmacodynamic and pharmacokinetic properties, and therapeutic use in hypertension and congestive heart failure. *Drugs*, **1988**, *35*, 646–669.

Page, I. H., and Bumpus, F. M. (eds.). *Angiotensin. Handbuch der Experimentellen Pharmakologie,* Vol. 37. Springer-Verlag, Berlin, **1974**.

Peach, M. J. Renin-angiotensin system: biochemistry and mechanisms of action. *Physiol. Rev.*, **1977**, *57*, 313–370.

———. Pharmacology of angiotensin II. In, *Kidney Hormones,* Vol. 3. (Fisher, J. W., ed.) Academic Press, Inc., London, **1986**, pp. 273–308.

———. Actions of angiotensin on elements of the vascular wall and myocardium. In, *Angiotensin and Blood Pressure Regulation.* (Harding, J. W.; Wright, J. W.; Speth, R. C.; and Barnes, C. D.; eds.) Academic Press, Inc., New York, **1988**, pp. 35–59.

Petrillo, E. W., Jr., and Ondetti, M. A. Angiotensin-converting enzyme inhibitors: medicinal chemistry and biological actions. *Med. Res. Rev.*, **1982**, *2*, 1–41.

Quinn, S. J., and Williams, G. H. Regulation of aldosterone secretion. *Annu. Rev. Physiol.*, **1988**, *50*, 409–426.

Regoli, D.; Park, W. K.; and Rioux, F. Pharmacology of angiotensin. *Pharmacol. Rev.*, **1974**, *26*, 69–123.

Romankiewicz, J. A.; Brogden, R. N.; Heel, R. C.; Speight, T. M.; and Avery, G. S. Captopril: an update review of its pharmacological properties and therapeutic efficacy in congestive heart failure. *Drugs*, **1983**, *25*, 6–40.

Ryan, J. W. Processing of the endogenous polypeptides by the lungs. *Annu. Rev. Physiol.*, **1982**, *44*, 241–255.

Schmieder, R. E.; Messerli, F. H.; Sturgill, D.; Garavaglia, G. E.; and Nunez, B. D. Cardiac performance after reduction of myocardial hypertrophy. *Am. J. Med.*, **1989**, *87*, 22–27.

Schwartz, A. B., and Chatterjee, K. Vasodilator therapy in chronic congestive heart failure. *Drugs*, **1983**, *26*, 148–173.

Smith, T. W., and Braunwald, E. The management of heart failure. In, *Heart Disease*, 2nd ed., Vol. I. (Braunwald, E., ed.) W. B. Saunders Co., Philadelphia, **1984**, pp. 503–559.

Symposium. (Various authors.) Captopril: worldwide clinical experience. *Br. J. Clin. Pharmacol.*, **1982**, *14*, Suppl. 2, 65S–252S.

Symposium. (Various authors.) The kidney in hypertension. *Am. J. Nephrol.*, **1983a**, *3*, 57–192.

Symposium. (Various authors.) Symposium on the renin–angiotensin–aldosterone system: treatment of hypertension and heart failure. (Murphy, B., ed.) *J. Hyperten.*, **1983b**, *1*, Suppl. 1, 1–157.

Symposium. (Various authors.) Regional hemodynamics following captopril therapy. *Am. J. Med.*, **1984**, *76*, Suppl. 5B, 1–119.

Symposium. (Various authors.) The National Heart, Lung, and Blood Institute Workshop on Antihypertensive Drug Treatment. *Hypertension*, **1989**, *13*, Suppl. I, 1–172.

Torretti, J. Sympathetic control of renin release. *Annu. Rev. Pharmacol. Toxicol.*, **1982**, *22*, 167–192.

CHAPTER

32 DRUGS USED FOR THE TREATMENT OF ANGINA: ORGANIC NITRATES, CALCIUM-CHANNEL BLOCKERS, AND β-ADRENERGIC ANTAGONISTS

Ferid Murad

Angina pectoris is the principal symptom of ischemic heart disease. Both the typical and variant forms of angina may be manifested by sudden, severe, pressing substernal pain that often radiates to the left shoulder and along the flexor surface of the left arm; however, the location and character of the pain may vary. The pain of typical angina is commonly induced by exercise, emotion, or eating and is often associated with depression of the S–T segment of the electrocardiogram (ECG). The underlying pathological process is usually advanced atherosclerosis of the coronary vasculature. In contrast, variant (Prinzmetal's) angina is caused by vasospasm of the coronary vessels and may not be associated with severe atherosclerosis. Patients with variant angina may develop chest pain while at rest and exhibit elevation of the S–T segment of the ECG.

Anginal attacks may recur for years or may rapidly increase in their frequency (unstable angina). They result from temporary ischemia of the myocardium, such that blood flow is insufficient to maintain adequate oxygenation. This can be due to a decrease in myocardial blood flow, an increase in the requirement of the myocardium for oxygen, or both.

This chapter deals with the pharmacological agents that are used in the treatment of angina pectoris. The primary drugs include organic nitrates, Ca^{2+}-channel blockers, and β-adrenergic antagonists. The strategy for pharmacological relief of angina is based on improvement of the balance between myocardial oxygen supply and demand. For typical exertional angina, this necessitates increasing the blood flow to the heart or decreasing its work load. Treatment of variant (Prinzmetal's) angina is directed at reduction of vasospasm of the coronary vessels.

Nitroglycerin has long been known to be useful to prevent or relieve acute anginal attacks. More recently, the efficacy of β-adrenergic antagonists and Ca^{2+}-channel blockers has been established. Although antianginal agents provide only symptomatic or prophylactic treatment, administration of β-adrenergic antagonists (and other agents) does appear to decrease the incidence of sudden death associated with myocardial ischemia and infarction (*see* Chapters 11 and 31). The uses of inhibitors of platelet aggregation, fibrinolytic agents, and cholesterol-lowering agents in these and related disorders are discussed particularly in Chapters 36 and 55. Percutaneous transluminal coronary angioplasty and coronary artery bypass graft surgery are alternatives to pharmacological treatment.

ORGANIC NITRATES

History. Nitroglycerin was first synthesized in 1846 by Sobrero, who observed that a small quantity of the oily substance placed on the tongue elicited a severe headache. Constantin Hering, in 1847, developed the sublingual dosage form for nitroglycerin, which he advocated for a number of diseases. The eminent English physician T. Lauder Brunton was unable to relieve severe recurrent anginal pain except when he bled his patient, and he believed that phlebotomy provided relief by lowering arterial blood pressure. The concept that reduced cardiac afterload and work are beneficial continues to the present day (*see* below). In 1857, Brunton administered amyl nitrite, a known vasodepressor, by inhalation, and he noted that anginal pain was relieved within 30 to 60 seconds. The action of amyl nitrite was transitory, however, and the dosage was difficult to adjust. In 1879, William Murrell decided that the action of nitroglycerin mimicked that of amyl nitrite, and he established the use of sublingual nitroglycerin for relief of the acute anginal attack and as a prophylactic agent to be taken prior to exertion. The empirical observation that organic nitrates could be used safely for the rapid, dramatic alleviation of the symptoms of angina pectoris led to their widespread acceptance by the medical profession.

Chemistry. Organic nitrates are polyol esters of nitric acid, whereas organic nitrites are esters of nitrous acid (Table 32–1). Nitrate esters (—C—O—NO_2) and nitrite esters (—C—O—NO) are characterized by a sequence of carbon–oxygen–nitrogen, whereas nitro compounds possess carbon–nitrogen bonds (C—NO_2). Thus, glyceryl trinitrate is not a nitro compound, and it is erroneously called nitroglycerin; however, this nomenclature is both widespread and official. Amyl nitrite is a highly volatile liquid that is administered by inhalation. Organic nitrates of low molecular weight (such as nitroglycerin) are moderately volatile, oily liquids, whereas the high-molecular-weight nitrate esters (*e.g.*, erythrityl tetranitrate, pentaerythritol tetranitrate, isosorbide dinitrate) are solids. The fully nitrated polyols are lipid soluble, whereas their incompletely nitrated metabolites are more soluble in water. In the pure form (without an inert carrier such as lactose), nitroglycerin is explosive. The organic nitrates and nitrites and several other compounds that are capable of conversion to nitric oxide (NO) have been collectively termed *nitrovasodilators*. Nitric oxide is thought to be the active intermediate in the action of this broad class of agents (*see* Murad, 1986).

PHARMACOLOGICAL PROPERTIES

Cardiovascular Effects. *Hemodynamic Effects.* The nitrovasodilators relax most smooth muscle, including that in arteries and veins. The mechanism of this effect is discussed below. Low concentrations

Table 32–1. ORGANIC NITRATES AVAILABLE FOR CLINICAL USE

NONPROPRIETARY NAME AND TRADE NAMES	CHEMICAL STRUCTURE	PREPARATIONS, USUAL DOSES, AND ROUTES OF ADMINISTRATION *	
Amyl nitrite (isoamyl nitrite)	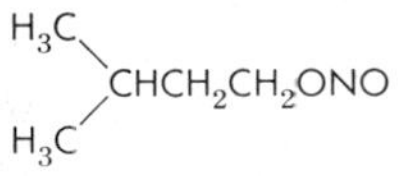	Inh:	0.18 or 0.3 ml, inhalation
Nitroglycerin (glyceryl trinitrate; NITRO-BID, NITROSTAT, others)	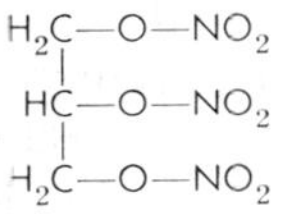	T: S: C: B: O: D: IV:	0.15 to 0.6 mg as needed 0.4 mg per spray as needed 2.5 to 9 mg two to four times daily 1 mg every 3 to 5 hr 1.25 to 5 cm (1/2 to 2 in.), topical to skin every 4 to 8 hr 1 disc (2.5 to 15 mg/24 hr) every 24 hr 5 μg/min; increments of 5 μg/min
Isosorbide dinitrate (ISORDIL, SORBITRATE, others)	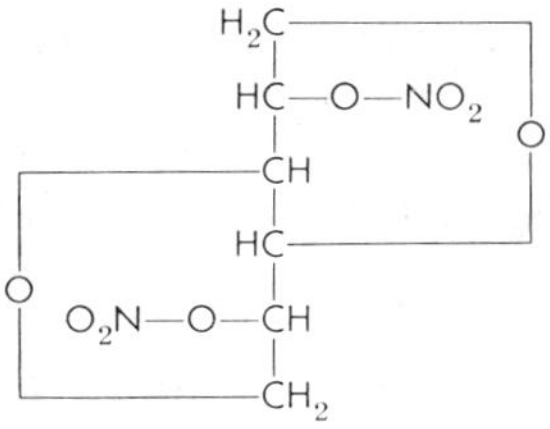	T: T (C): T (O): C:	2.5 to 10 mg every 2 to 3 hr 5 to 10 mg every 2 to 3 hr 10 to 40 mg every 6 hr 40 to 80 mg every 8 to 12 hr
Erythrityl tetranitrate (CARDILATE)	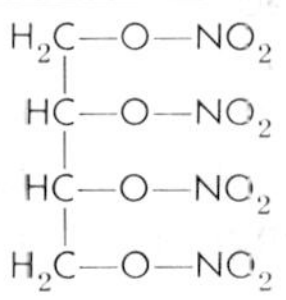	T: T (O):	5 to 10 mg as needed 10 mg three times daily
Pentaerythritol tetranitrate (PERITRATE, others)	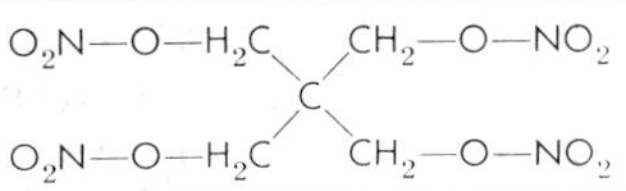	T (O): C:	10 to 40 mg four times daily 30 to 80 mg every 12 hr

* B = buccal (transmucosal) tablets; C = sustained-release capsule or tablet; D = transdermal disc; Inh = inhalant; IV = intravenous injection; O = ointment; S = lingual spray; T = tablet for sublingual use; T (C) = chewable tablet; T (O) = oral tablet or capsule.

of nitroglycerin produce dilatation of the veins that predominates over that of arterioles. The apparent selectivity of some nitrovasodilators for different vascular beds may relate to their bioavailability and differential cellular metabolism of the drugs to nitric oxide. Venodilatation results in decreased left and right ventricular end-diastolic pressures, which are greater on a percentage basis than is the decrease in systemic arterial pressure. Systemic vascular resistance is usually unaffected; heart rate is unchanged or slightly increased reflexly; and pulmonary vascular resistance and cardiac output are reduced (Ferrer *et al.*, 1966). Doses of nitroglycerin that do not alter systemic arterial pressure often produce arteriolar dilatation in the face and neck, resulting in a flush. The same doses may also cause headache because of dilatation of meningeal arterial vessels.

Rapid administration of high doses of organic nitrates decreases systolic and diastolic blood pressure and cardiac output, resulting in pallor, weakness, dizziness, and activation of compensatory sympathetic reflexes. The resultant tachycardia and peripheral arteriolar vasoconstriction tend to maintain systemic vascular resistance; this is superimposed on sustained venous pooling. Coronary blood flow increases transiently, owing to coronary vasodilatation, but subsequently falls as arterial blood pressure decreases and cardiac output falls. A marked hypotensive effect may occasionally follow sublingual administration of nitroglycerin. This effect is especially likely when the individual is in the upright position, which augments venous pooling and further decreases cardiac output. Repeated dosage at frequent intervals also precipitates hypotension.

Mechanism of Relief of Symptoms of Angina Pectoris. Typical attacks of angina are usually precipitated by exercise, stress, cold, or meals, all of which increase cardiac work and myocardial demand for oxygen. Drugs could correct the inadequacy of myocardial oxygenation by (1) increasing the supply of oxygen to ischemic myocardium by direct dilatation of the coronary vasculature, or (2) decreasing the oxygen demand secondary to a reduction of cardiac work. Brunton ascribed the relief of anginal pain afforded by nitrates to a decrease in cardiac work secondary to the fall in systemic blood pressure. After demonstration of direct coronary vasodilatation in experimental animals, it became generally accepted that nitrates relieved anginal pain by dilating coronary arteries and thereby increasing coronary blood flow. However, this hypothesis was questioned by Gorlin and associates (1959), who were unable to demonstrate increases in coronary blood flow in patients with coronary insufficiency following the administration of nitroglycerin. Although the mode of action of organic nitrates to relieve typical angina is not fully understood, the preponderance of evidence favors a reduction in myocardial work and the requirement for oxygen as the major action. In contrast, the ability of nitrates to dilate large coronary vessels selectively may be the primary mechanism by which they benefit patients with angina caused by coronary spasm (*see* below). The ability of nitrovasodilators to inhibit platelet aggregation may also contribute to the relief of pain in some forms of angina (Furlong *et al.*, 1987).

Effects on Total and Regional Coronary Blood Flow. Increases in the myocardial requirement for oxygen are normally met by increasing blood flow, rather than by more complete extraction of oxygen from the blood. Ischemia is a powerful stimulus to coronary vasodilatation, and regional blood flow is adjusted by autoregulatory mechanisms that alter the tone of small resistance vessels. In the presence of atherosclerotic coronary occlusion, ischemia distal to the lesion is a stimulus for vasodilatation, and, if the degree of occlusion is severe, much of the capacity to dilate is utilized to maintain resting blood flow to the compromised area. When situations arise that increase demand, further dilatation may not be possible.

As mentioned, organic nitrates do not increase total coronary blood flow in patients with typical angina due to atherosclerosis. However, these drugs do appear to cause redistribution of blood flow in the heart when the coronary circulation is partially occluded. Under these circumstances, there is a disproportionate reduction in blood flow to the subendocardial regions of the heart, which are subjected to the greatest extravascular compression during systole; organic nitrates tend to restore blood flow in these regions toward normal. For example, nitroglycerin increases the rate of washout of radioactive xenon injected directly into diseased regions of the ventricular wall of angina patients (Horwitz *et al.*, 1971), indicating that blood flow to regions of poorly perfused myocardium has been improved.

The hemodynamic mechanisms responsible for these effects are not entirely clear. Most hypotheses have focused on the ability of organic nitrates to cause dilatation of large epicardial vessels without impairing autoregulation in the small vessels, which are responsible for about 90% of the overall coronary vascular resistance. Experimental evidence in patients undergoing coronary bypass surgery indicates that nitrates do have a selective effect on large coronary vessels. Moreover, analyses of coronary angiograms in human subjects have shown that sublingual nitroglycerin can dilate epicardial stenoses and reduce the resistance to flow through such areas (Brown *et al.*, 1981; Feldman *et al.*, 1981). The resultant increase in blood flow would be distributed preferentially to ischemic myocardial regions as a consequence of vasodilatation induced by autoregulation. An important indirect mechanism for a preferential increase in subendocardial blood flow is the nitroglycerin-induced reduction in intracavitary systolic and diastolic pressures that oppose blood flow to the subendocardium (*see* below). To the extent that organic nitrates decrease myocardial requirements for oxygen (*see* below), the increased blood flow in ischemic regions could be balanced by decreased flow in nonischemic areas, and an overall increase in coronary blood flow need not occur. Redistribution of blood flow to subendocardial tissue is *not* typical of all vasodilators. Dipyridamole, for example, dilates resistance vessels nonselectively by distorting autoregulation; it is ineffective in patients with typical angina.

Effects on Myocardial Oxygen Requirements. By their effects on the systemic circulation, the organic nitrates can also reduce the requirement of the myocardium for oxygen. The major determinants of myocardial oxygen consumption include the stress on the ventricular wall during systole, the heart rate, and the state of contractility of the myocardium. The stress on the ventricular wall is affected by a number of factors that are generally considered under the categories of "preload" and "afterload." *Preload* is determined by the diastolic pressure that distends the relaxed ventricular wall (ventricular end-diastolic pressure). Increasing end-diastolic pressure and volume augment the ventricular tension required to eject blood (by the law of Laplace, tension = pressure × radius). Increasing venous capacitance decreases venous return to the heart, decreases ventricular end-diastolic pressure and volume, and thereby decreases oxygen consumption. An additional benefit of reducing preload is that it increases the pressure gradient for perfusion across the ventricular wall; this favors subendocardial perfusion (Parratt, 1979). *Afterload,* or ventricular systolic wall tension, is the force distributed in the ventricular wall during ejection of blood. It is related to the radius of the ventricle and to the intracavitary ventricular systolic pressure, which, in the absence of aortic valvular disease, is related to peripheral resistance. Decreasing peripheral arteriolar resistance reduces afterload and thus myocardial work and consumption of oxygen.

Organic nitrates do not directly alter the inotropic or chronotropic state of the heart. The drugs do decrease both preload and afterload as a result of respective dilatation of venous capacitance and arteriolar resistance vessels. Since the primary determinants of oxygen demand are reduced by the nitrates, their net effect usually is to decrease myocardial consumption of oxygen.

Paradoxically, however, high doses of organic nitrates may reduce blood pressure to such an extent that coronary flow is compromised; reflex tachycardia and adrenergic enhancement of contractility also occur. These effects may override the salutary action of the drugs on myocardial oxygen demand. The resultant negative effect on oxygen balance can aggravate ischemia and, potentially, initiate an anginal attack.

Relative Importance of the Actions of

Organic Nitrates. Of the two general mechanisms by which nitrates can reduce myocardial ischemia, their ability to reduce the demand for oxygen (by reducing preload and afterload) appears to be the most important for patients with typical angina. When nitroglycerin is injected or infused directly into the coronary circulation of patients with coronary artery disease, anginal attacks (induced by electrical pacing) are not aborted, even when coronary blood flow is increased. However, sublingual administration of nitroglycerin does relieve anginal pain in the same patients (Ganz and Marcus, 1972). Furthermore, venous phlebotomy that is sufficient to reduce left ventricular end-diastolic pressure can mimic the beneficial effect of nitroglycerin.

Patients are able to exercise for considerably longer periods after the administration of nitroglycerin. Nevertheless, angina occurs, with or without nitroglycerin, at the same value of the "triple product" (aortic pressure × heart rate × ejection time). The triple product can be determined experimentally and is proportional to the myocardial consumption of oxygen. The observation that angina occurs at the same level of myocardial oxygen consumption suggests that the beneficial effects of nitroglycerin are the result of a reduced cardiac oxygen demand, rather than the result of an increase in the delivery of oxygen to ischemic regions of myocardium. However, these results do not preclude the possibility that a favorable redistribution of blood flow to ischemic subendocardial myocardium contributes to the relief of pain in a typical anginal attack, nor do they preclude the possibility that direct coronary vasodilatation may *not* be the major effect of nitroglycerin in situations where vasospasm compromises myocardial blood flow.

Other Effects. The nitrovasodilators act on almost all smooth muscle. Bronchial smooth muscle is relaxed irrespective of the cause of the preexisting tone. The muscles of the biliary tract, including those of the gallbladder, biliary ducts, and sphincter of Oddi, are effectively relaxed. Smooth muscle of the gastrointestinal tract, including that of the esophagus, can be relaxed and its spontaneous motility decreased by nitrates both *in vivo* and *in vitro*. The effect may be transient and incomplete *in vivo*, but abnormal "spasm" is frequently reduced. Indeed, many incidences of atypical chest pain and "angina" are due to biliary or esophageal spasm that too can be relieved by nitrates. Similarly, nitrates can relax ureteral and uterine smooth muscle, but these effects are somewhat unpredictable.

Mechanism of Action. Nitrites, organic nitrates, nitroso compounds, and a variety of other nitrogen oxide–containing substances (including nitroprusside; *see* Chapter 33) can activate guanylate cyclase and increase the synthesis of guanosine 3′,5′-monophosphate (cyclic GMP) in smooth muscle and other tissues (*see* Rapaport and Murad, 1983; Murad, 1986). These agents all lead to the formation of the reactive free radical nitric oxide (NO), which interacts with and activates guanylate cyclase. A cyclic GMP–dependent protein kinase is thus stimulated, with resultant alteration of the phosphorylation of various proteins in smooth muscle. This eventually leads to the *de*phosphorylation of the light chain of myosin (Waldman and Murad, 1987). Phosphorylation of the myosin light chain regulates the maintenance of the contractile state in smooth muscle. The pharmacological and biochemical effects of the nitrovasodilators appear to be identical to those of the endothelial-derived relaxing factor (EDRF; *see* Chapter 5). EDRF may in fact be the "endogenous nitrovasodilator"; it may be nitric oxide itself or a precursor of nitric oxide (Murad, 1986; Moncada *et al.*, 1988).

Absorption, Fate, and Excretion. The biotransformation of organic nitrates is the result of reductive hydrolysis catalyzed by the hepatic enzyme glutathione–organic nitrate reductase. The enzyme converts the lipid-soluble organic nitrate esters into more water-soluble denitrated metabolites and inorganic nitrite. The partially denitrated metabolites are considerably less potent vasodilators than are the parent compounds. However, under certain conditions their activity may become important. Since the liver has an enormous capacity to catalyze the reduction of organic nitrates, their biotransformation is a major factor in determining oral bioavailability and duration of action. The pharmacokinetic properties of nitroglycerin and isosorbide dinitrate have been studied in the greatest detail.

Nitroglycerin. One molecule of nitroglycerin reacts with two molecules of reduced glutathione to release one inorganic nitrite ion from either the 2 or 3 position; the products are 1,3- or 1,2-glyceryl dinitrate and oxidized glutathione (Needleman, 1975). A comparison of the maximal velocities of metabolism of the clinically used nitrates by this reductase indicates that erythrityl tetranitrate is degraded three times faster than is nitroglycerin, while isosorbide dinitrate and pentaerythritol nitrate are denitrated at one-sixth and one-tenth the rate of nitroglycerin.

In man, peak concentrations of nitroglycerin are found in plasma within 4 minutes of sublingual administration; the compound has a half-life of 1 to 3 minutes. Dinitrate metabolites, which are about ten times less potent as vasodilators, appear to have a half-life of approximately 40 minutes (*see* Appendix II).

Isosorbide Dinitrate. The major route of metabolism of isosorbide dinitrate in man is by enzymatic denitration followed by formation of glucuronide conjugates. Sublingual administration produces maximal concentrations of the drug in plasma by 6 minutes, and the fall in concentration is rapid (half-life approximately 45 minutes). The primary initial metabolites, isosorbide-2-mononitrate and isosorbide-5-mononitrate, have longer half-lives (2 to 5 hours) and are presumed to be responsible, at least in part, for the therapeutic efficacy of isosorbide dinitrate. There is considerable interest in the therapeutic potential of isosorbide-5-mononitrate, since its bioavailability is excellent after oral administration and it has a significantly longer half-life than does isosorbide dinitrate.

Correlation of Plasma Concentrations of Drug and Biological Activity. Intravenous administration of nitroglycerin or the long-acting nitrates (isosorbide dinitrate, pentaerythritol tetranitrate, and erythrityl tetranitrate) in anesthetized animals produces the same transient (1 to 4 minutes) decrease in blood pressure. Relative to nitroglycerin, the potency of erythrityl tetranitrate as a vasodepressor in dogs is about 12%, and isosorbide dinitrate 3.5%. Since denitration markedly reduces the activity of the organic nitrates, their rapid clearance from blood indicates that the transient duration of action under these conditions correlates with the concentrations of the parent compounds. The kinetics of hepatic denitration is characteristic of each nitrate. In addition, it is influenced by hepatic blood flow or the presence of hepatic disease. In experimental animals, injection of moderate amounts of organic nitrates into the portal vein results in little or no vasodepressor activity, indicating that a substantial fraction of drug can be metabolized during its first circulation through the liver.

Routes of Administration. When relief of acute anginal pain is the objective, rapid onset of action is essential and duration of effect is less important. In contrast, for prevention of ischemia, duration of action and predictability of effect are the main issues. The rapidity of onset and the duration of action of any nitrate are directly related to the method of administration. Formulations are also available that permit sustained release of organic nitrate.

Sublingual Administration. The sublingual route of administration of organic nitrates is effective for the treatment of acute attacks of angina pectoris. Most of the drug bypasses the hepatic circulation initially, since only about 20% of the cardiac output is delivered to the liver. A transient but effective concentration of drug appears in the circulation. The onset of action is in 1 to 2 minutes, but the effects fall off rapidly and are undetectable within 1 hour.

The duration of action of the various nitrates is similar when relatively small doses are taken sublingually, since the capacity for their metabolism is high. Under this condition, their half-lives depend only on the rate at which they are delivered to the liver. Indeed, when equieffective doses of nitroglycerin and isosorbide dinitrate are given sublingually, there is no significant difference in their duration of action; effects on exercise tolerance wane with a half-time of about 20 minutes. Erythrityl tetranitrate is also able to prolong exercise tolerance and prevent depression of the S–T segment in the ECG when administered sublingually to patients with typical angina. However, the duration of action of this agent is also short when it is given in this way (10 to 45 minutes). Thus, the sublingual administration of organic nitrates is most appropriate to alleviate acute attacks of angina and for the immediate prophylaxis of such attacks.

Oral Administration. Organic nitrates have been administered orally in an attempt to provide convenient and prolonged prophylaxis against attacks of angina. Under these circumstances, the drugs must be given in sufficient dosage to saturate the liver's capacity to degrade them. These formulations generally have a slow onset of action because of efficient initial clearance. Peak effects occur at 60 to 90 minutes, and the duration of action is 3 to 6 hours.

There is little evidence for the efficacy of low doses of organic nitrates (*e.g.*, 5 mg of isosorbide dinitrate) given orally for the prophylaxis of angina. Relatively high doses of nitrates given orally can cause a small decrease in arterial blood pressure, a substantial decrease in left ventricular filling pressure, and an increase in the exercise tolerance of patients with angina. High doses of isosorbide dinitrate (30 mg orally, given four times daily) produce sustained hemodynamic and antianginal effects. Under these circumstances the activities of less potent metabolites may also contribute to the therapeutic effect. Chronic oral administration of isosorbide dinitrate (120 to 720 mg daily) results in persistence of the parent compound and higher concentrations of metabolites in plasma. However, such high doses are more likely to cause troublesome side effects and tolerance. Significant, prolonged (up to 4 hours) improvement of exercise tolerance can also be demonstrated in patients with angina pectoris who are given a sustained-release oral form of nitroglycerin. Again, high doses (6.5 mg) of nitroglycerin are required to elicit prolonged hemodynamic responses.

Intravenous Nitroglycerin. The intravenous administration of nitroglycerin permits rapid attainment of high concentrations of drug in the systemic circulation and prompt initiation of therapy. Because of its rapid degradation, the concentration can be titrated quickly and safely. The antianginal effects of intravenous nitroglycerin are useful in the treatment of coronary vasospasm and unstable angina pectoris, and this route of administration may become the preferred approach for the urgent treatment of congestive heart failure and acute ischemic syndromes (*see* Jaffe and Roberts, 1982). Intravenous nitroglycerin has been shown to be effective in the control of hypertension during and after coronary artery bypass surgery, and it may be efficacious in controlling pulmonary hypertension associated with acute respiratory failure.

Nitroglycerin Ointment and Discs. Administration of nitroglycerin to the skin in an ointment has been used to allow gradual absorption of the drug for prolonged prophylactic purposes. Effects are apparent within 60 minutes, and they last 4 to 8 hours. Doses of nitroglycerin ointment are large (often up to 30 mg), and absorption is quite variable. Patients with angina who used 2% nitroglycerin ointment (average dose of 5 mg) experienced improved and prolonged exercise capacity and showed decreased ischemic S–T segment changes in the ECG (Reichek *et al.,* 1974). Slow-release preparations of nitroglycerin for cutaneous use—for example, nitroglycerin discs (transdermal systems)—represent an alternative means to produce sustained concentrations of the drug in plasma. The preparations utilize a nitroglycerin reservoir (impregnated into a polymer bonded to an adhesive bandage) that permits gradual absorption over 24 hours. The onset of action is slow, and peak effects occur after 1 to 2 hours. If tolerance is avoided (*see* below), such therapy may provide a simple method for long-term prophylaxis of myocardial ischemia.

Transmucosal or Buccal Nitroglycerin. The patient inserts this formulation under the upper lip, adherent to the gingiva. Dissolution of the tablet proceeds in a gradual, uniform manner. This formulation appears to act as promptly as does sublingual nitroglycerin (hemodynamic alterations occur in 2 to 5 minutes), and it is therefore useful for short-term prophylaxis of angina. The tablet continues to release nitroglycerin into the circulation for a prolonged period, and exercise tolerance may be enhanced for up to 5 hours (Abrams, 1983).

Tolerance. Sublingual organic nitrates are usually taken by the patient at the time of an anginal attack or in anticipation of exercise or stress. Such intermittent treatment results in reproducible cardiovascular effects. However, frequently repeated exposure to high doses of organic nitrates leads to a decrease in the magnitude of most of their pharmacological effects. The therapeutic significance of this phenomenon is likely to increase as the oral and transdermal administration of higher doses of organic nitrates (and use of the sustained-release preparations) becomes prevalent. For example, the long-term oral use of isosorbide dinitrate (120 mg per day) led to the development of partial tolerance to the hemodynamic effects of the drug and to cross-tolerance to the venodilatation produced by sublingual nitroglycerin (Zelis and Mason, 1975). However, clinical experience with high-dose nitrate therapy is limited, and other studies have demonstrated undiminished therapeutic activity in response to the administration of long-acting nitrates for 10 months (Abrams, 1980). The magnitude of tolerance is a function of dosage and the frequency of administration of the preparation. Brief periods (hours or overnight) of no therapy may be sufficient to avoid the development of tolerance or to permit recovery.

A special aspect of tolerance has been observed among individuals exposed to nitroglycerin in the manufacture of explosives. If protection is inadequate, workers may experience severe headaches, dizziness, and postural weakness during the first several days of employment. Tolerance then develops, but headache and other symptoms may reappear after a few days away from the job, the "Monday disease." The most serious effect of chronic exposure is a form of organic nitrate dependence. Individuals without demonstrable organic vascular disease have died suddenly or developed myocardial infarctions after a few days' break in chronic exposure, and there are now well-documented cases with typical subjective and objective findings of severe myocardial ischemia, relieved by nitroglycerin, during withdrawal from long-term exposure to an organic nitrate. Coronary and digital arteriospasm during withdrawal and its relaxation by nitroglycerin have also been demonstrated radiographically. Because of the potential problem of nitrate dependence, it seems prudent not to withdraw nitrates abruptly from a patient who has received such therapy chronically.

The mechanism of initiation and maintenance of tolerance to these drugs is unclear. When blood vessels are removed from animals that have been made tolerant to organic nitrates, they too are hyposensitive to the effects of the agents, suggesting alteration in the activation of the guanylate cyclase–cyclic GMP system discussed above (Molina *et al.*, 1987; Bennett *et al.*, 1989). Induction of tolerance to nitroglycerin results in partial tolerance to other nitrovasodilators, as well as to endothelium-dependent vasodilators.

Toxicity and Untoward Responses. Untoward responses to the therapeutic use of organic nitrates are almost all secondary to actions on the cardiovascular system. Headache is common and can be severe. It usually decreases over a few days if treatment is continued, and often can be controlled by decreasing the dose. Transient episodes of dizziness, weakness, and other manifestations associated with postural hypotension may develop, particularly if the patient is standing immobile, and may occasionally progress to loss of consciousness. This reaction appears to be accentuated by alcohol. Even in the most severe nitrate syncope, positioning and other procedures to facilitate venous return are the only therapeutic measures required. It was widely believed that nitrates can increase intraocular pressure and precipitate glaucoma, but this fear appears to be completely unfounded. All the organic nitrates can occasionally produce drug rash, but it appears to occur most commonly with pentaerythritol tetranitrate.

Preparations and Dosage. Data for the nitrites and organic nitrates available for clinical use are given in Table 32–1. Sodium nitrite is obsolete except as an intravenous solution for use in the treatment of cyanide poisoning (*see* Chapter 67). Amyl nitrite acts very rapidly after inhalation and is occasionally used for very brief effects. Nitroglycerin is unstable and volatile. Although tablets of nitroglycerin are now stabilized, they should be dispensed in glass containers and protected from moisture, extremes of temperature, and light. Active tablets should produce a distinct burning sensation when placed under the tongue. Only nitroglycerin, erythrityl tetranitrate, and isosorbide dinitrate are available in sublingual tablets.

THERAPEUTIC USES

Angina. Diseases that predispose to angina should be treated as part of a comprehensive therapeutic program. Such conditions as hypertension, anemia, thyrotoxicosis, obesity, heart failure, cardiac arrhythmias, and chronic and acute anxiety can precipitate anginal symptoms in many patients. The patient should be asked to stop smoking, overeating, and exercising shortly after meals. Consumption of caffeine should be limited, and exposure to sympathomimetic agents (*e.g.*, those in nasal decongestants) should be avoided. The use of drugs that modify the perception of pain is a poor approach to the treatment of angina, since the underlying myocardial ischemia is not relieved.

Sublingual Administration. Because of its rapid action, long-established efficacy, and low cost, nitroglycerin is the most useful drug among the organic nitrates that can be given sublingually. An initial dose of 0.3 mg of nitroglycerin will often relieve pain within 3 minutes. Pain may be prevented when the drug is used prophylactically immediately prior to exercise or stress. The smallest effective dose should be prescribed. Patients should be taught to contact their physicians when more than three tablets taken over a 15-minute period do not relieve a sustained attack, since this situation may be indicative of myocardial infarction or another cause for the pain. The patient should be advised that there is no virtue in trying to avoid taking the sublingual nitroglycerin tablets for anginal pain. Other nitrates that can be taken sublingually do not appear to be longer acting or more effective than nitroglycerin, and are often more expensive.

Oral Administration. Oral nitrates employed at usual dose (*e.g.*, 5 to 10 mg of isosorbide dinitrate) are no more effective than placebo in decreasing the frequency of angina or increasing the patient's exercise tolerance. Clinical studies that have used higher doses either of isosorbide dinitrate (*e.g.*, 20 mg or more orally every 4 hours) or sustained-release preparations of nitroglycerin indicate that such regimens decrease the frequency of attacks of angina, improve exercise tolerance, and favorably alter the determinants of myocardial oxygen demand. However, these high doses increase the risk of hypotension, tachycardia, and tolerance.

Topical Administration. Application of nitroglycerin ointment can relieve angina for 4 hours or more. Usually 2% nitroglycerin ointment is applied to the skin (2.5 to 5 cm [1 to 2 in.] as it is squeezed from the tube; it is then spread in a uniform layer); the dosage must be adjusted for each patient. The ointment is particularly useful for controlling nocturnal angina, which commonly develops within 3 hours after the patient goes to sleep. A transdermal nitroglycerin disc applied once every 24 hours produces a continuous concentration of nitrate in blood. Although effective initially, long-term topical administration of nitroglycerin can lead to the rapid development of tolerance and loss of the therapeutic effect. Therapy should be interrupted for about 8 hours each day.

Congestive Heart Failure. The goal of treatment of congestive heart failure is to increase cardiac output and reduce pulmonary and peripheral edema. Conventional therapy of heart failure involves the use of positive inotropic agents and diuretics (*see* Chapters 28 and 34). Vasodilators can improve cardiovascular function in congestive heart failure, even in some patients who are unresponsive to conventional therapy (*see* Symposium, 1983, 1984).

Acute Heart Failure. The utility of vasodilators to relieve pulmonary congestion and to increase cardiac output in acute congestive heart failure is well established. The acceptance of these drugs for such treatment has been aided by the development of bedside techniques that allow frequent measurement of ventricular filling pressure and cardiac output. Thus, the effects of the drug can be objectively evaluated, and their doses and intervals of administration can be optimized to improve left ventricular performance. Initially, use of vasodilators was aimed at reduction of preload by producing venodilatation, which reduced end-diastolic pressure and relieved pulmonary congestion. More recently, reduction of afterload by dilatation of arterioles and reduction of peripheral resistance has also been utilized to increase cardiac output.

The response of the cardiovascular system to vasodilators is different in patients with congestive heart failure than in normal individuals. In normal subjects the administration of a venodilator decreases preload and results in decreased cardiac output, whereas drugs that reduce afterload cause only a small increase in stroke volume. The net effect of arteriolar and venous dilatation in a normal individual is a decrease in blood pressure and a reflex tachycardia.

Patients with congestive heart failure have elevated peripheral vascular resistance owing to compensatory increases in adrenergic tone and enhanced activity of the renin-angiotensin system. These factors act to maintain blood pressure and redistribute blood flow to vital organs, despite a low cardiac output. However, this increase in afterload is detrimental to cardiac performance and contributes to the reduction in cardiac output. Drugs that reduce peripheral resistance in patients with congestive heart failure significantly increase the ejection fraction, stroke volume, cardiac output, and tissue perfusion. The increase in cardiac output may counterbalance the fall in peripheral resistance, and little or no change in the patient's blood pressure and heart rate may occur. However, if the reduction of preload is excessive (to below-normal levels), the cardiac output will fall. The hemodynamic effects of the drugs must, therefore, be monitored carefully. When this is done, the treatment can be individualized such that preload and afterload are appropriately reduced and myocardial oxygen demand is lowered despite an increase in cardiac output. The use of conventional positive inotropic agents may allow a similar increase in cardiac output, but at the cost of increased consumption of oxygen.

Many of the vasodilators used in other clinical conditions (*e.g.*, angina and hypertension) have also been used to improve left ventricular function and provide relief of symptoms in acute heart failure. Classification of these drugs is usually based on their major site of action. Thus, agents such as nitroglycerin and isosorbide dinitrate are described as primarily relaxing venous smooth muscle. They would be expected to decrease venous return, lower ventricular filling pressures, and relieve pulmonary congestion. Small decreases in preload would result in little effect on cardiac output, but excessive decreases in preload would reduce cardiac output. A second group of agents (*e.g.*, hydralazine, minoxidil) is designated as primarily arterial vasodilators; these drugs decrease afterload and increase cardiac output with little change in filling pressure or preload. These agents are discussed in Chapter 33. Some drugs act on both arterial and venous beds to similar degrees. These include nitroprusside, α-adrenergic antagonists, and inhibitors of angiotensin converting enzyme. Termed "balanced" vasodilators, they tend to decrease both filling pressure and pulmonary congestion and increase cardiac output as a result of a decrease in arterial resistance. Although this description of the effects of these agents is useful clinically, it is clearly an oversimplification from the point of view of the pharmacological actions of the drugs and the physiological responses to arterial and venous dilatation in the heterogeneous conditions that are manifest as congestive heart failure. These agents are also discussed in Chapters 11, 31, and 33.

Some agents (nitrates, minoxidil, hydralazine, nitroprusside) cause arteriolar dilatation and/or venodilatation of all regional vascular beds rather uniformly. They require widely varying doses in different individuals, and these doses are usually higher than those necessary to treat angina or hypertension. In contrast, α-adrenergic blocking agents and inhibitors of angiotensin converting enzyme would be expected to reverse the inappropriately high vasoconstrictive effects of norepinephrine and angiotensin on specific vascular beds. Doses of these agents that produce vasodilatation in heart failure are comparable to those used in the treatment of hypertension (Packer, 1982).

Most of the adverse effects of vasodilator therapy in acute heart failure relate to excessive vasodilatation, which results in excessively reduced filling pressures, hypotension, decreased ventricular performance, and decreased perfusion of tissues. These problems can be avoided by careful attention to changes in ventricular filling pressures and cardiac output. In addition, the abrupt withdrawal of an infusion of nitroprusside from patients with severe heart failure may be associated with a rebound in hemodynamic effects that produce a transient deterioration in cardiac performance. Presumably, this is due to the activation of baroreceptor reflexes, and its magnitude is related to the degree of preservation of compensatory vasoconstrictive mechanisms in individual patients.

Chronic Heart Failure. In addition to their well-established efficacy in acute failure, vasodilators are effective for the treatment of chronic heart failure (Parmley, 1989). The objectives of long-term vasodilator therapy are to reduce morbidity and mortality, to produce sustained improvement of left ventricular function, and to improve exercise tolerance. Unfortunately, the initial improvement in left ventricular function produced by some vasodilators (*e.g.*, prazosin) does not persist in many patients. With arteriolar vasodilators such as hydralazine, even sustained increases in cardiac output have not been associated with demonstrable increases in exercise capacity or relief of symptoms (Packer, 1982). At present, neither the mechanisms that underlie the tolerance to some vasodilators nor the reasons why increases in cardiac output do not always correlate with increased exercise capacity are clearly understood. However, in contrast to the results obtained with arteriolar vasodilators, treatment with organic nitrate venodilators can improve exercise tolerance, even though cardiac output changes little. Concurrent administration of isosorbide dinitrate and an arteriolar dilator (hydralazine) not only improves exercise tolerance but can prolong life when the regimen for treatment of moderate congestive heart failure also includes digitalis and a diuretic (Cohn *et al.*, 1986). Inhibition of angiotensin converting enzyme reduces both preload and afterload (*see* Chapter 31). Although these drugs cause only a modest increase in cardiac output, they, too, improve exercise tolerance. When given together with digitalis and a diuretic, inhibitors of angiotensin converting enzyme prolong the life of patients with severe heart failure (Consensus Trial Study Group, 1987). Of interest, salutary effects of converting enzyme inhibitors on exercise tolerance are observed in patients with mild-to-moderate heart failure who also receive a diuretic but not digitalis. These findings indicate that there are alternatives to digitalis for the initial management of early cardiac failure (Captopril-Digoxin Multicenter Research Group, 1988; *see also* Chapters 31 and 34).

Myocardial Infarction. Some therapeutic maneuvers are directed at reducing the size of a myocardial infarction and preserving or retrieving viable tissue by reducing the oxygen demand of the myocardium. A drug that favorably alters the oxygen balance could decrease the area of myocardial damage if it were given soon after infarction.

In the past, nitroglycerin was considered to be contraindicated for use in patients with acute myocardial infarction. Its ability to induce hypotension and trigger a reflex tachycardia was feared. However, intravenous infusion of nitroglycerin in patients with acute myocardial infarction at doses that maintain or improve stroke work can relieve pulmonary congestion by decreasing left ventricular filling pressure; furthermore, myocardial oxygen demand is reduced. Nitroglycerin can also decrease the electrophysiological signs of ischemic injury in patients with acute myocardial infarction (Roberts, 1983). Nevertheless, there have been contradictory reports, and additional experience is required to define the utility of organic nitrates in myocardial infarction.

Variant (Prinzmetal's) Angina. Numerous studies in experimental animals have demonstrated that coronary blood flow can be modulated by neurogenic stimulation of the large coronary arteries. These vessels normally contribute little to coronary resistance. However, stimulation of the large vessels may cause marked coronary constriction, resulting in reduced blood flow and ischemic pain. Variant angina is believed to be the result of coronary vasospasm, possibly resulting from such stimulation. Transmitters that have been hypothesized to be involved in the initiation of vasospasm include catecholamines, 5-hydroxytryptamine, and histamine. It has also been postulated that endothelial-cell injury may promote contraction because of the deficiency of vasodilators that originate from these cells. Ergonovine maleate, a vasoconstrictor (*see* Chapter 39), has been utilized intravenously during coronary arteriography as a provocative diagnostic test to induce coronary artery vasospasm and identify patients with variant angina. Ergonovine-induced coronary artery spasm is reversed by nitroglycerin.

CALCIUM-CHANNEL BLOCKERS

Hass and Hartfelder reported in 1962 that verapamil, a putative coronary vasodilator, possessed negative inotropic and chronotropic effects that were not seen with other vasodilatory agents, such as nitroglycerin. Fleckenstein subsequently suggested that the negative inotropic effect resulted from inhibition of excitation–contraction coupling and that the mechanism involved reduction of the movement of Ca^{2+} into cardiac myocytes (Fleckenstein *et al.*, 1967).

Rougier, Coraboeuf, and colleagues subsequently presented definitive evidence that depolarization in atrial tissue was mediated by two inwardly directed ionic currents (Rougier *et al.*, 1969). When the transmembrane potential of a cardiac cell reaches threshold, the membrane permeability (conductance) for Na^+ increases rapidly and markedly. The so-called *fast channel* is responsible for this influx of Na^+, and it is blocked by tetrodotoxin (*see* Chapter 35). The time required for the second inward current to reach maximal values is much longer. This current is caused in large part by the movement of Ca^{2+} into the cell through a membrane pore that is thus termed the *slow channel* or *Ca^{2+} channel*. The movement of Ca^{2+} through this slow channel is inhibited by Mn^{2+}, but not by tetrodotoxin, and it contributes to the maintenance of the plateau phase of the cardiac action potential (Rougier *et al.*, 1969). A derivative of verapamil, D-600 (gallopamil), was subsequently shown to block the movement of Ca^{2+} through the slow channel and thereby alter the plateau phase of the cardiac action potential (Kohlhardt *et al.*, 1972).

Chemistry. The five Ca^{2+}-channel blockers that have been approved for clinical use in the United States, and others that are under development, have diverse chemical structures. Four classes of compounds have been extensively examined: phenylalkylamines, dihydropyridines, benzothiazepines, and diphenylpiperazines. At present diltiazem (a benzothiazepine); nicardipine, nifedipine, and nimodipine (dihydropyridines); and verapamil (a phenylalkylamine) are approved for clinical use in the United States. Their structures are shown in Table 32–2.

PHARMACOLOGICAL PROPERTIES

Increased concentrations of cytosolic Ca^{2+} cause increased contraction of the myocardium and vascular smooth muscle. The entry of extracellular Ca^{2+} is more important in initiating the contraction of myocardial cells, while the release of Ca^{2+} from intracellular storage sites also participates in vascular smooth muscle, particularly in some vascular beds. In addition, the entry of extracellular Ca^{2+} can trigger the release of additional Ca^{2+} from intracellular stores.

The extracellular concentration of Ca^{2+} is high; the intracellular concentration of free Ca^{2+} is approximately 10,000-fold lower (*see* Chapter 62). This gradient is established by membrane pumps and intracellular storage sites. The cytosolic Ca^{2+} concentration is increased by various contractile stimuli. Thus, many hormones and neurohormones increase Ca^{2+} influx through so-called "receptor operated" channels, while high external concentrations of K^+ and depolarizing electrical stimuli increase Ca^{2+} influx through voltage-sensitive or "potential-operated" channels. Some blood vessels also exhibit increased Ca^{2+} influx when stretched; they are said to contain "stretch-operated" channels (Bevan *et al.*, 1982).

Voltage-sensitive Ca^{2+} channels belong to a family of homologous proteins that also includes channels for Na^+ and K^+ (*see* Chapters 5 and 15). These channels contain domains of homologous sequence that are arranged in tandem within a single large subunit (Na^+ and Ca^{2+} channels) or multiple smaller subunits with homologous sequences (K^+ channels). These domains or subunits contain several hydrophobic regions that span the membrane and outline an internal pore. In addition to this major channel-forming subunit (termed α_1), Ca^{2+} channels contain several other associated subunits (termed α_2, β, γ, and δ) (*see* Catterall, 1988). The dihydropyridines bind only to the large α_1 subunit.

Table 32–2. RELATIVE CARDIOVASCULAR EFFECTS OF SOME Ca^{2+}-CHANNEL BLOCKERS *

COMPOUND AND STRUCTURE	VASODILATATION (CORONARY FLOW)	SUPPRESSION OF CARDIAC CONTRACTILITY	SUPPRESSION OF AUTOMATICITY (SA NODE)	SUPPRESSION OF CONDUCTION (AV NODE)
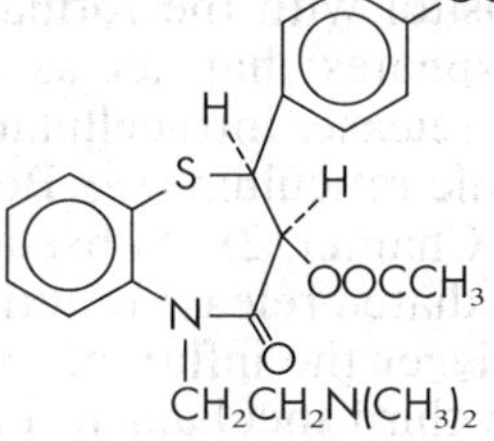 Diltiazem	3	2	5	4
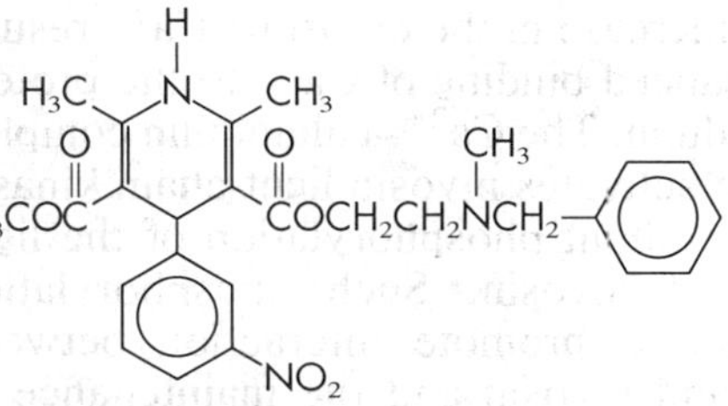 Nicardipine	5	0	1	0
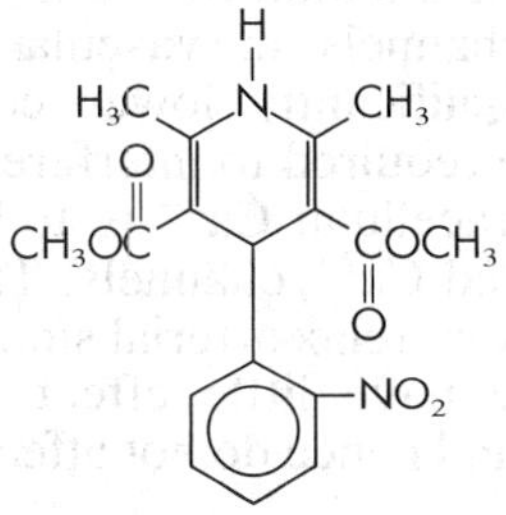 Nifedipine	5	1	1	0
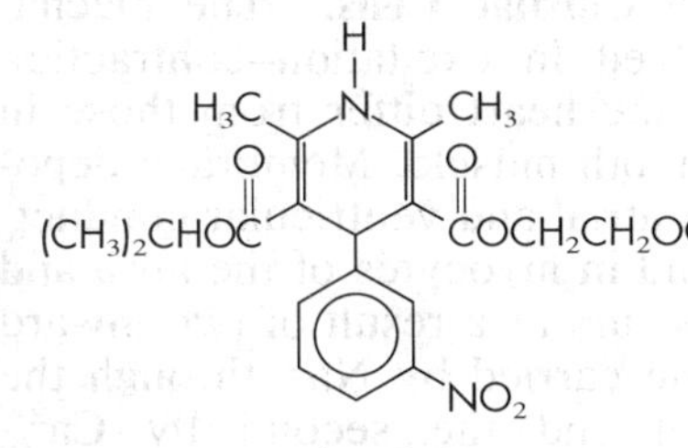 Nimodipine	5	1	1	0
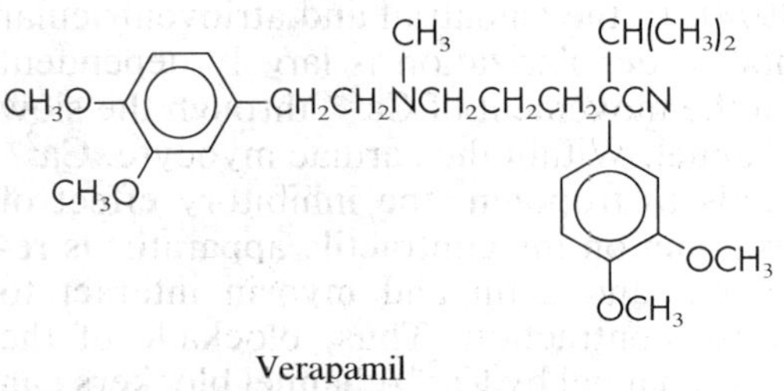 Verapamil	4	4	5	5

* The relative cardiovascular effects are ranked from no effect (0) to most prominent (5). (Adapted from Julian, 1987; Taira, 1987.)

Voltage-sensitive Ca^{2+} channels have been divided into three subtypes, termed *L, N,* and *T* based on their conductances and sensitivities to voltage (Schwartz *et al.*, 1988; Tsien *et al.,* 1988). Only the L-type channel is sensitive to the Ca^{2+}-channel blockers shown in Table 32–2. (Certain snail toxins from the genus *Conus* and large divalent cations such as Cd^{2+} and Mn^{2+} block a wider range of Ca^{2+} channels.) Although the dihydropyridines bind to a common site, Ca^{2+}-channel blockers of different structure bind to distinct sites on the L channel. The selectivity of the pharmacological effects of these Ca^{2+}-channel blockers appears to arise in particular because of the abundance of L channels in cardiac and smooth muscle. Pharmacokinetic factors and the enhanced affinity of the ligands for the channel when the membrane is depolarized also appear to contribute (Miller, 1987).

The dihydropyridines may also inhibit cyclic nucleotide phosphodiesterases. The dual capacity of the dihydropyridines to decrease cytosolic Ca^{2+} and to increase cyclic nucleotide concentrations may contribute to their greater effects on vascular relaxation.

The vascular and cardiac effects of some of the Ca^{2+}-channel blockers are summarized below and in Table 32–2.

Actions in Vascular Tissue. Although there is some involvement of Na^+ currents, depolarization of vascular smooth muscle cells is insensitive to tetrodotoxin and is primarily dependent on the inward movement of Ca^{2+} (Bolton, 1979). Furthermore, as mentioned, contraction of vascular smooth muscle is regulated by the cytoplasmic concentration of free Ca^{2+}. At least three distinct mechanisms appear to be responsible for contraction of vascular smooth muscle cells. The first of these is mediated by voltage-sensitive Ca^{2+} channels, which open in response to depolarization of the membrane. Extracellular Ca^{2+} moves down its electrochemical gradient into the cell to initiate the contractile process. After closure of the Ca^{2+} channels, a finite period of time is required before the channel can open again in response to a stimulus. The second mechanism involves an agonist-induced contraction that occurs without depolarization of the membrane. It results from the hydrolysis of membrane phosphatidylinositol with the formation of inositol trisphosphates that act as second messengers to release intracellular Ca^{2+} from sarcoplasmic reticulum (*see* Berridge, 1987; *see also* Chapter 2). Subsequently, this receptor-mediated release of intracellular Ca^{2+} may trigger the influx of extracellular Ca^{2+}. The third mechanism involves receptor-operated Ca^{2+} channels, but little is currently known about their structure.

An increase in the cytosolic Ca^{2+} results in enhanced binding of Ca^{2+} to the protein calmodulin. The Ca^{2+}–calmodulin complex in turn activates myosin light-chain kinase, with resultant phosphorylation of the light chain of myosin. Such phosphorylation appears to promote interaction between actin and myosin and the maintenance of contraction of smooth muscle. Ca^{2+}-channel blockers inhibit the voltage-dependent Ca^{2+} channels in vascular smooth muscle at significantly lower concentrations than are required to interfere with the release of intracellular Ca^{2+} or to block receptor-operated Ca^{2+} channels. The Ca^{2+}-channel blockers relax arterial smooth muscle, but they have little effect on most venous beds and hence do not affect cardiac preload.

Actions in Cardiac Cells. The mechanisms involved in excitation–contraction coupling in the heart differ from those in vascular smooth muscle. Membrane depolarization in atrial and ventricular conducting tissue and in myocytes of the atria and ventricles occurs as a result of two inward currents, one carried by Na^+ through the fast channel and the second by Ca^{2+} through the slow channel (Coraboeuf, 1978). In the sinoatrial and atrioventricular nodes, depolarization is largely dependent on the movement of Ca^{2+} through the slow channel. Within the cardiac myocyte, Ca^{2+} binds to troponin, the inhibitory effect of troponin on the contractile apparatus is relieved, and actin and myosin interact to cause contraction. Thus, blockade of the slow channel by Ca^{2+}-channel blockers can result in a negative inotropic effect.

The effect of a Ca^{2+}-channel blocker on

atrioventricular conduction and on the rate of the sinus node pacemaker appears to be dependent in part on whether the agent delays the recovery of the slow channel (Henry, 1983). Recovery is the process in repolarized membranes whereby a channel regains its capacity to carry Ca^{2+} in response to activation. Although nifedipine reduces the slow inward current in a dose-dependent manner, it does not affect the rate of recovery of the slow Ca^{2+} channel (Kohlhardt and Fleckenstein, 1977). The channel blockade caused by nifedipine and related dihydropyridines also shows little dependence on the frequency of stimulation. At doses used clinically, nifedipine does not affect conduction through the node. In contrast, verapamil not only reduces the magnitude of the Ca^{2+} current through the slow channel but also decreases the rate of recovery of the channel (Ehara and Kaufmann, 1978). In addition, channel blockade caused by verapamil (and to a lesser extent by diltiazem) is enhanced as the frequency of stimulation increases. Verapamil and diltiazem depress the rate of the sinus node pacemaker and slow AV conduction; the latter effect is the basis for their use in the treatment of supraventricular tachyarrhythmias (*see* Chapter 35).

Hemodynamic Effects. All of the Ca^{2+}-channel blockers that have been approved for clinical use decrease coronary vascular resistance and increase coronary blood flow. Nifedipine, nicardipine, and nimodipine are more potent vasodilators *in vivo* and *in vitro* than is verapamil, which is more potent than diltiazem. Since the hemodynamic effects of each of these agents vary depending on the route of administration and the extent of left ventricular dysfunction, each will be presented separately.

Nifedipine given intravenously increases forearm blood flow with little effect on venous pooling; this indicates a selective dilatation of arterial resistance vessels (Robinson *et al.,* 1980). The decrease in arterial blood pressure elicits sympathetic reflexes, with resultant tachycardia and positive inotropy. Nifedipine also has direct negative inotropic effects *in vitro*. However, nifedipine relaxes vascular smooth muscle at significantly lower concentrations than those required for prominent direct effects on the heart (Ono and Hashimoto, 1983). Thus, blood pressure is lowered, contractility and segmental ventricular function are improved, and heart rate and cardiac output are increased modestly (Serruys *et al.,* 1981; Visser *et al.,* in Symposium, 1987b). After oral administration of nifedipine, arterial dilatation increases peripheral blood flow; venous tone does not change (Robinson *et al.,* 1980). The increase in cardiac output is due to a decrease in arteriolar resistance coupled with the positive inotropic effect that results from the enhanced sympathetic reflex response (Theroux *et al.,* 1980).

The dihydropyridines nicardipine and nimodipine share many of the cardiovascular effects of nifedipine. There may be some selectivity of nicardipine for coronary vessels compared with peripheral vessels and somewhat less negative inotropic effects on the heart when compared with nifedipine. Intravenous or oral administration of nicardipine results in decreases in systolic and diastolic blood pressure that are accompanied by an increase in cardiac output because of the reduction in afterload and compensatory increases in heart rate and ejection fraction (*see* Symposium, 1987b). Nicardipine decreases the frequency of anginal attacks and improves exercise tolerance in patients with effort-induced angina (Hasegawa, 1988; Pepine and Lambert, 1988).

Verapamil is a less potent vasodilator *in vivo* than are the dihydropyridines. As with the latter agents, verapamil causes little effect on venous resistance vessels at concentrations that produce arteriolar dilatation (Robinson *et al.,* 1980). With doses of verapamil sufficient to produce peripheral arterial vasodilatation, there are more direct negative chronotropic, dromotropic, and inotropic effects than with the dihydropyridines. Intravenous verapamil causes a decrease in arterial blood pressure due to a decrease in vascular resistance, but the reflex tachycardia is blunted by the direct negative chronotropic effect of the drug. The intrinsic negative inotropic effect of verapamil is partially offset by both a decrease in afterload and the reflex increase in adrenergic tone. Thus, in patients without congestive heart failure, ventricular performance is not impaired and may actually improve (Hecht *et al.*, 1981). In contrast, in patients with congestive heart failure, intravenous verapamil can cause a marked decrease in contractility and left ventricular function (Chew *et al.*, 1981). Oral administration of verapamil results in reduction of peripheral vascular resistance and blood pressure with no change in heart rate (Theroux *et al.*, 1980).

Intravenous administration of diltiazem can result initially in a marked decrease in peripheral vascular resistance and arterial blood pressure, which elicits a reflex increase in heart rate and cardiac output. Heart rate then falls below initial levels because of the direct negative chronotropic effect of the agent. Oral administration of diltiazem results in a sustained fall in both heart rate and mean arterial blood pressure (Theroux *et al.*, 1980). Despite the fact that diltiazem and verapamil produce similar effects on the SA and AV nodes, the negative inotropic effect of diltiazem is more modest.

ABSORPTION, FATE, AND EXCRETION

Pharmacokinetic parameters for the Ca^{2+}-channel blockers are presented in Appendix II.

Although the absorption of these agents is nearly complete after oral administration, their bioavailability is reduced, in some cases markedly, because of first-pass hepatic metabolism. The effects of these drugs are evident within 30 to 60 minutes of an oral dose. Peak effects of verapamil occur within 15 minutes of its intravenous administration. All these agents are bound to plasma proteins to a significant extent (70 to 99%); their elimination half-lives range from 1.3 to 5 hours. During repeated oral administration bioavailability and half-life may increase because of saturation of hepatic metabolism. A major metabolite of diltiazem is desacetyldiltiazem, which has about one half of diltiazem's potency as a vasodilator. N-Demethylation of verapamil results in production of norverapamil, which is biologically active but much less potent than the parent compound. The half-life of norverapamil is about 10 hours. The metabolites of the dihydropyridines are inactive or weakly active. In patients with hepatic cirrhosis, the bioavailabilities and half-lives of the Ca^{2+}-channel blockers may be increased, and dosage should be decreased accordingly. The half-lives of these agents may also be longer in older patients.

Preparations, Routes of Administration, and Dosages. Many Ca^{2+}-channel blockers are currently being evaluated. Only those five agents currently approved for clinical use in the United States will be discussed below.

Nifedipine (PROCARDIA, ADALAT) is supplied in 10- and 20-mg capsules. The initial oral dosage is 10 mg three times daily; this dosage should then be titrated over a period of 7 to 14 days to control symptoms of angina. The usual effective dosage is 10 to 20 mg three times daily, but 20 to 30 mg taken three or four times daily may be necessary. The total daily dose should not exceed 180 mg.

Nicardipine hydrochloride (CARDENE) is available in 20- and 30-mg tablets for use in hypertension and angina. The recommended dosage is 20 to 40 mg three times a day. At least 3 days should elapse between adjustments of dosage.

Nimodipine (NIMOTOP) is available in 30-mg capsules. The approved indication for its use is to improve neurological deficits due to vasospasm following subarachnoid hemorrhage from ruptured congenital intracranial aneurysms. The recommended dosage is 60 mg every 4 hours for 21 days, beginning within 96 hours of the hemorrhage.

Verapamil hydrochloride (CALAN, ISOPTIN) is supplied as 40-, 80-, or 120-mg tablets, 240-mg extended-release tablets (for hypertension), and an injection (2.5 mg/ml). The drug is given intravenously to interrupt supraventricular arrhythmias, and arterial pressure and the ECG must be monitored. An initial intravenous dose of 5 to 10 mg (or 75 to 150 μg/kg) is given over at least 2 minutes. This can be repeated 30 minutes later if necessary. The usual oral dosage of verapamil for the treatment of angina is 80 to 120 mg three times daily. Dosage is titrated at daily or weekly intervals to a maximum of 480 mg per day.

Diltiazem hydrochloride (CARDIZEM) is supplied in tablets and sustained-release capsules. Oral administration of diltiazem tablets is initiated at a dosage of 30 mg four times daily, and the dose can be increased as necessary up to 360 mg daily. The sustained-release preparation is given twice daily.

TOXICITY AND UNTOWARD RESPONSES

The most common side effects caused by the Ca^{2+}-channel blockers, particularly the dihydropyridines, are due to excessive vasodilatation. These effects may be expressed as dizziness, hypotension, headache, flushing, digital dysesthesia, and nausea. Patients may also experience peripheral edema, coughing, wheezing, and pulmonary edema. Pedal edema may occur in 2 to 10% of patients and is related to dose. Less common side effects include rashes and somnolence. These side effects are usually benign and may abate with time or with adjustment of the dose. Aggravation of myocardial ischemia has been reported, possibly caused by excessive hypotension and decreased coronary perfusion, selective coronary vasodilatation in nonischemic regions of the myocardium (*i.e.*, coronary steal, since vessels perfusing ischemic regions may already be maximally dilated), or an increase in oxygen demand owing to excessive tachycardia. Because of their lower capacity to induce excessive peripheral arteriolar dilatation and tachycardia, verapamil and diltiazem are less likely at therapeutic doses to aggravate myocardial ischemia.

Although bradycardia, transient asystole, and exacerbation of heart failure have been reported, these responses have usually occurred after intravenous administration of verapamil, in patients with disease of the SA node or AV nodal conduction disturbances, or in the presence of β-adrenergic blockade. The use of intravenous verapamil with a β-adrenergic antagonist is contraindicated because of the increased propensity for atrioventricular block and/or severe depression of ventricular function. Patients with ventricular dysfunction, SA or AV nodal conduction disturbances, and systolic blood pressures below 90 mm Hg should not be treated with verapamil or diltiazem, particularly intravenously. Some Ca^{2+}-channel blockers can cause an increase in the concentration of digoxin in plasma, although toxicity from the cardiac glycoside rarely develops (Schwartz *et al.*, 1982). The use of verapamil to treat digitalis toxicity is thus contraindicated; AV nodal conduction disturbances may be exacerbated, particularly if paroxysmal atrial tachycardia with atrioventricular block is present.

THERAPEUTIC USES

The clinical uses of Ca^{2+}-channel blockers have been the subject of several recent symposia (1987a, 1987b, 1987c).

Variant Angina. Variant angina is a direct result of a reduction in flow, not the result of an increase in oxygen demand. Controlled clinical trials have demonstrated efficacy of the Ca^{2+}-channel blocking agents for the treatment of variant angina. These drugs can attenuate ergonovine-induced vasospasm in patients with variant angina, which suggests that protection in variant angina is due to coronary dilatation rather than to alterations in peripheral hemodynamics (Waters *et al.*, 1981). In a large multicenter study, nifedipine eliminated attacks of variant angina in 63% of patients. The incidence of attacks was greatly reduced in most of the remaining patients; in only 7% of those studied was the agent ineffective (Antman *et al.*, 1980). Although some reports indicate that verapamil is equally effective (Severi *et al.*, 1980), others have reported that verapamil is less effective than nifedipine (Kimura and Kishida, 1981). Nicardipine and diltiazem also appear to be effective.

Exertional Angina. Ca^{2+}-channel blockers are also effective in the treatment of exertional or exercise-induced angina. The utility of these agents could result from an increase in blood flow due to coronary arterial dilatation or from a decrease in myocardial oxygen demand, secondary to a decrease in arterial blood pressure, heart rate, or contractility. Numerous studies with double-blind, placebo-controlled protocols have shown that these drugs decrease the number of anginal attacks and attenuate exercise-induced depression of the S–T segment.

The double product, which is calculated as heart rate × systolic blood pressure, is an indirect measure of myocardial oxygen demand. Since these agents reduce the level of the double product (or oxygen demand) at a given external work load, and the value of the double product at peak exercise is not altered, the beneficial effect of Ca^{2+}-channel blockers is likely due to a decrease in oxygen demand rather than to an increase in nutritional coronary flow (Moskowitz *et al.*, 1979; Wagniart *et al.*, 1982; Rouleau *et al.*, 1983). The fixed obstruction present in the patient with exertional angina appears to be unresponsive to dilatation by any of the Ca^{2+}-channel blockers.

In some patients Ca^{2+}-channel blockers, particularly the dihydropyridines, may aggravate anginal symptoms. This may be caused by increased sympathetic tone secondary to peripheral vasodilatation, a marked decrease in coronary perfusion pressure, or coronary steal. This adverse effect is not prominent with verapamil or diltiazem because of their limited ability to induce marked peripheral vasodilatation and reflex tachycardia. Concurrent therapy with nifedipine and propranolol has proven more effective than either agent given alone in exertional angina, presumably because the β-adrenergic antagonist suppresses reflex tachycardia (Bassan *et al.*, 1982). This concurrent drug therapy is particularly attractive, since the dihydropyridines, unlike verapamil and diltiazem, do not delay atrioventricular conduction and will not enhance the negative dromotropic effects associated with β-adrenergic blockade. Although concurrent administration of verapamil or diltiazem with a β-adrenergic antagonist is also effective, the potential for atrioventricular block, severe bradycardia, and decreased left ventricular function requires that these combinations be used judiciously. This is particularly important if left ventricular function is compromised prior to therapy.

Unstable Angina. Although described by a number of terms, including preinfarction angina or crescendo angina, unstable angina can best be defined as recurrent angina associated with minimal exertion. It is prolonged and frequent; both elevation and depression of the S–T segment are observed, as is inversion of the T wave. Coronary flow is severely restricted, and it is likely that vasospasm also occurs in some patients (Hugenholtz *et al.*, 1981). Medical therapy for unstable angina involves administration of nitrates and β-adrenergic blocking agents, which are effective in controlling pain, and the long-term use of aspirin. However, mortality after 1 year is nearly 7%, and 20% of patients have a myocardial infarction (Multicenter Study, 1978). Ca^{2+}-channel blockers offer a unique approach to the treatment of unstable angina. These agents may be particularly effective if the underlying mechanism is vasospasm with S–T segment elevation. However, there is insufficient evidence to assess whether such treatment actually decreases mortality. By contrast, therapy directed toward reduction of platelet function and thrombotic episodes does appear to decrease morbidity and mortality in patients with unstable angina (*see* Chapters 26 and 55).

Other Uses. The use of Ca^{2+}-channel blockers as antiarrhythmic agents is discussed in Chapter 35, and their use for the treatment of hypertension is discussed in Chapter 33. Clinical trials are underway to evaluate the capacity of Ca^{2+}-channel blockers to slow the progression of renal failure. These agents are also being tested to ascertain whether they will minimize ischemia-reperfusion injury in the myocardium.

β-ADRENERGIC ANTAGONISTS

The β-adrenergic antagonists are effective in reducing the severity and frequency of attacks of exertional angina. In contrast, these agents are not useful for vasospastic angina and may, on occasion, worsen the condition. This deleterious effect is likely due to an increase in coronary resistance caused by the unopposed effects of catecholamines acting at α-adrenergic receptors. Although propranolol has been the agent evaluated most extensively in the treatment of angina, most β-adrenergic antagonists appear to be equally effective in the treatment of exertional angina (Thadani *et al.*, 1980). The effectiveness of β-adrenergic antagonists in the treatment of exertional angina is attributable to a fall in myocardial oxygen consumption at rest and during exertion. The decrease in myocardial oxygen consumption is due to a negative chronotropic effect (particularly during exercise), a negative inotropic effect, and a reduction in arterial blood pressure (particularly systolic pressure) during exercise. Not all the actions of β-adrenergic antagonists are beneficial. The decrease in heart rate and contractility causes an increase in the systolic ejection period and an increase in left ventricular end-diastolic volume; this tends to increase oxygen consumption. However, the net effect of β-adrenergic blockade is usually to decrease myocardial oxygen consumption, particularly during exercise. Nevertheless, in patients with limited cardiac reserve who are critically dependent on adrenergic stimulation, β-adrenergic blockade can result in profound decreases in left ventricular function.

There are numerous β-adrenergic blocking agents approved for clinical use in the United States. They are considered in detail in Chapter 11.

COMBINATION THERAPY

Since nitrates, Ca^{2+}-channel blockers, and β-adrenergic antagonists are each useful in the treatment of exertional angina and reduce oxygen consumption by different means, concurrent therapy has been advocated.

Nitrates and β-Adrenergic Antagonists. The concurrent use of organic nitrates and β-adrenergic antagonists can be very effective in the treatment of typical exertional angina. The additive efficacy is primarily a result of one drug blocking the adverse effects of the other agent on net myocardial oxygen consumption. β-Adrenergic antagonists can block the reflex tachycardia and positive inotropic effects that are sometimes associated with nitrates. Nitrates can attenuate the increase in left ventricular end-diastolic volume associated with β-adrenergic blockade by increasing venous capacitance. Concurrent administration of nitrates can also alleviate the increase in coronary vascular resistance associated with blockade of β-adrenergic receptors.

Ca^{2+}-Channel Blockers and β-Adrenergic Antagonists. In patients with exertional angina that is not controlled adequately with nitrates and β-adrenergic antagonists, the administration of a Ca^{2+}-channel blocker can provide improvement. Most studies to date have evaluated the combined use of nifedipine and a β-adrenergic blocker because the latter agent will attenuate the reflex increase in heart rate caused by nifedipine. During exercise, the combined use of propranolol and nifedipine results in a lower heart rate and blood pressure than are observed with either agent alone. As mentioned above, the dihydropyridines do not depress the SA node, AV nodal conduction, or ventricular inotropy *in vivo* and, therefore, do not enhance the adverse effects of propranolol. However, close monitoring is required during adjustment of dosage, since severe hypotension may ensue. Verapamil and diltiazem should be used cautiously, if at all, if a β-adrenergic blocking agent is being taken concurrently. Verapamil or diltiazem must not be administered intravenously under such circumstances.

Ca^{2+}-Channel Blockers and Nitrates. In severe vasospastic or exertional angina, the combination of a nitrate and a Ca^{2+}-channel blocker may provide additional relief over that obtained with either type of agent alone. Since nitrates reduce preload, whereas Ca^{2+}-channel blockers reduce afterload, the net effect on reduction of oxygen demand should be additive. However, excessive vasodilatation can occur. The concurrent administration of a nitrate and nifedipine has been advocated in particular for patients with exertional angina with heart failure, the sick sinus syndrome, or AV nodal conduction disturbances. The combined use of a Ca^{2+}-channel blocker and β-adrenergic antagonist would not be appropriate in such situations.

Ca^{2+}-Channel Blockers, β-Adrenergic Antagonists, and Nitrates. In patients with exertional angina that is not controlled by the administration of two types of antianginal agents, the use of all three may provide improvement. The dihydropyridines decrease afterload, nitrates decrease preload, and β-adrenergic antagonists decrease heart rate and myocardial contractility. Only dihydropyridines (and *not* verapamil or diltiazem) should be used in conjunction with a β-adrenergic antagonist under these circumstances.

DIPYRIDAMOLE

Dipyridamole (2,6-*bis*-[diethanolamino]-4,8-dipiperidinopyrimido-[5,4-*d*]-pyrimidine) is a vasodilator that usually produces only slight alteration of systemic blood pressure or peripheral blood flow. The drug does decrease coronary vascular resistance and increases coronary blood flow and oxygen tension in coronary sinus blood. However, dipyridamole appears to act predominantly on small resistance vessels of the coronary bed, and it alters transcapillary exchange in the same way as does severe hypoxemia. Thus, it appears to have little effect on vascular resistance in ischemic areas where small vessels are already maximally dilated.

The actions of dipyridamole seem to be linked, at least in part, to the metabolism and transport of adenosine and adenine nucleotides; in particular, dipyridamole inhibits the uptake of adenosine by erythrocytes and other cells. Adenosine, which is released from the hypoxic myocardium, is a coronary vasodilator and appears to be an important signal for the autoregulation of coronary blood flow.

In the doses usually employed clinically, dipyridamole is quite nontoxic. Gastrointestinal intolerance with nausea, vomiting, and diarrhea occurs occasionally, as do headache and vertigo. Excessive doses can cause peripheral vasodilatation and hypotension.

Dipyridamole has been used predominantly for the prophylaxis of angina pectoris. Although many conflicting observations have been reported, there is no convincing evidence that either acute or long-term administration decreases the frequency or severity of anginal attacks. There is no improvement of performance during standardized exercise tolerance tests. The effects of dipyridamole on platelets are described in Chapter 55.

VASODILATORS IN THE TREATMENT OF VASCULAR INSUFFICIENCY

Vasodilator drugs have been used in an attempt to increase peripheral blood flow to areas where perfusion is compromised by acute or chronic arterial obstruction or vasospasm. The drugs that have been used can be divided into agents that interfere with adrenergically mediated vasoconstriction (Chapter 11) and drugs that directly dilate vascular smooth muscle, such as papaverine, ethaverine, isoxsuprine, nylidrin, cyclandelate, and niacin derivatives. The pharmacological properties of this latter group are described in *earlier editions* of this textbook, although additional information on niacin and nicotinamide can be found in Chapters 36 and 63.

Despite the fact that these drugs continue to be promoted and widely prescribed for the treatment of chronic occlusive vascular diseases of skeletal muscle (arteriosclerosis obliterans, thromboangiitis obliterans), there is no acceptable evidence that they are efficacious (*Medical Letter,* 1978; Coffman, 1979). Likewise, the utility of vasodilators in reversing or delaying the deleterious effects of acute or chronic cerebrovascular insufficiency is controversial, and the case for clinical efficacy is unimpressive. Direct-acting vasodilators can increase blood flow in normal resting skeletal muscle and in brain. However, it is unlikely that any vasodilator drug can significantly increase blood flow distal to a physical occlusion. Autoregulatory mechanisms in skeletal muscle and cerebral vascular beds produce dilatation in response to ischemia; hence, vasodilators will increase blood flow primarily to nonischemic areas.

Vasospastic conditions affecting cutaneous circulation (*e.g.,* Raynaud's syndrome) may be responsive to α-adrenergic antagonists, but drug therapy is usually reserved for the most severe cases.

Although not a vasodilator, pentoxifylline increases blood flow in the ischemic limbs of some patients with intermittent claudication due to chronic occlusive arterial disease; the mechanism of this action has not been established (*see* Chapter 25).

Abrams, J. Nitrate tolerance and dependence. *Am. Heart J.*, **1980**, *99*, 113–123.

———. Nitroglycerin and long-acting nitrates in clinical practice. *Am. J. Med.*, **1983**, *74*, Suppl., 85–94.

Antman, E., and others. Nifedipine therapy for coronary-artery spasm: experience in 127 patients. *N. Engl. J. Med.*, **1980**, *302*, 1269–1273.

Bassan, M.; Weiler-Raveil, D.; and Shalev, O. The additive anti-anginal action of oral nifedipine in patients receiving propranolol. *Circulation*, **1982**, *66*, 710–716.

Bennett, B. M.; Leitman, D. C.; Schröder, H.; Kawamato, J. H.; Nakatsu, K.; and Murad, F. Relationship between biotransformation of glyceryl trinitrate and cyclic GMP accumulation in various cultured cell lines. *J. Pharmacol. Exp. Ther.*, **1989**, *250*, 316–323.

Bevan, J. A.; Bevan, R. D.; Huo, J. J.; Owen, M. P.; Tayo, F. M.; and Winquist, R. J. Calcium, extrinsic and intrinsic (myogenic) vascular tone. In, *International Symposium on Calcium Modulators.* (Godfraind, T.; Albertini, A.; and Paoletti, R.; eds.) Elsevier Biomedical Press, Amsterdam, **1982**, pp. 125–132.

Brown, B. G.; Bolson, E.; Petersen, R. B.; Pierce, C. D.; and Dodge, H. T. The mechanism of nitroglycerin action: stenosis vasodilation as a major component of the drug response. *Circulation*, **1981**, *64*, 1089–1097.

Captopril-Digoxin Multicenter Research Group. Comparative effects of therapy with captopril and digoxin in patients with mild to moderate heart failure. *J.A.M.A.*, **1988**, *259*, 539–544.

Catterall, W. A. Structure and function of voltage sensitive ion channels. *Science*, **1988**, *842*, 50–61.

Chew, C. Y. C.; Hecht, H. S.; Collett, J. T.; McAllister, R. G.; and Singh, B. N. Influence of severity of ventricular dysfunction on hemodynamic responses to intravenously administered verapamil in ischemic heart disease. *Am. J. Cardiol.*, **1981**, *47*, 917–922.

Cohn, J. N., and others. Effect of vasodilator therapy on mortality in chronic congestive heart failure: results of a Veterans Administration Cooperative Study (V-HEFT). *N. Engl. J. Med.*, **1986**, *314*, 1547–1552.

Consensus Trial Study Group. Effects of enalapril on mortality in severe congestive heart failure. *N. Engl. J. Med.*, **1987**, *316*, 1429–1435.

Coraboeuf, E. Ionic basis of electrical activity in cardiac tissues. *Am. J. Physiol.*, **1978**, *234*, H101–H116.

Ehara, T., and Kaufmann, R. The voltage- and time-dependent effects of (-)-verapamil on the slow inward current in isolated cat ventricular myocardium. *J. Pharmacol. Exp. Ther.*, **1978**, *207*, 49–55.

Feldman, R. L.; Pepine, C. J.; and Conti, C. R. Magnitude of dilation of large and small coronary arteries by nitroglycerin. *Circulation*, **1981**, *64*, 324–333.

Ferrer, M. I.; Bradley, S. E.; Wheeler, H. O.; Enson, Y.; Preiseg, R.; Brickner, P. W.; Conroy, R. J.; and Harvey, R. M. Some effects of nitroglycerin upon the splanchnic, pulmonary, and systemic circulations. *Circulation*, **1966**, *33*, 357–373.

Fleckenstein, J. A.; Kammermeier, H.; Doring, H.; and Freund, H. J. Zum Wirkungs—Mechanismus neuartiger Koronardilalatoren mit gleichzeitig Sauerstoff—einsparenden, myokard—Effekten, Prenylamin und Iproveratril. *Z. Kreislaufforsch*, **1967**, *56*, 716–744, 839–853.

Furlong, B. A.; Henderson, H.; Lewis, J.; and Smith, J. A. Endothelium-derived relaxing factor inhibits *in vitro* platelet aggregation. *Br. J. Pharmacol.*, **1987**, *90*, 687–692.

Ganz, W., and Marcus, H. S. Failure of intracoronary nitroglycerin to alleviate pacing-induced angina. *Circulation*, **1972**, *46*, 880–889.

Gorlin, R.; Brachfield, N.; MacLeod, C.; and Bopp, P. Effect of nitroglycerin on the coronary circulation in patients with coronary artery disease or increased left ventricular work. *Circulation*, **1959**, *19*, 705–718.

Hecht, H. S.; Chew, C. Y. C.; Burnam, M. H.; Hopkins, J.; Schnugg, S.; and Singh, B. N. Verapamil in chronic stable angina: amelioration of pacing-induced abnormalities of left ventricular ejection fraction, regional wall motion, lactate metabolism and hemodynamics. *Am. J. Cardiol.*, **1981**, *48*, 536–544.

Horwitz, L. D.; Gorlin, R.; Taylor, W. J.; and Kemp, H. G. Effects of nitroglycerin on regional myocardial blood flow in coronary artery disease. *J. Clin. Invest.*, **1971**, *50*, 1578–1584.

Hugenholtz, P. G.; Michels, H. R.; Serruys, P. W.; and Brower, R. W. Nifedipine in the treatment of unstable angina, coronary spasm and myocardial ischemia. *Am. J. Cardiol.*, **1981**, *47*, 163–173.

Jaffe, A. S., and Roberts, R. The use of intravenous nitroglycerin in cardiovascular disease. *Pharmacotherapy*, **1982**, *2*, 273–280.

Kimura, E., and Kishida, H. Treatment of variant angina with drugs: a survey of 11 cardiology institutes in Japan. *Circulation*, **1981**, *63*, 844–848.

Kohlhardt, M.; Bauer, B.; Krause, H.; and Fleckenstein, A. Differentiation of the transmembrane Na and Ca channels in mammalian cardiac fibres by the use of specific inhibitors. *Pflugers Arch.*, **1972**, *335*, 309–322.

Kohlhardt, M., and Fleckenstein, A. Inhibition of the slow inward current by nifedipine in mammalian ventricular myocardium. *Naunyn Schmiedebergs Arch. Pharmacol.*, **1977**, *298*, 267–272.

Medical Letter. Drugs for ischemic peripheral arterial disease. **1978**, *20*, 11.

Miller, R. J. Multiple calcium channels and neuronal function. *Science*, **1987**, *235*, 46–52.

Molina, C.; Andresen, J. W.; Rapoport, R. M.; Waldman, S. A.; and Murad, F. Effects of *in vivo* nitroglycerin therapy on endothelium-dependent and -independent relaxation and cyclic GMP accumulation in rat aorta. *J. Cardiovasc. Pharmacol.*, **1987**, *10*, 371–378.

Moskowitz, R. M.; Piccini, P. A.; Nacarelli, G.; and Zelis, R. Nifedipine therapy for stable angina pectoris: preliminary results of effects on angina frequency and treadmill exercise response. *Am. J. Cardiol.*, **1979**, *44*, 811–816.

Multicenter Study. Unstable angina pectoris: national cooperative study group to compare surgical and medical therapy. II. In-hospital experience and initial follow-up results in patients with one, two, and three vessel disease. *Am. J. Cardiol.*, **1978**, *42*, 839–848.

Pepine, C. J., and Lambert, C. R. Effects of nicardipine on coronary blood flow. *Am. Heart J.*, **1988**, *116*, 248–254.

Reichek, N.; Goldstein, R. E.; and Redwood, D. R. Sustained effects of nitroglycerin ointment in patients with angina pectoris. *Circulation*, **1974**, *50*, 348–352.

Roberts, R. Intravenous nitroglycerin in acute myocardial infarction. *Am. J. Med.*, **1983**, *74*, Suppl., 45–52.

Robinson, B. F.; Dobbs, R. J.; and Kelsey, C. R. Effects of nifedipine on resistance vessels, arteries and veins in man. *Br. J. Clin. Pharmacol.*, **1980**, *10*, 433–438.

Rougier, O.; Vossort, G.; Garnier, D.; Gargouil, Y. M.; and Coraboeuf, E. Existence and role of a slow inward current during the frog atrial action potential. *Pflugers Arch.*, **1969**, *308*, 91–110.

Rouleau, J.-L.; Chatterjee, K.; Ports, T. A.; Doyle, M. B.; Hiramatsu, B.; and Parmley, W. W. Mechanism of relief of pacing-induced angina with oral verapamil: reduced oxygen demand. *Circulation*, **1983**, *67*, 94–100.

Schwartz, A.; McKenna, E.; and Vaghy, P. L. Receptors

for calcium antagonists. *Am. J. Cardiol.*, **1988**, *62*, 3G–6G.
Schwartz, J. B.; Keefe, D.; Kates, R. E.; Kirsten, E. B.; and Harrison, D. C. Acute and chronic pharmacodynamic interaction of verapamil and digoxin in atrial fibrillation. *Circulation*, **1982**, *65*, 1163–1170.
Serruys, P. W.; Brower, R. W.; Ten Katen, H. J.; Bom, A. H.; and Hugenholtz, P. G. Regional wall motion from radiopaque markers after intravenous and intracoronary injections of nifedipine. *Circulation*, **1981**, *63*, 584–591.
Severi, S.; Davies, G.; Maseri, A.; Marzullo, P.; and L'Abbate, A. Long-term prognosis of "variant" angina with medical treatment. *Am. J. Cardiol.*, **1980**, *46*, 223–232.
Thadani, U.; Davidson, C.; Singleton, W.; and Taylor, S. H. Comparison of five beta-adrenoreceptor antagonists with different ancillary properties during sustained twice daily therapy in angina pectoris. *Am. J. Med.*, **1980**, *68*, 243–250.
Theroux, P.; Waters, D. D.; DeBaisieux, J. C.; Szlachcic, J.; Mizgala, H. F.; and Bourassa, M. G. Hemodynamic effects of calcium ion antagonists after acute myocardial infarction. *Clin. Invest. Med.*, **1980**, *3*, 81–85.
Tsien, R. W.; Lipscombe, D.; Madison, D. V.; Bley, K. R.; and Fox, A. P. Multiple types of neuronal calcium channels and their selective modulation. *Trends Neurosci.*, **1988**, *11*, 431–438.
Wagniart, P.; Ferguson, R. J.; Chaitmann, B. R.; Achard, F.; Benacerraf, A.; Delanguenhagen, B.; Morin, B.; Pasternac, A.; and Bourassa, M. G. Increased exercise tolerance and reduced electrocardiographic ischemia with diltiazem in patients with stable angina pectoris. *Circulation*, **1982**, *66*, 23–28.
Waters, D. D.; Theroux, P.; Szlachcic, J.; and Dauwe, F. Provocative testing with ergonovine to assess the efficacy of treatment with nifedipine, diltiazem and verapamil in variant angina. *Am. J. Cardiol.*, **1981**, *48*, 123–130.
Zelis, R., and Mason, D. T. Isosorbide dinitrate. Effect on the vasodilator response to nitroglycerin. *J.A.M.A.*, **1975**, *234*, 166–170.

Monographs and Reviews

Berridge, M. Inositol trisphosphate and diacylglycerol: two interacting second messengers. *Annu. Rev. Biochem.*, **1987**, *56*, 159–193.
Bolton, T. B. Mechanisms of action of transmitters and other substances on smooth muscle. *Physiol. Rev.*, **1979**, *59*, 606–718.
Coffman, J. D. Vasodilator drugs in peripheral vascular disease. *N. Engl. J. Med.*, **1979**, *300*, 713–717.
Hasegawa, G. R. Nicardipine, nitrendipine and bepridil: new calcium antagonists for cardiovascular disorders. *Clin. Pharm.*, **1988**, *7*, 97–108.
Henry, P. D. Mechanisms of action of calcium antagonists in cardiac and smooth muscle. In, *Calcium Channel Blocking Agents in the Treatment of Cardiovascular Disorders*. (Stone, P. H., and Antman, E. M., eds.) Futura Publishing Co., Mount Kisco, N.Y., **1983**, pp. 107–154.
Julian, D. G. Symposium—concluding remarks. *Am. J. Cardiol.*, **1987**, *59*, 37J.
Moncada, S.; Radomski, M. W.; and Palmer, R. M. Endothelium-derived relaxing factor. Identification as nitric oxide and role in the control of vascular tone and platelet function. *Biochem. Pharmacol.*, **1988**, *37*, 2495–2501.
Murad, F. Cyclic guanosine monophosphate as a mediator of vasodilation. *J. Clin. Invest.*, **1986**, *78*, 1–5.
Needleman, P. Biotransformation of organic nitrates. In, *Organic Nitrates*. (Needleman, P., ed.) *Handbuch der Experimentellen Pharmakologie*, Vol. 40. Springer-Verlag, Berlin, **1975**, pp. 57–96.
Ono, H., and Hashimoto, K. *In vitro* tissue effects of calcium flux inhibition. In, *Calcium Channel Blocking Agents in the Treatment of Cardiovascular Disorders*. (Stone, P. H., and Antman, E. M., eds.) Futura Publishing Co., Mount Kisco, N.Y., **1983**, pp. 155–175.
Packer, M. Selection of vasodilator drugs for patients with severe chronic heart failure: an approach based on a new classification system. *Drugs*, **1982**, *24*, 64–74.
Parmley, W. W. Pathophysiology and current therapy of congestive heart failure. *J. Am. Coll. Cardiol.*, **1989**, *13*, 771–785.
Parratt, J. R. Nitroglycerin—the first one hundred years: new facts about an old drug. *J. Pharm. Pharmacol.*, **1979**, *31*, 801–809.
Rapaport, R. M., and Murad, F. Endothelium-dependent and nitrovasodilator-induced relaxation of vascular smooth muscle: role for cyclic GMP. *J. Cyclic Nucleotide Protein Phosphorylation Res.*, **1983**, *9*, 281–296.
Symposium. (Various authors.) First North American conference on nitroglycerin therapy: perspectives and mechanisms. (Abrams, J., and Roberts, R., eds.) *Am. J. Med.*, **1983**, *74*, 1–93.
Symposium. (Various authors.) Second North American conference on nitroglycerin: perspectives and mechanisms. (Roberts, R., ed.) *Am. J. Med.*, **1984**, *76*, 1–83.
Symposium. (Various authors.) Calcium antagonists: emerging clinical opportunities. *Am. J. Cardiol.*, **1987a**, *59*, 1B-187B.
Symposium. (Various authors.) Nicardipine—a vasoselective calcium antagonist. *Am. J. Cardiol.*, **1987b**, *59*, 1J–37J.
Symposium. (Various authors.) The calcium antagonists. *J. Mol. Cell. Cardiol.*, **1987c**, Suppl. 2, 1–121.
Taira, N. Differences in cardiovascular profile among calcium antagonists. *Am. J. Cardiol.*, **1987**, *59*, 24B–29B.
Waldman, S. A., and Murad, F. Cyclic GMP synthesis and function. *Pharmacol. Rev.*, **1987**, *39*, 163–196.

CHAPTER

33 ANTIHYPERTENSIVE AGENTS AND THE DRUG THERAPY OF HYPERTENSION

John G. Gerber and Alan S. Nies

Hypertension, defined as an elevation of systolic and/or diastolic blood pressures to above 140/90 mm Hg, afflicts up to 60 million people in the United States; it is thus the most common cardiovascular disease. Hypertension has been classified as "malignant," when it results in arteriolitis, or "benign" ("essential"). Untreated, malignant hypertension causes the death of 90% of patients within a year. Adequate treatment of this condition can lead to long-term survival, and controlled clinical trials were not necessary to prove the benefit of treatment in this disease (Harrington *et al.*, 1959). Based on the elevation of the diastolic pressure, benign hypertension can be subdivided into mild (diastolic pressure, 90 to 104 mm Hg), moderate (diastolic pressure, 105 to 114 mm Hg), and severe (diastolic pressure, ≥ 115 mm Hg). The terms "benign" and "essential" as applied to hypertension were based on the mistaken impression that such elevation of blood pressure was not dangerous, since it did not cause symptoms in most patients, and might even be required for normal perfusion. It is now known that benign hypertension is a major risk factor for stroke, congestive heart failure, and coronary artery disease. Since 1972, the national age-adjusted mortality rate for stroke has fallen 50% and the mortality rate for coronary heart disease has fallen 35%; these changes have been associated with national programs for the detection and treatment of hypertension (Shea *et al.*, 1985; Joint National Committee, 1988). Clinical trials have shown that control of hypertension reverses the risk of stroke and congestive heart failure associated with high blood pressure; however, the risk of coronary disease is not reversed as readily (MacMahon *et al.*, 1986). Thus, these studies indicate that hypertension is neither benign nor essential in the usual sense of these terms.

Some of the earliest randomized, double-blind, controlled clinical trials of drug therapy for any disease were begun in the early 1960s for hypertension (*see* MacMahon *et al.*, 1986; Robertson, 1987). As a result of studies such as those by the Veterans Administration Cooperative Study Group on Antihypertensive Agents (1967, 1970), a substantial and unequivocal benefit of drug treatment to reduce serious cardiovascular morbidity was shown for patients with severe hypertension. The benefit was largely confined to events that were known to be direct results of elevated pressure, including cerebrovascular accidents (CVA), congestive heart failure, dissecting aneurysm, and nephropathy. The studies were all too small and of too short a duration to demonstrate a reduction of mortality, except for one study of patients who had recovered from a CVA, in which antihypertensive therapy enhanced survival related to a reduction of fatal cerebral reinfarction (Carter, 1970).

Subsequent studies of patients with mild-to-moderate hypertension have shown that antihypertensive therapy reduces the incidence of CVA; when the results from several trials were pooled, it was apparent that mortality from all causes was reduced, primarily because of a large decrease in the incidence of fatal stroke (MacMahon *et al.*, 1986). However, pooled data from all of the controlled studies suggest only a small trend to reduce the risk of coronary heart disease. The reasons for this are unknown but include the possibilities that 1) the study population was too small, 2) the follow-up period was too short, 3) active treatment in the "control" group of patients reduced the power of the studies, and 4) the drugs had adverse effects that contributed to the development of coronary disease and thus offset some of the benefits of reducing blood pressure (MacMahon *et al.*, 1986; Kaplan, 1988a). The drugs used for most of the trials were thiazide-like diuretics with the subsequent addition of a sympatholytic drug (in the United States usually reserpine). Various trials comparing β-adrenergic blocking agents with diuretics have produced mixed results, and the capacity of β-adrenergic antagonists to prevent coronary events in any group of hypertensive patients remains uncertain (The IPPPSH Collaborative Group, 1985; Medical Research Council Working Party, 1985,

1988; Wilhelmsen *et al.,* 1987; Wikstrand *et al.,* 1988).

In all of the studies of mild-to-moderate hypertension, the benefits of therapy were more obvious for patients with diastolic pressures ≥ 105 mm Hg than for those with diastolic pressures of 90 to 104 mm Hg; however, based on all of the data, it seems likely that antihypertensive drug therapy benefits all patients with diastolic pressures ≥ 95 mm Hg. Although patients with diastolic pressures of 90 to 94 mm Hg are certainly at higher risk of developing cardiovascular disease than are individuals with normal blood pressure, the benefit from drug therapy is less clear, and treatment must be individualized (*see* below). Increased mortality from coronary heart disease also appears to be caused by excessive lowering of arterial blood pressure, perhaps owing to the production of myocardial ischemia in patients who have a critical narrowing of the coronary arteries (Cruickshank, 1988). A challenge for future therapeutic trials is to determine whether the newer therapies are superior to previous approaches in reducing the risk of coronary heart disease in hypertensive patients, particularly in those with mild-to-moderate hypertension.

Table 33–1. CLASSIFICATION OF ANTIHYPERTENSIVE DRUGS BY THEIR PRIMARY SITE OR MECHANISM OF ACTION

A. *Diuretics* (Chapter 28)
  1. Thiazides and related agents (hydrochlorothiazide, chlorthalidone, *etc.*)
  2. Loop diuretics (furosemide, bumetanide, ethacrynic acid)
  3. Potassium-sparing diuretics (triamterene, spironolactone, amiloride)

B. *Sympatholytic Drugs* (Chapters 9, 11, 33)
  1. Centrally acting agents (methyldopa, clonidine, guanabenz, guanfacine)
  2. Ganglionic blocking agents (trimethaphan)
  3. Adrenergic neuron blocking agents (guanethidine, guanadrel, reserpine)
  4. β-Adrenergic antagonists (propranolol, metoprolol, *etc.*)
  5. α-Adrenergic antagonists (prazosin, phenoxybenzamine, phentolamine)
  6. Mixed antagonists (labetalol)

C. *Vasodilators* (Chapter 33)
  1. Arterial (hydralazine, minoxidil, diazoxide)
  2. Arterial and venous (nitroprusside)

D. *Calcium Channel Blockers* (Chapter 32) (verapamil, diltiazem, nifedipine, nicardipine, nitrendipine)

E. *Angiotensin Converting Enzyme Inhibitors* (Chapter 31) (captopril, enalapril, lisinopril)

I. Pharmacology of Specific Antihypertensive Agents

Drugs (and physiological control mechanisms) influence arterial blood pressure at four effector sites—the resistance vessels (arterioles), the capacitance vessels (veins), the heart, and the kidneys—and they do so by several mechanisms (Table 33–1). Many of the antihypertensive drugs that affect adrenergic receptors, autonomic ganglia, the renin–angiotensin system, Ca^{2+} channels, and Na^+ and water balance have been discussed in detail in Chapters 9, 11, 28, 31, and 32. The pharmacology of antihypertensive agents that are not discussed elsewhere is presented here; in addition, the properties of all of the major drugs that are particularly relevant to their use in hypertension are reviewed, and an overview of the therapy of hypertension is provided.

The hemodynamic consequences of long-term treatment with antihypertensive agents are presented in Table 33–2, which also provides a framework for potential complementary effects of concurrent therapy with two or more drugs. The simultaneous use of drugs with similar mechanisms of action and hemodynamic effects often produces little additional benefit. However, concurrent use of drugs from different classes is a common strategy to achieve effective control of blood pressure with a tolerable burden of adverse effects.

DIURETICS

One of the earliest strategies for the management of hypertension was to alter Na^+ balance by restriction of salt in the diet. Long-term alteration of Na^+ balance with drugs became practical in the 1950s with the development of the orally active benzothiadiazine (thiazide) diuretics (*see* Chapter 28). These agents and the related phthalimidine derivatives (*e.g.*, chlorthalidone) have become the mainstay of antihypertensive regimens. Not only do such diuretics have antihypertensive effects when used alone, they enhance the efficacy of virtually all other antihypertensive drugs.

The exact mechanism for reduction of arterial blood pressure by diuretics is not certain. The drugs first decrease extracellular volume and car-

Table 33–2. HEMODYNAMIC EFFECTS OF LONG-TERM ADMINISTRATION OF ANTIHYPERTENSIVE AGENTS *

	HEART RATE	CARDIAC OUTPUT	TOTAL PERIPHERAL RESISTANCE	PLASMA VOLUME	PLASMA RENIN ACTIVITY	RENAL BLOOD FLOW
Diuretics	↔	↔	↓	↧	↑	↧
Sympatholytic agents						
Centrally acting	↧	↧	↓	↥	↧	↧
Adrenergic neuron blockers	↧	↓	↓	↑	↥	↧
α Blockers	↥	↥	↓	↥	↔	↔
β Blockers No ISA †	↓	↓	↔	↥	↓	↧
ISA	↔	↔	↓	↥	↧	↧
Arteriolar vasodilators	↑	↑	↓	↑	↑	↥
Ca^{2+}-channel blockers	↓ or ↑	↥	↓	↔	↥	↥
Angiotensin converting enzyme inhibitors	↔	↔	↓	↔	↑	↥

* Changes are indicated as follows: ↑, increased; ↓, decreased; ↥, increased or no change; ↧, decreased or no change; ↔, unchanged.

† ISA, intrinsic sympathomimetic activity.

diac output. However, the hypotensive effect is maintained during long-term therapy because of reduced vascular resistance; cardiac output returns to pretreatment values and extracellular volume remains somewhat reduced. Because of the persistent reduction in vascular resistance, some investigators have postulated that the diuretics have a direct effect on vascular smooth muscle that is independent of their saluretic effect. However, substantial data indicate that this is not the case. Thus, anephric patients and nephrectomized animals do not show a reduction in blood pressure when given diuretics (Bennett *et al.*, 1977); a high salt intake or an infusion of saline (but not dextran) to counteract the net negative Na^+ balance produced by diuretics reverses the antihypertensive effect; during effective therapy plasma volume remains about 5% below pretreatment values and the plasma renin activity remains elevated, indicating a persistent small reduction in body Na^+ (Shah *et al.*, 1978); diuretics do not relax vascular smooth muscle *in vitro;* and the hemodynamic effects of the diuretics to reduce vascular resistance are reproduced by restriction of salt (Freis, 1983).

Potential mechanisms for reduction of vascular resistance by a persistent, albeit small, reduction in body Na^+ include a decrease in interstitial fluid volume; a fall in smooth muscle Na^+ concentration that may secondarily reduce intracellular Ca^{2+} concentration, such that the cells are more resistant to contractile stimuli; and a change in the affinity and response of cell surface receptors to vasoconstrictor hormones (Insel and Motulsky, 1984).

BENZOTHIADIAZINES AND RELATED COMPOUNDS

Thiazides and related compounds comprise the most frequently used antihypertensive agents in the United States. These drugs have a similar pattern of pharmacological effects and are generally interchangeable with appropriate adjustment of dosage (*see* Chapter 28). The hypotensive effect of thiazides occurs at low doses (*e.g.*, 25 mg of hydrochlorothiazide or equivalent) that produce a small natriuretic effect; increasing the dose above the equivalent of 50 mg of hydrochlorothiazide per day usually will not increase the antihypertensive effect unless the patient is on a high-salt diet, in which case the lower dose may not produce a net loss of Na^+ (Materson *et al.*, 1978; McVeigh *et al.*, 1988). Larger doses of the thiazides cause obvious diuresis, increased loss of K^+ in the urine, more metabolic abnormalities (hypokalemia, hyperuricemia, hyperlipoproteinemia, and hyperglycemia), and symptoms that can cause poor patient compliance. The need for large doses of the thiazides can be avoided by modest restriction of Na^+ to a daily intake of 70 to 100 mmol; strict salt restriction is not necessary or desirable. Since the degree of K^+ loss relates to the amount of Na^+ delivered to the distal tubule, modest restriction of Na^+ can also minimize the production of hypokalemic alkalosis. Thiazide-like drugs are not effective as diuretics or antihypertensive agents in patients who have a glomerular filtration rate below 30 ml/min. One exception is metolazone, which retains efficacy in patients with this degree of renal failure.

Most patients will respond to thiazides within 2 to 4 weeks, although a minority will not achieve maximal reduction of arterial pressure for up to 12 weeks on a given dose. Therefore, doses should not be increased more often than every 2 to 4 weeks. The average response to a thiazide is a reduction of blood pressure of 20/10 mm Hg, but this is variable among patients. Although the blood pressure of patients who have suppressed plasma renin activity is almost uniformly sensitive to a thiazide, many other patients also respond. There is no way to predict the antihypertensive response from the duration or severity of the hypertension in a given patient, although thiazides are less likely to be effective as sole therapy in patients with severe hypertension. Since the effect of a thiazide is additive with that of other antihypertensive drugs, combination regimens that include a thiazide are common and rational. Thiazides also have the advantage of minimizing the retention of salt and water that is commonly caused by vasodilators and some sympatholytic drugs. If thiazides are not effective at a low dose, it is more rational either to substitute a different drug or to add a second drug than to increase the dose of thiazide above the equivalent of 50 mg of hydrochlorothiazide per day (which enhances the probability of unwanted effects).

Toxicity and Precautions. The adverse effects of diuretics are discussed in Chapter 28. However, because antihypertensive therapy is continued for many years in patients who often have no symptoms of disease, the adverse effects are particularly important in determining patient compliance. In addition, metabolic effects that are of little consequence during short-term therapy cause concern in the long term. There is usually no obvious consequence of thiazide-induced hyperuricemia, although gout occurs on occasion. Similarly, hyperglycemia is often minimal, but an occasional patient with adult-onset diabetes may decompensate when exposed to a thiazide. More problematic are the consequences of hypokalemia and hyperlipoproteinemia. Concerns have been raised by studies showing that effective antihypertensive therapy with thiazides has not produced the expected benefit of a reduced incidence of coronary heart disease (Multiple Risk Factor Intervention Trial Research Group, 1982; Kaplan 1988a). Hypokalemia may cause arrhythmias, and the thiazide-induced increase of cholesterol in low-density lipoprotein (LDL) and very-low-density lipoprotein (VLDL) may enhance coronary atherosclerosis. Although these worries are appropriate, there is no substantial evidence to justify them (Freis, 1986). No study has shown hypokalemia to be closely linked to ventricular irritability in patients who have no evidence of overt heart disease other than left ventricular hypertrophy. However, this is not to suggest that hypokalemia is necessarily benign in hypertensive patients. Hypokalemia may account for some of the disturbances in glucose metabolism associated with thiazides, as well as symptoms of weakness and fatigue. Additionally, high-risk patients who have symptomatic coronary disease, congestive heart failure, and particularly those who are taking digitalis should be protected from hypokalemia. However, in the majority of otherwise healthy hypertensive patients, the mild hypokalemia that results from diuretics is of little clinical consequence.

Hypokalemia can be minimized in all patients by the use of low doses of the diuretic and modest dietary restriction of Na^+. In high-risk patients, supplementation with KCl or the use of a K^+-sparing diuretic in combination with a thiazide may be required. K^+-sparing diuretics are somewhat more effective than K^+ supplements in restoring plasma concentrations of K^+ to normal when hypokalemia already exists (Morgan and Davidson, 1980). The use of dietary means to replace K^+ has the disadvantages of high cost, the potential for excessive caloric intake, and the lack of sufficient Cl^- to correct the metabolic alkalosis. For instance, bananas, a frequently prescribed source of K^+, have only about 1 mmol of K^+ per 2.5 cm of banana, and the usual replacement dose of K^+ is from 20 to 40 mmol per day.

The increase in LDL- and VLDL-cholesterol caused by diuretics is about 5 to 10%, with considerable intersubject variability. Long-term studies have suggested that the increase in lipids wanes with time and may return to baseline after 1 to 2 years of therapy, but this is not entirely clear (Fries, 1986; Lardinois and Neuman, 1988). Because of apprehension about the potential cardiovascular toxicity of the thiazides and the availability of many newer effective antihypertensive drugs, recommendations for initial drug therapy for hypertensive patients now include many drugs other than diuretics. However, there are insufficient data to determine whether these other drugs provide any additional benefit to reduce the incidence of coronary heart disease in hypertensive patients.

All of the thiazide-like drugs cross the placenta, but they have not been found to have direct adverse effects on the fetus. However, if administration of a thiazide is begun during pregnancy, there is a risk of transient volume depletion that may result in placental hypoperfusion. Since the thiazides appear in breast milk, they should be avoided by nursing mothers.

Other Diuretic Antihypertensive Agents

The thiazide-type diuretics are more effective antihypertensive agents than are the loop diuretics, such as furosemide and bumetanide, in patients who have normal renal function (Ram *et al.*, 1981). This differential effect is most likely related to the short duration of action of loop diuretics, such that a single daily dose does not cause a significant net loss of Na^+ for an entire 24-hour period. The spectacular efficacy of the loop diuretics in producing a rapid and profound natriuresis is a potential detriment for the treatment of hypertension. When a loop diuretic is given twice daily, the amount of natriuresis can be excessive and lead to more side effects than does a slower-acting, milder thiazide diuretic. The loop diuretics produce hypercalciuria, rather than the hypocalciuria associated with the thiazides. However, the other metabolic consequences of the thiazides are shared with the loop diuretics, including hypokalemia, hyperuricemia, glucose intolerance, and potentially adverse effects on plasma concentrations of lipids. Loop diuretics may be particularly useful in patients with azotemia. Some hypertensive patients with refractory edema may require the concurrent use of a thiazide and a loop diuretic, but such combinations have the potential to produce severe derangements in electrolyte balance and must be used with extreme caution (Wollam *et al.*, 1982).

Although spironolactone in doses up to 100 mg per day is equivalent to hydrochlorothiazide in its hypotensive effect (Jeunemaitre *et al.*, 1988), higher doses produce an unacceptable incidence of side effects (Schrijver and Weinberger, 1979). Spironolactone may be particularly useful for individuals with clinically significant hyperuricemia, hypokalemia, or glucose intolerance, and it is the agent of choice for management of primary aldosteronism. In contrast to thiazide diuretics, spironolactone does not affect plasma concentrations of Ca^{2+} or glucose. The effects of spironolactone on plasma lipids have not been studied extensively, but data indicate that the changes in triglycerides, LDL-cholesterol, and total cholesterol are less than those seen with the thiazides. However, spironolactone may decrease the concentration of HDL-cholesterol (Falch and Schreiner, 1983). The other potassium-sparing diuretics, triamterene and amiloride, are used primarily to reduce the kaliuresis and potentiate the hypotensive effect of a thiazide (De Carvalho *et al.*, 1980; Multicenter Diuretic Cooperative Study Group, 1981). These agents should be used cautiously with frequent measurements of K^+ concentrations in plasma in patients predisposed to hyperkalemia and in patients receiving K^+ supplements or K^+-containing "salt substitutes." Renal insufficiency is a relative contraindication to the use of K^+-sparing diuretics.

Diuretic-Associated Drug Interactions. Since the antihypertensive effects of diuretics are frequently additive with those of other antihypertensive agents, a diuretic is commonly used in combination with other drugs. The K^+- and Mg^{2+}-depleting effects of the thiazide-like and loop diuretics can potentiate arrhythmias that arise from digitalis toxicity. Corticosteroids can amplify the hypokalemia produced by the diuretics. All diuretics can decrease the clearance of Li^+, resulting in increased plasma concentrations of Li^+ and potential toxicity (Amdisen, 1982). Nonsteroidal antiinflammatory drugs that inhibit the synthesis of prostaglandins reduce the antihypertensive effects of diuretics. It is not known if this interaction is due to Na^+ retention as a result of blockade of the natriuretic effect of the diuretic by the antiinflammatory agent or whether the effect is related to inhibition of vascular synthesis of prostaglandins (Webster, 1985). Nonsteroidal antiinflammatory drugs, β-adrenergic receptor antagonists, and angiotensin converting enzyme inhibitors reduce plasma concentrations of aldosterone and can potentiate the hyperkalemic effects of a K^+-sparing diuretic.

SYMPATHOLYTIC AGENTS

Since the demonstration in 1940 that bilateral excision of the thoracic sympathetic chain could lower blood pressure, the search for effective, chemical sympatholytic agents has been intensive. Many compounds were tolerated poorly because they produced symptomatic orthostatic hypotension, sexual dysfunction, diarrhea, and fluid retention with subsequent reduction of the antihypertensive effect. However, newer agents and rational combinations of these drugs with diuretics and vasodilators have overcome many of these difficulties. The subgroups of sympatholytic agents are shown in Table 33–1.

METHYLDOPA

Introduced to clinical medicine in 1963, methyldopa was originally synthesized as an analog of 3,4-dihydroxyphenylalanine (DOPA) that can inhibit L-aromatic amino acid (DOPA) decarboxylase, an enzyme required for the biosynthesis of catecholamines (*see* Chapter 5). The structural formula of methyldopa, which is marketed as the L-isomer, is as follows:

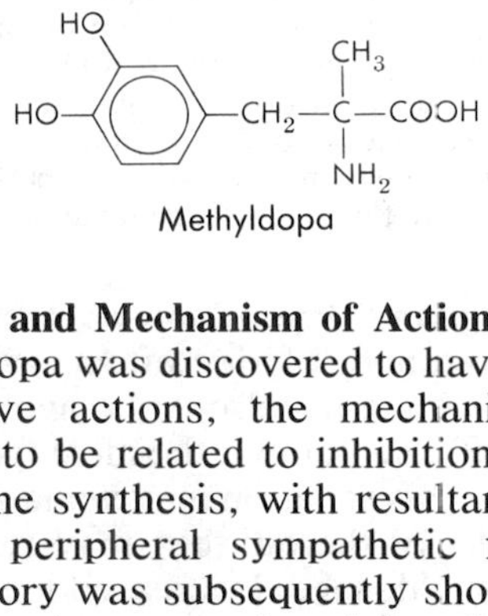

Methyldopa

Locus and Mechanism of Action. When methyldopa was discovered to have antihypertensive actions, the mechanism was thought to be related to inhibition of catecholamine synthesis, with resultant inhibition of peripheral sympathetic function. This theory was subsequently shown to be incorrect; it was replaced by the "false neurotransmitter" theory (*see* Chapter 10) after the finding that methyldopa was metabolized in adrenergic neurons to methyldopamine and methylnorepinephrine. According to this theory, a false transmitter (a substance not normally present in neurons) accumulates in the same sites as the physiological transmitter and is released by the same stimuli that release the true transmitter. Although methylnorepinephrine fulfills these requirements for a false neurotransmitter, it is nearly as potent as norepinephrine and thus could not produce sufficient diminution of peripheral sympathetic function to explain the antihypertensive effects of methyldopa. Subsequently, methyldopa was found to be metabolized to false transmitters in adrenergic neurons in the brain, and this central effect is now thought to be responsible for the antihypertensive effects of the drug (Bobik *et al.*, 1986; Reid, 1986).

In animals, the hypotensive effect of methyldopa is blocked by DOPA decarboxylase inhibitors that have access to the brain but not by inhibitors that are excluded from the central nervous system (CNS). The hypotensive action is also abolished by inhibitors of dopamine β-hydroxylase and by centrally acting α-adrenergic receptor antagonists. These findings have led to the conclusion that methyldopa must be metabolized in the CNS to methylnorepinephrine, which produces its antihypertensive effect by stimulating α_2-adrenergic receptors in the brainstem; such stimulation results in decreased sympathetic outflow from the CNS.

However, not all data support the hypothesis that methylnorepinephrine is the major mediator of hypotension after the administration of methyldopa, since neither concentrations of methylnorepinephrine in the CNS nor turnover of methylnorepinephrine is closely correlated with the fall in blood pressure. Epinephrine-containing neurons have recently been described in regions of the CNS that are apparently important for regulation of blood pressure (Ward-Routledge and Marsden, 1988). Methyldopa can be metabolized to methylepinephrine both in the adrenal medulla and in the brain, and methylepinephrine is more potent than methylnorepinephrine in reducing arterial pressure when injected into the cerebral ventricles of animals. However, the amount of methylepinephrine actually formed from methyldopa in the CNS is probably too small to have pharmacological effects. Nonetheless, methyldopa depletes epinephrine from brainstem nuclei, raising the possibility that this action may have some relationship to the antihypertensive effects of methyldopa (Tung *et al.*, 1988).

Pharmacological Effects. Methyldopa reduces vascular resistance without causing much change in cardiac output or heart rate in younger patients with uncomplicated essential hypertension. In older patients, however, cardiac output may be decreased as a result of a reduction in heart rate and stroke volume; this is secondary to relaxation of veins and a reduction in preload. The fall in arterial pressure is maximal

6 to 8 hours after an oral or intravenous dose. Although the decrease in supine blood pressure is less than that in the upright position, symptomatic orthostatic hypotension is less common with methyldopa than with drugs that act exclusively on peripheral adrenergic neurons or autonomic ganglia. Renal blood flow is maintained, and renal function is unchanged during treatment with methyldopa.

Plasma concentrations of norepinephrine fall in association with the reduction in arterial pressure, and this reflects the decrease in sympathetic tone. Renin secretion is also reduced by methyldopa, but this is not a major effect of the drug and is not necessary for its hypotensive effects. Salt and water are often gradually retained with prolonged use of methyldopa, and this tends to blunt the antihypertensive effect. This has been termed "pseudotolerance," and it can be overcome with concurrent use of a diuretic. Of interest, treatment with methyldopa may reverse left ventricular hypertrophy within 12 weeks without any apparent relationship to the degree of change of arterial pressure (Fouad *et al.*, 1982).

Absorption, Metabolism, and Excretion. Since methyldopa is a prodrug that is metabolized in the brain to the active form, its concentration in plasma has less relevance for its effects than is true for many other drugs. When administered orally, methyldopa is absorbed by an active amino acid transporter. Peak concentrations in plasma occur after 2 to 3 hours. The drug is distributed in a relatively small apparent volume (0.4 liter/kg) and is eliminated with a half-life of about 2 hours. The transport of methyldopa into the CNS is apparently also an active process (Bobik *et al.*, 1986). Methyldopa is excreted in the urine primarily as the sulfate conjugate (50 to 70%) and as the parent drug (25%). The remaining fraction is excreted as other metabolites, including methyldopamine, methylnorepinephrine, and O-methylated products of these catecholamines (Campbell *et al.*, 1985). The half-life of methyldopa is prolonged to 4 to 6 hours in patients with renal failure.

In spite of its rapid absorption and short half-life, the peak effect of methyldopa is delayed for 6 to 8 hours, even after intravenous administration, and the duration of action of a single dose is usually about 24 hours; this permits once or twice daily dosing (Wright *et al.*, 1982). The discrepancy between the effects of methyldopa and the measured concentrations of the drug in plasma is most likely related to the time required for transport into the CNS, conversion to the active metabolites, and removal of these metabolites from the brain. Patients with renal failure are more sensitive to the antihypertensive effect of methyldopa, but it is not known if this is due to alteration in excretion of the drug or to an increase in transport into the CNS.

Preparations, Routes of Administration, and Dosage. *Methyldopa* (ALDOMET, others) is available in oral tablets containing 125, 250, or 500 mg and in an oral suspension (50 mg/ml). The usual initial dose is 250 mg twice daily, and there is little additional effect with doses above 2 g per day. Administration of a single daily dose of methyldopa at bedtime minimizes sedative effects, but administration twice daily may be required for some patients. A parenteral preparation of the ethyl ester of methyldopa, *methyldopate hydrochloride* (ALDOMET ESTER HYDROCHLORIDE) is also available (50 mg/ml). It is usually given by intermittent intravenous infusion of 250 to 1000 mg every 6 hours. The rate of deesterification of the methyldopate is variable among patients, and the doses given intravenously may deliver less methyldopa to the circulation than the same dose given orally.

Toxicity and Precautions. Methyldopa shares a number of side effects with other centrally acting α_2-adrenergic agonists (*see* Chapter 10 and below); the most frequent is sedation. This sedation may wane after several weeks of therapy but may recur with increases in dosage. Decreased mental acuity and forgetfulness are more subtle problems with an insidious onset that can incapacitate individuals who require a high degree of mental alertness. Symptomatic postural hypotension may occur, especially in patients who are depleted of salt and water as a result of aggressive use of diuretics. Other side effects that are related to the pharmacological effects in the CNS include dry mouth, nasal stuffiness, headaches, sleep disturbances, impotence, diarrhea, blurred vision, parkinsonian signs, bradycardia, carotid sinus hypersensitivity, first-degree heart block, and depression.

In addition to these annoying side effects, methyldopa is unique in producing a constellation of less common side effects that can be serious and require prompt discontinuation of the drug. These include hemolytic anemia, leukopenia, thrombocytopenia, hepatitis, red-cell aplasia, lupus-like syndromes, and hyperthermia that can mimic sepsis. At least 20% of patients who receive methyldopa for a year develop a positive Coombs' test that is due to autoantibodies directed against the Rh locus on the patient's erythrocytes. The development of Coombs' positivity *per se* is not an indication to stop therapy with methyldopa; however, 1 to 5% of these patients will develop a hemolytic anemia, which requires prompt discontinuation of the drug. The Coombs' test may remain positive for as long as a year after discontinuation of methyldopa, but the hemolytic anemia usually resolves in a matter of weeks. Severe hemolysis may be limited by treatment with corticosteroids.

The incidence of methyldopa-induced hepatitis is unknown, but about 5% of patients will have transient increases in transaminase activities in plasma. The development of hepatitis is usually heralded by symptoms of fatigue and anorexia that are similar to symptoms of viral hepatitis. Histologically, acute hepatitis due to methyldopa may be indistinguishable from viral hepatitis. Hepatic dysfunction is usually reversible with prompt discontinuation of the drug, but it will recur if methyldopa is taken again, and a few cases of fatal hepatic necrosis have been reported. Hepatitis may occur after long-term therapy with methyldopa, but it usually appears within 2 months of starting the drug. All patients receiving methyldopa should have serum transaminase activity measured monthly for the first 2 months and at the first sign or symptom of hepatitis, regardless of the duration of therapy. It is advisable to avoid the use of methyldopa in patients with hepatic disease.

A variety of rare toxic reactions include lichenoid and granulomatous skin eruptions, myocarditis, retroperitoneal fibrosis, pancreatitis, colitis, malabsorption, and hyperprolactinemia with or without gynecomastia and galactorrhea.

Adverse drug interactions that involve methyldopa are uncommon. Hypotension can be increased by the concurrent administration of diuretics, other antihypertensive agents, and general anesthetics. In experimental animals, tricyclic antidepressants interfere with the antihypertensive effect of methyldopa, but this has not been confirmed in controlled studies in man.

Therapeutic Uses. Methyldopa is an effective antihypertensive agent when given in conjunction with a diuretic. However, frequent side effects and the potential for immunological abnormalities and organ toxicity limit its usefulness.

CLONIDINE, GUANABENZ, AND GUANFACINE

The detailed pharmacology of the α_2-adrenergic agonists, clonidine, guanabenz, and guanfacine, is discussed in Chapter 10. These drugs stimulate α_2-adrenergic receptors in the brainstem, resulting in a reduction in sympathetic outflow from the CNS (Sattler and van Zwieten, 1967; Langer *et al.*, 1980). The decrease in plasma concentrations of norepinephrine is correlated directly with the hypotensive effect (Goldstein *et al.*, 1985; Sorkin and Heel, 1986). Patients who have had a spinal cord transection above the level of the sympathetic outflow tracts do not display a hypotensive response to clonidine (Reid *et al.*, 1977). At doses higher than those required to stimulate central α_2-adrenergic receptors, these drugs can activate α_2 receptors on vascular smooth muscle cells. This effect accounts for the initial vasoconstriction that is seen when overdoses of these drugs are taken, and it has been postulated to be responsible for the loss of therapeutic effect that is observed with high doses of these drugs (Frisk-Holmberg *et al.*, 1984; Frisk-Holmberg and Wibell, 1986).

Pharmacological Effects. The α_2-adrenergic agonists lower arterial pressure by an effect on both cardiac output and peripheral resistance. In the supine position, when the sympathetic tone to the vasculature is low, the major effect is to reduce both heart rate and stroke volume; however, in the upright position, when sympathetic outflow to the vasculature is normally increased, these drugs reduce vascular resistance. Some degree of orthostatic hypotension always occurs because of a reduction in venous return (secondary to systemic venodilatation), but symptomatic postural hypotension is uncommon in the absence of volume depletion. Sympathetic reflexes are damped but not entirely inhibited, and the sympathetic responses that are associated with the use of arteriolar vasodilators such as hydralazine and minoxidil are blunted. However, the α_2-adrenergic agonists do not interfere with the hemodynamic response to exercise, and exercise-induced hypotension is unusual. These drugs do not reduce myocardial contractility directly, and the bradycardia that results from the decrease in cardiac sympathetic tone is rarely severe. Renal blood flow and glomerular filtration rate are maintained. Secretion of renin is often reduced, although it will respond to volume depletion or maintenance of an upright posture; there is no correlation between the hypotensive response and the effect on plasma renin activity. Retention of salt and water may occur with the α_2-adrenergic agonists, and it may be necessary to use a diuretic concurrently. Centrally acting α_2-adrenergic agonists have either no effect on plasma lipids or produce a slight reduction of total cholesterol, LDL-cholesterol, and triglycerides (Lardinois and Neuman, 1988).

When guanabenz was first introduced, there was considerable interest in observations that the drug could be natriuretic in experimental animals. However, studies in man have given variable results. With long-term therapy there is usually a small loss of weight with no clinically significant changes in salt and water balance, suggesting that the "pseudotolerance" (Na^+ retention) seen with methyldopa and guanethidine may not occur with guanabenz. Nonetheless, the antihypertensive effects of diuretics and guanabenz are additive. If individuals are given guanabenz after a salt load, the drug has a natriuretic effect, and a new steady-state of Na^+ balance is attained by 1 week. This short-term effect is thought to be related to a reduction in renal sympathetic stimulation, with a consequent reduction in Na^+ reabsorption in the proximal nephron (Gehr *et al.,* 1986). Guanabenz has also been shown to cause a water diuresis in some situations, which may be due to inhibition of the release and the renal actions of vasopressin (Strandhoy, 1985). Stimulation of renal α_2-adrenergic receptors by guanabenz may inhibit vasopressin-induced accumulation of cyclic AMP (Gellai and Edwards, 1988).

Toxicity and Precautions. Although the α_2-adrenergic agonists do not cause life-threatening adverse reactions, many patients experience annoying and sometimes intolerable side effects. Sedation and xerostomia occur in at least 50% of patients upon initiation of therapy with clonidine and guanabenz and in 25% of patients who receive guanfacine (Wilson *et al.,* 1986). Although these symptoms may diminish after several weeks of therapy, at least 10% of patients discontinue the drug because of persistence of these effects or because of impotence, nausea, or dizziness. The xerostomia may be accompanied by dry nasal mucosa, dry eyes, and parotid gland swelling and pain. Clonidine may produce a lower incidence of dry mouth and sedation when given transdermally, perhaps because high peak concentrations are avoided. Less common CNS side effects include sleep disturbances with vivid dreams or nightmares, restlessness, and depression. Cardiac effects related to the sympatholytic action of these drugs include symptomatic bradycardia in patients with dysfunction of the sinoatrial node and atrioventricular (AV) block in patients with AV nodal disease or in patients taking other drugs that depress the AV node. Fifteen to 20% of patients who receive transdermal clonidine may develop a contact dermatitis.

Sudden discontinuation of an α_2-adrenergic agonist may cause a withdrawal syndrome consisting of headache, apprehension, tremors, abdominal pain, sweating, and tachycardia. The arterial blood pressure may rise to levels above those that were present prior to treatment, but the syndrome may occur in the absence of an overshoot in pressure. Symptoms typically occur 18 to 36 hours after the drug is stopped, and they are associated with increased sympathetic discharge, as evidenced by elevated plasma and urine concentrations of catecholamines. The exact incidence of the withdrawal syndrome is not known, but it seems to be uncommon. It has been reported with all of the drugs of this class, but it may be milder with guanfacine, perhaps because of its longer half-life. Rebound hypertension has also been seen after discontinuation of transdermal administration of clonidine (Metz *et al.,*

1987). Patients who are maintained on a β-adrenergic antagonist after an α_2-adrenergic agonist is discontinued may have more severe hypertension during the withdrawal syndrome.

Treatment of the withdrawal syndrome depends on the urgency of reducing the arterial blood pressure. In the absence of hypertensive encephalopathy, patients can be treated with their usual dose of antihypertensive drug, which should reduce the pressure within 2 hours. If a more rapid effect is required, sodium nitroprusside or a combination of an α- and β-adrenergic blocker is appropriate. β-Adrenergic blocking agents should not be used alone in this setting, since they will accentuate the hypertension by allowing unopposed α-adrenergic vasoconstriction caused by the elevated circulating concentrations of epinephrine.

Because perioperative hypertension has been described in patients when clonidine was withdrawn the night before surgery, surgical patients who are being treated with an α_2-adrenergic agonist should either be switched to another drug prior to elective surgery or should receive their morning dose and/or transdermal clonidine prior to the procedure. All patients who receive one of these drugs should be apprised of the potential danger of discontinuing the drug abruptly, and patients known to be noncompliant with medications should not be given α_2-adrenergic agonists for hypertension.

Adverse drug interactions with α_2-adrenergic agonists are rare. Diuretics potentiate the hypotensive effect of these drugs in a predictable manner. A maximum effective dose of methyldopa will inhibit the hypotensive effect of clonidine, presumably because both drugs act in the same manner. Tricyclic antidepressants may inhibit the antihypertensive effect of clonidine, but the mechanism of this interaction is not known. It has been postulated that the α-adrenergic blocking effect of the antidepressants inhibits the action of clonidine in the CNS; this seems unlikely because the tricyclic antidepressants appear to have a low affinity for α_2-adrenergic receptors (U'Pritchard *et al.*, 1977).

Overdosage with an α_2-adrenergic agonist causes depression of the sensorium, transient hypertension followed by hypotension, bradycardia, and respiratory depression. The depressed respiration (with miosis) resembles the effects of an opioid. Treatment consists of ventilatory support, atropine or a sympathomimetic for bradycardia, and circulatory support with dopamine or dobutamine and intravenous fluids. Although systemic administration of an α-adrenergic antagonist that can enter the CNS may reverse the effects of the centrally-acting α_2 agonists, the use of supportive therapy seems more prudent.

Therapeutic Uses. The α_2-adrenergic agonists are usually used in conjunction with diuretics for the treatment of hypertension, but they may be effective when given alone; all of the drugs in this class are equally efficacious (Holmes *et al.*, 1983). These drugs are also effective in blunting the reflex increase in sympathetic activity produced by vasodilators, and they may be used instead of a β-adrenergic antagonist for this purpose.

Clonidine also has been used in hypertensive patients for the diagnosis of pheochromocytoma. The lack of suppression of the plasma concentration of norepinephrine to less than 500 pg/ml 3 hours after an oral dose of 0.3 mg of clonidine suggests the presence of such a tumor. A modification of this test, wherein overnight urinary excretion of norepinephrine and epinephrine is measured after administration of a 0.3-mg dose of clonidine at bedtime, may be useful when results based on plasma norepinephrine concentrations are equivocal (MacDougall *et al.*, 1988). Other uses for α_2-adrenergic agonists are discussed in Chapters 10, 14, and 22.

GANGLIONIC BLOCKING AGENTS

Ganglionic blocking agents are discussed in Chapter 9. These drugs are effective antihypertensive agents, but they are no longer used except for the short-term treatment of hypertension associated with dissecting aneurysm of the aorta and for the production of controlled hypotension during surgery. The most useful drug for aortic dissection is trimethaphan because it reduces both arterial blood pressure and the upslope of the arterial pressure wave in the aorta; the latter effect is important in slowing the propagation of the dissection. Trimethaphan camsylate is given by intravenous infusion at a rate of 0.3 to 5 mg/min. Hypotension is enhanced by having the patient in the Trendelenburg position; this increases venous pooling and results in reduced cardiac preload. The onset of the hypotensive effect is within 5 minutes, and the effect disappears within 15 minutes upon discontinuation of the infusion. Tachyphylaxis to the antihypertensive effect develops after 24 to 48 hours; this is partly due to expansion of plasma volume, and sensitivity can often be restored with diuresis. Trimethaphan produces a number of unwanted side effects related to ganglionic blockade, including paralytic ileus, bladder dysfunction, dry mouth, and blurred vision. Trimethaphan can produce respiratory arrest when given in doses greater than 5 mg/min, and such doses should be avoided.

GUANETHIDINE

Guanethidine is the prototype of drugs that specifically depress the activity of postganglionic sympathetic nerves. Guanethidine and related compounds contain a strongly basic moiety such as the guanidine group. The structure of guanethidine is as follows:

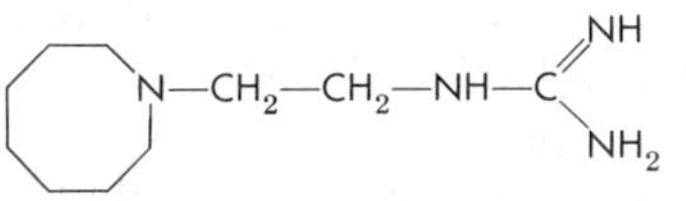

Guanethidine

Locus and Mechanism of Action. Guanethidine is uniquely targeted to the peripheral adrenergic neuron, where it inhibits sympathetic function. The drug reaches its site of action by active transport into the neuron, which is accomplished by the reuptake mechanism for norepinephrine (*see* Chapter 5). Once in the neuron guanethidine binds to storage vesicles. Initially, guanethidine produces sympathetic blockade by inhibiting the release of norepinephrine that normally follows nerve stimulation. Subsequently, guanethidine produces depletion of neuronal norepinephrine. In some ways guanethidine is reminiscent of a "false neurotransmitter," in that the drug is present in storage vesicles, it depletes the normal transmitter, and it can be released by stimuli that normally release norepinephrine. However, the fact that the sympathetic blockade is established well before significant depletion of norepinephrine takes place indicates that the false transmitter concept is not an adequate explanation for guanethidine's action (Shand *et al.,* 1973).

When given intravenously, guanethidine can initially release norepinephrine in an amount sufficient to increase arterial blood pressure. This does not occur with oral administration, since norepinephrine is released only slowly from the vesicles under this circumstance and is degraded within the neuron by monoamine oxidase. Nonetheless, because of the potential for norepinephrine release, guanethidine is contraindicated in patients with pheochromocytoma.

During adrenergic neuron blockade with guanethidine, effector cells become supersensitive to norepinephrine. The supersensitivity is similar to that produced by postganglionic sympathetic denervation.

Pharmacological Effects. Essentially all of the therapeutic and adverse effects of guanethidine result from sympathetic blockade (Woosley and Nies, 1976). A combination of venodilatation, which reduces cardiac preload, and inhibition of the cardiac sympathetic nerves results in a reduction in cardiac output. The arterioles do not respond to the reduction of cardiac output, since guanethidine blocks sympathetically mediated vasoconstriction. Thus, the arterial pressure is reduced modestly in the supine position when sympathetic activity is normally low, but the pressure can fall markedly during situations where sympathetic activation is increased, such as assumption of the upright posture, exercise, and depletion of plasma volume. Renal blood flow and glomerular filtration rate are modestly decreased during therapy with guanethidine, but this is without clinical consequence; renin secretion is not reduced. Plasma volume often becomes expanded, which may diminish the antihypertensive efficacy of guanethidine and require administration of a diuretic to restore the antihypertensive effect. Guanethidine does not enter the CNS and the drug does not affect brain function.

Absorption, Metabolism, and Excretion. The bioavailability of guanethidine is low and variable, and only 3 to 50% of an oral dose reaches the systemic circulation. The drug is rapidly transported to its intraneuronal site of action, from which it is eliminated with a half-life of 5 days. About 50% of the drug is metabolized, and the remainder is excreted unchanged in the urine. Because of its long half-life, guanethidine can be given once daily, and repeated daily doses will accumulate for at least 2 weeks.

Preparations, Routes of Administration, and Dosage. *Guanethidine monosulfate* (ISMELIN SULFATE) is available in 10- and 25-mg tablets for oral administration. The usual dose is 25 to 50 mg taken once daily, but the initial dose should be 10 mg per day. Guanethidine should always be given with a diuretic, and adjustments of dosage should be made no more often than every 2 weeks. Doses of up to 400 mg per day may be required. A loading regimen has been described for more rapid control of blood pressure in hospitalized patients (Shand *et al.,* 1975).

Toxicity and Precautions. Guanethidine produces undesirable effects that are related entirely to sympathetic blockade. Symptomatic hypotension during standing, exercise, ingestion of alcohol, and hot weather are the result of the lack of sympathetic compensation for these stresses. A general feeling of weakness is partially, but not entirely, related to postural hypotension. Rarely, guanethidine can precipitate congestive heart failure in patients with limited cardiac reserve as a result of the decrease in cardiac adrenergic tone and drug-induced fluid retention. Sexual dysfunction usually begins as delayed or retrograde ejaculation. Diarrhea may also occur and be sufficiently severe to limit the dose. Although diarrhea is commonly attributed to sympathetic blockade with parasympathetic predominance, the extent of the problem is not well correlated with the degree of sympathetic blockade, and other drugs that produce sympathetic blockade may cause less diarrhea.

Since guanethidine is actively transported to its site of action, drugs that block neuronal uptake of norepinephrine or displace norepinephrine from its storage sites will inhibit the effect of guanethidine. Such drugs include the tricyclic antidepressants, cocaine, chlorpromazine, ephedrine, phenylpropanolamine, and amphetamine (Michell *et al.*, 1970).

Therapeutic Uses. In the early 1970s guanethidine was a major antihypertensive drug for severely hypertensive patients; it was also used for patients who could not tolerate the CNS effects of methyldopa and reserpine. Many other drugs are now available that are as effective and that are much better tolerated than guanethidine; it is the rare patient who actually requires guanethidine.

GUANADREL

Guanadrel is another guanidine-containing adrenergic neuron blocking agent; its structure is as follows:

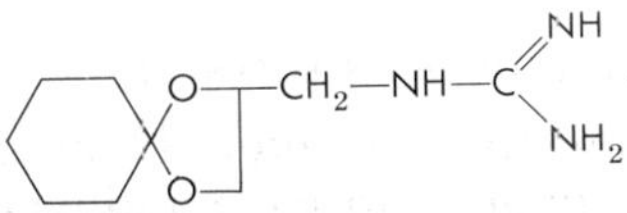

Guanadrel

Guanadrel and guanethidine act in the same way. The major difference between the two compounds is in their pharmacokinetic properties (Finnerty and Brogden, 1985). The bioavailability of guanadrel is high (85%), and the drug has an elimination half-life of 10 hours. Thus, guanadrel must be given twice daily to produce a sustained effect, and it accumulates to steady state rapidly. As a result of the short half-life and duration of action, claims have been made that the dose of guanadrel can be adjusted to avoid some of the side effects of guanethidine. In fact, most studies indicate that the efficacy and adverse effects of guanadrel and guanethidine are similar, with the exception of a lower incidence of diarrhea with guanadrel. Drug interactions with guanadrel are the same as with guanethidine.

Preparations, Routes of Administration, and Dosage. *Guanadrel sulfate* (HYLOREL) is available in 10- and 25-mg tablets for oral administration. The drug is given two or more times daily. The usual initial daily dose is 10 mg, and maintenance doses range from 20 to 75 mg per day.

RESERPINE

Reserpine is an alkaloid extracted from the root of *Rauwolfia serpentina* (Benth), a climbing shrub indigenous to India. Descriptions of the medicinal use of the root of this plant are present in ancient Hindu ayurvedic writings. "Modern" use of the whole root for the treatment of hypertension and psychoses was described in the Indian literature in 1931 (Sen and Bose, 1931). However, rauwolfia alkaloids were not used in Western medicine until the mid-1950s. Reserpine was the first drug that was found to interfere with the function of the sympathetic nervous system in man, and its use began the modern era of effective pharmacotherapy of hypertension. The structure of reserpine is as follows:

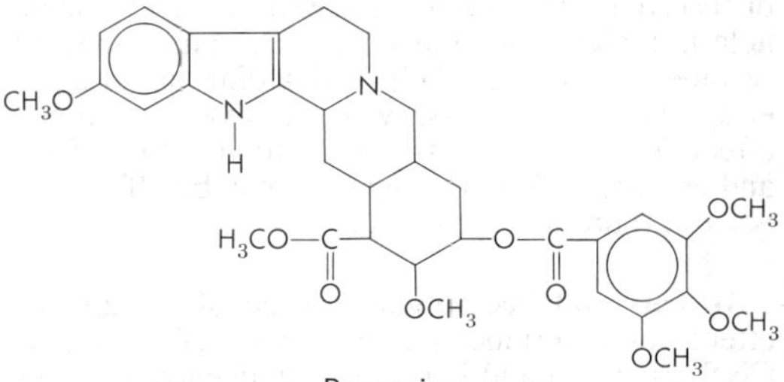

Reserpine

Locus and Mechanism of Action. Reserpine binds tightly to storage vesicles in central and peripheral adrenergic neurons, and the drug remains at such sites for prolonged periods of time (Giachetti and Shore, 1978). The storage vesicles are destroyed as a result of their interaction with reserpine, and nerve endings lose their ability to concentrate and store norepinephrine and dopamine. Catecholamines leak into the cytoplasm, where they are destroyed by intraneuronal monoamine oxidase, and little or no active transmitter is discharged from nerve endings when they are depolarized. A similar process occurs at storage sites for 5-hydroxytryptamine. Reserpine-induced depletion of biogenic amines correlates with evidence of sympathetic dysfunction and antihypertensive effects. Recovery of sympathetic function requires synthesis of new storage vesicles, which takes days to weeks after discontinuation of the drug. Since reserpine depletes amines in the CNS as well as in the peripheral adrenergic neuron, it is probable that its antihypertensive effects are related to both a central and a peripheral action; it is certain that many of the side effects of reserpine are related to its effects in the CNS.

Pharmacological Effects. Both cardiac output and peripheral vascular resistance are reduced during long-term therapy with reserpine. Orthostatic hypotension may occur but does not usually cause symptoms. Heart rate and renin secretion fall. Salt and water are retained, which commonly results in "pseudotolerance."

Absorption, Metabolism, and Excretion. Few data are available on the pharmacokinetic properties of reserpine because of the lack of an assay capable of detecting low concentrations of the drug or its metabolites. Reserpine that is bound to isolated storage vesicles cannot be removed by dialysis, indicating that the binding is not in equilibrium with the surrounding medium. Because of the irreversible nature of reserpine binding, the amount of drug in plasma is unlikely to bear any consistent relationship to drug concentration at the site of action. Reserpine is entirely metabolized, and none of the parent drug is excreted unchanged.

Preparations, Routes of Administration, and Dosage. Many preparations of rauwolfia and its derivatives are available. The powdered whole root of *Rauwolfia serpentina* (RAUDIXIN, others) is available in tablets containing 50 or 100 mg; 200 to 300 mg of this preparation is equivalent to 0.5 mg of reserpine. *Reserpine* (SERPASIL, others) is available in tablets containing 0.1, 0.25, and 1 mg. Reserpine is used once daily with a diuretic, and several weeks are necessary to achieve a maximum effect. The daily dose should be limited to 0.25 mg, and as little as 0.05 mg per day may be efficacious when a diuretic is also used.

Toxicity and Precautions. Most of the adverse effects of reserpine are due to its effect on the CNS. Sedation and inability to concentrate or perform complex tasks are the most common adverse effects. More serious is the occasional psychotic depression that can lead to suicide. Depression usually appears insidiously over many weeks or months and may not be attributed to the drug because of the delayed and gradual onset of symptoms. Reserpine must be discontinued at the first sign of depression, and the drug should never be given to patients with a history of depression. Depression appears to be uncommon, but not unknown, with doses of 0.25 mg per day or less. Other side effects include nasal stuffiness and exacerbation of peptic ulcer disease, which is uncommon with small oral doses. The literature contains epidemiological studies that link reserpine with breast cancer. It is nearly certain that these findings were the result of a bias in choosing patients, and recent data do not support the contention that reserpine is a risk factor for the development of breast cancer (Feinstein, 1988).

Therapeutic Uses. Reserpine was the sympatholytic drug used in the landmark Veterans Administration cooperative studies that demonstrated the beneficial effects of treatment of hypertension (Veterans Administration Cooperative Study Group on Antihypertensive Agents, 1967, 1970), but with the availability of newer drugs that are both effective and well tolerated, the use of reserpine has diminished because of its CNS side effects. However, in comparative studies, low doses of reserpine given concurrently with a diuretic were as well tolerated as combinations of a diuretic with propranolol or methyldopa. The major advantage of reserpine is that it is much less expensive than other antihypertensive drugs.

METYROSINE

Metyrosine is (−)-α-methyl-L-tyrosine. It has the following structure:

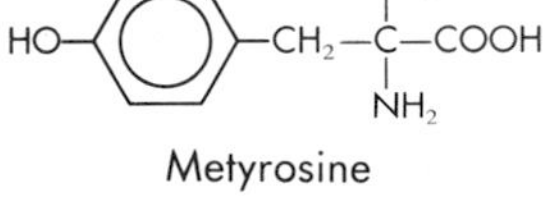

Metyrosine

Metyrosine is an inhibitor of tyrosine hydroxylase, the enzyme that catalyzes the conversion of tyrosine to DOPA; this is the rate-limiting step in catecholamine biosynthesis (*see* Chapter 5). At a dose of 1 to 4 g per day, metyrosine decreases catecholamine biosynthesis by 35 to 80% in patients with pheochromocytoma. The maximal decrease in synthesis occurs within several days, and the effect may be assessed by measurements of urinary catecholamines and their metabolites.

Metyrosine (DEMSER) has seen limited use as an adjuvant to phenoxybenzamine and other α-adrenergic blocking agents for the management of malignant pheochromocytoma (Brogden *et al.*, 1981). Metyrosine carries a risk of crystalluria, which can be minimized by maintaining a daily urine volume of more than 2 liters. Other adverse effects include sedation, extrapyramidal signs, diarrhea, anxiety, and psychic disturbances. Doses must be titrated carefully to achieve significant inhibition of catecholamine biosynthesis and yet minimize these substantive side effects.

β-ADRENERGIC ANTAGONISTS

β-Adrenergic receptor blocking drugs were not thought to have antihypertensive effects when they were first investigated. However, pronethalol, a drug that was never marketed, was found to reduce arterial blood pressure in hypertensive patients with angina pectoris. This antihypertensive effect was subsequently demonstrated for propranolol and all other β-adrenergic antagonists. The pharmacology of these drugs is discussed in Chapter 11; characteristics relevant to their use in hypertension will be described here.

Locus and Mechanism of Action. The precise mechanism for reduction of blood pressure by β-adrenergic antagonists is unknown, and it is likely that there are multiple modes of action. Among the theories that have been proposed are effects on renin secretion, cardiac output, adrenergic neuronal function, control of blood pressure in the CNS, baroreceptor sensitivity, and prostaglandin synthesis. Since all β-adrenergic antagonists are effective antihypertensive agents and since (+)-propranolol, which has little β-adrenergic receptor blocking activity, has no effect on blood pressure, the therapeutic effect is undoubtedly related to blockade of β-adrenergic receptors.

Pharmacological Effects. The β blockers vary in their lipid solubility, selectivity for the β_1-adrenergic receptor, presence of partial agonist or intrinsic sympathomimetic activity, and membrane-stabilizing properties. Regardless of these differences, all of the β-adrenergic antagonists are equally effective as antihypertensive agents. Drugs without intrinsic sympathomimetic activity produce an initial reduction in cardiac output and a rise in peripheral resistance with no net change in arterial pressure. In patients who respond with a reduction in blood pressure, peripheral resistance returns to pretreatment values in a few hours to a few days. It is this recovery of vascular resistance in the face of a persistently reduced cardiac output that accounts for the reduction in arterial pressure (van den Meiracker *et al.*, 1988). Drugs with intrinsic sympathomimetic activity produce less of an effect on resting heart rate and cardiac output, and the fall in arterial pressure is correlated with a fall in vascular resistance below pretreatment levels, probably because of stimulation of vascular β_2-adrenergic receptors that mediate vasodilatation.

Renal blood flow is reduced in the short term by most β-adrenergic antagonists, but reports of deterioration of renal function associated with long-term administration of these drugs are rare. Nevertheless, small reductions in renal plasma flow and glomerular filtration rate may persist, particularly with the nonselective drugs that block both β_1- and β_2-adrenergic receptors.

Toxicity and Precautions. The adverse effects of β-adrenergic blocking agents are discussed in Chapter 11. These drugs should be avoided in patients with reactive airway disease, congestive heart failure, or sinoatrial or atrioventricular nodal abnormalities. Patients with insulin-dependent diabetes are also better treated with other drugs. Although there have been concerns about the safety of the β-adrenergic antagonists for the treatment of hypertension during pregnancy, these drugs are effective and well tolerated, and controlled trials have not supported the initial fears about induction of premature labor, neonatal hypoglycemia, or small newborns.

β-Adrenergic antagonists without intrinsic sympathomimetic activity increase concentrations of triglycerides in plasma and lower those of HDL-cholesterol without changing total cholesterol concentrations. β-Adrenergic blocking agents with intrinsic sympathomimetic activity have little or no effect on blood lipids or increase HDL-cholesterol. The long-term consequences of these effects are unknown.

Sudden withdrawal of some β-adrenergic blockers can produce a withdrawal syndrome that is reminiscent of sympathetic hyperactivity; this can exacerbate the symptoms of coronary artery disease. Rebound hypertension to levels higher than those that existed before treatment has been noted with discontinuation of β-adrenergic antagonists in hypertensive patients (Houston and Hodge, 1988). Thus, β blockers should not be discontinued abruptly, except under close observation; dosage should be tapered over 10 to 14 days prior to discontinuation.

Nonsteroidal antiinflammatory drugs such as indomethacin can blunt the antihypertensive effect of propranolol and probably other β-adrenergic antagonists. This effect may be related to inhibition of vascular synthesis of prostacyclin, as well as to retention of Na^+ (Beckmann *et al.*, 1988).

Epinephrine can produce severe hypertension and bradycardia when a nonselective β-adrenergic receptor antagonist is present. This is due to the unopposed stimulation of α-adrenergic receptors when vascular β_2 receptors are blocked, and the bradycardia is the result of reflex vagal stimulation. Such "paradoxical" hypertensive responses to β-adrenergic antagonists have been observed in patients with hypoglycemia or pheochromocytoma or during withdrawal from clonidine or administration of epinephrine as a therapeutic agent.

Therapeutic Uses. The β-adrenergic receptor antagonists provide effective therapy for many cardiovascular and other diseases, and they are useful for all grades of hypertension. Despite marked differences in their pharmacokinetic properties, the antihypertensive effect of all the β blockers is of sufficient duration to permit once daily administration. Populations that have a lesser antihypertensive response to β blocking agents include the elderly and blacks, but some individuals in these groups may have an excellent response. Patients who smoke were recently shown to have a lesser antihypertensive response to propranolol than do nonsmokers, but this may not be the case with a selective β_1 receptor antagonist such as metoprolol (The IPPPSH Collaborative Group, 1985; Medical Research Council Working Party, 1985; Wikstrand *et al.,* 1988). The β-adrenergic receptor antagonists do not usually cause retention of salt and water, and administration of a diuretic is not necessary to avoid edema or the development of tolerance. However, diuretics do have additive antihypertensive effects when combined with β blockers. The combination of a β-adrenergic antagonist, a diuretic, and a vasodilator is particularly effective. When minoxidil is the vasodilator, this combination can control the arterial pressure of most patients, even if they are resistant to other regimens.

α-ADRENERGIC ANTAGONISTS

The development of drugs that selectively block α_1-adrenergic receptors without affecting α_2-adrenergic receptors has added another group of effective antihypertensive agents. The pharmacology of these drugs is discussed in detail in Chapter 11. Prazosin and terazosin are the two agents that are available for the treatment of hypertension, and several additional congeners (*e.g.,* trimazosin and doxazosin) are being developed. Additionally, investigational drugs such as ketanserin, indoramin, and urapidil may owe a major portion of their antihypertensive effects to blockade of α_1-adrenergic receptors (Cubeddu, 1988).

Pharmacological Effects. Initially, prazosin and terazosin reduce arteriolar resistance and increase venous capacitance; this causes a sympathetically mediated reflex increase in heart rate and plasma renin activity. During long-term therapy, vasodilatation persists but cardiac output, heart rate, and plasma renin activity return to normal. Renal blood flow is unchanged during therapy with an α_1-adrenergic antagonist. Prazosin and terazosin can cause a variable amount of postural hypotension, depending on the plasma volume. Retention of salt and water occurs in many patients during continued administration of prazosin or terazosin, and this attenuates the postural hypotension. Administration of an α_1-adrenergic antagonist may reduce plasma concentrations of triglycerides and total and LDL-cholesterol and increase HDL-cholesterol. These potentially favorable effects on lipids persist when a thiazide-type diuretic is given concurrently. The long-term consequences of these drug-induced changes in lipids are unknown.

Toxicity and Precautions. The major precaution to be remembered when prazosin or terazosin is used for hypertension is the so-called first-dose phenomenon—symptomatic orthostatic hypotension that occurs within 90 minutes of the initial dose of the drug or when the dosage is increased rapidly. This effect may be seen in up to 50% of patients, and it is particularly likely to occur in patients who are already receiving a diuretic or a β-adrenergic antagonist.

Therapeutic Uses. Prazosin and terazosin can be used to treat hypertension of any degree, but these agents are usually not effective by themselves except in patients with mild-to-moderate hypertension. Diuretics and β-adrenergic antagonists enhance the efficacy of the α_1 blockers. Prazosin has been used in patients with pheochromocytoma, but it is not the drug of choice, since it is a short-acting competitive antagonist; in addition, vasoconstriction can still result from activation of unblocked vascular α_2-adrenergic receptors.

COMBINED α- AND β-ADRENERGIC ANTAGONISTS

Labetalol (*see* Chapter 11) is an equimolar mixture of four stereoisomers. One isomer is an α_1-adrenergic antagonist (like prazosin), another is a nonselective β-adrenergic antagonist with partial agonist activity (like pindolol), and the other two isomers are inactive. The isomer that is the β-adrenergic antagonist is being developed as a separate drug (dilevalol) (Lund-Johansen, 1988). Labetalol lowers arterial pressure by reducing vascular resistance as a consequence of blockade of α_1-adrenergic receptors and stimulation of β_2 receptors. Cardiac output at rest is not reduced. Because of its capacity to block α_1 receptors, labetalol given intravenously can reduce pressure sufficiently rapidly to be useful for the treatment of hypertensive emergencies. Given over the long term, labetalol has efficacy and side effects similar to a combination of β- and α_1-adrenergic receptor antagonists; it also has the disadvantages that are inherent in fixed-dose combination products.

VASODILATORS

HYDRALAZINE

Hydralazine was one of the first orally active antihypertensive drugs to be marketed in the United States; however, the drug quickly lost its popularity because of unacceptable side effects and tachyphylaxis. With a better understanding of the compensatory cardiovascular responses that accompany use of arteriolar vasodilators, hydralazine was combined with sympatholytic agents and diuretics with greater therapeutic success. Numerous phthalazines have been synthesized in the hope of producing vasoactive agents, but only those with hydrazine moieties in the 1 or 4 position of the ring have vasodilatory activity (Reece, 1981). None of the analogs has any advantage over hydralazine. Hydralazine (1-hydrazinophthalazine) has the following structural formula:

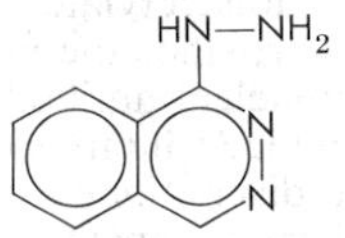

Hydralazine

Locus and Mechanism of Action. Hydralazine causes direct relaxation of arteriolar smooth muscle. The mechanism of this effect is unclear, and numerous hypotheses have been put forth. Part of the vascular relaxation caused by hydralazine is dependent on the presence of the endothelium (Spokas *et al.*, 1983). In addition, nitric oxide can be generated from hydralazine *in vitro* (Kruszyna *et al.*, 1987). Since nitric oxide may be liberated from endothelium-derived relaxing factor (EDRF) or may itself be EDRF, the mechanism of action of hydralazine is similar to the mechanisms of action of EDRF, organic nitrates, and sodium nitroprusside (*see* Chapter 32). Hydralazine can also cause hyperpolarization of isolated arteries and interfere with mobilization of Ca^{2+} in vascular smooth muscle (Kreye, 1984). Hydralazine-induced vasodilatation is associated with stimulation of the sympathetic nervous system, which results in increased heart rate and contractility, increased plasma renin activity, and fluid retention; all of these effects counteract the antihypertensive effect of hydralazine. Although most of the sympathetic activity is due to a baroreceptor-mediated reflex, hydralazine may stimulate the release of norepinephrine from sympathetic nerve terminals and augment myocardial contractility directly (Azuma *et al.*, 1987).

Pharmacological Effects. Most of the effects of hydralazine are confined to the cardiovascular system. The decrease in blood pressure after administration of hydralazine is associated with a selective decrease in vascular resistance in the coronary, cerebral, and renal circulation, with a smaller effect in skin and muscle. Because of preferential dilatation of arterioles over veins, postural hypotension is not a common problem. Hydralazine lowers peripheral vascular resistance equally in the supine and upright positions. Although hydralazine lowers pulmonary vascular resistance, the increase in cardiac output can cause mild pulmonary hypertension. It is difficult to predict which patients will respond in this manner, but the increase in cardiac output can be attenuated by the use of β-adrenergic blocking agents.

Absorption, Metabolism, and Excretion. Hydralazine is well absorbed through the gastrointestinal tract, but the systemic bioavailability is low (16% in fast acetylators and 35% in slow acetylators). Since the acetylated compound is inactive, the dose necessary to produce a systemic effect is larger in fast acetylators. N-acetylation of hydralazine occurs in the bowel and/or the liver, and the rate of acetylation is genetically determined; about half of the people in the United States acetylate rapidly and half do so slowly. The half-life of hydralazine is 1 hour and the systemic clearance of the drug is about 50 ml/kg · min. Since the systemic clearance exceeds hepatic blood flow, extrahepatic metabolism must occur. Indeed, hydralazine rapidly combines with circulating α keto acids to form hydrazones, and the major metabolite recovered from the plasma is hydralazine pyruvic acid hydrazone. This metabolite has a longer half-life than hydralazine, but it does not appear to be very active (Reece *et al.*, 1985). Although the rate of acetylation is an important determinant of the bioavailability of hydralazine, it does not play a role in the systemic elimination of the drug. This suggests that almost all acetylation of hydralazine occurs prior to the time that the drug reaches the systemic circulation. This pharmacokinetic profile is unusual, since other drugs that are metabolized by the genetically determined N-acetyltransferase (*e.g.*, isoniazid, dapsone, procainamide) have a rate of elimination that is dependent upon the acetylator phenotype.

The peak concentration of hydralazine in plasma and the peak hypotensive effect of the drug occur within 30 to 120 minutes of ingestion. Although its half-life in plasma is about an hour, the duration of the hypotensive effect can last as long as 12 hours. There is no clear explanation for this discrepancy.

Preparations, Routes of Administration, and Dosage. *Hydralazine hydrochloride* (APRESOLINE HYDROCHLORIDE, others) is available in 10-, 25-, 50-, and 100-mg tablets and in 1-ml ampules containing 20 mg of the drug. The usual oral dosage is 25 to 100 mg twice daily. Twice-daily administration of hydralazine is as effective as administration four times a day for control of blood pressure, regardless of acetylator phenotype. Hydralazine can be given intramuscularly or intravenously in doses of 20 to 40 mg when there is an urgent need to lower blood pressure.

Toxicity and Precautions. Two types of side effects occur after the use of hydralazine. The first, which are extensions of the pharmacological effects of the drug, includes headache, nausea, flushing, hypotension, palpitation, tachycardia, dizziness, and angina pectoris. In addition, if the drug is used alone, there may be salt retention with development of congestive heart failure. These symptoms were common during the early clinical use of hydralazine; because tachyphylaxis developed, the daily dose of the drug was frequently increased to 400 to 1000 mg. When combined with a β-adrenergic receptor blocker and a diuretic, hydralazine is better tolerated, although side effects such as headache are still commonly described and may necessitate discontinuation of the drug.

The second type of side effect is caused by immunological reactions, of which the drug-induced lupus syndrome is the most common. Administration of hydralazine can also result in an illness that resembles serum sickness, hemolytic anemia, vasculitis, and rapidly progressive glomerulonephritis. The mechanism of these autoimmune reactions is unknown, but hydralazine has recently been shown to inhibit methylation of DNA and induce self-reactivity in T cells (Cornacchia *et al.*, 1988).

The drug-induced lupus syndrome usually occurs after at least 6 months of continuous treatment with hydralazine, and its incidence is related to dose, sex, acetylator phenotype, and race (Perry, 1973). In one study, after three years of treatment with hydralazine drug-induced lupus occurred in 10.4% of patients who received 200 mg daily, 5.4% who received 100 mg daily, and none who received 50 mg daily (Cameron and Ramsay, 1984). The incidence is four times higher in women than in men, and the syndrome is seen more commonly in whites than in blacks. The rate of conversion to a positive antinuclear antibody test is faster in slow acetylators than in rapid acetylators, suggesting that the native drug or a nonacetylated metabolite is responsible. However, since the majority of patients with positive antinuclear antibody tests do not develop the drug-induced lupus syndrome, hydralazine need not be discontinued unless clinical features of the syndrome appear. These features are similar to those of other drug-induced lupus syndromes and consist mainly of arthralgia, arthritis, and fever. Pleuritis and pericarditis may be present, and pericardial effusion can occasionally cause cardiac tamponade. Discontinuation of the drug is all that is necessary for most patients with the hydralazine-induced lupus syndrome, but symptoms may persist in a few patients and administration of corticosteroids may be necessary.

Hydralazine can also produce a pyridoxine-responsive polyneuropathy. The mechanism appears to be related to the ability of hydralazine to combine with pyridoxine to form a hydrazone. This side effect is very unusual with doses up to 200 mg per day.

Therapeutic Uses. Hydralazine should be used for the treatment of hypertension only when the combination of a diuretic and a β-adrenergic antagonist does not control blood pressure adequately. Hydralazine should never be used as the sole drug for the long-term treatment of hypertension because of the development of tachyphylaxis secondary to an increase in cardiac output and fluid retention. In addition, the drug should be used with the greatest of caution in elderly patients and in patients with coronary artery disease because of the possibility of precipitation of myocardial ischemia. The maximum recommended dose of hydralazine is 200 mg per day in order to avoid the drug-induced lupus syndrome. Slow acetylators show a better response to this dosage than do fast acetylators because of the greater bioavailability of the drug.

Hydralazine has been used widely to treat hypertension that occurs during pregnancy. However, the drug should be used cautiously during early pregnancy, since hydralazine can combine with DNA and cause a positive Ames test (Williams *et al.*, 1980). Parenteral administration of hydralazine has been used for the treatment of hypertensive emergencies. However, the hypotensive response to hydralazine given intramuscularly or intravenously is very unpredictable, and prolonged hypotension is not unusual even with intravenous doses as low as 10 mg. The drug is contraindicated for the short-term production of hypotension in patients with dissecting aortic aneurysm or in those with symptomatic ischemic heart disease.

MINOXIDIL

The discovery in 1965 of the hypotensive action of minoxidil was a significant advance in the treatment of hypertension, since the drug has proven to be efficacious in patients with the most severe and drug-resistant forms of hypertension. The chemical structure of minoxidil is as follows:

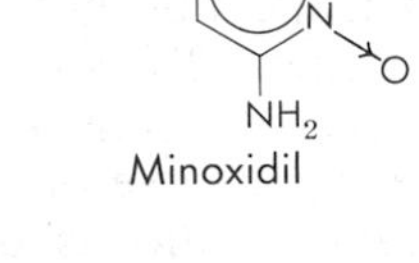

Minoxidil

Locus and Mechanism of Action. Minoxidil is not active *in vitro* but must be metabolized by hepatic sulfotransferase to the active molecule, minoxidil N-O sulfate (McCall *et al.*, 1983); the formation of this compound is a minor pathway in the metabolic disposition of minoxidil. Minoxidil sulfate relaxes vascular smooth muscle in isolated systems where the parent drug is inactive. The mechanism of this effect is incompletely understood, but there is mounting evidence that minoxidil sulfate increases the permeability of the cell membrane to K^+, with resultant hyperpolarization (Meisheri *et al.*, 1988).

Pharmacological Effects. Minoxidil produces arteriolar vasodilatation with essentially no effect on the capacitance vessels; the drug resembles hydralazine and diazoxide in this regard. Minoxidil increases blood flow to skin, skeletal muscle, the gastrointestinal tract, and the heart more than to the CNS. The disproportionate increase in blood flow to the heart may have a metabolic basis, in that administration of minoxidil is associated with a reflex increase in cardiac output and myocardial contractility. This compensatory increase in cardiac output can be as much as threefold to fourfold and is mediated by the sympathetic nervous system.

The effects of minoxidil on the kidney are complex. Minoxidil is a renal vasodilator, but systemic hypotension produced by the drug can occasionally decrease renal blood flow and worsen renal function. However, in the majority of patients who take minoxidil for the treatment of hypertension, renal function improves, especially if renal dysfunction is secondary to hypertension (Mitchell *et al.*, 1980). Minoxidil is a very potent stimulator of renin secretion; this effect is mediated by a combination of renal sympathetic stimulation and activation of the intrinsic renal mechanisms for regulation of renin release.

Absorption, Metabolism, and Excretion. Minoxidil is well absorbed from the gastrointestinal tract. Although peak concentrations of minoxidil in blood occur 1 hour after oral administration, the maximal hypotensive effect of the drug occurs later, possibly because formation of the active metabolite is delayed. Only about 20% of the absorbed drug is excreted unchanged in the urine, and the main route of elimination is by hepatic metabolism. The major metabolite of minoxidil is the glucuronide conjugate at the N-oxide position in the pyrimidine ring. This metabolite is less active than minoxidil, but it persists longer in the body. The extent of biotransformation of minoxidil to its active metabolite, minoxidil N-O sulfate, has not been evaluated in man. Minoxidil has a half-life in plasma of 3 to 4 hours, but its duration of action is 24 hours or occasionally even longer. It has been proposed that persistence of minoxidil in vascular smooth muscle is responsible for this discrepancy. However, without knowledge of the pharmacokinetic properties of the active metabolite, an explanation for the prolonged duration of action cannot be given.

Preparation, Routes of Administration and Dosage. *Minoxidil* (LONITEN, others) is supplied in 2.5- and 10-mg tablets. The initial daily dose is usually 5 mg, which can be increased gradually to 40 mg in one or two daily doses. Although daily doses of up to 100 mg have been used, most patients require 40 mg or less (Dormois *et al.*, 1975).

Toxicity and Precautions. Minoxidil is well tolerated, even though use of the drug is confined to patients with severe hypertension. The side effects of minoxidil are predictable and can be divided into three major categories: fluid and salt retention, cardiovascular effects, and hypertrichosis.

Retention of salt and water results from increased proximal renal tubular reabsorption, which is in turn secondary to reduced renal perfusion pressure and to reflex stimulation of renal tubular α-adrenergic receptors. Similar antinatriuretic effects can be observed with the other arteriolar dilators (*e.g.*, diazoxide and hydralazine). Although administration of minoxidil causes increased secretion of renin and aldosterone, this is not an important mechanism for retention of salt and water in this case. Fluid retention can usually be controlled by the administration of a diuretic. However, thiazides may not be sufficiently efficacious, and it may be necessary to use a loop diuretic. This is especially true if the patient has any degree of renal dysfunction.

The majority of the cardiovascular effects of minoxidil are secondary to baroreceptor-mediated activation of the sympathetic nervous system. Increased cardiac contractility can be effectively counteracted with adequate doses of a β-adrenergic antagonist, but some increase in heart rate may persist because tachycardia is mediated in part by withdrawal of parasympathetic tone. Pulmonary hypertension may result from increased cardiac output (despite decreased pulmonary vascular resistance) or from salt and water retention with consequent congestive heart failure. Minoxidil should thus be used with caution in patients with ischemic heart disease. However, with adequate blockade of β-adrenergic receptors, the decrease in blood pressure and heart size associated with reduction of afterload can favorably affect myocardial oxygen demand in hypertensive patients. The flattened and inverted T waves observed in the electrocardiogram during initial therapy with minoxidil are not ischemic in origin. Pericardial effusion is a real but rare complication of minoxidil. Although more commonly described in patients with renal failure and congestive heart failure, pericardial effusion can occur in patients with normal cardiovascular and renal function. Asymptomatic pericardial effusion is not an indication for stopping minoxidil, but the situation should be monitored closely to avoid progression to tamponade. The effusion usually clears when the drug is discontinued, but it will recur if treatment with minoxidil is resumed (Reichgott, 1981).

Hypertrichosis, which occurs in all patients who receive minoxidil for an extended period, is particularly offensive to women. Growth of hair occurs on the face, back, arms, and legs. The cause of this side effect is unclear, but it may be secondary to enhanced cutaneous blood flow. Similar side effects have been described during long-term oral administration of diazoxide. Frequent shaving or depilatory agents can be used to manage this problem. Topical minoxidil (ROGAINE 2% solution) is now marketed for the treatment of male-pattern baldness. The topical use of minoxidil can cause measurable cardiovascular effects in some individuals (Leenen *et al.*, 1988).

Other side effects of the drug are rare

and include rashes, Stevens–Johnson syndrome, glucose intolerance, serosanguinous bullae, formation of antinuclear antibodies, and thrombocytopenia.

Therapeutic Uses. Minoxidil is best reserved for the treatment of severe hypertension that responds poorly to other antihypertensive medications (Campese, 1981). It has been used successfully in the treatment of hypertension in both adults and children. Minoxidil should never be used alone; it must be given concurrently with a diuretic to avoid fluid retention and a sympatholytic drug (usually a β-adrenergic antagonist) to control reflex cardiovascular effects. The drug is usually administered either once or twice a day, but some patients may require more frequent dosage for adequate control of blood pressure.

SODIUM NITROPRUSSIDE

Although sodium nitroprusside has been known since 1850 and its hypotensive effect in man was described in 1929, its safety and usefulness for the short-term control of severe hypertension were not demonstrated until the mid 1950s. Several investigators subsequently demonstrated that sodium nitroprusside was also effective in improving cardiac function in patients with left ventricular failure. The structural formula of sodium nitroprusside is as follows:

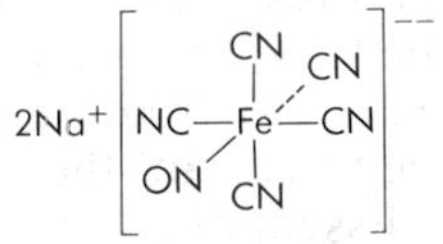

Sodium Nitroprusside

Locus and Mechanism of Action. The nitroso moiety of sodium nitroprusside is necessary for its vasodilatory action. When nitroprusside comes in contact with red blood cells, the molecule decomposes, releasing nitric oxide (Smith and Kruszyna, 1974). Nitric oxide is an unstable compound that causes vasodilatation and inhibits platelet aggregation by activating guanylate cyclase in vascular smooth muscle cells and platelets (*see* Chapter 32; Ignarro *et al.*, 1980). Recent evidence also suggests that nitric oxide is generated endogenously; as mentioned above, it may be the same as EDRF or be derived from EDRF (Moncada *et al.*, 1988).

Pharmacological Effects. Nitroprusside dilates both arterioles and venules, and the hemodynamic response to its administration results from a combination of venous pooling and reduced arterial impedance. Because of its effect on venules, sodium nitroprusside is a more effective hypotensive agent when the patient is upright. In subjects with normal left ventricular function, venous pooling affects cardiac output more than does the reduction of afterload; cardiac output thus tends to fall. In contrast, in patients with severely impaired left ventricular function and diastolic ventricular distention, the combination of venous pooling and the reduction of arterial impedance cause a rise in cardiac output.

Sodium nitroprusside is a nonselective vasodilator, and regional distribution of blood flow is little affected by the drug. In general, renal blood flow and glomerular filtration are maintained, and plasma renin activity increases. Unlike minoxidil, hydralazine, diazoxide, and other arteriolar vasodilators, administration of sodium nitroprusside usually causes only a modest increase in heart rate and an overall reduction in myocardial demand for oxygen.

Absorption, Metabolism, and Excretion. Sodium nitroprusside is an unstable molecule that decomposes under strongly alkaline conditions and when exposed to light. The drug must be given by continuous intravenous infusion to be effective. Its onset of action is within 30 seconds; the peak hypotensive effect occurs within 2 minutes, and when the infusion of the drug is stopped, the effect disappears within 3 minutes.

The breakdown of nitroprusside is probably initiated by its reduction. The ferrous ion of the drug reacts promptly with membrane-bound sulfhydryl groups of the vascular wall and erythrocytes to form an unstable nitroprusside radical, which then immediately dissociates into its components, cyanide and nitric oxide (Ivankovich *et al.*, 1978). Cyanide is further metabolized by liver rhodanase to thiocyanate, which is eliminated almost entirely in the urine. The mean elimination half-time for thiocyanate is 3 days in patients with normal renal function, and it can be much longer in patients with renal insufficiency.

Preparation, Route of Administration, and Dosage. *Sodium nitroprusside* (NIPRIDE, NITROPRESS) is available in 2- or 5-ml vials that contain 50 mg. The contents of the vial should be dissolved in 2 to 3 ml of 5% dextrose in water. Addition of this solution to 250 to 1000 ml of 5% dextrose in water produces a concentration of 50 to 200 μg/ml. Because the compound decomposes in light, only fresh solutions should be used and the bottle should be covered with an opaque wrapping. The drug must be administered as a controlled, continuous infusion and the patient must be closely observed. The majority of hypertensive patients respond to an infusion of 0.5 to 1.5 μg/kg per minute. Higher rates of infusion are necessary to produce controlled hypotension in normotensive patients under surgical anesthesia. High rates of infusion of nitroprusside over a prolonged period can cause cyanide and/or thiocyanate poisoning. Patients who are receiving other antihypertensive medications usually require less nitroprusside to lower blood pressure. If infusion rates of 10 μg/kg per minute do not produce adequate reduction of blood pressure within 10 minutes, administration of nitroprusside should be stopped to minimize potential toxicity.

Toxicity and Precautions. The short-term side effects of nitroprusside are due to excessive vasodilatation with hypotension and the consequences thereof. Close monitoring of blood pressure and the use of a continuously variable-rate infusion pump will prevent an excessive hemodynamic response to the drug in the majority of the cases. Less commonly, toxicity may result from conversion of nitroprusside to cyanide and thiocyanate. Accumulation of cyanide can occur if sodium nitroprusside is infused at a rate greater than 2 μg/kg per minute. The limiting factor in the metabolism of cyanide appears to be the availability of sulfur-containing substrates in the body (mainly thiosulfate). The concomitant administration of sodium thiosulfate can prevent accumulation of cyanide in patients who are receiving higher than usual doses of sodium nitroprusside; the efficacy of the drug is unchanged (Schulz, 1984). The risk of thiocyanate toxicity increases when sodium nitroprusside is infused for more than 24 to 48 hours, especially if renal function is impaired. Signs and symptoms of thiocyanate toxicity include anorexia, nausea, fatigue, disorientation, and toxic psychosis. The plasma concentration of thiocyanate should be monitored during prolonged infusions of nitroprusside and should not be allowed to exceed 0.1 mg/ml. Rarely, excessive concentrations of thiocyanate may cause hypothyroidism by inhibiting iodine uptake by the thyroid gland. In patients with renal failure, thiocyanate can be removed readily by hemodialysis.

Nitroprusside can worsen arterial hypoxemia in patients with chronic obstructive pulmonary disease because the drug interferes with hypoxic pulmonary vasoconstriction and therefore promotes mismatching of ventilation with perfusion. Rebound hypertension may occur after abrupt cessation of short-term nitroprusside infusions (Packer *et al.*, 1979); this may be caused by persistently elevated concentrations of renin in the plasma.

Therapeutic Uses. Sodium nitroprusside is used primarily to treat hypertensive emergencies, but the drug can be used in many situations when short-term reduction of cardiac preload and/or afterload is desired. Thus, nitroprusside has been used to lower blood pressure during acute aortic dissection, to increase cardiac output in congestive heart failure, and to decrease myocardial oxygen demand after acute myocardial infarction. In addition, nitroprusside is the drug most often used to induce controlled hypotension during anesthesia in order to reduce bleeding in surgical procedures. In the treatment of acute aortic dissection, it is important to administer a β-adrenergic antagonist with nitroprusside, since reduction of blood pressure with nitroprusside alone can increase the rate of development of force by the heart, thereby enhancing propagation of the dissection.

DIAZOXIDE

Diazoxide was initially developed as an oral antihypertensive drug, but early clinical trials revealed unacceptable toxicity. At least 50% of patients displayed hyperglycemia, and 20% developed hypertrichosis. The drug was then marketed for parenteral use for the treatment of hypertensive emergencies, but sodium nitroprusside soon replaced diazoxide as the drug of choice for this indication. Diazoxide maintains a place in the treatment of hypertensive emergencies in situations in which accurate infusion pumps are not available and close monitoring of blood pressure is not feasible. The drug is a benzothiadiazine derivative, like the thiazide diuretics, but it does not cause diuresis, apparently because it lacks a sulfonamido group. Its structural formula is as follows:

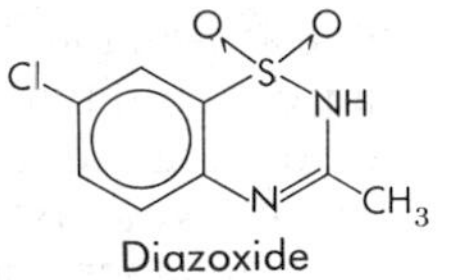

Diazoxide

Mechanism of Action and Pharmacological Effects. Diazoxide hyperpolarizes arterial smooth muscle cells by activating ATP-sensitive K^+ channels; this causes relaxation of the vascular smooth muscle (Standen *et al.*, 1989). The effect of the drug *in vivo* is exclusively arteriolar, with negligible effect on capacitance vessels. Reflex activation of the sympathetic nervous system and retention of salt and water occur. Cardiac output may double from stimulation of heart rate and myocardial contractility. The avid retention of salt and water was thought to be secondary to a direct effect of diazoxide on renal-tubular function. However, studies in animals have never substantiated these claims, and in fact, direct infusion of diazoxide into the renal artery causes renal vasodilatation and diuresis (Brouhard *et al.*, 1981). More likely, the salt and water retention is a result of stimulation of renal sympathetic nerves and changes in intrarenal hemodynamics, as with other arteriolar vasodilators. Diazoxide increases coronary blood flow, and cerebral and renal blood flows are maintained by autoregulation. Renin secretion is enhanced, and the combination of an increased cardiac output, salt and water retention, and elevated concentrations of angiotensin II counteract the antihypertensive effects of diazoxide.

Absorption, Metabolism, Excretion. Although well absorbed orally, diazoxide is administered only intravenously for the treatment of severe hypertension. Approximately 20 to 50% of the drug is eliminated as such by the kidney, and the rest is metabolized in the liver to the 3 hydroxymethyl and 3 carboxy derivatives (Pruitt *et al.*, 1974). Although the plasma half-life of diazoxide is 20 to 60 hours, the duration of the hypotensive response to the drug is variable and can be as short as 4 hours or as long as 20 hours.

Preparation, Route of Administration, Dosage, and Therapeutic Use. *Diazoxide* (HYPERSTAT I.V.) is available for intravenous use in solutions containing 15 mg/ml. The main indication is for the treatment of hypertensive emergencies. Injection of an intravenous bolus lowers blood pressure within 30 seconds, and a maximum effect is achieved within 3 to 5 minutes. Because of the ease of administration and the rapid response, the drug can be used in emergency situations in which close monitoring of blood pressure is not feasible. Although initial recommendations were to administer a 300-mg bolus of diazoxide, excessive hypotension with resultant cerebral and cardiovascular damage has resulted from this practice. Hypotension can be minimized by the administration of a "minibolus" of 50 to 100 mg at intervals of 10 to 15 minutes until the desired blood pressure is achieved (Wilson and Vidt, 1978). Diazoxide can also be given by slow intravenous infusion of the undiluted solution at a rate of 15 to 30 mg per minute (Garrett and Kaplan, 1982). Prior administration of a β-adrenergic antagonist will enhance the hypotensive effect of the drug. Diazoxide should not be used to treat hypertension associated with aortic coarctation, arteriovenous shunts, or aortic dissection. Similarly, risks outweigh benefits in its use for intracerebral hemorrhage, acute pulmonary edema, and acute ischemic heart disease.

Toxicity and Precautions. The two most common side effects caused by diazoxide are salt and water retention and hyperglycemia. Retention of fluid can be avoided by restriction of salt and water. The routine use of diuretic agents with diazoxide is not recommended because patients with malignant hypertension are frequently volume depleted. Hyperglycemia results from diazoxide's capacity to inhibit the secretion of insulin from pancreatic β cells. This effect also appears to result from stimulation of ATP-sensitive K^+ channels (Zünkler *et al.*, 1988). The drug does not alter the response to administration of insulin. Thus, hyperglycemia is mainly a problem in non-insulin-dependent diabetic patients who are being treated with oral hypoglycemic agents. Severe hyperglycemia with hyperosmolar, nonketotic coma has been described. Other side effects include tachycardia and myocardial and cerebral ischemia caused by excessive hypotension. Diazoxide relaxes uterine smooth muscle and may arrest labor when used to treat the hypertensive crisis of eclampsia. Rare side effects include gastrointestinal disturbances, flushing, local pain and inflammation after extravasation, altered ability to taste and smell, excessive salivation, and dyspnea. Long-term administration of diazoxide can cause hypertrichosis, as with minoxidil.

Ca^{2+}-CHANNEL BLOCKERS

Ca^{2+}-channel blocking agents are emerging as a very important group of drugs for the treatment of hypertension. The general pharmacology of these drugs is presented in Chapter 32. The antihypertensive effect of Ca^{2+}-channel blockers was demonstrated over 20 years ago, but these drugs have undergone rigorous evaluation for the treatment of hypertension only in the past decade. The logic behind their use for this purpose comes from the understanding that fixed hypertension is the result of increased peripheral vascular resistance. Since contraction of vascular smooth muscle is dependent on the free intracellular concentration of Ca^{2+}, inhibition of transmembrane movement of Ca^{2+} should decrease the total amount of Ca^{2+} that reaches intracellular sites. Indeed, all of the Ca^{2+}-channel blockers lower blood pressure by relaxing arteriolar smooth muscle and decreasing peripheral vascular resistance (Lehmann *et al.*, 1983). However, unlike other arteriolar dilators, Ca^{2+}-channel blockers do not cause fluid retention, and only the dihydropyridines (nifedipine, nitrendipine, and nicardipine) produce a mild-to-moderate reflex tachycardia (Frishman *et al.*, 1987). Because both verapamil and diltiazem have direct effects on the sinoatrial (SA) node to decrease heart rate, reflex tachycardia is usually not significant with these two drugs. All Ca^{2+}-channel blockers are equally effective when used alone for the treatment of mild-to-moderate hypertension, and in comparative trials, Ca^{2+}-channel blockers are as effective as β-adrenergic antagonists or diuretics (Doyle, 1983; Inouye *et al.*, 1984).

The Ca^{2+}-channel blockers are well tolerated, and only a small fraction of patients discontinue the drug because of an adverse reaction. The dihydropyridines cause the highest incidence of vascular side effects. Approximately 10% of patients develop headache, flushing, dizziness, and peripheral edema. However, edema is clearly not secondary to fluid retention; it most likely results from increased hydrostatic pressure in the lower extremities owing to precapillary dilatation and reflex postcapillary constriction. The most common side effect of verapamil is constipation, while bradycardia occurs most commonly with diltiazem (Russell, 1988).

Although some investigators have advocated the sublingual use of nifedipine for treatment of hypertensive emergencies, it is not readily absorbed from the buccal mucosa; nitroprusside remains the drug of choice because of the ability to titrate the response to the drug quickly. In situations in which close monitoring of blood pressure is not possible, ingestion of 10 to 20 mg of nifedipine can cause a hypotensive effect in 10 minutes, with a maximal effect in 30 to 40 minutes.

Ca^{2+}-channel blockers are versatile drugs with proven efficacy in all types of patients (Kiowski *et al.*, 1986). They seem to be especially efficacious in low-renin hypertension (*i.e.*, blacks and the elderly). The efficacy of Ca^{2+}-channel blockers is enhanced by the concomitant use of a β-adrenergic antagonist, an inhibition of angiotensin converting enzyme, or methyldopa. Diuretics may also enhance the efficacy of Ca^{2+}-channel blockers, but the data have not been consistent. There are significant drug–drug interactions to be recalled when Ca^{2+}-channel blockers are used to treat hypertension. Verapamil can increase plasma concentrations of digoxin (Pedersen *et al.*, 1981). When used with quinidine, Ca^{2+}-channel blockers may cause excessive hypotension, particularly in patients with idiopathic hypertrophic subaortic stenosis. Diltiazem and verapamil must be given with caution to patients who are also receiving a β blocker because of the possible development of AV block or heart failure.

Overall, Ca^{2+}-channel blockers are safe and effective in the treatment of hypertension. They should not be used in patients with SA or AV nodal abnormalities or in patients with overt congestive heart failure. These drugs are usually safe, however, in hypertensive patients with asthma, hyperlipidemia, diabetes mellitus, and renal dysfunction. Unlike β-adrenergic antagonists, Ca^{2+}-channel blockers do not alter exercise tolerance; nor do they alter plasma concentrations of lipids, uric acid, or electrolytes.

ANGIOTENSIN CONVERTING ENZYME INHIBITORS

The importance of the renin–angiotensin system for regulation of cardiovascular function has been appreciated for some time (*see* Chapter 31). The ability to inhibit the activity of the system with orally effective inhibitors of angiotensin converting enzyme is more recent. Captopril was the first such agent to be marketed for the treatment of hypertension. Since then, enalapril and lisinopril have also become available. These drugs have proven to be very useful for the treatment of hypertension because of their efficacy and their very favorable profile of side effects, which enhances compliance. Although elderly hypertensive patients tend to have lower plasma renin activity than do younger individuals, angiotensin converting enzyme inhibitors have equal antihypertensive efficacy in the two groups (Cooper *et al.*, 1987). Black hypertensive patients are somewhat resistant to the hypotensive effect of these drugs; however, the concurrent use of a diuretic overcomes this relative resistance. These drugs are discussed in detail in Chapter 31.

II. Therapy of Hypertension

NONPHARMACOLOGICAL THERAPY OF HYPERTENSION

Interest in nonpharmacological methods to lower blood pressure arises in part from the fact that about 70% of hypertensive subjects have a mild, asymptomatic elevation of blood pressure. To maintain compliance with a therapeutic regimen, the intervention should not lessen the quality of life. All drugs have side effects. If minor alterations of normal activity or diet can reduce blood pressure to a satisfactory level, the complications of drug therapy can be avoided. In addition, nonpharmacological methods to lower blood pressure allow the patient to participate actively in the management of his or her disease. Reduction of weight, restriction of salt, and moderation in the use of alcohol may reduce blood pressure and improve the efficacy of drug treatment. In addition, regular isotonic exercise, relaxation therapy, and increased consumption of K^+ may also lower blood pressure in hypertensive patients.

Smoking *per se* does not cause hypertension. However, smokers do have a higher incidence of malignant hypertension (Isles *et al.*, 1979), and smoking is a major risk factor for coronary heart disease. Hypertensive patients should stop smoking. Consumption of caffeine can raise blood pressure and elevate plasma concentrations of norepinephrine, but long-term consumption of caffeine causes tolerance to these effects and has not been associated with the development of hypertension. An increased intake of Ca^{2+} has been reported by some investigators to lower blood pressure. The mechanism of this effect is not understood, but suppression of the secretion of parathyroid hormone is apparently involved. However, supplemental Ca^{2+} does not lower blood pressure when populations of hypertensive subjects are studied. Although it is possible that there are some hypertensive patients who have a hypotensive response to Ca^{2+}, there is no easy way to identify such individuals. Supplemental use of Ca^{2+} for this purpose cannot be recommended at the present time (Kaplan, 1988b).

Reduction of Body Weight. Obesity and hypertension are closely associated, and the degree of obesity is positively correlated with the incidence of hypertension. Obese hypertensives may lower their blood pressure by losing weight regardless of a change in salt consumption (Maxwell *et al.*, 1984). The mechanism by which obesity causes hypertension is unclear, but increased secretion of insulin in obesity could result in insulin-mediated enhancement of renal tubular reabsorption of Na^+ and an expansion of extracellular volume. Obesity is also associated with increased activity of the sympathetic nervous system; this is reversed by weight loss. Maintenance of weight loss is difficult for many. A combination of aerobic physical exercise and dietary counseling may enhance compliance.

Sodium Restriction. High salt diets are associated with a high prevalence of hypertension (MacGregor, 1985). Severe restriction of salt will lower the blood pressure in most hospitalized hypertensive patients; this treatment method was advocated prior to the development of effective antihypertensive drugs (Kempner, 1948). However, severe salt restriction is not practical from a standpoint of compliance. Several studies have shown that moderate restriction of salt intake to approximately 5 g per day will, on average, lower blood pressure by 12 mm Hg systolic and 6 mm Hg diastolic. The higher the initial blood pressure, the greater the response. In addition, subjects over 40 years of age are more responsive to the hypotensive effect of moderate restriction of salt (Grobbee and Hofman, 1986). However, not all hypertensive patients respond to restriction of salt. Nonetheless, this intervention is benign and can easily be tried as an initial approach in all patients with mild hypertension. An additional benefit of salt restriction is improved responsiveness to some antihypertensive drugs.

Alcohol Restriction. Consumption of alcohol can raise blood pressure, but it is unclear how much alcohol must be consumed to observe this effect (MacMahon *et al.*, 1984). Heavy consumption of alcohol increases the risk of cerebrovascular accidents but not coronary heart disease (Kagan *et al.*, 1985). In fact, small amounts of ethanol have been found to protect against the development of coronary artery disease. The mechanism by which alcohol raises blood pressure is unknown, but it may involve increased transport of Ca^{2+} into vascular smooth muscle cells. Excessive intake of alcohol may also result in poor compliance with antihypertensive regimens. All hypertensive patients should be advised to restrict consumption of ethanol to no more than 30 ml per day.

Physical Exercise. Increased physical activity lowers rates of cardiovascular disease in men (Paffenbarger *et al.*, 1986). It is not known if this beneficial effect is secondary to an antihypertensive response to exercise. Lack of physical activity is associated with a higher incidence of hypertension (Blair *et al.*, 1984). Although consistent changes in blood pressure are not always observed, meticulously controlled studies have demonstrated that regular isotonic exercise reduces both systolic and diastolic blood pressures by approximately 10 mm Hg (Nelson *et al.*, 1986). The mechanism by which exercise can lower blood pressure is not clear, but several hemodynamic and humoral changes have been documented. Regular isotonic exercise reduces blood volume and plasma catecholamines and elevates plasma concentrations of atrial natriuretic factor. The beneficial effect of exercise can occur in subjects who demonstrate no change in body weight or salt intake during the training period.

Relaxation and Biofeedback Therapy. The fact that long-term stressful stimuli can cause sustained hypertension in animals has given credence to the possibility that relaxation therapy will lower blood pressure in some hypertensive patients. A few studies have generated positive results, but in general, relaxation therapy has inconsistent and modest effects on blood pressure (Jacob *et al.*, 1986). In addition, the long-term efficacy of such treatment has been difficult to demonstrate, presumably in part because patients must be highly motivated to respond to relaxation and biofeedback therapy. Only those few patients with mild hypertension who wish to use this method should be encouraged to try, and these patients should be closely followed and receive alternative treatment if necessary.

Potassium Therapy. There is a positive correlation between total body Na^+ and blood pressure and a negative correlation between total body K^+ and blood pressure in hypertensive patients (Lever *et al.*, 1981). In addition, dietary intake, plasma concentrations, and urinary excretion of K^+ are reduced in various populations of hypertensive subjects. Increased intake of K^+ might reduce blood pressure by increasing excretion of Na^+, suppressing renin secretion, causing arteriolar dilatation (possibly by stimulating Na^+, K^+–ATPase activity and decreasing intracellular concentrations of Ca^{2+}) and impairing responsiveness to endogenous vasoconstrictors. In hypertensive rats, supplementation with K^+ decreases blood pressure and reduces the incidence of stroke, irrespective of blood pressure (Tobian, 1986). In mildly hypertensive patients, oral K^+ supplements of 48 mmol per day reduce both systolic and diastolic blood pressure (Siana *et al.*, 1987). Supplementation with K^+ may also protect against ventricular ectopy and stroke (Khaw and Barrett-Connor, 1987). Based on all of these data, it seems prudent to use a high K^+ diet and moderate restriction of Na^+ in the treatment of hypertension.

DRUG THERAPY OF HYPERTENSION

Drug therapy is reserved for hypertensive patients in whom blood pressure cannot be maintained within the normal range by nonpharmacological means. Thus, patients with diastolic blood pressures consistently above 90 mm Hg and systolic blood pressures above 140 mm Hg should be considered for therapy. A casual blood pressure measurement in the physician's office may be elevated because of the artificial and stressful circumstances. Ambulatory measurements of blood pressure are much more satisfactory. In one study, 22% of patients with a diagnosis of borderline hypertension had normal ambulatory blood pressures (Pickering *et al.*, 1988).

The report of the Joint National Committee on Detection, Evaluation, and Treatment of High Blood Pressure (1988) suggests that patients with diastolic blood pressures that are consistently greater than 94 mm Hg should be treated and that individuals with diastolic blood pressures between 90 and 94 mm Hg who have other risk factors (*e.g.*, men, smokers, target-organ damage, diabetes mellitus, hyperlipidemia, or other major risk factors for cardiovascular disease) should also be treated. Patients with diastolic blood pressures between 90 and 94 mm Hg who have no other risk factors for developing cardiovascular disease can be treated nonpharmacologically, but they should be followed closely to be certain that blood pressure does not rise further. The desired goal of therapy is to reduce diastolic blood pressure to below 90 mm Hg.

Selection of Therapy. Until recently, initial therapy for hypertension consisted of either a thiazide diuretic or a β-adrenergic antagonist. However, numerous studies have shown that the Ca^{2+}-channel blockers and inhibitors of angiotensin converting enzyme are also effective as first-line treatment. In choosing initial drug therapy, issues such as side effects, quality of life, cost, and efficacy of drugs in certain subgroups of hypertensive patients should be considered. Thus, the simplified "stepped care approach," previously advocated by most investigators, has been replaced by a more individualized approach in which the patient's age, race, concomitant diseases and therapies, life style, and even, possibly, socioeconomic status are considered.

Thiazide diuretics are the least expensive of the first-line drugs and should be considered for the treatment of hypertension in the elderly and in patients with volume-dependent hypertension. Most black and obese hypertensives belong in the latter group. Thiazides should be avoided in patients with hyperuricemia, hyperglycemia, hyperlipidemia, and hypokalemia. Hypertensive individuals with left ventricular hypertrophy should not be treated with a thiazide diuretic alone, since these drugs have not been shown to reverse the hypertrophy, even though blood pressure is reduced (Drayer *et al.*, 1982).

β-Adrenergic antagonists should be considered for young hypertensive patients and patients with angina pectoris, a history of myocardial infarction, cardiac arrhythmias, or mitral-valve prolapse.

Ca^{2+}-channel blockers should be considered for patients who cannot tolerate diuretics or β-adrenergic antagonists. In general, hypertensive patients with low renin levels respond well to Ca^{2+}-channel blockers. Thus, elderly and black hypertensive patients who have underlying bronchospastic pulmonary disease are good candidates to receive one of these drugs. Patients with left ventricular hypertrophy and/or a history of cardiac arrhythmias and those with peripheral vascular disease can safely be given a Ca^{2+}-channel blocker.

Inhibitors of angiotensin converting enzyme can be used for initial therapy in patients who cannot tolerate diuretics or β blockers. These drugs are also appropriate in patients with congestive heart failure or diabetes mellitus and can be used safely in those with left ventricular hypertrophy and/or cardiac arrhythmias.

Patients who do not respond to a single drug can be switched to another drug with a different mechanism of action. If treatment with a single drug is not successful, addition of a second drug from a different class is appropriate. For example, diuretics will greatly enhance the hypotensive potency of converting enzyme inhibitors. Diuretics also add to the antihypertensive efficacy of β-adrenergic antagonists and Ca^{2+}-channel blockers. If two drugs do not control the blood pressure adequately a third drug of a different class can be added to the existing regimen. However, before proceeding to the next level of therapy, the physician should always consider certain explanations for the inadequate response. Noncompliance must be ruled out carefully, especially if the drug is causing side effects. Drug dosage may be inappropriate or the patient may metabolize the drug rapidly. The concomitant use of drugs that can reverse or alter the effect of antihypertensive agents should be evaluated. Volume overload should always be considered, since excessive retention of fluid can oppose the action of many antihypertensive drugs. Excess intake of alcohol can increase blood pressure, and people who consume alcohol excessively tend to be noncompliant with their therapeutic regimen. Progressive renal insufficiency or surgically correctable causes of hypertension should be evaluated in patients with refractory hypertension.

An attempt to withdraw drug therapy can be made with patients with mild hypertension who have had a satisfactory response to a drug for at least a year, but nonpharmacological means to reduce blood pressure should be continued. Although such patients may at first remain normotensive, the majority will eventually require drug therapy again; careful follow-up is thus of the utmost importance.

The effect of antihypertensive therapy on the quality of life has not been studied frequently, but the fact that more than 10% of patients in large studies stop taking antihypertensive medications because of side effects cannot be overlooked. Croog and coworkers (1986) compared the effects of captopril, methyldopa, and propranolol on the quality of life of hypertensive patients. Captopril was the least likely to interfere with everyday living in terms of side effects and measures of satisfaction; methyldopa was the least satisfactory, and propranolol fell in between these two. More such studies are needed.

Hypertensive Emergencies. Hypertensive emergencies are situations that require immediate intervention to lower the blood pressure. It is never the absolute blood pressure that defines the emergency, but the damage that is caused by the elevated pressure. Examples of emergencies include hypertensive encephalopathy, intracranial hemorrhage, acute left ventricular failure with pulmonary edema, unstable angina pectoris, acute myocardial infarction, dissecting aortic aneurysm, eclampsia, head trauma, and extensive burns. Patients with these conditions are best treated with parenteral drugs; sodium nitroprusside is most suitable because of the rapidity with which control can be achieved and the level of blood pressure adjusted. For the treatment of aortic dissection, a parenteral β-adrenergic antagonist is necessary prior to administration of nitroprusside. Aortic dissection can also be treated with trimethaphan. Although many hypertensive emergencies can also be treated with small intravenous doses of diazoxide, the drug is contraindicated in aortic dissection and in patients with ischemic cardiovascular disease. In the treatment of hypertensive encephalopathy, it is critical not to lower the blood pressure too quickly because of inadequate autoregulation of cerebral blood flow. It is reasonable to lower blood pressure by 15% quickly and then toward normal over the next 24 hours. Once parenteral antihypertensive therapy is initiated, it is important to begin oral treatment so that the parenteral drug can be discontinued as soon as possible.

Hypertensive urgencies are situations in which the blood pressure should be lowered within several hours, such as in patients with malignant hypertension and progressive renal insufficiency but without signs of encephalopathy. Accelerated administration of oral antihypertensive medications can result in adequate control of blood pressure in such conditions without resorting to parenteral drugs. Since many patients with hypertensive emergencies or malignant hypertension are somewhat volume depleted, the routine use of diuretics should be avoided.

Hypertensive crises in pediatric patients are generally treated with the same drugs that are used in adults, with appropriate modification of dose (Report of the Second Task Force on Blood Pressure Control in Children, 1987). Management of acute hypertension during pregnancy has been reviewed by Maikranz and Lindheimer (1987). Drugs to be avoided in pregnancy include angiotensin converting enzyme inhibitors and sodium nitroprusside.

Treatment of Isolated Systolic Hypertension. Isolated systolic hypertension (systolic blood pressure greater than 160 mm Hg and diastolic blood pressure less than 90 mm Hg) is a common finding in the elderly. When isolated systolic hypertension occurs in a young patient, it is usually indicative of a hyperdynamic circulation, and diastolic hypertension may develop later. An elevation of systolic blood pressure clearly increases the risk of cardiovascular morbidity and mortality in elderly patients. However, there are no definitive data to show that treatment of isolated systolic hypertension will reduce this risk. Definitive recommendations must await the conclusions of an ongoing study, the Systolic Hypertension in the Elderly Program. Until then, the physician should evaluate the risk–benefit ratio for each patient, keeping in mind the fact that the elderly are prone to develop complications from drugs. In the feasibility phase of the Systolic Hypertension in the Elderly Program, chlorthalidone was found to be effective for treatment of systolic hypertension with an acceptable incidence of side effects (Hulley *et al.*, 1985); Ca^{2+}-channel blockers are reasonable alternatives.

Azuma, J.; Sawamura, A.; Harada, H.; Awata, N.; Kishimoto, S.; and Sperelakis, N. Mechanism of direct cardiostimulating actions of hydralazine. *Eur. J. Pharmacol.*, **1987**, *135*, 137–144.

Beckmann, M. L.; Gerber, J. G.; Byyny, R. L.; LoVerde, M.; and Nies, A. S. Propranolol increases prostacyclin synthesis in patients with essential hypertension. *Hypertension*, **1988**, *12*, 582–588.

Bennett, W. M.; McDonald, W. J.; Kuehnel, E.; Hartnett, M. N.; and Porter, G. A. Do diuretics have antihypertensive properties independent of natriuresis? *Clin. Pharmacol. Ther.*, **1977**, *22*, 499–504.

Blair, S. N.; Goodyear, N. N.; Gibbons, L. W.; and Cooper, K. H. Physical fitness and incidence of hypertension in healthy normotensive men and women. *J.A.M.A.*, **1984**, *252*, 487–490.

Bobik, A.; Jennings, G.; Jackman, G.; Oddie, C.; and Korner, P. Evidence for a predominantly central hypotensive effect of alpha-methyldopa in humans. *Hypertension*, **1986**, *8*, 16–23.

Brouhard, B. H.; LaGrone, L.; Allen, W. R.; and Cunningham, R. J. Role of sympathetic nerve activity in antinatriuresis after diazoxide and sodium nitroprusside infusion. *J. Pharmacol. Exp. Ther.*, **1981**, *218*, 148–153.

Cameron, H. A., and Ramsay, L. E. The lupus syndrome induced by hydralazine: a common complication with low dose treatment. *Br. Med. J.* [*Clin. Res.*], **1984**, *289*, 410–412.

Campbell, N. R. C.; Sundaram, R. S.; Werness, P. G.; Van Loon, J.; and Weinshilboum, R. M. Sulfate and methyldopa metabolism: metabolite patterns and platelet phenol sulfotransferase activity. *Clin. Pharmacol. Ther.*, **1985**, *37*, 308–315.

Carter, A. B. Hypotensive therapy in stroke survivors. *Lancet*, **1970**, *1*, 485–489.

Cooper, W. D.; Glover, D. R.; and Kimber, G. R. Influence of age on blood pressure response to enalapril. *Gerontology*, **1987**, *33*, Suppl. 1, 48–54.

Cornacchia, E.; Golbus, J.; Maybaum, J.; Strahler, J.; Hanash, S.; and Richardson, B. Hydralazine and procainamide inhibit T cell DNA methylation and induce autoreactivity. *J. Immunol.*, **1988**, *140*, 2197–2200.

Croog, S. H.; Levine, S.; Testa, M. A.; Brown, B.; Bulpitt, C. J.; Jenkins, D.; Klerman, G. L.; and Williams,

G. H. The effects of antihypertensive therapy on the quality of life. *N. Engl. J. Med.*, **1986**, *314*, 1657–1664.

Cruickshank, J. M. Coronary flow reserve and the J curve relation between diastolic blood pressure and myocardial infarction. *Br. Med. J. [Clin. Res.]*, **1988**, *297*, 1227–1230.

De Carvalho, J. G. R.; Emery, A. C.; and Frohlich, E. D. Spironolactone and triamterene in volume-dependent essential hypertension. *Clin. Pharmacol. Ther.*, **1980**, *27*, 53–56.

Dormois, J. C.; Young, J. L.; and Nies, A. S. Minoxidil in severe hypertension. Value when conventional drugs have failed. *Am. Heart J.*, **1975**, *90*, 360–368.

Drayer, J. I.; Gardin, J. M.; Weber, M. A.; and Aronow, W. S. Changes in ventricular septal thickness during diuretic therapy. *Clin. Pharmacol. Ther.*, **1982**, *32*, 283–288.

Falch, D. K., and Schreiner, A. The effect of spironolactone on lipid, glucose and uric acid levels in blood during long-term administration to hypertensives. *Acta Med. Scand.*, **1983**, *213*, 27–30.

Fouad, F. M.; Nakashima, Y.; Tarazi, R. C.; and Salcedo, E. E. Reversal of left ventricular hypertrophy in hypertensive patients treated with methyldopa; lack of association with blood pressure control. *Am. J. Cardiol.*, **1982**, *49*, 795–801.

Frisk-Holmberg, M.; Paalzow, L.; and Wibell, L. Relationship between the cardiovascular effects and steady-state kinetics of clonidine in hypertension. *Eur. J. Clin. Pharmacol.*, **1984**, *26*, 309–313.

Frisk-Holmberg, M., and Wibell, L. Concentration-dependent blood pressure effects of guanfacine. *Clin. Pharmacol. Ther.*, **1986**, *39*, 169–172.

Garrett, B. N., and Kaplan, N. M. Efficacy of slow infusion of diazoxide in the treatment of severe hypertension without organ hypoperfusion. *Am. Heart J.*, **1982**, *103*, 390–394.

Gehr, M.; MacCarthy, E. P.; and Goldberg, M. Guanabenz: a centrally acting, natriuretic antihypertensive drug. *Kidney Int.*, **1986**, *29*, 1203–1208.

Gellai, M., and Edwards, R. M. Mechanism of α_2-adrenoceptor agonist-induced diuresis. *Am. J. Physiol.*, **1988**, *255*, F317–F323.

Giachetti, A., and Shore, P. A. The reserpine receptor. *Life Sci.*, **1978**, *23*, 89–92.

Goldstein, D. S.; Levinson, P. D.; Zimlichman, R.; Pitterman, A.; Stull, R.; and Keiser, H. R. Clonidine suppression testing in essential hypertension. *Ann. Intern. Med.*, **1985**, *102*, 42–48.

Harrington, M.; Kincaid-Smith, P.; and McMichael, J. Results of treatment in malignant hypertension: a seven-year experience in 94 cases. *Br. Med. J. [Clin. Res.]*, **1959**, *2*, 969–980.

Hulley, S. B.; Furberg, C. D.; Gurland, B.; McDonald, R.; Perry, H. M.; Schnaper, H. W.; Schoenberger, J. A.; Smith, W. M.; and Vogt, T. M. Systolic hypertension in the elderly program (SHEP). Antihypertensive efficacy of chlorthalidone. *Am. J. Cardiol.*, **1985**, *56*, 913–920.

Ignarro, L. J.; Edwards, J. C.; Gruetter, D. Y.; Barry, B. K.; and Gruetter, C. A. Possible involvement of S-nitrothiols in the activation of guanylate cyclase by nitroso compounds. *FEBS Lett.*, **1980**, *110*, 275–278.

Inouye, I. K.; Massie, B. M.; Benowitz, N.; Simpson, P.; and Loge, D. Antihypertensive therapy with diltiazem and comparison with hydrochlorothiazide. *Am. J. Cardiol.*, **1984**, *53*, 1588–1592.

IPPPSH Collaborative Group. Cardiovascular risk and risk factors in a randomized trial of treatment based on the beta-blocker oxprenolol: The International Prospective Primary Prevention Study in Hypertension (IPPPSH). *J. Hypertens.*, **1985**, *3*, 379–392.

Isles, C.; Brown, J. J.; Cumming, A. M. M.; Lever, A. F.; McAreavey, D.; Robertson, J. I. S.; Hawthorne, V. M.; Stewart, G. M.; Robertson, J. W. K.; and Wapshaw, J. Excess smoking in malignant-phase hypertension. *Br. Med. J. [Clin. Res.]*, **1979**, *1*, 579–581.

Jacob, R. G.; Shapiro, A. P.; Reeves, R. A.; Johnson, A. M.; McDonald, R. H.; and Coburn, P. C. Relaxation therapy for hypertension. Comparison of effects with concomitant placebo, diuretic, and β-blocker. *Arch. Intern. Med.*, **1986**, *146*, 2335–2340.

Jeunemaitre, X.; Charru, A.; Chatellier, G.; Degoulet, P.; Julien, J.; Plouin, P.-F.; Corvol, P.; and Menard, J. Long-term metabolic effects of spironolactone and thiazides combined with potassium-sparing agents for treatment of essential hypertension. *Am. J. Cardiol.*, **1988**, *62*, 1072–1077.

Kagan, A.; Popper, J. S.; Rhoads, G. G.; and Yano, K. Dietary and other risk factors for stroke in Hawaiian Japanese men. *Stroke*, **1985**, *16*, 390–396.

Kempner, W. Treatment of hypertensive vascular disease with rice diet. *Am. J. Med.*, **1948**, *4*, 545–577.

Khaw, K.-T., and Barrett-Connor, E. Dietary potassium and stroke associated mortality: a 12 year prospective population study. *N. Engl. J. Med.*, **1987**, *316*, 235–240.

Kruszyna, H.; Kruszyna, R.; Smith, R. P.; and Wilcox, D. E. Red blood cells generate nitric oxide from directly acting, nitrogenous vasodilators. *Toxicol. Appl. Pharmacol.*, **1987**, *91*, 429–438.

Leenen, F. H. H.; Smith, D. L.; and Unger, W. P. Topical minoxidil: cardiac effects in bald man. *Br. J. Clin. Pharmacol.*, **1988**, *26*, 481–485.

Lever, A. F.; Beretta-Piccoli, C.; Brown, J. J.; Davies, D. L.; Fraser, R.; and Robertson, J. I. S. Sodium and potassium in essential hypertension. *Br. Med. J. [Clin. Res.]*, **1981**, *283*, 463–468.

MacDougall, I. C.; Isles, C. G.; Stewart, H.; Inglis, G. C.; Finlayson, J.; Thomson, I.; Lees, K. R.; McMillan, N. C.; Morley, P.; and Ball, S. G. Overnight clonidine suppression test in the diagnosis and exclusion of pheochromocytoma. *Am. J. Med.*, **1988**, *84*, 993–1000.

MacGregor, G. A. Sodium is more important that calcium in essential hypertension. *Hypertension*, **1985**, *7*, 628–637.

MacMahon, S. W.; Blacket, R. B.; and MacDonald, G. J. Obesity, alcohol consumption and blood pressure in Australian men and women. The National Heart Foundation of Australia Risk Factor Prevalence Study. *J. Hypertens.*, **1984**, *2*, 85–91.

McCall, J. M.; Aiken, J. W.; Chidester, C. G.; DuCharme, D. W.; and Wendling, M. G. Pyrimidine and triazine 3-oxide sulfates: a new family of vasodilators. *J. Med. Chem.*, **1983**, *26*, 1791–1793.

McVeigh, G.; Galloway, D.; and Johnston, D. The case for low dose diuretics in hypertension: comparison of low and conventional doses of cyclopenthiazide. *Br. Med. J. [Clin. Res.]*, **1988**, *297*, 95–98.

Materson, B. J.; Oster, J. R.; Michael, U. F.; Bolton, S. M.; Burton, Z. C.; Stambaugh, J. E.; and Morledge, J. Dose response to chlorthalidone in patients with mild hypertension; efficacy of a lower dose. *Clin. Pharmacol. Ther.*, **1978**, *24*, 192–198.

Maxwell, M. H.; Kushiro, T.; Dornfeld, L. P.; Tuck, M. L.; and Waks, A. U. BP changes in obese hypertensive subjects during rapid weight loss; comparison of restricted v. unchanged salt intake. *Arch. Intern. Med.*, **1984**, *144*, 1581–1584.

Medical Research Council Working Party. MRC trial of treatment of mild hypertension: principal results. *Br. Med. J. [Clin. Res.]*, **1985**, *291*, 97–104.

———. Stroke and coronary heart disease in mild hypertension: risk factors and the value of treatment. *Br. Med. J. [Clin. Res.]*, **1988**, *296*, 1565–1570.

Meisheri, K. D.; Cipkus, L. A.; and Taylor, C. J. Mechanism of action of minoxidil sulfate-induced vasodilation: a role for increased K^+ permeability. *J. Pharmacol. Exp. Ther.*, **1988**, *245*, 751–760.

Metz, S.; Klein, C.; and Morton, N. Rebound hypertension after discontinuation of transdermal clonidine therapy. *Am. J. Med.*, **1987**, *82*, 17–19.

Mitchell, H. C.; Graham, R. M.; and Pettinger, W. A. Renal function during long-term treatment of hypertension with minoxidil. *Ann. Intern. Med.*, **1980**, *93*, 676–681.

Michell, J. R.; Cavanaugh, J. H.; Arias, L.; and Oates, J. A. Guanethidine and related agents. III. Antagonism by drugs which inhibit the norepinephrine pump in man. *J. Clin. Invest.*, **1970**, *49*, 1596–1604.

Moncada, S.; Radomski, M. W.; and Palmer, R. M. J. Endothelial-derived relaxing factor. Identification as nitric oxide and role in the control of vascular tone and platelet function. *Biochem. Pharmacol.*, **1988**, *37*, 2495–2501.

Multicenter Diuretic Cooperative Study Group. Multiclinic comparison of amiloride, hydrochlorothiazide, and hydrochlorothiazide plus amiloride in essential hypertension. *Arch. Intern. Med.*, **1981**, *141*, 482–486.

Multiple Risk Factor Intervention Trial Research Group. Multiple risk factor intervention trial: risk factor changes and mortality results. *J.A.M.A.*, **1982**, *248*, 1465–1477.

Nelson, L.; Jennings, G.; Esler, M. D.; and Korner, P. I. Effect of changing levels of physical activity on blood pressure and hemodynamics in essential hypertension. *Lancet*, **1986**, *2*, 473–476.

Packer, M.; Meller, J.; Medina, N.; Gorlin, R.; and Herman, M. V. Rebound hemodynamic events after the abrupt withdrawal of nitroprusside in patients with severe chronic heart failure. *N. Engl. J. Med.*, **1979**, *301*, 1193–1197.

Paffenbarger, R. S., Jr.; Hyde, R. T.; Wing, A. L.; and Hsieh, C.-C. Physical activity, all-cause mortality, and longevity of college alumni. *N. Engl. J. Med.*, **1986**, *314*, 605–613.

Pedersen, K. E.; Dorph-Pedersen, A.; Hvidt, S.; Klitgaard, N. A.; and Nielsen-Kudsk, F. Digoxin-verapamil interaction. *Clin. Pharmacol. Ther.*, **1981**, *30*, 311–316.

Pickering, T. G.; James, G. D.; Boddie, C.; Harshfield, G. A.; Blank, S.; and Laragh, J. H. How common is white coat hypertension? *J.A.M.A.*, **1988**, *259*, 225–228.

Pruitt, A. W.; Faraj, B. A.; and Dayton, P. G. Metabolism of diazoxide in man and experimental animals. *J. Pharmacol. Exp. Ther.*, **1974**, *188*, 248–256.

Ram, C. V. S.; Garrett, B. N.; and Kaplan, N. M. Moderate sodium restriction and various diuretics in the treatment of hypertension; effects of potassium wastage and blood pressure control. *Arch. Intern. Med.*, **1981**, *141*, 1015–1019.

Reece, P. A.; Stafford, I.; Prager, R. H.; Walker, G. J.; and Zacest, R. Synthesis, formulation, and clinical pharmacological evaluation of hydralazine pyruvic acid hydrazone in two healthy volunteers. *J. Pharm. Sci.*, **1985**, *74*, 193–196.

Reichgott, M. J. Minoxidil and pericardial effusion: an idiosyncratic reaction. *Clin. Pharmacol. Ther.*, **1981**, *30*, 64–70.

Reid, J. L.; Wing, L. M. H.; Mathias, C. J.; Frankel, H. L.; and Neill, E. The central hypotensive effect of clonidine. Studies in tetraplegic subjects. *Clin. Pharmacol. Ther.*, **1977**, *21*, 375–381.

Sattler, R. W., and van Zwieten, P. A. Acute hypotensive action of 2-(2,6-dichlorophenylamino)-2-imidazoline hydrochloride (St 155) after infusion into the cat's vertebral artery. *Eur. J. Pharmacol.*, **1967**, *2*, 9–13.

Schrijver, G., and Weinberger, M. H. Hydrochlorothiazide and spironolactone in hypertension. *Clin. Pharmacol. Ther.*, **1979**, *25*, 33–42.

Sen, G., and Bose, K. C. *Rauwolfia serpentina*, a new Indian drug for insanity and high blood pressure. *Indian Med. World*, **1931**, *2*, 194–201.

Shah, S.; Khatri, I.; and Freis, E. D. Mechanism of antihypertensive effect of thiazide diuretics. *Am. Heart J.*, **1978**, *95*, 611–618.

Shand, D. G.; Morgan, D. H.; and Oates, J. A. The release of guanethidine and bethanidine by splenic nerve stimulation: a quantitative evaluation showing dissociation from adrenergic blockade. *J. Pharmacol. Exp. Ther.*, **1973**, *184*, 73–80.

Shand, D. G.; Nies, A. S.; McAllister, R. G.; and Oates, J. A. A loading-maintenance regimen for more rapid initiation of the effect of guanethidine. *Clin. Pharmacol. Ther.*, **1975**, *18*, 139–144.

Shea, S.; Cook, E. F.; Kannel, W. B.; and Goldman, L. Treatment of hypertension and its effect on cardiovascular risk factors: data from the Framingham Heart Study. *Circulation*, **1985**, *71*, 22–30.

Siana, A.; Strazzullo, P.; Russo, L.; Guglielmi, S.; Iacoviello, L.; Ferrara, L. A.; and Mancinci, M. Controlled trial of long-term oral potassium supplements in patients with mild hypertension. *Br. Med. J.* [*Clin. Res.*], **1987**, *294*, 1453–1456.

Smith, R. P., and Kruszyna, H. Nitroprusside produces cyanide poisoning via a reaction with hemoglobin. *J. Pharmacol. Exp. Ther.*, **1974**, *191*, 557–563.

Spokas, E. G.; Folco, G.; Quilley, J.; Chander, P.; and McGiff, J. C. Endothelial mechanism in the vascular action of hydralazine. *Hypertension*, **1983**, *5*, Suppl. I, I107–I111.

Standen, N. B.; Quayle, J. M.; Davies, N. W.; Brayden, J. E.; Huang, Y.; and Nelson, M. T. Hyperpolarizing vasodilators activate ATP-sensitive K^+ channels in arterial smooth muscle. *Science*, **1989**, *245*, 177–180.

Tobian, L. High potassium diets markedly protect against stroke deaths and kidney disease in hypertensive rats, a possible legacy from prehistoric times. *Can. J. Physiol. Pharmacol.*, **1986**, *64*, 840–848.

Tung, C.-S.; Goldberg, M. R.; Hollister, A. S.; Sweetman, B. J.; and Robertson, D. Depletion of brainstem epinephrine stores by α-methyldopa: possible relation to attenuated sympathetic outflow. *Life Sci.*, **1988**, *42*, 2365–2371.

U'Pritchard, D. C.; Greenberg, D. A.; and Snyder, S. H. Binding characteristics of a radiolabelled agonist and antagonist at central nervous system alpha noradrenergic receptors. *Mol. Pharmacol.*, **1977**, *13*, 454–473.

van den Meiracker, A. H.; Man in't Veld, A. J.; Ritsema van Eck, H. J.; Boomsma, F.; and Schalekamp, M. A. D. H. Hemodynamic and hormonal adaptations to β-adrenoceptor blockade. A 24-hour study of acebutolol, atenolol, pindolol, and propranolol in hypertensive patients. *Circulation*, **1988**, *78*, 957–968.

Veterans Administration Cooperative Study Group on Hypertensive Agents. Effects of treatment on morbidity in hypertension: results in patients with diastolic blood pressure averaging 115 through 129 mm Hg. *J.A.M.A.*, **1967**, *202*, 1028–1034.

———. Effects of treatment on morbidity in hypertension. II. Results in patients with diastolic blood pressure averaging 90 through 114 mm Hg. *Ibid.*, **1970**, *213*, 1143–1152.

Wikstrand, J.; Warnold, I.; Olsson, G.; Tuomilehto, J.; Elmfeldt, D.; and Berglund, G. Primary prevention with metoprolol in patients with hypertension. Mortality results from the MAPHY study. *J.A.M.A.*, **1988**, *259*, 1976–1982.

Wilhelmsen, L.; Berglund, G.; Elmfeldt, D.; Fitzsimons, T.; Holzgreve, H.; Hosie, J.; Hörnkvist, P.-E.; Pennert, K.; Tuomilehto, J.; and Wedel, H. Beta-blockers versus diuretics in hypertensive men: main results from the HAPPHY trial. *J. Hypertens.*, **1987**, *5*, 561–572.

Williams, G. M.; Mazue, G.; McQueen, C. A.; and Shimdad, T. Genotoxicity of the antihypertensive drugs hydralazine and dihydralazine. *Science*, **1980**, *210*, 329–330.

Wilson, D. J., and Vidt, D. G. Control of severe hypertension with pulse doses of diazoxide. *Clin. Pharmacol. Ther.*, **1978**, *23*, 135–140.

Wilson, M. F., and others. Comparison of guanfacine versus clonidine for efficacy, safety and occurrence of withdrawal syndrome in step-2 treatment of mild to moderate essential hypertension. *Am. J. Cardiol.*, **1986**, *57*, 43E–49E.

Wollam, G. L.; Tarazi, R. C.; Bravo, E. L.; and Dustan, H. P. Diuretic potency of combined hydrochlorothiazide and furosemide therapy in patients with azotemia. *Am. J. Med.*, **1982**, *72*, 929–938.

Wright, J. M.; Orozco-Gonzalez, M.; Polak, G.; and Dollery, C. T. Duration of effect of single daily dose methyldopa therapy. *Br. J. Clin. Pharmacol.*, **1982**, *13*, 847–854.

Zünkler, B. J.; Lenzen, S.; Männer, K.; Panten, U.; and Trube, G. Concentration-dependent effects of tolbutamide, meglitinide, glipizide, glibenclamide and diazoxide on ATP-regulated K^+ currents in pancreatic B-cells. *Naunyn Schmiedebergs Arch. Pharmacol.*, **1988**, *337*, 225–230.

Monographs and Reviews

Amdisen, A. Lithium and drug interactions. *Drugs*, **1982**, *24*, 133–139.

Brogden, R. N.; Heel, R. C.; Speight, T. M.; and Averg, G. S. Alpha methyl-L-tyrosine: a review of its pharmacology and clinical use. *Drugs*, **1981**, *21*, 81–89.

Campese, V. M. Minoxidil: a review of its pharmacological properties and therapeutic use. *Drugs*, **1981**, *22*, 257–278.

Cubeddu, L. X. New $alpha_1$-adrenergic receptor antagonists for the treatment of hypertension: role of vascular alpha receptors in the control of peripheral resistance. *Am. Heart J.*, **1988**, *116*, 133–162.

Doyle, A. E. Comparison of beta-adrenoceptor blockers and calcium antagonists in hypertension. *Hypertension*, **1983**, *5*, II103–II108.

Feinstein, A. R. Scientific standards in epidemiologic studies of the menace of daily life. *Science*, **1988**, *242*, 1257–1263.

Finnerty, F. A., Jr., and Brogden, R. N. Guanadrel. A review of its pharmacodynamic and pharmacokinetic properties and therapeutic use in hypertension. *Drugs*, **1985**, *30*, 22–31.

Freis, E. D. How diuretics lower blood pressure. *Am. Heart J.*, **1983**, *106*, 185–187.

———. The cardiovascular risks of thiazide diuretics. *Clin. Pharmacol. Ther.*, **1986**, *39*, 239–244.

Frishman, W. H.; Stroh, J. A.; Greenberg, S. M.; Suarez, T.; Karp, A.; and Peled, H. B. Calcium channel blockers in systemic hypertension. *Curr. Probl. Cardiol.*, **1987**, *12*, 285–346.

Grobbee, D. E., and Hofman, A. Does sodium restriction lower blood pressure? *Br. Med. J.* [*Clin. Res.*], **1986**, *293*, 27–29.

Holmes, B.; Brogden, R. N.; Heel, R. C.; Speight, T. M.; and Avery, G. S. Guanabenz. A review of its pharmacodynamic properties and therapeutic efficacy in hypertension. *Drugs*, **1983**, *26*, 212–229.

Houston, M. C., and Hodge, R. Beta-adrenergic blocker withdrawal syndromes in hypertension and other cardiovascular diseases. *Am. Heart J.*, **1988**, *116*, 515–523.

Insel, P. A., and Motulsky, H. J. A hypothesis linking intracellular sodium, membrane receptors, and hypertension. *Life Sci.*, **1984**, *34*, 1009–1013.

Ivankovich, A. D.; Miletich, D. J.; and Tinker, J. H. Sodium nitroprusside: metabolism and general considerations. *Int. Anesthesiol. Clin.*, **1978**, *16*, 1–29.

Joint National Committee. The 1988 report of the Joint National Committee on Detection, Evaluation, and Treatment of High Blood Pressure. *Arch. Intern. Med.*, **1988**, *148*, 1023–1038.

Kaplan, N. M. Maximally reducing cardiovascular risk in the treatment of hypertension. *Ann. Intern. Med.*, **1988a**, *109*, 36–40.

———. Calcium and potassium in the treatment of essential hypertension. *Semin. Nephrol.*, **1988b**, *8*, 176–184.

Kiowski, W.; Bühler, F. R.; Fadyomi, M.; Erne, P.; Müller, F. B.; Hulthen, U. L.; and Bolli, P. Age, race, blood pressure and renin: predictors for antihypertensive treatment with calcium antagonists. *Am. J. Cardiol.*, **1986**, *56*, 81H–85H.

Kreye, V. A. W. Direct vasodilators with unknown modes of action: the nitro-compounds and hydralazine. *J. Cardiovasc. Pharmacol.*, **1984**, *6*, S646–S655.

Langer, S. Z.; Cavero, I.; and Massingham, R. Recent developments in noradrenergic neurotransmission and its relevance to the mechanism of action of certain antihypertensive agents. *Hypertension*, **1980**, *2*, 372–382.

Lardinois, C. K., and Neuman, S. L. The effects of antihypertensive agents on serum lipids and lipoproteins. *Arch. Intern. Med.*, **1988**, *148*, 1280–1288.

Lehmann, H.-V.; Hochrein, H.; Witt, E.; and Mies, H. W. Hemodynamic effects of calcium antagonists. Review. *Hypertension*, **1983**, *5*, II66–II73.

Lund-Johansen, P. Hemodynamic effects of β-blocking compounds possessing vasodilating activity: a review of labetalol, prizidilol, and dilevalol. *J. Cardiovasc. Pharmacol.*, **1988**, *11*, Suppl. 2, S12–S17.

MacMahon, S. W.; Cutler, J. A. Furberg, C. D.; and Payne, G. H. The effects of drug treatment for hypertension on morbidity and mortality from cardiovascular disease: a review of randomized controlled trials. *Prog. Cardiovasc. Dis.*, **1986**, *29*, Suppl. 1, 99–118.

Maikranz, P., and Lindheimer, M. D. Hypertension in pregnancy. *Med. Clin. North Am.*, **1987**, *71*, 1031–1043.

Morgan, D. B., and Davidson, C. Hypokalemia and diuretics: an analysis of publications. *Br. Med. J.* [*Clin. Res.*], **1980**, *280*, 905–908.

Perry, H. M. Late toxicity to hydralazine resembling systemic lupus erythematosus or rheumatoid arthritis. *Am. J. Med.*, **1973**, *54*, 58–72.

Reece, P. A. Hydralazine and related compounds: chemistry, metabolism, and mode of action. *Med. Res. Rev.*, **1981**, *1*, 73–96.

Reid, J. L. Alpha-adrenergic receptors and blood pressure control. *Am. J. Cardiol.*, **1986**, *57*, 6E–12E.

Report of the Second Task Force on Blood Pressure Control in Children—1987. *Pediatrics*, **1987**, *79*, 1–25.

Robertson, J. I. S. The large studies in hypertension: what have they shown? *Br. J. Clin. Pharmacol.*, **1987**, *24*, 3S–14S.

Russell, R. P. Side effects of calcium channel blockers. *Hypertension*, **1988**, *11*, II42–II44.

Schulz, V. Clinical pharmacokinetics of nitroprusside, cyanide, thiosulphate and thiocyanate. *Clin. Pharmacokinet.*, **1984**, *9*, 239–251.

Sorkin, E. M., and Heel, R. C. Guanfacine. A review of its pharmacodynamic and pharmacokinetic properties, and therapeutic efficacy in the treatment of hypertension. *Drugs*, **1986**, *31*, 301–336.

Strandhoy, J. W. Role of alpha-2 receptors in the regulation of renal function. *J. Cardiovasc. Pharmacol.*, **1985**, *7*, Suppl. 8, S28–S33.

Ward-Routledge, C., and Marsden, C. A. Adrenaline in the CNS and the action of antihypertensive drugs. *Trends Pharmacol. Sci.*, **1988**, *9*, 209–214.

Webster, J. Interactions of NSAIDs with diuretics and β-blockers. Mechanisms and clinical implications. *Drugs*, **1985**, *30*, 32–41.

Woosley, R. L., and Nies, A. S. Guanethidine. *N. Engl. J. Med.*, **1976**, *295*, 1053–1057.

CHAPTER

34 DIGITALIS AND ALLIED CARDIAC GLYCOSIDES

Brian F. Hoffman and J. Thomas Bigger, Jr.

Digitalis and certain other cardiac glycosides have in common a powerful action on the myocardium that traditionally has been relied upon for the treatment of heart failure. These drugs are found in a number of plants, and a few also are present in the venom of certain toads. In the following discussion, the term *digitalis* is used to designate the entire group of cardiac glycosides and aglycones. The general descriptions of the pharmacology and uses of digitalis apply to all related cardiac glycosides unless otherwise stated.

History. A large number of plant extracts containing cardiac glycosides have been used by natives in various parts of the world as arrow and ordeal poisons. *Squill* was known as a medicine to the ancient Egyptians. The Romans employed it as a diuretic, heart tonic, emetic, and rat poison. *Strophanthus* was introduced into medicine in 1890 by Sir Thomas Fraser, who discovered its digitalis-like action while studying African arrow poisons. The dried skin of the common toad has been used for centuries as a drug by the Chinese. Digitalis, or foxglove, was mentioned in 1250 in the writings of Welsh physicians. It was described botanically 300 years later by Fuchsius, who gave it the name *Digitalis purpurea*.

In 1785, William Withering published his famous book, entitled *An Account of the Foxglove and Some of Its Medical Uses: With Practical Remarks on Dropsy and Other Diseases*. Withering was aware that digitalis was effective only in certain forms of dropsy (edema) but apparently did not associate this with the cardiac actions of the drug. He recognized that the heart was affected, however, for he wrote, "It has a power over the motion of the heart to a degree yet unobserved in any other medicine, and this power may be converted to salutary ends." Apparently, John Ferriar in 1799 was the first to ascribe to digitalis a primary action on the heart and to relegate the diuretic effect to a position of secondary importance. Whereas Withering recorded the benefits to be derived from the proper use of foxglove, his advice was not always heeded. Even during the nineteenth century, digitalis was used indiscriminately for many disorders, often in toxic doses. During the early twentieth century, as a result of the work of Cushny, Mackenzie, Lewis, and others, the drug gradually came to be looked upon as specific for the treatment of atrial fibrillation. Only subsequently was it established that digitalis is also valuable for the therapy of congestive heart failure.

Sources and Composition of the Digitalis Principles. Official digitalis is the dried leaf of the foxglove plant, *Digitalis purpurea*. Seeds and leaves of a number of other digitalis species also contain active cardiac principles. *Digitalis lanata* leaves are used in Europe and are the source of certain purified preparations employed in the United States. Strophanthus is obtained from the seeds of the *Strophanthus Kombé* or *hispidus;* ouabain is derived from *Strophanthus gratus*. *Squill,* the dried, fleshy bulb of the "sea onion," comes from *Urginea (Scilla) maritima*. Other sources of cardiac glycosides are described in *earlier editions* of this textbook.

Chemical Nature and Properties of the Cardiac Glycosides. Each glycoside represents the combination of an aglycone, or genin, with from one to four molecules of sugar. Pharmacological activity resides in the aglycone, but the particular sugars attached to the aglycone modify water and lipid solubility, potency, and the pharmacokinetic properties of the resulting glycoside (*see* Chen and Henderson, 1954; Marshall, 1970).

The aglycones are chemically related to bile acids, sterols, and steroid hormones. The basic structure is a cyclopentanoperhydrophenanthrene nucleus to which is attached an unsaturated lactone ring at C 17. All the naturally occurring aglycones carry OH groups at position 14, and many have additional OH groups, particularly at position 3, where the sugar moieties usually are attached. The hydroxyl group at C 3 is highly reactive, and semisynthetic derivatives have been made by reaction of aglycones with organic acids, sugars, and other agents. Acetylstrophanthidin, one such semisynthetic derivative, is not employed clinically but is used experimentally because of its rapid onset and relatively short duration of action. The number and the position of other OH groups are important for determining aqueous versus lipid solubility, protein binding, metabolic disposition, and duration of action. In general, the aglycones have more transient and less potent myocardial actions than the glycosides but cause similar toxic effects.

The unsaturated lactone ring attached to C 17 possesses the $\Delta^{\alpha,\beta}$ structure, and may be five- or six-membered. Saturation of the lactone ring reduces activity by tenfold or more, and increases the speed of development of the cardiac actions; opening of the ring completely abolishes activity.

The structural formulas of digoxigenin and digitoxigenin are as follows:

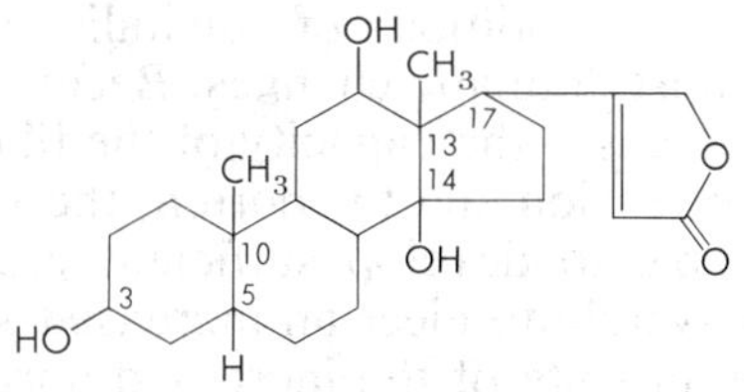

Digoxigenin

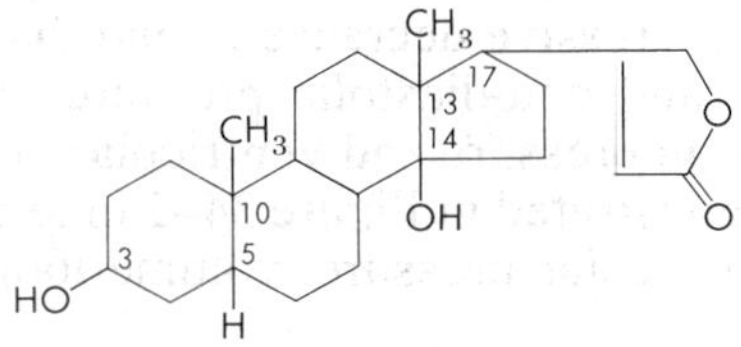

Digitoxigenin

Digoxin and digitoxin are the only cardiac glycosides used frequently; they consist of the corresponding aglycone with three molecules of digitoxose, a 2,6-dideoxyhexose, joined in glycosidic linkage and attached at position 3. The chemical constituents of various other glycosides are described in *earlier editions* of this textbook.

PHARMACODYNAMICS

Digitalis is used most frequently to improve circulation in patients with congestive heart failure and to slow the ventricular rate in the presence of atrial fibrillation and flutter. The main pharmacodynamic property of digitalis is its ability to increase the force of myocardial contraction. The beneficial effects of the drug in patients with heart failure—increased cardiac output; decreased heart size, venous pressure, and blood volume; diuresis and relief of edema—result mainly from the increased contractile force, a positive inotropic action. The second important action of digitalis is to slow the ventricular rate in atrial fibrillation or flutter.

The mechanisms responsible for the beneficial effects of digitalis are complex. Digitalis exerts direct effects on the heart that modify both its mechanical and electrical activity. It also acts directly on the smooth muscle of the vascular system. In addition, digitalis exerts a number of effects on neural tissue and thus indirectly influences the mechanical and electrical activity of the heart and modifies vascular resistance and capacitance. Finally, changes in the circulation brought about by digitalis often result in reflex alterations in autonomic activity and hormonal balance that indirectly influence cardiovascular function. In describing the effects of digitalis on the heart and circulation, it is convenient to discuss the direct and indirect actions on the heart before considering the integrated effects of digitalis on the entire cardiovascular system.

DIRECT EFFECTS

Myocardial Contractility. Digitalis increases the contractility of cardiac muscle in a dose-dependent manner—a positive inotropic effect. The effects are similar for both atrial and ventricular muscle and are qualitatively the same for muscle obtained from either normal or failing hearts. The effects of digitalis on mechanical activity can be demonstrated for both isometric and isotonic contractions. If an isolated preparation of cardiac muscle is studied under isometric conditions and the resting length is set at the peak of the length–tension relationship, an appropriate concentration of digitalis increases the peak force developed. In addition, digitalis increases the rate of development of force and decreases the time to peak tension. These changes occur without any alteration in resting tension. The effects are qualitatively similar at all points on the length–tension relationship.

The extent to which digitalis increases isometric tension depends strongly on the initial condition of the muscle. If the capacity to develop force is severely depressed, the effect is much larger than would occur in normal muscle (Figure 34–1).

If the preparation of cardiac muscle is studied under isotonic conditions, digitalis shifts the force–velocity curve upward. Both the maximal load and the rate of shortening increase. Digitalis thus increases not only the rate at which work can be done but also the maximal work that the muscle can perform. Concentrations of digitalis considerably higher than those needed to demonstrate the positive inotropic effect cause an increase in resting tension and

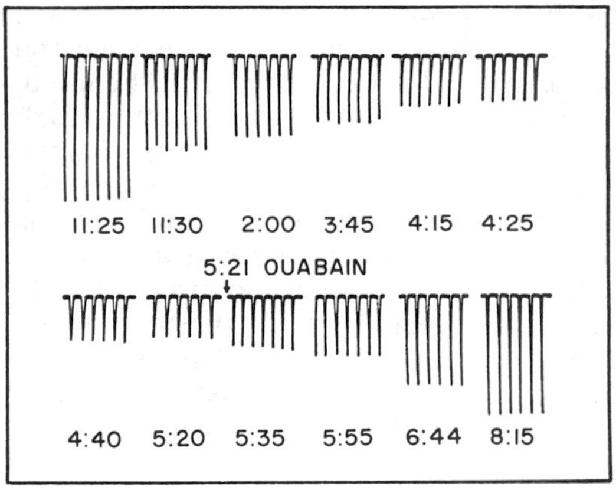

Figure 34–1. *The effect of ouabain on force of contraction of an isolated papillary muscle from the right ventricle of a cat heart.*

The muscle was prepared for isometric recording of contractions induced by rhythmic electrical stimulation. Systolic tension of the muscle, recorded as a downward deflection, decreased spontaneously during 6 hours of perfusion. The addition of ouabain in a concentration of 13 μg per liter (22 nM) restored the force of contraction. (After Gold and Cattell, 1940. Courtesy of the *Archives of Internal Medicine*.)

partial contracture. This toxic effect is associated with a decrease in shortening velocity and peak isometric tension.

When digitalis is studied in the isolated but intact mammalian heart, the drug increases the maximal rate of development of intraventricular pressure, decreases the duration of isovolumic contraction, increases ejection velocity, increases peak systolic pressure, and decreases the duration of contraction. Usually, stroke volume and aortic flow increase and, because the ventricle empties more completely during systole, end-systolic volume is reduced. Such a preparation can be induced to fail by increasing resistance to aortic flow. A sufficient increase in resistance reduces stroke volume; as a consequence, end-systolic volume is increased. With reasonably constant ventricular filling during diastole, end-diastolic pressure and volume increase. Because of the length–tension relationship, the increase in end-diastolic fiber length initially compensates for the elevated resistance to ejection. However, with time contraction weakens; there are progressive decreases in stroke volume and progressive increases in both end-diastolic pressure and volume. If heart rate is held constant, aortic flow necessarily decreases. Under these conditions, addition of digitalis brings about most dramatic changes. Because digitalis increases the capacity of the fibers to develop tension and to shorten, the ventricle is able to develop sufficient pressure during systole to eject an increased stroke volume in spite of the increased aortic resistance. The increased stroke volume results in a decrease in end-systolic volume and a progressive decrease in end-diastolic volume and end-diastolic pressure. These changes in pressure and ventricular volume are demonstrated in Figure 34–2 in terms of intraventricular pressure–volume loops.

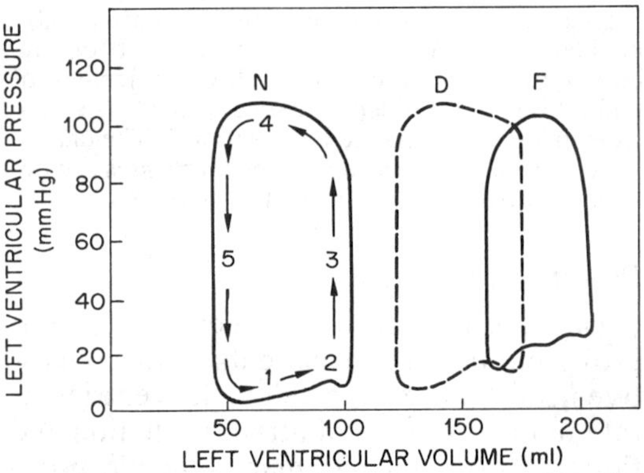

Figure 34–2. *Schematic representation of pressure–volume loops for the normal and failing left ventricle and the effects of digitalis.*

For the control loop (N), the arrows show the changes in ventricular pressure and volume with time during the single cardiac cycle. The numbers on the control loop indicate the phases of the cardiac cycle: 1 = diastasis, 2 = atrial systole, 3 = isovolumic contraction, 4 = ejection, 5 = isovolumic relaxation. End-diastolic pressure is relatively low, for the control curve pressure develops rapidly, and ejection is well maintained during systole. The loop labeled F shows the types of change that result from failure. End-systolic and end-diastolic volumes are greatly increased, as is end-diastolic pressure. During isovolumic contraction, pressure develops less rapidly and stroke volume is reduced. When digitalis has exerted its positive inotropic effect (D), the loop shifts to lower diastolic pressures and volumes and stroke volume increases.

Mechanism of Action. It appears that the positive inotropic effect of digitalis has two components: direct inhibition of the membrane-bound Na^+,K^+-activated adenosine triphosphatase (Na^+,K^+-ATPase), which leads to an increase in the intracellular concentration of Ca^{2+} ($[Ca^{2+}]_i$); and an associated increase in a slow inward Ca^{2+} current (i_{Ca}) during the action potential (AP). This current is the result of movement of Ca^{2+} into the cell, and it contributes to the plateau of the AP. Digitalis, in therapeutic concentrations, exerts no direct effect on the contractile proteins or on the interactions between them. Also, the positive inotropic effect of digitalis is not due to any action on the cellular mechanisms that provide the chemical energy for contraction. The hydrolysis of adenosine triphosphate (ATP) by the Na^+,K^+-ATPase drives the so-called Na^+ pump—the system in the sarcolemma of cardiac fibers that actively extrudes Na^+ and transports K^+ into the fibers. Digitalis glycosides bind specifically to the Na^+,K^+-ATPase, inhibit its enzymatic activity, and impair the active transport of these two monovalent cations. As a result, there is a gradual increase in intracellular Na^+ ($[Na^+]_i$) and a gradual small decrease in $[K^+]_i$ (Deitmer and Ellis, 1978; Eisner *et al.*, 1983). These changes are small at therapeutic concentrations of the drug. It is the increase in $[Na^+]_i$ that at present is judged to be crucially related to the positive inotropic effect of digitalis. This is so because in cardiac fibers intracellular Ca^{2+} is exchanged for extracellular Na^+ by a transport system that is driven by the concentration gradients for these ions and the transmembrane potential (Figure 34–3) (Eisner and Lederer, 1985; Noble, 1986). When $[Na^+]_i$ is increased because of inhibition of the pump by digitalis, the exchange of extracellular Na^+ for intracellular Ca^{2+} is diminished, and $[Ca^{2+}]_i$ increases (both prior to and during contraction) (Blinks *et al.*, 1982; Lee and Dagostino, 1982). The consequence of this is an increased store of Ca^{2+} in the sarcoplasmic reticulum (SR) and, with each AP, a greater release of Ca^{2+} to activate the contractile apparatus.

This exchange of ions results from the operation of a carrier in the membrane. Through such a mechanism either an increase in extracellular $[Ca^{2+}]$ ($[Ca^{2+}]_o$), a decrease in $[Na^+]_o$, or an increase in $[Na^+]_i$ would elevate $[Ca^{2+}]_i$ and cause a positive inotropic effect. This mechanism explains the well-known observation that force of cardiac contraction is roughly proportional to the extracellular ratio of $[Ca^{2+}]/[Na^+]^2$. The positive inotropic effect of a reduction in $[K^+]_o$ can also be explained, since a sufficient decrease in extracellular K^+ inhibits outward transport of Na^+ by the pump (Eisner *et al.*, 1983).

In addition, by mechanisms that are not clearly defined, the increase in $[Ca^{2+}]_i$ in-

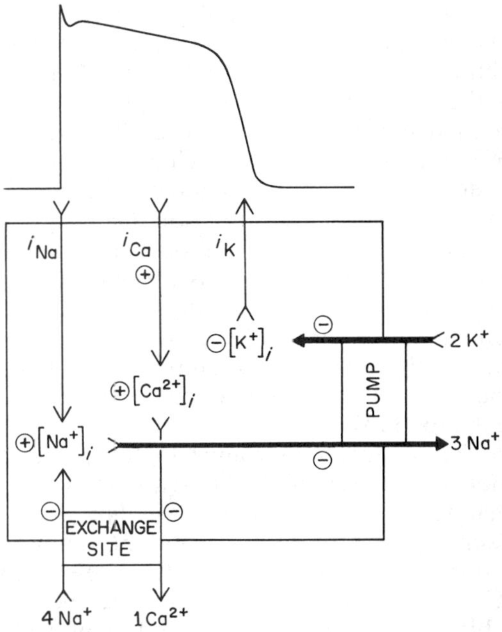

Figure 34–3. *Schematic representation of fluxes of Na^+, K^+, and Ca^{2+} across the cardiac cell membrane and the effects of digitalis thereon.*

During the transmembrane action potential, shown at the top, there is a net entry of Na^+ and Ca^{2+} and a net loss of K^+. The intracellular concentrations of Na^+ ($[Na^+]_i$) and K^+ ($[K^+]_i$) are maintained by the activity of the Na^+,K^+ pump, shown at the right. The intracellular concentration of calcium ($[Ca^{2+}]_i$) is in part regulated by exchange for Na^+ (exchange site). The effects of digitalis are shown as ⊕ or ⊖ next to the relevant process or parameter. Active extrusion of Na^+ is decreased; this leads to an increase in $[Na^+]_i$, which, in turn, causes an increase in $[Ca^{2+}]_i$. This, in turn, increases i_{Ca}.

creases the peak magnitude of i_{Ca}; this change parallels the positive inotropic action (Lederer and Eisner, 1982; Marban and Tsien, 1982). The change in i_{Ca} is a consequence of the increase in $[Ca^{2+}]_i$ and not of the increase in $[Na^+]_i$. Thus, more Ca^{2+} is delivered during the plateau of each AP to activate each contraction (*see* Figure 34–3). Contraction of most mammalian hearts is initiated by and is proportional to the influx of Ca^{2+} that occurs during the AP (Beeler and Reuter, 1970). This Ca^{2+} influx causes the release of additional Ca^{2+} from the sarcoplasmic reticulum (Fabiato and Fabiato, 1977).

The relative importance to the positive inotropic effect of the increase in $[Ca^{2+}]_i$ that results from reduction in Na^+–Ca^{2+} exchange on the one hand, and the augmentation of i_{Ca} that results from elevated $[Ca^{2+}]_i$ on the other, remains to be established. Both effects would contribute to the increased $[Ca^{2+}]_i$, whereas the latter might also directly influence excitation–contraction coupling. However, a positive inotropic effect can be demonstrated in the absence of an increase in i_{Ca} (Marban and Tsien, 1982).

Na^+–H^+ exchange also appears to play a role in amplifying the increase in $[Ca^{2+}]_i$ that results from inhibition of the Na^+ pump. The increase in $[Ca^{2+}]_i$ causes a fall in intracellular pH, and protons are exchanged for $[Na^+]_o$ to compensate. This further increases $[Na^+]_i$ (Kim *et al.*, 1987).

The mechanism described thus assumes that the Na^+,K^+-ATPase is the pharmacological receptor for digitalis and that when digitalis binds to this enzyme it induces a conformational change that decreases the active transport of Na^+. Many studies have provided evidence that digitalis binds to the ATPase in a specific and saturable manner, that the binding results in a conformational change of the enzyme, that the rate of binding is increased by $[Na^+]$ and decreased by $[K^+]$, and that the binding site for digitalis is probably on the external surface of the membrane (*see* Schwartz, 1976; Hess and Müller, 1982). Furthermore, the magnitude of the inotropic effect of digitalis is proportional to the degree of inhibition of the enzyme (Akera *et al.*, 1970; Hougen and Smith, 1978).

Electrical Activity. Because some of the therapeutic and most of the serious toxic effects of digitalis can be related to its effects on the electrophysiological properties of the heart, these actions of the drug have been studied extensively; nevertheless, there is still some uncertainty about the underlying mechanisms (*see* Weingart, 1981; Hoffman, 1983; Vassalle, 1986; Cranefield and Aronson, 1988). To a large extent, the consequences of digitalis-induced changes are intensified as the rate of generation of action potentials is increased.

Purkinje Fibers. Most attempts to explain the effects of digitalis on the electrical activity of the heart have been based on data obtained with Purkinje fibers. The effects of increasing frequency of stimulation and concentration of drug can be considered in three general categories: (1) decreased resting potential (RP) or maximal diastolic potential (MDP), which slows the rate of phase-0 depolarization and conduction velocity; (2) decreases in the action potential duration (APD), which result in an increased responsiveness of fibers to electrical stimuli; and (3) enhancement of automaticity, which results from an increase in the rate of phase-4 depolarization and from the appearance of delayed afterdepolarizations (Figure 34–4).

Changes in RP (MDP). Inhibition of the Na^+,K^+-ATPase increases $[Na^+]_i$ (and tends to increase $[K^+]_o$). At low concentrations of digitalis, the resulting depolarization (decrease in MPD) causes only a slight reduction in the rate of phase-0 depolarization; there is a small increase in conduction velocity because the fibers are closer to their threshold for firing and larger blocks of tissue can be excited simultaneously. At higher concentrations of drug (and/or greater frequency of stimulation), the decrease in MPD is larger and voltage-dependent inactivation of fast Na^+ channels becomes more significant. The decrease in the rate of phase-0 depolarization is now large enough to lower conduction velocity because the decreased amplitude of the action potential and the attenuated flow of electrotonic current excite a smaller block of tissue. The spread of current is also hampered by changes in the gap junctions between cells, caused by an increase in $[Ca^{2+}]_i$ (DeMello, 1975; Weingart, 1977). There may be an additional direct effect of digitalis to promote inactivation of Na^+ channels (Kassebaum, 1963). Ultimately the fibers become inexcitable because of the marked decrease in RP and inactivation of fast Na^+ channels.

Changes in APD. At low concentrations of digi-

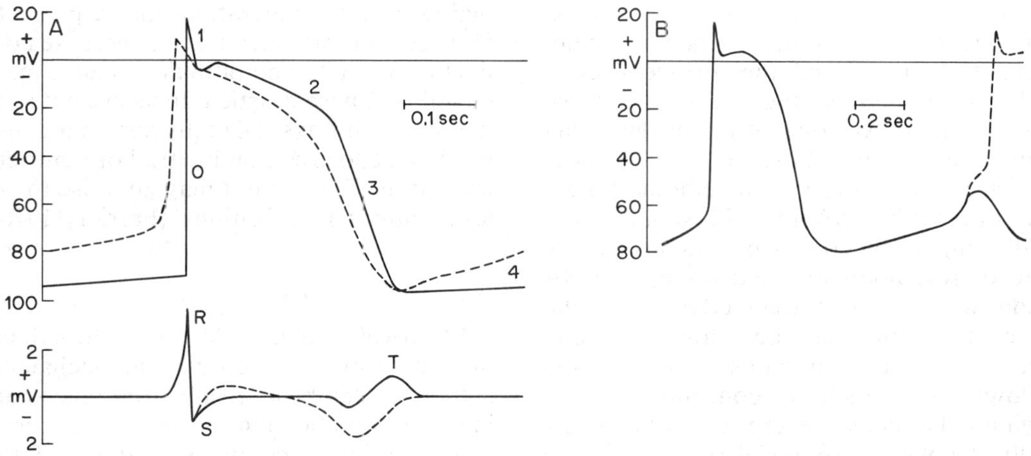

Figure 34–4. *Effects of digitalis on transmembrane potentials and electrograms.*

A. Schematic representation of a transmembrane action potential recorded from a cardiac Purkinje fiber (top trace) and a unipolar electrogram recorded from the same preparation (bottom trace) under control conditions (solid lines) and in the presence of digitalis (dashed lines). Phases 0, 1, 2, 3, and 4 have their usual meaning. After the effects of digitalis have developed, there is a decrease in maximal diastolic potential, an increase in the slope of phase-4 depolarization, and a decrease in action potential duration. Because of the increase in phase-4 depolarization, the fiber becomes automatic. Voltage at which activation occurs shifts to a more positive value, and the amplitude of the action potential decreases. Because of the change in the slope and duration of phases 2 and 3, there is a change in the S–T segment and T wave of the electrogram and a decrease in the R–T interval.

B. Schematic representation of the appearance of delayed afterdepolarizations caused by digitalis in the record of transmembrane potential from a Purkinje fiber. The delayed afterdepolarizations are shown as being subthreshold (solid line) and suprathreshold (dashed line); the latter initiates an extra action potential. *See* text for further explanation.

talis, the small increases in $[Ca^{2+}]_i$ (resulting from increased $[Na^+]_i$) lead to augmentation of i_{Ca} (*see* above); as a result, the plateau of the AP (phase 2) is shifted to more positive potentials and the APD is prolonged. Although this contributes importantly to inotropic effects, the impact on electrical properties of the heart is small. However, this prolongation of APD does tend to counteract the increased automaticity that results from the digitalis-induced rise in the rate of phase-4 depolarization (*see* below). As the frequency of stimulation or the concentration of digitalis is increased, the APD progressively shortens. Three factors contribute: (1) $[K^+]_o$ is increased, which accelerates the activation of a voltage-activated K^+ (repolarizing) current by an unknown mechanism; (2) the larger increase in $[Ca^{2+}]_i$ increases the function of a Ca^{2+}-dependent K^+ channel; and (3) the larger increase in $[Ca^{2+}]_i$ accelerates the inactivation of Ca^{2+} channels, thereby decreasing inward (depolarizing) current (Marban and Tsien, 1982). The decrease in APD can contribute to automaticity because the shortened refractory period increases the likelihood that fibers will respond to any spontaneous depolarization (*see* below).

Automaticity. Digitalis increases the tendency for the generation of spontaneous APs by two general mechanisms. First, the slope of phase-4 depolarization is increased, probably because the decrease in MDP enhances the rate of activation of the inward pacemaker current (i_f); this time- and voltage-dependent current is carried primarily by Na^+ (DiFrancesco, 1981). It is not known whether digitalis has any direct effects on this current. Second, delayed afterdepolarizations can appear, and these lead to the generation of propagated APs (*see* Figure 34–4; *see also* Chapter 35). The afterdepolarizations are promoted by any condition that enhances intracellular stores of Ca^{2+}, including increased frequency of contraction, β_1-adrenergic agonists, increases in $[Ca^{2+}]_o$, or digitalis, and they are suppressed by anything that reduces the influx of Ca^{2+}, such as blockade of Ca^{2+} channels. Evidence indicates that Ca^{2+} overload causes an oscillatory release and reuptake of Ca^{2+} by intracellular sites of storage, most likely the sarcoplasmic reticulum, and a coincidental transient inward current. This current may result from a special sarcolemmal conductance that is sensitive to changes in $[Ca^{2+}]_i$ or it may reflect alterations in electrogenic exchange of Na^+ for Ca^{2+}. The transient current, in turn, causes the afterdepolarizations. At present, it is often not possible to differentiate clinically between effects that result from enhanced phase-4 depolarization and those that are caused by promotion of delayed afterdepolarizations.

Other Specialized Fibers. Digitalis exerts direct effects on the fibers of the sinoatrial (SA) node and the atrioventricular (AV) node, and on the specialized atrial fiber system. At concentrations that may obtain during clinical use, digitalis has little direct effect on the transmembrane potentials of the rabbit SA node. Most of the clinically important effects of digitalis on the rate of formation of impulses by the SA node are due to indirect effects that the drug exerts through the parasympathetic and sympathetic nervous systems (*see* below). Nevertheless, concentrations of digitalis that cause severe toxicity can partially depolarize SA nodal fibers and stop the generation of impulses. High concentrations of digitalis directly depress conduction of impulses through the AV node. However, as for the SA node, the clinically important actions of cardiac glycosides on the AV node are mediated by the autonomic nervous system. The direct actions decrease conduction velocity, increase the effective refractory period (ERP), and ultimately cause complete AV block. These changes in conduction are associated with a decrease in MDP and in the rate of rise and amplitude of the AV nodal AP. The specialized atrial fibers respond to digitalis in much the same manner as do Purkinje fibers. Most importantly, digitalis causes not only an increase in automaticity owing to enhanced phase-4 depolarization but also generation of ectopic impulses because of production of delayed afterdepolarizations (*see* above).

Atrial and Ventricular Muscle Fibers. The changes in the duration of the AP in ventricular muscle fibers resemble those described for Purkinje fibers. The decrease in this value is not marked but probably accounts for the decrease in the Q–T interval of the ECG (*see* Figure 34–4 and below). The ventricular transmembrane APs also show an increase in slope of the plateau and a decrease in the slope of phase 3. These alterations in the transmembrane potential cause changes in the S–T segment and the T wave in the ECG (*see* Figure 34–4 and below). In sufficiently high concentration, digitalis decreases both the RP and the amplitude of the AP of atrial and ventricular fibers and decreases the maximal rate of depolarization during phase 0. High concentrations thus can decrease conduction velocity and ultimately cause inexcitability. These drastic effects are not seen in clinical settings. Digitalis does not cause phase-4 depolarization in atrial or ventricular muscle fibers, but it may give rise to delayed afterdepolarizations (Ferrier, 1976).

INDIRECT EFFECTS

Electrical Activity. Many of the effects of digitalis on the electrical and mechanical activity of the heart result from glycoside-induced modification of both autonomic neural activity and the sensitivity of the heart to the vagal and sympathetic neurotransmitters. The decrease in sinus rate in the presence of heart failure is caused in large part by a glycoside-induced increase in efferent vagal impulses and a reflexly induced decrease in sympathetic tone; these changes are associated with improvement of the circulation (Ferguson *et al.*, 1989). Other alterations of autonomic activity are more complex and less well understood (*see* Gillis and Quest, 1980; Vassalle, 1986).

The increase in vagal activity caused by digitalis appears to result from effects at several sites in the nervous system. The arterial baroceptors are sensitized, probably because of an effect of digitalis on active transport of cations in the afferent nerve terminals (Saum *et al.*, 1976). Digitalis affects the central vagal nuclei and the nodose ganglion (Chai *et al.*, 1967) and may modify the excitability of efferent vagal fibers (Ten Eick and Hoffman, 1969). Digitalis also increases the sensitivity of the sinus node to the negative chronotropic effect of acetylcholine (Toda and West, 1966). Most data indicate that administration of digitalis will intensify the effects of the vagus nerve on the heart through several or all of these mechanisms as well as by effects on the heart and circulation that modify input to the autonomic nervous system (*see* below).

Digitalis also changes activity in the sympathetic nervous system. Acute administration of therapeutic doses of a digitalis glycoside reduces sympathetic activity (Ferguson *et al.*, 1989). Sufficiently high concentrations of glycoside can decrease the sensitivity of the SA and AV nodes to catecholamines and efferent sympathetic impulses. However, efferent sympathetic activity is enhanced by toxic concentrations of digitalis (*see* Gillis and Quest, 1980). This may result from effects of digitalis that gains access to structures in the area postrema of the medulla oblongata via the choroid plexus (Mudge *et al.,* 1978). The role of increased effects of norepinephrine in causing digitalis-induced arrhythmias has been reviewed by Gillis and Quest (1980) and by Rosen (1981). The importance of norepinephrine in promoting arrhythmias caused by digitalis is suggested by studies on isolated cardiac Purkinje fibers (Tse and Han, 1978) and also by the capacity of β-adrenergic blocking drugs to attenuate or prevent some digitalis-induced disturbances of ventricular rhythm.

The combined effects of these indirect actions of digitalis on the normal heart and circulation are reasonably clear. However, when the circulation is abnormal, as in congestive heart failure, the net effects may be quite different. When the heart is normal, the augmented vagal activity typically decreases the rate of generation of impulses in the SA node; other effects of digitalis on this node probably are not significant with usual therapeutic concentrations of the drug. In normal man at rest, digitalis may not cause a decrease in sinus rate; however, the maximal heart rate achieved during exercise is significantly diminished (Horwitz *et al.,* 1977). If the sinus rate is increased, as in heart failure, the negative chronotropic effect of digitalis is usually quite prominent. Here, withdrawal of compensatory sympathetic activity contributes to the net effect.

Atrial fibers, both specialized and nonspecialized, are quite sensitive to the actions of acetylcholine. The indirect action of digitalis thus causes prominent changes in the electrical activity of the atrium. At what may be assumed to be therapeutic concentrations, vagally mediated indirect effects predominate over direct effects. The liberated acetylcholine causes an increase in RP, a decrease in latent automaticity of specialized atrial fibers, and a marked decrease in the duration of the atrial AP and ERP. If hyperpolarization is significant, conduction is slowed. Although such hyperpolarization is opposed by a directly induced decrease in RP, the most significant direct effects at therapeutic concentrations of digitalis are the decreases in atrial APD and ERP. These changes combine to permit the atria to respond to stimulation at much higher rates. Thus, if digitalis is given during atrial flutter or atrial fibrillation, the net rate of atrial impulses may increase (*see* below).

If the RP of human atrial muscle is significantly decreased because of disease, the vagotonic action of digitalis can cause hyperpolarization and improvement in APs and conduction (Hordof *et al.,* 1978). If there is phase-4 depolarization, automaticity is decreased.

The AV node is strongly influenced by the indirect actions of digitalis. The enhanced vagal activity and the decrease in sensitivity to catecholamines have pronounced effects on both the generation of the AV nodal AP and the transmission of impulses through the node. Acetylcholine causes some hyperpolarization of certain fibers in the AV node but, more importantly, decreases the rate of rise and amplitude of APs at these sites. Also, the recovery of excitability is delayed. Because of these changes, conduction is slowed and the ERP is greatly prolonged. The impairment of conduction may progress to complete heart block. The decreased sensitivity to norepinephrine intensifies these effects. In the AV node, therefore, the direct and indirect effects of digitalis bring about similar changes. The most important result is to diminish the rate at which atrial impulses can be transmitted to the ventricles. Thus, in atrial tachycardias, atrial flutter, and atrial fibrillation, administration of digitalis will decrease the ventricular rate because of block of an increased fraction of atrial impulses in the AV junction.

The effectiveness of the AV block due to the direct and indirect effects on the AV node is enhanced in atrial flutter and fibrillation because digitalis, through its indirect effect on the atria, usually *increases* the rate at which impulses enter the atrial margin of the node. Those impulses that enter the node but fail to propagate through it spread slowly and leave the tissue refractory in their wake (concealed conduction); this repetitive concealed conduction increases the fraction of time during which the node is effectively refractory (*see* below).

The His-Purkinje system is strongly influenced by the sympathetic nervous system but ordinarily is not particularly sensitive to changes in vagal activity. Thus, in contrast to the SA node, atria, and AV node, it is the sympathetic nervous system that mediates indirect effects of digitalis on the electrical activity of the specialized ventricular conducting system.

Enhanced efferent sympathetic activity may be important in relation to the drug-initiated arrhythmias that occur when the concentration of digitalis is high. If the heart is deprived of sympathetic innervation, toxic doses of digitalis usually cause cardiac arrest rather than ventricular arrhythmias and fibrillation (Erlij and Mendez, 1964; Ten Eick and Hoffman, 1969). It seems reasonable to conclude, therefore, that the indirect and direct effects may at times act synergistically to cause disturbances of rhythm.

The indirect effects of digitalis probably result in only minor changes in the electrical activity of ventricular fibers; only extremely high concentrations of acetylcholine affect canine ventricular transmembrane RPs and APs. Similarly, catecholamines cause only small changes in the duration of the ventricular AP.

In summary, the indirect effects of digitalis, mediated primarily through the vagus, result in prominent changes in the activity of the sinus node, the atria, and the AV node. At therapeutic concentrations, neurally mediated indirect effects on the functions of the specialized ventricular conducting system and the ventricles are much less important.

Mechanical Activity. The direct action of digitalis is primarily responsible for its positive inotropic effect on the heart. Nevertheless, certain of the drug's indirect effects do contribute to alterations of mechanical activity. For example, the decrease in heart rate caused by sinus slowing influences contractility because of a change in end-diastolic fiber length; there is also a direct inotropic effect due to the change in rate. A decrease in ventricular rate caused by partial AV block has similar effects. Enhanced vagal activity decreases the force of atrial contraction, but this negative inotropic effect, which might slightly reduce atrial transfer of blood, does not significantly attenuate the direct positive inotropic effect of digitalis on ventricular function. Interactions between digitalis and the sympathetic nervous system also are not crucially important in relation to the positive inotropic effect of digitalis. The glycoside can exert a strong positive inotropic effect after complete blockade of cardiac β-adrenergic receptors.

EFFECTS ON ELECTRICAL ACTIVITY OF THE HEART *IN SITU*

There is a reasonable correspondence between the toxic effects of digitalis on the canine and the human heart, and observations made on experimental animals have thus contributed importantly to our understanding of the therapeutic and toxic effects of digitalis in man.

The Canine Heart *in Situ*. Digitalis has a biphasic effect on the electrical excitability of both the atria and the ventricles. Low doses cause a slight increase in excitability, whereas higher doses decrease it. The enhanced excitability likely results from a small decrease in RP. The decreased excitability caused by very high concentrations of digitalis presumably results from the direct effect of digitalis on voltage-dependent inactivation of the fast inward Na^+ channel and also from a reduction in RP sufficient to cause partial inactivation of the fast inward channel. Sufficiently high concentrations of digitalis can cause inexcitability of all cardiac tissues. The atria are more sensitive than ventricular muscle, and Purkinje fibers are much more sensitive than ventricular muscle to these toxic actions of digitalis (*see* Hoffman and Singer, 1964).

The effects of digitalis on conduction velocity in the different cardiac tissues is variable. Conduction velocity depends, among other factors, not only on the level of the RP but also on the threshold potential, the degree of inactivation of the fast inward channel, the membrane resistance, and the resistance between cardiac cells at gap junctions. Since high concentrations of digitalis can decrease RP, shift the curve describing inactivation of the fast inward channel in a depolarizing direction, decrease membrane resistance, and perhaps increase the resistance of the gap junctions, toxic concentrations of the drug can decrease conduction velocity in atrial and ventricular muscle fibers and cardiac Purkinje fibers. In addition, the presence of delayed afterdepolarizations can slow and impair impulse propagation.

In the atrium, the direct effects of therapeutic concentrations of a cardiac glycoside usually are antagonized by the enhanced vagal effect (*see* above), although conduction slows with high toxic concentrations. In Purkinje fibers and ventricular muscle, low concentrations of glycoside slightly speed conduction, whereas very high concentrations cause slowing. Conduction in the Purkinje system is impaired at a lower concentration of drug than is required to affect ventricular muscle. Since digitalis typically does not prolong the QRS complex in the human ECG, the meaning of slowing of impulse propagation in the specialized conducting system of the canine heart is difficult to evaluate. The depression of conduction through the AV node has been described in the previous section. Prolongation of the P–R interval and the production of heart block are due primarily to actions on the AV node.

The effects of digitalis on the refractoriness of atrial muscle depend on the relative predominance of the indirect (vagal) effects and the direct effects. Ordinarily, because of the enhanced vagal effects, the atrial refractory period is shortened. This parallels a decrease in the duration of the atrial transmembrane AP. However, if the heart has been denervated or if atropine has been given, digitalis increases the duration of atrial refractory periods. The effects of digitalis on the ERP of the AV node have been described in detail. The vagal effect, the antiadrenergic effect, and the direct effect all increase the effective and functional refractory periods of the AV junction. In the ventricle, digitalis shortens the duration of refractoriness, in parallel with the decrease in duration of the transmembrane AP. The change is modest in magnitude and proportional to the change in the Q–T interval on the ECG. Digitalis also alters the response of ventricular muscle to a single stimulus applied after the end of the T wave, such that a single stimulus can elicit repetitive ventricular responses (Lown *et al.*, 1967).

The effects of digitalis on impulse generation and conduction in the canine heart *in situ* provide a reasonably good picture of the usual changes brought about by therapeutic and toxic concentrations of cardiac glycosides in man. Small doses of drug decrease the sinus rate, minimally increase the P–R interval, and prolong the ERP of the AV node. Also, if the vagus is stimulated to cause AV block, it can be seen that digitalis increases the automaticity of the specialized ventricular conducting system. This is evidenced by a decrease in the interval between the block and the first ventricular escape beat and by an increase in the rate of the escape rhythm as the dose of digitalis increases.

The Human Heart *in Situ*. Perhaps surprisingly, most studies of the human atrium have shown only minimal effects of digitalis on the duration of refractoriness. This is true of normal atria (Dhingra *et al.*, 1975; Wu *et al.*, 1975) and those that have been denervated by cardiac transplantation (Goodman *et al.*, 1975). Refractoriness of the AV node is increased, and AV nodal conduction is slowed. There is no significant change in refractoriness or conduction in the His-Purkinje system (Gomes *et al.*, 1978). In contrast, the functional and effective refractory periods of ventricular muscle are decreased slightly but significantly. This may increase the interval during which ventricular premature depolarizations can induce reentrant excitation through the specialized conducting system.

Mechanism of Cardiac Slowing in Atrial Fibrillation. In typical atrial fibrillation the impulse spreads through the atrium in a manner that may best be described as random reentry. Most atrial fibers are reexcited as soon as they recover sufficiently from refractoriness. The impulses arriving at the AV node are rapid (as many as 500 per minute) and random in time. Most of these impulses either fail to enter the AV node because it is refractory or propagate only partway through it and give rise to the phenomenon of concealed conduction. The concealed conduction of these impulses increases the time during which nodal tissues are partially or totally refractory. Longer ventricular cycles occur when one or more successive atrial impulses enter the node but fail to propagate to the His bundle. When atrial fibrillation is accompanied by congestive heart failure, the resulting reduction in vagal tone and increase in sympathetic tone increase the ventricular rate. In rapid atrial fibrillation, the ventricular rate is grossly irregular and stroke volume may be very small. The major effect of digitalis on ventricular rate during atrial fibrillation results from its capacity to increase the ERP of the AV node (described above). The effect is to decrease ventricular rate and, very often, to improve ventricular function.

In addition to its effects on AV transmission, digitalis reduces ventricular rate during atrial fibrillation by another mechanism that operates simultaneously. Through its indirect action on the atria, mediated by acetylcholine, digitalis decreases the duration of the atrial transmembrane AP and decreases the ERP of atrial fibers. Thus, there is an increase in the mean frequency at which atrial fibers are excited and at which impulses enter the atrial margin of the AV node; a greater proportion of impulses are extinguished as a result of concealed conduction and a smaller proportion propagate to the ventricles.

Action in Atrial Flutter. When atrial flutter is established in an animal in which the vagi have been blocked with atropine, the administration of digitalis slows the flutter frequency and eventually restores normal sinus rhythm. In similar preparations in which the vagus nerves are intact, digitalis often converts the atrial flutter to atrial fibrillation. Administration of atropine may now restore normal rhythm. The explanation of these results may be found in the direct and indirect effects of digitalis upon the atrial refractory period. When the vagi are blocked, digitalis prolongs the refractory period; however, when the nerves are not blocked, the ERP is abbreviated. The vagal effects are not uniformly distributed; the atrial refractory period is greatly reduced at some points and not at all at others. As a result, the flutter wave front becomes fractionated and fibrillation occurs.

Effect in Patients with the Wolff-Parkinson-White Syndrome. Effects of digitalis on conduction in and refractoriness of anomalous AV bypass tracts are variable. Wellens and Durrer (1973) found that ouabain *decreased* refractoriness of the accessory pathways but did not change refractoriness of atrial muscle. In contrast, Sellers and coworkers (1977) found variable effects among different subjects. The important point to remember is that digitalis can decrease the ERP of the bypass tract sufficiently so that more atrial impulses can be conducted to the ventricle. Thus, administration of digitalis to a patient with atrial fibrillation and the Wolff-Parkinson-White syndrome can trigger ventricular fibrillation. This decrease in refractoriness is seen in about 30% of patients with Wolff-Parkinson-White syndrome given the drug; it is an absolute contraindication to the use of digitalis.

Electrocardiographic Effects. Although digitalis has characteristic effects on the ECG, these cannot be used to estimate digitalis dosage or the degree of digitalization. Furthermore, the effects of digitalis are often superimposed on changes resulting from the basic cardiac disease. As mentioned previously, even toxic doses of digitalis typically do not cause an increase in the duration of the QRS complex.

Within 2 to 4 hours after a large oral dose of digitalis, definite alterations may appear in the ECG. Changes are first noted in the S–T segment or in the T wave itself. The normally upright T wave becomes diminished in amplitude, isoelectric, or inverted in one or more leads. The S–T segment may also show depression when the main QRS complex is upward; occasionally, the S–T segment is elevated by digitalis when the main QRS deflection is downward. The changes in the S–T segment and the T wave may occur alone or may coincide. In precordial leads, these changes can simulate those resulting from coronary artery disease or recent coronary occlusion. After exercise in digitalized patients the J point may show depression similar to that caused by myocardial ischemia.

Digitalis may prolong the P–R interval. This effect occurs somewhat later than the changes described above. The interval rarely becomes greater than 0.25 second, unless the conduction system is diseased. Atropine can abolish lower degrees of AV block produced by digitalis, but the direct (or antiadrenergic) actions of the drug are not overcome by atropine.

Digitalis shortens the Q–T interval because it accelerates ventricular repolarization. Large doses occasionally cause changes in the size and the shape of the P wave. Digitalis can widen the abnormal QRS complex in the Wolff-Parkinson-White syndrome, probably by slowing AV nodal propagation without affecting conduction time in the anomalous AV pathway. This effect may be reversed by atropine. Almost every type of ECG tracing associated with cardiac disorders can be simulated by the effects of digitalis on the heart. However, if QRS widening occurs during normal sinus rhythm, it almost certainly is the result of concurrent disease, since digitalis does not cause this change.

EFFECTS ON THE CARDIOVASCULAR SYSTEM

The overall effects of digitalis on the cardiovascular system not only are a composite of changes in the force of ventricular contraction and heart rate but also result from effects on the autonomic nervous system and on vascular smooth muscle; furthermore, reflex adjustments to the initial hemodynamic changes caused by the drug are also important. The effects of digitalis on cardiovascular function differ depending on whether the heart and circulation are normal or whether there is congestive heart failure.

The Normal Heart and Circulation. When a rapidly acting drug like ouabain is injected intravenously into a normal conscious dog, both systolic and mean arterial pressures increase; they reach their maxima in 5 minutes and decline slowly over 30 minutes (McRitchie and Vatner, 1976; Horwitz *et al.*, 1977). All indices of ventricular contractility increase, but not markedly. This clearly results from the direct positive inotropic effect of digitalis and does not depend on changes in fiber length or contributions from the sympathetic nervous system. Heart rate usually decreases moderately, stroke volume increases, end-systolic ventricular volume decreases somewhat, and cardiac output is diminished slightly (because of the change in rate). The major cause of the sinus slowing is a reflex response to both the rate of change and the extent of increase in arterial pressure.

Since mean systemic arterial pressure is elevated without an increase in cardiac output, there must be an increase in systemic vascular resistance. This increase results from a direct effect of digitalis to cause contraction of arterioles. Sympathetic outflow from the CNS is augmented, but this probably causes only minimal change in arterial resistance. Digitalis also acts directly on smooth muscle in veins to cause constriction (*see* McRitchie and Vatner, 1976; Horwitz *et al.*, 1977). The effects on normal human subjects are very similar (Smith and Haber, 1973). Cardiac glycosides can reduce exercise tolerance in normal subjects by limiting the maximum increase in heart rate.

Heart Failure. To understand the effects of digitalis in patients with congestive heart failure, it is important to consider the factors that regulate cardiac contractility and their alteration in this disease. Furthermore, it is essential to appreciate other changes that are secondary to heart failure, such as retention of salt and water and reflex adjustments to impaired cardiac function.

The force developed by the ventricles during systole is regulated by both extrinsic factors, such as the level of sympathetic tone, and intrinsic factors, which include the frequency of contraction and the length of the fibers just before the onset of systole. In addition, the external work done by the ventricles is determined by their volume and the interaction between the afterload (the impedance met by the ventricle during ejection) and the contracting ventricle.

To describe the effects of digitalis on the failed ventricle it is essential first to consider the pressure–volume relationship described by Patterson and Starling in 1914 and extended by others in the form of the cardiac function curve (Figure 34–5). For any given state of the ventricles, when end-

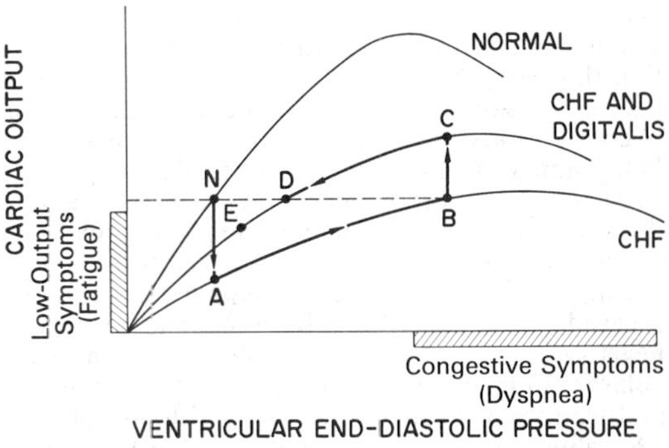

Figure 34–5. *Diagrammatic representation of the use of the Frank-Starling mechanism as a compensation for congestive heart failure.*

The three curves depict ventricular function in normal subjects and in those with congestive heart failure (CHF) and heart failure after treatment with digitalis. The points N through D represent in sequence: initial reduction of contractility due to congestive heart failure (N to A); use of Frank-Starling compensation to maintain cardiac output (A to B); increase in contractility when digitalis is administered (B to C); and reduction in the use of Frank-Starling compensation, which digitalis allows (C to D). Any factor that reduces ventricular filling pressure (decreased venous return) will lower cardiac output in spite of an inotropic effect (D to E). Of note is the fact that points N, B, and D all lie on the same line in the vertical axis and thus all represent the same cardiac output, but each is on a different end-diastolic pressure on the horizontal axis. The levels at which symptoms of congestion, such as dyspnea, and symptoms of low cardiac output, such as fatigue, occur are represented by the cross-hatched areas. (After Mason, 1973. Courtesy of *The American Journal of Cardiology*.)

diastolic fiber length and end-diastolic volume increase because of an increase in filling pressure, the force of ventricular contraction increases, up to a limit. Usually this results in an increase in the force developed during systole and in the stroke volume and stroke work. The absolute value of stroke volume or work for a given end-diastolic volume depends on the inotropic state of the ventricles. In the failing heart, the capacity to develop force during systole is reduced and thus a greater end-diastolic volume is needed to perform any given level of external work. In cardiac failure, therefore, one can imagine the following sequence of events. Reduced systolic ejection, caused by a mismatch of work capacity and load, results in decreased systolic ejection and an increased end-systolic volume. With constant filling, end-diastolic pressure and volume increase. If this sequence progresses, the ventricular volume will increase progressively. At the same time, because of the Laplace relationship, the effectiveness of increased wall tension in developing intraventricular pressure and the extent to which fiber shortening results in systolic ejection will both diminish. Further dilatation thus may be needed to maintain aortic flow. (At an excessive end-diastolic fiber length the force of contraction decreases; whether this occurs in the failed human heart *in situ* is uncertain.)

If, by means of the pressure–volume relation, the heart is unable to compensate for the load imposed, other mechanisms must be recruited; these usually include increased sympathetic and decreased vagal activity. These changes increase heart rate, myocardial contractility, systemic vascular resistance, and venous tone. Retention of salt and water may increase circulating blood volume. The retention of salt and water is due to several factors, including decreased renal blood flow (in part because of increased activity in efferent sympathetic nerves), increased activity of the renin–angiotensin–aldosterone system, and increased secretion of antidiuretic hormone. Salt and water retention occurs despite increased secretion of atrial natriuretic peptide from the heart. The increase in venous pressure is due in part to the venoconstriction, in part to the increased intravascular volume, and in part to the increase in end-diastolic right ventricular pressure.

If severe congestive heart failure involves both the right and left ventricles, the following changes from normal usually will be found. Heart rate is elevated, end-diastolic ventricular pressures and volumes are increased, stroke volume is diminished, and end-systolic volume is increased. Cardiac output is decreased at rest and increases minimally with exertion. Systemic arterial pressure is usually maintained by a substantial increase in systemic vascular resistance, which is elevated by increased sympathetic activity and by increased production of angiotensin. The increase in afterload further depresses cardiac output, resulting in a vicious cycle. Venous beds may also be constricted. Because of the elevated diastolic left ventricular pressure, pulmonary capillary pressure is increased; if this capillary pressure exceeds a critical value, pulmonary edema develops. Because of edema and venous congestion, the lungs become stiffened and the work of breathing is increased; this results in dyspnea, orthopnea, and tachypnea. Because of the elevated right ventricular diastolic pressure, systemic venous pressure is increased and peripheral congestion, hepatomegaly, and edema result. Renal retention of salt and water increases blood volume and contributes to the formation of edema. Because of the decrease in cardiac output, perfusion of tissues is inadequate. Reduced blood flow to skeletal muscle causes fatigue; hepatic and renal blood flow may be decreased enough to reduce the clearance of some drugs, and cerebral perfusion may be impaired and result in confusion and other abnormalities of function of the CNS. The alterations in distribution of arterial flow, increased blood volume, and edema change the volume of distribution of many drugs quite markedly.

When digitalis is administered to patients with heart failure, its beneficial effects are primarily due to its direct positive inotropic action. A second important effect is the indirect action to decrease sinus rate. Because of the direct positive inotropic effect, the ventricles shift from one ventricular function curve to another (*see* Figure 34–5). They are thus able to develop more tension, empty more adequately, and eject more blood against the existing afterload. The increased stroke volume causes a decrease in end-systolic volume; since the ventricles contain less blood at the onset of diastole, end-diastolic pressure and volume both decrease if filling is constant. In spite of the decrease in fiber length, the ventricles can still do enough work to increase stroke volume because of the improved inotropic state. The decrease in heart size and the increase in output occur in spite of the decrease in heart rate. The direct positive inotropic effect thus increases cardiac output, decreases cardiac filling pressures, and decreases heart size and venous and capillary pressures. The decrease in ventricular volume increases the efficiency of contraction. Because of the improvement in the circulation, the activities of the neural and humoral vasoconstrictor mechanisms are reduced (Ferguson *et al.*, 1989); this, in turn, results in a decrease in systemic arterial resistance and venous tone. The former change decreases the afterload on the left ventricle and permits a further improvement in cardiac function.

Digitalization relieves edema by improving cardiac output and renal blood flow. The improved hemodynamic state that follows the administration of digitalis causes a reduction in activities of the neural and humoral systems that cause retention of salt and water. In addition, the decrease in sympathetic impulses to the kidney may also result from a direct effect of digitalis on afferent nerve fiber endings in the heart. Acetylstrophanthidin applied to the ventricular epicardium or injected into the coronary circulation of dogs causes an almost immediate decrease in sympathetic nerve activity in the kidneys (Thames, 1979). This action appears to be mediated through neural receptors in the heart with vagal afferent connections. This mechanism might account for a number of other responses to digitalis that are manifest before the positive inotropic action is fully developed.

Effects on the Coronary Circulation. Digitalis glycosides constrict coronary arteries, presumably by a direct action on their smooth muscle. This effect may not be prominent at therapeutic concentrations of the drugs. Studies in man show no significant change in coronary blood flow or cardiac oxygen consumption in normal subjects or in those with heart failure given strophanthus glycosides intravenously. If the heart is dilated because of failure, it is likely that digitalis will improve the relationship between coronary flow and the needs of the myocardium for perfusion. The larger the heart during diastole, the greater the wall tension required to produce a given intraventricular pressure during systole. If digitalis decreases heart size during diastole, it is likely that this effect will more than compensate for any increase in oxygen consumption and requirement for perfusion that may result from the direct inotropic effect. If digitalis causes a decrease in heart rate and a decrease in the duration of systole, both of these changes will augment coronary perfusion. In summary, if the heart is dilated in failure, it seems most likely that the therapeutic effect of digitalis will improve the relationship between coronary flow and myocardial demand for perfusion.

PHARMACOKINETIC PROPERTIES

A detailed consideration of the pharmacokinetic properties of cardiac glycosides will be restricted to digoxin and digitoxin; these are the two most widely used preparations and have been studied most thoroughly in relation to clinical use. Pharmacokinetic data are summarized in Table 34–1 (*see also* Appendix II).

Table 34–1. DOSAGES, TIME OF EFFECT, AND FATE OF DIGOXIN AND DIGITOXIN IN MAN *

	DIGOXIN	DIGITOXIN
Average digitalizing dose		
Oral	0.75–1.25 mg	0.8–1.2 mg
IV	0.5–1.0 mg	
Average daily maintenance dose		
Oral	0.125–0.5 mg	0.05–0.3 mg
IV	0.25 mg	
Onset of action		
Oral	1.5–6 hr †	3–6 hr
IV	5–30 min	
Maximal effect		
Oral	4–6 hr	6–12 hr
IV	1.5–4 hr	
Intestinal absorption	< 40–100% ‡ (75%)	90–100%
Plasma protein binding	25%	95%
Disposition half-time	1.6 days	7 days
Route of elimination	Renal excretion of unchanged drug; limited hepatic metabolism	Hepatic degradation of molecule; renal excretion of metabolites
Enterohepatic circulation	Small	Large
"Therapeutic" plasma concentration	0.5–2.0 ng/ml	10–35 ng/ml

* *See also* Appendix II.

† Dependent on relationship of dose to meals, gastric emptying time, and type of preparation.

‡ Nearly 100% of encapsulated digoxin solution is absorbed from a normal enteric tract; about 75% of a tablet with high bioavailability is absorbed by a normal enteric tract. Absorption may be poor with certain tablets or when there is gastrointestinal malabsorption.

Absorption. Absorption of digoxin after oral administration is somewhat variable; the fraction of the administered dose that is absorbed is related to the rate and extent of dissolution of various dosage forms and therefore depends strongly on the preparation used. Absorption is close to 100% with the encapsulated preparation in a hydroalcoholic vehicle. Variation in bioavailability with tablets has been recognized as a significant clinical problem (Lindenbaum *et al.*, 1971; New York Heart Association Task Force on Digitalis Preparations, 1974). Absorption of some preparations may be as low as 40%; with others the fraction reaches 75%. It is advisable for physicians to use a preparation with which they are familiar and to indicate the commercial source if the drug is prescribed by a nonproprietary name. Absorption of digoxin tablets can also be retarded by the presence of food in the gastrointestinal tract, by delayed gastric emptying, and by malabsorption syndromes. In approximately 10% of patients, a substantial fraction of ingested digoxin is converted (prior to absorption) to inactive products, such as dihydrodigoxin, by the intestinal microorganism *Eubacterium lentum* (Lindenbaum *et al.*, 1981). This can be avoided by using encapsulated digoxin solution, which is absorbed in the upper small intestine, or it can be reversed with antibiotics. Neomycin can decrease absorption of digoxin, as can steroid-binding resins.

After oral administration, the concentration of digoxin in plasma typically reaches a peak in 2 to 3 hours; the maximal effect is apparent in 4 to 6 hours (*see* Table 34–1). If a loading dose of digoxin is not given, up to 1 week can elapse before steady-state plasma concentrations are attained, since the half-life of the drug in the body is 1 to 2 days.

Absorption of digitoxin tablets is much more complete (90 to 100%) than is that of digoxin tablets because digitoxin is more lipid soluble. No significant problems with bioavailability have been noted for digitoxin, but its rate of absorption is also influenced by the factors mentioned above for digoxin. Because of its long half-life, steady-state concentrations in plasma are attained slowly and recovery from toxicity is protracted.

Distribution. The glycosides are distributed slowly in the body, in part due to their relatively large volume of distribution. As for other drugs, the presence of congestive heart failure can slow the rate at which steady-state distribution is attained. About 25% of digoxin in the plasma is bound to proteins; in contrast, most (95% or more) digitoxin is so bound. These differences in binding account in part for the differences in apparent volume of distribution of the glycosides and in the concentrations in plasma that are associated with therapeutic effects. Digitalis glycosides are distributed to most body tissues. At equilibrium, the concentrations in cardiac tissue are 15 to 30 times those in the plasma; the concentration in skeletal muscle is about half that in the heart. Binding to tissue is decreased by an increase in extracellular concentration of K^+, and the volume of distribution may be altered in some disease states. The time required to attain peak concentrations of digitalis glycosides in the heart and plasma is usually less than the time required for maximal effect; peak effect may not occur until 1 hour or more after levels in the heart reach their maximal value.

Elimination. Digoxin is eliminated primarily by the kidney. The drug is both filtered at the glomerulus and secreted by the tubules. There is some reabsorption from the tubular lumen, and this may become significant when the rate of flow of tubular fluid is markedly reduced. A rare patient seems to form antibodies to digoxin, and this prevents its therapeutic effect. Digitoxin is actively metabolized by hepatic microsomal enzymes; one of the products is digoxin. Metabolism of digitoxin may be accelerated by drugs that induce microsomal enzymes, including phenylbutazone, phenobarbital, phenytoin, and rifampin; the magnitude of this effect is variable among patients.

The half-time for elimination of digoxin, which averages 1.6 days, is strongly dependent on renal function; in most instances, there is a close correlation between the decrease in creatinine clearance and the concentration of digoxin in plasma that is attained with any given maintenance dose. Interventions that change renal perfusion, such as the administration of vasodilators, may cause significant change in the rate of elimination of digoxin. The half-time for elimination of digitoxin is nearly 7 days and is *not* appreciably changed by hepatic disease; this probably reflects the huge reserve capacity of the liver for metabolic degradation of this drug. Digitoxin undergoes enterohepatic circulation, but only a minor fraction of unchanged drug is eliminated through the intestine.

Dosage and Administration. Digitalis is used almost exclusively for two purposes—to restore an adequate circulation in patients with congestive heart failure and to slow ventricular rate in patients with atrial fibrillation or flutter. Since both conditions require long-term therapy, it is necessary to establish and maintain an adequate concentration of digitalis in the heart. If there is no urgent need for an immediate effect, a maintenance dose can be given daily by mouth and its effect evaluated after appropriate intervals. A maximal effect will be achieved in approximately four elimination half-lives. On the other hand, if it is desired to achieve a full therapeutic effect fairly rapidly, it is necessary to give a large initial dose because of the relatively long half-time for elimination (*see* Table 34–1).

By tradition, the initial loading dose is called the *digitalizing dose*. The size of this dose may be difficult to estimate. In theory, it is the steady-state total body store sufficient to cause the desired therapeutic effect. However, the estimate of the loading dose must be adjusted for the condition of the individual patient. Depending on the state of the heart and the cause of the cardiac abnormality, the "digitalizing" dose may be much less than the dose that is likely to cause toxicity or it may be almost equal to it.

In practice, the digitalizing dose is selected from prior estimates (*see* Table 34–1), with consideration of factors that increase or decrease the requirement for the individual patient (*see* below). If the need for a partial effect of digitalis is urgent, the initial dose is often given intravenously. If it is certain that the patient has *not* been taking digitalis, 1.0 mg of digoxin can be given intravenously over a period of 5 minutes or longer. Very often the loading dose is divided into two doses of 0.5 mg, given 3 to 4 hours apart. After the initial dose, a maintenance dose is administered daily that, after an appropriate interval, may be increased or decreased as indicated by the therapeutic response and the concentration of drug in plasma. Because digitalis causes serious toxic effects so frequently and because digitalis toxicity may be lethal, it always is essential to observe the patient carefully, and it is frequently necessary to adjust the maintenance dose to achieve an optimal effect.

The maintenance dose must be equal to the daily loss. For digoxin, this is approximately 35% of the total body store (in patients with normal renal function); for digitoxin, approximately 10%. Regardless of the size of the initial dose, after a sufficient time (four to five times the $t_{1/2}$) the concentration in plasma and the total body store will be determined solely by the maintenance dose. Whether or not the desired effect has been obtained can be evaluated by careful and frequent observation of the patient. In patients with atrial fibrillation, the dose can be adjusted to produce the desired decrease in ventricular rate at rest and during exertion. Evaluation of effects in patients with heart failure is more difficult and should include quantification of changes in the signs and symptoms of failure, such as measurement of changes in body weight, venous pressure, systolic time intervals, and exercise tolerance. The ECG and measurement of the concentration of cardiac glycoside in plasma may be helpful in adjusting the dosage.

Choice of Preparations and Routes of Administration. These decisions are made with consideration of the desired speed of onset of the therapeutic effect, the suitability of various routes of administration for the individual patient, the need for a stable concentration in plasma, and the likelihood of toxicity. Digoxin can be given intravenously or orally; after intravenous administration an appreciable effect is noted in 5 to 30 minutes and a maximal effect in 1.5 to 4 hours. Digoxin should not be given intramuscularly because it causes severe pain and muscle necrosis. After oral administration, an effect usually will be evident in 1 to 2 hours and the peak effect will occur in 4 to 6 hours. Because of its relatively short $t_{1/2}$, the steady-state concentration of digoxin in plasma can be changed reasonably rapidly. The disadvantage of the use of this drug is that the therapeutic effect may be greatly diminished or lost if the patient fails to take several doses. Its advantage is that toxic effects disappear relatively rapidly after the drug is discontinued. Digitoxin is not associated with problems of bioavailability. Absorption is virtually complete after oral administration, and, compared with digoxin, concentrations in plasma are better maintained, particularly if a patient's compliance is sporadic. Elimination of the parent drug is ordinarily independent of renal function, and at times this may be an important consideration. On the other hand, because of the long $t_{1/2}$ of digitoxin, it may take many days after discontinuation of therapy for a sufficient fraction of the total body store to be eliminated if there is toxicity. The major active glycoside in digitalis leaf is digitoxin. The preparation is standardized by bioassay. Variability in the potency of the preparation is likely, and there is no compelling reason to use it.

Preparations Available for Clinical Use. *Digitoxin* (CRYSTODIGIN) is the pure glycoside obtained from *Digitalis purpurea*. Digitoxin tablets are available for oral use, each tablet containing 0.1 or 0.2 mg of drug.

Digoxin (LANOXIN) is a glycoside obtained from the leaves of *Digitalis lanata*. It is available for both oral and intravenous administration. Digoxin tablets contain 0.125, 0.25, or 0.5 mg each. Digoxin solution in capsules (LANOXICAPS) contains either 0.05, 0.1, or 0.2 mg of digoxin in stable solution in each capsule. Bioavailability is close to 100%, which is 25% greater than for tablets; the capsules are intended to be equivalent to 0.0625, 0.125, and 0.25 mg in tablet form. Digoxin elixir contains 0.05 mg/ml. Digoxin injection contains 0.1 mg/ml or 0.25 mg/ml; the appropriate dose can be diluted with 10 ml of sterile 0.9% sodium chloride solution before injection. The solution should be administered slowly (5 minutes or longer), and care should be taken to avoid extravenous injection.

THERAPEUTIC USES

Heart Failure. The most important use of digitalis is to treat heart failure. Digitalis is useful regardless of whether the failure is predominantly of the left or right ventricle or involves both. With some exceptions, the type of rhythm exhibited by the decompensated heart neither indicates nor contraindicates the use of digitalis. Nevertheless, arrhythmias may modify the response to the drug.

Although the treatment of heart failure frequently includes the administration of digitalis, a cardiac glycoside is not the only modality that is utilized (Williams and Fisch, 1983). Traditionally, treatment of chronic mild failure has included limitation of physical activity, restriction of salt intake, and the use of a diuretic. If these measures were not sufficient, digitalis was typically added. Currently, systemic vasodilators (including inhibitors of angiotensin converting enzyme) are used for both acute and long-term treatment of congestive failure in conjunction with a diuretic, digitalis, or both (Packer *et al.*, 1983; Alicandri *et al.*, 1986; Gheorghiade *et al.*, 1989; *see also* Chapters 31 and 32). A reduction in cardiac work, brought about by a reduction in afterload, coupled with elimination of excess salt and water and a reduction in ventricular filling pressures (caused by diuretics and venodilators), often is sufficient to relieve symptoms of heart failure. Digitalis is thus not *essential* for treatment of all cases of failure. Moreover, since long-term administration of digitalis is associated with significant toxicity (*see* below), the drug should not be used unless it is clearly indicated. The role of digitalis in treating heart failure is undergoing reevaluation (Mulrow *et al.*, 1984; Poole-Wilson, 1984).

The use of vasodilators and diuretics without digitalis may not be effective for long-term treatment because of development of tolerance to the effects of the vasodilator and progression of the underlying disease. At the same time, if diuretics and vasodilators result in a satisfactory hemodynamic and clinical response, long-term treatment without digitalis is reasonable. The use of drugs that inhibit angiotensin converting enzyme is becoming the first choice in many instances. Furthermore, the combination of a converting enzyme inhibitor with digoxin seems to provide greater benefits than does either drug alone, at least in acute heart failure (Gheorghiade *et al.*, 1989). If failure is associated with atrial fibrillation (*see* below), digitalis is still the drug of choice, although other means to control ventricular rate are available (*see* Chapter 35).

Effectiveness. The effectiveness of digitalis in treating heart failure depends in part on the cause of the failure and in part on the severity of the cardiac damage. Failure can result from an increase in the requirement for blood flow, as in patients with anemia or left-to-right shunts; from an increase in the impedance to flow, as in patients with hypertension or valvular stenosis; or from a decrease in the capacity of the heart to do work, as in patients with coronary artery disease. In the first two cases, digitalis might exert a strong positive inotropic effect but still not restore the circulation to normal. In the third case, even with a maximal inotropic effect, the performance of the heart may be limited. Patients who show the best response to digitalis have a dilated heart, a low ejection fraction, and a protodiastolic (S_3) gallop sound on physical examination (Parmley, 1989). Digitalis is usually of limited value in failure associated with anemia, thyrotoxicosis, or severe thiamine deficiency. Poor response to digitalis is also to be expected in cases of active rheumatic and other forms of infectious or toxic myocarditis, and in advanced cardiomyopathy. When shock and congestive failure exist together, as they may after myocardial infarction, digitalis may be indicated for therapy of the failure, in conjunction with drugs that decrease afterload. In the final analysis, improvement of cardiac function by digitalis depends on the cardiac reserve. In badly damaged hearts digitalis cannot provide much benefit.

Since it seems that toxic effects of digitalis on the heart are more likely if the heart is severely damaged, it is important to estimate the degree of improvement in the circulation that can be expected from an optimal concentration of drug in plasma and to recognize the need to correct abnormalities that increase the work required of the heart. During maintenance therapy changes may occur in the condition of the patient that increase the concentration of digitalis in plasma or increase the sensitivity of the heart to its therapeutic or toxic effects (*see* below); usually it is desirable to use the lowest maintenance dose that provides the desired results.

Once digitalis has restored compensation, its continued use has traditionally been thought to prevent the recurrence of heart failure. Usually digitalis is given chronically to patients with diminished cardiac reserve who previously have experienced an episode of failure, even though they are subsequently free of symptoms (unless the cause of failure has been eliminated). However, digitalis has not been shown to prolong the lives of patients with heart failure.

There are two major clinical problems associated with the use of diuretics to treat congestive heart failure. Many diuretics decrease total body stores of K^+, and this increases the likelihood of digitalis toxicity (*see* below). Furthermore, potent diuretics can cause such a large decrease in circulating blood volume that end-diastolic ventricular pressure may decrease markedly. If the heart requires an elevated filling pressure to perform its external work, this may further reduce cardiac output (*see* Figure 34–5). A similar problem may result from the use of vasodilators that decrease preload excessively.

Use of Digitalis to Prevent Heart Failure. It is possible that digitalization can decrease the rate of progression of cardiac damage in patients in whom the requirement for cardiac work, in relation to the work capacity of the heart, is such that a progressive increase in end-diastolic pressure and volume will occur. This may be particularly important in patients with inadequate coronary flow in whom the increase in ventricular volume and wall tension will decrease perfusion but increase the need for such perfusion. In all patients, if an increase in heart rate is needed to compensate for a diminished stroke volume, the energy requirement of the heart will be increased. Finally, it seems likely that marked overdistention of the ventricles causes structural changes that subsequently are not fully reversed by digitalization.

Atrial Fibrillation. Even in the absence of congestive heart failure, digitalis may be indicated in many cases of atrial fibrillation (*see* below). The inappropriately rapid ventricular rate in this disorder results in palpitation that may cause great discomfort, and a reduction in cardiac work capacity that may lead to heart failure. The aim of digitalis therapy in patients with atrial fibrillation is to reduce the ventricular rate. The mechanism of ventricular slowing by digitalis has been discussed. Digitalis rarely halts atrial fibrillation, and the drug should not be employed with this objective. The dosage should be adjusted to maintain the ventricular rate in the range of 60 to 80 per minute at rest, and not to exceed 100 with moderate exercise. If digitalis fails to cause a sufficient decrease in ventricular rate, verapamil or a β-adrenergic blocking drug such as propranolol may also be used (*see* Chapter 35). Digitalis occasionally may be indicated as a prophylactic agent in patients in whom atrial fibrillation is likely.

Atrial Flutter. Digitalis can be used to manage atrial flutter. As with atrial fibrillation, the primary effect of the drug is to increase the ERP of the AV node. This almost always decreases the ventricular rate by increasing the degree of AV block. Furthermore, digitalis prevents sudden increases in ventricular rate when exercise, excitement, or other factors decrease vagal and enhance sympathetic effects on AV transmission. Digitalis can terminate atrial flutter. However, quite large doses are usually required, and cardioversion is preferable. Digitalis also may convert atrial flutter to fibrillation, and this, too, facilitates control of ventricular rate. Finally, if such conversion to fibrillation occurs, withdrawal of digitalis may result in the return of sinus rhythm. The change from flutter to fibrillation and the conversion to normal sinus rhythm probably result from digitalis-induced changes in vagal effects. The use of digitalis prior to attempts to convert atrial flutter to sinus rhythm with quinidine increases the risk of digitalis toxicity (*see* below and Chapter 35).

Paroxysmal Tachycardia. Atrial and AV nodal paroxysmal tachycardia are the most common tachyarrhythmias next to atrial fibrillation. Attacks are often abruptly terminated by measures that enhance vagal activity. Digitalis is often successful, probably by virtue of its vagal effects; intravenous administration of a rapidly acting preparation may be required. It should be remembered that paroxysmal supraventricular tachycardia with partial AV block may be a *result* of serious intoxication with digitalis. It is extremely important to be certain of the diagnosis and etiology of the tachyarrhythmia before using digitalis.

Effects in Patients with the Sick Sinus Syndrome (Sinoatrial Dysfunction). In dogs, digoxin slows conduction into and out of the sinus node, increases the sinus escape interval after overdrive, and increases the likelihood of sinus node reentry. In normal man, however, digoxin decreases corrected sinus node recovery times and does not decrease sinus rate (Reiffel *et al.*, 1979). These findings suggest that digoxin does not have an adverse effect on the function of the sinus node in patients with the sick sinus syndrome. On the other hand, there has been one report of severe toxicity in this condition (Margolis *et al.*, 1975). It would seem appropriate, if digitalization of such patients is required, to evaluate the effects of digitalis either by electrophysiological testing or by careful clinical monitoring.

Anomalous Atrioventricular Pathway. In patients with an anomalous AV pathway, digitalis should *not* be used to treat atrial fibrillation or flutter unless it has been proven that digitalis will not increase the ventricular rate by shortening the ERP of the accessory pathway.

DIGITALIS INTOXICATION

Withering recognized many of the signs of digitalis toxicity: "The foxglove when given in very large and quickly repeated doses, occasions sickness, vomiting, purging, giddiness, confused vision, objects appearing green or yellow; increased secretion of urine, with frequent motions to part with it; slow pulse, even as low as 35 in a minute, cold sweats, convulsions, syncope, death."

Toxic effects of digitalis are frequent and can be severe or lethal. The overall incidence of digitalis toxicity is not certain, but it has been estimated that approximately 25% of hospitalized patients taking digitalis show some signs of toxicity (Beller *et al.*, 1971; Smith, 1975). The single most frequent cause of intoxication with digitalis is the concurrent administration of diuretics that cause depletion of K^+. As might be expected from the mode of action of digitalis, the manifestations of toxicity are varied and can involve most organ systems in the body. The most important toxic effects, in terms of risk to the patient, are those that involve the heart. If unrecognized or improperly treated, such reactions frequently are fatal.

Digitalis is one of the most commonly prescribed drugs, and the number of patients for whom it is prescribed may increase as the proportion of older individuals in the population increases. Furthermore, digoxin and digitoxin have comparably low margins of safety and can cause similarly severe toxic reactions. The only difference between them is the duration of toxicity; digoxin is more rapidly eliminated, and the duration of toxicity is thus comparatively short.

Toxic Effects on the Heart. Concentrations of digitalis in blood that are associated with toxicity typically cause abnormalities of cardiac rhythm and disturbances of AV conduction, including complete AV block. Ordinarily, abnormalities of conduction in the ventricular specialized conducting system and in the ventricles are not seen and, thus, digitalis does not directly prolong the QRS complex. Very high concentrations of the drug may impair conduction in the atria and prolong the P wave.

It is important to realize that all disturbances of rhythm associated with high concentrations of digitalis in plasma or tissues are not necessarily manifestations of digitalis toxicity and that low concentrations of the drug in plasma do not preclude the possibility of drug-induced arrhythmias or other toxicity. The concentrations measured in plasma serve only as crude, although useful, guides to the likelihood of efficacy and toxicity. Digitalis is used to treat patients with diseased hearts, and such hearts are likely to develop arrhythmias and conduction abnormalities. For example, an increase in the severity of heart failure is often itself a cause of atrial or ventricular arrhythmias. The demonstration that digitalis is the cause of such an arrhythmia or conduction abnormality primarily depends on noting the response when administration of the drug is stopped (Smith, 1975).

Although digitalis toxicity can mimic almost any arrhythmia or conduction disturbance, certain abnormalities are of special importance (Bigger, 1972; Bigger and Strauss, 1972). Digitalis can cause marked sinus bradycardia and can also bring about complete SA block. Both abnormalities probably result from a combination of enhanced vagal effects, a decreased sympathetic influence, and the direct effects of the drug. The likelihood is greater in patients with disease involving the sinus node. Toxicity can also be manifested as disturbances of atrial rhythm, including premature depolarizations and paroxysmal and nonparoxysmal supraventricular tachycardias. These arrhythmias are most likely caused by delayed afterdepolarizations or by reentrant excitation owing to depressed conduction in the AV and SA nodes, but enhancement of automaticity by digitalis is also a possible mechanism. Sufficiently precise tests are not yet available to identify each mechanism in patients.

The effects of digitalis on the AV junction are important in relation to both its therapeutic and toxic effects. Toxicity is manifested by high levels of AV block and by the appearance of accelerated AV junctional rhythms; the most typical disturbances appear as either escape beats or as a nonparoxysmal AV junctional tachycardia. This arrhythmia is almost always due to digitalis but occasionally can be caused by acute inferior myocardial infarction or acute myocarditis. The development of AV block is due in part to the vagal effects of digitalis and sometimes can be overcome by atropine; at other times the depression of AV conduction almost certainly results from the direct effect of digitalis on the AV node, perhaps intensified by its antiadrenergic action.

The accelerated rhythms originating in the AV junction were assumed to result from enhanced phase-4 depolarization, but more recent studies support delayed afterdepolarizations as a cause of some types of escape beats (Rosen *et al.*, 1980). An AV junctional tachycardia caused by toxic levels of digitalis may be quite difficult to recognize in patients with atrial fibrillation.

The disturbances of ventricular rhythm most frequently caused by digitalis are premature depolarizations that appear as coupled beats (bigeminy, trigeminy); these arrhythmias are not specific for digitalis. Digitalis toxicity also can cause ventricular tachycardia and ventricular fibrillation. The premature depolarizations usually are not caused by increased automaticity; some very likely are due to reentry and some to delayed afterdepolarizations. Persistent ventricular tachycardia probably results from increased automaticity of Purkinje fibers.

As mentioned above, digitalis decreases the ERP of human ventricular muscle but not that of the His-Purkinje system; it thus increases the interval during which reentrant excitation can be elicited (Gomes *et al.*, 1978). In addition, it has been shown in experiments with dogs that certain disturbances of rhythm caused by digitalis respond to alterations in the dominant heart rate and rhythm in a manner that suggests they are due to delayed afterdepolarizations (Wittenberg *et al.*, 1972). This finding makes it difficult to identify the mechanisms responsible for ventricular arrhythmias caused by digitalis. Sometimes, when digitalis causes a ventricular tachycardia, the polarity of the major QRS deflection in the ECG reverses for alternate complexes. This so-called *bidirectional tachycardia* was once thought to be a certain indication of excessive digitalis; however, the same ECG abnormality can be caused by other factors. The alternation in QRS polarity probably results from alternate excitation of the ventricles over one and then the other bundle branch.

Two further points about cardiac toxicity are of particular importance. First, the likelihood and probably also the severity of the arrhythmia are directly related to the severity of the underlying heart disease. If subjects with normal hearts ingest large but not lethal quantities of digitalis, either in an attempt at suicide or by accident, premature impulses and rapid arrhythmias are infrequent. The only typical findings are sinus bradycardia and AV block. These disturbances probably result in large part from the marked increase in the concentration of K^+ in plasma that is caused by severe, acute intoxication with digitalis. Second, infants and children seem to tolerate higher concentrations of digitalis in their plasma and myocardium than do adults. Studies on preparations isolated from canine hearts indicate that this results, at least in part, from real differences in sensitivity of the young specialized fibers to toxic effects of digitalis (Rosen *et al.*, 1975). Also, the volume of distribution and the half-time for elimination of digitalis may be age dependent (Glantz *et al.*, 1976; Berman *et al.*, 1977).

Other Untoward Effects. *Gastrointestinal Effects.* Anorexia is very common with digoxin, and this symptom is easily missed in the elderly or depressed patient. Vomiting may occasionally develop without preliminary anorexia or nausea. Nausea and vomiting may be transitory or entirely absent in some patients. Diarrhea may also be noted, and in rare cases it is the only gastrointestinal manifestation of digitalis toxicity. Abdominal discomfort or pain often accompanies the gastrointestinal symptoms. Once the drug is stopped, gastrointestinal symptoms disappear in a few days. The nausea and vomiting are primarily due to a direct action of digitalis to excite the chemoreceptor trigger zone (CTZ) in the area postrema of the medulla rather than to a direct irritant effect on the gastrointestinal tract.

Neurological Effects. Headache, fatigue, malaise, and drowsiness are common symptoms and can occur early in the course of digitalis intoxication; generalized muscle weakness and easy fatigability may be particularly prominent. Neuralgic pain, usually involving the lower third of the face and simulating trigeminal neuralgia, may be the earliest, most severe, and even the sole manifestation of digitalis intoxication; the extremities and lumbar area may also be involved, and paresthesias often accompany the pain. Mental symptoms include disorientation, confusion, aphasia, and even delirium and hallucinations ("digitalis delirium"); rarely, convulsions have occurred. Neuropsychiatric effects are especially likely to develop in elderly patients with atherosclerotic disease. The exact role played by digitalis is uncertain.

Vision. Vision is often blurred. White borders or halos may appear on dark objects ("white vision"), and objects may appear frosted. Color vision can be disturbed; chromatopsia is most common for yellow and green, but less frequently red, brown, and blue vision can occur. Transitory amblyopia, diplopia, and scotomata may also ensue. It has been reported that digitalis can affect the papillomacular fibers of the optic nerve and cause retrobulbar neuritis. In an epidemic of accidental digitoxin intoxication, 95% of 179 patients complained of visual disturbances; 95% complained of extreme fatigue and weakness. ECG signs considered characteristic of digitalis poisoning were observed in 70% of the subjects (Lely and van Enter, 1970).

Other Effects. Gynecomastia may be induced in men by digitalis therapy; it has been suggested that the drug, on the basis of its chemical similarity to the sex hormones, may exert estrogenic activity in certain cases.

Factors Influencing the Likelihood of Toxicity. The most obvious cause of digitalis toxicity is the ingestion of too large a maintenance dose. The most frequent cause is concurrent administration of a diuretic that decreases body stores of K^+. Overdosage may result from the physician's decision, from the patient independently increasing the dose, or from improved absorption of the drug. The last-named cause might result from a change to a formulation with greater bioavailability or the administration of an antibiotic to a patient whose intestinal bacteria metabolize and inactivate digoxin. A decreased rate of elimination also could increase the concentration of drug in plasma to the toxic range. For digoxin, this can result from a decrease in renal function. Even quite marked abnormalities of hepatic function do not significantly decrease the metabolism of digitoxin. However, since one metabolite of digitoxin is digoxin, changes in renal elimination of the latter might contribute to toxicity when a patient is taking digitoxin.

Many factors are important in modifying the sensitivity of the heart to digitalis. A decrease in the plasma concentration of K^+ is perhaps the most important cause of toxicity because many patients with congestive heart failure receive diuretics. Dialysis also can result in depletion of K^+. An abnormally high concentration of Ca^{2+} in plasma can also contribute to toxicity. This could result from prolonged bed rest, myeloma, or parathyroid disease. A low concentration of Mg^{2+} in plasma has effects similar to those of high Ca^{2+}. This change might result from diuretic therapy or dialysis. Hypothyroidism increases the likelihood of toxicity because elimination of digitalis is depressed and because in this condition the heart is more sensitive to cardiac glycosides. Conversely, hyperthyroid patients may require larger doses of digitalis to achieve a therapeutic effect. If hyperkalemia occurs in a patient taking maintenance doses of digitalis, complete AV block may result. Increased activity of the sympathetic nervous system and a number of pharmacological agents can increase the likelihood of arrhythmias due to digitalis intoxication; the latter are discussed in a subsequent section.

It is important to remember that almost any worsening of the condition of the heart or circulation may increase the sensitivity of the heart to toxic actions of digitalis. Cardiac ischemia has this effect, as does an increase in the severity of congestive heart failure. Severe impairment of ventilation or circulation will cause hypoxia and acidosis. The latter certainly contributes to toxicity, since a decrease in pH, like an increase in $[Ca^{2+}]_o$, depresses the Na^+,K^+ pump in cardiac tissues. With severe circulatory impairment, renal perfusion may be depressed. In addition, there likely will be an increase in heart rate in spite of the action of digitalis. The increase in rate can intensify the effects of digitalis by increasing the requirement for the pump to transport cations. Finally, with severe heart failure there may be either an increase in sympathetic activity or additional depletion of cardiac stores of norepinephrine. Both changes might contribute to toxicity.

Advanced age almost always decreases the required maintenance dose of digitalis, and, as suggested above, infants and children often require larger doses than would be estimated from body size. In contrast, premature infants may be unusually sensitive to digitalis. During the first 24 to 48 hours after the onset of myocardial infarction there may be an increased likelihood of toxic effects on rhythm and conduction.

Diagnosis of Digitalis Intoxication. Digitalis is often used in situations in which the toxic effects of the drug are difficult to distinguish from the effects of cardiac disease. The diagnostic problem arises most frequently with the hospital admission of a patient with serious arrhythmia and congestive failure from whom a history of recent digitalis therapy cannot be elicited. Administration of a loading dose of a cardiac glycoside to such a patient obviously could be lethal if the arrhythmia were caused by digitalis. Means to diagnose latent or overt toxicity have been suggested but not widely adopted. Introduction of a single electrical stimulus to the ventricles after the end of the T wave causes repetitive ventricular responses in patients who are marginally toxic (Lown *et al.*, 1967). The intravenous administration of edrophonium will cause AV block and the appearance of ventricular premature depolarizations in patients on the verge of overt toxicity. However, these tests are not without risk.

The concentration of digitalis glycosides in plasma can be measured with specific immunoassays, and this will show whether digitalis has been taken and, if it has, whether the concentration is in a therapeutic or toxic range. However, these ranges overlap. Careful and judicious clinical appraisal is still the most important diagnostic tool (Smith, 1975).

Treatment of Digitalis Intoxication. The treatment of digitalis toxicity is almost always successful if appropriate means are used (Bigger and Strauss, 1972; Smith and Haber, 1973; Smith, 1975; Williams and Fisch, 1983). Thus, it is vitally important to make the correct diagnosis. The patient should be admitted to an intensive care unit and the ECG should be monitored. No additional digitalis should be given. Diuretics that cause depletion of K^+ should be withheld. If severe arrhythmias are present, additional treatment is needed. Phenytoin, lidocaine, and potassium salts are the most effective agents. Administration of K^+, either orally or intravenously, decreases the binding of digitalis to the heart and directly antagonizes certain cardiotoxic effects of the glycoside. If intravenous infusions are utilized, the ECG must be monitored frequently. It is essential to measure the concentration of K^+ in plasma before and during the administration of K^+. If this value is low or normal, an increase will usually suppress many ectopic beats and abnormal rhythms caused by digitalis and improve depressed AV conduction. In contrast, if the initial concentration of K^+ in plasma is high (for example, in patients with renal failure or patients who have taken a massive overdose of digoxin), a further increase will *intensify* AV block and depress the automaticity of ventricular pacemakers. The result may be complete AV block and cardiac arrest. K^+ is contraindicated if AV block is severe.

Among the antiarrhythmic drugs, phenytoin and lidocaine are quite effective in suppressing ventricular arrhythmias caused by digitalis (*see* Chapter 35). Other antiarrhythmic drugs (quinidine, procainamide, propranolol) are effective at times but are associated with a higher probability of producing new arrhythmias and AV block. In addition, quinidine can increase the concentration of digitalis in plasma (*see* below). Atropine will sometimes diminish sinus bradycardia, SA arrest, and second- or third-degree AV block. The use of electrical countershock to treat arrhythmias in digitalized patients is hazardous, because it may cause severe conduction abnormalities and ventricular arrhythmias. If it must be used, the energy of the shock should be as low as possible.

When toxicity is life-threatening, it can be reversed with antibodies to the glycoside

(Smith *et al.*, 1982). Very high doses of digitalis cause inhibition of Na^+,K^+-ATPase in cells throughout the body sufficient to produce a progressive increase in the plasma concentration of K^+ that is uniformly lethal. This can be reversed by the timely administration of Fab fragments of digoxin-specific antibody (DIGIBIND). These fragments bind both digoxin and digitoxin effectively and decrease the concentration of free drug available to interact with the heart cell membrane. The total concentration of glycoside in plasma rises markedly because of binding to the antibody, but the fraction of drug in the plasma that is free is reduced to extremely low levels. The Fab-digitalis complex is eliminated readily in the urine.

Drug Interactions. The administration of quinidine results in an increase in the plasma concentration of the glycoside in over 90% of digitalized patients (*see* Bigger, 1982). The degree of change is proportional to the dose of quinidine; the average change is about twofold. The concentration of digoxin starts to rise within 24 hours after initiation of quinidine and reaches a new steady state in about 4 days. The initial effect of quinidine is due, in part, to the displacement of digoxin from binding sites in tissues, but the increased steady-state concentration is due to a reduction in renal clearance by 40 to 50%. When digoxin and quinidine are administered concurrently, the effects of the cardiac glycoside on the sinus and AV nodes are intensified, but effects on Na^+,K^+-ATPase activity in the ventricle are not. The digitalized patient who receives quinidine should be followed closely for signs of toxicity and changes in the ECG, and the concentration of digoxin in plasma should be monitored to make an appropriate adjustment of dosage. The use of antiarrhythmic drugs in conjunction with digitalis is discussed further in Chapter 35. In addition to quinidine, concentrations of digoxin in plasma are also increased by quinine, verapamil, propafenone, diltiazem, and amiodarone.

Interactions between cardiac glycosides and diuretics have been discussed above. Amphotericin B, which can also cause hypokalemia, may similarly provoke manifestations of digitalis intoxication. Administration of β-adrenergic agonists or succinylcholine may increase the likelihood of arrhythmias in digitalized patients. Several other drugs, including nifedipine, spironolactone, amiloride, and triamterene, have been reported to decrease renal clearance of digoxin. Phenylbutazone, phenobarbital, phenytoin, rifampin, and other drugs that increase hepatic microsomal enzyme activity may speed the metabolism of digitoxin. For other drug interactions, *see* the Index.

OTHER POSITIVE INOTROPIC AGENTS

Several drugs that exert a positive inotropic effect but that do not inhibit the sarcolemmal Na^+,K^+-ATPase have been evaluated as substitutes for digitalis in the treatment of heart failure. These agents can be grouped in classes based on their major mechanism of action. Most require further evaluation at both the basic and clinical levels, and most have not been approved for use in patients. The positive inotropic actions of the methylxanthines (*see* Chapter 25) and glucagon (*see* Chapter 61) are well known. The synthetic catecholamine dobutamine (*see* Chapter 10) increases the force of myocardial contraction at concentrations that cause only modest changes in sinus rate and peripheral vascular resistance. When administered acutely, dobutamine increases cardiac output and decreases systemic vascular resistance in patients with moderately severe heart failure (Colucci *et al.*, 1986). The dihydropyridine analog Bay K 8644 causes a strong positive inotropic effect; it interacts with *L*-type Ca^{2+} channels to augment i_{Ca}. However, it also causes peripheral vasoconstriction. A fairly large number of inhibitors of a phosphodiesterase that specifically hydrolyze adenosine 3′,5′-monophosphate (cyclic AMP) are undergoing clinical evaluation or have been released for general clinical use. These include enoximone, piroximone, and the bypyridines amrinone and milrinone.

AMRINONE AND MILRINONE

These two bipyridine derivatives have shown some promise for both acute and long-term treatment of heart failure (Farah *et al.*, 1984; Colucci *et al.*, 1986; Le Jemtel *et al.*, 1986; Erhardt, 1987). They have the following structural formulas:

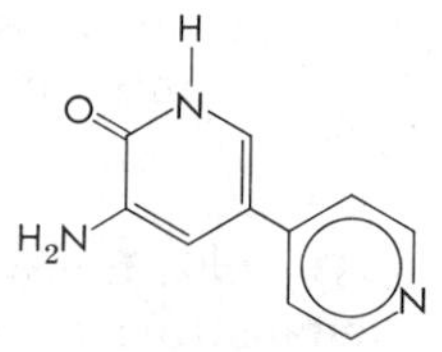

Amrinone

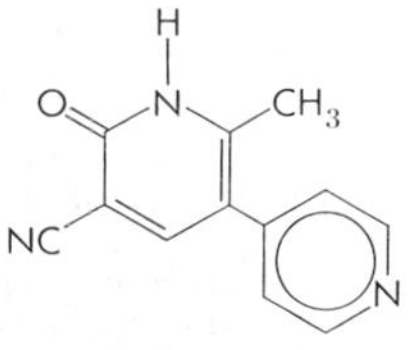

Milrinone

Both agents increase force of contraction and rate of shortening of cardiac muscle *in vitro;* milrinone is considerably more potent. Amrinone has no effects on transmembrane potentials of canine Purkinje fibers, but it augments slow responses. It is unlikely to cause afterdepolarizations but increases those caused by digitalis. The positive inotropy is not prevented by α- or β-adrenergic blockade or by depletion of catecholamines, and it is not associated with inhibition of the sarcolemmal Na^+,K^+-ATPase. Inotropic effects are additive to those of digitalis. Amrinone also relaxes vascular and tracheal smooth muscle. Both agents increase contractility of the normal canine heart *in situ* and cause a dose-dependent increase in heart rate and decrease in systemic vascular resistance.

Amrinone has been evaluated in a number of patients with severe heart failure. When given to digitalized subjects in heart failure, amrinone rapidly increases cardiac index and stroke work index; decreases left ventricular end-diastolic pressure, wedge pressure, and systemic vascular resistance; and causes only minor changes in sinus rate and systemic arterial pressure. Exercise performance is increased. The utility of amrinone for the long-term treatment of heart failure has not been demonstrated conclusively. On withdrawal of the drug, symptoms of failure reappear promptly. Toxicity includes gastrointestinal intolerance, hepatotoxicity, fever, and reversible thrombocytopenia in 20% of patients.

Amrinone is approved for use in the United States for the short-term management of congestive heart failure, and it is indicated for treatment of patients who have not responded adequately to digitalis, diuretics, or vasodilators. It is supplied as *amrinone lactate injection* (INOCOR) for intravenous administration. Therapy is initiated with a dose of 0.75 mg/kg given over 2 to 3 minutes, followed by a maintenance infusion of 5 to 10 μg/kg per minute. The recommended maximal daily dose is 10 mg/kg. The normal half-time for elimination of amrinone is 3 to 4 hours, but this value is increased to about 6 hours in patients with heart failure. The drug is excreted in the urine both as metabolites and the parent compound. Fluid balance, electrolyte concentrations, and renal function should be monitored carefully during treatment, and measurements of central venous pressure may also be useful.

Milrinone (COROTROPE) is not yet available for general use in the United States, but its marketing is anticipated. During short trials in a limited number of patients, milrinone has also been shown to be effective in the treatment of severe heart failure by increasing cardiac contractility and decreasing systemic vascular resistance (Maskin *et al.*, 1983). Its actions are like those of amrinone, and it does not seem to cause thrombocytopenia. However, in a recent study of patients with moderately severe cardiac failure, milrinone was less effective and was more arrhythmogenic than digoxin. Moreover, the combination of milrinone and digoxin was no more effective than digoxin alone (DiBianco *et al.*, 1989).

Akera, T.; Larsen, F. S.; and Brody, T. M. Correlation of cardiac sodium- and potassium-activated adenosine triphosphatase activity with ouabain-induced inotropic stimulation. *J. Pharmacol. Exp. Ther.*, **1970**, *173*, 145–151.

Alicandri, C.; Fariello, R.; Boni, E.; Zaninelli, A.; and Muiesen, G. Comparison of captopril and digoxin in mild to moderate heart failure. *Postgrad. Med. J.*, **1986**, *62*, 170–175.

Beeler, G. W., and Reuter, H. The relationship between membrane potential, membrane currents and activation of contraction in ventricular myocardial fibers. *J. Physiol. (Lond.)*, **1970**, *207*, 211–229.

Beller, G. A.; Smith, T. W.; Abelman, W. H.; Haber, E.; and Hood, W. B., Jr. Digitalis intoxication. A prospective clinical study with serum level correlations. *N. Engl. J. Med.*, **1971**, *284*, 989–997.

Berman, W., Jr.; Ravenscroft, P. J.; Sheiner, L. B.; Hayman, M. A.; Melmon, K. L.; and Rudolph, A. M. Differential effects of digoxin at comparable concentrations in tissues of fetal and adult sheep. *Circ. Res.*, **1977**, *41*, 635–642.

Bigger, J. T., Jr., and Strauss, H. C. Digitalis toxicity: drug interactions promoting toxicity and the management of toxicity. *Semin. Drug Treat.*, **1972**, *2*, 147–177.

Chai, C. Y.; Wang, H. H.; Hoffman, B. F.; and Wang, S. C. Mechanisms of bradycardia induced by digitalis substances. *Am. J. Physiol.*, **1967**, *212*, 26–34.

Deitmer, J. W., and Ellis, D. The intracellular sodium activity of cardiac Purkinje fibers during inhibition and reactivation of the Na-K pump. *J. Physiol. (Lond.)*, **1978**, *284*, 241–259.

DeMello, W. C. Effect of intracellular injection of calcium and strontium on cell communication in heart. *J. Physiol. (Lond.)*, **1975**, *250*, 231–245.

Dhingra, R. C.; Amat-y-Leon, F.; Wyndham, C.; Wu, D.; Denes, P.; and Rosen, K. The electrophysiological effects of ouabain on sinus node and atrium in man. *J. Clin. Invest.*, **1975**, *56*, 555–562.

DiBianco, R.; Shabetai, R.; Kostuk, W.; Moran, J.; Schlant, R. C.; and Wright, R. for the Milrinone Multicenter Trial Group. A comparison of oral milrinone, digoxin, and their combination in the treatment of patients with chronic heart failure. *N. Engl. J. Med.*, **1989**, *320*, 677–683.

DiFrancesco, D. A new interpretation of the pace-maker current in calf Purkinje fibres. *J. Physiol. (Lond.)*, **1981**, *314*, 359–376.

Eisner, D. A., and Lederer, W. J. Na-Ca exchange: stoichiometry and electrogenicity. *Am. J. Physiol.*, **1985**, *248*, C189–C202.

Eisner, D. A.; Lederer, W. J.; and Vaughan-Jones, R. D. The control of tonic tension by membrane potential and intracellular sodium activity in the sheep cardiac Purkinje fibre. *J. Physiol. (Lond.)*, **1983**, *335*, 723–743.

Erlij, D., and Mendez, R. The modification of digitalis intoxication by excluding adrenergic influences on the heart. *J. Pharmacol. Exp. Ther.*, **1964**, *144*, 97–103.

Fabiato, A., and Fabiato, F. Calcium release from the sarcoplasmic reticulum. *Circ. Res.*, **1977**, *40*, 119–129.

Farah, A. E.; Alousi, A. A.; and Schwarz, R. P., Jr. Positive inotropic agents. *Annu. Rev. Pharmacol. Toxicol.*, **1984**, *24*, 275–328.

Ferguson, D. W.; Berg, W. J.; Sanders, J. S.; Roach, P. J.; Kempf, J. S.; and Kienzle, M. G. Sympathoinhibitory responses to digitalis glycosides in heart failure patients. Direct evidence from sympathetic neural recordings. *Circulation*, **1989**, *80*, 65–77.

Ferrier, G. R. Effects of tension on acetylstrophanthidin-induced transient depolarizations and after-contractions in canine myocardial and Purkinje tissues. *Circ. Res.*, **1976**, *38*, 156–161.

Gheorghiade, M.; Hall, V.; Lakier, J. B.; and Goldstein, S. Comparative hemodynamic and neurohormonal effects of intravenous captopril and digoxin and their combinations in patients with severe heart failure. *J. Am. Coll. Cardiol.*, **1989**, *13*, 134–142.

Glantz, J. A.; Kernoff, R.; and Goldman, R. H. Age-related changes in ouabain pharmacology: ouabain exhibits a different volume of distribution in adult and young dogs. *Circ. Res.*, **1976**, *39*, 407–414.

Gold, H., and Cattell, M. Mechanism of digitalis action in abolishing heart failure. *Arch. Intern. Med.*, **1940**, *65*, 263–278.

Gomes, J. A. C.; Dhatt, M. S.; Akhtar, M.; Carambas, C. R.; Rubenson, D. S.; and Damato, A. Effects of digitalis on ventricular myocardial and His-Purkinje refractoriness and reentry in man. *Am. J. Cardiol.*, **1978**, *42*, 931–939.

Goodman, D. J.; Rossen, R. M.; Cannom, D. S.; Rider, A. K.; and Harrison, D. C. Effects of digoxin on atrioventricular conduction. Studies in patients with and without cardiac autonomic innervation. *Circulation*, **1975**, *51*, 251–256.

Hess, P., and Müller, P. Extracellular versus intracellular digoxin action on bovine myocardium, using a digoxin antibody and intracellular glycoside application. *J. Physiol. (Lond.)*, **1982**, *322*, 197–210.

Hordof, A. J.; Spotnitz, A.; Mary-Rabine, L.; Edie, R. N.; and Rosen, M. R. The cellular electrophysiologic effects of digitalis on human atrial fibers. *Circulation*, **1978**, *57*, 223–229.

Horwitz, L. D.; Atkins, J. M.; and Saito, M. Effects of digitalis on left ventricular function in exercising dogs. *Circ. Res.*, **1977**, *41*, 744–749.

Hougen, T. J., and Smith, T. W. Inhibition of myocardial cation active transport by subtoxic doses of ouabain in the dog. *Circ. Res.*, **1978**, *42*, 856–863.

Kassebaum, D. G. Electrophysiological effects of strophanthin in the heart. *J. Pharmacol. Exp. Ther.*, **1963**, *140*, 329–338.

Kim, D.; Cragoe, E. J., Jr.; and Smith, T. W. Relations among sodium pump inhibition, Na-Ca and Na-H exchange activities, and Ca-H interaction in cultured chick heart cells. *Circ. Res.*, **1987**, *60*, 185–193.

Lederer, W. J., and Eisner, D. A. The effects of sodium pump activity on the slow inward current in sheep cardiac Purkinje fibres. *Proc. R. Soc. Lond. [Biol.]*, **1982**, *214*, 249–262.

Lee, C. O., and Dagostino, M. Effect of strophanthidin on intracellular Na ion activity and twitch tension of constantly driven canine cardiac Purkinje fibers. *Biophys. J.*, **1982**, *40*, 185–198.

Le Jemtel, T. H.; Karan, G.; Reis, D.; and Sonnenblick, E. H. The role of novel inotropic agents in the treatment of heart failure. *J. Cardiovasc. Pharmacol.*, **1986**, *8*, Suppl. A, 547–554.

Lely, A. H., and van Enter, C. H. J. Large scale digitoxin intoxication. *Br. Med. J.*, **1970**, *3*, 737–740.

Lindenbaum, J.; Mellow, M. H.; Blackstone, M. O.; and Butler, V. P., Jr. Variability in biological availability of digoxin from four preparations. *N. Engl. J. Med.*, **1971**, *285*, 1344–1347.

Lindenbaum, J.; Rund, D. G.; Butler, V. P.; Tse-Eng, D.; and Saha, J. R. Inactivation of digoxin by the gut flora: reversal by antibiotic therapy. *N. Engl. J. Med.*, **1981**, *305*, 789–794.

Lown, B.; Cannon, R. L.; and Rossi, M. A. Electrical stimulation and digitalis drugs: repetitive response in diastole. *Proc. Soc. Exp. Biol. Med.*, **1967**, *126*, 698–701.

McRitchie, R. J., and Vatner, S. F. The role of the arterial baroceptors in mediating cardiovascular responses to cardiac glycosides in conscious dogs. *Circ. Res.*, **1976**, *38*, 321–326.

Marban, E., and Tsien, R. W. Enhancement of calcium current during digitalis inotropy in mammalian heart: positive feed-back regulation by intracellular calcium? *J. Physiol. (Lond.)*, **1982**, *329*, 589–614.

Margolis, J. R.; Strauss, H. C.; Miller, H. C.; Gilbert, M.; and Wallace, A. G. Digitalis and the sick sinus syndrome: clinical and electrophysiologic documentation of a severe toxic effect on sinus node function. *Circulation*, **1975**, *52*, 162–169.

Maskin, C. S.; Sinoway, L.; Chadwick, B.; Sonnenblick, E. H.; and LeJemtel, T. H. Sustained hemodynamic and clinical effects of a new cardiotonic agent, WIN 47203, in patients with severe congestive heart failure. *Circulation*, **1983**, *67*, 1065–1070.

Mason, D. T. Regulation of cardiac performance in clinical heart disease: interactions between contractile state mechanical abnormalities and ventricular compensatory mechanisms. *Am. J. Cardiol.*, **1973**, *32*, 437–448.

Mudge, G. H.; Lloyd, B. L.; Greenblatt, D. J.; and Smith, T. W. Inotropic and toxic effects of a polar cardiac glycoside derivative in the dog. *Circ. Res.*, **1978**, *43*, 847–854.

Mulrow, C. D.; Feussner, J. R.; and Velez, R. Reevaluation of digitalis efficacy: new light on an old lead. *Ann. Intern. Med.*, **1984**, *101*, 113–117.

New York Heart Association Task Force on Digitalis Preparations. What should the practicing physician know about digoxin bioavailability and how will FDA action affect him? *Circulation*, **1974**, *49*, 399–400.

Packer, M.; Medina, N.; Yushak, M.; and Meller, J. Hemodynamic patterns of response during long-term captopril therapy for severe chronic heart failure. *Circulation*, **1983**, *68*, 803–812.

Poole-Wilson, P. A. The role of digitalis in the future. *Br. J. Clin. Pharmacol.*, **1984**, *18*, 1513–1565.

Reiffel, J. A.; Bigger, J. T., Jr.; and Cramer, M. The effects of digoxin on sinus nodal function before and after vagal blockade in patients with sinus nodal dysfunction: a clue to the mechanisms of the action of digitalis on the sinus node. *Am. J. Cardiol.*, **1979**, *43*, 983–989.

Rosen, M. R.; Fisch, C.; Hoffman, B. F.; Danilo, P.; Lovelace, D. E.; and Knoebel, S. B. Can accelerated atrioventricular junctional escape rhythms be explained by delayed afterdepolarizations? *Am. J. Cardiol.*, **1980**, *45*, 1272–1284.

Rosen, M. R.; Hordof, A. J.; Hodess, A. B.; Verosky, M.; and Vulliemoz, Y. Ouabain-induced changes in electrophysiologic properties of neonatal, young and adult canine cardiac Purkinje fibers. *J. Pharmacol. Exp. Ther.*, **1975**, *194*, 255–263.

Saum, R. W.; Brown, A. M.; and Tuley, F. H. An electrogenic sodium pump and baroceptor function in normotensive and spontaneously hypertensive rats. *Circ. Res.*, **1976**, *39*, 497–505.

Schwartz, A. Is the cell membrane Na^{+},K^{+}-ATPase enzyme system the pharmacological receptor for digitalis? *Circ. Res.*, **1976**, *39*, 2–7.

Sellers, T. D., Jr.; Bashore, T. M.; and Gallagher, J. J. Digitalis in the preexcitation syndrome: analysis during atrial fibrillation. *Circulation*, **1977**, *56*, 260–270.

Smith, T. W. Digitalis toxicity: epidemiology and clinical use of serum concentration measurements. *Am. J. Med.*, **1975**, *58*, 470–476.

Smith, T. W.; Butler, V. P., Jr.; Haber, E.; Fozzard, H.; Marcus, F. I.; Bremner, F.; Schulman, I. C.; and Phillips, A. Treatment of life-threatening digitalis intoxication with digoxin-specific Fab antibody fragments. *N. Engl. J. Med.*, **1982**, *307*, 1357–1362.

Smith, T. W., and Haber, E. Digitalis. *N. Engl. J. Med.*, **1973**, *289*, 945–952, 1010–1015, 1063–1072, 1125–1129.

Ten Eick, R. E., and Hoffman, B. F. The effect of digitalis on the excitability of autonomic nerves. *J. Pharmacol. Exp. Ther.*, **1969**, *169*, 95–108.

Thames, M. D. Acetylstrophanthidin-induced reflex inhibition of canine renal sympathetic nerve activity mediated by cardiac receptors with vagal afferents. *Circ. Res.*, **1979**, *44*, 8–15.

Toda, N., and West, T. C. Influence of ouabain on cholinergic responses in the sinoatrial node. *J. Pharmacol. Exp. Ther.*, **1966**, *153*, 104–113.

Tse, W., and Han, J. Interaction of epinephrine and ouabain on automaticity of canine Purkinje fibers. *Circ. Res.*, **1978**, *34*, 777–782.

Weingart, R. The actions of ouabain on intercellular coupling and conduction velocity in mammalian ventricular muscle. *J. Physiol. (Lond.)*, **1977**, *264*, 341–365.

Wellens, H. J., and Durrer, D. Effect of digitalis on atrioventricular conduction and circus movement tachycardias in patients with Wolff-Parkinson-White syndrome. *Circulation*, **1973**, *47*, 1229–1233.

Wittenberg, S. M.; Gandel, P.; Hogan, P. M.; Kreuger, W.; and Klocke, F. J. Relationship of heart rate to ventricular automaticity in dogs during ouabain administration. *Circ. Res.*, **1972**, *30*, 167–176.

Wu, D.; Wyndham, C.; Amat-y-Leon, F.; Denes, P.; Dhingra, R.; and Rosen, K. The effects of ouabain on induction of atrioventricular nodal re-entrant paroxysmal supraventricular tachycardia. *Circulation*, **1975**, *52*, 201–207.

Monographs and Reviews

Bigger, J. T., Jr. Mechanisms of digitalis toxic arrhythmias and the clinical recognition of toxicity. In, *Controversies in Clinical Pharmacology and Drug Development.* (Palmer, W., ed.) Futura Publishing Co., Inc., Mount Kisco, N.Y., **1972.**

———. The quinidine-digoxin interaction. *Mod. Concepts Cardiovasc. Dis.*, **1982**, *51*, 73–78.

Blinks, J. R.; Wier, W. G.; Morgan, J. P.; and Hess, P. Regulation of intracellular [Ca^{2+}] by cardiotonic drugs. In, *Advances in Pharmacology and Therapeutics II.* Vol. 3, *Cardio-Renal and Cell Pharmacology.* (Xoshida, H.; Hagiwara, Y.; and Ebashi, S.; eds.) Pergamon Press, Ltd., Oxford, **1982**, pp. 205–216.

Chen, K. K., and Henderson, F. G. Pharmacology of sixty-four cardiac glycosides and aglycones. *J. Pharmacol. Exp. Ther.*, **1954**, *111*, 365–383.

Colucci, W. S.; Wright, R. F.; and Braunwald, E. New positive inotropic agents in the treatment of heart failure: mechanisms of action and recent clinical developments. *N. Engl. J. Med.*, **1986**, *314*, 290–299, 349–358.

Cranefield, P. F., and Aronson, R. S. *Cardiac Arrhythmias: The Role of Triggered Activity and Other Mechanisms.* Futura Publishing Co., Inc., Mount Kisco, N.Y., **1988.**

Erhardt, P. W. In search of a digitalis replacement. *J. Med. Chem.*, **1987**, *30*, 231–237.

Gillis, R. A., and Quest, J. A. The role of the central nervous system in the cardiovascular effects of digitalis. *Pharmacol. Rev.*, **1980**, *31*, 19–97.

Hoffman, B. F. The pharmacology of cardiac glycosides. In, *Cardiac Therapy.* (Rosen, M. R., and Hoffman, B. F., eds.) Martinus Nijhoff, Boston, **1983**, pp. 387–412.

Hoffman, B. F., and Singer, D. H. Effects of digitalis on electrical activity of cardiac fibers. *Prog. Cardiovasc. Dis.*, **1964**, *7*, 226–260.

Marshall, P. G. Steroids: cardiotonic glycosides and aglycones: toad poisons. In, *Rodd's Chemistry of Carbon Compounds*, 2nd ed., Vol. 2 D. (Coffey, S., ed.) Elsevier Publishing Co., Amsterdam, **1970**, pp. 360–421.

Noble, D. Sodium-calcium exchange and its role in generating electric current. In, *Cardiac Muscle: The Regulation of Excitation and Contraction.* (Nathan, R. D., ed.) Academic Press, Inc., New York, **1986**, pp. 121–200.

Parmley, W. W. Pathophysiology and current therapy of congestive heart failure. *J. Am. Coll. Cardiol.*, **1989**, *13*, 771–785.

Rosen, M. R. Interactions of digitalis with the autonomic nervous system and their relationship to cardiac arrhythmias. In, *Disturbances in Neurogenic Control of the Circulation.* (Abboud, F.; Fozzard, H.; Gilmore, J.; and Reis, D.; eds.) American Physiological Society, Bethesda, Md., **1981**, pp. 251–263.

Vassalle, M. Cardiac glycosides: regulation of force and rhythm. In, *Cardiac Muscle: The Regulation of Excitation and Contraction.* (Nathan, R. D., ed.) Academic Press, Inc., New York, **1986**, pp. 237–267.

Weingart, R. Influence of cardiac glycosides on electrophysiologic processes. In, *Cardiac Glycosides*, Pt. 1. *Handbook of Experimental Pharmacology*, Vol. 56/1. Springer-Verlag, Berlin, **1981**, pp. 221–254.

Williams, E. S., and Fisch, C. Treatment of cardiac failure. In, *Cardiac Therapy.* (Rosen, M. R., and Hoffman, B. F., eds.) Martinus Nijhoff, Boston, **1983**, pp. 453–480.

CHAPTER

35 ANTIARRHYTHMIC DRUGS

J. Thomas Bigger, Jr., and Brian F. Hoffman

Drug therapy for cardiac arrhythmias is based on knowledge of the mechanism, consequences, and natural history of the arrhythmia to be treated and on a clear understanding of the pharmacology of the drugs to be used. The latter includes knowledge of drug action on the electrophysiological properties of normal and abnormal cardiac tissues, of their effects on the mechanical properties of the heart and vasculature, and of their interactions with the autonomic nervous system and their effects on other organ systems. Optimal therapy of cardiac arrhythmias requires an appreciation of the pharmacokinetic properties of antiarrhythmic drugs and how they are affected by disease. Finally, a broad knowledge of adverse effects of the agents and their potential interactions with other drugs is necessary to monitor the course of therapy.

CARDIAC ELECTROPHYSIOLOGY

Resting Potential. There is a voltage difference across the surface membrane of all cardiac cells, the resting transmembrane voltage or potential (*Vm*). For most cardiac cells, the resting *Vm* is about −80 to −90 mV relative to the extracellular fluid. The resting transmembrane concentration gradients for ions such as Na^+ and K^+ are established by active transport. Typical values for concentrations of ions in myocardial cells (*i*) and in extracellular fluid (*o*) (in millimoles per liter of water) are $[K]_o = 4.0$, $[K]_i = 150$, $[Na]_o = 140$, and $[Na]_i = 6$ to 12. If there were no voltage gradient across the membrane and the membrane were semipermeable to an ion, such as K^+, K^+ would diffuse out of the cell until the concentrations inside and outside were equal. However, the Na^+–K^+ exchange pump counteracts diffusional forces. In addition, fixed negative charges in the cell attract K^+ and counteract the concentration gradient that promotes diffusion. When these forces are equal, no net flux of ions will occur. The Nernst equation can be solved for the voltage that will maintain the existing transmembrane concentration gradient for a particular cation at a constant value—the equilibrium voltage E_X for a monovalent cation X:

$$E_X = \frac{RT}{F} \ln \frac{[X]_o}{[X]_i},$$

where $[X]_o$ is the concentration of the ion in extracellular fluid, $[X]_i$ is the intracellular concentration, *R* is the gas constant, *T* is the absolute temperature, and *F* is the Faraday constant. Given the ion concentrations listed above, $E_K = -97$ mV and $E_{Na} = +65$ mV. Since the resting membrane is permeable primarily to K^+, the resting *Vm* is close to E_K. However, other ions, such as Na^+, make small contributions to the resting *Vm*, as does the Na^+–K^+ pump (because it exchanges 3 Na^+ for 2 K^+).

Action Potentials. When cardiac cells are excited a complex sequence of voltage changes occurs as a function of time, due to changes in ionic conductances across the membrane. A typical transmembrane action potential of a Purkinje fiber is diagrammed in Figure 35–1, *A*. The action potential is divided into phases for purposes of description and discussion. Phase 0 = rapid depolarization; phase 1 = rapid repolarization to the plateau level of voltage; phase 2 = the plateau of the action potential; phase 3 = rapid repolarization; and phase 4 = the diastolic voltage time course. A variety of action potentials are seen in the normal heart. Action potentials of sinus and atrioventricular (AV) nodal cells have a slowly rising phase 0, and phases 1, 2, and 3 are not clearly distinguished from one another. Also, many cells have a steady value of *Vm* during phase 4, whereas others depolarize spontaneously during this period. Automatic fibers in the sinus node and His–Purkinje system reach a maximal negative value of *Vm* at the end of phase-3 repolarization, which is followed by spontaneous depolarization; excitation occurs when the *Vm* achieves the critical threshold voltage. The firing rate of a normally automatic cell is determined by (1) the value of maximal diastolic voltage, (2) the slope of phase-4 depolarization, and (3) the value of the threshold voltage. When a cell or group of cells undergoes self-excitation by this process and initiates an impulse that propagates to the rest of the heart, it is known as a *pacemaker*.

The ionic basis for the cardiac action potential continues to be the subject of active study. Although the voltage clamp technique has revealed clearly the ionic basis of action potentials in nerves, there are serious technical problems in the application of this technique to cardiac muscle. It has been most successfully used in cardiac Purkinje fibers. More recently, ionic currents have been investigated by the voltage clamp technique using

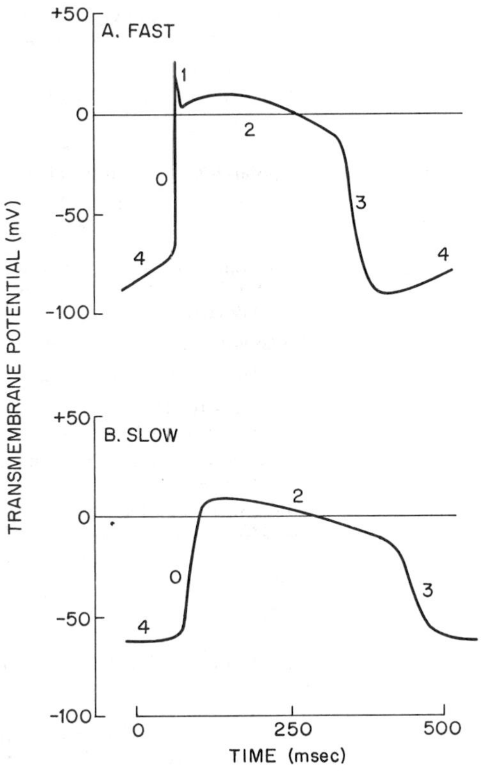

Figure 35–1. *Diagrammatic representation of fast and slow responses from mammalian cardiac Purkinje fibers.*

A. Fast Response. The phases of the normal fast response are shown: depolarization (*0*), repolarization (*1, 2, 3*), and the diastolic phase (*4*). Note the spontaneous phase-4 depolarization in this example. The rate of rise of phase 0 is rapid, and propagation will be rapid.

B. Slow Response. The slow response is initiated from a reduced (less negative) level of diastolic transmembrane voltage, shows slow depolarization, and has a long duration. Such an action potential propagates exceedingly slowly and leaves a long refractory wake.

single cardiac cells or isolated patches of plasma membrane (Grant and Starmer, 1987; Tseng *et al.*, 1987; Cohen *et al.*, 1989). Current concepts of the genesis of the cardiac action potential have been reviewed by Noble (1984), Baumgarten and Fozzard (1986), Brown and Yatani (1986), Cohen and colleagues (1986), and Pelzer and Trautwein (1987). A summary of the important ionic currents is given in Table 35–1.

Phase 0. In most cardiac cells, phase 0 is generated by the movement of Na^+ through selective channels that are activated in a voltage-dependent manner when the propagating cardiac impulse or spontaneous phase-4 depolarization causes the hypothetical *m* gate in the channel to open. The inward Na^+ current, i_{Na}, is very intense but very brief; it is terminated by a process called *inactivation*—rapid closure of a hypothetical gate (the *h* gate) in the Na^+ channel. After inactivation, the Na^+ channel does not open again until it has been reactivated by repolarization. Thus, the Na^+ channel can exist in one of three states: resting, active, or inactivated. Most of the Na^+ channels are closed during the plateau of the action potential, but a few are open, thereby permitting a small (inward) Na^+ current to flow.

Phase 1. Quick repolarization to the plateau of the action potential is brought about by several factors: the passive electrical properties of Purkinje fibers; inactivation of i_{Na}; and activation of i_{to1}, a transient outward (K^+) current (Tseng and Hoffman, 1989).

Phase 2. The plateau of the action potential is one of the most unusual features of the cardiac action potential. Membrane conductance is lower during the plateau than during diastole (phase 4). Although two Ca^{2+} channels, designated L and T, are activated on depolarization, the L channel (sensitive to Ca^{2+}-channel blockers) is primarily responsible for the current, i_{Ca}, that flows during the plateau (Bean, 1985). This current is inactivated in a manner analogous to the inactivation of i_{Na}, but the time constant for inactivation of i_{Ca} is much greater (50 msec as compared with 0.5 msec). Therefore, i_{Ca} declines slowly during the plateau. Because of low membrane conductance, small changes in any ionic current can have a marked effect on the time course of voltage during phase 2.

Phase 3. A time-dependent outward current that is carried primarily by K^+ (i_K) plays an important role in terminating the plateau and causing the fiber to repolarize to normal diastolic values of *Vm* (Gintant *et al.*, 1985). The i_K channel opens at about −40 mV, with a time constant of about 0.5 second. By the end of the plateau, i_K has waxed to a considerable value, while i_{Ca} has waned. Phase 3 is primarily the result of activated i_K in the presence of inactivating i_{Ca}. On repolarization, the i_K channel closes promptly and it remains closed at values of *Vm* more negative than −50 mV.

Phase 4. In many cells (*e.g.*, ordinary atrial or ventricular muscle), *Vm* is constant during diastole; these cells will rest indefinitely until activated by a propagating impulse or an external stimulus. However, as mentioned above, other cells exhibit spontaneous phase-4 depolarization and self-excitation (*i.e.*, automaticity; *see* Figure 35–1, *A*). This type of behavior is characteristic of the sinus node, AV node, and the His–Purkinje system. The main determinant of phase-4 depolarization is the pacemaker current (i_f) (DiFrancesco, 1981a, 1985). The i_f begins to activate when the *Vm* becomes more negative than −50 mV and progressively activates during diastole to depolarize the fiber. Both Na^+ and K^+ contribute to i_f (DiFrancesco, 1981b). Several other ionic currents modulate phase-4 depolarization. Electrogenic extrusion of Na^+ can be an important part of background outward current. Also, Ca^{2+} current flowing through T channels may be important during the latter part of phase 4 (Hagiwara *et al.*, 1988). Spontaneous activity of

Table 35–1. IONIC CURRENTS AND THE PURKINJE FIBER ACTION POTENTIAL

CURRENT	MAJOR ION RESPONSIBLE FOR THE CURRENT	PHASE OF ACTION POTENTIAL	REVERSAL VOLTAGE (mV)	DIRECTION OF CURRENT FLOW	PHYSIOLOGICAL ROLE
i_{Na}	Na^+	0	+65	Inward	Depolarizes fiber during phase 0
i_{to1}	K^+	1	−50 to −80	Outward	Rapid repolarization in phase 1
i_{to2}	K^+	1	?	Outward	Role uncertain
$i_{Ca,L}$ *	Ca^{2+}	1, 2	+60 to +80	Inward	Contributes to plateau of action potential; triggers the release of internal Ca^{2+}
$i_{Ca,T}$	Ca^{2+}	1, 2	+40	Inward	Physiological role uncertain
i_K	K^+	3	−70	Outward	Repolarizes fiber during phase 3
i_{K_1}	K^+	0, 1, 2, 3, 4	−90	Outward	Maintains resting potential, tends to repolarize fiber
i_f	Na^+	4	−10 to −20	Inward	Activation promotes spontaneous depolarization
i_{bi}	Na^+, Ca^{2+}	0, 1, 2, 3, 4	+40 †	Inward	Tends to depolarize fiber

* Referred to as i_{Ca} in text.
† Current is inward at voltages negative to E_K.

sinus nodal cells is faster than that of Purkinje fibers because i_f activates at a faster rate.

Fast and Slow Responses. Two categories of cardiac action potentials can be distinguished: *fast* and *slow* responses. Depolarization in the fast response (*see* Figure 35–1, *A*) is generated by an intense inward i_{Na}, has a large, fast-rising phase 0, propagates very rapidly, and has a large safety factor for conduction. Normal atrial, ventricular, and Purkinje fiber action potentials are examples of the fast response. The slow response has a slowly rising phase 0, propagates very slowly, and has a low safety factor for conduction (Figure 35–1, *B*). Action potentials of cells in the sinus and AV nodes are examples of slow responses seen under normal conditions. The main depolarizing current for slow responses is carried by Ca^{2+} and has the characteristics of the current that flows through L channels.

Excitability and Refractoriness. Excitability is traditionally measured in terms of the strength of an electrical pulse required to excite the heart. The functional significance of changes in excitability is difficult to determine. Therefore, little emphasis is placed here on the effects of antiarrhythmic drugs on excitability. Refractoriness has been defined in many different ways; in this discussion, refractoriness is used to refer to the duration of the effective refractory period (ERP), which is the minimal interval between two propagating responses. In cardiac cells with fast responses, the ERP is closely linked to action potential duration (APD), because recovery of Na^+ channels from inactivation closely parallels repolarization. In cardiac cells with slow responses, refractoriness can outlast full repolarization (*i.e.*, ERP is longer than APD) because i_{Ca} recovers only slowly from inactivation. Antiarrhythmic drugs prolong the ERP relative to the APD in many types of cardiac cells.

Responsiveness and Conduction. The term *membrane responsiveness* is used to describe the response of a cardiac fiber to a stimulus (*e.g.*, a propagating action potential or applied electrical pulse). Cardiac fibers do not regain their ability to develop a normal response until repolarization is complete. Changes in the maximal rate of depolarization during phase 0 ($\dot{V}_{max}$) provide an index of changes in availability of the Na^+ conductance system or the degree of recovery from inactivation of the Na^+ channel. Phase-0 $\dot{V}_{max}$ is an important determinant of conduction velocity and block of premature impulses. In cardiac Purkinje fibers, the $\dot{V}_{max}$ of a response is very strongly dependent on *Vm* at the instant of excitation (*see* Figure 35–2). In normal fibers, the time constant for recovery from inactivation of the Na^+ channel is quite short, such that recovery of $\dot{V}_{max}$ is primarily a function of transmembrane voltage as repolarization occurs. Consequently, $\dot{V}_{max}$ is similar when a cardiac fiber is stimulated at a given level of *Vm*, regardless of whether the fiber is stimulated during phase-3 repolarization or during phase-4 depolarization. The time constant for recovery of Na^+ channels is significantly longer: (1) at low (more positive) values of *Vm*; (2) during treatment with antiarrhythmic drugs; and (3) in membranes altered by disease. The S-shaped relationship between $\dot{V}_{max}$ and *Vm* is typical not only of cardiac Purkinje fibers but also of atrial and ventricular muscle. Cells of the sinus node and the AV node do not regain full responsiveness until well after repolarization is complete. There is a considerable safety factor in cardiac muscle (except in the sinus and AV nodes), since $\dot{V}_{max}$ must be reduced to half or less of normal before conduction velocity decreases.

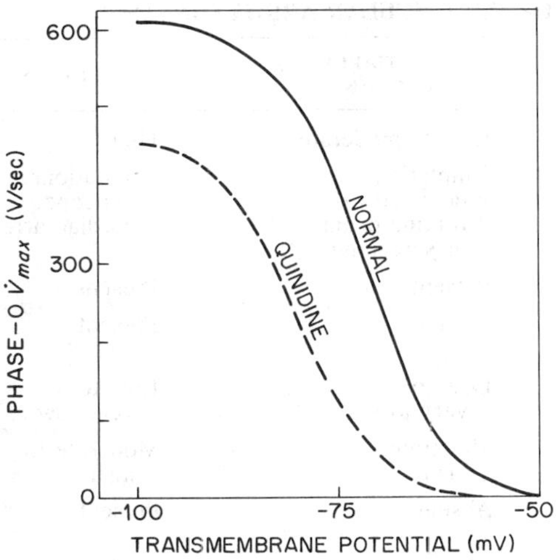

Figure 35–2. *Membrane responsiveness.*

Membrane responsiveness in a cardiac Purkinje fiber is depicted. The maximal rate of rise of depolarization during phase 0 is plotted as a function of transmembrane voltage at the time of activation. The solid line shows the relationship under normal conditions, and the dashed line depicts the effect of a moderate-to-high concentration of quinidine. Quinidine shifts the relationship on its voltage axis so that a reduced response is obtained at any given level of transmembrane voltage. Also, the maximal rate of depolarization is reduced.

MECHANISMS RESPONSIBLE FOR CARDIAC ARRHYTHMIAS

An arrhythmia is an abnormality of rate, regularity, or site of origin of the cardiac impulse or a disturbance in conduction that causes an alteration in the normal sequence of activation of the atria and ventricles. Clinically, ventricular arrhythmias are classified as benign, potentially malignant, or malignant based on the risk of their causing sudden death (*see* Table 35–2). Such arrhythmias may arise because of alterations in impulse generation, impulse conduction, or both.

Arrhythmias Due to Abnormalities of Impulse Generation

There are many examples of arrhythmias that arise because of either enhancement or failure of normal automaticity. Mechanisms of abnormal automaticity are also subjects of ongoing experimental interest.

Altered Normal Automaticity. When considering arrhythmias due to abnormalities of automaticity, it is important to recall that only a few types of cardiac cells frequently develop normal automaticity: sinus node, distal AV node, and the His–Purkinje system. Other cell types can develop automaticity as well, for example, specialized atrial fibers in the internodal tracts and fibers near the ostium of the coronary sinus.

Sinus Node. In the sinus node, rate can be altered by autonomic activity or intrinsic disease. Increased vagal activity can slow or stop sinus nodal pacemakers by increasing K^+ conductance (g_K); this increases outward K^+ currents, hyperpolarizes the pacemaker cells, and slows or stops their depolarization. Increased sympathetic traffic to the sinus node increases the rate of phase-4 depolarization, probably by a combination of effects (*e.g.*, increased rate of activation of the pacemaker current i_f; increased magnitude of i_{Ca}). Intrinsic disease of sinus nodal pacemaker cells seems to be responsible for faulty pacemaker activity in the sick sinus syndrome in man (Bigger and Reiffel, 1979; Kerr *et al.*, 1983). The precise mechanism and pathogenesis are still unknown.

Purkinje Fibers. Augmented automaticity in the His–Purkinje system is a common cause of arrhythmias in human subjects. Increased sympathetic nerve activity can cause a substantial increase in the rate of spontaneous firing. This increase is brought about by an ionic mechanism that is similar to the changes causing sinus tachycardia (DiFrancesco, 1981a). It is possible for AV junctional pacemakers to usurp control of the ventricles in the presence of a normal sinus node and normal AV conduction because of selectivity of traffic in sympathetic nerves (Randall, 1977). As a result, higher neural activity, including that associated with cardiovascular reflexes, can alter cardiac rate and produce disturbances of rhythm primarily by changing the pattern of firing of various subunits of the cardiac autonomic nerves (Levitt *et al.*, 1976). The effect of the vagus on the His–Purkinje system in man is not well understood. The response of Purkinje fibers to acetylcholine varies with species; acetylcholine slows normal pacemaker activity in the dog but accelerates it in sheep. In addition, many questions about functional vagal innervation of the His–Purkinje system are unsettled; it appears that vagal innervation of the proximal system may be significant, whereas that of the peripheral system is more sparse (Levy, 1977).

In disease, automaticity in the His–Purkinje system may become reduced. In the sick sinus syndrome it is typical for the ventricular pacemakers to be depressed as well as the sinus node (*see* Bigger and Reiffel, 1979). Thus, very long pauses in cardiac rhythm may occur when the sinus node fails as a pacemaker. In AV block due to widespread bundle-branch disease, the rate of ventricular pacemakers may also be abnormally slow. In neither of these examples has a mechanism been identified.

Abnormal Generation of Impulses. In addition to the arrhythmias caused by alterations of normal automaticity, numerous abnormal mechanisms for the generation of impulses have been observed in experimental preparations (*see* Cranefield and Aronson, 1988). Many of these mechanisms appear to fit into one of two categories—abnormal automaticity or triggered activity. Abnormal automatic-

Table 35–2. PROGNOSTIC CLASSIFICATION OF VENTRICULAR ARRHYTHMIAS *

	BENIGN	POTENTIALLY MALIGNANT	MALIGNANT
Risk for sudden death	Very Low	Low to moderate	High
Clinical presentation	Palpitations; detected by routine exam	Paliptations; detected by routine exam or screening	Palpitations; syncope; cardiac arrest
Heart disease	Usually absent	Present	Present
Cardiac scarring and/or hypertrophy	Absent	Present	Present
Left ventricular ejection fraction	Normal	Low to very low	Low to very low
Frequency of VPDs †	Low to moderate	Moderate to high	Moderate to high
Sustained ventricular tachycardia	Absent	Absent	Present
Hemodynamic effects of arrhythmia	Absent	Absent to mild	Moderate to severe

* The characteristics listed are typical, but there are exceptions (*e.g.*, benign ventricular arrhythmias can be frequent, and occasionally, repetitive).

† VPD = ventricular premature depolarization(s).

ity refers to spontaneous diastolic depolarization that occurs at a very low (relatively positive) value of *Vm* in a cell that normally has a much higher value of *Vm* in diastole. Triggered activity is the generation of impulses by afterdepolarizations that reach threshold (*see* below). Both of these mechanisms differ strikingly from those responsible for normal automaticity. Moreover, both of these mechanisms can cause the formation of impulses in fibers that ordinarily are incapable of automatic function (*e.g.*, ordinary atrial or ventricular muscle cells).

Abnormal Automaticity. Purkinje fibers, atrial cells, and ventricular cells can all show spontaneous diastolic depolarization and repetitive automatic firing when their resting *Vm* is reduced substantially (*e.g.*, to −60 mV or less negative values). The ionic mechanisms for such abnormal automaticity are not known, but i_K and i_{Ca} probably contribute to this behavior.

Early Afterdepolarizations. Early afterdepolarizations are secondary depolarizations that occur before repolarization is complete. Characteristically, the secondary depolarization commences at membrane potentials close to those present during the plateau of the action potential (*see* Figure 35–3, *A*). In isolated tissues, a burst of depolarizations often occurs, and is followed by a few damped oscillations, until, finally, *Vm* either rests at the range of the plateau voltage (about −20 to −40 mV) or returns to a relatively high resting value. Experimentally, early afterdepolarizations have been produced in cardiac Purkinje fibers by a number of maneuvers, including stretching, hypoxia, and chemical alterations. Early afterdepolarizations are promoted by (and may result from) (1) decreased background outward current (i_{K_1}), (2) increased background inward current (i_{bi}), (3) increased residual i_{Na} during the plateau, (4) increased magnitude and/or duration of i_{Ca}, and (5) reduced magnitude of i_K. When the *Vm* of cardiac muscle fibers is in the range of the plateau voltage, the membrane conductance is low and tiny inward currents cause substantial depolarization.

Delayed Afterdepolarizations. A delayed afterdepolarization is a secondary depolarization that occurs early in diastole, that is, after full repolarization has been achieved (*see* Figure 35–3, *B*). The delayed afterdepolarization is not self-initiated but is dependent on a prior action potential. Delayed afterdepolarizations may be seen when certain cell types are exposed to catecholamines, digitalis, low $[K]_o$, or perfusates containing low $[Na]_o$ and high $[Ca]_o$. Delayed afterdepolarizations can reach threshold and give rise to a single premature depolarization. If the premature depolarization is followed by another delayed afterdepolarization, a second impulse may result. In this way, delayed afterdepolarizations can cause either coupled extrasystoles or runs of tachyarrhythmias. Several factors increase the amplitude of delayed afterdepolarizations and promote triggered activity. They include increased heart rate, premature systoles, increased $[Ca]_o$, catecholamines, and other drugs, particularly digitalis. The mechanism for delayed afterdepolarizations that arise in digitalis toxicity is discussed in Chapter 34. Delayed afterdepolarizations can readily be induced by digitalis in the His–Purkinje system and, with more difficulty, in specialized atrial or ordinary ventricular cells. The delayed afterdepolarizations induced by digitalis in Purkinje fibers are associated with an

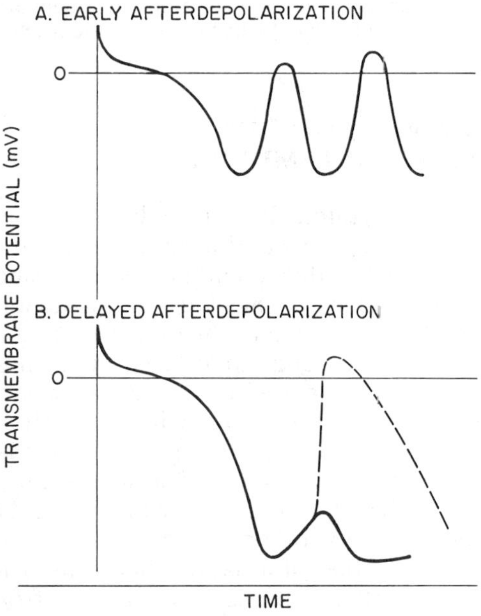

Figure 35–3. *Two forms of triggered activity in a cardiac Purkinje fiber.*

A. Early Afterdepolarization. Repolarization is interrupted by secondary depolarizations. Such responses may excite neighboring fibers and be propagated.

B. Delayed Afterdepolarization. After full repolarization is achieved, *Vm* again transiently depolarizes. If the delayed afterdepolarization reaches threshold, a propagating response can occur (dashed line).

abnormal transient inward current that is carried mainly by Na^+. It is reasonable to speculate that some clinical arrhythmias caused by digitalis (*e.g.*, coupled ventricular premature depolarizations and atrial or ventricular tachycardias) result from delayed afterdepolarizations. Also, some supraventricular tachycardias that arise in the absence of drug therapy may be triggered activity because of delayed afterdepolarizations.

Triggered Activity. As mentioned, when a delayed afterdepolarization reaches threshold, a single extrasystole may result or sustained repetitive firing may be triggered (Cranefield and Aronson, 1988). Activation by this mechanism must be initiated by an action potential; thus, it cannot arise *de novo,* as can a normal automatic rhythm. Although triggered activity cannot be self-initiated, it can be self-sustained. Triggered activity in cells that have delayed afterdepolarizations shares many characteristics with reentrant tachyarrhythmias (*see* below). As a result, it is difficult to know which mechanism is responsible for a given clinical tachyarrhythmia.

Arrhythmias Caused by Abnormalities of Impulse Conduction

Arrhythmias may arise by recirculating activation that is incited by an initiating depolarization. Such arrhythmias (often referred to as *reentrant arrhythmias*), like triggered rhythms, are self-sustained but not self-initiated. For reentry to be initiated, one-way block of conduction must occur, and there must be an anatomical or functional "barrier" to conduction that forms a circuit (*see* Bigger, 1973). Furthermore, the pathlength of the circuit must be greater than the wavelength of the cardiac impulse, where wavelength is the product of conduction velocity and the refractory period (*see* Figure 35–4). For reentry to occur, normal conduction must be greatly slowed, refractoriness markedly shortened, or both. Conduction is normally very slow in the sinus and AV nodes. Further slowing by premature activation or by disease easily creates conditions that permit reentry. Disease processes may also create conditions that permit reentry even in fibers that usually conduct the cardiac impulse at very rapid rates, such as cardiac Purkinje fibers. Usually, marked slowing of conduction is the abnormality that permits reentry. However, marked abbreviation of action potentials and of refractoriness can have a role as well. Con-

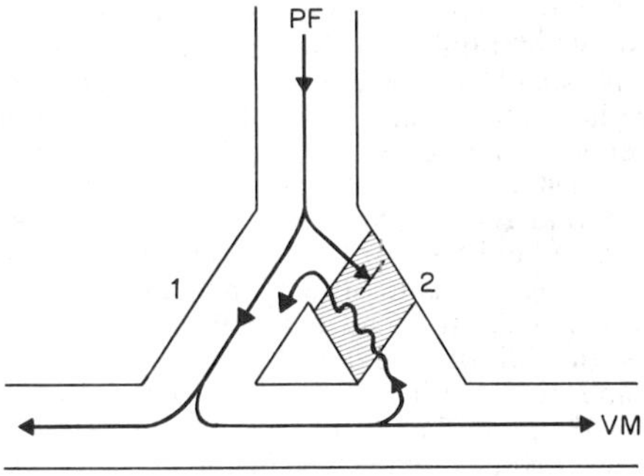

Figure 35–4. *Reentry.*

The diagram shows one of the forms of reentrant reexcitation in the ventricle (Schmitt and Erlanger, 1928–29). A branched Purkinje fiber (*PF*) terminates on a strip of ventricular muscle (*VM*). The shaded area in branch 2 represents a depolarized area that is the site of a one-way block; thus, orthograde sinus impulses are blocked in this area, but retrograde responses are propagated successfully. Retrograde conduction in branch 2 is slow enough for cells in branch 1 to recover and respond to the reentering impulse. A single reactivation of branch 1 will produce a single ventricular premature depolarization; continuous conduction around the circuit will cause ventricular tachycardia.

Antiarrhythmic drugs can abolish such reentrant activity by producing two-way block in branch 2 or by improving conduction in branch 2, that is, by removing the one-way block.

duction may be slowed because of alterations in the fast response or development of slow responses.

Altered Fast Response. When resting *Vm* is more depolarized than −75 mV (as with stretch or high $[K]_o$), $\dot{V}_{max}$ and conduction velocity decrease substantially because of voltage-dependent inactivation of the fast Na^+ channel (*see* Figure 35–2). When resting *Vm* is between −50 and −65 mV, conduction velocity is greatly reduced and abnormal "fast responses" can propagate slowly enough to permit reentry. If *Vm* is more positive than −50 mV or so, Na^+ channels will be almost totally inactivated and fast responses cannot be elicited. At such low values of *Vm*, fast responses may conduct decrementally; that is, the adequacy of the propagating response as a stimulus to resting tissue in its path lessens progressively as it propagates in depolarized tissues. Under such conditions, a delicate balance exists that determines whether conduction succeeds or fails.

Slow Responses and Very Slow Conduction. Slow action potentials appear in cardiac Purkinje fibers when they are exposed to increased $[K]_o$ and catecholamines. In the voltage range at which slow potentials emerge, i_{Na} is inactivated and the pacemaker current i_f is fully deactivated; thus, these currents are unlikely to have a role in the genesis of the slow response. The inward current that causes the slow potential is i_{Ca}. Because this current is relatively small in magnitude, slow responses are more likely to develop when background outward currents are decreased. Typically, slow responses are 40 to 80 mV in amplitude, depolarize at 1 to 2 V per second (*i.e.*, about 0.002 the rate of the fast response), and last for 0.4 to 1 second (*see* Figure 35–1, *B*). As a result, slow responses propagate so slowly that reentry can occur in very short pathways. In addition, the duration of the action potential and refractoriness may shorten dramatically just proximal to the site of block because of a repolarizing current provided by neighboring resting tissue. The short duration of the refractory period in tissue at the site of unidirectional block permits reentry of subsequent impulses even if the reentry pathway is short.

Significance of Reentry. Reentry may occur in many sites in the heart; it is relatively easy to elicit in the vicinity of the sinus or AV nodes by the use of premature stimulation to slow conduction and to produce a functional one-way block, even in normal hearts. Clinically, reentry is the usual cause of paroxysmal supraventricular tachycardia. Reentry in the His–Purkinje system is thought to be one cause of coupled ventricular premature depolarizations and ventricular tachycardia in man. This idea is supported by extensive study in both man and animals. For example, Durrer and coworkers (1971) and El-Sherif and associates (1977) have shown, in experiments with acute myocardial infarction in dogs, that the cardiac impulse can meander through the infarcted region and emerge much later to produce ventricular premature depolarizations, ventricular tachycardia, or ventricular fibrillation.

CLASSIFICATION OF ANTIARRHYTHMIC DRUGS

Antiarrhythmic drugs have been grouped together according to the pattern of electrophysiological effects that they produce and/or their presumed mechanisms of action. Classifications such as the one presented in Table 35–3 are commonly used in discussing antiarrhythmic drugs, and physicians should thus be acquainted with them. However, it should also be recognized that drugs within a class do differ significantly: one may be effective and safe in a particular patient while another may not.

Much of the information that is used to classify antiarrhythmic drugs comes from experimental studies in animals (Arnsdorf and Wasserstrom, 1986). For example, the classification in Table 35–3 relies heavily on observations made with preparations of rabbit atria and canine or bovine cardiac Purkinje fibers. The agents in class I directly alter membrane conductances of cations, particularly those of Na^+ and K^+. It is useful to subcategorize these drugs in terms of their relative ability to depress $\dot{V}_{max}$ (by blockade of fast Na^+ channels) and to slow membrane repolarization. Class II includes agents that have primarily indirect effects on electrophysiological parameters by virtue of their ability to block β-adrenergic receptors. The agents in class III are mechanistically the least well defined. They share the capacity to delay membrane repolarization (and thus prolong refractoriness) with relatively little effect on $\dot{V}_{max}$. Finally, class-IV agents have relatively selective depressant actions on Ca^{2+} channels, primarily those of the L type.

Such schemes can lead to ambiguities. Some drugs have multiple actions and therefore belong in more than one class. It may not be clear in a particular case which of the drug's actions is responsible for its efficacy. Moreover, when drugs are given to patients with heart disease and arrhythmias, their effects on the central and autonomic nervous systems, on hemodynamics, or on myocardial ischemia or metabolism may greatly influence their antiarrhythmic action.

Table 35–3. CLASSIFICATION OF ANTIARRHYTHMIC DRUGS ACCORDING TO THEIR MECHANISM OF ACTION

CLASS	ACTION	DRUGS
I.	*Sodium Channel Blockade*	
A.	Moderate phase-0 depression and slow conduction (2+) *; usually prolong repolarization	Quinidine, procainamide, disopyramide, moricizine
B.	Minimal phase-0 depression and slow conduction (0 to 1+); usually shorten repolarization	Lidocaine, mexiletine, phenytoin, tocainide
C.	Marked phase-0 depression and slow conduction (3+ to 4+); little effect on repolarization	Encainide, flecainide, propafenone, indecainide
II.	*β-Adrenergic Blockade*	Propranolol, acebutolol, esmolol, others
III.	*Prolong Repolarization*	Amiodarone, bretylium, sotalol
IV.	*Ca^{2+}-Channel Blockade*	Verapamil, diltiazem

* Relative magnitude of effect on conduction velocity indicated on a scale of 1+ to 4+.

USE-DEPENDENT BLOCKADE OF ION CHANNELS

An understanding of the effects of many antiarrhythmic drugs on the heart depends in part on knowledge of how those drugs interact with the gated channels that permit ionic currents across the sarcolemma (*see* Hondeghem and Katzung, 1977; Hille, 1978). This question has been evaluated in studies on single channels with the patch clamp technique (Ogden *et al.*, 1981) and on populations of channels by voltage clamping (Hondeghem and Katzung, 1980; Bean *et al.*, 1983; Gintant and Hoffman, 1983). The effects of local anesthetic antiarrhythmic agents on i_{Na} have been explained by assuming that the drugs bind to the Na^+ channel and block its function, with the result that Na^+ conductance remains at zero for as long as the drug is bound (*see* Hondeghem and Katzung, 1977; Hondeghem, 1987). The interaction of drug and channel can be represented as shown in Figure 35–5. *R, O,* and *I* represent the resting, open, and inactivated states of the channel, respectively; *D* is drug; and R^*, O^*, and I^* are the nonconducting forms of the channel to which drug is bound. *A* indicates the voltage- and time-dependent reactivation of the channel, and A^* is any modification of this process caused by drug. The diagram is greatly simplified

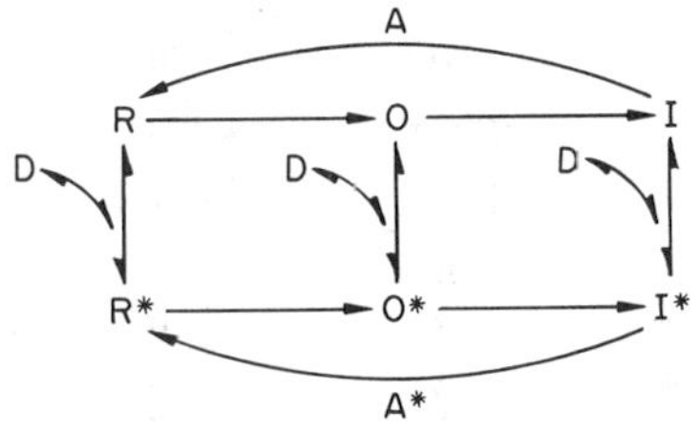

Figure 35–5. *Modulated-receptor hypothesis for the action of antiarrhythmic drugs.* (*See* text for explanation.)

and, in particular, ignores the fact that there are probably a number of transition states for the channel, as between *R* and *O*.

In terms of this diagram, a drug such as lidocaine could interact with any or all of the three states of the channel. However, the drug may preferentially combine with channels in the *R, O,* or *I* state. This preference may reflect state-dependent affinities of the channel for the drug (modulated receptor hypothesis) or may result from state-dependent access to and/or egress from the vicinity of the binding site (guarded receptor hypothesis) (Starmer and Grant, 1985). In addition, the drug-channel complex need not undergo voltage-dependent transitions in the usual way. A more negative transmembrane potential might be needed for the $I^* \rightarrow R^*$ transition than for $I \rightarrow R$ or, alternatively, the drug might have to dissociate from channels in the I^* state for the $I \rightarrow R$ transition to occur.

For many local anesthetic antiarrhythmic drugs, it appears as if channel blockade is most likely when the channel is in the *O* or *I* state and that reactivation is slowed or incomplete at usual transmembrane voltages. The consequences of this are important for the actions of antiarrhythmic drugs. A concentration of drug that exerted a minimal effect on a quiescent fiber at normal resting potential could block a significant fraction of channels during one action potential. Also, to the extent that the $I^* \rightarrow R^*$ (or $I^* \rightarrow R$) transition is slowed, channels would accumulate in the I^* state during repeated action potentials and i_{Na} for each action potential would decrease until a steady state had been attained. This is the phenomenon of use-dependent block, and it has been described for all local-anesthetic antiarrhythmic drugs and for some Ca^{2+}-channel blocking drugs (*see* below; *see also* Chapter 32). In addition, some antiarrhythmic drugs appear to cause "tonic" (*i.e.*, not use-dependent) block of i_{Na} through interaction with channels in the *R* state.

If the association of drug with channel and dissociation of drug from channel are both relatively rapid, use-dependent block will reach a steady state during the course of a few action potentials, and, if the interval between action potentials is reasonably long, little blockade will persist at the time of the upstroke of the action potential. If dissociation is quite slow, use-dependent block may not develop fully until there have been many action potentials, and a significant degree of block will be present at the time that each action potential is initiated. Finally, since a decrease in transmembrane voltage causes inactivation of fast channels, the effects of drugs on i_{Na} are enhanced in depolarized cells.

INDIVIDUAL ANTIARRHYTHMIC AGENTS

Discussion of the individual drugs is organized by class (*see* Table 35–3). The effects of each class of agent on the electrophysiological properties of specialized cardiac fibers are summarized in Table 35–4, while drug-induced alterations in the electrocardiogram (ECG) are listed in Table 35–5. The clinical usefulness of each agent is described in the text, and an overall estimate of their value in the management of specific arrhythmias is presented in Table 35–6. Pharmacokinetic parameters for the major agents are summarized in Appendix II.

CLASS I_A: QUINIDINE, PROCAINAMIDE, AND DISOPYRAMIDE

As noted above, class I_A antiarrhythmic drugs inhibit i_{Na}, depress phase-0 depolarization, and slow conduction velocity in myocardial Purkinje fibers to a moderate degree at normal resting values of *Vm* (*see* Table 35–3). These effects are intensified when the membrane is depolarized or when the frequency of excitation is increased. Although quinidine is often considered to be prototypical, procainamide does not have the capacity of quinidine and disopyramide to block muscarinic cholinergic receptors or the apparent ability of disopyramide to block Ca^{2+} channels. Some discussion of moricizine, an investigational agent, is included here even though it displays some of the characteristics of class I_B agents.

History. It was noted many years ago that patients with malaria who also had atrial fibrillation would occasionally be cured of the arrhythmia

Table 35–4. EFFECTS OF THERAPEUTIC CONCENTRATIONS OF ANTIARRHYTHMIC DRUGS ON ELECTROPHYSIOLOGICAL PROPERTIES OF SPECIALIZED CARDIAC FIBERS *

	CLASS OF ANTIARRHYTHMIC DRUG					
	I_A	I_B	I_C	*II*	*III*	*IV*
Sinus node						
Automaticity	0, ↑	0	0	↓	↓, ↑ †	↓
AV node						
Effective refractory period (ERP) ‡	↓, 0, ↑	0, ↓	↑	**↑**	↓, 0, ↑	**↑**
Purkinje fibers						
Action potential amplitude	↓	0, ↓, ↑	↓	0	0	0
Phase-0 $\dot{V}_{max}$	↓	0, ↓, ↑	**↓**	0, ↓	0, ↓	0
Action potential duration (APD)	↑, ↓	↓	↓	↓, 0, ↑	↑	0, ↓
Effective refractory period (ERP)	↑, ↓	↓	↓	↓, 0, ↑	↑	0, ↓
ERP/APD	↑	↑	↑	↑	0	0
Membrane responsiveness	↓	0, ↓	**↓**	↓	0	0
Automaticity	↓, 0	↓	↓	↓	↓, ↑ †	0, ↓

* Changes are indicated as follows: ↓, decreased; 0, no change; ↑, increased; where bidirectional arrows are shown, there is variability in the direction of change. Boldface arrows indicate effects of greater magnitude.

† Bretylium only; due to release of catecholamines on initial exposure to the drug.

‡ Due to a complex balance of direct and indirect autonomic effects.

Table 35–5. EFFECTS OF THERAPEUTIC CONCENTRATIONS OF ANTIARRHYTHMIC DRUGS ON SINUS RATE AND ELECTROPHYSIOLOGICAL AND ELECTROCARDIOGRAPHIC INTERVALS *

	CLASS OF ANTIARRHYTHMIC DRUG					
	I_A	I_B	I_C	*II*	*III*	*IV*
Sinus rate	0, ↑	0	0	↓	↓	↓
P–R	0, ↑	0	↑	↑	↑	↑
A–H	↓, 0, ↑	0, ↓	↑	↑	↑	↑
H–V	0, ↑	0	↑	0	0, ↑	0
QRS	↑	0	**↑**	0	0	0
Q–T_c †	↓, 0, ↑	↓	↑	↓, 0, ↑ ‡	**↑**	0
JT §	↓, 0, ↑	↓	↓	↓, 0, ↑ ‡	**↑**	0
Ventricular rate in atrial fibrillation	0, ↑	↓, 0, ↑	↓, 0, ↑	↓	↓	↓

* Changes are indicated as follows: ↓, decreased; 0, no change; ↑, increased; where bidirectional arrows are shown, there is variability in the direction of change. Boldface arrows indicate effects of greater magnitude.

† The Q–T_c interval is the Q–T interval corrected for heart rate.

‡ Depends on the drug (*e.g.*, propranolol shortens, sotalol lengthens).

§ J–T interval = Q–T_c – QRS.

when they were treated with cinchona. Perhaps the earliest recorded reference to the use of cinchona in atrial fibrillation is that by Jean-Baptiste de Sénac of Paris in 1749 (*see* Willius and Keys, 1942). Years later Wenckebach (1914) reported on the effect of quinine alkaloids in certain cardiac arrhythmias. Impressed by this report, Frey (1918) studied the use of cinchonine, quinine, and quinidine (an optical isomer of quinine) in patients with atrial fibrillation and found quinidine to be the most effective.

In 1936, Mautz demonstrated that application of procaine elevated the threshold of ventricular muscle to electrical stimulation. Extension of this observation by numerous workers established that the cardiac actions of procaine resemble those of quinidine. However, the therapeutic value of procaine is limited by rapid enzymatic hydrolysis and prominent adverse effects on the central nervous system (CNS). Procainamide was discovered as a result of a systematic study of congeners and metabolites of procaine to find a compound with clinically useful quinidine-like actions (Mark *et al.*, 1951).

Table 35–6. USEFULNESS OF ANTIARRHYTHMIC DRUGS IN THE TREATMENT OF SPECIFIC CARDIAC ARRHYTHMIAS *

ARRHYTHMIA	CLASS OF ANTIARRHYTHMIC DRUG					
	I_A	I_B	I_C	*II*	*III*	*IV*
Supraventricular						
Atrial fibrillation, conversion	2	0	—	1	1	1
Atrial fibrillation, prophylaxis	3	0	—	2	0	2
Atrial fibrillation, rate control	0	0	—	2	2	2
Paroxysmal supraventricular tachycardia	2	1	NI	3	NI	3
Atrial premature depolarizations	2	1	NI	2	NI	2
Ventricular						
Ventricular premature depolarizations	3	2	NI	2	NI	0
Ventricular tachycardia (unsustained)	3	2	NI	1	NI	0
Ventricular tachycardia (sustained)	3	2	2	1	1, 2 †	0
Digitalis-induced arrhythmias						
Atrial tachycardia with block	1	3	NI	2	NI	NI
Nonparoxysmal AV junctional tachycardia	1	3	NI	2	NI	NI
Ventricular arrhythmias	1	3	NI	2	NI	NI

* The utility score is based on an overall estimate of efficacy, convenience, and toxicity. The scale of relative utility is as follows: 0, none; 1, poor; 2, fair; 3, good; 4, excellent; —, insufficient data to give a score; NI, not indicated.

† Depends on the drug (*i.e.*, bretylium, 1, amiodarone 2).

The propensity of procainamide to produce a syndrome similar to systemic lupus erythematosus has encouraged the search for other agents with quinidine-like properties. Disopyramide was introduced in 1978, but it has significant antimuscarinic and negative inotropic actions. Moricizine, developed in the Soviet Union in the 1960s, is the most recent candidate; it is currently under clinical investigation.

Chemistry. The chemistry of the cinchona alkaloids is presented in the discussion of quinine (Chapter 41). Quinidine differs from quinine only in the steric configuration of the secondary alcohol group. Procainamide differs from procaine merely by the replacement of an amide for an ester linkage. The structures of procainamide, disopyramide, and moricizine (a phenothiazine) are as follows:

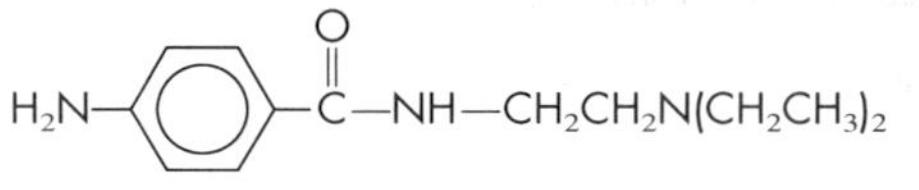

Procainamide

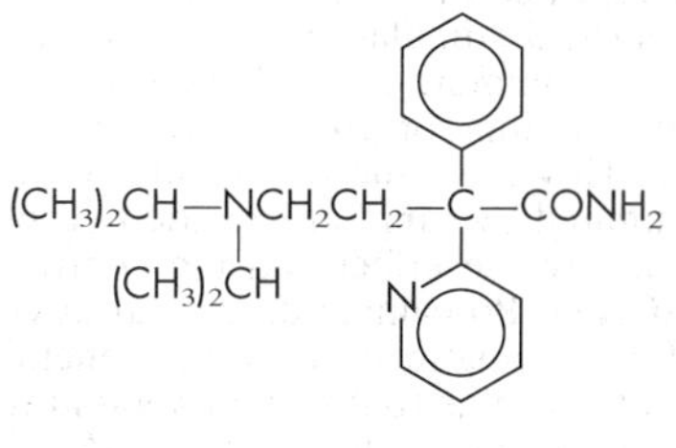

Disopyramide

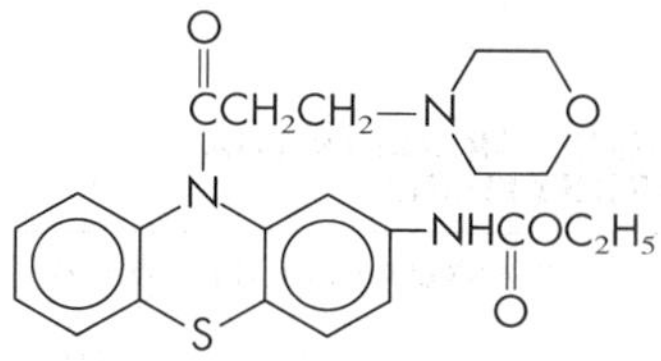

Moricizine

Cardiac Electrophysiological Effects. Antiarrhythmic agents in class I_A have powerful direct effects on most types of cells in the heart. Depending on the agent, the electrical properties of cardiac cells are also influenced indirectly by drug-induced alterations of autonomic regulation of the heart.

Automaticity. Although all the drugs in class I_A can cause severe depression of the sinus node in patients with the sick sinus syndrome (*see* Bigger and Reiffel, 1979), only disopyramide appreciably slows the denervated human heart. In normal man, quinidine can increase the sinus rate by cholinergic blockade or by reflexly increasing sympathetic activity; disopyramide usually causes little change in the sinus rate, apparently because its direct depressant effects are counterbalanced by its prominent anticholinergic actions. Therapeutic concentrations of quinidine, procainamide, and disopyramide substantially decrease the firing rate of cardiac Purkinje fibers by a direct action; they decrease the slope of phase-4 depolarization and shift the threshold voltage toward zero. The shift in threshold is due to use-dependent blockade of fast Na^+ channels and slowing of their rate of reactivation. The decrease in the slope of phase 4 has not yet been explained. This effect on the normal automaticity in the His–Purkinje system presents a hazard in the treatment of arrhythmias in the presence of AV block. Therapeutic concentrations of Class I_A agents have little effect on abnormal automaticity in markedly depolarized Purkinje fibers or on delayed afterdepolarizations. However, these agents may prevent triggered activity by preventing the premature depolarization that initiates the process or by shifting the threshold potential in a positive direction.

Excitability, Responsiveness, and Conduction. Class-I_A drugs increase the diastolic electrical current threshold in atrial and ventricular muscle and in Purkinje fibers; they also increase the fibrillation threshold in atria and ventricles. The amplitude, overshoot, and $\dot{V}_{max}$ of phase 0 in atrial, ventricular, and Purkinje cells is decreased in a dose-dependent fashion; however, these effects are not accompanied by a significant change in the resting *Vm*. The upstroke of premature responses is particularly depressed because the drugs cause changes in the voltage and time dependence of reactivation; for any steady-state value of *Vm*, $\dot{V}_{max}$ is reduced and, during dynamic changes in *Vm*, $\dot{V}_{max}$ takes longer to reach its steady-state value (*see* Figure 35–2). The time-dependent changes are most marked at low (less negative) values of *Vm*.

Duration of the Action Potential and Refractoriness. Quinidine, procainamide, and disopyramide cause small but significant increases in the duration of the action potential of ordinary atrial, ventricular, or

Purkinje cells. The effective refractory period (ERP) of these cell types increases much more than would be expected from the changes in the duration of the action potential because of the changes in responsiveness discussed above. By contrast, moricizine shortens the duration of action potentials in Purkinje fibers (*see* Symposium, 1987).

Effect on Reentrant Arrhythmias. Reentrant arrhythmias are abolished by class I_A agents because of their effects on ERP, responsiveness, and conduction. For example, when ventricular premature depolarizations are caused by reentry in loops of Purkinje fibers, one-way block can be converted to two-way block, thus making reentry impossible (*see* Figure 35–4).

The mechanisms of the antiarrhythmic actions of these drugs in atrial flutter or fibrillation are more complex.

Atrial Flutter. Prolongation of the ERP of the atrium is commonly cited as the one desirable attribute of an "antiflutter" drug. The situation is by no means simple, for the effects of antiarrhythmic drugs on ERP and on conduction velocity are inextricably linked. When quinidine or procainamide is administered to a dog in which a circus-movement flutter has been established, or to a patient with atrial flutter, the frequency invariably declines before reversion to sinus rhythm abruptly ensues. Conduction velocity slows in atrial muscle, which could account for the reduction of rate; but the atrial refractory period is also increased, which could reduce the rate by forcing the circulating impulse to travel in relatively refractory tissue. The two actions are opposed. If the predominant effect were a primary reduction of conduction velocity, reversion to sinus rhythm would not be expected to occur until the flutter frequency diminished to less than the prevailing rate of the sinus node. But if the action is primarily on the ERP, then the conduction velocity will be secondarily depressed until some minimal value is reached below which successful impulse propagation is no longer possible. This may well be the mechanism of action of class I_A agents in the experimental situation, but the details of the process are still not clearly defined.

Atrial Fibrillation. If atrial fibrillation were due to a single circus movement about an obstacle so limited in size that activation of the surrounding tissue is irregular and fractionated, then the circuit itself would be unstable. This mechanism seems unlikely, for fibrillation can be, and often is, a very stable arrhythmia. However, if fibrillation is due to the random reentry of numerous fractionated wavelets, changing in breadth, direction, and number from moment to moment, then the persistence of the arrhythmia is critically related to the mass and degree of inhomogeneity of the tissue and to the mean ERP. Vagal stimulation or cholinomimetic drugs should tend to perpetuate the arrhythmia by reducing the mean ERP and by increasing the range of variation of the ERPs. The action of quinidine or disopyramide here is twofold. By virtue of their direct and antivagal actions, they may increase the mean ERP and also reduce the inhomogeneity. Thus, the ability to reduce the number of wavelets possible in a given mass of tissue may be more important than the ability to snuff out a dominant circus movement.

Electrocardiographic Effects. At therapeutic concentrations in man, the agents in class I_A produce no change or only small increases in heart rate and in the P–R, H–V, and QRS intervals. The effects on the A–H interval are variable; quinidine is more apt to shorten this interval (and to increase heart rate) because of its effects on the autonomic regulation of the heart. Although moricizine shortens the Q–T interval, the other agents prolong the Q–T interval, reflecting more rapid and slowed rates of repolarization, respectively. Widening of the QRS complex is related to the plasma concentration of drug, and this effect is sometimes useful for monitoring therapy.

Autonomic Nervous System Effects. In experiments with animals, quinidine has a significant atropine-like action, blocking the effects of vagal stimulation or acetylcholine. Quinidine also has α-adrenergic blocking properties. This action can cause vasodilatation and, via baroreceptors, activate sympathetic efferent activity. Together, the cholinergic blockade and increased β-adrenergic activity caused by quinidine can increase sinus rate and enhance AV nodal conduction in some human subjects.

The anticholinergic action of procainamide is much weaker than that of quinidine. Procainamide does not produce α-adrenergic blockade, but, in dogs, it can block autonomic ganglia weakly and cause a measurable impairment of cardiovascular reflexes.

Disopyramide has cholinergic blocking properties about 10% as potent as atropine (Birkhead and Vaughan Williams, 1977; Mirro *et al.*, 1980). These properties usually nullify its direct depressant effects on the sinus and AV nodes. The drug is neither an α- nor a β-adrenergic antagonist.

Absorption, Distribution, and Elimination. *Quinidine.* When administered orally, quinidine sulfate is absorbed rapidly and peak concentrations in plasma are attained in 60 to 90 minutes. The absorption of quinidine gluconate is slower and perhaps less complete; peak concentrations in plasma are not reached until 3 or 4 hours after an oral dose. Although quinidine can be given intramuscularly, it causes pain at the injection site and a substantial increase in creatine kinase activity in plasma.

About 90% of quinidine in plasma is bound to proteins (α_1-acid glycoprotein and albumin). The drug is distributed rapidly to most tissues except brain, and the apparent volume of distribution is 2 to 3 liters per kilogram.

Quinidine is largely metabolized by the liver, and the metabolites and some of the parent drug (20%) are excreted in the urine; the elimination half-time is about 6 hours. Most urinary metabolites are hydroxylated at only one site, either on the quinoline ring or on the quinuclidine ring; small amounts of dihydroxy compounds are also found. The fraction of a dose of quinidine that is metabolized and the metabolic pathway appear to vary considerably from patient to patient. There is controversy about whether the concentration of quinidine in plasma rises in patients with renal failure or congestive heart failure (*see* Kessler *et al.*, 1974; Conrad *et al.*, 1977; Drayer *et al.*, 1977). The situation is complicated by the fact that some of quinidine's major metabolites are probably cardioactive.

Quinidine is both filtered at the glomerulus and secreted by the proximal renal tubule. Since quinidine is a weak base, its reabsorption is reduced and its excretion is enhanced if the urine is acidic. When the urinary pH is increased from the 6–7 range to the 7–8 range, renal clearance of quinidine decreases by as much as 50% and its concentration in the plasma increases. This situation rarely occurs clinically unless the patient takes sodium bicarbonate or acetazolamide concurrently or has renal tubular acidosis.

Procainamide. Procainamide is quickly and nearly completely absorbed after oral administration to normal subjects. The peak concentration in plasma is reached 45 to 75 minutes after ingestion of capsules, but somewhat later after administration of tablets. In the first week after acute myocardial infarction, oral absorption may be poor, the peak plasma concentration may be quite delayed, and concentrations of the drug may be inadequate to control arrhythmias. Sustained-release formulations of procainamide can increase the duration of action to about 8 hours or more, but these have lower bioavailability than do standard capsules.

About 20% of the procainamide in plasma is bound to proteins. Procainamide is rapidly distributed into most body tissues except the brain, and the apparent volume of distribution is about 2 liters per kilogram. However, this value can decrease substantially in patients with cardiac failure or shock. Compensation for this change should be made in calculating dosage.

Procainamide is eliminated by renal excretion and hepatic metabolism. The major metabolic pathway involves N-acetylation by a bimodally distributed N-acetyltransferase that metabolizes isoniazid, dapsone, and other drugs (Gibson *et al.*, 1975; Reidenberg *et al.*, 1975). However, there is another acetylase system that does not show such genetic variation and that also may contribute to the metabolism of procainamide (Giardina *et al.*, 1977). In fast acetylators or in renal insufficiency, 40% or more of a dose of procainamide may be excreted as N-acetylprocainamide (NAPA), and concentrations of NAPA in plasma may equal or exceed those of the parent drug. This compound, which has been assigned the nonproprietary name of *acecainide,* is a less potent antiarrhythmic agent than procainamide, and has qualitatively different cardiac actions. Although it also prolongs the duration of action potentials in Purkinje fibers, NAPA has little effect on $\dot{V}_{max}$ or automaticity. Hence, information should be available about the concentrations of both procainamide and NAPA in plasma for optimal case management.

Up to 70% of a dose of procainamide is eliminated unchanged in the urine. Procainamide is a weak base that is filtered, secreted by the proximal tubule, and reabsorbed by the distal tubule. Marked increases in the pH of the urine cause a decrease in the renal excretion of procainamide. When intrinsic renal function or renal perfusion decreases, the concentration of procainamide in plasma rises significantly. However, as the blood urea nitrogen rises, the fraction of a dose of procainamide that is excreted unchanged decreases, and NAPA can accumulate to dangerous levels.

Disopyramide. About 90% of an oral dose of disopyramide is absorbed, of which a small fraction is subject to first-pass metabolism by the liver. Concentrations in plasma peak at 1 to 2 hours after a dose.

At normal therapeutic concentrations (3 μg/ml) about 70% of disopyramide is bound to plasma proteins; the bound fraction varies inversely with the total concentration of drug in plasma. The apparent volume of distribution of disopyramide is about 0.6 liter per kilogram, but the value is dependent on dose because of the saturable binding to plasma protein.

About 50% of a dose of disopyramide is excreted by the kidney unchanged, 20% as the mono-N-dealkylated metabolite, and another 10% as unidentified metabolites. The monodealkylated metabolite has less antiarrhythmic and atropine-like activity than does the parent compound. The half-time for elimination is 5 to 7 hours, and this value is markedly prolonged in patients with renal insufficiency (up to 20 hours or more).

Preparations, Dosage, and Routes of Administration. *Quinidine.* For practical purposes, quinidine is only given orally, although it can be administered either intramuscularly or intravenously under special circumstances. The usual oral dose of quinidine sulfate is 200 to 300 mg three or four times a day for patients with premature atrial or ventricular contractions or for maintenance therapy. Higher and/or more frequent doses can be used for limited periods for treatment of paroxysmal ventricular tachycardia. During maintenance therapy, quinidine will usually reach a steady state within about 24 hours, and its concentration in plasma will fluctuate less than 50% between doses. Because of the large interindividual variation, drug interactions, and other causes of variability, it is wise to examine the ECG carefully after the initial dose of quinidine and to measure the plasma concentration of the drug at steady state (*see* Appendix II). Adjustment of dosage is often necessary.

Quinidine sulfate (CIN-QUIN) is available in tablets (100 to 300 mg) and capsules (200 and 300 mg); 300-mg sustained-release tablets (QUINIDEX) are available, as is an injection (200 mg/ml). Preparations of the gluconate and polygalacturonate salts are also marketed.

Procainamide. Procainamide hydrochloride (PRONESTYL, others) is available for oral administration as capsules and tablets (250 to 500 mg) and as sustained-release tablets (250 to 1000 mg). *Procainamide hydrochloride injection* contains 100 or 500 mg/ml and is suitable for intramuscular and intravenous injection.

Procainamide can be administered intravenously, intramuscularly, or orally. The concentration in plasma needed to produce antiarrhythmic effects is usually 3 to 10 μg/ml, and occasionally is much higher. The probability of toxicity becomes greater as the plasma concentration rises above 8 μg/ml. The cardiac effects of procainamide are enhanced if the concentration of K^+ in plasma is elevated.

In acute or unstable situations, intravenous administration of procainamide is desirable for speed (injection or rapid infusion), precision (constant infusion), and reliability of effect. The total loading dose is never given as a single intravenous injection because it can cause hypotension. One rapid and safe method to establish effective concentrations in plasma is intermittent intravenous administration: 100 mg is injected over 2 to 4 minutes, and this dose is repeated every 5 minutes until the arrhythmia is controlled, until adverse effects are seen, or until the total size of the dose (about 1000 mg) suggests that the arrhythmia under treatment is resistant. The 5-minute dosing interval permits examination of the blood pressure and ECG after each dose. Serious hypotension or excessive widening of the QRS interval can thus be avoided. Alternatively, the same dose can be given over a similar period by rapid intravenous infusion. For example, 600 mg can be infused at a rate of 20 mg per minute. The same precautions should be taken. When the arrhythmia is controlled, a constant-rate intravenous infusion is often used to maintain effective concentrations in plasma. The infusion rate can be estimated as the product of the desired concentration (3 to 10 μg/ml) and the estimated total clearance of procainamide (*see* Appendix II).

For long-term oral therapy, total daily doses of 3 to 6 g or more usually are required for therapeutic efficacy. Because its elimination half-life is short (about 3 hours in normal subjects and up to 5 to 8 hours in patients with cardiac disease), the drug must be given fairly frequently. However, most patients can take procainamide orally at intervals of 6 to 8 hours. A steady state is reached within 1 day without loading doses because of the short half-life of the drug. When changing from intravenous infusion to oral dosage, the infusion should be stopped and about one elimination half-time permitted to elapse before administration of the first oral dose; the oral dose can be chosen very precisely based on the previous intravenous dose and the resulting plasma concentrations.

Disopyramide. In the United States, disopyramide is approved only for oral administration. It is available as *disopyramide phosphate* in immediate- or controlled-release capsules containing 100 or 150 mg of the base (NAPAMIDE, NORPACE). The usual total daily dose is 400 to 800 mg. This amount can be divided into four doses (most often 100 to 150 mg four times daily) alternatively, 200 to 300 mg of a controlled-release preparation can be given every 12 hours. Although loading doses of 200 to 300 mg will rapidly produce effective concentrations, loading doses are not given to patients with cardiomyopathy or possible cardiac decompensation, and initial doses are limited to 100 mg every 6 to 8 hours. Therapy is never initiated with a controlled-release preparation. Maintenance doses must be carefully adjusted for patients with renal failure according to the creatinine clearance; efficacy, toxic manifestations, and plasma concentrations should be monitored in such patients.

Therapeutic Uses. The drugs in class I_A have a broad spectrum of action and are effective for short- and long-term treatment of supraventricular and ventricular arrhythmias. Although experience in Europe indicates that disopyramide is useful in the treatment of atrial arrhythmias, in the United States it is approved only for the treatment of ventricular arrhythmias in adults. Individualization of dosage is usually required at the outset of therapy because both plasma concentrations and antiarrhythmic responses will vary from patient to patient. Several 24-hour Holter ECG recordings are often required to ensure adequate control of arrhythmias. Vigilance must be maintained to detect toxic reactions.

Paroxysmal Supraventricular Tachycardia (PSVT). Quinidine, procainamide, and disopyramide can be effective against recurrent, aggravating PSVT, either the usual AV nodal reciprocating tachycardia or the PSVT seen in the Wolff–Parkinson–White syndrome. In the AV nodal form of PSVT, digitalis administration and other methods usually are tried before quinidine or other drugs in class I_A. The mode of action of these agents in PSVT is not certain. They may suppress the atrial premature depolarizations that trigger the PSVT, or alter conduction and refractoriness of the atrium and AV node so that PSVT no longer occurs. In the Wolff–Parkinson–White syndrome, these drugs slow conduction and increase refractoriness in the accessory AV connection and, therefore, prevent attacks of PSVT.

Atrial Flutter or Fibrillation. Quinidine was once used as the drug of choice for conversion of atrial flutter or atrial fibrillation to sinus rhythm. Since the advent of direct-current (DC) cardioversion, quinidine and procainamide have been relegated to supporting roles in the management of these two arrhythmias. Patients scheduled for cardioversion are given oral maintenance doses 1 or 2 days before the anticipated cardioversion. Perhaps one third of patients with atrial fibrillation and a similar proportion of patients with atrial flutter will convert to sinus rhythm before cardioversion, but the majority require DC shock. Maintenance therapy with quinidine or procainamide helps to prevent recurrence of atrial fibrillation. If atrial premature depolarizations occur soon after cardioversion, the dose of drug should be increased until they are abolished or drug toxicity is encountered. If uninterrupted sinus rhythm resumes after cardioversion, the concentration of drug in plasma should be adjusted to achieve optimal steady-state values (*e.g.*, between 2 and 5 μg of quinidine per milliliter).

Ventricular Premature Depolarizations and Unsustained Ventricular Tachycardia. Class-I_A drugs are effective for the long-term treatment of these arrhythmias or for the the prevention of ventricular fibrillation. Ventricular premature depolarization (VPD) is a very common rhythm disturbance. VPDs are treated when they cause discomfort (palpitations), impair hemodynamic performance, or increase the likelihood of death (*see* Table 35–2). When treating VPDs or brief recurrent bursts of ventricular tachycardia, the dosage of drug is adjusted and 24-hour Holter ECG recordings are used to establish drug efficacy. Usually, the dosage of drug is increased until complex forms (pairs or runs of VPDs) are abolished and the frequency of VPDs is reduced by 70 to 80%; this dosage is then maintained. When the arrhythmia is caused by an acute process, such as open-heart surgery, acute myocardial infarction, or acute myocarditis, the drug can be discontinued when the situation is resolved. If the arrhythmia treated was life threatening, the drug should be discontinued while the patient is being monitored.

Sustained Ventricular Tachycardia. The treatment of sustained ventricular tachycardia is quite different. Prior to the advent of DC cardioversion, heroic and skilled dosage with quinidine was used to convert ventricular tachycardia to sinus rhythm. The incidence of toxicity was high with this approach, and it has been abandoned. Although sustained ventricular tachycardia can be relatively resistant to treatment with drugs, it usually responds readily to DC conversion. After conversion, drug efficacy is evaluated by electrophysiological observations (Horowitz *et al.*, 1980; Swerdlow *et al.*, 1983).

Digitalis-Induced Arrhythmias. The complex rhythm disturbances that can attend digitalis toxicity are discussed in detail in Chapter 34. Although quinidine or other class I_A agents can be effective for the treatment of digitalis-induced arrhythmias, they are not the preferred drugs, because adverse effects on cardiac rhythm are more likely to occur with their use than with other effective treatments (*e.g.*, phenytoin, lidocaine, or anti-digoxin antibody).

Untoward Effects. *Quinidine.* About one third of the patients who receive quinidine will have immediate adverse effects that necessitate discontinuation of therapy.

If this initial hurdle is passed, few extracardiac adverse effects are encountered during long-term therapy. However, excessive concentration of the drug in plasma will cause adverse effects in any patient. Because quinidine has a low therapeutic ratio, constant vigilance is required in every patient taking this drug (*see* Woosley and Roden, 1987).

Cardiotoxicity. As the concentration of quinidine in plasma rises above 2 μg/ml, the QRS complex and the Q–T_c interval will widen progressively. These changes are useful in monitoring quinidine therapy. If the duration of the QRS complex increases by 50% or more, the dosage should be reduced. At high plasma concentrations of the drug, cardiac toxicity may become severe; SA block or arrest, high-grade AV block, ventricular tachyarrhythmias, or asystole may occur. Conduction is slowed tremendously in all parts of the heart. In addition, Purkinje fibers can become depolarized and develop abnormal automaticity. These changes are responsible for the bizarre arrhythmias seen in severe poisoning with quinidine. Quinidine can produce early afterdepolarizations and triggered activity in Purkinje fibers exposed to low concentrations of K^+ *in vitro* (Roden and Hoffman, 1985). Polymorphic ventricular tachycardia (*torsades de pointes*) caused by quinidine is a life-threatening event and must be treated with the utmost caution. The ECG must be closely monitored in an intensive care unit. Sodium lactate or bicarbonate, catecholamines, glucagon, and magnesium sulfate may be useful in counteracting ventricular tachyarrhythmias caused by quinidine. Quinidine and its hydroxy metabolites can be removed by dialysis (Conrad *et al.,* 1977).

Occasionally, patients taking quinidine experience syncope or sudden death. In some instances, this reaction may be the result of high concentrations of quinidine in plasma or the result of coexisting digitalis toxicity. However, *torsades de pointes* may occur in susceptible individuals while the concentrations of quinidine in plasma are below or within the therapeutic range. Individuals with the long Q–T syndrome or those who respond to low concentrations of quinidine with marked lengthening of the Q–T interval appear to be particularly at risk and should not be treated with this drug (Koster and Wellens, 1976). Bradycardia and hypokalemia are also risk factors for *torsades de pointes* (Morganroth, 1987).

A frequently mentioned complication of quinidine when the drug is used to treat atrial fibrillation is the so-called paradoxical increase in ventricular rate. Quinidine and other drugs in class I_A can cause a substantial decrease in the atrial rate in atrial fibrillation. If the atrial rate decreases sufficiently, the ventricular rate may increase abruptly because of the decrease in concealed conduction of atrial impulses in the AV node. In some patients, quinidine (or disopyramide) may be anticholinergic as well. A paradoxical increase in ventricular rate is not common in patients treated with these drugs. However, the effect can be so dramatic that it is traditional to digitalize patients with atrial fibrillation or flutter prior to administration of a class-I_A antiarrhythmic agent.

Blood Pressure. Quinidine can cause significant hypotension, particularly when given intravenously. This response is probably due to the α-adrenergic blocking effect of the drug. Hemodynamic studies indicate that hypotension due to quinidine is caused by vasodilatation without a significant decrease in cardiac output; therapeutic concentrations of quinidine have no significant adverse effects on myocardial performance.

Arterial Embolism. The risk of embolism after conversion of atrial fibrillation to sinus rhythm is a source of concern. The fibrillating atria do not contract, and thrombi often develop in the left atrium. After sinus rhythm resumes, atrial contraction may dislodge thrombi; stroke is the most dreaded sequela of the resultant arterial embolization. However, the long-term risk of systemic embolization is greater if atrial fibrillation persists than if conversion to sinus rhythm occurs. If cardioversion is performed as an elective procedure, patients are usually given anticoagulants for 1 to 2 weeks prior to conversion.

Cinchonism. Like other cinchona alkaloids and the salicylates, quinidine can cause cinchonism. Symptoms of mild cinchonism include tinnitus, loss of hearing, slight blurring of vision, and gastrointestinal upset. If toxicity is severe, headache, diplopia, photophobia, and altered color perception may occur, as can confusion, delirium, and psychosis. The skin may be hot and flushed; nausea, vomiting, diarrhea, and abdominal pain are likely.

Gastrointestinal Symptoms. The most common adverse reactions to quinidine occur in the gastrointestinal tract—nausea, vomiting, and diarrhea. Gastrointestinal symptoms often occur even when drug concentrations in plasma are low. This type of adverse reaction is apparent almost immediately after quinidine is started and forces early discontinuation of the drug in almost one third of patients so treated.

Hypersensitivity Reactions. Hypersensitivity to quinidine can cause fever; this reaction is rare and disappears when the drug is discontinued. Rarely, quinidine causes anaphylactic reactions, which require emergency measures. Thrombocytopenia is an uncommon but potentially lethal outcome of treatment with quinidine. Thrombocytopenia usually occurs after several weeks or months of therapy and is due to formation of drug–platelet complexes that evoke a circulating antibody. When quinidine, platelets, antibody, and complement are all present in the circulation, platelets agglutinate and lyse. Thrombocytopenia can be profound, and severe bleeding may ensue. If quinidine is stopped, the platelet count will return to near normal within days. Until the bleeding time is normal, patients should be kept in the hospital and, if necessary, treated with adrenocorticosteroids. Asthma-like respiratory difficulty or vascular collapse can occur as a result of hypersensitivity. Artificial ventilation and supportive measures are usually effective.

Procainamide. Cardiotoxicity. Excessive plasma concentrations of procainamide produce ECG changes very similar to those seen during quinidine therapy. The same rules and precautions for using and discontinuing quinidine (*see* above) pertain to procainamide. Interestingly, the syndrome of marked Q–T prolongation and *torsades de pointes* described for quinidine is less common with procainamide and usually occurs in renal failure when plasma concentrations of NAPA rise markedly. Procainamide, like quinidine, will slow the atria in atrial fibrillation and can thereby cause a "paradoxical" increase in the ventricular response.

Blood Pressure. If procainamide is administered intravenously, it can cause hypotension. Intermittent or continuous intravenous infusion can be adjusted so that significant hypotension is unusual, provided that doses do not exceed 600 mg over a period of 25 to 30 minutes. Toxic concentrations of procainamide can diminish myocardial performance and promote hypotension.

Extracardiac Adverse Effects. During oral administration of procainamide, gastrointestinal symptoms (anorexia, nausea, vomiting, and, rarely, diarrhea) may occur; these symptoms are much less common than with quinidine. Procainamide can produce adverse effects on the CNS, including giddiness, psychosis, hallucinations, and mental depression.

Hypersensitivity Reactions. Occasionally, fever occurs during the first few days of therapy and forces discontinuance of procainamide. Agranulocytosis may occur in the early weeks of therapy; fatal infections may follow (Meyers *et al.*, 1985). Leukocyte and differential blood counts should be done regularly during therapy, and complaints of sore throat should be promptly evaluated. Myalgias, angioedema, skin rashes, digital vasculitis, and Raynaud's phenomenon have all been attributed to procainamide.

Procainamide can cause a syndrome that superficially resembles authentic systemic lupus erythematosus (SLE). Arthralgia is the most common symptom; pericarditis, pleuropneumonic involvement, fever, and hepatomegaly are common signs. The most serious complication is hemorrhagic pericardial effusion with tamponade. Drug-induced SLE is different from the naturally occurring disease in that there is no predilection for females; the brain and kidney are spared; leukopenia, anemia, thrombocytopenia, and hyperglobulinemia are rare; and false-positive serologic tests for syphilis do not occur. The drug-induced syndrome is reversible when procainamide is discontinued. At least 60 to 70% of patients who receive procainamide will develop antinuclear antibodies after 1 to 12 months of therapy. These antibodies are directed against nuclear histones. Only 20 to 30% of patients with antinuclear antibodies will develop the clinical symptoms and signs of the SLE syndrome if treatment is continued. When symptoms occur, LE-cell preparations are often positive. The development of antinuclear antibodies alone is insufficient reason to discontinue therapy with procainamide. However, the benefits and risks of continued therapy should be assessed, and procainamide is usually stopped when patients become symptomatic. It is not yet clear if individuals who acetylate procainamide slowly have an increased risk of developing the SLE-like syndrome; however, antinuclear antibodies appear more rapidly in slow acetylators than in fast acetylators (Giardina *et al.*, 1977; Woosley *et al.*, 1978). The use of acecainide (NAPA) has only rarely been associated with the development of antinuclear antibodies.

Disopyramide. The anticholinergic action of disopyramide produces a significant incidence of dry mouth, constipation, blurred vision, urinary hesitancy, and, occasionally, urinary retention. These effects are more common than with other drugs in class I_A. Disopyramide can cause nausea, abdominal pain, vomiting, or diarrhea, but gastrointestinal symptoms are significantly less common than when quinidine is used. Disopyramide reduces cardiac output and left ventricular performance by a direct depressant effect and peripheral arteriolar constriction. The adverse effects on ventricular function can be striking in patients who have preexisting ventricular failure (Jensen *et al.*, 1975; Podrid *et al.*, 1980). Great caution should be exercised in treating such patients with disopyramide. The adverse hemodynamic effects are more marked than those of other antiarrhythmic drugs. The blood pressure usually increases transiently after intravenous administration of disopyramide, even though the cardiac output falls; total peripheral vascular resistance thus increases markedly (*see* Di Bianco *et al.*, 1987; Willis, 1987).

Drug Interactions. Drugs that induce drug-metabolizing enzymes in the liver, such as phenobarbital or phenytoin, may significantly shorten the duration of action of quinidine by increasing its rate of elimination. Since patients vary tremendously in their susceptibility to enzyme induction, it is difficult to predict which individuals will be affected. When quinidine is given to patients who have stable concentrations of digoxin in plasma, the digoxin concentration usually doubles because of a decrease in its clearance (Bigger, 1982). Occasionally, patients who are receiving warfarin or other oral anticoagulants will have an increase in prothrombin time after quinidine is begun; the mechanism of this reaction is not clear. Since quinidine is an α-adrenergic blocking agent, it can interact additively with drugs that cause vasodilatation or decreased blood volume. For example, nitroglycerin can cause severe postural hypotension in patients who are taking quinidine. The effect of any given concentration of any antiarrhythmic drug in class I_A on conduction in the heart is greater when the concentration of K^+ in plasma is increased.

CLASS I_B: LIDOCAINE, PHENYTOIN, TOCAINIDE, AND MEXILETINE

Antiarrhythmic drugs in class I_B produce only small changes in phase-0 depolarization and conduction velocity in myocardial Purkinje fibers when resting values of Vm are normal (*see* Table 35–3). However, the depressant effects of class-I_B drugs on these parameters are markedly intensified when the membrane is depolarized or when the frequency of excitation is increased. In contrast to drugs in class I_A, those in class I_B usually hasten membrane repolarization. Lidocaine is the prototypical agent, although it is the only member of this class that is not effective orally.

History. Lidocaine is widely used as a local anesthetic (*see* Chapter 15). It was introduced as an antiarrhythmic agent in 1962 for the emergency treatment of ventricular arrhythmias after cardiac surgery or acute myocardial infarction. Two orally effective relatives of lidocaine have recently become available—tocainide in 1984 and mexiletine in 1986.

Phenytoin has been used since 1938 for the treatment of seizures (*see* Chapter 19). In 1950, Harris and Kokernot found that phenytoin was therapeutically effective for ventricular tachycardia in experimental myocardial infarction in dogs. Clinical studies have demonstrated its usefulness for ventricular arrhythmias in man, especially those associated with digitalis toxicity.

Chemistry. The chemistry and structures of lidocaine and phenytoin are discussed in Chapters 15 and 19, respectively. The chemical structures of tocainide and mexiletine closely resemble that of lidocaine and are as follows:

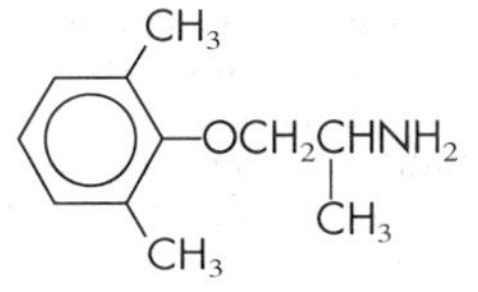

Mexiletine

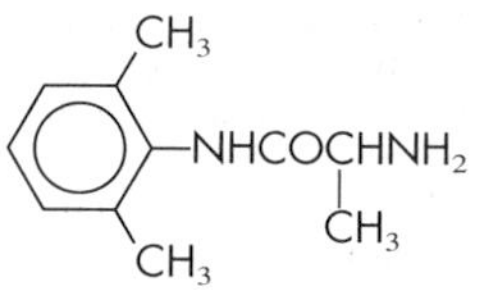

Tocainide

Cardiac Electrophysiological Effects. *Automaticity.* It is distinctly unusual for therapeutic concentrations of class-I_B drugs to depress the human sinus node, but it can occur in patients with preexisting disease of the sinus node (Bigger and Reiffel, 1979; Kerr *et al.*, 1983). Therapeutic concentrations of these agents decrease the slope of normal phase-4 depolarization in Purkinje fibers. This action is caused by a decrease in the pacemaker current (i_f) and an increase in time-independent outward current (i_{K_1}) (Weld and Bigger, 1976; Carmeliet and Saikawa, 1982). However, the capacity of tocainide and mexiletine to reduce the automaticity of Purkinje fibers is more reminiscent of quinidine, in that a shift of the threshold voltage for firing toward more positive values of *Vm* has an important role (Roden and Woosley, 1986b; Campbell, 1987). Lidocaine also can counteract automaticity in depolarized, stretched Purkinje fibers, and both lidocaine and phenytoin are effective in abolishing triggered activity due to digitalis-induced delayed afterdepolarizations (Rosen *et al.*, 1976; Peon *et al.*, 1978). These effects could result from an increase in i_{K_1} that overcomes small inward currents that cause depolarization or from a decrease in inward Na^+ current (Carmeliet and Saikawa, 1982; Colatsky, 1982).

Excitability and Threshold. Class-I_B agents cause an increase in the diastolic electrical current threshold in cardiac Purkinje fibers by increasing K^+ conductance (g_{K_1}) without changing resting *Vm* or the voltage threshold. They also increase the threshold for ventricular fibrillation.

Responsiveness and Conduction. The effects of lidocaine on membrane responsiveness are complex. The steady-state relationship between $\dot{V}_{max}$ and *Vm* is little altered in normal Purkinje fibers by therapeutic concentrations of lidocaine, but fast responses are prevented at low (less negative) values of *Vm*. This effect can be explained by a lidocaine-induced increase in i_{K_1}. The effect of lidocaine on responsiveness depends on $[K]_o$: at $[K]_o$ up to 4.5 mM, therapeutic concentrations have little effect; at $[K]_o$ of 5.6 or 6.0, therapeutic concentrations of lidocaine reduce $\dot{V}_{max}$ at any level of *Vm* (Obayashi *et al.*, 1975). Toxic concentrations shift responsiveness in much the same way as quinidine does. Lidocaine suppresses the responsiveness of abnormal ventricular muscle fibers that survive experimental infarction (Kupersmith *et al.*, 1975). The effect of lidocaine on responsiveness is use dependent and is increased at fast heart rates (*see* above) (Hondeghem and Katzung, 1980; Bean *et al.*, 1983).

Because of the large safety factor for conduction, lidocaine and the other drugs in class I_B usually have no effect on conduction velocity in normal tissues of the His–Purkinje system or ventricular muscle. Under abnormal circumstances, these agents may either decrease or increase conduction velocity in the His–Purkinje system or in ventricular muscle; in ischemic tissues, conduction velocity usually decreases substantially (Kupersmith *et al.*, 1975). In tissues depolarized by stretch or low $[K]_o$, lidocaine can cause hyperpolarization and significant increases in conduction velocity (Arnsdorf and Bigger, 1972). It is not known if other drugs in class I_B share this property with lidocaine.

Duration of the Action Potential and Refractoriness. Antiarrhythmic drugs in class I_B cause almost no change in the duration of the action potential of atrial fibers. They substantially decrease the duration of the action potential in Purkinje fibers and ventricular muscle; this effect is attributed to blockade of small Na^+ currents that flow during the plateau of the action potential (Colatsky, 1982). The greatest change is seen in the portions of the His–Purkinje system in which the duration of the action potential is normally longest (Wittig *et al.*, 1973). This tends to reduce the temporal and spatial dispersion of refractoriness. The effective refractory period shortens after exposure to drugs in this class.

Effect on Reentrant Arrhythmias. Class-I_B drugs can abolish ventricular reentry, either by causing two-way block or by improving conduction. If one-way block occurs in ischemic, depolarized elements of a reentry circuit, two-way block is the more likely mechanism. In patients with impaired AV nodal and ventricular conduction, tocainide and mexiletine may be more apt to reduce conduction velocities in the affected regions than is lidocaine (*see* Keefe *et al.*, 1981). Conduction can actually be improved by lidocaine if depolarization and slow conduction are due to decreased g_{K_1} (*e.g.*, stretch or low $[K]_o$).

The drugs in class I_B are much less effective than quinidine, procainamide, or disopyramide in slowing the atrial rate in atrial flutter or atrial fibrillation or in converting these arrhythmias to sinus rhythm. This is expected, since class-I_B agents have so little effect on either refractoriness or responsiveness in the atria.

Electrocardiographic Effects. In striking contrast to the drugs in class I_A, those in class I_B cause negligible change in the ECG; the Q–T interval may shorten, but the QRS does not widen. The refractory period of the AV node shortens or does not change; in patients with atrial flutter and who show substantial shortening of the AV nodal refractory period, a marked increase in ventricular response can result. Usually the ERP in the His–Purkinje system shortens substantially during treatment with these agents; however, it can lengthen in patients with preexisting bundle-branch disease.

Autonomic Nervous System Effects. Except for phenytoin, the agents in class I_B have no significant interaction with the autonomic nervous system. Most of the effects of phenytoin, if not all, arise from actions within the CNS; vagal efferent activity is modulated, and the efferent traffic in cardiac sympathetic nerves that is enhanced during digitalis intoxication is reduced by phenytoin.

Absorption, Distribution, and Elimination. *Lidocaine.* Although lidocaine is well absorbed after oral administration, it is subject to extensive first-pass hepatic metabolism, and only about one third of the drug reaches the general circulation. Many patients experience nausea, vomiting, and abdominal discomfort after oral administration of lidocaine; this route is not used. The drug is almost completely absorbed after intramuscular administration.

About 70% of lidocaine in plasma is bound to proteins, mostly α_1-acid glycoprotein. Distribution is rapid, and the apparent volume of distribution for lidocaine is normally about 1 liter per kilogram; this volume is substantially reduced in patients with heart failure.

Essentially no lidocaine is excreted unchanged in the urine. Deethylation in the liver results in the appearance of monoethylglycylxylidine and then glycine xylidide. The former metabolite has antiarrhythmic activity, while the latter has almost none (Burney *et al.*, 1974). Severe hepatic disease or reduced perfusion of the liver in heart failure decreases the rate of metabolism. The clearance of lidocaine approaches the rate of hepatic blood flow and is thus very sensitive to changes in this parameter (Nies *et al.*, 1976). The clearance of lidocaine also may decrease as a result of prolonged infusion (LeLorier *et al.*, 1977). The half-time for elimination is normally about 100 minutes.

Phenytoin. Only a few points that are crucial to the use of phenytoin as an antiarrhythmic drug will be discussed here. A more detailed discussion is presented in Chapter 19. Absorption of phenytoin from the gastrointestinal tract is slow and somewhat erratic. Absorption after intramuscular injection is also slow and may be incomplete. About 90% of phenytoin in plasma is bound to albumin; the fraction is less in patients with uremia. After intravenous administration, phenytoin is distributed to tissues rapidly. The drug is eliminated by hepatic hydroxylation. The major metabolites of phenytoin probably lack antiarrhythmic activity. Metabolism is relatively slow and is not substantially altered by changes in hepatic blood flow. The enzyme system that metabolizes phenytoin becomes saturated by concentrations of the drug in the therapeutic range; hence, the half-time for elimination is dose dependent, and unexpected toxicity can occur (*see* Chapter 19; Appendix II).

Tocainide. Tocainide is completely absorbed after oral administration; peak concentrations in plasma occur within 1 to 2 hours. About 40% of a dose of tocainide is excreted as such in the urine. The half-life in plasma is 11 to 15 hours, and this value may increase twofold in patients with renal or hepatic disease (*see* Holmes *et al.*, 1983; Hasegawa, 1985).

Mexiletine. Mexiletine is readily absorbed after oral administration, and its systemic bioavailability is about 90%. The drug is eliminated after hepatic metabolism; about 10% of a dose is found unchanged in the urine. The elimination half-life is approximately 10 hours (*see* Schrader and Bauman, 1986).

Preparations, Dosage, and Routes of Administration. *Lidocaine. Lidocaine hydrochloride injection* (XYLOCAINE) is available for intravenous administration in solutions for infusion (2, 4, or 8 mg/ml), for direct administration (10 or 20 mg/ml), and for dilution into admixtures (40, 100, or 200 mg/ml); solutions for intramuscular injection contain 100 mg/ml. These solutions contain no preservative, sympathomimetic, or other vasoconstrictor. Catastrophic arrhythmias can occur if preparations that contain sympathomimetic amines are used accidentally.

Lidocaine is only administered intravenously or intramuscularly. To achieve effective concentrations rapidly, intravenous administration of about 0.7 to 1.4 mg/kg of body weight is used. A second injection may be required in 5 minutes; no more than 200 to 300 mg should be given in 1 hour. Smaller doses should be used for patients who have heart failure. Rapid infusion may also be employed to administer a loading dose. A constant rate of intravenous infusion is used to maintain an effective concentration. Infusions in the range of 1 to 4 mg per minute produce therapeutic concentrations in plasma of 1 to 5 μg/ml in 7 to 10 hours; in patients with heart failure or shock, the same rate of infusion will produce plasma concentrations two or more times higher (*see* Appendix II). As the circulatory status changes, hepatic blood flow can change dramatically and shifts in the concentration of lidocaine in plasma will reflect these alterations (Nies *et al.*, 1976). An intramuscular dose of 4 to 5 mg/kg will produce an effective concentration of lidocaine within 15 minutes, and this therapeutic level is maintained for about 90 minutes.

Phenytoin. The preparations of phenytoin are presented in Chapter 19. Phenytoin should be given orally or by intermittent injection; the injectable preparation has a pH of about 12 and causes severe phlebitis if infused. Critical arrhythmias should not be treated by the intramuscular route because absorption is too unreliable. The schedule for intermittent intravenous injection of phenytoin is almost identical to that described above for procainamide: 100 mg of phenytoin is given every 5 minutes until the arrhythmia is controlled or until adverse effects are encountered (Bigger *et al.*, 1968). The rate of injection should not exceed 50 mg per minute. Usually about 700 mg is required; doses above 1000 mg are rarely needed. Oral treatment of arrhythmias usually is initiated with loading doses because of phenytoin's long elimination half-time. A dose of 15 mg/kg is given the first day, 7.5 mg/kg on the second day, and 4 to 6 mg/kg per day for long-term maintenance (most often 300 to 400 mg per day). The oral maintenance dose can be given once a day or divided into two portions.

Tocainide. Tocainide hydrochloride (TONOCARD) is available in 400- and 600-mg tablets. The usual oral dose is 400 to 600 mg every 8 hours up to a maximum of about 2400 mg per day; daily dosages should be reduced to less than 1200 mg in patients with renal or hepatic impairment.

Mexiletine. Mexiletine hydrochloride (MEXITIL) is supplied in 150-, 200-, and 250-mg capsules. The usual oral dosage is 200 to 300 mg (up to a maximum of 400 mg) given every 8 hours with food or antacids. For rapid response, an initial dose of 400 mg may be given. Reduced dosage may be required in patients with hepatic impairment.

Therapeutic Uses. *Lidocaine.* Lidocaine is used almost exclusively to treat ventricular arrhythmias, primarily in intensive care units. Lidocaine is effective against ventricular arrhythmias caused by acute myocardial infarction, open-heart surgery, and digitalis. Lidocaine tends to prevent primary ventricular fibrillation in the acute phase of myocardial infarction, but no beneficial effect on mortality has been demonstrated (DeSilva *et al.*, 1981; MacMahon *et al.*, 1988).

Phenytoin. Phenytoin is used to treat ventricular arrhythmias, paroxysmal atrial flutter or fibrillation, and supraventricular arrhythmias caused by digitalis. Phenytoin is effective against the ventricular arrhythmias seen after open-heart surgery and acute myocardial infarction, but lidocaine is equally effective and is easier to use. Phenytoin is relatively ineffective against recurrent, drug-resistant ventricular tachycardia in patients with chronic ischemic heart disease. Phenytoin reduces ventricular arrhythmias in the year after myocardial infarction if the concentration of the drug in plasma is kept above 10 μg/ml; such concentrations are readily attained with doses of 400 to 500 mg per day. Phenytoin is highly effective against multiform and complex ventricular premature depolarizations, ventricular tachycardia, and atrial tachycardia with AV block induced by digitalis; often, small doses are effective. It is somewhat less effective against nonparoxysmal AV junctional tachycardia; larger doses are needed, and a larger fraction of cases fails to respond. Phenytoin has been used effectively with electrophysiological guidance against sustained ventricular tachycardia in chronic coronary heart disease and against ventricular tachyarrhythmias in the long Q–T syndrome, in conjunction with a β-adrenergic blocking agent (Schwartz *et al.*, 1975). The effects of phenytoin on sinus arrest or sinoatrial block caused by digitalis in human subjects are unknown. Phenytoin is relatively ineffective against the common atrial arrhythmias, such as atrial flutter, atrial fibrillation, and supraventricular tachycardia (*see* Atkinson and Davison, 1974; Wit *et al.*, 1975).

Tocainide and Mexiletine. Tocainide and mexiletine are indicated for the oral treatment of ventricular arrhythmias; responsiveness to lidocaine is quite predictive of a response to tocainide. Long-term oral treatment of ventricular ectopic beats with either tocainide or mexiletine has met with variable success. The effectiveness of these drugs is less than that of procainamide or quinidine (*see* Holmes *et al.*, 1983). Mexiletine can suppress ventricular tachycardia in some patients who have not responded to quinidine or other drugs in class I_A.

Untoward Effects. Antiarrhythmic agents in class I_B have fewer adverse cardiac effects than do those in either class I_A or class I_C. They cause less serious proarrhythmic effects and are less likely to aggravate heart failure.

Lidocaine. Lidocaine has few undesirable cardiovascular effects. Its main adverse effects are on the CNS. At concentrations in plasma near 5 μg/ml, symptoms are often subtle, such as feelings of dissociation, paresthesias (often perioral), mild drowsiness, or agitation. Higher concentrations may cause decreased hearing, disorientation, muscle twitching, convulsions, or respiratory arrest. The minor CNS effects are not dangerous, but do severely disturb some patients. Such symptoms should prompt a decrease of the infusion rate. The more severe toxic manifestations are life threatening.

Phenytoin. The most prominent adverse effects of phenytoin during short-term treatment of arrhythmias are referable to the CNS and include drowsiness, nystagmus, vertigo, ataxia, and nausea. The progression of such symptoms shows an orderly relationship to increasing concentrations in plasma. In short-term treatment of arrhythmias, neurological signs usually indicate that plasma concentrations are in excess of 20 μg/ml. This information is useful; if an arrhythmia has not responded to phenytoin at concentrations of about 20 μg/ml, it is unlikely to respond at higher concentrations.

Tocainide and Mexiletine. Both tocainide and mexiletine cause CNS symptoms (*e.g.*, dizziness, light-headedness, and tremor) and gastrointestinal symptoms (*e.g.*, nausea, vomiting, and anorexia) (Roden and Woosley, 1986b; Campbell, 1987). The use of tocainide, but not of mexiletine, has been associated with agranulocytosis, bone marrow depression, and thrombocytopenia (Volosin *et al.*, 1985; Soff and Kadin, 1987). The sequelae of granulocytopenia have included serious infections, sepsis, and death. When the white blood cell count is less than 1000, the mortality rate is about 25%. Granulocytopenia usually occurs in the first 12 weeks of treatment; it is recommended that white blood cell, differential, and platelet counts be done weekly for the first 3 months of treatment. If abnormalities are detected, tocainide should be discontinued. The blood cell counts usually return to normal within a month. Because of the risk of agranulocytosis, tocainide should be used only when other drugs have been ineffective.

Drug Interactions. Few drug interactions have been reported with lidocaine. β-Adrenergic antagonists can decrease hepatic blood flow in patients with heart disease, causing a decrease in the rate of hepatic metabolism of lidocaine and an increase in its plasma concentration (Nies *et al.*, 1976). Other basic drugs can displace lidocaine from its binding sites on α_1-acid glycoprotein (Routledge *et al.*, 1980). Plasma concentrations of lidocaine are higher in patients who are receiving cimetidine concurrently. The mechanism of this interaction is complex, but the dose of lidocaine may require adjustment (Knapp *et al.*, 1983). Lidocaine can potentiate the effects of succinylcholine.

The hepatic metabolism of mexiletine can be accelerated by concurrent administration of phenytoin or rifampin. No clinically significant drug interactions have been reported for tocainide.

A large number of interactions with other drugs have been described during long-term administration of phenytoin; these are discussed in Chapter 19.

CLASS I_C: FLECAINIDE, ENCAINIDE, AND PROPAFENONE

Class-I_C drugs have a high affinity for sarcolemmal Na^+ channels; they are the most potent of the antiarrhythmic agents in slowing conduction of the cardiac impulse and in suppressing i_{Na} and spontaneous ventricular premature complexes (*see* Symposium, 1984c; Roden and Woosley, 1986a). The first drug in this class, flecainide, was introduced into clinical practice in the United States in 1986. Encainide is also available for general use, while propafenone and indecainide are being investigated. The role of these drugs in the treatment of supraventricular and ventricular arrhythmias is still being defined.

Chemistry. The structural formulas of flecainide, encainide, propafenone, and indecainide are as follows:

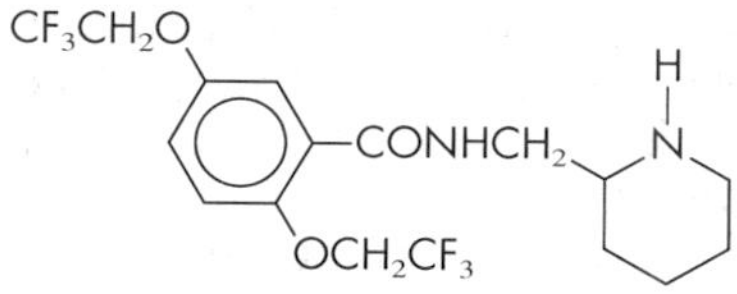

Flecainide

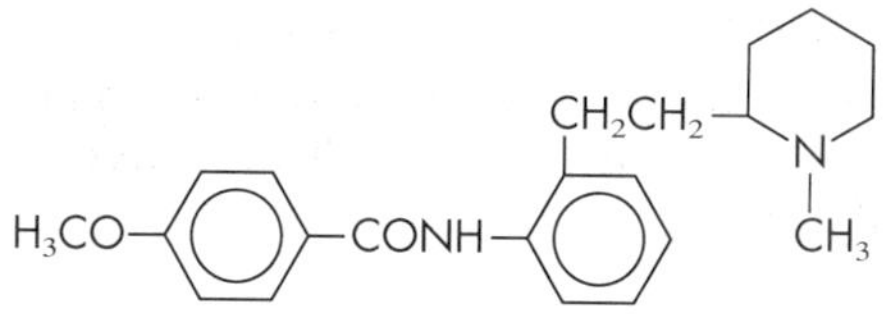

Encainide

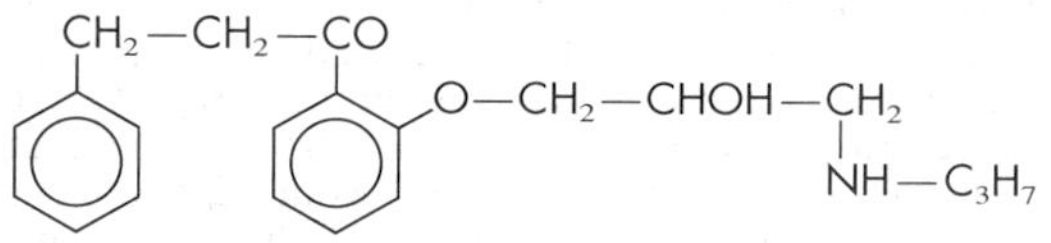

Propafenone

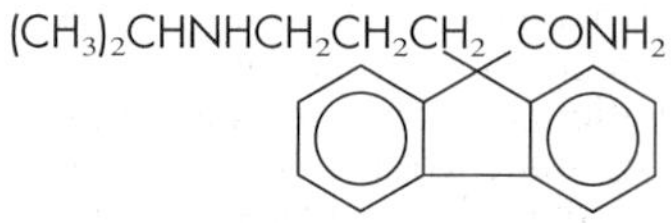

Indecainide

Cardiac Electrophysiological Effects. The drugs in class I_C bind tightly to and block fast Na^+ channels. Thus, they decrease the $\dot{V}_{max}$ and overshoot of action potentials in atrial, ventricular, and Purkinje fibers and slow conduction in these structures, most prominently in the His–Purkinje system (*see* Symposium, 1984c, 1984d, 1986). There are relatively small effects on repolarization, duration of action potentials, and the ERP in Purkinje fibers. The refractory period of the AV node is usually increased and refractory periods in accessory pathways are markedly prolonged by these drugs. In addition, propafenone has weak β-adrenergic blocking effects.

Electrocardiographic Effects. At therapeutic concentrations in man, class-I_C drugs have little effect on heart rate; however, they cause a substantial increase in the P–R interval and the duration of the QRS complex (Symposium, 1984c, 1984d, 1986). The P–R interval may increase to 0.30 second and the QRS complex may be prolonged to 0.18 second; the dose should be reduced if these values are exceeded. The Q–T_c interval may be prolonged due to marked widening of the QRS complex, but the J–T interval (from end of QRS to the end of the T wave) always shortens. Clinical electrophysiological studies reveal a substantial increase in the P–A, A–H, and H–V intervals; the latter may lengthen by 15 to 20 msec, more than that observed with any other class of antiarrhythmic drugs.

Absorption, Distribution, and Elimination. *Flecainide.* Flecainide is almost completely absorbed after oral administration; peak concentrations in plasma occur at about 3 hours. Flecainide is metabolized by the liver; about 40% is excreted in the urine unchanged. The metabolites have little or no antiarrhythmic activity. The average half-time of elimination is about 11 hours. Flecainide may accumulate in patients with renal failure, and its concentration in plasma and the ECG should be carefully monitored during treatment of such patients (Symposium, 1984c; Roden and Woosley, 1986a).

Encainide. Encainide is also almost completely absorbed after oral administration, but its bioavailability is reduced to about 30% by first-pass hepatic metabolism. Peak concentrations in plasma occur at 30 to 90 minutes. Encainide is metabolized by the hepatic cytochrome P_{450} system and has a half-life in plasma of 2 to 3 hours. About 10% of the population have a genetically determined deficiency in this

P_{450} system; the bioavailability increases to greater than 80% and the half-life is prolonged to 10 to 12 hours in such individuals. Two active metabolites are formed: O-desmethylencainide (half-life of 3 to 4 hours) and 3-methoxy-O-desmethylencainide (half-life of 6 to 12 hours). While the parent compound is responsible for the effects of the drug in the 10% of patients who metabolize encainide slowly, these metabolites account for most of the antiarrhythmic actions of encainide in the majority of patients. They accumulate in the plasma of patients with renal failure, thus necessitating a reduction in dosage (Symposium, 1986; Woosley *et al.*, 1988).

Propafenone. Although propafenone is almost completely absorbed from the gastrointestinal tract, its bioavailability is reduced by extensive first-pass hepatic metabolism and is dose dependent; values range from 5 to 40% for patients with normal hepatic function or up to 60% in those with severe liver disease (*see* Symposium, 1984d). Peak concentrations in plasma occur at about 3 hours. Propafenone is 97% bound to α_1-acid glycoprotein. The drug is almost completely metabolized in the liver before excretion, primarily in the feces. At least 11 metabolites have been detected; two compounds, 5-hydroxypropafenone and N-desalkylpropafenone, have electrophysiological effects similar to those of the parent drug. The steady-state concentrations of each of these metabolites in plasma is about 20% of that of propafenone. Like encainide, rates of hepatic metabolism of propafenone are bimodally distributed in the population. The elimination half-life of propafenone averages 5 to 6 hours in fast metabolizers and 17 hours in slow metabolizers; dosage should be reduced for the latter individuals. These values may increase up to twofold in patients with severe hepatic dysfunction. The pharmacokinetic properties of propafenone are dose dependent; for example, an increase in dose from 300 to 900 mg per day can result in as much as a tenfold increase in its concentration in plasma.

Indecainide. Indecainide is almost completely absorbed after oral administration; peak concentrations in plasma occur at about 1 to 2 hours. About 50% of the drug is bound to plasma proteins. Indecainide is eliminated with a half-time of around 8 hours, principally by renal excretion of the unchanged drug; the dosage should be reduced in patients with compromised renal function. The principal metabolite of indecainide, N-desalkylindecainide, has substantial antiarrhythmic activity; its concentration in plasma is usually about 20% of that of indecainide.

Preparations, Dosage, and Routes of Administration. *Flecainide. Flecainide acetate* (TAMBOCOR) is available for oral administration as 50-, 100-, and 150-mg tablets. The initial dose is 100 mg twice a day. Dosage may be increased every 4 days in increments of 100 mg per day to a maximum of 400 to 600 mg per day given in two or three portions. Therapeutic effects are usually achieved at concentrations of 0.2 to 1.0 μg of flecainide per milliliter of plasma; the probability of toxicity increases when the concentration exceeds 1.0 μg/ml.

Encainide. Encainide hydrochloride (ENKAID) is supplied for oral administration as 25-, 35-, and 50-mg capsules. The initial dose is 25 mg given three times a day; this can be increased every 3 to 5 days to a maximum of 50 mg four times a day. It may be necessary to adjust dosage in patients with renal or hepatic impairment.

Therapeutic Uses. Flecainide and encainide are indicated for life-threatening ventricular arrhythmias; propafenone and indecainide may eventually be found to be similarly useful. The use of these drugs should be initiated in hospital for patients with malignant ventricular arrhythmias, symptomatic congestive heart failure, bifascicular block, or sinus node dysfunction. These drugs are under investigation for the treatment of supraventricular tachycardia and paroxysmal atrial fibrillation (Symposium, 1988a, 1988b).

Untoward Effects. All drugs in class I_C produce similar adverse cardiac effects. Proarrhythmic effects occur in 8 to 15% of patients with malignant ventricular arrhythmias, but such effects were thought to be rare in patients with benign or potentially malignant ventricular arrhythmias (Morganroth *et al.*, 1986). However, encainide and flecainide have recently been shown to increase the risk of sudden death and cardiac arrest in patients who have had a myocardial infarction and who have asymptomatic unsustained ventricular arrhythmias (CAST Investigators, 1989). For this reason, these drugs are no longer indicated for benign or potentially malignant ventricular arrhythmias. All of these drugs can aggravate sinus mode dysfunction; heart failure can also be aggravated, but this effect seems most prominent for flecainide and indecainide. High therapeutic doses of flecainide and encainide cause visual disturbances; 10 to 15% of patients treated with flecainide have such symptoms, usually blurred or double vision on quick, far lateral gaze. Propafenone has been associated with granulocytopenia and with a SLE-like syndrome. The concentrations of flecainide, encainide, and propafenone in plasma increase during concurrent administration of cimetidine.

CLASS II: β-ADRENERGIC ANTAGONISTS

The pharmacology of the β-adrenergic blocking agents is discussed in Chapter 11. Only properties related to their use in the treatment of cardiac arrhythmias are considered here. Propranolol, acebutolol, and esmolol are indicated for the treatment of arrhythmias. Metoprolol, propranolol, and timolol are used prophylactically after myocardial infarction to reduce the incidence of sudden death in these patients.

Cardiac Electrophysiological Effects. Most of the antiarrhythmic effects of β-adrenergic antagonists can be explained by their selective blockade of β receptors. Propranolol is known to have two other direct actions that may be relevant to its antiarrhythmic activity: it increases background outward current (i_{K_1}) and, in high concentrations, it significantly depresses i_{Na} (membrane-stabilizing action).

Automaticity. β-Adrenergic stimulation causes a marked increase in the slope of phase-4 depolarization and in the spontaneous firing rate of the sinus node. This effect is competitively blocked by β-adrenergic antagonists. The effect on sinus rate is small when catecholamines are absent. However, blockade of β receptors can cause severe slowing of sinus rate in patients with preexisting sinus node disease (Strauss *et al.*, 1976). There are also significant inhibitory effects on automaticity in cardiac Purkinje fibers when their firing rate has been increased by catecholamines. Under some circumstances, cardiac Purkinje fibers require the action of catecholamines to sustain their spontaneous activity. In this case, β-adrenergic antagonists can totally abolish automaticity in the His–Purkinje system. At low concentrations, propranolol increases outward background current, i_{K_1}, in Purkinje fibers, as do lidocaine and phenytoin; this action decreases automaticity as well (Stagg and Wallace, 1974). Other β-adrenergic antagonists in clinical use appear to lack this action.

Excitability and Threshold. The electrical threshold of the atria and ventricles of normal dogs is not affected by β-adrenergic blockade, but the threshold for fibrillation after experimental infarction is increased (Gang *et al.*, 1984).

Responsiveness and Conduction. Only very high concentrations of propranolol (*e.g.*, 1000 to 3000 ng/ml) decrease responsiveness in Purkinje fibers (Davis and Temte, 1968). These concentrations are much higher than those needed for substantial β-adrenergic blockade (100 to 300 ng/ml). However, concentrations over 1000 ng/ml are sometimes required for control of ventricular arrhythmias (Woosley *et al.*, 1977). Low-amplitude premature responses are abolished by propranolol (Davis and Temte, 1968). These effects are similar to those seen with lidocaine or phenytoin and are probably due to an increase in g_{K_1}. Different effects may occur in abnormal fibers. In the dog heart *in situ*, propranolol causes slowing of intramyocardial conduction in muscle that is made acutely ischemic. It has no such effect on normal portions of the ventricle (Kupersmith *et al.*, 1976). Slow responses can be dependent on catecholamines, as can afterdepolarizations; β-adrenergic blockers ameliorate arrhythmias caused by these mechanisms.

Duration of the Action Potential and Refractoriness. Blockade of β receptors has little effect on the duration of action potentials in the sinus node, atrium, or AV node; the effect on action potentials in ventricular muscle or Purkinje fibers is variable. All β-adrenergic blocking drugs cause a substantial increase in the ERP of the AV node; this action is the basis for the major uses of these drugs as antiarrhythmic agents.

Effect on Reentrant Arrhythmias. In supraventricular tachycardia due to AV nodal reentry, the β-adrenergic antagonists abolish reentry by increasing AV nodal refractoriness. In the ventricles, these drugs abolish slow responses that are dependent on catecholamines. In addition, propranolol can repolarize tissues that have been depolarized by stretch or low $[K]_o$, and thus enhances fast responses in ischemic ventricular muscle. In higher concentration, propranolol and acebutolol have "quinidine-like" effects on phase-0 depolarization and responsiveness of Purkinje fibers. In addition, β-adrenergic antagonists may favorably influence arrhythmias by decreasing myocardial oxygen utilization, thereby reducing myocardial ischemia.

Electrocardiographic Effects. β-Adrenergic blockade causes a small increase in the P–R interval but has no effect on the duration of the QRS complex. Effects on the Q–T_c interval vary with individual drugs. In man, β-adrenergic blockade causes a substantial increase in the ERP of the AV node, but there is no increase in the H–V interval (Seides *et al.,* 1974).

Autonomic Nervous System Effects. All β-adrenergic blocking drugs that are used to treat arrhythmias leave vagal and α-adrenergic mechanisms intact. Propranolol blocks both β_1- and β_2-adrenergic receptors and has substantial local anesthetic (membrane-stabilizing) actions, but it exhibits no intrinsic sympathomimetic activity. Both acebutolol and esmolol are relatively selective β_1-adrenergic antagonists; the former drug possesses significant intrinsic sympathomimetic activity and membrane-stabilizing actions, while the latter does not. A detailed discussion of β-adrenergic antagonists is presented in Chapter 11.

Absorption, Distribution, and Elimination. *Propranolol.* Intestinal absorption of propranolol is excellent, but extensive first-pass metabolism reduces bioavailability to about 25% (*see* Chapter 11; Appendix II). Its half-time for elimination is about 4 hours. As with lidocaine, the hepatic extraction of propranolol is very high and elimination is significantly reduced when hepatic blood flow decreases. Propranolol may decrease its own elimination rate by decreasing cardiac output and hepatic blood flow, particularly in patients with left ventricular dysfunction.

Acebutolol. Like propranolol, acebutolol is well absorbed from the gastrointestinal tract, and its oral bioavailability is less than 50%; substantially higher values occur in elderly patients, and reduction of dosage may be required. The principal metabolite is N-acetylacebutolol (diacetolol), which is equipotent as a β blocker and even more selective for β_1 receptors as compared with the parent drug. The elimination half-time of acebutolol is about 3 hours and that of diacetolol is 8 to 12 hours. Diacetolol is eliminated largely by urinary excretion; lower doses of acebutolol are thus required for patients with renal failure.

Esmolol. Esmolol is given only by intravenous infusion; it distributes to tissues with a half-time of 2 minutes. The ester bond of esmolol is hydrolyzed rapidly by esterases in red blood cells. The elimination half-time is about 8 minutes and the metabolites are inactive.

Dosage and Routes of Administration. *Propranolol.* Propranolol is primarily given orally for long-term treatment of cardiac arrhythmias. Concentrations in plasma that are associated with therapeutic effects vary widely (20 to 1000 ng/ml) and depend on the arrhythmia being treated. The dosage ranges from 30 to 320 mg per day for treatment of arrhythmias that are sensitive to effects of the drug. As much as 1000 mg a day may be needed to suppress some ventricular arrhythmias. Propranolol is effective when given three to four times a day. The duration of action can be prolonged by the administration of large doses, since β-adrenergic blocking agents have a greater margin of safety than do most antiarrhythmic drugs. For emergency use, propranolol can be injected intravenously; 1 to 3 mg is given over several minutes with careful monitoring of the ECG, arterial blood pressure, and pulmonary arterial pressure (by means of a Swan–Ganz catheter); this dose may be repeated after a few minutes if necessary. Much lower doses are needed to achieve a given plasma concentration when given intravenously than after oral administration because first-pass hepatic extraction is avoided.

Acebutolol. Acebutolol is given orally for the treatment of cardiac arrhythmias. The usual initial dose is 200 mg taken twice a day. The dosage is gradually increased to a maximum daily dose of 600 to 1200 mg given in two portions.

Esmolol. Esmolol is administered intravenously for short-term or emergency treatment of supraventricular tachycardias. Dosage regimens are discussed in Chapter 11. After control of ventricular rate is achieved, long-term oral therapy is instituted with an appropriate drug.

Therapeutic Uses. *Supraventricular Arrhythmias.* Propranolol is used primarily to treat supraventricular tachyarrhythmias such as atrial fibrillation, atrial flutter, or paroxysmal supraventricular tachycardia. For these arrhythmias, the objective of therapy usually is to slow the ventricular rate rather than to abolish the arrhythmia. Propranolol accomplishes this objective by blocking β-adrenergic influences on the AV node, thereby increasing refractoriness of the AV node. Only rarely does propranolol convert these supraventricular arrhythmias to sinus rhythm. Not infrequently, propranolol and digitalis will successfully control the ventricular rate in patients with atrial fibrillation or flutter when maximal doses of digitalis alone do not; this additive effect may result from the fact that digitalis increases vagal tone, while propranolol blocks β-adrenergic influences on the AV node.

Combination therapy with quinidine and propranolol probably improves the likelihood of converting atrial fibrillation to sinus rhythm. Propranolol has been helpful in preventing paroxysmal supraventricular tachycardia due to AV nodal reciprocation and the paroxysmal supraventricular tachycardia of the Wolff–Parkinson–White syndrome alone or in combination with quinidine. In the latter condition, quinidine increases the refractoriness of the accessory AV connection and propranolol can be relied upon to increase AV nodal refractoriness. Esmolol is indicated for rapid control of ventricular rate in patients with atrial flutter or fibrillation in postoperative or other emergency circumstances in which control with a short-acting agent is desirable (Angaran *et al.*, 1986).

Ventricular Arrhythmias. Doses of propranolol of as much as 320 mg per day are not likely to be effective against ventricular arrhythmias except in special circumstances. Propranolol is an excellent choice for treatment of symptomatic ventricular premature depolarizations in patients without structural heart disease; the drug often markedly reduces symptoms, even when the arrhythmia is not greatly affected. When ventricular arrhythmias are triggered by exercise or emotion, smaller doses of propranolol (*e.g.*, 80 to 160 mg per day) are very likely to prevent them. In patients with ischemic heart disease, propranolol may ameliorate ventricular arrhythmias by preventing or reducing ischemia. However, most ventricular arrhythmias respond incompletely or not at all to conventional doses of propranolol. Large doses of propranolol (500 to 1000 mg a day) may be required to control ventricular arrhythmias (Woosley *et al.*, 1979). Acebutolol is indicated for the management of ventricular premature complexes (Singh *et al.*, 1986). Propranolol is the drug of choice for severe ventricular arrhythmias in the prolonged Q–T syndrome; when propranolol fails, removal of the left stellate ganglion may be effective (Schwartz, 1984; Moss *et al.*, 1985; Moss, 1986).

Three large, randomized, placebo-controlled trials with timolol (10 mg twice a day), propranolol (60 or 80 mg three times a day), and metoprolol (100 mg twice a day) showed that treatment with these β-adrenergic antagonists was effective for reducing death and nonfatal myocardial infarction in the year after acute myocardial infarction (Beta-Blocker Heart Attack Study Group, 1981; Norwegian Multicenter Study Group, 1981; Symposium, 1984a).

Digitalis-Induced Arrhythmias. Propranolol abolishes ventricular arrhythmias induced by digitalis by effects both directly on the heart and, probably, on the CNS. However, the incidence of adverse effects (*e.g.*, sinus bradycardia or AV block) during treatment of digitalis-induced arrhythmias with propranolol is higher than with phenytoin or lidocaine.

Untoward Effects. In patients with ventricular failure, the level of sympathetic activity is high and can provide significant support to the ventricle. Therefore, when β-adrenergic antagonists are used as antiarrhythmic drugs, significant hypotension or left ventricular failure can occur. However, many patients who have ventricular failure can tolerate long-term oral therapy with propranolol if digitalis, vasodilators, or diuretics are used concomitantly. The potent effect of β-adrenergic blockade on conduction in the AV node can also lead to serious adverse effects, such as AV block or asystole. Sudden withdrawal of β-adrenergic antagonists in patients with angina pectoris can precipitate worsening of angina, cardiac arrhythmias, and acute myocardial infarction. Other untoward effects are described in Chapter 11.

CLASS III: BRETYLIUM, AMIODARONE, AND SOTALOL

The drugs in class III possess diverse pharmacological properties. However, they all share the capacity to prolong the duration of action potentials and refractoriness in Purkinje and ventricular muscle fibers. All of these drugs have significant interactions with the autonomic nervous system. Bretylium was approved in 1978 for emergency treatment of drug-resistant ventricular fibrillation or sustained ventricular tachycardia. Amiodarone was approved in 1986 for the treatment of recurrent ventricular fibrillation or sustained ventricular tachycardia that is resistant to other drugs. Sotalol is under investigation for treatment of life-threatening or symptomatic ventricular arrhythmias.

Chemistry. Bretylium, amiodarone, and sotalol have the following structural formulas.

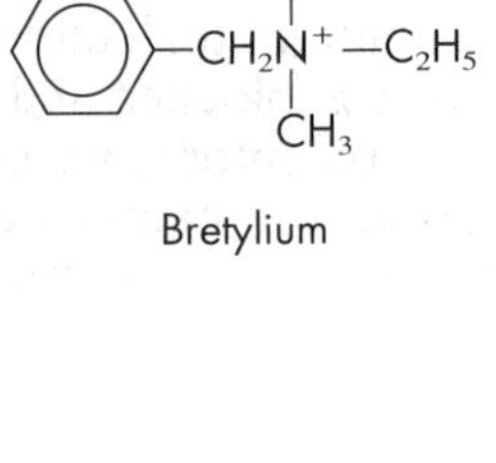

Bretylium

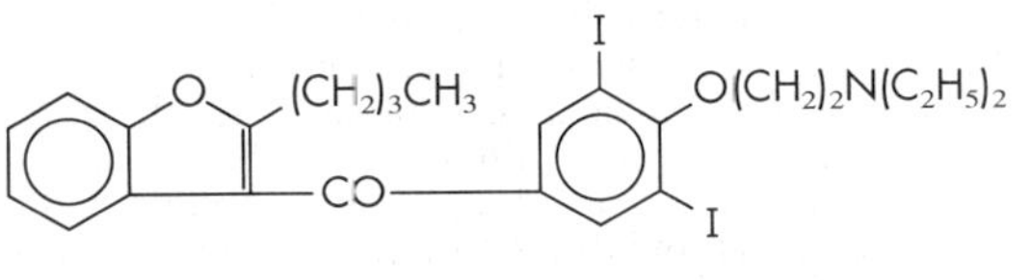

Amiodarone

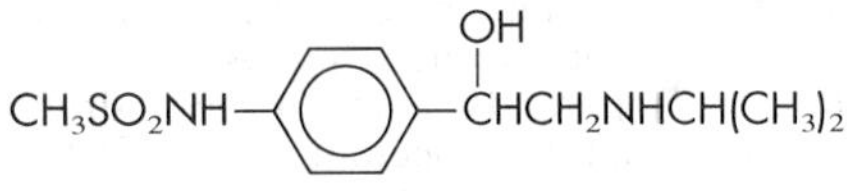

Sotalol

Cardiac Electrophysiological Effects. *Duration of the Action Potential and Refractoriness.* All class-III drugs prolong the action potential duration and the ERP of Purkinje fibers and ventricular muscle cells. Except for bretylium, these drugs produce similar but less intense effects on these parameters in atrial and AV nodal cells.

Automaticity. There is little direct effect of the drugs in class III or automaticity in the sinus node and the His–Purkinje system. Bretylium briefly increases automaticity immediately after its injection by releasing norepinephrine from sympathetic nerve terminals. These effects can be prevented experimentally by prior depletion of catecholamines with reserpine or clinically by β-adrenergic blockade (Bigger and Jaffe, 1971). Amiodarone substantially decreases the automaticity of the sinus node and the His–Purkinje system by mechanisms that are not understood; the drug (or its metabolites) may possess noncompetitive β-adrenergic blocking actions. Sotalol decreases automaticity, presumably because it is a β-adrenergic antagonist (Carmeliet, 1985).

Excitability and Threshold. The class-III drugs have little effect on diastolic electrical current threshold. However, they substantially increase the threshold for ventricular fibrillation (Kniffen *et al.*, 1975; Symposium, 1983; Lynch *et al.*, 1984).

Responsiveness and Conduction. Bretylium and sotalol have no significant effect on membrane responsiveness or conduction in cardiac Purkinje fibers. Amiodarone binds to inactivated Na^+ channels and decreases membrane responsiveness and conduction in Purkinje fibers (Mason *et al.*, 1984). Conduction through the AV node is decreased significantly by sotalol and amiodarone, but is little affected by bretylium.

Effect on Reentrant Arrhythmias. Amiodarone, bretylium, and sotalol are thought to terminate reentrant arrhythmias by markedly prolonging refractoriness without affecting propagation of the cardiac impulse (Singh and Nademanee, 1985). In addition, bretylium may cause repolarization and increased rate of conduction in abnormal depolarized regions by releasing catecholamines.

Electrocardiographic Effects. At therapeutic concentrations in man, amiodarone and sotalol decrease heart rate; bretylium causes little change. During long-term treatment with amiodarone, symptomatic sinus bradycardia can develop. Amiodarone and sotalol, but not bretylium, cause a substantial increase in the P–R interval. All three drugs prolong the Q–T_c, J–T, P–A, and A–H intervals. Only amiodarone increases the H–V interval and the duration of the QRS complex (Mason, 1987).

Autonomic Nervous System Effects. None of these three drugs alters vagal reflexes or the responsiveness of cardiac cholinergic receptors. Sotalol is a β-adrenergic antagonist, while amiodarone causes some noncompetitive α- and β-adrenergic blockade. Like guanethidine, bretylium is taken up and concentrated in adrenergic nerve terminals (*see* Chapter 33). Initially, bretylium releases norepinephrine from nerve terminals; later, it prevents release of the transmitter. It does not depress conduction in sympathetic nerves, impair transmission across ganglia, deplete the adrenergic neuron of norepinephrine, or decrease the responsiveness of adrenergic receptors. During long-term treatment with bretylium, adrenergic receptors show increased responsiveness to circulating catecholamines.

Hemodynamic Effects. None of the three drugs in class III directly decreases the contractility of the mammalian myocardium. However, β-adrenergic blockade with sotalol can reduce cardiac function in patients who are dependent upon the sympathetic nervous system to maintain a normal cardiac output. Although bretylium can increase myocardial contractility transiently by releasing catecholamines, it can also cause orthostatic hypotension by blockade of sympathetic cardiovascular reflexes (Chatterjee *et al.*, 1973). Amiodarone can decrease myocardial oxygen demand and enhance cardiac performance because it relaxes vascular smooth muscle and decreases systemic and coronary vascular resistance.

Absorption, Distribution, and Elimination. *Bretylium.* Oral absorption of bretylium is poor, as would be expected of a quaternary amine. After intramuscular administration, bretylium is eliminated almost entirely by renal excretion, without significant metabolism. The average half-time for elimination is about 9 hours; half-times of 15 to 30 hours occur in patients with renal insufficiency (*see* Heissenbuttel and Bigger, 1979).

Amiodarone. Oral doses of amiodarone are poorly and slowly absorbed; the bioavailability is about 45%, with marked interindividual variability. Peak concentrations in plasma occur about 5 to 6 hours after an oral dose. Amiodarone is extensively bound to tissues and is metabolized slowly in the liver. The elimination of the drug displays complex pharmacokinetic properties, but the half-time of its elimination is estimated to be about 25 to 60 days. During long-term treatment with amiodarone, the active desethyl derivative accumulates in plasma, and its concentration may exceed that of the parent compound.

Sotalol. Oral doses of sotalol are readily absorbed, and the bioavailability is nearly 100%. Maximum concentrations in plasma are reached 2 to 3 hours after administration, and only a small fraction of the drug is bound to plasma proteins. The half-life of elimination from plasma is about 10 to 15 hours. The elimination of sotalol is almost entirely by urinary excretion of unchanged drug, and dosage must be reduced in patients with renal failure.

Preparations, Dosage, and Routes of Administration. *Bretylium.* Bretylium is available as *bretylium tosylate* (BRETYLOL) in a solution containing 50 mg/ml. The drug is diluted to a concentration of 10 mg/ml or less, and a dose of 5 to 10 mg/kg is infused over 10 to 30 minutes; subsequent doses can be given at intervals of 1 to 2 hours if the arrhythmia persists or every 6 hours for maintenance. The dosing interval should be increased in patients with impaired renal function. In emergencies, such as during cardiac resuscitation, a dose of 5 mg/kg of the undiluted solution can be injected intravenously; if ventricular fibrillation persists, the dose may be increased to 10 mg/kg and repeated as necessary. For intramuscular administration, undiluted bretylium tosylate should be used, and the dose of 5 to 10 mg/kg is repeated every 1 to 2 hours if the arrhythmia persists or every 6 to 8 hours for maintenance.

Amiodarone. *Amiodarone hydrochloride* (CORDARONE) is supplied as 200-mg tablets. Because it can take several months to reach full effect, loading doses of 800 to 1600 mg per day are given for 1 to 3 weeks in hospital, with continuous electrocardiographic monitoring. Then, daily doses of 600 to 800 mg are given (usually for 4 weeks) before maintenance treatment is started with 400 to 600 mg per day. Treatment is evaluated after 2 to 8 weeks, usually with programmed ventricular stimulation. The drug is continued if the sustained ventricular arrhythmia becomes noninducible or is slowed enough to be asymptomatic. Long-term effective treatment has been associated with plasma concentrations of 1.0 to 2.5 μg/ml.

Sotalol. Sotalol is not yet available for general use in the United States, and its formulation has not been finalized. Doses of 80 to 320 mg twice a day have been used to treat ventricular arrhythmias. The initial dose is usually 80 mg twice a day and is increased as needed every 3 or 4 days. Efficacy is evaluated either by 24-hour ECG recordings or by programmed ventricular stimulation.

Therapeutic Uses. Bretylium is currently recommended only for treatment of life-threatening ventricular arrhythmias that fail to respond to adequate doses of a first-line antiarrhythmic drug such as lidocaine or procainamide. Use of bretylium should be limited to intensive care facilities. The response of severe, refractory ventricular fibrillation has been impressive (*see* Heissenbuttel and Bigger, 1979; Symposium, 1984b). Ventricular tachycardia usually responds only after some time—6 hours or more after administration of a dose.

Because of its long half-life and life-threatening adverse effects (*see* below), amiodarone is indicated only for recurrent ventricular fibrillation and recurrent, hemodynamically unstable sustained ventricular tachycardia. Treatment should always be started in hospital, and efficacy must be assessed with a provocative approach (usually programmed ventricular stimulation). Thus, amiodarone should be used only in hospitals with electrocardiographic monitoring and clinical electrophysiological facilities. Intravenous use of amiodarone is under investigation for the emergency treatment of persistent or frequently recurring, life-threatening ventricular arrhythmias.

Sotalol is apparently a much safer drug than amiodarone, and it may become a good first choice for the treatment of malignant ventricular arrhythmias, as well as for benign or potentially malignant ventricular arrhythmias. Sotalol appears to be effective for the treatment of paroxysmal supraventricular tachycardia and atrial fibrillation, but comparative studies have not yet firmly positioned it relative to alternative modes of treatment.

Untoward Effects. Hypotension is the principal undesirable effect of bretylium when it is used intravenously to treat acute arrhythmias. Orthostatic hypotension is usually significant, and supine hypotension is common. Rapid intravenous administration may cause nausea and vomiting. Tricyclic antidepressant drugs can prevent uptake of bretylium by adrenergic nerve terminals.

Adverse effects of amiodarone are common and increase markedly after a year of treatment; they affect many organ systems, and some cause death (Mason, 1987). More than 75% of patients treated for 1 to 2 years experience adverse effects and 25 to 33% discontinue treatment because of them. Symptomatic pulmonary toxicity occurs in 10 to 15% of those treated for 1 to 3 years and can cause death in about 10% of those so affected. Hepatic injury is common but is rarely fatal. Aggravation of arrhythmias occurs in 2 to 5% of patients receiving the drug. Asymptomatic corneal microdeposits occur in all. Cutaneous photosensitivity occurs in 10 to 15% and blue discoloration in about 5% during long-term therapy. Amiodarone inhibits the peripheral conversion of thyroxine to triiodothyronine; although symptomatic hypothyroidism occurs in 5% and hyperthyroidism in 2% of patients, abnormal tests of thyroid function are much more common. Substantial increases in LDL-cholesterol concentrations are frequently observed.

Sotalol has the typical adverse effects of a β-adrenergic blocking agent (*see* Chapter 11). In a large controlled trial, treatment with the drug was discontinued because of the development of heart failure (1%), proarrhythmias (2.5%), and bradycardia (3%). *Torsades de pointes* occurs in about 2% of the patients treated with sotalol for malignant ventricular arrhythmias, usually in the first week of treatment and after the $Q-T_c$ interval is substantially prolonged. The $Q-T_c$ interval should be monitored during treatment and consideration given to decreasing the dosage of sotalol if it exceeds 0.50 second.

Drug Interactions. Amiodarone increases the plasma concentrations and effects of digoxin, warfarin, quinidine, procainamide, phenytoin, encainide, flecainide, and diltiazem. Amiodarone increases the likelihood of bradycardia, sinus arrest, and AV block when β-adrenergic antagonists or Ca^{2+}-channel blockers are administered concurrently. Because of its slow elimination, the potential for interactions and other adverse effects persists for many weeks after amiodarone is discontinued.

CLASS IV: VERAPAMIL AND DILTIAZEM

The antiarrhythmic agents in Class IV are Ca^{2+}-channel blockers. The clinically important consequences of this action for the treatment of arrhythmias are depression of Ca^{2+}-dependent action potentials and slowing of conduction in the AV node. Verapamil is the only Ca^{2+}-channel blocker that is currently marketed as an antiarrhythmic drug; the efficacy and safety of diltiazem for the treatment of supraventricular arrhythmias are being evaluated.

Verapamil, a derivative of papaverine, blocks Ca^{2+} channels (principally L channels) in the membranes of smooth and cardiac muscle cells. In 1981, verapamil was approved in the United States for treatment of angina pectoris and supraventricular arrhythmias. The general discussion of Ca^{2+}-channel blockers appears in Chapter 32. Discussion here is confined to their use in treating arrhythmias.

Cardiac Electrophysiological Effects. Verapamil and diltiazem have direct effects on the electrical and mechanical properties of heart muscle and vascular smooth muscle cells.

Impulse Formation. Verapamil and diltiazem slow the spontaneous firing of pacemaker cells in the sinus node *in vitro*. However, in intact animals and in man the heart rate slows only minimally because this direct effect is counteracted by increased reflex sympathetic activity resulting from arterial vasodilatation.

Verapamil decreases the rate of phase-4 spontaneous depolarization in cardiac Purkinje fibers (Danilo *et al.*, 1980) and can block the delayed afterdepolarizations and triggered activity seen in experimental digitalis toxicity (Rosen and Danilo, 1980).

Effect on Reentrant Arrhythmias. The most marked effect of verapamil or diltiazem is to decrease the conduction velocity through the AV node and increase its functional refractory period. The effect on AV nodal conduction is presumably a direct result of Ca^{2+}-channel blockade, but it is not prominent at concentrations of certain other Ca^{2+}-channel blockers (*e.g.*, nifedipine) that are achieved clinically. Depression of the AV node is responsible for slowing the ventricular response to atrial flutter or fibrillation and termination of paroxysmal supraventricular tachycardia.

Electrocardiographic Effects. Verapamil and diltiazem increase the P–R interval in sinus rhythm and slow the ventricular rate substantially in patients with atrial fibrillation.

Autonomic Nervous System Effects. Neither verapamil nor diltiazem has cholinergic or β-adrenergic blocking properties. However, verapamil does have appreciable α-adrenergic blocking activity.

Absorption, Distribution, and Elimination. The pharmacokinetic properties of verapamil and diltiazem are discussed in Chapter 32 (*see also* Appendix II).

Dosage and Routes of Administration. To convert PSVT to sinus rhythm, a dose of 5 to 10 mg of verapamil is given intravenously over at least 2 to 3 minutes. To obtain rapid control of the ventricular rate in atrial fibrillation or atrial flutter, 10 mg of verapamil can be given intravenously over 2 to 5 minutes, and this dose can be repeated in 30 minutes if necessary. To prevent recurrences of PSVT or to control the ventricular response to atrial fibrillation, oral doses of 240 to 480 mg per day are given in three to four divided portions.

Although not yet an approved indication, oral doses of 60 to 90 mg of diltiazem given every 6 hours have been used for prophylaxis against PSVT.

Therapeutic Uses. *Supraventricular Arrhythmias.* Verapamil has become the drug of first choice for abolishing acute episodes of paroxysmal supraventricular tachycardia due to AV nodal reentry or due to anomalous AV connections. Verapamil is also very useful for immediate reduction of the ventricular response to atrial fibrillation or atrial flutter unless the arrhythmia is associated with the Wolff–Parkinson–White syndrome. In man, intravenous verapamil (75 μg/kg) slows the ventricular response to atrial fibrillation by about 30%. Atrial tachycardia with AV block caused by digitalis toxicity may be a manifestation of delayed afterdepolarizations and triggered activity. Verapamil could be effective in abolishing this arrhythmia, but its use is too risky because it can cause additional AV block and suppress automaticity in the His–Purkinje system. Diltiazem has similar effects but is not yet approved for this use.

Ventricular Arrhythmias. Verapamil and diltiazem do not have a major role in the treatment of ventricular arrhythmias. Verapamil and diltiazem are used to treat ventricular tachycardia and ventricular fibrillation caused by coronary artery spasm; they prevent spasm and improve the tolerance of ventricular tissues to ischemia, rather than having a significant direct antiarrhythmic effect.

Untoward Effects. The principal adverse effects of verapamil and diltiazem are cardiac and gastrointestinal. Intravenous use of these drugs is contraindicated in patients who have hypotension, severe heart failure, sick sinus syndrome, AV block, atrial fibrillation, Wolff–Parkinson–White syndrome, or ventricular tachycardia (McGovern *et al.*, 1986). Verapamil can increase the ventricular rate when given intravenously to patients with the Wolff–Parkinson–White syndrome and atrial fibrillation. This is due to reflex increases in sympathetic nervous activity (Gulamhusein *et al.*, 1982); in some patients, a reduction of the ERP in the bundle of Kent also contributes to the increase in the ventricular rate. Verapamil can also cause severe hypotension or ventricular fibrillation in patients with ventricular tachycardia (Rankin *et al.*, 1987). Unexpected sinus bradycardia, AV block, left ventricular failure, or hypotension can occur in elderly patients after intravenous administration of verapamil. Lower doses and a slower rate of injection should thus be used in patients over the age of 60. The major gastrointestinal adverse effect of verapamil is constipation, but gastric upset and other upper gastrointestinal symptoms can occur as well. Diltiazem is better tolerated in this regard.

Drug Interactions. Concurrent use of verapamil and β-adrenergic blocking agents or digitalis can lead to significant bradycardia or AV block. The main reason for this is the additive effects of these drugs on the sinus or AV nodes. In addition, verapamil interacts with digoxin in a manner similar to the quinidine–digoxin interaction (*see* Chapter 34). Concomitant use of verapamil or diltiazem with antihypertensive drugs that depress the sinus node (*e.g.*, reserpine or methyldopa) can intensify sinus bradycardia.

Angaran, D. M.; Schultz, N. J.; and Tschida, V. H. Esmolol hydrochloride: an ultrashort-acting, beta-adrenergic blocking agent. *Clin. Pharm.*, **1986**, *5*, 288–303.

Arnsdorf, M. F., and Bigger, J. T., Jr. Effect of lidocaine hydrochloride on membrane conductance in mammalian cardiac Purkinje fibers. *J. Clin. Invest.*, **1972**, *51*, 2252–2263.

Arnsdorf, M. F., and Wasserstrom, J. A. Mechanisms of action of antiarrhythmic drugs: a matrical approach. In, *The Heart and Cardiovascular System. Scientific Foundations*, Vol. 2. (Fozzard, H. A.; Haber, E.; Jennings, R. B.; Katz, A. M.; and Morgan, H. E.; eds.) Raven Press, New York, **1986**, pp. 1259–1316.

Atkinson, A. J., and Davison, R. Diphenylhydantoin as an antiarrhythmic drug. *Annu. Rev. Med.*, **1974**, *25*, 99–113.

Bean, B. P. Two kinds of calcium channels in canine atrial cells: differences in kinetics, selectivity, and pharmacology. *J. Gen. Physiol.*, **1985**, *86*, 1–30.

Bean, B. P.; Cohen, C. J.; and Tsien, R. W. Lidocaine block of cardiac sodium channels. *J. Gen. Physiol.*, **1983**, *81*, 613–642.

Beta-Blocker Heart Attack Study Group. The beta-blocker heart attack trial. *J.A.M.A.*, **1981**, *246*, 2073–2074.

Bigger, J. T., Jr., and Jaffe, C. C. The effect of bretylium tosylate on the electrophysiologic properties of ventricular muscle and Purkinje fibers. *Am. J. Cardiol.*, **1971**, *27*, 82–92.

Bigger, J. T., Jr.; Schmidt, D. H.; and Kutt, H. Relationship between the plasma level of diphenylhydantoin sodium and its cardiac antiarrhythmic effects. *Circulation*, **1968**, *38*, 363–374.

Birkhead, J. S., and Vaughan Williams, E. M. Dual effect of disopyramide on atrial and atrioventricular conduction and refractory periods. *Br. Heart J.*, **1977**, *39*, 657–660.

Burney, R. G.; DiFazio, C. A.; Peach, M. J.; Petrie, K. A.; and Silvester, M. J. Antiarrhythmic effects of lidocaine metabolites. *Am. Heart J.*, **1974**, *88*, 765–769.

Carmeliet, E. Electrophysiologic and voltage clamp analysis of the effects of sotalol on isolated cardiac muscle and Purkinje fibers. *J. Pharmacol. Exp. Ther.*, **1985**, *232*, 817–825.

Carmeliet, E., and Saikawa, T. Shortening of the action potential and reduction of pacemaker activity by lidocaine, quinidine, and procainamide in sheep cardiac Purkinje fibers. An effect on Na or K currents? *Circ. Res.*, **1982**, *50*, 257–272.

CAST Investigators. (The Cardiac Arrhythmia Suppression Trial Investigators.) Preliminary report: effect of encainide and flecainide on mortality in a randomized trial of arrhythmia suppression after myocardial infarction. *N. Engl. J. Med.*, **1989**, *321*, 406–412.

Chatterjee, K.; Mandel, W. J.; Vyden, J. K.; Parmley, W. W.; and Forrester, J. S. Cardiovascular effects of bretylium tosylate in acute myocardial infarction. *J.A.M.A.*, **1973**, *223*, 757–760.

Cohen, I. S.; DiFrancesco, D.; Mulrine, N. K.; and Pennefather, P. Internal and external K^+ help gate the inward rectifier. *Biophys. J.*, **1989**, *55*, 197–202.

Colatsky, T. J. Mechanisms of action of lidocaine and quinidine on action potential duration in rabbit cardiac Purkinje fibers. An effect on steady state sodium currents? *Circ. Res.*, **1982**, *50*, 17–27.

Conrad, K. A.; Molk, B. L.; and Chidsey, C. A. Pharmacokinetic studies of quinidine in patients with arrhythmias. *Circulation*, **1977**, *55*, 1–7.

Danilo, P., Jr.; Hordof, A. J.; Reder, R. F.; and Rosen, M. R. Effects of verapamil on electrophysiologic properties of blood superfused cardiac Purkinje fibers. *J. Pharmacol. Exp. Ther.*, **1980**, *213*, 222–227.

Davis, L. D., and Temte, J. V. Effects of propranolol on the transmembrane potentials of ventricular muscle and Purkinje fibers of the dog. *Circ. Res.*, **1968**, *22*, 661–667.

DeSilva, R. A.; Lown, B.; Hennekens, C. H.; and Casscells, W. Lignocaine prophylaxis in acute myocardial infarction: an evaluation of randomized trials. *Lancet*, **1981**, *3*, 855–858.

DiFrancesco, D. A new interpretation of the pace-maker current in calf Purkinje fibers. *J. Physiol. (Lond.)*, **1981a**, *314*, 359–376.

———. A study of the ionic nature of the pace-maker current in calf Purkinje fibers. *Ibid.*, **1981b**, *314*, 377–393.

Drayer, D. E.; Restivo, K.; and Reidenberg, M. M. Specific determination of quinidine and (3S)-3-hydroxyquinidine in human serum by high pressure liquid chromatography. *J. Lab. Clin. Med.*, **1977**, *90*, 816–822.

Durrer, D.; Van Dam, R. T.; Freud, G. E.; and Janse, M. J. Reentry and ventricular arrhythmias in local ischemia and infarction in the intact dog heart. *Proc. K. Ned. Akad. Wet. [Biol. Med.]*, **1971**, *74*, 321–334.

El-Sherif, N.; Scherlag, B. J.; Lazzara, R.; and Hope, R. R. Reentrant ventricular arrhythmias in the late myocardial infarction period. 1. Conduction characteristics in the infarction zone. *Circulation*, **1977**, *55*, 686–702.

Frey, W. Weitere Erfährungen mit Chinidin bei absoluter Herzunregelmässigkeit. *Wien Klin. Wochenschr.*, **1918**, *55*, 849–853.

Gang, E. S.; Bigger, J. T., Jr.; and Uhl, E. W. Effects of timolol and propranolol on inducible sustained ventricular tachyarrhythmias in dogs with subacute myocardial infarction. *Am. J. Cardiol.*, **1984**, *53*, 275–281.

Giardina, E. G. V.; Stein, R. M.; and Bigger, J. T., Jr. The relationship between the metabolism of procainamide and sulfamethazine. *Circulation*, **1977**, *55*, 388–394.

Gibson, T. P.; Matusik, J.; Matusik, E.; Nelson, H. A.; Wilkinson, J.; and Briggs, W. A. Acetylation of procainamide in man and its relationship to isonicotinic acid hydrazide acetylation phenotype. *Clin. Pharmacol. Ther.*, **1975**, *17*, 395–399.

Gintant, G.; Datyner, N.; and Cohen, I. S. Gating of delayed rectification in acutely isolated canine cardiac Purkinje myocytes. *Biophys. J.*, **1985**, *48*, 1059–1064.

Gintant, G. A., and Hoffman, B. F. The influence of molecular form of local anesthetic-type antiarrhythmic agents on the maximum upstroke velocity of canine cardiac Purkinje fibers. *Circ. Res.*, **1983**, *52*, 735–746.

Grant, A. O., and Starmer, C. F. Mechanisms of closure of cardiac sodium channels in rabbit ventricular myocytes. *Circ. Res.*, **1987**, *60*, 897–913.

Gulamhusein, S.; Ko, P.; Carruthers, S. G.; and Klein, G. J. Acceleration of the ventricular response during atrial fibrillation in the Wolff–Parkinson–White syndrome after verapamil. *Circulation*, **1982**, *65*, 348–354.

Hagiwara, N.; Irisawa, H.; and Kameyama, M. Contribution of two types of calcium currents to the pacemaker potentials of rabbit sino-atrial node cells. *J. Physiol. (Lond.)*, **1988**, *395*, 233–253.

Heissenbuttel, R. H., and Bigger, J. T., Jr. Bretylium tosylate: a newly available antiarrhythmic drug for ventricular arrhythmias. *Ann. Intern. Med.*, **1979**, *90*, 229–238.

Hondeghem, L. M., and Katzung, B. G. Test of a model of antiarrhythmic drug action. Effect of quinidine and lidocaine on myocardial conduction. *Circulation*, **1980**, *61*, 1217–1224.

Horowitz, L. N.; Josephson, M. E.; and Kastor, J. A. Intracardiac electrophysiologic studies as a method for the optimization of drug therapy in chronic ventricular arrhythmia. *Prog. Cardiovasc. Dis.*, **1980**, *23*, 81–98.

Jensen, G.; Sigurd, B.; and Uhrenholt, A. Hemodynamic effects of intravenous disopyramide in heart failure. *Eur. J. Clin. Pharmacol.*, **1975**, *8*, 167–173.

Kerr, C. R.; Grant, A. O.; Wenger, T. L.; and Strauss, H. C. Sinus node dysfunction. *Cardiol. Clin.*, **1983**, *1*, 187–207.

Kessler, K. M.; Lowenthal, D. T.; Warner, H.; Gibson, T.; Briggs, W.; and Reidenberg, M. M. Quinidine elimination in patients with congestive heart failure or poor renal function. *N. Engl. J. Med.*, **1974**, *290*, 706–709.

Knapp, A. B.; Maguire, W.; Keren, G.; Karmen, A.; Levitt, B.; Miura, D. S.; and Somberg, J. C. The cimetidine–lidocaine interaction. *Ann. Intern. Med.*, **1983**, *98*, 174–177.

Kniffen, F. J.; Lomas, T. E.; Counsell, R. E.; and Lucchesi, B. R. The antiarrhythmic and antifibrillatory actions of bretylium and its *o*-iodobenzyl trimethylammonium analog, UM-360. *J. Pharmacol. Exp. Ther.*, **1975**, *192*, 120–128.

Koster, R. W., and Wellens, H. J. J. Quinidine-induced ventricular flutter and fibrillation without digitalis therapy. *Am. J. Cardiol.*, **1976**, *38*, 519–523.

Kupersmith, J.; Antman, E. M.; and Hoffman, B. F. *In vivo* electrophysiological effects of lidocaine in canine acute myocardial infarction. *Circ. Res.*, **1975**, *36*, 84–91.

Kupersmith, J.; Shiang, H.; Litwak, R. S.; and Herman, M. V. Electrophysiological and antiarrhythmic effects of propranolol in canine acute myocardial ischemia. *Circ. Res.*, **1976**, *38*, 302–307.

LeLorier, J.; Moisan, R.; Gagne, J.; and Caille, G. Effect of the duration of infusion on the disposition of lidocaine in dogs. *J. Pharmacol. Exp. Ther.*, **1977**, *203*, 507–511.

Levitt, B.; Cagin, N.; Kleid, J.; Somberg, J.; and Gillis, R. A. Role of the nervous system in the genesis of cardiac rhythm disorders. *Am. J. Cardiol.*, **1976**, *37*, 1111–1113.

Levy, M. N. Parasympathomimetic control of the heart. In, *Neural Regulation of the Heart.* (Randall, W. C., ed.) Oxford University Press, New York, **1977**, pp. 95–130.

Lynch, J. J.; Wilber, D. J.; Montgomery, D. G.; Hsieh, T. M.; Patterson, E.; and Lucchesi, B. R. Antiarrhythmic and antifibrillatory actions of the levo- and dextrorotatory isomers of sotalol. *J. Cardiovasc. Pharmacol.*, **1984**, *6*, 1132–1141.

MacMahon, S.; Collins, R.; Peto, R.; Koster, R. W.; and Yusuf, S. Effects of prophylactic lidocaine in suspected acute myocardial infarction: an overview of results from the randomized, controlled trials. *J.A.M.A.*, **1988**, *260*, 1910–1916.

McGovern, B.; Garan, H.; and Ruskin, J. N. Precipitation of cardiac arrest by verapamil in patients with Wolff–Parkinson–White syndrome. *Ann. Intern. Med.*, **1986**, *104*, 791–794.

Mark, L. C.; Kayden, H. J.; Steele, J. M.; Cooper, J. R.; Berlin, I.; Rovenstine, E. A.; and Brodie, B. B. The physiological disposition and cardiac effects of procaine amide. *J. Pharmacol. Exp. Ther.*, **1951**, *102*, 5–15.

Mason, J. W.; Hondeghem, L. M.; and Katzung, B. G. Block of inactivated sodium channels and of depolarization-induced automaticity in guinea pig papillary muscle by amiodarone. *Circ. Res.*, **1984**, *55*, 277–285.

Meyers, D. G.; Gonzalez, E. R.; Peters, L. L.; Davis, R. B.; Feagler, J. R.; Egan, J. D.; and Nair, C. K. Severe neutropenia associated with procainamide: comparison of sustained release and conventional preparations. *Am. Heart J.*, **1985**, *109*, 1393–1395.

Mirro, M. J.; Watanabe, A. M.; and Bailey, J. C. Electrophysiological effects of disopyramide and quinidine on guinea-pig atria and canine cardiac Purkinje fibers. Dependence on underlying cholinergic tone. *Circ. Res.*, **1980**, *46*, 660–668.

Morganroth, J. Risk factors for the development of proarrhythmic events. *Am. J. Cardiol.*, **1987**, *59*, 32E–37E.

Morganroth, J.; Anderson, J. L.; and Gentzkow, G. D. Classification by type of ventricular arrhythmias predicts frequency of adverse cardiac events from flecainide. *J. Am. Coll. Cardiol.*, **1986**, *8*, 607–615.

Moss, A. J.; Schwartz, P. J.; Crampton, R. S.; Locati, E.; and Carleen, E. The long QT syndrome: a prospective international study. *Circulation*, **1985**, *71*, 17–21.

Nies, A. S.; Shand, D. G.; and Wilkinson, G. R. Altered hepatic blood flow and drug disposition. *Clin. Pharmacokinet.*, **1976**, *1*, 135–155.

Norwegian Multicenter Study Group. Timolol-induced reduction in mortality and reinfarction in patients surviving acute myocardial infarction. *N. Engl. J. Med.*, **1981**, *304*, 801–807.

Obayashi, K.; Hayakawa, H.; and Mandel, W. J. Interrelationships between external potassium concentration and lidocaine: effects on canine Purkinje fiber. *Am. Heart J.*, **1975**, *89*, 221–226.

Ogden, D. C.; Siegelbaum, S.; and Colquhoun, D. Block of acetylcholine activated ion channels by an uncharged local anesthetic. *Nature*, **1981**, *289*, 596–598.

Peon, J.; Ferrier, G. R.; and Moe, G. K. The relationship of excitability to conduction velocity in canine Purkinje tissue. *Circ. Res.*, **1978**, *43*, 125–135.

Podrid, P. J.; Schoenberger, A.; and Lown, B. Congestive heart failure caused by oral disopyramide. *N. Engl. J. Med.*, **1980**, *302*, 614–617.

Randall, W. C. Sympathetic control of the heart. In, *Neural Regulation of the Heart*. (Randall, W. C., ed.) Oxford University Press, New York, **1977**, pp. 43–94.

Rankin, A. C.; Rae, A. P.; and Cobbe, S. M. Misuse of intravenous verapamil in patients with ventricular tachycardia. *Lancet*, **1987**, *2*, 472–474.

Reidenberg, M. M.; Drayer, D. E.; Levy, M.; and Warner, H. Polymorphic acetylation of procainamide in man. *Clin. Pharmacol. Ther.*, **1975**, *17*, 722–730.

Roden, D. M., and Hoffman, B. F. Action potential prolongation and induction of abnormal automaticity by low quinidine concentrations in canine Purkinje fibers. Relationship to potassium and cycle length. *Circ. Res.*, **1985**, *56*, 857–867.

Rosen, M. R., and Danilo, P., Jr. Effects of tetrodotoxin, lidocaine, verapamil and AHR-2666 on ouabain-induced delayed afterdepolarizations in canine Purkinje fibers. *Circ. Res.*, **1980**, *46*, 117–124.

Rosen, M. R.; Danilo, P., Jr.; Alonso, M. B.; and Pippenger, C. E. Effects of therapeutic concentrations of diphenylhydantoin on transmembrane potentials of normal and depressed Purkinje fibers. *J. Pharmacol. Exp. Ther.*, **1976**, *197*, 594–604.

Routledge, P. A.; Barchowsky, A.; Bjornsson, T. D.; Kitchell, B. B.; and Shand, D. G. Lidocaine plasma protein binding. *Clin. Pharmacol. Ther.*, **1980**, *27*, 347–351.

Schmitt, F. O., and Erlanger, J. Directional differences in the conduction of the impulse through heart muscle and their possible relation to extrasystolic and fibrillary contractions. *Am. J. Physiol.*, **1928–29**, *87*, 326–347.

Schwartz, P. J.; Periti, M.; and Malliani, A. The long Q–T syndrome. *Am. Heart J.*, **1975**, *89*, 378–390.

Seides, S. F.; Josephson, M. E.; Batsford, W. P.; Weisfogel, G. M.; Lau, S. H.; and Damato, A. N. The electrophysiology of propranolol in man. *Am. Heart J.*, **1974**, *88*, 733–741.

Singh, B. N., and Nademanee, K. Control of cardiac arrhythmias by selective lengthening of repolarization: theoretic considerations and clinical observations. *Am. Heart J.*, **1985**, *109*, 421–430.

Soff, G. A., and Kadin, M. E. Tocainide-induced reversible agranulocytosis and anemia. *Arch. Intern. Med.*, **1987**, *147*, 598–599.

Stagg, A. L., and Wallace, A. G. The effect of propranolol on membrane conductance in canine cardiac Purkinje fibers. *Circulation*, **1974**, *50*, Suppl. III, 145.

Starmer, C. F., and Grant, A. O. Phasic ion channel block: a kinetic model and parameter estimation procedure. *Mol. Pharmacol.*, **1985**, *28*, 348–356.

Strauss, H. C.; Gilbert, M.; Svenson, R. H.; Miller, H.; and Wallace, A. G. Electrophysiological effects of propranolol on sinus node function in patients with sinus node dysfunction. *Circulation*, **1976**, *54*, 452–459.

Swerdlow, C. D.; Winkle, R. A.; and Mason, J. W. Determinants of survival in patients with ventricular tachyarrhythmias. *N. Engl. J. Med.*, **1983**, *308*, 1436–1442.

Tseng, G. N., and Hoffman, B. F. Two components of transient outward current in canine ventricular myocytes. *Circ. Res.*, **1989**, *64*, 633–647.

Tseng, G. N.; Robinson, R. B.; and Hoffman, B. F. Passive properties and membrane currents of canine ventricular myocytes. *J. Gen. Physiol.*, **1987**, *90*, 671–701.

Volosin, K.; Greenberg, R. M.; and Greenspon, A. J. Tocainide associated agranulocytosis. *Am. Heart J.*, **1985**, *109*, 1392–1393.

Weld, F. M., and Bigger, J. T., Jr. The effect of lidocaine on diastolic transmembrane currents determining pacemaker depolarization in cardiac Purkinje fibers. *Circ. Res.*, **1976**, *38*, 203–208.

Wenckebach, K. F. *Die unregelmässige Herztätigkeit und ihre klinische Bedeutung*. W. Engelmann, Leipzig, **1914**.

Willius, F. A., and Keys, T. E. Cardiac clinics. XCIV. A remarkably early reference to the use of cinchona in cardiac arrhythmia. *Proc. Staff Meet. Mayo Clin.*, **1942**, *17*, 294–296.

Wit, A. L.; Rosen, M. R.; and Hoffman, B. F. Electrophysiology and pharmacology of cardiac arrhythmias. VIII. Cardiac effects of diphenylhydantoin. *Am. Heart J.*, **1975**, *90*, 265–272, 397–404.

Wittig, J.; Harrison, L. A.; and Wallace, A. G. Electrophysiological effects of lidocaine on distal Purkinje fibers of canine heart. *Am. Heart J.*, **1973**, *86*, 69–78.

Woosley, R. L.; Drayer, D. E.; Reidenberg, M. M.; Nies, A. S.; Carr, K.; and Oates, J. A. Effect of acetylator phenotype on the rate at which procainamide induces antinuclear antibodies and the lupus syndrome. *N. Engl. J. Med.*, **1978**, *298*, 1157–1159.

Woosley, R. L.; Kornhauser, D.; Smith, R.; Reele, S.; Higgins, S. B.; Nies, A. S.; Shand, D. G.; and Oates, J. A. Suppression of chronic ventricular arrhythmias with propranolol. *Circulation*, **1979**, *60*, 819–827.

Woosley, R. L., and Roden, D. M. Pharmacologic causes of arrhythmogenic actions of antiarrhythmic drugs. *Am. J. Cardiol.*, **1987**, *59*, 19E–25E.

Woosley, R. L.; Shand, D.; Kornhauser, D.; Nies, A. S.; and Oates, J. A. Relation of plasma concentration and dose of propranolol to its effect on resistant ventricular arrhythmias. *Clin. Res.*, **1977**, *25*, 262A.

Monographs and Reviews

Baumgarten, C. M., and Fozzard, H. A. The resting and pacemaker potentials. In, *The Heart and Cardiovascular System. Scientific Foundations*, Vol. 1. (Fozzard, H. A.; Haber, E.; Jennings, R. B.; Katz, A. M.; and Morgan, H. E.; eds.) Raven Press, New York, **1986**, pp. 601–626.

Bigger, J. T., Jr. Electrical properties of cardiac muscle and possible causes of cardiac arrhythmias. In, *Cardiovascular Arrhythmias*. (Dreifus, L. S., and Likoff, W., eds.) Grune & Stratton, New York, **1973**, pp. 13–34.

———. The quinidine-digoxin interaction. *Mod. Concepts Cardiovasc. Dis.*, **1982**, *51*, 73–78.

Bigger, J. T., Jr., and Reiffel, J. A. Sick sinus syndrome. *Annu. Rev. Med.*, **1979**, *30*, 91–118.

Brown, A. M., and Yatani, A. Ca and Na channels in the heart. In, *The Heart and Cardiovascular System. Scientific Foundations*, Vol. 1. (Fozzard, H. A.; Haber, E.; Jennings, R. B.; Katz, A. M.; and Morgan, H. E.; eds.) Raven Press, New York, **1986**, pp. 627–636.

Campbell, R. W. Mexiletine. *N. Engl. J. Med.*, **1987**, *316*, 29–34.

Cohen, I. S.; Datyner, N. B.; Gintant, G. A.; and Kline, R. P. Time-dependent outward currents in the heart. In, *The Heart and Cardiovascular System. Scientific Foundations*, Vol. 1. (Fozzard, H. A.; Haber, E.; Jennings, R. B.; Katz, A. M.; and Morgan, H. E.; eds.) Raven Press, New York, **1986**, pp. 637–670.

Cranefield, P. F., and Aronson, R. S. *The Role of Triggered Activity and Other Mechanisms*. Futura Press, Mount Kisco, New York, **1988.**

Di Bianco, R.; Gottdiener, J. S.; Singh, S. N.; and Fletcher, R. D. A review of the effects of disopyramide phosphate on left ventricular function and the peripheral circulation. *Angiology*, **1987**, *38*, 174–183.

DiFrancesco, D. The cardiac hyperpolarizing-activated current i_f. Origins and developments. *Prog. Biophys. Mol. Biol.*, **1985**, *46*, 163–183.

Hasegawa, G. R. Tocainide: a new oral antiarrhythmic. *Drug Intell. Clin. Pharm.*, **1985**, *19*, 514–517.

Hille, B. Local anesthetic action on inactivation of the Na channel in nerve and skeletal muscle: possible mechanisms for antiarrhythmic agents. In, *Biophysical Aspects of Cardiac Muscle*. (Morad, M., ed.) Academic Press, Inc., New York, **1978**, pp. 55–74.

Holmes, B.; Brogden, R. N.; Heel, R. C.; Speight, T. M.; and Avery, G. S. Tocainide: a review of its pharmacological properties and therapeutic efficacy. *Drugs*, **1983**, *26*, 93–123.

Hondeghem, L. M. Antiarrhythmic agents: modulated receptor applications. *Circulation*, **1987**, *75*, 514–520.

Hondeghem, L. M., and Katzung, B. G. Time- and voltage-dependent interactions of antiarrhythmic drugs with cardiac sodium channels. *Biochim. Biophys. Acta*, **1977**, *472*, 373–398.

Keefe, D. L. D.; Kates, R. E.; and Harrison, D. C. New antiarrhythmic drugs: their place in therapy. *Drugs*, **1981**, *22*, 363–400.

Mason, J. W. Amiodarone. *N. Engl. J. Med.*, **1987**, *316*, 455–466.

Moss, A. J. Prolonged QT-interval syndromes. *J.A.M.A.*, **1986**, *256*, 2985–2987.

Noble, D. The surprising heart: a review of recent progress in cardiac electrophysiology. *J. Physiol. (Lond.)*, **1984**, *353*, 1–50.

Pelzer, D., and Trautwein, W. Currents through ionic channels in multicellular cardiac tissue and single heart cells. *Experientia*, **1987**, *43*, 1153–1162.

Roden, D. M., and Woosley, R. L. Flecainide. *N. Engl. J. Med.*, **1986a**, *315*, 36–41.

———. Tocainide. *N. Engl. J. Med.*, **1986b**, *315*, 41–45.

Schrader, B. J., and Bauman, J. L. Mexiletine: a new type I antiarrhythmic agent. *Drug Intell. Clin. Pharm.*, **1986**, *20*, 255–260.

Schwartz, P. J. The rationale and the role of left stellectomy for the prevention of malignant arrhythmias. *Ann. N.Y. Acad. Med.*, **1984**, *427*, 199–220.

Singh, B. N.; Thoden, W. R.; and Wahl, J. Acebutolol: a review of its pharmacology, pharmacokinetics, clinical uses, and adverse effects. *Pharmacotherapy*, **1986**, *6*, 45–63.

Symposium. (Various authors.) Amiodarone: basic concepts and clinical applications. (Singh, B. N., and Zipes, D. P., eds.) *Am. Heart J.*, **1983**, *106*, 787–964.

Symposium. (Various authors.) The Göteborg metoprolol trial in acute myocardial infarction. (Roberts, W. C., ed.) *Am. J. Cardiol.*, **1984a**, *53*, 1D–50D.

Symposium. (Various authors.) Symposium on the management of ventricular dysrhythmias. (Roberts, W. C., ed.) *Am. J. Cardiol.*, **1984b**, *54*, 1A–36A.

Symposium. (Various authors.) Symposium on flecainide acetate. (Bigger, J. T., Jr., ed.) *Am. J. Cardiol.*, **1984c**, *53*, 1B–122B.

Symposium. (Various authors.) Recent advances in antiarrhythmic therapy: symposium on propafenone. (Zipes, D. P., ed.) *Am. J. Cardiol.*, **1984d**, *54*, 1D–73D.

Symposium. (Various authors.) A symposium: encainide. (Harrison, D. H., and Morganroth, J., eds.) *Am. J. Cardiol.*, **1986**, *58*, 1C–116C.

Symposium. (Various authors.) A symposium: ethmozine (moricizine HCl)—a new antiarrhythmic agent. (Lown, B., ed.) *Am. J. Cardiol.*, **1987**, *60*, 1F–89F.

Symposium. (Various authors.) International symposium on supraventricular arrhythmias: focus on flecainide. (Anderson, J. L., and Pritchett, E. L. C., eds.) *Am. J. Cardiol.*, **1988a**, *62*, 1D–67D.

Symposium. (Various authors.) A symposium: the use of encainide in supraventricular tachycardias. (Naccarelli, G. V., and Wellens, H. J. J., eds.) *Am. J. Cardiol.*, **1988b**, *62*, 1L–84L.

Willis, P. W. The clinical scope of disopyramide seven years after introduction—an overview. *Angiology*, **1987**, *38*, 165–173.

Woosley, R. L.; Wood, A. J.; and Roden, D. M. Encainide. *N. Engl. J. Med.*, **1988**, *318*, 1107–1115.

CHAPTER 36 DRUGS USED IN THE TREATMENT OF HYPERLIPOPROTEINEMIAS

Michael S. Brown and Joseph L. Goldstein

The *hyperlipoproteinemias* are traditionally defined as conditions in which the concentration of cholesterol- or triglyceride-carrying lipoproteins in plasma exceeds an arbitrary normal limit, typically defined as the ninety-fifth percentile of a random population. Clinical concern arises because an elevated concentration of lipoproteins can accelerate the development of atherosclerosis, with its dual sequelae of thrombosis and infarction. About half of the deaths in the United States are a result of such events. However, an increased risk of myocardial infarction does not require classical hyperlipoproteinemia as defined above. Such risk begins at concentrations of cholesterol in plasma that were previously considered to be normal. When defined in this way, nearly half the adults in the United States have concentrations of cholesterol in plasma that are above the optimal range, and these individuals should also be considered to have hyperlipoproteinemia.

Recent studies have demonstrated conclusively that reduction of the concentration of cholesterol-carrying lipoproteins in plasma can diminish the risk of myocardial infarction (Lipid Research Clinics Program, 1984a, 1984b; Helsinki Heart Study, 1987). Therapy for hypercholesterolemia is thus recommended particularly for individuals with a family history of premature atherosclerosis and for individuals with other risk factors, such as smoking, hypertension, or diabetes mellitus. Certain types of hypertriglyceridemia can also cause life-threatening pancreatitis, and in this case a reduction of lipoprotein concentrations has also been shown to be beneficial

NORMAL PATHWAYS OF LIPOPROTEIN TRANSPORT

Plasma cholesterol and triglycerides are transported in lipoproteins, which are large, globular particles that contain an oily core of nonpolar lipid (cholesteryl esters or triglycerides) surrounded by a polar coat of phospholipids, free (*i.e.*, unesterified) cholesterol, and apoproteins. There are six classes of lipoproteins that differ from one another in size and density, in the relative proportions of triglycerides and cholesteryl esters in the core, and in the nature of the apoproteins on the surface (Table 36–1). Each class of lipoproteins has a specific tissue (or tissues) of origin and catabolism, and each plays a defined role in the transport of lipids. The pathway for transport of lipoproteins, shown schematically in Figure 36–1, can be divided into two components: one for transport of exogenous lipids (*i.e.*, lipids that enter the circulation from the intestine), and another for the transport of endogenous lipids (*i.e.*, lipids that enter the circulation from the liver and tissues other than the intestine) (Goldstein *et al.*, 1983; Brown and Goldstein, 1986; Havel, 1987).

Exogenous Pathway. Exogenous lipid transport begins with intestinal incorporation of dietary triglycerides and cholesterol into large lipoprotein particles called *chylomicrons* (diameter, 80 to 500 nm), which are secreted into the lymph and subsequently enter the bloodstream. When chylomicrons reach the capillaries of adipose tissue and muscle, they are digested by an enzyme, lipoprotein lipase, that is bound to the surface of the endothelial cells. Lipoprotein lipase hydrolyzes the triglycerides in the core of the chylomicrons, and the liberated fatty acids cross the endothelium and enter the underlying adipocytes or muscle cells; they are then either esterified again to form triglycerides for storage or oxidized to provide energy.

After most of the triglycerides have been removed in this fashion, the chylomicron dissociates from the capillary endothelium and enters the circulation again. Its size has been reduced and its content of triglycerides diminished, but its cholesteryl esters remain intact. The particle is now designated as a *chylomicron remnant* (diameter, 30 to 50 nm). When the remnant reaches the liver, it is cleared from the circulation by a receptor that recognizes two of its protein components, apoproteins E and B-48. The receptor-bound remnant is taken

Table 36–1. CHARACTERISTICS OF THE MAJOR CLASSES OF LIPOPROTEINS IN HUMAN PLASMA

LIPOPROTEIN CLASS *	MAJOR CORE LIPIDS	MAJOR APOPROTEINS	ORIGIN OF APOPROTEINS	TRANSPORT FUNCTION	MECHANISM OF LIPID DELIVERY
Chylomicrons	Dietary triglycerides	A-1, A-2, A-4, B-48	Small intestine	Dietary triglyceride	Hydrolysis by lipoprotein lipase
Chylomicron remnants	Dietary cholesteryl esters	B-48, E	Chylomicrons	Dietary cholesterol	Receptor-mediated endocytosis in liver
VLDL	Endogenous triglycerides	B-100, C, E	Liver and small intestine	Endogenous triglyceride	Hydrolysis by lipoprotein lipase
IDL	Endogenous cholesteryl esters and triglycerides	B-100, E	VLDL	Endogenous cholesterol	Receptor-mediated endocytosis in liver (50%) or conversion to LDL (50%)
LDL	Endogenous cholesteryl esters	B-100	IDL	Endogenous cholesterol	Receptor-mediated endocytosis in liver or extrahepatic tissues
HDL	Endogenous cholesteryl esters	A-1, A-2	Liver and small intestine	Facilitates removal of cholesterol from extrahepatic tissues	Cholesteryl ester transfer to IDL and LDL

* VLDL denotes very-low-density lipoprotein; IDL, intermediate-density lipoprotein; LDL, low-density lipoprotein; HDL, high-density lipoprotein.

into the hepatic cell by a process termed *receptor-mediated endocytosis*. Within the cell the remnant is digested in lysosomes, and the cholesteryl esters are cleaved to generate free cholesterol. The free cholesterol has several fates: it can be used for membrane synthesis, it can be stored by the liver cell as cholesteryl esters, it can be excreted into the bile either as cholesterol or after conversion to bile acids, or it can be used to form endogenous lipoproteins that are secreted into plasma.

Endogenous Pathway. Endogenous lipid transport begins when the liver secretes triglycerides and cholesterol into the plasma in *very-low-density lipoproteins* (VLDL; diameter, 30 to 80 nm). The major stimulus for such secretion is a high-calorie intake (especially a high-carbohydrate intake), which induces the liver to assemble triglycerides for export and storage in adipose tissue. The triglycerides of VLDL are cleaved in capillaries by the same lipoprotein lipase that digests chylomicrons. Digestion produces a VLDL remnant (analogous to the chylomicron remnant) that is designated as *intermediate-density lipoprotein* (IDL; diameter, 25 to 35 nm). After release from the endothelium, the IDL particles have two metabolic fates. Some of the particles are cleared rapidly by the liver, again by receptor-mediated endocytosis. The receptor that acts on the IDL particle is called the *low-density lipoprotein* (LDL) receptor. It binds lipoproteins that contain apoprotein E or B-100, and it therefore interacts with both IDL and LDL particles (*see* below).

About half of the IDL particles are not cleared rapidly by the liver. Rather, they remain in the circulation, where most of the remaining triglycerides are removed, and the density of the particle increases further, until it becomes LDL (diameter, 18 to 28 nm). LDL circulates for a relatively long time in man (half-life of about 1.5 days). The particles are eventually degraded by binding to LDL receptors in liver and certain extrahepatic tissues. Circulating LDL constitutes the major reservoir of cholesterol in human plasma, accounting for 60 to 70% of the total. When liver or extrahepatic tissues require cholesterol for the synthesis of new membranes, steroid hormones, or bile acids, they synthesize LDL receptors and obtain cholesterol by the receptor-mediated endocytosis of LDL. Conversely, when tissues no longer require cholesterol for cell growth or metabolic purposes, they decrease the synthesis of LDL receptors. This phenomenon of feedback regulation can be exploited in the design of drugs that reduce plasma concentrations of LDL by stimulating production of LDL receptors (*see* below).

As cells of the body die and as cell membranes undergo turnover, free cholesterol is continually released into the plasma. This cholesterol is immediately adsorbed onto *high-density lipoproteins* (HDL; diameter, 5 to 12 nm), and in this location it is esterified with a long-chain fatty acid by an enzyme in plasma, lecithin:cholesterol acyltransferase (LCAT). The newly formed cholesteryl esters are rapidly transferred from HDL to VLDL or IDL particles by a cholesteryl ester transfer protein in

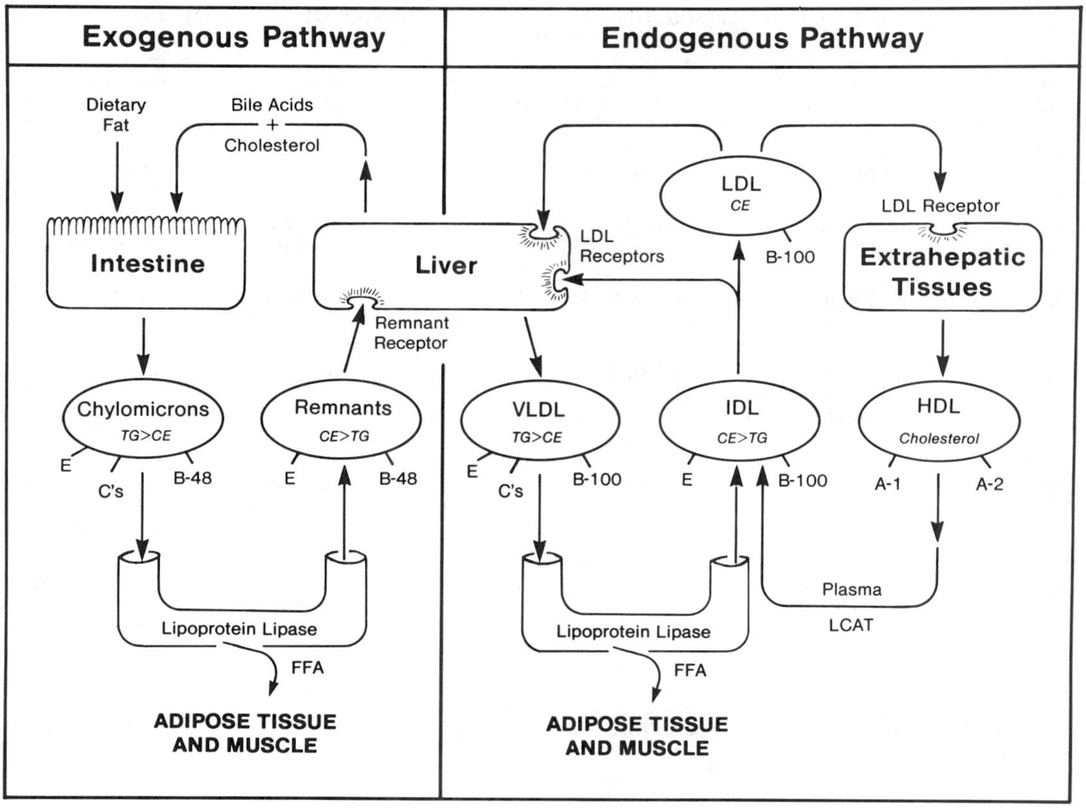

Figure 36–1. *Model for the metabolism of plasma lipoproteins, showing the separate pathways for transport of endogenous and exogenous lipids.*

CE denotes cholesteryl esters; *FFA*, free fatty acids; *TG*, triglycerides; *HDL*, high-density lipoprotein; *IDL*, intermediate-density lipoprotein; *LCAT*, lecithin:cholesterol acyltransferase; *LDL*, low-density lipoprotein; and *VLDL*, very-low-density lipoprotein. *A-1, A-2, B-48, B-100, C's,* and *E* represent the apoproteins associated with the indicated lipoprotein particle. For further explanation, *see* the text. (Modified from Goldstein, Kita, and Brown, 1983.)

plasma. The IDL particles are ultimately taken up by the liver or converted to LDL. The process by which HDL promotes the removal of cholesterol from peripheral cells and facilitates its delivery back to the liver is referred to as *reverse cholesterol transport*. This transport is facilitated by the synthesis and secretion of apoprotein E by peripheral tissues (Mahley, 1988).

In addition to degradation by specific receptors, lipoproteins are also disposed of by less specific pathways, some of which operate in macrophages and other scavenger cells. When the plasma concentration of a lipoprotein rises, the rate of its degradation by such pathways increases. This contributes to the deposition of cholesterol in macrophages of arterial walls (producing atheromas) and macrophages of tendons and skin (producing xanthomas) (Brown and Goldstein, 1983).

Recent evidence has implicated oxidized LDL as a major source of cholesterol in macrophages within atheromas (Steinberg *et al.*, 1989). Macrophages and endothelial cells possess few LDL receptors, but they do produce a "scavenger receptor" that recognizes LDL only after its lysine residues have been chemically modified (Brown and Goldstein, 1983). When LDL is oxidized in the presence of a heavy metal, such as copper or iron, the lysine residues are modified by reaction with oxidation products of fatty acids. This modified particle is taken up rapidly by macrophages through the scavenger receptor. Such oxidation is likely to occur locally when LDL penetrates into arterial walls, and this event may be responsible for much of the deposition of cholesterol in atherosclerotic plaques (Steinberg *et al.*, 1989).

DISEASES THAT CAUSE HYPERLIPOPROTEINEMIA

The hyperlipoproteinemias can be designated as either primary or secondary. Secondary hyperlipoproteinemias are complications of a more generalized metabolic disturbance, such as diabetes mellitus, hypothyroidism, or excessive intake of ethanol (Table 36–2). The primary hyperlipoproteinemias can be divided into two major groups: those that are caused by an inherited single-gene defect (so-called *monogenic hyperlipoproteinemias*) and those that appear to be caused by a combination of multiple subtle genetic factors that act together with environmental insults (so-called *multifactorial* or *polygenic hyperlipoproteinemias*) (Table 36–3). The monogenic disorders are inherited in a predictable Mendelian fashion; each family member can be classified as either affected or unaffected. In multifactorial hyperlipoproteinemia, the plasma lipid concentrations of an entire family are shifted toward the upper range of normal, and those relatives with values at the high end of the family spectrum are in the high-risk range for atherosclerosis. Diets high in saturated fats and cholesterol contribute to the elevated cholesterol concentrations in these individuals. Of all people in the population with hyperlipoproteinemia, the vast majority have the multifactorial type. Individuals with the monogenic forms of hyperlipoproteinemia generally have much higher concentrations of lipid than do those with the polygenic type.

Tables 36–2 and 36–3 summarize the characteristics of the diseases that cause hyperlipoproteinemia. The monogenic disorders range from extremely common autosomal dominant diseases, such as the heterozygous forms of familial hypercholesterolemia (population prevalence of 1 in 500) and multiple lipoprotein–type hyperlipoproteinemia (population prevalence of 1 in 250), to rare diseases, such as familial lipoprotein lipase deficiency (prevalence of 1 in 1,000,000). The mutant gene product has been identified in three of the monogenic disorders. In familial lipoprotein lipase deficiency, affected homozygotes fail to produce lipoprotein lipase, and they are thus unable to catabolize dietary triglyceride contained within chylomicrons. In familial hypercholesterolemia, the gene for the LDL receptor is defective; thus LDL and IDL cannot be removed from the circulation at a normal rate (Goldstein and Brown, 1989). In type-III hyperlipoproteinemia, patients inherit two mutant genes at the locus for apo E, the apoprotein

Table 36–2. THE MAJOR SECONDARY FORMS OF HYPERLIPOPROTEINEMIA

DISORDER	PLASMA LIPOPROTEIN ELEVATION	PROPOSED MECHANISM	TYPICAL PLASMA LIPID CONCENTRATIONS *T = Triglyceride* *C = Cholesterol* *mg/dl (mM)*	TYPICAL CLINICAL FINDINGS *
Diabetes mellitus	VLDL (occasionally chylomicrons)	Increased secretion and delayed catabolism of VLDL	T: 300–10,000 (3.4–113) C: 200–300 (5.2–7.8)	X, P, A
Hypothyroidism	LDL	Decreased catabolism of LDL, owing to suppressed LDL receptors	T: 100–400 (1.1–4.5) C: 300–400 (7.8–10.3)	A
Nephrotic syndrome	VLDL and LDL	Increased secretion of VLDL and LDL; decreased catabolism of VLDL and LDL	T: 100–500 (1.1–5.6) C: 300–500 (7.8–12.9)	A
Uremia	VLDL	Decreased catabolism of VLDL	T: 300–800 (3.4–9.0) C: 200–300 (5.2–7.8)	A
Primary biliary cirrhosis	Lipoprotein X (↑ cholesterol and phospholipid)	Diversion of biliary cholesterol and phospholipids into bloodstream	T: 100 (1.1) C: 300–2000 (7.8–52)	X, A
Alcoholic hyperlipidemia	VLDL (usually chylomicrons)	Increased secretion of VLDL in individuals genetically predisposed to hypertriglyceridemia	T: 300–10,000 (3.4–113) C: 200–300 (5.2–7.8)	X, P
Oral contraceptives	VLDL (occasionally chylomicrons)	Increased secretion of VLDL in individuals genetically predisposed to hypertriglyceridemia	T: 300–10,000 (3.4–113) C: 200–300 (5.2–7.8)	X, P

* X = xanthomas; P = pancreatitis; A = premature atherosclerosis.

Table 36–3. THE MAJOR PRIMARY FORMS OF HYPERLIPOPROTEINEMIA

DISORDER AND PATTERN OF INHERITANCE *	BIOCHEMICAL DEFECT	PLASMA LIPOPROTEIN ELEVATION	PROPOSED MECHANISM	TYPICAL PLASMA LIPID CONCENTRATIONS: *T = Triglyceride C = Cholesterol mg/dl (mM)*	TYPICAL CLINICAL FINDINGS †	DRUG THERAPY: *First Choice*	DRUG THERAPY: *Other*
Monogenic							
Familial lipoprotein lipase deficiency; R	Deficiency of lipoprotein lipase	Chylomicrons	Decreased hydrolysis of triglycerides in chylomicrons	T: 10,000 (113) C: 500 (12.9)	X, P	None	None
Familial type-III hyperlipoproteinemia (dysbetalipoproteinemia); R ‡	Abnormal form of apo E	Chylomicron remnants and IDL	Decreased catabolism of chylomicron remnants and IDL	T: 350 (4.0) C: 350 (9.1)	X, A	Gemfibrozil	Nicotinic acid; clofibrate
Familial hypercholesterolemia (heterozygous form); D	Deficiency of LDL receptor	LDL	Decreased catabolism of LDL; decreased catabolism of IDL with increased conversion to LDL	T: 100 (1.1) C: 350 (9.1)	X, A	Lovastatin ± bile acid resin	Probucol or nicotinic acid ± bile acid resin
Familial hypertriglyceridemia; D	Unknown	VLDL (rarely chylomicrons)	Decreased catabolism or increased production of VLDL	T: 500 (5.6) C: 200 (5.2)	X, A, P	Nicotinic acid; gemfibrozil	Clofibrate
Multiple lipoprotein–type hyperlipidemia (familial combined hyperlipidemia); D	Unknown	VLDL and LDL (rarely chylomicrons)	Increased production of VLDL	T: 100–500 (1.1–5.6) C: 250–400 (6.5–10.3)	X, A, P	Nicotinic acid; gemfibrozil	Clofibrate; bile acid resin
Multifactorial							
Polygenic hypercholesterolemia; complex	Unknown	LDL	Unknown	T: 100 (1.1) C: 280 (7.2)	A	Bile acid resin; lovastatin	Probucol; β-sitosterol; neomycin
Hypertriglyceridemia; complex	Unknown	VLDL	Unknown	T: 500 (5.6) C: 200 (5.2)	—	Gemfibrozil	Nicotinic acid; clofibrate

* All of the monogenic disorders are autosomal. R = recessive; D = dominant.
† X = xanthomas; P = pancreatitis; A = premature atherosclerosis.
‡ Requires homozygosity for apo-E abnormality plus additional factor(s) for clinical expression.

necessary for binding of chylomicron remnants and IDL to hepatic receptors (Mahley and Rall, 1989). The defective molecules of apoprotein E fail to bind to either chylomicron remnant receptors or LDL receptors. Surprisingly, homozygosity for the abnormal apo E gene is necessary, but not sufficient, to produce hyperlipoproteinemia. In addition to such homozygosity (which occurs in 1 in 100 individuals), the development of hyperlipoproteinemia (which occurs in only 1 in 100 homozygotes) requires another aggravating factor, such as hypothyroidism or the simultaneous inheritance of a second genetic defect in lipoprotein metabolism.

The causes of the multifactorial hyperlipoproteinemias are not established. The postulated subtle genetic abnormalities that predispose to these forms of disease are often aggravated by obesity and by diets that are high in saturated fats and cholesterol. For this reason, patients with the multifactorial diseases often respond better to dietary manipulation than do patients with the monogenic defects (*see* below).

EVALUATION OF HYPERLIPOPROTEINEMIA

The definition of hypercholesterolemia has been changing rapidly in recent years as the concept of optimal lipoprotein concentrations has evolved. A variety of national and international panels have formulated guidelines for the interpretation of plasma cholesterol concentrations. The most influential of these in the United States is the National Cholesterol Education Panel (*see* Report, 1988); its guidelines for classification of blood cholesterol in adults are given in Table 36–4. The panel defined cholesterol concentrations of less than 200 mg/dl (5.2 mM) as desirable; 200 to 239 mg/dl (5.2 to 6.2 mM) as borderline; and values of 240 mg/dl (6.2 mM) or higher as elevated. The recommended follow-up for borderline hypercholesterolemia depends on the presence of other risk factors, which include definite evidence of coronary artery disease, male sex, family history of premature coronary artery disease, cigarette smoking, a low plasma concentration of HDL-cholesterol (below 35 mg/dl [0.9 mM]), diabetes mellitus, and severe obesity. A similar consensus has not evolved with respect to hypertriglyceridemia as it might relate to coronary artery disease.

Knowledge of the plasma concentrations of cholesterol and triglyceride usually reveals the class of lipoprotein that is elevated, and this in turn is useful in making a genetic diagnosis. An elevated concentration of cholesterol in the presence of a normal value for triglyceride is almost always due to an excessive concentration of LDL. If one defines hypercholesterolemia as in Table 36–4, then the vast majority of individuals with an elevation of LDL will have polygenic hypercholesterolemia. About 1 in 100 of such individuals will have the heterozygous form of familial hypercholesterolemia. This disease can usually be diagnosed by a constellation of clinical findings: an extremely high concentration of plasma cholesterol (typically 350 to 450 mg/dl [9.1 to 11.6 mM]), the presence of tendon xanthomas (present in 75% of affected adults), and a strong family history of hypercholesterolemia and premature heart disease. Heterozygotes express about one half the normal number of LDL receptors and manifest hypercholesterolemia from the time of birth. This is in contrast to the polygenic form of hypercholesterolemia, which does not usually become manifest until adulthood. About 1 in 1,000,000 individuals in the population inherits two abnormal genes for the LDL receptor. Such homozygotes have a distinct syndrome that is characterized by severe hypercholesterolemia of 600 to 1000 mg/dl (about 15 to 25 mM) (LDL concentrations eight to ten times normal), a unique form of cutaneous planar xanthomas, and clinical signs of coronary atherosclerosis beginning as early as 5 years of age and typically ending in death from myocardial infarction by 20 to 30 years of age (Goldstein and Brown, 1989).

A triglyceride concentration in the range of 200 to 800 mg/dl (2.3 to 9.0 mM) with a normal or near-normal cholesterol concentration almost always

Table 36–4. GUIDELINES FOR CLASSIFICATION AND FOLLOW-UP BASED ON TOTAL PLASMA CHOLESTEROL CONCENTRATION

TOTAL CHOLESTEROL *mg/dl (mM)*	CLASSIFICATION	RECOMMENDED FOLLOW-UP
< 200 (< 5.2)	Desirable blood cholesterol	Repeat blood test within 5 years
200 to 239 (5.2 to 6.2)	Borderline high blood cholesterol	*Without* CAD * or CAD risk factors—provide dietary information and recheck annually
		With CAD or CAD risk factors—obtain lipoprotein analysis; further action based on LDL-cholesterol value
≥ 240 (≥ 6.2)	High blood cholesterol	Obtain lipoprotein analysis; further action based on LDL-cholesterol value

* CAD, coronary artery disease.

Adapted from Guidelines of the National Cholesterol Education Panel (*see* Report, 1988).

indicates a simple elevation of VLDL. Triglyceride concentrations greater than 1000 mg/dl (11.3 mM) usually indicate the presence of chylomicrons, either alone or in addition to elevated VLDL. This distinction can be made by allowing such severely hyperlipemic plasma (which is usually either turbid or milky) to stand in the refrigerator at 4° C overnight. If chylomicrons are present, a creamy layer will form on top. If the plasma below the creamy layer is turbid, then VLDL is also elevated. If the plasma below the creamy layer is clear, then the VLDL is not elevated. The distinction between a primary and a secondary form of hypertriglyceridemia is often a difficult one, especially since many hypertriglyceridemic individuals with a genetically determined predisposition (*see* Table 36–3) can have their disease aggravated by the simultaneous presence of one of several common conditions, such as diabetes mellitus, excessive intake of alcohol, or use of oral contraceptives (*see* Table 36–2).

A moderate elevation of both cholesterol and triglyceride usually indicates that an individual has an elevation of both LDL and VLDL; this occurs frequently in familial multiple lipoprotein-type hyperlipoproteinemia and less commonly in familial hypercholesterolemia. Such a combined elevation might also be a sign of familial dysbetalipoproteinemia. The latter disease can be suspected if tuberous or palmar xanthomas are found. If doubt exists, the presence of dysbetalipoproteinemia can be confirmed by ultracentrifugation and electrophoretic techniques in specialized laboratories (Mahley and Rall, 1989).

INDICATIONS FOR TREATMENT OF HYPERLIPOPROTEINEMIA

Abundant evidence indicates that treatment of hyperlipoproteinemia will diminish or prevent atherosclerotic complications. Numerous population studies have shown that an elevated concentration of total cholesterol or LDL-cholesterol in plasma constitutes a major risk factor for the occurrence of atherosclerotic events (Goldstein *et al.*, 1973; Keys, 1975). Moreover, in the monogenic disorders, family studies have documented a markedly increased risk of vascular disease among affected members (Stone *et al.*, 1974; Brunzell *et al.*, 1976). Nevertheless, treatment of hyperlipoproteinemia was, until recently, a controversial issue, mainly because the lowering of plasma lipids had not been shown prospectively to prolong life or diminish the clinical complications of atherosclerosis. In 1984, the results of the Lipid Research Clinics Coronary Primary Prevention Trial, a multicenter, randomized, double-blind study, provided strong evidence that a reduction in plasma concentrations of LDL-cholesterol can reduce the risk of coronary artery disease (Lipid Research Clinics Program, 1984a, 1984b).

The design of this major study was as follows. A large number (3806) of asymptomatic middle-aged men with primary forms of hypercholesterolemia were divided into control and treatment groups. The treatment group received cholestyramine, a bile acid–binding resin, and the control group received a placebo for an average of 7.4 years. Both groups followed a moderate cholesterol-lowering diet. In the cholestyramine group, plasma LDL-cholesterol concentrations were reduced by 20%, which was 13% greater than that obtained in the control group ($p < 0.001$). The cholestyramine group experienced a 24% reduction in death by myocardial infarction and a 19% reduction in nonfatal myocardial infarction ($p < 0.05$). In addition, the incidence of newly positive exercise tests (indicative of myocardial ischemia), angina pectoris, and coronary bypass surgery was reduced in the cholestyramine group by 25%, 20%, and 21%, respectively. No serious adverse effects of cholestyramine were noted. One or more gastrointestinal symptoms (*e.g.*, gas, heartburn, bloating, and constipation) were noted in 29% of the cholestyramine group and 26% of the placebo group.

These results provided the long-sought evidence that reduction of LDL-cholesterol concentrations can diminish the incidence of morbidity and mortality of coronary artery disease. These conclusions were confirmed in 1987 by the Helsinki Heart Study, which showed that treatment of men with more moderate hypercholesterolemia (mean total cholesterol of 289 mg/dl [7.5 mM]) could reduce the incidence of coronary events. The drug used was gemfibrozil (*see* below), and the clinical benefits were correlated with a fall in LDL-cholesterol, an increase in HDL-cholesterol, and a decrease in plasma triglycerides.

Analysis of the relationship between cholesterol and coronary artery disease suggests that a 25% reduction of the total cholesterol in plasma would reduce the incidence of coronary events by nearly 50% (Lipid Research Clinics Program, 1984b).

The role of hypertriglyceridemia (in the range of 300 to 1000 mg/dl; 3.4 to 11 mM) as an independent risk factor for coronary atherosclerosis has not been established unequivocally, although several epidemiological studies have revealed a correlation (Carlson and Bottiger, 1981). The decision about drug treatment in this group of patients should be influenced by the presence of other risk factors for coronary artery disease (*see* below) and a family history of premature atherosclerosis. Patients with triglyceride concentrations approaching 1000 mg/dl (11 mM) are subject to sudden and precipitous increases in plasma VLDL and chylomicrons, which can lead to acute pancreatitis. Drug treatment is clearly indicated for this group.

Epidemiological studies have revealed a negative correlation between the plasma concentration of HDL, which normally accounts for 20 to 30% of the total plasma cholesterol, and the risk of coronary artery disease (Miller, 1980). The basis of this association is not yet clear. It is not known whether high concentrations of HDL are themselves protective or whether they are an indication of some other beneficial aspect of lipid metabolism. For example, hypertriglyceridemic individuals frequently have a low concentration of HDL-cholesterol. When these patients are treated with drugs that lower VLDL concentrations, the HDL will often return to the normal range. The fibric acids and the inhibitors of 3-hydroxy-3-methylglutaryl coenzyme A (HMG CoA) reductase raise HDL and lower LDL. This combination of action is considered ideal in the prevention of atherosclerosis (*see* below).

THERAPEUTIC STRATEGIES

Diet. The first principle for treatment of all hyperlipoproteinemias is the provision of a diet that maintains a normal body weight and that minimizes concentrations of lipids in plasma. Individuals who are overweight should initially consume a weight-reducing diet. They should be placed on a diet that is low in cholesterol (< 300 mg/day), low in total fats (< 30% of calories), and low in saturated fats (< 10% of calories). For specific details of such diets, *see* the report of the National Cholesterol Education Program (Report, 1988) and an article by Connor and Connor (1982). Rare individuals with extreme sensitivity to dietary triglycerides (*i.e.*, those with familial lipoprotein lipase deficiency) must be placed on a diet that is severely reduced in total fat.

Elimination of Aggravating Factors. If an individual has a hyperlipoproteinemia that is exacerbated by some other illness (such as diabetes mellitus, alcoholism, or hypothyroidism), the exacerbating disease must be treated. In addition, individuals with hyperlipoproteinemia should be encouraged to reduce all other risk factors that might potentiate the development of atherosclerosis. Such a regimen would include cessation of smoking, treatment of hypertension, maintenance of a good exercise and physical fitness program, and careful control of blood glucose in diabetics.

Drugs. The final aspect of therapy for hyperlipoproteinemia involves the administration of drugs that lower plasma concentrations of lipoproteins, either by diminishing the production of lipoproteins or by enhancing the efficiency of their removal from plasma. The drugs that exist for this purpose are reviewed below. The concept has now arisen that a combination of drugs may have synergistic effects in lowering plasma lipid concentrations, especially that of LDL. The first successful combination was one of *nicotinic acid* and a *bile acid–binding resin,* which effectively lowers LDL concentrations in patients with heterozygous familial hypercholesterolemia (Kane *et al.*, 1981). *Probucol* (Kuo *et al.*, 1988) and *lovastatin* (Illingworth and Bacon, 1987) have also been given concurrently with bile acid–binding resins for their effect on LDL.

DRUGS THAT LOWER CONCENTRATIONS OF PLASMA LIPOPROTEINS

HMG CoA Reductase Inhibitors: Lovastatin and Related Drugs

An encouraging development in the treatment of hypercholesterolemia has been the introduction of a new class of fungal-derived compounds that are potent competitive inhibitors of HMG CoA reductase, the rate-controlling enzyme in the biosynthetic pathway for cholesterol. These drugs are extremely effective in lowering plasma concentrations of LDL-cholesterol. Four HMG CoA reductase inhibitors have been studied in humans; their structures are shown in Table 36–5. *Mevastatin* (originally called compactin), the first such inhibitor, was isolated in Japan by Endo in 1976. The compound was obtained from cultures of *Penicillium* species (Endo *et al.,* 1976) and was shown to inhibit cholesterol synthesis in cultured human cells (Brown *et al.*, 1978). Several years later, a structurally related compound, *lovastatin* (also called mevinolin or monacolin K), was isolated from cultures of *Aspergillus* and *Monascus* species independently by workers at the Merck Sharp and Dohme Research Laboratories and by Endo. Chemically modified versions of these compounds (*pravastatin* and *simvastatin*) have recently become available for clinical investigation.

Table 36–5. STRUCTURAL FORMULAS OF HMG CoA REDUCTASE INHIBITORS

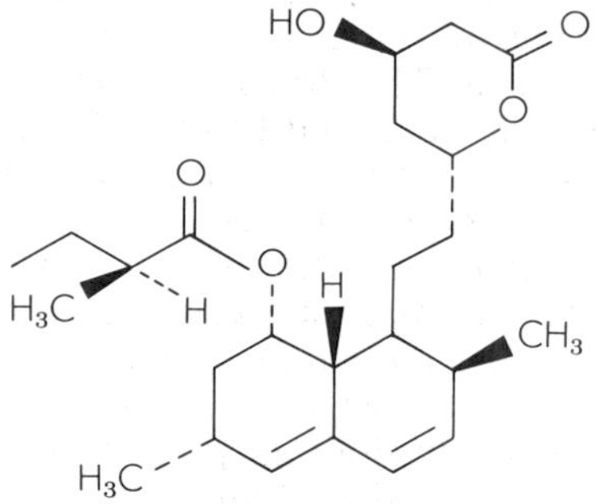

Lovastatin

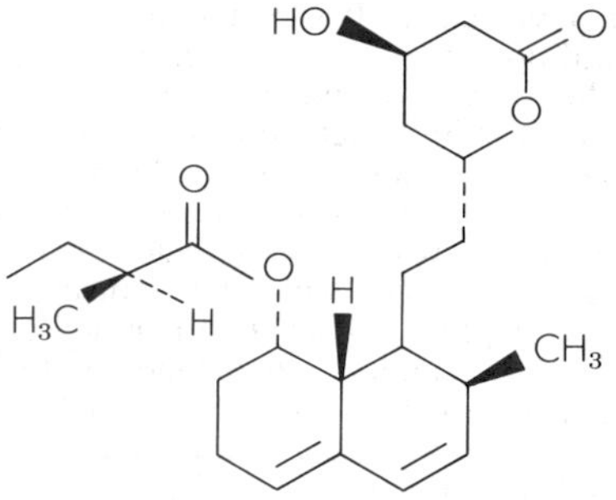

Mevastatin

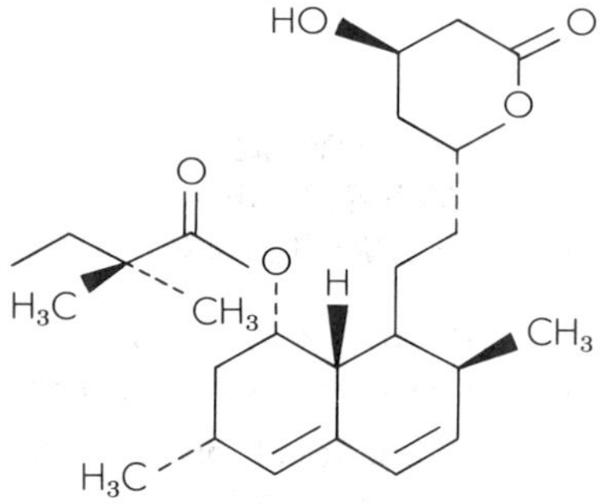

Simvastatin

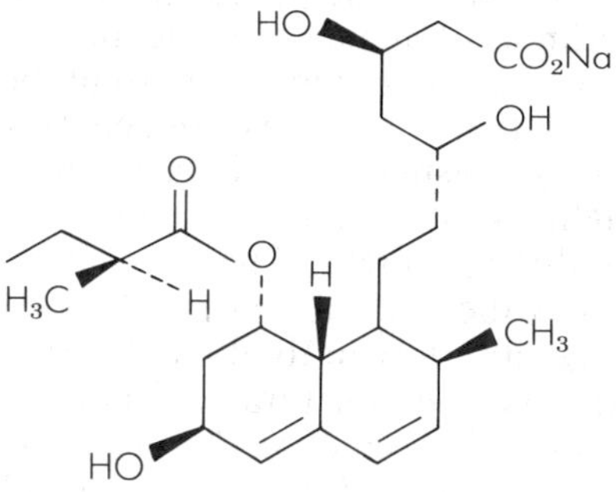

Pravastatin

Chemistry. Each of the microbial HMG CoA reductase inhibitors is composed of a hexahydronaphthalene ring system with two appendages: a methylbutyrate ester and a hydroxy acid that can form a six-membered lactone ring. The hydroxy acid is a structural analog of the half-reduced intermediate in the HMG CoA reductase reaction, as shown in Figure 36–2. Inhibition of the enzyme is reversible and competitive with respect to the substrate, HMG CoA. The drugs have inhibitory constants in the range of 1 nM, which is three orders of magnitude lower than the dissociation constant for HMG CoA. These data suggest that the inhibitors act as transition state analogs. Lovastatin and simvastatin are administered as prodrugs in the lactone form. The lactone ring is opened in the liver by chemical or enzymatic hydrolysis (or both) and the active inhibitor is generated. Pravastatin is administered as the acid and does not require activation (*see* Grundy, 1988; Alberts *et al.*, 1989).

Effects on Plasma Lipids and Lipoproteins. All the inhibitors of HMG CoA reductase have similar effects on plasma lipids. Lovastatin has been studied most extensively and will be described in detail. When given as a single agent to patients consuming a diet moderately low in cholesterol, lovastatin produces a dose-related decrease in the concentration of LDL-cholesterol in plasma. Typical decreases range from 20% at 10 mg per day to 40% at 80 mg per day (*see* Symposium, 1988b). This change can be attributed primarily to a decrease in the total number of LDL particles. There is also a slight decrease in the mean content of cholesterol of each LDL particle. The amount of cholesterol in VLDL also declines, possibly due to a decrease in the cholesterol content of secreted VLDL. Triglyceride concentrations decline up to 25%. The concentration of HDL-cholesterol typically rises 10 to 13%. The drug has similar effects in patients with heterozygous familial hypercholesterolemia and polygenic hypercholesterolemia. It is also effective in patients with hypercho-

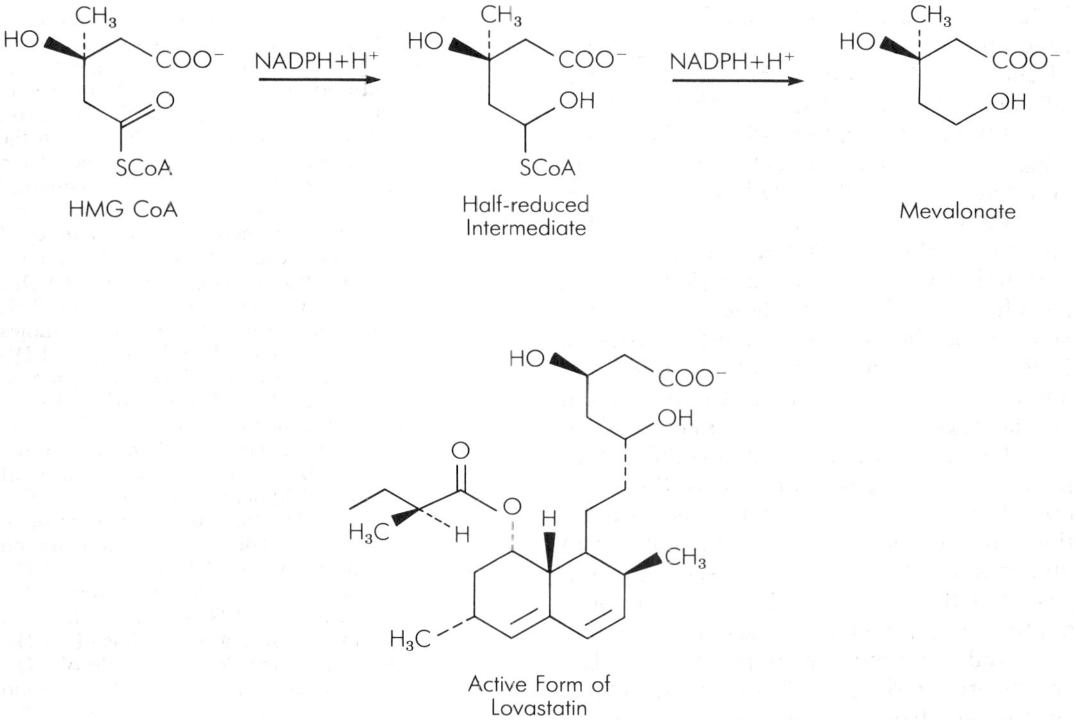

Figure 36–2. *The conversion of HMG CoA to mevalonate by HMG CoA reductase.*

HMG CoA is reduced in two stages by two molecules of reduced nicotinamide adenine dinucleotide phosphate (NADPH) to form mevalonate. The half-reduced intermediate is a structural analog of the active form of lovastatin.

lesterolemia associated with diabetes mellitus or with the nephrotic syndrome (Grundy, 1988).

Lovastatin acts in an additive fashion with bile acid–binding resins such as cholestyramine and colestipol. Patients with heterozygous familial hypercholesterolemia given 20 g of colestipol and 80 mg of lovastatin daily show decreases of approximately 50% in both total cholesterol and LDL-cholesterol (Illingworth and Bacon, 1987). Heretofore, such changes were obtainable only with the combination of nicotinic acid and a bile acid–binding resin—a regimen that causes many unpleasant side effects (Malloy *et al.*, 1987).

Mechanism of Action. Inhibitors of HMG CoA reductase block synthesis of cholesterol in the liver, thereby triggering compensatory reactions that lead to a reduction in plasma LDL. Much of the information about the mechanism for this reduction comes from studies in cell culture and in experimental animals. Cultured human fibroblasts respond to an inhibition of HMG CoA reductase by accumulating increased amounts of the enzyme (Brown *et al.*, 1978). The increase is attributable to an increase in the rate of transcription of the HMG CoA reductase gene, an increase in the rate of translation of the messenger RNA, and a decrease in the rate of degradation of the protein. Through these compensatory mechanisms, cultured cells can increase the amount of HMG CoA reductase sufficiently to restore rates of cholesterol synthesis almost to normal, even in the presence of relatively high concentrations of the inhibitor. An increase in HMG CoA reductase also occurs in the livers of rabbits, rats, and hamsters treated with these inhibitors. A similar adaptation is presumed to occur in man. Studies of sterol balance suggest that therapeutic concentrations of lovastatin reduce rates of total-body cholesterol synthesis by less than 20%. No correlation is observed between the magnitude of change in the rate of cholesterol synthesis and the decrease in plasma LDL (Grundy and Bilheimer, 1984). These data suggest that human subjects may be able to compensate at least partially for the inhibitory effect of the drug by increasing the amount of HMG CoA reductase.

If inhibitors of the reductase do not cause a profound inhibition of cholesterol synthesis, how do they lower the concentration of LDL? Observations in cultured cells and animals suggest a mechanism that is based on the regulation (enhanced synthesis) of the LDL receptor. Although it is difficult to prove such a mechanism in man, the available data are consistent with this formulation. Studies of lipoprotein metabolism in human subjects treated with lovastatin suggest that the fall in LDL results predominantly from an increase in the receptor-mediated clearance from plasma of LDL and its precursor IDL. This increased clearance results from an increase in the number of LDL receptors in the liver; it may also be a consequence of a change in the composition of IDL particles, such that they bind more efficiently to hepatic LDL receptors (Kovanen *et al.*, 1981; Alberts *et al.*, 1989).

Reductase inhibitors increase the concentration of LDL receptors by relieving the sterol-mediated suppression that normally regulates the transcription of the LDL receptor gene. This suppression is mediated by a short DNA sequence that is part of the promoter in the 5′-flanking region of the gene. A similar sequence, designated the sterol regulatory element, occurs in the promoters of the genes for HMG CoA synthase and HMG CoA reductase, sequential enzymes in the cholesterol biosynthetic pathway (Smith *et al.*, 1988). When sterols accumulate within cells, they act upon the sterol regulatory elements to repress transcription of all three genes. Teleologically, this repression seems designed to protect cells against an overaccumulation of cholesterol by limiting the uptake of LDL-cholesterol and by reducing synthesis of endogenous cholesterol. Reductase inhibitors relieve this repression by causing the intracellular concentration of sterol to fall, and this leads to increased transcription of all three genes. Although the increase in HMG CoA reductase is sufficient to offset somewhat the inhibition of cholesterol synthesis, this compensation can be maintained only as long as transcription of the reductase gene is driven at a high rate. The same mechanism that drives transcription of this gene also drives transcription of the gene for the LDL receptor. Therefore, the concentration of receptors increases and plasma LDL falls (*see* Goldstein and Brown, 1984).

At present, there is no evidence to suggest that reductase inhibitors reduce the rate of either synthesis or secretion of apoprotein B-100; however, they may reduce the amount of cholesterol in the secreted VLDL particles. The IDL formed from this cholesterol-poor VLDL may have an increased affinity for the LDL receptor. An increase in this affinity coupled with an increase in the number of LDL receptors would cause an enhanced clearance of IDL and a reduction in its conversion to LDL. Thus, the rate of LDL production would slow. This mechanistic formulation is consistent with studies of the rates of catabolism of radiolabeled VLDL and LDL in patients treated with reductase inhibitors (Bilheimer *et al.*, 1983; Uauy *et al.*, 1988).

The strongest evidence that supports this model comes from the ineffectiveness of lovastatin in patients with the LDL receptor–negative form of homozygous familial hypercholesterolemia (Uauy *et al.*, 1988). Even when treated with high doses of lovastatin, these subjects do not exhibit a reduction in either concentrations of LDL or rates of LDL production or catabolism. The only detectable effect is a lowering of VLDL-cholesterol. Even though lovastatin can cause a remodeling of VLDL in these patients, it cannot lower the rate of LDL production because there are no receptors to bind the resultant IDL.

The additivity of the effects of lovastatin and bile acid–binding resins results, hypothetically, from the capacity of both agents to lower the level of hepatic cholesterol by independent mechanisms; therefore, they reinforce each other in inducing LDL receptors (*see* Brown and Goldstein, 1986). This mechanism has been shown to operate in dogs given this combination of agents (Kovanen *et al.*, 1981). In addition, treatment with a bile acid–binding resin results in an increase in hepatic HMG CoA reductase activity (*see* below). Concurrent administration of a reductase inhibitor would blunt the effect of this compensatory mechanism.

Absorption, Fate, and Excretion. In several animal species, approximately 30% of an oral dose of lovastatin is absorbed. Although data are not available for human subjects, the extent of absorption is probably similar. Much of the drug is extracted from the blood during the first pass through the liver. Thereafter, lovastatin is extensively metabolized, and active as well as inactive metabolites accumulate in plasma. More than 95% of the drug and its metabolites are protein-bound. Most of the degradation products are excreted in the feces; less than 10% appears in the urine (*see* Alberts *et al.*, 1989).

Peak plasma concentrations of lovastatin and its active metabolites are observed 2 to 4 hours after a single oral dose. After 3 days of once-daily therapy, steady-state concentrations of drug approach 1.5 times the peak values seen after a single dose. Higher concentrations of the drug are achieved in plasma when lovastatin is given with food. There is no evidence that lovastatin induces cytochrome P_{450} drug-metabolizing enzymes.

Adverse Effects and Drug Interactions. Lovastatin became widely available in the United States in September, 1987. By December, 1988, more than 750,000 individuals in the United States were taking the drug on a daily basis. Thus far, the drug has been generally well tolerated and no unexpected toxicity has been reported (*see* Symposium, 1988b; Alberts *et al.*, 1989). A small percentage of patients (< 10%) develop various gastrointestinal symptoms, headache, or rash, but these symptoms rarely necessitate discontinuation of therapy. Asymptomatic elevations of serum transaminases derived from liver occur in approximately 2% of patients. Although frank jaundice is rare, it is recommended that patients be monitored every 4 to 6 weeks during the first 15 months of therapy and periodically thereafter. The drug should be discontinued in the face of persistently high or rising transaminase activity. Discontinuation is usually followed by a slow return of these values to normal.

Asymptomatic elevations of the plasma concentration of the muscle isozyme of creatine phosphokinase occur in up to 11% of patients taking lovastatin. In general, this is not a reason for discontinuation of the drug unless the creatine phosphokinase is persistently greater than three times normal or unless there are symptoms of myopathy. In patients with uncomplicated medical histories who are receiving lovastatin as a single drug, the incidence of myopathy is less than 0.2%. However, myopathy is much more frequent and severe in patients with complex histories who are taking other drugs, such as immunosuppressive agents (cyclosporine) or other lipid-lowering drugs (nicotinic acid or gemfibrozil). Some of these patients have experienced rhabdomyolysis with myoglobinuria and renal failure. Lovastatin should be used with care in these settings, and the daily dose should probably be limited to 20 mg (*see* Reaven and Witztum, 1988; Symposium, 1988b). Clinical experience with the other inhibitors of HMG CoA reductase has not been sufficient to determine the frequency of these side effects.

Extremely high doses of lovastatin produce cataracts in dogs. Because of the cataractogenic action of an earlier cholesterol-lowering drug (triparanol), particular attention has been paid to the potential occurrence of cataracts in patients treated with lovastatin. These studies have revealed a high incidence (about 30%) of minor lens opacities in hypercholesterolemic patients prior to the initiation of therapy with lovastatin. There is no evidence that the drug increases the incidence or accelerates the progression of these opacities; nevertheless, physicians are advised to monitor patients by slit-lamp examination of the eyes (*see* Symposium, 1988b; Alberts *et al.*, 1989).

Preparations, Dosage, and Therapeutic Uses. *Lovastatin* (MEVACOR) is the only inhibitor of HMG CoA reductase currently available for general use in the United States. It is available in tablets of 20 and 40 mg. Dosage is begun at 20 to 40 mg per day, given with food. If necessary, the dosage is increased at 4-week intervals to a maximum of 80 mg per day. The drug is slightly more effective when administered in divided doses, but this marginal benefit is outweighed by the inconvenience. When given once daily, the drug is more effective when taken in the evening, possibly due to a diurnal rhythm in the synthesis of cholesterol. Lovastatin can be given together with a bile acid–binding resin. The combination of lovastatin and gemfibrozil is extremely effective in certain patients, but it should be used with caution because of the possibility of myopathy (*see* above). Lovastatin (and all other drugs for hypercholesterolemia) should be used only after the patient has failed to respond to a diet that is low in cholesterol and saturated fat. All clinical trials of the reductase inhibitors have been performed in patients who are consuming such a diet.

Lovastatin is indicated as first-line therapy for patients who are at high risk of myocardial infarction attributable to hypercholesterolemia. This includes individuals with total cholesterol concentrations in plasma greater than 300 mg/dl (7.8 mM) or those with values greater than 240 mg/dl (6.2 mM) who also have documented coronary artery disease or one of the other risk factors discussed above. For other patients, the physician should consider the risk of myocardial infarction as balanced against the degree of uncertainty about the long-term side effects that accompanies the introduction of any new drug. As clinical experience with lovastatin increases, the indications for its use may expand. In addition to its effects in primary hypercholesterolemia, lovastatin is also effective in secondary hypercholesterolemia associated with diabetes mellitus and the nephrotic syndrome. The drug has teratogenic effects in animals; it is contraindicated in pregnant women or women of childbearing age who may become pregnant.

FIBRIC ACIDS: GEMFIBROZIL, CLOFIBRATE, AND FENOFIBRATE

As a result of screening tests in rats, Thorp and Waring (1962) found that a series of aryloxyisobutyric acids was effective in reducing plasma concentrations of triglyceride and cholesterol. The first compound that combined maximal effectiveness with minimal toxicity was *clofibrate,* and subsequently this drug was used widely for the treatment of hypertriglyceridemia. However, its use has become increasingly circumscribed because it has not been proven to be effective for the prevention of atherosclerosis (Coronary Drug Project, 1975; Oliver *et al.*, 1978); furthermore, awareness of latent adverse effects has grown (Oliver *et al.*, 1978; Palmer, 1978).

Several chemical relatives of clofibrate, collectively referred to as *fibric acids,* have proven to be less toxic and more effective for the treatment of hypertriglyceridemia and hypercholesterolemia than has clofibrate itself. One of these drugs, *gemfibrozil,* has been used extensively in the United States and Europe since the mid 1970s and was approved for use in the United States in 1982. A related experimental compound, *fenofibrate*, is widely prescribed in Europe (Brown, 1987).

Chemistry. Clofibrate, the ethyl ester of p-chlorophenoxyisobutyric acid, is the prototype of the fibric acids. The structural formulas of clofibrate and the related fibric acid derivatives are shown in Table 36–6. Gemfibrozil, fenofibrate, bezafibrate, and ciprofibrate all are more potent than clofibrate and can be used in lower doses (*see* Carlson and Olsson, 1979; Brown, 1987; Monk and Todd, 1987).

Effects on Plasma Lipids and Lipoproteins. Clofibrate characteristically reduces plasma triglycerides by lowering the concentration of VLDL within 2 to 5 days after initiation of therapy. In most patients, total cholesterol and LDL-cholesterol concentrations in plasma fall slightly. Some patients who exhibit a large fall in VLDL may show a paradoxical rise in LDL, such that the net effect on total cholesterol is minimal. The mean value of plasma cholesterol was reduced only 6% in men treated chronically with clofibrate (1.8 g per day) during the Coronary Drug Project (1975); the reduction in plasma triglyceride was 22%.

In a similar trial of primary prevention involving asymptomatic men with hypercholesterolemia, clofibrate lowered the plasma cholesterol concentration by only 6 to 11% (Oliver *et al.*, 1978). This very modest effect in unselected patients can be contrasted with that seen in patients with familial type-III hyperlipoproteinemia, in whom concentrations of cholesterol and triglycerides were lowered by approximately 50% and by as much as 80%, respectively (Levy *et al.*, 1972). In such patients, administration of clofibrate results in the mobilization of deposits of cholesterol in tissues, accompanied by regression and disappearance of xanthomas. Clofibrate has no effect on hyperchylomicronemia, nor does it affect concentrations of HDL. Thus, clofibrate appears to have specific efficacy only in patients with familial type-III hyperlipoproteinemia.

The clinical evidence for the efficacy of clofibrate in preventing deaths from coronary artery disease is not encouraging. A number of clinical trials have been completed, and none has shown a clear-cut beneficial effect. A double-blind study conducted by the World Health Organization compared clofibrate with placebo in 10,000 men in the upper third of the distribution of plasma cholesterol concentrations (Oliver *et al.*, 1978). Patients treated with clofibrate had a decrease in nonfatal myocardial infarctions but not in fatal myocardial infarctions. Moreover, clofibrate-treated patients had a higher noncardiac mortality rate than did control subjects, owing mainly to an increased incidence of malignant neoplasms and complications of cholecystectomy.

Gemfibrozil characteristically decreases plasma triglycerides by 40 to 55% by lowering the concentration of VLDL. A maximal effect is usually achieved within 3 to 4 weeks. The drug also lowers VLDL-cholesterol concentrations to a comparable de-

Table 36-6. STRUCTURAL FORMULAS OF FIBRIC ACIDS

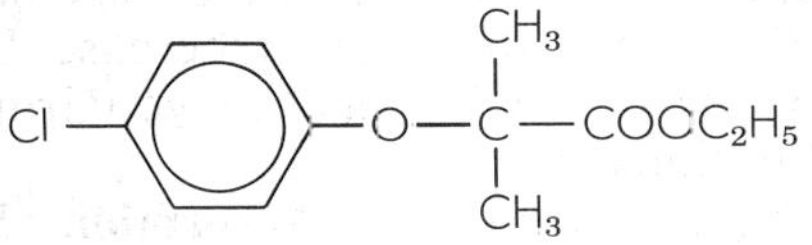

Clofibrate

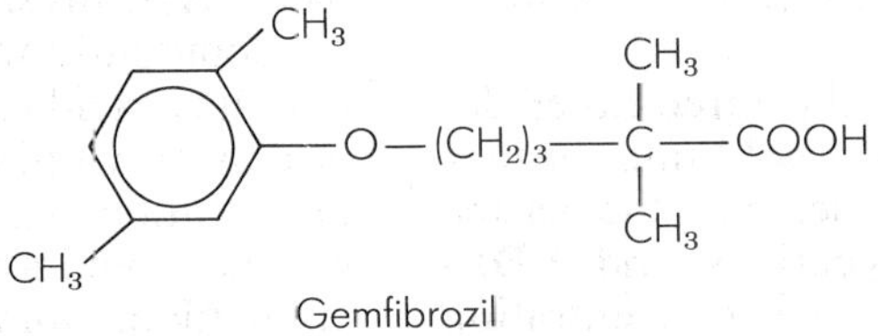

Gemfibrozil

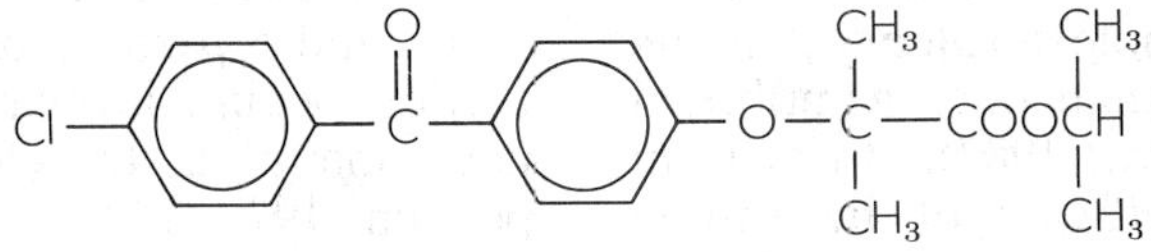

Fenofibrate

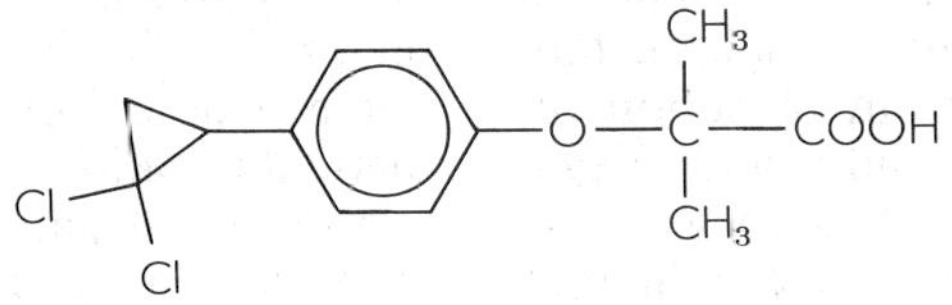

Ciprofibrate

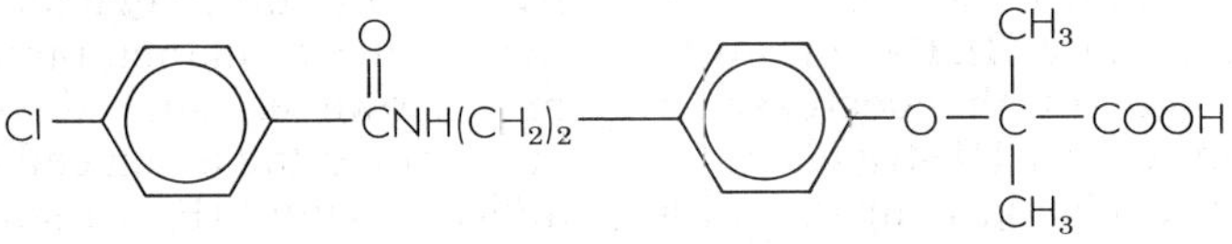

Bezafibrate

gree. This reduction is accompanied by a significant increase (10 to 25%) in the plasma concentrations of HDL-cholesterol (Samuel, 1983; Helsinki Heart Study, 1987). The drug is much less effective in lowering LDL, and it reduces plasma LDL-cholesterol by about 10% in hypercholesterolemic patients. Like clofibrate, gemfibrozil is extremely effective in normalizing the concentration of lipoproteins in patients with familial type-III hyperlipoproteinemia. Regression of xanthomas was observed in one study of 8 patients treated for 2.5 to 3 years (Kuo *et al.*, 1988).

A recent large-scale prospective clinical trial of gemfibrozil demonstrated a striking efficacy in reducing the manifestations of coronary artery disease. In this trial, 4081 middle-aged Finnish men who had hypercholesterolemia with or without mild hypertriglyceridemia were treated for 5 years with gemfibrozil or placebo (Helsinki Heart

Study, 1987). Gemfibrozil reduced total cholesterol by 11%, LDL-cholesterol by 10%, and triglycerides by 43%, and it increased HDL-cholesterol by 10%. Fatal and nonfatal myocardial infarctions were reduced by 34%, which was highly significant statistically. The beneficial effect of gemfibrozil was not evident until the last 2 years of the trial, when the reduction in coronary events in the treated group was about 50%.

As with gemfibrozil, the three other derivatives of clofibrate—fenofibrate, bezafibrate, and ciprofibrate—decrease the plasma concentration of triglycerides and LDL-cholesterol and raise the concentration of HDL-cholesterol. Several multicenter studies suggest that fenofibrate lowers LDL-cholesterol in hypercholesterolemic patients to a greater degree than does gemfibrozil or clofibrate (Brown, 1987). Long-term clinical trials of the efficacy of these three drugs in decreasing coronary artery disease have not been reported.

Mechanism of Action. The sites of action of the fibric acids are only partially established, and their mechanism of action remains controversial (Grundy and Vega, 1987). Their primary effect is to increase the activity of lipoprotein lipase, which in turn promotes the catabolism of the triglyceride-rich lipoproteins, VLDL and IDL. The drugs may also decrease the hepatic synthesis and secretion of VLDL. Fibric acids are believed to raise HDL-cholesterol indirectly as a result of the decrease in the concentration of VLDL-triglyceride. VLDL normally exchanges lipids with HDL, the triglycerides of VLDL moving to HDL and the cholesteryl esters of HDL moving to VLDL. When VLDL concentrations are reduced, this exchange is slowed. Cholesteryl esters remain in HDL and thus the concentration of HDL-cholesterol increases. Gemfibrozil may also stimulate the synthesis of apo A-1, the major apoprotein of HDL (Grundy and Vega, 1987).

The mechanism by which fibric acids lower LDL-cholesterol is not known, but it may involve enhanced hepatic clearance of VLDL and IDL, which would reduce the production of LDL (*see* Figure 36–1). Some patients taking a fibric acid derivative do not show a decrease in LDL-cholesterol; occasionally, LDL-cholesterol may even increase, but usually not to the abnormal range (Grundy and Vega, 1987).

Absorption, Fate, and Excretion. The fibric acid esters are rapidly and completely absorbed from the gastrointestinal tract, particularly when administered with a meal. Hydrolysis of the ester bond occurs concomitantly with absorption, and the active fibric acid reaches peak concentrations in plasma within several hours of oral administration. The active acids are bound to plasma albumin and undergo enterohepatic circulation. Administration of a single dose of gemfibrozil (600 mg) results in a plasma concentration of about 15 μg/ml after 2 hours and 5 μg/ml after 9 hours. Final excretion occurs primarily through the kidneys, mainly as the glucuronide (*see* Symposium, 1976, 1987).

Adverse Effects and Drug Interactions. The fibric acids are generally well tolerated. Mild gastrointestinal distress (abdominal pain, diarrhea, nausea) is the most frequent side effect and occurs in 2 to 5% of patients. Skin rash, alopecia, blurred vision, weight gain, impotence, leukopenia, and anemia have been reported occasionally. Atrial and ventricular arrhythmias have been noted only for clofibrate. Clofibrate has been shown to potentiate the effect of oral anticoagulants and to displace these drugs from their binding sites on albumin. However, such displacement cannot account for the enhanced effect of the oral anticoagulants (Bjornsson *et al.*, 1979). Possible mechanisms of this clinically significant drug interaction include a clofibrate-induced alteration in the synthesis of clotting factors, disposition of vitamin K, or characteristics of the warfarin receptor. A reduction in the dosage of the oral anticoagulant and frequent determination of prothrombin time are usually required in patients who are receiving both medications. Other fibric acid drugs also are highly bound to plasma albumin, but clinically significant interactions with oral anticoagulants have not been reported. An infrequent although disturbing effect of the fibric acids is a myositis or flu-like syndrome, associated with severe muscle cramps and tenderness, stiffness, and weakness. The syndrome recurs whenever the drug is taken and is associated with elevated plasma activities of creatine phosphokinase and glutamic-oxaloacetic transaminase. These enzymatic activities are sometimes elevated even in asymptomatic patients who are receiving one of the fibric acids.

The fibric acids increase the lithogenicity of bile, and they have been associated with an increased incidence of cholelithiasis and cholecystitis (Palmer, 1978). Several studies in which patients were treated for 1 year or longer have shown a 1 to 1.5% incidence of new or enlarged gallstones, a frequency that is slightly higher than in untreated controls. The drugs promote gallstone formation by increasing the hepatic secretion of cholesterol into the bile and by decreasing the conversion of cholesterol into bile acids in the liver (Grundy and Vega, 1987). Both of these changes increase the saturation, or lithogenicity, of bile. There is no evidence that the fibric acids differ in their lithogenic potential. All the fibric acids are contraindicated in patients with impaired renal or hepatic function and in pregnant or nursing women. The safety and effectiveness of fibric acids in children have not been established. The administration of high doses of clofibrate to mice and rats increases the frequency of benign and malignant hepatic tumors. In man, the long-term use of clofibrate may be associated with a slightly increased incidence of various tumors (Oliver *et al.*, 1978).

Preparations, Dosage, and Therapeutic Uses. *Clofibrate* (ATROMID-S) is available as 500-mg capsules. The drug is administered orally to adults in a dose of 2 g daily, in two or four portions. An increase in dosage above 2 g per day does not appear to produce greater effects on lipids but markedly increases the incidence of side effects. In all cases, its effects on lipids are enhanced by a low fat diet. Clofibrate is indicated only in subjects with increased concentrations of VLDL and IDL (such as patients with familial type-III hyperlipoproteinemia) who have failed to respond adequately to gemfibrozil or nicotinic acid. Because clofibrate has only a modest effect on LDL and more effective agents are available for lowering the concentration of LDL, the drug is of limited utility for patients with either familial hypercholesterolemia or polygenic hypercholesterolemia.

Gemfibrozil (LOPID) is available as 300-mg capsules and 600-mg tablets. The usual recommended dosage (for adults only) is 600 mg twice daily, taken 30 minutes before the morning and evening meals. Gemfibrozil is the drug of choice for patients with hypertriglyceridemia with or without hypercholesterolemia. It is particularly effective in patients with familial type-III hyperlipoproteinemia. The drug is also effective in most patients with severe hypertriglyceridemia associated with elevated chylomicrons (type-V hyperlipoproteinemia) who are at risk for developing acute pancreatitis (Garg and Grundy, 1989). Gemfibrozil is not effective for the treatment of hyperchylomicronemia due to familial lipoprotein lipase deficiency. It is not as effective as HMG CoA reductase inhibitors or bile acid–binding resins in reducing LDL-cholesterol concentrations, and thus it should not be used as primary therapy in patients with isolated hypercholesterolemia without hypertriglyceridemia. Its HDL-elevating action may make it useful in patients with mild hypercholesterolemia who have low HDL-cholesterol concentrations, but the benefit of elevating HDL in these patients has not been established.

Fenofibrate is not available for general use in the United States but is widely used in Europe. The usual dosage is 100 mg orally after each meal. Administration of the drug with meals reduces the gastric irritation that occurs in a few patients. Fenofibrate has the same indications as gemfibrozil (*see* above).

BILE ACID–BINDING RESINS: CHOLESTYRAMINE AND COLESTIPOL

The first of these agents, *cholestyramine*, was originally used to control pruritus in patients with elevated concentrations of plasma bile acid due to cholestasis. While this remains a valid use of the drug, greater interest now centers on the ability of this and similar agents to lower concentrations of plasma LDL-cholesterol (Hashim and Van Itallie, 1965). Inasmuch as the bile acid–binding resins are not absorbed from the gastrointestinal tract, they are perhaps the safest drugs currently available for the treatment of hyperlipoproteinemia.

Chemistry. Cholestyramine is the chloride salt of a basic anion-exchange resin. The ion-exchange sites are provided by trimethylbenzylammonium groups in a large copolymer of styrene and divinylbenzene. The average polymeric molecular weight is greater than 10^6. Cholestyramine has the following structural formula:

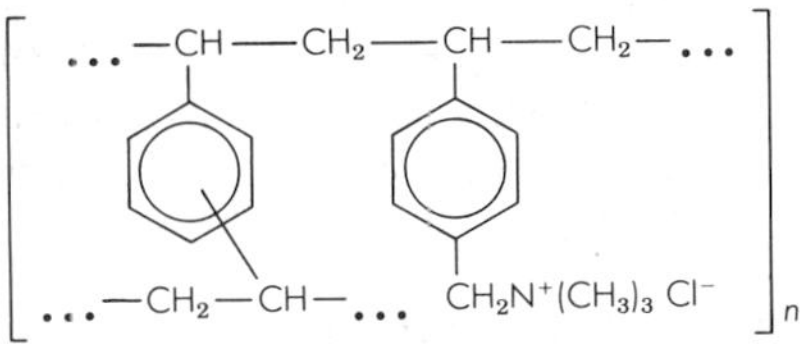

Cholestyramine

A second resin, colestipol hydrochloride, is a copolymer of diethyl pentamine and epichlorohydrin. The structural formula of colestipol is as follows:

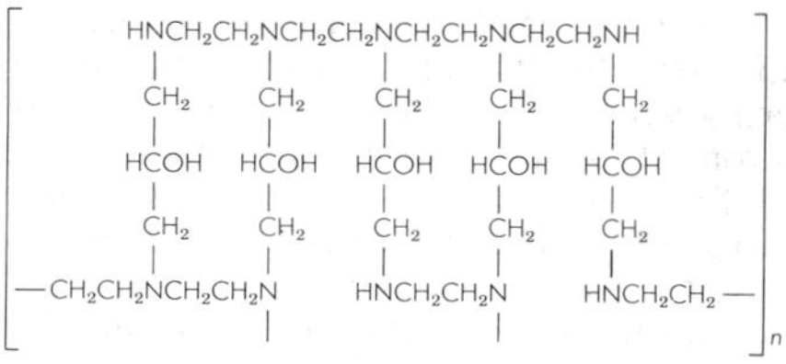

Colestipol

These agents are hydrophilic but insoluble in water. They are unaffected by digestive enzymes, remain unchanged in the gastrointestinal tract, and are not absorbed.

Effects on Plasma Lipids and Lipoproteins. The bile acid–binding resins characteristically reduce the concentration of cholesterol in plasma by lowering the level of LDL. The fall in the concentration of LDL is usually apparent in 4 to 7 days and approaches 90% of the maximal effect within 2 weeks. The magnitude of the effect on LDL is related to the dose and is usually in the range of 20%. In most patients, concentrations of triglyceride in plasma (VLDL) increase by 5 to 20% during the first weeks of therapy with a bile acid–binding resin; this increase usually then disappears gradually, and, within 4 weeks, concentrations of VLDL and triglyceride return to pretreatment values. In patients with elevated concentrations of VLDL and IDL, the increase of triglycerides that follows the initiation of therapy with these agents may be greater and the increase in VLDL and IDL may be more sustained. For these reasons, bile acid–binding resins are most effective when only LDL is in excess, as in familial hypercholesterolemia or polygenic hypercholesterolemia. Bile acid–binding resins have no predictable effect on the concentration of HDL. When therapy with the resin is discontinued, plasma concentrations of lipids rise rapidly and then slowly approach the pretreatment values over a period of 3 to 4 weeks. The efficacy of bile acid–binding resins is markedly increased when they are given with inhibitors of HMG CoA reductase (*see* above).

Mechanism of Action. These resins, administered orally, are not absorbed. They bind bile acids in the intestine, and there is thus a large increase in the fecal excretion of the acids. Since bile acids suppress the microsomal hydroxylase that catalyzes the rate-limiting step in the conversion of cholesterol to bile acids, their removal increases production of bile acids from cholesterol (Grundy *et al.*, 1971). Furthermore, since bile acids are required for the intestinal absorption (and enterohepatic reabsorption) of cholesterol, there is some additional fecal loss of neutral sterol. The net loss of bile acids and neutral sterol from the liver leads to two compensatory changes in hepatic metabolism: an increase in the number of cell-surface LDL receptors and an increase in the activity of HMG CoA reductase, the rate-controlling enzyme in cholesterol synthesis (Brown and Goldstein, 1986). Both of these compensatory changes restore homeostasis to the liver by providing increased amounts of cholesterol for conversion to bile acid. The increased number of hepatic LDL receptors leads to an increased uptake of LDL from plasma, resulting in a lower plasma LDL-cholesterol concentration (Shepherd *et al.*, 1980; Kovanen *et al.*, 1981). The effectiveness of the resin depends on the ability of hepatic cells to increase the number of active LDL receptors. Thus, individuals with the homozygous form of familial hypercholesterolemia, who lack LDL functional receptors, do not respond to such therapy (Goldstein and Brown, 1989). However, heterozygotes, who have one normal gene for the receptor, do respond. Body pools of cholesterol are decreased after long-term therapy with bile acid–binding resins, and tendon xanthomas also regress.

Adverse Effects and Drug Interactions. These preparations often have an unpleasant sandy or gritty quality, and patients may complain of this. Nausea, abdominal discomfort, indigestion, and constipation are frequent difficulties. Impaction may occur, and hemorrhoids are frequently aggravated. The addition of bran cereal to the diet is usually sufficient to minimize the constipation. Besides increasing concentrations of triglycerides in plasma, the bile acid–binding resins often transiently increase activities of alkaline phosphatase and hepatic transaminases. Since cholestyramine is a chloride form of an anion-exchange resin, hyperchloremic acidosis can occur, especially in younger and smaller patients in whom the relative dose is higher.

With high doses of resins steatorrhea may occur, and preexisting steatorrhea is aggravated by conventional doses. In such cases, the absorption of fat-soluble vitamins is also impaired and vitamin supplementation is recommended. Hypoprothrombinemia has been observed.

The resins may also bind other compounds in the intestine, including drugs administered concurrently. This has been noted particularly with chlorothiazide, phenylbutazone, phenobarbital, anticoagulants, thyroxine, and various digitalis preparations. As a general rule, it is recommended that other drugs taken orally should be ingested at least 1 hour before or 4 hours after the resin.

Bile acid–binding resins should probably not be administered during pregnancy. Children with heterozygous familial hypercholesterolemia should not begin therapy with resins until 6 years of age (Kane and Malloy, 1982).

Preparations, Dosage, and Therapeutic Uses. *Cholestyramine resin* (QUESTRAN) is available in packets that contain 9 g of powder (equivalent to 4 g of resin) or in cans that contain 378 g; it is also available in chewable bars containing 4 g of anhydrous resin (CHOLYBAR). *Colestipol hydrochloride* (COLESTID) is available in packets containing 5 g of resin and in bottles containing 500 g of drug. One level teaspoonful of drug is roughly equivalent to one packet of resin (4 g of cholestyramine or 5 g of colestipol). Both resins must be mixed with water or other fluids or pulpy fruits before ingestion. They should never be swallowed in the dry form. They are usually administered in daily dosages of 12 to 16 g (cholestyramine) or 15 to 30 g (colestipol), divided into two to four portions to be taken either before or during meals and at bedtime.

Cholestyramine and colestipol are useful in patients with elevated concentrations of LDL (heterozygous familial hypercholesterolemia and polygenic hypercholesterolemia). When administered with a diet low in both cholesterol and saturated fats, the resins lower plasma LDL by 15 to 20%. When cholestyramine or colestipol is administered in conjunction with either an inhibitor of HMG CoA reductase (lovastatin) or nicotinic acid, a reduction of LDL concentrations in the range of 50 to 60% can be achieved (Kane *et al.*, 1981; Bilheimer *et al.*, 1983; Illingworth and Bacon, 1987). The bile acid–binding resins are of no known benefit to patients with excessive concentrations of chylomicrons, VLDL, or IDL, and they may indeed exacerbate the excess of triglycerides. Thus, they should not be used to treat disorders characterized primarily by hypertriglyceridemia.

A long-term prospective study, the Lipid Research Clinics Coronary Primary Prevention Trial, has provided conclusive evidence for the efficacy and safety of cholestyramine in lowering LDL-cholesterol concentrations and in reducing the morbidity and mortality of coronary heart disease (Lipid Research Clinics Program, 1984a, 1984b). A summary of the results of this study is reviewed above.

PROBUCOL

Probucol is a synthetic lipophilic antioxidant related structurally to butylated hydroxytoluene. It was discovered empirically to lower plasma cholesterol in animals (Barnhart *et al.*, 1970); in man it causes a slight reduction in LDL-cholesterol and has been used therapeutically for the past decade. Enthusiasm for the drug has been limited because probucol reduces HDL-cholesterol even more than LDL-cholesterol. However, interest in probucol has been rekindled recently because of the possibility that it may retard atherosclerosis by antioxidant mechanisms that extend beyond its effects on plasma cholesterol concentrations.

Chemistry. Probucol has no structural similarity to other agents that lower cholesterol concentrations. It consists of two butylated hydroxytoluene molecules connected by a sulfur-carbon-sulfur bridge and has the following structural formula:

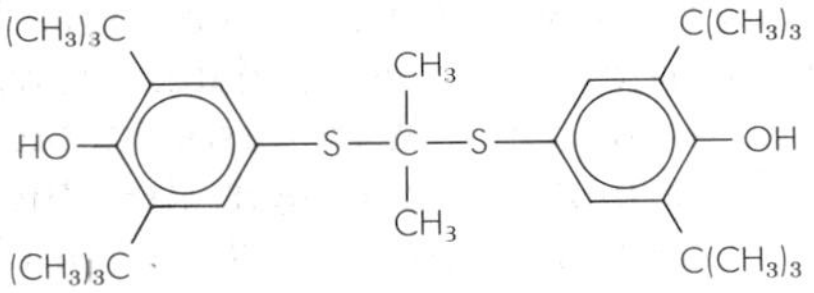

Probucol

Effects on Plasma Lipids and Lipoproteins. Probucol usually reduces total plasma cholesterol by 10 to 15% when given to patients who are already consuming a low-fat, low-cholesterol diet. The reduction in LDL-cholesterol is usually less than 10%, but the reduction in HDL-cholesterol is in the range of 30%. The effects of probucol on VLDL and triglycerides are minimal. In most studies, the maximal effect on plasma cholesterol (LDL plus HDL) occurs after 1 to 3 months of treatment (Atmeh *et al.*, 1983; Symposium, 1988a).

In two studies of patients with homozygous familial hypercholesterolemia, probucol caused a marked reduction of cutaneous and tendon xanthomas that was greater than would be expected from the modest lowering of cholesterol (Baker *et al.*, 1982; Yamamoto *et al.*, 1986). Although direct evidence for regression of atheromas was not sought, a few patients showed improvement of angina pectoris and in the electrocardiographic manifestations of ischemia (Baker *et al.*, 1982). It should be noted that probucol did not lower HDL-cholesterol in these homozygous individuals as it does in other hypercholesterolemic patients.

Two research groups have administered probucol to Watanabe heritable-hyperlipidemic (WHHL) rabbits, a strain that is homozygous for a mutation in the LDL receptor gene; thus, these animals have a defect that is analogous to that found in one class of homozygous patients with familial hypercholesterolemia (Carew *et al.*, 1987; Kita *et al.*, 1987). Probucol was started at 2 months of age and continued for several months. Plasma cholesterol concentrations fell slightly but remained in the range of 600 mg/dl (15.5 mM). At autopsy, the probucol-treated animals had a marked reduction in atherosclerotic lesions in the thoracic and abdominal aorta; the coronary arteries were not examined.

Absorption, Fate, and Excretion. Despite its lipid solubility, less than 10% of an oral dose of probucol is absorbed. Peak concentrations in blood are higher and less variable when the drug is taken with food. Probucol is transported in plasma in the hydrophobic core of LDL and other lipoprotein particles. It accumulates slowly in adipose tissue, and it persists in fat and blood for 6 months or longer after the last dose is taken. The major pathway of elimination is via the bile and feces; renal clearance is negligible.

Mechanism of Action. The effect of probucol on LDL concentrations is too small to allow any study of the mechanism. The drug does not cause a significant change in the rate of either synthesis or catabolism of LDL (Atmeh *et al.*, 1983). Probucol reduces the light fraction of HDL (HDL_2) as well as the heavy fraction (HDL_3). The content of both protein and cholesterol of these fractions declines; however, the decrease in cholesterol is greater than the decrease in protein, indicating that probucol causes the production of HDL that is relatively poor in cholesterol. The fall in HDL protein is attributable to a decline in the rate of production of both apo A-1 and apo A-2. The mechanism for these effects is unknown.

The probucol-mediated reduction of xanthomas in homozygous patients with familial hypercholesterolemia and of atheromas in WHHL rabbits is hypothesized to result from inhibition of the oxidation of LDL. Incubation of LDL *in vitro* with endothelial cells, or with heavy metals such as copper, leads to the oxidation of fatty acids in the phospholipids of LDL (Steinberg *et al.*, 1989). The oxidized fatty acids then attack the lysine residues of apo B-100; their positive charge is lost and the protein becomes fragmented. This oxidatively modified LDL is recognized by a cell-surface receptor on macrophages, and the resultant uptake converts the macrophages into foam cells. Probucol prevents this oxidation when added with LDL to cultured endothelial cells, presumably because of its antioxidant activity. LDL isolated from probucol-treated WHHL rabbits is resistant to oxidation by cupric ions (Kita *et al.*, 1987; Steinberg *et al.*, 1989), and the aortas of the treated animals accumulate only half as much proteolytically degraded LDL as do those of untreated WHHL rabbits when radiolabeled LDL is administered intravenously (Steinberg *et al.*, 1989). These data are consistent with the hypothesis that the antioxidant effects of probucol are responsible for its anti-atherogenic effect in WHHL rabbits, but more direct evidence is not yet available. Because of these observations, it is of obvious importance to determine whether therapeutic doses of probucol can decrease atherosclerosis in man.

Adverse Effects. Probucol is well tolerated, and there is little short-term toxicity. Diarrhea, flatulence, abdominal pain, and nausea are the most troublesome side effects, occurring in about 10% of patients. Occasional adverse effects include eosinophilia, paresthesias, and angioneurotic edema. The safety of probucol has not been established for children or during pregnancy. Because of its persistence in the body, it is recommended that women discontinue probucol and practice contraception for at least 6 months before attempting to become pregnant.

Probucol has caused fatal cardiac arrhythmias in monkeys that received a diet high in cholesterol and saturated fat; however, no adverse effects were observed in monkeys fed a low-fat diet who were treated continuously for 8 years at doses 3 to 30 times the human dose. Although prolongation of the Q–T interval occurs occasionally in patients treated with the drug, there have been no reports of other arrhythmias or of unexplained syncope. Nevertheless, patients should be advised to adhere to a low-cholesterol, low-fat diet throughout treatment, and an ECG should be obtained prior to therapy, 6 months later, and every year thereafter. Probucol should not be given to patients with evidence of recent myocardial damage or with ECG findings suggestive of ventricular irritability.

Preparations, Dosage, and Therapeutic Uses. *Probucol* (LORELCO) is available in 250-mg and 500-mg tablets. The recommended dosage (for adults only) is 250 to 500 mg twice daily, taken with morning and evening meals. As a sole LDL-lowering agent, probucol is less effective than lovastatin, nicotinic acid, or bile acid–binding resins, and hence its use should be restricted to hypercholesterolemic patients who require combined therapy, such as probucol plus a bile acid–binding resin or an HMG CoA reductase inhibitor. The drug is of no benefit in patients with hypertriglyceridemia. On the basis of recent studies *in vitro* and in WHHL rabbits showing that probucol may retard the formation of cholesterol-rich foam cells, it may be appropriate to combine probucol with other LDL-lowering drugs in the treatment of severely hypercholesterolemic patients. Despite the enthusiasm generated by these recent studies, there are as yet no data on the efficacy of probucol for prevention or control of atherosclerosis or its clinical sequelae in human subjects.

NICOTINIC ACID

Nicotinic acid was discovered as a hypolipidemic drug in 1955 (Altschul *et al.*, 1955). The lipid-lowering property of nicotinic acid is not shared by nicotinamide and has nothing to do with the role of these substances as vitamins. Pharmacological doses of nicotinic acid are useful in the treatment of most forms of hyperlipoproteinemia, but this usefulness is limited by the frequent occurrence of side effects. The chemistry of nicotinic acid and its function as a vitamin are discussed in Chapter 63.

Effects on Plasma Lipids and Lipoproteins. Large doses of nicotinic acid rapidly reduce the concentrations of triglycerides in plasma by lowering concentrations of VLDL; effects are noted in 1 to 4 days. Plasma concentrations of triglycerides may be reduced by 20% to over 80%; the degree of reduction is directly related to the initial concentration of VLDL (Carlson and Olsson, 1979). Concentrations of LDL-cholesterol fall more slowly, but a drop is clearly apparent within 5 to 7 days of the initiation of therapy. The magnitude of the fall in LDL is related to the dose, and the maximal effect is usually achieved 3 to 5 weeks after an appropriate dosage regimen has been established. When nicotinic acid is used alone, a 10 to 15% reduction in plasma LDL-cholesterol is typically seen; when it is used in combination with a bile acid–binding resin, a 40 to 60% reduction may occur (Kane *et al.*, 1981). In a recent study, nicotinic acid was used in combination with a bile acid–binding resin (colestipol) plus an HMG CoA reductase inhibitor (lovastatin) for treatment of patients with heterozygous familial hypercholesterolemia; this regimen produced a 69% reduction in LDL-cholesterol, and mean LDL-cholesterol values decreased from 323 to 103 mg/dl (8.4 to 2.7 mM) (Malloy *et al.*, 1987). Administration of nicotinic acid usually results in a mild-to-moderate increase in the concentration of HDL-cholesterol. Eruptive, tuboeruptive, tuberous, and tendon xanthomas regress after prolonged therapy.

Mechanism of Action. Nicotinic acid decreases the production of VLDL, which in turn results in a decreased production of its daughter particles, IDL and LDL (Grundy *et al.*, 1981). The mechanism by which nicotinic acid lowers VLDL production remains uncertain, but it is likely related to several of the drug's diverse actions, including inhibition of lipolysis in adipose tissue, decreased esterification of triglycerides in the liver, and increased activity of lipoprotein lipase (Gey and Carlson, 1971). Nicotinic acid does not produce any detectable change in total body synthesis of cholesterol, nor does it significantly alter excretion of bile acids (Grundy *et al.*, 1981).

Adverse Effects. Nicotinic acid produces an intense cutaneous flush and pruritus, involving the face and the upper part of the body. While these reactions decrease in intensity in most individuals after they have been on therapy for several weeks, they are unpleasant and may result in poor patient compliance. One aspirin (325 mg) taken 30 minutes before the nicotinic acid can markedly reduce the flushing, which appears to be mediated by a prostaglandin. Slow upward adjustment of dosage also appears to ameliorate this problem. Gastrointestinal disturbances such as vomiting, diarrhea, and dyspepsia are also common, and peptic ulceration has been reported. In rare instances, hyperpigmentation, acanthosis nigricans, and dry skin may occur after prolonged therapy.

Abnormalities of hepatic function occur in patients taking large doses of nicotinic acid. These include jaundice, a decrease in the excretion of bromosulfophthalein, and increases of plasma transaminase activities. Hyperglycemia and abnormal glucose tolerance occur in many nondiabetic patients taking nicotinic acid. Plasma concentrations of uric acid may also be elevated, and the incidence of acute gouty arthritis is increased. The drug should therefore be used with extreme caution, if at all, in patients who have hepatic disease, diabetes mellitus, or gout. The abnormalities of plasma glucose and uric acid and hepatic function are reversible when the drug is discontinued. Nicotinic acid may increase the vasodilatation and postural hypotension caused by antihypertensive agents. Toxic amblyopia (one case) and reversible cystoid edema of the macula (three cases) have also been reported. Nicotinic acid should not be used during pregnancy unless it is absolutely essential to prevent life-threatening pancreatitis owing to hypertriglyceridemia.

Preparations, Dosage, and Therapeutic Uses. Preparations of *nicotinic acid* (*niacin*) are described in Chapter 63. The usual daily dose of nicotinic acid is 2 to 6 g, divided into three portions and taken orally with or just after meals. Other preparations of nicotinic acid produce sustained concentrations of the drug in blood, but they appear to cause gastrointestinal irritation and hepatotoxicity. To reduce gastric irritation and to enhance absorption of nicotinic acid, the drug is best given at mealtimes, initially in small doses (three 100- or 200-mg tablets per day). Over a 1- to 3-week period, additional tablets are added to the regimen until the maintenance dose is reached.

By virtue of its actions in decreasing VLDL and LDL and in raising HDL, nicotinic acid is useful in the management of all types of hyperlipoproteinemia except familial lipoprotein lipase deficiency. Because of the variety of troublesome side effects associated with its use, most patients tolerate the drug poorly. In general, most hyperlipidemia can be effectively controlled by drugs with fewer side effects, such as gemfibrozil for hypertriglyceridemia and lovastatin for hypercholesterolemia. The one clinical situation in which nicotinic acid is especially useful is in patients with severe hypertriglyceridemia associated with elevated chylomicrons (type-V hyperlipoproteinemia) who do not respond to gemfibrozil. A maintenance dosage of 3 g of nicotinic acid per day can prevent the recurrent bouts of pancreatitis and eruptive xanthomas that occur in this disorder.

In one trial, the long-term use of nicotinic acid significantly decreased the incidence of recurrent myocardial infarction (Coronary Drug Project, 1975) and lowered the mortality rate 9 years after the study ended (Canner *et al.*, 1986). In another study, men with previous coronary bypass surgery who were treated for 2 years with nicotinic acid plus colestipol showed significantly more regression of atherosclerotic lesions in both native arteries and grafts than did a placebo-treated group (Blankenhorn *et al.*, 1987).

OTHER DRUGS

The antibiotic *neomycin* (*see* Chapter 47) has a hypolipidemic effect only when administered orally. The effect is not dependent on its antimicrobial activity but appears to be secondary to the formation of insoluble complexes with bile acids in the intestine. Its mechanism of action might thus be similar to that of the sequestrants of bile acids. Small doses of neomycin reduce the plasma concentration of LDL; effects on VLDL are variable. Neomycin is administered in divided doses of 0.5 to 2 g per day. While the drug is absorbed only to a minor extent, ototoxicity and nephrotoxicity may occur in patients with impaired renal function. Diarrhea and malabsorption are other complications. Neomycin should be considered only for patients with familial hypercholesterolemia or polygenic hypercholesterolemia who are unable or unwilling to follow other regimens.

β-Sitosterol is a plant sterol with a structure similar to that of cholesterol, except for the substitution of an ethyl group at C 24 of its side chain. Like most plant sterols, it is not absorbed by man. β-Sitosterol lowers plasma concentrations of LDL but has no effect on VLDL. Its mechanism of action is not known but may relate to an inhibition of the absorption of dietary cholesterol. It is indicated only for treatment of excess LDL in patients with polygenic hypercholesterolemia who appear to be extremely sensitive to small amounts of dietary cholesterol (Kane and Malloy, 1982). The long-term effects of β-sitosterol are unknown. Adverse reactions include a mild laxative effect and occasional nausea and vomiting. The recommended dose is 6 g (usually mixed with coffee, tea, fruit juice, or milk to increase palatability), taken 30 minutes before meals and at bedtime.

Dextrothyroxine (CHOLOXIN), the optical isomer of the naturally occurring hormone L-thyroxine, lowers plasma concentrations of LDL modestly. However, use of this drug may cause serious cardiac toxicity, and it is not recommended. For additional information on dextrothyroxine, *see* previous editions of this textbook.

Alberts, A. W.; MacDonald, J. S., Till, A. E.; and Tobert, J. A. Lovastatin. *Cardiol. Drug Rev.*, **1989**, *7*, 89–109.

Altschul, R.; Hoffer, A.; and Stephen, J. D. Influence of nicotinic acid on serum cholesterol in man. *Arch. Biochem. Biophys.*, **1955**, *54*, 558–559.

Atmeh, R. F.; Stewart, J. M.; Boag, D. E.; Packard, C. J.; Lorimer, A. R.; and Shepherd, J. The hypolipidemic action of probucol: a study of its effects on high and low density lipoproteins. *J. Lipid Res.*, **1983**, *24*, 588–595.

Baker, S. G.; Joffe, B. I.; Mendelsohn, D.; and Seftel, H. C. Treatment of homozygous familial hypercholesterolaemia with probucol. *S. Afr. Med. J.*, **1982**, *62*, 7–11.

Barnhart, J. W.; Sefranka, J. A.; and McIntosh, D. D. Hypocholesterolemic effect of 4,4′-(isopropylidenedithio)-*bis*(2,6-di-*t*-butylphenol) (probucol). *Am. J. Clin. Nutr.*, **1970**, *23*, 1229–1233.

Bilheimer, D. W.; Grundy, S. M.; Brown, M. S.; and Goldstein, J. L. Mevinolin and colestipol stimulate receptor-mediated clearance of low density lipoprotein from plasma in familial hypercholesterolemia heterozygotes. *Proc. Natl. Acad. Sci. U.S.A.*, **1983**, *80*, 4124–4128.

Bjornsson, T. D.; Meffin, P. J.; Swezey, S.; and Blaschke, T. F. Clofibrate displaces warfarin from plasma proteins in man: an example of a pure displacement interaction. *J. Pharmacol. Exp. Ther.*, **1979**, *210*, 316–321.

Blankenhorn, D. H.; Nessim, S. A.; Johnson, R. L.; Sanmarco, M. F.; Azen, S. P.; and Cashin-Hemphill, L. Beneficial effects of combined colestipol-niacin therapy on coronary atherosclerosis and coronary venous bypass grafts. *J.A.M.A.*, **1987**, *257*, 3233–3240.

Brown, M. S.; Faust, J. R.; Goldstein, J. L.; Kaneko, I.; and Endo, A. Induction of 3-hydroxy-3-methylglutaryl coenzyme A reductase activity in human fibroblasts incubated with compactin (ML-236B), a competitive inhibitor of the reductase. *J. Biol. Chem.*, **1978**, *253*, 1121–1128.

Brown, W. V. Potential use of fenofibrate and other fibric acid derivatives in the clinic. *Am. J. Med.*, **1987**, *83*, Suppl. 5B, 85–89.

Brunzell, J. D.; Schrott, H. G.; Motulsky, A. G.; and Bierman, E. L. Myocardial infarction in the familial forms of hypertriglyceridemia. *Metabolism*, **1976**, *25*, 313–320.

Canner, P. L.; Berge, K. G.; Wenger, N. K.; Stamler, J.; Friedman, L.; Prineas, R. J.; and Friedewald, W. Fifteen year mortality in coronary drug project patients:

long-term benefit with niacin. *J. Am. Coll. Cardiol.*, **1986**, *8*, 1245–1255.

Carew, T. E.; Schwenke, D. C.; and Steinberg, D. Antiatherogenic effect of probucol unrelated to its hypocholesterolemic effect: evidence that antioxidants *in vivo* can selectively inhibit low density lipoprotein degradation in macrophage-rich fatty streaks and slow the progression of atherosclerosis in the Watanabe heritable hyperlipidemic rabbit. *Proc. Natl. Acad. Sci. U.S.A.*, **1987**, *84*, 7725–7729.

Carlson, L. A., and Bottiger, L. E. Serum triglycerides, to be or not to be a risk factor for ischaemic heart disease? *Atherosclerosis*, **1981**, *39*, 287–291.

Coronary Drug Project. Clofibrate and niacin in coronary heart disease. *J.A.M.A.*, **1975**, *231*, 360–381.

Endo, A.; Kuroda, M.; and Tanzawa, K. Competitive inhibition of 3-hydroxy-3-methylglutaryl coenzyme A reductase by ML-236A and ML-236B, fungal metabolites having hypocholesterolemic activity. *F.E.B.S. Lett.*, **1976**, *72*, 323–326.

Garg, A., and Grundy, S. M. Gemfibrozil alone and in combination with lovastatin for treatment of hypertriglyceridemia in NIDDM. *Diabetes*, **1989**, *38*, 364–372.

Goldstein, J. L.; Schrott, H. G.; Hazzard, W. R.; Bierman, E. L.; and Motulsky, A. G. Hyperlipidemia in coronary heart disease. II. Genetic analysis of lipid levels in 176 families and delineation of a new inherited disorder, combined hyperlipidemia. *J. Clin. Invest.*, **1973**, *52*, 1544–1568.

Grundy, S. M.; Ahrens, E. H., Jr.; and Salen, G. Interruption of the enterohepatic circulation of bile acids in man: comparative effects of cholestyramine and ileal exclusion on cholesterol metabolism. *J. Lab. Clin. Med.*, **1971**, *78*, 94–121.

Grundy, S. M., and Bilheimer, D. W. Inhibition of 3-hydroxy-3-methylglutaryl-CoA reductase by mevinolin in familial hypercholesterolemia heterozygotes: effects on cholesterol balance. *Proc. Natl Acad. Sci. U.S.A.*, **1984**, *81*, 2538–2542.

Grundy, S. M.; Mok, H. Y. I.; Zech, L.; and Berman, M. Influence of nicotinic acid on metabolism of cholesterol and triglycerides in man. *J. Lipid Res.*, **1981**, *22*, 24–36.

Hashim, S. A., and Van Itallie, T. B. Cholestyramine resin therapy for hypercholesterolemia: clinical and metabolic studies. *J.A.M.A.*, **1965**, *192*, 289–293.

Helsinki Heart Study. Primary-prevention trial with gemfibrozil in middle-aged men with dyslipidemia. *N. Engl. J. Med.*, **1987**, *317*, 1237–1245.

Illingworth, D. R., and Bacon, S. Hypolipidemic effects of HMG-CoA reductase inhibitors in patients with hypercholesterolemia. *Am. J. Cardiol.*, **1987**, *60*, 33G–42G.

Kane, J. P., and Malloy, M. J. Treatment of hypercholesterolemia. *Med. Clin. North Am.*, **1982**, *66*, 537–550.

Kane, J. P.; Malloy, M. J.; Tun, P.; Phillips, N. R.; Freedman, D. D.; Williams, M. L.; Rowe, J. S.; and Havel, R. J. Normalization of low-density-lipoprotein levels in heterozygous familial hypercholesterolemia with a combined drug regimen. *N. Engl. J. Med.*, **1981**, *304*, 251–258.

Kita, T.; Nagano, Y.; Yokode, M.; Ishii, K.; Kume, N.; Ooshima, A.; Yoshida, H.; and Kawai, C. Probucol prevents the progression of atherosclerosis in Watanabe heritable hyperlipidemic rabbit, an animal model for familial hypercholesterolemia. *Proc. Natl. Sci. U.S.A.*, **1987**, *84*, 5928–5931.

Kovanen, P. T.; Bilheimer, D. W.; Goldstein, J. L.; Jaramillo, J. J.; and Brown, M. S. Regulatory role for hepatic low density lipoprotein receptors *in vivo* in the dog. *Proc. Natl. Acad. Sci. U.S.A.*, **1981**, *78*, 1194–1198.

Kuo, P. T.; Wilson, A. C.; Kostis, J. B.; Moreyra, A. E.; and Dodge, H. T. Treatment of type III hyperlipoproteinemia with gemfibrozil to retard progression of coronary artery disease. *Am. Heart J.*, **1988**, *116*, 85–90.

Levy, R. I.; Fredrickson, D. S.; Shulman, R.; Bilheimer, D. W.; Breslow, J. L.; Stone, N. J.; Lux, S. E.; Sloan, H. R.; Kraus, R. M.; and Herbert, P. N. Dietary and drug treatment of primary hyperlipoproteinemia. *Ann. Intern. Med.*, **1972**, *77*, 267–294.

Lipid Research Clinics Program. The Lipid Research Clinics Coronary Primary Prevention Trial Results. I. Reduction in incidence of coronary heart disease. *J.A.M.A.*, **1984a**, *251*, 351–364.

———. The lipid research clinics coronary primary prevention trial results. II. The relationship of reduction in incidence of coronary heart disease to cholesterol lowering. *Ibid.*, **1984b**, *251*, 365–374.

Malloy, M. J.; Kane, J. P.; Kunitake, S. T.; and Tun, P. Complementarity of colestipol, niacin, and lovastatin in treatment of severe familial hypercholesterolemia. *Ann. Intern. Med.*, **1987**, *107*, 616–623.

Oliver, M. F.; Heady, J. A.; Morris, J. N.; and Cooper, M. J. A co-operative trial in the primary prevention of ischaemic heart disease using clofibrate. *Br. Heart J.*, **1978**, *40*, 1069–1118.

Palmer, R. H. Prevalence of gallstones in hyperlipidemia and incidence during treatment with clofibrate and/or cholestyramine. *Trans. Assoc. Am. Physicians*, **1978**, *91*, 424–432.

Reaven, P., and Witztum, J. L. Lovastatin, nicotinic acid, and rhabdomyolysis. *Ann. Intern. Med.*, **1988**, *109*, 597–598.

Report. Report of the national cholesterol education program expert panel on detection, evaluation, and treatment of high blood cholesterol in adults. *Arch. Intern. Med.*, **1988**, *148*, 36–69.

Samuel, P. Effects of gemfibrozil on serum lipids. *Am. J. Med.*, **1983**, *74*, 23–27.

Shepherd, J.; Packard, C. J.; Bicker, S.; Lawrie, T. D. V.; and Morgan, H. G. Cholestyramine promotes receptor-mediated low-density-lipoprotein catabolism. *N. Engl. J. Med.*, **1980**, *302*, 1219–1222.

Smith, J. R.; Osborne, T. F.; Brown, M. S.; Goldstein, J. L.; and Gil, G. Multiple sterol regulatory elements in promoter for hamster 3-hydroxy-3-methylglutaryl coenzyme A synthase. *J. Biol. Chem.*, **1988**, *263*, 18480–18487.

Stone, N. J.; Levy, R. I.; Fredrickson, D. S.; and Verter, J. Coronary artery disease in 116 kindred with familial type II hyperlipoproteinemia. *Circulation*, **1974**, *49*, 476–488.

Thorp, J. M., and Waring, W. S. Modification and distribution of lipids by ethyl chlorophenoxyisobutyrate. *Nature*, **1962**, *194*, 948–949.

Uauy, R.; Vega, G. L.; Grundy, S. M.; and Bilheimer, D. M. Lovastatin therapy in receptor-negative homozygous familial hypercholesterolemia: lack of effect on low-density lipoprotein concentrations or turnover. *J. Pediatr.*, **1988**, *113*, 387–392.

Yamamoto, A.; Matsuzawa, Y.; Yokoyama, S.; Funahashi, T.; Yamamura, T.; and Kishino, B.-I. Effects of probucol on xanthomata regression in familial hypercholesterolemia. *Am. J. Cardiol.*, **1986**, *27*, 29H–35H.

Monographs and Reviews

Brown, M. S., and Goldstein, J. L. Lipoprotein metabolism in the macrophage: implications for cholesterol deposition in atherosclerosis. *Annu. Rev. Biochem.*, **1983**, *52*, 223–261.

———. A receptor-mediated pathway for cholesterol homeostasis. *Science*, **1986**, *232*, 34–47.

Carlson, L. A., and Olsson, A. G. Effect of drugs on lipoprotein metabolism. *Prog. Biochem. Pharmacol.*, **1979**, *15*, 238–257.

Connor, W. E., and Connor, S. L. The dietary treatment of hyperlipidemia: rationale, technique and efficacy. *Med. Clin. North Am.*, **1982**, *66*, 485–518.

Gey, K. F., and Carlson, L. A. (eds.). *Metabolic Effects of Nicotinic Acid and Its Derivatives*. Hans Huber Publishers, Bern, **1971.**

Goldstein, J. L., and Brown, M. S. Progress in understanding the LDL receptor and HMG CoA reductase, two membrane proteins that regulate the plasma cholesterol. *J. Lipid Res.*, **1984,** *25,* 1450–1461.

———. Familial hypercholesterolemia. In, *The Metabolic Basis of Inherited Disease*, 6th ed. (Scriver, C. R.; Beaudet, A. L.; Sly, W. S.; and Vallee, D.; eds.) McGraw-Hill Book Co., New York, **1989,** pp. 1215–1250.

Goldstein, J. L.; Kita, T.; and Brown, M. S. Defective lipoprotein receptors and atherosclerosis: lessons from an animal counterpart of familial hypercholesterolemia. *N. Engl. J. Med.*, **1983,** *309,* 288–295.

Grundy, S. M. HMG-CoA reductase inhibitors for treatment of hypercholesterolemia. *N. Engl. J. Med.*, **1988,** *319,* 24–32.

Grundy, S. M., and Vega, G. L. Fibric acids: effects on lipids and lipoprotein metabolism. *Am. J. Med.*, **1987,** *83,* Suppl. 5B, 9–20.

Havel, R. J. Lipid transport function of lipoproteins in blood plasma. *Am. J. Physiol.*, **1987,** *253,* E1–E5.

Keys, A. Coronary heart disease: the global picture. *Atherosclerosis*, **1975,** *22,* 149–192.

Mahley, R. W. Apolipoprotein E: cholesterol transport protein with expanding role in cell biology. *Science*, **1988,** *240,* 622–630.

Mahley, R. W., and Rall, S. C. Type III hyperlipoproteinemia (dysbetalipoproteinemia): the role of apolipoprotein E in normal and abnormal lipoprotein metabolism. In, *The Metabolic Basis of Inherited Disease*, 6th ed. (Scriver, C. R.; Beaudet, A. L.; Sly, W. S.; and Vallee, D.; eds.) McGraw-Hill Book Co., New York, **1989,** pp. 1195–1213.

Miller, G. J. High density lipoproteins and atherosclerosis. *Annu. Rev. Med.*, **1980,** *31,* 97–108.

Monk, J. P., and Todd, P. A. Bezafibrate: a review. *Drugs*, **1987,** *33,* 539–576.

Steinberg, D.; Parthasarathy, S.; Carew, T. E.; Khoo, J. C.; and Witztum, J. L. The role of post-secretory structural modification of low density lipoproteins in atherogenesis. *N. Engl. J. Med.*, **1989,** *320,* 915–924.

Symposium. (Various authors.) Gemfibrozil: a new lipid lowering agent. *Proc. R. Soc. Med.*, **1976,** *69,* Suppl. 2, 1–120.

Symposium. (Various authors.) Fenofibrate, a third-generation fibric acid derivative. *Am. J. Med.*, **1987,** *83,* Suppl. 5B, 1–89.

Symposium. (Various authors.) Second International Conference on Hypercholesterolemia—Examining New Data on Probucol After a Decade of Use. *Am. J. Cardiol.*, **1988a,** *62,* 1B–81B.

Symposium. (Various authors.) HMG CoA reductase inhibitors—a new therapeutic class. *Am. J. Cardiol.*, **1988b,** *62,* 1J–49J.

SECTION

VIII

Drugs Affecting Gastrointestinal Function

CHAPTER

37 AGENTS FOR CONTROL OF GASTRIC ACIDITY AND TREATMENT OF PEPTIC ULCERS

Laurence L. Brunton

Dyspepsia, in its many forms, has been mankind's companion since the advent of bad cooking, overindulgence, and anxiety. Since one "is not altogether fit for the battle of life who is in perpetual contention with his dinner" (Meredith, 1859), considerable energy has gone into relieving the symptoms of gastric upset and peptic ulcer disease.

For centuries, neutralization of gastric acid with antacids provided the only relief from the pain of ulcers. More recent studies of the physiological control of acid secretion demonstrated that anticholinergic agents would blunt this process. The development by Black and colleagues of antagonists that act at H_2-histaminergic receptors provided a more specific class of inhibitors of gastric acid secretion. The more recent advent of substituted benzimidazole inhibitors of the H^+,K^+-ATPase offers a very effective means of selectively blocking the proton pump that is responsible for acid secretion by the parietal cell. Although gastric acid has dominated thinking about peptic ulcer disease, appreciation of the means by which the gastric mucosa normally protects itself from damage has suggested additional therapeutic approaches (Hornick, 1987; Talley and Ormand, 1989).

The rationale for the use of agents that reduce gastric acidity is best understood in terms of the physiological regulation of acid secretion. A model of the functions of the oxyntic gland in the fundus and corpus of the stomach is shown in Figure 37–1. Although all the anatomical and functional relationships have not been precisely defined, the central role of histamine is evident from the ability of H_2 antagonists to suppress secretory responses to food, gastrin, and vagal stimulation (*see* Black and Shankley, 1987; Wolfe and Soll, 1988). Although mast cells are present in the gastric mucosa, the histamine that is responsible for stimulation of acid secretion appears to arise from endocrine or paracrine cells in the oxyntic gland; these cells express receptors for both muscarinic cholinergic agonists and gastrin, and they secrete histamine in response to activation of these receptors. Gastrin secretion (primarily from the antrum) is stimulated by food, both directly and indirectly (by elevation of gastric pH and by reflexes mediated by the vagus). Although parietal cells also have receptors for gastrin, their response to gastrin is greatly potentiated when H_2 receptors are activated concomitantly. Thus, histamine both transmits and facilitates the stimulation of acid secretion by gastrin.

Histamine plays a similar dual role in acid secretion evoked by stimulation of the vagus, but the anatomical relationships are less clearly defined. In addition to the effects that are mediated by gastrin, vagal stimulation produces an increased secretion of histamine and gastric acid that can be blocked by either nicotinic or M_1-muscarinic antagonists (*e.g.*, pirenzepine). Moreover, cholinergic agonists can exert powerful stimulatory effects on acid secretion in the presence of H_2 antagonists through interaction with muscarinic receptors on parietal cells; the receptor subtype that mediates this response has not been firmly established (*see* Chapters 5 and 6). Evidently, endogenous ACh has only limited access to parietal cells, apparently because it is released from postganglionic neurons that are closer to endocrine than to parietal cells. It is not clear how transmission from the vagus to these postganglionic neurons is accomplished; the potent blocking effects of pirenzepine are also unexplained, in part because the type of muscarinic receptor on the endocrine cells has not been defined.

Stimulation of H_2 receptors on parietal cells causes activation of adenylyl cyclase (*see* Chapter 2), and a complex array of morphological and biochemical changes ensues (*see* Sachs *et al.*, 1988; Forte *et al.*, 1989). Although the sequence of events is not completely known, mediation by adenosine 3′,5′-monophosphate (cyclic AMP) has been established. An increase in the concentration of cytosolic Ca^{2+} is also involved, and stimulation of parietal cells by cholinergic agonists elevates intracellular Ca^{2+} and stimulates nearly maximal rates of acid secretion (without a change in cyclic AMP). Ultimately, the most important consequence of these early events is the activation of a unique H^+,K^+-ATPase and its insertion into the membrane of the apical canaliculus of the parietal cell. This enzyme catalyzes the exchange of intracellular H^+ for extracellular K^+, and, with the concomitant increase in the permeability of the apical membrane to K^+ and Cl^-, about 0.1 N HCl accumulates in the lumen of the canaliculus. The human stomach is capable of producing 20 to 40 mEq of HCl per hour; this capacity accounts for the use of 960 mEq of antacid per day in many therapeutic regimens. Inhibitors of the H^+,K^+-ATPase, such as omeprazole, can virtually eliminate acid secretion.

Stimuli for acid secretion also enhance the secretion of mucus and bicarbonate, which serve to pro-

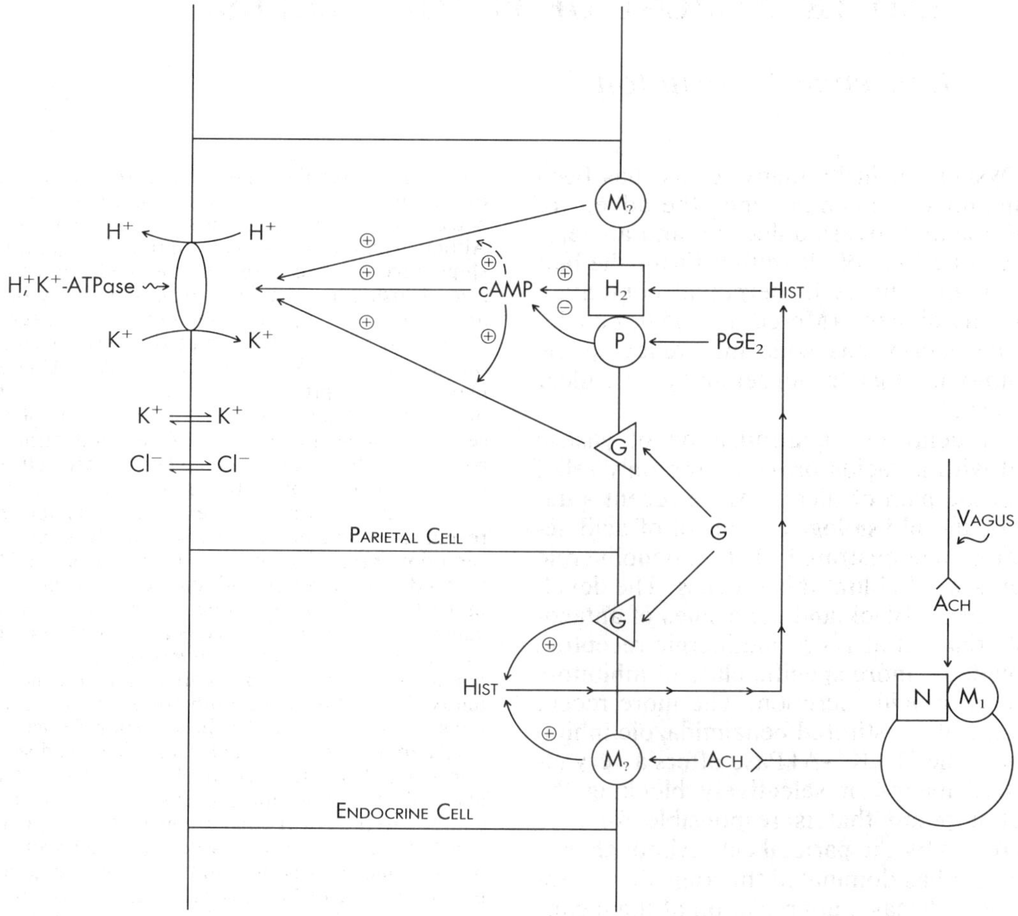

Figure 37–1. *Regulation of acid secretion by the parietal cell.*

ACH = acetylcholine; G = gastrin; HIST = histamine; cAMP = cyclic AMP; PGE_2 = prostaglandin E_2; ⊕ = stimulation; ⊖ = inhibition; [H₂] = H_2 histamine receptor; ◁G = gastrin receptor; P = prostaglandin receptor; [N] = nicotinic cholinergic receptor; (M) = muscarinic cholinergic receptor. The muscarinic receptors in parietal and endocrine cells have not been fully characterized. *See* text for detailed description.

tect the gastric mucosa from damage. To an important degree, this "cytoprotective" function is mediated by the elaboration of prostaglandins such as PGE_2, which also participate in feedback regulation of acid secretion by inhibition of both adenylyl cyclase activity and the release of gastrin. Interference with the protective functions of prostaglandins by inhibition of their synthesis is thought to account for much of the ulcerogenic effect of aspirin-like drugs. Although enhancement of cytoprotection might provide an alternative method for treatment of peptic ulcers, such use of analogs of PGE_2 (*e.g.*, misoprostol) appears to be effective only when there is substantial inhibition of the secretion of acid.

H_2-RECEPTOR ANTAGONISTS

The inability of H_1 antagonists to inhibit gastric acid secretion, including that elicited by histamine, has long been known. However, the development in the 1970s of H_2 antagonists provided incontrovertible evidence for the importance of endogenous histamine in the physiological control of gastric secretion (*see* Figure 37–1; *see also* Chapter 23).

Chemistry. The H_2 antagonists in clinical use are analogs of histamine that contain a bulky side chain in place of the ethylamine moiety. Early representatives of the group, such as burimamide (Black *et al.*, 1972) and cimetidine (the first compound released for general use) retain the imidazole ring of histamine. This ring is replaced in more recently developed compounds by a furan (ranitidine) or a thiazole (famotidine, nizatidine). The structures of H_2 antagonists that are currently available are presented in Table 37–1. As a group, these drugs are more hydrophilic than are the H_1 antagonists, and they reach the central nervous system (CNS) to only a limited extent.

Pharmacological Properties. H_2 antagonists inhibit competitively the interaction of histamine with H_2 receptors. They are highly selective and have little or no effect on H_1 or other receptors. Although H_2 receptors are present in numerous tissues, including vascular and bronchial smooth muscle, H_2 antagonists interfere remarkably little with physiological functions other than gastric secretion. Nevertheless, they measurably inhibit effects on the cardiovascular and other systems that are elicited through H_2 receptors by exogenous or endogenous histamine (*see* Brogden *et al.*, 1982; Ganellin and Parsons, 1982).

Table 37–1. STRUCTURES OF H_2 ANTAGONISTS

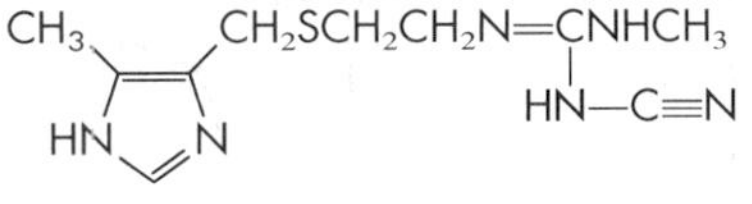

Cimetidine

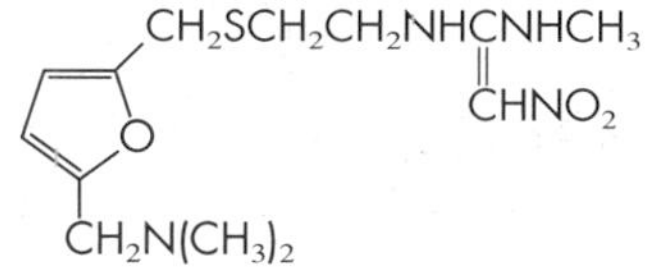

Ranitidine

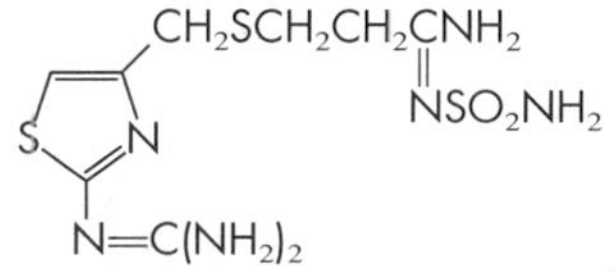

Famotidine

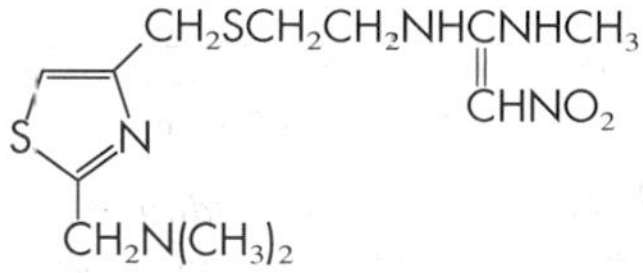

Nizatidine

Gastric Secretion. H_2 antagonists inhibit gastric acid secretion elicited by histamine and other H_2 agonists in a dose-dependent, competitive manner; the degree of inhibition parallels the concentration of the drug in plasma over a wide range (Figure 37–2). The H_2 antagonists also inhibit acid secretion elicited by gastrin and, to a lesser extent, by muscarinic agonists. Importantly, these drugs inhibit basal (fasting) and nocturnal acid secretion and that stimulated by food, sham feeding, fundic distention, and various pharmacological agents; this property reflects the vital role of histamine in mediating the effects of diverse stimuli (*see* Figure 37–1). The H_2 antagonists reduce both the volume of gastric juice secreted and its H^+ concentration. The output of pepsin, which is secreted by the chief cells of gastric glands (mainly under cholinergic control), generally falls in parallel with the reduction in volume of gas-

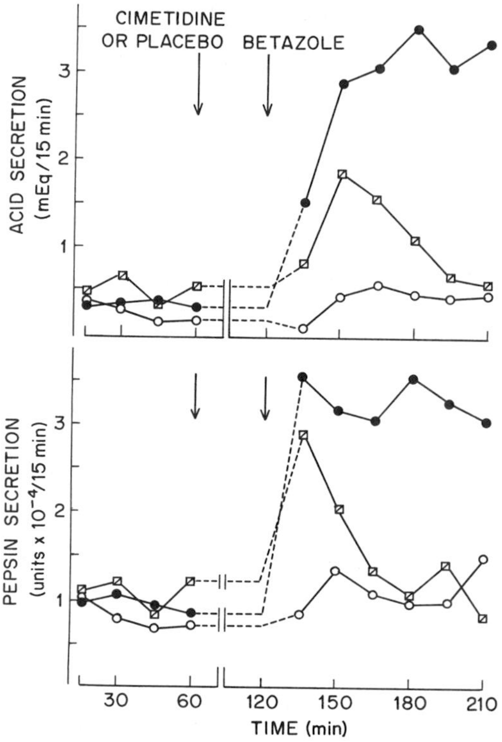

Figure 37–2. *Effect of cimetidine on betazole stimulation of secretion of acid (upper panel) and of pepsin (lower panel) in man.*

A placebo (•) or cimetidine (200 mg, ⊠; 300 mg, ○) was given orally 1 hour before the subcutaneous administration of betazole (1.5 mg/kg). (Modified from Binder and Donaldson, 1978.)

tric juice (*see* Figure 37–2). Secretion of intrinsic factor is also reduced; however, since this protein is normally secreted in great excess, absorption of vitamin B_{12} is usually adequate even during long-term therapy with H_2 antagonists. The concentration of gastrin in plasma is not significantly altered under fasting conditions, although the normal prandial elevation may be augmented; this increase is apparently a consequence of reduction of the feedback inhibition of gastrin secretion that is normally provided by H^+.

H_2 antagonists protect experimental animals from gastric ulceration induced by stress, pyloric ligation, aspirin, H_2 agonists, or cholinomimetics. H_2 antagonists also counter peptic ulceration in man, as described below. They have no consistent effect on the rate of gastric emptying, the pressure of the lower esophageal sphincter, or pancreatic secretion.

Absorption, Fate, and Excretion. As a group, H_2 antagonists are rapidly and well absorbed after oral administration; peak concentrations in plasma are attained within 1 or 2 hours. The oral bioavailability of nizatidine approximates 90%, whereas first-pass hepatic metabolism limits the bioavailability of the other compounds to about 50%. The half-time for elimination of cimetidine, ranitidine, and famotidine is 2 to 3 hours, while that of nizatidine is somewhat shorter—about 1.3 hours. These drugs are in large part excreted in the urine without being metabolized. However, the half-life of ranitidine is significantly prolonged in patients with hepatic dysfunction.

Adverse Effects. A variety of adverse reactions have been ascribed to cimetidine and ranitidine, reflecting, in part, the very large number of patients who have been treated with these drugs. The incidence of reactions is low, and they are generally minor. The low incidence is attributable in part to the limited function of H_2 receptors in organs other than the stomach and to the poor penetration of these agents across the normal blood–brain barrier. The profoundly hypochlorhydric stomach favors the formation of bezoars and the survival of microorganisms; the latter may explain rare cases of candidal peritonitis. Reduction of gastric acidity by H_2 antagonists can also impair the absorption of nonheme dietary iron, but this effect is generally without significance.

The incidence of adverse effects with cimetidine is about 5%; reactions are usually less intense with the other drugs, and some are not produced at all. The most common side effects of cimetidine are altered laxation, headache, dizziness and nausea, myalgia, skin rashes, and itching. The incidence of symptoms related to the CNS appears to be higher in the elderly and in patients with impaired renal function. Loss of libido, impotence, and gynecomastia are sometimes observed in patients who receive long-term therapy with high doses of cimetidine. These effects are presumably related to the ability of the drug to enhance the secretion of prolactin and to bind to androgen receptors. In addition, cimetidine inhibits the cytochrome P_{450}–catalyzed hydroxylation of estradiol and increases the plasma concentration of estradiol in men (Gailbraith and Michnovicz, 1989). These effects on male sexual function are not shared by the other agents. Case reports suggest that cimetidine occasionally causes hematological effects (various cytopenias) and altered function of the immune system. Rarely, the use of cimetidine has been associated with reversible bone marrow depression, hepatitis, or anaphylaxis. Cimetidine appears to inhibit competitively the renal tubular secretion of creatinine and causes a small increase in its plasma concentration. Rapid intravenous infusion of H_2 antagonists has caused bradycardia and release of histamine. (For reviews of the adverse effects of H_2 antagonists, *see* Zeldis *et al.*, 1983; Powell and Donn, 1984; and Aymard *et al.*, 1988.)

Drug Interactions. All agents that inhibit gastric acid secretion may alter the bioavailability and rate of absorption of certain drugs secondary to changes in gastric pH (*see* below).

Cimetidine (but not the other H_2 blockers) inhibits the activity of cytochrome P_{450}, thereby slowing the metabolism of many drugs that are substrates for hepatic mixed-function oxidases. Thus, the concurrent administration of cimetidine will prolong the half-life of a host of drugs, including warfarin, phenytoin, theophylline, phenobarbital, many benzodiazepines, propranolol, nifedipine, digitoxin, quinidine, mexiletine, and tricyclic antidepressants such as imipramine. Such interactions may require either reduction of dosage or alteration of the regimen. (The drug interactions of H_2 antagonists have been reviewed by Sedman, 1984; Nazario, 1986; and Aymard *et al.*, 1988.)

Preparations, Routes of Administration, and Dosage. H_2 antagonists are well tolerated and can be administered in doses well in excess of those needed to produce an effect. Thus, despite their short half-lives in plasma, these drugs can often be taken only once or twice daily (the "maximal dose" strategy).

Cimetidine (TAGAMET) is available for oral use as tablets containing 200, 300, 400, or 800 mg and as a liquid containing 300 mg/5 ml. For treatment of active duodenal or benign gastric ulcers, the recommended dosage is 800 mg at bedtime. Alternatively, 300 mg four times a day or 400 mg twice daily may be used. Treatment is usually continued for 4 to 8 weeks; however, a dose of 400 mg may be given at bedtime for prevention of recurrence of duodenal ulcers. Solutions of the hydrochloride salt of cimetidine (6 or 150 mg/ml) are available for intramuscular or intravenous administration.

Ranitidine hydrochloride (ZANTAC) is available in tablets (150 or 300 mg) and as a syrup (15 mg/ml) for oral use. The usual dosage schedule for treatment of active duodenal ulcer is 150 mg twice daily or 300 mg at bedtime. Injectable solutions (0.5 or 25 mg/ml) are also available; 50 mg can be given intramuscularly or by intravenous infusion every 6 to 8 hours.

Famotidine (PEPCID) is available in tablets (20 or 40 mg), an oral suspension (40 mg/5 ml), and a solution (10 mg/ml) for intravenous injection. For acute duodenal ulcer, 40 mg at bedtime or 20 mg twice daily is recommended.

Nizatidine (AXID) is supplied as 150-mg and 300-mg capsules for oral use. The recommended dosage for active duodenal ulcer is 300 mg at bedtime or 150 mg twice a day.

Therapeutic Uses. The clinical use of H_2 antagonists stems largely from their capacity to inhibit gastric acid secretion, especially in patients with peptic ulceration. In appropriate doses, the various H_2 antagonists appear to produce equivalent therapeutic responses, although they differ in their propensity to cause adverse reactions.

Duodenal Ulcer. H_2 antagonists profoundly lower basal and nocturnal secretion of acid and that stimulated by meals and other factors; they reduce both the pain of duodenal ulcer and the consumption of antacids, and they hasten healing. Duodenal ulcers usually heal within 4 to 6 weeks of treatment, but 8 weeks is sometimes required. About 10% of patients do not respond in this period of time, and more prolonged treatment with H_2 antagonists is then of questionable value. Although similar rates of healing can be achieved by the vigorous administration of antacids, H_2 antagonists are more conveniently administered and lack pronounced effects on bowel motility. After successful treatment, ulcers recur within a year in about 50% of patients; this rate can be reduced to about 20% by the administration of maintenance doses of an H_2 antagonist once daily at bedtime.

Gastric Ulcer. H_2 antagonists also accelerate the healing of benign gastric ulcers; treatment for 8 weeks is sufficient for 50 to 75% of patients. The drugs also markedly reduce the rate of relapse when given in maintenance doses at bedtime.

Zollinger–Ellison Syndrome. In this disease, a non–beta cell tumor of the pancreatic islets may produce gastrin in a quantity sufficient to stimulate secretion of gastric acid to life-threatening levels;

H_2 antagonists provide valuable treatment. However, very high doses of these agents are necessary, and adequate suppression of acid secretion may not be achieved (Jensen *et al.*, 1983). Newly developed inhibitors of the H^+,K^+-ATPase appear to be of particular value in this condition (*see* below).

Other Conditions. H_2 antagonists may be useful whenever it is appropriate to reduce gastric acid secretion. Such conditions include reflux esophagitis, stress ulcers, short-bowel (anastomosis) syndrome, and hypersecretory states associated with systemic mastocytosis or basophilic leukemia with hyperhistaminemia. They are also used as a preanesthetic medication in emergency operations to reduce the danger of aspiration of acidic gastric contents (Baron, 1981; Brogden *et al.*, 1982; Riley and Salmon, 1982; Zeldis *et al.*, 1983).

Most patients with acute urticaria respond well to administration of H_1 histaminergic antagonists (*see* Chapter 23). However, a small number of these individuals develop chronic urticaria that is refractory to both H_1 antagonists and to all efforts to eliminate exposure to potential allergens. An ill-defined percentage of these patients appears to respond well to the concurrent administration of both an H_1 and an H_2 antagonist (Bleehen *et al.*, 1987). This effect is presumed to reflect some contribution to the condition from H_2 receptors in the cutaneous microvasculature.

INHIBITORS OF H^+,K^+-ATPASE

The ultimate mediator of acid secretion is the H^+,K^+-ATPase ("proton pump") of the apical membrane of the parietal cell (*see* Figure 37–1). A number of specific inhibitors of this unique enzyme have been developed; a family of substituted benzimidazoles were discovered first, and one of these compounds, omeprazole, has been released for clinical use (*see* Sachs *et al.*, 1988). These agents offer a means to inhibit acid secretion to any desired level. They are especially useful in patients with hypergastrinemia and may be valuable in those

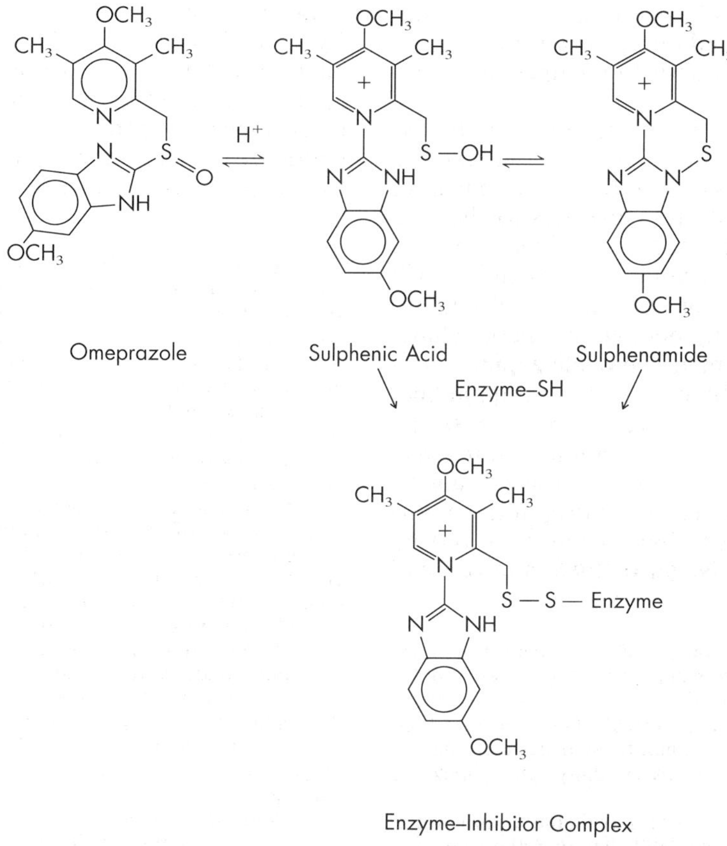

Figure 37–3. *Chemical reactions of omeprazole that lead to inhibition of H^+,K^+-ATPase. See* text for explanation.

whose peptic ulcer disease is not well controlled by H_2 antagonists.

Chemistry and Mechanism of Action. The prototypical compound, omeprazole, contains a sulfinyl group in the bridge that links substituted benzimidazole and pyridine rings (Figure 37–3). Omeprazole is chemically stable and devoid of inhibitory activity at neutral pH. However, the compound is protonated at pH 5 and below and rapidly rearranges to two species, a sulphenic acid and a sulphenamide, that react with sulfhydryl groups in the enzyme. Complete inhibition occurs when two reactive molecules derived from omeprazole are bound to each molecule of enzyme through disulfide linkages.

The selective distribution of the H^+,K^+-ATPase and the requirement for an acidic environment to generate the active forms of omeprazole lend a high degree of specificity to its action. The active species are permanent cations, and they are concentrated within the highly acidic lumen of the parietal cell canaliculi, adjacent to the luminal face of the target enzyme. The reaction shown in Figure 37–3 results in permanent inhibition of enzyme activity *in vivo,* and secretion of acid resumes only after insertion of new molecules of H^+,K^+-ATPase into the luminal membrane (*see* Lindberg *et al.,* 1987; Sachs *et al.,* 1988; Forte *et al.,* 1989).

Pharmacological Properties. The pharmacological effects of omeprazole are largely confined to inhibition of gastric acid secretion and effects that result therefrom. Omeprazole produces only small and inconsistent changes in the volume of gastric juice or in the secretion of pepsin and intrinsic factor; gastric motility is not affected.

Omeprazole produces a dose-related inhibition of gastric acid secretion that persists after the drug disappears from the plasma (Figure 37–4). Given in sufficient dosage (*e.g.,* 30 mg per day for 7 days), omeprazole can reduce the daily production of acid by more than 95%; pretreatment values are not achieved until 4 or 5 days after withdrawal of the drug, presumably reflecting the time required to synthesize the protein. One consequence of profound reduction in gastric acidity is increased secretion of gastrin, and patients who take the usual therapeutic dose of omeprazole have a modest hypergastrinemia. Prolonged administration of very high doses of omeprazole to experimental animals causes hyperplasia of oxyntic mucosal cells, presumably because of trophic effects of gastrin on these cells; carcinoid

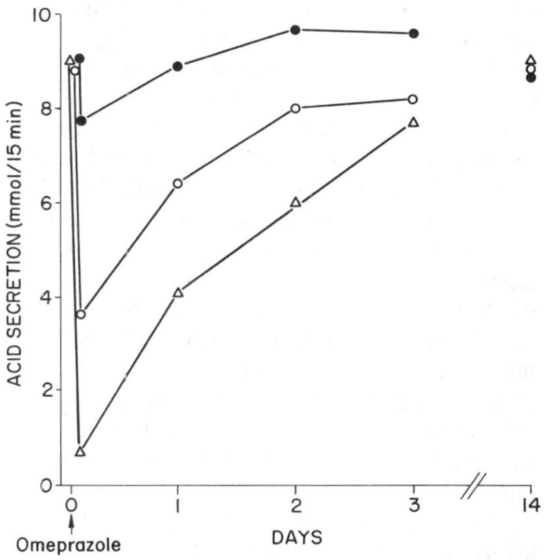

Figure 37–4. *Inhibitory effect of omeprazole on secretion of gastric acid in man.*

Maximal secretory responses were elicited in six healthy human subjects by infusing pentagastrin (91 μg) over a 1-hour period before and at various intervals after a single oral dose of omeprazole (○, 20 mg; △, 40 mg) or placebo (●). Note the profound and prolonged inhibition. (Modified from Lind *et al.,* 1983.)

tumors are also produced in rats. Although no evidence of mucosal proliferation has been found in human subjects, many clinicians are unwilling to administer omeprazole for longer than 8 weeks if suitable alternative therapy is available. The pharmacological properties of omeprazole have been reviewed by Clissold and Campoli-Richards (1986) and by Adams and coworkers (1988).

Absorption and Fate. Orally administered omeprazole is absorbed rapidly but to a variable extent; its bioavailability depends upon dose and gastric pH, and it may reach 70% with repeated administration. These properties presumably reflect the lability of the drug in acid and its impact on gastric pH. It is extensively (more than 95%) bound to plasma protein. Omeprazole is cleared from the circulation by hepatic metabolism with a half-time of 30 to 90 minutes; most of the metabolites are excreted in the urine (*see* Clissold and Campoli-Richards, 1986).

Adverse Effects. Omeprazole is generally well tolerated, and treatment of patients with Zollinger–Ellison syndrome with doses of 180 to 360 mg per day for up to 4 years has not caused serious side effects (*see* Adams *et al.*, 1988). About 3% of patients experience gastrointestinal effects, including nausea, diarrhea, and abdominal colic; CNS effects (*e.g.*, headache, dizziness, somnolence) have been reported less frequently. Skin rash, leukopenia, and transient elevations of plasma activities of hepatic aminotransferases have been observed occasionally. Although not yet noted with omeprazole, bacterial overgrowth in the gastrointestinal tract and development of nosocomial pneumonia are potential risks of long-term elevation of gastric pH.

Drug Interactions. Since omeprazole interacts with cytochrome P_{450} *in vitro*, inhibition of hepatic metabolism of certain drugs may be of potential importance. Although the clearance of diazepam is reduced by about 50%, omeprazole has only minor effects on the elimination of single oral doses of phenytoin.

Preparations and Dosage. Omeprazole (LOSEC) is supplied in 20-mg tablets for oral use. The dosage for the treatment of gastric or duodenal ulcers or reflux esophagitis is 20 to 40 mg given once daily in the morning for up to 8 weeks. The long-term management of patients with Zollinger–Ellison syndrome may require more than 120 mg of omeprazole per day given in two or three divided doses.

Therapeutic Uses. Omeprazole promotes healing of ulcers in the stomach, duodenum, and esophagus. It is of particular value in the treatment of patients who do not respond adequately to H_2 antagonists, especially those with Zollinger–Ellison syndrome (*see* Adams *et al.*, 1988).

Peptic Ulcers and Reflux Esophagitis. The administration of 20 to 30 mg of omeprazole per day produces about the same rate of healing of benign gastric ulcers as do usual therapeutic doses of either cimetidine or ranitidine; daily doses of 40 mg produce faster rates of healing and reduced rates of relapse (Walan *et al.*, 1989). Although relief of pain may occur more rapidly, most studies of patients with duodenal ulcers indicate that omeprazole (20 to 40 mg daily) is equivalent to the H_2 antagonists in rates of healing and relapse. By contrast, omeprazole is appreciably more effective than H_2 antagonists in the treatment of reflux esophagitis.

Zollinger–Ellison Syndrome. The peptic and esophageal ulceration associated with gastrin-producing tumors is often difficult to treat. Long-term studies indicate that chronic administration of omeprazole promotes healing and suppresses recurrence of ulcers in patients with this condition. The goal of therapy is to reduce the basal secretion of acid to below 10 mEq per hour. This usually requires administration of 60 to 70 mg of omeprazole per day; 90% of patients are controlled with daily doses of 120 mg.

ANTACIDS

Antacids are basic compounds that neutralize acid in the gastric lumen. The substantial incidence of placebo effects in individuals with minor gastrointestinal upsets, and even with peptic ulcer, deludes the self-medicating laity and often the physician into inappropriate use of antacids. Even when indicated, antacids are frequently used in quantities insufficient for optimal effect.

Chemistry. Antacids are compared quantitatively in terms of their acid-neutralizing capacity, defined as the quantity of 1 N HCl (expressed in milliequivalents) that can be brought to pH 3.5 in 15 minutes. The time limit reflects the fact that some formulations may react with acid so slowly that a negligible amount is neutralized during the sojourn of the preparation in the stomach.

Although the basic anions used in antacids include carbonate, bicarbonate, citrate, phosphate, and trisilicate, hydroxide is the most commonly employed. The antacid properties and therapeutic suitability of a product are also greatly influenced by the metallic cation. Aluminum and magnesium hydroxides are the usual preparations. The hydroxides of the alkali metals are completely ionized in water and are thus too strongly basic for clinical use. The solubility of $Mg(OH)_2$ is very low; consequently, OH^- does not accumulate to a concentration that would be corrosive. Nevertheless, $Mg(OH)_2$ is quite reactive with H^+, and it is the most rapidly acting of the insoluble antacids. $MgCO_3$ is much more soluble, yet it reacts less rapidly with acid because of its crystalline structure. Magnesium trisilicate is a relatively poor antacid that reacts only slowly with HCl to form silicon dioxide hydrate. Thus, the stomach may empty before significant neutralization occurs.

$Al(OH)_3$ is also relatively insoluble. The rate of neutralization of acid by $Al(OH)_3$ is considerably slower than that achieved with $Mg(OH)_2$, $MgCO_3$, or $CaCO_3$, and it varies with the method of preparation. Because of complexities of the chemistry of hydrated Al^{3+}, even the most reactive $Al(OH)_3$ cannot elevate the pH much above 4.5. An important chemical property of Al^{3+} in the intestinal milieu is its capacity to form insoluble salts with dietary phosphate.

$CaCO_3$ neutralizes HCl rapidly and effectively; the rate depends on the particle size and crystal structure of the preparation. The liberated Ca^{2+}

may enter into other chemical reactions in the duodenum and in the more alkaline environment of the small intestine, including the formation of insoluble calcium phosphates and calcium soaps.

PHARMACOLOGICAL PROPERTIES

Gastrointestinal Effects. *Intragastric pH.* The acid-neutralizing properties of antacids in the stomach roughly parallel those observed *in vitro*. The pH achieved depends on the form and dosage of the antacid and on whether the stomach is full or empty. The presence of food alone elevates gastric pH to about 5 for approximately 1 hour. Meals prolong the neutralizing effects of antacids for about 2 hours; the compounds are cleared from the empty stomach in about 30 minutes.

Mucoproteins and other substances tend to slow the rate of neutralization and decrease the acid-neutralizing capacity, especially of $Al(OH)_3$. In addition, the rate of neutralization of gastric acid by $Al(OH)_3$ is usually too slow relative to gastric emptying time to neutralize gastric acid when the stomach is empty. The concurrent use of $Mg(OH)_2$ and $Al(OH)_3$ provides both a fast-acting component, which can achieve neutralization within a few minutes, and a more sustained effect. Food in the stomach delays emptying and allows more time for $Al(OH)_3$ to react.

Antipeptic Effects. Partial neutralization of human gastric juice can *increase* its peptic activity. At pH 2, peptic activity is nearly four times that at pH 1.3. Its activity declines as the pH rises further, but active proteolysis occurs until the pH exceeds 5. Pepsin becomes irreversibly inactivated as the pH approaches neutrality. In addition, the autocatalytic activation of pepsin from pepsinogen is initiated by acid. Thus, reduction of gastric acidity will also suppress activation of pepsin. In addition, Al^{3+}-containing antacids may have direct antipeptic effects because of the reversible adsorption of pepsin to particles of $Al(OH)_3$ above pH 3 (*see* Berstad, 1982a).

Effects on Acid Secretion. Elevation of the pH in the gastric antrum increases the secretion of gastrin and causes a compensatory secretion of acid and pepsin. In normal individuals, the effect of gastric alkalinization on acid secretion after a meal appears to be small. In patients with duodenal ulcer, the effect of $NaHCO_3$ may be quite pronounced; maintenance of a continuous pH over 5.5 may double the acid secretion caused by a meal.

Once intragastric pH has been increased by antacids, gastric acid secretion persists even after the pH has returned to a value that normally terminates the antral secretion of gastrin. This "rebound" secretion is brief and of a low degree after ingestion of $Al(OH)_3$, $Mg(OH)_2$, or $NaHCO_3$, but it is prolonged and relatively intense after large doses (*e.g.*, more than 1 g) of $CaCO_3$. The greater acid rebound after $CaCO_3$ probably results from stimulatory effects of Ca^{2+} on the secretion of gastrin and HCl (*see* Holtermüller and Dehdaschti, 1982).

Gastrointestinal Motor Activity. Alkalinization of the gastric contents increases gastric motility through the action of gastrin. However, Al^{3+} can relax the smooth muscle of the stomach and delay gastric emptying, effects that are diminished by Mg^{2+}. Thus, $Al(OH)_3$ and $Mg(OH)_2$ taken concurrently have relatively little effect on gastric emptying (Lux *et al.*, 1982). Alkalinization of the gastric contents also increases lower esophageal pressure and esophageal clearance.

Antacids affect bowel motility and secretions. Magnesium salts cause laxation and are frequently used for that effect (*see* Chapter 38). Laxation is sometimes attributed to an osmotic effect, but Mg^{2+} also stimulates the secretion of cholecystokinin, which may contribute to the increased motor activity. Aluminum compounds cause constipation. Most commercial antacids contain mixtures of aluminum and magnesium compounds and usually do not change bowel function drastically. Nevertheless, the ratio of components varies considerably among individual products and the outcome is often unpredictable. Because of its capacity to enhance secretion and to form insoluble compounds, $CaCO_3$ has complex effects; it is variously described as causing laxation or constipation (*see* Clemens and Feinstein, 1977; Holtermüller and Dehdaschti, 1982; Ström, 1982).

Miscellaneous Gastrointestinal Effects. Al^{3+} may stimulate mucus secretion, an effect that would enhance the mucosal barrier to acid (*see* Caspary, 1982). In the gut, antacids form insoluble compounds with numerous substances, thereby interfering with their absorption. For example, Al^{3+} and Ca^{2+} form insoluble phosphates and Ca^{2+} forms insoluble CaF_2, thereby decreasing the bioavailability of dietary phosphate and fluoride. Ingestion of large amounts of Ca^{2+}-containing antacids can contribute to the milk-alkali syndrome (*see* below).

Al^{3+}-containing antacids adsorb bile acids, lysolecithin, and various proteins, such as pepsin (*see* above). Furthermore, Al^{3+} is strongly astringent, precipitates many proteins, and can react with fatty acids to form hydrophobic soaps. $CaCO_3$ and $Mg(OH)_2$ have weaker adsorptive activity than $Al(OH)_3$, and Ca^{2+} and Mg^{2+} are also less astringent than Al^{3+}.

Absorption, Distribution, and Excretion. *Effect of Absorption on Acid–Base Balance.* Antacids vary in the extent to which they are absorbed. Unneutralized $NaHCO_3$ and sodium citrate are completely absorbed and cause transient metabolic alkalosis. Antacids that are neutralized in the stomach may also disturb systemic acid–base balance. Normally, gastric HCl is neutralized by enteric $NaHCO_3$, such that there is no net effect on the overall acid–base balance. Exogenous antacid upsets this cycle by neutralizing the HCl and permitting absorption of the spared enteric $NaHCO_3$.

Antacids that contain aluminum, calcium, or magnesium are less completely absorbed than those that contain $NaHCO_3$ or sodium citrate. Unreacted insoluble antacids pass through the intestines largely as such and are eliminated in the feces. When the products from reacted antacids enter the intestine, some of the cations are absorbed. Unabsorbed cation may not spare enteric $NaHCO_3$, because an equivalent amount of HCO_3^- or CO_3^{2-} is consumed in the formation of insoluble hydroxides or carbonates. For example, Ca^{2+} reacts with CO_3^{2-} in the small intestine to form $CaCO_3$. The equivalent of $2HCO_3^-$ is thus retained in the gut, and there is no net change in overall acid–base balance. Al^{3+} may be excreted as aluminum carbonates, aluminum hydroxide, and oxyaluminum hydroxide. Mg^{2+} is eliminated in the feces as $Mg(OH)_2$ and as soluble salts, such as the chloride and bicarbonate. Small amounts of the cations from the insoluble antacids are eliminated as soaps, phosphates, and sundry other insoluble compounds.

Aluminum-Containing Antacids. Dietary intake of Al^{3+} is normally in the range of 10 mg daily, of which about 0.1% is absorbed. Use of antacids considerably increases this load, and about 0.1 to 0.5 mg of the cation may be absorbed from a standard daily dose of an Al^{3+}-containing antacid, depending on dietary factors (Weberg and Berstad, 1986). In persons with normal renal function, ingestion of Al^{3+}-containing antacids leads to about a doubling of the average concentration of Al^{3+} in plasma. Since Al^{3+} is eliminated in the urine, plasma concentrations rise in renal failure and toxicity can occur (*see* below). The absorption, distribution, and excretion of aluminum have been reviewed in detail by Alfrey (1983).

Calcium-Containing Antacids. The fraction of Ca^{2+} absorbed from $CaCO_3$ averages 15% in normal patients and seems to vary in proportion to gastric acid secretion. A dose–absorption relationship has not been established for $CaCO_3$; however, by analogy with other forms of Ca^{2+}, the amount absorbed probably reaches a plateau at a daily dose of about 20 g of Ca^{2+}. Dietary factors such as the content of fat alter Ca^{2+} absorption, and it is also regulated by several hormones (*see* Chapter 62).

Hypercalcemia is only transient after a single dose of a Ca^{2+}-containing antacid. A normal individual can ingest 20 g per day without developing chronic hypercalcemia, but clinically dangerous hypercalcemia may follow the administration of as little as 3.4 g per day to patients with uremia. Bicarbonate that accompanies the absorption of Ca^{2+} from $CaCO_3$ causes a slight-to-moderate metabolic alkalosis after each dose; a clinically significant and persistent alkalosis develops only slowly during a maintenance regimen.

The main route of elimination of absorbed Ca^{2+} is by urinary excretion, which varies with the creatinine clearance. With long-term use of Ca^{2+}-containing antacids, absorption exceeds excretion for many weeks and it may take months to achieve a new steady state (*see* Makoff *et al.*, 1969; *see also* Chapter 62).

Magnesium-Containing Antacids. The chronic ingestion of antacid doses of $Mg(OH)_2$ causes only slight increases in plasma concentrations of Mg^{2+} in persons with normal renal function. Since renal excretion is the principal route of elimination, toxic concentrations may occur in persons with renal failure (*see* Chapter 27).

Adverse Effects. Adverse effects of antacids may be classified into those that are dependent on the magnitude of change in pH or acid–base balance and those that are dependent upon a particular chemical entity.

pH-Dependent Effects. Distortions of acid–base balance by absorbed cations from antacids are usually transient and clinically insignificant in persons with normal renal function. In the past, when large doses of $NaHCO_3$ and/or $CaCO_3$ were commonly administered with milk or cream for the management of peptic ulcer, the milk-alkali syndrome occurred relatively frequently. This syndrome results from the ingestion of large quantities of Ca^{2+} and absorbable alkali; effects consist of hypercalcemia, reduced secretion of parathyroid hormone, retention of phosphate, precipitation of calcium salts in the kidney, and renal insufficiency. In general, alkaluria from the long-term use of any antacid predisposes to nephrolithiasis by favoring precipitation of calcium phosphate.

Composition-Dependent Effects. Antacids affect bowel habits. $Al(OH)_3$ causes constipation in rough proportion to the dose. The effect is greater in elderly patients. The most frequent side effect of $Mg(OH)_2$ is loose stools or diarrhea. With preparations that contain both $Al(OH)_3$ and $Mg(OH)_2$ the net effect depends on the ratio of the two components and the quantity used; if the dose of $Mg(OH)_2$ is large enough (in excess of 8.5 g per day), diarrhea will prevail. Magnesium trisilicate and $MgCO_3$ also cause laxation. The effects of $CaCO_3$ are variable, but constipation has been reported more frequently than laxation.

The release of CO_2 from carbonate-containing antacids causes belching, abdominal distention, flatulence, and occasional nausea. Bicarbonate is usually neutralized in the stomach or absorbed, such that only belching results. Gastroesophageal reflux may be exacerbated during episodes of belching.

Al^{3+}-containing antacids rarely cause adverse effects in persons with normal renal function, although severe hypophosphatemia can sometimes occur. In persons with renal impairment, long-term administration of Al^{3+} either in medications or as a contaminant of fluids used for dialysis or alimentation can exacerbate or even initiate osteodystrophy, proximal myopathy, and encephalopathy; the latter may take the form of dementia or seizures. Hyperaluminumemia results, in part, from diminished renal clearance of Al^{3+} and may be exacerbated by increased absorption of Al^{3+} as a result of hyperparathyroidism associated with uremia; however, some investigators attribute the hyperparathyroidism to hyperaluminumemia. The osteodystrophy is thought to result in part from deposition of Al^{3+} in bone. The use of Al^{3+}-containing compounds as the major method to decrease intestinal absorption of phosphate in uremic patients seems hazardous and inappropriate. Suitable doses of $CaCO_3$ similarly reduce phosphate absorption and suppress concentrations of phosphate and parathyroid hormone in plasma without causing hypercalcemia (*see* Bournerias *et al.*, 1983; Gokal *et al.*, 1983; Coburn and Salusky, 1989). For reviews of Al^{3+} toxicity, *see* Mayor and Burnatowska-Hledin (1986), Sherrard (1986), Mach and colleagues (1988), and Monteagudo and coworkers (1989).

Knowledge of the Na^+ content of antacids can be important, particularly for patients with heart failure or hypertension who should limit Na^+ intake. Numerous preparations are suitably low in Na^+ (*see* Table 37–2).

Drug Interactions. Chiefly by altering gastric and urinary pH, antacids may alter rates of dissolution and absorption, bioavailability, and renal elimination of a number of drugs. Thus, it is prudent to avoid concurrent use of antacids and drugs intended for systemic absorption (*see* Hurwitz, 1977; Ritschel, 1984). Most interactions can be avoided by taking antacids 2 hours before or after ingestion of other drugs.

The interactions of antacids with other drugs may be complex, in part because the chemical properties and physiological effects of the compounds vary. Compounds containing Al^{3+} delay gastric emptying, thereby slowing the entry of drugs to the absorptive surface of the small intestine and hence the rate of absorption. However, there may be no effect on bioavailability, particularly if additional time for dissolution in the stomach makes later absorption more rapid. Generally, unless bioavailability is also affected, altered rates of absorption have little clinical significance when drugs are given chronically in multiple doses. In combination products, compounds that contain Mg^{2+} can partially offset the effects of Al^{3+} on gastric motility. Magnesium trisilicate and Al^{3+} compounds are notable for their propensity to adsorb drugs and to form insoluble complexes that are not absorbed. Thus, through a combination of factors many antacids decrease the bioavailability of iron, tetracyclines, isoniazid, ethambutol, some antimuscarinic drugs, benzodiazepines, phenothiazines, ranitidine, indomethacin, phenytoin, nitrofurantoin, vitamin A, fluoride, and phosphate. Antacids reportedly decrease the bioavailability of atenolol and propranolol and increase that of metoprolol. Antacids increase the dissolution and absorption of the acidic forms of sulfonamides and the rate of absorption of levodopa.

Alkalinization of the urine affects renal clearance of drugs that are weak acids or bases (*see* Chapter 1). Concurrent antacid therapy increases the rate of elimination of salicylates and phenobarbital and decreases the elimination of amphetamine, ephedrine, mecamylamine, pseudoephedrine, and quinidine.

Antacids decrease the hepatic metabolism of ranitidine and reduce the efficacy of nitrofurantoin in the therapy of urinary tract infections. Thiazide diuretics cause retention of Ca^{2+}, and may thus exacerbate hypercalcemia from $CaCO_3$.

PREPARATIONS AND DOSAGE

Antacid products vary widely in their chemical composition, acid-neutralizing capacity, and Na^+ content. Table 37–2 provides a comparison of the common oral suspensions. Comparable data on solid dosage forms can be found below. In general, the composition and neutralizing capacity of a tablet are close to those of 5 ml of the corresponding oral suspension.

Both dosage forms frequently contain simethicone, a surface-active agent that is included to disperse foam. This effect may be helpful in reducing gastroesophageal reflux, but simethicone does not have antacid or ulcer-healing properties. Some preparations contain alginic acid, which is thought to protect against the irritating effect of HCl during periods of esophageal reflux; it has no beneficial effects in the treatment of ulcers.

Aluminum Compounds. *Aluminum Hydroxide Gel.* As sold in antacids, "aluminum hydroxide" is actually a mixture of $Al(OH)_3$ and aluminum oxide hydrates, often containing some carbonate. Aluminum hydroxide is marketed mostly in combination with $Mg(OH)_2$ (*see* Table 37–2). During storage, $Al(OH)_3$ loses acid neutralizing capacity; the loss from solid dosage forms exceeds that from suspensions.

Table 37–2. COMPOSITION AND NEUTRALIZING CAPACITY OF REPRESENTATIVE PROPRIETARY ANTACID SUSPENSIONS *

PRODUCT	CONTENT (mg/5 ml)					ACID-NEUTRALIZING CAPACITY ‡ (per 5 ml)
	$Al(OH)_3$	$Mg(OH)_2$	$CaCO_3$	Simeth †	Na	
MAALOX TC §	600	300	0	0	0.8	27
MYLANTA-II	400	400	0	40	1.1	25
KUDROX DOUBLE STRENGTH	565	180	0	0	<15	25
GELUSIL-II	400	400	0	30	1.3	24
CAMALOX	225	200	250	0	1.2	18
DI-GEL	200	200	0	20	<5	—
MARBLEN	400 $MgCO_3$ + 520 $CaCO_3$ ‖			0	3	18
ALTERNAGEL	600	0	0	—	<2.5	16
SILAIN-GEL	282	285	0	25	4.4	15
RIOPAN	540 magaldrate ‖			0	<0.1	15
GELUSIL-M §	300	200	0	25	1.2	15
milk of magnesia	0	390	0	0	0.12	14
MAALOX	225	200	0	0	1.4	13
MYLANTA	200	200	0	20	0.7	13
ALUDROX	307	103	0	—	2.3	12
BASALJEL	$Al(OH)CO_3$ equivalent to 400 $Al(OH)_3$ ‖			—	2.9	12
GELUSIL	200	200	0	25	0.7	12
WINGEL	180	160	0	0	—	10
KOLANTYL GEL	150	150	0	0	<5	10
AMPHOJEL	320	0	0	—	<2.3	10
GAVISCON	31.7 $Al(OH)_3$ + 137 $MgCO_3$ + Na alginate ‖			0	13	4

* Many of these preparations are also available in solid dosage forms. Although the composition of these forms is often similar to that of the suspension, there are variations.
† Simeth = simethicone.
‡ In milliequivalents. In some cases, a 60-minute rather than a 15-minute test was performed.
§ TC = therapeutic concentrate; M = medium strength.
‖ Indicated composition is in lieu of $Al(OH)_3$, $Mg(OH)_2$, and/or $CaCO_3$.

Basic Aluminum Carbonate Gel. The chemical composition of this substance is indefinite and is represented by $Al(OH)CO_3$ in Table 37–2. It is marketed as a suspension that contains the equivalent of 400 mg of $Al(OH)_3$ per 5 ml or as tablets or capsules, each of which contains 500 mg.

Dihydroxyaluminum Sodium Carbonate. This product, a combination of $Al(OH)_3$ and $NaHCO_3$, provides the rapid effect of carbonate and the slower, more sustained effect of the dihydroxyaluminum moiety. Each tablet (ROLAIDS ANTACID) contains 334 mg of the compound, including 53 mg of Na^+, and has the capacity to neutralize 7.5 mEq of acid.

Aluminum Phosphate Gel. This compound, marketed as PHOSPHALJEL, has an insignificant capacity to act as an antacid.

Magnesium Compounds. *Magnesium Hydroxide.* The only single-entity preparation of $Mg(OH)_2$ is *milk of magnesia*. $Mg(OH)_2$ is frequently combined with $Al(OH)_3$.

Magaldrate. Magaldrate is a complex hydroxymagnesium aluminate with the approximate formula $[Mg(OH)^+]_4\ [Al_2(OH)_{10}{}^{4-}] \cdot 2H_2O$. In the presence of HCl, the hydroxymagnesium is relatively rapidly converted to Mg^{2+} and the aluminate to hydrated $Al(OH)_3$; the $Al(OH)_3$ then reacts more slowly to give a sustained antacid effect. Magaldrate (RIOPAN) is available as a suspension and as tablets either to chew or to swallow; each tablet contains 480 mg of magaldrate and not more than 0.1 mg of Na^+, and has an acid-neutralizing capacity of 13.5 mEq.

Sodium Compounds. *Sodium Bicarbonate.* $NaHCO_3$ is available in tablets that contain 325 to 650 mg. One gram neutralizes 12 mEq of acid. For continuous nasogastric irrigation during surgery or in intensive care, a 0.05-N solution may be used.

Sodium Citrate. As an antacid, sodium citrate is used in the form of a 0.3-M solution, which can be made as needed in hospital pharmacies. Modified Shohl's solution (BICITRA) contains citric acid and sodium citrate and has about the same neutralizing capacity.

Calcium Compounds. *Calcium carbonate* is available as a single-entity preparation under a variety of proprietary names (*e.g.*, TUMS). Tablets contain from 350 to 1250 mg and have an acid-neutralizing capacity of approximately 10 mEq per 500-mg tablet.

Antacid Mixtures. Antacids are used in combination to give both immediate and sustained action, to minimize undesirable effects by using a lower dose of each component, and to use one component to antagonize side effects of another (*e.g.*, laxation versus constipation). The most common combination is that of $Al(OH)_3$ and $Mg(OH)_2$ (*see* Table 37–2). Most preparations are also available as tablets with composition and neutralizing capacities similar to those of 5 ml of the corresponding suspension. Other combinations include $CaCO_3$ and $Mg_2Si_3O_8$.

Dosage. Recent studies of the efficacy of antacids in healing duodenal ulcers have demonstrated a significant placebo effect, the ineffectiveness of very low doses of antacids, and the lack of need for extremely high doses (greater than 1000 mEq per day). A popular dosage regimen is based on the attempt to neutralize the maximum capacity for production of acid by the stomach (*see* Peterson *et al.*, 1977). Thus, antacids are administered 1 and 3 hours after eating and at bedtime, for a total of 1000 mEq of neutralizing capacity per day. This regimen takes advantage of the postprandial delay in gastric emptying and stresses the value of lowering gastric acid as the neutralizing effect of food begins to wane (*see* Lam, 1988; Soll, 1989). However, this scheme provides little nocturnal protection, since antacids are neutralized or removed rapidly from the empty stomach. More recent studies indicate that smaller doses are equally effective (*see* Kumar *et al.*, 1984). A total daily dose of 400 mEq of neutralizing capacity, taken in portions an hour after meals and at bedtime, appears adequate. This regimen is more convenient and should promote improved patient compliance.

Daily doses of antacid as low as 180 mEq of acid-neutralizing capacity may also be effective, suggesting that factors other than simple neutralization may contribute to the healing effects. Nevertheless, more than 1000 mEq per day may be required in the treatment of patients with Zollinger–Ellison syndrome, even in conjunction with antisecretory drugs.

THERAPEUTIC USES

The clinical status of antacids is in a state of flux.

Peptic Ulcer. In the treatment of duodenal ulcers, antacids and the H_2 antagonists generally produce equivalent effects on the incidence of healing after a 4- to 8-week course of therapy and on the frequency of relapse thereafter. Effective daily doses of antacids have ranged from 120 to 1000 mEq (*see* Berstad, 1982b; Ippoliti *et al.*, 1983; Isenberg *et al.*, 1983; Kumar *et al.*, 1984; Lam, 1988; Soll, 1989). Results in the treatment of gastric ulcers have been less consistent, and in some instances antacids have been no more effective than placebo. In addition to simpler dosing schedules, therapeutic regimens using H_2 antagonists usually result in a lower incidence of side effects. Thus, antacids are not the agents of choice for the treatment of peptic ulcer disease. Moreover, continuous use of antacids for prophylaxis is not recommended for the reasons itemized above. However, high doses of antacids may be useful adjuncts in combination with H_2 antagonists or inhibitors of the H^+,K^+-ATPase for the treatment of giant duodenal ulcers and the Zollinger–Ellison syndrome.

Gastroesophageal Reflux. Changes in lifestyle and eating habits are of primary importance in treating this condition. To reduce gastric acidity and hence the acidity of the refluxate, H_2 antagonists or omeprazole are preferred; if the tone of the lower esophageal sphincter is reduced or esophageal peristalsis is impaired, these may be supplemented by pirenzepine or so-called prokinetic agents, such as bethanechol, metoclopramide, or cisapride. Antacids may still be useful adjuncts for this condition, since they neutralize acidic secretions that are not susceptible to H_2 antagonists and they increase the pressure of the lower esophageal sphincter.

The alginate-containing product GAVISCON reportedly decreases acidic reflux and increases esophageal clearance of acid. This compound has no demonstrable effect on lower esophageal sphincter pressure and is not a potent antacid. The alginate component may protect the mucosa and mechanically impair reflux by forming a viscous layer on the surface of the gastric contents. The efficacy of this product in managing gastroesophageal reflux has not been demonstrated unequivocally. Nonetheless, it is widely used in the treatment of mild-to-moderate reflux esophagitis.

Miscellaneous Uses. During anesthesia, coma, cesarean section, or endoscopy, aspiration of gastric contents may occur and cause pneumonitis or pneumonia. Prior neutralization of gastric acid provides some protection. The aim should be to keep the pH above 3.5 (possibly as high as 5, to suppress peptic activity). Antacids may be given just prior to and during the procedure. However, if aspirated, the particulate antacids themselves can cause pulmonary damage, which makes the use of sodium citrate (15 ml of a 0.3 M solution) attractive (*see* Wrobel *et al.*, 1982). Because conventional antimuscarinic drugs decrease the competency of the lower-esophageal sphincter, their use is not advised.

Antacids and H_2 antagonists are both effective in the prophylaxis of stress ulceration and consequent acute upper-gastrointestinal hemorrhage (*see* Schiessel, 1989). The management of upper-gastrointestinal bleeding has been reviewed by Peterson (1989).

MUSCARINIC ANTAGONISTS

Muscarinic cholinergic antagonists can reduce basal secretion of gastric acid by 40 to 50%; stimulated secretion is inhibited to a lesser extent. Selective antagonists of M_1 receptors are as effective as atropine or other nonselective muscarinic antagonists, but they are less likely to produce the adverse effects that are characteristic of cholinergic blockade (*e.g.*, dry mouth, tachycardia). Two such drugs currently in clinical trial in the United States are pirenzepine and telenzepine. These agents have relatively low affinities for M_2 and M_3 receptors (*see* Chapter 8). Since the muscarinic receptors on histamine-containing cells have not been characterized, it is not clear where the M_1 antagonists act.

Nor is it known whether blockade of M_1 receptors on intramural cholinergic neurons will interrupt transmission of vagal impulses. M_1 antagonists may also inhibit the secretion of gastrin, mucous, and HCO_3^-, which is regulated by acetylcholine acting at M_1 receptors.

Although pirenzepine is less effective than cimetidine in reducing acid secretion, it has produced comparable rates of healing of duodenal ulcers in several clinical trials. Used in maintenance dosage, it also appears to equal cimetidine for preventing the recurrence of ulcers. Both pirenzepine and the more potent telenzepine are quite hydrophilic and penetrate the blood–brain barrier poorly (*see* Carmine and Brogden, 1985). The effective dosage of pirenzepine is 50 mg two or three times daily. The pharmacological properties of muscarinic antagonists are described in Chapter 8.

SUCRALFATE

Sucralfate is a complex formed from sucrose octasulfate and polyaluminum hydroxide. Its primary unit may be represented as $C_{12}H_6O_{11}$-$[SO_3^-Al_2(OH)_5^+]_8 \cdot nH_2O$. When the pH is below 4, there is extensive polymerization and cross-linking of sucralfate. The condensed polymer is a very sticky, viscid, yellow-white gel. Continued reaction with acid gradually consumes $Al_2(OH)_5^+$ until some sucrose octasulfate moieties are entirely freed of Al^{3+}. The reaction is very slow and is incomplete during the sojourn of the substance in the stomach. Sucralfate has no practical acid-neutralizing capacity. Even though the pH in the duodenum is well above 4, the gel retains its viscid, demulcent properties. The gel adheres strongly to epithelial cells and to the base of ulcer craters. The affinity for the crater base is much higher than that for the epithelial surface, and it is difficult to wash the gel from the crater. In man, the gel remains adherent to ulcerated epithelium for longer than 6 hours, and it is more adherent to duodenal than to gastric ulcers. This binding to ulcer craters probably represents the main therapeutic action of sucralfate. Antacids and food do not appear to affect the integrity of the adherent gel, but proteins in foodstuffs adsorb to its luminal surface, thus adding an additional layer. The gel interacts very little with mucin. Investigations *in vitro* show that the gel coating on the mucosa is considerably less permeable to H_3O^+ than are mucin and aluminum hydroxide. It has been proposed that sucralfate stimulates the formation of prostaglandins by the gastric mucosa, thereby exerting a "cytoprotective" effect (Ligumsky *et al.*, 1984).

The incidence and severity of side effects from sucralfate are very low; only constipation (2%) and a sense of dry mouth (less than 1%) appear significant, although diarrhea, nausea, gastric distress, rash, pruritus, and dizziness have also been reported. Sherman and coworkers (1983) found that sucralfate lowers concentrations of phosphate in plasma toward normal in uremic patients. The use of sucralfate also results in elevated plasma concentrations of Al^{3+} in uremic patients (*see* Leung *et al.*, 1983). Studies in laboratory animals indicate that sucralfate can adsorb and thereby reduce the bioavailability of a number of drugs, including tetracycline, phenytoin, digoxin, and cimetidine.

Sucralfate (CARAFATE) is available as 1-g tablets. The dosage is one tablet 1 hour before each meal and at bedtime. Treatment should be continued for 4 to 8 weeks unless healing has been proven. Since the preparation is activated by acid, antacids should not be taken for 30 minutes before or after sucralfate.

There have been a number of prospective trials of sucralfate in the treatment of peptic ulcer. In all studies sucralfate has been effective against both duodenal and gastric ulcers. Administration before meals was found to be distinctly more effective than after meals. In several trials in which sucralfate and cimetidine were compared, the percentage of healed ulcers after sucralfate treatment was about the same as that after cimetidine. After remission, continued treatment with sucralfate postpones relapse more effectively than does cimetidine. However, after discontinuation of treatment, relapses occur sooner with sucralfate than with cimetidine. The rate of healing of gastric ulcer is less than for duodenal ulcer. For additional information about sucralfate, *see* Brogden and colleagues (1984) and Symposium (1989a).

BISMUTH COMPOUNDS

Suspensions of various bismuth colloids have long been self-administered by the laity for gastrointestinal upsets. However, their potential utility in the treatment of peptic ulcers has recently come under scrutiny. Although these compounds have no substantial acid-neutralizing capacity, they inhibit the activity of pepsin, increase secretion of mucus, and interact with proteins in the necrotic ulcer crater, presumably forming a barrier to the diffusion of acid. Bismuth colloids also cause detachment of *Campylobacter pylori* from the gastric epithelium with subsequent lysis of the bacteria. The therapeutic importance of this action is uncertain, but a growing body of evidence indicates a relationship between colonization by *C. pylori* and a variety of gastric diseases (*see* Hornick, 1987; Talley and Ormand, 1989).

The available colloids are bismuth subgallate, subnitrate, subcitrate, and subsalicylate (PEPTO-BISMOL). They are not currently approved as treatments for peptic ulcer disease in the United States but are under active investigation. In studies with bismuth subcitrate, four daily doses of one tablet or 5 ml containing 120 mg of the drug (taken before meals and at bedtime) are about as effective as cimetidine for the treatment of gastric and duodenal ulcers. Although relatively little of the colloid is absorbed, plasma concentrations of Bi^{3+} rise with prolonged therapy; the long-term use of other bismuth salts produces higher concentrations of Bi^{3+}, which can cause encephalopathy and osteodystrophy. Other potential problems include darkening of the oral cavity. The results of recent clinical studies with bismuth colloids appear in several reviews (*see* Baron *et al.*, 1986; Bianchi Porro *et al.*, 1986; Elder, 1986).

PROSTAGLANDINS

Prostaglandins E_2 and I_2, the predominant prostaglandins synthesized by the gastric mucosa, inhibit the secretion of acid and stimulate the secretion of mucus and bicarbonate (*see* Chapters 24 and 26). The ulcerogenic properties of aspirin-like drugs that inhibit the synthesis of prostaglandins suggest a role for these autacoids in normal gastric function. Because the administration of prostaglandins can protect the gastric mucosa of animals against various ulcerogenic insults, a number of slowly metabolized analogs have been developed and tested in man. These include misoprostol, an analog of PGE_1, which has recently been released for general use in the United States (*see* Chapter 24). Clinical studies indicate that misoprostol is about as effective as H_2 antagonists in promoting the healing of duodenal ulcers. Although the drug displays distinct cytoprotective effects in animals, clinical efficacy appears to require doses of misoprostol (200 μg four times daily) that produce marked suppression of acid secretion. By contrast, such doses do not appear to be as effective as H_2 antagonists in healing gastric ulcers or in relieving the symptoms of reflux esophagitis. Current investigation is focused on the use of misoprostol to prevent gastric ulceration in patients who use large doses of aspirin-like drugs for the treatment of arthritis. Although early results have been encouraging, it is not yet clear whether the prophylactic use of misoprostol offers advantages over other therapeutic strategies in such patients.

Effective oral doses of misoprostol and related agents cause diarrhea and some abdominal cramping. Although these side effects are experienced frequently, they are usually self-limiting and rarely interfere with therapy. These compounds are potential abortifacients and should not be used in women in whom conception is a possibility. The actions and therapeutic use of misoprostol have been reviewed by Monk and Clissold (1987) and in Symposia (1988, 1989b).

MISCELLANEOUS DRUGS FOR PEPTIC ULCER DISEASE

A number of other drugs are in use or under investigation as antiulcer agents. Carbenoxolone, a liquorice extract in general use as an antiulcer drug in Europe since 1962, is an oleandane derivative obtained from glycyrrhiza. The drug has a steroid-like structure and possesses significant mineralocorticoid activity. While other mineralocorticoids do not have antiulcer properties, the concurrent administration of spironolactone interferes with the therapeutic effect of carbenoxolone.

Carbenoxolone alters the composition of mucus and enhances the mucosal barrier to diffusion of acid. Suggested (but unproven) therapeutic effects of carbenoxolone include augmentation of glycoprotein synthesis, inhibition of enzymes that inactivate prostaglandins, and suppression of the activation of pepsinogen. Although in some trials carbenoxolone has appeared to be as effective as cimetidine for peptic ulcers, adverse effects result fairly frequently from its mineralocorticoid actions. These adverse reactions include hypokalemia, fluid retention, and hypertension; impaired glucose tolerance is also observed. These adverse effects constitute major deterrents to the use of carbenoxolone (*see* Barrowman and Pfeiffer, 1982).

Deglycyrrhizinized liquorice is marketed outside the United States as an antiulcer agent. Its actions on the gastroduodenal mucosae are like those of carbenoxolone, but the drug lacks mineralocorticoid activity. Metoclopramide, a prokinetic agent, has been used in the treatment of peptic ulcer with the intention of augmenting normal peristalsis and abolishing the enterogastric reflux of bile, which is thought to be a factor in the pathogenesis of many gastric and some duodenal ulcers. It is of some value in the treatment of gastric ulcer, but its efficacy has been poor in duodenal ulcer. Metoclopramide reduces gastroesophageal reflux and is used in the management of reflux esophagitis; it is discussed in Chapter 38.

PROMOTERS OF GASTRIC SECRETION

To evaluate gastric secretory problems, it may be useful to determine whether parietal cell function is normal. Use of histamine (with an H_1 antagonist), H_2 agonists, or muscarinic agonists is limited by adverse effects. Gastrin and its analogs cause fewer and less severe side effects and are more useful for this purpose.

Pentagastrin. Gastrin, a heptadecapeptide, is a potent physiological gastric secretagogue that is released from the pyloric antrum by vagal stimuli and in response to feeding. Smaller fragments of the peptide are also fully active, and a synthetic pentapeptide, pentagastrin, is available to test gastric function; its structure is as follows:

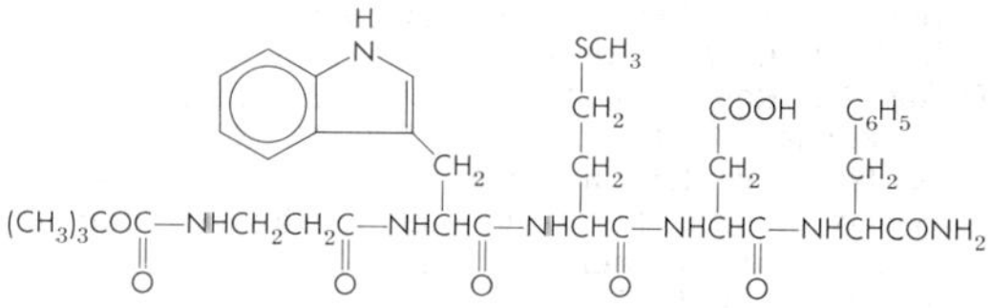

Pentagastrin

The most prominent action of pentagastrin is to stimulate the secretion of gastric acid, pepsin, and intrinsic factor. It also stimulates pancreatic secretion, inhibits absorption of water and electrolytes from the ileum, relaxes the sphincter of Oddi, and increases blood flow in the gastric mucosa. Although it contracts the smooth muscle of the lower esophageal sphincter and the stomach, pentagastrin delays gastric emptying. The half-life of pentagastrin in the circulation is about 10 minutes.

After subcutaneous injection, pentagastrin elicits reproducible gastric secretory responses comparable to those induced by histamine or betazole. Side effects are usually minor and transient; these may include nausea, borborygmi, the urge to defecate, flushing, tachycardia, faintness, and dizziness. Allergic reactions are rare. Gastric secretion begins within 10 minutes, peaks within 20 to 30 minutes, and lasts about an hour (*see* Baron, 1972).

Pentagastrin (PEPTAVLON) is marketed in ampuls containing 0.25 mg/ml. The diagnostic dose is 6 μg/kg, administered by subcutaneous injection.

Baron, J. H.; Barr, J.; Batten, J.; Sidebotham, R.; and Spencer, J. Acid, pepsin and mucus secretion in patients with gastric and duodenal ulcer before and after colloidal bismuth subcitrate. *Gut*, **1986**, *27*, 486–490.

Berstad, A. Antacids and pepsin. *Scand. J. Gastroenterol.*, **1982a**, *17*, Suppl. 75, 13–15.

———. Antacid therapy of duodenal ulcer. Effects of smaller doses. *Ibid.*, **1982b**, *17*, Suppl. 75, 97–99.

Bianchi Porro, G.; Parente, F.; Lazzaroni, M.; and Pace, F. Colloidal bismuth subcitrate and two different dosages of cimetidine in the treatment of resistant duodenal ulcer. *Scand. J. Gastroenterol.*, **1986**, *21*, Suppl. 122, 39–41.

Binder, H. J., and Donaldson, R. M., Jr. Effect of cimetidine on intrinsic factor and pepsin secretion in man. *Gastroenterology*, **1978**, *74*, 371–375.

Black, J. W.; Duncan, W. A. M.; Durant, C. J.; Ganellin, C. R.; and Parsons, E. M. Definition and antagonism of histamine H_2 receptors. *Nature*, **1972**, *236*, 385–390.

Bleehen, S. S., and others. Cimetidine and chlorpheniramine in the treatment of chronic idiopathic urticaria: a multi-centre randomized double-blind study. *Br. J. Dermatol.*, **1987**, *117*, 81–88.

Bournerias, F.; Monnier, N.; and Reveillaud, R. J. Risk of orally administered aluminum hydroxide and results of withdrawal. *Proc. Eur. Dial. Transplant Assoc.*, **1983**, *20*, 207–212.

Caspary, W. F. Measurement of intragastric potential difference. In, *Antacids in the Eighties*. (Halter, F., ed.) Urban & Schwarzenberg, Munich, **1982**, pp. 64–69.

Coburn, J. W., and Salusky, I. B. Control of serum phosphorus in uremia. *N. Engl. J. Med.*, **1989**, *320*, 1140–1142.

Elder, J. B. Recent experimental and clinical studies on the pharmacology of colloidal bismuth subcitrate. *Scand. J. Gastroenterol.*, **1986**, *21*, Suppl. 122, 14–16.

Gailbraith, R. A., and Michnovicz, J. J. The effects of cimetidine on the oxidative metabolism of estradiol. *N. Engl. J. Med.*, **1989**, *321*, 269–274.

Gokal, R.; Ramos, J. M.; Ellis, H. A.; Parkinson, I.; Sweetman, V.; Dewar, J.; Ward, M. K.; and Kerr, D. N. Histological renal osteodystrophy and 25-hydroxycholecalciferol and aluminum levels in patients on continuous ambulatory peritoneal dialysis. *Kidney Int.*, **1983**, *23*, 15–21.

Hornick, R. B. Peptic ulcer disease: a bacterial infection? *N. Engl. J. Med.*, **1987**, *316*, 1518.

Ippoliti, A.; Elashoff, J.; Valenzuela, J.; Cano, R.; Frankl, H.; Samloff, M.; and Koretz, R. Recurrent ulcer after successful treatment with cimetidine or antacid. *Gastroenterology*, **1983**, *85*, 875–880.

Isenberg, J. I.; Peterson, W. L.; Elashoff, J. D.; Sanderfeld, M. A.; Reedy, T. J.; Ippoliti, A. F.; Van Deventer, G. M.; Frankl, H.; Longstreth, G. F.; and Anderson, D. S. Healing of benign gastric ulcer with low-dose antacid or cimetidine: a double-blind, randomized, placebo-controlled trial. *N. Engl. J. Med.*, **1983**, *308*, 1319–1324.

Jensen, R. T.; Collen, M. J.; Pandol, S. J.; Allende, H. D.; Raufman, J.-P.; Bissonette, B. M.; Duncan, W. C.; Durgan, P. L.; Gillin, J. C.; and Gardner, J. D. Cimetidine-induced impotence and breast changes in patients with gastric hypersecretory states. *N. Engl. J. Med.*, **1983**, *308*, 883–887.

Kumar, N.; Vij, J. C.; Karol, A.; and Anand, B. S. Controlled therapeutic trial to determine the optimum dose of antacids in duodenal ulcer. *Gut*, **1984**, *25*, 1199–1202.

Leung, A. C.; Henderson, I. S.; Halls, D. J.; and Dobbie, J. W. Aluminum hydroxide versus sucralfate as a phosphate binder in uraemia. *Br. Med. J.*, **1983**, *30*, 1379–1381.

Ligumsky, M.; Karmski, F.; and Rochmilewitz, D. Sucralfate stimulation of gastric PGE synthesis: possible mechanism to explain its effective cytoprotective mechanism. *Gastroenterology*, **1984**, *86*, 1164.

Lind, T.; Cederberg, C.; Ekenved, G.; Hagland, U.; and Olbe, L. Effect of omeprazole—a gastric proton pump inhibitor—on pentagastrin stimulated acid secretion in man. *Gut*, **1983**, *24*, 270–276.

Lux, G.; Hartog, C.; Ruppin, H.; and Rösch, W. Combined acid secretion and gastric emptying under antacid and pirenzepine. In, *Antacids in the Eighties*. (Halter, F., ed.) Urban & Schwarzenberg, Munich, **1982**, pp. 57–63.

Makoff, D. L.; Gordon, A.; Franklin, A. S.; and Gerstein, A. R. Chronic calcium carbonate therapy in uremia. *Arch. Intern. Med.*, **1969**, *123*, 15–21.

Peterson, W. L.; Sturdevant, R. A. L.; Frankl, H. D.; Richardson, C. T.; Isenberg, J. I.; Elashoff, J. D.; Sones, J. Q.; Gross, R. A.; McCallum, R. W.; and Fordtran, J. S. Healing of a duodenal ulcer with antacid regimen. *N. Engl. J. Med.*, **1977**, *297*, 341–345.

Sherman, R. A.; Hwang, E. R.; Walker, J. A.; and Eisinger, R. P. Reduction in serum phosphorus due to sucralfate. *Am. J. Gastroenterol.*, **1983**, *78*, 210–211.

Walan, A.; Bader, J.; Classen, M.; Lamers, C. B. H. W.; Piper, D. W.; Rutgersson, K.; and Eriksson, S. Effect of omeprazole and ranitidine on ulcer healing and relapse rates in patients with benign gastric ulcer. *N. Engl. J. Med.*, **1989**, *320*, 69–75.

Weberg, R., and Berstad, A. Gastrointestinal absorption of aluminum from single doses of aluminum containing antacids in man. *Eur. J. Clin. Invest.*, **1986**, *16*, 428–432.

Wrobel, J.; Koh, T. C.; and Saunders, J. M. Sodium citrate: an alternative antacid for prophylaxis against aspiration pneumonitis. *Anaesth. Intensive Care*, **1982**, *10*, 116–119.

Monographs and Reviews

Adams, M. H.; Ostrosky, J. D.; and Kirkwood, C. F. Therapeutic evaluation of omeprazole. *Clin. Pharm.*, **1988**, *7*, 725–745.

Alfrey, A. C. Aluminum. *Adv. Clin. Chem.*, **1983**, *23*, 69–91.

Aymard, J.; Aymard, B.; Netter, P.; Bannwarth, B.; Trechot, P.; and Streiff, F. Haematological adverse effects of histamine H_2-receptor antagonists. *Med. Toxicol. Adverse Drug Exp.*, **1988**, *3*, 430–448.

Baron, J. H. Gastric function tests. In, *Chronic Duodenal Ulcer*. (Wastell, C., ed.) Appleton-Century-Crofts, New York, **1972**, pp. 82–114.

———. (ed.). *Cimetidine in the 80's*. Churchill Livingstone, Edinburgh, **1981.**

Barrowman, J. A., and Pfeiffer, C. J. Carbenoxolone: a critical analysis of its clinical value in peptic ulcer. In, *Drugs and Peptic Ulcer*, Vol. 1. (Pfeiffer, C. J., ed.) CRC Press, Boca Raton, Fla., **1982**, pp. 123–132.

Black, J. W., and Shankley, N. P. How does gastrin act to stimulate oxyntic cell secretion? *Trends Pharmacol. Sci.*, **1987**, *8*, 486–490.

Brogden, R. N.; Carmine, A. A.; Heel, R. C.; Speight, T. M.; and Avery, G. S. Ranitidine: a review of its pharmacology and therapeutic use in peptic ulcer disease and other allied diseases. *Drugs,* **1982,** *24,* 267–303.

Brogden, R. N.; Heel, R. C.; Speight, T. M.; and Avery, G. S. Sucralfate: a review of its pharmacodynamic properties and therapeutic use in peptic ulcer disease. *Drugs,* **1984,** *27,* 194–209.

Carmine, A. A., and Brogden, R. N. Pirenzepine: a review of its pharmacodynamic and pharmacokinetic properties and therapeutic efficacy in peptic ulcer disease and other allied diseases. *Drugs,* **1985,** *30,* 85–126.

Clemens, J. D., and Feinstein, A. R. Calcium carbonate and constipation: an historical review of medical mythopoeia. *Gastroenterology,* **1977,** *72,* 957–961.

Clissold, S. P., and Campoli-Richards, D. M. Omeprazole: a preliminary review of its pharmacodynamic and pharmacokinetic properties, and therapeutic potential in peptic ulcer disease and Zollinger–Ellison syndrome. *Drugs,* **1986,** *32,* 15–47.

Forte, J. G.; Hanzel, D. K.; and Urushidani, T. Mechanisms of parietal cell function. In, *Advances in Drug Therapy of Gastrointestinal Ulceration.* (Garner, A., and Whittle, B. J. R., eds.) John Wiley & Sons, Ltd., New York, **1989**, pp. 33–52.

Ganellin, C. R., and Parsons, M. E. (eds.). *Pharmacology of Histamine Receptors.* John Wright & Sons, Ltd., Bristol, England, **1982.**

Holtermüller, K. H., and Dehdaschti, M. Antacids and hormones. *Scand. J. Gastroenterol.,* **1982,** *17,* Suppl. 75, 24–31.

Hurwitz, A. Antacid therapy and drug kinetics. *Clin. Pharmacokinet.,* **1977,** *2,* 269–280.

Lam, S. K. Antacids: the past, the present, and the future. *Baillieres Clin. Gastroenterol.,* **1988,** *2,* 641–654.

Lindberg, P.; Brandstrom, A.; and Wallmark, B. Structure–activity relationships of omeprazole analogues and their mechanism of action. *Trends Pharmacol. Sci.,* **1987,** *8,* 399–402.

Mach, J. R., Jr.; Korchik, W. P.; and Mahowald, M. W. Dialysis dementia. *Clin. Geriatr. Med.,* **1988,** *4,* 853–867.

Mayor, G. H., and Burnatowska-Hledin, M. The metabolism of aluminum and aluminum-related encephalopathy. *Semin. Nephrol.,* **1986,** *6,* Suppl. 1, 1–4.

Meredith, G. A. *The Ordeal of Richard Feverel.* (**1859;** revised in **1878.**) New American Library of World Literature, New York, **1961,** p. 13.

Monk, J. P., and Clissold, S. P. Misoprostol: a preliminary review of its pharmacodynamic and pharmacokinetic properties, and therapeutic efficacy in the treatment of peptic ulcer disease. *Drugs,* **1987,** *33,* 1–30.

Monteagudo, F. S.; Cassidy, M. J.; and Folb, P. I. Recent developments in aluminum toxicology. *Med. Toxicol. Adverse Drug Exp.,* **1989,** *4,* 1–16.

Nazario, M. The hepatic and renal mechanisms of drug interactions with cimetidine. *Drug Intell. Clin. Pharm.,* **1986,** *20,* 342–348.

Peterson, W. L. Gastrointestinal bleeding. In, *Gastrointestinal Disease,* 4th ed. (Sleisenger, M. H., and Fordtran, J. S., eds.) W. B. Saunders Co., Philadelphia, **1989,** pp. 397–427.

Powell, J. R., and Donn, K. H. Histamine H_2-antagonist drug interactions in perspective: mechanistic concepts and clinical implications. *Am. J. Med.,* **1984,** *77,* Suppl. 5B, 57–84.

Riley, A. J., and Salmon, P. R. (eds.). *Ranitidine.* Excerpta Medica, Amsterdam, **1982.**

Ritschel, W. A. Antacids. In, *Antacids and Other Drugs in Gastrointestinal Diseases.* Drug Intelligence Publications, Inc., Hamilton, Ill., **1984,** pp. 41–124.

Sachs, G.; Carlsson, E.; Londberg, P.; and Wallmark, B. Gastric H^+,K^+-ATPase as therapeutic target. *Annu. Rev. Pharmacol. Toxicol.,* **1988,** *28,* 269–284.

Schiessel, R. Stress ulceration and mucosal acid–base balance. In, *Advances in Drug Therapy of Gastrointestinal Ulceration.* (Garner, A., and Whittle, B. J. R., eds.) John Wiley & Sons, Ltd., New York, **1989,** pp. 221–230.

Sedman, A. J. Cimetidine—drug interactions. *Am. J. Med.,* **1984,** *76,* 109–114.

Sherrard, D. J. Aluminum and renal osteodystrophy. *Semin. Nephrol.,* **1986,** *6,* Suppl. 1, 5–11.

Soll, A. H. Duodenal ulcer and drug therapy. In, *Gastrointestinal Disease,* 4th ed. (Sleisenger, M. H., and Fordtran, J. S., eds.) W. B. Saunders Co., Philadelphia, **1989,** pp. 814–879.

Ström, M. Antacid side-effects on bowel habits. *Scand. J. Gastroenterol.,* **1982,** *17,* Suppl. 75, 54–56.

Symposium. (Various authors.) International Symposium on Gastroenterology. Focus on misoprostol. *Postgrad. Med. J.,* **1988,** *64,* Suppl. 1, 1–88.

Symposium. (Various authors.) The 5th International Sucralfate Research Conference. *Am. J. Med.,* **1989a,** *86,* 1–152.

Symposium. (Various authors.) Ulcer epidemiology. *Gastroenterology,* **1989b,** *96,* Suppl., 559–681.

Talley, N. J., and Ormand, J. E. Is antibacterial therapy against *Campylobacter pylori* useful in the treatment of indigestion and chronic peptic ulceration? *Trends Pharmacol. Sci.,* **1989,** *10,* 36–40.

Wolfe, M., and Soll, A. H. The physiology of gastric acid secretion. *N. Engl. J. Med.,* **1988,** *319,* 1707–1715.

Zeldis, J. B.; Friedman, L. S.; and Isselbacher, K. J. Drug therapy: ranitidine—a new H_2-receptor antagonist. *N. Engl. J. Med.,* **1983,** *309,* 1368–1373.

CHAPTER

38 AGENTS AFFECTING GASTROINTESTINAL WATER FLUX AND MOTILITY, DIGESTANTS, AND BILE ACIDS

Laurence L. Brunton

The proper flux of nutrients, wastes, electrolytes, and water through the intestines depends on an appropriate balance of absorption and secretion of water and electrolytes by the intestinal epithelium. Normally, there is net absorption of water in the intestine in response to osmotic gradients that result from the uptake and secretion of ions and the absorption of nutrients (mainly sugars and amino acids). Neurohumoral mechanisms, pathogens, and drugs (*see* Tables 38–1 and 38–3) can alter these uptake and secretory processes and the osmotic gradients for water flux such that excessive absorption or net secretion of water occurs, contributing to constipation or diarrhea, respectively. Additionally, drugs can stimulate or reduce intestinal motility and thereby alter the transit time of compounds through the intestine. Since the extent of absorption generally parallels transit time, altered motility also contributes to diarrhea or constipation. Gastrointestinal motility is also an important component of vomiting, and enhanced gastric emptying is a significant aspect of the actions of some antiemetic agents.

Most agents considered in this chapter are used to control gastrointestinal symptoms. However, the physician must remember that there may often be important underlying causes of altered intestinal motility and absorption that require attention.

GENERAL CONSIDERATIONS

Intestinal Fluxes of Water and Electrolytes. Normally about 9 liters of fluid enter the small intestine daily—2 liters from ingestion and the remainder from intestinal secretions (Figure 38–1). The small intestine absorbs about 80% of this load. Since the gastrointestinal tract lacks significant concentrating mechanisms, the osmolarity of the fluid that traverses the upper jejunum is adjusted toward that of plasma, and fluid that enters the middle portion of the small intestine is mainly in the form of an isotonic salt solution. All but about 1 to 1.5 liters of this fluid is absorbed by the ileum. The colon absorbs nearly all of the remainder, and about 0.1 liter of water is passed into the stool. Thus, the small bowel normally absorbs roughly 8 liters per day, which is about 50% of its capacity. Any reduction in absorption by the small intestine adds to the burden of the colon, which can absorb 4 to 5 liters of water per day. The presentation to the colon of fluid in excess of this amount or of a load of impermeant solutes will increase the passage of isosmotic fluid through the anal sphincter.

The causes of diarrhea are legion, but the overall alterations in intestinal function are similar. The intestine ceases, at least along a part of its length, to be an organ of net absorption of water and electrolytes, and to the extent that the fluid produced exceeds the absorptive capacity of the remaining intestine, water passes into the stool. The aim of the treatment of diarrhea is to enhance intestinal absorption of water by reducing the content of luminal electrolytes (by increasing active absorption of Na^+ or decreasing secretion of anions) or by decreasing intestinal motility (thereby favoring absorption). The aims of therapies for constipation are, conversely, to increase the water content of the feces (thereby softening them) and to encourage intestinal motility. (For detailed discussion of the fluxes of intestinal electrolytes and water, *see* Binder, 1989; Fine *et al.*, 1989.)

Colonic Function. The absorption of fluid by the colon is secondary to active transport of Na^+; the luminal equilibrium concentration for net uptake of Na^+ is 25 to 30 mM. The mechanism responsible for colonic absorption of Na^+ is primarily electrogenic Na^+ transport, which relies on a Na^+,K^+-ATPase activity in the basolateral membrane of the colonic epithelium; neutral absorption of NaCl may also be involved. The colon absorbs Cl^- by an electrically neutral mechanism that involves exchange of Cl^- for HCO_3^- and by neutral uptake of NaCl. Agents that elevate intracellular concentrations of adenosine 3′,5′-monophosphate (cyclic AMP) in colonic enterocytes apparently stimulate electrogenic secretion of Cl^- and may inhibit neutral NaCl uptake. This causes net fluid secretion. The colon also secretes K^+, probably by means of an active mechanism that is stimulated by cyclic AMP.

The colon absorbs relatively few nutrients; it does, however, absorb short-chain fatty acids (two

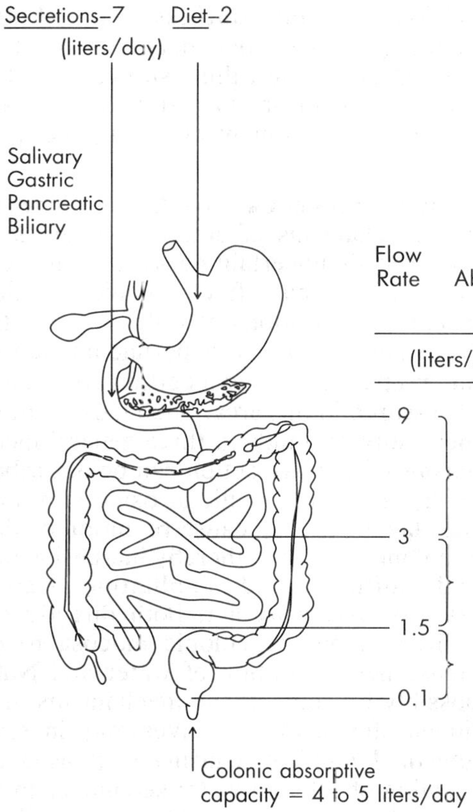

Flow Rate	H_2O Absorbed	Ion Concentrations Na^+	K^+	Cl^-	HCO_3^-	Osmolality
(liters/day)		(mEq/liter)				(mOsm/kg)
9		60	15	60	15	Variable
	6					
3		140	6	100	30	Isotonic
	1.5					
1.5		140	8	60	70	Isotonic
	1.4					
0.1		40	90	15	30	Isotonic

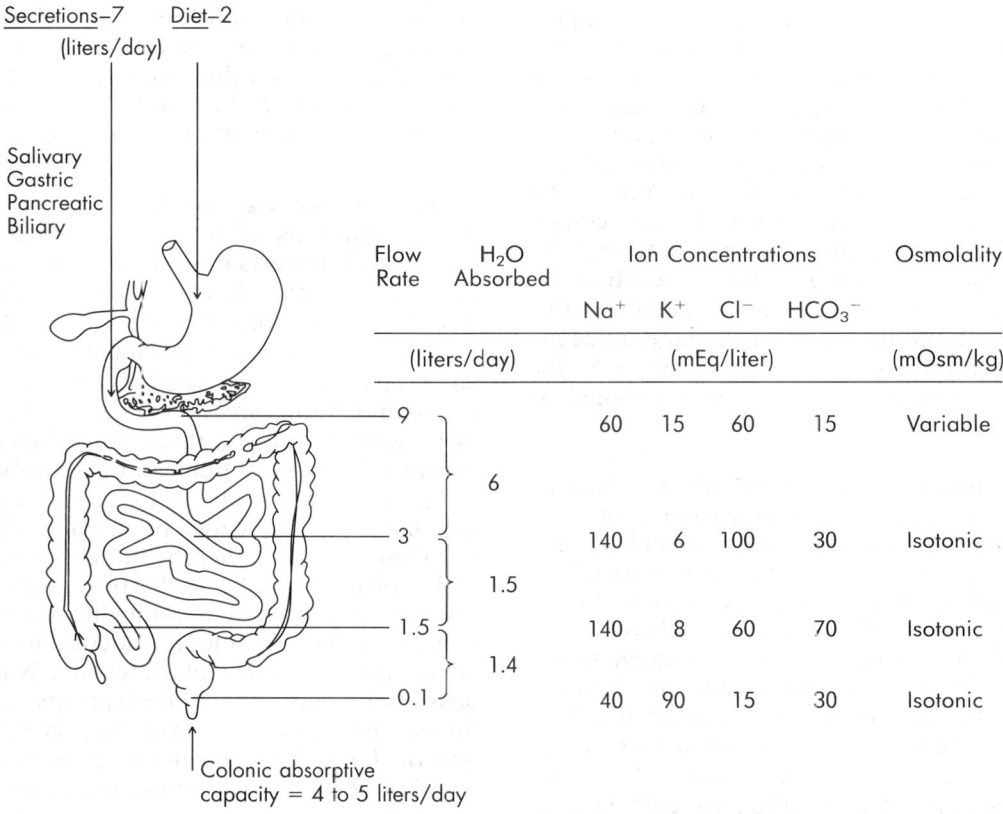

Figure 38–1. *The approximate volume and composition of fluid that traverses the small and large intestines daily.* (Adapted from Binder, 1989; Fine *et al.*, 1989.)

to four carbon atoms in length) by diffusion. The absorption of these fatty acids increases that of fluid and electrolytes. This effect is in contrast to the effects of longer-chain fatty acids (≥ 12 carbons) and dihydroxy bile acids (*see* below; *see also* Binder, 1989).

Colonic function is subject to complex sets of regulatory influences. In contrast to the small intestine, electrolyte transport in the colon is susceptible to regulation by mineralocorticoids. The response of the colon to aldosterone is similar to that of the kidney: uptake of Na^+ and H_2O is enhanced, while K^+ is secreted. Other hormones and neurotransmitters that influence colonic fluxes of water and electrolyte include somatostatin, opioids, antidiuretic hormone, and dopaminergic and adrenergic agonists, all of which enhance absorption or inhibit secretion; vasoactive intestinal peptide (VIP) and prostaglandins, which are secretagogues; and cholinergic agonists, which cause net secretion of NaCl and H_2O (*see* Bridges *et al.*, 1983; Donowitz *et al.*, 1983; Binder, 1989). In some systems, these agents act to inhibit adenylyl cyclase (somatostatin and opiate peptides) or to stimulate the enzyme (prostaglandins E and I_2 and VIP). Some of their effects may thus be due to cyclic AMP–dependent regulation of Cl^- secretion. Cholera toxin, "the ultimate laxative," clearly stimulates intestinal secretion in the small intestine and the colon by its ability to activate adenylyl cyclase in the mucosa. The effects of adrenergic and cholinergic agents do not fit well with such a theory, however; both α_2- and β-adrenergic agonists cause net uptake of fluid, whereas muscarinic cholinergic stimulation causes net fluid secretion. Coordinate adrenergic and cholinergic control of colonic function likely involves the integration of cyclic AMP– and Ca^{2+}–dependent pathways (*see* Chapter 2), and several cellular loci are probably involved, including enterocytes, components of the enteric nervous system, smooth muscle, and mucus-secreting goblet cells. Superposed on local hormonal regulation of fluid and electrolyte fluxes are the effects of neurohumors and sensory and reflex pathways that involve the lumbar spinal cord, pelvic nerves, and higher inhibitory centers, through which poorly quantifiable factors such as stress and other psychological variables affect colonic function.

LAXATIVES

Laxatives promote defecation. Their zealous overuse by a self-prescribing public, fostered by advertising, reflects a misconception of what frequency of bowel movement is normal, desirable, or necessary. Although there are valid indications for the use of laxatives, constipation can generally be resolved by increasing the fiber content of the diet, exercise, and bowel training. In some instances, constipation may result from important underlying causes, such as adverse reactions to drugs or toxins (Table 38–1), metabolic disorders, and disorders of the large intestine (*see* Devroede, 1989); in these cases the cause rather than the symptom should be treated.

Defecation and Constipation. Normal size, frequency, and consistency of fecal output are difficult to quantify and are subject to personal variation and to sociological patterning, of which the makers of laxatives take full advantage. There is no distinct advantage in having frequent bowel movements. While once daily may be average, between three times weekly and three times daily may be considered normal (*see* Devroede, 1989). Patients' fears of "autointoxication" by retention of colonic contents are unfounded if hepatic function is normal.

Reduced frequency and bulk and increased hardness of feces surely do occur, mainly owing to dehydration of material that stays too long in the colon before expulsion. The bulk, softness, and hydration of feces are very dependent on the fiber content of the diet; thus, sufficient dietary fiber and water are mainstays in any regimen for the treatment of constipation.

Table 38–1. SOME COSTIVE (CONSTIPATING) AGENTS

Analgesics (inhibitors of prostaglandin synthesis)
Antacids (containing calcium carbonate or aluminum hydroxide)
Anticholinergic agents
Antidiarrheal agents
Antihistamines (H_1 blockers; anticholinergic effect)
Antiparkinsonian drugs (anticholinergic effect)
Barium sulfate
Diuretics that cause hypokalemia
Ganglionic blocking agents
Heavy metals (especially lead)
Iron
Laxatives (used chronically)
Monoamine oxidase inhibitors
Muscle relaxants
Opioids
Phenothiazines (anticholinergic effect)
Polystyrene resins
Tricyclic antidepressants (anticholinergic effect)
Verapamil

Mechanisms of Laxative Action. The precise mechanisms of action of many laxatives remain uncertain because of the complex factors that affect colonic function, prominent variations of water and electrolyte transport among experimental species and preparations, and a certain costiveness of research in this area. Such lack of movement notwithstanding, three general mechanisms of laxative action can be described. (1) By their hydrophilic or osmotic properties, laxatives may cause retention of fluid in colonic contents, thereby increasing bulk and softness and facilitating transit. (2) Laxatives may act, both directly and indirectly, on the colonic mucosa to decrease net absorption of water and NaCl, possibly by some of the mechanisms mentioned above. (3) Laxatives may increase intestinal motility, causing decreased absorption of salt and water secondary to decreased transit time. Abnormal colonic motility is thought to be a contributing factor in constipation, and the interactions of motility with absorptive and secretory functions are topics of current research. More detailed information on putative mechanisms of action of individual agents appears below.

Classification and Choice of Laxatives. In this chapter, laxatives are classified by their general mechanisms of action. However, commonly used agents may also be arranged according to the pattern of laxative effects produced by the usual clinical dosage (Table 38–2). Note that the latency and effect of all laxatives vary with dosage. In sufficiently high dosage, many laxatives promote catharsis, which implies purgation and a more fluid evacuation. Although the major group of agents (*e.g.*, bulk-forming agents, docusates) frequently have distinguishing characteristics that limit or indicate their usefulness in a particular patient, agents within each group usually share utility and limitations.

Table 38–2. CLASSIFICATION AND COMPARISON OF REPRESENTATIVE LAXATIVES

LAXATIVE EFFECT AND LATENCY IN USUAL CLINICAL DOSAGE		
Softening of Feces, 1 to 3 Days	*Soft or Semifluid Stool, 6 to 8 Hours*	*Watery Evacuation, 1 to 3 Hours*
Bulk-forming laxatives Bran Psyllium preparations Methylcellulose	Diphenylmethane derivatives Phenolphthalein Bisacodyl	Saline cathartics * Sodium phosphates Magnesium sulfate Milk of magnesia
Docusates	Anthraquinone derivatives Senna Cascara sagrada	Castor oil
Lactulose		

* Also employed in lower dosage for laxative effect.

DIETARY FIBER AND BULK-FORMING LAXATIVES

The most satisfactory prophylactic and therapeutic agent for functional constipation is a diet rich in fiber. Dietary fiber will also benefit patients who need to avoid straining at the stool and patients with irritable bowel disease and diverticular disease of the colon. There are various bulk-forming agents that can be utilized as supplements to dietary fiber; these include both natural and semisynthetic polysaccharides and celluloses derived from grains, seed husks, or kelp, including bran, psyllium, methylcellulose, and carboxymethylcellulose, as well as the synthetic resin polycarbophil.

Dietary fiber is plant cell wall that escapes digestion by the secretions of the gastrointestinal tract. Usual sources of dietary fiber are whole grains, bran, vegetables, and fruit. Plant cell walls consist of varying quantities of fibrillar polysaccharides (mainly cellulose), matrix polysaccharides (pectins, hemicelluloses), lignins, cutin, waxes, and some glycoproteins (*see* Selvendran, 1984). Dietary fiber may act as a laxative by several mechanisms. It can bind water and ions in the colonic lumen, thereby softening the feces and increasing their bulk. Some components of dietary fiber (*e.g.*, pectins) are digested by colonic bacteria to metabolites that contribute to laxative action by adding to the osmotic activity of the luminal fluid. Dietary fiber can also support the growth of colonic bacteria, thereby increasing fecal mass. It is also possible that bacterial fermentation of dietary fiber produces metabolites that directly influence colonic mechanisms of fluid and electrolyte transport. Dietary fibers and bulk-forming agents from different sources vary in their composition, and thus in their water-holding capacity, and in the relative contribution of these different modes of action (*see* Cummings, 1984). The fiber contents of common foods are now listed in numerous textbooks and diet plans. On the basis of satisfactory laxation as judged from patients' comments, 20 to 60 g of dietary fiber daily is sufficient (*see* Mendeloff, 1977; Bingham *et al.*, 1979).

Effects on the Intestinal Tract; Systemic Effects. Dietary fiber and bulk-forming agents increase the mass of stool, its water content, and the rate of colonic transit. These effects are usually apparent within 24 hours and, with repeated administration, reach a maximum after several days. Dietary fiber alone, in the form of a diet rich in fruit, vegetables, and whole grains, can increase the daily fecal mass markedly. The lignin and pectin in dietary fibers will bind bile acids, thereby reducing their reabsorption and protecting them from bacterial degradation, which increases their excretion in the feces. The consequent enhancement of hepatic synthesis of bile acids from cholesterol may reduce plasma concentrations of cholesterol in low-density lipoproteins. The effects of dietary fiber on plasma cholesterol and lipoproteins are variable and depend on the type of fiber studied (*see* Anderson and Chen, 1979; Symposium, 1983). Refined gums and pectin, for instance, are hypocholesterolemic in man, primarily by reducing the plasma low-density lipoprotein fraction, whereas cellulose is not (Behall *et al.*, 1984). The mechanisms of such effects may be similar to those responsible for the effects of bile acid–binding resins (*see* Chapter 36).

When used over several months, bran and other bulk-forming agents reduce intraluminal rectosigmoid pressure and relieve symptoms in patients with irritable bowel disease and diverticular disease of the colon (*see* Brodribb, 1977). Whether a lack of dietary fiber contributes to disorders of the large bowel and other diseases remains to be established (*see* Painter and Burkitt, 1975; Mendeloff, 1977).

Their ability to absorb water and to provide an emollient intestinal mass makes the bulk-forming laxatives useful for the symptomatic relief of acute diarrhea and for regulation of the effluent in patients with an ileostomy or colostomy. However, loss of Na^+, K^+, and H_2O may be increased in such patients. The alleged effectiveness of the bulk-forming agents as appetite suppressants in the management of obesity has not been substantiated. The beneficial effects of dietary fiber notwithstanding, representations of bran as a panacea for the ills of Western civilization are very likely exaggerated.

Adverse Effects. Bulk-forming laxatives have few side effects and minimal systemic effects. Allergic reactions may occur, especially with use of plant gums. Flatulence and borborygmi occur occasionally. Possible alterations in Ca^{2+} metabolism are incompletely defined, as are effects on glucose tolerance. The latter may be related to the dextrose content of some preparations and should be considered in the treatment of diabetic patients. Cellulose can bind and reduce the intestinal absorption of many drugs, including cardiac glycosides, salicylates, and nitrofurantoin; psyllium may bind coumarin derivatives. Although specific information is sparse, the potential for such interactions is great and warrants monitoring and discussion with the patient. Ingestion of drugs and laxatives should be separated in time as much as possible. Carboxymethylcellulose sodium and psyllium husk may contain significant quantities of Na^+ and should not be used when systemic retention of Na^+ and H_2O could be a problem.

Intestinal obstruction and impaction may occur after the administration of bulk-forming agents, especially in patients with preexisting gastrointestinal disease, and individuals with stenosis, ulceration, or adhesions should avoid these agents. Esophageal and intestinal obstruction can occur when these substances are taken dry. Patients may avoid these problems by drinking a glass of water concurrently.

Preparations and Dosages. *Bran, Whole Grains, and Other Dietary Fiber.* Bran contains more than 40% dietary fiber and is a convenient source of intestinal bulk. Bran-rich cereals contain 25% dietary fiber. Crude bran may be added to cereals, salads, and baked goods. Approximately 6 g of crude miller's bran daily produces a noticeable enhancement in the bulk and softness of stools (*see* Editorial, 1987). Fresh fruits, vegetables, and legumes contribute generously to dietary fiber. Burkitt and Meisner (1979) have provided a helpful guide to the fiber content of foods. *Malt soup extract* (MALTSUPEX), 12 g daily in four divided doses (as tablets), provides an adult with a fiber and maltose supplement derived from barley.

Psyllium Husk. *Plantago seed* has been replaced by refined preparations from psyllium seeds that are enriched in mucilloid, a hydrophilic substance that forms a gelatinous mass when mixed with water. Typical brand-name preparations are EFFER-SYLLIUM, KONSYL, METAMUCIL, and MODANE BULK. Some of these preparations contain dextrose or sucrose. The usual dose is 2.5 to 4 g, once to thrice daily, in 250 ml of fruit juice, water, or other liquid. Long-term administration of the psyllium preparations may produce modest reduction of plasma cholesterol concentration, apparently by interference with reabsorption of bile acids. Sensitization, with asthmatic symptoms upon inhalation of psyllium powder, has been reported in atopic individuals chronically exposed to the powder during its manufacture.

Semisynthetic Celluloses and Gums. *Methylcellulose* (CITRUCEL, COLOGEL) and *carboxymethylcellulose sodium* are hydrophilic derivatives of cellulose. These indigestible and unabsorbable compounds form a bulky colloid when mixed with water, leading to a softening of the stool within 1 to 3 days. Such celluloses have also been used to increase the bulk and consistency of stools in patients who suffer from chronic watery diarrhea. Capsules (which also contain other ingredients) and oral solutions of these agents are available; all should be administered with ample water, and the usual dose is 2 to 6 g daily in two or three portions.

Other Bulk-Forming Agents. *Polycarbophil* and *calcium polycarbophil* (MITROLAN, others) are nonabsorbed hydrophilic polyacrylic resins with more water-binding capacity than the aforementioned agents. They absorb 60 to 100 times their weight in water and thereby add soft bulk to feces. These preparations have the advantage of a low content of Na^+. Calcium polycarbophil releases Ca^{2+} in the gastrointestinal tract and should thus be avoided by patients who must restrict their intake of Ca^{2+} or who are taking tetracyclines. Calcium polycarbophil is available as chewable tablets that contain the equivalent of 500 mg of polycarbophil. The recommended adult dose is 1 g, one to four times daily; each dose should be taken with 250 ml of water.

SALINE AND OSMOTIC LAXATIVES

These agents include various Mg^{2+} salts; the sulfate, phosphate, and tartrate salts of Na^+ or K^+; the disaccharide lactulose; glycerin; and sorbitol. They are poorly and slowly absorbed and act by their osmotic properties in the luminal fluid. Mg^{2+} salts may, in addition, cause duodenal secretion of cholecystokinin (Harvey and Read, 1975), a hormone whose pharmacological actions include stimulation of fluid secretion and motility; it is possible that this mechanism contributes to their laxative activity. The primary osmotic effect of lactulose, which is not absorbed in the upper intestine, may be augmented in the distal ileum and colon by bacterial metabolism of the disaccharide to lactate and other organic acids that are only partially absorbed. There is speculation that the concomitant reduction in luminal pH enhances motility and secretion.

Effects on the Intestinal Tract. Full cathartic doses of saline laxatives (15 g of $MgSO_4$ or the equivalent with 250 ml of water) produce a thorough, semifluid or water evacuation in 3 hours or less. Lower doses produce a laxative effect with a latency of 6 to 8 hours. The cathartic effect is most prominent if the laxative is taken when the stomach is empty. These agents are useful for emptying the bowel prior to surgical, radiological, and colonoscopic procedures and can help eliminate parasites following appropriate therapy (*see* Chapter 40).

The increased osmotic activity in the lumen that follows administration of lactulose results in modest accumulation of fluid and passage of soft, formed feces in 1 to 3 days. Another important aspect of the action of lactulose is reduction of intestinal absorption of ammonia, in part because of reduced production and increased utilization of ammonia by intestinal bacteria. In addition, fecal excretion of ammonia is enhanced because bacterial metabolism of lactulose lowers the pH of luminal contents and traps ammonia as NH_{4^+}. These effects account for the efficacy of lactulose in lowering concentrations of ammonia in blood in 75% of patients with portal hypertension and hepatic encephalopathy associated with chronic liver disease. With a latency of 1 to 7 days, lactulose reduces blood ammonia in these patients by 25 to 50% (Avery *et al.*, 1972; Conn, 1978).

Adverse Effects. Some absorption of the component ions of the saline laxatives does occur, and in certain instances they may produce systemic toxicity. In an individual with impaired renal function, the accumulation of Mg^{2+} in the body fluids may be sufficient to cause intoxication (*see* Chapters 27 and 37). Laxatives that contain Mg^{2+} should thus be administered only if renal function is adequate. Similarly, Na^+ salts may be contraindicated in patients with congestive heart failure or renal disease, and phosphate salts may reduce the concentration of Ca^{2+} in plasma. Hypertonic solutions of the saline laxatives can produce significant dehydration. For this reason, these salts should be administered with sufficient water by mouth to ensure that no net loss of body water occurs.

Lactulose may cause flatulence, cramps, and abdominal discomfort, especially when therapy is initiated; these symptoms occur in about 20% of patients receiving full doses of the drug. Nausea and vomiting have also been reported, particularly with higher dosage. Excessive dosage can cause diarrhea, loss of fluid and K^+, and exacerbation of hepatic encephalopathy. Since lactulose is a disaccharide of galactose and fructose, its use is contraindicated in patients who require a galactose-free diet, and it must be used cautiously in diabetics. The preparation also contains some lactose.

Preparations and Dosages. *Magnesium Salts.* The usual dose of *magnesium sulfate* (*Epsom salt*) is 10 to 15 g, but 5 g (about 40 mEq of Mg^{2+}) produces a significant laxative effect when administered in dilute solution to a fasting individual or to a child. The intensely bitter taste may induce nausea and should be masked by taking the salt in citrus juices. *Milk of magnesia* is a 7.0 to 8.5% aqueous suspension of $Mg(OH)_2$. The usual adult dose is 15 to 40 ml (about 40 to 110 mEq of Mg^{2+}). *Magnesium hydroxide* is also available as tablets. The usual dose is 1.8 to 3.6 g (62 to 124 mEq). Other Mg^{2+} salts commonly employed as gastric antacids have similar laxative properties (*see also* Chapter 37). *Magnesium citrate oral solution* provides the equivalent of 4 g of $Mg(OH)_2$ in the usual 240-ml dose.

Sodium Phosphates. Phosphate salts are relatively pleasant tasting. The most frequently employed preparation is *sodium phosphates oral solution* (FLEET PHOSPHO-SODA), which contains 1.8 g of dibasic sodium phosphate and 4.8 g of monobasic sodium phosphate in 10 ml. The usual dose is 20 to 30 ml, taken with ample water. *Sodium phosphates enema,* in a dose of 118 ml, is employed for rectal administration.

Other Saline Laxatives. Polyethylene glycol–electrolyte solutions (COLYTE, GOLYTELY) are mixtures of sodium sulfate, sodium bicarbonate, sodium chloride, and potassium chloride in an isotonic solution that contains 60 g of polyethylene glycol per liter. Patients drink 4 liters of this solution over 3 to 4 hours prior to colonoscopy. The large volume of nonabsorbable fluid results in copious watery diarrhea and the efficient removal of solid wastes from the gastrointestinal tract. Dehydration does not occur, because the solution is isotonic. This preparation should not be used in patients with intestinal obstruction, perforation, or toxic megacolon. Other saline laxatives, such as *sodium sulfate* (*Glauber's salt*) and *potassium sodium tartrate* (*Rochelle salt*), are now little used and have no advantage over the preparations listed above.

Lactulose. This agent is a semisynthetic disaccharide with the following structure:

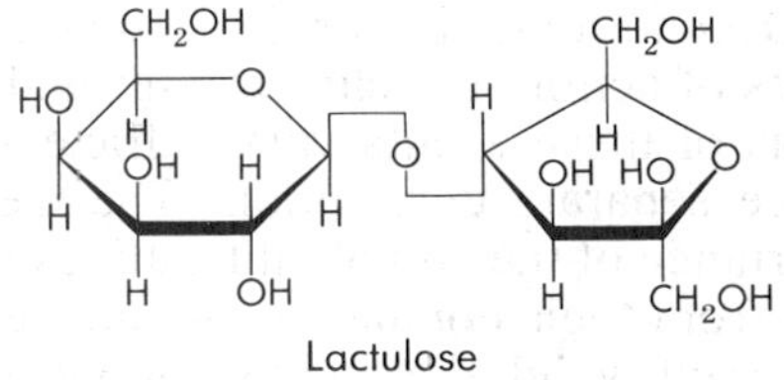

Lactulose

Lactulose (CEPHULAC, CHRONULAC, others) is available as a syrup; each 15 ml contains 10 g of lactulose and less than 2.2 g of galactose, 1.2 g of lactose, and 1.2 g of other sugars. The sweet taste can be masked by mixing the syrup with fruit juice.

The daily maintenance dose for management of constipation varies widely but may be as low as 7 to 10 g, as a single dose or divided. Larger doses (up to 40 g) are sometimes required, and the full effect of lactulose may not be attained for a few days.

For management of chronic portal hypertension and hepatic encephalopathy, the usual maintenance dose is 20 to 30 g (30 to 45 ml), three or four times daily; this is adjusted such that there are two or three soft stools daily and a fecal pH of 5 to 5.5. Therapy can be initiated with hourly doses of 20 to 30 g if indicated. Lactulose can also be given rectally if necessary. Maintenance of the proper fecal pH is essential for appropriate effects on intestinal elimination of ammonia. Excessive diarrhea must be avoided. To avoid inadequate acidification of the stool, other laxatives should not be used concurrently. For additional aspects of the management of this disease, *see* Avery and colleagues (1972).

Glycerin. This agent acts mainly by its osmotic effect to soften and lubricate the passage of inspissated feces. It may also stimulate rectal contraction. Rectal suppositories promote colonic evacuation in 30 minutes. A rectal liquid is available for children.

Sorbitol. Sorbitol (D-glucitol), a polyalcohol of sorbose, acts as an osmotic agent when administered rectally as an enema (120 ml of a 25 to 30% solution for adults; 30 to 60 ml for children). It can also be given orally (*e.g.*, 30 ml of a 70% solution). When sodium polystyrene sulfonate is utilized in the therapy of hyperkalemia, sorbitol is frequently included to combat the constipating effect of the cation-exchange resin. Similarly, sorbitol is often mixed with activated charcoal in the management of poisonings or drug overdoses.

STIMULANT LAXATIVES

These agents stimulate accumulation of water and electrolytes in the colonic lumen, and they also enhance intestinal motility. Included in this group are diphenylmethane derivatives, anthraquinones, and castor oil, as well as the surfactants, docusates, poloxamers, and bile acids. Docusates and poloxamers are also known as stool softeners. Despite some similarities in their mechanisms of action, the clinical uses and limitations of these agents vary sufficiently to require separate description. The medical importance of the stimulant laxatives stems more from their popularity and abuse than from their valid therapeutic applications.

The effects of the stimulant laxatives on intestinal fluxes of electrolytes and water are readily demonstrated *in vitro* or *in situ* under conditions in which effects on motility are excluded. Concentrations of these agents that reduce net absorption of electrolytes and water also increase the permeability of the mucosa, possibly by making tight junctions leaky. The stimulant laxatives may inhibit intestinal Na^+,K^+-ATPase; this action could account for at least a portion of their laxative effect (*see* above). Many of the stimulant laxatives also increase the synthesis of prostaglandins and cyclic AMP, and this action may contribute to increased secretion of water and electrolytes. Inhibition of prostaglandin synthesis with indomethacin does reduce the effects of many of these agents on net water flux (*see* Symposium, 1983). Fairbairn and Moss (1970) have summarized structure–activity relationships among the stimulant laxatives.

Diphenylmethane Derivatives. The primary diphenylmethane laxatives are phenolphthalein and bisacodyl. These agents have similar pharmacological characteristics and clinical uses. Their structures are as follows:

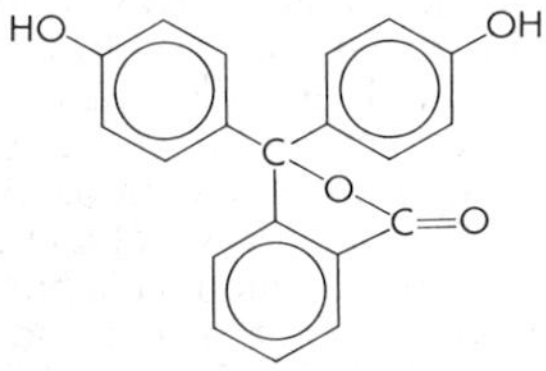

Phenolphthalein

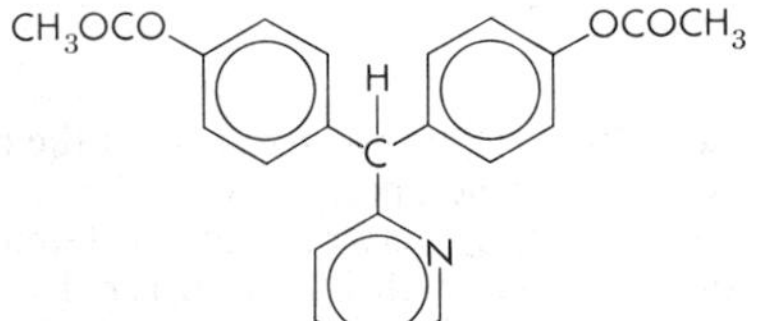

Bisacodyl

The laxative effect of phenolphthalein was discovered in 1902 by Vamossy, during a study undertaken for the Hungarian government to determine its safety as an additive for identification of artificial wines. It has since been widely used as a laxative, fortunately not as an additive to wines. Bisacodyl—4,4′-(2-pyridylmethylene) diphenol diacetate—was introduced as a laxative in 1953 on the basis of structure–activity studies of compounds related to phenolphthalein.

Laxative Effects. Individual effective doses of the diphenylmethane derivatives vary as much as fourfold to eightfold. Consequently, recommended doses that promote laxation in the majority of patients may be relatively ineffective in some patients but may produce griping and excessively fluid evacuation in others. Since the diphenylmethane derivatives act primarily on the colon, laxative effects are not usually produced in less than 6 hours.

They are frequently taken at bedtime to produce their effect the next morning. Use of these agents should be limited to 10 consecutive days (*see* below).

Absorption and Excretion. As much as 15% of a therapeutic dose of phenolphthalein is absorbed and eliminated by the kidney, most of it in conjugated form. The urine becomes pink or red if it is sufficiently alkaline. Some absorbed drug is also excreted in the bile, and the resulting enterohepatic cycle may contribute to prolongation of the laxative effect.

Bisacodyl is rapidly converted by intestinal and bacterial enzymes to its active desacetyl metabolite. As much as 5% of an orally administered dose is absorbed and excreted in the urine as the glucuronide. This inactive metabolite is also excreted in the bile and may be hydrolyzed to active drug in the colon.

Adverse Effects. The major dangers of overdosage of the diphenylmethane derivatives are fluid and electrolyte deficits resulting from excessive laxative effect. Moreover, allergic reactions, including fixed-drug eruption, Stevens–Johnson syndrome, a syndrome that resembles lupus erythematosus, osteomalacia, and protein-losing gastroenteropathy, have been reported to follow the use of phenolphthalein. Laxatives containing phenolphthalein are additionally undesirable because of their potential for abuse (*see* below).

Preparations and Dosages. Phenolphthalein (MODANE, others) is available as tablets and in numerous proprietary preparations. The usual dose is 30 to 200 mg for adults and 15 to 60 mg for children. Phenolphthalein usually acts in 6 to 8 hours. The patient should be warned of possible pink coloring of the urine and feces.

Bisacodyl (DULCOLAX, others) is available as 5-mg enteric-coated tablets for oral administration and as 10-mg suppositories and in suspension (10 mg/30 ml) for rectal administration. It is also supplied in kits, sometimes with other agents, for evacuation of the bowel prior to diagnostic procedures or surgery. The usual oral dose is 10 to 15 mg for adults and 5 to 10 mg for children (0.3 mg/kg). To avoid gastric irritation, patients should swallow tablets without chewing or crushing and should not take bisacodyl within 1 hour of milk or antacid medication. One or two soft, formed stools are usually produced within 6 to 12 hours. Recommended rectal dosage is 10 mg for adults and for children over 2 years, and 5 mg for children under 2 years. After rectal administration, the drug usually acts in 15 to 60 minutes. Bisacodyl suppositories may produce a burning sensation in the rectum; mild proctitis and sloughing of epithelium have been reported after use of the suppositories for several weeks. Hence, prolonged use should be discouraged.

Anthraquinone Laxatives. The anthraquinone laxatives include the glycosides of derivatives of 1,8-dihydroxyanthraquinone (danthron) that are contained in senna, cascara, rheum (rhubarb), and aloe (and other members of the *Liliaceae*). The structural formula of danthron is as follows:

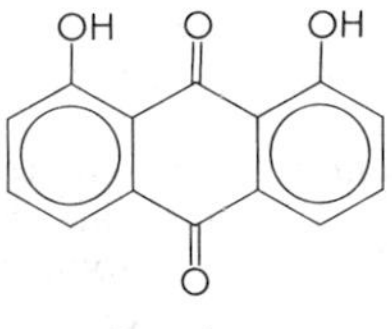

Danthron

Preparations that contain danthron itself have been withdrawn from the market because of the association of danthron with the appearance of hepatic and intestinal tumors in laboratory animals (Mori *et al.*, 1985, 1986). Although the naturally occurring glycosides may differ in this regard, their chronic use is not recommended (*see* Dufour and Gendre, 1988). The clinical uses and limitations of cascara and senna are similar to those of derivatives of diphenylmethane.

Absorption, Metabolism, and Excretion. Following an oral dose, the naturally occurring anthraquinone glycosides are poorly absorbed from the small intestine. After removal of the sugar (D-glucose or L-rhamnose) and reduction to the anthrol by colonic bacteria, the agents are absorbed to a moderate degree. Absorbed material may be excreted in the bile, with possible effects on the small bowel, and in saliva, breast milk, and urine.

Laxative Effects. The effects of the individual preparations vary, depending on their anthraquinone content and the ease of liberation of the active constituents from their precursor glycosides by the intestinal microflora. These agents do increase colonic motility, an effect attributed to stimulation of Auerbach's plexus by anthraquinone derivatives. The galenical preparations often employed may contain other active ingredients. Since the laxative effect of the anthraquinone is limited mainly to the large intestine, these agents are generally effective 6 hours or more after oral administration.

Adverse Effects. The undesirable properties of anthraquinone laxatives are mainly an excessive laxative effect and abdominal pain. Following a normal laxative dose, the quantity appearing in milk during lactation may be sufficient to affect a nursing infant; nursing mothers should be warned to avoid these agents. Renal excretion of the compounds may cause abnormal color of the urine (yellowish brown turning red with increasing pH). Large doses may produce nephritis. A melanotic pigmentation of the colonic mucosa (melanosis coli) has been observed in individuals who have taken anthraquinone laxatives over extended periods. The pigmentation is benign and is usually reversible within 4 to 12 months after medication is discontinued. Its presence may help confirm a suspicion of laxative abuse.

Preparations and Dosages. Senna is obtained from the dried leaflets or pods of *Cassia acutifolia* or *Cassia angustifolia*. Preparations of senna leaf—*senna, senna fluid extract,* and *senna syrup*—usually produce a single, thorough bowel evacuation within 6 hours, but with considerable griping.

Griping reflects the effect of the drug on colonic motility. *Concentrates of senna pods,* standardized by chemical or biological assay, are usually preferred. They are more stable and more reliable than the preparations of senna leaf and are alleged to cause less cramping and griping than does crude senna. Preparations of senna pods are available as granules, syrup, suppositories, and tablets. The dosage is as labeled.

Cascara sagrada (*sacred bark*) is obtained from the bark of the buckthorn tree, *Rhamnus purshiana.* The most commonly employed preparation is *aromatic cascara fluid extract.* A 5-ml dose usually causes a single soft or semifluid evacuation of the bowel in approximately 8 hours. Proprietary preparations that contain the anthranol glycosides from cascara sagrada (*casanthranol*) are also available. The adult dose is 30 mg.

Castor Oil. The bean of the castor plant, *Ricinus communis,* contains two well-known noxious ingredients: an extremely toxic protein, ricin, and an oil composed chiefly of the triglyceride of ricinoleic acid (12-hydroxyoleic acid). The objectionable taste and purgative qualities of the oil, ascribable to the ricinoleic acid, have been dreaded by children since the time of the early Egyptians. The cathartic effect is too strong to warrant use of this agent for common constipation.

Metabolism, Catharsis, and Adverse Effects. Used externally, castor oil is a bland emollient. Within the small intestine, however, pancreatic lipases hydrolyze the oil to glycerol and ricinoleic acid. Ricinoleate, like other anionic surfactants, reduces net absorption of fluid and electrolytes and stimulates intestinal peristalsis. Ricinoleic acid is also absorbed and metabolized like other fatty acids.

Because ricinoleate acts in the small intestine, accumulation of fluid and evacuation are prompt and thorough, such as desired before radiological examination. Colonic emptying is so complete that several days may pass before feces do.

The altered intestinal permeability caused by castor oil may reflect grosser morphological damage to the intestinal mucosa. The strong purgative action can cause colic as well as dehydration with electrolyte imbalance. For these reasons and because of possible reduction of the absorption of nutrients, long-term use of castor oil must be avoided. The stimulant effects of this agent are reportedly sufficient to cause uterine contraction in pregnant women, who should, therefore, avoid using castor oil.

Preparations and Dosage. Castor oil is usually administered when the stomach is empty. As little as 4 ml may produce a laxative effect in the fasting adult. However, the usual dose for a cathartic effect is 15 to 60 ml for adults. Full doses of castor oil cause the evacuation of one or two copious, semifluid stools within 1 to 6 hours; thus, this laxative should not be taken late in the day with the expectation of sleeping. Flavored castor oil emulsions are somewhat more palatable than is castor oil itself.

Docusates. Docusate sodium, the prototype for this group of anionic surfactants, is widely employed in the pharmaceutical industry as an emulsifying, wetting, and dispersing agent. It has the following structural formula:

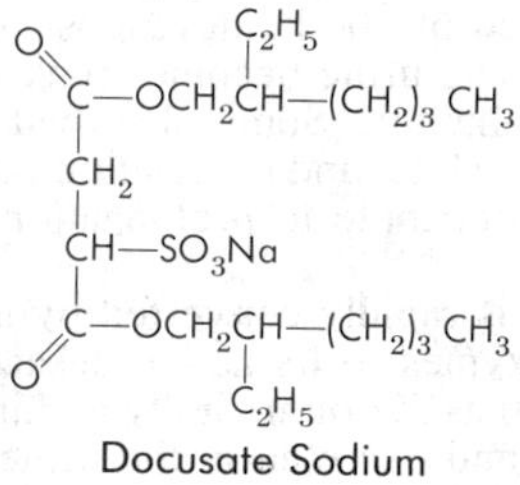

Docusate Sodium

In recommended dosage, the docusates have minimal laxative effects; their clinical usefulness is limited to keeping the feces soft such that straining at the stool can be avoided. Many details of their pharmacology remain uncertain.

Laxative Effects. In recommended oral dosage, the docusates produce minimal softening of the feces with a latency of 1 to 3 days. These surfactants apparently hydrate and soften the stool by emulsifying feces, water, and fat. *In vitro* and *in situ,* docusate sodium also alters net intestinal absorption of electrolytes and water and has effects on the intestinal mucosa similar to those of other stimulant laxatives (Donowitz, 1979).

Adverse Effects. The docusates are well tolerated. Cramping pains have been reported occasionally, and the liquid preparations sometimes cause nausea. Docusates increase the intestinal absorption of other drugs administered concurrently and may increase their toxicity. Of particular concern are the observations that docusate sodium is absorbed, appears in the bile in significant concentration, and has cytotoxic effects on liver cells in tissue culture.

Preparations and Dosage. Docusate sodium (*dioctyl sodium sulfosuccinate;* COLACE, DOXINATE, others), *docusate calcium* (*dioctyl calcium sulfosuccinate;* SURFAK, others), and *docusate potassium* (*dioctyl potassium sulfosuccinate;* KASOF, others) are available as capsules. Docusate sodium is also available in tablets and solution and as a syrup. The usual oral dose of docusate sodium for adults is 50 to 500 mg daily. The solutions should be administered in milk or fruit juice to mask the bitter taste. The usual rectal dose of the liquid is 50 to 100 mg, as a 0.1% solution.

Poloxamers. Poloxamers are polyoxyethylene-polyoxypropylene polymers that are nonionic surfactants and, when ingested, have many of the properties of the docusates. Poloxamer 188 is a water-soluble powder with an average molecular weight of 8350. A dosage of 240 to 480 mg of poloxamer 188, once daily, softens the stool in 3 to 5 days.

Dehydrocholic Acid. Bile acids have effects on the intestine that are similar to those of other anionic surfactants and stimulant laxatives; they reduce net absorption of water and electrolytes and cause diarrhea if they escape ileal absorption. *Dehydrocholic acid* (DECHOLIN, others) is considered safe and effective as an oral laxative when administered to adults in a dosage of 750 mg to 1.5 g daily in three divided doses. Dehydrocholate is also an effective hydrocholeretic in this dosage range (*see* below).

OTHER LAXATIVES

Mineral Oil. Mineral oil is a mixture of aliphatic hydrocarbons obtained from petroleum. The oil is indigestible and absorbed only to a limited extent. When taken for 2 or 3 days, it penetrates and softens the stool and may also interfere with absorption of water. The adverse effects that may result from the use of mineral oil as a laxative argue against its use. These include interference with the absorption of essential fat-soluble substances, elicitation of foreign-body reactions in the intestinal mucosa and in other tissues, and leakage of the oil past the anal sphincter. Lipid pneumonitis can also follow oral ingestion of mineral oil.

Mixtures and Combinations. There is no evidence that mixtures of several laxatives have advantages over single agents used judiciously. Indeed, the use of a mixture of laxatives can have serious drawbacks, for instance, the enhanced absorption of other agents by docusates. It is prudent to avoid these mixtures.

USES AND ABUSES OF LAXATIVES

In otherwise healthy patients, laxatives are of secondary importance to a fiber-rich diet and other nonpharmacological means for the prevention and treatment of constipation. Laxatives have no role in the management of constipation that results from intestinal pathology. Valid uses of these agents include maintenance of soft feces, prevention of straining at the stool (especially in the elderly and in patients with cardiac disease or hernia), and evacuation of the bowel prior to diagnostic or surgical procedures. All laxatives are contraindicated in a patient with cramps, colic, nausea, vomiting, or other symptoms of appendicitis or any undiagnosed abdominal pain.

Constipation. Many of the causes of functional constipation are simple to correct without the use of drugs. A fiber-rich diet, bowel training, the reminder that "haste does not make waste," adequate fluid intake, appropriate physical activity, reassurance to overcome emotional factors, and similar measures are often successful. Correction of underlying disease must not be neglected. In cases of drug-induced constipation, correction by readjustment of drug dosage or by use of alternative drugs should be attempted before resorting to concurrent laxative medication.

If nonpharmacological measures alone are inadequate or unrealistic due to age or infirmity, they may be supplemented by the bulk-forming agents. Stimulant laxatives should be used only in refractory cases. When laxatives are employed in the treatment of constipation, they should be administered in the lowest effective dosage as infrequently as possible, and they should be discontinued promptly and completely upon termination of the need.

Other Valid Uses. Laxatives are frequently indicated, both before and after surgery, to maintain soft feces in patients with hemorrhoids and other anorectal disorders. For these purposes, dietary fiber or the bulk-forming agents are generally satisfactory and should be preferred. A fiber-rich diet and related drugs also have an established role in the management of diverticular disease of the colon and irritable bowel disease.

Stimulant or saline laxatives at cathartic doses are frequently used prior to radiological examination of the gastrointestinal tract, kidneys, or other abdominal or retroperitoneal structures and prior to elective bowel surgery. Saline laxatives, taken orally, have largely replaced enemas for emptying the large bowel prior to colonoscopy or proctological examination.

In the treatment of oral poisoning, cathartic doses of saline laxatives (*e.g.*, sodium phosphate, 16 g; magnesium sulfate, 30 g) may be administered with the hope of facilitating the removal of the poison from the intestine (*see* Chapter 3). Stimulant laxatives must be avoided.

Cathartic Colon (Laxative Abuse). The prolonged and habitual use of laxatives is unhealthy. Many individuals have unusual notions regarding the frequency, quantity, and consistency of stools necessary for health, and they readily resort to self-prescribed laxatives to achieve these goals. Abuse of laxatives now extends to their misuse in controlling weight. Even the casual use of these drugs can develop into the cathartic habit. After a thorough evacuation of the colon by a laxative, several days may elapse before a normal bowel movement can again occur. In the interim, the patient becomes convinced of constipation and again turns to the favorite remedy. After a time, bowel habits become so abnormal that the patient is totally reliant on a daily dose of a laxative for a bowel movement.

The patient suffering from cathartic colon presents a difficult therapeutic problem. Initially, all laxatives should be discontinued, and the patient should be informed not to expect a bowel movement for several days. The underlying cause for constipation, if one exists, must be found and eliminated, and the patient's misconceptions pertaining to bowel function must be corrected. Proper diet, exercise, and bowel training must be undertaken. A bulk-forming laxative in minimally effective dosage may be employed during the period in which reestablishment of normal colonic function and defecatory reflexes is being attempted (*see* Devroede, 1989).

Dangers of Laxative Abuse. In addition to perpetuating dependence upon drugs, the laxative habit may provide the basis for serious gastrointestinal disturbances. Spastic colitis and other functional ills have been traced to the habitual use of stimulant laxatives; after prolonged abuse, the appearance of the digestive tract by x-ray examination may resemble that of enterocolitis. Surreptitious ingestion of laxatives can cause signs and symptoms that are mistaken for gastrointestinal disease and may lead to unnecessary surgery.

Repeated misuse of stimulant laxatives may also result in excessive loss of water and electrolytes; secondary aldosteronism may occur if volume depletion is prominent. Steatorrhea and protein-losing gastroenteropathy with hypoalbuminemia have been observed, as have excessive excretion of Ca^{2+} in the stools and osteomalacia of the vertebral column.

Much more dangerous than the laxative habit is the practice of taking a laxative for the relief of abdominal pain. An inflamed appendix can be ruptured by the resulting intestinal motor activity, and the mortality rate of the condition is vastly increased.

ANTIDIARRHEAL AGENTS

The excessive fecal loss of fluid and electrolytes that characterizes diarrhea is an important aspect of many infectious and noninfectious gastrointestinal disorders (*see* Fine *et al.*, 1989; Gorbach, 1989). Although acute-onset diarrhea is most often of infectious origin, it is usually self-limited, and specific chemotherapy is seldom warranted or effective unless there is evidence of gastrointestinal erosion or systemic disease. Hence, the treatment of diarrhea is generally nonspecific and is usually aimed at reducing the discomfort and inconvenience of frequent bowel movements; in some instances the oral or parenteral replenishment of fluid and electrolytes may also be necessary and even life saving.

Several drugs are among the common causes of acute, chronic, or recurrent diarrhea (Table 38–3). Adjustment of dosage or change in medication is much preferred to the concurrent administration of an antidiarrheal agent, especially on a long-term basis. Although avoidance of laxatives seems all too obvious, surreptitious abuse of stimulant laxatives is a surprisingly frequent cause of chronic diarrhea of unknown origin (*see* Fine *et al.*, 1989). Avoidance of alcoholic or methylxanthine-containing beverages is also a useful adjunct in the therapy of diarrhea, but stopping the ingestion of nonabsorbable hexitols such as sorbitol is a less obvious maneuver; diabetic patients are especially likely to eat foods sweetened with these agents and to suffer from diarrhea as a result.

Table 38–3. SOME AGENTS CAUSING DIARRHEA

Adrenergic neuron blocking agents (reserpine, guanethidine)
Antimicrobials (*e.g.*, sulfonamides, tetracyclines, most broad-spectrum agents)
Bile acids
Carcinoid tumor secretions (*e.g.*, 5-hydroxytryptamine, vasoactive intestinal peptide)
Cholinergic agonists and cholinesterase inhibitors
Fatty acids
Osmotic laxatives (sorbitol, saline cathartics)
Prokinetic agents (metoclopramide, domperidone)
Prostaglandins
Quinidine
Stimulant laxatives

The mainstay of nonspecific drug therapy for diarrhea continues to be the opioid agonists. These agents reduce the amount of fluid presented to the colon by the small bowel, mainly by slowing transit time; the absorption of water and electrolytes is thus promoted. A more direct action to enhance absorption and/or reduce secretion by enterocytes may also be involved. The most effective over-the-counter agent is bismuth subsalicylate, which can provide substantial relief in mild-to-moderate diarrhea and is useful in the prophylaxis of travelers' diarrhea caused by a variety of infectious agents; its mode of action is poorly understood (*see* below).

Opioids. The pharmacological properties, clinical toxicity, and preparations of opioids are described in Chapter 22. Although hydroalcoholic solutions of opium powder (opium tincture; paregoric), have long been used to treat diarrhea, synthetic opioids (diphenoxylate; loperamide) are now preferred. Opioid agonists that act at μ (and possibly δ) receptors on enteric neurons increase gastrointestinal contractions but disrupt aboral peristaltic movement, thereby increasing the transit time of intestinal contents; the tone of the rectal sphincter is also increased. Actions within the spinal cord and at supraspinal sites produce similar effects but are not required for therapeutic responses. The prolonged transit time facilitates absorption of fluid and solutes throughout the intestinal tract. In addition, active absorption of NaCl in the ileum is stimulated (*see* Binder, 1989). Although opioids are effective in the treatment of moderate-to-severe diarrhea, they should not be used in patients with chronic ulcerative colitis or acute bacillary or amoebic dysentery, since they appear to potentiate ulcerating processes in the colon and can provoke the development of toxic megacolon (*see* Binder, 1989).

Diphenoxylate. Diphenoxylate is a piperidine opioid that is structurally related to meperidine. Although its salts are poorly soluble in water, the compound is readily absorbed after oral administration and it can produce systemic effects if used in doses greater than those recommended for diarrhea (5 to 20 mg per day). After absorption, diphenoxylate is rapidly converted to diphenoxylic acid (difenoxin), an active metabolite that is eliminated with a half-time of about 12 hours. *Diphenoxylate hydrochloride* is available in preparations that also contain 25 μg of atropine sulfate per 2.5 mg of diphenoxylate (LOMOTIL, others); its adverse effects include those caused by both μ-opioid agonists and nonselective muscarinic antagonists (*see* Chapters 8 and 22). Atropine is included to discourage abuse of the preparation. Difenoxin hydrochloride is available in 1-mg tablets that contain 25 μg of atropine sulfate (MOTOFEN). The usual dosage is 1 tablet every 3 to 4 hours as needed.

Loperamide. Loperamide is also a piperidine opioid. It is slowly and incompletely absorbed after oral administration, and a large proportion of the drug is excreted in the feces. In addition, loperamide apparently enters the brain relatively slowly, since the administration of doses greatly in excess of those recommended for treatment of diarrhea (4 to 8 mg per day to a maximum of 16 mg per day) produce only modest effects on the central nervous system. *Loperamide hydrochloride* (IMODIUM) is available in 2-mg capsules and as a liquid (1 mg per 5 ml).

Bismuth Subsalicylate. Although the basis of the effectiveness of bismuth subsalicylate in the treatment of mild-to-moderate diarrhea is poorly understood, it is thought that local antiinflammatory actions of salicylate are primarily involved. This notion is supported by observations of the antimotility and antisecretory effects of inhibitors of cyclooxygenase (*e.g.*, indomethacin) and the promotion of diarrhea by prostaglandins. Antibacterial actions of Bi^{3+} may also be involved, especially in the prevention of travelers' diarrhea (*see* Gorbach, 1989). The ready availability of a relatively inexpensive preparation (PEPTO-BISMOL) may facilitate overuse of the drug and toxicity due to both salicylate and Bi^{3+} (*see* Chapters 26 and 37). A regimen of eight doses of 520 mg each (30 ml or two tablets), taken every 30 minutes, provides relief from the symptoms of mild diarrhea (Ericsson *et al.*, 1986); four 520-mg doses per day is effective for the prevention of travelers' diarrhea (Gorbach, 1989).

Oral Rehydration Therapy. Although an otherwise healthy adult may not be harmed by dietary abstinence during an episode of mild-to-moderate diarrhea, the ingestion of soft, easily digested foods and/or noncarbonated beverages such as fruit juices is advocated. Dehydration can thus be prevented or treated by providing readily absorbed sugars and amino acids that enhance the absorption of water by the small intestine. Although severe diarrhea may require parenteral replenishment of fluid and electrolytes, especially in patients unable to take fluids by mouth, the oral administration of solutions that contain electrolytes, glucose, and amino acids usually suffices. Such solutions are readily available (PEDIALYTE, REHYDRALYTE, others), and their use has saved many lives, especially in the developing countries of the World (*see* Pierce and Hirschhorn, 1977; World Health Organization, 1984).

Other Agents. Many traditional remedies have little or no value in the treatment of acute infectious diarrhea; these include kaolin, pectin, lactobacilli, and muscarinic antagonists (*see* Gorbach, 1989). The use of a number of other drugs such as nonsteroidal antiinflammatory agents and analogs of somatostatin is under investigation, and the potential utility of an inhibitor of Cl^- secretion has been emphasized (Donowitz *et al.*, 1986). Of particular note are the antisecretory effects of α_2-adrenergic agonists; clonidine is effective in the treatment of diabetic patients with watery diarrhea syndrome (*see* Binder, 1989).

ANTIEMETIC AND PROKINETIC AGENTS

Nausea and vomiting can follow the administration of many drugs, particularly cancer chemotherapeutic agents. These symptoms may occur upon emergence from general anesthesia and often accompany infectious and noninfectious gastrointestinal disorders. They are also encountered all too frequently during early pregnancy or as a result of motion sickness.

Emesis is a complicated process that requires coordination by the vomiting center in the lateral reticular formation of the medulla. This center receives input from the chemoreceptor trigger zone (CTZ) in the area postrema in the floor of the fourth ventricle; from the vestibular apparatus; from higher brainstem and cortical structures; and from visceral afferents that originate in such peripheral structures as the heart, testes, and various sites in the gastrointestinal tract. The blood–brain barrier is poorly developed in the area postrema, and the CTZ is readily accessible to emetic substances in the circulation (*e.g.*, emetine, apomorphine, cardiac glycosides, opioids, nicotine, *etc.*). In some instances, however, emesis that is mediated by visceral afferents can be induced by the oral administration of emetic substances even after ablation of the CTZ. Moreover, emesis is promoted by conditions that slow gastric emptying.

Following stimulation of the vomiting center, emesis is mediated by various efferent pathways, including the vagus, the phrenic nerves, and the spinal innervation of the abdominal musculature. The initial manifestations of the response often involve nausea, in which gastric tone is reduced, gastric peristalsis is reduced or absent, and the tone of the duodenum and upper jejunum is increased, such that their contents reflux. Ultimately, the upper portion of the stomach relaxes while the pylorus constricts, and the coordinated contraction of the diaphragm and abdominal muscles leads to expulsion of gastric contents.

The neuropharmacology of the vomiting center and its afferent and efferent connections is not known in any detail. However, the CTZ is richly endowed with receptors for dopamine, histamine, and acetylcholine; dopaminergic agonists such as apomorphine are emetic, while dopaminergic, muscarinic, and H_1 antagonists have antiemetic properties to varying degrees. Dopaminergic receptors in the stomach appear to mediate the inhibition of gastric motility that occurs during nausea and vomiting, and these receptors may provide an additional site of action for antiemetic dopaminergic antagonists such as metoclopramide. These receptors also participate in reflexes that result in relaxation of the upper portion of the stomach and delayed gastric emptying in response to gastric distention by food; this forms the basis for the use of metoclopramide as a so-called prokinetic agent (*see* below). Cholinergic and histaminergic fibers are thought to be involved in transmission from the vestibular apparatus to the vomiting center, in large part because of the efficacy of muscarinic and H_1 antagonists in the treatment of motion sickness (*see* Chapters 8 and 23). The utility of benzodiazepines and glucocorticoids as adjuncts in antiemetic regimens may in part reflect actions of these agents on cortical and other higher inputs to the vomiting center.

ANTIEMETIC AGENTS

The important role of dopamine in the function of the CTZ and as a mediator of motor reflexes in the stomach is presumably the primary basis for the fact that a number of drugs with prominent dopaminergic antagonistic properties are useful in the treatment of vomiting. These drugs include certain neuroleptic phenothiazines and butyrophenones; their uses as antipsychotic agents are discussed in Chapter 18. Metoclopramide, a benzamide, is another dopaminergic antagonist with important antiemetic uses. Although the underlying mechanisms are unknown, cannabinoids, including Δ^9-tetrahydrocannabinol (THC), can reduce the emesis caused by cancer chemotherapeutic agents in some patients who are refractory to other antiemetic therapy (McCabe *et al.*, 1988); their pharmacological properties are discussed in Chapter 22. The preparations and dosages of the principal agents that are effective in the treatment of nausea and vomiting are listed in Table 38–4.

Although used more frequently in the prevention of motion sickness (*see* Chapter 23), H_1 antagonists with prominent anticholinergic properties are often included in antiemetic regimens, in part to reduce the extrapyramidal side effects of neuroleptics; they can also reduce the incidence of nausea and vomiting in ambulatory patients following the administration of drugs such as morphine. Benzodiazepines, especially lorazepam, can enhance the effectiveness of antiemetic regimens and are thought to be beneficial in the prevention of anticipatory emesis; their amnestic actions may be an important factor in these effects (*see* Triozzi *et al.*, 1988; *see also* Chapter 17). Dexamethasone and other glucocorticoids appear to have antiemetic effects and may improve the efficacy of antiemetic regimens in some cancer patients; the underlying mechanisms are poorly understood (*see* Cersosimo and Karp, 1986).

Neuroleptic Drugs. Chlorpromazine, in relatively low nonsedative doses, can prevent vomiting from certain causes. The potent and selective antiemetic action of the drug is useful in various disorders in which vomiting is prominent, including uremia, gastroenteritis, carcinomatosis, radiation sickness, and emesis caused by drugs including estrogens, tetracyclines, opioid analgesics, cancer chemotherapeutic agents, and disulfiram. Chlorpromazine has also been used to treat nausea and vomiting during pregnancy, but pregnant women should not be given the drug for this purpose (*see* Morselli, 1977; Goldberg and DiMascio, 1978). Chlorpromazine does not appear to control motion sickness. Although prochlorperazine is a potent antiemetic agent, it produces a high incidence of dystonias, especially when given intramuscularly, and hence should be used cautiously. The use of phenothiazines to control nausea and vomiting may mask diagnostic symptoms in acute surgical conditions or neurological syndromes. Not all the phenothiazines are equally effective as antiemetics, and thioridazine is a notable exception to the general rule that most neuroleptic agents have antiemetic effects.

Butyrophenones, especially those available for parenteral administration (*e.g.*, haloperidol and droperidol) have been used as alternatives to phenothiazines in antiemetic regimens for patients receiving cancer chemotherapy (*see* Triozzi and Laszlo, 1987). The butyrophenones may cause less sedation and hypotension than do chlorpromazine and triflupromazine.

Benzamides. *Metoclopramide.* This drug was developed in France during the early 1960s as an antiemetic agent for potential use during pregnancy. Its structural formula is as follows:

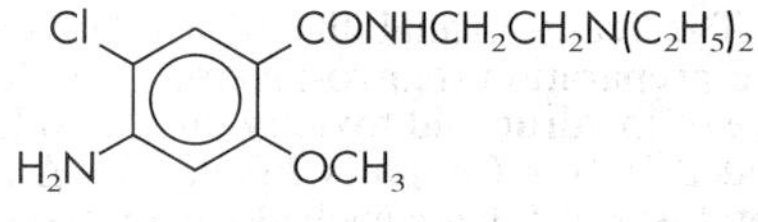

Metoclopramide

Although structurally related to procainamide, metoclopramide lacks significant local anesthetic or antiarrhythmic actions. The history and pharmacological properties of metoclopramide have been reviewed by Pinder and colleagues (1976) and by McCallum and Albibi (1983).

Table 38–4. SOME AGENTS USED IN THE TREATMENT OF NAUSEA AND VOMITING

CLASS	NONPROPRIETARY NAME (REPRESENTATIVE TRADE NAME)	ROUTE, DOSAGE FORM, AND ADULT DOSAGE		
		Oral *	*Suppository*	*Parenteral*
Phenothiazines	Chlorpromazine (THORAZINE)	O, SR, L 10–25 mg every 4–6 hr	50–100 mg every 6–8 hr	25–50 mg IM every 3–4 hr
	Perphenazine (TRILAFON)	O, L 8–16 mg daily	—	5 mg IM every 6 hr
	Prochlorperazine (COMPAZINE)	O, L 5–10 mg 3–4 times daily SR 10 mg every 12 hr	25 mg every 12 hr	5–10 mg IM every 3–4 hr (up to 40 mg daily)
	Promethazine † (PHENERGAN)	O, L 12.5–25 mg every 4–6 hr	12.5–25 mg every 4–6 hr	12.5–25 mg IM every 4 hr
	Thiethylperazine (TORECAN)	O 10 mg 1–3 times daily	10 mg 1–3 times daily	10 mg IM 1–3 times daily
	Triflupromazine (VESPRIN)	—	—	5–15 mg IM every 4 hr (up to 60 mg daily)
Butyrophenones	Droperidol (INAPSINE)	—	—	2.5–5 mg IM or IV
Benzamides	Metoclopramide (REGLAN)	O, L 5–20 mg 3–4 times daily	—	1.2 mg/kg IV every 2–3 hr beginning 30 min prior to chemotherapy
	Trimethobenzamide (TIGAN)	O 250 mg every 6–8 hr	200 mg every 6–8 hr	200 mg IM every 6–8 hr
Cannabinoids	Dronabinol (Δ^9-THC) (MARINOL)	O 5–7.5 mg/m^2 1–3 hr before and every 2–4 hr after chemotherapy	—	—
	Nabilone (CESAMET)	O 1–2 mg 1–3 hr before and every 8–12 hr after chemotherapy	—	—

* Oral dosage forms: O = solid; SR = sustained release; L = liquid.
† Promethazine is not known to have antipsychotic effects, but it does have relatively strong anticholinergic and antihistaminic actions.

Pharmacological Effects. Metoclopramide causes most of the CNS effects that are characteristic of dopaminergic blockade. These include antagonism of emesis induced by apomorphine and ergotamine, and hyperprolactinemia, which can lead to galactorrhea, breast tenderness, and menstrual irregularities in women. Although metoclopramide does not have useful antipsychotic effects, it can cause significant extrapyramidal symptoms, especially at high intravenous doses; symptoms can usually be prevented or treated by the administration of diphenhydramine or benztropine. Other adverse CNS effects are fairly common and include drowsiness, dizziness, and anxiety.

In the gastrointestinal tract, metoclopramide enhances the motility of smooth muscle from the esophagus through the proximal small bowel and accelerates gastric emptying and the transit of intestinal contents from the duodenum to the ileocecal valve. These actions are important in its use as a prokinetic agent (*see* below), but they may contribute to bowel disturbances that are sometimes observed during antiemetic therapy. Although metoclopramide can accelerate the absorption of many drugs, the shortened transit time may decrease the bioavailability of others, most notably digoxin. In addition, the delivery of food to the intestine may be altered sufficiently in diabetic patients to require adjustment of insulin dosage.

Pharmacokinetic Properties. Metoclopramide is rapidly and completely absorbed after oral administration, but hepatic first-pass metabolism reduces its bioavailability to about 75%. The drug is distributed rapidly into most tissues and readily crosses the blood–brain barrier and the placenta; the concentration of the drug in breast milk may exceed that in plasma. Up to 30% of metoclopramide is excreted unchanged in the urine, and the remainder is eliminated in the urine and the bile after conjugation with sulfate or glucuronic acid. The half-life of the drug in the circulation is about 4 to 6 hours, but it may be as much as 24 hours in patients with impaired renal function.

Therapeutic Uses. The oral administration of metoclopramide may be of value in the prevention of nausea and vomiting from a variety of causes, including pregnancy. Although significant effects on fetal development have not been evident in animal studies, no well-controlled studies have been performed in pregnant women, and the drug should be used during pregnancy only when the expected benefits outweigh the unknown potential hazards to the fetus. Because it is well tolerated in high intravenous doses, metoclopramide is widely used to control emesis during cancer chemotherapy, especially when highly emetogenic agents such as cisplatin or cyclophosphamide are used (*see* Triozzi and Laszlo, 1987). Although metoclopramide is usually combined with diphenhydramine, the concomitant intravenous administration of lorazepam may also reduce the incidence of dystonic symptoms; the amnesia and marked sedation caused by lorazepam may be desirable in this setting (Gordon *et al.*, 1989). Regimens that are effective in countering vomiting induced by cisplatin or cyclophosphamide include those that utilize the intravenous administration of metoclopramide and dexamethasone in combination with lorazepam plus benztropine or droperidol plus diphenhydramine (Sridhar and Donnelly, 1988; Marshall *et al.*, 1989).

Trimethobenzamide. Trimethobenzamide has the following structural formula:

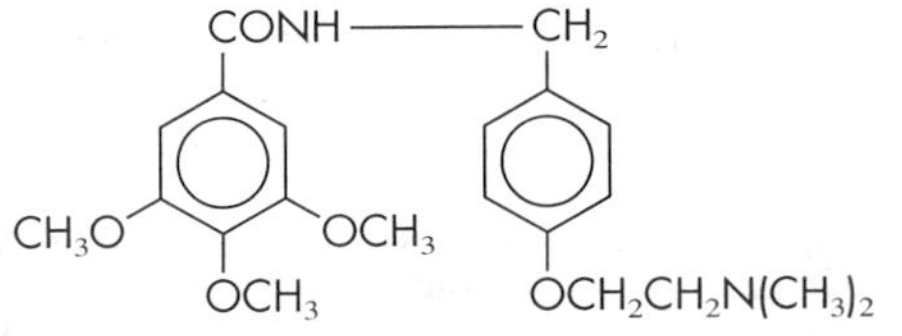

Trimethobenzamide

Although its mechanism of action is obscure, the relatively weak antiemetic effects of trimethobenzamide appear to result from blockade of dopaminergic receptors; dystonic symptoms may follow its parenteral administration. Trimethobenzamide is not as effective as the phenothiazines or metoclopramide, but it can be given intramuscularly to combat nausea and vomiting induced by cancer chemotherapeutic agents with mild or moderate emetogenic potential (*e.g.*, vincristine or procarbazine) (*see* Triozzi and Laszlo, 1987). Adverse effects other than pain at the site of injection are uncommon, but drowsiness, dizziness, allergic-type skin eruptions, extrapyramidal symptoms, and convulsions have been reported.

PROKINETIC AGENTS

Gastric hypomotility with delayed emptying of liquid and/or solid contents is a component of a number of gastrointestinal disorders (*see* McCallum, 1989). The symptoms of such disorders may include nausea, vomiting, heartburn, postprandial discomfort, and indigestion. Gastroesophageal reflux is often evident and can give rise to esophageal ulceration; there may also be respiratory symptoms or intense substernal pain that can be confused with asthma or myocardial infarction, respectively. Although the cause is unknown in the majority of patients, gastric stasis or hypomotility is frequently a consequence of diabetic neuropathy; this condition is also often present in patients with anorexia nervosa or achlorhydria or following gastric surgery.

The medical management of patients with gastric hypomotility usually includes the administration of a prokinetic agent. Although antiemetic phenothiazines or bethanechol may provide some relief, these drugs do not accelerate gastric emptying in the vast majority of patients and often produce unacceptable side effects. At present, the only available prokinetic agent is metoclopramide, but several others (*e.g.*, domperidone; cisapride) are being evaluated.

Metoclopramide. Metoclopramide decreases receptive relaxation in the upper portion of the stomach and increases antral contractions. The pylorus and duodenum are relaxed, while the tone of the lower esophageal sphincter is enhanced. These effects combine to accelerate the emptying of gastric contents and to reduce reflux from the duodenum and the stomach into the esophagus. In addition, the transit time of material from the duodenum to the ileocecal valve is reduced as a result of increased jejunal peristalsis. Metoclopramide has little effect on gastric secretion or colonic motility. In general, dopaminergic agonists produce the opposite pattern of effects, and these are mediated by D_2 receptors that are located, at least in part, within the gastrointestinal tract.

The mechanism of action of metoclopramide is poorly understood, even though it is clearly a dopaminergic antagonist and can block the gastrointestinal effects caused by the local or systemic administration of dopaminergic agonists. Although vagotomy does not abolish the effects of metoclopramide, its prokinetic actions can be blocked by atropine or other muscarinic antagonists. Moreover, not all dopaminergic antagonists speed gastric emptying. It is thought that the drug promotes the release of acetylcholine from myenteric neurons, although direct evidence of this action is lacking. Since bethanechol can enhance the effects of metoclopramide, enhanced responsiveness to acetylcholine may also be involved.

Metoclopramide hydrochloride (REGLAN, others) is available as tablets (5 and 10 mg), a syrup (5 mg/5 ml), and in injectable solutions (5 and 10 mg/ml). For esophageal reflux, 10 to 15 mg is generally taken 30 minutes prior to meals and at bedtime. Similar doses are taken for diabetic gastroparesis. (For additional discussion of metoclopramide, *see* above.)

Domperidone. Domperidone is a derivative of benzimidazole that possesses both prokinetic and antiemetic properties. Its structural formula is as follows:

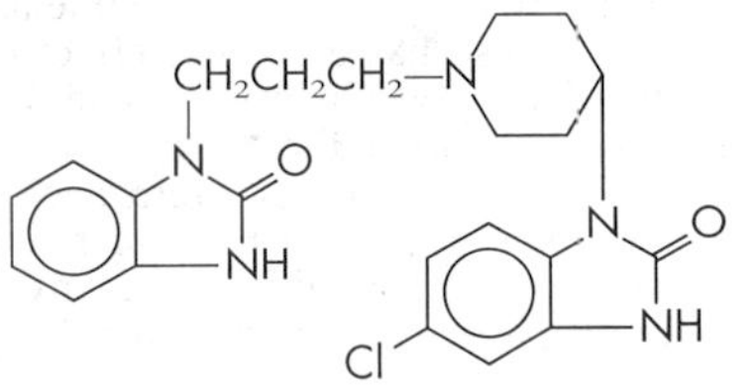

Domperidone

Domperidone is a dopaminergic antagonist, and it produces marked hyperprolactinemia; its effects on gastrointestinal motility also closely resemble those of metoclopramide (*see* above). However, unlike metoclopramide, these effects are not antagonized by atropine; an explanation for this difference has not yet been advanced. Domperidone crosses the blood–brain barrier to only a limited extent, and it causes extrapyramidal side effects only rarely. As a result, it does not interfere with the treatment of Parkinson's disease, and it may be useful in counteracting the gastrointestinal disturbances caused by levodopa and bromocriptine. Thus far, the drug appears to have the same therapeutic utility as metoclopramide in the treatment of patients with gastric hypomotility (*see* Brogden *et al.*, 1982; McCallum, 1989). However, it has less antiemetic activity.

Domperidone appears to be rapidly absorbed after oral administration, but its bioavailability is only about 15%; most of the drug and its metabolites are excreted in the feces. The half-time for its elimination from plasma is about 7 to 8 hours.

Domperidone is not generally available in the United States; it is available elsewhere as MOTILIUM. Optimal dosage has not been established, but daily oral doses of 40 to 120 mg have been utilized in the treatment of gastric hypomotility.

Cisapride. Cisapride is a benzamide with the following structural formula:

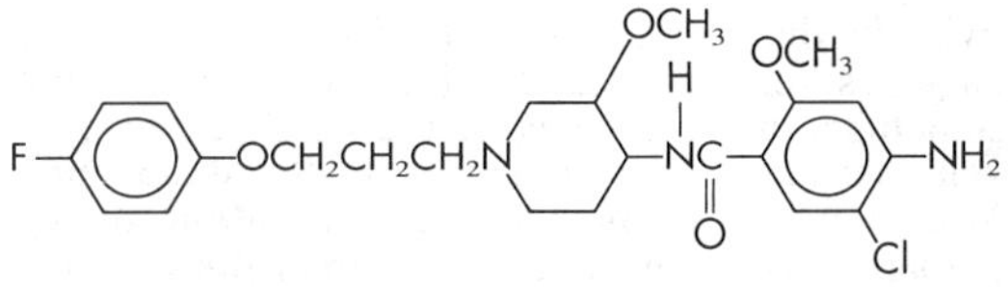

Cisapride

The effects of cisapride on the motility of the stomach and small bowel closely resemble those of metoclopramide and domperidone; however, unlike these drugs, it also increases colonic motility and can cause diarrhea (*see* McCallum *et al.*, 1988; McCallum, 1989). The mechanism of its gastrointestinal actions is poorly understood. Like metoclopramide, these actions are blocked by atropine and may involve the release of myenteric acetylcholine (Schuurkes *et al.*, 1988). Cisapride appears to be devoid of dopaminergic blocking activity, and it does not influence the concentration of prolactin in plasma or cause extrapyramidal symptoms. The drug binds to and blocks 5-HT_2 tryptaminergic receptors in the rat ileum (Moriarty *et al.*, 1987), but the relationship of this action to its effects in man has not been established.

Cisapride is not generally available in the United States. Thus far the efficacy of the drug in the treatment of disorders of gastric hypomotility appears to equal those of metoclopramide and domperidone without the side effects that result from dopaminergic blockade (*see* McCallum *et al.*, 1988). In addition, cisapride may be useful in the treatment of patients with chronic idiopathic constipation or with colonic hypomotility due to spinal cord injury (Muller-Lissner, 1987; Binnie *et al.*, 1988).

DIGESTANTS

Digestants are drugs that supposedly promote the process of digestion in the gastrointestinal tract in conditions characterized by a lack of one or more of the specific substances that function in the digestion of food. Although a number of products are marketed, including many bizarre mixtures of components, the only preparations that merit consideration here are those of pancreatic enzymes.

PANCREATIC ENZYMES

The enzymes of the pancreas are obtainable in preparations known as pancreatin and pancrelipase. They contain principally amylase, trypsin (protease), and lipase. Pancrelipase is of porcine origin and has relatively more lipase activity than does pancreatin. Pancreatin is prepared from porcine or bovine pancreas. These preparations are employed for the treatment of conditions in which the secretion of pancreatic juice is deficient, for example, pancreatitis and mucoviscidosis. Their administration can significantly reduce the nitrogen and fat content of the stool, and these parameters can be monitored as a guide to dosage, which should be individualized. Since acid and peptic activity in the stomach can destroy the pancreatic enzymes, enteric-coated tablets or capsules are sometimes used. However, the coating may prevent delivery of the enzymes in the duodenum. Moreover, in recommended doses, enteric-coated preparations often contain less than one-half the lipase activity of conventional preparations (*see* Marotta *et al.*, 1989). Supplementation of the regimen with an H_2-blocking agent may help to overcome gastric inactivation, but usually only in patients with relatively high maximal acid secretion. Adverse effects of pancreatic enzymes are few. High doses may cause nausea and diarrhea; the administration of these preparations may also cause hyperuricemia.

BILE ACIDS

The bile acids and their conjugates are important constituents of bile. The important bile acids in human bile are cholic acid (3,7,12-trihydroxycholanic acid), chenodeoxycholic acid (3α,7α-dihydroxycholanic acid; chenodiol), and ursodeoxycholic acid (3α,7β-dihydrocholanic acid; ursodiol). These are mainly present as the glycine and taurine conjugates, the salts of which are often referred to as the bile salts. The structure of cholanic acid is as follows:

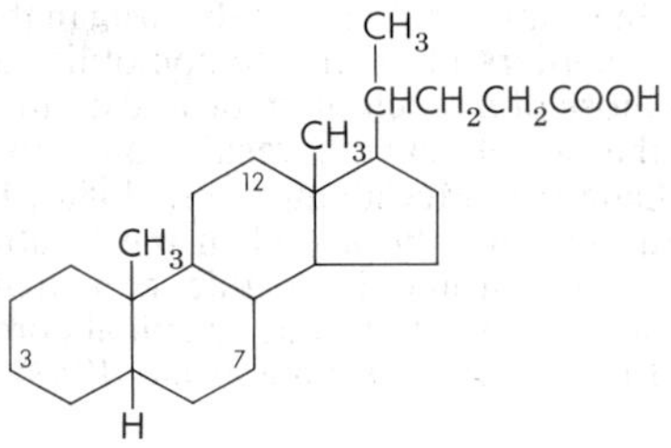

Cholanic Acid

Bile salts are strongly amphophilic and, with the aid of biliary phospholipids, they readily form micelles with and emulsify lipids. They are important not only for the emulsification of cholesterol and other lipids in bile but also for the emulsification of dietary lipids preparatory to digestion and absorption.

Pharmacological and Toxic Effects. Bile acids increase the output of bile and hence are called *choleretic* drugs; the bile salts have little choleretic activity. Dehydrocholic acid, a semisynthetic cholate, is especially active and evokes the secretion of a bile of low specific gravity; it is therefore called a *hydrocholeretic drug.* The increase in bile flow is not the result of true cholepoiesis, since the augmented flow is only that necessary to secrete the increased load of bile acid imposed by that administered. Dehydrocholate decreases the excretion of bilirubin. Therefore, bile acids are ineffective in attenuating jaundice.

Chenodiol and ursodiol, but not cholic acid, decrease the cholesterol content of bile. Several mechanisms are involved (*see* Tint *et al.*, 1986). (1) Ursodiol sharply reduces hepatic secretion of cholesterol into the bile; chenodiol reduces secretion only after prolonged administration. (2) Chenodiol reduces the synthesis of cholesterol by inhibition of hydroxymethylglutaryl-CoA reductase; the effects of ursodiol are variable but may be more prominent with prolonged administration. (3) The administration of ursodiol reduces the fractional reabsorption of cholesterol by the intestine, but chenodiol does not. The decrease in cholesterol concentration in bile may halt the formation of cholesterolic gallstones; it can also promote their dissolution during sustained treatment. Although chenodiol decreases the synthesis of bile acids by inhibition of cholesterol 7α-hydroxylase, the compound readily enters the bile and causes an increase in the concentration of total bile acids, thereby enhancing the solubility of cholesterol. Ursodiol has little effect on the synthesis of bile acids, and it has less impact on the total concentration of bile acids because it enters the bile less efficiently. Ursodiol also has a smaller effect on cholesterol solubility; nevertheless, it can mobilize cholesterol by promoting the formation of liquid crystals (*see* Tint *et al.*, 1986). Both agents have little effect on calcified stones or on radiolucent bile pigment stones. In addition, therapy is successful only in patients with functional gallbladders.

Full therapeutic doses of chenodiol cause diarrhea and elevation of aminotransferases in plasma in 25 to 50% of patients; these side effects are rarely observed with ursodiol, perhaps because lower doses are used (*see* Rosenbaum and Cluxton, 1988). Withdrawal of chenodiol is required in about 2% of patients because of marked increases in plasma aminotransferases. Hepatotoxicity of chenodiol may be due, at least in part, to its conversion by intestinal microorganisms to the hepatotoxin lithocholic acid. The extent of formation of lithocholic acid from ursodiol appears to be smaller, even though there is microbial interconversion of ursodiol and chenodiol in the intestine. Chenodiol causes fetal abnormalities in primates at doses only slightly greater than those utilized clinically, and pregnancy is a contraindication to its use; the teratogenic potential of ursodiol is unknown.

Preparations and Dosage. *Dehydrocholic acid* (DECHOLIN, others) is available in tablets. The usual dose is 244 to 500 mg, three times daily after meals. *Chenodiol* (CHENIX) is available in 250-mg tablets. It is given initially in divided doses that total 8 to 10 mg/kg per day; this is then adjusted upward to 13 to 16 mg/kg. Chronic administration of chenodiol in daily doses of less than 10 mg/kg is usually ineffective and may increase the risk of cholecystectomy. The drug is contraindicated in women who are or may become pregnant. *Ursodiol* (ACTIGALL) is available in 300-mg capsules; the recommended daily dosage is 8 to 10 mg/kg in two or three divided doses. Ursodiol is not indicated for use by children or pregnant women.

Therapeutic Uses. Because of their physiological role in the absorption of dietary lipids, the bile salts were once used widely for so-called replacement therapy in pathological conditions in which the concentration of bile acids in the upper intestine is low (such as biliary fistula, disease or resection of the ileum, and hepatic or extrahepatic cholestasis). However, the usual preparations are generally ineffective and sometimes harmful. They are little used today. Hydrocholeretic drugs are sometimes used after gallbladder surgery to facilitate T-tube drainage.

The National Cooperative Gallstone Study established the safety and efficacy of chenodiol for the dissolution of gallstones (*see* Schoenfield *et al.*, 1981). However, the overall response rate was not high and appropriate selection of patients for such treatment is thus important. At a daily dose of 750 mg of chenodiol (the highest dose tested), complete dissolution of radiolucent gallstones was confirmed in only 13% of patients during 2 years of treatment. Partial or complete dissolution occurred in 41% of this group. Therapy was most successful in women, in thin patients, and in those with small or floating gallstones or with plasma cholesterol concentrations above 227 mg/dl (5.9 mM). In addition to the side effects listed above, the mean plasma cholesterol concentration was elevated slightly. Ursodiol may be more effective than chenodiol, and complete dissolution may eventually occur in up to 50% of compliant patients with radiolucent gallstones no greater than 15 mm in diameter (*see* Rosenbaum and Cluxton, 1988). Combined therapy with chenodiol and ursodiol (5 mg/kg of each per day) may cause more rapid dissolution of gallstones than with ursodiol alone (10 mg/kg per day) (Podda *et al.*, 1989). When combined with extracorporeal lithotripsy, the use of similar regimens has resulted in the complete dissolution of much larger stones in up to 90% of patients (Sackmann *et al.*, 1988; Ponchon *et al.*, 1989). Studies indicate that gallstones will recur in a relatively high percentage of patients after cessation of treatment with bile acids.

Anderson, J. W., and Chen, W.-J. L. Plant fiber: carbohydrate and lipid metabolism. *Am. J. Clin. Nutr.*, **1979**, *32*, 346–363.

Behall, K. M.; Lee, K. H.; and Moser, P. B. Blood lipids and lipoproteins in adult men fed four refined fibers. *Am. J. Clin. Nutr.*, **1984**, *39*, 209–214.

Bingham, S.; Cummings, J. H.; and McNeil, N. I. Intakes and sources of dietary fiber in the British population. *Am. J. Clin. Nutr.*, **1979**, *32*, 1313–1319.

Binnie, N. R.; Creasey, G. H.; Edmond, P.; and Smith, A. N. The action of cisapride on the chronic constipation of paraplegia. *Paraplegia*, **1988**, *26*, 151–158.

Bridges, R. J.; Nell, G.; and Rummel, W. Influence of vasopressin and calcium on electrolyte transport across isolated colonic mucosa of the rat. *J. Physiol. (Lond.)*, **1983**, *338*, 463–475.

Brodribb, A. J. M. Treatment of symptomatic diverticular disease with a high-fibre diet. *Lancet*, **1977**, *1*, 664–666.

Burkitt, D. P., and Meisner, P. How to manage constipation with high-fiber diet. *Geriatrics*, **1979**, *34*, No. 2, 33–40.

Conn, H. O. Lactulose: a drug in search of a modus operandi. *Gastroenterology*, **1978**, *74*, 624–626.

Cummings, J. H. Constipation, dietary fibre and the control of large bowel function. *Postgrad. Med. J.*, **1984**, *60*, 811–819.

Donowitz, M. Current concepts of laxative action: mechanisms by which laxatives increase stool water. *J. Clin. Gastroenterol.*, **1979**, *1*, 77–84.

Donowitz, M.; Elta, G.; Battisti, L; Fogel, R.; and Label-Schwartz, E. Effect of dopamine and bromocriptine on rat ileal and colonic transport. *Gastroenterology*, **1983**, *84*, 516–523.

Dufour, P., and Gendre, P. Long-term mucosal alterations by sennosides and related compounds. *Pharmacology*, **1988**, *36*, Suppl. 1, 194–202.

Editorial. The bran wagon. *Lancet*, **1987**, *1*, 782–783.

Fairbairn, J. W., and Moss, M. J. R. The relative purgative activities of 1,8-dihydroxyanthracene derivatives. *J. Pharm. Pharmacol.*, **1970**, *22*, 584–593.

Gordon, C. J.; Pazdur, R.; Ziccarelli, A.; Cummings, G.; and Al-Sarraf, M. Metoclopramide versus metoclopramide and lorazepam: superiority of combined therapy in the control of cisplatin-induced emesis. *Cancer*, **1989**, *63*, 578–582.

Harvey, R. F., and Read, A. E. Mode of action of the saline purgatives. *Am. Heart J.*, **1975**, *89*, 810–812.

McCabe, M.; Smith, F. P.; Macdonald, J. S.; Woolley, P. V.; Goldberg, D.; and Schein, P. S. Efficacy of tetrahydrocannabinol in patients refractory to standard antiemetic therapy. *Invest. New Drugs*, **1988**, *6*, 243–246.

Marshall, G.; Kerr, S.; Vowels, M.; O'Gorman-Hughes, D.; and White, L. Antiemetic therapy for chemotherapy-induced vomiting: metoclopramide, benztropine, dexamethasone, and lorazepam regimen compared with chlorpromazine alone. *J. Pediatr.*, **1989**, *115*, 156–160.

Mendeloff, A. I. Dietary fiber and human health. *N. Engl. J. Med.*, **1977**, *297*, 811–814.

Mori, H.; Sugie, S.; Niwa, K.; Takahashi, M.; and Kawai, K. Induction of intestinal tumours in rats by chrysazin. *Br. J. Cancer*, **1985**, *52*, 781–783.

Mori, H.; Sugie, S.; Niwa, K.; Yoshimi, N.; Tanaka, T.; and Hirono, I. Carcinogenicity of chrysazin in large intestine and liver of mice. *Jpn. J. Cancer Res.*, **1986**, *77*, 871–876.

Moriarty, K. J.; Higgs, N. B.; Woodford, M.; Warhurst, G.; and Turnberg, L. A. Inhibition of the effect of serotonin on rat ileal transport by cisapride: evidence in favour of the involvement of 5-HT_2 receptors. *Gut*, **1987**, *28*, 844–848.

Muller-Lissner, S. A. Treatment of chronic constipation with cisapride and placebo. *Gut*, **1987**, *28*, 1033–1038.

Painter, N. S., and Burkitt, D. P. Diverticular disease of the colon, a 20th century problem. *Clin. Gastroenterol.*, **1975**, *4*, 3–21.

Podda, M.; Zuin, M.; Battezzati, P. M.; Ghezzi, C.; de Fazio, C.; and Dioguardi, M. L. Efficacy and safety of a combination of chenodeoxycholic acid and ursodeoxycholic acid for gallstone dissolution: a comparison with ursodeoxycholic acid alone. *Gastroenterology*, **1989**, *96*, 222–229.

Ponchon, T.; Barkun, A. N.; Pujol, B.; Mestas, J. L.; and Lambert, R. Gallstone disappearance after extracorporeal lithotripsy and oral bile acid dissolution. *Gastroenterology*, **1989**, *97*, 457–463.

Sackmann, M., and others. Shock-wave lithotripsy of gallbladder stones: the first 175 patients. *N. Engl. J. Med.*, **1988**, *318*, 393–397.

Schoenfield, L. J., and others. Chenodiol (chenodeoxycholic acid) for dissolution of gallstones: The National Cooperative Gallstone Study. *Ann. Intern. Med.*, **1981**, *95*, 257–282.

Schuurkes, J. A.; Van Bergen, P. J.; and Van Nueten, J. M. Prejunctional muscarinic (M_1)-receptor interactions on guinea-pig ileum: lack of effect of cisapride. *Br. J. Pharmacol.*, **1988**, *94*, 228–234.

Selvendran, R. R. The plant cell wall as a source of dietary fiber: chemistry and structure. *Am. J. Clin. Nutr.*, **1984**, *39*, 320–337.

Sridhar, K. S., and Donnelly, E. Combination antiemetics for cisplatin chemotherapy. *Cancer*, **1988**, *61*, 1508–1517.

Monographs and Reviews

Avery, G. S.; Davies, E. F.; and Brogden, R. N. Lactulose: a review of its therapeutic and pharmacological properties with particular reference to ammonia metabolism and its mode of action in portal systemic encephalopathy. *Drugs*, **1972**, *4*, 7–48.

Binder, H. J. Absorption and secretion of water and electrolytes by small and large intestine. In, *Gastrointestinal Disease*, 4th ed. (Sleisenger, M. H., and Fordtran, J. S., eds.) W. B. Saunders Co., Philadelphia, **1989**, pp. 1022–1045.

Brogden, R. N.; Carmine, A. A.; Heel, R. C.; Speight, T. M.; and Avery, G. S. Domperidone: a review of its pharmacological activity, pharmacokinetics and therapeutic efficacy in the symptomatic treatment of chronic dyspepsia and as an antiemetic. *Drugs*, **1982**, *24*, 360–400.

Cersosimo, R. J., and Karp, D. D. Adrenal corticosteroids as antiemetics during cancer chemotherapy. *Pharmacotherapy*, **1986**, *6*, 118–127.

Devroede, G. Constipation. In, *Gastrointestinal Disease*, 4th ed. (Sleisenger, M. H., and Fordtran, J. S., eds.) W. B. Saunders Co., Philadelphia, **1989**, pp. 331–368.

Donowitz, M.; Wicks, J.; and Sharp, G. W. G. Drug therapy for diarrheal diseases: a look ahead. *Rev. Infect. Dis.*, **1986**, *8*, Suppl. 2, S188–S201.

Ericsson, C. D.; DuPont, H. L.; and Johnson, P. C. Nonantibiotic therapy for travelers' diarrhea. *Rev. Infect. Dis.*, **1986**, *8*, S202–S206.

Fine, K. D.; Krejs, G. J.; and Fordtran, J. S. Diarrhea. In, *Gastrointestinal Disease*, 4th ed. (Sleisenger, M. H., and Fordtran, J. S., eds.) W. B. Saunders Co., Philadelphia, **1989**, pp. 290–316.

Goldberg, H. L., and DiMascio, A. Psychotropic drugs in pregnancy. In, *Psychopharmacology: A Generation of Progress*. (Lipton, M. A.; DiMascio, A.; and Killam, K. F.; eds.) Raven Press, New York, **1978**, pp. 1047–1055.

Gorbach, S. L. Infectious diarrhea. In, *Gastrointestinal Disease*, 4th ed. (Sleisenger, M. H., and Fordtran, J. S., eds.) W. B. Saunders Co., Philadelphia, **1989**, pp. 1191–1232.

McCallum, R. W. Motor function of the stomach in health and disease. In, *Gastrointestinal Disease*, 4th ed. (Sleisenger, M. H., and Fordtran, J. S., eds.) W. B. Saunders Co., Philadelphia, **1989**, pp. 675–713.

McCallum, R. W., and Albibi, R. Metoclopramide: pharmacology and clinical application. *Ann. Intern. Med.*, **1983**, *98*, 86–95.

McCallum, R. W.; Prakash, C.; Campoli-Richards, D. M.; and Goa, K. L. Cisapride: a preliminary review of its pharmacodynamic and pharmacokinetic properties, and therapeutic use as a prokinetic agent in gastrointestinal motility disorders. *Drugs*, **1988**, *36*, 652–681.

Marotta, F.; O'Keefe, S. J. D.; Marks, I. N.; Girdwood, A.; and Young, G. Pancreatic enzyme replacement therapy: importance of gastric acid secretion, H_2-antagonists, and enteric coating. *Dig. Dis. Sci.*, **1989**, *34*, 456–461.

Morselli, P. L. Psychotropic drugs. In, *Drug Disposition during Development*. (Morselli, P. L., ed.) Spectrum Publications, Inc., New York, **1977**, pp. 431–474.

Pierce, N. F., and Hirschhorn, N. Oral fluid—a simple weapon against dehydration in cholera. *WHO Chron.*, **1977**, *31*, 87–93.

Pinder, R. M.; Brogden, R. N.; Sawyer, P. R.; Speight, T. M.; and Avery, G. S. Metoclopramide: a review of its pharmacological properties and clinical use. *Drugs*, **1976**, *12*, 81–131.

Rosenbaum, C. L., and Cluxton, R. J., Jr. Ursodiol: a cholesterol gallstone solubilizing agent. *Drug Intell. Clin. Pharm.*, **1988**, *22*, 941–945.

Symposium. (Various authors.) Symposia of the Giovanni Lorenzini Foundation. In, *New Trends in Pathophysiology and Therapy of the Large Bowel*, Vol. 17. (Barbara, L.; Miglioli, M.; and Phillips, S. F.; eds.) Elsevier Science Publishers, Amsterdam, **1983.**

Tint, G. S.; Salen, G.; and Shefer, S. Effect of ursodeoxycholic acid and chenodeoxycholic acid on cholesterol and bile acid metabolism. *Gastroenterology*, **1986**, *91*, 1007–1018.

Triozzi, P. L., and Laszlo, J. Optimum management of nausea and vomiting in cancer chemotherapy. *Drugs*, **1987**, *34*, 136–149.

Triozzi, P. L.; Goldstein, D.; and Laszlo, J. Contributions of benzodiazepines to cancer therapy. *Cancer Invest.*, **1988**, *6*, 103–111.

World Health Organization. *A Manual for the Treatment of Acute Diarrhea*. World Health Organization, Geneva, **1984.**

SECTION

IX

Drugs Affecting Uterine Motility

In this section, only the uterine-stimulating (or oxytocic) and uterine-relaxing (or tocolytic) agents are discussed. The effects of estrogens, androgens, and anterior pituitary hormones on the reproductive system are presented in Section XV.

CHAPTER

39 OXYTOCIN, PROSTAGLANDINS, ERGOT ALKALOIDS, AND OTHER DRUGS; TOCOLYTIC AGENTS

Theodore W. Rall

Drugs that modify the progress of labor and delivery have obvious utility in modern obstetrics. Historically, the ergot alkaloids (now represented by *ergonovine* and *methylergonovine*) were the first agents to be used to initiate or accelerate parturition. In modern practice, *oxytocin* has displaced these drugs for this purpose, and their use is now confined to the postpartum period. The utility of oxytocin and the ergot alkaloids in obstetrics, as well as their general pharmacological properties, will be described below. The prostaglandins are the most recent group of uterine-stimulating agents to be studied. Discussion in this chapter will be limited to the effects of prostaglandins of the E and F types on the uterus and their potential for use as abortifacients and to facilitate delivery at term. The general discussion of the prostaglandins appears in Chapter 24.

Several classes of drugs, notably β_2-adrenergic agonists and alcohol, have been used to inhibit uterine contractility and to delay parturition. The general discussion of the pharmacology of these compounds appears in Chapters 10 and 17, respectively. This chapter discusses only their therapeutic use in obstetrics.

Physiological and Anatomical Considerations. Uterine smooth muscle is characterized by a high degree of spontaneous electrical and contractile activity (*see* Kao, 1977). Waves of decreased membrane potential with superimposed spike activity are associated with contraction. Cell-to-cell spread of excitation occurs, but electrical conduction is slow and decremental in nature. Low-resistance contacts between cells (gap junctions) greatly facilitate the spread of excitation. The number of such junctions is regulated by steroid hormones and increases in the later stages of pregnancy. Increased frequency and duration of spike activity in "pacemaker" areas and more extensive spread of excitation are associated with increases in force of contraction. In most species (including the human female), the influx of Na^+ appears to play the primary role in depolarization. However, the duration of spike potentials is relatively long, and depolarization is not affected by tetrodotoxin. This fact indicates the lack of participation of so-called fast Na^+ channels in this process.

Even in those species in which most of the depolarizing current appears to be carried by Ca^{2+}, the amount of Ca^{2+} that crosses the plasma membrane during excitation is insufficient to cause contraction directly. It is sufficient, however, to trigger the release of much larger amounts of Ca^{2+} from the sarcoplasmic reticulum (*see* Huszar and Roberts, 1982; van Breemen and Saida, 1989). Hence, the availability of extracellular Ca^{2+} (or the presence of blockers of Ca^{2+} channels) strongly influences the response of uterine smooth muscle to various physiological and pharmacological stimuli. As in cardiac and skeletal muscle, the interaction of actin and myosin that results in muscle contraction is instigated by Ca^{2+}. However, the anatomical arrangement and biochemical properties of contractile proteins are much different in smooth muscle, including that of the uterus. Of particular importance in smooth muscle is the fact that contraction is initiated by the relatively slow process of phosphorylation of the light chains of myosin, a reaction that is catalyzed by myosin light chain kinase, a calcium- and calmodulin-dependent enzyme (*see* Hai and Murphy, 1989).

The uterus has parasympathetic and sympathetic innervation, the former by way of the pelvic nerve and the latter by way of postganglionic fibers from the inferior mesenteric and hypogastric ganglia. Both can elicit increased activity in the mature human uterus, but denervation causes little change in uterine motor activity. Both α_1- (excitatory) and β_2- (inhibitory, hyperpolarizing) adrenergic receptors are clearly demonstrable in the myometrium of mammals. As in other smooth muscles, the inhibitory effects of β_2-adrenergic agonists on uterine contractility are thought to be mediated by adenosine 3′,5′-monophosphate (cyclic AMP). Although the cyclic nucleotide promotes an inhibitory phosphorylation of myosin light chain kinase and can hasten the uptake and extrusion of cytoplasmic Ca^{2+}, these mechanisms are not yet established as important for myometrial relaxation (*see* Carsten and Miller, 1987; Kamm and Stull, 1989; van Breemen and Saida, 1989). Relaxin, a small peptide hormone produced by the corpus luteum and the placenta, also inhibits uterine contractility (*see* Weiss, 1987). Excitatory receptors for oxytocin have been demonstrated. Prostaglandins E_2 and $F_{2\alpha}$ and, in some species, 5-hydroxytryptamine (5-HT) increase uterine contractile activity.

Uterine smooth muscle is unusually susceptible to endocrine influence, especially that of the estrogens. Thus, spontaneous activity, as well as responsiveness to neurogenic, hormonal, and pharmacological stimulation, increases greatly at puberty and varies thereafter with the ovulatory cycle. In some species, progesterone markedly inhibits uterine activity. Whether progesterone has an important physiological role in regulating the motor activity of the human uterus has yet to be clearly demonstrated.

In addition to such factors as endocrinological status, contractile responses of uterine smooth muscle are strongly influenced by variables such as the period of gestation, the degree of stretch, and the region of the uterus under consideration. Thus, it is not surprising that there are many conflicting reports of the effects of drugs on this organ. Unless otherwise stated, the effects of the drugs to be discussed here are those that have been confirmed in the human female.

Human Parturition. The physiological processes that are involved in the onset and progression of labor in human beings are complex and have been defined only to a limited degree; it has been particularly difficult to establish the sequence of events that leads to the initiation of labor. The views of most investigators have centered on the complementary and sometimes synergistic actions of oxytocin and the prostaglandins, and the changes in their capacity to exert effects that can result from developmental events in the fetus, placenta, and fetal membranes (*see* Fuchs, 1987; Angle and Johnston, 1990).

Oxytocin has stimulatory effects on the smooth muscle of the uterus that are so potent and selective as to suggest that the polypeptide serves a true hormonal function at this site. Oxytocin elicits contractions of the fundus that are indistinguishable in amplitude, duration, and frequency from those seen in late pregnancy and during spontaneous labor. However, a direct link between endogenous oxytocin and the onset of labor has been difficult to establish. Parturition still occurs in the complete absence of oxytocin; however, labor is prolonged. Although the concentration of oxytocin in plasma rises progressively throughout gestation, only small increases can be detected at the onset of spontaneous labor. In addition, mechanical stimulation of the fetal membranes or the cervix—manipulations that can induce labor—produce little change in plasma oxytocin (De Geest *et al.*, 1985). However, the sensitivity of the uterus to oxytocin increases as pregnancy progresses (*see* below), and the number of receptors for oxytocin in the myometrium and decidua is markedly elevated in the later stages of pregnancy. While maternal oxytocin may not trigger the onset of labor, it can be considered, at least, to play an important facilitatory role in parturition.

Prostaglandins also appear to have important functions in human parturition. Inhibitors of prostaglandin synthesis can delay the onset of or prolong spontaneous labor (*see* Chapter 26). Although uterine sensitivity to the prostaglandins changes relatively little during pregnancy, the specific activity of phospholipases that catalyze the rate-limiting step in the formation of prostaglandins increases in human amnion late in gestation. This fetal membrane also possesses large amounts of both cyclooxygenase and phospholipids that contain arachidonic acid. The formation of prostaglandins by the amnion may increase progressively during the later stages of pregnancy as a result of the accumulation of substances derived from the fetus, especially platelet activating factor (PAF). In addition to causing the elaboration of prostaglandins, PAF can initiate uterine contraction directly. Since PAF hydrolase in the maternal plasma declines during the last trimester, it is possible that the amounts of PAF and prostaglandins that reach the myometrium may be sufficient to initiate labor (*see* Angle and Johnston, 1990).

The views just presented are not mutually exclusive, and it is likely that both oxytocin and prostaglandins play direct roles in the initiation and maintenance of uterine contractions during labor. In addition, the entire process of human parturition is under the influence of steroidal hormones. Most attention has been focused on the increasing concentrations of estrogens in the plasma and amniotic fluid during the later stages of pregnancy, especially the marked changes in the final 2 to 3 weeks. Progesterone concentrations may decrease at the same time; furthermore, a progesterone-binding protein accumulates in the fetal membranes and may serve to decrease the effective concentration of the hormone in these structures. In any event, the progressive domination by estrogen has been held responsible for the increases in myometrial excitability (owing to increases in slow Na^+ channels and gap junctions), the myometrial sensitivity to oxytocin, and the capacity to elaborate prostaglandins in the fetal membranes. The changing hormonal milieu may also be responsible for the so-called ripening of the uterine cervix during pregnancy; among other changes, a marked, progressive decrease occurs in the content of collagen (Uldbjerg *et al.*, 1983). These alterations are thought to be crucial in preparation for the softening, dilatation, and effacement that occur during normal labor and delivery. (*See* Huszar *and also* Challis and Mitchell, in Symposium, 1981; Liggins, in Symposium, 1983.)

OXYTOCIN

The structure, formation, storage, and release of the neurohypophyseal hormones—oxytocin and antidiuretic hormone (ADH)—and a comparison of their biological activities have been presented in Chapter 29. The following discussion will deal in more detail with the physiological and pharmacological properties of oxytocin. This hormone has slight, but not insignificant, antidiuretic and vascular activity that may become manifest when large doses are used (*see* below).

Biosynthesis and Physiological Role of Oxytocin. Oxytocin is synthesized in the supraoptic and paraventricular nuclei of the hypothalamus within neurons that are distinct from those that contain ADH. It is formed by the processing of a larger precursor molecule that also contains a specific binding protein for the hormone, termed oxytocin-neurophysin. Oxytocin-neurophysin contains a sequence of more than 90 amino acid residues that is identical with a region in ADH-neurophysin (Land *et al.*, 1983). The two neurophysins can bind either hormone (Rholam *et al.*, 1982). The dimeric complex of oxytocin and its neurophysin is stored in and released from secretory granules in nerve endings, especially in the neurohypophysis.

Sensory stimuli arising from the cervix and vagina can induce secretion of oxytocin from the posterior pituitary; ovarian relaxin is inhibitory (Dayanithi *et al.*, 1987). Stimulation of the breast also results in secretion of oxytocin. The hormone causes contraction of the myoepithelium that surrounds aveolar channels in the mammary gland. This milk-ejection reflex fails to occur in the complete absence of oxytocin. The secretion of both ADH and oxytocin is provoked by increases in the osmolality of plasma and is suppressed by ethanol; the latter effect forms the basis for the use of ethanol as a tocolytic agent (*see* below). Although the peripheral actions of oxytocin appear to play no significant role in responses to dehydration or hypovolemia, neurons that contain oxytocin project to regions in the hypothalamus, brainstem, and spinal cord that are known to be involved in the regulation of the autonomic nervous system (*see* Buijs, 1983). Thus, such release from the neurohypophysis might reflect activation of oxytocinergic neurons that may participate in the central regulation of blood pressure. Indeed, the stress-induced release of oxytocin is associated with reduced sensitivity of the baroreflex (*see* Petty, 1987).

Oxytocin has also been implicated in the modulation of memory, primarily on the basis of the amnestic effects that follow its injection into the cerebral ventricles. Studies of such phenomena have revealed the capacity of synaptic membranes to convert oxytocin to a specific peptide fragment that has greatly enhanced amnestic potency but is devoid of uterine-stimulating properties (Burbach *et al.*, 1983).

The genes that encode both oxytocin and ADH are also expressed in tissues outside the brain, including the ovary and placenta (*see* Fuchs, 1987). In certain nonprimate species, oxytocin may participate in uterine influences on the lifespan of the corpus luteum; in primates, a paracrine function to regulate the synthesis of progesterone is suspected.

PHARMACOLOGICAL PROPERTIES

Uterus. Oxytocin stimulates both the frequency and force of contractile activity in uterine smooth muscle. With higher concentrations, sustained decreases in resting membrane potential occur. At threshold concentrations, where there is no change in membrane potential, oxytocin initiates spike discharges, increases the frequency and number of spikes in a burst discharge, and increases the amplitude of spike discharges (*see* Kao, 1977). These effects are highly dependent on the presence of estrogen, and the immature uterus is quite resistant. Although progesterone antagonizes the stimulant effect of oxytocin *in vitro*, the corresponding effect in the pregnant human uterus has been difficult to demonstrate.

A very low level of motor activity prevails in the human uterus during the first and second trimesters of pregnancy. During the third trimester, spontaneous motor activity increases progressively until the sharp rise that constitutes the initiation of labor and delivery. The responsiveness of the uterus to oxytocin roughly parallels the increase in spontaneous activity. Oxytocin can initiate or enhance rhythmic contractions at any time, but in early pregnancy only very high doses elicit a response. Approximately an eightfold increase in responsiveness occurs between the twentieth and thirty-ninth week. Most of this increase takes place during the last 9 weeks. Thus, slow intravenous infusion of a few units of oxytocin usually is effective in initiating labor at term. However, individuals vary considerably in their response to oxytocin, and labor has been initiated by the infusion of as little as 25 milliunits (0.05 μg) of oxytocin (*see* below).

Mechanism of Action. The demonstration of specific receptors for oxytocin in human myometrium and the progressive increase in their number that occurs during pregnancy have been discussed above. Such sites may well mediate the actions of oxytocin, but the mechanism for translation of receptor binding into increased frequency and force of contraction is poorly understood. Although there is evidence for oxytocin-induced hydrolysis of phosphoinositides (*see* Fuchs, 1987), the marked inhibitory effects of Ca^{2+}-channel blockers on contractile responses suggest that release of intracellular Ca^{2+} by inositol-1,4,5-trisphosphate plays a relatively minor role. Direct or depolarization-induced activation of voltage-sensitive Ca^{2+} channels by oxytocin may be of greater importance. Oxytocin causes the release of prostaglandins in several species; however, it is unclear whether this effect is primary or is a result of uterine contraction. Reports conflict as to whether inhibitors of prostaglandin synthesis can alter the contractile effect of oxytocin on the human myometrium *in vitro* (Garrioch, 1978; Wikland *et al.*, 1982). The effects of prostaglandins on uterine muscle are discussed below.

Mammary Gland. The alveolar ramifications of the mammary gland are surrounded by a network of modified smooth muscle, the myoepithelium. Contraction of these cells forces milk from the alveolar channels into the large sinuses, where it is easily available to the suckling infant. This function is known as milk ejection (milk letdown, in domestic animals). The myoepithelium is highly responsive to oxytocin. Although the catecholamines inhibit milk ejection, the contraction of the myoepithelium is not believed to be dependent on autonomic innervation, but is considered to be under the control of oxytocin and the reflex pathways that initiate the release of the hormone. Oxytocin is occasionally used to promote milk ejection when this component of lactation appears to be inefficient in nursing mothers.

Cardiovascular System. Oxytocin causes a marked but transient relaxation of vascular smooth muscle when large amounts are administered to man. A decrease in systolic and especially diastolic blood pressure, flushing, reflex tachycardia, and an increase in limb blood flow are observed. In addition to direct actions on blood vessels, inhibitory effects of oxytocin on sympathetic preganglionic neurons and on neurons in the caudal medulla may also be involved (*see* Petty, 1987). The amounts of oxytocin administered for most obstetrical purposes are insufficient to produce marked alterations of blood pressure. However, large doses may produce a marked fall in arterial pressure, particularly in deeply anesthetized patients.

When studied *in vitro*, oxytocin has a weak constricting effect on renal, splanchnic, and skeletal muscle arteries of various species, including man; however, relaxation will often occur if the vessel is first constricted by another agent. By contrast, oxytocin is a powerful constrictor of umbilical arteries and veins; its potency on human vessels is sufficient to suggest a role for oxytocin in effecting their closure at birth (*see* Altura and Altura, 1984).

Other Actions. Oxytocin usually produces an increase in Na^+ excretion in experimental animals, although this effect may depend on the presence of ADH in the circulation. Such effects are minor in man. However, when large doses of oxytocin are administered for therapeutic purposes, an antidiuretic effect can occur, and signs of water intoxication have been observed when excessive volumes of intravenous fluids have been administered concurrently. Oxytocin can suppress the secretion of ACTH (Legros *et al.*, 1984).

Absorption, Fate, and Excretion. Oxytocin is effective after administration by any parenteral route. A less efficient but convenient route is intranasal application of a spray. The ready absorption of oxytocin from buccal lozenges also permits the use of the oral mucosa as a route of administration. The nasal route of administration is reserved for uses post partum.

The distribution and fate of oxytocin in the body are much like those of ADH (*see* Chapter 29). While there is evidence for passage of oxytocin through the primate placenta, the extent to which the hormone crosses the human placenta is not certain (*see* Roy and Karim, 1983). Oxytocin is found in increasing concentrations in the fetal circulation and the amniotic fluid during the later stages of pregnancy and labor, but the relative fetal and maternal contribution has not been determined. Estimates of the half-life of oxytocin have varied from less than 5 to more than 12 minutes. The higher values are more consistent with the 30 to 60 minutes usually required to achieve maximal steady-state contractile effects during infusions of the hormone (Curtis and Safransky, 1988). The removal of oxytocin from plasma is accomplished largely by the kidney and the liver. During pregnancy, the concentration of an aminopeptidase (oxytocinase or cystyl-aminopeptidase) in plasma increases about tenfold (Majkić-Singh *et al.*, 1982). This enzyme is capable of degrading both oxytocin and ADH and is apparently derived from the placenta, where it may serve to regulate the local concentration of oxytocin in the uterus. This enzyme evidently has little to do with the disappearance of oxytocin from plasma because the half-life of the hormone is similar in females during labor and in males (Amico *et al.*, 1984).

Bioassay and Unitage. The uterine-stimulating potency of posterior pituitary extracts is determined by bioassay of their avian vasodepressor activity, which parallels uterine-stimulating activity. Activity is expressed in terms of USP units. The strength of the preparations of synthetic oxytocin now in use is still expressed in these units, each unit being the equivalent of approximately 2 μg of the pure hormone.

Preparations and Routes of Administration. *Oxytocin injection* (PITOCIN, SYNTOCINON) contains 10 USP units per milliliter and may be administered intravenously or intramuscularly. All commercial preparations of oxytocin are now synthetic. Oxytocin is also available in the form of a nasal spray, containing 40 USP units per milliliter.

Therapeutic Uses

The uses of oxytocin in obstetrics are discussed below.

Use during Lactation. Theoretically, oxytocin should be of value for the relief of engorgement of the breasts during lactation and in cases of inadequacy of breast-feeding in which insufficient milk ejection is felt to be a contributing factor. The hormone is administered most conveniently by the intranasal route. In cases of inadequacy of breast-feeding, it is given by a single burst of the nasal spray in one or both nostrils 2 to 3 minutes before a feeding is to begin. The procedure is often not successful. However, it is simple and without risk to the patient, and when effective it resolves a frustrating and sometimes painful problem. Oxytocin is not useful when inadequate production of milk is the underlying problem.

PROSTAGLANDINS

The sources, chemistry, and physiological actions of this ubiquitous group of autacoids are presented in Chapter 24. In the female reproductive system, prostaglandins are found in the ovary, myometrium, and menstrual fluid in concentrations that vary with the ovulatory cycle. Following coitus, accessible portions of the female reproductive tract are also exposed to prostaglandins, which occur in high concentrations in seminal fluid. The fetal membranes are an important source of these and other products of the metabolism of arachidonic acid in the pregnant uterus. At term and during labor, prostaglandin concentrations rise in amniotic fluid, umbilical cord blood, and maternal blood. The physiological role of the prostaglandins in human parturition has been discussed above.

In spite of the clearly demonstrable effectiveness of the prostaglandins in stimulating (or, in a few instances, relaxing) smooth muscle in reproductive organs, their physiological role in menstruation and conception remains debatable. The semen of a number of mammalian species is devoid of prostaglandins. Although the widely used drugs aspirin and indomethacin profoundly depress prostaglandin synthesis, their use has not yet been clearly shown to influence menstruation or reproduction in patients receiving therapeutic doses. However, aspirin-like drugs are effective in the treatment of uterine hypercontractility and cramping pain in women with primary dysmenorrhea (*see* Owen, 1984; *see also* Chapters 26 and 58). These agents can also delay the onset of or prolong spontaneous labor (*see* below).

Pharmacological Properties

The prostaglandins can be considered to be local hormones since, with few exceptions, they exert their effects and are inactivated principally in the tissues or organs in which they are synthesized. Those found most abundantly in the uterus, and in the menstrual and amniotic fluid, are of the E and F types. Prostacyclin (PGI_2) is confined largely to the uterine, umbilical, and fetal vasculature, where it may serve to ensure an adequate flow of blood and a patent ductus arteriosus. Clinical investigation for obstetrical use has been limited almost entirely to PGE_2, $PGF_{2\alpha}$, and the synthetic derivative, 15-methyl $PGF_{2\alpha}$.

Myometrium. During the last two trimesters of pregnancy, the administration of either PGE_2 or $PGF_{2\alpha}$ causes strong uterine contractions and can induce delivery of the fetus (*see* Andersson *et al.*, in Symposium, 1983). As with oxytocin, the sensitivity of the uterus to prostaglandins increases as gestation progresses. However, the changes are less pronounced, and prostaglandins are much more effective than is oxytocin in inducing contractions in the earlier months. The higher doses that are required to produce abortion in the first few weeks after conception result in serious systemic effects. No information is available on alterations in the number or function of myometrial receptors for the prostaglandins during pregnancy, and the increasing sensitivity may primarily reflect changes in the excitability of uterine smooth muscle that are induced by steroids (*see* above).

When studied *in vitro*, $PGF_{2\alpha}$ consistently stimulates contractions of myometrial tissue from both pregnant and nonpregnant women, while PGE_2 often causes relaxation. As a result, the formation of disproportionately large amounts of $PGF_{2\alpha}$ has generally been held responsible for the uterine hypercontractility that occurs in primary dysmenorrhea. However, PGE_2 is as effective as $PGF_{2\alpha}$ for the induction of labor at term. This apparent discrepancy between observations *in vivo* and *in vitro* may be explained by the biphasic effects of PGE_2 on strips of uterine muscle from women late in pregnancy; low concentrations of PGE_2 regularly increase contractions, while higher concentrations produce a brief or weak excitatory response followed by a long period of quiescence (Wikland *et al.*, 1982). Since PGI_2 consistently inhibits myometrial contractions *in vitro*, the effects of high doses of PGE_2 may reflect interaction with receptors for PGI_2, a circumstance that has been observed elsewhere (*e.g.*, in platelets; *see* Chapter 24).

Cervix. The local instillation of prostaglandins can induce cervical ripening at doses that do not affect uterine motility (*see* Symposium, 1983; Brindley and Sokol, 1988). These agents can also produce softening of the cervix late in the first trimester of pregnancy, by which time a major change in the structure of cervical collagen has occurred. The mechanisms underlying these effects are not known, and the role of endogenous prostaglandins in cervical ripening during normal, spontaneous labor is yet to be established. However, it is likely that they are important in the ripening that is produced by the insertion of various devices (*e.g.*, bougies) into the cervix to induce such changes.

Toxicity. The principal side effects that attend the use of the prostaglandins are caused by their stimulatory action on the smooth muscle of the alimentary tract. Hence, antiemetic and antidiarrheal drugs are usually administered concurrently. In addition, many patients who have received PGE_2 or 15-methyl $PGF_{2\alpha}$ experience transient pyrexia. This is probably due to actions on thermoregulatory centers in the hypothalamus. Large doses of $PGF_{2\alpha}$ or 15-methyl $PGF_{2\alpha}$ may cause hypertension by constricting vascular smooth muscle, while large doses of PGE_2 may produce vasodilatation.

Preparations and Routes of Administration. *Dinoprostone* (PROSTIN E2) is available in vaginal suppositories containing 20 mg of PGE_2. It is used to induce abortion, to evacuate the uterus in the management of missed abortion, and to treat benign hydatidiform mole. *Carboprost tromethamine* (HEMABATE) is a solution containing 0.25 mg of carboprost (15-methyl $PGF_{2\alpha}$) per milliliter for intramuscular administration. It is used to induce abortion, to aid in the expulsion of the fetus during the course of abortion by another method, or to treat postpartum hemorrhage owing to uterine atony. Dosage of these preparations is discussed below.

THERAPEUTIC USES

The major use of PGE_2 and 15-methyl $PGF_{2\alpha}$ that is currently approved in the United States is for the performance of midtrimester abortions. This use is discussed below. 15-Methyl $PGF_{2\alpha}$ may also be used as an alternative to ergonovine or oxytocin in the treatment of postpartum hemorrhage. In addition, there have been numerous investigations of the potential use of prostaglandins as cervical ripening agents to facilitate normal or induced labor (*see* Symposium, 1983; Lange *et al.*, 1984); also under investigation is the use of these agents to soften the cervix prior to performance of first-trimester abortions by the method of dilatation and evacuation (Kent *et al.*, 1983; Arias, 1984).

ERGOT AND THE ERGOT ALKALOIDS

The dramatic effect of ergot ingested during pregnancy has been recognized for over 2000 years, and it was first used by physicians as a uterine-stimulating agent almost 400 years ago. In the early years of this century, the isolation and chemical identification of the active principles of ergot were accomplished, and detailed study of their biological activity was begun. The elucidation of the constituents of ergot and their complex actions comprises a most important chapter in the evolution of modern pharmacology. The ergot alkaloids are therefore discussed in some detail in this and other chapters, even though the very complexity of their actions limits their therapeutic uses.

Source. *Ergot* is the product of a fungus (*Claviceps purpurea*) that grows upon rye and other grains. Rye is the most susceptible. The parasite can be found in the grainfields of North America and Europe. Rye destined for commercial sale is subject to government inspection and is rejected if it contains more than 0.3% infected grain. In dry years the rejection rate is usually less than 1%, but in other years it has been as high as 36%.

The spores are carried by insects or the wind to the ovaries of young rye, where they germinate into hyphal filaments. As the hyphal filaments penetrate deep into the ovary of the rye, a dense tissue forms. This tissue gradually consumes the entire substance of the grain and hardens into a purple, curved body called the *sclerotium*. This sclerotium is still a major commercial source of ergot alkaloids.

History. The contamination of an edible grain by a poisonous, parasitic fungus spread death and destruction for centuries. As early as 600 B.C., an Assyrian tablet alluded to a "noxious pustule in the ear of grain"; and in one of the sacred books of the Parsees (400 to 300 B.C.) the following pertinent passage occurs, "Among the evil things created by Angro Maynes are noxious grasses that cause pregnant women to drop the womb and die in childbed." It was fortunate for the ancient Greeks that they objected to the "black malodorous product of Thrace and Macedonia," and therefore did not eat rye. Rye was also comparatively unknown to the early Romans, for it was not introduced into Southwest Europe until after the beginning of the Christian era. Consequently, there is no undisputed reference to ergot poisoning in the early Greek and Roman literature. It was not until the Middle Ages that written descriptions of ergot poisoning first appeared, although it is probable that the disease was prevalent long before this time. Strange epidemics were described in which the characteristic symptom was gangrene of the feet, legs, hands, and arms. In severe cases, the tissue became dry and black and the mummified limbs separated off without loss of blood. Limbs were said to be consumed by the Holy Fire and blackened like charcoal. Mention was also made of agonizing burning sensations in the extremities. The disease was called Holy Fire or St. Anthony's fire, the latter name being in honor of the saint at whose shrine relief was said to be obtained. The relief that followed migration to the shrine of St. Anthony was probably real, for the sufferers received a diet free of contaminated grain during their sojourn at the shrine. The symptoms of ergot poisoning were not restricted to the limbs. Indeed, a frequent complication of ergot poisoning was abortion. A convulsive type of ergotism was also known. The effects of ergot poisoning were described most effectively in paintings and woodcuts during the late Middle Ages (*e.g.*, Grünewald's altar paintings, now located in the museum at Colmar, France).

Ergot was known as an obstetrical herb before it was identified as the cause of St. Anthony's fire. It was mentioned as early as 1582 by Lonicer as a proven means of producing pains in the womb. It was used by midwives long before it was recognized by the medical profession. The first physician to employ ergot was Desgranges, but he did not publish his observations until 1818. Ten years before, a letter published by John Stearns in the *Medical Repository* of New York, entitled "Account of the Pulvis Parturiens, a Remedy for Quickening Childbirth," marked the official introduction of ergot into medicine (Thoms, 1931). This communication is of sufficient historical interest to quote certain pertinent portions of it:

> It [pulvis parturiens] expedites lingering parturition and saves to the accoucheur a considerable portion of time, without producing any bad effects on the patient. . . . Previous to its exhibition it is of the utmost consequence to ascertain the presentation . . . as the violent and almost incessant action which it induces in the uterus precludes the possibility of turning. . . . If the dose is large it will produce nausea and vomiting. In most cases you will be surprised with the suddenness of its operation; it is, therefore, necessary to be completely ready before you give the medicine. . . . Since I have adopted the use of this powder I have seldom found a case that detained me more than three hours. . . .

The use of ergot spread rapidly in the United States, but its adoption in Europe was delayed, perhaps because the Old World had suffered too much from the poisonous properties of ergot. The dangers attending the use of the drug, however, were soon recognized. In 1824, Hosack wrote that the number of stillborn children had increased so greatly since the introduction of ergot that the Medical Society of New York instituted an inquiry. Said Hosack, "The ergot has been called . . . *pulvis ad partum;* as it regards the child, it may, with almost equal truth be denominated the *pulvis ad mortem.*" This astute observer recommended that the drug be used only to control postpartum hemorrhage. Thus, more than a century and a half ago, the indications and contraindications of ergot were accurately defined.

Chemistry. The ergot alkaloids can all be considered to be derivatives of the tetracyclic compound 6-methylergoline. The naturally occurring alkaloids contain a substituent in the β configuration at position 8 and a double bond in ring D (Table 39–1). The natural alkaloids of therapeutic interest are amide derivatives of *d-lysergic acid;* these compounds contain a double bond between C 9 and C 10 and thus belong to the family of 9-ergolene compounds. Many alkaloids, containing either a methyl or a hydroxymethyl group at position 8, are present in ergot in small quantities. These have been called *clavine alkaloids* and consist principally of both 9-ergolenes (*e.g., lysergol*) and 8-ergolenes (*e.g., elymoclavine,* the 8-ergolene isomer of lysergol). A crystalline, pharmacologically active preparation was first isolated from ergot in 1906 by Barger, Carr, and Dale as well as by Kraft. This material was called *ergotoxine.* It is now known to be a mixture of four alkaloids: *ergocornine, ergocristine, α-ergocryptine,* and *β-ergocryptine.* The first pure ergot alkaloid, *ergotamine,* was obtained by Stoll in 1920. Moir reported the discovery of the "water soluble uterotonic principle of ergot" in 1932. This was subsequently determined to be *ergonovine* (also designated *ergometrine*).

The chemical structures of the alkaloids of ergot have been elucidated primarily by Stoll and associates and by Jacobs and Craig and their coworkers (*see* Rutschmann and Stadler, 1978). Optical isomerism is due to the presence of two asymmetrical carbon atoms (positions 5 and 8) in the lysergic acid portion of the molecule. Derivatives of *l*-lysergic acid (the epimer at position 5) and of *d*-isolysergic acid (the epimer at position 8) display relatively little biological activity. The latter derivatives include *ergotaminine,* which constitutes 40% of clinical preparations of ergotamine tartrate as a result of spontaneous epimerization (*see* Tfelt-Hansen, 1986). Upon hydrolysis, ergonovine and its derivatives yield lysergic acid and an amine; consequently they are designated as *amine alkaloids.* The alkaloids of higher molecular weight yield lysergic acid, ammonia, pyruvic acid (or a derivative thereof), proline, and one other amino acid (either phenylalanine, leucine, isoleucine, or valine) and are thus known as *amino acid alkaloids* or *ergopeptines.*

Numerous semisynthetic derivatives of the ergot alkaloids have been prepared, and several are of therapeutic interest (*see* Rutschmann and Stadler, 1978). The earliest derivatives were prepared by the catalytic hydrogenation of the natural alkaloids, yielding a series of compounds that are saturated in ring D of lysergic acid. These have been designated *dihydroergotamine, dihydroergocristine,* and so forth, and possess somewhat different pharmacological properties than do the parent alkaloids. Another ergopeptine derivative is *bromocriptine* (2-bromo-α-ergocryptine). In addition, it is possible to prepare different amides of lysergic acid. Two products of this series, lysergic acid diethylamide (LSD; Chapter 22) and lysergic acid hydroxybutylamide (*methylergonovine*), are of pharmacological interest. Methylation of the indole nitrogen of the latter compound yields 1-methylmethylergonovine (*methysergide*). A large number of related compounds that are not derivatives of lysergic acid have also been prepared. These include *lisuride* (Chapter 20), *lergotrile* (2-chloro-6-methyl-8β-cyanomethyl-ergoline), and *metergoline* (1,6-dimethyl-8β-carbobenzoxyaminomethyl-ergoline).

PHARMACOLOGICAL PROPERTIES

The pharmacological actions of the ergot alkaloids are varied and complex; some actions are completely unrelated, and some are even mutually antagonistic. The marked effects of ergotamine on the cardiovascular system, for example, are due to simultaneous peripheral vasoconstriction, depression of vasomotor centers, and peripheral adrenergic blockade. The following presentation will be concerned primarily with the responses of the smooth muscle of the uterus and blood vessels. The actions on adrenergic receptors and vasomotor reflexes are discussed in Chapter 11; CNS effects are discussed in Chapters 20 and 22. The use of bromocriptine to control the secretion of prolactin is described in Chapter 56. A summary of the actions of representative ergot alkaloids is presented in Table 39–2.

The stimulation of vascular and uterine smooth muscle by ergot alkaloids was once thought to reflect an action that was exerted independently of receptors for other substances that cause such contractile responses. However, convincing evidence now indicates that mediation by α-adrenergic receptors, tryptaminergic receptors, or both is involved (*see* Berde and Stürmer, 1978; Müller-Schweinitzer and Weidmann, 1978). In general, the effects of all the ergot alkaloids appear to result from their actions as partial agonists or antagonists at adrenergic, dopaminergic, and tryptaminergic receptors (*see* Table 39–2). The spectrum of effects depends on the agent, dosage, species, tissue, and experimental or physiological conditions. However, some aspects of the actions of ergot alkaloids are not entirely compatible with this view: (1) while

Table 39–1. NATURAL AND SEMISYNTHETIC ERGOT ALKALOIDS

A. AMINE ALKALOIDS AND CONGENERS

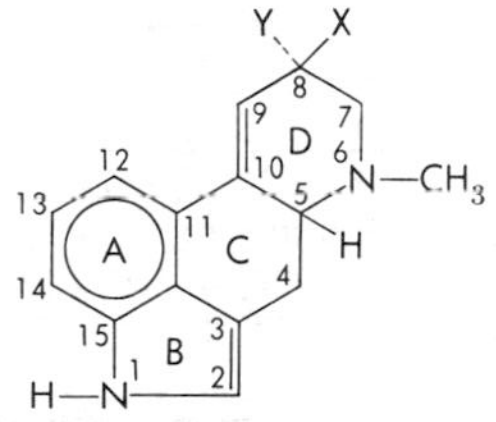

ALKALOID	X	Y
d-Lysergic acid	$-COOH$	$-H$
d-Isolysergic acid	$-H$	$-COOH$
d-Lysergic acid diethylamide (LSD)	$-C(=O)-N(CH_2CH_3)_2$	$-H$
Ergonovine (ergometrine)	$-C(=O)-NH-CH(CH_3)CH_2OH$	$-H$
Methylergonovine	$-C(=O)-NH-CH(CH_2CH_3)(CH_2OH)$	$-H$
Methysergide *	$-C(=O)-NH-CH(CH_2CH_3)(CH_2OH)$	$-H$
Lisuride	$-H$	$-NH-C(=O)-N(CH_2CH_3)_2$
Lysergol	$-CH_2OH$	$-H$
Lergotrile †,‡	$-CH_2CN$	$-H$
Metergoline *,†	$-CH_2-NH-C(=O)-O-CH_2-$phenyl	$-H$

B. AMINO ACID ALKALOIDS

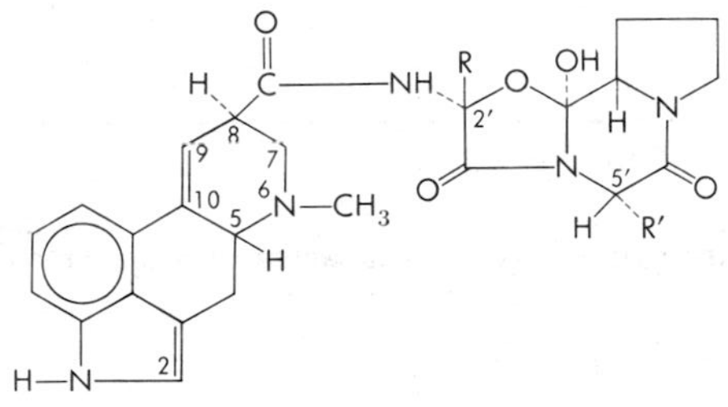

ALKALOID §	R(2′)	R′(5′)
Ergotamine	$-CH_3$	$-CH_2-$phenyl
Ergosine	$-CH_3$	$-CH_2CH(CH_3)_2$
Ergostine	$-CH_2CH_3$	$-CH_2-$phenyl
Ergotoxine group:		
Ergocornine	$-CH(CH_3)_2$	$-CH(CH_3)_2$
Ergocristine	$-CH(CH_3)_2$	$-CH_2-$phenyl
α-Ergocryptine	$-CH(CH_3)_2$	$-CH_2CH(CH_3)_2$
β-Ergocryptine	$-CH(CH_3)_2$	$-CH(CH_3)CH_2CH_3$
Bromocriptine ¶	$-CH(CH_3)_2$	$-CH_2CH(CH_3)_2$

* Contains methyl substitution at N 1.
† Contains hydrogen atoms at C 9 and C 10.
‡ Contains chlorine atom at C 2.
§ Dihydro derivatives contain hydrogen atoms at C 9 and C 10.
¶ Contains bromine atom at C 2.

Table 39–2. PHARMACOLOGICAL ACTIONS OF SELECTED ERGOT ALKALOIDS

COMPOUND	PHARMACOLOGICAL ACTIONS			
	Interactions with Tryptaminergic Receptors	*Interactions with Dopaminergic Receptors*	*Interactions with α-Adrenergic Receptors*	*Uterine Stimulation*
Ergotamine	Partial agonist in certain blood vessels; nonselective antagonist in various smooth muscles; poor agonist/antagonist in CNS	No notable actions on central or peripheral structures, but high emetic potency after intravenous administration	Partial agonist and antagonist in blood vessels and various smooth muscles; mainly antagonist in peripheral and central nervous systems	Highly active
Dihydroergotamine	Partial agonist and antagonist in a few smooth muscles; may be agonist in lateral geniculate nucleus	Nonselective antagonist in sympathetic ganglia; low emetic potency	Partial agonist in veins; antagonist in blood vessels, various smooth muscles, and peripheral and central nervous systems	Active on pregnant human uterus
Bromocriptine	Only a few weak antagonistic actions reported	Partial agonist and antagonist in various areas of CNS; presumed agonist in inhibiting secretion of prolactin; less emetic potency than ergotamine	No agonistic effects; somewhat less potent antagonist than dihydroergotamine in various tissues	Inactive
Ergonovine and methylergonovine	Partial agonists in human umbilical and placental blood vessels; selective and fairly potent antagonists in various smooth muscles; partial agonists and antagonists in some areas of CNS	Weak antagonists in certain blood vessels; partial agonists and antagonists in various areas of CNS; less potent than bromocriptine in producing emesis or inhibiting secretion of prolactin	Partial agonists in blood vessels (less than ergotamine); little antagonistic action	Very highly active
Methysergide	Partial agonist in certain blood vessels and areas of CNS; selective and very potent antagonist in many tissues and areas of CNS	Little evidence for agonistic or antagonistic activity; no emetic activity	Little or no agonistic or antagonistic action	Very little activity

agonistic effects are generally apparent only at concentrations that are lower than those required to observe antagonism, this is not always the case (*e.g.*, the action of methysergide on cerebral blood vessels); (2) the effects of full agonists (*e.g.*, norepinephrine) are usually augmented by low concentrations of ergot alkaloids, even those with weak efficacy as partial agonists (*e.g.*, the action of ergonovine on arterioles); and (3) the contractile responses to other agents, such as acetylcholine or angiotensin, are sometimes also augmented by low concentrations of ergot alkaloids, and such synergistic effects are not always prevented by adrenergic or tryptaminergic blocking agents. These and other observations emphasize the importance of the physiological or pathophysiological state in determining the spectrum and intensity of effects produced in animals or patients. An emerging body of biochemical data suggests that ergot alkaloids and chemically related compounds interact to varying degrees with subtypes of receptors for the biogenic amines (Gundlach *et al.*, 1983; McPherson and Beart, 1983; Markstein *et al.*, 1983). This type of information may eventually provide more complete explanations for the complex patterns of effects produced by these agents.

Aside from the stereochemical considerations mentioned above, few rules governing structure–activity relationships have emerged. In general, small amide derivatives of lysergic acid are potent and relatively selective antagonists of 5-HT, while the amino acid alkaloids are usually less selective and show similar affinities as blocking agents at α-adrenergic and tryptaminergic receptors. Dihydrogenated derivatives usually have fewer and less intense agonistic actions than do the parent alkaloids. Finally, insertion of a methyl group at position 1 usually results in compounds with less affinity for receptors for catecholamines and with more selective ability to block tryptaminergic receptors.

Uterus. All the natural alkaloids of ergot markedly increase the motor activity of the uterus. After small doses, contractions are increased in force or frequency, or both, but are followed by a normal degree of relaxation. As the dose is increased, contractions become more forceful and prolonged, resting tonus is markedly increased, and sustained contracture can result. Although this characteristic precludes their use for induction or facilitation of labor, it is quite compatible with their use post partum or post abortion to control bleeding and maintain uterine contraction. The sensitivity of the uterus to ergot alkaloids varies, especially with the degree of maturity and the stage of gestation, but even an immature uterus is stimulated. The gravid uterus is very sensitive, and small doses of ergot alkaloids can be given immediately post partum to obtain a marked uterine response, usually without significant side effects.

Although all natural ergot alkaloids have qualitatively the same effect on the uterus, they exhibit marked differences in potency. Ergonovine is the most active and is less toxic than ergotamine, the most potent of the amino acid alkaloids; unlike ergotamine, ergonovine is also effective after oral administration. For these reasons, ergonovine and its semisynthetic derivative, methylergonovine, have replaced other ergot preparations as uterine-stimulating agents in obstetrics.

Methylergonovine differs little from ergonovine in its uterine actions. The dihydrogenated alkaloids do not have the uterine-stimulating properties of the parent alkaloids when tested in experimental animals. However, they are capable of exerting a marked uterine-stimulating action on the pregnant human uterus at term.

The uterine-stimulating effect of ergot alkaloids apparently involves interactions with receptors for biogenic amines, in that cyproheptadine blocks the effects of both 5-HT and ergonovine in the rat uterus (Hashimoto *et al.*, 1977), while phentolamine blocks the effects of both norepinephrine and ergotamine, but not of oxytocin, in the rabbit uterus (*see* Berde and Stürmer, 1978).

Cardiovascular System. Ergotamine, the other natural amino acid alkaloids, and the dihydrogenated derivatives exert complex actions on the cardiovascular system. These are discussed further in Chapter 11.

The natural amino acid alkaloids, particularly ergotamine, constrict both arteries and veins. While dihydroergotamine retains appreciable vasoconstrictor activity, it is far more effective on capacitance than on resistance vessels. This property is the basis for investigation of its usefulness in the treatment of postural hypotension. The dihydrogenated derivatives of the ergotoxine group are considerably less active and usually produce hypotension because of effects in the CNS. In doses used in the treatment of migraine, the rectal administration of ergotamine produces little change in blood pressure but does cause a slowly progressing increase in peripheral vascular resistance that persists for up to 24 hours (Bülow *et al.*, 1986). Presumably, this reflects constriction of arteries mediated by stimulation of tryptaminergic receptors. Dihydroergotamine has relatively little capacity to produce such effects in man (Andersen *et al.*, 1987). At the higher plasma concentrations achieved by intravenous administration, both ergotamine and dihydroergotamine cause a rapid increase in blood pressure that dissipates in a few hours (Andersen *et al.*, 1987). This is thought to reflect action on arterioles, which in the rat results from stimulation of α_2-adrenergic receptors (Roquebert and Grenié, 1986). With the notable exception of the cerebrum, the prolonged increase in vascular resistance is accompanied by decreased blood flow in various organs. This results in part from reduced flow through nonnutritive arteriovenous anastomoses (*see* Saxena, 1978). While less potent than ergotamine, the amine alkaloids can also raise blood pressure slightly and decrease blood flow in the extremities when administered in therapeutic doses. The intensity of pressor effects is greater when the blood pressure is elevated.

Ergot alkaloids that produce peripheral vasoconstriction can also damage the capillary endothelium. The mechanism of this toxic action is not clearly understood. Vascular stasis, thrombosis, and gangrene result and are prominent features of ergot poisoning. The propensity of these alkaloids to cause gangrene appears to parallel their vasoconstrictor activity.

Vascular Responses Related to the Therapy of Migraine. Ergotamine is effective in relieving migraine headaches, even though it is neither a sedative nor an analgesic. The etiology of migraine is complex and poorly understood, and there are multiple forms of the syndrome that may involve different pathophysiological processes. Those attacks that are associated with a subjective "aura" or objective prodromal neurological signs and symptoms have been classified as "classical" migraine. For 40 years, the dominant view has been that the prodromal signs of classical migraine were caused by cerebral vasospasm with resultant localized ischemia, perhaps as a consequence of the release of 5-HT from platelets (*see* Wolff, 1987). Attacks without prodromal symptoms (classified as "common" migraine) were thought to begin in a similar, but less intense, fashion. This scenario is now disputed (*see* below), but there is less controversy over subsequent events, especially the prolonged period of increased blood flow in both intracerebral and extracranial vessels (Sakai and Meyer, 1978). The resultant increased amplitude of pulsations of the cranial arteries, chiefly the meningeal branches of the external carotid, is believed to be at least one source of the pain. Factors that decrease the amplitude of pulsation (*e.g.*, digital pressure on the carotid artery) reduce the intensity of the headache, and a parallel decline occurs in arterial pulsation when ergotamine provides relief from pain. In addition to reducing extracranial blood flow, ergotamine can decrease hyperperfusion of regions served by the basilar artery without decreasing cerebral hemispheric flow (Sakai and Meyer, 1978). There is also some evidence that opening of arteriovenous anastomoses during an attack contributes to the marked decrease in resistance to flow in areas served by the carotid artery (*see* Saxena, 1978). In experimental animals, therapeutic doses of ergotamine, acting perhaps as a tryptaminergic agonist, cause decreased shunting of blood from the carotid artery to the jugular vein. Indeed, agents that are selective agonists for a certain subtype of 5-HT_1 receptor in cephalic veins also abort migraine attacks (*see* Saxena and Ferrari, 1989).

Although no single unifying hypothesis has emerged, a number of observations appear to contradict important elements of the view described above. First, studies that employed sophisticated techniques for the measurement of regional cerebral blood flow have not detected areas of reduced flow at the onset of attacks of common migraine; moreover, they showed that attacks of classical migraine begin with a spreading wave of reduced blood flow that is usually preceded by focal hyperemia at some site (*see* Lauritzen, 1987). The pattern and progression of the oligemia are not consistent with a vasospastic episode in a major cerebral vessel, and the degree of hypoperfusion is not sufficient to produce signs and symptoms of ischemia. Hence, both the prodromal symptoms and the oligemia of classical migraine are thought to be separate consequences of unknown events in adjacent brain tissue. Second, dilatation of cranial noncerebral blood vessels alone cannot account for the intensity of the pain of migraine (*see* Spierings, 1988a). Neurogenic activation of pain fibers in the dura mater is thought to occur independent of vascular events during attacks, leading to a sterile inflammatory response and potentiation of subsequent painful stimuli. In animal models, both ergotamine and dihydroergotamine can block extravasation of plasma into the dura mater produced by electrical stimulation of the trigeminal nerve; this property is not exhibited by various other vasoconstrictor agents (Markowitz *et al.*, 1988; Saito *et al.*, 1988). Thus, the therapeutic effects of ergot alkaloids in migraine may not be a consequence of their vascular actions.

Absorption, Fate, and Excretion. The pharmacokinetic properties of ergotamine have been reviewed by Perrin (1985). Owing to extensive first-pass hepatic metabolism, the oral administration of ergotamine by itself results in undetectable concentrations of the drug systemically. The bioavailability after sublingual administration is also poor and is often inadequate for therapeutic purposes. Although the concurrent administration of caffeine (50 to 100 mg per 1 mg of ergotamine) improves both the rate and extent of absorption, the oral bioavailability of ergotamine in such preparations is probably still less than 1%, and peak concentrations in plasma of about 20 pg/ml are produced 70 minutes after a 2-mg dose. The bioavailability after administration of rectal suppositories is greater, and maximal plasma concentrations of ergotamine of over 400 pg/ml can be achieved following a 2-mg dose (Sanders *et al.*, 1986). However, there is little correspondence between the concentration of ergotamine in plasma and the intensity or duration of therapeutic or toxic effects. For example, although the bioavailability of ergotamine given intramuscularly averages nearly 50%, more than 50-fold the value for oral administration, the oral dose of ergotamine effective in producing uterine contractions is only about 10-fold the intramuscular dose. Ergotamine may be rapidly sequestered at its sites of action, or unidentified active substances may result from its hepatic metabolism.

Ergotamine is metabolized in the liver by largely undefined pathways, and 90% of the metabolites are excreted in the bile. Only traces of unmetabolized drug can be found in urine and feces. Despite a half-time of about 2 hours for its disappearance from plasma, ergotamine produces vasoconstriction that endures for 24 hours or longer (*see* above).

Bromocriptine is absorbed more completely after oral administration and is eliminated more slowly than is ergotamine. Dihydroergotamine and dihydroergotoxine are much less completely absorbed and are eliminated more rapidly than is ergotamine. The low bioavailability of dihydroergotamine is also apparently due primarily to rapid hepatic clearance (Little *et al.*, 1982). The amine alkaloids are rapidly and virtually completely absorbed after oral administration and reach peak concentrations in plasma within 60 to 90 minutes that are more than tenfold those achieved with an equivalent dose of ergotamine. A uterotonic effect can be observed within 10 minutes after oral administration of 0.2 mg of ergonovine to women post partum. Judging from the relative duration of action, ergonovine is metabolized and/or eliminated more rapidly than is ergotamine. The half-life of methylergonovine in plasma ranges between 0.5 and 2 hours (Mantyla and Kanto, 1981). Studies in animals indicate that the principal metabolites of the amine alkaloids are hydroxylated in the A ring, while the metabolism of the amino acid alkaloids primarily involves alterations in the tricyclopeptide moiety. Nearly all the metabolites recovered after the administration of methysergide to human subjects are devoid of the methyl group at position 1.

Toxicity. The ergot alkaloids are highly toxic and may cause acute or chronic poisoning. At present, however, the epidemic form of chronic ergot poisoning arising from the ingestion of contaminated grain is seldom seen. (For a description, *see previous editions* of this textbook.) Furthermore, when ergotamine is prescribed in correct dosage in the absence of contraindications, it is a safe and useful drug; few serious complications have been reported from its use in the migraine syndrome.

Nausea and vomiting occur in approximately 10% of patients after oral administration and in about twice that number after parenteral administration; the drug has a direct effect on CNS emetic centers. However, severe nausea is common during attacks of migraine regardless of treatment. Weakness in the legs is common, and muscle pains, which occasionally are quite severe, may occur in the extremities. Numbness and tingling of the fingers and toes are other reminders of the ergotism that this alkaloid may cause. Precordial distress and pain suggestive of angina pectoris, as well as transient tachycardia or bradycardia, have also been noted, presumably as a result of coronary vasospasm induced by ergotamine. At least one case of sudden death has been reported. Localized edema and itching may occur in an occasional hypersensitive patient. Most of these effects are not alarming and ordinarily do not necessitate interruption of ergotamine therapy. Contraindications to the use of ergot alkaloids are described below.

Treatment. The treatment of ergotism consists in complete withdrawal of the offending drug and symptomatic measures. The latter include attempts to maintain an adequate circulation to the affected parts. Pharmacological agents that have been employed include anticoagulants, low-molecular-weight dextran, and potent vasodilator drugs, especially the intravenous infusion of sodium nitroprusside. Nausea and vomiting may be relieved by atropine or by antiemetic compounds of the phenothiazine type.

Preparations and Routes of Administration. Only a few of the purified ergot alkaloids are available for therapeutic application. *Ergotamine tartrate* (ERGOMAR, others) is available in sublingual tablets that contain 2 mg of the salt. The drug is also available as a suspension for oral inhalation; each dose delivers 0.36 mg of the salt. Preparations containing mixtures of *ergotamine tartrate and caffeine* (CAFERGOT, others) are also available; tablets contain 1 mg of ergotamine tartrate and 100 mg of caffeine, and the corresponding suppositories contain 2 mg and 100 mg, respectively. *Dihydroergotamine mesylate* (D.H.E. 45) is supplied as a solution (1 mg/ml) for injection. *Methysergide maleate* (SANSERT) is available as oral tablets containing 2 mg.

Ergonovine maleate (ERGOTRATE MALEATE) is available in solution for injection (0.2 mg/ml) and in 0.2-mg oral tablets. *Methylergonovine maleate* (METHERGINE) is marketed for injection (0.2 mg/ml) and in 0.2-mg oral tablets.

Ergoloid mesylates (*dihydrogenated ergot alkaloids;* HYDERGINE, others) are available in 0.5- and 1.0-mg tablets. Each 0.5-mg tablet contains 0.167 mg each of dihydroergocornine, dihydroergocristine, and dihydroergocryptine (dihydro-α-ergocryptine and dihydro-β-ergocryptine in the proportion of 2:1) as the mesylates. A liquid containing 1 mg/ml and liquid-filled 1-mg capsules are also available.

Bromocriptine mesylate (PARLODEL) is supplied in 2.5-mg tablets and in 5-mg capsules.

THERAPEUTIC USES

The major therapeutic uses of the ergot alkaloids fall into two categories: (1) applications in obstetrics (discussed later in this chapter), and (2) treatment of migraine. The use of bromocriptine in the treatment of Parkinson's disease is discussed in Chapter 20, while the uses related to the suppression of the secretion of prolactin are presented in Chapter 56.

Migraine. Ergotamine remains an important agent for symptomatic relief of the pain of migraine, particularly in those patients for whom naproxen or other aspirin-like drugs provide incomplete relief (*see* Diamond and Millstein, 1988; Diamond and Solomon, 1988; Edmeads, 1988; Pradalier *et al.*, 1988). However, before reliance is placed on ergotamine or other medications, it is important that the physician attempt to assess and correct any underlying emotional or physical stresses, dietary or hormonal factors, or ingestion of drugs that may influence the incidence and severity of attacks.

Dosage and Route of Administration. Ergotamine is usually administered orally (in combination with caffeine) or sublingually; the dose is 2 mg, given as soon as the headache starts. Doses of 2 mg may be given at intervals of 30 minutes thereafter, if necessary, until a total of 6 mg has been taken. No more than 10 mg should be ingested per week.

Ergotamine may also be administered by oral inhalation. A single inhalation (0.36 mg) is used at the onset of an attack, and may be repeated at intervals of 5 minutes to a total of six doses in 24 hours. The maximal dosage in 1 week is 5.4 mg (about 15 inhalations).

If a patient cannot tolerate ergotamine orally, rectal administration of a mixture of caffeine and ergotamine tartrate may be attempted. At the onset of an attack, one suppository (2 mg) may be used, and another suppository may be used in 1 hour, if necessary. No more than two suppositories per attack or five suppositories per week should be administered.

Dihydroergotamine mesylate can be administered by intramuscular injection (1 mg, repeated at 1-hour intervals to a total of 3 mg) or, in some circumstances, intravenously (2 mg, maximum). No more than 6 mg should be given parenterally in 1 week.

Since overdosage is the chief cause of untoward effects from ergotamine, the smallest amount effective for relief of the headache should be used. The speed and thoroughness of the relief from pain are directly proportional to the promptness with which medication is started after the onset of an attack. If the drug is given early, the dose may be decreased considerably. If the headache has reached its peak, larger amounts of ergotamine are needed. Not only is a longer time then required for effective action but also unpleasant side effects from medication are more pronounced.

Efficacy. Ergotamine is effective in the vast majority of cases. The specificity of the drug for migraine is indicated by the fact that only occasionally are other types of headaches influenced. Relief is often dramatic. After parenteral injection of dihydroergotamine, the headache may disappear in 15 minutes, but sometimes only after 2 hours or more. Oral medication is much slower in bringing relief, an average of 5 hours being required, and it may fail in severe attacks. The drug is not useful in preventing attacks. Observance of the specified maximal weekly doses is important, not only to minimize the untoward effects of the drug but also to avoid possible dependence. Patients who take ergotamine daily for prolonged periods may require increased dosage to achieve relief and may experience rebound attacks of migraine.

Caffeine enhances the action of the ergot alkaloids in the treatment of migraine, a discovery that must be credited to the sufferers from the disease who observed that strong coffee gave symptomatic relief, especially when combined with the ergot alkaloids. As mentioned, caffeine increases the oral and rectal absorption of ergotamine, and it is widely believed that this accounts for its enhancement of therapeutic effects.

Contraindications. Because ergotamine-induced gangrene has occurred in a number of patients with infection, sepsis is a definite contraindication. It should not be used in patients with vascular disease, and diseases of the liver or kidney are also contraindications. Serious toxicity has been reported from the use of ergotamine in patients with pruritus, especially when the symptom is secondary to hepatic disease. Although very large amounts of ergotamine are required to produce abortion, pregnancy constitutes an objection to use.

Other Uses. The mixture of ergoloid mesylates has been widely used in the treatment of senile dementias. In a few apparently well-controlled studies, patients treated with dihydroergotoxine have displayed slight improvement in some behavioral or other psychological measures (*see* Loew and Weil, 1982). In one study, treatment with ergoloid mesylates for 8 weeks improved the perfusion of hypoxic brain regions (Hartmann and Tsuda, 1988); greater improvement in behavioral symptoms and cerebral blood flow was noted following the administration of pentoxifylline, an agent used to treat intermittent claudication (*see* Chapter 25). Nevertheless, the mechanisms that underlie any beneficial responses are poorly understood, and the subject remains controversial.

Ergonovine has been used as a provocative agent during coronary arteriography to aid in the diagnosis of angina pectoris secondary to coronary artery spasm (Prinzmetal's variant angina) (*see* Chapter 32).

Prophylaxis of Migraine. Because of the putative role of 5-HT in the genesis of attacks of migraine, attention was focused initially on tryptaminergic antagonists for use in prophylactic treatment. However, only a few such antagonists (notably methysergide) have been found to be effective. In recent years, there has been a proliferation of agents that either are, or appear to be, effective in reducing the number and/or severity of attacks. One of the most important problems in making such a judgment is the occurrence of a prominent placebo response. In addition, studies often do not make a distinction between effects in classical migraine and those in common migraine.

Propranolol. Propranolol is currently the preferred drug for the prophylaxis of migraine (*see* Diamond and Millstein, 1988). Its beneficial effects were first noted incidental to its use in the treatment of angina (*see* Chapter 11). About 70% of patients with either classical or common migraine experience fewer or less intense attacks during the administration of 80 to 160 mg of propranolol per day; the level of benefit remains constant for up to 12 months and often is maintained for 1 to 2 months after tapered discontinuation of the medication. The mechanisms that underlie this effect are not known, and the relevance of β-adrenergic blockade has been questioned (*see* Edmeads, 1988). While some other β-adrenergic antagonists (*e.g.*, atenolol, nadolol, and timolol) also appear to be effective, those with intrinsic sympathomimetic activity (*e.g.*, pindolol) are not.

Methysergide. Although methysergide is not useful for the treatment of acute attacks of migraine, it was the first agent found to be effective prophylactically. The proportion of patients who respond to methysergide (4 to 8 mg per day) is somewhat less than that for propranolol (*see* Saper, 1978). The major disadvantage to therapy with this drug is the danger of retroperitoneal fibrosis; drug-free periods of 3 to 4 weeks are recommended every 6 months. The relevance of tryptaminergic blockade to the beneficial effects of methysergide has been questioned because, with the exception of pizotyline, no other such antagonist has been found to be effective. On the other hand, it has been proposed that β-adrenergic antagonists with prophylactic actions also interact with certain tryptaminergic receptors in the CNS (*see* Edmeads, 1988).

Tricyclic Antidepressants. Amitriptyline, doxepin, and protriptyline appear to be about as effective as methysergide for the prophylaxis of migraine (*see* Diamond and Millstein, 1988). This effect seems relatively independent of antidepressant responses to the drugs since nondepressed patients with severe migraine have experienced improvement most frequently. The mechanisms that underlie this effect are not known. Patients who fail to respond to these agents or who are unable to tolerate them may respond to inhibitors of monoamine oxidase, such as phenelzine.

Aspirin-like Drugs. Several aspirin-like drugs have been evaluated for their effectiveness, both in aborting attacks of migraine and as prophylactic agents (*see* Pradalier *et al.*, 1988). These include aspirin, naproxen, ibuprofen, mefenamic acid, flufenamic acid, and tolfenamic acid. In general, this class of agents is especially effective in treating attacks of so-called menstrual migraine, and appear to be as effective as ergotamine in the treatment of common migraine, especially when metoclopramide is administered concurrently to combat gastric stasis during attacks. The results in classical migraine have been less consistent. Similarly, in the majority of trials that compared these drugs with agents such as propranolol, aspirin-like drugs were equally effective in reducing the number and severity of attacks. However, the doses employed were sometimes quite high (*e.g.*, 1100 mg of naproxen sodium per day), and it remains to be seen whether lower, less toxic doses will be as effective.

Ca^{2+}-Channel Blockers. Among this group of drugs are several agents that have shown promise for the prophylactic treatment of migraine and a related syndrome known as cluster headaches (*see* Greenberg, 1986; Olesen, 1986; Spierings, 1988b). Newer agents, such as flunarizine and nimodipine, appear to be more useful than verapamil and nifedipine. Of these, flunarizine has undergone the most extensive evaluation, and it may reduce the frequency of either classical or common migraine attacks by as much as 90%. It may also be effective in preventing more complicated syndromes, such as childhood hemiplegic migraine (*see* Caers *et al.*, 1987). It is of interest that maximal effects require 1 to 2 months of treatment. While their potential for combating vasospastic episodes prompted the initial trials of Ca^{2+}-channel blockers, it is not at all clear that actions on blood vessels are of importance in their efficacy as prophylactic agents. Flunarizine, for example, has anticonvulsant actions in man and can antagonize the production of spreading depression in the cerebral cortex of experimental animals. These observations have been used to support hypotheses regarding the neuronal origins of migraine. A general discussion of the pharmacology of Ca^{2+}-channel blockers appears in Chapter 32.

THE CLINICAL USE OF DRUGS THAT STIMULATE UTERINE MOTILITY

There are many indications for, and contraindications to, the clinical use of agents that stimulate uterine contractions (*see* Kruse, 1986; Brindley and Sokol, 1988; Curtis and Safransky, 1988). In brief, the clearest indications are (1) to induce or augment labor in *selected* individuals, (2) to control postpartum uterine atony and hemorrhage, (3) to cause uterine contraction after cesarean section or during other uterine surgery, and (4) to induce therapeutic abortion.

Induction of Labor. Although some physicians are less conservative when they utilize modern techniques to monitor the fetus during labor, the use of uterine-stimulating agents for the induction of labor is usually reserved for those cases where continuation of the pregnancy is considered to be a greater risk to the mother or fetus than the concomitant risks of pharmacological induction.

When it is determined that a medical indication exists for the termination of pregnancy (*e.g.*, maternal diabetes, isoimmunization, hypertensive states, anemia, prolonged pregnancy with placental insufficiency), a careful assessment of the clinical variables must be made. Objective determination of fetal maturity must also be made, and the possibility of fetopelvic disproportion should be considered. Other potential contraindications to induction of labor include abnormal fetal position, evidence of fetal distress, placental abnormalities, and previous uterine surgery.

The drug of choice for the induction of labor is oxytocin. For all antepartum indications except abortion, oxytocin should be given by intravenous infusion of a dilute solution, preferably by means of a variable-speed infusion pump. A suitable concentration for use in induction of labor at term is 10 milliunits per milliliter. Although there is continuing debate concerning the optimal procedure for the administration of oxytocin (*see* Brindley and Sokol, 1988; Curtis and Safransky, 1988), many physicians advocate the protocol developed by Seitchik and Castillo (1982, 1983). This involves an initial dose of 1 milliunit per minute, escalation of the dose at a rate no greater than 1 milliunit per minute every 30 minutes, and maintenance of a dose of 4 milliunits per minute (if attained) for at least 1 hour before increasing the dose further. In their hands, no patient has required a dose greater than 9 milliunits per minute. A more aggressive protocol has been recommended by O'Driscoll and Meagher (1986) for the *augmentation* (not *induction*) of labor in nulliparous patients, in whom the risk of uterine rupture is extremely low.

During the entire procedure, trained personnel must be present and uterine activity should be carefully monitored. If contractions become too forceful or frequent or resting tone is elevated, the infusion should be immediately discontinued. Changes in fetal heart rate are useful indicators of fetal distress. Occasionally, even the cautious use of oxytocin will stimulate the uterus to a sustained tetanic contraction, which may so interfere with the placental circulation that it may be necessary to administer a general anesthetic to effect uterine relaxation. As labor progresses, it may be necessary to decrease the dosage of oxytocin or to terminate the infusion. The infusion should be maintained at the lowest possible rate that will allow adequate progression of labor (Baxi *et al.*, 1980).

When employed at term, oxytocin induces labor in the majority of cases. If amniotomy is also used, as it is by many obstetricians, successful induction occurs in most cases (80 to 90%).

The prostaglandins are potential alternatives to oxytocin for the induction of labor. However, these agents have proven to be more valuable as adjunctive therapy in the management of spontaneous or induced labor for their effects on cervical ripening (*see* Symposium, 1983; Lange *et al.*, 1984; Brindley and Sokol, 1988). Although such use of prostaglandins is currently investigational in the United States, suitable preparations are under development.

The prostaglandins have the potential advantage of stimulating uterine contractions at any stage of pregnancy; thus, they are useful for the treatment of most cases of missed abortion, late intrauterine death, molar gestation, and premature rupture of the membranes (*see* Thiery and Amy, 1977).

Augmentation of Labor. In most circumstances, oxytocin should not be used for the augmentation of labor if labor is progressing, albeit slowly. The type of contraction produced often is too forceful and sustained to be compatible with the safety of mother and fetus. When the uterus, under the stimulus of a drug, contracts too forcibly against an incompletely dilated and rigid cervix, the following accidents may occur: (1) the force of the contraction may drive the presenting part through the incompletely dilated cervical tissues and cause severe laceration of the mother and trauma to the infant; (2) if the soft tissues are unyielding, the uterus may rupture; and (3) the forceful tetanic contraction of the uterus may compromise placental exchange and fetal oxygenation.

There are occasions, however, when oxytocin can be used advantageously by the experienced obstetrician to manage *dysfunctional labor*. Some authorities believe that prolongation of labor beyond 10 to 12 hours imposes unnecessary hazards on both the fetus and the mother (*see* O'Driscoll and Meagher, 1986). Since nulliparous patients frequently appear to benefit from treatment with oxytocin and are at little risk from uterine rupture, early intervention can be considered. Nevertheless, because the injudicious use of oxytocin can induce dysfunctional labor, cases should be selected carefully and dosage regulated continuously. Oxytocin is usually effective in patients with a very prolonged latent phase of cervical dilatation as well as in those cases where there is a significant arrest of dilatation or descent. When there is protracted dilatation or descent without actual arrest, a response to uterine-stimulating agents will generally not be obtained (*see* Friedman, 1978). In patients who are receiving epidural anesthesia, the reflexly stimulated release of oxytocin during the second stage of labor may be impaired (Goodfellow *et al.*, 1983). The cautious use of oxytocin may reduce the need to employ forceps for delivery under these circumstances.

Third Stage of Labor and Puerperium. After delivery of the fetus, it is desirable to have the uterus firm and active. This reduces greatly the incidence and extent of postpartum hemorrhage. However, the use of uterine-stimulating agents for this purpose has declined in recent years, in part because of the decreased utilization of general anesthetics during delivery. Indeed, there is little objective evidence for reduction of postpartum bleeding by the administration of either oxytocin or ergonovine in patients who have undergone normal vaginal deliveries (Pedrón *et al.*, 1987). With current obstetrical practices, there is little justification for the *routine* use of uterine-stimulating agents, especially since ergonovine may intensify uterine pain after delivery and may occasionally cause more serious side effects (Taylor and Cohen, 1985). When the decision is made to use uterine-stimulating agents, the usual procedure is to await delivery of the placenta before their administration. In any case, it is necessary to exclude the possibility of a multiple pregnancy before the drug is given. Ergonovine (or methylergonovine) is usually preferred for this use because of its sustained duration of action. The intramuscular injection of 0.2 mg produces a rapid and lasting response. Either alkaloid may also be given intravenously in a dose of 0.2 mg if immediate action is desirable. Alternatively, intramuscular injection of carboprost (250 μg) may be used; if necessary, additional doses can be administered at intervals of 15 to 90 minutes up to a maximal total dose of 2 mg.

In the normal individual, the period of uterine involution is 8 to 10 weeks, but the process is most rapid during the first 10 days. If involution is delayed, stimulation of the uterus is definitely helpful because delayed involution is usually associated with uterine atony. Under such conditions, either ergonovine (0.2 to 0.4 mg, two to four times daily) or methylergonovine (0.2 mg, three to four times daily) may be given orally for as long a period as is necessary to accomplish the desired results (usually 2 to 7 days). If infection develops in the postpartum uterus, the use of ergonovine may limit its spread. Caution must be observed in the use of ergonovine for an extended period of time. The possibility of interference with lactation must be considered with the use of either alkaloid.

Therapeutic Abortion. Abortion during the first trimester is most commonly accomplished by means of suction curettage. No satisfactory form of drug-induced abortion during this period is yet available. Beyond the first few weeks of the second trimester several alternative procedures for abortion are available. Intraamniotic injection of a hypertonic (20%) solution of sodium chloride has been used, but numerous failures occur and the procedure entails serious potential hazards for the patient. Vaginal suppositories of dinoprostone (PGE_2) inserted at intervals of 3 to 5 hours have been used effectively. In other circumstances, especially when the uterine contents have not been eliminated but the membranes are ruptured, the intramuscular administration of 0.25 mg of carboprost tromethamine (15-methyl $PGF_{2\alpha}$) has been effective; subsequent doses of up to 0.5 mg may be administered at approximately 2-hour intervals. Nausea, vomiting, and diarrhea are frequent side effects of the use of these prostaglandins. The intraamniotic instillation of low doses (5 to 10 mg) of $PGF_{2\alpha}$ in combination with a hyperosmolar solution of urea has been investigated and compared with the widely used method of dilatation and evacuation (Kafrissen *et al.*, 1984). The principal conclusion was that dilatation and evacuation remains the safest and most effective procedure available for abortion at 13 to 20 weeks' gestation.

After spontaneous or therapeutic abortion or premature delivery, the postpartum indications for ergonovine, oxytocin, and carboprost to control bleeding and maintain uterine tone are similar to those after delivery at term.

Oxytocin-Challenge Test. Oxytocin has been used for an antepartum test of uteroplacental insufficiency in high-risk pregnancies. Oxytocin is infused initially at the rate of 0.5 milliunit per minute; this rate is increased slowly until uterine contractions occur every 3 to 4 minutes. Concurrent monitoring of the pattern of the fetal heart rate indicates whether the contractions result in signs of fetal distress. The outcome of the oxytocin-challenge test is helpful in determining the presence of adequate placental reserve for continuation of a high-risk pregnancy (Freeman, 1975).

THE CLINICAL USE OF DRUGS THAT INHIBIT UTERINE MOTILITY

There are several indications for, and contraindications to, the clinical use of agents that inhibit uterine contractions. The clearest indications are (1) to delay or prevent premature parturition in selected individuals and (2) to slow or arrest delivery for brief periods in order to undertake other therapeutic measures. Tocolytic agents that are currently in use include β_2-adrenergic agonists (*see* Chapter 10), magnesium sulfate (*see* Chapter 27), and ethanol (*see* Chapter 17). The use of tocolytic agents has been reviewed in several symposia (Symposium, 1981, 1982) and by Caritis (1983).

Premature Labor. Premature births account for a large fraction of perinatal morbidity and mortality. Despite major advances in neonatal care, retention of the fetus *in utero* is preferred in most instances. It is often difficult to determine whether premature birth is imminent, and 50% or more of patients who present with regular uterine contractions will respond to bed rest and hydration. If this fails, a tocolytic agent may be administered. However, the desire to prolong intrauterine development must be balanced against the risks of continued pregnancy to both the mother and fetus, as well as the risks of pharmacological intervention. In general, the use of tocolytic agents is reserved for those pregnancies where the gestational age is greater than 20 weeks and less than 34 to 36 weeks; at the more advanced gestational ages, definite evidence for immaturity of the fetus is usually sought. When the decision to use a tocolytic agent is made, therapeutic success is most likely if cervical dilatation is less than 4 cm and cervical effacement is less than 80%; tocolysis is usually not attempted if the membranes have ruptured, since there is risk of infection. Other contraindications for tocolysis include eclampsia or severe preeclampsia, chorioamnionitis, premature detachment of the placenta, and fetal distress.

β_2-Adrenergic Agonists. These agents are preferred for the treatment of premature labor. Currently, only *ritodrine* is approved for this use in the United States. *Ritodrine hydrochloride* (YUTOPAR) is available in a solution (10 or 15 mg/ml) for intravenous administration and in 10-mg oral tablets. Treatment is initiated by the intravenous infusion of a solution of ritodrine (0.3 mg/ml) at the rate of 0.1 mg per minute. If tolerated, the dose is gradually increased (0.05 mg per minute every 10 minutes) to a maximum of 0.35 mg per minute or until labor is controlled. Once contractions cease, the infusion is usually continued for at least 12 hours at the rate attained. Oral therapy is begun 30 minutes before termination of the infusion by the administration of 10 mg every 2 hours for the first 24 hours,

followed by 10 to 20 mg every 4 to 6 hours; the total daily dose should not exceed 120 mg.

As might be expected, the administration of ritodrine or other β_2-adrenergic agonists produces a number of cardiovascular and metabolic side effects in the mother (*see* Chapter 10). Although mean arterial pressure changes very little, a dose-related tachycardia and increase in cardiac output occurs that probably results from a reflex response to the lowered diastolic blood pressure combined with direct actions on β_1-adrenergic receptors in the heart. The secretion of renin is enhanced, and this presumably contributes to the decreased renal excretion of Na^+, K^+, and water that occurs. If hydration during therapy is overly vigorous, pulmonary edema may result, either with or without evidence of myocardial failure. Total fluid intake should be restricted to less than 2 liters in 24 hours, and noninvasive monitoring of cardiovascular parameters, including pulmonary capillary pressure, has been advocated (Hadi *et al.*, 1987). Evidence of cardiac disease is a contraindication to the use of these agents.

Ritodrine and similar drugs can cause marked hyperglycemia. While this usually does not require treatment, persistent hyperglycemia (>200 mg/dl) may result in reactive hypoglycemia in the infant should parturition proceed. The use of β_2-adrenergic agonists in patients with insulin-dependent diabetes is hazardous and is usually considered to be contraindicated. In most cases, the concomitant infusion of insulin is required to prevent the development of diabetic ketoacidosis. Hypokalemia is another consequence of the administration of ritodrine. Since this reflects the movement of K^+ into the intracellular compartment, total body stores are not reduced and treatment is not indicated.

A number of other selective β_2-adrenergic agonists have also been employed for the management of preterm labor, including *terbutaline, fenoterol,* and *albuterol.* The indications, contraindications, and side effects associated with the use of any of these agents are similar to those for ritodrine.

Magnesium Sulfate. The major indication for the administration of magnesium sulfate to pregnant women is for the prevention or control of seizures associated with eclampsia or severe preeclampsia. At doses somewhat higher than those useful in these conditions, uterine contractions can be effectively inhibited. In the presence of normal renal function, magnesium sulfate may be a useful alternative when the use of a β_2-adrenergic agonist is contraindicated. A variety of protocols has been used. The regimen recommended by Petrie (Symposium, 1981) involves the intravenous administration of a loading dose of 6 g of magnesium sulfate over a period of 20 minutes, followed by an infusion at the rate of 2 g per hour until the frequency of uterine contractions is reduced to less than 1 every 10 minutes. Thereafter, the rate of infusion is reduced to 1 g per hour, and therapy is continued for 24 to 72 hours. More prolonged infusions (up to 6 weeks) have also been employed (Wilkins *et al.*, 1986; Dudley *et al.*, 1989). Oral therapy with magnesium gluconate (1 g every 2 to 4 hours) may prove to be of value in patients whose labor has been arrested by intravenous tocolysis (Martin *et al.*, 1987, 1988). If cervical dilatation progresses beyond 5 cm, the administration of magnesium sulfate is discontinued. Effective inhibition of uterine contractions has been associated with concentrations of Mg^{2+} in plasma of 4 to 8 mg/dl (3.3 to 6.6 mEq/liter). Higher concentrations produce progressive inhibition of cardiac conduction and neuromuscular transmission and can lead to respiratory depression and cardiac arrest (*see* Chapter 27). Neonatal depression can also occur; this may be alleviated by the administration of a calcium salt. The prolonged administration of magnesium salts may produce congenital rickets, perhaps by suppression of the fetal parathyroid gland (Lamm *et al.*, 1988).

The concurrent administration of magnesium sulfate and ritodrine is without demonstrable benefit over the use of a single agent and increases the incidence of cardiovascular side effects, especially myocardial ischemia (Ferguson *et al.*, 1984, 1987; Wilkins *et al.*, 1988).

Ethanol. Ethanol has been used for nearly 2 decades in the prevention of premature labor. While ethanol may be nearly as effective as ritodrine in prolonging gestation, it does not produce a corresponding reduction in the incidence of fetal respiratory distress (*see* Fuchs and Fuchs, in Symposium, 1981). As a result, it has been largely supplanted by β_2-adrenergic agonists. Nevertheless, circumstances remain in which other agents are contraindicated (*e.g.*, cardiac disease) and in which ethanol may be useful. Inhibition of uterine contractions is associated with concentrations of ethanol in plasma of 0.12 to 0.18%. These are achieved by the intravenous infusion of a 10% solution at a rate of 7.5 ml/kg per hour for 2 hours and maintained by infusion at a rate of 1.5 ml/kg per hour for up to 10 hours.

Other Agents. Ca^{2+}-Channel blockers are known to relax the myometrium *in vitro* and to inhibit markedly the amplitude (but not the frequency) of oxytocin-induced contractions. Despite indications of clinical efficacy, observations in experimental animals suggest that Ca^{2+}-channel blockers may reduce placental perfusion to the extent that fetal hypoxemia and acidosis are produced (Ducsay *et al.*, 1987; Holbrook *et al.*, 1987). Although inhibitors of prostaglandin synthesis, such as indomethacin, can prolong gestation in both term and preterm pregnancies, their use in the management of premature labor has been curtailed because of concern for their potential to cause adverse effects in the fetus. Of particular importance is the possibility of premature closure of the ductus arteriosus and the production of pulmonary hypertension. However, fetal echocardiography can detect early signs of constriction of the ductus arteriosus, and its use may permit the continued administration of indomethacin or related agents in those instances where evidence of ductal constriction is absent (Moise *et al.*, 1988).

Other Uses. There are a number of circumstances in which inhibition of uterine contractions for brief periods would provide the opportunity to initiate other therapeutic measures under more favorable conditions. Among the more obvious of these is the alleviation of fetal distress during transport of the mother to hospital or during preparation for operative delivery that might be necessitated by such complications as a breech presentation, prolapsed cord, or partial premature detachment of the placenta (*see* Lipshitz, in Symposium, 1981). Both β_2-adrenergic agonists and magnesium sulfate have been used successfully for the management of these and other complications of both spontaneous and induced labor.

Amico, J. A.; Seitchik, J.; and Robinson, A. G. Studies of oxytocin in plasma of women during hypocontractile labor. *J. Clin. Endocrinol. Metab.*, **1984**, *58*, 274–279.

Andersen, A. R.; Tfelt-Hansen, P.; and Lassen, N. A. The effect of ergotamine and dihydroergotamine on cerebral blood flow in man. *Stroke*, **1987**, *18*, 120–123.

Arias, F. Efficacy and safety of low-dose 15-methyl prostaglandin $F_{2\alpha}$ for cervical ripening in the first trimester of pregnancy. *Am. J. Obstet. Gynecol.*, **1984**, *149*, 100–101.

Barger, G.; Carr, F. H.; and Dale, H. H. An active alkaloid from ergot. *Br. Med. J.*, **1906**, *2*, 1792.

Baxi, L. V.; Petrie, R. H.; and Caritis, S. N. Induction of labor with low-dose prostaglandin $F_{2\alpha}$ and oxytocin. *Am. J. Obstet. Gynecol.*, **1980**, *136*, 28–31.

Bülow, P. M.; Ibraheem, J. J.; Paalzow, G.; and Tfelt-Hansen, P. Comparison of pharmacodynamic effects and plasma levels of oral and rectal ergotamine. *Cephalalgia*, **1986**, *6*, 107–111.

Burbach, J. P. H.; Bohus, B.; Kovacs, G. L.; Van Nispen, J. W.; Greven, H. M.; and De Wied, D. Oxytocin is a precursor of potent behaviourally active neuropeptides. *Eur. J. Pharmacol.*, **1983**, *94*, 125–131.

Dayanithi, G.; Cazalis, M.; and Nordmann, J. J. Relaxin affects the release of oxytocin and vasopressin from the neurohypophysis. *Nature*, **1987**, *325*, 813–816.

De Geest, K.; Thiery, M.; Piron-Possuyt, G.; and Vanden Driessche, R. Plasma oxytocin in human pregnancy and parturition. *J. Perinat. Med.*, **1985**, *13*, 3–13.

Ducsay, C. A.; Thompson, J. S.; Wu, A. T.; and Novy, M. J. Effects of calcium entry blocker (nicardipine) tocolysis in rhesus macaques: fetal plasma concentrations and cardiorespiratory changes. *Am. J. Obstet. Gynecol.*, **1987**, *157*, 1482–1486.

Dudley, D.; Gagnon, D.; and Varner, M. Long-term tocolysis with intravenous magnesium sulfate. *Obstet. Gynecol.*, **1989**, *73*, 373–378.

Ferguson, J. E., II; Hensleigh, P. A.; and Kredenster, D. Adjunctive use of magnesium sulfate with ritodrine for preterm labor tocolysis. *Am. J. Obstet. Gynecol.*, **1984**, *148*, 166–171.

Ferguson, J. E., II; Holbrook, R. H., Jr.; Stevenson, D. K.; Hensleigh, P. A.; and Kredenster, D. Adjunctive magnesium sulfate infusion does not alter metabolic changes associated with ritodrine tocolysis. *Am. J. Obstet. Gynecol.*, **1987**, *156*, 103–107.

Freeman, R. K. The use of the oxytocin challenge test for antepartum clinical evaluation of uteroplacental respiratory function. *Am. J. Obstet. Gynecol.*, **1975**, *121*, 481–489.

Fuchs, A.-R. Prostaglandin F2alpha and oxytocin interactions in ovarian and uterine function. *J. Steroid Biochem.*, **1987**, *27*, 1073–1080.

Garrioch, D. B. The effect of indomethacin on spontaneous activity in the isolated human myometrium and on the response to oxytocin and prostaglandin. *Br. J. Obstet. Gynaecol.*, **1978**, *85*, 47–52.

Goodfellow, C. F.; Hull, M. G. R.; Swaab, D. F.; Dogterom, J.; and Buijs, R. M. Oxytocin deficiency at delivery with epidural analgesia. *Br. J. Obstet. Gynaecol.*, **1983**, *90*, 214–219.

Gundlach, A. L.; Krstich, M.; and Beart, P. M. Guanine nucleotides reveal differential actions of ergot derivatives at D-2 receptors labelled by [^{3}H]spiperone in striatal homogenates. *Brain Res.*, **1983**, *278*, 155–163.

Hadi, H. A.; Abdulla, A. M.; Fadel, H. E.; Stefadouros, M. A.; and Metheny, W. P. Cardiovascular effects of ritodrine tocolysis: a new noninvasive method to measure pulmonary capillary pressure during pregnancy. *Obstet. Gynecol.*, **1987**, *70*, 608–612.

Hartmann, A., and Tsuda, Y. A controlled study on the effect of pentoxifylline and an ergot alkaloid derivative on regional cerebral blood flow in patients with chronic cerebrovascular disease. *Angiology*, **1988**, *39*, 449–457.

Hashimoto, H.; Hayashi, M.; Nakahara, Y.; Niwaguchi, T.; and Ishii, H. Actions of D-lysergic acid diethylamide (LSD) and its derivatives on 5-hydroxytryptamine receptors in the isolated uterine smooth muscle of the rat. *Eur. J. Pharmacol.*, **1977**, *45*, 341–348.

Holbrook, R. H., Jr.; Lirette, M.; and Katz, M. Cardiovascular and tocolytic effects of nicardipine HCl in the pregnant rabbit: comparison with ritodrine HCl. *Obstet. Gynecol.*, **1987**, *69*, 83–87.

Kafrissen, M. E.; Schulz, K. F.; Grimes, D. A.; and Cates, W., Jr. Midtrimester abortion. Intra-amniotic instillation of hyperosmolar urea and prostaglandin $F_{2\alpha}$ *v* dilatation and evacuation. *J.A.M.A.*, **1984**, *251*, 916–919.

Kent, D. R.; Goldstein, A. I.; and Milokovich, D. Preoperative cervical dilatation with a single long-acting prostaglandin analog suppository. *J. Reprod. Med.*, **1983**, *28*, 778–780.

Kraft, F. Über das Mutterkorn. *Arch. Pharm.*, **1906**, *244*, 336–359.

Lamm, C. I.; Norton, K. I.; Murphy, R. J.; Wilkins, I. A.; and Rabinowitz, J. G. Congenital rickets associated with magnesium sulfate infusion for tocolysis. *J. Pediatr.*, **1988**, *113*, 1078–1082.

Land, H.; Grez, M.; Ruppert, S.; Schmale, H.; Rehbain, M.; Richter, D.; and Schütz, G. Deduced amino acid sequence from the bovine oxytocin—neurophysin I precursor cDNA. *Nature*, **1983**, *302*, 342–344.

Lange, I. R.; Collister, C.; Johnson, J.; Cote, D.; Torchia, M.; Freund, G.; and Manning, F. A. The effect of vaginal prostaglandin E_2 pessaries on induction of labor. *Am. J. Obstet. Gynecol.*, **1984**, *148*, 621–629.

Legros, J. J.; Chiodera, P.; Geenen, V.; Smitz, S.; and von Frenckell, R. Dose-response relationship between plasma oxytocin and cortisol and adrenocorticotropin concentrations during oxytocin infusion in normal men. *J. Clin. Endocrinol. Metab.*, **1984**, *58*, 105–109.

Little, P. J.; Jennings, G. L.; Skews, H.; and Bobik, A. Bioavailability of dihydroergotamine in man. *Br. J. Clin. Pharmacol.*, **1982**, *13*, 785–790.

McPherson, G. A., and Beart, P. M. The selectivity of some ergot derivatives for α_1 and α_2-adrenoceptors of rat cerebral cortex. *Eur. J. Pharmacol.*, **1983**, *91*, 363–369.

Majkić-Singh, N.; Vuković, A.; Spasić, S.; Ruzic, A.; Stojanov, M.; and Berkés, I. Oxytocinase (CAP) activity in serum during normal pregnancy. *Clin. Biochem.*, **1982**, *15*, 152–153.

Mantyla, R., and Kanto, J. Clinical pharmacokinetics of methylergometrine (methylergonovine). *Int. J. Clin. Pharmacol. Ther. Toxicol.*, **1981**, *19*, 386–391.

Markowitz, S.; Saito, K.; and Moskowitz, A. Neurogenically mediated plasma extravasation in dura mater: effect of ergot alkaloids. *Cephalalgia*, **1988**, *8*, 83–91.

Markstein, R.; Closse, A.; and Frick, W. Interaction of ergot alkaloids and their combination (co-dergocrine) with α-adrenoceptors in the CNS. *Eur. J. Pharmacol.*, **1983**, *93*, 159–168.

Martin, R. W.; Gaddy, D. K.; Martin, J. N., Jr.; Lucas, J. A.; Wiser, W. L.; and Morrison, J. C. Tocolysis with oral magnesium. *Am. J. Obstet. Gynecol.*, **1987**, *156*, 433–434.

Martin, R. W.; Martin, J. N., Jr.; Pryor, J. A.; Gaddy, D. K.; Wiser, W. L.; and Morrison, J. C. Comparison of oral ritodrine and magnesium gluconate for ambulatory tocolysis. *Am. J. Obstet. Gynecol.*, **1988**, *158*, 1440–1445.

Moir, C. The action of ergot preparations on the puerperal uterus. *Br. Med. J.*, **1932**, *1*, 1119–1122.

Moise, K. J., Jr.; Huhta, J. C.; Sharif, D. S.; Ou, C.-N.; Kirshon, B.; Wasserstrum, N.; and Cano, L. Indomethacin in the treatment of premature labor. *N. Engl. J. Med.*, **1988**, *319*, 327–331.

Pedrón, N.; Mondragón, H.; Marcushamer, B.; Aznar, R.; and Gallegos, A. J. Estimates of postpartum bleeding. *Contraception*, **1987**, *35*, 339–344.

Rholam, M.; Nicolas, P.; and Cohen, P. Binding of neurohypophyseal peptides to neurophysin dimer promotes formation of compact and spherical complexes. *Biochemistry*, **1982**, *21*, 4968–4973.

Roquebert, J., and Grenié, B. α_2-Adrenergic agonist and α_1-adrenergic antagonist activity of ergotamine and dihydroergotamine in rats. *Arch. Int. Phramacodyn. Ther.*, **1986**, *284*, 30–37.

Saito, K.; Markowitz, S.; and Moskowitz, M. A. Ergot alkaloids block neurogenic extravasation in dura mater: proposed action in vascular headaches. *Ann. Neurol.*, **1988**, *24*, 732–737.

Sakai, F., and Meyer, J. S. Regional cerebral hemodynamics during migraine and cluster headaches measured by the ^{133}Xe inhalation method. *Headache*, **1978**, *18*, 122–132.

Sanders, S. W.; Haering, N.; Mosberg, H.; and Jaeger, H. Pharmacokinetics of ergotamine in healthy volunteers following oral and rectal dosing. *Eur. J. Clin. Pharmacol.*, **1986**, *30*, 331–334.

Seitchik, J., and Castillo, M. Oxytocin augmentation of dysfunctional labor. I. Clinical data. *Am. J. Obstet. Gynecol.*, **1982**, *144*, 899–905.

———. Oxytocin augmentation of dysfunctional labor. III. Multiparous patients. *Ibid.*, **1983**, *145*, 777–780.

Spierings, E. L. H. Clinical and experimental evidence for a role of calcium entry blockers in the treatment of migraine. *Ann. N.Y. Acad. Sci.*, **1988b**, *522*, 676–689.

Stoll, A. Zur Kenntnis der Mutterkornalkaloide. *Verh. Naturf. Ges. (Basel)*, **1920**, *101*, 190–191.

Taylor, G. J., and Cohen, B. Ergonovine-induced coronary artery spasm and myocardial infarction after normal delivery. *Obstet. Gynecol.*, **1985**, *66*, 821–822.

Thoms, H. John Stearns and pulvis parturiens. *Am. J. Obstet. Gynecol.*, **1931**, *22*, 418–423.

Uldbjerg, N.; Ekman, G.; Malmström, A.; Olsson, K.; and Ulmsten, U. Ripening of the human uterine cervix related to changes in collagen, glycosaminoglycans, and collagenolytic activity. *Am. J. Obstet. Gynecol.*, **1983**, *147*, 662–666.

Wikland, M.; Lindblom, B.; Wilhelmsson, L.; and Wiqvist, N. Oxytocin, prostaglandins, and contractility of the human uterus at term pregnancy. *Acta Obstet. Gynecol. Scand.*, **1982**, *61*, 467–472.

Wilkins, I. A.; Goldberg, J. D.; Phillips, R. N.; Bacall, C. J.; Chervenak, F. A.; and Berkowitz, R. L. Long-term use of magnesium sulfate as a tocolytic agent. *Obstet. Gynecol.*, **1986**, *67*, Suppl. 3, 38S–40S.

Wilkins, I. A.; Lynch, L.; Mehalek, K. E.; Berkowitz, G. S.; and Berkowitz, R. L. Efficacy and side effects of magnesium sulfate and ritodrine as tocolytic agents. *Am. J. Obstet. Gynecol.*, **1988**, *159*, 685–689.

Monographs and Reviews

Altura, B. M., and Altura, B. T. Actions of vasopressin, oxytocin, and synthetic analogs on vascular smooth muscle. *Fed. Proc.*, **1984**, *43*, 80–86.

Angle, M. J., and Johnston, J. M. Fetal tissues in autacoid biosynthesis in relation to the initiation of parturition and implantation. In, *The Cellular Basis of Uterine Function.* (Carsten, M., ed.) Plenum Press, New York, **1990**, In Press.

Berde, B., and Stürmer, E. Introduction to the pharmacology of ergot alkaloids and related compounds as a basis of their therapeutic application. In, *Ergot Alkaloids and Related Compounds.* (Berde, B., and Schild, H. O., eds.) *Handbuch der Experimentellen Pharmakologie*, Vol. 49. Springer-Verlag, Berlin, **1978**, pp. 1–28.

Brindley, B. A., and Sokol, R. J. Induction and augmentation of labor: basis and methods for current practice. *Obstet. Gynecol. Surv.*, **1988**, *43*, 730–743.

Buijs, R. M. Vasopressin and oxytocin—their role in neurotransmission. *Pharmacol. Ther.*, **1983**, *22*, 127–141.

Caers, L. I.; De Beukelaar, F.; and Amery, W. K. Flunarizine, a calcium-entry blocker, in childhood migraine, epilepsy, and alternating hemiplegia. *Clin. Neuropharmacol.*, **1987**, *10*, 162–168.

Caritis, S. N. Treatment of preterm labour: a review of the therapeutic options. *Drugs*, **1983**, *26*, 243–261.

Carsten, M. E., and Miller, J. D. A new look at uterine muscle contraction. *Am. J. Obstet. Gynecol.*, **1987**, *157*, 1303–1315.

Curtis, P., and Safransky, N. Rethinking oxytocin protocols in the augmentation of labor. *Birth*, **1988**, *15*, 199–202.

Diamond, S., and Millstein, E. Current concepts of migraine therapy. *J. Clin. Pharmacol.*, **1988**, *28*, 193–199.

Diamond, S., and Solomon, G. D. Pharmacologic treatment of migraine. *Ration. Drug Ther.*, **1988**, *22*, 1–6.

Edmeads, J. G. Migraine. *Can. Med. Assoc. J.*, **1988**, *138*, 107–113.

Friedman, E. A. *Labor: Clinical Evaluation and Management*, 2nd ed. Appleton-Century-Crofts, New York, **1978.**

Greenberg, D. A. Calcium channel antagonists and the treatment of migraine. *Clin. Neuropharmacol.*, **1986**, *9*, 311–328.

Hai, C.-M., and Murphy, R. A. Ca^{2+}, Crossbridge phosphorylation, and contraction. *Annu. Rev. Physiol.*, **1989**, *51*, 285–298.

Huszar, G., and Roberts, J. M. Biochemistry and pharmacology of the myometrium and labor: regulation at the cellular and molecular levels. *Am. J. Obstet. Gynecol.*, **1982**, *142*, 225–237.

Kamm, K. E., and Stull, J. T. Regulation of smooth muscle contractile elements by second messengers. *Annu. Rev. Physiol.*, **1989**, *51*, 299–313.

Kao, C. Y. Electrophysiological properties of the uterine smooth muscle. In, *Biology of the Uterus.* (Wynn, R. M., ed.) Plenum Press, New York, **1977**, pp. 423–496.

Kruse, J. Oxytocin: pharmacology and clinical application. *J. Fam. Pract.*, **1986**, *23*, 473–479.

Lauritzen, M. Cerebral blood flow in migraine and cortical spreading depression. *Acta Neurol. Scand.* [*Suppl.*], **1987**, *113*, 1–40.

Loew, D. M., and Weil, C. Hydergine in senile mental impairment. *Gerontology*, **1982**, *28*, 54–74.

Müller-Schweinitzer, E., and Weidmann, H. Basic pharmacological properties. In, *Ergot Alkaloids and Related Compounds.* (Berde, B., and Schild, H. O., eds.) *Handbuch der Experimentellen Pharmakologie*, Vol. 49. Springer-Verlag, Berlin, **1978**, pp. 87–232.

O'Driscoll, K. M., and Meagher, D. J. *Active Management of Labour: The Dublin Experience*, 2nd ed. Balliere Tindall, London, **1986.**

Olesen, J. Role of calcium entry blockers in the prophylaxis of migraine. *Eur. Neurol.*, **1986**, *25*, Suppl. 1, 72–79.

Owen, P. R. Prostaglandin synthetase inhibitors in the treatment of primary dysmenorrhea. *Am. J. Obstet. Gynecol.*, **1984**, *148*, 96–103.

Perrin, V. L. Clinical pharmacokinetics of ergotamine in migraine and cluster headache. *Clin. Pharmacokinet.*, **1985**, *10*, 334–352.

Petty, M. A. The cardiovascular effects of the neurohypophysial hormone oxytocin. *J. Auton. Pharmacol.*, **1987**, *7*, 97–104.

Pradalier, A.; Clapin, A.; and Dry, J. Treatment review: non-steroid anti-inflammatory drugs in the treatment and long-term prevention of migraine attacks. *Headache*, **1988**, *28*, 550–557.

Roy, A. C., and Karim, S. M. M. Significance of the inhibition by prostaglandins and cyclic GMP of oxytocinase activity in human pregnancy and labour. *Prostaglandins*, **1983**, *25*, 55–70.

Rutschmann, J., and Stadler, P. A. Chemical background. In, *Ergot Alkaloids and Related Compounds*. (Berde, B., and Schild, H. O., eds.) *Handbuch der Experimentellen Pharmakologie*, Vol. 49. Springer-Verlag, Berlin, **1978**, pp. 29–85.

Saper, J. R. Migraine. II. Treatment. *J.A.M.A.*, **1978**, *239*, 2480–2484.

Saxena, P. R. Arteriovenous shunting and migraine. *Res. Clin. Stud. Headache*, **1978**, *6*, 89–102.

Saxena, P. R., and Ferrari, M. D. 5-HT_1-Like receptor agonists and the pathophysiology of migraine. *Trends Pharmacol. Sci.*, **1989**, *10*, 200–204.

Spierings, E. L. H. Recent advances in the understanding of migraine. *Headache*, **1988a**, *28*, 655–658.

Symposium. (Various authors.) Preterm parturition. (Creasy, R. K., ed.) *Semin. Perinatol.*, **1981**, *5*, 191–302.

Symposium. (Various authors.) Beta-receptor agonists in obstetrics. (Ingemarsson, I., ed.) *Acta Obstet. Gynecol. Scand.*, **1982**, *108*, Suppl. 1, 13–72.

Symposium. (Various authors.) The forces of labor: uterine contractions and the resistance of the cervix. (Ulmsten, U., and Ueland, K., eds.) *Clin. Obstet. Gynecol.*, **1983**, *26*, 1–106.

Tfelt-Hansen, P. The effect of ergotamine on the arterial system in man. *Acta Pharmacol. Toxicol.*, **1986**, *59*, Suppl. 3, 1–29.

Thiery, M., and Amy, J. Spontaneous and induced labor: two roles for the prostaglandins. *Obstet. Gynecol. Annu.*, **1977**, *6*, 127–171.

van Breemen, C., and Saida, K. Cellular mechanisms regulating $[Ca^{2+}]_i$ smooth muscle. *Annu. Rev. Physiol.*, **1989**, *51*, 315–329.

Weiss, G. The production and function of ovarian relaxin. In, *The Primate Ovary*. (Stouffer, R. L., ed.) Plenum Press, New York, **1987**, pp. 223–236.

Wolff, H. G. *Wolff's Headache and Other Head Pain*, 5th ed. (Dalessio, D. J., ed.) Oxford University Press, New York, **1987**.

SECTION

X

Chemotherapy of Parasitic Infections

INTRODUCTION

Leslie T. Webster, Jr.

Parasitic infections are a major worldwide health problem; this is particularly true in less-developed countries, where these diseases also cause a substantial economic burden. The global prevalence of human parasitic infections already exceeds 50% and is increasing. Diverse factors are responsible, including population crowding; poor sanitation and health education; inadequate control of parasite vectors and reservoirs of infection; introduction of agricultural water control and supply systems; increased world travel, population migration, and military operations; and development of resistance to agents used for chemotherapy or control of vectors. A few parasitic infections, such as malaria, attract attention and resources because, without treatment, they cause high morbidity and mortality. But most, such as those caused by the majority of pathogenic helminths, remain neglected because their effects on human health are more subtle.

Despite encouraging progress in identifying promising molecular targets for intervention with vaccines, chemotherapy remains the single most effective, efficient, and inexpensive method to control most parasitic infections. For optimal results, such therapies must be combined with other public health measures appropriate for the particular infection, environment, and host population. Safe and effective drugs for the treatment of certain serious parasitic infections, such as leishmaniasis and trypanosomiasis, have yet to be discovered. The development of resistance to currently effective agents, such as the antimalarials, also poses an ongoing challenge. Basic research and the development and surveillance of promising pharmaceuticals must continue to ensure the availability of improved antiparasitic compounds and to detect possible long-term toxicity, rare but life-threatening reactions, and drug resistance.

To be used for mass chemotherapy, an ideal antiparasitic agent should be safe at high therapeutic doses; easily given, preferably by the oral route in a single dose or divided doses on the same day; chemically stable for long periods under climatic conditions of use; ineffective as an inducer of drug resistance; and inexpensive. Few antiparasitic drugs meet all of these criteria.

Most antiparasitic agents have been discovered by screening many natural products and synthetic compounds for efficacy against pathogenic parasites in appropriate animal models. This traditional strategy is now complemented by research aimed at elucidating aspects of parasite and host biology that can be selectively exploited to chemotherapeutic advantage. The latter approach demands increased understanding of the basic biochemistry, physiology, and cell and molecular biology of parasites and of their interactions with their hosts. Improved methods to maintain parasites *in vitro* and to screen compounds *in vitro* and *in vivo* for antiparasitic activity are also needed to accelerate this process. However, the crucial test remains the demonstration of efficacy and safety of a given drug in man.

Table X–1. DRUGS FOR CHEMOTHERAPY OF PARASITIC INFECTIONS

The recommendations presented here represent the best judgment not only of the author but also of several authorities in the United States and abroad. However, this field is a dynamic one; in time, certain of these recommendations will require modification not only in the order of choice but also in the specific drugs that are recommended.

INFECTION AND PARASITE	DRUG ORDER OF CHOICE 1st	2nd	COMMENTS
I. PROTOZOAN INFECTIONS			
Amebiasis			
Entamoeba histolytica Asymptomatic and noninvasive intestinal amebiasis	Diloxanide furoate *	—	Although effective, iodoquinol and dehydroemetine * are *not* recommended because of potential toxicity (*see* Chapter 42)
Invasive intestinal and systemic amebiasis, including amebic abscesses	Metronidazole plus diloxanide furoate * subsequently	Tinidazole † plus diloxanide furoate * subsequently	
Balantidiasis			
Balantidium coli	Tetracycline ‡	—	—
Giardiasis			
Giardia lamblia	Metronidazole ‡ or quinacrine	—	Tinidazole †, in a single dose of 2 g for adults, is also effective
Leishmaniasis			
Leishmania braziliensis and *L. mexicana* American mucocutaneous and cutaneous leishmaniasis	Stibogluconate sodium *	Amphotericin B	Amphotericin B is used when antimonials are ineffective or contraindicated
L. donovani Visceral leishmaniasis (kala azar)	Stibogluconate sodium *	Pentamidine isethionate ‡	Pentamidine is used when antimonials are ineffective or contraindicated
L. tropica Cutaneous leishmaniasis (oriental sore)	Stibogluconate sodium *	—	Topical heat may be effective
Malaria			
Infections with chloroquine-sensitive *Plasmodium falciparum; P. malariae; P. ovale; P. vivax*	Chloroquine phosphate	—	Used for both prophylaxis and treatment of uncomplicated attacks; chloroquine HCl can be used parenterally when oral medication cannot be taken
Infections with *P. vivax* and *P. ovale*	Primaquine phosphate after or with chloroquine phosphate	—	Used to prevent attacks after departure from an endemic area or to effect a "radical" cure
Infections with chloroquine-resistant or multidrug-resistant *P. falciparum*			
a. Prophylaxis	Chloroquine; carry a self-treatment dose of pyrimethamine-sulfadoxine or chloroguanide † with or without chloroquine or doxycycline ‡	Mefloquine *	Choice of regimen depends on geographical area; consult Centers for Disease Control

Table X–1. DRUGS FOR CHEMOTHERAPY OF PARASITIC INFECTIONS (Continued)

INFECTION AND PARASITE	DRUG ORDER OF CHOICE		COMMENTS
	1st	*2nd*	
b. Treatment	Quinine sulfate orally or quinine dihydrochloride * intravenously	Quinine plus doxycycline ‡ or mefloquine *	Quinidine gluconate ‡ may be substituted for quinine dihydrochloride; mefloquine * can only be given orally (*see* Chapter 41)
Pneumocystosis			
Pneumocystis carinii	Trimethoprim–sulfamethoxazole	Pentamidine isethionate	Aerosolized pentamidine isethionate is used for prophylaxis of *P. carinii* pneumonia
Trichomoniasis			
Trichomonas vaginalis	Metronidazole	—	Both sexual partners should be treated
Trypanosomiasis			
Trypanosoma cruzi South American trypanosomiasis (Chagas' disease)	Nifurtimox *	Benznidazole †	More effective in acute than in chronic infection
T. rhodesiense; T. gambiense African trypanosomiasis (sleeping sickness)			
a. No CNS involvement (early stage)	Suramin *	Pentamidine isethionate ‡	Pentamidine ‡ is used only for *T. gambiense*
b. CNS involvement (late stage)	Suramin * followed by melarsoprol *	—	
II. METAZOAN (HELMINTH) INFECTIONS			
A. NEMATODE (ROUNDWORM) INFECTIONS			
Ascariasis			
Ascaris lumbricoides	Mebendazole, pyrantel pamoate, or ivermectin *,‡,§	Piperazine citrate	Choice influenced by spectrum of polyparasitic infections
Capillariasis			
Capillaria philippinensis	Mebendazole ‡	—	—
Dracunculiasis			
Dracunculus medinensis (guinea worm infection)	Metronidazole ‡	—	—
Enterobiasis			
Enterobius (Oxyuris) vermicularis (pinworm infection)	Pyrantel pamoate or mebendazole	Ivermectin *,‡,§	Choice influenced by spectrum of polyparasitic infections

Table X–1. **DRUGS FOR CHEMOTHERAPY OF PARASITIC INFECTIONS (Continued)**

INFECTION AND PARASITE	DRUG ORDER OF CHOICE		COMMENTS
	1st	*2nd*	
Filariasis			
Wuchereria bancrofti, Brugia (W.) malayi, Dipetalonema perstans, Loa loa	Diethylcarbamazine †	—	—
Onchocerca volvulus	Ivermectin *,‡	Diethylcarbamazine †	—
Hookworm Infections			
Necator americanus Ancylostoma duodenale	Mebendazole or pyrantel pamoate ‡	—	Mebendazole is preferred for polyparasitic infections
Cutaneous larva migrans	Thiabendazole	—	—
Strongyloidiasis			
Strongyloides stercoralis	Thiabendazole or ivermectin *,‡,§	—	Immunosuppressed patients are especially at risk
Toxocariasis			
Toxocara species Visceral larva migrans	Thiabendazole or diethylcarbamazine †,‡	—	Efficacy is questionable
Trichinosis			
Trichinella spiralis	Thiabendazole	—	In man, efficacy is questionable, particularly against larvae in tissues
Trichuriasis			
Trichuris trichiura (whipworm infection)	Mebendazole or ivermectin *,‡,§	Oxantel pamoate † or thiabendazole	Mebendazole is preferred for polyparasitic infections
B. CESTODE (TAPEWORM) INFECTIONS			
Taeniasis			
Taenia saginata (beef tapeworm)	Niclosamide or praziquantel ‡	—	—
Taenia solium (pork tapeworm)	Praziquantel ‡	Niclosamide ‡	Praziquantel is preferred for *T. solium* because of the danger of cysticercosis
Diphyllobothriasis			
Diphyllobothrium latum (fish tapeworm)	Niclosamide or praziquantel ‡	—	—
Hymenolepiasis			
Hymenolepis nana (dwarf tapeworm)	Niclosamide or praziquantel ‡	—	—

Table X–1. DRUGS FOR CHEMOTHERAPY OF PARASITIC INFECTIONS (Continued)

INFECTION AND PARASITE	DRUG ORDER OF CHOICE		COMMENTS
	1st	*2nd*	
Echinococcosis			
Echinococcus granulosus Cystic hydatid disease or hydatidosis	Mebendazole ‡,§	—	Treatment by surgical resection is recommended; albendazole †,§ may be superior to mebendazole but efficacy is marginal
Echinococcus multilocularis Alveolar hydatid disease	Mebendazole ‡,§	—	Surgical resection is recommended first; mebendazole is *not* larvicidal, and efficacy is questionable
C. TREMATODE (FLUKE) INFECTIONS			
Blood Fluke Infections (Schistosomiasis)			
Schistosoma haematobium	Praziquantel	Metrifonate †	—
S. japonicum	Praziquantel	—	
S. mansoni	Praziquantel	Oxamniquine	
S. mekongi	Praziquantel	—	
S. intercalatum	Praziquantel ‡	—	
Intestinal Fluke Infections			
Fasciolopsis buski, Heterophyes heterophyes, Metagonimus yokogawai	Praziquantel ‡,§	—	—
Liver Fluke Infections			
Clonorchis sinensis, Opisthorchis felineus, Opisthorchis viverrini	Praziquantel ‡	—	—
Fasciola hepatica	—	—	Praziquantel may not be effective
Lung Fluke Infections (Paragonimiasis)			
Paragonimus species, *P. westermani, P. kellicotti*	Praziquantel ‡	—	—

* Available from the Center for Infectious Disease, Centers for Disease Control, Atlanta, Georgia 30333. *Telephone:* 404-639-3670 (8:00 A.M. to 4:30 P.M., EST) and 404-639-2888 (emergencies).
† Not available in the United States.
‡ Considered investigational for this use in the United States.
§ Limited data.

Careful clinical pharmacological and pharmacokinetic studies of relatively few patients in major endemic areas of infection should be conducted to determine the feasibility and optimal dosage regimens for chemotherapy. Population-based chemotherapy would ideally be instituted only after appropriate parasitological and epidemiological studies have been conducted to determine patterns of transmission and both the age-specific prevalence and intensity of infection as these variables relate to disease. Analysis of such patterns after periodic follow-up observations should improve the chemotherapy of parasitic infections.

The major parasitic infections of man and the agents currently favored for their prophylaxis or treatment are listed in Table X–1; the pharmacology of anthelmintic and antiprotozoal drugs is presented in Chapters 40 to 43. Treatment of infections with ectoparasites is not considered here, nor is comprehensive or exhaustive coverage of the chemotherapy of human parasitic infections intended. In addition to the current medical and scientific literature, authoritative information about this subject can be obtained from the Centers for Disease Control, Atlanta, Georgia 30333, and the World Health Organization.

CHAPTER 40 DRUGS USED IN THE CHEMOTHERAPY OF HELMINTHIASIS

Leslie T. Webster, Jr.

Anthelmintics are drugs used to rid the body of worms known as helminths. The term anthelmintic applies to agents that act either locally to expel worms from the gastrointestinal tract or systemically to eradicate species and developmental forms of helminths that invade organs and tissues. Such drugs are extremely important because helminthiasis afflicts over 2 billion people and its prevalence is rising. For example, schistosomiasis is an increasingly common problem because greater agricultural use of land and artificial irrigation has enhanced the multiplication of the freshwater snails that serve as intermediate hosts for species of schistosomes that infect man. Simultaneous infection with more than one type of parasitic helminth is common in many tropical regions. Moreover, due to human travel and migration, worms can spread to geographical locations that previously had been free of these organisms.

Worms parasitic for man are Metazoa that belong to widely different zoological species; they vary with respect to life cycle, bodily structure, physiology, development, habitat within the human host, and susceptibility to chemotherapy. Immature forms of these parasites infect humans, where they evolve into well-differentiated adults that characteristically are large enough to be seen by the naked eye. With rare exceptions such as *Strongyloides*, helminths cannot complete their life cycle, *i.e.*, replicate themselves, within the definitive human host. Therefore, the extent of human exposure to these organisms relates to the severity of the infection, and reduction in the number of adult parasites by chemotherapy is sustained unless reinfection takes place. Because of substantial progress in the discovery and development of drugs, particularly in veterinary medicine, the physician now has effective agents that will cure or control most human infections caused by intestinal helminths. However, improved drugs are still badly needed to combat several types of systemic infections, for example, echinococcosis, filariasis, and trichinosis that are caused by tissue-dwelling helminths. The availability of more selective and safer anthelmintics places greater responsibility on the physician to make an accurate diagnosis and prescribe proper therapy.

In the following presentation, specific anthelmintics are presented in alphabetical order, without regard to their relative importance or therapeutic application. Treatment of certain common helminthic infections is then discussed briefly.

ANTIMONY COMPOUNDS

Trivalent antimonial compounds, such as antimony potassium tartrate, are no longer recommended for the treatment of helminth infections because of their unacceptable toxicity and difficulty of administration. Sodium stibogluconate, a pentavalent antimonial used to treat leishmaniasis, is discussed in Chapter 43.

DIETHYLCARBAMAZINE

During World War II, over 15,000 cases of filariasis occurred in American military personnel quartered on the islands of the Western Pacific. This stimulated the search for effective filaricides. The most promising group of antifilarial compounds to emerge were piperazine derivatives, of which diethylcarbamazine is the most important (Hewitt *et al.*, 1948; Hawking, 1979; Mackenzie and Kron, 1985).

Chemistry. Diethylcarbamazine has the following structural formula:

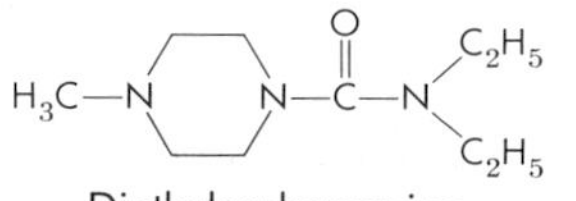

Diethylcarbamazine

The drug is used as the citrate salt, which is highly soluble in water.

Anthelmintic Action. Diethylcarbamazine causes rapid disappearance of microfilariae of *Wuchereria bancrofti, W.* (*Brugia*) *malayi,* and *Loa loa* from the blood of man. The drug causes microfilariae of *Onchocerca volvulus* to disappear from the skin but does not kill microfilariae in nodules that contain the adult (female) worms. It does not affect the microfilariae of *W. bancrofti* in a hydrocele, despite penetration into the fluid. The drug has two types of action on susceptible microfilariae. The first is to decrease the muscular activity and eventually immobilize the organisms; this may result from a hyperpolarizing effect of the piperazine moiety, and it causes dislocation of the parasites from their normal habitats in the host (Langham and Kramer, 1980). The second action is to produce alterations in the microfilarial surface membranes, thereby rendering them more susceptible to destruction by host defense mechanisms (*see* Hawking, 1979; Mackenzie and Kron, 1985). There is evidence that diethylcarbamazine kills adult worms of *Loa loa* and presumptive evidence that it kills adult *W. bancrofti* and *W. malayi.* However, it has little action against adult *O. volvulus.* The mechanism of the filaricidal action of diethylcarbamazine is unknown (*see* Hawking, 1979). However, studies with mammalian cells suggest that diethylcarbamazine may compromise intracellular processing and transport of certain macromolecules to the plasma membrane (Spiro *et al.*, 1986). The drug may also affect specific immune and inflammatory responses of the host by as yet undefined mechanisms (*see* Mackenzie and Kron, 1985; Ottesen, 1987).

Absorption, Fate, and Excretion. Diethylcarbamazine is rapidly absorbed from the gastrointestinal tract. After a single oral dose, the concentration in plasma peaks in 1 to 2 hours; the plasma half-life is about 10 to 12 hours. The apparent volume of distribution in an adult is 200 to 240 liters—well in excess of total body water (Edwards *et al.*, 1981a). Metabolism of diethylcarbamazine is both rapid and extensive (Faulkner and Smith, 1972). Excretion is by urinary and extraurinary routes; over 50% of an oral dose appears in acidic urine as the unchanged drug; this value is decreased when the urine is alkaline (Edwards *et al.*, 1981b).

Route of Administration and Dosage. The dosage of *diethylcarbamazine citrate* used to treat filarial disease is derived empirically and has varied considerably. Suggested dosage regimens may be modified effectively according to local experience.

Wuchereria bancrofti, W. malayi. For mass treatment with the objective of reducing microfilaremia to subinfective levels for mosquitoes, the dose is 2 mg/kg, three times daily after meals, for 5 to 7 days; for treatment directed toward possible cure, this dosage regimen is carried out for 10 to 30 days. Much experience has shown that, if people take an adequate total dose of diethylcarbamazine (about 72 to 126 mg/kg of the citrate salt), the microfilariae and probably some of the adult worms will be destroyed. The period over which this amount is taken has varied from area to area; spaced, low weekly doses of 6 mg/kg for prolonged periods produce as good an effect as high daily or monthly doses, and are less likely to cause adverse reactions (World Health Organization, 1967; Partono *et al.*, 1981; Jain *et al.*, 1988). Retreatment may be necessary to kill the adult worms (Ottesen, 1985).

Loa loa. After a test dose of 25 to 50 mg on the first day, a dose of 2 mg/kg should be given three times daily after meals for 3 to 4 weeks. If repeated courses are required to produce cure, they should be separated by periods of 3 to 4 weeks.

Onchocerca volvulus. Because of its adverse effects, diethylcarbamazine has severe limitations in the treatment of onchocerciasis. Treatment is effective in removing microfilariae from the skin, but they usually return after some weeks because the adult worms are not killed. In heavy infections or when lesions of the eye are present, the initial test dose of diethylcarbamazine should not exceed 0.5 mg/kg. This is given once on the first day and twice on the second. The dose is then increased to 1 mg/kg, three times daily for the third day, and therapy is continued up to a total of 14 days with a dose of 2 to 3 mg/kg in two divided doses each day.

In patients infected with *O. volvulus* or *W. malayi*, and to a lesser extent in those infected with *W. bancrofti* and *Loa loa*, the initial systemic reactions provoked by the massive destruction of microfilariae, macrofilariae, or both during treatment may be severe. In such cases the dosage should be lowered or the drug discontinued temporarily. Relief of these symptoms in heavily infected individuals may be afforded by pretreatment with corticosteroids (Awadzi *et al.*, 1982). Once the initial reactions have subsided, continued treatment should not provoke a further series of reactions.

Toxicity and Side Effects. Untoward direct reactions to diethylcarbamazine, although fairly frequent, are not severe and usually disappear within a few days despite continuation of therapy. These include anorexia, nausea, headache, and, at high doses, vomiting. The major adverse effects result directly or indirectly from destruction of the parasites. These are especially severe in patients heavily infected with *O. volvulus*. In *W. malayi* or *Loa loa* infections, reactions are usually milder, although the drug may induce severe encephalitis in *Loa loa*. In patients with onchocerciasis, there is usually a typical reaction (termed a Mazzotti reaction) that occurs within a few hours after the first oral dose. This consists of intense itching and skin rashes, enlargement and tenderness of the lymph nodes, sometimes a fine papular rash, fever, tachycardia, arthralgia, and headache. These symptoms persist for 3 to 7 days and then subside, after which quite high doses can be tolerated. Ocular complications include limbitis, punctate keratitis, uveitis, and atrophy of the retinal pigment epithelium (Rivas-Alcala *et al.*, 1981; Dominguez-Vazquez *et al.*, 1983). In patients with bancrofian or brugian filariasis, nodular swellings may occur along the course of the lymphatics, and there is often an accompanying lymphadenitis. This reaction also subsides within a few days. Almost all patients receiving therapy exhibit a leukocytosis, first evident on the second day, reaching its peak on the fourth or fifth day, and gradually subsiding over a period of a few weeks. Reversible proteinuria may occur, and the eosinophilia frequently observed in patients with filariasis can be intensified by drug therapy. Diethylcarbamazine appears to be safe for use during pregnancy.

Precautions and Contraindications. Low doses of diethylcarbamazine should be used for initial therapy, especially in onchocerciasis and infection due to *Loa loa* (to minimize adverse reactions to destruction of the parasites). As mentioned, pretreatment with corticosteroids may be undertaken to minimize such reactions. These may be especially severe in patients with mixed infections due to *O. volvulus* and *Loa loa*.

Therapeutic Uses. Diethylcarbamazine can be used effectively to treat infections caused by *W. bancrofti, W. malayi, Loa loa*, and *O. volvulus*. In the first three, radical cure can be achieved by either single or multiple courses of treatment. In onchocerciasis, radical cure is unlikely because the drug fails to kill the adult worms. Control can be achieved by short periodic courses of treatment, but diethylcarbamazine can cause serious adverse reactions in heavily infected individuals. The drug is now being replaced by ivermectin for treatment of this condition. Diethylcarbamazine has been used effectively to treat filariasis due to *Tetrapetalonema perstans* or *T. streptocerca*. In patients with eosinophilic lung (tropical eosinophilia), treatment with this compound causes a rapid disappearance of symptoms. This, and the finding of microfilariae in lung biopsies, suggest an association between filariasis and certain pulmonary syndromes. Diethylcarbamazine is also effective in clearing *Ascaris* infections, but other agents are used clinically for this purpose.

IVERMECTIN

In the mid-1970s, a survey of natural products for antinematodal activity revealed that a fermentation broth of a soil actinomycete (*Streptomyces avermitilis*) ameliorated infection with *Nematospiroides dubius* in mice (Burg *et al.*, 1979; Egerton *et al.*, 1979; Miller *et al.*, 1979). Isolation of the active components from cultures of this organism led to the discovery of the avermectins, a novel class of macrocyclic lactones (*see* review by Campbell *et al.*, 1983). *Ivermectin,* a mixture of about 80% component B_{1a} and 20% component B_{1b}, is formed by selective catalytic hydrogenation of avermectin B_1. This semisynthetic agent is used extensively in veterinary medicine to treat and control a wide variety of infections caused by parasitic nematodes (roundworms) and arthropods (insects, ticks, and mites) that plague livestock and domestic animals (*see* Campbell and Benz, 1984). In humans, ivermectin is now the drug of choice to treat and control onchocerciasis, the filarial infection responsible for river blindness.

Chemistry. The structures of ivermectin components B_{1a} and B_{1b} are as follows:

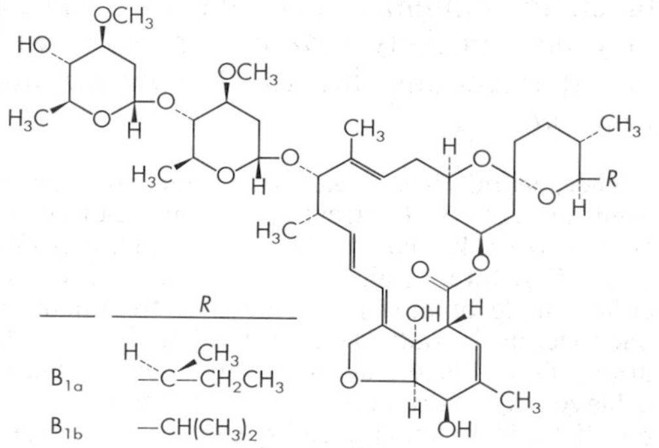

Ivermectin

Homologs with either a *sec*-butyl (B_{1a}) or an isopropyl (B_{1b}) group at position 25 appear to be equiactive.

Antiparasitic Activity. Ivermectin is effective and highly potent against at least some developmental stages of many parasitic nematodes that infect animals and man. The drug causes immobilization of affected organisms by producing a tonic paralysis of the peripheral musculature. The mechanism of this action is not well understood, although potentiation of the release and binding of gamma-aminobutyric acid (GABA) at certain synapses is thought to be involved (Wang and Pong, 1982). Lack of GABA-mediated neural control of peripheral muscles in cestodes and trematodes may explain why ivermectin is ineffective against these organisms.

In humans infected with *Onchocerca volvulus,* ivermectin causes a rapid and marked decrease in microfilarial counts in the skin and ocular tissues that lasts for 6 to 12 months (Greene *et al.*, 1985, 1987; Newland *et al.*, 1988). The drug causes little discernible harm to adult parasites but seems to affect developing larvae and to block egress of microfilariae from the uterus of the adult female worm (Awadzi *et al.*, 1985; Court *et al.*, 1985). Ivermectin may decrease transmission of *O. volvulus* microfilariae to its *Simulium* vector (Cupp *et al.*, 1986, 1989). The agent has microfilaricidal activity in brugian filariasis that may prove clinically useful (Diallo *et al.*, 1987). Moreover, certain gastrointestinal nematodes that infect man are also susceptible to ivermectin. Thus, the drug appears highly effective in strongyloidiasis, ascariasis, trichuriasis, and enterobiasis; hookworms are also affected but to a lesser extent (Naquira *et al.*, 1989).

Absorption, Fate, and Excretion. In humans, peak concentrations of ivermectin in plasma are achieved within 4 hours of oral administration; the half-life of the drug is about 10 hours. Animal studies reveal that only 1 to 2% of an orally administered dose of ivermectin appears in the urine; the remainder is found in the feces, nearly all as the unchanged drug. The highest tissue concentrations occur in the liver and fat. Extremely low levels of ivermectin are found in the brain, the site of GABA-containing neurons in mammals. This probably accounts for the paucity of central nervous system (CNS) side effects and the relative safety of this agent in man.

Preparation, Route of Administration, and Dosage. *Ivermectin* is an investigational drug in the United States. It is available from the Centers for Disease Control as MECTIZAN tablets, each containing 6 mg. Data indicate that a single oral dose of 0.15 to 0.20 mg/kg in adults causes a rapid and marked reduction of *O. volvulus* microfilaria in the skin and ocular tissues. This effect is noted within a few days and lasts for 6 to 12 months; the dose should then be repeated.

Toxicity and Side Effects. Ivermectin is well tolerated by uninfected humans and other mammals. In animals, signs of CNS toxicity including lethargy, ataxia, mydriasis, tremors, and eventually death occur only at very high doses; dogs are particularly susceptible to such toxicity (Campbell and Benz, 1984). In humans with *O. volvulus* infection, side effects last just a few days and are usually limited to mild itching, swollen lymph glands, and rarely, dizziness and postural hypotension. Notably, lesions of ocular tissues are not exacerbated by this agent (Newland *et al.,* 1988; Taylor *et al.,* 1989). The significance of minor changes in the electrocardiogram that occur 2 days after initiation of therapy is unclear (Awadzi *et al.,* 1985). There is no evidence that ivermectin is carcinogenic or teratogenic.

Therapeutic Uses. Single doses of ivermectin (0.15 to 0.20 mg/kg) given every 6 to 12 months are considered effective, safe, and practical for the control of onchocerciasis in man. Most important, such treatment results in reversal of lymphadenopathy and acute inflammatory changes in ocular tissues and arrests the development of further ocular pathology due to microfilariae. Cure is not attained, because this agent does not affect adult *O. volvulus.* Insufficient data are available to evaluate the clinical utility of ivermectin in brugian filariasis. If confirmed, the finding that a single dose of 150 to 200 mg of ivermectin can cure human *strongyloidiasis* represents a significant advance, particularly because the drug is also effective against coexisting ascariasis, trichuriasis, and enterobiasis (Naquira *et al.,* 1989).

MEBENDAZOLE

Mebendazole was introduced for the treatment of roundworm infections as a result of research carried out by Brugmans and collaborators (1971). It is representative of a number of benzimidazole derivatives, including albendazole and flubendazole, which were developed as broad-spectrum anthelmintics for animal and human use (*see* review by Van den Bossche *et al.,* 1982). Mebendazole has the following structural formula:

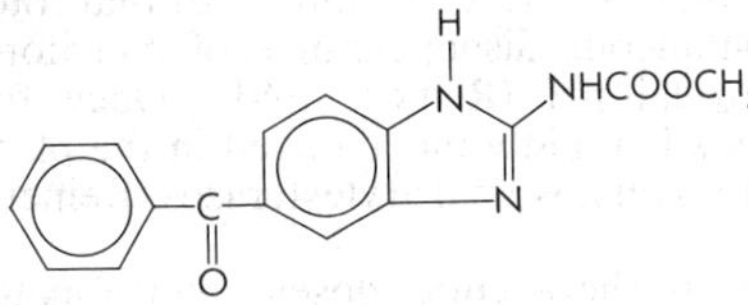

Mebendazole

Anthelmintic Action. Mebendazole is a versatile anthelmintic agent, particularly against gastrointestinal nematodes where its action is independent of its systemic concentration. It is highly effective in ascariasis, intestinal capillariasis, enterobiasis, trichuriasis, and hookworm (*Ancylostoma duodenale* and *Necator americanus*) infection as single or mixed infections. The drug is active against both larval and adult stages of the nematodes that cause these infections, and it is ovicidal for *Ascaris* and *Trichuris* (Keystone and Murdoch, 1979; Van den Bossche *et al.,* 1982). Immobilization and death of susceptible gastrointestinal organisms occur slowly, and clearance from the gastrointestinal tract may not be complete until a few days after treatment with mebendazole. Marginal results have been obtained against *Strongyloides stercoralis*. Together with albendazole, mebendazole has shown some promise in the treatment of hydatid disease (Wilson *et al.,* 1987). Efficacy against filariases due to *Loa loa* or *Mansonella perstans* has also been reported (Van Hoegaerden *et al.,* 1987). The drug causes selective disappearance of cytoplasmic microtubules in the tegumental and intestinal cells of affected worms. Secretory substances accumulate in Golgi areas, secretion of acetylcholinesterase and uptake of glucose are impaired, and glycogen is depleted. These effects of mebendazole are not noted in host cells. Mebendazole has a high affinity for parasite tubulin *in vitro,* but it also binds to host tubulin. The biochemical basis for its selective action is thus unclear (*see* Van den Bossche, 1981; Watts *et al.,* 1982).

Absorption, Fate, and Excretion. Tablet formulations of mebendazole are poorly and erratically absorbed, and concentrations of the drug in plasma are low and do not reflect the dosage taken (Witassek *et al.,* 1981). The low systemic bioavailability of mebendazole results from a combination of poor absorption and rapid first-pass hepatic metabolism. Mebendazole is about 95% bound to plasma proteins and is extensively metabolized. Two major metabolites, methyl 5-(α-hydroxybenzyl)-2-benzimidazole carbamate and 2-amino-5-benzoylbenzimidazole, have lower rates of clearance than does mebendazole itself (Braithwaite *et al.,* 1982); conjugates of mebendazole and its metabolites have been found in bile (Witassek *et al.,* 1983). Little unchanged mebendazole appears in the urine.

Preparation, Route of Administration, and Dosage. *Mebendazole* (VERMOX) is available as chewable tablets, each containing 100 mg of the drug. Mebendazole is given orally, and the same dosage schedule applies to adults and children more than 2 years old. For control of enterobiasis, a single 100-mg tablet is given; a second should be given after 2 weeks. For control of ascariasis, trichuriasis, and hookworm infection, 100 mg is administered morning and evening on 3 consecutive days. If the patient is not cured 3 weeks after treatment, a second course should be given. Fasting or purging is not required.

Infections with *Capillaria philippinensis* are more resistant to treatment; 400 mg of the drug has been given per day in two divided doses for at least 20 days. Mebendazole has been used to treat cystic hydatid disease, although surgery should be performed first and chemotherapy with albendazole is preferable. The usual regimen is 400 to 600 mg of mebendazole three times a day for 21 to 30 days or longer.

Toxicity and Side Effects. Probably as a result of its poor absorption, mebendazole does not cause significant systemic toxicity in routine clinical use, even in the presence of anemia and malnutrition. Transient symptoms of abdominal pain and diarrhea have occurred in cases of massive infestation and expulsion of worms. Rare side effects in patients treated with high doses include allergic reactions, alopecia, reversible neutropenia, agranulocytosis, and hypospermia. Embryotoxic and teratogenic effects may occur in pregnant rats at single oral doses as low as 10 mg/kg.

Precautions and Contraindications. Mebendazole should not be given to pregnant women, nor is it advised in children less than 2 years old. It should not be used in patients who have experienced allergic reactions to the agent.

Therapeutic Uses. Mebendazole is an excellent drug for the treatment of *Trichuris trichiura*. It produces a large proportion of cures and, in those not cured with a first course of treatment, a marked reduction in egg production. It is also highly effective for infection with *Ancylostoma duodenale*. Mebendazole is particularly valuable in the treatment of double or triple infections because it also has high activity, and is a good alternative to pyrantel pamoate against ascariasis, enterobiasis, and *Necator americanus* infection (Chavarria *et al.*, 1973; Sargent *et al.*, 1974). In the Philippines, mebendazole has been used successfully in high dosage to treat intestinal capillariasis (Singson *et al.*, 1975). In even higher dosage successful cure of hydatid disease has been reported, but surgery is often required and additional clinical evaluation of both mebendazole and albendazole is necessary for this refractory condition. Although drugs of the benzimidazole class are being tested clinically for treatment of *onchocerciasis*, superior agents are available.

METRIFONATE

Metrifonate (BILARCIL) is an organophosphorus inhibitor of cholinesterases, used first as an insecticide (DIPTEREX, DYLOX) and later as an anthelmintic. The original trials in man arose from the hope that the anticholinesterase activity of organophosphorus compounds in arthropods would extend to other invertebrates, including the helminths. Metrifonate was selected for trial on the basis of *in-vitro* tests carried out with *Ascaris lumbricoides*. In 1962 it was shown to have high anthelmintic activity in several different human infections. The substance has the following structural formula:

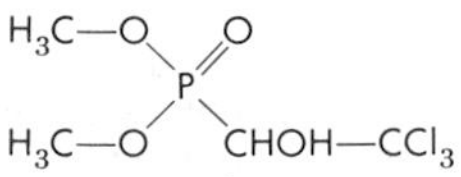

Metrifonate

Metrifonate undergoes extensive metabolism *in vivo*, and it also rearranges spontaneously at physiological pH to form dichlorvos (2,2-dichlorovinyl dimethyl phosphate, DDVP); this metabolite is probably responsible for inhibition of acetylcholinesterase (Reiner *et al.*, 1975; Symposium, 1981b). However, this effect alone is unlikely to explain the antischistosomal properties of metrifonate (Bloom, 1981). *In vitro*, the drug is about equipotent as an inhibitor of acetylcholinesterase in *S. mansoni* and *S. haematobium*, yet clinically it is effective only against infection with *S. haematobium*. Location of *S. haematobium* in the vesical plexus rather than in the mesenteric venous plexus in man may be an important determinant of the clinical efficacy of metrifonate (Omer and Teesdale, 1978; Feldmeier *et al.*, 1982; Doehring *et al.*, 1986).

Peak concentrations in plasma of metrifonate (30 μM) and of dichlorvos (0.3 μM) are reached within an hour after a single oral dose of metrifonate (10 mg/kg). The half-life of both compounds in plasma is about 1.5 hours (Nordgren *et al.*, 1981); this value is similar to that found for the spontaneous disappearance of metrifonate at physiological pH (Reiner, 1981). Once formed, dichlorvos is rapidly metabolized in the plasma as well as by schistosomal arylesterases (Reiner *et al.*, 1980).

Given in therapeutic doses, metrifonate produces rapid and almost complete inhibition of plasma cholinesterase activity of the host; this recovers to almost normal levels within a few weeks of stopping treatment. Erythrocyte acetylcholinesterase is inhibited to a lesser degree but recovers more slowly (Nordgren *et al.*, 1981). Despite these changes, the drug is well tolerated. Side effects such as mild vertigo, lassitude, nausea, and colic are dose related and occur infrequently. Treated individuals should be free from recent exposure to insecticides that might add to the anticholinesterase effect and not receive depolarizing neuromuscular blocking agents for at least 48 hours after treatment.

Metrifonate is now recommended only for the treatment of *S. haematobium* infection. Its low cost, effectiveness, and ready acceptance have given it an important role in the treatment of urinary schistosomiasis in Africa. The dose is 7.5 to 10 mg/kg, given orally three times at intervals of 2 weeks. Successful prophylaxis has been carried out in a highly endemic area with a dosage of 7.5 mg/kg, given once every 4 weeks (Jewsbury *et al.*, 1977). Metrifonate is not available in the United States.

NICLOSAMIDE

Niclosamide is a halogenated salicylanilide derivative that was introduced as a taeniacide after laboratory trials in rats infected with *Hymenolepis diminuta* (Gönnert and Schraufstätter, 1960). Impressive evidence of its high activity and safety has accumulated, and it is generally regarded as a very effective agent for treating most infections with cestodes in animals and man (Keeling 1968). Niclosamide has the following structural formula:

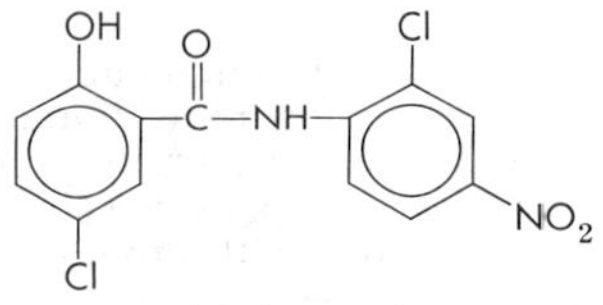

Niclosamide

Anthelmintic Action. Niclosamide has prominent activity against most of the cestodes that infect man; *Enterobius* (*Oxyuris*) *vermicularis* is also susceptible. At low concentrations, niclosamide stimulates oxygen uptake by *H. diminuta*, but at higher concentrations respiration is inhibited and glucose uptake is blocked. The principal action of the drug may be to inhibit anaerobic phosphorylation of adenosine diphosphate (ADP) by the mitochondria of the parasite, an energy-producing process that is dependent on CO_2 fixation (Scheibel and Saz, 1966; Scheibel *et al.*, 1968). Worms affected by the drug either in the gut or *in vitro* deteriorate, such that the scolex and segments may be partially digested and become unrecognizable.

Preparation, Route of Administration, and Dosage. *Niclosamide* (NICLOCIDE) is supplied in 500-mg chewable tablets. The drug is given orally in a single dose, usually after a light meal; those with chronic constipation should first be given a laxative. The recommended dose for an adult is 2 g, the tablets to be chewed thoroughly and washed down with a small amount of water. The dosage for children who weigh between 11 and 34 kg is 1 g and for children under 2 years, 0.5 g. For small children it is advisable to grind the tablets as finely as possible and to mix the powder with a little water. A purge may be given 2 hours after the dose in the hope of obtaining less damaged lengths of the worm and an identifiable scolex.

In infections with *H. nana*, which are usually multiple, the recommended dose of 2 g should be taken once daily for 7 days after a light meal. Discharge of intestinal mucus can be promoted by the administration of sour fruit juices. Worms lodging under accumulations of mucus thus become more readily accessible to the drug.

Toxicity and Side Effects. Niclosamide is quite free of undesirable effects other than very occasional gastrointestinal upset. Very little is absorbed from the gastrointestinal tract, and the drug has no direct irritant effect. No side effects were observed when niclosamide was given to debilitated or pregnant patients (Gönnert and Schraufstätter, 1960). Follow-up studies showed no alteration in hepatic or renal function or in blood counts of treated patients (Abdallah and Saif, 1961).

Precautions and Contraindications. There are no contraindications to the use of niclosamide as a taeniacide. However, it is important to note that the lethal action of the drug against the adult worm does not extend to the ova. Thus, use of niclosamide in *Taenia solium* infections may expose the patient to the risk of cysticercosis, since, following digestion of the dead segments, viable ova will be liberated into the lumen of the gut. It is desirable to give an adequate purge within 3 to 4 hours after the drug has been given, to clear the bowel of all dead segments before they can be digested. In *T. saginata* infections in which there is no risk of cysticercosis, purging is unnecessary unless immediate proof of cure by finding the scolex is desired.

Therapeutic Uses. Niclosamide can be considered an agent of choice in the treatment of *Diphyllobothrium latum*, *H. nana*, *T. saginata*, and most other human intestinal cestode infections (Brown, 1968; Jones, 1979). It is also very effective in the treatment of *T. solium* infection, but the danger of cysticercosis following its administration makes praziquantel the preferred drug for this condition. The ready acceptance of niclosamide by patients, together with the fact that fasting is not necessary, makes it valuable, particularly in the treatment of children.

OXAMNIQUINE

Oxamniquine is a metabolite of the most active of a novel series of 2-aminomethyltetrahydroquinoline compounds that showed promising schistosomicidal activity and low toxicity in laboratory animals (*see* Foster, 1973). It is prepared by microbial (*Aspergillus sclerotiorum*) hydroxylation of its synthetic precursor. Oxamniquine has the following structural formula:

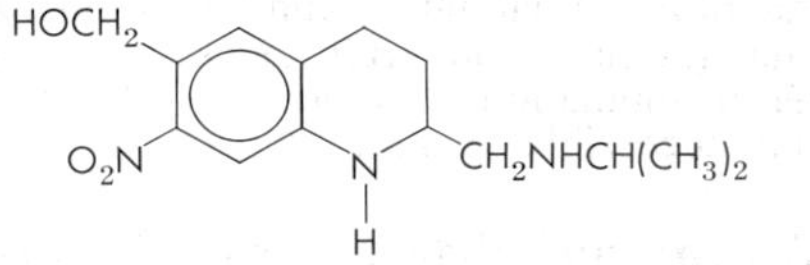

Oxamniquine

Anthelmintic Action. *Schistosoma mansoni* is highly susceptible to oxamniquine, but *S. haematobium* and *S. japonicum* are virtually unaffected by therapeutic doses. Adult male *S. mansoni* worms are more vulnerable to the action of oxamniquine than are the female worms. The males preferentially concentrate the drug and die without leaving the liver. Surviving unpaired females may return to the mesentery but do not lay eggs. Although oxamniquine exhibits anticholinergic properties, its primary mode of action is unknown. An intriguing possibility is that the compound is converted by susceptible parasites to an unstable ester, which dissociates to yield chemically reactive electrophiles. These intermediates then alkylate essential macromolecules such as DNA (Archer, 1985; Cioli *et al.*, 1985; Pica-Mattoccia and Cioli, 1985). Direct evidence for this hypothesis is lacking, but it is consistent with the species selectivity of oxamniquine for *S. mansoni*, the high resistance of certain strains of *S. mansoni* to oxamniquine and a structurally related drug, hycanthone, and the inheritance of such resistance as an autosomal recessive trait.

Absorption, Fate, and Excretion. Oxamniquine is readily absorbed following oral ingestion, and peak concentrations in plasma occur within 0.5 to 3 hours. The presence of food retards absorption and limits the concentration achieved in plasma; bioavailability is about 50 to 70% when compared to intramuscular administration. About 70% of an administered dose is excreted in the urine, mostly as a 6-carboxyl metabolite, and there are traces of unchanged drug and a 2-carboxylic acid metabolite. The major 6-carboxyl metabolite is formed in the intestine during absorption and is present in the plasma at concentrations more than tenfold greater than those of oxamniquine. It is excreted predominantly in the first 12 hours and is devoid of schistosomicidal activity (Kaye and Woolhouse, 1976; Kaye and Roberts, 1980; Kaye, 1984).

Preparation, Route of Administration, and Dosage. *Oxamniquine* (VANSIL) is available as capsules, each of which contains 250 mg of the drug. Because of severe local pain following intramuscular injection, oxamniquine is taken orally; the dosage depends on the geographical location. For the treatment of all forms of *S. mansoni* infections in Brazil, the recommended dose is 15 mg/kg, given as a single dose. For children weighing less than 30 kg, the dose is 20 mg/kg (in two doses of 10 mg/kg with an interval of 2 to 8 hours between them). In Africa, the recommended total dose may range from 15 to 60 mg/kg, given over 1 to 3 days. The most appropriate regimen within this range is determined by the geographical location and the particular strain of *S. mansoni*. Intrinsic differences in the susceptibility of parasites to the drug rather than pharmacokinetic factors seem to account for most of the variation in dosage (Kaye, 1984; Daneshmend and Homeida, 1987).

Toxicity and Side Effects. Occasional headache, dizziness, drowsiness, nausea, and diarrhea have been reported after the administration of oxamniquine. Neuropsychiatric disturbances and convulsions are rare. Minor and transient elevation of transaminase activities may be of little clinical significance, since oxamniquine has been used safely in patients with severe hepatosplenic disease. The mild eosinophilia that occurs after treatment is likely due to the host's reaction to dead and dying worms. Orange-to-red discoloration of the urine may follow therapy.

Therapeutic Uses. Oxamniquine is currently used only for the treatment of infections with *S. mansoni*. Its value as an orally administered, readily accepted, and inexpensive schistosomicide has been proven, both for the treatment of individual patients and in mass-treatment and control programs (*see* Katz *et al.*, 1977; Bassily *et al.*, 1978; Omer, 1978; Sleigh *et al.*, 1986). It is effective in all stages of infection and in patients with hepatosplenic involvement. Recommended dosages differ in various geographical areas (*see* above). Oxamniquine has been used successfully in combination with metrifonate for the treatment of mixed infections with *S. mansoni* and *S. haematobium*.

PIPERAZINE

The discovery of the anthelmintic properties of piperazine is usually credited to Fayard (1949), but these were first observed by Boismare, a Rouen pharmacist, whose recipe is quoted in Fayard's thesis. Clinically, the drug is highly effective against both *Ascaris lumbricoides* and *Enterobius* (*Oxyuris*) *vermicularis*. A large number of substituted piperazine derivatives exhibit anthelmintic activity, but apart from diethylcarbamazine none has found a place in human therapeutics (*see* Standen, 1963). Piperazine has the following structural formula:

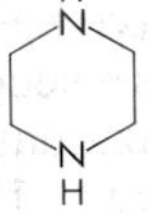

Piperazine

It is available as the hexahydrate, which contains about 44% of base, and as various salts.

Anthelmintic Action. The predominant effect of piperazine on *Ascaris* is to cause a flaccid paralysis that results in expulsion of the worm by peristalsis. Affected worms recover if incubated in drug-free medium. Piperazine blocks the response of *Ascaris* muscle to acetylcholine, apparently by altering the permeability of the cell membrane to ions that are responsible for the maintenance of the resting potential. The drug causes hyperpolarization and suppression of spontaneous spike potentials with accompanying paralysis (*see* Saz and Bueding, 1966). The basis for its selectivity of action is not clear.

Absorption, Fate, and Excretion. Piperazine is rapidly absorbed after an oral dose. About 20% is excreted unchanged in the urine (Fletcher *et al.*, 1982). Accurate pharmacokinetic studies of piperazine in man have been impeded by the lack of appropriate analytical methods; this has now been developed (Skarping *et al.*, 1986).

Preparations, Route of Administration, and Dosage. Piperazine salts are available as tablets, each containing 250 mg, and as syrups containing 100 mg/ml, calculated as the hexahydrate. The various preparations are probably equivalent, but the liquid formulations are more acceptable for children. *Piperazine citrate* is the salt available in the United States (VERMIZINE).

Piperazine preparations are always given orally. Prior fasting or supplementary treatment with cathartics or enemas is unnecessary. Many different dosage schedules have been investigated, and all have resulted in a considerable measure of success. In ascariasis, accepted therapy is to give 75 mg/kg (maximum of 3.5 g) as a single daily dose for 2 consecutive days. Children should be treated in the same way. This dosage schedule will cure nearly all patients. A single dose of 4 g has been shown to cure about 50% of patients and to reduce markedly the worm burden in the remainder (Goodwin and Standen, 1958). In oxyuriasis, single daily doses of 65 mg/kg, with a maximum of 2.5 g, given for 7 days, will result in 95 to 100% cure. One study in hospital patients showed that a single dose of 4 g of piperazine cured more than 90% of patients (White and Scopes, 1960). Because of the possibility of autoinfection, a second dose should be given to ambulatory patients 1 to 2 weeks after the first.

Toxicity and Side Effects. There is a large difference between effective therapeutic and overtly toxic doses of piperazine. Laboratory studies on patients receiving treatment for several days have showed no abnormality. Very occasionally gastrointestinal upset, transient neurological effects, and urticarial reactions have attended its use. Piperazine has been used without ill effect during pregnancy. Lethal doses cause convulsions and respiratory depression.

Precautions and Contraindications. Piperazine is contraindicated in patients with a history of epilepsy. Neurotoxic effects have occurred in individuals with renal dysfunction because urinary excretion is the main route of elimination of the drug.

Therapeutic Uses. Piperazine is particularly useful in treating combined ascariasis and oxyuriasis. In the treatment of ascariasis, piperazine has the advantage of greatly reducing the motility of the worms, thereby reducing the hazard of migration. Since the worms are usually alive when passed, there is little chance of absorption of disintegration products. Where partial intestinal obstruction is a complication of infection, conservative management together with the administration of piperazine syrup through a drainage tube may obviate the need for surgical intervention.

Treatment of oxyuriasis is complicated by the readiness with which reinfection may occur. Many authorities advocate the simultaneous treatment of the entire household with piperazine in lieu of investigation of each member by anal swabs. The palatability of the various preparations, ease of administration to children, and low toxicity make piperazine a good agent for pinworm infections. Its main disadvantage is the requirement for multiple doses over a prolonged period.

PRAZIQUANTEL

Praziquantel is a pyrazinoisoquinoline derivative that was developed after this class of compounds was discovered to have anthelmintic activity in 1972. It is clinically effective against a wide spectrum of cestode and trematode infections in animals and humans; in contrast, parasitic nematodes are relatively unaffected by the compound (*see* Symposium, 1981a, and reviews by Andrews *et al.*, 1983; Wegner, 1984; Andrews, 1985; and Mahmoud, 1987). Praziquantel has the following structural formula:

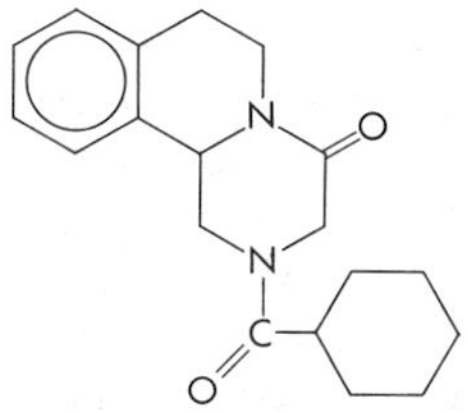

Praziquantel

The (−) isomer is responsible for most of the drug's anthelmintic activity.

Anthelmintic Action. Praziquantel is rapidly and reversibly taken up but not metabolized by helminths *in vitro*. The compound exerts two prompt actions in susceptible organisms. At the lowest effective concentrations it causes increased muscular activity, followed by contraction and spastic paralysis. This effect probably causes the worms to lose their attachment to host tissues, resulting, for example, in the rapid shift of *Schistosoma mansoni* and *S. japonicum* from the mesenteric veins to the liver or in the expulsion of intestinal cestodes into the environment. At slightly higher but still therapeutic concentrations, praziquantel causes vacuolization and vesiculation of the tegument of susceptible parasites. If sufficiently pronounced, this effect activates host defense mechanisms and results in destruction of the worms. Comparisons of stage-specific susceptibility of *S. mansoni* to praziquantel *in vitro* and *in vivo* indicate that the clinical efficacy of this drug correlates better with its tegumental action (Xiao *et al.*, 1985).

The molecular basis of the actions of praziquantel is unknown. The drug causes increased membrane permeability to certain monovalent and divalent cations, particularly Ca^{2+} (Pax *et al.*, 1978). Drug-induced muscular contraction and tegumental damage of *S. mansoni* are both dependent on extracellular Ca^{2+}, but praziquantel acts differently than do K^+, Ca^{2+} ionophores, or many agonists that are active in mammalian systems. Other biochemical effects have been observed, but it is likely that they are secondary to the principal action of praziquantel (*see* Andrews *et al.*, 1983; Andrews, 1985).

Absorption, Fate, and Excretion. In man, praziquantel is readily absorbed after oral administration. Maximal concentrations in plasma occur in 1 to 2 hours. Rapid first-pass metabolism to many hydroxylated and conjugated products limits bioavailability of praziquantel; its half-life in plasma is 1.5 hours, and only traces of unchanged drug are recovered in the urine. Plasma concentrations of metabolites are at least 100-fold that of praziquantel. About 80% of a dose of praziquantel is recovered as metabolites in the urine after 4 days; 90% of this amount is excreted within 24 hours.

Preparation, Route of Administration, and Dosage. To date, *praziquantel* (BILTRICIDE) is approved in the United States only for the treatment of all species of human schistosomiasis. The same preparation is used elsewhere to treat other infections with trematodes (*see* Table X–1). Although dosage schedules may vary, a single oral dose of 40 mg/kg or three oral doses of 20 mg/kg each given 4 to 6 hours apart produce good results for single or mixed infections with *S. mansoni* and *S. haematobium*. Two oral doses of 30 mg/kg several hours apart are recommended for *S. japonicum* infections. Praziquantel, given in three oral doses of 25 mg/kg per day for 1 or 2 days, has allowed high rates of cure of infections with the liver flukes, *Clonorchis sinensis* and *Opisthorchis viverrini*. Whether *Fasciola hepatica* would respond to more prolonged treatment is questionable; this trematode is quite refractory to praziquantel in animal hosts and *in vitro*. Infections with the lung fluke, *Paragonimus westermani*, have responded to three doses per day of praziquantel at 25 mg/kg for 2 days. Three oral doses of 25 mg/kg each on the same day have produced good results in infections with the intestinal flukes, *Fasciolopsis buski*, *Heterophyes heterophyes*, and *Metagonimus yokogawai*. Lower doses are recommended for treatment of infections with adult cestodes, for example, a single dose of 25 mg/kg for *Hymenolepis nana* and 10 to 20 mg/kg for *Diphyllobothrium latum*, *Taenia saginata*, or *T. solium*. Although low doses of praziquantel are effective in eliminating juvenile and adult stages of *Echinococcus granulosus* and *E. multilocularis* from dogs and cats, these infections and hydatid disease in man appear quite resistant to the drug. The use of prolonged high-dose therapy with praziquantel for human cysticercosis is promising but still investigational; moreover, albendazole may prove to be a useful alternative for this purpose (*see* Sotelo *et al.*, 1984, 1988).

Toxicity and Side Effects. Abdominal discomfort, particularly pain and nausea, and malaise, headache, and dizziness may occur shortly after administration of the drug; these effects are transient and appear to be dose related. Fever, eosinophilia, and skin rashes are noted occasionally. Extensive tests for mutagenesis, carcinogenesis, and teratogenicity have been essentially negative (*see* review by Frohberg and Schencking, 1981).

Therapeutic Uses. Praziquantel is well tolerated, safe, and effective when given in one to three doses during the same day for single or mixed infections with all species of schistosomes that infect man. It thus appears to have ideal properties for individual or population-based chemotherapy. With the exception of fascioliasis, the drug also appears to be extremely useful against infections with other trematodes and cestodes that affect man; this even includes previously untreatable *Clonorchis sinensis* infections and cysticercosis caused by the larval stage of *Taenia solium*.

PYRANTEL PAMOATE

Pyrantel pamoate was introduced first into veterinary practice as a broad-spectrum anthelmintic directed against pinworm, roundworm, and hookworm (Austin *et al.*, 1966). Its effectiveness and lack of toxicity led to its trial against related intestinal helminths in man (Bumbalo *et al.*, 1969). Successful clinical trials have resulted in its acceptance for the treatment of infections with various intestinal nematodes. Oxantel pamoate, an *m*-oxyphenol analog of pyrantel, is effective for single-dose treatment of trichuriasis. Pyrantel is employed as the pamoate salt. It has the following structural formula:

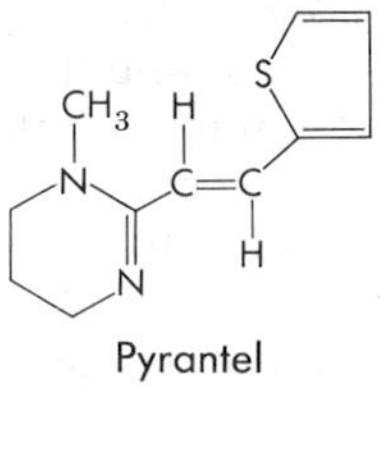

Pyrantel

Anthelmintic Action. Pyrantel and its analogs are depolarizing neuromuscular blocking agents. They induce marked, persistent nicotinic activation, which results in spastic paralysis of the worm. Pyrantel also inhibits cholinesterases. It causes a slowly developing contracture of preparations of *Ascaris* at 1% of the concentration of acetylcholine required to produce the same effect. In single muscle cells of this helminth, pyrantel causes depolarization and increased spike-discharge frequency, accompanied by increase in tension. In contrast, piperazine causes hyperpolarization with reduction in spike-discharge frequency and relaxation. Thus pyrantel and piperazine are mutually antagonistic in *Ascaris* preparations (Aubry *et al.*, 1970; Eyre, 1970). Pyrantel is effective against hookworm, pinworm, and roundworm; unlike its analog oxantel, it is ineffective against *Trichuris trichiura*.

Absorption, Fate, and Excretion. Pyrantel pamoate is poorly absorbed from the gastrointestinal tract, a property that contributes to its selective action on gastrointestinal nematodes. Less than 15% is excreted in the urine as parent drug and metabolites. The major proportion of an administered dose is recovered in the feces.

Preparation, Route of Administration, and Dosage. *Pyrantel pamoate* (ANTIMINTH) is supplied as a suspension (50 mg of the base per milliliter). The drug is given orally without regard to ingestion of food or beverages. A single dose of 11 mg/kg, to a maximum of 1 g, should be used to treat infections with *Ascaris lumbricoides, Enterobius (Oxyuris) vermicularis, Ancylostoma duodenale, Necator americanus,* or *Trichostrongylus*. In the case of pinworm, it is wise to repeat the treatment after an interval of 2 weeks.

Toxicity and Side Effects. When given parenterally, pyrantel can produce complete neuromuscular blockade in animals; if given orally, toxic effects are produced only by very large doses. Transient and mild gastrointestinal symptoms are occasionally observed in man, as are headache, dizziness, rash, and fever.

Precautions and Contraindications. Pyrantel pamoate has not been studied in pregnant women. Thus, its use in pregnant patients and children less than 2 years of age is not recommended. Because pyrantel pamoate and piperazine are mutually antagonistic, the two should not be used together.

Therapeutic Uses. Pyrantel pamoate is an agent of choice in the treatment of ascariasis and enterobiasis. High cure rates have been achieved after single-dose treatment. Similarly, high rates of cure have been obtained against *Ancylostoma, Necator americanus,* and *Trichostrongylus.* The drug should be used in combination with oxantel for mixed infections with *Trichuris trichiura.*

THIABENDAZOLE

Thiabendazole was the product of investigation of several hundred substituted benzimidazole compounds. Some of these are among the most potent chemotherapeutic agents known, complete larvicidal activity being manifested *in vitro* at 10 pg/ml. This potency, coupled with the absence of activity toward other microorganisms and relatively low mammalian toxicity, suggests an interference with metabolic pathways essential to a variety of helminths (Brown *et al.,* 1961). The drug has been reviewed extensively (*see* Symposium, 1969). Thiabendazole has the following structural formula:

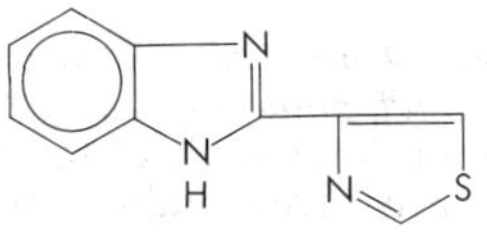

Thiabendazole

Anthelmintic Action. Thiabendazole is highly active against a wide range of nematodes that infect the gastrointestinal tract of domestic animals; it is also larvicidal and ovicidal *in vitro* at very low concentrations (Brown *et al.,* 1961; Egerton, 1961; Standen, 1963). Its primary mechanism of action is unknown, although the compound inhibits the helminth-specific mitochondrial fumarate reductase system, possibly by interacting with an endogenous quinone (Kohler and Bachmann, 1978). In *Strongyloides,* thiabendazole may suppress assembly of microtubules, leading to inhibition of secretion of parasite acetylcholinesterase and dislodgement of the worm (Watts *et al.,* 1982). Although the drug appears to be effective against intestinal stages of *Trichinella spiralis* in man, larvae in tissues appear relatively unaffected. Thiabendazole has no effect on filariasis. It is active *in vitro* against a variety of saprophytic and pathogenic fungi, particularly against strains of *Trichophyton* and *Microsporum.* Clinically, however, response to treatment of superficial fungal infections has been equivocal.

Absorption, Fate, and Excretion. Thiabendazole is rapidly absorbed after oral administration. Peak concentrations in plasma occur about 1 hour after treatment. Most of the drug is excreted in the urine within 24 hours as 5-hydroxythiabendazole, conjugated either as the glucuronide or as the sulfate.

Preparations, Route of Administration, and Dosage. *Thiabendazole* (MINTEZOL) is available as an oral suspension containing 500 mg/5 ml and in 500-mg chewable tablets. The drug is preferably given after meals. The maximal daily recommended dose is 3 g. The standard dose for treating roundworm infection is 25 mg/kg taken twice a day for 2 days. A 2-day course is required in treating cutaneous larva migrans and may be repeated in 2 days if active lesions are still present; the condition has been treated successfully by topical application of thiabendazole. In early trichinosis infection, treatment may be continued for a total of 5 days, according to the response of the patient. Treatment with thiabendazole for disseminated strongyloidiasis should be continued for at least 5 days. Thiabendazole may be tried in the treatment of visceral larva migrans at the usual dosage until either the symptoms subside or toxic effects intervene. Because this is usually a self-limiting disease, treatment should be restricted to severe cases.

Toxicity and Side Effects. Side effects frequently encountered are anorexia, nausea, vomiting, and dizziness. Less frequently, diarrhea, weariness, drowsiness, giddiness, and headache occur. Occasional fever, rashes, erythema multiforme, hallucinations, sensory disturbances, and Stevens–Johnson syndrome have been reported. Angioneurotic edema, shock, tinnitus, convulsions, and intrahepatic cholestasis are rare complications of therapy. Some patients may excrete a metabolite that imparts an odor to urine, much like that occurring in some after ingestion of asparagus. Crystalluria without hematuria has been reported on occasion; it promptly subsides with discontinuation of therapy. Transient leukopenia has been noted in a few patients on thiabendazole therapy.

The clinical utility of thiabendazole is compromised by its toxicity. Up to one third of patients treated with the recommended dosage have been incapacitated for several hours by one or more symptoms; half were incapacitated for as long as 24 hours by doses of about 50 mg/kg.

Precautions and Contraindications. There are no absolute contraindications to the use of thiabendazole. Because CNS side effects occur quite frequently, activities requiring mental alertness should be prohibited during therapy. Thiabendazole has hepatotoxic potential, and it should be used with caution in patients with hepatic disease or decreased hepatic function.

Therapeutic Uses. The introduction of thiabendazole was a major advance in the therapy of cutaneous larva migrans and *S. stercoralis* infections. The majority of patients experience marked relief of symptoms of creeping eruption. Progression of the disease should cease after 2 successive days of treatment. If active lesions persist after a 2-day interval, a second course of treatment is recommended. A 2- to 5-day course of treatment produces a better-than-90% cure rate in strongyloidiasis. There is circumstantial evidence that the drug is also beneficial in the treatment of visceral larva migrans. Although thiabendazole is effective against trichinosis in animals, its value in the human disease remains unproven. It seems to allay symptoms and to reduce eosinophilia early in the infection, but its effect on larvae that have migrated to muscle is open to doubt. An advantage of thiabendazole had been its effectiveness against mixed infections with *Ascaris, Enterobius, Strongyloides,* and *Trichuris;* however, it is being replaced by less toxic agents for this purpose.

TREATMENT OF HELMINTH INFECTIONS

NEMATODES (ROUNDWORMS)

Ascaris lumbricoides. *Ascaris lumbricoides,* known as the "roundworm," is cosmopolitan and affects about 25% of the world's population. Although cases of ascariasis are not infrequent in temperate climates, the parasite flourishes best in warm localities. In tropical countries, from 70 to 90% of a population may be infected. In the rural southern United States, the incidence of ascariasis is high in the children of poorer families.

Treatment. The older, less efficient, and more toxic ascaricides have largely been replaced by more effective, less toxic compounds. Both mebendazole and pyrantel pamoate are preferred agents. Piperazine is effective but used less often because of occasional neurotoxicity and hypersensitivity reactions. Cure with any of these drugs can be achieved in nearly 100% of cases. If ascariasis complicates hookworm infection, great care should be taken in treating the latter to avoid promoting unusual activity of the ascarids. Under such circumstances, the roundworms may block the lumen of the appendix and produce symptoms of appendicitis. They can occlude the common bile duct and occasionally invade the hepatic parenchyma. Perforation of the intestinal wall with subsequent peritonitis may rarely occur. If the worms are unusually active, they may form a tangled mass and cause intestinal obstruction. In the treatment of such mixed infections the advantage lies with pyrantel pamoate and mebendazole, because these agents are effective against *Ascaris* and both species of hookworms. Preference should probably be given to pyrantel pamoate because single-dose treatment is effective and it does not possess the teratogenic potential of mebendazole. However, mebendazole offers an advantage in that it is also effective against *Trichuris*. Ivermectin has recently shown promise in the treatment of single or mixed infections with *Ascaris, Strongyloides, Trichuris,* and *Oxyuris;* reduction in hookworm infestation was also reported (Naquira *et al.,* 1989).

Hookworm: *Necator americanus, Ancylostoma duodenale.* *N. americanus* predominates in the United States, whereas *A. duodenale* occurs nearly exclusively in other parts of the world. These related species affect over 20% of the human population and flourish chiefly between latitudes 30° south and 40° north. Distribution much further north, into areas where a similar environment prevails, has been brought about by carriers. Such conditions occur in mines and large mountain tunnels, hence the terms miner's disease and tunnel disease.

Treatment. Treatment of hookworm disease involves two related objectives. The first is to restore the blood values to normal, and the second is to expel the intestinal parasites. Proper diet and treatment with iron are usually sufficient for the first objective, but blood transfusion may occasionally be required. Mebendazole and pyrantel pamoate are now agents of first choice against both *A. duodenale* and *N. americanus,* and have the advantage of effectiveness against other roundworms when there is multiple infection. Thiabendazole is the drug of choice for treating *larva migrans* or "creeping eruption," due most commonly to penetration of the skin of man by larvae of the dog hookworm, *Ancylostoma braziliense*.

Trichuris trichiura. *Trichuris* (whipworm) infection is encountered throughout the world, especially in warm, humid climates. It is frequently found along with *Ascaris* and hookworms. The worm does not usually cause problems except in heavily infected young children, who may exhibit mild toxicity and some degree of anemia. Rarely, worms may lodge in the appendix or may penetrate the bowel wall and give rise to peritonitis.

Treatment. Mebendazole in a dosage of 100 mg twice daily for 3 days is considered the safest and most effective treatment against whipworm, either alone or in combination with *Ascaris* and hookworm. Although quite toxic, thiabendazole is also effective in an appreciable proportion of cases. Ivermectin shows promise in the treatment of this infection.

Strongyloides stercoralis. *S. stercoralis,* sometimes called the threadworm or dwarf threadworm, is frequently found in tropical and subtropical regions, often together with other intestinal helminths. Infection with this worm is common in parts of the southern United States. Similar environmental conditions often exist underground in mines, even in temperate zones, where the worm is occasionally found. Multiplication of the parasite in the host and autoinfection account for persistence of the infection.

Treatment. Thiabendazole is highly effective and has been considered to be the drug of choice. A 2-day course of therapy is normally prescribed; in disseminated strongyloidiasis, thiabendazole should be taken for at least 5 days. Ivermectin (0.1 to 0.2 mg/kg per day for 2 days) may prove an excellent alternative for therapy of this infection.

Enterobius (Oxyuris) vermicularis. *Oxyuris,* the pinworm, is cosmopolitan and the most common helminthic infection in the United States, especially in schoolchildren. This parasite rarely causes serious complications; pruritus in the perianal and perineal regions, however, can be severe, and scratching may cause secondary infection. In female patients, worms may wander into the genital tract and penetrate into the peritoneal cavity. Salpingitis or even peritonitis may ensue. Because the infection is easily distributed throughout members of a family, a school, or an institution, the physician must decide whether to treat all individuals in close contact with an infected person, and more than one course of therapy may be required.

Treatment. Both mebendazole and pyrantel pamoate are highly effective, and ivermectin also shows great promise. When their use is allied with rigid standards of personal hygiene, a very high proportion of cures can be obtained. Treatment is simple and almost devoid of side effects. Mebendazole should not be used during pregnancy because of its teratogenic potential. Daily doses of piperazine for 1 week are also effective but less convenient. Pyrantel pamoate, mebendazole, ivermectin, and piperazine have the added advantage of successfully clearing concurrent *Ascaris* infection.

Trichinella spiralis. The trichina worm is ubiquitous, regardless of climate, and does live outside a host. It is found frequently in Canada, Eastern Europe, and the United States. The infection results from eating raw, or insufficiently cooked, flesh of trichinous animals. All pork, including pork sausages, should be thoroughly cooked before being eaten. The encysted larvae are killed by exposure to heat of 60°C for 5 minutes.

Treatment. Thiabendazole, in well-tolerated doses, has been shown to kill *Trichinella* larvae in the muscle of experimental animals. In human cases, results have been variable. The drug may allay symptoms and reduce eosinophilia in early infections, but its effect on larvae that have migrated to muscle is questionable. Corticosteroids may be of considerable value in controlling the acute and dangerous manifestations of established infection.

Filariae. Infection with *Wuchereria bancrofti* is especially a risk in Central Africa, South America, India, and southern China, although it is also widely distributed throughout the tropics. *W. (Brugia) malayi* is restricted to Indonesia, the Malay peninsula, Vietnam, southern China, central India, and Sri Lanka. The migrating filaria, *Loa loa,* is a purely African species. It is found chiefly in the large river regions of western Central Africa, from Sierra Leone to Angola. The causative agent of "river blindness," *Onchocerca volvulus,* is very common in all parts of West and Central

Africa. It was presumably imported from there into Mexico, northeastern Venezuela, and Guatemala.

Treatment. Although other drugs may have therapeutic potential, diethylcarbamazine is now the only agent used for both suppression and cure of infections with *W. bancrofti, W. malayi,* and *Loa loa*. It is advisable to start with a small initial dose to diminish host reactions that result from destruction of microfilariae, particularly those of *Loa loa*. Corticosteroids may be required to control acute reactions. In rare instances, serious cerebral reactions occur in the treatment of loiasis, probably due to destruction of microfilariae in the brain. If headache is severe and there is other evidence of an adult *Loa loa* near the orbit, extra care is advisable in initial dosing. The most satisfactory results are achieved in *W. bancrofti* and *W. malayi* infections if chemotherapy is started early, before obstructive lesions of the lymphatics have occurred. Even in late cases, however, improvement may result. In longstanding elephantiasis, surgical measures are required to improve lymph drainage and remove redundant tissue.

Ivermectin, given as a single oral dose of 0.15 to 0.20 mg/kg every 6 to 12 months to adults, has replaced diethylcarbamazine as the drug of choice for the control and treatment of onchocerciasis. Both agents only kill microfilaria of *O. volvulus,* but ivermectin produces far milder systemic reactions and few, if any, ocular complications. With diethylcarbamazine, such reactions are likely to be even more severe than those encountered in the treatment of *Loa loa*; great care must be exercised in initial dosing, particularly in cases where there are lesions of the eye. Although suramin (*see* Chapter 43) is lethal to adult *O. volvulus,* treatment with this relatively toxic agent is probably unwarranted when good control of onchocerciasis can be achieved with ivermectin. Nonetheless, the search for less toxic macrofilariacides should continue.

Dracunculus medinensis. Known as the guinea, dragon, or Medina worm, this parasite occurs in East and West Africa, India, Pakistan, Bangladesh, Arabia, and Iraq, where it produces dracunculiasis.

Treatment. Traditional treatment for this disabling condition is to draw the adult female worm out alive. Natives do this by rolling it onto a small piece of wood, drawing it out slowly day by day. If the worm is ruptured, severe secondary infections may occur. Therefore, the site at which the worm has broken through should be continuously washed with water to cause the worm to discharge all the larvae. After this it may be more easily extracted. Alternatively the worm may be removed under local anesthesia by incisions along its course. Satisfactory healing with either extrusion of the worm or, if no worm is extruded, complete symptomatic and functional relief has been obtained by the administration of metronidazole (Chapter 42). The oral dose for adults is 250 mg given three times a day for 10 days. No local reactions occur if the worm is ruptured on extrusion. Suppression of host responses rather than a direct effect on the parasite probably accounts for the action of metronidazole.

CESTODES (FLATWORMS)

Taenia saginata. Man is the definitive host for *T. saginata,* known as the beef tapeworm. This most common form of tapeworm is usually detected after passage of proglottids from the intestine. It is cosmopolitan and rarely produces serious clinical disease. However, the infection must be distinguished from that produced by *T. solium*.

Treatment. Niclosamide and praziquantel are the drugs of choice for treatment of infection by *T. saginata*. Both are very effective, simple to administer, and comparatively free from side effects. Assessment of cure can be difficult because the worm, segments as well as scolex, is usually passed in a partially digested state. Cure can be assumed only if no further segments are detected by the end of 4 months. If parasitological diagnosis is uncertain, praziquantel is the preferred drug because of the danger of cysticercosis (*see* below).

Taenia solium. *T. solium,* or pork tapeworm, is also cosmopolitan. A danger unique to *T. solium* infection is cysticercosis, the harboring of the cysticerci (larvae) in the tissues of the human host. This autoinfection by parasite eggs usually results either from ingestion of fecally contaminated infected material or from eggs, liberated from a gravid segment, passing upward into the duodenum, where the outer layers are digested. In either case, the free larvae gain access to the circulation and the tissues exactly as in their cycle in the intermediate host, the pig. The seriousness of the disease that results depends upon the particular tissue invaded. The usual sites are the brain, orbit, muscles, liver, and lungs.

Treatment. Praziquantel is preferred over niclosamide in the treatment of infection with *T. solium* because the drug is also efficacious in combating cysticercosis. Repeated therapy may be required if parasitological cure is not obtained.

Diphyllobothrium latum. *D. latum,* the fish tapeworm, is a common parasite in many European countries, the Near East, Siberia, northern Manchuria, Japan, and the lake regions of Canada and the United States. In North America the pike is the most common second intermediate host. The eating of inadequately cooked infested fish introduces the larvae into the human intestine. The tasting of foods containing fish during their preparation is another common cause of infection. In countries where infection with fish tapeworm is common, there is a high incidence of megaloblastic anemia, which resembles addisonian pernicious anemia in all respects. This syndrome, which has been termed "bothriocephalus anemia," is especially prevalent in Finland, where in the past, 90% of the population of certain provinces harbored worms. The deficiency of vitamin B_{12} results from use of the vitamin by the worm, and expulsion of the worm results in a hematological remission.

Treatment. Treatment is again the same as that for *T. saginata,* that is, niclosamide or praziquantel. The presence of eggs in the stool 18 or more days after treatment is indicative of drug failure or reinfection.

Hymenolepis nana. *H. nana,* the dwarf tapeworm, is the smallest of the tapeworms found in the small intestine of man. Children are infected more often than adults. The infection is cosmopolitan but is more common in warm climates. It is the most frequently occurring tapeworm disease in the southern United States. *H. nana* can develop from ovum to mature adult in man without an intermediate host. The cysticerci develop in the villi of the intestine for 3 to 4 days and then regain access to the intestinal lumen. Treatment must therefore be adapted to this form of development.

Treatment. Niclosamide or praziquantel is the agent of choice in North America. Failure of treatment or reinfection is indicated by the appearance of eggs in the stool about 4 weeks after the last dose.

TREMATODES (FLUKES)

Schistosoma haematobium, S. mansoni, S. japonicum. These are the main species of blood flukes that cause human schistosomiasis; less common species are *S. intercalatum* and *S. mekongi.* The infection affects over 200 million people, and more than 500 million are considered at risk. Geographically, schistosomiasis is widely distributed over the South American continent and certain Caribbean islands (*S. mansoni*), much of the Arabian Peninsula and Africa (*S. mansoni* and *S. haematobium*), and China, the Philippines, and Indonesia (*S. japonicum*). Infected snails act as intermediate hosts for fresh-water transmission of the infection, which continues to spread as the development of agricultural and water resources increases. Schistosomal disease, which generally correlates with the intensity of infection, primarily involves the liver, spleen, and gastrointestinal tract (*S. mansoni* and *S. japonicum*) or the genitourinary tract (*S. haematobium*).

Treatment. Praziquantel is now considered to be the drug of choice for treating all species of schistosomes that infect man. The drug is safe and effective when it is given in single or divided oral doses on the same day. These properties make praziquantel particularly suitable for population-based chemotherapy. Although not effective clinically against *S. haematobium* and *S. japonicum,* oxamniquine has proven to be effective for treatment of *S. mansoni* infections, particularly in South America, where the sensitivity of most strains may permit single-dose therapy. However, resistance has been reported, in both the field and the laboratory, and higher doses of the drug are required to treat African than Brazilian strains of *S. mansoni.* Metrifonate has been used with considerable success in the treatment of *S. haematobium* infections, but the drug is not effective against *S. mansoni* and *S. japonicum.* Metrifonate is relatively inexpensive and can be used in conjunction with oxamniquine for treatment of mixed infections with *S. haematobium* and *S. mansoni.*

Paragonimus westermani, P. kellicotti. Called lung flukes, a number of *Paragonimus* species are pathogenic for man and carnivores. Found in the Far East and on the African and South American continents, these parasites have two intermediate hosts—snails and crustaceans. Man becomes infected by eating raw or undercooked crabs or crayfish.

Treatment. Although rather refractory to the drug *in vitro,* preliminary clinical results with praziquantel are encouraging. Three doses of 25 mg/kg each are recommended daily for two consecutive days, but an optimal dosage schedule is still to be established.

Clonorchis sinensis, Opisthorchis viverrini, O. felineus, Fasciola hepatica. These parasites are all liver flukes. *C. sinensis,* the Chinese liver fluke, and *Opisthorchis* species inhabit the biliary system of man, where they may produce disease. Snails and fish serve as primary and secondary hosts, respectively, for these parasites. *F. hepatica,* the large liver fluke, primarily infects herbivorous ruminants but incidentally infects the biliary system of man. Snails and fresh-water plants, such as watercress, serve as primary and secondary hosts for this parasite.

Treatment. Praziquantel has largely replaced older, rather ineffective drugs for treatment of infections with *C. sinensis* and *O. viverrini.* These respond well to doses of 25 mg/kg given three times during a single day. Unlike infections with other flukes, fascioliasis probably does not respond to praziquantel.

Fasciolopsis buski, Heterophyes heterophyes, Metagonimus yokogawai. *F. buski,* the giant intestinal fluke, occurs chiefly in Southeast Asia, whereas the other smaller intestinal flukes occur in various parts of the world. These parasites generally cause clinical symptoms only if infection is massive. As is the case for infections with other trematodes, praziquantel is emerging as the drug of choice for these infections.

Abdallah, A., and Saif, M. The efficacy of N-2′-chloro-4′-nitrophenyl-5-chlorosalicylamide in the treatment of taeniasis. *J. Egypt. Med. Assoc.,* **1961,** *44,* 379–381.

Aubry, M. L.; Cowell, P.; Davey, M. J.; and Shevde, S. Aspects of the pharmacology of a new anthelmintic: pyrantel. *Br. J. Pharmacol.,* **1970,** *38,* 332–344.

Austin, W. C.; Courtney, W.; Danilewicz, J. C.; Morgan, D. H.; Conover, L. H.; Howes, H. L., Jr.; Lynch, J. E.; McFarland, J. W.; Cornwall, R. L.; and Theodorides, V. J. Pyrantel tartrate, a new anthelmintic effective against infections of domestic animals. *Nature,* **1966,** *212,* 1273–1274.

Awadzi, K.; Dadzie, K. Y.; Schulz-Key, H.; Haddock, D. R. W.; Gilles, H. M.; and Aziz, M. A. The chemotherapy of onchocerciasis. X. An assessment of four single-dose treatment regimens of MK-933 (ivermectin) in human onchocerciasis. *Ann. Trop. Med. Parasitol.,* **1985,** *79,* 63–78.

Awadzi, K.; Orme, M. L.; Breckenridge, A. M.; and Gilles, H. M. The chemotherapy of onchocerciasis. VII. The effect of prednisone on the Mazzotti reaction. *Ann. Trop. Med. Parasitol.,* **1982,** *76,* 331–338.

Bassily, S.; Farid, Z.; Higashi, G. I.; and Watten, R. H. Treatment of complicated schistosomiasis mansoni with oxamniquine. *Am. J. Trop. Med. Hyg.,* **1978,** *27,* 1284–1286.

Bloom, A. Studies of the mode of action of metrifonate and DDVP in schistosomes—cholinesterase activity and the hepatic shift. *Acta Pharmacol. Toxicol. (Copenh.),* **1981,** *49,* Suppl. V, 109–113.

Braithwaite, P. A.; Roberts, M. S.; Allan, R. J.; and Watson, T. R. Clinical pharmacokinetics of high dose mebendazole in patients treated for hydatid disease. *Eur. J. Clin. Pharmacol.,* **1982,** *22,* 161–169.

Brown, H. D.; Matzuk, A. R.; Ilves, I. R.; Peterson, L. H.; Harris, S. A.; Sarett, L. H.; Egerton, J. R.; Yakstis, J. J.; Campbell, W. C.; and Cuckler, A. C. Antiparasitic drugs. IV. 2-(4′-thiazolyl)-benzimidazole, a new anthelmintic. *J. Am. Chem. Soc.,* **1961,** *83,* 1764–1765.

Brugmans, J. P.; Thienpont, D. C.; van Wijngaarden, I.; Vanparijs, O. F.; Schuermans, V. L.; and Lauwers, H. L. Mebendazole in enterobiasis. Radiochemical and pilot clinical study in 1278 subjects. *J.A.M.A.,* **1971,** *217,* 313–316.

Bumbalo, T. S.; Fugazzoto, D. J.; and Wyczalek, J. V. Treatment of enterobiasis with pyrantel pamoate. *Am. J. Trop. Med. Hyg.,* **1969,** *18,* 50–52.

Burg, R. A., and others. Avermectins, new family of potent anthelmintic agents: producing organism and fermentation. *Antimicrob. Agents Chemother.,* **1979,** *15,* 361–367.

Chavarria, A. P.; Swartzwelder, J. C.; Villarejos, V. M.; and Zeledon, R. Mebendazole, an effective broad-spectrum anthelmintic. *Am. J. Trop. Med. Hyg.,* **1973,** *22,* 592–595.

Cioli, D.; Pica-Mattoccia, L.; Rosenberg, L.; and Archer, S. Evidence for the mode of antischistosomal action of hycanthone. *Life Sci.,* **1985,** *37,* 161–167.

Court, J. P.; Bianco, A. E.; Townson, S.; Ham, P. J.; and Friedheim, E. Study on the activity of antiparasitic agents against *Onchocerca lienalis* third stage larvae *in vitro. Trop. Med. Parasitol.,* **1985,** *36,* 117–119.

Cupp, E. W.; Bernardo, M. J.; Kiszewski, A. E.; Collins, R. C.; Taylor, H. R.; Aziz, M. A.; and Greene, B. M. The effects of ivermectin on transmission of *Onchocerca volvulus. Science,* **1986,** *231,* 740–742.

Cupp, E. W.; Ochoa-A., O.; Collins, R. C.; Ramberg, F. R.; and Zea-F., G. The effect of multiple ivermectin treatments on infection of *Simulium ochraceum* with *Onchocerca volvulus. Am. J. Trop. Med. Hyg.,* **1989,** *40,* 501–506.

Daneshmend, T. K., and Homeida, M. Oxamniquine pharmacokinetics in hepatosplenic schistosomiasis in Sudan. *J. Antimicrob. Chemother.,* **1987,** *19,* 87–93.

Diallo, S.; Aziz, M. A.; Ndir, O.; Badiane, S.; Bah, I. B.; and Gaye, O. Dose-ranging study of ivermectin in treatment of filariasis due to *Wuchereria bancrofti. Lancet,* **1987,** *1,* 1030.

Doehring, E.; Poggensee, U.; and Feldmeier, H. The effect of metrifonate in mixed *Schistosoma haematobium* and *Schistosoma mansoni* infections in humans. *Am. J. Trop. Med. Hyg.,* **1986,** *35,* 323–329.

Dominguez-Vazquez, A.; Taylor, H. R.; Greene, B. M.; Ruvalcaba-Macias, A. M.; Rivas-Alcala, A. R.; Murphy, R. P.; and Beltran-Hernandez, F. Comparison of flubendazole and diethylcarbamazine in treatment of onchocerciasis. *Lancet,* **1983,** *1,* 137–143.

Edwards, G.; Awadzi, K.; Breckenridge, A. M.; Gilles, H. M.; Orme, M. L.; and Ward, S. A. Diethylcarbamazine disposition in patients with onchocerciasis. *Clin. Pharmacol. Ther.,* **1981a,** *30,* 551–557.

Edwards, G.; Breckenridge, A. M.; Adjepon-Yamoah, K. K.; Orme, M. L.; and Ward, S. A. The effect of variations in urinary pH on the pharmacokinetics of diethylcarbamazine. *Br. J. Clin. Pharmacol.,* **1981b,** *12,* 807–812.

Egerton, J. R. The effect of thiabendazole upon *Ascaris* and *Stephanurus* infections. *J. Parasitol.,* **1961,** *47,* Sect. 2, 37.

Egerton, J. R.; Ostlind, D. A.; Blair, L. S.; Eary, C. H.; Suhayda, D.; Cifelli, S.; Reik, R. F.; and Campbell, W. C. Avermectins, new family of potent anthelmintic agents: efficacy of the B_{1a} component. *Antimicrob. Agents Chemother.,* **1979,** *15,* 372–378.

Eyre, P. Some pharmacodynamic effects of the nematocides: methyridine, tetramisole and pyrantel. *J. Pharm. Pharmacol.,* **1970,** *22,* 26–36.

Faulkner, J. K., and Smith, K. J. Dealkylation and N-oxidation in the metabolism of 1-diethyl-carbamyl-4-methylpiperazine in the rat. *Xenobiotica*, **1972**, *2*, 59–68.

Fayard, C. Ascaridiose et piperazine. Thesis, Paris, **1949**. (Quoted from *Sem. Hop. Paris*, **1949**, *35*, 1778.)

Feldmeier, H.; Doehring, E.; Daffala, A. A.; Omer, A. H. S.; and Dietrich, M. Efficacy of metrifonate in urinary schistosomiasis: comparison of reduction of *Schistosoma haematobium* and *S. mansoni* eggs. *Am. J. Trop. Med. Hyg.*, **1982**, *31*, 1188–1194.

Fletcher, K. A.; Evans, D. A. P.; and Kelly, J. A. Urinary piperazine excretion in healthy Caucasians. *Ann. Trop. Med. Parasitol.*, **1982**, *76*, 77–82.

Foster, R. The preclinical development of oxamniquine. *Rev. Inst. Med. Trop. Sao Paulo*, **1973**, *15*, 1–9.

Gönnert, R., and Schraufstätter, E. Experimentelle Untersuchungen mit N-(2′-chlor-4′-nitrophenyl)-5-Chlorsalicylamid, einen neuen Bandwurmmitel. I. Mitterlung: Chemotherapeutische Versuche. *Arzneim. Forsch.*, **1960**, *10*, 881–884.

Goodwin, L. G., and Standen, O. D. Treatment of ascariasis with various salts of piperazine. *Br. Med. J.*, **1958**, *1*, 131–133.

Greene, B. M., and others. Comparison of ivermectin and diethylcarbamazine in the treatment of onchocerciasis. *N. Engl. J. Med.*, **1985**, *313*, 133–138.

Greene, B. M.; White, A. T.; Newland, H. S.; Keyvan-Larijani, E.; Dukuly, Z. D.; Gallin, M. Y.; Aziz, M. A.; Williams, P. N.; and Taylor, H. R. Single dose therapy with ivermectin for onchocerciasis. *Trans. Assoc. Am. Physicians*, **1987**, *100*, 131–138.

Jain, D. C.; Sethumadhavan, K. V.; Babu, C. S.; Johney, V. M.; and Ghosh, T. K. Practical and effective dose schedule of diethylcarbamazine (DEC) against bancroftian filariasis for mass therapy campaigns. *J. Commun. Dis.*, **1988**, *23*, 61–69.

Jewsbury, J. M.; Cooke, M. J.; and Weber, M. C. Field trial of metrifonate in the treatment and prevention of schistosomiasis infection in man. *Ann. Trop. Med. Parasitol.*, **1977**, *71*, 67–83.

Jones, W. Niclosamide as a treatment for *Hymenolepis diminuta* and *Dipylidium caninum* infection in man. *Am. J. Trop. Med. Hyg.*, **1979**, *28*, 300–302.

Katz, N.; Zicker, F.; and Pereira, J. P. Field trials with oxamniquine in a schistosomiasis mansoni–endemic area. *Am. J. Trop. Med. Hyg.*, **1977**, *26*, 234–237.

Kaye, B. Oxamniquine: metabolism, pharmacokinetics and mode of action. *WHO Scientific Working Group on the Biochemistry and Chemotherapy of Schistosomiasis*. WHO, Geneva, **1984**, pp. 1–19.

Kaye, B., and Roberts, D. W. The metabolism of oxamniquine in gut wall. *Xenobiotica*, **1980**, *10*, 97–101.

Kaye, B., and Woolhouse, N. M. The metabolism of oxamniquine, a new schistosomicide. *Ann. Trop. Med. Parasitol.*, **1976**, *70*, 323–328.

Keystone, J. S., and Murdoch, J. K. Mebendazole. *Ann. Intern. Med.*, **1979**, *91*, 582–586.

Kohler, P., and Bachmann, R. The effects of the antiparasitic drugs levamisole, thiabendazole, praziquantel, and chloroquine on mitochondrial electron transport in muscle tissue from *Ascaris suum*. *Mol. Pharmacol.*, **1978**, *14*, 155–158.

Langham, M. E., and Kramer, T. R. The *in vitro* effect of diethylcarbamazine on the motility and survival of *Onchocerca volvulus* microfilariae. *Tropenmed. Parasitol.*, **1980**, *31*, 59–66.

Miller, T. W., and others. Avermectins, new family of potent anthelmintic agents: isolation and chromatographic properties. *Antimicrob. Agents Chemother.*, **1979**, *15*, 368–371.

Naquira, C.; Jimenez, G.; Guerra, J. G.; Bernal, R.; Nalin, D. R.; Neu, D.; and Aziz, M. Ivermectin for human strongyloidiasis and other intestinal helminths. *Am. J. Trop. Med. Hyg.*, **1989**, *40*, 304–309.

Newland, H. S.; White, A. T.; Greene, B. M.; D'Anna, S. A.; Keyvan-Larijani, E.; Aziz, M. A.; Williams, P. N.; and Taylor, H. R. Effect of single-dose ivermectin therapy on human *Onchocerca volvulus* infection with onchocercal ocular involvement. *Br. J. Ophthalmol.*, **1988**, *72*, 561–569.

Nordgren, I.; Bengtsson, E.; Holmstedt, B.; and Pettersson, B. M. Levels of metrifonate and dichlorvos in plasma and erythrocytes during treatment of schistosomiasis with BILARCIL. *Acta Pharmacol. Toxicol. (Copenh.)*, **1981**, *49*, Suppl. V, 79–86.

Omer, A. H. S. Oxamniquine for treating *Schistosoma mansoni* infection in Sudan. *Br. Med. J.*, **1978**, *2*, 163–165.

Omer, A. H. S., and Teesdale, C. H. Metrifonate trial in the treatment of various presentations of *Schistosoma haematobium* and *S. mansoni* infections in the Sudan. *Ann. Trop. Med. Parasitol.*, **1978**, *72*, 145–150.

Partono, F.; Purnomo, O. S.; Oemijati, S.; and Soewarta, A. The long term effects of repeated diethylcarbamazine administration with special reference to microfilaremia and elephantiasis. *Acta Trop. (Basel)*, **1981**, *38*, 217–225.

Pax, R.; Bennet, J. L.; and Fetterer, R. A benzodiazepine derivative and praziquantel: effects on musculature of *Schistosoma mansoni* and *Schistosoma japonicum*. *Naunyn Schmiedebergs Arch. Pharmacol.*, **1978**, *304*, 309–315.

Pica-Mattoccia, L., and Cioli, D. Studies on the mode of action of oxamniquine and related schistosomicidal drugs. *Am. J. Trop. Med. Hyg.*, **1985**, *34*, 112–118.

Reiner, E. Esterases in schistosomes. Reaction with substrates and inhibitors. *Acta Pharmacol. Toxicol. (Copenh.)*, **1981**, *49*, Suppl. V, 72–78.

Reiner, E.; Krauthacker, B.; Simeon, V.; and Skrinjaric-Spoljar, M. Mechanism of inhibition *in vitro* of mammalian acetylcholinesterase and cholinesterase in solutions of O,O-dimethyl-2,2,2-trichloro-1-hydroxyethyl phosphonate (TRICHLORPHON). *Biochem. Pharmacol.*, **1975**, *24*, 717–722.

Reiner, E.; Simeon, V.; and Skrinjaric-Spoljar, M. Hydrolysis of O,O-dimethyl-2,2-dichlorovinyl phosphate (DDVP) by esterases in parasitic helminths, and in vertebrate plasma and erythrocytes. *Comp. Biochem. Physiol. [C]*, **1980**, *66C*, 149–152.

Rivas-Alcala, A. R.; Greene, B. M.; Taylor, H. R.; Dominguez-Vazquez, A.; Ruvalcaba-Macias, A. M.; Lugo-Pfeiffer, C.; Mackenzie, C. D.; and Beltran, H. F. Chemotherapy of onchocerciasis: a controlled comparison of mebendazole, levamisole, and diethylcarbamazine. *Lancet*, **1981**, *2*, 485–490.

Sargent, R. G.; Savory, A. M.; Mina, A.; and Lee, P. R. A clinical evaluation of mebendazole in the treatment of trichuriasis. *Am. J. Trop. Med. Hyg.*, **1974**, *23*, 375–377.

Scheibel, L. W., and Saz, H. J. The pathway for anaerobic carbohydrate dissimilation in *Hymenolepis diminuta*. *Comp. Biochem. Physiol.*, **1966**, *18*, 151–162.

Scheibel, L. W.; Saz, H. J.; and Bueding, E. The anaerobic incorporation of ^{32}P into adenosine triphosphate by *Hymenolepis diminuta*. *J. Biol. Chem.*, **1968**, *243*, 2229–2235.

Singson, C. N.; Banzon, T. C.; and Cross, J. H. Mebendazole in the treatment of intestinal capillariasis. *Am. J. Trop. Med. Hyg.*, **1975**, *24*, 932–934.

Skarping, G.; Bellander, T.; and Mathiasson, L. Determination of piperazine in working atmosphere and in human urine using capillary gas chromatography with nitrogen and mass-selective detection. *J. Chromatogr.*, **1986**, *370*, 245–258.

Sleigh, A. C.; Hoff, R.; Mott, K. E.; Maguire, J. H.; and da Franca Silva, J. T. Manson's schistosomiasis in Brazil: 11-year evaluation of successful disease control with oxamniquine. *Lancet*, **1986**, *1*, 635–637.

Sotelo, J.; Escobedo, F.; and Penagos, P. Albendazole

versus praziquantel for therapy for neurocysticercosis. A controlled trial. *Arch. Neurol.*, **1988**, *45*, 532–534.

Sotelo, J.; Escobedo, F.; Rodriguez-Carbajal, J.; Torres, B.; and Rubio-Donnadieu, F. Therapy of parenchymal brain cysticercosis with praziquantel. *N. Engl. J. Med.*, **1984**, *310*, 1001–1007.

Spiro, R. C.; Parsons, W. G.; Perry, S. K.; Caulfield, J. P.; Hein, A.; Reisfeld, R. A.; Harper, J. R.; Austen, K. F.; and Stevens, R. L. Inhibition of post-translational modification and surface expression of a melanoma-associated chondroitin sulfate proteoglycan by diethylcarbamazine or ammonium chloride. *J. Biol. Chem.*, **1986**, *261*, 5121–5129.

Taylor, H. R.; Semba, R. D.; Newland, H. S.; Keyvan-Larijani, E.; White, A.; Dukuly, Z.; and Greene, B. M. Ivermectin treatment of patients with severe ocular onchocerciasis. *Am. J. Trop. Med. Hyg.*, **1989**, *40*, 494–500.

Van Hoegaerden, M.; Ivanoff, B.; Flocard, F.; Salle, A.; and Chabaud, B. The use of mebendazole in the treatment of filariases due to *Loa loa* and *Mansonella perstans*. *Ann. Trop. Med. Parasitol.*, **1987**, *81*, 275–282.

Watts, S. D. M.; Rapson, E. B.; Atkins, A. M.; and Lee, D. L. Inhibition of acetylcholinesterase secretion from *Nippostrongylus brasiliensis* by benzimidazole anthelmintics. *Biochem. Pharmacol.*, **1982**, *31*, 3035–3040.

White, R. H. R., and Scopes, J. W. A single-dose treatment of threadworms in children. *Lancet*, **1960**, *1*, 256–258.

Wilson, J. F.; Rausch, R. L.; McMahon, B. J.; Schantz, P. M.; Trujillo, D. E.; and O'Gorman, M. A. Albendazole therapy in alveolar hydatid disease: a report of favorable results in two patients after short-term therapy. *Am. J. Trop. Med. Hyg.*, **1987**, *37*, 162–168.

Witassek, F.; Allan, R. J.; Watson, T. R.; Woodtli, W.; Ammann, R.; and Bircher, J. Preliminary observations on the biliary elimination of mebendazole and its metabolites in patients with echinococcosis. *Eur. J. Clin. Pharmacol.*, **1983**, *25*, 81–84.

Witassek, F.; Burkhardt, B.; Eckert, J.; and Bircher, J. Chemotherapy of alveolar echinococcosis: comparison of plasma mebendazole concentrations in animals and man. *Eur. J. Clin. Pharmacol.*, **1981**, *20*, 427–433.

Xiao, S.; Catto, B. A.; and Webster, L. T., Jr. Effects of praziquantel on different stages of *Schistosoma mansoni in vitro* and *in vivo*. *J. Infect. Dis.*, **1985**, *151*, 1130–1137.

Monographs and Reviews

Andrews, P. Praziquantel: mechanisms of anti-schistosomal activity. *Pharmacol. Ther.*, **1985**, *29*, 129–156.

Andrews, P.; Thomas, H.; Pohlke, R.; and Seubert, J. Praziquantel. *Med. Res. Rev.*, **1983**, *3*, 147–200.

Archer, S. The chemotherapy of schistosomiasis. *Annu. Rev. Pharmacol. Toxicol.*, **1985**, *25*, 485–508.

Brown, H. W. Anthelmintics, new and old. *Clin. Pharmacol. Ther.*, **1968**, *10*, 5–21.

Campbell, W. C., and Benz, G. W. Ivermectin: a review of efficacy and safety. *J. Vet. Pharmacol. Ther.*, **1984**, *7*, 1–16.

Campbell, W. C.; Fisher, M. H.; Stapley, E. O.; Albers-Schönberg, G.; and Jacob, T. A. Ivermectin: a potent new antiparasitic agent. *Science*, **1983**, *221*, 823–828.

Frohberg, H., and Schencking, M. S. Toxicological profile of praziquantel, a new drug against cestode and schistosome infections, as compared to some other schistosomicides. *Arzneimittelforsch.*, **1981**, *31*, 555–565.

Hawking, F. Diethylcarbamazine and new compounds for the treatment of filariasis. *Adv. Pharmacol. Chemother.*, **1979**, *16*, 129–194.

Hewitt, R. I.; White, D. E.; Kushner, S.; Wallace, W. S.; Stuart, M. W.; and Subba Row, Y. Parasitology of piperazines in the treatment of filariasis. *Ann. N.Y. Acad. Sci.*, **1948**, *50*, 128–140.

Keeling, J. E. D. The chemotherapy of cestode infections. *Adv. Chemother.*, **1968**, *3*, 109–152.

Mackenzie, C. D., and Kron, M. A. Diethylcarbamazine: a review of its action in onchocerciasis, lymphatic filariasis and inflammation. *Trop. Dis. Bull.*, **1985**, *82*, R1–R37.

Mahmoud, A. A. F. Praziquantel for the treatment of helminthic infections. *Adv. Intern. Med.*, **1987**, *32*, 193–206.

Ottesen, E. A. Efficacy of diethylcarbamazine in eradicating infection with lymphatic-dwelling filariae in humans. *Rev. Infect. Dis.*, **1985**, *7*, 341–356.

———. Description, mechanisms and control of reactions to treatment in the human filariases. In, *Filariasis.* Ciba Foundation Symposium 127. John Wiley & Sons Ltd., Chichester, England, **1987**, pp. 265–283.

Saz, H. J., and Bueding, E. Relationships between anthelmintic effects and biochemical and physiological mechanisms. *Pharmacol. Rev.*, **1966**, *18*, 871–894.

Standen, O. D. Chemotherapy of helminthic infections. In, *Experimental Chemotherapy*, Vol. I. (Schnitzer, R. J., and Hawking, F., eds.) Academic Press, Inc., New York, **1963**, pp. 701–892.

Symposium. (Various authors.) Thiabendazole. *Tex. Rep. Biol. Med.*, **1969**, *27*, 533–708.

Symposium. (Various authors.) Biltricide symposium on African schistosomiasis. (Classen, H. G., and Schramm, V., eds.) *Arzneimittelforsch.*, **1981a**, *31*, 535–618.

Symposium. (Various authors.) Metrifonate and dichlorvos: theoretical and practical aspects. *Acta Pharmacol. Toxicol. (Copenh.)*, **1981b**, *49*, Suppl. V, 7–113.

Van den Bossche, H. A look at the mode of action of some old and new antifilarial compounds. *Ann. Soc. Belg. Med. Trop.*, **1981**, *61*, 287–296.

Van den Bossche, H.; Rochette, F.; and Horig, C. Mebendazole and related anthelmintics. *Adv. Pharmacol. Chemother.*, **1982**, *19*, 67–128.

Wang, C. C., and Pong, S. S. Actions of avermectin B_{1a} on GABA nerves. *Prog. Clin. Biol. Res.*, **1982**, *97*, 373–395.

Wegner, D. H. G. The profile of the trematodicidal compound, praziquantel. *Arzneimittelforschung*, **1984**, *35*, 1132–1136.

World Health Organization. *Report of the Expert Committee on Filariasis*. Technical Report No. 359, WHO, Geneva, **1967**.

CHAPTER

41 DRUGS USED IN THE CHEMOTHERAPY OF PROTOZOAL INFECTIONS

Malaria

Leslie T. Webster, Jr.

Malaria remains the world's most devastating human infection, affecting over 200 million people and causing more than 2 million deaths each year. Much of this mortality is caused by infection with *Plasmodium falciparum,* which poses the greatest risk to nonimmune individuals and children less than 5 years of age. Although the mosquito-borne infection has been virtually eradicated from the United States, emigration from and travel to endemic regions constitute a continuing health problem. Practical, effective, and safe drugs, insecticides, and vaccines are still needed to combat malaria. In the 1950s, attempts to eradicate this scourge from most parts of the world failed, primarily because of the development of resistance to insecticides and antimalarial drugs. Since 1960, transmission of malaria has risen in most tropical areas where the infection is endemic, chloroquine-resistant and multidrug-resistant strains of *P. falciparum* have spread, and the degree of resistance to drugs of this most prevalent and dangerous plasmodial species has increased.

Most antimalarial drugs were developed on the basis of their action against asexual erythrocytic forms of malarial parasites, which are responsible for the clinical illness. Highly effective chemotherapeutic agents in this category are chloroquine, quinine, quinidine, and mefloquine. Pyrimethamine, sulfonamides, sulfones, and tetracyclines share this property but are slower acting, less effective, and nearly always used in combination with other antimalarial compounds. Primaquine is the only antimalarial that is employed clinically to eradicate tissue forms of plasmodia that cause relapses. Compounds that are being evaluated for use against chloroquine-resistant and multidrug-resistant strains of *P. falciparum* include mefloquine, a 4-quinolinemethanol derivative, and halofantrine, a 9-phenanthrenemethanol; both of these compounds are related to quinine. Derivatives of qinghaosu, a novel sesquiterpene lactone discovered in China, are also being tested. The advent of techniques for continuous maintenance of human malarial parasites *in vitro* has been of fundamental importance for the development of chemotherapeutic agents and vaccines (Trager and Jensen, 1976). A related advance has been the establishment of practical methods to assess the susceptibility of human malarial strains to drugs *in vitro* (Rieckmann *et al.,* 1978; Desjardins *et al.,* 1979a). The opportunity for experimental chemotherapy of human malarias in a nonhuman primate host has been provided by the successful passage of both falciparum and vivax malarias in the owl monkey (*see* World Health Organization, 1973; Schmidt, 1978).

The biology of malarial infection must be appreciated in order to understand the actions and uses of antimalarial drugs.

BIOLOGY OF MALARIAL INFECTION

Human malaria is caused by four species of obligate intracellular Protozoa of the genus *Plasmodium;* they reproduce asexually in man, but sexually in female mosquitoes (genus *Anopheles*). Each species has distinguishing morphological features, and the disease caused by each is also distinctive. (1) *P. falciparum* causes malignant tertian malaria, the most dangerous form of human malaria. Because of its potential to invade erythrocytes of any age, this species can produce an overwhelming parasitemia and fulminating infection in the nonimmune patient that, if untreated, may rapidly cause death. Delay in treatment until after demonstration of parasitemia may lead to an irreversible state of shock, and death may ensue even after the peripheral blood is free of parasites. If treated early, the infection usually responds readily to appropriate antimalarial drugs and relapses will not occur. If treatment is inadequate, however, recrudescence of infection may result from multiplication of parasites that persist in the blood. (2) *P. vivax* causes benign tertian malaria and produces milder clinical attacks than those of *P. falciparum*. *P. vivax* infection has a low mortality rate in untreated adults and is characterized by relapses that occur as long as 2 years after primary infection. (3) *P. ovale* causes a rare malarial infection with a periodicity and relapses similar to those of *P. vivax,* but it is milder and more readily cured. (4) *P. malariae* causes quartan malaria, an infection that is common in localized areas of the tropics. Clinical attacks may occur years after infection but are much rarer than after infection with *P. vivax*.

Although malaria can be transmitted by transfusion of infected blood, man is naturally infected by sporozoites injected by the bite of infected female anopheline mosquitoes. The parasites rapidly leave the circulation and localize in hepatic parenchymal cells, where they multiply and develop into tissue schizonts. This asymptomatic tissue (preerythrocytic or exoerythrocytic) stage of infection lasts for 5 to 16 days, depending on the species of plasmodium. The tissue schizonts then rupture, each releasing thousands of merozoites; these enter the circulation, invade erythrocytes, and initiate the erythrocytic stage or cycle of infection. In *P. falciparum* and *P. malariae* infections, tissue schizonts burst more or less simultaneously, leaving no forms of the parasite in the liver. But in *P. vivax* and *P. ovale* infections, some tissue parasites persist and proliferate only later to produce relapses of erythrocytic infection months to years after the primary attack. The origin of such tissue forms is unclear (Schmidt, 1986). One hypothesis is that they are derived from a minor fraction of released hepatic merozoites that invade uninfected hepatic cells to establish yet another generation of tissue stages (Shortt and Garnham, 1948). A second, more recent, concept is that they arise from subpopulations of sporozoites that develop within the liver into latent forms termed *hypnozoites*. The hypnozoites are programmed to resume differentiation and multiplication after various time intervals, thereby accounting for the relapses (Bray and Garnham, 1982; Krotoski, 1985). In any case, once human plasmodia enter the erythrocytic cycle, they cannot invade other tissues; thus, there is no tissue stage of infection for human malarias that are contracted by transfusion. In erythrocytes, most parasites undergo asexual development from young ring forms to trophozoites and finally to mature schizonts. Schizont-containing erythrocytes rupture, each releasing 6 to 24 merozoites, and it is this process that produces the febrile clinical attack. The released merozoites then invade more erythrocytes to continue the cycle, which proceeds until death of the host or modulation by drugs or acquired immunity. The periodicity of parasitemia and febrile clinical manifestations in tertian or quartan malaria thus depends on the timing of schizogony of a generation of erythrocytic parasites.

Some erythrocytic parasites differentiate into sexual forms known as gametocytes. After blood is ingested by a female mosquito, exflagellation of the male gametocyte is followed by male gametogenesis and fertilization of the female gametocyte in the gut of the insect. The resulting zygote, which develops in the gut wall as an oocyst, eventually gives rise to the infective sporozoite, which invades the salivary gland of the mosquito. The insect then can infect another human host by taking a blood meal.

CLASSIFICATION OF ANTIMALARIAL AGENTS

Antimalarials can be categorized according to the stage of the parasite that they affect.

Tissue Schizontocides Used for Causal Prophylaxis. These agents act on primary tissue forms of plasmodia within the liver that are destined within a month or less to initiate the erythrocytic stage of infection. Invasion of erythrocytes and further transmission of malaria to mosquitoes is thereby prevented. Pyrimethamine is extensively used for causal prophylaxis of falciparum malaria. Primaquine also has causal prophylactic activity but is not used for this purpose because of its toxicity.

Tissue Schizontocides Used to Prevent Relapse. These compounds act on the hepatic forms of *P. vivax* and *P. ovale* that produce relapses after the primary attack. Together with an appropriate blood schizontocide, these agents can achieve a radical cure of *P. vivax* and *P. ovale* infections. Primaquine is the prototypical drug to prevent relapse, and pyrimethamine also displays some of this type of activity against *P. vivax*.

Schizontocides (Blood Schizontocides) Used for Clinical or Suppressive Cure. These important drugs act on asexual erythrocytic stages of malarial parasites to interrupt erythrocytic schizogony and thereby terminate clinical attacks (clinical cure). The term suppressive cure refers to the complete elimination of malarial parasites from the body by continued suppressive treatment.

Blood schizontocides can be divided roughly into two groups according to their clinical efficacy and mechanisms of action. The first group includes the classical antimalarial alkaloids chloroquine, quinine, and related derivatives such as quinidine, mefloquine, and halofantrine. These weak bases concentrate in erythrocytes infected with sensitive plasmodia, cause characteristic damage to the parasites, and produce rapid clinical improvement when given alone. Their mechanisms of action are poorly understood, and resistance of *P. falciparum* to their action develops relatively slowly (*see* discussion under Chloroquine). The second group includes pyrimethamine, chloroguanide, and their derivatives that inhibit dihydrofolate reductase; it also includes the sulfonamides and sulfones, which interfere with dihydropteroic acid synthesis and thus with folate biosynthesis (a process that does not occur in mammals) (*see* Chapter 45), and the tetracyclines, which inhibit protein synthesis (*see* Chapter 48). Clinically, such compounds are slower acting, less effective, and nearly always given together with another blood schizontocide. Resistance of *P. falciparum* to these agents is common in the field and is readily elicited in the laboratory.

Gametocytocides. An agent of this type acts by destroying sexual erythrocytic forms of plasmodia, thereby preventing transmission of malaria to the mosquito. Primaquine has this type of activity, particularly against *P. falciparum*. Chloroquine and quinine show such activity against *P. vivax* and *P. malariae* but lack it against *P. falciparum*.

Sporontocides. These drugs ablate transmission of malaria by preventing or inhibiting formation of malarial oocysts and sporozoites in infected mosquitoes. Primaquine and chloroguanide are the major antimalarials with this type of action.

ACQUIRED RESISTANCE TO ANTIMALARIAL DRUGS

The chief obstacle to successful chemotherapy of malaria is the development of resistance to available drugs, particularly chloroquine. Acquired drug resistance should not be confused with insensitivity or natural refractoriness to antimalarials.

Of the plasmodial species that infect man, acquired drug resistance poses a serious clinical problem only with *P. falciparum*. However, this species accounts for over 85% of the cases and much of the mortality of human malaria. Resistance to chloroquine, first documented in Thailand and Columbia in 1959 to 1960, now affects large regions of South America, the Western Pacific, East Asia, India, and, most recently, Africa south of the Sahara. This situation is further complicated by the development of resistance of *P. falciparum* to pyrimethamine and sulfadoxine, a combination of antifolate drugs that had been used extensively as an alternative to chloroquine for chemoprophylaxis of falciparum malaria. There now is considerable overlap in the geographical distribution of resistance to pyrimethamine–sulfadoxine and to chloroquine. Prophylaxis and treatment of infections caused by such multidrug-resistant strains have necessitated a return to effective but more toxic schizontocides, such as quinine, quinidine, and most recently, mefloquine. However, even when used in combination with a tetracycline, the effectiveness of quinine has become limited because of resistance to this agent in areas where the use of antimalarial drugs has been intensive. Increasing tolerance of *P. falciparum* to the current battery of antimalarials dramatically illustrates the need for improved chemotherapeutic agents that act by different mechanisms and that are not subject to cross-resistance.

Because resistant parasites can be selected in the presence of antimalarial agents *in vivo* or *in vitro* and studied in laboratory models, progress is being made in defining the biochemical basis of acquired drug resistance. Particularly with the antimalarial alkaloids, investigation is complicated by considerable variation in the infectious behavior of malarial parasites from the same species and the presence of genetically distinct clones of parasites in field isolates of *P. falciparum*. Moreover, testing of *P. falciparum* for susceptibility *in vitro* to antimalarial drugs has yet to predict clinical outcome with much accuracy. Recent studies suggest that chloroquine-resistant strains of *P. falciparum* do not accumulate high concentrations of the drug and that sensitivity to chloroquine can be restored partially by concurrent administration of Ca^{2+} channel blockers (Martin *et al.*, 1987; Bitonti *et al.*, 1988). The simultaneous acquisition of resistance to several chemically unrelated compounds is reminiscent of that described for multidrug-resistant neoplastic cells (Fojo *et al.*, 1985; Krogstad *et al.*, 1988). The ability to characterize the molecular basis of antimalarial drug resistance should eventually have beneficial implications for the chemotherapy of this devastating infection.

CHLOROQUINE AND ITS CONGENERS

History. Chloroquine is one of a large series of 4-aminoquinolines investigated as part of the extensive cooperative program of antimalarial research in the United States during World War II. The objective was to discover more effective and less toxic suppressive agents than quinacrine, an acridine derivative abandoned for antimalarial chemotherapy because of its toxicity and inability to cure vivax malaria or to act as a causal prophylactic. Although the 4-aminoquinolines had been described as potential antimalarials by Russian investigators, serious attention was not paid to this chemical class until the French reported that one derivative (SONTOCHIN, SONTOQUIN) was well tolerated and had high activity in human malarias. Beginning in 1943, thousands of these compounds were synthesized and tested for activity. Chloroquine eventually proved most promising and was released for field trial. When hostilities ceased, it was discovered that the chemical had been synthesized and studied under the name of RESOCHIN by the Germans as early as 1934.

Chemistry and Structure–Activity Relationship. Chloroquine has the following structural formula:

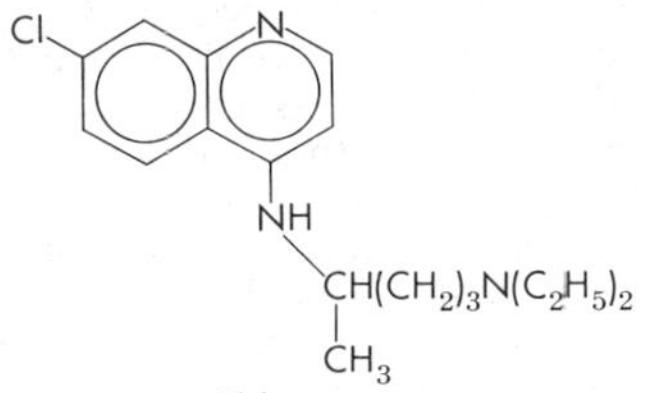

Chloroquine

Chloroquine contains the same alkyl side chain as quinacrine (*see* Chapter 42); it differs from the latter in having a quinoline instead of an acridine nucleus and in lacking the methoxy moiety. Chloroquine also closely resembles pamaquine and pentaquine (obsolete 8-aminoquinoline antimalarials). The *d*, *l*, and *dl* forms of chloroquine are indistinguishable in potency tests in duck malaria, but the *d* isomer is somewhat less toxic than the *l* isomer in mammals. The 4-aminoquinolines with the greatest antimalarial activity in both avian and human malarias have a chlorine atom in position 7 of the quinoline. The details of the structure–activity relationship of chloroquine and its congeners are given by Berliner and coworkers (1948) and Coatney and colleagues (1953).

Amodiaquine is a congener of chloroquine that is used much less frequently than chloroquine for the treatment of overt malarial attacks and for suppression. Although it may be more active than chloroquine against certain strains of *P. falciparum* with decreased susceptibility to chloroquine, amodiaquine is no longer recommended for chemoprophylaxis because its use is associated with hepatic toxicity and agranulocytosis. Hydroxychloroquine, in which one of the N-ethyl substituents of chloroquine is β-hydroxylated, is considered to be essentially equivalent to the parent molecule. Hydroxychloroquine has been used successfully in place of chloroquine against normally sensitive strains. Because of lesser toxicity, high doses of hydroxychloroquine have an advantage over chloroquine for the treatment of rheumatoid arthritis and lupus erythematosus.

Pharmacological Effects. Although chloroquine was developed primarily as an antimalarial agent, it possesses several other pharmacological properties. Its use to treat extraintestinal amebiasis is described in Chapter 42. The anti-inflammatory effects of chloroquine are well known. The drug has been used occasionally in the treatment of rheumatoid arthritis and more frequently for discoid lupus erythematosus; its efficacy in the latter condition is controversial (*see* Dubois, 1978). Chloroquine has been employed with success to treat porphyria cutanea tarda, solar urticaria, and polymorphous light eruption. Treatment of these conditions requires much larger doses than are used for malaria, which mandates caution about the toxicity of this agent (*see* Isaacson *et al.*, 1982).

Antimalarial Actions. Chloroquine, even in massive doses, exerts no significant activity against the exoerythrocytic tissue stages of plasmodia. The drug is thus not a causal prophylactic agent and does not prevent the establishment of infection. However, it is highly effective against the asexual erythrocytic forms of *P. vivax* and sensitive strains of *P. falciparum*, and gametocytes of *P. vivax*. It is superior to quinine in suppressing vivax malaria. In the acute malarial attack, chloroquine rapidly controls clinical symptoms and parasitemia; most patients become completely afebrile within 24 to 48 hours after receiving therapeutic doses, and thick smears of peripheral blood are generally negative for parasites by 48 to 72 hours. Except for certain chloroquine-resistant or multidrug-resistant strains, the drug completely cures falciparum malaria. Chloroquine, like quinine, does not prevent relapses in vivax malaria, but it substantially lengthens the interval between relapses. Chloroquine is well tolerated and is thus more reliably administered than quinine. It differs from quinine in that no therapeutic or toxic synergism is manifested when it is given with primaquine.

Mechanism of Antimalarial Action. The primary mechanisms of action of chloroquine, quinine, and related blood schizontocides remain obscure. A 1960s postulate that chloroquine acts by interference with nucleic acid synthesis, possibly by intercalating with plasmodial DNA, seems unlikely because of the rapid onset of morphological changes that are induced by low concentrations of this drug in infected erythrocytes. A more recent hypothesis is that ferriprotoporphyrin IX (haemin), released during degradation of hemoglobin in parasitized erythrocytes, serves as a receptor for chloroquine and other antimalarial alkaloids and that the resulting drug–haemin complexes have deleterious effects on membranous structures of plasmodia and erythrocytes (Chou *et al.*, 1980). However, studies of the interactions between haemin and a series of such antimalarial compounds do not support this concept fully (*see* Aikawa, 1972; *see also* Warhurst, 1987; and Schlesinger *et al.*, 1988).

In part because they are weak bases, the current view is that the antimalarial alkaloid blood schizontocides concentrate in and raise the pH of acidic vesicles within sensitive malarial parasites. There, they interfere with lysosomal degradation of hemoglobin and cause histological abnormalities characteristic of the particular drug class; these include rapid chloroquine-induced clumping of pigment or the more delayed and subtle pigment changes produced by aryl amino alcohols like quinine, mefloquine, or halofantrine (*see* Warhurst, 1987; Schlesinger *et al.*, 1988). The unique sensitivity of intraerythrocytic plasmodia to these drugs appears in part related to their ability to concentrate them selectively. Furthermore, the uptake of chloroquine by infected erythrocytes and the subsequent clumping of pigment can be blocked competitively by quinine and related antimalarial blood schizontocides. These findings suggest that drug transport by plasmodia is an energy-dependent, carrier-mediated process. Beyond the alteration of lysosomal pH, the molecular mechanisms by which these blood schizontocides act are unknown; however, inhibition of the functions of Ca^{2+}-dependent proteins such as calmodulin has been implicated (Scheibel *et al.*, 1987).

Absorption, Fate, and Excretion. Chloroquine is absorbed well (about 90%) from the gastrointestinal tract and is absorbed rapidly from intramuscular or subcutaneous sites. The drug distributes relatively slowly into a very large apparent volume (over 100 liters/kg) (*see* White, 1988; Appendix II). This is due to extensive sequestration of chloroquine in tissues, particularly liver, spleen, kidney, lung, melanin-containing tissues, and, to a lesser extent, brain and spinal cord. Chloroquine undergoes appreciable biotransformation. The major metabolite, monodesethylchloroquine, has antimalarial activity and reaches plasma concentrations that approximate 20 to 35% of those of the parent compound. The renal clearance of chloroquine is about half of its total systemic clearance. Unchanged chloroquine and its major metabolite account for over 50% and 20% of the urinary drug products, respectively.

Chloroquine exhibits complex pharmacokinetic properties; these are similar in adults and children (*see* White, 1988; White *et al.*, 1988). Because of extensive tissue binding, a loading dose is required to achieve effective concentrations in plasma. Rapid entry together with relatively slow exit of chloroquine from the central compartment can result in transiently high and even toxic concentrations of the drug in plasma after parenteral administration; hence, the drug is given either slowly by constant intravenous infusion or in small divided doses at frequent intervals by the intramuscular or subcutaneous routes (White *et al.*, 1988).

If chloroquine is discontinued after daily dosage for 2 weeks, plasma concentrations and urinary excretion both decrease with a half-life of about 9 days during the next 4 weeks; subsequently, the half-time for urinary excretion is markedly prolonged, and small amounts may be found in the urine for several years. In an adult, daily oral dosage of 300 mg of chloroquine base results in a steady-state concentration in plasma of about 125 μg per liter. With a weekly 0.5-g dose, the peak concentration in plasma varies between 150 and 250 μg per liter; just before the succeeding dose, the range is between 20 and 40 μg per liter. This compares to therapeutic concentrations of about 30 μg per liter for drug-sensitive *P. falciparum* and 15 μg per liter for *P. vivax*. After single or weekly doses, the half-life of the drug in plasma is about 3 days. Congeners of chloroquine (such as amodiaquine) interfere with its metabolism; with their concurrent use, plasma concentrations of chloroquine are elevated for prolonged periods.

Preparations. *Chloroquine phosphate* (ARALEN PHOSPHATE) is available as tablets containing either 250 or 500 mg of the diphosphate. Approximately 60% of the diphosphate represents the base. *Chloroquine hydrochloride* is available as an injection (50 mg/ml; equivalent to 40 mg/ml of the base). Chloroquine phosphate is also combined in tablets with primaquine for prophylactic use only.

Hydroxychloroquine sulfate (PLAQUENIL SULFATE) is available in 200-mg tablets, equivalent to 155 mg of the base. For purposes of dosage, 400 mg of hydroxychloroquine sulfate is equivalent to 500 mg of chloroquine phosphate.

Routes of Administration and Dosage. Chloroquine phosphate is given orally with food. The hydrochloride salt of chloroquine may be employed for parenteral administration if necessary.

For chemoprophylaxis or suppressive therapy an oral dose of 500 mg of the phosphate is given to adults once each week starting 2 weeks before and continuing for 8 weeks after the last exposure in an endemic area. Usual pediatric doses are 5 mg/kg of the base weekly. These regimens may not be sufficient to control infection with certain chloroquine-resistant or multidrug-resistant strains of *P. falciparum,* a topic discussed below.

For the treatment of the acute attack of malaria caused by chloroquine-susceptible plasmodia, an initial loading dose of 1 g of chloroquine phosphate is given; this is followed by an additional 500 mg after 6 to 8 hours and a single dose of 500 mg on each of 2 consecutive days, such that a total of 2.5 g is given in 3 days. This dosage is usually sufficient to cure completely most chloroquine-sensitive *P. falciparum* infections and to terminate promptly fever and parasitemia in acute *P. vivax* infections. Freedom from clinical attacks in vivax malaria may then be maintained by suppressive doses of 500 mg weekly.

Chloroquine can safely be given parenterally to comatose or vomiting patients until the drug can be taken orally. However, standard dosage schedules for parenteral administration must be revised because of the risk of acute chloroquine toxicity. Although more information is needed, a recent study showed that a regimen of 0.83 mg of base/kg per hour for 30 hours (continuous intravenous infusion) or 3.5 mg of base/kg every 6 hours (subcutaneous or intramuscular administration) was safe and effective (White *et al.,* 1988).

Dosages administered to infants or children, orally or intramuscularly, should not exceed 10 mg of chloroquine base per kilogram of body weight per day; the usual dose is 5 mg of the base per kilogram.

Toxicity and Side Effects. The amounts of chloroquine employed for oral therapy of the acute malarial attack may cause gastrointestinal upset, pruritus, mild and transient headache, and visual disturbances. Prolonged medication for suppressive purposes causes few significant untoward effects, and only rarely must the drug be discontinued because of intolerance. All symptoms readily disappear when the drug is withheld. Chloroquine may cause discoloration of nailbeds and mucous membranes.

Prolonged treatment with chloroquine may cause a lichenoid skin eruption in a few patients; the condition is mild and subsides promptly when the drug is discontinued. Readministration of chloroquine usually does not result in reappearance of the lesion. Large doses given for a year to a group of healthy volunteers occasionally caused some visual symptoms (blurring of vision, diplopia), bleaching of the hair, T-wave abnormalities in the ECG, mild skin eruptions, headache, and slight weight loss; the observed toxic effects caused no incapacity and were reversible upon withdrawal of the drug (Alving *et al.,* 1948). These findings emphasize the relative safety of chloroquine in the usual dose range. High daily doses (>250 mg) of chloroquine, used for long-term treatment of diseases other than malaria, can result in irreversible retinopathy. This complication is presumably related to deposition of drug in melanin-rich tissues (Bernstein *et al.,* 1963) and can be avoided if the daily dose is 250 mg or less (*see* Dubois, 1978; Olansky, 1982). Prolonged daily therapy with high doses of chloroquine or hydroxychloroquine can also cause toxic myopathy, cardiomyopathy, and peripheral neuropathy; these reactions are reversible if the drug is discontinued promptly (Estes *et al.,* 1987). Rarely, neuropsychiatric disturbances, including suicide, may be related to overdosage (*see* Good and Shader, 1982). There is no convincing evidence that chloroquine given during pregnancy causes fetal abnormalities.

Manifestations of severe acute chloroquine toxicity relate primarily to the cardiovascular system; these include hypotension, vasodilatation, suppressed myocardial function, electrocardiographic abnormalities, and eventual cardiac arrest. Doses of more than 5 g are usually fatal. Prompt treatment with mechanical ventilation, epinephrine, and diazepam may be lifesaving (Riou *et al.,* 1988).

Precautions and Contraindications. Chloroquine should be used cautiously (or not at all) in the presence of hepatic disease or severe gastrointestinal, neurological, or blood disorders. If such disorders occur during the course of therapy, the drug should be discontinued. Concomitant use of gold or phenylbutazone with chloroquine should be avoided because of the tendency of all three agents to produce dermatitis. For patients on long-term, large-dose therapy, ophthalmological examination is recommended before and periodically during treatment (Good and Shader, 1982).

Therapeutic Uses. Chloroquine has neither prophylactic nor radically curative value in human vivax malarias. However, in well-tolerated doses it is highly effective in terminating acute attacks, and when administered in the long term it acts as an effective suppressive agent. When medication is discontinued, relapses may occur but the intervals between their appearance are prolonged. In falciparum malaria, the drug is very effective in controlling acute attacks caused by sensitive strains, and as a rule it completely cures the infection. Chloroquine is superior to quinine in that it is more potent and less toxic and it need be given only once weekly as a suppressive agent. It is the most generally useful of the antimalarial drugs except in parts of the world where strains of *P. falciparum* occur that are relatively or completely insensitive to the drug.

CHLOROGUANIDE

History. Known internationally as proguanil, chloroguanide is a biguanide derivative that emerged in 1945 as a product of British antimalarial research. The compound serves as a prodrug that is converted in mammals to a cyclic triazine metabolite that acts as an inhibitor of plasmodial dihydrofolate reductase. Its use as a safe and well-tolerated antimalarial prophylactic is severely compromised by the development of chloroguanide-resistant strains of *P. falciparum*. Nonetheless, there is renewed interest in this drug, particularly for the prophylaxis of strains of *P. falciparum* in sub-Saharan Africa that are resistant to chloroquine, pyrimethamine, and sulfadoxine (Fogh *et al.*, 1988). Moreover, research on this drug and its active metabolite, cycloguanil pamoate (chloroguanide triazine pamoate; CAMOLAR), opened the field for the development of other antimalarial dihydrofolate reductase inhibitors such as pyrimethamine. This may also lead to the discovery of compounds that act on other stages of malarial parasites (*see* below).

Chemistry. Chloroguanide has the following structural formula:

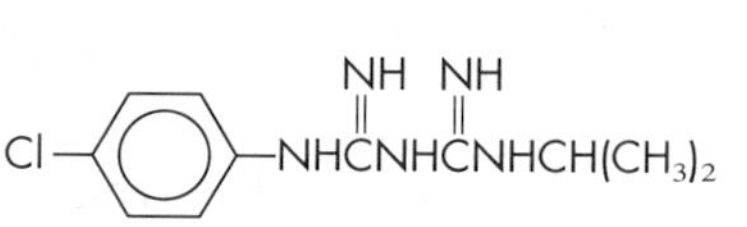

Chloroguanide

Chloroguanide has the widest margin of safety of a large series of plasmodicidal biguanide analogs examined. Dihalogen substitution in positions 3 and 4 of the benzene ring yields chlorproguanil (LAPUDRINE), which is a more potent prodrug than chloroguanide and is also used clinically. The structure of the active cyclic triazine metabolite of chloroguanide bears some resemblance to pyrimethamine.

Pharmacological Effects. *Antimalarial Actions.* Chloroguanide exerts causal prophylactic and suppressive activity in sporozoite-induced falciparum malaria, adequately controls the acute clinical attack, and usually eradicates the infection. The drug exhibits suppressive activity against *P. vivax* infections and controls the acute clinical attack. However, it is not fully prophylactic against mosquito-induced vivax malaria because it does not affect the exoerythrocytic tissue stage of this infection. Also, erythrocytic forms of *P. vivax* often reappear in the blood shortly after suppressive doses of chloroguanide are withdrawn. Its action on the erythrocytic forms of all malarial parasites is slow as compared with that of the 4-aminoquinolines. Gametocytes are not destroyed, but the development of fertilized gametes encysted in the gut wall of the mosquito is usually prevented. Chloroguanide and quinine do not act synergistically in the prevention of relapse in vivax malaria, in contrast to the combination of an 8-aminoquinoline antimalarial and quinine.

Mechanism of Antimalarial Action. The triazine metabolite of chloroguanide acts as a selective inhibitor of plasmodial dihydrofolate reductase. Inhibition of this enzyme is consistent with the morphological appearance of affected parasites; nuclear division is prevented and schizogony stops at an early stage. For this reason, chloroguanide acts slowly in the treatment of acute malaria, and relief of symptoms occurs only after all the plasmodia have developed to a stage where extensive synthesis of nuclear material is essential for further development. The fact that the drug acts not only on the erythrocytic stage of plasmodia but also on the exoerythrocytic tissue stage, especially of *P. falciparum*, may aid in the discovery of causal prophylactic and curative antimalarial agents. Also of interest is the finding that chloroguanide does not destroy gametocytes in the human host but usually renders them noninfectious for mosquitoes.

Absorption, Fate, and Excretion. Chloroguanide is slowly but adequately absorbed from the gastrointestinal tract. After single oral doses, peak concentrations of the drug in plasma are usually attained within 5 hours; the mean plasma elimination half-time is about 16 to 20 hours. The two major metabolites of chloroguanide, the active triazine and the inactive 4-chlorophenylbiguanide, constitute about 30% and 23% of the total drug concentration in plasma, respectively (Bygbjerg *et al.*, 1987). Chloroguanide does not accumulate significantly in tissues during long-term administration, although its concentration in erythrocytes is about four times that in plasma. In man, from 40 to 60% of the absorbed chloroguanide is excreted in the urine as either the parent drug or the active metabolite.

Preparations, Route of Administration, and Dosage. *Chloroguanide hydrochloride* (PALUDRINE) is not available in the United States. The drug is formulated in tablets, each containing 100 mg for oral administration. The adult dosage for long-term prophylaxis of falciparum malaria is 200 mg daily; this is taken in addition to a weekly prophylactic dose of chloroquine.

Toxicity and Side Effects. In prophylactic doses of 200 to 300 mg daily, chloroguanide causes few untoward effects except occasional nausea and diarrhea. Large doses (1 g daily or more) may cause vomiting, abdominal pain, diarrhea, hematuria, and the transient appearance of epithelial cells and casts in the urine. Gross accidental or deliberate overdosage (as much as 15 g) has been followed by complete recovery. Doses as high as 700 mg twice daily have been taken for over 2 weeks without serious toxicity. Chloroguanide is considered safe for use during pregnancy.

Therapeutic Uses. Because of its relative safety, chloroguanide is currently used as an alternative to pyrimethamine and sulfadoxine for the long-term prophylaxis of chloroquine-resistant falciparum malaria in East Africa; its utility in West Africa requires further study. Limited data suggest that chloroguanide by itself or with chloroquine is not effective for the long-term prophylaxis of multi-drug-resistant falciparum malaria in Thailand and New Guinea; whether the drug will prove more effective for this purpose when given together with a short-acting sulfonamide is under investigation.

DIAMINOPYRIMIDINES

History. Of the many 2,4-diaminopyrimidines synthesized and tested for antimicrobial activity, two stand out. The first, pyrimethamine, was developed and used almost solely as an antimalarial agent; the second, trimethoprim, was developed as an antibacterial agent and found later to have antimalarial properties. Several 2,4-diaminopyrimidines were found to antagonize competitively folic and folinic acids in the growth of *Lactobacillus casei*. The prediction was made that *L. casei* would not be unique in its sensitivity to these substances; this was borne out by the successful treatment of malaria in experimental animals with diaminopyrimidines. Several members of the series had high antimalarial activity; the most active, pyrimethamine, was later found to be highly effective against the plasmodia infecting man (*see* Falco *et al.*, 1951; Symposium, 1952), and has since been used widely for prophylaxis and suppression. Pyrimethamine has the following structural formula:

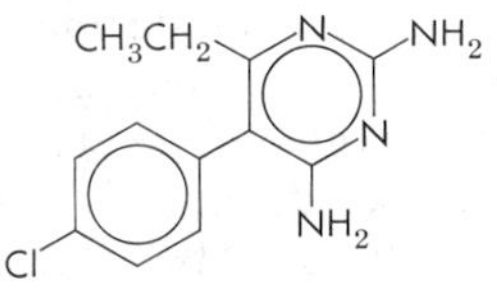

Pyrimethamine

Pharmacological Effects. *Antimalarial Actions.* The antimalarial effects of pyrimethamine are similar to those of chloroguanide. Its potency *in vivo*, however, is considerably greater, undoubtedly because it acts directly and its half-life is much longer than that of the active metabolite of chloroguanide. The major use of pyrimethamine is in prophylaxis, suppression, and combined chemotherapy of chloroquine-resistant strains of falciparum malaria. Suppressive cure of some vivax infections may be achieved by continuing prophylactic medication for 10 weeks after leaving a malarious area, and some causal prophylactic activity may occur in vivax infections. The antimalarial effects of both chloroguanide and pyrimethamine have been reviewed by Davey (1963) and Hill (1963).

Mechanisms of Antimalarial Action. In an elegant series of investigations, the 2,4-diaminopyrimidines were shown to act by inhibiting dihydrofolate reductase of plasmodia at concentrations far lower than required to produce comparable inhibition of the mammalian enzymes (Ferone *et al.*, 1969) (*see* Table 41–1). Dihydrofolate reductase catalyzes the reduction of dihydrofolate to tetrahydrofolate, which is in turn required for the biosynthesis of purines, pyrimidines, and certain amino acids (*see* Chapter 54). Inhibition of dihydrofolate reductase by pyrimethamine is manifested in the malarial parasite by failure of nuclear division at the time of schizont formation in erythrocytes and liver.

The concept of inhibiting two steps in an essential metabolic pathway with separate drugs to produce a supra-additive effect explains the synergistic action of the 2,4-diaminopyrimidines with the sulfonamides or sulfones (*see* Hitchings and Burchall, 1965). The two steps involved are the utilization of para-aminobenzoic acid (PABA) in the synthesis of dihydropteroic acid, inhibited by sulfonamides, and the reduction of dihydrofolate to tetrahydrofolate, inhibited by pyrimethamine. The value of pyrimethamine–sulfonamide or pyrimethamine–sulfone combinations lies in preventing or delaying strains of plasmodia from

Table 41–1. INHIBITION OF DIHYDROFOLATE REDUCTASES BY PYRIMETHAMINE AND TRIMETHOPRIM *

	CONCENTRATION (nM) FOR 50% INHIBITION OF DIHYDROFOLATE REDUCTASES FROM VARIOUS SOURCES		
INHIBITOR	*Mammalian* (*rat liver*)	*Bacterial* (E. coli)	*Protozoal* (P. berghei)
Pyrimethamine	700	2500	~0.5
Trimethoprim	260,000	5	70

* Modified from Ferone, Burchall, and Hitchings, 1969.

developing resistance to these drugs. Such strains have arisen readily when small doses of pyrimethamine alone were used for long periods of time. Suitable combinations, particularly that of pyrimethamine and sulfadoxine, have shown their value in the treatment and suppression of some multiresistant strains (World Health Organization, 1981). Combinations of trimethoprim, the related diaminopyrimidine, with sulfamethoxazole are of particular value in the treatment of bacterial infections (*see* Chapter 45).

Absorption, Fate, and Excretion. Pyrimethamine is slowly but completely absorbed after oral administration. The compound accumulates mainly in kidneys, lungs, liver, and spleen and is eliminated slowly with a half-life in plasma of about 80 to 95 hours. Concentrations that are suppressive for drug-sensitive strains remain in the blood for 2 weeks (*see* Brooks *et al.*, 1969; Stickney *et al.*, 1973). Several metabolites of pyrimethamine appear in the urine, but few data are available on either their structure or their antimalarial activity. Pyrimethamine is also excreted in the milk of nursing mothers.

Preparations, Route of Administration, and Dosage. Although pyrimethamine (DARAPRIM) is still marketed by itself in tablets each containing 25 mg, the drug is nearly always used together with a sulfonamide or sulfone for the chemotherapy of malaria due to chloroquine-resistant strains of *P. falciparum*. Known as FANSIDAR, a fixed-combination tablet containing pyrimethamine (25 mg) and sulfadoxine (500 mg) is available for this purpose. Sulfadoxine is a sulfonamide with a particularly long half-life (7 to 9 days). For treatment of an acute malarial attack, three pyrimethamine–sulfadoxine tablets (a total of 75 mg of pyrimethamine and 1500 mg of sulfadoxine) are taken orally as a single dose. Pediatric doses range as follows: 2 to 11 months, one-quarter tablet; 1 to 3 years, one-half tablet; 4 to 8 years, one tablet; and 9 to 14 years, two tablets. Because of potential severe toxicity (*see* below), pyrimethamine–sulfadoxine is no longer recommended for long-term prophylaxis except where medical care is unavailable and where prolonged, high exposure to chloroquine-resistant falciparum malaria is likely to occur. In this case, the regimen should start 1 week before and continue for 6 weeks after possible exposure. The Centers for Disease Control now recommends that travelers to areas of chloroquine-resistant falciparum malaria take chloroquine prophylaxis weekly and carry a therapeutic dose of pyrimethamine–sulfadoxine to use for presumptive treatment of febrile illness if professional medical care is unavailable. Prompt medical evaluation should then be obtained. Pyrimethamine (12.5 mg) is also available in combination with dapsone (100 mg) as MALOPRIM, which has been given weekly for prophylaxis and suppressive therapy.

Toxicity, Precautions, and Contraindications. At a dosage of 25 mg once weekly, pyrimethamine alone causes no significant clinical toxicity except occasional skin rashes and depression of hematopoiesis. Excessive doses do produce a megaloblastic anemia resembling that of folic acid deficiency; this reverses readily on discontinuation of treatment or on administration of leucovorin (folinic acid). At very high doses pyrimethamine is teratogenic in animals, but there is no evidence for this complication in humans.

In rare cases, weekly prophylactic doses of pyrimethamine (25 mg) taken together with sulfadoxine (500 mg) cause severe and even fatal cutaneous reactions, such as erythema multiforme, Stevens–Johnson syndrome, and toxic epidermal necrolysis. This combination has also been associated with serum-sickness-type reactions, urticaria, exfoliative dermatitis, and hepatitis (Miller *et al.*, 1986). These adverse effects are due to the sulfonamide component of the mixture. If prophylaxis with pyrimethamine–sulfadoxine is prescribed, it should be discontinued immediately if lesions of the skin or mucous membranes appear or if there is itching or sore throat. Such medication is contraindicated for persons with histories of reactions to sulfonamides and for infants less than 2 months old. Administration of the combination of pyrimethamine and dapsone has occasionally been associated with agranulocytosis (Cook and Kish, 1985).

Therapeutic Uses. Pyrimethamine is now used almost exclusively in combination with sulfonamides or sulfones. The drug by itself has little value in the treatment of the acute primary attack of malaria. It is slow in clearing parasitemia, but it prevents development of the fertilized gamete and has some causal prophylactic activity. In combination with a short-acting sulfonamide (*e.g.*, sulfadiazine) or a sulfone, pyrimethamine is useful for the treatment of acute attacks of uncomplicated chloroquine-resistant *P. falciparum* malaria. Quinine is generally included in such regimens to ensure a prompt schizontocidal effect. Pyrimethamine–sulfadoxine is no longer recommended for routine prophylaxis of chloroquine-resistant strains of *P. falciparum,* but this medication is advised for presumptive treatment of febrile illness due to such strains when medical evaluation is unavailable (*see* above). The combination is not radically curative in vivax malaria.

Pyrimethamine given concurrently with sulfadiazine is useful in the treatment of toxoplasmosis, which can be particularly severe in immunologically compromised states such as acquired immunodeficiency syndrome (AIDS) (*see* Feldman, 1968; McCabe and Remington, 1984; Leport *et al.*, 1988). Leucovorin calcium (10 mg daily) should be given concurrently to obviate the hematological toxicity that may occur with continued daily use of pyrimethamine.

MEFLOQUINE

History. Based on the U.S. Army research program in malaria during World War II (Wiselogle, 1946), *mefloquine* was identified during the war in Viet Nam as part of a search for compounds with antimalarial activity against multidrug-resistant strains of *P. falciparum*. Because such strains are at least partially responsive to quinine, substances with some structural resemblance to that alkaloid were selected for evaluation. Of the many compounds that were then tested, derivatives of 4-quinoline-methanol showed the most promise. One of these, mefloquine, emerged from eventual clinical trial as a readily tolerated antimalarial drug that is highly active against both the usual and the multidrug-resistant strains of *P. falciparum* (*see* Schmidt *et al.*, 1978; World Health Organization, 1983, 1984). Promising alternatives to mefloquine, such as halofantrine, were also identified but require further clinical evaluation (Cosgriff *et al.*, 1982). Mefloquine has the following structural formula:

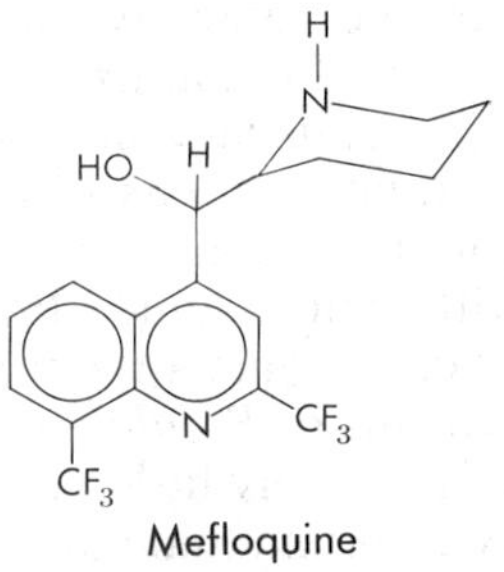

Mefloquine

Pharmacological Effects. *Antimalarial Actions.* Mefloquine in single, well-tolerated doses was shown in early studies to eliminate fever and parasitemia rapidly in nonimmune volunteers or patients in endemic areas infected with either chloroquine-sensitive or highly chloroquine-resistant strains of *P. falciparum* and to effect a radical cure. It was also shown to effect suppressive cure against all strains of *P. falciparum* and suppression of *P. vivax*. In *P. vivax* infections, however, malarial attacks recurred some time after the end of treatment (Rieckmann *et al.*, 1974; Trenholme *et al.*, 1975; Clyde *et al.*, 1976). Unfortunately, however, mefloquine-resistant strains of *P. falciparum* have been detected by more recent studies *in vitro* (Boudreau *et al.*, 1982; Bygbjerg *et al.*, 1983; Hoffman *et al.*, 1985) and therapeutic failures have been encountered. Development of resistance to mefloquine is probably fostered by the long sojourn of this drug at subtherapeutic concentrations in the blood (*see* below).

Mechanism of Antimalarial Action. The mechanism of action of mefloquine is unknown. In many respects, mefloquine behaves like quinine, but it does not intercalate with DNA (Davidson *et al.*, 1977). Mefloquine and quinine produce similar morphological changes in early ring stages of *P. falciparum* and *P. vivax* (Schmidt *et al.*, 1978); the major ultrastructural abnormality produced by mefloquine in *P. falciparum* is swelling of secondary lysosomes (Jacobs *et al.*, 1987). Like chloroquine, low extracellular concentrations of mefloquine raise the intravesicular pH of plasmodia in excess of that predicted from the passive distribution of a weak base (Schlesinger *et al.*, 1988). This suggests that there is a mechanism for concentration of mefloquine that has yet to be characterized. Mefloquine probably affects membranes of malarial parasites (Brown *et al.*, 1979). Like quinine, mefloquine competes for accumulation of chloroquine by infected erythrocytes and inhibits chloroquine-induced clumping of pigment in the parasite (Fitch *et al.*, 1979; Warhurst, 1987).

Absorption, Fate, and Excretion. Mefloquine is available for oral administration only; the bioavailability of commercial preparations exceeds 85%. The drug is absorbed reasonably rapidly and is extensively bound (98%) to plasma proteins. Peak concentrations in plasma are attained in a few hours and decline slowly with an elimination half-time of 2 to 3 weeks (Desjardins *et al.*, 1979b; Karbwang *et al.*, 1987). In rats, the gastrointestinal system serves as an important compartment for the drug as it undergoes a continuous enterohepatic and enterogastric circulation (Mu *et al.*, 1975). Concentrations in tissues, particularly liver and lungs, are relatively high for extended periods of time. Excretion is mainly in the feces, and only very small amounts of drug appear in the urine. These findings are consistent with the large volume of distribution and low clearance of mefloquine in human volunteers (Karbwang *et al.,* 1987). Several metabolites are formed.

Preparation, Route of Administration, and Dosage. *Mefloquine* is available as LARIAM in 250-mg tablets and as FANSIMET in tablets that contain 250 mg of mefloquine together with 25 mg of pyrimethamine and 500 mg of sulfadoxine. A single therapeutic dose (1000 to 1500 mg of base for adults and 25 mg of base/kg for children) has been recommended for treatment of multidrug-resistant falciparum malaria. The drug may be used as an alternative for prophylaxis of multidrug-resistant falciparum malaria. The optimal prophylactic dose needs to be established. However, a schedule of 250 mg of mefloquine base weekly for 4 weeks, followed by 125 mg of the base weekly has been used successfully for adults. Current information should be obtained from the Centers for Disease Control.

Toxicity and Side Effects. Mefloquine, given orally in single doses up to 1500 mg or in 500-mg doses each week for 1 year, is generally well tolerated. Side effects such as nausea, vomiting, abdominal pain, and dizziness are dose related, self-limiting, and uncommon with single doses of 1 g or less. Rarely, manifestations of CNS toxicity such as disorientation, hallucinations, seizures, and depression may occur, but these respond to symptomatic therapy. Studies of mutagenicity, carcinogenicity, and teratogenicity have been negative. However, because of lack of adequate information, the use of mefloquine in women of child-bearing age and infants is not yet recommended.

Therapeutic Uses. Mefloquine is indicated for the treatment and prevention of chloroquine-resistant falciparum malaria. Currently, it is the only agent that, when used alone, is capable of ensuring suppression and cure of infections due to multi-drug-resistant strains of *P. falciparum*. The drug should be used *only* for the treatment and prevention of infections with such strains, because its misuse could result in the development of mefloquine-resistant plasmodia. As in the case of chloroquine, the use of mefloquine in combination with pyrimethamine and sulfadoxine is not recommended for routine prophylaxis because of potentially serious toxicity (Miller *et al.,* 1986).

PRIMAQUINE

History. In 1891, Ehrlich discovered that methylene blue exhibited weak plasmodicidal activity. Later it was shown that 8-aminoquinoline had weak schizontocidal activity and also that the slight antimalarial potency of methylene blue could be intensified by substitution of a dialkylaminoalkyl group for one of the N-methyl groups of the dye. Because the methoxy group on the quinoline ring, as in quinine, was believed important for antimalarial activity, a large series of quinoline derivatives was synthesized in which both the methoxy and substituted 8-amino groups were present. Pamaquine was the first of the 8-aminoquinoline antimalarials to be introduced into medicine (Mühlens, 1926). During World War II, several hundred derivatives of 8-aminoquinoline were examined in an attempt to discover compounds more potent and less toxic than pamaquine (*see* Elderfield *et al.,* 1946; Wiselogle, 1946). Of these, three agents—pentaquine, isopentaquine, and primaquine—were selected for further study; only primaquine, which received extensive field trials with United Nations forces in Korea, is widely used now. Quinocide, a substance very similar in structure to primaquine, is employed in some parts of the world. Primaquine has the following structural formula:

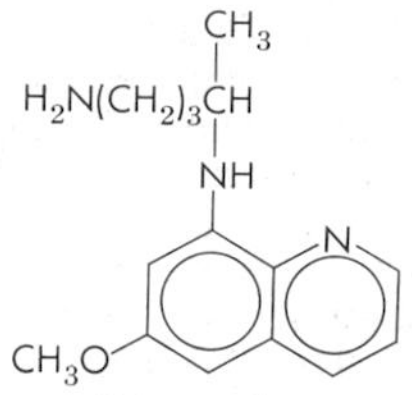

Primaquine

Pharmacological Effects. *Antimalarial Actions.* The great clinical value of primaquine lies in the radically curative treatment of vivax and ovale (relapsing) malarias and, in unusual situations where chloroquine treatment has proven unsatisfactory, in its use as a supplement to suppression with chloroquine. Primaquine is also highly active against the primary exoerythrocytic forms of *P. falciparum*, but this activity is of relatively little practical value. The activity of primaquine against erythrocytic stages of *P. vivax* also has little clinical application; the drug is almost completely ineffective against the asexual blood forms of *P. falciparum,* and it is for this reason that primaquine is almost always used in conjunction with a blood schizontocide. The 8-aminoquinolines exert a marked gametocytocidal effect against all four species of plasmodia that infect man, especially *P. falciparum*.

Although resistance of *P. vivax* to primaquine has not yet become a major clinical problem, resistance to 8-aminoquinoline compounds can be developed in experimental animal models, and various strains of *P. vivax* do show different susceptibilities to the action of primaquine in man. Thus, it is of the utmost importance that this drug not be misused and that new drugs of this type be developed.

Mechanism of Antimalarial Action. Little is known of the mode of action of 8-aminoquinolines, especially why they are far more active against tissue forms and gametes than asexual blood forms of plasmodia. There is some evidence that primaquine itself accounts for the antimalarial activity, whereas metabolites of primaquine may be more active than the parent compound in causing hemolysis (*see* Symposium, 1987).

Absorption, Fate, and Excretion. The absorption of primaquine is nearly complete after oral administration. After a single dose the plasma concentration reaches a maximum within 3 hours and then falls with an apparent elimination half-time of 6 hours (Fletcher *et al.*, 1981). The apparent volume of distribution of primaquine is several times that of total body water.

Primaquine is rapidly metabolized; only a small fraction of an administered dose is excreted as the parent drug. The three oxidative metabolites of primaquine identified to date are 8-(3-carboxyl-1-methyl-propylamino)-6-methoxyquinoline, 5-hydroxy primaquine, and 5-hydroxy-6-desmethylprimaquine. The carboxyl derivative is the major metabolite found in human plasma (Baker *et al.*, 1982; Mihaly *et al.*, 1984). After a single dose it reaches concentrations in plasma more than 10 times those of primaquine; this nontoxic metabolite is also eliminated more slowly and accumulates with multiple doses (Ward *et al.*, 1985). The three metabolites of primaquine appear to have appreciably less antimalarial activity than does primaquine. However, except for the carboxyl derivative, their hemolytic activity, as assessed by formation of methemoglobin *in vitro*, is greater than that of the parent compound (Symposium, 1987).

Tarlov and coworkers (1962) outlined a scheme for primaquine metabolism modeled after an earlier proposal for the degradation of pentaquine. In this scheme, the 6-methoxy group of primaquine is converted to a hydroxy moiety, a second hydroxy group is added in the 5 position, and the resultant compound is converted to a quinonimine by way of the 5,6-quinone derivative of the parent compound. Such a derivative is, or may be, transformed into a resonating compound capable of acting as an oxidation-reduction mediator. Such an agent may accelerate the oxidation of essential substances in sensitive erythrocytes by acting as an electron acceptor and thereby promote hemolysis. This redox behavior could also contribute to antimalarial activity by interfering with parasite electron-transfer pathways or by generating reactive oxygen species, such as superoxide free radical.

Preparation, Route of Administration, and Dosage. *Primaquine phosphate* is supplied in tablets containing 26.3 mg of the salt, equivalent to 15 mg of base. The dosage is usually expressed in terms of the base.

Primaquine is always given orally. When combined with standard chloroquine therapy, a dose of 15 mg daily of primaquine for 14 days is effective for the radical cure of infections with primaquine-sensitive strains of *P. vivax*. The recommended therapy for patients infected with intrinsically resistant strains of vivax malaria is 600 mg of chloroquine, followed 6 hours later by 300 mg of chloroquine combined with 45 mg of primaquine in one dose. Thereafter 300 mg of chloroquine combined with 45 mg of primaquine should be given as a single dose at weekly intervals for 7 additional weeks.

Toxicity and Side Effects. In the usual therapeutic doses, primaquine is fairly innocuous when given to Caucasians. Mild-to-moderate abdominal cramps and occasional epigastric distress occur in some individuals given the larger doses, and mild anemia, cyanosis (methemoglobinemia), and leukocytosis have been observed. Higher doses (60 to 240 mg of primaquine daily) accentuate the abdominal symptoms and cause methemoglobinemia and cyanosis in most subjects and leukopenia in some. Methemoglobinemia can occur even with usual doses of primaquine, chloroquine, or dapsone and can be severe in individuals with congenital deficiency of nicotinamide adenine dinucleotide (NADH) methemoglobin reductase (Cohen *et al.*, 1968). Hepatic function is unaffected. Abdominal distress can be alleviated by taking the drug at mealtime. Granulocytopenia and agranulocytosis are rare complications of therapy and are usually associated with overdosage. Also rare are hypertension, arrhythmias, and symptoms referable to the central nervous system (CNS).

The toxicity of primaquine in most blacks is as described above; however, in a fraction of the black population with glucose-6-phosphate dehydrogenase (G6PD) deficiency (about 10% of black males in the United States) anemia develops, due to intravascular hemolysis at daily doses of 15 mg (base) and higher. Such primaquine sensitivity of erythrocytes can be even more severe in some darker-hued Caucasian ethnic groups, including Sardinians, Sephardic Jews, Greeks, and Iranians. Since primaquine sensitivity is inherited by a gene on the X chromosome, the hemolysis is often of intermediate severity in heterozygous females who have two populations of red cells, one normal and the other deficient in G6PD. Because of "variable penetrance," such females may be less frequently affected than predicted.

The incidence of hemolysis (and of the sickle trait) in general follows the same geographical pattern as the distribution of falciparum malaria; erythrocytes that reflect these genetic changes are less subject to malarial infection. A decreased activity of G6PD in primaquine-sensitive erythrocytes is the major abnormality responsible for hemolysis. In normal erythrocytes there are several enzymatic and nonenzymatic mechanisms involving reduced glutathione (GSH) that protect cellular enzymes, hemoglobin, and cellular membranes from damage by chemical insults in the form of oxidants, peroxides, and free radicals. The net result of these protective reactions is to convert GSH to oxidized glutathione (GSSG). This in turn activates GSSG reductase, which oxidizes NADPH to $NADP^+$ and regenerates GSH. This process normally triggers G6PD to replenish NADPH. In G6PD-deficient erythrocytes, however, failure to replenish NADPH at an adequate rate results in accumulation of GSSG, in addition to altered forms of hemoglobin, membrane proteins, and lipids. This causes abnormal cellular transport, deformation of erythrocytes, and overt hemolysis. Certain metabolites of primaquine are capable of redox cycling within erythrocytes, leading to formation of oxidized and mixed disulfide forms of hemoglobin, generation of radicals and peroxides, and accumulation of GSSG. Such oxidative stress is poorly tolerated by G6PD-deficient cells (*see* Fletcher *et al.*, 1988). Brewer and colleagues (1960) devised a simple test for detecting such primaquine sensitivity based on the observation that the rate of methemoglobin reduction by erythrocytes from these individuals is markedly slower than normal in the presence of methylene blue. Results from this test correlate very well with the severity of hemolysis. The World Health Organization (1967) and Beutler and Mitchell (1968) have described other simple tests.

Primaquine is the prototype of more than 50 drugs and other substances that are known to be capable of inducing hemolysis in individuals deficient in glucose-6-phosphate dehydrogenase. These include antimalarials, sulfonamides, nitrofurans, antipyretics, analgesics, sulfones, vitamin K analogs, fava beans (favism), and certain other vegetables.

The severity of the hemolysis is dependent on the dose of drug used. In blacks, if the initial dose is not too large, the hemolysis is self-limited even when the same dose of drug is continued. This is because older erythrocytes are most susceptible, and, after their destruction, the remaining younger cells and newly produced reticulocytes are relatively resistant to hemolysis. However, in enzyme-deficient individuals of Mediterranean origin, red cells of all ages are susceptible, and the hemolysis is more severe. In addition, the severity of hemolysis can be enhanced or mitigated by many factors and is often unpredictable. For this reason the administration of primaquine or other potentially hemolytic drugs should be discontinued immediately if marked darkening of the urine or a sudden decrease in hemoglobin concentration occurs.

Precautions and Contraindications. Because of the possibility of hemolytic reactions (*see* above), one should watch for suggestive signs. If a daily dose of more than 30 mg of primaquine base (more than 15 mg daily in possibly sensitive patients such as blacks) is administered, repeated peripheral blood counts and at least gross examination of the urine should be performed during therapy. If the drug is used in schemes for mass administration, supervision is required.

Primaquine is contraindicated in acutely ill patients suffering from systemic disease characterized by a tendency to granulocytopenia, such as very active forms of rheumatoid arthritis and lupus erythematosus. It should not be given to subjects receiving, at the same time, other potentially hemolytic drugs or agents capable of depressing the myeloid elements of the bone marrow.

Therapeutic Uses. Primaquine is used mainly for the radical cure of vivax and other relapsing malarias. If it is administered during the long-term latent period of the infection, radical cure can be achieved. Its use during an acute clinical attack will prevent subsequent recrudescences. Primaquine should always be given in conjunction with full doses of a 4-aminoquinoline schizontocide, preferably chloroquine, in order to reduce the possibility of developing drug-resistant strains. In appropriate circumstances it may be used in combination with a 4-aminoquinoline for prophylaxis or for the interruption of transmission, especially of *P. falciparum*.

QUININE AND THE CINCHONA ALKALOIDS

History. Quinine is the chief alkaloid of cinchona, the bark of the cinchona tree indigenous to certain regions of South America. The bark is also called Peruvian, Jesuit's, or Cardinal's bark. The first written record of the use of cinchona occurs in a religious book written in 1633 and published in Spain in 1639. The author, an Augustinian monk named Calancha, of Lima, Peru, wrote: "A tree grows which they call 'the fever tree' in the country of Loxa, whose bark, the color of cinnamon, is made into powder amounting to the weight of two small silver coins and given as a beverage, cures the fevers and tertians; it has produced miraculous results in Lima." A variety of colorful and fanciful versions of the discovery of the fever bark exist. A popular and persistent version is that the bark was employed in 1638 to treat Countess Anna del Chinchón, wife of the viceroy to Peru, and that her miraculous cure resulted in the introduction of cinchona into Spain in 1639 for the treatment of ague. There is no evidence that the countess ever used the bark; yet for many years the drug was called *los Polvos de la Condesa*. However, the viceroy did bring a large shipment of cinchona to Spain. By 1640, the bark was being employed for fevers in Europe. Its use was first mentioned in European medical literature in 1643 by a Belgian, Herman van der Heyden.

The term *cinchona* was chosen by Linné (who accidentally misspelled it) for the species of trees yielding the bark. Although this term is probably derived from the name of the countess whose alleged cure led to its wide use, some believe that it comes from a word of Incan origin, *kinia*, which means "bark." The Jesuit fathers were the main importers and distributors of cinchona in Europe, and the name Jesuit bark soon became attached to the drug. It was sponsored in Rome chiefly by the eminent philosopher Cardinal de Lugo; hence the drug came to be called Cardinal's bark. The conservative medical groups viewed the new antipyretic with disdain because its use did not conform to the teachings of Galen. Others looked upon it with suspicion because the Jesuits used it. For these reasons, the drug was dispensed for many years predominantly by charlatans and in the form of secret remedies. The first official recognition of cinchona came in 1677, when it was included in an edition of the *London Pharmacopoeia* as "Cortex Peruanus."

For almost two centuries the bark was employed for medicine as a powder, extract, or infusion. In 1820, Pelletier and Caventou isolated quinine and cinchonine from cinchona, and the use of the alkaloids as such gained favor rapidly.

Chemistry. Although quinine has been synthesized, the procedure is complex; quinine and the other alkaloids are, therefore, still obtained entirely from natural sources. Cinchona contains a mixture of more than 20 alkaloids. The most important of these are two pairs of optical isomers, quinine and quinidine, and cinchonidine and cinchonine. Quinine and cinchonidine are levorotatory.

Quinine has the following structural formula:

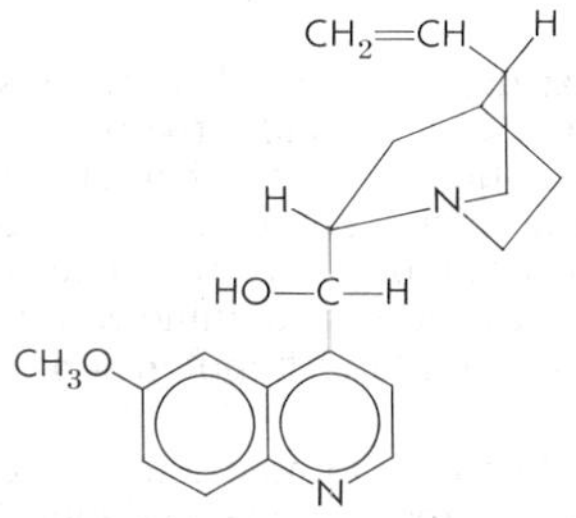

Quinine

Quinine contains a quinoline group attached through a secondary alcohol linkage to a quinuclidine ring. A methoxy side chain is attached to the quinoline ring and a vinyl to the quinuclidine. Quinidine has the same structure as quinine except for the steric configuration of the secondary alcohol group. Stereoisomerism at this position is a relatively unimportant factor in the structure–activity relationship. Quinidine is both more potent as an antimalarial and more toxic than quinine (*see* White, 1988). The many natural alkaloids related to quinine and the semisynthetic chemicals derived from quinine differ mainly in the nature of the substitutions on the side chain. Each alteration in the chemical structure of quinine causes corresponding quantitative but not qualitative changes in the pharmacological actions of the resulting compounds. Details of the structure–activity relationship of the cinchona alkaloids may be found elsewhere (*see* Oettingen, 1933; Wiselogle, 1946). Historically, this important field has provided the necessary background for the search for more effective and less toxic antimalarials, for example, *mefloquine*.

PHARMACOLOGICAL PROPERTIES

Antimalarial Actions. Quinine acts primarily as a blood schizontocide; it has little effect on sporozoites or preerythrocytic forms of malarial parasites. The alkaloid is also gametocidal for *P. vivax* and *P. malariae* but not for *P. falciparum*. As both a suppressive and therapeutic agent, quinine is more toxic and less effective than chloroquine, possibly because its activity stems primarily from its properties as a weak base (*see* above; *see also* Schlesinger *et al.*, 1988). However, quinine is especially valuable for the treatment of severe illness due to chloroquine-resistant and multidrug-resistant strains of *P. falciparum*.

Central Nervous System. Therapeutic doses of quinine have few effects on the CNS other than to cause analgesia and antipyresis. The discovery that cinchona lowered the fever of malarial patients quickly led to its use in all forms of febrile illnesses. However, quinine is not a potent or particularly effective antipyretic.

Cardiovascular System. The actions of quinine on cardiac muscle are qualitatively similar to those of its isomer, quinidine (*see* Chapter 35). Therapeutic doses of quinine have little, if any, effect on the normal heart or blood pressure in man. When given as a bolus intravenously, quinine causes sometimes alarming and even fatal hypotension.

Skeletal Muscle. Quinine and related cinchona alkaloids exert effects on skeletal muscle that have clinical implications. Quinine increases the tension response to a single maximal stimulus delivered to the muscle directly or through the nerve, but it also increases the refractory period of muscle so that the response to tetanic stimulation is diminished. The excitability of the motor end-plate region decreases so that responses to repetitive nerve stimulation and to acetylcholine are reduced. Thus, quinine can antagonize the actions of physostigmine on skeletal muscle as effectively as does curare. Quinine may cause symptomatic relief of myotonia congenita. This disease is the pharmacological antithesis of myasthenia gravis, such that drugs effective in one syndrome aggravate the other. Thus, quinine may produce alarming respiratory distress and dysphagia in patients with myasthenia.

Gastrointestinal Tract. The irritant properties of the cinchona alkaloids cause considerable gastric distress. Nausea, vomiting, and diarrhea are prominent when large doses are taken orally. Toxic amounts also produce vomiting by a central action on the medulla. The musculature of the intestinal tract is not stimulated by concentrations of the drug reached clinically.

Pancreas. Therapeutic doses of quinine and quinidine may lower blood glucose concentrations by stimulating insulin secretion (Looareesuwan *et al.*, 1985; Phillips *et al.*, 1986; Okitolonda *et al.*, 1987). Recurrent hyperinsulinemic hypoglycemia can be particularly serious when these alkaloids are used during pregnancy or when there is severe infection.

Absorption, Fate, and Excretion. Quinine and its congeners are readily absorbed when given orally or intramuscularly. In the former case absorption occurs mainly from the upper small intestine and is over 80% complete, even in patients with marked diarrhea. Peak plasma concentrations of cinchona alkaloids occur within 1 to 3 hours after a single oral dose. After termination of quinine therapy, the plasma concentration falls with a half-time of about 11 hours. Plasma concentrations of quinine between 8 and 15 mg per liter are effective clinically and are generally nontoxic; such values are usually achieved with standard therapeutic doses. Quinine has an apparent volume of distribution of about 2 liters/kg. In acute malaria, however, the volume of distribution contracts, the clearance is reduced, and the elimination half-life increases in proportion to the severity of the illness. On a given dosage regimen, concentrations of quinine in plasma are thus elevated during the acute illness and return toward the usual values only as the patient improves. About 90% of plasma quinine is bound to proteins. The concentration of the alkaloid in cerebrospinal fluid is only about 2 to 5% of that in the plasma. Quinine readily reaches the tissues of the fetus.

The cinchona alkaloids are extensively metabolized, especially in the liver, so that only about 10% of an administered dose is excreted unaltered in the urine. There is no accumulation of the drugs in the body upon continued administration; metabolites are excreted in the urine. Renal excretion of quinine is twice as rapid when the urine is acidic as when it is alkaline. The pharmacokinetic properties of quinine have been studied in patients with cerebral and uncomplicated falciparum malaria (White *et al.*, 1982; *see also* White, 1988.)

Toxicity and Side Effects. The fatal oral dose of quinine for adults is approximately 2 to 8 g. When quinine is repeatedly given in full therapeutic doses, a typical dose-related cluster of symptoms occurs, termed cinchonism. In mild form this consists of ringing in the ears, headache, nausea, and disturbed vision; however, when medication is continued or after large single doses, gastrointestinal, cardiovascular, and dermal manifestations may appear.

Hearing and vision are particularly disturbed. Functional impairment of the eighth nerve results in tinnitus, decreased auditory acuity, and vertigo. Visual signs consist of blurred vision, disturbed color perception, photophobia, diplopia, night blindness, constricted visual fields, scotomata, mydriasis, and, very rarely, even blindness (Bateman and Dyson, 1986). The visual and auditory effects are probably the result of direct neurotoxicity, although secondary vascular changes may have a role. Marked spastic constriction of the retinal vessels occurs; the retina is ischemic, the discs are pale, and retinal edema may ensue. In severe cases, optic atrophy results. Degenerative changes in the spiral ganglion cells similar to those noted in the ganglion cells of the retina support the notion that cellular injury from quinine is direct.

Gastrointestinal symptoms are also prominent in cinchonism. Nausea, vomiting, abdominal pain, and diarrhea result from the local irritant action of quinine, but the nausea and emesis also have a central basis. The skin is often hot and flushed, and sweating is prominent. Rashes frequently appear. Angioedema, especially of the face, is occasionally observed.

Central nervous system symptoms are noted in more severe grades of poisoning, particularly headache, fever, vomiting, apprehension, excitement, confusion, delirium, and syncope. Respiration is first stimulated and is then shallow and depressed. The skin becomes cold and cyanotic as poisoning progresses, the body temperature and the blood pressure fall, weakness is extreme, the pulse is feeble, coma ensues, and death occurs from respiratory arrest. If the patient recovers, symptoms usually disappear completely except for variable degrees of residual optic and auditory damage in some cases.

At times, renal damage may be caused by quinine, and anuria and uremia may ensue. The triad of massive hemolysis, hemoglobinemia, and hemoglobinuria is a rare complication of quinine therapy in pregnant women or in patients with malaria. Quinine is capable of causing hypoprothrombinemia; the simultaneous administration of vitamin K counteracts the prolongation of the prothrombin time. Rarely, quinine may cause symptomatic thrombocytopenic purpura by an immune mechanism that involves the participation of antibody and compliment. This may even occur with ingestion of tonic water (cocktail purpura). In a few instances, the drug appears to have caused agranulocytosis. Abortion may result from quinine overdosage, but this is not necessarily due to an oxytocic action of the drug. The alkaloid may cause asthma in hypersensitive individuals. Transient ventricular tachycardia may rarely be observed after massive acute overdosage.

When small doses of cinchona alkaloids cause toxic manifestations, the individual is usually hypersensitive to the drug. Cinchonism may appear after a single dose of quinine, but it is usually mild. Cutaneous flushing, pruritus, skin rashes, fever, gastric distress, dyspnea, ringing in the ears, and visual impairment are the usual expressions of hypersensitivity; extreme flushing of the skin accompanied by intense, generalized pruritus is the most common form. Hemoglobinuria and asthma from quinine may occur more rarely.

Precautions and Contraindications. Quinine must be used with considerable caution, if at all, in patients who manifest hypersensitivity to the drug, especially when this takes the form of cutaneous, angioedematous, visual, or auditory symptoms. Quinine should be discontinued immediately if evidence of hemolysis appears. The drug should not be used in patients with tinnitus or optic neuritis. In patients with atrial fibrillation, the administration of quinine requires the same precautions as outlined for quinidine (*see* Chapter 35).

Preparations, Routes of Administration, and Dosages. There are numerous preparations of cinchona alkaloids available, particularly in tropical communities where malaria is endemic and where inexpensive medication is essential. In the United States, the pure alkaloids are employed rather than the galenical preparations.

The most commonly used salt of quinine is the sulfate, which is available in tablets and capsules. When given alone, the usual oral dose of quinine sulfate for adults is 650 mg three times daily for 7 to 10 days. This regimen may be shortened to 3 to 7 days when quinine is administered together with other antimalarial agents such as sulfadiazine, a tetracycline, or pyrimethamine and sulfadoxine. The drug is given after meals, preferably in capsules, to minimize gastric irritation.

Totaquine contains approximately 75% of the total anhydrous crystallizable cinchona alkaloids, of which 20% is quinine. The drug is cheaper than quinine and available in abundance in parts of the world where quinine is expensive or limited in supply. In proper doses, it is as effective as quinine in malaria inasmuch as it contains cinchona alkaloids with approximately the same order of antimalarial potency as quinine. The usual dosage of totaquine for malaria is 600 mg three times daily after meals.

Quinine should be given orally whenever possible. Intravenous infusion of the drug is reserved for critical situations such as severe or cerebral malaria; the dihydrochloride salt is employed. An appropriate dosage regimen for adults consists of a loading dose of 20 mg of the salt/kg in 300 to 500 ml of normal saline infused over the first 4 hours, followed by 10 mg/kg given as a 4-hour infusion every 8 hours (White *et al.*, 1983). A maximum daily dose of 1800 mg of the salt (1500 mg of base) should not be exceeded. Quinine dihydrochloride is available in the United States only from the Centers for Disease Control.

Quinidine is a practical alternative to quinine for the chemotherapy of severe malaria, even though this use is considered investigational in the United States. Quinidine gluconate is given by continuous intravenous infusion. The Centers for Disease Control currently recommends a schedule for adults of 10 mg of the salt/kg over 1 to 2 hours, followed by 0.02 mg of salt/kg per minute; nevertheless, up-to-date information should be sought (Miller *et al.*, 1989).

THERAPEUTIC USES

Quinine currently has two valid therapeutic applications: the treatment of malaria and the relief of nocturnal leg cramps.

Status as an Antimalarial. The prompt use of intravenous quinine (or quinidine) as a rapidly acting schizontocidal drug to treat severe forms of chloroquine-resistant or multidrug-resistant falciparum malaria is mandatory and can be lifesaving. Combinations of quinine either with pyrimethamine and a sulfonamide or with a tetracycline have been used successfully to effect suppressive cure of patients with multidrug-resistant falciparum malaria (*see* Symposium, 1987; and reviews by Krogstad *et al.*, 1988; and White, 1988).

Nocturnal Leg Cramps. Recumbency leg muscle cramps (night cramps) are reportedly relieved by quinine. The dose is 200 to 300 mg before retiring. In some individuals, only a brief period of quinine therapy is required to provide relief; even large doses of the drug are ineffective in others.

ANTIBACTERIAL AGENTS IN ANTIMALARIAL CHEMOTHERAPY

Shortly after their introduction into therapeutics, the sulfonamides were shown to possess antimalarial activity. The sulfones were also shown to be effective; the first trial of dapsone was against *P. falciparum* in 1943. Current interest stems from their use, usually along with quinine or in combination with pyrimethamine, against chloroquine-resistant strains of *P. falciparum*. The activity of tetracyclines against drug-resistant malarial parasites is also proving useful, although their schizontocidal action is slow.

Sulfonamides and Sulfones. Much of the important work on sulfonamides was carried out during the intensive antimalarial program during World War II. This and later work focused attention on sulfadiazine, because of its relatively high activity. It was found, however, to be active only against the asexual blood forms of the human malarial parasites, and to act slowly. Today, sulfadiazine is used together with quinine to treat acute attacks of malaria due to multidrug-resistant strains of *P. falciparum*. The oral dose for adults is 500 mg of sulfadiazine every 6 hours for 5 days. The combination of a long-acting sulfonamide, sulfadoxine, and pyrimethamine had been used extensively for the prophylaxis of chloroquine-resistant strains of *P. falciparum*. The utility of this combination has been severely compromised, however, by the increased prevalence of multidrug-resistant strains and the potential toxicity of the sulfonamides (*see* above). The danger of producing resistant strains, not only of malarial parasites but also of pathogenic bacteria, by the use of combinations containing sulfonamides or sulfones is a matter of continuing concern. Neither sulfonamides nor sulfones are as active against *P. vivax* as they are against *P. falciparum*.

Tetracyclines. Tetracyclines are particularly useful for the treatment of the acute malarial attack due to multiresistant strains of *P. falciparum* that also show partial resistance to quinine (Chongsuphajaisiddhi *et al.*, 1986). Their relative slowness of action makes concurrent treatment with quinine mandatory for rapid control of parasitemia. Several tetracyclines appear equivalent; most data have accumulated for tetracycline itself, and tetracycline or doxycycline is usually recommended. The dosage for adults is 250 mg every 6 hours for 7 to 10 days. Although tetracycline has shown marked activity against primary tissue schizonts of chloroquine-resistant strains of *P. falciparum*, its long-term use as a prophylactic agent is not advised. However, doxycycline can be used by travelers as an alternative to sulfadoxine–pyrimethamine for short-term prophylaxis against multidrug-resistant strains. The usual oral dose is 100 mg daily. Because of their adverse effects on bones and teeth, tetracyclines should not be given to pregnant women or children less than 8 years old. Photosensitivity reactions or drug-induced superinfections may mandate discontinuation of therapy or prophylaxis with these agents.

PRINCIPLES OF ANTIMALARIAL PROPHYLAXIS AND CHEMOTHERAPY

Due primarily to the increasing resistance of *P. falciparum* to antimalarial drugs, the prophylaxis and chemotherapy of the most dangerous form of human malaria has become more complex and less satisfactory. By 1984, varying degrees of resistance to chloroquine had been identified in well over 30 countries in Asia, South America, and Africa. The incidence of resistance to the combination of pyrimethamine and sulfadoxine has risen appreciably in areas of use, and this preparation has become ineffective for the prophylaxis and treatment of chloroquine-resistant strains of *P. falciparum* malaria in certain parts of southeast Asia. Lack of responsiveness to the usual doses of quinine has even posed a problem in these regions. Only broad guidelines for the prophylaxis and treatment of malaria are presented here, because specific chemotherapeutic regimens change. The

Malaria Branch of the Centers for Disease Control is a reliable source of current information about this subject.

With a few important exceptions, the chemotherapy of an acute attack of human malaria is the same for all species of plasmodia; only subsequent treatment is dependent on species. The acute attack requires prompt treatment with a rapidly acting schizontocide; chloroquine is the drug of choice for *P. vivax, P. ovale, P. malariae,* and chloroquine-sensitive strains of *P. falciparum*. The oral route of administration should be used whenever possible, but chloroquine can be given intramuscularly or even intravenously if suitable precautions are taken. For acute attacks with chloroquine-resistant or multidrug resistant strains of *P. falciparum,* the preferred schizontocide is quinine, despite its toxicity. Quinine can be given together with other effective but slower acting blood schizontocides such as a sulfonamide or a tetracycline for multidrug-resistant strains. Quinine is given by the oral route whenever possible, but intravenous preparations are used when oral medication cannot be taken. If intravenous quinine dihydrochloride is not immediately available, quinidine gluconate should be substituted; exchange transfusion may be of additional benefit in severe malaria (*see* White, 1988; Miller *et al.*, 1989). When the diagnosis of chloroquine-resistant falciparum malaria is suspected from a travel history and clinical findings, treatment with quinine (or quinidine) should be instituted promptly. It is inadvisable to wait for a definitive diagnosis by hematological findings in nonimmune patients because the clinical status of the patient may deteriorate rapidly.

Attacks of malaria may recur during or after a course of antimalarial chemotherapy, even in the absence of reinfection. Recurrent attacks of *P. vivax, P. ovale,* or *P. malariae* are usually well controlled by another course of chloroquine, combined with primaquine in the case of *P. vivax* and *P. ovale*. Some patients with vivax infection may require more than one course to effect a radical cure. Recrudescence of falciparum malarial attacks or parasitemia after appropriate treatment with chloroquine usually denotes infection with chloroquine-resistant plasmodia (for clinical classification, *see* World Health Organization, 1981). Treatment with a course of quinine usually suffices to solve this problem. However, some multidrug-resistant strains, particularly in Southeast Asia, fail to respond adequately to the usual therapeutic doses of quinine. Several options must be considered in this difficult situation. Quinine has been used successfully together with a slower acting schizontocide such as doxycycline in Southeast Asia or with an antifolate in East Africa. Quinidine can be substituted for quinine; this is an effective choice in some instances. Mefloquine provides an excellent alternative, especially in geographic areas where resistance to this alkaloid has not been encountered; however, the drug cannot be administered parenterally.

In areas where malaria is endemic, chloroquine remains the drug of choice for the prophylaxis and control of infections due to *P. vivax, P. ovale, P. malariae,* or chloroquine-sensitive strains of *P. falciparum*. Attempts at radical cure of vivax malaria by administration of primaquine should be delayed until the patient leaves an endemic area. In areas where chloroquine-resistant *P. falciparum* is endemic, pyrimethamine–sulfadoxine had been given for the most effective prophylaxis, but this is no longer recommended because of the potential toxicity of sulfadoxine. Instead, travelers are advised to take chloroquine weekly and carry a therapeutic dose of pyrimethamine–sulfadoxine for treatment of a presumed malarial illness if a physician is not immediately available. In Africa south of the Sahara, chloroguanide may be used along with chloroquine for effective prophylaxis of chloroquine-resistant falciparum malaria. However, chloroquine with pyrimethamine–sulfadoxine or chloroguanide may fail to abort attacks with highly chloroquine-resistant or multidrug-resistant strains of *P. falciparum* such as those found in Southeast Asia; prophylaxis with doxycycline or mefloquine may prove more successful. However, the physician may have no alternative but to treat the acute attack. Quinine alone or together with sulfadiazine or a tetracycline is used for this purpose and more than one course of chemotherapy may be required.

Prophylaxis and chemotherapy of malaria in children and pregnant women present special problems. With appropriate dosage adjustments and safety precautions, the treatment of children is generally the same as in adults, except that tetracyclines should not be given to children less than 8 years old. Malarial infection, particularly with *P. falciparum,* tends to be especially severe in infants and in pregnant women. The latter should be urged to avoid travel to endemic areas, if at all possible. While chloroquine and quinine may be used during pregnancy, antifolates, tetracyclines, and primaquine should be avoided. The exception here is chloroguanide, which is considered to be quite safe during pregnancy.

Aikawa, M. High-resolution autoradiography of malarial parasites treated with ^{3}H-chloroquine. *Am. J. Pathol.*, **1972**, *67*, 277–280.

Alving, A. S.; Eichelberger, L.; Craige, B., Jr.; Jones, R., Jr.; Whorton, C. M.; and Pullman, T. N. Studies on the chronic toxicity of chloroquine (SN-7618). *J. Clin. Invest.*, **1948**, *27*, 60–65.

Baker, J. K.; McChesney, J. D.; Hufford, C. D.; and Clark, A. M. High-performance liquid chromatographic analysis of the metabolism of primaquine and the identification of a new mammalian metabolite. *J. Chromatogr.*, **1982**, *230*, 69–77.

Berliner, R. W.; Earle, D. P., Jr.; Taggart, J. V.; Zubrod, C. G.; Welch, W. J.; Conan, N. J.; Bauman, E.; Scudder, S. T.; and Shannon, J. A. Studies on the chemotherapy of the human malarias. VI. The physiological disposition, antimalarial activity, and toxicity of several derivatives of 4-aminoquinoline. *J. Clin. Invest.*, **1948**, *27*, 98–107.

Bernstein, H. N.; Svaifler, N. J.; Rubin, M.; and Mausour, A. M. The ocular deposition of chloroquine. *Invest. Ophthalmol. Visual Sci.*, **1963**, *2*, 384–392.

Beutler, E., and Mitchell, M. Special modifications of the fluorescent screening method for glucose-6-phosphate dehydrogenase deficiency. *Blood*, **1968**, *32*, 816–818.

Bitonti, A. J.; Sjoerdsma, A.; McCann, P. P.; Kyle, D. E.; Oduola, A. M. J.; Rossan, R. N.; Milhous, W. K.; and Davidson, D. E., Jr. Reversal of chloroquine resistance in malaria parasite *Plasmodium falciparum* by desipramine. *Science,* **1988,** *242,* 1301–1303.

Boudreau, E. F.; Webster, H. K.; Pavanand, K.; and Thosingha, L. Type II mefloquine resistance in Thailand. *Lancet,* **1982,** *2,* 1335.

Brewer, G. J.; Tarlov, A. R.; and Alving, A. S. Methemoglobin reduction test: a new simple, *in vitro* test for identifying primaquine-sensitivity. *Bull. W.H.O.,* **1960,** *22,* 633–640.

Brooks, M. H.; Malloy, J. P.; Bartelloni, P. J.; Sheehy, T. W.; and Barry, K. G. Quinine, pyrimethamine, and sulphorthodimethoxine: clinical response, plasma levels, and urinary excretion during the initial attack of naturally acquired *falciparum* malaria. *Clin. Pharmacol. Ther.,* **1969,** *10,* 85–91.

Brown, R. E.; Stancatto, F. A.; and Wolfe, A. D. The effects of mefloquine on *Escherichia coli. Life Sci.,* **1979,** *25,* 1857–1864.

Bygbjerg, I. C.; Schapira, A.; Flachs, H.; Gomme, G.; and Jepsen, S. Mefloquine resistance of falciparum malaria from Tanzania enhanced by treatment. *Lancet,* **1983,** *1,* 774–775.

Bygbjerg, I.; Ravn, P.; Flachs, H.; and Hvidberg, E. F. Human pharmacokinetics of proguanil and its metabolites. *Trop. Med. Parasitol.,* **1987,** *38,* 77–80.

Chou, A. C.; Chevli, R.; and Fitch, C. D. Ferriprotoporphyrin IX fulfills the criteria for identification as the chloroquine receptor of malaria parasites. *Biochemistry,* **1980,** *19,* 1543–1549.

Clyde, D. F.; McCarthy, V. C.; Miller, R. M.; and Hornick, R. B. Suppressive activity of mefloquine in sporozoite-induced human malaria. *Antimicrob. Agents Chemother.,* **1976,** *9,* 384–386.

Cohen, R. J.; Sachs, J. R.; Wicker, D. J.; and Conrad, M. E. Methemoglobinemia provoked by malarial chemoprophylaxis in Vietnam. *N. Engl. J. Med.,* **1968,** *279,* 1127–1131.

Cook, I. F., and Kish, M. Y. Haematological safety of long-term malarial prophylaxis with dapsone pyrimethamine. *Med. J. Aust.,* **1985,** *143,* 139–141.

Cosgriff, T. M.; Boudreau, E. F.; Pamplin, C. L.; Doberstyn, E. B.; Desjardins, R. E.; and Canfield, C. J. Evaluation of the antimalarial activity of the phenanthrene methanol halofantrine (WR 171669). *Am. J. Trop. Med. Hyg.,* **1982,** *31,* 1075–1079.

Davidson, M. W.; Griggs, B. G., Jr.; Boykin, D. W.; and Wilson, W. D. Molecular structural effects involved in the interaction of quinolinemethanolamines with DNA. Implications for antimalarial action. *J. Med. Chem.,* **1977,** *20,* 1117–1122.

Desjardins, R. E.; Canfield, C. J.; Haynes, J. D.; and Chulay, J. D. Quantitative assessment of antimalarial activity *in vitro* by a semiautomated microdilution technique. *Antimicrob. Agents Chemother.,* **1979a,** *16,* 710–718.

Desjardins, R. E.; Pamplin, C. L.; von Bredow, J.; Barry, K. G.; and Canfield, C. J. Kinetics of a new antimalarial, mefloquine. *Clin. Pharmacol. Ther.,* **1979b,** *26,* 372–379.

Elderfield, R. C., and others. Alkylaminoalkyl derivatives of 8-aminoquinoline. *J. Am. Chem. Soc.,* **1946,** *68,* 1524–1529.

Estes, M. L.; Ewing-Wilson, D.; Chou, S. M.; Mitsumoto, H.; Hanson, M.; Shirey, E.; and Ratliff, N. B. Chloroquine neuromyotoxicity: clinical and pathologic perspective. *Am. J. Med.,* **1987,** *82,* 447–455.

Falco, E. A.; Goodwin, L. G.; Hitchings, G. H.; Rollo, I. M.; and Russell, P. B. 2:4-Diaminopyrimidines—a new series of antimalarials. *Br. J. Pharmacol. Chemother.,* **1951,** *6,* 185–200.

Ferone, R.; Burchall, J. J.; and Hitchings, G. H. *Plasmodium berghei* dihydrofolate reductase: isolation, properties, and inhibition by antifolates. *Mol. Pharmacol.,* **1969,** *5,* 49–59.

Fitch, C. D.; Chan, R. L.; and Chevli, R. Chloroquine resistance in malaria: accessibility of drug receptors to mefloquine. *Antimicrob. Agents Chemother.,* **1979,** *15,* 258–262.

Fletcher, K. A.; Barton, P. F.; and Kelly, J. A. Studies on the mechanisms of oxidation in the erythrocyte by metabolites of primaquine. *Biochem. Pharmacol.,* **1988,** *37,* 2683–2690.

Fletcher, K. A.; Price Evans, D. A.; Gilles, H. M.; Greaves, J.; Bunnag, D.; and Harinasuta, T. Studies on the pharmacokinetics of primaquine. *Bull. W.H.O.,* **1981,** *59,* 407–412.

Fogh, S.; Schapira, A.; Bygbjerg, I. C.; Jepsen, S.; Mordhorst, C. H.; Kuijlen, K.; Ravn, P.; Rønn, A.; and Gøtzsche, P. C. Malaria chemoprophylaxis in travelers to east Africa: a comparative prospective study of chloroquine plus proguanil with chloroquine plus sulfadoxine-pyrimethamine. *Br. Med. J.* [*Clin. Res.*], **1988,** *296,* 820–822.

Fojo, A.; Akiyama, S.-I.; Gottesman, M. M.; and Pastan, I. Reduced drug accumulation in multiply drug-resistant human KB carcinoma cell lines. *Cancer Res.,* **1985,** *45,* 3002–3007.

Hoffman, S. L.; Rustama, D.; Dimpudus, A. J.; Punjabi, N. H.; Campbell, J. R.; Oetomo, H. S.; Marwoto, H. A.; Harun, S.; Sukri, N.; and Heizmann, P. RII and RIII type resistance of *Plasmodium falciparum* to combination of mefloquine and sulfadoxine/pyrimethamine in Indonesia. *Lancet,* **1985,** *2,* 1039–1040.

Jacobs, G. H.; Aikawa, M.; Milhous, W. K.; and Rabbege, J. R. An ultrastructural study of the effects of mefloquine on *Plasmodium falciparum. Am. J. Trop. Med. Hyg.,* **1987,** *36,* 9–14.

Karbwang, J.; Bunnag, D.; Breckenridge, A. M.; and Back, D. J. The pharmacokinetics of mefloquine when given alone or in combination with sulphadoxine and pyrimethamine in Thai male and female subjects. *Eur. J. Clin. Pharmacol.,* **1987,** *32,* 173–177.

Leport, C.; Raffi, F.; Matheron, S.; Katlama, C.; Regnier, B.; Saimot, A. G.; Marche, C.; Vendrenne, C.; and Vilde, J. L. Treatment of central nervous system toxoplasmosis with pyrimethamine/sulfadiazine combination in 35 patients with the acquired immunodeficiency syndrome. Efficacy of long-term therapy. *Am. J. Med.,* **1988,** *84,* 94–100.

Looareesuwan, S.; Phillips, R. E.; White, N. J.; Kietinun, S.; Karbwang, J.; Rackow, C.; Turner, R. C.; and Warrell, D. A. Quinine and severe falciparum malaria in late pregnancy. *Lancet,* **1985,** *2,* 4–8.

Martin, S. K.; Oduola, A. M. J.; and Milhous, W. K. Reversal of chloroquine resistance in *Plasmodium falciparum* by verapamil. *Science,* **1987,** *235,* 899–901.

Mihaly, G. W.; Ward, S. A.; Edwards, G.; Orme, M. L.; and Breckenridge, A. M. Pharmacokinetics of primaquine in man: identification of the carboxylic acid derivative as a major plasma metabolite. *Br. J. Clin. Pharmacol.,* **1984,** *17,* 441–446.

Miller, K. D.; Lobel, H. D.; Satriale, R. F.; Kuritsky, J. N.; Stern, R.; and Campbell, C. C. Severe cutaneous reactions among American travelers using pyrimethamine-sulfadoxine (FANSIDAR) for malaria prophylaxis. *Am. J. Trop. Med. Hyg.,* **1986,** *35,* 451–458.

Miller, K. D.; Greenberg, A. E.; and Campbell, C. C. Treatment of severe malaria in the United States with a continuous-infusion of quinidine gluconate and exchange transfusion. *N. Engl. J. Med.,* **1989,** *321,* 65–70.

Mu, J. Y.; Israili, Z. H.; and Dayton, P. G. Studies of the disposition and metabolism of mefloquine HCl (WR 142490), a quinolinemethanol antimalarial, in the rat. *Drug Metab. Dispos.,* **1975,** *3,* 198–210.

Mühlens, P. Die Behandlung der naturlichen menschli-

chen Malaria-Infektion mit Plasmochin. *Naturwissenschaften*, **1926**, *14*, 1162–1166.
Okitolonda, W.; Delacollette, C.; Mallengrean, M.; and Henquin, J. C. High incidence of hypoglycaemia in African patients treated with intravenous quinine for severe malaria. *Br. Med. J.* [*Clin. Res.*], **1987**, *295*, 716–718.
Phillips, R. E.; Looareesuwan, S.; White, N. J.; Chanthavanich, P.; Karbwang, J.; Supanaranond, W.; Turner, R. C.; and Warrell, D. A. Hypoglycaemia and antimalarial drugs: quinidine and release of insulin. *Br. Med. J.* [*Clin. Res.*], **1986**, *292*, 1319–1321.
Rieckmann, K. H.; Campbell, G. H.; Sax, L. J.; and Mrema, J. E. Drug sensitivity of *Plasmodium falciparum*. An *in vitro* microtechnique. *Lancet*, **1978**, *2*, 22–23.
Rieckmann, K. H.; Trenholme, G. M.; Williams, R. L.; Carson, P. E.; Frischer, H.; and Desjardins, R. E. Prophylactic activity of mefloquine hydrochloride (WR 142490) in drug-resistant malaria. *Bull. W.H.O.*, **1974**, *51*, 375–377.
Riou, B.; Barriot, P.; Rimailho, A.; and Baud, F. J. Treatment of severe chloroquine poisoning. *N. Engl. J. Med.*, **1988**, *318*, 1–6.
Scheibel, L. W.; Colombani, P. M.; Hess, A. D.; Aikawa, M.; Atkinson, C. T.; and Milhous, W. K. Calcium and calmodulin antagonists inhibit human malaria parasites (*Plasmodium falciparum*): implications for drug design. *Proc. Natl. Acad. Sci. U.S.A.*, **1987**, *84*, 7310–7314.
Schmidt, L. H. *Plasmodium falciparum* and *Plasmodium vivax* infections in the owl monkey (*Aotus trivirgatus*). *Am. J. Trop. Med. Hyg.*, **1978**, *27*, 671–737.
———. Compatibility of relapse patterns of *Plasmodium cynomolgi* infections in rhesus monkeys with continuous cyclical development and hypnozoite concepts of relapse. *Am. J. Trop. Med. Hyg.*, **1986**, *35*, 1077–1099.
Schmidt, L. H.; Crosby, R.; Rasco, J.; and Vaughan, D. Antimalarial activities of various 4-quinolinemethanols with special attention to WR-142,490 (mefloquine). *Antimicrob. Agents Chemother.*, **1978**, *13*, 1011–1030.
Shortt, H. E., and Garnham, P. C. C. Demonstration of a persisting exo-erythrocytic cycle in *Plasmodium cynomolgi* and its bearing on the production of relapses. *Br. J. Med.* [*Clin. Res.*], **1948**, *1*, 1225–1228.
Stickney, D. R.; Simmons, W. S.; De Angelis, R. L.; Rundles, R. W.; and Nichol, C. A. Pharmacokinetics of pyrimethamine (PRM) and 2,4-diamino-5-(3′,4′-dichlorophenyl)-6-methyl pyrimidine (DMP) relevant to meningeal leukemia. *Proc. Am. Assoc. Cancer Res.*, **1973**, *14*, 52.
Trager, W., and Jensen, J. B. Human malaria parasites in continuous culture. *Science*, **1976**, *193*, 673–675.
Trenholme, G. M.; Williams, R. L.; Desjardins, R. E.; Frischer, H.; Carson, P. E.; and Rieckmann, K. H. Mefloquine (WR 142,490) in the treatment of human malaria. *Science*, **1975**, *190*, 792–794.
Ward, S. A.; Mihaly, G. W.; Edwards, G. Looareesuwan, S.; Phillips, R. E.; Chanthavanich, P.; Warrell, D. A.; Orme, M. L.; and Breckenridge, A. M. Pharmacokinetics of primaquine in man. II. Comparison of acute vs chronic dosage in Thai subjects. *Br. J. Clin. Pharmacol.*, **1985**, *19*, 751–755.
White, N. J.; Looareesuwan, S.; Warrell, D. A.; Warrell, M. J.; Bunnag, D.; and Harinasuta, T. Quinine pharmacokinetics and toxicity in cerebral and uncomplicated falciparum malaria. *Am. J. Med.*, **1982**, *73*, 564–572.
White, N. J.; Looareesuwan, S.; Warrell, D. A.; Warrell, M. J.; Chanthavanich, P.; Bunnag, D.; and Harinasuta, T. Quinine loading dose in cerebral malaria. *Am. J. Trop. Med. Hyg.*, **1983**, *32*, 1–5.
White, N. J.; Miller, K. D.; Churchill, F. C.; Berry, C.; Brown, J.; Williams, S. B.; and Greenwood, B. M. Chloroquine treatment of severe malaria in children. Pharmacokinetics, toxicity and new dosage recommendations. *N. Engl. J. Med.*, **1988**, *319*, 1493–1500.

Monographs and Reviews

Bateman, D. N., and Dyson, E. H. Quinine toxicity. *Adverse Drug React. Acute Poisoning Rev.*, **1986**, *4*, 215–233.
Bray, R. S., and Garnham, P. C. C. The life-cycle of primate malaria parasites. *Br. Med. Bull.*, **1982**, *38*, 117–122.
Chongsuphajaisiddhi, T., and others. Severe and complicated malaria. *Trans. R. Soc. Trop. Med. Hyg.*, **1986**, *80*, Suppl., 1–50.
Coatney, G. R.; Cooper, W. C.; Eddy, N. B.; and Greenberg, J. *Survey of Antimalarial Agents: Chemotherapy of Plasmodium gallinaceum Infections; Toxicity; Correlation of Structure and Action.* Public Health Service Monograph No. 9, U.S. Government Printing Office, Washington, D.C., **1953**.
Davey, D. G. Chemotherapy of malaria. Part 1. Biological basis of testing methods. In, *Experimental Chemotherapy*, Vol. 1. (Schnitzer, R. J., and Hawking, F., eds.) Academic Press, Inc., New York, **1963**, pp. 487–511.
Dubois, E. L. Antimalarials in the management of discoid and systemic lupus erythematosus. *Semin. Arthritis Rheum.*, **1978**, *8*, 33–51.
Feldman, H. A. Toxoplasmosis. *N. Engl. J. Med.*, **1968**, *279*, 1370–1375, 1431–1437.
Good, M. I., and Shader, R. I. Lethality and behavioral side effects of chloroquine. *J. Clin. Psychopharmacol.*, **1982**, *2*, 40–47.
Hill, J. Chemotherapy of malaria. Part 2. The antimalarial drugs. In, *Experimental Chemotherapy*, Vol. 1. (Schnitzer, R. J., and Hawking, F., eds.) Academic Press, Inc., New York, **1963**, pp. 513–601.
Hitchings, G. H., and Burchall, J. J. Inhibition of folate biosynthesis and function as a basis for chemotherapy. *Adv. Enzymol.*, **1965**, *27*, 417–468.
Isaacson, D.; Elgart, M.; and Turner, M. L. Antimalarials in dermatology. *Int. J. Dermatol.*, **1982**, *21*, 379–395.
Krogstad, D. J.; Schlesinger, P. H.; and Herwaldt, B. L. Antimalarial agents: mechanism of chloroquine resistance. *Antimicrob. Agents Chemother.*, **1988**, *32*, 799–801.
Krotoski, W. A. Discovery of the hypnozoite and a new theory of malarial relapse. *Trans. R. Soc. Trop. Med. Hyg.*, **1985**, *79*, 1–11.
McCabe, R. E., and Remington, J. S. Toxoplasmosis. In, *Tropical and Geographical Medicine*. (Warren, K. S., and Mahmoud, A. A. F., eds.) McGraw-Hill Book Company, New York, **1984**, pp. 281–292.
Oettingen, W. F. von. *The Therapeutic Agents of the Quinoline Group*. Chemical Catalog Co., New York, **1933**.
Olansky, A. J. Antimalarials and ophthalmologic safety. *J. Am. Acad. Dermatol.*, **1982**, *6*, 19–23.
Schlesinger, P. H.; Krogstad, D. J.; and Herwaldt, B. L. Antimalarial agents: mechanisms of action. *Antimicrob. Agents Chemother.*, **1988**, *32*, 793–798.
Symposium on DARAPRIM. (Various authors.) *Trans. R. Soc. Trop. Med. Hyg.*, **1952**, *46*, 467–508.
Symposium. (Various authors.) *Primaquine: Pharmacokinetics, Metabolism, Toxicity, and Activity*. Proceedings of a meeting of the Scientific Working Group on the Chemotherapy of Malaria. (Wernsdorfer, W. H., and Trigg, P. I., eds.) John Wiley & Sons, Inc., New York, **1987**.
Tarlov, A. R.; Brewer, G. J.; Carson, P. E.; and Alving, A. S. Primaquine sensitivity. *Arch. Intern. Med.*, **1962**, *109*, 209–234.

Warhurst, D. C. Cinchona alkaloids and malaria. *Acta Leiden.*, **1987**, *55*, 53–64.
White, N. J. Drug treatment and prevention of malaria. *Eur. J. Clin. Pharmacol.*, **1988**, *34*, 1–14.
Wiselogle, F. Y. (ed.). *A Survey of Antimalarial Drugs, 1941–1945*. J. W. Edwards, Publisher, Inc., Ann Arbor, Mich., **1946**. (Two volumes.)
World Health Organization. *Standardization of Procedures for the Study of Glucose-6-Phosphate Dehydrogenase*. Technical Report No. 366, WHO, Geneva, **1967**.
———. *Chemotherapy of Malaria and Resistance to Antimalarials*. Technical Report No. 529, WHO, Geneva, **1973**.
———. *Chemotherapy of Malaria*, 2nd ed. WHO Monograph Series No. 27, WHO, Geneva, **1981**.
———. Development of mefloquine as an antimalarial drug. *Bull. W.H.O.*, **1983**, *61*, 169–178.
———. *Report of the Steering Committees of the Scientific Working Groups on Malaria*. WHO, Geneva, **1984**.

CHAPTER

42 DRUGS USED IN THE CHEMOTHERAPY OF PROTOZOAL INFECTIONS [*Continued*]

Amebiasis, Giardiasis, and Trichomoniasis

Leslie T. Webster, Jr.

Anaerobic protozoa of the genera *Entamoeba, Giardia,* and *Trichomonas* are the causative agents, respectively, of *amebiasis, giardiasis,* and *trichomoniasis,* three parasitic infections of man commonly encountered in the United States and other temperate and tropical climates. These disorders are described briefly here, along with the specific drugs used for their treatment. More details about the diagnosis and clinical management of these conditions are given in the specialized literature and reviews cited at the end of this chapter.

Amebiasis, caused by *Entamoeba histolytica,* has a cosmopolitan distribution, but it is most severe in subtropical and tropical regions. Although endemic amebiasis is relatively rare among the general population of the United States, the infection still has a prevalence of 2 to 4%. It is transmitted by the fecal–oral route and is particularly common under poor hygienic conditions in lower socioeconomic groups, institutionalized individuals, and male homosexuals. Ingested amebic *cysts* from contaminated material change into *trophozoites* that reside in the human colon. There they multiply, encyst, and pass into the environment, thereby completing the cycle. Trophozoites usually exist as commensals in the large intestine; that is, they produce cysts but otherwise cause little harm to the host. However, trophozoites may change into pathogenic forms that invade tissues. In this case, they produce a variety of local and systemic manifestations, most commonly colitis, hepatitis, and abscesses of the liver. The diagnosis of amebiasis and its persistence is made by appropriate examination of rectal scrapings or of the stool. However, a skilled microscopist may be required to distinguish *E. histolytica* from nonpathogenic amebae or white blood cells.

Drugs used to treat amebiasis (amebicides) can be categorized as *luminal, systemic,* or *mixed.* Luminal amebicides, exemplified by *diloxanide furoate* and other *dichloroacetamide derivatives,* are active only against intestinal forms of amebae. These compounds can be used successfully by themselves to treat asymptomatic or mild intestinal forms of amebiasis or, in conjunction with a systemic or mixed amebicide, to eradicate the infection. Systemic amebicides are effective only in invasive forms of amebiasis. These agents have been employed primarily to treat severe amebic dysentery (*dehydroemetine*) or hepatic abscesses (*dehydroemetine* or *chloroquine*), but they are rarely used now unless other drugs fail or cause unacceptable side effects. Mixed amebicides are active against both intestinal and systemic forms of amebiasis. *Metronidazole,* a nitroimidazole derivative, is the prototypical mixed amebicide, and its use has revolutionized the treatment of this protozoal infection. Because it is well absorbed and therefore may fail to reach the large intestine in therapeutic concentrations, this compound is likely to be more effective against systemic than intestinal amebiasis. Antibiotics such as the amebicidal aminoglycoside *paromomycin* or *tetracycline* can be used in conjunction with metronidazole to treat severe forms of intestinal amebiasis. Treatment with metronidazole is often followed by a luminal amebicide to effect a cure.

Giardiasis, caused by the flagellated protozoan *Giardia lamblia,* is the most commonly reported intestinal protozoal infection in developed countries, including the United States. Most infected individuals are asymptomatic. However, these organisms may produce either isolated cases or epidemics of diarrhea; this can be transient or persistent, and it occasionally results in malabsorption, manifested by steatorrhea and weight loss. Travelers, campers, children and adults living under crowded unhygienic conditions, and male homosexuals are especially at risk. *Cysts,* in feces or in contaminated food or water, transmit the infection, and the organism does not require an intermediate host. However, animals other than man can carry the parasite and contaminate water supplies. Ingested cysts change into active *trophozoites* that eventually reside and proliferate in the upper small intestine, where they may or may not produce disease. The diagnosis of giardiasis is made by identification of cysts or trophozoites in fecal specimens. Chemotherapy with *metronidazole* or *quinacrine* is usually successful.

Trichomoniasis is caused by the flagellated protozoan *Trichomonas vaginalis.* This organism inhabits the genitourinary tract of the human host, where it can produce vaginitis in women and urethritis in men. Transmission of the infection occurs primarily by sexual contact, and over 200 million people worldwide become affected each year. Only *trophozoite* forms of the parasite have been identified in infected secretions, which are routinely examined for diagnostic purposes. Proper treatment of both partners with either *metronidazole* or related *nitroimidazole compounds* is nearly always successful.

CHLOROQUINE

History. The unique therapeutic value of chloroquine in *extraintestinal amebiasis* in man was first reported by Conan (1948, 1949) and Murgatroyd and Kent (1948). *In-vitro* studies with trophozoites of *E. histolytica* had revealed that chloroquine possesses amebicidal activity greater than that of the halogenated 8-hydroxyquinolines but less than that of emetine. This discovery, combined with the knowledge that chloroquine localizes in the liver in a concentration several hundred times greater than that in the plasma, suggested its use in *hepatic amebiasis*. Clinical trial then revealed that the signs and the symptoms of amebic hepatitis disappeared within a few days after initiating chloroquine therapy and that this aspect of amebic disease was adequately controlled and often cured.

Pharmacological Properties. The pharmacology and the toxicology of chloroquine are presented in Chapter 41. Only those features of the drug pertinent to its use in amebiasis are described here.

Chloroquine is now used as a systemic amebicide to treat hepatic amebiasis only when treatment with metronidazole is unsuccessful or contraindicated. The clinical response to chloroquine in patients with hepatic amebiasis is often prompt, and there is no evidence that amebae develop resistance to this agent. The drug is much less effective in amebiasis of the colon, partly because it attains a much lower concentration in the intestinal wall than in the liver and partly because it is almost completely absorbed from the small bowel. Because colonic infection with *E. histolytica* is always the source of extraintestinal amebiasis, a drug effective in intestinal amebiasis is routinely given to all patients receiving chloroquine for hepatic amebiasis; such therapy reduces the relapse rate. Conversely, because of the difficulty of determining whether individuals with colonic amebiasis also have hepatic involvement, it is often wise to administer metronidazole or chloroquine when a luminal amebicide is prescribed.

The conventional course of treatment with chloroquine phosphate for extraintestinal amebiasis in adults is 1 g daily for 2 days, followed by 500 mg daily for at least 2 to 3 weeks. Because of the low toxicity of the drug, this dose schedule can be increased if necessary. Treatment with chloroquine may be repeated. Extended courses of therapy with chloroquine (10 weeks) have also been recommended (Cohen and Reynolds, 1975).

DILOXANIDE FUROATE

History. *Diloxanide* is a dichloroacetamide derivative that was introduced by Bristow and associates (1956) as a result of the examination of a series of substituted acetanilides for amebicidal activity. Clinical trials showed diloxanide to be effective in cyst-passing patients, but to be relatively ineffective in the treatment of acute intestinal amebiasis. This was attributed to the presence of inadequate concentrations of the drug at the sites of infection. Of the many derivatives of diloxanide prepared in attempts to solve this problem, the furoate ester proved to be appreciably more active than the parent compound in experimentally infected rats (Main *et al.,* 1960). The results of clinical trials showed it to be effective in cases of acute intestinal amebiasis. *Teclozan* and *etofamide* are other dichloroacetamide derivatives that have been used with success as intraluminal amebicides (*see* Neal, 1983).

Chemistry and Preparation. *Diloxanide furoate* (FURAMIDE) has the following structural formula:

Diloxanide Furoate

After oral ingestion the ester is hydrolyzed to diloxanide and furoic acid. In the United States diloxanide furoate is available from the Centers for Disease Control.

Pharmacological Effects. Diloxanide is directly amebicidal when tested *in vitro*. The furoate ester is active at 0.01 to 0.1 μg/ml, and it is thus considerably more potent than emetine. Little is known of its mechanism of action.

Absorption, Fate, and Excretion. In experimental animals, 60 to 90% of an oral dose of diloxanide furoate is excreted in the urine within 48 hours. More than half of this appears within 6 hours. Excretion in the feces accounts for 4 to 9% of the dose. Peak concentrations appear in the blood within 1 hour but fall to a fraction of this within 6 hours. The ester is largely hydrolyzed in the lumen or mucosa of the intestine, so that only diloxanide appears in the systemic circulation. The drug appears in the urine largely as the glucuronide.

Route of Administration and Dosage. Diloxanide furoate is given only orally. The recommended dosage is 500 mg, three times daily for 10 days. If necessary, a second course may be given immediately following the first. Children should be given 20 mg/kg per day in three divided doses for 10 days.

Toxicity and Side Effects. Side effects are mild. Flatulence is most commonly reported; vomiting, pruritus, and urticaria occur occasionally (*see* Wolfe, 1973).

Therapeutic Uses. Given alone, diloxanide furoate is the drug of choice in the treatment of asymptomatic passers of cysts (Krogstad *et al.*, 1978). It is ineffective when administered alone in the treatment of extraintestinal amebiasis, and its efficacy when used alone in the treatment of acute amebiasis with frank dysentery is controversial. Although good results have been reported from some areas, other trials have been less successful (*see* Suchak *et al.*, 1962; Wilmot *et al.*, 1962). In trials carried out primarily on asymptomatic subjects passing trophozoites or cysts, or on patients with nondysenteric, symptomatic intestinal amebiasis, treatment with diloxanide furoate resulted in a high percentage of cures (Woodruff and Bell, 1960; Wolfe, 1973). Diloxanide furoate is used along with an appropriate systemic or mixed amebicide to effect a cure of invasive and extraintestinal amebiasis. In all cases the drug has been well tolerated. The relatively low cost of this compound is also an advantage, particularly in underdeveloped countries.

EMETINE AND DEHYDROEMETINE

Emetine is an alkaloid obtained from ipecac ("Brazil root"); it is also prepared semisynthetically by methylation of cephaëline, another alkaloid in ipecac. The use of this compound as a direct-acting systemic amebicide dates from 1912, when Vedder showed that the drug killed amebae *in vitro*. Since then, emetine has been one of the most widely used agents in the treatment of severe invasive *intestinal amebiasis, amebic hepatitis,* and *amebic abscesses*. Dehydroemetine has similar pharmacological properties, but it is considered to be less toxic. Both drugs have largely been replaced by mixed amebicides of the *nitroimidazole class,* which are as effective but far safer (*see* below). Thus, emetine and dehydroemetine should not be used unless the nitroimidazoles are ineffective or contraindicated. Disadvantages of these alkaloids are as follows: (1) Both compounds require parenteral administration by subcutaneous or deep intramuscular injection; local reactions ranging from pain to abscess formation are not uncommon. (2) Particularly after prolonged administration, both agents may produce systemic toxic reactions, some of which can be serious or even fatal; adverse effects primarily involve the heart and cardiovascular system, the neuromuscular system, the central nervous system, and the gastrointestinal tract. (3) Although their use can occasionally be lifesaving because of direct amebicidal action, neither compound can be used alone for curative purposes. (4) Patients receiving either agent should remain sedentary, and they require close medical supervision (including electrocardiographic monitoring). (5) Use of either drug is contraindicated in patients who are pregnant or who have cardiac, renal, or neuromuscular disease.

Details of the pharmacology and toxicology of emetine and dehydroemetine are presented in the *fifth and earlier editions* of this textbook (*see also* Yang and Dubick, 1980; Harries, 1982). The dosage for injectable dehydroemetine in adults is 1 to 1.5 mg/kg per day, to a maximal daily dose of 90 mg. This regimen is continued for up to 5 days. The daily pediatric dose is the same, except that one half of it is given every 12 hours. Dehydroemetine (MEBADIN) is available from the Centers for Disease Control.

8-HYDROXYQUINOLINES

A number of halogenated 8-hydroxyquinolines have been synthesized and used clinically as luminal amebicides, particularly to treat asymptomatic passers of cysts. Such direct-acting amebicidal agents have also been used in combination with metronidazole to treat intestinal forms of amebiasis. *Iodoquinol* (*diiodohydroxyquin*) and *clioquinol* (*iodochlorhydroxyquin*) are the best known of this class of compounds. They have been widely and all too often indiscriminately employed for the treatment of diarrhea. The use of these drugs, particularly at doses exceeding 2 g per day for long periods, is unfortunately associated with significant risk. The most important toxic reaction, which has been ascribed primarily to clioquinol, is *subacute myelo-optic neuropathy* (SMON). This disease is a myelitis-like illness that was first described in epidemic form (thousands of afflicted patients) in Japan; only sporadic cases have been reported elsewhere, but the actual prevalence is undoubtedly higher. Although SMON in Japan was apparently caused by clioquinol, similar toxic effects have been noted in other countries with other 8-hydroxyquinolines (*see* Oakley, 1973). Administration of iodoquinol in high doses to children with chronic diarrhea, for example, has been associated with optic atrophy and permanent loss of vision. Clioquinol has not been used in Japan since 1970, and severe restrictions were imposed on its sale in other countries, including the United States. Iodoquinol is thought to be safer than clioquinol (probably because the former is less well absorbed after oral administration), and it remains available as YODOXIN and MOEBIQUIN in the United States. *However, routine use of either compound is not recommended* because members of the less toxic *dichloroacetamide class* of luminal amebicides (*e.g.*, diloxanide furoate) are available. The dosage of iodoquinol is 650 mg three times daily after meals for 20 days in adults or 40 mg/kg per day for 20 days in children. The pharmacology and toxicology of the 8-hydroxyquinolines is described in greater detail in the *fifth and previous editions* of this textbook (*see also* review by Clifford and Gawel, 1984).

METRONIDAZOLE

History. The discovery of *azomycin* (2-nitroimidazole) by Nakamura in 1955 and the demonstration of its trichomonacidal properties led to the chemical synthesis and biological testing of many nitroimidazoles. One compound, 1-(β-hydroxyethyl)-2-methyl-5-nitroimidazole, now called *metronidazole,* was found to have particularly high activity *in vitro* and *in vivo* against *T. vaginalis* and *E. histolytica* (Cosar and Julou, 1959; Cosar *et al.*, 1961). Durel and associates (1960) reported that oral doses of the drug imparted trichomonacidal activity to semen and urine and that a high cure rate could be obtained in both male and female patients suffering from trichomoniasis. Metronidazole has an extremely broad spectrum of protozoal and antimicrobial activity, which is used to clinical advantage (*see* below). Other clinically effective 5-nitroimidazoles closely related in structure and activity to metronidazole are available outside the United States. These include *tinidazole* (FASIGYN, others), *nimorazole* (NAXOGIN, others), and *ornidazole* (TIBERAL, others). *Benznidazole* (ROCHAGAN) is another 5-nitroimidazole derivative that is unusual in that it is effective in acute Chagas' infection (*see* Chapter 43). Metronidazole has the following structural formula:

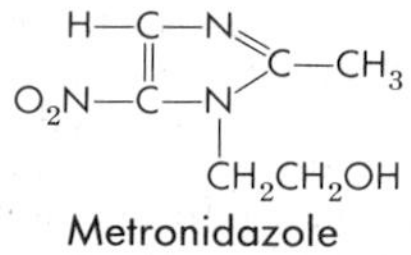

Metronidazole

Antiparasitic and Antimicrobial Effects. Metronidazole is directly trichomonacidal. Sensitive isolates of *T. vaginalis* are killed by <0.05 μg/ml of the drug under anaerobic conditions; higher concentrations are required when 1% oxygen is present or with isolates from patients who displayed a poor therapeutic response to metronidazole (Lumsden *et al.*, 1988). The drug is also potent against *E. histolytica* under either xenic or axenic culture conditions (*see* Burchard and Mirelman, 1988). Trophozoites of *G. lamblia* are probably also directly affected by metronidazole at concentrations of 1 to 50 μg/ml *in vitro* (Jokipii and Jokipii, 1980).

Metronidazole also displays antibacterial activity against all anaerobic cocci and both anaerobic gram-negative bacilli, including *Bacteroides* species, and anaerobic spore-forming gram-positive bacilli. Nonsporulating gram-positive bacilli are often resistant, as are aerobic and facultatively anaerobic bacteria (*see* Symposium, 1977; Oldenburg and Speck, 1983).

Metronidazole is clinically effective in *trichomoniasis, amebiasis,* and *giardiasis,* as well as in a variety of infections caused by obligate anaerobic bacteria, including *Bacteroides fragilis*. Other effects of nitroimidazoles include suppression of cellular immunity, mutagenesis, carcinogenesis, and sensitization of hypoxic cells to radiation (*see* Miller, 1980; Voogd, 1981; Brown *et al.*, 1984). Several reviews of the nitroimidazoles are available (Goldman, 1980; Molavi *et al.*, 1982; Oldenburg and Speck, 1983).

The mechanism of action of the nitroimidazoles is reflected in a selective toxicity to anaerobic or microaerophilic microorganisms and for anoxic or hypoxic cells. The nitro group of metronidazole accepts electrons from electron-transport proteins such as flavoproteins in mammalian cells and ferredoxins or their equivalent in bacteria and diverts them from normal energy-yielding pathways. In the former case, a nitro reductase catalyzes the reaction of the flavin radical with the nitro compound; in the latter case, the reduction is catalyzed by iron–sulfur complexes. The source of electrons for the reduction may be a number of endogenous reduced substrates, such as reduced nicotinamide adenine dinucleotide phosphate (NADPH) or sulfide. It is currently thought that chemically reactive reduced forms of the drug lead to the formation of cytotoxic products that destroy the cell. Although earlier work had established that the drug inhibits DNA synthesis in *T. vaginalis* and *Clostridium bifermentans* and causes degradation of existing DNA in the latter microorganism, further studies with mammalian DNA indicate that reduced metronidazole causes a loss of the helical structure of DNA, strand breakage, and an accompanying impairment of its function. Such findings are consistent with the antimicrobial and mutagenic effects of metronidazole and its ability to potentiate the effects of radiation on hypoxic tumor cells (*see* LaRusso *et al.,* 1977; Adams *et al.,* 1980; Edwards, 1980; Moreno and Docampo, 1985; Yarlett *et al.,* 1985).

Absorption, Fate, and Excretion. The pharmacokinetic properties of metronidazole and its two major metabolites have been investigated intensively (*see* review by Ralph, 1983; *see also* Jensen and Gugler, 1983; Loft *et al.,* 1986, 1987, 1988). The drug is usually completely and promptly absorbed after oral administration, reaching concentrations in plasma of about 10 μg/ml approximately 1 hour after a single 500-mg dose. (Mean effective concentrations of the compound are 8 μg/ml or less for most susceptible protozoa and bacteria.) A linear relationship between dose and plasma concentration pertains for doses between 200 and 2000 mg. Repeated doses every 6 to 8 hours result in some accumulation of the drug. The half-life of metronidazole in plasma is about 8 hours, and its volume of distribution is approximately that of total body water. About 10% of the drug is bound to plasma proteins. Metronidazole penetrates well into body tissues and fluids, including vaginal secretions, seminal fluid, saliva, and breast milk. Therapeutic concentrations are also achieved in cerebrospinal fluid.

Both unchanged metronidazole and several metabolites are excreted in various proportions in the urine after oral administration of the parent compound (Ralph, 1983). The liver is the main site of metabolism, and this accounts for over 50% of the systemic clearance of metronidazole. The two principal metabolites result from oxidation of side chains; both have antitrichomonal activity. Formation of glucuronides is also observed. Small quantities of reduced metabolites, including ring-cleavage products, are formed by the gut flora (Koch *et al.,* 1981). The urine of some patients may be reddish-brown due to the presence of unidentified pigments derived from the drug. Oxidative metabolism of metronidazole is inducible by phenobarbital and possibly by ethanol.

Preparations, Routes of Administration, and Dosage. *Metronidazole* (FLAGYL, others) is formulated as 250- and 500-mg tablets for oral administration. The drug is also available in forms for intravenous infusion. *Benzoyl metronidazole,* a tasteless form of metronidazole, can be obtained in some countries as an oral suspension for children.

Many different dosage schedules have been used in the treatment of trichomoniasis. However, the currently accepted regimen for adults is one 250-mg tablet, given orally three times daily for 7 days. Some prefer a single 2-g dose of metronidazole, which may be as effective. When repeated courses and higher doses of the drug are required for stubborn infections, it is recommended that intervals of 4 to 6 weeks elapse between courses. In such cases, leukocyte counts should be carried out before, during, and after each course of treatment. Lack of satisfactory response may be due to chronic infection of the cervical glands or of Skene's and Bartholin's glands. Although metronidazole-resistant strains of *T. vaginalis* exist, these are not common and probably only occasionally account for failure of treatment (Müller *et al.,* 1980; Lumsden *et al.,* 1988; Robertson *et al.,* 1988).

Reinfection by an infected male partner may also cause an unsatisfactory response. Trichomonads are demonstrated in the urogenital tract in over 30% of male partners of infected women. The male may be treated by the oral administration of 250 mg, three times daily for 7 days or with a single 2-g dose. Both partners should be treated over the same 7-day period.

For amebiasis, in all geographical areas and regardless of the virulence of the strains or the form of infection being treated, it is recommended that patients receive 750 mg of metronidazole, three times daily for 5 to 10 days. The daily dose for children is 35 to 50 mg/kg, given in three divided doses for 10 days. Treatment with metronidazole is least effective when the drug is administered to the *asymptomatic* passer of cysts. While metronidazole is still effective, fewer failures result from the use of purely luminal amebicides; the latter are thus preferred alone or in combination with metronidazole. Despite considerable clinical use over the past several years, resistance of *E. histolytica* to metronidazole has not occurred. Indeed, attempts to produce resistance to the drug *in vitro* have been unsuccessful. *Mass treatment* with a large dose of metronidazole once monthly for a few months and then in alternate months has resulted in a marked decrease in the incidence of amebic dysentery in relatively isolated communities with a high degree of endemicity.

Metronidazole is a drug of choice in the treatment of giardiasis. It is effective at the same or lower doses than those used for trichomoniasis; the usual regimen is 250 mg three times a day for 5 to 7 days. A daily dose of 2 g for 3 successive days has also been used successfully. Metronidazole is considered to be helpful for the elimination of the guinea worm in dracunculiasis, even though it has no direct effect on the parasite (Padonu, 1973; Sharma *et al.*, 1979). Recommended dosage is 250 mg of the drug, given three times daily for 10 days. Both of these uses are investigational in the United States.

Metronidazole is also extremely useful for treatment of serious infections due to susceptible anaerobic bacteria, including *Bacteroides, Clostridium, Fusobacterium, Peptococcus, Peptostreptococcus,* and *Eubacterium*. The drug may also be used along with appropriate antimicrobial agents for concomitant infections with aerobic microorganisms. Under these circumstances, metronidazole is usually given intravenously. The recommended intravenous dosage regimen for anaerobic infections includes a loading dose (15 mg/kg), followed 6 hours later by a maintenance dose of 7.5 mg/kg every 6 hours, usually for 7 to 10 days.

Toxicity and Drug Interactions. The toxicity of metronidazole has been reviewed by Roe (1977). Side effects are only rarely sufficiently severe to cause discontinuation of treatment. The most common are headache, nausea, dry mouth, and a metallic taste. Vomiting, diarrhea, and abdominal distress are occasionally experienced. Furry tongue, glossitis, and stomatitis may occur during therapy and be associated with a sudden intensification of moniliasis. Neurotoxic effects of metronidazole have also been observed. Dizziness, vertigo, and, very rarely, encephalopathy, convulsions, incoordination, and ataxia may appear. Numbness or paresthesia of an extremity occurs occasionally, and the drug should be discontinued when this happens. Reversal of serious sensory neuropathies may be slow or incomplete (Coxon and Pallis, 1976). Urticaria, flushing, pruritus, dysuria, cystitis, and a sense of pelvic pressure have also been reported. Metronidazole has a well-documented disulfiram-like effect, such that some patients experience abdominal distress, vomiting, flushing, or headache if they drink alcoholic beverages during a course of treatment. Confusional and psychotic states may also occur during concurrent administration of metronidazole and disulfiram.

Although related chemicals have caused blood dyscrasias, only a temporary neutropenia, which reverses after therapy, occurs with metronidazole (*see* Lefebvre and Hesseltine, 1965; Goldman, 1980).

Treatment should be discontinued promptly if ataxia, convulsions, or any other symptom of central nervous system (CNS) involvement occurs. Metronidazole is contraindicated in patients with active disease of the CNS. The dosage should be reduced in patients with severe obstructive hepatic disease, alcoholic cirrhosis, or severe renal dysfunction (*see* Lau *et al.*, 1987; Plaisance *et al.*, 1988).

After prolonged, high oral doses, metronidazole is carcinogenic in rodents; it is also mutagenic in bacteria (*see* review by Voogd, 1981). Furthermore, mutagenic activity is associated with metronidazole and several of its metabolites, which are found in the urine of patients treated with therapeutic doses of the drug (Speck *et al.*, 1976). Two relatively short-term studies of human subjects treated with metronidazole failed to reveal an increased risk of carcinogenesis, but long-term surveillance is needed (Beard *et al.*, 1979; Goldman, 1980). This evidence should compel the prudent use of the drug. While metronidazole has been given with no apparent adverse effects during all stages of pregnancy (Peterson *et al.*, 1966; Voogd, 1981), its use during the first trimester is not recommended.

Therapeutic Uses. The clinical uses of metronidazole have been the subject of several reviews (Goldman, 1980; Molavi *et al.*, 1982; Oldenburg and Speck, 1983). Metronidazole cures genital infections with *T. vaginalis* in both males and females in a high percentage of cases. This efficacy and a probable low incidence of comparatively minor side effects have led to its adoption as the agent of choice. Only in a few cases has resistance to metronidazole constituted a proven therapeutic problem (Lumsden *et al.*, 1988). There is also no doubt that persistent reinfection of the female can be prevented if the male partner harboring the parasite is treated concurrently.

Metronidazole is an effective amebicide and has become the agent of choice for the treatment of all symptomatic forms of amebiasis. The drug also kills *G. lamblia* and has been shown to be effective in treating giardiasis. Its use in the treatment of dracunculiasis may facilitate removal of the female worm (*see* Chapter 40).

Many studies have indicated that metronidazole may be useful for the treatment of infections with various anaerobic bacteria, particularly *B. fragilis*. The drug is an alternative to clindamycin, certain beta-lactam antibiotics, and chloramphenicol for this purpose. Metronidazole has been employed for the prophylaxis of postsurgical abdominal and pelvic infections and for the treatment of endocarditis caused by *B. fragilis* (*see* Roe, 1977; Symposium, 1977; Galgiani *et al.*, 1978). The drug is useful for the treatment of brain abscesses that are not uncommonly caused by such microorganisms. Metronidazole can also be used to treat pseudomembranous colitis caused by *Clostridium difficile*.

Nitroimidazoles have been used to sensitize hypoxic tumor cells to the effects of ionizing radiation but metronidazole should not be used clinically for this purpose.

QUINACRINE

Quinacrine is an acridine derivative widely used during World War II as an antimalarial agent. Other drugs with more desirable properties have now replaced quinacrine as an antimalarial and for the treatment of infestations with tapeworms. Currently, the major indication for the administration of quinacrine is for the treatment of *giardiasis* (Wolfe, 1975). For a fuller description of its properties, the *fifth and earlier editions* of this textbook should be consulted. Quinacrine has the following structural formula:

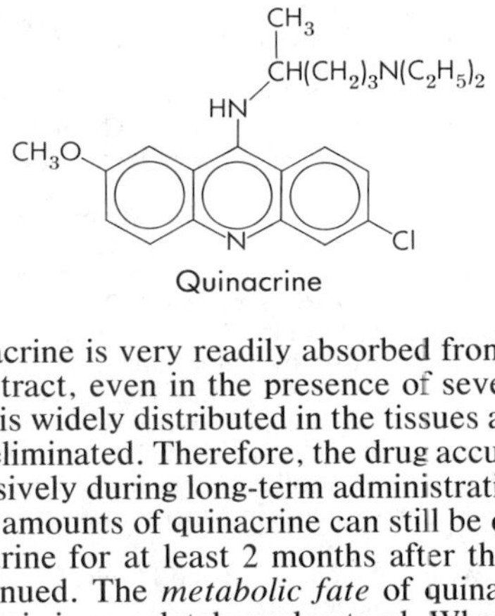

Quinacrine

Quinacrine is very readily absorbed from the intestinal tract, even in the presence of severe diarrhea. It is widely distributed in the tissues and very slowly eliminated. Therefore, the drug accumulates progressively during long-term administration. Significant amounts of quinacrine can still be detected in the urine for at least 2 months after therapy is discontinued. The *metabolic fate* of quinacrine in the body is incompletely understood. Whether this agent exerts its antiparasitic actions *per se* or after metabolic transformation remains to be determined. However, its ready intercalation into DNA suggests that the parent drug is the active substance and that its selective toxicity is a function of relative distribution rather than specificity of action.

Quinacrine is available as the dihydrochloride, designated *quinacrine hydrochloride* (*mepacrine hydrochloride;* ATABRINE). It contains approximately 80% quinacrine base and is supplied as tablets containing 100 mg of the dihydrochloride.

For treatment of *giardiasis*, 100 mg should be given three times daily for 5 to 7 days. A second course of treatment may be given, if necessary, 2 weeks later. The daily dosage for children is 7 mg/kg to a maximum of 300 mg. The microorganisms disappear from the stools, and symptoms referable to the infection clear rapidly.

Because of its widespread use as an antimalarial drug, the toxic effects of quinacrine are well documented. (*See* review by Findlay, 1951.) The drug frequently causes headache, dizziness, and vomiting. Blood dyscrasias, urticaria, and exfoliative dermatitis may also follow its administration. The skin may acquire a yellow stain from deposition of the drug, and blue or black pigmentation of the nails can occur. Ocular toxicity, similar to that caused by chloroquine, occurs occasionally. The relatively large doses formerly used in the treatment of cestode infection may cause the transitory *toxic psychosis* that is seen in a small proportion of patients receiving lower doses. The duration of the drug-induced psychosis is usually 2 to 4 weeks, and the course is relatively benign. Only symptomatic therapy is indicated.

Great caution should be exercised in administering quinacrine (and other antimalarial compounds) to patients with *psoriasis*, since pronounced exacerbation occurs frequently and exfoliative lesions sometimes develop. Quinacrine is contraindicated in patients receiving antimalarial therapy with primaquine. Concurrent administration of the two drugs results in a markedly elevated concentration of primaquine (or other 8-aminoquinolines) in plasma and greatly enhances its toxicity. Quinacrine should not be given to pregnant women because the drug readily passes the placenta and reaches the fetus.

ANTIBIOTIC AMEBICIDES

A number of antibiotics have been found to be of value in the treatment of intestinal amebiasis, especially *paromomycin*, some of the *tetracyclines*, and *erythromycin*. Paromomycin is discussed briefly here because it is the only one that is directly amebicidal. Other antibiotics act by interfering with the enteric flora essential for the proliferation of pathogenic amebae. The older tetracyclines, for example tetracycline itself, are the most frequently used, and their efficacy probably depends on the relatively large proportion of the administered dose that escapes absorption in the bowel. The better-absorbed agents are much less effective. If a tetracycline is used, it should be given together with the appropriate drugs for either intestinal or extraintestinal amebic infections.

Paromomycin. This aminoglycoside antibiotic, isolated from cultures of *Streptomyces rimosus*, is amebicidal both *in vitro* and *in vivo*. Many of its properties are similar to those of other antibiotics in this class (*see* Chapter 47). Paromomycin acts directly on amebae but also has antibacterial activity against normal and pathogenic microorganisms in the gastrointestinal tract. Its structural formula is as follows:

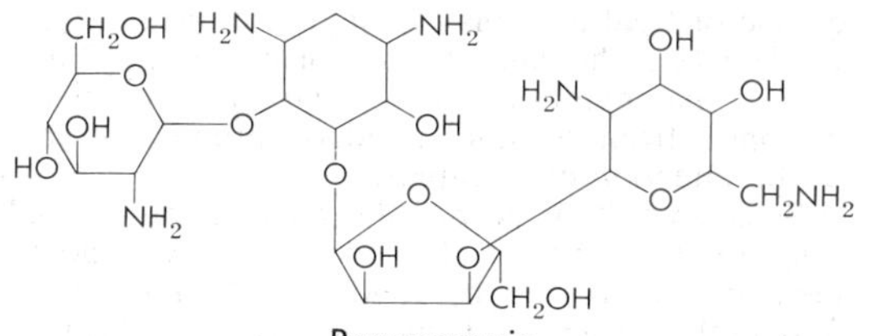

Paromomycin

Paromomycin sulfate (HUMATIN) is supplied in capsules, each containing 250 mg. The recommended dosage for intestinal amebiasis is 25 to 35 mg/kg each day, orally in three divided doses at mealtimes, for 7 days. Higher doses, up to 66 mg/kg, have been used by some investigators. After oral administration, little of the drug is absorbed into the systemic circulation. Side effects are mainly limited to gastrointestinal upset and diarrhea. Marked renal damage occurs in animals treated parenterally with the drug. Experience has shown paromomycin to be effective, but by no means infallible, in the treatment of *intestinal amebiasis;* it is ineffective against extraintestinal forms of the disease (*see* Woolfe, 1965). Paromomycin is also effective in the treatment of infections with various tapeworms.

Adams, G. E.; Stratford, I. J.; Wallace, I. G.; Wardman, P.; and Watts, M. E. Toxicity of nitrocompounds towards hypoxic mammalian cells *in vitro;* dependence on reduction potential. *J. Natl. Cancer Inst.*, **1980**, *64*, 555–560.

Beard, C. M.; Noller, K. L.; O'Fallon, W. M.; Kurland, L. T.; and Dockerty, M. B. Lack of evidence for cancer due to use of metronidazole. *N. Engl. J. Med.*, **1979**, *301*, 519–522.

Bristow, N. W.; Oxley, P.; Williams, G. A. H.; and Woolfe, G. ENTAMIDE, a new amoebicide; preliminary note. *Trans. R. Soc. Trop. Med. Hyg.*, **1956**, *50*, 182.

Burchard, G. D., and Mirelman, D. *Entamoeba histolytica:* virulence potential and sensitivity to metronidazole and emetine of four isolates possessing nonpathogenic zymodemes. *Exp. Parasitol.*, **1988**, *66*, 231–242.

Cohen, H. G., and Reynolds, T. B. Comparison of metronidazole and chloroquine for the treatment of amebic liver abscess: a controlled trial. *Gastroenterology*, **1975**, *69*, 35–41.

Conan, N. J., Jr. Chloroquine in amebiasis. *Am. J. Trop. Med. Hyg.*, **1948**, *28*, 107–110.

———. The treatment of hepatic amebiasis with chloroquine. *Am. J. Med.*, **1949**, *6*, 309–320.

Cosar, C.; Ganter, P.; and Julou, L. Etude expérimentale du métronidazole, 8823 R.P., activités trichomonacide et amoebicide. Toxicité et propriétés pharmacologiques générales. *Presse Med.*, **1961**, *69*, 1069–1972.

Cosar, C., and Julou, L. Activité de l'(hydroxy-2′ ethyl)-1 méthyl-2 nitro-5 imidazole (8,823 R.P.) vis-à-vis des infections expérimentales à *Trichomonas vaginalis*. *Ann. Inst. Pasteur (Paris)*, **1959**, *96*, 238–241.

Coxon, A., and Pallis, C. A. Metronidazole neuropathy. *J. Neurol. Neurosurg. Psychiatry*, **1976**, *39*, 403–405.

Durel, P.; Roiron, V.; Siboulet, H.; and Borel, L. J. Systemic treatment of human trichomoniasis with a derivative of nitroimidazole, 8823 R.P. *Br. J. Vener. Dis.*, **1960**, *36*, 21–26.

Galgiani, J. N.; Busch, D. F.; Brass, C.; Rumans, L. W.; Mangels, J. I.; and Stevens, D. A. *Bacteroides fragilis* endocarditis, bacteremia and other infections treated with oral or intravenous metronidazole. *Am. J. Med.*, **1978**, *65*, 284–289.

Jensen, J. C., and Gugler, R. Single and multiple-dose metronidazole kinetics. *Clin. Pharmacol. Ther.*, **1983**, *34*, 481–487.

Jokipii, L., and Jokipii, A. M. M. *In vitro* susceptibility of *Giardia lamblia* trophozoites to metronidazole and tinidazole. *J. Infect. Dis.*, **1980**, *141*, 317–325.

Koch, R. L.; Beaulieau, B. B., Jr.; Chrystal, E. J. T.; and Goldman, P. A metronidazole metabolite in urine and its risk. *Science*, **1981**, *211*, 398–400.

LaRusso, N. F.; Tomasz, M.; Müller, M.; and Lipman, R. Interaction of metronidazole with nucleic acids *in vitro*. *Mol. Pharmacol.*, **1977**, *13*, 872–882.

Lau, A. H.; Evans, R.; Chang, C.-H.; and Seligsohn, R. Pharmacokinetics of metronidazole in patients with alcoholic liver disease. *Antimicrob. Agents Chemother.*, **1987**, *31*, 1662–1664.

Lefebvre, I., and Hesseltine, H. C. The peripheral white blood cells and metronidazole. *J.A.M.A.*, **1965**, *194*, 15–18.

Loft, S.; Dossing, M.; Poulsen, H. E.; Sonne, J.; Olesen, K.-L.; Simonsen, K.; and Andreasen, P. B. Influence of dose and route of administration on disposition of metronidazole and its major metabolites. *Eur. J. Clin. Pharmacol.*, **1986**, *30*, 467–473.

Loft, S.; Poulsen, H. E.; Sonne, J.; and Dossing, M. Metronidazole clearance: a one-sample method and influencing factors. *Clin. Pharmacol. Ther.*, **1988**, *43*, 420–428.

Loft, S.; Sonne, J.; Poulsen, H. E.; Petersen, K. T.; Jorgensen, B. G.; and Dossing, M. Inhibition and induction of metronidazole and antipyrine metabolism. *Eur. J. Clin. Pharmacol.*, **1987**, *32*, 35–41.

Lumsden, W. H. R.; Harrison, C.; and Robertson, D. H. H. Treatment failure in *Trichomonas vaginalis* infections in females. II. *In-vitro* estimation of the sensitivity of the organism to metronidazole. *J. Antimicrob. Chemother.*, **1988**, *21*, 555–564.

Main, P. T.; Bristow, N. W.; Oxley, P.; Watkins, T. I.; Williams, G. A. H.; Wilmshurst, E. C.; and Woolfe, G. ENTAMIDE. *Ann. Biochem. Exp. Med.*, **1960**, *20*, 441–448.

Müller, M.; Meingassner, J. G.; Miller, W. A.; and Ledger, W. J. Three metronidazole-resistant strains of *Trichomonas vaginalis* from the United States. *Am. J. Obstet. Gynecol.*, **1980**, *138*, 808–812.

Murgatroyd, F., and Kent, R. P. Refractory amoebic liver abscess treated by chloroquine. *Trans. R. Soc. Trop. Med. Hyg.*, **1948**, *42*, 15–16.

Oakley, G. P., Jr. The neurotoxicity of the halogenated hydroxyquinolines. *J.A.M.A.*, **1973**, *225*, 395–397.

Padonu, K. O. A controlled trial of metronidazole in the treatment of dracontiasis in Nigeria. *Am. J. Trop. Med. Hyg.*, **1973**, *22*, 42–44.

Peterson, W. F.; Stauch, J. E.; and Ryder, C. D. Metronidazole in pregnancy. *Am. J. Obstet. Gynecol.*, **1966**, *94*, 343–349.

Plaisance, K. I.; Quintiliani, R.; and Nightingale, C. H. The pharmacokinetics of metronidazole and its metabolites in critically ill patients. *J. Antimicrob. Chemother.*, **1988**, *21*, 195–200.

Robertson, D. H. H.; Heyworth, R.; Harrison, C.; and Lumsden, W. H. R. Treatment failure in *Trichomonas vaginalis* infections in females. I. Concentrations of metronidazole in plasma and vaginal content during normal and high dosage. *J. Antimicrob. Chemother.*, **1988**, *21*, 373–378.

Sharma, V. P.; Rathmore, H. S.; and Sharma, M. M.

Efficacy of metronidazole in dracunculiasis. *Am. J. Trop. Med. Hyg.*, **1979**, *28*, 658–660.

Speck, W. T.; Stein, A. B.; and Rosenkranz, H. S. Mutagenicity of metronidazole: presence of several active metabolites in human urine. *J. Natl. Cancer Inst.*, **1976**, *56*, 283–284.

Suchak, N. G.; Satoskar, R. S.; and Sheth, U. K. ENTAMIDE FUROATE in the treatment of intestinal amoebiasis. *Am. J. Trop. Med. Hyg.*, **1962**, *11*, 330–332.

Wilmot, A. J.; Powell, S. J.; McLeod, I.; and Elsdon-Dew, R. Some newer amoebicides in acute amoebic dysentery. *Trans. R. Soc. Trop. Med. Hyg.*, **1962**, *56*, 85–86.

Wolfe, M. S. Nondysenteric intestinal amebiasis. Treatment with diloxanide furoate. *J.A.M.A.*, **1973**, *224*, 1601–1604.

Woodruff, A. W., and Bell, S. Clinical trials with ENTAMIDE FUROATE and related compounds. I. In a non-tropical environment. *Trans. R. Soc. Trop. Med. Hyg.*, **1960**, *54*, 389–395.

Yarlett, N.; Gorrell, T. E.; Marczak, R.; and Müller, M. Reduction of nitroimidazole derivatives by hydrogenosomal extracts of *Trichomonas vaginalis*. *Mol. Biochem. Parasitol.*, **1985**, *14*, 29–40.

Monographs and Reviews

Brown, J.; Biaglow, J.; Hall, E.; Kinsella, T.; Phillips, R. C.; Urtasun, R.; Utley, J.; and Yuhas, J. Sensitizers and protectors to radiation and chemotherapeutic drugs. In, *The Interdisciplinary Program for Radiation Oncology Research*. (Wittes, R. E., ed.) *Cancer Treatment Symposia*, Vol. 1. U.S. Government Printing Office, Washington, D.C., **1984**, pp. 85–102.

Clifford, R. F., and Gawel, M. Clioquinol neurotoxicity: an overview. *Acta Neurol. Scand.* [*Suppl.*], **1984**, *100*, 137–145.

Edwards, D. I. Mechanisms of selective toxicity of metronidazole and other nitroimidazole drugs. *Br. J. Vener. Dis.*, **1980**, *56*, 285–290.

Findlay, G. M. *Recent Advances in Chemotherapy*, Vol. II. J. & A. Churchill, Ltd., London, **1951**.

Goldman, P. Metronidazole. *N. Engl. J. Med.*, **1980**, *303*, 1212–1218.

Harries, J. Amoebiasis: a review. *J. R. Soc. Med.*, **1982**, *75*, 190–197.

Krogstad, D. J.; Spencer, H. C., Jr.; and Healy, G. R. Amebiasis. *N. Engl. J. Med.*, **1978**, *298*, 262–265.

Miller, J. J. The imidazoles as immunosuppressive agents. *Transplant. Proc.*, **1980**, *12*, 300–303.

Molavi, A.; LeFrock, J. L.; and Prince, R. A. Metronidazole. *Med. Clin. North Am.*, **1982**, *66*, 121–133.

Moreno, S. N. J., and Docampo, R. Mechanism of toxicity of nitro compounds used in the chemotherapy of trichomoniasis. *Environ. Health Perspect.*, **1985**, *64*, 199–208.

Neal, R. A. Experimental amoebiasis and the development of anti-amoebic compounds. *Parasitology*, **1983**, *86*, 175–191.

Oldenburg, B., and Speck, W. T. Metronidazole. *Pediatr. Clin. North Am.*, **1983**, *30*, 71–75.

Ralph, E. D. Clinical pharmacokinetics of metronidazole. *Clin. Pharmacokinet.*, **1983**, *8*, 43–62.

Roe, F. J. C. Metronidazole: review of uses and toxicity. *J. Antimicrob. Chemother.*, **1977**, *3*, 205–212.

Symposium. (Various authors.) *Proceedings of the International Metronidazole Conference*, International Congress Series No. 438. (Finegold, S. M., ed.) Excerpta Medica, Amsterdam, **1977**.

Voogd, C. E. On the mutagenicity of nitroimidazoles. *Mutat. Res.*, **1981**, *86*, 243–277.

Wolfe, M. S. Giardiasis. *J.A.M.A.*, **1975**, *233*, 1362–1365.

Woolfe, G. The chemotherapy of amoebiasis. In, *Progress in Drug Research*, Vol. 8. (Jucker, E., ed.) Birkhaüser Verlag, Basel, **1965**, pp. 11–52.

Yang, W. C. T., and Dubick, M. Mechanism of emetine cardiotoxicity. *Pharmacol. Ther.*, **1980**, *10*, 15–26.

CHAPTER

43 DRUGS USED IN THE CHEMOTHERAPY OF PROTOZOAL INFECTIONS

[*Continued*]

Leishmaniasis, Trypanosomiasis, and Other Protozoal Infections

Leslie T. Webster, Jr.

Two protozoal infections other than malaria are particularly devastating to inhabitants of tropical regions. Caused by members of the order *Kinetoplastida, trypanosomiasis* and *leishmaniasis* in their protean forms can be especially difficult to prevent or cure. Recent substantial progress in understanding the natural course of these illnesses and identifying distinctive features of the parasites that would permit chemotherapeutic intervention has yet to be turned to practical advantage. Effective drugs are simply not available to treat some forms of these infections. Moreover, agents with established clinical efficacy are either too toxic or impractical for wide-scale administration.

This chapter provides brief descriptions of trypanosomiasis, leishmaniasis, and certain other protozoal infections of man. Specific drugs traditionally employed for chemoprophylaxis and therapy of these diseases are then presented in alphabetical order. One of these agents, pentamidine, is also used extensively to control infections with *Pneumocystis carinii*.

Trypanosomiasis. *African trypanosomiasis* is transmitted by tsetse flies of the genus *Glossinia* and is caused by subspecies of the hemoflagellate *Trypanosoma brucei*. The parasite is detectable in the blood, lymph, and spinal fluid of the human host. Two main types of human African trypanosomal disease exist, the *Rhodesian* and the *Gambian*. *T. brucei rhodesiense* produces a progressive and usually fatal form of disease marked by early involvement of the central nervous system (CNS) and terminal cardiac failure; *T. brucei gambiense* causes so-called sleeping sickness, characterized by later involvement of the CNS and a more long-term course. Treatment with standard but toxic agents such as *suramin, pentamidine,* and *melarsoprol* is inadequate; therapy must be given parenterally over extended periods and is often unsuccessful (Apted, 1980). *T. brucei* does offer a number of attractive biochemical targets for selective pharmacological intervention (*see* Opperdoes, 1985). Most promising of these appears to be inhibition of polyamine biosynthesis by the antitumor drug *eflornithine* (α-difluoromethylornithine) (Bacchi, 1981; Fairlamb *et al.,* 1985; McCann *et al.,* 1986). Initial clinical studies have indicated that this site-directed irreversible inhibitor of ornithine decarboxylase can be employed successfully to treat late-stage Gambian trypanosomiasis (Van Nieuwenhove *et al.,* 1985; Doua *et al.,* 1987; Taelman *et al.,* 1987; Petru *et al.,* 1988). However, pharmacokinetic and logistic problems may limit the widespread use of this agent, even if it proves to be safe and effective (Gutteridge, 1987).

American trypanosomiasis or *Chagas' disease,* a zoonosis caused by *T. cruzi,* affects about 24 million people from Southern California to Argentina and Chile (Schofield, 1985), where the chronic form of the disease in adults is a major cause of cardiomyopathy, megaesophagus, megacolon, and death. Transmitted by bloodsucking *triatomid bugs,* metacyclic *trypomastigotes* enter host cells and proliferate as intracellular *amastigotes*. These forms then differentiate intracellularly into *trypomastigotes,* which are released into the circulation. Trypomastigotes in the bloodstream do not multiply until they invade other cells or are ingested by an insect vector during a blood meal. Transfusion of blood containing these organisms can also transmit the infection in about 10% of cases. Chronic disease of the heart and gastrointestinal tract eventually results from destruction of myocardial cells and neurons of the myenteric plexus. Although nitroheterocyclic drugs such as *nifurtimox* and *benznidazole* can suppress parasitemia and possibly cure or ameliorate the acute phase of Chagas' infection, they have little effect on the chronic disease (Brener, 1979). *T. cruzi* is especially vulnerable to drugs that form intracellular free radicals. Both nifurtimox and benznidazole have this capability, and other agents with similar potential are being evaluated as antitrypanosomal agents (*see* Marr and Docampo, 1986; Morello, 1988).

Leishmaniasis. Human *leishmaniasis* is caused by protozoal species and subspecies of the genus

Leishmania and family *Trypanasomatidae*. The infection occurs on all continents except Australia and probably affects at least 100 million people; the annual incidence is estimated at over 12 million cases. Nonhuman mammals are the reservoirs for this infection, which is transmitted to man most often by the bites of infected female phlebotamine sandflies. Flagellated extracellular, free *promastigotes,* which live in the gastrointestinal tract and saliva of the insect vector, are injected into the host, where they become phagocytized by tissue monocytes. Inside these cells they are transformed into rounder *amastigotes,* which reside in intracellular phagolysosomes. The occurrence of localized or systemic disease depends on the species or subspecies of infecting parasite, the distribution of infected macrophages, and the host's immunological response. In increasing order of systemic involvement and clinical severity, human leishmaniasis can be classified into *cutaneous, mucocutaneous,* and *visceral* (*kala azar*) forms.

The natural course and chemotherapy of leishmaniasis, as well as the biochemical properties of leishmania pertinent to selective therapeutic intervention, have been reviewed by Berman (1988). It now appears that the cutaneous forms of leishmaniasis are self-limiting, whereas the mucocutaneous and visceral forms are not. Initial treatment with pentavalent antimonials according to regimens based on collective empirical experience appears safe and effective in over 90% of cases. Second-line drugs, such as pentamidine and amphotericin B, are less satisfactory because of unacceptable toxicity at effective therapeutic doses. Other experimental agents such as allopurinol ribonucleoside, certain pyrazolopyrimidines, the 8-aminoquinoline WR 6026, and itraconazole (an inhibitor of sterol biosynthesis) show promise and are in various stages of evaluation.

Other Protozoal Infections. *Toxoplasmosis,* caused by the intracellular protozoan *Toxoplasma gondii,* is a zoonosis that is a common cause of latent human infection worldwide. Acute infection is particularly threatening to the fetus and the immunocompromised host. The treatment of choice for this infection is pyrimethamine and a sulfonamide (*see* Chapter 45). Pneumonia caused by *Pneumocystis carinii* is an opportunistic protozoal infection that also occurs in immunocompromised individuals. About 70 to 80% of patients with the acquired immunodeficiency syndrome (AIDS) develop this serious complication; despite treatment, the mortality rate is about 20% per episode. Standard therapy for this condition is either trimethoprim–sulfamethoxazole (Chapter 45) or parenteral pentamidine. Inhalation of aerosolized pentamidine for prophylaxis and for treatment of mild-to-moderate cases or those unresponsive to other drugs has also been used successfully. Examples of less common protozoal infections affecting man are *babesiosis, balantidiasis,* and *coccidiosis.* While balantidiasis responds to *tetracyclines,* the two other infections are quite refractory to specific chemotherapy.

MELARSOPROL

In 1940, Friedheim described trypanocidal activity of an organic compound of arsenic containing the melamine nucleus. Two compounds made subsequently, the pentavalent melarsen and the trivalent melarsen oxide, were effective in advanced cases of trypanosomiasis but were also more toxic than tryparsamide, an older pentavalent arsenical. In 1949, Friedheim demonstrated that a dimercaprol derivative of melarsen oxide could be used effectively and with greater safety in the treatment of such cases; this compound was named *Mel B* and is now known as *melarsoprol.* Of considerable importance was the finding that trypanocidal arsenicals of the melamine type were effective against tryparsamide-resistant strains of trypanosomes (Van-Hoof, 1947).

Chemistry and Preparation. Melarsoprol has the following structural formula:

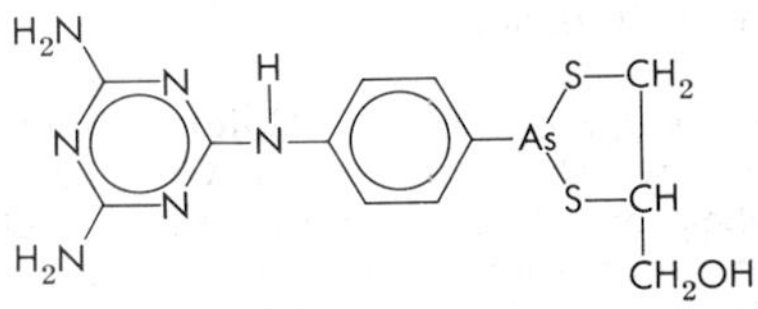

Melarsoprol

Melarsoprol (*Mel B;* ARSOBAL) is provided as a 3.6% (w/v) solution in propylene glycol. It is available in the United States only from the Centers for Disease Control. The dosage regimens below refer to the 3.6% solution.

Antiprotozoal Effects. It is the arsenoxide form of an organic arsenical that accounts for both its rapid lethal effect on African trypanosomes and its toxicity to the host (*see* Albert, 1979). Arsenoxides react avidly and reversibly with sulfhydryl groups, including those of proteins, and thereby inactivate a great number and variety of enzymes. The same nonspecific mechanism by which melarsoprol is lethal to parasites is probably responsible for its toxicity to host tissues. However, trypanosomes susceptible to arsenicals actively concentrate these compounds; so-called arsenic-resistant parasites may resemble host cells in that they concentrate organic arsenicals to a lesser extent. Once inside the trypanosome, arsenical drugs act differently upon the terminal glycolytic enzyme, pyruvate kinase, depending on whether the source of the enzyme is trypanosomal or mammalian (Flynn and Bowman, 1969). Mammalian tissues also oxidize melarsoprol to nontoxic and readily excreted pentavalent compounds more rapidly than does the protozoan.

Absorption, Fate, and Excretion. Melarsoprol is usually administered intravenously. A small but therapeutically significant amount of the drug enters the cerebrospinal fluid and has a lethal effect on trypanosomes infecting the CNS. The substance is excreted quite quickly, and its prophylactic action lasts no more than a few days (*see* Hawking, 1963).

Route of Administration and Dosage. Melarsoprol is administered by slow intravenous injection, and care must be taken to avoid leakage into surrounding tissues because it is intensely irritating. Patients with advanced meningoencephalitis, or those who are febrile or wasted, should receive preliminary treatment with suramin (two to four doses of 250 to 500 mg on alternate days). Adults in good condition weighing 50 kg or more and whose cerebrospinal fluid contains less than 40 mg of protein per 100 ml should be given up to 3.6 mg/kg of melarsoprol daily for 3 or 4 days; this course should be repeated after an interval of at least 7 days. A third course may be given if required after 10 to 21 days. Lesser doses should be given to children and debilitated patients. Following such regimens, about 80 to 90% of patients are cured. A proportion of those who relapse will be refractory to further treatment with melarsoprol.

Toxicity and Side Effects. Unfortunately, toxicity is common during treatment with melarsoprol (*see* Robertson, 1962). A febrile reaction often occurs soon after drug injection, particularly if parasitemia is high. The most serious complications involve the nervous system. A reactive encephalopathy occurs in about 5% of patients, usually between the first two courses of therapy, and is fatal in 50 to 75% of cases. Manifestations include convulsions associated with acute cerebral edema, rapidly progressive coma, or acute nonlethal mental disturbances without neurological signs. This reaction may occur in the early hemolymphatic stage as well as in the later CNS stage of illness. Its cause is unknown; a delayed drug-related immunological response, rather than a direct effect of the drug, has been proposed to account for most cases (*see* Haller *et al.*, 1986). Hypersensitivity reactions may occur, particularly during the second or subsequent course of treatment. After recovery, a small dose provokes a lesser reaction, and desensitization may be carried out by starting with a small dose and increasing this slightly, allowing time for recovery, until it is possible to give a final 3- or 4-day course in full dosage. Corticosteroids may be used to control the symptoms during such a procedure. Peripheral neuropathy may be noted. Hypertension and myocardial damage are not uncommon, although shock is rare. Albuminuria occurs frequently, and occasionally the appearance of numerous casts in the urine or evidence of hepatic disturbance may necessitate modification of treatment. Vomiting and abdominal colic are also frequent, but their incidence can be reduced by injecting the drug slowly in the supine, fasting patient. The patient should remain in bed and not eat for several hours after the injection is given.

Precautions and Contraindications. Melarsoprol should be given only to patients under hospital supervision so that the dosage regimen may be modified if necessary. It is most important that the initial dosage be based upon clinical assessment of the general condition of the patient, rather than on body weight. Initiation of therapy during a febrile episode has been associated with an increased incidence of reactive encephalopathy (Haller *et al.*, 1986). Administration of melarsoprol to leprous patients may precipitate erythema nodosum. The use of the drug is contraindicated during epidemics of influenza. Severe hemolytic reactions have been reported in patients with deficiency of glucose-6-phosphate dehydrogenase.

Therapeutic Uses. Because of its ability to enter the cerebrospinal fluid, melarsoprol is the drug of choice for treatment of the meningoencephalitic stage of African trypanosomiasis. It is effective in both Gambian and Rhodesian varieties of the disease. Its value lies in its prompt action against both early and late stages of trypanosomiasis, its effectiveness against tryparsamide-resistant strains of trypanosomes, and its failure to produce ocular toxicity. For these reasons, it has largely superseded tryparsamide. Melarsoprol is also effective in the treatment of the early hemolymphatic stage of the disease. Because of early CNS involvement and a relatively rapid clinical course, treatment with melarsoprol is usually initiated shortly after the diagnosis of Rhodesian trypanosomiasis. However, because of its toxicity, melarsoprol is usually reserved for treatment of the late stage of Gambian trypanosomiasis. For this reason also, it has no place in prophylaxis.

NIFURTIMOX

Nitrofurans were known to be effective in experimental infections with *T. cruzi*, and numerous congeners have been investigated for their chemotherapeutic usefulness. Of these, one drug, 3-methyl-4(5′-nitrofurfurylidene-amino)-tetrahydro-4H-1,4-thiazine-1,1-dioxide, is quite effective clinically in acute Chagas' infection (Brener, 1979).

Chemistry and Preparation. *Nifurtimox* (*Bayer 2502;* LAMPIT) has the following structural formula:

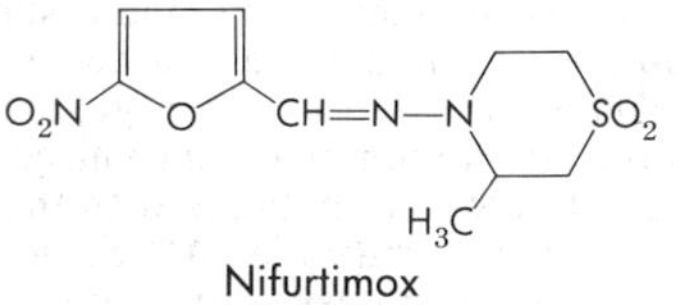

Nifurtimox

Nifurtimox is marketed in tablets that contain 100 mg of the drug; it is available in the United States only from the Centers for Disease Control.

Antiprotozoal Effects. Nifurtimox is trypanocidal against both the trypomastigote and the amastigote forms of *T. cruzi*. Concentrations of 1 μM damage intracellular amastigotes *in vitro* and inhibit their development. Continuous exposure to this concentration of the drug lengthens considerably the intracellular cycle. Trypomastigotes are less sensitive; 10-μM concentrations of nifurtimox inhibit penetration of vertebrate cells by the parasites but do not eliminate this process (*see* Dvorak and Howe, 1977). The trypanocidal action of nifurtimox appears to be related to its ability to undergo partial reduction to form chemically reactive radicals that cause production of toxic, partially reduced products of oxygen, for example, superoxide, hydrogen peroxide, and hydroxyl radicals (*see* Docampo and Moreno, 1984, 1986; Morello, 1988). *T. cruzi* apparently has low levels of reduced glutathione and lacks both catalase and glutathione peroxidase, making the parasite extremely vulnerable to hydrogen peroxide and hydrogen peroxide-related free radicals (Boveris *et al.*, 1980). Reaction of free radicals with cellular macromolecules results in lipid peroxidation and membrane injury, enzyme inactivation, damage to DNA, and mutagenesis. Nifurtimox may also produce damage to mammalian tissues by formation of radicals and redox cycling (Moreno *et al.*, 1980).

Absorption, Fate, and Excretion. Nifurtimox is well absorbed after oral administration. Despite this, only low concentrations of the drug (10 to 20 μM) are present in plasma and little is present in the tissues or urine. High concentrations of several unidentified metabolites are found, however, and it is obvious that biotransformation occurs rapidly. The effect of biotransformation on trypanocidal activity is unknown.

Route of Administration and Dosage. The drug is given orally. Children 1 to 10 years of age with acute Chagas' disease should receive 15 to 20 mg/kg per day in four divided doses for 90 days; for individuals 11 to 16 years old the daily dose is 12.5 to 15 mg/kg given according to the same schedule. Adults with acute disease should receive 8 to 10 mg/kg daily in four divided doses for 120 days. Although nifurtimox is used to treat chronic Chagas' infection, its efficacy is questionable for this condition. Gastric upset and weight loss are not uncommon during treatment. If the latter occurs, dosage should be reduced. The ingestion of alcohol should be avoided during treatment, since the incidence of side effects may increase.

Toxicity and Side Effects. Drug-related side effects are common. They range from hypersensitivity reactions, such as dermatitis, fever, icterus, pulmonary infiltrates, and anaphylaxis, to dose- and age-dependent complications primarily referable to the gastrointestinal tract and both the peripheral and central nervous systems (*see* Wegner and Rohwedder, 1972; Brener, 1979). Nausea and vomiting are common, as are myalgia and weakness. Peripheral neuropathy and gastrointestinal symptoms are particularly common after prolonged treatment; the latter complication may lead to weight loss and preclude further therapy. Headache, psychic disturbances, paresthesias, polyneuritis, and CNS excitation are less frequent. Leukopenia and decreased sperm counts have also been reported. The compound may suppress cell-mediated immune reactions, both *in vivo* and *in vitro* (Lelchuk *et al.*, 1977a, 1977b). Children appear to tolerate nifurtimox better than do adults. Because of the seriousness of the disease and the lack of superior drugs, there are no absolute contraindications to the use of nifurtimox.

Therapeutic Uses. Nifurtimox is employed in the treatment of *trypanosomiasis* caused by *T. cruzi* (Chagas' disease). It is effective in the acute and, to a questionable extent, in the chronic stages of the infection (*see* Brener, 1979). Treatment with nifurtimox has no effect on irreversible organ lesions brought about by the disease process. In the acute stage, drug therapy results in disappearance of parasitemia, amelioration of symptoms, and cure in over 80% of those treated. In the chronic stage, cure rates of over 90% were achieved in trials in Argentina, southern Brazil, Chile, and Venezuela, but much poorer results were obtained in the middle section of Brazil, where the character of the infection is somewhat different. Differences in the susceptibility of various strains of *T. cruzi* to nifurtimox have been described in animal models (*see* Brener, 1979), but whether these account for the variable clinical results is not known.

PENTAMIDINE

The discovery of antiprotozoal activity in the diamidine group of drugs, of which pentamidine is a member, was quite fortuitous (*see* King *et al.*, 1938; Lourie and Yorke, 1939). Of the compounds of this type, three were found to possess outstanding activity: 4,4'-diamidinostilbene (*stilbamidine*), 4,4'-diamidinophenoxy pentane (*pentamidine*), and 4,4'-diamidinophenoxy propane (*propamidine*). Despite its toxicity, *pentamidine* is the most useful clinically because of its relative stability, lower toxicity, and ease of administration. Although it is effective clinically against a number of pathogenic protozoa, pentamidine is now used primarily for the treatment and prophylaxis of *pneumocystosis*. *Hydroxystilbamidine isethionate* (2-hydroxy-4,4'-diamidinostilbene diisethionate) is preferred by some for the therapy of kala azar in East Africa (Manson-Bahr, 1959).

Chemistry and Preparation. Pentamidine has the following structural formula:

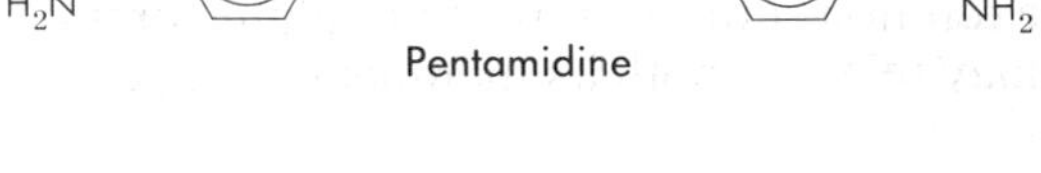

Pentamidine

Pentamidine isethionate, the preparation that is used, is marketed in vials containing 300 mg of the drug for injection (PENTAM 300) or for use as an aerosol (NEBUPENT). Solutions should be used promptly after preparation.

Antiprotozoal Effects. The aromatic diamidines are toxic to a number of different protozoa, yet show rather marked selectivity of action. For example, the drugs are curative against *T. rhodesiense* and *T. congolense* infections in experimental animals but are ineffective in curing mice infected with *T. cruzi*. They are also capable of curing *Babesia canis* infections in puppies and *Leishmania donovani* infections in hamsters. These findings provide the basis for diamidine treatment of African trypanosomiasis and leishmaniasis in man. At approximate therapeutic concentrations, pentamidine exerts a direct lethal effect on nonreplicating forms of *P. carinii* in culture (Pesanti, 1980; Pesanti and Cox, 1981; Pifer *et al.*, 1983). This presumably relates to the well-documented clinical efficacy of the drug in pneumocystosis.

The diamidines are also fungicidal. This can be readily demonstrated *in vitro* against *Blastomyces dermatitidis,* and has led to the successful therapeutic trial of the drugs in systemic blastomycosis. The use of *amphotericin B,* however, has reduced the value of the diamidines in the treatment of this disease.

Mechanism of Action. The mechanism of action of the diamidines has not been established; it is probably specific for individual parasites, and more than one action may be involved (*see* Sands *et al.*, 1985). The diamidines are concentrated by *T. brucei* via an energy-dependent, high-affinity uptake system, which operates more rapidly in drug-sensitive than in drug-resistant strains (Damper and Patten, 1976a, 1976b). Their trypanocidal activity may emanate from interactions of these cationic compounds with DNA or nucleotides and their derivatives; another suggestion is that these agents interfere with the uptake or function of polyamines (*see* Bacchi, 1981; Meshnick, 1984). The mechanism by which pentamidine inhibits glucose metabolism in nonreplicating *P. carinii* is unknown (Pesanti and Cox, 1981).

Absorption, Fate, and Excretion. Pentamidine isethionate is fairly well absorbed from parenteral sites of administration. Following a single dose to patients with AIDS, the drug disappears from plasma with an apparent half-life of about 6 hours. However, pentamidine is eliminated much more slowly in the urine as unchanged drug; its renal clearance accounts for only about 2% of its plasma clearance (Conte *et al.*, 1987). Extensive accumulation in tissues and slow excretion during repeated administration may relate to both its therapeutic properties and its prophylactic efficacy in African trypanosomiasis and pneumocystosis. After multiple parenteral doses, the liver, kidney, adrenal, and spleen of patients with AIDS contain the highest concentrations of drug, whereas only traces are found in the brain (Donnelly *et al.*, 1988). Lungs of such patients contain intermediate but therapeutic concentrations after five daily doses of 4 mg/kg. Higher pulmonary concentrations should be achieved by inhalation of pentamidine aerosols for prophylaxis or as adjunctive treatment of mild-to-moderate *P. carinii* pneumonia; delivery of drug by this route results in little systemic absorption and toxicity (Montgomery *et al.*, 1988; O'Doherty *et al.*, 1988).

Therapeutic Uses, Routes of Administration, and Dosage. Pentamidine isethionate is usually given parenterally by intramuscular injection or by slow intravenous infusion (60 minutes) in single daily doses of 4 mg per kilogram of body weight. In the treatment of *early African trypanosomiasis,* a course of ten injections should be given. Pentamidine is far less effective in treating *T. rhodesiense* than *T. gambiense* infections because of the rapidity with which *T. rhodesiense* invades the CNS. Treatment with pentamidine is no longer recommended for infection with *T. rhodesiense*. It is also ineffective in *T. gambiense* infections once the CNS is involved.

In the treatment of *visceral leishmaniasis* (*L. donovani* leishmaniasis, or *kala azar*), pentamidine has been used successfully in courses of 12 to 15 doses. A second course, given after an interval of 1 to 2 weeks, may be necessary in areas where the infection is known to respond less well to treatment. The drug is particularly useful in cases that have failed to respond to antimonials—for example, in the Sudan, where the disease responds only to high doses of antimonials, and in China, where many patients with kala azar are hypersensitive to antimonials. Some success has followed the use of pentamidine in the treatment of *cutaneous* (*L. tropica*) *leishmaniasis* (Oriental sore), but the drug is not routinely employed for this condition (*see* Berman, 1988).

Along with trimethoprim–sulfamethoxazole, pentamidine is a drug of choice for the treatment of *P. carinii* pneumonia, the most common opportunistic infection of patients with AIDS. Patients with *P. carinii* pneumonia should be treated daily with 4 mg/kg intramuscularly or intravenously for 14 days. The drug should be infused intravenously in 50 to 250 ml of 5% dextrose over 60 minutes to avoid immediate toxic reactions (Navin and Fontaine, 1984). If treatment is effective, clinical improvement will occur usually 4 to 6 days after the first injection. A high proportion of cures can be expected, depending on supportive therapy and, if possible, elimination of predisposing conditions.

The prognosis is less favorable in debilitated patients with altered immunity or neoplastic disease who may require more than one course of therapy. Treatment failures, relapses, and drug toxicity and intolerance are especially prevalent in patients with AIDS. Pentamidine can also be inhaled as an aerosol directly into the lungs; this strategy is used for both prophylaxis and second-line therapy of mild-to-moderate cases of *P. carinii* pneumonia (Conte *et al.*, 1987; Armstrong and Bernard, 1988; Montgomery *et al.*, 1989). Optimal dosage regimens have yet to be established. Successful prophylaxis has been achieved by monthly inhalation of 300 mg of the drug in a 5 to 10% nebulized aqueous solution over 30 to 45 minutes (*see* Armstrong and Bernard, 1988; Golden *et al.*, 1989). For adjunctive therapy, the total dose can be increased to 600 mg per administration (Montgomery *et al.*, 1989). Both the particle size (less than 4 μm diameter) and the design and operation of the equipment are important to achieve uniform distribution of the aerosol throughout the lungs (Montgomery *et al.*, 1988; O'Doherty *et al.*, 1988). The use of pentamidine has also markedly reduced mortality in the epidemic form of *P. carinii* infection found in debilitated and premature infants. However, trimethoprim–sulfamethoxazole is the preferred treatment for the last-named condition.

Toxicity and Side Effects. The major complications of pentamidine therapy have been well reviewed (Walzer *et al.*, 1974; Sands *et al.*, 1985). Intravenous injection of pentamidine (and other diamidines) can be followed quickly by alarming and sometimes dangerous reactions. These include breathlessness, tachycardia, dizziness or fainting, headache, and vomiting. These reactions are probably connected with the sharp fall in blood pressure that follows too rapid intravenous administration of the drug, and they may be due in part to the release of histamine. If solutions of pentamidine cannot be given slowly by the intravenous route, the drug is well tolerated after intramuscular injection, even though sterile abscesses may develop. Pentamidine does not appear to cause late neuropathies such as have been reported frequently after courses of stilbamidine. Pancreatitis and hypoglycemia and, paradoxically, hyperglycemia and insulin-dependent diabetes have been well documented following administration of pentamidine; the hypoglycemia may be life threatening or even fatal if not recognized (*see* Sands *et al.*, 1985; Waskin *et al.*, 1988; Collins *et al.*, 1989). Reversible renal dysfunction has been associated with the use of the drug in a small proportion of treated patients (*see* DeVita *et al.*, 1969; Sands *et al.*, 1985).

SODIUM STIBOGLUCONATE

The history of the development of leishmanicidal antimonial compounds evolved in three distinct phases. At first, the use of *antimony potassium tartrate* (*tartar emetic*) in the treatment of trypanosomiasis was followed by its successful use against cutaneous leishmaniasis and, shortly afterward, in cases of kala azar. Inconvenient administration of this drug, however, led to the trial of several other trivalent antimonial compounds, notably *antimony sodium tartrate, stibophen,* and *anthiolimine.* These were found to be as effective as and less toxic than tartar emetic. During this period, the successful syntheses of pentavalent antimonial derivatives of phenylstibonic acid were followed by the introduction of a variety of drugs that were as effective as and much less toxic than tartar emetic, thus permitting the use of larger doses and reduction in the period of treatment. Subsequent syntheses reverted to the "tartar-emetic" type of compound in which trivalent antimony was replaced by pentavalent antimony. An early member of this type of compound was *sodium stibogluconate.* This drug is widely used today and, together with *meglumine antimonate* (GLUCANTIME), a compound of the same type that is preferred in French-speaking countries, is the mainstay of the treatment of leishmaniasis by antimony. Full details of the investigations of leishmanicides can be found in the reviews of Findlay (1950), Beveridge (1963), and Berman (1988).

Chemistry. Sodium stibogluconate has the following structural formula:

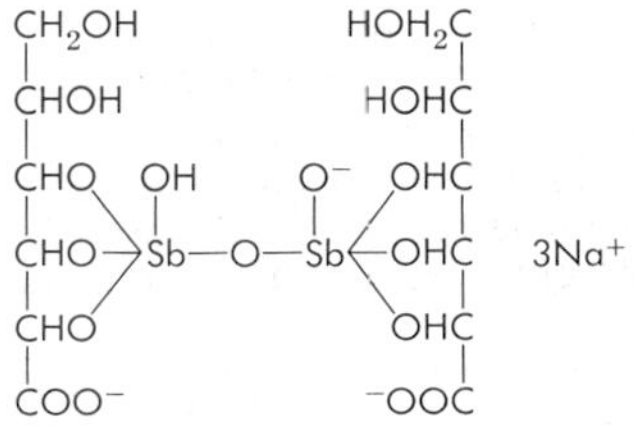

Sodium Stibogluconate

However, clinical formulations of sodium stibogluconate consist of multiple uncharacterized molecular forms, some of which have higher molecular weights than the compound shown (Berman, 1988). The preparation contains 30 to 34% pentavalent antimony.

Antiprotozoal Effects. Sodium stibogluconate appears to interfere with the bioenergetics of leishmania amastigotes (*see* Berman, 1988). Both glycolysis and fatty acid oxidation, processes primarily localized in unusual organelles termed glycosomes, are inhibited; this is accompanied by a net reduction in the generation of ATP and GTP. Other mechanisms may also be involved, such as nonspecific binding of antimony to the sulfhydryl groups of amastigote proteins. It is not known if reduction of pentavalent antimony to the trivalent form is required for the drug's antileishmanial action. Liposome-encapsulated antimonials have been used successfully to treat *L. donovani* infections in hamsters. In this form, the drug is selectively taken up by endocytosis and reaches the phagolysosomes of macrophages where the parasites reside (*see* Steck, 1981; Chang, 1983).

Absorption, Distribution, and Excretion. The pentavalent antimonials attain much higher concentrations in plasma than do the trivalent compounds. Consequently, most of a single dose of sodium stibogluconate is excreted in the urine within 24 hours. Its pharmacokinetic behavior is similar whether the drug is given intravenously or intramuscularly (Rees *et al.*, 1980; Pamplin *et al.*, 1981; Chulay *et al.*, 1988). The agent is rapidly absorbed, distributed in an apparent volume of about 0.22 liter/kg, and eliminated in two phases. The first has a rapid half-life of about 2 hours, and the second is much slower ($t_{1/2}$ = 33 to 76 hours). The terminal elimination phase may reflect conversion of the pentavalent antimonial to the trivalent form; this could also account for accumulation and slow release of the drug during multiple dosing (Chulay *et al.*, 1988).

Toxicity. Untoward reactions to pentavalent antimonials are qualitatively similar to those that follow the administration of trivalent compounds, but they are far less frequent and rarely as severe. In general, sodium stibogluconate is tolerated relatively well. Specific reactions commonly noted include pain at the injection site after intramuscular administration, gastrointestinal symptoms, delayed muscle pain, and stiffness of the joints. Changes in the electrocardiogram, which may occur later, include T-wave flattening and inversion and prolongation of the Q–T interval; these are usually reversible but may precede serious arrhythmias. Elevations of hepatic transaminases have been noted, but these are reversible after cessation of therapy. Rarely, there is shock and sudden death.

Preparation. *Sodium stibogluconate* (*sodium antimony gluconate;* PENTOSTAM) is available in aqueous solution for parenteral administration. Each milliliter contains drug equivalent to 100 mg of pentavalent antimony. It is available in the United States only from the Centers for Disease Control.

Routes of Administration, Dosage, and Therapeutic Uses. Although sodium stibogluconate may be given either intravenously or intramuscularly, uniform guidelines for the chemotherapy of various forms of leishmaniasis have not been established.

Based on an analysis by Berman (1988), certain earlier proposals should probably be modified, while others are retained (*see* WHO, 1984). For cutaneous leishmaniasis, a daily dose of sodium stibogluconate (20 mg of Sb/kg) should be given for 20 days. If a cure rate of 95% or higher is achieved, lower doses or a shorter period of time may be tried. For mucocutaneous leishmaniasis, the WHO recommendation of 20 mg of Sb/kg for 30 days seems appropriate. The identical regimen is also advised for systemic leishmaniasis. Children usually tolerate the drug well, and the dose per kilogram is the same as that given to adults. If unfavorable reactions occur in particularly debilitated individuals shortly after therapy is begun, the drug may be administered on alternate days or at longer intervals. Cure rates are high if the above recommendations are followed; increasing the daily dose from 10 to 20 mg of Sb/kg ordinarily causes minimal added risk for the patient. Despite certain reports, resistance to pentavalent antimonials has yet to be established rigorously. Sodium stibogluconate remains the "drug of choice" for leishmaniasis. Its main disadvantages are the long courses of therapy required, the necessity for parenteral administration, and its relatively high cost. For the 15% of cases of East African kala azar that are unresponsive to pentavalent antimonials, therapy with pentamidine should be considered. Similarly, amphotericin B is an excellent albeit toxic alternative for the treatment of mucosal leishmaniasis.

SURAMIN

Based on the observed trypanocidal activity of the dyestuffs *trypan red, trypan blue,* and *afridol violet,* several years of research in Germany resulted in the introduction of *suramin* into therapy in 1920. Today the drug is used primarily for treatment of *African trypanosomiasis*. Although suramin is effective in clearing adult filariae in *onchocerciasis,* ivermectin has largely replaced suramin for treatment of that infection (*see* Chapter 40). Because suramin is an inhibitor of retroviral reverse transcriptase, it was recently tested unsuccessfully in a multicenter clinical trial for treatment of patients with AIDS (de Clercq, 1979; Mitsuya *et al.*, 1984; Cheson *et al.*, 1987). Drug-associated adrenal insufficiency noted in such clinical studies and in animal models has also stimulated interest in the efficacy of suramin in metastatic adrenocortical carcinoma and adrenocortical hyperfunction. The pertinent clinical pharmacology of this agent has been reviewed (*see* Hawking, 1978; Broder *et al.*, 1985; Collins *et al.*, 1986; Cheson *et al.*, 1987).

Chemistry and Preparation. *Suramin sodium* (GERMANIN, others) has the structural formula shown below. Only freshly prepared solutions of suramin should be employed. Suramin is available in the United States only from the Centers for Disease Control.

Antiprotozoal Effects. The primary mechanism of action of suramin is not established, which is not surprising in view of its general toxicity. However, there is considerable specificity in the structure of this polyanionic drug, since removal of the two methyl groups results in complete loss of antitrypanosomal activity. Suramin inhibits many trypanosomal enzymes (*see* Meshnick, 1984). Inhibi-

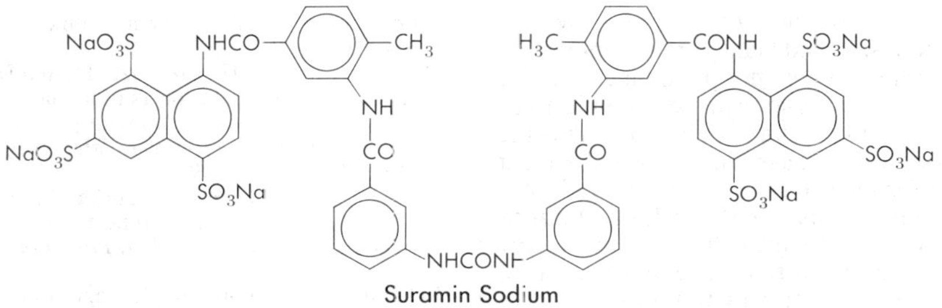

Suramin Sodium

tion of glycerol phosphate oxidase, a parasite enzyme involved in energy metabolism, correlates with the antitrypanosomal activity of several derivatives of suramin (Fairlamb and Bowman, 1977). Furthermore, energy metabolism of trypanosomes obtained from suramin-treated animals is reduced. The delayed onset of drug activity may be due to slow endocytic uptake by the parasite of a suramin–plasma protein complex (Fairlamb and Bowman, 1980). Williamson and Macadam (1965) observed changes in suramin-treated trypanosomes characterized by damage to intracellular membranous structures other than lysosomes.

Absorption, Fate, and Excretion. Suramin must be given parenterally. Following its intravenous administration, the concentration in plasma falls fairly rapidly for a few hours, then more slowly for a few days, with a half-life of about 48 hours, and finally very slowly, with a terminal elimination half-life of about 50 days. The persistence of suramin in the circulation is due to extremely tight binding to plasma protein. The drug is not metabolized to any extent, and its renal clearance of 0.3 ml/min accounts for elimination of about 80% of the compound from the body. Although the apparent volume of distribution of suramin in an adult is about 40 liters, this large polar anion does not enter cells readily, and tissue concentrations are uniformly lower than those in the plasma. In experimental animals, however, the kidneys have been found to contain considerably more suramin than other organs. This retention may account for the fairly frequent occurrence of albuminuria following injection of the drug in man. Very little suramin penetrates into the cerebrospinal fluid, consistent with its lack of efficacy once the CNS has been invaded. The persistence of suramin in the circulation explains why the drug has proven valuable in the prophylaxis of trypanosomiasis.

Route of Administration and Dosage. Suramin is usually given by slow intravenous injection in 10% aqueous solution. Treatment of active *African trypanosomiasis* should not be started until 24 hours after diagnostic lumbar puncture, and caution is required if the patient has onchocerciasis. The normal single dose for adults is 1 g. It is advisable to employ a small test dose of 200 mg initially to detect sensitivity, after which the normal dose is given on days 1, 3, 7, 14, and 21; weekly doses may be given for an additional 5 weeks. The pediatric dose is 20 mg/kg, given according to the same schedule. Patients in poor condition should be treated cautiously during the first week.

Toxicity and Side Effects. Suramin can cause a variety of untoward reactions that vary in intensity and frequency and tend to be more severe in debilitated patients. The most serious immediate reaction consists of nausea, vomiting, shock, and loss of consciousness. Fortunately, the incidence is low (0.1 to 0.3%). Malaise, nausea, and fatigue are common immediate reactions. Fever, erythematous skin rashes, and neurological complications (including headache, metallic taste, paresthesias, and peripheral neuropathy) are also common. These complications occur somewhat later and nearly always disappear spontaneously despite continued therapy. Other less prevalent reactions include vomiting, diarrhea, stomatitis, chills, abdominal pain, and edema. Laboratory abnormalities noted in 12 to 26% of patients with AIDS include leukopenia and occasional agranulocytosis, thrombocytopenia, proteinuria, and elevations of plasma creatinine, transaminases, and bilirubin. These abnormalities are also reversible. Unexpected findings that were described recently in patients with AIDS are adrenal insufficiency and vortex keratopathy.

Precautions and Contraindications. Patients receiving suramin should be followed closely. Therapy should not be continued in patients who show intolerance to initial doses, and the drug should be employed with great caution in individuals with renal insufficiency. Moderate albuminuria is common during control of the acute phase, but persisting, heavy albuminuria calls for caution as well as modification of the schedule of treatment. If casts appear, treatment with suramin should be discontinued. The occurrence of palmar–plantar hyperesthesia necessitates caution since it may presage peripheral neuritis.

Therapeutic Uses. Suramin is used to treat *African trypanosomiasis* but is of no value in South American trypanosomiasis caused by *T. cruzi*. Because only small amounts of the drug enter the cerebrospinal fluid, suramin is more effective in treating infections with *T. gambiense* than those with *T. rhodesiense*. In contrast to *T. rhodesiense*, *T. gambiense* organisms invade the CNS relatively late in the course of illness. Of currently approved drugs, only the toxic arsenicals are quite effective in both types of African trypanosomiasis once the

CNS is involved. Suramin is effective for the prophylaxis of Rhodesian and Gambian trypanosomiasis. Chemoprophylaxis is not recommended for travelers on occasional brief visits to endemic areas since the risk of serious drug toxicity outweighs the risk of acquiring the disease. Suramin is the most effective drug for clearing the adult filariae in *onchocerciasis*, but because of the risk of Mazzotti reactions in addition to drug toxicity, it is now rarely used for this condition. The single dose of 1 g is repeated weekly for 5 or 6 weeks.

Boveris, A.; Sies, H.; Martino, E. E.; Docampo, R.; Turrens, J. F.; and Stoppani, A. O. M. Deficient metabolic utilization of hydrogen peroxide in *Trypanosoma cruzi*. *Biochem. J.*, **1980**, *188*, 643–648.

Broder, S., and others. Effects of suramin on HTLV-III/LAV infection presenting as Kaposi's sarcoma or AIDS-related complex: suppression of virus replication *in vivo*. *Lancet*, **1985**, *2*, 627–630.

Cheson, B. D., and others. Suramin therapy in AIDS and related disorders. Report of the U.S. Suramin Working Group. *J.A.M.A.*, **1987**, *258*, 1347–1351.

Chulay, J. D.; Fleckenstein, L.; and Smith, D. H. Pharmacokinetics of antimony during treatment of visceral leishmaniasis with sodium stibogluconate or meglumine antimoniate. *Trans. R. Soc. Trop. Med. Hyg.*, **1988**, *82*, 69–72.

Collins, J. M.; Klecker, R. W., Jr.; Yarchoan, R.; Lane, H. C.; Fauci, A. S.; Redfield, R. R.; Broder, S.; and Myers, C. E. Clinical pharmacokinetics of suramin in patients with HTLV-III/LAV infection. *J. Clin. Pharmacol.*, **1986**, *26*, 22–26.

Collins, R. J.; Pien, F. D.; and Houk, J. H. Case report: insulin-dependent diabetes mellitus associated with pentamidine. *Am. J. Med. Sci.*, **1989**, *297*, 174–175.

Conte, J. E., Jr.; Upton, R. A.; and Lin, E. T. Pentamidine pharmacokinetics in patients with AIDS with impaired renal function. *J. Infect. Dis.*, **1987**, *156*, 885–890.

de Clercq, E. Suramin: a potent inhibitor of the reverse transcriptase of RNA tumor viruses. *Cancer Lett.*, **1979**, *8*, 9–22.

DeVita, V. T.; Emmer, M.; Levine, A.; Jacobs, B.; and Berard, C. *Pneumocystis carinii* pneumonia. *N. Engl. J. Med.*, **1969**, *280*, 287–291.

Donnelly, H.; Bernard, E. M.; Rothkotter, H.; Gold, J. W. M.; and Armstrong, D. Distribution of pentamidine in patients with AIDS. *J. Infect. Dis.*, **1988**, *157*, 985–989.

Doua, F.; Boa, F. Y.; Schechter, P. J.; Miezan, T. W.; Diai, D.; Sanon, S. R.; De Raadt, P.; Haegele, K. D.; Sjoerdsma, A.; and Konian, K. Treatment of human late stage Gambiense trypanosomiasis with α-difluoromethylornithine (eflornithine): efficacy and tolerance in 14 cases in Cote d'Ivoire. *Am. J. Trop. Med. Hyg.*, **1987**, *37*, 525–533.

Dvorak, J. A., and Howe, C. L. The effects of LAMPIT (Bayer 2502) on the interaction of *Trypanosoma cruzi* with vertebrate cells *in vitro*. *Am. J. Trop. Med. Hyg.*, **1977**, *26*, 58–63.

Fairlamb, A. H.; Blackburn, P.; Urich, P.; Chait, B. T.; and Cerami, A. Trypanothione: a novel bis(glutathionyl)spermidine cofactor for glutathione reductase in trypanosomatids. *Science*, **1985**, *227*, 1485–1487.

Flynn, I. W., and Bowman, I. B. R. Further studies on the mode of action of arsenicals on trypanosome pyruvate kinase. *Trans. R. Soc. Trop. Med. Hyg.*, **1969**, *63*, 121.

Golden, J. A.; Chernoff, D.; Hollander, H.; Feigal, D.; and Conte, J. E. Prevention of *Pneumocystis carinii* pneumonia by inhaled pentamidine. *Lancet*, **1989**, *1*, 654–657.

Haller, L.; Adams, H.; Merouze, F.; and Dago, A. Clinical and pathological aspects of human African trypanosomiasis (*T. b. gambiense*) with particular reference to reactive arsenical encephalopathy. *Am. J. Trop. Med. Hyg.*, **1986**, *35*, 94–99.

King, H.; Lourie, E. M.; and Yorke, W. Studies in chemotherapy. XIX. Further report on new trypanocidal substances. *Ann. Trop. Med. Parasitol.*, **1938**, *32*, 177–192.

Lelchuk, R.; Cardoni, R. L.; and Fuks, A. S. Cell-mediated immunity in Chagas' disease: alterations induced by treatment with a trypanocidal drug (nifurtimox). *Clin. Exp. Immunol.*, **1977a**, *30*, 434–438.

Lelchuk, R.; Cardoni, R. L.; and Lewis, S. Nifurtimox-induced alterations in the cell-mediated immune response to PPD in guinea pigs. *Clin. Exp. Immunol.*, **1977b**, *30*, 469–473.

Lourie, E. M., and Yorke, W. Studies in chemotherapy. XXI. The trypanocidal action of certain aromatic diamidines. *Ann. Trop. Med. Parasitol.*, **1939**, *33*, 289–304.

Manson-Bahr, P. E. C. East African kala-azar with special reference to the pathology, prophylaxis and treatment. *Trans. R. Soc. Trop. Med. Hyg.*, **1959**, *53*, 123–137.

Mitsuya, H.; Popovic, M.; Yarchoan, R.; Matsushita, S.; Gallo, R. C.; and Broder, S. Suramin protection of T cells *in vitro* against infectivity and cytopathic effect of HTLV-III. *Science*, **1984**, *226*, 172–174.

Montgomery, A. B.; Debs, R. J.; Luce, J. M.; Corkery, K. J.; Turner, J.; Brunette, E. N.; Lin, E. T.; and Hopewell, P. C. Selective delivery of pentamidine to the lung by aerosol. *Am. Rev. Respir. Dis.*, **1988**, *137*, 477–478.

Montgomery, A. B.; Debs, R. J.; Luce, J. M.; Corkery, K. J.; Turner, J.; and Hopewell, P. C. Aerosolized pentamidine as second line therapy in patients with AIDS and *Pneumocystis carinii* pneumonia. *Chest*, **1989**, *95*, 747–750.

Moreno, S. N. J.; Palmero, D. J.; de Palmero, K. E.; Docampo, R.; and Stoppani, A. O. M. Stimulation of lipid peroxidation and ultrastructural alterations induced by nifurtimox in mammalian tissues. *Medicina (B. Aires)*, **1980**, *40*, 553–559.

Navin, T. R., and Fontaine, R. E. Intravenous versus intramuscular administration of pentamidine. *N. Engl. J. Med.*, **1984**, *311*, 1701–1702.

O'Doherty, M. J.; Thomas, S.; Page, C.; Barlow, D.; Bradbeer, C.; Nunan, T. O.; and Bateman, N. T. Differences in relative efficiency of nebulisers for pentamidine administration. *Lancet*, **1988**, *2*, 1283–1286.

Pamplin, C. L.; Desjardins, R.; Chulay, J.; Tramont, E.; Hendricks, L.; and Canfield, C. Pharmacokinetics of antimony during sodium stibogluconate therapy for cutaneous leishmaniasis. *Clin. Pharmacol. Ther.*, **1981**, *29*, 270–271.

Pesanti, E. *In vitro* effects of antiprotozoan drugs and immune serum on *Pneumocystis carinii*. *J. Infect. Dis.*, **1980**, *141*, 775–780.

Pesanti, E., and Cox, C. Metabolic and synthetic activities of *Pneumocystis carinii in vitro*. *Infect. Immun.*, **1981**, *34*, 908–914.

Petru, A. M.; Azimi, P. H.; Cummins, S. K.; and Sjoerdsma, A. African sleeping sickness in the United States. Successful treatment with eflornithine. *Am. J. Dis. Child.*, **1988**, *142*, 224–228.

Pifer, L. L.; Pifer, D. D.; and Woods, D. R. Biological profile and response to anti-pneumocystis agents of *Pneumocystis carinii* in cell culture. *Antimicrob. Agents Chemother.*, **1983**, *24*, 674–678.

Taelman, H.; Schechter, P. J.; Marcelis, L.; Sonnet, J.; Kazyumba, G.; Dasnoy, J.; Haegele, K. D.; Sjoerdsma, A.; and Wery, M. Difluoromethylornithine, an effective new treatment of Gambian trypanosomiasis. *Am. J. Med.*, **1987**, *82*, 607–614.

VanHoof, L. M. J. J. Observations on trypanosomiasis in Belgian Congo. *Trans. R. Soc. Trop. Med. Hyg.*, **1947**, *40*, 728–761.

Van Nieuwenhove, S.; Schechter, P. J.; de Clercq, J.; Bone, G.; Burke, J.; and Sjoerdsma, A. Treatment of *gambiense* sleeping sickness in the Sudan with DFMO (DL-α-difluoromethylornithine), an inhibitor of ornithine decarboxylase: first field trial. *Trans. R. Soc. Trop. Med. Hyg.*, **1985**, *79*, 692–698.

Walzer, P. D.; Perl, D. P.; Krogstad, D. J.; Rawson, P. G.; and Schultz, M. G. *Pneumocystis carinii* pneumonia in the United States. *Ann. Intern. Med.*, **1974**, *80*, 83–93.

Waskin, H.; Stehr-Green, J. K.; Helmick, C. G.; and Sattler, F. R. Risk factors for hypoglycemia associated with pentamidine therapy for pneumocystis pneumonia. *J.A.M.A.*, **1988**, *260*, 345–347.

Wegner, D. H. G., and Rohwedder, R. W. Experience with nifurtimox in chronic Chagas' infection. Preliminary report. *Arzneimittelforsch.*, **1972**, *22*, 1635–1641.

Williamson, J., and Macadam, R. F. Effect of trypanocidal drugs on the fine structure of *Trypanosoma rhodesiense*. *Trans. R. Soc. Trop. Med. Hyg.*, **1965**, *59*, 367–368.

Monographs and Reviews

Albert, A. *Selective Toxicity: The Physico-Chemical Basis of Therapy*, 6th ed. Chapman & Hall, Ltd., London, **1979.**

Apted, F. I. C. Present status of chemotherapy and chemoprophylaxis of human trypanosomiasis in the eastern hemisphere. *Pharmacol. Ther.*, **1980**, *11*, 391–413.

Armstrong, D., and Bernard, E. Aerosol pentamidine. *Ann. Intern. Med.*, **1988**, *109*, 852–854.

Bacchi, C. J. Content, synthesis and function of polyamines in trypanosomatids: relationship to chemotherapy. *J. Protozool.*, **1981**, *28*, 20–27.

Berman, J. D. Chemotherapy for leishmaniasis: biochemical mechanisms, clinical efficacy, and future strategies. *Rev. Infect. Dis.*, **1988**, *10*, 560–586.

Beveridge, E. Chemotherapy of leishmaniasis. In, *Experimental Chemotherapy*, Vol. I. (Schnitzer, R. J., and Hawking, F., eds.) Academic Press, Inc., New York, **1963**, pp. 257–287.

Brener, Z. Present status of chemotherapy and chemoprophylaxis of human trypanosomiasis in the Western Hemisphere. *Pharmacol. Ther.*, **1979**, *7*, 71–90.

Chang, K.-P. Cellular and molecular mechanisms of intracellular symbiosis in leishmaniasis. *Int. Rev. Cytol.*, **1983**, *14*, Suppl., 267–305.

Damper, D., and Patten, C. L. Pentamidine transport and sensitivity in *brucei*-group trypanosomes. *J. Protozool.*, **1976a**, *23*, 349–356.

———. Pentamine transport in *Trypanosoma brucei*—kinetics and specificity. *Biochem. Pharmacol.*, **1976b**, *25*, 271–276.

Docampo, R., and Moreno, S. N. J. Free radical metabolites in the mode of action of chemotherapeutic agents and phagocytic cells on *Trypanosoma cruzi*. *Rev. Infect. Dis.*, **1984**, *6*, 223–238.

———. Free radical metabolism of antiparasitic agents in free radical metabolites of toxic chemicals. *Fed. Proc.*, **1986**, *45*, 2471–2476.

Fairlamb, A. H., and Bowman, I. B. R. *Trypanosoma brucei:* suramin and other trypanocidal compounds: effects on sn-glycerol-3-phosphate oxidase. *Exp. Parasitol.*, **1977**, *43*, 353–361.

Fairlamb, A. H., and Bowman, I. B. R. Uptake of the trypanocidal drug suramin by bloodstream forms of *Trypanosoma brucei* and its effect on respiration and growth rate *in vivo*. *Mol. Biochem. Parasitol.*, **1980**, *1*, 315–333.

Findlay, G. M. *Recent Advances in Chemotherapy*, Vol. I. J. & A. Churchill, Ltd., London, **1950.**

Gutteridge, W. E. New anti-protozoal agents. *Int. J. Parasitol.*, **1987**, *17*, 121–129.

Hawking, F. Chemotherapy of trypanosomiasis. In, *Experimental Chemotherapy*, Vol. I. (Schnitzer, R. J., and Hawking, F., eds.) Academic Press, Inc., New York, **1963**, pp. 129–256.

———. Suramin: with special reference to onchocerciasis. *Adv. Pharmacol. Chemother.*, **1978**, *15*, 289–322.

McCann, P. P.; Bacchi, C. J.; Clarkson, A. B., Jr.; Bey, P.; Sjoerdsma, A.; Schechter, P. J.; Walzer, P. D.; and Barlow, J. L. R. Inhibition of polyamine biosynthesis by difluoromethylornithine in African trypanosomes and *Pneumocystis carinii* as a basis of chemotherapy: biochemical and clinical aspects. *Am. J. Trop. Med. Hyg.*, **1986**, *35*, 1153–1156.

Marr, J. J., and Docampo, R. Chemotherapy for Chagas' disease: a perspective of current therapy and considerations for future research. *Rev. Infect. Dis.*, **1986**, *8*, 884–903.

Meshnick, S. R. The chemotherapy of African trypanosomiasis. In, *Parasitic Diseases*, Vol. 2. (Mansfield, J. M., ed.) Marcel Dekker, Inc., New York, **1984**, pp. 165–199.

Morello, A. The biochemistry of the mode of action of drugs and the detoxication mechanisms in *Trypanosoma cruzi*. *Comp. Biochem. Physiol. [C]*, **1988**, *90C*, 1–12.

Opperdoes, F. R. Biochemical peculiarities of trypanosomes, African and South American. *Br. Med. Bull.*, **1985**, *41*, 130–136.

Rees, P. H.; Keating, M. I.; Kager, P. A.; and Hockmeyer, W. T. Renal clearance of pentavalent antimony (sodium stibogluconate). *Lancet*, **1980**, *2*, 226–229.

Robertson, D. H. H. Chemotherapy of African trypanosomiasis. *Practitioner*, **1962**, *188*, 80–83.

Sands, M.; Kron, M. A.; and Brown, R. B. Pentamidine: a review. *Rev. Infect. Dis.*, **1985**, *7*, 625–634.

Schofield, C. J. Control of Chagas' disease vectors. *Br. Med. Bull.*, **1985**, *41*, 187–194.

Steck, E. A. The chemotherapy of protozoal infections: whither? *J. Protozool.*, **1981**, *28*, 30–35.

WHO. The leishmaniases. *WHO Tech. Rep. Series*, **1984**, *701*, 99–109.

SECTION

XI

Chemotherapy of Microbial Diseases

CHAPTER

44 ANTIMICROBIAL AGENTS

General Considerations

Merle A. Sande, Joan E. Kapusnik-Uner, and Gerald L. Mandell

Historical Aspects and Introduction. The first investigators to recognize the clinical potential of microorganisms as therapeutic agents were Pasteur and Joubert, who recorded their observations and speculations in 1877. They noted that anthrax bacilli grew rapidly when inoculated into sterile urine but failed to multiply and soon died if one of the "common" bacteria of the air was introduced in the urine at the same time. The same type of experiment in animals produced similar results. They commented on the fact that life destroys life among the lower species even more than among higher animals and plants, and came to the astonishing conclusion that anthrax bacilli could be administered to an animal in large numbers, and it would not sicken, provided that "ordinary" bacteria were given at the same time. They stated that this observation might hold great promise for therapeutics. During the latter part of the nineteenth century and the early years of the twentieth century, several antimicrobial substances were demonstrated in bacterial cultures, and some were even tested clinically but discarded because they proved to be highly toxic.

The modern era of the chemotherapy of infection started with the clinical use of sulfanilamide in 1936. The "golden age" of antimicrobial therapy began with the production of penicillin in 1941, when this compound was mass-produced and first made available for limited clinical trial. At least 30% of all hospitalized patients now receive one or more courses of therapy with antibiotics, and millions of potentially fatal infections have been cured. However, at the same time, these pharmaceutical agents have become among the most misused of those available to the practicing physician. One result of widespread use of antimicrobial agents has been the emergence of antibiotic-resistant pathogens, which in turn has created an ever-increasing need for new drugs. Many of these agents have also contributed significantly to the rising costs of medical care.

The history of antimicrobial agents has thus been dynamic, characterized by the constant emergence of new challenges followed by investigation, discovery, and the production of new drugs. The following pages present both a philosophical and a practical approach to the appropriate use of antimicrobial agents, as well as a discussion of the factors that influence the outcome of such treatment.

Definition and Characteristics. Antibiotics are chemical substances produced by various species of microorganisms (bacteria, fungi, actinomycetes) that suppress the growth of other microorganisms and may eventually destroy them. However, common usage often extends the term *antibiotics* to include synthetic antibacterial agents, such as the sulfonamides and quinolones, that are not products of microbes. The number of antibiotics that has been identified now extends into the hundreds, and many of these have been developed to the stage where they are of value in the therapy of infectious diseases. Antibiotics differ markedly in physical, chemical, and pharmacological properties, antibacterial spectra, and mechanisms of action. In recent years, knowledge of molecular mechanisms of bacterial, fungal, and viral replication has greatly facilitated rational development of compounds that can interfere with the life cycles of these microorganisms.

Classification and Mechanism of Action. There are several methods used to classify and group antimicrobial agents, and all are hampered by exceptions and overlaps. Historically, the most common classification has been based on chemical structure and proposed mechanism of action, as follows: (1) agents that inhibit synthesis of or activate enzymes that disrupt bacterial cell walls to cause loss of viability and, often, cell lysis; these include the penicillins and cephalosporins, which are structurally similar, and dissimilar agents such as cycloserine, vancomycin, bacitracin, and the imidazole antifungal agents (miconazole, ketoconazole, and clotrimazole); (2) agents that act directly on the cell membrane of the microorganism, affecting permeability and leading to leakage of intracellular compounds; these include the detergents, polymyxin and colistimethate, and the polyene antifungal agents, nystatin and amphotericin B, that bind to cell-wall sterols; (3) agents that affect the function of bacterial ribosomes to cause a reversible inhibition of protein synthesis; these bacteriostatic drugs include chloramphenicol, the tetracyclines, erythromycin, and clindamycin; (4) agents that bind to the 30 S ribosomal subunit and alter protein synthesis, which eventually leads to cell death; these include the aminoglycosides; (5) agents that affect nucleic acid metabolism, such as the rifamycins (*e.g.*, rifampin), which inhibit DNA-dependent RNA polymerase, and the quinolones, which inhibit DNA supercoiling and DNA synthesis; (6) the antimetabolites, including trimethoprim and the sulfonamides, which block specific metabolic steps that are essential to microorganisms; (7) nucleic acid analogs, such as zidovudine, ganciclovir, vidarabine, and acyclovir, which bind to viral enzymes that are essential for DNA synthesis, thus halting viral replication. Additional categories will likely emerge as more complex mechanisms are elucidated; at the present time, the precise mechanism of action of some antimicrobial agents is unknown.

Factors That Determine the Susceptibility and Resistance of Microorganisms to Antimicrobial Agents. When antibiotics are used to treat an infection, a favorable therapeutic outcome is influenced by numerous factors. However, in simple terms, success is dependent on achieving a level of antibacterial activity at the site of infection that is sufficient to inhibit the bacteria in a manner that tips the balance in favor of the host. When host defenses are maximally effective, the antibacterial effect required may be minimal, for example, that provided by bacteriostatic agents that slow protein synthesis or prevent microbial cell division. On the other hand, when host defenses are impaired, complete antibiotic-mediated killing or lysis of the bacteria may be required to achieve a successful outcome. The dose of drug utilized must be sufficient to produce the necessary effect on the microorganisms; however, concentrations of the agent in plasma and tissues must remain below those that are toxic to human cells. If this can be achieved, the microorganism is considered to be susceptible to the antibiotic. If the concentration of drug required to inhibit or kill the organism is greater than the concentration that can safely be achieved, the microorganism is considered to be resistant to the antibiotic.

The precise information required to make accurate decisions about concentrations of drugs in various tissues or body fluids is frequently unavailable. Thus, determination of antibiotic sensitivity of microorganisms is at best an inexact science. For example, group-A beta-hemolytic streptococci are exquisitely sensitive to penicillin G and are inhibited and killed by low concentrations (0.01 μg/ml), yet very high concentrations of penicillin (20 to 100 μg/ml) can be safely achieved in plasma. There is thus a very large "therapeutic window." On the other hand, many gram-negative aerobic bacilli, such as *Pseudomonas aeruginosa,* may require 2 to 4 μg/ml of gentamicin or tobramycin to be inhibited. Such bacilli are considered to be susceptible to these antimicrobials, although peak concentrations in plasma above 6 to 10 μg/ml may result in ototoxicity or nephrotoxicity. Thus, the ratio of toxic to therapeutic concentrations is very low and such agents are more difficult to use. Furthermore, concentrations of these drugs at certain sites of infection (such as vitreous fluid or cerebrospinal fluid) may be much lower than those in plasma. Thus, the drug may be only marginally effective or ineffective in such cases even though standardized *in-vitro* tests would likely report the microorganism as "sensitive." Conversely, concentrations of drug in urine may be much higher than those in plasma. Microorganisms reported as "resistant" may thus respond to therapy when infection is limited to the urinary tract. Most *in-vitro* sensitivity tests are standardized on the basis of the drug concentrations that can be safely achieved in plasma. They do *not* reflect concentrations that can be attained at sites of infection, nor do they consider any local factors that may affect the activity of the drug. Hence, it is most important to understand the limitations of such *in-vitro* tests.

There are multiple factors that determine the relative antimicrobial activity of a drug against a specific microorganism. For an antibiotic to be effective, it must bind to target sites of action on or in the bacterial cell. Bacteria can develop resistance to specific antimicrobial agents by preventing their access to these sites (Vaudaux, 1981). Some bacteria produce enzymes that reside at or within the cell surface that inactivate the drug. Others possess impermeable cell membranes that prevent influx of the drug. Hydrophilic antibiotics traverse the outer membrane of microbial cells via aqueous channels (pores) comprised of specific proteins (porins). Bacteria deficient in these channels can be resistant to such drugs (Jaffe *et. al.,* 1983). Still others lack the transport systems that are required for entrance of the drug into the bacterial cell (Dickie *et al.,* 1978). Since many antibiotics are organic acids, their penetration may be pH dependent (Bryant, 1987); in addition, permeation may be altered by osmolality or by various cations in the external milieu (Zimilis and Jackson, 1973). The transport mechanisms for certain drugs are energy dependent and are not operative in an anaerobic environment (Verklin and Mandell, 1977). Once the drug has gained access to the target site, it must exert an effect that is deleterious to the microorganism. Natural variation or acquired changes in the target sites that prevent drug binding or action are additional mechanisms of resistance.

Acquired Resistance to Antimicrobial Agents. When the antimicrobial activity of a new agent is first tested, a pattern of "sensitivity" and "resistance" is usually defined. Unfortunately, this spectrum of activity can subsequently change to a remarkable degree, because microorganisms have evolved the array of ingenious alterations discussed above that allow them to survive in the presence of antibiotics. The mechanism of drug resistance varies from microorganism to microorganism and from drug to drug. For example, strains of *Staphylococcus aureus* that were resistant to penicillin G appeared shortly after this antibiotic was introduced. This resistance was the result of elaboration, by the bacteria, of beta-lactamase, an enzyme that hydrolyzes and inactivates penicillin G. The frequency has increased such that over 80% of both hospital- and community-acquired strains of this bacterium are now resistant. In recent years, other strains of *Staph. aureus* have appeared that are highly resistant to all beta-lactam antibiotics. These so-called methicillin-resistant organisms are prominent in hospitals, especially in intensive care units, where antibiotic use is great (Chambers, 1988). Emergence of resistance in some other species has occurred more slowly. The gonococcus gradually acquired low-level resistance to penicillin G (*i.e.,* higher doses became necessary for cure) over a period of 20 years, especially in areas where this drug was used excessively. This was due to an alteration in an outer-membrane porin protein that prevents access of drug to its target site. However, in 1974 many gonococcal strains suddenly emerged that produce a penicillinase that inactivates the drug (Judson, 1989). These strains are highly resistant to penicillin G, and infections produced by them are not cured even with high doses of the drug. The pneumococcus (*Streptococcus pneumoniae*) has also historically been exquisitely sensitive to penicillin G; however, in 1978, strains resistant to this drug emerged in South Africa (Jacobs *et al.*, 1978). Several similar strains have subsequently been isolated in the United States. These strains have altered their target sites for penicillin G—penicillin-binding proteins 1 and 3 (Handwerger and Tomasz, 1986).

The development of resistance to antibiotics usually involves a stable genetic change, heritable from generation to generation. Any of the mechanisms that result in alteration of bacterial genetic composition can operate. While mutation is frequently the cause, resistance to antimicrobial agents may be acquired through transfer of genetic material from one bacterium to another by transduction, transformation, or conjugation.

Mutation. Any large population of antibiotic-susceptible bacteria is likely to contain some mutants that are relatively resistant to the drug. Such variants can be isolated when the microorganisms are grown in medium containing the antibiotic, and analysis indicates that these strains have undergone a stable genetic change that may persist in the absence of the drug. There is, however, no evidence that these mutations are actually a result of exposure to the particular drug. Strains of some bacterial species isolated long before certain antibacterial agents were developed have subsequently been found to be naturally highly resistant to these drugs; such was the case with penicillinase-producing *Staph. aureus*. Such mutations are random events, and the resultant alteration is usually specific for a single drug or class of drugs.

Microorganisms that acquire resistance to a particular antimicrobial agent become important clinically, particularly when the use of an individual drug is widespread. Sensitive strains are suppressed and resistant ones multiply unimpaired; in time, resistant microorganisms predominate. This process is called *selection*.

The acquisition of resistance to antimicrobial agents can follow different temporal patterns. In some instances, a single-step mutation results in a high degree of resistance. For example, when *Escherichia coli* or *Staph. aureus* is exposed to rifampin, highly resistant mutants emerge that contain an altered DNA-dependent RNA polymerase that does not bind the drug (Wehrli, 1983). In other cases the emergence of resistant mutants may be a slow stepwise process, with each step conferring only slight alterations in susceptibility. As mentioned, this has occurred with the gonococcus, where there has been a gradual reduction in accessibility of penicillin G to target sites (penicillin-binding proteins) in the cell envelope of the organism.

Mutational changes that confer resistance to a drug may simultaneously alter virulence factors that affect the pathogenicity of the microorganism. For example, some strains of *Staph. aureus* that spontaneously develop resistance to rifampin also produce less catalase and are less virulent in animals. These resistant strains do not persist well in the environment. Strains of *Neisseria gonorrhoeae* that have acquired stepwise, low-level resistance to penicillin G are less pathogenic and rarely disseminate from the genital sites of primary infection. Such dissemination is more common with their penicillin-sensitive counterparts. Unfortunately, all antibiotic-resistant mutants are *not* less virulent—for example, penicillinase-producing *Staph. aureus*.

Transduction. This process occurs by the intervention of a bacteriophage (a virus that infects bacteria) that can carry bacterial DNA incorporated within its protein coat. If this genetic material includes a gene for drug resistance, a newly infected bacterial cell may become resistant to the agent and capable of passing the trait on to its progeny. Transduction is particularly important in the transfer of antibiotic resistance among strains of *Staph. aureus*, where some phages can carry plasmids (autonomously replicating pieces of extrachromosomal DNA) that code for penicillinase, while others transfer genetic information for resistance to erythromycin, tetracycline, or chloramphenicol.

Transformation. This method of transferring genetic information involves incorporation of DNA that is free in the environment into bacteria. Although some bacterial cells are capable of excreting transforming DNA during certain phases of growth, the importance of this method of transfer remains unknown.

Conjugation. The passage of genes from cell to cell by direct contact through a sex pilus or bridge is termed conjugation. This is now recognized as an extremely important mechanism for spread of antibiotic resistance, since DNA that codes for resistance to multiple drugs may be so transferred. Conjugation was first recognized in Japan in 1959 after an outbreak of bacillary dysentery caused by *Shigella flexneri* that was resistant to four different classes of antibiotics (Watanabe, 1966). Resistance could be easily transferred to sensitive strains of both *Shigella* and other Enterobacteriaceae. The transferable genetic material consists of two differ-

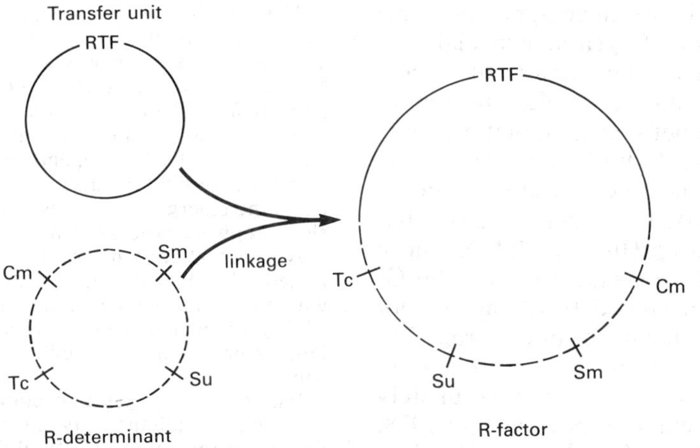

Figure 44–1. *Formation of an R-factor that contains genetic information for conferring resistance to tetracycline (Tc), sulfonamide (Su), streptomycin (Sm), and chloramphenicol (Cm).*

See text for description. (After Pratt and Fekety, 1986. Courtesy of Oxford University Press.)

ent sets of DNA sequences contained in plasmids (Figure 44–1). The first set of sequences codes for the actual resistance and is termed the R-determinant plasmid. For example, in the case of resistance to aminoglycosides or chloramphenicol, the R-determinant codes for the synthesis of drug-inactivating enzymes (Davies *et al.*, 1971). The second plasmid, termed the resistance transfer factor or RTF, contains information necessary for bacterial conjugation (Datta and Nugent, 1984). Each of these two plasmids can exist independently or they can combine to form a complete R factor, which can be disseminated by bacterial conjugation. Some genes that encode proteins that confer resistance to antimicrobial agents have the ability to "jump" from place to place in the bacterial genome (from plasmid to plasmid, from plasmid to chromosome, or vice versa) if the gene is flanked by so-called insertion sequences. A gene or genes with an insertion sequence at each end is termed a *transposon*. Such genes can be spread widely and quickly.

Transfer of such information by conjugation occurs predominantly among gram-negative bacilli, and resistance is conferred on a susceptible cell as a single event. Conjugation can take place in the intestinal tract between nonpathogenic and pathogenic microorganisms. While the efficiency of transfer is low *in vitro* and still lower *in vivo*, antibiotics can exert a powerful selective pressure to allow emergence of the resistant strain. The proportion of enteric bacteria that carry plasmids for multiple-drug resistance has thus risen slowly in the past 30 years. In some studies, more than 50% of persons have been found to carry multiply-resistant coliform bacilli containing R factors, and such bacteria have been isolated in large numbers from rivers containing untreated sewage. Multiply-resistant Enterobacteriaceae have become a problem worldwide, taxing the physician and creating a constant need for new antibiotics. In several situations where antibiotic usage has been controlled, the rate of emergence of these resistant strains was slowed; in some instances their incidence was actually reduced.

The worldwide emergence of *Haemophilus* and gonococci that produce beta-lactamase is a major therapeutic problem. The gene for production of this enzyme is carried on small plasmids. At least some of the gonococcal plasmids are similar in size to the *H. influenzae* gene, and a *Haemophilus* plasmid has been transferred to gonococci by conjugation *in vitro* (Sparling, 1978). Likewise, many gonococcal strains carry a conjugative plasmid that enables sexual transfer to other *Neisseria* and to *E. coli*. It is thus likely that beta-lactamase-producing gonococci initially obtained their plasmid from a *Haemophilus* species and may maintain the potential to transfer it to penicillin-sensitive species such as *N. meningitidis*. Fortunately, some of these genes are unstable, which may explain the reduction in the incidence of these resistant strains in England and their failure to become predominant in the United States.

SELECTION OF AN ANTIMICROBIAL AGENT

Optimal and judicious selection of antimicrobial agents for the therapy of infectious diseases is a complex procedure that requires clinical judgment and detailed knowledge of pharmacological and microbiological factors. Unfortunately, the decision to use antibiotics is frequently made lightly, without regard to the potential infecting microorganism or to the pharmacological features of the drug. Antibiotics are used in two general ways—as empiric therapy and as definitive therapy. When used as empiric, or initial, therapy, the antibiotic must "cover" all of the likely pathogens, since the infecting organism(s) has not yet been defined. Combination therapy or treatment with a single broad-spectrum agent is often employed. However, once the infecting microorganism is identified, definitive antimicrobial therapy is instituted—a narrow-spectrum, low-toxicity regimen to complete the course of treatment. When an antimicrobial agent is indicated, the goal is to choose a drug that is selectively active for the most likely infecting microorganism(s) and that has the least potential to cause toxicity or allergic reactions in the individual being treated (*see* Table 44–1).

The first decision to be made is whether administration of an antimicrobial agent is truly indicated. Many physicians reflexly associate fever with treatable infections and prescribe antimicrobial therapy without further evaluation. This practice is irrational and dangerous, since the diagnosis may be masked if cultures are not obtained prior to therapy and all antibiotics can cause serious toxicity. As noted above, injudicious use of antimicrobial agents can also result in the selection of resistant microorganisms. Of course, one does not always have the luxury of a definitive identification of a bacterial infection before treatment must be initiated. In the absence of a clear indication, antibiotics may often be used if disease is severe and if it seems likely that withholding therapy will result in failure to manage a potentially life-threatening infection.

Initiation of optimal empiric antibiotic therapy requires a knowledge of the most likely infecting microorganisms and their susceptibilities to antimicrobial drugs. A number of techniques are helpful in the selection of an antibiotic regimen. Importantly, the clinical picture may suggest the specific microorganism: the therapist must know the microorganisms most likely to cause specific infections in a given host. In addition, simple and rapid laboratory techniques are available for the examination of infected tissues. The most valuable and time-tested method for immediate identification of bacteria is the examination of the infected secretion or body fluid with Gram's stain. Tests such as this one help to narrow the list of potential pathogens and permit more rational selection of initial antibiotic therapy. However, in most situations, identification of the morphology of the infecting organism is not adequate to arrive at a specific bacteriological diagnosis, and the selection of a single narrow-spectrum antibiotic may be inappropriate, particularly if the infection is life threatening. Broad antimicrobial coverage is then indicated, pending isolation and identification of the microorganism. *Whenever the clinician is faced with initiating therapy on a presumptive bacteriological diagnosis, cultures of blood and certain other body fluids should be taken prior to the institution of drug therapy.* If the patient has been receiving antibiotics, then beta-lactamase should be added to the culture media or other mechanisms for removal of antibiotics ("antibiotic removal devices") should be employed. Definitive therapy most often requires that the regimen be changed to a more specific (narrow-spectrum) antimicrobial agent. Many factors need to be considered before this change is made.

Testing for Microbial Sensitivity to Antimicrobial Agents. There may be wide variations in the susceptibility of different strains of the same bacterial species to antibiotics. Essential to the choice of drug is information about the pattern of sensitivity of the infecting microorganism. Several tests are now available for determination of bacterial sensitivity to antimicrobial agents.

The most commonly used test of sensitivity to antimicrobial agents is the Kirby–Bauer or disc diffusion technique (Bauer *et al.*, 1966). Although it is simple to perform and relatively inexpensive, it provides only qualitative or semiquantitative information on the susceptibility of a given microorganism to a given antibiotic. The test is performed by applying commercially available filter-paper discs impregnated with specific quantities of the drug onto the surface of agar plates over which a culture of the microorganism has been streaked. After 18 hours of incubation, the size of a clear zone of inhibition around the disc is determined; this is related to the activity of the drug against the test strain.

Table 44–1. CURRENT USE OF ANTIMICROBIAL AGENTS IN THE THERAPY OF INFECTIONS

The presentation of choices of specific agents for the treatment of various infections is always provocative of discussion and disagreement because such choices often represent the distillate of personal experiences that may not duplicate those of others. In addition, the current availability of a number of drugs that are approximately equally effective makes an order of choice very difficult, if not impossible. To complicate matters, patterns of sensitivity of a number of microorganisms often vary with the hospital or clinic in which they are isolated; in some instances, this reflects a varying degree of exposure to specific agents. The material presented in this table represents not only the practice of the authors, based on their experience with the management of these infections, but also that of other experts in the United States. These drug selections represent initial therapy only. Each choice must be verified by testing the etiological isolate for sensitivity to antibiotics. It is important to stress that, as more information accumulates, as recently introduced drugs are used for longer periods, and as entirely new agents are developed, some of the recommendations will require modification not only in the order of choice but even in the specific drugs that are suggested.

I. GRAM-POSITIVE COCCI	DISEASES		DRUG ORDER OF CHOICE		
			First	*Second* [1]	*Third* [1]
Staphylococcus aureus *	Abscesses Bacteremia Endocarditis Pneumonia Meningitis Osteomyelitis Cellulitis Other	Pencillin G–sensitive [2]	Pencillin G	A cephalosporin (G1) [3] Vancomycin	Clindamycin [4,5] Erythromycin [4,5] Trimethoprim-sulfamethoxazole + rifampin [6] Ciprofloxacin + rifampin [6]
		Pencillin G–resistant	A penicillinase-resistant penicillin	A cephalosporin (G1) [3] Vancomycin	
		Methicillin-resistant	Vancomycin [7]	Ciprofloxacin + rifampin	Trimethoprim-sulfamethoxazole + rifampin [6]
Streptococcus pyogenes (group A)	Pharyngitis Scarlet fever Otitis media, sinusitis Cellulitis Erysipelas Pneumonia Bacteremia Other systemic infections		Penicillin G Penicillin V	A cephalosporin (G1) [3,8] Erythromycin	Vancomycin [8]
Streptococcus * (viridans group)	Endocarditis (bacteremia)		Penicillin G [9] ± gentamicin or streptomycin	A cephalosporin (G1) [3]	Vancomycin
Streptococcus agalactiae (group B)	Bacteremia		Ampicillin or penicillin G [10] ± an aminoglycoside	A cephalosporin (G1) [3]	Erythromycin
	Meningitis			A cephalosporin (G3) [3]	Chloramphenicol [11]

Streptococcus bovis	Endocarditis Bacteremia	*See* viridans streptococci	—	—
Streptococcus * (anaerobic species)	Bacteremia Endocarditis Brain and other abscesses Sinusitis	Penicillin G [10]	A cephalosporin (G1) [3] Clindamycin [4,5]	Chloramphenicol [11] Erythromycin [4,5]
Streptococcus pneumoniae * (pneumococcus)	Pneumonia Arthritis Sinusitis Otitis	Penicillin G or V	A cephalosporin (G1) [3] Erythromycin	Chloramphenicol Clindamycin Trimethoprim-sulfamethoxazole
	Meningitis or other serious infections	Penicillin G [10]	Cefuroxime or a third-generation cephalosporin	Chloramphenicol [11]
Enterococcus	Endocarditis or other serious infections (bacteremia)	Gentamicin or streptomycin + penicillin G or ampicillin	Vancomycin + gentamicin	—
	Urinary tract infection	Ampicillin or penicillin G	Vancomycin	Ciprofloxacin or norfloxacin Nitrofurantoin
II. GRAM-NEGATIVE COCCI				
Neisseria gonorrhoeae [12] (gonococcus)	Penicillinase-producing	Ceftriaxone	Cefuroxime or cefoxitin Spectinomycin	Ciprofloxacin
	Penicillin-sensitive	Ampicillin + probenecid or amoxicillin + probenecid Penicillin G + probenecid	Ceftriaxone A tetracycline	Erythromycin Spectinomycin Ciprofloxacin

* All strains must be examined *in vitro* for sensitivity to various antimicrobial agents.

[1] Drugs included for second and third choices are (a) indicated in patients hypersensitive to equally or more effective agents, (b) potentially more dangerous than equally active drugs, (c) less likely to produce the desired therapeutic response, or (d) in need, in some cases, of further study to allow a valid evaluation of their efficacy.

[2] Minimal inhibitory concentration (MIC) is less than 0.2 μg/ml.

[3] G1 and G3 designate first- and third-generation cephalosporins, respectively. If no generation is specified, certain agents may be preferable to others (*see* Chapter 46). Therapeutic concentrations of most cephalosporins may not be achieved in the cerebrospinal fluid (CSF) (exceptions include cefotaxime, ceftriaxone, and ceftizoxime), and alternative agents should be used to treat infections of the central nervous system (CNS).

[4] Therapeutic concentrations are not achieved in the CSF, and alternative agents should be used to treat infections of the CNS.

[5] Not indicated for endocarditis; only bactericidal drugs should be used.

[6] Rifampin is highly active against most strains of *S. aureus*, including some that are resistant to methicillin. Since resistance develops rapidly (one-step mutation) during therapy, a second active drug, such as trimethoprim-sulfamethoxazole or ciprofloxacin, should be used concurrently.

[7] Vancomycin is the only antimicrobial agent proven to be effective for treatment of serious infections due to methicillin-resistant *S. aureus*.

[8] Especially for bacteremia and endocarditis.

[9] Therapy depends on host and bacteria: (a) age > 65 years: penicillin G (4 weeks); (b) age < 65 years, with normal auditory and renal function: penicillin G (2 weeks) + streptomycin or gentamicin (2 weeks); (c) nutritionally deficient strains of viridans streptococci: penicillin G (4 weeks) + streptomycin or gentamicin (2 weeks).

[10] Large doses of penicillin G may be required.

[11] Chloramphenicol is effective for infection of the CNS in patients who are allergic to beta-lactam antibiotics.

Table 44–1. CURRENT USE OF ANTIMICROBIAL AGENTS IN THE THERAPY OF INFECTIONS (Continued)

II. GRAM-NEGATIVE COCCI	DISEASES	DRUG ORDER OF CHOICE		
		First	*Second* [1]	*Third* [1]
Neisseria meningitidis (meningococcus)	Meningitis Bacteremia	Penicillin G	Cefuroxime or a third-generation cephalosporin	Chloramphenicol [11]
	Carrier state (posttreatment)	Rifampin	Ceftriaxone	Minocycline Ciprofloxacin
Branhamella catarrhalis	Otitis Sinusitis Pneumonia	A beta-lactamase inhibitor + ampicillin or amoxicillin	Trimethoprim-sulfamethoxazole Cefuroxime Cefaclor	Ciprofloxacin Tetracycline Erythromycin
III. GRAM-POSITIVE BACILLI				
Bacillus anthracis *	"Malignant pustule" Pneumonia	Penicillin G	Erythromycin A tetracycline	A cephalosporin (G1) [3] Chloramphenicol
Corynebacterium diphtheriae [13]	Pharyngitis Laryngotracheitis Pneumonia Other local lesions	Penicillin G	Erythromycin	A cephalosporin (G1) [3] Clindamycin Rifampin
	Carrier state	Erythromycin	Penicillin G	—
Corynebacterium species *, aerobic and anaerobic (diphtheroids)	Endocarditis Infected foreign bodies Bacteremia	Penicillin G ± an aminoglycoside Vancomycin	Rifampin + penicillin G Ampicillin-sulbactam	—
Listeria monocytogenes	Meningitis	Ampicillin or penicillin G [10] ± gentamicin	Trimethoprim-sulfamethoxazole	—
	Bacteremia			A tetracycline Erythromycin Chloramphenicol
Erysipelothrix rhusiopathiae	Erysipeloid	Penicillin G	Erythromycin A tetracycline	Chloramphenicol
Clostridium perfringens * and other species	Gas gangrene [14]	Penicillin G	Cefoxitin A cephalosporin (G3) [3] Clindamycin	Imipenem Chloramphenicol A tetracycline
Clostridium tetani	Tetanus [14]	Penicillin G [15]	A tetracycline	Erythromycin
Clostridium difficile	Antibiotic-associated colitis	Vancomycin (oral) Metronidazole (oral)	Bacitracin (oral)	—

IV. GRAM-NEGATIVE BACILLI				
Escherichia coli *	Urinary tract infection [16]	Trimethoprim-sulfamethoxazole Ampicillin + an aminoglycoside	A cephalosporin [3] A penicillin + a penicillinase inhibitor [17] An aminoglycoside Norfloxacin or ciprofloxacin A sulfonamide	Aztreonam Nitrofurantoin A tetracycline
	Other infections Bacteremia	Ampicillin + an aminoglycoside A cephalosporin [3,18]	An aminoglycoside A penicillin + a penicillinase inhibitor [17] Aztreonam	Trimethoprim-sulfamethoxazole
Enterobacter species	Urinary tract [19] and other infections	A cephalosporin (G3) [3] An aminoglycoside [20]	A broad-spectrum penicillin [21] Aztreonam	Trimethoprim-sulfamethoxazole Imipenem
Proteus mirabilis *	Urinary tract [19] and other infections	Ampicillin or amoxicillin	A cephalosporin [3] An aminoglycoside [20]	—
Proteus, other species *	Urinary tract [19] and other infections	An aminoglycoside [20] A cephalosporin (G3) [3]	A broad-spectrum penicillin [21] A penicillin + a penicillinase inhibitor [17]	Aztreonam Imipenem
Pseudomonas aeruginosa *	Urinary tract infection [19]	A broad-spectrum penicillin [21] Norfloxacin or ciprofloxacin	An aminoglycoside [20] Aztreonam	—
	Pneumonia [22] Bacteremia [22]	A broad-spectrum penicillin [21] + an aminoglycoside	An antipseudomonal cephalosporin [23] + an aminoglycoside Ticarcillin	Aztreonam Imipenem

[12] All strains of gonococci should be considered to be penicillinase-producers until proven otherwise.

[13] Antibiotics alone do not alter the clinical course of diphtheria, but drugs can eradicate the carrier state.

[14] Adequate debridement is absolutely essential.

[15] Ten to 20 million units of penicillin G daily, with debridement and adsorbed tetanus toxoid.

[16] Trimethoprim-sulfamethoxazole, quinolones, and urinary tract antiseptics are useful for acute urinary tract infections, especially cystitis, in the patient without obstructive uropathy or in whom the disease has not become chronic. These agents also prove useful for chronic suppressive therapy in patients with recurrent urinary tract infection. Some clinicians prefer to reserve the antibiotics, such as ampicillin and aminoglycosides, for cases in which there are systemic manifestations—particularly in acute pyelonephritis. In some areas, 20 to 40% of *E. coli* infections acquired in the community are resistant to ampicillin.

[17] Amoxicillin-clavulanate or ampicillin-sulbactam or ticarcillin-clavulanate.

[18] An increasing number of strains are becoming resistant to the first- and second-generation cephalosporins.

[19] Urinary tract infections caused by microorganisms other than *E. coli* are less usual and frequently occur in the setting of obstructive uropathy or an indwelling urinary catheter, or following recurrent infections and the use of antibiotics. Therapy must be individualized but is frequently unsuccessful unless the underlying condition is corrected.

[20] Gentamicin, tobramycin, amikacin, or netilmicin only.

[21] Ticarcillin, piperacillin, mezlocillin, or azlocillin.

[22] Although single-drug therapy with an antipseudomonal beta-lactam antibiotic or an aminoglycoside is adequate for some infections caused by *P. aeruginosa*, the combination of the two classes of drug is recommended for therapy of serious infections, especially in the neutropenic patient or in the individual with pneumonia.

Table 44–1. CURRENT USE OF ANTIMICROBIAL AGENTS IN THE THERAPY OF INFECTIONS (Continued)

IV. GRAM-NEGATIVE BACILLI	DISEASES	DRUG ORDER OF CHOICE		
		First	*Second* [1]	*Third* [1]
Klebsiella pneumoniae *	Urinary tract infection [19]	A cephalosporin [3]	An aminoglycoside Mezlocillin or piperacillin	Trimethoprim-sulfamethoxazole
	Pneumonia	A cephalosporin [3,18] + an aminoglycoside	Mezlocillin or piperacillin ± an aminoglycoside Aztreonam	A penicillin + a penicillinase inhibitor [17] Imipenem
Salmonella *	Typhoid fever Paratyphoid fever Bacteremia	Trimethoprim-sulfamethoxazole Chloramphenicol	Cefoperazone or ceftriaxone	Ampicillin [24]
	Acute gastroenteritis	Norfloxacin or ciprofloxacin	No therapy or trimethoprim-sulfamethoxazole	—
Shigella *	Acute gastroenteritis	Ciprofloxacin or norfloxacin	Trimethoprim-sulfamethoxazole	Ampicillin [24]
Serratia *	Variety of nosocomial and opportunistic infections	Imipenem Cefoxitin, cefotetan, or a third-generation cephalosporin	A broad-spectrum penicillin [21] Aztreonam	Ticarcillin-clavulanate
Acinetobacter *	Various nosocomial infections	Imipenem An aminoglycoside [20]	A cephalosporin (G3) [3]	—
Haemophilus influenzae *	Otitis media Sinusitis Bronchitis	Trimethoprim-sulfamethoxazole Amoxicillin-clavulanate	Cefaclor or cefuroxime axetil Amoxicillin or ampicillin [24]	Ciprofloxacin
	Epiglottitis Pneumonia Meningitis	Cefuroxime or a third-generation cephalosporin Chloramphenicol	Ampicillin [24] Ampicillin-sulbactam [25]	Trimethoprim-sulfamethoxazole
Haemophilus ducreyi	Chancroid	Trimethoprim-sulfamethoxazole Erythromycin	Ceftriaxone Rifampin	A sulfonamide A tetracycline
Brucella	Brucellosis	Doxycycline + rifampin	Trimethoprim-sulfamethoxazole ± gentamicin [26]	Chloramphenicol
Yersinia pestis	Plague	Streptomycin ± a tetracycline	A tetracycline	Chloramphenicol
Yersinia enterocolitica	Yersiniosis	No treatment or trimethoprim-sulfamethoxazole [27]	A cephalosporin (G3) [3,28]	—
	Sepsis	An aminoglycoside Chloramphenicol		

Francisella tularensis	Tularemia	Streptomycin	A tetracycline	Chloramphenicol Ciprofloxacin
Pasturella multocida	Wound infection (animal bites) Abscesses Bacteremia Meningitis	Penicillin G	A tetracycline [4] A first-generation cephalosporin or ceftriaxone	Amoxicillin-clavulanate
Vibrio cholerae	Cholera	A tetracycline	Trimethoprim-sulfamethoxazole	Chloramphenicol Ciprofloxacin
Flavobacterium meningosepticum	Meningitis	Vancomycin	Trimethoprim-sulfamethoxazole	Rifampin
Pseudomonas mallei	Glanders	Streptomycin + a tetracycline	Streptomycin + chloramphenicol	—
Pseudomonas pseudomallei	Melioidosis	Trimethoprim-sulfamethoxazole	Chloramphenicol	—
Campylobacter jejuni *	Enteritis	Ciprofloxacin or norfloxacin	Erythromycin	A tetracycline Clindamycin
Bacteroides species [29] (oral, pharyngeal)	Oral disease Sinusitis Brain abscess Lung abscess	Penicillin G [24,30] Clindamycin [4]	Metronidazole [30] Cefoxitin, cefotetan, or ceftizoxime	Chloramphenicol [30] Erythromycin A tetracycline
Bacteroides fragilis	Brain abscess Lung abscess Intraabdominal abscess Empyema Bacteremia Endocarditis	Metronidazole [30,31] Clindamycin [4]	Cefoxitin or cefotetan Ticarcillin-clavulanate or ampicillin-sulbactam	Chloramphenicol [30] Imipenem
Fusobacterium nucleatum	Ulcerative pharyngitis Lung abscess, empyema Genital infections Gingivitis	Penicillin G Clindamycin	Metronidazole A cephalosporin (G1) [3]	Erythromycin A tetracycline Chloramphenicol Cefoxitin

[23] Cephalosporins that are most active against *P. aeruginosa* include ceftazidime and cefoperazone, but resistance may develop during therapy.
[24] Many strains are now resistant to ampicillin, amoxicillin, and penicillin G.
[25] Experience with ampicillin-sulbactam in the treatment of meningitis is limited.
[26] Gentamicin added to therapy for approximately first 5 days.
[27] Data on treatment are sparse, but therapy with trimethoprim-sulfamethoxazole has been successful in some cases.
[28] Activity *in vitro* is good.
[29] Isolates should be checked for beta-lactamase production.
[30] Preferred antibiotic for CNS infections.
[31] Metronidazole is bactericidal against *B. fragilis* and is thus recommended in endocarditis.

Table 44–1. CURRENT USE OF ANTIMICROBIAL AGENTS IN THE THERAPY OF INFECTIONS (Continued)

IV. GRAM-NEGATIVE BACILLI	DISEASES	DRUG ORDER OF CHOICE		
		First	*Second* [1]	*Third* [1]
Calymmatobacterium granulomatis	Granuloma inguinale	A tetracycline	Trimethoprim-sulfamethoxazole	—
Streptobacillus moniliformis	Bacteremia Arthritis Endocarditis Abscesses	Penicillin G	Streptomycin A tetracycline	Erythromycin Chloramphenicol
Legionella pneumophila	Legionnaires' disease	Erythromycin ± rifampin	Ciprofloxacin Trimethoprim-sulfamethoxazole	—
V. ACID-FAST BACILLI				
Mycobacterium tuberculosis [32]	Pulmonary, miliary, renal, meningeal, and other tuberculous infections (*see* Chapter 49)	Isoniazid + rifampin + pyrazinamide [33]	Isoniazid + rifampin + ethambutol	Rifampin + ethambutol ± streptomycin
Mycobacterium leprae	Leprosy (*see* Chapter 49)	Dapsone + rifampin	Clofazimine	—
VI. SPIROCHETES				
Treponema pallidum	Syphilis	Penicillin G	Ceftriaxone	A tetracycline
Treponema pertenue	Yaws	Penicillin G Streptomycin	A tetracycline	—
Borrelia burgdorferi (Lyme disease)	Erythema chronica migrans—skin	A tetracycline	Penicillin G	Ceftriaxone
	Stage 2—neurological, cardiac, arthritis	Penicillin G [10]	Ceftriaxone	Tetracycline
Borrelia recurrentis	Relapsing fever	A tetracycline	Erythromycin	Penicillin G
Leptospira	Weil's disease Meningitis	Penicillin G [10]	A tetracycline [34]	—

VII. ACTINOMYCETES				
Actinomyces israelii	Cervicofacial, abdominal, thoracic, and other lesions	Penicillin G [10] Ampicillin	A tetracycline	Erythromycin
Nocardia asteroides *	Pulmonary lesions Brain abscess Lesions of other organs	Trimethoprim-sulfamethoxazole A sulfonamide	Minocycline ± a sulfonamide	—
VIII. MISCELLANEOUS AGENTS				
Ureaplasma urealyticum	Nonspecific urethritis	A tetracycline [35]	Erythromycin	—
Mycoplasma pneumoniae	"Atypical pneumonia"	Erythromycin A tetracycline	—	—
Rickettsia	Typhus fever Murine typhus Brill's disease Rocky Mountain spotted fever Q fever Rickettsialpox	Chloramphenicol A tetracycline	—	—
Chlamydia psittaci	Psittacosis (ornithosis)	A tetracycline	Chloramphenicol	—
Chlamydia trachomatis	Lymphogranuloma venereum	A tetracycline	Erythromycin A sulfonamide	—
	Trachoma	Doxycycline [36]	Erythromycin	A sulfonamide
	Inclusion conjunctivitis (blennorrhea)	Doxycycline	Erythromycin	A sulfonamide
	Nonspecific urethritis	A tetracycline	Erythromycin	A sulfonamide
Chlamydia pneumoniae	Pneumonia	A tetracycline	Erythromycin	—
Pneumocystis carinii	Pneumonia in impaired host	Trimethoprim-sulfamethoxazole	Pentamidine (parenteral)	Dapsone + trimethoprim Pentamidine (aerosolized)

[32] Second- and third-choice drugs are available for the treatment of disease caused by *M. tuberculosis*; their use, which is complex, is discussed in Chapter 49. The choice of drugs for treatment of infections with atypical mycobacteria is also discussed in Chapter 49.

[33] Use isoniazid, rifampin, and pyrazinamide plus ethambutol when primary resistance is likely.

[34] Some physicians favor a tetracycline over penicillin G as the drug of first choice.

[35] Six to 10% of ureaplasma are resistant to tetracycline.

[36] A tetracycline may be given orally alone, or it may be applied locally in the conjunctival sac while a sulfonamide is being administered orally.

Table 44–1. CURRENT USE OF ANTIMICROBIAL AGENTS IN THE THERAPY OF INFECTIONS (Continued)

IX. FUNGI	DISEASES	DRUG ORDER OF CHOICE		
		First	*Second* [1]	*Third* [1]
Candida species	Cutaneous or vaginal thrush	An imidazole [37] Nystatin [37]	Ketoconazole or fluconazole	—
	Oral thrush	Clotrimazole Nystatin	Ketoconazole or fluconazole	—
	Deep infection	Amphotericin B ± flucytosine	—	—
Coccidioides immitis	Disseminated (nonmeningeal)	Amphotericin B	Ketoconazole or itraconazole	—
	Meningitis	Amphotericin B [38]	Miconazole [38]	—
Histoplasma capsulatum	Chronic pulmonary disease	Ketoconazole or itraconazole	Amphotericin B	—
	Disseminated	Amphotericin B	Ketoconazole	—
Blastomyces dermatitidis	All	Ketoconazole or itraconazole	Amphotericin B	—
Paracoccidioides brasiliensis	All	Ketoconazole or itraconazole	Amphotericin B followed by a sulfonamide	—
Sporothrix schenckii	Cutaneous	Iodide	Itraconazole	—
	Extracutaneous	Amphotericin B	—	—
Aspergillus species	Invasive	Amphotericin B	Itraconazole	—
Agents of mucormycosis	All	Amphotericin B	—	—
Cryptococcus neoformans	Pulmonary	None or amphotericin B	—	—
	Meningitis	Amphotericin B ± flucytosine	Fluconazole	—

X. VIRUSES				
Herpes simplex virus	Genital disease Mucocutaneous HSV in immunocompromised host	Acyclovir	—	—
	Keratoconjunctivitis	Trifluridine	Vidarabine	Idoxuridine
	Encephalitis	Acyclovir	Vidarabine	—
	Neonatal HSV	Vidarabine	Acyclovir	—
	Mucocutaneous HSV in immunocompromised host	Acyclovir	—	—
Varicella zoster virus	Herpes zoster or varicella in immunocompromised host	Acyclovir	Vidarabine	—
	Herpes zoster in normal host	Acyclovir	—	—
Cytomegalovirus	Retinitis in patients with AIDS	Ganciclovir	Foscarnet	—
Human immunodeficiency virus	AIDS HIV antibody positive and CD4 count less than 200/mm^3	Zidovudine	—	—
Influenza A	Influenza	Amantadine	Rimantadine	—
Respiratory syncytial virus	Pneumonia and bronchiolitis of infancy	Ribavirin	—	—
Human papilloma virus	Genital papilloma	Inteferon alfa	—	—

[37] Topical application.
[38] Intrathecal.

Standards for sensitivity vary for each microorganism, and they are based on the concentration of drug that can safely be achieved in plasma without producing toxicity. Even though the concentration of the antibiotic in plasma is the standard used for these tests, it may not always reflect the drug concentration at the site of the infection. There are several notable exceptions where the Kirby–Bauer disc diffusion test does not accurately predict therapeutic effectiveness: (1) methicillin-resistant *Staph. aureus,* which may appear to be sensitive to cephalosporins; (2) enterococci, which may appear to be sensitive to cephalosporins and trimethoprim–sulfamethoxazole; and (3) *Shigella* species, which may appear to be sensitive to cephalosporins. These drugs have been proven *not* to be useful in such infections.

Tests that are quantitatively more reliable involve serial dilutions of antibiotics in solid agar or broth media containing a culture of the test microorganism. The lowest concentration of the agent that prevents visible growth after 18 to 24 hours of incubation is known as the minimal inhibitory concentration (MIC), and the lowest concentration that sterilizes the medium or results in a 99.9% decline in bacterial numbers is known as the minimal bactericidal concentration (MBC). The latter test is used only in special instances where very precise knowledge of the ability of a given antimicrobial agent to kill a specific clinical isolate is required, as in the therapy of bacterial endocarditis.

In addition to tests of antimicrobial activity *in vitro,* it would be valuable to have a test to predict efficacy of antimicrobial treatment. One test that has been used for many years is a measure of the bactericidal activity of the patient's serum against the infecting microorganism. This test has been used extensively to monitor therapy in patients with bacterial endocarditis and, more recently, in neutropenic patients with disseminated infections (Klastersky and Staquet, 1982). The test simply estimates the dilution of the patient's serum that produces a bactericidal effect. Interpretation is controversial because standardized methods have only recently been discussed (Wolfson and Swartz, 1985). Some physicians strive to achieve a bactericidal titer in serum of 1:8, taken at the peak of the drug concentration *in vivo,* in patients with endocarditis or neutropenia. However, attempts to correlate efficacy with this titer have not always supported this concept (Coleman *et al.,* 1982; Hackbarth *et al.,* 1986).

Pharmacokinetic Factors. Although the knowledge that an antibiotic is active *in vitro* against the infecting microorganism is critical, it is not the only factor to be considered. Successful therapy depends upon achieving antibacterial activity at the site of the infection without significant toxicity to the host. To accomplish this, several pharmacokinetic and host factors must be evaluated.

The location of the infection may, to a large extent, dictate the choice of drug and the route of administration. The minimal drug concentration achieved at the infected site should be at least equal to the MIC for the infecting organism, although in most instances it is advisable to achieve multiples of this concentration if possible. However, there is evidence to suggest that even subinhibitory concentrations of antibiotics may enhance phagocytosis (Yourtee and Root, 1984) and tip the balance in favor of the host. Although these and related observations may explain why some infections are cured even when inhibitory concentrations are not achieved, it should be the aim of antimicrobial therapy to produce antibacterial concentrations of drug at the site of infection during the dosing interval. This can only be achieved if the pharmacokinetic and pharmacodynamic principles presented in Chapters 1 and 2 are understood and employed.

Access of antibiotics to sites of infection depends on multiple factors. If the infection is in the cerebrospinal fluid (CSF), the drug must pass the blood–brain barrier, and many antimicrobial agents that are polar at physiological pH do so poorly; some, such as penicillin G, are actively transported out of the CSF by an anion transport mechanism in the choroid plexus. For example, the concentrations of penicillins and cephalosporins in the CSF are usually only 0.5 to 5% of steady-state concentrations determined simultaneously in plasm. However, the integrity of the blood–brain barrier is diminished during active bacterial infection; tight junctions in cerebral capillaries open, leading to a marked increase in the penetration of even polar drugs (Quagliarello *et al.,* 1986). As the infection is eradicated and the inflammatory reaction subsides, penetration reverts toward normal. Since this may occur while viable microorganisms persist in the CSF, drug dosage should not be reduced as the patient improves until the CSF is presumed or proven to be sterile.

Penetration of drugs into infected loci almost always depends on passive diffusion. The rate of penetration is thus proportional to the concentration of free drug in the plasma or extracellular fluid. Drugs that

are extensively bound to protein thus may not penetrate to the same extent as do congeners that are bound to a lesser extent.

As a practical matter, it seems reasonable to attempt to achieve antibacterial activity at the site of infection for a major portion of the dosing interval. However, controversy exists as to whether the therapeutic effect achieved from relatively constant antibacterial activity is superior to that from high peak concentrations followed by periods of subinhibitory activity. Knowledge of the time required for bacteria to begin to divide after the concentration of drug has dropped below the MIC is required, and this varies from drug to drug and microorganism to microorganism. While studies in animals with meningitis suggest that pulse dosing (intermittent administration) of beta-lactam antibiotics may be more efficient (equivalent efficacy from less drug) (Täuber *et al.*, 1989), it appears that constant activity is superior in other experimental infections. Recent experimental studies suggest that aminoglycosides are at least as efficacious and are less toxic when given in a single, large daily dose than when given more frequently (Kapusnik *et al.*, 1988; Wood *et al.*, 1988). Studies in patients also suggest that continuous administration of aminoglycosides may cause unnecessary toxicity (Keating *et al.*, 1979).

Knowledge of the status of the individual patient's mechanisms for elimination of drugs is also essential, especially when excessive plasma or tissue concentrations of the drugs cause serious toxicity. Most antimicrobial agents and their metabolites are eliminated primarily by the kidneys. Specific nomograms are available to facilitate adjustment of dosage of many such agents in patients with renal insufficiency. These are discussed in the chapters dealing with the individual drugs and in Appendix II. One must be particularly careful when using aminoglycosides, vancomycin, or flucytosine in patients with impaired renal function, since these drugs are completely eliminated by renal mechanisms and their toxicity appears to correlate with their concentrations in plasma and tissue. Furthermore, a vicious cycle may ensue if care is not exercised, since the toxicity of certain of these drugs is particularly manifested on the kidney.

For drugs that are metabolized or excreted by the liver (erythromycin, chloramphenicol, metronidazole, clindamycin), dosages must be reduced in patients with hepatic failure. Rifampin and isoniazid also have prolonged half-lives in patients with cirrhosis. If there is infection in the biliary tract, hepatic disease or biliary obstruction may reduce the access of the drug to the site of infection. This has been shown to occur with ampicillin and other drugs that are normally excreted into the bile.

Route of Administration. The discussion of choice of routes of administration that appears in Chapter 1 of course applies to antimicrobial agents. While oral administration is preferred whenever possible, parenteral administration of antibiotics is usually recommended in seriously ill patients in whom predictable concentrations of drug must be achieved. Specific factors that govern the choice of route of administration for individual agents are discussed in the chapters that follow.

Host Factors. Innate host factors, which may appear to be completely unrelated to the infectious disorder being treated, are often the prime determinants not only of the type of drug selected but also of its dosage, route of administration, risk and nature of untoward effects, and therapeutic effectiveness.

Host Defense Mechanisms. An important determinant of the therapeutic effectiveness of antimicrobial agents is the functional state of the host's defense mechanisms. Both humoral and cellular immunity are important. Inadequacy of type, quality, and quantity of the immunoglobulins, alteration of the cellular immune system, or either a qualitative or, most important, a quantitative defect in phagocytic cells may result in therapeutic failure despite the use of otherwise appropriate and effective drugs. Frequently, successful treatment of infection with antimicrobial agents may be achieved by merely halting multiplication of the microorganisms (a bacteriostatic effect). When the defenses of the host are impaired, this action may be inadequate. In infections where host defenses have been shown to be inefficient, rapidly bactericidal antimicrobial agents have been shown to be essential for cure. Examples include bacterial endocarditis, where phagocytic cells are excluded from the infected site; bacterial meningitis, where phagocytic cells are ineffective because of lack of opsonins; and disseminated gram-negative bacillary infections, especially pseudomonal infections in neutropenic patients, where the total mass of phagocytic cells is reduced. Patients with acquired immunodeficiency syndrome (AIDS) have impaired cellular immune responses, and therapy for various opportunistic infections in these patients is usually suppressive but not curative. For example, most patients with bacteremia due to *Salmonella* will respond to conventional therapy; however, most AIDS patients with this infection will relapse even after prolonged treatment (Jacobson *et al.,* 1989).

Local Factors. Cure of an infection with antibiotics depends on an understanding of how local factors at the site of infection affect the antimicrobial activity of the drug. Pus, which consists of phagocytes, cellular debris, fibrin, and protein, binds aminoglycosides and vancomycin, resulting in a reduction in their antimicrobial activity (Bryant, 1987). Large accumulations of hemoglobin in infected hematomas can bind penicillins and tetracyclines and may thus reduce their effectiveness (Craig and Kunin, 1976). The pH in abscess cavities and in other confined infected sites (pleural space, CSF, and urine) is usually low, resulting in a marked loss of antimicrobial activity of aminoglycosides, erythromycin, and clindamycin (Strausbaugh and Sande, 1978). However, some drugs, such as chlortetracycline, nitrofurantoin, and methenamine, are more active in such an acidic environment. The anaerobic conditions found in abscess cavities may also impair activity of the aminoglycosides (Verklin and Mandell, 1977). Penetration of antimicrobial agents into infected areas such as abscess cavities is impaired, since the vascular supply is reduced. Successful therapy of abscesses usually requires drainage.

The presence of a foreign body in an infected site markedly reduces the likelihood of effective antimicrobial therapy. This factor has become increasingly important in the present era of prosthetic cardiac valves, prosthetic joints, pacemakers, vascular prostheses, and various vascular and central nervous system (CNS) shunts. The prosthesis is apparently perceived by the phagocytic cells as foreign. In an attempt to phagocytize and destroy it, degranulation occurs, resulting in the depletion of intracellular bactericidal substances. Thus, these phagocytes are relatively inefficient in killing bacterial pathogens; in fact, microbes may even reside within phagocytes, protected from most antimicrobial agents (Zimmerli *et al.,* 1984). In addition, microbes may attach to foreign bodies by elaboration of a glycocalyx substrate. When embedded in this substrate, they are often relatively resistant to the actions of antimicrobial agents. Infections associated with foreign bodies are thus characterized by frequent relapses and failure, even with long-term, high-dose therapy with antibiotics. Successful therapy usually requires removal of the foreign material. Other infectious agents that reside within phagocytic cells (intracellular parasites) may also be relatively resistant to the action of antimicrobial agents, since many of these drugs penetrate into cells only poorly. This may be a problem in infections with *Salmonella, Brucella, Toxoplasma, Listeria,* and *Mycobacterium,* and, in some instances, even in infections caused by *Staph. aureus*. Rifampin is one drug that is very soluble in lipid, penetrates cells well, and can kill many intraleukocytic microbes.

Another interesting twist that may influence the efficacy of antimicrobial therapy is the adverse effect of some of these agents on various host immune responses; these include leukocyte chemotaxis, lymphocyte and monocyte transformation, antibody production, phagocytosis, and the microbicidal action of polymorphonuclear leukocytes (Mandell, 1982). While the clinical significance of this immunosuppression is not known, these observations should help discourage the indiscriminate use of antibiotics.

Age. The age of the patient is an important determinant of pharmacokinetic properties of antimicrobial agents (*see* Chapter 1). Mechanisms of elimination, especially renal excretion and hepatic biotransformation, are poorly developed in the newborn; this is particularly true of the premature infant. Failure to make adjustments for such differences can have disastrous consequences (*e.g.*, *see* discussion of the "gray baby syndrome," caused by chloramphenicol, in Chapter 48). Elderly patients may also have significantly reduced rates of creatinine clearance and drug metabolism. Also, elderly patients are particularly susceptible to the ototoxic effects of aminoglycosides.

Developmental factors may also determine the *type* of untoward response to a drug. Tetracyclines bind avidly to developing teeth and bones, and their use in young children can result in retardation of bone growth and discoloration or hypoplasia of tooth enamel. Kernicterus may follow the use of sulfonamides in newborn infants because this class of drugs competes effectively with bilirubin for binding sites on plasma albumin. Achlorhydria in young children and in the elderly (or antacid therapy) may alter absorption of orally administered antimicrobial agents (*e.g.*, increased absorption of penicillin G and decreased absorption of ketoconazole).

Genetic Factors. Certain genetic or metabolic abnormalities must be considered when prescribing antibiotics. A number of drugs, including the sulfonamides, nitrofurantoin, chloramphenicol, and nalidixic acid, may produce acute hemolysis in patients with glucose-6-phosphate dehydrogenase deficiency; more common in black males, the defect is also occasionally found in Caucasians. Patients who acetylate isoniazid rapidly may have suboptimal concentrations of the drug in plasma.

Pregnancy. Pregnancy imposes an increased risk of reaction to some antimicrobial agents for both mother and fetus. For example, hearing loss in the child has been associated with administration of streptomycin to the mother during pregnancy. Tetracyclines can affect the bones and teeth of the fetus and can also be particularly toxic to the pregnant female. Pregnant women receiving these drugs may develop fatal acute fatty necrosis of the liver, pancreatitis, and associated renal damage. Pregnancy may also affect the pharmacokinetics of various antibiotics.

The lactating female can pass antimicrobial agents to her nursing child. Both nalidixic acid and sulfonamides in breast milk have been associated with hemolysis in children with glucose-6-phosphate dehydrogenase deficiency. In addition, sulfonamides, even in the small amounts received from breast milk, may predispose the nursing child to kernicterus (Vorherr, 1974).

Drug Allergy. Antibiotics, especially the beta-lactam derivatives and their degradation products, are notorious for provoking allergic reactions in man. Patients with a history of atopic allergy seem particularly susceptible to the development of these reactions. The sulfonamides, trimethoprim, nitrofurantoin, and erythromycin have particularly been associated with hypersensitivity reactions, especially rash. Certain viral infections, especially that caused by the Epstein–Barr virus (mononucleosis), dramatically increase the frequency of rash in response to ampicillin and amoxicillin, but this does not imply true allergy to these drugs. When use of a penicillin is contemplated, a history of anaphylaxis (immediate reaction) or hives and laryngeal edema (accelerated reaction) precludes the use of the drug in all but extreme, life-threatening situations. Skin testing, particularly of the penicillins, has some value in predicting the life-threatening reactions. However, the controversy over the utility of such tests is only partly resolved (*see* Chapter 46). It should also be noted that antimicrobial agents and other drugs can cause "drug fever," which can be mistaken for a sign of continued infection.

Disorders of the Nervous System. Patients with diseases of the nervous system that predispose them to seizures are prone to developing localized or major motor seizures while taking high doses of penicillin G. Neurotoxicity of penicillin and other beta-lactam antibiotics correlates with high concentrations of drug in the CSF and usually occurs in patients with renal insufficiency who are receiving large doses of these drugs. Decreased renal function increases concentrations of penicillin in CSF by two mechanisms: reduction of renal elimination of penicillin from plasma, which results in a higher concentration gradient for passive diffusion into CSF; and accumulation of organic acids (in the uremic state), which competitively inhibit the transport mechanism in the choroid plexus that removes penicillin and other organic acids from the CSF. Patients with myasthenia gravis or other neuromuscular problems appear to be particularly susceptible to the neuromuscular blocking effect of the aminoglycosides, polymyxins, and colistin. Patients undergoing general anesthesia who receive a neuromuscular blocking agent are also particularly susceptible to such antibiotic toxicity.

THERAPY WITH COMBINED ANTIMICROBIAL AGENTS

The simultaneous use of two or more antimicrobial agents has a certain rationale and is recommended in specifically defined situations (Table 44–1). However, selection of an appropriate combination requires an understanding of the potential for interaction between the antimicrobial agents. Such interactions may have consequences for both the microorganism and the host. Since the various classes of antimicrobial agents exert different actions on the microorganism, one drug has the potential to either enhance or inhibit the effect of the second. Similarly, combinations of drugs that might rationally be used to cure infections may have additive or supra-additive toxicities. For example, vancomycin when given alone usually has minimal nephrotoxicity, as does tobramycin; however, when the drugs are given in combination they may cause marked impairment of renal function (Farber and Moellering, 1983).

Methods of Testing Antimicrobial Activity of Drug Combinations. To predict the potential therapeutic efficacy of combinations of antibiotics, methods have been developed to quantitate their effects on bacterial growth *in vitro*. Two distinctly different methods are used. The first employs serial twofold dilutions of antibiotics in broth inoculated with a standard number of the test microorganism in a checkerboard fashion, so that a large number of antibiotic concentrations in different proportions can be tested simultaneously (Figure 44–2). Inhibition of bacterial growth is quantified after 18 hours of incubation. This test determines whether the MIC of one drug is reduced, unchanged, or increased in the presence of another drug. Synergism is defined as inhibition of growth with a combination of drugs when their concentrations are less than or equal to 25% of the MIC of each drug acting alone. This implies that one drug is affecting the microorganism in such a way that it becomes more sensitive to the inhibitory effect of the other. If one half of the inhibitory concentration of each drug is required to produce inhibition, the result is called additive (fractional inhibitory concentration [FIC] index = 1; *see* Figure 44–2), suggesting that the two drugs are working independently of each other. If more than one half of the MIC of each drug is necessary to produce the inhibitory effect, the drugs are said to be antagonistic (FIC index >1). When the drugs are tested for a variety of proportionate drug concentrations, such as with the checkerboard technique, an isobologram may be constructed (Figure 44–2). Synergism is shown by a concave curve, the additive effect by a straight line, and antagonism by a convex curve.

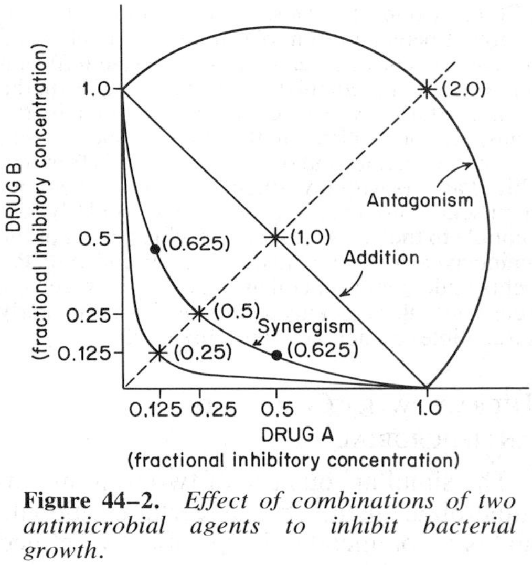

Figure 44–2. *Effect of combinations of two antimicrobial agents to inhibit bacterial growth.*

The effects are expressed as isobols and fractional inhibitory concentration (FIC) indices. The FIC index is equal to the sum of the values of FIC for the individual drugs:

$$\text{FIC index} = \frac{\text{MIC of A with B}}{\text{MIC of A alone}} + \frac{\text{MIC of B with A}}{\text{MIC of B alone}}$$

Points on concave isobols (FIC index < 1) are indicative of synergistic interaction between the two agents, and points on convex isobols (FIC index > 1) represent antagonism. The nature of the interaction is adequately revealed by testing combinations lying along the dotted line (marked +). *See* text for further explanation.

The second method for evaluating drug combinations involves quantitation of their rate of bactericidal action. Identical cultures are incubated simultaneously with antibiotics added singly or in combination. If a combination of antibiotics is more rapidly bactericidal than either drug alone, the result is termed *synergism*. Moellering (1985) has recommended that the minimal criterion for synergism should be the observation of a 100-fold additional decrease in the number of microorganisms counted at any one time. If the bactericidal rate of the combination is less than that for either drug alone, *antagonism* is said to occur. If the bactericidal rate is as rapid as that for the more bactericidal drug, the result is called *indifference*. Comparative evaluation of these two distinctly different laboratory techniques has, in general, demonstrated a good correlation between the results (Rahal, 1978).

There have been various attempts to predict synergism and antagonism from a knowledge of the action of the two drugs involved. Jawetz and Gunnison (1952) devised a simple scheme that is still useful. They observed that bacteriostatic antibiotics frequently antagonize the action of a bactericidal drug and that two bactericidal drugs may exhibit synergism. An updated grouping of these bactericidal and bacteriostatic drugs was proposed by Rahal (1978), as follows. Group-1 drugs, which are primarily bactericidal, include the penicillins, cephalosporins, aminoglycosides, and vancomycin. Group-2 agents, which are primarily bacteriostatic, include the tetracyclines, clindamycin, chloramphenicol, and erythromycin. There is frequent antagonism between the drugs of group 1 and those in group 2 because most of the bactericidal agents require active cell division or protein synthesis for expression of their bactericidal activity, and many of the bacteriostatic drugs in group 2 inhibit these processes. However, drugs in group 1 may exhibit synergism by combination of their bactericidal actions. For example, the uptake of streptomycin into *Enterococcus faecalis* is increased markedly following exposure of the organism to penicillin G. The action of penicillin on the cell wall of the bacterium may accelerate the uptake of the aminoglycoside, thereby allowing higher concentrations of the latter drug to reach the ribosome.

The efficacy of the combination of trimethoprim and sulfamethoxazole is relatively unique, in that synergism results from sequential inhibition of two steps in the pathway of biosynthesis of tetrahydrofolate (*see* Chapter 45).

Indications for the Clinical Use of Combinations of Antimicrobial Agents. Numerous reasons have been given to justify the use of combinations of antimicrobial agents. These will be considered individually.

Treatment of Mixed Bacterial Infections. Some infections are caused by two or more microorganisms. These include intra-abdominal, hepatic, and brain abscesses and many of the genital tract infections. In such situations it may be necessary to administer different antibiotics with different antimicrobial spectra to obtain the necessary breadth of activity.

Following perforation of a viscus such as the colon, one can expect contamination and, frequently, infection with aerobic Enterobacteriaceae, anaerobic and aerobic gram-positive cocci (streptococci), anaerobic bacilli such as *Bacteroides fragilis,* and anaerobic gram-positive rods such as *Clostridium* species. Since a single drug may be ineffective against this mixed infection, a rational combination would be an aminoglycoside for the Enterobacteriaceae, and either clindamycin or metronidazole for the anaerobic microorganisms, including *B. fragilis*. Such combinations may be replaced by some of the newer, broad-spectrum beta-lactam antibiotics (Clissold *et al.,* 1987). In most intra-abdominal infections, therapy with antibiotics alone is rarely successful unless there is adequate drainage. The importance of combined therapy has been demonstrated in an animal model of intraperitoneal infection produced by artificial contamination with stool (Joiner *et al.,* 1982). Animals not treated with antimicrobial agents rapidly died of sepsis due to *E. coli*. Those receiving gentamicin alone were protected from the septic complications of the Enterobacteriaceae, but abscesses containing *B. fragilis* developed in the majority of cases. Treatment with clindamycin alone prevented abscess formation, but animals were again killed by the *E. coli*. When both drugs were used in combination, the majority of animals survived without formation of abscesses. While such studies lend support to the use of combination therapy in mixed microbial infections, not all such infections need to be treated with multiple drugs. For example, cellulitis due to the combination of *Staph. aureus* and group-A streptococci can be treated with a penicillinase-resistant penicillin alone. A drug of this type has antimicrobial activity against both microorganisms. Once results of cultures of aspirated material are known, the minimal number of drugs that will be effective should be used.

Therapy of Severe Infections in Which a Specific Cause Is Unknown. Combination chemotherapy is probably most frequently used in the empiric therapy of infections in which the causative agent has not been or cannot be identified. In these situations, the goal of treatment is to select antibiotic "coverage" for microorganisms that are most likely involved. This selection of antimicrobials must be based on the physician's clinical judgment, which reflects a knowledge of the signs and symptoms of the various infectious diseases and of the microbiology of these diseases and an understanding of the antibiotic spectrum of available drugs. The breadth of the antibiotic blanket that is used is inversely related to one's ability to narrow the list of potential infectious agents.

Prolonged administration of broad-spectrum or multiple antibiotics may lead to overuse of toxic and expensive drugs. This problem most often arises when the physician fails to obtain adequate cultures prior to the initiation of therapy or fails to discontinue the combination chemotherapy after identifying the microorganism and determining sensitivities. There is an understandable reluctance to change antimicrobial agents when a favorable clinical response has occurred. However, the goal of chemotherapy should always be to use the most selectively active drug that produces the fewest adverse effects.

Enhancement of Antibacterial Activity in the Treatment of Specific Infections. As mentioned above, when two antimicrobial agents are administered together, they may produce a synergistic effect. This may permit a reduction in the dosage of one or both drugs with achievement of a similar therapeutic effect. Alternatively, the combination may produce a more rapid or complete bactericidal effect than could be achieved with either drug alone. There are specific clinical indications for the use of combinations of antimicrobial agents, and they are based on documented proof of efficacy (Sande and Scheld, 1980).

Perhaps the best-documented need for a synergistic combination of antimicrobial agents is in the treatment of enterococcal endocarditis. *In vitro,* a combination of penicillin and streptomycin or gentamicin is bactericidal, while penicillin alone is bacteriostatic against most strains of *Enterococcus faecalis*. Treatment of enterococcal endocarditis with penicillin alone frequently results in relapses, while combination therapy is curative at rates that are comparable to those achieved with endocarditis caused by streptococci that are more sensitive to penicillin (Wilson *et al.*, 1984). This is a clear-cut case where combination therapy produces superior clinical results. Antibiotic therapy of endocarditis caused by strains of penicillin-sensitive viridans streptococci may also be improved and the duration of treatment shortened when two drugs are used. Penicillin and streptomycin are synergistic *in vitro* against the vast majority of these strains. In animal models of endocarditis, this combination produces more rapid eradication of bacteria from infected vegetations on heart valves than does penicillin G alone. Wilson and associates (1978) reported a 100% cure rate for patients with this condition who received a short course (2 weeks) of combination chemotherapy; those who advocate treatment with penicillin G alone recommend treatment for 4 weeks (Bisno *et al.*, 1981).

Synergism *in vitro* and in experimental models *in vivo* by a combination of a penicillin and an aminoglycoside has also been demonstrated with *Staph. aureus*. Patients with endocarditis caused by *Staph. aureus* have been treated successfully with nafcillin and a low dose of tobramycin. This combination was administered for a total of 2 weeks, instead of the 4 to 6 weeks traditionally used to treat this disease (Chambers *et al.*, 1988).

Synergistic antibiotic combinations have been recommended in the therapy of infections with *Pseudomonas* in neutropenic patients. *In vitro*, antipseudomonal penicillins plus an aminoglycoside are synergistic against most strains of *Pseud. aeruginosa*. Studies in animals support the superiority of the combination over either drug alone, and clinical studies suggest improved survival with the combination. Despite the fact that the microorganism is sensitive to gentamicin *in vitro*, administration of gentamicin alone frequently does not cure the infection and may even allow sustained bacteremia. The addition of an antipseudomonal beta-lactam antibiotic such as ticarcillin markedly increases the cure rate, a phenomenon that correlates with a more rapid bactericidal effect *in vitro*. This success may be a reflection of the importance of the use of antibiotics that produce bactericidal effects rapidly when infection occurs in the neutropenic patient (Klastersky and Staquet, 1982).

Sulfonamides combined with trimethoprim are synergistic *in vitro* and are effective against infections caused by microorganisms that may be resistant to sulfonamides alone. A fixed combination of trimethoprim and sulfamethoxazole is available for clinical use and has emerged as an effective treatment of recurrent urinary tract infections, *Pneumocystis carinii* pneumonia, typhoid fever, shigellosis, and certain infections due to ampicillin-resistant *H. influenzae*.

There is considerable interest in the application of a new concept in combination chemotherapy—the use of an inhibitor of beta-lactamase, which has little or no intrinsic antimicrobial activity, in combination with a beta-lactam antibiotic that is susceptible to beta-lactamase (amoxicillin, ampicillin, or ticarcillin). The prototypical enzyme inhibitors are clavulanate and sulbactam (Neu, 1985). This approach may allow successful treatment of infections by microorganisms that produce beta-lactamase. For example, infections caused by beta-lactamase-producing *H. influenzae* may be treatable with ampicillin plus a beta-lactamase inhibitor. Thus, the utility of time-tested antibiotics (*e.g.*, penicillin G and ampicillin) may be restored in infections for which they had become ineffective.

Advances have also been made by combination of synergistic agents in the antimicrobial therapy of fungal infections. A combination of flucytosine and amphotericin B has been shown to be synergistic *in vitro* and in animal models of infection. In the therapy of cryptococcal meningitis a combination of flucytosine and a low dose of amphotericin B for 6 weeks was as effective as therapy with a higher dose of amphotericin B for 10 weeks and caused less renal toxicity (Bennett *et al.*, 1979).

Prevention of the Emergence of Resistant Microorganisms. The use of combinations of antimicrobial agents was first proposed as a method to prevent the emergence of resistant mutants during therapy. If spontaneous mutation were the predominant means by which microorganisms acquired resistance to antibiotics, combination chemotherapy would, in theory, be an effective means of prevention. For example, if the frequency of mutation for the acquisition of resistance to one drug is 10^{-7} and that for a second drug 10^{-6}, the probability of independent mutation to resistance to both drugs in a single cell is the product of the two frequencies, 10^{-13}. This makes the emergence of such mutant resistant strains statistically unlikely. In practice, however, this method has received extensive use only in the treatment of tuberculosis, where the concomitant use of two or more appropriate agents strikingly reduces the development of drug resistance by the tubercle bacillus.

Disadvantages of Combinations of Antimicrobial Agents. It is important that physicians understand the potential negative aspects of the use of combinations of antimicrobial agents. The most obvious are the risk of toxicity from two or more agents, the selection of microorganisms that are resistant to antibiotics that may not have been necessary, and increased cost to the patient. In addition, as noted above, antagonism of antibacterial effect may result when bacteriostatic and bactericidal agents are given concurrently. The clinical significance of antibiotic antagonism is not fully understood. Although antagonism of one antibiotic by another has been a frequent observation *in vitro,* well-documented clinical examples are relatively rare. The most notable of these involves the therapy of pneumococcal meningitis.

In 1951, Lepper and Dowling reported that the fatality rate among patients with pneumococcal meningitis who were treated with penicillin alone was 21%, while patients who received the combination of penicillin and chlortetracycline had a fatality rate of 79%. This conclusion was supported by Mathies and colleagues (1967), who treated children with bacterial meningitis of multiple causes with either ampicillin alone or with the combination of ampicillin, chloramphenicol, and streptomycin. The mortality rate among those treated with ampicillin was 4.3%, while those treated with the combination was significantly greater—10.5%.

Antagonism between antibiotics is probably relatively unimportant in most infections. If an antagonistic interaction between two antibiotics is to occur, both agents must be active against the infecting microorganism. The addition of a bacteriostatic to a bactericidal drug frequently results in only a bacteriostatic effect. In many infections where host defenses are adequate, this may still be sufficient to tip the balance in favor of the host. Where host defenses are impaired, as in patients with neutropenia, or with special infections, such as endocarditis and meningitis, the bactericidal effect may become more important. In clinical trials in man, the more rapidly bactericidal combinations of antibiotics have in general been more effective than less rapidly bactericidal or purely bacteriostatic drugs in the therapy of gram-negative infections in neutropenic patients.

THE PROPHYLAXIS OF INFECTION WITH ANTIBIOTICS

A large percentage (from 30 to 50%) of antibiotics administered in the United States are given to prevent infection rather than to treat established disease. This practice accounts for some of the most flagrant misuses of these drugs.

Clinical studies have demonstrated that there are some situations in which chemoprophylaxis is highly effective and others in which it is totally without value and may in fact be deleterious. There are still numerous situations where the attempt to use antimicrobial compounds to prevent bacterial infections is controversial. *In general, if a single effective drug is used to prevent infection by a specific microorganism or to eradicate infection immediately or soon after it has become established, then chemoprophylaxis is frequently successful. On the other hand, if the aim of prophylaxis is to prevent colonization or infection by any or all microorganisms present in the environment of a patient, then prophylaxis often fails.*

Chemoprophylaxis has been employed primarily for three purposes. (1) Prophylaxis may be used to protect healthy persons from acquisition of or invasion by specific microorganisms to which they are exposed. Successful examples of this practice include the following: the use of penicillin G to prevent infection by group-A streptococci; prevention of gonorrhea or syphilis after contact with an infected person; the intermittent use of trimethoprim–sulfamethoxazole to prevent recurrent urinary tract infections usually caused by *E. coli;* and the use of rifampin, minocycline, or sulfadiazine to prevent meningococcal disease. (2) Attempts are often made to prevent secondary bacterial infection in patients who are ill with other diseases. Certain centers have reported a decrease in the incidence of bacterial infections in neutropenic patients given trimethoprim–sulfamethoxazole, although increased numbers of fungal infections were noted in some series. Fluoroquinolones also show promise as prophylactic agents for neutropenic patients. The normal microbial flora of the host represents an important defense in the prevention of colonization and infection with various pathogens (Sanders and Sanders, 1984). "Shotgun" chemoprophylaxis disrupts this barrier and may be self-defeating. Elaborate techniques involving sterile food, life islands, and nonabsorbable antibiotics have shown modest success in decreasing infections in neutropenic patients with hematological malignancies. (3) Chemoprophylaxis *should* be performed to prevent endocarditis in patients with valvular or other structural lesions of the heart who are undergoing dental, surgical, or other procedures that produce a high incidence of bacteremia. Endocarditis results from the bacterial colonization of the endocardium, particularly the cardiac valves. The area of colonization is probably a deposit of fibrin and platelets on a damaged valve associated with areas of turbulent blood flow. Any procedure that injures a mucous membrane where there are large numbers of bacteria (such as in the oropharyngeal or gastrointestinal tract) will produce transient bacteremia. Streptococci from the mouth, enterococci from the gastrointestinal or genitourinary tract, and staphylococci from the skin have a propensity to produce endocarditis, and chemoprophylaxis directed against these microorganisms is recommended (*Medical Letter*, 1984). Therapy should not begin until immediately before the procedure, since prolonged administration of antibiotics can lead to colonization by resistant strains. Criteria have been established for the selection of specific drugs and patients who should receive chemoprophylaxis for various procedures (*see* Chapter 46).

Chemoprophylaxis to prevent wound infections after various surgical procedures is much more controversial. There are several well-controlled clinical studies that support the use of prophylactic antimicrobial agents in certain surgical procedures. The first such demonstration was by Bernard and Cole (1964), who showed the effectiveness of prophylactic antibiotics in patients undergoing operations involving the stomach, pancreas, and bowel. Wound infection results when a critical number of bacteria are present in the wound at the time of closure. Several factors determine the size of this critical inoculum, and these include the virulence of the bacteria, the presence of devitalized or poorly vascularized tissue, the presence of a foreign body, and the status of the host. Antimicrobial agents directed against the invading microorganisms may reduce the number of viable bacteria below the critical level and thus prevent infection.

Several factors are important to the effective and judicious use of antibiotics in this situation (Kaiser, 1990). First, antimicrobial activity must be present at the wound site at the time of its closure. This has led to the recommendation that the drug be given immediately preoperatively and, perhaps, intraoperatively. Second, the antibiotic must be active against the most likely contaminating microorganisms. This has prompted the wide use of first-generation cephalosporins in this form of chemoprophylaxis. Third, there is mounting evidence that the continued use of drugs after the surgical procedure is unwarranted. There are no data to suggest that the incidence of wound infections is lower if antimicrobial treatment is continued after the day of surgery (Rowlands *et al.*, 1982). Prolongation of use beyond 24 to 72 hours does, however, lead to the development of more resistant flora and of wound infections caused by antibiotic-resistant strains. The risk of toxicity and unnecessary expense are, of course, additional disadvantages. In practice, however, this guideline is frequently broken. In a survey of the usage of antibiotics in Pennsylvania, where one third of all antimicrobial agents used were given for chemoprophylaxis, the median duration of such use was 7 days.

Chemoprophylaxis should be used only in selected operative procedures. A number of studies indicate that it can be justified in dirty and contaminated surgical procedures (*e.g.*, resection of the colon), where the incidence of wound infections is high. These include less than 10% of all operations. In clean surgical procedures, which account for approximately 75% of the total, the expected incidence of wound infection is less than 5%, and antibiotics should not be used routinely. Exceptions are rational when the surgical procedure involves insertion of a prosthetic implant. Although clear-cut data are not available to support the use of antibiotics during placement of prosthetic cardiac valves or artificial orthopedic devices, the complications of infection are so drastic that most authorities currently agree to chemoprophylaxis with this indication. Of course, the use of systemic antibiotics for chemoprophylaxis during surgical procedures does not reduce the need for sterile and skilled surgical technique.

SUPERINFECTIONS

The untoward reactions produced by anti-infective agents include toxic effects and hypersensitivity reactions. These are discussed for individual agents in the chapters that follow. Antibiotics also cause unique reactions that result from alterations in the microbial flora of the host.

All individuals who receive therapeutic doses of these agents undergo alterations in the normal microbial population of the intestinal, upper respiratory, and genitourinary tracts; some develop *superinfection* as a result of such changes. This phenomenon may be defined as the appearance of bacteriological and clinical evidence of a new infection during the chemotherapy of a primary one. It is relatively common and potentially very dangerous because the microorganisms responsible for the new infection are, in many cases, Enterobacteriaceae, *Pseudomonas,* and *Candida* or other fungi; these may be very difficult to eradicate with the presently available anti-infective drugs. Superinfection by these microorganisms is due to removal of the inhibitory influence of the flora that normally inhabits the oropharynx and other body orifices. Many members of the normal flora appear to produce antibacterial substances (bacteriocins), and they also presumably compete for essential nutrients. The more "broad" the effect of an antibiotic on microorganisms, the greater is the alteration in the normal microflora and the greater is the possibility that a single microorganism will become predominant, invade the host, and produce infection. Thus, the incidence of superinfection is lowest with penicillin G, higher with tetracyclines and chloramphenicol, and highest with combinations of broad-spectrum antimicrobials and the expanded-spectrum third-generation cephalosporins. It can be expected that further production of agents with increased breadth of antimicrobial activity will lead to more extensive alterations in the normal flora and, thus, more superinfections. The development of agents that kill pathogens selectively while carefully preserving the normal flora would be beneficial. The most specific antimicrobial agent to treat a given infection should be chosen whenever possible. The incidence of superinfection also increases when administration of antibiotics is prolonged.

The fact that harmful effects may follow the therapeutic or the prophylactic use of anti-infective agents must never discourage the physician from their administration in any situation in which they are definitely indicated. It should, however, make the physician very careful in their use when they are required, and very hesitant to employ them in instances in which indications for their application are either entirely lacking or, at most, only suggestive. To do otherwise is to run the risk, at times, of converting a simple, benign, and self-limited disease into one that may be serious or even fatal.

MISUSES OF ANTIBIOTICS

The purpose of this introductory chapter has been to lay the groundwork for the maximally effective utilization of antimicrobial drugs. Unfortunately, in reality, these agents are frequently misused and overused (Symposium, 1978).

Treatment of Untreatable Infections. A common misuse of these agents is in infections that have been proved by experimental and clinical observation to be untreatable. The majority of the diseases caused by viruses will not respond to any of the presently available anti-infective compounds. Thus, antimicrobial therapy of measles, chickenpox, mumps, and at least 90% of infections of the upper respiratory tract is totally ineffective and, therefore, worse than useless.

Therapy of Fever of Undetermined Origin. Fever of undetermined etiology may be of two types: one that is present for only a few days to a week and another that persists for an extended period. Both of these are frequently treated with antimicrobial agents. Most instances of pyrexia of short duration, in the absence of localizing signs, are probably associated with undefined viral infections, often of the upper respiratory tract, and do not respond to antibiotics. In the bulk of these cases, defervescence takes place spontaneously within a week or less. Studies of prolonged fever have shown that three common infectious causes are tuberculosis, often of the disseminated variety, hidden pyogenic intra-abdominal abscess, and infectious endocarditis. Also, the so-called collagen-vascular disorders and various neoplasms, especially lymphoma, are frequently responsible for prolonged and significant degrees of fever. Various types of cancer, metabolic disorders, hepatitis, asymptomatic regional enteritis, atypical rheumatoid arthritis, and a number of other noninfectious disorders may present themselves as cases of fever of unknown etiology (Larson *et al.,* 1982).

It must be stressed that the anti-infective agents are not antipyretics. The most rational approach to the problem of fever of unknown etiology is not one that concentrates on the elevated temperature alone but one that involves a thorough search for its cause. The patient should not be unnecessarily exposed to chemotherapy in the hope, often in vain, that, if one agent is not effective, another one or a combination of drugs will be helpful.

Improper Dosage. Erroneous dosage of antimicrobial agents is of two types: administration of excessive amounts and use of suboptimal quantities. There is little doubt that harm may be produced by overdoses of most antimicrobial agents. The difficulties that may arise from drug overdosage in patients with impairment of drug elimination have already been discussed. It is, however, critical that adequate dosage be given to achieve the desired effects. Drugs such as aminoglycosides are frequently administered in insufficient quantities, probably because of fear of toxicity; the potential for clinical failures is thus increased (Lesar *et al.,* 1982).

Reliance on Chemotherapy with Omission of Surgical Drainage. To rely on anti-infective agents alone to cure some types of infections is to place a demand on them that they cannot always satisfy. The conditions in which this is a problem are usually those with appreciable quantities of purulent exudate or necrotic or avascular infected tissues. Two of many possible examples will be cited. The patient with pneumonia and empyema often fails to be cured by the administration of large doses of an effective drug until drainage of the involved area is established. The patient with renal lithiasis will frequently suffer recurrent episodes of acute pyelonephritis, regardless of the number of times he is treated with antimicrobial agents, until the stones are removed. As a generalization, it may be said that, when an appreciable quantity of pus, necrotic tissue, or a foreign body is present, the most effective treatment is a combination of an antimicrobial agent given in adequate dose plus a properly performed surgical procedure.

Lack of Adequate Bacteriological Information. One half of the courses of antimicrobial therapy administered to hospitalized patients appear to be given in the absence of support from the microbiological laboratory. It is clear that the great bulk of the use of these drugs in hospitals is based on clinical judgment alone. A high proportion of the use is for chemoprophylaxis of questionable value. Bacterial cultures and gram stains of infected material are obtained too infrequently, and the results, when available, are often disregarded in the selection and application of drug therapy. Frequent use of drug combinations or drugs with the broadest spectra is a cover for diagnostic imprecision. The agents selected are more likely to be those of habit rather than for specific indications, and the dosages employed are routine. Antimicrobial drug therapy must be individualized on the basis of the clinical situation, microbiological information, and the pharmacological considerations presented in this chapter and the subsequent chapters of this section. (For discussions of patterns of antibiotic administration by physicians, *see* Symposium, 1978.)

Bauer, A. W.; Kirby, W. M. M.; Sherris, J. C.; and Turck, M. Antibiotic susceptibility testing by a standardized single disc method. *Am. J. Clin. Pathol.,* **1966,** *45,* 493–496.

Bennett, J. E., and others. Amphotericin B–flucytosine in cryptococcal meningitis. *N. Engl. J. Med.,* **1979,** *301,* 126–131.

Bernard, H. R., and Cole, W. R. The prophylaxis of surgical infections: the effect of prophylactic antimicrobial drugs on the incidence of infection following potentially contaminated operations. *Surgery,* **1964,** *56,* 151–157.

Bisno, A. L.; Dismukes, W. E.; Durack, D. T.; Kaplan, E. L.; Karchmer, A. W.; Kaye, D.; Sande, M. A.; Sanford, J. P.; and Wilson, W. R. Treatment of infective endocarditis due to *viridans* streptococci. *Circulation,* **1981,** *63,* 730A–733A.

Bryant, R. E. Pus: friend or foe? In, *Contemporary Issues in Infectious Diseases,* Vol. 6. *New Surgical and Medical Approaches in Infectious Diseases.* (Root, R. K.; Trunkey, D.D.; and Sande, M. A.; eds.) Churchill Livingstone, Inc., New York, **1987,** pp. 31–48.

Chambers, H. F. Methicillin-resistant staphylococci. *Clin. Microbiol. Rev.,* **1988,** *1,* 173–186.

Chambers, H. F.; Miller, R. T.; and Newman, M. D. Right-sided *Staphylococcus aureus* endocarditis in intravenous drug abusers: two-week combination therapy. *Ann. Intern. Med.*, **1988**, *109*, 619–624.

Clissold, S. P.; Todd, P. A.; and Campoli-Richards, D. M. Imipenem/cilastatin. *Drugs*, **1987**, *33*, 183–241.

Coleman, D. L.; Horwitz, R. I.; and Andriole, V. T. Association between serum inhibitory and bactericidal concentrations and therapeutic outcome in bacterial endocarditis. *Am. J. Med.*, **1982**, *73*, 260–267.

Datta, N., and Nugent, M. E. Bacterial variation. In, *Topley and Wilson's Principles of Bacteriology, Virology, and Immunity*, 7th ed., Vol. 1. (Wilson, G. S., and Dick, H. M., eds.) The Williams & Wilkins Co., Baltimore, **1984**, pp. 145–176.

Davies, J.; Brzezinska, M.; and Benveniste, R. R factors: biochemical mechanisms of resistance to aminoglycoside antibiotics. *Ann. N.Y. Acad. Sci.*, **1971**, *182*, 226–233.

Dickie, P.; Bryan, L. E.; and Pichard, M. A. Effect of enzymatic adenylation on dihydrostreptomycin accumulation in *Escherichia coli* carrying an R-factor: model explaining aminoglycoside resistance by inactivating mechanisms. *Antimicrob. Agents Chemother.*, **1978**, *14*, 569–580.

Farber, B., and Moellering, R. C., Jr. Retrospective study of the toxicity of preparations of vancomycin from 1974–1981. *Antimicrob. Agents Chemother.*, **1983**, *23*, 138–141.

Hackbarth, C. J.; Chambers, H. F.; and Sande, M. A. Serum bactericidal titer as a predictor of outcome in endocarditis. *Eur. J. Clin. Microbiol.*, **1986**, *5*, 93–97.

Handwerger, S., and Tomasz, A. Alterations in kinetic properties of penicillin-binding proteins of penicillin-resistant *Streptococcus pneumoniae*. *Antimicrob. Agents Chemother.*, **1986**, *30*, 57–63.

Jacobs, M. R.; Koornhof, H. J.; Robins-Browne, R. M.; Stevenson, C. M.; Vermaak, Z. A.; Freiman, I.; Miller, G. B.; Witcomb, M. A.; Isaäcson, M.; Ward, J. I.; and Austrian, R. Emergence of multiply resistant pneumococci. *N. Engl. J. Med.*, **1978**, *299*, 735–740.

Jacobson, M. A.; Hahn, S. M.; Gerberding, J. L.; Lee, B.; and Sande, M. A. Ciprofloxacin therapy for salmonella bacteremia in patients with acquired immunodeficiency syndrome. *Ann. Intern. Med.*, **1989**, *110*, 1027–1029.

Jaffe, A.; Chabbert, Y. A.; and Derlot, E. Selection and characterization of betalactam-resistant *Escherichia coli* K-12 mutants. *Antimicrob. Agents Chemother.*, **1983**, *23*, 622–625.

Jawetz, E., and Gunnison, J. B. Studies on antibiotic synergism and antagonism: the scheme of combined antimicrobial activity. *Antibiot. Chemother.*, **1952**, *2*, 243–248.

Joiner, K.; Lowe, B.; Dzink, J.; and Bartlett, J. G. Comparative efficacy of ten antimicrobial agents in experimental infections with *B. fragilis*. *J. Infect. Dis.*, **1982**, *145*, 561–568.

Judson, F. N. Management of antibiotic-resistant *Neisseria gonorrhoeae*. *Ann. Intern. Med.*, **1989**, *110*, 5–7.

Kaiser, A. Postoperative infections and antimicrobial prophylaxis. In, *Principles and Practice of Infectious Diseases*, 3rd ed. (Mandell, G. L.; Douglas, R. G., Jr.; and Bennett, J. E.; eds.) Churchill Livingstone, Inc., New York, **1990**, pp. 2245–2257.

Kapusnik, J. E.; Hackbarth, C. J.; Chambers, H. F.; Carpenter, T.; and Sande, M. A. Single, large, daily dosing versus intermittent dosing of tobramycin for treating experimental pseudomonas pneumonia. *J. Infect. Dis.*, **1988**, *158*, 7–12.

Keating, M. J.; Bodey, G. P.; Valdivieso, M.; and Rodriguez, V. A randomized comparative trial of three aminoglycosides—comparison of continuous infusions of gentamicin, amikacin, and sisomicin combined with carbenicillin in the treatment of infections in neutropenic patients with malignancies. *Medicine (Baltimore)*, **1979**, *58*, 159–170.

Larson, E. B.; Featherstone, H. J.; and Petersdorf, R. G. Fever of undetermined origin: diagnosis and follow-up of 105 cases, 1970–1980. *Medicine (Baltimore)*, **1982**, *61*, 269–292.

Lepper, M. H., and Dowling, H. F. Treatment of pneumococcic meningitis with penicillin plus AUREOMYCIN: studies including observations on apparent antagonism between penicillin and AUREOMYCIN. *Arch. Intern. Med.*, **1951**, *88*, 489–494.

Lesar, T. S.; Rotschafer, J. C.; Strand, L. M.; Solem, L. D.; and Zaske, D. E. Gentamicin dosing errors with four commonly used nomograms. *J.A.M.A.*, **1982**, *248*, 1190–1193.

Mandell, L. A. Effects of antimicrobial and antineoplastic drugs on the phagocytic and microbicidal function of the polymorphonuclear leukocyte. *Rev. Infect. Dis.*, **1982**, *4*, 683–697.

Mathies, A. W., Jr.; Leedom, J. M.; Ivler, D.; Wehrle, P. F.; and Portnoy, B. Antibiotic antagonism in bacterial meningitis. *Antimicrob. Agents Chemother.*, **1967**, *7*, 218–224.

Medical Letter. Prevention of bacterial endocarditis. **1984**, *26*, 3–4.

Neu, H. C. Beta-lactamase inhibition: therapeutic advances. *Am. J. Med.*, **1985**, *79*, Suppl. 5B, 1–12.

Pasteur, L., and Joubert, J. Charbonne et septicemie. *C. R. Acad. Sci. [D]*, **1877**, *85*, 101–115.

Pratt, W. B., and Fekety, R. *The Antimicrobial Drugs*. Oxford University Press, New York, **1986**.

Quagliarello, V. J.; Long, W. J.; and Scheld, W. M. Morphologic alterations of the blood–brain barrier with experimental meningitis in the rat. *J. Clin. Invest.*, **1986**, *77*, 1084–1095.

Rahal, J., Jr. Antibiotic combinations: the clinical relevance of synergy and antagonism. *Medicine (Baltimore)*, **1978**, *57*, 179–195.

Rowlands, B. J.; Clark, R. G.; and Richards, D. G. Single-dose intraoperative antibiotic prophylaxis in emergency abdominal surgery. *Arch. Surg.*, **1982**, *117*, 195–199.

Sande, M. A., and Scheld, W. M. Combination antibiotic therapy of bacterial endocarditis. *Ann. Intern. Med.*, **1980**, *92*, 390–395.

Sanders, W. E., Jr., and Sanders, C. C. Modification of normal flora by antibiotics: effects on individuals and the environment. In, *New Dimensions in Antimicrobial Therapy*. (Root, R. K., and Sande, M. A., eds.) Churchill Livingstone, Inc., New York, **1984**, pp. 217–241.

Sparling, F. P. Current problems in sexually transmitted diseases. *Adv. Intern. Med.*, **1978**, *24*, 203–228.

Strausbaugh, L. J., and Sande, M. A. Factors influencing the therapy of experimental *Proteus mirabilis* meningitis in rabbits. *J. Infect. Dis.*, **1978**, *137*, 251–260.

Täuber, M. G.; Kunz, S.; Zak, O.; and Sande, M. A. Influence of antibiotic dose, dosing interval and duration of therapy on outcome in experimental pneumococcal meningitis in rabbits. *Antimicrob. Agents Chemother.*, **1989**, *33*, 418–423.

Vaudaux, P. Peripheral inactivation of gentamicin. *J. Antimicrob. Chemother.*, **1981**, *8*, Suppl. A, S17–S25.

Verklin, R. M., Jr., and Mandell, G. L. Alteration of effectiveness of antibiotics by anaerobiosis. *J. Lab. Clin. Med.*, **1977**, *89*, 65–71.

Vorherr, H. Drug excretion in breast milk. *Postgrad. Med.*, **1974**, *56*, 97–104.

Watanabe, T. Infectious drug resistance in enteric bacteria. *N. Engl. J. Med.*, **1966**, *275*, 888–894.

Wehrli, W. Rifampin: mechanisms of action and resistance. *Rev. Infect. Dis.*, **1983**, *5*, Suppl., S407–S411.

Wilson, W. R.; Geraci, J. E.; Wilkowske, C. J.; and Washington, J. A., II. Short-term intramuscular therapy with procaine penicillin plus streptomycin for infective endocarditis due to *viridans* streptococci. *Circulation*, **1978**, *57*, 1158–1161.

Wilson, W. R.; Wilkowske, C. J.; Wright, A. J.; Sande, M. A.; and Geraci, J. E. Treatment of streptomycin-susceptible and streptomycin-resistant enterococcal endocarditis. *Ann. Intern. Med.*, **1984**, *100*, 816–823.

Wolfson, J. S., and Swartz, M. N. Serum bactericidal activity as a monitor of antibiotic therapy. *N. Engl. J. Med.*, **1985**, *312*, 968–975.

Wood, C. A.; Norton, D. R.; Kohlhepp, S. J.; Kohven, P. W.; Porter, G. A.; Houghton, D. C.; Brummett, R. E.; Bennett, W. M.; and Gilbert, D. N. The influence of tobramycin dosage regimens on nephrotoxicity, ototoxicity, and antibacterial efficacy in a rat model of subcutaneous abscess. *J. Infect. Dis.*, **1988**, *158*, 13–22.

Yourtee, E. L., and Root, R. K. Effect of antibiotics on phagocyte-microbe interactions. In, *New Dimensions in Antimicrobial Therapy*. (Root, R. K., and Sande, M. A., eds.) Churchill Livingstone, Inc., New York, **1984**, pp. 243–275.

Zimilis, V. M., and Jackson, G. G. Activity of aminoglycoside antibiotics against *Pseudomonas aeruginosa:* specificity and site of calcium and magnesium antagonism. *J. Infect. Dis.*, **1973**, *127*, 663–669.

Zimmerli, W.; Lew, P. D.; and Waldvogel, F. A. Pathogenesis of foreign body infection. *J. Clin. Invest.*, **1984**, *73*, 1191–1200.

Monographs and Reviews

Calderwood, S. B., and Moellering, R. C., Jr. Principles of anti-infective therapy. In, *Internal Medicine*, 3rd ed. (Stein, J. H., ed.) Little, Brown & Co., Boston, **1990**, pp. 1202–1218.

Conte, J. E., Jr., and Barriere, S. L. *Manual of Antibiotics and Infectious Diseases*, 6th ed. Lea & Febiger, Philadelphia, **1988.**

Craig, W. A., and Kunin, D. M. Significance of serum protein and tissue binding of antimicrobial agents. *Annu. Rev. Med.*, **1976**, *27*, 287–300.

Klastersky, J., and Staquet, M. J. (eds.). *Combination Antibiotic Therapy in the Compromised Host*. Vol. 9, *Monograph Series of the European Organization for Research on Treatment of Cancer*. Raven Press, New York, **1982.**

Kucers, A., and Bennett, N. McK. *The Use of Antibiotics. A Comprehensive Review with Clinical Emphasis*, 4th ed. J. B. Lippincott Co., Philadelphia, **1987.**

Moellering, R. C., Jr. Principles of anti-infective therapy. In, *Principles and Practice of Infectious Diseases*, 2nd ed. (Mandell, G. L.; Douglas, R. G., Jr.; and Bennett, J. E.; eds.) John Wiley & Sons, Inc., New York, **1985**, pp. 153–164.

Peterson, P. K., and Verhoef, J. (eds.). *The Antimicrobial Agents Annual 3*. Elsevier Science Publishing Co., Amsterdam, **1988.**

Sande, M. A., and Volberding, P. A. (eds.). *The Medical Management of AIDS*. W. B. Saunders Co., Philadelphia, **1988.**

Sanford, J. P. *Guide to Antimicrobial Therapy 1989*. Sanford, Bethesda, **1989.**

Symposium. (Various authors.) The impact of infections on medical care in the United States. (Kunin, C., and Edelman, R., eds.) *Ann. Intern. Med.*, **1978**, *89*, Suppl., Pt. 2, 737–866.

CHAPTER

45 ANTIMICROBIAL AGENTS

[*Continued*]

Sulfonamides, Trimethoprim–Sulfamethoxazole, Quinolones, and Agents for Urinary Tract Infections

Gerald L. Mandell and Merle A. Sande

SULFONAMIDES

The sulfonamide drugs were the first effective chemotherapeutic agents to be employed systemically for the prevention and cure of bacterial infections in man. The considerable medical and public health importance of their discovery and their subsequent widespread use were quickly reflected in the sharp decline in morbidity and mortality figures for the treatable infectious diseases. The advent first of penicillin and subsequently of other antibiotics has diminished the usefulness of the sulfonamides, and they presently occupy a relatively small place in the therapeutic armamentarium of the physician. However, the introduction in the mid-1970s of the combination of trimethoprim and sulfamethoxazole has resulted in increased use of sulfonamides for the treatment of specific microbial infections.

History. Investigations at the I. G. Farbenindustrie resulted, in 1932, in a German patent to Klarer and Mietzsch, covering PRONTOSIL and several other azo dyes containing a sulfonamide group. Domagk, a research director of the I. G. working with Klarer and Mietzsch, was aware of the fact that synthetic azo dyes had been studied for their action against streptococci, which prompted him to test the new compounds. He quickly observed that mice with streptococcal and other infections could be protected by PRONTOSIL (Domagk, 1935). To Domagk belongs the credit for the discovery of the chemotherapeutic value of PRONTOSIL, for which he was awarded the Nobel Prize in Medicine for 1938. In 1933, the first clinical case study was reported by Foerster, who gave PRONTOSIL to a 10-month-old infant with staphylococcal septicemia and obtained a dramatic cure. However, no great attention was paid elsewhere to these epoch-making advances in chemotherapy until the interest of English investigators was aroused. Colebrook and Kenny (1936) as well as Buttle and coworkers (1936) reported their favorable clinical results with PRONTOSIL and its active metabolite, sulfanilamide, in puerperal sepsis and meningococcal infections. These two reports awakened the medical profession to the new field of antibacterial chemotherapy, and experimental and clinical articles soon appeared in great profusion. Anyone interested in the history of sulfonamides is referred to *earlier editions* of this textbook and the references therein.

Chemistry. The term *sulfonamide* is employed herein as a generic name for derivatives of para-aminobenzenesulfonamide (sulfanilamide); the structural formulas of selected members of this class are shown in Table 45–1. Most of them are relatively insoluble in water, but their sodium salts are readily soluble. The minimal structural prerequisites for antibacterial action are all embodied in sulfanilamide itself. The $—SO_2NH_2$ group is not essential as such, but the important feature is that the sulfur is directly linked to the benzene ring. The para-NH_2 group (the N of which has been designated as N^4) is essential and can be replaced only by such radicals as can be converted *in vivo* to a free amino group. Substitutions made in the amide NH_2 group (the N of which has been designated as N^1) have variable effects on antibacterial activity of the molecule. However, substitution of heterocyclic aromatic nuclei at N^1 yields highly potent compounds.

EFFECTS ON MICROBIAL AGENTS

Sulfonamides have a wide range of antimicrobial activity against both gram-positive and gram-negative bacteria. However, resistant strains have become common in recent years, and the usefulness of these agents has diminished correspondingly. In general, the sulfonamides exert only a bacteriostatic effect, and cellular and humoral defense mechanisms of the host are essential for the final eradication of the infection.

Antibacterial Spectrum. Among the microorganisms usually susceptible *in vitro* to sulfonamides are *Streptococcus pyogenes, Strep. pneumoniae, Haemophilus influenzae, H. ducreyi, Nocardia, Actinomyces, Calymmatobacterium granulomatis,*

Table 45–1. STRUCTURAL FORMULAS OF SELECTED SULFONAMIDES AND PARA-AMINOBENZOIC ACID *

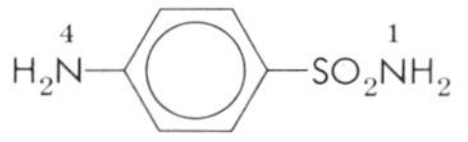

Sulfanilamide

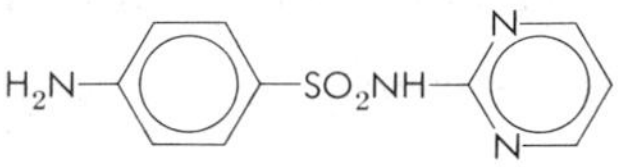

Sulfadiazine

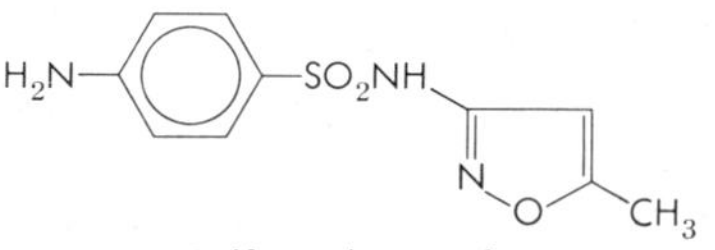

Sulfamethoxazole

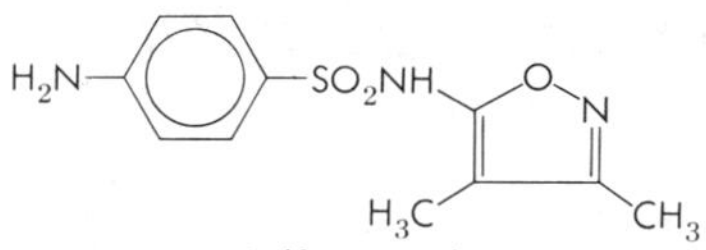

Sulfisoxazole

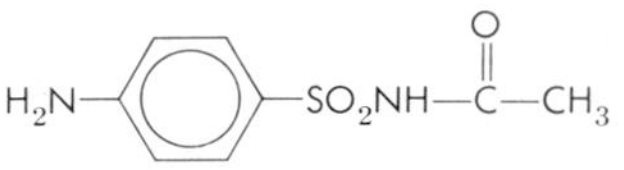

Sulfacetamide

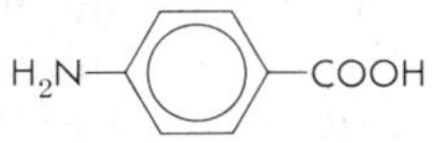

Para-aminobenzoic Acid

* The N of the para-NH_2 group is designated as N^4; that of the amide NH_2, as N^1.

and *Chlamydia trachomatis*. Minimal inhibitory concentrations range from 0.1 μg/ml for *C. trachomatis* to 4 to 64 μg/ml for *Escherichia coli*. Peak plasma drug concentrations achievable *in vivo* are approximately 100 to 200 μg/ml.

Although sulfonamides were used successfully for the management of meningococcal infections for many years, the majority of isolates of *N. meningitidis* of serogroups B and C in the United States and group-A isolates from other countries are now resistant. A similar situation prevails with respect to *Shigella*. Strains of *E. coli* isolated from patients with urinary tract infections (community acquired) are often resistant to sulfonamides, such that they are no longer the therapy of choice for such infections.

Mechanism of Action. Sulfonamides are structural analogs and competitive antagonists of para-aminobenzoic acid (PABA), and thus prevent normal bacterial utilization of PABA for the synthesis of folic acid (pteroylglutamic acid) (*see* Fildes, 1940; Woods, 1940). More specifically, sulfonamides are competitive inhibitors of dihydropteroate synthase, the bacterial enzyme responsible for the incorporation of PABA into dihydropteroic acid, the immediate precursor of folic acid. Sensitive microorganisms are those that must synthesize their own folic acid; bacteria that can utilize preformed folate are not affected. Bacteriostasis induced by sulfonamides is counteracted by PABA competitively. Sulfonamides do not affect mammalian cells by this mechanism, since they require preformed folic acid and cannot synthesize it. They are, therefore, comparable to sulfonamide-insensitive bacteria that utilize preformed folate.

The mechanism presented above does not explain all the known facts concerning the action of sulfonamides on bacteria. Brown (1962), using cell-free extracts of *E. coli*, found that sulfonamides can also be used as alternative substrates by the enzyme system to form products that are probably analogs of reduced forms of pteroic acid. The synthesis of sulfonamide-containing analogs of folate by intact bacteria has also been demonstrated. These analogs could then exert inhibitory effects. The development of knowledge concerning the mode of action of the sulfonamides has been reviewed by Woods (1962).

Synergists and Antagonists of Sulfonamides. One of the most active agents that exerts a synergistic effect when used with a sulfonamide is trimethoprim (*see* Bushby and Hitchings, 1968). This compound is a potent and selective competitive inhibitor of microbial dihydrofolate reductase, the enzyme that reduces dihydrofolate to tetrahydrofolate. It is this reduced form of folic acid that is required for one-carbon transfer reactions. The simultaneous administration of a sulfonamide and trimethoprim thus introduces sequential blocks in the pathway by which microorganisms synthesize tetrahydrofolate from precursor molecules. The expectation that such a combination would yield synergistic antimicrobial effects has been realized both *in vitro* and *in vivo* (*see* below).

PABA is the most prominent sulfonamide antagonist. Certain local anesthetics, such as procaine, that are esters of PABA antagonize these drugs *in vitro* and *in vivo*. PABA may be added to cultures of blood or body fluids in order to block the inhibitory effect of sulfonamides on microbial growth; sensitivity to sulfonamides must be determined in media that are free of PABA. The antibacterial action of these drugs is also inhibited by blood, pus, and tissue breakdown products because the bacterial requirement for folic acid is reduced in media that contain purines and thymidine.

Acquired Bacterial Resistance to Sulfonamides. Bacteria resistant to sulfonamides are presumed to originate by random mutation and selection or by transfer of resistance by plasmids (Chapter 44). Such resistance, once it is maximally developed, is usually persistent and irreversible, particularly when produced *in vivo*. Acquired resistance to sulfonamide usually does not imply cross-resistance to chemotherapeutic agents of other classes. The *in-vivo* acquisition of resistance has little or no effect either on virulence or on antigenic characteristics of microorganisms.

Resistance to sulfonamide is probably the consequence of an altered enzymatic constitution of the bacterial cell; the alteration may be characterized by (1) an alteration in the enzyme that utilizes PABA, dihydropteroate synthase, (2) an increased capacity to destroy or inactivate the drug, (3) an alternative metabolic pathway for synthesis of an essential metabolite, or (4) an increased production of an essential metabolite or drug antagonist. The latter possibility has received most attention. For example, some resistant staphylococci may synthesize 70 times as much PABA as do the susceptible parent strains. Nevertheless, an increased production of PABA is not a constant finding in sulfonamide-resistant bacteria, and resistant mutants may possess enzymes for folate biosynthesis that are less readily inhibited by sulfonamides.

Absorption, Fate, and Excretion

Except for sulfonamides especially designed for their local effects in the bowel, this class of drugs is rapidly absorbed from the gastrointestinal tract. Approximately 70 to 100% of an oral dose is absorbed, and sulfonamide can be found in the urine within 30 minutes of ingestion. The small intestine is the major site of absorption, but some of the drug is absorbed from the stomach. Absorption from other sites, such as the vagina, respiratory tract, or abraded skin, is variable and unreliable, but a sufficient amount may enter the body to cause toxic reactions in susceptible persons or to produce sensitization.

All sulfonamides are bound in varying degree to plasma proteins, particularly to albumin. The extent to which this occurs is determined by the hydrophobicity of a particular drug and its pK_a; at physiological pH, drugs with a high pK_a exhibit a low degree of protein binding, and vice versa.

Sulfonamides are distributed throughout all tissues of the body. The diffusible fraction of sulfadiazine is uniformly distributed throughout the total body water, while sulfisoxazole is largely confined to the extracellular space. The sulfonamides readily enter pleural, peritoneal, synovial, ocular, and similar body fluids, and may reach concentrations therein that are 50 to 80% of the simultaneously determined concentration in blood. Since the protein content of such fluids is usually low, the drug is present in the unbound active form.

After systemic administration of adequate doses, sulfadiazine and sulfisoxazole attain concentrations in cerebrospinal fluid that may be effective in meningeal infections. At steady state, the concentration ranges between 10 and 80% of that in the blood. However, because of the emergence of sulfonamide-resistant microorganisms, these drugs are now used only rarely for the treatment of meningitis.

Sulfonamides readily pass through the placenta and reach the fetal circulation. The concentrations attained in the fetal tissues are sufficient to cause both antibacterial and toxic effects.

The sulfonamides undergo metabolic alterations *in vivo*, especially in the liver. The major metabolic derivative is the N^4-acetylated sulfonamide. Acetylation, which occurs to a different extent with each agent, is disadvantageous because the resulting products have no antibacterial activity and yet retain the toxic potentialities of the parent substance.

Sulfonamides are eliminated from the body partly as the unchanged drug and partly as metabolic products. The largest fraction is excreted in the urine, and the half-life of sulfonamides in the body is thus dependent on renal function. Small amounts are eliminated in the feces and in bile, milk, and other secretions.

Pharmacological Properties, Preparations, and Dosage of Individual Sulfonamides

The sulfonamides may be classified into four groups on the basis of the rapidity with which they are absorbed and excreted: (1) agents absorbed rapidly and excreted rapidly, such as sulfisoxazole and sulfadiazine; (2) agents absorbed very poorly when administered orally and hence active in the bowel lumen, such as sulfasalazine; (3) sulfonamides employed mainly for topical use, such as sulfacetamide, mafenide, and silver sulfadiazine; and (4) long-acting sulfonamides, such as sulfadoxine, which are absorbed rapidly but excreted slowly.

Rapidly Absorbed and Rapidly Eliminated Sulfonamides. *Sulfisoxazole.* Early studies of sulfisoxazole established that it was a rapidly absorbed and rapidly excreted sulfonamide with excellent antibacterial activity. Since its high solubility eliminates much of the renal toxicity inherent in the use of older sulfonamides, it has essentially replaced the less-soluble agents.

Sulfisoxazole is extensively bound to plasma proteins. Following an oral dose of 2 to 4 g, peak concentrations in plasma of 110 to 250 μg/ml are found in 2 to 4 hours. From 28 to 35% of sulfisoxazole in the blood and about 30% in the urine is in the acetylated form. Approximately 95% of a single dose is excreted by the kidney in 24 hours. Concentrations of the drug in urine thus greatly exceed those in blood and may be bactericidal. The cerebrospinal fluid concentration averages about a third of that in the blood.

The recommended daily oral dosage of sulfisoxazole for children is 150 mg/kg of body weight; one half of this is given initially, followed by one fourth or one sixth of the daily dose every 6 or 4 hours (not to exceed 6 g in 24 hours). The oral dosage for adults is 2 to 4 g initially, followed by 4 to 8 g daily, in four to six divided doses. The areas of clinical usefulness of sulfisoxazole are discussed below.

Less than 0.1% of patients receiving sulfisoxazole suffer serious toxic reactions. The untoward effects produced by this agent are similar to those that follow the administration of other sulfonamides, as discussed below. Because of its relatively high solubility in the urine as compared to sulfadiazine, sulfisoxazole only infrequently produces hematuria or crystalluria (0.2 to 0.3%). Despite this, patients taking this drug should ingest an adequate quantity of water. Sulfisoxazole and all sulfonamides that are absorbed must be used with caution in patients with impaired renal function. Like all other sulfonamides, sulfisoxazole may produce hypersensitivity reactions, some of which are potentially lethal. Sulfisoxazole is presently preferred over other sulfonamides by most clinicians, when a rapidly absorbed and rapidly excreted sulfonamide is indicated.

Sulfisoxazole (GANTRISIN, others) is available in 500-mg tablets for oral use. Preparations of sulfisoxazole suitable for parenteral administration are no longer marketed in the United States. *Sulfisoxazole diolamine* is available in 4% solution or ointment prepared for topical use in the eye. *Sulfisoxazole acetyl* is tasteless and hence preferred for oral use in children; it is available as a flavored syrup and pediatric suspension (100 mg/ml). The compound is deacetylated by the enzymes in the small intestine, and this results in a relatively slow absorption of the active form of the drug. Sulfisoxazole is also marketed in a fixed-dose combination with phenazopyridine (sulfisoxazole, 500 mg; phenazopyridine, 50 mg; AZO GANTRISIN, others) as a urinary tract antiseptic and analgesic. The urine becomes orange-red soon after ingestion of this mixture because of the presence of phenazopyridine, an orange-red dye. Sulfisoxazole acetyl (600 mg/5 ml) is also marketed in combination with erythromycin ethylsuccinate (200 mg/5 ml) as PEDIAZOLE or ERYZOLE for use in children with otitis media. The dose is 50 mg/kg per day of the erythromycin component, given in divided doses four times daily.

Sulfamethoxazole. *Sulfamethoxazole* (GANTANOL, others) is a close congener of sulfisoxazole, but its rates of enteric absorption and urinary excretion are slower. It is employed for both systemic and urinary tract infections. Precautions must be observed to avoid sulfamethoxazole crystalluria because of the high percentage of the acetylated, relatively insoluble form of the drug in the urine. Sulfamethoxazole is available for oral use, as 500-mg and 1-g tablets and as a suspension (100 mg/ml). The dosage of sulfamethoxazole for children is 50 to 60 mg/kg initially, followed by 25 to 30 mg/kg morning and evening thereafter. The dosage for adults with mild infections is 2 g, followed by 1 g every 12 hours; for severe disease, the initial dose is 2 g and then 1 g every 8 hours. The half-life of sulfamethoxazole in babies during the first 10 days of life is considerably longer than in adults. It falls rapidly, being about 9 hours at 3 weeks of age and 4 to 5 hours at 1 year. It then increases toward the half-life characteristic for adults, namely, 6 to 12 hours. The clinical uses of sulfamethoxazole are the same as those for sulfisoxazole. It is presently marketed in fixed-dose combinations with phenazopyridine (AZO GANTANOL) as a urinary antiseptic and analgesic, and with trimethoprim (*see* below).

Sulfadiazine. Sulfadiazine given orally is rapidly absorbed from the gastrointestinal tract, and peak blood concentrations are reached within 3 to 6 hours after a single dose. Following an oral dose of 3 g, peak concentrations in plasma are 50 μg/ml. About 55% of the drug is bound to plasma protein at a concentration of 100 μg/ml when plasma protein levels are normal. Therapeutic concentrations are attained in cerebrospinal fluid within 4 hours after a single oral dose of 60 mg/kg.

Sulfadiazine is excreted quite readily by the kidney in both the free and the acetylated form, rapidly at first and then more slowly over a period of 2 to 3 days. It can be detected in the urine within 30 minutes after oral ingestion. About 15 to 40% of the excreted sulfadiazine is in the acetylated form. This form of the drug is excreted more readily than the free fraction, and the administration of alkali accelerates the renal clearance of both forms by further diminishing their tubular reabsorption.

In adults who are being treated with sulfadiazine, the initial dose for oral administration is 2 to 4 g, followed by 2 to 4 g per day in three to six divided doses. Children over 2 months of age should receive one half of a calculated daily dose to initiate therapy and then 150 mg/kg (to a maximum of 6 g) daily in four to six divided doses. Every precaution must be taken to ensure fluid intake adequate to produce a urine output of at least 1200 ml in adults and a corresponding quantity in children. If this cannot be accomplished, sodium bicarbonate may be given to reduce the risk of crystalluria. *Sulfadiazine* is available as tablets that contain 500 mg of the drug.

Sulfacytine. *Sulfacytine* (RENOQUID) is a rapidly excreted sulfonamide for the oral treatment of acute urinary tract infections. The half-life in plasma is shorter than that of sulfisoxazole (4 hours vs. 7 hours). Concentrations in blood are lower than those achieved with sulfisoxazole, and this agent should be used only for the treatment of urinary tract infections. A loading dose of 500 mg should be given, followed by 250 mg four times per day. Sulfacytine is supplied in 250-mg tablets.

Sulfamethizole. *Sulfamethizole* (PROKLAR, THIOSULFIL) is a rapidly eliminated sulfonamide; concentrations of the drug in blood are thus low after the administration of conventional doses. It is used for the treatment of urinary tract infections in a dosage of 500 to 1000 mg, given three or four times daily. Sulfamethizole is available in tablets containing 500 mg.

Poorly Absorbed Sulfonamides. *Sulfasalazine* (AZALINE, AZULFIDINE) is very poorly absorbed from the gastrointestinal tract. It is used in the therapy of ulcerative colitis and regional enteritis, but relapses tend to occur in about one third of patients who experience a satisfactory initial response. Sulfasalazine is preferred to corticosteroids by some gastroenterologists for treatment of patients mildly or moderately ill with ulcerative colitis (Riis *et al.*, 1973). The drug is also being employed as the first approach to treatment of relatively mild cases of regional enteritis and granulomatous colitis (Singleton, 1977; Summers *et al.*, 1979; Peppercorn, 1984). Sulfasalazine is broken down by intestinal bacteria to sulfapyridine, an active sulfonamide that is absorbed and eventually excreted in the urine, and 5-aminosalicylate, which reaches high levels in the feces. There is convincing evidence that this latter compound is the effective agent in inflammatory bowel disease, whereas the sulfapyridine is responsible for most of the toxicity (Klotz *et al.*, 1980). Toxic reactions include Heinz-body anemia, acute hemolysis in patients with glucose-6-phosphate dehydrogenase deficiency, and agranulocytosis. Nausea, fever, arthralgias, and rashes occur in up to 20% of patients treated with the drug; desensitization has been effective (Taffet and Das, 1982). The usual total daily dose is 3 to 4 g initially, followed by 500 mg four times daily for maintenance. There is no evidence that the compound alters the intestinal microflora of persons with ulcerative colitis. Sulfasalazine is available in 500-mg tablets and in a suspension (250 mg/5 ml).

Sulfonamides for Topical Use. *Sulfacetamide.* Sulfacetamide is the N^1-acetyl-substituted derivative of sulfanilamide. Its aqueous solubility (1:140) is approximately 90 times that of sulfadiazine. Solutions of the sodium salt of the drug are employed extensively in the management of ophthalmic infections. Although topical sulfonamide for most purposes is discouraged because of lack of efficacy and a high risk of sensitization, sulfacetamide has certain advantages. Very high aqueous concentrations are nonirritating to the eye and are effective against susceptible microorganisms. A 30% solution of the sodium salt has a pH of 7.4, whereas the solutions of sodium salts of other sulfonamides are highly alkaline. The drug penetrates into ocular fluids and tissues in high concentration. Sensitivity reactions to sulfacetamide are rare, but the drug should not be used in patients with known hypersensitivity to sulfonamides.

The usual dose of sodium sulfacetamide solution applied topically to the eye is 1 or 2 drops of a 10 to 30% solution every 2 hours for severe infections and the same amount three or four times a day for chronic conditions. An ophthalmic ointment may be used instead of the solution, provided there is no wound of the cornea; as a rule, the ointment is reserved for application at bedtime.

Sulfacetamide sodium (ISOPTO CETAMIDE, SULAMYD SODIUM) is available for topical application to the eye, as an ophthalmic solution (10, 15, and 30%) and an ophthalmic ointment (10%).

Silver Sulfadiazine (SILVADENE, others). This drug inhibits the growth *in vitro* of nearly all pathogenic bacteria and fungi, including some species resistant to sulfonamides. The compound is used topically to reduce microbial colonization and the incidence of infections of wounds from burns. It should not be used to treat an established deep infection. Silver is released slowly from the preparation in concentrations that are selectively toxic to the microorganisms. However, bacteria may develop resistance to silver sulfadiazine. While little silver is absorbed, the plasma concentration of sulfadiazine may approach therapeutic levels if a large surface area is involved. Adverse reactions are infrequent and include burning, rash, and itching. Silver sulfadiazine is considered by most authorities to be one of the agents of choice for the prevention of infection of burns. It is available as a cream (10 mg/g) to be applied once or twice daily (Pruitt, 1987).

Mafenide. This sulfonamide (α-amino-*p*-toluenesulfonamide) is marketed as *mafenide acetate cream* (SULFAMYLON), which contains 85 mg/g. It is effective, when applied topically, for the prevention of colonization of burns by a large variety of gram-negative and gram-positive bacteria. It should not be used in treatment of an established deep infection. Superinfection with *Candida* may occasionally be a problem. The cream is applied once or twice daily to a thickness of 1 to 2 mm over the burned skin. Cleansing of the wound and removal of debris should be carried out before each application of the drug. Therapy is continued until skin grafting is possible. Mafenide is rapidly absorbed systemically and converted to para-carboxybenzenesulfonamide. Studies of absorption from the burn surface indicate that peak plasma concentrations are reached in 2 to 4 hours. Adverse effects include intense pain at sites of application, allergic reactions, and loss of fluid by evaporation from the burn surface, since occlusive dressings are not used. The drug and its primary metabolite inhibit carbonic anhydrase, and the urine becomes alkaline. A metabolic acidosis with compensatory tachypnea and hyperventilation may ensue (White and Asch, 1971).

Long-Acting Sulfonamides. Sulfadoxine (N^1-[5,6-dimethoxy-4-pyrimidinyl] sulfanilamide) is a sulfonamide with a particularly long half-life (7 to 9 days). It is utilized in combination with pyrimethamine (500 mg of sulfadoxine plus 25 mg of pyrimethamine as FANSIDAR) for the prophylaxis and treatment of malaria caused by chloroquine-resistant strains of *Plasmodium falciparum* (*see* Chapter 41) (Pearson and Hewlett, 1987). Because of severe and sometimes fatal reactions, including the Stevens–Johnson syndrome, the drug should be used for prophylaxis only where the risk of resistant malaria is high (Zitelli *et al.*, 1987). The combination of sulfadoxine and pyrimethamine has also been used for prophylaxis of *Pneumocystis carinii* pneumonia in patients with acquired immunodeficiency syndrome (AIDS), but experience is limited and side effects may be severe.

UNTOWARD REACTIONS TO SULFONAMIDES

The untoward effects that follow the administration of sulfonamides are numerous and varied; the overall incidence of reactions is about 5% (*see* Weinstein *et al.*, 1960). Certain forms of toxicity may be related to individual differences in sulfonamide metabolism (Shear *et al.*, 1986).

Disturbances of the Urinary Tract. Although the risk of crystalluria was relatively high with the older, less soluble sulfonamides, the incidence of this problem is very low with more soluble agents such as sulfisoxazole. Crystalluria has occurred in dehydrated patients with AIDS who were receiving sulfadiazine for toxoplasma encephalitis. Fluid intake should be such as to ensure a daily urine volume of at least 1200 ml (in adults). Alkalinization of the urine may be desirable if urine volume or pH is unusually low, since the solubility of sulfisoxazole increases greatly with slight elevations of pH.

Disorders of the Hematopoietic System. *Acute Hemolytic Anemia.* The mechanism of the acute hemolytic anemia produced by sulfonamides is not always readily apparent. In some cases, it has been thought to be a sensitization phenomenon. In other instances, the hemolysis is related to an erythrocytic deficiency of glucose-6-phosphate dehydrogenase activity. Hemolytic anemia is rare after sulfadiazine (0.05%); its exact incidence following therapy with sulfisoxazole is unknown.

Agranulocytosis. Agranulocytosis occurs in about 0.1% of patients who receive sulfadiazine; it also can follow the use of other sulfonamides. Although return of granulocytes to normal levels may be delayed for weeks or months after sulfonamide is withdrawn, most patients recover spontaneously with supportive care.

Aplastic Anemia. Complete suppression of bone-marrow activity with profound anemia, granulocytopenia, and thrombocytopenia is an extremely rare occurrence with sulfonamide therapy. It probably results from a direct myelotoxic effect, and may be fatal. However, reversible suppression of the bone marrow is quite common in patients with limited bone marrow reserve (*e.g.*, patients with AIDS or those receiving myelosuppressive chemotherapy).

Hypersensitivity Reactions. The incidence of other hypersensitivity reactions to sulfonamides is quite variable. Among the skin and mucous-membrane manifestations attributed to sensitization to sulfonamide are morbilliform, scarlatinal, urticarial, erysipeloid, pemphigoid, purpuric, and petechial rashes; and erythema nodosum, erythema multiforme of the Stevens–Johnson type, Behçet's syndrome, exfoliative dermatitis, and photosensitivity. Drug eruptions occur most often after the first week of therapy, but may appear earlier in previously sensitized individuals. Fever, malaise, and pruritus are frequently present simultaneously. The incidence of untoward dermal effects is about 2% with sulfisoxazole. A syndrome similar to serum sickness may appear after several days of sulfonamide therapy. Drug fever is a common untoward manifestation of sulfonamide treatment; the incidence approximates 3% with sulfisoxazole.

Focal or diffuse necrosis of the liver due to direct drug toxicity or sensitization occurs in less than 0.1% of patients. Headache, nausea, vomiting, fever, hepatomegaly, jaundice, and laboratory evidence of hepatocellular dysfunction usually appear 3 to 5 days after sulfonamide administration is started, and the syndrome may progress to acute yellow atrophy and death.

Miscellaneous Reactions. Anorexia, nausea, and vomiting occur in 1 to 2% of persons receiving sulfonamides, and these manifestations are probably central in origin. The administration of sulfonamides to premature infants may lead to the displacement of bilirubin from plasma albumin. Sulfonamides should not be given to pregnant women near term.

Drug Interactions. The most important interactions of the sulfonamides involve those with the oral anticoagulants, the sulfonylurea hypoglycemic agents, and the hydantoin anticonvulsants. In each case sulfonamides can potentiate the effects of the other drug by mechanisms that appear to involve primarily inhibition of metabolism and, possibly, displacement from albumin. Dosage adjustment may be necessary when a sulfonamide is given concurrently.

SULFONAMIDE THERAPY

The number of conditions for which the sulfonamides are therapeutically useful and constitute drugs of first choice has been sharply reduced by the development of more effective antimicrobial agents and by the gradual increase in the resistance of a number of bacterial species to this class of drugs. However, the use of sulfonamides has undergone a revival as a result of the introduction of the combination of trimethoprim and sulfamethoxazole (*see* below).

Urinary Tract Infections. Since a significant percentage of urinary tract infections in many parts of the world are caused by sulfonamide-resistant microorganisms, these drugs are no longer a therapy of first choice. Trimethoprim–sulfamethoxazole, a quinolone, or ampicillin are the preferred agents. However, sulfisoxazole may be used effectively in areas where the prevalence of resistance is not high or when the organism is known to be sensitive. The usual dosage is 2 g initially followed by 1 g, orally, four times a day for 5 to 10 days. Patients with acute pyelonephritis with high fever and other severe constitutional manifestations are at risk of bacteremia and shock and should not be treated with a sulfonamide. Most physicians prefer to administer an antibiotic parenterally, selected on the basis of the anticipated antimicrobial sensitivities and later modified, if necessary, by knowledge of the laboratory data.

Bacillary Dysentery (Shigella Diarrhea). Because of the frequency of resistant strains, the sulfonamides are now only infrequently useful in the management of this disease. Trimethoprim–sulfamethoxazole appears to be effective when given orally, although resistance to this combination is developing in some geographical areas. The usual oral dosage for adults is 160 mg of trimethoprim plus 800 mg of sulfamethoxazole every 12 hours for 5 days (Nelson *et al.*, 1976; DuPont *et al.*, 1982a).

Meningococcal Infections. Resistance to sulfonamides is now common in the various serological groups of *N. meningitidis*. All forms of disease produced by meningococci should now be treated with large doses of penicillin G or ampicillin, a third-generation cephalosporin, or chloramphenicol.

Chemoprophylaxis should be considered for close contacts of patients with meningococcal disease. Rifampin is now considered the prophylactic agent of choice. However, if the strain of *N. meningitidis* is known to be sensitive to sulfonamides, sulfisoxazole (1 g every 12 hours for four doses) may be given. One half of this dosage is administered to children 1 to 12 years of age. Minocycline is also effective, but its use is not recommended because of a high incidence of vestibular toxicity. Preliminary data suggest that ciprofloxacin is also efficacious. Penicillin G and several other antibiotics are not effective for prophylaxis.

Nocardiosis. Sulfonamides are of value in the treatment of infections due to *Nocardia* species. A number of instances of complete recovery from the disease after adequate treatment with a sulfonamide have been recorded. Sulfisoxazole or sulfadiazine may be given in dosages of 6 to 8 g daily. Concentrations of sulfonamide in plasma should be 80 to 160 μg/ml. This schedule is continued for several months after all manifestations have been controlled. The administration of sulfonamide together with an antibiotic has been recommended, especially for advanced cases, and ampicillin, erythromycin, or streptomycin has been suggested for this purpose. The clinical response and the results of sensitivity testing may be helpful in choosing a companion drug. It should be emphasized, however, that there are no clinical data to show that combination therapy is better than therapy with a sulfonamide alone. Trimethoprim–sulfamethoxazole has also been effective, and some authorities consider it to be the drug of choice (*see* below).

Trachoma and Inclusion Conjunctivitis. Systemic therapy with a tetracycline (Hoshiwara *et al.*, 1973) or erythromycin for 3 weeks appears to be the most effective treatment for trachoma. A sulfonamide may also be used. While the topical use of such agents will often suppress signs of infection, it will not eradicate the microorganism. Therapeutic results are best when therapy is initiated early, but even chronic cicatricial cases may respond. The local symptoms may disappear in a few days. Pannus, keratitis, conjunctival granulations, entropion, trichiasis, iritis, and corneal ulcerations improve and may even disappear. Corneal lesions respond more rapidly than do those of the conjunctivae. Blindness may be prevented. Inclusion conjunctivitis should be treated like trachoma.

Lymphogranuloma Venereum and Chancroid. Oral administration of tetracycline (500 mg four times daily for 21 days) or a sulfonamide (1 g of sulfisoxazole four times daily for 21 days) has been successful for the treatment of lymphogranuloma venereum. A similar schedule is recommended for chancroid.

Toxoplasmosis. The combination of pyrimethamine and sulfadiazine is the treatment of choice for toxoplasmosis (McCabe and Remington, 1990). In patients with severe chorioretinitis, it is advisable to add a corticosteroid to the therapeutic regimen (*see* Remington and Desmonts, 1976).

Use of Sulfonamides for Prophylaxis. The sulfonamides exhibit a degree of effectiveness equal to that of oral penicillin in preventing streptococcal infections and recurrences of rheumatic fever among susceptible subjects. Despite the efficacy of sulfonamides for long-term prophylaxis of rheumatic fever, their toxicity and the possibility of infection by drug-resistant streptococci make them less desirable than penicillin for this purpose. They should be used, however, without hesitation in patients who are hypersensitive to penicillin. The recommended dosage of sulfisoxazole is 1 g twice daily; for children under 27 kg (60 lb), the dose is halved. If untoward responses occur, they usually do so during the first 8 weeks of therapy; serious reactions after this time are rare. White-cell counts should be carried out once weekly during the first 8 weeks.

TRIMETHOPRIM–SULFAMETHOXAZOLE

The introduction of trimethoprim in combination with sulfamethoxazole constitutes an important advance in the development of clinically effective antimicrobial agents and represents the practical application of a theoretical consideration; that is, if two drugs act on sequential steps in the pathway of an obligate enzymatic reaction in bacteria, the result of their combination will be synergistic (*see* Hitchings, 1961). In much of the world the combination is known as co-trimoxazole. (*See* Wormser *et al.*, 1982, for an extensive review.)

Chemistry. Sulfamethoxazole has been discussed on page 1050, and its structural formula is shown in Table 45–1. The history of trimethoprim, a diaminopyrimidine, is discussed in Chapter 41. Its structural formula is as follows:

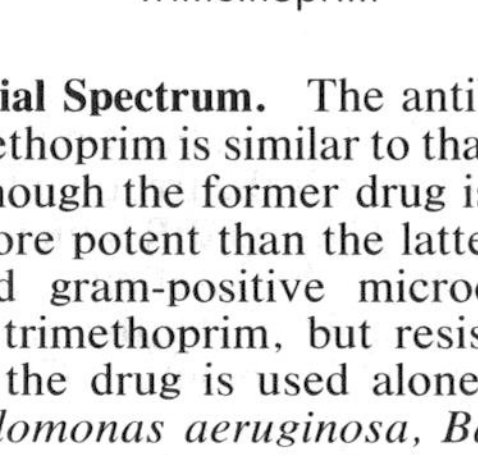

Trimethoprim

Antibacterial Spectrum. The antibacterial spectrum of trimethoprim is similar to that of sulfamethoxazole, although the former drug is usually 20 to 100 times more potent than the latter. Most gram-negative and gram-positive microorganisms are sensitive to trimethoprim, but resistance can develop when the drug is used alone (Ward *et al.*, 1982). *Pseudomonas aeruginosa, Bacteroides fragilis,* and enterococci are usually resistant. There is significant variation in the susceptibility of Enterobacteriaceae in different geographical locations to trimethoprim because of the spread of resistance mediated by plasmids and transposons (Goldstein *et al.*, 1986). The data presented below refer to the antimicrobial activity of the combination of trimethoprim and sulfamethoxazole.

Streptococcus pneumoniae, C. diphtheriae, and *N. meningitidis* are sensitive to trimethoprim–sulfamethoxazole. From 50 to 95% of strains of *Staphylococcus aureus, Staph. epidermidis, Strep. pyogenes,* the viridans group of streptococci, *E. coli, Proteus mirabilis, Pr. morganii, Pr. rettgeri, Enterobacter* species, *Salmonella, Shigella, Pseud. pseudomallei, Serratia,* and *Alcaligenes* species are inhibited. Also sensitive are *Klebsiella* species, *Brucella abortus, Pasteurella haemolytica, Yersinia pseudotuberculosis, Y. enterocolitica,* and *Nocardia asteroides.* Methicillin-resistant strains of *Staph. aureus,* although also resistant to trimethoprim or sulfamethoxazole alone, may be susceptible to the combination. A synergistic interaction between the components of the preparation is apparent even when microorganisms are resistant to sulfonamide or resistant to sulfonamide and moderately resistant to trimethoprim. However, a maximal degree of synergism occurs when microorganisms are sensitive to both components. The activity of trimethoprim–sulfamethoxazole *in vitro* depends on the medium in which it is determined; for example, low concentrations of thymidine almost completely abolish the antibacterial activity (*see* Symposium, 1969, 1973; Pelton *et al.*, 1977).

Mechanism of Action. The antimicrobial activity of the combination of trimethoprim and sulfamethoxazole results from its actions on two steps of the enzymatic pathway for the synthesis of tetrahydrofolic acid. Sulfonamide inhibits the incorporation of PABA into folic acid, and trimethoprim prevents the reduction of dihydrofolate to tetrahydrofolate. The latter is the form of folate essential for one-carbon transfer reactions, for example, the synthesis of thymidylate from deoxyuridylate. Selective toxicity for microorganisms is achieved in two ways. Mammalian cells utilize preformed folates from the diet and do not synthesize the compound. Furthermore, trimethoprim is a highly selective inhibitor of dihydrofolate reductase of lower organisms (*see* Chapter 41). This is vitally important, since this enzymatic function is a crucial one in all species.

The synergistic interaction between sulfonamide and trimethoprim is thus predictable from their respective mechanisms. There is an optimal ratio of the concentrations of the two agents for synergism, and this is equal to the ratio of the minimal inhibitory concentrations of the drugs acting independently. While this ratio varies for different bacteria, the most effective ratio for the greatest number of microorganisms is 20 parts of sulfamethoxazole to one part of trimethoprim. The combination is thus formulated to achieve a sulfamethoxazole concentration *in vivo* 20 times greater than that of trimethoprim. (*See* articles by Hitchings, Burchall, and Bushby, in Symposium, 1973.) The pharmacokinetic properties of the sulfonamide chosen to be in combination with trimethoprim are thus important, since relative constancy of the concentrations of the two compounds in the body is desired.

Examination of the sensitivity pattern of a typical isolate of *E. coli* illustrates the extent of synergism. The minimal inhibitory concentration for sulfamethoxazole alone is 3 μg/ml, while that for trimethoprim is 0.3 μg/ml. When the combination is tested at a ratio of 20:1, inhibitory concentrations are 1.0 μg/ml and 0.05 μg/ml, respectively. The combination is actually bactericidal for some microorganisms.

Bacterial Resistance. The frequency of development of bacterial resistance to trimethoprim–sulfamethoxazole is lower than it is to either of the agents alone. This is logical, since a microorganism that has acquired resistance to one of the components may still be killed by the other. Trimethoprim-resistant microorganisms may arise by mutation. Resistance in gram-negative bacteria is often associated with the acquisition of a plasmid that codes for an altered dihydrofolate reductase (Burchall *et al.,* 1982; Houvinen, 1987). Resistance to trimethoprim in *Staph. aureus* appears to be determined by a chromosomal gene rather than by a plasmid (Nakhla, 1973). The development of resistance to the combination also occurs *in vivo*. Resistance of *Staph. aureus* increased from 0.4% to 12.6% during one 5-year period of use. In New York, 10 to 20% of gram-negative microorganisms were found to be resistant (Wormser *et al.,* 1982).

Absorption, Distribution, and Excretion. The pharmacokinetic profiles of sulfamethoxazole and trimethoprim are closely but not perfectly matched to achieve a constant ratio of 20:1 in their concentrations in blood and tissues. The ratio in blood is often greater than 20:1, and that in tissues is frequently less. After a single oral dose of the combined preparation, trimethoprim is absorbed more rapidly than sulfamethoxazole. The concurrent administration of the drugs appears to slow the absorption of sulfamethoxazole. Peak blood concentrations of trimethoprim usually occur by 2 hours in most patients, while peak concentrations of sulfamethoxazole occur by 4 hours after a single oral dose. The half-lives of trimethoprim and sulfamethoxazole are approximately 11 and 10 hours, respectively.

When 800 mg of sulfamethoxazole is given with 160 mg of trimethoprim (the conventional 5:1 ratio) twice daily, the peak concentrations of the drugs in plasma are approximately 40 and 2 μg/ml, the optimal ratio. Peak concentrations are similar (46 and 3.4 μg/ml) after intravenous infusion of 800 mg of sulfamethoxazole and 160 mg of trimethoprim over a period of 1 hour.

Trimethoprim is rapidly distributed and concentrated in tissues, and about 40% is bound to plasma protein in the presence of sulfamethoxazole. The volume of distribution of trimethoprim is almost nine times that of sulfamethoxazole. The drug readily enters cerebrospinal fluid and sputum. High concentrations of each component of the mixture are also found in bile. About 65% of sulfamethoxazole is bound to plasma protein.

About 60% of administered trimethoprim and from 25 to 50% of sulfamethoxazole are excreted in the urine in 24 hours. Two thirds of the sulfonamide is unconjugated. Metabolites of trimethoprim are also excreted. The rates of excretion and the concentrations of both compounds in the urine are significantly reduced in patients with uremia.

Preparations, Routes of Administration, and Dosage. *Sulfamethoxazole and trimethoprim tablets* (BACTRIM, SEPTRA) are available in two sizes: 400 mg of sulfamethoxazole plus 80 mg of trimethoprim, and 800 mg of sulfamethoxazole plus 160 mg of trimethoprim. An oral suspension of 200 mg of sulfamethoxazole plus 40 mg of trimethoprim per 5 ml is also available, as is a preparation for intravenous use (400 mg of sulfamethoxazole plus 80 mg of trimethoprim per 5 ml). The usual adult dose is 800 mg of sulfamethoxazole plus 160 mg of trimethoprim every 12 hours for 10 to 14 days for management of most infections. Larger quantities have been given in special circumstances in patients with serious or life-threatening disease. Dosage must be reduced in patients with renal insufficiency (*see* Appendix II), and the preparation should not be administered if creatinine clearance is less than 15 ml per minute.

The recommended daily dose for children for treatment of urinary tract infections and otitis media is 8 mg/kg of trimethoprim and 40 mg/kg of sulfamethoxazole, given in two divided doses every 12 hours for 10 days; the same regimen is followed for 5 days to treat shigellosis.

The combination should not be used in infants under 2 months of age, during pregnancy (at term), and during the nursing period.

Trimethoprim is also available as a single-entity preparation (PROLOPRIM, TRIMPEX) in 100- and 200-mg tablets.

Untoward Effects. There is no evidence that trimethoprim–sulfamethoxazole, when given in the recommended doses, induces folate deficiency in normal persons. However, the margin between toxicity for bacteria and that for man may be relatively narrow when the cells of the patient are deficient in folate. In such cases, trimethoprim–sulfamethoxazole may cause or precipitate megaloblastosis, leukopenia, or thrombocytopenia. In routine use, the combination appears to exert little toxicity. About 75% of the untoward effects involve the skin. These are typical of those known to be produced by sulfonamides, as already described. However, trimethoprim–sulfamethoxazole has been reported to cause up to three times as many dermatological reactions as does sulfisoxazole when given alone (5.9% vs. 1.7%; Arndt and Jick, 1976). Exfoliative dermatitis, Stevens–Johnson syndrome, and toxic epidermal necrolysis (Lyell's syndrome) are rare, occurring primarily in older individuals. Nausea and vomiting constitute the bulk of gastrointestinal reactions; diarrhea is rare. Glossitis and stomatitis are relatively common. Mild and transient jaundice has been noted and appears to have the histological features of allergic cholestatic hepatitis. Central nervous system reactions consist of headache, depression, and hallucinations, manifestations known to be produced by sulfonamides. Hematological reactions, in addition to those mentioned above, are various types of anemia (including aplastic, hemolytic, and macrocytic), coagulation disorders, granulocytopenia, agranulocytosis, purpura, Henoch–Schönlein purpura, and sulfhemoglobinemia. Permanent impairment of renal function may follow the use of trimethoprim–sulfamethoxazole in patients with renal disease (Kalowski *et al.*, 1973), and a reversible decrease in creatinine clearance has been noted in patients with normal renal function (Symposium, 1973; Shouval *et al.*, 1978).

Patients with AIDS frequently react adversely when trimethoprim–sulfamethoxazole is administered to treat infection due to *P. carinii* (Gordin *et al.*, 1984). Fever, malaise, rash, and/or pancytopenia were noted in 8 of 18 patients in one series (Jaffe *et al.*, 1983); the incidence was 90% in another (Wharton *et al.*, 1984). It may be possible to continue therapy if the dose of the combination is lowered and concentrations of trimethoprim in plasma are monitored (Sattler *et al.*, 1988). Renal allograft recipients may suffer from severe hematological toxicity (Bradley *et al.*, 1980).

Therapeutic Uses. *Urinary Tract Infections.* Treatment of uncomplicated lower urinary tract infections with trimethoprim–sulfamethoxazole is often highly effective, even when the infecting agent is resistant to the sulfonamides alone. A dose of 800 mg of sulfamethoxazole plus 160 mg of trimethoprim every 12 hours for 10 days produces cure in the vast majority of cases. The preparation has been shown to produce a better therapeutic effect than does either of its components given separately when the infecting microorganisms are of the family Enterobacteriaceae. Single-dose therapy (320 mg of trimethoprim plus 1600 mg of sulfamethoxazole) has also been effective for the treatment of acute uncomplicated urinary tract infections (Harbord and Grüneberg, 1981; Counts *et al.*, 1982). Fihn and colleagues (1988) suggest a 3-day course of therapy.

The combination appears to have special efficacy in chronic and recurrent infections of the urinary tract (*see* Gleckman, 1975). Small doses (200 mg of sulfamethoxazole plus 40 mg of trimethoprim per day, or two to four times these amounts once or twice per week) appear to be effective in reducing the number of recurrent urinary tract infections in females (Stamm *et al.*, 1980). This effect may be related to the presence of therapeutic concentrations of trimethoprim in vaginal secretions (Stamey and Condy, 1975). Enterobacteriaceae surrounding the urethral orifice may be eliminated or markedly reduced in number, thus diminishing the chance of an ascending reinfection (*see* Stamey *et al.*, 1977). Trimethoprim is also found in therapeutic concentrations in prostatic secretions, and trimethoprim–sulfamethoxazole is often effective for the treatment of bacterial prostatitis (Dabhiolwala *et al.*, 1976).

Trimethoprim given alone has also been effective for urinary tract infections (Lacey *et al.*, 1980; Iravani *et al.*, 1981), but the development of resistant organisms limits the usefulness of this treatment. The usual dose for adults is 100 mg every 12 hours for 10 days.

Bacterial Respiratory Tract Infections. Trimethoprim–sulfamethoxazole is effective for acute exacerbations of chronic bronchitis. Administration of 800 to 1200 mg of sulfamethoxazole plus 160 to 240 mg of trimethoprim twice a day appears to be effective in decreasing fever, purulence and volume of sputum, and sputum bacterial count. The microorganisms involved were *H. influenzae* and *Strep. pneumoniae* (*see* Carroll *et al.*, 1977; Tandon, 1977). Trimethoprim–sulfamethoxazole should *not* be used to treat streptococcal pharyngitis, since it does not eradicate the microorganism. It is effective for acute otitis media in children and acute maxillary sinusitis in adults caused by susceptible strains of *H. influenzae* and *Strep. pneumoniae* (*see* Cameron *et al.*, 1975; Willner *et al.*, 1978; Hamory *et al.*, 1979). However, bacteremia with resistant pneumococci has been reported (Markman *et al.*, 1982).

Gastrointestinal Infections. The combination is useful for treatment of shigellosis, since many strains of the causative agent are now resistant to ampicillin (*see* Chang *et al.*, 1977); however, resistance to trimethoprim–sulfamethoxazole has now been reported. It is also effective for typhoid fever, but there is some difference of opinion concerning the precise role of trimethoprim–sulfamethoxazole for the management of this disease. The experience of Scragg and Rubidge (1971) suggests that, in children, this drug is not as effective as chloramphenicol. In adults, trimethoprim–sulfamethoxazole appears to be effective when the dose is 800 mg of sulfamethoxazole plus 160 mg of trimethoprim every 12 hours for 15 days. Chloramphenicol remains the drug of choice for typhoid fever in areas where the incidence of strains that are resistant to the drug is low (*see* Ramachandran *et al.*, 1978). Initial experience indicates that cefoperazone and ceftriaxone are also very effective in this disease (*see* Chapter 46).

Trimethoprim–sulfamethoxazole appears to be effective in the management of carriers of *S. typhi* and other species of *Salmonella*. One proposed schedule is the administration of 800 mg of sulfamethoxazole plus 160 mg of trimethoprim twice a day for 3 months; however, failures have occurred. The presence of chronic disease of the gallbladder may be associated with a high incidence of failure to clear the carrier state (*see* Symposium, 1969, 1973; Geddes, 1975). Acute diarrhea due to enteropathogenic *E. coli* can be treated or prevented with either trimethoprim or trimethoprim plus sulfamethoxazole (DuPont *et al.*, 1982a, 1982b).

Infection by Pneumocystis carinii. High-dose therapy (trimethoprim, 20 mg/kg per day, plus sulfamethoxazole, 100 mg/kg per day, in three or four divided doses) is effective for this severe infection in patients with AIDS. This combination compares favorably to pentamidine for treatment of this disease. However, the incidence of side effects is high for both regimens (Sattler and Remington, 1983; Wharton *et al.*, 1984). Lower dose, oral therapy with 800 mg of sulfamethoxazole plus 160 mg of trimethoprim (given twice daily) has been used successfully in AIDS patients with less severe pneumonia ($pO_2 > 60$ mm Hg) (Medina *et al.*, 1990). Prophylaxis with 800 mg of sulfamethoxazole and 160 mg of trimethoprim twice daily is effective in preventing pneumonia caused by this organism in patients with AIDS (Fischl *et al.*, 1988). However, adverse reactions (usually rash) occur in half the patients, and it is often necessary to stop treatment.

Prophylaxis in Neutropenic Patients. Several studies have demonstrated the effectiveness of low-dose therapy (150 mg/m^2 of body-surface area of trimethoprim and 750 mg/m^2 of body-surface area of sulfamethoxazole) for the prophylaxis of infection by *Pneumocystis carinii* (*see* Hughes *et al.*, 1977). In addition, significant protection against sepsis caused by gram-negative bacteria was noted when 800 mg of sulfamethoxazole plus 160 mg of trimethoprim was given twice daily to severely neutropenic patients (Enno *et al.*, 1978; Gurwith *et al.*, 1979; Kauffman *et al.*, 1983). The emergence of fungi and resistant bacteria may limit the usefulness of trimethoprim–sulfamethoxazole for prophylaxis (Gualtieri *et al.*, 1983).

Genital Infections. Chancroid is treated effectively with either erythromycin (500 mg orally four times daily for 10 days) or trimethoprim–sulfamethoxazole (160 mg plus 800 mg orally twice daily for 10 days). Because of bacterial resistance, trimethoprim–sulfamethoxazole is no longer recommended for the treatment of gonorrhea (Centers for Disease Control, 1987).

Miscellaneous Infections. Nocardia infections have been treated successfully with the combination (Smego *et al.*, 1983), but failures have also been reported (Stamm *et al.*, 1983). Although a combination of doxycycline and rifampin is now considered to be the treatment of choice for brucellosis, trimethoprim–sulfamethoxazole may be effective. Doses of trimethoprim–sulfamethoxazole have ranged from one tablet (800 mg/160 mg) three times a day for 1 week followed by one tablet a day for 2 weeks to two to four tablets per day for 2 months. Most patients recover, particularly when the latter dosage schedule is employed; however, relapse has occurred in 4% of cases even with this regimen. Hassan and associates (1971) have suggested that such therapy (one to two tablets per day) be continued for an additional 6 weeks to minimize the risk of relapse.

Intravenous administration of trimethoprim–sulfamethoxazole plus carbenicillin has been used effectively in the treatment of infections in neutropenic patients (Stuart *et al.*, 1980). Trimethoprim–sulfamethoxazole has also been useful in a variety of serious infections in children (Ardati and Dajani, 1979) and adults (Sattler and Remington, 1983; Symposium, 1987). Strains of methicillin-resistant *Staph. aureus* may be susceptible, and the combination with or without rifampin has been effective oral therapy for mild infections. Vancomycin remains the drug of choice for serious infections caused by methicillin-resistant *Staph. aureus*.

THE QUINOLONES

Older members of this class of synthetic antimicrobial agents, particularly nalidixic acid, have been available for the treatment of urinary tract infections for many years. These drugs are of relatively minor significance because of their limited therapeutic utility and the rapid development of bacterial resistance. Against this backdrop, the more recent introduction of fluorinated 4-quinolones such as norfloxacin and ciprofloxacin represents a particularly important therapeutic advance, since these agents have broad antimicrobial activity and are effective after oral administration for the treatment of a wide variety of infectious diseases. Relatively few side effects appear to accompany the use of these fluoroquinolones, and microbial resistance to their action does not develop rapidly (*see* Andriole, 1988, 1990a).

Chemistry. The compounds that are currently available for clinical use in the United States are 4-quinolones that all contain a carboxylic acid moiety in the 3 position of the basic ring structure (Table 45–2). The newer fluoroquinolones also contain a fluorine substituent at position 6, and many of these compounds contain a piperazine moiety at position 7. Other fluoroquinolones that are under

Table 45–2. STRUCTURAL FORMULAS OF SELECTED QUINOLONES AND FLUOROQUINOLONES

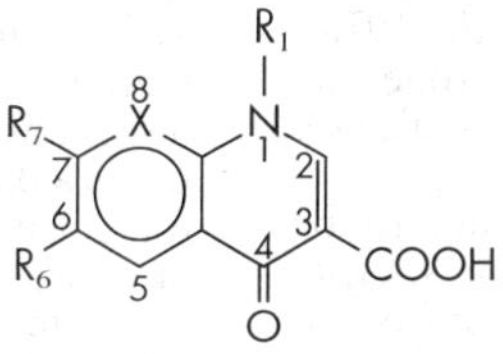

CONGENER	R1	R6	R7	X
Nalidixic acid	$—C_2H_5$	—H	$—CH_3$	—N—
Cinoxacin *	$—C_2H_5$	[Fused dioxolo ring] †		—CH—
Norfloxacin	$—C_2H_5$	—F	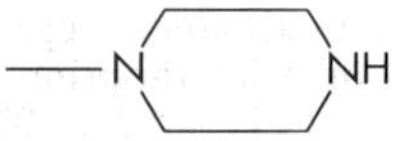	—CH—
Ciprofloxacin	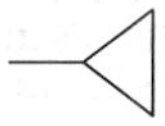	—F	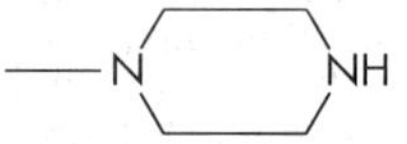	—CH—

* An N replaces C-2 in the basic ring structure of cinoxacin.

† 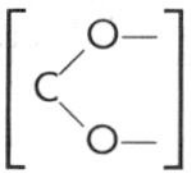

investigation include pefloxacin, ofloxacin, enoxacin, and fleroxacin.

Mechanism of Action. The two strands of double-helical DNA must be separated to permit DNA replication or transcription. However, anything that separates the strands results in "overwinding" or excessive positive supercoiling of the DNA in front of the point of separation. To combat this mechanical obstacle, the bacterial enzyme DNA gyrase is responsible for the continuous introduction of negative supercoils into DNA. This is an ATP-dependent reaction that requires that both strands of the DNA be cut to permit passage of a segment of DNA through the break; the break is then resealed.

The DNA gyrase of *E. coli* is composed of two 105,000-dalton A subunits and two 95,000-dalton B subunits. The A subunits, which carry out the strand-cutting function of the gyrase, are the site of action of the quinolones. The drugs inhibit gyrase-mediated DNA supercoiling at concentrations that correlate well with those required to inhibit bacterial growth (0.1 to 10 μg/ml). Mutations of the gene that encode the A subunit polypeptide can confer resistance to these drugs (Hooper *et al.*, 1987). Eukaryotic cells do not contain DNA gyrase. However, they do contain a conceptually and mechanistically similar type-II DNA topoisomerase that removes positive supercoils from eukaryotic DNA to prevent its tangling during replication. Quinolones inhibit eukaryotic type-II topoisomerase only at much higher concentrations (100 to 1000 μg/ml).

Antibacterial Spectrum. Although nalidixic acid and cinoxacin are bactericidal to most of the common gram-negative bacteria that cause urinary tract infections, their intrinsic activity is limited. Concentrations of nalidixic acid that approach 20 μg/ml are required to kill most enteric gram-negative bacilli; *Pseudomonas aeruginosa* is resistant. By contrast, the fluoroquinolones are rapidly bactericidal *in vitro* and are considerably more potent against *E. coli* and various species of *Salmonella*, *Shigella*, *Enterobacter*, *Campylobacter*, and *Neisseria* (*see* Sanders, 1988). Minimal inhibitory concentrations of ciprofloxacin and norfloxacin for 90% of these strains (MIC_{90}) are usually less than 0.2 μg/ml (*see* Norris and Mandell, 1988). These drugs are somewhat less active against *Pseud. aeruginosa*, enterococci, and pneumococci; values of MIC_{90} range from 0.5 to 2 μg/ml. Ciprofloxacin also has good activity against staphylococci, including methicillin-resistant strains (MIC_{90} = 1 μg/ml). Several intracellular bacteria are inhibited by ciprofloxacin at concentrations that can be achieved in plasma; these include species of *Chlamydia*, *Mycoplasma*, *Legionella*, *Brucella*, and *Mycobacterium* (including *Mycobacterium tuberculosis*) (Leysen *et al.*, 1989). However, clinical experience with these pathogens remains limited. Most anaerobic microorganisms are resistant to the fluoroquinolones. Resistance to these drugs may develop during therapy, especially with *Pseud. aeruginosa*; there is cross resistance among the members of the group. However, the frequency of selection of spontaneous single-step mutants of

E. coli that are resistant to quinolones is 100-fold lower with ciprofloxacin than with nalidixic acid.

Absorption, Fate, and Excretion. The quinolones are well absorbed after oral administration and are widely distributed in body tissues. A significant fraction of each drug is excreted unchanged in the urine; hepatic metabolism also takes place.

Norfloxacin. Norfloxacin is absorbed rapidly, although only 40% of an oral dose reaches the systemic circulation. Peak concentrations in plasma average 1.5 μg/ml after the usual dose of 400 mg. Food and antacids delay the absorption of the drug (Wolfson and Hooper, 1988). Norfloxacin is excreted by the kidney by both glomerular filtration and tubular secretion; approximately 30% of an administered dose is recovered in the urine as the parent drug. The drug is also metabolized and excreted in the bile. Concentrations of norfloxacin in urine may exceed 200 μg/ml 2 to 3 hours after administration and remain above 300 μg/ml for 12 hours in patients with normal renal function. The half-life of the drug in plasma is 5 hours.

Ciprofloxacin. The bioavailability of ciprofloxacin is approximately 60%, and peak concentrations in plasma average 2.4 μg/ml after a 500-mg oral dose. Antacids reduce the bioavailability of ciprofloxacin significantly. One half of an oral dose is recovered unchanged in the urine; renal clearance occurs by both filtration and tubular secretion. The remainder of the dose is recovered unaltered in the feces and as urinary metabolites. The half-time for elimination of ciprofloxacin is 3 to 4 hours when renal function is normal.

Nalidixic Acid. Almost all of orally administered nalidixic acid is absorbed. Plasma concentrations of 20 to 50 μg/ml may be achieved, but the drug is 93 to 97% bound to plasma proteins. In the body some nalidixic acid is converted to an active metabolite, hydroxynalidixic acid, and both are excreted into the urine. Very high concentrations of nalidixic acid plus its active metabolite are achieved in the urine—100 to 500 μg/ml. Some nalidixic acid is conjugated in the liver. The plasma half-life is normally about 8 hours, but it may be as long as 21 hours in the presence of renal failure.

Cinoxacin. Cinoxacin is completely absorbed after oral administration, and peak concentrations in plasma of 15 μg/ml are achieved after a 500-mg dose. About 50% of the drug is excreted unchanged in the urine; 30% is found as inactive metabolites. The half-time for elimination of cinoxacin from plasma is 2 hours.

Preparations and Dosage. *Norfloxacin* (NOROXIN) is supplied in 400-mg tablets. The dose for uncomplicated urinary tract infections is 400 mg, twice daily for 7 to 10 days; treatment for complicated urinary tract infections should be extended to 10 to 21 days. Tablets should be taken 1 hour before or 2 hours after a meal. Dosage should be halved for patients with creatinine clearances of less than 30 ml/min · 1.73 m^2 of body-surface area. Norfloxacin should not be administered to children or pregnant women.

Ciprofloxacin (CIPRO) is available as tablets containing 250, 500, or 750 mg of the drug. The usual oral dosage for adults with urinary tract infections is 250 mg twice daily. Respiratory tract, skin, bone, and joint infections should be treated with 500 mg every 12 hours, or, if severe, with 750 mg twice daily. Therapy is usually continued for 7 to 14 days; bone and joint infections may require treatment for 4 to 6 weeks or more. Dosage should be reduced for patients with severely impaired renal function. Ciprofloxacin should not be given to children or pregnant women.

Nalidixic acid (NEGGRAM) is available in tablets containing 250, 500, or 1000 mg of the drug and in an oral suspension containing 250 mg/5 ml. The recommended dosage for adults is 1 g four times a day for 1 to 2 weeks; thereafter a daily dose of 2 g is suggested. The recommended daily dosage for children is 55 mg/kg of body weight, given in four divided doses. The drug should not be used in infants under 3 months of age.

Cinoxacin (CINOBAC) is available in 250- and 500-mg capsules; the usual dosage for adults is 1 g daily in two to four divided portions for 7 to 14 days. This dosage should be reduced for patients with impaired renal function.

Adverse Effects. Quinolones and fluoroquinolones are generally well tolerated. The most common adverse reactions are nausea, abdominal discomfort, headache, and dizziness. Rashes, including photosensitivity reactions, can also occur. All of these agents can produce arthropathy in several species of immature animals. Although such lesions have not been reported in man, these drugs are not recommended for use in prepuberal children or pregnant women. Ciprofloxacin inhibits the metabolism of theophylline, and toxicity from elevated concentrations of the methylxanthine may occur when the two drugs are administered concurrently (Schwartz *et al.*, 1988).

Clinical Uses. Nalidixic acid and cinoxacin are useful only for urinary tract infections caused by susceptible microorganisms. The fluoroquinolones are significantly more potent and have a much broader spectrum of antimicrobial activity. Although norfloxacin is approved for use in the United States only for urinary tract infections, other indications (*e.g.*, prostatic and gastrointestinal infections) are being explored. Comparative clinical trials indicate that norfloxacin and trimethoprim–sulfamethoxazole are equally efficacious for the treatment of urinary tract infections (Stein *et al.*, 1987; Urinary Tract Infection Study Group, 1987).

Ciprofloxacin has been demonstrated to be very effective for the treatment of urinary tract infections and prostatitis (Weidner *et al.*, 1987) and for acute diarrheal disease caused by *E. coli*, *Shigella*, *Salmonella*, and *Campylobacter* (Ericsson *et al.*, 1987; Neighbor *et al.*, 1989). Bone and soft-tissue infections caused by staphylococci and gram-negative microorganisms have been treated effectively with ciprofloxacin (Greenberg *et al.*, 1987), as have infections caused by methicillin-resistant staphylococci (Piercy *et al.*, 1989). Ciprofloxacin and rifampin should probably be given concurrently for the treatment of serious staphylococcal infections. Fluoroquinolones also show promise in reducing the incidence of infections in neutropenic patients (Young, 1987) and in reducing meningococcal (Renkonen *et al.*, 1987) and typhoid (Gotuzzo *et al.*, 1988) carrier rates. Although ciprofloxacin has been effective in treating infections of the upper and lower respiratory tract, including some in patients with cystic fibrosis, the drug should not be used for pneumococcal respiratory tract infections or streptococcal cellulitis; beta-lactam antibiotics are preferred in these situations. Fluoroquinolones are not indicated for treatment of infections caused by anaerobes.

AGENTS FOR URINARY TRACT INFECTIONS

The urinary tract antiseptics inhibit the growth of many species of bacteria. They cannot be used to treat systemic infections because effective concentrations are not achieved in plasma with safe doses. However, because they are concentrated in the renal tubules, they can be used to treat infections of the urinary tract. Furthermore, effective antibacterial concentrations reach the renal pelves and the bladder. Treatment with such drugs can be thought of as local therapy in that only in the kidney and bladder, with the rare exceptions mentioned below, are adequate therapeutic levels achieved (*see* Andriole, 1990b).

Methenamine. Methenamine is a urinary tract antiseptic that owes its activity to formaldehyde.

Chemistry. Methenamine is hexamethylenetetramine (hexamethyleneamine). It has the following structure:

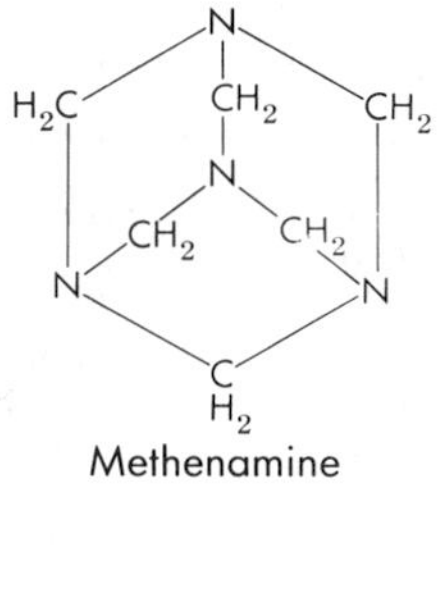

Methenamine

The compound decomposes in water to generate formaldehyde, according to the following reaction:

$$N_4(CH_2)_6 + 6H_2O + 4H^+ \rightarrow 4NH_4^+ + 6HCHO.$$

At pH 7.4 almost no decomposition occurs; however, 6% of the theoretical amount of formaldehyde is yielded at pH 6 and 20% at pH 5. Thus, acidification of the urine promotes the formaldehyde-dependent antibacterial action. The reaction is fairly slow, and 3 hours are required to reach 90% of completion.

Antimicrobial Activity. Nearly all bacteria are sensitive to free formaldehyde at concentrations of about 20 μg/ml. Urea-splitting microorganisms (*e.g.*, *Proteus* species) tend to raise the pH of the urine and thus inhibit the release of formaldehyde. Microorganisms do not develop resistance to formaldehyde.

Pharmacology and Toxicology. Methenamine is absorbed orally, but 10 to 30% decomposes in the gastric juice unless the drug is protected by an enteric coating. Because of the ammonia produced, methenamine is contraindicated in hepatic insufficiency. Excretion into the urine is nearly quantitative. When the urine pH is 6 and the daily urine volume is 1000 to 1500 ml, a daily dose of 2 g will yield a concentration of 18 to 60 μg/ml of formaldehyde; this is more than the minimal inhibitory concentration for most urinary tract pathogens. Various poorly metabolized acids can be used to acidify the urine. Low pH alone is bacteriostatic, so that acidification serves a double function. The acids commonly used are mandelic acid and hippuric acid.

Gastrointestinal distress frequently is caused by doses greater than 500 mg four times a day, even with enteric-coated tablets. Painful and frequent micturition, albuminuria, hematuria, and rashes may result from doses of 4 to 8 g a day given for longer than 3 to 4 weeks. Once the urine is sterile, a high dose should be reduced. Because systemic methenamine is nontoxic, renal insufficiency does not constitute a contraindication to the use of methenamine alone, but the acids given concurrently may be detrimental. Methenamine mandelate is contraindicated in renal insufficiency. Crystalluria from the mandelate moiety can occur. Methenamine combines with sulfamethizole and perhaps other sulfonamides in the urine, which results in mutual antagonism.

Preparations and Dosage. Methenamine mandelate (MANDELAMINE) is given in an oral suspension or as tablets or granules in a dose of 1 g, four times a day, for adults. *Methenamine hippurate* (UREX) is usually given in a dose of 1 g, twice a day.

Therapeutic Uses and Status. Methenamine is not a primary drug for the treatment of acute urinary tract infections, but it is of value for chronic suppressive treatment (Freeman *et al.*, 1975). The agent is most useful when the causative organism is *E. coli*, but it can usually suppress the common gram-negative offenders and often *Staph. aureus* and *Staph. epidermidis* as well. *Enterobacter aerogenes* and *Proteus vulgaris* are usually resistant. Urea-splitting bacteria (mostly *Proteus*) make it difficult to control the urine pH. The physician should strive to keep the pH below 5.5.

Nitrofurantoin. Nitrofurantoin is a synthetic nitrofuran that is used for the prevention and treatment of infections of the urinary tract. Its structural formula is as follows:

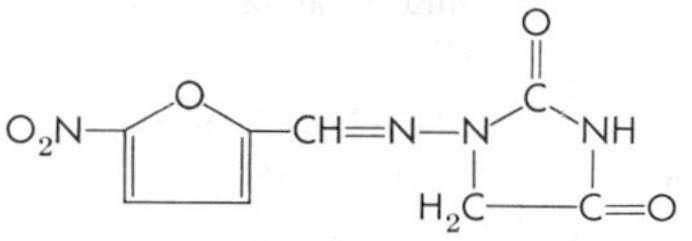

Nitrofurantoin

Antimicrobial Activity. Enzymes capable of reducing nitrofurantoin appear to be crucial for its activation. Highly reactive intermediates are formed, and these seem responsible for the observed capacity of the drug to damage DNA. Bacteria reduce nitrofurantoin more rapidly than do mammalian cells, and this is thought to account for the selective antimicrobial activity of the compound. Bacteria that are susceptible to the drug rarely become resistant during therapy. Nitrofurantoin is active against many strains of *E. coli* and enterococci. However, most species of *Proteus* and *Pseudomonas* and many of *Enterobacter* and *Klebsiella* are resistant. Nitrofurantoin is bacteriostatic for most susceptible microorganisms at concentrations of 32 μg/ml or less. The antibacterial activity is higher in an acidic urine.

Pharmacology and Toxicity. Nitrofurantoin is rapidly and completely absorbed from the gastrointestinal tract. The macrocrystalline form of the drug is absorbed and excreted more slowly. Antibacterial concentrations are not achieved in plasma following ingestion of recommended doses, because the drug is rapidly eliminated. The plasma half-life is 0.3 to 1 hour; about 40% is excreted unchanged into the urine. The average dose of nitrofurantoin yields a concentration in urine of approximately 200 μg/ml. This amount is soluble at pH values above 5, but the urine should not be alkalinized because this reduces antimicrobial activity. The rate of excretion is linearly related to the creatinine clearance, so that in patients with impaired glomerular function the efficacy of the drug may be decreased and the systemic toxicity increased. Nitrofurantoin colors the urine brown.

The most common untoward effects are nausea, vomiting, and diarrhea; the macrocrystalline preparation is better tolerated. Various hypersensitivity reactions occasionally occur. These include chills, fever, leukopenia, granulocytopenia, hemolytic anemia (associated with glucose-6-phosphate dehydrogenase deficiency), cholestatic jaundice, and hepatocellular damage. Chronic active hepatitis is an uncommon but serious side effect (Black *et al.*, 1980; Tolman, 1980). Acute pneumonitis with fever, chills, cough, dyspnea, chest pain, pulmonary infiltration, and eosinophilia may occur within hours to days of the initiation of therapy; it usually resolves within hours after discontinuation of the drug. More insidious subacute reactions may also be noted, and interstitial pulmonary fibrosis can occur in patients on chronic medication. Elderly patients are especially susceptible to the pulmonary toxicity of nitrofurantoin (*see* Holmberg *et al.*, 1980). Megaloblastic anemia is rare. Various neurological disorders are occasionally observed. Headache, vertigo, drowsiness, muscular aches, and nystagmus are readily reversible, but severe polyneuropathies with demyelination and degeneration of both sensory and motor nerves have been reported; signs of denervation and muscle atrophy result. Neuropathies are most likely to occur in patients with impaired renal function and in persons on long-continued treatment. Nitrofurantoin-induced polyneuropathy has been reviewed by Toole and Parrish (1973). Certain adverse reactions may be caused by toxic reactive metabolites (Spielberg and Gordon, 1981).

Nitrofurantoin (FURADANTIN, others) is available in tablets and capsules containing 50 or 100 mg of the drug and in an oral suspension containing 25 mg/5 ml. Nitrofurantoin macrocrystals (MACRODANTIN) are available in 25-, 50-, and 100-mg capsules. The oral dosage for adults is 50 to 100 mg four times a day, with meals and at bedtime. Alternatively, the daily dosage is better expressed as 5 to 7 mg/kg in four divided doses (not to exceed 400 mg). A single 50- to 100-mg dose at bedtime may be sufficient to prevent recurrences (Stamey *et al.*, 1977). The daily dose for children is 5 to 7 mg/kg, but it may be as low as 1 mg/kg for long-term therapy (Lohr *et al.*, 1977). A course of therapy should not exceed 14 days, and repeated courses should be separated by rest periods. Pregnant women, individuals with impaired renal function (creatinine clearance less than 40 ml per minute), and children less than 1 month of age should not receive nitrofurantoin.

Nitrofurantoin is approved only for the treatment of urinary tract infections caused by microorganisms that are known to be susceptible to the drug. It has been used to prevent recurrent infections and for the prevention of bacteriuria after prostatectomy (Matthew *et al.*, 1978).

Phenazopyridine. *Phenazopyridine hydrochloride* (PYRIDIUM) is *not* a urinary antiseptic. However, it does have an analgesic action on the urinary tract and alleviates symptoms of dysuria, frequency, burning, and urgency. Phenazopyridine is supplied in tablets containing 100 or 200 mg of the drug for oral administration. The usual dose is 200 mg three times daily. The compound is an azo dye, and the urine is colored orange or red; the patient should be so informed. Gastrointestinal upset is seen in up to 10% of patients; overdosage may result in methemoglobinemia. Phenazopyridine is also marketed in combination with sulfisoxazole (AZO GANTRISIN) and sulfamethoxazole (AZO GANTANOL) (*see* above).

Ardati, K. O., and Dajani, A. S. Intravenous trimethoprim–sulfamethoxazole in the treatment of serious infections in children. *J. Pediatr.*, **1979**, *95*, 801–806.

Arndt, K. A., and Jick, H. Rates of cutaneous reactions to drugs. *J.A.M.A.*, **1976**, *235*, 918–923.

Black, M.; Rabin, L.; and Schatz, N. Nitrofurantoin-induced chronic active hepatitis. *Ann. Intern. Med.*, **1980**, *92*, 62–64.

Bradley, P. P.; Warden, G. D.; Maxwell, J. G.; and Rothstein, G. Neutropenia and thrombocytopenia in renal allograft recipients treated with trimethoprim–sulfamethoxazole. *Ann. Intern. Med.*, **1980**, *93*, 560–562.

Brown, G. M. The biosynthesis of folic acid. II. Inhibition by sulfonamides. *J. Biol. Chem.*, **1962**, *237*, 536–540.

Burchall, J. J.; Elwell, L. P.; and Fling, M. E. Molecular mechanisms of resistance to trimethoprim. *Rev. Infect. Dis.*, **1982**, *4*, 246–254.

Bushby, S. R. M., and Hitchings, G. H. Trimethoprim, a sulphonamide potentiator. *Br. J. Pharmacol. Chemother.*, **1968**, *33*, 72–90.

Buttle, G. A. H.; Gray, W. H.; and Stephenson, D. Protection of mice against streptococcal and other infections by *p*-aminobenzenesulphonamide and related substances. *Lancet*, **1936**, *1*, 1286–1290.

Cameron, G. G.; Pomahac, A. C.; and Johnston, M. T. Comparative efficacy of ampicillin and trimethoprim–sulfamethoxazole in otitis media. *Can. Med. Assoc. J.*, **1975**, *112*, 87S–88S.

Carroll, P. G.; Krejci, S. P.; Mitchell, J.; Puranik, V.; Thomas, R.; and Wilson, B. A comparative study of co-trimoxazole and amoxycillin in the treatment of acute bronchitis in general practice. *Med. J. Aust.*, **1977**, *2*, 286–287.

Centers for Disease Control. Antibiotic-resistant strains of *Neisseria gonorrhoeae*: policy guidelines for detection, management, and control. *M.M.W.R.*, **1987**, *36*, Suppl., 1S–18S.

Chang, M. J.; Dunkle, L. M.; Van Reken, D.; Anderson, D.; Wong, M. L.; and Feigin, R. D. Trimethoprim–sulfamethoxazole compared to ampicillin in the treatment of shigellosis. *Pediatrics*, **1977**, *51*, 726–729.

Colebrook, L., and Kenny, M. Treatment of human puerperal infections, and of experimental infections in mice, with PRONTOSIL. *Lancet*, **1936**, *1*, 1279–1286.

Counts, G. W.; Stamm, W. E.; McKevitt, M.; Running, K.; Holmes, K. K.; and Turck, M. Treatment of cystitis in women with a single dose of trimethoprim–sulfamethoxazole. *Rev. Infect. Dis.*, **1982**, *4*, 484–490.

Dabhiolwala, N. F.; Bye, A.; and Claridge, M. A study of concentrations of trimethoprim–sulfamethoxazole in the human prostate gland. *Br. J. Urol.*, **1976**, *48*, 77–81.

Domagk, G. Ein Beitrag zur Chemotherapie der Bakteriellen Infektionen. *Dtsch. Med. Wochenschr.*, **1935**, *61*, 250–253.

DuPont, H. L.; Evans, D. G.; Rios, N.; Cabada, F. J.; Evans, D. J., Jr.; and DuPont, M. W. Prevention of travelers' diarrhea with trimethoprim–sulfamethoxazole. *Rev. Infect. Dis.*, **1982a**, *4*, 533–539.

DuPont, H. L.; Reves, R. R.; Galindo, E.; Sullivan, P. S.; Wood, L. V.; and Mendiola, J. G. Treatment of travelers' diarrhea with trimethoprim/sulfamethoxazole and with trimethoprim alone. *N. Engl. J. Med.*, **1982b**, *307*, 841–844.

Enno, A.; Catovsky, D.; Darrell, J.; Goldman, J. M.; Hows, J.; and Galton, D. A. G. Co-trimoxazole for prevention of infection in acute leukemia. *Lancet*, **1978**, *1*, 395–398.

Ericsson, C. D.; Johnson, P. C.; DuPont, H. L.; Morgan, D. R.; Birsura, J. A. M.; and De La Cabada, F. J. Ciprofloxacin or trimethoprim–sulfamethoxazole as initial therapy for travelers' diarrhea. *Ann. Intern. Med.*, **1987**, *106*, 216–220.

Fihn, S. D.; Johnson, C.; Roberts, P. L.; Running, K.; and Stamm, W. E. Trimethoprim–sulfamethoxazole for acute dysuria in women: a single-dose or 10-day course. *Ann. Intern. Med.*, **1988**, *108*, 350–357.

Fildes, P. A rational approach to research in chemotherapy. *Lancet*, **1940**, *1*, 955–957.

Fischl, M. A.; Dickinson, G. M.; and La Voie, L. Safety and efficacy of sulfamethoxazole and trimethoprim chemoprophylaxis for *Pneumocystis carinii* pneumonia in AIDS. *J.A.M.A.*, **1988**, *259*, 1185–1189.

Freeman, R. B.; Smith, W. M.; and Richardson, J. A. Long-term therapy for chronic bacteriuria in men: U.S. Public Health Service Cooperative Study. *Ann. Intern. Med.*, **1975**, *83*, 133–147.

Geddes, A. M. Trimethoprim–sulfamethoxazole in the treatment of gastrointestinal infections, including enteric fever and typhoid carriers. *Can. Med. Assoc. J.*, **1975**, *112*, 35S–36S.

Gleckman, R. A. Trimethoprim–sulfamethoxazole vs. ampicillin in chronic urinary tract infections. *J.A.M.A.*, **1975**, *233*, 427–431.

Goldstein, F. W.; Papdopoulou, B.; and Acar, J. R. The changing pattern of trimethoprim resistance in Paris, with a review of worldwide experience. *Rev. Infect. Dis.*, **1986**, *8*, 725–737.

Gordin, F. M.; Simon, G. L.; Wofsy, C. B.; and Mills, J. Adverse reactions to trimethoprim–sulfamethoxazole in patients with acquired immuno-deficiency syndrome. *Ann. Intern. Med.*, **1984**, *100*, 495–499.

Gotuzzo, E.; Guerra, J. G.; Benavente, L.; Palomino, J. C.; Carrillo, C.; Lopera, J.; Delgado, F.; Nalin, D. R.; and Sabbaj, J. Use of norfloxacin to treat chronic typhoid carriers. *J. Infect. Dis.*, **1988**, *157*, 1221–1225.

Greenberg, R. N.; Kennedy, D. J.; Reilly, P. M.; Luppen, K. L.; Weinandt, W. J.; Bollinger, M. R.; Aguirre, F.; Kodesch, F.; and Saeed, A. M. Treatment of bone, joint, and soft-tissue infections with oral ciprofloxacin. *Antimicrob. Agents Chemother.*, **1987**, *31*, 151–155.

Gualtieri, R. J.; Donowitz, G. R.; Kaiser, D. L.; Hess, C. E.; and Sande, M. A. Double-blind randomized study of prophylactic trimethoprim/sulfamethoxazole in granulocytopenic patients with hematologic malignancies. *Am. J. Med.*, **1983**, *74*, 934–940.

Gurwith, M. J.; Brunton, J. L.; Lank, B. A.; Harding, G. K. M.; and Ronald, A. R. A prospective controlled investigation of prophylactic trimethoprim–sulfamethoxazole in hospitalized granulocytic patients. *Am. J. Med.*, **1979**, *66*, 248–256.

Hamory, B. H.; Sande, M. A.; Sydnor, A.; and Gwaltney, J. M. Etiology and antimicrobial therapy of acute maxillary sinusitis. *J. Infect. Dis.*, **1979**, *139*, 197–202.

Harbord, R. D., and Grüneberg, R. N. Treatment of urinary tract infection with a single dose of amoxycillin, co-trimoxazole or trimethoprim. *Br. Med. J.*, **1981**, *283*, 1301–1302.

Hassan, A.; Erian, M. M.; Farid, Z.; Hathout, S. D.; and Sorensen, K. Trimethoprim–sulphamethoxazole in acute brucellosis. *Br. Med. J.*, **1971**, *3*, 159–160.

Hitchings, G. H. A biochemical approach to chemotherapy. *Ann. N.Y. Acad. Sci.*, **1961**, *23*, 700–708.

Holmberg, L.; Boman, G.; Bottiger, L. E.; Eriksson, B. A.; Spross, R.; and Wessling, A. Adverse reactions to nitrofurantoin. *Am. J. Med.*, **1980**, *69*, 733–738.

Hooper, D. C.; Wolfson, J. S.; Ng, E. Y.; and Swartz, M. N. Mechanisms of action of and resistance to ciprofloxacin. *Am. J. Med.*, **1987**, *82*, Suppl. 4A, 12–20.

Hoshiwara, J.; Oster, B.; Hana, L.; Cignett, F.; Colema, V. R.; and Jawetz, E. Doxycycline treatment of chronic trachoma. *J.A.M.A.*, **1973**, *224*, 220–223.

Houvinen, P. Trimethoprim resistance. *Antimicrob. Agents Chemother.*, **1987**, *31*, 1451–1456.

Hughes, W. T.; Kuhn, S.; Chaudhary, S.; Feldman, S.; Verzosa, M.; Aur, J. A. R.; Pratt, C.; and George, S. L. Successful chemoprophylaxis for *Pneumocystis carinii* pneumonitis. *N. Engl. J. Med.*, **1977**, *297*, 1419–1426.

Iravani, A.; Richard, G. A.; and Baer, H. Treatment of uncomplicated urinary tract infection with trimethoprim versus sulfisoxazole with special reference to antibody-coated bacteria and faecal flora. *Antimicrob. Agents Chemother.*, **1981**, *19*, 824–850.

Jaffe, H. S.; Abrams, D. I.; Ammann, A. J.; Lewis, B. J.; and Golden, J. A. Complications of co-trimoxazole in treatment of AIDS-associated *Pneumocystis carinii* pneumonia in homosexual men. *Lancet*, **1983**, *2*, 1109–1111.

Kalowski, S.; Nanra, R. S.; Mathew, T. H.; and Kincaid-Smith, P. Deterioration in renal function in association with co-trimoxazole therapy. *Lancet*, **1973**, *2*, 394–397.

Kauffman, C. A.; Liepman, M. K.; Bergman, A. G.; and Mioduszewski, J. Trimethoprim/sulfamethoxazole prophylaxis in neutropenic patients. *Am. J. Med.*, **1983**, *74*, 599–607.

Klotz, U.; Maier, K.; Fischer, C.; and Heinkel, K. Therapeutic efficacy of sulfasalazine and its metabolites in patients with ulcerative colitis and Crohn's disease. *N. Engl. J. Med.*, **1980**, *303*, 1499–1502.

Lacey, R. W.; Lord, V. L.; Gunasekera, H. K.; Leiberman, P. J.; and Luxton, D. E. Comparison of trimethoprim alone with trimethoprim–sulphamethoxazole in the treatment of respiratory and urinary infections with particular reference to selection of trimethoprim resistance. *Lancet*, **1980**, *1*, 1270–1273.

Leysen, D. C.; Haemers, A.; and Pattyn, S. R. Mycobacteria and the new quinolones. *Antimicrob. Agents Chemother.*, **1989**, *33*, 1–5.

Lohr, J. A.; Nunley, D. H.; Howards, S. S.; and Ford, R. F. Prevention of recurrent urinary tract infections in girls. *Pediatrics*, **1977**, *59*, 562–565.

Markman, M.; Mannisi, J.; Dick, J. D.; Filburn, B.; Santos, G. W.; and Rein, S. Sulfamethoxazole–trimethoprim-resistant pneumococcal sepsis. *J.A.M.A.*, **1982**, *248*, 3011–3012.

Matthew, A. D.; Gonzalez, R.; Jeffords, D.; and Pinto, M. H. Prevention of bacteriuria after transurethral prostatectomy with nitrofurantoin macrocrystals. *J. Urol.*, **1978**, *120*, 442–443.

Medina, I. L.; Mills, J.; Leoung, G.; Hopewell, P. C.; Feigal, D. W., Jr.; and Wofsy, C. B. Oral therapy for *Pneumocystis carinii* pneumonia (PCP) in AIDS: a randomized, double-blind trial comparing trimethoprim and sulfamethoxazole with dapsone and trimethoprim. *N. Engl. J. Med.*, **1990**. In press.

Nakhla, L. S. Genetic determinants of trimethoprim resistance in a strain of *Staphylococcus aureus*. *J. Clin. Pathol.*, **1973**, *26*, 712–715.

Neighbor, M. L.; Cohen, P. T.; Siegel, D.; Newman, M. D.; Hadley, W. K.; Yajko, D. M.; Feigal, D. W., Jr.; Larkin, H.; and Sande, M. A. Ciprofloxacin in the treatment of acute infectious diarrhea. *Ann. Emerg. Med.*, **1989**, *18*, 464.

Nelson, J. D.; Kusmiesz, H.; and Jacobson, L. H. Comparison of trimethoprim–sulfamethoxazole and ampicillin therapy for shigellosis in ambulatory patients. *J. Pediatr.*, **1976**, *89*, 491–493.

Pearson, R. D., and Hewlett, E. L. Use of pyrimethamine-sulfadoxine (FANSIDAR) in prophylaxis against chloroquine-resistant *Plasmodium falciparum* and *Pneumocystis carinii*. *Ann. Intern. Med.*, **1987**, *106*, 714–718.

Pelton, S. I.; Shurin, P. A.; Klein, J. O.; and Finland, M. Quantitative inhibition of *Haemophilus influenzae* by trimethoprim–sulfamethoxazole. *Antimicrob. Agents Chemother.*, **1977**, *12*, 649–654.

Peppercorn, M. A. Sulfasalazine: pharmacology, clinical use, toxicity, and related new drug development. *Ann. Intern. Med.*, **1984**, *3*, 377–384.

Piercy, E. A.; Barbaro, D.; Luby, J. P.; and Mackowiak, P. A. Ciprofloxacin for methicillin-resistant *Staphylococcus aureus* infections. *Antimicrob. Agents Chemother.*, **1989**, *33*, 128–130.

Ramachandran, S.; Godfrey, J. J.; and Lionel, N. D. W. A comparative trial of co-trimoxazole and chloramphenicol in typhoid and paratyphoid fever. *J. Trop. Med. Hyg.*, **1978**, *81*, 36–39.

Remington, J. S., and Desmonts, G. Toxoplasmosis. In, *Infectious Diseases of the Fetus and Newborn Infant*. (Remington, J. S., and Klein, J. O., eds.) W. B. Saunders Co., Philadelphia, **1976**, pp. 191–332.

Renkonen, O. V.; Sivonen, A.; and Visadorpi, R. Effect of ciprofloxacin on carrier rates of *Neisseria meningitidis* in army recruits in Finland. *Antimicrob. Agents Chemother.*, **1987**, *31*, 962–963.

Riis, P.; Anthonisen, P.; Wulff, R.; Folkenborg, O.; Bonnevie, O.; and Binder, V. The prophylactic effect of salicylazosulphapyridine in ulcerative colitis during long-term treatment. *Scand. J. Gastroenterol.*, **1973**, *8*, 71–74.

Sanders, C. C. Ciprofloxacin: *in vitro* activity, mechanism of action, and resistance. *Rev. Infect. Dis.*, **1988**, *10*, 516–527.

Sattler, F. R., and Remington, J. R. Intravenous trimethoprim–sulfamethoxazole therapy for *Pneumocystis carinii* pneumonia. *Arch. Intern. Med.*, **1983**, *143*, 1709–1712.

Sattler, F. R.; Cowan Robert Nielson, D. M.; and Ruskin, J. Trimethoprim–sulfamethoxazole compared with pentamidine for treatment of *Pneumocystis carinii* pneumonia in the acquired immunodeficiency syndrome. *Ann. Intern. Med.*, **1988**, *109*, 280–287.

Schwartz, J.; Jauregui, L.; Lettieri, J.; and Bachmann, K. Impact of ciprofloxacin on theophylline clearance and steady-state concentrations in serum. *Antimicrob. Agents Chemother.*, **1988**, *32*, 75–77.

Scragg, J. N., and Rubidge, C. J. Trimethoprim and sulphamethoxazole in typhoid fever in children. *Br. Med. J.*, **1971**, *3*, 738–741.

Shear, N. H.; Spielberg, S. P.; Grant, D. M.; Tang, B. K.; and Kalow, W. Differences in metabolism of sulfonamides predisposing to idiosyncratic toxicity. *Ann. Intern. Med.*, **1986**, *105*, 179–184.

Shouval, D.; Ligumsky, M.; and Ben-Ishay, D. Effect of co-trimoxazole on normal creatinine clearance. *Lancet*, **1978**, *2*, 244–245.

Singleton, J. W. National Cooperative Crohn's Disease Study (NCCDS). Results of drug treatment. *Gastroenterology*, **1977**, *72*, A110/1133.

Smego, R. A.; Moeller, M. B.; and Gallis, H. A. Trimethoprim–sulfamethoxazole therapy for *Nocardia* infections. *Arch. Intern. Med.*, **1983**, *143*, 711–718.

Spielberg, S. P., and Gordon, G. B. Nitrofurantoin cytotoxicity. *J. Clin. Invest.*, **1981**, *67*, 37–71.

Stamey, T. A., and Condy, M. The diffusion and concentration of trimethoprim in human vaginal fluid. *J. Infect. Dis.*, **1975**, *131*, 261–266.

Stamey, T. A.; Condy, M.; and Mihara, G. Prophylactic efficacy of nitrofurantoin macrocrystals and trimethoprim–sulfamethoxazole in urinary infections: biologic effects on the vaginal and rectal flora. *N. Engl. J. Med.*, **1977**, *296*, 780–783.

Stamm, A. M.; McFall, D. W.; and Dismukes, W. E. Failure of sulfonamides and trimethoprim in the treatment of nocardiosis. *Arch. Intern. Med.*, **1983**, *143*, 383–385.

Stamm, W. E.; Counts, G. W.; Wagner, K. F.; Martin, D.; Gregory, D.; McKevitt, M.; Turck, M.; and Holmes, K. K. Antimicrobial prophylaxis or recurrent urinary tract infections. *Ann. Intern. Med.*, **1980**, *92*, 770–775.

Stein, G. E.; Mummaw, N.; Goldstein, E. J. C.; Boyko, E. J.; Reller, L. B.; Kurtz, T. O.; Miller, K.; and Cox, C. E. A multicenter comparative trial of three-day norfloxacin *vs* ten-day sulfamethoxazole and trimethoprim for the treatment of uncomplicated urinary tract infections. *Arch. Intern. Med.*, **1987**, *147*, 1760–1762.

Stuart, R. K.; Braine, H. G.; Lietman, P. S.; Saral, R.; and Fuller, D. J. Carbenicillin–trimethoprim/sulfamethoxazole versus carbenicillin–gentamicin as empiric therapy of infection in granulocytopenic patients. *Am. J. Med.*, **1980**, *68*, 876–885.

Summers, R. W.; Switz, D. M.; Sessions, J. T., Jr.; Becktel, J. M.; Best, W. R.; Kern, F., Jr.; and Singleton, J. W. National Cooperative Crohn's Disease Study: results of drug treatment. *Gastroenterology*, **1979**, *77*, 847–869.

Taffet, S. L., and Das, K. M. Desensitization of patients with inflammatory bowel disease to sulfasalazine. *Am. J. Med.*, **1982**, *73*, 520–524.

Tandon, M. K. A comparative trial of co-trimoxazole and amoxycillin in the treatment of acute exacerbations of chronic bronchitis. *Med. J. Aust.*, **1977**, *2*, 281–284.

Tolman, K. G. Nitrofurantoin and chronic active hepatitis. *Ann. Intern. Med.*, **1980**, *92*, 119–120.

Toole, J. F., and Parrish, M. L. Nitrofurantoin polyneuropathy. *Neurology (Minneap.)*, **1973**, *23*, 554–559.

Urinary Tract Infection Study Group. Coordinated multicenter study of norfloxacin versus trimethoprim–sulfamethoxazole treatment of symptomatic urinary tract infections. *J. Infect. Dis.*, **1987**, *155*, 170–177.

Ward, L. R.; Rowe, B.; and Threlfall, E. J. Incidence of trimethoprim resistance in salmonellae isolated in Britain: a twelve year study. *Lancet*, **1982**, *2*, 705–706.

Weidner, W.; Schifer, H. G.; and Dalhoff, A. Treatment of chronic bacterial prostatitis with ciprofloxacin. *Am. J. Med.*, **1987**, *82*, Suppl. 4A, 280–283.

Wharton, M.; Coleman, D. L.; Fitz, G.; Golden, J.; Wofsy, C.; Luce, J.; and Hopewell, P. Prospective, randomized trial of trimethoprim–sulfamethoxazole versus pentamidine for *Pneumocystis carinii* pneumonia in the acquired immunodeficiency syndrome. *Am. Rev. Respir. Dis.*, **1984**, *129*, A–188.

White, M. G., and Asch, M. J. Acid–base effects of topical mafenide acetate in the burned patient. *N. Engl. J. Med.*, **1971**, *284*, 1281–1286.

Willner, M. M.; Dull, T. A.; and McDonald, H. Comparison of trimethoprim–sulfamethoxazole and ampicillin in the treatment of acute bacterial otitis media in children. In, *Current Chemotherapy: Proceedings of the Tenth International Congress of Chemotherapy*, Vol. I. (Siegenthaler, W., and Lüthy, R., eds.) American Society for Microbiology, Washington, D. C., **1978**, pp. 125–127.

Wolfson, J. S., and Hooper, D. C. Norfloxacin: a new targeted fluoroquinolone antimicrobial agent. *Ann. Intern. Med.*, **1988**, *108*, 238–251.

Woods, D. D. Relation of *p*-aminobenzoic acid to mechanism of action of sulphanilamide. *Br. J. Exp. Pathol.*, **1940**, *21*, 74–90.

———. The biochemical mode of action of the sulphonamide drugs. *J. Gen. Microbiol.*, **1962**, *29*, 687–702.

Young, L. S. The new fluorinated quinolones for infection prevention in acute leukemia. *Ann. Intern. Med.*, **1987**, *106*, 144–146.

Zitelli, B. J.; Alexander, J.; Taylor, S.; Miller, K. D.; Howrie, D. L.; Kuritsky, J. N.; Perez, T. H.; and Van Thiel, D. H. Fatal hepatic necrosis due to pyrimethamine-sulfadoxine (FANSIDAR). *Ann. Intern. Med.*, **1987**, *106*, 393–395.

Monographs and Reviews

Andriole, V. T. (ed.). *The Quinolones*. Academic Press, Inc., New York, **1988.**

———. Quinolones. In, *Principles and Practice of Infectious Diseases*, 3rd ed. (Mandell, G. L.; Douglas, R. G., Jr.; and Bennett, J. E.; eds.) Churchill Livingstone, Inc., New York, **1990a**, pp. 334–345.

———. Urinary tract agents: nitrofurantoin and methenamine. In, *Principles and Practice of Infectious Diseases*, 3rd ed. (Mandell, G. L.; Douglas, R. G., Jr.; and Bennett, J. E.; eds.) Churchill Livingstone, Inc., New York, **1990b**, pp. 345–349.

McCabe, R. E., and Remington, J. S. *Toxoplasma gondii*. In, *Principles and Practice of Infectious Diseases*, 3rd ed. (Mandell, G. L.; Douglas, R. G., Jr.; and Bennett, J. E.; eds.) Churchill Livingstone, Inc., New York, **1990**, pp. 2090–2103.

Norris, S., and Mandell, G. L. The quinolones: history and overview. In, *The Quinolones*. (Andriole, V. T., ed.) Academic Press, Inc., New York, **1988.**

Pruitt, B. A. Opportunistic infections in burn patients: diagnosis and treatment. In, *New Surgical and Medical Approaches in Infectious Diseases*. (Root, R.; Trunkey, R.; and Sande, M. A.; eds.) Churchill Livingstone, Inc., New York, **1987**, pp. 245–261.

Symposium. (Various authors.) The synergy of trimethoprim and sulphonamides. *Postgrad. Med. J.*, **1969**, *45*, Suppl., 3–104.

Symposium. (Various authors.) Trimethoprim–sulfamethoxazole. *J. Infect. Dis.*, **1973**, *128*, Suppl., 425–816.

Symposium. (Various authors.) Update and advances in intravenous therapy with trimethoprim–sulfamethoxazole. (Remington, J. S., ed.) *Rev. Infect. Dis.*, **1987**, *9*, Suppl. 2, S153–S229.

Weinstein, L.; Madoff, M. A.; and Samet, C. A. The sulfonamides. *N. Engl. J. Med.*, **1960**, *263*, 793–800, 842–849, 900–907.

Wormser, G. P.; Keusch, G. T.; and Rennie, C. H. Co-trimoxazole (trimethoprim–sulfamethoxazole): an updated review of its antibacterial activity and clinical efficacy. *Drugs*, **1982**, *24*, 459–518.

CHAPTER

46 ANTIMICROBIAL AGENTS [*Continued*]

Penicillins, Cephalosporins, and Other Beta-Lactam Antibiotics

Gerald L. Mandell and Merle A. Sande

THE PENICILLINS

The penicillins constitute one of the most important groups of antibiotics. Although numerous other antimicrobial agents have been produced since the first penicillin became available, these are still widely used, major antibiotics, and new derivatives of the basic penicillin nucleus are being produced every year. Many of these have unique advantages, such that members of this group of antibiotics are presently the drugs of choice for a large number of infectious diseases.

History. The history of the brilliant research that led to the discovery and development of penicillin has been recorded by the chief participants. (*See* Fleming, 1946; Florey, 1946, 1949; Abraham, 1949; Chain, 1954.) In 1928, while studying staphylococcus variants in the laboratory at St. Mary's Hospital in London, Alexander Fleming observed that a mold contaminating one of his cultures caused the bacteria in its vicinity to undergo lysis. Broth in which the fungus was grown was markedly inhibitory for many microorganisms. Because the mold belonged to the genus *Penicillium*, Fleming named the antibacterial substance *penicillin*.

A decade later penicillin was developed as a systemic therapeutic agent by the concerted research of a group of investigators at Oxford University headed by Florey, Chain, and Abraham. By May 1940 the crude material then available was found to produce dramatic therapeutic effects when administered parenterally to mice with experimentally produced streptococcal infections. Despite great obstacles to its laboratory production, enough penicillin was accumulated by 1941 to conduct therapeutic trials in several patients desperately ill with staphylococcal and streptococcal infections refractory to all other therapy. At this stage, the crude amorphous penicillin was only about 10% pure and it required nearly 100 liters of the broth in which the mold had been grown to obtain enough of the antibiotic to treat one patient for 24 hours. Herrell (1945) records that bedpans were actually used by the Oxford group for growing cultures of *P. notatum*. Case 1 in the 1941 report from Oxford was that of a policeman who was suffering from a severe mixed staphylococcal and streptococcal infection. He was treated with penicillin, some of which had been recovered from the urine of other patients who had been given the drug. It is said that an Oxford professor referred to penicillin as a remarkable substance, grown in bedpans and purified by passage through the Oxford Police Force.

A vast research program was soon initiated in the United States. During 1942, 122 million units of penicillin were made available, and the first clinical trials were conducted at Yale University and the Mayo Clinic, with dramatic results. By the spring of 1943, 200 patients had been treated with the drug. The results were so impressive that the surgeon general of the U.S. Army authorized trial of the antibiotic in a military hospital. Soon thereafter, penicillin was adopted throughout the medical services of the U.S. Armed Forces.

The deep-fermentation procedure for the biosynthesis of penicillin marked a crucial advance in the large-scale production of the antibiotic. From a total production of a few-hundred-million units a month in the early days, the quantity manufactured rose to over 200 trillion units (nearly 150 tons) by 1950. The first marketable penicillin cost several dollars per 100,000 units; today, the same dose costs only a few cents.

Chemistry. The basic structure of the penicillins, as shown in Figure 46–1, consists of a thiazolidine ring (A) connected to a beta-lactam ring (B), to which is attached a side chain (R). The penicillin nucleus itself is the chief structural requirement for biological activity; metabolic transformation or chemical alteration of this portion of the molecule causes loss of all significant antibacterial activity. The side chain (*see* Table 46–1, page 1076) determines many of the antibacterial and pharmacological characteristics of a particular type of penicillin. Several natural penicillins can be produced, depending on the chemical composition of the fermentation medium used to culture *Penicillium*. Penicillin G (benzylpenicillin) has the greatest antimicrobial activity of these and is the only natural penicillin used clinically.

Semisynthetic Penicillins. The discovery that 6-aminopenicillanic acid could be obtained from cultures of *P. chrysogenum* that were depleted of side-chain precursors led to the development of the semisynthetic penicillins. Side chains can be added

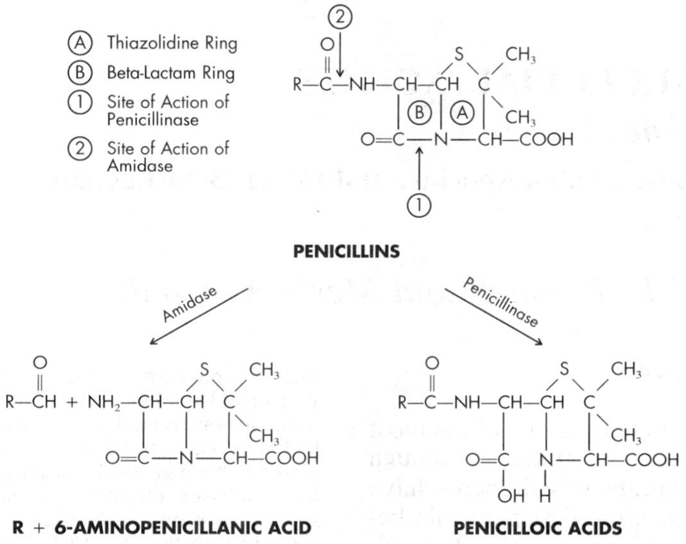

Figure 46–1. *Structure of penicillins and products of their enzymatic hydrolysis.*

that alter the susceptibility of the resultant compounds to inactivating enzymes (beta-lactamases) and that change the antibacterial activity and the pharmacological properties of the drug. 6-Aminopenicillanic acid is now produced in large quantities with the aid of an amidase from *P. chrysogenum* (Figure 46–1). This enzyme splits the peptide linkage by which the side chain of penicillin is joined to 6-aminopenicillanic acid.

Unitage of Penicillin. The international unit of penicillin is the specific penicillin activity contained in 0.6 μg of the crystalline sodium salt of penicillin G. One milligram of pure penicillin G sodium thus equals 1667 units; 1.0 mg of pure penicillin G potassium represents 1595 units. The dosage and the antibacterial potency of the semisynthetic penicillins are expressed in terms of weight.

Mechanism of Action of the Penicillins and Cephalosporins. The beta-lactam antibiotics can kill susceptible bacteria. Although knowledge of the mechanism of this action is incomplete, numerous researchers have supplied information that allows understanding of the basic phenomenon (*see* Neu, 1976, 1983; Yocum *et al.*, 1980; Tomasz, 1986).

The cell walls of bacteria are essential for their normal growth and development. Peptidoglycan is a heteropolymeric component of the cell wall that provides rigid mechanical stability by virtue of its highly cross-linked latticework structure. In gram-positive microorganisms, the cell wall is 50 to 100 molecules thick, but it is only 1 or 2 molecules thick in gram-negative bacteria. The peptidoglycan is composed of glycan chains, which are linear strands of two alternating amino sugars (N-acetylglucosamine and N-acetylmuramic acid), that are cross-linked by peptide chains. The composition of the peptide cross-links is characteristic of individual microbial species. In *Staphylococcus aureus,* tetrapeptide units are bonded to the acetylmuramic acid residues, and pentaglycine chains bridge between the tetrapeptide moieties on adjacent strands (Figure 46–2).

The biosynthesis of the peptidoglycan involves about 30 bacterial enzymes and may be considered in three stages. The first stage, precursor formation, takes place in the cytoplasm. The product, uridine diphosphate (UDP)–acetylmuramyl-pentapeptide, called a "Park nucleotide" after its discoverer (Park and Strominger, 1957), accumulates in cells when subsequent synthetic stages are inhibited. The last reaction in the synthesis of this compound is the addition of a dipeptide, D-alanyl-D-alanine. Synthesis of the dipeptide involves prior racemization of L-alanine and condensation catalyzed by D-alanyl-D-alanine synthetase. D-Cycloserine is a structural analog of D-alanine and acts as a competitive inhibitor of both the racemase and the synthetase (*see* Chapter 49).

During reactions of the second stage, UDP-acetylmuramyl-pentapeptide and UDP-acetylglucosamine are linked (with the release of the uridine nucleotides) to form a long polymer. To form this species, the sugar pentapeptide is first attached by a pyrophosphate bridge to a phospholipid in the cell membrane. The second sugar is then added, followed by the addition of five glycine residues as a branch of the heteropentapeptide. The first half of the pentaglycine cross-link is thus formed. The molecule is then assumed to "flip" across the cell membrane, such that the peptidoglycan precursor faces the periplasm. The completed unit is then cleaved from the membrane-bound phospholipid, a reaction that is inhibited by vancomycin (Chapter 48).

The third and final stage involves the completion of the cross-link. This is accomplished by a transpeptidation reaction that occurs outside the cell

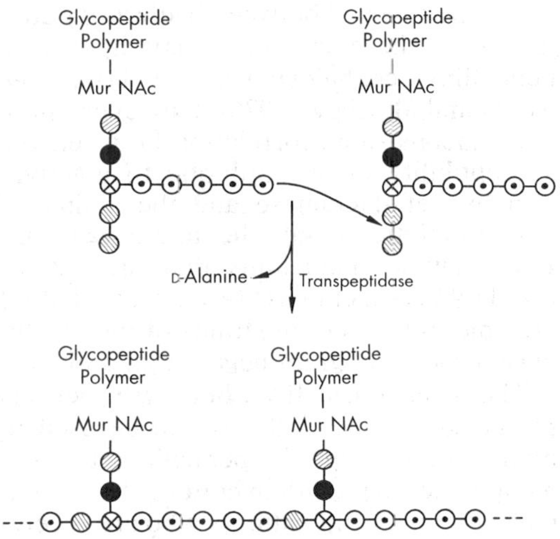

Figure 46–2. *The transpeptidase reaction in* Staphylococcus aureus *that is inhibited by penicillins and cephalosporins.*

See text for details. Mur NAc = N-acetylmuramic acid; ⊘ = L-alanine; ● = D-glutamate; ⊗ = L-lysine; ◍ = D-alanine; ⊙ = glycine.

membrane. The transpeptidase itself is membrane bound. The terminal glycine residue of the pentaglycine bridge is linked to the fourth residue of the pentapeptide (D-alanine), releasing the fifth residue (also D-alanine) (Figure 46–2). It is this last step in peptidoglycan synthesis that is inhibited by the beta-lactam antibiotics. Stereomodels reveal that the conformation of penicillin is very similar to that of D-alanyl-D-alanine (Waxman *et al.*, 1980; Kelley *et al.*, 1982). The transpeptidase is probably acylated by penicillin; that is, penicilloyl enzyme is apparently formed, with cleavage of the —CO—N— bond of the beta-lactam ring.

Although inhibition of the transpeptidase described above is demonstrably important, there are additional, related targets for the actions of penicillins and cephalosporins; these are collectively termed penicillin-binding proteins (PBPs) (Spratt, 1975, 1980). All bacteria have several such entities; for example, *Staph. aureus* has four PBPs, while *E. coli* has at least seven. The PBPs vary in their affinities for different beta-lactam antibiotics, although the interactions eventually become covalent. The higher molecular weight PBPs of *E. coli* (PBP 1a and 1b) include the transpeptidases responsible for synthesis of the peptidoglycan. Other PBPs in *E. coli* include those that are necessary for maintenance of the rodlike shape of the bacterium and for septum formation at division. Inhibition of the transpeptidases causes spheroplast formation and rapid lysis. However, inhibition of the activities of other PBPs may cause delayed lysis (PBP 2) or the production of long filamentous forms of the bacterium (PBP 3).

The lysis of bacteria that usually follows their exposure to beta-lactam antibiotics is ultimately dependent on the activity of cell-wall autolytic enzymes—autolysins or murein hydrolases. Although the natural role of these enzymes remains to be defined in detail, they may function normally in processes related to cell division. The relationship between inhibition of PBP activity and activation of autolysins is unclear. Interference with peptidoglycan assembly in the face of ongoing autolysin activity might well lead to cell lysis, but the mechanism appears to be more complex. Some evidence suggests that exposure of bacteria to beta-lactam antibiotics results in loss of an inhibitor of the autolysins. Whatever the explanation, the growth of autolysin-deficient bacteria can be arrested by beta-lactam antibiotics, but lysis does not occur and the bacteria remain viable. These bacteria are said to be "penicillin-tolerant," and such strains of streptococci and staphylococci have been isolated from patients with persistent infections (*see* Tomasz and Holtje, 1977; Tomasz, 1979; *see also* Pratt and Fekety, 1986).

Mechanisms of Bacterial Resistance to Penicillins and Cephalosporins. Although most or all bacteria contain PBPs, beta-lactam antibiotics cannot kill or even inhibit all bacteria, and various mechanisms of bacterial resistance to these agents are operative. The microorganism may be intrinsically resistant because of structural differences in the PBPs that are the targets of these drugs. Furthermore, it is possible for a sensitive strain to acquire resistance of this type by mutation. This mechanism for the acquisition of resistance, while uncommon, has been described for gram-positive cocci (Malouin and Bryan, 1986).

Other instances of bacterial resistance to the beta-lactam antibiotics are caused by the inability of the agent to penetrate to its site of action (Jaffe *et al.*, 1982; Kobayashi *et al.*, 1982). In gram-positive bacteria the peptidoglycan polymer is very near the cell surface. Only surface macromolecules (capsule) are external to the peptidoglycan. The small beta-lactam antibiotic molecules can easily penetrate to the outer layer of the cytoplasmic membrane and the penicillin-binding proteins, where the final stages of the synthesis of the peptidoglycan take place. The situation is different with gram-negative bacteria. Their surface structure is more complex, and the inner membrane (which is analogous to the cytoplasmic membrane of gram-positive bacteria) is covered by the outer membrane, lipopolysaccharide, and capsule. The outer membrane functions as an impenetrable barrier for some antibiotics (*see* Nakae, 1986). However, some small, hydrophilic antibiotics diffuse through aqueous channels in the outer membrane that are formed by proteins called *porins*. Broader-spectrum penicillins, such as ampicillin and amoxicillin, and most of the cephalosporins diffuse through the pores in the *E. coli* outer membrane significantly more rapidly than can penicillin G. The number and size of pores in the outer membrane are variable among different gram-negative bacteria.

Bacteria can destroy beta-lactam antibiotics enzymatically. While amidohydrolases may be present, these enzymes are relatively inactive and do not protect the bacteria. Beta-lactamases, however, are capable of inactivating certain of these antibiotics and may be present in large quantities (*see* Figure 46–1). Different microorganisms elaborate a number of distinct beta-lactamases, although most bacteria produce only one form of the enzyme. The substrate specificities of some of these enzymes are relatively narrow, and these are often described as either penicillinases or cephalosporinases. Other "broad-spectrum" enzymes are less discriminant and can hydrolyze a variety of beta-lactam antibiotics. Individual penicillins and cephalosporins vary in their susceptibility to these enzymes.

In general, gram-positive bacteria produce a large amount of beta-lactamase that is secreted extracellularly. Most of these enzymes are penicillinases. The information for staphylococcal penicillinase is encoded in a plasmid, and this may be transferred by bacteriophage to other bacteria. The enzyme is inducible by substrates, and 1% of the dry weight of the bacterium can be penicillinase. In gram-negative bacteria, beta-lactamases are found in relatively small amounts but are located in the periplasmic space between the inner and outer cell membranes. Since the enzymes of cell-wall synthesis are on the outer surface of the inner membrane, these beta-lactamases are strategically located for maximal protection of the microbe. Beta-lactamases of gram-negative bacteria are encoded either in chromosomes or plasmids, and they may be constitutive or inducible. The plasmids can be transferred between bacteria by conjugation. These enzymes may hydrolyze penicillins, cephalosporins, or both (*see* Sykes and Matthew, 1976). However, there is an inconsistent correlation between the susceptibility of an antibiotic to inactivation by beta-lactamase and the ability of that antibiotic to kill the microorganism. For example, penicillins that are hydrolyzed by beta-lactamase (*e.g.*, carbenicillin) are able to kill certain strains of beta-lactamase-producing gram-negative microbes.

The penicillinase from *Bacillus* species is produced commercially. It can be used to hydrolyze susceptible penicillins to augment bacterial growth in cultures from samples obtained from patients who are receiving the drug.

Other Factors That Influence the Activity of Beta-Lactam Antibiotics. The density of the bacterial population and the age of an infection influence the activity of beta-lactam antibiotics. The drugs may be several thousand times more potent when tested against small bacterial inocula as compared to their activity against a dense culture. Many factors are involved. Among these are the greater number of relatively resistant microorganisms in a large population, the amount of beta-lactamase produced, and the phase of growth of the culture. The clinical significance of this effect of inoculum size is uncertain. The intensity and the duration of penicillin therapy needed to abort or cure experimental infections in animals increase with the duration of the infection. The reason is primarily that the bacteria are no longer multiplying as rapidly as they do in a fresh infection. These antibiotics are most active against bacteria in the logarithmic phase of growth and have little effect on microorganisms in the stationary phase, when there is no need to synthesize components of the cell wall.

The presence of proteins and other constituents of pus, low pH, or low oxygen tension does not appreciably decrease the ability of beta-lactam antibiotics to kill bacteria. However, bacteria that survive inside viable cells of the host are protected from the action of the beta-lactam antibiotics.

Classification of the Penicillins and Summary of Their Pharmacological Properties

It is useful to classify the penicillins according to their spectrum of antimicrobial activity (*see* Table 46–1, page 1076; Neu, 1985).

1. Penicillin G and its close congener penicillin V are highly active against gram-positive cocci, but they are readily hydro-

lyzed by penicillinase. Thus, they are ineffective against most strains of *Staph. aureus*.

2. The penicillinase-resistant penicillins (methicillin, nafcillin, oxacillin, cloxacillin, and dicloxacillin) have less potent antimicrobial activity against microorganisms that are sensitive to penicillin G, but they are effective against penicillinase-producing *Staph. aureus*.

3. Ampicillin, amoxicillin, cyclacillin, bacampicillin, and others comprise a group of penicillins whose antimicrobial activity is extended to include such gram-negative microorganisms as *Haemophilus influenzae, Escherichia coli,* and *Proteus mirabilis*. Unfortunately, these drugs and the others listed below are readily hydrolyzed by broad-spectrum beta-lactamases that are found with increasing frequency in clinical isolates of these gram-negative bacteria.

4. The antimicrobial activity of carbenicillin and its indanyl ester (carbenicillin indanyl), ticarcillin, and azlocillin is extended to include *Pseudomonas, Enterobacter,* and *Proteus* species.

5. Other extended-spectrum penicillins include mezlocillin and piperacillin, which have useful antimicrobial activity against *Pseudomonas, Klebsiella,* and certain other gram-negative microorganisms.

While the pharmacological properties of the individual drugs are discussed in detail below, certain generalizations are useful. Following absorption, penicillins are widely distributed throughout the body. Therapeutic concentrations of these agents are readily achieved in tissues and in such secretions as joint fluid, pleural fluid, pericardial fluid, and bile. However, only low concentrations of these drugs are found in prostatic secretions, brain tissue, and intraocular fluid, and penicillins do not penetrate living phagocytic cells to a significant extent. Concentrations of penicillins in cerebrospinal fluid (CSF) are variable but are less than 1% of those in plasma when the meninges are normal. When there is inflammation, concentrations in CSF may increase to as much as 5% of the plasma value. Penicillins are rapidly eliminated, particularly by glomerular filtration and renal tubular secretion, such that their half-lives in the body are short; values of 30 to 60 minutes are typical. Concentrations of these drugs in urine are thus high.

PENICILLIN G AND PENICILLIN V

Antimicrobial Activity. The antimicrobial spectra of penicillin G (benzylpenicillin) and penicillin V (the phenoxymethyl derivative) are very similar for aerobic gram-positive microorganisms. However, penicillin G is five to ten times more active against gram-negative microorganisms, especially *Neisseria* species, and certain anaerobes.

Penicillin G is highly effective *in vitro* against many, but not all, species of gram-positive and gram-negative cocci. Streptococci (but not enterococci) are very susceptible to the drug; concentrations of less than 0.01 μg/ml are usually effective. Whereas most strains of *Staph. aureus* were highly sensitive to similar concentrations of penicillin G when this agent was first employed therapeutically, more than 90% of strains of staphylococci isolated from individuals inside or outside of hospitals are now resistant to penicillin G. Most strains of *Staph. epidermidis* are also resistant to penicillin. Although gonococci are generally sensitive to penicillin G, continued exposure of this microorganism to the antibiotic has led to a general decrease in sensitivity. Unfortunately, penicillinase-producing strains of gonococci that are highly resistant to penicillin G have also become widespread. With rare exceptions, meningococci are quite sensitive to penicillin G. Pneumococci of all serological types are, in general, highly susceptible to penicillin G; however, some highly resistant strains have now been described.

Although the vast majority of strains of *Corynebacterium diphtheriae* are sensitive to penicillin G, some are highly resistant. This is also true for *Bacillus anthracis*. Most anaerobic microorganisms, including *Clostridium* species, are highly sensitive. *Bacteroides fragilis* is an exception; many strains are now resistant because of elaboration of beta-lactamase. Some strains of *Bacteroides melaninogenicus* have also acquired this trait. *Actinomyces israelii, Streptobacillus moniliformis, Pasteurella multocida,* and *Listeria monocytogenes* are inhibited by penicillin G. Most species of *Leptospira* are moderately susceptible to the drug. One of the most exquisitely sensitive microorganisms is *Treponema pallidum. Borrelia burgdorferi*, the organism responsible for Lyme disease, is also susceptible. None of the penicillins is effective against amebae, plasmodia, rickettsiae, fungi, or viruses.

Although many species of gram-negative bacilli are resistant to penicillin G, some are affected by moderate-to-high concentrations. The majority of strains of *Pr. mirabilis* are inhibited by 10 μg/ml or less of the drug. Many strains of *E. coli* are also susceptible to high concentrations of penicillin G.

Absorption. *Oral Administration of Penicillin G.* About one third of an orally administered dose of penicillin G is absorbed from the intestinal tract under favorable conditions. Gastric juice at pH 2 rapidly destroys the antibiotic. The decrease in gastric acid production with aging accounts for better absorption of penicillin G from the gastrointestinal tract of older individuals. Absorption is rapid, and maximal concentrations in blood are attained in 30 to 60 minutes. The peak value is approximately 0.5 unit/ml (0.3 μg/ml) after an oral dose of 400,000 units (about 250 mg) in an adult. Ingestion of food interferes with enteric absorption of all penicillins, perhaps by adsorption of the antibiotic onto food particles. Thus, oral penicillin G should be administered at least 30 minutes before a meal or 2 hours after. Despite the convenience of oral administration of penicillin G, this route should be used only in infections in which clinical experience has proven its efficacy.

Oral Administration of Penicillin V. The sole virtue of penicillin V in comparison with penicillin G is that it is more stable in an acidic medium, and therefore is better absorbed from the gastrointestinal tract. On an equivalent oral-dose basis, the compound yields plasma concentrations two to five times greater than those provided by penicillin G. The peak concentration in the blood of an adult after an oral dose of 500 mg is nearly 3 μg/ml. Once absorbed, penicillin V is distributed in the body and excreted by the kidney in the same manner as penicillin G.

Parenteral Administration of Penicillin G. After intramuscular injection, peak concentrations in plasma are reached within 15 to 30 minutes. This value declines rapidly, since the half-life of penicillin G is 30 minutes.

Many means for prolonging the sojourn of the antibiotic in the body and thereby reducing the frequency of injections have been explored. Probenecid blocks renal tubular secretion of penicillin, but it is rarely used for this purpose (*see* below and Chapter 30). More commonly, repository preparations of penicillin G are employed. The two such compounds currently favored are penicillin G procaine and penicillin G benzathine (*see* section on preparations). Such agents release penicillin G slowly from the area in which they are injected and produce relatively low but persistent concentrations of antibiotic in the blood.

The injection of 300,000 units of penicillin G procaine produces a peak concentration in plasma of about 0.9 μg/ml within 1 to 3 hours; after 24 hours the concentration is reduced to 0.1 μg/ml, and by 48 hours it has fallen to 0.03 μg/ml. A larger dose (600,000 units) yields somewhat higher values that are maintained for as long as 4 to 5 days.

Penicillin G benzathine is very slowly absorbed from intramuscular depots and produces the longest duration of detectable antibiotic of all the available repository penicillins. For example, in adults, a dose of 1.2 million units given intramuscularly produces a concentration in plasma of 0.09 μg/ml on the first, 0.02 μg/ml on the fourteenth, and 0.002 μg/ml on the thirty-second day after injection. The average duration of demonstrable antimicrobial activity in the plasma is about 26 days. Similar pharmacokinetic data are available for newborn infants (Kaplan and McCracken, 1973).

Intrathecal administration of any of the penicillins is no longer recommended. Penicillin is a potent convulsant when given by this route. Bactericidal concentrations of the drug can be attained in the brain and meninges by the use of other parenteral routes.

Distribution. Penicillin G is widely distributed throughout the body, but the concentrations in various fluids and tissues differ widely. Its apparent volume of distribution is about 0.35 l/kg. Approximately 60% of the penicillin G in plasma is reversibly bound to albumin. Significant amounts appear in liver, bile, kidney, semen, joint fluid, lymph, and intestine.

While probenecid markedly decreases the tubular secretion of the penicillins, this is not the only factor responsible for the elevated plasma concentrations of the antibiotic that follow its administration. Probenecid also produces a significant decrease in the apparent volume of distribution of the penicillins.

Cerebrospinal Fluid. Penicillin does not readily enter the CSF when the meninges are normal. However, when the meninges are acutely inflamed, penicillin penetrates into the CSF more easily. Although the concentrations attained vary and are unpredictable, they are usually in the range of 5% of the value in plasma and are therapeutically effective against susceptible microorganisms.

Penicillin and other organic acids are rapidly secreted from the CSF into the bloodstream by an active transport process. Probenecid competitively inhibits this transport and thus elevates the concentration of penicillin in CSF (Dacey and Sande, 1974). In uremia, other organic acids accumulate in the CSF and compete with penicillin for secretion; the drug occasionally reaches toxic concentrations in brain and can produce convulsions.

Excretion. Under normal conditions, penicillin G is rapidly eliminated from the body, mainly by the kidney but in small part in the bile and by other routes. Approximately 60 to 90% of an intramuscular dose of penicillin G in aqueous solution is eliminated in the urine, largely within the first hour after injection. The half-time for elimination is about 30 minutes in normal adults. Approximately 10% of the drug is eliminated by glomerular filtration and 90% by tubular secretion. Renal clearance approximates the total renal plasma flow. The maximal tubular secretory capacity for penicillin in the normal male adult is about 3 million units (1.8 g) per hour.

Clearance values are considerably lower in neonates and infants, because of incomplete development of renal function; as a result, after doses proportionate to surface area, the persistence of penicillin in the blood is several times as long in premature infants as in children and adults. The half-life of the antibiotic in children less than 1 week old is 3 hours; by 14 days of age it is 1.4 hours. After renal function is fully established in young children, the rate of renal excretion of penicillin G is considerably more rapid than in adults.

Anuria increases the half-life of penicillin G from a normal value of 0.5 hour to about 10 hours. When renal function is impaired, 7 to 10% of the antibiotic may be inactivated each hour by the liver. Patients with renal shutdown who require high-dose therapy with penicillin can be treated adequately with 3 million units of aqueous penicillin G followed by 1.5 million units every 8 to 12 hours. The dose of the drug must be readjusted during dialysis and the period of progressive recovery of renal function. If, in addition to renal failure, hepatic insufficiency is also present, the half-life will be prolonged even further.

Preparations and Dosage. Preparations of penicillin G that are available for parenteral use include aqueous solutions and repository forms that are slowly absorbed from intramuscular depots. In addition, there are many preparations of penicillin G and penicillin V for oral administration. Details of dosage of these preparations are presented in the discussions of the treatment of specific infections.

Penicillin G in Aqueous Solution for Parenteral Use. This preparation can be utilized for intravenous or intramuscular injection. It can be given as an infusion over 20 to 30 minutes or by constant drip. The potassium salts are most frequently used; each million units of penicillin G potassium contains about 1.7 mEq of potassium. Usual doses of intravenous penicillin G for adults are 6 to 20 million units per day in four to six portions or by continuous infusion. Severe infections, such as meningitis, should be treated either by continuous infusion or with high doses every 2 to 3 hours. Children should receive 100,000 to 250,000 units/kg per day in four to six portions. Newborns up to 1 week of age should receive 50,000 to 150,000 units/kg per day in two or three portions.

Repository Forms of Penicillin G. Repository penicillin preparations are designed for deep intramuscular injection, to provide a tissue depot from which the drug is slowly absorbed over a period of 12 hours to several days. The objective is to maintain therapeutic concentrations in plasma with as few injections as possible. Repository penicillin should never be injected intravenously or subcutaneously or into body cavities.

Penicillin G procaine suspension (DURACILLIN A.S., WYCILLIN, others) is an aqueous preparation of the crystalline salt that is only 0.4% soluble in water. Procaine combines with penicillin mol for mol; a dose of 300,000 units thus contains approximately 120 mg of procaine. When large doses of penicillin G procaine are given (*e.g.*, 4.8 million units), procaine may reach toxic concentrations in the plasma. If the patient is believed to be hypersensitive to procaine, 0.1 ml of 1% solution of procaine should be injected intradermally as a test. The anesthetic effect of the procaine accounts in part for the fact that injections of penicillin G procaine are virtually painless.

Penicillin G benzathine suspension (BICILLIN L-A, PERMAPEN) is the aqueous suspension of the salt obtained by the combination of 1 mol of an ammonium base and 2 mol of penicillin G to yield N,N′-dibenzylethylenediamine dipenicillin G. The salt itself is only 0.02% soluble in water. The long persistence of penicillin in the blood after a suitable intramuscular dose reduces cost, need for repeated injections, and local trauma. The local anesthetic effect of penicillin G benzathine is comparable to that of penicillin G procaine. Penicillin G benzathine should be used only for treatment or prophylaxis of group-A beta-hemolytic streptococcal pharyngitis, treatment of group-A beta-hemolytic streptococcal pyoderma, or treatment of syphilis outside the central nervous system.

Preparations of Penicillin G and Penicillin V for Oral Use. The oral preparations of penicillin G are *penicillin G potassium tablets, penicillin G potassium for oral solution,* and *penicillin G benzathine tablets.* They are marketed as tablets containing from 200,000 to 800,000 units. Dry salts of penicillin G mixed with flavoring material are available for pediatric use.

Penicillin V potassium (PEN-VEE K, V-CILLIN K, others) is supplied for oral use as tablets (125, 250, or 500 mg each) and powders for solution (125 or 250 mg/5 ml).

Therapeutic Uses. Penicillin G is the antibiotic of choice for a wide variety of infectious diseases (*see* Table 44–1, page 1024).

Pneumococcal Infections. Penicillin G remains the agent of choice for the management of infections of all types caused by *Strep. pneumoniae.* However, rare strains of pneumococci resistant to usual doses of penicillin G have been encountered in several countries, including the United States (*see* Jacobs *et al.,* 1978).

Pneumococcal Pneumonia. For parenteral therapy, penicillin G or penicillin G procaine are favored, and 600,000 units of procaine penicillin G, given intramuscularly every 12 hours, is adequate therapy for uncomplicated cases. Although oral treatment with 500 mg of penicillin V given every 6 hours has been used with success in this disease, it cannot be recommended for routine initial use. Therapy should be continued for 7 to 10 days, including 3 to 5 days after the temperature has returned to normal.

Pneumococcal Meningitis. Penicillin has reduced the death rate in this disease from nearly 100% to about 25%. The recommended therapy is 20 to 24 million units of penicillin G daily by constant intravenous infusion or divided into boluses given every 2 to 3 hours. The usual duration of therapy is 14 days.

Other Pneumococcal Infections. Penicillin G provides excellent therapy for suppurative arthritis, osteomyelitis, acute suppurative mastoiditis, endocarditis, peritonitis, and pericarditis due to the pneumococcus. Because of poor penetration of the drug into purulent exudate, the plasma and tissue-fluid concentrations must be high; this is best accomplished by the intravenous administration of large doses of aqueous penicillin G. Doses on the order of 12 to 20 million units per day may be required for cure. Oral and repository penicillins should not be used. The shortest period of treatment for any of these disorders should be 2 weeks. Infections in the middle ear and paranasal sinuses caused by the pneumococcus may be treated with 300,000 to 600,000 units of procaine penicillin G intramuscularly every 12 hours or with 250 to 500 mg of oral penicillin V every 6 hours.

Streptococcal Infections. Streptococcal Pharyngitis (Including Scarlet Fever). This is the most common disease produced by *Strep. pyogenes* (group-A beta-hemolytic streptococcus). The preferred oral therapy is with penicillin V, 500 mg every 6 hours for 10 days. Equally good results are produced by the administration of 600,000 units of penicillin G procaine intramuscularly, once daily for 10 days, or by a single injection of 1.2 million units of penicillin G benzathine. Parenteral therapy is preferred if there are questions of patient compliance. Penicillin therapy of streptococcal pharyngitis reduces the risk of subsequent acute rheumatic fever; however, current evidence suggests that the incidence of glomerulonephritis that follows streptococcal infections is not reduced to a significant degree by treatment with penicillin.

Streptococcal Pneumonia, Arthritis, Meningitis, and Endocarditis. While uncommon, these conditions should be treated with penicillin G when they are caused by *Strep. pyogenes;* daily doses of 12 to 20 million units are administered intravenously for 2 to 4 weeks. Such treatment of endocarditis should be continued for a full 4 weeks.

Streptococcal Otitis Media and Sinusitis. Treatment with an oral preparation, such as 250 to 500 mg of penicillin V every 6 hours for 2 weeks, is usually adequate. Streptococcal mastoiditis is now an uncommon complication of otitis media; it should be treated with high doses of parenteral penicillin G for at least 2 weeks.

Infections Due to Other Streptococci. Group-B (*Strep. agalactiae*) streptococcal infections, including meningitis and bacteremia, are frequent in neonates and should be treated with high doses of penicillin G given parenterally (150,000 to 250,000 units/kg per day).

The viridans streptococci are the most common cause of infectious endocarditis. These are nongroupable alpha-hemolytic microorganisms that are usually highly sensitive to penicillin G (minimal inhibitory concentration less than 0.1 μg/ml). Since enterococci may also be beta-hemolytic and certain other alpha-hemolytic strains may be relatively resistant to penicillin, it is important to determine quantitative microbial sensitivities to penicillin G in patients with endocarditis. Patients with penicillin-sensitive viridans-group streptococcal endocarditis can be successfully treated with 1.2 million units of procaine penicillin G, given four times daily for 2 weeks, or with daily doses of 12 to 20 million units of intravenous penicillin G for 2 weeks, both regimens in combination with streptomycin, 500 mg intramuscularly every 12 hours or gentamicin (1 mg/kg every 8 hours). Some physicians prefer a 4-week course of treatment with penicillin G alone (Bisno *et al.,* 1981).

Enterococcal endocarditis is one of the few diseases that is optimally treated with two antibiotics. The recommended therapy is 20 million units of penicillin G or 12 grams of ampicillin daily, administered intravenously in combination with an aminoglycoside. Some physicians prefer to initiate treatment with streptomycin (500 mg intramuscularly every 12 hours) in combination with penicillin. Others prefer to initiate treatment with gentamicin (1 mg/kg every 8 hours) plus penicillin, since up to 40% of enterococcal strains are highly resistant to streptomycin *in vitro.* If synergism between penicillin and streptomycin is demonstrated (*see* Chapter 44), then therapy with penicillin and streptomycin can be used. Therapy should usually be continued for 6 weeks, but selected patients with a short duration of illness (less than 3 months) have been treated successfully in 4 weeks (Wilson *et al.*, 1984). An increasing number of isolates have been found that produce beta-lactamase and/or aminoglycoside-inactivating enzymes. These strains have proven difficult to treat with conventional regimens (*see* Chapter 47).

Infections with Anaerobes. Many anaerobic infections are caused by mixtures of microorganisms. The majority are sensitive to penicillin G. An exception is *B. fragilis,* in which 20 to 50% of strains may be resistant to high concentrations of this antibiotic. Pulmonary and periodontal infections usually respond well to penicillin G, although a multicenter study indicated that clindamycin is more effective than penicillin for therapy of lung abscess (Levison *et al.*, 1983). Mild-to-moderate infections at these sites may be treated with oral medication (either penicillin G or penicillin V, 400,000 units four times daily). More severe infections should be treated with 12 to 20 million units of penicillin G intravenously. Anaerobic infections involving the gastrointestinal tract and certain pelvic infections may be due in part to *B. fragilis*. The most serious infections should be treated with either clindamycin, chloramphenicol, or metronidazole; other alternatives are one of the beta-lactam antibiotics with good activity against anaerobes, such as imipenem (plus cilastatin) or ticarcillin (plus clavulanate). Because aerobic gram-negative bacteria may also be involved, an aminoglycoside or third-generation cephalosporin should be included for the treatment of anaerobic infections originating from the gastrointestinal tract. Brain abscesses also frequently contain several species of anaerobes, and most authorities prefer to treat such disease with high doses of penicillin G (20 million units per day) plus chloramphenicol (2 to 4 g per day, intravenously) or metronidazole (2 to 4 g per day, intravenously). Some physicians add a third-generation cephalosporin for activity against aerobic gram-negative bacilli.

Staphylococcal Infections. The vast majority of staphylococcal infections are caused by microorganisms that produce penicillinase. A patient with a staphylococcal infection who requires treatment with an antibiotic should receive one of the penicillinase-resistant penicillins—for example, nafcillin, oxacillin, or methicillin. Concurrent administration of an aminoglycoside for the first five days of treatment may hasten the clinical and bacteriological response.

So-called methicillin-resistant staphylococci are resistant to penicillin G, all of the penicillinase-resistant penicillins, and the cephalosporins. Isolates may occasionally appear to be sensitive to various cephalosporins *in vitro,* but resistant populations arise during therapy and lead to failure (Chambers *et al.*, 1984). Vancomycin is the drug of choice for infections caused by these bacteria. Ciprofloxacin is also effective.

Meningococcal Infections. Penicillin G remains the drug of choice for meningococcal disease. Patients should be treated with high doses of penicillin given intravenously, as described for pneumococcal meningitis. It should be remembered that penicillin G does not eliminate the meningococcal carrier state, and its administration is thus ineffective as a prophylactic measure.

Gonococcal Infections. Gonococci have gradually become more resistant to penicillin G, and penicillins are no longer the therapy of first choice unless it is known that gonococcal strains in a particular geographical area are susceptible. Uncomplicated gonococcal urethritis is the most common infection and a single intramuscular injection of 250 mg of ceftriaxone is the recommended treatment (Handsfield, 1990). For patients in areas where resistance to penicillin is not a significant problem, the oral administration of amoxicillin (3 g) plus probenecid (1 g) or ampicillin (3.5 g) plus probenecid is recommended. A total of 4.8 million units of penicillin G procaine injected into two sites, combined with oral probenecid (1 g), is equally efficacious. Treatment of contacts of known cases of gonorrhea is the same as is that for gonococcal urethritis.

Gonococcal arthritis, disseminated gonococcal infections with skin lesions, and gonococcemia should be treated with ceftriaxone, 1 g daily given either intramuscularly or intravenously for 7 to 10 days. Ophthalmia neonatorum should also be treated with ceftriaxone for 7 to 10 days (25 to 50 mg/kg per day intramuscularly or intravenously).

Syphilis. Therapy of syphilis with penicillin G is highly effective. Primary, secondary, and latent syphilis of less than 1 year's duration may be treated with penicillin G procaine (2.4 million units per day intramuscularly) plus probenecid (1.0 g per day orally) for 10 days or with a single intramuscular dose of 2.4 million units of penicillin G benzathine. Patients with late latent syphilis, neurosyphilis, or cardiovascular syphilis may be treated with a variety of regimens. Since these diseases are potentially lethal and their progression can be halted (but not reversed), intensive therapy with 20 million units of penicillin G daily for 10 days is recommended.

Infants with congenital syphilis discovered at birth or during the postnatal period should be treated for at least 10 days with 50,000 units/kg daily of aqueous penicillin G in two divided doses or 50,000 units/kg of procaine penicillin G in a single daily dose (*see* Tramont, 1990).

The majority (70 to 90%) of patients with secondary syphilis develop the Jarisch–Herxheimer reaction. This may also be seen in patients with other forms of syphilis. Several hours after the first injection of penicillin, chills, fever, headache, myalgias, and arthralgias may develop. The syphilitic cutaneous lesions may become more prominent, edematous, and brilliant in color. Manifestations usually persist for a few hours, and the rash begins to fade within 48 hours. It does not recur with the second or subsequent injections of penicillin. This reaction is thought to be due to release of spirochetal antigens, with subsequent host reactions to the products. Aspirin gives symptomatic relief, and therapy with penicillin should not be discontinued.

Actinomycosis. Penicillin G is the agent of choice for the treatment of all forms of actinomycosis. The dose should be 12 to 20 million units of penicillin G intravenously per day for 6 weeks. Some physicians continue therapy for 2 to 3 months with oral penicillin V (500 mg four times daily). Surgical drainage or excision of the lesion may be necessary before cure is accomplished.

Diphtheria. There is no evidence that penicillin or any other antibiotic alters the incidence of complications or the outcome of diphtheria; specific antitoxin is the only effective treatment. However, penicillin G eliminates the carrier state. The parenteral administration of 2 to 3 million units per day in divided doses for 10 to 12 days, eliminates the diphtheria bacilli from the pharynx and other sites in practically 100% of cases. A single daily injection of penicillin G procaine for the same period produces about the same results. Erythromycin is as effective, and some consider it to be preferable.

Anthrax. Penicillin G is the agent of choice in the treatment of all clinical forms of anthrax. However, strains of *B. anthracis* resistant to this antibiotic have been recovered from human infections. When penicillin G is used, the dose should be 12 to 20 million units per day.

Clostridial Infections. Penicillin G is the agent of choice for gas gangrene; the dose is in the range of 12 to 20 million units per day, given parenterally. Adequate debridement of the infected areas is essential. Antimicrobial drugs probably have no effect on the ultimate outcome of tetanus. Debridement and administration of human tetanus immune globulin may be indicated. Penicillin is administered, however, to eradicate the vegetative forms of the bacteria that may persist.

Fusospirochetal Infections. Gingivostomatitis, produced by the synergistic action of *Leptotrichia buccalis* and spirochetes that are present in the mouth, is readily treatable with penicillin. For simple "trench mouth," 500 mg of penicillin V given every 6 hours for several days is usually sufficient to clear the disease.

Rat-Bite Fever. The two microorganisms responsible for this infection, *Spirillum minus* in the Orient and *Streptobacillus moniliformis* in America and Europe, are sensitive to penicillin G, the therapeutic agent of choice. Since most cases due to streptobacillus are complicated by bacteremia and, in many instances, by metastatic infections especially of the synovia and endocardium, the dose should be large; a daily dose of 12 to 15 million units given parenterally, for 3 to 4 weeks, has been recommended.

Listeria Infections. Penicillin G or ampicillin with or without gentamicin are regarded as the drugs of choice in the management of infections due to *List. monocytogenes*. The recommended dose of penicillin G is 15 to 20 million units parenterally per day, for at least 2 weeks. When endocarditis is the problem, the dose is the same, but the duration of treatment should be no less than 4 weeks.

Pasteurella Infections. The only species of *Pasteurella* highly susceptible to penicillin is *Past. multocida*. Soft-tissue infection, bacteremia, and meningitis are the most common forms of the disease produced by this microorganism in man, and often occur following animal bites. Penicillin G, 4 to 6 million units per day parenterally for at least 2 weeks, is effectively curative.

Lyme Disease. Although tetracycline is the usual drug of choice for early disease, penicillin V is effective; the dose is 500 mg four times daily for 10 to 21 days. Severe disease is treated with 20 million units of intravenous penicillin G daily for 14 days.

Erysipeloid. The causative agent of this disease, *Erysipelothrix rhusiopathiae*, is sensitive to penicillin. The uncomplicated infection responds well to a single injection of 1.2 million units of penicillin G benzathine. When endocarditis is present, penicillin G, 12 to 20 million units per day, has been found effective; therapy should be continued for 4 to 6 weeks.

Prophylactic Uses of the Penicillins. Demonstration of the effectiveness of penicillin in eradicating microorganisms was quickly, and quite naturally, followed by attempts to prove that it was also effective in preventing infection in susceptible hosts. As a result, the antibiotic has been administered in almost every situation in which a risk of bacterial invasion has been present. As prophylaxis has been investigated under controlled conditions, it has become clear that penicillin is highly effective in some situations, useless and potentially dangerous in others, and of questionable value in still others (*see* Chapter 44).

Streptococcal Infections. The administration of penicillin to individuals exposed to *Strep. pyogenes* affords protection from infection. The oral ingestion of 200,000 units of penicillin G or penicillin V twice a day or a single injection of 1.2 million units of penicillin G benzathine is effective. Indications for this type of prophylaxis include outbreaks of streptococcal disease in closed populations, such as boarding schools or military bases. Patients with extensive deep burns are at high risk of severe wound infections with *Strep. pyogenes;* several days of "low-dose" prophylaxis appears to be effective in reducing the incidence of this complication.

Recurrences of Rheumatic Fever. The oral administration of 200,000 units of penicillin G or penicillin V every 12 hours produces a striking decrease in the incidence of recurrences of rheumatic fever in susceptible individuals. Because of the difficulties of compliance, parenteral administration is preferable, especially in children. The intramuscular injection of 1.2 million units of penicillin G benzathine once a month yields excellent results. In cases of hypersensitivity to penicillin, sulfisoxazole or sulfadiazine, 1 g twice a day for adults, is also effective; for children weighing under 27 kg, the dose is halved. Prophylaxis must be continued throughout the year. The duration of such treatment is an unsettled question. It has been suggested that prophylaxis should be continued for life, because instances of acute rheumatic fever have been observed in the fifth and sixth decades. However, the necessity for such prolonged prophylaxis has not been established.

Gonorrhea. Sexual contacts of patients with gonorrhea should receive a course of antibiotics identical to that described for the treatment of gonococcal urethritis.

Syphilis. Prophylaxis for a contact with syphilis consists of a course of therapy as described for primary syphilis. A serological test for syphilis should be performed at monthly intervals for at least 4 months thereafter.

Surgical Procedures in Patients with Valvular Heart Disease. About 25% of cases of subacute bacterial endocarditis follow dental extractions. This observation, together with the fact that up to 80% of persons who have teeth removed experience a transient bacteremia, emphasizes the potential importance of chemoprophylaxis for those who have congenital or acquired valvular heart disease of any type and need to undergo dental procedures. Since transient bacterial invasion of the bloodstream occurs occasionally after surgical procedures (*e.g.*, tonsillectomy and genitourinary and gastrointestinal procedures) and during childbirth, these too are indications for prophylaxis in patients with valvular heart disease. Bacteremia is not eliminated by the use of penicillin. Whether the incidence of bacterial endocarditis is actually altered by this type of chemoprophylaxis remains to be determined.

Detailed recommendations for both adults and children with valvular heart disease have been formulated (*see* American Heart Association, 1984; *Medical Letter,* 1986; Durack, 1990).

THE PENICILLINASE-RESISTANT PENICILLINS

The penicillins described in this section are resistant to hydrolysis by staphylococcal penicillinase. Their appropriate use should be restricted to the treatment of infections that are known or suspected to be caused by staphylococci that elaborate the enzyme—the vast majority of strains of this bacterium that are encountered in the hospital or in the general community. These drugs are less active than is penicillin G against other penicillin-sensitive microorganisms, including non-penicillinase-producing staphylococci.

The penicillinase-resistant penicillins remain the agents of choice for most staphylococcal disease despite the increasing incidence of isolates of so-called methicillin-resistant microorganisms. As commonly used, this latter term denotes resistance of these bacteria to all of the penicillinase-resistant penicillins and cephalosporins. Such strains are usually resistant as well to the aminoglycosides, tetracyclines, erythromycin, and clindamycin. Vancomycin is considered to be the drug of choice for such infections. Some physicians use a combination of vancomycin and rifampin, especially for life-threatening infections and those involving foreign bodies. Altered penicillin-binding proteins have been found in some methicillin-resistant strains. From 40 to 60% of strains of *Staph. epidermidis* are also resistant to the penicillinase-resistant penicillins. As with methicillin-resistant *Staph. aureus,* these strains may appear to be susceptible to cephalosporins on disc sensitivity testing, but there is usually a significant population of microbes that is resistant to cephalosporins and that emerges during such therapy. Vancomycin is also the drug of choice for serious infection caused by methicillin-resistant *Staph. epidermidis*; rifampin is given concurrently when a foreign body is involved.

Methicillin. This semisynthetic penicillin is prepared from 6-aminopenicillanic acid. Its structural formula is shown in Table 46–1. The drug is highly resistant to cleavage by penicillinase.

Pharmacological Properties. Methicillin is bactericidal for susceptible strains of *Staph. aureus* at concentrations of 1 to 6 μg/ml. Microorganisms that are inhibited only by concentrations in excess of 12.5 μg/ml are considered to be resistant. Penicillinase-producing strains are from 15 to 80 times more susceptible to methicillin than to penicillin G, although methicillin is not as effective as penicillin G against other gram-positive microorganisms. Methicillin is not effective against gram-negative bacteria, some of which may even inactivate it.

Methicillin is not employed by the oral route because it is poorly absorbed and readily destroyed by the acidic gastric contents. When the drug is given intramuscularly, peak concentrations in plasma are reached in about 30 minutes to 1 hour. A 2-g dose provides a peak concentration over 20 μg/ml, and approximately 8 μg/ml is still present after 4 hours. About 40% of the methicillin in plasma is bound to protein. The distribution and excretion of methicillin and penicillin G are essentially identical (*see* above).

Preparations and Routes of Administration. The available preparation is *methicillin sodium for*

Table 46–1. CHEMICAL STRUCTURES AND MAJOR PROPERTIES OF VARIOUS PENICILLINS

SIDE CHAIN *	NONPROPRIETARY NAME	MAJOR PROPERTIES		
		Absorption after Oral Administration	*Resistance to Penicillinase*	*Useful Antimicrobial Spectrum*
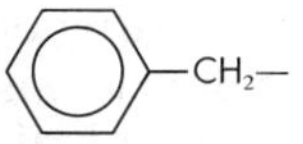	Penicillin G	Variable (poor)	No	*Streptococcus* species, *Neisseria* species, many anaerobes, spirochetes, others
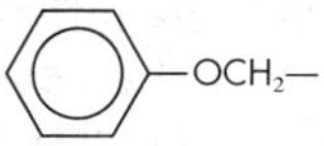	Penicillin V	Good	No	
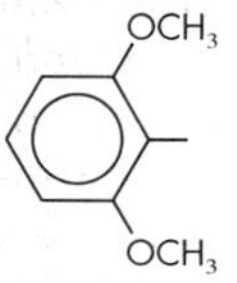	Methicillin	Poor (not given orally)	Yes	
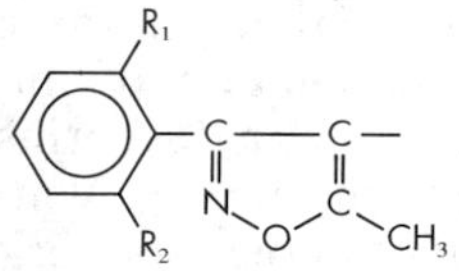	Oxacillin ($R_1 = R_2 = H$) Cloxacillin ($R_1 = Cl$; $R_2 = H$) Dicloxacillin ($R_1 = R_2 = Cl$)	Good	Yes	*Staphylococcus aureus*
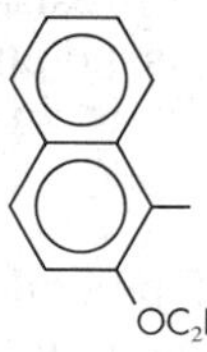	Nafcillin	Variable	Yes	
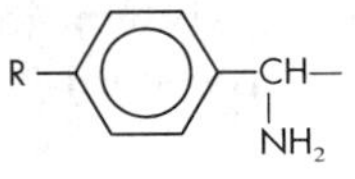	Ampicillin † (R = H) Amoxicillin (R = OH)	Good Excellent	No	*Haemophilus influenzae*, *Proteus mirabilis*, ‡ *Escherichia coli*,‡ *Neisseria* species
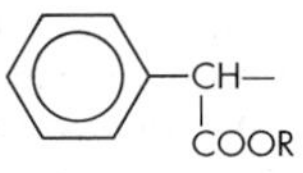	Carbenicillin (R = H) Carbenicillin indanyl (R = 5-indanol)	Poor (not given orally) Good	No	Above plus *Pseudomonas* species, *Enterobacter* species, and *Proteus* (indole positive)
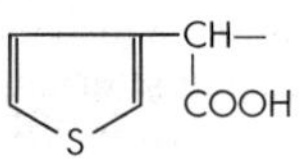	Ticarcillin	Poor (not given orally)	No	
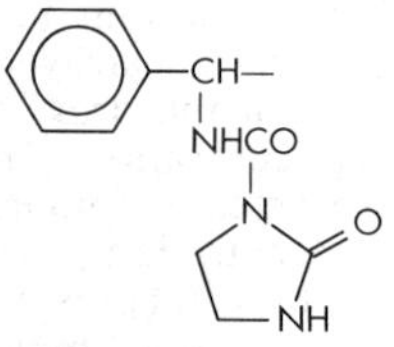	Azlocillin	Poor (not given orally)	No	*Pseudomonas* species

Table 46–1. CHEMICAL STRUCTURES AND MAJOR PROPERTIES OF VARIOUS PENICILLINS

SIDE CHAIN *	NONPROPRIETARY NAME	MAJOR PROPERTIES		
		Absorption after Oral Administration	*Resistance to Penicillinase*	*Useful Antimicrobial Spectrum*
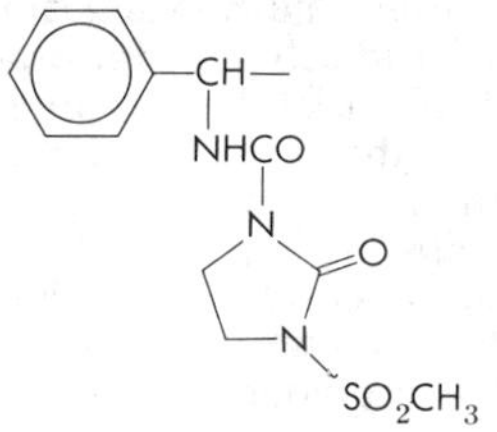	Mezlocillin	Poor (not given orally)	No	*Pseudomonas* species, *Enterobacter* species, many *Klebsiella*
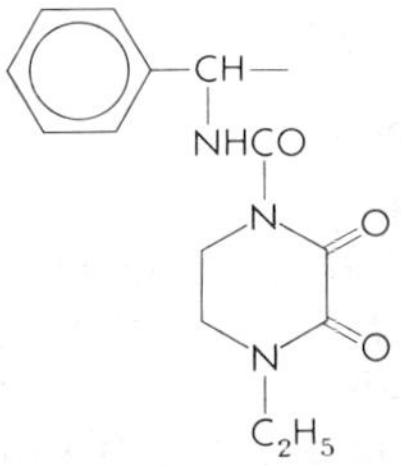	Piperacillin	Poor (not given orally)	No	*Pseudomonas* species, *Enterobacter* species, many *Klebsiella*

* Equivalent to R in Figure 46–1 (page 1066).
† There are other congeners of ampicillin; *see* the text.
‡ Up to 30% of strains may be resistant to ampicillin.

injection (STAPHCILLIN); it is administered intravenously or intramuscularly. The usual dose is 6 to 12 g per day for adults and 100 to 300 mg/kg per day for children, given in four or six portions intravenously.

The Isoxazolyl Penicillins: Oxacillin, Cloxacillin, and Dicloxacillin. These three congeneric semisynthetic penicillins are similar pharmacologically and are thus conveniently considered together. Their structural formulas are shown in Table 46–1. All are relatively stable in an acidic medium and are adequately absorbed after oral administration. All are markedly resistant to cleavage by penicillinase. These drugs are not substitutes for penicillin G in the treatment of diseases amenable to it. Furthermore, because of variability in intestinal absorption, oral administration is not a substitute for the parenteral route in the treatment of serious staphylococcal infections that require a penicillin unaffected by penicillinase.

Pharmacological Properties. The isoxazolyl penicillins are potent inhibitors of the growth of most penicillinase-producing staphylococci. This is their valid clinical use. Dicloxacillin is the most active, and most strains of *Staph. aureus* are inhibited by concentrations of 0.05 to 0.8 μg/ml. Comparable values for cloxacillin and oxacillin are 0.1 to 3 μg/ml and 0.4 to 6 μg/ml, respectively. These differences may have little practical significance, however, since dosages are adjusted accordingly. These agents are, in general, less effective against microorganisms susceptible to penicillin G, and they are not useful against gram-negative bacteria.

These agents are rapidly but incompletely (30 to 80%) absorbed from the gastrointestinal tract. Absorption of the drugs is more efficient when they are taken on an empty stomach. Peak concentrations in plasma are attained by 1 hour and approximate 5 to 10 μg/ml after the ingestion of 1 g of oxacillin. Slightly higher concentrations are achieved after the administration of 1 g of cloxacillin, while the same oral dose of dicloxacillin yields peak plasma concentrations of 15 μg/ml. There is little evidence that these differences are of clinical significance. Since absorption is less than complete, higher plasma concentrations are achieved following intramuscular injection. For example, a 500-mg dose of oxacillin given intramuscularly results in peak concentrations in plasma of approximately 15 μg/ml after 30 to 60 minutes. All these congeners are bound to plasma albumin to a great extent (approximately 90 to 95%); none is removed from the circulation to a significant degree by hemodialysis.

The isoxazolyl penicillins are rapidly excreted by the kidney. Normally, about one half of any of these drugs is excreted in the urine in the first 6 hours after a conventional oral dose. There is also significant hepatic elimination of these agents in the bile. The half-lives for all are between 30 and 60 minutes. Intervals between doses of oxacillin, cloxacillin, and dicloxacillin do not have to be altered for patients with renal failure. The above-noted differences in plasma concentrations produced by the isoxazolyl penicillins are related mainly to differences in rate of urinary excretion and degree of resistance to degradation in the liver.

Preparations and Routes of Administration. *Oxacillin sodium* (BACTOCILL, PROSTAPHLIN) is available for oral use in capsules containing 250 or 500 mg of drug, and as *oxacillin sodium for oral solution* (250 mg/5 ml). The drug is preferably administered 1 hour before or 2 hours after meals, to ensure better absorption. The daily oral dose of oxacillin for adults is 2 to 4 g, divided into four portions; for children, 50 to 100 mg/kg per day is administered similarly. An injectable form of the drug is also available. For adults a total of 2 to 12 g per day, and for children 100 to 300 mg/kg per day, may be given intravenously or intramuscularly, injections being given every 4 to 6 hours.

Cloxacillin sodium (CLOXAPEN, TEGOPEN) is available in capsules (250 and 500 mg) and as a powder for oral solution (125 mg/5 ml). The dosage for adults is 250 mg orally every 6 hours for mild-to-moderate infections; for severe infections, it is 500 mg or more every 6 hours. The dose for children is 50 to 100 mg/kg per day, divided into equal quantities and given every 6 hours; for those weighing more than 20 kg, adult doses are recommended.

Dicloxacillin sodium (DYNAPEN, others) is available for oral use in capsules (125, 250, and 500 mg) and as a powder for oral suspension (62.5 mg/5 ml). The dosage for adults and for children weighing more than 40 kg is 250 mg or more every 6 hours; for children weighing less than 40 kg, the recommended daily dose is 25 mg/kg, given in four equal portions at intervals of 6 hours. Dicloxacillin should be taken 1 to 2 hours before meals. The drug should not be given to newborn infants.

Nafcillin. This semisynthetic penicillin is highly resistant to penicillinase and has proven effective against infections caused by penicillinase-producing strains of *Staph. aureus*. Its structural formula is shown in Table 46–1.

Pharmacological Properties. Nafcillin is slightly more active than oxacillin against penicillin G–resistant *Staph. aureus* (most strains are inhibited by 0.06 to 2 μg/ml). While it is the most active of the penicillinase-resistant penicillins against other microorganisms, it is not as potent as penicillin G.

Nafcillin is inactivated to a variable degree in the acidic medium of the gastric contents. Its absorption after oral administration is irregular, regardless of whether the drug is taken with meals or on an empty stomach. The peak plasma concentration is about 8 μg/ml 60 minutes after a 1-g intramuscular dose. Nafcillin is about 90% bound to plasma protein. Peak concentrations of nafcillin in bile are well above those found in plasma. Concentrations of the drug in CSF appear to be adequate for therapy of staphylococcal meningitis.

Preparations and Routes of Administration. *Nafcillin sodium* (UNIPEN, others) is available for oral and parenteral use. Capsules and tablets contain 250 or 500 mg of the drug, and powders for solution are also marketed for injection or for oral use. However, because of its variable absorption from the gastrointestinal tract, the injectable preparation should be used. Serious staphylococcal infections should be treated with 6 to 9 g of the drug daily, given in divided doses every 4 hours. Children should receive 100 to 200 mg/kg per day in divided doses given every 4 to 6 hours.

THE AMINOPENICILLINS: AMPICILLIN, AMOXICILLIN, AND THEIR CONGENERS

These agents have similar antibacterial activity and a spectrum that is broader than the antibiotics heretofore discussed. They are all destroyed by beta-lactamase (from both gram-positive and gram-negative bacteria) and thus are ineffective for most staphylococcal infections.

Antimicrobial Activity. Ampicillin and the related aminopenicillins are bactericidal for both gram-positive and gram-negative bacteria. They are somewhat less active than penicillin G against gram-positive cocci sensitive to the latter agent. The meningococcus, pneumococcus, gonococcus, and *List. monocytogenes* are sensitive to the drug. *Haemophilus influenzae* and the viridans group of streptococci are usually inhibited by very low concentrations of ampicillin. However, strains of type-b *H. influenzae* that are highly resistant to ampicillin have been recovered from children with meningitis. It is estimated that 25 to 30% of cases of *H. influenzae* meningitis are now caused by ampicillin-resistant strains. Enterococci are about twice as sensitive to ampicillin, on a weight basis, as they are to penicillin G (minimal inhibitory concentration for ampicillin averages 1.5 μg/ml). Although most strains of *E. coli, Pr. mirabilis, Salmonella,* and *Shigella* were highly susceptible when ampicillin was first used in the early 1960s, an increasing percentage of these species is now resistant. From 30 to 50% of *E. coli,* a significant number of *Pr. mirabilis,* and practically all species of *Enterobacter* are presently insensitive. Resistant strains of *Salmonella* (plasmid mediated) have been recovered with increasing frequency in various parts of the world. Most strains of *Shigella* are now resistant. Most strains of *Pseudomonas, Klebsiella, Serratia, Acinetobacter,* and indole-positive *Proteus* are also resistant to this group of penicillins; these antibiotics are less active against *B. fragilis* than is penicillin G. However, concurrent administration of a beta-lactamase inhibitor such as clavulanate or sulbactam markedly expands the spectrum of activity of these drugs (*see* below).

Ampicillin. This drug is the prototypical agent of the group. Its structural formula is shown in Table 46–1.

Pharmacological Properties. Ampicillin is stable in acid and is well absorbed after oral administration. An oral dose of 0.5 g produces peak concentrations in plasma of about 3 μg/ml at 2 hours. Intake of food prior to ingestion of ampicillin results in less complete absorption. Intramuscular injection of 0.5 or 1 g of sodium ampicillin yields peak plasma concentrations of about 7 or 10 μg/ml, respectively, at 1 hour; these decline exponentially, with a half-time of approximately 80 minutes. Severe renal impairment markedly prolongs the persistence of ampicillin in the plasma. Peritoneal dialysis is ineffective in removing the drug from the blood, but hemodialysis removes about 40% of the body store in about 7 hours. Adjustment of the dose of ampicillin is required in the presence of renal dysfunction (*see* Appendix II). Ampicillin appears in the bile, undergoes enterohepatic circulation, and is excreted in appreciable quantities in the feces.

Preparations and Routes of Administration. Ampicillin (AMCILL, OMNIPEN, POLYCILLIN, others) is available for oral use in capsules containing 250 or 500 mg; for parenteral use, as the sodium salt; for oral suspension (125 to 500 mg/5 ml); and in pediatric drops (100 mg/ml). The dose varies with the type and the severity of the infection being treated, with renal function, and with age. Newborns (up to 1 week of age) should receive 25 to 50 mg/kg every 12 hours. Infants (1 to 4 weeks of age) should receive 100 to 200 mg/kg per day in three portions, while older children should receive the same daily dose in four portions. For mild-to-moderate disease, the oral dose for adults is 1 to 4 g per day, divided and given every 6 hours. For severe infections, it is best to administer the drug parenterally in doses ranging from 6 to 12 g per day. The treatment of meningitis requires the use of large doses, up to 400 mg/kg per day parenterally (in equally divided portions given every 4 hours) for children, and 12 g per day for adults.

Amoxicillin. This drug, a penicillinase-susceptible semisynthetic penicillin, is a close chemical and pharmacological relative of ampicillin (*see* Table 46–1). The drug is stable in acid and is designed for oral use. It is more rapidly and completely absorbed from the gastrointestinal tract than is ampicillin, which is the major difference between the two. The antimicrobial spectrum of amoxicillin is essentially identical to that of ampicillin, with the important exception that amoxicillin appears to be less effective than ampicillin for shigellosis (Neu, 1979).

Peak concentrations of amoxicillin in plasma are two to two and one-half times greater for amoxicillin than for ampicillin after oral administration of the same dose; they are reached at 2 hours and average about 4 μg/ml when 250 mg is administered. Food does not interfere with absorption. Perhaps because of more-complete absorption of this congener, the incidence of diarrhea with amoxicillin is less than that following administration of ampicillin. The incidence of other adverse effects appears to be similar. While the half-life of amoxicillin is similar to that for ampicillin, effective concentrations of orally administered amoxicillin are detectable in the plasma for twice as long as with ampicillin, again because of the more-complete absorption. About 20% of amoxicillin is protein bound in plasma, a value similar to that for ampicillin. Most of a dose of the antibiotic is excreted in an active form in the urine. Probenecid delays excretion of the drug. (*See* Gordon *et al.*, 1972; *see also* Appendix II.)

Preparations and Dosage. Amoxicillin (AMOXIL, others) is available for oral use in tablets and capsules (125 to 500 mg), as a powder for oral suspension (125 or 250 mg/5 ml), and as pediatric drops (50 mg/ml). Usual dosages are 0.75 to 1.5 g per day in three divided portions for adults and 20 to 40 mg/kg per day in three portions for children.

Bacampicillin. This agent is the 1-ethoxy-carbonyloxyethyl ester of ampicillin. It is absorbed well after oral administration and is hydrolyzed to ampicillin during absorption from the gastrointestinal tract. Concentrations in blood are about 50% higher than those achieved with amoxicillin, and the drug has been effective when given twice daily. *Bacampicillin hydrochloride* (SPECTROBID) is available in tablets (400 mg; chemically equivalent to 280 mg of ampicillin) and as a powder for oral suspension. The usual dose for adults is 800 to 1600 mg per day divided into two portions (Scheife and Neu, 1982). Children should receive 25 to 50 mg/kg per day.

Other Congeners. *Pivampicillin* is the pivaloyloxymethyl ester of ampicillin. It too is active only after conversion to ampicillin *in vivo*. Absorption after oral administration is similar to that for amoxicillin. There is no indication that the use of this drug will offer any advantage. *Talampicillin* is another similar ester of ampicillin. *Epicillin* and *cyclacillin* are aminopenicillins that are also similar to ampicillin and have little or no advantage over the parent compound. None of these drugs, with the exception of cyclacillin (CYCLAPEN-W), is currently available in the United States.

Therapeutic Indications for the Aminopenicillins. *Upper Respiratory Infections.* Ampicillin and amoxicillin are active against *Strep. pneumoniae, Strep. pyogenes,* and most strains of *H. influenzae,* which are the major upper respiratory bacterial pathogens. The drugs constitute effective therapy for sinusitis, otitis media, acute exacerbations of chronic bronchitis, and epiglottitis. Ampicillin-resistant *H. influenzae* may be a problem in some areas. Bacterial pharyngitis should be treated with penicillin G or penicillin V, since *Strep. pyogenes* is the major pathogen.

Urinary Tract Infections. Most uncomplicated urinary tract infections are caused by Enterobacteriaceae, and *E. coli* is the most common species; ampicillin is usually an effective agent. Enterococcal urinary tract infections are treated effectively with ampicillin alone.

Meningitis. Acute bacterial meningitis in children is most frequently due to *H. influenzae, Strep. pneumoniae,* or *Neisseria meningitidis.* Ampicillin is still frequently used for therapy. Since 20 to 30% of strains of *H. influenzae* may now be resistant to this antibiotic, chloramphenicol should be given concurrently until the microorganism is identified and its sensitivities are determined. Alternatives that may now offer the most rational approach include the use of cefuroxime, ceftriaxone, cefotaxime, or ceftizoxime.

Salmonella Infections. Disease associated with bacteremia, disease with metastatic foci, and the enteric fever syndrome (including typhoid fever) respond favorably to antibiotics. Chloramphenicol is considered by some to be the drug of choice, but the administration of trimethoprim–sulfamethoxazole, a third-generation cephalosporin, or high doses of ampicillin (12 g per day for adults) is also effective. In some geographical areas resistance to chloramphenicol and/or ampicillin is common. The typhoid carrier state has been successfully eliminated in patients without gallbladder disease with ampicillin, trimethoprim–sulfamethoxazole, or ciprofloxacin.

Other Infections. The dual administration of ampicillin and an aminoglycoside may be used to treat sepsis caused by gram-negative bacteria acquired in the general community. After sensitivities of infecting microorganisms are known, it is advisable to treat with a beta-lactam antibiotic and to discontinue the aminoglycoside, if possible. Thus, ampicillin may be used alone to treat a variety of serious gram-negative infections once the bacterial sensitivities have been determined.

ANTIPSEUDOMONAL PENICILLINS: THE CARBOXYPENICILLINS AND THE UREIDOPENICILLINS

The carboxypenicillins, carbenicillin and ticarcillin and their close relatives, are active against most isolates of *Pseudomonas aeruginosa* and certain indole-positive *Proteus* species that are resistant to ampicillin and its congeners. They are ineffective against most strains of *Staph. aureus. Bacteroides fragilis* is susceptible to high concentrations of these drugs, but penicillin G is actually more active on the basis of weight (Maki *et al.,* 1978). The ureidopenicillins, azlocillin, mezlocillin, and piperacillin, are also active against *Pseud. aeruginosa.* In addition, mezlocillin and piperacillin are useful for treatment of infections with *Klebsiella.*

Carbenicillin and Carbenicillin Indanyl. *Carbenicillin.* This drug is a penicillinase-susceptible derivative of 6-aminopenicillanic acid. Its structural formula is shown in Table 46–1. The major advantage of this agent is that it often cures serious infections caused by *Pseudomonas* species, *Proteus* strains resistant to ampicillin, and certain other gram-negative microorganisms.

Low concentrations of carbenicillin inhibit the growth of *Pr. mirabilis* and many microorganisms sensitive to penicillin G. *E. coli, Enterobacter,* and *Salmonella* are less sensitive. The majority of strains of *Pr. vulgaris* and *Pseud. aeruginosa* are sensitive to 25 μg/ml or less of the drug; 70 to 80% of *Pseudomonas* are inhibited by 100 μg/ml. Penicillin G–resistant staphylococci, *Klebsiella,* and *Serratia* are resistant to carbenicillin. Enterococci are suppressed in the range of 50 to 100 μg/ml. Bacterial resistance may appear *in vivo* during treatment with suboptimal doses of carbenicillin.

Carbenicillin is not absorbed from the gastrointestinal tract, and therefore must be given parenterally. Large doses are often necessary. Intramuscular injection of 1 g produces peak concentrations in plasma of 15 to 20 μg/ml in 0.5 to 2 hours. Maximal plasma concentrations are about four times higher after intravenous than after intramuscular administration of the antibiotic. Intravenous infusion at a rate of 1 g per hour results in average plasma concentrations of approximately 150 μg/ml. Intravenous infusion of 4 to 5 g over a 2-hour period every 4 hours will maintain drug concentrations in blood above 100 μg/ml. About 50% of the antibiotic in plasma is protein bound. The distribution of carbenicillin is similar to that of other penicillins. The half-life of carbenicillin in individuals with normal renal function is about 1 hour; it is prolonged to about 2 hours in the presence of hepatic dysfunction. Hemodialysis reduces the concentration of the antibiotic in plasma. Carbenicillin is excreted primarily by the renal tubules. About 75 to 85% of a dose is recoverable in active form in the urine in 9 hours.

Preparations of carbenicillin may cause adverse effects in addition to those that follow use of the other penicillins (*see* below). Congestive heart failure may result from the administration of excessive Na^+. Hypokalemia may occur because of obligatory excretion of cation with the large amount of nonreabsorbable anion (carbenicillin) presented to the distal renal tubule. The drug interferes with platelet function, and bleeding may occur because of abnormal aggregation of platelets (*see* Shattil *et al.*, 1980).

Carbenicillin is available for parenteral injection as the disodium salt (GEOPEN). The daily dose for adults with serious infections is 30 to 40 g in divided doses given every 4 to 6 hours or by continuous infusion. Daily doses up to 600 mg/kg have been used to treat children with life-threatening infection. In patients with severe renal failure, the dose should not exceed 2 g every 12 hours; during hemodialysis, the interval between doses may be reduced to 4 to 6 hours. Available preparations of carbenicillin contain approximately 5 mEq of Na^+ per gram.

Carbenicillin Indanyl. This congener is the indanyl ester of carbenicillin; it is acid stable and is suitable for oral administration. After absorption, the ester is rapidly converted to carbenicillin by hydrolysis of the ester linkage. The antimicrobial spectrum of the drug is therefore that of carbenicillin. Although relatively low concentrations of carbenicillin are achieved in plasma, the active moiety is excreted rapidly in the urine. Thus, the only use of this drug is for the management of urinary tract infections caused by *Proteus* species other than *Pr. mirabilis* and by *Pseud. aeruginosa.*

Carbenicillin indanyl sodium (GEOCILLIN) is available in tablets containing 500 mg of the drug (equivalent to 382 mg of carbenicillin). The recommended daily doses are 2 to 4 g, given in four divided portions. The higher end of this range is preferred for treatment of chronic infections or those caused by *Pseudomonas.*

Carbenicillin phenyl sodium is very similar to carbenicillin indanyl.

Ticarcillin. This semisynthetic penicillin (Table 46–1) is very similar to carbenicillin, but it is two to four times more active against *Pseud. aeruginosa.* Doses are thus usually smaller, and, hopefully, the incidence of toxicity may be decreased. Ticarcillin is now the preferred carboxypenicillin for the treatment of serious infections caused by *Pseudomonas.*

Ticarcillin disodium (TICAR) is available for parenteral injection. Daily doses of the drug are 200 to 300 mg/kg, given in four to six divided portions. These doses must be adjusted for patients with impaired renal function. Ticarcillin disodium contains about 5 mEq of Na^+ per gram (*see* Parry and Neu, 1976, 1978).

Azlocillin. Azlocillin sodium (Table 46–1) is a newer penicillin that is about ten times more active than carbenicillin against *Pseudomonas.* It is also more active against streptococci and resembles ampicillin in this regard (Fu and Neu, 1978). The half-life of azlocillin is 60 minutes in normal subjects but is extended to 6 hours when the creatinine clearance is less than 10 ml per minute. Peak concentrations in blood are about 300 μg/ml after the intravenous administration of 4 g; these values are not directly proportional to doses (Bergen, 1983; Neu *et al.,* 1983). *Azlocillin sodium* (AZLIN) is available as a powder to be dissolved for injection. The preparation contains about 2 mEq of Na^+ per gram. The usual dose is 8 to 18 g per day, given in divided portions four to six times daily.

Mezlocillin. This ureidopenicillin is more active against *Klebsiella* than is carbenicillin; its activity against *Pseudomonas in vitro* is similar to that of ticarcillin. The pharmacokinetic properties of mezlocillin resemble those of azlocillin (*see* McCloskey *et al.,* 1982). *Mezlocillin sodium* (MEZLIN) is available as a powder to be dissolved for injection and contains about 2 mEq of Na^+ per gram. The usual dose for adults is 6 to 18 g per day, divided into four to six portions.

Piperacillin. Piperacillin is another similar derivative with activity against *Klebsiella* that resembles that of mezlocillin and activity against *Pseudomonas* similar to that of azlocillin. Pharmacokinetic properties are reminiscent of the other ureidopenicillins (*see* Eliopoulos and Moellering, 1982). The usual doses are 6 to 18 g per day, given in three to six equal portions. *Piperacillin sodium* (PIPRACIL) is available as a powder for solubilization and injection and contains about 2 mEq of Na^+ per gram.

Therapeutic Indications. These penicillins are important agents for the treatment of patients with serious infections caused by gram-negative bacteria. Such patients frequently have impaired immunological defenses, and their infections are often acquired in the hospital. Many authorities feel that a beta-lactam agent, often in combination with an aminoglycoside, should be employed for all such infections. Therefore, these penicillins find their greatest use in treating bacteremias, pneumonias, infections following burns, and urinary tract infections due to microorganisms resistant to penicillin G and ampicillin; the bacteria especially responsible include *Pseud. aeruginosa,* indole-positive strains of *Proteus,* and *Enterobacter* species. Since *Pseudomonas* infections are common in neutropenic patients, therapy for severe bacterial infections in such individuals should include a beta-lactam antibiotic with good activity against these microorganisms.

UNTOWARD REACTIONS TO PENICILLINS

Hypersensitivity Reactions. Hypersensitivity reactions are by far the most common adverse effects noted with the penicillins, and these agents are probably the most common cause of drug allergy. There is no convincing evidence that any single penicillin differs from the group in its potential for causing true allergic reactions. In approximate order of decreasing frequency, manifestations of allergy to penicillins include maculopapular rash, urticarial rash, fever, bronchospasm, vasculitis, serum sickness, exfoliative dermatitis, Stevens–Johnson syndrome, and anaphylaxis (*see* Levine, 1972; Saxon *et al.*, 1987; *Medical Letter*, 1988). The overall incidence of such reactions to the penicillins varies from 0.7 to 10% in different studies (Idsøe *et al.*, 1968).

Hypersensitivity reactions may occur with any dosage form of penicillin; allergy to one penicillin exposes the patient to a greater risk of reaction if another is given. On the other hand, the occurrence of an untoward effect does not necessarily imply repetition on subsequent exposures. Hypersensitivity reactions may appear in the absence of a previous known exposure to the drug. This may be caused by unrecognized prior exposure to penicillin in the environment (*e.g.*, in foods of animal origin or from the fungus producing penicillin). Although elimination of the antibiotic usually results in rapid clearing of the allergic manifestations, they may persist for 1 or 2 weeks or longer after therapy has been stopped. In some cases, the reaction is mild and disappears even while the use of penicillin is continued; in others, it necessitates immediate cessation of penicillin treatment. In a few instances, it is necessary to interdict the future use of penicillin because of the risk of death, and the patient should be so warned. It must be stressed that fatal episodes of anaphylaxis have followed the ingestion of very small doses of this antibiotic or skin testing with minute quantities of the drug.

Penicillins and breakdown products of penicillins act as haptens after their covalent reaction with proteins. The most important antigenic intermediate of penicillin appears to be the penicilloyl moiety, which is formed when the beta-lactam ring is opened. This is considered to be the major (predominant) determinant of penicillin allergy. In addition, minor determinants of allergy to penicillins are present. These include the intact molecule itself and penicilloate. These products are formed *in vivo* and can also be found in solutions of penicillin prepared for administration. The terms *major determinant* and *minor determinant* refer to the frequency with which antibodies to these haptens appear to be formed. They do *not* describe the severity of the reaction that may result.

Antipenicillin antibodies are detectable in virtually all patients who have received the drug and in many who have never knowingly been exposed to it (Klaus and Fellner, 1973). Recent treatment with the antibiotic induces an increase in major-determinant-specific antibodies that are skin sensitizing. The incidence of positive skin reactors is three to four times higher in atopic than in nonatopic individuals. Clinical and immunological studies suggest that immediate allergic reactions are mediated by skin-sensitizing or IgE antibodies, usually of minor-determinant specificities. Accelerated and late urticarial reactions are usually mediated by major-determinant-specific, skin-sensitizing antibodies. The recurrent-arthralgia syndrome appears to be related to the presence of skin-sensitizing antibodies of minor-determinant specificities. Some maculopapular and erythematous reactions may be due to toxic antigen–antibody complexes of major-determinant-specific IgM antibodies. Accelerated and late urticarial reactions to penicillin may terminate spontaneously because of the development of blocking antibodies (*see* Levine *et al.*, 1966).

Skin rashes of all types may be caused by allergy to penicillin. Scarlatiniform, morbilliform, urticarial, vesicular, and bullous eruptions may develop. Purpuric lesions are uncommon and are usually the result of a vasculitis; thrombocytopenic purpura may occur very rarely. Henoch–Schönlein purpura with renal involvement has been a rare complication. Contact dermatitis is observed occasionally in pharmacists, nurses, and physicians who prepare penicillin solutions. Fixed-drug reactions have also occurred. More severe reactions involving the skin are exfoliative dermatitis and exudative erythema multiforme of either the erythematopapular or vesiculobullous type; these lesions may be very severe and atypical in distribution and constitute the characteristic Stevens–Johnson syndrome. The incidence of skin rashes appears to be highest following the use of ampicillin, being about 9%; rashes follow the administration of ampicillin in nearly all patients with infectious mononucleosis.

When allopurinol and ampicillin are administered concurrently, the incidence of rash also increases. Ampicillin-induced skin eruptions in such patients may represent a "toxic" rather than a truly allergic reaction. Positive skin reactions to the major and minor determinants of penicillin sensitization may be absent. The rash may clear even while administration of the drug is continued.

The most serious hypersensitivity reactions produced by the penicillins are angioedema and anaphylaxis. Angioedema with marked swelling of the lips, tongue, face, and periorbital tissues, frequently accompanied by asthmatic breathing and "giant hives," has been observed after topical, oral, or systemic administration of penicillins of various types.

Acute anaphylactic or anaphylactoid reactions induced by various preparations of penicillin constitute the most important immediate danger connected with their use. Among all drugs, the penicillins are most often responsible for this type of untoward effect. Anaphylactoid reactions may occur at any age. Their incidence is thought to be 0.04 to 0.2% in persons treated with penicillins. About 0.001% of patients treated with these agents die from anaphylaxis. It has been estimated that there are at least 300 deaths per year due to this complication of therapy. About 15% of those who succumb have had other types of allergy; 70% have had penicillin previously, and one third of these reacted to it on a prior occasion (Idsøe *et al.*, 1968). Anaphylaxis has most often followed the injection of penicillin, although it has also been observed after oral ingestion of the drug, and has even resulted from the intradermal instillation of a very small quantity for the purpose of testing for the presence of hypersensitivity. The clinical pictures that develop vary in severity. The most dramatic is sudden, severe hypotension and rapid death. In other instances, bronchoconstriction with severe asthma, or abdominal pain, nausea, and vomiting, or extreme weakness and a fall in blood pressure, or diarrhea and purpuric skin eruptions have characterized the anaphylactic episodes.

Serum sickness varies from mild fever, rash, and leukopenia to severe arthralgia or arthritis, purpura, lymphadenopathy, splenomegaly, mental changes, electrocardiographic abnormalities suggestive of myocarditis, generalized edema, albuminuria, and hematuria. It is mediated by IgG antibodies. This reaction usually appears after penicillin treatment has been continued for 1 week or more; it may be delayed, however, until 1 or 2 weeks after the drug has been stopped. Serum sickness caused by penicillin may persist for a week or longer.

Vasculitis of the skin or other organs may be related to hypersensitivity to penicillin. The Coombs' reaction frequently becomes positive during prolonged therapy with a penicillin or cephalosporin, but hemolytic anemia is rare. Reversible neutropenia may occur. It is not known if this is truly a hypersensitivity reaction; it has been noted with all of the penicillins and has been seen in up to 30% of patients treated with 8 to 12 g of nafcillin for longer than 21 days. The bone marrow shows an arrest of maturation.

Fever may be the only evidence of a hypersensitivity reaction to the penicillins. It may reach high levels and be maintained, remittent, or intermittent; chills occasionally occur. The febrile reaction usually disappears within 24 to 36 hours after administration of the drug is stopped, but may persist for days.

Eosinophilia is an occasional accompaniment of other allergic reactions to penicillin. At times, it may be the sole abnormality, and eosinophils may reach levels of 10 to 20% or more of the total number of circulating white blood cells.

Interstitial nephritis may rarely be produced by the penicillins; methicillin has been implicated most frequently. Hematuria, albuminuria, pyuria, renal-cell and other casts in the urine, elevation of serum creatinine, and even oliguria have been noted. Biopsy shows a mononuclear infiltrate with eosinophilia and tubular damage. IgG is present in the interstitium (*see* Ditlove *et al.*, 1977; Kancir *et al.*, 1978). This reaction is usually reversible.

Management of the Patient Potentially Allergic to Penicillin. Evaluation of the patient's history is the most practical way to avoid the use of penicillin in patients who are at the greatest risk of adverse reaction.

The majority of patients who give a history of allergy to penicillin should be treated with a different type of antibiotic. In the unusual instance where treatment with a penicillin is essential, skin tests may be of some help (Solley *et al.,* 1982). Lack of a response to benzylpenicilloyl polylysine (PRE-PEN) makes it very unlikely that a patient will develop an immediate or accelerated reaction to penicillin; this preparation is not immunogenic, nor is it likely to provoke severe reactions. Furthermore, only 3% of such patients will develop a delayed reaction (usually rash). Patients with a positive response to benzylpenicilloyl polylysine are at significant risk of serious reaction, and in two thirds of these patients some form of allergic reaction will develop. In order to reduce the likelihood of an immediate severe reaction further, sensitivity to the minor antigenic determinants probably should also be tested. Unfortunately, mixtures of the minor antigenic determinants are not commercially available. A scratch test with a very dilute (5 units/ml) solution of the penicillin to be administered, followed by a scratch test with a more concentrated solution (10,000 units/ml), can be performed; if this is negative, an intradermal test with 0.02 ml of a solution of 100 units/ml should also be done. If these are negative, penicillin may be administered cautiously. Administration of epinephrine is the therapy of choice for an immediate or accelerated reaction to penicillin.

''Desensitization'' is occasionally recommended for patients who are allergic to penicillin and who must receive the drug. This procedure consists of administering gradually increasing doses of penicillin in the hope of avoiding a severe reaction. This may result in a subclinical anaphylactic discharge and the binding of all IgE before full doses are administered. Penicillin may be given in doses of 1, 5, 10, 100, and 1000 units intradermally in the lower arm, with 60-minute intervals between doses. If this is well tolerated, then 10,000 units and 50,000 units may be given subcutaneously. Desensitization may also be accomplished by the oral administration of penicillin (Sullivan *et al.,* 1982). When full doses are reached, penicillin should not be discontinued and then restarted, since immediate reactions may recur (*see* Weiss and Adkinson, 1990, for details). The patient should be observed constantly during the procedure, an intravenous line must be in place, and epinephrine and equipment and expertise for artificial ventilation must be on hand. It must be emphasized that this procedure may be dangerous and its efficacy is unproven.

Patients with life-threatening infections (*e.g.,* endocarditis or meningitis) may be continued on penicillin despite the development of a maculopapular rash. The rash often clears as therapy is continued. This is thought to be due to the development of blocking antibodies of the IgG class. The rash may be treated with antihistamines or adrenocorticosteroids, although there is no evidence that this therapy is efficacious. Rarely, exfoliative dermatitis with or without vasculitis develops in these patients if therapy with penicillin is continued. Therefore, alternative antimicrobial agents should be used whenever possible.

Other Adverse Reactions. The penicillins have minimal direct toxicity (*see* Parker, 1975). Apparent toxic effects that have been reported include bone-marrow depression, granulocytopenia, and hepatitis. The last-named effect is rare but is most commonly seen following the administration of oxacillin and nafcillin (Onorato and Axelrod, 1978; Kirkwood *et al.*, 1983). The administration of penicillin G, carbenicillin, or ticarcillin has been associated with a potentially significant defect of hemostasis that appears to be due to an impairment of platelet aggregation; this may be caused by interference with the binding of aggregating agents to platelet receptors (Fass *et al.*, 1987).

Most common among the irritative responses to penicillin are pain and sterile inflammatory reactions at the sites of intramuscular injections, reactions that are related to concentration. Serum transaminases and lactic dehydrogenase may be elevated as a result of local damage to muscle. In some individuals who receive penicillin intravenously phlebitis or thrombophlebitis develops. Many persons who take various penicillin preparations by mouth experience nausea, with or without vomiting, and some have mild-to-severe diarrhea. These manifestations are often related to the dose of the drug.

When penicillin is injected accidentally into the sciatic nerve, severe pain occurs and dysfunction in the area of distribution of this nerve develops and persists for weeks. Intrathecal injection of penicillin G may produce arachnoiditis or severe and fatal encephalopathy. Because of this, intrathecal or intraventricular administration of penicillins should be avoided. The parenteral administration of large doses of penicillin G (greater than 20 million units per day, or less with renal insufficiency) may produce lethargy, confusion, twitching, multifocal myoclonus, or localized or generalized epileptiform seizures. These are most apt to occur in the presence of renal insufficiency, localized CNS lesions, or hyponatremia. When the concentration of penicillin G in CSF exceeds 10 μg/ml, significant dysfunction of the CNS is frequent. The injection of 20 million units of penicillin G potassium, which contains 34 mEq of K^+, may lead to severe or even fatal hyperkalemia in persons with renal dysfunction.

Injection of penicillin G procaine may result in an immediate reaction, characterized by dizziness, tinnitus, headache, hallucinations, and sometimes seizures. This is due to the rapid liberation of toxic concentrations of procaine. It has been reported to occur in 1 of 200 patients receiving 4.8 million units of penicillin G procaine to treat their venereal disease.

Reactions Unrelated to Hypersensitivity or Toxicity. Regardless of the route by which the drug is administered, but most strikingly when it is given by mouth, penicillin changes the composition of the microflora by eliminating sensitive microorganisms. This phenomenon is usually of no clinical significance and the normal microflora is reestablished shortly after therapy is stopped. In some persons, however, superinfection results from the changes in flora. Pseudomembranous colitis, related to overgrowth and production of a toxin by *Clostridium difficile*, has followed oral and, less commonly, parenteral administration of penicillins.

THE CEPHALOSPORINS

History and Source. *Cephalosporium acremonium*, the first source of the cephalosporins, was isolated in 1948 by Brotzu from the sea near a sewer outlet off the Sardinian coast. Crude filtrates from cultures of this fungus were found to inhibit the *in-vitro* growth of *Staph. aureus* and to cure staphylococcal infections and typhoid fever in man. Culture fluids in which the Sardinian fungus was cultivated were found to contain three distinct antibiotics, which were named cephalosporin P, N, and C. With the isolation of the active nucleus of cephalosporin C, 7-aminocephalosporanic acid, and with the addition of side chains, it became possible to produce semisynthetic compounds with antibacterial activity very much greater than that of the parent substance. (For a historical review and discussion of the biochemistry of the cephalosporins, *see* Abraham, 1962; Flynn, 1972.)

Chemistry. Cephalosporin C contains a side chain derived from D-α-aminoadipic acid, which is condensed with a dihydrothiazine beta-lactam ring system (7-aminocephalosporanic acid). Compounds containing 7-aminocephalosporanic acid are relatively stable in dilute acid and highly resistant to penicillinase, regardless of the nature of their side chains and their affinity for the enzyme.

Cephalosporin C can be hydrolyzed by acid to 7-aminocephalosporanic acid. This compound has been subsequently modified by the addition of different side chains to create a whole family of cephalosporin antibiotics. It appears that modifications at position 7 of the beta-lactam ring are associated with alteration in antibacterial activity and that substitutions at position 3 of the dihydrothiazine ring are associated with changes in the metabolism and the pharmacokinetic properties of the drugs (*see* Huber *et al.*, 1972).

The cephamycins are similar to the cephalosporins, but have a methoxy group at position 7 of the beta-lactam ring of the 7-aminocephalosporanic acid nucleus. The structural formulas of representative cephalosporins and cephamycins are shown in Table 46–2.

Mechanism of Action. Cephalosporins and cephamycins inhibit bacterial cell-wall synthesis in a manner similar to that of penicillin. This is discussed in detail above (*see* page 1066).

Classification. The explosive growth of the cephalosporins during the past decade has taxed the best of memories and makes a system of classification most desirable. Although cephalosporins may be classified by their chemical structure, clinical pharmacology, resistance to beta-lactamase, or antimicrobial spectrum, the well-accepted system of classification by "generations" is very useful, although admittedly somewhat arbitrary (Table 46–2).

Classification by generations is based on general features of antimicrobial activity (*see* Donowitz and Mandell, 1990). The first-generation cephalosporins, epitomized by cephalothin and cefazolin, have good activity against gram-positive bacteria and relatively modest activity against gram-negative microorganisms. Most gram-positive cocci (with the exception of enterococci, methicillin-resistant *Staph. aureus*, and *Staph. epidermidis*) are susceptible. Activity against *E. coli, Klebsiella pneumoniae*, and *Pr. mirabilis* is good. The second-generation cephalosporins have somewhat increased activity against gram-negative microorganisms but are much less active than the third-generation agents. Third-generation cephalosporins are generally less active than first-generation agents against gram-positive cocci, but they are much more active against the Enterobacteriaceae, including beta-lactamase-producing strains. A subset of third-generation agents is also active against *Pseud. aeruginosa* (Donowitz and Mandell, 1988).

Table 46–2. NAMES, STRUCTURAL FORMULAS, DOSAGE, AND DOSAGE FORMS OF SELECTED CEPHALOSPORINS AND RELATED COMPOUNDS

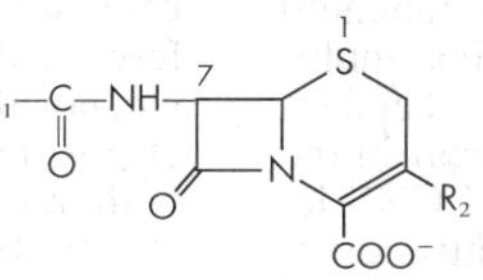

COMPOUND (TRADE NAMES)	R_1	R_2	DOSAGE FORMS, * ADULT DOSAGE FOR SEVERE INFECTION, AND HALF-LIVES
First Generation			
Cephalothin (KEFLIN)	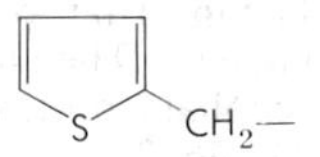	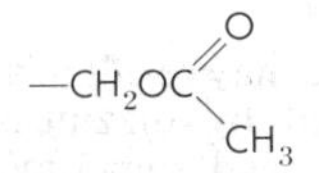	I: 1 to 2 g every 4 hours $T_{1/2}$ = 0.6 hour
Cephapirin (CEFADYL)	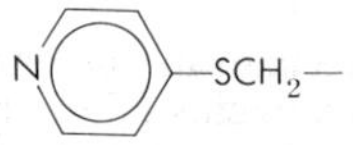	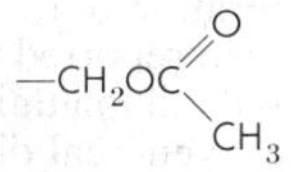	I: 1 to 2 g every 4 hours $T_{1/2}$ = 0.7 hours
Cefazolin (ANCEF, KEFZOL, others)	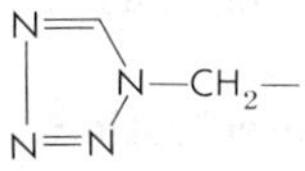	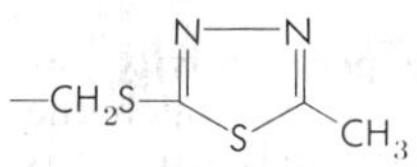	I: 1 to 1.5 g every 6 hours $T_{1/2}$ = 1.8 hours
Cephalexin (KEFLET, KEFLEX)	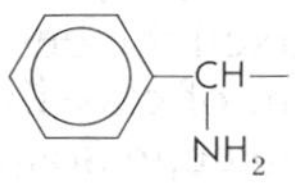	—CH_3	C,T,O: 1 g every 6 hours $T_{1/2}$ = 0.9 hour
Cephradine (ANSPOR, VELOSEF)	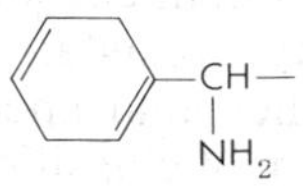	—CH_3	C,O: 1 g every 6 hours I: 2 g every 6 hours $T_{1/2}$ = 0.8 hour
Cefadroxil (DURICEF, ULTRACEF)	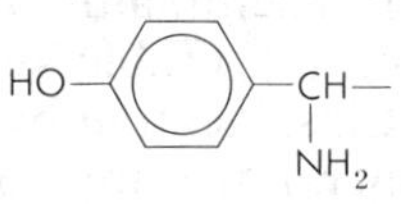	—CH_3	C,T,O: 1 g every 12 hours $T_{1/2}$ = 1.1 hours
Second Generation			
Cefamandole (MANDOL)	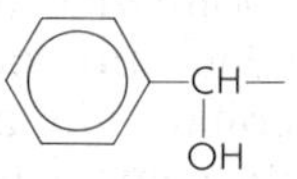	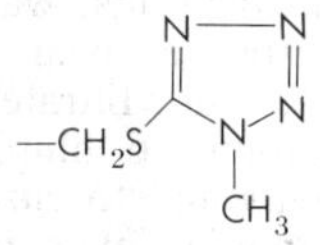	I: 2 g every 4 to 6 hours $T_{1/2}$ = 0.8 hour
Cefoxitin† (MEFOXIN)	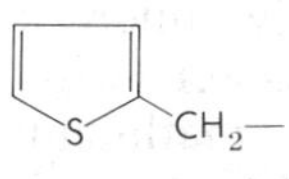	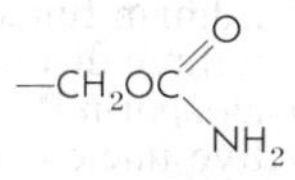	I: 2 g every 4 hours or 3 g every 6 hours $T_{1/2}$ = 0.7 hour
Cefaclor (CECLOR)	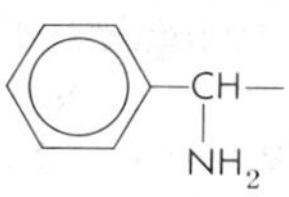	—Cl	C,O: 1 g every 8 hours $T_{1/2}$ = 0.7 hour
Cefuroxime (KEFUROX, ZINACEF)	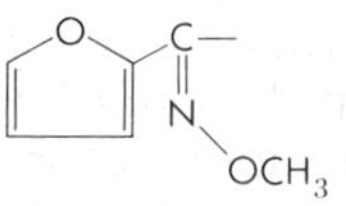	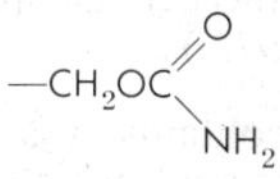	I: up to 3 g every 8 hours $T_{1/2}$ = 1.7 hours
Cefuroxime axetil ‡ (CEFTIN)			T: 500 mg every 12 hours
Cefonicid (MONOCID)	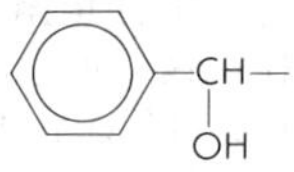	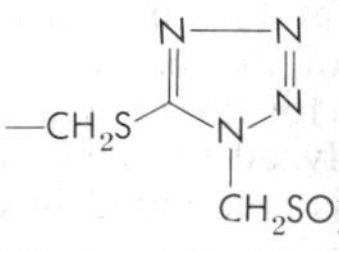	I: 2 g every 24 hours $T_{1/2}$ = 4.4 hours

Table 46–2. NAMES, STRUCTURAL FORMULAS, DOSAGE, AND DOSAGE FORMS OF SELECTED CEPHALOSPORINS AND RELATED COMPOUNDS (Continued)

COMPOUND (TRADE NAMES)	R_1	R_2	DOSAGE FORMS, * ADULT DOSAGE FOR SEVERE INFECTION, AND HALF-LIVES
Cefotetan (CEFOTAN)	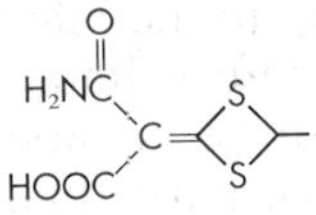	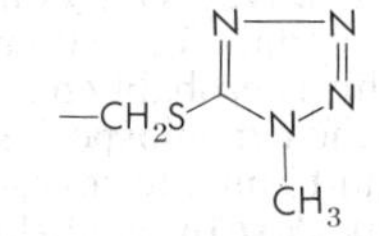	I: 2 to 3 g every 12 hours $T_{1/2}$ = 3.3 hours
Ceforanide (PRECEF)	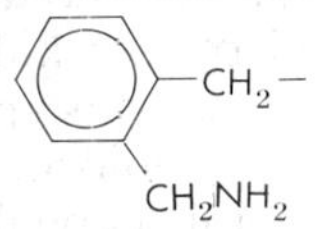	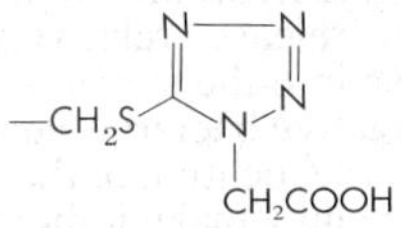	I: 1 g every 12 hours $T_{1/2}$ = 2.6 hours
Third Generation Cefotaxime (CLAFORAN)	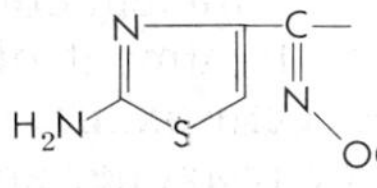	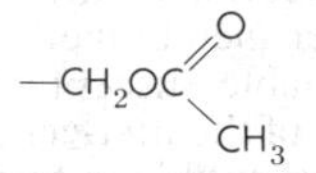	I: 2 g every 4 to 8 hours $T_{1/2}$ = 1.1 hours
Ceftizoxime (CEFIZOX)	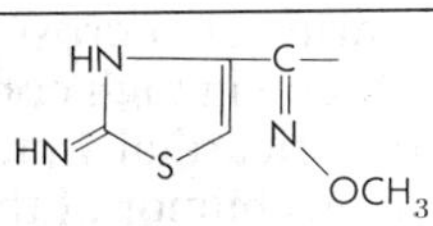	—H	I: 3 to 4 g every 8 hours $T_{1/2}$ = 1.8 hours
Ceftriaxone (ROCEPHIN)	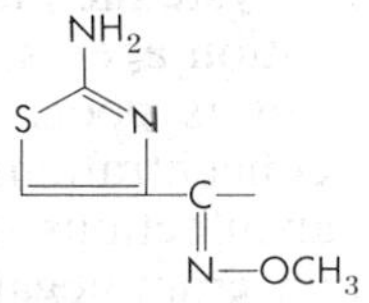	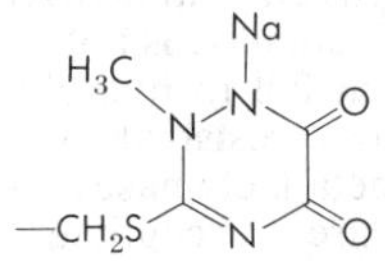	I: 2 g every 12 to 24 hours $T_{1/2}$ = 8 hours
Cefoperazone (CEFOBID)	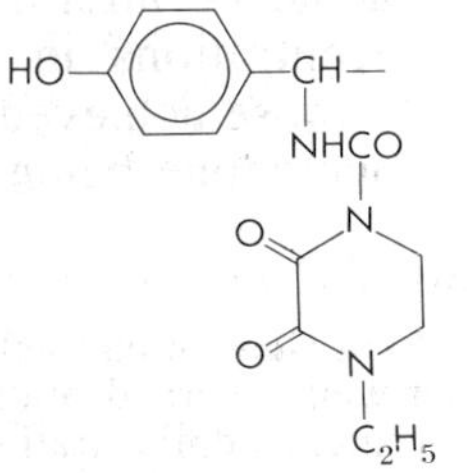	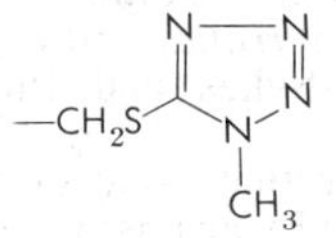	I: 1.5 to 4 g every 6 or 8 hours $T_{1/2}$ = 2.1 hours
Ceftazidime (FORTAZ, others)	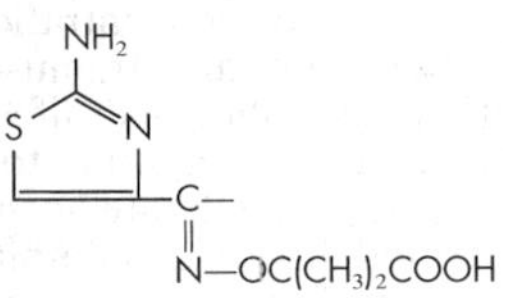	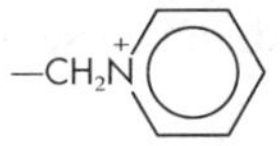	I: 2 g every 8 hours $T_{1/2}$ = 1.8 hours

* T = tablet, C = capsule, O = oral suspension, I = injection.
† Cefoxitin, a cephamycin, has a $—OCH_3$ residue at position 7.
‡ Cefuroxime axetil is the acetyloxyethyl ester of cefuroxime.

Mechanisms of Bacterial Resistance to the Cephalosporins. Resistance to the cephalosporins may be related to inability of the antibiotic to reach its sites of action, alterations in the antibiotic-binding proteins such that interaction does not take place, or bacterial enzymes (beta-lactamases) that can hydrolyze the beta-lactam ring and inactivate the cephalosporin.

If the antibiotic binds to and inactivates only one enzyme, a mutation in the gene coding for that enzyme may lead to resistance. This is probably not a common cause of resistance to the cephalosporins, since most of these agents appear to bind to several different proteins. Bacteria may destroy cephalosporins by hydrolysis of the beta-lactam ring. Many gram-positive microorganisms release relatively large amounts of beta-lactamase into the surrounding medium. Although gram-negative bacteria seem to produce less beta-lactamase, the location of their enzyme in the periplasmic space may make it more effective in destroying cephalosporins as they diffuse to their targets on the inner membrane.

The cephalosporins have variable susceptibility to beta-lactamase. For example, of the first-generation agents, cefazolin is more susceptible to hydrolysis by beta-lactamase from *Staph. aureus* than is cephalothin. Cefoxitin, cefuroxime, and the third-generation cephalosporins are the most resistant to hydrolysis by the beta-lactamases produced by gram-negative bacteria (Sykes and Bush, 1983). However, the correlation between antimicrobial activity and resistance to beta-lactamase is not perfect. Some bacterial strains that fail to hydrolyze the antibiotics are nevertheless resistant. Conversely, some bacteria with beta-lactamases that can destroy cephalosporins are susceptible to them. Although most of the third-generation cephalosporins are relatively resistant to hydrolysis by bacterial beta-lactamases, there have been reports of the development of resistance to the third-generation agents by *Enterobacter, Serratia,* and especially *Pseudomonas* species (Sykes and Bush, 1983).

It is important to remember that none of the cephalosporins has reliable activity against the following microorganisms: penicillin-resistant *Strep. pneumoniae,* methicillin-resistant *Staph. aureus,* methicillin-resistant *Staph. epidermidis, Enterococcus, List. monocytogenes, Legionella pneumophila, Legionella micdadei, Clostridium difficile, Pseud. maltophilia, Pseud. putida, Campylobacter jejuni, Acinetobacter* species, and, of course, *Candida albicans.*

General Features of the Cephalosporins. Cephalexin, cephradine, cefaclor, cefadroxil, and cefuroxime axetil are absorbed after oral administration and can be given by this route. Cephalothin and cephapirin cause pain when given by intramuscular injection and thus are usually used only intravenously. The other agents can be administered intramuscularly or intravenously.

Cephalosporins are primarily excreted by the kidney; dosage should thus be altered in patients with renal insufficiency. Probenecid slows the tubular secretion of most cephalosporins, but not moxalactam (DeSante *et al.,* 1982). Cefoperazone is an exception, since it is excreted predominantly in the bile. Cephalothin, cephapirin, and cefotaxime are deacetylated *in vivo,* and these metabolites have less antimicrobial activity than the parent compounds. The deacetylated metabolites are also excreted by the kidneys. None of the other cephalosporins appears to undergo appreciable metabolism.

Several cephalosporins penetrate into CSF in sufficient concentration to be useful for the treatment of meningitis. These include cefuroxime, moxalactam, cefotaxime, ceftriaxone, and ceftizoxime. Cephalosporins also cross the placenta, and they are found in high concentrations in synovial and pericardial fluid. Penetration into the aqueous humor of the eye is relatively good after systemic administration of third-generation agents, but penetration into the vitreous is poor. There is some evidence that concentrations sufficient for therapy of ocular infections due to gram-positive and certain gram-negative microorganisms can be achieved after systemic administration. Concentrations in bile are usually high, with those achieved after administration of cefoperazone being the highest.

SPECIFIC AGENTS

First-Generation Cephalosporins. Cephalothin is not well absorbed orally and is available only for parenteral administration. Because of pain on intramuscular injection, it is usually given intravenously. Peak concentrations in plasma are about 20 μg/ml after an intramuscular dose of 1 g. Cephalothin has a short half-life (30 to 40 minutes) and is metabolized in addition to being excreted. The deacetylated metabolite accounts for 20 to 30% of the excreted drug. Cephalothin does not enter the CSF to a significant extent, and this drug should obviously not be used for the treatment of meningitis. Since among the cephalosporins cephalothin is the most impervious to attack by staphylococcal beta-lactamase, it is very effective in severe staphylococcal infections, such as endocarditis.

Cephapirin is very similar to cephalothin (Renzini *et al.,* 1975).

The antibacterial spectrum of cefazolin is similar to that of cephalothin. Although cefazolin is more active against *E. coli* and *Klebsiella* species, it is somewhat more sensitive to staphylococcal beta-lactamase than is cephalothin (Fong *et al.*, 1976a; Byrant, 1984). Cefazolin is relatively well tolerated after either intramuscular or intravenous administration, and concentrations of the drug in plasma are higher after intramuscular (64 μg/ml after 1 g) or intravenous injection than are concentrations of cephalothin. The half-life is also appreciably longer—1.8 hours. The renal clearance of cefazolin is lower than that of cephalothin; this is presumably related to the fact that cefazolin is excreted by glomerular filtration, whereas cephalothin is also secreted by the kidney tubule. Cefazolin is bound to plasma proteins to a great extent (about 85%). Cefazolin is usually preferred among the first-generation cephalosporins, since it can be administered less frequently because of its longer half-life (Quintiliani and Nightingale, 1978).

Cephalexin is available for oral administration, and it has the same antibacterial spectrum as the other first-generation cephalosporins. However, it is somewhat less active against penicillinase-producing staphylococci. Oral therapy with cephalexin results in peak concentrations in plasma of 16 μg/ml after a dose of 0.5 g; this is adequate for the inhibition of many gram-positive and gram-negative pathogens that are sensitive to cephalothin. The drug is not metabolized, and more than 90% is excreted in the urine.

Cephradine is similar in structure to cephalexin, and its activity *in vitro* is almost identical. Cephradine is not metabolized and, after rapid absorption from the gastrointestinal tract, is excreted unchanged in the urine. Cephradine can be administered orally, intramuscularly, or intravenously. When administered orally, it is difficult to distinguish cephradine from cephalexin; some authorities feel that these two drugs can be used interchangeably. Because cephradine is so well absorbed, the concentrations in plasma are nearly equivalent after oral or intramuscular administration (about 10 to 18 μg/ml after 0.5 g orally or intramuscularly) (Neiss, 1973).

Cefadroxil is the para-hydroxy analog of cephalexin. Concentrations of cefadroxil in plasma and urine are at somewhat higher levels than are those with cephalexin. The drug may be used once or twice a day for the treatment of urinary tract infections. Its activity *in vitro* is similar to that of cephalexin (Hartstein *et al.*, 1977).

Second-Generation Cephalosporins. Cefamandole is more active than the first-generation cephalosporins against certain gram-negative microorganisms. This is especially evident for *H. influenzae*, *Enterobacter* species, indole-positive *Proteus* species, *E. coli*, and *Klebsiella* species (Meyers and Hirschman, 1978). Heavy inocula of bacteria show decreased susceptibility, and this appears to be related to destruction of the antibiotic by beta-lactamase. Most gram-positive cocci are sensitive to cefamandole. The half-life of the drug is 45 minutes, and it is excreted unchanged in the urine. Concentrations in plasma are 20 to 36 μg/ml after a dose of 1 g is given intramuscularly (Fong *et al.*, 1976b; Neu, 1978).

Cefoxitin is a cephamycin produced by *Streptomyces lactamdurans*. It is highly resistant to beta-lactamases produced by gram-negative rods (Kass and Evans, 1979). This antibiotic is more active than cephalothin against certain gram-negative microorganisms, although it is less active than cefamandole against *Enterobacter* species and *H. influenzae*. It is also less active than both cefamandole and the first-generation cephalosporins against gram-positive bacteria. Cefoxitin is more active than other first- or second-generation agents (except cefotetan) against anaerobes, especially *B. fragilis*. This activity is similar to that of moxalactam and better than that of other third-generation cephalosporins. After an intramuscular dose of 1 g, concentrations in plasma are about 22 μg/ml. The half-life is approximately 40 minutes. Cefoxitin's special role seems to be for treatment of certain anaerobic and mixed aerobic–anaerobic infections, such as pelvic inflammatory disease and lung abscess (Sutter and Finegold, 1975; Bach *et al.*, 1977; Chow and Bednorz, 1978). It is an effective agent for gonorrhea caused by penicillinase-producing *Neisseria* (Greaves *et al.*, 1983).

Cefaclor is used orally. The concentrations in plasma after oral administration are about 50% of those achieved after an equivalent oral dose of cephalexin. However, cefaclor is more active against *H. influenzae*, although some beta-lactamase-producing strains of *H. influenzae* may be resistant (Silver *et al.*, 1977).

Cefuroxime is very similar to cefamandole in structure and antibacterial activity *in vitro* (Smith and LeFrock, 1983), although it is somewhat more resistant to beta-lactamases. The half-life is longer than that of cefamandole (1.7 hours vs. 0.8 hour), and the drug can be given every 8 hours. Concentrations in CSF are about 10% of those in plasma, and the drug is effective for meningitis due to *H. influenzae* (including strains resistant to ampicillin), *N. meningitidis*, and *Strep. pneumoniae* (Johansson *et al.*, 1982). However, relapses have occurred after therapy.

Cefuroxime axetil is the 1-acetyloxyethyl ester of cefuroxime. Thirty to fifty percent of an oral dose is absorbed, and the drug is then hydrolyzed to cefuroxime; resultant concentrations in plasma are variable.

Cefonicid has antimicrobial activity *in vitro* similar to that of cefamandole. The half-life of the drug is about 4 hours, and administration once daily has been effective for certain infections caused by susceptible microorganisms (Gremillion *et al.*, 1983).

Cefotetan is a cephamycin, and, like cefoxitin, it has good activity against *B. fragilis*. It is also effective against several other species of *Bacteroides*, and it is slightly more active than cefoxitin against gram-negative aerobes. After an intramuscular dose of 1 g, peak plasma concentrations of cefotetan average 70 μg/ml. It has a half-life of 3.3 hours (Phillips *et al.*, 1983; Wexler and Finegold, 1988). Hypoprothrombinemia with bleeding has occurred in malnourished patients receiving cefotetan; this is preventable if vitamin K is also administered.

Ceforanide is similar in structure and antimicrobial activity to cefamandole; however, it is less active against strains of *H. influenzae* (Barriere and Mills, 1982). Its half-life is about 2.6 hours and it is administered parenterally every 12 hours.

Third-Generation Cephalosporins. Cefotaxime was the first of the third-generation cephalosporins to become available in the United States. The drug is highly resistant to bacterial beta-lactamases and has good activity against many gram-positive and gram-negative aerobic bacteria. However, activity against *B. fragilis* is poor as compared to agents such as clindamycin and metronidazole (Neu *et al.*, 1979). Cefotaxime has a half-life in plasma of about 1 hour, and the drug should be administered every 4 to 8 hours for serious infections. The drug is metabolized *in vivo* to desacetylcefotaxime, which is less active against most microorganisms than is the parent compound. However, the metabolite acts synergistically with the parent compound against certain microbes (Neu, 1982). Cefotaxime has been utilized effectively for meningitis caused by gram-negative bacteria (Landesman *et al.*, 1981; Cherubin *et al.*, 1982; Mullaney and John, 1983).

Moxalactam has a unique structure (designated oxa-beta-lactam), which is created by the substitution of an oxygen for the sulfur atom in the cephem nucleus. Moxalactam has the broad antimicrobial activity characteristic of the third-generation cephalosporins (Symposium, 1982). Clinically significant (and sometimes fatal) bleeding has been described after administration of moxalactam, and it appears that moxalactam can interfere with hemostasis as a result of either hypoprothrombinemia, platelet dysfunction, or, more rarely, immunologically mediated thrombocytopenia (Pakter *et al.*, 1982; Weitekamp and Aber, 1983). Because of this toxicity, moxalactam is not recommended for clinical use.

Ceftizoxime has a spectrum of activity *in vitro* very similar to that of cefotaxime. The half-life is somewhat longer, 1.8 hours, and the drug can thus be administered every 8 to 12 hours for serious infections. Ceftizoxime is not metabolized and is excreted in the urine (Neu *et al.*, 1982).

Ceftriaxone has activity *in vitro* very similar to that of ceftizoxime and cefotaxime. A half-life of about 8 hours is the outstanding feature. Administration of the drug once or twice daily has been effective for patients with meningitis (Del Rio *et al.*, 1983; Brogden and Ward, 1988), while dosage once a day has been effective for other infections (Baumgartner and Glauser, 1983). About half of the drug can be recovered from the urine; the remainder appears to be eliminated by biliary secretion. A single dose of ceftriaxone (250 mg) is effective in the treatment of gonorrhea, including disease caused by penicillinase-producing microorganisms (Rajan *et al.*, 1982; Handsfield and Murphy, 1983).

Third-Generation Cephalosporins with Good Activity against Pseudomonas. Cefoperazone is less active than cefotaxime against gram-positive microorganisms and less active than cefotaxime or moxalactam against many species of gram-negative bacteria. However, it is more active than both of these agents against *Pseud. aeruginosa*. Unfortunately, resistant strains may emerge on treatment. Activity against *B. fragilis* is similar to that of cefotaxime. Cefoperazone is slightly less stable with beta-lactamases than are the cefotaxime-like or 7-methoxycephem drugs (Klein and Neu, 1983). Only 25% of a dose of cefoperazone can be recovered from the urine, and most of the drug is eliminated by biliary excretion. The half-life is about 2 hours. Concentrations of cefoperazone in bile are higher than those achieved with other cephalosporins; concentrations in blood are two to three times higher than those found with cefotaxime. The dose of cefoperazone does not have to be altered in patients with renal insufficiency, but hepatic dysfunction or biliary obstruction affects clearance. Cefoperazone can cause bleeding due to hypoprothrombinemia; this can be reversed by administration of vitamin K. A disulfiram-like reaction has been reported in patients who drink alcohol while taking cefoperazone.

Ceftazidime is one quarter to one half as active by weight against gram-positive microorganisms as is cefotaxime. Its activity against the Enterobacteriaceae is very similar, but its major distinguishing feature is good activity against *Pseudomonas*. Ceftazidime has poor activity against *B. fragilis* (Hamilton-Miller and Brumfitt, 1981). Its half-life in plasma is about 1.5 hours, and the drug is not metabolized. Ceftazidime was found to be more active *in vitro* against *Pseudomonas* than was cefoperazone or piperacillin (Neu, 1981; Neu and Labthavikul, 1982).

Adverse Reactions. Hypersensitivity reactions to the cephalosporins are the most common side effects (*see* Petz, 1978), and there is no evidence that any single cephalosporin is more or less likely to cause such sensitization. The reactions appear to be identical to those caused by the penicillins, and this may be related to the shared beta-lactam structure of both groups of antibiotics (Bennett *et al.*, 1983). Immediate reactions such as anaphylaxis, bronchospasm, and urticaria are observed. More commonly, maculopapular rash develops, usually after several days of therapy; this may or may not be accompanied by fever and eosinophilia.

Because of the similarity in structure of the penicillins and cephalosporins, patients who are allergic to one class of agents may manifest cross-reactivity when a member of the other class is administered. Immunological studies have demonstrated cross-reactivity in as many as 20% of patients who are allergic to penicillin (*see* Levine, 1973), but clinical studies indicate a much lower frequency (about 1%) of such reactions (Saxon *et al.*, 1987). There are no skin tests that can reliably predict whether a patient will manifest an allergic reaction to the cephalosporins.

Patients with a history of a mild or a temporally distant reaction to penicillin appear to be at low risk of rash or other allergic reaction following the administration of a cephalosporin. However, patients who have had a recent severe, immediate reaction to a penicillin should be given a cephalosporin with great caution, if at all. A positive Coombs' reaction appears frequently in patients who receive large doses of a cephalosporin. Hemolysis is not usually associated with this phenomenon, although it has been reported. Cephalosporins have produced rare instances of bone-marrow depression, characterized by granulocytopenia (Kammer, 1984).

The cephalosporins have been implicated as potentially nephrotoxic agents, although they are not nearly as toxic to the kidney as are the aminoglycosides or the polymyxins (Barza, 1978). Renal tubular necrosis has followed the administration of cephaloridine in doses greater than 4 g per day; this agent is no longer available in the United States. Other cephalosporins are much less toxic, and in recommended doses, rarely produce significant renal toxicity when used by themselves. High doses of cephalothin have produced acute tubular necrosis in certain instances, and usual doses (8 to 12 g per day) have caused nephrotoxicity in patients with preexisting renal disease (Pasternack and Stephens, 1975). There is good evidence that the concurrent administration of cephalothin and gentamicin or tobramycin causes nephrotoxicity synergistically (Wade *et al.*, 1978). This is especially marked in patients over 60 years of age. Diarrhea can result from the administration of cephalosporins and may be more frequent with cefoperazone, perhaps because of its greater biliary excretion. Intolerance of alcohol (a disulfiram-like reaction) has been noted with cefamandole, cefotetan, moxalactam, and cefoperazone. Serious bleeding related either to hypoprothrombinemia, thrombocytopenia, and/or platelet dysfunction has been reported with several beta-lactam antibiotics (Bank and Kammer, 1983; Sattler *et al.*, 1986). This appears to be a particular problem with certain patients (elderly, poorly nourished, or those with renal insufficiency) who are receiving moxalactam.

Therapeutic Uses. The cephalosporins are widely used antibiotics. Unfortunately they are often overused for conditions in which much less expensive antibiotics would provide adequate therapy. Clinical studies have shown them to be effective as both therapeutic and prophylactic agents (Donowitz and Mandell, 1988). Cephalosporins, either with or without aminoglycosides, have been considered to be the drugs of choice for serious infections caused by *Klebsiella, Enterobacter, Proteus, Providencia, Serratia,* and *Haemophilus* species. Ceftriaxone is now the therapy of choice for all forms of gonorrhea, unless strains in a given geographical area are known to be sensitive to penicillin (*see* page 1073). Prophylaxis during and after surgery is another area where cephalosporins have found wide use; there are numerous instances where first-generation cephalosporins have been shown to be safe and effective for this purpose. Some of the third-generation cephalosporins are currently the drugs of choice for meningitis caused by gram-negative enteric bacteria because of their antimicrobial activity, good penetration into CSF, and record of clinical successes. Therapy with some second- or third-generation cephalosporins is equivalent or superior to treatment with a combination of ampicillin and chloramphenicol for meningitis caused by *H. influenzae* (Jacobs *et al.*, 1985; Barson *et al.*, 1986).

Cephalosporins are still useful as alternatives to penicillins for a variety of infections in patients who cannot tolerate penicillins. These include streptococcal and staphylococcal infections.

Infections with anaerobes are often treated with combinations of antibiotics, since aerobic microorganisms are usually also present. Cefoxitin and cefotetan have good activity against anaerobes and are useful alternatives to combination therapy under certain conditions. The spectrum of activity of cefuroxime, cefotaxime, ceftriaxone, and ceftizoxime appears to be excellent for the treatment of pneumonias acquired in the community, *i.e.*, those caused by pneumococci, *H. influenzae* (including strains that produce beta-lactamase), or staphylococci.

Cefoperazone and ceftriaxone have been used effectively for the treatment of typhoid fever (Pape *et al.*, 1986; Farid *et al.*, 1987). If clinical experience supports the results of these initial reports, these agents may become drugs of first choice for this disease.

Nosocomial infections are frequently caused by microorganisms that are resistant to many of the commonly used agents, such as the first-generation cephalosporins, ampicillin, and some of the aminoglycosides. Third-generation cephalosporins and imipenem have been useful additions to therapy in these situations. Patients who are severely neutropenic have been treated successfully with either a third-generation cephalosporin plus an aminoglycoside or, for selected patients, a third-generation cephalosporin that is active against *Pseudomonas* (*e.g.*, ceftazidime) without an aminoglycoside (Pizzo *et al.*, 1986). However, resistant strains frequently emerge during treatment of severe infections with *Pseudomonas* when single agents are used.

OTHER BETA-LACTAM ANTIBIOTICS

Agents with a beta-lactam structure that are neither penicillins nor cephalosporins have been developed recently.

IMIPENEM

Imipenem is the most active agent available (*in vitro*) against a wide variety of bacteria. It is marketed in combination with cilastatin, a drug that inhibits the degradation of imipenem by a renal tubular dipeptidase.

Source and Chemistry. Imipenem is derived from a compound produced by *Streptomyces cattleya*. The compound, thienamycin, is unstable, but the N-formimidoyl derivative, imipenem, is stable. The structural formula of imipenem is as follows:

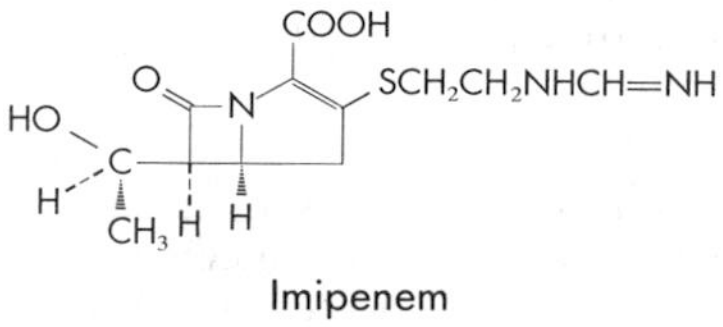

Imipenem

Antimicrobial Activity. Imipenem, like other beta-lactam antibiotics, binds to penicillin-binding proteins, disrupts bacterial cell wall synthesis, and causes death of susceptible microorganisms. It is very resistant to hydrolysis by most beta-lactamases.

The activity of imipenem is excellent *in vitro* for a wide variety of aerobic and anaerobic microorganisms. Streptococci, enterococci, staphylococci (including penicillinase-producing strains), and *Listeria* are all susceptible. Although some strains of methicillin-resistant staphylococci are susceptible, many strains are not. Activity against the Enterobacteriaceae is excellent. Most strains of *Pseudomonas* and *Acinetobacter* are inhibited. *Pseud. maltophilia* is resistant. Anaerobes, including *B. fragilis*, are highly susceptible. *Clostridium difficile*, the cause of pseudomembranous colitis, is inhibited by concentrations of 6 to 8 μg/ml (Cullman *et al.*, 1982; Blumenthal *et al.*, 1983; Barza, 1985).

Pharmacokinetics and Adverse Reactions. Imipenem is not absorbed orally. The drug is rapidly hydrolyzed by a dipeptidase found in the brush border of the proximal renal tubule (Kropp *et al.*, 1982). Because concentrations of active drug in urine were low, an inhibitor of the dehydropeptidase was synthesized. This compound is called cilastatin. A preparation has been developed that contains equal amounts of imipenem and cilastatin (PRIMAXIN).

After the intravenous administration of 500 mg of imipenem (as PRIMAXIN), peak concentrations in plasma average 33 μg/ml. Both imipenem and cilastatin have a half-life of about 1 hour. When administered concurrently with cilastatin, approximately 70% of administered imipenem is recovered in the urine as the active drug.

Nausea and vomiting are the most common adverse reactions (1 to 2%). Seizures have also been noted, especially when high doses are given to patients with CNS lesions and to those with renal insufficiency. Patients who are allergic to other beta-lactam antibiotics may have hypersensitivity reactions when given imipenem.

Preparation, Dosage, and Clinical Use. *Imipenem–cilastatin* is given intravenously. The preparation (PRIMAXIN) contains equivalent amounts of the two drugs. The usual dose for severe infections is 500 mg of imipenem every 6 hours; this can be doubled, if necessary, to treat infections caused by less susceptible microorganisms. Dosage should be modified for patients with renal insufficiency.

Imipenem–cilastatin is effective for a wide variety of infections (Eron *et al.*, 1983), including urinary tract and lower respiratory infections; intra-abdominal and gynecological infections; and skin, soft-tissue, bone, and joint infections. The drug combination appears to be especially useful for the treatment of mixed infections caused by nosocomial organisms.

AZTREONAM

Aztreonam is a monocyclic beta-lactam compound (a monobactam) isolated from *Chromobacterium violaceum* (Sykes *et al.*, 1981). Its structural formula is as follows:

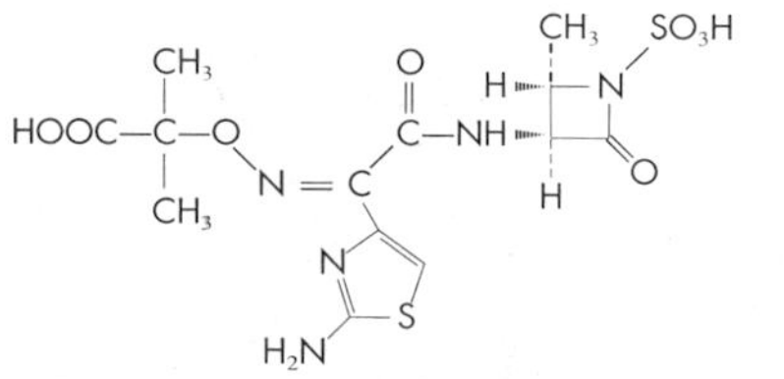

Aztreonam

Aztreonam interacts with penicillin-binding proteins of susceptible microorganisms and induces the formation of long filamentous bacterial structures. The compound is resistant to the beta-lactamases that are elaborated by most gram-negative bacteria.

The antimicrobial activity of aztreonam differs from those of other beta-lactam antibiotics and more closely resembles that of an aminoglycoside. Gram-positive bacteria and anaerobic organisms are resistant. However, activity against Enterobacteriaceae is excellent, as is that against *Pseud. aeruginosa*. It is also highly active *in vitro* against *H. influenzae* and gonococci.

Aztreonam is administered either intramuscularly or intravenously. Peak concentrations of aztreonam in plasma average nearly 50 μg/ml after a 1-g intramuscular dose. The half-time for elimination is 1.7 hours, and most of the drug is recovered unaltered in the urine. The half-life is prolonged to about 6 hours in anephric patients.

Aztreonam is generally well tolerated. Interestingly, patients who are allergic to penicillins or cephalosporins appear not to react to aztreonam (Saxon *et al.*, 1984).

The usual dose of *aztreonam* (AZACTAM) for severe infections is 2 g every 6 to 8 hours. This should be reduced for patients with renal insufficiency. Although aztreonam has been used successfully for the therapy of a variety of infections, its place in the treatment of infectious diseases remains to be defined. In selected instances, it can be used in place of an aminoglycoside.

BETA-LACTAMASE INHIBITORS

Certain molecules can bind to beta-lactamases and inactivate them, thus preventing the destruction of beta-lactam antibiotics that are substrates for these enzymes.

Clavulanic acid is produced by *Streptomyces clavuligerus;* its structural formula is as follows:

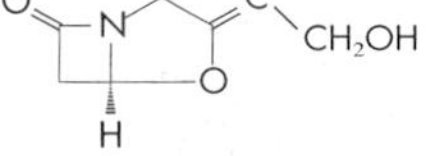

Clavulanic Acid

It has poor intrinsic antimicrobial activity but is a "suicide" inhibitor of beta-lactamases produced by a wide range of gram-positive and gram-negative microorganisms (Neu and Fu, 1978). Clavulanic acid is well absorbed by mouth and can also be given parenterally. It has been combined with amoxicillin as an oral preparation (AUGMENTIN) and with ticarcillin as a parenteral preparation (TIMENTIN).

AUGMENTIN is currently available in the United States as tablets and as powders for oral suspension. Amoxicillin plus clavulanate is effective *in vitro* and *in vivo* for beta-lactamase-producing strains of staphylococci, *H. influenzae,* gonococci, and *E. coli* (Ball *et al.*, 1980; Yogev *et al.*, 1981).

The addition of clavulanate to ticarcillin extends its spectrum such that it resembles imipenem and includes aerobic gram-negative bacilli, *Staph. aureus,* and *Bacteroides* species. There is no increased activity against *Pseudomonas* species (Bansal *et al.*, 1985). The commercial preparation (TIMENTIN) contains 3 g of ticarcillin (as the disodium salt) and 100 mg of clavulanate (as the potassium salt) per vial. The usual intravenous dosage for adults with serious infections is 3 g of ticarcillin every 4 to 6 hours. This dosage should be adjusted for patients with renal insufficiency. The combination is especially useful for mixed nosocomial infections and is often used with an aminoglycoside.

Sulbactam is another beta-lactamase inhibitor similar in structure to clavulanic acid. It may be given orally or parenterally along with a beta-lactam antibiotic. It is available for intravenous or intramuscular use combined with ampicillin (UNASYN). The usual dose for adults is 1 to 2 g of ampicillin plus 0.5 to 1 g of sulbactam every 6 hours. Dosage must be adjusted for patients with impaired renal function. The combination has good activity against gram-positive cocci, including beta-lactamase-producing strains of *Staph. aureus,* gram-negative aerobes (but not *Pseudomonas*), and anaerobes; it has also been used effectively for the treatment of mixed intra-abdominal and pelvic infections (Reinhardt *et al.*, 1986).

American Heart Association Committee on Rheumatic Fever and Infectious Endocarditis. Prevention of bacterial endocarditis. *Circulation,* **1984**, *70,* 1123a.

Bach, V. T.; Roy, I.; and Thadepalli, H. Susceptibility of anaerobic bacteria to cefoxitin and related compounds. *Antimicrob. Agents Chemother.,* **1977**, *11,* 912–913.

Ball, A. P.; Geddes, A. M.; Davey, P. G.; Farrell, I. D.; and Brookes, G. R. Clavulanic acid and amoxycillin: a clinical, bacteriological, and pharmacological study. *Lancet,* **1980**, *1,* 620–623.

Bansal, M. B.; Chuah, S. K.; and Thadepalli, H. *In vitro* activity and *in vivo* evaluation of ticarcillin plus clavulanic acid against aerobic and anaerobic bacteria. *Am. J. Med.,* **1985**, *79,* Suppl. 5B, 33–38.

Barriere, S. L., and Mills, J. Ceforanide: antibacterial activity, pharmacology, and clinical efficacy. *Pharmacotherapy,* **1982**, *2,* 322–327.

Barson, W. J.; Miller, M. A.; Brady, M. T.; and Powell, D. A. Prospective comparative trial of ceftriaxone *vs* conventional therapy for treatment of bacterial meningitis in children. *Pediatr. Infect. Dis. J.,* **1986**, *4,* 362–368.

Barza, M. The nephrotoxicity of cephalosporins: an overview. *J. Infect. Dis.,* **1978**, *137,* 560–573.

———. Imipenem: first of a new class of beta-lactam antibiotics. *Ann. Intern. Med.*, **1985**, *103*, 552–560.

Baumgartner, J., and Glauser, M. P. Single daily dose treatment of severe refractory infections with ceftriaxone. *Arch. Intern. Med.*, **1983**, *143*, 1868–1881.

Bennett, S.; Wise, R.; Weston, D.; and Dent, J. Pharmacokinetics and tissue penetration of ticarcillin combined with clavulanic acid. *Antimicrob. Agents Chemother.*, **1983**, *23*, 831–834.

Bisno, A. L.; Dismukes, W. E.; Durack, D. T.; Kaplan, E. L.; Karchmer, A. W.; Kaye, D.; Sande, M. A.; Sanford, J. P.; and Wilson, W. R. Treatment of infective endocarditis due to *viridans* streptococci. *Circulation*, **1981**, *63*, 730A–733A.

Blumenthal, R. M.; Raeder, R.; Takemotoa, C. D.; and Freimer, E. H. Occurrence and expression of imipemide (N-formimidoyl thienamycin) resistance in clinical isolates of coagulase-negative staphylococci. *Antimicrob. Agents Chemother.*, **1983**, *24*, 61–69.

Brogden, R. N., and Ward, A. Ceftriaxone: a reappraisal of its antibacterial activity and pharmacokinetic properties, and an update on its therapeutic use with particular reference to once-daily administration. *Drugs*, **1988**, *35*, 604–645.

Bryant, R. E. Effect of the suppurative environment on antibiotic activity. In, *New Dimensions in Antimicrobial Therapy*. (Root, R. K., and Sande, M. A., eds.) Churchill Livingstone, Inc., New York, **1984**, pp. 313–337.

Chain, E. B. The development of bacterial chemotherapy. *Antibiot. Chemother.*, **1954**, *4*, 215–241.

Chambers, H. F.; Hackbarth, C. J.; Drake, T. A.; Rusnak, M. G.; and Sande, M. A. Endocarditis due to methicillin-resistant *Staphylococcus aureus* in rabbits: expression of resistance to beta-lactam antibiotics *in vivo* and *in vitro*. *J. Infect. Dis.*, **1984**, *149*, 894–903.

Chow, A. W., and Bednorz, D. Comparative *in vitro* activity of newer cephalosporins against anaerobic bacteria. *Antimicrob. Agents Chemother.*, **1978**, *14*, 668–671.

Cullman, W.; Opferkuch, W.; Stieglitz, M.; and Werkmeister, U. A comparison of the antibacterial activities of N-formimidoyl thienamycin (MK0787) with those of other recently developed β-lactam derivatives. *Antimicrob. Agents Chemother.*, **1982**, *22*, 302–307.

Dacey, R. G., and Sande, M. A. Effect of probenecid on cerebrospinal fluid concentrations of penicillin and cephalosporin derivatives. *Antimicrob. Agents Chemother.*, **1974**, *6*, 437–441.

Del Rio, M. A.; Chrane, D.; Shelton, S.; McCracken, G. H.; and Nelson, J. D. Ceftriaxone versus ampicillin and chloramphenicol for treatment of bacterial meningitis in children. *Lancet*, **1983**, *1*, 1241–1244.

DeSante, K. A.; Israel, K. S.; Brier, G. L.; Wolny, J. D.; and Hatcher, B. L. Effect of probenecid on the pharmacokinetics of moxalactam. *Antimicrob. Agents Chemother.*, **1982**, *21*, 58–61.

Ditlove, J.; Weidmann, P.; Bernstein, M.; and Massry, S. G. Methicillin nephritis. *Medicine (Baltimore)*, **1977**, *56*, 483–491.

Eliopoulos, G. M., and Moellering, R. C. Azlocillin, mezlocillin, and piperacillin: new broad-spectrum penicillins. *Ann. Intern. Med.*, **1982**, *97*, 755–760.

Eron, L. J.; Hixon, D. L.; Choong, H. P.; Goldenberg, R. I.; and Poretz, D. M. Imipenem versus moxalactam in the treatment of serious infections. *Antimicrob. Agents Chemother.*, **1983**, *24*, 841–846.

Farid, Z.; Girgis, N.; and El Ella, A. A. Successful treatment of typhoid fever in children with parenteral ceftriaxone. *Scand. J. Infect. Dis.*, **1987**, *19*, 467–468.

Fass, R. J.; Copelan, E. A.; Brandt, J. T.; Moeschberger, M. L.; and Ashton, J. J. Platelet-mediated bleeding caused by broad-spectrum penicillins. *J. Infect. Dis.*, **1987**, *155*, 1242–1248.

Fong, I. W.; Engelking, E. R.; and Kirby, W. M. M. Relative inactivation by *Staphylococcus aureus* of eight cephalosporin antibiotics. *Antimicrob. Agents Chemother.*, **1976a**, *9*, 939–944.

Fong, I. W.; Ralph, E. D.; Engelking, E. R.; and Kirby, W. M. M. Clinical pharmacology of cefamandole as compared with cephalothin. *Antimicrob. Agents Chemother.*, **1976b**, *9*, 65–69.

Fu, K. P., and Neu, H. C. Azlocillin and mezlocillin—new ureido penicillins. *Antimicrob. Agents Chemother.*, **1978**, *13*, 930–938.

Gordon, R. C.; Regamey, C.; and Kirby, W. M. M. Comparative clinical pharmacology of amoxicillin and ampicillin administered orally. *Antimicrob. Agents Chemother.*, **1972**, *1*, 504–507.

Greaves, W. L.; Kraus, S. J.; McCormack, W. M.; Biddle, J. W.; Zaidi, A.; Fiumara, N. J.; and Guinan, M. E. Cefoxitin vs penicillin in the treatment of uncomplicated gonorrhea. *Sex. Transm. Dis.*, **1983**, *10*, 53–55.

Gremillion, D. H.; Winn, R. E.; and Vandenbout, E. Clinical trial of cefoxicid for treatment of skin infections. *Antimicrob. Agents Chemother.*, **1983**, *23*, 944–946.

Hamilton-Miller, J. M. T., and Brumfitt, W. Activity of ceftazidime (GR20263) against nosocomially important pathogens. *Antimicrob. Agents Chemother.*, **1981**, *19*, 1067–1069.

Handsfield, H. H., and Murphy, V. L. Comparative study of ceftriaxone and spectinomycin for treatment of uncomplicated gonorrhoea in men. *Lancet*, **1983**, *2*, 67–70.

Hartstein, A. I.; Patrick, K. E.; Jones, S. R.; Miller, M. J.; and Bryant, R. E. Comparison of pharmacological and antimicrobial properties of cefadroxil and cephalexin. *Antimicrob. Agents Chemother.*, **1977**, *12*, 93–97.

Huber, F. M.; Chauvette, R. R.; and Jackson, B. G. Preparative methods for 7-aminocephalosporanic acid and 6-aminopenicillanic acid. In, *Cephalosporins and Penicillins*. (Flynn, E. H., ed.) Academic Press, Inc., New York, **1972**, p. 27.

Idsøe, O.; Guthe, T.; Willcox, R. R.; and DeWeck, A. L. Nature and extent of penicillin side-reactions, with particular reference to fatalities from anaphylactic shock. *Bull. WHO*, **1968**, *38*, 159–188.

Jacobs, M. R.; Koornhof, H. J.; Robins-Browne, R. M.; Stevenson, C. M.; Vermaak, Z. A.; Freiman, I.; Miller, G. B.; Witcomb, M. A.; Isaacson, M.; Ward, J. I.; and Austrian, R. Emergence of multiply resistant pneumococci. *N. Engl. J. Med.*, **1978**, *299*, 735–740.

Jacobs, R. F.; Wells, T. G.; Steele, R. W.; and Yamauchi, T. A prospective randomized comparison of cefotaxime *vs* ampicillin and chloramphenicol for bacterial meningitis in children. *J. Pediatr.*, **1985**, *107*, 129–133.

Jaffe, A.; Chabbert, Y. A.; and Semonin, O. Role of porin proteins OmpF and OmpC in the permeation of beta-lactams. *Antimicrob. Agents Chemother.*, **1982**, *22*, 942–948.

Johansson, O., and others. Cefuroxime versus ampicillin and chloramphenicol for the treatment of bacterial meningitis. *Lancet*, **1982**, *1*, 295–298.

Kancir, L. M.; Tuazon, C. U.; Cardella, T. A.; and Sheagren, J. H. Adverse reactions to methicillin and nafcillin during treatment of serious *Staphylococcus aureus* infections. *Arch. Intern. Med.*, **1978**, *138*, 909–911.

Kaplan, J. M., and McCracken, G. H., Jr. Clinical pharmacology of benzathine penicillin G in neonates with regard to its recommended use in congenital syphilis. *J. Pediatr.*, **1973**, *82*, 1069–1072.

Kelley, J. A.; Moews, P. C.; Know, J. R.; Frere, J.; and Ghuysen, J. Penicillin target enzyme and the antibiotic binding site. *Science*, **1982**, *218*, 479–481.

Kirkwood, C. F.; Smith, L. L.; Rustagi, P. K.; and Schentag, J. J. Neutropenia associated with β-lactam antibiotics. *Clin. Pharm.*, **1983**, *2*, 569–578.

Klaus, M. V., and Fellner, M. J. Penicilloyl-specific serum antibodies in man. Analysis in 592 individuals from the newborn to old age. *J. Gerontol.*, **1973**, *28*, 312–316.

Klein, J. O., and Neu, H. C. Empiric therapy for bacterial infections: evaluation of cefoperazone. *Rev. Infect. Dis.*, **1983**, *5*, S1–S209.

Kobayashi, Y.; Takahashi, T.; and Nakae, T. Diffusion of beta-lactam antibiotics through liposome membranes containing purified porins. *Antimicrob. Agents Chemother.*, **1982**, *22*, 775–780.

Kropp, H.; Sundelof, J. G.; Hajdu, R.; and Kahan, F. M. Metabolism of thienamycin and related carbapenem antibiotics by the renal dipeptidase, dehydropeptidase-I. *Antimicrob. Agents Chemother.*, **1982**, *22*, 62–70.

Landesman, S. H.; Corrado, M. S.; Shah, P. M.; Armengaud, M.; Barza, M.; and Cherubin, M. D. Past and current roles for cephalosporin antibiotics in treatment of meningitis. *Am. J. Med.*, **1981**, *71*, 693–703.

Levine, B. B. Skin rashes with penicillin therapy: current management. *N. Engl. J. Med.*, **1972**, *286*, 42–43.

———. Antigenicity and cross reactivity of penicillins and cephalosporins. *J. Infect. Dis.*, **1973**, *128*, S364–S366.

Levine, B. B.; Redmond, A. P.; Fellner, M. J.; Voss, H. E.; and Levytska, V. Penicillin allergy and the heterogeneous immune responses of man. *J. Clin. Invest.*, **1966**, *45*, 1895–1906.

Levison, M. E.; Mangura, C. T.; Lorber, B.; Abrutyn, E.; Pesanti, E. L.; Levy, R. S.; MacGregor, R. R.; and Schwartz, A. R. Clindamycin compared with penicillin for the treatment of anaerobic lung abscess. *Ann. Intern. Med.*, **1983**, *98*, 466–471.

McCloskey, R. V.; LeFrock, J. L.; Smith, B. R.; and Aronoff, G. R. Microbiology, pharmacology and clinical use of mezlocillin sodium. *Pharmacotherapy*, **1982**, *2*, 300–310.

Maki, D. G.; Karzynski, T. A.; and Agger, W. A. Carbenicillin for treatment of *Bacteroides fragilis* infections: why not penicillin? *J. Infect. Dis.*, **1978**, *138*, 859–864.

Malouin, F., and Bryan, L. E. Modification of penicillin-binding proteins as mechanisms of β-lactam resistance. *Antimicrob. Agents Chemother.*, **1986**, *30*, 1–5.

Medical Letter. Prevention of bacterial endocarditis. **1986**, *28*, 22.

———. Penicillin allergy. **1988**, *30*, 79–80.

Meyers, B. R., and Hirschman, S. Z. Antibacterial activity of cefamandole *in vitro*. *J. Infect. Dis.*, **1978**, *137*, 525–531.

Mullaney, D. T., and John, J. F. Cefotaxime therapy. *Arch. Intern. Med.*, **1983**, *143*, 1705–1708.

Neiss, E. Cephradine—summary of preclinical studies and clinical pharmacology. *J. Ir. Med. Assoc.*, **1973**, *44*, S1–S12.

Neu, H. C. Mecillinam, a novel penicillanic acid and derivative with unusual activity against gram-negative bacteria. *Antimicrob. Agents Chemother.*, **1976**, *9*, 793–799.

———. Comparison of the pharmacokinetics of cefamandole and other cephalosporin compounds. *J. Infect. Dis.*, **1978**, *137*, S80–S87.

———. Amoxicillin. *Ann. Intern. Med.*, **1979**, *90*, 356–360.

———. *In-vitro* activity of ceftazidime, a beta-lactamase stable cephalosporin. *J. Antimicrob. Chemother.*, **1981**, *8*, Suppl. B, 131–134.

———. Antibacterial activity of desacetylcefotaxime alone and in combination with cefotaxime. *Rev. Infect. Dis.*, **1982**, *4*, Suppl. 3, S374–S378.

Neu, H. C.; Aswapokee, N.; Aswapokee, P.; and Fu, K. P. HR756, a new cephalosporin active against gram-positive and gram-negative aerobic and anaerobic bacteria. *Antimicrob. Agents Chemother.*, **1979**, *15*, 273–281.

Neu, H. C., and Fu, K. P. Clavulanic acid, a novel inhibitor of β-lactamases. *Antimicrob. Agents Chemother.*, **1978**, *14*, 650–655.

Neu, H. C., and Labthavikul, P. Antibacterial activity and beta-lactamase stability of ceftazidime, an aminothiazolyl cephalosporin potentially active against *Pseudomonas aeruginosa*. *Antimicrob. Agents Chemother.*, **1982**, *21*, 11–18.

Neu, H. C.; Reeves, D. S.; and Leigh, D. A. (eds.). Azlocillin—an antipseudomonas penicillin. *J. Antimicrob. Chemother.*, **1983**, *11*, Suppl. B, 1–235.

Neu, H. C.; Turck, M.; and Phillips, I. Ceftizoxime, a broad-spectrum beta-lactamase stable cephalosporin. *J. Antimicrob. Chemother.*, **1982**, *10*, Suppl. C, 1–355.

Onorato, I. M., and Axelrod, J. L. Hepatitis from intravenous high-dose oxacillin therapy. Findings in an adult inpatient population. *Ann. Intern. Med.*, **1978**, *89*, 497–500.

Pakter, R. L.; Russel, T. R.; Mielke, H.; and West, D. Coagulopathy associated with the use of moxalactam. *J.A.M.A.*, **1982**, *248*, 1100.

Pape, J. W.; Gerdes, H.; Oriol, L.; and Johnson, W. D. Typhoid fever: successful therapy with cefoperazone. *J. Infect. Dis.*, **1986**, *153*, 272–276.

Park, J. T., and Strominger, J. L. Mode of action of penicillin. *Science*, **1957**, *125*, 99–101.

Parry, M. F., and Neu, H. C. Ticarcillin for treatment of serious infections with gram-negative bacteria. *J. Infect. Dis.*, **1976**, *134*, S476–S485.

———. A comparative study of ticarcillin plus tobramycin versus carbenicillin plus gentamicin for the treatment of serious infections due to gram-negative bacilli. *Am. J. Med.*, **1978**, *64*, 961–966.

Pasternack, D. P., and Stephens, B. G. Reversible nephrotoxicity associated with cephalothin therapy. *Arch. Intern. Med.*, **1975**, *135*, 599–602.

Petz, L. D. Immunologic cross-reactivity between penicillins and cephalosporins: a review. *J. Infect. Dis.*, **1978**, *137*, S74–S79.

Phillips, I.; Wise, R.; and Leigh, D. A. Cefotetan: a new cephamycin. *J. Antimicrob. Chemother.*, **1983**, *11*, Suppl. A, 1–303.

Pizzo, P. A., and others. A randomized trial comparing ceftazidime alone with combination antibiotic therapy in cancer patients with fever and neutropenia. *N. Engl. J. Med.*, **1986**, *315*, 552–558.

Quintiliani, R., and Nightingale, C. H. Cefazolin—diagnosis and treatment. *Ann. Intern. Med.*, **1978**, *89*, 650–656.

Rajan, V. S.; Sng, E. H.; Thirumoorthy, T.; and Goh, C. L. Ceftriaxone in the treatment of ordinary and penicillinase-producing strains of *Neisseria gonorrhoeae*. *Br. J. Vener. Dis.*, **1982**, *58*, 314–316.

Reinhardt, J. F., and others. A randomized, double-blind comparison of sulbactam/ampicillin and clindamycin for the treatment of aerobic and aerobic-anaerobic infections. *Rev. Infect. Dis.*, **1986**, *8*, Suppl. 5, S569–S592.

Renzini, G.; Ravagnan, G.; and Oliva, B. *In vitro* and *in vivo* microbiological evaluation of cephapirin, a new antibiotic. *Chemotherapy*, **1975**, *21*, 289–296.

Sattler, F. R.; Weitekamp, M. R.; and Ballard, J. O. Potential for bleeding with the new beta-lactam antibiotics. *Ann. Intern. Med.*, **1986**, *105*, 924–931.

Saxon, A.; Beall, G. N.; Rohr, A. S.; and Adelman, D. C. Immediate hypersensitivity reactions to beta-lactam antibiotics. *Ann. Intern. Med.*, **1987**, *107*, 204–215.

Saxon, A.; Hassner, A.; Swabb, E. A.; Wheller, B.; and Adkinson, N. F., Jr. Lack of cross-reactivity between aztreonam, a monobactam antibiotic, and penicillin in penicillin-allergic subjects. *J. Infect. Dis.*, **1984**, *149*, 16–22.

Scheife, R. T., and Neu, H. C. Bacampicillin hydrochloride: chemistry, pharmacology, and clinical use. *Pharmacotherapy,* **1982,** *2,* 313–320.

Shattil, J. S.; Bennett, J. S.; McDonough, M.; and Turnbull, J. Carbenicillin and penicillin G inhibit platelet functions *in vitro* by impairing the interaction of agonists with the platelet surface. *J. Clin. Invest.,* **1980,** *65,* 329–337.

Silver, M. S.; Counts, G. W.; Zeleznik, D.; and Turck, M. Comparison of *in vitro* antibacterial activity of three oral cephalosporins: cefaclor, cephalexin, and cephradine. *Antimicrob. Agents Chemother.,* **1977,** *12,* 591–596.

Smith, B. R., and LeFrock, J. L. Cefuroxime: antimicrobial activity, pharmacology, and clinical efficacy. *Ther. Drug Monit.,* **1983,** *5,* 149–160.

Solley, G. O.; Gleich, G. J.; and Van Dellen, R. G. Penicillin allergy: clinical experience with a battery of skin-test reagents. *J. Allergy Clin. Immunol.,* **1982,** *69,* 238–244.

Spratt, B. G. Distinct penicillin binding proteins involved in the division, elongation and shape of *Escherichia coli,* K 12. *Proc. Natl Acad. Sci. U.S.A.,* **1975,** *72,* 2999–3003.

———. Biochemical and genetical approaches to the mechanism of action of penicillin. *Philos. Trans. R. Soc. Lond.* [*Biol.*], **1980,** *289,* 273–283.

Sullivan, T. J.; Yecies, L. D.; Shatz, G. S.; Parker, C. W.; and Wedner, H. J. Desensitization of patients allergic to penicillin using orally administered β-lactam antibiotics. *J. Allergy Clin. Immunol.,* **1982,** *69,* 275–282.

Sutter, V. L., and Finegold, S. M. Susceptibility of anaerobic bacteria to carbenicillin, cefoxitin, and related drugs. *J. Infect. Dis.,* **1975,** *131,* 417–422.

Sykes, R. B., and Bush, K. Interaction of new cephalosporins with beta-lactamases and beta lactamase-producing gram-negative bacilli. *Rev. Infect. Dis.,* **1983,** *5,* S356–S366.

Sykes, R. B., and Matthew, M. β-lactamases of gram-negative bacteria and their role in resistance to β-lactam antibiotics. *J. Antimicrob. Chemother.,* **1976,** *2,* 115–157.

Sykes, R. B., and others. Monocyclic β-lactam antibiotics produced by bacteria. *Nature,* **1981,** *291,* 489–491.

Tomasz, A. Penicillin-binding proteins and the antibacterial effectiveness of β-lactam antibiotics. *Rev. Infect. Dis.,* **1986,** *8,* Suppl. 3, S270-S278.

Tomasz, A., and Holtje, J. V. Murein hydrolases and the lytic and killing action of penicillin. In, *Microbiology—1977.* (Schlessinger, D., ed.) American Society for Microbiology, Washington, D. C., **1977,** pp. 209–215.

Wade, J. C.; Smith, C. R.; Petty, B. G.; Lipsky, J. J.; Conrad, G.; Ellner, J.; and Leitman, P. S. Cephalothin plus an aminoglycoside is more nephrotoxic than methicillin plus an aminoglycoside. *Lancet,* **1978,** *2,* 604–606.

Waxman, D. J.; Yocum, R. R.; and Strominger, J. L. Penicillins and cephalosporins are active site-directed acylating agents: evidence in support of the substrate analogue hypothesis. *Philos. Trans. R. Soc. Lond.* [*Biol.*], **1980,** *289,* 257–271.

Weitekamp, M. R., and Aber, R. C. Prolonged bleeding times and bleeding diathesis associated with moxalactam administration. *J.A.M.A.,* **1983,** *249,* 69–71.

Wexler, J. M., and Finegold, S. M. *In vitro* activity of cefotetan compared with that of other antimicrobial agents against anaerobic bacteria. *Antimicrob. Agents Chemother.,* **1988,** *32,* 601–604.

Wilson, W. R.; Wilkowske, C. J.; Wright, A. J.; Sande, M. A.; and Geraci, J. E. Treatment of streptomycin-susceptible and streptomycin-resistant enterococcal endocarditis. *Ann. Intern. Med.,* **1984,** *100,* 816–823.

Yocum, R. R.; Waxman, D. W.; and Strominger, J. L. The mechanism of action of penicillin. *J. Biol. Chem.,* **1980,** *255,* 3977–3986.

Yogev, R.; Melick, C.; and Kabat, W. J. *In vitro* and *in vivo* synergism between amoxicillin and clavulanic acid against ampicillin-resistant *Haemophilus influenzae* type b. *Antimicrob. Agents Chemother.,* **1981,** *19,* 993–996.

Monographs and Reviews

Abraham, E. P. The action of antibiotics on bacteria. In, *Antibiotics,* Vol. II. (Florey, H. W., *et al.,* authors.) Oxford University Press, New York, **1949,** pp. 1438–1496.

———. The cephalosporins. *Pharmacol. Rev.,* **1962,** *14,* 473–500.

Bank, N. U., and Kammer, R. B. Hematologic complications associated with beta-lactam antibiotics. *Rev. Infect. Dis.,* **1983,** *5,* Suppl. 2, S380–S398.

Bergen, T. Review of the pharmacokinetics and dose dependency of azlocillin in normal subjects and patients with renal insufficiency. *J. Antimicrob. Chemother.,* **1983,** *11,* Suppl. B, 101–114.

Cherubin, C. E.; Neu, H. C.; and Turck, M. Current status of cefotaxime sodium: a new cephalosporin. *Rev. Infect. Dis.,* **1982,** *4,* S281–S488.

Donowitz, G. R., and Mandell, G. L. Beta-lactam antibiotics. *N. Engl. J. Med.,* **1988,** *318,* 419–426 and 490–500.

———. Cephalosporins. In, *Principles and Practice of Infectious Diseases,* 3rd ed. (Mandell, G. L.; Douglas, R. G., Jr.; and Bennett, J. E.; eds.) Churchill Livingstone, Inc., New York, **1990,** pp. 246–257.

Durack, D. T. Prophylaxis in infective endocarditis. In, *Principles and Practice of Infectious Diseases,* 3rd ed. (Mandell, G. L.; Douglas, R. G., Jr.; and Bennett, J. E.; eds.) Churchill Livingstone, Inc., New York, **1990,** pp. 716–721.

Fleming, A. History and development of penicillin. In, *Penicillin: Its Practical Application.* (Fleming, A., ed.) The Blakiston Co., Philadelphia, **1946,** pp. 1–33.

Florey, H. W. The use of micro-organisms for therapeutic purposes. *Yale J. Biol. Med.,* **1946,** *19,* 101–118.

———. Historical introduction. In, *Antibiotics,* Vol. I. (Florey, H. W., *et al.,* authors.) Oxford University Press, New York, **1949,** pp. 1–73.

Flynn, E. H. (ed.). *Cephalosporins and Penicillins: Chemistry and Biology.* Academic Press, Inc., New York, **1972.**

Handsfield, H. Neisseria gonorrhoeae. In, *Principles and Practice of Infectious Diseases,* 3rd ed. (Mandell, G. L.; Douglas, R. G., Jr.; and Bennett, J. E.; eds.) Churchill Livingstone, Inc., New York, **1990,** pp. 491–509.

Herrell, W. E. *Penicillin and Other Antibiotic Agents.* W. B. Saunders Co., Philadelphia, **1945.**

Kammer, R. B. Host effects of beta-lactam antibiotics. In, *Contemporary Issues in Infectious Diseases.* Vol. 1, *New Dimensions in Antimicrobial Therapy.* (Root, R. K., and Sande, M. A., eds.) Churchill Livingstone, Inc., New York, **1984,** pp. 101–119.

Kass, E. H., and Evans, D. A. (eds.). Future prospects and past problems in antimicrobial therapy: the role of cefoxitin. *Rev. Infect. Dis.,* **1979,** *1,* 1–244.

Nakae, T. Outer-membrane permeability of bacteria. *CRC Crit. Rev. Microbiol.,* **1986,** *13,* 1–62.

Neu, H. C. Structure-activity relations of new β-lactam compounds and *in vitro* activity against common bacteria. *Rev. Infect. Dis.,* **1983,** *5,* Suppl. 2, S319–S336.

———. Penicillins. *In, Principles and Practice of Infectious Diseases.* (Mandell, G. L.; Douglas, R. G., Jr.; and Bennett, J. E.; eds.) John Wiley & Sons, Inc., New York, **1985,** pp. 166–180.

Parker, C. W. Drug allergy. *N. Engl. J. Med.,* **1975,** *292,* 957–960.

Pratt, W. B., and Fekety, R. *The Antimicrobial Drugs.* Oxford University Press, New York, **1986,** pp. 85–112.

Symposium. (Various authors.) Moxalactam international symposium. (Moellering, R. C., and Young, L. S., eds.) *Rev. Infect. Dis.*, **1982,** *4,* S489–S726.

Tomasz, A. From penicillin-binding proteins to the lysis and death of bacteria: a 1979 view. *Rev. Infect. Dis.*, **1979,** *1,* 434–467.

Tramont, E. C. Treponema pallidum. In, *Principles and Practice of Infectious Diseases,* 3rd ed. (Mandell, G. L.; Douglas, R. G., Jr.; and Bennett, J. E.; eds.) Churchill Livingstone, Inc., New York, **1990,** pp. 1794–1808.

Weiss, M. E., and Adkinson, N. F. Beta-lactam allergy. In, *Principles and Practice of Infectious Diseases,* 3rd ed. (Mandell, G. L.; Douglas, R. G., Jr.; and Bennett, J. E.; eds.) Churchill Livingstone, Inc., New York, **1990,** pp. 264–269.

CHAPTER

47 ANTIMICROBIAL AGENTS

[*Continued*]

The Aminoglycosides

Merle A. Sande and Gerald L. Mandell

The aminoglycoside antibiotics—gentamicin, tobramycin, amikacin, netilmicin, kanamycin, streptomycin, and neomycin—are discussed in this chapter. As the group name implies, all these drugs contain amino sugars linked to an aminocyclitol ring by glycosidic bonds. They are polycations, and their polarity is in part responsible for pharmacokinetic properties shared by all members of the group. For example, none is adequately absorbed after oral administration, inadequate concentrations are found in cerebrospinal fluid, and all are excreted relatively rapidly by the normal kidney.

The aminoglycosides are used primarily to treat infections caused by aerobic gram-negative bacteria; they act to interfere with protein synthesis in susceptible microorganisms. Although most inhibitors of microbial protein synthesis are bacteriostatic, the aminoglycosides are bactericidal. Mutations affecting proteins in the bacterial ribosome, the target for these drugs, can confer marked resistance to their action. Resistance can also result from the acquisition of plasmids that contain genes that encode aminoglycoside-metabolizing enzymes. Bacteria that acquire resistance to one aminoglycoside may exhibit resistance to others.

Serious toxicity is a major limitation to the usefulness of the aminoglycosides, and the same spectrum of toxicity is shared by all members of the group. Most notable are ototoxicity, which can involve both the auditory and vestibular functions of the eighth cranial nerve, and nephrotoxicity.

History and Source. The development of streptomycin was the result of a well-planned, scientific search for antibacterial substances. Stimulated by the discovery of penicillin, Waksman and coworkers examined a number of soil actinomycetes between 1939 and 1943. In 1943, a strain of *Streptomyces griseus* was isolated that elaborated a potent antimicrobial substance. The first public announcement of the discovery of this new antibiotic—*streptomycin*—was made by Schatz, Bugie, and Waksman early in 1944, and it was soon shown to inhibit the growth of the tubercle bacillus and a number of aerobic gram-positive and gram-negative microorganisms. In less than 2 years, extensive bacteriological, chemical, and pharmacological investigations of streptomycin had been carried out, and its clinical usefulness was established (Waksman, 1949). However, streptomycin-resistant gram-negative bacilli and gram-positive cocci (enterococci) have emerged, limiting its clinical usefulness. It is now rarely used except for the treatment of certain types of streptococcal bacterial endocarditis, tularemia, plague, and as a second- or third-line agent for tuberculosis.

In 1949, Waksman and Lechevalier isolated a soil organism, *Streptomyces fradiae,* which produced a group of antibacterial substances that were named "neomycin." One component, neomycin B, is still used. However, it is only employed topically or given orally for its local effect on bowel flora because it causes severe renal toxicity and ototoxicity when administered parenterally.

Kanamycin, an antibiotic elaborated by *Streptomyces kanamyceticus,* was first produced and isolated by Umezawa and coworkers at the Japanese National Institutes of Health in 1957. It was shown to be active against a variety of microorganisms and, for several years, was an important antibiotic for the treatment of serious infections due to aerobic gram-negative bacilli. Because of toxicity and the emergence of resistant microorganisms, kanamycin has largely been replaced by the newer aminoglycosides.

Gentamicin and netilmicin are both broad-spectrum antibiotics derived from species of the actinomycete *Micromonospora*. The difference in spelling (*-micin*) as compared with that of the other aminoglycoside antibiotics (*-mycin*) reflects this difference in origin. Gentamicin was first studied and described by Weinstein and coworkers in 1963; it was isolated, purified, and characterized by Rosselot and colleagues (1964). It has a broader spectrum of activity than kanamycin and is currently widely used. Tobramycin and amikacin were introduced into clinical practice in the 1970s. Tobramycin is one of several components of an aminoglycoside complex (nebramycin) that is produced by *Streptomyces tenebrarius* (Higgins and Kastners, 1967). It is most similar in antimicrobial activity and toxicity to gentamicin. In contrast to the other aminoglycosides, amikacin and netilmicin are semisynthetic products. Amikacin, which is a derivative of kanamycin, was described by Kawaguchi and coworkers (1972); netilmicin is a derivative of sisomicin. The development of newer aminoglycoside antibiotics continues (Price, 1986).

Chemistry. The aminoglycosides all consist of two or more amino sugars joined in glycosidic linkage to a hexose nucleus, which is usually in a central position (*see* Figure 47–1). This hexose, or aminocyclitol, is either streptidine (found in streptomycin) or 2-deoxystreptamine (characteristic of all other available aminoglycosides). These compounds are thus aminoglycosidic aminocyclitols, although the simpler term *aminoglycoside* is commonly used to describe them. An additional drug, spectinomycin, is an aminocyclitol that does not contain amino sugars; it is discussed in Chapter 48.

The aminoglycoside families are distinguished by the amino sugars attached to the aminocyclitol. In the neomycin family, which includes neomycin B and paromomycin, an aminoglycoside used orally for the treatment of amebiasis (Sullam *et al.*, 1986; *see* Chapter 42), there are three amino sugars attached to the central 2-deoxystreptamine. This is in contrast to the kanamycin and gentamicin families, which have only two such amino sugars. Neomycin B has the following structural formula:

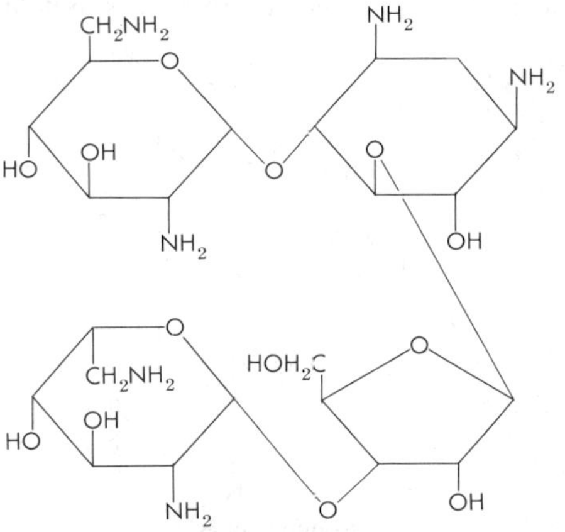

Neomycin B

In the kanamycin family, which includes kanamycins A and B, amikacin, and tobramycin, two amino sugars are linked to a centrally located 2-deoxystreptamine moiety; one of these is a

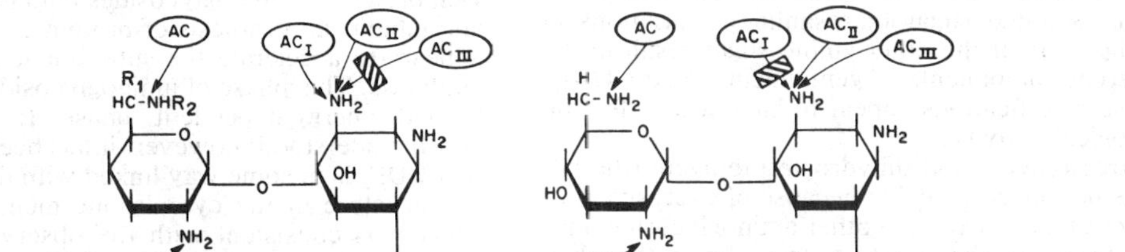

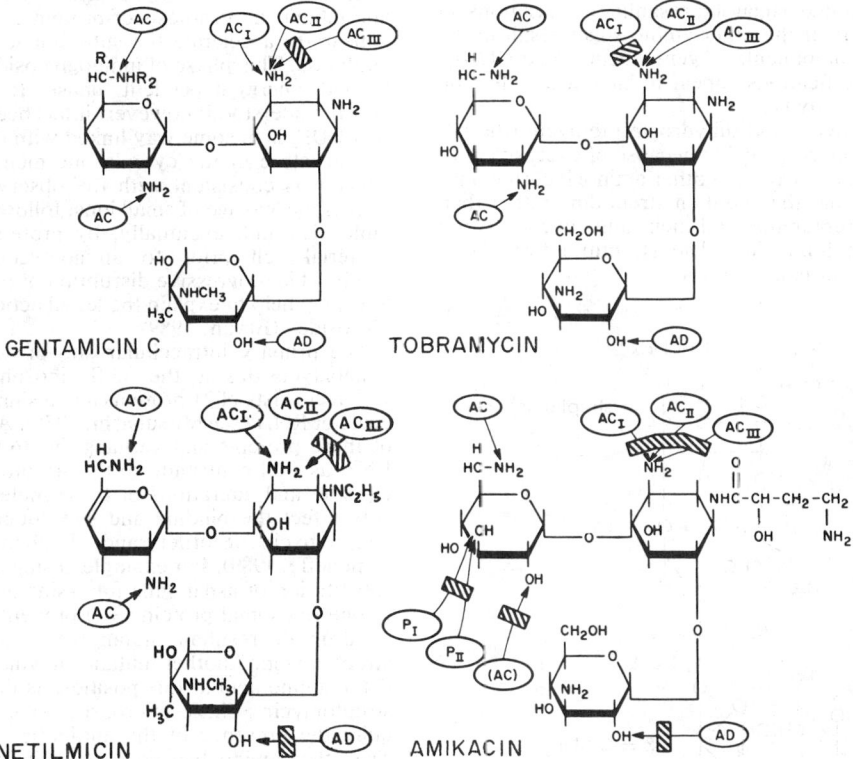

Figure 47–1. *Sites of activity of various plasmid-mediated enzymes capable of inactivating aminoglycosides.*

The symbol ▨ indicates regions of the molecule that are protected from the designated enzyme (AC = acetylase; AD = adenylylase; P = phosphorylase). In gentamicin C_1, $R_1 = R_2 = CH_3$; in gentamicin C_2, $R_1 = CH_3$, $R_2 = H$; in gentamicin C_{1a}, $R_1 = R_2 = H$. (Modified from Moellering, 1977. Courtesy of the *Medical Journal of Australia.*)

3-aminohexose (*see* Figure 47–1). The structural formula of kanamycin A, which is the major component of the commercial product, is as follows:

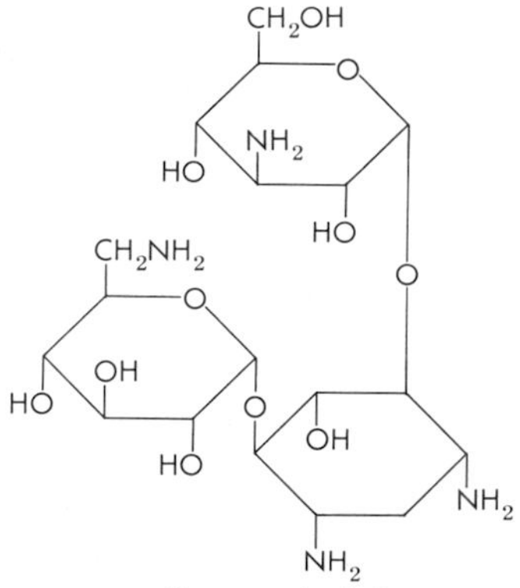

Kanamycin A

Amikacin is a semisynthetic derivative prepared from kanamycin A by acylation of the 1-amino group of the 2-deoxystreptamine moiety with 2-hydroxy-4-aminobutyric acid.

The gentamicin family, which includes gentamicin C_1, C_{1a}, and C_2, sisomicin, and netilmicin (the 1-N-ethyl derivative of sisomicin), contains a different 3-amino sugar (garosamine). Variations in methylation of the other amino sugar result in the different components of gentamicin (Figure 47–1). These modifications appear to have little effect on biological activity.

Streptomycin and dihydrostreptomycin (the latter is no longer available because of excessive ototoxicity) differ from the other aminoglycoside antibiotics in that they contain streptidine rather than 2-deoxystreptamine, and their aminocyclitol is not in a central position. The structural formula of streptomycin is as follows:

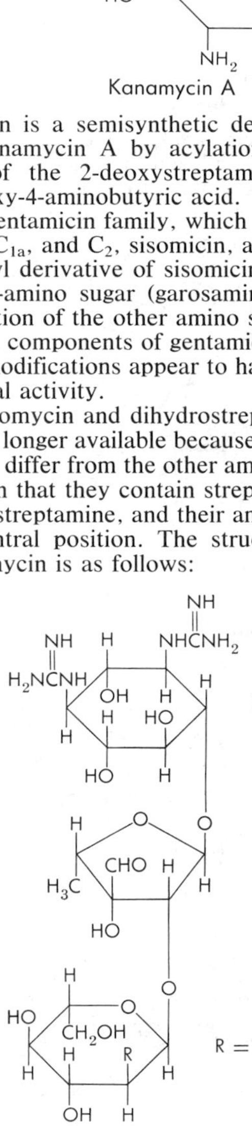

Streptomycin

Mechanism of Action. The aminoglycoside antibiotics are rapidly bactericidal. Although much is known about their capacity to inhibit protein synthesis and decrease the fidelity of translation of mRNA at the ribosome (Shannon and Phillips, 1982), this does not provide an obvious explanation for their rapidly lethal effect.

Aminoglycosides diffuse through aqueous channels formed by porin proteins in the outer membrane of gram-negative bacteria and thereby enter the periplasmic space (Nakae and Nakae, 1982). Subsequent transport of aminoglycosides across the cytoplasmic (inner) membrane is dependent on electron transport, in part because of a requirement for a membrane potential (interior negative) to drive permeation of these antibiotics (Bryan and Kwan, 1981, 1983; Mates *et al.*, 1983). This phase of transport has been termed energy-dependent phase I. It is rate limiting and can be blocked or inhibited by divalent cations (*e.g.*, Ca^{2+} and Mg^{2+}), hyperosmolarity, a reduction in pH, and anaerobiasis. The last two of these conditions impair the ability of the bacteria to maintain the driving force necessary for transport (membrane potential). Thus, for example, the antimicrobial activity of aminoglycosides is markedly reduced in the anaerobic environment of an abscess, in hyperosmolar acidic urine, and so forth (Bryan and Kwan, 1981). Following transport across the cytoplasmic membrane, the aminoglycosides bind to polysomes and inhibit the synthesis of proteins. This process appears to accelerate the subsequent transport of antibiotic. This phase of aminoglycoside transport, termed energy-dependent phase II (EDP_2), is poorly understood; however, it has been suggested that EDP_2 is in some way linked with disruption of the structure of the cytoplasmic membrane. This concept is consistent with the observed progression of the leakage of small ions, followed by larger molecules and, eventually, by proteins from the bacterial cell prior to aminoglycoside-induced death. This progressive disruption of the cell envelope may help to explain the lethal action of aminoglycosides (Bryan, 1989).

The primary intracellular site of action of the aminoglycosides is the 30 S ribosomal subunit, which consists of 21 proteins and a single 16 S molecule of RNA (*see* Mitsuhashi, 1975). At least three of these proteins and perhaps the 16 S ribosomal RNA as well contribute to the streptomycin binding site, and alterations of these molecules markedly affect the binding and subsequent action of streptomycin (Stöffler and Tischendorf, 1975; Cundlieffe, 1989). For example, a single amino acid substitution of asparagine for lysine at position 42 of one ribosomal protein (S_{12}) prevents binding of the drug; the resultant mutant is totally resistant to streptomycin. Another mutant, in which glutamine is the amino acid at this position, is dependent on streptomycin. These microorganisms actually require the presence of the antibiotic for survival. The other aminoglycosides also bind to the 30 S ribosomal subunit; however, they also appear to bind to several sites on the 50 S ribosomal subunit as well (Davies, 1988).

Aminoglycosides disrupt the normal cycle of ribosomal function by interfering, at least in part, with the initiation of protein synthesis, leading to the accumulation of abnormal initiation complexes or "streptomycin monosomes" (Luzzatto *et al.*, 1969). Another effect of the aminoglycosides is their capacity to induce misreading of the mRNA template, and incorrect amino acids are incorporated into the growing polypeptide chains (*see* Tai *et al.*, 1978). The aminoglycosides vary in their capacity to cause misreading, and this property presumably depends on differences in their affinities for specific ribosomal proteins. Although there appears to be a strong correlation between bactericidal activity and the ability to induce misreading (Hummel and Böck, 1989), it remains uncertain if this is the primary mechanism of aminoglycoside-induced cell death. The mutation to dependence on streptomycin is thought to result from misreading of the genetic code (*see* Stöffler and Tischendorf, 1975). Thus, if there is a mutation at some other site in the bacterial genome that would effectively prevent growth (*e.g.*, an amino acid substitution in a protein essential for normal metabolism), streptomycin-induced misreading of the mutation could result in an acceptable correction of the defect (phenotypic suppression). Bacteria could then resume growth only in the presence of the aminoglycoside. While this is a fascinating phenomenon, it is not of apparent clinical significance.

Microbial Resistance to the Aminoglycosides. Appreciation of the mechanisms of resistance to aminoglycosides is essential to understanding their spectra of antibacterial activity (Bryan, 1988). Bacteria may be resistant to the antimicrobial activity of the aminoglycosides because of failure of permeation of the antibiotic, low affinity of the drug for the bacterial ribosome, or inactivation of the drug by microbial enzymes. The last-named mechanism is by far the most important explanation for the acquired microbial resistance to aminoglycosides that is encountered in clinical practice.

Penetration of drug through the pores in the outer membrane of gram-negative microorganisms into the periplasmic space may be retarded; resistance of this type is unimportant clinically. Once the aminoglycoside does reach the periplasmic space, it may be altered by microbial enzymes that phosphorylate, adenylate, or acetylate specific hydroxyl or amino groups (Figure 47–1). The genetic information for these enzymes is acquired primarily by conjugation and the transfer of DNA as plasmids and resistance transfer factors (*see* Chapter 44). These plasmids have become widespread in nature (especially in hospital environments), and they code for a large number of enzymes (more than 20) that have markedly reduced the clinical usefulness of kanamycin and, more recently, of gentamicin and tobramycin. Amikacin is less vulnerable to these inactivating enzymes because of protective molecular side chains (Figure 47–1); thus, this drug may have a particularly important role in certain hospital settings. Unfortunately, these plasmids may also spread resistance to other antibiotics simultaneously. The metabolites of the aminoglycosides may compete with the unaltered drug for intracellular transport, but they are incapable of binding effectively to ribosomes and interfering with protein synthesis.

Plasmid-mediated elaboration of aminoglycoside-inactivating enzymes has become a source of concern with regard to treatment of enterococcal infections. In several centers, a significant percentage of clinical isolates of these organisms (both *E. faecalis* and *E. faecium*) are highly resistant to all aminoglycosides because of this mechanism (Zervos *et al.*, 1987; Eliopoulos *et al.*, 1988). Although there is usually a synergistic bactericidal effect of certain beta-lactam antibiotics and aminoglycosides on enterococci, this too is lost. An additional complicating factor is the recently recognized ability of enterococci to acquire plasmids that code for beta-lactamases (Murray and Mederski-Samaroj, 1983). These factors could make serious enterococcal infections, such as endocarditis, extremely difficult to treat.

Another common form of natural resistance to aminoglycosides is caused by failure of the drug to penetrate the cytoplasmic (inner) membrane. As mentioned above, the transport of aminoglycosides across the cytoplasmic membrane is an oxygen-dependent, active process. Strictly anaerobic bacteria are thus resistant to these drugs, since they lack the necessary transport system. Similarly, facultative bacteria are generally much more resistant when they are grown under anaerobic conditions (Mates *et al.*, 1983). The significance of this so-called permeability barrier as an explanation for resistance to aminoglycosides among aerobic gram-negative bacilli is not known. Natural resistance to amikacin by *Pseudomonas maltophilia* and certain other microorganisms appears to have a similar basis, as does the low-level resistance of some gram-positive cocci to aminoglycosides. The addition of antibiotics, such as the beta-lactams, that alter the structure of the cell wall can markedly increase the entrance of aminoglycosides into these bacteria. Although this has been extremely useful in the treatment of enterococcal infections, newly resistant strains (discussed above) are not susceptible to this synergistic effect. The combination of oxacillin and streptomycin has such a synergistic effect on *Staphylococcus aureus* (Zenilman *et al.*, 1986).

Resistance that results from alterations in ribosomal structure is less relevant clinically for most bacterial infections. Single-step mutations in *Escherichia coli* that result in the substitution of a single amino acid in a crucial ribosomal protein may prevent binding of the drug. Although such strains of *E. coli* are highly resistant to streptomycin (Stöffler and Tischendorf, 1975), they are not widespread in nature. Similarly, only 5% of strains of *Pseud. aeruginosa* exhibit such ribosomal resistance to streptomycin. However, up to 50% of strains of enterococci isolated from patients with endocarditis are resistant to high concentrations of streptomycin, and ribosomes from these strains fail to bind the antibiotic. For this reason there is no synergistic effect of penicillin and streptomycin against these strains demonstrable *in vitro*. However, because ribosomal resistance is often specific for a single aminoglycoside, the vast majority of these strains of enterococci are sensitive to a combination of penicillin and gentamicin *in vitro*.

Antibacterial Activity of the Aminoglycosides. The antibacterial activity of gentamicin, tobramycin, kanamycin, netilmicin, and amikacin is primarily directed against aerobic, gram-negative bacilli. As noted above, these antibiotics have little activity against anaerobic microorganisms or facultative bacteria under anaerobic conditions. Their action against most gram-positive bacteria is limited. *Streptococcus pneumoniae* and *Strep. pyogenes* are highly resistant, and, in fact, gentamicin has been added to blood-agar plates to aid in the isolation of these microorganisms from sputum and pharyngeal secretions. Streptomycin and gentamicin are active against "sensitive" strains of enterococci and streptococci at concentrations that can be achieved clinically only when combined with a penicillin. Such combinations result in a more rapid bactericidal effect than is produced by either drug alone. Both gentamicin and tobramycin are active *in vitro* against more than 90% of strains of *Staph. aureus* and 75% of strains of *Staph. epidermidis*. However, resistance that is mediated by conjugatively transferable plasmids that code for aminoglycoside-modifying enzymes is increasing worldwide (Kucers and Bennett, 1987). The clinical efficacy of aminoglycosides in the treatment of serious staphylococcal infections has not been documented, and they should not be used alone in such situations. Gentamicin-resistant mutant strains of staphylococci emerge rapidly during exposure to the drug.

The aerobic gram-negative bacilli vary in their susceptibility to the aminoglycosides. "Sensitive" microorganisms are defined as those inhibited by concentrations that can be achieved clinically in plasma without a high incidence of toxicity; these therapeutic peak values are 4 to 8 μg/ml for gentamicin, tobramycin, and netilmicin and 8 to 16 μg/ml for amikacin and kanamycin. In general, gentamicin, tobramycin, netilmicin, and amikacin are more active than kanamycin. Tobramycin and gentamicin exhibit similar activity against most gram-negative bacilli, although tobramycin is usually more active against *Pseud. aeruginosa* and against some strains of *Proteus* species. Most gram-negative bacilli (except *Pseud. aeruginosa*) that are resistant to gentamicin because of plasmid-mediated inactivating enzymes will also inactivate tobramycin. However, approximately 50% of *Pseud. aeruginosa* that are resistant to gentamicin remain sensitive to tobramycin (Symposium, 1976b). In some hospitals, the nosocomial flora have undergone considerable alterations in susceptibility to antibiotics during the past 20 years, with a gradual increase in resistance to gentamicin and tobramycin. The relative frequency of these changes varies dramatically—even in different units within a single hospital (Cross *et al.*, 1983). Fortunately, amikacin (Betts *et al.*, 1984) and, in some instances, netilmicin have retained their activity in this setting, a phenomenon attributed to resistance of the drugs to the aminoglycoside-inactivating enzymes. These agents thus have a broad spectrum of activity and are particularly valuable in treating nosocomial infections.

ABSORPTION, DISTRIBUTION, AND ELIMINATION OF THE AMINOGLYCOSIDES

Absorption. The aminoglycosides are highly polar cations; they are thus very poorly absorbed from the gastrointestinal tract. Less than 1% of a dose is absorbed following either oral or rectal administration. The drugs are not inactivated in the intestine, and they are eliminated quantitatively in the feces. Absorption of gentamicin from the gastrointestinal tract may be increased by gastrointestinal disease (ulcers, inflammatory bowel disease) (Cox, 1970; Breen *et al.*, 1972). However, long-term oral or rectal administration may result in accumulation of aminoglycosides to toxic concentrations in patients with renal impairment. Instillation of these drugs into body cavities with serosal surfaces may result in rapid absorption and unexpected toxicity. Similarly, intoxication may occur when aminoglycosides are applied topically for long periods to large wounds, burns, or cutaneous ulcers, particularly if there is renal insufficiency.

All of the aminoglycosides are absorbed rapidly from intramuscular sites of injection. Peak concentrations in plasma occur after 30 to 90 minutes and are similar to those observed 30 minutes after completion of an intravenous infusion of an equal dose over a 30-minute period. In critically ill patients, especially those in shock, absorption of drug may be reduced from intramuscular sites because of poor perfusion.

Distribution. Because of their polar nature, the aminoglycosides are largely excluded from most cells, from the central nervous system, and from the eye. Except for streptomycin, there is negligible binding of aminoglycosides to plasma albumin. The apparent volume of distribution of these drugs is 25% of lean body weight and approximates the volume of extracellular fluid (Barza *et al.*, 1975).

As would be expected, concentrations of aminoglycosides in secretions and tissues are low. High concentrations are found only in the renal cortex and in the endolymph and perilymph of the inner ear; this may contribute to the nephrotoxicity and ototoxicity caused by these drugs (Davies *et al.,* 1984). Concentrations in bile approach 30% of those found in plasma as a result of active hepatic secretion, but this represents a very minor excretory route for the aminoglycosides. Penetration into respiratory secretions is poor (Levy, 1986). Diffusion into pleural and synovial fluid is relatively slow, but concentrations that approximate those in the plasma may be achieved after repeated administration. Inflammation increases the penetration of aminoglycosides into peritoneal and pericardial cavities.

Concentrations of aminoglycosides that can be safely achieved in cerebrospinal fluid (CSF) are very limited. In experimental animals and man, concentrations in CSF are less than 10% of those in plasma in the absence of inflammation; this value may approach 20% when there is meningitis (Strausbaugh *et al.,* 1977). The concentrations achieved are therefore inadequate for the treatment of gram-negative bacillary meningitis in adults. Intrathecal or intraventricular administration of aminoglycosides was utilized frequently in the past, but the availability of third-generation cephalosporins has now made this rare. Therapeutic results of systemic administration of aminoglycosides to neonates with meningitis indicate no additional benefit of either intrathecal or intraventricular injection of these drugs, perhaps because of the immaturity of the blood–brain barrier (McCracken *et al.,* 1980; McCracken, 1985). Penetration of aminoglycosides into ocular fluids is so poor that effective therapy of bacterial endophthalmitis requires periocular injections of the drugs (Barza, 1978).

Administration of aminoglycosides to women late in pregnancy may result in accumulation of drug in fetal plasma and amniotic fluid. Streptomycin can cause hearing loss in children born to women who receive the drug during pregnancy (Warkang, 1979). Insufficient data are available regarding the other aminoglycosides; it is thus recommended that they be used with caution in pregnancy and only for strong clinical indications in the absence of suitable alternatives (*Medical Letter,* 1987).

Elimination. The aminoglycosides are excreted almost entirely by glomerular filtration, and concentrations in the urine of 50 to 200 μg/ml are achieved. A large fraction of a parenterally administered dose is excreted unchanged during the first 24 hours, with most of this appearing in the first 12 hours. The half-lives of the aminoglycosides in plasma are similar and vary between 2 and 3 hours in patients with normal renal function. Renal clearance of aminoglycosides is approximately two thirds of the simultaneous creatinine clearance; this observation suggests some tubular reabsorption of these drugs.

Following a single dose of an aminoglycoside, disappearance from the plasma exceeds renal excretion by 10 to 20%; however, after 1 to 2 days of therapy, nearly 100% of subsequent doses is eventually recovered in the urine. This lag period probably represents saturation of binding sites in tissues. The rate of elimination of drug from these sites is considerably longer than from plasma; the half-life for tissue-bound aminoglycoside has been estimated to range from 30 to 700 hours (Schentag and Jusko, 1977). For this reason, small amounts of aminoglycosides can be detected in the urine for 10 to 20 days after drug administration is discontinued. Aminoglycoside bound to renal tissue appears to exhibit antibacterial activity and protects experimental animals against bacterial infections of the kidney, even when the drug can no longer be detected in serum (Bergeron *et al.,* 1982).

The concentration of aminoglycoside in plasma produced by the initial or loading dose is dependent only on the volume of distribution of the drug. Since the elimination of aminoglycosides is almost entirely dependent on the kidney, a linear relationship exists between the concentration of creatinine in plasma and the half-life of all aminoglycosides in patients with moderately compromised renal function. In anephric patients, the half-life varies from 20 to 40 times that determined in normal individuals. *Since the incidence of nephrotoxicity and ototoxicity is related to the concentration to which an aminoglycoside accumulates, it is critical to reduce the maintenance dosage of these drugs in patients with impaired renal function.* This must be done with precision, since the concentration in plasma that is associated with toxicity is not much greater than that required for treatment of many bacterial infections. The size of the individual dose, the interval between doses, or both can be altered. There is no conclusive information on the best approach. A variety of specific recommendations and nomograms may be found in the literature (*e.g.*, Hull and Sarubbi, 1976). The most consistent plasma concentrations are achieved when the loading dose is given in milligrams per kilogram of body weight, and, since aminoglycosides are minimally distributed in fatty tissue, the lean or expected body weight should be used. Methods for calculation of dosage are described in Appendix II.

However, there are obvious difficulties in utilizing any of these approaches for ill patients with rapidly changing renal function (Lesar *et al.*, 1982). In addition, even when known factors are taken into consideration, concentrations of aminoglycosides achieved in plasma after a given dose vary widely between patients (Barza *et al.*, 1975). If the extracellular volume is expanded, concentrations will be reduced. For unknown reasons the clearances are increased and the half-lives of the aminoglycosides are reduced in patients with cystic fibrosis; the volume of distribution is increased in patients with leukemia (Rosenthal *et al.*, 1977; Spyker *et al.*, 1978). Patients with anemia (hematocrit <25%) have a concentration in plasma that is higher than expected, probably because of a reduction in the number of binding sites on red blood cells (Siber *et al.*, 1975).

Determination of the concentration of drug in plasma is an essential guide to the proper administration of aminoglycosides. Ideally, a plasma concentration at the trough of the fluctuating curve, collected just prior to a dose, and a peak concentration, collected 30 minutes after a 30-minute infusion of the dose, should be obtained to ensure adequacy of the antimicrobial activity (peak) and to detect accumulation of drug (trough). In patients with life-threatening systemic infections, aminoglycoside concentrations should be determined several times per week (more frequently if renal function is changing) and should always be determined within 24 hours after a change in dosage.

Aminoglycosides are removed from the body by either hemodialysis or peritoneal dialysis. Approximately 50% of the administered dose is removed in 12 hours by hemodialysis, and this technique has been used for the treatment of overdosage (Alexander and Gambertoglio, 1985). As a general rule, a dose equal to half the loading dose administered after each hemodialysis should maintain the plasma concentration in the desired range; however, a number of variables make this a rough approximation at best. Frequent monitoring of drug concentrations in plasma is again crucial.

Peritoneal dialysis is less effective than hemodialysis in removing aminoglycosides. Clearance rates are approximately 5 to 10 ml per minute for the various drugs, but are highly variable (Appel and Neu, 1977). If a patient who requires dialysis has bacterial peritonitis, a therapeutic concentration of the aminoglycoside will probably not be achieved in the peritoneal fluid, since the ratio of the concentration in plasma to that in peritoneal fluid may be 10 to 1 (Smithivas *et al.*, 1971). It is thus recommended that antibiotic be added to the dialysate to achieve concentrations equal to those desired in plasma (*i.e.*, 4 μg/ml for gentamicin, tobramycin, and netilmicin; 15 μg/ml for amikacin and kanamycin). This should be preceded by the parenteral administration of a loading dose.

Although excretion of aminoglycosides is similar in adults and children over 6 months of age, half-lives of the drugs may be significantly prolonged in the newborn. Newborn infants who weigh less than 2 kg have half-lives for aminoglycosides of 8 to 11 hours during the first week of life, while those who weigh over 2 kg eliminate these drugs with half-lives of about 5 hours (Yow, 1977). It is thus critically important to monitor concentrations of aminoglycosides during treatment of neonates (Phillips *et al.*, 1982).

Aminoglycosides can be inactivated by various penicillins *in vitro* (Konishi *et al.*, 1983) and in patients with end-stage renal failure (Blair *et al.*, 1982), thus making dosage recommendations even more difficult. Special care must be taken when obtaining serum for determinations of concentrations of these drugs, since inactivation of the aminoglycoside may continue *in vitro* unless the penicillin has been inactivated with beta-lactamase or the specimen has been frozen (Pickering and Gearhart, 1979). Amikacin appears to be the least affected by this interaction.

UNTOWARD EFFECTS OF THE AMINOGLYCOSIDES

All aminoglycosides have the potential to produce reversible and irreversible vestibular, cochlear, and renal toxicity. These side effects complicate the use of these compounds and make their proper administration difficult (Appel and Neu, 1977).

Ototoxicity. Both vestibular and auditory dysfunction can follow the administration of any of the aminoglycosides. Studies of both animals and man have documented progressive accumulation of these drugs in the perilymph and endolymph of the inner ear (Huy *et al.*, 1983). Accumulation occurs predominantly when concentrations in plasma are high and diffusion back into the bloodstream is slow; the half-lives of the aminoglycosides are five to six times longer in the otic fluids than in plasma. Back diffusion is facilitated when the concentration of drug in plasma reaches a trough. Thus, ototoxicity is more evident in patients with persistently elevated concentrations of drug in plasma. However, even a single dose of tobramycin has been reported to produce slight temporary cochlear dysfunction during periods when the concentration in plasma is at its peak (Wilson and Ramsden, 1977). The relationship of this observation to permanent loss of hearing is not known.

Ototoxicity is the result of progressive destruction of vestibular or cochlear sensory cells, which are highly sensitive to damage by aminoglycosides (Brummett and Fox, 1982). Studies in guinea pigs exposed to large doses of gentamicin reveal degeneration of the type-I sensory hair cells in the central part of the crista ampullaris (vestibular organ) and fusion of individual sensory hairs into giant hairs (Wersäll *et al.*, 1973). Similar studies with gentamicin and tobramycin also demonstrate loss of hair cells in the cochlea of the organ of Corti (Theopold, 1977). With increasing dosage and prolonged exposure, damage progresses from the base of the cochlea, where high-frequency sounds are processed, to the apex, which is necessary for the perception of low frequencies. While these histological changes correlate with the ability of the cochlea to generate an action potential in response to sound, the biochemical mechanism for ototoxicity is poorly understood. Early changes induced by aminoglycosides have been shown in experimental ototoxicity to be reversible by Ca^{2+}. Once sensory cells are lost, however, regeneration does not occur; retrograde degeneration of the auditory nerve follows, resulting in irreversible hearing loss (Lietman, 1990). It has been suggested that aminoglycosides interfere with the active transport system essential for the maintenance of the ionic balance of the endolymph (Neu and Bendush, 1976); this would lead to alteration in the normal concentrations of ions in the labyrinthine fluids, with impairment of electrical activity and nerve conduction. Eventually, the electrolyte changes, or perhaps the drugs themselves, damage the hair cells irreversibly. Interest has also centered on the interaction of aminoglycosides with membrane phospholipids, particularly phosphatidylinositol and its phosphorylated derivatives, which are the precursors of the intracellular second messengers inositol 1,4,5-trisphosphate and diacylglycerol.

The degree of permanent dysfunction correlates with the number of destroyed or altered sensory hair cells and is thought to be related to sustained exposure to the drug. Repeated courses of aminoglycosides, each resulting in the loss of more cells, can lead to deafness. Since there appears to be a decrease in the number of cells with age, older patients may be more susceptible to ototoxicity. Drugs such as ethacrynic acid and furosemide potentiate the ototoxic effects of the aminoglycosides in animals (Brummett, 1983); data implicating furosemide are less convincing in man (Moore *et al.*, 1984a). Hearing loss is also more likely to develop in patients with preexisting auditory impairment following exposure to these agents.

Although all of the aminoglycosides are capable of affecting both cochlear and vestibular function, some preferential toxicity is evident. Streptomycin and gentamicin produce predominantly vestibular effects, whereas amikacin, kanamycin, and neomycin primarily affect auditory function; tobramycin affects both equally. The incidence of ototoxicity is extremely difficult to determine. Data from audiometry suggest that the incidence may be as high as 25% (Moore *et al.*, 1984a). The relative incidence appears to be equal for tobramycin, gentamicin, and amikacin. Initial studies in laboratory animals and man suggested that netilmicin is less ototoxic than other aminoglycosides (Brummett and Fox, 1982; Lerner *et al.*, 1983); however, the incidence of ototoxicity from netilmicin is not negligible—such complications developed in 10% of patients in one clinical trial of netilmicin (Trestman *et al.*, 1978). A definitive statement on relative ototoxicity awaits further clinical evaluation.

The incidence of vestibular toxicity is particularly high in patients receiving streptomycin; nearly 20% of individuals who received 500 mg twice daily for 4 weeks for enterococcal endocarditis developed clinically detectable, irreversible vestibular damage (Wilson *et al.*, 1984). In addition, up to 75% of patients who received 2 g of streptomycin for more than 60 days showed evidence of nystagmus or postural imbalance.

It is recommended that patients receiving high doses and/or prolonged courses of aminoglycosides be carefully monitored for ototoxicity, since the initial symptoms may be reversible; however, deafness may occur several weeks after therapy is discontinued.

Clinical Symptoms of Cochlear Toxicity. A high-pitched tinnitus is often the first symptom of impending difficulty. If the drug is not discontinued, auditory impairment may develop after a few days. The tinnitus may persist for several days to 2 weeks after therapy is stopped. Since perception of sound in the high-frequency range (outside the conversational range) is lost first, the affected individual is not aware of the difficulty; it will not be detected unless careful audiometric examination is carried out. If the loss of hearing progresses, the lower sound ranges are affected, and conversation becomes difficult.

Clinical Symptoms of Vestibular Toxicity. Moderately intense headache lasting 1 or 2 days may precede the onset of labyrinthine dysfunction. This is immediately followed by an acute stage, in which nausea, vomiting, and difficulty with equilibrium develop and persist for 1 to 2 weeks. Vertigo in the upright position, inability to perceive termination of movement ("mental past pointing"), and difficulty in sitting or standing without visual cues are prominent symptoms. Drifting of the eyes at the end of a movement so that focusing and reading are difficult, positive Romberg test, and rarely, pendular trunk movement and spontaneous nystagmus are outstanding signs. The acute stage ends suddenly and is followed by the appearance of manifestations consistent with chronic labyrinthitis, in which, although symptomless while in bed, the patient has difficulty when he attempts to walk or make sudden movements; ataxia is the most prominent feature. The chronic phase persists for approximately 2 months; it is gradually superseded by a compensatory stage, in which symptoms are latent and appear only when the eyes are closed. Adaptation to the impairment of labyrinthine function is accomplished by the use of visual cues and deep proprioceptive sensation for determining movement and position; it is more adequate in the young than in the old, but may not be sufficient to permit the high degree of coordination required in many special trades. Recovery from this phase may require 12 to 18 months, and most patients have some permanent residual damage. Although there is no specific treatment for the vestibular deficiency, early discontinuation of the drug may permit recovery prior to irreversible damage of the hair cells.

Nephrotoxicity. Approximately 8 to 26% of patients who receive an aminoglycoside for more than several days will develop mild renal impairment that is almost always reversible (Smith *et al.,* 1977, 1980). The toxicity is apparently a result of marked accumulation and avid retention of aminoglycoside in the proximal tubular cells (Aronoff *et al.,* 1983; Lietman and Smith, 1983). The initial damage at this site is manifested by the excretion of enzymes of the renal tubular brush border (Patel *et al.,* 1975). After several days there is a defect in renal concentrating ability, mild proteinuria, and the appearance of hyaline and granular casts; the glomerular filtration rate is reduced after several additional days (Schentag *et al.,* 1979). The nonoliguric phase of renal insufficiency has been postulated to be due to the effects that aminoglycosides exert on the distal portion of the nephron. They are thought by some investigators to decrease the sensitivity of the collecting-duct epithelium to endogenous antidiuretic hormone (Appel, 1982). While severe acute tubular necrosis may occur rarely, the most common significant finding is a mild rise in plasma creatinine (0.5 to 2.0 mg/dl; 40 to 175 μM); hypokalemia, hypocalcemia, and hypophosphatemia are seen very infrequently. The impairment in renal function is almost always reversible, since the proximal tubular cells have the capacity to regenerate.

Several variables appear to influence nephrotoxicity from aminoglycosides. Toxicity correlates with the total amount of drug administered. Continuous infusion is more nephrotoxic in dogs and rats than is intermittent dosing (Reiner *et al.,* 1978; Powell *et al.,* 1983), and constant concentrations of drug in plasma above a critical level appear to correlate with toxicity in man (Keating *et al.,* 1979). Recent studies in animals indicate that there is less nephrotoxicity with no reduction in efficacy when aminoglycosides are given once daily (Kapusnik *et al.,* 1988; Woods *et al.,* 1988). There have been few clinical studies on this point (Gilbert, 1990).

The nephrotoxic potential varies among individual aminoglycosides. The relative toxicity correlates with the concentration of drug found in the renal cortex in experimental animals; however, clinical studies have not consistently supported this notion. Neomycin, which concentrates to the greatest degree, is highly nephrotoxic in man and should not be administered systemically. Streptomycin does not concentrate in the renal cortex and is the least nephrotoxic. Most of the controversy has concerned the relative toxicities of gentamicin and tobramycin. Gentamicin is concentrated in the kidney to a greater degree than is tobramycin, but several controlled clinical trials have given different estimates of their relative nephrotoxicities (Smith *et al.,* 1977, 1980; Fong *et al.,* 1981; Keys *et al.,* 1981). If differences between the renal toxicity of these two aminoglycosides do exist in man, they appear to be slight. Comparative studies with amikacin, sisomicin, and netilmicin are not conclusive. Other drugs, such as amphotericin B, vancomycin, cisplatin, and cyclosporine, may potentiate aminoglycoside-induced nephrotoxicity (Woods *et al.*, 1986). Several studies suggest that cephalothin aggravates the nephrotoxicity produced by aminoglycosides (Klastersky *et al.*, 1975; Wade *et al.*, 1978). Furosemide enhances the nephrotoxicity of aminoglycosides in rats if concurrent depletion of fluid is not corrected (Mitchell *et al.*, 1977), and it has been suggested that the diuretic-induced loss of K^+ might be responsible for this toxicity. Studies in man have not conclusively proven furosemide to aggravate nephrotoxicity (Smith and Lietman, 1983); however, both volume depletion and wasting of K^+ have been incriminated.

Although advanced age, liver disease, and septic shock have been suggested as risk factors for the development of nephrotoxicity from aminoglycosides, data are not convincing (Moore *et al.*, 1984b). However, in the elderly patient renal function is overestimated from measurement of creatinine concentration in plasma, and overdosing will occur if this value is used as the only guide.

Thus, while aminoglycosides consistently alter the structure and function of renal proximal tubular cells, these effects are usually reversible. The most important result of this toxicity may be reduced excretion of the drug, which in turn will lead to ototoxicity. Monitoring drug concentrations in plasma is useful, particularly during prolonged and/or high-dose therapy. However, it has never been proven that toxicity can be prevented by avoiding excessive peak or trough concentrations of aminoglycosides.

The biochemical events leading to tubular cell damage and glomerular dysfunction are poorly understood, but they may involve perturbations of the structure of cellular membranes. Aminoglycosides inhibit various phospholipases, sphingomyelinases, and ATPases, and they alter the function of mitochondria and ribosomes (Silverblatt, 1982; Queener *et al.*, 1983; Humes *et al.*, 1984). Because of the ability of cationic aminoglycosides to interact with anionic phospholipids, these drugs may impair the generation of membrane-derived autacoids and intracellular second messengers such as prostaglandins, inositol phosphates, and diacylglycerol. Derangements of prostaglandin metabolism might explain the relationship between tubular damage and reduction in glomerular filtration rate. Others have observed morphological changes in glomerular endothelial cells (decreased number of endothelial fenestrations) in animals receiving aminoglycosides (Luft and Evans, 1980) and drug-induced reduction in the glomerular capillary ultrafiltration coefficient (Baylis *et al.*, 1977).

Ca^{2+} has been shown to inhibit the uptake and binding of aminoglycosides to the renal brush-border luminal membrane *in vitro*, and supplementary dietary Ca^{2+} attenuates experimental nephrotoxicity (Bennett *et al.*, 1982; Humes *et al.*, 1984; Quarum *et al.*, 1984). Aminoglycosides are eventually internalized by pinocytosis; morphologically there is clear evidence of accumulation of drug in liposomes. Aminoglycosides are thereby trapped, concentrated (up to 50 times the plasma concentration) (Aronoff *et al.*, 1983), and prepared for extrusion into the urine as multilamellar, phospholipid structures called "myeloid bodies" (Silverblatt, 1982).

Neuromuscular Blockade. A rather unique toxic reaction of acute neuromuscular blockade and apnea has been attributed to the various aminoglycosides. A review of 83 reports of prolonged muscular paralysis implicated neomycin as the most frequent cause (Pittinger *et al.*, 1970). In experimental systems the order of decreasing potency is neomycin, kanamycin, amikacin, gentamicin, and tobramycin.

In man, neuromuscular blockade has generally occurred after intrapleural or intraperitoneal instillation of large doses of an aminoglycoside; however, the reaction has followed the intravenous, intramuscular, and even the oral administration of these agents (Holtzman, 1976). Most episodes have occurred in association with anesthesia or the administration of other neuromuscular blocking agents. Patients with myasthenia gravis are particularly susceptible to this effect.

Animal studies indicate that the aminoglycosides inhibit prejunctional release of acetylcholine while also reducing postsynaptic sensitivity to the transmitter (Pittinger and Adamson, 1972; Sokoll and Gergis, 1981). Ca^{2+} overcomes the effect of the aminoglycoside at the neuromuscular junction, and the intravenous administration of a calcium salt is the preferred treatment for this toxicity (Singh *et al.*, 1978). Inhibitors of cholinesterase (edrophonium, neostigmine) have also been used with varying degrees of success. Since physicians have become aware of this complication, it is now relatively uncommon.

Other Effects on the Nervous System. The administration of streptomycin in particular may produce dysfunction of the optic nerve. Scotomas, presenting as enlargement of the blind spot, have been associated with the drug.

Among the less common toxic reactions to streptomycin is peripheral neuritis. This may be due either to accidental injection of a nerve during the course of parenteral therapy or to toxicity involving nerves remote from the site of antibiotic administration. Paresthesia, most commonly perioral but also present in other areas of the face or in the hands, occasionally follows the use of the antibiotic and usually appears within 30 to 60 minutes after injection of the drug; it may persist for several hours.

Other Untoward Effects. In general, the aminoglycosides have little allergenic potential; both anaphylaxis and rash are unusual. Rare hypersensitivity reactions, including skin rashes, eosinophilia, fever, blood dyscrasias, angioedema, exfoliative dermatitis, stomatitis, and anaphylactic shock, have been reported. Other reactions that have been attributed to individual drugs are discussed below.

STREPTOMYCIN

Streptomycin is used today for the treatment of certain unusual infections, generally in combination with other antimicrobial agents. It is also occasionally administered for tuberculosis (*see* Chapter 49).

Preparations, Routes of Administration, and Dosage. *Streptomycin sulfate* is supplied for intramuscular injection either as a powder or in solution (400 mg/ml).

Streptomycin is administered by intermittent, deep intramuscular injection. These injections are often painful; hot tender masses may develop at sites of injection. The total daily dose usually varies from 1 to 2 g (15 to 25 mg/kg); 500 mg to 1 g is injected every 12 hours. In plague or other severe fulminating infections, up to 4 g per day may be given in two to four divided doses. In adults, 1 g given intramuscularly produces a peak plasma concentration of 25 to 30 μg/ml. Children should receive 20 to 40 mg/kg daily, in two to four divided doses. Except in tuberculosis and subacute bacterial endocarditis, it is rarely necessary to give streptomycin for more than 7 to 10 days. Dosage schedules for tuberculosis are described in Chapter 49.

Therapeutic Uses. *Bacterial Endocarditis.* Streptomycin and penicillin produce a synergistic bactericidal effect *in vitro* and in animal models of infection against strains of enterococci, group-D streptococci, and the various oral streptococci of the viridans group. Many authorities administer such antibiotics concurrently for treatment of endocarditis caused by these microorganisms. Penicillin G alone is ineffective in the therapy of enterococcal endocarditis, and either streptomycin (500 mg twice daily) or gentamicin (1 mg/kg three times daily) must also be given to ensure cure. Gentamicin is preferred when the strain shows complete (ribosomal) resistance to streptomycin (minimal inhibitory concentration [MIC] > 2000 μg/ml). Both penicillin G and the aminoglycoside are administered for 4 to 6 weeks. Treatment for 4 weeks has been successful in patients who had symptoms for less than 3 months prior to therapy (Wilson *et al.,* 1984). Some authorities recommend gentamicin for all cases of enterococcal endocarditis, since its toxicity is primarily renal and reversible while that of streptomycin is vestibular and irreversible; however, streptomycin has been effective in many patients with enterococcal endocarditis and many other clinicians prefer to use it when microorganisms are susceptible. Unfortunately, strains of enterococci have now appeared that produce enzymes that inactivate all aminoglycosides (Eliopoulos *et al.,* 1988).

Endocarditis caused by penicillin-sensitive streptococci (MIC < 0.1 μg/ml) has been successfully treated with penicillin G alone for 4 weeks (relapse rate 1 to 2%; Karchmer *et al.,* 1979), penicillin G plus streptomycin (0.5 g twice a day) for 2 weeks (relapse rate 1 to 2%, Wilson *et al.,* 1978), or penicillin G for 4 weeks combined with streptomycin for the first 2 weeks of therapy (relapse rate 0%; Wolfe and Johnson, 1974). The clinician thus has several options, one of which can be chosen based on the needs of the individual patient. For example, the elderly patient with streptococcal endocarditis due to a penicillin-sensitive strain should probably receive penicillin alone because of the increased toxicity from streptomycin in this age group. The short, 2-week course of therapy is now recommended for uncomplicated cases (Bisno *et al.,* 1989). However, if the infection is on a prosthetic valve, or is caused by a relatively resistant strain (MIC of penicillin > 0.2 μg/ml), or is caused by nutritionally deficient (pyridoxal-requiring) streptococci, a longer duration of therapy is prudent (Sande, 1983).

Tularemia. Patients with tularemia benefit dramatically from the administration of streptomycin (Evans *et al.,* 1985). The best results are obtained when therapy is instituted early; however, chronicity does not exclude the possibility of complete cure. Most cases respond to the administration of 1 to 2 g of streptomycin per day for 7 to 10 days. The tetracyclines are also highly effective in tularemia and are preferred by some physicians for milder forms of the disease.

Plague. Streptomycin is one of the most effective agents for the treatment of all forms of plague. The tetracyclines and chloramphenicol are also beneficial in this disease. When streptomycin is used, a dose of 1 to 4 g per day is given for 7 to 10 days.

GENTAMICIN

Gentamicin is an important agent for the treatment of many serious gram-negative bacillary infections. However, emergence of resistant microorganisms in some hospitals has become a serious problem and may limit the future use of this agent.

Preparations, Routes of Administration, and Dosage. *Gentamicin sulfate* (GARAMYCIN) is available in various forms: vials and prefilled syringes containing 40 mg/ml (or 10 mg/ml for pediatric use), an intrathecal injection (without preservatives) containing 2 mg/ml, an ointment and cream (0.1%), an ophthalmic ointment (0.3%), and ophthalmic solution (0.3%). The recommended intramuscular or intravenous dose for adults is 3 to 5 mg/kg per day, one third being given every 8 hours. Several dosage schedules have been suggested for infants: 2 to 2.5 mg/kg every 8 hours has been found to be safe for children up to 2 years of age; 5 mg/kg daily, divided into two equally spaced injections, has been recommended for neonates with severe infections.

While the peak concentration in plasma is approximately 2 to 3 μg/ml after the intramuscular administration of 1 mg/kg, careful studies by a number of investigators have emphasized that the recommended doses of gentamicin do not always yield desired concentrations. Periodic determinations of the plasma concentration of aminoglycosides are strongly recommended, especially in seriously ill patients, to confirm that drug concentrations are therapeutic. Although it has not yet been established exactly what plasma concentration is toxic, "trough" (predose) concentrations that exceed 2 μg/ml for longer than 10 days have been associated with toxicity.

The presence of any significant degree of renal insufficiency imposes additional difficulty in establishing a regimen of therapy that will yield maximal therapeutic benefit with minimal or no risk of toxic reactions. This problem has been discussed above.

Penicillins and aminoglycosides must never be mixed in the same bottle because the penicillin inactivates the aminoglycoside to a significant degree; similar incompatibilities exist *in vitro* to different degrees between gentamicin and heparin, amphotericin B, and the various cephalosporins.

Gentamicin is very slowly absorbed when applied in an ointment, but absorption may be more rapid when a cream is used topically. When the antibiotic is applied to large areas of denuded body surface, as may be the case in burned patients, plasma concentrations can reach 1 μg/ml, and 2 to 5% of the drug used may appear in the urine.

Untoward Effects. The untoward effects of gentamicin are similar to those of other aminoglycosides. The most important and serious side effects of the use of gentamicin are nephrotoxicity and irreversible ototoxicity. Intrathecal or intraventricular administration may cause local inflammation and can result in radiculitis and other complications and therefore is rarely used (*see* above).

Therapeutic Uses of Gentamicin and Other Aminoglycosides. Gentamicin, tobramycin, amikacin, and netilmicin can be used interchangeably for the treatment of most of the following infections and will be discussed together. For most indications, gentamicin is the preferred agent because of long experience with its use and its low cost. Specific usages will be reviewed under each drug heading. A large variety of infections has been treated successfully with these aminoglycosides; however, due to their toxicities, prolonged use *must* be restricted to the therapy of life-threatening infections and those for which a less toxic antimicrobial agent is less effective. These antibiotics are frequently used (often in combination with a penicillin or a cephalosporin) for the therapy of proven or suspected serious gram-negative microbial infections, especially those due to *Pseud. aeruginosa, Enterobacter, Klebsiella, Serratia,* and other species resistant to less toxic antibiotics. Among these are urinary tract infections, bacteremia, infected burns, osteomyelitis, pneumonia, peritonitis, and otitis.

Urinary Tract Infections. Aminoglycosides are not usually indicated for the treatment of uncomplicated urinary tract infections, although a single intramuscular dose of gentamicin (5 mg/kg) or kanamycin (500 mg) has been effective in curing over 90% of uncomplicated infections of the lower urinary tract (Ronald *et al.*, 1976; Varese *et al.*, 1980). In the seriously ill patient with pyelonephritis, an aminoglycoside alone or in combination with a beta-lactam antibiotic offers broad and effective initial coverage. Once the microorganism is isolated and its sensitivities to antibiotics are determined, the aminoglycoside should be discontinued if the infecting microorganism is sensitive to less toxic antibiotics. The antibacterial activity of aminoglycosides is markedly reduced by low pH (Strausbaugh and Sande, 1978) and hyperosmolarity (Papapetropoulou *et al.*, 1983); however, the very high concentrations achieved in urine in patients with normal renal function are usually sufficient to eradicate sensitive microorganisms. The prolonged release of gentamicin from the renal cortex following discontinuation of therapy has been shown to produce a therapeutic effect for several months in experimental pyelonephritis in rats (Bergeron *et al.*, 1982).

Pneumonia. The frequency of pneumonia caused by various gram-negative bacilli is increasing, especially in hospitalized patients, patients on respirators, and those with impaired defenses (especially granulocytopenia). Selection of an antibiotic depends on the sensitivity of the microorganism. The aminoglycosides are widely used in this setting, but most authorities administer a penicillin or a cephalosporin concurrently, since therapy with an aminoglycoside alone is not very effective. One of the aminoglycosides given concurrently with an antipseudomonal penicillin or cephalosporin constitutes effective treatment of pneumonia caused by *Pseud. aeruginosa*. An aminoglycoside plus a broad-spectrum cephalosporin or penicillin (*e.g.*, mezlocillin, piperacillin) is used for sensitive strains of *Klebsiella;* an aminoglycoside plus ampicillin is preferred for pneumonia caused by sensitive strains of *E. coli* or *Proteus mirabilis*. All empiric selections should be based on institution-specific patterns of sensitivity.

Gentamicin- and tobramycin-resistant strains of *Klebsiella, Enterobacter, Serratia, Proteus,* and *Pseudomonas* have emerged in many hospitals. The major reservoirs for these microorganisms are burn units and intensive care units, where these drugs are used extensively. Critically ill patients with tracheostomies and impaired host defenses and those with indwelling intravenous and urinary catheters all appear to acquire resistant bacteria frequently.

Aminoglycosides are ineffective for treatment of pneumonia due to anaerobes or *Strep. pneumoniae,* which are common causes of community-acquired pneumonia. They should not be considered as effective single-drug therapy for any aerobic gram-positive cocci (including *Staph. aureus* or streptococci), the microorganisms commonly responsible for suppurative pneumonia or lung abscess. Thus, gentamicin (or other aminoglycosides) should never be used as the sole agent to treat pneumonia acquired in the community or as the initial treatment for pneumonia acquired in the hospital (Kunin, 1977).

Meningitis. Meningitis caused by gram-negative microorganisms presents a grave therapeutic problem. Development of the newer cephalosporins (especially cefuroxime, cefotaxime, and ceftriaxone) has reduced the need for treatment with aminoglycosides in most cases, except for rare isolates that are resistant to beta-lactam antibiotics (*e.g.,* species of *Pseudomonas* and *Acinetobacter*). If therapy with an aminoglycoside is necessary, it must usually be administered intrathecally. Rahal and associates (1974) have recommended parenteral administration of gentamicin in combination with intrathecal injection of 4 to 12 mg every 18 hours for 5 to 10 days. However, even this regimen is associated with a significant number of treatment failures, probably because of coexistent ventriculitis. In such instances, direct administration of gentamicin (or other aminoglycosides) into the cerebral ventricles with an Ommaya reservoir has been suggested. However, in one study children with gram-negative bacillary meningitis failed to show a beneficial effect from such treatment. (For discussion, *see* Kaiser and McGee, 1975).

Other Infections. Patients who develop peritonitis as a result of peritoneal dialysis may benefit from therapy with an aminoglycoside. Since suboptimal intraperitoneal concentrations of the antibiotic may follow intramuscular or intravenous administration in patients undergoing dialysis, the procedure should be continued with fluids containing an appropriate concentration of the aminoglycoside (*see* page 1104).

While there are very few indications for the use of aminoglycosides for gram-positive bacterial infections, it may at times be necessary and lifesaving. In cases of enterococcal endocarditis, up to 50% of isolates of enterococci are not killed by penicillin plus streptomycin; these strains are nearly always sensitive to penicillin plus gentamicin (page 1072). However, this is not revealed by testing for sensitivity to a standard dose of gentamicin.

When a patient has granulocytopenia and infection (sepsis) with *Pseud. aeruginosa* is suspected, the administration of an antipseudomonal penicillin in combination with gentamicin, tobramycin, amikacin, or netilmicin is recommended. Treatment of gram-negative bacillary sepsis, especially in neutropenic patients, has been improved by the use of such synergistic combinations (Klastersky, 1987).

TOBRAMYCIN

The antimicrobial activity and pharmacokinetic properties of tobramycin are very similar to those of gentamicin.

Preparations, Routes of Administration, and Dosage. *Tobramycin* (NEBCIN) is available as the sulfate salt for parenteral administration in solutions containing 40 mg/ml. A pediatric injection (10 mg/ml) is also available. Tobramycin may be given either intramuscularly or intravenously. Dosages are identical to those for gentamicin. When doses of 1 mg/kg are given intravenously or intramuscularly every 8 hours, peak concentrations in plasma are typically 5 to 8 μg/ml and minimal concentrations are 1 to 2 μg/ml. Toxicity is most common at minimal ("trough") concentrations that exceed 2 μg/ml for a prolonged period. The latter observation usually suggests impairment of renal function and requires reduction of dosage.

Tobramycin (TOBREX) is also available in ophthalmic ointments and solutions at concentrations of 3 mg/g or 3 mg/ml, respectively.

Untoward Effects. Tobramycin, like other aminoglycosides, causes both nephrotoxicity and ototoxicity, as discussed above. Studies in experimental animals suggest that tobramycin may be less toxic to hair cells in the cochlear and vestibular end organs and cause less renal tubular damage than does gentamicin (Symposium, 1976b). However, clinical data are less convincing.

Therapeutic Uses. Indications for the use of tobramycin are essentially identical to those for gentamicin. The superior activity of tobramycin against *Pseud. aeruginosa* may make it desirable in the treatment of bacteremia, osteomyelitis, and pneumonia caused by *Pseudomonas* species; it should usually be used concurrently with an antipseudomonal penicillin, aztreonam, or ceftazidime.

In contrast to gentamicin, tobramycin shows poor activity in combination with penicillin against enterococci; a large percentage of strains of *Enterococcus faecium* are highly resistant (Moellering *et al.,* 1979). Tobramycin is ineffective against mycobacteria, although most other aminoglycosides are active against these microorganisms (Gangadharam *et al.,* 1977).

AMIKACIN

The spectrum of antimicrobial activity of amikacin is the broadest of the group, and, because of its unique resistance to the aminoglycoside-inactivating enzymes, it has a special role in hospitals where gentamicin- and tobramycin-resistant microorganisms are prevalent. Amikacin is similar to kanamycin in dosage and pharmacokinetic properties.

Preparations, Routes of Administration, and Dosage. *Amikacin* (AMIKIN) is available as the sulfate in vials containing 100, 500, or 1000 mg of the drug. The recommended dose is 15 mg/kg per day, divided into two or three equal portions. The individual dose or the interval between doses must be altered in patients with renal failure. The drug is rapidly absorbed after intramuscular injection, and peak concentrations in plasma approximate 20 μg/ml after injection of 7.5 mg/kg. An intravenous infusion of the same dose over a 30-minute period produces a peak concentration in plasma of nearly 40 μg/ml at the end of the infusion; this falls to about 20 μg/ml 30 minutes later.

Untoward Effects. Like the other aminoglycosides, amikacin causes both ototoxicity and nephrotoxicity. Auditory deficits are most commonly produced, as discussed above.

Therapeutic Uses. Amikacin has become the preferred agent for initial treatment of serious nosocomial gram-negative bacillary infections in hospitals where resistance to gentamicin and tobramycin has become a significant problem. Some hospitals have restricted its use to avoid emergence of resistant strains, although some suggest that this is not likely (Betts *et al.*, 1984).

Because of its unique resistance to aminoglycoside-inactivating enzymes, amikacin is active against the vast majority of aerobic gram-negative bacilli in both the community and the hospital (Symposium, 1976a). This includes most strains of *Serratia, Proteus,* and *Pseud. aeruginosa*. It is active against nearly all strains of *Klebsiella, Enterobacter,* and *E. coli* that are resistant to gentamicin and tobramycin. Most resistance to amikacin is found among strains of *Acinetobacter, Providencia,* and *Flavobacter* and strains of *Pseudomonas* other than *Pseud. aeruginosa;* these are all unusual pathogens. While amikacin is not active against the majority of gram-positive anaerobic bacteria, it is effective against *Mycobacterium tuberculosis* (99% of strains inhibited by 4 μg/ml) and certain atypical mycobacteria (Gangadharam *et al.*, 1977).

NETILMICIN

Netilmicin is the latest of the aminoglycosides to be marketed. It is similar to gentamicin and tobramycin in its pharmacokinetic properties and dosage. Its antibacterial activity is broad against aerobic gram-negative bacilli; like amikacin, it is not metabolized by the majority of the aminoglycoside-inactivating enzymes, and it may be active against certain bacteria that are resistant to gentamicin.

Preparations, Routes of Administration, and Dosage. *Netilmicin* (NETROMYCIN) is available as the sulfate salt in vials containing 100 mg/ml; the drug may be given intravenously or intramuscularly.

The recommended dose of netilmicin for complicated urinary tract infections in adults is 1.5 to 2 mg/kg every 12 hours. For other serious systemic infections, a total daily dose of 4 to 6.5 mg/kg is divided into two or three portions. Children should receive 5.5 to 8 mg/kg per day in two to three divided doses; neonates receive 4 to 6.5 mg/kg per day in two divided doses. The distribution and elimination of netilmicin, gentamicin, and tobramycin are very similar. When given intramuscularly, peak concentrations of netilmicin in plasma approximate 5 μg/ml 30 to 60 minutes after a dose of 2 mg/kg (Humbert *et al.*, 1978). An intravenous infusion of the same dose, given over a 60-minute period, results in a peak plasma concentration of approximately 11 μg/ml (Luft *et al.*, 1978). The half-time for elimination is usually 2.0 to 2.5 hours in adults and increases with renal insufficiency.

Untoward Effects. Netilmicin may also produce ototoxicity and nephrotoxicity. Although studies in animals have suggested that netilmicin may be less toxic (Luft *et al.*, 1976), this remains to be proven in man (Trestman *et al.*, 1978; Bock *et al.*, 1980).

Therapeutic Uses. Netilmicin is a useful antibiotic for the treatment of serious infections due to susceptible Enterobacteriaceae and other aerobic gram-negative bacilli. It has been shown to be effective against certain gentamicin-resistant pathogens (Panwalker *et al.*, 1978).

KANAMYCIN

The use of kanamycin has declined markedly because its spectrum of activity is limited compared to those of other aminoglycosides.

Preparations, Routes of Administration, and Dosage. *Kanamycin sulfate* (KANTREX) is available as injections (250 or 333 mg/ml), a pediatric injection (75 mg/2 ml), and for oral use in capsules containing 500 mg. The parenteral dose for adults is 15 mg/kg per day (two to four equally divided and spaced doses) with a maximum of 1.5 g per day. Children may be given up to 15 mg/kg per day.

Untoward Effects. The untoward effects of the oral administration of aminoglycosides are considered under Neomycin, below.

Therapeutic Uses. There are few indications for the parenteral use of kanamycin. In the past, kanamycin was employed to treat tuberculosis in combination with other effective drugs. Since the therapy of this disease is protracted and involves the administration of large total doses of the drug, with the risk of ototoxicity and nephrotoxicity, kanamycin should be used only to treat patients who harbor microorganisms that are resistant to the more commonly used agents (*see* Chapter 49).

Prophylactic Uses. Kanamycin can be administered orally as adjunctive therapy in cases of hepatic coma. The rationale for such therapy is described under Neomycin (*see* below). The dose usually employed for these purposes is 6 to 8 g per day; quantities as large as 12 g per day have been given. The effect on intestinal bacteria may not be sustained even when such large doses of kanamycin are administered.

NEOMYCIN

Antibacterial Activity. Neomycin is a broad-spectrum antibiotic. Susceptible microorganisms are usually inhibited by concentrations of 5 to 10 μg/ml or less. Gram-negative species that are highly sensitive are *E. coli, Enterobacter aerogenes, Klebsiella pneumoniae,* and *Pr. vulgaris;* gram-positive microorganisms that are inhibited include *Staph. aureus* and *E. faecalis. M. tuberculosis* is also sensitive to neomycin. Strains of *Pseud. aeruginosa* are resistant to neomycin.

Preparations, Routes of Administration, and Dosage. *Neomycin sulfate* (MYCIFRADIN, MYCIGUENT) is available for topical and oral administration. Neomycin sulfate is marketed as 500-mg oral tablets, in an oral solution (125 mg/5 ml), and in dermatological ointments and creams. Ointments or creams contain 5 mg of neomycin sulfate per gram, and should be applied two or three times a day. *Neomycin and polymyxin B sulfates solution for irrigation* (NEOSPORIN G.U. IRRIGANT) contains 40 mg of neomycin and 200,000 units of polymyxin B per milliliter. One milliliter of this preparation is added to 1000 ml of 0.9% sodium chloride solution and is used for continuous irrigation of the urinary bladder through appropriate catheter systems. The goal is to prevent bacteriuria and bacteremia associated with the use of indwelling catheters. The bladder is usually irrigated at the rate of 1000 ml every 24 hours. Oral therapy with neomycin sulfate (usually in combination with erythromycin base) either for "preparation" of the bowel for surgery or for the management of hepatic coma requires the ingestion of 4 to 12 g daily, in divided doses.

Neomycin is presently available in many brands of creams, ointments, and other products both alone and in combination with polymyxin, bacitracin, other antibiotics, and a variety of corticosteroids. There is no evidence that these topical preparations shorten the time required for healing of wounds or that those containing a steroid are more effective.

Absorption and Excretion. Neomycin is poorly absorbed from the gastrointestinal tract and is excreted by the kidney, as are the other aminoglycosides. An oral dose of 3 g produces a peak plasma concentration of only 1 to 4 μg/ml; a total daily intake of 10 g for 3 days yields a blood concentration below that associated with systemic toxicity if renal function is normal. About 97% of an oral dose of neomycin escapes absorption and is eliminated unchanged in the feces. Although neomycin can be given orally to very young children, in doses as high as 100 mg/kg per day, its use in such patients for longer than 3 weeks should be avoided because of partial absorption from the intestinal tract, especially if it is the site of disease.

Untoward Effects. Hypersensitivity reactions, primarily skin rashes, occur in 6 to 8% of patients when neomycin is applied topically. Individuals sensitive to this agent may develop cross-reactions when exposed to other aminoglycosides. The most important toxic effects of neomycin are renal damage and nerve deafness. These were most frequent when relatively large quantities of the antibiotic were used parenterally and are the reason the drug is no longer used in this way. Toxicity has even occurred in patients with normal renal function following topical application or irrigation of wounds with 0.5% neomycin solution. Neuromuscular blockade with respiratory paralysis has also occurred after irrigation of wounds or serosal cavities.

The most important adverse effects resulting from the oral administration of neomycin are intestinal malabsorption and superinfection. Individuals treated with 4 to 6 g of the drug by mouth per day sometimes develop a spruelike syndrome with diarrhea, steatorrhea, and azotorrhea. The outstanding example of drug-induced malabsorption is that caused by neomycin. In man, the drug produces a moderate malabsorption syndrome for a variety of substances, including fat, protein, cholesterol, carotene, glucose, lactose, Na^+, Ca^{2+}, cyanocobalamin, and iron. This effect may be produced by as little as 3 g of the drug per day but is more marked with a dose of 12 g per day. Neomycin produces mild morphological changes of intestinal villi; precipitates bile salts within the lumen of the intestine; inhibits intraluminal hydrolysis of long-chain triglycerides, presumably by inhibition of pancreatic lipase activity; increases the fecal bile acid excretion, presumably by decreasing bile acid absorption; and reduces intestinal lactase activity. The antibiotic causes a marked decrease in plasma cholesterol concentrations and has been used therapeutically for this effect (*see* Chapter 36). The drug has been shown to produce intestinal crypt-cell necrosis, and, since cholesterol synthesis may occur at these sites, this may account for the effect. Overgrowth of yeasts in the intestine may also occur; this is not associated with diarrhea or other symptoms in most cases. The oral administration of even large doses of neomycin usually has no effect on blood levels of prothrombin.

Therapeutic Uses. Neomycin has been widely used for topical application in a variety of infections of the skin and mucous membranes caused by microorganisms susceptible to the drug. These include burns, wounds, ulcers, and infected dermatoses. However, such treatment does not eradicate bacteria from the lesions.

The oral administration of neomycin has been employed primarily for preparation of the bowel for surgery and as an adjunct to the therapy of hepatic coma. In a controlled study, concurrent administration of neomycin and erythromycin base to prepare the bowel for surgery was found to reduce the incidence of postoperative wound infections significantly (Clarke *et al.*, 1977).

While the importance of reducing the number of bacteria in the intestine in patients with hepatic coma has not been proven, general clinical experience suggests strongly that this may have an important role in producing a satisfactory outcome in this disease. Blood concentrations of ammonia are reduced during therapy. A daily dose of 4 to 12 g by mouth can be given without difficulty to such patients, provided renal function is normal. Because severe renal insufficiency may develop in the late stages of hepatic failure, treatment with neomycin must be followed with the greatest care and stopped if evidence of ototoxicity or further injury to the kidney appears.

Appel, G. B. Aminoglycoside nephrotoxicity: physiologic studies of the sites of nephron damage. In, *The Aminoglycosides: Microbiology, Clinical Use, and Toxicity.* (Whelton, A., and Neu, H. C., eds.) Marcel Dekker, Inc., New York, **1982,** pp. 269–282.

Appel, G. B., and Neu, H. C. Nephrotoxicity of antimicrobial agents. *N. Engl. J. Med.,* **1977,** *296,* 722–728.

Aronoff, G. R.; Pottratz, S. T.; Brier, M. E.; Walker, N. E.; Fineberg, N. S.; Glant, M. D.; and Luft, F. C. Aminoglycoside accumulation kinetics in rat renal parenchyma. *Antimicrob. Agents Chemother.,* **1983,** *23,* 74–78.

Barza, M. Factors affecting the intraocular penetration of antibiotics, the influence of route, inflammation, animal species, and tissue pigmentation. *Scand. J. Infect. Dis.,* **1978,** *14,* 151–159.

Barza, M.; Brown, R. B.; Shen, D.; Gibaldi, M.; and Weinstein, L. Predictability of blood levels of gentamicin in man. *J. Infect. Dis.,* **1975,** *132,* 165–174.

Baylis, C.; Rennke, H. R.; and Brenner, B. M. Mechanisms of the defect in glomerular ultrafiltration associated with gentamicin administration. *Kidney Int.,* **1977,** *12,* 344–353.

Bennett, W. M.; Elliott, W. C.; Houghton, D. C.; Gilbert, D. N.; DeFehr, J.; and McCarron, D. A. Reduction of experimental gentamicin nephrotoxicity in rats by dietary calcium loading. *Antimicrob. Agents Chemother.,* **1982,** *22,* 508–512.

Bergeron, M. G.; Bastille, A.; Lessard, C.; and Gagnon, P. M. Significance of intrarenal concentrations of gentamicin for the outcome of experimental pyelonephritis in rats. *J. Infect. Dis.,* **1982,** *146,* 91–96.

Betts, R. F.; Valenti, W. M.; Chapmen, S. W.; Chonmaitree, T.; Mowrer, G.; Pincus, P.; Messner, M.; and Robertson, R. Five-year surveillance of aminoglycoside usage in a university hospital. *Ann. Intern. Med.,* **1984,** *100,* 219–222.

Bisno, A. L., and others. Antimicrobial treatment of infective endocarditis due to viridans streptococci, enterococci, and staphylococci. *J.A.M.A.,* **1989,** *261,* 1471–1477.

Blair, D. C.; Duggan, D. O.; and Schroeder, E. T. Inactivation of amikacin and gentamicin by carbenicillin in patients with end-stage renal failure. *Antimicrob. Agents Chemother.,* **1982,** *22,* 376–379.

Bock, B. V.; Edelstein, P. H.; and Meyer, R. D. Prospective comparative study of efficacy and toxicity of netilmicin and amikacin. *Antimicrob. Agents Chemother.,* **1980,** *17,* 217–225.

Breen, K. J.; Bryant, R. E.; Levinson, J. D.; and Schenker, S. Neomycin absorption in man. *Ann. Intern. Med.,* **1972,** *76,* 211–218.

Brummett, R. Animal models of aminoglycoside antibiotic ototoxicity. *Rev. Infect. Dis.,* **1983,** *5,* Suppl. 2, S294–S303.

Brummett, R. E., and Fox, K. E. Studies of aminoglycoside ototoxicity in animal models. In, *The Aminoglycosides: Microbiology, Clinical Use, and Toxicity.* (Whelton, A., and Neu, H. C., eds.) Marcel Dekker, Inc., New York, **1982,** pp. 419–451.

Bryan, L. E. General mechanisms of resistance to antibiotics. *J. Antimicrob. Chemother.,* **1988,** *22,* Suppl. A, 1–15.

Bryan, L. E., and Kwan, S. Mechanisms of aminoglycoside resistance of anaerobic bacteria and facultative bacteria grown anaerobically. *J. Antimicrob. Chemother.,* **1981,** *8,* Suppl. D, 1–8.

———. Roles of ribosomal binding, membrane potential, and electron transport in bacterial uptake of streptomycin and gentamicin. *Antimicrob. Agents Chemother.,* **1983,** *23,* 835–845.

Clarke, J. S.; Condon, R. E.; Bartlett, J. G.; Gorbach, S. L.; Nichols, R. L.; and Ochi, S. Preoperative oral antibiotics reduce septic complications of colon operations: results of prospective, randomized, double-blind clinical study. *Ann. Surg.,* **1977,** *186,* 251–259.

Cox, C. E. Gentamicin. *Med. Clin. North Am.,* **1970,** *54,* 1305–1315.

Cross, A. S.; Opal, S.; and Kopecko, D. J. Progressive increase in antibiotic resistance of gram-negative bacterial isolates. *Arch. Intern. Med.,* **1983,** *143,* 2075–2080.

Cundlieffe, E. Methylation of RNA and resistance to antibiotics. In, *Microbial Resistance to Drugs.* (Bryan, L. E., ed.) Springer-Verlag, Berlin, **1989,** pp. 291–312.

Davies, B. D. The lethal action of aminoglycosides. *J. Antimicrob. Chemother.,* **1988,** *22,* 1–3.

Davies, B. D.; Brummett, R. E.; Bendrick, T. W.; and Himes, D. L. Dissociation of maximum concentration of kanamycin in plasma and perilymph from ototoxic effect. *J. Antimicrob. Chemother.,* **1984,** *14,* 291–302.

Eliopoulos, G. M.; Wennersten, C.; Zighelboim-Daum, S.; Reiszner, E.; Goldmann, D.; and Moellering, R. C., Jr. High-level resistance to gentamicin in clinical isolates of *Streptococcus* (enterococcus) *faecium. Antimicrob. Agents Chemother.,* **1988,** *32,* 1528–1532.

Evans, M. E.; Gregory, D. W.; Schaffner, W.; and McGee, Z. A. Tularemia: a 30-year experience with 88 cases. *Medicine,* **1985,** *64,* 251–269.

Fong, I. W.; Fenton, R. S.; and Bird, R. Comparative toxicity of gentamicin versus tobramycin: a randomized prospective study. *J. Antimicrob. Chemother.,* **1981,** *7,* 81–88.

Gangadharam, P. R. J.; Candler, E. R.; and Ramakrishna, P. V. *In vitro* anti-mycobacterial activity of some new aminoglycoside antibiotics. *J. Antimicrob. Chemother.,* **1977,** *3,* 285–286.

Gilbert, D. N. Mini-review: once-daily aminoglycoside therapy. *Antimicrob. Agents Chemother.,* **1990.** In Press.

Higgins, C. E., and Kastners, R. E. Nebramycin, a new broad-spectrum antibiotic complex. II. Description of *Streptomyces tenebrarius. Antimicrob. Agents Chemother.,* **1967,** *7,* 324–331.

Holtzman, J. L. Gentamicin neuromuscular blockade. *Ann. Intern. Med.,* **1976,** *84,* 55.

Hull, J. H., and Sarubbi, F. A., Jr. Gentamicin serum concentrations: pharmacokinetic predictions. *Ann. Intern. Med.,* **1976,** *85,* 183–189.

Humbert, G.; Leroy, A.; Fillastre, J. P.; and Oksenhendler, G. Pharmacokinetics of netilmicin in the presence of normal or impaired renal function. *Antimicrob. Agents Chemother.,* **1978,** *14,* 40–44.

Humes, H. D.; Sastrasinh, M.; and Weinberg, J. M. Calcium is a competitive inhibitor of gentamicin–renal membrane binding interactions, and dietary calcium supplementation protects against gentamicin nephrotoxicity. *J. Clin. Invest.,* **1984,** *73,* 134–147.

Hummel, H., and Böck, A. Ribosomal changes resulting in antibiotic resistance. In, *Microbial Resistance to Drugs*. (Bryan, L. E., ed.) *Handbook of Experimental Pharmacology*, Vol. 91. Springer-Verlag, Berlin, **1989**, pp. 235–262.

Huy, P. T. B.; Meulemans, A.; Wassef, M.; Manuel, C.; Sterkers, O.; and Amiel, C. Gentamicin persistence in rat endolymph and perilymph after a two-day constant infusion. *Antimicrob. Agents Chemother.*, **1983**, *23*, 344–346.

Kaiser, A. B., and McGee, Z. A. Aminoglycoside therapy of gram-negative bacillary meningitis. *N. Engl. J. Med.*, **1975**, *293*, 1215–1220.

Kapusnik, J. E.; Hackbarth, C. J.; Chambers, H. F.; Carpenter, T.; and Sande, M. A. Single, large, daily dosing versus intermittent dosing of tobramycin for treating experimental pseudomonas pneumonia. *J. Infect. Dis.*, **1988**, *158*, 7–12.

Karchmer, A. W.; Moellering, R. C.; Maki, D. G.; and Swartz, M. N. Single-antibiotic therapy for streptococcal endocarditis. *J.A.M.A.*, **1979**, *241*, 1801–1806.

Kawaguchi, H.; Naito, T.; Nakagowa, S.; and Fugijawa, K. BBK8, a new semisynthetic aminoglycoside antibiotic. *J. Antibiot.* (*Tokyo*), **1972**, *25*, 695.

Keating, M. J.; Bodey, G. P.; Valdivieso, M.; and Rodriguez, V. A randomized comparative trial of three aminoglycosides—comparison of continuous infusions of gentamicin, amikacin, and sisomicin combined with carbenicillin in the treatment of infections in neutropenic patients with malignancies. *Medicine* (*Baltimore*), **1979**, *58*, 159–170.

Keys, T. F.; Kurtz, S. B.; Jones, J. D.; and Muller, S. M. Renal toxicity during therapy with gentamicin or tobramycin. *Mayo Clin. Proc.*, **1981**, *56*, 556–559.

Klastersky, J.; Hensgens, C.; and Debusscher, L. Empiric therapy for cancer patients: comparative study of ticarcillin-tobramycin, ticarcillin-cephalothin, and cephalothin-tobramycin. *Antimicrob. Agents Chemother.*, **1975**, *7*, 640–645.

Konishi, H.; Goto, M.; Nakamoto, Y.; Yamamoto, I.; and Yamashina, H. Tobramycin inactivation by carbenicillin, ticarcillin, and piperacillin. *Antimicrob. Agents Chemother.*, **1983**, *23*, 653–657.

Kunin, C. M. Blunder drug for pneumonia. *N. Engl. J. Med.*, **1977**, *297*, 113–114.

Lerner, A. M.; Cone, L. A.; Jansen, W.; Reyes, M.; Blair, D. C.; Wright, G. E.; and Lorber, R. R. Randomized controlled trial of the comparative efficacy, auditory toxicity, and nephrotoxicity of tobramycin and netilmicin. *Lancet*, **1983**, *1*, 1123–1126.

Lesar, T. S.; Rotschafer, J. C.; Strand, L. M.; Solem, L. D.; and Zaske, D. E. Gentamicin dosing errors with four commonly used nomograms. *J.A.M.A.*, **1982**, *248*, 1190–1193.

Levy, J. Antibiotic activity in sputum. *J. Pediatr.*, **1986**, *108*, 841–846.

Lietman, P. S., and Smith, C. R. Aminoglycoside nephrotoxicity in humans, *J. Infect. Dis.*, **1983**, *5*, Suppl. 2, S284–S292.

Luft, F. C.; Brannon, D. R.; Stropes, L. L.; Costello, R. J.; Sloan, R. S.; and Maxwell, D. R. Pharmacokinetics of netilmicin in patients with renal impairment and in patients on dialysis. *Antimicrob. Agents Chemother.*, **1978**, *14*, 403–407.

Luft, F. C., and Evans, A. P. Comparative effects of tobramycin and gentamicin on glomerular ultrastructure. *J. Infect. Dis.*, **1980**, *142*, 910–914.

Luft, F. C.; Yum, M. N.; and Kleit, S. Comparative nephrotoxicities of netilmicin and gentamicin in rats. *Antimicrob. Agents Chemother.*, **1976**, *10*, 845–849.

Luzzatto, L.; Apirion, D.; and Schlessinger, D. Polyribosome depletion and blockage of the ribosome cycle by streptomycin in *Escherichia coli*. *J. Mol. Biol.*, **1969**, *42*, 315–335.

McCracken, G. H., Jr.; Mize, S. G.; and Threlkeld, N. Intraventricular gentamicin therapy in gram-negative bacillary meningitis of infancy. *Lancet*, **1980**, *1*, 787–791.

Mates, S. M.; Patel, L.; Kaback, H. R.; and Miller, M. H. Membrane potential in anaerobically growing *Staphylococcus aureus* and its relationship to gentamicin uptake. *Antimicrob. Agents Chemother.*, **1983**, *23*, 526–530.

Medical Letter. Safety of antimicrobial drugs in pregnancy. **1987**, *29*, 61–63.

Mitchell, C. J.; Bullocks, S.; and Ross, B. D. Renal handling of gentamicin and other antibiotics by the isolated perfused rat kidney: mechanism of nephrotoxicity. *Antimicrob. Agents Chemother.*, **1977**, *3*, 593–600.

Moellering, R. C. Microbiological considerations in the use of tobramycin and related aminoglycosidic aminocyclitol antibiotics. *Med. J. Aust.*, **1977**, *2*, Suppl., 4–8.

Moellering, R. C.; Korzeniowski, O. M.; Sande, M. A.; and Wennersten, C. B. Species-specific resistance to antimicrobial synergism among enterococci. *J. Infect. Dis.*, **1979**, *140*, 203–208.

Moore, R. D.; Smith, C. R.; and Lietman, P. S. Risk factors for the development of auditory toxicity in patients receiving aminoglycosides. *J. Infect. Dis.*, **1984a**, *149*, 23–30.

Moore, R. D.; Smith, C. R.; Lipsky, J. J.; Mellits, D.; and Lietman, P. S. Risk factors for nephrotoxicity in patients with aminoglycosides. *Ann. Intern. Med.*, **1984b**, *100*, 352–357.

Murray, B. E., and Mederski-Samaroj, B. Transferable beta-lactamase: a new mechanism for *in vitro* penicillin resistance in *Streptococcus faecalis*. *J. Clin. Invest.*, **1983**, *72*, 1168–1171.

Nakae, R., and Nakae, T. Diffusion of aminoglycoside antibiotics across the outer membrane of *Escherichia coli*. *Antimicrob. Agents Chemother.*, **1982**, *22*, 554–559.

Neu, H. C., and Bendush, C. L. Ototoxicity of tobramycin: a clinical overview. *J. Infect. Dis.*, **1976**, *134*, S206–S218.

Panwalker, A. P.; Malon, J. B.; Zimelis, V. M.; and Jackson, G. G. Netilmicin: clinical efficacy, tolerance, and toxicity. *Antimicrob. Agents Chemother.*, **1978**, *13*, 170–176.

Papapetropoulou, M.; Papavassiliou, J.; and Legakis, N. J. Effect of the pH and osmolality of urine on the antibacterial activity of gentamicin. *J. Antimicrob. Chemother.*, **1983**, *12*, 571–575.

Patel, V.; Luft, F. C.; Yum, M. N.; Patel, B.; Zeman, W.; and Kleit, S. H. Enzymuria in gentamicin-induced kidney damage. *Antimicrob. Agents Chemother.*, **1975**, *7*, 364–369.

Phillips, J. B.; Satterwhite, C.; Dworsky, M. E.; and Cassady, G. Recommended amikacin doses in newborns often produce excessive serum levels. *Pediatr. Pharmacol.* (*New York*), **1982**, *2*, 121–125.

Pickering, L. K., and Gearhart, P. Effect of time and concentration upon interaction between gentamicin, tobramycin, netilmicin, or amikacin and carbenicillin or ticarcillin. *Antimicrob. Agents Chemother.*, **1979**, *15*, 592–596.

Pittinger, C., and Adamson, R. Antibiotic blockade of neuromuscular function. *Annu. Rev. Pharmacol.*, **1972**, *12*, 169–184.

Pittinger, C. B.; Eryasa, Y.; and Adamson, R. Antibiotic-induced paralysis. *Anesth. Analg.*, **1970**, *49*, 487–501.

Powell, S. H.; Thompson, W. L.; Luthe, M. A.; Stern, R. C.; Grossniklaus, D. A.; Bloxham, D. D.; Groden, D. L.; Jacobs, M. R.; Discenna, A. O.; Cash, H. A.; and Klinger, J. D. Once-daily versus continuous aminoglycoside dosing: efficacy and toxicity in animal and clinical studies of gentamicin, netilmicin, and tobramycin. *J. Infect. Dis.*, **1983**, *147*, 918–932.

Quarum, M. L.; Houghton, D. C.; Gilbert, D. N.; McCarron, D. A.; and Bennett, W. M. Increasing dietary calcium moderates experimental gentamicin nephrotoxicity. *J. Lab. Clin. Med.*, **1984**, *103*, 104–114.

Queener, S. F.; Luft, F. C.; and Hamel, F. G. Effect of gentamicin treatment on adenylate cyclase and Na^+,K^+-ATPase activities in renal tissues of rats. *Antimicrob. Agents Chemother.*, **1983**, *24*, 815–818.

Rahal, J. J., Jr.; Hyams, P. S.; Simberkoff, M. S.; and Rubenstein, E. Intrathecal and intramuscular gentamicin for gram-negative meningitis: pharmacologic study of 21 patients. *N. Engl. J. Med.*, **1974**, *290*, 1394–1398.

Reiner, N. E.; Bloxham, D. D.; and Thompson, W. L. Nephrotoxicity of gentamicin and tobramycin given once daily or continuously in dogs. *J. Antimicrob. Chemother.*, **1978**, *4*, Suppl. A, 85–101.

Ronald, A. R.; Boutros, P.; and Mourtada, H. Bacteriuria localization and response to single-dose therapy in women. *J.A.M.A.*, **1976**, *235*, 1854–1856.

Rosenthal, A.; Button, L. N.; and Khaw, K. T. Blood volume changes in patients with cystic fibrosis. *Pediatrics*, **1977**, *59*, 588–594.

Rosselot, J. P.; Marquez, J.; Meseck, E.; Murawski, A.; Hamdan, A.; Joyner, C.; Schmidt, R.; Migliore, D.; and Herzog, H. L. Isolation, purification, and characterization of gentamicin. In, *Antimicrobial Agents and Chemotherapy—1963*. (Sylvester, J. C., ed.) American Society for Microbiology, Ann Arbor, Mich., **1964**, pp. 14–16.

Schentag, J. J.; Gengo, F. M.; Plant, M. E.; Danner, D.; Mangione, A.; and Jusko, W. J. Urinary casts as an indicator of renal tubular damage in patients receiving aminoglycosides. *Antimicrob. Agents Chemother.*, **1979**, *16*, 468–474.

Schentag, J. J., and Jusko, W. J. Renal clearance and tissue accumulation of gentamicin. *Clin. Pharmacol. Ther.*, **1977**, *22*, 364–370.

Siber, G. R.; Echeverria, P.; Smith, A. L.; Paisley, J. W.; and Smith, D. H. Pharmacokinetics of gentamicin in children and adults. *J. Infect. Dis.*, **1975**, *132*, 637–651.

Silverblatt, F. J. Pathogenesis of nephrotoxicity of cephalosporins and aminoglycosides: a review of current concepts. *Rev. Infect. Dis.*, **1982**, *4*, Suppl., S360–S365.

Singh, Y. N.; Harvey, A. L.; and Marshall, I. G. Antibiotic-induced paralysis of the mouse phrenic nerve—hemidiaphragm preparation and reversibility by calcium and by neostigmine. *Anesthesiology*, **1978**, *48*, 418–424.

Smith, C. R.; Baughman, K. L.; Edwards, C. Q.; Rogers, J. F.; and Lietman, P. S. Controlled comparison of amikacin and gentamicin. *N. Engl. J. Med.*, **1977**, *296*, 349–353.

Smith, C. R., and Lietman, P. S. Effect of furosemide on aminoglycoside-induced nephrotoxicity and auditory toxicity in humans. *Antimicrob. Agents Chemother.*, **1983**, *23*, 133–137.

Smith, C. R.; Lipsky, J. J.; Laskin, O. L.; Hellman, D. B.; Mellits, E. D.; Longstreth, J.; and Lietman, P. S. Double-blind comparison of the nephrotoxicity and auditory toxicity of gentamicin and tobramycin. *N. Engl. J. Med.*, **1980**, *302*, 1106–1109.

Smithivas, T.; Hyams, P. J.; Matalon, R.; Simberkoff, M. S.; and Rahal, J. J. The use of gentamicin in peritoneal dialysis. I. Pharmacologic results. *J. Infect. Dis.*, **1971**, *124*, Suppl., S77–S83.

Sokoll, M. D., and Gergis, S. D. Antibiotics and neuromuscular function. *Anesthesiology*, **1981**, *55*, 148–159.

Spyker, D. A.; Sande, M. A.; and Mandell, G. L. Tobramycin pharmacokinetics in patients with cystic fibrosis and leukemia. In, *Eighteenth Interscience Conference on Antimicrobial Agents and Chemotherapy*. American Society for Microbiology, Washington, D.C., **1978**, p. 345.

Stöffler, G., and Tischendorf, G. W. Antibiotic receptor-sites in *E. coli* ribosomes. In, *Drug Receptor Interactions in Antimicrobial Chemotherapy*. Vol. I, *Topics in Infectious Diseases*. (Drews, J., and Hahn, F. E., eds.) Springer-Verlag, New York, **1975**.

Strausbaugh, L. J.; Mandaleris, C. D.; and Sande, M. A. Comparison of four aminoglycoside antibiotics in the therapy of experimental *E. coli* meningitis. *J. Lab. Clin. Med.*, **1977**, *89*, 692–701.

Strausbaugh, L. J., and Sande, M. A. Factors influencing the therapy of experimental *Proteus mirabilis* meningitis. *J. Infect. Dis.*, **1978**, *137*, 251–260.

Sullam, P. M.; Slutkin, G.; Gottlieb, A. B.; and Mills, J. Paromomycin therapy of endemic amebiasis in homosexual men. *Sex. Transm. Dis.*, **1986**, *13*, 151–155.

Tai, P.-C.; Wallace, B. J.; and Davis, B. D. Streptomycin causes misreading of natural messenger by interacting with ribosomes after initiation. *Proc. Natl Acad. Sci. U.S.A.*, **1978**, *75*, 275–279.

Theopold, H. M. Comparative surface studies of ototoxic effects of various aminoglycoside antibiotics on the organ of Corti in the guinea pig. A scanning electron microscopic study. *Acta Otolaryngol. (Stockh.)*, **1977**, *84*, 57–64.

Trestman, I.; Parsons, J.; Santoro, J.; Goodhart, G.; and Kaye, D. Pharmacology and efficacy of netilmicin. *Antimicrob. Agents Chemother.*, **1978**, *13*, 832–836.

Varese, L. A.; Graziolo, F.; Viretto, A.; and Antoniola, P. Single-dose (bolus) therapy with gentamicin in management of urinary tract infection. *Int. J. Pediatr. Nephrol.*, **1980**, *1*, 104–105.

Wade, J. C.; Smith, C. R.; Petty, B. G.; Lipsky, J. J.; Conrad, G.; Ellner, J.; and Lietman, P. S. Cephalothin plus an aminoglycoside is more nephrotoxic than methicillin plus an aminoglycoside. *Lancet*, **1978**, *2*, 604–606.

Warkang, J. Antituberculous drugs. *Teratology*, **1979**, *20*, 133–138.

Wersäll, J.; Bjorkroth, B.; Flock, A.; and Lundquist, P.-G. Experiments on the ototoxic effects of antibiotics. *Adv. Otorhinolaryngol.*, **1973**, *20*, 14–41.

Wilson, P., and Ramsden, R. T. Immediate effects of tobramycin on human cochlea and correlation with serum tobramycin levels. *Br. Med. J.*, **1977**, *1*, 259–261.

Wilson, W. R.; Geraci, J. E.; Wilkowske, C. J.; and Washington, J. A., II. Short-term intramuscular therapy with procaine penicillin plus streptomycin for infective endocarditis due to *viridans* streptococci. *Circulation*, **1978**, *57*, 1158–1161.

Wilson, W. R.; Wilkowske, C. J.; Wright, A. J.; Sande, M. A.; and Geraci, J. E. Treatment of streptomycin-susceptible and streptomycin-resistant enterococcal endocarditis. *Ann. Intern. Med.*, **1984**, *100*, 816–823.

Wolfe, J. C., and Johnson, W. D., Jr. Penicillin-sensitive streptococcal endocarditis. *Ann. Intern. Med.*, **1974**, *81*, 178–181.

Woods, C. A.; Kohlhepp, S. J.; Houghton, D. C.; and Gilbert, D. N. Vancomycin enhancement of experimental tobramycin nephrotoxicity. *Antimicrob. Agents Chemother.*, **1986**, *30*, 20–24.

Woods, C. A.; Norton, D. R.; Kohlhepp, S. J.; Kohnen, P. W.; Porter, G. A.; Houghton, D. C.; Brummett, R. E.; Bennett, W. M.; and Gilbert, D. N. The influence of tobramycin dosage regimens on nephrotoxicity, ototoxicity, and antibacterial efficacy in a rat model of subcutaneous abscess. *J. Infect. Dis.*, **1988**, *158*, 13–22.

Yow, M. O. An overview of pediatric experience with amikacin. *Am. J. Med.*, **1977**, *62*, 954–958.

Zenilman, J. M.; Miller, M. H.; and Mandel, L. J. *In vitro* studies simultaneously examining effects of oxacillin on radiolabeled streptomycin and on associated bacterial lethality in *Staphylococcus aureus*. *Antimicrob. Agents Chemother.*, **1986**, *30*, 877–882.

Zervos, M. J.; Kaufman, C. A.; Therasse, P. M.; Bergman, A. G.; Mikesell, T. S.; and Schaberg, D. R. Nosocomial infection by gentamicin-resistant *Streptococcus faecalis*. *Ann. Intern. Med.*, **1987**, *106*, 687–691.

Monographs and Reviews

Alexander, D. P., and Gambertoglio, J. G. Drug overdose and pharmacologic considerations in dialysis. In,

Introduction to Dialysis. (Cogan, M. G., and Garovoy, M. R., eds.) Churchill Livingstone, Inc., New York, **1985**, pp. 261–292.

Bryan, L. E. Cytoplasmic membrane transport and antimicrobial resistance. In, *Microbial Resistance to Drugs*. (Bryan, L. E., ed.) *Handbook of Experimental Pharmacology*, Vol. 91. Springer-Verlag, Berlin, **1989**, pp. 35–57.

Klastersky, J. A. Fever in the compromised host. In, *Internal Medicine*, 2nd ed. (Stein, J. H., ed.) Little, Brown & Co., Boston, **1987**, pp. 1467–1472.

Kucers, A., and Bennett, N. McK. Gentamicin. In, *The Use of Antibiotics*, 4th ed. (Kucers, A., and Bennett, N. McK., eds.) J. B. Lippincott Co., Philadelphia, **1987**, pp. 619–674.

Lietman, P. S. Aminoglycosides and spectinomycin: aminocyclitols. In, *Principles and Practice of Infectious Diseases*, 3rd ed. (Mandell, G. L.; Douglas, R. G., Jr.; and Bennett, J. E.; eds.) Churchill Livingstone, Inc., New York, **1990**, pp. 269–284.

McCracken, G. H., Jr. New developments in the management of neonatal meningitis. In, *Contemporary Issues in Infectious Diseases*. Vol. 3, *Bacterial Meningitis*. (Sande, M. A.; Smith, A. L.; and Root, R. K.; eds.) Churchill Livingstone, Inc., New York, **1985**, pp. 159–166.

Mitsuhashi, S. (ed.). *Drug Action and Drug Resistance in Bacteria*. Vol. 2, *Aminoglycoside Antibiotics*. University Park Press, Baltimore, **1975**.

Price, K. E. Mini-review: aminoglycoside research 1975–1985: prospects for development of improved agents. *Antimicrob. Agents Chemother.*, **1986**, *29*, 543–548.

Sande, M. A. Infective endocarditis. In, *Internal Medicine*. (Stein, J. H., ed.) Little, Brown & Co., Boston, **1983**, pp. 537–547.

Shannon, K., and Phillips, I. Mechanisms of resistance to aminoglycosides in clinical isolates. *J. Antimicrob. Chemother.*, **1982**, *9*, 91–102.

Symposium. (Various authors.) Advances in aminoglycoside therapy: amikacin. *J. Infect. Dis.*, **1976a**, *134*, S235–S460.

Symposium. (Various authors.) Tobramycin. *J. Infect. Dis.*, **1976b**, *134*, S1–S234.

Waksman, S. A. (ed.). *Streptomycin, Nature, and Practical Applications*. The Williams & Wilkins Co., Baltimore, **1949**.

CHAPTER

48 ANTIMICROBIAL AGENTS

[*Continued*]

Tetracyclines, Chloramphenicol, Erythromycin, and Miscellaneous Antibacterial Agents

Merle A. Sande and Gerald L. Mandell

TETRACYCLINES

History. The development of the tetracycline antibiotics was the result of a systematic screening of soil specimens collected from many parts of the world for antibiotic-producing microorganisms. The first of these compounds, chlortetracycline, was introduced in 1948. Soon after their initial development, the tetracyclines were found to be highly effective against rickettsiae, a number of gram-positive and gram-negative bacteria, and the chlamydial species responsible for lymphogranuloma venereum, inclusion conjunctivitis, and psittacosis, and hence became known as "broad-spectrum" antibiotics. With establishment of their *in-vitro* antimicrobial activity, effectiveness in experimental infections, and pharmacological properties, the tetracyclines rapidly became widely used in therapy. (*See* Dowling, 1955; Lepper, 1956.)

Although there are specific and useful differences between the tetracyclines currently available in the United States, they are sufficiently similar to permit discussion of these drugs as a group.

Source and Chemistry. Chlortetracycline and oxytetracycline are elaborated by *Streptomyces aureofaciens* and *Strep. rimosus,* respectively. Tetracycline is produced semisynthetically from chlortetracycline; demeclocycline is the product of a mutant strain of *Strep. aureofaciens;* and methacycline, doxycycline, and minocycline are all semisynthetic derivatives.

The tetracyclines are closely congeneric derivatives of the polycyclic naphthacenecarboxamide. Their structural formulas are shown in Table 48–1.

Table 48–1. STRUCTURAL FORMULAS OF THE TETRACYCLINES

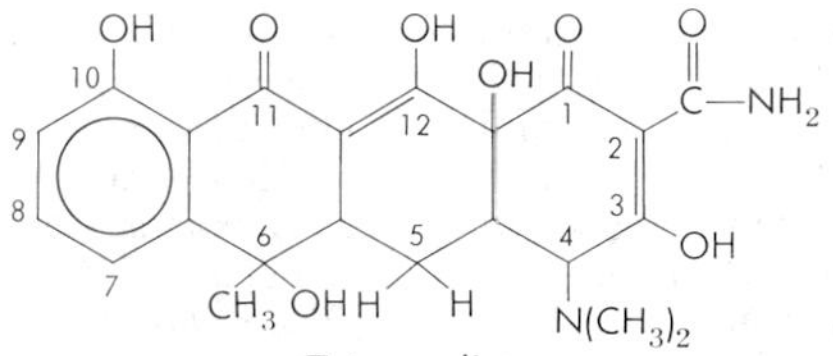

Tetracycline

CONGENER	SUBSTITUENT(S)	POSITION(S)
Chlortetracycline	—Cl	(7)
Oxytetracycline	—OH,—H	(5)
Demeclocycline	—OH,—H; —Cl	(6; 7)
Methacycline	—OH,—H; $=CH_2$	(5; 6)
Doxycycline	—OH,—H; $—CH_3$,—H	(5; 6)
Minocycline	—H,—H; $—N(CH_3)_2$	(6; 7)

Effects on Microorganisms. The tetracyclines possess a wide range of antimicrobial activity against gram-positive and gram-negative bacteria, which overlaps that of many other antimicrobial drugs. They are also effective against some microorganisms that are resistant to agents that exert their effects on the bacterial cell wall, such as *Rickettsia, Mycoplasma, Chlamydia* (the agents of urethritis, lymphogranuloma venereum, psittacosis, inclusion conjunctivitis, and trachoma), *Ureaplasma,* some atypical mycobacteria, and amebae. They have little activity against fungi.

In vitro, these drugs are primarily bacteriostatic. Only multiplying microorganisms are affected. The sensitivity or resistance of a particular microorganism to each of the congeners is similar. However, minocycline is usually the most active, followed by doxycycline. Tetracycline and oxytetracycline are the least active. Strains inhibited by 2 μg/ml or less of a tetracycline are considered sensitive.

Bacteria. In general, gram-positive microorganisms are affected by lower concentrations of tetracycline than are gram-negative species. However, these agents are rarely indicated for infections caused by gram-positive bacteria because of problems of resistance and the availability of superior antimicrobial agents. Most strains of group-B and group-D streptococci are not susceptible to tetracycline, while strains of *Staphylococcus aureus* remain mostly susceptible (Atkinson, 1986). Both tetracycline and doxycycline are quite active against most strains of pneumococci (minimal inhibitory concentration for 90% of strains [MIC 90] = 0.4 to

0.8 μg/ml). Although as many as 30% of pneumococcal strains have been found to be resistant in some geographical areas, the prevalence of such resistance to tetracyclines is low in most regions (Neu, 1978).

Neisseria gonorrhoeae and many strains of *N. meningitidis* are inhibited by tetracyclines (MIC 90 = 1 to 2 μg/ml), but resistance may develop if a tetracycline is used as sole therapy for gonorrhea (Knapp *et al.*, 1987).

Although the tetracyclines were initially useful for treatment of infections with aerobic gram-negative bacilli, many species are now relatively resistant. However, more than 90% of strains of *Haemophilus influenzae* may still be sensitive to either tetracycline or doxycycline (Ringertz and Dornbusch, 1988). Although all strains of *Pseudomonas aeruginosa* are resistant, 90% of strains of *Pseud. pseudomallei* (the cause of melioidosis) are sensitive. Nearly 80% of strains of *Campylobacter* are sensitive, but clinical studies demonstrating efficacy have not been reported. Most strains of *Brucella* are also susceptible. Tetracyclines are particularly useful for infections caused by *H. ducreyi* (chancroid), *Brucella*, and *Vibrio cholerae*. These drugs also inhibit the growth of *Yersinia pestis* (plague), *Y. enterocolitica, Francisella tularensis* (tularemia), and *Pasteurella multocida*. The tetracyclines are active against many anaerobic and facultative microorganisms, and their activity against *Actinomyces* is particularly relevant. A variable number of anaerobic bacteria are sensitive to doxycycline, the most active congener of tetracycline. Only 40 to 50% of strains of *Bacteroides fragilis* are inhibited by 2 μg/ml of doxycycline or tetracycline. Tetracyclines are much less active against *B. fragilis* than is chloramphenicol, clindamycin, metronidazole, or certain beta-lactam antibiotics, and these agents have replaced the tetracyclines for the therapy of most anaerobic infections (Sanford, 1989).

Rickettsiae. Like chloramphenicol, all the tetracyclines are highly effective against the rickettsiae responsible for Rocky Mountain spotted fever, murine typhus, epidemic typhus, scrub typhus, rickettsialpox, and Q fever.

Miscellaneous Microorganisms. The tetracyclines are active against many spirochetes, including *Borrelia recurrentis, Bor. burgdorferi* (Lyme disease), *Treponema pallidum* (syphilis), and *T. pertenue*. The activity of tetracyclines against *Chlamydia* and *Mycoplasma* has become particularly relevant. Strains of *Mycobacterium marinum* are also susceptible.

Effects on Intestinal Flora. Since many of the tetracyclines are incompletely absorbed from the gastrointestinal tract, high concentrations are reached in the intestinal contents. Within 48 hours after daily administration of conventional doses of these agents, the enteric flora is markedly altered. Many aerobic and anaerobic coliform microorganisms and gram-positive spore-forming bacteria are sensitive and may be markedly suppressed during long-term medication regimens before resistant strains reappear. The stools become softer and odorless and acquire a yellow-green color. However, as the fecal coliform count declines, tetracycline-resistant microorganisms, particularly yeasts, enterococci, *Proteus*, and *Pseudomonas*, overgrow and the total fecal microbial count may actually increase. Tetracycline occasionally produces so-called antibiotic-associated colitis (pseudomembranous colitis). Normal intestinal flora is restored several days after antibiotic medication is withdrawn.

Mechanism of Action. Tetracyclines inhibit bacterial protein synthesis. Their site of action is the bacterial ribosome, but at least two processes appear to be required for these antibiotics to gain access to the ribosomes of gram-negative bacteria (Chopra and Howe, 1978). The first is passive diffusion through the hydrophilic channels formed by the porin proteins in the outer cell membrane. Minocycline and perhaps doxycycline are more lipophilic than the other congeners and pass directly through the lipid bilayer. The second process involves an energy-dependent active transport system that pumps all tetracyclines through the inner cytoplasmic membrane. Such transport may require a periplasmic protein carrier. Although permeation of these drugs into gram-positive bacteria is less well understood, it too requires an energy-dependent system. Once the tetracyclines gain access to the bacterial cell, they bind principally to the 30 S subunits of bacterial ribosomes. They appear to prevent access of aminoacyl tRNA to the acceptor site on the mRNA–ribosome complex. This prevents the addition of amino acids to the growing peptide chain. Only a small portion of the drug is irreversibly bound, and the inhibitory effects of the tetracyclines are reversible when the drug is removed. At high concentrations, these compounds also impair protein synthesis in mammalian cells; however, the host cells lack the active transport system found in bacteria. Differences in sensitivity at the ribosomal level are also presumed to be important determinants of the selective action of tetracyclines. Tetracyclines, even in subinhibitory concentrations, have been shown to reduce the ability of *Escherichia coli* to adhere to mammalian epithelial cells *in vitro*. The details of the extensive studies in this field have been reviewed by Pratt and Fekety (1986).

Resistance to the Tetracyclines. Resistance to the tetracyclines produced *in vitro* appears slowly in a graded, stepwise fashion similar to that observed with penicillin. Microorganisms that have become resistant to one tetracycline frequently exhibit resistance to the others. Resistance to the tetracyclines in *E. coli* and probably in other bacterial species is mediated by plasmids and is an inducible trait; that is, the bacteria become resistant only after exposure to the drug. A number of transferable resistance determinants for tetracycline have been identified (Park *et al.*, 1987), and at least two mechanisms of resistance have been detected. Many resistant microorganisms display decreased accumulation of tetracycline as a result of either decreased influx of the antibiotic or the acquisition of an energy-dependent efflux pathway; a decreased effect of tetracycline on the ribosome may also be evident.

Absorption, Distribution, and Excretion. *Absorption.* Most of the tetracyclines are adequately but incompletely absorbed from the gastrointestinal tract. The percentage of an oral dose that is absorbed (when the stomach is empty) is lowest for chlortetracycline (30%); intermediate for oxytetracycline, demeclocycline, and tetracycline (60 to 80%); and high for doxycycline (95%) and minocycline (100%) (Barza and Scheife, 1977). The percentage that is not absorbed rises as the dose increases. Most absorption takes place from the stomach and upper small intestine and is greater in the fasting state; it is much less complete from the lower portions of the intestinal tract. Absorption of tetracyclines is impaired by the concurrent ingestion of dairy products; aluminum hydroxide gels; calcium, magnesium, and iron salts; and bismuth subsalicylate (Ericsson *et al.,* 1982). The mechanism responsible for the decreased absorption appears to be chelation of divalent and trivalent cations.

The wide range of plasma concentrations present in different individuals following the oral administration of the various tetracyclines is related in large measure to the irregularity of their absorption from the gastrointestinal tract. These drugs can be divided into three groups based on the dosage and frequency of oral administration required to produce effective plasma concentrations.

Oxytetracycline and tetracycline are incompletely absorbed. After a single oral dose peak plasma concentrations are attained in 2 to 4 hours. These drugs have half-lives in the range of 6 to 12 hours, and they are frequently administered two to four times daily. The administration of 250 mg every 6 hours produces peak plasma concentrations of 2 to 2.5 μg/ml. Increasing the dosage above 1 g every 6 hours does not produce significantly higher concentrations of the drugs in plasma.

Demeclocycline and methacycline are usually administered in lower daily dosages than are the above-mentioned congeners. Their absorption is also incomplete, but their half-lives are about 16 hours and effective plasma concentrations may thus persist for 24 to 48 hours. This is particularly true for demeclocycline. Poor absorption of methacycline may lead to lower plasma concentrations than with recommended doses of tetracycline, despite the difference in half-life. The peak concentration of methacycline is approximately 2 μg/ml after an oral dose of 500 mg.

Doxycycline and minocycline should be administered in even lower daily dosages by the oral route, since their half-lives are long (16 to 18 hours) and they are well absorbed. After an oral dose of 200 mg of doxycycline, plasma concentrations of the drug reach a maximum of 3 μg/ml at 2 hours and are maintained above 1 μg/ml for 8 to 12 hours. Plasma concentrations are equivalent when doxycycline is given by the oral or parenteral route. Food does not interfere with the absorption of doxycycline or minocycline.

Distribution. The apparent volume of distribution of many of the tetracyclines is larger than that of the body water. They are bound to plasma proteins in varying degrees. The approximate values are as follows: doxycycline, 80 to 95%; demeclocycline, 65 to 90%; methacycline, about 80%; minocycline, about 75%; tetracycline, about 65%; and oxytetracycline, 20 to 40%. However, the values reported in the literature are highly variable (*see* Appendix II).

All the tetracyclines are concentrated in the liver and excreted, by way of the bile, into the intestine, from which they are partially reabsorbed. Decreased hepatic function or obstruction of the common bile duct results in reduction in the biliary excretion of these agents and their consequent persistence in the blood. Because of their enterohepatic circulation, the tetracyclines may be present in the blood for a long time after cessation of therapy.

Inflammation of the meninges is not a prerequisite for the passage of tetracyclines into the cerebrospinal fluid (CSF); route and duration of treatment are major determinants. The intravenous injection of a tetracycline results in the gradual appearance of the drug in the spinal fluid over a period of 6 hours. Oral dosage yields very low concentrations in spinal fluid.

Penetration of these drugs into most other fluids and tissues is excellent. Concentrations in synovial fluid and the mucosa of the maxillary sinus approach that of plasma. Minocycline reaches a concentration in tears and saliva sufficient to eradicate the meningococcal carrier state; this characteristic is unique to minocycline among the tetracyclines and has been attributed to its greater lipid solubility. The tetracyclines are stored in the reticuloendothelial cells of the liver, spleen, and bone marrow, and in bone and the dentine and enamel of unerupted teeth (*see* below). Tetracyclines cross the placenta and enter the fetal circulation and amniotic fluid. Concentrations of tetracycline in umbilical-cord plasma reach 60% and in amniotic fluid 20% of those in the circulation of the mother. Relatively high concentrations of these drugs are also found in breast milk.

Excretion. All the tetracyclines are excreted in the urine and the feces; the primary route for most is the kidney. Since renal clearance of these drugs is by glomerular filtration, their excretion is significantly affected by the state of renal function (*see* below). Twenty to sixty percent of an intravenous dose of 0.5 g of tetracycline is excreted in the urine during the first 24 hours; from 20 to 55% of an oral dose is excreted by this route. Ten to thirty-five percent of a dose of oxytetracycline is excreted in active form in the urine, in which it is detectable within 30 minutes and reaches a peak concentration about 5 hours after it is administered. The rate of renal clearance of demeclocycline is less than half that of tetracycline. About 50% of methacycline is excreted unchanged in the urine.

Minocycline is recoverable from both urine and feces in significantly lower amounts than are the other tetracyclines, and it appears to be metabolized to a considerable extent. Renal clearance of minocycline is low. The drug persists in the body after its administration is stopped; this may be due to retention in fatty tissues. The half-life of minocycline is apparently not prolonged in patients with hepatic failure.

An important distinction should be made in the case of doxycycline. It is clear that, with conventional doses, doxycycline is not eliminated via the same pathways as are other tetracyclines, and it does not accumulate significantly in the blood of patients with renal failure. It is thus one of the safest of the tetracyclines for the treatment of extrarenal infections in such individuals. The drug is excreted in the feces, largely as an inactive conjugate or perhaps as a chelate; for this reason it has relatively less impact on the intestinal microflora (Nord and Heimdahl, 1988). The half-life of doxycycline may be shortened from approximately 16 to 7 hours in patients who are receiving long-term treatment with barbiturates or phenytoin.

As mentioned, the intestine is an important avenue of elimination of the tetracyclines. Because these agents are incompletely absorbed from the bowel when given orally or when excreted into the intestine in the bile, they are present in varying concentrations in the feces. Elimination from the intestinal tract occurs even when the drugs are given parenterally, as a result of excretion in the bile.

Preparations, Routes of Administration, and Dosage. *Oxytetracycline* (TERRAMYCIN, others), *tetracycline* (ACHROMYCIN, others), *demeclocycline* (DECLOMYCIN), *methacycline* (RONDOMYCIN), *doxycycline* (VIBRAMYCIN, others), and *minocycline* (MINOCIN) are available in a wide variety of forms for oral, topical, and parenteral administration.

The tetracyclines are usually prescribed for oral use, but most may be administered by intravenous injection. Topical administration is best avoided because of the high risk of sensitization, except for use in the eye. The tetracyclines should never be injected intrathecally, and they are rarely given intramuscularly.

Preparations for Oral Administration. All the tetracyclines listed above are available for oral administration, usually as capsules and occasionally in tablet form, in appropriate single doses ranging from 50 to 500 mg, depending on the preparation. Some of the tetracyclines are also marketed as oral suspensions, flavored powders for oral suspension, and syrups for pediatric use.

The oral dose of the tetracyclines varies with the nature and the severity of the disease. For tetracycline and oxytetracycline, it ranges from 1 to 2 g per day in adults. Children over 8 years of age should receive 25 to 50 mg/kg daily in two to four divided doses. The recommended doses of demeclocycline and methacycline are somewhat lower, being 150 mg every 6 hours or 300 mg every 12 hours for adults. The daily doses for children over 8 years of age are 6 to 12 mg/kg in two to four divided portions. The dose of doxycycline for adults is 100 mg every 12 hours during the first 24 hours, followed by 100 mg once a day, or twice daily when severe infection is present. Children over 8 years of age should receive 4 to 5 mg/kg per day, divided into two equal doses given at a 12-hour interval during the first day, after which a single daily dose of half this amount is administered; in serious disease, the same quantity is given every 12 hours. The dose of minocycline for adults is 200 mg initially, followed by 100 mg every 12 hours; for children it is 4 mg/kg initially, followed by 2 mg/kg every 12 hours.

Because the incidence of gastrointestinal distress and particularly of tetracycline-resistant bacterial enteritis rises as the dose of the antibiotic is increased, the minimal dose compatible with the desired therapeutic response is recommended. Gastrointestinal distress, nausea, and vomiting can be minimized by administration of the tetracyclines with food (but not dairy products). Milk, antacids containing aluminum or magnesium hydroxide or silicate, and bismuth subsalicylate interfere with the absorption of the drugs and should not be ingested at the same time as is a tetracycline.

Preparations for Parenteral Administration. Injectable preparations of oxytetracycline, tetracycline, doxycycline, and minocycline are designed for intravenous use, while preparations of tetracycline and oxytetracycline for intramuscular injection are also available. Preparations designed for intramuscular injection contain a local anesthetic.

Intravenous administration of the tetracyclines can be used in severe illness in which an appropriately large dose may cause nausea and vomiting if given orally, in patients unable to ingest medication, and when the response to oral therapy is inadequate. However, it should be emphasized that there are currently very few indications for intravenous administration of these drugs, since better alternatives are usually available; thrombophlebitis is also a problem (*see* below). The total daily intravenous dose of oxytetracycline or tetracycline for most acute infections is 500 mg to 1 g, usually administered in two equal portions at 12-hour intervals. Up to 2 g per day may be given in severe infections, but this dose may cause difficulty in some patients (*see* below); quantities larger than 2 g per day must not be given parenterally. The recommended daily intravenous dose for children over 8 years of age is 10 to 20 mg/kg of body weight. Because of local irritation and poor absorption, intramuscular administration of these tetracyclines is generally unsatisfactory and is rarely indicated. The usual intravenous dose of doxycycline is 200 mg in one or two infusions on the first day and 100 to 200 mg on subsequent days. The dose for children who weigh less than 45 kg is 4.4 mg/kg on the first day, and this is then reduced correspondingly. The intravenous dose of minocycline for adults is 200 mg, followed by 100 mg every 12 hours. Children over 8 years of age should receive an initial dose of 4 mg/kg, followed by 2 mg/kg every 12 hours.

Preparations for Local Application. Except for local use in the eye, topical use of the tetracyclines is not recommended. Ophthalmic preparations include *chlortetracycline hydrochloride ophthalmic ointment, tetracycline hydrochloride ophthalmic ointment,* and *tetracycline hydrochloride ophthalmic suspension.* One or two drops are instilled in the conjunctival sac two to six times daily, or more. The usual concentration of a tetracycline for ophthalmic use is 1%.

UNTOWARD EFFECTS

Toxic Effects. *Gastrointestinal.* The tetracyclines all produce gastrointestinal irritation to varying degrees in some but not all individuals; such effects are more common after oral administration of the drugs. Epigastric burning and distress, abdominal discomfort, nausea, and vomiting may occur. The larger the dose, the greater is the likelihood of an irritative reaction. If troublesome, gastric distress can be controlled by administration of the tetracyclines with food (not dairy products). Nausea and vomiting often subside as medication continues and can often be controlled by temporary reduction in dose or by the use of smaller amounts at more frequent intervals. Esophagitis and esophageal ulcers have been reported (Winckler, 1981; Amendola and Spera, 1985), as has an association with pancreatitis (Elmore and Rogge, 1981). Diarrhea may also result from the irritative effects of the tetracyclines given orally; although frequent and fluid, the stools do not contain blood or leukocytes. *It is imperative that this type of diarrhea be promptly distinguished from that which results from pseudomembranous colitis caused by overgrowth of* Clostridium difficile, *a potentially life-threatening complication* (*see* below).

Phototoxicity. Demeclocycline, doxycycline, and, to a lesser extent, other derivatives may produce mild-to-severe reactions in the skin of treated individuals exposed to sunlight; this phenomenon is a phototoxic reaction, and it may be found in 1 to 2% of patients treated with demeclocycline. Onycholysis and pigmentation of the nails may develop simultaneously.

Hepatic Toxicity. Hepatic toxicity due to tetracycline was first observed by Lepper in 1951 in patients receiving large doses of tetracycline orally or intravenously. Microscopic study of the liver reveals cytoplasmic changes, such as the appearance of small vacuoles, and an increase in fat (Zimmerman and Lewis, 1984). Oxytetracycline and tetracycline appear to be less hepatotoxic than are the other drugs of this group. Most reactions of this type develop in patients receiving 2 g or more of drug per day parenterally; however, this effect may also occur when large quantities are administered orally. Pregnant women appear to be particularly susceptible to severe, tetracycline-induced hepatic damage. Jaundice appears first, and azotemia, acidosis, and irreversible shock may follow. The liver is diffusely infiltrated with fat; although hepatic fat is increased during pregnancy, the quantity appears to be even greater after exposure to a tetracycline.

Renal Toxicity. Tetracyclines may aggravate uremia in patients with renal disease by inhibiting protein synthesis and provoking a catabolic effect; azotemia is thereby increased from metabolism of amino acids (Shils, 1963). Doxycycline has been reported to produce fewer renal side effects than do other tetracyclines; however, a possible association between this drug and the production of renal failure has been suggested (Orr *et al.,* 1978). Nephrogenic diabetes insipidus has been observed in some patients receiving demeclocycline, and this phenomenon has been exploited for the treatment of chronic, inappropriate secretion of antidiuretic hormone (Forrest *et al.*, 1978; *see* Chapter 29).

A clinical picture characterized by nausea, vomiting, polyuria, polydipsia, proteinuria, acidosis, glycosuria, and gross aminoaciduria—a form of the Fanconi syndrome—has been observed in patients ingesting outdated and degraded tetracycline because of a toxic effect on proximal renal tubules.

Effects on Calcified Tissues. Children receiving long- or short-term therapy with a tetracycline may develop brown discoloration of the teeth. The larger the dose of drug relative to body weight, the more intense the discoloration of enamel. The duration of therapy appears to be less important than the total quantity of antibiotic administered. The risk of this untoward effect is highest when the tetracycline is given to neonates and babies prior to the first dentition. However, pigmentation of the permanent dentition may develop if the drug is given between the ages of 2 months and 5 years, when these teeth are being calcified. An early characteristic of this defect is a yellow fluorescence of the dental pigment, which has an ultraviolet spectrum with an absorption peak at 270 nm. The deposition of the drug in the teeth and bones is probably due to its chelating property and the formation of a tetracycline–calcium orthophosphate complex. As time progresses, the yellow fluorescence is replaced by a nonfluorescent brown color that may represent an oxidation product of the antibiotic, the formation of which is hastened by light. This discoloration is permanent.

Treatment of pregnant patients with tetracyclines may produce discoloration of the teeth in their children. The period of greatest danger to the teeth is from midpregnancy to about 4 to 6 months of the postnatal period for the deciduous anterior teeth, and from a few months to 5 years of age for the permanent anterior teeth, the periods when the crowns of the teeth are being formed. However, children up to 8 years old may be susceptible to this complication of tetracycline therapy.

Tetracyclines are deposited in the skeleton during gestation and throughout childhood. A 40% depression of bone growth, as determined by measurement of fibulas, has been demonstrated in premature infants treated with these agents (Cohlan *et al.*, 1963). This is readily reversible if the period of exposure to the drug is short.

Miscellaneous Effects. The intravenous administration of the tetracyclines is frequently followed by thrombophlebitis, especially when a single vein is used for repeated infusion. The highly irritative effects of these agents are emphasized by the severe pain that they produce when injected intramuscularly without a local anesthetic.

Long-term therapy with tetracyclines may produce changes in the peripheral blood. Leukocytosis, atypical lymphocytes, toxic granulation of granulocytes, and thrombocytopenic purpura have been observed.

The tetracyclines may cause increased intracranial pressure and tense bulging of the fontanels (pseudotumor cerebri) in young infants, even when given in the usual therapeutic doses. Except for the elevated pressure, the spinal fluid is normal. Discontinuation of therapy results in prompt return of the pressure to normal. This complication may occur rarely in older individuals (Walters and Gubbay, 1981).

Patients receiving minocycline may experience vestibular toxicity, manifested by dizziness, ataxia, nausea, and vomiting. The symptoms occur soon after the initial dose and generally disappear within 24 to 48 hours after drug administration is stopped. The frequency of this side effect is directly related to the dose and has been noted more often in women than in men (Fanning *et al.*, 1977).

Hypersensitivity Reactions. Various skin reactions, including morbilliform rashes, urticaria, fixed drug eruptions, and generalized exfoliative dermatitis, may follow the use of any of the tetracyclines, but they are rare. Among the more severe allergic responses are angioedema and anaphylaxis; anaphylactoid reactions can occur even after the oral use of these agents. Other effects that have been attributed to hypersensitivity are burning of the eyes, cheilosis, atrophic or hypertrophic glossitis, pruritus ani or vulvae, and vaginitis; these effects often persist for weeks or months after cessation of tetracycline therapy. The exact cause of these reactions is unknown. Fever of varying degrees and eosinophilia may occur when these agents are administered. Asthma has also been observed.

It should be emphasized that cross-sensitization among the various tetracyclines is common.

Biological Effects Other Than Allergic or Toxic. Like all antimicrobial agents, the tetracyclines administered orally or parenterally may lead to the development of superinfections that are usually due to strains of bacteria or yeasts resistant to these agents. Vaginal, oral, pharyngeal, and even systemic infections with yeasts and fungi are observed. The incidence of these infections appears to be much higher with the tetracyclines than with the penicillins.

Among the most important superinfections associated with the administration of the tetracyclines are those that involve the intestinal tract; they may occur with either oral or parenteral therapy. The possibility that drug-induced diarrhea may be due to active infection of the bowel merits serious consideration in every instance.

Pseudomembranous colitis is characterized by severe diarrhea, fever, and stools containing shreds of mucous membrane and a large number of neutrophils. It has been attributed to the overgrowth of toxin-producing bacteria (*Clostridium difficile*). The toxin is cytotoxic to mucosal cells and causes shallow ulcerations that can be seen by sigmoidoscopy. Discontinuation of the drug, combined in some instances with the oral administration of metronidazole or vancomycin, is usually curative, but relapses do occur (Lyerly *et al.*, 1988).

To decrease the incidence of toxic effects, the following precautions should be observed in the use of the tetracyclines. They should not be given to pregnant patients; they should not be employed for treatment of the common infections in children under the age of 8 years, and unused supplies of these antibiotics should be discarded.

THERAPEUTIC USES

The tetracyclines have been used extensively both for the treatment of infectious diseases and as an additive to animal feeds to facilitate growth. Both uses have resulted in increasing bacterial resistance to these drugs. Because of this and the development of new, less toxic antimicrobial agents that are more effective for specific infections, the number of indications for the use of tetracyclines has declined. These agents are especially useful in diseases caused by *Rickettsia, Mycoplasma,* and *Chlamydia*. The status of the tetracyclines for the therapy of various infections is given in Table 44–1.

Rickettsial Infections. The tetracyclines and chloramphenicol are effective and may be lifesaving in rickettsial infections, including Rocky Mountain spotted fever, recrudescent epidemic typhus (Brill's disease), murine typhus, scrub typhus, rickettsialpox, and Q fever. Fever usually subsides in 1 to 3 days, and the rash disappears in 3 to 5 days; striking clinical improvement is often evident within 24 hours after initiation of therapy.

Mycoplasma Infections. *Mycoplasma pneumoniae* is sensitive to the tetracyclines. Treatment of pneumonia with either tetracycline or erythromycin results in a shorter duration of fever, cough, malaise, fatigue, pulmonary rales, and radiological changes in the lungs. Mycoplasma may persist in the sputum following cessation of therapy, despite rapid resolution of the active infection.

Chlamydia. *Lymphogranuloma Venereum.* The tetracyclines are currently the treatment of choice in this infection. Tetracycline should be given in oral doses of 500 mg four times a day for at least 2 weeks; longer treatment may be required in more chronic cases. Doxycycline, 100 mg orally twice daily for 2 weeks, may be as effective but has not been extensively studied. Decided reduction in the size of buboes is observed within 4 days, and inclusion and elementary bodies entirely disappear from the lymph nodes within 1 week. Lymphogranulomatous proctitis is promptly improved. Rectal pain, discharge, and bleeding are markedly decreased. When relapses occur, treatment is resumed with full doses and is continued for longer periods.

Chlamydia pneumoniae is a newly described infectious agent that causes pneumonia. While erythromycin may be an alternative to tetracycline for treatment, tetracycline should probably be used for recurrent infections.

Psittacosis. The tetracyclines are also of value in cases of psittacosis. Drug therapy for 12 to 14 days is usually adequate.

Inclusion Conjunctivitis. This disease responds clinically to topical administration of a tetracycline (doxycycline), in ointment or liquid form, four times a day for 3 weeks. However, this treatment does not always eradicate the microorganisms. Systemic therapy with tetracycline or a sulfonamide for 3 weeks is preferred in adults. In infants, erythromycin has been used systemically, but experience with it is limited (Bowie and Holmes, 1985).

Trachoma. Although the sulfonamides are preferred by some for the treatment of trachoma, the tetracyclines have proven very effective. While topical therapy has been used, oral administration of an antimicrobial agent is now recommended. The most effective regimen has been doxycycline given once daily for 40 days in a dose of 2.5 to 4 mg/kg (Hoshiwara *et al.*, 1973).

Nonspecific Urethritis. Nonspecific urethritis is thought in most instances to be caused by *Chlamydia trachomatis*. This microorganism is sensitive to tetracycline; oral administration of 500 mg of tetracycline every 6 hours or 100 mg of doxycycline every 12 hours for 7 days is recommended.

Sexually Transmitted Diseases. Although penicillin G is still useful for the treatment of gonorrhea in some geographic areas, it cannot be used in some patients because of hypersensitivity and it is not recommended in regions where there is a high prevalence (> 1.0%) of penicillinase-producing strains of *N. gonorrhoeae*. Tetracycline given orally every 6 hours for 7 days (or doxycycline, 100 mg orally twice daily for 7 days) is usually effective for uncomplicated gonococcal infections. However, resistance of *N. gonorrhoeae* to tetracycline has now emerged, especially in areas where this drug has been used as the sole therapy (Knapp *et al.*, 1987). Tetracycline may still be useful in treating disseminated gonococcal infections, gonococcal salpingitis (pelvic inflammatory disease), and epididymitis in men less than 35 years of age in regions where resistance to tetracycline is not prevalent. However, ceftriaxone has emerged as the drug of choice for gonorrhea in many areas (*see Medical Letter,* 1988; Chapter 46). A tetracycline should also be administered empirically to treat coexistent infection with *Chl. trachomatis,* which is present in up to 45% of women and 25% of heterosexual men with gonorrhea (Centers for Disease Control, 1985). A diagnosis of gonorrhea has become an indication to treat chlamydia as well.

Tetracyclines have been used for treatment of syphilis in patients unable to tolerate beta-lactam antibiotics. A dose of 500 mg of tetracycline given every 6 hours for 15 days is recommended for early syphilis (less than 1 year's duration), but therapy should be continued for 30 days if the disease has been present for longer than 1 year. Erythromycin should be used for treatment of pregnant women who are allergic to beta-lactam antibiotics. Tetracyclines are also effective in chancroid and granuloma inguinale, but their use in these diseases entails the risk of masking a syphilitic infection that may have been contracted at the same time. If they are employed, the dose and duration of treatment should be the same as those used to treat syphilis.

Endocervical or rectal infections caused by *Chlamydia* should be treated with either tetracycline, 500 mg orally four times daily for 7 days, or doxycycline, 100 mg twice daily for 7 days. When disease occurs in pregnant women, erythromycin, 500 mg orally four times daily for 7 days, should be used. *Chlamydia* is commonly a coexistent pathogen in acute pelvic inflammatory disease (endometritis, salpingitis, parametritis, and/or peritonitis), and doxycycline, 100 mg intravenously twice daily, is recommended for at least 4 days or 48 hours after defervescence, followed by oral therapy at the same dosage to complete a 10-day course. Doxycycline is usually combined with cefoxitin (2 g intravenously four times daily) to cover microorganisms that may be resistant to doxycycline (anaerobes, facultative aerobes, and some strains of penicillinase-producing *N. gonorrhoeae*). Acute epididymo-orchitis is caused by either *Chl. trachomatis* or *N. gonorrhoeae* in men less than 35 years of age. Effective regimens include a single injection of ceftriaxone (250 mg) plus either tetracycline, 500 mg orally four times daily for at least 10 days, or doxycycline, 100 mg orally twice daily for at least 10 days. Sexual partners of patients with any of the above conditions should also be treated.

Bacillary Infections. *Brucellosis.* Treatment with the tetracyclines is effective for infections caused by *Brucella melitensis, suis,* and *abortus.* Both acute and chronic forms of the disease respond dramatically. Combination therapy with doxycycline, 200 mg, plus rifampin, 600 to 900 mg, daily for 6 weeks is currently recommended by the World Health Organization for the treatment of acute brucellosis (World Health Organization, 1986). Good results have also been obtained with full doses of a tetracycline for 3 weeks. Clinical and bacteriological relapses are not the result of the development of resistant strains of *Brucella* and usually respond to a second course of therapy. The combination of a tetracycline given with streptomycin (1 g daily, intramuscularly) has also provided prompt results in patients severely ill with acute brucellosis.

Tularemia. Although streptomycin is preferable, treatment with the tetracyclines also produces prompt results in tularemia (Evans *et al.*, 1985). Both the ulceroglandular and typhoidal types of the disease respond well. Fever, toxemia, and clinical signs and symptoms are all improved; the bacteria rapidly disappear from blood, sputum, and pleural fluid; and complications are usually prevented.

Cholera. In a controlled trial of the effects of oral antibiotics in the management of cholera in children in Pakistan, Lindebaum and associates (1967) found that tetracycline was the most effective of the agents studied in reducing stool volume, intravenous fluid requirement, and the duration of diarrhea and positive stool cultures. Only 1% of the children given tetracycline had diarrhea for more than 4 days. Treatment with tetracycline was significantly more effective than intravenous fluid therapy alone, regardless of the severity of the disease. When oral drug therapy was given for only 48 hours, bacteriological relapse developed in 20% of the cases despite a good clinical response. It must be emphasized that antimicrobial agents are not substitutes for fluid and electrolyte replacement in this disease. The effectiveness of tetracycline as a prophylactic agent in families of cholera patients was demonstrated by McCormack and coworkers (1968). They noted that the administration of the drug for 5 days was effective in preventing infection in contacts.

Other Bacillary Infections. Therapy with the tetracyclines is not uniformly effective in infections caused by *Shigella, Salmonella,* or other Enterobacteriaceae. Doxycycline has been used successfully to reduce the incidence of traveler's diarrhea, especially that caused by enterotoxin-producing strains of *E. coli* (Sack *et al.*, 1978). Emergence of resistant strains and the potential for an increased incidence of salmonellosis will likely limit the usefulness of this approach.

Coccal Infections. The tetracyclines are no longer indicated for infections caused by staphylococci, streptococci, or meningococci. Although minocycline (given in a dose of 100 mg every 12 hours for 5 days) has been found to prevent the development of meningococcal disease and to lower the carrier rate, its use for this purpose is not recommended because of the vestibular disturbances that this drug can cause (*see* above).

Urinary Tract Infections. The usefulness of tetracyclines for urinary tract infections has also been reduced appreciably by the increase in the number of drug-resistant microorganisms. As a rule, these drugs are not active against *Proteus* and *Pseud. aeruginosa*. Treatment of urinary tract infections with a tetracycline should be undertaken only if the infecting strain is sensitive. Treatment is usually continued for 7 to 10 days. For severe acute pyelonephritis, tetracyclines should be used only in the unlikely event that no other antimicrobial agent is effective. The acute urethral syndrome in women has been effectively treated with doxycycline (100 mg twice daily for 10 days) (Stamm *et al.*, 1981). While doxycycline may be given to patients with renal dysfunction, the drug concentration in the urine may not be sufficient for treatment of urinary tract infections.

Other Infections. Actinomycosis, although most responsive to penicillin G, may be successfully treated with a tetracycline; in severe infections, intravenous therapy for 1 week, followed by oral administration of drug for a month or more, may be required. Minocycline has been suggested for the treatment of nocardiosis, but a sulfonamide should be used concurrently. Yaws and relapsing fever respond favorably to the tetracyclines and penicillin (Salih and Mustafa, 1977). Although either tetracycline or penicillin G is used to treat leptospirosis, evidence of efficacy is not convincing with these or any other antimicrobial agent. Lyme disease, caused by *Bor. burgdorferi,* is characterized by fever, skin lesions, arthritis, and aseptic meningitis. It responds to either penicillin G or a tetracycline, although tetracycline has been observed to be ineffective in advanced *Bor. burgdorferi* infection (Dattwyler *et al.*, 1987). The tetracyclines have been used to treat atypical mycobacterial diseases, including those caused by *Mycobacterium marinum* (Izumi *et al.*, 1977).

Intestinal Disease. Patients with Whipple's disease may respond to tetracycline, although relapses may occur more frequently than after therapy with penicillin G. The administration of tetracycline to some patients with tropical sprue may be associated with repletion of folate, a favorable hematological response, decrease in diarrhea, improvement in the enzymatic activity and morphology of the superficial epithelium of the jejunal mucosa, gain in weight, and reversal of the abnormal pattern of lipid distribution. Tetracyclines may also be of value in the blind-loop syndrome.

Acne. Tetracyclines have been used for the treatment of acne, and good results have been reported by some investigators. Benefit has been produced by small doses. It has been suggested that these drugs may act by inhibiting propionibacteria, which reside in sebaceous follicles and metabolize lipids into irritating free fatty acids. Although it is generally accepted that the tetracyclines or other antibiotics have a beneficial effect in acne, some placebo crossover studies raise doubt concerning the value of this kind of therapy. Use of tetracycline seems to be associated with few side effects when given in doses of 250 mg orally twice a day.

CHLORAMPHENICOL

History and Source. Chloramphenicol is an antibiotic produced by *Streptomyces venezuelae,* an organism first isolated in 1947 from a soil sample collected in Venezuela (Bartz, 1948). When the relatively simple structure of the crystalline material was determined, the antibiotic was prepared synthetically. Late in 1947, the small amount of available chloramphenicol was employed in an outbreak of epidemic typhus in Bolivia, with dramatic results. It was then tried with excellent success in cases of scrub typhus on the Malay peninsula. By 1948, chloramphenicol was produced in amounts sufficient for general clinical use. By 1950, however, it became evident that the drug could cause serious and fatal blood dyscrasias. For this reason, use of the drug is reserved for certain patients with serious infections, such as meningitis, typhus, and typhoid fever; it is also a first-line agent for Rocky Mountain spotted fever. An awareness of its activity against anaerobic bacteria, especially *B. fragilis,* has resulted in an increased use of chloramphenicol in recent years (Cuchural *et al.*, 1988).

Chemistry. Chloramphenicol has the following structural formula:

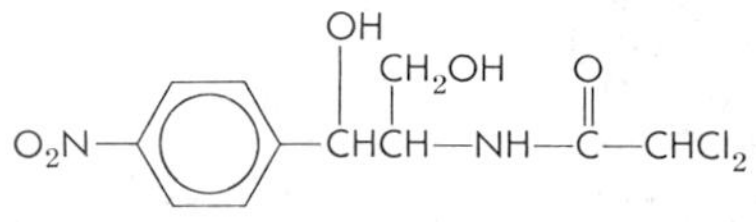

Chloramphenicol

The antibiotic is unique among natural compounds in that it contains a nitrobenzene moiety and is a derivative of dichloroacetic acid. The biologically active form is levorotatory.

Mechanism of Action. Chloramphenicol inhibits protein synthesis in bacteria and, to a lesser extent, in eukaryotic cells. The drug readily penetrates into bacterial cells, probably by a process of facilitated diffusion. Chloramphenicol acts primarily by binding reversibly to the 50 S ribosomal subunit (near the site of action of the macrolide antibiotics and clindamycin, which it inhibits competitively). Although binding of tRNA at the codon recognition site on the 30 S ribosomal subunit is thus undisturbed, the drug appears to prevent the binding of the amino acid–containing end of aminoacyl tRNA to the acceptor site on the 50 S ribosomal subunit. The interaction between peptidyl transferase and its amino acid substrate cannot occur, and peptide bond formation is inhibited (*see* Pratt and Fekety, 1986).

Chloramphenicol can also inhibit mitochondrial protein synthesis in mammalian cells, perhaps because mitochondrial ribosomes resemble bacterial ribosomes (both are 70 S) more than they do the 80 S cytoplasmic ribosomes of mammalian cells. The peptidyl transferase of bovine mitochondrial ribosomes, but not cytoplasmic ribosomes, is susceptible to the inhibitory action of chloramphenicol. Mammalian erythropoietic cells seem to be particularly sensitive to the drug.

Effects on Microbial Agents. Chloramphenicol possesses a fairly wide spectrum of antimicrobial activity. Strains are considered sensitive if they are inhibited by concentrations of 12.5 μg/ml or less. It is primarily bacteriostatic, although it may be bactericidal to certain species, such as *H. influenzae*. More than 95% of strains of the following gram-negative bacteria are inhibited *in vitro* by 8.0 μg/ml or less of chloramphenicol: *H. influenzae, N. meningitidis, N. gonorrhoeae, Salmonella typhi, Brucella* species, and *Bordetella pertussis*. Likewise, most anaerobic bacteria, including gram-positive cocci and *Clostridium* species and gram-negative rods including *B. fragilis*, are inhibited by this concentration of the drug. Some aerobic gram-positive cocci, including *Strep. pyogenes, Strep. agalactiae* (group-B streptococci), and *Strep. pneumoniae*, are sensitive to 8 μg/ml, while fourfold higher concentrations are required to inhibit more than 95% of strains of *Staph. aureus* (Standiford, 1990).

The Enterobacteriaceae have a variable sensitivity to chloramphenicol. Although 95% of strains of *E. coli* are inhibited by 12.5 μg/ml, only 75% of *Klebsiella pneumoniae*, 50% of *Enterobacter*, and 33% of *Serratia marcescens* are inhibited. Ninety percent of strains of *Proteus mirabilis* are inhibited by 12.5 μg/ml. All strains of *Pseud. pseudomallei* are inhibited by this concentration; however, *Pseud. aeruginosa* is resistant to even very high concentrations of chloramphenicol. Eighty-four percent of *V. cholerae* are inhibited by 6.3 μg/ml, as are 90% of *Shigella*. Chloramphenicol exerts marked prophylactic and therapeutic effects in experimental infections produced by all rickettsiae. The drug, as a rule, only suppresses rickettsial growth. Chloramphenicol is also effective against *Chlamydia* and *Mycoplasma*.

Resistance to Chloramphenicol. The resistance of gram-positive and gram-negative microorganisms to chloramphenicol *in vivo* is a problem of increasing clinical importance. Resistance of gram-negative bacteria to the drug is usually caused by a plasmid acquired by conjugation and is due to the presence of a specific acetyltransferase that inactivates the drug. At least three types of enzyme have been characterized (Gaffney and Foster, 1978). Acetylated derivatives of chloramphenicol fail to bind to bacterial ribosomes (Piffaretti and Froment, 1978). Strains of *H. influenzae* that are resistant to chloramphenicol contain plasmids that code not only for the production of acetyltransferase, but also invariably for resistance to tetracyclines; they may also code for a beta-lactamase that mediates resistance to ampicillin (Doern *et al.*, 1988). Plasmid-mediated resistance to chloramphenicol in *S. typhi* emerged as a significant problem during the epidemic of 1972–1973 in Mexico and the United States (Baine *et al.*, 1977). However, the prevalence of resistance of *S. typhi* to chloramphenicol is negligible today, except in some areas of Southeast Asia (Ling *et al.*, 1988). The prevalence of resistance of staphylococci to this antibiotic has also increased; it varies from one hospital to another and is as high as 50% or more in some. Resistant strains of *Staph. aureus* contain one of several related forms of chloramphenicol acetyltransferase that are inducible (Sands and Shaw, 1973). Although loss of sensitivity to chloramphenicol is usually due to acetylation of the drug, both decreased permeability of the microorganisms (which has been found in *E. coli* and *Pseudomonas*) and mutation to ribosomal insensitivity have also been described (Sompolinsky and Samra, 1968; Baughman and Fahnestock, 1979).

Absorption, Distribution, Fate, and Excretion. Chloramphenicol is available for oral administration in two dosage forms: the active drug itself and the inactive prodrug, chloramphenicol palmitate (which is used to prepare an oral suspension). Hydrolysis of the ester bond of chloramphenicol palmitate is accomplished rapidly and almost completely by pancreatic lipases in the duodenum under normal physiological conditions (Kauffman *et al.*, 1981). Chloramphenicol is then absorbed from the gastrointestinal tract, and peak concentrations of 10 to 13 μg/ml occur within 2 to 3 hours after the administration of a 1-g dose. In patients with gastrointestinal disease or in newborns, the bioavailability is greater for chloramphenicol than for chloramphenicol palmitate, probably due to the incomplete hydrolysis of the latter (Smith and Weber, 1983). The preparation of chloramphenicol for parenteral use is the water-soluble, inactive sodium succinate preparation. Absorption after intramuscular injection was previously thought to be highly unpredictable; however, a more recent study demonstrated comparable concentrations of chloramphenicol succinate in plasma after intravenous and intramuscular administration (Shann *et al.*, 1985). It is unclear where the hydrolysis of chloramphenicol succinate occurs *in vivo*, but esterases of the liver, kidneys, and lungs may all be involved. Chloramphenicol succinate itself is rapidly cleared from plasma by the kidneys. This renal clearance of the prodrug may affect the overall bioavailability of chloramphenicol, because excretion of up to 20 to 30% of the dose may occur prior to hydrolysis. Poor renal function in the neonate and other states of renal insufficiency result in increased plasma concentrations of chloramphenicol succinate and of chloramphenicol (Slaughter *et al.*, 1980b; Mulhall *et al.*, 1983). Decreased esterase activity has been observed in the plasma of neonates and infants. This results in a prolonged period to reach peak concentrations of active chloramphenicol (up to 4 hours) and a longer period over which renal clearance of chloramphenicol succinate can occur (Kauffman *et al.*, 1981).

Chloramphenicol is well distributed in body fluids and readily reaches therapeutic concentrations in CSF, where values are approximately 60% of those in plasma (range, 45 to 99%) in the presence or absence of meningitis (Friedman *et al.*, 1979). The drug may actually accumulate in brain tissue (Kramer *et al.*, 1969). Chloramphenicol is present in bile, is secreted into milk, and readily traverses the placental barrier. It also penetrates into the aqueous humor after subconjunctival injection.

The major route of elimination of chloramphenicol is hepatic metabolism to the inactive glucuronide. This metabolite, as well as chloramphenicol itself, is excreted in the urine by filtration and secretion. Over a 24-hour period, 75 to 90% of an orally administered dose is so excreted; about 5 to 10% is in the biologically active form. Patients with hepatic cirrhosis have decreased metabolic clearance, and dosage should be adjusted in these individuals. The half-life of chloramphenicol has been correlated with plasma bilirubin concentrations (Koup *et al.*, 1979). About 50% of chloramphenicol is bound to plasma proteins; such binding is reduced in cirrhotic patients and in neonates (*see* Appendix II). The half-life of the active drug (4 hours) is not significantly changed in patients with renal failure as compared with those with normal renal function. Full doses of chloramphenicol must still be given to achieve therapeutic concentrations of the active drug in uremia. The extent to which hemodialysis removes chloramphenicol from plasma does not appear to be sufficient to warrant adjustment of dosage (Blouin *et al.*, 1980). However, when patients undergoing dialysis have other complications, such as cirrhosis, the clearance due to dialysis may become important. In such cases it may be best to administer the maintenance dose at the end of hemodialysis to minimize this effect (Slaughter *et al.*, 1980a). The variability in the metabolism and pharmacokinetic parameters of chloramphenicol in neonates, infants, and children necessitates monitoring of drug concentrations in plasma, especially when phenobarbital, phenytoin, or rifampin are administered concomitantly (McCracken *et al.*, 1987).

Preparations, Routes of Administration, and Dosage. *Chloramphenicol* (CHLOROMYCETIN) is marketed in capsules containing 250 and 500 mg for oral use. *Chloramphenicol palmitate* is a water-insoluble powder; 1.7 g of this preparation is equivalent to 1 g of chloramphenicol base. *Chloramphenicol palmitate oral suspension* contains an amount of chloramphenicol palmitate equivalent to 150 mg of chloramphenicol base, mixed with suitable dispersing and flavoring agents, in each 5 ml. *Chloramphenicol sodium succinate* is marketed as the dry powder; it is intended for solution for intravenous use.

Chloramphenicol may be administered orally or intravenously. Dosage schedules for the therapy of specific infections are presented below. Adjustment in dose must be made when chloramphenicol palmitate is used, as indicated above.

Untoward Effects. Chloramphenicol inhibits the synthesis of proteins of the inner mitochondrial membrane that are synthesized within mitochondria, probably by inhibition of the ribosomal peptidyl transferase. These include subunits of cytochrome *c* oxidase, ubiquinone-cytochrome *c* reductase, and the proton-translocating ATPase. Much of the toxicity observed with this drug can be attributed to these effects (Smith and Weber, 1983).

Hypersensitivity Reactions. Although relatively uncommon, macular or vesicular skin rashes occur as a result of hypersensitivity to chloramphenicol. Fever may appear simultaneously or be the sole manifestation. Angioedema is a rare complication. Herxheimer reactions have been observed shortly after institution of chloramphenicol therapy for syphilis, brucellosis, and typhoid fever.

Hematological Toxicity. The most important adverse effect of chloramphenicol is on the bone marrow; of all the drugs that may be responsible for pancytopenia, chloramphenicol is the most common cause (Wallerstein *et al.*, 1969). Changes in peripheral blood include leukopenia, thrombocytopenia, and aplasia of the marrow with fatal pancytopenia. These reactions are thought to be idiosyncratic. The incidence is not related to dose; however, it seems to occur more commonly in individuals who undergo prolonged therapy and especially in those who are exposed to the drug on more than one occasion. A genetic predisposition is suggested by the occurrence of pancytopenia in identical twins. Although the incidence of the reaction is low, 1 in approximately 30,000 or more courses of therapy, the fatality rate is high when bone-marrow aplasia is complete, and there is a higher risk of acute leukemia in those who recover (Shu *et al.*, 1987).

A compilation of 576 cases of blood dyscrasia due to chloramphenicol indicates that aplastic anemia was the most common type reported, accounting for about 70% of the cases; hypoplastic anemia, agranulocytosis, thrombocytopenia, and bone-marrow inhibition made up the remainder. Among the patients with pancytopenia the outcome was apparently unrelated to the dose of chloramphenicol taken. However, the longer the interval between the last dose of chloramphenicol and the appearance of the first sign of the blood dyscrasia, the greater was the mortality rate; nearly all patients in whom this interval was longer than 2 months died.

Holt (1967) noted the absence of reported instances of aplastic anemia following parenteral administration of chloramphenicol and suggested that absorption of a toxic breakdown product from the gastrointestinal tract might be responsible. Subsequently, a few cases of aplastic anemia have been described in patients who received parenteral chloramphenicol. However, some of these patients had also received other drugs known to affect the bone marrow (phenylbutazone and glutethimide). The issue thus remains unsettled (Kucers and Bennett, 1987). The structural feature of chloramphenicol that is responsible for aplastic anemia is hypothesized to be the nitro group, which might be metabolized by intestinal bacteria to a toxic intermediate (Jimenez *et al.*, 1987). However, the exact biochemical mechanism has not yet been elucidated.

The risk of aplastic anemia does not contraindicate the use of chloramphenicol in situations in which it is necessary; however, it emphasizes that the drug should never be employed in undefined situations or in diseases readily, safely, and effectively treatable with other antimicrobial agents.

A second hematological effect of chloramphenicol is a common and predictable (but reversible) erythroid suppression of the bone marrow that is probably due to its inhibitory action on mitochondrial protein synthesis. A result is a reduction of uptake of ^{59}Fe by normoblasts and of the incorporation of this isotope into heme (Ward, 1966). The clinical picture is marked initially by reticulocytopenia, which occurs 5 to 7 days after the initiation of therapy, followed by a decrease in hemoglobin, an increase in plasma iron, cytoplasmic vacuolation of early erythroid forms and and granulocyte precursors, and normoblastosis with a shift to early erythrocyte forms (Scott *et al.*, 1965). Leukopenia and thrombocytopenia may also occur. The incidence and severity of this syndrome are related to dose. It occurs regularly when plasma concentrations are 25 μg/ml or higher and is observed during the use of large doses of chloramphenicol, prolonged treatment with the antibiotic, or both. Dose-related suppression of the bone marrow has been reported to progress to fatal aplasia, but this does not occur predictably (Daum *et al.*, 1979).

The administration of chloramphenicol in the presence of hepatic disease frequently results in depression of erythropoiesis; this is most intense when ascites and jaundice are present (Suhrland and Weisberger, 1963). About one third of patients with severe renal insufficiency exhibit the same reaction.

Toxic and Irritative Effects. Nausea, vomiting, unpleasant taste, diarrhea, and perineal irritation may follow the oral administration of chloramphenicol. Among the rare toxic effects produced by this antibiotic are blurring of vision and digital paresthesias. Optic neuritis occurs in 3 to 5% of children with mucoviscidosis who are given chloramphenicol; there is symmetrical loss of ganglion cells from the retina and atrophy of the fibers in the optic nerve (Godel *et al.*, 1980).

Fatal chloramphenicol toxicity may develop in neonates, especially premature babies, when they are exposed to excessive doses of the drug. The illness, the "gray syndrome," usually begins 2 to 9 days (average, 4 days) after treatment is started. The manifestations in the first 24 hours are vomiting, refusal to suck, irregular and rapid respiration, abdominal distention, periods of cyanosis, and passage of loose, green stools. All the children are severely ill by the end of the first day and, in the next 24 hours, become flaccid, turn an ashen-gray color, and become hypothermic. Metabolic acidosis has been observed as an early sign of the gray syndrome, especially in patients with liver disease (Evans and Kleiman, 1986). Potentially reversible alterations in myocardial function have also been noted (Fripp *et al.,* 1983). Death occurs in about 40% of patients. Those who recover usually exhibit no sequelae.

Two mechanisms are apparently responsible for this toxic effect in neonates (Craft *et al.,* 1974): (1) failure of the drug to be conjugated with glucuronic acid, due to inadequate activity of glucuronyl transferase in the liver, which is characteristic of the first 3 to 4 weeks of life; and (2) inadequate renal excretion of unconjugated drug in the newborn. At the time of onset of the clinical syndrome, the chloramphenicol concentrations in plasma usually exceed 100 μg/ml, although they may be as low as 75 μg/ml. Excessive plasma concentrations of the glucuronide conjugate are also present, despite its low rate of formation, because tubular secretion, the pathway of excretion of this compound, is underdeveloped in the neonate. Children 2 weeks of age or younger should receive chloramphenicol in a daily dose no larger than 25 mg/kg of body weight; after this age, full-term infants may be given daily quantities up to 50 mg/kg. Toxic effects have not been observed in the newborn when as much as 1 g of the antibiotic has been given every 2 hours to women in labor.

Chloramphenicol is removed from the blood to only a very small extent by either peritoneal dialysis or hemodialysis. However, both exchange transfusion and charcoal hemoperfusion have been used to treat overdose with chloramphenicol in infants (Freundlich *et al.,* 1983).

Other organ systems that have a high rate of oxygen consumption may also be affected by the action of chloramphenicol on mitochondrial enzyme systems; encephalopathic changes have been observed (Levine *et al.,* 1970), and cardiomyopathy has also been reported (Biancaniello *et al.,* 1981).

Drug Interactions. Chloramphenicol irreversibly inhibits hepatic microsomal enzymes of the cytochrome P_{450} complex (Halpert, 1982), and thus may prolong the half-life of drugs that are metabolized by this system. Such drugs include dicumarol, phenytoin, chlorpropamide, and tolbutamide. Severe toxicity and death have occurred because of failure to recognize such effects. The inhibitory effect of chloramphenicol on hepatic enzymes may protect the liver from the toxic effects of carbon tetrachloride, since metabolism is apparently necessary to convert carbon tetrachloride to toxic products.

Conversely, other drugs may alter the elimination of chloramphenicol. Chronic administration of phenobarbital or acute administration of rifampin shortens the half-life of the antibiotic, presumably because of enzyme induction, and may result in subtherapeutic concentrations of the drug (Powell *et al.,* 1981; Prober, 1985).

Therapeutic Uses. *Therapy with chloramphenicol must be limited to infections for which the benefits of the drug outweigh the risks of the potential toxicities. When other antimicrobial drugs are available that are equally effective but potentially less toxic than chloramphenicol, they should be used* (*see* Kucers and Bennett, 1987; Standiford, 1990).

Typhoid Fever. Although chloramphenicol is still an important drug for the treatment of typhoid fever and other types of systemic salmonella infections, other drugs are also effective. Epidemics in some parts of the world have been due to strains of *S. typhi* highly resistant to chloramphenicol. Ampicillin and amoxicillin are also effective in the management of such infections (DuPont and Pickering, 1980). There appear to be fewer carriers and fewer relapses after ampicillin than after chloramphenicol (Snyder *et al.,* 1976). However, the increasing prevalence of resistance to the drug makes it necessary to determine the sensitivity of the microorganisms recovered from patients with these diseases. Trimethoprim–sulfamethoxazole is also very effective for the treatment of typhoid fever, including disease caused by chloramphenicol-resistant *S. typhi* (Gilman *et al.,* 1975). More recently, cefoperazone and ceftriaxone have emerged as candidates for drugs of choice for the treatment of this disease (*see* Chapter 46).

Within a few hours after chloramphenicol is administered, *S. typhi* disappears from the blood. Stool cultures frequently become negative in a few days. Clinical improvement is often evident within 48 hours, and fever and other signs of the disease commonly abate within 3 to 5 days. The patient usually becomes afebrile before the intestinal lesions heal; as a result, intestinal hemorrhage and perforation may occur at a time when the clinical condition is rapidly improving. The incidence and the duration of the carrier state are not altered. The dose of chloramphenicol employed in adults with typhoid fever is 1 g every 6 hours for 4 weeks. Although both intravenous and oral routes have been used, the response is more rapid with oral administration. Relapses usually respond satisfactorily to re-treatment; microorganisms isolated during recurrences are usually still sensitive to the antibiotic *in vitro*.

Bacterial Meningitis. Treatment with chloramphenicol produces excellent results in *H. influenzae* meningitis that are equal to or better than those achieved with ampicillin (Jones and Hanson, 1977; Koskinniemi *et al.*, 1978). The total daily dose for children should be 50 to 75 mg/kg of body weight, divided into four equal doses given intravenously every 6 hours for 2 weeks. Such therapy is still recommended for the 25 to 40% of strains of *H. influenzae* that are resistant to ampicillin; furthermore, dual administration of ampicillin and chloramphenicol is still recommended by some authorities for initial treatment of bacterial meningitis in children prior to evaluation of the results of cultures. Excellent results have also been obtained with several cephalosporins, including cefotaxime, ceftriaxone, cefuroxime, and ceftizoxime (Freedman *et al.*, 1983; Bryant, 1984). These drugs will likely replace chloramphenicol as initial therapy for meningitis when *H. influenzae* is suspected. Although chloramphenicol is bacteriostatic against most microorganisms, it is bactericidal for many meningeal pathogens, such as *H. influenzae* (Rahal and Simberkoff, 1979). There is no evidence of antagonism *in vivo* when it is combined with ampicillin, and, in fact, an additive or synergistic effect may result (Feldman, 1978). However, antagonism between chloramphenicol and beta-lactam antibiotics has been observed *in vitro* with other gram-negative bacilli (*e.g.*, *Klebsiella* and *Proteus*) (Asmar *et al.*, 1988). Rare strains of *H. influenzae* resistant to chloramphenicol have produced meningitis (Centers for Disease Control, 1984), and sensitivity tests should be obtained on all isolates; approximately 0.6% of clinical isolates in the United States are resistant (Doern *et al.*, 1988). Chloramphenicol remains an alternative drug for the treatment of meningitis caused by *N. meningitidis* and *Strep. pneumoniae* in patients who are allergic to penicillin. The newer cephalosporins listed above have also been shown to be efficacious, and they may replace chloramphenicol for this indication as well (*see* Bryan, 1984; *see also* Chapter 46). Since some strains of *Strep. pneumoniae* may be inhibited but not killed by chloramphenicol, lumbar puncture should be repeated 2 to 3 days after treatment has been initiated to ensure that an adequate response has occurred (Scheld *et al.*, 1979). Higher doses of chloramphenicol (100 mg/kg per day) may be required in some instances.

Anaerobic Infections. Chloramphenicol is quite effective against most anaerobic bacteria, including *Bacteroides* species (Cuchural *et al.*, 1988). It may be used instead of metronidazole or clindamycin in patients with serious anaerobic infections originating from foci in the bowel or pelvis. Chloramphenicol, together with penicillin, is used for the treatment of brain abscesses. However, many authorities now recommend penicillin plus metronidazole. Most of these infections are caused by anaerobic or mixed aerobic–anaerobic bacteria, including *B. fragilis*. Although chloramphenicol and metronidazole both concentrate in brain tissue, clindamycin is largely excluded from the brain and CSF. Chloramphenicol may also be used in conjunction with a penicillin and an aminoglycoside for the treatment of intra-abdominal or pelvic abscesses, which are frequently caused by anaerobic bacteria (especially *B. fragilis*). However, either clindamycin or metronidazole can be substituted for chloramphenicol. Antimicrobial therapy should be accompanied by surgical drainage whenever possible.

Rickettsial Diseases. The tetracyclines are usually the preferred agents for the treatment of rickettsial diseases. However, in patients sensitized to these drugs, in those with reduced renal function, in pregnant women, and in certain patients who require parenteral therapy because of severe illness, chloramphenicol is the drug of choice. Either tetracycline or chloramphenicol produces a favorable clinical response early in the course of Rocky Mountain spotted fever (Woodward, 1984). Epidemic, murine, scrub, and recrudescent typhus as well as Q fever respond well to chloramphenicol. The same dose schedule is applicable in all the rickettsial diseases. For adults, 50 mg/kg per day is recommended. Oral therapy is preferable, whenever possible. The daily dose of chloramphenicol for children with these diseases is 75 mg/kg of body weight, divided into equal portions and given every 6 to 8 hours; if chloramphenicol palmitate is used, the daily maintenance dose may be as high as 100 mg/kg, given at the same intervals. Therapy should be continued until the general condition has improved and fever has been absent for 24 to 48 hours. The duration of illness and the incidence of relapses and complications are greatly reduced.

Brucellosis. Chloramphenicol is not as effective as the tetracyclines in the treatment of brucellosis. In cases in which the use of a tetracycline is contraindicated, 750 mg to 1 g of chloramphenicol orally every 6 hours may produce a beneficial effect in both the acute and chronic forms of the disease. Relapses usually respond to retreatment.

Miscellaneous Uses. Rarely, chloramphenicol (1 g intravenously every 6 hours) may be useful therapy for infections caused by strains of *K. pneumoniae* resistant to beta-lactam antibiotics and aminoglycosides. Although chloramphenicol therapy is quite effective in lymphogranuloma venereum, psittacosis, and infections caused by *Mycoplasma pneumoniae* and *Y. pestis*, other antimicrobial agents are preferred.

ERYTHROMYCIN

History and Source. Erythromycin is an orally effective antibiotic, discovered in 1952 by McGuire and coworkers in the metabolic products of a strain of *Streptomyces erythreus*, originally obtained from a soil sample collected in the Philippine Archipelago. These investigators also carried out the initial *in-vitro* observations, determined the range of toxicity, and demonstrated the effectiveness of the drug in experimental and naturally occurring infections due to gram-positive cocci.

Chemistry. Erythromycin is one of the macrolide antibiotics, so named because they contain a many-membered lactone ring to which are attached one or more deoxy sugars. The structural formula of erythromycin is as follows:

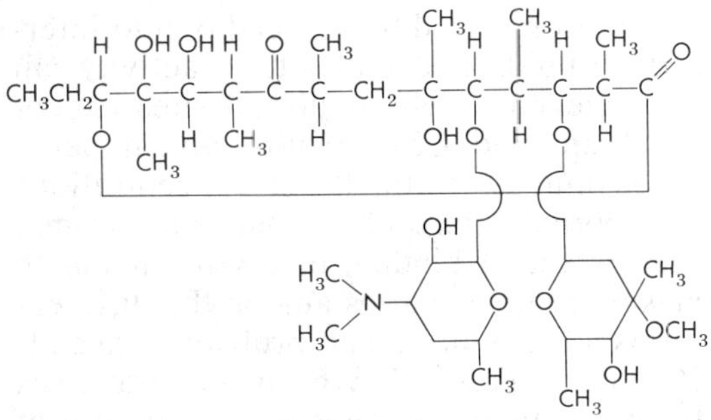

Erythromycin

Antibacterial Activity. Erythromycin may be either bacteriostatic or bactericidal, depending on the microorganism and the concentration of the drug. The bactericidal activity is greatest against a small number of rapidly dividing microorganisms and increases markedly as the pH of the medium is raised over the range of 5.5 to 8.5. The antibiotic is most effective *in vitro* against gram-positive cocci such as *Strep. pyogenes* and *Strep. pneumoniae*, for which the MIC is from 0.001 to 0.2 μg/ml (Steigbigel, 1990). Resistant strains of these bacteria are rare and are usually isolated from populations of people who have been recently exposed to macrolide antibiotics. Strains of *Strep. pneumoniae* and *Strep. pyogenes* that have been selected for resistance to erythromycin are often also resistant to clindamycin. Viridans streptococci are often inhibited by 0.02 to 3.1 μg/ml. Although some staphylococci are sensitive to erythromycin, the range of inhibitory concentrations is great (MIC for *Staph. epidermidis*, 0.2 to 100 μg/ml; for *Staph. aureus*, 0.005 to 100 μg/ml). Erythromycin-resistant strains of *Staph. aureus* are frequently encountered in hospitals, and resistance may emerge during treatment of an individual patient; cross-resistance with other macrolide antibiotics and with clindamycin is common. Many other gram-positive bacilli are also sensitive to erythromycin; values of MIC are from <0.1 to 8 μg/ml for *Cl. perfringens*, from <0.01 to 3 μg/ml for *Corynebacterium diphtheriae*, and from 0.1 to 0.3 μg/ml for *Listeria monocytogenes*.

Erythromycin is not active against most aerobic gram-negative bacilli. However, it has moderate activity *in vitro* against *H. influenzae* (MIC, 0.1 to 6 μg/ml) and *N. meningitidis* (MIC, 0.1 to 1.6 μg/ml), and excellent activity against most strains of *N. gonorrhoeae* (MIC, 0.005 to 0.4 μg/ml). Useful antibacterial activity is also observed against *Past. multocida*, *Borrelia*, *Bord. pertussis*, and less than half of the strains of *B. fragilis* (the MIC ranging from 0.1 to 100 μg/ml). It is quite active against over 90% of strains of *Campylobacter jejuni* (Vanhoof *et al.*, 1980). Erythromycin is effective against *M. pneumoniae* (MIC, 0.001 to 0.02 μg/ml) and the agent of legionnaires' disease, *Legionella pneumophila* (MIC, <0.5 μg/ml). Most strains of *C. trachomatis* are inhibited by 0.1 to 0.5 μg/ml of erythromycin. Some of the atypical mycobacteria are sensitive to erythromycin *in vitro*, where approximately 85% of strains of *Mycobacterium scrofulaceum* and nearly all of *M. kansasii* are sensitive to 0.5 to 2 μg/ml of the drug; the remainder are inhibited by 4 to 16 μg/ml. Nearly all strains of *M. fortuitum* are resistant, while strains of *M. intracellulare* vary in sensitivity (Molavi and Weinstein, 1971). Erythromycin has no effect on viruses, yeasts, and fungi.

Mechanism of Action. Erythromycin and other macrolide antibiotics inhibit protein synthesis by binding reversibly to 50 S ribosomal subunits of sensitive microorganisms (*see* Brisson-Noël *et al.*, 1988). Erythromycin can interfere with the binding of chloramphenicol, which also acts at this site. Certain resistant microorganisms with mutational changes in components of this ribosomal subunit fail to bind the drug. It is believed that erythromycin does not inhibit peptide bond formation directly but rather inhibits the translocation step wherein a newly synthesized peptidyl tRNA molecule moves from the acceptor site on the ribosome to the peptidyl (or donor) site.

Gram-positive bacteria accumulate about 100 times more erythromycin than do gram-negative microorganisms. The nonionized form of the drug is considerably more permeable to cells, and this probably explains the increased antimicrobial activity that is observed at alkaline pH (Sabath *et al.*, 1968; Vogel *et al.*, 1971).

Resistance to erythromycin results from at least three plasmid-mediated alterations: a decrease in the permeability of the drug through the cell envelope, as occurs with *Staph. epidermidis* (Lampson *et al.*, 1986); a modification of the target sites on the ribosome, which occurs with both gram-positive and gram-negative organisms, including *Legionella* species (Dowling *et al.*, 1985); and hydrolysis of erythromycin by an esterase produced by Enterobacteriaceae (Barthélémy *et al.*, 1984).

Absorption, Distribution, and Excretion. Erythromycin base is incompletely but adequately absorbed from the upper part of the small intestine; it is inactivated by gastric juice, and the drug is thus administered as protected tablets or capsules containing enteric-coated pellets that dissolve in the duodenum. Food in the stomach delays its ultimate absorption. Peak concentrations in plasma are only 0.3 to 0.5 μg/ml 4 hours after oral administration of 250 mg of the base and are 0.3 to 1.9 μg/ml after a single dose of 500 mg. Various esters of erythromycin have been prepared to attempt to improve stability and facilitate absorption. However, concentrations of erythromycin in plasma are little different if the stearate is given orally, and its bioavailability is decreased when administered with food. Erythromycin estolate is less susceptible to acid than is the parent compound; it is better absorbed than other forms of the drug, and this is not appreciably altered by food. A single, oral 250-mg dose of the estolate produces peak concentrations in plasma of approximately 1.5 μg/ml after 2 hours, and a 500-mg dose produces peak concentrations of 4 μg/ml. These peak values include both the ester and the free base, the latter comprising 20 to 35% of the total. Thus, the actual concentration of erythromycin base in plasma may be similar for the three preparations.

The actual antibacterial activity of the estolate ester of erythromycin is difficult to measure *in vitro*. Only the free base binds to bacterial ribosomes. However, strains of *Staph. aureus* are more susceptible to the estolate ester than to the base if bacteria are exposed for short periods (10 minutes). This suggests that the estolate penetrates into the bacterial cell more rapidly and is hydrolyzed by bacterial enzymes to the active component. Such esterases have been isolated from various species of bacteria.

Erythromycin ethylsuccinate is another ester that is adequately absorbed after oral administration, particularly when the stomach is empty. Peak concentrations in plasma are 1.5 μg/ml (0.5 μg/ml of base) 1 to 2 hours after administration of a 500-mg dose.

High concentrations of erythromycin can be achieved by intravenous administration. Values are approximately 10 μg/ml 1 hour after intravenous administration of 500 to 1000 mg of erythromycin lactobionate or gluceptate.

Only 2 to 5% of orally administered erythromycin is excreted in active form in the urine and from 12 to 15% after intravenous infusion. The antibiotic is concentrated in the liver and excreted in active form in the bile, which may contain as much as 250 μg/ml when plasma concentrations are very high. Some of the drug may be inactivated by demethylation in the liver. The plasma half-life of erythromycin is approximately 1.6 hours. Although some reports suggest a prolonged half-life in patients with anuria, reduction of dosage is not routinely recommended. The drug is not removed significantly by either peritoneal dialysis or hemodialysis.

Erythromycin diffuses readily into intercellular fluids, and antibacterial activity can be achieved at essentially all sites except the brain and CSF. Erythromycin penetrates into prostatic fluid; concentrations are approximately 40% of those in plasma. The extent of binding of erythromycin to plasma proteins varies among the different forms of the drug but probably exceeds 70% in all cases. Erythromycin traverses the placental barrier, and concentrations of the drug in fetal plasma are about 5 to 20% of those in the maternal circulation.

Preparations, Routes of Administration, and Dosage. *Erythromycin* (E-MYCIN, ILOTYCIN, others), *erythromycin stearate* (ERYPAR, others), *erythromycin estolate* (ILOSONE), and *erythromycin ethylsuccinate* (E.E.S., PEDIAMYCIN, others) are available in a wide variety of preparations for oral administration, including tablets, chewable tablets, capsules, oral suspensions, and drops. *Erythromycin gluceptate* (ILOTYCIN GLUCEPTATE) and *erythromycin lactobionate* (ERYTHROCIN LACTOBIONATE–I.V.) are available for intravenous injection in the form of sterile dry powders.

The usual oral dose of erythromycin for adults ranges from 1 to 2 g per day, in equally divided and spaced amounts, usually given every 6 hours, depending on the nature and severity of the infection. Daily doses of erythromycin as large as 8 g orally, given for 3 months, have been well tolerated. Food should be avoided, if possible, immediately before or after oral administration of erythromycin base or the stearate; this precaution need not be taken when the estolate or ethylsuccinate is administered. The oral dose of erythromycin for children is 30 to 50 mg/kg per day, divided into four portions; this dose may be doubled for severe infections. Intramuscular administration of erythromycin is not recommended because of pain upon injection. Intravenous administration is used infrequently and is reserved for the therapy of severe infections, such as legionellosis. The usual dose is 0.5 to 1 g every 6 hours; 1 g of erythromycin gluceptate has been given intravenously every 6 hours for as long as 4 weeks with no difficulty except for thrombophlebitis at the site of injection.

Untoward Effects. Serious untoward effects are only rarely caused by erythromycin. Among the allergic reactions observed are fever, eosinophilia, and skin eruptions, which may occur alone or in combination; each disappears shortly after therapy is stopped. Cholestatic hepatitis is the most striking side effect. It is caused primarily by erythromycin estolate and only rarely by the ethylsuccinate or the stearate (*see* Ginsburg and Eichenwald, 1976). The illness starts after about 10 to 20 days of treatment and is characterized initially by nausea, vomiting, and abdominal cramps. The pain often mimics that of acute cholecystitis, and unnecessary surgery has been performed. These symptoms are followed shortly thereafter by jaundice, which may be accompanied by fever, leukocytosis, eosinophilia, and elevated activities of transaminases in plasma. Biopsy of the liver reveals cholestasis, periportal infiltration by neutrophils, lymphocytes, and eosinophils, and, occasionally, necrosis of neighboring parenchymal cells. All manifestations usually disappear within a few days after cessation of drug therapy and rarely are prolonged. The syndrome may represent a hypersensitivity reaction to the estolate ester (*see* Tolman *et al.*, 1974).

Mild elevations of serum aspartate aminotransferase activity were noted in 16 of 161 pregnant women who received 250 mg of erythromycin estolate orally four times a day for 3 to 6 weeks during the second trimester. In 4 of the 16 pregnant women, aminotransferase activities had returned to normal by the last day of treatment. Three of 97 patients treated with erythromycin stearate reacted similarly (McCormack *et al.*, 1977).

Oral administration of erythromycin, especially of large doses, is very frequently accompanied by epigastric distress, which may be quite severe; intravenous administration may occasionally cause similar symptoms. Abdominal cramps, nausea, vomiting, and diarrhea are dose-related and occur more commonly in children and young adults (Seifert *et al.*, 1989). Intravenous infusion of 1-g doses, even when dissolved in a large volume, is often followed by thrombophlebitis; this can be minimized by slow rates of infusion.

Transient auditory impairment is a potential complication of treatment with erythromycin that has been observed to follow intravenous administration of large doses of the gluceptate or lactobionate (4 g per day) or oral ingestion of large doses of the estolate (Karmody and Weinstein, 1977). Hypertrophic pyloric stenosis was observed in five infants during administration of erythromycin estolate (Filippo, 1976).

Erythromycin has been reported to potentiate the effects of carbamazepine, corticosteroids, cyclosporine, digoxin, and warfarin probably by interfering with their cytochrome P_{450}–mediated metabolism (Ludden, 1985; Martell *et al.*, 1986). In addition, high and potentially toxic concentrations of theophylline may result when erythromycin is administered concomitantly.

Therapeutic Uses. Extensive studies of the clinical application of erythromycin have demonstrated its usefulness in a variety of infections, but it is currently the preferred drug for only a few (Modai, 1988).

Mycoplasma pneumoniae *Infections.* Erythromycin (given orally in doses of 500 mg four times daily, or, if oral administration is not tolerated, given intravenously) reduces the duration of fever caused by *M. pneumoniae*. In addition, the rate of clearing as noted in the chest x-ray is accelerated (Rasch and Mogabgab, 1965). Tetracycline is just as effective.

Legionnaires' Disease. Erythromycin is currently recommended for the treatment of pneumonia caused by *Legionella pneumophila, L. micdadei,* or other *Legionella* species (Skerrett and Locksley, 1986). The antibiotic may be given orally (0.5 to 1 g four times daily) or intravenously (1 to 4 g per day) for 3 weeks. Some recommend the concurrent administration of rifampin for severe disease, but there are no controlled trials to support this practice. Both trimethoprim–sulfamethoxazole and ciprofloxacin are active *in vitro* and in animal models of infection, but clinical experience is limited.

Chlamydia Infections. *Chlamydia* infections can be treated effectively with erythromycin. It is specifically recommended as an alternative to tetracycline in patients with uncomplicated urethral, endocervical, rectal, or epididymal infections (500 mg orally every 6 hours for at least 7 days). During pregnancy, erythromycin is the drug of choice for chlamydial urogenital infections; it is also preferred for chlamydial pneumonia of infancy (50 mg/kg per day in four divided doses for 14 days), when tetracyclines are contraindicated because of their effects on tissues that are calcifying (Centers for Disease Control, 1985).

Chlamydia pneumoniae, a newly described agent that causes pneumonia, appears to respond to treatment with erythromycin (500 mg orally every 6 hours for 14 days, or 250 mg orally every 6 hours for 21 days). However, tetracycline, when not contraindicated, may prove to be a better choice. Dosage regimens for tetracycline are the same as for erythromycin (Grayston, 1989).

Diphtheria. Erythromycin is very effective in eradicating the acute or chronic diphtheria bacillus carrier state. Erythromycin estolate (250 mg four times daily for 7 days) was found to be effective in 90% of adults. Most of the failures were due to lack of patient compliance (McClosky *et al.*, 1971). It must be remembered, however, that neither erythromycin nor any other antibiotic alters the course of an acute infection with the diphtheria bacillus or the risk of complications.

Pertussis. If administered early in the course of whooping cough, erythromycin may shorten the duration of illness. The drug has little influence on the disease once the paroxysmal stage is reached, although it may eliminate the microorganisms from the nasopharynx (*see* Bass *et al.*, 1969). Erythromycin can prevent whooping cough in susceptible individuals who are exposed to the disease.

Streptococcal Infections. Pharyngitis, scarlet fever, and erysipelas produced by *Strep. pyogenes* respond to erythromycin. The oral administration of 250 to 500 mg every 6 hours or 20 to 50 mg/kg per day (of the estolate) or 30 mg/kg per day (for other forms of erythromycin) for 10 days cures these diseases, prevents the appearance of suppurative complications, and suppresses the formation of antistreptococcal antibodies. Higher rates of eradication of streptococci and fewer side effects were noted in children who received erythromycin estolate, as compared with those who received the ethylsuccinate preparation (Ginsburg *et al.*, 1984). Treatment with erythromycin appears to produce a rate of cure about equal to that obtained with penicillin G (Shapera *et al.*, 1973). Pneumococcal pneumonia responds to oral therapy with 250 to 500 mg of erythromycin every 6 hours. Erythromycin is thus a valuable alternative for the treatment of streptococcal infections in patients who are allergic to penicillin.

Staphylococcal Infections. Erythromycin is an alternative agent for the treatment of relatively minor infections caused by either penicillin-sensitive or penicillin-resistant *Staph. aureus*. However, the emergence of appreciable numbers of strains that are resistant to erythromycin limits the use of the drug. The availability of the penicillinase-resistant penicillins and the cephalosporins has reduced the need to use erythromycin for the treatment of serious staphylococcal disease. The oral administration of 500 mg of erythromycin every 6 hours for 7 to 10 days is effective treatment for staphylococcal infections of the skin or of wounds in patients who are allergic to penicillins and cephalosporins.

Campylobacter Infections. The treatment of gastroenteritis caused by *Campylobacter jejuni* with erythromycin (250 to 500 mg orally four times a day for 7 days) has been shown to hasten the eradication of the microorganism from the stools, and early treatment of children reduces the duration of symptoms (Salazar-Lindo *et al.*, 1986). However, erythromycin had no detectable benefit in infants in Thailand, where resistance to the drug is prevalent (Taylor *et al.*, 1987). The current availability of quinolone antimicrobials, which are highly active against *Campylobacter* species and other enteric pathogens, has largely replaced the need for erythromycin for this disease in adults (*see* Chapter 45).

Tetanus. Erythromycin (500 mg orally every 6 hours for 10 days) may be given to eradicate *Cl. tetani* in patients with tetanus who are allergic to penicillin. The mainstays of therapy are debridement, physiological support, tetanus antitoxin, and drug control of convulsions.

Syphilis. Erythromycin in doses of 2 to 4 g per day for 10 to 15 days has been employed successfully in the treatment of early syphilis in patients who are allergic to penicillin (*Medical Letter*, 1988).

Gonorrhea. Both erythromycin estolate and the base have been used in the therapy of gonococcal urethritis. However, the relapse rate is nearly 25% after the oral administration of 9 g over a 4-day period; this is unacceptably high for routine use. Erythromycin may be useful for disseminated gonococcal disease in pregnant patients who are allergic to beta-lactam antibiotics (since tetracyclines should be avoided during pregnancy). Patients who are treated with 500 mg of erythromycin estolate or stearate, given orally every 6 hours for 5 days, show rapid clinical and bacteriological responses. Ceftriaxone is now the drug of choice for the treatment of all forms of gonorrhea (*see* Chapter 46).

Prophylactic Uses. Although penicillin is the drug of choice for the prophylaxis of recurrences of rheumatic fever, another antistreptococcal agent must be used in individuals who are allergic to this antibiotic. The sulfonamides are cheap and effective for this purpose. In some instances, however, it may be preferable to use erythromycin, which is also efficacious.

Erythromycin is recommended as an alternative to penicillin in allergic patients for prevention of bacterial endocarditis following dental or respiratory-tract procedures. The dose is 1 g orally 1 hour before the procedure, followed by a single dose of 500 mg 6 hours later (American Heart Association Committee, 1984).

LINCOMYCIN

Lincomycin is elaborated by an actinomycete, *Streptomyces lincolnensis,* so named because it was isolated from soil collected near Lincoln, Nebraska; it was the first lincosamide antibiotic to be used clinically. Clindamycin, the 7-deoxy,7-chloro derivative of lincomycin, is more active and causes fewer unwanted effects. There are thus few, if any, valid reasons to use lincomycin (LINCOCIN). Its properties are discussed in the *fifth edition* of this textbook.

CLINDAMYCIN

Chemistry. Clindamycin is a derivative of the amino acid trans-L-4-*n*-propylhygrinic acid, attached to a sulfur-containing derivative of an octose. As mentioned above, it is a congener of lincomycin. The structural formula of clindamycin is as follows:

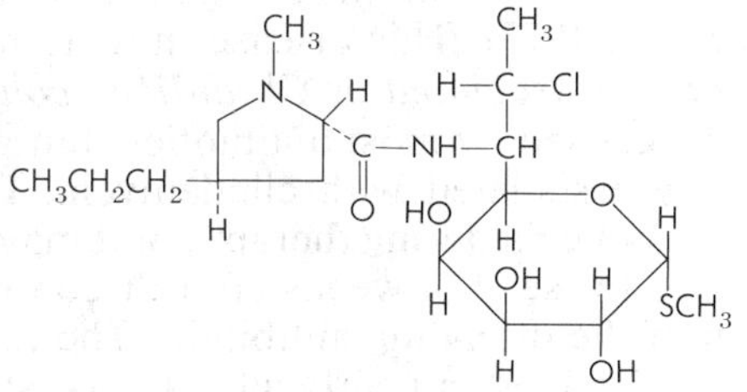

Clindamycin

Mechanism of Action. Clindamycin and lincomycin bind exclusively to the 50 S subunit of bacterial ribosomes and suppress protein synthesis. Although clindamycin, erythromycin, and chloramphenicol are not structurally related, they all act at this site, and the binding of one of these antibiotics to the ribosome may inhibit the interaction of the other. There are no clinical indications for the concurrent use of these antibiotics. Plasmid-mediated resistance to clindamycin (and erythromycin) has been found in *B. fragilis* (Tally *et al.*, 1979); it may be due to methylation of bacterial RNA found in the 50 S ribosomal subunit (Steigbigel, 1990). Other mechanisms of resistance are similar to those discussed above for erythromycin.

Antibacterial Activity. In general, clindamycin is similar to erythromycin in its activity *in vitro* against pneumococci, *Strep. pyogenes,* and viridans streptococci. Almost all such bacterial strains are inhibited by concentrations of 0.04 μg/ml (Steigbigel, 1990), although resistant microorganisms are encountered (Maruyama *et al.,* 1979; Linares *et al.,* 1983). It is also active against many strains of *Staph. aureus,* but not methicillin-resistant strains. Strains that are resistant to clindamycin are often also resistant to erythromycin. In some hospitals, such resistance has been found in 20% of isolates. Clindamycin is inactive against enterococci and *N. meningitidis* in concentrations that can be achieved clinically.

Clindamycin is more active than erythromycin against many anaerobic bacteria, especially *B. fragilis;* some strains are inhibited by <0.1 μg/ml and over 90% of strains are inhibited by 2 μg/ml. A recent survey in the United States found a stable rate of resistance (3 to 9%) over 5 years among strains of *B. fragilis* (MIC >4 μg/ml) (Cuchural *et al.,* 1988). Minimal inhibitory concentrations for other anaerobes are as follows: *B. melaninogenicus,* 0.1 to 1 μg/ml; *Fusobacterium,* < 0.5 μg/ml (although most strains of *F. varium* are resistant); *Peptostreptococcus,* < 0.1 to 0.5 μg/ml; *Peptococcus,* 1 to 100 μg/ml (with 10% of strains resistant); and *Cl. perfringens,* < 0.1 to 8 μg/ml. Ten to twenty percent of clostridial species, other than *Cl. perfringens,* are resistant (Bartlett, 1982). Strains of *Actinomyces israelii* and *Nocardia asteroides* are sensitive. Essentially all aerobic gram-negative bacilli are resistant, as is *Mycoplasma pneumoniae.* Strains of *Toxoplasma gondii* have been inhibited by clindamycin in experimental infections (Hofflin and Remington, 1987). Clindamycin has some activity against both chloroquine-sensitive and chloroquine-resistant strains of *Plasmodium falciparum* and *P. vivax,* but a cure rate of only 50% of patients with malaria was observed in one study (Hall *et al.,* 1975; *see also* Seaberg *et al.,* 1984).

Absorption, Fate, and Excretion. Clindamycin is nearly completely absorbed following oral administration, and peak plasma concentrations of 2 to 3 μg/ml are attained within 1 hour after the ingestion of 150 mg. The presence of food in the stomach does not reduce absorption significantly. The half-life of the antibiotic is about 2.7 hours, and modest accumulation of drug is thus expected if it is given at 6-hour intervals.

Clindamycin palmitate, an oral preparation for pediatric use, is an inactive prodrug, but the ester is hydrolyzed rapidly *in vivo.* Its rate and extent of absorption are similar to those of clindamycin. After several oral doses at 6-hour intervals, children attain plasma concentrations of 2 to 4 μg/ml with the administration of 8 to 16 mg/kg.

The phosphate ester of clindamycin, which is given parenterally, is also rapidly hydrolyzed *in vivo* to the active parent compound. After intramuscular injection, peak concentrations in plasma are not attained until 3 hours in adults and 1 hour in children; these values approximate 6 μg/ml after a 300-mg dose and 9 μg/ml after a 600-mg dose in adults.

While clindamycin is widely distributed in many fluids and tissues, including bone, significant concentrations are not attained in CSF, even when the meninges are inflamed. The drug readily crosses the placental barrier. Ninety percent or more of clindamycin is bound to plasma proteins (*see* Panzer *et al.,* 1972). Clindamycin accumulates in polymorphonuclear leukocytes and alveolar macrophages; the clinical relevance of this phenomenon is unknown. Clindamycin is also concentrated in abscesses in experimental animals (Joiner *et al.*, 1981).

Only about 10% of the clindamycin administered is excreted unaltered in the urine, and small quantities are found in the feces. However, antimicrobial activity persists in feces for 5 or more days after parenteral therapy with clindamycin is stopped; growth of sensitive microorganisms in colonic contents remains suppressed for up to 2 weeks (Kager *et al.*, 1981). Most of the drug is inactivated by metabolism to N-demethylclindamycin and clindamycin sulfoxide, which are excreted in the urine and bile. Accumulation of clindamycin can occur in patients with severe hepatic failure unless dosage is adjusted.

Preparations, Routes of Administration, and Dosage. *Clindamycin hydrochloride* (CLEOCIN HCL) is supplied for oral administration in capsules containing 75, 150, or 300 mg. *Clindamycin palmitate hydrochloride* (CLEOCIN PEDIATRIC) is a preparation of flavored granules for solution to a concentration of 75 mg/5 ml. *Clindamycin phosphate* (CLEOCIN PHOSPHATE) is available for intramuscular or intravenous use and as a topical solution or gel (CLEOCIN T).

The oral dose of clindamycin for adults is 150 to 300 mg every 6 hours; for severe infections, 300 to 450 mg every 6 hours. Children should receive 8 to 12 mg/kg per day of the palmitate hydrochloride in three or four divided doses; for severe infections, 13 to 25 mg/kg per day. However, children weighing 10 kg or less should receive ½ teaspoonful of clindamycin palmitate hydrochloride (37.5 mg) three times daily as a minimal dose.

For serious infections due to aerobic gram-positive cocci and the more sensitive anaerobes (not generally including *B. fragilis, Peptococcus,* and *Clostridium* species other than *Cl. perfringens*), intravenous or intramuscular administration is recommended in dosages of 600 to 1200 mg per day, divided into two to four equal portions for adults. For more severe infections, particularly those proven or suspected to be caused by *B. fragilis, Peptococcus,* or *Clostridium* species other than *Cl. perfringens,* parenteral administration of 1200 to 2700 mg per day of clindamycin is suggested. In life-threatening situations due to aerobes or anaerobes, these doses may be increased. Daily doses as high as 4800 mg have been given intravenously to adults. Children should receive 10 to 40 mg/kg per day in three or four divided doses; in severe infections, a minimal daily dose of 300 mg is recommended, regardless of body weight.

Untoward Effects. The reported incidence of diarrhea associated with the administration of clindamycin ranges from 2 to 20%; the average appears to be about 8%. A number of patients (variously reported as 0.01 to 10%) have developed pseudomembranous colitis, characterized by diarrhea, abdominal pain, fever, and mucus and blood in the stools. Proctoscopic examination reveals white-to-yellow plaques on the mucosa of the colon. *This syndrome may be lethal.* It is caused by a toxin secreted by strains of *Cl. difficile* (Rifkin *et al.*, 1977). This disease, now termed *antibiotic-associated* or *Cl. difficile colitis,* can be caused by most antibiotics, but was initially associated with clindamycin. Disease may begin during therapy, or it may be delayed for several weeks after discontinuation of the offending antibiotic. The toxin can be detected in nearly all patients' stool by a cytotoxicity assay. If significant diarrhea or colitis occurs during therapy, the drug should be discontinued immediately; vancomycin, given orally in doses of 125 to 500 mg every 6 hours for 7 to 10 days, is effective in reducing the frequency of diarrhea (Tedesco, 1977). Oral metronidazole and bacitracin also appear to be effective. Cholestyramine (4 g, given three or four times daily) has proven beneficial in some instances but should not be administered simultaneously with oral vancomycin. Agents that inhibit peristalsis, such as opioids, may prolong and worsen the condition. Although the incidence of this problem is unknown, it is clear that the therapeutic indications for clindamycin should be considered very seriously before it is given.

Skin rashes occur in approximately 10% of patients treated with clindamycin. Other reactions, which are uncommon, include exudative erythema multiforme (Stevens–Johnson syndrome), reversible elevation of aspartate aminotransferase and alanine aminotransferase, granulocytopenia, thrombocytopenia, and anaphylactic reactions. Local thrombophlebitis may follow intravenous administration of the drug. Clindamycin can inhibit neuromuscular transmission and may potentiate the effect of a neuromuscular blocking agent administered concurrently (Fogdall and Miller, 1974).

Therapeutic Uses. Although a number of infections with gram-positive cocci will respond favorably to clindamycin, the high incidence of diarrhea and the occurrence of colitis require limitation of its use to infections in which it is clearly superior to other agents. Clindamycin is particularly valuable for the treatment of infections with anaerobes, especially those due to *B. fragilis* (Bartlett, 1982). It has been used successfully in combination with an aminoglycoside for infections resulting from fecal spillage (intra-abdominal or pelvic abscesses and peritonitis), and this regimen is superior to combinations of an aminoglycoside and penicillin or cephalothin (DiZerega *et al.*, 1979). Other drugs that are effective against anaerobes, such as metronidazole, cefoxitin, cefotetan, chloramphenicol, ticarcillin plus clavulanate, ampicillin plus sulbactam, or imipenem–cilastatin appear to be as efficacious as clindamycin in this setting (Harding *et al.*, 1980; Bartlett, 1982; Solomkin *et al.*, 1985). Clindamycin is not predictably useful for the treatment of brain abscesses, since penetration into the central nervous system (CNS) is poor; either metronidazole or chloramphenicol in combination with penicillin is preferred (Thadepalli *et al.*, 1973).

A prospective study has demonstrated that parenteral clindamycin (600 mg intravenously every 8 hours) was superior to penicillin (1 million units intravenously every 4 hours) for the treatment of lung abscesses (Levison *et al.*, 1983). Although questions have been raised (Bartlett and Gorbach, 1983), this study may reflect the increasing rate of isolation of penicillin-resistant (beta-lactamase-producing) strains of various species of *Bacteroides* from bronchopulmonary infections. The therapeutic role of clindamycin in the treatment of aspiration pneumonia, postobstructive pneumonia, or lung abscesses has yet to be settled, but it appears to be a reasonable alternative to penicillin. Although clindamycin is effective topically or orally in acne vulgaris (Dhawan and Thadepalli, 1982), less toxic forms of therapy are preferred (Leyden *et al.*, 1987).

Clindamycin (1200 mg given intravenously every 6 hours) in combination with pyrimethamine (75 mg orally each day) may be effective for treatment of encephalitis caused by *Toxoplasma gondii* in patients with acquired immunodeficiency syndrome (AIDS) (Luft and Remington, 1988). Lower-dose, oral suppressive therapy is also being tested in an attempt to prevent relapse (Israelski and Remington, 1988).

SPECTINOMYCIN

Source and Chemistry. Spectinomycin is an antibiotic produced by *Streptomyces spectabilis*. The drug is an aminocyclitol; its structural formula is as follows:

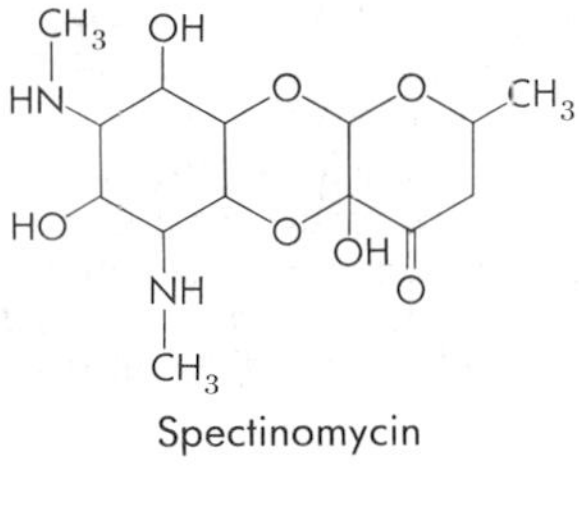

Spectinomycin

Antibacterial Activity and Mechanism. While spectinomycin is active against a number of gram-negative bacterial species, it is inferior to other drugs to which such microorganisms are susceptible (Schoutens *et al.*, 1972). Its only use is in the treatment of gonorrhea, and it inhibits gonococci at concentrations of 7 to 20 μg/ml; these concentrations are achieved in plasma by the administration of recommended doses.

Spectinomycin selectively inhibits protein synthesis in gram-negative bacteria. The antibiotic binds to and acts on the 30 S ribosomal subunit. There are similarities in its action to that of the aminoglycosides; however, spectinomycin is not bactericidal and does not cause misreading of polyribonucleotides. A high degree of bacterial resistance may develop as a result of mutation.

Absorption, Distribution, and Excretion. Spectinomycin is rapidly absorbed after intramuscular injection. A single dose of 2 g produces peak concentrations in plasma of 100 μg/ml at 1 hour; after an injection of 4 g, 160 μg/ml is achieved. Eight hours after injection of 2 or 4 g, the concentrations in plasma are 15 μg/ml or 30 μg/ml, respectively. The drug is not significantly bound to plasma protein, and all of an administered dose is recovered in the urine within 48 hours after injection.

Preparations. *Spectinomycin hydrochloride* (TROBICIN) is supplied as a sterile powder for reconstitution. This solution is for intramuscular injection only.

Untoward Effects. Spectinomycin, when given as a single intramuscular injection, produces few significant untoward effects (Duncan *et al.*, 1972). Urticaria, chills, and fever have been noted after single doses, as have dizziness, nausea, and insomnia. The injection may be painful.

Therapeutic Uses. The most recent recommendations from the Centers for Disease Control (1987) for the treatment of gonorrhea include ceftriaxone (250 mg intramuscularly) as the drug of choice for this disease. However, spectinomycin can be recommended for the treatment of uncomplicated gonococcal infections (*i.e.*, acute genital and rectal gonorrhea) in patients who are allergic to beta-lactam antibiotics. The recommended dose for both men and women is a single deep intramuscular injection of 2 to 4 g. The rate of cure for these forms of gonorrhea is about 95%. Spectinomycin is the preferred drug for patients with such infections who have not been cured by other treatment regimens. High rates of failure (50%) have followed single-dose treatment with spectinomycin for gonococcal pharyngitis. Multiple doses of spectinomycin (2 g intramuscularly, twice a day for 3 to 5 days) can be used for the treatment of disseminated gonococcal infections (arthritis–dermatitis syndrome) caused by penicillinase-producing strains of *N. gonorrhoeae* (*see* Center for Disease Control, 1979). It must be emphasized that spectinomycin has no effect on incubating or established syphilis, and it is not active against *Chlamydia*.

POLYMYXIN B AND COLISTIN

Because of the extreme nephrotoxicity associated with parenteral administration of these drugs, they are now rarely used. Information regarding parenteral administration of these agents can be found in the *fifth edition* of this textbook.

Source and Chemistry. The polymyxins, discovered in 1947, are a group of closely related antibiotic substances elaborated by various strains of *Bacillus polymyxa*, an aerobic spore-forming rod found in soil. Colistin (polymyxin E) is produced by *Bacillus (Aerobacillus) colistinus*, a microorganism isolated from a soil sample obtained from Fukushima Prefecture, Japan. These drugs, which are cationic detergents, are relatively simple, basic peptides with molecular weights of about 1000. The structural formula for polymyxin B, which is itself a mixture of polymyxins B_1 and B_2, is as follows:

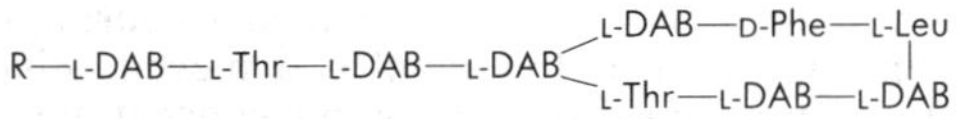
L-DAB—D-Phe—L-Leu
R—L-DAB—L-Thr—L-DAB—L-DAB
L-Thr—L-DAB—L-DAB

Polymyxin B_1: R = (+)-6-Methyloctanoyl
Polymyxin B_2: R = 6-Methylheptanoyl
DAB = α,γ-Diaminobutyric Acid

Colistin is polymyxin E, and it has a similar structure; it is available for clinical use as colistin sulfate, for oral use, and as colistimethate sodium, a parenteral preparation.

Antibacterial Activity and Mechanism of Action. The antimicrobial activity of polymyxin B and colistin are similar and are restricted to gram-negative bacteria, including *Enterobacter, E. coli, Klebsiella, Salmonella, Pasteurella, Bordetella*, and *Shigella*, which are usually sensitive to concentrations of 0.05 to 2.0 μg/ml. Most strains of *Pseud. aeruginosa* are inhibited by less than 8 μg/ml *in vitro*.

Polymyxins are surface-active, amphipathic agents (containing both lipophilic and lipophobic groups within the molecule). They interact strongly with phospholipids and penetrate into and disrupt the structure of cell membranes. The permeability of the bacterial membrane changes immediately on contact with the drug. Sensitivity to polymyxin B is apparently related to the phospholipid content of the cell wall–membrane complex (Brown and Wood, 1972). The cell wall of certain resistant bacteria may prevent access of the drug to the cell membrane.

The binding of polymyxin B to the lipid A portion of endotoxin (the lipopolysaccharide of the outer membrane of gram-negative bacteria) inactivates this molecule; polymyxin B also prevents most of the pathophysiological consequences of the release of endotoxin in several experimental systems (Shenep *et al.*, 1984; Täuber *et al.*, 1987). Since many antibiotics, especially the beta-lactam compounds, lyse gram-negative bacteria with resultant release of endotoxin, strategies to neutralize this harmful material may prove useful. Antiendotoxin antibodies are also being tested in this way.

Absorption, Distribution, and Excretion. Neither polymyxin B nor colistin is absorbed when given orally. They are also poorly absorbed from mucous membranes and the surface of large burns.

Preparations, Routes of Administration, and Dosage. *Polymyxin B sulfate* is available for ophthalmic, otic, and topical use in combination with a variety of other compounds. Although parenteral preparations are still marketed, they are not recommended. *Colistin sulfate* (COLY-MYCIN S) is marketed as a powder to be suspended in distilled water. It has been administered orally to infants and children with diarrhea caused by bacteria susceptible to the drug; the dose is 5 to 15 mg/kg daily, in three divided portions. *Colistimethate sodium*, a parenteral preparation, is seldom used.

Untoward Effects. Polymyxin B applied to intact or denuded skin or mucous membranes produces no systemic reactions because of its almost complete lack of absorption from these sites. Hypersensitization is uncommon when the antibiotic is used in this way. Nausea, vomiting, and diarrhea are produced by large doses (600 mg) taken orally. Adverse effects that follow the parenteral administration of these drugs are discussed in the *fifth edition* of this textbook.

Therapeutic Uses. Infections of the skin, mucous membranes, eye, and ear due to polymyxin B–sensitive microorganisms respond to local application of the antibiotic in solution or ointment. External otitis, frequently due to *Pseudomonas*, may be cured by the topical use of the drug. *Pseud. aeruginosa* is a common cause of infection of corneal ulcers; local application or subconjunctival injection of polymyxin B is often curative.

VANCOMYCIN

History and Source. Vancomycin is an antibiotic produced by *Strep. orientalis*, an actinomycete isolated from soil samples obtained in Indonesia and India. Purification of the antibiotics was accomplished and its antimicrobial properties were described within a short time after its discovery (McCormick *et al.*, 1956).

Chemistry. Vancomycin is a complex and unusual tricyclic glycopeptide with a molecular weight of about 1500. Its structural formula was determined by x-ray analysis (Sheldrick *et al.*, 1978).

Antibacterial Activity. Vancomycin is primarily active against gram-positive bacteria. Strains of *Staph. aureus*, including those resistant to methicillin, are inhibited by concentrations of 0.8 to 1.6 μg/ml (Atkinson, 1986). Rare strains of *Staph. aureus* are resistant to concentrations of the antibiotic that can be achieved clinically, but there has been no increase in the incidence of such resistance during the 30 years of the drug's use. Synergism between vancomycin and gentamicin or tobramycin has been demonstrated *in vitro* against *Staph. aureus*, including methicillin-resistant strains

(Watanakunakorn and Tisone, 1982). The minimal inhibitory concentrations of vancomycin for *Staph. epidermidis* range from 0.4 to 1.5 μg/ml; for *Strep. pyogenes*, from 0.15 to 2 μg/ml; for *Strep. pneumoniae*, from 0.1 to 0.3 μg/ml; for the viridans streptococci, from 0.3 to 1.5 μg/ml; and for *Enterococcus faecalis*, from 0.3 to 2.5 μg/ml. Vancomycin is not generally bactericidal for *Ent. faecalis;* however, 40 to 70% of susceptible strains are sensitive to a synergistic bactericidal effect when vancomycin and streptomycin are used concurrently, and nearly all strains are killed by a combination of vancomycin and gentamicin (Harwick *et al.*, 1973). *Corynebacterium* species (diphtheroids) are inhibited by less than 0.04 to 3.1 μg/ml of vancomycin, most species of *Actinomyces* by 5 to 10 μg/ml, and *Clostridium* species by 0.39 to 6 μg/ml. Several strains of *Staph. hemolyticus* and *Lactobacillus*, as well as enterococci, that have high-level resistance to vancomycin have now been isolated (Schwalbe *et al.*, 1987). Unfortunately, this trait is plasmid-mediated and thus transferable between strains. This probably explains the recent isolation of clinically significant, vancomycin-resistant enterococci (Uttley *et al.*, 1988), which may foretell a serious, emerging problem. Essentially all species of gram-negative bacilli and mycobacteria are resistant to vancomycin (*see* Cunha and Ristuccia, 1983).

Mechanism of Action. Vancomycin inhibits the synthesis of the cell wall in sensitive bacteria by binding with high affinity to precursors of this structure. The D-alanyl-D-alanine portion of the cell-wall precursor units appears to be a crucial site of attachment (*see* Figure 46–2, page 1067; Nieto and Perkins, 1971a, 1971b). The drug is rapidly bactericidal for dividing microorganisms (Watanakunakorn, 1981). The resistance to vancomycin (discussed above) that is emerging among enterococci is associated with expression of a unique cytoplasmic protein that appears to reduce access of vancomycin to its site of action (Shlaes *et al.*, 1989).

Absorption, Distribution, and Excretion. Vancomycin is poorly absorbed after oral administration, and large quantities are excreted in the stool. For parenteral therapy, the drug should be administered intravenously. A single intravenous dose of 1 g in adults produces plasma concentrations of 15 to 30 μg/ml 1 hour after a 1- to 2-hour infusion. The drug has a half-life in the circulation of about 6 hours (Matzke *et al.*, 1986). Approximately 30% of vancomycin is bound to plasma protein. Vancomycin appears in various body fluids, including the CSF when the meninges are inflamed; bile; and pleural, pericardial, synovial, and ascitic fluids (Levine, 1987). Up to 90% of an injected dose is excreted by glomerular filtration. Dangerously high concentrations may accumulate if renal function is impaired, and dosage adjustments must be made under these circumstances (Cunha *et al.*, 1981; Moellering *et al.*, 1981). The drug can be rapidly cleared from plasma with the newer, high-flux methods of hemodialysis (Lanese *et al.*, 1989). Patients with impaired hepatic function also eliminate vancomycin more slowly than normal, and dosage adjustments may be necessary (Brown *et al.*, 1983).

Preparations, Routes of Administration, and Dosage. *Vancomycin hydrochloride* (VANCOCIN HCL, others) is marketed for *intravenous* use as a sterile powder for solution. The desired dose is preferably diluted and injected intravenously over at least a 60-minute period. The dose of vancomycin for adults is 500 mg every 6 hours or 1 g every 12 hours; this will yield an average steady-state concentration of 15 μg/ml (*see* Moellering *et al.*, 1981). The following dosage schedules are recommended for pediatric patients: for newborns during the first week of life, 15 mg/kg every 12 hours; for infants 8 to 30 days old, 15 mg/kg every 8 hours; for older infants and children, 10 mg/kg every 6 hours (Schaad *et al.*, 1980). Alteration of dosage is required for patients with impaired renal function (*see* Appendix II). The drug has been used effectively in functionally anephric patients (who are being dialyzed) by the administration of 1 g (approximately 15 mg/kg) each week. When 1 g is given intravenously to such patients, the peak concentration in plasma is 40 to 50 μg/ml; this falls to a value of 15 μg/ml in 3 to 5 hours. After 7 days, concentrations in plasma are usually still in the therapeutic range (5 to 7 μg/ml). Close monitoring of plasma drug concentrations is recommended.

Vancomycin can be administered orally to patients with "antibiotic-associated" colitis (*see* discussion of clindamycin, above). The dose for adults is 125 to 500 mg every 6 hours; the total daily dose for children is 40 mg/kg, given in three to four divided doses. *Vancomycin hydrochloride for oral solution* is available for this purpose, as are capsules.

Untoward Effects. Among the hypersensitivity reactions produced by vancomycin are macular skin rashes and anaphylaxis. Phlebitis and pain at the site of intravenous injection are relatively uncommon. Chills, rash, and fever may occur. A shocklike state (so-called red-neck or red-man syndrome) may develop during the course of a rapid intravenous infusion (Newfield and Roizen, 1979; Davis *et al.*, 1986), and appears to be due to release of histamine (Polk *et al.*, 1988). The most significant untoward reactions have been ototoxicity and nephrotoxicity. Auditory impairment, which is frequently although not always permanent, may follow the use of this drug. Ototoxicity is associated with excessively high concentrations of the drug in plasma (80 to 100 μg/ml). Nephrotoxicity was formerly quite common but has become an unusual side effect when appropriate doses are used, as judged by renal function and determinations of the concentration of the antibiotic in blood. Caution must be exercised when other ototoxic or nephrotoxic drugs such as aminoglycosides are administered concurrently (Farber and Moellering, 1983), or in patients with impaired renal function.

Therapeutic Uses. Vancomycin should be employed only to treat serious infections and is particularly useful in the management of infections due to methicillin-resistant staphylococci, including pneumonia, empyema, endocarditis, osteomyelitis, and soft-tissue abscesses (Sorrell *et al.*, 1982). The drug is also extremely valuable in severe staphylococcal infections in patients who are allergic to penicillins and cephalosporins (Geraci, 1977). Treatment with vancomycin is effective and convenient when there is disseminated staphylococcal infection or localized infection of a shunt in a patient with irreversible renal disease who is being maintained by hemodialysis or peritoneal dialysis (Nolan *et al.*, 1980; Krothapalli *et al.*, 1983). Intraventricular administration of vancomycin (via a shunt or reservoir) has been necessary in a few cases of CNS infections due to susceptible microorganisms that did not respond to intravenous therapy alone (Visconti and Peter, 1979; Sutherland *et al.*, 1981).

Administration of vancomycin is an effective alternative for the treatment of endocarditis caused by viridans streptococci in patients who are allergic to penicillin. In combination with an aminoglycoside, it may be used for endocarditis caused by *Enterococcus faecalis*. Vancomycin is also effective for the treatment of infections caused by *Flavobacterium* and *Corynebacterium* species. As an oral agent, vancomycin benefits patients with colitis caused by toxin-producing bacteria such as *Cl. difficile*.

BACITRACIN

History and Source. Bacitracin is an antibiotic produced by the Tracy-I strain of *Bacillus subtilis*, isolated in 1943 from the damaged tissue and street dirt debrided from a compound fracture in a young girl named Tracy; hence the name bacitracin. The history, properties, and uses of bacitracin have been reviewed by Meleney and Johnson (1949).

Chemistry. The bacitracins are a group of polypeptide antibiotics; multiple components have been demonstrated in the commercial products. The major constituent is bacitracin A. Its probable structural formula is as follows:

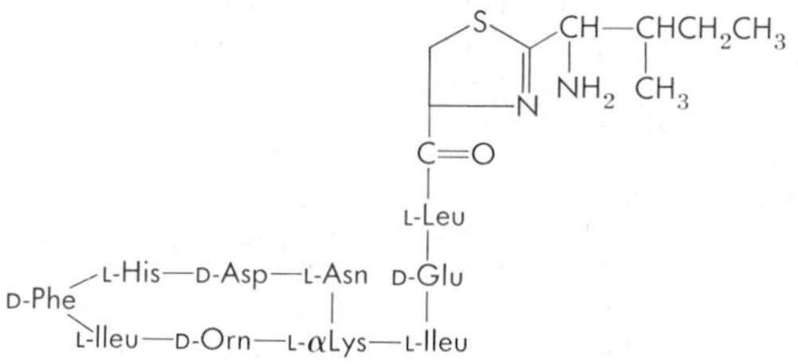

Bacitracin

A unit of the antibiotic is equivalent to 26 μg of the USP standard.

Antibacterial Activity. A variety of gram-positive cocci and bacilli, *Neisseria*, *H. influenzae*, and *T. pallidum* are sensitive to 0.1 unit or less of bacitracin per milliliter. *Actinomyces* and *Fusobacterium* are inhibited by concentrations of 0.5 to 5 units/ml. Enterobacteriaceae, *Pseudomonas*, *Candida* species, and *Nocardia* are resistant to the drug. Bacitracin inhibits bacterial cell-wall synthesis.

Absorption, Fate, and Excretion. While bacitracin has been employed parenterally in the past, current use is restricted to topical application. The reader is referred to *earlier editions* of this textbook for descriptions of the pharmacokinetics of this antibiotic.

Preparations, Route of Administration, and Dosage. Only information pertinent to topical application will be presented. *Bacitracin* (AK-TRACIN, BACIGUENT) is available in ophthalmic and dermatological ointments; the antibiotic is also available in the form of a powder for the preparation of topical solutions. The ointments are applied directly to the involved surface one or more times daily. A number of topical preparations of bacitracin to which neomycin or polymyxin or both have been added are available, and some contain the three antibiotics plus hydrocortisone.

Untoward Effects. Serious nephrotoxicity results from the parenteral use of this antibiotic. Hypersensitivity reactions result from topical application, but this is uncommon.

Therapeutic Uses. Topical bacitracin alone or in combination with other antimicrobial agents has no established value in the treatment of furunculosis, pyoderma, carbuncle, impetigo, and superficial and deep abscesses. For open infections such as infected eczema and infected dermal ulcers, the local application of the antibiotic may be of some help in eradicating sensitive bacteria. Bacitracin has an advantage over other antibiotics in that topical administration, even in an ointment, rarely produces hypersensitivity. Suppurative conjunctivitis and infected corneal ulcer respond well to the topical use of bacitracin when they are caused by susceptible bacteria. Oral bacitracin has been used with some success for the treatment of antibiotic-associated diarrhea caused by *Cl. difficile* (Dudley *et al.*, 1986).

Amendola, M. A., and Spera, T. D. Doxycycline-induced esophagitis. *J.A.M.A.*, **1985**, *253*, 1009–1011.

American Heart Association Committee. Prevention of bacterial endocarditis. *Circulation*, **1984**, *70*, 1123A–1127A.

Asmar, B. I.; Prainito, M.; and Dajani, A. S. Antagonistic effect of chloramphenicol in combination with cefotaxime or ceftriaxone. *Antimicrob. Agents Chemother.*, **1988**, *32*, 1375–1378.

Atkinson, B. A. Species incidence and trends of susceptibility to antibiotics in the United States and other countries: MIC and MBC. In, *Antibiotics in Laboratory Medicine*, 2nd ed. (Lorian, V., ed.) The Williams & Wilkins Co., Baltimore, **1986**, pp. 995–1162.

Baine, W. B.; Farmer, J. J.; Gangarosa, E. J.; Hermann, G. T.; Thornsberry, C.; and Rice, P. A. Typhoid fever in the United States associated with the 1972–1973 epidemic in Mexico. *J. Infect. Dis.*, **1977**, *135*, 649–653.

Barthélémy, P.; Autissier, D.; Gerbaud, G.; and Courvain, P. Enzymatic hydrolysis of erythromycin by a strain of *Escherichia coli*. *J. Antibiot. (Tokyo)*, **1984**, *37*, 1692–1696.

Bartlett, J. G. Anti-anaerobic antibacterial agents. *Lancet*, **1982**, *2*, 478–481.

Bartlett, J. G., and Gorbach, S. L. Penicillin or clindamycin for primary lung abscesses? *Ann. Intern. Med.*, **1983**, *98*, 546–548.

Bartz, Q. R. Isolation and characterization of CHLOROMYCETIN. *J. Biol. Chem.*, **1948**, *172*, 445–450.

Barza, M., and Scheife, R. T. Antimicrobial spectrum, pharmacology, and therapeutic use of antibiotics. *J. Maine Med. Assoc.*, **1977**, *68*, 194–210.

Bass, J. W.; Klenk, E. L.; Klotheimer, J. B.; Linnemann, C. C.; and Smith, M. H. D. Antimicrobial treatment of pertussis. *J. Pediatr.*, **1969**, *75*, 768–781.

Baughman, G. A., and Fahnestock, S. F. Chloramphenicol resistance mutation in *Escherichia coli* which maps in the major ribosomal protein gene cluster. *J. Bacteriol.*, **1979**, *137*, 1315–1323.

Biancaniello, T.; Meyer, R. A.; and Kaplan, S. Chloramphenicol and cardiotoxicity. *J. Pediatr.*, **1981**, *98*, 828–830.

Blouin, R. A.; Erwin, W. G.; Dutro, M. P.; Bustrack, J. A.; and Rowse, K. L. Chloramphenicol hemodialysis clearance. *Ther. Drug Monit.*, **1980**, *2*, 351–354.

Brisson-Noël, A.; Trieu-Cuot, P.; and Courvalis, P. Mechanism of action of spiramycin and other macrolides. *J. Antimicrob. Chemother.*, **1988**, *22*, Suppl. B, 13–23.

Brown, M. R. W., and Wood, S. M. Relation between cation and lipid content of cell walls of *Pseudomonas aeruginosa*, *Proteus vulgaris* and *Klebsiella aerogenes* and their sensitivity to polymyxin B and other antibacterial agents. *J. Pharm. Pharmacol.*, **1972**, *24*, 215–228.

Brown, N.; Ho, D. H. W.; Fong, K.-L. L.; Bogerd, L.; Maksymiuk, A.; Bolivar, R.; Fainstein, V.; and Bodey, G. P. Effects of hepatic function on vancomycin clinical pharmacology. *Antimicrob. Agents Chemother.*, **1983**, *23*, 603–609.

Bryan, L. E. Mechanisms of action of aminoglycoside antibiotics. In, *Contemporary Issues in Infectious Diseases*. Vol. 1, *New Dimensions in Antimicrobial Therapy*. (Root, R. K., and Sande, M. A., eds.) Churchill Livingstone, Inc., New York, **1984**, pp. 17–36.

Center for Disease Control. Gonorrhea. Recommended treatment schedules, 1979. *Ann. Intern. Med.*, **1979**, *90*, 809–811.

Centers for Disease Control. Ampicillin and chloramphenicol resistance in systemic *Haemophilus influenzae* disease. *M.M.W.R.*, **1984**, *33*, 35–37.

———. *Chlamydia trachomatis* infections. *M.M.W.R.*, **1985**, *34*, Suppl. 3, 53S–74S.

———. Antibiotic-resistant strains of *Neisseria gonorrhoeae*. *M.M.W.R.*, **1987**, *36*, 1S–18S.

Cohlan, S. Q.; Bevelander, G.; and Tiamsic, T. Growth inhibition of prematures receiving tetracycline: clinical and laboratory investigation. *Am. J. Dis. Child.*, **1963**, *105*, 453–461.

Craft, A. W.; Brocklebank, J. T.; Hey, E. N.; and Jackson, R. H. The "grey toddler": chloramphenicol toxicity. *Arch. Dis. Child.*, **1974**, *49*, 235–237.

Cuchural, G. J., Jr., and others. Susceptibility of the *Bacteroides fragilis* group in the United States: analysis by site of isolation. *Antimicrob. Agents Chemother.*, **1988**, *32*, 717–722.

Cunha, B. A.; Quintiliani, R.; Deglin, J. M.; Izard, M. W.; and Nightingale, C. H. Pharmacokinetics of vancomycin in anuria. *Rev. Infect. Dis.*, **1981**, *3*, Suppl., S269–S272.

Cunha, B. A., and Ristuccia, A. M. Clinical usefulness of vancomycin. *Clin. Pharm.*, **1983**, *2*, 417–424.

Dattwyler, R. J.; Halperin, J. J.; Pass, H.; and Luft, B. J. Ceftriaxone as effective therapy in refractory Lyme disease. *J. Infect. Dis.*, **1987**, *155*, 1322–1325.

Daum, R. S.; Cohen, D. L.; and Smith, A. L. Fatal aplastic anemia following apparent "dose-related" chloramphenicol toxicity. *J. Pediatr.*, **1979**, *94*, 403–405.

Davis, R. L.; Smith, A. L.; and Koup, J. R. The "red man's syndrome" and slow infusion of vancomycin. *Ann. Intern. Med.*, **1986**, *104*, 285–286.

Dhawan, V. K., and Thadepalli, H. Clindamycin: a review of fifteen years of experience. *Rev. Infect. Dis.*, **1982**, *4*, 1133–1153.

DiZerega, G.; Yonekura, L.; Roy, S.; Nakamura, R. M.; and Ledger, W. J. A comparison of clindamycin–gentamicin and penicillin–gentamicin in the treatment of post-cesarean section endometritis. *Am. J. Obstet. Gynecol.*, **1979**, *134*, 238–242.

Doern, G. V.; Jorgensen, J. H.; Thornsberry, C.; Preston, D. A.; Tubert, T.; Redding, J. S.; and Maher, L. A. National collaborative study of prevalence of antimicrobial resistance among clinical isolates of *Haemophilus influenzae*. *Antimicrob. Agents Chemother.*, **1988**, *32*, 180–185.

Dowling, J. N.; McDevitt, D. A.; and Pasculle, A. W. Isolation and preliminary characterization of erythromycin-resistant variants of *Legionella pneumophilia*. *Antimicrob. Agents Chemother.*, **1985**, *27*, 272–274.

Dudley, M. N.; McLaughlin, J. C.; Carrington, G.; Frick, J.; Nightingale, C. H.; and Quintiliani, R. Oral bacitracin vs. vancomycin therapy for *Clostridium difficile*–induced diarrhea. *Arch. Intern. Med.*, **1986**, *146*, 1101–1104.

Duncan, W. C.; Holder, W. R.; Roberts, D. P.; and Know, J. M. Treatment of gonorrhea with spectinomycin hydrochloride: comparison with standard penicillin schedules. *Antimicrob. Agents Chemother.*, **1972**, *1*, 210–214.

DuPont, H. L., and Pickering, L. K. Salmonellosis. In, *Current Topics in Infectious Disease*. (Greenough, W. B., III, and Merigan, T. C., eds.) Vol. 2, *Infections of the Gastrointestinal Tract: Microbiology, Pathophysiology, and Clinical Features*. Plenum Medical Book Co., New York, **1980**, pp. 83–128.

Elmore, M. F., and Rogge, J. D. Tetracycline induced pancreatitis. *Gastroenterology*, **1981**, *81*, 1134–1136.

Ericsson, C. D.; Feldman, S.; Pickering, L. K.; and Cleary, T. G. Influence of subsalicylate bismuth on absorption of doxycycline. *J.A.M.A.*, **1982**, *247*, 2266–2267.

Evans, L. S., and Kleiman, M. B. Acidosis as a presenting feature of chloramphenicol toxicity. *J. Pediatr.*, **1986**, *108*, 475–477.

Evans, M. E.; Gregory, D. W.; Schaffner, W.; and McGee, Z. A. Tularemia: a 30-year experience with 88 cases. *Medicine (Baltimore)*, **1985**, *64*, 251–269.

Fanning, W. L.; Gump, D. W.; and Safferman, R. A. Side effects of minocycline: a double-blind study. *Antimicrob. Agents Chemother.*, **1977**, *11*, 712–717.

Farber, B. F., and Moellering, R. C., Jr. Retrospective study of the toxicity of preparations of vancomycin from 1974 to 1981. *Antimicrob. Agents Chemother.*, **1983**, *23*, 138–141.

Feldman, W. E. Effect of ampicillin and chloramphenicol against *Haemophilus influenzae*. *Pediatrics*, **1978**, *61*, 406–409.

Filippo, J. A. Infantile hypertrophic pyloric stenosis related to ingestions of erythromycin estolate: a report of five cases. *J. Pediatr. Surg.*, **1976**, *11*, 177–180.

Fogdall, R. P., and Miller, R. D. Prolongation of a pancuronium-induced neuromuscular blockade by clindamycin. *Anesthesiology*, **1974**, *41*, 407–408.

Forrest, J. N.; Cox, M.; Hong, C.; Morrison, G.; Bia, M.; and Singer, I. Superiority of demeclocycline over lithium in the treatment of chronic syndrome of inappropriate secretion of antidiuretic hormone. *N. Engl. J. Med.*, **1978**, *298*, 173–177.

Freedman, J. M.; Hoffman, S. H.; Scheld, W. M.; Lynch, M. A.; da Silva, H. R.; and Sande, M. A. Moxalactam for the treatment of bacterial meningitis in children. *J. Infect. Dis.*, **1983**, *148*, 886–891.

Freundlich, M.; Cyanmon, H.; Tamer, A.; Steele, B.; Zilleruelo, G.; and Strauss, J. Management of chloramphenicol intoxication in infancy by charcoal perfusion. *J. Pediatr.*, **1983**, *103*, 485–486.

Friedman, C. A.; Lovejoy, F. C.; and Smith, A. L. Chloramphenicol disposition in infants and children. *J. Pediatr.*, **1979**, *95*, 1071–1077.

Fripp, R. R.; Carter, M. C.; Werner, J. C.; Schuler, H. G.; Rannels, A. M.; Whitman, V.; and Nelson, N. M. Cardiac function and acute chloramphenicol toxicity. *J. Pediatr.*, **1983**, *103*, 487–490.

Gaffney, D. F., and Foster, T. J. Chloramphenicol acetyltransferase determined by R plasmids from gram-negative bacteria. *J. Gen. Microbiol.*, **1978**, *109*, 351–358.

Geraci, J. E. Vancomycin. *Mayo Clin. Proc.*, **1977**, *52*, 631–634.

Gilman, R. H.; Terminel, M.; Levine, M. M.; Hernandez-Mendosa, P.; Calderone, E.; Vasquez, V.; Martinez, E.; Snyder, M. J.; and Hornick, R. B. Comparison of trimethoprim-sulfamethoxazole and amoxicillin in therapy of chloramphenicol-resistant and chloramphenicol-sensitive typhoid fever. *J. Infect. Dis.*, **1975**, *132*, 630–636.

Ginsburg, C. M., and Eichenwald, H. F. Erythromycin: a review of its uses in pediatric practice. *J. Pediatr.*, **1976**, *86*, 272A.

Ginsburg, C. M.; McCracken, G. H., Jr.; Crow, S. D.; Dildy, B. R.; Morchower, G.; Steinberg, J. B.; and Lancaster, K. Erythromycin therapy for Group A streptococcal pharyngitis. Results of a comparative study of the estolate and ethyl succinate formulation. *Am. J. Dis. Child.*, **1984**, *138*, 536–539.

Godel, V.; Nemet, P.; and Lazar, M. Chloramphenicol optic neuropathy. *Arch. Ophthalmol.*, **1980**, *98*, 1417–1421.

Grayston, J. T. *Chlamydia pneumoniae*, strain TWAR. *Chest*, **1989**, *95*, 664–669.

Hall, A. P.; Doberstyn, E. B.; Nanakorn, A.; and Sonkom, P. Falciparum malaria semiresistant to clindamycin. *Br. Med. J.*, **1975**, *2*, 12–14.

Halpert, J. Further studies of the suicide inactivation of purified rat liver cytochrome P-450 by chloramphenicol. *Mol. Pharmacol.*, **1982**, *21*, 166–172.

Harding, G. K. M.; Buckwold, F. J.; Ronald, A. R.; Marrie, T. J.; Brunton, J. L.; Koss, J. C.; Gurwith, M. J.; and Albritton, W. L. Prospective, randomized comparative study of clindamycin, chloramphenicol, and ticarcillin, each in combination with gentamicin, in therapy for intraabdominal and female genital tract sepsis. *J. Infect. Dis.*, **1980**, *142*, 384–393.

Harwick, H. J.; Kalmanson, G. M.; and Guze, L. B. *In vitro* activity of ampicillin or vancomycin combined with gentamicin or streptomycin against enterococci. *Antimicrob. Agents Chemother.*, **1973**, *4*, 383–387.

Hofflin, J. M., and Remington, J. S. Clindamycin in a murine model of toxoplasmic encephalitis. *Antimicrob. Agents Chemother.*, **1987**, *31*, 492–496.

Holt, R. The bacterial degradation of chloramphenicol. *Lancet*, **1967**, *1*, 1259–1260.

Hoshiwara, I.; Ostler, B.; Hanna, L.; Cignetti, F.; Coleman, V. R.; and Jawetz, E. Doxycycline treatment of chronic trachoma. *J.A.M.A.*, **1973**, *224*, 220–223.

Israelski, D. M., and Remington, J. S. Toxoplasmic encephalitis in patients with AIDS. In, *The Medical Management of AIDS*. (Sande, M. A., and Volberding, P. A., eds.) W. B. Saunders Co., Philadelphia, **1988**, pp. 193–211.

Izumi, A. K.; Hanke, C. W.; and Higaki, M. *Mycobacterium marinum* infections treated with tetracycline. *Arch. Dermatol.*, **1977**, *113*, 1067–1068.

Jimenez, J. J.; Hrimura, G. K.; Abon-Khalil, W. H.; Isildar, M.; and Yunis, A. A. Chloramphenicol-induced bone marrow injury: possible role of bacterial metabolites of chloramphenicol. *Blood*, **1987**, *70*, 1180–1185.

Joiner, K. A.; Lowe, B. R.; Dzink, J. L.; and Bartlett, J. G. Antibiotic levels in infected and sterile subcutaneous abscesses in mice. *J. Infect. Dis.*, **1981**, *143*, 487–494.

Jones, F. E., and Hanson, D. R. *H. influenzae* meningitis treated with ampicillin or chloramphenicol, and subsequent hearing loss. *Dev. Med. Child Neurol.*, **1977**, *19*, 593–597.

Kager, L.; Liljeqvist, L.; Malmborg, A. S.; and Nord, C. E. Effect of clindamycin prophylaxis on the colonic microflora in patients undergoing colorectal surgery. *Antimicrob. Agents Chemother.*, **1981**, *20*, 736–740.

Karmody, C. S., and Weinstein, L. Reversible sensorineural hearing loss with intravenous erythromycin lactobionate. *Ann. Otol. Rhinol. Laryngol.*, **1977**, *86*, 9–11.

Kauffman, R. E.; Thirumoorthi, M. C.; Buckley, J. A.; Aravind, M. K.; and Dajani, A. S. Relative bioavailability of intravenous chloramphenicol succinate and oral chloramphenicol palmitate in infants and children. *J. Pediatr.*, **1981**, *99*, 963–967.

Knapp, J. S.; Zenilman, J. M.; Biddle, J. W.; Perkins, G. H.; DeWitt, W. E.; Thomas, M. L.; Johnson, S. R.; and Morse, S. A. Frequency and distribution in the United States of strains of *Neisseria gonorrhoeae* with plasmid-mediated, high-level resistance to tetracycline. *J. Infect. Dis.*, **1987**, *155*, 819–822.

Koskinniemi, M.; Pettay, O.; Raivio, M.; and Sarna, S. *Haemophilus influenzae* meningitis. A comparison between chloramphenicol and ampicillin therapy with special reference to impaired hearing. *Acta Paediatr. Scand.*, **1978**, *67*, 17–24.

Koup, J. R.; Lau, A. H.; Brodsky, B.; and Slaughter, R. L. Chloramphenicol pharmacokinetics in hospitalized patients. *Antimicrob. Agents Chemother.*, **1979**, *15*, 651–657.

Kramer, P. W.; Griffith, R. S.; and Campbell, R. L. Antibiotic penetration of the brain: a comparative study. *J. Neurosurg.*, **1969**, *31*, 295–302.

Krothapalli, R. K.; Senekjian, H. O.; and Ayus, J. C. Efficacy of intravenous vancomycin in the treatment of gram-positive peritonitis in long-term peritoneal dialysis. *Am. J. Med.*, **1983**, *75*, 345–348.

Kucers, A., and Bennett, N. McK. Chloramphenicol and thiamphenicol. In, *The Use of Antibiotics*, 4th ed. J. B. Lippincott Co., Philadelphia, **1987**, pp. 757–807.

Lampson, B. C.; von David, W.; and Parisi, J. T. Novel

mechanism for plasmid-mediated erythromycin resistance by pNE24 from *Staphylococcus epidermidis*. *Antimicrob. Agents Chemother.*, **1986**, *30*, 653–658.

Lanese, D. M.; Alfrey, P. S.; and Moliforis, B. A. Rapid vancomycin removal during high flux hemodialysis necessitates supplementation to maintain therapeutic levels. *Kidney Int.*, **1989**, *35*, 254.

Levine, J. F. Vancomycin: a review. *Med. Clin. North Am.*, **1987**, *71*, 1135–1145.

Levine, P. H.; Regelson, W.; and Holland, J. F. Chloramphenicol associated encephalopathy. *Clin. Pharmacol. Ther.*, **1970**, *11*, 194–199.

Levison, M. E.; Mangura, C. T.; Lorber, B.; Abrutyn, E.; Pesanti, E. L.; Levy, R. S.; Macgregor, R. R.; and Schwartz, A. R. Clindamycin compared with penicillin for the treatment of anaerobic lung abscesses. *Ann. Intern. Med.*, **1983**, *98*, 466–471.

Leyden, J. J.; Shalita, A. R.; Saatjian, G. D.; and Sefton, J. Erythromycin 2% gel in comparison with clindamycin phosphate 1% solution in acne vulgaris. *J. Am. Acad. Dermatol.*, **1987**, *16*, 822–827.

Linares, J.; Garau, J.; Dominquez, C.; and Perez, J. L. Antibiotic resistance and serotypes of *Streptococcus pneumoniae* from patients with community-acquired pneumococcal disease. *Antimicrob. Agents Chemother.*, **1983**, *23*, 545–547.

Lindebaum, J.; Greenough, W. B.; and Islam, M. R. Antibiotic therapy of cholera in children. *Bull. W.H.O.*, **1967**, *37*, 529–538.

Ling, J.; Kam, K. M.; Lam, A. W.; and French, G. L. Susceptibilities of Hong Kong isolates of multiply resistant *Shigella spp.* to 25 antimicrobial agents, including ampicillin plus sulbactam and new 4-quinolones. *Antimicrob. Agents Chemother.*, **1988**, *32*, 20–23.

Ludden, T. M. Pharmacokinetic interactions of the macrolide antibiotics. *Clin. Pharmacokinet.*, **1985**, *10*, 63–79.

Luft, B. J., and Remington, J. S. Toxoplasmic encephalitis. *J. Infect. Dis.*, **1988**, *157*, 1–6.

Lyerly, D. M.; Krivan, H. C.; and Wilkins, T. D. *Clostridium difficile*: its disease and toxins. *Clin. Microbiol. Rev.*, **1988**, *1*, 1–18.

McClosky, R. V.; Eller, J. J.; Green, M.; Mauney, C. U.; and Richards, S. E. M. The 1970 epidemic of diphtheria in San Antonio. *Ann. Intern. Med.*, **1971**, *75*, 495–503.

McCormack, W. M.; Chowdhury, A. M.; Jahangir, N.; Fariduddin Ahmed, A. B.; and Mosley, W. H. Tetracycline prophylaxis in families of cholera patients. *Bull. W.H.O.*, **1968**, *38*, 787–792.

McCormack, W. M.; Donner, G. H.; Kodgis, L. F.; Alpert, S.; Lower, E. W.; and Kass, E. H. Hepatotoxicity of erythromycin estolate during pregnancy. *Antimicrob. Agents Chemother.*, **1977**, *12*, 630–635.

McCormick, M. H.; Stark, W. M.; Pittenger, G. E.; Pittenger, R. C.; and McGuire, J. M. Vancomycin, a new antibiotic. I. Chemical and biologic properties. In, *Antibiotics Annual, 1955–1956*. Medical Encyclopedia, Inc., New York, **1956**, pp. 606–611.

McCracken, G. H., Jr.; Nelson, J. D.; Kaplan, S. L.; Overturf, G. D.; Rodriquez, W. J.; and Steele, R. W. Consensus report: antimicrobial therapy for bacterial meningitis in infants and children. *Pediatr. Infect. Dis. J.*, **1987**, *6*, 501–505.

Martell, R.; Heinrichs, D.; Stiller, C. R.; Jenner, M.; Keown, P. A.; and Dupre, J. The effects of erythromycin in patients treated with cyclosporin. *Ann. Intern. Med.*, **1986**, *104*, 660–661.

Maruyama, S.; Yoshioka, H.; Fujita, K.; Takimoto, M.; and Satake, Y. Sensitivity of group A streptococci to antibiotics. *Am. J. Dis. Child.*, **1979**, *133*, 1143–1145.

Matzke, G. R.; Zhanel, G. G.; and Guay, D. R. P. Clinical pharmacokinetics of vancomycin. *Clin. Pharmacokinet.*, **1986**, *11*, 257–282.

Medical Letter. Treatment of sexually transmitted diseases. **1988**, *35*, 5–10.

Meleney, F. L., and Johnson, B. A. Bacitracin. *Am. J. Med.*, **1949**, *7*, 794–806.

Moellering, R. C.; Krogstad, D. J.; and Greenblatt, D. J. Vancomycin therapy in patients with impaired renal function: a nomogram for dosage. *Ann. Intern. Med.*, **1981**, *94*, 343–346.

Modai, J. The clinical use of macrolides. *J. Antimicrob. Chemother.*, **1988**, *22*, Suppl. B, 145–153.

Molavi, A., and Weinstein, L. *In vitro* activity of erythromycin against atypical mycobacteria. *J. Infect. Dis.*, **1971**, *123*, 216–219.

Mulhall, A.; de Louvois, J.; and Hurley, R. The pharmacokinetics of chloramphenicol in the neonate and young infant. *J. Antimicrob. Chemother.*, **1983**, *12*, 629–639.

Neu, H. C. A symposium on tetracyclines: a major appraisal. Introduction. *Bull. N.Y. Acad. Med.*, **1978**, *54*, 141–155.

Newfield, P., and Roizen, M. F. Hazards of rapid administration of vancomycin. *Ann. Intern. Med.*, **1979**, *91*, 581.

Nieto, M., and Perkins, H. R. Physicochemical properties of vancomycin and iodovancomycin and their complexes with diacetyl-L-lysyl-D-alanyl-D-alanine. *Biochem. J.*, **1971a**, *123*, 773–787.

———. The specificity of combination between ristocetins and peptides related to bacterial cell wall mucopeptide precursors. *Ibid.*, **1971b**, *124*, 845–852.

Nolan, C. M.; Flanigan, W. J.; Rastogi, S. P.; and Brewer, T. E. Vancomycin penetration into CSF during treatment of patients receiving hemodialysis. *South. Med. J.*, **1980**, *73*, 1333–1334.

Nord, C. E., and Heimdahl, A. Impact of different antimicrobial agents on the colonization resistance in the intestinal tract with special reference to doxycycline. *Scand. J. Infect. Dis.*, **1988**, Suppl. 53, 50–58.

Orr, L. H., Jr.; Rudisill, E., Jr.; Brodkin, R.; and Hamilton, R. W. Exacerbation of renal failure associated with doxycycline. *Arch. Intern. Med.*, **1978**, *138*, 793–794.

Panzer, J. D.; Brown, D. C.; Epstein, W. L.; Lipson, R. L.; Mahaffrey, H. W.; and Atkinson, W. H. Clindamycin levels in various body tissues and fluids. *J. Clin. Pharmacol.*, **1972**, *12*, 259–262.

Park, B. H.; Hendricks, M.; Malamy, M. H.; Tally, F. P.; and Levy, S. B. Cryptic tetracycline resistance determinant (class F) from *Bacteroides fragilis*–mediated resistance in *Escherichia coli* by actively reducing tetracycline accumulation. *Antimicrob. Agents Chemother.*, **1987**, *31*, 1739–1743.

Piffaretti, J. C., and Froment, Y. Binding of chloramphenicol and its acetylated derivatives to *Escherichia coli* ribosomal subunits. *Chemotherapy*, **1978**, *24*, 24–28.

Polk, R. E.; Healy, D. P.; Schwartz, L. B.; Rock, D. T.; Garson, M. L.; and Roller, K. Vancomycin and the red-man syndrome: pharmacodynamics of histamine release. *J. Infect. Dis.*, **1988**, *157*, 502–507.

Powell, D. A.; Nahata, M. C.; Darrell, D. C.; Durrell, D. C.; Glazer, J. P.; and Hilty, M. D. Interactions among chloramphenicol, phenytoin, and phenobarbital in a pediatric patient. *J. Pediatr.*, **1981**, *98*, 1001–1003.

Pratt, W. B., and Fekety, R. *The Antimicrobial Drugs*. Oxford University Press, New York, **1986**, pp. 205–208.

Prober, C. G. Effect of rifampin on chronic chloramphenicol levels. *N. Engl. J. Med.*, **1985**, *312*, 788–789.

Rahal, J. J., Jr., and Simberkoff, M. S. Bactericidal and bacteriostatic action of chloramphenicol against meningeal pathogens. *Antimicrob. Agents Chemother.*, **1979**, *16*, 13–18.

Rasch, J. R., and Mogabgab, W. J. Therapeutic effect of erythromycin on *Mycoplasma pneumoniae* pneumonia. *Antimicrob. Agents Chemother.*, **1965**, *5*, 693–699.

Rifkin, G. D.; Fekety, F. R.; and Silva, J. Antibiotic-induced colitis: implication of a toxin neutralized by *Clostridium sordellii* antitoxin. *Lancet*, **1977**, *2*, 1103–1106.

Ringertz, S., and Dornbusch, K. *In vitro* susceptibility to tetracycline and doxycycline in clinical isolates of *Haemophilus influenzae*. *Scand. J. Infect. Dis.*, **1988**, Suppl. 53, 7–11.
Sabath, L. D.; Gerstein, D. A.; Loder, P. B.; and Finland, M. Excretion of erythromycin and its enhanced activity in urine against gram-negative bacilli with alkalinization. *J. Lab. Clin. Med.*, **1968**, *72*, 916–923.
Sack, D. A.; Kaminsky, D. C.; Sack, R. B.; Itotja, J. N.; Arthur, R. R.; Kapikian, A. Z.; Orskov, F.; and Orskov, I. Prophylactic doxycycline for travelers' diarrhea: results of a prospective double-blind study of Peace Corps volunteers in Kenya. *N. Engl. J. Med.*, **1978**, *298*, 758–763.
Salazar-Lindo, E.; Sack, R. B.; Chea-Woo, E.; Kay, B. A.; Piscoya, Z. A.; Leon-Barua, R.; and Yi, A. Early treatment with erythromycin of *Campylobacter jejuni*–associated dysentery in children. *J. Pediatr.*, **1986**, *109*, 355–360.
Salih, S. Y., and Mustafa, D. Louse-borne relapsing fever. II. Combined penicillin and tetracycline therapy in 160 Sudanese patients. *Trans. R. Soc. Trop. Med. Hyg.*, **1977**, *71*, 49–51.
Sands, L. C., and Shaw, W. V. Mechanism of chloramphenicol resistance in staphylococci: characterization and hybridization of variants of chloramphenicol acetyltransferase. *Antimicrob. Agents Chemother.*, **1973**, *3*, 299–305.
Sanford, J. P. *Guide to Antimicrobial Therapy 1989*. Antimicrobial Therapy, Inc., West Bethesda, Md., **1989**, p. 36.
Schaad, U. B.; McCracken, G. H., Jr.; and Nelson, J. D. Clinical pharmacology and efficacy of vancomycin in pediatric patients. *J. Pediatr.*, **1980**, *96*, 119–126.
Scheld, W. M.; Brown, R. S., Jr.; Fletcher, D. D.; and Sande, M. A. Bactericidal versus bacteriostatic antibiotic therapy of experimental pneumococcal meningitis. *Ann. Clin. Res.*, **1979**, *27*, 355a.
Schoutens, E.; Peromet, M.; and Yourassowsky, E. Microbiological and clinical study of spectinomycin in urinary tract infections: reevaluation with hospital strains. *Curr. Ther. Res.*, **1972**, *14*, 349–357.
Schwalbe, R. S.; Stapleton, J. T.; and Gilligan, P. H. Emergence of vancomycin resistance in coagulase-negative staphylococci. *N. Engl. J. Med.*, **1987**, *316*, 927–931.
Scott, J. L.; Finegold, S. M.; Belkin, G. A.; and Lawrence, J. S. A controlled double-blind study of the hematologic toxicity of chloramphenicol. *N. Engl. J. Med.*, **1965**, *272*, 1137–1142.
Seaberg, L. S.; Parquette, A. R.; Gluzman, I. Y.; Phillips, G. W., Jr.; Brodasky, T. F.; and Krogstad, D. J. Clindamycin activity against chloroquine-resistant *Plasmodium falciparum*. *Antimicrob. Agents Chemother.*, **1984**, *150*, 904–911.
Seifert, C. F.; Swaney, R. J.; and Bellanger-McCleery, R. A. Intravenous erythromycin lactobionate-induced severe nausea and vomiting. *Drug Intell. Clin. Pharm.*, **1989**, *23*, 40–44.
Shann, F.; Linneman, V.; MacKenzie, A.; Barker, J.; Gratten, M.; and Crinis, N. Absorption of chloramphenicol sodium succinate after intramuscular administration in children. *N. Engl. J. Med.*, **1985**, *313*, 410–414.
Shapera, R. M.; Hable, K. A.; and Matsen, J. M. Erythromycin therapy twice daily for streptococcal pharyngitis. Controlled comparison with erythromycin or penicillin phenoxymethyl four times daily or penicillin G benzathine. *J.A.M.A.*, **1973**, *226*, 531–555.
Sheldrick, G. M.; Jones, P. G.; Kennard, O.; Williams, D. H.; and Smith, G. A. Structure of vancomycin and its complex with acyl-D-alanyl-D-alanine. *Nature*, **1978**, *271*, 223–225.
Shenep, J. L.; Barton, R. P.; and Morgan, K. A. Role of antibiotic class in the rate of liberation of endotoxin during therapy for experimental gram-negative bacterial sepsis. *J. Infect. Dis.*, **1984**, *150*, 380–388.
Shils, M. E. Renal disease and the metabolic effects of tetracycline. *Ann. Intern. Med.*, **1963**, *58*, 389–408.
Shlaes, D. M.; Bouvet, A.; Devine, C.; Shlaes, J. H.; Al-Obeid, S.; and Williamson, R. Inducible, transferable resistance to vancomycin in *Enterococcus faecalis* A256. *Antimicrob. Agents Chemother.*, **1989**, *33*, 198–203.
Shu, X. O.; Linet, M. S.; Gao, R. N.; Gao, Y. T.; Brinton, L. A.; Jin, F.; and Fraumeni, J. F., Jr. Chloramphenicol use and childhood leukemia in Shanghai. *Lancet*, **1987**, *2*, 934–937.
Skerrett, S. J., and Locksley, R. M. Legionellosis: ecology and pathogenesis. In, *Contemporary Issues in Infectious Diseases*. Vol. 5, *Respiratory Infections*. (Sande, M. A.; Hudson, L. D.; and Root, R. K.; eds.) Churchill Livingstone, Inc., New York, **1986**, pp. 161–190.
Slaughter, R. L.; Cerra, F. B.; and Koup, J. R. Effect of hemodialysis on total body clearance of chloramphenicol. *Am. J. Hosp. Pharm.*, **1980a**, *37*, 1083–1086.
Slaughter, R. L.; Pieper, J. A.; Cerra, F. B.; Brodsky, B.; and Koup, J. R. Chloramphenicol sodium succinate kinetics in critically ill patients. *Clin. Pharmacol. Ther.*, **1980b**, *28*, 69–77.
Smith, A. L., and Weber, A. Pharmacology of chloramphenicol. *Pediatr. Clin. North Am.*, **1983**, *30*, 209–236.
Snyder, M. J.; Gonzalez, O.; Palomino, C.; Music, S. I.; Hornick, R. B.; Perroni, J.; Woodward, W. E.; Gonzalez, C.; DuPont, H. R.; and Woodward, L. E. Comparative efficacy of chloramphenicol, ampicillin, and co-trimoxazole in the treatment of typhoid fever. *Lancet*, **1976**, *2*, 1155–1157.
Solomkin, J. S.; Fant, W. K.; Rivera, J. O.; and Alexander, J. W. Randomized trial of imipenem/cilastatin versus gentamicin and clindamycin in mixed flora infections. *Am. J. Med.*, **1985**, *78*, Suppl. 6A, 85–91.
Sompolinsky, D., and Samra, Z. Mechanism of high-level resistance to chloramphenicol in different *Escherichia coli* variants. *J. Gen. Microbiol.*, **1968**, *50*, 55–66.
Sorrell, T. C.; Packham, D. R.; Shanker, S.; Foldes, M.; and Munro, R. Vancomycin therapy for methicillin-resistant *Staphylococcus aureus*. *Ann. Intern. Med.*, **1982**, *97*, 344–350.
Stamm, W. E.; Running, K.; McKevitt, M.; Counts, G. W.; Turck, M.; and Holmes, K. K. Treatment of the acute urethral syndrome. *N. Engl. J. Med.*, **1981**, *304*, 956–958.
Standiford, H. C. Tetracyclines and chloramphenicol. In, *Principles and Practice of Infectious Diseases*, 3rd ed. (Mandell, G. L.; Douglas, R. G., Jr.; and Bennett, J. E.; eds.) John Wiley & Sons, Inc., New York, **1990**, pp. 284–295.
Steigbigel, N. H. Erythromycin, lincomycin, and clindamycin. In, *Principles and Practice of Infectious Diseases*, 3rd ed. (Mandell, G. L.; Douglas, R. G., Jr.; and Bennett, J. E.; eds.) John Wiley & Sons, Inc., New York, **1990**, pp. 308–317.
Suhrland, L. F., and Weisberger, A. S. Chloramphenicol toxicity in liver and renal disease. *Arch. Intern. Med.*, **1963**, *112*, 747–754.
Sutherland, G. E.; Palitang, E. G.; Marr, J. J.; and Luedke, S. L. Sterilization of Ommaya reservoir by instillation of vancomycin. *Am. J. Med.*, **1981**, *71*, 1068–1070.
Tally, F. P.; Snydman, D. R.; Gorbach, S. L.; and Malamy, M. H. Plasmid-mediated transferable resistance to clindamycin and erythromycin in *Bacteroides fragilis*. *J. Infect. Dis.*, **1979**, *139*, 83–88.
Täuber, M. G.; Shibl, A. M.; Hackbarth, C. J.; Larrick, J. W.; and Sande, M. A. Antibiotic therapy, endotoxin concentration in cerebrospinal fluid, and brain edema in

experimental *Escherichia coli* meningitis in rabbits. *Antimicrob. Agents Chemother.*, **1987**, *156*, 456–462.

Taylor, D. N.; Blaser, M. J.; Echeverria, P.; Pitarangsi, C.; Bodhidatta, L.; and Wang, W.-L. L. Erythromycin-resistant *Campylobacter* infections in Thailand. *Antimicrob. Agents Chemother.*, **1987**, *31*, 438–442.

Tedesco, F. J. Clindamycin and colitis: a review. *J. Infect. Dis.*, **1977**, *135S*, 95–98.

Thadepalli, H.; Gorbach, S. L.; Broido, P. W.; Norsen, J.; and Nyhus, L. Abdominal trauma, anaerobes, and antibiotics. *Surg. Gynecol. Obstet.*, **1973**, *137*, 270–276.

Tolman, K. G.; Sannella, J. J.; and Freston, J. W. Chemical structure of erythromycin and hepatotoxicity. *Ann. Intern. Med.*, **1974**, *81*, 58–60.

Uttley, A. H. C.; Collins, C. H.; Naidodo, J.; and George, R. C. Vancomycin-resistant enterococci. *Lancet*, **1988**, *1*, 57–58.

Vanhoof, R.; Gordts, B.; Dierickx, R.; Coignau, H.; and Butzler, J. D. Bacteriostatic and bactericidal activities of 24 antimicrobial agents against *Campylobacter fetus* subs. *jejuni*. *Antimicrob. Agents Chemother.*, **1980**, *18*, 118–121.

Visconti, E. B., and Peter, G. Vancomycin treatment of cerebrospinal fluid shunt infections. *J. Neurosurg.*, **1979**, *51*, 245–246.

Vogel, Z.; Vogel, T.; and Elson, D. The effect of erythromycin on peptide bond formation and the termination reaction. *FEBS Lett.*, **1971**, *15*, 249–253.

Wallerstein, R. O.; Condit, P. K.; Kasper, C. K.; Brown, J. W.; and Morrison, F. R. Statewide study of chloramphenicol therapy and fatal aplastic anemia. *J.A.M.A.*, **1969**, *208*, 2045–2050.

Walters, B. N. J., and Gubbay, S. S. Tetracycline and benign intracranial hypertension: report of five cases. *Br. Med. J.*, **1981**, *282*, 19–20.

Ward, H. P. The effect of chloramphenicol on RNA and heme synthesis in bone marrow cultures. *J. Lab. Clin. Med.*, **1966**, *68*, 400–410.

Watanakunakorn, C. The antibacterial action of vancomycin. *Rev. Infect. Dis.*, **1981**, *3*, Suppl., S210–S215.

Watanakunakorn, C., and Tisone, J. C. Synergism between vancomycin and gentamicin or tobramycin for methicillin-susceptible and methicillin-resistant *Staphylococcus aureus* strains. *Antimicrob. Agents Chemother.*, **1982**, *22*, 903–905.

Winckler, K. Tetracycline ulcers of the oesophagus; endoscopy, histology, and roentgenology in two cases, and review of the literature. *Endoscopy*, **1981**, *13*, 225–228.

Woodward, T. E. Rocky Mountain spotted fever: epidemiological and early clinical signs are keys to treatment and reduced mortality. *J. Infect. Dis.*, **1984**, *150*, 465–468.

World Health Organization. Joint FAO/WHO Expert Committee on Brucellosis. *World Health Organization Technical Report Series*, 6th Report. **1986**, *740*, 1–128.

Zimmerman, H. J., and Lewis, J. H. Hepatic toxicity of antimicrobial agents. In, *Contemporary Issues in Infectious Diseases*. Vol. 1, *New Dimensions in Antimicrobial Therapy*. (Root, R. K., and Sande, M. A., eds.) Churchill Livingstone, Inc., New York, **1984**, pp. 153–202.

Monographs and Reviews

Bowie, W., and Holmes, K. K. *Chlamydia* trachomatis (trachoma, inclusion conjunctivitis, lymphogranuloma venereum). In, *Principles and Practice of Infectious Diseases*, 2nd ed. (Mandell, G. L.; Douglas, R. G., Jr.; and Bennett, J. E.; eds.) John Wiley & Sons, Inc., New York, **1985**, pp. 1464–1476.

Bryant, R. E. Effect of the suppurative environment on antibiotic activity. In, *Contemporary Issues in Infectious Diseases*. Vol. 1, *New Dimensions in Antimicrobial Therapy*. (Root, R. K., and Sande, M. A., eds.) Churchill Livingstone, Inc., New York, **1984**, pp. 313–338.

Chopra, I., and Howe, T. G. B. Bacterial resistance to the tetracyclines. *Microbiol. Rev.*, **1978**, *42*, 707–724.

Dowling, H. F. *Tetracycline*. Medical Encyclopedia, Inc., New York, **1955**.

Lepper, M. H. AUREOMYCIN (*Chlortetracycline*). Medical Encyclopedia, Inc., New York, **1956**.

CHAPTER

49 ANTIMICROBIAL AGENTS

[*Continued*]

Drugs Used in the Chemotherapy of Tuberculosis and Leprosy

Gerald L. Mandell and Merle A. Sande

The pharmacological characteristics and the therapeutic use of each class of compounds employed in the chemotherapy of tuberculosis and leprosy are discussed in this chapter. The treatment of mycobacterial infections in man has become an even more important and challenging problem because of the acquired immunodeficiency syndrome (AIDS) pandemic, which has been associated with a marked increase in tuberculosis and infection caused by the *Mycobacterium avium* complex. Since the microorganisms grow slowly and the diseases are often chronic, patient compliance, drug toxicity, and the development of microbial resistance present special therapeutic problems.

I. Drugs for Tuberculosis

Drugs used in the treatment of tuberculosis can be divided into two major categories. ''First-line'' agents combine the greatest level of efficacy with an acceptable degree of toxicity; these include isoniazid, rifampin, ethambutol, streptomycin, and pyrazinamide. The large majority of patients with tuberculosis can be treated successfully with these drugs. Administration of rifampin in combination with isoniazid for 9 months is effective therapy for all forms of disease caused by sensitive strains of *M. tuberculosis*. Excellent results can also be obtained with a shorter, 6-month course of treatment; for the first 2 months, isoniazid, rifampin, and pyrazinamide are given, followed by isoniazid and rifampin for the remaining 4 months. In areas where primary resistance to isoniazid is high, therapy is usually initiated with four drugs—rifampin, isoniazid, pyrazinamide, and ethambutol (or streptomycin)—until sensitivity tests are completed. Occasionally, however, because of microbial resistance or patient-related factors, it may be necessary to resort to a ''second-line'' drug; this category of agents includes ethionamide, aminosalicylic acid, cycloserine, amikacin, kanamycin, and capreomycin (*see* Des Prez and Heim, 1990).

ISONIAZID

Isoniazid is still considered to be the primary drug for the chemotherapy of tuberculosis, and all patients with disease caused by isoniazid-sensitive strains of the tubercle bacillus should receive the drug if they can tolerate it.

History. The discovery of isoniazid was somewhat fortuitous. In 1945, Chorine reported that nicotinamide possesses tuberculostatic action. Examination of the compounds related to nicotinamide revealed that many pyridine derivatives possess tuberculostatic activity; among these are congeners of isonicotinic acid. Because the thiosemicarbazones were known to inhibit *M. tuberculosis*, the thiosemicarbazone of isonicotinaldehyde was synthesized and studied. The starting material for this synthesis was the methyl ester of isonicotinic acid, and the first intermediate was isonicotinylhydrazide (isoniazid). The interesting history of these chemical studies has been reviewed by Fox (1953).

Chemistry. Isoniazid is the hydrazide of isonicotinic acid; the structural formula is as follows:

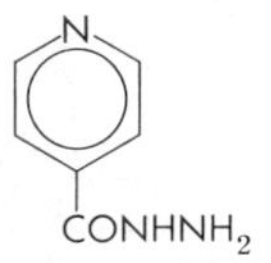

Isoniazid

The isopropyl derivative of isoniazid, iproniazid (1-isonicotinyl-2-isopropylhydrazide), also inhibits the multiplication of the tubercle bacillus. This compound, which is a potent inhibitor of monoamine oxidase, is too toxic for use in man. However, its study led to the use of monoamine oxidase inhibitors for the treatment of depression (*see* Chapter 18).

Antibacterial Activity. Isoniazid is bacteriostatic for "resting" bacilli but is bactericidal for rapidly dividing microorganisms. The minimal tuberculostatic concentration is 0.025 to 0.05 μg/ml. The bacteria undergo one or two divisions before multiplication is arrested. The drug is remarkably selective for mycobacteria, and concentrations in excess of 500 μg/ml are required to inhibit the growth of other microorganisms.

Isoniazid is highly effective for the treatment of experimentally induced tuberculosis in animals and is strikingly superior to streptomycin. Unlike streptomycin, isoniazid penetrates cells with ease and is just as effective against bacilli growing within cells as it is against those growing in culture media.

Among the various nontuberculous (atypical) mycobacteria, only *M. kansasii* is usually susceptible to isoniazid. However, sensitivity must always be tested *in vitro*, since the inhibitory concentration required may be rather high.

Bacterial Resistance. When tubercle bacilli are grown *in vitro* in increasing concentrations of isoniazid, mutants are readily selected that are resistant to the drug, even when the drug is present in enormous concentrations. However, cross-resistance between isoniazid and other agents used to treat tuberculosis does not occur. Current evidence suggests that the mechanism of resistance is related to failure of the drug to penetrate or to be taken up by the microorganisms.

As with the other agents described, treatment with isoniazid alone leads to the emergence *in vivo* of resistant strains. The shift from primarily sensitive to mainly insensitive microorganisms occasionally occurs within a few weeks after therapy is started; however, the time of appearance of this phenomenon varies considerably from one case to another. Approximately one in 10^6 tubercle bacilli will be genetically resistant to isoniazid; since tuberculous cavities may contain as many as 10^7 to 10^9 microorganisms, it is not surprising that treatment with isoniazid alone results in the selection of these resistant bacteria. The incidence of primary resistance to isoniazid in the United States appears to be fairly stable at 2 to 5% of isolates of *M. tuberculosis*, but it may be much higher in certain populations, including Asians and Hispanics (Carpenter *et al.*, 1982; Centers for Disease Control, 1983).

Mechanism of Action. While the mechanism of action of isoniazid is unknown, several hypotheses have been proposed. These include effects on lipids, nucleic acid biosynthesis, and glycolysis (Herman and Weber, 1980). Takayama and associates (1975) have suggested a primary action of isoniazid to inhibit the biosynthesis of mycolic acids, important constituents of the mycobacterial cell wall. Low concentrations of isoniazid may prevent elongation of the very-long-chain fatty acid precursor of the molecule, and the drug inhibits the mycobacterial desaturase that catalyzes the first reaction that is specific to mycolic acid synthesis (Davidson and Takayama, 1979). Since mycolic acids are unique to mycobacteria, this action would explain the high degree of selectivity of the antimicrobial activity of isoniazid. Exposure to isoniazid leads to a loss of acid fastness and a decrease in the quantity of methanol-extractable lipid of the microorganisms. Only isoniazid-sensitive tubercle bacilli take up the drug. This uptake appears to be an active process, although most of the drug within the bacilli is the inactive isonicotinic acid metabolite (Jenne and Beggs, 1973).

Absorption, Distribution, and Excretion. Isoniazid is readily absorbed when administered either orally or parenterally. Aluminum-containing antacids may interfere with absorption (Hurwitz and Schlozman, 1974). Peak plasma concentrations of 3 to 5 μg/ml develop 1 to 2 hours after oral ingestion of usual doses.

Isoniazid diffuses readily into all body fluids and cells. The drug is detectable in significant quantities in pleural and ascitic fluids; concentrations in the cerebrospinal fluid (CSF) are similar to those in the plasma (Holdiness, 1985). Isoniazid penetrates well into caseous material. The concentration of the agent is initially higher in the plasma and muscle than in the infected tissue, but the latter retains the drug for a long time in quantities well above those required for bacteriostasis.

From 75 to 95% of a dose of isoniazid is excreted in the urine within 24 hours, mostly as metabolites. The main excretory products in man are the result of enzymatic acetylation (acetylisoniazid) and enzymatic hydrolysis (isonicotinic acid). Small quantities of an isonicotinic acid conjugate (probably isonicotinyl glycine), one or more isonicotinyl hydrazones, and traces of N-methylisoniazid are also detectable in the urine.

Human populations show genetic heterogeneity with regard to the rate of acetylation of isoniazid (Evans *et al.*, 1960). The distribution of slow and rapid inactivators of the drug is bimodal owing to differences in the activity of an acetyltransferase. The rate of acetylation significantly alters the concentrations of the drug that are achieved in plasma and its half-life in the circulation. The half-life of the drug may be prolonged in the presence of hepatic insufficiency.

The frequency of each acetylation phenotype is dependent upon race but is not influenced by sex or age. Fast acetylation is found in Eskimos and Japanese. Slow acetylation is the predominant phenotype in most Scandinavians, Jews, and North African Caucasians. The incidence of "slow acetylators" among the various racial types in the United States is about 50% (La Du, 1972). Since high acetyltransferase activity (fast acetylation) is inherited as an autosomal dominant trait, "fast acetylators" of isoniazid are either heterozygous or homozygous. The average concentration of active isoniazid in the circulation of fast acetylators is about 30 to 50% of that present in persons who acetylate the drug slowly. In the whole population, the half-life of isoniazid varies from less than 1 to more than 3 hours. The mean half-life in fast acetylators is approximately 70 minutes, while 3 hours is characteristic of slow acetylators. However, because isoniazid is relatively nontoxic, a sufficient amount of drug can be administered to fast acetylators to achieve a therapeutic effect equal to that seen in slow acetylators.

The clearance of isoniazid is dependent to only a small degree on the status of renal function, but patients who are slow inactivators of the drug may accumulate toxic concentrations if their renal function is impaired. Bowersox and colleagues (1973) have suggested that 300 mg per day of the drug can be administered safely to individuals in whom the plasma creatinine concentration is less than 12 mg/dl (1.1 mM).

Preparations, Routes of Administration, and Dosage. *Isoniazid* (*isonicotinic acid hydrazide;* NYDRAZID, others) is available in tablets containing 50, 100, and 300 mg; as a syrup containing 10 mg/ml; and as an injection in a concentration of 100 mg/ml. The commonly used total daily dose of the drug is 5 mg/kg, with a maximum of 300 mg; oral and intramuscular doses are identical. Isoniazid is usually given orally in a single daily dose but may be given in two divided doses. While doses of 10 mg/kg with a maximum of 600 mg are occasionally used in severely ill patients, there is no evidence that this regimen is more effective. Children should receive 10 to 20 mg/kg per day (300 mg maximum). Isoniazid may be used as intermittent therapy for tuberculosis. After a minimum of 2 months of daily therapy with isoniazid, rifampin, and pyrazinamide, patients may be treated with twice-weekly doses of isoniazid (15 mg/kg, orally) plus rifampin (10 mg/kg, up to 600 mg per dose) for 4 months.

Pyridoxine (15 to 50 mg per day) should be administered with isoniazid to minimize adverse reactions (*see* below) in malnourished patients and those predisposed to neuropathy (*e.g.*, the elderly, pregnant women, diabetics, alcoholics, and uremics) (Snider, 1980).

Untoward Effects. The incidence of adverse reactions to isoniazid was estimated to be 5.4% among more than 2000 patients treated with the drug; the most prominent of these reactions were rash (2%), fever (1.2%), jaundice (0.6%), and peripheral neuritis (0.2%) (Pitts, 1977). Hypersensitivity to isoniazid may result in fever, various skin eruptions, hepatitis, and morbilliform, maculopapular, purpuric, and urticarial rashes. Hematological reactions may also occur (agranulocytosis, eosinophilia, thrombocytopenia, anemia). Vasculitis associated with antinuclear antibodies may appear during treatment but disappears when the drug is stopped (Rothfield *et al.*, 1978). Arthritic symptoms (back pain, bilateral proximal interphalangeal joint involvement, arthralgia of the knees, elbows, and wrists, and the "shoulder–hand" syndrome) have been attributed to this agent.

If pyridoxine is not given concurrently, peripheral neuritis is the most common reaction to isoniazid and occurs in about 2% of patients receiving 5 mg/kg of the drug daily. Higher doses may result in peripheral neuritis in 10 to 20% of patients. The prophylactic administration of pyridoxine prevents the development not only of peripheral neuritis but also of most other nervous system disorders in practically all instances, even when therapy lasts as long as 2 years.

Isoniazid may precipitate convulsions in patients with seizure disorders and, rarely, in patients with no history of seizures. Optic neuritis and atrophy have also occurred during therapy with the drug. Muscle twitching, dizziness, ataxia, paresthesias, stupor, and toxic encephalopathy that may be fatal are other manifestations of the neurotoxicity of isoniazid. A number of mental abnormalities may appear during the use of this drug; among these are euphoria, transient impairment of memory, separation of ideas and reality, loss of self-control, and florid psychoses.

Isoniazid is known to inhibit the parahydroxylation of phenytoin, and signs and symptoms of toxicity occur in approximately 27% of patients given both drugs, particularly in those who are slow acetylators (Miller *et al.*, 1979). Concentrations of phenytoin in plasma should be monitored and adjusted if necessary. The dosage of isoniazid should not be changed.

Although jaundice has been known for some time to be an untoward effect of exposure to isoniazid, it was not until the early 1970s that it became apparent that severe hepatic injury leading to death may occur in some individuals receiving this drug (Garibaldi *et al.,* 1972). Additional studies in adults and children have confirmed this observation; the characteristic pathological process is bridging and multilobular necrosis. Continuation of the drug after symptoms of hepatic dysfunction have appeared tends to increase the severity of damage. The mechanisms responsible for this toxicity are unknown, although acetylhydrazine, which is a metabolite of isoniazid, causes hepatic damage in adults (Mitchell *et al.,* 1976). A contributory role of alcoholic hepatitis has been noted (Gronhagen-Riska *et al.,* 1978), but chronic carriers of hepatitis B virus tolerate isoniazid (McGlynn *et al.,* 1986). Age appears to be the most important factor in determining the risk of isoniazid-induced hepatotoxicity. Hepatic damage is rare in patients less than 20 years old; the complication is observed in 0.3% of those 20 to 34 years old, and the incidence increases to 1.2% and 2.3% in individuals 35 to 49 and older than 50 years of age, respectively (Public Health Service, 1974). The incidence of hepatotoxicity also appears to be greater in slow acetylators. Up to 12% of patients receiving isoniazid may have elevated plasma transaminase activities (Bailey *et al.,* 1974). Patients receiving isoniazid should be carefully evaluated at monthly intervals for symptoms of hepatitis (anorexia, malaise, fatigue, nausea, and jaundice). Some clinicians also prefer to determine serum aspartate aminotransferase activities at monthly intervals (Byrd *et al.,* 1979) and recommend that an elevation greater than five times normal is cause for discontinuation of the drug. Most hepatitis occurs 4 to 8 weeks after the start of therapy. Isoniazid should be administered with great care to those with preexisting hepatic disease. (*See* Maddrey and Boitnott, 1973.)

Among miscellaneous reactions associated with isoniazid therapy are dryness of the mouth, epigastric distress, methemoglobinemia, tinnitus, and urinary retention. In persons predisposed to pyridoxine-deficiency anemia, the administration of isoniazid may result in its appearance in full-blown form. Treatment with large doses of the vitamin gradually returns the blood to normal in such cases (*see* Goldman and Braman, 1972). A drug-induced syndrome resembling systemic lupus erythematosus has been reported (Rothfield *et al.,* 1978). Overdose of isoniazid, as in attempted suicide, may result in coma, seizures, metabolic acidosis, and hyperglycemia. Pyridoxine is an antidote in this setting; it should be given in a dose that approximates the amount of isoniazid ingested.

Therapeutic Status. Isoniazid is still the most important drug for the treatment of all types of tuberculosis. Toxic effects can be minimized by prophylactic therapy with pyridoxine and careful surveillance of the patient. The drug must be used concurrently with another agent for treatment, although it is used alone for prophylaxis.

Details of the use of isoniazid in the chemotherapy of tuberculosis are given below.

RIFAMPIN

The rifamycins are a group of structurally similar, complex macrocyclic antibiotics produced by *Streptomyces mediterranei;* rifampin is a semisynthetic derivative of one of these—rifamycin B.

Chemistry. Rifampin is soluble in organic solvents and in water at acidic pH. It has the following structure:

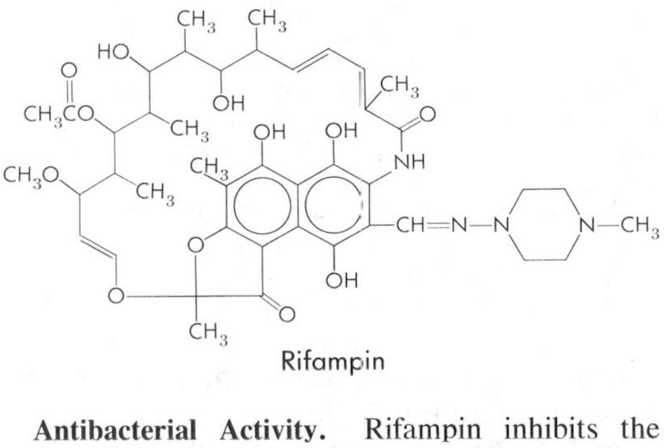

Rifampin

Antibacterial Activity. Rifampin inhibits the growth of most gram-positive bacteria, as well as many gram-negative microorganisms such as *Esch-*

erichia coli, Pseudomonas, indole-positive and indole-negative *Proteus,* and *Klebsiella.* Rifampin is very active against *Staphylococcus aureus* and coagulase-negative staphylococci; bactericidal concentrations range from 3 to 12 ng/ml. The drug is also highly active against *Neisseria meningitidis* and *Haemophilus influenzae;* minimal inhibitory concentrations range from 0.1 to 0.8 μg/ml. Rifampin is very inhibitory to *Legionella* species in cell culture and in animal models (Thornsberry *et al.,* 1983).

Rifampin in concentrations of 0.005 to 0.2 μg/ml inhibits the growth of *M. tuberculosis in vitro.* Among nontuberculous mycobacteria, *M. kansasii* is inhibited by 0.25 to 1 μg/ml. The majority of strains of *M. scrofulaceum, M. intracellulare,* and *M. avium* are suppressed by concentrations of 4 μg/ml, but certain strains may be resistant to 16 μg/ml. *M. fortuitum* is highly resistant to the drug. Rifampin increases the *in-vitro* activity of streptomycin and isoniazid, but not that of ethambutol, against *M. tuberculosis* (Hobby and Lenert, 1972).

Bacterial Resistance. Microorganisms, including mycobacteria, may develop resistance to rifampin rapidly *in vitro* as a one-step process, and one of every 10^7 to 10^8 tubercle bacilli is resistant to the drug. This also appears to be the case *in vivo,* and therefore the antibiotic must not be used alone in the chemotherapy of tuberculosis. When rifampin has been used for eradication of the meningococcal carrier state, failures have been due to the appearance of drug-resistant bacteria after treatment for as little as 2 days (Devine *et al.,* 1971). Microbial resistance to rifampin is due to an alteration of the target of this drug, DNA-dependent RNA polymerase. Certain rifampin-resistant bacterial mutants have decreased virulence. Tuberculosis caused by rifampin-resistant mycobacteria has been described in patients who had not received prior chemotherapy, but this is very rare (usually less than 1%) (Cauthen *et al.,* 1988).

Mechanism of Action. Rifampin inhibits DNA-dependent RNA polymerase of mycobacteria and other microorganisms, leading to suppression of initiation of chain formation (but not chain elongation) in RNA synthesis. More specifically, the β subunit of this complex enzyme is the site of action of the drug, although rifampin binds only to the holoenzyme. Nuclear RNA polymerase from a variety of eukaryotic cells does not bind rifampin, and RNA synthesis is correspondingly unaffected. While rifampin can inhibit RNA synthesis in mammalian mitochondria, considerably higher concentrations of the drug are required than for the inhibition of the bacterial enzyme. Rifampin is bactericidal for both intracellular and extracellular microorganisms. (*See* Wehrli, 1983.)

Absorption, Distribution, and Excretion. The oral administration of rifampin produces peak concentrations in plasma in 2 to 4 hours; after ingestion of 600 mg this value is about 7 μg/ml, but there is considerable variability. Aminosalicylic acid may delay the absorption of rifampin, and adequate plasma concentrations may not be reached. If these agents are used concurrently, they should be given separately at an interval of 8 to 12 hours (*see* Radner, 1973).

Following absorption from the gastrointestinal tract, rifampin is rapidly eliminated in the bile, and an enterohepatic circulation ensues. During this time the drug is progressively deacetylated, such that after 6 hours nearly all of the antibiotic in the bile is in the deacetylated form. This metabolite retains essentially full antibacterial activity. Intestinal reabsorption is reduced by deacetylation (as well as by food), and metabolism thus facilitates elimination of the drug. The half-life of rifampin varies from 1.5 to 5 hours and is increased in the presence of hepatic dysfunction; it may be decreased in patients receiving isoniazid concurrently who are slow inactivators of this drug. The half-life of rifampin is progressively shortened by about 40% during the first 14 days of treatment, owing to induction of hepatic microsomal enzymes with acceleration of deacetylation of the drug. Up to 30% of a dose of the drug is excreted in the urine; less than half of this may be unaltered antibiotic. Adjustment of dosage is not necessary in patients with impaired renal function.

Rifampin is distributed throughout the body and is present in effective concentrations in many organs and body fluids, including the CSF (Sippel *et al.,* 1974). This is perhaps best exemplified by the fact that the drug may impart an orange-red color to the urine, feces, saliva, sputum, tears, and sweat; patients should be so warned. (For various aspects of rifampin metabolism, *see* Furesz, 1970; Jenne and Beggs, 1973; Farr and Mandell, 1990.)

Preparations, Route of Administration, and Dosage. *Rifampin* (RIFADIN, RIMACTANE) is supplied in capsules containing 150 or 300 mg. The drug is also available as a fixed-dose combination with isoniazid (150 mg of isoniazid, 300 mg of rifampin; RIFAMATE). The dose for therapy of tuberculosis in adults is 600 mg, given once daily, either 1 hour before or 2 hours after a meal. Children should receive 10 mg/kg, with a daily maximum of 600 mg, given in the same way. Doses of 15 mg/kg or higher are associated with increased hepatotoxicity in children (3.2%) (Centers for Disease Control, 1980). Higher doses are reserved for other (short-term) uses. To prevent meningococcal disease (*see* below), adults may be treated with 600 mg once daily for 4 days; children should receive 10 to 20 mg/kg, to a maximum of 600 mg. For prophylaxis of *H. influenzae* (type-B) meningitis, some authorities recommend a dose of 20 mg/kg daily for 4 days (Broome *et al.*, 1987).

Untoward Effects. Rifampin is generally well tolerated. When given in usual doses, less than 4% of patients with tuberculosis have significant adverse reactions; the most common are rash (0.8%), fever (0.5%), and nausea and vomiting (1.5%) (*see* Grosset and Leventis, 1983). The most notable problem is the development of jaundice (Scheuer *et al.*, 1974). Sixteen deaths associated with this reaction have been recorded in 500,000 treated patients. Hepatitis from rifampin rarely occurs in patients with normal hepatic function; likewise, the combination of isoniazid and rifampin appears generally safe in such patients (Gangadharam, 1986). However, chronic liver disease, alcoholism, and old age appear to increase the incidence of severe hepatic problems when rifampin is given alone or concurrently with isoniazid (Gronhagen-Riska *et al.*, 1978).

Administration of rifampin on an intermittent schedule (less than twice weekly) and/or daily doses of 1200 mg or greater is associated with frequent side effects, and the drug should not be used in this manner. A flu-like syndrome with fever, chills, and myalgias develops in 20% of patients so treated. The syndrome may also include eosinophilia, interstitial nephritis, acute tubular necrosis, thrombocytopenia, hemolytic anemia, and shock (Flynn *et al.*, 1974; Girling and Hitze, 1979).

Since rifampin is a potent inducer of hepatic microsomal enzymes (Ohnhaus *et al.*, 1979), its administration results in a decreased half-life for a number of compounds, including prednisone, digitoxin, quinidine, ketoconazole, propranolol, metoprolol, clofibrate, and the sulfonylureas. There is a similar and significant interaction between rifampin and oral anticoagulants of the coumarin type, which leads to a decrease in efficacy of the latter agents. This effect appears about 5 to 8 days after rifampin administration is started and persists for 5 to 7 days after it is stopped (O'Reilly, 1975). Rifampin also appears to enhance the catabolism of a variety of steroids (Buffington *et al.*, 1976); for this reason it decreases the effectiveness of oral contraceptives (Skolnick *et al.*, 1976). Methadone metabolism is also increased, and the precipitation of withdrawal syndromes has been reported. Rifampin may reduce biliary excretion of contrast media used for visualization of the gallbladder (*see* Baciewicz *et al.*, 1987).

Gastrointestinal disturbances produced by rifampin (epigastric distress, nausea, vomiting, abdominal cramps, diarrhea) have occasionally required discontinuation of the drug. Various symptoms related to the nervous system have also been noted, including fatigue, drowsiness, headache, dizziness, ataxia, confusion, inability to concentrate, generalized numbness, pain in the extremities, and muscular weakness. Among hypersensitivity reactions are fever, pruritus, urticaria, various types of skin eruptions, eosinophilia, and soreness of the mouth and tongue. Hemolysis, hemoglobinuria, hematuria, renal insufficiency, and acute renal failure have been observed rarely; these are also thought to be hypersensitivity reactions. Thrombocytopenia, transient leukopenia, and anemia have occurred during therapy. Since the potential teratogenicity of rifampin is unknown, and the drug is known to cross the placenta, it is best to avoid the use of this agent during pregnancy.

Graber and associates (1973) have noted immunoglobulin light-chain proteinuria (either kappa, lambda, or both) in about 85% of patients with tuberculosis treated with rifampin. None of the patients had symptoms or electrophoretic patterns compatible with myeloma. However, renal failure has been associated with light-chain proteinuria (Warrington *et al.*, 1977).

Rifampin suppresses the transformation of antigen-sensitized lymphocytes by the antigen. The administration of rifampin in conventional doses has been noted to suppress T-cell function (Gupta *et al.*, 1975) and cutaneous hypersensitivity to tuberculin (Mukerjee *et al.*, 1973). Rifampin also causes immunosuppression in animal models (Bassi *et al.*, 1973); this effect may be related to inhibition of protein synthesis by cells involved in the immune process (Buss *et al.*, 1978). However, rifampin does not suppress the antibody response to influenza vaccine (Albert *et al.*, 1978), and there is no evidence that rifampin-induced immunosuppression causes deleterious effects in patients receiving the drug (Farr and Mandell, 1982).

Therapeutic Status. Rifampin and isoniazid are the most effective drugs available for the treatment of tuberculosis. Rifampin (like isoniazid) should never be used alone for this disease because of the rapidity with which resistance may develop. Despite the long list of untoward effects from rifampin, their incidence is low and treatment seldom has to be interrupted.

The use of rifampin in the chemotherapy of tuberculosis is detailed below.

Rifampin is a drug of choice for chemoprophylaxis of meningococcal disease and meningitis due to *H. influenzae* in household contacts of patients with such infections. The drug also shows promise in the treatment of certain nonmycobacterial diseases (Symposium, 1983). Combined with a beta-lactam antibiotic or vancomycin, rifampin may be useful for therapy in selected cases of staphylococcal endocarditis (on both natural and prosthetic valves) or osteomyelitis, especially those caused by staphylococci "tolerant" to penicillin (Kapusnik *et al.*, 1984). Rifampin may be indicated for therapy of infections in patients with inadequate leukocytic bactericidal activity and for eradication of the staphylococcal nasal carrier state in patients with chronic furunculosis (Wheat *et al.*, 1983). Rifampin can also be used in combination with trimethoprim–sulfamethoxazole in patients who are allergic to beta-lactam antibiotics for the treatment of infections with methicillin-resistant staphylococci.

ETHAMBUTOL

Chemistry. Ethambutol is a water-soluble and heat-stable compound. The structural formula is as follows:

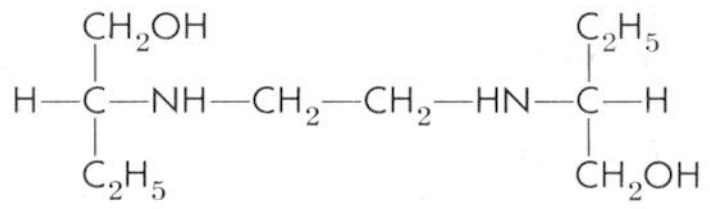

Ethambutol

Antibacterial Activity. Nearly all strains of *M. tuberculosis* and *M. kansasii* as well as a number of strains of *M. avium* complex are sensitive to ethambutol. The sensitivities of other nontuberculous organisms are variable. Ethambutol has no effect on other bacteria. It suppresses the growth of most isoniazid- and streptomycin-resistant tubercle bacilli. Resistance to ethambutol develops very slowly *in vitro*.

Mycobacteria take up ethambutol rapidly when the drug is added to cultures that are in the exponential growth phase. However, growth is not significantly inhibited before about 24 hours; the drug is tuberculostatic. Although the precise mechanism of action of ethambutol is unknown, the drug has been shown to inhibit the incorporation of mycolic acid into the mycobacterial cell wall (Takayama *et al.*, 1979). Bacterial resistance to the drug develops *in vivo* when it is given in the absence of another effective agent.

Absorption, Distribution, and Excretion. About 75 to 80% of an orally administered dose of ethambutol is absorbed from the gastrointestinal tract. Concentrations in plasma are maximal in man 2 to 4 hours after the drug is taken and are proportional to the dose. A single dose of 15 mg/kg produces a plasma concentration of about 5 μg/ml at 2 to 4 hours. The drug has a half-life of 3 to 4 hours.

Within 24 hours, two thirds of an ingested dose of ethambutol is excreted unchanged in the urine; up to 15% is excreted in the form of two metabolites, an aldehyde and a dicarboxylic acid derivative (Peets *et al.*, 1965). Renal clearance of ethambutol is approximately 7 $ml \cdot min^{-1} \cdot kg^{-1}$, and thus it is evident that the drug is excreted by tubular secretion in addition to glomerular filtration.

Preparation, Route of Administration, and Dosage. *Ethambutol hydrochloride* (MYAMBUTOL) is available in tablets containing 100 or 400 mg of the *d* isomer. The usual adult dose is 15 mg/kg, given once a day. Some physicians prefer to institute therapy with a dose of 25 mg/kg per day for the first 60 days and then to reduce the dose to 15 mg/kg per day, particularly for those who have received previous therapy.

Ethambutol accumulates in patients with impaired renal function, and adjustment of dosage is necessary (*see* Appendix II). Ethambutol is not recommended for children under 5 years of age, in part because of concern about the ability to test their visual acuity reliably (*see* below).

Untoward Effects. Ethambutol produces very few reactions. Daily doses of 15 mg/kg are minimally toxic. Less than 2% of nearly 2000 patients who received 15 mg/kg of ethambutol had adverse reactions; 0.8% experienced diminished visual acuity, 0.5% had a rash, and 0.3% developed drug fever (Pitts, 1977). Other side effects that have been observed are pruritus, joint pain, gastrointestinal upset, abdominal pain, malaise, headache, dizziness, mental confusion, disorientation, and possible hallucination. Numbness and tingling of the fingers owing to peripheral neuritis are infrequent. Anaphylaxis and leukopenia are rare.

The most important side effect is optic neuritis, resulting in decrease of visual acuity and loss of ability to differentiate red from green. The incidence of this reaction is proportional to the dose of ethambutol and is observed in 15% of patients receiving 50 mg/kg per day, in 5% of patients receiving 25 mg/kg per day, and in less than 1% of patients receiving daily doses of 15 mg/kg. The intensity of the visual difficulty is related to the duration of therapy after the decrease in visual acuity first becomes apparent, and it may be unilateral or bilateral. Tests of visual acuity and red–green discrimination prior to the start of therapy and periodically thereafter are thus recommended. Recovery usually occurs when ethambutol is withdrawn; the time required is a function of the degree of visual impairment.

Therapy with ethambutol results in an increased concentration of urate in the blood in about 50% of patients, owing to decreased renal excretion of uric acid. The effect may be detectable as early as 24 hours after a single dose or as late as 90 days after treatment is started. This untoward effect is possibly enhanced by isoniazid and pyridoxine (Postlethwaite *et al.*, 1972).

Therapeutic Status. Ethambutol has been used with notable success in the therapy of tuberculosis of various forms when given concurrently with isoniazid. Because of a lower incidence of toxic effects and better acceptance by patients, it has essentially replaced aminosalicylic acid (*see* Bobrowitz, 1974).

The use of ethambutol in the chemotherapy of tuberculosis is described below.

STREPTOMYCIN

A discussion of the pharmacology of streptomycin, including its adverse effects and its uses in infections other than tuberculosis, is presented in Chapter 47. Only features of the drug related to its antibacterial activity and therapeutic effects in the management of diseases caused by mycobacteria are considered here.

History. Streptomycin was the first clinically effective drug to become available for the treatment of tuberculosis. At first, it was given in large doses, but problems related to toxicity and the development of resistant microorganisms seriously limited its usefulness. The antibiotic was then administered in smaller quantities, but streptomycin administered alone still proved to be far from the ideal agent for the management of all forms of the disease. However, the discovery of other compounds that, given concurrently with the antibiotic, reduced the rate at which microorganisms became drug resistant enabled physicians to treat tuberculosis effectively with streptomycin. It is now the least used of the "first-line" agents in the therapy of tuberculosis.

Antibacterial Activity. Streptomycin is bactericidal for the tubercle bacillus *in vitro*. Concentrations as low as 0.4 μg/ml may inhibit growth. The vast majority of strains of *M. tuberculosis* are sensitive to 10 μg/ml. *M. kansasii* is frequently sensitive, but other nontuberculous mycobacteria are only occasionally susceptible.

The activity of streptomycin *in vivo* is essentially suppressive. When the antibiotic is administered to experimental animals prior to inoculation with the tubercle bacillus, the development of disease is not prevented. Infection progresses until the animals' immunological mechanisms respond. The presence of viable microorganisms in abscesses and in the regional lymph nodes adds support to the concept that the activity of streptomycin *in vivo* is to suppress, not to eradicate, the tubercle bacillus. This property of streptomycin may be related to the observation that the drug does not readily enter living cells and thus cannot kill intracellular microbes.

Bacterial Resistance. Large populations of all strains of tubercle bacilli include a number of cells that are markedly resistant to streptomycin because of mutation. However, primary resistance to the antibiotic is found in only 2 to 3% of isolates of *M. tuberculosis*.

Selection for resistant tubercle bacilli occurs *in vivo* as it does *in vitro*. In general, the longer therapy is continued, the greater is the incidence of resistance to streptomycin. When streptomycin was used alone, as many as 80% of patients harbored insensitive tubercle bacilli after 4 months of treatment; many of these microorganisms were not inhibited by concentrations of drug as high as 1000 μg/ml.

Preparations, Route of Administration, and Dosage. The preparations and route of administration of streptomycin are considered in detail in Chapter 47. The dosage schedules used in the treatment of various forms of tuberculosis are discussed below.

Untoward Effects. Untoward effects of streptomycin are considered in detail in Chapter 47. Of 515 patients with tuberculosis who were treated with this aminoglycoside, 8.2% had adverse reactions; half of these involved the auditory and vestibular functions of the eighth cranial nerve. Other relatively frequent problems included rash (in 2%) and fever (in 1.4%) (Pitts, 1977).

Therapeutic Status. Since other effective agents have become available, the use of streptomycin for the treatment of pulmonary tuberculosis has been sharply reduced. Many clinicians prefer to give three drugs, of which streptomycin may be one, for the most serious forms of tuberculosis, such as disseminated disease or meningitis.

The use of streptomycin in the chemotherapy of tuberculosis is described below.

PYRAZINAMIDE

Chemistry. Pyrazinamide is the synthetic pyrazine analog of nicotinamide. It has the following structural formula:

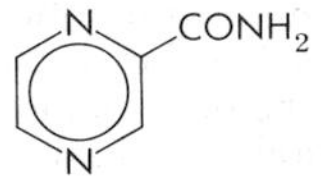

Pyrazinamide

Antibacterial Activity. Pyrazinamide exhibits bactericidal activity *in vitro* only at a slightly acidic pH. Tubercle bacilli within monocytes *in vitro* are killed by the drug at a concentration of 12.5 μg/ml. Resistance develops rapidly if pyrazinamide is used alone. The mechanism of action of the drug is not known.

Absorption, Distribution, and Excretion. Pyrazinamide is well absorbed from the gastrointestinal tract, and it is widely distributed throughout the body. The oral administration of 1 g produces plasma concentrations of about 45 μg/ml at 2 hours and 10 μg/ml at 15 hours. The drug is excreted primarily by renal glomerular filtration; urinary concentrations are 50 to 100 μg/ml for several hours after a single dose. Pyrazinamide is hydrolyzed to pyrazinoic acid and subsequently hydroxylated to 5-hydroxypyrazinoic acid, the major excretory product (Weiner and Tinker, 1972).

Preparation, Route of Administration, and Dosage. *Pyrazinamide* is marketed in tablets containing 500 mg. The daily dose for adults is 20 to 35 mg/kg orally, given in three or four equally spaced doses. Although not approved in the United States, therapy with a single daily dose has been safe and effective in a number of studies. The maximum quantity to be given is 3 g per day, regardless of weight.

Untoward Effects. Injury to the liver is the most common and serious side effect of pyrazinamide. When a dose of 3 g per day (40 to 50 mg/kg) is administered orally, signs and symptoms of hepatic disease appear in about 15% of patients, with jaundice in 2 to 3% and death due to hepatic necrosis in rare instances. Elevations of the plasma alanine and aspartate aminotransferases are the earliest abnormalities produced by the drug. Regimens employed currently (20 to 35 mg/kg per day) are much safer (Girling, 1978; Zierski and Bek, 1980; Pilheu *et al.*, 1981). All patients who are being treated with pyrazinamide should undergo studies of hepatic function before the drug is administered; these studies should be repeated at frequent intervals during the entire period of treatment. If evidence of significant hepatic damage becomes apparent, therapy must be stopped. Pyrazinamide should not be given to individuals with any degree of hepatic dysfunction, unless this is absolutely unavoidable.

The drug inhibits excretion of urate, resulting in hyperuricemia in nearly all patients; acute episodes of gout have occurred. Other untoward effects that have been observed with pyrazinamide are arthralgias, anorexia, nausea and vomiting, dysuria, malaise, and fever.

Therapeutic Status. Pyrazinamide has become an important component of short-term (6-month) multiple-drug therapy of tuberculosis (Zierski and Bek, 1980; Dutt and Stead, 1982; British Thoracic Association, 1983; American Thoracic Society, 1986).

ETHIONAMIDE

Chemistry. Synthesis and study of a variety of congeners of thioisonicotinamide revealed that an alpha-ethyl derivative—ethionamide—is considerably more effective than the parent compound. It has the following structural formula:

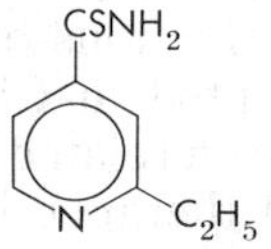

Ethionamide

Antibacterial Activity. The multiplication of *M. tuberculosis* is suppressed by concentrations of ethionamide ranging from 0.6 to 2.5 μg/ml. Resistance can develop rapidly *in vitro*. A concentration of 10 μg/ml or less will inhibit approximately 75% of photochromogenic mycobacteria; the scotochromogens are more resistant. Ethionamide is very effective in the treatment of experimental tuberculosis in animals, although its activity varies greatly with the animal model studied.

Absorption, Distribution, and Excretion. The oral administration of 1 g of ethionamide yields peak concentrations in plasma of about 20 μg/ml in 3 hours; the concentration at 9 hours is 3 μg/ml. The half-life of the drug is about 2 hours. Approximately 50% of patients are unable to tolerate a single dose larger than 500 mg because of gastrointestinal disturbance. Ethionamide is rapidly and widely distributed; the concentrations in the blood and various organs are approximately equal. Significant concentrations are present in CSF. Ethionamide, like aminosalicylic acid, inhibits the acetylation of isoniazid *in vitro*. Less than 1% of ethionamide is excreted in active form in the urine; there are several metabolites.

Preparation, Route of Administration, and Dosage. *Ethionamide* (TRECATOR-SC) is administered only orally. Tablets containing 250 mg of the drug are available. The initial dosage for adults is 250 mg twice daily; it is increased by 125 mg per day every 5 days until a dose of 15 to 20 mg/kg per day is achieved. The maximal dose is 1 g daily. The drug is best taken with meals in order to minimize gastric irritation.

Untoward Effects. The most common reactions to ethionamide are anorexia, nausea, and vomiting. A metallic taste may also be noted. Severe postural hypotension, mental depression, drowsiness, and asthenia are common. Convulsions and peripheral neuropathy are rare. Other reactions referable to the nervous system include olfactory disturbances, blurred vision, diplopia, dizziness, paresthesias, headache, restlessness, and tremors. Severe allergic skin rashes, purpura, stomatitis, gynecomastia, impotence, menorrhagia, acne, and alopecia have also been observed. Hepatitis has been associated with the use of the drug in about 5% of cases (Simon *et al.,* 1969). The signs and symptoms of hepatotoxicity clear when treatment is stopped. Hepatic function should be assessed at regular intervals in patients receiving ethionamide. The concomitant use of pyridoxine is recommended for patients being treated with ethionamide.

Therapeutic Status. Ethionamide is a secondary agent, to be used concurrently with other drugs only when therapy with primary agents is ineffective or contraindicated. (*See* Schwartz, 1966.)

AMINOSALICYLIC ACID

Chemistry. The structural formula of aminosalicylic acid is as follows:

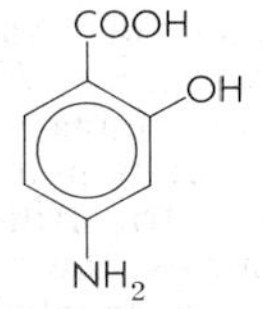

Aminosalicylic Acid

Antibacterial Activity. Aminosalicylic acid is bacteriostatic. *In vitro,* most strains of *M. tuberculosis* are sensitive to a concentration of 1 μg/ml. The antimicrobial activity of aminosalicylic acid is highly specific, and microorganisms other than *M. tuberculosis* are unaffected. Most nontuberculous mycobacteria are not inhibited by the drug.

Studies of the treatment of experimental *M. tuberculosis* infections indicate that aminosalicylic acid exerts a beneficial effect on the disease. However, the doses required are relatively large, and the compound must be present continuously. Aminosalicylic acid alone is of little value in the treatment of tuberculosis in man.

Bacterial Resistance. Strains of tubercle bacilli insensitive to several hundred times the usual bacteriostatic concentration of aminosalicylic acid can be produced *in vitro*. Resistant strains of tubercle bacilli also emerge in patients treated with aminosalicylic acid, but much more slowly than with streptomycin.

Mechanism of Action. Aminosalicylic acid is a structural analog of paraaminobenzoic acid, and its mechanism of action appears to be very similar to that of the sulfonamides (*see* Chapter 45). Since the sulfonamides are ineffective against *M. tuberculosis*, and aminosalicylic acid is inactive against sulfonamide-susceptible bacteria, it is probable that the enzymes responsible for folate biosynthesis in various microorganisms may be quite exacting in their capacity to distinguish various analogs from the true metabolite.

Absorption, Distribution, and Excretion. Aminosalicylic acid is readily absorbed from the gastrointestinal tract. A single oral dose of 4 g of the free acid produces maximal concentrations in plasma of about 75 μg/ml within 1.5 to 2 hours. The sodium salt is absorbed even more rapidly. The drug appears to be distributed throughout the total body water and reaches high concentrations in pleural fluid and caseous tissue. However, values in CSF are low, perhaps because of active outward transport (Spector and Lorenzo, 1973).

The drug has a half-life of about 1 hour, and concentrations in plasma are negligible within 4 to 5 hours after a single conventional dose. Over 80% of the drug is excreted in the urine; more than 50% is in the form of the acetylated compound. The largest portion of the remainder is made up of the free acid. Excretion of aminosalicylic acid is greatly retarded in the presence of renal dysfunction, and the use of the drug is not recommended in such patients. Probenecid decreases the renal excretion of this agent.

Preparation, Route of Administration, and Dosage. *Aminosalicylate sodium* (TEEBACIN) is available in tablets containing 500 or 1000 mg. The drug is administered orally in a daily dose of 14 to 16 g. Because it is a gastric irritant, the drug is best administered after meals, the daily dose being divided into three or four equal-sized portions.

Untoward Effects. The incidence of untoward effects associated with the use of aminosalicylic acid is approximately 10 to 30%. Gastrointestinal problems, including anorexia, nausea, epigastric pain, abdominal distress, and diarrhea, are predominant (Pitts, 1977), and patients with peptic ulcer tolerate the drug poorly. Compliance is often poor because of gastrointestinal distress. Hypersensitivity reactions to aminosalicylic acid are seen in 5 to 10% of patients. High fever may develop abruptly, with intermittent spiking, or it may appear gradually and be low-grade. Generalized malaise, joint pains, or sore throat may be present at the same time. Skin eruptions of various types appear as isolated reactions or accompany the fever. Among the hematological abnormalities that have been observed are leukopenia, agranulocytosis, eosinophilia, lymphocytosis, an atypical mononucleosis syndrome, and thrombocytopenia. Acute hemolytic anemia may appear in some instances.

Therapeutic Status. Aminosalicylic acid is a "second-line" agent. Its importance in the management of pulmonary and other forms of tuberculosis has markedly decreased since more active and better-tolerated drugs, such as rifampin and ethambutol, have been developed (*see* discussion of chemotherapy of tuberculosis, below).

CYCLOSERINE

Cycloserine is a broad-spectrum antibiotic produced by *Streptomyces orchidaceus*. It was first isolated from a fermentation brew in 1955 and was later synthesized.

Chemistry. Cycloserine is D-4-amino-3-isoxazolidone; the structural formula is as follows:

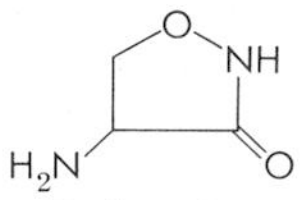

Cycloserine

The drug is stable in alkaline solution but is rapidly destroyed when exposed to neutral or acidic pH.

Antibacterial Activity and Mechanism of Action. Cycloserine is inhibitory for *M. tuberculosis* in concentrations of 5 to 20 μg/ml *in vitro*. There is no cross-resistance between cycloserine and other tuberculostatic agents. While the antibiotic is effective in experimental infections caused by other microorganisms, studies *in vitro* reveal no suppression of growth in cultures made in conventional media, which contain D-alanine; this amino acid blocks the antibacterial activity of cycloserine. The two compounds are structural analogs, and cycloserine inhibits reactions in which D-alanine is involved in bacterial cell-wall synthesis (*see* Chapter 46). The use of media free of D-alanine reveals that the antibiotic inhibits the growth *in vitro* of enterococci, paracolon strains, *Escherichia coli, Staphylococcus aureus, Nocardia* species, and *Chlamydia*.

Absorption, Distribution, and Excretion. When given orally, cycloserine is rapidly absorbed. Peak concentrations in plasma are reached 3 to 4 hours after a single dose and are in the range of 20 to 35 μg/ml in children who receive 20 mg/kg; only small quantities are present after 12 hours. Cycloserine is distributed throughout body fluids and tissues. There is no appreciable blood–brain barrier to the drug, and CSF concentrations in all patients are approximately the same as those in plasma. About 50% of a parenteral dose of cycloserine is excreted unchanged in the urine in the first 12 hours; a total of 65% is recoverable in the active form over a period of 72 hours. Approximately 35% of the antibiotic is metabolized. The drug may accumulate to toxic concentrations in patients with renal insufficiency; it may be removed from the circulation by dialysis.

Preparation, Route of Administration, and Dosage. *Cycloserine* (SEROMYCIN) is available in capsules containing 250 mg for oral administration. The usual dose for adults is 15 to 20 mg/kg per day or up to 500 mg twice a day.

Untoward Effects. Reactions to cycloserine most commonly involve the central nervous system. They tend to appear within the first 2 weeks of therapy and usually disappear when the drug is withdrawn. Among the central manifestations are somnolence, headache, tremor, dysarthria, vertigo, confusion, nervousness, irritability, psychotic states with suicidal tendencies, paranoid reactions, catatonic and depressed reactions, twitching, ankle clonus, hyperreflexia, visual disturbances, paresis, and tonic–clonic or absence seizures. Large doses of cycloserine or the ingestion of ethyl alcohol increases the risk of seizures. Cycloserine is contraindicated in individuals with a history of epilepsy.

Therapeutic Status. Cycloserine should be used only when retreatment is necessary or when microorganisms are resistant to other drugs. When cycloserine is employed to treat tuberculosis, it must be given together with other effective agents.

OTHER DRUGS

The agents grouped in this section are similar in several aspects. They are all "second-line" drugs that are used only for treatment of disease caused by resistant microorganisms or by nontuberculous mycobacteria. They all must be given parenterally, and they have similar pharmacokinetics and toxicity. Since these agents are potentially ototoxic and nephrotoxic, no two drugs from this group should be employed simultaneously, and these drugs should not be used in combination with streptomycin.

Kanamycin, an aminoglycoside that is discussed in Chapter 47, inhibits the growth of *M. tuberculosis in vitro* in a concentration of 10 μg/ml or less. Small groups of patients with tuberculosis have been treated with 1 g of kanamycin daily; toxic effects have been common.

Amikacin is also an aminoglycoside (*see* Chapter 47). It is extremely active against several mycobacterial species, and may become an important drug for treatment of disease caused by nontuberculous mycobacteria (*see* Sanders *et al.*, 1976; Dalovisio and Pankey, 1978).

Capreomycin is an antimycobacterial cyclic peptide elaborated by *Streptomyces capreolus*. It consists of four active components—capreomycins IA, IB, IIA, and IIB—the structures of which have largely been elucidated by Bycroft and associates (1971). The agent used clinically contains primarily IA and IB. The drug is effective both *in vitro* and in experimental tuberculosis (Wilson, 1967). Bacterial resistance to capreomycin develops when it is given alone; such microorganisms show cross-resistance with kanamycin.

Capreomycin must be given intramuscularly. The recommended daily dose is 15 to 30 mg/kg per day or up to 1 g for 60 to 120 days, followed by 1 g two to three times a week. Capreomycin should be administered together with other effective agents. It has proven to be of value in the therapy of "resistant," or treatment-failure, tuberculosis when given with ethambutol or isoniazid (Wilson, 1967; Donomae, 1968). *Capreomycin sulfate* (CAPASTAT SULFATE) is supplied in vials containing 1 g of the drug.

The reactions associated with the use of capreomycin are hearing loss, tinnitus, transient proteinuria, cylindruria, and nitrogen retention. Severe renal failure is rare. Eosinophilia is common. Leukocytosis, leukopenia, rashes, and fever have also been observed. Injections of the drug may be painful.

CHEMOTHERAPY OF TUBERCULOSIS

The availability of effective agents has so altered the treatment of tuberculosis that most patients are now treated in the ambulatory setting, often after diagnosis and initial therapy in a general hospital. Prolonged bed rest is not necessary or even helpful in speeding recovery. Patients must be seen at frequent intervals to follow the course of their disease and treatment. The local health department must be notified of all cases. Contacts should be investigated for the possibility of disease and for the appropriateness of prophylactic therapy with isoniazid.

The vast majority of cases of previously untreated tuberculosis in the United States is caused by microorganisms that are sensitive to isoniazid, rifampin, ethambutol, and streptomycin. To prevent the development of resistance to these agents that frequently occurs during the course of therapy of the individual patient, *treatment must include at least two drugs to which the bacteria are sensitive*. The standard 6-month treatment program is usually preferred for adults and children and consists of isoniazid, rifampin, and pyrazinamide for 2 months, followed by isoniazid and rifampin for 4 additional months. The combination of isoniazid and rifampin for 9 months is equally effective. In life-threatening disease, large cavitary disease, or renal tuberculosis, three drugs should be used initially to be certain that the mycobacteria are sensitive to at least two of them.

Patients infected with the human immunodeficiency virus (HIV) should receive more intensive therapy. The Centers for Disease Control (1989) advises treatment of such individuals for a minimum of 9 months: 2 months with isoniazid, rifampin, and pyrazinamide followed by at least 7 months with isoniazid and rifampin. Ethambutol is added to the initial treatment regimen for patients with central nervous system or disseminated tuberculosis, or when mycobacterial resistance to isoniazid is suspected. Treatment should be continued for at least 6 months after three negative cultures have been obtained. If isoniazid or rifampin cannot be used, therapy should be continued for at least 18 months (12 months after cultures become negative). Chemoprophylaxis (*see* below) should be undertaken if a patient with HIV infection has a positive tuberculin test.

Therapy of Specific Types of Tuberculosis. Therapy for uncomplicated pulmonary tuberculosis consists of isoniazid (5 mg/kg, up to 300 mg per day), rifampin (600 mg once daily), and pyrazinamide (25 mg/kg). Pyridoxine, 15 to 50 mg per day, should also be included for most adults to minimize adverse reactions to isoniazid. Isoniazid, rifampin, and pyrazinamide are given for 2 months; isoniazid and rifampin are then continued for 4 additional months. Children are treated similarly; doses are isoniazid, 10 to 20 mg/kg per day (300 mg maximum); rifampin, 10 to 20 mg/kg per day (600 mg maximum); pyrazinamide, 15 to 30 mg/kg per day (American Thoracic Society, 1986; Des Prez and Heim, 1990). Surgery is rarely indicated (Des Prez and Heim, 1990).

Certain patients should receive four drugs initially to ensure that the microorganisms will be susceptible to at least two of the agents. These patients include (1) those known to have been exposed to drug-resistant microorganisms; (2) Asians and Hispanics, especially if they are recent immigrants; (3) those with miliary tuberculosis or other extrapulmonary disease; (4) those with meningitis; and (5) those with extensive pulmonary disease. The microorganisms should be cultured for determination of their sensitivity to antimicrobial agents, but results will not be available for several weeks. The fourth agent may be either ethambutol or streptomycin (1 g daily). The dosage of streptomycin is reduced to 1 g twice weekly after 2 months.

Clinical improvement is readily discernible in the vast majority of patients with pulmonary tuberculosis if the treatment is appropriate. Efficacy usually becomes obvious within the first 2 weeks of therapy and is evidenced by a reduction of fever, decrease in cough, gain in weight, and increase in the sense of well-being. Progressive radiological improvement is also evident. Over 90% of patients who receive optimal treatment will have negative cultures within 3 to 6 months, depending on the severity of the disease. Cultures that remain positive after 6 months frequently yield resistant microorganisms; the value of using an alternative therapeutic program should then be considered.

Failure of chemotherapy may be due to (1) irregular or inadequate therapy (resulting in persistent or resistant mycobacteria) caused by poor patient compliance during the protracted therapeutic regimen; (2) the use of a single drug, with interruption necessitated by toxicity or hypersensitivity; (3) an inadequate initial regimen; or (4) the primary resistance of the microorganism.

Problems in Chemotherapy. *Bacterial Resistance to Drugs.* One of the more important problems in the chemotherapy of tuberculosis is bacterial resistance. For this reason all patients with active tuberculous disease should receive two or more drugs concurrently.

A spate of publications has appeared on the incidence of resistance of bacilli isolated from untreated patients. Results depend on the population studied (*e.g.*, patients in Veterans Administration hospitals harbor more resistant microorganisms than do those in the United States as a whole), geographical location, and ethnic and socioeconomic factors. At present, most observers believe that the frequency of bacterial resistance is not rising at a rate sufficient to threaten the effectiveness of programs of concurrent drug therapy (Centers for Disease Control, 1983). However, the physician must obtain sensitivity data at the beginning of therapy to ensure the selection of a proper combination of drugs. Disease caused by strains of *M. tuberculosis* that are found to be resistant to the drugs being used should be treated with two or three drugs to which the microorganisms are known to be susceptible.

Where drug resistance is suspected but sensitivities are not yet known (such as in patients who have undergone several courses of treatment), therapy should be instituted with five or six drugs, including two or three that the patient has not received in the past. Such a program might include isoniazid, rifampin, ethambutol, streptomycin, pyrazinamide, and ethionamide. Some physicians include isoniazid in the therapeutic regimen even if microorganisms are resistant, because of some evidence that disease with isoniazid-resistant mycobacteria does not "progress" during such therapy. Others prefer to discontinue isoniazid to lessen the possibility of toxicity. Therapy should be continued for at least 24 months.

Nontuberculous (Atypical) Mycobacteria. These microorganisms have been recovered from a variety of lesions in man. Because they frequently are resistant to many of the commonly used agents, they must be examined for sensitivity *in vitro* and drug therapy selected on this basis. In some instances, surgical removal of the infected tissue followed by long-term treatment with effective agents is necessary.

M. kansasii causes disease similar to that caused by *M. tuberculosis*, but it may be milder. The microorganisms may be resistant to isoniazid. Therapy with isoniazid, rifampin, and ethambutol has been successful (Davidson, 1976; Nicholson, 1976; Pezzia *et al.*, 1981). *M. avium* complex can cause a disease with symptoms that resemble chronic bronchitis. Cavities are found in the lungs of most patients. The microorganisms are often highly resistant to drugs *in vitro*. Therapy with isoniazid, rifampin, streptomycin, ethambutol, and cycloserine has been successful (*see* Sanders and Horowitz, 1990). Patients with AIDS present a special problem, since they develop disseminated disease with large numbers of microorganisms (Young, 1988). Ansamycin (rifabutin), an experimental rifamycin, and clofazimine (*see* below) plus other drugs have been used, but results of therapy have been poor (Sanfilippo *et al.*, 1980; Greene *et al.*, 1982; Masur *et al.*, 1987). *M. marinum* causes skin lesions. A combination of rifampin and ethambutol is probably effective; minocycline (Loria, 1976) or tetracycline is active *in vitro* and is used by some physicians (Izumi *et al.*, 1977). *M. scrofulaceum* causes cervical lymphadenitis, especially in children. Surgical excision still seems to be the therapy of choice (Lincoln and Gilberg, 1972). Microbes of the *M. fortuitum* complex (including *M. chelonei*) are usually saprophytes, but they may cause chronic lung disease and infections of skin and soft tissues. The microorganisms are highly resistant to most drugs, but amikacin, cefoxitin, and tetracyclines are active *in vitro* (Sanders *et al.*, 1977; Sanders, 1982).

Chemoprophylaxis of Tuberculosis. Prophylactic therapy can effectively prevent the development of active tuberculosis in certain instances (Des Prez and Heim, 1990). There are three categories of patients for whom prophylactic therapy should be considered: those exposed to tuberculosis but who have no evidence of infection; those with infection (positive tuberculin test; more than 10 mm of induration to 5 units of PPD) and no apparent disease; and those with a history of tuberculosis but in whom the disease is presently "inactive" (*see* Edwards, 1977; Snider and Farer, 1978; American Thoracic Society, 1986).

Household contacts and other close associates of patients with tuberculosis who have negative tuberculin tests should receive isoniazid for at least 6 months after the contact has been broken. This is especially important for children. If the tuberculin skin test becomes positive, therapy should be continued for 12 months.

Persons without apparent disease whose skin test has converted from negative to positive within the preceding 2 years should probably receive isoniazid for 12 months. These patients are considered to be "infected" but not to have clinical disease. Some authorities believe that persons with positive skin tests, no matter when they became so, who are under 35 years of age, or who are at risk of infection because of such factors as infection with the human immunodeficiency virus, immunosuppressive therapy, leukemia, lymphoma, or silicosis should receive isoniazid for 1 year (Comstock, 1981; American Thoracic Society, 1986). For individuals over 35 years of age, the risk of isoniazid toxicity may outweigh the potential benefit of therapy.

Patients with old "inactive" tuberculosis who have not received adequate chemotherapy in the past should be considered for 1 year of treatment with isoniazid (*see* Comstock, 1983).

Prophylaxis with isoniazid is contraindicated for patients who have active hepatic disease or who have had reactions to the drug. There are insufficient data on the advisability of prophylaxis with alternative drugs, such as rifampin. In pregnant women, prophylaxis should usually be delayed until after delivery. For prophylaxis, isoniazid is generally given to adults in a daily dose of 300 mg. Children should receive 10 mg/kg to a maximal daily dose of 300 mg.

II. Drugs for Leprosy

Although leprosy (Hansen's disease) is rarely seen in the United States, it is estimated that 12 million patients worldwide have this disease. The development of effective chemotherapy for leprosy has allowed most patients to be managed outside of hospitals.

SULFONES

The sulfones, as a class, are derivatives of 4,4′-diaminodiphenylsulfone (dapsone), all of which have certain pharmacological properties in common. They are discussed here as a class; only dapsone and sulfoxone will be considered individually.

History. The sulfones first attracted interest because of their chemical relationship to the sulfonamides. In the 1940s sulfones were found to be effective in suppressing experimental infections with the tubercle bacillus and for rat leprosy; this finding was soon followed by successful clinical trials in human leprosy. The sulfones are currently the most important drugs for the treatment of this disorder.

Chemistry. All the sulfones of clinical value are derivatives of dapsone. Despite the study and development of a large variety of sulfones, this drug remains the agent most useful clinically. The structures of dapsone and sulfoxone sodium are as follows:

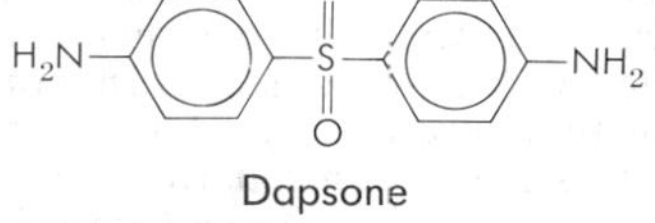

Dapsone

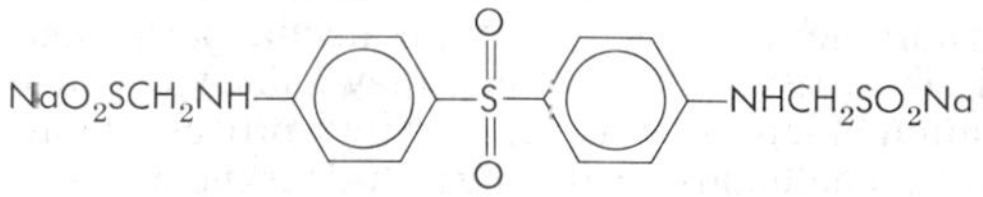

Sulfoxone Sodium

Antibacterial Activity. Because *M. leprae* does not grow on artificial media, conventional methods cannot be applied to determine its susceptibility to potential therapeutic agents *in vitro*. Crude sensitivities *in vivo* can be determined by injecting microorganisms into the foot pads of mice and treating them with the agents to be tested. After 6 to 8 months the mice are killed, the foot pads are homogenized, and microscopic counts are made of acid-fast microorganisms (Shepard *et al.*, 1976). Dapsone is bacteriostatic, but not bactericidal, for *M. leprae*, and the estimated sensitivity to the drug is between 1 and 10 ng/ml for microorganisms recovered from untreated patients (Levy and Peters, 1976). *M. leprae* may become resistant to the drug during therapy.

The mechanism of action of the sulfones is the same as that of the sulfonamides. Both possess approximately the same range of antibacterial activity and both are antagonized by paraaminobenzoic acid.

Dapsone-resistant strains of *M. leprae* are termed "secondary" if they emerge during therapy. Secondary resistance is usually seen in lepromatous (multibacillary) patients treated with a single drug. The incidence is as high as 19% (WHO Study Group, 1982). Partial-to-complete primary resistance (seen in previously untreated patients) has been described in from 2.5 to 40% of patients, depending on geographical location (Centers for Disease Control, 1982).

Untoward Effects. The reactions induced by various sulfones are very similar. The most common untoward effect is hemolysis of varying degree. This develops in almost every individual treated with 200 to 300 mg of dapsone per day. Doses of 100 mg or less in normal healthy persons and 50 mg or less in healthy individuals with a glucose-6-phosphate dehydrogenase deficiency do not cause hemolysis (DeGowin, 1967). Methemoglobinemia is also common, and Heinz-body formation may occur. A genetic deficiency in the NADH-dependent methemoglobin reductase can result in severe methemoglobinemia after administration of dapsone. While diminished red-cell survival usually occurs during the use of sulfones, and is presumed to be a dose-related effect of their oxidizing activity, hemolytic anemia is unusual unless the patient also has a disorder either of the erythrocytes or of the bone marrow (Pengelly, 1963). The hemolysis may be so severe that manifestations of hypoxia become striking.

Anorexia, nausea, and vomiting may follow the oral administration of sulfones. Isolated instances of headache, nervousness, insomnia, blurred vision, paresthesia, reversible peripheral neuropathy (thought to be due to axonal degeneration), drug fever, hematuria, pruritus, psychosis, and a variety of skin rashes have been reported (Rapoport and Guss, 1972). An infectious mononucleosis–like syndrome, which may be fatal, occurs occasionally (Leiker, 1956). The sulfones may induce an exacerbation of lepromatous leprosy by a process thought to be analogous to the Jarisch–Herxheimer reaction. This "sulfone syndrome" may develop 5 to 6 weeks after initiation of treatment in malnourished people. Its manifestations include fever, malaise, exfoliative dermatitis, jaundice with hepatic necrosis, lymphadenopathy, methemoglobinemia, and anemia (DeGowin, 1967).

The sulfones may be given safely for many years in doses adequate for the successful therapy of leprosy if proper precautions are observed. Treatment should be initiated with a small dose and the quantity then increased gradually. Patients must be under consistent and prolonged laboratory and clinical supervision. The reactions induced by the sulfones, especially those related to exacerbation of the leprosy, may be very severe and may require the cessation of treatment as well as the institution of specific measures to reduce the threat to life.

Absorption, Distribution, and Excretion. Dapsone is slowly and nearly completely absorbed from the gastrointestinal tract. The disubstituted sulfones, such as sulfoxone, are incompletely absorbed when administered orally, and large amounts are excreted in the feces. Peak concentrations of dapsone in plasma are reached within 1 to 3 hours after administration; the mean half-life of elimination is about 22 hours. Twenty-four hours after oral ingestion of 100 mg, plasma concentrations range from 0.4 to 1.2 μg/ml (Shepard *et al.*, 1976), and a dose of 100 mg of dapsone per day produces an average of 2 μg of "free" dapsone per gram of blood or nonhepatic tissue. About 70% of the drug is bound to plasma protein. Concentrations in plasma following conventional doses of sulfoxone sodium are 10 to 15 μg/ml. These values fall relatively rapidly; however, appreciable quantities are still present at 8 hours.

The sulfones are distributed throughout the total body water and are present in all tissues. They tend to be retained in skin and muscle, and especially in liver and kidney; traces of the drug are present in these organs up to 3 weeks after therapy is stopped. The sulfones are retained in the circulation for a long time because of intestinal reabsorption from the bile; periodic interruption of treatment is advisable for this reason. Dapsone is acetylated in the liver, and the rate of acetylation is genetically determined; the same enzyme carries out the acetylation of isoniazid.

The urinary excretion of sulfones varies with the type of drug; about 70 to 80% of a dose of dapsone is so excreted. The drug is present in urine as an acid-labile mono-N-glucuronide and mono-N-sulfamate in addition to an unknown number of unidentified metabolites (Shepard, 1969). Probenecid decreases the urinary excretion of the acid-labile dapsone metabolites significantly and that of free dapsone to a lesser extent (Goodwin and Sparell, 1969).

Preparation, Route of Administration, and Dosage. *Dapsone* is available for oral administration in tablets containing 25 or 100 mg. Several dosage schedules have been recommended (*see* Trautman, 1965; Bullock, 1990). Daily therapy with 50 mg has been successful in adults. If the clinical response is not adequate, the daily dose may be increased to 100 mg. Therapy is usually begun with smaller amounts, and doses are increased to those recommended over 1 to 2 months. Therapy should be continued for at least 2 years and may be necessary for the lifetime of the patient (*see* below).

Sulfoxone sodium may be substituted for dapsone in patients in whom the latter drug produces sufficient gastric distress to impede effective therapy. The recommended daily dose is 330 mg.

The use of sulfones in malaria resistant to the usual antimalarial drugs is discussed in Chapter 41.

RIFAMPIN

Rifampin has been discussed above with regard to its use in tuberculosis. This antibiotic is rapidly bactericidal for *M. leprae,* and the minimal inhibitory concentration is less than 1 μg/ml. Infectivity of patients is rapidly reversed by therapy that includes rifampin (Bullock, 1983). Because of the prevalence of resistance to dapsone, the WHO Study Group (1982) now recommends a regimen of multiple drugs, including rifampin.

CLOFAZIMINE

Clofazimine is a phenazine dye with the following structural formula:

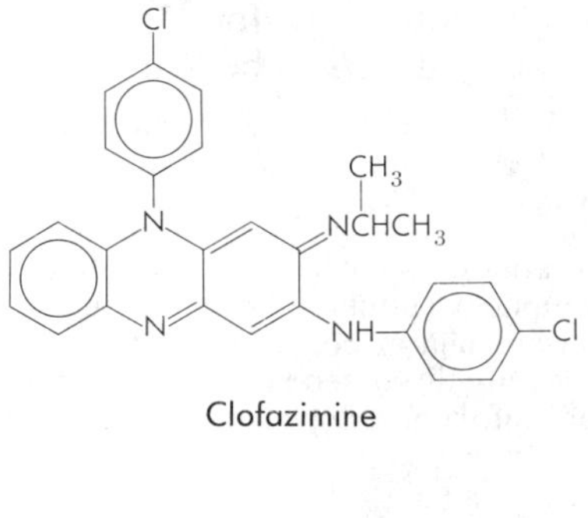

Clofazimine

Clofazimine may inhibit the template function of DNA by binding to it (Morrison and Marley, 1976). It is weakly bactericidal against *M. leprae*. The drug also exerts an antiinflammatory effect and prevents the development of erythema nodosum leprosum. Clofazimine is now recommended as a component of multiple-drug therapy for leprosy (*see* below). The compound is also useful for treatment of chronic skin ulcers (Buruli ulcer) produced by *M. ulcerans*, and it has some activity against the *M. avium* complex (*Medical Letter*, 1987).

Clofazimine is absorbed by the oral route and appears to accumulate in tissues. Human leprosy from which dapsone-resistant bacilli have been recovered has been treated with clofazimine with good results. However, unlike dapsone-sensitive microorganisms, in which killing occurs immediately after dapsone is administered, dapsone-resistant strains do not exhibit an appreciable effect until 50 days after initiation of therapy with clofazimine. The daily dose of clofazimine is usually 100 mg. (*See* Levy *et al.*, 1972.) Patients treated with clofazimine may develop red discoloration of the skin, which may be very distressing to light-skinned individuals. Eosinophilic enteritis has also been described as an adverse reaction to the drug (Mason *et al.*, 1977). *Clofazimine* (LAMPRENE) is available in 50- and 100-mg capsules.

MISCELLANEOUS AGENTS

Thalidomide seems to be effective for the treatment of erythema nodosum leprosum (Iyer *et al.*, 1971). Doses of 100 to 300 mg per day have been effective. The marked teratogenicity of thalidomide limits its use; it is not available in the United States.

Ethionamide has been discussed above as an agent for treatment of tuberculosis. It can be used as a substitute for clofazimine in oral doses of 250 to 375 mg per day.

CHEMOTHERAPY OF LEPROSY

Few physicians, other than specialists in the field, are called upon to treat leprosy. Consultation is available with physicians at the National Hansen's Disease Center, Carville, Louisiana 70721, or at regional centers. Therefore, the following discussion will serve mainly to familiarize the reader with the progress that has been made in the treatment of this chronic bacterial disease that has proven very resistant to chemotherapy.

Five clinical types of leprosy are recognized. At one end of the spectrum is *tuberculoid leprosy*. This form of the disease is characterized by skin macules with clear centers and well-defined margins; these are invariably anesthetic. *M. leprae* is rarely found in smears made from quiescent lesions, but may appear during activity. Virchow cells are not demonstrable. Noncaseating foci with giant cells of the Langhans variety are present. The patient's cell-mediated immune responses are normal, and the lepromin test (intradermal injection of a suspension of heat-killed, bacillus-laden tissue) is invariably positive. The disease is characterized by prolonged remissions with periodic reactivation.

At the other end of the spectrum is the widely disseminated *lepromatous* form of the disease. Patients with this disease have markedly impaired cell-mediated immunity and are frequently anergic; the lepromin test causes no reaction. Lepromatous disease is characterized by diffuse or ill-defined localized infiltration of the skin, which becomes thickened, glossy, and corrugated; areas of decreased sensation may appear. *M. leprae* is demonstrable in smears, and granulomas containing bacteria-laden histiocytes (Virchow cells) are present. As the disease progresses, large nerve trunks are involved and anesthesia, atrophy of skin and muscle, absorption of small bones, ulceration, and spontaneous amputations may occur. Three intermediate forms of the disease are recognized: borderline tuberculoid disease, borderline lepromatous disease, and borderline disease (Bullock, 1990).

Patients with tuberculoid leprosy may develop "reversal reactions," which are manifestations of delayed hypersensitivity to antigens of *M. leprae*. Cutaneous ulcerations and deficits of peripheral nerve function may occur. Early therapy with corticosteroids or clofazimine is effective.

Reactions in the lepromatous form of the disease (erythema nodosum leprosum) are characterized by the appearance of raised, tender, intracutaneous nodules, severe constitutional symptoms, and high fever. This reaction may be triggered by several conditions but is often associated with therapy. It is thought to be an Arthus-type reaction related to release of microbial antigens in patients harboring large numbers of bacilli. Treatment with clofazimine or thalidomide is effective.

The outlook for persons with leprosy has been remarkably altered by successful chemotherapy, surgical procedures that help to restore function and repair disfigurement, and a striking change in the attitude of the public toward patients who have this infection. The social stigma based on ignorance and Biblical castigation of individuals with this affliction is gradually being replaced by the attitude that considers leprosy a disease, not a social stigma. Patients with leprosy can be classified as "infectious" or "noninfectious" on the basis of the type, duration, and effects of therapy. Thus, even "infectious" patients need not be hospitalized, provided adequate medical supervision and therapy are maintained, the home environment meets specific conditions, and the local health officer concurs in the disposition of the case.

Therapy, when effective, heals ulcers and mucosal lesions in months. Cutaneous nodules respond more slowly, and it may take years to eradicate bacteria from mucous membranes, skin, and nerves. The degree of residual pigmentation or depigmentation, atrophy, and scarring depends upon the extent of the initial involvement. Severe ocular lesions show little response to the sulfones. If treatment is initiated before ocular disease is evident, it may be prevented. Keratoconjunctivitis and corneal ulceration may be secondary to nerve involvement.

The World Health Organization now recommends therapy with multiple drugs for all patients with leprosy (WHO Study Group, 1982). The reasons for using combinations of agents include reduction in the development of resistance, the need for adequate therapy when primary resistance already exists, and reduction in the duration of therapy. Dosage recommendations for control programs take a number of practical constraints into account. For patients with large populations of bacteria (multibacillary forms), including lepromatous disease, borderline lepromatous disease, and borderline disease, the following regimen is suggested: dapsone, 100 mg daily, plus clofazimine, 100 mg daily, plus rifampin, 600 mg once a month under supervision. Some prefer to give a daily dose of rifampin (450 to 600 mg) (Jacobson, 1982). All drugs are given orally. The minimal duration of therapy is 2 years, and treatment should continue until acid-fast bacilli are not detected in lesions.

Patients with a small population of bacteria (paucibacillary disease), including those with tuberculoid, borderline tuberculoid, and indeterminate disease, should be treated with dapsone, 100 mg daily, plus rifampin, 600 mg once monthly (under supervision), for 6 months. Relapses are treated by repeating the regimen.

More prolonged treatment programs are recommended for patients in the United States (*see* Hastings and Franzblau, 1988).

Albert, R. K.; Lakshminarayan, S.; and Miller, W. T. Long-term therapy with rifampin and the secondary antibody response to killed influenza vaccine. *Am. Rev. Respir. Dis.*, **1978**, *117*, 605–607.

Baciewicz, A. M.; Self, T. H.; and Bekemeyer, W. B. Update on rifampin drug interactions. *Arch. Intern. Med.*, **1987**, *147*, 565.

Bailey, W. C.; Weill, H.; DeRouen, T. A.; Ziskind, M. M.; Jackson, H. A.; and Greenberg, H. B. The effect of isoniazid on transaminase levels. *Ann. Intern. Med.*, **1974**, *81*, 200–202.

Bassi, L.; DiBerardino, L.; Arioli, V.; Silvestri, L. G.; and Cherie Ligniere, E. L. Conditions for immunosuppression by rifampicin. *J. Infect. Dis.*, **1973**, *128*, 736–744.

Bobrowitz, I. D. Ethambutol–isoniazid versus streptomycin–ethambutol–isoniazid in original treatment of cavitary tuberculosis. *Am. Rev. Respir. Dis.*, **1974**, *109*, 548–553.

Bowersox, D. W.; Winterbauer, R. H.; Stewart, G. L.; Orme, B.; and Barron, E. Isoniazid dosage in patients with renal failure. *N. Engl. J. Med.*, **1973**, *289*, 84–87.

British Thoracic Association. A controlled trial of six months chemotherapy in pulmonary tuberculosis. Second report: results during the twenty-four months after the end of chemotherapy. *Am. Rev. Respir. Dis.*, **1983**, *126*, 460–462.

Broome, C. V.; Mortimer, E. A.; Katz, S. L.; Fleming, D. W.; and Hightower, A. W. Use of chemoprophylaxis to prevent the spread of *Hemophilus influenzae* b in day-care facilities. *N. Engl. J. Med.*, **1987**, *316*, 1226–1228.

Buffington, G. A.; Dominguez, J. H.; Piering, W. F.; Hebert, L. A.; Kouffman, H. M.; and Lemann, J. Interaction of rifampin and glucocorticoids. *J.A.M.A.*, **1976**, *236*, 1958–1960.

Buss, W. C.; Morgan, R.; Guttman, J.; Barela, T.; and Stalter, K. Rifampicin inhibition of protein synthesis in mammalian cells. *Science*, **1978**, *200*, 432–434.

Bycroft, B. W.; Cameron, D.; Croft, L. R.; Hassanali-Walji, A.; Johnson, A. W.; and Webb, T. Total structure of capreomycin 1B, a tuberculostatic peptide antibiotic. *Nature*, **1971**, *231*, 301–302.

Byrd, R. B.; Horn, B. R.; Solomon, D. A.; and Griggs, G. W. Toxic effects of isoniazid in tuberculosis chemoprophylaxis. *J.A.M.A.*, **1979**, *241*, 1239–1241.

Carpenter, J. L.; Covelli, H. D.; Avant, M. E.; McAllister, C. K.; Higbee, J. W.; and Ognibene, A. J. Drug-resistant *Mycobacterium tuberculosis* in Korean isolates. *Am. Rev. Respir. Dis.*, **1982**, *126*, 1092–1095.

Cauthen, G. M.; Kilburn, J. O.; Kelly, G. D.; and Good, R. C. Resistance to anti-tuberculosis drugs in patients with and without prior treatment: survey of 31 state and large city laboratories, 1982–1986. *Am. Rev. Respir. Dis.*, **1988**, *137*, Suppl., 260.

Centers for Disease Control. Adverse drug reactions among children treated for tuberculosis. *M.M.W.R.*, **1980**, *29*, 589–591.

———. Increase in prevalence of leprosy caused by dapsone-resistant *Mycobacterium leprae*. *Ibid.*, **1982**, *30*, 637–638.

———. Primary resistance to antituberculosis drugs. *Ibid.*, **1983**, *32*, 521–523.

———. Tuberculosis and human immunodeficiency virus infection. Recommendations of the Advisory Committee for the Elimination of Tuberculosis (ACET). *Ibid.*, **1989**, *38*, 236–250.

Comstock, G. W. Evaluating isoniazid preventive therapy: the need for more data. *Ann. Intern. Med.*, **1981**, *94*, 817–819.

———. New data on preventive treatment with isoniazid. *Ibid.*, **1983**, *98*, 663–665.

Dalovisio, J. R., and Pankey, G. A. *In vitro* susceptibility of *Mycobacterium fortuitum* and *Mycobacterium chelonei* to amikacin. *J. Infect. Dis.*, **1978**, *137*, 318–321.

Davidson, L. A., and Takayama, K. Isoniazid inhibition of the synthesis of monosaturated long-chain fatty acids in *Mycobacterium tuberculosis* H37Ra. *Antimicrob. Agents Chemother.*, **1979**, *16*, 104–105.

Davidson, P. T. Treatment and long-term follow-up of patients with atypical mycobacterial infections. *Bull. Int. Union Tuberc.*, **1976**, *51*, 257–261.

Devine, L. F.; Johnson, D. P.; Rhode, S. L., III; Hagerman, C. R.; Pierce, W. E.; and Peckinpaugh, R. D. Rifampin—effect of two-day treatment on the meningococcal carrier state and the relationship to the levels of the drug in sera and saliva. *Am. J. Med. Sci.*, **1971**, *26*, 74–83.

Donomae, I. The combined use of capreomycin and ethambutol in re-treatment of pulmonary tuberculosis. *Am. Rev. Respir. Dis.*, **1968**, *98*, 699–702.

Dutt, A. K., and Stead, W. W. Present chemotherapy for tuberculosis. *J. Infect. Dis.*, **1982**, *146*, 698–704.

Edwards, P. Q. Tuberculosis, now and the future: short-term therapy, preventive therapy, and bacillus Calmette–Guérin. *Bull. N.Y. Acad. Med.*, **1977**, *53*, 526–531.

Evans, D. A. P.; Manley, K. A.; and McKusick, V. A. Genetic control of isoniazid metabolism in man. *Br. Med. J.*, **1960**, *2*, 485–491.

Flynn, C. T.; Rainford, D. J.; and Hope, E. Acute renal failure and rifampicin: danger of unsuspected intermittent dosage. *Br. Med. J.*, **1974**, *2*, 482.

Fox, H. H. The chemical attack on tuberculosis. *Trans. N.Y. Acad. Sci.*, **1953**, *15*, 234–242.

Furesz, S. Chemical and biological properties of rifampicin. *Antibiot. Chemother.*, **1970**, *16*, 316–351.

Gangadharam, P. R. J. Isoniazid, rifampin, and hepatotoxicity. *Am. Rev. Respir. Dis.*, **1986**, *133*, 963–965.

Garibaldi, R. A.; Drusin, R. E.; Ferebee, S. H.; and

Gregg, M. B. Isoniazid-associated hepatitis. Report of an outbreak. *Am. Rev. Respir. Dis.*, **1972**, *106*, 357–365.
Girling, D. J. The hepatic toxicity of antituberculous regimens containing isoniazid, rifampicin and pyrazinamide. *Tubercle*, **1978**, *59*, 13–32.
Girling, D. J., and Hitze, H. L. Adverse reactions to rifampicin. *Bull. W.H.O.*, **1979**, *57*, 45–49.
Goodwin, C. S., and Sparell, G. Inhibition of dapsone excretion by probenecid. *Lancet*, **1969**, *2*, 884–885.
Graber, C. D.; Jebaily, J.; Galphin, R. L.; and Doering, E. Light chain proteinuria and humoral immunocompetence in tuberculous patients treated with rifampin. *Am. Rev. Respir. Dis.*, **1973**, *107*, 713–717.
Greene, J. B., and others. *Mycobacterium avium-intracellulare:* a cause of disseminated life-threatening infection in homosexuals and drug abusers. *Ann. Intern. Med.*, **1982**, *97*, 539–546.
Gronhagen-Riska, C.; Hellstrom, P. E.; and Froseth, B. Predisposing factors in hepatitis induced by isoniazid–rifampin treatment of tuberculosis. *Am. Rev. Respir. Dis.*, **1978**, *118*, 461–466.
Grosset, J., and Leventis, S. Adverse effects of rifampin. *Rev. Infect. Dis.*, **1983**, *5*, Suppl. 3, S440–S446.
Gupta, S.; Grieco, M. H.; and Siegel, I. Suppression of T-lymphocyte rosettes by rifampin. *Ann. Intern. Med.*, **1975**, *82*, 484–488.
Herman, R. P., and Weber, M. M. Site of action of isoniazid on the electron transport chain and its relationship to nicotinamide adenine dinucleotide regulation in *Mycobacterium phlei*. *Antimicrob. Agents Chemother.*, **1980**, *17*, 450–454.
Hobby, G. L., and Lenert, T. F. Observations on the action of rifampin and ethambutol alone and in combination with other antituberculous drugs. *Am. Rev. Respir. Dis.*, **1972**, *105*, 292–295.
Holdiness, M. R. Cerebrospinal fluid pharmacokinetics of antituberculosis antibiotics. *Clin. Pharmacokinet.*, **1985**, *10*, 532–534.
Hurwitz, A., and Schlozman, D. L. Effect of antacids on gastrointestinal absorption of isoniazid in rat and man. *Am. Rev. Respir. Dis.*, **1974**, *109*, 41–47.
Iyer, C. G. S.; Languillon, J.; and Ramanujam, K. WHO coordinated short-term double-blind trial with thalidomide in the treatment of acute lepra reactions in male lepromatous patients. *Bull. W.H.O.*, **1971**, *45*, 719–732.
Izumi, A. K.; Hanke, E. W.; and Higaki, M. *M. marinum* infections treated with tetracycline. *Arch. Dermatol.*, **1977**, *113*, 1067–1068.
Jenne, J. W., and Beggs, W. H. Correlation of *in vitro* and *in vivo* kinetics with clinical use of isoniazid, ethambutol and rifampin. *Am. Rev. Respir. Dis.*, **1973**, *107*, 1013–1021.
La Du, B. N. Isoniazid and pseudocholinesterase polymorphisms. *Fed. Proc.*, **1972**, *31*, 1276–1285.
Leiker, D. L. The mononuclear syndrome in leprosy patients treated with sulfones. *Int. J. Lepr.*, **1956**, *24*, 402–405.
Levy, L., and Peters, J. H. Susceptibility of *Mycobacterium leprae* to dapsone as a determinant of patient response to acedapsone. *Antimicrob. Agents Chemother.*, **1976**, *9*, 102–112.
Levy, L.; Shepard, C. C.; and Fasal, P. Clofazimine therapy of lepromatous leprosy caused by dapsone-resistant *Mycobacterium leprae*. *Am. J. Trop. Med. Hyg.*, **1972**, *21*, 315–321.
Lincoln, E. M., and Gilberg, L. A. Disease in children due to mycobacteria other than *M. tuberculosis*. *Am. Rev. Respir. Dis.*, **1972**, *105*, 683–714.
Loria, P. R. Minocycline hydrochloride treatment for atypical acid-fast infection. *Arch. Dermatol.*, **1976**, *112*, 517–519.
McGlynn, K. A.; Lustabader, E. D.; Sharrar, R. G.; Murphy, E. C.; and London, W. T. Isoniazid prophylaxis in hepatitis B carriers. *Am. Rev. Respir. Dis.*, **1986**, *134*, 666–668.
Maddrey, W. C., and Boitnott, J. K. Isoniazid hepatitis. *Ann. Intern. Med.*, **1973**, *79*, 1–12.
Mason, G. H.; Ellis-Pegler, R. B.; and Arthur, J. F. Clofazimine and eosinophilic enteritis. *Lepr. Rev.*, **1977**, *48*, 175–180.
Masur, H.; Tuazon, C.; Gill, V.; Grimes, G.; Baird, B.; Fauci, A. S.; and Lane, H. C. Effect of combined clofazimine and ansamycin therapy on *Mycobacterium avium–Mycobacterium intracellulare* bacteremia in patients with AIDS. *J. Infect. Dis.*, **1987**, *155*, 127–129.
Medical Letter. Clofazimine for leprosy and *Mycobacterium avium* complex infections. **1987**, *29*, 77–78.
Miller, R. R.; Porter, J.; and Greenblatt, D. J. Clinical importance of the interaction of phenytoin and isoniazid. *Chest*, **1979**, *75*, 356–358.
Mitchell, J. R.; Zimmerman, H. J.; Ishak, K. G.; Thorgeirsson, U. P.; Timbrell, J. A.; Snodgrass, W. R.; and Nelson, S. D. Isoniazid liver injury: clinical spectrum, pathology, and probable pathogenesis. *Ann. Intern. Med.*, **1976**, *84*, 181–192.
Morrison, N. E., and Marley, G. M. Clofazimine binding studies with deoxyribonucleic acid. *Int. J. Lepr.*, **1976**, *44*, 475–481.
Mukerjee, P.; Schuldt, S.; and Kasik, J. E. Effect of rifampin on cutaneous hypersensitivity to purified protein derivatives in humans. *Antimicrob. Agents Chemother.*, **1973**, *4*, 607–611.
Nicholson, D. P. Atypical tuberculosis: features and therapy. *Br. J. Dis. Chest*, **1976**, *70*, 217–218.
Ohnhaus, E. E.; Kirchhof, B.; and Peheim, E. Effect of enzyme induction on plasma lipids using antipyrine, phenobarbital, and rifampicin. *Clin. Pharmacol. Ther.*, **1979**, *25*, 591–597.
O'Reilly, R. A. Interaction of chronic daily warfarin therapy and rifampin. *Ann. Intern. Med.*, **1975**, *83*, 506–508.
Peets, E. A.; Sweeney, W. M.; Place, V. A.; and Buyske, D. A. The absorption, excretion and metabolic fate of ethambutol in man. *Am. Rev. Respir. Dis.*, **1965**, *91*, 51–58.
Pengelly, C. D. R. Dapsone-induced hemolysis. *Br. Med. J.*, **1963**, *2*, 662–664.
Pezzia, W.; Raleigh, J. W.; Bailey, M. C.; Toth, E. A.; and Silverblatt, J. Treatment of pulmonary disease due to *Mycobacterium kansasii:* recent experience with rifampin. *Rev. Infect. Dis.*, **1981**, *3*, 1035–1039.
Pilheu, J. A.; De Salvo, M. C.; and Koch, O. Liver alterations in antituberculosis regimens containing pyrazinamide. *Chest*, **1981**, *80*, 720–724.
Postlethwaite, A. E.; Bartel, A. G.; and Kelley, W. N. Hyperuricemia due to ethambutol. *N. Engl. J. Med.*, **1972**, *286*, 761–762.
Public Health Service, U.S. Department of Health, Education, and Welfare. Isoniazid-associated hepatitis: summary of the report of the Tuberculosis Advisory Committee and special consultants to the Director, Center for Disease Control. *M.M.W.R.*, **1974**, *23*, 97–98.
Radner, D. B. Toxicologic and pharmacologic aspects of rifampin. *Chest*, **1973**, *64*, 213–216.
Rapoport, A. M., and Guss, S. B. Dapsone-induced peripheral neuropathy. *Arch. Neurol.*, **1972**, *27*, 184–186.
Rothfield, N. F.; Bierer, W. F.; and Garfield, J. W. Isoniazid induction of antinuclear antibodies. *Ann. Intern. Med.*, **1978**, *88*, 650–652.
Sanders, W. E., Jr. Lung infection caused by rapidly growing mycobacteria. *J. Respir. Dis.*, **1982**, *3*, 30–38.
Sanders, W. E., Jr.; Cacciatore, R.; Valdez, H.; Schneider, N.; and Hartwig, C. Activity of amikacin against mycobacteria *in vitro* and in experimental infections with *M. tuberculosis*. *Am. Rev. Respir. Dis.*, **1976**, *113*, 59.
Sanders, W. E., Jr.; Hartwig, E. C.; Schneider, N. J.; Cacciatore, R.; and Valdez, H. Susceptibility of organisms in the *Mycobacterium fortuitum* complex to antitu-

berculous and other antimicrobial agents. *Antimicrob. Agents Chemother.*, **1977**, *12*, 295–297.

Sanfilippo, A.; Della Bruna, C.; Marsili, L.; Morvillo, E.; Pasqualucci, C. R.; Schioppacassi, G.; and Ungheri, D. Biological activity of a new class of rifamycins, spiropiperidyl-rifamycins. *J. Antibiot. (Tokyo)*, **1980**, *33*, 1193–1198.

Scheuer, P. J.; Summerfield, J. A.; Lal, S.; and Sherlock, S. Rifampin hepatitis. *Lancet*, **1974**, *1*, 421–425.

Schwartz, W. S. Comparison of ethionamide with isoniazid in original treatment cases of pulmonary tuberculosis. XIV. A report of the Veterans Administration–Armed Forces Cooperative Study. *Am. Rev. Respir. Dis.*, **1966**, *93*, 685–692.

Shepard, C. C.; Ellard, G. A.; Levy, L.; Opromolla, V.; Pattyn, S. R.; Peters, J. H.; Rees, R. J. W.; and Waters, M. F. R. Experimental chemotherapy of leprosy. *Bull. W.H.O.*, **1976**, *53*, 425–433.

Simon, E.; Veres, E.; and Banki, G. Changes in SGOT activity during treatment with ethionamide. *Scand. J. Respir. Dis.*, **1969**, *50*, 314–322.

Sippel, J. E.; Mikhail, I. A.; Girgis, N. I.; and Youssef, H. H. Rifampin concentrations in cerebrospinal fluid of patients with tuberculous meningitis. *Am. Rev. Respir. Dis.*, **1974**, *109*, 579–580.

Skolnick, J. L.; Stoler, B. S.; Katz, D. B.; and Anderson, W. H. Rifampin, oral contraceptives, and pregnancy. *J.A.M.A.*, **1976**, *236*, 1382.

Snider, D. E., Jr. Pyridoxine supplementation during isoniazid therapy. *Tubercle*, **1980**, *61*, 191–196.

Snider, D. E., and Farer, L. S. Preventive therapy with isoniazid for "inactive" tuberculosis. *Chest*, **1978**, *73*, 4–5.

Spector, R., and Lorenzo, W. V. The active transport of para-aminosalicylic acid from the cerebrospinal fluid. *J. Pharmacol. Exp. Ther.*, **1973**, *185*, 642–648.

Takayama, K.; Armstrong, E. L.; Kunugi, K. A.; and Kilburn, J. O. Inhibition by ethambutol of mycolic acid transfer into the cell wall of *Mycobacterium smegmatis*. *Antimicrob. Agents Chemother.*, **1979**, *16*, 240.

Takayama, K.; Schnoes, H. K.; Armstrong, E. L.; and Boyle, R. W. Site of inhibitory action of isoniazid in the synthesis of mycolic acids in *Mycobacterium tuberculosis*. *J. Lipid Res.*, **1975**, *16*, 308–317.

Thornsberry, C.; Hill, B. C.; Swenson, J. M.; and McDougal, L. K. Rifampin: spectrum of antibacterial activity. *Rev. Infect. Dis.*, **1983**, *5*, Suppl. 3, S412–S417.

Trautman, J. R. The management of leprosy and its complications. *N. Engl. J. Med.*, **1965**, *273*, 756–758.

Warrington, R. J.; Hogg, G. R.; Paraskevas, F.; and Tse, K. S. Insidious rifampin-associated renal failure with light-chain proteinuria. *Arch. Intern. Med.*, **1977**, *137*, 927–930.

Wehrli, W. Rifampin: mechanisms of action and resistance. *Rev. Infect. Dis.*, **1983**, *5*, Suppl. 3, S407–S411.

Weiner, I. M., and Tinker, J. P. Pharmacology of pyrazinamide: metabolic and renal function studies related to the mechanism of drug-induced urate retention. *J. Pharmacol. Exp. Ther.*, **1972**, *180*, 411–434.

Wheat, L. J.; Kohler, R. B.; Luft, F. C.; and White, A. Long-term studies of the effect of rifampin on nasal carriage of coagulase-positive staphylococci. *Rev. Infect. Dis.*, **1983**, *5*, Suppl. 3, S459–S462.

WHO Study Group. Chemotherapy of leprosy for control programmes. WHO Technical Report Series No. 675, WHO, Geneva, **1982**, 7–33.

Wilson, T. M. Current therapeutics. CCXL. Capreomycin and ethambutol. *Practitioner*, **1967**, *199*, 817–824.

Young, L. S. *Mycobacterium avium* complex infection. *J. Infect. Dis.*, **1988**, *157*, 863–867.

Zierski, M., and Bek, E. Side effects of drug regimens used in short course chemotherapy for pulmonary tuberculosis. A controlled study. *Tubercle*, **1980**, *61*, 41–49.

Monographs and Reviews

American Thoracic Society. Treatment of tuberculosis and tuberculosis infections in adults and children. *Am. Rev. Respir. Dis.*, **1986**, *134*, 363–368.

Bullock, W. E. Rifampin in the treatment of leprosy. *Rev. Infect. Dis.*, **1983**, *5*, S606–S613.

———. *Mycobacterium leprae* (leprosy). In, *Principles and Practice of Infectious Diseases*, 3rd ed. (Mandell, G. L.; Douglas, R. G., Jr.; and Bennett, J. E.; eds.) Churchill Livingstone, Inc., New York, **1990**, pp. 1906–1914.

DeGowin, R. L. A review of the therapeutic and hemolytic effects of dapsone. *Arch. Intern. Med.*, **1967**, *120*, 242–248.

Des Prez, R. M., and Heim, C. R. *Mycobacterium tuberculosis*. In, *Principles and Practice of Infectious Diseases*, 3rd ed. (Mandell, G. L.; Douglas, R. G., Jr.; and Bennett, J. E.; eds.) Churchill Livingstone, Inc., New York, **1990**, pp. 1877–1906.

Farr, B. F., and Mandell, G. L. Rifampin. *Med. Clin. North Am.*, **1982**, *66*, 157–168.

———. Rifamycins. In, *Principles and Practice of Infectious Diseases*, 3rd ed. (Mandell, G. L.; Douglas, R. G., Jr.; and Bennett, J. E.; eds.) Churchill Livingstone, Inc., New York, **1990**, pp. 295–303.

Goldman, A. L., and Braman, S. S. Isoniazid: a review with emphasis on adverse effects. *Chest*, **1972**, *62*, 71–77.

Hastings, R. C., and Franzblau, S. G. Chemotherapy of leprosy. *Annu. Rev. Pharmacol. Toxicol.*, **1988**, *28*, 231–245.

Jacobson, R. R. The treatment of leprosy (Hansen's disease). *Hosp. Formulary*, **1982**, *17*, 1076–1091.

Kapusnik, J. E.; Parenti, F.; and Sande, M. The use of rifampicin in staphylococcal infections—a review. *J. Antimicrob. Chemother.*, **1984**, *13*, 61–66.

Pitts, F. W. Tuberculosis: prevention and therapy. In, *Current Concepts of Infectious Diseases*. (Hook, E. W.; Mandell, G. L.; Gwaltney, J. M., Jr.; and Sande, M. A.; eds.) John Wiley & Sons, Inc., New York, **1977**, pp. 181–194.

Sanders, W. E., Jr., and Horowitz, E. A. Other *Mycobacterium* species. In, *Principles and Practice of Infectious Diseases*, 3rd ed. (Mandell, G. L.; Douglas, R. G., Jr.; and Bennett, J. E.; eds.) Churchill Livingstone, Inc., New York, **1990**, pp. 1914–1926.

Shepard, C. C. Chemotherapy of leprosy. *Annu. Rev. Pharmacol.*, **1969**, *9*, 37–50.

Symposium. (Various authors.) The use of rifampin in treatment of nontuberculous infections. *Rev. Infect. Dis.*, **1983**, *5*, Suppl., S399–S632.

CHAPTER

50 ANTIMICROBIAL AGENTS

[*Continued*]

Antifungal Agents

John E. Bennett

Although options for the treatment of fungal infections have increased substantially over the past three decades, the pharmacological principles of antifungal therapy are only partially understood (*see* Trinci and Riley, 1984; Symposium, 1988). A major difficulty is that *in-vitro* testing of fungi for either primary or secondary resistance to chemotherapeutic agents does not provide clinically useful information. There is extreme variation in the results obtained with different methods for testing susceptibility to drugs; there is even significant variation between laboratories when the same method is used. No single assay is generally accepted (*see* Galgiani, 1989). Without a firm grasp on concentrations of drugs necessary to inhibit fungal growth *in vitro,* it is obviously difficult to estimate what concentration of drug might be therapeutic.

The tissue distribution of antifungal agents correlates variably with the clinical outcome. For example, systemic treatment of cutaneous mycoses has been enhanced by drugs such as griseofulvin and ketoconazole, which are concentrated in the stratum corneum, either because of partitioning into cutaneous lipids or binding to keratinocytes. Unfortunately, interpretation of the utility of drug concentrations that are achieved in cerebrospinal fluid has been more problematic.

Fungal infections are traditionally divided into two distinct classes—superficial and systemic. Accordingly, the major antifungal agents are described in this chapter under two major headings—systemic antifungal agents and topical antifungal agents. It should be noted, however, that this distinction is becoming arbitrary. Some of the drugs (imidazoles and triazoles; polyenes) may be used in either manner, and many superficial mycoses may be treated either systemically or topically.

I. Systemic Antifungal Agents

AMPHOTERICIN B

History and Source. Amphotericin B was discovered by Gold and coworkers (1956), who were studying a strain of *Streptomyces nodosus,* an aerobic actinomycete, obtained from the Orinoco River Valley of Venezuela. The antibiotic was isolated by Vandeputte and associates (1956).

Chemistry. Amphotericin B is one of a family of some 200 polyene macrolide antibiotics. Those studied to date share the characteristics of four to seven conjugated double bonds, an internal cyclic ester, poor aqueous solubility, substantial toxicity on parenteral administration, and a common mechanism of antifungal action. Amphotericin B (*see* below) is a heptaene macrolide, containing seven conjugated double bonds in the trans position, and 3-amino-3,6-dideoxymannose (mycosamine) connected to the main ring by a glycosidic bond. The amphoteric behavior for which the drug is named derives from the presence of a carboxyl group on

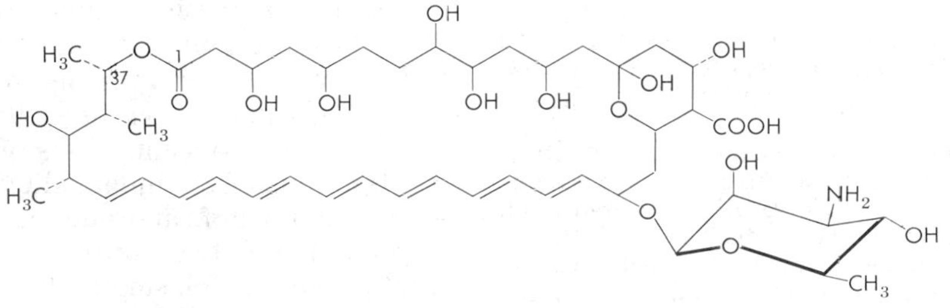

Amphotericin B

the main ring and a primary amino group on mycosamine; these groups confer aqueous solubility at extremes of pH. X-ray crystallography has shown the molecule to be rigid and rod-shaped, with the hydrophilic hydroxyl groups of the macrolide ring forming an opposing face to the lipophilic polyenic portion (Kerridge and Whelan, 1984).

Aqueous insolubility of amphotericin B at neutral pH renders intravenous infusion difficult. Bartner and coworkers (1958) found that amphotericin B could be solubilized as a colloidal dispersion in deoxycholate. Although this formulation has been in clinical use for more than 30 years, toxicity of the deoxycholate complex has prompted attempts to develop other formulations. N-acyl derivatives of amphotericin B or esters of the carboxyl group are generally less active *in vitro* but can be formulated as water-soluble salts. For example, the methyl ester has been administered intravenously as the hydrochloride, ascorbate, or aspartate salt (*see* Hoeprich *et al.*, in Symposium, 1988). The amphipathic property of amphotericin B also permits incorporation of the drug into liposomes. Preliminary clinical experience with two liposomal preparations indicated that neither caused azotemia, but the two differed profoundly in the drug concentrations that were achieved in plasma (*see* Lopez-Berestein, and *see also* Meunier *et al.*, in Symposium, 1988). Formulations in lipid emulsions and as complexes with cholesterol have also been tested; there is reason to hope for improved formulations of this useful drug.

Current regulations in the United States require that amphotericin B for intravenous use be at least 75% pure and have no more than 5% amphotericin A, a tetraene. The amount of amphotericin A and of amphotericin X in the commercial product depends upon the strain of *Streptomyces* used for production and the purification process. Differences in pyrogenicity between lots of the drug and between manufacturers are probably attributable to variable composition and to technical problems in measuring contamination of preparations with endotoxin.

Antifungal Activity. Amphotericin B has useful clinical activity against *Candida* species, *Cryptococcus neoformans, Blastomyces dermatitidis, Histoplasma capsulatum, Torulopsis glabrata, Coccidioides immitis, Paracoccidioides braziliensis, Aspergillus* species, and the agents of mucormycosis. Methods for determination of susceptibility of fungi to amphotericin B are still controversial, although efforts at standardization are in progress.

Amphotericin B has limited activity against the protozoa, *Leishmania braziliensis,* and *Naegleria fowleri.* The drug has no antibacterial activity.

Mechanism of Action. The antifungal activity of amphotericin B is at least in part dependent on its binding to a sterol moiety, primarily ergosterol, present in the membrane of sensitive fungi. By virtue of their interaction with the sterols of cell membranes, polyenes appear to form pores or channels. The result is an increase in the permeability of the membrane, allowing leakage of a variety of small molecules (*see* Hamilton-Miller, 1974). Additional mechanisms of action may include oxidative damage to fungal cells, at least *in vitro* (Sokol-Anderson *et al.*, 1986), and some capability to enhance cell-mediated immunity in the host (Medoff *et al.*, 1983).

Fungal Resistance. Mutants with decreased susceptibility to amphotericin B have been isolated from several fungal species by passage in culture medium containing the drug. Many but not all of these mutants have decreased concentrations of ergosterol in their cell membranes. Some resistant strains have elevated concentrations of precursors of ergosterol with lower affinity for the polyene antibiotics. Isolation from blood or deep tissues of strains with decreased susceptibility has been reported (Powderly *et al.*, 1988). More commonly, species of *Candida* with decreased susceptibility have been isolated only from the throat, stool, or urine, with no evidence that infection with drug-resistant organisms has occurred.

Absorption, Distribution, and Excretion. Absorption of amphotericin B from the gastrointestinal tract is negligible. Repeated daily intravenous infusions to adults of 0.5 mg/kg results in concentrations in plasma of about 1.0 to 1.5 μg/ml at the end of the infusion, which falls to about 0.5 to 1.0 μg/ml 24 hours later (Bindschadler and Bennett, 1969). The drug is released from its complex with deoxycholate in the bloodstream, and the amphotericin B that remains in plasma is more than 90% bound to proteins, largely β-lipoprotein. Approximately 2 to 5% of each dose appears in the urine when patients are on daily therapy. Elimination of the drug appears to be unchanged in anephric patients and in patients receiving hemodialysis. In dogs, biliary occlusion results in elevated concentrations of amphotericin B in blood (Craven *et al.*, 1979), but hepatic or biliary disease have no known effect on metabolism of the drug in man. At least a third of the injected doses can be recovered unchanged by methanolic extraction of tissue at autopsy; the highest concentrations are found in liver and spleen, with lesser amounts in kidney and lung (Christiansen *et al.*, 1985; Collette *et al.*, 1989). Concentrations of amphotericin B in fluids from inflamed pleura, peritoneum, synovium, and aqueous humor are approximately two thirds of trough concentrations in plasma. The drug probably crosses the placenta readily (Bennett,

1990). Little amphotericin B penetrates into cerebrospinal fluid (CSF), vitreous humor, or normal amniotic fluid. Because of extensive binding to tissues, there is a terminal phase of elimination with a half-time of about 15 days.

Preparations, Routes of Administration, and Dosage. *Amphotericin B* (FUNGIZONE) is available for injection. The sterile, lyophilized powder is marketed in vials containing 50 mg of amphotericin B plus 41 mg of sodium deoxycholate and sodium phosphate buffer. The contents of the vial should be dissolved, with shaking, in 10 ml of sterile water and then added to 5% dextrose in water. Solutions of some electrolytes, acidic solutions, or solutions with preservatives should not be used because they cause precipitation of this antifungal agent (Jurgens *et al.*, 1981). If fever and chills in response to administration of the drug are severe, the addition of 0.7 mg/kg of hydrocortisone may alleviate the symptoms in some patients. Meperidine is also effective (Burks *et al.*, 1980). Topical preparations of amphotericin B are also marketed (*see* below).

Opinions vary as to the most effective dosage for administration of amphotericin B. To a certain extent, the dosage is dependent on the type and severity of infection. Most physicians agree that a small test dose (1 mg dissolved in 20 ml of 5% dextrose solution) should first be administered intravenously over 20 to 30 minutes. The temperature, pulse, respiratory rate, and blood pressure should be recorded every 30 minutes for 4 hours. Fever, chills, hypotension, and dyspnea are common. A patient with a severe, rapidly progressing fungal infection, good cardiopulmonary function, and a mild reaction to the test dose can immediately receive 0.3 mg/kg of amphotericin B intravenously over a period of 2 to 4 hours (Bennett, 1990). If the patient has a severe reaction to the test dose or cardiopulmonary impairment, a smaller dose is recommended—for example, 0.1 mg/kg, or 5 to 10 mg. This dose may then be increased by 5 to 10 mg per day. In severe or fulminant infections, dosage should be escalated rapidly until the patient is receiving 0.5 to 1.0 mg/kg daily. Incremental doses can be given every 6 to 8 hours if reactions in a fragile patient make immediate advancement to full dosage inadvisable. For example, a severe reaction to a 1-mg dose could be followed by 5, 15, and 25 mg given at 8-hour intervals, followed by 40 mg 24 hours later. The recommended maintenance dose for most deep mycoses is 0.4 to 0.6 mg/kg per day, infused over 2 to 4 hours. Adult doses of 10 to 15 mg daily can be sufficient in *Candida* esophagitis. When used with flucytosine, the daily dose of amphotericin B is 0.3 mg/kg.

The febrile reactions associated with the administration of amphotericin B usually subside despite continued use of the drug, and the concurrent use of hydrocortisone frequently can be stopped. Amphotericin B may be administered every other day by doubling the recommended daily dose without sacrifice of therapeutic efficacy. The individual dose should not exceed 70 mg in the alternate-day regimen, even if the daily dose was greater than 35 mg. There is a greater chance for toxicity and no proof of additional efficacy above this dose. Although this schedule decreases the number of venipunctures and allows more ambulation, the incidence of nephrotoxicity is not reduced, and the severity of febrile reactions may increase.

Intrathecal infusion of amphotericin B is necessary in patients with meningitis caused by *Coccidioides*. The drug can be injected into the CSF of the lumbar spine, cisterna magna, or lateral cerebral ventricle. Irrespective of site, the treatment is begun with 0.05 to 0.1 mg and increased on a three-times-a-week schedule to 0.5 mg, as tolerance permits. Therapy is then continued on a twice-a-week schedule. Fever and headache are common reactions and may be decreased by administration of 10 to 15 mg of hydrocortisone. Less common but more serious problems attend the use of intrathecal injections; the nature of the problem depends on the injection site chosen. Local injections of amphotericin B into a joint or peritoneal dialysate fluid commonly produce irritation and pain. Intraocular injection following pars plana vitrectomy has been used successfully for fungal endophthalmitis, but retinal damage can occur.

Untoward Effects. Intravenous administration of amphotericin B can cause a large number of adverse effects; the two most common are fever and azotemia. Fever and chills are most common at the beginning of therapy; they tend to subside later in the course. The reaction often begins an hour or two after start of the infusion and lasts 2 to 4 hours. Dyspnea and tachycardia may precede fever. Bronchospasm and true anaphylaxis are rare. The capacity of the drug to release interleukin 1 and tumor necrosis factor from human monocytes and murine macrophages *in vitro* suggests a mechanism for pyrogenicity. Although administration of amphotericin B following leukocyte transfusion was, at one time, thought to cause pulmonary infiltrates and hypoxemia, this observation has not been confirmed. Amphotericin B can, however, cause leukocyte aggregation *in vitro,* an action that could lead to trapping of leukocytes in the pulmonary capillary bed if it occurred *in vivo*.

Azotemia occurs in 80% of patients who receive amphotericin B for deep mycoses. Toxicity is dose-dependent, transient, and increased by concomitant therapy with other nephrotoxic agents such as aminoglycosides or cyclosporine (Kennedy *et al.*,

1983). Although permanent histologic damage to renal tubules occurs even during short courses, permanent functional defects are uncommon in patients whose renal function was normal prior to treatment unless a total dose in excess of 3 to 4 g is given (to an adult). Renal tubular acidosis and renal wasting of K^+ and Mg^{2+} may also be seen during and for several weeks after therapy. Supplemental K^+ is required in a third of patients on prolonged therapy. An increase in intrarenal vascular resistance is the major cause of nephrotoxicity in amphotericin B–treated rats (Tolins and Raij, 1988). In patients and experimental animals, loading with sodium chloride has decreased nephrotoxicity, even in the absence of water or salt deprivation. Administration of 1 liter of saline intravenously on the day that amphotericin B is to be given has been recommended for adults who are able to tolerate the Na^+ load and who are not already receiving that amount in intravenous fluids (Branch, 1988).

Hypochromic, normocytic anemia is usual; the average hematocrit declined to 27% in one study. Decreased production of erythropoietin is the probable mechanism. Anemia reverses slowly following therapy. Headache, nausea, vomiting, malaise, weight loss, and phlebitis at peripheral infusion sites are common side effects. Thrombocytopenia or mild leukopenia is observed rarely.

Therapeutic Uses. Intravenous administration of amphotericin B is the treatment of choice for mucormycosis, invasive aspergillosis, extracutaneous sporotrichosis, and cryptococcosis. Although imidazoles or triazoles are useful in many patients with blastomycosis, histoplasmosis, coccidioidomycosis, and paracoccidioidomycosis, amphotericin B is preferred when these mycoses are rapidly progressive, occur in an immunosuppressed host, or involve the central nervous system. Amphotericin B can also be useful in selected patients with profound neutropenia and fever that is unresponsive to broad-spectrum antibacterial agents. Amphotericin B given once weekly has been used to prevent relapse in patients with acquired immunodeficiency syndrome (AIDS) who have been treated successfully for cryptococcosis or histoplasmosis. Topical amphotericin B is useful only in cutaneous candidiasis. Oral tablets are commercially available in Europe for decreasing colonization of the intestine by *Candida*.

FLUCYTOSINE

Chemistry. *Flucytosine* is a fluorinated pyrimidine related to fluorouracil and floxuridine. It is 5-fluorocytosine, the formula of which is as follows:

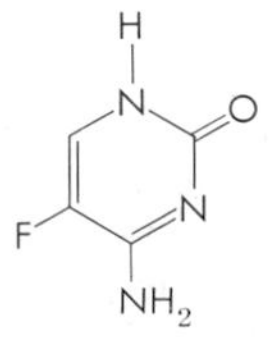

Flucytosine

Antifungal Activity. Flucytosine has clinically useful activity against *Cryptococcus neoformans*, *Candida* species, *Torulopsis glabrata*, and the agents of chromomycosis. Within these species, determination of susceptibility *in vitro* has been extremely dependent on the method employed and, when performed on isolates obtained prior to treatment, has not correlated with clinical outcome.

Fungal Resistance. Drug resistance that arises during therapy (secondary resistance) is an important cause of therapeutic failure when flucytosine is used alone in cryptococcosis and candidiasis. In chromomycosis, resurgence of lesions after an initial response has led to the presumption of secondary drug resistance. In isolates of *Cryptococcus* and *Candida* species, secondary drug resistance has been accompanied by a change in the minimal inhibitory concentration from less than 2.5 μg/ml to more than 360 μg/ml. The mechanism for this resistance can be loss of the permease necessary for cytosine transport or decreased activity of either uridine monophosphate (UMP) pyrophosphorylase or cytosine deaminase (*see* Mechanism of Action, below; *see also* Kerridge and Whelan, 1984). In *Candida albicans*, a diploid fungus, partial resistance can occur because of heterozygous deficiency of UMP pyrophosphorylase. The clinical significance of partial resistance is unknown.

Mechanism of Action. All susceptible fungi are capable of deaminating flucytosine to 5-fluorouracil, a potent antimetabolite (*see* Chapter 52). Fluorouracil is metabolized first to 5-fluorouridylic acid by the enzyme UMP pyrophosphorylase. It can then either be incorporated into RNA (via synthesis of 5-fluorouridine triphosphate) or be metabolized to 5-fluorodeoxyuridylic acid, a potent inhibitor of thymidylate synthetase. DNA synthesis is impaired as the ultimate result of this latter reaction (*see* Kerridge and Whelan, 1984). Mammalian cells do not convert flucytosine to fluorouracil. This fact is crucial for the selective action of this compound.

Absorption, Distribution, and Excretion. Flucytosine is rapidly and well absorbed from the gastrointestinal tract. It is widely distributed in the body, with a volume of distribution that approximates total body water. The drug is minimally bound to plasma proteins. The peak plasma concentration in patients with normal renal function is approximately 70 to 80 μg/ml 1 to 2 hours after a dose of 37.5 mg/kg (Bennett *et al.*, 1979). Approximately 80% of a given dose is excreted in the urine in unchanged form; concentrations in the urine range from 200 to 500 μg/ml. The half-life of the drug is 3 to 6 hours in normal individuals. In renal failure, the half-life may be as long as 200 hours. The clearance of flucytosine is approximately equivalent to that of creatinine. Because of the obligate renal excretion of the drug, modification of dosage is necessary in patients with decreased renal function (*see* Appendix II). It is recommended that concentrations of drug in plasma be measured periodically in patients with renal insufficiency. Peak concentrations should range between 50 and 100 μg/ml. Flucytosine is cleared by hemodialysis, and patients undergoing such treatment should receive a single dose of 37.5 mg/kg after dialysis (Block *et al.*, 1974); the drug is also removed by peritoneal dialysis.

Flucytosine is present in CSF at a concentration about 65 to 90% of that simultaneously present in the plasma. The drug also appears to penetrate into the aqueous humor.

Preparations, Route of Administration, and Dosage. *Flucytosine* (ANCOBON) is supplied in capsules containing either 250 or 500 mg for oral administration. An intravenous formulation is no longer available. The usual daily dose is 100 to 150 mg/kg, divided into four portions. This dosage must be altered, as described above, for patients with renal insufficiency.

Untoward Effects. Flucytosine may depress the function of bone marrow and lead to the development of leukopenia and thrombocytopenia; patients are more prone to the appearance of this complication if they have an underlying hematological disorder, are being treated with radiation or drugs that injure the bone marrow, or have a history of treatment with such agents. Other untoward effects, including rash, nausea, vomiting, diarrhea, and severe enterocolitis, have been noted. In approximately 5% of patients elevation of hepatic enzymes in plasma has occurred, but this is reversible when therapy is stopped. Toxicity is more frequent in patients with AIDS or azotemia (including those who are receiving amphotericin B concurrently), and when concentrations of the drug in plasma exceed 100 μg/ml (Stamm *et al.*, 1987). Toxicity may be the result of conversion of flucytosine to 5-fluorouracil by the microbial flora in the intestinal tract of the host (Harris *et al.*, 1986).

Therapeutic Uses. Amphotericin B remains the most effective therapeutic agent for the management of infections due to yeasts and fungi; flucytosine is used predominantly in combination with amphotericin B. Except in the treatment of chromoblastomycosis, rapid emergence of flucytosine-resistant strains has restricted its use as a single drug. Flucytosine may be useful for treatment of infections of the urinary tract with *Candida*, but not if a catheter is in the bladder. The concurrent administration of amphotericin B (0.3 mg/kg per day) and flucytosine (100 to 150 mg/kg per day) has become the treatment of choice for cryptococcal meningitis and that caused by *Candida* (Bennett *et al.*, 1979; Smego *et al.*, 1984).

IMIDAZOLES AND TRIAZOLES

Imidazoles and the structurally related N-substituted triazoles are considered together because they share the same antifungal spectrum and mechanism of action. The systemic triazoles are more slowly metabolized and have less effect on human sterol synthesis than do the imidazoles. Because of these advantages, new congeners under development are mostly triazoles, not imidazoles. Of the drugs now on the market in the United States, clotrimazole, miconazole, ketoconazole, econazole, butoconazole, oxiconazole, and sulconazole are imidazoles. Terconazole is the only triazole that is currently available, but itraconazole and fluconazole are likely to be marketed in the near future. The topical use of these drugs is described in the second section of this chapter.

Antifungal Activity. Testing *in vitro* has shown these agents to be highly active against a broad spectrum of fungi. However, the results of such tests have been very dependent upon the methods employed, and they correlate poorly with clinical results. For unexplained reasons, inhibition of germ tube formation in *Candida albicans* occurs at much lower concentrations than does inhibition of blastosporulation. These drugs do not appear to have any useful antibacterial or antiparasitic activity, with the possible exception of antiprotozoal effects against *Leishmania major*.

Mechanism of Action. At concentrations achieved during systemic use, the major effect of imidazoles and triazoles on fungi is inhibition of sterol 14-α-demethylase, a microsomal cytochrome P_{450}–dependent enzyme system. Imidazoles and triazoles thus impair the biosynthesis of ergosterol for the cytoplasmic membrane and lead to the accumulation of 14-α-methyl sterols (Vanden Bossche *et al.*, 1986). These methyl sterols may disrupt the close packing of acyl chains of phospholipids, impairing the functions of certain membrane-bound enzyme systems and inhibiting growth.

Creation of drug-resistant mutants has proven difficult *in vitro*. The rare drug-resistant mutants that have been obtained from patients were not isolated from deep sources, making it unclear whether these mutants retained the potential to cause deeply invasive disease.

KETOCONAZOLE

Ketoconazole, administered orally, has broad therapeutic potential for the treatment of a number of superficial and systemic fungal infections. Its structural formula is as follows:

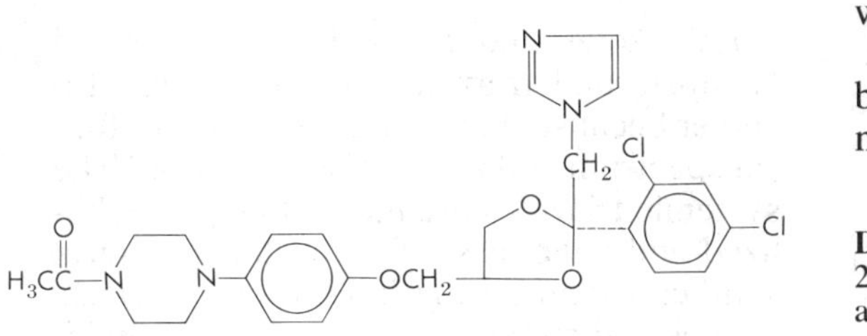

Ketoconazole

Absorption, Distribution, and Excretion. Oral absorption of ketoconazole is variable between individuals. Since an acidic environment is required for the dissolution of ketoconazole, bioavailability is markedly depressed in patients taking H_2 histaminergic receptor blocking agents such as cimetidine, ranitidine, or famotidine. Simultaneous administration of antacids may also impair absorption, but ingestion of food has no significant effect on the maximal concentration of the drug achieved in plasma. After oral doses of 200, 400, and 800 mg, peak plasma concentrations of ketoconazole are approximately 4, 8, and 20 μg/ml. The half-life of the drug increases with dose, and it may be as long as 7 to 8 hours when the dose is 800 mg. Ketoconazole is extensively metabolized, and the inactive products appear in the feces. Concentrations of active drug in urine are very low. In blood, 84% of ketoconazole is bound to plasma proteins, largely albumin; 15% is bound to erythrocytes; and 1% is free. Metabolism of the drug is unchanged by azotemia, hemodialysis, or peritoneal dialysis. Moderate hepatic dysfunction has no effect on the concentration of ketoconazole in blood.

Ketoconazole reaches keratinocytes efficiently, and its concentration in vaginal fluid approaches that in plasma. The concentration of ketoconazole in the CSF of patients with fungal meningitis is less than 1% of the total drug concentration in plasma.

Induction of hepatic microsomal enzymes by rifampin accelerates the metabolic clearance of ketoconazole, and concentrations of the antifungal agent may be reduced by more than 50%. Ketoconazole appears to compete with cyclosporine for hepatic metabolism; plasma concentrations of the latter drug are increased, leading to nephrotoxicity. The anticoagulant effect of warfarin may also be enhanced.

The pharmacology of ketoconazole has been reviewed by Daneshmend and Warnock (1988).

Preparations, Route of Administration, and Dosage. *Ketoconazole* (NIZORAL) is available as 200-mg scored tablets. A 2% topical cream is also available. The usual adult dose is 400 mg, taken once daily. Children over the age of 2 may receive 3.3 to 6.6 mg/kg as a single daily dose. For chronic suppression of mucocutaneous candidiasis, lower doses may be sufficient for adults. Doses up to 800 mg per day have been used in refractory cases of histoplasmosis, coccidioidomycosis, and blastomycosis, but there is little evidence of improved efficacy. The duration of therapy is 5 days for acute vulvovaginitis caused by *Candida*, 10 to 14 days for esophageal candidiasis, and 6 to 12 months for histoplasmosis and blastomycosis.

Untoward Effects. The most common side effects of ketoconazole are dose-dependent nausea, anorexia, and vomiting, which occur in about 20% of patients receiving 400 mg daily. Administration of the drug with food, at bedtime, or in divided doses may improve tolerance. An allergic rash occurs in about 4% of ketoconazole-treated patients, and pruritus without rash in about 2%.

Ketoconazole inhibits steroid biosynthesis in patients, as it does in fungi, by inhibition of cytochrome P_{450}–dependent enzyme systems (Loose *et al.*, 1983). Several endocrinological abnormalities may thus be evident. Approximately 10% of females report menstrual irregularities. A variable number of males experience gynecomastia and decreased libido and potency. At high doses, azoospermia has been reported, but sterility has not been permanent. Doses of ketoconazole as low as 400 mg can cause a transient drop in the plasma concentrations of free testosterone and estradiol C-17β (De Coster *et al.*, 1985). Similar doses can also cause a transient decrease in the ACTH-stimulated plasma cortisol response. Daily doses of 800 to 1200 mg of ketoconazole have been used to suppress plasma cortisol in patients with Cushing's disease. Similar doses were evaluated in patients with prostatic carcinoma. Hypertension and fluid retention have been reported and are associated with elevated concentrations of deoxycorticosterone, corticosterone, and 11-deoxycortisol. Although reports of Addison's disease due to ketoconazole are not convincing, it would seem prudent to discontinue the drug prior to major surgical procedures and to avoid the use of high doses in patients with trauma, severe burns, or other stressful conditions.

Mild, asymptomatic elevation of aminotransferase activity in plasma is common, occurring in 5 to 10% of patients; these values revert to normal spontaneously. Symptomatic drug-induced hepatitis is rare but is potentially fatal. Hepatitis may occur after a few days of treatment or it may be delayed for many months. The earliest symptoms are anorexia, malaise, nausea, and vomiting, with or without dull abdominal pain. Liver function tests usually mimic the pattern seen with hepatitis A, but a cholestatic or mixed picture can occur (Lewis *et al.*, 1984). Patients should be alerted to the symptoms and asked to return for liver function tests should this toxicity be suspected. Ketoconazole is teratogenic in animals, causing syndactyly in rats. Its use during pregnancy is not recommended, and because of secretion of the drug into breast milk, its use in nursing mothers is also unwise.

Therapeutic Uses. Ketoconazole is the current drug of choice for the treatment of nonmeningeal blastomycosis, histoplasmosis, coccidioidomycosis, pseudoallescheriasis, and paracoccidioidomycosis in patients who are *not* gravely ill and who *are* immunologically competent (NIAID Mycoses Study Group, 1985). It is also the preferred agent for treatment of chronic mucocutaneous candidiasis. Ketoconazole is effective therapy for oral and esophageal candidiasis. However, attempts to prevent deep candidiasis in immunosuppressed patients by the prophylactic administration of ketoconazole have been disappointing. Although oral dosage with ketoconazole is more convenient than intravaginal therapy of acute *Candida* vulvovaginitis, the possibility of hepatitis and contraindication during pregnancy relegate ketoconazole to management of recurrent symptomatic cases. Ketoconazole is also useful in griseofulvin-resistant ringworm of the glabrous skin and in patients with widespread tinea versicolor. The efficacy of ketoconazole is variable but usually inadequate in lymphocutaneous sporotrichosis, pulmonary cryptococcosis, chromomycosis, and eumycetoma. Ketoconazole is not indicated in mucormycosis and fungal meningitis.

MICONAZOLE

The topical use of miconazole is discussed below. A parenteral formulation in polyethoxylated castor oil is available for intravenous or intrathecal administration. Indications for the use of this preparation have become rare with the advent of newer agents.

ITRACONAZOLE

This investigational triazole is closely related to ketoconazole; its structural formula is as follows:

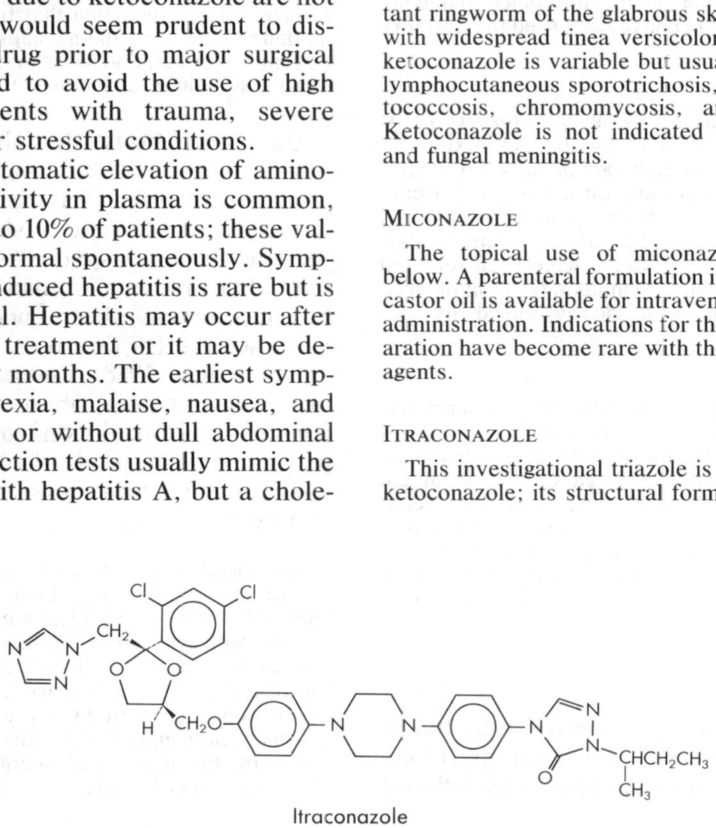

Itraconazole

Itraconazole is administered orally; it appears to have fewer adverse effects than does ketoconazole, and it may have a slightly expanded spectrum of activity.

Absorption, Distribution, and Excretion. The extent of absorption of itraconazole in the fasting state is 30% of that when the drug is taken with food. Peak concentrations in blood rise during the first 13 days of successive dosing and, for unknown reasons, are much higher when a bioassay is used rather than a direct assay. Using the latter technique, peak concentrations in plasma after 15 days of dosing (with food) are approximately 0.5 μg/ml per 100 mg daily dose (Hardin *et al.*, 1988). The elimination half-life of the drug is about 36 hours (after 15 days of dosing). Although concentrations of itraconazole in plasma are much lower than are provided by the same doses of ketoconazole, concentrations of itraconazole in tissues are high. Active drug is usually not detectable in urine and CSF. Concurrent administration of rifampin decreases concentrations of itraconazole in plasma substantially. The effect of itraconazole on cyclosporine concentrations appears to be modest or nil.

Preparation, Route of Administration, and Dosage. It is anticipated that itraconazole (SPORANOX) will be available in 100-mg capsules. No parenteral formulation is available. The usual oral dose is 200 mg taken once daily, but daily doses of up to 400 mg have been used in refractory mycoses.

Untoward Effects. Itraconazole appears to be well tolerated at a dose of 200 mg. Approximately 10 to 15% of patients complain of nausea or vomiting, but symptoms usually do not require discontinuation of therapy. Rash, pruritus, weakness, dizziness, vertigo, pedal edema, paresthesias, impotence, and loss of libido have been reported occasionally. To date, symptomatic drug-induced hepatitis has not been clearly linked to itraconazole.

Therapeutic Uses. Early clinical experience has been favorable for most of the same indications as ketoconazole, including blastomycosis, histoplasmosis, coccidioidomycosis, paracoccidioidomycosis, oral and esophageal thrush, and tinea versicolor. Unlike ketoconazole, itraconazole may have some therapeutic effect in lymphocutaneous sporotrichosis and selected cases of aspergillosis. (For additional information, *see* Symposium, 1987.)

FLUCONAZOLE

Fluconazole is an experimental, fluorinated bis-triazole with novel pharmacological properties. Its structure is as follows:

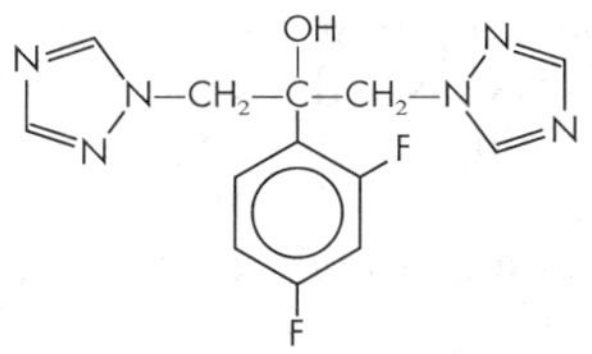

Fluconazole

Absorption, Distribution, and Excretion. Fluconazole is almost completely absorbed from the gastrointestinal tract. Concentrations in plasma are essentially the same when the drug is given orally or intravenously, and bioavailability is not altered by food or gastric acidity. Peak plasma concentrations are 4 to 8 μg/ml after repetitive doses of 100 mg (Tucker *et al.*, 1988). Renal excretion accounts for over 90% of elimination, and the elimination half-time is 25 hours. Fluconazole diffuses readily into body fluids, including sputum and saliva; concentrations in CSF are 50 to 90% of the simultaneous values in plasma.

Preparations, Routes of Administration, and Dosage. It is anticipated that fluconazole will be marketed in 50- and 100-mg capsules and as an intravenous formulation containing 2 mg/ml. Daily dosages for adults have ranged from 100 to 400 mg.

Untoward Effects. Initial studies suggest that fluconazole is well tolerated. The most common side effect has been gastrointestinal distress. Allergic rash, eosinophilia, Stevens–Johnson syndrome, transient abnormalities of hepatic function, and thrombocytopenia have been encountered in patients with AIDS (Stern *et al.*, 1988; Sugar and Saunders, 1988). Endocrine abnormalities have not been observed. Concurrent administration of fluconazole can increase plasma concentrations of phenytoin, sulfonylureas, and, to a lesser extent, warfarin and cyclosporine.

Therapeutic Uses. Fluconazole has been effective for oral and esophageal candidiasis in patients with AIDS. The drug is clearly efficacious in some patients with cryptococcal meningitis, although it is not yet known which patients should be selected for this therapy. Preliminary evidence indicates that fluconazole is useful in preventing relapse of cryptococcal meningitis in patients with AIDS following treatment with amphotericin B (Stern *et al.*, 1988; Sugar and Saunders, 1988).

GRISEOFULVIN

History and Source. Griseofulvin was first isolated from *Penicillium griseofulvum dierckx* by Oxford and coworkers in 1939. Because it was ineffective against bacteria, no further attention was paid to it for some time. In 1946, Brian and associates found a substance in *Penicillium janczewski* that produced shrinking and stunting of fungal hyphae; they named this the *curling factor,* and it was later found to be griseofulvin. During the next 10 years, the antibiotic was widely employed in the treatment of a variety of fungal diseases in plants and of ringworm of cattle. The search for potential therapeutic compounds for the management of fungal infections of the feet of Scottish miners led Gentles in 1958 to observe that griseofulvin cured experimentally produced mycotic disease of guinea pigs. Soon thereafter, the drug was subjected to clinical trials and became available for general use.

Chemistry. The structural formula of griseofulvin is as follows:

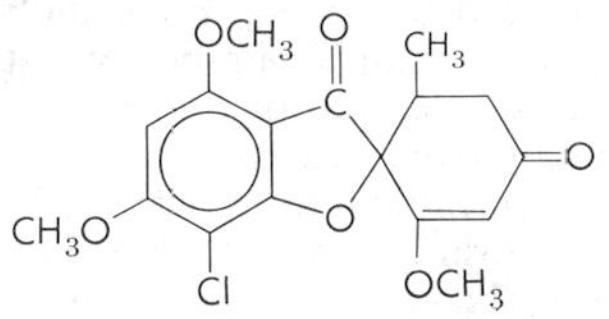

Griseofulvin

The drug is practically insoluble in water. It is remarkably thermostable.

Antifungal Activity. Griseofulvin is fungistatic *in vitro* for various species of the dermatophytes *Microsporum, Epidermophyton,* and *Trichophyton.* The drug has no effect on bacteria or on other fungi, yeasts, *Actinomyces,* or *Nocardia.* Young, actively metabolizing cells may be killed by the drug, but older, more dormant elements are only inhibited.

Fungal Resistance. *Trichophyton, Epidermophyton,* and *Microsporum* can be made resistant to griseofulvin *in vitro,* and such strains remain fully virulent as infectious agents in animals. Isolates from patients receiving the antibiotic appear, with a few exceptions, to retain their sensitivity to the drug when examined *in vitro.* Dermatophytes concentrate griseofulvin by an energy-dependent process, and such uptake is correlated with the sensitivity of the fungi to the antibiotic (*see* El-Nakeeb and Lampen, 1965).

Mechanism of Action. A prominent morphological manifestation of the action of griseofulvin is the production of multinucleate cells as the drug inhibits fungal mitosis (Gull and Trinci, 1973). An explanation for this phenomenon appears to come from studies of the effects on mammalian cells of higher concentrations of the antibiotic. Griseofulvin causes disruption of the mitotic spindle by interacting with polymerized microtubules. Although the effects of the drug are thus similar to those of colchicine and the vinca alkaloids, its binding sites on the microtubular protein are distinct. (*See* Malawista *et al.,* 1968; Grisham *et al.,* 1973.)

Absorption, Distribution, and Excretion. The oral administration of a 0.5-g dose of griseofulvin produces peak plasma concentrations of approximately 1 μg/ml in about 4 hours. These values are quite variable because of the insolubility of griseofulvin. Absorption may be increased if the drug is taken with a fatty meal. Since the rates of dissolution and disaggregation limit the bioavailability of griseofulvin, microsized and ultramicrosized powders are now used in preparations. Although the bioavailability of the ultramicrocrystalline preparation is said to be 50% greater than that of the conventional microsized powder, this may not always be true (Aoyagi *et al.,* 1982). Griseofulvin has a half-life in plasma of about 1 day, and approximately 50% of the oral dose can be detected in the urine within 5 days, mostly in the form of metabolites. The primary metabolite is 6-methylgriseofulvin. Barbiturates decrease the absorption of griseofulvin from the gastrointestinal tract.

The drug is deposited in keratin precursor cells. The antibiotic present in such cells when they differentiate is tightly bound to, and persists in, keratin and makes this substance resistant to fungal invasion. For this reason, the new growth of hair or nails is the first to become free of disease. As the fungus-containing keratin is shed, it is replaced by normal tissue. Griseofulvin is detectable in the stratum corneum of the skin within 4 to 8 hours of oral administration. Sweat and transepidermal fluid loss play an important role in the transfer of the drug in the stratum corneum (Shah *et al.,* 1974). Only a very small fraction of a dose of the drug is present in body fluids and tissues.

Preparations, Routes of Administration, and Dosage. *Griseofulvin* microsize (FULVICIN-U/F, GRIFULVIN V, GRISACTIN) is marketed in capsules containing 125 or 250 mg and in tablets containing 250 or 500 mg; it is also available as an oral suspension (125 mg/5 ml). The recommended daily dose for children is 10 mg/kg; for adults, 500 mg to 1 g. Larger doses (1.5 to 2 g per day) may be used for a short time in severe and extensive infections, but the amount should be reduced to 500 mg to 1 g per day when the lesions begin to respond. Best results may be obtained when medication is given at 6-hour intervals. Tablets incorporating an ultramicrosized preparation (FULVICIN P/G, GRISACTIN ULTRA, GRIS-PEG) contain 125 to 330 mg of griseofulvin.

Treatment with griseofulvin must continue until uninfected skin, hair, or nails replaces the infected tissue; at least 1 month for scalp and hair infections and 6 to 9 months for infections of the fingernails. Infections of toenails may require at least 1 year of continuous treatment and may never respond.

Untoward Effects. The incidence of serious reactions associated with the use of griseofulvin is very low. One of the minor effects is headache; it is sometimes severe and usually disappears as therapy is continued. The incidence of headache may be as high as 15%. Other nervous system manifestations include peripheral neuritis, lethargy, mental confusion, impairment of performance of routine tasks, fatigue, syncope, vertigo, blurred vision, transient macular edema, and augmentation of the effects of alcohol. Among the side effects involving the alimentary tract are nausea, vomiting, diarrhea, heartburn, flatulence, dry mouth, and angular stomatitis. Hepatotoxicity has also been observed. Hematological effects include leukopenia, neutropenia, punctate basophilia, and monocytosis; these often disappear despite continuation of therapy. Blood studies should be carried out at least once a week during the first month of treatment or longer. Common renal effects include albuminuria and cylindruria, without evidence of renal insufficiency. Reactions involving the skin are cold and warm urticaria, photosensitivity, lichen planus, erythema, erythema multiforme–like rashes, and vesicular and morbilliform eruptions. Serum-sickness syndromes and severe angioedema develop rarely during treatment with griseofulvin. Estrogen-like effects have been observed in children. A moderate but inconsistent increase of fecal protoporphyrins has been noted when the drug is used for a long time.

Griseofulvin induces hepatic microsomal enzymes, thus increasing the rate of metabolism of warfarin; adjustment of the dosage of the latter agent may be necessary in some patients. The drug may reduce the efficacy of some oral contraceptive agents, probably by a similar mechanism.

Therapeutic Uses. Mycotic disease of the skin, hair, and nails due to *Microsporum, Trichophyton,* or *Epidermophyton* responds to griseofulvin therapy. Infections that are readily treatable with this agent include infections of the hair (tinea capitis) caused by *M. canis, M. audouini, T. schoenleinii,* and *T. verrucosum;* "ringworm" of the glabrous skin; tinea cruris and tinea corporis caused by *M. canis, T. rubrum, T. verrucosum,* and *E. floccosum;* and tinea of the hands (*T. rubrum, T. mentagrophytes*) and beard (*Trichophyton* species). Griseofulvin is also highly effective in "athlete's foot" or epidermophytosis involving the skin and nails, the vesicular form of which is most commonly due to *T. mentagrophytes* and the hyperkeratotic type to *T. rubrum*. However, topical therapy is preferred (*see* below). *Trichophyton rubrum* and *T. mentagrophytes* infections may require higher-than-conventional doses. Since very high doses of griseofulvin are carcinogenic and teratogenic in laboratory animals, the drug should not be used to treat trivial infections that respond to topical therapy. (For a review of griseofulvin therapy, *see* Symposium, 1960; Goldman, 1970.)

THERAPY OF SYSTEMIC FUNGAL INFECTIONS

Infections with pathogenic fungi that are initiated after inhalation may resolve spontaneously. Acute histoplasmosis, coccidioidomycosis, and blastomycosis, as well as subacute cases of cryptococcosis that are confined to the lungs of previously normal persons, may not require treatment. Chemotherapy may be prudent if the pneumonia is severe, the infection already appears to be chronic, the physician is uncertain whether dissemination has occurred, or if the consequences of dissemination are formidable. Patients with AIDS or other forms of immunosuppression should ordinarily receive chemotherapy for fungal pneumonia of any cause.

Aspergillosis. Invasive pulmonary aspergillosis occurs in seriously immunocompromised patients and responds poorly to treatment with antifungal agents. The drug of choice is amphotericin B, given in daily intravenous doses of 0.5 to 1.0 mg/kg; the higher doses are used for patients with rapidly progressive disease.

Blastomycosis. Ketoconazole (400 mg per day orally for 6 to 12 months) is currently the drug of choice for most patients with blastomycosis. Itraconazole (200 to 400 mg once daily) has also been effective in a small number of patients. Amphotericin B is reserved for those who should not receive ketoconazole, who have a profound or rapidly progressive infection, or who have blastomycosis in the central nervous system. The usual regimen is 0.4 mg/kg daily for 10 weeks. Surgery is generally not necessary except to drain large collections of pus around bone lesions.

Candidiasis. Retrograde candidiasis of the urinary tract acquired by catheterization or instrumentation may require therapy in patients with kidney stones, urinary tract obstruction, renal transplantation, or poorly controlled diabetes mellitus. In the absence of invasion of the renal parenchyma, irrigation with amphotericin B (50 μg/ml in sterile water for 5 to 7 days) may be sufficient. Parenchymal disease acquired by the hematogenous or retrograde route is treated with intravenous amphotericin B, as is deep candidiasis of other organs.

Flucytosine has been used in combination with amphotericin B in patients with *Candida* meningitis, endophthalmitis, arthritis, and some other deep infections. Flucytosine diffuses into some infected sites better than does amphotericin B; it seems to have an additive effect with amphotericin B, permitting use of lower doses of the latter agent.

Coccidioidomycosis. Chronic disease caused by *Coccidioides immitis* and characterized by single pulmonary cavities or fibrocavitary infiltrates does not respond well to chemotherapy and may require resection. When there is extrapulmonary dissemination, intravenous amphotericin B is useful as initial therapy in seriously ill or immunosuppressed patients, including those with AIDS. Ketoconazole has been useful in the long-term suppression of skin, bone, and soft-tissue lesions in patients with normal immune function. In initial studies itraconazole (200 to 400 mg once daily) has appeared to be useful for the same indications. The drug of choice for coccidioidal meningitis is amphotericin B given intrathecally.

Cryptococcosis. Amphotericin B is the drug of choice for cryptococcosis; the daily intravenous dose is 0.4 to 0.5 mg/kg. The duration of therapy depends upon the rapidity with which cultures become negative. Addition of flucytosine to the regimen permits use of a lower daily dose of amphotericin B (0.3 mg/kg). Toxicity caused by flucytosine has been a particular problem in patients with AIDS, which is an underlying condition in more than half the patients. Relapse after therapy has been so frequent in patients with AIDS that lifetime suppressive therapy with amphotericin B (1 mg/kg weekly) is commonly used. Fluconazole appears to be useful for suppressive therapy in patients with AIDS and may also be useful as primary treatment for some of the more indolent meningeal infections.

Histoplasmosis. Ketoconazole (400 mg daily) can be used to treat most patients with chronic pulmonary histoplasmosis or the less severe, nonmeningeal disseminated infections that occur in patients with normal immunological systems. Itraconazole (200 to 400 mg once daily) also appears to be effective, but experience with this agent is limited. Other patients should receive amphotericin B intravenously. The usual duration of treatment is 6 to 12 months with ketoconazole and 10 weeks with amphotericin B. Relapse of disseminated histoplasmosis in patients with AIDS has prompted the administration of weekly intravenous doses of amphotericin B following an initial intensive course of treatment with the drug.

Mucormycosis. Craniofacial mucormycosis is treated with intravenous amphotericin B, aggressive surgical debridement, and control of diabetes mellitus (the usual concomitant disease). Although pulmonary mucormycosis is usually fatal despite treatment, the drug of choice is also amphotericin B.

Paracoccidioidomycosis. Ketoconazole (400 mg daily) is the drug of choice. Seriously ill patients should receive amphotericin B initially. Treatment is continued for at least 6 to 12 months.

Sporotrichosis. Oral administration of a saturated solution of potassium iodide is the treatment of choice for lymphocutaneous sporotrichosis. About 40 drops are given three times daily in a small amount of water or juice for about a month after inflammation has resolved. Iodides are not effective for pulmonary or osteoarticular sporotrichosis; amphotericin B is the drug of choice for these conditions, but failures are common. Resection of small, well-localized pulmonary lesions should be considered.

II. Topical Antifungal Agents

Topical treatment is useful in many superficial fungal infections—that is, those confined to the stratum corneum, squamous mucosa, or cornea. Such diseases include dermatophytosis (ringworm), candidiasis, tinea versicolor, piedra, tinea nigra, and fungal keratitis. Topical administration of antifungal agents is usually not successful for mycoses of the nails (onychomycosis) and hair (tinea capitis) and has no place in the treatment of subcutaneous mycoses, such as sporotrichosis and chromomycosis. The efficacy of topical agents in the superficial mycoses depends not only on the type of lesion and mechanism of action of the drug but also upon the viscosity, hydrophobicity, and acidity of the formulation. Irrespective of formulation, penetration of topical drugs into hyperkeratotic lesions is often poor. Removal of thick, infected keratin is sometimes a useful adjunct to therapy; this is, for example, the principal mode of action of Whitfield's ointment.

A plethora of topical agents are available for the treatment of superficial mycoses. Many of the older drugs, including gentian violet, carbol-fuchsin, acrisorcin, triacetin, sulfur, iodine, and aminacrine, are now rarely indicated and will not be discussed here (*see previous editions* of this textbook). Among the topical agents to be discussed, the preferred formulation for cutaneous application is usually a cream or solution. Ointments are messy and are too occlusive for macerated or fissured intertriginous lesions. The use of powders, whether applied by shake containers or aerosols, is largely confined to the feet and moist lesions of the groin and other intertriginous areas.

The systemic agents that are used for the treatment of superficial mycoses are discussed in the first section of this chapter. Some of these agents are also administered topically; these uses will be described here.

IMIDAZOLES AND TRIAZOLES

As discussed above, these closely related classes of drugs are synthetic antifungal agents that are used both topically and systemically. Indications for their topical use include ringworm, tinea versicolor, and mucocutaneous candidiasis. Resistance to imidazoles or triazoles is very rare among the fungi that cause these superficial mycoses. Selection of one of these agents should be based upon cost and availability, since testing *in vitro* for fungal susceptibility to these drugs has not been standardized and is not predictive of clinical responses.

Cutaneous Application. The preparations for cutaneous use described below are effective for tinea corporis, tinea pedis, tinea cruris, tinea versicolor, and cutaneous candidiasis. They should be applied twice a day for 3 to 6 weeks. Despite some activity *in vitro* against bacteria, this effect is not clinically useful. The cutaneous formulations are not suitable for oral, vaginal, or ocular use.

Vaginal Application. The vaginal creams, suppositories, and tablets are the preparations of choice for vaginal candidiasis. None is useful in trichomoniasis, despite some activity *in vitro*. They are all used once a day, preferably at bedtime to facilitate retention. All vaginal creams are administered in 5-g amounts. Two vaginal formulations, clotrimazole tablets and miconazole suppositories, come in both low- and high-dose preparations. A shorter duration of therapy is recommended for the higher dose of each. Except for the 500-mg, single-dose clotrimazole tablet, these preparations are administered for 3 to 7 days.

Some imidazoles are embryotoxic in rats or mice, a finding that has raised concern about adverse effects during the first trimester of pregnancy. Approximately 5 to 10% of the vaginal dose is absorbed. However, no adverse effects on the fetus have been attributed to the vaginal use of imidazoles or triazoles. The most common side effect is vaginal burning or itching. A male sexual partner may experience mild penile irritation. Cross-allergenicity among these compounds is assumed, based upon their structural similarities.

Oral Use. Use of the oral troche of clotrimazole is properly considered as topical therapy. The only indication for this 10-mg troche is oropharyngeal candidiasis. Antifungal activity is due entirely to the local concentration of the drug; there is no systemic effect. The patient should be told to suck on the troche until it dissolves.

Clotrimazole. Clotrimazole has the following structure:

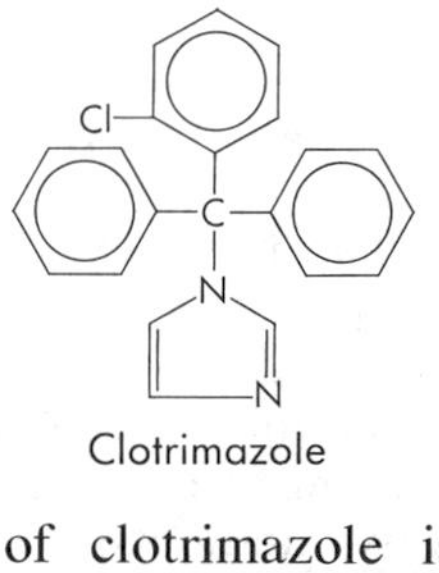

Clotrimazole

Absorption of clotrimazole is less than 0.5% after application to the intact skin; from the vagina, it is 3 to 10%. Fungicidal concentrations remain in the vagina for as long as 3 days after application of the drug (Ritter *et al.*, 1982). The small amount absorbed is metabolized in the liver and excreted in bile. In adults, an oral dose of 200 mg per day will give rise to plasma concentrations of 0.2 to 0.35 μg/ml.

In a small fraction of recipients, clotrimazole on the skin may cause stinging, erythema, edema, vesication, desquamation, pruritus, and urticaria. Applied to the vagina, about 1.6% of recipients complain of a mild burning sensation and, rarely, of lower abdominal cramps, slight increase in urinary frequency, or skin rash. Occasionally, the sexual partner may experience penile or urethral irritation. By the oral route, clotrimazole can cause mild gastrointestinal irritation. In patients using troches, the incidence is about 5%.

Preparations, Dosage, and Therapeutic Uses. Clotrimazole is available as a 1% cream, lotion, and solution (LOTRIMIN, MYCELEX), 1% vaginal cream, 100-mg and 500-mg vaginal tablets (GYNE-LOTRIMIN, MYCELEX-G), and 10-mg troches (MYCELEX). On the skin, applications are made twice a day. For the vagina, the standard regimens are one 100-mg tablet once a day at bedtime for 7 days, one 500-mg tablet inserted only once, or 5 g of cream once a day for 7 to 14 days. For nonpregnant females, two 100-mg tablets may be used once a day for 3 days. Troches are to be dissolved slowly in the mouth five times a day for 14 days.

Clotrimazole has been reported to cure dermatophyte infections in 60 to 100% of cases. From a number of studies, the cure rates in cutaneous candidiasis are 80 to 100%. In vulvovaginal candidiasis, the cure rate is usually above 80% when the 7-day regimen is used. A 3-day regimen of 200 mg once a day appears to be similarly effective, as does single-dose treatment (500 mg) (*see* Goormans *et al.*, 1982; Krause, 1982; Milsom and Forssman, 1982). Recurrences are common after all regimens. The cure rate with oral troches for oral and pharyngeal candidiasis may be as high as 100% in the immunocompetent host.

The details of the pharmacology and clinical uses of clotrimazole may be found in a symposium (Symposium, 1974) and in the review by Sawyer and associates (1975b).

Econazole. Econazole, the deschloro derivative of miconazole, has the following structure:

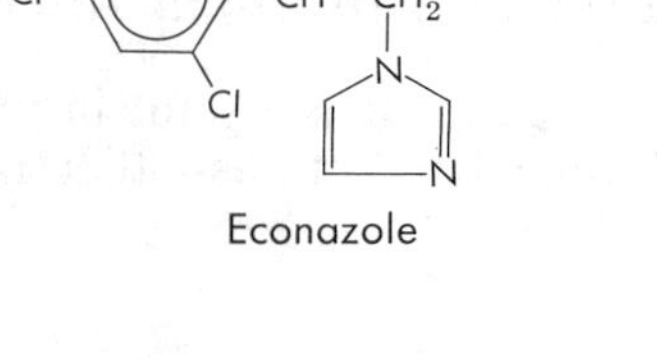

Econazole

Econazole readily penetrates the stratum corneum and is found in effective concentrations down to the mid dermis. However, less than 1% of an applied dose appears to be absorbed into the blood. Approximately 3% of recipients have local erythema, burning, stinging, or itching.

Econazole nitrate (SPECTAZOLE) is available as a water-miscible cream (1%) to be applied twice a day.

Miconazole. Miconazole is a very close chemical congener of econazole, with the following structure:

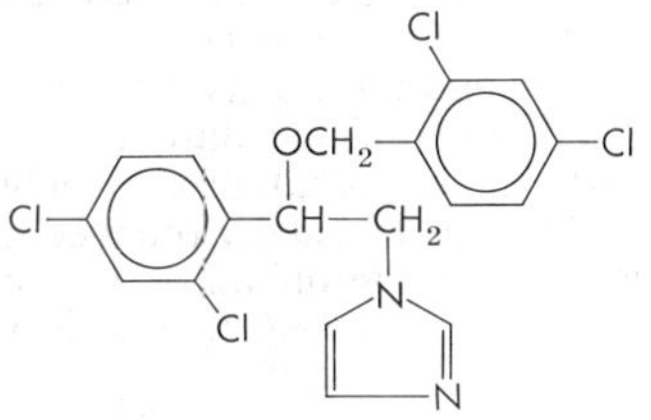

Miconazole

Miconazole readily penetrates the stratum corneum of the skin and persists there for more than 4 days after application. Less than 1% is absorbed into the blood. Absorption is no more than 1.3% from the vagina.

Adverse effects from topical application to the vagina include burning, itching, or irritation in about 7% of recipients, and, infrequently, pelvic cramps (0.2%), headache, hives, or skin rash. Irritation, burning, and maceration are rare after cutaneous application. Miconazole is considered safe for use during pregnancy, although some authors believe that its vaginal use should be avoided during the first trimester.

Preparations, Dosage, and Therapeutic Uses. Miconazole nitrate is available as a 2% dermatological cream, spray, powder, or lotion (MICATIN, MONISTAT-DERM). To avoid maceration, only the lotion should be applied to intertriginous areas. It is available as a 2% vaginal cream, 100-mg suppositories (MONISTAT 7), to be applied high in the vagina at bedtime for 7 days, and 200-mg vaginal suppositories (MONISTAT 3) for 3-day therapy.

In the treatment of tinea pedis, tinea cruris, and tinea versicolor the cure rate may be over 90%. In the treatment of vulvovaginal candidiasis, the mycological cure rate at the end of 1 month is about 80 to 95%. In one double-blind study, the cure rates with miconazole and clotrimazole were almost identical (Lebherz *et al.*, 1983). Pruritus sometimes is relieved after a single application. Some vaginal infections caused by *Trichophyton glabrata* also respond. The actions and uses of miconazole have been reviewed by Sawyer and associates (1975a), Kobayashi and Medoff (1977), and Heel and associates (1980).

Terconazole and Butoconazole. Terconazole is a ketal triazole with structural similarities to ketoconazole. Its structure is as follows:

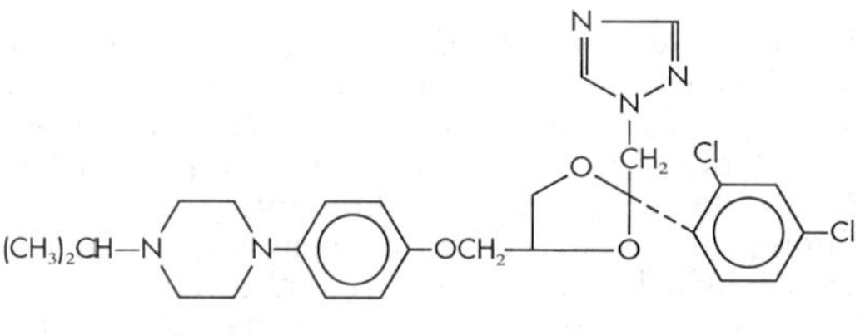

Terconazole

The mechanism of action of terconazole is similar to that of the imidazoles (Isaacson *et al.*, 1988). The 80-mg vaginal suppository (TERAZOL 3) is inserted at bedtime for 3 days, while the 0.4% vaginal cream (TERAZOL 7) is used for 7 days. Clinical efficacy and patient acceptance of both preparations are at least as good as for clotrimazole in patients with vaginal candidiasis (Kjaeldgaard, 1986).

Butoconazole is an imidazole quite comparable to clotrimazole (Hajman, 1988). Its structural formula is as follows:

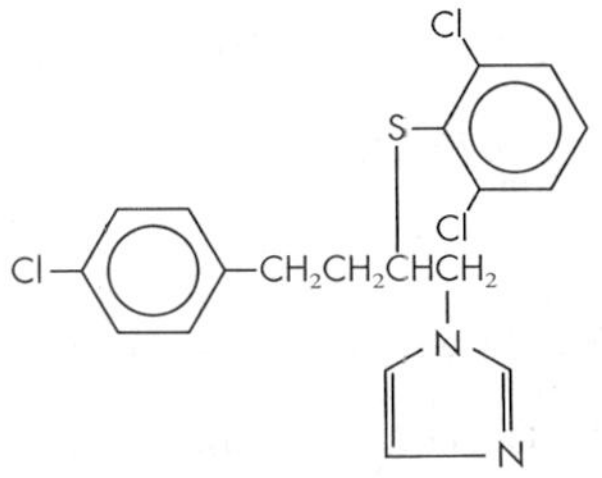

Butoconazole

Butoconazole nitrate (FEMSTAT) is available as a 2% vaginal cream; it is used at bedtime for 3 days in nonpregnant females. Because of the slower response during pregnancy, a 6-day course is recommended (during the second and third trimester).

Oxiconazole and Sulconazole. Oxiconazole and sulconazole are two new imidazole derivatives that are used for the topical treatment of infections caused by the common pathogenic dermatophytes. *Oxiconazole nitrate* (OXISTAT) is available as a 1% cream; *sulconazole nitrate* (EXELDERM) is supplied as a 1% solution.

CICLOPIROX OLAMINE

Ciclopirox olamine (LOPROX) has broad-spectrum antifungal activity. The chemical structure is:

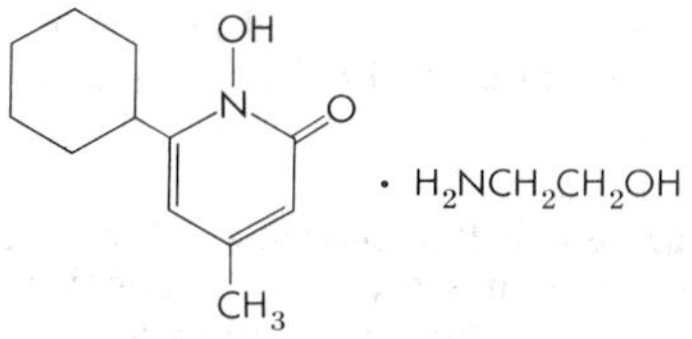

Ciclopirox Olamine

It is fungicidal to *Candida albicans, Epidermophyton floccosum, Microsporum canis, Trichophyton mentagrophytes,* and *T. rubrum*. It also inhibits the growth of *Pityrosporum obiculare* (*Malassezia furfur*). After application to the skin, it penetrates through the epidermis into the dermis, but even under occlusion less than 1.5% is absorbed into the systemic circulation. Since the half-life is 1.7 hours, no systemic accumulation occurs. The drug penetrates into hair follicles and sebaceous glands. It can sometimes cause hypersensitivity. It is available as a 1% cream and lotion for the treatment of cutaneous candidiasis and tinea corporis, cruris, pedis, and versicolor. Cure rates in the dermatomycoses and candidal infections have been variously reported to be 81 to 94%. No topical toxicity has been noted.

HALOPROGIN

Haloprogin is a halogenated phenolic ether with the following structure:

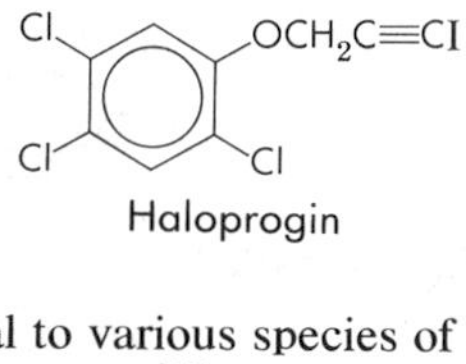

Haloprogin

It is fungicidal to various species of *Epidermophyton, Pityrosporum, Microsporum, Trichophyton,* and *Candida*. During treatment with this drug, irritation, pruritus, burning sensations, vesiculation, increased maceration, and "sensitization" (or exacerbation of the lesion) occasionally occur, especially on the foot if occlusive footgear is worn. It is possible that the sensitization indicates a rapid therapeutic response in which the release of toxins makes the lesion temporarily worse. Haloprogin is poorly absorbed through the skin; it is converted to trichlorophenol in the body. The systemic toxicity from topical application appears to be low.

Haloprogin (HALOTEX) is available as a 1% cream or solution. It is applied twice a day for 2 to 4 weeks. Its principal use is against tinea pedis, for which the cure rate is about 80%; it is thus approximately equal in efficacy to tolnaftate (*see* below). It is also used against tinea cruris, tinea corporis, tinea manuum, and tinea versicolor.

TOLNAFTATE

Tolnaftate is a thiocarbamate with the following structure:

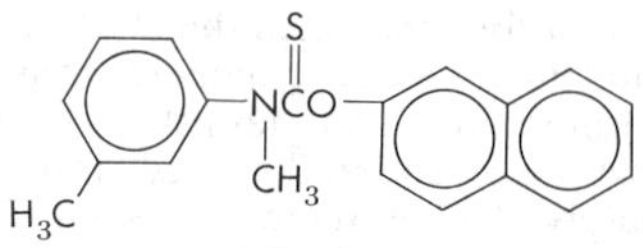

Tolnaftate

Tolnaftate is effective in the treatment of the majority of cutaneous mycoses caused by *T. rubrum, T. mentagrophytes, T. tonsurans, E. floccosum, M. canis, M. audouini, M. gypseum,* and *P. obiculare,* but it is ineffective against *Candida*. In tinea pedis the cure rate is around 80%, compared with about 95% for miconazole. Toxic or allergic reactions to tolnaftate have not been reported.

Tolnaftate (AFTATE, TINACTIN, others) is available in a 1% concentration as a cream, gel, powder, aerosol powder, and topical solution, or as a topical aerosol liquid. The preparations are applied locally twice a day. Pruritus is usually relieved in 24 to 72 hours. Involution of interdigital lesions due to susceptible fungi is very often complete in 7 to 21 days.

NAFTIFINE

Naftifine is an allylamine with the following structure:

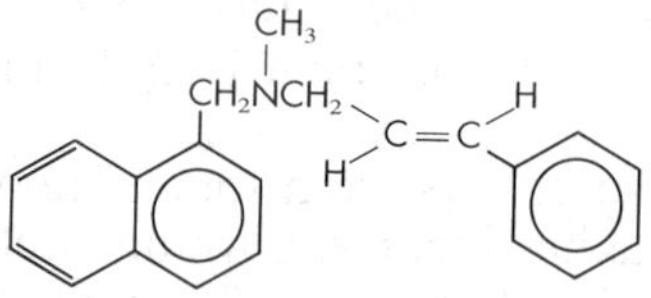

Naftifine

Naftifine is representative of a class of synthetic agents that inhibit squalene-2,3-epoxidase and thus inhibit fungal biosynthesis of ergosterol. The drug has broad-spectrum fungicidal activity *in vitro*. *Naftifine hydrochloride* (NAFTIN) is available as a 1% cream. It is effective for the topical treatment of tinea cruris and tinea corporis (Millikan *et al.*, 1988); twice daily application is recommended. The drug is well tolerated, although local irritation has been observed in 3% of treated patients. Allergic contact dermatitis has also been reported. Naftifine may also be efficacious for cutaneous candidiasis and tinea versicolor, although the drug has not been approved for these uses.

POLYENE ANTIFUNGAL ANTIBIOTICS

Nystatin. Nystatin was discovered in the New York State Health Laboratory and was named accordingly; it is a tetraene macrolide produced by *Streptomyces noursei*. Although nystatin is structurally similar to amphotericin B and has the same mechanism of action, it is more toxic and is not used systemically. Nystatin is not absorbed from the gastrointestinal tract, skin, or vagina.

Nystatin (MYCOSTATIN, NILSTAT, others) is useful only for candidiasis and is supplied in preparations intended for cutaneous, vaginal, or oral administration for this purpose. Infections of the nails and hyperkeratinized or crusted skin lesions do not respond. Topical preparations include ointments, creams, and powders, all of which contain 100,000 units per gram. Powders are preferred for moist lesions and are applied two or three times a day. Creams or ointments are used twice daily. Combinations of nystatin with antibacterial agents or corticosteroids are also available. Allergic reactions to nystatin are very uncommon.

Vaginal tablets containing 100,000 units of the drug are inserted once daily for 2 weeks. Although the tablets are well tolerated, imidazoles or triazoles are more effective agents for vaginal candidiasis.

An oral suspension that contains 100,000 units of nystatin per milliliter is given four times a day. Premature and low-birth-weight neonates should receive 1 ml of this preparation, infants 2 ml, and children or adults 4 to 6 ml per dose. Older children and adults should be instructed to swish the drug around the mouth and then swallow. If not otherwise instructed, the patient may expectorate the bitter liquid and fail to treat the infected mucosa in the posterior pharynx or esophagus. Nystatin suspension is usually effective for oral candidiasis of the immunocompetent host. Other than the bitter taste and occasional complaints of nausea, adverse effects are uncommon. Oral tablets containing 500,000 units have been used to decrease gastrointestinal colonization with *Candida* in the hope of preventing relapse of vaginal candidiasis or of protecting the neutropenic patient from gastrointestinal candidiasis. Careful studies have failed to document efficacy for these indications.

Amphotericin B. Topical amphotericin B (FUNGIZONE) is also used for cutaneous and mucocutaneous candidiasis. A lotion, cream, and ointment are marketed; these preparations all contain 3% amphotericin B and are applied to the lesion two to four times daily.

Natamycin. *Natamycin* (NATACYN) is a pentaenic macrolide. It is much less irritating to the eye than is the complex of amphotericin B and deoxycholate and hence is used to treat fungal keratitis. It is the drug of choice in infections caused by *Fusarium solani*. However, it penetrates poorly and may not reach deep corneal mycoses. It is used as a 5% suspension.

MISCELLANEOUS ANTIFUNGAL AGENTS

Undecylenic Acid. Undecylenic acid is 10-undecenoic acid, an 11-carbon, unsaturated compound. It is a yellow liquid with a characteristic rancid odor. It is primarily fungistatic, although fungicidal activity may be observed with long exposure to high concentrations of the agent. The drug is active against a variety of fungi, including those that cause ringworm. *Undecylenic acid* (DESENEX) is available in a foam, ointment, cream, powder, soap, and liquid. *Zinc undecylenate* is marketed in combination with other ingredients. The zinc provides an astringent action that aids in the suppression of inflammation. *Compound undecylenic acid ointment* (DESENEX, UNDOGUENT) contains both undecylenic acid (about 5%) and zinc undecylenate (about 20%). *Calcium undecylenate* (CALDESENE, CRUEX) is available as a powder.

Undecylenic acid preparations are used in the treatment of various dermatomycoses, especially tinea pedis. Concentrations of the acid as high as 10%, as well as in the compound ointment, may be applied to the skin. The preparations as formulated are usually not irritating to tissue, and sensitization to them is uncommon. It is of undoubted benefit in retarding fungal growth in tinea pedis, but the infection frequently persists despite intensive treatment with preparations of the acid and the zinc salt. At best, the clinical "cure" rate is about 50% (Smith *et al.*, 1977) and is thus much lower than that obtained with the imidazoles, haloprogin, or tolnaftate. The efficacy in the treatment of tinea capitis is marginal, and the drug is no longer used for that purpose. Undecylenic acid preparations are also approved for use in the treatment of diaper rash, tinea cruris, and other minor dermatological conditions.

Benzoic Acid and Salicylic Acid. Benzoic and salicylic acids ointment is known as *Whitfield's ointment*. It combines the fungistatic action of benzoate with the keratolytic action of salicylate. It contains benzoic acid and salicylic acid in a ratio of 2:1 (usually 6%:3%). It is used mainly in the treatment of tinea pedis. Since benzoic acid is only fungistatic, eradication of the infection occurs only after the infected stratum corneum is shed, and continuous medication is required for several weeks to months. The salicylic acid accelerates the desquamation. The ointment is also sometimes used to treat tinea capitis. Mild irritation may occur at the site of application.

Propionic Acid and Caprylic Acid. Propionic acid and sodium propionate are promoted for the treatment of the dermatomycoses. Both their low efficacy and exaggerated price make them irrational choices for treatment. They may be compounded together or with sodium caprylate or other agents. Sodium propionate is used in proprietary preparations in concentrations of 1 to 5%.

Aoyagi, N.; Ogata, H.; Kaniwa, N.; Koibuchi, M.; Shibazaki, T.; and Ejima, A. Bioavailability of griseofulvin from tablets in humans and the correlation with its dissolution rate. *J. Pharm. Sci.*, **1982**, *71*, 1165–1169.

Bennett, J. E., and others. A collaborative study: amphotericin B–flucytosine in cryptococcal meningitis. *N. Engl. J. Med.*, **1979**, *301*, 126–131.

Bindschadler, D. D., and Bennett, J. E. A pharmacologic guide to the clinical use of amphotericin B. *J. Infect. Dis.*, **1969**, *120*, 427–436.

Block, E. R.; Bennett, J. E.; Livoti, L. G.; Klein, W. J.; Brandriss, M. W.; MacGregor, R. R.; and Henderson, L. Flucytosine and amphotericin B: hemodialysis effects on the plasma concentration and clearance. *Ann. Intern. Med.*, **1974**, *80*, 613–617.

Branch, R. A. Prevention of amphotericin B-induced renal impairment. *Arch. Intern. Med.*, **1988**, *148*, 2389–2394.

Burks, L. C.; Aisner, J.; Fortner, C. L.; and Wiernik, P. H. Meperidine for the treatment of shaking chills and fever. *Arch. Intern. Med.*, **1980**, *140*, 483–484.

Christiansen, K. J.; Bernard, E. M.; Gold, J. W. M.; and Armstrong, D. Distribution and activity of amphotericin B in humans. *J. Infect. Dis.*, **1985**, *152*, 1037–1043.

Collette, N.; van der Auwere, P.; Lopez, A. P.; Heymans, C.; and Meunier, F. Tissue concentrations and bioactivity of amphotericin B in cancer patients treated with amphotericin B deoxycholate. *Antimicrob. Agents Chemother.*, **1989**, *33*, 362–368.

Craven, P. C.; Ludden, T. M.; Drutz, D. J.; Rogers, W.; Haegele, K. A.; and Skrdlant, H. B. Excretion pathways of amphotericin B. *J. Infect. Dis.*, **1979**, *140*, 329–341.

De Coster, R.; Caers, I.; Haelterman, C.; and Debroye, M. Effect of a single administration of ketoconazole on total and physiologically free plasma testosterone and 17-beta-oestradiol levels in healthy male volunteers. *Eur. J. Clin. Pharmacol.*, **1985**, *29*, 489–493.

El-Nakeeb, M. A., and Lampen, J. O. Uptake of griseofulvin by microorganisms and its correlation with sensitivity to griseofulvin. *J. Gen. Microbiol.*, **1965**, *39*, 285–293.

Galgiani, J. N. Progress on standardizing antifungal susceptibility tests. *Clin. Lab. Med.*, **1989**, *9*, 269–277.

Goormans, E.; Bergstein, N. A.; Loendersloot, E. W.; and Branolte, J. H. One-dose therapy of *Candida* vaginitis. I. Results of an open multicentre trial. *Chemotherapy*, **1982**, *28*, Suppl. 1, 106–109.

Grisham, L. M.; Wilson, L.; and Bensch, K. Antimitotic action of griseofulvin does not involve disruption of microtubules. *Nature*, **1973**, *244*, 294–296.

Gull, K., and Trinci, A. P. J. Griseofulvin inhibits fungal mitosis. *Nature*, **1973**, *244*, 292–294.

Hajman, A. J. Vulvovaginal candidosis: comparison of 3-day treatment with 2% butoconazole nitrate cream and 6-day treatment with 1% clotrimazole cream. *J. Int. Med. Res.*, **1988**, *16*, 367–375.

Hamilton-Miller, J. M. T. Fungal sterols and the mode of action of the polyene antibiotics. *Adv. Appl. Microbiol.*, **1974**, *17*, 109–134.

Hardin, T. C.; Graybill, J. R.; Fetchick, R.; Woestenborghs, R.; Rinaldi, M. G.; and Kuhn, J. G. Pharmacokinetics of itraconazole following oral administration to normal volunteers. *Antimicrob. Agents Chemother.*, **1988**, *32*, 1310–1313.

Harris, B. E.; Manning, B. W.; Federle, T. W.; and Diasio, R. B. Conversion of 5-fluorocytosine to 5-fluorouracil by human intestinal flora. *Antimicrob. Agents Chemother.*, **1986**, *29*, 44–48.

Isaacson, D. M.; Tolman, E. L.; Tobia, A. J.; Rosenthale, M. E.; McGuire, J. L.; Vanden Bossche, H.; and Janssen, P. A. Selective inhibition of 14 alpha-desmethyl sterol synthesis in *Candida albicans* by terconazole, a new triazole antimycotic. *J. Antimicrob. Chemother.*, **1988**, *21*, 333–343.

Jurgens, R. W., Jr.; DeLuca, P. P.; and Papadimitriou, D. Compatibility of amphotericin B with certain large-volume parenterals. *Am. J. Hosp. Pharm.*, **1981**, *38*, 377–378.

Kennedy, M. S.; Deeg, H. J.; Siegel, M.; Crowley, J. J.; Storb, R.; and Thomas, E. D. Acute renal toxicity with combined use of amphotericin B and cyclosporine after marrow transplantation. *Transplantation*, **1983**, *35*, 211–215.

Kjaeldgaard, A. Comparison of terconazole and clotrimazole vaginal tablets in the treatment of vulvovaginal candidosis. *Pharmatherapeutica*, **1986**, *4*, 525–531.

Krause, U. Results of a single-dose treatment of vaginal mycoses with 500 mg CANESTEN vaginal tablets. *Chemotherapy*, **1982**, *28*, Suppl. 1, 99–105.

Lebherz, T. B.; Goldman, L.; Wiesmeier, E.; Mason, D.; and Ford, L. C. A comparison of the efficacy of two vaginal creams for vulvovaginal candidiasis, and correlations with the presence of *Candida* species in the perianal area and oral contraceptive use. *Clin. Ther.*, **1983**, *5*, 409–416.

Lewis, J. H.; Zimmerman, H. J.; Benson, G. D.; and Ishak, K. G. Hepatic injury associated with ketoconazole therapy. *Gastroenterology*, **1984**, *86*, 503–513.

Loose, D. S.; Kan, P. B.; Hirst, M. A.; Marcus, R. A.; and Feldman, D. Ketoconazole blocks adrenal steroidogenesis by inhibiting cytochrome P450-dependent enzymes. *J. Clin. Invest.*, **1983**, *71*, 1495–1499.

Malawista, S. E.; Sato, H.; and Bensch, K. G. Vinblastine and griseofulvin reversibly disrupt the living mitotic spindle. *Science*, **1968**, *160*, 770–772.

Millikan, L. E.; Galen, W. K.; Gewirtzman, G. B.; Horwitz, S. N.; Landow, R. K.; Nesbitt, L. T., Jr.; Roth, H. L.; Sefton, J.; and Day, R. M. Naftifine cream 1% versus econazole cream 1% in the treatment of tinea cruris and tinea corporis. *J. Am. Acad. Dermatol.*, **1988**, *18*, 52–56.

Milsom, I., and Forssman, L. Treatment of vaginal candidosis with a single 500-mg clotrimazole pessary. *Br. J. Vener. Dis.*, **1982**, *58*, 124–126.

NIAID Mycoses Study Group. Treatment of blastomycosis and histoplasmosis with ketoconazole. *Ann. Intern. Med.*, **1985**, *103*, 861–872.

Powderly, W. G.; Kobayashi, G. S.; Herzig, G. P.; and Medoff, G. Amphotericin B-resistant yeast infection in severely immunocompromised patients. *Am. J. Med.*, **1988**, *84*, 826–832.

Ritter, W.; Patzschke, K.; Krause, U.; and Stettendorf, S. Pharmacokinetic fundamentals of vaginal treatment with clotrimazole. *Chemotherapy*, **1982**, *28*, Suppl. 1, 37–42.

Shah, V. P.; Epstein, W. L.; and Riegelman, S. Role of sweat in accumulation of orally administered griseofulvin in skin. *J. Clin. Invest.*, **1974**, *53*, 1673–1678.

Smego, R. A.; Perfect, J. R.; and Durack, D. T. Combined therapy with amphotericin B and 5-fluorocytosine for *Candida* meningitis. *Rev. Infect. Dis.*, **1984**, *6*, 791–801.

Smith, E. B.; Powell, R. F.; Graham, J. L.; and Ulrich, J. A. Topical undecylenic acid in tinea pedis: a new look. *Int. J. Dermatol.*, **1977**, *16*, 52–56.

Sokol-Anderson, M. L.; Brajtburg, J.; and Medoff, G. Amphotericin B-induced oxidative damage and killing of *Candida albicans*. *J. Infect. Dis.*, **1986**, *154*, 76–83.

Stamm, A. M.; Diasio, R. B.; Dismukes, W. E.; Shadomy, S.; Cloud, G. C.; Bowles, C. A.; Karam, G. H.; and Espinel-Ingroff, A. Toxicity of amphotericin B plus flucytosine in 194 patients with cryptococcal meningitis. *Am. J. Med.*, **1987**, *83*, 236–242.

Stern, J. J.; Hartman, B. J.; Sharkey, P.; Rowland, V.; Squires, K. E.; Murray, H. W.; and Graybill, J. R. Oral fluconazole therapy for patients with acquired immunodeficiency syndrome. *Am. J. Med.*, **1988**, *297*, 178–179.

Sugar, A. M., and Saunders, C. Oral fluconazole as suppressive therapy of disseminated cryptococcosis in patients with acquired immunodeficiency syndrome. *Am. J. Med.*, **1988**, *85*, 481–489.

Tucker, R. M.; Williams, P. L.; Arathoon, R. G.; Levine, B. E.; Harstein, A. I.; Hanson, L. H.; and Stevens, D. A. Pharmacokinetics of fluconazole in cerebrospinal fluid and serum in human coccidioidal meningitis. *Antimicrob. Agents Chemother.*, **1988**, *32*, 369–373.

Vanden Bossche, H., and others. Cytochrome P-450: target of itraconazole. *Drug Dev. Res.*, **1986**, *8*, 287–298.

Monographs and Reviews

Bartner, E.; Zinnes, H.; Moe, R. A.; and Kulesza, J. S. Studies on a new solubilized preparation of amphotericin B. In, *Antibiotics Annual, 1957–1958*. Medical Encyclopedia, Inc., New York, **1958,** pp. 53–57.

Bennett, J. E. Antifungal agents. In, *Principles and Practice of Infectious Diseases,* 3rd ed. (Mandell, G. L.; Douglas, R. G., Jr.; and Bennett, J. E.; eds.) Churchill Livingstone, Inc., New York, **1990,** pp. 361–370.

Daneshmend, T. K., and Warnock, D. W. Clinical pharmacokinetics of ketoconazole. *Clin. Pharmacokinet.,* **1988,** *14,* 13–34.

Gold, W.; Stout, H. A.; Pagano, J. F.; and Donovick, R. Amphotericins A and B, antifungal antibiotics produced by a Streptomycete. I. *In vitro* studies. In, *Antibiotics Annual, 1955–1956.* Medical Encyclopedia, Inc., New York, **1956,** pp. 579–586.

Goldman, L. Griseofulvin. *Med. Clin. North Am.,* **1970,** *54,* 1339–1345.

Heel, R. C.; Brogden, R. N.; Pakes, G. E.; Speight, T. M.; and Avery, G. S. Miconazole: a preliminary review of its therapeutic efficacy in systemic fungal infections. *Drugs,* **1980,** *19,* 7–30.

Kerridge, D., and Whelan, W. L. The polyene macrolide antibiotics and 5-fluorocytosine: molecular actions and interactions. In, *Mode of Action of Antifungal Agents.* (Trinci, A. P. J., and Riley, J. R., eds.) British Mycological Society, London, **1984,** pp. 343–375.

Kobayashi, G. S., and Medoff, G. Antifungal agents: recent developments. *Annu. Rev. Microbiol.,* **1977,** *31,* 291–308.

Medoff, G.; Brajtburg, J.; Koragrashi, G.; and Bolard, J. Antifungal agents useful in the therapy of systemic fungal infection. *Annu. Rev. Pharmacol. Toxicol.,* **1983,** *23,* 303–330.

Sawyer, P. R.; Brogden, R. N.; Pinder, R. M.; Speight, T. M.; and Avery, G. S. Miconazole: a review of its antifungal activity and therapeutic efficacy. *Drugs,* **1975a,** *9,* 406–423.

———. Clotrimazole: a review of its antifungal activity and therapeutic efficacy. *Ibid.,* **1975b,** *9,* 424–447.

Symposium. (Various authors.) Griseofulvin and dermatomycoses. *Arch. Dermatol.,* **1960,** *81,* 650–882.

Symposium. (Various authors.) Clotrimazole. *Postgrad. Med. J.,* **1974,** *50,* Suppl. 1, 1–108.

Symposium. (Various authors.) First international symposium on itraconazole. (Kass, E. H., ed.) *Rev. Infect. Dis.,* **1987,** *9,* S1–S152.

Symposium. (Various authors.) Antifungal drugs. (St. Georgiev, V., ed.) *Ann. N.Y. Acad. Sci.,* **1988,** *544,* 1–590.

Tolins, J. P., and Raij, L. Adverse effect of amphotericin B administration on renal hemodynamics in the rat. Neurohumoral mechanisms and influence of calcium channel blockade. *J. Pharmacol. Exp. Ther.,* **1988,** *245,* 594–599.

Trinci, A. P. J., and Riley, J. F. (eds.). *Mode of Action of Antifungal Agents.* British Mycological Society, London, **1984.**

Vandeputte, J.; Wachtel, J. L.; and Stiller, E. T. Amphotericins A and B, antifungal antibiotics produced by a streptomycete. II. The isolation and properties of the crystalline amphotericins. In, *Antibiotics Annual, 1955–1956.* Medical Encyclopedia, Inc., New York, **1956,** pp. 587–591.

CHAPTER

51 ANTIMICROBIAL AGENTS

[*Continued*]

Antiviral Agents

R. Gordon Douglas, Jr.

The development of compounds useful for the prophylaxis and therapy of viral disease has been more difficult than the search for drugs effective in disorders caused by other microorganisms. This is so because, in contrast to most other infectious agents, viral replication depends primarily on the metabolic processes of the invaded cell. Thus, agents that may inhibit or cause the death of viruses are also very likely to injure the host cells that harbor them. The challenge has been to discover drugs that inhibit processes that are specific to a given virus, such as attachment, uncoating, replication, or virus-directed macromolecular synthesis.

Concomitant with the elucidation of molecular targets for antiviral therapy and the development of specific antiviral agents has been a rapidly increasing need for such drugs. This need arises from the increasing incidence of diseases such as cytomegalovirus infections in immunocompromised patients, recurrent genital herpes simplex virus infections, and most importantly, acquired immunodeficiency syndrome (AIDS), the most important microbial epidemic of the decade, if not the century.

Understanding of the mechanisms of action of the antiviral agents is the basis for new drug development, as well as for avoiding antagonism between drugs and for improving synergy of other drug combinations. As with other antimicrobial therapy, viral resistance to chemotherapeutic agents is an increasing problem clinically; however, study of the mechanisms of resistance to drugs often permits identification of their sites of action. A number of antiviral agents are now available for clinical use. These drugs, their molecular sites of action, and their uses in therapy are described in this chapter (*see also* Crumpacker, 1989; Hayden and Douglas, 1990).

ZIDOVUDINE (AZIDOTHYMIDINE; AZT)

Zidovudine, first synthesized in a search for anticancer drugs (Horwitz *et al.*, 1964), was rediscovered a decade later as an antiviral agent by Ostertag and coworkers (1974), who showed that it inhibited replication of the Friend leukemia virus. Mitsuya and associates (1985) described the capacity of zidovudine to inhibit the infectivity *in vitro* and the cytopathic effects of human immunodeficiency virus type 1 (HIV-1), the causative agent of AIDS. Since the acute toxicity of the drug appeared to be low, they cautiously suggested that zidovudine might be useful clinically. In the short time that has followed, zidovudine has become the most important agent available for the palliation of this devastating disease.

Chemistry and Antiviral Activity. Zidovudine (3′-azido-3′-deoxythymidine; AZT) is a thymidine analog in which the 3′ hydroxyl of the deoxyribose moiety has been replaced by an azido group. Its structural formula is as follows:

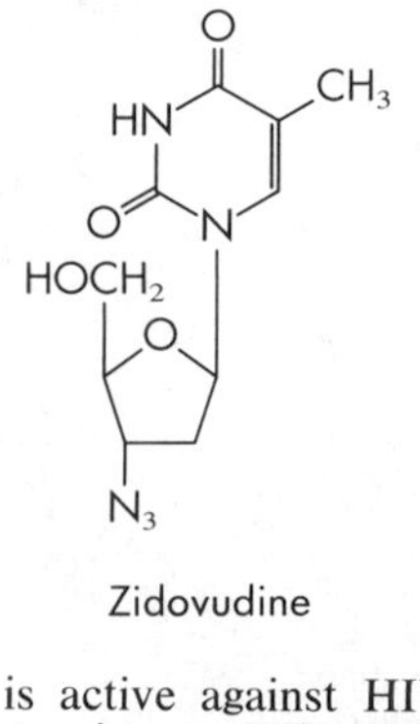

Zidovudine

Zidovudine is active against HIV-1 and other mammalian retroviruses (Mitsuya *et al.*, 1985;

Mitsuya and Broder, 1987). Concentrations of 0.013 μg/ml decrease reverse transcriptase activity in cultured infected cells, and concentrations of 0.02 to 1.3 μg/ml inhibit the replication of HIV-1 in exogenously infected cells. Much higher concentrations of the drug are required to block replication in chronically infected cells. Zidovudine also inhibits human lymphotrophic virus type 1 (HTLV-1), which is associated with T-cell leukemias, but it is less active against HIV-2. The drug inhibits Epstein–Barr virus in concentrations of 1.4 to 2.7 μg/ml, but not herpes simplex or varicella–zoster virus. Many Enterobacteriaceae and *Giardia lamblia* are also inhibited.

Mechanism of Action and Resistance. Zidovudine is phosphorylated *in vivo* by cellular enzymes to the corresponding deoxynucleoside triphosphate derivative. In this form the drug inhibits viral RNA-dependent DNA polymerase (reverse transcriptase) (Furman *et al.*, 1986; Yarchoan and Broder, 1987). Its antiviral selectivity is due to its greater affinity for reverse transcriptase than for human DNA polymerases. As an important part of its mechanism of action, zidovudine also causes chain termination during DNA synthesis. Thus, if azidothymidine triphosphate is incorporated into a growing strand of DNA, additional nucleotides cannot be added because of the modification in the 3′ position of the drug.

The antiviral activity of zidovudine is enhanced by acyclovir, interferon, dideoxyadenosine, granulocyte–macrophage colony-stimulating factor, and neutralizing antibody, but it is antagonized by thymidine and ribavirin (Hammer and Gillis, 1987). Antagonism probably results from competition for phosphorylation, reducing intracellular concentrations of zidovudine triphosphate.

Resistant strains of HIV-1 have been developed in the laboratory, and significant resistance has also been encountered in clinical isolates from patients with AIDS who have been treated with zidovudine for 6 months or more. These resistant strains have remained sensitive to dideoxycytidine and foscarnet (Larder *et al.*, 1989).

Absorption, Distribution, and Excretion. The oral bioavailability of zidovudine is 60 to 65% (Klecker *et al.*, 1987). It is rapidly absorbed, and peak concentrations in plasma are achieved after 30 to 90 minutes. When doses of 250 mg are taken orally every 4 hours, maximal and minimal concentrations in plasma are 0.6 to 1.0 μg/ml and 0.1 to 0.2 μg/ml, respectively. Only about 25% of the drug is bound to plasma proteins, and concentrations in cerebrospinal fluid are close to those in plasma. Concentrations of zidovudine in semen vary widely but may be 1.3- to 20-fold higher than those observed in plasma. In children, continuous infusion of zidovudine (0.5 to 1.8 mg/kg per hour) results in concentrations in blood above 1 μM (0.3 μg/ml), the optimal virostatic concentration *in vitro*. This concentration can be achieved with a lower daily dose of the drug than that used in the usual intermittent regimen (Balis *et al.*, 1989).

Zidovudine is eliminated from plasma rather rapidly ($t_{1/2}$, about 1 hour) (Surbone *et al.*, 1988). The drug is metabolized quickly to the 5′ glucuronide, which has no antiviral activity. The parent drug and the glucuronide are filtered at the glomerulus; renal tubular secretion of the glucuronide also takes place. Most of the drug is recovered in the urine, of which 85% is the glucuronide.

Preparation, Route of Administration, and Dosage. Zidovudine (RETROVIR) is supplied as 100-mg capsules for oral administration. The usual dosage is 200 mg every 4 hours *continuously*. Interruption or reduction of dosage may be necessary if there is significant anemia or granulocytopenia. There is no preparation available for parenteral use.

Untoward Effects. The major toxicities of zidovudine have been granulocytopenia and anemia, which occur in up to 45% of treated patients (Gill *et al.*, 1987; Richman *et al.*, 1987; Walker *et al.*, 1988). The risk is directly related to the numbers of CD4 lymphocytes and granulocytes present at the time therapy is initiated, as well as to the hemoglobin concentration. Far advanced disease and deficiency of vitamin B12 are also risk factors. Anemia may occur as early as 2 to 4 weeks after starting treatment, but is more commonly seen after 6 weeks; granulocytopenia usually occurs after 6 to 8 weeks. Anemia is associated with erythroid hypoplasia or aplasia and megaloblastic changes in the bone marrow. Macrocytosis is common but does not predict the extent of anemia. Careful hematological monitoring should be performed at 2-week intervals. Transfusions are required by 30% of patients; recombinant human erythropoietin is being evaluated as an alternative (*see* Chapter 54). Granulocytopenia is controlled only by reduction of dosage or interruption of therapy.

Other untoward effects include severe headache, nausea, insomnia, and myalgias. Progressive pigmentation of the nails may occur in black patients. Severe neurotoxicity is also observed. Seizures may occur as soon as 48 hours after initiation of therapy; Wernicke's encephalopathy and a polymyositis-like syndrome, which may be delayed for 6 to 17 months, have also been observed (Davtyan and Vinters, 1987).

Drugs that inhibit glucuronyl transferase reactions increase the risks of hematological toxicity and therefore should be avoided; these include acetaminophen, aspirin, indomethacin, and probenecid. Probenecid also reduces the renal excretion of zidovudine. Nephrotoxic or other cytotoxic drugs should also be used with great caution, as should those that affect leukocytes or erythrocytes.

Zidovudine causes transformation of cultured mammalian cells and chromosomal abnormalities in cultured human lymphocytes; however, the potential carcinogenicity and teratogenicity of the drug have not yet been adequately evaluated.

Therapeutic Uses. The efficacy of zidovudine in patients with AIDS (who also have a recent documented pneumonia caused by *Pneumocystis carinii*) and in symptomatic patients with AIDS-related complex (ARC) is well established (Fischl *et al.*, 1987). Over the short term, the quality of life is enhanced; mortality and the incidence of opportunistic infections are reduced dramatically. Concentrations of viral proteins (p24 antigen) in blood decrease (Jackson *et al.*, 1988). Patients gain weight, and certain immunological responses are restored. Neurological disease associated with AIDS also appears to improve, although adequately controlled studies have not been performed (Yarchoan *et al.*, 1987; Dalakas *et al.*, 1988). Dementia and peripheral neuropathy respond rapidly, and up to 50% of patients show sustained neurological improvement for many months. AIDS-associated thrombocytopenia, psoriasis, and lymphocytic interstitial pneumonia may also improve. The estimated mortality from AIDS after 1 year is about 10% of patients who are treated with zidovudine, as compared with more than 50% of untreated patients. Survival is improved if treatment with zidovudine is initiated soon after diagnosis of *P. carinii* pneumonia and if there is concurrent prophylaxis against this infection. Zidovudine also appears to delay the development of signs and symptoms of AIDS in patients who are asymptomatic but have seropositive tests for HIV.

ACYCLOVIR

Chemistry and Antiviral Activity. *Acyclovir* is a synthetic purine nucleoside analog, 9-[(2-hydroxyethoxy)methyl]guanine, in which a linear side chain has been substituted for the cyclic sugar of the naturally occurring guanosine molecule. Its structural formula is as follows:

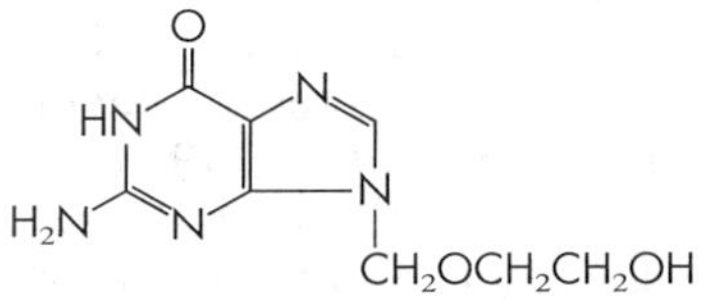

Acyclovir

Acyclovir has antiviral activity that is essentially confined to the herpesviruses (Dorsky and Crumpacker, 1987); it is particularly active against herpes simplex type 1 (concentrations of 0.02 to 0.2 μg/ml will reduce viral plaque formation *in vitro* by 50%) and herpes simplex type 2 (corresponding values are 0.03 to 0.5 μg/ml). Varicella–zoster virus is less sensitive but is inhibited by concentrations that can be achieved clinically (0.8 to 1.2 μg/ml) (Biron and Elion, 1980), while Epstein–Barr virus may be inhibited only at concentrations of at least 1.6 μg/ml (Colby *et al.*, 1980). Cytomegalovirus is inhibited when concentrations of acyclovir are greater than or equal to 23 μg/ml (Lang and Cheung, 1982; Dorsky and Crumpacker, 1987; Hayden and Douglas, 1990). *In vitro,* acyclovir is more than 100 times more active than vidarabine and 10 times more active then idoxuridine against herpes simplex type 1, but it has activity similar to that of vidarabine against varicella–zoster virus. In addition, acyclovir enhances inhibition of HIV-1 *in vitro* by zidovudine. Uninfected mammalian cells are not affected by acyclovir until concentrations exceed 70 μg/ml (Mitsuya and Broder, 1987).

Mechanism of Action and Resistance. Acyclovir inhibits viral replication by inhibiting DNA synthesis. Selectivity in this action comes from two distinct interactions of the drug with viral proteins. In order to inhibit DNA synthesis, acyclovir must be phosphorylated, first by viral thymidine kinase. The affinity of acyclovir for herpesvirus-encoded thymidine kinase is 200 times greater than for the mammalian enzyme, and phosphorylation of acyclovir by the mammalian enzyme proceeds at a negligible rate. After synthesis of acyclovir monophosphate (acyclo-GMP) in virally infected cells, normal cellular enzymes catalyze the sequential synthesis of acyclo-GDP and acyclo-GTP. The amount of acyclo-GTP formed in herpesvirus-infected cells is 40 to 100 times greater than that in uninfected cells. Acyclo-GTP then selectively inhibits the viral DNA polymerase by competing with deoxyguanosine triphosphate and, to a much lesser extent, the cellular polymerases. In addition, acyclo-GTP is incorporated into the elongating viral DNA, where it causes termination of biosynthesis of the viral DNA strand (*see* McGuirt and Furman, 1982; Furman *et al.*, 1984; Elion, 1986).

Resistant herpes simplex viruses have been recovered *in vitro*, in animal models of infection, and in certain clinical situations (Corey and Holmes, 1983). Alterations in either the viral thymidine kinase or the DNA polymerase are responsible. Most such mutant viruses are deficient in thymidine kinase, and concentrations of acyclovir in excess of 3 μg/ml are required for inhibition (Schnipper and Crumpacker, 1980; Coen and Schaffer, 1982). Although these mutant strains are less virulent in animal models of infection, the virulence of resistant clinical isolates has not been established. However, in AIDS patients, acyclovir-resistant strains of herpes simplex virus have caused problematic mucocutaneous infections; these strains are also resistant to ganciclovir, although they have remained sensitive to vidarabine and foscarnet (Erlich *et al.*, 1989b). Resistance of varicella–zoster virus to acyclovir has not yet been a clinical problem.

Absorption, Distribution, and Excretion. Commonly used intravenous doses of acyclovir in adults (5 mg/kg) result in peak concentrations in plasma of 10 μg/ml; these values decline to an average of 0.7 μg/ml by 8 hours. Comparable concentrations are achieved in pediatric patients after intravenous administration of 250 mg/m^2 (Blum *et al.*, 1982; Laskin, 1983). The volume of distribution of acyclovir corresponds to total body water, and the drug is generally well distributed; however, concentrations in cerebrospinal fluid and aqueous humor are only one third to one half of those in plasma. The elimination half-life of acyclovir is about 2.5 hours in patients with normal renal function; this value is about 4 hours in neonates and increases to 20 hours in anuric patients (Hintz *et al.*, 1982; Laskin *et al.*, 1982; Laskin, 1983). Acyclovir is predominantly eliminated as such by glomerular filtration and tubular secretion, and only about 15% or less of an administered dose is recovered in the urine as an inactive metabolite, 9-carboxymethoxymethylguanine (De Miranda *et al.*, 1982). Acyclovir may decrease the renal clearance of other drugs, such as methotrexate, that are eliminated by active tubular secretion.

The bioavailability of acyclovir is only 15 to 30% when the drug is given orally. An 800-mg dose results in peak concentrations in plasma of 1.7 μg/ml after approximately 1.5 hours (McKindrick *et al.*, 1986). *Desciclovir* is a prodrug that is absorbed efficiently and rapidly and is then converted to acyclovir; it is not yet available for clinical use. Percutaneous absorption of acyclovir is poor, and only very low concentrations are detected in the plasma of patients with herpes zoster who have received topical therapy (Corey and Holmes, 1983).

Preparations, Routes of Administration, and Dosage. *Acyclovir sodium* (ZOVIRAX) is available in 200-mg capsules, as an ointment (5%) in a polyethylene glycol base, and as a powder to be reconstituted for intravenous use. For initial treatment of genital herpes, 200 mg of acyclovir is given orally every 4 hours (five times a day) for 10 days. Higher doses have been used to treat herpes simplex proctitis and for herpes zoster infections. Dosage for long-term suppressive therapy of recurrent disease is 200 mg three to five times daily for up to 6 months. Topical treatment of lesions caused by herpes simplex should be initiated as early as possible by application (with a fresh finger cot) of a 1.25-cm (½-in.) ribbon of ointment per 25 cm^2 [4 sq in.] of affected surface area. Ointment is applied every 3 hours, six times daily, for 7 days. Care should be taken to prevent autoinoculation. The ointment is for cutaneous use only and is not to be used in the eye or the vagina. Since acyclovir is concentrated in breast milk it should not be given to nursing mothers. Acyclovir should be given slowly by the intravenous route. The usual dose for treatment of infections of the skin and mucous membranes in adults is 5 mg/kg every 8 hours for 5 to 7 days; for encephalitis caused by herpes simplex virus, the dose is 10 mg/kg every 8 hours. The infusion is given over a 1-hour period.

Untoward Effects. The toxicity of topical acyclovir is limited to local irritation and a transient burning when the preparation is applied to genital lesions (Corey and

Holmes, 1983); this may be caused by the polyethylene glycol base.

The intravenous preparation of acyclovir is usually tolerated quite well. Rarely, infusions have been associated with local phlebitis, rash, diaphoresis, nausea, hematuria, and hypotension (Keeney *et al.*, 1983; Laskin, 1983; Sylvester *et al.*, 1986). However, encephalopathy develops in about 1% of patients (Keeney *et al.*, 1983; Wade and Meyers, 1983; Bean and Aeppli, 1985). This is associated with renal insufficiency and unexpectedly high concentrations of acyclovir in plasma. Encephalopathy is also more common when patients are being treated concurrently with interferon or with methotrexate (intrathecally) (Bean *et al.*, 1982; Balfour *et al.*, 1983). Obstructive nephropathy has also occurred with high, intravenous doses of acyclovir (Sawyer *et al.*, 1988).

Little toxicity has been reported to date with the oral administration of acyclovir, with the exception of occasional nausea, emesis, or headaches (Balfour *et al.*, 1983; Douglas *et al.*, 1988).

Therapeutic Uses. Acyclovir is effective in the treatment of many types of herpes simplex virus type-1 and type-2 infections, including chronic and recurrent mucocutaneous herpes in the immunologically impaired host (Shepp *et al.*, 1986), primary and secondary genital herpes (Gold and Corey, 1987; Mertz, 1987), neonatal herpes, and herpes simplex encephalitis (Whitley *et al.*, 1986). The drug is useful in varicella–zoster infections, especially in patients whose cellular immune responses are impaired (Balfour *et al.*, 1983; Shepp *et al.*, 1986; Feldman and Lott, 1987). It is not effective in cytomegalovirus infections, and its use in infections caused by the Epstein–Barr virus is experimental. Therapeutic uses are discussed in more detail below. (*See also* Hayden and Douglas, 1990.)

GANCICLOVIR

Ganciclovir is mechanistically similar to acyclovir and differs from it structurally only by the addition of a hydroxymethyl group. Its structural formula is as follows:

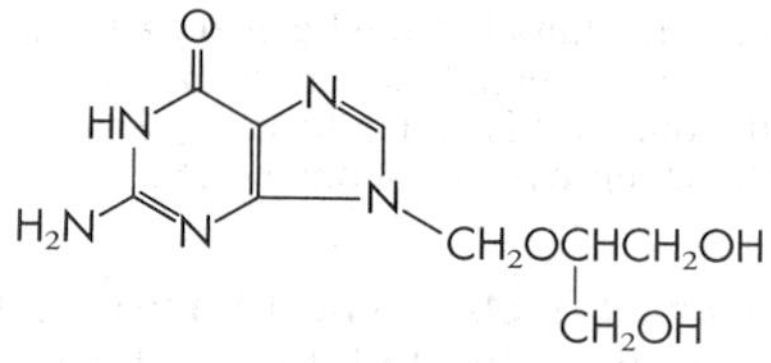

Ganciclovir

Antiviral Activity, Mechanism of Action, and Resistance. Ganciclovir is active *in vitro* against all herpesviruses, including cytomegalovirus (Hayden and Douglas, 1990). It is 100 times more active against cytomegaloviral infections in cell culture than is acyclovir. Strains of herpes simplex virus types 1 and 2 are inhibited by 0.05 to 0.6 μg/ml, cytomegalovirus by 0.3 to 2.8 μg/ml, varicella–zoster virus by 0.4 to 10 μg/ml, and Epstein–Barr virus by 1 to 5 μg/ml (Field *et al.*, 1983). Ganciclovir inhibits viral DNA synthesis (Biron *et al.*, 1985; Smee *et al.*, 1985). It is phosphorylated initially to the monophosphate derivative by both viral and cellular kinases and then to the diphosphate and triphosphate by cellular enzymes. Intracellular concentrations of the triphosphate are higher than those achieved with acyclovir, and they decline slowly. As the triphosphate, ganciclovir is a competitive inhibitor of the incorporation of deoxyguanosine triphosphate into DNA, and it inhibits viral DNA polymerase selectively. The incorporation of the phosphorylated drug into viral DNA also prevents chain elongation.

Strains of herpes simplex that are resistant to acyclovir because of deficiency of thymidine kinase are also somewhat resistant to ganciclovir. Mutations in the viral DNA polymerase can also cause resistance. Progressive disease caused by ganciclovir-resistant cytomegalovirus has been a problem in immunocompromised patients (Erice *et al.*, 1989).

Absorption, Distribution, and Excretion. The oral bioavailability of ganciclovir is very low, and the drug is not administered by this route. After a one-hour intravenous infusion of 5 mg/kg of ganciclovir, plasma concentrations average 8 to 11 μg/ml. Values then decline with a half-time of 3 to 4 hours. The drug is reasonably well distributed into the central nervous system and elsewhere. Most ganciclovir is eliminated unchanged in the urine, and its half-life is prolonged to about 30 hours in severe renal failure.

Preparation, Routes of Administration, and Dosage. Ganciclovir has been administered intravenously; the usual initial daily doses have been 10 mg/kg in 2 or 3 divided portions. Lower doses (5 mg/kg given once daily for 5 days) have been used for suppressive or maintenance therapy. Intravitreal injection of ganciclovir has also been used to achieve high intraocular concentrations and to avoid systemic toxicity. Ganciclovir is not available for general use in the United States.

Untoward Effects. In man, the most common adverse effect of ganciclovir is bone marrow suppression. Neutropenia (less than 1000 cells/mm^3) occurs in 40% or more of treated patients, and thrombocytopenia (less than 50,000 platelets/mm^3) is observed in 20% (Kotler *et al.*, 1986; Laskin *et al.*, 1987a). Neutropenia usually occurs during the second week of therapy and is most often reversible. Central nervous system (CNS) effects, including headache, behavioral changes, psychosis, convulsions, and coma, have been described in

5 to 15% of patients. Anemia, rash, fever, hepatic abnormalities, azotemia, nausea, vomiting, eosinophilia, and phlebitis at the infusion site may also occur. Ganciclovir is teratogenic and mutagenic in experimental animals.

Therapeutic Uses. Because of its toxicity, the use of ganciclovir has been limited to life- or sight-threatening infections with cytomegalovirus. In patients with AIDS and cytomegalovirus retinitis, the use of intravenous doses of 10 mg/kg per day results in clinical improvement or stabilization of 85% of cases (Henderly *et al.*, 1987; Laskin *et al.*, 1987a; Jacobson and Mills, 1988). Viral cultures become negative or viral titers fall dramatically prior to clinical improvement. Historical controls indicate that 90% of untreated patients in this population have progressive disease that leads to blindness. Patients are usually treated for 3 weeks; almost all relapse 2 to 5 weeks later. Suppressive doses of ganciclovir (5 mg/kg per day for 5 days each week) prevent relapse in up to 60% of patients for at least 120 days. Lower doses are not effective. Ganciclovir may be effective in other syndromes in AIDS patients that are caused by cytomegalovirus, such as colitis, wasting syndrome, pneumonia, and esophagitis, but there is less evidence to support its use in these cases.

The combined use of ganciclovir and anti-cytomegalovirus immune globulin to treat pneumonia caused by cytomegalovirus in recipients of bone marrow transplants has been associated with improved survival (52 to 70%) as compared with historical controls (0 to 22%); ganciclovir alone is not effective (Emanuel *et al.*, 1988; Reed *et al.*, 1988).

VIDARABINE

Vidarabine (adenine arabinoside, ara-A) is an analog of adenosine (arabinose is the 2′-epimer of ribose). Its structural formula is as follows:

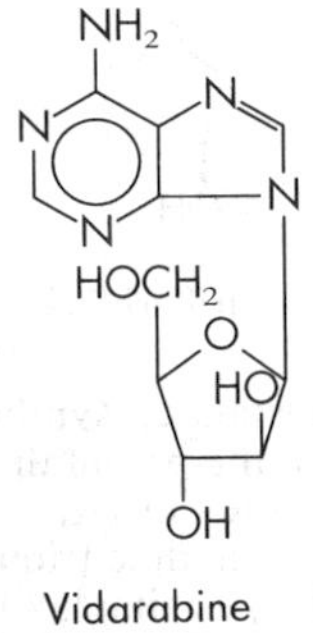

Vidarabine

Antiviral Activity and Mechanism of Action. Vidarabine is phosphorylated to the corresponding nucleotides within the cell, and it acts by inhibiting viral DNA polymerase; mammalian DNA synthesis is inhibited to a lesser extent. Vidarabine triphosphate is incorporated into both cellular and viral DNA, where it acts to terminate the extension of newly synthesized strands of nucleic acid (Pelling *et al.*, 1981). Vidarabine is also metabolized rapidly by adenosine deaminase to the less active hypoxanthine arabinoside, which may act synergistically with the parent compound to enhance its antiviral activity (Gephart and Lerner, 1981). *Cyclaradine*, the carbocyclic analog of vidarabine, is resistant to the action of adenosine deaminase. Vidarabine is active *in vitro* against vaccinia virus, herpes simplex virus types 1 and 2, varicella–zoster virus, variola virus, rhabdoviruses, and some RNA tumor viruses; activity against cytomegalovirus is variable. Most strains of herpes simplex and varicella–zoster virus are inhibited by 3 μg/ml or less; strains of these viruses that are resistant to acyclovir are sensitive to vidarabine (Field *et al.*, 1981; Erlich *et al.*, 1989b). The drug is not active against other DNA viruses, such as adenoviruses or papovaviruses, or against RNA viruses.

Absorption, Distribution, and Excretion. During a constant 12-hour infusion of 10 mg/kg of vidarabine, the drug itself is undetectable in plasma. However, concentrations of hypoxanthine arabinoside peak at 3 to 6 μg/ml as a result of the rapid deamination of vidarabine by adenosine deaminase (Whitley *et al.*, 1980). The half-life of hypoxanthine arabinoside in plasma is 3.5 hours. About 50% of the total dose is recovered in the urine as hypoxanthine arabinoside and a very small amount as the parent drug.

Preparations, Routes of Administration, and Dosage. *Vidarabine* (VIRA-A) is available for injection in 5-ml vials that contain 200 mg/ml of the monohydrate in a suspension (equivalent to 187 mg of vidarabine). The drug is also supplied as a 3% ophthalmic ointment. The recommended daily dose of vidarabine for treatment of encephalitis caused by herpes simplex virus is 15 mg/kg. Since vidarabine is only slightly soluble in water, large volumes of fluid are needed to dissolve the compound (*e.g.*, 2.5 liters). The drug should be given intravenously at a constant rate over a 12- to 24-hour period, daily for 10 days. Herpes simplex keratoconjunctivitis is treated with a 3% ophthalmic ointment, which is administered topically every 3 hours (five times daily).

Untoward Effects. Vidarabine causes relatively few side effects, but these can include rash, weakness, thrombophlebitis at the site of drug administration, hypokalemia, and inappropriate secretion of antidiuretic hormone (Whitley *et al.*, 1980). Effects on the CNS, such as hallucinations, psychoses, ataxia, tremor, pain syndrome, and dizziness, have been noted, as have megaloblastic anemia, leukopenia, and thrombocytopenia (Friedman and Grasela, 1981; Feldman *et al.*, 1986). Side effects are intensified if interferon is given concurrently or if there is renal or hepatic disease. The dosage should be reduced in patients with renal insufficiency. There is evidence that vidarabine is mutagenic and carcinogenic.

Therapeutic Uses. Vidarabine is effective in the treatment of herpes simplex encephalitis, but acyclovir is superior (Skoldenberg *et al.*, 1984;

Whitley *et al.*, 1986). In neonates, vidarabine reduces the mortality of herpes simplex virus infections that are complicated by visceral dissemination or involvement of the CNS; acyclovir is not superior to vidarabine in this condition. Vidarabine is also effective in mucocutaneous infections caused by herpes simplex virus in immunocompromised hosts, but it is less effective than acyclovir (Whitley *et al.*, 1984).

In herpes zoster infections in immunocompromised patients, vidarabine is effective in reducing the formation of new vesicles; it also accelerates the clearance of virus from vesicles, reduces pain, decreases the risk of dissemination, and decreases the total duration of postherpetic neuralgia (Whitley *et al.*, 1982b). Similar results have been observed in immunocompromised patients with varicella infections (Whitley *et al.*, 1982a). The drug should not be used to treat unimpaired hosts with uncomplicated herpes zoster; neither is it useful for treatment of recurrent or primary herpes genitalis (Hayden and Douglas, 1990). It is also not effective in cytomegalovirus infections. In some patients with chronic hepatitis B infections, use of vidarabine is associated with reductions in titers of viral antigens and viral DNA polymerase activity (Bassendine *et al.*, 1981).

Vidarabine applied topically is better tolerated and is as effective as idoxuridine for herpes simplex keratoconjunctivitis (Pavan-Langston, 1984; Kaufman, 1988).

IDOXURIDINE

Idoxuridine is 5-iodo-2′-deoxyuridine. Its structure is as follows:

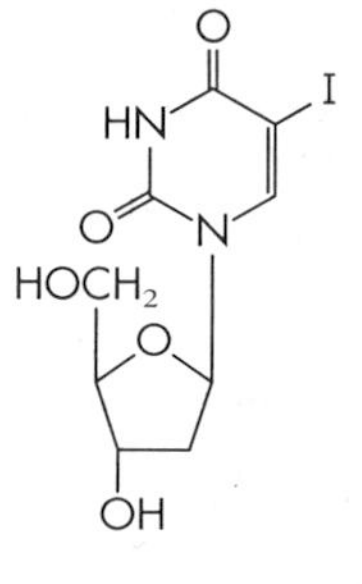

Idoxuridine

Idoxuridine resembles thymidine. It is phosphorylated within cells, and the triphosphate derivative is incorporated into both viral and mammalian DNA. Such DNA is more susceptible to breakage, and altered viral proteins may result from faulty transcription (Prusoff, 1988). Thus, the activity of idoxuridine is largely limited to DNA viruses, primarily herpesviruses and poxviruses. Most strains of herpes simplex virus are inhibited by concentrations of 10 μg/ml or less. Resistance of viruses to the drug develops readily *in vitro* and has also been documented in man (Field, 1983).

The primary clinical use of idoxuridine has been in the treatment of herpes simplex keratitis. In reporting on 1500 cases, Maxwell (1963) noted a correlation between the type of infection and the response to therapy. Epithelial infections, especially initial attacks in which a dendritic figure is present, respond best. The results are less favorable when the stroma is involved. In recurrent episodes, the acute disease is often controlled. Other localized herpesvirus infections, such as those caused by herpes simplex virus type 2 and varicella–zoster do not respond to the drug. When applied topically to the conjunctiva, irritation, pain, pruritus, inflammation or edema of the eyelids, and photophobia may develop. Punctate areas may appear in the cornea after several days of therapy; they disappear when idoxuridine is discontinued (Pavan-Langston, 1984; Kaufman, 1988).

Idoxuridine (HERPLEX, STOXIL) is supplied as an ophthalmic ointment (0.5%) and an ophthalmic solution (0.1%). The dosage of the 0.1% solution is 1 drop in the conjunctival sac every hour during the day and every 2 hours during the night until definite improvement is apparent, after which the same dose is applied every 2 hours during the day and every 4 hours at night. When the 0.5% ointment is used, it is applied every 4 hours during the day and once before bedtime. Therapy is continued for 3 to 5 days after healing is complete, as demonstrated by fluorescein staining.

TRIFLURIDINE

Trifluridine (5-trifluoromethyl-2′-deoxyuridine, trifluorothymidine) is a fluorinated pyrimidine deoxynucleoside that inhibits viral DNA synthesis. Its structural formula is as follows:

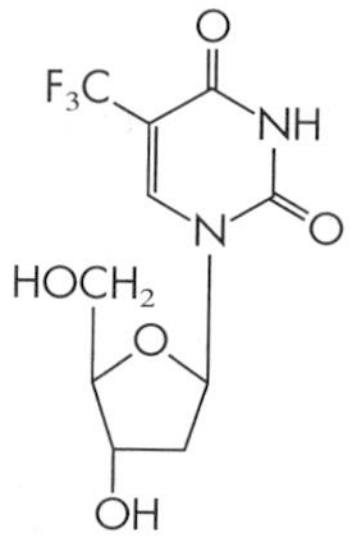

Trifluridine

Trifluridine triphosphate, synthesized *in vivo* by phosphorylation of the parent drug, is incorporated into viral and, to a lesser extent, cellular DNA in competition with thymidine triphosphate. The drug is active against herpes simplex virus types 1 and 2 (including thymidine kinase–deficient strains), cytomegalovirus, vaccinia, and some strains of adenovirus. Viral resistance has not been reported (Spector *et al.*, 1983; Prusoff, 1988).

Trifluridine exhibits mutagenic, teratogenic, and antineoplastic activities in experimental systems. Its use is limited to topical treatment of primary and recurrent keratoconjunctivitis caused by herpes simplex virus types 1 and 2. It is more active than idoxuridine, but comparable in efficacy to topical vidarabine for this purpose. It may be effective in patients who have not responded to idoxuridine, as well as in those who have experienced ocular toxicity from idoxuridine or hypersensitivity to the drug. It has not been proven effective in ocular infections caused by vaccinia virus or adenovirus. Adverse reactions include discomfort, irritation, palpebral edema, and uncommonly, hypersensitivity reactions.

Trifluridine (VIROPTIC) is supplied as a 1% aqueous ophthalmic solution. The usual dosage for herpes simplex keratitis is 1 drop onto the cornea every 2 hours while awake, with a maximum daily dose of 9 drops. After reepithelialization of the cornea, the dosage is reduced to 1 drop every 4 hours while awake, with a minimum of 5 drops per day for an additional 7 days.

FOSCARNET

Foscarnet sodium (trisodium phosphonoformate) is a simple inorganic phosphonate analog. It is not available for general use in the United States. Its structural formula is as follows:

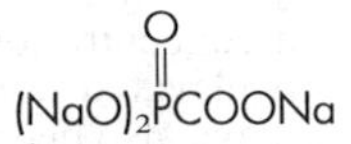

Foscarnet Sodium

Foscarnet inhibits viral DNA polymerase and reverse transcriptase. The drug interacts with the pyrophosphate binding sites on these enzymes, which are distinct from the loci of action of acyclovir (on DNA polymerase) and zidovudine (on reverse transcriptase). Foscarnet is active against herpesviruses, including cytomegalovirus, and HIV at concentrations of 3 μg/ml. Resistance has not been detected (Hayden and Douglas, 1990). Strains of herpes simplex that are resistant to acyclovir and ganciclovir are sensitive to foscarnet (Erlich *et al.*, 1989b), and foscarnet has been used successfully to treat patients with mucocutaneous infections caused by acyclovir-resistant strains of herpes simplex (Chatis *et al.*, 1989).

To date, foscarnet has been administered intravenously. After an initial bolus of 20 mg/kg over 30 minutes, a continuous infusion of 230 mg/kg per day is given for 2 to 3 weeks. Intermittent dosage of 60 mg/kg every 8 hours has also been employed for 12 to 50 days (Erlich *et al.*, 1989a). Foscarnet penetrates the CNS well. Unlike zidovudine, it also enters macrophages and inhibits the replication of HIV within these cells. Foscarnet is eliminated by the kidney; small amounts accumulate in bone. Dosage must be reduced for patients with impaired renal function.

The most common untoward effect of foscarnet is reduced renal function, and the risk of renal insufficiency increases with the severity and duration of infection with HIV. The drug markedly increases both fluid intake and urine output. It has also been associated with malaise, nausea, vomiting, fatigue, and headaches. Anemia is common, but granulocytopenia does not occur. Tremor, seizures, irritability, and hypocalcemia have been observed, and the latter may be accentuated by the concurrent administration of pentamidine.

Foscarnet has been used to treat retinitis due to cytomegalovirus in patients with AIDS (Bloom and Palestine, 1988; Walmsley *et al.*, 1988). Clinical responses occur in most patients and are similar to those seen with ganciclovir. Relapses also occur after cessation of treatment in most patients, as they do after ganciclovir. Treatment with foscarnet of severe, acyclovir-resistant herpes simplex virus type-2 infections in patients with AIDS has been effective (Erlich *et al.*, 1989a). The drug has also been used in place of or in addition to zidovudine for the treatment of HIV infections. A decline in the concentration of HIV antigens in plasma has been observed in several studies. However, additional data are needed to assess the potential of foscarnet for the treatment of AIDS or infections with cytomegalovirus.

HUMAN INTERFERON

Interferons are glycoproteins that have a variety of biological actions; they are potent cytokines that possess complex antiviral, immunomodulating, and antiproliferative effects (Pestka *et al.*, 1987). Endogenous production and release of interferon occur in response to viruses, especially double-stranded RNA viruses, and other inducers, including bacterial exotoxins, polyanions, certain low-molecular-weight compounds, and microorganisms capable of intracellular growth. There are three major types of human interferons, officially designated alpha (alfa), beta, and gamma (Pestka *et al.*, 1987; Zoon, 1987). Interferon alfa and beta are produced by most cells in response to viral infection, whereas synthesis of interferon gamma is restricted to T lymphocytes. Most studies of interferon have used purified proteins produced by recombinant DNA technology, but earlier work was performed with human leukocyte interferon.

Interferon alfa-2a and alfa-2b (the preparations currently available; *see* below) are highly purified proteins with molecular weights of approximately 19,000; they each contain 165 amino acid residues, are produced in *Escherichia coli,* and are essentially identical to one another (differing in only one amino acid residue).

The effects of interferon on viral infections are complex and may depend on the immunomodulating as well as the antiviral activities of the proteins. Interferon appears at the site of infection at the time that peak titers of virus are detectable (or just after) and before the appearance of humoral antibody (Hayden and Douglas, 1990). The appearance of interferon correlates with reduction of viral titers, suggesting an important host defense mechanism. Administration of interferon can prevent, but not cure, certain viral infections. By contrast, there are situations in which interferon may be harmful and in which the presence of the protein correlates with the progression of disease. It has also been suggested that endogenous interferon may be responsible for the symptomatology that is common to many viral infections (*e.g.*, fever, malaise, and myalgia).

Antiviral Activity and Mechanism of Action. Most RNA and DNA viruses are sensitive to the antiviral activity of the interferons, but the mechanisms and degree of effect vary with virus and cell type (Greenberg, 1987; Whitaker-Dowling and Youngner, 1987). Interferons produce their antiviral effect by binding to specific cell-surface receptors and inhibiting viral penetration or uncoating, synthesis or methylation of messenger RNA, translation of viral proteins, or viral assembly and release (Whitaker-Dowling and Youngner, 1987). For most viruses, the major effect is to inhibit viral protein synthesis. Evidence shows that interference with protein synthesis may involve the induction by interferons of an enzyme that synthesizes a series of short 2′-5′-linked oligoadenylates; the oligoadenylates in turn activate a latent ribonuclease that degrades messenger RNAs. Interferons also appear to induce a protein kinase that phosphorylates and inactivates one of the proteins necessary for initiation of protein synthesis (eIF-2).

Absorption, Distribution, and Excretion. Interferons are not absorbed orally. After intramuscular or subcutaneous injection of interferon alfa, concentrations in plasma peak by 4 to 8 hours. Interferon is inactivated rapidly in body fluids and in various tissues; the protein disappears from plasma with an initial half-time of about 40 minutes and a terminal half-time of about 5 hours (*see* Appendix II). Negligible amounts are excreted by the kidney. By contrast, intramuscular or subcutaneous injection of interferon beta or gamma results in negligible concentrations in plasma; however, there is evidence of effects of these interferons on peripheral-blood leukocytes.

After an intramuscular dose of interferon alfa (1.8×10^7 I.U.), the activity of 2′-5′ oligoadenylate synthase in peripheral-blood mononuclear cells increases and remains elevated for 4 days. These cells display antiviral activity after 1 hour; this peaks at 24 hours and wanes over 6 days. Biological effects of interferon outlive elevated concentrations in plasma.

Preparation, Routes of Administration, and Dosage. *Interferon alfa-2a* (ROFERON-A) is available in solution or as a powder for injection after reconstitution. The protein may be given subcutaneously or intramuscularly. The subcutaneous route should be used for patients who are thrombocytopenic.

Interferon alfa-2b (INTRON A) is also available as a powder for reconstitution. It may be administered subcutaneously, intramuscularly, or intralesionally.

The doses of interferon alfa that have been used to treat herpesvirus infections are high—usually 36×10^6 I.U. per day for 5 to 7 days. Lower doses have been used to treat hepatitis B—3 to 20×10^6 I.U. per day, three times per week for several weeks. In condylomata acuminata (papillomavirus infection), intralesional interferon alfa has been employed at a dosage of 1×10^6 I.U. per lesion three times weekly for 3 weeks. For the prophylaxis of respiratory viral infections, interferon alfa has been given intranasally (5×10^6 I.U.) once daily for 7 days. High parenteral doses of interferon alfa and interferon gamma have been tested for treatment of HIV infections.

Untoward Effects. An influenza-like illness follows the systemic administration of 10^4 to 10^5 I.U./kg of interferon alfa; manifestations include fever (up to 40°C), chills, headache, myalgias, nausea, vomiting, and diarrhea. The same syndrome may also follow intralesional therapy (Hayden and Douglas, 1990). The reaction is diminished by pretreatment with antipyretics (Dinarello *et al.*, 1988).

Bone marrow suppression with granulocytopenia and thrombocytopenia is common. Leukopenia is maximal at the end of the second week. Neurotoxicity characterized by somnolence, confusion, behavioral changes, electroencephalographic changes, and seizures is another result of therapy with interferon alfa. During long-term treatment, neurasthenia with profound fatigue, anorexia, weight loss, and myalgias may occur (McDonald *et al.*, 1987). Plasma concentrations of hepatic enzymes are commonly elevated. Renal insufficiency and cardiac toxicity have also been reported. Interferons reduce metabolism of other drugs by the hepatic cytochrome P_{450} system (Williams *et al.*, 1987).

Antibodies to interferons develop with continued use and may result in decreased antiviral activity. Local tenderness and erythema occur frequently after subcutaneous injection. Prolonged intranasal administration of interferon is associated with mucosal friability, ulcerations, and bleeding in up to 50% of recipients, as well as complaints of dryness and stuffiness.

Therapeutic Uses. Interferon alfa is currently approved for use in hairy-cell leukemia, AIDS-related Kaposi's sarcoma, and condylomata acuminata (genital warts).

In cancer patients with localized herpes zoster, early treatment with high doses of interferon alfa given intramuscularly reduces progression of localized zoster, prevents cutaneous or visceral dissemination, and diminishes the severity of postherpetic neuralgia (Greenberg, 1987; Ho, 1987). Parenteral administration of interferon alfa also prevents visceral dissemination of varicella in immunocompromised children.

Topical administration of interferon alfa combined with other antiviral agents (acyclovir, trifluridine) is more effective than any single agent alone in the treatment of herpes keratoconjunctivitis. Consistent effects have not been observed in herpes genitalis infections.

Interferon alfa is not effective in treating established infections caused by cytomegalovirus. Although the drug may prevent cytomegaloviral disease in renal transplant recipients, it is not effective in patients with bone marrow transplants (Meyers *et al.*, 1987).

Interferon alfa reduces markers of hepatitis B virus in patients with chronic infections (Davis and Hoofnagle, 1986; Alexander *et al.*, 1987). Long-term administration (2 to 4 months) of very low doses of interferon alfa (2.5 to 5 × 10^6 I.U. per day) is associated with permanent disappearance of viral DNA polymerase activity in up to one third of patients. However, clinical responses are infrequent. This has led to trials of combinations of interferon alfa with vidarabine, acyclovir, or prednisone.

In papillomavirus infections, interferon alfa has been used topically, intralesionally, and parenterally (Weck *et al.*, 1986; Greenberg, 1987). Intralesional therapy eradicates genital warts in 36 to 62% of patients who are refractory to conventional therapy (Eron *et al.*, 1986; Friedman-Kien *et al.*, 1988). Involution of lesions occurs by 4 weeks and is maximal by 4 to 12 weeks. In juvenile laryngeal papillomatosis, the clinical and virological response to systemic interferon alfa is variable; however, the adult form of the disease appears to respond more favorably.

Interferon alfa is very effective (90%) in preventing colds caused by rhinoviruses but not by other viruses (Douglas *et al.*, 1986; Hayden *et al.*, 1986a). It is not effective in treating established colds. Antiviral effects against HIV, cytomegalovirus, or herpes simplex virus have not been observed consistently when patients with AIDS have been given interferon alfa for treatment of Kaposi's sarcoma (Groopman and Scadden, 1989).

AMANTADINE

Amantadine (1-adamantanamine) is a water-soluble, tricyclic amine; its unusual structure is not related to that of any of the other antimicrobial agents. Its structural formula is as follows:

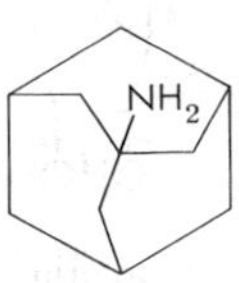

Amantadine

Antiviral Activity, Mechanism of Action, and Resistance. Amantadine appears to block a late stage in the assembly of the influenza A virus, but its detailed mechanism of action remains unclear. Attachment of the virus to cells, penetration, and RNA-dependent RNA polymerase activity are not affected by the drug (Couch and Six, 1986). Using a sensitive plaque-reduction assay, most strains of influenza A viruses, including H3N2, H2N2, and H1N1 subtypes, are inhibited by 0.4 μg/ml of amantadine or less. Higher concentrations (25 to 50 μg/ml) are required to inhibit influenza B, rubella, and other viruses (Hayden *et al.*, 1980; Hayden and Douglas, 1990).

Resistance to amantadine is readily achieved in the laboratory by serial passage of virus *in vitro* or in animals in the presence of the drug. Resistant strains have been recovered from treated as well as untreated patients (Pemberton *et al.*, 1986); their significance remains to be determined.

Absorption, Distribution, and Excretion. Amantadine is well absorbed from the gastrointestinal tract. Peak concentrations in plasma are 0.3 to 0.6 μg/ml after ingestion of a 200-mg dose. Almost all of the absorbed drug is excreted in the urine unchanged; the drug is not metabolized (Aoki and Sitar, 1985; Hayden *et al.*, 1985). The half-time for elimination is about 16 hours; this value is increased in elderly persons and in patients with impaired renal function.

Preparations, Route of Administration, and Dosage. *Amantadine hydrochloride* (SYMADINE, SYMMETREL) is available in capsules containing 100 mg and as a syrup (50 mg/5 ml). The daily dose for children 1 to 9 years of age is 4.4 to 8.8 mg/kg, but it should not exceed a total of 150 mg per day. For older children and adults, the dose is 200 mg once daily or 100 mg twice daily. For those over 65 years of age, the dose should be reduced to 100 mg once daily.

Untoward Effects. Plasma concentrations of amantadine of 1 to 5 μg/ml are associated with CNS toxicity, including nervousness, confusion, hallucinations, seizures, and coma. One to 5% of patients with normal renal function who receive amantadine (200 mg once daily) report minor neurological symptoms, including insomnia and difficulty in concentrating (Dolin *et al.*, 1982; Tominack and Hayden, 1987). Symptoms may be reduced by administration of 100 mg twice a day. Persons with cerebral atherosclerosis, psychiatric disorders, or a history of epilepsy must be observed closely when taking this drug. It should not be administered to pregnant women and nursing mothers.

Prophylactic and Therapeutic Uses. A number of clinical studies have demonstrated the effectiveness of amantadine in preventing infection with influenza A viruses (Dolin *et al.*, 1982; World Health

Organization, 1985; Tominack and Hayden, 1987). The efficacy of amantadine in preventing such illness varies from 50 to over 90%; these rates are comparable to those achieved with influenza vaccines. The drug is valuable in both nosocomial and community settings (*see* Atkinson *et al.*, 1986; Arden *et al.*, 1988; Hayden and Douglas, 1990). In double-blind, placebo-controlled studies of amantadine in patients with naturally occurring infections due to influenza A virus, the drug has been found to produce a therapeutic effect even when given within 48 hours after the onset of illness (Younkin *et al.*, 1983; World Health Organization, 1985; Tominack and Hayden, 1987). There is a more rapid defervescence of illness, the duration is shortened by 50%, the frequency and quantity of shedding of virus decreases, and peripheral airway resistance is reduced more rapidly. The development of specific antibody is not suppressed.

Influenza virus vaccine is the preferred method of prophylaxis. However, in the presence of a documented influenza A virus epidemic, amantadine is recommended for unimmunized patients of all ages who have a high risk of developing complications from influenza. Prophylactic administration of amantadine to high-risk patients should be initiated as soon as influenza A activity is documented in the community and continued for the duration of the epidemic (usually 5 to 6 weeks). Since the drug does not impair the immune response to influenza vaccine, patients can be vaccinated at the same time and amantadine discontinued after 2 weeks. Patients who acquire a typical clinical picture of acute influenza during the influenza season should be treated with amantadine. Under this circumstance the drug is given for 5 days (Hayden and Douglas, 1990).

The discovery that amantadine is also useful in the treatment of parkinsonism was an act of serendipity. This therapeutic application is discussed in Chapter 20.

RIMANTADINE

Rimantadine is a structural analog of amantadine, and it shares its antiviral specificity, mechanism of action, and potential for development of resistant viral strains (Hayden *et al.*, 1980; Browne *et al.*, 1983; Webster *et al.*, 1985; Hayden and Douglas, 1990). The structural formula of rimantadine is as follows:

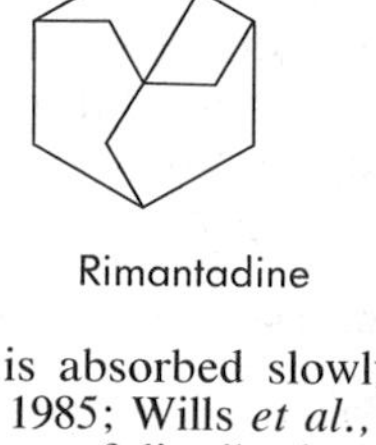

Rimantadine

Rimantadine is absorbed slowly but efficiently (Hayden *et al.*, 1985; Wills *et al.*, 1987). The drug has a large volume of distribution, and higher relative concentrations are achieved in respiratory secretions as compared with amantadine. In contrast to amantadine, rimantadine is extensively metabolized, and less than 15% is excreted unchanged in the urine. The half-time for elimination is 24 to 36 hours.

Rimantadine is as effective as amantadine in preventing naturally occurring infections with influenza A and in treating established illness (World Health Organization, 1985; Betts *et al.*, 1987; Tominack and Hayden, 1987). At doses of 200 or 300 mg per day, CNS side effects are significantly less frequent with rimantadine than with amantadine.

Rimantadine (FLUMADINE) is not yet available for general use in the United States. If it is marketed, it may offer certain advantages over amantadine. These include a decrease in the frequency of CNS side effects and the lack of dependence on the kidney for elimination of the drug.

RIBAVIRIN

Ribavirin is a purine nucleoside analog that inhibits the replication *in vitro* of a wide range of RNA and DNA viruses, including myxoviruses, paramyxoviruses, arenaviruses, bunyaviruses, retroviruses, herpesviruses, adenoviruses, and poxviruses. Its structural formula is as follows:

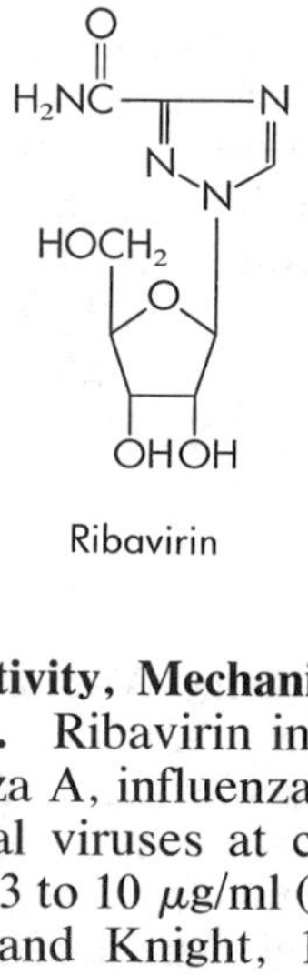

Ribavirin

Antiviral Activity, Mechanism of Action, and Resistance. Ribavirin inhibits replication of influenza A, influenza B, and respiratory syncytial viruses at concentrations in the range of 3 to 10 μg/ml (Hruska *et al.*, 1980; Gilbert and Knight, 1986; Hayden and Douglas, 1990). It is generally not active against viruses that contain single-stranded RNA acting as messenger RNA, such as the picornaviruses.

Although ribavirin most resembles guanosine structurally, it also mimics adenosine in certain conformations. The drug is first phosphorylated to ribavirin 5′-monophosphate (RMP) by adenosine kinase.

RMP is a strong inhibitor of inosine monophosphate dehydrogenase; this prevents the conversion of inosine monophosphate to xanthosine monophosphate and, ultimately, the synthesis of guanine nucleotides. Intracellular concentrations of GTP are thus lowered. After further phosphorylation to ribavirin 5′-triphosphate (RTP), the drug inhibits viral RNA polymerase by competing with both GTP and ATP for substrate sites on the enzyme. Interestingly, RTP also inhibits GTP-dependent viral enzymes that are necessary for "capping" of viral messenger RNA (*see* Wray *et al.*, 1985). Thus, ribavirin appears to have multiple sites of action, and some of these effects (*e.g.*, inhibition of GTP synthesis) may potentiate others (*e.g.*, competitive inhibition of GTP-dependent enzymes). Perhaps because of its multiplicity of effects, resistance to ribavirin has not been encountered experimentally or clinically. Unfortunately, ribavirin antagonizes the activity of zidovudine against HIV-1 (Baba *et al.*, 1987).

Absorption, Distribution, and Excretion. The oral bioavailability of ribavirin is about 45%. Peak concentrations in plasma occur after 1 to 2 hours, and these average 1.3 and 2.5 μg/ml after single oral doses of 600 and 1200 mg, respectively (Laskin *et al.*, 1987b). High plasma concentrations of the drug can be achieved by intravenous administration; the drug can also be given as an aerosol (Connor *et al.*, 1984).

The initial half-time for elimination of ribavirin from plasma is approximately 2 hours, but there is a prolonged phase of elimination with a half-time of 36 hours. Ribavirin triphosphate accumulates in erythrocytes, where it persists with a $t_{1/2}$ of about 40 days (Knight *et al.*, 1988).

Preparations, Routes of Administration, and Dosage. Ribavirin (VIRAZOLE) is administered by aerosol using a specific nebulizer. The estimated dose that is delivered to infants is 1.4 mg/kg per hour. Treatment is carried out for 12 to 18 hours per day for 3 to 7 days.

Intravenous and oral dosage forms of ribavirin are available for investigational purposes. Oral treatment regimens for adults have varied between 600 and 1800 mg per day, usually in divided doses. Intravenous divided doses of 4000 mg per day have been used in patients with hemorrhagic fevers and a high risk of death.

Untoward Effects. When administered orally or intravenously, ribavirin causes anemia due to extravascular hemolysis and suppression of the bone marrow (Roberts *et al.*, 1987). Plasma concentrations of bilirubin, iron, and uric acid become elevated. Reticulocytosis commonly occurs after cessation of therapy. Long-term oral therapy is associated with both gastrointestinal and CNS symptoms. Ribavirin is teratogenic and mutagenic in small animals.

Aerosolized ribavirin is generally well tolerated (Hall *et al.*, 1983; Rodriguez *et al.*, 1987). Conjunctival irritation and rash, transient wheezing, and reversible deterioration in pulmonary function may occur occasionally.

Therapeutic Uses. Aerosolized ribavirin shortens the duration of shedding of virus and improves arterial oxygen saturation in infants with respiratory syncytial viral pneumonia and bronchiolitis; the drug is approved for such use (Hall *et al.*, 1983; Rodriguez *et al.*, 1987). Improvement has been documented in children with congenital heart disease or bronchopulmonary dysplasia, as well as in otherwise normal children (Hall *et al.*, 1985).

Some, but not all, studies indicate that aerosolized ribavirin causes clinical and virological improvement in young adults with influenza A or B viral infection (Knight and Gilbert, 1987; Bernstein *et al.*, 1988). Oral ribavirin is not effective in such cases. In patients with life-threatening Lassa fever, large doses of ribavirin given orally or intravenously reduce mortality significantly if given during the first 6 days of illness (McCormick *et al.*, 1986). Positive effects are also observed in Korean and Argentinian hemorrhagic fevers. Oral administration of ribavirin (800 mg per day) may delay the progression from ARC to AIDS, but this observation has not yet been confirmed. Patients with AIDS may show transient clinical improvement when treated with ribavirin (Crumpacker *et al.*, 1987).

THERAPY OF VIRAL INFECTIONS

Human Immunodeficiency Virus. All patients with a clinical diagnosis of AIDS and patients who are seropositive for antibody to HIV and have CD4 lymphocyte counts below 200 cells/mm^3 should receive long-term therapy with zidovudine, 200 mg orally every 4 hours. Significant reduction in mortality has been demonstrated with this regimen (Fischl *et al.*, 1987; Richman *et al.*, 1987). The time to 50% mortality before the availability of zidovudine was under 12 months; with zidovudine the time is approximately 24 months. The prognosis can be enhanced further (one-year mortality less than 10%) with concomitant prophylaxis for *P. carinii* pneumonia; such regimens include sulfadoxine and pyrimethamine (FANSIDAR), dapsone, or aerosolized pentamidine. Hematological toxicity may require modification of dosage or interruption of treatment. The minimal effective dose of zidovudine is being studied, as are regimens that involve less frequent administration of the drug.

In addition to prolongation of life, benefits of therapy include reduction in opportunistic infections, return of cutaneous delayed-hypersensitivity reactions, weight gain, and stabilization or improvement of functional status (Fauci, 1988). Decreases in titers of HIV p24 antigens may also occur (Jackson *et al.*, 1988). Uncontrolled studies also suggest a beneficial response of associated neurological signs and symptoms (Yarchoan *et al.*, 1987, 1988). Dementia and peripheral neuropathy often improve within 8 weeks, and this may be sustained for 5 to 10 months. Other manifestations of HIV infection such as thrombocytopenia (Oksenhendler *et al.*, 1989), psoriasis, and lymphocytic interstitial pneumonia also benefit from treatment with zidovudine.

Important initial results indicate that significantly fewer patients with early AIDS-related complex (ARC) progress to advanced ARC and AIDS when treated with zidovudine. It may be possible to treat such patients with relatively low doses of the drug (*e.g.*, 500 mg per day) that cause only minor side effects.

Therapy with combinations of zidovudine and acyclovir, foscarnet, or interferon alfa is being tested for treatment of HIV infections. Dextran sulfate (*see* Chapter 27), a drug that blocks the binding of HIV to target cells, is well tolerated by man and is undergoing clinical trials (Abrams *et al.*, 1989). Dideoxycytidine, an inhibitor of reverse transcriptase, reduces circulating concentrations of HIV p24 antigen in patients with AIDS, but it causes peripheral neuropathy (Merigan *et al.*, 1989). Dideoxyinosine is being evaluated for its efficacy in the treatment of AIDS and is being used (at a uniquely early stage of its development) as an alternative to zidovudine for patients who have displayed unacceptable side effects with the latter drug. The adverse effects of dideoxyinosine have not been evaluated in detail, but pancreatitis and severe pain in the extremities have been observed in initial (phase 1) trials. Kaposi's sarcoma in patients with AIDS responds to interferon alfa (Groopman and Scadden, 1989).

Several other molecular targets for antiviral therapy are under active investigation. The *pol* gene in HIV-1 encodes three proteins—the reverse transcriptase, a self-cleaving protease that is required for processing the reverse transcriptase, and a nuclease that is essential for integration of viral DNA into the genome of the host cell. The *pol* gene is adjacent to a *gag* gene, and the products of the two genes are first expressed as a fusion protein. This fusion protein must be cleaved by the HIV protease. Inhibitors of the HIV protease have been developed with the aid of a crystal structure of the protein (Navia *et al.*, 1989); this protease represents a unique target for antiviral therapy. Other potential targets include the glycosylated envelope protein of HIV and the receptor protein (CD4) on the surface of lymphocytes to which the virus binds. A soluble form of CD4 can bind to the viral envelope protein and prevent the virus from entering cells. Alternatively, a conjugate of CD4 and a toxin might be used to attack HIV-infected cells, since such cells express the envelope protein on their surface (*see* Crumpacker, 1989).

Herpesviruses. Infection with herpes simplex virus type 1 causes disease of the mouth, face, skin, esophagus, or brain. Herpes simplex type 2 usually causes infections of the rectum, genital area, skin of the lower body, or meninges. In either case, the infection may be a primary one or disease can result from activation of a latent infection.

Herpes Simplex Virus 1. Primary, severe oral-labial herpes infections respond to acyclovir given orally or intravenously (Raborn *et al.*, 1987). Recurrent oral-labial lesions (fever blisters) may show moderate improvement when acyclovir is given orally (Spruance *et al.*, 1982).

Both vidarabine and acyclovir are effective in herpes simplex virus encephalitis (Skoldenberg *et al.*, 1984; Whitley *et al.*, 1986). Intravenous acyclovir (10 mg/kg every 8 hours for 10 days) was found to be superior to intravenous vidarabine (15 mg/kg per day for 10 days) in preventing death; survival rates were 81% and 46%, respectively. Acyclovir is now the preferred therapy, and vidarabine is reserved for patients who are unable to tolerate acyclovir. In addition to antiviral therapy, the age of the patient and the depth of coma at the time of initiation of therapy are correlated with the outcome.

Herpes simplex type-1 infections are usually more severe in patients whose cellular immune functions are impaired; a simple fever blister of the lip may progress to an invasive oral–pharyngeal necrotizing lesion, esophagitis, pneumonia, or disseminated disease. In such situations, intravenous acyclovir (5 to 10 mg/kg every 8 hours for 5 to 7 days) has been shown to be effective in severe chronic and recurrent mucocutaneous herpes. Healing time is shortened, as is the duration of pain and local symptoms and the period of time during which virus is shed (Wade *et al.*, 1982; Gold and Corey, 1987). Intravenous acyclovir can prevent the occurrence of herpes simplex infections in patients who have received bone marrow transplants (Saral *et al.*, 1981; Lundgren *et al.*, 1985); oral acyclovir may prevent subsequent recurrences of herpes simplex infections in such patients (Gluckman *et al.*, 1983; Wade *et al.*, 1984).

Herpes simplex virus type 1 also causes keratoconjunctivitis, a serious infection of the eye that can result in blindness. Trifluridine (one drop of a 1% solution every 2 hours), vidarabine (a 1.25-cm [½-in.] ribbon of 3% ointment five times daily), and idoxuridine (one drop of a 0.1% solution every 1 to 2 hours) are all effective when applied topically. Trifluridine is preferred because of greater efficacy and decreased toxicity (Kaufman, 1988).

Herpes Simplex Virus 2. This type of herpesvirus most commonly causes genital disease, but it may also be responsible for meningitis and extensive mucocutaneous disease in immunocompromised patients, particularly those with AIDS. Primary genital herpes can be treated with acyclovir. Therapy results in more rapid healing, reduction in viral titers, and more rapid disappearance of pain.

Topical application (5% ointment, five or six times daily for 10 days) can be used for mild-to-moderate disease (Corey *et al.*, 1982). Oral therapy (200 mg five times daily for 10 days) is much more effective and is currently the best regimen for initial treatment of genital herpes simplex viral infections (Bryson *et al.*, 1982; Nilsen *et al.*, 1982). There is a reduction in the formation of new lesions, a decrease in the duration of viral shedding, and a marked abatement of clinical symptoms in both sexes. Higher doses (400 mg five times daily for 10 days) are similarly effective for proctitis caused by herpes simplex virus (Rompalo *et al.*, 1988). Parenteral treatment is very effective but is reserved for severely ill patients who require hospitalization (Mindel *et al.*, 1982; Corey *et al.*, 1983).

Recurrence of genital herpes is not prevented by treatment of the primary disease with acyclovir. In recurrent herpes simplex genitalis, topical therapy is completely ineffective, whereas oral acyclovir has a beneficial effect on healing and the shedding of virus (Nilsen *et al.*, 1982; Reichman *et al.*, 1983). Oral administration of acyclovir (200 mg two to five times daily) has also been shown to prevent 90% of recurrences of genital herpes for up to 1 year, but infections recur at their former frequency when the drug is stopped (Douglas *et al.*, 1984; Gold and Corey, 1987; Mertz *et al.*, 1988).

Neonatal infections with herpes simplex virus are often severe and are characterized by progressive dissemination and death. Vidarabine (15 mg/kg per day for 10 days) decreases morbidity and mortality from 74% to 38%. Intravenous acyclovir (10 mg/kg every 8 hours for 10 days) also appears to be effective, but it is no more effective than vidarabine. There are as yet no data on the treatment of meningitis caused by herpes simplex type 2.

Varicella–Zoster Virus. In most children, varicella (chickenpox) is a mild disease that does not require therapy with an antiviral agent. Occasionally, it may be severe, especially in patients with immunological deficiencies. Both vidarabine (10 mg/kg intravenously per day for 5 days) and acyclovir (500 mg/m^2 for children or 10 mg/kg for adults intravenously every 8 hours for 7 days) cause a reduction in cutaneous lesions and fever and lower the incidence of visceral complications (Prober *et al.*, 1982; Nyerges *et al.*, 1988). Shingles, caused by varicella–zoster virus, is usually confined to one dermatome, and routine antiviral therapy is not recommended. Several studies have demonstrated that intravenous acyclovir (15 mg/kg per day) will reduce the duration of viral shedding, decrease erythema and pain, and accelerate healing (Bean *et al.*, 1982). However, there is no apparent effect on postherpetic neuralgia. High doses of acyclovir given orally (800 mg five times daily for 7 to 10 days) reduce pain and hasten healing, but this regimen also has no effect on postherpetic neuralgia (Cobo *et al.*, 1986; McKindrick *et al.*, 1986). Thus, use of acyclovir for varicella–zoster in the normal host should probably be reserved for patients with severe disease or involvement of the eye.

In patients with impaired cellular immune responses, varicella–zoster infection may be severe, with widespread dissemination to skin and vital organs. Studies have demonstrated that both vidarabine (10 mg/kg per day for 5 days) and acyclovir (10 mg/kg every 8 hours for 7 days or 500 mg/m^2 every 8 hours for 7 days) produce similar local beneficial effects and prevent dissemination to distant cutaneous and visceral sites (Peterslund *et al.*, 1981; Whitley *et al.*, 1982b; McGill *et al.*, 1983; Hayden and Douglas, 1990). One study found acyclovir to be superior to vidarabine in this regard (Shepp *et al.*, 1986). Interferon alfa is also effective (Ho, 1987). Sufficient data have now accumulated to recommend that acyclovir or vidarabine be administered intravenously to immunocompromised patients who are suffering from infections with varicella–zoster virus.

Cytomegalovirus. Infections with cytomegalovirus, although tolerated well by normal hosts, are common problems among immunocompromised patients, particularly recipients of transplants and patients with AIDS (Jacobson and Mills, 1988). Clinical manifestations include febrile states, leukopenia, myalgias, pneumonia, gastritis, hepatitis, colitis, retinitis, and adrenal necrosis.

Cytomegalovirus retinitis in patients with AIDS has been particularly troublesome, and it usually causes blindness (Bloom and Palestine, 1988). Both ganciclovir (5 mg/kg every 12 hours) and foscarnet (230 mg/kg daily) are effective in stabilizing or improving this condition in more than 85% of patients when administered for 2 weeks, although there has been considerably more experience with ganciclovir (Collaborative DHPG Treatment Study Group, 1986; Laskin *et al.*, 1987c; Walmsley *et al.*, 1988). The effectiveness of both drugs is limited by toxic effects: ganciclovir by leukopenia and foscarnet by renal insufficiency. As in most opportunistic infections in patients with AIDS, most relapse within 1 month; maintenance therapy is thus necessary.

Uncontrolled studies in patients with AIDS and colitis, wasting syndrome, pneumonia, or especially esophagitis suggest that these syndromes also respond to the intravenous administration of ganciclovir. By contrast, patients who have received bone marrow transplants and who have pneumonia caused by cytomegalovirus do not respond to ganciclovir. However, the combined use of ganciclovir and anticytomegalovirus immune globulin enhanced survival in two studies (Emanuel *et al.*, 1988; Reed *et al.*, 1988). Cytomegalovirus infections in renal transplant recipients have been prevented with interferon alfa (Spruance *et al.*, 1982).

Epstein–Barr Virus. Infectious mononucleosis is a self-limited infection, and antiviral drug therapy is not required. Several drugs are effective *in vitro* against Epstein–Barr virus, including acyclovir, vidarabine, and ganciclovir. Some, but not all, patients with severe infections caused by Epstein–Barr virus have responded to acyclovir given intravenously (Sullivan *et al.*, 1982). Oral hairy leukoplakia related to Epstein–Barr virus responds to acyclovir given orally (Resnick *et al.*, 1988). Chronic fatigue syndrome, which in some cases may be due to chronic infection with Epstein–Barr virus, does not respond to intravenous acyclovir (Straus *et al.*, 1988).

Hepatitis B. Chronic infection with hepatitis B virus may progress to cirrhosis and hepatic failure. Acyclovir, vidarabine, corticosteroids, and interferon alfa, alone and in combination, have been tested in clinical trials. Low doses of interferon alfa given for several months may produce a virological response, but clinical responses are observed only after therapy with combinations of interferon alfa plus corticosteroids or acyclovir (Hayden *et al.*, 1986b; Steele and Charlton, 1987). Further studies are needed.

Papillomavirus. Human papillomaviruses are responsible for laryngeal papillomas and genital warts, as well as the common wart and, probably, cervical cancer. Interferon alfa-2b given intralesionally is effective in about 60% of patients with condylomata acuminata (genital warts) that are refractory to conventional therapy (Knight *et al.*, 1981; Hall *et al.*, 1983; Taber *et al.*, 1983), and the drug is approved for such use. In extensive disease, intramuscular or subcutaneous therapy with interferon alfa may be required (Rodriguez *et al.*, 1987). At present, treatment with interferon alfa should be reserved for patients who do not respond adequately to conventional therapy, such as topical podophyllum or cryosurgery. Laryngeal papillomatosis also responds to the intramuscular or subcutaneous administration of interferon alfa. Adult-onset disease appears to respond better than does disease in children.

Influenza. Influenza viruses produce epidemics of severe respiratory and systemic diseases during the winter months of almost every year; these are most commonly due to a subtype of influenza A virus. Amantadine, given orally in doses of 200 mg daily, prevents both infection and illness from influenza A. It also results in reduction of fever and respiratory tract symptoms and shortens the duration of illness by about 50% when administered up to 48 hours after the onset of symptoms. The drug is not effective against influenza B virus.

Influenza virus vaccine remains the mainstay for prevention of this disease. Amantadine should be reserved for individuals at high risk who cannot receive vaccine because it is contraindicated or not available (Advisory Committee on Immunization Practices, 1988; Hayden and Douglas, 1990). In such cases, amantadine should be administered in daily doses of 200 mg (100 mg for those over 65 years of age) for the winter season or, preferably, for the duration of the epidemic (5 to 7 weeks) if public health information concerning epidemic influenza A is available. It should also be used for short-term prophylaxis (14 days) in conjunction with vaccine to provide prophylaxis during an epidemic until protective antibodies develop. Amantadine can abort nosocomial outbreaks of influenza if given to both patients and staff (Shields *et al.*, 1985; Atkinson *et al.*, 1986).

Treatment of established infection is especially important in patients at high risk for complications, including those with chronic cardiac or pulmonary disease, persons over 65 years of age, children receiving long-term therapy with aspirin (to prevent possible development of Reye's syndrome), and those with other underlying conditions. However, any person with acute symptomatic influenza A may benefit from treatment with amantadine (Kantor *et al.*, 1980).

Respiratory Syncytial Virus. Respiratory syncytial virus is the most important cause of pneumonia and bronchiolitis in infants. Treatment with ribavirin given in an aerosol results in a more rapid improvement in illness (*see* "Ribavirin," above). Because of the cost and difficulty in administration of the aerosol, this treatment should be reserved for hospitalized patients with moderately severe disease. More trials are needed to determine whether this treatment reduces mortality, duration of hospitalization, or the necessity for intubation.

Hemorrhagic Fevers. In patients with Lassa fever who are at high risk of death (high-titer viremia or elevated plasma activity of aspartate aminotransferase), administration of ribavirin (4 g per day intravenously) significantly reduces mortality, particularly if treatment is begun during the first 6 days of illness. Oral ribavirin is less effective. Ribavirin may also be effective in Korean and Argentinian hemorrhagic fevers.

Common Colds. Approximately 240 serologically distinct viruses cause common colds; the rhinoviruses, which are RNA picornaviruses, are common offenders. These are among the simplest viruses structurally, and the nucleotide sequence and three dimensional structure of one rhinovirus have been determined. Discrete hydrophobic pockets to which specific experimental drugs bind have been identified. These agents block disassembly of the virus and expression of viral RNA (Smith *et al.*, 1986).

There is no specific antiviral treatment for established colds. However, interferon alfa can prevent the acquisition of an infection with a rhinovirus (Colby *et al.*, 1980; Lin *et al.*, 1983). Other respiratory viral infections are not prevented, and long-term prophylaxis cannot be given because of local toxicity.

Abrams, D. I.; Kuno, S.; Wong, R.; Jeffords, K.; Nash, M.; Molaghan, J. B.; Gorter, R.; and Ueno, R. Oral dextran sulfate (UA001) in the treatment of the acquired immunodeficiency syndrome (AIDS) and AIDS-related complex. *Ann. Intern. Med.*, **1989**, *110*, 183–188.

Advisory Committee on Immunization Practices. Prevention and control of influenza. *MMWR*, **1988**, *37*, 361–373.

Alexander, G. J. M.; Fagan, E. A.; Daniels, H. M.; Brahm, J.; Smith, H. M.; Eddleston, A. L.; and Williams, R. Loss of HBsAg with interferon therapy in chronic hepatitis B virus infection. *Lancet,* **1987**, *2,* 66–69.

Aoki, F. Y., and Sitar, D. S. Amantadine kinetics in healthy elderly men: implications for influenza prevention. *Clin. Pharmacol. Ther.,* **1985**, *37,* 137–144.

Arden, N. H.; Patriarca, P. A.; Fasano, M. B.; Lui, K.-J.; Harmon, M. W.; Kendal, A. P.; and Rimland, D. The roles of vaccination and amantadine prophylaxis in controlling an outbreak of influenza A (H3N2) in a nursing home. *Arch. Intern. Med.,* **1988**, *148,* 865–868.

Atkinson, W. L.; Arden, N. H.; Patriarca, P. A.; Leslie, N.; Lui, K.-J.; and Gohd, R. Amantadine prophylaxis during an institutional outbreak of type A (H1N1) influenza. *Arch. Intern. Med.,* **1986**, *146,* 1751–1756.

Baba, M.; Pauwels, R.; Balzarini, J.; Herdewijn, P.; DeClercq, E.; and Dysmyter, J. Ribavirin antagonizes inhibitory effects of pyrimine 2′,3′-dideoxynucleosides but enhances inhibitory effects of purine 2′,3′-dideoxynucleosides on replication of human immunodeficiency virus *in vitro. Antimicrob. Agents Chemother.,* **1987**, *31,* 1613–1617.

Balfour, H. H., Jr., and others; Burroughs Wellcome Collaborative Acyclovir Study Group. Acyclovir halts progression of herpes zoster in immunocompromised patients. *N. Engl. J. Med.,* **1983**, *308,* 1448–1453.

Balis, F. M.; Pizzo, P. A.; Murphy, R. F.; Eddy, J.; Jarosinski, P. F.; Falloon, J.; Broder, S.; and Poplack, D. G. The pharmacokinetics of zidovudine administered by continuous infusion in children. *Ann. Intern. Med.,* **1989**, *110,* 279–285.

Bassendine, M. F.; Chadwick, R. G.; Salmeron, J.; Shipton, U.; Thomas, H. C.; and Sherlock, S. Adenine arabinoside therapy in HB_sAg-positive chronic liver disease: a controlled study. *Gastroenterology,* **1981**, *80,* 1016–1022.

Bean, B., and Aeppli, D. Adverse effects of high-dose intravenous acyclovir in ambulatory patients with acute herpes zoster. *J. Infect. Dis.,* **1985**, *151,* 362–364.

Bean, B.; Braun, C.; and Balfour, H. H., Jr. Acyclovir therapy for acute herpes zoster. *Lancet,* **1982**, *2,* 118–121.

Bernstein, D. I.; Reuman, P. D.; Sherwood, J. R.; Young, E. C.; and Schiff, G. M. Ribavirin small-particle-aerosol treatment of influenza B virus infection. *Antimicrob. Agents Chemother.,* **1988**, *32,* 761–764.

Betts, R. F.; Treanor, J. J.; Graman, P. S.; Bentley, D. W.; and Dolin, R. Antiviral agents to prevent or treat influenza in the elderly. *J. Resp. Dis.,* **1987**, *8,* Suppl. 11A, S56–S59.

Biron, K. K., and Elion, G. B. *In vitro* susceptibility of varicella-zoster virus to acyclovir. *Antimicrob. Agents Chemother.,* **1980**, *18,* 443–447.

Biron, K. K.; Stanat, S. C.; Sorrell, J. B.; Fyfe, J. A.; Keller, P. M.; Lambe, C. U.; and Nelson, D. J. Metabolic activation of the nucleoside analog 9-[2-hydroxy-1-(hydroxymethyl)ethoxy]methyl guanine in human diploid fibroblasts infected with human cytomegalovirus. *Proc. Natl. Acad. Sci. U.S.A.,* **1985**, *82,* 2473–2477.

Bloom, J. N., and Palestine, A. G. The diagnosis of cytomegalovirus retinitis. *Ann. Intern. Med.,* **1988**, *109,* 963–969.

Blum, R. M.; Liao, S. H. T.; and De Miranda, P. Overview of acyclovir pharmacokinetic disposition in adults and children. *Am. J. Med.,* **1982**, *73,* Suppl., 186–192.

Browne, M. J.; Moss, M. Y.; and Boyd, M. R. Comparative activity of amantadine and ribavirin against influenza virus *in vitro*: possible clinical relevance. *Antimicrob. Agents Chemother.,* **1983**, *23,* 503–505.

Bryson, Y. J.; Dillon, M.; Lovett, M.; Acuna, G.; Taylor, S.; Cherry, J. D.; Johnson, B. L.; Weismeier, E.; Growdon, W.; Creagh-Kirk, T.; and Keeney, R. Treatment of first episodes of genital herpes simplex virus infection with oral acyclovir: a randomized double-blind controlled trial in normal subjects. *N. Engl. J. Med.,* **1982**, *308,* 916–921.

Chatis, P. A.; Miller, C. H.; Schrager, L. E.; and Crumpacker, C. S. Successful treatment with foscarnet of an acyclovir-resistant mucocutaneous infection with herpes simplex virus in a patient with acquired immunodeficiency syndrome. *N. Engl. J. Med.,* **1989**, *320,* 297–300.

Cobo, L. M.; Foulks, G. N.; Liesegang, T.; Lass, J.; Sutphin, J. E.; Wilhelmus, K.; Jones, D. B.; Chapman, S.; Segretti, A. C.; and King, D. H. Oral acyclovir in the treatment of acute herpes zoster ophthalmicus. *Ophthalmology,* **1986**, *93,* 763–770.

Coen, D., and Schaffer, P. A. Two distinct loci confer resistance to acycloguanosine in herpes simplex virus type 1. *Am. J. Med.,* **1982**, *73* Suppl., 2265–2269.

Colby, B. M.; Shaw, J. E.; Elion, G. B.; and Pagano, J. S. Effect of acyclovir [9-(2-hydroxyethoxymethyl)-guanine] on Epstein-Barr virus DNA replication. *J. Virol.,* **1980**, *34,* 560–568.

Collaborative DHPG Treatment Study Group. Treatment of serious cytomegalovirus infections with 9-(1,3-dihydroxy-2-propoxymethyl) guanine in patients with AIDS and other immunodeficiencies. *N. Engl. J. Med.,* **1986**, *314,* 801–805.

Connor, J. D.; Hintz, M.; Van Dyke, R.; McCormick, J. B.; and McIntosh, K. Ribavirin pharmacokinetics in children and adults during therapeutic trials. In, *Clinical Applications of Ribavirin.* (Smith, R. A.; Knight, V.; and Smith, J. A. D.; eds.) Academic Press, Orlando, Fla., **1984**, pp. 107–123.

Corey, L.; Fife, K. H.; Benedetti, J. K.; Winter, C. A.; Fahnlander, A.; Connor, J. D.; Hintz, M. A.; and Holmes, K. K. Intravenous acyclovir for the treatment of primary genital herpes. *Ann. Intern. Med.,* **1983**, *93,* 914–921.

Corey, L., and Holmes, K. K. Genital herpes simplex virus infections: current concepts in diagnosis, therapy, and prevention. *Ann. Intern. Med.,* **1983**, *98,* 973–983.

Corey, L.; Nahmias, A. J.; Guinan, M. E.; Benedetti, J. K.; Critchlow, C. W.; and Holmes, K. K. A trial of topical acyclovir in genital herpes simplex virus infections. *N. Engl. J. Med.,* **1982**, *306,* 1313–1319.

Couch, R. B., and Six, H. R. The antiviral spectrum and mechanism of action of amantadine and rimantadine. In, *Antiviral Chemotherapy: New Directions for Clinical Applications and Research.* (Mills, J., and Corey, L., eds.) Elsevier, New York, **1986**, pp. 50–57.

Crumpacker, C., and others. Ribavirin treatment of the acquired immunodeficiency syndrome (AIDS) and the acquired-immunodeficiency-syndrome-related complex (ARC). A phase 1 study shows transient clinical improvement associated with suppression of the human immunodeficiency virus and enhanced lymphocyte proliferation. *Ann. Intern. Med.,* **1987**, *107,* 664–674.

Dalakas, M. C.; Yarchoan, R.; Spitzer, R.; Elder, G.; and Sever, J. L. Treatment of human immunodeficiency virus-related polyneuropathy with 3′-azido-2′,3′-dideoxythymidine. *Ann. Neurol.,* **1988**, *23,* S92–S94.

Davis, G. L., and Hoofnagle, J. H. Interferon in viral hepatitis: role in pathogenesis and treatment. *Hepatology,* **1986**, *6,* 1038–1041.

Davtyan, D. G., and Vinters, H. V. Wernicke's encephalopathy in AIDS patient treated with zidovudine. *Lancet,* **1987**, *1,* 919–920.

De Miranda, P.; Good, S. S.; Krasny, H. C.; Connor, J. D.; Laskin, O. L.; and Lietman, P. S. Metabolic fate of radioactive acyclovir in humans. *Am. J. Med.,* **1982**, *73,* Suppl., 215–220.

Dinarello, C. A.; Cannon, J. G.; and Wolff, S. M. New concepts on the pathogenesis of fever. *Rev. Infect. Dis.,* **1988**, *10,* 168–189.

Dolin, R.; Reichman, R. C.; Madore, H. P.; Maynard, R.; Linton, P. N.; and Webber-Jones, J. A controlled trial of amantadine and rimantadine in the prophylaxis of influenza A infection. *N. Engl. J. Med.*, **1982**, *307*, 580–584.

Dorsky, D. I., and Crumpacker, C. S. Drugs five years later: acyclovir. *Ann. Intern. Med.*, **1987**, *107*, 859–874.

Douglas, J. M.; Crichlow, C.; Benedetti, J.; Mertz, G. J.; Connor, J. D.; Hintz, M. A.; Fahnlander, A.; Remington, M.; Winter, C.; and Corey, L. A double-blind study of oral acyclovir for suppression of recurrences of genital herpes simplex virus infection. *N. Engl. J. Med.*, **1984**, *310*, 1551–1556.

Douglas, J. M., Jr.; Davis, L. G.; Remington, M. L.; Paulsen, C. A.; Perrin, E. B.; Goodman, P.; Connor, J. D.; King, D.; and Corey, L. A double-blind, placebo-controlled trial of the effect of chronically administered oral acyclovir on sperm production in men with frequently recurrent genital herpes. *J. Infect. Dis.*, **1988**, *157*, 588–593.

Douglas, R. B.; Moore, B. W.; Miles, H. B.; Davies, L. M.; Graham, N. M. H.; Ryan, P.; Worswick, D. A.; and Albrecht, J. K. Prophylactic efficacy of intranasal $alpha_2$-interferon against rhinovirus infections in the family setting. *N. Engl. J. Med.*, **1986**, *314*, 65–70.

Emanuel, D., and others. Cytomegalovirus pneumonia after bone marrow transplantation successfully treated with the combination of ganciclovir and high-dose intravenous immune globulin. *Ann. Intern. Med.*, **1988**, *109*, 777–782.

Erice, A.; Chou, S.; Biron, K. K.; Stanat, S. C.; Balfour, H. H.; and Jordan, M. C. Progressive disease due to ganciclovir-resistant cytomegalovirus in immunocompromised patients. *N. Engl. J. Med.*, **1989**, *320*, 289–293.

Erlich, K. S.; Jacobson, M. A.; Koehler, J. E.; Follansbee, S. E.; Drennan, D. P.; Gooze, L.; Safrin, S.; and Mills, J. Foscarnet therapy for severe acyclovir-resistant herpes simplex virus type-2 infections in patients with the acquired immunodeficiency syndrome (AIDS): an uncontrolled trial. *Ann. Intern. Med.*, **1989a**, *110*, 710–713.

Erlich, K. S.; Mills, J.; Chatis, P.; Mertz, G. J.; Busch, D. F.; Follansbee, S. E.; Grant, B. S.; and Crumpacker, C. S. Acyclovir-resistant herpes simplex virus infections in patients with the acquired immunodeficiency syndrome. *N. Engl. J. Med.*, **1989b**, *320*, 293–296.

Eron, L. J., and others. Interferon therapy for condylomata acuminata. *N. Engl. J. Med.*, **1986**, *315*, 1059–1064.

Feldman, S., and Lott, L. Varicella in children with cancer: impact of antiviral therapy and prophylaxis. *Pediatrics*, **1987**, *80*, 465–472.

Feldman, S.; Robertson, P. K.; Lott, L.; and Thornton, D. Neurotoxicity due to adenine arabinoside therapy during varicella-zoster virus infections in immunocompromised children. *J. Infect. Dis.*, **1986**, *154*, 889–893.

Field, A. K.; Davies, M. E.; DeWitt, C.; Perry, H. C.; Liou, R.; Germershausen, J.; Karkas, J. D.; Ashton, W. T.; Johnston, D. B. R.; and Tolman, R. L. 9-[2-Hydroxy-1-(hydroxymethyl)ethoxy]methyl guanine: a selective inhibitor of herpes group virus replication. *Proc. Natl. Acad. Sci. U.S.A.*, **1983**, *80*, 4139–4143.

Field, H.; McMillan, A.; and Darby, G. The sensitivity of acyclovir-resistant mutants of herpes simplex virus to other antiviral drugs. *J. Infect. Dis.*, **1981**, *143*, 281–284.

Field, H. J. The problem of drug-induced resistance in viruses. In, *Problems of Antiviral Therapy: The Fifth Beecham Colloquium*. (Stuart-Harris, C. H., and Oxford, J. S., eds.) Academic Press, London, **1983**, pp. 71–107.

Fischl, M. A., and others. The efficacy of azidothymidine (AZT) in the treatment of patients with AIDS and AIDS-related complex. *N. Engl. J. Med.*, **1987**, *317*, 185–191.

Friedman, H. M., and Grasela, T. Adenine arabinoside and allopurinol—possible adverse drug interaction. *N. Engl. J. Med.*, **1981**, *304*, 423.

Friedman-Kien, A. E.; Eron, L. J.; Conant, M.; Growdon, W.; Badiak, H.; Bradstreet, P. W.; Fedorczyk, D.; Trout, J. R.; and Plasse, T. F. Natural interferon alfa for treatment of condylomata acuminata. *J.A.M.A.*, **1988**, *259*, 533–538.

Furman, P. A., and others. Phosphorylation of 3′-azido-3′-deoxythymidine and selective interaction of the 5′-triphosphate with human immunodeficiency virus reverse transcriptase. *Proc. Natl. Acad. Sci. U.S.A.*, **1986**, *83*, 8333–8337.

Furman, P. A.; St. Clair, M. H.; and Spector, T. Acyclovir triphosphate is a suicidal inactivator of the herpes simplex virus DNA polymerase. *J. Biol. Chem.*, **1984**, *259*, 9575–9579.

Gephart, J. F., and Lerner, A. M. Comparison of the effects of arabinosyladenine, arabinosylhypoxanthine, and arabinosyladenine 5′-monophosphate against herpes simplex virus, varicella-zoster virus, and cytomegalovirus with their effects on cellular deoxyribonucleic acid synthesis. *Antimicrob. Agents Chemother.*, **1981**, *19*, 170–178.

Gilbert, B. E., and Knight, V. Minireview: biochemistry and clinical applications of ribavirin. *Antimicrob. Agents Chemother.*, **1986**, *30*, 201–205.

Gill, P. S.; Rarick, M.; Brynes, R. K.; Causey, D.; Loureiro, C.; and Levine, A. M. Azidothymidine associated with bone marrow failure in the acquired immunodeficiency syndrome (AIDS). *Ann. Intern. Med.*, **1987**, *107*, 502–505.

Gluckman, E.; Devergie, A.; Melo, R.; Nebout, T.; Lotsberg, J.; Zhao, X. M.; Gomez-Morales, M.; Mazeron, M. C.; and Perol, Y. Prophylaxis of herpes infections after bone-marrow transplantation by oral acyclovir. *Lancet*, **1983**, *2*, 706–708.

Gold, D., and Corey, L. Acyclovir prophylaxis for herpes simplex virus infections. *Antimicrob. Agents Chemother.*, **1987**, *31*, 361–367.

Greenberg, S. B. Human interferon in viral diseases. *Infect. Dis. Clin. North Am.*, **1987**, *1*, 383–423.

Groopman, J. E., and Scadden, D. T. Interferon therapy for Kaposi sarcoma associated with the acquired immunodeficiency syndrome (AIDS). *Ann. Intern. Med.*, **1989**, *110*, 335–337.

Hall, C. B.; McBride, J. T.; Gala, C. L.; Hildreth, S. W.; and Schnabel, K. C. Ribavirin treatment of respiratory syncytial infection in infants with underlying cardiopulmonary disease. *J.A.M.A.*, **1985**, *254*, 3047–3051.

Hall, C. B.; McBride, J. T.; Walsh, E. E.; Bell, D. M.; Gala, C.; Hildreth, S.; TenEyck, L. G.; and Hall, W. J. Aerosolized ribavirin treatment of infants with respiratory syncytial viral infection. *N. Engl. J. Med.*, **1983**, *308*, 1443.

Hammer, S. M., and Gillis, J. M. Synergistic activity of granulocyte-macrophage colony-stimulating factor and 3′-azido-3′-deoxythimidine against human immunodeficiency virus *in vitro*. *Antimicrob. Agents Chemother.*, **1987**, *31*, 1046–1050.

Hayden, F. G.; Albrecht, J. K.; Kaiser, D. L.; and Gwaltney, J. M., Jr. Prevention of natural colds by contact prophylaxis with intranasal $alpha_2$-interferon. *N. Engl. J. Med.*, **1986a**, *314*, 71–75.

Hayden, F. G.; Cote, K. M.; and Douglas, R. G., Jr. Plaque inhibition assay for drug susceptibility testing of influenza viruses. *Antimicrob. Agents Chemother.*, **1980**, *17*, 865–870.

Hayden, F. G.; Minocha, A.; Spyker, D. A.; and Hoffman, H. E. Comparative single-dose pharmacokinetics of amantadine hydrochloride and rimantadine hydrochloride in young and elderly adults. *Antimicrob. Agents Chemother.*, **1985**, *28*, 216.

Henderly, D. E.; Freeman, W. R.; Causey, D. M.; and Rao, N. A. Cytomegalovirus retinitis and response to therapy with ganciclovir. *Ophthalmology*, **1987**, *94*, 425–434.

Hintz, M.; Connor, J. D.; Spector, S. A.; Blum, M. R.; Keeney, R. E.; and Yeager, A. S. Neonatal acyclovir pharmacokinetics in patients with herpes virus infections. *Am. J. Med.*, **1982**, *73*, Suppl., 210–214.

Ho, M. Interferon for the treatment of infections. *Annu. Rev. Med.*, **1987**, *38*, 51–59.

Horwitz, J. P.; Chua, J.; and Noel, M. Nucleosides 5. The monomesylates of 1-(2′-deoxy-β-D-lyxofuranosyl)thymine. *J. Org. Chem.*, **1964**, *29*, 2076–2080.

Hruska, J. F.; Bernstein, J. M.; Douglas, R. G., Jr.; and Hall, C. B. Effects of ribavirin on respiratory syncytial virus *in vitro*. *Antimicrob. Agents Chemother.*, **1980**, *17*, 770–775.

Jackson, G. G.; Paul, D. A.; Falk, L. A.; Rubenis, M.; Despotes, J. C.; Mack, D.; Knigge, M.; and Emeson, E. E. Human immunodeficiency virus (HIV) antigenemic (p24) in the acquired immunodeficiency syndrome (AIDS) and the effect of treatment with zidovudine (AZT). *Ann. Intern. Med.*, **1988**, *108*, 175–180.

Jacobson, M. A., and Mills, J. Serious cytomegalovirus disease in the acquired immunodeficiency syndrome (AIDS). *Ann. Intern. Med.*, **1988**, *108*, 585–594.

Kantor, R. J.; Stevens, D.; Potts, D. W.; and Noble, G. R. Prevention of influenza A/USSR/77 (H1N1): an evaluation of the side effects and efficacy of amantadine in recruits at Fort Sam Houston. *Milit. Med.*, **1980**, *145*, 312–315.

Kaufman, H. E. The treatment of herpetic eye infections with trifluridine and other antivirals. In, *Clinical Use of Antiviral Drugs*. (DeClercq, E., ed.) Martinus Nijhoff, Norwell, Mass., **1988**, pp. 25–38.

Keeney, R. E.; Kirk, L. E.; and Bridgen, D. Acyclovir tolerance in humans. *Am. J. Med.*, **1983**, *75*, Suppl., 176–181.

Klecker, R. W., Jr.; Collins, J. M.; Yarchoan, R.; Thomas, R.; Jenkins, J. F.; Broder, S.; and Myers, C. E. Plasma and cerebrospinal fluid pharmacokinetics of 3′-azido-3′-deoxythymidine: a novel pyrimidine analog with potential application for the treatment of patients with AIDS and related diseases. *Clin. Pharmacol. Ther.*, **1987**, *41*, 407–412.

Knight, V., and Gilbert, B. E. Ribavirin aerosol treatment of influenza. *Infect. Dis. Clin. North Am.*, **1987**, *1*, 441–457.

Knight, V.; Wilson, S. Z.; Quarles, J. M.; Greggs, S. E.; McClung, H. W.; Waters, B. K.; Cameron, R. W.; Zerwas, J. M.; and Couch, R. B. Ribavirin small-particle aerosol treatment of influenza. *Lancet*, **1981**, *2*, 945–949.

Knight, V.; Yu, C. P.; Gilbert, B. E.; and Divine, G. W. Estimating the dosage of ribavirin aerosol according to age and other variables. *J. Infect. Dis.*, **1988**, *158*, 443–448.

Kotler, D. P.; Culpepper-Morgan, J. A.; Tierney, A. R.; and Klein, E. B. Treatment of disseminated cytomegalovirus infection with 9-(1,3 dihydroxy-2-propoxymethyl)guanine: evidence of prolonged survival in patients with acquired immunodeficiency syndrome. *AIDS Res.*, **1986**, *2*, 299–308.

Lang, D. J., and Cheung, K.-S. Effectiveness of acycloguanosine and trifluorothymidine as inhibitors of cytomegalovirus infection *in vitro*. *Am. J. Med.*, **1982**, *73*, Suppl., 49–53.

Larder, B. A.; Darby, G.; and Richman, D. D. HIV with reduced sensitivity to zidovudine (AZT) isolated during prolonged therapy. *Science*, **1989**, *243*, 1731–1734.

Laskin, O. L. Clinical pharmacokinetics of acyclovir. *Clin. Pharmacokinet.*, **1983**, *8*, 187–201.

Laskin, O. L.; Cederberg, D. M.; Mills, J.; Eron, L. J.; Mildvan, D.; and Spector, S. A. Ganciclovir for the treatment and suppression of serious infections caused by cytomegalovirus. *Am. J. Med.*, **1987a**, *83*, 201–207.

Laskin, O. L.; Longstreth, J. A.; Hart, C. C.; Scavuzzo, D.; Kalman, C. M.; Connor, J. D.; and Roberts, R. B. Ribavirin disposition in high-risk patients for acquired immunodeficiency syndrome. *Clin. Pharmacol. Ther.*, **1987b**, *41*, 546–555.

Laskin, O. L.; Longstreth, J. A.; Whelton, A.; Krasny, H. C.; Keeney, R. E.; Rocco, L.; and Lietman, P. S. Effect of renal failure on the pharmacokinetics of acyclovir. *Am. J. Med.*, **1982**, *73*, Suppl., 197–201.

Laskin, O. L.; Stahl-Bayliss, C. M.; Kalman, C. M.; and Rosecan, L. R. Use of ganciclovir to treat serious cytomegalovirus infections in patients with AIDS. *J. Infect. Dis.*, **1987c**, *155*, 323–327.

Lin, J.-C.; Smith, M. C.; Cheng, Y. C.; and Pagano, J. S. Epstein–Barr virus: inhibition of replication by three new drugs. *Science*, **1983**, *221*, 578–579.

Lundgren, G.; Wilczek, H.; Lonnqvist, B.; Lindholm, A.; Wahren, B.; and Ringden, O. Acyclovir prophylaxis in bone marrow transplant recipients. *Scand. J. Infect. Dis.*, **1985**, *47*, 137–144.

McCormick, J. B.; King, I. J.; Webb, P. A.; Scribner, C. L.; Craven, R. B.; Johnson, K. M.; Elliott, L. H.; and Belmont-Williams, R. Lassa fever: effective therapy with ribavirin. *N. Engl. J. Med.*, **1986**, *314*, 20–26.

McDonald, E. M.; Mann, A. H.; and Thomas, H. C. Interferons as mediators of psychiatric morbidity. *Lancet*, **1987**, *2*, 1175–1178.

McGill, J.; MacDonald, D. R.; Fall, C.; McKendrick, G. D. W.; and Copplestone, A. Intravenous acyclovir in acute herpes zoster infection. *J. Infect.*, **1983**, *6*, 157–161.

McGuirt, P. V., and Furman, P. A. Acyclovir inhibition of viral DNA chain elongation in herpes simplex virus-infected cells. *Am. J. Med.*, **1982**, *73*, Suppl., 67–71.

McKindrick, M. W.; McGill, J. I.; White, J. E.; and Wood, M. J. Oral acyclovir in acute herpes zoster. *Br. Med. J.* [*Clin. Res.*], **1986**, *293*, 1529–1532.

Maxwell, E. Treatment of herpes keratitis with 5-iodo-2-deoxyuridine (IDU): a clinical evaluation of 1500 cases. *Am. J. Ophthalmol.*, **1963**, *56*, 571–573.

Merigan, T. C., and others. Circulating p24 antigen levels and responses to dideoxycytidine in human immunodeficiency virus (HIV) infections. *Ann. Intern. Med.*, **1989**, *110*, 189–194.

Mertz, G. J. Diagnosis and treatment of genital herpes infections. *Infect. Dis. Clin. North Am.*, **1987**, *1*, 341–366.

Mertz, G. J.; Jones, C. C.; Mills, J.; Fife, K. H.; Lemon, S. M.; Stapleton, J. T.; Hill, E. L.; Davis, G.; and the Acyclovir Study Group. Long-term acyclovir suppression of frequently recurring genital herpes simplex virus infection. *J.A.M.A.*, **1988**, *260*, 201–206.

Meyers, J. D., and others. Prophylactic use of human leukocyte interferon after allogeneic marrow transplantation. *Ann. Intern. Med.*, **1987**, *107*, 809–816.

Mindel, A.; Adler, M. W.; Sutherland, S.; and Fiddian, A. P. Intravenous acyclovir treatment for primary genital herpes. *Lancet*, **1982**, *1*, 697–700.

Mitsuya, H., and Broder, S. Strategies for antiviral therapy in AIDS. *Nature*, **1987**, *325*, 773–778.

Mitsuya, H.; Weinhold, K. J.; Furman, P. A.; St. Clair, M. H.; Lehrman, S. N.; Gallo, R. C.; Bolognesi, D.; Barry, D. W.; and Broder, S. 3′-Azido-3′-deoxythymidine (BW A509U): an antiviral agent that inhibits the infectivity and cytopathic effect of human T-lymphotrophic virus type III/lymphadenopathy-associated virus *in vitro*. *Proc. Natl. Acad. Sci. U.S.A.*, **1985**, *82*, 7096–7100.

Navia, M. A.; Fitzgerald, P. M.; McKeever, B. M.; Leu, C. T.; Heimbach, J. C.; Herber, W. K.; Sigal, I. S.;

Darke, P. L.; and Springer, J. P. Three-dimensional structure of aspartyl protease from human immunodeficiency virus HIV-1. *Nature,* **1989,** *337,* 615–620.
Nilsen, A. E.; Aasen, T.; Halsos, A. M.; Kinge, B. R.; Tiotta, E. A.; Wikström, K.; and Fiddian, A. P. Efficacy of oral acyclovir in the treatment of initial and recurrent genital herpes. *Lancet,* **1982,** *2,* 571–573.
Nyerges, G.; Meszner, Z.; Gyarmati, E.; and Kerpel-Fronius, S. Acyclovir prevents dissemination of varicella in immunocompromised children. *J. Infect. Dis.,* **1988,** *157,* 309–313.
Oksenhendler, E.; Bierling, P.; Ferchal, F.; Clauvel, J. P.; and Seligmann, M. Zidovudine for thrombocytopenic purpura related to human immunodeficiency virus (HIV) infection. *Ann. Intern. Med.,* **1989,** *110,* 365–368.
Ostertag, W.; Roesler, G.; Krieg, C. J.; Kind, J.; Cole, T.; Crozier, T.; Gaedicke, G.; Steinheider, G.; Kluge, N.; and Dube, S. Induction of endogenous virus and of thymidine kinase by bromodeoxyuridine in cell cultures transformed by Friend virus. *Proc. Natl. Acad. Sci. U.S.A.,* **1974,** *71,* 4980–4985.
Pavan-Langston, D. R. Ocular viral diseases. In, *Antiviral Agents and Viral Diseases of Man,* 2nd ed. (Galasso, G. J.; Merigan, T. C.; and Buchanan, R. A.; eds.) Raven Press, New York, **1984,** pp. 207–245.
Pelling, J. C.; Drach, J. C.; and Shipman, C., Jr. Internucleotide incorporation of arabinosyladenine into herpes simplex virus and mammalian cell DNA. *Virology,* **1981,** *109,* 323–335.
Pemberton, R. M.; Jennings, R.; Potter, C. W.; and Oxford, J. S. Amantadine resistance in clinical influenza A (H3N2) and (H1N1) virus isolates. *J. Antimicrob. Chemother.,* **1986,** *18,* Suppl. B, 135–140.
Pestka, S.; Langer, J. A.; Zoon, K. C.; and Samuel, S. A. Interferons and their actions. *Annu. Rev. Biochem.,* **1987,** *56,* 727–777.
Peterslund, N. A.; Ipsen, J.; Schonheyder, H.; Seyer-Hansen, K.; Esmann, V.; and Juhl, H. Acyclovir in herpes zoster. *Lancet,* **1981,** *2,* 827–830.
Prober, C. G.; Kirk, L. E.; and Keeney, R. E. Acyclovir therapy of chickenpox in immunosuppressed children—a collaborative study. *J. Pediatr.,* **1982,** *101,* 622–625.
Prusoff, W. H. Idoxuridine or how it all began. In, *Clinical Use of Antiviral Drugs.* (DeClercq, E., ed.) Martinus Nijhoff, Norwell, Mass., **1988,** pp. 15–24.
Raborn, G. W.; McGaw, W. T.; Grace, M.; Tyrrell, L. D.; and Samuels, S. M. Oral acyclovir and herpes labialis: a randomized, double-blind, placebo-controlled study. *J. Am. Dent. Assoc.,* **1987,** *115,* 38–42.
Reed, E. C.; Bowden, R. A.; Dandliker, P. S.; Lilleby, K. E.; and Meyers, J. D. Treatment of cytomegalovirus pneumonia with ganciclovir and intravenous cytomegalovirus immunoglobin in patients with bone marrow transplants. *Ann. Intern. Med.,* **1988,** *109,* 783–788.
Reichman, R. C., and others. Patient-initiated therapy of recurrent herpes simplex genitalis with orally administered acyclovir. *Clin. Res.,* **1983,** *31,* 373A.
Resnick, L.; Herbst, J. S.; Ablashi, C. V.; Atherton, S.; Frank, B.; Rosen, L.; and Horwitz, S. N. Regression of oral hairy leukoplakia after orally administered acyclovir therapy. *J.A.M.A.,* **1988,** *259,* 384–388.
Richman, D. D., and others. The toxicity of azidothymidine (AZT) in the treatment of patients with AIDS and AIDS-related complex. *N. Engl. J. Med.,* **1987,** *317,* 192–197.
Roberts, R. B.; Laskin, O. L.; Laurence, J.; Scavuzzo, D.; Murray, H. W.; Kim, Y. T.; and Connor, J. D. Ribavirin pharmacodynamics in high-risk patients for acquired immunodeficiency syndrome. *Clin. Pharmacol. Ther.,* **1987,** *42,* 365–373.
Rodriguez, W. J.; Kim, H. W.; Brandt, C. D.; Fink, R. J.; Getson, P. R.; Arrobio, J.; Murphy, T. M.; McCarthy, V.; and Parrott, R. H. Aerosolized ribavirin in the treatment of patients with respiratory syncytial virus disease. *Pediatr. Infect. Dis. J.,* **1987,** *6,* 159–163.
Rompalo, A. M.; Mertz, G. J.; Davis, L. G.; Benedetti, J.; Critchlow, C.; Stamm, W. E.; and Corey, L. Oral acyclovir for treatment of first-episode herpes simplex virus proctitis. *J.A.M.A.,* **1988,** *259,* 2879–2881.
Saral, R.; Burns, W. H.; Laskin, O. L.; Santos, G. W.; and Lietman, P. S. Acyclovir prophylaxis of herpes simplex virus infections. *N. Engl. J. Med.,* **1981,** *305,* 63–67.
Sawyer, M. H.; Webb, D. E.; Balow, J. E.; and Straus, S. E. Acyclovir-induced renal failure: clinical course and histology. *Am. J. Med.,* **1988,** *84,* 1067–1071.
Schnipper, L. E., and Crumpacker, C. S. Resistance of herpes simplex virus to acycloguanosine: role of viral thymidine kinase and DNA polymerase loci. *Proc. Natl. Acad. Sci. U.S.A.,* **1980,** *77,* 2270–2273.
Shepp, D. H.; Dandliker, P. S.; and Meyers, J. D. Treatment of varicella–zoster virus infection in severely immunocompromised patients. *N. Engl. J. Med.,* **1986,** *314,* 208–212.
Shields, W. D.; Lake, J. L.; and Chugani, H. T. Amantadine in the treatment of refractory epilepsy in childhood: an open trial in 10 patients. *Neurology,* **1985,** *35,* 579.
Skoldenberg, B., and others. Acyclovir versus vidarabine in herpes simplex encephalitis. *Lancet,* **1984,** *2,* 707–711.
Smee, D. F.; Boehme, R.; Chernow, M.; Binko, B.; and Matthews, T. R. Intracellular metabolism and enzymatic phosphorylation of 9-(1,3-dihydroxy-2-propoxymethyl) guanine and acyclovir in herpes simplex virus-infected and uninfected cells. *Biochem. Pharmacol.,* **1985,** *34,* 1049–1056.
Smith, T. J.; Kremer, M. J.; Luo, M.; Vriend, G.; Arnold, E.; Kamer, G.; Rossmann, M. G.; McKinlay, M. A.; Diana, G. D.; and Otto, M. J. The site of attachment in human rhinovirus 14 for antiviral agents that inhibit uncoating. *Science,* **1986,** *233,* 1286–1293.
Spector, S. A.; Tyndall, M.; and Kelly, E. Inhibition of human cytomegalovirus by trifluorothymidine. *Antimicrob. Agents Chemother.,* **1983,** *23,* 133.
Spruance, S. L., and others. Treatment of herpes simplex labialis with topical acyclovir in polyethylene glycol. *J. Infect. Dis.,* **1982,** *146,* 85.
Steele, R. W., and Charlton, R. K. Immune modulators as antiviral agents. In, *Clinics in Laboratory Medicine,* Vol. 7. (Drew, W. L., ed.) W. B. Saunders, Philadelphia, **1987,** pp. 911–924.
Straus, S. E.; Dale, J. K.; Tobi, M.; Lawley, T.; Preble, O.; Blaese, M.; Hallahan, C.; and Henle, W. Acyclovir treatment of the chronic fatigue syndrome: lack of efficacy in a placebo-controlled trial. *N. Engl. J. Med.,* **1988,** *319,* 1692–1698.
Sullivan, J. L.; Bryon, K. S.; Brewster, F. E.; Sakamoto, K.; Shaw, J. E.; and Pagano, J. S. Treatment of life-threatening Epstein-Barr virus infections with acyclovir. *Am. J. Med.,* **1982,** *73,* Suppl., 262–266.
Surbone, A., and others. Treatment of the acquired immunodeficiency syndrome (AIDS) and AIDS-related complex with a regimen of 3′-azido-2′,3′-dideoxythymidine (azidothymidine or zidovudine) and acyclovir. *Ann. Intern. Med.,* **1988,** *108,* 534–540.
Sylvester, R. K.; Ogden, W. B.; Draxler, C. A.; and Lewis, F. B. Vesicular eruption. *J.A.M.A.,* **1986,** *255,* 385–386.
Taber, L. H.; Knight, V.; Gilbert, B. E.; McClung, H. W.; Wilson, S. Z.; Norton, J.; Thurson, J. M.; Gordon, W. H.; Atmar, R. L.; and Schlaudt, W. R. Ribavirin aerosol treatment of bronchiolitis associated with respiratory syncytial virus infection in infants. *Pediatrics,* **1983,** *72,* 613.
Tominack, R. L., and Hayden, F. G. Rimantadine hydro-

chloride and amantadine hydrochloride use in influenza A virus infections. *Infect. Dis. Clin. North Am.*, **1987**, *1*, 459–478.
Wade, J. C., and Meyers, J. D. Neurologic symptoms associated with parenteral acyclovir treatment after marrow transplantation. *Ann. Intern. Med.*, **1983**, *98*, 921–925.
Wade, J. C.; Newton, B.; Flournoy, N.; and Meyers, J. D. Oral acyclovir for prevention of herpes simplex virus reactivation after marrow transplantation. *Ann. Intern. Med.*, **1984**, *100*, 823–828.
Wade, J. C.; Newton, B.; McLaren, C.; Flournoy, N.; Keeney, R. E.; and Meyers, J. D. Intravenous acyclovir to treat mucocutaneous herpes simplex virus infection after marrow transplantation. *Ann. Intern. Med.*, **1982**, *96*, 265.
Walker, R. E.; Parker, R. I.; Kovacs, J. A.; Masur, H.; Lane, H. C.; Carleton, S.; Kirk, L. E.; Gralnick, H. R.; and Fauci, A. S. Anemia and erythropoiesis in patients with the acquired immunodeficiency syndrome (AIDS) and Kaposi sarcoma treated with zidovudine. *Ann. Intern. Med.*, **1988**, *108*, 372–376.
Walmsley, S. L.; Chew, E.; Read, S. E.; Vellend, H.; Salit, I.; Rachlis, A.; and Fanning, M. M. Treatment of cytomegalovirus retinitis with trisodium phosphonoformate hexahydrate (foscarnet). *J. Infect. Dis.*, **1988**, *157*, 569–572.
Webster, R. G.; Kawaoka, Y.; Bean, W. J.; Beard, C. W.; and Brugh, M. Chemotherapy and vaccination: a possible strategy for the control of highly virulent influenza virus. *J. Virol.*, **1985**, *55*, 173–176.
Weck, P. K.; Brandsma, J. L.; and Whisnant, J. K. Interferons in the treatment of human papillomavirus diseases. *Cancer Metastasis Rev.*, **1986**, *5*, 139–165.
Whitaker-Dowling, P., and Youngner, J. S. Antiviral effects of interferon in different virus-host cell systems. In, *Mechanisms of Interferon Actions*, Vol. 1. (Pfeffer, L. M., ed.) CRC Press, Boca Raton, Fla., **1987**, pp. 83–98.
Whitley, R.; Alford, C.; Hess, F.; and Buchanan, R. Vidarabine: a preliminary review of its pharmacological properties and therapeutic use. *Drugs*, **1980**, *20*, 267–282.
Whitley, R. J., and others and the NIAID Collaborative Antiviral Study Group. Vidarabine therapy of varicella in immunosuppressed patients. *J. Pediatr.*, **1982a**, *101*, 125–131.
———. Early vidarabine therapy to control the complications of herpes zoster in immunosuppressed patients. *N. Engl. J. Med.*, **1982b**, *307*, 971–975.
———. Vidarabine therapy of mucocutaneous herpes simplex virus infections in the immunocompromised host. *J. Infect. Dis.*, **1984**, *149*, 1.
———. Vidarabine versus acyclovir therapy in herpes simplex encephalitis. *N. Engl. J. Med.*, **1986**, *314*, 144–149.
WHO. Current status of amantadine and rimantadine as anti-influenza-A agents. Bull. WHO, **1985**, *63*, 51.
Williams, S. J.; Baird-Lambert, J. A.; and Farrell, G. C. Inhibition of theophylline metabolism by interferon. *Lancet*, **1987**, *2*, 939–941.
Wills, R. J.; Farolino, D. A.; Choma, N.; and Keigher, N. Rimantadine pharmacokinetics after single and multiple doses. *Antimicrob. Agents Chemother.*, **1987**, *31*, 826–828.
Wray, S. K.; Gilbert, B. E.; and Knight, V. Effect of ribavirin triphosphate on primer generation and elongation during influenza virus transcription *in vitro*. *Antiviral Res.*, **1985**, *5*, 39–48.
Yarchoan, R., and Broder, S. Development of antiretroviral therapy for the acquired immunodeficiency syndrome and related disorders. *N. Engl. J. Med.*, **1987**, *316*, 557–564.
Yarchoan, R., and others. Response of human-immunodeficiency-virus-associated neurological disease to 3′-azido-3′-deoxythymidine. *Lancet*, **1987**, *1*, 132–135.
———. Long-term administration of 3′-azido-2′,3′-dideoxythymidine to patients with AIDS-related neurological disease. *Ann. Neurol.*, **1988**, *23*, Suppl., S82–S87.
Younkin, S. W.; Betts, R. F.; Roth, F. K.; and Douglas, R. G., Jr. Reduction in fever and symptoms in young adults with influenza A/Brazil/78 H1N1 infection after treatment with aspirin or amantadine. *Antimicrob. Agents Chemother.*, **1983**, *23*, 577–582.
Zoon, K. C. Human interferons: structure and function. In, *Interferon 9*. Academic Press, London, **1987**, pp. 1–12.

Monographs and Reviews

Crumpacker, C. S. Molecular targets of antiviral therapy. *N. Engl. J. Med.*, **1989**, *321*, 163–172.
Elion, G. B. History, mechanism of action, spectrum and selectivity of nucleoside analogs. In, *Antiviral Chemotherapy: New Directions for Clinical Application and Research*. (Mills, J., and Corey, L., eds.) Elsevier, New York, **1986**, pp. 118–137.
Fauci, A. S. The human immunodeficiency virus: infectivity and mechanisms of pathogenesis. *Science*, **1988**, *239*, 617–622.
Hayden, F. G., and Douglas, R. G., Jr. Antiviral agents. In, *Principles and Practice of Infectious Diseases*, 3rd ed. (Mandell, G. L.; Douglas, R. G., Jr.; and Bennett, J. E.; eds.) Churchill Livingstone, Inc., New York, **1990**, pp. 370–393.
Hayden, F. G.; Laskin, O. L.; and Douglas, R. G., Jr. Antiviral agents. In, *Antibiotics in Laboratory Medicine*, 2nd ed. (Lourian, V., ed.) Williams and Wilkins, Baltimore, **1986b**, pp. 359–380.

SECTION

XII

Chemotherapy of Neoplastic Diseases

INTRODUCTION

Paul Calabresi and Bruce A. Chabner

Fundamental advances continue in the chemotherapy of neoplastic diseases. The greatest progress in recent years has been not in the discovery of new, superior chemotherapeutic agents but in conceptual therapeutic developments. These include (1) the design of more effective regimens for concurrent administration of drugs, including combinations of antineoplastic agents with so-called "biologic-response modifiers"; (2) the acquisition of knowledge of the mechanisms of action of many antitumor agents, which facilitates the design of new methods to prevent or minimize drug toxicity; (3) greater insight into mechanisms of resistance to antineoplastic drugs; (4) the increased use of adjuvant chemotherapy (*e.g.*, the design of chemotherapeutic approaches to destroy micrometastases and prevent the development of secondary neoplasms after removal or destruction of the primary tumor by surgery or irradiation) and "neo-adjuvant" chemotherapy (*e.g.*, the administration of drugs before surgery or radiotherapy in order to diminish the volume of large primary neoplasms); and (5) increased knowledge about such vital processes as tumor initiation and the dissemination, implantation, and growth of metastases.

Of great importance is recognition of the problems imposed by the heterogeneity of tumors, with the realization that individual tumors may contain many subpopulations of neoplastic cells that differ in crucial characteristics, such as karyotype, morphology, immunogenicity, rate of growth, the capacity to metastasize, and, significantly, responsiveness to antineoplastic agents. Tumors may fail to respond to chemotherapeutic agents *de novo* or they may become resistant to treatment after an initial response. An understanding of drug resistance is important in the search for new agents and in the design of more effective regimens. Various biochemical changes that are usually specific for the selecting agent characterize resistant tumor-cell populations in experimental systems. These changes include alterations in drug transport, an increased concentration of the target enzyme or changes in its affinity for an inhibitor, and increased capacity to inactivate the drug. Some changes may lead to resistance to more than one agent, and this may profoundly limit the range of potentially effective drugs. An example includes amplification of the multidrug resistance gene, which encodes the so-called P-glycoprotein; this protein appears to be responsible for the transport of a broad range of toxic substances, including certain antineoplastic agents, out of cells. In the design of new regimens, oncologists seek to avoid simultaneous use of drugs to which cells can become resistant by a common mechanism, since a single mutation could lead to resistance to more than one agent in the combination; this defeats the rationale for combination chemotherapy. In the search for new drugs, compounds are sought that evade specific mechanisms of resistance and that demonstrate activity against resistant tumor cells.

Accumulating information in the fields of molecular and cellular biology has resulted in a greater understanding of cellular division and differentiation, tumor immunology, and viral and chemical carcinogenesis. Particularly significant are recent discoveries of the role of oncogenes in carcinogenesis. These genes are activated forms of normal cellular proto-oncogenes that have been altered by chromosomal translocation or by mutation. Although the exact functions of the proteins encoded by proto-oncogenes (and their activated, oncogenic forms) are still being elucidated, they are important in various cellular processes, including regulation of proliferation. For example, certain of these proteins are related to cellular growth factors or their receptors. Thus, striking homology has been shown between the protein encoded by the v-*erb-B* oncogene of the avian erythroblastosis virus and the receptor for epidermal growth factor; the protein encoded by the v-*sis* oncogene is homologous with platelet-derived growth factor. It is hoped that these discoveries will provide new targets for therapy.

To appreciate the progress made in the field during the past half century one need only examine *earlier editions* of this textbook. The first edition, published in 1941, does not have a chapter that discusses the chemotherapy of neoplasia. Indeed, the rubric "cancer" does not appear in the index. Significantly, in the years between the appearance of the first and second editions, the original authors, Louis S. Goodman and Alfred Gilman, initiated the clinical investigation of the first major antineoplastic agent, nitrogen mustard, a drug that continues to have an important place in therapeutics. Shortly thereafter came the development of antimetabolite chemotherapy, with the introduction of antifolate compounds by Sidney Farber and colleagues, as well as the synthesis and study of a remarkable series of purine analogs by George Hitchings and Gertrude Elion. By 1965, significant palliative results had been achieved with chemotherapy for a number of human neoplasms, and the first indications had emerged that choriocarcinoma in women could be cured by treatment with methotrexate. Today, we can list a substantial number of neoplastic diseases that can be cured if treated with chemotherapeutic agents alone or with these drugs in combination with other methods. These include choriocarcinoma in women; acute leukemia, Wilms' tumor, Ewing's sarcoma, rhabdomyosarcoma, and retinoblastoma in children; and Hodgkin's disease, several types of non-Hodgkin's lymphoma, and testicular carcinoma. Despite these impressive advances, there is the sobering realization that many of the most prevalent forms of human cancer still resist effective chemotherapeutic intervention.

The entire population of neoplastic cells must be eradicated in order to obtain these desired results. The concept of "total cell-kill" applies to chemotherapy as it does to other means of treatment; total excision of tumor is necessary for surgical cure, and complete destruction of all cancer cells is required for a cure with radiation therapy. By investigating a model tumor system, the L1210 leukemia of mice, Skipper and colleagues established a number of important principles that have guided and redirected modern cancer chemotherapy. These may be briefly summarized as follows.

(1) A single clonogenic malignant cell can give rise to sufficient progeny to kill the host; to achieve cure it is thus necessary to destroy every such cell. Since the doubling time of most tumors is relatively constant during logarithmic growth, the life span of the host is inversely related to the number of malignant cells that are inoculated or that survive therapeutic measures.

(2) In antimicrobial chemotherapy, in most instances there are major contributions by the immune mechanisms and other host defenses. However, these play a negligible role in the therapy of neoplastic disease unless only a small number of malignant cells is present.

(3) The cell-kill caused by antineoplastic agents follows first-order kinetics; that is, a constant percentage, rather than a constant number, of cells is killed by a given therapeutic maneuver. This finding has had a profound impact on clinical cancer chemotherapy. For example, a patient with advanced acute lymphocytic leukemia might harbor 10^{12} or about 1 kg of malignant cells. A drug capable of killing 99.99% of these cells would reduce the tumor mass to about 100 mg, and this would be apparent as a complete clinical remission. However, 10^8 malignant cells would remain, any one of which could cause a relapse in the

disease. The logical outgrowth of these concepts has been the attempt to achieve total cell-kill by the use of several chemotherapeutic agents concurrently or in rational sequences. The resulting prolonged survival of patients with acute lymphocytic leukemia through the use of such multiple-drug regimens has encouraged the application of these principles to the treatment of other neoplasms.

An understanding of cell-cycle kinetics is essential for the proper use of the current generation of antineoplastic agents. Many of the most potent cytotoxic agents act at specific phases of the cell cycle and, therefore, have activity only against cells that are in the process of division. Accordingly, human neoplasms that are currently most susceptible to chemotherapeutic measures are those with a large growth fraction, that is, a high percentage of cells in the process of division. Similarly, normal tissues that proliferate rapidly (bone marrow, hair follicles, and intestinal epithelium) are subject to damage by some of these potent antineoplastic drugs, and such toxicity often limits the usefulness of drugs. On the other hand, slow-growing tumors with a small growth fraction (for example, carcinomas of the colon or lung) are often unresponsive to cytotoxic drugs. Although differences in the duration of the cell cycle occur between cells of various types, all cells display a similar pattern during the division process. This may be characterized as follows: (1) there is a presynthetic phase (G_1); (2) the synthesis of DNA occurs (S); (3) an interval follows the termination of DNA synthesis, the postsynthetic phase (G_2); and (4) mitosis (M) ensues—the G_2 cell, containing a double complement of DNA, divides into two daughter G_1 cells. Each of these may immediately reenter the cell cycle or pass into a nonproliferative stage, referred to as G_0. The cells of certain specialized tissues may differentiate into functional cells that are no longer capable of division. On the other hand, many cells, especially those in slow-growing tumors, may remain in the G_0 state for prolonged periods, only to be recruited into the division cycle again at a much later time. Most antineoplastic agents act specifically on processes such as DNA synthesis, transcription, or the function of the mitotic spindle and, therefore, are regarded as cell-cycle specific. Some agents may act during several or all stages of the cell cycle; while not cell-cycle specific, their cytotoxic effects may still be dependent on proliferation. It is obvious that further understanding of the cell cycle and of the factors that regulate the recruitment of G_0 cells into the cycle should prove of great value in future attempts to develop chemotherapeutic measures for slow-growing tumors.

A great variety of compounds has been investigated in experimental animals, and a few have proven sufficiently useful in the clinical treatment of human neoplasms, at acceptable levels of toxicity, to deserve the designation of chemotherapeutic agents. It should be emphasized that the compounds selected for discussion represent, for the most part, those that are generally available and have withstood the test of time, although a few have been included either because they illustrate special circumstances or because they are representative of newer developments.

The emphasis in Chapter 52 is placed upon the drugs themselves. Although this is appropriate in a textbook of pharmacology, it is also essential to point out the importance of the role played by the patient. It is generally agreed that patients in good nutritional state and without severe metabolic disturbances, infections, or other complications are better candidates for significant improvement from antineoplastic therapy than are severely debilitated individuals. Ideally, the patient also should have adequate renal, hepatic, and bone-marrow function, uncompromised by tumor invasion, previous chemotherapy, or radiation (particularly of the spine or pelvis). Nevertheless, even patients with advanced disease have improved dramatically with chemotherapy. Although methods that would enable accurate prediction of the responsiveness of a particular tumor to a given agent are still investigational, efforts are being made to establish better clinical and laboratory criteria for the rational selection of patients prior to therapy. Despite efforts to anticipate the development of complications, anticancer agents, like many other potent drugs with only moderate selectivity, may cause severe toxicity. In such circumstances, the physician must have at his disposal adequate facilities for vigorous supportive therapy; some of these, including plate-

Table XII–1. CHEMOTHERAPEUTIC AGENTS USEFUL IN NEOPLASTIC DISEASE

CLASS	TYPE OF AGENT	NONPROPRIETARY NAMES (OTHER NAMES)	DISEASE *
Alkylating Agents	Nitrogen Mustards	Mechlorethamine (HN_2)	Hodgkin's disease, non-Hodgkin's lymphomas
		Cyclophosphamide Ifosfamide	Acute and chronic lymphocytic leukemias, Hodgkin's disease, non-Hodgkin's lymphomas, multiple myeloma, neuroblastoma, breast, ovary, lung, Wilms' tumor, cervix, testis, soft-tissue sarcomas
		Melphalan (L-sarcolysin)	Multiple myeloma, breast, ovary
		Chlorambucil	Chronic lymphocytic leukemia, primary macroglobulinemia, Hodgkin's disease, non-Hodgkin's lymphomas
	Ethylenimines and Methylmelamines	Hexamethylmelamine	Ovary
		Thiotepa	Bladder, breast, ovary
	Alkyl Sulfonates	Busulfan	Chronic granulocytic leukemia
	Nitrosoureas	Carmustine (BCNU)	Hodgkin's disease, non-Hodgkin's lymphomas, primary brain tumors, multiple myeloma, malignant melanoma
		Lomustine (CCNU)	Hodgkin's disease, non-Hodgkin's lymphomas, primary brain tumors, small-cell lung
		Semustine (methyl-CCNU)	Primary brain tumors, stomach, colon
		Streptozocin (streptozotocin)	Malignant pancreatic insulinoma, malignant carcinoid
	Triazenes	Dacarbazine (DTIC; dimethyltriazenoimidazolecarboxamide)	Malignant melanoma, Hodgkin's disease, soft-tissue sarcomas
Antimetabolites	Folic Acid Analogs	Methotrexate (amethopterin)	Acute lymphocytic leukemia, choriocarcinoma, mycosis fungoides, breast, head and neck, lung, osteogenic sarcoma
	Pyrimidine Analogs	Fluorouracil (5-fluorouracil; 5-FU) Floxuridine (fluorodeoxyuridine; FUdR)	Breast, colon, stomach, pancreas, ovary, head and neck, urinary bladder, premalignant skin lesions (topical)
		Cytarabine (cytosine arabinoside)	Acute granulocytic and acute lymphocytic leukemias
	Purine Analogs and Related Inhibitors	Mercaptopurine (6-mercaptopurine; 6-MP)	Acute lymphocytic, acute granulocytic, and chronic granulocytic leukemias
		Thioguanine (6-thioguanine; TG)	Acute granulocytic, acute lymphocytic, and chronic granulocytic leukemias
		Pentostatin (2′-deoxycoformycin)	Hairy cell leukemia, mycosis fungoides, chronic lymphocytic leukemia

* Neoplasms are carcinomas unless otherwise indicated.

Table XII–1. CHEMOTHERAPEUTIC AGENTS USEFUL IN NEOPLASTIC DISEASE (Continued)

CLASS	TYPE OF AGENT	NONPROPRIETARY NAMES (OTHER NAMES)	DISEASE *
Natural Products	Vinca Alkaloids	Vinblastine (VLB)	Hodgkin's disease, non-Hodgkin's lymphomas, breast, testis
		Vincristine	Acute lymphocytic leukemia, neuroblastoma, Wilms' tumor, rhabdomyosarcoma, Hodgkin's disease, non-Hodgkin's lymphomas, small-cell lung
	Epipodophyllotoxins	Etoposide Teniposide	Testis, small-cell lung and other lung, breast, Hodgkin's disease, non-Hodgkin's lymphomas, acute granulocytic leukemia, Kaposi's sarcoma
	Antibiotics	Dactinomycin (actinomycin D)	Choriocarcinoma, Wilms' tumor, rhabdomyosarcoma, testis, Kaposi's sarcoma
		Daunorubicin (daunomycin; rubidomycin)	Acute granulocytic and acute lymphocytic leukemias
		Doxorubicin	Soft-tissue, osteogenic, and other sarcomas; Hodgkin's disease, non-Hodgkin's lymphomas, acute leukemias, breast, genitourinary, thyroid, lung, stomach, neuroblastoma
		Bleomycin	Testis, head and neck, skin, esophagus, lung, and genitourinary tract; Hodgkin's disease, non-Hodgkin's lymphomas
		Plicamycin (mithramycin)	Testis, malignant hypercalcemia
		Mitomycin (mitomycin C)	Stomach, cervix, colon, breast, pancreas, bladder, head and neck
	Enzymes	L-Asparaginase	Acute lymphocytic leukemia
	Biological Response Modifiers	Interferon alfa	Hairy cell leukemia, Kaposi's sarcoma, melanoma, carcinoid, renal cell, ovary, bladder, non-Hodgkin's lymphomas, mycosis fungoides, multiple myeloma, chronic granulocytic leukemia
Miscellaneous Agents	Platinum Coordination Complexes	Cisplatin (*cis*-DDP) Carboplatin	Testis, ovary, bladder, head and neck, lung, thyroid, cervix, endometrium, neuroblastoma, osteogenic sarcoma
	Anthracenedione	Mitoxantrone	Acute granulocytic leukemia, breast
	Substituted Urea	Hydroxyurea	Chronic granulocytic leukemia, polycythemia vera, essential thrombocytosis, malignant melanoma
	Methyl Hydrazine Derivative	Procarbazine (N-methylhydrazine, MIH)	Hodgkin's disease
	Adrenocortical Suppressant	Mitotane (*o,p'*-DDD)	Adrenal cortex
		Aminoglutethimide	Breast

Table XII–1. CHEMOTHERAPEUTIC AGENTS USEFUL IN NEOPLASTIC DISEASE (Continued)

CLASS	TYPE OF AGENT	NONPROPRIETARY NAMES (OTHER NAMES)	DISEASE *
Hormones and Antagonists	Adrenocorticosteroids	Prednisone (several other equivalent preparations available; *see* Chapter 60)	Acute and chronic lymphocytic leukemias, non-Hodgkin's lymphomas, Hodgkin's disease, breast
	Progestins	Hydroxyprogesterone caproate Medroxyprogesterone acetate Megestrol acetate	Endometrium, breast
	Estrogens	Diethylstilbestrol Ethinyl estradiol (other preparations available; *see* Chapter 58)	Breast, prostate
	Antiestrogen	Tamoxifen	Breast
	Androgens	Testosterone propionate Fluoxymesterone (other preparations available; *see* Chapter 59)	Breast
	Antiandrogen	Flutamide	Prostate
	Gonadotropin-releasing hormone analog	Leuprolide	Prostate

* Neoplasms are carcinomas unless otherwise indicated.

let transfusions, the administration of allopurinol to prevent the complications of hyperuricemia, and the empirical use of broad-spectrum antibiotics in the febrile neutropenic patient, have been widely adopted; others, including the use of bone marrow transplantation and hematopoietic growth factors, are the subject of intensive investigation (*see* Chapter 54).

Drugs currently used in chemotherapy of neoplastic diseases may be divided into several classes, as shown in Table XII–1. This somewhat arbitrary classification is used in Chapter 52 as a convenient framework for describing the various types of agents. The major clinical indications for the drugs are listed in Table XII–1 in order to facilitate rapid reference. Dosage regimens, which are often complex, are discussed under the individual drugs.

Mechanistic classification of these agents is increasingly important, particularly as investigators attempt to use this information to design "rational" regimens for chemotherapy. A simplified overview of the sites of action of many of the drugs described in Chapter 52 is shown in Figure XII–1.

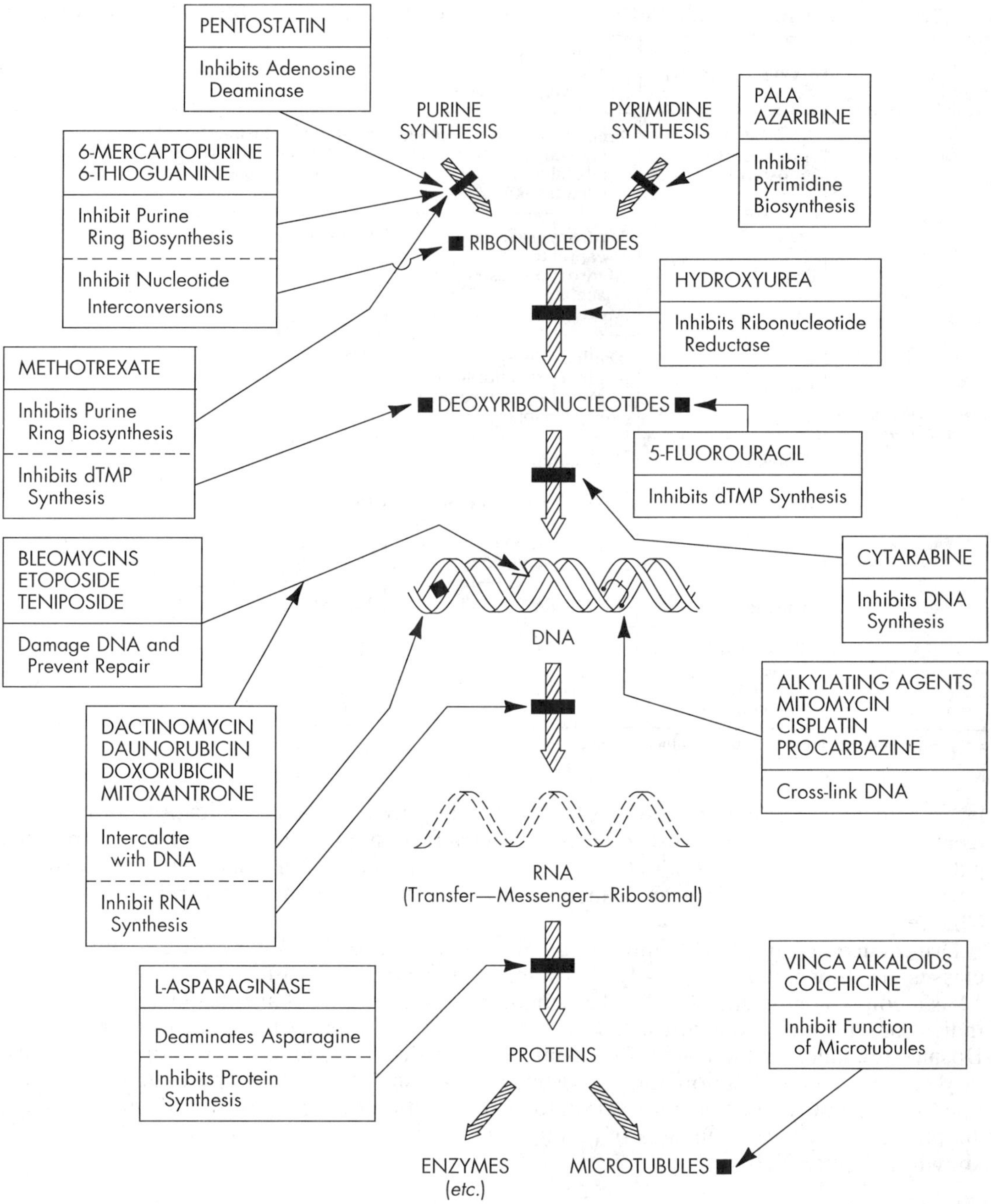

Figure XII–1. *Summary of the mechanisms and sites of action of chemotherapeutic agents useful in neoplastic disease.*

PALA = N-phosphonoacetyl-L-aspartate.

CHAPTER

52 ANTINEOPLASTIC AGENTS

Paul Calabresi and Bruce A. Chabner

I. Alkylating Agents

History. Although synthesized in 1854, the vesicant properties of sulfur mustard were not described until 1887. During World War I, medical attention was first focused on the vesicant action of sulfur mustard on the skin, eyes, and respiratory tract. It was appreciated later, however, that serious systemic toxicity also follows exposure. In 1919, Krumbhaar and Krumbhaar made the pertinent observation that the poisoning caused by sulfur mustard is characterized by leukopenia and, in cases that came to autopsy, by aplasia of the bone marrow, dissolution of lymphoid tissue, and ulceration of the gastrointestinal tract.

In the interval between World Wars I and II, extensive studies of the biological and chemical actions of the *nitrogen mustards* were conducted. The marked cytotoxic action on lymphoid tissue prompted Gilman, Goodman, and T. F. Dougherty to study the effect of nitrogen mustards on transplanted lymphosarcoma in mice, and in 1942 clinical studies were initiated. This launched the era of modern cancer chemotherapy (Gilman, 1963).

In their early phases, all these investigations were conducted under secrecy restrictions imposed by the use of classified chemical-warfare agents. At the termination of World War II, however, the nitrogen mustards were declassified and a general review was presented by Gilman and Philips (1946). Other reviews include those by Colvin (1982), Wheeler (1982), and Ludlum and Tong (1985).

Thousands of variants of the basic chemical structure of the nitrogen mustards have been prepared, but only a few of these agents have proven more useful than the original compound in specific clinical circumstances (*see* below). At present five major types of alkylating agents are used in the chemotherapy of neoplastic diseases: (1) the nitrogen mustards, (2) the ethylenimines, (3) the alkyl sulfonates, (4) the nitrosoureas, and (5) the triazenes.

Chemistry. The chemotherapeutic alkylating agents have in common the property of becoming strong electrophiles through the formation of carbonium ion intermediates or of transition complexes with the target molecules. These reactions result in the formation of covalent linkages by alkylation of various nucleophilic moieties such as phosphate, amino, sulfhydryl, hydroxyl, carboxyl, and imidazole groups. The chemotherapeutic and cytotoxic effects are directly related to the alkylation of DNA. The 7 nitrogen atom of guanine is particularly susceptible to the formation of a covalent bond with both monofunctional and bifunctional alkylating agents and may well represent the key target that determines the biological effects of these agents. It must be appreciated, however, that other atoms in the purine and pyrimidine bases of DNA—for example, the 1 or 3 nitrogens of adenine, the 3 nitrogen of cytosine, and the 6 oxygen of guanine—may also be alkylated to a lesser degree, as are the phosphate atoms of the DNA chains and the proteins associated with DNA.

To illustrate the actions of alkylating agents, possible consequences of the reaction of mechlorethamine (nitrogen mustard) with guanine residues in DNA chains are shown in Figure 52–1. First, one 2-chloroethyl side chain undergoes a first-order (S_N1) intramolecular cyclization, with release of Cl^- and formation of a highly reactive ethyleniminium intermediate. By this reaction the tertiary amine is converted to a quaternary ammonium compound. The ethyleniminium intermediates can react avidly, through formation of a carbonium ion or transition complex intermediate, with a large number of inorganic ions and organic radicals by reactions that resemble a second-order (S_N2) nucleophilic substitution reaction (Price, 1975). Alkylation of the 7 nitrogen of guanine residues in DNA, a highly favored reaction, may exert several effects of considerable biological importance, as illustrated in Figure 52–1. Normally, guanine residues in DNA exist predominantly as the keto tautomer and readily make Watson–Crick base pairs by hydrogen bonding with cytosine residues. However, when the 7 nitrogen of guanine is alkylated (to become a quaternary ammonium nitrogen), the guanine residue is more acidic and the enol tautomer is favored. The modified guanine can form base pairs with thymine residues, thus leading to possible miscoding and the ultimate substitution of an adenine–thymine base pair for a guanine–cytosine base pair. Second, alkylation of the 7 nitrogen labilizes the imidazole ring, making possible the opening of the imidazole ring or depurination by excision of guanine residues. Either of these reactions can result in serious damage to the DNA molecule (Shapiro, 1968). Third, with bifunctional alkylating agents, such as nitrogen mustard, the second 2-chloroethyl side chain can undergo a similar cyclization reaction and alkylate a second guanine residue or another nucleophilic moiety, such as an amino group or a sulfhydryl radical of a protein. This can result in the cross-linking of two nucleic acid chains or the linking of a nucleic acid to a protein by covalent bonds, alterations that would cause a major disruption in nucleic acid function. Any of these effects could adequately explain both the mutagenic and the cytotoxic effects of alkylating agents.

In addition to the formation of covalent bonds

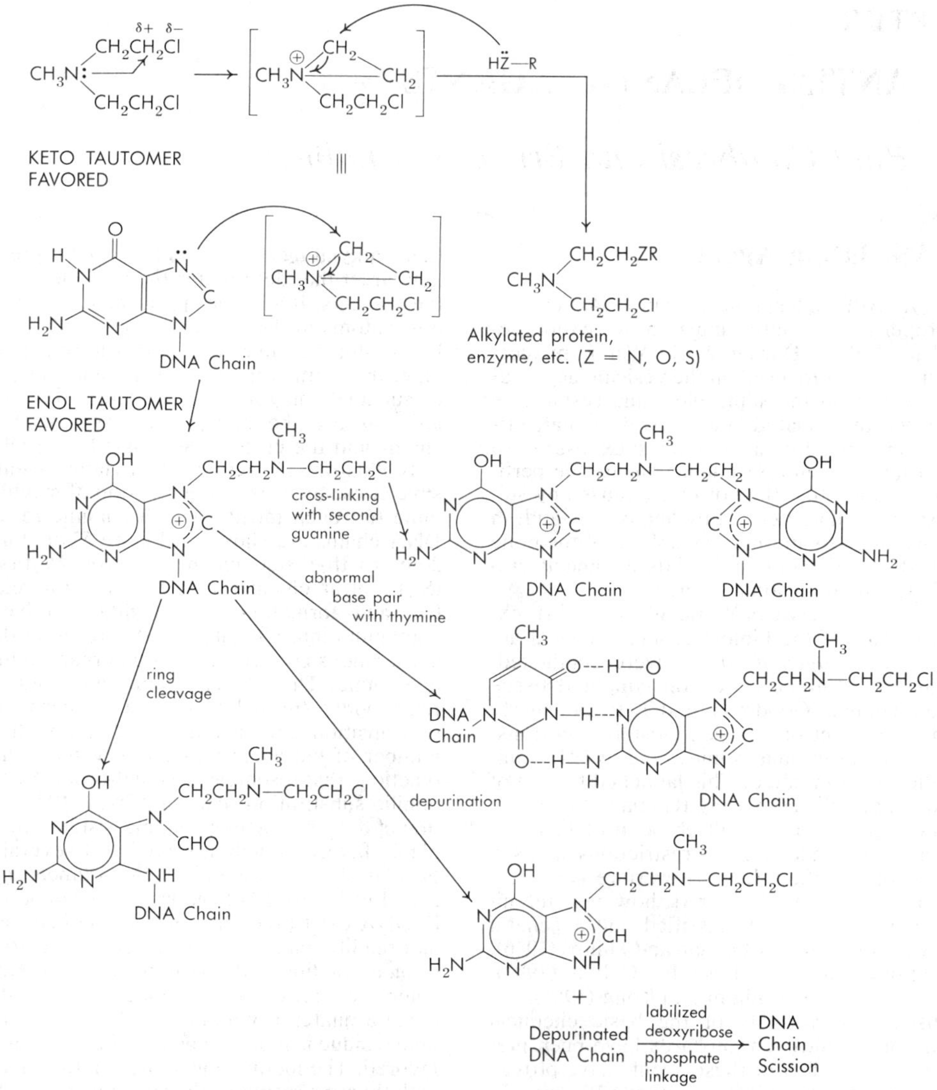

Figure 52–1. *Mechanism of action of alkylating agents.*

with purine or pyrimidine residues of DNA, alkylation of other biological molecules may result in important effects on cellular function and viability.

All nitrogen mustards are chemically unstable but vary greatly in their degree of instability. Therefore, the specific chemical properties of each member of this class of drugs must be considered individually in therapeutic applications. For example, mechlorethamine is very unstable, and it reacts almost completely in the body within a few minutes of its administration. By contrast, agents such as chlorambucil are sufficiently stable to permit oral administration, and cyclophosphamide requires biochemical activation by the cytochrome P_{450} system of the liver before its cytotoxicity becomes evident.

The ethylenimine derivatives react by an S_N2 reaction; however, since the opening of the ethylenimine ring is acid catalyzed, they are more reactive at acidic pH. Busulfan is an atypical alkylating agent with unusual biological properties that differ significantly from substituted nitrogen mustards and ethylenimines (Fox, 1975).

Structure–Activity Relationship. The alkylating agents used in chemotherapy encompass a diverse group of chemicals that have in common the capacity to contribute, under physiological conditions, alkyl groups to biologically vital macromolecules such as DNA. In most instances, physical and chemical parameters, such as lipophilicity, capacity to cross biological membranes, acid dissociation constants, stability in aqueous solution, and so forth, rather than similarity to cellular constituents, have proven crucial to biological activity. With several of the most valuable agents (for example, cyclophosphamide and the nitrosoureas) the active alkylating moieties are generated *in vivo* after complex degradative reactions, some of which are enzymatic. Since many of these physicochemical factors and activation reactions are still unclear, most alkylating agents in use today were discovered by empirical rather than by rational approaches.

The nitrogen mustards may be regarded as nitrogen analogs of sulfur mustard. The biological activity of both types of compounds is based upon the presence of the *bis*-(2-chloroethyl) grouping. Although a very large number of alkylating agents have been synthesized and evaluated, the methyl derivative, mechlorethamine, has received wide clinical use and has been accepted generally as a standard of reference. Various structural modifications have been made in order to achieve greater selectivity and, therefore, less toxicity. *Bis*-(2-chloroethyl) groups have been linked to amino acids (phenylalanine), substituted phenyl groups (aminophenyl butyric acid, as in chlorambucil), pyrimidine bases (uracil), and several other substances, including a cyclic phosphamide ester. Although none of these modifications has produced an agent highly selective for malignant cells, some of the compounds exhibit notable differences in their secondary pharmacological properties and are used clinically more often than is mechlorethamine. The structural formulas of some of the more commonly used nitrogen mustards are shown in Table 52–1.

The addition of substituted phenyl groups has produced a series of derivatives that retain the ability to react by an S_N1 mechanism; however, the electron-withdrawing capacity of the aromatic ring greatly reduces the rate of carbonium ion formation, and these compounds can therefore reach distant sites in the body before reacting with components of blood and other tissues. Chlorambucil is the most successful example of such aromatic mustards. Compounds such as chlorambucil are better tolerated by patients than is mechlorethamine and can be administered orally if desired.

A classical example of the role of host metabolism in the activation of an alkylating agent is seen with cyclophosphamide—now the most widely used agent of this class. The original rationale that guided design of this molecule was twofold. First, if a cyclic phosphamide group replaced the N-methyl of mechlorethamine, the compound might be relatively inert, presumably because the *bis*-(2-chloroethyl) group of the molecule could not ionize until the cyclic phosphamide was cleaved at the phosphorus–nitrogen linkage. Second, it was hoped that neoplastic tissues might possess high phosphatase or phosphamidase activity capable of accomplishing this cleavage, thus resulting in the selective production of an activated nitrogen mustard in the malignant cells. In accord with these predictions, cyclophosphamide displays only weak cytotoxic, mutagenic, or alkylating activity and is relatively stable in aqueous solution. However, when administered to experimental animals or patients bearing susceptible tumors, marked chemotherapeutic effects, as well as mutagenicity and carcinogenicity, are seen. Although a role for phosphatases or phosphamidases in the mechanism of action of cyclophosphamide has not been demonstrated, it has been clearly established that the drug initially undergoes metabolic activation by the cytochrome P_{450} mixed-function oxidase system of the liver, with subsequent transport of the activated intermediate to sites of action, as discussed below. It also appears that the selectivity of cyclophosphamide against certain malignant tissues may result in part from the capacity of normal tissues, such as liver, to protect themselves against cytotoxicity by further degrading the activated intermediates.

Ifosfamide is an oxazaphosphorine, similar to cyclophosphamide. Cyclophosphamide has two chloroethyl groups on the exocyclic nitrogen atom, whereas one of the two chloroethyl groups of ifosfamide is on the cyclic phosphamide nitrogen of the oxazaphosphorine ring. Ifosfamide is also activated in the liver by oxidation to 4-hydroxyifosfamide.

Although initially considered as an antimetabolite, the triazene derivative 5-(3,3-dimethyl-1-

Table 52–1. NITROGEN MUSTARDS EMPLOYED IN THERAPY

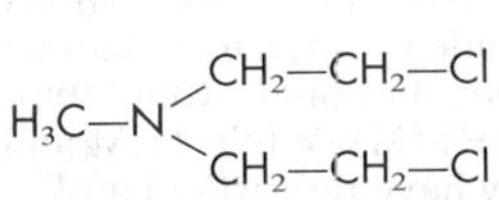

Mechlorethamine

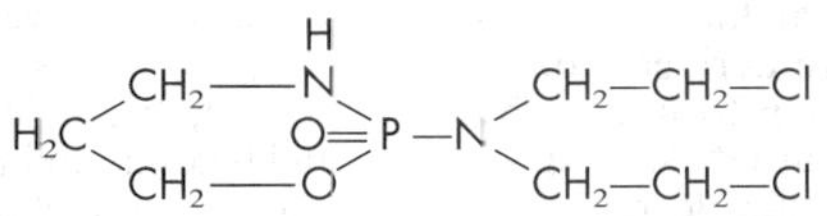

Cyclophosphamide

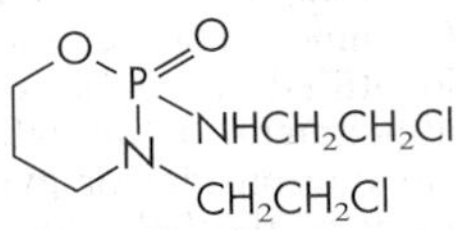

Ifosfamide

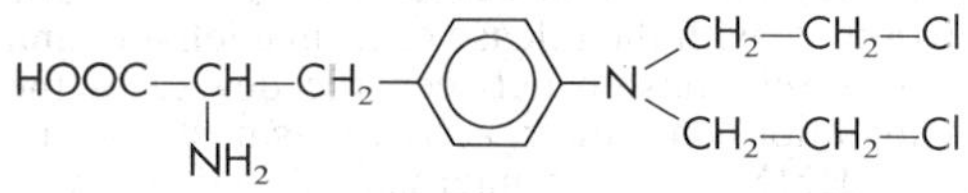

Melphalan

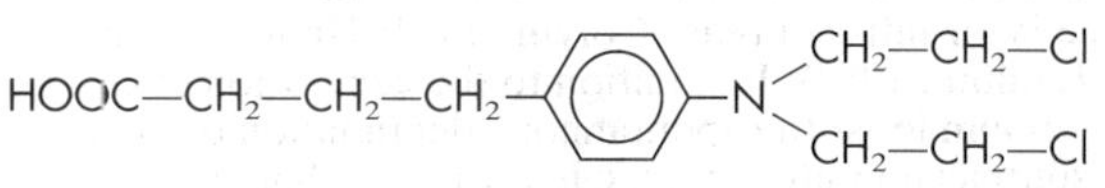

Chlorambucil

triazeno)-imidazole-4-carboxamide, usually referred to as dacarbazine or DTIC, is now known to function through alkylation. Its structural formula is as follows:

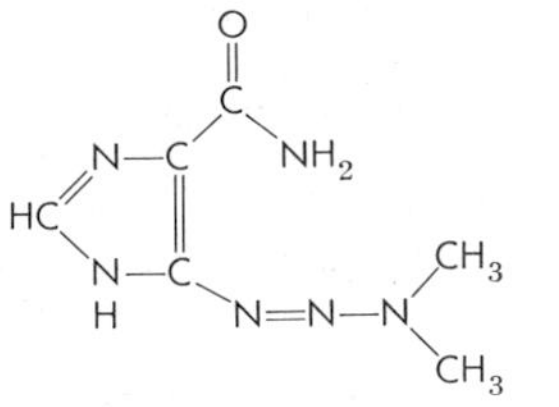

Dacarbazine

This compound bears a striking resemblance to the known metabolite 5-aminoimidazole-4-carboxamide (AIC), which is capable of conversion to inosinic acid by enzymes of purine synthesis. Thus, it was suspected that dacarbazine acts by inhibiting purine metabolism and nucleic acid synthesis. This resemblance to AIC appears to be fortuitous, since, for chemotherapeutic effectiveness, dacarbazine requires initial activation by the cytochrome P_{450} system of the liver through an N-demethylation reaction. In the target cell, there then occurs a spontaneous cleavage liberating AIC and an alkylating moiety, presumably diazomethane (Chabner, 1982).

Although the mechanism of action is not yet fully established, it is generally assumed that the nitrosoureas, which include compounds such as 1,3-*bis*-(2-chloroethyl)-1-nitrosourea (carmustine, BCNU), 1-(2-chloroethyl)-3-cyclohexyl-1-nitrosourea (lomustine, CCNU), and its methyl derivative (semustine, methyl-CCNU), as well as the antibiotic streptozocin (streptozotocin), exert their cytotoxicity through the liberation of alkylating and carbamoylating moieties. Their structural formulas are shown in Table 52–2.

Table 52–2. CLASSIFICATION AND STRUCTURES OF SOME ANTINEOPLASTIC NITROSOUREAS

METHYLNITROSOUREAS (MNU)

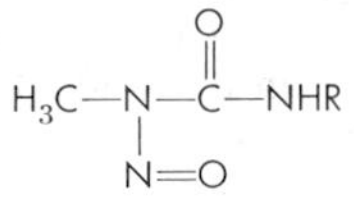

Streptozocin
R = 2-substituted glucose

2-CHLOROETHYLNITROSOUREAS (CNU)

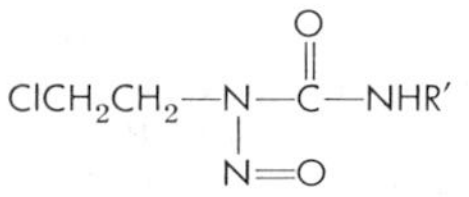

Carmustine (BCNU)
$R' = —CH_2CH_2Cl$

Lomustine (CCNU)

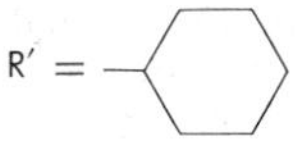

Semustine (Methyl-CCNU)

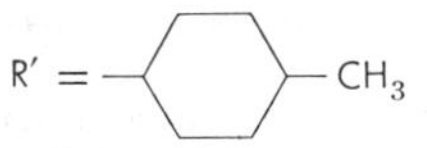

Chlorozotocin
R′ = 2-substituted glucose

The antineoplastic nitrosoureas have in common the capacity to undergo spontaneous, nonenzymatic degradation with the formation of a variety of products. Of these, the methyl carbonium ion (from MNU compounds) and the 2-chloroethyl carbonium ion (from CNU compounds) are strongly electrophilic and can alkylate a variety of substances, including the purine and pyrimidine bases of DNA. Guanine, cytidine, and adenine adducts have been identified; a number of these are derived from the attachment of the haloethyl group to nucleophilic sites on purines or pyrimidines in DNA. Displacement of the halogen atom can then lead to interstrand or intrastrand cross-linking of the DNA. The formation of the cross-links after the initial alkylation reaction is a relatively slow process and can be interrupted by a DNA repair enzyme. As with the nitrogen mustards, it is generally agreed that interstrand cross-linking is associated with the cytotoxicity of nitrosoureas (Colvin, 1982; Hemminki and Ludlum, 1984). In addition to the generation of carbonium ions, the spontaneous degradation of nitrosoureas liberates organic isocyanates that are capable of carbamoylating lysine residues of proteins. This reaction can apparently inactivate certain of the DNA repair enzymes. The reactions of the nitrosoureas with macromolecules are shown in Figure 52–2. (For reviews of the nitrosoureas, *see* Colvin, 1982; Ludlum and Tong, 1985.)

Since the formation of the ethyleniminium ion constitutes the initial reaction of the nitrogen mustards, it is not surprising that other ethylenimine derivatives or compounds that can produce related structures have antitumor activity. Several agents of this type have been discussed in *earlier editions* of this textbook; these include triethylenemelamine (TEM), triethylene thiophosphoramide (thiotepa), and hexamethylmelamine (HMM). While TEM and thiotepa are cytotoxic, they have no particular clinical advantage over the other alkylating agents for most purposes. Although there is no evidence that the methylmelamines function as alkylating agents, HMM is mentioned here because of its chemical similarity to the ethylenimine melamines. The methylmelamines are N-demethylated by hepatic microsomes, with the release of formaldehyde, and there is a relationship between the degree of the demethylation and their activity against murine tumors. HMM requires microsomal activation to display cytotoxicity. The drug appears to have activity against a number of neoplasms that are resis-

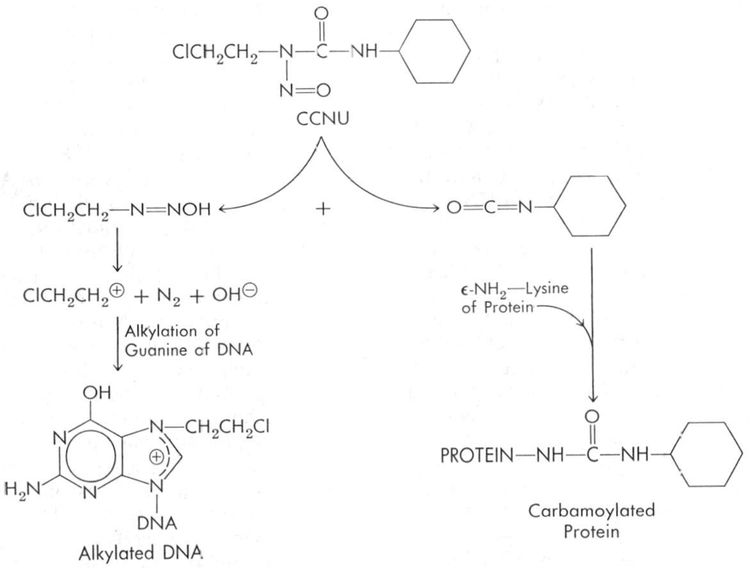

Figure 52–2. *Degradation of lomustine (CCNU) with generation of alkylating and carbamoylating intermediates.*

tant to other alkylating agents. Among these are carcinomas of the ovary, breast, and lung (small cell) and certain lymphomas (Chabner, 1982).

Several interesting compounds have emerged from a large group of esters of alkanesulfonic acids. One of these, busulfan, is of great value in the treatment of chronic granulocytic leukemia; its structural formula is as follows:

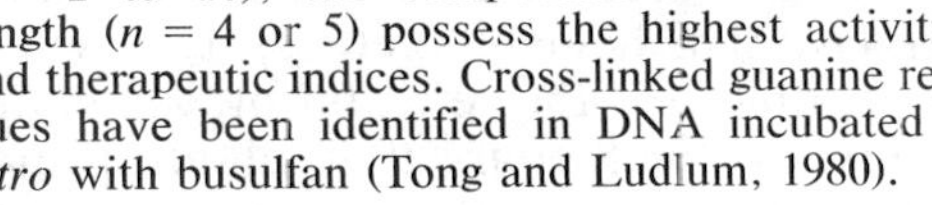

Busulfan

Busulfan is a member of a series of symmetrical *bis*-substituted methanesulfonic acid esters with varying lengths of a bridge of methylene groups ($n = 2$ to 10); the compounds of intermediate length ($n = 4$ or 5) possess the highest activities and therapeutic indices. Cross-linked guanine residues have been identified in DNA incubated *in vitro* with busulfan (Tong and Ludlum, 1980).

Pharmacological Actions

The pharmacological actions of the various groups of alkylating agents are considered together in the following discussion. Although there are many similarities, some notable differences are also evident. Primary consideration will be given to the cytotoxic actions that follow the administration of a sublethal dose.

Cytotoxic Actions. The most important pharmacological actions of the alkylating agents are those that disturb the fundamental mechanisms concerned with cell growth, mitotic activity, differentiation, and function. The capacity of these drugs to interfere with normal mitosis and cell division in all rapidly proliferating tissues provides the basis for their therapeutic applications and for many of their toxic properties. Whereas certain alkylating agents may have damaging effects on tissues with normally low mitotic indices—for example, liver, kidney, and mature lymphocytes—they are most cytotoxic to rapidly proliferating tissues in which a large proportion of the cells are in division. These compounds may readily alkylate nondividing cells, but cytotoxicity is markedly enhanced if such cells are stimulated to divide. Thus, the process of alkylation itself may not be a lethal event if the DNA repair enzymes can correct the lesions in DNA prior to the next cellular division.

In contrast to many other antineoplastic agents, the effects of the alkylating drugs, although dependent on proliferation, are not cell-cycle specific, and the drugs may act on cells at any stage of the cycle. However, the toxicity is usually expressed when the cell enters the S phase and progression through the cycle is blocked at the G_2 (premitotic) phase (*see* Wheeler, 1967). While not strictly cell-cycle specific, quantitative differences may be detected when nitrogen mustards are applied to synchronized cells at different phases of the cycle. Cells appear more sensitive in late G_1 or S than in G_2, mitosis, or early G_1. Polynucleotides are more susceptible to alkylation in the unpaired state than in the helical form; during replication of DNA, portions of the molecule are unpaired.

The cells accumulating behind the block at G_2 may have a double complement of DNA while continuing to synthesize other cellular components, such as protein and RNA. This can result in unbalanced growth, with the formation of enlarged or giant cells that can continue to synthesize DNA, making as much as four or five times the normal complement. Lethal cytotoxic action may occur by so-called interphase death and mitotic death; on the other hand, relatively undifferentiated cells of mammalian germinal tissues may remain nonproliferative during exposure and may later undergo nuclear and cytoplasmic hypertrophy, differentiating without further mitosis into more adult cell types. Interphase death is generally regarded as the result of damage to many cellular sites. Nevertheless, this may not be the case; certainly it occurs without any evidence of mitotic activity. For detailed reviews of the cytotoxic and biochemical effects of alkylating agents, *see* Colvin (1982).

Biochemical Actions. The great preponderance of evidence indicates that the primary target of pharmacological doses of alkylating agents is the DNA molecule, as illustrated in Figure 52–1. A crucial distinction that must be emphasized is between the bifunctional agents, in which cytotoxic effects predominate, and the monofunctional methylating agents, which have much greater capacity for mutagenesis and carcinogenesis. This suggests that biochemical events such as the cross-linking of DNA strands, only possible with bifunctional agents, represent a much greater threat to cellular survival than do other effects, such as depurination and chain scission. On the other hand, the latter reactions may cause permanent modifications in DNA structure that are compatible with continued life of the cell and are transmissible to subsequent generations; such modifications may result in mutagenesis or carcinogenesis (Colvin, 1982; Ludlum and Tong, 1985).

The remarkable DNA repair systems found in most cells appear to have a key, if not determining, role in the relative resistance of nonproliferating tissues, the selectivity of action against particular cell types, and acquired resistance to alkylating agents. Although alkylation of a single strand of DNA may often be repaired with relative ease, interstrand cross-linkages, such as those produced by the bifunctional alkylating agents, require more complex mechanisms for repair. Many of the cross-links formed in DNA by these agents at low doses may also be corrected; higher doses cause extensive cross-linkage, and DNA breakdown occurs.

Detailed information is lacking on mechanisms of cellular uptake of alkylating agents. Mechlorethamine appears to enter murine tumor cells by means of an active transport system, the natural substrate of which is choline. Melphalan, an analog of phenylalanine, is taken up by at least two active transport systems that normally react with leucine and other neutral amino acids. The highly lipophilic nitrosoureas, carmustine and lomustine, diffuse into cells passively (Colvin, 1982).

Mechanisms of Resistance to Alkylating Agents. Acquired resistance to alkylating agents is a common event, and the acquisition of resistance to one alkylating agent may impart cross-resistance to others. While definitive information on the biochemical mechanisms of resistance is lacking, several biochemical mechanisms have been implicated in the development of such resistance by tumor cells. In contrast to the development of resistance to antimetabolites, where single-step mutations can result in almost complete resistance to drug effects, the acquisition of resistance to alkylating agents is usually a slower process, not resulting from single biochemical changes. Resistance of this type may represent the summation of a series of changes, none of which by itself can confer significant resistance. Among the biochemical changes identified in cells resistant to alkylating agents are decreased permeation of the drugs and increased production of nucleophilic substances that can compete with the target DNA for alkylation. The administration of cysteine can considerably reduce the antitumor effects of alkylating agents, and there are several examples of animal tumors with acquired resistance that have greater concentrations of free thiol groups than do the sensitive tumor lines from which they were derived. There has been much speculation about the possibility that increased activity of the DNA repair system may permit cells to acquire resistance to alkylating agents. It has been suggested that cellular resistance to cyclophosphamide may result from increased rates of metabolism of the activated forms of the drug to the inactive keto and carboxy metabolites (*see* Figure 52–3, page 1217). In addition, pleiotropic drug resistance has been documented in experimental and human tumor cell lines; such cells have become resistant to agents with different chemical structures and mechanisms of action (Colvin, 1982).

Hematological and Immunosuppressive Actions. The hematopoietic system is very susceptible to the effects of alkylating agents. Within 8 hours after administration of a sublethal dose of a nitrogen mustard, cessation of mitosis and disintegration of formed elements may be evident in the marrow and lymphoid tissues. Lymphocytes are more sensitive to the destructive action of the mustards and relatively resistant to the effects of busulfan, an action that is considered responsible for the immunosuppressive effects observed with the former group, particularly cyclophosphamide. Busulfan is more toxic to granulocytes, and suitable combinations of busulfan and chlorambucil, an aromatic mustard, can simulate closely the hematological effects of whole-body x-radiation. The effects of chlorambucil are followed by rapid recovery, except in lymphoid organs, whereas depression of hematopoiesis after busulfan occurs more gradually. In patients treated with mechlorethamine, lymphocytopenia is apparent within 24 hours and becomes more severe for 6 to 8 days; within a few days, granulocytopenia is evident and lasts for 10 days to 3 weeks. Variable depression of platelet and erythrocyte counts may occur during the second or third week after therapy; with ensuing regeneration, hematological recovery is complete at the end of 4 to 6 weeks and rebound hyperplasia may be present from the fifth to the seventh week.

Actions on Epithelial Tissues. The intestinal mucosa can be damaged by the parenteral administration of minimal lethal doses of a nitrogen mustard in experimental animals; mitotic arrest, cellular hypertrophy, pyknosis, disintegration, and desquamation of the epithelium are evident. Damage to the hair follicles is much more pronounced with cyclophosphamide than with other mustards and frequently results in alopecia; this effect is usually reversible, even with continued therapy.

Sulfur mustard and the nitrogen mustards are powerful local vesicants. Either direct contact with the compounds or exposure to vapors can lead to serious local reactions. The susceptible tissues are skin, eyes, and respiratory tract. The vesicant properties of the nitrogen mustards are of concern to the clinician in that local reactions can occur if certain precautions are not observed during the course of administration (*see* below).

Actions on Reproductive Tissues. In women, amenorrhea of several months' duration sometimes follows a course of therapy with alkylating agents. Impairment of spermatogenesis may be noted in men.

Actions on the Nervous System. All nitrogen mustards have effects on the central nervous system (CNS). Nausea and vomiting are prominent side effects, particularly of mechlorethamine, and are presumably the result of CNS stimulation. Convulsions, progressive muscular paralysis, and various cholinomimetic effects have been observed. These effects and a poorly understood "delayed-death" syndrome reported in animals indicate that the cytotoxicity of the alkylating agents extends to cellular functions unrelated to proliferative activity. More detailed descriptions and references appear in the *fourth* and *earlier editions* of this textbook.

NITROGEN MUSTARDS

The chemistry and the pharmacological actions of the alkylating agents as a group, and of the nitrogen mustards, have been presented above. Only the unique pharmacological characteristics of the individual agents are considered below.

MECHLORETHAMINE

Mechlorethamine was the first of the nitrogen mustards to be introduced into clinical medicine and is the most rapidly acting of the drugs in this class.

Absorption and Fate. Severe local reactions of exposed tissues necessitate intravenous injection of mechlorethamine for most clinical uses. In either water or body fluids, at rates affected markedly by pH, mechlorethamine rapidly undergoes chemical transformation and combines with either water or reactive compounds of cells, so that the drug is no longer present in active form after a few minutes. Indeed, it is possible to protect a given tissue from the effects of the agent by interrupting the blood supply to the area for a few minutes during and immediately after injection of the drug. Conversely, it is possible, but not always feasible, to localize the action of mechlorethamine or related agents to a large extent in a given tissue by injecting the drug into the arterial bloodstream supplying that tissue.

Preparation, Dosage, and Routes of Administration. *Mechlorethamine hydrochloride* (MUSTARGEN) is supplied in 10-mg vials. The solution for injection must be freshly prepared before each administration; gloves are worn to protect the hands. The solution is injected into the tubing of a rapidly flowing intravenous infusion.

A course of therapy with mechlorethamine consists of the injection of a total dose of 0.4 mg/kg of body weight or 10 mg/m^2. Although this total dose may be given in either two or four daily consecutive injections, a single administration is preferable; the therapeutic response is equal, and the patient is spared an additional 2 or 3 days of anorexia, nausea, and vomiting. In the presence of extensive infiltration of bone marrow by neoplastic cells, as is often the case in diffuse lymphoma, it is wise to reduce the dose to 0.3 or even 0.2 mg/kg, at least for the first course of therapy. A course of mechlorethamine may be repeated only after bone-marrow function has recovered. Usually, at least 6 weeks should elapse between courses of this agent.

Direct intracavitary administration of the drug (0.2 to 0.4 mg/kg) for malignant effusions, particularly of pleural origin, provides valuable palliation.

Therapeutic Uses and Clinical Toxicity. The beneficial results of mechlorethamine in Hodgkin's disease and, less predictably, in other lymphomas have been extensively confirmed. Although the drug has been effective alone, current practice favors its use in combination with other agents. In generalized Hodgkin's disease (stages III and IV), the so-called MOPP regimen (the combination of mechlorethamine, vincristine [ONCOVIN], procarbazine, and prednisone) is considered the treatment of choice (DeVita *et al.*, 1972). In patients with generalized mycosis fungoides, very dilute solutions (0.02%) of mechlorethamine may be painted on the involved cutaneous areas with marked beneficial results. Although palliative results have been observed in carcinomas of the bronchus, ovary, breast, and other solid tumors, alkylating agents of intermediate or slower reactivity are preferable. (*See* Lane, 1977; Colvin, 1982; Calabresi *et al.*, 1985.)

The major toxic manifestations of mechlorethamine include nausea and vomiting, as well as myelosuppression. Leukopenia and thrombocytopenia constitute the major limitation on the amount of drug that can be given in a single course. Rarely, hemorrhagic complications of nitrogen mustard therapy may be due to hyperheparinemia; in such a circumstance, specific therapy with protamine corrects the hemorrhagic diathesis (Chapter 55).

On rare occasions, a maculopapular skin eruption may follow therapy with mechlorethamine. The reaction apparently is not due to hypersensitivity; neither does it necessarily recur with subsequent administration of the drug. Herpes zoster is frequently associated with nitrogen mustard therapy. A latent viral infection is not uncommon in patients with malignant lymphoma, and therapy with either a nitrogen mustard or radiation may be followed by overt manifestations of the viral disease.

Women should be warned that menstrual irregularities may be produced by mechlorethamine, and, since fetal abnormalities can be induced, the drug should not be used if pregnancy exists or is suspected. Breast feeding should be terminated before therapy with mechlorethamine is initiated. After a course of therapy, catamenia may be delayed or several consecutive menstrual periods may be missed. The effect is presumably the result of arrest of maturation of the graafian follicles, but there appears to be no permanent damage to ovarian function.

Local reactions to extravasation of mechlorethamine into the subcutaneous tissue result in a severe, brawny, tender induration that may persist for a long time. If the local reaction is unusually severe, a slough may result. If it is obvious that extravasation has occurred, the involved area should be promptly infiltrated with an isotonic solution of sodium thiosulfate (1/6 M); an ice compress then should be applied intermittently for 6 to 12 hours. Thiosulfate provides an ion that reacts avidly with the nitrogen mustard and thereby protects tissue constituents. Thrombophlebitis is a potential complication of therapy with mechlorethamine; it rarely occurs if the drug is injected into the tubing during the course of an intravenous infusion.

CYCLOPHOSPHAMIDE

Pharmacological and Cytotoxic Actions. Although the general cytotoxic action of this drug is similar to that of other alkylating agents, some notable differences have been observed. When compared with mechlorethamine, damage to the megakaryocytes and thrombocytopenia are less common. Another unusual manifestation of selectivity is more prominent damage to the hair follicles, resulting frequently in alopecia. None of the severe acute CNS manifestations reported with the typical nitrogen mustards has been noted with cyclophosphamide. Nausea and vomiting, however, may occur. The drug is not a vesicant, and there is no local irritation.

Absorption, Fate, and Excretion. Cyclophosphamide is well absorbed orally. As mentioned above, the drug is activated by the hepatic cytochrome P_{450} system (*see* Colvin, 1982; *see also* Figure 52–3). Cyclophosphamide is first converted to 4-hydroxycyclophosphamide, which is in a steady state with the acyclic tautomer, aldophosphamide. These compounds may be oxidized further by hepatic aldehyde oxidase and perhaps by other enzymes, yielding the metabolites carboxyphosphamide and 4-ketocyclophosphamide, neither of which possesses significant biological activity. It appears that hepatic damage is minimized by these secondary reactions,

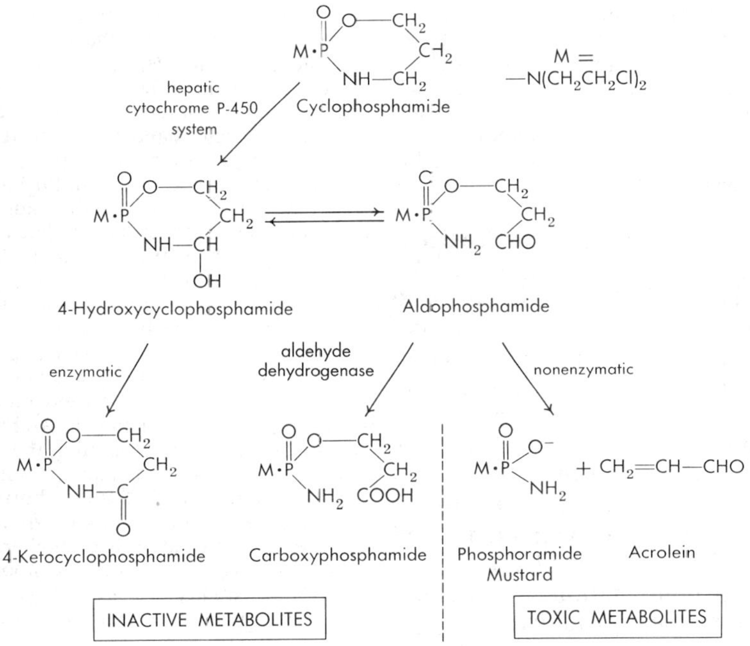

Figure 52–3. *Metabolism of cyclophosphamide.*

whereas significant amounts of the activated metabolites, such as aldophosphamide, are transported to the target sites by the circulatory system. In cells that are susceptible to cytolysis, the aldophosphamide may be cleaved by a β-elimination reaction, generating stoichiometric amounts of phosphoramide mustard and acrolein. The latter compound may be responsible for the hemorrhagic cystitis seen during therapy with cyclophosphamide. This can be reduced in intensity or prevented by the parenteral administration of acetylcysteine or other sulfhydryl compounds; acrolein reacts readily with sulfhydryl groups (Colvin, 1982).

If the cytochrome P_{450} system is induced by pretreatment of an animal with phenobarbital or inhibited by administration of proadifen (SK&F 525-A), the antitumor activity and therapeutic index of cyclophosphamide are not significantly modified (Sladek, 1972). The explanation proposed for this unexpected finding illustrates important pharmacological principles. Cyclophosphamide, which is biologically relatively inactive, is eliminated from the body very slowly. The activated metabolites (*e.g.*, 4-hydroxycyclophosphamide) either generate phosphoramide mustard, which alkylates target sites in susceptible cells, or are detoxified by the formation of inactive metabolites, which are rapidly excreted by the kidneys. The cytotoxic effects are related to the total amount rather than to the velocity of generation of the activated metabolites. Thus, it seems likely that the biological actions of cyclophosphamide may be affected more drastically by alterations in the rates of detoxification and elimination than by changes in the rate of generation of the activated metabolites.

Urinary and fecal recovery of unchanged cyclophosphamide is minimal after intravenous administration. Maximal concentrations in plasma are achieved 1 hour after oral administration, and the half-life of cyclophosphamide in plasma is about 7 hours. Prior treatment with allopurinol significantly prolongs this value.

Preparations, Dosage, and Routes of Administration. *Cyclophosphamide* (CYTOXAN, NEOSAR) is supplied as 25- and 50-mg tablets and as a powder for injection.

The drug has been administered orally, intravenously, intramuscularly, intrapleurally, and intraperitoneally. A conservative daily dose of 2 to 3 mg/kg, orally or intravenously, has been recommended for patients with more susceptible neoplasms such as lymphomas and leukemias or with compromised bone-marrow function. A higher daily dosage of 4 to 8 mg/kg intravenously for 6 days, followed by an oral maintenance dose of 1 to 5 mg/kg daily, 3 to 5 mg/kg intravenously twice weekly, or 10 to 15 mg/kg intravenously every 7 to 10 days, has been used for the treatment of carcinomas and more resistant neoplasms. Large single doses of 30 mg/kg (750 to 1000 mg/m^2) have been very effective in patients with lymphomas and cause a rapid response approaching that seen with mechlorethamine; in patients without complications or previous therapy, the recommended total initial loading dose is 40 to 50 mg/kg (1500 to 1800 mg/m^2), administered intravenously over a period of 2 to 5 days. Careful evaluation of bone-marrow function is imperative, and prolonged therapy is guided by keeping the total leukocyte count between 2500 and 4000 cells/mm^3 or by obtaining the desired response by the tumor.

Therapeutic Uses and Clinical Toxicity. The clinical spectrum of activity for cyclophosphamide is very broad and is similar to that of nitrogen mustard. It is an essential component of many effective drug combinations. Cyclophosphamide is effective in Hodgkin's disease and other lymphomas. Complete remissions and presumed cures have been reported in Burkitt's lymphoma and in acute lymphoblastic leukemia of childhood when cyclophosphamide is used concurrently with other agents. It is frequently used in combination with methotrexate and fluorouracil as adjuvant therapy after surgery for carcinoma of the breast when there is involvement of axillary nodes (Bonadonna and Valagussa, 1983).

Notable advantages of this drug are the availability of oral as well as parenteral routes of administration and the possibility of giving fractionated doses over prolonged periods. For these reasons it possesses a versatility of action that allows an intermediate range of use, between that of the highly reactive intravenous mechlorethamine and that of oral chlorambucil. Beneficial results have been obtained in multiple myeloma; chronic lymphocytic leukemia; carcinomas of the lung, breast, cervix, and ovary; and neuroblastoma, retinoblastoma, and other neoplasms of childhood. In addition to the combination mentioned above, it is also often used in combination with doxorubicin, vincristine, and prednisone. (*See* Holland and Frei, 1982.)

Because of its potent immunosuppressive properties, cyclophosphamide has received considerable attention for the control of organ rejection after transplantation and in nonneoplastic disorders associated with altered immune reactivity, including Wegener's granulomatosis, rheumatoid arthritis, and the nephrotic syndrome in children. Caution is advised when the drug is considered for use in these conditions, not only because of its acute toxic effects but also because of its high potential for inducing sterility, teratogenic effects, mutations, and cancer. The drug should not be used during pregnancy or breast feeding.

The clinical toxicity of cyclophosphamide differs from that of other nitrogen mustards in that significant degrees of thrombocytopenia are much less common, but there is frequent occurrence of alopecia. Patients should be forewarned of this possible event, which is usually reversible even without interruption of therapy. Nausea and vomiting are common and occur with equal frequency whether the drug is given by the oral or the intravenous route. Mucosal ulcerations, dizziness of short duration, transverse ridging of the nails, increased skin pigmentation, interstitial pulmonary fibrosis, and hepatic toxicity have been reported. Extravasation of the drug into subcutaneous tissues does not produce local reactions, and thrombophlebitis does not complicate intravenous administration. The occurrence of sterile, hemorrhagic cystitis has been reported in 5 to 10% of patients. This has been attributed to chemical irritation produced by reactive metabolites of cyclophosphamide. Its incidence has been reduced by administration of acetylcysteine (*see* above) or mesna (sodium 2-mercaptoethanesulfonate) (Brock and Pohl, 1986). For routine clinical use, ample fluid intake and frequent voiding are recommended. Administration of the drug should be interrupted at the first indication of dysuria or hematuria. The syndrome of inappropriate secretion of antidiuretic hormone (ADH) has been observed in patients receiving cyclophosphamide, usually at doses higher than 50 mg/kg (DeFronzo *et al.*, 1973). It is important to be aware of the possibility of water intoxication, since these patients are usually vigorously hydrated.

IFOSFAMIDE

As mentioned above, ifosfamide is an analog of cyclophosphamide that is also activated by hydroxylation in the liver. Severe urinary tract toxicity limited the use of ifosfamide when it was first introduced in the early 1970s. However, alterations of dosage regimens, adequate hydration, and the concomitant administration of mesna now permit the administration of effective doses of ifosfamide with a markedly decreased incidence of hemorrhagic cystitis. Mesna acts in the urine to detoxify the metabolites of ifosfamide that cause this untoward effect.

Ifosfamide is currently approved for use in combination with other drugs for germ cell testicular cancer. Clinical trials have also shown ifosfamide to be active against carcinomas of the cervix and lung, Hodgkin's and non-Hodgkin's lymphomas, and certain sarcomas. In addition to hemorrhagic cystitis, ifosfamide causes nausea, vomiting, anorexia, leukopenia, nephrotoxicity, and CNS disturbances (especially somnolence or confusion) (*see* Brade *et al.*, 1987).

Ifosfamide (IFEX) is available as a powder in 1-g vials. The drug is usually infused intravenously over at least 30 minutes at a dose of 1.2 g/m^2 per day for 5 days. Intravenous mesna (MESNEX) is given concomitantly and again 4 and 8 hours later at a dose of 240 mg/m^2 with each dose of ifosfamide. Patients should also receive at least 2 liters of oral or intravenous fluid daily. Treatment cycles are usually repeated every 3 weeks.

MELPHALAN

Pharmacological and Cytotoxic Actions. The general pharmacological and cytotoxic actions of melphalan, the phenylalanine derivative of nitrogen mustard, are similar to those of other nitrogen mustards (*see* Colvin, 1982; Wheeler, 1982). The drug is not a vesicant.

Absorption, Fate, and Excretion. When given orally, melphalan is absorbed in an incomplete and variable manner, and 20 to 50% of the drug is recovered in the stool. The drug has a half-life in plasma of approximately 90 minutes, and 10 to 15% of an administered dose is excreted unchanged in the urine (Tattersall *et al.*, 1978; Alberts *et al.*, 1979b; Colvin, 1982).

Preparation, Dosage, and Route of Administration. *Melphalan* (ALKERAN) is available in 2-mg tablets. The usual oral dose for multiple myeloma is 6 mg daily for a period of 2 to 3 weeks, during which time the blood count should be carefully observed. A rest period of up to 4 weeks should then intervene. When the leukocyte and platelet counts are rising, maintenance therapy, ordinarily 2 to 4 mg daily, is begun. It is usually necessary to maintain a significant degree of bone-marrow depression (total leukocyte count in the range of 3000 to 3500 cells per cubic millimeter) in order to achieve optimal results.

Therapeutic Uses and Clinical Toxicity. Although the general spectrum of action of melphalan seems to resemble that of other nitrogen mustards, the advantages of a gradual but continuous administration by the oral route have made the drug useful in the treatment of multiple myeloma (Bergsagel, 1972). Beneficial effects have also been reported in malignant melanoma and in carcinoma of the breast and ovary. The clinical toxicity of melphalan is mostly hematological and is similar to that of other alkylating agents. Nausea and vomiting are infrequent. Alopecia does not occur, and changes in renal or hepatic function have not been observed.

CHLORAMBUCIL

Pharmacological and Cytotoxic Actions. The cytotoxic effects of chlorambucil on the bone marrow, lymphoid organs, and epithelial tissues are similar to those observed with the nitrogen mustards. Although CNS side effects can occur, these have been observed only with large doses. Nausea and vomiting may result from single oral doses of 20 mg or more.

Absorption, Fate, and Excretion. Oral absorption of chlorambucil is adequate and reliable. The drug has a half-life in plasma of approximately 1 hour, and it is almost completely metabolized (Alberts *et al.*, 1979a).

Preparation, Dosage, and Route of Administration. *Chlorambucil* (LEUKERAN) is available in 2-mg tablets for oral administration. The standard initial daily dosage is 0.1 to 0.2 mg/kg, continued for at least 3 to 6 weeks. The total daily dose, usually 4 to 10 mg, is given at one time. With a fall in the peripheral total leukocyte count or clinical improvement, the dosage is reduced; maintenance therapy (usually 2 mg daily) is feasible and may be required, depending on the nature of the disease. More recently, high intermittent doses of chlorambucil (16 mg/m^2 daily for 5 days once each month) have been used effectively for the treatment of lymphoma (Portlock *et al.*, 1987).

Therapeutic Uses and Clinical Toxicity. At the recommended dosages, chlorambucil is the slowest-acting nitrogen mustard in clinical use. It is the treatment of choice in chronic lymphocytic leukemia and in primary (Waldenström's) macroglobulinemia.

In chronic lymphocytic leukemia, chlorambucil may be given orally for long periods, achieving its effects gradually and often without toxicity to a precariously compromised bone marrow. Its spectrum of action is similar to that of other alkylating agents, and remissions may be expected in Hodgkin's disease and lymphomas, and sometimes in solid tumors. Clinical improvement comparable to that with melphalan or cyclophosphamide has been observed in some patients with plasma-cell myeloma. Beneficial results have also been reported in disorders with altered immune reactivity, such as vasculitis associated with rheumatoid arthritis and autoimmune hemolytic anemia with cold agglutinins (Knospe *et al.*, 1974).

Although it is possible to induce marked hypoplasia of the bone marrow with excessive doses of chlorambucil administered over long periods, its myelosuppressive action is usually moderate, gradual, and rapidly reversible. Gastrointestinal discomfort, azoospermia, amenorrhea, pulmonary fibrosis, seizures, dermatitis, and hepatotoxicity may be encountered. A marked increase in the incidence of leukemia and other tumors has been noted in a large controlled study of its use for the treatment of polycythemia vera by the National Polycythemia Vera Study Group, as well as in patients with breast cancer receiving long-term adjuvant chemotherapy (Lerner, 1978).

ETHYLENIMINES AND METHYLMELAMINES

TRIETHYLENEMELAMINE (TEM), THIOTEPA (TRIETHYLENE THIOPHOSPHORAMIDE), AND HEXAMETHYLMELAMINE (HMM)

Status. Although nitrogen mustards have largely replaced ethylenimines in general clinical practice, this class of agents continues to have specific use. Thiotepa is active as an intravesicular agent in bladder cancer (Nissenkorn *et al.*, 1985), and hexamethylmelamine (HEXASTAT) is an integral part of combination regimens for the treatment of advanced ovarian cancer. Their pharmacological properties are described in the *third edition* of this textbook.

ALKYL SULFONATES

BUSULFAN

Pharmacological and Cytotoxic Actions. Busulfan is unique in that it exerts virtually no pharmacological action other than myelosuppression. At low doses, selective depression of granulocytopoiesis is evident. Platelets are also affected by relatively small amounts of drug, and erythroid elements may be suppressed as the dosage is raised; eventually, a pancytopenia results. Cytotoxic action does not appear to extend to either the lymphoid tissues or the gastrointestinal epithelium.

Absorption, Fate, and Excretion. Busulfan is well absorbed after oral administration, and it disappears from the blood with a half-time of 2 to 3 hours. Almost all of the drug is excreted in the urine as methanesulfonic acid.

Preparation, Dosage, and Route of Administration. *Busulfan* (MYLERAN) is available in 2-mg tablets. The initial oral dose varies with the total leukocyte count and the severity of the disease; daily doses from 2 to 8 mg are recommended to initiate therapy and are adjusted appropriately to subsequent hematological and clinical responses. It has been reported that reduction of the total leukocyte count to 10,000 or fewer cells/mm^3 before discontinuing the drug results in longer remissions. If maintenance doses are required to keep the hematological status under control, 1 to 3 mg may be given daily.

Therapeutic Uses and Clinical Toxicity. The beneficial effects of busulfan in chronic granulocytic leukemia are well established, and remissions may be expected in 85 to 90% of patients after the initial course of therapy.

Reduction in morbidity is readily apparent with symptomatic response, characterized by increased appetite and sense of well-being, which may occur within a few days. Reduction of the leukocyte count is noted during the second or third week, and regression of splenomegaly follows. Beneficial results have been reported in other myeloproliferative disorders, including polycythemia vera and myelofibrosis with myeloid metaplasia. High doses of busulfan (16 mg/kg) have been used effectively in combination with high doses of cyclophosphamide to prepare patients with acute myelogenous leukemia for bone marrow transplantation (Santos *et al.*, 1983).

The major toxic effects of busulfan are related to its myelosuppressive properties, and thrombocytopenia may be a hazard. Occasional instances of nausea, vomiting, diarrhea, impotence, sterility, amenorrhea, and fetal malformation have been reported. The drug may be carcinogenic and leukemogenic (Stott *et al.*, 1977). Hyperuricemia, resulting from extensive purine catabolism accompanying the rapid cellular destruction, and renal damage from precipitation of urates have been noted. The concurrent use of allopurinol is recommended to avoid this complication. A number of unusual complications have been observed in patients receiving busulfan, but their relation to the drug is poorly understood; these include generalized skin pigmentation, cataracts, gynecomastia, cheilosis, glossitis, anhidrosis, and pulmonary and endocardial fibrosis (Colvin, 1982).

NITROSOUREAS

The nitrosoureas are important antitumor agents that have demonstrated activity against a wide spectrum of human malignancies; they appear to function chemotherapeutically as bifunctional alkylating agents. Since their introduction by investigators at the Southern Research Institute (Johnston *et al.*, 1963; Schabel, 1973), many nitrosoureas have been synthesized. Certain of these agents, particularly carmustine (BCNU) and lomustine (CCNU), have attracted special interest because of their high lipophilicity and, thus, their capacity to cross the blood–brain barrier; this enables their use in the treatment of meningeal leukemias and brain tumors. Unfortunately, the nitrosoureas used in the clinic to date, with the exception of streptozocin, cause profound, cumulative myelosuppression that restricts their therapeutic value. In addition, long-term treatment with the nitrosoureas, especially semustine (methyl-CCNU), has resulted in renal failure with lesions that resemble radiation-induced nephritis. As with other alkylating agents, the nitrosoureas are both carcinogenic and mutagenic (Colvin, 1982).

Streptozocin, originally discovered as an antibiotic, is of special interest. This compound has a methylnitrosourea (MNU) moiety attached to the 2 carbon of glucose (*see* Table 52–2). It has special affinity for beta cells of the islets of Langerhans and is employed as a diabetogenic agent in experimental animals. Streptozocin is useful in the treatment of human pancreatic islet-cell carcinoma and malignant carcinoid tumors, as well as other human malignancies (Schein *et al.*, 1974). Although MNU, the active moiety of streptozocin, is cytotoxic to selected human tumors, it also produces powerful and delayed myelosuppression. Furthermore, MNU is particularly prone to cause carbamoylation of lysine residues of proteins (*see* Figure 52–2). Streptozocin is not myelosuppressive and displays little carbamoylating activity. Thus, the nitrosourea-type moiety has been attached to various carrier molecules, with alterations in crucial properties such as tissue specificity, distribution, and toxicity. Chlorozotocin, an agent in which the 2 carbon of glucose is substituted by the chloronitrosourea group (CNU), was developed and subjected to clinical testing (Green *et al.*, 1982). This compound, unlike streptozocin, is not diabetogenic and, unlike many other nitrosoureas, causes little myelosuppression or carbamoylation.

CARMUSTINE (BCNU)

Pharmacological and Cytotoxic Actions. Carmustine is capable of inhibiting the synthesis of DNA, RNA, and protein in a manner similar but not identical to that of other alkylating agents. Although bone-marrow suppression is observed, this drug characteristically causes an unusually delayed onset of leukopenia and thrombocytopenia. The nadir of the leukocyte and platelet counts may not be reached until 6 weeks after treatment. Cytotoxic effects on the liver, kidneys, and CNS have been reported (Oliverio, 1976).

Absorption, Fate, and Excretion. Although carmustine is rapidly absorbed by the oral route, it is administered intravenously because tissue uptake and metabolism occur quickly; disappearance from the plasma takes place with a half-life of 90 minutes. Approximately 80% of the drug appears in the urine within 24 hours as degradation products. The pharmacokinetic properties of the drug may be affected by the lipid content of the plasma and the other tissues. Active metabolites may be responsible for the delayed bone-marrow toxicity. Their entry into the cerebrospinal fluid (CSF) is rapid, and their concentrations in the CSF of man are 15 to 30% of the concurrent plasma values (Oliverio, 1976; Levin *et al.*, 1978).

Preparation, Dosage, and Route of Administration. *Carmustine* (BICNU) is a powder at 4°C; it melts to an oily liquid at 31°C and is stable in the anhydrous state. It is available in vials containing 100 mg. Carmustine is usually administered intravenously at doses of 150 to 200 mg/m^2, given by infusion over 1 to 2 hours, and it is not repeated for 6 weeks. When used in combination with other chemotherapeutic agents, the dose is usually reduced by 25 to 50%.

Therapeutic Uses and Clinical Toxicity. The spectrum of activity of carmustine is similar to that of other alkylating agents, with significant responses observed in Hodgkin's disease and to a lesser extent in other lymphomas and myeloma. Because of its ability to cross the blood–brain barrier, it has been used in meningeal leukemia and in primary and metastatic tumors of the brain, with encouraging results. Beneficial responses have been reported in melanomas, as well as in gastrointestinal, breast, bronchogenic, and renal-cell carcinomas (Young *et al.*, 1971; Walker, 1973; Wilson *et al.*, 1976; Moertel, 1978).

The most significant clinical toxicity is the characteristically delayed hematopoietic depression described above. The drug is not a vesicant, but local burning pain has been reported after intravenous administration. Nausea and vomiting occur approximately 2 hours after injection, and flushing of the skin and conjunctiva, CNS toxicity, esophagitis, diarrhea, dyspnea, interstitial pulmonary fibrosis, and renal and hepatic toxicity have been reported (Young *et al.*, 1971; Wiemann and Calabresi, 1985).

LOMUSTINE (CCNU) AND SEMUSTINE (METHYL-CCNU)

Pharmacological and Cytotoxic Actions. The cytotoxic effects of these compounds are similar to those of carmustine, as is their clinical toxicity. Delayed bone-marrow depression, reflected by leukopenia and thrombocytopenia, is characteristic and similar to that caused by carmustine

(Wasserman *et al.*, 1975; Wasserman, 1976).

Absorption, Fate, and Excretion. Lomustine and semustine are rapidly absorbed from the gastrointestinal tract and are administered orally. Although lomustine is rapidly and completely metabolized, prolonged plasma half-life of its metabolites, ranging from 16 to 48 hours, has been reported. Approximately 50% of the administered dose is detectable in the urine within 24 hours and 75% within 4 days. Semustine is not detectable in either plasma or urine. The chloroethyl moiety has a half-life of 36 hours, while the cyclohexyl portion has a biphasic disappearance curve with an early half-life of 24 hours and a slower secondary phase with a half-life of 72 hours. Although neither drug can be detected intact in the CSF, active metabolites appear in significant concentrations within 30 minutes (Oliverio, 1976).

Preparations, Dosage, and Route of Administration. *Lomustine* (CEENU) is available in 10-mg, 40-mg, and 100-mg capsules. Semustine is available only for investigational use. The usual oral dose of lomustine is 130 mg/m^2, while the recommended oral dose of semustine is 200 mg/m^2. Both drugs are administered as a single dose, which is not repeated for 6 weeks. When used concurrently with other antineoplastic drugs, the dose is usually reduced by 25 to 50% (Wasserman, 1976).

Therapeutic Uses and Clinical Toxicity. These agents have a wide spectrum of activity. Lomustine appears to be more effective than carmustine in Hodgkin's disease. Beneficial results of therapy with lomustine and particularly semustine, alone and concurrently with other agents, have been reported in patients with malignant gliomas, adenocarcinomas of the gastrointestinal tract, Hodgkin's disease and other lymphomas, carcinoma of the breast, malignant melanoma, hypernephromas, multiple myeloma, and various squamous-cell carcinomas (Wilson *et al.*, 1976; Moertel, 1978).

The clinical toxicity of both drugs is similar, with the characteristically delayed bone-marrow suppression described above being the dose-limiting effect. Nausea and vomiting are frequently encountered. Nephrotoxicity may occur, particularly when semustine is administered at total doses greater than 1500 mg/m^2. The earliest manifestation of this toxic effect may be a decrease in renal size. Both drugs are mutagenic, carcinogenic, and leukemogenic (Green *et al.*, 1982; Calabresi, 1983).

STREPTOZOCIN

This naturally occurring nitrosourea is an antibiotic derived from *Streptomyces acromogenes*. It has been particularly useful in treating functional, malignant pancreatic islet-cell tumors. The drug is capable of inhibiting synthesis of DNA in microorganisms and mammalian cells; it affects all stages of the mammalian cell cycle.

Absorption, Fate, and Excretion. Streptozocin is administered parenterally. After intravenous infusions of 200 to 1600 mg/m^2, peak concentrations in the plasma are 30 to 40 μg/ml; the half-life of the drug is approximately 15 minutes. Only 10 to 20% of a dose is recovered in the urine (Schein *et al.*, 1973).

Preparation, Dosage, and Route of Administration. *Streptozocin* (ZANOSAR) is available in 1-g vials as a powder for injection. The intravenous dose is 500 mg/m^2 once daily for 5 days; this course is repeated every 6 weeks. Alternatively, 1000 mg/m^2 can be given weekly for 2 weeks, and the weekly dose can then be increased to a maximum of 1500 mg/m^2.

Therapeutic Uses and Clinical Toxicity. Streptozocin has been used primarily in patients with metastatic pancreatic islet-cell carcinoma, and beneficial responses are translated into a significant increase in 1-year survival rate and a doubling of median survival time for the responders. It has also been found to be active in Hodgkin's disease, other lymphomas, and occasionally in melanoma and malignant carcinoid tumors (Schein *et al.*, 1974). Broder and Carter (1973) noted nausea and vomiting in almost all of 52 patients treated for islet-cell carcinoma. Renal or hepatic toxicity occurs in approximately two thirds of cases; although usually reversible, renal toxicity may be fatal, and proximal tubular damage is the most important toxic effect. Serial determinations of urinary protein are most valuable in detecting early renal effects. Hematological toxicity—anemia, leukopenia, or thrombocytopenia—occurs in 20% of patients.

TRIAZENES

DACARBAZINE (DTIC)

Dacarbazine functions as an alkylating agent after metabolic activation in the liver. It appears to inhibit the synthesis of RNA and protein more than it inhibits the synthesis of DNA. It kills cells slowly, and there appears to be no phase of the cell cycle in which sensitivity is increased (Bono, 1976).

Absorption, Fate, and Excretion. Dacarbazine is administered intravenously; after an initial rapid phase of disappearance ($t_{1/2}$ of about 20 minutes), the drug is removed from plasma with a half-time of about 5 hours (Loo *et al.*, 1976). The half-life is prolonged in the presence of hepatic or renal disease. Almost one half of the compound is excreted intact in the urine by tubular secretion. Elevated urinary concentrations of 5-aminoimidazole-4-carboxamide (AIC) are derived from the catabolism of dacarbazine, rather than by inhibition of *de-novo* purine biosynthesis. Concentrations of dacarbazine in CSF are approximately 14% of those in plasma (Chabner, 1982).

Preparation, Dosage, and Route of Administration. *Dacarbazine* (DTIC-DOME) is available in vials that contain 100, 200, or 500 mg. The recommended regimen is to give 3.5 mg/kg per day, intravenously, for a 10-day period; this is repeated every 28 days. Alternatively, 250 mg/m^2 can be given daily for 5 days and repeated every 3 weeks. Extravasation of the drug may cause tissue damage and severe pain.

Therapeutic Uses and Clinical Toxicity. At present, dacarbazine is employed principally for the treatment of malignant melanoma; the overall response rate is about 20%. Beneficial responses have also been reported in patients with Hodgkin's disease, particularly when the drug is used concurrently with doxorubicin, bleomycin, and vinblastine (Santora and Bonadonna, 1979), as well as in various sarcomas when used with doxorubicin (Costanzi, 1976; Gottlieb *et al.*, 1976). Toxicity includes nausea and vomiting in more than 90% of patients; this usually develops 1 to 3 hours after treatment. Myelosuppression, with both leukopenia and thrombocytopenia, is usually mild to moderate. A flu-like syndrome, consisting of chills, fever, malaise, and myalgias, may occur during treatment. Hepatotoxicity, alopecia, facial flushing, neurotoxicity, and dermatological reactions have also been reported.

II. Antimetabolites

FOLIC ACID ANALOGS

METHOTREXATE

Antifolates occupy a special place in antineoplastic chemotherapy, in that they produced the first striking, although temporary, remissions in leukemia (Farber *et al.*, 1948) and the first cure of a solid tumor, choriocarcinoma (Hertz, 1963). The attainment of a high percentage of permanent remissions in choriocarcinoma provided great impetus to investigations into chemotherapeutics. Interest in folate antagonists has increased greatly with the introduction of high-dose regimens with "rescue" of host toxicity by leucovorin (folinic acid, citrovorum factor). These methods extend the usefulness of methotrexate to tumors such as osteogenic sarcoma that do not respond to lower doses.

Methotrexate has also been used with benefit in the therapy of psoriasis, a non-neoplastic disease of the skin characterized by abnormally rapid proliferation of epidermal cells (McDonald, 1981). Additionally, folate antagonists are potent inhibitors of cell-mediated immune reactions and have been employed as immunosuppressive agents, for example, in organ transplantation and for the treatment of rheumatoid arthritis and Wegener's granulomatosis (Jackson, 1984; Chabner *et al.*, 1985).

Structure–Activity Relationship. Folic acid is an essential dietary factor from which is derived a series of tetrahydrofolate cofactors that provide single carbon groups for the synthesis of precursors of DNA (thymidylate and purines) and RNA (purines). A detailed description of the biological functions and therapeutic applications of folic acid appears in Chapter 54.

The enzyme dihydrofolate reductase (DHFR) is the primary site of action of most folate analogs studied to date (*see* Figure 54–6). Inhibition of DHFR leads to partial depletion of the tetrahydrofolate cofactors that are required for the synthesis of purines and thymidylate (Chabner *et al.*, 1985). Differences in the specificity for inhibitors among the DHFRs from different species have enabled the identification of important therapeutic agents for the treatment of bacterial and parasitic infections (*see* discussions of trimethoprim, Chapter 45; pyrimethamine, Chapter 41). These inhibitors have much greater activity against the bacterial and protozoal DHFRs than they do against the mammalian enzyme. By contrast, methotrexate is an effective inhibitor of DHFR in virtually all species. Crystallographic studies have revealed the atomic basis for the high affinity of methotrexate for DHFR (Kraut and Matthews, 1987) and the differences in amino acid sequences in the active centers of the various DHFRs that are responsible for the high species specificity of the agents used in antimicrobial chemotherapy (Matthews *et al.*, 1985).

Because folic acid and many of its analogs are very polar, they cross the blood–brain barrier poorly and require specific transport mechanisms to enter mammalian cells (Elwood, 1989). Once in the cell, additional glutamyl residues are added to the molecule by the enzyme folylpolyglutamate synthetase (Cichowicz and Shane, 1987). Intracel-

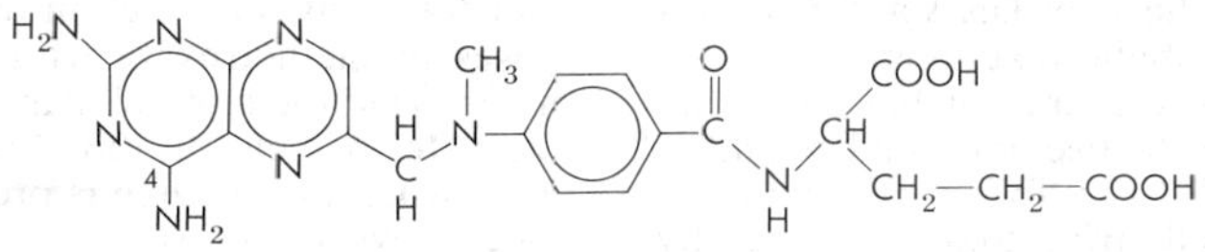

Methotrexate

lular methotrexate polyglutamates have been identified with as many as five glutamyl residues. Since these polyglutamates cross cellular membranes poorly, if at all, this serves as a mechanism of entrapment and may account for the prolonged retention of methotrexate in tissues such as liver. Evidence indicates that polyglutamylated folates have substantially greater affinity than the monoglutamate form for folate-dependent enzymes that are required for purine and thymidylate synthesis, but not for DHFR.

Novel folate antagonists have been identified that exploit differences in the folate influx system in certain tumors in comparison with normal tissues (*e.g.*, bone marrow). The analog 10-deaza,10-ethyl aminopterin is transported into some tumor cells much more efficiently than into normal tissues and is an excellent inhibitor of DHFR. This promising new compound is undergoing clinical evaluation (Sirotnak *et al.*, 1984; Shum *et al.*, 1988). In efforts to bypass the obligatory membrane transport system and facilitate penetration of the blood–brain barrier, lipid-soluble folate antagonists have also been synthesized. The most important of these, trimetrexate, has clinical activity in carcinoma of the colon and, interestingly, against *Pneumocystis carinii* (Allegra *et al.*, 1987). (For a recent review, *see* Allegra, 1990.)

Mechanism of Action. To understand the mechanism of action of folate analogs such as methotrexate, it is necessary to appreciate the complexities of the metabolism of folate cofactors and their multiplicity of functions; this is discussed in Chapter 54. To function as a cofactor in one-carbon transfer reactions, folate must first be reduced by DHFR to tetrahydrofolate (FH_4). Single-carbon fragments are added enzymatically to FH_4 in various configurations and may then be transferred in specific synthetic reactions. A key metabolic event is catalyzed by thymidylate synthase and involves the conversion of 2′-deoxyuridylate (dUMP) to thymidylate, an essential component of DNA. The methyl group transferred to the uracil moiety of dUMP is donated by N^{5-10}-methylene FH_4. Significantly, this carbon atom is transferred to the pyrimidine ring at the oxidation level of formaldehyde and is reduced to methyl by hydrogen atoms donated from the pteridine ring of the folate coenzyme; in the process, the reduced folate cofactor is converted to dihydrofolate (FH_2). To function again as a cofactor, FH_2 must first be reduced to FH_4 by DHFR. Inhibitors with a high affinity for DHFR prevent the formation of FH_4, producing an acute intracellular deficiency of folate coenzymes and a vast accumulation of the toxic substrate, FH_2 polyglutamates. The one-carbon transfer reactions crucial for the *de-novo* synthesis of purine nucleotides and thymidylate cease, with the subsequent interruption of the synthesis of DNA and RNA (as well as other vital metabolic reactions).

Understanding of these events enables appreciation of the rationale for the use of thymidine and/or leucovorin (N^5-formyl FH_4; folinic acid) in the "rescue" of normal cells from toxicity caused by drugs such as methotrexate. Leucovorin is a fully reduced folate coenzyme that enters cells via the specific carrier-mediated transport system and is converted to other active folate cofactors. It does not require reduction by DHFR. On the other hand, thymidine may be converted to thymidylate by thymidine kinase, thus bypassing the reaction catalyzed by thymidylate synthase and providing the necessary precursor for DNA synthesis.

An important feature of the binding of active folate antagonists with DHFRs is their very high affinity for the enzyme (K_i = 0.01 nM). Binding requires the participation of NADPH as an obligatory cofactor in a ternary complex with enzyme and inhibitor (Kamen *et al.*, 1983).

As with most antimetabolites, methotrexate is only partially selective for tumor cells and is toxic to rapidly dividing normal cells, such as those of the intestinal epithelium and bone marrow. Folate antagonists kill cells during the S phase of the cell cycle, and evidence indicates that methotrexate is much more effective when the cellular population is in the logarithmic phase of growth, rather than in the plateau phase. Because it is also capable of inhibiting RNA and protein synthesis, however, methotrexate slows the entry of cells into S phase and its cytotoxic action has been referred to as "self-limiting" (Skipper and Schabel, 1982).

Mechanism of Resistance to Antifolates. Several biochemical mechanisms of acquired resistance to methotrexate have been demonstrated: (1) impaired transport of methotrexate into cells (Assaraf and Schimke, 1987), (2) production of altered forms of DHFR that have decreased affinity for the inhibitor (Thillet *et al.*, 1988), (3) increased concentrations of intracellular DHFR, (4) decreased ability to synthesize methotrexate polyglutamates, and (5) decreased thymidylate synthase activity (Curt *et al.*, 1985). Marked increases in the activity of leukemic cell DHFR appear within days after treatment of patients with methotrexate; this likely reflects induction of new enzyme synthesis. Over longer periods of treatment, tumor-cell populations appear that contain markedly increased levels of DHFR. These cells have amplified their original single copy of the DHFR gene, and they contain multiple gene copies either in mitotically unstable double-minute chromosomes or in stable, homogeneously staining regions of the tumor cell chromosomes. First identified as an explanation for resistance to methotrexate (Schimke *et al.*, 1978), gene amplification has since been implicated in the resistance to many antitumor agents, including fluorouracil and pentostatin (2′-deoxycoformycin) (Stark and Wahl, 1984). Evidence supports the conclusion that gene amplification is a clinically significant phenomenon (Curt *et al.*, 1983).

Various therapeutic tactics have been recommended to avoid selection of resistant cells. High doses of methotrexate with leucovorin "rescue" may permit the intracellular accumulation of methotrexate in concentrations that inactivate DHFR even when the enzyme is present at markedly elevated levels. Alternation of methotrexate with other active agents that function by different mechanisms is another way to prevent the outgrowth of resistant cells.

General Toxicity and Cytotoxic Action. The actions of 4-amino analogs of folate in animals have been studied extensively. Animals given a lethal dose survive for at least 48 hours and usually die within 3 to 5 days. Anorexia, progressive weight loss, bloody diarrhea, leukopenia, depression, and coma are the outstanding features of fatal intoxication. The major lesions occur in the intestinal tract and bone marrow. Swelling and cytoplasmic vacuolization of the mucosal cells of the intestinal epithelium are evident within 6 hours. These changes are followed by desquamation of epithelial cells, extrusion of plasma into the lumen of the bowel, and leukocytic infiltration of the submucosa. Terminally, the entire intestinal tract exhibits a severe hemorrhagic enteritis. Loss of proliferating cells from the bone marrow begins within 24 hours, and within a few days the bone marrow becomes aplastic. The disturbance in hematopoiesis is reflected in the circulating blood by a marked thrombocytopenia, granulocytopenia, and reticulocytopenia and a moderate lymphopenia.

Folic acid antagonists are highly toxic to developing embryos and induce abortion in pregnant subjects, especially during the first trimester.

Absorption, Fate, and Excretion. Methotrexate is readily absorbed from the gastrointestinal tract at doses of less than 25 mg/m^2, but larger doses are absorbed incompletely and are routinely administered intravenously. Peak concentrations in the plasma of 1 to 10 μM are obtained after doses of 25 to 100 mg/m^2, and concentrations of 0.1 to 1 mM are achieved after high-dose infusions of 1.5 g/m^2 or more (Allegra, 1990). A direct relationship exists between dose and plasma concentrations. After intravenous administration, the drug disappears from plasma in a triphasic fashion (Huffman *et al.*, 1973). The rapid distributive phase is followed by a second phase, which reflects renal clearance ($t_{1/2}$ of about 2 hours). The final phase has a half-time of approximately 8 hours. This terminal half-life, if unduly prolonged by renal failure, may be responsible for major toxic effects of the drug on the marrow and gastrointestinal tract. Distribution of methotrexate into body spaces, such as the pleural or peritoneal cavities, occurs slowly. However, if such spaces are expanded (*e.g.*, by ascites or pleural effusion), they may act as a site of storage and release of drug with resultant prolonged elevation of plasma concentrations and more severe toxicity.

Approximately 35% of methotrexate is bound to plasma proteins and may be displaced from plasma albumin by a number of drugs, including sulfonamides, salicylates, tetracycline, chloramphenicol, and phenytoin; caution should be used if these are given concomitantly. Of the drug absorbed, from 40 to 50% of a small dose (2.5 to 15 μg/kg) to about 90% of a larger dose (150 μg/kg) is excreted unchanged in the urine within 48 hours, mostly within the first 8 hours. A small amount of methotrexate is also excreted in the stool, probably through the biliary tract. Metabolism of methotrexate in man is usually minimal. After high doses, however, metabolites do accumulate; these include 7-hydroxymethotrexate, which is potentially nephrotoxic (*see* Allegra, 1990). The portion of each dose of methotrexate that normally is excreted rapidly gains access to the urine by a combination of glomerular filtration and active tubular secretion. Therefore, the concurrent use of drugs that reduce renal blood flow (*e.g.*, nonsteroidal anti-inflammatory agents), that are nephrotoxic (*e.g.*, cisplatin), or that are weak organic acids (*e.g.*, aspirin or piperacillin) can delay drug excretion and lead to severe myelosuppression (Stoller *et al.*, 1977; Iven and Brasch, 1988). Particular caution must be exercised in treating patients with renal insufficiency.

Methotrexate is retained in cells as polyglutamates for long periods, for example, for weeks in the kidneys and for several months in the liver. There is also evidence for enterohepatic recirculation.

It is important to emphasize that concentrations of methotrexate in cerebrospinal fluid are only 3% of those in the systemic circulation at steady state; hence, neoplastic cells in the CNS are probably not killed by standard dosage regimens. When high doses of methotrexate are given (greater than 1.5 g/m^2), followed by leucovorin "rescue" (*see* below), cytotoxic concentrations of methotrexate may be attained in the CNS.

Preparations, Dosage, and Routes of Administration. *Methotrexate sodium* (*amethopterin*; FOLEX, MEXATE, others) is provided in 2.5-mg tablets and as preparations for injection.

Although the standard daily oral dosage of methotrexate ordinarily employed in patients with acute lymphocytic leukemia has been 2.5 to 5 mg for children and 2.5 to 10 mg for adults, newer therapeutic concepts have emerged involving revised dosage schedules and the use of multiple drugs sequentially and concurrently. Methotrexate induces remission slowly, probably because the cells in acute lymphocytic leukemia are not in the logarithmic phase of growth. For induction of remission it has been superseded by more rapid and effective therapy with vincristine plus prednisone, with or without daunorubicin. Methotrexate is of great value in the maintenance of remissions, particularly when administered intermittently at doses of 30 mg/m^2, intramuscularly, twice a week, or by intensive 2-day "pulses" of 175 to 525 mg/m^2 at monthly intervals.

The intrathecal administration of methotrexate has been employed for treatment or prophylaxis of meningeal leukemia or lymphoma or for treatment of meningeal carcinomatosis. This route of administration achieves high concentrations of methotrexate in the CSF and is effective also in patients whose systemic disease has become resistant to methotrexate, since the leukemic cells in the CNS beyond the blood–brain barrier have survived in a pharmacological sanctuary and retain their original degree of sensitivity to the drug. The recommended intrathecal dose is 12 mg/m^2 up to a maximum total dose of 12 mg (Bleyer, 1978). The dose is repeated every 4 days until malignant cells are no longer evident in the CSF. Leucovorin may be administered intramuscularly to counteract the toxicity of methotrexate that escapes into the systemic circulation.

In the treatment of choriocarcinoma with methotrexate, 1 mg/kg is administered intramuscularly every other day for four doses, alternating with leucovorin (0.1 mg/kg every other day). Courses are repeated at 3-week intervals, toxicity permitting, and urinary gonadotropin titers are used as a guide for persistence of disease.

Methotrexate has been used in the treatment of severe, disabling psoriasis in doses of 2.5 mg orally for 5 days, followed by a rest period of at least 2 days, or 10 to 25 mg intravenously weekly. An initial parenteral test dose of 5 to 10 mg is recommended to detect any possible idiosyncrasy. It is also used intermittently at low dosage to induce remission in refractory rheumatoid arthritis (Hoffmeister, 1983). Complete awareness of the pharmacology and toxic potential of methotrexate is a prerequisite for its use in these nonneoplastic disorders (Weinstein, 1977).

Continuous infusion of relatively large amounts of methotrexate may be employed (from 250 mg to 7.5 g/m^2, or more, weekly), but only when leucovorin "rescue" is used. The rationale for the administration of high doses is to achieve an excess of intracellular unbound drug, such that resistance due to deficiency of transport or amplification of DHFR is overcome. In addition, such regimens produce cytotoxic concentrations of drug in the CSF and protect against leukemic meningitis. After infusion of methotrexate for 6 hours, leucovorin is injected at a dose of 15 mg/m^2 every 6 hours for seven doses; the goal is to rescue normal cells and thereby prevent toxicity. The administration of methotrexate in high dosage may be extremely dangerous and should be performed only by experienced chemotherapists who are able to monitor concentrations of methotrexate in plasma. If values measured 48 hours after drug administration remain above 1 μM, higher doses and more prolonged administration of leucovorin must be undertaken (Stoller *et al.*, 1977). With appropriate precautions, these investigational schedules are surprisingly free of toxicity. It is imperative to maintain the output of a large volume of alkaline urine, since methotrexate precipitates in the renal tubules in acidic urine. In the presence of malignant effusions, delayed clearance may cause severe toxicity. Although the use of methotrexate in high doses with leucovorin "rescue" has been studied clinically for several years with promising results in osteosarcoma, childhood leukemia, and non-Hodgkin's lymphoma, the optimal timing, dose of leucovorin required, and proof of enhanced therapeutic efficacy remain to be established.

Therapeutic Uses and Clinical Toxicity. Methotrexate is a useful drug in the management of acute lymphoblastic leukemia in children. However, methotrexate is of very limited value in the types of leukemia seen in adults, except for treatment and prevention of leukemic meningitis. It is of established value in choriocarcinoma and related trophoblastic tumors of women; cure is achieved in approximately 75% of advanced cases treated sequentially with methotrexate and dactinomycin, and in over 90% when early diagnosis is made. In addition, many women with nonmetastatic trophoblastic disease, hydatidiform mole, and chorioadenoma destruens have been treated successfully with methotrexate. Beneficial effects are also observed in patients with osteosarcoma and mycosis fungoides and when methotrexate is used as part of the combination therapy of Burkitt's and other non-Hodgkin's lymphomas and carcinomas of the breast, head and neck, ovary, and bladder. High-dose methotrexate, with leucovorin "rescue," can cause substantial tumor regression in osteosarcoma and in combination therapy of leukemias and non-Hodgkin's lymphomas. (For references, *see* Calabresi *et al.*, 1985.) Striking improvement has been observed with the use of methotrexate in the treatment of severe psoriasis. Furthermore, methotrexate is an effective immunosuppressive agent and has been used for prevention of graft-versus-host reactions that result from marrow transplantation, as well as in the management of dermatomyositis, rheumatoid arthritis, Wegener's granulomatosis, and pityriasis rubra pilaris.

The primary toxic effects of methotrexate are exerted on the bone marrow and the intestinal epithelium; blood cell counts are depressed and there is mucosal ulceration. Such patients may be at risk for spontaneous hemorrhage or life-threatening infection, and they require prophylactic transfusion of platelets to maintain the count above 20,000 cells/mm^3 and broad-spectrum antibiotics if febrile. Side effects usually disappear within 2 weeks, but prolonged suppression of the bone marrow may occur in patients with compromised renal function who have delayed excretion of the drug. The dosage of methotrexate must be reduced in proportion to any reduction in creatinine clearance, and high-dose regimens should not be administered to patients with impaired renal function. Such regimens can cause renal failure because of precipitation of drug in the renal tubules and should be used only in vigorously hydrated patients (Stoller *et al.*, 1977).

Additional toxicities of methotrexate include alopecia, dermatitis, interstitial pneumonitis, nephrotoxicity, defective oogenesis or spermatogenesis, abortion, and teratogenesis. Hepatic dysfunction is usually reversible but sometimes leads to cirrhosis after long-term administration. Intrathecal administration of methotrexate often causes meningismus and an inflammatory response in the CSF. Seizures, coma, and death may occur rarely. Leucovorin does not reverse neurotoxicity.

PYRIMIDINE ANALOGS

This class of agents encompasses a diverse and interesting group of drugs that have in common the capacity to inhibit the biosynthesis of pyrimidine nucleotides or to mimic these natural metabolites to such an extent that they interfere with vital cellular functions, such as the synthesis of nucleic acids. Analogs of deoxycytidine and thymidine have been synthesized as inhibitors of DNA synthesis, and an analog of uracil, 5-fluorouracil, is an effective inhibitor of both RNA function and the synthesis of thymidylate. Drugs in this group are employed in the treatment of a variety of afflictions, including neoplastic diseases, psoriasis, and infections caused by fungi and DNA-containing viruses. The metabolic activation and degradation of these compounds and the interactions of their active metabolites with intracellular targets have been studied in great detail; these drugs present opportunities for the development of synergistic combination therapies that are under clinical investigation (Wasternack and Hause, 1987).

General Mechanism of Action. The best-characterized agents in this class are the halogenated pyrimidines, a group that includes such compounds as fluorouracil (5-fluorouracil or 5-FU), floxuridine (5-fluoro-2′-deoxyuridine or 5-FUdR), and idoxuridine (an antiviral agent; *see* Chapter 51). If one compares the van der Waals radii of the various substituents (Table 52–3), the dimension of the fluorine atom resembles that of hydrogen, whereas the bromine and iodine atoms are close in size to the methyl group. Thus, idoxuridine behaves as an analog of thymidine, and its primary biological action results from its phosphorylation and ultimate incorporation into DNA in place of thymidylate. If the hydrogen on position 5 of the pyrimidine ring is replaced with fluorine to produce 5-FU, the molecule mimics uracil biochemically. Fluorine has an inductive (electron-withdrawing) effect, which is reflected in a much lower pK_a of fluorouracil-containing compounds than with the natural compounds. Thus, substitution of a halogen atom of the correct dimensions can produce a molecule that sufficiently resembles a natural pyrimidine to interact with enzymes of pyrimidine metabolism but at the same time interferes drastically with certain other aspects of pyrimidine action.

Nucleotides in RNA and DNA contain ribose and 2′-deoxyribose, respectively. Among the various modifications of the sugar moiety that have been attempted, the replacement of the ribose of cytidine with arabinose has yielded a useful chemotherapeutic agent, cytarabine (AraC). As may be seen in Table 52–3, the hydroxyl group in this molecule is attached to the 2′-carbon in the β or upward configuration, as compared with the α or downward position of the 2′-hydroxyl in ribose. The arabinose analog is recognized enzymatically as a 2′-deoxyriboside; it is phosphorylated to a nucleoside triphosphate that competes with dCTP for incorporation into DNA (Chabner, 1990).

Several agents are available that inhibit different steps in the synthesis of pyrimidines and that exert synergistic cytotoxicity when used concurrently with a pyrimidine analog such as AraC or 5-FU. N-phosphonoacetyl-L-aspartate (PALA; sparfosate) is a "transition-state" inhibitor of the enzyme aspartate transcarbamylase, which catalyzes an early step in pyrimidine biosynthesis (Stark and Bartlett, 1983). Three other agents are potent inhibitors of a later step in pyrimidine nucleotide synthesis, the coupled enzymatic reactions by which orotate is converted first to the 5′-monophosphate nucleotide (orotidylate) and then decarboxylated to form uridylate. The compounds 5-azacytidine, 6-azauridine, and pyrazofuran, after being converted to the corresponding 5′-monophosphate nucleotides, are potent inhibitors of orotidylate decarboxylase. Azacytidine is being studied clinically for its usefulness in the treatment of refractory acute myelogenous leukemia; the drug can produce profound myelosuppression. Two other agents, 3-deazauridine and the glutamine antagonist acivicin, block the conversion of uridine triphosphate (UTP) to cytidine triphosphate (CTP). Use of these various agents in combination with cytosine arabinoside has resulted in increased for-

Table 52–3. STRUCTURAL FORMULAS OF PYRIMIDINE ANALOGS

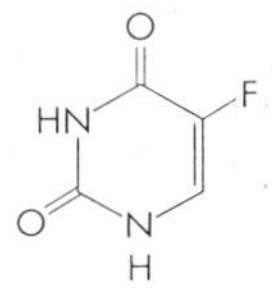

Fluorouracil
(pK_a 8.1)

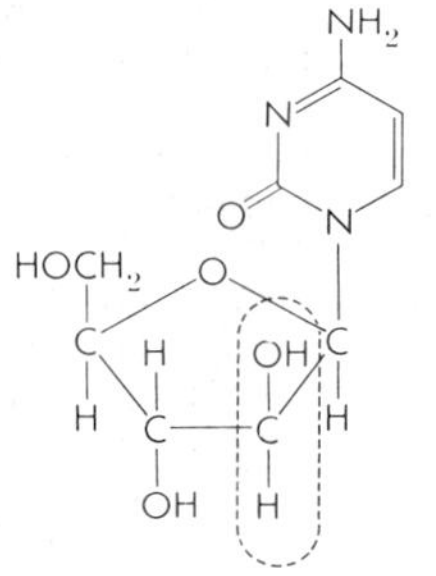

Cytarabine
(Cytosine Arabinoside)
(pK_a 4.5)

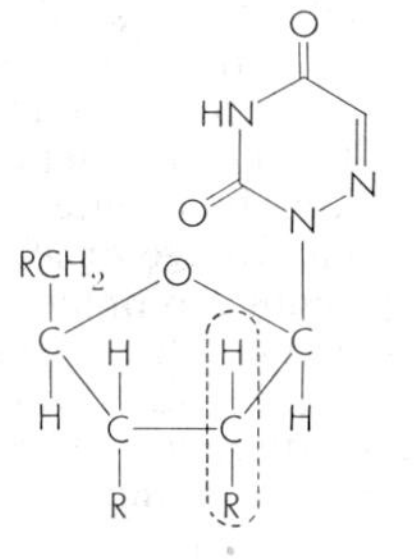

Azauridine: R = —OH

Azaribine: R = —O—C(=O)—CH_3
(pK_a 6.7)

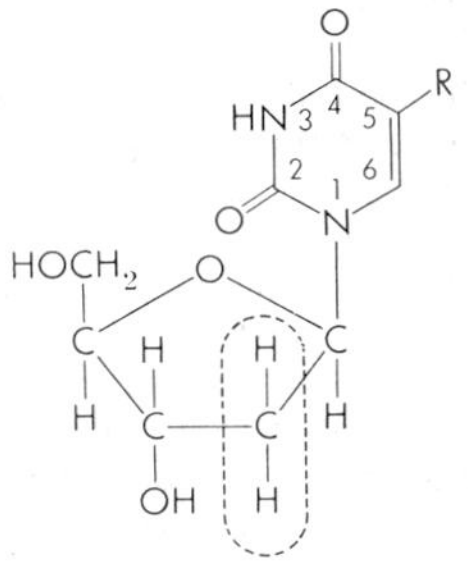

R	*van der Waals Radii (Å)*	*Compound*	pK_a
H	1.20	Deoxyuridine	9.3
F	1.35	Floxuridine (fluorodeoxyuridine)	7.6
Cl	1.80	Chlorodeoxyuridine	7.9
Br	1.95	Bromodeoxyuridine	7.9
CH_3	2.00	Thymidine	9.8
I	2.15	Idoxuridine (iododeoxyuridine)	8.25
CF_3	2.44	Trifluoromethyldeoxyuridine	7.35

mation of intracellular AraCTP and synergistic cytotoxicity.

FLUOROURACIL AND FLOXURIDINE (FLUORODEOXYURIDINE)

Mechanism of Action. 5-FU requires enzymatic conversion to the nucleotide in order to exert its cytotoxic activity. Several routes are available for the formation of the 5′-monophosphate nucleotide (F-UMP) in animal cells. 5-FU may be converted to fluorouridine by uridine phosphorylase and then to F-UMP by uridine kinase or it may react directly with 5-phosphoribosyl-1-pyrophosphate (PRPP), catalyzed by the enzyme orotate phosphoribosyl transferase, to form F-UMP. 5-FU may also be converted directly to 5-FUdR by the enzyme thymidine phosphorylase. Many metabolic pathways are available to F-UMP, including incorporation into RNA. A reaction sequence crucial for antineoplastic activity involves reduction of the diphosphate nucleotide by the enzyme ribonucleotide diphosphate reductase to the deoxynucleotide level and the eventual formation of 5-fluoro-2′-deoxyuridine-5′-phosphate (F-dUMP). This complex metabolic pathway for the generation of the actual growth inhibitor, F-dUMP, may be bypassed through use of the deoxyribonucleoside of fluorouracil—floxuridine (fluorodeoxyuridine, FUdR)—which is converted directly to F-dUMP by thymidine kinase. However, FUdR is a good substrate for both thymidine and uridine phosphorylases, and it can also be degraded to 5-FU.

There have been notable advances in our understanding of the interaction between F-dUMP and the enzyme thymidylate synthase, which is an important site of the cytotoxic action of the drug. The folate cofactor, $N^{5\text{-}10}$-methylenetetrahydrofolate, and F-dUMP form a covalently bound ternary complex with the enzyme. This inhibitory complex resembles the transition state formed during the normal enzymatic reaction when dUMP is converted to thymidylate. Although the physiological complex progresses to the synthesis of thymidylate by transfer of the methylene group and two hydrogen atoms from folate to dUMP, this reaction is blocked in the inhibitory complex by the fluorine atom on F-dUMP; sustained inhibition of the enzyme results (Santi *et al.*, 1974; Danenberg and Lockshin, 1981.)

5-FU is incorporated into both RNA and DNA. Incorporation into RNA has been associated with toxicity and has major effects on both the processing and functions of RNA. The significance of the incorporation of FUdR into DNA is unclear.

Although it has been shown that 5-FU is much more lethal to logarithmically growing cells than to stationary cells, there is no clearly demonstrated effect at a definite stage of the cell cycle. The phenomenon of "thymineless death" has been invoked to explain the cytotoxic effects of 5-FU and its derivatives. The blockade of the thymidylate synthase reaction inhibits DNA synthesis, while cellular production of both RNA and protein continues. An imbalance in growth occurs that is not compatible with cell survival. In accord with this proposal, the administration of thymidine can reverse the toxicity of low concentrations of 5-FU, presumably through bypass of the block at thymidylate synthase.

A number of biochemical mechanisms have been identified that are associated with resistance to the cytotoxic effects of 5-FU or floxuridine. These mechanisms include loss or decreased activity of the enzymes necessary for activation of 5-FU, decreased pyrimidine monophosphate kinase (which decreases incorporation into RNA), amplification of thymidylate synthase, and altered thymidylate synthase that is not inhibited by F-dUMP. Some malignant cells appear to have insufficient concentrations of N^{5-10}-methylene tetrahydrofolate and, thus, cannot form maximal levels of the inhibited ternary complex with thymidylate synthase. Addition of exogenous folate in the form of N^5-formyltetrahydrofolate (leucovorin) increases formation of the complex in both laboratory and clinical experiments and has enhanced responses to 5-FU in clinical trials (Ullman *et al.*, 1978). It is not established which (if any) of these mechanisms is associated with clinical resistance to 5-FU and its derivatives (Grem *et al.*, 1987).

General Toxicity and Cytotoxic Action. The major sites of action of 5-FU and floxuridine on normal tissues are the bone marrow and the epithelium of the gastrointestinal and oral mucosa. These are described in detail under "Therapeutic Uses and Clinical Toxicity" below.

Absorption, Fate, and Excretion. 5-FU and floxuridine are administered parenterally, since absorption after ingestion of the drugs is unpredictable and incomplete. Metabolic degradation occurs, particularly in the liver. Floxuridine is converted by thymidine or deoxyuridine phosphorylases into 5-FU. 5-FU is inactivated by reduction of the pyrimidine ring; this reaction is carried out by dihydrouracil dehydrogenase, which is found in liver, intestinal mucosa, and other tissues. Inherited deficiency of this enzyme leads to greatly increased sensitivity to the drug. The product of this reaction, 5-fluoro-5,6-dihydrouracil is ultimately degraded to α-fluoro-β-alanine (Heidelberger, 1975; McDermott *et al.*, 1982).

Rapid intravenous administration of 5-FU produces plasma concentrations of 0.1 to 1.0 mM; plasma clearance is rapid ($t_{1/2}$ = 10 to 20 minutes). Urinary excretion of a single dose of 5-FU given intravenously amounts to only 11% in 24 hours. Although the liver contains high concentrations of dihydrouracil dehydrogenase, dosage does not have to be modified in patients with hepatic dysfunction, presumably because of degradation of the drug at extrahepatic sites. Given by continuous intravenous infusion for 24 hours, plasma concentrations in the range of 0.5 to 3.0 μM are obtained and the urinary excretion of 5-FU is only 4%. 5-FU readily enters the CSF, and concentrations of about 7 μM are reached within 30 minutes after intravenous administration; values are sustained for approximately 3 hours and subside slowly over a period of 9 hours (Fraile *et al.*, 1980).

Preparations, Dosage, and Routes of Administration. *Fluorouracil* (*5-FU*; ADRUCIL) is available as a solution (50 mg/ml) for intravenous administration. The recommended dose for average-risk patients in good nutritional status with adequate hematopoietic function is 12 mg/kg daily for 4 days, by rapid injection, followed by 6 mg/kg on alternate succeeding days for four doses if no toxicity is observed. The maximal daily dose has been established arbitrarily at 800 mg. Other regimens use daily doses of 500 mg/m^2 for 5 days, repeated in monthly cycles. When used with leucovorin, daily doses of 5-FU must be reduced to 375 mg/m^2 for 5 days because of mucositis and diarrhea. With any of these regimens, treatment should be discontinued at the earliest manifestation of toxicity (usually stomatitis or diarrhea) because the maximal effects of bone-marrow suppression will not be evident until the ninth to fourteenth day. The first course of therapy should be administered either in the hospital or under extremely close supervision in order to establish the tolerance of the individual patient. After a period of 30 days from the last injection of the preceding course, a new course of therapy is initiated; the dosage is adjusted on the basis of the previous response and is repeated at monthly intervals. It is usually necessary to produce significant toxicity in order to achieve an antineoplastic effect, and there is a clear relationship of dose to response in treatment of carcinoma of the colon (Hryniuk, 1987).

In the selection of patients, the roles of nutritional deficiencies and protein depletion have been stressed, particularly in relation to surgery. Reduced tolerance of the hematopoietic system may be present in elderly patients or may be the result of invasion of the bone marrow by either neoplastic cells or myelofibrosis. Patients with compromised bone-marrow function as a result of previous therapy either with alkylating agents or x-ray to the pelvis or vertebrae are particularly sensitive to the myelosuppressive action of these compounds.

Topical 5-FU as a 1% or 5% cream or a 1 to 5% solution in propylene glycol (EFUDEX, FLUOROPLEX) is used to treat basal cell carcinomas and premalignant keratoses.

Floxuridine (*fluorodeoxyuridine;* FUDR) is available in preparations for injection. Its primary use is by continuous infusion into the hepatic artery for treatment of metastatic carcinoma of the colon; the response rate to such infusion is 40 to 50%, or double that observed with intravenous administration. Intrahepatic arterial infusion for 14 to 21 days may be used with minimal systemic toxicity. However, there is a significant risk of biliary sclerosis if this route is used for multiple cycles of therapy (Ansfield *et al.*, 1971; Ensminger *et al.*, 1978). Continuous infusion of floxuridine into the arterial blood supply of tumors at other sites, such as in the head and neck region, may provide beneficial clinical effects. Intraarterial infusions, at doses of 0.1 to 0.6 mg/kg per 24 hours, are administered continuously until local toxicity is encountered (Fraile *et al.*, 1980).

Therapeutic Uses and Clinical Toxicity. Accumulated experience with 5-FU indicates that the drug produces partial or complete responses in 10 to 30% of patients with metastatic carcinomas of the breast and the gastrointestinal tract; beneficial effects have also been reported in hepatoma, as well as in carcinoma of the ovary, cervix, urinary bladder, prostate, pancreas, and oropharyngeal areas. Higher response rates are seen when 5-FU is used in combination with other agents, such as cyclophosphamide and methotrexate (breast cancer) and cisplatin (ovary and head and neck cancer). The use of 5-FU in combination regimens has improved survival in the adjuvant treatment of breast cancer (Early Breast Cancer Trialists, 1988) and colorectal cancer (Wolmark *et al.*, 1988). 5-FU is widely used with very favorable results for the topical treatment of premalignant keratoses of the skin and multiple superficial basal cell carcinomas. It is also effective in severe recalcitrant psoriasis (Alper *et al.*, 1985).

Adjuvant treatment of colorectal carcinoma with a combination of 5-FU and levamisole reduces the rate of recurrence of disease after surgical resection when compared with levamisole alone or with no adjuvant therapy (Laurie *et al.*, 1989). Overall improvements in survival exceeded those observed during previous studies with 5-FU alone or in combination with other chemotherapeutic agents. Levamisole was a widely used anthelminthic agent (*see* the *seventh edition* of this textbook); its side effects are minimal. The immunostimulatory activity of levamisole provided the impetus for such study.

The clinical manifestations of toxicity caused by 5-FU and floxuridine are similar and may be difficult to anticipate because of their delayed appearance. The earliest untoward symptoms during a course of therapy are anorexia and nausea; these are followed by stomatitis and diarrhea, which constitute reliable warning signs that a sufficient dose has been administered. Mucosal ulcerations occur throughout the gastrointestinal tract and may lead to fulminant diarrhea, shock, and death, particularly in patients who are receiving continuous infusions of 5-FU or in those receiving 5-FU with leucovorin. The major toxic effects of bolus-dose regimens result from the myelosuppressive action of these drugs. The nadir of leukopenia is usually between the ninth and fourteenth day after the first injection of drug. Thrombocytopenia and anemia may also occur. Loss of hair, occasionally progressing to total alopecia, nail changes, dermatitis, and increased pigmentation and atrophy of the skin may be encountered. Neurological manifestations, including an acute cerebellar syndrome, have been reported, and myelopathy has been observed after the intrathecal administration of 5-FU. Cardiac toxicity, particularly acute chest pain with evidence of ischemia in the electrocardiogram, may also occur. The low therapeutic indices of these agents emphasize the need for very skillful supervision by physicians familiar with the action of the fluorinated pyrimidines and the possible hazards of chemotherapy.

CYTARABINE (CYTOSINE ARABINOSIDE)

Cytarabine (1-β-D-arabinofuranosylcytosine; AraC) is the most important antimetabolite used in the therapy of acute myelocytic leukemia. It is the single most effective agent for induction of remission in this disease. (For review, *see* Chabner, 1990.)

Mechanism of Action. This compound is an analog of 2′-deoxycytidine with the 2′-hydroxyl in a position *trans* to the 3′-hydroxyl of the sugar, as shown in Table 52–3. The 2′-hydroxyl causes steric hindrance to the rotation of the pyrimidine base around the nucleosidic bond. The bases of polyarabinonucleotides cannot stack normally, as do the bases of polydeoxynucleotides.

As with most purine and pyrimidine antimetabolites, cytarabine must be "activated" by conversion to the 5′-monophosphate nucleotide (AraCMP), in this case catalyzed by deoxycytidine kinase. AraCMP can then react with appropriate nucleotide kinases to form the diphosphate and triphosphate nucleotides (AraCDP and AraCTP). Accumulation of AraCTP causes potent inhibition of DNA synthesis in many cells. Previously, this was thought to result from competitive inhibition of DNA polymerase by AraCTP. However, studies now indicate that inhibition of DNA synthesis by mammalian cells occurs at AraCTP concentrations 1/100 or less than those required for inhibition of DNA polymerase, and the incorporation of AraC molecules into alkali-labile internucleotide linkages in DNA has been implicated. There is a significant relationship between inhibition of DNA synthesis and the total amount of AraC incorporated into DNA (Kufe and Major, 1982). Thus, the incorporation of about five molecules of AraC per 10^4 bases in DNA decreases cellular clonogenicity by about 50%. There is also evidence that AraC acts by slowing both chain elongation and the movement of newly replicated DNA through the matrix-bound replication apparatus. In addition, AraC inhibits β-DNA polymerase, an enzyme involved in DNA repair.

AraC and other cytidine analogs are potent inducers of tumor cell differentiation. In an attempt to exploit this potential, low-dose regimens of AraC (20 mg/m^2 per day) have been used to induce remission in acute myelocytic leukemia. However, the mechanism by which such regimens work is uncertain, and severe myelosuppression occurs.

Despite a wealth of observation, the precise mechanism of cellular death caused by AraC is not understood. Fragmentation of DNA is observed in AraC-treated cells. Potentially important is the phenomenon of "unbalanced growth," which results from prolonged suppression of macromolecular syntheses. Thus, inhibition of DNA synthesis by AraC without concomitant inhibition of protein and RNA syntheses can result in marked increases in cellular volume and in cellular death. It is likely that continued inhibition of DNA synthesis for at least one cell cycle is necessary. This mechanism may thus be important when AraC is administered by continuous prolonged infusion. A number of investigations have indicated that the optimal interval between bolus doses of AraC is about 8 to 12 hours. This interval may be determined by the need to maintain intracellular concentrations of AraCTP at inhibitory levels for at least one cell cycle. The mean cycle time of acute myelocytic leukemia cells is 1 to 2 days. Typical schedules for administration of AraC employ bolus doses every 12 hours or continuous infusion for 7 days.

Mechanisms of Resistance to Cytarabine. A crucial factor in determining the response to AraC is the relative activities of anabolic and catabolic enzymes that influence the conversion of AraC to AraCTP. The rate-limiting enzyme is deoxycytidine kinase, which produces AraCMP. An important degradative enzyme is cytidine deaminase, which deaminates AraC to a nontoxic metabolite, arauridine. This enzyme is found in high activity in many tissues, including some human tumors. A second degradative enzyme, dCMP deaminase, converts AraCMP to the inactive metabolite, AraUMP. Thus, the balance between the anabolic and catabolic enzymes determines the concentrations of AraCTP achieved. Clear relationships have been shown between the synthesis and retention of AraCTP and the duration of complete remission in patients with acute myeloblastic leukemia (Preisler *et al.*, 1985). The ability of cells to transport AraC also appears to be an important determinant of the clinical response (Wiley *et al.*, 1985).

Several biochemical mechanisms have been identified in AraC-resistant subpopulations in various murine and human tumor cell lines. Most commonly encountered is deficiency of deoxycytidine kinase (Kees *et al.*, 1989). Another mechanism of resistance is marked expansion of the dCTP pool due to increased CTP synthase activity. The increased concentrations of intracellular dCTP presumably can block the actions of AraCTP on DNA synthesis. Other mechanisms include increased cytidine deaminase activity and reduced affinity of DNA polymerase for AraCTP.

Tetrahydrouridine, a relatively potent inhibitor of cytidine deaminase, can enhance net synthesis of AraCTP and increase the cytotoxicity of AraC in several cell lines that have high activities of cytidine deaminase. Unfortunately, when the combination of tetrahydrouridine and AraC was subjected to clinical evaluation, marked increases in myelotoxicity were observed, suggesting that the therapeutic index was not improved.

Absorption, Fate, and Excretion. Cytarabine is poorly and unpredictably absorbed after oral administration, with only about 20% of the drug reaching the circulation. Peak concentrations of 2 to 50 μM are measurable in plasma after injection of 30 to 300 mg/m^2 intravenously. After intravenous administration there is a rapid phase of disappearance of cytarabine ($t_{1/2}$ = 10 minutes), followed by elimination with a half-time of about 2.5 hours. Only about 10% of the injected dose is excreted unchanged in the urine within 12 to 24 hours, while most appears as the inactive, deaminated product, arabinosyl uracil. Higher concentrations of cytarabine are found in CSF after continuous infusion than after rapid intravenous injection. After intrathecal administration of the drug at a dose of 50 mg/m^2, relatively little deamination occurs, even after 7 hours, and peak concentrations of 1 to 2 μM are achieved. The half-life of cytarabine in CSF is approximately 2 hours after intrathecal injection (Ho and Frei, 1971).

Preparation, Dosage, and Routes of Administration. *Cytarabine* (CYTOSAR-U) is marketed as a powder for injection for the treatment of acute leukemias in children and adults. Two dosage schedules are recommended: (1) rapid intravenous injection of 100 to 200 mg/m^2 every 12 hours for 5 to 7 days; or (2) continuous intravenous infusion of

100 to 200 mg/m^2 daily for 5 to 7 days. In general, children seem to tolerate higher doses than do adults. Maintenance therapy with subcutaneous injections of 1 mg/kg, weekly or every other week, can be used, although the drug appears more effective for the induction of remissions in acute leukemia. Intrathecal doses of 30 mg/m^2 every 4 days have been used to treat meningeal leukemia.

Therapeutic Uses and Clinical Toxicity. Cytarabine is indicated for induction of remission in acute leukemia in children and adults. When used alone, remission rates of 20 to 40% have been reported. The drug is particularly useful in acute myelocytic leukemia in adults. Cytarabine is more effective when used with other agents, particularly daunorubicin, mitoxantrone, or amsacrine (m-AMSA; an acridine dye derivative), complete remission rates of greater than 50% are to be expected. The drug is also used in combination therapy for non-Hodgkin's lymphomas in adults and in children, and for treatment of relapses of acute lymphocytic leukemia in both age groups. For relapses of leukemia, high doses of AraC (3 g/m^2 every 12 hours for 12 doses) yield a high rate of complete responses, but severe leukopenia and neurotoxicity are produced (Barnett *et al.*, 1985).

Cytarabine is primarily a potent myelosuppressive agent capable of producing severe leukopenia, thrombocytopenia, and anemia with striking megaloblastic changes. Other toxic manifestations include gastrointestinal disturbances and, less frequently, stomatitis, conjunctivitis, hepatic dysfunction, thrombophlebitis at the site of injection, fever, and dermatitis. Seizures and other manifestations of neurotoxicity may occur after intrathecal administration when high doses are administered intravenously (*e.g.*, 36 g/m^2 over 6 days) (Herzig *et al.*, 1987).

AZARIBINE

Azaribine is the triacetyl derivative and prodrug form of azauridine; it was synthesized in order to achieve better absorption after oral administration and to prevent metabolism of azauridine to azauracil by intestinal microorganisms, a factor that contributes to CNS toxicity from azauridine. Azaribine has marked therapeutic activity in psoriasis, mycosis fungoides, and polycythemia vera (McDonald and Calabresi, 1971; Skoda, 1975). Unfortunately, when the drug became available for clinical usage, thromboembolic disorders developed in some patients with psoriasis; since psoriasis itself is associated with an increased incidence of this complication, it is questionable whether this problem should be attributed to the drug or to the disease (McDonald and Calabresi, 1978; Shubin, 1979).

PURINE ANALOGS

Since the pioneering studies of Hitchings and associates, begun in 1942, many analogs of natural purine bases, nucleosides, and nucleotides have been examined in a wide variety of biological and biochemical systems. These extensive investigations have led to the development of several drugs, not only of use in the treatment of malignant diseases (mercaptopurine, thioguanine) but also for immunosuppressive (azathioprine) and antiviral (acyclovir, vidarabine, zidovudine) therapy. The hypoxanthine analog allopurinol, a potent inhibitor of xanthine oxidase, is an important by product of this effort (*see* Chapter 26). A promising development has been the discovery of powerful inhibitors of adenosine deaminase, for example, erythro-9-(2-hydroxy-3-nonyl)-adenine (EHNA) and pentostatin (2′-deoxycoformycin). Recent studies have confirmed that pentostatin has clinical activity against certain leukemias and lymphomas. In experimental systems these inhibitors of adenosine deaminase have produced marked synergistic effects in combination with various analogs of adenosine, such as vidarabine (arabinosyladenine; AraA); they also show promise as immunosuppressive agents. (*See* reviews by Elion and Hitchings, 1965; McCormack and Johns, 1982.)

Structure–Activity Relationship. Mercaptopurine and thioguanine, both established clinical agents for the therapy of human leukemias, are analogs of the natural purines hypoxanthine and guanine, in which the keto group on carbon 6 of the purine ring is replaced by a sulfur atom. Substitution in this position by chlorine or selenium also yields antineoplastic compounds. Cytotoxicity is also observed with the β-D-ribonucleoside and β-D-2′-deoxyribonucleoside derivatives. Because these nucleoside analogs are excellent substrates for purine nucleoside phosphorylase, a highly active enzyme in many tissues, the analog nucleosides act as prodrugs and generate respective hypoxanthine or guanine analogs in tissues. With several important exceptions, analogs of purine bases or nucleosides must undergo enzymatic conversion to the nucleotide to display cytotoxic activity.

Many attempts have been made to modify the structures of such analogs in order to improve their therapeutic indices or selectivity. Azathioprine (Table 52–4) was developed to decrease the rate of inactivation of 6-mercaptopurine by enzymatic S-methylation, nonenzymatic oxidation, or conversion to thiourate by xanthine oxidase. Azathioprine can react with sulfhydryl compounds such as glutathione (apparently nonenzymatically) and thus serves as a prodrug, permitting the slow liberation

Table 52–4. STRUCTURAL FORMULAS OF ADENOSINE AND VARIOUS PURINE ANALOGS

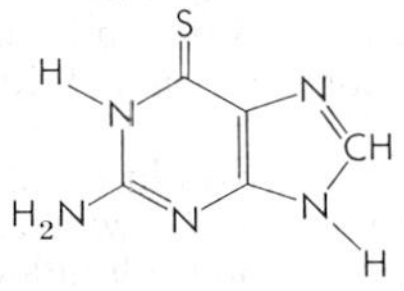

Thioguanine

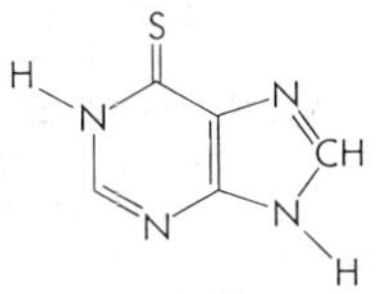

Mercaptopurine

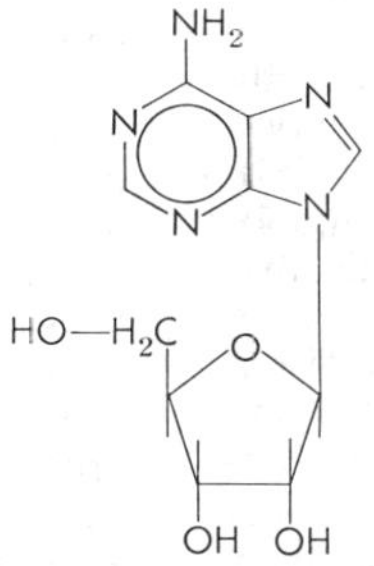

Adenosine

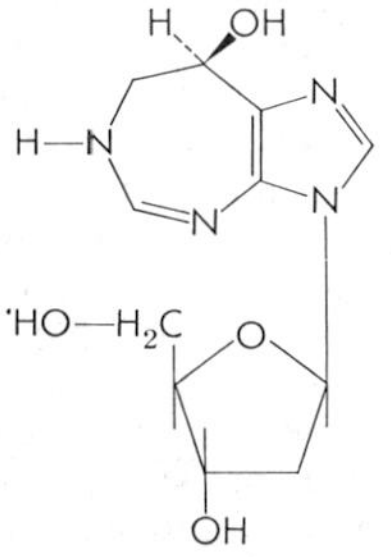

Pentostatin
(2′-Deoxycoformycin)

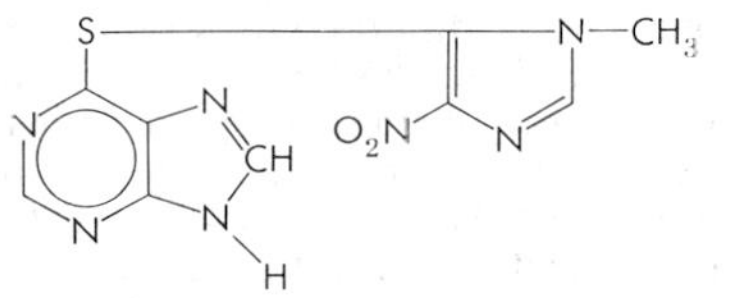

Azathioprine

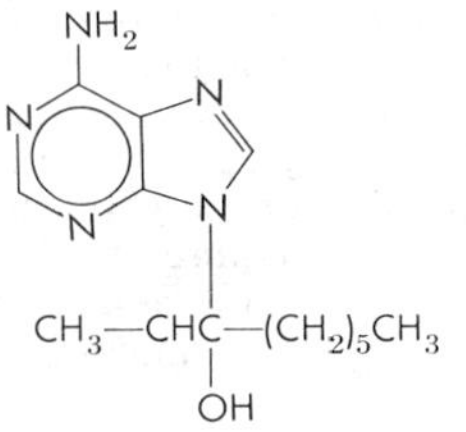

Erythrohydroxynonyladenine
(EHNA)

of mercaptopurine in tissues. Superior immunosuppressive activity is achieved in comparison with mercaptopurine (Elion, 1967).

An important development has been the discovery of potent inhibitors of adenosine deaminase such as pentostatin (2′-deoxycoformycin; K_i = 2.5 pM) and erythro-9-(2-hydroxy-3-nonyl)-adenine (EHNA; K_i = 2 nM). Pentostatin (Table 52–4) is a natural product derived from *Streptomyces*. Structurally, the drug resembles the transition state of adenosine as it is hydrolyzed by adenosine deaminase. As a result, the drug has an affinity for the enzyme that is 10^7-fold greater than that of the natural substrate. The enzyme–inhibitor complex is very stable and dissociates with a $t_{1/2}$ of about 25 to 30 hours (Agarwal *et al.*, 1977; Agarwal, 1982). Thus, pentostatin blocks not only the deamination of natural nucleosides but also that of many analogs used in chemotherapy.

Mechanism of Action. Although animal tissues have nucleoside kinases that are capable of converting adenosine or the 2′-deoxyribonucleosides of guanine, hypoxanthine, adenine, and many of their analogs to the corresponding 5′-monophosphates, similar reactions do not occur with inosine, guanosine, or their analogs. The latter compounds must first undergo phosphorolysis by purine nucleoside phosphorylase, which is present in high activity in many human tissues. The liberated bases may then be converted to the corresponding nucleotide by hypoxanthine-guanine phosphoribosyltransferase (HGPRT). Similarly, 2′-deoxyguanosine, 2′-deoxyinosine, and many related analogs may react with purine nucleoside phosphorylase, and the product of this reaction—a purine base or analog—may then be converted to the corresponding ribonucleoside 5′-monophosphate.

Both thioguanine and mercaptopurine are excellent substrates for HGPRT and are converted to the ribonucleotides 6-thioguanosine-5′-phosphate (6-thioGMP) and 6-thioinosine-5′-phosphate (T-IMP), respectively. Because T-IMP is a poor substrate for guanylyl kinase, the enzyme that converts GMP to GDP, T-IMP accumulates intracellularly. Careful studies have demonstrated, however, that mercaptopurine can be incorporated into cellular DNA in the form of thioguanine deoxyribonucleotide, indicating that slow reactions catalyzed by enzymes of guanine metabolism can operate. The accumulation of T-IMP may inhibit several vital metabolic reactions, such as the conversion of inosinate (IMP) to adenylosuccinate (AMPS) and then to adenosine-5′-phosphate (AMP) and the oxidation of IMP to xanthylate (XMP) by inosinate dehydrogenase. These reactions are crucial steps in the conversion of IMP to adenine and guanine nucleotides. On the other hand, in cells incubated with thioguanine,

6-thioGMP first accumulates; it is a poor, but definite, substrate for guanylyl kinase. Thus, there is slow conversion to 6-thioGDP and 6-thioGTP and entry of thioguanine nucleotides into the nucleic acids of the cell. In addition, the concentrations of 6-thioGMP achieved are sufficient to cause progressive and irreversible inhibition of inosinate dehydrogenase, presumably through the formation of disulfide bonds. Furthermore, both 6-thioGMP and T-IMP, as well as a number of other 5′-monophosphate derivatives of purine nucleoside analogs, can cause "pseudofeedback inhibition" of the first committed step in the *de-novo* pathway of purine biosynthesis, the reaction of glutamine and PRPP to form ribosylamine-5-phosphate. This enzyme is a major control point in the biosynthesis of purine nucleotides, and its activity is regulated by the intracellular concentrations of 5′-mononucleotides (natural, as well as analogs). The synthesis of PRPP is also powerfully inhibited by ADP and ATP or related analogs.

Despite extensive investigations, it is still not possible to assess precisely the role of incorporation of thioguanine or mercaptopurine into cellular DNA in the production of either the therapeutic or toxic effects of these drugs. These compounds can cause marked inhibition of the coordinated induction of various enzymes required for DNA synthesis, as well as potentially critical alterations in the synthesis of polyadenylate-containing RNA (Carrico and Sartorelli, 1977).

Other studies indicate that disruption of the synthesis of membrane glycoproteins may be caused by brief exposure to 6-thioguanine. These effects, which are potentially lethal to cellular survival, are likely mediated by depletion of guanosine diphosphate sugars. In view of these diverse biochemical actions, which involve vital systems such as purine biosynthesis, nucleotide interconversions, DNA and RNA synthesis, chromosomal replication, and glycoprotein synthesis, it is not possible to pinpoint a single biochemical event as the cause of thiopurine cytotoxicity. It seems likely that this class of drugs acts by multiple mechanisms (McCormack and Johns, 1982).

Of many adenosine analogs studied experimentally, *vidarabine* (arabinosyladenine, AraA) is used for the treatment of herpetic infections (*see* Chapter 51); its testing as an antineoplastic agent in combination with inhibitors of adenosine deaminase is under way. Vidarabine is converted enzymatically to AraATP. This analog nucleotide can inhibit DNA polymerases by competing with dATP and, in fact, may be incorporated into DNA. In this regard vidarabine resembles the analogous pyrimidine nucleoside antimetabolite cytarabine (AraC). By contrast, vidarabine, when administered alone, is relatively nontoxic and causes minimal immunosuppression. A related compound that has recently been in clinical trial is the analog nucleotide, 2-fluoro-9-β-D-arabinosyladenine-5′-phosphate (2-F-AraAMP). This analog serves as a prodrug; 2-F-AraA is released by cell membrane–associated 5′-ectonucleotidases. Both 2-F-AraAMP and 2-F-AraA are resistant to enzymatic deamination, which inactivates the parent analog, AraA. Although the drug has substantial activity in patients with refractory leukemia, sporadic but sometimes fatal neurotoxicity may limit its further development. (For additional discussion and references, *see* Bloch, 1975; McCormack and Johns, 1982; Chun *et al.*, 1986.)

As mentioned above, pentostatin is a potent inhibitor of adenosine deaminase. However, the relationship between this effect and drug-induced cytotoxicity is not clear. Alterations of the usual intracellular concentrations of adenosine-containing compounds appear to cause feedback inhibition of S-adenosylhomocysteine hydrolase; as a result, cellular methylation reactions are impaired. The drug interferes with the synthesis of nicotinamide adenine dinucleotide. The nucleoside triphosphate analog of pentostatin can be incorporated into DNA, resulting in strand breakage (Siaw and Coleman, 1984; Johnston *et al.*, 1986; Begleiter *et al.*, 1987).

Genetic deficiency of adenosine deaminase is associated with malfunction of both T and B lymphocytes, with little effect on other normal tissues (Giblett *et al.*, 1972). Thus, animals treated with pentostatin display marked immunosuppression. Severe and sometimes fatal opportunistic infections have also been associated with the clinical use of pentostatin. Treatment with pentostatin alone has induced remissions in T-lymphocyte–related diseases, such as T-cell leukemia and mycosis fungoides. These initial trials were predicated on the observation that malignant T cells have high levels of adenosine deaminase. However, encouraging results have also been obtained in B-cell disease; 25% of patients with refractory chronic lymphocytic leukemia have responded to the drug, as have 90% of patients with hairy cell leukemia (Cheson and Martin, 1987; Golomb and Ratain, 1987; O'Dwyer *et al.*, 1988). (*See* Symposium, 1984; Tritsch, 1985.)

Mechanisms of Resistance to the Purine Antimetabolites. As with other tumor-inhibiting antimetabolites, acquired resistance is a major obstacle to the successful use of the purine analogs. The most commonly encountered mechanism observed *in vitro* is deficiency or complete lack of the enzyme HGPRT. In addition, resistance can result from decreases in the affinity of this enzyme for its substrates. Cells that are resistant because of these mechanisms usually show cross-resistance to analogs such as mercaptopurine, thioguanine, and 8-azaguanine.

Another mechanism of resistance identified in cells from leukemic patients is an increase in particulate alkaline phosphatase activity. Other mechanisms include (1) decreased drug transport, (2) increased rates of degradation of the drugs or their intracellular "activated" analogs, (3) alteration in allosteric inhibition of ribosylamine 5-phosphate synthase, and (4) loss or alterations of the enzymes adenine phosphoribosyltransferase or adenosine kinase (for adenine or adenosine analogs). However, the most important determinants of resistance to these drugs in the clinical setting remains uncertain. (For reviews, *see* Brockman, 1974; McCormack and Johns, 1982.)

MERCAPTOPURINE

The introduction of mercaptopurine by Elion and coworkers represents a landmark in the history of antineoplastic and immunosuppressive therapy. Today mercaptopurine and its derivative, azathioprine, are among the most important and most clinically useful drugs of the class. The structure–activity relationship and the mechanism of action and of drug resistance are discussed above. The structural formula of mercaptopurine is presented in Table 52–4.

Absorption, Fate, and Excretion. Absorption of mercaptopurine is incomplete after oral ingestion and is affected by first-pass metabolism by the liver. Oral bioavailability is only 10 to 15%, with great interpatient variability. Measurements of drug concentrations in plasma may be necessary to optimize therapy with oral mercaptopurine. After an intravenous dose, the half-life of the drug in plasma is relatively short (about 50 minutes) due to uptake by cells, renal excretion, and rapid metabolic degradation. There are two main pathways for the metabolism of mercaptopurine. The first involves methylation of the sulfhydryl group and subsequent oxidation of the methylated derivatives. Low levels of erythrocyte thiopurine methyltransferase activity are associated with increased drug toxicity in individual patients. The formation of nucleotides of 6-methylmercaptopurine has been shown to occur after administration of mercaptopurine or mercaptopurine ribonucleoside. Substantial amounts of the mono-, di-, and triphosphate nucleotides of 6-methylmercaptopurine ribonucleoside (6-MMPR) have been identified in the blood and bone marrow of patients treated with mercaptopurine or azathioprine. Desulfuration of thiopurines can occur, and relatively large percentages of the administered sulfur are excreted as inorganic sulfate. The second major pathway for mercaptopurine metabolism involves the enzyme xanthine oxidase, which is present in relatively large amounts in the liver. Mercaptopurine is a good substrate for this enzyme, which oxidizes it to 6-thiouric acid, a noncarcinostatic metabolite.

An attempt to modify the metabolic inactivation of mercaptopurine by xanthine oxidase led to the development of allopurinol. This analog of hypoxanthine is a powerful inhibitor of xanthine oxidase, and not only blocks the conversion of mercaptopurine to 6-thiouric acid but also interferes with the production of uric acid from hypoxanthine and xanthine (*see* Chapter 26). Because of its ability to interfere with the enzymatic oxidation of mercaptopurine and related derivatives, allopurinol increases the exposure of cells to the action of these compounds. Although it greatly potentiates the antineoplastic action of mercaptopurine in tumor-bearing mice, allopurinol increases the toxicity as well, and there is no apparent improvement in the therapeutic index (McCormack and Johns, 1982; Zinner and Klastersky, 1985).

Preparation, Dosage, and Route of Administration. *Mercaptopurine (6-mercaptopurine;* PURINETHOL) is marketed as 50-mg tablets. The initial average daily oral dose is 2.5 mg/kg. Starting doses usually range from 100 to 200 mg per day; with hematological and clinical improvement, the dose is diminished to an appropriate multiple of 25 mg and, in general, maintenance therapy of 1.5 to 2.5 mg/kg per day is continued. If beneficial effects have not been noted after 4 weeks, the daily dose may be increased gradually up to 5 mg/kg until evidence of toxicity is encountered. The total dose required to produce depression of the bone marrow in patients with nonhematological malignancies is about 45 mg/kg and may range from 18 to 106 mg/kg.

Hyperuricemia with hyperuricosuria may occur during treatment; the accumulation of uric acid presumably reflects the destruction of cells with release of purines that are oxidized by xanthine oxidase, as well as an inhibition of the conversion of inosinic acid to precursors of nucleic acids. This circumstance may be an indication for the use of allopurinol. Special caution must be employed if mercaptopurine or its imidazolyl derivative, azathioprine, is used with allopurinol, for reasons presented above. Patients treated simultaneously with both drugs should receive approximately 25% of the usual dose of mercaptopurine (*see* Appendix II).

Therapeutic Uses and Clinical Toxicity. In the early studies with mercaptopurine, bone-marrow remissions were described in more than 40% of children with acute leukemia. In adults with acute leukemia, the results have been much less impressive, but occasional remissions have been obtained.

The drug has contributed to the treatment of lymphoblastic leukemia more by maintaining than by inducing remissions. Cross-resistance does not occur between mercaptopurine and other classes of antileukemic agents.

In the treatment of chronic granulocytic leukemia, maintenance therapy with mercaptopurine can be useful. Mercaptopurine has not been of value in chronic lymphocytic leukemia, Hodgkin's disease and related lymphomas, and a wide variety of carcinomas, even at unusually high doses. Although active as an immunosuppressive agent, it has been superseded by its imidazolyl derivative, azathioprine.

The principal toxic effect of mercaptopurine is bone-marrow depression, although, in general, this develops more gradually than with folic acid antagonists; accordingly, thrombocytopenia, granulocytopenia, or anemia may not be encountered for several weeks. When depression of normal bone-marrow elements occurs, cessation of therapy with the drug usually results in prompt recovery. Anorexia, nausea, or vomiting is seen in approximately 25% of adults, but stomatitis and diarrhea are rare; manifestations of gastrointestinal effects are less frequent in children than in adults. The occurrence of jaundice in about one third of adult patients treated with mercaptopurine has been reported; although the pathogenesis of this manifestation is obscure, it usually clears upon discontinuation of therapy. Its appearance has been associated with bile stasis and hepatic necrosis. Dermatological manifestations have been reported. The long-term complications associated with the use of mercaptopurine and its derivative, azathioprine, for immunosuppressive therapy are discussed by Schein and Winokur (1975).

AZATHIOPRINE

Azathioprine, a derivative of 6-mercaptopurine, is used as an immunosuppressive agent; its structural formula is shown in Table 52–4. The rationale that led to its synthesis and its mechanism of action and metabolic degradation have been discussed above. Additional information is presented in Chapter 53.

THIOGUANINE

The synthesis of thioguanine was first described by Elion and Hitchings in 1955. It is of particular value in the treatment of acute granulocytic leukemia when given with cytarabine. The structural formula of thioguanine is shown in Table 52–4, and its mechanism of action is discussed above.

Absorption, Fate, and Excretion. Absorption of thioguanine is incomplete and erratic, and concentrations of the drug in plasma may vary more than tenfold after oral administration. Peak concentrations in the blood are reached 2 to 4 hours after ingestion. When thioguanine is administered to man, the S-methylation product, 2-amino-6-methylthiopurine, rather than free thioguanine appears in the urine; inorganic sulfate is also a major urinary metabolite. Lesser amounts of 6-thiouric acid are formed, suggesting that deamination catalyzed by the enzyme guanase does not have a major role in the metabolic inactivation of thioguanine. Accordingly, it may be administered concurrently with allopurinol without reduction in dosage, unlike mercaptopurine and azathioprine.

Preparation, Dosage, and Route of Administration. *Thioguanine* (*6-thioguanine, TG*) is available in 40-mg tablets. The average daily dose is 2 mg/kg. If there is no clinical improvement or toxicity after 4 weeks, the dosage may be cautiously increased to 3 mg/kg daily.

Therapeutic Uses and Clinical Toxicity. Clinically, thioguanine has been used in the treatment of acute leukemia and, in conjunction with cytarabine, is one of the most effective agents for induction of remissions in acute granulocytic leukemia; it has not been useful in the treatment of patients with solid tumors. This compound has been used as an immunosuppressive agent, particularly in patients with nephrosis and with collagen–vascular disorders. Toxic manifestations include bone-marrow depression and gastrointestinal effects, although the latter may be less pronounced than with mercaptopurine.

III. Natural Products

VINCA ALKALOIDS

History. The beneficial properties of the periwinkle plant (*Vinca rosea* Linn.), a species of myrtle, have been described in medicinal folklore for many years in various parts of the world. While exploring claims that extracts of the periwinkle might have beneficial effects in diabetes mellitus, Noble and coworkers (1958) observed granulocytopenia and bone-marrow suppression in rats, effects that led to purification of an active alkaloid. Other investigations by Johnson and associates demonstrated activity of certain alkaloidal fractions against an acute lymphocytic neoplasm in mice. Fractionation of these extracts yielded four active dimeric alkaloids: vinblastine, vincristine, vinleurosine, and vinrosidine. Two of these, vinblastine and vincristine, are important clinical agents (*see* Bender *et al.*, 1990).

Chemistry. The vinca alkaloids are asymmetrical dimeric compounds; the structures of vincristine and vinblastine are as follows:

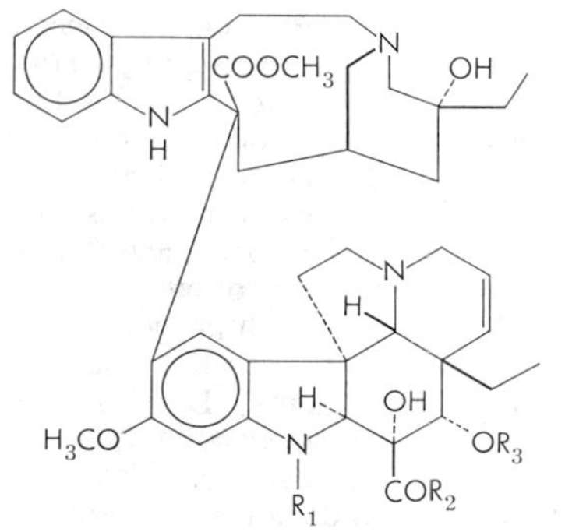

	Vincristine	Vinblastine
R_1:	$-CHO$	$-CH_3$
R_2:	$-OCH_3$	$-OCH_3$
R_3:	$-COCH_3$	$-COCH_3$

Structure–Activity Relationship. Minor differences in structure result in notable differences in toxicity and antitumor spectra among the vinca alkaloids. A number of related dimeric alkaloids are without biological activity. Removal of the acetyl group at C4 of one portion of vinblastine destroys its antileukemic activity, as does acetylation of the hydroxyl groups. Either hydrogenation of the double bond or reductive formation of carbinols reduces or destroys activity of these compounds.

Mechanism of Action. The vinca alkaloids are cell-cycle–specific agents and, in common with other drugs such as colchicine and podophyllotoxin, block mitosis and produce metaphase arrest. It seems likely that most of the biological activities of these drugs can be explained by their ability to bind specifically to tubulin and to block the ability of the protein to polymerize into microtubules. When cells are incubated with vinblastine, dissolution of the microtubules occurs, and highly regular crystals are formed that contain 1 mol of bound vinblastine per mol of tubulin. Colchicine and podophyllotoxin also can bind specifically with tubulin, but apparently at a site on the protein different from that bound by vinblastine. Through disruption of the microtubules of the mitotic apparatus, cell division is arrested in metaphase. In the absence of an intact mitotic spindle, the chromosomes may disperse throughout the cytoplasm (exploded mitosis) or may occur in unusual groupings, such as balls or stars. The inability to segregate chromosomes correctly during mitosis presumably leads to cell death.

In addition to their key role in the formation of mitotic spindles, microtubules are involved in many other cellular functions. Some types of cellular movements, phagocytosis, and axonal transport of subcellular organelles are dependent on microtubules, which explains some of the other effects of vinca alkaloids.

Drug Resistance. Despite their structural similarity, only a certain degree of cross-resistance is seen between the individual vinca alkaloids. Recently, however, attention has been drawn to the phenomenon of pleiotropic drug resistance, in which tumor cells become cross-resistant to a wide range of chemically dissimilar agents after exposure to a single (natural product) drug. Such multidrug-resistant tumor cells display cross-resistance to vinca alkaloids, the epipodophyllotoxins, anthracyclines, dactinomycin, and colchicine. Chromosomal abnormalities consistent with gene amplification have been observed, and the cells contain markedly increased levels of the P-glycoprotein that participates in the transport of these drugs from the cells (*see* Endicott and Ling, 1989). Ca^{2+}-channel blockers, such as verapamil, can reverse resistance of this type. Another frequent form of resistance to vinca alkaloids involves mutations in tubulin that prevent their effective binding.

Cytotoxic Actions. Despite their antiproliferative effects, vincristine and vinblastine have markedly different patterns of host toxicity. Vinblastine is strongly myelosuppressive and causes epithelial ulceration. The relatively low toxicity of vincristine for normal marrow cells and epithelial cells makes this agent unusual among antineoplastic drugs, and it is often included in combination chemotherapy with other myelosuppressive agents. However, loss of hair secondary to effects on the epithelial cells of the hair follicles appears to occur more frequently with vincristine than with vinblastine. No definite explanation is available for the striking differences in the toxicities of these closely related chemical structures.

Neurological Actions. Although neurotoxicity may occasionally be encountered with vinblastine, particularly at high dosage levels, neuromuscular abnormalities are more frequently observed with vincristine. Indeed, this untoward effect most frequently proves to be the limiting factor during therapy with vincristine. Several types of manifestations have been recognized. Peripheral neuropathy is the most common at usual clinical doses. Numbness and tingling of the extremities, followed by weakness, loss of reflexes, foot-drop, ataxia, muscular cramps, and neuritic pains, have also been observed frequently. Clinical neurophysiological studies have demonstrated that depression of deep tendon reflexes is the earliest and most consistent sign of vincristine-induced neuropathies. However, these symptoms do not warrant reduction of dosage. Weakness of limb musculature is a more serious, dose-limiting toxicity. Muscular weakness involving the larynx and the extrinsic muscles of the eye also has been noted. An effect on the autonomic nervous system may be responsible for severe, and even obstructive, constipation that frequently may develop with prolonged administration of vincristine, but it is seen only rarely with vinblastine. Temporary mental depression, occurring on the second or third day after treatment, especially with vinblastine, may be of clinical significance. In rare instances, vincristine causes a syndrome of inappropriate secretion of antidiuretic hormone.

Absorption, Fate, and Excretion. Unpredictable absorption has been reported after oral administration of vinblastine or vincristine. At the usual clinical doses the peak concentration of each drug in plasma is approximately 0.4 μM (Owellen *et al.*, 1977b). Vinblastine and vincristine bind to plasma proteins. They are extensively concentrated in platelets and to a lesser extent in leukocytes and erythrocytes.

After intravenous injection, vinblastine has a multiphasic pattern of clearance from the plasma; after distribution, drug disappears from plasma with half-lives of approximately 1 and 20 hours (Owellen *et al.*, 1977a). Vinblastine is metabolized in the liver to the biologically active derivative desacetylvinblastine. Approximately 15% of an administered dose is detected intact in the urine, and about 10% is recovered in the feces after biliary excretion. Vincristine also has a multiphasic pattern of clearance from the plasma; the terminal half-life is about 24 hours (Bender *et al.*, 1977). The drug is metabolized in the liver, but no biologically active derivatives have been identified. Both vinca alkaloids should be used with caution and doses should be reduced in patients with hepatic dysfunction. At least a 50% reduction in dosage is indicated if the concentration of bilirubin in plasma is greater than 3 mg/dl (about 50 μM).

VINBLASTINE

Preparations, Dosage, and Route of Administration. *Vinblastine sulfate* (VELBAN, others) is available in preparations for injection. The drug is given intravenously; special precautions must be taken against subcutaneous extravasation, since this may cause painful irritation and ulceration. The drug should not be injected into an extremity with impaired circulation. After a single dose of 0.3 mg/kg of body weight, myelosuppression reaches its maximum in 7 to 10 days. If a moderate level of leukopenia (approximately 3000 cells/mm^3) is not attained, the weekly dose may be increased gradually by increments of 0.05 mg/kg of body weight. In regimens designed to cure testicular cancer, vinblastine is used in doses of 0.3 mg/kg every 3 weeks irrespective of blood cell counts or toxicity.

Therapeutic Uses and Clinical Toxicity. The most important clinical use of vinblastine is with bleomycin and cisplatin (*see* below) in the curative therapy of metastatic testicular tumors (Williams and Einhorn, 1985). Beneficial responses have been reported in various lymphomas, particularly Hodgkin's disease, where significant improvement may be noted in 50 to 90% of cases. The effectiveness of vinblastine in a high proportion of lymphomas is not diminished when the disease is refractory to alkylating agents. It is also active in Kaposi's sarcoma, neuroblastoma, and Letterer–Siwe disease (histiocytosis X), as well as in carcinoma of the breast and choriocarcinoma in women.

The nadir of the leukopenia that follows the administration of vinblastine usually occurs within 7 to 10 days, after which recovery ensues within 7 days. Other toxic effects of vinblastine include neurological manifestations as described above. Gastrointestinal disturbances, including nausea, vomiting, anorexia, and diarrhea, may be encountered. The syndrome of inappropriate secretion of antidiuretic hormone (ADH) has been reported, and ischemic cardiac toxicity has also been noted. Loss of hair, mucositis of the mouth, and dermatitis may occur infrequently. Extravasation during injection may lead to cellulitis and phlebitis. Local injection of hyaluronidase and application of moderate heat to the area may be of help by dispersing the drug.

VINCRISTINE

Preparations, Dosage, and Route of Administration. *Vincristine sulfate* (ONCOVIN, VINCASAR PFS) is available as a solution (1 mg/ml) for intravenous injection. Vincristine used together with corticosteroids is presently the treatment of choice to induce remissions in childhood leukemia; the optimal dosages for these drugs appear to be vincristine, intravenously, 2 mg/m^2 of body-surface area, weekly, and prednisone, orally, 40 mg/m^2, daily. Adult patients with Hodgkin's disease or non-Hodgkin's lymphomas usually receive vincristine as part of a complex protocol. When used in the MOPP regimen (*see* below), the recommended dose of vincristine is 1.4 mg/m^2. High doses of vincristine seem to be tolerated better by children with leukemia than by adults, who may experience severe neurological toxicity. Administration of the drug more frequently than every 7 days or at higher doses seems to increase the toxic manifestations without proportional improvement in the response rate. Maintenance therapy with vincristine is not recommended in children with leukemia. Precautions should also be used to avoid extravasation during intravenous administration of vincristine. Vincristine (and vinblastine) can be infused into the arterial blood supply of tumors in doses several times larger than those that can be administered intravenously with comparable toxicity, but inadvertent intrathecal administration of vincristine has been lethal (Gaidys *et al.*, 1983; Williams *et al.*, 1983).

Therapeutic Uses and Clinical Toxicity. Vincristine has a spectrum of clinical activity that is similar to that of vinblastine, but there are some notable differences. An important feature is the incomplete cross-resistance between these agents, a remarkable finding in view of the very close similarity of their chemical structures and their common mechanism of action. Vincristine is effective in Hodgkin's disease and other lymphomas. Although it appears to be somewhat less beneficial than vinblastine when used alone in Hodgkin's disease, when used with mechlorethamine, prednisone, and procarbazine (the so-called MOPP regimen), it is the preferred treatment for the advanced stages (III and IV) of this disease (DeVita, 1981). In non-Hodgkin's lymphomas, vincristine is an important agent, particularly when used with cyclophosphamide, bleomycin, doxorubicin, and prednisone. As mentioned previously, vincristine is more useful than vinblastine in lymphocytic leukemia. Beneficial responses have been reported in patients with a variety of other neoplasms, particularly Wilms' tumor, neuroblastoma, brain tumors, rhabdomyosarcoma, and carcinomas of the breast, bladder, and the male and female reproductive systems (Calabresi *et al.,* 1985).

The clinical toxicity of vincristine is mostly neurological, as described above. The more severe neurological manifestations may be avoided or reversed by either suspending therapy or reducing the dosage upon occurrence of motor dysfunction. Severe constipation, sometimes resulting in colicky abdominal pain and obstruction, may be prevented by a prophylactic program of laxatives and hydrophilic agents.

Alopecia occurs in about 20% of patients given vincristine; however, it is always reversible, frequently without cessation of therapy. Although less common than with vinblastine, leukopenia may occur with vincristine, and thrombocytopenia, anemia, polyuria, dysuria, fever, and gastrointestinal symptoms have been reported occasionally. Ischemic cardiac toxicity has been reported. The syndrome of hyponatremia associated with high urinary concentration of Na^+ and inappropriate secretion of antidiuretic hormone has been occasionally observed during vincristine therapy. In view of the rapid action of the vinca alkaloids, it is advisable to take appropriate precautions to prevent the complication of hyperuricemia. This can be accomplished by the administration of allopurinol (*see* above).

TAXOL

Taxol is an experimental antimitotic agent, isolated from the bark of the ash tree, *Taxus brevifolia*. It binds to tubulin (at a site distinct from that used by the vinca alkaloids) and promotes the assembly of microtubules (Schiff *et al.,* 1979). Cells resistant to vinca alkaloids because of mutations in tubulin remain sensitive to taxol, but multidrug-resistant cells that overexpress the P-glycoprotein are resistant to the drug (Racker *et al.,* 1986). Taxol is currently being evaluated clinically; it has activity against malignant melanoma and carcinoma of the ovary. Maximal doses are 30 mg/m^2 per day for 5 days or 210 to 250 mg/m^2 given once every 3 weeks. The primary toxicity of taxol is myelosuppression and a sensory neuropathy (Wiernik *et al.,* 1987).

EPIPODOPHYLLOTOXINS

Podophyllotoxin, extracted from the mandrake plant (or May apple), *Podophyllum peltatum,* was used as a folk remedy by the American Indians and early colonists for its emetic, cathartic, and anthelmintic effects. Two semisynthetic glycosides of the active principle, podophyllotoxin, have been developed that show significant therapeutic activity in several human neoplasms, including small-cell carcinomas of the lung, testicular tumors, Hodgkin's disease, and diffuse histiocytic lymphoma. These derivatives are referred to as etoposide (VP-16-213) and teniposide (VM-26). Although podophyllotoxin binds to tubulin at a site distinct from that for interaction with the vinca alkaloids, etoposide and teniposide have no effect on microtubular structure or function at usual concentrations. (For reviews of the epipodophyllotoxins, *see* Doyle, 1984; O'Dwyer *et al.,* 1985.)

Chemistry. The chemical structures of etoposide and teniposide are shown below:

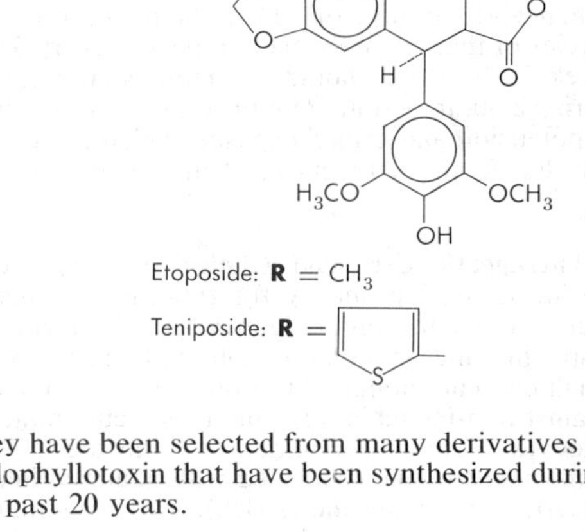

Etoposide: **R** = CH_3

Teniposide: **R** =

They have been selected from many derivatives of podophyllotoxin that have been synthesized during the past 20 years.

Mechanism of Action. Although the biochemical mechanisms of action are not yet understood, it appears that etoposide and teniposide are similar in their actions and in the spectrum of human tumors affected. Unlike podophyllotoxin, they do not cause mitotic arrest by binding to microtubules. Rather, at low concentrations, they block cells at the S–G_2 interface of the cell cycle and, at higher concentrations, they cause G_2 arrest. The greatest lethality is seen in the S and G_2 phases. Single-strand DNA breaks are observed in intact cells but not with purified DNA, suggesting that cellular enzymes are in some way involved. Growing evidence indicates that the epipodophyllotoxins stimulate DNA topoisomerase II to cleave DNA (Bender *et al.*, 1990). Resistant cells demonstrate either amplification of the P-glycoprotein that promotes drug efflux or alterations of topoisomerase II (Gupta, 1983; Pommier *et al.*, 1986).

ETOPOSIDE

Absorption, Fate, and Excretion. Oral administration of etoposide results in absorption of about 50% of the drug. After intravenous injection, peak plasma concentrations of 30 μg/ml are achieved; there is a biphasic pattern of clearance, with a terminal half-life of about 8 hours in patients with normal renal function. Approximately 40% of an administered dose of etoposide is excreted as such in the urine. Dosage should be reduced in proportion to reductions in creatinine clearance. Concentrations of etoposide in CSF range from 1 to 10% of the simultaneous value in plasma (Creaven and Allen, 1975; Wiemann and Calabresi, 1985).

Preparations, Dosage, and Routes of Administration. *Etoposide* (VEPESID) is available as a solution (20 mg/ml) for intravenous administration and as 50-mg, liquid-filled capsules for oral use. The intravenous dose for testicular cancer (in combination therapy) is 50 to 100 mg/m^2 daily for 5 days, or 100 mg/m^2 on alternate days, for three doses. For small-cell carcinoma of the lung, the intravenous dose (in combination therapy) is 35 mg/m^2, daily for 4 days, to 50 mg/m^2, daily for 5 days. When given orally, the dose should be doubled. Cycles of therapy are usually repeated every 3 to 4 weeks. The drug should be administered slowly during a 30- to 60-minute infusion in order to avoid hypotension and bronchospasm, which are probably due to the solvents used in the formulation.

Therapeutic Uses and Clinical Toxicity. Etoposide is used primarily for treatment of testicular tumors, in combination with bleomycin and cisplatin, and in combination with cisplatin for small-cell carcinoma of the lung. It is also active against non-Hodgkin's lymphomas, acute nonlymphocytic leukemia, carcinoma of the breast, and Kaposi's sarcoma associated with acquired immunodeficiency syndrome (AIDS). The dose-limiting toxicity of etoposide is leukopenia, with a nadir at 10 to 14 days and recovery by 3 weeks. Thrombocytopenia occurs less often and is usually not severe. Nausea, vomiting, stomatitis, and diarrhea occur in approximately 15% of patients treated intravenously, and in about 55% of patients who receive the drug orally. Alopecia is common but reversible. Fever, phlebitis, dermatitis, and allergic reactions including anaphylaxis have been observed. Hepatic toxicity is particularly evident after experimental high doses are given. Peripheral neuropathy is usually mild.

TENIPOSIDE

Teniposide is usually administered intravenously and has a multiphasic pattern of clearance from plasma. After distribution, half-lives of 4 hours and 10 to 40 hours are observed. Approximately 45% of the drug is excreted in the urine but, in contrast to etoposide, as much as 80% is recovered as metabolites. Dosage need not be reduced for patients with impaired renal function (Sinkule *et al.*, 1984). Less than 1% of the drug crosses the blood–brain barrier.

Teniposide is available for investigational use, and it has orphan drug status for treatment of refractory acute lymphoblastic leukemia in children. It is administered by intravenous infusion in doses that range from 50 mg/m^2 per day for 5 days to 165 mg/m^2 per day twice weekly. The clinical spectrum of activity includes acute leukemia in children, particularly monocytic leukemia in infants. Myelosuppression, nausea, and vomiting are its primary toxic effects.

ANTIBIOTICS

DACTINOMYCIN (ACTINOMYCIN D)

History. The first crystalline antibiotic agent to be isolated from a culture broth of a species of *Streptomyces* was actinomycin A (Waksman and Woodruff, 1940). Many related antibiotics, including actinomycin D, have subsequently been obtained (Waksman Conference on Actinomycins, 1974). Dactinomycin has beneficial effects in the treatment of a number of tumors, particularly certain neoplasms of childhood and choriocarcinoma.

Chemistry and Structure–Activity Relationship. The actinomycins are chromopeptides, and most of them contain the same chromophore, the planar phenoxazone actinocin, which is responsible for the yellow-red color of the compounds. The differences among naturally occurring actinomycins are confined to the peptide side chains, and the variations are in the structure of the constituent amino acids. By varying the amino acid content of the growth medium it is possible to alter the types of actinomycins produced and the biological activity of the molecule (Crooke, 1983). The chemical structure of dactinomycin is as follows:

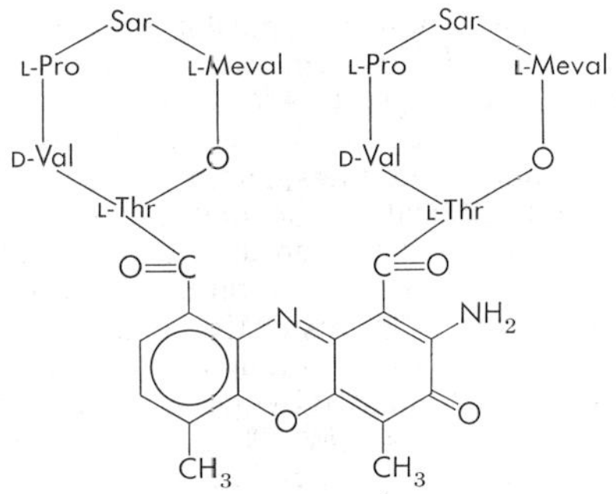

Dactinomycin

(Sar = sarcosine
Mevcl = N-methylvaline)

Mechanism of Action. The capacity of actinomycins to bind with double-helical DNA is responsible for their biological activity and cytotoxicity. X-ray studies of a crystalline complex between dactinomycin and deoxyguanosine permitted formulation of a model that appears to explain the binding of the drug to DNA (Sobell, 1973). The planar phenoxazone ring intercalates between adjacent guanine–cytosine base pairs of DNA, where the guanine moieties are on opposite strands of the DNA, while the polypeptide chains extend along the minor groove of the helix. The summation of these interactions provides great stability to the dactinomycin–DNA complex, and, as a result of the binding of dactinomycin, the transcription of DNA by RNA polymerase is blocked. The DNA-dependent RNA polymerases are much more sensitive to the effects of dactinomycin than are the DNA polymerases. In addition, dactinomycin causes single-strand breaks in DNA, possibly through a free-radical intermediate or as a result of the action of topoisomerase II. (*See* Waksman Conference on Actinomycins, 1974; Goldberg *et al.*, 1977)

Cytotoxic Action. Dactinomycin inhibits rapidly proliferating cells of normal and neoplastic origin and, on a molar basis, is among the most potent antitumor agents known. Atrophy of thymus, spleen, and other lymphatic tissues occurs in experimental animals. It may produce alopecia, and, when extravasated subcutaneously, the drug causes marked local inflammation. Erythema sometimes progressing to necrosis has been noted in areas of the skin exposed to x-radiation either before, during, or after administration of dactinomycin.

Absorption, Fate, and Excretion. Dactinomycin is much less potent when given orally than when administered by parenteral injection. The drug is excreted both in bile and in the urine, and disappears from plasma with a terminal half-life of 36 hours. Metabolism of the drug is minimal. Dactinomycin does not cross the blood–brain barrier.

Preparation, Dosage, and Route of Administration. *Dactinomycin* (*actinomycin D;* COSMEGEN) is supplied as a lyophilized powder (0.5 mg in each vial). The usual daily dose is 10 to 15 μg/kg; this is given intravenously for 5 days; if no manifestations of toxicity are encountered, additional courses may be given at intervals of 3 to 4 weeks. Daily injections of 100 to 400 μg have been given to children for 10 to 14 days; in other regimens, 3 to 6 μg/kg, for a total of 125 μg/kg, and weekly maintenance doses of 7.5 μg/kg have been used. Although it is safer to administer the drug into the tubing of an intravenous infusion, direct intravenous injections have been given, with the precaution of discarding the needle used to withdraw the drug from the vial in order to avoid subcutaneous reaction.

Therapeutic Uses and Clinical Toxicity. The most important clinical use of dactinomycin is in the treatment of rhabdomyosarcoma and Wilms' tumor in children, where it is curative in combination with primary surgery, radiotherapy, and other drugs, particularly vincristine and cyclophosphamide (Pinkel and Howarth, 1985). Antineoplastic activity has been noted in Ewing's tumor, Kaposi's sarcoma, and soft-tissue sarcomas. Dactinomycin can be effective in women with advanced cases of choriocarcinoma. It also produces consistent responses in combination with chlorambucil and methotrexate in patients with metastatic testicular carcinomas, but this regimen is not as effective as those that incorporate vinblastine, cisplatin, and bleomycin. It is of limited value in other neoplastic diseases of adults, although a response may sometimes be observed in patients with Hodgkin's disease and non-Hodgkin's lymphomas. Dactinomycin has also been used to inhibit immunological responses, particularly the rejection of renal transplants.

Toxic manifestations include anorexia, nausea, and vomiting, usually beginning a few hours after administration. Hematopoietic suppression with pancytopenia may occur in the first week after completion of therapy. Proctitis, diarrhea, glossitis, cheilitis, and ulcerations of the oral mucosa are common; dermatological manifestations include alopecia, as well as erythema, desquamation, and increased inflammation and pigmentation in areas previously or concomitantly subjected to x-radiation. Severe injury may occur as a result of local toxic extravasation.

DAUNORUBICIN AND DOXORUBICIN

These anthracycline antibiotics and their derivatives are among the most important of the newer antitumor agents. They are produced by the fungus *Streptomyces peucetius* var. *caesius*. Although they differ only slightly in chemical structure, daunorubicin has been used primarily in the acute leukemias, whereas doxorubicin displays broader activity against human neoplasms, including a variety of solid tumors. The clinical value of both agents is limited by an unusual cardiomyopathy, the occurrence of which is related to the total dose of the drug; it is often irreversible. In a search for agents with high antitumor activity but reduced cardiac toxicity, hundreds of anthracycline derivatives and related compounds have been prepared. Several of these have shown promise in the early stages of clinical study, including epirubicin and the synthetic compound mitoxantrone, which is an amino anthracenedione. (For review, *see* Myers, 1990.)

Chemistry. The anthracycline antibiotics have tetracycline ring structures with an unusual sugar, daunosamine, attached by glycosidic linkage. Cytotoxic agents of this class all have quinone and hydroquinone moieties on adjacent rings that permit them to function as electron-accepting and -donating agents. Although there are marked differences in the clinical use of daunorubicin and doxorubicin, their chemical structures differ only by a single hydroxyl group on C14. The chemical structures of daunorubicin and doxorubicin are as follows:

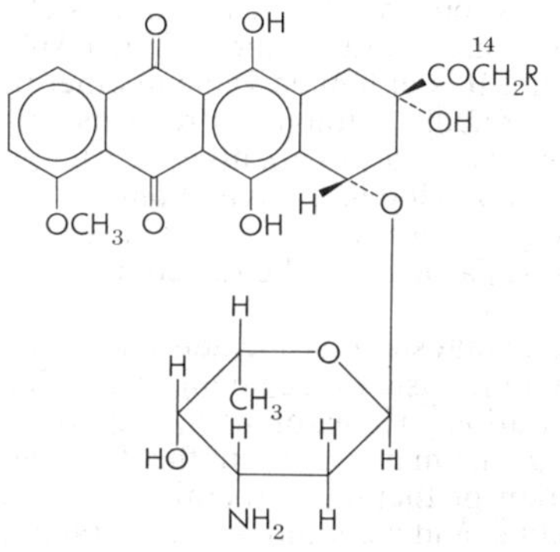

Daunorubicin: R = H
Doxorubicin: R = OH

Mechanism of Action. A number of important biochemical effects have been described for the anthracyclines and anthracenediones, any one or all of which could have a role in the therapeutic and toxic effects of such drugs. These compounds can intercalate with DNA. Many functions of DNA are affected, including DNA and RNA synthesis. Single- and double-strand breaks occur, as does sister chromatid exchange. Thus, the anthracyclines are both mutagenic and carcinogenic. Scission of DNA is believed to be mediated either by the action of topoisomerase II (Tewey *et al.*, 1984) or by the generation of free radicals. The anthracyclines react with cytochrome P_{450} reductase in the presence of reduced nicotinamide adenine dinucleotide phosphate (NADPH) to form semiquinone radical intermediates, which in turn can react with oxygen to produce superoxide anion radicals. These can generate both hydrogen peroxide and hydroxyl radicals (·OH), which are highly destructive to cells. The production of free radicals is significantly stimulated by the interaction of doxorubicin with iron (Myers, 1988). In addition, intramolecular electron-transfer reactions of the semiquinone intermediates result in the generation of other radicals and, thus, of potent alkylating agents. Enzymatic defenses such as superoxide dismutase and catalase are believed to have an important role in protecting cells against the toxicity of the anthracyclines, and these defenses can be augmented by exogenous antioxidants such as alpha tocopherol or by an iron chelator, ADR-529 (formerly called ICRF-187), which protects against cardiac toxicity (Speyer *et al.*, 1988). The anthracyclines can also interact with cell membranes and alter their functions; this may play an important part in both the antitumor actions and the cardiac toxicity caused by these drugs (Tritton *et al.*, 1978).

As might be expected of compounds that inhibit DNA function, maximal toxicity occurs during the S phase of the cell cycle. At low concentrations of drug, cells will proceed through the S phase and die in G_2.

As discussed above, the phenomenon of pleiotropic drug resistance is observed with the anthracyclines. This appears to result from acceleration of the efflux of anthracyclines and other agents from the cell. The P-glycoprotein, synthesized in high quantity as a result of gene amplification, has been implicated (Endicott and Ling, 1989). Other biochemical changes in resistant cells include increased glutathione peroxidase activity (Sinha *et al.*, 1989) and decreased activity of topoisomerase II (Deffie *et al.*, 1989).

Absorption, Fate, and Excretion. Daunorubicin and doxorubicin are usually administered intravenously, and they are then cleared rapidly from the plasma. The disappearance curve for doxorubicin is multiphasic, with elimination half-lives of 3 hours and about 30 hours. There is rapid uptake of the drugs in the heart, kidneys, lungs, liver, and spleen. They do not cross the blood–brain barrier.

Daunorubicin and doxorubicin are both eliminated by metabolic conversion to a variety of less active or inactive products. Daunorubicin is metabolized primarily to daunorubicinol. Doxorubicin is converted to doxorubicinol, to aglycones, and to other derivatives. Precise guidelines for reduction of dosage in patients with impaired hepatic function have not been defined, but some initial reduction should be considered in patients with significantly elevated concentrations of bilirubin in plasma.

Daunorubicin. *Preparation, Dosage, and Route of Administration.* *Daunorubicin hydrochloride* (*daunomycin, rubidomycin;* CERUBIDINE) is available as a powder in 20-mg vials. The recommended dosage is 30 to 60 mg/m^2 daily for 3 days. The agent is administered intravenously with appropriate care to prevent extravasation, since severe local vesicant action may result. Patients should be advised that the drug may impart a red color to the urine.

Therapeutic Uses and Clinical Toxicity. Daunorubicin is very useful in the treatment of acute lymphocytic and acute granulocytic leukemias. It is among the most active drugs for treatment of acute nonlymphoblastic leukemia in adults and, given with cytarabine, is the treatment of choice in these conditions. The drug has some activity against solid tumors in children and in lymphomas; its activity against solid tumors in adults appears to be minimal.

The toxic manifestations of daunorubicin include bone-marrow depression, stomatitis, alopecia, gastrointestinal disturbances, and dermatological manifestations. Cardiac toxicity is a peculiar adverse effect observed with this agent. It is characterized by tachycardia, arrhythmias, dyspnea, hypotension, pericardial effusion, and congestive failure unresponsive to digitalis (*see* below).

Doxorubicin. *Preparation, Dosage, and Route of Administration.* *Doxorubicin hydrochloride* (ADRIAMYCIN, RUBREX) is supplied as a red-orange powder and as a solution (2 mg/ml) for injection. The recommended dose is 60 to 75 mg/m^2, administered as a single rapid intravenous infusion, and is repeated after 21 days. Care should be taken to avoid extravasation, since severe local vesicant action and tissue necrosis may result. Patients should be advised that the drug may impart a red color to the urine.

Therapeutic Uses and Clinical Toxicity. Doxorubicin is effective in acute leukemias and malignant lymphomas; however, in contrast to daunorubicin, it is also active in a number of solid tumors, particularly breast cancer. Used concurrently with cyclophosphamide, vincristine, procarbazine, and other agents, it is an important ingredient for the successful treatment of Hodgkin's disease and non-Hodgkin's lymphomas. Together with cyclophosphamide and cisplatin, it has considerable activity against carcinoma of the ovary. It is a valuable component of various regimens of chemotherapy for carcinoma of the breast and small-cell carcinoma of the lung. The drug is also particularly beneficial in a wide range of sarcomas, including osteogenic, Ewing's, and soft-tissue sarcomas. In metastatic thyroid carcinoma, doxorubicin is probably the best available agent. The drug has demonstrated activity in carcinomas of the endometrium, testes, prostate, cervix, and head and neck, and in plasma cell myeloma (Calabresi *et al.,* 1985).

The toxic manifestations of doxorubicin are similar to those of daunorubicin. Myelosuppression is a major dose-limiting complication, with leukopenia usually reaching a nadir during the second week of therapy and recovering by the fourth week; thrombocytopenia and anemia follow a similar pattern but are usually less pronounced. Stomatitis, gastrointestinal disturbances, and alopecia are common but reversible. Erythematous streaking near the site of infusion ("ADRIAMYCIN flare") is a benign local allergic reaction and should not be confused with extravasation. Facial flushing, conjunctivitis, and lacrimation may occur rarely. The drug may produce severe local toxicity in irradiated tissues (*e.g.,* the skin, heart, lung, esophagus, and gastrointestinal mucosa). Such reactions may occur even when the two therapies are not administered concomitantly.

Cardiomyopathy is a unique characteristic of the anthracycline antibiotics. Two types of cardiomyopathies may occur. (1) An acute form is characterized by abnormal electrocardiographic changes, including ST–T-wave alterations and arrhythmias. This is brief and rarely a serious problem. Cineangiographic studies have shown an acute, reversible reduction in ejection fraction 24 hours after a single dose. An exaggerated manifestation of acute myocardial damage, the "pericarditis–myocarditis syndrome," may be characterized by severe disturbances in impulse conduction and frank congestive heart failure, often associated with pericardial effusion. (2) Chronic, cumulative dose-related toxicity is manifested by congestive heart failure that is unresponsive to digitalis. The mortality rate is in excess of 50%. Total dosage of doxorubicin as low as 250 mg/m^2 can cause myocardial toxicity, as demonstrated by subendocardial biopsies. Nonspecific alterations, including a decrease in the number of myocardial fibrils, mitochondrial changes, and cellular degeneration, are visible by electron microscopy. The most promising noninvasive technique used to detect the early development of drug-induced congestive heart failure is radionuclide cineangiography. Although no completely practical and reliable predictive tests are available, the frequency of serious cardiomyopathy is 1 to 10% at total doses below 450 mg/m^2. The risk increases markedly (to > 20% of patients) at total doses higher than 550 mg/m^2, and this total dosage should be exceeded only under exceptional circumstances. Cardiac irradiation or administration of high doses of cyclophosphamide or another anthracycline may increase the risk of cardiotoxicity. There is evidence that cardiac damage is reduced by the concomitant administration of the iron chelator ADR-529, an experimental agent that is not generally available for clinical use (Speyer *et al.,* 1988).

Several promising analogs of doxorubicin have shown impressive clinical activity in initial studies and may cause less cardiac toxicity; these include epirubicin (4′-epidoxorubicin) and idarubicin (4-demethoxydaunorubicin). A related anthracenedione, mitoxantrone, has been approved for use in acute nonlymphocytic leukemias. Its structural formula is as follows:

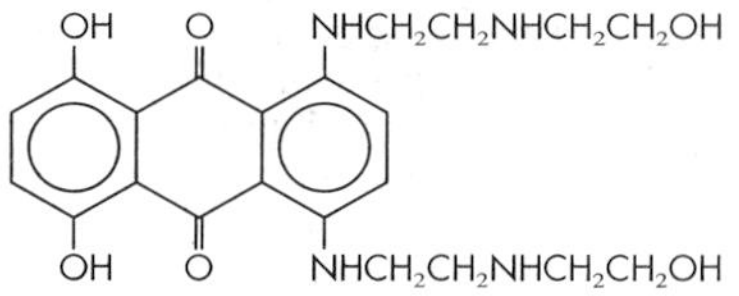

Mitoxantrone

Mitoxantrone lacks the ability to produce quinone-type free radicals and causes less cardiac toxicity than does doxorubicin. Mitoxantrone exerts its antitumor action by stimulating the formation of strand breaks in DNA; this is mediated by topoisomerase II; it also intercalates with DNA. Its range of antitumor activity is confined to leukemias and breast cancer (Shenkenberg and Von Hoff, 1986), but it produces somewhat lower response rates than does doxorubicin when used as a single agent for metastatic breast cancer. Mitoxantrone produces acute myelosuppression and mucositis as its major toxicities; the drug causes less nausea and vomiting and alopecia than does doxorubicin.

Mitoxantrone (NOVANTRONE) is supplied as a solution (2 mg/ml) for intravenous infusion. To induce remission in acute nonlymphocytic leukemia in adults, the drug is given in a daily dose of 12 mg/m^2 for 3 days as a component of a regimen that also includes cytosine arabinoside.

BLEOMYCINS

The bleomycins are an important group of antitumor agents discovered by Umezawa and colleagues as fermentation products of *Streptomyces verticillus*. The drug that is currently employed clinically is a mixture of copper-chelating glycopeptides that consists predominantly of two closely related agents, bleomycin A_2 and bleomycin B_2. The various bleomycins differ only in their terminal-amine moiety (*see* below), and the addition of various amines to fermentation broths have made possible the preparation of more than 200 different congeners. Both the toxic effects and the antitumor spectrum can be modified by such changes.

Bleomycins have attracted great interest because of their activity in a variety of human tumors, including squamous carcinomas of skin, head, neck, and lungs, in addition to lymphomas and testicular tumors. In comparison with many other antineoplastic agents, the bleomycins have minimal myelosuppressive and immunosuppressive activities. They do, however, cause unusual cutaneous and pulmonary toxicity. Since the toxic manifestations of the bleomycins do not overlap significantly with those of most other drugs and since their apparent mechanism of action is also unique (*see* below), the bleomycins have an important place in multidrug chemotherapy. (*See* Twentyman, 1984.)

Chemistry. The bleomycins are water-soluble, basic glycopeptides that differ from one another in their terminal-amine moieties. The structures of bleomycin A_2 and B_2 are shown on page 1245 (Oppenheimer *et al.*, 1979). The core of the bleomycin molecule is a complex metal-binding structure containing a pyrimidine chromophore linked to propionamide, a β-aminoalanine amide side chain, and the sugars L-gulose and 3-O-carbamoyl-D-mannose. Attached to this core is a tripeptide chain and a terminal bithiazole carboxylic acid; this latter segment binds to DNA. The bleomycins form equimolar complexes with Cu^{2+} and Fe^{2+}.

Mechanism of Action. Although the bleomycins have a number of interesting biochemical properties, their cytotoxic action results from their ability to cause fragmentation of DNA. Studies *in vitro* indicate that bleomycin causes accumulation of cells in the G_2 phase of the cell cycle, and many of these cells display chromosomal aberrations, including chromatid breaks, gaps, and fragments, as well as translocations.

Bleomycin appears to cause scission of DNA by interacting with O_2 and Fe^{2+}. In the presence of O_2 and a reducing agent, such as dithiothreitol, the metallobleomycin complex becomes activated and functions mechanistically as a ferrous oxidase, transferring electrons from Fe^{2+} to molecular oxygen to produce activated species of oxygen (Caspary *et al.*, 1979). It has also been shown that metallobleomycin complexes can be activated by reaction with the flavin enzyme, NADPH–cytochrome P_{450} reductase (Kilkuskie *et al.*, 1984). Bleomycin binds to DNA through its amino terminal peptide, and the activated complex generates free radicals that are responsible for scission of the DNA chain (*see* Grollman *et al.*, 1985; Burger *et al.*, 1986; Keller and Oppenheimer, 1987).

Bleomycin is degraded by a hydrolase that is found in a variety of normal tissues, including liver; however, this enzymatic activity is low in skin and lung (Sebti *et al.*, 1987). Some, but not all, bleomycin-resistant cells contain high levels of hydrolase activity (Brabbs and Ware, 1979). This suggests that mechanisms of resistance other than increased drug degradation, such as enhanced capacity to repair DNA, are also operative (*see* Lazo *et al.*, 1982; Twentyman, 1984; Zuckerman *et al.*, 1986).

Absorption, Fate, and Excretion. Bleomycin is usually administered parenterally,

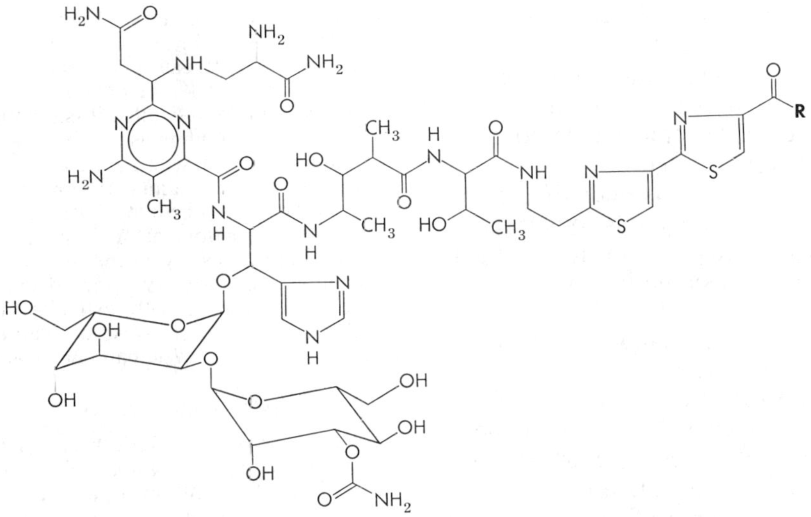

Bleomycinic Acid: **R** = OH

Bleomycin A_2: **R** = $NHCH_2CH_2CH_2—\overset{+}{S}(CH_3)_2$

Bleomycin B_2: **R** = $NHCH_2CH_2CH_2CH_2NHC(=NH)NH_2$

and data on oral absorption are lacking. Relatively high concentrations of the drug are detected in the skin and lungs of experimental animals, the major sites of toxicity. Bleomycin does not cross the blood–brain barrier. In man, bleomycin localizes in various tumors, suggesting a lower level of inactivating enzyme at these sites.

After intravenous administration of a bolus dose of 15 units/m^2, peak concentrations of 1 to 10 mU/ml are achieved in plasma. The half-time for elimination is approximately 3 hours. The average steady-state concentration of bleomycin in plasma of patients receiving continuous intravenous infusions of 30 units daily for 4 to 5 days is approximately 0.15 mU/ml, and there is little bound to plasma proteins. Nearly two thirds of the drug is normally excreted in the urine, probably by glomerular filtration. Concentrations in plasma are greatly elevated if usual doses are given to patients with renal impairment, and such patients are at high risk of developing pulmonary toxicity. Doses of bleomycin should be reduced in the presence of severe renal failure (*see* Dalgleish *et al.*, 1984).

Preparation, Dosage, and Routes of Administration. *Bleomycin sulfate* (BLENOXANE) is available as a powder in 15-unit vials. The recommended dose is 10 to 20 units/m^2, weekly or twice weekly, and the drug is most commonly administered intravenously or intramuscularly. It may also be given by subcutaneous, intrapleural, intraperitoneal, or intraarterial injection. Total courses exceeding 400 units should be given with great caution because of a marked increase in the incidence of pulmonary toxicity; this may occur at lower doses when bleomycin is used concomitantly with other antineoplastic agents.

Therapeutic Uses and Clinical Toxicity. Bleomycin is effective in the treatment of testicular carcinomas. The overall response rate to bleomycin given alone is approximately 30%, and this is increased to 90% when the drug is used with vinblastine. With the addition of cisplatin to this regimen, the majority of patients can be cured (Williams and Einhorn, 1985). Bleomycin is also useful in the treatment of squamous-cell carcinomas of the head, neck, esophagus, skin, and the genitourinary tract, including the cervix, vulva, scrotum, and penis. It is active in Hodgkin's disease and in other lymphomas (*see* Calabresi *et al.*, 1985).

In contrast to most other antineoplastic agents, bleomycin causes minimal bone-marrow toxicity. The most commonly encountered adverse effects are fever and mucocutaneous reactions, including stomatitis and alopecia, as well as hyperpigmentation, hyperkeratosis, pruritic erythema, ulceration, and vesiculation of the skin. These changes may begin with swelling and hyperesthesia of the hands or erythematous, ulcerating lesions over elbows, knuckles, and other pressure areas of the body. Recrudescence of mucocutaneous complications has been reported when other antineoplastic agents are used within 6 weeks after a course of bleomycin. The most serious adverse reaction to this drug is pulmonary toxicity, which begins with fine rales, cough, and diffuse basilar infiltrates and progresses to severe, and sometimes fatal, pulmonary fibrosis. Approximately 5 to 10% of patients receiving bleomycin develop this severe complication, and about 1% of all individuals treated with the drug have died of pulmonary toxicity. In most patients who recover from pulmonary toxicity, pulmonary function returns to pretreatment levels (Van Barneveld *et al.*, 1987). Pulmonary function studies have not been of predictive value. The risk is related to the total dose, with a significant increase in the incidence of pulmonary fibrosis noted at total doses higher than 400 units and in patients over 70 years of age or with underlying pulmonary disease; single doses above 30 mg/m^2 are also associated with an increased risk of pulmonary toxicity. Such toxicity of bleomycin may be potentiated by the administration of oxygen during anesthesia or postoperatively (Toledo *et al.*, 1982), by combination chemotherapy (Bauer *et al.*, 1983), and by previous radiation to the thorax. The use of corticosteroids has been advocated, but their value in reversing or preventing this complication remains to be established.

Other toxic reactions to bleomycin include hyperthermia, headache, nausea, and vomiting, as well as a peculiar, acute fulminant reaction observed in patients with lymphomas. This is characterized by profound hyperthermia, hypotension, and sustained cardiorespiratory collapse; it does not appear to be a classical anaphylactic reaction and may possibly be related to release of an endogenous pyrogen. Because this reaction has occurred in approximately 1% of patients with lymphomas and has resulted in deaths, it is recommended that patients with lymphomas receive a 1-unit test dose of bleomycin, followed by a 24-hour period of observation, before administration of the drug on standard dosage schedules. Unexplained exacerbations of rheumatoid arthritis have also been reported during bleomycin therapy. Raynaud's phenomenon and coronary artery disease have been reported in patients with testicular tumors treated with bleomycin in combination with other chemotherapeutic agents (Wiemann and Calabresi, 1985).

PLICAMYCIN (MITHRAMYCIN)

This cytotoxic antibiotic was isolated from cultures of *Streptomyces tanashiensis* by Rao and associates in 1962. Although the drug is highly toxic, it has some clinical value in the treatment of advanced embryonal tumors of the testes. Plicamycin appears to have a relatively specific effect on osteoclasts and lowers the plasma Ca^{2+} concentrations in hypercalcemic patients, including those with various types of cancer and metastatic tumors in bone. The drug has been used experimentally in the treatment of symptomatic Paget's disease, and striking reductions in plasma alkaline phosphatase activity with concomitant relief of bone pain have been observed. For a discussion of the chemistry of plicamycin and related antibiotics, *see* Umezawa (1979). The structural formula of plicamycin is as shown.

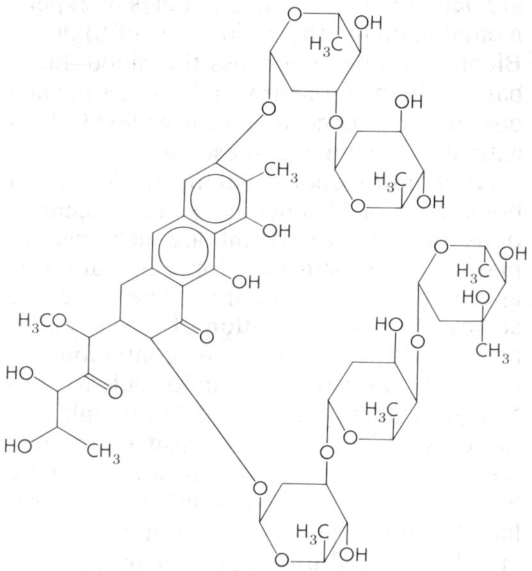

Plicamycin

Mechanism of Action. Plicamycin intercalates into DNA in a manner similar to that of dactinomycin, with preferential binding to guanine–cytosine base pairs. In fact, these two drugs compete for the same binding sites on DNA. Inhibition of RNA, DNA, and protein synthesis is observed.

The relatively specific effect of plicamycin on plasma concentrations of Ca^{2+} suggests that the drug may have a direct action on bone (Robins and Jowsey, 1973). Studies with a tissue culture system of embryonic rat bone showed that the release of Ca^{2+} caused by the addition of parathyroid hormone can be abolished by simultaneous treatment with low concentrations of plicamycin (Cortes *et al.*, 1972). These effects are thought to be the result of a direct action on osteoclasts.

Absorption, Fate, and Excretion. Plicamycin is much less potent when administered orally than when given intravenously. Studies of its clinical pharmacology are lacking, and information on distribution, metabolic fate, and excretion is incomplete.

Preparation, Dosage, and Route of Administration. *Plicamycin* (*mithramycin;* MITHRACIN) is available as a powder in vials containing 2.5 mg of drug. The recommended dosage for treatment of testicular tumors is 25 to 30 μg/kg daily or on alternate days for eight to ten doses or until toxicity intervenes. The drug is usually diluted in 1 liter of 5% dextrose in water or saline and administered by slow intravenous infusion over a period of 4 to 6 hours. Extravasation can cause local irritation and cellulitis. For the treatment of hypercalcemia or hypercalciuria, 25 μg/kg has been given daily for up to four doses; this is repeated at intervals of 1 week or more.

Therapeutic Uses and Clinical Toxicity. Plicamycin is of limited value in the treatment of neoplastic disease because of its severe toxicity. It has been beneficial in patients with disseminated testicular carcinomas, especially of the embryonal-cell type, but has been largely superseded by other drug regimens, particularly vinblastine, cisplatin, and bleomycin. The drug is useful in treating patients with severe hypercalcemia or hypercalciuria, particularly when associated with advanced or metastatic carcinoma that involves bone or produces parathyroid hormone–like substances. Its effectiveness in severe Paget's disease is encouraging but still considered investigational. Plicamycin is toxic to the bone marrow, liver, and kidneys. It produces a severe hemorrhagic diathesis, which may be the result of impaired synthesis of various clotting factors in addition to thrombocytopenia. Characteristically, this begins with epistaxis and may proceed to generalized hemorrhagic complications and even death. Adverse gastrointestinal, cutaneous, and neurological manifestations are also frequently observed. At the lower total dose recommended above for the treatment of hypercalcemia, toxicity is less severe.

MITOMYCIN

This antibiotic was isolated from *Streptomyces caespitosus* by Wakaki and associates in 1958. Mitomycin contains a urethane and a quinone group in its structure, as well as a mitosane ring, and each of these can participate in covalent reactions with DNA. Its structural formula is as follows:

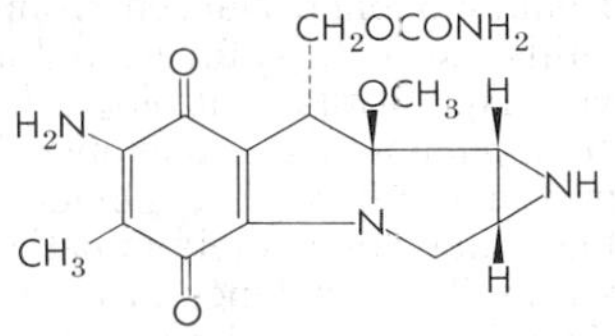

Mitomycin

Mechanism of Action. After intracellular enzymatic reduction of the quinone and loss of the methoxy group, mitomycin becomes a bifunctional or trifunctional alkylating agent; it can also be activated nonenzymatically. The drug inhibits DNA synthesis and cross-links DNA at the N^6 position of adenine and at the O^6 and N^2 positions of guanine (Dorr *et al.*, 1985). In addition, single-strand breakage of DNA is caused by reduced mitomycin; this can be prevented by free radical scavengers. Its action is most prominent during the late G_1 and early S phases of the cell cycle. Mitomycin is teratogenic and carcinogenic in rodents, but its immunosuppressive properties are relatively weak (Crooke and Bradner, 1976).

Absorption, Fate, and Excretion. Mitomycin is absorbed inconsistently from the gastrointestinal tract, and it is therefore administered intravenously. It disappears rapidly from the blood after injection. Peak concentrations in plasma are 0.4 μg/ml after doses of 20 mg/m^2. Mitomycin is cleared from plasma with a half-time of approximately 1 hour (den Hartigh *et al.*, 1983). The drug is widely distributed throughout the body but is not detected in the brain. Inactivation occurs by metabolism, but the products have not been identified. It is metabolized primarily in the liver, and less than 10% of the active drug is excreted in the urine or the bile.

Preparation, Dosage, and Route of Administration. *Mitomycin* (*mitomycin C;* MUTAMYCIN) is available as deep blue-violet crystals in vials containing 5, 20, or 40 mg. It is administered by intravenous infusion; extravasation may result in severe local injury. The usual dose (10 to 20 mg/m^2) may be administered intravenously as a single bolus infusion and is usually given as part of a combination regimen for treatment of carcinoma of the colon or stomach.

Therapeutic Uses and Clinical Toxicity. Mitomycin is useful for the palliative treatment of gastric adenocarcinoma, in conjunction with 5-FU and doxorubicin. It has produced temporary beneficial effects in carcinomas of the cervix, colon, rectum, pancreas, breast, bladder, head and neck, and lung, and in melanomas. It has also shown activity against lymphomas and leukemias, particularly chronic granulocytic leukemia, but not in myeloma. All responses have been of brief duration and are complicated by toxicity. The major toxic effect is myelosuppression, characterized by marked leukopenia and thrombocytopenia; this may be delayed and cumulative, with recovery only after 6 to 8 weeks of pancytopenia. Nausea, vomiting, diarrhea, stomatitis, dermatitis, fever, and malaise are also observed. Hemolysis, neurological abnormalities, interstitial pneumonia, and glomerular damage resulting in renal failure (the hemolytic–uremic syndrome) may develop acutely in patients treated with mitomycin. The incidence of renal failure increases to 28% in patients who receive total doses of 70 mg/m^2 or higher (Valavaara and Nordman, 1985). The hemolytic–uremic syndrome is exacerbated by blood transfusion, which may cause pulmonary edema. Mitomycin may potentiate the cardiotoxicity of doxorubicin when used in conjunction with this drug (Bachur *et al.,* 1978).

ENZYMES

L-ASPARAGINASE

History. Guinea pig serum was noted to have antileukemic cell activity, and L-asparaginase, which is present in high concentrations in this serum, was ultimately found to be responsible for this effect (Kidd, 1953). The enzyme was introduced into cancer chemotherapy in an effort to exploit what was thought to be a distinct, qualitative biochemical difference between normal and certain malignant cells. Although this difference is now known to be a quantitative one, L-asparagine occupies an important place in the treatment of acute lymphoblastic leukemia.

Mechanism of Action. Most normal tissues synthesize L-asparagine in amounts sufficient for protein synthesis. Certain neoplastic tissues, however, including acute lymphoblastic leukemic cells in children, require an exogenous source of this amino acid. L-Asparaginase, by catalyzing the hydrolysis of asparagine to aspartic acid and ammonia, deprives these malignant cells of the asparagine available from extracellular fluid, which results in a cessation of protein synthesis and cellular death. There may be striking synergistic effects when asparaginase is used in combination with other drugs, such as methotrexate or cytarabine. The sequence of drug administration is crucial. For example, synergistic cytotoxicity is seen when methotrexate is administered before asparaginase. When the reverse sequence is used, the toxicity of methotrexate is attenuated. Several patients with refractory acute leukemias have responded favorably to such combinations. (For further discussion, *see* Capizzi and Handschumacher, 1982.)

Absorption, Fate, and Excretion. L-Asparaginase is given parenterally. The rate of clearance from plasma varies considerably with different preparations; the half-life of EC-2 (*see* below) is from 14 to 22 hours (Broome, 1981).

Preparation, Dosage, and Route of Administration. *Escherichia coli* produces two L-asparaginase isozymes, only one of which (EC-2) has antileukemic activity. The *E. coli* enzyme has been purified to homogeneity and is available for therapeutic use. *Asparaginase* (ELSPAR) is a dry powder in vials containing 10,000 international units (I.U.) per vial. The molecular weight of the enzyme is about 130,000, and it consists of four equivalent subunits (*see* Patterson, 1975). These preparations have weak glutaminase activity that may play a role in certain of the biological effects.

L-Asparaginase is administered intravenously or intramuscularly. The suggested dosage for the induction of remission in acute lymphoblastic leukemia is 1000 I.U./kg daily for 10 to 20 days. Intermittent dosage regimens are used infrequently because of the increased risk of anaphylaxis. The concentration of L-asparagine in plasma falls to immeasurable levels immediately after drug administration and remains depressed for 1 to 3 weeks after therapy.

Therapeutic Uses and Clinical Toxicity. Unfortunately, L-asparaginase has not fulfilled its early promise of high tumoricidal activity with minimal toxicity in the treatment of human neoplasms. However, complete remissions have been observed in acute lymphoblastic leukemia refractory to other antileukemic agents, and the drug is a useful component of certain regimens for the treatment of this type of leukemia. Transient remissions have also been observed in other forms of leukemia, and occasional beneficial responses have been reported in a few patients with malignant melanoma and T-cell lymphomas. Objective responses have not been seen with most solid tumors.

In contrast to most other antitumor drugs, L-asparaginase has minimal effects on the bone marrow and does not damage oral or intestinal mucosa or the hair follicles. On the other hand, severe toxicity may result from inhibition of the synthesis of clotting factors (both thrombosis and, later, hemorrhage), insulin (hyperglycemia), and albumin (hypoalbuminemia). Pancreatitis, abnormalities of mental status, and, rarely, coma occur in occasional patients and may cause fatalities (Bezeaud *et al.,* 1986; Homans *et al.,* 1987). Most patients display a substantial elevation of blood ammonia (as high as 7 to 9 μg/ml [about 400 to 500 μM]). L-Asparaginase has immunosuppressive activity, as seen by inhibition of antibody synthesis, delayed hypersensitivity, lymphocyte transformation, and graft rejection. Thus, both T- and B-lymphocyte functions are affected. Since L-asparaginase is a relatively large, foreign protein, it is antigenic, and hypersensitivity phenomena ranging from mild allergic reactions to anaphylactic shock have been reported in 5 to 20% of patients (Wiemann and Calabresi, 1985).

BIOLOGICAL RESPONSE MODIFIERS

So-called biological response modifiers include agents or approaches that affect the patient's biological response to a neoplasm beneficially. Included are agents that act indirectly to mediate their antitumor effects (*e.g.*, by enhancing the immunological response to neoplastic cells) or directly on the tumor cells (*e.g.*, differentiating agents). Recombinant DNA technology has greatly facilitated the identification and production of a number of human proteins with potent effects on the function and growth of both normal and neoplastic cells. Proteins that are currently in clinical trials include the interferons, interleukins (especially interleukin-2), hematopoietic growth factors such as erythropoietin (*see* Chapter 54), tumor necrosis factor, and epidermal growth factor. Most of these proteins have not yet been approved for general use.

Interleukin-2 (IL-2) is a cytokine that is secreted by T-cells; it causes a number of immunological effects, including induction of T-cell cytotoxicity and enhancement of natural killer cell activity. It is currently undergoing extensive clinical study by itself and in combination with delivery of lymphokine-activated killer (LAK) cells for the treatment of various malignancies; such treatment induces partial or complete remissions in approximately 25% of patients with melanoma or renal cell cancer.

The interferons are discussed in Chapter 51. All three types of interferon (alpha, beta, and gamma) have been tested clinically and have activity against certain neoplasms. Only the alpha interferons (interferon alfa 2a and 2b) have been approved for use. These uses include hairy cell leukemia, Kaposi's sarcoma in patients with acquired immunodeficiency syndrome (AIDS), and condylomata acuminata.

IV. Miscellaneous Agents

PLATINUM COORDINATION COMPLEXES

The platinum coordination complexes are cytotoxic agents that were first identified by Rosenberg and coworkers in 1965. Growth inhibition of *E. coli* was observed when electrical current was delivered between platinum electrodes. The inhibitory effects on bacterial replication were subsequently shown to be due to the formation of inorganic platinum-containing compounds in the presence of ammonium and chloride ions (Rosenberg *et al.*, 1965, 1967). *cis*-Diamminedichloroplatinum (II) (cisplatin) was found to be the most active of these substances in experimental tumor systems and has proven to be of clinical value (Rosenberg *et al.*, 1969; Rosenberg, 1973). More than 1000 platinum-containing compounds have subsequently been synthesized and tested. One of these, carboplatin, was approved for treatment of ovarian cancers in 1989; others are still being evaluated. Cisplatin has broad activity as an antineoplastic agent and the drug is especially useful in the treatment of epithelial malignancies. It has been the foundation for development of curative regimens for advanced testicular cancer. The drug also has predictable activity against ovarian cancer, cancer of the head and neck, bladder cancer, and small-cell cancer of the lung (Rozencweig *et al.*, 1977; Zwelling and Kohn, 1982; Hacker *et al.*, 1984).

Chemistry. *cis*-Diamminedichloroplatinum (II) (cisplatin) is an inorganic water-soluble, platinum-containing complex. The II indicates the valence of platinum. In carboplatin, platinum is incorporated into a more complex carbon-containing molecule. The structural formulas of cisplatin and carboplatin are as follows:

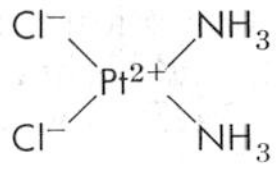

Cisplatin

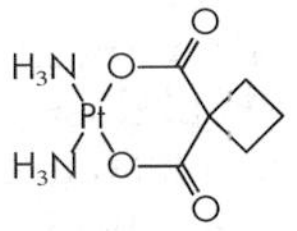

Carboplatin

Mechanism of Action. Cisplatin appears to enter cells by diffusion. The chloride atoms may be displaced directly by reaction with nucleophiles such as thiols; hydrolysis of chloride is probably responsible for formation of the activated species of the drug, which reacts with nucleic acids and proteins. Hydrolysis is favored at low concentrations of chloride. High concentrations of the anion inhibit activation of the drug; this is presumed to explain the effectiveness of chloride diuresis in preventing nephrotoxicity (*see* below). Hydrolysis of carboplatin removes the bidentate cyclobutanedicarboxylato group; this activation reaction occurs more slowly with carboplatin than with cisplatin.

The platinum complexes can react with DNA, forming both intrastrand and interstrand cross-links. The N(7) of guanine is very reactive, and platinum cross-links between adjacent guanines on the same DNA strand are the most readily demonstrated. The formation of interstrand cross-links is a relatively slow process and occurs to a much smaller extent. The covalent binding of proteins to DNA has also been demonstrated. At present, there is no conclusive association between a single type of biochemical lesion and cytotoxicity. (*See* Zwelling and Kohn, 1982; Eastman, 1985; Reed *et al.,* 1986.)

The specificity of cisplatin with regard to phase of the cell cycle appears to differ among cell types, although the effects on cross-linking are most pronounced during the S phase. Even though cisplatin is mutagenic, teratogenic, and carcinogenic, an increased incidence of second tumors, which has been observed with certain of the alkylating agents, has yet to be reported.

In addition to its reactivity with DNA, cisplatin can react with other nucleophiles, such as sulfhydryl groups of proteins. It is speculated that certain of the toxic effects of the drug, such as nephrotoxicity, ototoxicity, and intense emesis, may result from such reactions. This has led to the experimental testing of "rescue" techniques that employ molecules with high affinity for heavy metals. For example, infusions of sodium thiosulfate have permitted the administration of higher doses of cisplatin. Another compound, diethyldithiocarbamate (DDTC), a metabolite of disulfiram, has also shown promise. When administered to animals 2 hours after treatment with cisplatin, renal and gastrointestinal toxicity is ameliorated, while the antileukemic effects are not prevented. This compound is under consideration for introduction into clinical use (Zwelling and Kohn, 1982; Borch *et al.,* 1984; Pfeifle *et al.,* 1985; Bodenner *et al.,* 1986).

Cisplatin. *Absorption, Fate, and Excretion.* Cisplatin is not effective when administered orally. After rapid intravenous administration of usual doses, the drug has an initial half-life in plasma of 25 to 50 minutes; concentrations decline subsequently, with a half-life of 58 to 73 hours. The half-life of the drug is longer in patients who receive high doses of cisplatin. More than 90% of the platinum in the blood is bound to plasma proteins. High concentrations of cisplatin are found in the kidney, liver, intestine, and testes, but there is poor penetration into the CNS. Only a small portion of the drug is excreted by the kidney during the first 6 hours; after 5 days up to 43% of the administered dose is recovered in the urine. When given by infusion instead of rapid injection, the plasma half-life is shorter and the amount of drug excreted is greater. Biliary or intestinal excretion of cisplatin appears to be minimal (*see* Zwelling and Kohn, 1982; Shelley *et al.,* 1985; Wiemann and Calabresi, 1985).

Preparation, Dosage, and Route of Administration. Cisplatin (PLATINOL) is available as a lyophilized powder and in solution (1 mg/ml) for injection. When used alone for ovarian tumors, the usual intravenous dose is 100 mg/m^2, given once every 4 weeks. Doses of 40 mg/m^2 daily for 5 consecutive days have recently been used together with cyclophosphamide for the treatment of patients with advanced ovarian cancer. Cisplatin is frequently used with other drugs in chemotherapy, and the dosage is usually reduced in such situations to 50 mg/m^2 once every 3 weeks (when given with doxorubicin or cyclophosphamide for ovarian neoplasms) or to 20 mg/m^2 daily, for 5 consecutive days, every 3 weeks (when used in combination with bleomycin and vinblastine for testicular tumors). In order to prevent renal toxicity, hydration of the patient by the infusion of 1 to 2 liters of fluid prior to treatment is recommended. The appropriate amount of cisplatin is then diluted in a solution of dextrose, saline, and mannitol and administered intravenously over a period of 6 to 8 hours. Continued hydration to ensure adequate urinary output is recommended for 24 hours thereafter. Since aluminum reacts with and inactivates cisplatin, it is important not to use needles or other equipment that contain aluminum when preparing or administering the drug.

Therapeutic Uses and Clinical Toxicity. Combination chemotherapy with cisplatin, bleomycin, and vinblastine is curative for 85% of patients with advanced, non-seminomatous testicular cancer (Garnick, 1985; Williams and Einhorn, 1985; Einhorn, 1986). The drug is also beneficial in carcinoma of the ovary, particularly when used with cyclophosphamide or doxorubicin (Durant and Omura, 1985; Ozols, 1985). Cisplatin causes reproducible responses in cancers of the bladder, head and neck, and endometrium; small cell carcinoma of the lung; lymphomas; and some neoplasms of childhood. Interestingly, the drug also sensitizes cells to the cytotoxic effects of radiation therapy (*see* Einhorn and Williams, 1979; Batist *et al.,* 1986; Pearson and Raghavan, 1985; Slotman *et al.,* 1986).

Cisplatin-induced nephrotoxicity has been largely abrogated by the routine use of hydration and diuresis. However, ototoxicity caused by cisplatin is unaffected by diuresis and is manifested by tinnitus and hearing loss in the high-frequency range (4000 to 8000 Hz). The ototoxicity can be unilateral or bilateral, tends to be more frequent and severe with repeated doses, and may be more pronounced in children. Interestingly, fosfomycin, an antibacterial antibiotic, appears to protect against ototoxicity induced by cisplatin (Schwatzer *et al.,* 1986). Marked nausea and vomiting occur in almost all patients and can usually be controlled with antiemetic agents. At higher doses, cisplatin causes peripheral neuropathy, which may worsen after discontinuation of the drug. Mild-to-moderate myelosuppression may occur with transient leukopenia and thrombocytopenia. Electrolyte disturbances, including hypomagnesemia, hypocalcemia, hypokalemia, and hypophosphatemia are common. Hypocalcemia and tetany secondary to hypomagnesemia have been observed, and routine measurement of Mg^{2+} concentrations in plasma is recommended. Hyperuricemia, seizures, hemolytic anemia, and cardiac abnormalities have been reported. Anaphylactic-like reactions, characterized by facial edema, bronchoconstriction, tachycardia, and hypotension, may occur within minutes after administration and should be treated by intravenous injection of epinephrine and with corticosteroids or antihistamines (Wiemann and Calabresi, 1985).

Carboplatin. The mechanism of action and spectrum of clinical activity of carboplatin (CBDCA, JM-8) are similar to those of cisplatin (*see* above). However, there are significant differences in the chemical, pharmacokinetic, and toxicological properties of the two drugs (*see* Von Hoff, 1987; Muggia, 1989; Ozols, 1989).

Carboplatin is less reactive than cisplatin, and the drug is not bound to plasma proteins to a significant extent. As a result, there are no appreciable quantities of low-molecular-weight platinum-containing species (other than carboplatin itself) in plasma, and most of the drug is eliminated in the urine as such with a half-time of 3 to 6 hours. Platinum from the drug does become irreversibly bound to plasma proteins, and this fraction of the metal disappears slowly (half-time of 5 days or more).

Carboplatin is relatively well tolerated clinically. There is less nausea, neurotoxicity, ototoxicity, and nephrotoxicity than with cisplatin. Instead, the dose-limiting toxicity is myelosuppression, primarily evident as thrombocytopenia. Assessment of the relative roles of carboplatin and cisplatin in the treatment of specific cancers awaits the results of ongoing comparative trials. However, carboplatin is an effective alternative for patients with responsive tumors who are unable to tolerate cisplatin because of impaired renal function, refractory nausea, significant hearing impairment, or neuropathy.

Carboplatin (PARAPLATIN) is available as a powder in vials of 50, 150, and 450 mg. It is administered as an intravenous infusion over at least 15 minutes. The usual dose is 360 mg/m^2, given once every 28 days. Carboplatin is currently approved for the treatment of patients with ovarian cancer that has recurred after chemotherapy, including those who have received cisplatin.

HYDROXYUREA

First synthesized in 1869 by Dresler and Stein, hydroxyurea was found to produce leukopenia, anemia, and megaloblastic changes in the bone marrow of rabbits. It was later shown to have antineoplastic activity against sarcoma 180. Studies of its biological activity and assessments of clinical efficacy have been reviewed (Donehower, 1982). The structural formula of hydroxyurea is as follows:

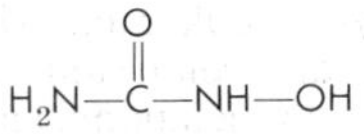

Hydroxyurea

Cytotoxic Action. Hydroxyurea is representative of a group of compounds that have as their primary site of action the enzyme ribonucleoside diphosphate reductase. A striking correlation has been observed between the relative growth rate of a series of rat hepatomas and the activity of ribonucleoside diphosphate reductase. This enzyme, which catalyzes the reductive conversion of ribonucleotides to deoxyribonucleotides, is a crucial and probably rate-limiting step in the biosynthesis of DNA, and it represents a logical target for the design of chemotherapeutic agents. Hydroxyurea destroys a tyrosyl free radical that is formed in the catalytic center of the enzyme. The drug is specific for the S phase of the cell cycle and causes cells to arrest at the G_1–S interface. Since cells are highly sensitive to irradiation in the G_1 phase of the cycle, combinations of hydroxyurea and irradiation cause synergistic toxicity *in vitro* (Agrawal and Sartorelli, 1975; Donehower, 1990).

Two mechanisms of resistance to hydroxyurea have been proposed: the acquisition of ribonucleotide reductases with decreased sensitivity to hydroxyurea and marked increases in ribonucleotide reductase, due to gene amplification.

Absorption, Fate, and Excretion. In man, hydroxyurea is readily absorbed from the gastrointestinal tract, and peak plasma concentrations of 0.3 to 2.0 μM are reached in 1 to 2 hours; the plasma half-life is about 2 hours. Hydroxyurea readily crosses the blood–brain barrier. Approximately 80% of the drug is recovered in the urine within 12 hours after either oral or intravenous administration (Donehower, 1990).

Preparation, Dosage, and Route of Administration. *Hydroxyurea* (HYDREA) is available for oral use in 500-mg capsules. Two dosage schedules are recommended: (1) intermittent therapy with 80 mg/kg, administered orally as a single dose every third day, and (2) continuous therapy with 20 to 30 mg/kg, administered orally as a single daily dose. Dosage should be adjusted according to the number of leukocytes in the peripheral blood. Treatment should be continued for a period of 6 weeks in order to determine its effectiveness; if satisfactory antineoplastic results are obtained, therapy can be continued indefinitely, although leukocyte counts at weekly intervals are advisable.

Therapeutic Uses and Clinical Toxicity. At present, the primary role of hydroxyurea in chemotherapy appears to be in the management of myeloproliferative disorders, including chronic granulocytic leukemia, polycythemia vera, and essential thrombocytosis. It has also been effective in the hypereosinophilic syndrome (Parrillo *et al.*, 1978) and in achieving rapid reductions of markedly elevated blast cells in the peripheral blood of patients with acute granulocytic leukemia. Hydroxyurea has produced temporary remissions in patients with metastatic malignant melanoma and occasionally in those with other solid tumors, including carcinomas of the head and neck and genitourinary systems. Because of its ability to synchronize neoplastic cells *in vitro* in a radiation-sensitive phase of the cell cycle (G_1), it has been used in combination with radiotherapy in carcinomas of the cervix, head and neck, and lung.

Hematopoietic depression, involving leukopenia, megaloblastic anemia, and occasionally thrombocytopenia, is the major toxic effect; recovery of the bone marrow is usually prompt if the drug is discontinued for a few days. Other adverse reactions include gastrointestinal disturbances and mild dermatological reactions; more rarely, stomatitis, alopecia, and neurological manifestations have been encountered. Inflammation and increased pigmentation may occur in areas previously exposed to radiation.

PROCARBAZINE

A group of antitumor agents, the methylhydrazine derivatives, was discovered among a large number of substituted hydrazines, which had been originally synthesized as potential monoamine oxidase inhibitors. Antineoplastic effects in experimental tumors have been reported with several compounds in this series (Bollag, 1963), including procarbazine, an agent useful clinically in Hodgkin's disease. Comprehensive descriptions of the effects of procarbazine have been published (Oliverio, 1982; Weinkam *et al.*, 1982). The structural formula of procarbazine is as follows:

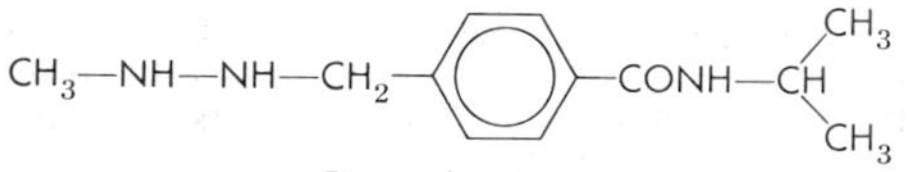

Procarbazine

Cytotoxic Action. Procarbazine itself is inert as a cytotoxic and mutagenic agent, and it must undergo metabolic activation to generate the proximal cytotoxic reactants. The activation pathways are complex and not yet fully understood. The first step involves oxidation of the hydrazine function with formation of the azo analog. This can occur spontaneously in neutral solution by reaction with molecular oxygen and can also occur enzymatically by reaction with the cytochrome P_{450} system of the liver. Further oxidations can generate the methylazoxy and benzylazoxy intermediates. It is postulated that the methylazoxy compound can react further to liberate an entity resembling diazomethane, a potent methylating reagent. Free-radical intermediates may also be involved in cytotoxicity. Activated procarbazine can produce chromosomal damage, including chromatid breaks and translocations, that are consistent with its mutagenic and carcinogenic actions. Antimitotic effects have been described in a number of cell types; cells in the G_1 phase of the cell cycle are most susceptible. Inhibition of DNA, RNA, and protein synthesis has been detected both *in vitro* and *in vivo*. Although resistance to procarbazine develops rapidly, there is no clear notion of the mechanism. The highly lipophilic drug enters cells readily by diffusion (*see* Averbuch, 1990).

Absorption, Fate, and Excretion. Procarbazine is absorbed almost completely from the gastrointestinal tract. After parenteral administration, the drug is readily equilibrated between the plasma and the CSF. It is rapidly metabolized in man, and its half-life in the blood after intravenous injection is approximately 7 minutes. Oxidation of procarbazine produces the corresponding azo compound and hydrogen peroxide. Further metabolism, presumably in the liver, yields azoxy derivatives that circulate in the bloodstream and have potent cytotoxic activity (Erickson *et al.*, 1989). Induction of microsomal enzymes by phenobarbital and other agents enhances the rate of conversion of procarbazine to its active metabolites; the potential for drug interaction thus exists when procarbazine is administered with other agents that are metabolized by microsomal enzymes. From 25 to 70% of an oral or parenteral dose given to man is recovered from the urine during the first 24 hours after administration; less than 5% is excreted as the unchanged compound, and the rest is mostly in the form of a metabolite, N-isopropylterephthalanic acid (Averbuch, 1990).

Preparation, Dosage, and Route of Administration. *Procarbazine hydrochloride* (MATULANE) is marketed in 50-mg capsules. The recommended oral daily dose for adults is 100 mg/m^2 for 10 days in combination regimens. The drug is rarely used alone.

Therapeutic Uses and Clinical Toxicity. The therapeutic effectiveness of procarbazine is greatest in Hodgkin's disease, particularly when given with mechlorethamine, vincristine, and prednisone (the MOPP regimen) (DeVita, 1981). Of major importance is the apparent lack of cross-resistance with other antineoplastic agents. When used with various other agents, procarbazine has also demonstrated activity against brain tumors, small-cell carcinoma of the lung, non-Hodgkin's lymphomas, myeloma, and melanoma.

The most common toxic effects include leukopenia, thrombocytopenia, nausea, and vomiting, which occur in 50 to 90% of patients. Myelosuppression may begin during the second week of therapy, and its severity is dose dependent. Other gastrointestinal symptoms as well as neurological and dermatological manifestations have been noted in 5 to 10% of cases; psychic disturbances have also been reported. Because of augmentation of sedative effects, the concomitant use of CNS depressants should be avoided. The ingestion of alcohol by patients receiving procarbazine may cause intense warmth and reddening of the face, as well as other effects resembling the acetaldehyde syndrome produced by disulfiram. Since procarbazine is a weak monoamine oxidase inhibitor, hypertensive reactions may result from its use concurrently with sympathomimetic agents, tricyclic antidepressants, and foods with high tyramine content. Procarbazine is highly carcinogenic, mutagenic, and teratogenic, and its use in MOPP therapy is associated with a 5 to 10% risk of acute leukemia; the greatest risk is for patients who also receive radiation therapy (Tucker *et al.*, 1988). Procarbazine is also a potent immunosuppressive agent and it causes infertility, particularly in males.

MITOTANE (*o,p'*-DDD)

The principal application of mitotane, a compound chemically similar to the insecticides DDT and DDD, is in the treatment of neoplasms derived from the adrenal cortex. In studies of the toxicology of related insecticides in dogs, it was noted that the adrenal cortex was severely damaged, an effect caused by the presence of the *o,p'* isomer of DDD. Its structural formula is as follows:

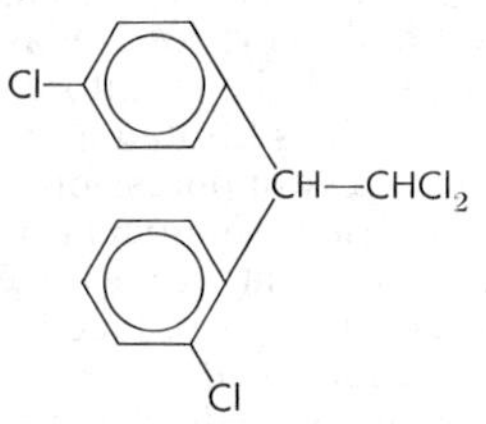

Mitotane

Cytotoxic Action. The mechanism of action of mitotane has not been elucidated, but its relatively selective attack on adrenocortical cells, normal or neoplastic, is well established. Thus, administration of the drug causes a rapid reduction in the levels of adrenocorticosteroids and their metabolites in blood and urine, a response that is useful both in guiding dosage and in following the course of hyperadrenocorticism (Cushing's syndrome) resulting from an adrenal tumor or hyperplasia. Damage to the liver, kidneys, or bone marrow has not been encountered.

Absorption, Fate, and Excretion. Clinical studies indicate that approximately 40% of mitotane is absorbed after oral administration. After daily doses of 5 to 15 g, concentrations of 10 to 90 μg/ml of unchanged drug and 30 to 50 μg/ml of a metabolite are present in the blood. After discontinuation of therapy, plasma concentrations of mitotane are still measurable for 6 to 9 weeks. Although the drug is found in all tissues, fat is the primary site of storage. A water-soluble metabolite of mitotane is found in the urine; approximately 25% of an oral or parenteral dose is recovered in this form. About 60% of an oral dose is excreted unchanged in the stool.

Preparation, Dosage, and Route of Administration. *Mitotane* (*o,p'*-DDD; LYSODREN) is supplied in 500-mg scored tablets. Initial daily oral doses of 2 to 6 g are usually given in three or four divided portions, but the maximal tolerated dose may vary from 2 to 16 g per day. Treatment should be continued for at least 3 months; if beneficial effects are observed, therapy should be maintained indefinitely. Spironolactone should not be administered concomitantly, since it interferes with the adrenal suppression produced by mitotane (Wortsman and Soler, 1977).

Therapeutic Uses and Clinical Toxicity. Treatment with mitotane is indicated for the palliation of inoperable adrenocortical carcinoma. Hutter and Kayhoe (1966) have reported on treatment in 138 patients, and 115 have been studied by Lubitz and associates (1973). Clinical effectiveness has been reported in 34 to 54% of these cases. Apparent cures have been reported in some patients with metastatic disease (Becker and Schumacher, 1975; Ostumi and Roginsky, 1975). Although the administration of mitotane produces anorexia and nausea in approximately 80% of patients, somnolence and lethargy in about 34%, and dermatitis in 15 to 20%, these effects do not contraindicate the use of the drug at lower doses. Since this drug damages the adrenal cortex, administration of adrenocorticosteroids is indicated, particularly in patients with evidence of adrenal insufficiency, shock, or severe trauma (Hogan *et al.*, 1978).

V. Hormones and Related Agents

ADRENOCORTICOSTEROIDS

The pharmacology, major therapeutic uses, and toxic effects of the adrenocorticosteroids are discussed in Chapter 63. Only the applications of the hormones in the treatment of neoplastic disease will be considered here. Because of their lympholytic effects and their ability to suppress mitosis in lymphocytes, the greatest value of these steroids is in the treatment of acute leukemia in children and of malignant lymphoma. They are especially effective in the management of frank hemolytic anemia and the hemorrhagic complications of thrombocytopenia that frequently accompany malignant lymphomas and chronic lymphocytic leukemia.

In acute lymphoblastic or undifferentiated leukemia of childhood, adrenocorticosteroids may produce prompt clinical improvement and objective hematological remissions in 30 to 50% of children. Although these responses frequently are characterized by complete disappearance of all detectable leukemic cells from the peripheral blood and bone marrow, the duration of remission is extremely variable (2 weeks to 9 months) and relapse of the disease invariably occurs. Remissions occur more rapidly with corticosteroids than with antimetabolites, and there is no evidence of cross-resistance to unrelated agents. For these reasons, therapy is often initiated with a steroid and other agents, usually vincristine and an anthracycline, with or without methotrexate or asparaginase, in order to induce remissions. This approach, followed by continuous maintenance treatment with various agents, yields more prolonged remissions (*see* section on Methotrexate). Adult leukemia seldom responds to glucocorticoid therapy, but many symptoms of the disease, including the hemorrhagic manifestations of thrombocytopenia, may be controlled effectively, albeit temporarily, without demonstrable changes in platelet counts.

The adrenocorticosteroids are used in conjunction with x-ray therapy to reduce the occurrence of radiation edema in critical areas such as the superior mediastinum, brain, and spinal cord. These drugs are particularly useful in the symptomatic palliation of patients with severe hematopoietic depression secondary to bone-marrow involvement or previous radiation or chemotherapy. They may produce rapid symptomatic improvement in critically ill patients by temporarily suppressing fever, sweats, and pain, and by restoring, to some degree, appetite, lost weight, strength, and sense of well-being. The symptoms tend to recur after the hormone is withdrawn, which indicates that the effects of the disease, but not necessarily the disease process itself, have been affected. Therefore, the value of this type of therapy is to provide the patient with a relatively asymptomatic period during which the general physical condition may improve sufficiently to permit further definitive therapy.

Several preparations are available and at appropriate dosages exert similar effects (*see* Chapter 60). Prednisone, for example, is usually administered orally in doses as high as 60 to 100 mg, or even higher, for the first few days and gradually reduced to levels of 20 to 40 mg per day. A continuous attempt should be made to lower the dosage required to control the manifestations of the disease.

AMINOGLUTETHIMIDE

Originally developed as an anticonvulsant, aminoglutethimide was subsequently found to inhibit the synthesis of adrenocortical steroids (*see* Chapter 60). Aminoglutethimide inhibits the conversion of cholesterol to pregnenolone, the first step in the synthesis of cortisol. Inhibition of cortisol synthesis, however, results in a compensatory rise in the secretion of ACTH sufficient to overcome the adrenal blockade. Administration of dexamethasone does not prevent the increase in ACTH secretion because aminoglutethimide accelerates the metabolism of dexamethasone. Since the metabolism of hydrocortisone (cortisol) is not affected by aminoglutethimide, this combination produces reliable inhibition of the synthesis of cortisol (Santen *et al.*, 1980). Aminoglutethimide has been used to treat patients with adrenocortical carcinoma and Cushing's syndrome.

Although aminoglutethimide effectively blocks the secretion of cortisol, the production of other adrenal steroids, such as testosterone, dihydrotestosterone, androstenedione, progesterone, and 17-hydroxyprogesterone, is only partially inhibited. In certain tissues, including fat, muscle, and liver, androstenedione is converted by aromatization to estrone and estradiol. In postmenopausal and castrated women, the adrenal gland does not produce estrogens, but it is the most important source of precursors of estrogens. By inhibiting cytochrome P_{450}-dependent hydroxylation reactions that are necessary for aromatization reactions, aminoglutethimide is a potent inhibitor of the conversion of androgens to estrogens in extra-adrenal tissues. Patients treated with aminoglutethimide and cortisol thus experience a lowering of plasma and urinary concentrations of estradiol that is equivalent to that observed in patients treated by surgical adrenalectomy (Santen *et al.*, 1982).

Therapeutic Uses and Clinical Toxicity. When it is used to treat patients with metastatic breast cancer, aminoglutethimide is administered orally at a dose of 250 mg four times a day, together with 40 mg of hydrocortisone (cortisol) in divided doses. The largest dose of hydrocortisone, 20 mg, is given at night. When used to control Cushing's syndrome, aminoglutethimide is given in the same dosage but without hydrocortisone. Plasma concentrations of cortisol should be monitored, and the dose of aminoglutethimide is titrated as necessary (up to 2 g per day) to achieve suppression of adrenal function. In some patients, significant inhibition of adrenal function occurs at doses of 250 to 500 mg daily, and toxicity is thus reduced.

A major indication for the use of aminoglutethimide is to produce "medical adrenalectomy" in patients with advanced carcinoma of the breast, when the tumor contains estrogen receptors. If women are selected for therapy without regard to the status of estrogen receptors in the tumor, the response rate is 37%; patients whose tumor cells contain estrogen receptors experience a 50% response rate. Skin, soft tissue, and bone lesions respond more frequently than do other sites of metastasis. Such treatment is equal or superior to surgical adrenalectomy or hypophysectomy (Harvey *et al.*, 1979).

Early toxic effects of aminoglutethimide include lethargy, visual blurring, drowsiness, and ataxia. These symptoms usually resolve after 4 to 6 weeks of treatment. A pruritic, maculopapular rash usually appears 10 days after treatment is initiated and resolves after approximately 5 days without withdrawal of the drug. Since the adrenal gland recovers normal secretory activity and the response to stress 36 hours after aminoglutethimide and hydrocortisone are withdrawn, it is not necessary to taper the administration of these drugs.

PROGESTINS

Progestational agents (*see* Chapter 58) are useful in the management of endometrial carcinoma previously treated by surgery and radiotherapy. These compounds were tried initially because of the concept that carcinoma of the endometrium results from the prolonged, unopposed overstimulation by estrogen. This led to the use of progesterone, which would correct this situation because of its physiological effect in producing maturation and secretory activity of the normal endometrium. Apparently a portion of neoplastic cells arising from this tissue is still influenced by normal hormonal controls.

There are several preparations available. Hydroxyprogesterone caproate is usually administered intramuscularly in doses of 1000 mg, one or more times weekly; medroxyprogesterone acetate can be administered intramuscularly in doses of 400 to 1000 mg weekly. An alternative oral agent is megestrol acetate (40 to 320 mg daily, in divided doses). Beneficial effects, usually characterized by regression of pulmonary metastases, have been observed in approximately one third of patients. Responses to progestational agents have also been reported in metastatic carcinomas of the breast and prostate, and in hypernephromas.

ESTROGENS AND ANDROGENS

A discussion of the pharmacology of the estrogens and androgens appears in Chapters 58 and 59. Their use in the treatment of certain neoplastic diseases will be discussed here. They are of value in this connection because certain organs that are often the primary site of growth, notably the prostate and the mammary gland, are dependent upon hormones for their growth, function, and morphological integrity. Carcinomas arising from these organs often retain some of the hormonal requirements of their normal counterparts for varying periods of time. By changing the hormonal environment of such tumors it is possible to alter the course of the neoplastic process.

Androgen-Control Therapy of Prostatic Carcinoma. The development of the androgen-control regimen for the treatment of prostatic carcinoma is largely the contribution of Huggins and associates (1941). Although the hormonal treatment of metastatic prostate carcinoma is palliative, life expectancy is increased and thousands of patients have enjoyed the benefit of its ameliorating effects.

Localized prostate cancer is curable with surgery or radiation therapy. However, when distant metastases are already present, hormonal therapy becomes the primary treatment. Standard approaches to achieve reduction in the concentrations of endogenous androgens or in their effects include bilateral orchiectomy, estrogen therapy, and the administration of gonadotropin-releasing hormone (GnRH) agonists with or without antiandrogens (*see* below).

The choice of estrogen is largely determined by cost and convenience. Diethylstilbestrol or a related synthetic compound is usually the preparation of choice. There is no evidence that survival is improved with excessively large doses, and, in fact, high doses substantially increase the risk of cardiovascular complications. An average daily dose of diethylstilbestrol is 1 to 3 mg. The dose of other estrogens is in proportion to their potency.

Subjective and objective improvements rapidly follow the institution of androgen-control therapy of prostatic carcinoma. From the patient's point of view the most gratifying of these is relief of pain. This is associated with an increase in appetite, weight gain, and a feeling of well-being. Objectively, there are regressions of the primary tumor and soft-tissue metastases, but neoplastic cells do not disappear completely. Plasma acid phosphatase activity and the concentrations of prostate-specific antigens are useful markers of disease. There is often an associated recovery from anemia. Eventually prostatic tumors become insensitive to the lack of androgen or the presence of estrogen; however, it is now well established that effective palliation is afforded by the therapeutic regimen and that the life expectancy of the treated patient is significantly increased.

Androgen-control therapy is one of the safest forms of cancer chemotherapy. The psychic trauma of orchiectomy is not inconsequential, but is often tempered by the age of the patient. After orchiectomy alone, hot flashes are common; these can be controlled by the administration of estrogen. Estrogens are capable of producing the untoward responses described in detail in Chapter 58. Mild gastrointestinal disturbances may be noted; occasionally, these may be severe enough to require discontinuation of the drug. There may be some expansion of extracellular fluid volume in patients with poor cardiac function. There is also significant mortality from cardiac and cerebrovascular complications. Gynecomastia is frequent and may be a disturbing feature in some patients. For this reason, many oncologists will radiate the breasts prophylactically prior to initiating therapy with an estrogen. In rare instances, carcinoma of the male breast has occurred in patients given estrogen for prolonged periods of time.

Estrogens and Androgens in the Treatment of Mammary Carcinoma. Because of the paucity of side effects and the equivalence of response, the use of antiestrogens such as tamoxifen has largely replaced treatment with estrogens or androgens as the initial approach to the hormonal therapy of breast cancer. However, since approximately half of women who develop progressive disease after response to tamoxifen will still respond to additional hormonal therapy, estrogens and androgens continue to have a role in the palliation of this disease.

Although the choice of regimen for the treatment of carcinoma of the breast is largely empirical, progress in endocrinology has led to the development of methods that are very useful for the selection of patients who are likely to respond to hormonal manipulation. Tissues that are responsive to estrogens contain receptors for the hormones that can be detected by either ligand-binding techniques or monoclonal antibodies. Carcinomas that lack specific estrogen-binding capacity rarely respond to hormonal therapy. The tumors that contain receptors usually do respond and, furthermore, are associated with a better overall prognosis independent of the type of therapy. Other predictors for response to hormonal therapy include the presence of progesterone receptors and the confinement of disease to bone or subcutaneous tissues.

Hormonal therapy uses doses much larger than those needed for physiological replacement. Androgen therapy with oral agents is preferable; a common regimen is fluoxymesterone, 10 to 40 mg daily in divided doses. Parenteral androgen therapy may be given as testosterone propionate, 50 to 100 mg intramuscularly three times weekly.

Numerous compounds have estrogenic activity. Oral diethylstilbestrol is the most frequently used; it is given initially in doses of 5 mg daily. This dose is gradually increased to a maintenance dose of 5 mg three times daily over a 1- to 2-week period. Other preparations may be used if diethylstilbestrol causes intolerable gastrointestinal effects. Ethinyl estradiol is also commonly used, the dosage being gradually increased from 0.5 mg orally once daily to the customary maintenance dose of 3 mg daily, given in three portions. Progestational therapy (medroxyprogesterone acetate, 100 mg intramuscularly three times weekly; megestrol acetate, 160 mg orally once a day) is also effective, particularly when tumors have high concentrations of androgen receptors.

The onset of action of the hormones is slow, and it is necessary to continue therapy for 8 to 12 weeks before a decision can be reached as to effectiveness. If a favorable response is obtained, hormonal treatment should be continued until an exacerbation of symptoms occurs. Withdrawal of the hormone at this time is followed by remission of disease in 30% of cases. The duration of an induced remission averages about 6 months to 1 year; however, some patients may receive benefit for several years.

All the untoward effects that commonly accompany estrogen and androgen therapy have been observed in the use of these agents in the treatment of mammary carcinoma; these effects are described in Chapters 58 and 59. Two toxic manifestations require emphasis. With either hormone, the combined effect of a steroid and osteolytic metastases may result in marked hypercalcemia. The chief dangers are ectopic calcification, particularly in the urinary tract, and the physiological disturbances that may accompany an increase in the concentration of Ca^{2+} in the extracellular fluid, including neurological changes, polyuria, and cardiac arrhythmias. Patients who show an elevation in plasma Ca^{2+} should have high fluid intakes. Severe hypercalcemia, whether spontaneous or drug induced, is a true medical emergency. If an estrogen or androgen is being used, it should be discontinued. Forced hydration is mandatory. Further measures may be necessary; these include saline diuresis, adrenocorticosteroids in large doses, or the intravenous administration of plicamycin (*see* above; *see also* Chapter 62). When drug-induced hypercalcemia is corrected, further therapy may be cautiously attempted. Plasma concentrations of Ca^{2+} should be determined routinely in patients receiving hormonal therapy.

Rarely, either estrogen or androgen therapy may cause exacerbation of the neoplastic process; this occurs more frequently as a result of estrogen administration.

ANTIESTROGENS

TAMOXIFEN

The introduction of effective antiestrogenic agents that block the actions of estrogens on target tissues has been a relatively recent development (*see* Chapter 58). Of various compounds tested, tamoxifen is in particular use in the United States (*see* Chapter 58). Tamoxifen provides effective, palliative treatment for certain patients with advanced breast cancer; it can also be used effectively as an adjuvant in the treatment of estrogen receptor–containing breast tumors (Lippman, 1986). Estrogen receptors can be detected in tumor cells of 50% of premenopausal women with breast cancer and 75% of postmenopausal women.

Absorption, Fate, and Excretion. After oral administration, peak concentrations of tamoxifen are found in blood after 4 to 7 hours. The decline in plasma concentration is biphasic; the initial $t_{1/2}$ is 7 to 14 hours, and the terminal $t_{1/2}$ is 4 to 7 days. Repeated administration of tamoxifen results in accumulation of the drug, and steady-state concentrations are achieved in 4 weeks. The principal metabolite of tamoxifen is N-desmethyltamoxifen. Concentrations of this metabolite in blood are approximately twice those of the parent compound at steady state. After enterohepatic circulation, glucuronides and other metabolites are excreted in the stool; excretion in the urine is minimal (Jordan, 1982).

Preparation, Dosage, and Route of Administration. *Tamoxifen citrate* (NOLVADEX) is marketed in 10-mg tablets. The recommended dose is 20 to 40 mg daily, administered orally in two divided doses. Objective responses usually occur in 4 to 10 weeks but may be delayed for several months in patients with bone metastases.

Therapeutic Uses and Clinical Toxicity. Because toxicity associated with the use of tamoxifen is rarely severe, it has become the drug of choice for the initial endocrine management of breast cancer. Tamoxifen is useful in both the palliative treatment of advanced carcinoma of the breast in postmenopausal women and the adjuvant therapy of this disease. Patients who have tumors that contain estrogen receptors are most likely to respond to the drug; those without receptor-binding activity are unlikely to benefit. Although a few premenopausal women have responded to this agent, it is more effective in patients who are several years postmenopausal, have metastases to soft tissues rather than to bone, and have derived beneficial effects from previous hormone therapy.

The most frequent adverse reactions include hot flashes, nausea, and vomiting. These may occur in approximately 25% of patients and are rarely severe enough to necessitate discontinuation of therapy. Menstrual irregularities, vaginal bleeding and discharge, pruritus vulvae, and dermatitis have occurred less frequently. The occurrence of pain in tumors, particularly bone metastases, as well as local flare of disease, characterized by increase in size and marked erythema of the lesions, is sometimes associated with good responses. Other infrequent adverse effects include hypercalcemia, peripheral edema, anorexia, depression, pulmonary embolism, light-headedness, headache, mild-to-moderate thrombocytopenia, leukopenia, cataracts, corneal changes, and retinopathy. Tamoxifen is said to be carcinogenic and teratogenic in animals. (For additional information, *see* Legha *et al.*, 1978; Furr and Jordan, 1984.)

GONADOTROPIN-RELEASING HORMONE ANALOGS

A recent development of considerable interest is the synthesis of various analogs of gonadotropin-releasing hormone (GnRH) (*see* Chapter 56). A marked decrease in circulating concentrations of gonadotropins and testosterone can be induced in patients with prostatic carcinoma treated with leuprolide, a nonapeptide analog with high agonist activity. This compound has biphasic effects on the pituitary. Initially, it stimulates the secretion of both follicle-stimulating hormone (FSH) and luteinizing hormone (LH). However, with long-term administration cell-surface receptors for GnRH become desensitized and down-regulated. As a result, there is inhibition of the secretion of LH and FSH, and the concentration of testosterone falls to castration levels in men and the concentrations of estrogens fall to postmenopausal values in women. Recent randomized trials in patients with prostatic carcinomas have shown that leuprolide produces responses that are equivalent to those achieved with diethylstilbestrol, with significantly less toxicity. One important side effect, a transient flare of disease, may result from the initial capacity of leuprolide to stimulate the pituitary, and it is not a cause for discontinuation of therapy. Flare of disease can be prevented by the concurrent administration of leuprolide and an anti-androgen such as flutamide (*see* Chapter 59). Flutamide blocks the actions of both testicular and adrenal androgens. Clinical trials are now under way to determine whether such combination therapy offers any advantage over leuprolide alone. Leuprolide cannot be administered orally. However, a depot form of the peptide that can be administered once monthly has been marketed recently.

Agarwal, R. P. Inhibitors of adenosine deaminase. *Pharmacol. Ther.*, **1982**, *17*, 399–430.

Agarwal, R. P.; Spector, T.; and Parks, R. E., Jr. Tight-binding inhibitors. IV. Inhibition of adenosine deaminases by various inhibitors. *Biochem. Pharmacol.*, **1977**, *26*, 359–367.

Alberts, D. S.; Chang, S. Y.; Chen, H. S. G.; Larcom, B. J.; and Jones, S. E. Pharmacokinetics and metabolism of chlorambucil in man: a preliminary report. *Cancer Treat. Rev.*, **1979a**, *6*, 9.

Alberts, D. S.; Chang, S. Y.; Chen, H. S. G.; Moon, T. E.; Evans, T. L.; Furner, R L.; Himmelstein, K.; and Gross, J. F. Kinetics of intravenous melphalan. *Clin. Pharmacol. Ther.*, **1979b**, *26*, 73–80.

Allegra, C. J., and others. Trimetrexate, a novel and effective agent for the treatment of *Pneumocystis carinii* pneumonia in patients with acquired immunodeficiency syndrome. *N. Engl. J. Med.*, **1987**, *79*, 478–482.

Alper, J. C.; Wiemann, M. C.; Rueckl, F. S.; McDonald, C. J.; and Calabresi, P. Rationally designed combination chemotherapy for the treatment of patients with recalcitrant psoriasis. *J. Am. Acad. Dermatol.*, **1985**, *12*.

Ansfield, F.; Ramirez, G.; Skibba, J. L.; Davis, H. L.; and Wirtanen, G. W. Intrahepatic arterial infusion with 5-fluorouracil. *Cancer*, **1971**, *28*, 1147–1151.

Assaraf, Y. G., and Schimke, R. T. Identification of methotrexate transport deficiency in mammalian cells using fluoresceinated methotrexate and flow cytometry. *Proc. Natl. Acad. Sci. U.S.A.*, **1987**, *84*, 7154–7157.

Bachur, R.; Gordon, S. L.; and Gee, R. V. A general mechanism for microsomal activation of quinone anticancer agents to free radicals. *Cancer Res.*, **1978**, *38*, 1745–1750.

Barnett, M. J.; Waxman, J. H.; Richards, M. A.; Ganesan, T. S.; Bragman, K. S.; Rohatiner, A. Z. S.; and Lister, T. A. High-dose cytosine arabinoside in the initial treatment of acute leukemia. *Semin. Oncol.*, **1985**, *12*, 133–138.

Batist, G.; Carney, D. N.; Cowan, K. H.; Veach, S. R.; Bunn, P. A.; and Ihde, D. C. Etoposide (VP-16) and cisplatinum in previously treated small cell lung cancer: clinical trials and *in vitro* correlates. *J. Clin. Oncol.*, **1986**, *4*, 982–989.

Bauer, K. A.; Skarin, A. T.; Balikian, J. P.; Garnick, M. B.; Rosenthal, D. S.; and Canellos, G. P. Pulmonary complications associated with combination chemotherapy programs containing bleomycin. *Am. J. Med.*, **1983**, *74*, 557–663.

Becker, D., and Schumacher, O. P. *o,p'*-DDD therapy in invasive adrenocortical carcinoma. *Ann. Intern. Med.*, **1975**, *82*, 677–679.

Begleiter, A.; Glazer, R. I.; Israels, L. G.; Pugh, L.; and Johnston, J. B. Deduction of DNA strand breaks in chronic lymphocytic leukemia following treatment with 2′-deoxycoformycin *in vivo* and *in vitro*. *Cancer Res.*, **1987**, *47*, 2498–2503.

Bender, R. A.; Castle, M. C.; Margileth, D. A.; and Oliverio, V. T. The pharmacokinetics of [^{3}H]-vincristine in man. *Clin. Pharmacol. Ther.*, **1977**, *22*, 430–438.

Bezeaud, A.; Drouet, L.; Leverger, G.; Griffin, J. H.; and Guillin, M. C. Effect of L-asparaginase therapy for acute lymphoblastic leukemia on plasma vitamin K-dependent coagulation factors and inhibitors. *J. Pediatr.*, **1986**, *108*, 698–701.

Bloch, A. (ed.). Chemistry, biology, and clinical uses of nucleoside analogs. *Ann. N.Y. Acad. Sci.*, **1975**, *255*, 1–610.

Bodenner, D. L.; Dedon, P. C.; Keng, P. C.; and Borch, R. F. Effect of diethyldithiocarbomate on cis-diammine dichloroplatinum (II)-induced cytotoxicity, DNA cross linking and γ-glutamyl transpeptidase inhibition. *Cancer Res.*, **1986**, *46*, 2745–2750.

Bollag, W. The tumor-inhibitory effects of the methylhydrazine derivative Ro 4-6467/1 (NSC-77213). *Cancer Chemother. Rep.*, **1963**, *33*, 1–4.

Bonadonna, G., and Valagussa, P. Chemotherapy of breast cancer: current views and results. *Int. J. Radiat. Oncol. Biol. Phys.*, **1983**, *3*, 279–297.

Bono, V. H., Jr. Studies on the mechanism of action of DTIC (NSC-45388). *Cancer Treat. Rep.*, **1976**, *60*, 141–148.

Brabbs, S., and Ware, J. R. Isolation and characterization of bleomycin-resistant clones of CHO cells. *Genet. Res.*, **1979**, *34*, 269–279.

Brock, N., and Pohl, J. Prevention of urotoxic side effects by regional detoxification with increased selectivity of oxazophosphorine cystostatics. *IARC Sci. Publ.*, **1986**, *78*, 269–279.

Broder, L. E., and Carter, S. K. Pancreatic islet cell carcinoma. II. Results of therapy with streptozotocin in 52 patients. *Ann. Intern. Med.*, **1973**, *79*, 108–118.

Burger, R. M.; Projan, S. J.; Horwitz, S. B.; and Peisach, J. The DNA cleavage mechanism of iron-bleomycin. *J. Biol. Chem.*, **1986**, *261*, 15955–15959.

Calabresi, P. Leukemia after cytotoxic chemotherapy—a pyrrhic victory? *N. Engl. J. Med.*, **1983**, *309*, 1118–1119.

Carrico, C. K., and Sartorelli, A. C. Effects of 6-thioguanine on macromolecular events in regenerating rat liver. *Cancer Res.*, **1977**, *37*, 1868–1875.

Caspary, W. J.; Niziak, C.; Lanzo, D. A.; Friedman, R.; and Bachur, N. R. Bleomycin A_2: a ferrous oxidase. *Mol. Pharmacol.*, **1979**, *16*, 256–260.

Cheson, B. D., and Martin, A. Clinical trials in hairy cell leukemia: current status and future directions. *Ann. Intern. Med.*, **1987**, *106*, 871–878.

Chun, H. G.; Leland-Jones, B. R.; Caryk, S. M.; and Hoth, D. F. Central nervous system toxicity of fludarabine phosphate. *Cancer Treat. Rep.*, **1986**, *70*, 1225.

Cichowicz, D. J., and Shane, B. Mammalian folyl-γ-polyglutamate synthetase. 1. Purification and general properties of the hog liver enzyme. *Biochemistry*, **1987**, *26*, 504–512.

Cortes, E. P.; Holland, J. F.; Moskowitz, R.; and Depoli, E. Effects of mithramycin on bone resorption *in vitro*. *Cancer Res.*, **1972**, *32*, 74–76.

Costanzi, J. J. Studies in the Southwest Oncology Group. *Cancer Treat. Rep.*, **1976**, *60*, 189–192.

Curt, G. A.; Carney, D. N.; Cowan, K. H.; Kao-Shan, C. S.; Minna, J. D.; and Chabner, B. A. Unstable methotrexate resistance in human small-cell carcinoma associated with double minute chromosomes. *N. Engl. J. Med.*, **1983**, *308*, 199–202.

Curt, G. A.; Jolivet, J.; Carney, D. N.; Bailey, B. D.; Drake, J. C.; Clendeninn, N. J.; and Chabner, B. A. Determinants of the sensitivity of human small-cell lung cancer cell lines to methotrexate. *J. Clin. Invest.*, **1985**, *76*, 1323–1329.

Dalgleish, A. G.; Woods, R. L.; and Levi, J. A. Bleomycin pulmonary toxicity: its relationship to renal dysfunction. *Med. Pediatr. Oncol.*, **1984**, *12*, 313–317.

Deffie, A. M.; Batra, J. K.; and Goldenberg, G. G. Direct correlation between DNA topoisomerase II activity and cytotoxicity in adriamycin-sensitive and -resistant P388 leukemia cell lines. *Cancer Res.*, **1989**, *49*, 58–62.

DeFronzo, R. A.; Braine, H.; and Colvin, O. M. Water intoxication in man after cyclophosphamide therapy. Time course and relation to drug activation. *Ann. Intern. Med.*, **1973**, *78*, 861–869.

den Hartigh, J.; McVie, J. G.; Van Oort, W. J.; and Pinedo, H. M. Pharmacokinetics of mitomycin C in humans. *Cancer Res.*, **1983**, *43*, 5017–5021.

Dorr, R. T.; Bowdan, G. T.; Alberts, D. S.; and Liddil, J. D. Interactions of mitomycin C with mammalian DNA detected by alkaline elution. *Cancer Res.*, **1985**, *45*, 3510–3516.

Early Breast Cancer Trialists' Collaborative Group. Effects of adjuvant tamoxifen and of cytotoxic therapy on mortality in early breast cancer: an overview of 61 randomized trials among 28,896 women. *N. Engl. J. Med.*, **1988**, *319*, 1681–1690.

Eastman, A. Intrastrand cross-links and sequence specificity in the reaction of cis-dichloro (ethylene-diamine) platinum (II) with DNA. *Biochemistry*, **1985**, *24*, 5027–5032.

Einhorn, L. H. Have new aggressive chemotherapy regimens improved results in advanced germ cell tumors? *Eur. J. Cancer Clin. Oncol.*, **1986**, *22*, 1289–1293.

Einhorn, L. H., and Williams, S. D. The role of *cis*-platinum in solid tumor therapy. *N. Engl. J. Med.*, **1979**, *300*, 289–291.

Elwood, P. C. Molecular cloning and characterization of the human folate binding protein cDNA from placenta and malignant tissue culture (KB) cells. *J. Biol. Chem.*, **1989**, *264*, 14893–14901.

Ensminger, W. D.; Rosowsky, A.; Raso, V.; Levin, D. C.; Glode, M.; Come, S.; Steele, G.; and Frei, E., III. A clinical-pharmacological evaluation of hepatic arterial infusions of 5-fluoro-2′-deoxyuridine and 5-fluorouracil. *Cancer Res.*, **1978**, *38*, 3784–3792.

Erickson, J. M.; Tweedie, D. J.; Ducore, J. M.; and Prough, R. A. Cytotoxicity and DNA damage caused by the azoxy metabolites of procarbazine in L1210 tumor cells. *Cancer Res.*, **1989**, *49*, 127–133.

Farber, S.; Diamond, L. K.; Mercer, R. D.; Sylvester, R. F.; and Wolff, V. A. Temporary remissions in acute leukemia in children produced by folic antagonist 4-amethopteroylglutamic acid (aminopterin). *N. Engl. J. Med.*, **1948**, *238*, 787–793.

Fraile, R. J.; Baker, L. H.; Buroker, T. R.; Horwitz, J.; and Vaitkevicius, V. K. Pharmacokinetics of 5-fluorouracil administered orally, by rapid intravenous and slow infusion. *Cancer Res.*, **1980**, *40*, 2223–2228.

Furr, B. J. A., and Jordan, V. C. Pharmacology and clinical uses of tamoxifen. *Pharmacol. Ther.*, **1984**, *25*, 127–206.

Gaidys, W. G.; Dickerman, J. D.; Walters, C. L.; and Young, P. C. Intrathecal vincristine. *Cancer*, **1983**, *52*, 799–801.

Garnick, M. B. Advanced testicular cancer: treatment choices in the "land of plenty." *J. Clin. Oncol.*, **1985**, *3*, 294–297.

Giblett, E. R.; Anderson, J. E.; Cohen, F.; Pollara, B.; and Meuwissen, H. J. Adenosine-deaminase deficiency in two patients with severely impaired cellular immunity. *Lancet*, **1972**, *2*, 1067–1069.

Gilman, A. The initial clinical trial of nitrogen mustard. *Am. J. Surg.*, **1963**, *105*, 574–578.

Golomb, H. M., and Ratain, M. J. Recent advances in the treatment of hairy cell leukemia. *N. Engl. J. Med.*, **1987**, *316*, 870–871.

Gottlieb, J. A., and others. Role of DTIC (NSC-45388) in the chemotherapy of sarcomas. *Cancer Treat. Rep.*, **1976**, *60*, 199–203.

Green, D.; Tew, K. D.; Hisamatsu, T.; and Schein, P. S. Correlation of nitrosourea murine bone marrow toxicity with deoxyribonucleic acid alkylation and chromatin binding sites. *Biochem. Pharmacol.*, **1982**, *31*, 1671–1679.

Grollman, A. P.; Takeshita, M.; Pillai, K. M.; and Johnson, F. Origin and cytotoxic properties of base propenals derived from DNA. *Cancer Res.*, **1985**, *45*, 1127–1131.

Gupta, R. S. Genetic, biochemical, and cross-resistance studies with mutants of Chinese hamster ovary cells resistant to the anticancer drugs VM-26 and VP16-213. *Cancer Res.*, **1983**, *43*, 1568–1574.

Harvey, H. A.; Santen, R. J.; Osterman, J.; Samojlik, E.; White, D. S.; and Lipton, A. A comparative trial of transphenoidal hypophysectomy and estrogen suppression with aminoglutethimide in advanced breast cancer. *Cancer*, **1979**, *43*, 2207–2214.

Hemminki, K., and Ludlum, D. B. Covalent modification of DNA by antineoplastic agents. *J. Natl. Cancer Inst.*, **1984**, *73*, 1021–1028.

Hertz, R. Folic acid antagonists: effects on the cell and the patient. Clinical staff conference at N.I.H. *Ann. Intern. Med.*, **1963**, *59*, 931–956.

Herzig, R. H.; Hines, J. D.; and Herzig, G. P. Cellular

toxicity with high-dose cytosine arabinoside. *J. Clin. Oncol.*, **1987**, *5*, 927–932.

Ho, D. H. W., and Frei, E., III. Clinical pharmacology of 1-beta-D-arabinofuranosylcytosine. *Clin. Pharmacol. Ther.*, **1971**, *12*, 944–954.

Hoffmeister, R. T. Methotrexate therapy in rheumatoid arthritis: 15 years experience. *Am. J. Med.*, **1983**, *30*, 69–73.

Hogan, T. F.; Citrin, D. L.; Johnson, B. M.; Nakamura, S.; Davis, T. E.; and Borden, E. C. *o,p'*-DDD (mitotane) therapy of adrenal cortical carcinoma. *Cancer*, **1978**, *42*, 2177–2181.

Homans, A. C.; Rybak, M. E.; Baglini, R. L.; and Forman, E. N. Effect of L-asparaginase administration on coagulation and platelet function in children with leukemia. *J. Clin. Oncol.*, **1987**, *5*, 811–817.

Huffman, D. H.; Wan, S. H.; Azarnoff, D. L.; and Hoogotraten, B. Pharmacokinetics of methotrexate. *Clin. Pharmacol. Ther.*, **1973**, *14*, 572–579.

Huggins, C.; Stevens, R. E., Jr.; and Hodges, C. V. Studies on prostatic cancer: effects of castration on advanced carcinoma of prostate gland. *Arch. Surg.*, **1941**, *43*, 209–223.

Iven, H., and Brasch, H. The effects of antibiotics and uricosuric drugs on the renal elimination of methotrexate and 7-hydroxymethotrexate in rabbits. *Cancer Chemother. Pharmacol.*, **1988**, *21*, 337–342.

Johnston, J. B.; Begleiter, A.; Pugh, L.; Leith, M. K.; Wilkins, J. A.; Cavers, D. J.; and Israels, L. G. Biochemical changes induced in hairy cell leukemia following treatment with the adenosine deaminase inhibitor 2'-deoxycoformycin. *Cancer Res.*, **1986**, *46*, 2179–2184.

Johnston, T. P.; McCaleb, G. S.; and Montgomery, J. A. The synthesis of antineoplastic agents. XXXII. N-Nitrosoureas. *J. Med. Chem.*, **1963**, *6*, 669–681.

Kamen, B. A.; Whyte-Bauer, W.; and Bertino, J. B. A mechanism of resistance to methotrexate: NADPH but not NADH stimulation of methotrexate binding to dihydrofolate reductase. *Biochem. Pharmacol.*, **1983**, *32*, 1837–1840.

Keller, T. J., and Oppenheimer, N. J. Enhanced bleomycin-mediated damage of DNA opposite charged nicks. A model for bleomycin-directed double strand scission of DNA. *J. Biol. Chem.*, **1987**, *262*, 15144–15150.

Kees, U. R.; Ford, J.; Dawson, V. M.; Piall, E.; and Aherne, G. W. Development of resistance to 1-β-D-arabinofuranosylcytosine after high-dose treatment in childhood lymphoblastic leukemia: analysis of resistance mechanism in established cell lines. *Cancer Res.*, **1989**, *49*, 3015–3019.

Kidd, J. G. Regression of transplanted lymphomas induced *in vivo* by means of normal guinea pig serum. I. Course of transplanted cancers of various kinds in mice and rats given guinea pig serum, horse serum, or rabbit serum. *J. Exp. Med.*, **1953**, *98*, 565–582.

Kilkuskie, R. E.; Macdonald, T. L.; and Hecht, S. M. Bleomycin may be activated for DNA cleavage by NADPH cytochrome P-450 reductase. *Biochemistry*, **1984**, *23*, 6165–6171.

Knospe, W. H.; Loeb, V.; and Huguley, C. M. Biweekly chlorambucil treatment of chronic lymphocytic leukemia. *Cancer*, **1974**, *33*, 555–562.

Laurie, J. A., and others. Surgical adjuvant therapy of large-bowel carcinoma: an evaluation of levamisole and the combination of levamisole and fluorouracil. *J. Clin. Oncol.*, **1989**, *7*, 1447–1456.

Lazo, J. S.; Boland, C. J.; and Schwartz, P. E. Bleomycin hydrolase activity and cytotoxicity in human tumors. *Cancer Res.*, **1982**, *42*, 4026–4031.

Lerner, H. J. Acute myelogenous leukemia in patients receiving chlorambucil as long-term adjuvant chemotherapy for stage II breast cancer. *Cancer Treat. Rep.*, **1978**, *62*, 1135–1143.

Levin, V. A.; Hoffman, W.; and Weinkam, R. J. Pharmacokinetics of BCNU in man: a preliminary study of 20 patients. *Cancer Treat. Rep.*, **1978**, *62*, 1305–1312.

Loo, T. L.; Housholder, G. E.; Gerulath, A. H.; Saunders, P. H.; and Farquhar, D. Mechanism of action and pharmacology studies with DTIC (NSC-45388). *Cancer Treat. Rep.*, **1976**, *60*, 149–157.

Lubitz, J. A.; Freeman, L.; and Okun, R. Mitotane use in inoperable adrenal cortical carcinoma. *J.A.M.A.*, **1973**, *223*, 1109–1112.

McDonald, C. J. The uses of systemic chemotherapeutic agents in psoriasis. *Pharmacol. Ther.*, **1981**, *14*, 1–24.

McDonald, C. J., and Calabresi, P. Azaribine for mycosis fungoides. *Arch. Dermatol.*, **1971**, *103*, 158–167.

———. Psoriasis and occlusive vascular disease. *Br. J. Dermatol.*, **1978**, *99*, 469–475.

McDermott, B. J.; van der Berg, H. W.; and Murphy, R. F. Nonlinear pharmacokinetics for the elimination of 5-fluorouracil after intravenous administration in cancer patients. *Cancer Chemother. Pharmacol.*, **1982**, *9*, 173–178.

Matthews, D. A., and others. Refined crystal structures of *Escherichia coli* and chicken liver dihydrofolate reductase containing bound trimethoprim. *J. Biol. Chem.*, **1985**, *260*, 381–391.

Nissenkorn, I.; Servadio, C.; Vilikowsky, E.; and Glanz, I. Long-term intravesicular thiotepa treatment in patients with superficial bladder tumors and vesicoureteral reflux. *J. Urol.*, **1985**, *132*, 198–199.

Noble, R. L.; Beer, C. T.; and Cutts, J. H. Further biological activities of vincaleukoblastine—an alkaloid isolated from *Vinca rosea* (L.). *Biochem. Pharmacol.*, **1958**, *1*, 347–348.

O'Dwyer, P. J.; Wagner, B.; Leyland-Jones, B.; Wittes, R. J.; Cheson, B. D.; and Hoth, D. F. 2'-Deoxycoformycin (pentostatin) for lymphoid malignancies. *Ann. Intern. Med.*, **1988**, *106*, 733–743.

Oppenheimer, N. J.; Rodrigues, L. O.; and Hecht, S. M. Proton nuclear magnetic resonance study of the structure of bleomycin and the zinc bleomycin complex. *Biochemistry*, **1979**, *18*, 3439–3445.

Ostumi, J. A., and Roginsky, M. S. Metastatic adrenal cortical carcinoma. *Arch. Intern. Med.*, **1975**, *139*, 1257–1258.

Owellen, R. J.; Hartke, C. A.; and Hains, F. O. Pharmacokinetics and metabolism of vinblastine in humans. *Cancer Res.*, **1977a**, *37*, 2597–2602.

Owellen, R. J.; Root, M. A.; and Hains, F. O. Pharmacokinetics of vindesine and vincristine in humans. *Cancer Res.*, **1977b**, *37*, 2603–2607.

Ozols, R. F. The case for combination chemotherapy in the treatment of advanced ovarian cancer. (Editorial.) *J. Clin. Oncol.*, **1985**, *3*, 1445–1447.

———. Optimal dosing with carboplatin. *Semin. Oncol.*, **1989**, *16*, 14–18.

Parrillo, J. E.; Fauci, A. S.; and Wolff, S. M. Therapy of the hypereosinophilic syndrome. *Ann. Intern. Med.*, **1978**, *89*, 167–172.

Pearson, B. S., and Raghavan, D. First line intravenous cisplatin for deeply invasive bladder cancer: update on 70 cases. *Br. J. Urol.*, **1985**, *57*, 690–693.

Pfeifle, C. E.; Howell, S. B.; Felthouse, R. D.; Woliver, T. B. S.; Andrews, P. A.; Markman, M.; and Murphy, M. D. High-dose cisplatin with sodium thiosulfate protection. *J. Clin. Oncol.*, **1985**, *3*, 237–244.

Pommier, Y.; Kerrigan, D.; Schwartz, R.; Swack, J. A.; and McCurdy, A. Altered DNA topoisomerase II activity in Chinese hamster cells resistant to topoisomerase II inhibitors. *Cancer Res.*, **1986**, *46*, 3075–3081.

Portlock, C. S.; Fischer, D. S.; Cadman, E.; Lundberg, W. B.; Levy, A.; Babrow, S.; Bertino, J. R.; and Faber, L. High-dose chlorambucil in advanced, low-grade, non-Hodgkins lymphoma. *Cancer Treat. Rep.*, **1987**, *71*, 1029–1031.

Preisler, H. D.; Rustum, Y.; and Priore, R. L. Relationship between leukemic cell retention of cytosine arabinoside triphosphate and the duration of remission in patients with acute nonlymphocytic leukemia. *Eur. J. Cancer Clin. Oncol.*, **1985**, *21*, 23–30.

Racker, E.; Wu, L. T.; and Westcott, D. Use of slow Ca^{2+} channel blockers to enhance inhibition by taxol of growth of drug-sensitive and -resistant Chinese hamster ovary cells. *Cancer Treat. Rep.*, **1986**, *70*, 275.

Reed, E.; Yupsa, S. H.; Zwelling, L. A.; Ozols, R. F.; and Poirier, M. C. Quantitation of cis-diamminedichloroplatinum II (cisplatin)-DNA-intrastrand adducts in testicular and ovarian cancer patients receiving cisplatin chemotherapy. *J. Clin. Invest.*, **1986**, *77*, 545–550.

Rosenberg, B. Platinum coordination complexes in cancer chemotherapy. *Naturwissenschaften*, **1973**, *60*, 399–406.

Rosenberg, B.; VanCamp, L.; Grimley, E. B.; and Thomson, A. J. The inhibition of growth or cell division in *Escherichia coli* by different ionic species of platinum (IV) complexes. *J. Biol. Chem.*, **1967**, *242*, 1347–1352.

Rosenberg, B.; VanCamp, L.; and Krigas, T. Inhibition of cell division in *Escherichia coli* by electrolysis products from a platinum electrode. *Nature*, **1965**, *205*, 698–699.

Rosenberg, B.; VanCamp, L.; Trosko, J. E.; and Mansour, V. H. Platinum compounds: a new class of potent antitumour agents. *Nature*, **1969**, *222*, 385–386.

Santen, R. J.; Samojlik, E.; and Wells, S. A. Resistance of the ovary to blockade of aromatization with aminoglutethimide. *J. Clin. Endocrinol. Metab.*, **1980**, *51*, 473–477.

Santen, R. J.; Worgul, T. J.; Lipton, A.; Harvey, H. A.; Boucher, A.; Samojlik, E.; and Wells, S. A. Aminoglutethimide as treatment of postmenopausal women with advanced breast carcinoma. *Ann. Intern. Med.*, **1982**, *96*, 94–101.

Santi, D. V.; McHenry, C. S.; and Somer, H. Mechanism of interaction of thymidylate synthetase with 5-fluorodeoxyuridylate. *Biochemistry*, **1974**, *13*, 471–481.

Santora, A., and Bonadonna, G. Prolonged disease-free survival in MOPP-resistant Hodgkin's disease after treatment with ADRIAMYCIN, bleomycin, vinblastine and dacarbazine (ABVD). *Cancer Chemother. Pharmacol.*, **1979**, *2*, 101–105.

Santos, G. W., and others. Marrow transplantation for acute non-lymphocytic leukemia after treatment with busulfan and cyclophosphamide. *N. Engl. J. Med.*, **1983**, *309*, 1347–1353.

Schein, P.; Kahn, R.; Gorden, P.; Wells, S.; and DeVita, V. T. Streptozotocin for malignant insulinomas and carcinoid tumor. *Arch. Intern. Med.*, **1973**, *132*, 555–561.

Schein, P. S.; O'Connell, M. J.; Blom, J.; Hubbard, S.; Magrath, I. T.; Bergevin, P.; Wiernick, P. H.; Ziegler, J. L.; and DeVita, V. T. Clinical antitumor activity and toxicity of streptozotocin (NCS-86998). *Cancer*, **1974**, *34*, 993–1000.

Schein, P. S., and Winokur, S. H. Immunosuppressive and cytotoxic chemotherapy: long-term complications. *Ann. Intern. Med.*, **1975**, *82*, 84–95.

Schiff, P. B.; Fant, J.; and Horwitz, S. B. Promotion of microtubule assembly *in vitro* by taxol. *Nature*, **1979**, *277*, 665–667.

Schwatzer, V. G.; Dolan, D. F.; and Snyder, R. Amelioration of cisplatin-induced cytotoxicity by fosfomycin. *Laryngoscope*, **1986**, *96*, 948.

Sebti, S. M.; DeLeon, J. C.; and Luzo, J. S. Purification, characterization, and amino acid composition of rabbit pulmonary bleomycin hydrolase. *Biochemistry*, **1987**, *26*, 4213–4219.

Shelley, M. D.; Fish, R. G.; and Adams, M. Biliary excretion of platinum in a patient treated with cis-dichlorodiammineplatinum (II). *Antimicrob. Agents Chemother.*, **1985**, *27*, 275–276.

Shubin, S. TRIAZURE and public drug policies. *Perspect. Biol. Med.*, **1979**, *22*, 185–204.

Shum, K. Y.; Kris, M. G.; Gralla, R. J.; Burke, M. T.; Marks, L. D.; and Heeland, R. T. Phase II study of 10-ethyl-10-deaza-aminopterin in patients with Stage III and IV non-small lung cancer. *J. Clin. Oncol.*, **1988**, *6*, 446–450.

Siaw, M. F., and Coleman, M. S. *In vitro* metabolism of deoxycoformycin in human T lymphoblastoid cells. Phosphorylation of deoxycoformycin and incorporation into cellular DNA. *J. Biol. Chem.*, **1984**, *259*, 9426–9433.

Sinha, B. K.; Mimnaugh, E. G.; Rajagopalan, S.; and Myers, C. E. Adriamycin activation and oxygen free radical formation in human breast tumor cells: protective role of glutathione peroxidase in adriamycin resistance. *Cancer Res.*, **1989**, *49*, 3844–3848.

Sinkule, J. A.; Stewart, C. F.; Crom, W. R.; Melton, E. T.; Dahl, G. V.; and Evans, W. E. Teniposide (VM-26) disposition in children with leukemia. *Cancer Res.*, **1984**, *44*, 1235–1237.

Sirotnak, F. M.; DeGraw, J. L.; Schmid, F. A.; Goutas, L. J.; and Moccio, D. M. New folate analogs of the 10-deaza-aminopterin series. Further evidence for markedly increased antitumor efficacy compared with methotrexate in ascitic and solid murine tumor models. *Cancer Chemother. Pharmacol.*, **1984**, *12*, 26–30.

Sladek, N. E. Therapeutic efficacy of cyclophosphamide as a function of its metabolism. *Cancer Res.*, **1972**, *32*, 535–542.

Speyer, J., and others. Protective effect of the bispiperazinedione ICRF-187 against doxorubicin-induced cardiac toxicity in women with advanced breast cancer. *N. Engl. J. Med.*, **1988**, *319*, 745–752.

Stark, G. R., and Bartlett, P. A. Design and use of potent, specific enzyme inhibitors. *Pharmacol. Ther.*, **1983**, *23*, 45–78.

Stoller, R. G.; Hande, K. R.; Jacobs, S. A.; Rosenberg, S. A.; and Chabner, B. A. Use of plasma pharmacokinetics to predict and prevent methotrexate toxicity. *N. Engl. J. Med.*, **1977**, *297*, 630–634.

Stott, H.; Fox, W.; Girling, D. J.; Stephans, R. J.; and Galton, D. A. Acute leukemia after busulphan. *Br. Med. J.* [*Clin. Res.*], **1977**, *2*, 1513–1517.

Tattersall, M. H. N.; Jarman, M.; Newlands, E. S.; Holyhead, L.; Milstead, R. A. V.; and Weinberg, A. Pharmaco-kinetics of melphalan following oral or intravenous administration in patients with malignant disease. *Eur. J. Cancer*, **1978**, *14*, 507–513.

Tewey, K. M.; Chen, G. L.; Nelson, E. M.; and Liu, L. F. Intercalative anticancer drugs interfere with the breakage-reunion reaction of mammalian DNA topoisomerase II. *J. Biol. Chem.*, **1984**, *259*, 9182–9187.

Thillet, J.; Absil, J.; Stone, S. R.; and Pictet, R. Site-directed mutagenesis of mouse dihydrofolate reductase: mutants with increased resistance to methotrexate and trimethoprim. *J. Biol. Chem.*, **1988**, *263*, 12500–12508.

Toledo, C. H.; Ross, W. E.; Hood, C. I.; and Block, E. R. Potentiation of bleomycin toxicity by oxygen. *Cancer Treat. Rep.*, **1982**, *66*, 359–362.

Tong, W. P., and Ludlum, D. B. Crosslinking of DNA by busulfan. Formation of diguanyl derivatives. *Biochim. Biophys. Acta*, **1980**, 19, 643–647.

Tritsch, G. L. (ed.). Role of adenosine deaminase in disorders of purine metabolism and in immune deficiency. *Ann. N.Y. Acad. Sci.*, **1985**, *451*.

Tritton, T. R.; Murphee, S. A.; and Sartorelli, A. C. ADRIAMYCIN: a proposal on the specificity of drug action. *Biochem. Biophys. Res. Commun.*, **1978**, *84*, 802–808.

Tucker, M. A.; Coleman, C. N.; Cox, R. S.;

Varghese, A.; and Rosenberg, S. A. Risk of second cancers after treatment for Hodgkin's disease. *N. Engl. J. Med.*, **1988**, *318*, 76–81.

Twentyman, P. R. Bleomycin—mode of action with particular reference to the cell cycle. *Pharmacol. Ther.*, **1984**, *23*, 417–441.

Ullman, B.; Lee, M.; Martin, D. W.; and Santi, D. V. Cytotoxicity of 5-fluoro-2′-deoxycoformycin: requirement for reduced folate cofactors and antagonism by methotrexate. *Proc. Natl. Acad. Sci. U.S.A.*, **1978**, *75*, 980–983.

Valavaara, R., and Nordman, E. Renal complications of mitomycin C therapy with special reference to the total dose. *Cancer*, **1985**, *55*, 47–50.

Van Barneveld, P. W.; Sleijfer, D. T.; van der Mark, T. W.; Mulder, N. H.; Koops, H. S.; Sluiter, H. J.; and Peset, R. Natural course of bleomycin-induced pneumonitis: a follow-up study. *Am. Rev. Respir. Dis.*, **1987**, *135*, 48–51.

Waksman, S. A., and Woodruff, H. B. Bacteriostatic and bactericidal substances produced by a soil actinomyces. *Proc. Soc. Exp. Biol. Med.*, **1940**, *45*, 609–614.

Wasserman, T. H. The nitrosoureas: an outline of clinical schedules and toxic effects. *Cancer Treat. Rep.*, **1976**, *60*, 709–711.

Wasserman, T. H.; Slavik, M.; and Carter, S. H. Clinical comparison of the nitrosoureas. *Cancer*, **1975**, *36*, 1258–1268.

Weinstein, G. D. Methotrexate. *Ann. Intern. Med.*, **1977**, *86*, 199–204.

Wiernik, P. K.; Schwartz, E. L.; Einzig, A.; Strausman, J. J.; Lipton, R. B.; and Dutcher, J. P. Phase I trial of taxol given as a 24-hour infusion every 21 days: responses observed in metastatic melanoma. *J. Clin. Oncol.*, **1987**, *5*, 1232–1239.

Wiley, J. S.; Taupin, J.; Jamieson, G. P.; Snook, M.; Sawyer, W. H.; and Finch, L. R. Cytosine arabinoside transport and metabolism in acute leukemias and T-cell lymphoblastic lymphoma. *J. Clin. Invest.*, **1985**, *75*, 632–642.

Williams, M. E.; Walker, A. M.; Bracikowski, J. P.; Garner, L.; Wilson, K. D.; and Carpenter, J. T. Ascending myeloencephalopathy due to intrathecal vincristine sulfate. A fatal chemotherapeutic error. *Cancer*, **1983**, *51*, 2041–2147.

Wilson, C. B.; Gutin, P.; Boldrey, E. B.; Crafts, D.; Levin, V. A.; and Enot, K. J. Single-agent chemotherapy of brain tumors. *Arch. Neurol.*, **1976**, *33*, 739–744.

Wolmark, N., and others. Postoperative adjuvant chemotherapy or BCG for colon cancer: results from NSABP protocol C-01. *J.N.C.I.*, **1988**, *80*, 30–36.

Wortsman, J., and Soler, N. G. Mitotane-spironolactone antagonism in Cushing's syndrome. *J.A.M.A.*, **1977**, *238*, 2527–2529.

Young, R. C.; DeVita, V. T., Jr.; Serpick, A. A.; and Canellos, G. P. Treatment of advanced Hodgkin's disease with [1,3 *bis*(2-chloroethyl)-1-nitrosourea] BCNU. *N. Engl. J. Med.*, **1971**, *285*, 475–479.

Zuckerman, J. E.; Raffin, T. A.; Brown, J. M.; Newman, R. A.; Etiz, B. B.; and Sikic, B. I. *In vitro* selection and characterization of a bleomycin-resistant subline of B16 melanoma. *Cancer Res.*, **1986**, *46*, 1748–1753.

Monographs and Reviews

Agrawal, K. C., and Sartorelli, A. C. α-(N)-heterocyclic carboxaldehyde thiosemicarbazones. In, *Antineoplastic and Immunosuppressive Agents*, Pt. II. (Sartorelli, A. C., and Johns, D. G., eds.) *Handbuch der Experimentellen Pharmakologie*, Vol. 38. Springer-Verlag, Berlin, **1975**, pp. 793–807.

Allegra, C. J. Antifolates. In, *Cancer Chemotherapy: Principles and Practice*. (Chabner, B. A., and Collins, J. M., eds.) J. B. Lippincott Co., Philadelphia, **1990**, pp. 110–153.

Averbuch, S. Non-classic alkylating agents. In, *Cancer Chemotherapy: Principles and Practice*. (Chabner, B. A., and Collins, J. M., eds.) J. B. Lippincott Co., Philadelphia, **1990**, pp. 314–340.

Bender, R. A.; Hamel, E.; and Hande, K. R. The plant alkaloids. In, *Cancer Chemotherapy: Principles and Practice*. (Chabner, B. A., and Collins, J. M., eds.) J. B. Lippincott Co., Philadelphia, **1990**, pp. 253–275.

Bergsagel, D. E. Plasma cell myeloma. An interpretive review. *Cancer*, **1972**, *30*, 1588–1594.

Bleyer, W. A. The clinical pharmacology of methotrexate. *Cancer*, **1978**, *41*, 36–51.

Borch, R. F.; Bodenner, D. L.; and Katz, J. C. Diethyldithiocarbamate and cis-platinum toxicity. In, *Platinum Coordination Complexes in Cancer Chemotherapy*. (Hacker, M. P.; Douple, E. B.; and Krakoff, I. H.; eds.) Martinus Nijhoff, Boston, **1984**, pp. 154–164.

Brade, W. P.; Nagel, G. A.; and Seeber, S. (eds.). *Ifosfamide in Tumor Therapy*. S. Karger, New York, **1987**.

Brockman, R. W. Resistance to purine analogs. Clinical pharmacology symposium. *Biochem. Pharmacol.*, **1974**, *23*, Suppl. 2, pp. 107–117.

Broome, J. D. L-Asparaginase: discovery and development as a tumor-inhibitory agent. *Cancer Treat. Rep.*, **1981**, *65*, Suppl. 4, 111–114.

Calabresi, P.; Schein, P. S.; and Rosenberg, S. A. (eds.). *Medical Oncology*. Macmillan Publishing Co., New York, **1985**.

Capizzi, R. L., and Handschumacher, R. E. Asparaginase. In, *Cancer Medicine*, 2nd ed. Lea & Febiger, Philadelphia, **1982**, pp. 920–932.

Chabner, B. A. Nonclassical alkylating agents. In, *Pharmacologic Principles of Cancer Treatment*. (Chabner, B. A., ed.) W. B. Saunders Co., Philadelphia, **1982**, pp. 340–362.

———. Cytidine analogs. In, *Cancer Chemotherapy: Principles and Practice*. (Chabner, B. A., and Collins, J. M., eds.) J. B. Lippincott Co., Philadelphia, **1990**, pp. 154–179.

Chabner, B. A.; Allegra, C. J.; Curt, G. A.; Clendeninn, N. J.; Baram, J.; Koizumi, S.; Drake, J. C.; and Jolivet, J. Polyglutamation of methotrexate. Is methotrexate a pro-drug? *J. Clin. Invest.*, **1985**, *76*, 907–912.

Colvin, M. The alklylating agents. In, *Pharmacologic Principles of Cancer Treatment*. (Chabner, B. A., ed.) W. B. Saunders Co., Philadelphia, **1982**, pp. 276–308.

Creaven, P. J., and Allen, L. M. EPEG, a new antineoplastic epipodophyllotoxin. *Clin. Pharmacol. Ther.*, **1975**, *18*, 221–226.

Crooke, S. T. Antitumor antibiotics II: actinomycin D, bleomycin, mitomycin C and other antibiotics. In, *The Cancer Pharmacology Annual*. (Chabner, B. A., and Pinedo, H. M., eds.) Excerpta Medica, Amsterdam, **1983**, pp. 69–79.

Crooke, S. T., and Bradner, W. T. Mitomycin C: a review. *Cancer Treat. Rev.*, **1976**, *3*, 121–139.

Danenberg, P. V., and Lockshin, A. Fluorinated pyrimidines as tight-binding inhibitors of thymidylate synthetase. *Pharmacol. Ther.*, **1981**, *13*, 69–90.

DeVita, V. T., Jr. Consequences of the chemotherapy of Hodgkin's disease. *Cancer*, **1981**, *47*, 1–13.

DeVita, V. T., Jr.; Canellos, G. P.; and Moxley, J. H., III. A decade of combination chemotherapy of advanced Hodgkin's disease. *Cancer*, **1972**, *30*, 1495–1504.

Donehower, R. C. Hydroxyurea. In, *Pharmacologic Principles of Cancer Treatment*. (Chabner, B. A., ed.) W. B. Saunders Co., Philadelphia, **1982**, pp. 269–275.

———. Hydroxyurea. In, *Cancer Chemotherapy: Principles and Practice*. (Chabner, B. A., and Collins, J. M., eds.) J. B. Lippincott Co., Philadelphia, **1990**, pp. 225–233.

Doyle, T. W. The chemistry of etoposide. In, *Etoposide (VP-16), Current Status and New Developments*. (Issel,

B. F.; Muggia, F. M.; and Carter, S. K.; eds.) Academic Press, Orlando, Fla., **1984**, pp. 15–32.

Durant, J. R., and Omura, G. A. Gynecologic neoplasms. In, *Medical Oncology*. (Calabresi, P.; Schein, P. S.; and Rosenberg, S. A.; eds.) Macmillan Publishing Co., New York, **1985**, pp. 1004–1044.

Elion, G. B. Biochemistry and pharmacology of purine analogs. *Fed. Proc.*, **1967**, *26*, 898–904.

Elion, G. B., and Hitchings, G. H. Metabolic basis for the actions of analogs of purines and pyrimidines. *Adv. Chemother.*, **1965**, *2*, 91–177.

Endicott, J. A., and Ling, V. The biochemistry of P-glycoprotein-mediated multidrug resistance. *Ann. Rev. Biochem.*, **1989**, *58*, 137–172.

Fox, B. W. Mechanism of action of methanesulfonates. In, *Antineoplastic and Immunosuppressive Agents*, Pt. II. (Sartorelli, A. C., and Johns, D. G., eds.) *Handbuch der Experimentellen Pharmakologie*, Vol. 38. Springer-Verlag, Berlin, **1975**, pp. 35–46.

Gilman, A., and Philips, F. S. The biological actions and therapeutic applications of the β-chlorethylamines and sulfides. *Science*, **1946**, *103*, 409–415.

Goldberg, I. H.; Beerman, T. A.; and Poon, R. Antibiotics: nucleic acids as targets in chemotherapy. In, *Cancer 5: A Comprehensive Treatise*. (Becker, F. F., ed.) Plenum Press, New York, **1977**, pp. 427–456.

Grem, J. L.; Hoth, D. F.; Hamilton, J. M.; King, S. A.; and Leyland-Jones, B. Overview of current status and future directions of clinical trials with 5-fluororuacil in combination with folinic acid. *Cancer Treat. Rep.*, **1987**, *71*, 1249–1264.

Hacker, M. P.; Douple, E. B.; and Krakoff, I. H. (eds.). *Platinum Coordination Complexes in Cancer Chemotherapy*. Martinus Nijhoff, Boston, **1984.**

Heidelberger, C. Fluorinated pyrimidines and their nucleosides. In, *Antineoplastic and Immunosuppressive Agents*, Pt. II. (Sartorelli, A. C., and Johns, D. G., eds.) *Handbuch der Experimentellen Pharmakologie*, Vol. 38. Springer-Verlag, Berlin, **1975**, pp. 193–231.

Holland, J. F., and Frei, E., III (eds.). *Cancer Medicine*, 2nd ed. Lea & Febiger, Philadelphia, **1982.**

Hryniuk, W. The impact of dose intensity on the design of clinical trials. *Semin. Oncol.*, **1987**, *14*, 65–74.

Hutter, A. M., Jr., and Kayhoe, D. E. Adrenal cortical carcinoma: clinical features of 138 patients. *Am. J. Med.*, **1966**, *41*, 572–592.

Kraut, J., and Matthews, D. A. Dihydrofolate reductase. In, *Biological Macromolecules and Assemblies*, Vol. 3. (Jurnak, F., and McPherson, A., eds.) John Wiley & Sons, New York, **1987**, pp. 1–21.

Jackson, R. C. Biological effects of folic acid antagonists with antineoplastic activity. *Pharmacol. Ther.*, **1984**, *25*, 61–82.

Jordan, V. C. Metabolites of tamoxifen in animals and man: identification, pharmacology, and significance. *Breast Cancer Res. Treat.*, **1982**, *2*, 123–138.

Kufe, D. W., and Major, P. P. Studies on the mechanism of action of cytosine arabinoside. *Med. Pediatr. Oncol.*, **1982**, Suppl. 1, 49–67.

Lane, M. Chemotherapy of cancer. In, *Cancer*, 5th ed. (del Regato, J. A., and Spjut, H. J., eds.) C. V. Mosby Co., St. Louis, **1977**, pp. 105–130.

Legha, S. S.; Davis, H. L.; and Muggia, F. M. Hormonal therapy of breast cancer: new approaches and concepts. *Ann. Intern. Med.*, **1978**, *88*, 69–77.

Lippman, M. E. The NIH Consensus Development Conference for Breast Cancer. *NCI Monogr.*, **1986**, *1*.

Ludlum, D. B., and Tong, W. P. DNA modification by the nitrosoureas: chemical nature and cellular repair. In, *Cancer Chemotherapy*, Vol. II. (Muggia, E. M., and Nishoff, M., eds.) Martinus Nijhoff, Boston, **1985**, pp. 141–154.

McCormack, J. J., and Johns, D. G. Purine antimetabolites. In, *Pharmacologic Principles of Cancer Treatment*. (Chabner, B. A., ed.) W. B. Saunders Co., Philadelphia, **1982**, pp. 213–228.

Moertel, C. G. Current concepts in chemotherapy of gastrointestinal cancer. *N. Engl. J. Med.*, **1978**, *299*, 1049–1052.

Muggia, F. M. Overview of carboplatin: replacing, complementing, and extending the therapeutic horizons of cisplatin. *Semin. Oncol.*, **1989**, *15*, 7–13.

Myers, C. E. Role of iron in anthracycline action. In, *Organ-Directed Toxicities of Anticancer Drugs*. (Hacker, M. P.; Lazo, J. S.; and Tritton, T. R.; eds.) Martinus Nijhoff Publishing, Boston, **1988**, pp. 17–30.

Myers, C. E., and Chabner, B. A. Anthracyclines. In, *Cancer Chemotherapy: Principles and Practice*. (Chabner, B. A., and Collins, J. M., eds.) J. B. Lippincott Co., Philadelphia, **1990**, pp. 356–381.

O'Dwyer, P. J.; Leyland-Jones, B.; Alonso, M. T.; Marsoni, S.; and Wittes, R. E. Etoposide (VP-16-213). Current status of an active anticancer drug. *N. Engl. J. Med.*, **1985**, *312*, 692–700.

Oliverio, V. T. Pharmacology of the nitrosoureas: an overview. *Cancer Treat. Rep.*, **1976**, *60*, 703–707.

———. Derivatives of triazanes and hydrazines. In, *Cancer Medicine*, 2nd ed. (Holland, J. F., and Frei, E., III, eds.) Lea & Febiger, Philadelphia, **1982**, pp. 850–860.

Patterson, M. K., Jr. L-Asparaginase: basic aspects. In, *Antineoplastic and Immunosuppressive Agents*, Pt. II. (Sartorelli, A. C., and Johns, D. G., eds.) *Handbuch der Experimentellen Pharmakologie*, Vol. 38. Springer-Verlag, Berlin, **1975**, pp. 695–722.

Pinkel, D., and Howarth, C. B. Pediatric neoplasms. In, *Medical Oncology*. (Calabresi, P.; Schein, P. S.; and Rosenberg, S. A.; eds.) Macmillan Publishing Co., New York, **1985**, pp. 1226–1258.

Price, C. C. Chemistry of alkylation. In, *Antineoplastic and Immunosuppressive Agents*, Pt. II. (Sartorelli, A. C., and Johns, D. G., eds.) *Handbuch der Experimentellen Pharmakologie*, Vol. 38. Springer-Verlag, Berlin, **1975**, pp. 1–5.

Robins, P. R., and Jowsey, J. Effect of mithramycin on normal and abnormal bone turnover. *J. Lab. Clin. Med.*, **1973**, *82*, 576–586.

Rozencweig, M.; Von Hoff, D. D.; Slavik, M.; and Muggia, F. M. *Cis*-diammine dichloroplatinum (II)—a new cancer drug. *Ann. Intern. Med.*, **1977**, *86*, 803–812.

Schabel, F. M., Jr. Historical development and future promise of the nitrosoureas as anticancer agents. *Cancer Chemother. Rep.*, **1973**, *4*, Part 3, No. 3, 3–6.

Schimke, R. T.; Kaufman, R. J.; Alt, F. W.; and Kellems, R. F. Gene amplification and drug resistance in cultured murine cells. *Science*, **1978**, *202*, 1051–1055.

Shapiro, R. Chemistry of guanine and its biologically significant derivatives. *Prog. Nucleic Acid Res. Mol. Biol.*, **1968**, *8*, 73–112.

Shenkenberg, T. D., and Von Hoff, D. D. Mitoxanthrone: a new anti-cancer drug with significant clinical activity. *Ann. Intern. Med.*, **1986**, *105*, 67–81.

Skipper, H. T., and Schabel, F. M., Jr. Quantitative and cytokinetic studies in experimental tumor models. In, *Cancer Medicine*, 2nd ed. (Holland, J. F., and Frei, E., III, eds.) Lea & Febiger, Philadelphia, **1982**, pp. 663–684.

Skoda, J. Azapyrimidine nucleosides. In, *Antineoplastic and Immunosuppressive Agents*, Pt. II. (Sartorelli, A. C., and Johns, D. G., eds.) *Handbuch der Experimentellen Pharmakologie*, Vol. 38. Springer-Verlag, Berlin, **1975**, pp. 348–372.

Slotman, G. J.; Cummings, F. J.; Glicksman, A. R.; Doolittle, C. L.; and Leone, L. A. Preoperative simultaneously administered cis-platinum plus radiation therapy for advanced squamous cell cancer of the head and neck. *Head Neck Surg.*, **1986**, *8*, 159–164.

Sobell, H. M. The stereochemistry of actinomycin binding to DNA and its implications in molecular biology. *Prog. Nucleic Acid Res. Mol. Biol.*, **1973**, *13*, 153–190.

Stark, G. R., and Bartlett, P. A. Design and use of potent, specific enzyme inhibitors. *Pharmacol. Ther.*, **1983**, *23*, 45–78.

Stark, G. R., and Wahl, G. M. Gene amplification. *Annu. Rev. Biochem.*, **1984**, *53*, 447–491.

Symposium. (Various authors.) Proceedings of the conference on 2′-deoxycoformycin: current status and future directions. *Cancer Treatment Symposia*, Vol. 2, National Cancer Institute, Washington, D.C., **1984**, pp. 1–104.

Umezawa, H. Cancer drugs of microbial origin. In, *Methods in Cancer Research, XVI: Cancer Drug Development*, Pt. A. (DeVita, V. T., Jr., and Busch, H., eds.) Academic Press, Inc., New York, **1979**, pp. 43–72.

Von Hoff, D. D. Whither carboplatin? A replacement for or an alternative to cisplatin. *J. Clin. Oncol.*, **1987**, *5*, 169–170.

Waksman Conference on Actinomycins: their potential for cancer chemotherapy. *Cancer Chemother. Rep.*, **1974**, *58*, 1–123.

Walker, M. D. Nitrosoureas in central nervous system tumors. *Cancer Chemother. Rep.*, **1973**, *4*, 21–26.

Wasternack, C., and Hause, B. Thirty years of 5-fluorouracil. *Pharmazie*, **1987**, *42*, 73–79.

Weinkam, R. J.; Shiba, D. A.; and Chabner, B. A. Nonclassical alkylating agents. In, *Pharmacologic Principles of Cancer Treatment*. (Chabner, B. A., ed.) W. B. Saunders Co., Philadelphia, **1982**, pp. 340–362.

Wheeler, G. P. Some biochemical effects of alkylating agents. *Fed. Proc.*, **1967**, *26*, 885–892.

———. Alkylating agents. In, *Cancer Medicine*, 2nd ed. (Holland, J. F., and Frei, E., III, eds.) Lea & Febiger, Philadelphia, **1982**, pp. 824–842.

Wiemann, M. C., and Calabresi, P. Pharmacology of antineoplastic agents. In, *Medical Oncology*. (Calabresi, P.; Schein, P. S.; and Rosenberg, S. A.; eds.) Macmillan Publishing Co., New York, **1985**, pp. 292–362.

Williams, S. D., and Einhorn, L. H. Neoplasms of the testis. In, *Medical Oncology*. (Calabresi, P.; Schein, P. S.; and Rosenberg, S. A.; eds.) Macmillan Publishing Co., New York, **1985**, pp. 1077–1088.

Zinner, S. H., and Klastersky, J. Infectious considerations in cancer. In, *Medical Oncology*. (Calabresi, P.; Schein, P. S.; and Rosenberg, S. A.; eds.) Macmillan Publishing Co., New York, **1985**, pp. 1327–1357.

Zwelling, L. A., and Kohn, K. W. Platinum complexes. In, *Pharmacologic Principles of Cancer Treatment*. (Chabner, B. A., ed.) W. B. Saunders Co., Philadelphia, **1982**, pp. 309–339.

SECTION
XIII
Drugs Used for Immunosuppression

CHAPTER
53 IMMUNOSUPPRESSIVE AGENTS

Robert E. Handschumacher

INTRODUCTION

Targets for the Actions of Immunosuppressive Drugs. Modification of immune function by pharmacological agents is emerging as a major area of therapeutics. The primary objective in the past has been to suppress the immune system to permit allotransplantation. However, the recent elucidation of the role of interleukins and related cytokines in a variety of other pathophysiological states has suggested new applications for agents that affect the production or action of these mediators.

A summary of the principal elements in the cellular and molecular cascades that are responsible for activation of the immune response is depicted in Figure 53–1 (for a detailed review, *see* Paul, 1989). Each element may be considered a potential site for pharmacological intervention. Activation of the immune system by "non-self" antigens (alloantigens) or "self" antigens (autoantigens) is generally believed to require processing of the antigen by phagocytic cells such as macrophages, monocytes, or related cells. The processing and subsequent presentation of the antigen to one of the subsets of lymphocytes is associated with the elaboration and secretion of a number of small proteins by the phagocytes. Prominent among these is interleukin 1 (IL-1). This initial series of reactions is blocked by the adrenocorticosteroids (*see* Chapter 60).

Activated phagocytic cells then communicate with thymus-derived lymphocytes (T cells), particularly helper T cells. Receptor sites on T cells are complex, in that they detect both the processed antigen in question and major histocompatibility complex (MHC) proteins on the antigen-presenting cell (*see* Perlmutter, 1989). A complex of at least five other transmembrane proteins, known collectively as the *cell differentiation complex 3* (CD3), is associated with the T-cell receptor. The role of this complex is incompletely understood, but it is essential to the activation process. The monoclonal antibody OKT3 is specific for epitopes in the CD3 complex, and it affords a means of inhibiting the functional interaction between antigen-presenting cells and T cells. T cells are commonly divided into two major subsets on the basis of their expression of either CD4, which recognizes MHC II–associated antigens (helper cells), or CD8, which recognizes MHC I–associated antigens (suppressor–cytolytic cells). The phenotypic characterization of these subsets of T cells is even more complex as a result of their expression of a variety of other surface proteins.

In response to these concerted stimuli, T

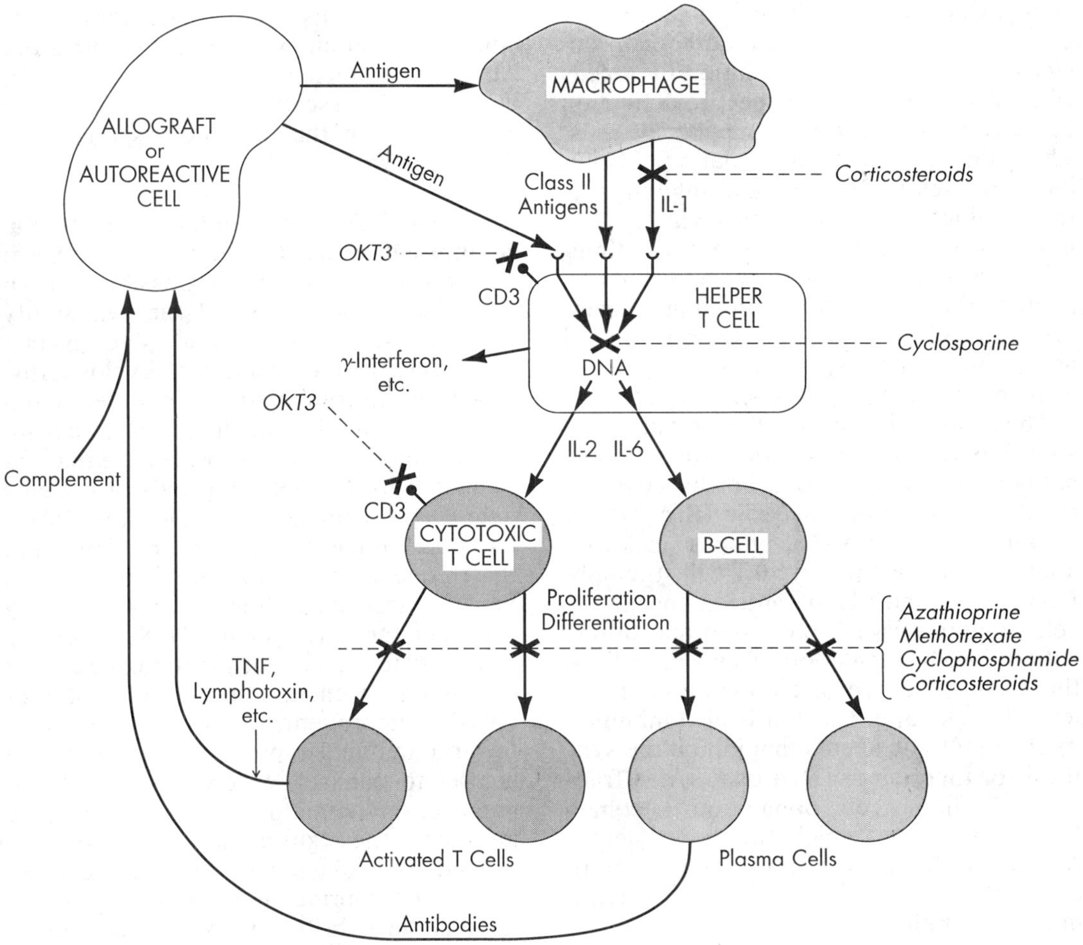

Figure 53–1. *Potential targets for immunosuppressive agents.*

The figure depicts the salient features of cellular and humoral immune responses and indicates the apparent sites of action of various immunosuppressive agents (*see* text for details). Abbreviations are: IL, interleukin; CD3, cell differentiation complex 3; OKT3, murine monoclonal antibody directed against an epitope in CD3; and TNF, tumor necrosis factor.

cells undergo clonal expansion, a proliferation process that requires both the expression of receptors for a growth factor, interleukin 2 (IL-2), and the production of IL-2 by T cells. Classical cytotoxic immunosuppressants such as methotrexate, azathioprine, and cyclophosphamide act by inhibiting the synthesis of DNA, thereby thwarting the stimulus for proliferation. The role of IL-1 in the activation of mature T cells is not clearly established, but it is an essential factor in the proliferation and differentiation of certain stem cells in the thymus that result in the emergence of mature T cells. Another consequence of the activation of helper T cells is the synthesis and release of a variety of cytokines that control both the cellular and humoral arms of the immune response (*see* Hamblin, 1988; Mizel, 1989; O'Garra *et al.*, 1988). It is this step in the activation of T cells that is exquisitely sensitive to cyclosporine and FK-506.

Cellular immunity is expressed as cytotoxicity toward target cells by activation of cytotoxic or "killer" T cells. Cytotoxicity is mediated both by direct cell–cell interactions and by secreted peptides, such as lymphotoxin, interferon, and tumor necrosis factor. The actions of the cytotoxic T cells (which are facilitated by accessory cells) are also inhibited by adrenocorticosteroids. Another subpopulation of T cells can balance the antigen-specific activation process; these are termed suppressor cells. Their function results in regulation of cellular responses to antigens and inhibition of the production of antibodies via the humoral arm of the immune response. Stimulation of suppressor activity represents an additional means of achieving immunosuppression, but it has not yet been identified as an important aspect of the action of available immunosuppressant drugs.

The humoral arm of the immune response is responsible for the production of antibodies; this is carried out by cells derived from the bone marrow (B cells). In response to a battery of lymphokines that are primarily elaborated by T cells (notably IL-4, IL-5, and IL-6), antigen-specific B cells undergo clonal expansion and differentiate into a population of plasma cells—the primary source of circulating antibodies. This clonal expansion is also inhibited by the cytotoxic agents that inhibit the synthesis or function of DNA or RNA. A fraction of the B-cell population becomes "memory" cells, which can subsequently respond to the specific antigen more rapidly and with greater production of specific immunoglobulins.

Since certain autoimmune diseases, such as rheumatoid arthritis, nephrosis, uveitis, thyroiditis, and early stages of insulin-dependent diabetes mellitus, appear to involve responses to autoantigens, a potential role for immunosuppressive drugs has been recognized. Similarly, psoriasis and inflammatory bowel disease may reflect activation of cellular elements by some of the lymphokines that are essential for immune function (Gottlieb, 1988). For example, IL-1 is a potent endogenous pyrogen and is a growth factor for endothelial cells, synovial cells, and fibroblasts. IL-3 and IL-4 serve as growth factors for mast cells and as co-mitogens for hematopoietic cells (Mizel, 1989). Excess production of these substances as a consequence of inappropriate activation of immune cells can cause secondary effects by the release of a spectrum of inflammatory mediators (*e.g.*, histamine, eicosanoids, kinins). The agents discussed in this chapter are thought to ameliorate autoimmune and inflammatory states by reducing the elaboration and/or function of these trophic molecules at an early stage in the immune response (*see* Bach, 1989b).

Principal Uses and Limitations of Immunosuppressive Agents. Successful allograft transplantation has been possible for almost 30 years because of the availability of cytotoxic immunosuppressive agents. However, the introduction of cyclosporine and its use in combination with older immunosuppressants has made organ transplantation a more successful procedure that extends life for tens of thousands of patients every year (Bennett and Norman, 1986). Although renal transplants predominate, the frequency and success of cardiac and hepatic transplantations are increasing (Metzger and Hoffman, 1988; O'Grady *et al.*, 1988). The transplantation of other organs has been less successful, but progressive improvement has been evident. Several immunosuppressant drugs can also be used to manage a wide variety of autoimmune or inflammatory diseases. In some instances, these drugs are among the approved methods for treatment; these include azathioprine and methotrexate for rheumatoid arthritis, cyclophosphamide for nephrotic conditions of immune origin, and methotrexate for psoriasis. In other instances, clinical improvement has been demonstrated in experimental protocols. Examples include the beneficial effects of azathioprine in the treatment of nephrotic conditions, antibody-mediated thrombocytopenia, and autoimmune hemolytic anemia and of cyclosporine in patients with rheumatoid arthritis, uveitis, early-onset insulin-dependent diabetes mellitus, psoriasis, nephrotic syndrome, and aplastic anemia.

Modification of the immune response by pharmacological agents is most effective if therapy is begun before exposure to the antigen has an opportunity to generate a primary response (*e.g.*, pretreatment of allograft recipients). The secondary or anamnestic response is much less sensitive to the classical cytotoxic agents, but it can be suppressed with large doses of corticosteroids.

The latter agents are thus an important element in the treatment of acute graft rejection.

Fortunately, the sensitivity of lymphoid elements to the classical cytotoxic agents is somewhat greater than is that of other stem cells in the marrow, at least during the initial step of antigen recognition and during establishment of memory cells. However, the therapeutic index is narrow. When cytotoxic drugs are given for cancer chemotherapy, they are often given in large doses intermittently; this strategy is designed to permit lymphoid and other cellular elements to recover between courses. These drugs are given more continuously but in lower doses to produce immunosuppression.

Despite recent therapeutic advances, nonspecific suppression of the immune response to either autoantigens or alloantigens engenders an increased risk of infection by viral, bacterial, and fungal organisms (Bach, 1989a; Boitard and Bach, 1989). The same opportunistic pathogens that afflict patients with acquired immunodeficiency syndrome frequently limit therapy with immunosuppressive agents. The profound depression of immune surveillance by all of these drugs also greatly increases the incidence (3- to 100-fold) of malignant neoplasms in patients after allograft transplantation (Penn, 1986; Boitard and Bach, 1989). However, the use of these agents in patients with autoimmune disease has been associated with only a minimal increase in the incidence of cancer, perhaps because lower doses and shorter periods of treatment have usually been employed. Lymphomas and related neoplasms comprise a much larger fraction of all cancers in transplant patients than in the general population. This may result from stimulation of feedback mechanisms and hyperproliferation of stem cells that serve to restore immune function.

CYCLOSPORINE

Chemistry. Cyclosporine is one of a family of cyclic peptides produced by the fungus *Tolypocladium inflatum Gams;* it is comprised of 11 amino acid residues (*see* below). Cyclosporine is a very hydrophobic molecule with a unique 9-carbon amino acid in position 1 and a remarkable lack of other functional groups (Wenger, 1986). All amide nitrogens are either hydrogen bonded or methylated, and biological activity is very sensitive to alterations in stereochemical configuration and to modification of the residues at positions 1, 2, 3, 10, and 11. Cyclosporine contains a single D-amino acid residue in position 8, and the methyl amide between residues 9 and 10 is in the *cis* configuration; all other methyl amide moieties are in the *trans* form.

Pharmacological Effects and Mechanism of Action. The introduction of cyclosporine has provided an entirely new ap-

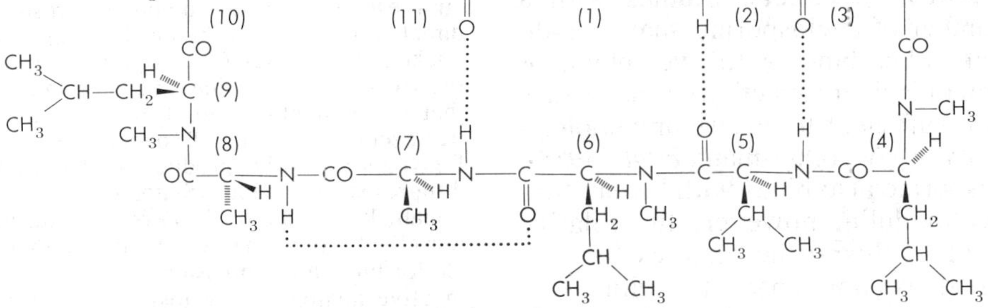

Cyclosporine

proach to immunosuppression by virtue of its highly selective ability to inhibit activation of T cells (Borel *et al.*, 1976; Borel, 1983; Shevach, 1985; Kahan and Bach, 1988). Unlike cytotoxic immunosuppressants, therapeutic concentrations of cyclosporine do not cause myelosuppression. Although its site of action has not been defined precisely, cyclosporine inhibits an early cellular response to antigenic and regulatory stimuli, primarily in populations of helper T cells (Kay and Benzie, 1984). Blockade of the pathways that effect the responsiveness of lymphocytes results in a spectrum of secondary changes in cellular function that generate both the therapeutic and unwanted effects of the drug (Drugge and Handschumacher, 1988).

The molecular targets for cyclosporine appear to be a family of proteins called *cyclophilins* (Handschumacher *et al.*, 1984; Harding *et al.*, 1986). These small proteins selectively bind cyclosporine and its active analogs with high affinity. Cyclophilins are abundant in lymphoid tissue, but isoforms of the protein are also found in varying proportions in most mammalian tissues (Koletsky *et al.*, 1986). Proteins with structures that are highly homologous to cyclosporine are present in essentially all eukaryotic organisms. The major isoform of cyclophilin has recently been shown to be identical to peptidyl proline *cis–trans* isomerase from porcine kidney (Fischer *et al.*, 1989; Takahashi *et al.*, 1989). This enzyme participates in the folding of proteins, presumably by assisting in the establishment of specific types of turns as nascent proteins assume their functional conformation. Thus far, all isoforms of this enzyme are inhibited by cyclosporine and its active analogs at concentrations that correlate with those required for their immunosuppressive effects. Studies with a large number of cyclosporine analogs indicate that either binding to cyclophilin or inhibition of isomerase activity is necessary but is not sufficient to ensure immunological activity *in vivo* (Quesniaux *et al.*, 1988).

Cyclosporine also binds with lower affinity to calmodulin; however, the relative affinity of cyclosporine analogs for calmodulin does not correlate with their immunosuppressive activity (Colombani *et al.*, 1985; LeGrue *et al.*, 1986; Foxwell *et al.*, 1988b). Nevertheless, this interaction with calmodulin may be responsible for some of the side effects of cyclosporine (*e.g.*, inhibition of protein phosphorylation) when plasma concentrations of the drug are elevated (Gschwendt *et al.*, 1987).

A direct connection has not yet been made between these molecular targets and the rapid and profound inhibition by cyclosporine of the production of IL-2 by helper T cells (Elliot *et al.*, 1984; Kronke *et al.*, 1984). Cyclosporine also causes a general reduction in the production and release of other lymphokines in response to an antigenic stimulus. At higher concentrations, cyclosporine inhibits expression of receptors for IL-2 (Herold *et al.*, 1986). Although cyclosporine can inhibit the activation of helper T cells, it does not prevent the stimulation of their clonal expansion by IL-2. It is potentially significant that cyclosporine allows the expression of suppressor cell activity at concentrations that inhibit the induction of cytotoxic T cells (Hess and Tutschka, 1980).

Pleotropic cellular responses to the administration of cyclosporine are well documented (Kahan and Bach, 1988). These include increased secretion of prolactin from the pituitary and reduced binding of prolactin to receptors on lymphocytes (Russell *et al.*, 1985; Larson, 1986). Patients treated with cyclosporine often have significantly increased concentrations of prolactin in the circulation. Variable effects on eicosanoid metabolism and Ca^{2+} fluxes have also been observed (Metcalf, 1984; Gelfand *et al.*, 1987). The relationship of these effects to cyclosporine-sensitive signal transduction mechanisms or to the role of cyclophilin is not at all clear.

Cyclosporine and its active analogs have other properties that seem quite unrelated to their actions on T cells and that may reflect in part the ubiquitous distribution of cyclophilins. A variety of parasitic infections including schistosomiasis and malaria respond to these compounds, presumably by a direct action on the parasite (Bueding *et al.*, 1981; Nickell *et al.*, 1982). Cyclosporine can also restore the sensitivity of cell lines and experimental tumors that are resistant to several cancer chemotherapeutic agents because of overexpression of the P-glycoprotein (the product of the MDR [multidrug-resistance] gene) (Slater *et al.*, 1986; Twentyman, 1988; Hait *et al.*, 1989). The mechanism of this effect is presumably unrelated to that responsible for immunosuppression, since both active and inactive analogs of cyclosporine can cause this effect.

Absorption, Fate, and Excretion. The oral bioavailability of cyclosporine varies from 20 to 50%; peak concentrations in plasma are achieved within 3 to 4 hours. About 60 to 70% of the drug in whole blood is contained in erythrocytes. Despite their small contribution to blood volume, leukocytes contain 10 to 20% of circulating cyclosporine. This concentration in leukocytes apparently reflects their content of cyclophilin; binding becomes saturated at plasma concentrations of cyclosporine in excess of 100 ng/ml (Foxwell, 1988a). The remainder of the drug circulates largely in association with plasma lipoproteins. Cyclosporine is also sequestered in tissues, and its apparent volume of distribution is rather large. It is cleared from blood with a half-life of about 6 hours, although wide variations in all pharmacokinetic parameters have been observed (Vine and Bowers, 1988; Kahan and Grevel, 1988).

Very little cyclosporine, or its metabolites, appears in the urine; most of the drug is excreted in the bile after metabolism in the liver (Maurer, 1985; Burckart *et al.*, 1986; Maurer and LeMaire, 1986). The cyclic peptide structure of cyclosporine is relatively resistant to attack, but cytochrome P_{450}–mediated oxidation of side chains is extensive (Aoyama *et al.*, 1989); hepatic dysfunction or concomitant administration of agents that affect the activity of cytochrome P_{450} causes dramatic changes in the elimination of cyclosporine (McMillan, 1989). Some of the metabolites have immunosuppressive activity, but their role in the therapeutic or toxic effects of the drug remains to be established (Freed *et al.*, 1987).

Drug Interactions. There have been many descriptions of effects of other drugs on the disposition of cyclosporine, but only a few of these interactions appear to be clinically significant. These reports are often difficult to evaluate because the methods used most commonly to analyze cyclosporine in whole blood detect both active and inactive metabolites (Vine and Bowers, 1988; McMillan, 1989). Accelerated clearance of cyclosporine has been demonstrated in patients receiving phenytoin, phenobarbital, trimethoprim–sulfamethoxazole, and rifampin, presumably as a result of induction of hepatic P_{450} systems. Administration of these drugs for the treatment of infections, seizures, or tuberculosis has caused rejection of transplanted organs because of reduced concentrations of cyclosporine in blood (McMillan, 1989). Decreased clearance of cyclosporine has been associated with concurrent administration of erythromycin, ketoconazole, or amphotericin B; this engenders a higher risk of toxicity from cyclosporine if its concentration in blood is not carefully monitored.

Clinical Toxicity. The major toxic manifestations of cyclosporine are renal, and nephrotoxicity occurs in 25 to 75% of patients treated with the drug. Although dose-related and usually reversible, nephrotoxicity frequently mandates cessation or modification of therapy (Mihatsch *et al.*, 1988; Racusen and Solez, 1988). The ultimate consequence is a reduction in glomerular filtration rate and renal plasma flow, but there is evidence of early damage to proximal tubules and to the endothelial and smooth muscle cells of small blood vessels. Plasma concentrations of creatinine and urea are used to guide dosage, but incipient rejection of a transplanted kidney will cause similar changes. Hypertension (10 to 15% elevation in blood pressure) is seen in more than 30% of patients with renal, hepatic, or cardiac transplants who receive cyclosporine (Bennett and Porter, 1988). Neurological toxicity is also common, especially in recipients of hepatic transplants (Walker and Brochstein, 1988); tremor occurs in over 50% of such patients and seizures in 5%. About 50% of patients who receive cyclosporine have elevated hepatic transaminase activities or concentrations of bilirubin in plasma; these abnormalities generally disappear if dosage is reduced or the drug is discontinued (Lorber *et al.*, 1987).

Treatment with cyclosporine is associated with an increased incidence of infections, but this problem is generally less prominent than with other immunosuppressant drugs (Kim and Perfect, 1989). There is a relatively low incidence of malignancies in patients who are treated with cyclosporine alone; however, when used in combination with other agents, the drug causes malignant lymphomas with an unusually high incidence of brain metastases (Boitard and Bach, 1989).

Hirsutism and gingival hyperplasia are seen in 10 to 30% of patients who receive cyclosporine, but these reactions rarely affect therapy. Headache, paresthesias, flushing, sinusitis, gynecomastia, conjunctivitis, and tinnitus are observed occasionally. Although the drug is embryotoxic in animals, and its use should be avoided in pregnant women, many successful childbirths have occurred during therapy with regimens that include cyclosporine.

Therapeutic Uses. Cyclosporine is used primarily in combination with prednisone to sustain renal, hepatic, and cardiac transplants (Fowler and Schroeder, 1986; Kahan *et al.,* 1987; O'Grady *et al.,* 1988). The 1-year survival rate of grafts with cadaveric kidneys ranges from 70 to 85%; more than 60% of hepatic grafts currently function for at least 1 year. The 1-year survival rate after cardiac transplantation is higher than 80% in some centers. Success in pancreatic transplantation has improved significantly (Sutherland *et al.,* 1989); experience with the small bowel is limited.

Transplantation of allogeneic bone marrow has become a preferred treatment for many patients with aplastic anemia, acute nonlymphocytic leukemia, and severe combined immunodeficiency syndrome. Cyclosporine is used as an alternative to methotrexate to prevent the evolution of graft-versus-host disease in these patients; some protocols employ both agents (Storb *et al.,* 1989). Clinical trials indicate that cyclosporine may be useful in the treatment of a variety of autoimmune and related disorders, including rheumatoid arthritis (Shand and Richardson, 1988), glomerulonephritis, red cell aplasias (Totterman *et al.,* 1989), uveitis (Nussenblatt *et al.,* 1985), inflammatory bowel disease (Brynskov *et al.,* 1989; Sachar, 1989), and psoriasis (Bos, 1988; Van Joost *et al.,* 1988; von Graffenried, 1989). Rapid and dramatic results are seen in many patients at doses of cyclosporine (3 to 5 mg/kg) that rarely cause serious toxicity. However, disease relapses in a significant proportion of patients when therapy is terminated. Thus, cyclosporine cannot be considered curative, but may be most useful for acute exacerbations of these diseases when they have become refractory to conventional agents. In insulin-dependent diabetes mellitus, the administration of cyclosporine within the first 6 weeks of onset can reverse the condition temporarily, presumably by inhibition of an autoimmune reaction (Feutren *et al.,* 1986; Bach *et al.,* 1988). However, the prospects for long-term therapy are not encouraging.

Preparations and Dosage. *Cyclosporine* (SANDIMMUNE) is available for oral administration as a solution containing 100 mg/ml of vehicle (12.5% ethanol in oil); this solution is mixed with milk or orange juice immediately before administration. The intravenous formulation contains 50 mg of cyclosporine/ml of vehicle (33% ethanol in polyoxyethylated castor oil); it is diluted with 0.9% sodium chloride or 5% dextrose immediately prior to infusion. Oral treatment is initiated 4 to 24 hours prior to transplantation with a dose of 15 mg/kg; this dose (given once daily) is continued for 1 to 2 weeks postoperatively. Thereafter, the dosage is reduced each week until a maintenance dose of 3 to 10 mg/kg per day is reached. Dosage is generally guided by signs of renal toxicity, as judged from changes in creatinine clearance. Care must be taken in patients with renal transplants not to confuse rejection with the renal toxicity of cyclosporine. For this reason, biopsies of grafts are generally performed to provide definitive evidence of potential rejection. The concentration of cyclosporine in the circulation is monitored 24 hours after single oral daily doses. The commonly employed methods measure both intact cyclosporine and a number of its metabolites (Vine and Bowers, 1988; McMillan, 1989); some of these have immunosuppressive activity (Freed *et al.,* 1987). Values of 250 to 800 ng/ml in whole blood or 50 to 300 ng/ml in plasma are generally acceptable. A more accurate estimation of intact cyclosporine can be achieved by methods that employ monoclonal antibodies (Quesniaux *et al.,* 1987) or high-performance liquid chromatography (HPLC). With HPLC, concentrations of intact cyclosporine in whole blood of 100 to 150 ng/ml are considered to be in the therapeutic range.

In patients who are unable to tolerate cyclosporine orally, the diluted intravenous formulation is infused slowly over a period of 2 to 6 hours or longer. The daily dose (usually 5 to 6 mg/kg) should be only one-third the oral dose. Because frequent reactions occur to the vehicle in the intravenous formulation of cyclosporine, intravenous administration should be discontinued as soon as the patient is able to tolerate oral medication. Some patients who are to receive liver transplants have compromised renal function from the hepatorenal syndrome. Immunosuppressive treatment of such patients may be started with azathioprine and prednisone and changed to a combination of cyclosporine and prednisone after renal function has improved (usually 1 week).

CYTOTOXIC AGENTS

AZATHIOPRINE

Many cancer chemotherapeutic agents cause bone marrow toxicity and consequent immunosuppression. This prompted attempts to use some of these agents for the prevention of allograft rejection. Azathioprine (combined with prednisone) has been the mainstay of attempts to suppress rejection of transplanted organs for 2 decades and has made renal transplantation an acceptable procedure (Elion and Hitchings, 1975).

In the body, nucleophiles such as glutathione cleave the prodrug azathioprine to mercaptopurine; this purine analog is subsequently converted into mercaptopurine-containing nucleotides that exert effects on the synthesis and utilization of precursors of RNA and DNA (*see* Chapter 52). Although experiments *in vitro* indicate that the immunosuppressive potency of azathioprine is greater than that of mercaptopurine, results *in vivo* are less clear (Wolberg, 1988). As compared with mercaptopurine, the apparently more favorable therapeutic effect of azathioprine may reflect differences in pharmacokinetic properties and local conversion of azathioprine to mercaptopurine at sites that are more conducive to specific effects on the immune system.

Concomitant administration of allopurinol and azathioprine engenders the hazard of overdosage with azathioprine because oxidation of mercaptopurine to inactive metabolites by xanthine oxidase is greatly reduced by allopurinol (*see* Chapter 26). Reduction of the normal dosage of azathioprine by 65 to 75% is recommended for patients who are also receiving allopurinol.

A regimen of azathioprine combined with both cyclosporine and prednisone is employed for suppression of organ rejection in some centers. Because of evidence that this regimen causes a high incidence of malignancies and infectious complications, physicians in other centers reserve this combination of drugs for patients who do not respond adequately to cyclosporine and prednisone (Salaman and Griffin, 1985). Azathioprine has also been approved for the treatment of severe refractory rheumatoid arthritis in nonpregnant adults (Hunter *et al.*, 1975).

Hematological toxicity manifested as leukopenia and thrombocytopenia must be monitored carefully to guide dosage of azathioprine. Nausea and vomiting are common, but generally do not limit treatment. Although hepatic toxicity is rare, a severe hepatic veno-occlusive disease has been seen in some patients with transplants.

Preparations and Dosage. *Azathioprine* (IMURAN) is supplied for oral administration in 50-mg tablets and in vials that contain the equivalent of 100 mg as the Na^+ salt for intravenous injection. Prophylactic therapy is usually initiated with daily doses of 3 to 10 mg/kg, 1 or 2 days prior to renal transplantation or on the day of the operation; the usual daily maintenance dose is 1 to 3 mg/kg. Treatment of rheumatoid arthritis is initiated at daily doses of 1 mg/kg, given in one or two portions. After 6 to 9 weeks, the daily dose is escalated slowly to a maximum of 2.5 mg/kg.

METHOTREXATE

In addition to its use as an antineoplastic agent (*see* Chapter 52), methotrexate is employed alone or in combination with cyclosporine for prophylaxis of graft-versus-host disease in bone marrow transplantation. It is also useful in selected forms of autoimmune and inflammatory disease. Methotrexate is a potent inhibitor of dihydrofolate reductase, with consequent effects on folate-requiring reactions in the biosynthesis of thymidylate and purines. The immunosuppressive activity of methotrexate presumably reflects inhibition of the replication and function of T cells and possibly B cells because of a relatively selective action on DNA synthesis. In leukemic patients who receive bone marrow transplants, there is some evidence that recurrence of disease is reduced in those given methotrexate as compared with those treated with cyclosporine, presumably because of the intrinsic antileukemic effect of methotrexate (*see* International Bone Marrow Transplant Registry, 1989).

Methotrexate has recently been approved for the treatment of severe, active rheumatoid arthritis in adults (Tugwell *et al.*, 1987; Weinblatt and Kremer, 1988) and of psoriasis that is refractory to other therapy (Roenigk *et al.*, 1988). For rheumatoid arthritis, the usual dose of methotrexate is 7.5 mg given once a week; this amount can be taken in three divided portions at 12-hour intervals. The dose may be increased slowly to a maximum of 20 mg per week. Similar dosage schedules are used to treat psoriasis (*see* Chapters 52 and 65).

The toxicities that result from the long-term administration of low doses of methotrexate are distinct from those associated with its use as an antineoplastic agent. Hepatic fibrosis and cirrhosis have been reported in as many as 30 to 40% of patients with psoriasis who were treated with the drug (Roenigk *et al.,* 1988); however, a lower incidence was found in a group of 210 patients with rheumatoid arthritis (Shergy *et al.*, 1988). In both diseases there was evidence of progressive dose-related hepatic changes during extended periods of treatment with methotrexate; these were correlated with ingestion of ethanol. Both acute and chronic nonseptic pneumonitis also occur in patients with rheumatoid arthritis. This toxic manifestation is generally reversible, but the mechanism and risk factors associated with this complication are not known. Patients with psoriasis have a much lower incidence of pulmonary toxicity.

CYCLOPHOSPHAMIDE

Details of the activation, mechanism of action, and antineoplastic activity of cyclophosphamide are presented in Chapter 52. Cyclophosphamide is activated by a cytochrome P_{450}–catalyzed reaction in the liver and other tissues to form alkylating species that interact with DNA. Cyclophosphamide is the primary agent used to ablate lymphoid elements in patients who are to receive bone marrow transplants. Very large single doses are employed, as compared with those used conventionally in cancer chemotherapy; toxic effects, especially chemical cystitis and cardiomyopathy, must be monitored carefully.

ANTIBODIES

Several preparations of antibodies have been approved as immunosuppressive agents. Some of these antibodies interact with lymphoid cells, leading either to blockade of their function (OKT3) or to their destruction (antithymocyte globulin). Most currently available preparations are from nonhuman sources and, hence, incur the potential for the development of anti-idiotypic antibodies, even in an immunosuppressed host. Nevertheless, their ability to lower the number and suppress the function of selected types of normal lymphoid cells has provided an important means to treat acute episodes of rejection in recipients of transplanted organs, as well as to prevent (and treat) graft-versus-host reactions in recipients of bone marrow transplants (*see* Seaman and Wofsy, 1988).

LYMPHOCYTE IMMUNE GLOBULIN

Several preparations of antithymocyte or antilymphocyte sera have been employed on an experimental basis. The preparation currently marketed (prepared in horses) can sharply lower the number of thymus-derived lymphocytes and inhibit normal responses of T cells. Since patients who receive this agent are also being treated with other immunosuppressive agents, allergic reactions to the equine protein are not as frequent or severe as would be expected. The half-life of the preparation ranges from 3 to 9 days in patients who are receiving other immunosuppressants. Chills and fever, leukopenia, thrombocytopenia, and skin reactions are seen in about 5% of patients. Anaphylaxis is a potentially serious reaction, although it occurs in only 1% of patients. The primary use of these preparations (in conjunction with other immunosuppressive agents) has been in acute graft rejection; they are also used for the treatment of severe aplastic anemia.

Preparation and Dosage. *Lymphocyte immune globulin* (antithymocyte globulin, equine; ATGAM) is available as a solution (50 mg/ml) for intravenous injection. The usual daily dose for adults is 10 to 30 mg/kg infused in saline through an in-line filter over a period of 4 or more hours. A central or other large vein is used to minimize the incidence of phlebitis.

ANTIBODIES AGAINST THE CD3 COMPLEX

Monoclonal antibodies provide a selective approach to immunosuppression; they also permit the administration of a homogeneous protein rather than a crude fraction of serum (Kung *et al.*, 1979). The primary focus has been on the receptor site for antigens on T cells and on a 20,000-dalton glycoprotein in the CD3 complex (*see* above). The commercially available preparation is a murine immunoglobulin (IgG_{2a}) termed OKT3. When complexed with its antigen (CD3), this monoclonal antibody blocks the function of all T cells that bear this receptor, presumably by preventing the initiation of signal transduction that is essential for cellular activation. When administered to patients, OKT3 causes a rapid decrease in the expression of the CD3 antigen on peripheral lymphocytes (Chatenoud *et al.*, 1982), but changes in the expression of CD3 are not apparent in lymphocytes within the graft.

Monoclonal antibody to CD3 is indicated as an adjuvant to other immunosuppressants in patients who are experiencing acute rejection of a renal allograft (Ortho Multicenter Group Transplant Study, 1985) or in prophylactic regimens (Filipovich *et al.*, 1985). When this antibody is used, the dosage of glucocorticoids and azathioprine should be reduced, and treatment with cyclosporine should probably be stopped. A large fraction of patients experience chills, fever, and other adverse effects, including dyspnea, chest pain, wheezing, gastrointestinal disturbances, and tremor. Potentially fatal pulmonary edema occurs in about 1% of patients after the first dose, and a reversible central nervous system syndrome that is characterized by fever, headache, photophobia, and neck stiffness is common; seizures occur rarely. These signs and symptoms may be caused by the release from the affected T cells of several lymphokines that are known to elicit similar reactions. Infections occur at a rate comparable to that seen during treatment with full doses of glucocorticoids. Lymphoproliferative syndromes or lymphomas have also occurred.

Preparation and Dosage. *Muromonab-CD3* (ORTHOCLONE OKT3) is available as a solution (1 mg/ml); the solution is filtered before use and is injected intravenously as a bolus. The total daily dose is 5 mg, and treatment is continued for 10 to 14 days. In order to minimize acute reactions, the first dose should be preceded by the intravenous administration of methylprednisolone (1 mg/kg), followed by 100 mg of hydrocortisone 30 minutes later. Patients are monitored at intervals for the appearance of anti-idiotypic antibodies in the event that additional courses of therapy are necessary.

RH_o(D) IMMUNE GLOBULIN

A highly specific form of immunological therapy is employed in Rh_o(D)-negative mothers whose immune system is exposed to Rh_o(D)-positive blood as a result of fetomaternal hemorrhage during abortions, amniocentesis, abdominal trauma, or even full-term deliveries. Administration of concentrated human antibodies against this erythrocyte antigen to the mother blocks the immune response, thus eliminating the risk of hemolytic disease in infants during subsequent pregnancies (Bowman, 1985; Thornton *et al.*, 1989). Large amounts of Rh_o(D) immune globulin can also be given to patients after accidental transfusion with mismatched blood. Several preparations of concentrated human IgG antibodies directed against the Rh_o(D) antigen on red cells are available for intramuscular administration at the time of a prenatal incident or prophylactically postpartum. These preparations should *not* be used in the infant, in mothers who have been sensitized previously, or in Rh_o(D)-positive patients. Minor reactions at the site of injection and mild fever have been observed.

Preparations and Dosage. *Rh_o(D) immune globulin* (RHOGAM, GAMULIN RH, others) is available for intramuscular injection in vials or syringes, each of which is capable of neutralizing approximately 15 ml of packed Rh_o(D)-positive erythrocytes. Larger doses are used in proportion to the amount of mismatched blood transfused or the estimated degree of fetal–maternal hemorrhage. Rh_o(D) immune globulin is best administered within 72 hours of delivery; postpartum treatment may be omitted if delivery occurs within 3 weeks of the last dose, unless the fetal–maternal hemorrhage is greater than the equivalent of 15 ml of packed erythrocytes.

Rh_o(D) immune globulin is also available in reduced dosage preparations (MICRHOGAM, MINI-GAMULIN RH, others). Each vial or syringe is capable of neutralizing 2.5 ml of packed Rh_o(D)-positive red cells. This preparation is used prophylactically in Rh_o(D)-negative women after termination of pregnancies up to and including 12 weeks' gestation unless either the father or fetus is Rh_o(D) negative. The full-strength preparation is employed at or beyond 13 weeks of gestation.

OTHER IMMUNOSUPPRESSIVE AGENTS

Adrenocorticosteroids. The lympholytic and antiinflammatory actions of adrenocorticosteroids are frequently used to advantage in immunosuppressive regimens (*see* Chapter 50). As a prophylactic measure to prevent rejection, prednisone is given for about 4 days in doses of 0.5 to 2.0 mg/kg; the dose is then tapered for maintenance to 5 to 10 mg per day. These doses can be reduced somewhat when cyclosporine is administered concomitantly. During episodes of acute organ rejection, 500 to 1500 mg of methylprednisolone is given intravenously for several days; lower doses are used for acute graft-versus-host disease after bone marrow transplantation. Glucocorticoids are commonly given intravenously before and after administration of lymphocyte immune globulin or monoclonal antibodies to minimize the incidence of reactions to these preparations. Because of the high dosage of glucocorticoids required for immunosuppression, major side effects are common; these include cushingoid reactions, psychoses, glucose intolerance, infections, hypertension, cataracts, skin fragility, bone dissolution, and impaired growth in children.

Sulfasalazine. Sulfasalazine was originally designed as a combination of an antimicrobial sulfonamide (sulfapyridine) and an antiinflammatory salicylate (5-aminosalicylic acid; mesalamine) for the treatment of ulcerative colitis and other inflammatory bowel diseases. Its usefulness in the treatment of rheumatoid arthritis has been investigated more recently (Pinals, 1988; Pullar, 1989). Although the therapeutic effects of sulfasalazine in ulcerative colitis have been attributed to the liberation of mesalamine in the colon, it would appear that sulfapyridine is responsible for its beneficial effects in rheumatoid arthritis. The mechanism of its therapeutic action has not been established, but there is evidence for suppression of the activity of natural killer cells (Gibson and Jewell, 1985) and impairment of lymphocyte transformation (Sheldon *et al.*, 1987).

FK-506. FK-506 is a newly described macrocyclic lactone–lactam antibiotic with immunosuppressive properties that are similar to those of cyclosporine (Starzl *et al.*, 1987; Tocci *et al.*, 1989; Todo *et al.*, 1989). It is between 50 and 100 times more potent than cyclosporine *in vitro*. FK-506 binds to a small protein with peptidyl proline isomerase activity that closely resembles cyclophilin; however, the specificity of binding is very different (Harding *et al.*, 1989; Siekierka *et al.*, 1989). Preliminary results from clinical studies are very encouraging and suggest that its therapeutic usefulness may be similar to that of cyclosporine, but with less toxicity. It must be appreciated, however, that the spectrum of problems engendered by immunosuppression with FK-506 is likely to be similar to that with cyclosporine. FK-506 has caused serious vasculitis and renal damage in some animal species.

Methoxsalen. A novel treatment method termed *extracorporeal photophoresis* causes beneficial effects in the majority of patients with the erythrodermic form of cutaneous T-cell lymphoma when disease is resistant to conventional therapy (Edelson *et al.*, 1987). Methoxsalen is given orally 2 hours before the removal of whole blood, which is then irradiated with ultraviolet light after it has been diluted in an appropriate medium. The irradiated cells, including the target T cells, are returned to the patient, and the process is repeated the next day. These 2-day courses are repeated at 4- to 8-week intervals. It has been postulated that photosensitization of the malignant T cells occurs and that this facilitates a further immune reaction against the neoplastic population of cells in the body. This approach is being extended to autoimmune and related diseases based on preliminary results in experimental systems (Perez *et al.*, 1989).

Thalidomide. Thalidomide is being investigated as an immunosuppressant for use in bone marrow transplantation. Despite its teratogenic properties, this sedative was shown to have immunosuppressive properties in experimental systems, as well as antiinflammatory activity in lepromatous leprosy (Barnhill and McDougall, 1982). Clinical trials are in progress (Vogelsang *et al.*, 1988).

Aoyama, T.; Yamano, S.; Waxman, D. J.; Lapenson, D. P.; Meyer, W. A.; Fischer, V.; Tyndale, R.; Inaba, T.; Kalow, W.; and Golboin, H. V. Cytochrome P-450 hPCN3, a novel cytochrome P-450 IIIA gene product that is differentially expressed in adult human liver. cDNA and deduced amino acid sequence and distinct specificities of cDNA-expressed hPCN1 and hPCN3 for the metabolism of steroid hormones and cyclosporine. *J. Biol. Chem.*, **1989**, *264*, 10388–10395.

Brynskov, J., and others. A placebo-controlled, double-blind, randomized trial of cyclosporine therapy in active chronic Crohn's disease. *N. Engl. J. Med.*, **1989**, *321*, 845–850.

Bueding, E.; Hawkins, J.; and Cha, Y. N. Antischistosomal effects of cyclosporin A. *Agents Actions*, **1981**, *11*, 380–383.

Burckart, G. J., and others. Excretion of cyclosporine and its metabolites in human bile. *Transplant. Proc.*, **1986**, *18*, Suppl. 5, 46–49.

Chatenoud, L.; Baudrihaye, M. F.; Kreis, H.; Goldstein, G.; Schindler, J.; and Bach, J. F. Human *in vivo* antigenic modulation induced by the anti-t-cell OKT3 monoclonal antibody. *Eur. J. Immunol.*, **1982**, *12*, 979–982.

Colombani, P. M.; Robb, A.; and Hess, A. D. Cyclosporin A binding to calmodulin: a possible site of action on T-lymphocytes. *Science*, **1985**, *228*, 337–339.

Edelson, R., and others. Treatment of cutaneous T-cell lymphoma by extracorporeal photochemotherapy. *N. Engl. J. Med.*, **1987**, *316*, 297–303.

Elliot, J. F.; Lin, Y.; Mizel, S. B.; Bleackley, R. C.; Harnish, D. G.; and Paettian, V. Induction of interleukin 2 messenger RNA inhibited by cyclosporin A. *Science*, **1984**, *226*, 1439–1441.

Feutren, G., and others. Cyclosporin increases the rate and length of remissions in insulin-dependent diabetes of recent onset. Results of a multicentre double-blind trial. *Lancet*, **1986**, *2*, 119–124.

Filipovich, A. H.; Krawczak, C. L.; Kersey, J. H.; McGlave, P.; Ramsay, N. K. C.; Goldman, A.; and Goldstein, G. Graft-vs-host disease prophylaxis with anti-T-cell monoclonal antibody OKT3, prednisone and methotrexate in allogeneic bone-marrow transplantation. *Br. J. Haematol.*, **1985**, *60*, 143–152.

Fischer, G.; Wittmann-Liebold, B.; Lang, K.; Kiefhaber, T.; and Schmid, F. X. Cyclophilin and peptydyl-prolyl cis-trans isomerase are probably identical proteins. *Nature*, **1989**, *337*, 476–478.

Fowler, M. B., and Schroeder, J. S. Current status of cardiac transplantation. *Mod. Concepts Cardiovasc. Dis.*, **1986**, *55*, 37–41.

Foxwell, B. M. J.; Frazer, G.; Winters, M.; Hiestand, P.; Wenger, R.; and Ryffel, B. Identification of cyclophilin as the erythrocyte ciclosporin-binding protein. *Biochim. Biophys. Acta*, **1988a**, *938*, 447–455.

Foxwell, B. M. J.; Hiestand, P. D.; Wenger, R. M.; and Ryffel, B. A comparison of cyclosporine-binding by cyclophilin and calmodulin and the identification of a novel 45 Kd binding phosphoprotein. *Transplantation*, **1988b**, *46*, Suppl. 2, 35–40.

Freed, B. M.; Rosano, T. G.; and Lempert, N. *In vitro* immunosuppressive properties of cyclosporine metabolites. *Transplantation*, **1987**, *43*, 123–127.

Gelfand, E. W.; Cheung, R.; and Mills, G. B. The cyclosporins inhibit lymphocyte activation at more than one site. *J. Immunol.*, **1987**, *138*, 1115–1120.

Gibson, P. R., and Jewell, D. P. Sulphasalazine and derivatives, natural killer activity and rheumatoid arthritis. *Clin. Sci.*, **1985**, *69*, 177–184.

Gschwendt, M.; Kittstein, W.; and Marks, F. Cyclosporin A inhibits phorbol ester-induced cellular proliferation and tumor promotion as well as phosphorylation of a 100-kd protein in mouse epidermis. *Carcinogenesis*, **1987**, *8*, 203–207.

Hait, W. M.; Stein, J. M.; Koletsky, A. J.; Harding, M. W.; and Handschumacher, R. E. Activity of cyclosporin A and a non-immunosuppressive cyclosporin against multidrug resistant leukemic cell lines. *Cancer Commun.*, **1989**, *1*, 35–43.

Handschumacher, R. E.; Harding, M. W.; Rice, J.; Drugge, R. J.; and Speicher, D. W. Cyclophilin: a specific cytosolic binding protein for cyclosporin A. *Science*, **1984**, *226*, 544–547.

Harding, M. W.; Galat, A.; Uehling, D. E.; and Schreiber, S. L. Fujiphilin: the receptor for the immunosuppressant FK-506 is a cis-trans peptidyl-prolyl isomerase (rotamase). *Nature*, **1989**, *341*, 758–760.

Harding, M. W.; Handschumacher, R. E.; and Speicher, D. W. Isolation and amino acid sequence of cyclophilin. *J. Biol. Chem.*, **1986**, *261*, 8547–8555.

Herold, K. C.; Lancki, D. W.; Moldwin, R. L.; and Fitch, F. W. Immunosuppressive effects of cyclosporin A on cloned T Cells. *J. Immunol.*, **1986**, *136*, 1315–1321.

Hess, A. D., and Tutschka, P. J. Effect of cyclosporine A on human lymphocyte responses *in vitro*. I. CsA allows for the expression of alloantigen activated suppressor cells which preferentially inhibit the induction of cytolytic-effector lymphocytes in MLR. *J. Immunol.*, **1980**, *124*, 2601–2608.

Hunter, T.; Urowitz, M. B.; Gordon, D. A.; Smythe, H. A.; and Ogryzlo, M. A. Azathioprine in rheumatoid arthritis. A long-term follow-up study. *Arthritis Rheum.*, **1975**, *18*, 15–20.

International Bone Marrow Transplant Registry. Effect of methotrexate on relapse after bone-marrow transplantation for acute lymphoblastic leukaemia. *Lancet*, **1989**, *1*, 535–537.

Kahan, B. D.; Mickey, R.; Flechner, S. M.; Lorber, M. I.; Wideman, C. A.; Kerman, R. H.; Tersaki, P.; and Van Buren, C. T. Multivariate analysis of risk factors impacting on immediate and eventual cadaver allograft survival in cyclosporine-treated recipients. *Transplantation*, **1987**, *43*, 65–70.

Kahan, B. D., and Grevel, J. Optimization of cyclosporine therapy in renal transplantation by a pharmacokinetic strategy. *Transplantation*, **1988**, *46*, 631–644.

Kay, J. E., and Benzie, C. R. Rapid loss of sensitivity of mitogen-induced lymphocyte activation to inhibition by cyclosporin A. *Cell. Immunol.*, **1984**, *87*, 217–224.

Koletsky, A. J.; Harding, M. W.; and Handschumacher, R. E. Cyclophilin: distribution and variant properties in normal and neoplastic tissues. *J. Immunol.*, **1986**, *137*, 1054–1059.

Kronke, M.; Leonard, W. J.; Depper, J. M.; Arya, S. K.; Wong-Staal, F.; Waldmann, T. A.; and Green, W. C. Cyclosporin A inhibits T cell growth factor gene expression at the level of mRNA transcription. *Proc. Natl. Acad. Sci. U.S.A.*, **1984**, *81*, 5214–5218

Kung, P. C.; Goldstein, G.; Reinherz, E. L.; and Schlossman, S. F. Monoclonal antibodies defining distinctive human T cell surface antigens. *Science*, **1979**, *206*, 347–349.

LeGrue, S. J.; Turner, R.; Weisbrodt, N.; and Dedman, J. R. Does the binding of cyclosporine to calmodulin result in immunosuppression? *Science*, **1986**, *234*, 68–71.

Lorber, M. I.; Van Buren, C. T.; Flechner, S. M.; Williams, C.; and Kahan, B. D. Hepatobiliary and pancreatic complications of cyclosporine therapy in 466 renal transplant recipients. *Transplantation*, **1987**, *43*, 35–40.

Maurer, G. Metabolism of cyclosporine. *Transplant. Proc.*, **1985**, *17*, Suppl. 5, 19–26.

Maurer, G., and LeMaire, M. Biotransformation and distribution in blood of cyclosporine and its metabolites. *Transplant. Proc.*, **1986**, *18*, Suppl. 5, 25–34.

Metcalf, S. Cyclosporine does not prevent cytoplasmic calcium changes associated with lymphocyte activation. *Transplantation*, **1984**, *38*, 161–164.

Nickell, S. P.; Scheibel, L. W.; and Cole, G. A. Inhibition by cyclosporin A of rodent malaria *in vivo* and human malaria *in vitro*. *Infect. Immun.*, **1982**, *37*, 1093–1100.

Nussenblatt, R. B.; Palestine, A. G.; and Chan, C. C. Cyclosporine therapy for uveitis: long-term follow-up. *J. Ocul. Pharmacol.*, **1985**, *1*, 369–382.

O'Grady, J. G.; Forbes, A.; Rolles, K.; Calne, R. Y.; and Williams, R. An analysis of cyclosporine efficacy and toxicity after liver transplantation. *Transplantation*. **1988**, *45*, 575–579.

Ortho Multicenter Transplant Study Group. A randomized clinical trial of OKT3 monoclonal antibody for acute rejection of cadaveric renal transplants. *N. Engl. J. Med.*, **1985**, *313*, 337–342.

Perez, M.; Edelson, R.; Laroche, L.; and Berger, C. Inhibition of anti-skin allograft immunity by infusions with syngeneic photoinactivated effector lymphocytes. *J. Invest. Dermatol.*, **1989**, *92*, 669–676.

Quesniaux, V. F.; Schreier, M. H.; Wenger, R. M.; Hiestand, P. C.; Harding, M. W.; and Van Regenmortel, M. H. V. Molecular characteristics of cyclophilin-cyclosporine interaction. *Transplantation*, **1988**, *46*, Suppl., S23–S27.

Quesniaux, V.; Tees, R.; Schreier, M. H.; Maurer, G.; and Van Regenmortel, M. H. V. Potential of monoclonal antibodies to improve therapeutic monitoring of cyclosporine. *Clin. Chem.*, **1987**, *33*, 32–37.

Russell, D.; Kibler, R.; Matrisian, L.; Larson, D.; Poulos, B.; and Magun, B. Prolactin receptors on human T and B lymphocytes: antagonism of prolactin binding by cyclosporine. *J. Immunol.*, **1985**, *134*, 3027–3031.

Salaman, J. R., and Griffin, P. J. A. Immunosuppression with a combination of cyclosporin, azathioprine, and prednisolone may be unsafe. *Lancet*, **1985**, *2*, 1066–1067.

Shand, N., and Richardson, B. Sandimmun (cyclosporin A): mode of action and clinical results in rheumatoid arthritis. *Scand. J. Rheumatol.* [*Suppl.*], **1988**, *76*, 265–278.

Sheldon, P. J.; Webb, C.; and Grindulis, K. A. Sulphasalazine in rheumatoid arthritis: pointers to a gut mediated immune effect. *Br. J. Rheumatol.*, **1987**, *26*, 318–319.

Shergy, W. J.; Polisson, R. P.; Caldwell, D. S.; Rice, J. R.; Piestesky, D. S.; and Allen, N. B. Methotrexate-associated hepatotoxicity: retrospective analysis of 210 patients with rheumatoid arthritis. *Am. J. Med.*, **1988**, *85*, 771–774.

Siekierka, J. J.; Hung, S. H. Y.; Poe, M.; Lin, C. S.; and Sigal, N. H. A cytosolic binding protein for the immunosuppressant FK506 has peptidyl-prolyl isomerase activity but is distinct from cyclophilin. *Nature*, **1989**, *341*, 755–757.

Slater, L. M.; Sweet, P.; Stupecky, M.; and Gupta, S. Cyclosporin A reverses vincristine and daunorubicin resistance in acute lymphatic leukemia *in vitro*. *J. Clin. Invest.*, **1986**, *77*, 1405–1408.

Storb, R., and others. Graft-versus-host disease prevention by methotrexate combined with cyclosporin compared to methotrexate alone in patients given marrow grafts for severe aplastic anaemia: long-term follow-up of a controlled trial. *Br. J. Haematol.*, **1989**, *72*, 567–572.

Sutherland, D. E. R.; Moudry, K. C.; and Fryd, D. S. Results of pancreas-transplant registry. *Diabetes*, **1989**, *38*, 46–54.

Takahashi, N.; Hayano, T.; and Masanori, S. Peptidyl-prolyl cis-trans isomerase is the cyclosporin A-binding protein cyclophilin. *Nature*, **1989**, *337*, 473–475.

Tocci, M. J.; Matkovich, D. A.; Collier, K. A.; Kwok, P.; Dumont, F.; Lin, S.; Degudicibus, S.; Siekierka, J. J.; Chin, J.; and Hutchinson, N. I. The immunosuppressant FK506 selectively inhibits expression of early T cell activation genes. *J. Immunol.*, **1989**, *143*, 718–726.

Todo, S.; Demetris, A.; Ueda, Y.; Mventarza, O.; Cadoff, E.; Zeevi, A.; and Starzl, T. E. Renal transplantation in baboons under FK 506. *Surgery*, **1989**, *106*, 444–451.

Totterman, T. H.; Hoglund, M.; Bengtsson, M.; Simonsson, B.; Almqvist, D.; and Killander, A. Treatment of pure red-cell aplasia and aplastic anaemia with ciclosporin: long-term clinical effects. *Eur. J. Haematol.*, **1989**, *42*, 126–133.

Tugwell, P.; Bennett, K.; and Gent, M. Methotrexate in rheumatoid arthritis. *Ann. Intern. Med.*, **1987**, *107*, 358–366.

Van Joost, T.; Bos, J. D.; Heule, F.; and Meinardi, M. M. Low-dose cyclosporin A in severe psoriasis: a double-blind study. *Br. J. Dermatol.*, **1988**, *118*, 183–190.

Monographs and Reviews

Bach, J. F. The risk/benefit ratio in immunointervention for autoimmune diseases. In, *Immunointervention in Autoimmune Diseases*. (Bach, J. F., ed.) Academic Press Ltd., London, **1989a**, pp. 215–224.

——— (ed.). *Immunointervention in Autoimmune Diseases*. Academic Press Ltd., London, **1989b**.

Bach, J. F.; Feutren, G.; and Boitard, C. The prospects of immunosuppression in Type I diabetes. *Adv. Neurol.*, **1988**, *17*, 321–340.

Barnhill, R. L., and McDougall, A. C. Thalidomide: use and possible mode of action in reactional lepromatous leprosy and in various other conditions. *J. Am. Acad. Dermatol.*, **1982**, *7*, 317–323.

Bennett, W. M., and Norman, D. J. Action and toxicity of cyclosporine. *Annu. Rev. Med.*, **1986**, *37*, 215–224.

Bennett, W. M., and Porter, G. A. Cyclosporine-associated hypertension. *Am. J. Med.*, **1988**, *85*, 131–138.

Boitard, C., and Bach, J. F. Long-term complications of conventional immunosuppressive treatment. *Adv. Nephrol.*, **1989**, *18*, 335–354.

Borel, J. F. Cyclosporine: historical perspectives. *Transplant. Proc.*, **1983**, *15*, 3–13.

Borel, J. F.; Feurer, C.; Gubler, H. U.; and Stahelin, H. Biological effect of cyclosporin A: a new antilymphocytic agent. *Agents Actions*, **1976**, *6*, 468–475.

Bos, J. D. The pathomechanisms of psoriasis: the skin immune system and cyclosporin. *Br. J. Dermatol.*, **1988**, *118*, 141–155.

Bowman, J. M. Who needs Rh immune globulin and when should it be given? *Am. J. Obstet. Gynecol.*, **1985**, *151*, 289–294.

Drugge, R. J., and Handschumacher, R. E. Cyclosporine—mechanism of action. *Transplant. Proc.*, **1988**, *20*, 301–309.

Elion, G. B., and Hitchings, G. H. Azathioprine. In, *Antineoplastic and Immunosuppressive Agents*. (Sartorelli, A. C., and Johns, D. G., eds.) *Handbuch der Experimentellen Pharmakologie*, Vol. 38. Springer-Verlag, Berlin, **1975**, pp. 403–425.

Gottlieb, A. B. Immunologic mechanisms in psoriasis. *J. Am. Acad. Dermatol.*, **1988**, *18*, 1376–1380.

Hamblin, A. S. Lymphokines. JRL Press, Oxford, **1988**.

Kahan B. D., and Bach, J. F. (eds.). Proceedings of the Second International Congress on Cyclosporine. *Transplant. Proc.*, **1988**, *20*, Suppl. 3, 1–1131.

Kim, J. H., and Perfect, J. R. Infection and cyclosporine. *Rev. Infect. Dis.*, **1989**, *2*, 677–690.

Larson, D. F. Cyclosporin—mechanism of action: antagonism of the prolactin receptor. *Prog. Allergy*, **1986**, *38*, 222–238.

McMillan, M. A. Clinical pharmacokinetics of cyclosporin. *Pharmacol. Ther.*, **1989**, *42*, 135–156.

Metzger, J. T., and Hoffman, L. A. Cardiac transplantation: the changing faces of immunosuppression. *Heart Lung*, **1988**, *17*, 414–425.

Mihatsch, M. J.; Thiel, G.; and Ryffel, B. Cyclosporine nephrotoxicity. *Adv. Nephrol.*, **1988**, *17*, 303–320.

Mizel, S. G. The interleukins. *FASEB J.*, **1989**, *3*, 2379–2388.

O'Garra, A.; Umland, S.; De France, T.; and Christiansen, J. β-Cell factors are pleiotropic. *Immunol. Today*, **1988**, *2*, 46–54.

Paul, W. E. *Fundamental Immunology*, 2nd ed. Raven Press, New York, **1989**.

Penn, I. Cancer is a complication of severe immunosuppression. *Surg. Gynecol. Obstet.*, **1986**, *162*, 603–610.

Perlmutter, R. M. T cell signaling. *Science*, **1989**, *245*, 344.

Pinals, R. S. Sulfasalazine in the rheumatic disease. *Semin. Arthritis Rheum.*, **1988**, *17*, 246–259.

Pullar, T. Sulphasalazine and related drugs in rheumatoid arthritis. *Pharmacol. Ther.*, **1989**, *42*, 459–468.

Racusen, L. C., and Solez, K. Cyclosporine nephrotoxicity. *Int. Rev. Exp. Pathol.*, **1988**, *30*, 107–157.

Roenigk, H. H., Jr.; Auerbach, R.; Maibach, H. I.; and Weinstein, G. D. Methotrexate in psoriasis: revised guidelines. *J. Am. Acad. Dermatol.*, **1988**, *19*, 145–156.

Sachar, D. B. Cyclosporine treatment for inflammatory bowel disease. *N. Engl. J. Med.*, **1989**, *321*, 894–896.

Seaman, W. E., and Wofsy, D. Selective manipulation of the immune response *in vivo* by monoclonal antibodies. *Ann. Rev. Med.*, **1988**, *39*, 231–241.

Shevach, E. M. The effects of cyclosporine A on the immune system. *Annu. Rev. Immunol.*, **1985**, *3*, 397–423.

Starzl, T. E.; Makowka, L.; and Todo, S. FK506: a potential breakthrough in immunosuppression. *Transplant. Proc.*, **1987**, *19*, 3–104.

Thornton, J. G.; Page, C.; Foote, G.; Arthur, G. R.; Tovey, L. A. D.; and Scott, J. S. Efficacy and long term effects of antenatal prophylaxis with anti-D immunoglobulin. *Br. Med. J.* [*Clin. Res.*], **1989**, *298*, 1671–1673.

Twentyman, P. R. A possible role for cyclosporins in cancer chemotherapy. *Anticancer Res.*, **1988**, *8*, 985–994.

Vine, W., and Bowers, L. D. Cyclosporine: structure, pharmacokinetics, and therapeutic drug monitoring. *CRC Crit. Rev. Clin. Lab. Sci.*, **1988**, *25*, 275–311.

Vogelsang, G. B.; Hess, A. D.; and Santos, G. W. Thalidomide for therapy of graft-versus-host disease. *Bone Marrow Transplant.*, **1988**, *3*, 393–398.

von Graffenried, B. Sandimmun (ciclosporin) in autoimmune diseases. *Am. J. Nephrol.*, **1989**, *9*, 51–56.

Walker, R. W., and Brochstein, J. A. Neurologic complications of immunosuppressive agents. *Neurol. Clin.*, **1988**, *6*, 261–278.

Weinblatt, M. E., and Kremer, J. M. Methotrexate in rheumatoid arthritis. *J. Am. Acad. Dermatol.*, **1988**, *19*, 126–128.

Wenger, R. M. Synthesis of ciclosporin and analogues: structural and conformational requirements for immunosuppressive activity. *Prog. Allergy*, **1986**, *38*, 46–64.

Wolberg, G. Antipurines and purine metabolism. In, *The Pharmacology of Lymphocytes*. (Bray, M. A., and Morley, J., eds.) *Handbook of Experimental Pharmacology*, Vol. 85. Springer-Verlag, Berlin, **1988**, pp. 517–533.

SECTION

XIV Drugs Acting on the Blood and the Blood-Forming Organs

A number of drugs, including hormonal growth factors, vitamins, and minerals, affect the blood and the blood-forming organs, either directly or indirectly. The first to be discussed in this section are the growth factors that control the proliferation and differentiation of hematopoietic stem cells. Their uses as therapeutic agents are under active investigation. Agents effective in specific anemias include iron, copper, vitamin B_{12}, folic acid, pyridoxine, and riboflavin; these substances are also described in the following chapter. In the second chapter of this section, attention is devoted chiefly to heparin and the oral anticoagulants, thrombolytic agents, and drugs that affect platelet function.

CHAPTER

54 HEMATOPOIETIC AGENTS: GROWTH FACTORS, MINERALS, AND VITAMINS

Robert S. Hillman

I. Hematopoietic Growth Factors

The relatively short lifespan of mature blood cells requires their continuous replacement, a process termed *hematopoiesis*. Furthermore, new cell production must be responsive to both basal needs and situations of increased demand. For example, the rate of red cell production, erythropoiesis, can vary over more than a fivefold range with increasingly severe anemia or hypoxia. The regulation of hematopoiesis is complex and involves cell–cell interactions within the microenvironment of the bone marrow, as well as both hematopoietic and lymphopoietic growth factors. Several of these proteins have now been identified and characterized; using recombinant DNA technology, their genes have been cloned and the proteins produced in quantities sufficient for use as therapeutic agents. A number of applications of these new agents have been and are being developed, ranging from treatment of primary hematological diseases to uses as adjunctive agents in the treatment of severe infections and in the management of patients who are undergoing chemotherapy.

History. Modern concepts of hematopoietic cell growth and differentiation began in the 1950s with the work of Jacobsen, Osgood, Ford, and others (Jacobsen *et al.*, 1949; Lindsley *et al.*, 1955; Ford *et al.*, 1956; Osgood, 1957). These investigators demonstrated the role cells from the spleen and bone marrow play in the restoration of hematopoietic tissue in irradiated animals. In 1961, Till and McCulloch were able to show that individual hematopoietic cells could form macroscopic hematopoietic nodules in the spleens of irradiated mice. Their work led to the concept of *colony-forming stem cells* (those found in the spleen are termed *CFU-S*). It also led to the subsequent proof that stem cells present in human bone marrow are pluripotent—that is, they give rise to granulocytes, monocytes, lymphocytes, megakaryocytes, and erythrocytes (Wu *et al.*, 1967).

The role of growth factors in hematopoiesis was not elucidated until the development of bone marrow culture techniques by Bradley, Metcalf, and others (Bradley and Metcalf, 1966; Pluznik and Sachs, 1966; Axelrad *et al.*, 1974). Their use made it possible to study the influence of conditioned media obtained from a variety of tissues and to isolate individual growth factors (Metcalf, 1985, 1986; Clark and Kamen, 1987). The target cells of these factors have also been characterized (*see* Figure 54–1). The pluripotent stem cell gives rise to committed progenitors, which can be identified as single colony-forming units, and to cells of increasing differentiation.

The existence of a circulating growth factor that controls erythropoiesis was first suggested by experiments carried out by Paul Carnot in 1906 (Carnot and Deflandre, 1906). He observed an increase in the red cell count in rabbits injected with serum obtained from anemic animals and postulated the existence of a factor that he called *hemapoietine*. However, it was not until the 1950s that Reissmann (1950), Erslev (1953), and Jacobsen and coworkers (1957) defined the origin and actions of the hormone, now called *erythropoietin*. Subsequently, extensive studies of erythropoietin were carried out in patients with anemia and polycythemia, culminating in 1977 with the purification of erythropoietin from urine by Miyake and colleagues. The gene that encodes the protein has now been cloned and expressed at a high level in a mammalian cell system (Jacobs *et al.*, 1985; Lin *et al.*, 1985); a recombinant hormone that is indistinguishable from human urinary erythropoietin is thus available. Similarly, complementary DNA and genomic clones for granulocyte and macrophage colony-stimulating factors (GM-CSF, G-CSF, and others) have been isolated, and sufficient quantities of biologically active growth factors have been produced for clinical investigation (Kawasaki *et al.*, 1985; Lee *et al.*, 1985; Wong *et al.*, 1985; Yang *et al.*, 1986).

Growth Factor Physiology. Steady-state hematopoiesis involves the production of

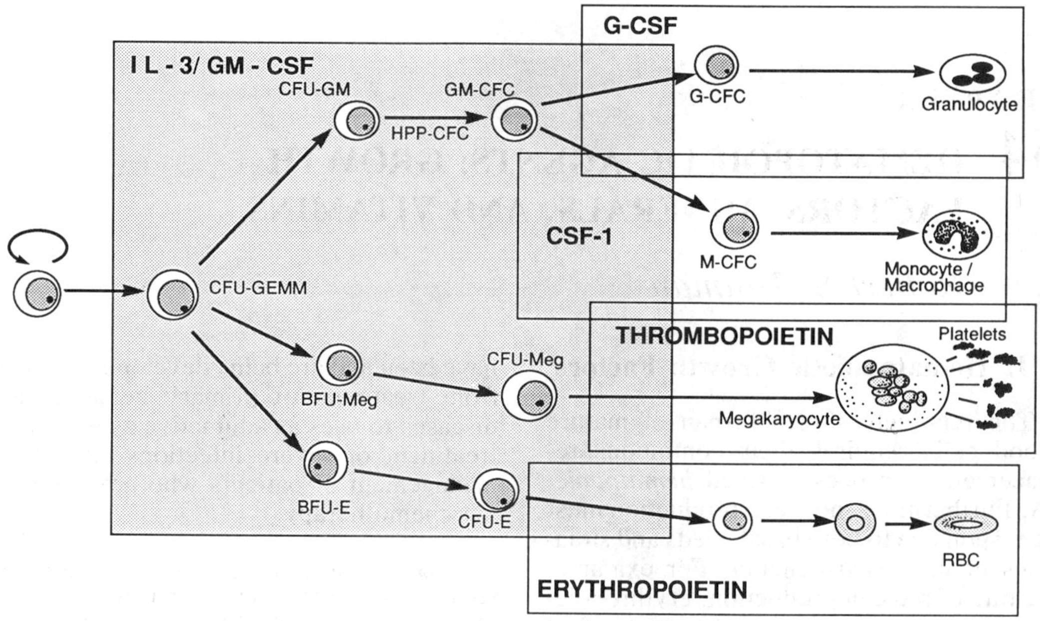

Figure 54–1. *Sites of Action of Hematopoietic Growth Factors in the Differentiation and Maturation of Marrow Cell Lines.*

A self-sustaining pool of marrow stem cells differentiates under the influence of specific hematopoietic growth factors to form a variety of hematopoietic and lymphopoietic cells. Interleukin-3 (IL-3) and granulocyte/macrophage colony-stimulating factor (GM-CSF), together with cell-cell interactions in the marrow stimulate stem cells to form a series of burst-forming units (BFU) and colony-forming units (CFU)—CFU-GEMM, CFU-GM, BFU-MEG, BFU-E, and CFU-E (GEMM = granulocyte, erythrocyte, monocyte, and megakaryote; GM = granulocyte and macrophage; MEG = megakaryocyte; E = erythrocyte). After considerable proliferation, further differentiation is stimulated by synergistic interactions with growth factors for each of the major cell lines—granulocyte colony-stimulating factor (G-CSF); monocyte/macrophage stimulating factor (CSF-1); thrombopoietin, and erythropoietin. Each of these factors also influences the proliferation, maturation, and, in some cases, the function of the derivative cell line (*see* Table 54–1).

more than 200 billion (2×10^{11}) blood cells each day. This production is under delicate control, and, with increased demand, the rate can increase severalfold. The hematopoietic organ is also unique in that several mature cell types are derived from a much smaller number of pluripotent stem cells that are formed in early embryonic life. These stem cells are capable of both maintaining their own number and differentiating to produce a variety of hematopoietic and lymphopoietic cells. A scheme for the differentiation of stem cells to form the major hematopoietic cell lines is shown in Figure 54–1. Marrow stem cells are also capable of differentiation into lymphopoietic cell lines (not shown in Figure 54–1).

Under the influence of cellular and humoral factors, a pluripotent stem cell is able to divide asymmetrically to produce a daughter cell that becomes a committed progenitor for one or another cell line. This latter process can be described as a series of steps in differentiation and proliferation (Quesenberry and Levitt, 1979). The first step involves the appearance of cells that produce so-called burst-forming units (BFU) or colony-forming units (CFU) for each of the major cell lines (colony-forming unit-granulocyte/macrophage, CFU-GM; burst-forming unit-erythrocyte, BFU-E, *etc.*). Although these cells are still not morphologically recognizable as precursors of a specific cell line, they are capable of further proliferation and differentiation, increasing their number by some 30-fold. This process requires both interleukin 3 (IL-3) and granulocyte/macrophage colony-stimulating factor (GM-CSF) as growth factors. Subsequently, these progenitors form colony-forming cells or units (G-CFC, M-CFC, CFU-E, *etc.*) under the control of an overlapping set of additional growth factors. Proliferation and gradual maturation of these now morphologically distinct cells can amplify the resulting mature cell product by another 30-fold or more, resulting in greater than 1000 mature cells produced from each committed stem cell (Lajtha *et al.*, 1969; Axelrad *et al.*, 1974). Several of the hematopoietic growth factors and their principal actions are listed in Table 54–1. A number of lymphopoietic factors have also been identified, and their roles in hematopoiesis and in the development and function of T and B lymphocytes are being defined.

In general, hematopoietic and lymphopoietic growth factors are produced by a number of marrow cells and peripheral tissues. The growth factors are glycoproteins and are active at very low concentrations, usually on more than one committed cell lineage. Most show synergistic interactions with other factors, as well as "networking," wherein stimulation of a cell line by one growth factor induces the production of additional growth factors. Finally, growth factors generally exert actions at several points in the processes of cell proliferation and differentiation and in mature cell function (Metcalf, 1985, 1986; Clark and Kamen, 1987). Some of the overlapping effects of the more important hematopoietic growth factors are illustrated in Figure 54–1 and listed in Table 54–1.

ERYTHROPOIETIN

Kinetic measurements of red cell production and survival demonstrate a clear relationship between anemia or hypoxia and the rate of erythropoiesis (Finch *et al.*, 1970). This finding led investigators to postulate a highly responsive feedback system involving a sensor (a kidney cell sensitive to blood oxygen content), rapid secretion of a growth factor (erythropoietin produced by the kidney), and a responsive cell factory capable of rapid expansion (erythroid marrow—BFU-E and CFU-E) (Erslev, 1953). Although erythropoietin is not the sole growth factor responsible for erythropoiesis (*see* Figure 54–1), it is the most important regulator of the proliferation of committed progenitors, maturation of erythroblasts, and release of reticulocytes into the circulation. In its absence, severe anemia is invariably present.

Erythropoietin is produced primarily by the peritubular cells in the proximal tubule of the kidney (Powell *et al.*, 1986; Bauer and Kurtz, 1989; Eckardt and Bauer, 1989), although a small amount of the protein is also synthesized in the liver. The primary gene product is a protein of 193 amino-acid residues, of which the first 27 are cleaved during secretion (Jacobs *et al.*, 1985; Lin

Table 54–1. HEMATOPOIETIC GROWTH FACTORS

INTERLEUKIN-3 (IL-3 or Multi-CSF)
- —Stimulates colony formation of most hematopoietic cell lines
- —Acts synergistically with GM-CSF to increase number of neutrophils, monocytes, and eosinophils in blood
- —Acts with erythropoietin to expand the BFU-E compartment and stimulate CFU-E proliferation
- —Directly stimulates pulmonary macrophages to proliferate and, with CSF-1, stimulates high proliferation potential forming cells (HPP-CFC), blood monocytes, and peritoneal macrophages
- —Influences functions of eosinophils and basophils

GRANULOCYTE/MACROPHAGE COLONY-STIMULATING FACTOR (GM-CSF)
- —Acts synergistically with IL-3 to stimulate colony formation and proliferation of granulocytes, monocytes/macrophages, and megakaryocytes
- —With erythropoietin, promotes formation of BFU-E
- —Increases phagocytic and cytotoxic potential of mature granulocytes, but reduces motility and clearance from circulation
- —Increases cytotoxicity of eosinophils and leukotriene synthesis
- —Stimulates proliferation of small cell carcinoma in culture

GRANULOCYTE COLONY-STIMULATING FACTOR (G-CSF)
- —Stimulates granulocyte colony formation and production of neutrophils
- —Acts synergistically with CSF-1 to stimulate HPP-CFC, with GM-CSF to stimulate granulocyte/macrophage colonies, and with IL-3 to induce formation of megakaryocytes
- —Induces release of granulocytes from marrow
- —Enhances phagocytic and cytotoxic activities of mature granulocytes
- —Stimulates proliferation of small cell carcinoma in culture

COLONY STIMULATING FACTOR (CSF-1 or M-CSF)
- —Stimulates monocyte/macrophage colony formation alone and synergistically with GM-CSF and IL-3
- —Induces synthesis of G-CSF and IL-1 and enhances the production of interferon and tumor necrosis factor
- —Enhances functions of monocytes and macrophages

ERYTHROPOIETIN
- —Stimulates proliferation, maturation, and hemoglobin formation by committed erythroid progenitors (CFU-E)
- —Acts synergistically with IL-3 and GM-CSF to expand the BFU-E compartment
- —Stimulates the early release of reticulocytes from marrow into the circulation

THROMBOPOIETIN
- —Acts in conjunction with megakaryocyte colony-stimulating factor to regulate megakaryocytopoiesis and hence production of platelets

et al., 1985). The final mature protein is heavily glycosylated and has a molecular weight of about 34,000. Glycosylation is important for prolonging the lifetime of erythropoietin in the circulation, but not for its biological activity. Measurable amounts of erythropoietin are always detectable in plasma, suggesting that it is an absolute requirement for red cell production. With anemia or hypoxemia, renal synthesis and secretion of erythropoietin can rapidly increase by 100-fold or more (Garcia *et al.,* 1982). This wave of hormone acts on both early (BFU-E) and late (CFU-E) progenitor cells to stimulate a dramatic recruitment of precursors into a programmed series of cell divisions and terminal maturation. Once initiated, a much lower concentration of erythropoietin is necessary to sustain the response. At the same time, the feedback loop can be interrupted at any point—by renal disease, structural damage of the marrow, or iron deficiency. An inadequate supply of iron (owing either to absolute iron deficiency or to reduced delivery of iron secondary to an inflammatory state) will suppress the marrow's response to even high concentrations of erythropoietin.

Erythropoietin binds to a receptor on the surface of erythroid precursor cells (McCaffery *et al.,* 1989). This protein appears to have a single membrane-spanning domain, but no obvious relationship with other cell-surface receptors that have been characterized to date (D'Andrea *et al.,* 1989). Changes in intracellular phosphorylation and increases in intracellular concentrations of Ca^{2+} and arachidonate are associated with activation of the receptor, but details of the signal transduction process are not understood.

Therapeutic Uses. Administered parenterally, erythropoietin is highly effective for the treatment of the anemia of chronic renal failure. In the initial clinical trial, erythropoietin was administered intravenously to transfusion-dependent patients who were undergoing hemodialysis. The drug alleviated the requirement for transfusions over a period of weeks and eventually normalized the hematocrit (Eschbach *et al.*, 1987; Eschbach and Adamson, 1988). The minimal effective dose was between 15 and 50 units/kg of body weight, given three times weekly. A dose of 50 to 150 units/kg, given intravenously or subcutaneously three times weekly, normalized the hematocrit in essentially anephric patients over a 3- to 4-month period (*see* Eschbach *et al.*, 1987). Subsequent experience with more than 1000 anemic dialysis patients suggests that the average dose necessary to maintain the hematocrit between 30 and 36% is 50 units/kg given three times each week. However, some patients require less than this amount, and 10% or more of patients require a dose as high as 200 units/kg three times weekly to maintain their hematocrit above 30%. Treatment with erythropoietin also corrects the anemia of patients with progressive renal failure who do not require dialysis (Eschbach *et al.*, 1989). The rate of response is similar to that observed in dialysis patients, although the dosage required for maintenance may be lower (25 to 75 units/kg three times a week).

Erythropoietin is also effective in the treatment of other forms of anemia, including the amelioration of the anemia of patients with acquired immunodeficiency syndrome (AIDS) who are being treated with zidovudine (AZT) (Fischl *et al.*, 1990) and the anemia associated with cancer chemotherapy. For patients who are to undergo elective surgery, erythropoietin can be used preoperatively to increase red cell production; this permits the storage of larger volumes of blood for autologous transfusion (Goodnough *et al.*, 1989).

Preparations and Dosage. Recombinant human erythropoietin is available as *epoetin alfa* (EPOGEN, EPREX). It is supplied in buffered saline containing human albumin in single-use vials of 2000, 4000, or 10,000 units of erythropoietin for intravenous or subcutaneous injection. When administered intravenously, epoetin alfa is cleared from plasma with a half-life of approximately 10 hours in patients with chronic renal failure. Following subcutaneous injection, peak concentrations in plasma occur within 5 to 24 hours. However, the drug need not be given more often than three times a week to achieve an adequate response. The recommended initial dose is 50 to 100 units/kg three times a week in patients with chronic renal failure. Care must be taken to titrate the dose to avoid an excessively rapid increase in the hematocrit early in treatment or a rise in hematocrit to values greater than 36% during maintenance therapy. The hematocrit should be determined at least once each week to measure the initial response. An increase of more than 4 percentage points in a 2-week period mandates a reduction in dose. Once the hematocrit exceeds 30%, the weekly dosage should be reduced and the hematocrit monitored at regular intervals.

The initial response to epoetin alfa may be delayed for 2 to 6 weeks in some patients. If the hematocrit does not increase by at least 5 percentage points after 2 months of therapy, the dosage of epoetin alfa can be increased, usually by increments of 25 units/kg at monthly intervals. The response to epoetin alfa requires adequate stores of iron, since the rate of red cell production correlates with the supply of iron to the erythroid marrow. Patients with chronic renal failure and elevated stores of iron show a predictable response to epoetin alfa; the response is blunted in patients with minimal iron stores or iron deficiency. In the latter case it may be necessary to administer an oral iron supplement or iron dextran injection; oral iron alone may not meet the needs of the rapidly proliferating marrow. Inflammation can also interfere with the supply of iron to the erythroid marrow and delay or prevent a rise in hematocrit. No other major restricting factors have been identified. Aluminum intoxication, elevated concentrations of parathyroid hormone, and osteitis fibrosa do not prevent a response, although higher doses of erythropoietin may be needed (Eschbach and Adamson, 1988).

Untoward Effects. No significant allergic reactions have been associated with the intravenous or subcutaneous administration of epoetin alfa, and antibodies to the growth factor have not been detected, even with prolonged administration. Complications associated with the administration of epoetin alfa to patients with renal disease include increased clotting of the dialyzer and exacerbation of or new onset of hypertension and seizures. The latter problems appear to be related to the rapidity of expansion of the red cell mass and the impact of such expansion on blood volume and viscosity. Increases in peripheral vascular resistance and blood pressure have been observed in anemic patients with renal disease in whom the hematocrit was increased suddenly. This response can be avoided by using a lower dose of erythropoietin to stimulate a more gradual increase in hematocrit and to allow time for physiological adaptation to the increase in red cell mass. The patient's blood pressure should be monitored closely throughout treatment to help titrate the dose of epoetin alfa; patients who are receiving antihypertensive medications may require adjustment of their dosage.

MYELOID GROWTH FACTORS

The myeloid growth factors or colony stimulating factors are glycoproteins that stimulate the proliferation and differentiation of several types of hematopoietic precursor cells. They also enhance the function of mature leukocytes. The genes for four human colony-stimulating factors have been cloned, and the recombinant forms of the glycoproteins have been synthesized; these include granulocyte/macrophage colony-stimulating factor, (GM-CSF) (Lee *et al.*, 1985), granulocyte colony-stimulating factor (G-CSF) (Wong *et al.*, 1985), interleukin 3 (IL-3) (Yang *et al.*, 1986), and macrophage colony-stimulating factor (M-CSF or CSF-1) (Kawasaki *et al.*, 1985). GM-CSF and IL-3 are normally synthesized by T lymphocytes, while GM-CSF, G-CSF, and M-CSF are produced by monocytes, fibroblasts, and endothelial cells. The actions of these growth factors are summarized in Table 54–1 (*see also* Groopman *et al.*, 1989).

GM-CSF has undergone clinical trials to define its value in the treatment of patients with relative or absolute neutropenia secondary to neoplasia, congenital cyclic neutropenia, aplastic anemia, myelodysplasia, and AIDS (Groopman *et al.*, 1987, 1989; Vadhan-Raj *et al.*, 1987). Another clear application is the blunting or prevention of the neutropenia associated with chemotherapy and autologous bone marrow transplantation (Bronchurd *et al.*, 1987; Brandt *et al.*, 1988; Gabrilove *et al.*, 1988; Groopman *et al.*, 1989).

Administration of GM-CSF produces rapid increases in bone marrow cellularity and a shift in the erythroid/granulocyte cell ratio (E/G ratio) in the marrow, indicative of increases in the proliferation of granulocyte/macrophage cell lines. This response is followed by dramatic elevations in the number of circulating neutrophils, eosinophils, and monocytes; GM-CSF also has a demonstrable effect on neutrophil mobility, delaying the exit of neutrophils from the circulation.

The hematological response to G-CSF consists predominantly of an increase in the number of circulating neutrophils; there is little eosinophilia. Clinical trials of G-CSF have largely been directed toward attempts to reduce neutropenia following cytotoxic chemotherapy. The response to the growth factor in this setting is consistently beneficial. The extent and duration of neutropenia are reduced, febrile episodes are fewer, and a higher percentage of patients are able to complete an entire course of chemotherapy. G-CSF has also shown promise in the treatment of idiopathic neutropenias and neutropenia associated with malignant infiltration of the bone marrow (*see* Glaspy and Golde, 1989; Groopman *et al.*, 1989).

Side effects are relatively prominent after the administration of GM-CSF. Local induration is seen after subcutaneous administration, and thrombophlebitis occurs at sites of infusion. Patients often exhibit fever, myalgias, fatigue, skin rashes, and gastrointestinal distress. Bone pain is a common complaint, and this increases in severity with higher doses. Pericarditis, pleuritis, pleural effusions, and pulmonary emboli represent dose-limiting toxicities. Administration of G-CSF is associated with fewer untoward effects. Mild-to-moderate bone pain, vasculitis, and worsening of psoriasis have been reported.

Despite these untoward effects, these growth factors show considerable promise as therapeutic agents. Generally, four major areas of clinical utility are apparent: restoration of normal hematopoiesis in patients with malignancies or nonneoplastic diseases that interfere with marrow production; reduction in the morbidity of chemotherapy by shortening the duration of severe neutropenia; augmentation of host defenses against infection; and, perhaps, adjunct roles in chemotherapeutic regimens by improving cytotoxicity against tumor cells or by diminishing self-renewal of leukemic cells by promoting cell maturation. However, it should also be recognized that the myeloid growth factors may, in themselves, have oncogenic potential. A clear relationship exists between the receptor for M-CSF and the v-*fms* oncogene product, and cotransfection of cells with the genes for the M-CSF receptor and M-CSF itself causes transformation of fibroblasts (Nicola, 1989).

II. Drugs Effective in Iron Deficiency and Other Hypochromic Anemias

IRON AND IRON SALTS

Iron deficiency is the most common cause of nutritional anemia in man. When severe, it results in a characteristic microcytic, hypochromic anemia secondary to a reduction in the synthesis of hemoglobin. However, the impact of iron deficiency is not limited to the erythron (Dallman, 1982). Iron is also an essential component of myoglobin; heme enzymes such as the cytochromes, catalase, and peroxidase; and the metalloflavoprotein enzymes, including xanthine oxidase and the mitochondrial enzyme α-glycerophosphate oxidase. Iron deficiency can affect metabolism in muscle independently of the effect of anemia on oxygen delivery. This may well reflect a reduction in the activity of iron-dependent mitochondrial enzymes. Iron deficiency has also been associated with behavioral and learning problems in children and with abnormalities in catecholamine metabolism and, possibly, heat production (Pollit and Leibel, 1982; Martinez-Torres *et al.*, 1984). Awareness of this ubiquitous role of iron has stimulated considerable interest in the early and accurate detection of iron deficiency and in its prevention.

History. Iron was used by European physicians through the Middle Ages and the Renaissance, but with little rationale. In the sixteenth century the role of iron deficiency in the then-prevalent "green sickness" or chlorosis of adolescent women began to be recognized, but Sydenham is properly credited with identifying iron as a specific remedy to take the place of bleedings and purgings. In 1681, he wrote (*see* Latham, 1850): ". . . I comfort the blood and the spirit belonging to it by giving a chalybeate [containing or charged with iron] 30 days running. This is sure to do good. To the worn out or languid blood it gives a spur or fillip, whereby the animal spirits which before lay prostrate and sunken under their own weight are raised and excited. Clear proof of this is found in the effect of steel in chlorosis. The pulse gains strength, the face (no longer pale and deathlike) a fresh ruddy color." In 1713, Lemery and Geoffry provided more direct evidence of the relationship by showing that iron was present in blood (ash) (*see* Christian, 1903). In 1832, the French physician Pierre Blaud recognized that failure in the treatment of chlorosis had been due to the use of too-small doses of iron and reported the rapid cure of 30 patients given a mixture of equal parts of ferrous sulfate and potassium carbonate in dosage increasing to as much as 770 mg of elemental iron daily. For many years Blaud's nephew distributed the "veritable pills of Blaud" throughout the world (Neuroth and Lee, 1941). The treatment of anemia with iron followed the principles enunciated by Sydenham and Blaud until the last decade of the nineteenth century. At that time, however, the teachings of Bunge, Quincke, von Noorden, and others cast doubt on this straightforward approach to the treatment of chlorosis. The dose of iron employed was reduced, and the resulting inefficacy of smaller doses brought discredit on the therapy. It was not until the third and fourth decades of the present century, through the efforts of Faber and Gram, Bloomfield, Heath and associates, and Reimann and coworkers, that the lessons taught by the earlier physicians were relearned (*see* Haden, 1939).

The past half century has brought a clearer understanding of many aspects of iron metabolism in man. In 1937, McCance and Widdowson reported on studies of iron balance that suggested a limited daily absorption and excretion of the element. At the same time, Heilmeyer and Plotner (1937) measured the concentration of iron in plasma and proposed its function in transport. Laurell in 1947 presented similar information concerning the plasma iron transport protein, which he called *transferrin*. Hahn and coworkers (1943) introduced the use of radioactive isotopes of iron as a means to quantitate absorption and demonstrated the capacity of the intestinal mucosa to regulate this function. In the next decade, Huff and associates (1950) initiated isotopic studies of internal iron exchange. Practical clinical measurements of the degree of saturation of transferrin and red-cell protoporphyrin were also developed to a point that permits the detection of iron-deficient erythropoiesis, while quantitation of iron in plasma ferritin and in marrow reveals the status of the body's stores (*see* Bothwell *et al.*, 1979).

Iron and the Environment. Iron exists in the environment largely as ferric oxide or hydroxide or as polymers. In this state, its biological availability is limited unless solubilized by acid or chelates. For example, to meet their needs, bacteria and some plants produce high-affinity chelating agents that extract iron from the surrounding environment (Neilands, 1974). In alkaline or high-phosphate soils, many plants develop an iron-deficiency disease, chlorosis, manifest by yellowness or blanching of normally green parts. Most mammals have little difficulty in acquiring iron; this ability is explained by a more ample iron intake and perhaps also by the animal's greater efficiency in absorbing iron. Man, however, appears to be an exception. Although total dietary intake of elemental iron exceeds requirements, the bioavailability of the iron in the diet is limited.

Iron Metabolism in Man. The body store of iron is divided between essential iron-containing compounds and excess iron, which is held in storage. From a quantitative standpoint, hemoglobin dominates the essential fraction (Table 54–2). This protein, with a molecular weight of 64,500, contains four atoms of iron per molecule, amounting to 1.1 mg of iron per milliliter of red blood cells (20 mM). Other forms of essential iron include myoglobin and a variety of heme and nonheme iron-dependent enzymes (Sigel, 1977). Ferritin is the protein of iron storage, and it exists as individual molecules or in an aggregated form. Apoferritin has a molecular weight of about 450,000 and is composed of 24 polypeptide subunits; these form an outer shell within which resides a storage cavity for polynuclear hydrous ferric oxide phosphate (Harrison, 1977). Over 30% of the weight of ferritin may be iron (4000 atoms of iron per ferritin molecule). Aggregated ferritin, referred to as *hemosiderin* and visible by light microscopy, constitutes about one third of normal stores, a fraction that increases as stores enlarge (Wixom *et al.*, 1979). The two predominant sites of iron storage are the reticuloendothelial system and the hepatocytes, although some storage also occurs in muscle (Bothwell *et al.*, 1979).

Table 54–2. THE BODY CONTENT OF IRON

	MALE	FEMALE
	mg/kg of body weight	
Essential iron		
Hemoglobin	31	28
Myoglobin and enzymes	6	5
Storage iron	13	4
Total	50	37

Internal exchange of iron is accomplished by the plasma protein transferrin (Aisen and Brown, 1977). This β_1-glycoprotein has a molecular weight of about 76,000 and two binding sites for ferric iron. Iron is delivered from transferrin to intracellular sites by means of specific transferrin receptors in the plasma membrane. The iron–transferrin complex binds to the receptor and the ternary complex is taken up by receptor-mediated endocytosis. Iron subsequently dissociates in a pH-dependent fashion in an acidic, intracellular vesicular compartment (the endosomes), and the receptor returns the apotransferrine to the cell surface, where it is released into the extracellular environment to function once again (*see* Brown *et al.*, 1983; Klausner, 1988).

Human cells regulate their expression of transferrin receptors and intracellular ferritin in response to the iron supply. When iron is plentiful, the synthesis of transferrin receptors is reduced and ferritin production is increased. Conversely, with iron deficiency, cells express a greater number of transferrin receptors and reduce ferritin concentrations to maximize uptake and prevent diversion of iron to stores. Isolation of the genes for the human transferrin receptor and ferritin has permitted a better definition of the molecular basis of this regulation. Iron acts in opposing directions to control the rates of translation and stabilities of the messenger RNAs (mRNAs) that encode both ferritin and the transferrin receptor (Casey *et al.*, 1988; Klausner, 1988).

The flow of iron through the plasma amounts to a total of 30 to 40 mg per day in the adult (about 0.46 mg/kg of body weight) (Finch and Huebers, 1982). The major internal circulation of iron involves the erythron and the reticuloendothelial cell (Figure 54–2). About 80% of the iron in plasma goes to the erythroid marrow to be packaged into new erythrocytes; these normally circulate for about 120 days before being catabolized by the reticuloendothelium. At that time a portion of the iron is immediately returned to the plasma bound to transferrin, while another portion is incorporated into the ferritin stores of the reticuloendothelial cell and is returned to the circulation more gradually. Isotopic studies indicate some degree of iron wastage in this process, wherein defective cells or unused portions of their iron are transferred to the reticuloendothelial cell during maturation, bypassing the circulating blood. When there are abnormalities in maturation of red cells, the predominant portion of iron assimilated by the erythroid marrow may be rapidly localized in the reticuloendothelial cell as defective red-cell precursors are broken down; this is termed *ineffective erythropoiesis*. With red-cell aplasia, the rate of turnover of iron in plasma may be reduced by one half or more, with all the iron now going to the hepatocyte for storage.

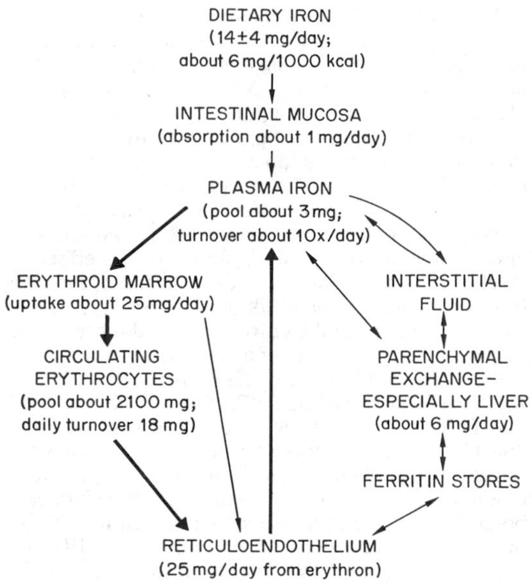

Figure 54–2. *Pathways of iron metabolism in man (excretion omitted).* (*See* text for explanation.)

The most remarkable feature of iron metabolism in man is the degree to which the body store is conserved. Only 10% of the total is lost per year from normal men, that is, about 1 mg per day (Green *et al.*, 1968). Two thirds of this iron is excreted from the gastrointestinal tract as extravasated red cells, iron in bile, and iron in exfoliated mucosal cells. The other third is accounted for by small amounts of iron in desquamated skin and in the urine. Physiological losses of iron in the male vary over a narrow range, from 0.5 mg in the iron-deficient individual to 1.5 to 2 mg per day when excessive iron is consumed. Additional losses of iron occur in the female due to menstruation (Hallberg *et al.*, 1966a). While the average loss is about 0.5 mg per day, 10% of normal menstruating females lose over 2 mg per day. Pregnancy imposes a requirement for iron of even greater magnitude (Table 54–3). Other causes of iron loss include the donation of blood, the use of anti-inflammatory drugs that cause bleeding from the gastric mucosa, gastrointestinal disease with associated bleeding, and so forth (Fairbanks *et al.*, 1971). Much rarer are the hemosiderinuria that follows intravascular hemolysis and pulmonary siderosis, wherein iron is deposited in the lungs and becomes unavailable to the rest of the body.

The limited physiological losses of iron point to the primary importance of absorption as the determinant of the body's iron content. Unfortunately, the biochemical nature of the absorptive process is understood only in general terms (Bothwell *et al.*, 1979). After acidification and partial digestion of food in the stomach, its content of iron is presented to the intestinal mucosa as either inorganic or heme iron. These fractions are taken up by the absorptive cells of the duodenum and upper small intestine, and the iron is either transported directly into the plasma or is stored as mucosal ferritin (Figure 54–3). Absorption is regulated by the relative activity of these two pathways, which is in some manner determined by the internal state of iron metabolism. The amount of a specific transferrin-like

Table 54–3. IRON REQUIREMENTS FOR PREGNANCY

	AVERAGE *mg*	RANGE *mg*
External iron loss	170	150–200
Expansion of red-blood-cell mass	450	200–600
Fetal iron	270	200–370
Iron in placenta and cord	90	30–170
Blood loss at delivery	150	90–310
Total requirement *	980	580–1340
Cost of pregnancy †	680	440–1050

* Blood loss at delivery not included.
† Iron lost to the mother; expansion of red-cell mass not included.
(After Council on Foods and Nutrition, 1968. Courtesy of the *Journal of the American Medical Association*.)

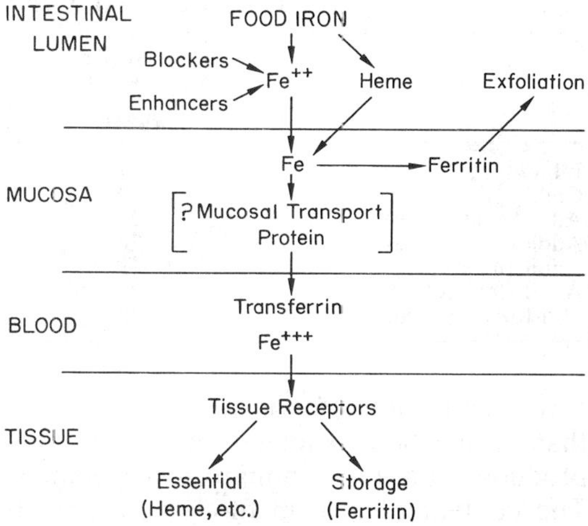

Figure 54–3. *Pathway of iron absorption.* (*See* text for explanation.)

mucosal protein may influence absorption (Huebers *et al.*, 1983). Normal absorption is about 1 mg per day in the adult male and 1.4 mg per day in the adult female. Increased uptake and delivery of iron into the circulation occur when iron intake is deficient, when iron stores are depleted, or when erythropoiesis is increased (Heinrich, 1983). However, 3 to 4 mg of dietary iron is the most that can be absorbed.

Iron Requirements and the Availability of Dietary Iron. Iron requirements are determined by obligatory physiological losses and the needs imposed by growth. Thus, the adult male has a requirement of only 13 μg/kg per day (about 1 mg), whereas the menstruating female requires about 21 μg/kg per day (about 1.4 mg). In the last two trimesters of pregnancy, requirements increase to about 80 μg/kg per day (5 to 6 mg), and the infant has similar requirements due to its rapid growth (Finch, 1976). These requirements (Table 54–4) must be considered in the context of the amount of dietary iron available for absorption.

The dietary content of iron in developed countries is about 6 mg/1000 kcal; this amount places the average daily iron intake of the adult male between 12 and 20 mg and that of the adult female between 8 and 15 mg. Foods high in iron (greater than 5 mg/100 g) include organ meats such as liver and heart, brewer's yeast, wheat germ, egg yolks, oysters, and certain dried

Table 54–4. DAILY IRON INTAKE AND ABSORPTION

SUBJECT	IRON REQUIREMENT ($\mu g/kg$)	AVAILABLE IRON IN POOR DIET–GOOD DIET ($\mu g/kg$)	SAFETY FACTOR (*Available Iron/Requirement*)
Infant	67	33–66	0.5–1
Child	22	48–96	2–4
Adolescent (male)	21	30–60	1.5–3
Adolescent (female)	20	30–60	1.5–3
Adult (male)	13	26–52	2–4
Adult (female)	21	18–36	1–2
Mid-to-late pregnancy	80	18–36	0.22–0.45

beans and fruits; foods low in iron (less than 1 mg/100 g) include milk and milk products and most nongreen vegetables. The content of iron in food is further affected by the manner of its preparation, since iron may be added through contamination with dirt and from cooking in iron pots.

Although the iron content of the diet is obviously important, of greater nutritional significance is the bioavailability of iron in food (Hallberg, 1981). Heme iron is far more available, and its absorption is independent of the composition of the diet. This is illustrated by the study carried out by Björn-Rasmussen and associates (1974) in which subjects were fed a diet that contained 17.4 mg of iron per day, of which 16.4 mg was nonheme iron and 1 mg was contained in heme; 37% of the heme iron but only 5% of the nonheme iron was absorbed. Thus, heme iron, which constituted only 6% of the dietary iron, represented 30% of iron absorbed. Nevertheless, it is the availability of the nonheme fraction that deserves the greatest attention, since it represents by far the largest amount of dietary iron that is ingested by the economically underprivileged. In a vegetarian diet, nonheme iron is absorbed very poorly because of the inhibitory action of a variety of components, particularly phosphates (Layrisse and Martinez-Torres, 1971). Two substances are known to facilitate the absorption of nonheme iron—ascorbic acid and meat. Ascorbate forms complexes with and/or reduces ferric to ferrous iron. While meat facilitates the absorption of iron by stimulating production of gastric acid, it is possible that some other effect, not yet identified, is also involved. Either of these substances can increase availability severalfold. Thus, assessments of available dietary iron should include not only the amount of iron ingested but also an estimate of its availability based on the intake of substances that enhance or inhibit its absorption (Monsen *et al.,* 1978) (Figure 54–4).

A comparison of iron requirements with available dietary iron is made in Table 54–4. Obviously, pregnancy and infancy represent periods of negative balance. The menstruating woman is also at risk, whereas iron balance in the adult male and nonmenstruating female is reasonably secure. The difference between dietary supply and requirements is reflected in the size of iron stores. These will be low or absent when iron balance is precarious and high when iron balance is favorable. Thus, in the infant after the third month of life and in the

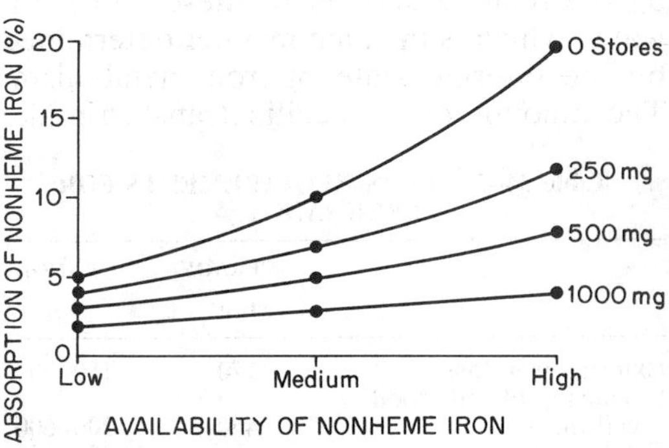

Figure 54–4. *Effect of iron status on the absorption of nonheme iron in food.*

The percentages of iron absorbed from diets of low, medium, and high bioavailability in individuals with iron stores of 0, 250, 500, and 1000 mg are portrayed. (After Monsen *et al.,* 1978. © *American Journal of Clinical Nutrition.* Courtesy of American Society for Clinical Nutrition.)

pregnant woman after the first trimester, stores of iron are negligible (Beaton, 1974). Menstruating females have approximately one third the stored iron found in the adult male, indicative of the extent to which the additional average daily loss of about 0.5 mg of iron affects balance (Finch *et al.*, 1977).

Iron Deficiency. The prevalence of iron-deficiency anemia depends on the economic status of the population and on the methods used for evaluation. In developing countries as many as 20 to 40% of infants and pregnant women may be affected (WHO Joint Meeting, 1975), while studies in the United States suggest that the current prevalence in adult men and women is as low as 0.2 to 3% (Cook *et al.*, 1986). The difficulty experienced by a substantial proportion of the population in achieving iron balance is recognized by the current practice of fortification of flour, by the use of iron-fortified formulas for infants, and by the prescription of medicinal iron supplements in pregnancy.

Iron-deficiency anemia results from a dietary intake of iron that is inadequate to meet normal requirements (nutritional iron deficiency), blood loss, or some interference with iron absorption. Most nutritional iron deficiency in the United States is mild. Moderate-to-severe iron deficiency is usually the result of blood loss, either from the gastrointestinal tract or, in the female, from the uterus. *In such patients, no effort should be spared in determining the cause of the bleeding.* Infrequently, impaired absorption of the iron in food results from partial gastrectomy or sprue.

The recognition of iron deficiency rests on an appreciation of the sequence of events that occurs with iron depletion (Cook, 1982; Hillman and Finch, 1985). A negative balance first results in a reduction of iron stores and, eventually, a parallel decrease in red-cell iron and iron-related enzymes (Figure 54–5). In adults, depleted stores may be recognized by a plasma ferritin of less than 12 μg per liter and the absence of reticuloendothelial hemosiderin in the marrow aspirate. Iron-deficient erythropoiesis, defined as a suboptimal supply of iron to the erythron, is identified by a decreased saturation of transferrin to less than 16% and/or by an increase above normal in red-cell protoporphyrin. Iron-deficiency anemia is associated with a recognizable decrease in the concentration of hemoglobin in blood. However, the physiological variation in the concentration of hemoglobin is so great that only about half the individuals with iron-deficient erythropoiesis are identified by signs of recognizable anemia (Cook *et al.*, 1976). Moreover, hemoglobin and iron values in infancy and childhood are different, owing to the more restricted supply of iron normally present in plasma at that age (Dallman *et al.*, 1980).

The importance of mild iron deficiency lies more in identifying the underlying cause of the deficiency than in any symptoms related to the deficient state. Because of the frequency of iron deficiency in infancy and in the menstruating or pregnant woman, the need for exhaustive evaluation of such individuals is usually determined by the severity of the anemia. However, iron deficiency in the male or postmenopausal female necessitates a search for a site of bleeding.

The diagnosis of iron deficiency is more accurately established by laboratory tests than by a therapeutic trial, particularly when the deficiency is mild. The presence of microcytic anemia is the most commonly recognized indicator of iron deficiency. Other laboratory tests, such as quantitation of transferrin saturation, red-cell protoporphyrin, or plasma ferritin, are required to distinguish iron deficiency from other causes of microcytosis. Such measurements are particularly useful when circulating red cells are not yet microcytic because of the recent nature of blood loss, but iron supply is nonetheless limiting erythropoiesis. More difficult is the differentiation of true iron deficiency from iron-deficient erythropoiesis due to inflammation (Finch, 1978). In the latter condition, the stores of iron are actually increased, but the release of iron from the reticuloendothelial cell is blocked; the concentration of iron in plasma is decreased, and the supply of iron to the erythroid marrow becomes inadequate. The increased stores of iron in this condition may be demonstrated directly by examination of an aspirate of marrow or

	Normal	Iron Depletion	Iron-Deficient Erythropoiesis	Iron-Deficiency Anemia

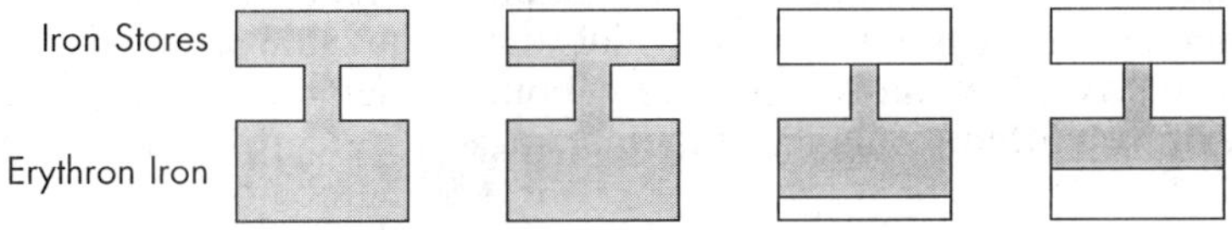

	Normal	Iron Depletion	Iron-Deficient Erythropoiesis	Iron-Deficiency Anemia
RE marrow Fe	2–3+	0–1+	0	0
Transferrin IBC μg/100 ml (μM)	330±30 (59±5)	360 (64)	390 (70)	410 (73)
Plasma ferritin (μg/l)	100±60	20	10	<10
Iron absorption (%)	5–10	10–15	10–20	10–20
Plasma iron μg/100 ml (μM)	115±50 (21±9)	115 (21)	<60 (<11)	<40 (<7)
Transferrin saturation (%)	35±15	30	<15	<10
Sideroblasts (%)	40–60	40–60	<10	<10
RBC protoporphyrin μg/100 ml RBC (μmol per liter RBC)	30 (0.53)	30 (0.53)	100 (1.8)	200 (3.5)
Erythrocytes	Normal	Normal	Normal	Microcytic/ Hypochromic

Figure 54–5. *Sequential changes (from left to right) in the development of iron deficiency in the adult.*

Rectangles enclose the first appearance of the indicated abnormal test results. IBC = iron-binding capacity. (After Hillman and Finch, 1985, as modified from Bothwell and Finch, 1962. Courtesy of F. A. Davis Co.)

may be inferred from determination of an elevated concentration of ferritin in plasma (Lipschitz *et al.*, 1974).

TREATMENT OF IRON DEFICIENCY

General Therapeutic Principles. The response of iron-deficiency anemia to treatment is influenced by several factors, including the cause and severity of the iron-deficient state, the presence of other complicating illnesses, and the ability of the patient to tolerate and absorb medicinal iron. Effective therapy is followed by an increased rate of production of red cells, and the increase is proportional to the severity of the anemia and the amount of iron made available to the marrow. Some idea of the importance of the relationship of iron delivery to marrow production is found in the studies of Hillman and Henderson (1969). When normal subjects were phlebotomized, erythropoiesis was reduced to less than one third the normal rate when the concentration of iron in plasma was below 12.5 μM (70 μg/dl). In contrast, production increased to more than three times the basal rate when the plasma iron concentration was between 13.4 and 26.9 μM (75 and 150 μg/dl). The highest rates of erythropoiesis occurred in subjects with increased destruction of red cells and elevated concentrations of iron in plasma; this situation is observed in patients with ineffective erythropoiesis and/or hemolysis of mature red cells (Hillman and Giblett, 1965).

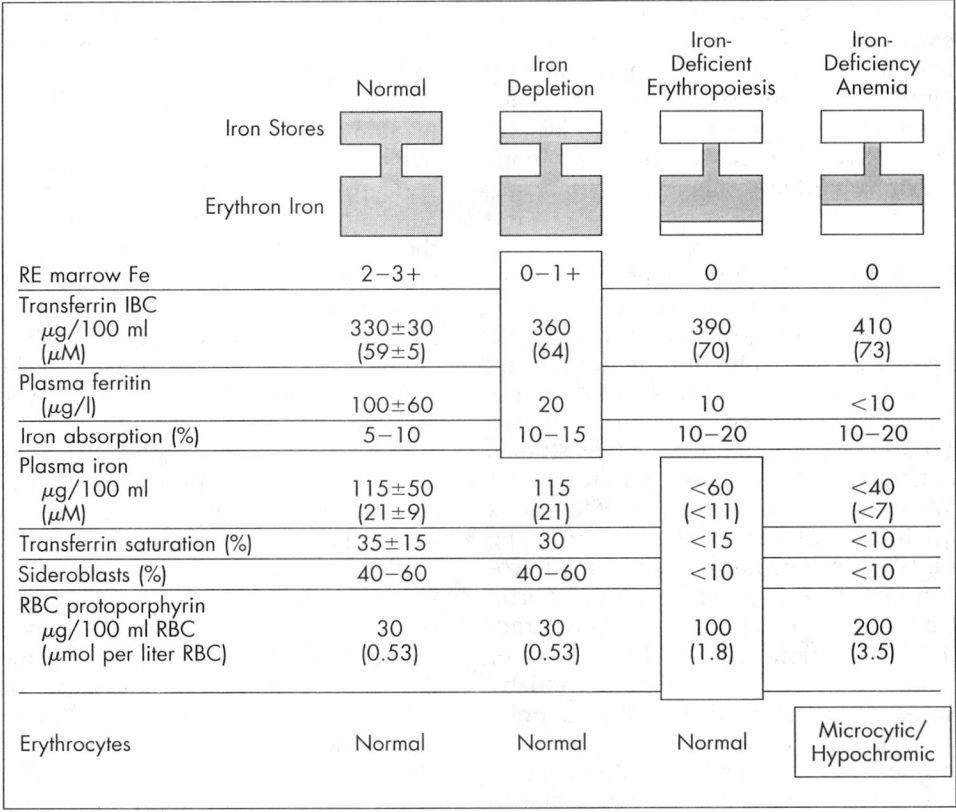

The level of response of the marrow is also a reflection of the severity of the anemia, and, by inference, the degree of stimulation of marrow precursors by erythropoietin. This assumes, of course, that the marrow can respond normally. An intrinsic disease of the marrow or, more commonly, a complicating illness (such as an inflammatory disorder) can blunt the response to therapy. Continued bleeding will also interfere with the response in terms of hemoglobin, although reticulocytes will increase in number. The ability of the patient to tolerate and absorb administered iron is another important factor in determining the rate of response. There are clear limits to the gastrointestinal tolerance for iron. In addition, the small intestine regulates absorption and prevents the entry of overwhelming amounts of iron into the bloodstream. This property places a ceiling on how much iron can be provided by oral therapy. In the patient with moderately severe anemia, maximal doses of oral iron will supply 40 to 60 mg of iron per day to the erythroid marrow, an amount sufficient for production of red cells at a rate that is two to three times normal.

The response to iron therapy can be evaluated with the reticulocyte production index and the rate of rise in the level of hemoglobin or the hematocrit. A modest increase in the reticulocyte index may be observed as early as 4 to 7 days after beginning therapy. A measurable increase in the hemoglobin or hematocrit should be evident after 1 week of therapy. If the concentration of hemoglobin before treatment is reduced by more than 30 g per liter, an average increment of hemoglobin of 2 g per liter per day is observed with the usual therapeutic doses of iron, administered either orally or parenterally. It should be noted that this amount is less than the 6 g per liter per day (three times basal) that the erythroid marrow can achieve when the supply of iron is optimal, which indicates that neither route of administration can provide sufficient iron for maximal erythropoiesis. A decision about the effectiveness of the treatment should not be made for 3 to 4 weeks. An increase of 20 g per liter or more in the concentration of hemoglobin by that time should be considered a positive response to iron, assuming no other change in the patient's clinical status can account for the improvement. It also assumes that the patient has not been transfused during this time.

If the response to oral iron is inadequate, the diagnosis must be reconsidered. A full laboratory evaluation should be carried out, and such factors as the presence of a concurrent inflammatory disease or poor compliance by the patient must be assessed. A source of continued bleeding should obviously be sought. If no other explanation can be found, an evaluation of the patient's ability to absorb oral iron should be considered. There is no justification for merely continuing oral iron therapy beyond 3 to 4 weeks if a favorable response has not occurred.

Once a response to oral iron is demonstrated, therapy should be continued until the hemoglobin returns to normal. Treatment may then be extended if it is desirable to establish iron stores. This may require a considerable period of time, since the rate of absorption of iron by the intestine will decrease markedly as iron stores are reconstituted. The prophylactic use of oral iron should be reserved for patients at high risk, including pregnant women, women with excessive menstrual blood loss, blood donors, and infants. Iron supplements may also be of value for rapidly growing infants who are consuming substandard diets and for adults with a recognized cause of chronic blood loss. Except for infants, in whom the use of supplemented formulas is routine, the use of "over-the-counter" mixtures of vitamins and minerals to prevent iron deficiency is to be discouraged. Also to be discouraged are multicomponent preparations, since the availability of their iron for absorption may be reduced.

Therapy with Oral Iron; Preparations, Dosage, and Untoward Effects. Orally administered ferrous sulfate, the least expensive of iron preparations, is the treatment of choice for iron deficiency (Fairbanks *et al.*, 1971; Callender, 1974; Bothwell *et al.*, 1979). Ferrous salts are absorbed about three times as well as ferric salts, and the discrepancy becomes even greater at high dosage (Brise and Hallberg, 1962). Variations in the particular ferrous salt have relatively little effect on bioavailability, and the sulfate, fumarate, succinate, gluconate, and other ferrous salts are absorbed to approximately the same extent.

Preparations and Dosage. Ferrous sulfate (*iron sulfate;* FEOSOL, others) is the hydrated salt, $FeSO_4 \cdot 7H_2O$, which contains 20% iron. It is available as tablets, timed-release preparations, syrups, elixirs, and drops. *Dried ferrous sulfate* (30% elemental iron) is also available in a variety of dosage forms. *Ferrous fumarate* (FEOSTAT, others) contains 33% iron and is moderately soluble in water, stable, and almost tasteless. It is available in tablets, controlled-release capsules, drops, and suspensions. *Ferrous gluconate* (FERGON, others) has also been successfully used in the therapy of iron-deficiency anemia. The gluconate contains 12% iron, and is available in tablets, capsules, and elixirs. The effective dose of all of these preparations is based on iron content.

Other iron compounds have utility in fortification of foods. Reduced iron (metallic iron, elemental iron) is considered as effective as ferrous sulfate, provided the material employed has a small particle size (Elwood, 1968; Cook *et al.*, 1973). Large-particle *ferrum reductum* and iron phosphate salts have a much lower bioavailability (Cook *et al.*, 1973), and their use for the fortification of foods is undoubtedly responsible for some of the confusion concerning effectiveness. Ferric edetate has been shown to have a suitable bioavailability and to have advantages for maintenance of the normal appearance and taste of food (Viteri *et al.*, 1978).

The amount of iron, rather than the mass of the total salt in iron tablets, is important. It is also essential that the coating of the tablet dissolves rapidly in the stomach. Enteric-coated tablets are virtually worthless but are still being marketed. Surprisingly, since iron is usually absorbed in the upper small intestine, certain delayed-release preparations have been reported to be effective and have been said to be even more effective than ferrous sulfate when taken with meals. However, reports of absorption from such preparations vary. Because a number of different forms of delayed-release preparations are on the market and information on their bioavailability is limited, the effectiveness of most such preparations must be considered questionable.

A variety of substances designed to enhance the absorption of iron have been marketed, including surface-acting agents, carbohydrates, inorganic salts, amino acids, and vitamins. One of the more popular of these is ascorbic acid. When present in an amount of 200 mg or more, ascorbic acid increases the absorption of medicinal iron by at least 30% (Brise and Hallberg, 1962). However, the increased uptake is associated with a significant increase in the incidence of side effects (Hallberg *et al.*, 1966b), and, therefore, the addition of ascorbic acid seems to have little advantage over increasing the amount of iron administered. These compounded preparations confer no practical benefit. It is particularly undesirable to use preparations that contain other compounds with therapeutic actions of their own, such as vitamin B_{12}, folate, or cobalt, since the patient's response to the combination cannot be easily interpreted. Despite the straightforward nature of therapy with iron, it is discouraging to see the frequency with which expensive preparations with worthless additives are prescribed.

The usual therapeutic dose of iron is about 200 mg per day (2 to 3 mg/kg), based on the iron content of the preparation. In selecting the optimal dose for adults, allowance should be made for body size. Children weighing 15 to 30 kg can take half the average adult dose, and smaller children and infants can tolerate relatively larger doses of iron—for example, 5 mg/kg. The dose used is a practical compromise between the therapeutic action desired and the toxic effects. Prophylaxis and mild nutritional iron deficiency may be managed with modest doses. When the object is the prevention of iron deficiency in pregnant patients, for example, doses of 15 to 30 mg of iron per day, if not taken with meals, are adequate to meet the 3- to 6-mg daily requirement of the last two trimesters. When the purpose is to treat iron-deficiency anemia, but the circumstances do not demand haste, a total dose of about 100 mg (35 mg three times daily) may be used. The average dose for the treatment of iron-deficiency anemia is about 200 mg of iron per day, given in three equal doses of 65 mg.

Table 54–5. AVERAGE RESPONSE TO ORAL IRON

TOTAL DOSE *mg of iron per day*	ESTIMATED ABSORPTION %	ESTIMATED ABSORPTION *mg*	INCREASE IN HEMOGLOBIN *g/l of blood per day*
35	40	14	0.7
105	24	25	1.4
195	18	35	1.9
390	12	45	2.2

The responses expected for different dosage regimens of oral iron are given in Table 54–5. However, these effects are modified by the severity of the iron-deficiency anemia and by the time of ingestion of iron relative to meals. Absorption is optimal when the ferrous salt is taken when fasting. As noted previously, food variably reduces the availability of an iron salt, depending on the composition of the diet. Bioavailability of iron ingested with food is probably one half or one third of that seen in the fasting subject (Grebe *et al.*, 1975; Ekenved, 1976). Antacids also reduce the absorption of iron if given concurrently. It is always preferable to administer iron in the fasting state, even if the dose must be reduced because of gastrointestinal side effects. For patients who require maximal therapy to encourage a rapid response or to counteract continued bleeding, as much as 120 mg of iron may be administered four times a day. The timing of the dose is important. Sustained high rates of red-cell production require an uninterrupted supply of iron. Oral doses should be spaced equally in order to maintain a continuous high concentration of iron in plasma.

The duration of treatment is governed by the recovery of hemoglobin and the desire to create iron stores (Norrby, 1974). The former depends on the severity of the anemia. With a daily rate of repair of 2 g of hemoglobin per liter of whole blood, the red-cell mass is usually reconstituted within 1 to 2 months. Thus, the individual with a hemoglobin of 50 g per liter may achieve a normal complement of 150 g per liter in about 50 days, whereas the individual with a hemoglobin of 100 g per liter may take only half that time. The creation of stores of iron is a different matter, requiring many months of oral iron administration. The rate of absorption decreases rapidly after recovery from anemia and, after 3 to 4 months of treatment, stores may be increasing at a rate of not much more than 100 mg per month. Much of the strategy of continued therapy depends on the estimated future iron balance of the individual. The person with an inadequate diet may require continued therapy with low doses of iron. The individual whose bleeding has stopped will require no further therapy after the hemoglobin has returned to normal. For the individual with continued bleeding, long-term therapy is clearly indicated.

Untoward Effects of Oral Preparations of Iron. Contrary to many advertisements, intolerance to oral preparations of iron is primarily a function of the amount of soluble iron in the upper gastrointestinal tract and of psychological factors. Side effects include heartburn, nausea, upper gastric discomfort, constipation, and diarrhea. A good policy, particularly if there has been previous intolerance to iron, is to initiate therapy at a small dosage, to demonstrate freedom from symptoms at that level, and then gradually to increase the dosage to that desired. With a dose of 200 mg of iron per day divided into three equal portions, symptoms occur in approximately 25% of individuals, compared with an incidence of 13% among those receiving placebos; this increases to approximately 40% when the dosage of iron is doubled. Nausea and upper abdominal pain are increasingly common manifestations at high dosage (Sölvell, 1970). Constipation and diarrhea, perhaps related to iron-induced changes in the intestinal bacterial flora, are not more prevalent at higher dosage, nor is heartburn. If a liquid is given, one can place the iron solution on the back of the tongue with a dropper to prevent transient staining of teeth.

Toxicity caused by the long-continued administration of iron with the resultant production of iron overload (hemochromatosis) has been the subject of a number of case reports (*see* Bothwell *et al.*, 1979); this condition is the result of inappropriate therapy. Available evidence suggests that the normal individual is able to control absorption of iron despite high intake, and it is only individuals with underlying disorders that augment the absorption of iron who run the hazard of developing hemochromatosis. However, recent data indicate that hemochromatosis may be a relatively common genetic disorder, present in 0.5% of the population.

Iron Poisoning. Large amounts of ferrous salts of iron are toxic but, in adults, fatalities are rare and almost exclusively suicidal. Most deaths occur in childhood and particularly between the ages of 12 and 24 months (Fairbanks *et al.*, 1971; Bothwell *et al.*, 1979). As little as 1 to 2 g of iron may cause death, but 2 to 10 g is usually ingested in fatal cases. The frequency of iron poisoning relates to its availability in the household, particularly the supply that remains after a pregnancy. The colored sugar coating of many of the commercially available tablets gives them the appearance of candy. All iron preparations should be kept in childproof bottles.

Signs and symptoms of severe poisoning may occur within 30 minutes or may be delayed for several hours after ingestion. They consist largely of abdominal pain, diarrhea, or vomiting brown or bloody stomach contents containing pills. Of particular concern are pallor or cyanosis, lassitude, drowsiness, hyperventilation due to acidosis, and cardiovascular collapse. If death does not occur within 6 hours, there may be a transient period of apparent recovery, followed by death in 12 to 24 hours. The corrosive injury to the stomach may result in subsequent pyloric stenosis or gastric scarring. Hemorrhagic gastroenteritis and hepatic damage are prominent findings at autopsy. In the evaluation of the child who is thought to have ingested iron, a color test for iron in the gastric contents and an emergency determination of the concentration of iron in plasma can be performed. If the latter is less than 63 μM (3.5 mg per liter), the child is not in immediate danger. However, vomiting should be induced when there is iron in the stomach, and an x-ray should be taken to evaluate the number of pills remaining in the small bowel (iron tablets are radioopaque). Iron in the upper gastrointestinal tract can be precipitated by lavage with sodium bicarbonate or phosphate solution, although the clinical benefit is questionable. When the plasma concentration of iron is greater than the total iron binding capacity (63 μM; 3.5 mg per liter), deferoxamine should be administered; dosage and routes of administration are detailed in Chapter 66. Shock, dehydration, and acid–base abnormalities should be treated in the conventional manner. Most important is the speed of diagnosis and therapy. With earlier and more effective treatment, the mortality from iron poisoning has been reduced from as high as 45% to about 1% at the present time.

Therapy with Parenteral Iron; Preparations, Dosage, and Untoward Effects. Parenteral administration of iron is the alternative to the use of oral preparations (Fairbanks *et al.*, 1971; Callender, 1974; Bothwell *et al.*, 1979). The rate of response to parenteral therapy is similar to that which follows usual oral doses (Pritchard, 1966; Strickland *et al.*, 1977). One advantage is that iron stores may be created rapidly, something that would take months to achieve by the oral route. Its most important indications are in patients with a disease such as sprue, which prevents absorption of iron from the gastrointestinal tract, and in patients who are receiving parenteral nutrition. Parenteral iron may also be indicated when oral administration has an adverse effect on inflammatory disease of the bowel and, on rare occasions, when intolerance to oral iron prevents effective therapy. In chronic disease states, such as rheumatoid arthritis, the utilization of parenteral iron can be suboptimal because of the inflammatory block in reticuloendothelial iron transport. Other indications have been suggested that do not seem to be soundly based. These include the unsubstantiated beliefs that the response to parenteral iron is faster than that to oral iron and that patients undergoing dialysis (who absorb oral iron perfectly well) are better managed by the parenteral route. An exception to this may well be the need to use parenteral iron initially in patients with renal disease who are receiving erythropoietin. Otherwise, the supply of iron may become the rate-limiting factor in the response of the marrow to the hormone (Eschbach *et al.*, 1987).

Iron dextran injection (IMFERON, others) is the parenteral preparation currently in general use in the United States. It is a complex of ferric oxyhydroxide with dextrans of 5000 to 7000 daltons in a viscous solution containing 50 mg/ml of iron. Iron dextran is available in vials containing 0.5% phenol for intramuscular use and in ampuls for intramuscular or intravenous administration. When given intramuscularly, a variable portion (10 to 50%) may become fixed locally for many months. The remainder enters the blood, mostly through the lymphatic circulation, and elevates the concentration of iron in plasma for days or 1 or 2 weeks due to the presence of the iron–dextran complex. During this time determination of plasma iron does not indicate the amount of iron present on transferrin. The iron dextran must first be phagocytized by reticuloendothelial cells and the iron released from the sugar molecule of the dextran before it becomes available to the body. A portion of the processed iron is rapidly returned to the plasma and made available to the erythroid marrow; however, an even greater portion remains temporarily trapped within the reticuloendothelial cell (Henderson and Hillman, 1969). These iron dextran deposits are very gradually converted into a usable form of iron. While all iron is eventually used (Kernoff *et al.*, 1975), many months are required before this is complete, and, in the interim, iron dextran within the reticuloendothelial cell can confuse the physician who attempts to evaluate the iron status of the patient.

Intramuscular injection of iron dextran can be carried out with an initial test dose of 0.5 ml, followed by the administration of as much as 5 ml at a time, half the dose in each buttock. However, local reactions, including long-continued discomfort at the site of injection and local discoloration of the skin, and the concern about malignant change at the site of injection (Weinbren *et al.*, 1978), make intramuscular administration inappropriate except when the intravenous route is inaccessible.

Intravenous administration of iron dextran avoids the deposition of iron in muscle and local reactions at the site of injection. The technique of intravenous administration involves first the injection of 0.5 ml of iron dextran over a period of 5 minutes; the patient is then observed for 1 hour for signs or symptoms of anaphylaxis. Daily doses of 2 ml are then administered until the total calculated dose is reached. It is essential to administer the drug slowly and to stop the infusion immediately if the patient complains of perioral numbness, tingling, back pain, or chest pain. Alternatively, the total dose needed to reconstitute red-cell mass and tissue stores may be diluted in 250 to 1000 ml of 0.9% sodium chloride solution and administered in one infusion over several hours, although this technique is not approved in the United States. Such a dose (in milligrams) may be calculated from the following formula: 0.23 × bodyweight in kilograms × (150 − patient's hemoglobin in grams per liter) + 500 mg (to reconstitute iron stores). However, such calculations do not take into consideration the delay in the utilization of the material injected or the possibility of continued loss of iron.

Reactions to intravenous iron include headache, malaise, fever, generalized lymphadenopathy, arthralgias, urticaria, and, in some patients with rheumatoid arthritis, exacerbation of the disease. Phlebitis may occur with prolonged infusions of a concentrated solution or when an intramuscular preparation containing 0.5% phenol is used in error. Of greatest concern, however, is the rare anaphylactic reaction, which may be fatal in spite of treatment. While only a few such deaths have been reported, it remains a deterrent to the use of iron dextran. Thus, there must be specific indications for the parenteral administration of iron.

COPPER

Deficiency of copper is extremely rare in man (Underwood, 1971; Evans, 1973). The amount present in food is more than adequate to provide the needed body complement of slightly over 100 mg. There is no evidence that copper ever needs to be added to a normal diet, either prophylactically or therapeutically. Even in clinical states associated with hypocupremia (sprue, celiac disease, nephrotic syndrome), effects of copper deficiency are usually not demonstrable. However, anemia due to copper deficiency has been described in individuals who have undergone intestinal bypass surgery (Zidar *et al.*, 1977), in those who are receiving parenteral nutrition (Karpel and Peden, 1972; Dunlap *et al.*, 1974), in malnourished infants (Holtzman *et al.*, 1970; Graham and Cordano, 1976), and in patients ingesting excessive amounts of zinc (Hoffman *et al.*, 1988). While an inherited disorder affecting the transport of copper in man (Menkes' disease; steely hair syndrome) is associated with reduced activity of several copper-dependent enzymes, this disease is not associated with hematological abnormalities.

Copper deficiency in experimental animals interferes with the absorption of iron and its release from reticuloendothelial cells (Lee *et al.*, 1976). The associated microcytic anemia is related both to a decrease in the availability of iron to the normoblasts and, perhaps even more importantly, to a decreased mitochondrial production of heme. It may be that the specific defect in the latter case is a decrease in the activity of cytochrome oxidase. Other pathological effects involving the skeletal, cardiovascular, and nervous systems have been observed in deficient experimental animals (O'Dell, 1976). In man, the outstanding findings have been leukopenia, particularly granulocytopenia, and anemia. Concentrations of iron in plasma are variable, and the anemia is not always microcytic. When a low plasma copper concentration is determined in the presence of leukopenia and anemia and in a setting conducive to a deficiency of the element, a therapeutic trial with copper is appropriate. Daily doses up to 0.1 mg/kg of cupric sulfate have been given by mouth, or 1 to 2 mg per day may be added to the solution of nutrients for parenteral administration. Copper deficiency usually occurs concurrently with multiple nutritional deficiencies, so that its specific role in the production of anemia is usually difficult to ascertain.

COBALT

The administration of cobalt can produce polycythemia in experimental animals and man (Berk *et al.*, 1949). The same effect may be observed in patients with hematological disorders where the underlying proliferative capacity of the marrow is unimpaired (sickle-cell anemia, thalassemia, chronic infection, and renal disease) (Symposium, 1955). In the 1950s cobalt was used in doses as high as 200 to 300 mg of cobaltous chloride daily, given in divided doses by mouth to patients with various types of anemia. While beneficial effects did not occur in those with aplastic anemia, a response was observed in two patients with pure red-cell aplasia (Voyce, 1963). Cobalt deficiency has not been reported in man.

It is thought that cobalt acts by inhibition of enzymes involved in oxidative metabolism, resulting in tissue hypoxia and an increase in the secretion of erythropoietin. More specifically, cobalt blocks the conversion of pyruvate to acetyl coenzyme A and of α-ketoglutarate to succinate (Webb, 1962). Large amounts of cobaltous chloride depress the production of erythrocytes. Accidental intoxication in children may produce cyanosis, coma, and death.

PYRIDOXINE

The first case of pyridoxine-responsive anemia was described in 1956 by Harris and associates. Subsequent reports suggested that the vitamin might improve hematopoiesis in up to 50% of patients with either hereditary or acquired sideroblastic anemias (Horrigan and Harris, 1968; Harris and Kellermeyer, 1970). Characteristically, these patients show an impairment in hemoglobin synthesis and an accumulation of iron in the perinuclear mitochondria of erythroid precursor cells, so-called ringed sideroblasts. Hereditary sideroblastic anemia is an X-linked recessive trait with variable penetrance and expression. Affected males typically show a dual population of normal red cells and microcytic, hypochromic cells in the circulation. In contrast, idiopathic acquired sideroblastic anemia and the sideroblastosis seen in association with a number of drugs, inflammatory states, neoplastic disorders, and preleukemic syndromes show a variable morphological picture. Moreover, erythrokinetic studies demonstrate a spectrum of abnormalities, from a hypoproliferative defect with little tendency to accumulate iron to marked ineffective erythropoiesis with iron overload of the tissues (Solomon and Hillman, 1979a).

Oral therapy with pyridoxine is of proven benefit in correcting the sideroblastic anemias associated with the antituberculosis drugs isoniazid and pyrazinamide, which act as vitamin B_6 antagonists. A daily dose of 50 mg of pyridoxine completely corrects the defect without interfering with treatment, and routine supplementation of pyridoxine is often recommended (*see* Chapter 49). In contrast, if pyridoxine is given to counteract the sideroblastic abnormality associated with administration of levodopa, the effectiveness of levodopa in controlling Parkinson's disease is decreased. Pyridoxine therapy does not correct the sideroblastic abnormalities produced by chloramphenicol and lead.

Patients with idiopathic acquired sideroblastic anemia generally fail to respond to oral pyridoxine, and those individuals who appear to have a pyridoxine-responsive anemia require prolonged therapy with large doses of the vitamin, 50 to 500 mg per day. Unfortunately, the early enthusiasm for such treatment with pyridoxine was not reinforced by later studies (Chillar *et al.*, 1976; Solomon and Hillman, 1979a). Moreover, even when a patient responds, the improvement is only partial, since both the ring sideroblasts and the red-cell defect persist and the hematocrit rarely returns to normal. However, in view of the low toxicity of oral pyridoxine, a therapeutic trial with the agent is appropriate.

As shown in studies of normal man, oral pyridoxine in a dosage of 100 mg three times daily produces a maximal increase in red-cell pyridoxine kinase and the major pyridoxal phosphate–dependent enzyme glutamic-aspartic aminotransferase (Solomon and Hillman, 1978). For an adequate therapeutic trial, the drug must be administered for at least 3 months, while monitoring the response by means of the reticulocyte index and the concentration of hemoglobin. It has been suggested that the occasional patient who is refractory to oral pyridoxine will respond to parenteral administration of pyridoxal phosphate (Hines and Love, 1975). However, oral pyridoxine in doses of 200 to

300 mg per day produces intracellular concentrations of pyridoxal phosphate equal to or greater than those generated by therapy with the phosphorylated vitamin (Solomon and Hillman, 1979b). Pyridoxine is discussed further in Chapter 63.

RIBOFLAVIN

A pure red-cell aplasia that responded to the administration of riboflavin was reported in patients with protein depletion and complicating infections (Foy *et al.*, 1961). Lane and associates (1964) induced riboflavin deficiency in man and demonstrated that a hypoproliferative anemia resulted within a month. The spontaneous appearance in man of red-cell aplasia due to riboflavin deficiency is undoubtedly rare, if, in fact, it occurs at all. It has been described in combination with infection and protein deficiency, both of which are capable of producing a hypoproliferative anemia. However, it seems reasonable to include riboflavin in the nutritional management of patients with gross, generalized malnutrition. Riboflavin is discussed further in Chapter 63.

III. Vitamin B_{12}, Folic Acid, and the Treatment of Megaloblastic Anemias

Vitamin B_{12} and folic acid are dietary essentials for man. A deficiency of either vitamin results in defective synthesis of DNA in any cell that attempts chromosomal replication and division. Since tissues with the greatest rate of cell turnover show the most dramatic changes, the hematopoietic system is especially sensitive to deficiencies of these vitamins. Clinically, the earliest sign of deficiency is a megaloblastic anemia, where the derangement in DNA synthesis results in a characteristic morphological abnormality of the precursor cells in the bone marrow. Abnormal macrocytic red blood cells are the product, and the patient becomes severely anemic. Recognition of this pattern of abnormal hematopoiesis—more than 100 years ago—permitted the initial diagnostic classification of such patients as having "pernicious anemia" and the investigations that subsequently led to the discovery of the clinical value of vitamin B_{12} and folic acid. Even today, the characteristic abnormality in morphology is used both for diagnosis and as a therapeutic guide for administration of the vitamins.

History. The discovery of vitamin B_{12} and folic acid is a dramatic story that starts more than 150 years ago and includes two Nobel prize–winning discoveries (*see* Castle, 1961; Kass, 1976). The first descriptions of what must have been megaloblastic anemias are credited to Combe and Addison, who published several case reports between 1824 and 1855. Although Combe suggested that the disorder might have some relationship to digestion, it was Austin Flint who, in 1860, first described the severe gastric atrophy and called attention to its possible relationship to the anemia. The name *progressive pernicious anemia* was coined in 1872 by Biermer, and this colorful term has persisted: it is still common practice to describe the condition as Addisonian pernicious anemia.

Following the observation by Whipple in 1925 that liver is a source of a potent hematopoietic substance for iron-deficient dogs, Minot and Murphy carried out their Nobel prize–winning experiments that demonstrated the effectiveness of the feeding of liver in pernicious anemia. Within a few years, Castle defined the need for both an intrinsic factor, a substance secreted by the parietal cells of the gastric mucosa, and an extrinsic factor, the vitamin-like material provided by crude liver extracts. However, nearly 20 years passed before Rickes and coworkers and Smith and Parker isolated and crystallized vitamin B_{12}; Dorothy Hodgkin then determined its crystal structure by x-ray diffraction and subsequently received the Nobel prize for this work.

As attempts were being made to purify extrinsic factor, Wills and her associates described a macrocytic anemia in women in India that responded to a factor present in crude liver extracts but not in the purified fractions known to be effective in pernicious anemia (Wills and Bilimoria, 1932; Wills *et al.*, 1937). This factor, first called Wills' factor and later vitamin M, is now known to be folic acid. The actual term *folic acid* was coined by Mitchell and coworkers in 1941, following its isolation from leafy vegetables.

More recent work has shown that neither vitamin B_{12} nor folic acid as purified from foodstuffs is the active coenzyme for man. During extraction procedures, active, labile forms are converted to stable congeners of vitamin B_{12} and folic acid, cyanocobalamin and pteroylglutamic acid, respectively. These congeners must then be modified *in vivo* to be effective. While much has been learned of the intracellular metabolic pathways in which these vitamins participate, many questions remain to be answered, especially the relationship of vitamin B_{12} deficiency to the neurological abnormalities that occur with this disorder (Chanarin *et al.*, 1985).

Relationships between Vitamin B_{12} and Folic Acid. The major roles of vitamin B_{12} and folic acid in intracellular metabolism are summarized in Figure 54–6. Intracellular vitamin B_{12} is maintained as two active coenzymes: methylcobalamin and deoxyadenosylcobalamin (Stahlberg, 1967; Lin-

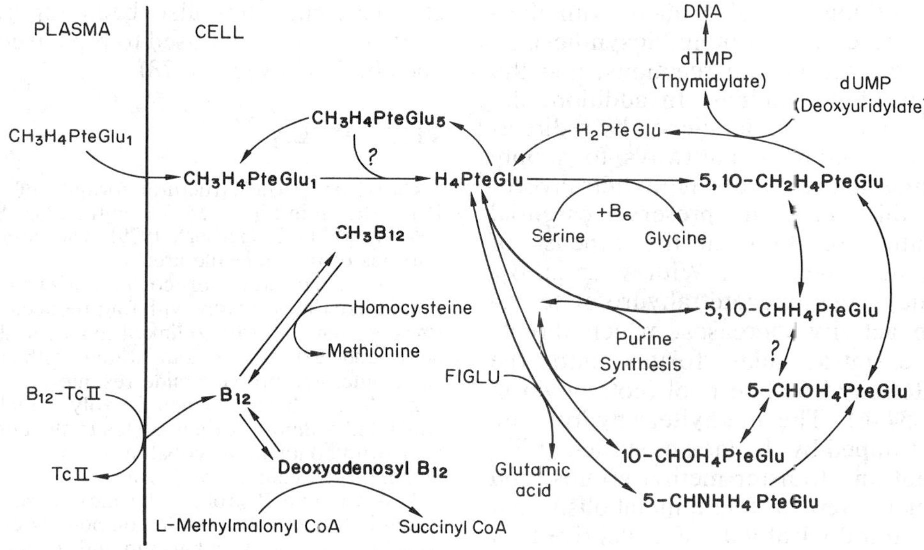

Figure 54–6. *Interrelationships and metabolic roles of vitamin B_{12} and folic acid.*

See text for explanation and Figure 54–9 for structures of the various folate coenzymes. *FIGLU* is formiminoglutamic acid, which arises from the catabolism of histidine.

nell *et al.*, 1971). Deoxyadenosylcobalamin is a cofactor for the mitochondrial mutase enzyme that catalyzes the isomerization of L-methylmalonyl CoA to succinyl CoA, an important reaction in both carbohydrate and lipid metabolism (Huennekens, 1968; Weissbach and Taylor, 1968). This reaction has no direct relationship to the metabolic pathways that involve folate. In contrast, methylcobalamin supports the methionine synthetase reaction, which is essential for normal metabolism of folate (Weir and Scott, 1983). Methyl groups contributed by methyltetrahydrofolate ($CH_3H_4PteGlu_1$) are used to form methylcobalamin, which then acts as a methyl group donor for the conversion of homocysteine to methionine. This folate–cobalamin interaction is pivotal for normal synthesis of purines and pyrimidines and, therefore, of DNA. The methionine synthetase reaction is largely responsible for the control of the recycling of folate cofactors; the maintenance of intracellular concentrations of folylpolyglutamates; and, through the synthesis of methionine and its product, S-adenosylmethionine, the maintenance of a number of methylation reactions.

Since methyltetrahydrofolate is the principal folate congener supplied to cells, the transfer of the methyl group to cobalamin is essential for the adequate supply of tetrahydrofolate ($H_4PteGlu_1$), the substrate for a number of metabolic steps. Tetrahydrofolate is a precursor for the formation of intracellular folylpolyglutamates; it also acts as the acceptor of a one-carbon unit in the conversion of serine to glycine, with the resultant formation of 5,10-methylenetetrahydrofolate (5,10-CH_2H_4PteGlu). The latter derivative donates the methylene group to deoxyuridylate for the synthesis of thymidylate—an extremely important reaction in DNA synthesis. In the process, the 5,10-CH_2H_4PteGlu is converted to dihydrofolate (H_2PteGlu). The cycle is then completed by the reduction of the H_2PteGlu to H_4PteGlu by dihydrofolate reductase, the step that is blocked by folate antagonists such as methotrexate (*see* Chapter 52). As shown in Figure 54–6, several other pathways also lead to the synthesis of 5,10-methylenetetrahydrofolate. These pathways are important in the metabolism of formiminoglutamic acid (FIGLU) and both purines and pyrimidines. (*See* reviews by Weir and Scott, 1983; Chanarin *et al.*, 1985).

In the presence of a deficiency of either vitamin B_{12} or folate, the decreased synthesis of methionine and S-adenosylmethionine interferes with protein biosynthesis, a number of methylation reactions, and the synthesis of polyamines. In addition, the cell responds to the deficiency by redirecting folate metabolic pathways to supply increasing amounts of methyltetrahydrofolate; this tends to preserve essential methylation reactions at the expense of nucleic acid synthesis. With vitamin B_{12} deficiency, methylenetetrahydrofolate reductase activity increases, which directs available intracellular folates into the methyltetrahydrofolate pool (not shown in Figure 54–6). The methyltetrahydrofolate is then trapped by the lack of sufficient B_{12} to accept and transfer methyl groups, and subsequent steps in folate metabolism that require tetrahydrofolate are deprived of substrate. This process provides a common basis for the development of a megaloblastic anemia with deficiency of either vitamin B_{12} or folic acid.

The mechanisms responsible for the neurological lesions of vitamin B_{12} deficiency are less well understood (Herbert and Tisman, 1973; Reynolds, 1976; Weir and Scott, 1983). Damage to the myelin sheath is the most obvious lesion in this neuropathy. This observation led to the early suggestion that the deoxyadenosyl B_{12}-dependent methylmalonyl CoA mutase reaction, a step in propionate metabolism, is related to the abnormality. However, more recent evidence suggests that the deficiency of methionine synthetase and the block of the conversion of methionine to S-adenosylmethionine is more likely to be responsible (Scott *et al.*, 1981).

Nitrous oxide (N_2O) can cause megaloblastic changes in the marrow and a neuropathy that resemble those of vitamin B_{12} deficiency (*see* Hoffbrand and Wickremasinghe, 1982; Chanarin *et al.*, 1985). Studies with N_2O in experimental animals and man have demonstrated a reduction in methionine synthetase and reduced concentrations of methionine and S-adenosylmethionine. The latter is necessary for methylation reactions, including those required for the synthesis of phospholipids and myelin. Significantly, the neuropathy induced with N_2O can be partially prevented by feeding methionine. A neuropathy similar to that occurring with vitamin B_{12} deficiency has also been reported in dentists who are exposed to N_2O used as an anesthetic (Layzer, 1978).

VITAMIN B_{12}

Chemistry. The structural formula of vitamin B_{12} is shown in Figure 54–7 (Smith, 1965; Skeggs, 1967; Pratt, 1972; Herbert, 1979). The three major portions of the molecule are:

1. A planar group or corrin nucleus—a porphyrin-like ring structure with four reduced pyrrole rings (designated *A* to *D*) linked to a central cobalt atom and extensively substituted with methyl, acetamide, and propionamide residues.
2. A 5,6-dimethylbenzimidazolyl nucleotide, which links almost at right angles to the corrin nucleus with bonds to the cobalt atom and to the propionate side chain of the D ring.
3. A variable R group—the most important of which is found in the stable compounds cyanocobalamin and hydroxocobalamin and the active coenzymes methylcobalamin and 5-deoxyadenosylcobalamin.

The terms *vitamin B_{12}* and *cyanocobalamin* are used interchangeably as generic terms for all the cobamides active in man. Preparations of vitamin B_{12} for therapeutic use contain either cyanocobalamin or hydroxocobalamin, since only these derivatives are stable with storage.

Metabolic Functions. The active coenzymes, methylcobalamin and 5-deoxyadenosylcobalamin, are essential for cell growth and replication. Methylcobalamin is required for the formation of methionine and its derivative S-adenosylmethionine from homocysteine. In addition, when concentrations of vitamin B_{12} are inadequate, folate becomes "trapped" as methyltetrahydrofolate to cause a functional deficiency of other vital intracellular forms of folic acid (*see* Figure 54–6 and discussion above). The hematological abnormalities that are observed in vitamin B_{12}–deficient patients are the result of this process (Herbert and Zalusky, 1962; Weir and Scott, 1983). 5-Deoxyadenosylcobalamin is required for the isomerization of L-methylmalonyl CoA to succinyl CoA.

Sources in Nature. Man depends on exogenous sources of vitamin B_{12} (Herbert, 1973). In nature, the only original source is certain microorganisms that grow in soil, sewage, water, or the intestinal lumen, and that synthesize the vitamin. Vegetable products are free of vitamin B_{12} unless they

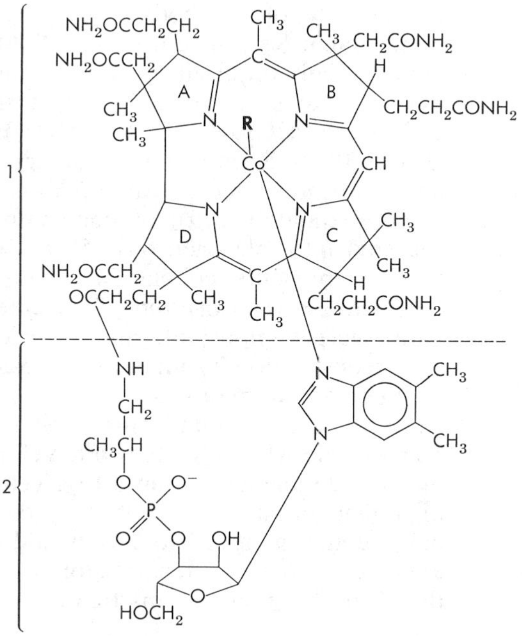

VITAMIN B_{12} CONGENERS

Permissive Name	R Group
Cyanocobalamin (Vitamin B_{12})	—CN
Hydroxocobalamin	—OH
Methylcobalamin	—CH_3
5′-Deoxyadenosyl-cobalamin	—5′-Deoxyadenosyl

Figure 54–7. *The structure and nomenclature of vitamin B_{12} congeners.* (*See* text for explanation.)

are contaminated with such microorganisms, so that animals are dependent on synthesis in their own alimentary tract or the ingestion of animal products containing vitamin B_{12}. In man, the daily nutritional requirement of 3 to 5 μg must be obtained from animal byproducts in the diet. At the same time, strict vegetarians rarely develop vitamin B_{12} deficiency. A certain amount of vitamin B_{12} is available from legumes, which are contaminated with bacteria capable of synthesizing vitamin B_{12}, and vegetarians generally fortify their diets with a wide range of vitamins and minerals.

Absorption, Distribution, Elimination, and Daily Requirements. The development of vitamin B_{12} deficiency during adult life is not usually the result of a deficient diet; rather, it reflects some defect in gastrointestinal absorption (*see* Figure 54–8). Classical Addisonian pernicious anemia is caused by a loss of gastric parietal-cell function and production of the glycoprotein gastric intrinsic factor, often called the intrinsic factor of Castle in recognition of his major contributions to the field (*see* Castle, 1953). The parietal cells may fail because of the presence of cytotoxic autoantibodies (de Aizpurua *et al.*, 1983). Dietary vitamin B_{12}, in the presence of gastric acid and pancreatic proteases, is released from a salivary binding protein and is immediately bound to intrinsic factor, a glycoprotein with a molecular weight of 59,000. The vitamin B_{12}–intrinsic factor complex then reaches the ileum, where it interacts with a specific receptor on ileal mucosal cells and is transported to the circulation. Intrinsic factor, bile, and sodium bicarbonate (a suitable pH) are required for ileal transport of vitamin B_{12} (Allen and Mehlman, 1973; Herzlich and Herbert, 1984).

Any of a number of intestinal diseases or defects can interfere with the absorption of the intrinsic factor–B_{12} complex (Beck, 1985). The combination of gastric achlorhydria and decreased secretion of intrinsic factor secondary to gastric atrophy or gastric surgery is a common cause of vitamin B_{12} deficiency in adults. The requirement for pancreatic proteases to release vitamin B_{12} from binding proteins, such that it can then bind to intrinsic factor, explains the malabsorption of the vitamin in pancreatic disorders (Allen *et al.*, 1978; Herzlich and Herbert, 1984). Antibodies to intrinsic factor or to the intrinsic factor–B_{12} complex may also play a role in impaired uptake by ileal cells. Bacterial overgrowth or certain

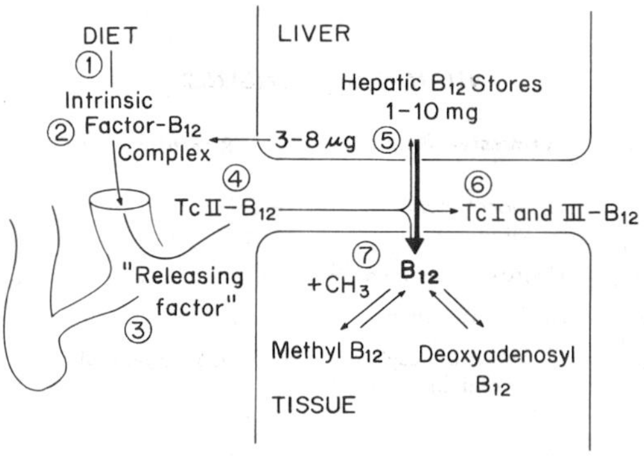

Figure 54–8. *The absorption and distribution of vitamin B_{12}.*

Deficiency of vitamin B_{12} can result from a congenital or acquired defect in any one of the following: (*1*) inadequate dietary supply; (*2*) inadequate secretion of intrinsic factor (classical pernicious anemia); (*3*) ileal disease: (*4*) congenital absence of transcobalamin II (Tc II); or (*5*) rapid depletion of hepatic stores by interference with reabsorption of vitamin B_{12} excreted in bile. The utility of measurements of the concentration of vitamin B_{12} in plasma to estimate supply available to tissues can be compromised by liver disease and (*6*) the appearance of abnormal amounts of transcobalamins I and III (Tc I and III) in plasma. Finally, the formation of methylcobalamin requires (*7*) normal transport into cells and an adequate supply of folic acid as $CH_3H_4PteGlu_1$.

intestinal parasites can prevent an adequate supply of B_{12} from reaching the ileum. Finally, any damage to ileal mucosal cells by disease or surgical procedures can interfere with absorption.

Once absorbed, vitamin B_{12} binds to transcobalamin II, a plasma β-globulin, for transport to tissues. Two other transcobalamins (I and III) are also present in plasma; their concentrations are related to the rate of turnover of granulocytes. They may represent intracellular storage proteins that are released with cell death (Scott *et al.*, 1974). Vitamin B_{12} bound to transcobalamin II is rapidly cleared from plasma and is preferentially distributed to hepatic parenchymal cells. The liver is thus a storage depot for other tissues. In the normal adult, as much as 90% of the body's stores of vitamin B_{12}, from 1 to 10 mg, is in the liver (Chanarin *et al.*, 1966). Vitamin B_{12} is stored as the active coenzyme with a turnover rate of 0.5 to 8 μg per day, depending on the size of the body stores (Heyssel *et al.*, 1966; Reizenstein *et al.*, 1966). The minimal daily requirement of the vitamin is estimated to be as little as 1 μg (Sullivan and Herbert, 1965; FAO/WHO Expert Group, 1970). Recommended dietary allowances are presented in Table XVI–1.

Approximately 3 μg of cobalamins are secreted into bile each day, 50 to 60% of which represents cobalamin analogs not destined for reabsorption. This enterohepatic cycle is important, since interference with reabsorption by intestinal disease can result in a continuous depletion of hepatic stores of the vitamin. This process may help explain why patients will develop vitamin B_{12} deficiency within 3 to 4 years following major gastric surgery even though a daily requirement of 1 to 2 μg would not be expected to deplete hepatic stores of more than 2 to 3 mg during this time.

The supply of vitamin B_{12} available for tissues is directly related to the size of the hepatic storage pool and the amount of vitamin B_{12} bound to transcobalamin II. Since vitamin B_{12} in liver cannot be easily measured, the concentration of vitamin B_{12} in plasma is the best routine measure of B_{12} deficiency. Normal individuals have plasma concentrations of the vitamin ranging from 150 to 660 pM (about 200 to 900 pg/ml), while a deficiency should be suspected whenever the value falls below 150 pM. The correlation is excellent except when the concentrations of transcobalamin I and III in the plasma increase—for example, as a result of hepatic disease or a myeloproliferative disorder. Inasmuch as the vitamin B_{12} bound to these transport proteins has a very slow turnover and, therefore, is relatively unavailable to cells, tissues can become deficient at a time when the concentration of vitamin B_{12} in plasma is normal or even high (Retief *et al.*, 1967). A congenital absence of transcobalamin II has been observed in at least two families (Hakami *et al.*, 1971; Hitzig *et al.*, 1974). In the children, megaloblastic anemia was present despite relatively normal concentrations of vitamin B_{12} in plasma. At the same time, the children responded to doses of parenteral vitamin B_{12} that were sufficient to exceed renal clearance.

Defects in intracellular metabolism of vitamin B_{12} have been reported in children with methylmalonic aciduria and homocystinuria. Mechanisms involved may include an incapacity of cells to transport vitamin B_{12} or accumulate the vitamin because of a failure to synthesize an intracellular acceptor, a defect in the formation of deoxyadenosylcobalamin, or a congenital lack of methylmalonyl CoA isomerase (Cooper, 1976).

Vitamin B_{12} Deficiency. Vitamin B_{12} deficiency is recognized clinically by its impact on both the hematopoietic and the nervous systems. The sensitivity of the hematopoietic system relates to its high rate of turnover of cells. Other tissues with high rates of cell turnover (*e.g.*, mucosa and cervical epithelium) have similar high requirements for the vitamin.

As a result of an inadequate supply of vitamin B_{12}, DNA replication becomes highly abnormal. Once a hematopoietic stem cell is committed to enter a programmed series of cell divisions, the defect in chromosomal replication results in an inability of maturing cells to complete nuclear divisions while cytoplasmic maturation continues at a relatively normal rate. This results in the production of morphologically abnormal cells or death of cells during maturation, a phenomenon referred to as ineffective hematopoiesis (Finch *et al.*, 1956). From the clinical viewpoint, these abnormalities are readily identified by examination of the bone marrow and peripheral blood. Usually, the changes are most marked for the red-cell series. The marrow shows proliferation of red-cell precursors that is appropriate to the severity of the anemia, but maturation is highly abnormal (megaloblastic erythropoiesis). Those cells that do leave the marrow are also abnormal, and many cell fragments, poikilocytes, and macrocytes appear in the peripheral blood. The mean red-cell volume increases to values greater than 110 fl (μm^3). When deficiency is marked, all cell lines may be affected, and a pronounced pancytopenia results.

The diagnosis of a vitamin B_{12}–deficiency state can be made by determination of the concentration of vitamin B_{12} in plasma and by tests of gastric function. Measurements of gastric acidity provide only indirect evidence of a defect in parietal-cell function, while the Schilling test can be used to quantitate ileal absorption of vitamin B_{12}. In addition, the Schilling test performed after the oral administration of intrinsic factor can help to delineate the mechanism of the abnormality of absorption (Schilling, 1953). A less commonly used index of vitamin B_{12} deficiency is the measurement of methylmalonate in serum or urine. Finally, the observation of reticulocytosis following a therapeutic trial of vitamin B_{12} confirms the diagnosis.

Vitamin B_{12} deficiency can result in irreversible damage to the nervous system. Progressive swelling of myelinated neurons, demyelination, and cell death are seen in the spinal column and cerebral cortex. This causes a wide range of neurological signs and symptoms, including paresthesias of the hands and feet, diminutions of vibration and position senses with resultant unsteadiness, decreased deep-tendon reflexes, and, in the later stages, loss of memory, confusion, moodiness, and even a loss of central vision. The patient may exhibit delusions, hallucinations, or even an overt psychosis. Since the neurological damage can be dissociated from the changes in the hematopoietic system, vitamin B_{12} deficiency must be considered as a possibility in elderly patients with dementia and psychiatric disorders, even if they are not anemic (Lindenbaum *et al.*, 1988). The ease of measurement of the concentration of vitamin B_{12} in plasma and the awareness of the medical profession of the causes of vitamin B_{12} deficiency make possible an earlier and more accurate diagnosis of B_{12}-deficient states, earlier therapy, and, hence, avoidance of irreversible neurological complications.

Preparations, Dosage, and Routes of Administration. Vitamin B_{12} is available in pure form for injection or oral administration or in combination with other vitamins and minerals for oral or parenteral administration. The choice of a preparation must always be made with recognition of the cause of the deficiency. Although oral preparations may be used to supplement deficient diets, they are of little value in the treatment of patients with deficiency of intrinsic factor or ileal disease. Even though small amounts of vitamin B_{12} may be absorbed by simple diffusion, the oral route of administration cannot be relied upon for effective therapy in the patient with a marked deficiency of B_{12} and abnormal hematopoiesis or neurological deficits. Therefore, the preparation of choice for treatment of a vitamin B_{12}–deficiency state is cyanocobalamin, and it should be given by intramuscular or deep subcutaneous injection.

Cyanocobalamin injection (REDISOL, RUBRAMIN PC, others) is a clear aqueous solution with a characteristic red color. The aqueous solution is available in concentrations of 30, 100, and 1000 $\mu g/ml$. Cyanocobalamin injection is extremely safe when given by the intramuscular or deep subcutaneous route, but it should never be given intravenously. There have been rare reports of transitory exanthema and anaphylaxis following injection. Therefore, if a patient reports a previous sensitivity to injections of vitamin B_{12}, an intradermal skin test should be carried out before the full dose is administered.

Cyanocobalamin is administered in doses of 1 to 1000 μg. Tissue uptake, storage, and utilization depend on the availability of transcobalamin II (*see* above). Doses in excess of 100 μg are rapidly cleared from plasma into the urine, and administration of larger amounts of vitamin B_{12} will not result in greater retention of the vitamin. Administration of 1000 μg is of value, however, in the performance of the Schilling test. After isotopically labeled vitamin B_{12} is administered orally, the compound that is absorbed can be quantitatively recovered in the urine if 1000 μg of cyanocobalamin is administered intramuscularly. This unlabeled material saturates the transport system and tissue binding sites, so that more than 90% of the labeled and unlabeled vitamin is excreted during the next 24 hours.

A number of multivitamin preparations are marketed either as nutritional supplements or for the treatment of anemia. Many of these contain up to 80 μg of cyanocobalamin without or with intrinsic factor concentrate prepared from the stomachs of hogs or other domestic animals. Purified preparations of intrinsic factor are standardized according to their ability to promote vitamin B_{12} absorption in patients with pernicious anemia. One oral unit of intrinsic factor is defined as that amount of material that will bind and transport 15 μg of cyanocobalamin. Most multivitamin preparations supplemented with intrinsic factor contain 0.5 oral unit per tablet. While the combination of oral vitamin B_{12} and intrinsic factor would appear to be ideal for patients with an intrinsic factor deficiency, such preparations are not reliable. Antibodies to human intrinsic factor may effectively counteract absorption of vitamin B_{12}. With prolonged therapy, some patients develop refractoriness to oral intrinsic factor, perhaps related to production of an intraluminal antibody against the hog protein (Ramsey and Herbert, 1965). Patients taking such preparations must be reevaluated at periodic intervals for recurrence of pernicious anemia.

Hydroxocobalamin given in doses of 100 μg intramuscularly has been reported to have a more sustained effect than cyanocobalamin, with a single dose maintaining plasma vitamin B_{12} concentrations in the normal range for up to 3 months. However, some patients show reductions of the concentration of B_{12} in plasma within 30 days, similar to that seen after cyanocobalamin. Furthermore, the administration of hydroxocobalamin has resulted in the formation of antibodies to the transcobalamin II–vitamin B_{12} complex (Skouby *et al.*, 1971). *Hydroxocobalamin* (CODROXOMIN, others) is therefore not recommended.

General Principles of Therapy. Vitamin B_{12} has an undeserved reputation as a health tonic and has been used for a number of diverse disease states. Effective use of the vitamin depends on accurate diagnosis and an understanding of the following general principles of therapy:

1. Vitamin B_{12} should be given prophylactically only when there is a reasonable indication. Dietary deficiency in the strict vegetarian, the predictable malabsorption of vitamin B_{12} in patients who have had a gastrectomy, and certain diseases of the small intestine constitute such indications. When gastrointestinal function is normal, an oral prophylactic supplement of vitamins and minerals, including vitamin B_{12}, may be indicated. Otherwise, the patient should receive monthly injections of cyanocobalamin.

2. The relative ease of treatment with vitamin B_{12} should not prevent a full investigation of the etiology of the disease. The initial diagnosis is usually suggested by a macrocytic anemia or an unexplained neuropsychiatric disorder. Full understanding of the etiology of the disease state involves studies of dietary supply, gastrointestinal absorption, and transport.

3. Therapy should always be as specific as possible. While a large number of multivitamin preparations are available, the use of "shotgun" vitamin therapy in the treatment of vitamin B_{12} deficiency can be dangerous. With such therapy, there is the danger that sufficient folic acid will be given to result in a hematological recovery. This can mask continued vitamin B_{12} deficiency and permit neurological damage to develop or progress.

4. Although a classical therapeutic trial with small amounts of vitamin B_{12} can help confirm the diagnosis, the acutely ill, elderly patient may not be able to tolerate the delay in the correction of a severe anemia. Such patients require supplemental blood transfusions and immediate therapy with both folic acid and vitamin B_{12} to guarantee rapid recovery.

5. Long-term therapy with vitamin B_{12} must be evaluated at intervals of 6 to 12 months in patients who are otherwise well. If there is an additional illness or a condition that may increase the requirement for the vitamin (*e.g.*, pregnancy), reassessment should be performed more frequently.

Treatment of the Acutely Ill Patient. The therapeutic approach depends on the severity of the patient's illness. The individual with uncomplicated pernicious anemia, in which the abnormality is restricted to a mild or moderate anemia without leukopenia, thrombocytopenia, or neurological signs or symptoms, will respond quite well to the administration of vitamin B_{12} alone. Moreover, therapy may be delayed until other causes of megaloblastic anemia have been ruled out and sufficient studies of gastrointestinal function have been performed to reveal the underlying cause of the disease. In this situation, a therapeutic trial with small amounts of parenteral vitamin B_{12} (1 to 10 μg per day) can confirm the presence of an uncomplicated vitamin B_{12} deficiency.

In contrast, patients with neurological changes or severe leukopenia or thrombocytopenia associated with infection or bleeding require emergency treatment. The older individual with a severe anemia (hematocrit less than 20%) is likely to have tissue hypoxia, cerebrovascular insufficiency, and congestive heart failure. Effective therapy must not wait for detailed diagnostic tests. Once the megaloblastic erythropoiesis has been confirmed and sufficient blood collected for later measurements of concentrations of vitamin B_{12} and folic acid, the patient should receive intramuscular injections of 100 μg of cyanocobalamin and 1 to 5 mg of folic acid. For the next 1 to 2 weeks the patient should receive daily intramuscular injections of 100 μg of cyanocobalamin, together with a daily oral supplement of 1 to 2 mg of folic acid. Since an effective increase in red-cell mass will not occur for 10 to 20 days, the patient with a markedly depressed hematocrit and tissue hypoxia should also receive a transfusion of 2 to 3 units of packed red cells. If congestive heart failure is present, phlebotomy to remove an equal volume of whole blood can be performed or diuretics can be administered to prevent volume overload.

The therapeutic response to vitamin B_{12} is characterized by a number of subjective and objective changes. Patients usually report an increased sense of well-being within the first 24 hours after the initiation of therapy. Objectively, memory and orientation can show dramatic improvement, although full recovery of mental function may take months or, in fact, may never occur. In addition, even before an obvious hematological response is apparent, the patient may report an increase in strength, a better appetite, and an improvement in the soreness of the mouth and tongue.

The first objective hematological change is the disappearance of the megaloblastic morphology of the bone marrow. As the ineffective erythropoiesis is corrected, the concentration of iron in plasma falls dramatically as the metal is used in the formation of hemoglobin. This usually occurs within the first 48 hours. Full correction of precursor maturation in marrow with production of an increased number of reticulocytes begins about the second or third day and reaches a peak 3 to 5 days later. When the anemia is moderate to severe, the maximal reticulocyte index will be between three and five times the normal value—that is, a reticulocyte count of 20 to 40% (Hillman *et al.*, 1968). The ability of the marrow to sustain a high rate of production determines the rate of recovery of the hematocrit. Patients with complicating iron deficiency, an infection or other inflammatory state, or renal disease may be unable to correct their anemia. It is important, therefore, to monitor the reticulocyte index over the first several weeks. If it does not continue at elevated levels while the hematocrit is less than 35%, plasma concentrations of iron and folic acid should again be determined and the patient reevaluated for an illness that could inhibit the response of the marrow.

During recovery from a vitamin B_{12}–related thrombocytopenia, the platelet count rises within 10 days to values that exceed normal. This overshoot is a typical response to the correction of an ineffective thrombocytopoietic state. The recovery of the white blood cells is less dramatic. In the absence of infection, the granulocyte count reverts to normal within the first 2 weeks, and large multilobed polymorphonuclear leukocytes gradually disappear from the circulation. Even though the turnover of circulating granulocytes is less than 8 to 12 hours, the continued presence of multilobed polymorphonuclear leukocytes in the peripheral blood reflects continued entry of abnormal cells from the granulocytic pool of the marrow.

Usually, the degree and rate of improvement of neurological signs and symptoms depend on the severity and the duration of the abnormalities. Those that have been present for only a few months disappear quite rapidly. When a defect has been present for months or years, full return to normal function may never occur.

Long-term Therapy with Vitamin B_{12}. Once begun, vitamin B_{12} therapy must be maintained for life. This fact must be impressed upon the patient and family, and a system should be established to guarantee continued monthly injections of cyanocobalamin. An intramuscular injection of 100 μg of cyanocobalamin every 2 to 4 weeks is sufficient to maintain a normal concentration of vitamin B_{12} in plasma and an adequate supply for tissues. Patients with severe neurological symptoms and signs may be treated with larger doses of vitamin B_{12} in the period immediately following the diagnosis. Doses of 100 μg per day or several times per week may be given for several months with the hope of encouraging faster and more complete recovery, although whether recovery is more rapid has not been proven. It is important to monitor vitamin B_{12} concentrations in plasma and to obtain peripheral blood counts at intervals of 3 to 6 months to confirm the adequacy of therapy. Since refractoriness to therapy can develop at any time, evaluation must continue throughout the patient's life.

Other Therapeutic Uses of Vitamin B_{12}. Vitamin B_{12} has been used in the therapy of a number of conditions, including trigeminal neuralgia, multiple sclerosis and other neuropathies, various psychiatric disorders, poor growth or nutrition, and as a "tonic" for patients complaining of tiredness or easy fatigability. There is no evidence for the validity of such therapy in any of these conditions. Maintenance therapy with vitamin B_{12} has been used with some apparent success in the treatment of children with methylmalonic aciduria (Cooper, 1976).

FOLIC ACID

Chemistry and Metabolic Functions. The structural formula of pteroylglutamic acid ($PteGlu_1$) is shown in Figure 54–9. Major portions of the molecule include a pteridine ring linked by a methylene bridge to paraaminobenzoic acid, which is joined by an amide linkage to glutamic acid. While pteroylglutamic acid is the common pharmaceutical form of folic acid, it is neither the principal folate congener in food nor the active coenzyme for intracellular metabolism. Following absorption, $PteGlu_1$ is rapidly reduced at the 5, 6, 7, and 8 positions to tetrahydrofolic acid ($H_4PteGlu_1$), which then acts as an acceptor of a number of one-carbon units. These are attached at either the 5 or the 10 position of the pteridine ring or bridge these atoms to form a new five-membered ring. The most important forms of the coenzyme that are synthesized by these reactions are listed in Figure 54–9. Each plays a specific role in intracellular metabolism, summarized as follows (*see also* previous section on Relationships between Vitamin B_{12} and Folic Acid, as well as Figure 54–6):

1. *Conversion of homocysteine to methionine.* This reaction requires $CH_3H_4PteGlu$ as a methyl donor and utilizes vitamin B_{12} as a cofactor.

2. *Conversion of serine to glycine.* This reaction requires tetrahydrofolate as an acceptor of a methylene group from serine and utilizes pyridoxal phosphate as a cofactor. It results in the formation of 5,10-$CH_2H_4PteGlu$, an essential coenzyme for the synthesis of thymidylate.

3. *Synthesis of thymidylate.* $CH_3H_4PteGlu$ donates a methyl group to deoxyuridylate for the synthesis of thymidylate—a rate-limiting step in DNA synthesis.

4. *Histidine metabolism.* $H_4PteGlu$ also acts as an acceptor of a formimino group in the conversion of formiminoglutamic acid to glutamic acid.

5. *Synthesis of purines.* Two steps in the synthesis of purine nucleotides require the participation of derivatives of folic acid. Glycinamide ribonucleotide is formylated by 5,10-$CHH_4PteGlu$; 5-aminoimidazole-4-carboxamide ribonucleotide is formylated by 10-$CHOH_4PteGlu$. By these reactions carbon atoms at positions 8 and 2, respectively, are incorporated into the growing purine ring.

6. *Utilization or generation of formate.* This reversible reaction utilizes $H_4PteGlu$ and 10-$CHOH_4PteGlu$.

Daily Requirements. Virtually all food sources are rich in folates, especially fresh green vegetables, liver, yeast, and some fruits. However, protracted cooking can destroy up to 90% of the folate content of such food (Herbert, 1973). Generally, a standard U.S. diet provides 50 to 500 μg of absorbable folate per day, although individuals with high intakes of fresh vegetables and meats will ingest as much as 2 mg per day. In the normal adult, the minimal daily requirement has been estimated at 50 μg, while the pregnant or lactating female and patients with high rates of cell turnover (such as patients with a hemolytic anemia) may require as much as 100 to 200 μg or

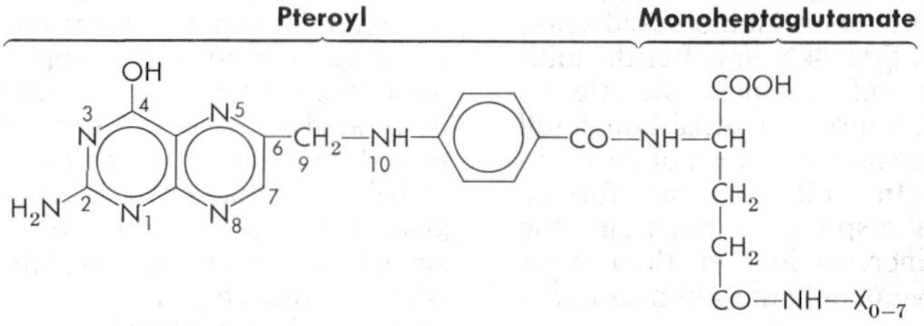

Position	Radical	Congener	
N^5	$—CH_3$	$CH_3H_4PteGlu$	Methyltetrahydrofolate
N^5	—CHO	5-$CHOH_4PteGlu$	Folinic acid (Citrovorum Factor)
N^{10}	—CHO	10-$CHOH_4PteGlu$	10-Formyltetrahydrofolate
N^{5-10}	—CH—	5,10-$CHH_4PteGlu$	5,10-Methenyltetrahydrofolate
N^{5-10}	$—CH_2—$	5,10-$CH_2H_4PteGlu$	5,10-Methylenetetrahydrofolate
N^5	—CHNH	$CHNHH_4PteGlu$	Formiminotetrahydrofolate
N^{10}	$—CH_2OH$	$CH_2OHH_4PteGlu$	Hydroxymethyltetrahydrofolate

Figure 54–9. *The structures and nomenclature of pteroylglutamic acid (folic acid) and congeners.*

See text for explanation. *X* represents additional residues of glutamate; polyglutamates are storage forms of the vitamin. The subscript that designates the number of residues of glutamate is frequently omitted because this number is variable.

more per day. Recommended dietary allowances of folate are presented in Table XVI–1.

Absorption, Distribution, and Elimination. As with vitamin B_{12}, diagnosis and management of deficiencies of folic acid depend on an understanding of the transport pathways and intracellular metabolism of the vitamin (Figure 54–10). Folates present in food are largely in the form of reduced polyglutamates (Tamura and Stokstad, 1973), and absorption requires transport and the action of a pteroyl-γ-glutamyl carboxypeptidase associated with mucosal cell membranes (Rosenberg, 1976). The mucosae of the duodenum and upper part of the jejunum are rich in dihydrofolate reductase and are capable of methylating most, if not all, absorbed, reduced folate. Since most absorption occurs in the proximal portion of the small intestine, it is not unusual for folate deficiency to occur when the jejunum is diseased.

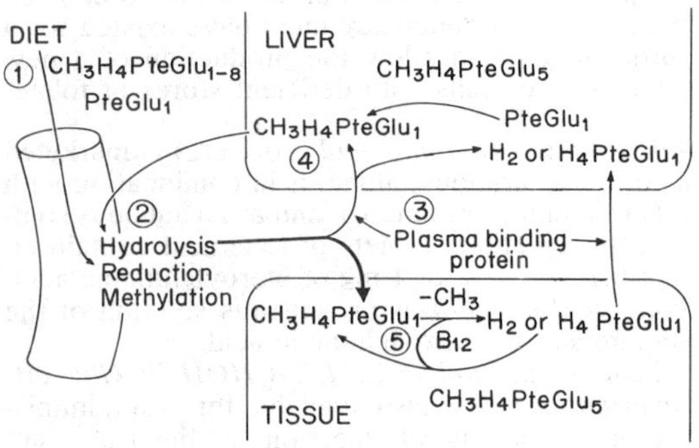

Figure 54–10. *Absorption and distribution of folate derivatives.*

Dietary sources of folate polyglutamates are hydrolyzed to the monoglutamate, reduced, and methylated to $CH_3H_4PteGlu_1$ during gastrointestinal transport. Folate deficiency commonly results from *(1)* inadequate dietary supply and *(2)* small intestinal disease. In patients with uremia, alcoholism, or hepatic disease there may be defects in *(3)* the concentration of folate binding proteins in plasma and *(4)* the flow of $CH_3H_4PteGlu_1$ into bile for reabsorption and transport to tissue (the folate enterohepatic cycle). Finally, vitamin B_{12} deficiency will *(5)* "trap" folate as $CH_3H_4PteGlu$, thereby reducing the availability of $H_4PteGlu_1$ for its essential roles in purine and pyrimidine synthesis.

Nontropical and tropical sprue are common causes of folate deficiency and megaloblastic anemia (Wellcome Trust Collaborative Study, 1971).

Once absorbed, folate is rapidly transported to tissues as $CH_3H_4PteGlu_1$. While certain plasma proteins do bind folate derivatives, they have a greater affinity for nonmethylated analogs. The role of such binding proteins in folate homeostasis is not well understood (Rothenberg *et al.*, 1977). An increase in binding capacity is detectable during deficiency of folate and in certain disease states, such as uremia, cancer, and alcoholism, but how binding affects transport and tissue supply requires further investigation.

A constant supply of $CH_3H_4PteGlu_1$ is maintained by food and by an enterohepatic cycle of the vitamin. The liver actively reduces and methylates $PteGlu_1$ (and H_2 or $H_4PteGlu_1$) and then transports the $CH_3H_4PteGlu_1$ into bile for reabsorption by the gut and subsequent delivery to tissues (Steinberg *et al.*, 1979). This pathway may provide as much as 200 μg or more of folate each day for recirculation to tissues. The importance of the enterohepatic cycle is suggested by studies in animals that show a rapid reduction of the concentration of folate in plasma following either drainage of bile or ingestion of alcohol, which apparently block the release of $CH_3H_4PteGlu_1$ from hepatic parenchymal cells (Hillman *et al.*, 1977).

Following uptake into cells by a process of receptor-mediated endocytosis (Kamen *et al.*, 1988), $CH_3H_4PteGlu$ acts as a methyl donor for the formation of methylcobalamin and as a source of $H_4PteGlu$ and other folate congeners, as described above. Folate is stored within cells as polyglutamates (Baugh and Krumdieck, 1969; Hoffbrand *et al.*, 1977).

Folate Deficiency. Folate deficiency is a common complication of diseases of the small intestine, which interfere with the absorption of folate from food and the recirculation of folate through the enterohepatic cycle. In acute or chronic alcoholism, daily intake of folate in food may be severely restricted, and the enterohepatic cycle of the vitamin may be impaired by the toxic effect of alcohol on hepatic parenchymal cells; this is perhaps the most common cause of folate-deficient megaloblastic erythropoiesis. However, it is also the most amenable to therapy, inasmuch as the reinstitution of a normal diet is sufficient to overcome the effect of alcohol. Disease states characterized by a high rate of cell turnover, such as hemolytic anemias, may also be complicated by deficiency of folate (Lindenbaum, 1977). Additionally, drugs that inhibit dihydrofolate reductase (*e.g.*, methotrexate, trimethoprim) or that interfere with the absorption and storage of folate in tissues (*e.g.*, certain anticonvulsants, oral contraceptives) are capable of lowering the concentration of folate in plasma and at times may cause a megaloblastic anemia (Stebbins *et al.*, 1973; Stebbins and Bertino, 1976).

Folate deficiency is recognized by its impact on the hematopoietic system. As with vitamin B_{12}, this fact reflects the increased requirement associated with high rates of cell turnover. The megaloblastic anemia that results from folate deficiency cannot be distinguished from that caused by a deficiency of vitamin B_{12}. This finding is to be expected, because of the final common pathway of the major intracellular metabolic roles of the two vitamins. At the same time, folate deficiency is rarely if ever associated with neurological abnormalities. Thus, the observation of characteristic abnormalities in vibratory and position sense and in motor and sensory pathways rules against the presence of an isolated deficiency of folic acid.

The appearance of megaloblastic anemia following deprivation of folate is much more rapid than that caused by the interruption of the absorption of vitamin B_{12} (*e.g.*, gastric surgery). This observation reflects the fact that stores of folate are quite limited *in vivo*. In Herbert's classical study of a single normal individual maintained on a diet low in folate for several months, megaloblastic erythropoiesis appeared after approximately 10 to 12 weeks (Herbert, 1962). Subsequent studies have shown that the rate of induction of megaloblastic erythropoiesis varies according to the population studied and the dietary background of the individual (Eichner *et al.*, 1971). A folate deficiency state may appear in 1 to 4 weeks, depending on the individual's dietary habits and stores of the vitamin.

Folate deficiency is best diagnosed from measurements of folate in plasma and in red cells by use of a microbiological assay or a competitive binding technique. The concentration of folate in plasma is extremely sensitive to changes in dietary intake of the vitamin and the influence of inhibitors of folate metabolism or transport, such as alcohol. Normal folate concentrations in plasma range from 9 to 45 nM (4 to 20 ng/ml). A deficiency state may be considered to be present whenever the value is below 9 nM. In the case of the alcoholic, the plasma folate concentration falls rapidly to values indicative of deficiency within 24 to 48 hours of steady ingestion of alcohol, while megaloblastic erythropoiesis becomes apparent after 1 to 2 weeks (Eichner and Hillman, 1971, 1973). At the same time, the plasma folate concentration will quickly revert to normal once such ingestion is stopped, even while the marrow is still megaloblastic. Such rapid fluctuations tend to detract from the clinical utility of the plasma folate concentration. Measurement of folate in red cells or the adequacy of stores in lymphocytes (by use of the deoxyuridine suppression test) may be employed to diagnose a longstanding deficiency of folic acid (Herbert *et al.*, 1973). (In this test, deoxyuridine fails to suppress the synthesis of DNA if normal amounts of folate are present in the cells.) For either test to be positive, a state of deficiency must have existed for a sufficient time to allow the production of a new population of cells with deficient stores of folate.

Preparations. *Folic acid* (FOLVITE) is marketed as oral preparations, alone or in combination with other vitamins or minerals, and as an aqueous solution for injection. Tablets of folic acid contain either 0.1, 0.4, 0.8, or 1 mg of pteroylglutamic acid. *Folic acid injection* is an aqueous solution of the sodium salt of pteroylglutamic acid.

Leucovorin (*folinic acid, 5-CHOH$_4$PteGlu, citrovorum factor*) is also available for oral administration or parenteral injection as the Ca^{2+} salt (WELLCOVORIN). Tablets contain either 5, 10, 15, or 25 mg of leucovorin. The principal indication for the use of folinic acid is to circumvent the action of inhibitors of dihydrofolate reductase, such as methotrexate (*see* Chapter 52). It is not indicated for use in the treatment of folic acid deficiency. Certainly, leucovorin should never be used for the treatment of pernicious anemia or other megaloblastic anemias secondary to a deficiency of vitamin B_{12}. Just as with folic acid, its use can result in an apparent response of the hematopoietic system, but neurological damage may occur or progress if already present.

Untoward Effects. There have been rare reports of reactions to parenteral injections of both folic acid and leucovorin. If a patient describes a history of a reaction before the drug is given, caution should be exercised. Oral folic acid is not toxic for man. Even with doses as high as 15 mg per day, there have been no substantiated reports of side effects. Folic acid in large amounts may counteract the antiepileptic effect of phenobarbital, phenytoin, and primidone and increase the frequency of seizures in susceptible children (Reynolds, 1968). While some studies have not supported these contentions, the U.S. Food and Drug Administration has recommended that oral tablets of folic acid be limited to strengths of 1 mg or less.

General Principles of Therapy. The therapeutic use of folic acid is limited to the prevention and treatment of deficiencies of the vitamin. As with vitamin B_{12} therapy, effective use of the vitamin depends on accurate diagnosis and an understanding of the mechanisms that are operative in a specific disease state. The following general principles of therapy should be respected:

1. Prophylactic administration of folic acid should be undertaken only when there is a clear indication. Dietary supplementation is necessary when there is an increased requirement that is not satisfied by normal dietary sources. Pregnancy, with the increased demands of the fetus, or lactation, where as much as 50 μg of folate is lost each day in the breast milk, is an indication for supplementation with folate. The most popular form of supplementation for this situation is a multivitamin preparation that contains 400 to 500 μg of pteroylglutamic acid. Patients with a disease state characterized by high levels of cell turnover (*e.g.*, a hemolytic anemia) should also receive folic acid prophylactically, usually one or two 1-mg tablets of folic acid each day. Patients receiving total parenteral nutrition should also receive a daily folic acid supplement.

2. As with vitamin B_{12} deficiency, any patient with folate deficiency and a megaloblastic anemia should be carefully evaluated to determine the underlying cause of the deficiency state. This should include evaluation of the effects of medications, the amount of alcohol intake, the patient's history of travel, and the function of the gastrointestinal tract.

3. Therapy should always be as specific as possible. Multivitamin preparations should be avoided unless there is good reason to suspect deficiency of several vitamins.

4. The potential of mistreating a patient who has vitamin B_{12} deficiency with folic acid must be kept in mind. The administration of large doses of folic acid can result in an apparent improvement of the megaloblastic anemia, inasmuch as PteGlu is converted by dihydrofolate reductase to $H_4PteGlu_1$; this circumvents the methylfolate "trap." However, folate therapy does not prevent or alleviate the neurological defects of vitamin B_{12} deficiency, and these may progress and become irreversible.

Treatment of the Acutely Ill Patient. As described in detail in the section on vitamin B_{12}, treatment of the patient who is acutely ill with megaloblastic anemia should begin with intramuscular injections of both vitamin B_{12} and folic acid. Inasmuch as the patient requires therapy before the exact cause of the disease has been defined, it is important to avoid the potential problem of a combined deficiency of both vitamin B_{12} and folic acid. When both are present, therapy with only one vitamin will not provide an optimal response. Longstanding nontropical sprue is one example of a disease in which combined deficiency of B_{12} and folate is common. When indicated, both vitamin B_{12} (100 μg) and folic acid (1 to 5 mg) should be administered intramuscularly, immediately, and the patient should then be maintained on daily oral supplements of 1 to 2 mg of folic acid for the next 1 to 2 weeks. Recommendations for administration of vitamin B_{12} are described above.

Oral administration of folate is generally satisfactory for all patients who are not acutely ill, regardless of the cause of the deficiency state. Even the patient with tropical or nontropical sprue and a demonstrable defect in absorption of folic acid will respond adequately to such therapy. Abnormalities in the activity of pteroyl-γ-glutamyl carboxypeptidase and the function of mucosal cells will not prevent passive diffusion of sufficient amounts of PteGlu across the mucosal barrier if dosage is adequate, and continued ingestion of alcohol or other drugs will also not prevent an adequate therapeutic response. The effect of most inhibitors of folate transport or dihydrofolate reductase is easily overcome by administration of pharmacological doses of the vitamin. Perhaps the only situation in which this tenet is not true is when vitamin C is severely deficient. The patient with scurvy may suffer from a megaloblastic anemia despite increased intake of folate and normal or high concentrations of the vitamin in plasma and cells.

The therapeutic response may be monitored by study of the hematopoietic system in a fashion identical to that described for vitamin B_{12}. Within 48 hours of the initiation of appropriate therapy, megaloblastic erythropoiesis disappears and, as efficient erythropoiesis begins, the concentration of iron in plasma falls to normal or below-normal values. The reticulocyte count begins to rise on the second or third day and reaches a peak by the fifth to seventh day; the reticulocyte index reflects the proliferative state of the marrow. Finally, the hematocrit begins to rise during the second week.

It is possible to use this reliable pattern of recovery as the basis for a therapeutic trial. For this purpose, the patient should receive a daily parenteral injection of 50 to 100 μg of folic acid. Administration of doses in excess of 100 μg per day entails the risk of inducing a hematopoietic response in patients who are deficient in vitamin B_{12}, while oral administration of the vitamin may be unreliable because of intestinal malabsorption. A number of other complications may also interfere with the therapeutic trial. The patient with sprue and deficiencies of other vitamins or iron may fail to respond because of these inadequacies. In cases of alcoholism, the presence of hepatic disease, inflammation, or iron deficiency can act to blunt the proliferative response of the marrow and to prevent the correction of the anemia. For these reasons, the therapeutic trial for the evaluation of the patient with a potential deficiency of folic acid has not gained great popularity.

Allen, R. H., and Mehlman, C. S. Isolation of gastric vitamin B_{12}–binding proteins using affinity chromatography. I. Purification and properties of human intrinsic factor. *J. Biol. Chem.*, **1973**, *248*, 3660–3669.

Allen, R. H.; Seetharam, B.; Allen, N. C.; Podell, E. R.; and Alpers, D. H. Correction of cobalamin malabsorption in pancreatic insufficiency with a cobalamin analogue that binds with high affinity to R protein but not to intrinsic factor. *J. Clin. Invest.*, **1978**, *61*, 1628–1634.

Baugh, C. M., and Krumdieck, C. L. Naturally occurring folates. *Ann. N.Y. Acad. Sci.*, **1969**, *186*, 7–28.

Berk, L.; Burchenal, J. H.; and Castle, W. B. Erythropoietic effect of cobalt in patients with or without anemia. *N. Engl. J. Med.*, **1949**, *240*, 754–761.

Björn-Rasmussen, E.; Hallberg, L.; Isaksson, B.; and Arvidsson, B. Food iron absorption in man. Applications of the two-pool extrinsic tag method to measure haem and non-haem iron absorption from the whole diet. *J. Clin. Invest.*, **1974**, *53*, 247–255.

Blaud, P. Sur les maladies chlorotiques, et sur un mode de traitement, spécifique dans ces affections. *Rev. Med. Fr. Etrang.*, **1832**, *1*, 337–367.

Bradley, T. R., and Metcalf, D. The growth of mouse bone marrow cells *in vitro*. *Aust. J. Exp. Biol. Med. Sci.*, **1966**, *44*, 287–300.

Brandt, S. J.; Peters, W. P.; Atwater, S. K.; Kurtzberg, J.; Borowitz, M. J.; Jones, R. B.; Shpall, E. J.; Bast, R. C., Jr.; Gilbert, C. J.; and Oette, D. H. Effect of recombinant human granulocyte-macrophage colony-stimulating factor on hematopoietic reconstitution after high-dose chemotherapy and autologous bone marrow transplantation. *N. Engl. J. Med.*, **1988**, *318*, 869–876.

Brise, H., and Hallberg, L. Absorbability of different iron compounds. *Acta Med. Scand.*, **1962**, *171*, Suppl. 376, 23–38. (*See also* related articles by these authors, pp. 7–22 and 51–58.)

Bronchurd, M. H.; Scarffe, J. H.; Thatcher, N.; Crowther, D.; and Dexter, M. Phase I/II study of recombinant human granulocyte colony stimulating factor in patients receiving intensive chemotherapy for small cell lung cancer. *Br. J. Cancer*, **1987**, *56*, 807–813.

Carnot, P., and Deflandre, C. Sur l'activité hémopoiétique de sérum au cours de la régenération du sang. *C.R. Acad. Sci. (III)*, **1906**, *143*, 384–386.

Casey, J. L., and others. Iron responsive elements: regulatory RNA elements control RNA levels and translation. *Science*, **1988**, *240*, 924–928.

Chanarin, I.; Hutchinson, M.; MacLean, N.; and Moule, M. Hepatic folate in man. *Br. Med. J.*, **1966**, *1*, 396–399.

Chillar, R. K.; Johnson, C. S.; and Beutler, E. Erythrocyte pyridoxine kinase levels in patients with sideroblastic anemia. *N. Engl. J. Med.*, **1976**, *295*, 881–883.

Christian, H. A. A sketch of the history of the treatment of chlorosis with iron. *Med. Lib. Hist. J.*, **1903**, *1*, 176–180.

Cook, J. D.; Finch, S. A.; and Smith, N. Evaluation of the iron status of a population. *Blood*, **1976**, *48*, 449–455.

Cook, J. D.; Minnich, V.; Moore, C. V.; Rasmussen, A.; Bradley, W. B.; and Finch, C. A. Absorption of fortification iron in bread. *Am. J. Clin. Nutr.*, **1973**, *26*, 861–872.

Cook, J. D.; Skikne, B. S.; Lynch, S. R.; and Reusser, M. E. Estimates of iron sufficiency in the U.S. population. *Blood*, **1986**, *68*, 726–731.

Dallman, P. R.; Siimes, M. A.; and Stekel, A. Iron deficiency in infancy and childhood. *Am. J. Clin. Nutr.*, **1980**, *33*, 86–118.

D'Andrea, A. D.; Lodish, H. F.; and Wong, G. G. Expression cloning of the murine erythropoietin receptor. *Cell*, **1989**, *57*, 277–285.

de Aizpurua, H. J.; Cosgrove, L. H.; Ungar, B.; and Tah, B. H. Autoantibodies cytotoxic to gastric parietal cells in serum of patients with pernicious anemia. *N. Engl. J. Med.*, **1983**, *309*, 625–629.

Dunlap, W. M.; James, G. W., III; and Hume, D. M. Anemia and neutropenia caused by copper deficiency. *Ann. Intern. Med.*, **1974**, *80*, 470–476.

Eckardt, K.-U. and Bauer, C. Erythropoietin in health and disease. *Eur. J. Clin. Invest.*, **1989**, *19*, 117–127.

Eichner, E. R., and Hillman, R. S. The evolution of anemia in alcoholic patients. *Am. J. Med.*, **1971**, *50*, 218–232.

———. The effect of alcohol on the serum folate level. *J. Clin. Invest.*, **1973**, *52*, 584–591.

Eichner, E. R.; Pierce, I.; and Hillman, R. S. Folate balance in dietary induced megaloblastic anemia. *N. Engl. J. Med.*, **1971**, *284*, 933–938.

Ekenved, G. Iron absorption studies: studies on oral iron preparations using serum iron and different radioiron isotope techniques. *Scand. J. Haematol.*, **1976**, Suppl. 28, 7–97.

Eschbach, J. W.; Egrie, J. C.; Downing, M. R.; Browne, J. K.; and Adamson, J. W. Correction of the anemia of end stage renal disease with recombinant human erythropoietin: results of a combined phase I and II clinical trial. *N. Engl. J. Med.*, **1987**, *316*, 73–78.

Eschbach, J. W.; Kelly, M. R.; Haley, N. R.; Abels, R. I.; and Adamson, J. W. Treatment of the anemia of progressive renal failure with recombinant human erythropoietin. *N. Engl. J. Med.*, **1989**, *321*, 158–162.

FAO/WHO Expert Group. Requirements of ascorbic acid, vitamin D, vitamin B_{12}, folate and iron. *WHO Tech. Rep. Ser.*, **1970**, *452*, 3–75.

Finch, C. A. Iron metabolism. In, *Nutrition Reviews' Present Knowledge in Nutrition*, 4th ed. (Hegsted, D. M., ed.) The Nutrition Foundation, Inc., New York, **1976**, pp. 280–289.

———. Anemia of chronic disease. *Postgrad. Med.*, **1978**, *64*, 107–113.

Finch, C. A.; Colman, D. H.; Motulsky, A. G.; Donohue, D. M.; and Reiff, R. H. Erythrokinetics in pernicious anemia. *Blood,* **1956,** *11,* 807–820.

Finch, C. A.; Cook, J. D.; Labbe, R. F.; and Culala, M. Effect of blood donation on iron stores as evaluated by serum ferritin. *Blood,* **1977,** *50,* 441–447.

Fischl, M., and others. Recombinant human erythropoietin therapy for AIDS patients treated with AZT: a double-blind, placebo-controlled clinical study. *N. Engl. J. Med.,* **1990,** In Press.

Ford, C. E.; Hamerton, J. L.; Barnes, D. W. H.; and Loutit, J. T. Cytological identification of radiation chimeras. *Nature,* **1956,** *177,* 452–454.

Foy, H.; Kondi, A.; and MacDougall, L. Pure red-cell aplasia in marasmus and kwashiorkor treated with riboflavin. *Br. Med. J.,* **1961,** *1,* 937–941.

Gabrilove, J. L., and others. Effect of granulocyte colony-stimulation factor on neutropenia and associated morbidity of chemotherapy for transitional cell carcinoma of the urethelium. *N. Engl. J. Med.,* **1988,** *318,* 1414–1422.

Garcia, J. F.; Ebbe, S. N.; Hollander, L.; Cutting, H. O.; Miller, M. E.; and Cronkite, E. P. Radioimmunoassay of erythropoietin: circulatory levels in normal and polycythemic human beings. *J. Lab. Clin. Med.,* **1982,** *99,* 624–635.

Goodnough, L.T., and others. Increased preoperative collection of autologous blood with recombinant human erythropoietin therapy. *N. Engl. J. Med.,* **1989,** *321,* 1163–1168.

Grebe, C.; Martinez-Torres, C.; and Layrisse, M. Effect of meals and ascorbic acid on the absorption of a therapeutic dose of iron as ferrous and ferric salts. *Curr. Ther. Res.,* **1975,** *17,* 382–397.

Green, R.; Charlton, R. W.; Seftel, H.; Bothwell, T.; Mayet, F.; Adams, B.; Finch, C.; and Layrisse, M. Body iron excretion in man. A collaborative study. *Am. J. Med.,* **1968,** *45,* 336–353.

Groopman, J. E.; Mitsuyasu, R. T.; DeLeo, M. J.; Oette, D. H.; and Golde, D. Effect of recombinant human granulocyte macrophage colony stimulating factor on myelopoiesis in the acquired immunodeficiency syndrome. *N. Engl. J. Med.,* **1987,** *317,* 593–598.

Groopman, J.E.; Molina, J.-M.; and Scadden, D. T. Hematopoietic growth factors. Biology and clinical applications. *N. Engl. J. Med.,* **1989,** *321,* 1449–1459.

Haden, R. J. Historical aspects of iron therapy in anemia. *J.A.M.A.,* **1939,** *111,* 1059–1061.

Hahn, P. F.; Bale, W. F.; Ross, J. F.; Balfour, W. M.; and Whipple, G. H. Radioactive iron absorption by the gastrointestinal tract: influence of anemia, anoxia and antecedent feeding; distribution in growing dogs. *J. Exp. Med.,* **1943,** *78,* 169–188.

Hakami, N.; Nieman, P. E.; Canellos, G. P.; and Lazerson, J. Neonatal megaloblastic anemia due to inherited transcobalamin II deficiency in two siblings. *N. Engl. J. Med.,* **1971,** *285,* 1163–1170.

Hallberg, L.; Hogdahl, A. M.; Nilsson, L.; and Rybo, G. Menstrual blood loss and iron deficiency. *Acta Med. Scand.,* **1966a,** *180,* 639–650.

Hallberg, L.; Ryttinger, L.; and Sölvell, L. Side effects of oral iron therapy. A double blind study of different iron compounds in tablet form. *Acta Med. Scand.,* **1966b,** *181,* Suppl. 459, 3–10.

Henderson, P. A., and Hillman, R. S. Characteristics of iron dextran utilization in man. *Blood,* **1969,** *34,* 357–375.

Herbert, V. Experimental nutritional folate deficiency in man. *Trans. Assoc. Am. Physicians,* **1962,** *75,* 307–320.

Herbert, V.; Tisman, G.; Go, L. T.; and Brenner, L. The dU suppression test using ^{125}I-UdR to define biochemical megaloblastosis. *Br. J. Haematol.,* **1973,** *24,* 713–723.

Herbert, V., and Zalusky, R. Interrelations of vitamin B_{12} and folic acid metabolism: folic acid clearance studies. *J. Clin. Invest.,* **1962,** *41,* 1263–1276.

Heyssel, R. M.; Bozian, R. C.; Darby, W. J.; and Bell, M. C. Vitamin B_{12} turnover in man: the assimilation of vitamin B_{12} from natural foodstuff by man and estimates of minimal daily dietary requirements. *Am. J. Clin. Nutr.,* **1966,** *18,* 176–184.

Hillman, R. S.; Adamson, J.; and Burka, E. Characteristics of B_{12} correction of the abnormal erythropoiesis of pernicious anemia. *Blood,* **1968,** *31,* 419–432.

Hillman, R. S., and Giblett, E. R. Red cell membrane alteration associated with marrow stress. *J. Clin. Invest.,* **1965,** *44,* 1730–1736.

Hillman, R. S., and Henderson, P. A. Control of marrow production by relative iron supply. *J. Clin. Invest.,* **1969,** *48,* 454–460.

Hillman, R. S.; McGuffin, R.; and Campbell, C. Alcohol interference with the folate enterohepatic cycle. *Trans. Assoc. Am. Physicians,* **1977,** *90,* 145–156.

Hines, J. D., and Love, D. L. Abnormal vitamin B_6 metabolism in sideroblastic anemia: effect of pyridoxal phosphate (PLP) therapy. *Clin. Res.,* **1975,** *23,* 403A.

Hitzig, W. H.; Dohmann, U.; Pluss, H. J.; and Vischer, D. Hereditary transcobalamin II deficiency: clinical findings in a new family. *J. Pediatr.,* **1974,** *85,* 622–628.

Hoffbrand, A. V.; Tripp, E.; and Lavoie, A. Folate polyglutamate synthesis and breakdown in cells. In, *Folic Acid: Proceedings of a Workshop on Human Folate Requirements, 1975.* National Academy of Sciences, Washington, D. C., **1977,** pp. 110–121.

Hoffman, H. N.; Phyliky, R. L.; and Fleming, C. R. Zinc-induced copper deficiency. *Gastroenterology,* **1988,** *94,* 508–512.

Holtzman, N. A.; Charache, P.; Cordano, A.; and Graham, G. G. Distribution of serum copper in copper deficiency. *Johns Hopkins Med. J.,* **1970,** *126,* 34–42.

Huebers, H.; Huebers, E.; Csiba, E.; Rummel, W.; and Finch, C. A. The significance of transferrin for intestinal iron absorption. *Blood,* **1983,** *61,* 283–290.

Huennekens, F. M. Folate and B_{12} coenzymes. In, *Biological Oxidation.* (Singer, T. P., ed.) John Wiley & Sons, Inc., New York, **1968,** pp. 439–513.

Huff, R. L.; Hennessy, T. G.; Austin, R. E.; Garcia, J. F.; Roberts, B. M.; and Lawrence, J. H. Plasma and red cell iron turnover in normal subjects and in patients having various hematopoietic disorders. *J. Clin. Invest.,* **1950,** *29,* 1041–1052.

Jacobs, K., and others. Isolation and characterization of genomic and cDNA clones of human erythropoietin. *Nature,* **1985,** *313,* 806–810.

Jacobsen, L. O.; Goldwasser, E.; Freed, W.; and Plzak, L. Role of the kidney in erythropoiesis. *Nature,* **1957,** *179,* 633–634.

Jacobsen, L. O.; Marks, E. K.; Gaston, E. O.; Robinson, M.; and Zirkle, R. E. The role of the spleen in radiation injury. *Proc. Soc. Exp. Biol. Med.,* **1949,** *70,* 740–742.

Kamen, B. A.; Wang, M.-T.; Streckfuss, A. J.; Peryea, X.; and Anderson, R. G. W. Delivery of folates to the cytoplasm of MA104 cells is mediated by a surface membrane receptor that recycles. *J. Biol. Chem.,* **1988,** *263,* 13602–13609.

Karpel, J. T., and Peden, V. H. Copper deficiency in long-term parenteral nutrition. *J. Pediatr.,* **1972,** *80,* 32–36.

Kawasaki, E. S., and others. Molecular cloning of a complementary DNA encoding human macrophage-specific colony-stimulating factor (CSF-l). *Science,* **1985,** *230,* 291–296.

Kernoff, L. M.; Dommisse, J.; and du Toit, E. D. Utilization of iron dextran in recurrent iron deficiency anaemia. *Br. J. Haematol.,* **1975,** *30,* 419–424.

Lane, M.; Alfrey, C. P.; Megel, C. E.; Doherty, M. A.;

and Doherty, J. The rapid induction of human riboflavin deficiency with galactoflavin. *J. Clin. Invest.*, **1964**, *43*, 357–373.

Latham, R. G. *The Works of Thomas Sydenham, M.D.*, Vol. 2. C. & J. Adlard, London, **1850**, p. 97.

Layzer, R. B. Myeloneuropathy after prolonged exposure to nitrous oxide. *Lancet*, **1978**, *2*, 1227–1230.

Lee, F.; Yokota, T.; Otsuka, T.; Gemmell, L.; Larson, N.; Luh, J.; Arai, K.; and Rennick, D. Isolation of cDNA for a human granulocyte-macrophage colony-stimulating factor by functional expression in mammalian cells. *Proc. Natl. Acad. Sci. U.S.A.*, **1985**, *82*, 4360–4364.

Lin, F. K., and others. Cloning and expression of the human erythropoietin gene. *Proc. Natl. Acad. Sci. U.S.A.*, **1985**, *82*, 7580–7585.

Lindenbaum, J. Folic acid requirement in situations of increased need. In, *Folic Acid: Proceedings of a Workshop on Human Folate Requirements, 1975*. National Academy of Sciences, Washington, D. C., **1977**, pp. 256–276.

Lindenbaum, J.; Healton, E. B.; Savage, D. G.; Brust, J. C.; Garrett, T. J.; Podell, E. R.; Marcell, P. D.; Stabler, S. P.; and Allen, R. H. Neuropsychiatric disorders caused by cobalamin deficiency in the absence of anemia or macrocytosis. *N. Engl. J. Med.*, **1988**, *318*, 1720–1728.

Lindsley, D. L.; Odell, T. T.; and Tausche, F. G. Implantation of functional erythropoietic elements following total body irradiation. *Proc. Soc. Exp. Biol. Med.*, **1955**, *90*, 512–515.

Linnell, J. C.; Hoffbrand, A. V.; Peters, T. T.; and Matthews, D. M. Chromatographic and bioautographic estimation of plasma cobalamins in various disturbances of vitamin B_{12} metabolism. *Clin. Sci.*, **1971**, *40*, 1–16.

Lipschitz, D. A.; Cook, J. D.; and Finch, C. A. A clinical evaluation of serum ferritin as an index of iron stores. *N. Engl. J. Med.*, **1974**, *290*, 1213–1216.

McCaffery, P. J.; Fraser, J. K.; Liu, F.-K.; and Berridge, M. V. Subunit structure of the erythropoietin receptor. *J. Biol. Chem.*, **1989**, *264*, 10507–10512.

Monsen, E. R.; Hallberg, L.; Layrisse, M.; Hegsted, D. M.; Cook, J. D.; Mertz, W.; and Finch, C. A. Estimation of available dietary iron. *Am. J. Clin. Nutr.*, **1978**, *31*, 134–141.

Neuroth, M. L., and Lee, C. O. A history of Blaud's pills. *J. Am. Pharm. Assoc., Sci. Ed.*, **1941**, *30*, 60–63.

Norrby, A. Iron absorption studies in iron deficiency. *Scand. J. Haematol.*, **1974**, Suppl. 20, 5–125.

Osgood, E. E. A unifying concept of the etiology of the leukaemias, lymphomas and cancers. *J. Natl. Cancer Inst.*, **1957**, *18*, 155–166.

Pluznik, D. H., and Sachs, L. The induction of clones of normal mast cells by a substance from conditioned medium. *Exp. Cell Res.*, **1966**, *43*, 553–563.

Powell, J. S.; Berkner, K. L.; Lebo, R. V.; and Adamson, J. W. Human erythropoietin gene: high level expression in stably transfected mammalian cells and chromosome localization. *Proc. Natl. Acad. Sci. U.S.A.*, **1986**, *83*, 6465–6469.

Pritchard, J. A. Hemoglobin regeneration in severe iron deficiency anemia. Response to orally and parenterally administered iron preparations. *J.A.M.A.*, **1966**, *195*, 717–720.

Ramsey, C., and Herbert, V. Dialysis assay for intrinsic factor and its antibody: demonstration of species specificity of antibodies to human and hog intrinsic factor. *J. Lab. Clin. Med.*, **1965**, *65*, 143–152.

Reissmann, K. R. Studies on the mechanism of erythropoietic stimulation in parabiotic rats during hypoxia. *Blood*, **1950**, *5*, 372–380.

Reizenstein, P.; Ek, G.; and Matthews, C. M. E. Vitamin B_{12} kinetics in man. Implications of total-body B_{12} determinations, human requirements and normal and pathological cellular B_{12} uptake. *Phys. Med. Biol.*, **1966**, *11*, 295–306.

Retief, F. P.; Gottlieb, C. W.; and Herbert, V. Delivery of $Co^{57}B_{12}$ to erythrocytes from alpha to beta globulin of normal, B_{12}-deficient, and chronic myeloid leukemia serum. *Blood*, **1967**, *29*, 837–851.

Reynolds, E. H. Mental effects of anticonvulsants and folic acid metabolism. *Brain*, **1968**, *91*, 197–214.

Rothenberg, S. P.; DaCosta, M.; and Fischer, C. Use and significance of folate binders. In, *Folic Acid: Proceedings of a Workshop on Human Folate Requirements, 1975*. National Academy of Sciences, Washington, D. C., **1977**, pp. 82–97.

Schilling, R. F. Intrinsic factor studies. II. The effect of gastric juice on the urinary excretion of radioactivity after the oral administration of radioactive vitamin B_{12}. *J. Lab. Clin. Med.*, **1953**, *42*, 860–866.

Scott, J. M.; Bloomfield, F. J.; Stebbins, R.; and Herbert, V. Studies on derivation of transcobalamin III from granulocytes. *J. Clin. Invest.*, **1974**, *53*, 228–239.

Scott, J. M.; Dinn, J. J.; Wilson, P.; and Weir, D. G. Pathogenesis of subacute combined degeneration: a result of methyl group deficiency. *Lancet*, **1981**, *2*, 334–337.

Skouby, A. P.; Hippe, E.; and Olesen, H. Antibody to transcobalamin II and B_{12} binding capacity in patients treated with hydroxycobalamin. *Blood*, **1971**, *38*, 769–774.

Solomon, L. R., and Hillman, R. S. Vitamin B_6 metabolism in human red blood cells. I. Variation in normal subjects. *Enzyme*, **1978**, *23*, 262–273.

———. Vitamin B_6 metabolism in idiopathic sideroblastic anaemia and related disorders. *Br. J. Haematol.*, **1979a**, *42*, 239–253.

———. Vitamin B_6 metabolism in anaemic and alcoholic man. *Ibid.*, **1979b**, *41*, 343–356.

Sölvell, L. Oral iron therapy—side effects. In, *Iron Deficiency: Pathogenesis, Clinical Aspects, Therapy*. (Hallberg, L.; Harwerth, H.-G.; and Vannotti, A.; eds.) Academic Press, Inc., New York, **1970**, pp. 573–583.

Stahlberg, K. G. Studies on methyl-B_{12} in man. *Scand. J. Haematol.*, **1967**, Suppl. 1, 3–99.

Stebbins, R.; Scott, J.; and Herbert, V. Drug-induced megaloblastic anemias. *Semin. Hematol.*, **1973**, *10*, 235–251.

Steinberg, S.; Campbell, C.; and Hillman, R. S. Kinetics of the normal folate enterohepatic cycle. *J. Clin. Invest.*, **1979**, *64*, 83–89.

Strickland, I. D.; DeSaintouge, C.; Boulton, F. E.; Francis, B.; Ronbikova, J.; and Waters, J. I. The therapeutic equivalence of oral and intravenous iron in renal dialysis patients. *Clin. Nephrol.*, **1977**, *7*, 55–57.

Sullivan, L. W., and Herbert, V. Studies on the minimum daily requirement for vitamin B_{12}: hematopoietic responses to 0.1 microgm. of cyanocobalamin or coenzyme B_{12} and comparison of their relative potency. *N. Engl. J. Med.*, **1965**, *272*, 340–346.

Tamura, T., and Stokstad, E. L. R. The availability of food folate in man. *Br. J. Haematol.*, **1973**, *25*, 513–532.

Vadhan-Raj, S.; Keating, M.; LeMaistre, A.; Hiltelman, W. W.; McCudie, K.; Tryillo, J. M.; Broxmeyer, H. E.; Herney, C.; and Gulterman, J. U. Effects of recombinant human granulocyte macrophage colony-stimulating factor in patients with myelodysplastic syndromes. *N. Engl. J. Med.*, **1987**, *317*, 1545–1552.

Viteri, F. E.; Garcia-Ibanez, R.; and Torun, B. Sodium iron NaFeEDTA as an iron fortification compound in Central America. Absorption studies. *Am. J. Clin. Nutr.*, **1978**, *31*, 961–971.

Voyce, M. A. A case of pure red-cell aplasia successfully treated with cobalt. *Br. J. Haematol.*, **1963**, *9*, 412–418.

Weinbren, K.; Salm, R.; and Greenberg, G. Intramuscular injections of iron compounds and oncogenesis in man. *Br. Med. J.*, **1978**, *1*, 683–685.

Weissbach, H., and Taylor, R. T. Metabolic role of vitamin B_{12}. *Vitam. Horm.*, **1968**, *26*, 395–412.

Wills, L., and Bilimoria, H. S. Studies in pernicious anaemia of pregnancy: production of macrocytic anaemia in monkeys by deficient feeding. *Indian J. Med. Res.*, **1932**, *20*, 391–402.

Wills, L.; Clutterbuck, P. W.; and Evans, P. D. F. A new factor in the production and cure of macrocytic anaemias and its relation to other haemopoietic principles curative in pernicious anaemia. *Biochem. J.*, **1937**, *31*, 2136–2147.

Wong, G. G., and others. Human GM-CSF: molecular cloning of the complementary DNA and purification of the natural recombinant proteins. *Science*, **1985**, *228*, 810–815.

Wu, A. M.; Till, J. E.; Siminovitch, L.; and McCulloch, E. A. A cytological study of the capacity for differentiation of normal haemopoietic colony forming cells. *J. Cell. Physiol.*, **1967**, *69*, 177–184.

Yang, Y. C., and others. Human IL-3 (multi-CSF): identification by expression cloning of a novel hematopoietic growth factor related to murine IL-3. *Cell*, **1986**, *47*, 3–10.

Zidar, B. L.; Shadduck, R. K.; Zeigler, Z.; and Winkelstein, A. Observations on the anemia and neutropenia of human copper deficiency. *Am. J. Hematol.*, **1977**, *3*, 177–185.

Monographs and Reviews

Aisen, P., and Brown, E. B. The iron-binding function of transferrin in iron metabolism. *Semin. Hematol.*, **1977**, *14*, 31–53.

Axelrad, A. A.; McLeod, D. L.; Shreeve, M. M.; and Heath, D. S. Properties of cells that produce erythrocytic colonies *in vitro*. In, *Hemopoiesis in Culture*. (Robinson, W. A., ed.) Department of Health, Education, and Welfare Publication No. (NIH) 74-205, Washington, D. C., **1974**, pp. 226–237.

Bauer, C. and Kurtz, A. Oxygen sensing in the kidney and its relation to erythropoietin formation. *Ann. Rev. Physiol.*, **1989**, *51*, 845–856.

Beaton, G. H. Epidemiology of iron deficiency. In, *Iron in Biochemistry and Medicine*. (Jacobs, A., and Worwood, M., eds.) Academic Press, Inc., New York, **1974**, pp. 477–528.

Beck, W. S. Megaloblastic anemias. In, *Cecil–Loeb Textbook of Medicine*, 17th ed. (Wyngaarden, J. B., and Smith L. H., eds.) W. B. Saunders Co., Philadelphia, **1985**, pp. 893–900.

Bothwell, T. H.; Charlton, R. W.; Cook, J. D.; and Finch, C. A. *Iron Metabolism in Man*. Blackwell Scientific Publications, Oxford, **1979**.

Bothwell, T. H., and Finch, C. A. *Iron Metabolism*. Little, Brown & Co., Boston, **1962**.

Brown, M. S.; Anderson, R. G. W.; and Goldstein, J. L. Recycling receptors: the round-trip itinerary of migrant membrane proteins. *Cell*, **1983**, *32*, 663–667.

Callender, S. T. Treatment of iron deficiency. In, *Iron in Biochemistry and Medicine*. (Jacobs, A., and Worwood, M., eds.) Academic Press, Inc., New York, **1974**, pp. 529–542.

Castle, W. B. Development of knowledge concerning the gastric intrinsic factor and its relation to pernicious anemia. *N. Engl. J. Med.*, **1953**, *249*, 603–614.

———. A century of curiosity about pernicious anemia. *Trans. Am. Clin. Climatol. Assoc.*, **1961**, *73*, 54–80.

Chanarin, I.; Deacon, R.; Lumb, M.; Muir, M.; and Perry, J. Cobalamin-folate interrelationships: a critical review. *Blood*, **1985**, *66*, 479–489.

Clark, S. C., and Kamen, R. The human hematopoietic colony-stimulating factors. *Science*, **1987**, *236*, 1229–1237.

Cook, J. D. Clinical evaluation of iron deficiency. *Semin. Hematol.*, **1982**, *19*, 6–18.

Cooper, B. A. Megaloblastic anaemia and disorders affecting utilization of vitamin B_{12} and folate in childhood. *Clin. Haematol.*, **1976**, *5*, 631–659.

Council on Foods and Nutrition. Iron deficiency in the United States. *J.A.M.A.*, **1968**, *203*, 119–124.

Dallman, P. R. Manifestations of iron deficiency. *Semin. Hematol.*, **1982**, *19*, 19–20.

Elwood, P. A. Radioactive studies of the absorption by human subjects of various iron preparations from bread. In, *Iron in Flour*. Ministry of Health Reports on Public Health and Medicine, Subject 117. Her Majesty's Stationery Office, London, **1968**, pp. 1–50.

Erslev, A. J. Humoral regulation of red cell production. *Blood*, **1953**, *8*, 349–387.

Eschbach, J. W., and Adamson, J. W. Recombinant human erythropoietin: implications for nephrology. *Am. J. Kidney Dis.*, **1988**, *11*, 203–209.

Evans, G. W. Copper homeostasis in the mammalian system. *Physiol. Rev.*, **1973**, *53*, 535.

Fairbanks, V. F.; Fahey, J. L.; and Beutler, E. *Clinical Disorders of Iron Metabolism*, 2nd ed. Grune & Stratton, Inc., New York, **1971**.

Finch, C. A., and Huebers, H. Perspectives in iron metabolism. *N. Engl. J. Med.*, **1982**, *306*, 1520–1528.

Finch, C. A., and others. Ferrokinetics in man. *Medicine (Baltimore)*, **1970**, *40*, 17–53.

Glaspy, J. A. and Golde, D. W. Clinical applications of the myeloid growth factors. *Semin. Hematol.*, **1989**, *26*, 5–8.

Graham, G. G., and Cordano, A. Copper deficiency in human subjects. In, *Trace Elements in Human Health and Disease*. Vol. 1, *Zinc and Copper*. (Prasad, A. S., and Oberleas, D., eds.) Academic Press, Inc., New York, **1976**, pp. 363–372.

Hallberg, L. Bioavailability of dietary iron in man. *Annu. Rev. Nutr.*, **1981**, *1*, 123–147.

Harris, J. W., and Kellermeyer, R. W. *The Red Cell*, rev. ed. Harvard University Press, Cambridge, Mass., **1970**.

Harrison, P. M. Ferritin: an iron-storage molecule. *Semin. Hematol.*, **1977**, *14*, 55–70.

Heilmeyer, L., and Plotner, K. *Das Serumeisen und die Eisenmangelkrankheit*. Gustav Fischer Verlag, Jena, **1937**.

Heinrich, H. C. Diagnostik Atiologie und Therapie des Eisenmangels unter besonderer Berucksichtigung der 59 Fe retentionsmessung im Gesamtkorperradioaktivitatsdetektor. *Nuklearmedizin*, **1983**, *1*, 137–269.

Herbert, V. Folic acid and vitamin B_{12}. In, *Modern Nutrition in Health and Disease*, 5th ed. (Goodhart, R. S., and Shils, M. E., eds.) Lea & Febiger, Philadelphia, **1973**, pp. 221–244.

———. Megaloblastic anemias. In, *Cecil–Loeb Textbook of Medicine*, 15th ed. (Beeson, P. B.; McDermott, W.; and Wyngaarden, J. B.; eds.) W. B. Saunders Co., Philadelphia, **1979**, pp. 1719–1729.

Herbert, V., and Tisman, G. Effects of deficiencies of folic acid and vitamin B_{12} on central nervous system function and development. In, *Biology of Brain Dysfunction*, Vol. 1. (Gaull, G., ed.) Plenum Press, New York, **1973**, pp. 373–392.

Herzlich, B., and Herbert, V. The role of the pancreas in cobalamin (Vitamin B_{12}) absorption. *Am. J. Gastroenterol.*, **1984**, *79*, 489–493.

Hillman, R. S., and Finch, C. A. *Red Cell Manual*, 5th ed. F. A. Davis Co., Philadelphia, **1985**.

Hoffbrand, A. V., and Wickremasinghe, R. G. Megaloblastic anemia. In, *Recent Advances in Haematology*. (Hoffbrand, A. V., ed.) Churchill-Livingstone, Ltd., Edinburgh, **1982**, pp. 25–44.

Horrigan, D. L., and Harris, J. W. Pyridoxine-responsive anemias in man. *Vitam. Horm.*, **1968**, *26*, 549.

Kass, L. *Pernicious Anemia*, Vol. II. W. B. Saunders Co., Philadelphia, **1976**.

Klausner, R. D. From receptors to genes—insights from

molecular iron metabolism. *Clin. Res.*, **1988**, *36*, 494–500.

Lajtha, L. G.; Pozzi, L. V.; Schofield, R.; and Fox, M. Kinetic properties of haemopoietic stem cells. *Cell Tissue Kinet.*, **1969**, *2*, 39–49.

Laurell, C. B. Studies on the transportation and metabolism of iron in the body. *Acta Physiol. Scand.*, **1947**, *14*, Suppl. 46, 1–129.

Layrisse, M., and Martinez-Torres, C. Iron absorption from food. *Prog. Hematol.*, **1971**, *6*, 137–160.

Lee, G. R.; Williams, D. M.; and Cartwright, G. E. Role of copper in iron metabolism and heme biosynthesis. In, *Trace Elements in Human Health and Disease*. Vol. 1, *Zinc and Copper*. (Prasad, A. S., and Oberleas, D., eds.) Academic Press, Inc., New York, **1976**, pp. 373–390.

Martinez-Torres, C.; Cobeddu, L.; Dillmann, E.; Brengelmann, G. L.; Leets, I.; Layrisse, M.; Johnson, P. G.; and Finch, C. A. Effect of exposure to low temperature on normal and iron deficient subjects. *Am. J. Physiol.*, **1984**, *246*, R380–R383.

Metcalf, D. The granulocyte-macrophage colony-stimulating factors. *Science*, **1985**, *229*, 16–22.

———. The molecular biology and functions of the granulocyte-macrophage colony-stimulating factors. *Blood*, **1986**, *67*, 257–267.

Neilands, J. B. (ed.). *Microbial Iron Metabolism: A Comprehensive Treatise*. Academic Press, Inc., New York, **1974.**

Nicola, N. A. Hemopoietic cell growth factors and their receptors. *Ann. Rev. Biochem.*, **1989**, *58*, 45–78.

O'Dell, B. L. Biochemistry of copper. *Med. Clin. North Am.*, **1976**, *60*, 687–703.

Pollit, E., and Leibel, R. L. (eds.). *Iron Deficiency: Brain Biochemistry and Behavior*. Raven Press, New York, **1982.**

Pratt, J. M. *Inorganic Chemistry of Vitamin B_{12}*. Academic Press, Inc., New York, **1972.**

Quesenberry, P., and Levitt, L. Hematopoietic stem cells. *N. Engl. J. Med.*, **1979**, *301*, 755–760; 819–823.

Reynolds, E. H. Neurological aspects of folate and vitamin B_{12} metabolism. *Clin. Haematol.*, **1976**, *5*, 661–696.

Rosenberg, I. Absorption and malabsorption of folates. *Clin. Haematol.*, **1976**, *5*, 589–618.

Sigel, H. *Metal Ions in Biological Systems*. Vol. 7, *Iron in Model and Natural Compounds*. Marcel Dekker, Inc., New York, **1977**, pp. 1–417.

Skeggs, H. R. Vitamin B_{12}. In, *The Vitamins: Chemistry, Physiology, Pathology, Methods*, 2nd ed., Vol. VII. (Gyorgy, P., and Pearson, W. N., eds.) Academic Press, Inc., New York, **1967**, pp. 277–301.

Smith, E. L. *Vitamin B_{12}*, 3rd ed. Methuen & Co., London; John Wiley & Sons, Inc., New York, **1965.**

Stebbins, R., and Bertino, J. R. Megaloblastic anemia produced by drugs. *Clin. Haematol.*, **1976**, *5*, 619–630.

Symposium. (Various authors.) The use of cobalt and cobalt-iron preparations in the therapy of anemia. *Blood*, **1955**, *10*, 852–861.

Underwood, E. J. *Trace Elements in Human and Animal Nutrition*, 3rd ed. Academic Press, Inc., New York, **1971.**

Webb, M. The biological action of cobalt and other metals. *Biochim. Biophys. Acta*, **1962**, *65*, 47.

Weir, D. G., and Scott, J. M. Interrelationships of folates and cobalamins. In, *Nutrition in Hematology*. Vol. 5, *Contemporary Issues in Clinical Nutrition*. (Lindenbaum, J., ed.) Churchill Livingstone, New York, **1983**, pp. 121–142.

Wellcome Trust Collaborative Study. *Tropical Sprue and Megaloblastic Anaemia*. Churchill Livingstone, Ltd., Edinburgh, **1971.**

WHO Joint Meeting. Control of nutritional anaemia with special reference to iron deficiency. World Health Organization Technical Report Series No. 580, WHO, Geneva, **1975.**

Wixom, R. L.; Rutkin, L.; and Munro, H. N. Hemosiderin: nature, formation and significance. *Int. Rev. Exp. Pathol.*, **1979**, *22*, 193–225.

CHAPTER

55 ANTICOAGULANT, THROMBOLYTIC, AND ANTIPLATELET DRUGS

Philip W. Majerus, George J. Broze, Jr., Joseph P. Miletich, and Douglas M. Tollefsen

OVERVIEW OF HEMOSTASIS

Hemostasis permits the cessation of blood loss from a damaged vessel. Platelets first adhere to macromolecules in the subendothelial regions of the injured blood vessel; they then aggregate to form the primary hemostatic plug. The platelets stimulate local activation of plasma coagulation factors, leading to generation of a fibrin clot that reinforces the platelet aggregate. Later, as wound healing occurs, the platelet aggregate and fibrin clot are degraded. Thrombosis is a pathological process in which a platelet aggregate and/or a fibrin clot occludes a blood vessel. Arterial thrombosis may result in ischemic necrosis of the tissue supplied by the artery (*e.g.*, myocardial infarction due to thrombosis of a coronary artery). Venous thrombosis may cause tissues drained by the vein to become edematous and inflamed. Thrombosis of a deep vein may be complicated by pulmonary embolism.

Coagulation *In Vitro*. Blood clots in 4 to 8 minutes when placed in a glass tube. Clotting is prevented if a chelating agent such as ethylenediaminetetraacetic acid (EDTA) or citrate is added to bind Ca^{2+}. Recalcified plasma clots in 2 to 4 minutes. The clotting time after recalcification is shortened to 26 to 33 seconds by the addition of negatively charged phospholipids and a particulate substance such as kaolin (aluminum silicate); this is termed the *activated partial thromboplastin time* (aPTT). Alternatively, recalcified plasma will clot in 12 to 14 seconds after addition of ''thromboplastin'' (a saline extract of brain that contains tissue factor and phospholipids); this is termed the *prothrombin time* (PT).

Intrinsic and Extrinsic Coagulation Pathways. Two pathways of coagulation are recognized. An individual with a prolonged aPTT and a normal PT is considered to have a defect in the intrinsic coagulation pathway, because all of the components of the aPTT test (except kaolin) are intrinsic to the plasma. A patient with a prolonged PT and a normal aPTT has a defect in the extrinsic coagulation pathway, since thromboplastin is extrinsic to the plasma. Prolongation of both the aPTT and the PT suggests a defect in a common pathway.

BIOCHEMISTRY OF COAGULATION

Coagulation involves a series of zymogen activation reactions, as shown in Figure 55–1. At each stage a precursor protein, or zymogen, is converted to an active protease by cleavage of one or more peptide bonds in the precursor molecule (Davie *et al.*, 1986). The components that can be involved at each stage include a protease from the preceding stage, a zymogen, a nonenzymatic protein cofactor, Ca^{2+}, and an organizing surface that is provided by a phospholipid emulsion *in vitro* or by platelets *in vivo*. The final protease to be generated is thrombin (factor IIa).

Conversion of Fibrinogen to Fibrin. Fibrinogen is a 330-kilodalton protein that consists of three pairs of polypeptide chains (designated Aα, Bβ, and γ) covalently linked by disulfide bonds. Thrombin converts fibrinogen to fibrin monomers by cleaving fibrinopeptides A (16 amino-acid residues) and B (14 amino-acid residues) from the amino-terminal ends of the Aα and Bβ chains, respectively. Removal of the fibrinopeptides allows the fibrin monomers

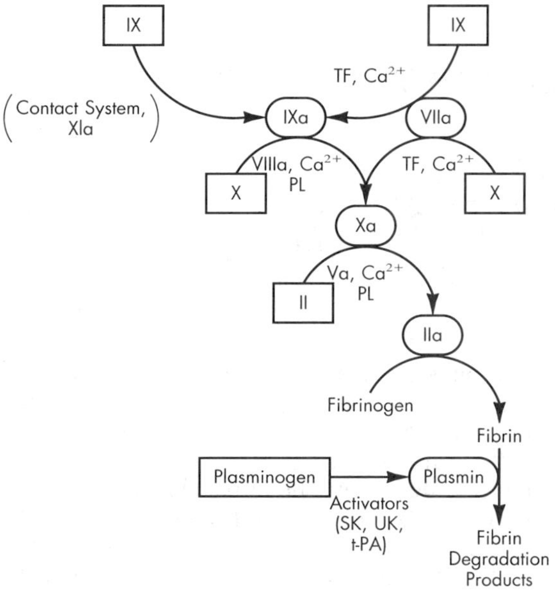

Figure 55–1. *Major reactions of blood coagulation and fibrinolysis.*

Boxes enclose the coagulation factor zymogens and the ovals the active proteases. PL = platelets or phospholipids; TF = tissue factor; Va = activated factor V; VIIIa = activated factor VIII; SK = streptokinase; UK = urokinase; t-PA = tissue plasminogen activator.

to form a gel, which constitutes the end point of the aPTT and PT tests. Initially, the fibrin monomers are bound to each other noncovalently. Subsequently, factor XIIIa catalyzes an interchain transglutamination reaction that cross-links adjacent fibrin monomers to enhance the strength of the clot.

Structure of Coagulation Protease Zymogens. The protease zymogens involved in coagulation include factors II (prothrombin), VII, IX, X, XI, XII, and prekallikrein. About 200 amino acid residues at the carboxyl-terminal end of each zymogen are homologous to trypsin and contain the active site of the protease. In addition, 9 to 12 glutamate residues near the amino-terminal ends of factors II, VII, IX, and X are converted to γ-carboxyglutamate (Gla) residues during biosynthesis in the liver (*see* Chapter 64). The Gla residues bind Ca^{2+} and are necessary for the coagulant activities of these proteins.

Nonenzymatic Protein Cofactors. Factors V and VIII are homologous 350-kilodalton proteins. Factor VIII circulates in plasma bound to von Willebrand factor, while factor V is present both free in plasma and as a component of platelets. Thrombin cleaves V and VIII to yield activated factors (Va and VIIIa) that have at least 50 times the coagulant activity of the precursor forms. Factors Va and VIIIa have no enzymatic activity themselves but serve as cofactors that increase the proteolytic efficiency of Xa and IXa, respectively. Tissue factor is a nonenzymatic lipoprotein cofactor that greatly increases the proteolytic efficiency of VII and VIIa. It is present on the surface of cells that are not normally in contact with plasma (*e.g.*, fibroblasts and smooth muscle cells) and initiates coagulation outside a broken blood vessel. Monocytes and endothelial cells may also express tissue factor when exposed to a variety of stimuli, such as endotoxin, tumor necrosis factor, and interleukin-1. Thus, these cells may be involved in thrombus formation under pathological circumstances. High-molecular-weight kininogen is a plasma protein that serves as the cofactor for XIIa when clotting is initiated *in vitro* in the aPTT test.

Activation of Prothrombin. Factor Xa cleaves two peptide bonds in prothrombin to form thrombin. Activation of prothrombin by Xa is accelerated by Va, phospholipids, and Ca^{2+}. When all these components are present, prothrombin is activated nearly 20,000 times faster than the rate achieved by Xa and Ca^{2+} alone. The maximal rate of activation occurs only when prothrombin and Xa both contain Gla residues and, therefore, have the ability to bind to phospholipids. Purified platelets can substitute for phospholipids and Va to facilitate activation of prothrombin *in vitro*, provided that the platelets are stimulated to release endogenous platelet factor Va or that factor Va is added exogenously to unstimulated platelets. The surface of platelets that are aggregated at the site of hemostasis concentrates the factors required for activation of prothrombin.

Initiation of Coagulation. Clotting by the intrinsic pathway is initiated *in vitro* when XII, prekallikrein, and high-molecular-weight kininogen interact with kaolin, glass, or another surface to generate small amounts of XIIa. Activation of XI to XIa and IX to IXa follow. IXa then activates X in a reaction that is accelerated by VIIIa, phospholipids, and Ca^{2+}. Activation of factor X by IXa appears to occur by a mechanism similar to that for activation of prothrombin and may also be accelerated by platelets *in vivo*. Activation of factor XII is not required for hemostasis, since patients with deficiency of XII, prekallikrein, and high-molecular-weight kininogen do not bleed, even though their aPTT values are prolonged. Bleeding sometimes occurs in patients with factor XI deficiency; the reason is unclear, since XIIa is the only known activator of XI.

Coagulation is initiated *in vivo* by the extrinsic pathway. In this pathway, factor VII is activated by its product, factor Xa. However, VII itself possesses proteolytic activity; although this is less than 1% that of VIIa, it is sufficient to initiate coagulation in the presence of tissue factor. Tissue factor accelerates activation of factor X by VIIa (or VII), phospholipids, and Ca^{2+} about 30,000-fold. It is likely that the availability of tissue factor at sites of injury plays a major role in the initiation of hemostasis. VIIa can also activate IX in the presence of tissue factor, providing a crossover point between the extrinsic and intrinsic pathways.

Natural Anticoagulant Mechanisms. Platelet activation and coagulation normally do not occur within an intact blood vessel. Thrombosis is prevented by several regulatory mechanisms that require a normal vascular endothelium (Esmon, 1987). Prostacyclin (PGI_2), a metabolite of arachidonic acid, is synthesized by endothelial cells, and it inhibits platelet aggregation and secretion (*see* Chapter 24). Antithrombin is a plasma protein that inhibits coagulation factors of the intrinsic and common pathways (*see* below). Heparan sulfate proteoglycans found on the endothelial surface stimulate the activity of antithrombin. Protein C is a plasma zymogen that is homologous to II, VII, IX, and X; its activity depends on the binding of Ca^{2+} to Gla residues within its amino-terminal domain. Activated protein C in combination with its nonenzymatic Gla-containing cofactor (protein S) degrades cofactors Va and VIIIa and thereby greatly diminishes the rates of activation of prothrombin and factor X. Protein C is activated by thrombin only in the presence of thrombomodulin, an integral membrane protein of endothelial cells. Like antithrombin, protein C appears to exert an anticoagulant effect in the vicinity of intact endothelial cells. Lipoprotein-associated coagulation inhibitor (LACI) is found in the lipoprotein fraction of plasma. When bound to factor Xa, LACI inhibits factor Xa and the factor VII–tissue factor complex. By this mechanism, factor Xa may regulate its own production.

HEPARIN

History. In 1916 a medical student named McLean, while investigating the nature of ether-soluble procoagulants, made the serendipitous finding of a phospholipid anticoagulant. Soon thereafter, a water-soluble mucopolysaccharide, named *heparin* because of its abundance in liver, was discovered by Howell (1922), in whose laboratory McLean had been working (*see* Jaques, 1978). The use of heparin *in vitro* to prevent the clotting of shed blood eventually led to its use *in vivo* to treat venous thrombosis.

BIOCHEMISTRY AND MECHANISM OF ACTION

Structure. The structure of heparin is best understood by considering its biosynthesis. Heparin is a complex linear polysaccharide of 60,000 to 100,000 daltons, covalently attached to a core protein that is found in mast cell secretory granules. It is synthesized from UDP-sugar precursors as a polymer of alternating D-glucuronic acid and N-acetyl-D-glucosamine residues (Figure 55–2; Lindahl *et al.,* 1986). The polymer then undergoes a series of modifications, which include the following: N-deacetylation and N-sulfation of glucosamine residues, epimerization of D-glucuronic acid to L-iduronic acid, O-sulfation of iduronic and glucuronic acid residues at the C-2 position, and O-sulfation of glucosamine residues at the C-3 and C-6 positions. Each of these modification reactions is incomplete, yielding a large variation of oligosaccharide structures within the glycosaminoglycan chain.

Heparan sulfate is a closely related glycosaminoglycan found on the surface of most eukaryotic cells and in the extracellular matrix. It is synthesized from the same repeating disaccharide precursor (D-glucuronic acid linked to N-acetyl-D-glucosamine) as is heparin. However, heparan sulfate undergoes less modification of the polymer than does heparin and therefore contains higher proportions of glucuronic acid and N-acetylglucosamine and fewer sulfate groups. Heparan sulfate produces an anticoagulant effect when added to plasma *in vitro,* although a higher concentration is required in comparison to heparin.

Dermatan sulfate is a repeating polymer of L-iduronic acid and N-acetyl-D-galactosamine. O-sulfation of iduronic acid residues at the C-2 position and of galactosamine residues at the C-4 and C-6 positions occurs to a variable extent. Like heparan sulfate, dermatan sulfate is a component of the cell surface and the extracellular matrix. Dermatan sulfate also produces an anticoagulant effect *in vitro.*

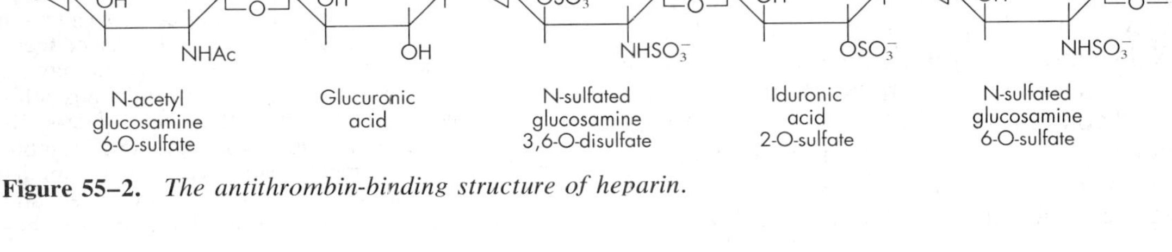

Figure 55–2. *The antithrombin-binding structure of heparin.*

Source. Heparin for therapeutic use is commonly extracted from porcine intestinal mucosa or bovine lung. During the isolation of heparin from these sources, the core protein is removed and the glycosaminoglycan chains become degraded slightly to yield a heterogeneous mixture of large fragments (5,000 to 30,000 daltons; mean, approximately 12,000 daltons). These preparations may also contain small amounts of other glycosaminoglycans. Despite the heterogeneity in composition among different commercial preparations of heparin, their biological activities are similar.

Low-molecular-weight heparins (< 7,000 daltons) are isolated from standard heparin by gel filtration chromatography or differential precipitation with ethanol. Alternatively, they can be produced by partial depolymerization with nitrous acid and other chemical reactions. Low-molecular-weight heparins differ from standard heparin in both their pharmacokinetic properties and mechanism of action.

Physiological Function. Heparin occurs intracellularly in tissues that contain mast cells. Its function within the secretory granules of these cells is unknown. When released from mast cells, heparin is rapidly ingested and destroyed by macrophages. Heparin cannot be detected in plasma under normal circumstances. However, patients with systemic mastocytosis who undergo massive degranulation of mast cells may have a mild prolongation of the aPTT, presumably resulting from the release of heparin into the circulation.

Heparan sulfate molecules present on the luminal surface of vascular endothelial cells interact with circulating antithrombin to provide a natural antithrombotic mechanism (Marcum and Rosenberg, 1987). Patients with malignancies may experience bleeding related to circulating heparan sulfate–like material that probably originates from lysis of the tumor cells.

Mechanism of Action. Antithrombin (or antithrombin III) is a glycosylated, single-chain polypeptide with a mass of about 58,000 daltons that rapidly inhibits thrombin only in the presence of heparin (Bjork and Danielsson, 1986). The protein is homologous to the α_1-antitrypsin family of protease inhibitors. Antithrombin is synthesized in the liver and circulates at an approximate concentration in plasma of 2.6 μM. It inhibits activated coagulation factors of the intrinsic and common pathways, including thrombin, Xa, IXa, XIa, XIIa, and kallikrein; however, it has little or no activity against factor VIIa. Inhibition of thrombin and factor Xa probably accounts for most of the anticoagulant effect of heparin. Antithrombin is a "suicide substrate" for these proteases; inhibition occurs when the protease attacks a specific Arg-Ser peptide bond in the reactive site of antithrombin and becomes trapped as a stable 1:1 complex.

Heparin increases the rate of the thrombin–antithrombin reaction at least 1000-fold by serving as a catalytic template to which both the inhibitor and the protease bind. Binding of heparin also induces a conformational change in antithrombin that makes the reactive site more accessible to the protease. Once a protease has become bound to antithrombin, the heparin molecule is released from the complex. The binding site for antithrombin on heparin is a specific pentasaccharide sequence that contains a 3-O-sulfated glucosamine residue (*see* Figure 55–2). This structure occurs in about 30% of heparin molecules and less abundantly in heparan sulfate. Other glycosaminoglycans (*e.g.,* dermatan sulfate, chondroitin-4-sulfate, and chondroitin-6-sulfate) lack the antithrombin-binding structure and do not stimulate antithrombin. Heparin molecules containing fewer than 18 monosaccharide units (3000 to 4000 daltons) do not catalyze inhibition of thrombin by antithrombin. Molecules of this length or greater are required to bind thrombin and antithrombin simultaneously. In contrast, the pentasaccharide shown in Figure 55–2 catalyzes inhibition of factor Xa by antithrombin. In this case, catalysis may occur solely by induction of a conformational change in antithrombin that facilitates reaction with the protease. Low-molecular-weight heparin preparations that are of insufficient length to catalyze inhibition of thrombin produce an anticoagulant effect mainly through inhibition of Xa by antithrombin.

When the concentration of heparin in plasma is 0.1 to 1.0 unit/ml, thrombin and factor Xa are inhibited rapidly by antithrombin (half-life less than 0.1 second). This effect results in prolongation of the aPTT and the thrombin time (*i.e.,* the time required for plasma to clot when exogenous thrombin is added); the prothrombin time is affected to a lesser degree. The anticoagulant effect of higher concentrations of heparin (> 5.0 units/ml), which may be present transiently after a bolus intravenous infusion, is mediated in part by heparin cofactor II. Heparin cofactor II is homologous to antithrombin and has a similar mechanism of action. It inhibits thrombin but not other coagulation proteases, and it binds heparin with a lower affinity than does antithrombin. In contrast to antithrombin, the activity of heparin cofactor II is stimulated approximately 1000-fold by dermatan sulfate. Addition of dermatan sulfate to plasma *in vitro* causes prolongation of the thrombin time and the aPTT, and intravenous infusion of dermatan sulfate into experimental animals produces an antithrombotic effect.

Several proteins interfere with catalysis of the thrombin–antithrombin reaction *in vitro* by inhibiting competitively the binding of antithrombin to heparin. These include two plasma proteins that are present in micromolar concentrations—histidine-rich glycoprotein and S-protein (vitronectin). Further studies are needed to determine whether variations in the concentrations of these proteins affect the dosage of heparin required to produce an anticoagulant effect *in vivo*. Platelet factor 4, released from the α-granules during platelet aggregation, also blocks binding of antithrombin to heparin or heparan sulfate and promotes local clot formation at the site of hemostasis.

Miscellaneous Effects. High doses of heparin can interfere with platelet aggregation and thereby prolong the bleeding time. It is unclear to what extent the antiplatelet effect of heparin contributes to the hemorrhagic complications of treatment with the drug. Heparin "clears" lipemic plasma *in vivo* by causing the release of lipoprotein lipase into the circulation. Lipoprotein lipase hydrolyzes triglycerides to glycerol and free fatty acids. The clearing of lipemic plasma may occur at concentrations of heparin below those necessary to produce an anticoagulant effect. Rebound hyperlipemia may occur after administration of heparin is stopped.

CLINICAL USE

Unitage and Preparations. The USP unit of heparin is the quantity that prevents 1.0 ml of citrated sheep plasma from clotting for 1 hour after the addition of 0.2 ml of 1% $CaCl_2$. The drug is available as *heparin sodium injection* from porcine intestinal mucosa (LIQUAEMIN SODIUM) or bovine lung at concentrations of 1000 to 40,000 USP units/ml. *Heparin calcium injection* from porcine intestinal mucosa (CALCIPARINE), widely used in Europe in a low-dose regimen for prophylaxis of thromboembolism, is reported to cause a lower incidence of local hematoma. It is available at a concentration of 25,000 USP units/ml. *Low-molecular-weight heparin* preparations, which are currently being evaluated clinically, are extremely heterogeneous in their chemical composition and molecular weight and are not standardized. In general, they produce a minimal effect on tests of clotting *in vitro*. In clinical trials, low-molecular-weight heparin is usually prescribed in units of anti-Xa activity; however, it cannot be assumed that the same anti-Xa dose of two preparations of low-molecular-weight heparin will produce equivalent antithrombotic effects.

Absorption and Pharmacokinetics. Heparin is not absorbed through the gastrointestinal mucosa and is therefore given parenterally. Administration is by continuous intravenous infusion, intermittent intravenous injection, or deep subcutaneous injection. Heparin has an immediate onset of action when given intravenously. In contrast, there is considerable variation in the bioavailability of heparin given subcutaneously, and the onset of action is delayed 20 to 60 minutes.

The anticoagulant activity of heparin disappears from the blood with apparent first-order kinetics. However, the half-life of the drug is dependent on the dose administered. When 100, 400, or 800 units/kg of heparin is injected intravenously, the half-life of the anticoagulant activity is approximately 1, 2.5, and 5 hours, respectively (*see* Appendix II). Heparin appears to be cleared and degraded primarily by the reticuloendothelial system; a small amount of undegraded heparin also appears in the urine. The half-life of heparin may be shortened somewhat in patients with pulmonary embolism and prolonged in patients with hepatic cirrhosis or end-stage renal disease. Low-molecular-weight heparins have longer biological half-lives than do standard preparations of the drug.

Administration and Dosage. So-called full-dose heparin therapy is administered by continuous intravenous infusion because of a reduced incidence of bleeding complications when compared with administration by intermittent infusion (Hyers *et al.*, 1986). Treatment is initiated with a bolus injection of 5000 units, followed by 700 to 2000 units per hour delivered by an infusion pump. Therapy is routinely monitored by the aPTT. A clotting time of 1.5 to 2.0 times the normal mean aPTT value (usually 50 to 70 seconds) is therapeutic. Initially, the aPTT should be measured and the infusion rate adjusted every 4 hours. Once a steady dosage schedule is established, daily monitoring is sufficient.

Subcutaneous administration of heparin can be used for the long-term management of patients in whom warfarin is contraindicated (*e.g.*, during pregnancy). A dose of 7500 to 15,000 units given every 12 hours is usually sufficient to achieve an aPTT of 1.5 times the control value (measured midway between doses). Monitoring is generally unnecessary once a steady dosage schedule is established.

Low-dose heparin therapy may prevent thromboembolism in certain patients. A current regimen for such treatment is 5000 units of heparin given subcutaneously every 8 to 12 hours. Laboratory monitoring is unnecessary, since this regimen does not prolong the aPTT. European trials suggest that low-molecular-weight heparin may be as effective as standard heparin for prophylaxis of thromboembolism postoperatively or in patients with stroke (Levine and Hirsh, 1988). Low-molecular-weight heparin did not cause less bleeding than standard heparin in these studies. However, the fact that it need be given subcutaneously only once a day (because of its long half-life) is a potential advantage.

Heparin Resistance. Occasionally a patient's aPTT will not be prolonged to 1.5 times the normal mean unless very high doses of heparin (> 50,000 units per day) are administered. Such patients may have "therapeutic" concentrations of heparin in plasma at the usual dose when values are measured by other tests (*e.g.*, anti-Xa activity or protamine sulfate titration). Many of these patients have very short aPTT values prior to treatment because of the presence of an increased concentration of factor VIII and may not be truly resistant to heparin. Other patients may require large doses of heparin because of accelerated clearance of the drug, as may occur with massive pulmonary embolism. Patients with inherited antithrombin deficiency ordinarily have 40 to 60% of the normal plasma concentration of this inhibitor and respond normally to intravenous heparin. However, acquired deficiency of antithrombin (concentration less than 25% of normal) may occur in patients with hepatic cirrhosis, nephrotic syndrome, or disseminated intravascular coagulation; large doses of heparin may not prolong the aPTT in these individuals.

Toxicity. Bleeding is the primary untoward effect of heparin. Major bleeding occurs in 1 to 33% of patients who receive various forms of heparin therapy, and in one study there were three fatal bleeding episodes among 647 patients (Levine and Hirsh, 1986). The number of bleeding episodes increases with the total daily dose of heparin and with the degree of prolongation of the aPTT and other clotting tests. Four randomized studies have compared the incidence of bleeding during intermittent and continuous intravenous infusion of heparin. Two of the studies demonstrated a significantly lower incidence of bleeding in the patients who received continuous intravenous infusions (0 to 1% versus 9 to 33%), and a third study reported a similar trend. However, the total dose of heparin administered by intermittent infusion was higher than that administered by continuous infusion. When the same doses were used, the incidence of bleeding was the same; this finding implies that toxicity is related to the dosage and not to the route of administration.

Two forms of acute, heparin-induced thrombocytopenia have been reported. Mild thrombocytopenia occurs in 2 to 5% of patients, 2 to 15 days after initiation of full-dose heparin therapy (Bell, 1988). The platelet count usually remains above 100,000/μl, and treatment can be continued without undue risk of bleeding. Severe thrombocytopenia occurs much less frequently, 7 to 14 days after initiation of full-dose or low-dose heparin therapy; the thrombocytopenia is reversible after discontinuation of the drug. Paradoxically, the severe form of heparin-induced thrombocytopenia has been associated with thrombotic complications, including arterial thrombosis with platelet-fibrin clots (so-called white clots) that may cause myocardial infarction or stroke or necessitate amputation of a limb. Tests for heparin-dependent, anti-platelet IgG in the serum of patients with the severe form of thrombocytopenia may be positive, but it is uncertain whether these tests can predict the recurrence of thrombocytopenia during subsequent administration of heparin. Thrombocytopenia appears to be less common with porcine heparin than with bovine heparin (Warkentin and Kelton, 1989).

In contrast to warfarin, heparin does not cross the placenta and has not been associated with fetal malformations; therefore, heparin is used for anticoagulation during pregnancy. However, fetal mortality or prematurity occurs about one third of the time when heparin is administered during pregnancy.

Abnormalities of hepatic function tests occur frequently in patients who are receiving heparin intravenously or subcutaneously. Mild elevations of the activities of hepatic transaminases in plasma occur without an increase in bilirubin or alkaline phosphatase. Osteoporosis and spontaneous vertebral fractures occur infrequently in patients who have received full therapeutic doses of heparin (greater than 20,000 units per day) for 3 to 6 months. Heparin can inhibit the synthesis of aldosterone by the adrenal glands and occasionally causes hyperkalemia, even when low doses are given. Allergic reactions to heparin (other than thrombocytopenia) are rare.

Antagonists. The anticoagulant effect of heparin disappears within hours after discontinuation of the drug. Mild bleeding due to heparin can usually be controlled without administration of an antagonist. If life-threatening hemorrhage occurs, the effect of heparin can be reversed quickly by the intravenous infusion of protamine sulfate. The protamines are low-molecular-weight, basic proteins that are isolated from fish sperm. They bind tightly to heparin *in vitro* and thereby neutralize its anticoagulant effect. *In vivo,* protamine also interacts with platelets, fibrinogen, and other plasma proteins and may cause an anticoagulant effect of its own. Therefore, one should give the minimal amount of protamine required to neutralize the heparin present in the plasma. This amount is approximately 1 mg of protamine for every 100 units of heparin remaining in the patient; the amount of heparin present can be estimated from its half-life and the amount most recently administered. Protamine sulfate must be given intravenously at a slow rate (not more than 50 mg over a 10-minute period), since more rapid infusion can cause dyspnea, flushing, bradycardia, hypotension, or anaphylaxis.

ORAL ANTICOAGULANTS

History. Sweet clover was planted in the Dakota plains and Canada at the turn of the century because it flourished on poor soil and substituted for corn in silage. In 1924, Schofield reported a previously undescribed hemorrhagic disorder in cattle that resulted from the ingestion of spoiled sweet clover silage. After Roderick traced the cause to a toxic reduction of plasma prothrombin, Campbell and Link, in 1939, identified the hemorrhagic agent as bishydroxycoumarin (dicumarol) (Link, 1959). In 1948, a more potent synthetic congener was introduced as an extremely effective rodenticide; the compound was named warfarin as an acronym derived from the name of the patent holder, Wisconsin Alumni Research Foundation, plus the cou*marin*-derived suffix. Potential for the use of warfarin as a therapeutic agent for thromboembolic disease was recognized but not widely accepted, partly due to fear of unacceptable toxicity. However, in 1951, an army inductee uneventfully survived an attempted suicide with massive dosages of a preparation of warfarin intended for rodent control. Since then, these anticoagulants have become a mainstay for prevention of thromboembolic disease, and they are administered to hundreds of thousands of patients annually. Warfarin is the prototypical oral anticoagulant and by far the most frequently prescribed. However, the anticoagulant action of all the drugs in this class is similar, differing mainly in potency and duration of action.

Chemistry. Numerous anticoagulants have been synthesized as derivatives of 4-hydroxycoumarin and of the related compound, indan-1,3-dione (Table 55–1). Only the coumarin derivatives are widely used; the 4-hydroxycoumarin residue, with a nonpolar carbon substituent at the 3 position, is the minimal structural requirement for activity. This carbon is asymmetrical in warfarin (and in phenprocoumon and acenocoumarol). The enantiomers differ in anticoagulant potency, metabolism, elimination, and interactions with some other drugs (O'Reilly, 1987). Commercial preparations of these anticoagulants are racemic mixtures, and any advantage of administering a single enantiomer has not yet been established.

PHARMACOLOGICAL PROPERTIES

Mechanism of Action. The oral anticoagulants are antagonists of vitamin K (*see* Chapter 64). Coagulation factors II, VII, IX, and X and the anticoagulant proteins C and S are biologically inactive unless certain glutamic acid residues (9 to 12 in number) are carboxylated by a microsomal enzyme system that utilizes reduced vitamin K as a cofactor. The modified γ-carboxyglutamyl (Gla) residues confer Ca^{2+}-binding properties on these proteins that are essential for their assembly into an efficient catalytic complex. Factors II, VII, IX, and X and protein C (and possibly protein S) are synthesized mainly in the liver. The glutamic acid carboxylase probably acts cotranslationally, and deficiency or antagonism of vitamin K decreases the rate of synthesis of the proteins.

A vitamin K epoxidase oxidizes reduced vitamin K, and this reaction is somehow coupled to the carboxylase reaction (Figure 55–3). A number of different enzymes can reduce vitamin K *in vitro* to make it available for subsequent carboxylation reactions. The oral anticoagulants block the regeneration of reduced vitamin K and thereby induce a state of functional vitamin K deficiency (Suttie, 1987). The mechanism of the inhibition of reductase(s) by the coumarin drugs is not known. There exist reductases that are less sensitive to these drugs but that act only at relatively high concentrations of oxidized vitamin K; this

Table 55–1. STRUCTURAL FORMULAS OF THE ORAL ANTICOAGULANTS *

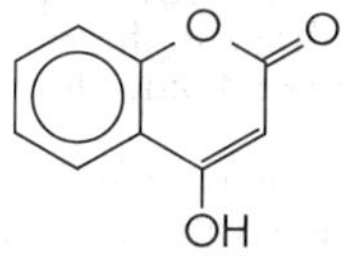

4-Hydroxycoumarin

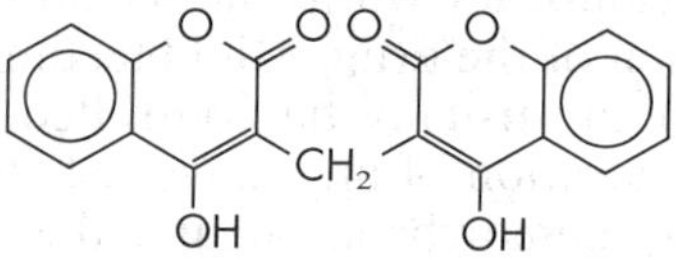

Dicumarol

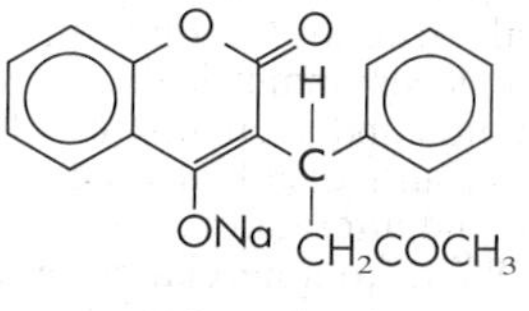

Warfarin Sodium

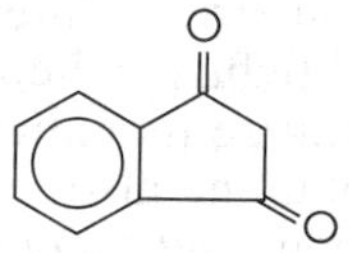

Indan-1,3-dione

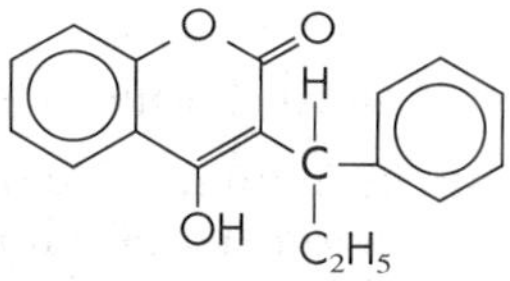

Phenprocoumon

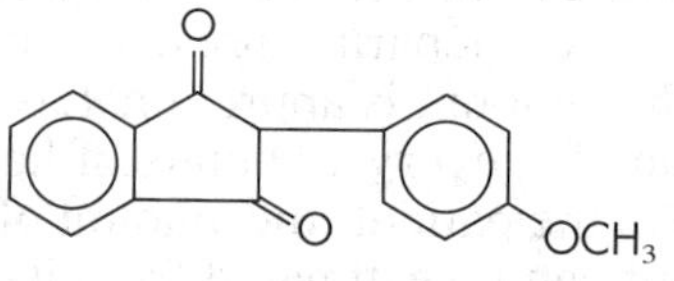

Anisindione

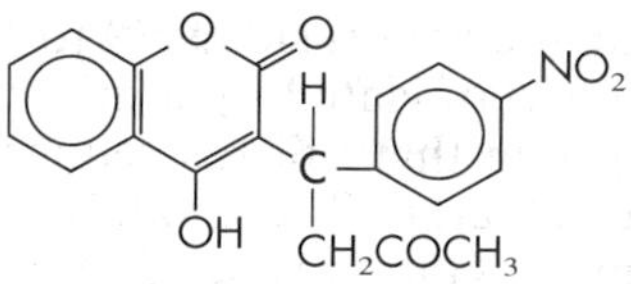

Acenocoumarol

* 4-Hydroxycoumarin and indan-1,3-dione are included to indicate the parent molecules from which the oral anticoagulants are derived. The asymmetrical carbon atoms in the coumarins are shown in bold face type.

property may explain the observation that administration of sufficient vitamin K can counteract even large doses of oral anticoagulants.

Therapeutic doses of warfarin decrease the total amount of each vitamin K–dependent coagulation factor made by the liver by 30 to 50%; in addition, the secreted molecules are under-carboxylated, resulting in diminished biological activity (10 to 40% of normal). Congenital deficiencies of the procoagulant proteins to these levels cause mild bleeding disorders. Oral anticoagulants have no effect on the activity of fully carboxylated molecules in the circulation. Thus, the time required for the activity of each factor in plasma to reach a new steady state after therapy is initiated or adjusted depends on its individual rate of clearance. The approximate half-lives (in hours) are as follows: factor VII, 6; factor IX, 24; factor X, 36; factor II, 50; protein C, 8; and protein S, 30. There is no selectivity of the effect of warfarin on any particular vitamin K–dependent coagulation factor, nor is the antithrombotic benefit or hemorrhagic risk of therapy correlated with any particular activity. Vitamin K–dependent carboxylase activity occurs in many tissues, and other proteins have Gla residues. Bone contains a group of low-molecular-weight vitamin K–dependent proteins (osteocalcin, bone Gla protein, matrix Gla protein), which are believed to play a role in mineralization. Surfactant-associated proteins containing Gla residues have also been identified, and their concentrations are correlated with the activity of a vitamin

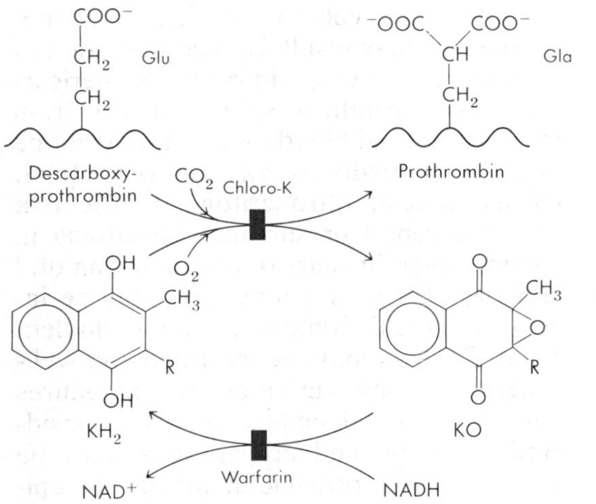

Figure 55–3. *Vitamin K cycle: metabolic interconversions of vitamin K associated with the modification of vitamin K–dependent clotting factors.*

Vitamin K_1 or K_2 is reduced to the hydroquinone form (KH_2). Stepwise oxidation to vitamin K epoxide (KO) is coupled to protein carboxylation, wherein descarboxyprothrombin (descarboxy-II) is converted to prothrombin (II) by carboxylation of glutamate residues (Glu) to γ-carboxyglutamate (Gla). Enzymatic reduction of the epoxide with reduced nicotinamide adenine dinucleotide (NADH) as a cofactor regenerates vitamin KH_2. The oxidation of vitamin K is inhibited by the chloro analog of vitamin K (Chloro-K), whereas the reduction of vitamin K epoxide is the warfarin-sensitive step (Warfarin). The R on the vitamin K molecule represents a 20-carbon phytyl side chain in vitamin K_1 and a 5- to 65-carbon prenyl side chain in vitamin K_2.

K–dependent carboxylase in developing fetal lung.

Absorption. The bioavailability of solutions of racemic sodium warfarin is nearly complete when the drug is administered orally, intramuscularly, intravenously, or rectally. In fact, bleeding has occurred from repeated contact of the skin with solutions of warfarin used as a rodenticide. However, different commercial preparations of warfarin tablets vary in their rate of dissolution, and this causes some variation in the rate and extent of absorption. Food in the gastrointestinal tract can also decrease the rate of absorption. Warfarin is usually detectable in plasma within 1 hour of its oral administration, and concentrations peak in 2 to 8 hours.

Distribution. Warfarin is almost completely (99%) bound to plasma proteins, principally albumin, and the drug distributes rapidly into a volume equivalent to the albumin space (0.14 liter/kg). Concentrations in fetal plasma approach the maternal values, but active warfarin is not found in milk (unlike other coumarins and indandiones).

Biotransformation and Elimination. Warfarin is transformed into inactive metabolites by the liver and kidneys, and these are excreted in urine and stool. The average rate of clearance from plasma is 0.045 ml $\cdot$ $min^{-1} \cdot kg^{-1}$. The half-life ranges from 20 to 60 hours, with a mean of about 40 hours; the duration of action of warfarin is 2 to 5 days.

Preparations, Routes of Administration, and Dosage. *Warfarin sodium* (COUMADIN, PANWARFIN, others) is available in tablets containing 2, 2.5, 5, 7.5, and 10 mg of the drug. The usual adult dose is 10 to 15 mg per day for 2 to 4 days, followed by 2 to 15 mg per day as indicated by PT measurements (*see* below). It should be taken at the same time each day; bedtime is often convenient and permits monitoring of a peak effect on morning blood samples. Large loading doses of warfarin are not indicated, since they do little to shorten the time required for an antithrombotic effect but increase toxicity. *Warfarin sodium for injection* (COUMADIN) is available in 50-mg vials, but parenteral use does not alter the speed of anticoagulation.

Drug and Other Interactions. The list of drugs and other factors that may affect the action of oral anticoagulants is prodigious and expanding (*see* Griffin *et al.,* 1988). Any substance or condition is potentially dangerous if it alters (1) the uptake or metabolism of the oral anticoagulant or vitamin K; (2) the synthesis, function, or clearance of any factor or cell involved in hemostasis or fibrinolysis; or (3) the integrity of any epithelial surface. Patients must be educated to report the addition or deletion of any medication (including nonprescription drugs and food supplements). Some of the more commonly described factors that cause a decreased effect of oral anticoagulants include reduced absorption of drug caused by binding to cholestyramine in the gastrointestinal tract; increased volume of distribution and a short half-life secondary to hypoproteinemia, as in nephrotic syndrome; increased metabolic clearance of drug secondary to induction of hepatic enzymes by barbiturates, rifampin, phenytoin, or chronic ingestion of alcohol; ingestion of large amounts of vitamin K–rich foods or supplements; and increased levels of coagulation factors during pregnancy. The PT will be shortened in most of these cases. Hereditary resistance to oral anticoagulants has been reported in three kindreds. The defect is probably in the microsomal vitamin K reductase. This defect also causes an increase in the daily requirement for the vitamin, possibly because alternative reductases that are not inhibited by oral anticoagulants are less efficient in recycling vitamin K.

Frequently cited interactions that enhance the risk of hemorrhage in patients taking oral anticoagulants include decreased metabolism and/or displacement from protein binding sites caused by phenylbutazone, sulfinpyrazone, metronidazole, disulfiram, allopurinol, cimetidine, amiodarone, or acute intake of ethanol. Relative deficiency of vitamin K may result from inadequate diet (*e.g.*, postoperative patients on parenteral fluids), especially when coupled with the elimination of intestinal flora by antimicrobial agents. Cephalosporins containing heterocyclic side chains inhibit the vitamin K epoxidase (and thereby the carboxylase). Low concentrations of coagulation factors may result from impaired hepatic function, congestive heart failure, or hypermetabolic states. Generally, these factors increase the prolongation of the PT. Serious interactions that do not alter the PT include inhibition of platelet function by agents such as aspirin and gastritis or frank ulceration induced by antiinflammatory drugs. Agents may have more than one effect; for example, clofibrate increases the rate of turnover of coagulation factors and inhibits platelet function. Age is correlated with increased sensitivity to oral anticoagulants.

Toxicity. Bleeding is the major toxicity of oral anticoagulant drugs. Especially serious episodes involve sites where irreversible damage may result from compression of vital structures (*e.g.*, intracranial, pericardial, nerve sheath, or spinal cord) or from massive internal blood loss that may not be diagnosed rapidly (*e.g.*, gastrointestinal, intraperitoneal, retroperitoneal). The risk of intracerebral or subdural hematoma in patients over 50 years of age taking an oral anticoagulant over a long term may be increased 10-fold (Verstraete and Vermylen, 1988). Patients must be informed and well-supervised; any activities or procedures that may cause bleeding must be considered carefully, and preparations must be made to treat possible hemorrhagic episodes. If a patient shows any sign of bleeding, the next dose of anticoagulant should be withheld and the PT measured. If bleeding is minor or self-limited, therapy may be continued after adjusting the dosage and/or correcting the reason for the altered response.

For continued or serious bleeding, vitamin K_1 (phytonadione) is an effective antidote. Other synthetic derivatives of vitamin K are less consistent in reversing the effects of oral anticoagulants and should not be used (Griminger, 1966). Since reversal of anticoagulation by vitamin K_1 requires synthesis of fully carboxylated coagulation proteins, significant improvement in hemostasis does not occur for several hours, regardless of the route of administration, and 24 hours or longer may be needed for maximal effect. If immediate hemostatic competence is necessary, adequate concentrations of vitamin K–dependent coagulation factors can be restored by transfusion of fresh frozen plasma (10 to 20 ml/kg). Concentrates prepared from plasma that are highly enriched in vitamin K–dependent proteins are available, but their use is not recommended in this setting because they are mainly intended for therapy of congenital deficiency of factor IX and are only standardized with respect to that activity. In most circumstances, vitamin K_1 should be given at the same time as plasma, since the transfused factors, particularly factor VII, are cleared from the circulation more quickly than is the residual oral anticoagulant. This will decrease the need for repeated transfusions. Usually, 5 to 10 mg of vitamin K_1 is sufficient, but some patients require much larger amounts. Repeated administration of vitamin K_1 may also be necessary, particularly in cases of overdose or if the oral anticoagulant has a long half-life in the patient. The use of vitamin K_1 can make the subsequent response to oral anticoagulants erratic for days or even weeks; thus, anticoagulation after resolution of a bleeding episode may require the short-term use of heparin or other agents. Partial reversal of oral anticoagulation for minor or elective procedures using smaller doses of vitamin K_1 is possible but should be attempted only by experienced clinicians. Given the variability in half-lives of the drugs and proteins involved, careful monitoring for evidence of bleeding or thrombosis and frequent measurements of the PT are essential.

Administration of warfarin during pregnancy is a cause of birth defects and abortion. A syndrome characterized by nasal hypoplasia and stippled epiphyseal calcifications that resemble chondrodysplasia punctata may result from maternal ingestion of warfarin during the first trimester. Central nervous system abnormalities have been reported following exposure during the second and third trimesters. Fetal or neonatal hemorrhage and intrauterine death may occur, even when maternal PT values are in the therapeutic range. Oral anticoagulants should not be used during pregnancy.

Coumarin-induced skin necrosis is a rare complication of oral anticoagulant therapy. First noted in 1943, this syndrome is characterized by the appearance of skin lesions 3 to 10 days after treatment is initiated. This unusual reaction has been observed with different congeners of coumarin and indandione. Patients who develop the lesions during one course of therapy often (but not always) can be treated later without a similar reaction. The severity of the skin lesions may not be affected by stopping as compared with continuing the drug. The lesions are most common on the extremities, but the female breast, adipose tissue, and the penis may be involved. Lesions are characterized by widespread thrombosis of the microvasculature and can spread rapidly, sometimes becoming necrotic and requiring disfiguring debridement or occasionally amputation. At least five cases have been reported recently in subjects heterozygous for protein C deficiency. Since protein C has a shorter half-life than do the other vitamin K–dependent coagulation factors (except factor VII), its functional activity falls more rapidly in response to the initial dose of vitamin K antagonist. It has been proposed that the skin necrosis is a manifestation of a temporal imbalance between the anticoagulant protein C and one or more of the procoagulant factors and is exaggerated in patients who are partially deficient in protein C. The thrombosis of small vessels is consistent with the notion that they are the principal site of activation of protein C, since the ratio of endothelial cell surface (and therefore of thrombomodulin) to plasma is greatest in small vessels. However, not all patients with heterozygous deficiency of protein C develop skin necrosis when treated with oral anticoagulants, and patients with normal activity of protein C can also be affected. Morphologically similar lesions can occur without oral anticoagulant therapy, especially in patients with vitamin K deficiency.

A reversible, sometimes painful, blue-tinged discoloration of the plantar surfaces and sides of the toes that blanches with pressure and fades with elevation of the legs (purple toe syndrome) may develop 3 to 8 weeks after initiation of therapy with coumarin anticoagulants. Other infrequent reactions include alopecia, urticaria, dermatitis, fever, nausea, diarrhea, abdominal cramps, and anorexia.

LABORATORY EVALUATION OF COAGULATION AND ANTICOAGULANT THERAPY

Prior to initiation of therapy, laboratory tests are used in conjunction with the patient's history and physical examination to uncover hemostatic defects that might make the use of oral anticoagulant drugs more dangerous (congenital coagulation factor deficiency, thrombocytopenia, hepatic or renal insufficiency, vascular abnormalities, *etc.*). Thereafter, the PT is used to monitor efficacy and compliance. Therapeutic ranges for various clinical indications have been established empirically and reflect dosages that reduce the morbidity from thromboembolic disease while increasing as little as possible the risk of serious hemorrhage.

Usually, the patient's PT is determined along with that for a control sample of plasma, and the two values are often reported as a ratio. The PT is prolonged when the functional levels of fibrinogen, factor V, or the vitamin K–dependent factors II, VII, or X are decreased. The sensitivity to changes in each of these proteins depends on the testing method and the thromboplastin used. Reduced levels of factor IX or proteins C or S have no effect on the PT. The prolongation of a given patient's PT over the control can vary widely between laboratories. Sources of the variability in results include (1) methods of sample collection, transport, and storage prior to testing; (2) thromboplastin reagent; (3) method of clot detection; and (4) source of control plasma. Ideally, a fasting blood sample is obtained 8 to 14 hours after the last dose. Renewed efforts to standardize testing between laboratories have been made recently, especially in Europe. An International Normalized Ratio (INR) system of reporting has been proposed; conceptually, it is the ratio of the patient PT to a control PT that would have been obtained by a standard method using a World Health Organization primary standard (human) thromboplastin. This system has not gained widespread acceptance in the United States. The major practical consequence from these efforts at standardization is an appreciation that the commercial thromboplastins from rabbit tissue (used especially in North America) are relatively insensitive to small reductions in the activities of coagulation factors. This property has led to administration of larger doses of oral anticoagulants than were considered optimal in many of the original clinical trials (where more sensitive human brain thromboplastins are usually used). The notion of maintaining good control by prolonging the PT to 1.4 to 2.5 times normal has been replaced by more specific recommendations, based both on indications and type of thromboplastin used for monitoring. Clinical indications are discussed below in the section on therapeutic uses. In most situations, the target range for the PT ratio is 1.2 to 1.5 if rabbit tissue thromboplastin is used or 2.0 to 3.0 for human thromboplastin; in long-term therapy for recurrent thromboembolic disease or when mechanical heart valves are present, the target ratio is increased to 1.5 to 2.0 (rabbit) or 3.0 to 4.5 (human). At the start of therapy (and especially if heparin is also administered), the significance of the PT can only be interpreted based on experience with both the laboratory and the treatment protocol. The prolongation of the PT is not a direct indication of the antithrombotic effect of therapy, which may be delayed for several days. Daily PTs are indicated initially to guard against excessive anticoagulation in the unusually sensitive patient; the testing interval can be gradually lengthened to weekly and then monthly for patients on long-term therapy in whom test results have been stable.

Other Oral Anticoagulants

Dicumarol. Dicumarol is the original oral anticoagulant isolated and the first used clinically, but it is now seldom used because it is absorbed slowly and erratically and frequently causes gastrointestinal side effects. It is available in 25- and 50-mg tablets and is usually given in maintenance doses of 25 to 200 mg daily. Its onset of action as monitored by the PT is 1 to 5 days, and its effect lasts 2 to 10 days after withdrawal.

Phenprocoumon, Acenocoumarol, and Ethyl Biscoumacetate. These agents are not generally available in the United States but are prescribed in Europe and elsewhere. *Phenprocoumon* (MARCUMAR) has a longer plasma half-life (5 days) than warfarin, as well as a somewhat slower onset of action and a longer duration of action (7 to 14 days). It is administered in daily maintenance doses of 0.75 to 6.0 mg. By contrast, *acenocoumarol* (NICOUMALONE; SINTHROME) has a shorter half-life (10 to 24 hours), a more rapid effect on the PT, and a shorter duration of action (2 days). The maintenance dose is 1 to 8 mg daily. *Ethyl biscoumacetate* (TROMEXANE, others) is seldom used; it is difficult to achieve stable anticoagulation even when given in divided doses because of its very short half-life (2 to 3 hours).

Indandione Derivatives. *Anisindione* (MIRADON) is available for clinical use in the United States. It is similar to warfarin in its kinetics of action; however, it offers no clear advantages and may cause a higher frequency of untoward effects. Phenindione was popular at one time and is still available in some countries. Serious hypersensitivity reactions, occasionally fatal, can occur within a few weeks of starting therapy with this drug, and its use can no longer be recommended. Diphenadione is a very long-acting agent (prolongation of the PT may persist for 20 days), which is of interest only because it is used as a rodenticide.

THROMBOLYTIC DRUGS

Fibrinolysis and Thrombolysis

The fibrinolytic system dissolves intravascular clots as a result of the action of plasmin, an enzyme that digests fibrin (*see* Figure 55–1). Plasminogen, an inactive precursor, is converted to plasmin by cleavage of a single peptide bond. Plasmin is a relatively nonspecific protease; it digests fibrin clots and other plasma proteins, including several coagulation factors. Therapy with thrombolytic drugs tends to dissolve both pathological thrombi and also fibrin deposits at sites of vascular injury. Therefore, the drugs are toxic, producing hemorrhage as a major side effect.

The fibrinolytic system is regulated such that unwanted fibrin thrombi are removed, while fibrin in wounds persists to maintain hemostasis (Collen and Lijnen, 1987). Tissue plasminogen activator (t-PA) is released from endothelial cells in response to various signals, including stasis produced by vascular occlusion. It is rapidly cleared from blood or inhibited by a circulating inhibitor, plasminogen activator inhibitor-1, and thus exerts little effect on circulating plasminogen. t-PA binds to fibrin and converts plasminogen, which also binds to fibrin, to plasmin. Plasminogen and plasmin bind to fibrin at binding sites located near their amino termini that are rich in lysine residues (*see* below). These sites are also required for binding of plasmin to α_2-antiplasmin. Therefore, fibrin-bound plasmin is protected from inhibition. Any plasmin that escapes this local milieu is rapidly inhibited. Some α_2-antiplasmin is bound covalently to fibrin and thereby protects fibrin from premature lysis. When plasminogen activators are administered for thrombolytic therapy, massive fibrinolysis is initiated, and the inhibitory controls just described are overwhelmed.

Plasminogen. Plasminogen is a single-chain glycoprotein that contains 790 amino acid residues; it is converted to an active protease by cleavage at arginine 560. The molecule contains high affinity, amino-terminal lysine-containing binding sites that mediate the binding of plasminogen (or plasmin) to fibrin; this enhances fibrinolysis. These sites are in the amino-terminal "kringle" domain between amino acids 80 and 165, and they also promote formation of complexes of plasmin with α_2-antiplasmin, the major physiological plasmin inhibitor. Plasminogen concentrations in human plasma average 2 μM. A degraded form of plasminogen termed lys-plasminogen binds to fibrin much more rapidly than does intact plasminogen. Lys-plasminogen has been used as an adjunctive fibrinolytic agent with streptokinase or urokinase in uncontrolled studies.

α_2-Antiplasmin. α_2-Antiplasmin is a glycoprotein composed of 452 amino acid residues. It forms a covalent complex with plasmin, thereby inactivating it. The complex results from the formation of an ester bond between the active-site serine of plasmin and an arginine residue in α_2-antiplasmin. A carboxyl-terminal peptide (approximately 8000 daltons) is released from α_2-antiplasmin in the process of formation of the ester. Plasma concentrations of α_2-antiplasmin (1 μM) are sufficient to inhibit about 50% of potential plasmin. When massive activation of plasminogen occurs, the inhibitor is depleted and free plasmin causes a "systemic lytic state," in which hemostasis is impaired. In this state, fibrinogen is destroyed and fibrinogen degradation products impair formation of fibrin and therefore increase bleeding from wounds. α_2-Antiplasmin inactivates plasmin nearly instantaneously, as long as the lysine binding sites on plasmin are unoccupied by fibrin or other antagonists, such as aminocaproic acid (ϵ-aminocaproic acid; *see* below).

Streptokinase. Streptokinase is a 47,000-dalton protein produced by β-hemolytic streptococci. It has no intrinsic enzymatic activity, but it forms a stable, noncovalent 1:1 complex with plasminogen. This produces a conformational change that exposes the active site on plasminogen that cleaves arginine 560 on free plasminogen molecules to form free plasmin.

A loading dose of streptokinase (250,000 units; 2.5 mg) must be given intravenously to overcome plasma antibodies that are directed against the protein. These inactivating antibodies result from prior streptococcal infections. The half-life of streptokinase (once antibodies are depleted) is about 80 minutes (Grierson and Bjornsson, 1987). The streptokinase–plasminogen complex is not inhibited by α_2-antiplasmin. Levels of antibodies differ greatly among individuals, but this factor is probably of little clinical significance when streptokinase is given in the large doses currently used for coronary thrombolysis. Adverse reactions (other than the bleeding problems that are common to all fibrinolytic agents) include allergic reactions, rarely anaphylaxis, and fever. Streptokinase (STREPTASE) is supplied in vials containing 250,000, 750,000, or 1,500,000 IU of the protein.

A streptokinase–plasminogen complex (*anistreplase;* EMINASE) in which lys-plasminogen is acylated at its active-site serine is currently being used in Europe for coronary thrombolysis (AIMS, 1988). The acyl group is hydrolyzed *in vivo,* allowing the complex to bind to fibrin prior to activation, and this modification may confer some specificity toward clots on the fibrinolytic process. However, when this agent is given as a bolus injection at the dose recommended for coronary thrombolysis (30 U), marked systemic fibrinolysis occurs.

Tissue Plasminogen Activator (t-PA). t-PA is a serine protease that contains 527 amino-acid residues. It is a poor plasminogen activator in the absence of fibrin (Collen and Lijnen, 1987). t-PA binds to fibrin via lysine binding sites at its amino terminus and activates bound plasminogen several hundred-fold more rapidly than it activates plasminogen in the circulation. The lysine binding sites on t-PA are in a "finger" domain that is homologous to similar sites on fibronectin. Under physiological conditions (t-PA concentrations of 5 to 10 ng/ml), the specificity of t-PA for fibrin limits systemic formation of plasmin and induction of a systemic lytic state. During therapeutic infusions of t-PA, however, concentrations rise to 300 to 3000 ng/ml.

Clearance of t-PA is primarily by hepatic metabolism, and the half-life of the protein is about 3 minutes. t-PA is effective in lysing thrombi during treatment of acute myocardial infarction. The human protein is produced by recombinant DNA technology and is supplied in 20- and 50-mg vials as *alteplase, recombinant* (ACTIVASE). The current recommended regimen for coronary thrombolysis is a 10-mg intravenous bolus, followed by a continuous infusion for 3 hours (50 mg the first hour, then 20 mg per hour). Adverse effects include hemorrhage, as discussed below. t-PA is expensive, costing considerably more than streptokinase per therapeutic dose (*Medical Letter,* 1987).

Urokinase. This two-chain serine protease contains 411 amino-acid residues. Urokinase is isolated from cultured human cells and is available in vials containing 250,000 IU (ABBOKINASE). Urokinase has a half-life of 15 minutes and is metabolized by the liver. Recommended dosage regimens include an intravenous loading dose of 1000 to 4500 U/kg, followed by continuous infusion of 4400 U/kg per hour for varying time periods. Current interest in urokinase is limited, since it has the disadvantages of both of the other available thrombolytic agents. Like streptokinase, it lacks fibrin specificity and therefore readily induces a systemic lytic state; like t-PA, it is very expensive. Saruplase (prourokinase; single chain urokinase) does display selectivity for clots by binding to fibrin before activation, and it is currently under investigation as a thrombolytic agent.

Hemorrhagic Toxicity of Thrombolytic Therapy. The major toxicity of all thrombolytic agents is hemorrhage, which results from two factors: (1) the lysis of fibrin in "physiological thrombi" at sites of vascular injury; and (2) a systemic lytic state that results from systemic formation of plasmin, which produces fibrinogenolysis and destruction of other coagulation factors (especially factors V and VIII). The actual toxicity of streptokinase, urokinase, and t-PA is difficult to assess. In early clinical trials, many bleeding episodes resulted from the extensive invasive monitoring of therapy that was required by the protocol. In the TIMI trial, which employed intravenous streptokinase and t-PA, over two thirds of bleeding episodes were at catheterization sites. Most studies to evaluate thrombolysis involve concurrent systemic heparinization, which also contributes to bleeding complications.

The contraindications to fibrinolytic therapy are listed in Table 55–2. Patients with the indicated conditions should not receive such treatment, and invasive procedures (*e.g.,* cardiac catheterization, arterial blood gases) should be avoided. If heparin is used concurrently with either streptokinase or t-PA, serious hemorrhage will occur in 2 to 4% of patients. Intracranial hemorrhage is by far the most serious problem; it occurs in approximately 1% of cases, and the frequency is the same with all three thrombolytic agents. Despite the fact that t-PA is relatively fibrin-specific, hemorrhage is just as common with this agent as with the others, possibly because t-PA is more effective at dissolving "physiological thrombi" than are the other two drugs and thus, despite less systemic lysis, bleeding at sites of injury may be more severe. Patients in the recent large streptokinase trials that did not routinely use heparin had very low incidences of serious hemorrhage (less than 1%). When streptokinase is used as in these regimens, the toxicity may be low enough to relax the contraindications listed in Table 55–2 (*e.g.,* hypertension). To date, t-PA has not been extensively evaluated in protocols that avoid heparin.

It is clear that the frequency of hemorrhage is less when thrombolytic agents are utilized to treat myocardial infarction compared with pulmonary embolism or venous thrombosis. A major difference in these regimens is the duration of therapy. A thrombolytic agent is infused for 1 to 3 hours for myocardial infarction; infusions of 12 to 72 hours have been used for venous disease. Such prolonged treatment should probably not be used. In the UPET trial, in

Table 55–2. CONTRAINDICATIONS TO THROMBOLYTIC THERAPY

1. Surgery within 10 days, including organ biopsy, puncture of noncompressible vessels, serious trauma, cardiopulmonary resuscitation
2. Serious gastrointestinal bleeding within 3 months
3. History of hypertension (diastolic pressure > 110 mm Hg)
4. Active bleeding or hemorrhagic disorder
5. Previous cerebrovascular accident or active intracranial process

which 12- to 24-hour infusions of streptokinase or urokinase were employed, 50% of patients had significant bleeding (Urokinase, 1974). Recent studies suggest that the concurrent administration of low doses of aspirin improves the efficacy of thrombolytic therapy of myocardial infarction. The role of other antiplatelet drugs and systemic anticoagulants in these treatments is currently under investigation.

Aminocaproic Acid. Aminocaproic acid is a lysine analog that binds to lysine binding sites on plasminogen and plasmin, thus blocking the binding of plasmin to target fibrin. Aminocaproic acid is thereby a potent inhibitor of fibrinolysis and can reverse states that are associated with excessive fibrinolysis. Although it has been used in a variety of bleeding conditions, it is without clearcut benefit (Marder *et al.*, 1987). The main problem with its use is that thrombi that form during treatment with the drug are not lysed. For example, in patients with hematuria, ureteral obstruction by clots may lead to renal failure after treatment with aminocaproic acid. Aminocaproic acid has been used to reduce bleeding after prostatic surgery or after tooth extractions in hemophiliacs. The clinical significance of reduced bleeding in these settings is uncertain. Use of aminocaproic acid to treat a variety of other bleeding disorders has been unsuccessful, either because of limited benefit or because of thrombosis (*e.g.*, after subarachnoid hemorrhage). Aminocaproic acid is rapidly absorbed after oral administration, and 50% is excreted unchanged in the urine within 12 hours. Usually, a loading dose of 4 to 5 g is given over 1 hour, followed by an infusion of 1 g per hour until bleeding is controlled. No more than 30 g should be given in a 24-hour period. Rarely, the drug causes myopathy and muscle necrosis.

ANTIPLATELET DRUGS

Platelets provide the initial hemostatic plug at sites of vascular injury. They also participate in reactions that lead to atherosclerosis and pathological thrombosis in numerous animal studies. Antagonists of platelet function have thus been used in attempts to prevent thrombosis and to alter the natural history of atherosclerotic vascular disease.

Aspirin. Processes including thrombosis, inflammation, wound healing, and allergy are modulated by oxygenated metabolites of arachidonate and related polyunsaturated fatty acids that are collectively termed eicosanoids. Interference with the synthesis of eicosanoids is the basis for the effects of many therapeutic agents, including analgesics, antiinflammatory drugs, and antithrombotic agents (*see* Chapters 24 and 26).

In platelets, the major eicosanoid is thromboxane A_2, a labile inducer of platelet aggregation and a potent vasoconstrictor. Aspirin blocks production of thromboxane A_2 by a unique mechanism: it covalently acetylates the active site of cyclooxygenase, the enzyme that produces the cyclic endoperoxide precursor of thromboxane A_2 (Majerus, 1983). Since platelets do not synthesize new proteins, the action of aspirin on platelet cyclooxygenase is permanent, lasting for the life of the platelet (7 to 10 days). Thus, repeated doses of aspirin produce a cumulative effect on platelet function. Complete inactivation of platelet cyclooxygenase is achieved when 160 mg of aspirin is taken daily. Therefore, aspirin is maximally effective as an antithrombotic agent at doses much lower than required for other actions of the drug. Numerous trials indicate that aspirin, when used as an antithrombotic drug, is maximally effective at doses of 160 to 320 mg per day. Higher doses do not improve efficacy, but they definitely increase toxicity, especially bleeding.

Other inhibitors of eicosanoid biosynthesis have been evaluated as potential antithrombotic agents, especially inhibitors of thromboxane synthetase. These drugs have the theoretical advantage of inhibiting production of thromboxane A_2 without blocking the synthesis of prostacyclin, an antithrombotic eicosanoid produced by the vascular endothelium. However, these drugs allow cyclic endoperoxide intermediates to accumulate, which themselves stimulate platelet aggregation. Thus, these agents have been relatively ineffective and do not measure up well against the cost, safety, and efficacy of aspirin.

Dipyridamole. This drug is a vasodilator that, in combination with warfarin, inhibits embolization from prosthetic heart valves and, in combination with aspirin, reduces thrombosis in patients with thrombotic diseases. Dipyridamole by itself has little or no benefit; in fact, in trials where a regimen of dipyridamole plus aspirin was compared with aspirin alone, dipyridamole provided no additional beneficial effect (Antiplatelet Trialists Collaboration, 1988). Dipyridamole interferes with platelet function by increasing the cellular concentration of adenosine 3′,5′-monophosphate (cyclic AMP). This effect is mediated by inhibition of cyclic nucleotide phosphodiesterase and/or by blockade of uptake of adenosine, which acts at A_2 receptors for adenosine to stimulate platelet adenylyl cyclase. The only current recommended use of dipyridamole is for primary prophylaxis of thromboemboli in patients with prosthetic heart valves; the drug is given in combination with warfarin. Dipyridamole is available in 25-, 50-, and 75-mg tablets (PERSANTINE).

Ticlopidine. This drug is a thienopyridine that inhibits platelet function by inducing a thrombasthenia-like state (DiMinno *et al.*, 1985). It interacts with platelet glycoprotein IIb/IIIa in an unknown way to inhibit the binding of fibrinogen to activated platelets. Glycoprotein IIb/IIIa is a fibrinogen receptor that links platelets via fibrinogen to form an aggregated plug; this action allows clot retraction. Thus, ticlopidine inhibits platelet aggregation and clot retraction. Ticlopidine prolongs the template bleeding time, with a maximal effect seen only after several days of therapy; abnormal platelet function persists for several days after treatment is discontinued. It is possible that some metabolite of ticlopidine is the active antithrombotic agent, since the drug is relatively ineffective in inhibiting platelet aggregation when added to platelets *in vitro* compared with its effects on platelets taken from patients who are ingesting the drug. The drug has no effect on eicosanoid metabolism, and it should act independently of aspirin; to date, however, these two agents have not been tested in combination. Ticlopidine currently is being tested for its efficacy in prevention of thrombosis in cerebral vascular and coronary artery disease. The drug is available in Europe and is being used experimentally in the United States and elsewhere. The dose is 250 mg, given twice daily. Side effects include bleeding, nausea, and diarrhea in 10% of patients, and severe neutropenia in approximately 1% of patients.

Sulfinpyrazone. This drug is used for its uricosuric properties (*see* Chapter 30). Sulfinpyrazone also inhibits a number of platelet functions, including the release reaction and adherence to subendothelial cells, and inhibits synthesis of prostaglandins. In large, randomized clinical trials in which 200 mg of sulfinpyrazone was taken four times a day, a reduction in the incidence of sudden death after myocardial infarction was described (ANTURANE Reinfarction Trial Research Group, 1978, 1980); however, the study was subsequently criticized for statistical and methodological reasons (*see* Hampton, 1982). The drug has not been approved by the United States Food and Drug Administration as an antithrombotic agent.

THERAPEUTIC USES OF ANTICOAGULANT, THROMBOLYTIC, AND ANTIPLATELET DRUGS

The information required to direct therapy in specific thromboembolic diseases is frequently nonexistent, incomplete, or conflicting. In the case of prophylactic treatment for arterial thrombotic disease, the relatively low frequency of end-point events (myocardial infarction, stroke, death) requires that studies utilize very large numbers of patients to achieve statistically significant results. Use of many of the drugs discussed in this chapter, in particular the thrombolytic agents and anticoagulants, carries a substantial risk of hemorrhage and a significant risk of death. Thus, the perceived risk/benefit assessment of a particular regimen depends upon the characteristics of the individual patient and may not concur with what is recommended for the population as a whole (American College, 1986). *Where treatment with warfarin is discussed in this section, the PT ratios given reflect use of rabbit thromboplastin, which is common in the United States* (*see* above).

Venous Thromboembolism. *Treatment.* The goal in the treatment of deep venous thrombosis and pulmonary embolism is the prevention of recurrent, fatal pulmonary embolism. Clinical experience suggests that heparin is efficacious, although convincing randomized studies have not been performed. Heparin is used for initial treatment because of the rapid onset of its anticoagulant effect. Heparin therapy is usually continued for 7 to 10 days and overlaps with warfarin treatment for 4 to 5 days. A study in which warfarin was begun early (after 1 day of heparin therapy) suggests that a shorter course of heparin (mean of 4 days) may suffice and would allow more rapid discharge of patients from hospital (Gallus *et al.*, 1986).

Streptokinase also has been used to treat pulmonary embolism and deep venous thrombosis. In these conditions therapy is given as a prolonged intravenous infusion of 100,000 U per hour for 12 to 72 hours. Thus far, no studies have shown reduced mortality after streptokinase therapy for pulmonary embolism. The rationale for use of thrombolytic therapy in venous thrombosis is that lysis of the clot may allow preservation of venous valves and therefore decrease the occurrence of postphlebitic signs in the legs (ulcers, edema). The efficacy of thrombolysis in preventing venous insufficiency and postphlebitic signs and symptoms remains to be established.

Anticoagulant therapy should be continued beyond the initial 7 to 10 days of treatment with heparin. This view is consistent with the results of two clinical trials. Following initial treatment with heparin, low-dose heparin (for proximal leg vein thrombosis) and no further therapy (for calf vein thrombosis) were shown to be less effective than warfarin in preventing recurrent thrombosis (Hull *et al.*, 1979; Lagerstedt *et al.*, 1985). Warfarin is most often used for long-term anticoagulation, although adjusted-dose, subcutaneous heparin appears to be equally efficacious (Hull *et al.*, 1982). A consensus panel has recommended 3 months of anticoagulation (PT ratio of 1.2 to 1.5) following an initial episode of pulmonary embolism or proximal deep venous thrombosis (American College, 1986). Six weeks of anticoagulant therapy may suffice for localized calf vein thrombosis. In patients with recurrent thromboembolism or with a persistent risk factor (*e.g.*, immobilization), more prolonged anticoagulation is appropriate.

Prevention. Due to the morbidity and mortality associated with the treatment of established venous thrombosis, and because routine screening of patients at risk to identify those who may develop thrombosis is prohibitively expensive, considerable effort has been spent to identify effective methods of prevention. The appropriate prophylactic therapy is based on the risk for thromboembolism and the cost and morbidity associated with the use of the preventive intervention itself (Hull *et al.*, 1986). The incidence of venous thromboembolism in low-risk patients (minor surgery in patients older than 40 or uncomplicated surgery in patients younger than 40 without other risk factors for thrombosis) is such that only graduated compression stockings and early ambulation are indicated. Low-dose subcutaneous heparin is effective in preventing thromboembolism in moderate-risk patients (general surgery lasting more than 30 minutes in patients older than 40, myocardial infarction, congestive heart failure) and has not been associated with a significantly increased risk of bleeding in general surgical patients. External pneumatic intermittent compression of the legs is preferred in open urological surgery, operations for gynecological malignancy, neurosurgery, and other situations associated with a high risk of hemorrhage (*e.g.*, eye surgery, spinal anesthesia), except in patients with significant peripheral arteriosclerosis and overt ischemia.

Prevention of thromboembolism is difficult in high-risk patients (general surgery in patients older than 40 with deep venous thrombosis or pulmonary embolism, extensive pelvic or abdominal surgery for malignant disease, major orthopedic surgery of lower limbs). Few regimens have been studied extensively or compared in randomized, controlled trials. Further, although these prophylactic methods decrease the incidence of thromboembolism compared with no treatment or placebo, the risk of thromboembolism remains substantial. Some investigators advise routine screening for deep venous thrombosis (repeated impedance plethysmography or doppler testing, or venography prior to hospital discharge) in addition to prophylactic therapy for high-risk patients.

Myocardial Infarction. One of the earliest trials of antithrombotic therapy utilized warfarin after myocardial infarction. It was not until recently, however, with the advent of thrombolytic agents, that antithrombotic treatment of acute myocardial infarction has been shown to be efficacious in both preserving cardiac function and reducing mortality.

Streptokinase has been given by intracoronary and intravenous routes for lysis of coronary thrombi in patients with myocardial infarction. When given by the intracoronary route, wherein patency of the vessel can be monitored, adequate reperfusion is obtained in 50 to 90% of patients (Ludbrook and Rentrop, 1987). Intracoronary thrombolysis is complex and expensive; it causes delays in therapy and requires facilities for catheterization. The practical advantages and proven efficacy of intravenous therapy have supplanted intracoronary therapy.

Streptokinase has been shown to be efficacious in two large studies when given intravenously for myocardial infarction. In "GISSI," 11,800 patients admitted to coronary care units within 12 hours after the onset of symptoms were randomized to receive streptokinase or no thrombolytic therapy (GISSI, 1986). Treated patients received 1.5 million units of streptokinase in 100 ml of physiological saline over 1 hour. In-hospital mortality (14 to 21 days) was 628 of 5860 (11%) in the treated group versus 758 of 5852 (13%) in the control group. Benefit was greatest in patients who were treated within 3 hours of the onset of symptoms, although statistically significant reduction in mortality was seen in patients treated within 6 hours.

In the second study, "ISIS 2," patients were randomized to receive aspirin, streptokinase, streptokinase plus aspirin, or placebo (ISIS-2, 1988). Approximately 4300 patients admitted to hospitals for treatment of acute myocardial infarction were assigned to each group. Both aspirin and streptokinase were beneficial in reducing mortality at 5 weeks. The deaths were placebo, 568 (13%); aspirin, 461 (11%); streptokinase, 448 (10%); and streptokinase plus aspirin, 343 (8%). The dose of streptokinase was 1.5 million units intravenously over 1 hour, and enteric-coated aspirin (160 mg per day) was given for 5 weeks. The benefits of treatment were sustained over a median follow-up of 15 months. Toxicity was very low; fatal intracerebral hemorrhages occurred in 0.1% of patients receiving streptokinase, and 2 to 3% of patients had some evidence of hemorrhage. Aspirin did not appear to increase the bleeding caused by streptokinase. The effects of aspirin and streptokinase appear to be independent and additive. This regimen underscores the fact that low doses of aspirin are effective and nontoxic in preventing thrombosis.

Intravenous t-PA and intravenous streptokinase have been compared in two studies that showed greater patency of vessels after t-PA (Verstraete *et al.*, 1985; Chesebro *et al.*, 1987). The combined results of these studies indicate that 113 of 174 patients (65%) treated with t-PA had patent vessels, compared with 71 of 181 (39%) treated with streptokinase. t-PA plus heparin also improved survival when compared with heparin alone in a total of 5000 patients (Wilcox *et al.*, 1988). Deaths with heparin alone were 245 (10%) versus 182 (8%) for t-PA plus heparin. Current trials are designed to compare survival in patients randomized to receive either streptokinase or t-PA.

Unstable Angina. Patients with stable angina have an annual mortality rate of 4% and a rate of myocardial infarction of 5%; in patients with unstable angina the risks are 10% and 8 to 10%, respectively. In a study of 1200 men with unstable angina, a 12-week course of aspirin (325 mg per day) was shown to reduce the risk of acute myocardial infarction by 51% and to reduce total mortality by 51% (Lewis *et al.*, 1983). A subsequent trial in which patients were followed for up to 2 years has confirmed these results. A recent study that compared heparin and aspirin in the acute treatment of unstable angina (first 6 days) found that both reduced the incidence of fatal and nonfatal myocardial infarction when compared with placebo. Heparin treatment was also associated with a reduced incidence of refractory angina (Theroux *et al.*, 1988).

Saphenous Vein Bypass Grafts. Occlusion of the saphenous grafts is an important cause of morbidity and mortality following coronary artery bypass surgery; antiplatelet therapy can reduce this risk. A low dose of aspirin (325 mg per day) is as effective as a higher dose (975 mg per day) or the combination of aspirin and dipyridamole in preventing occlusion of bypass graft. When aspirin is begun preoperatively, the incidence of hemorrhage is increased compared with that observed in untreated patients or in patients who received dipyridamole preoperatively and aspirin postoperatively. This finding suggests that the postoperative initiation of aspirin alone is a reasonable therapy. Ticlopidine also reduces the incidence of occlusion of bypass grafts.

Cerebral Embolism. Although systemic embolization from a cardiac thrombus is usually clinically silent, cerebral embolism is frequently devastating. Approximately 10 to 20% of all ischemic strokes are believed to be due to emboli, although the clinical diagnosis of embolic stroke is difficult, since many patients have both cerebrovascular atherosclerosis and a cardiac source of emboli.

The dilemma in cases of acute cerebral embolism is the timing of anticoagulant therapy. Although the risk of recurrent emboli is great (12% within 2 weeks), the early use of anticoagulants is associated with hemorrhagic transformation of the infarct. In the absence of specific data bearing on this question, a consensus panel has recommended the following: (1) in small- or moderate-sized embolic strokes in patients without significant hypertension, initiate anticoagulant therapy if a CT scan performed more than 24 hours after the onset of the stroke documents the absence of hemorrhage; (2) in large embolic strokes or in patients with significant hypertension, initiate anticoagulant therapy 5 to 7 days after onset if there is no hemorrhagic transformation; and (3) postpone the initiation of anticoagulation for 8 to 10 days in patients with embolic strokes complicated by hemorrhagic transformation (Sherman *et al.*, 1986). Anticoagulant therapy is begun with heparin (without an initial bolus) and, because of the persistent high risk of recurrent embolism, should be followed indefinitely with warfarin (PT ratio 1.2 to 1.5).

Acute Transmural Anterior Myocardial Infarction. The incidence of cerebral embolism in acute myocardial infarction is 3 to 4%, and more than 90% of these strokes occur in patients with transmural anterior myocardial infarctions (a large proportion of which develop mural thrombi). Other risk factors for embolism include large size of the infarct, heart failure, ventricular aneurysm, and atrial fibrillation. The risk of embolic stroke in patients with otherwise uncomplicated inferior myocardial infarctions is quite low. Thus, it is recommended that patients with anterior transmural myocardial infarctions be treated with full doses of heparin, followed by treatment with warfarin (PT ratio 1.3 to 1.5) for 3 months, during which time the majority of emboli occur in untreated patients.

Atrial Fibrillation. More than 50% of patients with cerebral embolism have atrial fibrillation. In the majority of these patients, the underlying cardiac disease is nonvalvular. Atrial fibrillation is common, and therefore only subgroups of patients have a frequency of cerebral embolism high enough to warrant anticoagulant therapy: patients with valvular heart disease, cardiomyopathy, or thyrotoxic heart disease or those undergoing elective cardioversion. The risk of ischemic stroke in patients with atrial fibrillation has been estimated to be 5% per year, with a cumulative risk of 35% during their lifetime (Sherman *et al.*, 1986). Only a portion of these strokes, however, are embolic; the rest are due to cerebrovascular atherosclerosis. Coexistent congestive heart failure and recent onset of atrial fibrillation may identify patients with a greater risk of emboli, and anticoagulant therapy is frequently considered for these patients. Some investigators believe that an enlarged left atrium (greater than 55 mm) is an additional risk factor, but studies have yet to document this theory. The incidence of atrial fibrillation in patients with thyrotoxicosis is 10 to 30%. Although the rate of embolism in hyperthyroid patients with normal sinus rhythm is low, it complicates the course of 8 to 39% of patients with concomitant atrial fibrillation. Although no clinical trial has documented efficacy, anticoagulant therapy is advised for thyrotoxic patients with atrial fibrillation. Patients who are undergoing elective cardioversion for atrial fibrillation should be treated with anticoagulants. The incidence of emboli in untreated patients is 5.3%, versus an incidence of 0.8% in those receiving anticoagulant therapy (Bjerkelund and Orning, 1969). Present recommendations usually exclude patients with very recent onset of atrial fibrillation (< 7 days) but dictate oral anticoagulant treatment (PT ratio 1.2 to 1.5) in the remainder, beginning 2 to 3 weeks prior to cardioversion and extending for several weeks thereafter.

Prosthetic Heart Valves. The risk of embolism associated with mechanical heart valves is 2 to 6% per patient per year despite anticoagulation. The embolic risk may be somewhat higher for the ball valve (Starr Edwards) than for the tilting disc valves (Lillehei–Kaster, Bjork–Shiley), and it is lowest for the bileaflet valve (St. Jude). The embolic risk for valves in the mitral area is significantly greater than that for aortic prostheses. Long-term oral anticoagulant therapy (PT ratio 1.5 to 2.0) is recommended in patients with mechanical valves, and the concurrent administration of dipyridamole (100 mg four times daily) may further reduce the risk of thromboembolism. The thrombogenicity of bioprosthetic valves is considerably less than their mechanical counterparts, although the valves are less durable. Because of an increased thromboembolic risk directly following their insertion, most patients with bioprosthetic valves are treated with oral anticoagulants (PT ratio 1.2 to 1.5) for 3 months postoperatively.

Valvular Heart Disease. Rheumatic mitral valve disease is associated with thromboembolic complications at reported rates of 1.5 to 4.7% per year; the incidence in patients with mitral stenosis is approximately 1.5 to 2 times that in patients with mitral regurgitation. The presence of atrial fibrillation is the single most important risk factor for thromboembolism in valvular disease, increasing the incidence of thromboembolism in both mitral stenosis and regurgitation four- to sevenfold. Additional risk factors are old age and heart failure. Patients with rheumatic mitral disease and atrial fibrillation should receive oral anticoagulant therapy (PT ratio 1.2 to 1.5). Some cardiologists suggest that patients with mitral disease but sinus rhythm should receive anticoagulant therapy if they have a large left atrium (greater than 55 mm), since the risk for the development of atrial fibrillation is high in these patients.

Prolapse of the mitral valve is a common entity, occurring in 4 to 6% of the population. Recent evidence has established a relationship between mitral valve prolapse and systemic embolism, most frequently presenting as transient ischemic attacks or partial stroke (Barnett *et al.*, 1980). However, the embolic risk in an individual with mitral valve prolapse is small. Attempts to identify a subset of such patients at particular risk of thromboembolism have been unsuccessful, and in most patients with embolic phenomena, the mitral valve prolapse was silent by auscultatory examination. It is presently recommended that patients with mitral valve prolapse and transient ischemic attacks be treated with aspirin; patients with concurrent atrial fibrillation and those with recurrent ischemic episodes despite treatment with aspirin should receive long-term oral anticoagulant therapy.

Cardiomyopathy. The cumulative risk of systemic embolism in patients with dilated cardiomyopathy is about 18%, and the presence of intracardiac thrombi as detected by echocardiography increases this risk. Prophylactic oral anticoagulant therapy (PT ratio 1.2 to 1.5) is advised for patients with dilated cardiomyopathy. By contrast, such drugs are usually withheld in patients with hypertrophic cardiomyopathy unless atrial fibrillation, which is most frequently associated with severe heart failure, develops.

Transient Ischemic Attacks. Early studies suggested that oral anticoagulant therapy reduced the incidence of transient ischemic attacks and subsequent stroke. Later, small trials that compared anticoagulants with aspirin failed to detect a difference between treatment groups in the frequencies of transient ischemic attacks, stroke, or mortality, but noted that the risk of hemorrhage was greater in those receiving anticoagulant therapy. Several studies of the use of aspirin for transient ischemic attacks have now been completed (Antiplatelet Trialists Collaboration, 1988). In sum, they show a beneficial effect of aspirin on the frequency of transient ischemic attacks, incidence of stroke, and mortality.

Peripheral Vascular Disease. Antithrombotic therapy for acute peripheral occlusive disease is largely empirical. Systemic thrombolytic therapy produces complete or partial lysis of both embolic and thrombotic occlusions in 40% of patients. Such treatment is most likely to be beneficial when initiated within 72 hours after the onset of the occlusion. Local/regional lytic therapy appears to produce a somewhat greater rate of lysis, possibly with a lower incidence of hemorrhagic complications, but the risk of hemorrhage remains substantial. Furthermore, rethrombosis occurs frequently (in about 40% of patients). In practice, thrombolytic therapy has been reserved for patients in whom the occlusion is not amenable to surgery and for those in whom a possible delay between the initiation of therapy and thrombolysis would not jeopardize the viability of the limb. Empirical treatment with heparin is routinely given to patients after lytic or surgical intervention and to otherwise untreated patients, although its efficacy in these settings has not been documented.

Secondary Prevention of Arterial Thromboembolism. Aspirin and other antiplatelet drugs have been used in several studies to examine their effect in patients with a history of myocardial infarction, stroke, transient ischemic attacks, or unstable angina. In most instances, there has been a trend favoring aspirin versus control in terms of total vascular mortality (and total mortality), although the trends have failed to reach statistical significance. In view of this and because a trial encompassing an enormous number of patients would be required to establish a benefit, meta-analysis has been used to evaluate the results of the 25 trials that have already been completed (Antiplatelet Trialists Collaboration, 1988). These trials included more than 29,000 patients, 3000 of whom died. This analysis showed that antiplatelet treatment had no effect on nonvascular mortality but reduced vascular mortality by 15% and nonfatal vascular events (stroke, myocardial infarction) by 30%. Furthermore, no combination of antiplatelet agents was found to be superior to low doses of aspirin (150 to 300 mg per day) alone. This type of analysis, although not accepted by all, is the basis for the recommendation that patients who have suffered an occlusive vascular event be given long-term therapy with a low dose of aspirin.

Primary Prevention of Arterial Thromboembolism. In view of the perceived benefit of aspirin in the secondary prevention of stroke and myocardial infarction, two large trials involving physicians as subjects were initiated to study aspirin's effect in the primary prevention of arterial thrombosis. In the American study, 22,000 volunteers (age 40 to 84 years) were randomly assigned to take 325 mg of aspirin every other day or placebo (Steering Committee, 1989). The trial was halted early, after a mean follow-up of 5 years, when a 45% reduction in the incidence of myocardial infarction and a 72% reduction in the incidence of fatal myocardial infarction was noted with aspirin treatment. However, total mortality was reduced only 4% in the aspirin group, a difference that was not statistically significant. Thus, the prophylactic use of aspirin in an apparently healthy population is not recommended at this time unless there are risk factors for myocardial infarction.

Miscellaneous Uses. Antithrombotic agents are routinely used to prevent the occlusion of extracorporeal devices: intravascular cannulas (heparin), vascular access shunts in hemodialysis patients (aspirin), hemodialysis machines (heparin), and cardiopulmonary bypass machines (heparin). In addition, they have been utilized in the treatment of certain renal diseases (heparin/warfarin) and small-cell lung cancer (warfarin). The appropriate use of heparin in acute disseminated intravascular coagulation remains controversial; anecdotal reports suggest that heparin rather than warfarin or antiplatelet drugs is the preferred therapy for chronic disseminated intravascular coagulation (Trousseau's syndrome) (Bell *et al.*, 1985).

AIMS. Effect of intravenous APSAC on mortality after acute myocardial infarction: preliminary report of a placebo-controlled clinical trial. *Lancet,* **1988,** *1,* 545–549.

ANTURANE Reinfarction Trial Research Group. Sulfinpyrazone in the prevention of cardiac death after myocardial infarction. *N. Engl. J. Med.,* **1978,** *298,* 289–295.

———. Sulfinpyrazone in the prevention of sudden death after myocardial infarction. *Ibid.,* **1980,** *302,* 250–256.

Barnett, H. J. M.; Boughner, D. R.; and Taylor, D. W. Further evidence relating mitral valve prolapse to cerebral ischemic events. *N. Engl. J. Med.,* **1980,** *302,* 139–144.

Bell, W. R. Heparin-associated thrombocytopenia and thrombosis. *J. Lab. Clin. Med.,* **1988,** *111,* 600–605.

Bell, W. R.; Starksen, N. F.; Tong, S.; and Porterfield, J. K. Trousseau's syndrome: devastating coagulopathy in the absence of heparin. *Am. J. Med.,* **1985,** *79,* 423–430.

Bjerkelund, C. J., and Orning, O. M. The efficacy of anticoagulant therapy in preventing embolism related to DC electrical conversion of atrial fibrillation. *Am. J. Cardiol.,* **1969,** *23,* 208–216.

Chesebro, J. H., and others. Thrombolysis in myocardial infarction (TIMI) trial: a comparison between intravenous tissue plasminogen activator and intravenous streptokinase. *Circulation,* **1987,** *76,* 142–154.

Davie, E. W.; Ichinose, A.; and Leytus, S. P. Structural features of the proteins participating in blood coagulation and fibrinolysis. *Cold Spring Harbor Symp. Quant. Biol.,* **1986,** *51,* 509–514.

DiMinno, G.; Cerbone, A. M.; Mattioli, P. L.; Turco, S.; Iovine, C.; and Mancini, M. Functionally thrombasthenic state in normal platelets following administration of ticlopidine. *J. Clin. Invest.,* **1985,** *75,* 328–338.

Gallus, A.; Jackaman, J.; Tillett, J.; Mills, W.; and Wycherleg, A. Safety and efficacy of warfarin started early after submassive venous thrombosis or pulmonary embolism. *Lancet,* **1986,** *2,* 1293–1296.

GISSI. Effectiveness of intravenous thrombolytic treatment in acute myocardial infarction. *Lancet,* **1986,** *1,* 397–402.

Grierson, D. S., and Bjornsson, T. D. Pharmacokinetics of streptokinase in patients based on amidolytic activator complex activity. *Clin. Pharmacol. Ther.,* **1987,** *41,* 304–313.

Hampton, J. R. The secondary prevention of heart attacks. *J. Ir. Colleges Physicians Surgeons,* **1982,** *11,* 143–150.

Howell, W. H. Heparin, an anticoagulant: preliminary communication. *Am. J. Physiol.,* **1922,** *63,* 434–435.

Hull, R.; Delmore, T.; Carter, C.; Hirsh, J.; Genton, E.; Gent, M.; Turpie, G.; and McLaughlin, D. Adjusted subcutaneous heparin vs warfarin sodium in the long-term treatment of venous thrombosis. *N. Engl. J. Med.,* **1982,** *306,* 189–194.

Hull, R.; Delmore, T.; Genton, E.; Hirsh, J.; Gent, M.; Sackett, D.; McLaughlin, D.; and Armstrong, P. Warfarin sodium versus low dose heparin in long-term treatment of venous thrombosis. *N. Engl. J. Med.,* **1979,** *301,* 855–858.

ISIS-2. Randomized trial of intravenous streptokinase, oral aspirin, both, or neither among 17,187 cases of suspected acute myocardial infarction. *Lancet,* **1988,** *2,* 349–360.

Jaques, L. B. Addendum: the discovery of heparin. *Semin. Thromb. Hemostas.,* **1978,** *4,* 350–353.

Lagerstedt, C. I.; Olsson, C. G.; Fagher, B. O.; Oquist, B. W.; and Albrechtsson, U. Need for long-term anticoagulant treatment in symptomatic calf-vein thrombosis. *Lancet,* **1985,** *2,* 515–518.

Lewis, H. D., Jr., and others. Protective effects of aspirin against acute myocardial infarction and death in men with unstable angina. *N. Engl. J. Med.,* **1983,** *309,* 396–403.

Lindahl, U.; Feingold, D. S.; and Roden, L. Biosynthesis of heparin. *Trends Biochem. Sci.,* **1986,** *11,* 221–225.

Link, K. P. The discovery of dicumarol and its sequels. *Circulation,* **1959,** *19,* 97–107.

Ludbrook, P. A., and Rentrop, P. Thrombolysis and the heart. *Cardiology Clin.,* **1987,** *5,* 79–90.

Marcum, J. A., and Rosenberg, R. D. Anticoagulantly active heparin sulfate proteoglycan and the vascular endothelium. *Semin. Thromb. Hemost.,* **1987,** *13,* 464–474.

Medical Letter. Tissue-type plasminogen activator for acute coronary thrombolysis. **1987,** *29,* 107–109.

O'Reilly, R. A. Warfarin metabolism and drug–drug interactions. *Adv. Exp. Med. Biol.,* **1987,** *214,* 205–212.

Sherman, D. G.; Dyken, M. L.; Fisher, M.; Harrison, M. J. G.; and Hart, R. G. Cerebral embolism. *Chest,* **1986,** *89,* Suppl., 82S–98S.

Steering Committee of the Physicians' Health Study Research Group. Final report: findings from the aspirin component of the ongoing physicians' health study. *N. Engl. J. Med.,* **1989,** *321,* 128–135.

Theroux, P., and others. Aspirin, heparin, or both to treat acute unstable angina. *N. Engl. J. Med.,* **1988,** *319,* 1105–1111.

Urokinase–Streptokinase Embolism Trial. Phase 2 results. A cooperative study. *J.A.M.A.,* **1974,** *229,* 1606–1613.

Verstraete, M., and others. Randomized trial of intravenous recombinant tissue-type plasminogen activator vs. intravenous streptokinase in acute myocardial infarction. *Lancet,* **1985,** *1,* 842–847.

Wilcox, R. G.; Olsson, C. G.; Skene, A. M.; Lippe, G.; Jensen, G.; and Hampton, J. R. Trial of t-PA for mortality reduction in acute myocardial infarction. *Lancet,* **1988,** *2,* 525–530.

Monographs and Reviews

American College of Chest Physicians and the National Heart, Lung, and Blood Institute. National Conference on Antithrombotic Therapy. *Chest,* **1986,** *89,* Suppl., 1S–106S.

Antiplatelet Trialists Collaboration. Secondary prevention of vascular disease by prolonged antiplatelet treatment. *Br. Med. J.* [*Clin. Res.*], **1988,** *296,* 320–331.

Bjork, I., and Danielsson, A. Antithrombin and related

inhibitors of coagulation proteinases. In, *Proteinase Inhibitors*. (Barrett, A. J., and Salveson, G., eds.) Elsevier Science Publishing Co., Inc., Amsterdam, **1986**, pp. 439–504.

Collen, D., and Lijnen, H. R. Fibrinolysis and the control of hemostasis. In, *The Molecular Basis of Blood Diseases*. (Stamatoyannopoulos, G.; Nienhuis, A. W.; Leder, P.; and Majerus, P. W.; eds.) W. B. Saunders Co., Philadelphia, **1987**, pp. 662–668.

Esmon, C. T. The regulation of natural anticoagulant pathways. *Science*, **1987**, *235*, 1348–1352.

Griffin, J. P.; D'Arcy, P. F.; and Speirs, C. J. Anticoagulants. In, *A Manual of Adverse Drug Interactions*, 4th ed. John Wright, London, **1988**, pp. 137–158.

Griminger, P. Biological activity of the various vitamin K forms. *Vitam. Horm.*, **1966**, *24*, 605–618.

Hull, R. D.; Raskob, G. E.; and Hirsh, J. Prophylaxis of venous thromboembolism: an overview. *Chest*, **1986**, *89*, Suppl., 374S–383S.

Hyers, T. M.; Hull, R. D.; and Weg, J. G. Antithrombotic therapy for venous thromboembolic disease. *Chest*, **1986**, *89*, Suppl., 26S–35S.

Levine, M. N., and Hirsh, J. Hemorrhagic complications of anticoagulant therapy. *Semin. Thromb. Hemost.*, **1986**, *12*, 39–57.

———. Clinical use of low molecular weight heparins and heparinoids. *Ibid.*, **1988**, *14*, 116–125.

Majerus, P. W. Arachidonate metabolism in vascular disorders. *J. Clin. Invest.*, **1983**, *72*, 1521–1525.

Marder, V. J.; Butler, F. A.; and Barlow, G. H. Antifibrinolytic therapy. In, *Hemostasis and Thrombosis: Basic Principles and Clinical Practice*, 2nd ed. (Colman, R. W.; Hirsh, J.; Marder, V. J.; and Salsman, E. W.; eds.) J. B. Lippincott Co., Philadelphia, **1987**, pp. 380–394.

Suttie, J. W. The biochemical basis of warfarin therapy. *Adv. Exp. Med. Biol.*, **1987**, *214*, 3–16.

Verstraete, M., and Vermylen, J. Drugs affecting blood coagulation and hemostasis. In, *Side Effects of Drugs*, Annual 12. (Dukes, M. N. G., and Beeley, L., eds.) Elsevier Science Publishing Co., Inc., Amsterdam, **1988**, pp. 309–315.

Warkentin, T. E., and Kelton, J. G. Heparin-induced thrombocytopenia. *Ann. Rev. Med.*, **1989**, *40*, 31–44.

SECTION

XV

Hormones and Hormone Antagonists

INTRODUCTION

Ferid Murad

Preparations that contain the active principles of the endocrine glands are utilized as drugs. Whereas most drugs are considered to be substances foreign to the body, the hormones are natural secretions of the endocrine glands and exert important functional effects upon other tissues. Consequently, the tendency has been to place hormones in a different category, although there is really no valid reason for doing so; indeed, some endocrine preparations have unobtrusively broken down this arbitrary distinction. For example, epinephrine is much more frequently viewed as a powerful sympathomimetic drug than as a hormone of the adrenal medulla.

Pharmacological studies on the actions of drugs of endocrine origin have contributed greatly to an understanding of the normal functions of the endocrine glands. Conversely, much can be learned about the effects of a hormonally active drug by observing the consequences of a deficiency or an excess of the hormone in question. The diverse actions of cortisol and its congeners, for instance, are strikingly illustrated by the changes from the normal shown by patients suffering from adrenal deficiency on the one hand and by patients with oversecretion on the other.

Analogs of the hormones—synthetic compounds resembling the natural products but differing from them in some important respects—have often proven more useful in therapeutics than have the hormones themselves. One aim in endocrinology is the isolation, identification, and synthesis of the active principles of each of the endocrine glands. Sometimes, when these formidable efforts have been successful, the product has been found to be of little use in therapy. It may prove inactive when given by mouth, as are the catecholamines and most peptides or proteins, or it may be so rapidly degraded that unless injected frequently little effect can be achieved, as in the case of the natural sex hormones. The design of synthetic analogs, compounds altered enough to outwit degradative enzymes but not enough to confuse the receptor sites, is one of the major contributions to endocrine therapy. In a number of instances the synthetic analogs, by their more desirable properties, represent improvements upon nature. A striking example was the discovery, 50 years ago, of diethylstilbestrol, a cheap synthetic substance that duplicates the actions of estrogen when given orally. Important challenges for the future include the design and synthesis of small molecules with reasonable oral bioavailability that mimic or antagonize the effects of peptide hormones. Innovative systems for the regional or targeted delivery of drugs can also influence the therapeutic efficacy of a hormone or analog by allowing control of its site or rate of delivery or its metabolism.

A number of useful drugs can influence the synthesis or secretion of hormones or antagonize their cellular actions. Most endocrine tissues store their hormones or precursors thereof intracellularly, often in granules that contain a prohormone or the biologically active compound itself. Secretion is frequently accomplished by exocytosis of the packaged products, and this process, stimulus-secretion coupling, generally requires Ca^{2+}. Synthesis, storage, and secretion of hormones are regulated at numerous steps. The antithyroid drugs provided the initial example of drugs that selectively inhibit hormone synthesis, and this action makes them effective in the treatment of hyperthyroidism. Equally specific substances have been developed to block one or another step in the synthesis of the hormones of the adrenal cortex.

Direct inhibition of the action of a hormone upon its receptor sites has been achieved experimentally in several instances and has been put to good use in isolated cases. Inhibition of the action of estrogen accounts for the therapeutic efficacy of clomiphene in reproductive disorders in women. By relieving the inhibitory influence of estrogen upon the pituitary, the substance acts to promote the secretion of gonadotropins.

Usually, when considering the clinical applications of the hormones, one thinks first of their use in replacement therapy—treatment of Addison's disease, myxedema, and so forth, with the appropriate drug. However, if the normal regulatory interactions of an endocrine system are understood, hormones and their antagonists can be exploited for a variety of additional therapeutic and diagnostic purposes. Regulation of the endocrine systems characteristically takes place on a multitude of levels. Many systems are ultimately responsive to neural or neuroendocrine control of either a stimulatory or inhibitory nature or both. A change in the magnitude of such control results in an appropriate alteration of secretion in a dependent target, and this secretion may serve as the immediate regulator of yet another endocrine organ. Any of the intermediate products, but more commonly the final hormonal secretion in such a chain, may "feed back" at any level to regulate the intensity of a controlling signal. Such feedback is predominantly negative; thus, a hormone can inhibit its own synthesis and secretion when its critical concentration is exceeded. Positive feedback systems are, however, occasionally utilized. Blood-borne chemicals, the concentrations of which are subject to hormonal regulation, are also used extensively as feedback regulators in such control systems. This knowledge is useful clinically, and it must be applied in the interpretation of a patient's basal laboratory data and in the performance of a variety of provocative tests of endocrine function. Similarly, therapeutic maneuvers also depend on these regulatory interactions. For example, the activity of the adrenal cortex can be suppressed by an adrenocorticosteroid through inhibition of the secretion of corticotropin; ovulation, if unwanted, can be abolished by ovarian hormones that suppress the secretion of hypophyseal gonadotropins.

The past 30 years have witnessed an explosive increase in our knowledge of the mechanisms of hormone action, and this is understood in detail for many endocrine secretions. The mechanisms of signal transduction that are used by hormones overlap broadly with those of other regulators of cell function, such as neurotransmitters and autacoids (*see* Chapter 2). To recapitulate briefly, many hormones interact with specific receptors in cellular plasma membranes that are linked via guanine nucleotide binding-regulatory proteins (G proteins) to the enzyme adenylyl cyclase, discovered by Sutherland and Rall. This enzyme is stimulated or inhibited by the hormone-receptor complex, and the result is an altered rate of synthesis of adenosine 3′,5′-monophosphate (cyclic AMP) from adenosine triphosphate (ATP). Cyclic AMP then acts as an intracellular mediator for the hormone, and the system thus functions as a mechanism for transferring and amplifying the information inherent in the extracellular hormone. Cyclic AMP regulates a variety of intracellular processes, and the ultimate effects are dependent on the cell's capacity to respond—its differentiated repertoire. The mechanism of cyclic AMP action involves the activation of protein kinases (protein kinases A) that phosphorylate cellular constituents and alter the rates at which processes involving these constituents proceed. The hormones discussed in the following chapters that appear to use this mechanism include the trophic hormones of the adenohypophysis, the melanocyte-stimulating hormones, some of the hypothalamic releasing hormones, glucagon, parathyroid hormone, and calcitonin. Many hormones appear to act by altering the uptake, release, and intracellular distribution of Ca^{2+}. Frequently this is accomplished through the receptor- and G protein-mediated stimulation of a membrane-associated phospholipase C that hydrolyzes polyphosphoinositides with the formation of inositol phosphates and a family of diacylglycerols. Of the inositol phosphates that are synthesized, inositol 1,4,5-trisphosphate in particular raises intracellular concentrations of Ca^{2+} by stimulating release of the ion from the endoplasmic reticulum. Diacylglycerols, like cyclic AMP, act by enhancing the catalytic activity of a group of related protein kinases, collectively referred to as protein kinase C. There are many situations in which these systems are interactive. These include instances in which diacylglycerols and/or Ca^{2+} modify the accumulation or action of cyclic AMP or in which cyclic AMP influences the distribution of Ca^{2+}. Other molecules are also utilized as intracellular messengers; candidates include guanosine 3′,5′-monophosphate (cyclic GMP).

Other hormones, particularly insulin, and certain growth factors act at plasma membrane-bound receptors that are themselves protein kinases. In contrast to the protein kinases A and C, which phosphorylate serine and threonine residues on substrate proteins, the insulin receptor and related molecules specifically phosphorylate tyrosine residues in their targets. Although the full significance of this activity remains to be elucidated, its mechanistic importance is well established.

The steroid hormones utilize an entirely different mechanism of information transfer. They gain access to the intracellular compartment and bind to cytoplasmic or nuclear receptor proteins. Following this interaction the cytosolic hormone-receptor complex migrates to sites of action within the nucleus. The complex then binds to specific regulatory elements in DNA and acts as a regulator (usually an enhancer) of transcription (synthesis of messenger RNA).

Mention should also be made of methodological advances that have greatly facilitated research and clinical applications in endocrine pharmacology. Foremost, perhaps, is the immunoassay, pioneered by Berson and Yalow. Using this sensitive and specific technique, the physician has rapid access to a wealth of analytical information about an individual patient. Advances in peptide and protein chemistry are also outstanding. The techniques for determination of amino acid sequences developed by Edman and for automated peptide synthesis developed by Merrifield have made the clinical use of various peptides a reality. Recent years have also witnessed spectacular advances in molecular biology. Recombinant DNA technology has permitted the incorporation of cloned genes that code for the synthesis of specific human hormones into the genome of bacterial or eukaryotic cells. The objective is the large-scale synthesis of the human protein. These techniques are making a major impact upon the availability of scarce hormones, such as human growth hormone, and help to overcome the immunological difficulties that are encountered with the clinical use of animal products such as insulin. These techniques have also allowed detailed structural analysis of many hormones and their receptors, which in turn will lead to the design of novel and improved therapeutic agents.

CHAPTER 56 ADENOHYPOPHYSEAL HORMONES AND RELATED SUBSTANCES

Jeffrey A. Kuret and Ferid Murad

The peptide hormones of the anterior pituitary are critical for the regulation of growth, reproduction, and metabolism. Their secretion is not only controlled by stimulatory and inhibitory peptides of hypothalamic origin, but also is influenced by hormones of the peripheral endocrine glands, by disease, and by many drugs. The interrelationships between the pituitary and its target tissues represent elegant examples of feedback regulation. These interactions have been exploited for many years in the diagnosis and treatment of clinical disorders in endocrinology. In addition, with the development of modern techniques for peptide synthesis and production of recombinant macromolecules, the peptide and protein hormones of the pituitary and hypothalamus have themselves emerged as important therapeutic agents.

Among the vertebrates, ten adenohypophyseal hormones are recognized: growth hormone, prolactin, two gonadotropins, thyrotropin, corticotropin, two melanocyte-stimulating hormones, and two lipotropins. Of these, the first six are demonstrably important in man. Nevertheless, it would be premature to deny the possible existence of others, since the pituitary gland is rich in polypeptides.

Elucidation of the amino acid sequences of the recognized adenohypophyseal hormones (and certain of their placental relatives) has clarified their evolutionary relationships, such that three groups of hormones are now apparent: the somatomammotropic hormones, the glycoprotein hormones, and the peptides derived from pro-opiomelanocortin (Table 56–1). The pharmacological properties of these adenohypophyseal hormones and their hypothalamic regulatory peptides are described in this chapter.

History. The name *pituitary* comes from the Latin *pituita,* meaning "phlegm." The gland was first thought to be a source of phlegm to moisten the membranes of the nose. In 1887, Minkowski associated the features of acromegaly with a tumor of the gland. Although the cause-and-effect relationship was by no means clear at first, by 1900 Hutchinson was able to conclude that ". . . in the pituitary body we appear to have a sort of growth-regulating centre for the entire body, the disturbance of which in early life will produce the phenomena of gigantism, and in later life those of acromegaly."

The induction of growth by the injection of pituitary extract was first accomplished in rats by Evans and Long in 1921; concurrently they noted for the first time the gonadotropic effect. Hypophysectomy as an experimental approach was introduced by Aschner in 1909. However, it was not until 1927 that the true consequences of hypophysectomy in mammals were clarified by Smith's classical experiments in the rat (Smith, 1927, 1930). The failure of growth and the atrophy of the gonads, thyroid, and adrenals that followed hypophysectomy were correctable by hypophyseal implants. This work had been anticipated 10 years earlier by parallel studies on the hypophysectomized tadpole wherein the several functions of the three parts of the pituitary were correctly assigned (*see* Allen, 1917). Smith's work in the rat was quickly followed by the definition of a thyrotropic hormone by Aron and by Loeb and Bassett in 1929, the preparation of an adrenotropic extract by Collip and coworkers in 1933, and the preparation and naming of prolactin by Riddle and associates in the same year. The year 1933 was further notable for the publication by Fevold and coworkers of the separate identity of a follicle-stimulating and a luteinizing hormone.

During the 1950s and 1960s, the development of better techniques for protein purification and analysis improved the quality of hormone preparations available for biological investigation. This led to the realization that growth hormone activity was species-specific, and culminated in the first successful treatment of a growth hormone–deficient child with human pituitary extracts in 1958 by Raben.

When it was recognized in the early 1940s that the major vascular supply to the anterior pituitary was made up of blood that had already traversed the capillaries of the median eminence of the hypothalamus, the proper setting for the neurohumoral control of the gland was evident. It is now recognized that hypothalamic cells transmit to the anterior lobe via the hypothalamicoadenohypophyseal portal system individual factors that regulate the secretion of each of its hormones, and this continues to be an area of intense research activity. It is now recognized that five different cell types in the anterior pituitary function independently to synthesize and release one or more hormones. These are the somatotroph, lactotroph, thyrotroph, gonadotroph, and corticotroph-lipotroph.

Hypopituitarism. Typically in endocrinology the functions of a gland and its secretions can be surmised from alterations that occur when it is congenitally absent or when the gland is destroyed or removed. A great deal has been learned from the consequences of pituitary deficiency.

Hypopituitarism in the Adult. Postpartum pituitary necrosis, described by Simmonds (1914) and by Sheehan (*see* Sheehan and Summers, 1949), can amount to complete destruction of the anterior lobe, and the patient may die from adrenal deficiency. If she survives, recovery of strength and well-being is slow and incomplete. The infant cannot be nursed, as there is no milk; the pubic hair, if shaved, does not grow back, and axillary and other body hair later fall out; the menstrual periods do not resume; and the genital tract atrophies. The skin becomes thin, soft, and finely wrinkled, assuming a waxy pallor from the mild anemia and the loss of dermal pigment. Libido is lost. Thyroid function is reduced, with sensitivity to cold, lack of sweating, low rate of metabolism, poor accumulation of radioiodine by the thyroid, and increased plasma cholesterol. Various indices of adrenocorti-

Table 56–1. PROPERTIES OF THE PROTEIN HORMONES OF THE HUMAN ADENOHYPOPHYSIS AND PLACENTA

HORMONE	APPROXIMATE MOLECULAR WEIGHT	PEPTIDE CHAINS	AMINO ACID RESIDUES	CARBO-HYDRATE	COMMENTS
Group 1					
Growth hormone (GH)	22,000	1	191	0	Human GH, Prl, and PL have considerably less homology of amino acid sequence, in contrast to the striking degree that is observed in other species
Prolactin (Prl)	22,500	1	198	0	
Placental lactogen (PL)	22,300	1	191	0	
Group 2					
Luteinizing hormone (LH or ICSH)	29,400	2	α-89 β-115	23%	Glycoproteins with nonidentical subunits (α and β); biological specificity is in β subunit
Follicle-stimulating hormone (FSH)	32,600	2	α-89 β-115	28%	The α subunits of LH, FSH, TSH, and CG are nearly identical and interchangeable
Chorionic gonadotropin (CG)	38,600	2	α-92 β-145	33%	Although carbohydrate sequences are incomplete, data suggest heterogeneity, even within each hormone
Thyroid-stimulating hormone (TSH)	30,500	2	α-89 β-112	22%	The physical properties of the glycoprotein hormones are discussed by Ryan and colleagues (1988)
Group 3					
Corticotropin (ACTH)	4500	1	39	0	This group of peptides is derived from a common precursor, pro-opiomelanocortin
α-Melanocyte-stimulating hormone (α-MSH)	1650	1	13	0	Group shares a common heptapeptide: Met-Glu-His-Phe-Arg-Trp-Gly
β-Melanocyte-stimulating hormone (β-MSH)	2100	1	18	0	ACTH (1-13) = α-MSH
β-Lipotropin (β-LPH)	9500	1	91	0	β-LPH (1-58) = γ-LPH β-LPH (41-58) = β-MSH
γ-Lipotropin (γ-LPH)	5800	1	58	0	β-LPH (61-91) = β-Endorphin β-LPH (61-65) = Met-Enkephalin

cal function also show a profound deficit. There is sensitivity to physical stress and to the stress of infection, and frequent episodes of collapse or severe illnesses may occur. Body weight is not grossly altered, but patients tend toward plumpness. Sometimes one or more of these clinical features are not present, presumably because destruction of the pituitary is not complete.

Hypopituitarism from local tumors often seems to affect the secretion of some hormones before others. The menstrual cycle may stop several years before the thyroid or adrenals are affected, or failure of growth may be the first manifestation. There may be features of advanced hypopituitarism at a time when the thyroid seems still to be normal. By contrast, the consequences of hypophysectomy in man resemble the complete picture of Sheehan's syndrome.

When hypopituitarism in the adult is treated by replacement with a glucocorticoid, thyroid hormone, and the appropriate sex hormone, complete clinical recovery is apparently achieved. The individual still lacks growth hormone, prolactin, and all other factors that have been detected in the adenohypophysis. However, such patients look like normal people, and they feel well and are capable of normal activities. Gametogenesis is lacking but can be corrected with human gonadotropins. Other deficits are by no means obvious.

Hypopituitary Dwarfism. Failure of the pituitary to develop during embryogenesis is, surprisingly, compatible with almost normal longevity. The most striking feature of the condition is, as the name implies, failure to grow normally. At the age of earliest recognition the child is small, with the deviation from the normal becoming more pronounced with advancing years. The dwarfism affects all parts of the body, and the individual comes to resemble a very small version of a normal child. Although growth is very slow, it does not cease; indeed, because it is not arrested by puberty as it is in the normal case, it continues throughout life.

During the years of childhood, the defect in gonadotropic function cannot be recognized clinically, although it can be detected by sensitive immunoassays of the blood for gonadotropic hormones. In the absence of these hormones sexual development does not occur in later years. Although there may be no thyrotropin or corticotropin, there is a small but important amount of activity on the part of the thyroid gland and the adrenal cortex. The dwarfing and retarded osseous development are not as extreme as in cretinism, nor does the hypopituitary dwarf show the mental retardation, the changes of the skin, or the facies of the cretin. However, thyroid function tests indicate hypoactivity, and the thyroid is easily stimulated by thyrotropin. The adrenal cortex is usefully functional also, for quite apart from secretion of aldosterone, which does not require corticotropin, some capacity to make glucocorticoids remains. Addisonian crises are not a feature of the condition, and the subjects withstand the stresses of life and of illness rather well. However, it can be shown that adrenocortical secretions are subnormal. The detection of such thyroid and adrenal deficiency helps to differentiate hypopituitarism from the host of other causes of dwarfism, including the isolated deficiency of secretion of growth hormone by the adenohypophysis.

Hypersecretion of Pituitary Hormones. In acromegaly, the most prominent features are those of excessive action of growth hormone, but it is possible that other hormones are also secreted in excess. One form of Cushing's syndrome is caused by an oversecretion of corticotropin, and in this condition, as in acromegaly, a tumor of the pituitary is often responsible. Increased secretion of prolactin from microadenomata of the pituitary is more common than initially suspected. This disorder in women can result in amenorrhea, galactorrhea, and infertility; in men, it can cause impotence. Precocious sexual development in association with tumors at the base of the brain appears to be due to isolated hypersecretion of the gonadotropins. Pituitary tumors that secrete one or both gonadotropins or thyrotropin are extremely rare. Excessive secretion of the several trophic hormones follows impaired function of the individual target glands, owing to the operation of the normal servomechanism. For example, with ovarian failure of the menopause, concentrations of the gonadotropins are markedly elevated. Similarly, primary disorders of the adrenal or thyroid result in decreased "feedback inhibition" of the pituitary and increases in the rates of secretion of the corresponding trophic hormones.

Assays and Standards. The biological potency of most clinically relevant peptide hormones is standardized in international units (I.U.) by the World Health Organization (WHO), working through its Expert Committee on Biological Standardization. After rigorous analysis in different laboratories throughout the world, WHO establishes a hormone preparation as an International Standard for calibrating a specific assay method (bioassay for potency; immunoassay or receptor binding assay for content). The results of the Committee's studies are summarized in the *WHO Technical Report Series*, and complete details are published in various journals. The committee also recommends specifications for product quality. The assays used to estimate protein purity, microheterogeneity, and immunogenicity have been reviewed in a monograph (Marshak and Liu, 1988).

SOMATOMAMMOTROPINS

The members of the somatomammotropic family of hormones (*see* Table 56–1)—growth hormone, prolactin, and placental lactogen—are related structurally and presumably arose as a result of the evolution of a single ancestral gene. These hormones coordinate the distribution of nutrients in the body, supporting general or selective tissue growth (Bauman *et al.*, 1982).

GROWTH HORMONE

Chemistry. Human growth hormone secreted from somatotrophs *in vivo* or cultured pituitary cells *in vitro* consists of a heterogeneous mixture of peptides that differ in their primary structure. The principal form of human growth hormone is a single-chain, 191-amino acid protein; it lacks covalently bound carbohydrate, contains two intrachain disulfide bonds, and has an unblocked amino terminus. This form of growth hormone is produced biosynthetically by recombinant DNA technology and is marketed as synthetic growth hormone (*somatropin*). The identical protein but containing an additional amino-terminal methionine residue is marketed as synthetic methionyl-growth hormone (*somatrem*). About 5% of the growth hormone secreted *in vitro* has a molecular weight of 20,000. This form arises from alternative splicing of growth hormone messenger RNA (mRNA), which results in the loss of 15 amino acid residues near the amino terminus (residues 32–46). Additional acidic forms, which represent deamidated or acetylated growth hormone, are recognized, but they comprise less than 5% of growth hormone secreted *in vitro*. High-molecular-weight forms of growth hormone represent aggregated monomers, linked noncovalently in some cases and by disulfide bonds in others. Because these oligomers are cleared more slowly from plasma than is the monomer, they can accumulate and comprise up to 45% of the total circulating growth hormone. A similar spectrum of forms of growth hormone is seen in acromegaly. It appears that all circulating growth hormone is derived from alternative splicing and posttranslational modification of a single gene product, encoded on chromosome 17. A second growth hormone gene, also on chromosome 17, is apparently inactive.

Physiological Actions. The concept of a growth hormone sprang from clinical observations on gigantism and acromegaly and was strengthened by the finding that crude extracts of the pituitary gland of the ox, when injected into dogs and rats, elicited increased growth.

Growth. The stimulus to growth provided by growth hormone administered to the rat affects nearly every organ and tissue of the body, the possible exceptions being the brain and the eye. Organs and tissues of the body respond to growth hormone by a proportional increase in size that is in keeping with the total increase in body weight. The growth of bones is reflected in increased body length; the skin and appendages grow, and the skeletal muscles enlarge. Growth of the thymus is a sensitive index of the action of growth hormone; like that of the lymph nodes, it can be countered by a direct action of the corticosteroids. Enlargement of the liver and increased cellular proliferation therein follow brief treatment with growth hormone, and accumulation of fat may augment somewhat the increase in weight. There is also slight enlargement of the gonads, adrenals, and thyroid, probably attributable to growth hormone itself rather than to specific trophic hormones that contaminated some early preparations.

In most tissues, growth hormone acts by increasing cell number rather than cell size. Growth responses in man to human growth hormone have been studied largely in dwarfs, and particularly in hypopituitary dwarfs, in whom striking effects can be achieved. The growth is at first normally proportioned. However, continued administration of growth hormone to hypogonadal dwarfs can eventually produce classical eunuchoid proportions (long limbs and short trunk), because sex steroids are responsible for promoting growth of the vertebral bodies.

Effects on Nitrogen Metabolism. Growth connotes increased protoplasm. It is thus mandatory that growth be associated with the accumulation of protein and nitrogen. Growth hormone causes a retention of nitrogen, and this property can be equated with its anabolic effect. However, since only 0.3 g of nitrogen need be retained daily to support rapid growth during puberty in man, the positive nitrogen balance caused by growth hormone can be difficult to measure. In fact, when growth hormone is given to human subjects in doses of 5 to 10 mg a day, a total of 3 to 5 g of nitrogen is retained daily—many times the amount needed for a normal rate of growth. Although prolonged balances have not been measured, evidently the effect is evanescent, and the site of storage of this extra nitrogen is unknown. Growth hormone increases the transport of amino acids into tissues and accelerates their incorporation into protein. Thus, in man, one of the early effects of growth hormone is a decrease in the concentration of urea in the blood, evidently because of diversion of amino acids into anabolic pathways.

In addition to nitrogen, growth hormone promotes the accretion of other tissue constituents, including Ca^{2+}, Mg^{2+}, K^+, Na^+, and phosphate. In the case of Ca^{2+}, a paradoxical increase in urinary loss is balanced by a greater increase in its intestinal absorption. In connective tissue, there is an increase in collagen synthesis, resulting in elevated urinary hydroxyproline levels, and an increase in the synthesis of chondroitin sulfate and hyaluronic acid. A variety of anabolic effects can also be observed with isolated tissues incubated *in vitro,* and in this respect the hormone mimics the action of insulin.

Effects on Metabolism of Carbohydrate and Lipid. Growth hormone has a number of important and complex effects on carbohydrate and lipid metabolism (*see* Davidson, 1987). A large number of hormones, notably growth hormone, insulin, glucocorticoids, catecholamines, and glucagon, play important roles in lipid, carbohydrate, and nitrogen homeostasis. As a first approximation, insulin and growth hormone can be viewed as the major anabolic influences, with the glucocorticoids and catecholamines as their catabolic antagonists. However, the details are not that simple. Each hormone in fact exerts a number of effects at different sites. Although an oversimplification of the facts, it might be said that growth hormone seems to switch over the source of fuel for the body from carbohydrate to fat. Thus, while insulin favors the use of sugar and its conversion to fat, growth hormone has just the opposite effect.

In patients suffering from diabetes mellitus, growth hormone exerts a clear-cut diabetogenic effect that can be offset by a larger dose of insulin. The diabetogenic effects of growth hormone are most apparent when it is administered to hypophysectomized patients with diabetes. For example, patients with severe diabetes who have been hypophysectomized for the palliation of ocular or renal lesions are sometimes exquisitely sensitive to growth hormone. A small fraction of the therapeutic dose for promotion of growth can lead to severe intensification of hyperglycemia and ketosis. However, in the nondiabetic patient with normal pancreatic reserve, the administration of growth hormone has little effect on concentrations of glucose and insulin in plasma.

The prominent metabolic actions of growth hormone resemble those brought about by fasting, and during fasting increased secretion of the hormone may be of central importance in adaptation to lack of food. With fasting there is increasing intolerance to carbohydrate (hunger diabetes), inhibited lipogenesis, mobilization of fat, and ketosis—responses that can be evoked by growth hormone. Circulating growth hormone also increases with exercise, and hypoglycemia is a particularly potent stimulus. In teleological terms it is difficult to understand this response, because growth, in the sense of building of protoplasm, cannot take place without food. However, one can imagine that, without growth hormone, tissue might be broken down during fasting and used indiscriminately for fuel. Growth hormone appears to hinder this response by enforcing the use of fat instead.

Although the effects of fasting mimic some of the actions of growth hormone and may in fact be thus mediated, the analogy by itself cannot be indefinitely extrapolated. On the one hand, growth hormone causes retention of nitrogen, increased assimilation of amino acids by tissue, and growth, whereas starvation has the reverse effects; on the other, growth hormone intensifies those very manifestations of the diabetic state that are ameliorated by fasting. It is difficult to escape the conclusion that the action of growth hormone is closely tied to the action of insulin and that the two hormones work against one another as well as together. When they work together, anabolic effects are dominant. In the fasting state, insulin is inconspicuous but not entirely lacking, and growth hormone then further depresses the use of carbohydrate and promotes the mobilization of fat and mild ketosis; in diabetes, when insulin is lacking or has decreased effectiveness, anabolism is impossible and growth hormone assumes the role of a diabetogenic agent. When growth hormone is lacking, insulin acts unopposed, carbohydrate is burned or converted to fat too quickly, and fasting becomes a major stress because, among other defects, there is difficulty in mobilizing fat for fuel.

Mechanism of Action. The metabolic and growth-promoting activities of growth hormone are the ultimate results of its binding to a specific cell-surface receptor that is distributed widely throughout the body. This transmembrane glycoprotein contains 620 amino acid residues and is similar in structure to the prolactin receptor, through which growth hormone can exert a lactogenic activity (Leung *et al.*, 1987; Boutin *et al.*, 1988). The intracellular events that follow the binding of growth hormone to receptors for either growth hormone or prolactin are unknown, but they do not appear to involve changes in cyclic nucleotides, intracellular Ca^{2+}, or any other well-documented mechanism of signal transduction discussed in Chapter 2.

Although growth hormone stimulates the differentiation of some cell types directly (Isaksson *et al.*, 1987), most of its proliferative and metabolic effects are mediated by extracellular factors, as first demonstrated in hypophysectomized rats. Serum from normal experimental animals or man increases the incorporation of sulfate into the constituents of cartilage incubated *in vitro,* while serum from hypophysectomized animals or hypopituitary patients is ineffective (Daughaday *et al.*, 1959). However, if growth hormone is injected into the hypophysectomized animals, their sera become endowed with the stimulating property. Added directly to the cartilage or admixed with serum, growth hormone is ineffectual. The activity in serum that appears in response to the action of growth hormone was initially referred to as *sulfation factor,* and later as *somatomedin* in recognition of its diverse actions. Thus, the concept emerged that growth hormone acts by stimulating the accumulation of somatomedins (*see* Daughaday, 1977).

It is now apparent that the major somatomedins are identical to polypeptides that had been termed insulin-like growth factors (IGF) 1 and 2. These proteins, which are 70 and 67 amino acid residues in length, respectively, share homology with each other and with insulin. Although the physiological role of IGF-2 is not clear, IGF-1 appears to function as the principal mediator of the action of growth hormone. Thus, administration of IGF-1 to hypophysectomized rats restores growth; enhances sulfate incorporation into proteoglycans; increases the synthesis of protein, RNA, and DNA; promotes the transport of amino acids and glucose into muscle; increases lipogenesis in adipose tissue; and increases renal plasma flow and glomerular filtration rate (Froesch *et al.,* 1985; Hirschberg and Kopple, 1989). Moreover, low plasma concentrations of IGF-1 are correlated with dwarfism in humans (African pygmies) and animals (toy poodles). Receptors selective for IGF-1, but also capable of binding insulin and IGF-2, are present in all tissues studied thus far and are similar in structure to insulin receptors. Like the insulin receptor, the IGF-1 receptor possesses intrinsic tyrosine-specific protein kinase activity that is responsible for transduction of the hormonal message (Roth, 1988).

Experiments in hypophysectomized rats suggest that the liver is the major source of circulating IGFs. They are synthesized and secreted in response to growth hormone, but they are not stored. IGFs are also synthesized by kidney, muscle, and many other tissues, where they act locally as paracrine factors. Circulating IGFs bind tightly to large carrier proteins in plasma, which reduces their rate of clearance (elimination half-life of 3 to 4 hours) and maintains a total plasma concentration that is higher than that of insulin.

The model of IGF-1–mediated growth hormone action just described clarifies the defect in Laron-type dwarfism. In this disease, there is an abundance of circulating growth hormone that is biologically active, but receptors for growth hormone and IGF-1 activity are lacking. Although these subjects are insensitive to exogenous growth hormone, they do respond to exogenous IGF-1, suggesting a possible therapy for this form of dwarfism (Laron *et al.,* 1988).

Secretion of Growth Hormone. Of all the active principles of the anterior pituitary, growth hormone is easily the most abundant, amounting to 10 to 15% of the gland's dry weight. Growth hormone is synthesized and stored in specific acidophilic cells referred to as *somatotrophs,* which comprise up to 50% of all pituicytes; these cells are probably derived from stem cells similar to those for prolactin-containing cells, or *lactotrophs.*

Growth hormone secretion is normally pulsatile; each day approximately 0.5 mg of growth hormone is released in six to eight discrete but irregular bursts. Between these pulses, the concentration of growth hormone in plasma is almost undetectable. The velocity of growth of prepubertal children is more closely correlated with the amplitude of growth hormone pulses than with their frequency (Brook *et al.,* 1988). The most pronounced secretory burst occurs shortly after the onset of deep sleep. This is not just a reflection of circadian rhythm; if the subject is kept awake all night or has frequent short naps, the rise does not take place until after he or she falls fast asleep the next day. Prepubertal children secrete 50 to 75% of their growth hormone during sleep, while secretion during waking hours becomes more significant in adolescents.

For these reasons, measurement of plasma concentrations of growth hormone during the day or over short periods of time is of little value in the diagnosis of growth-hormone deficiency in prepubertal children. Instead, measurement of spontaneous release over 24 hours or of the stimulation of the release by provocative testing (*see* below) is useful for this purpose (Rose *et al.,* 1988).

The control of the secretion of growth hormone by the central nervous system (CNS) is mediated by two hypothalamic factors—growth hormone–releasing hormone (GHRH) and growth hormone release–inhibiting hormone (somatostatin). The pulsatility of growth hormone secretion results from the asynchronous, episodic release of these mediators (Müller, 1987). Various drugs, neurotransmitters, hormones, metabolites, and other stimuli alter growth hormone secretion by acting at the hypothalamic level and influencing the secretion of GHRH and somatostatin. These include dopamine, 5-hydroxytryptamine (5-HT), and α-adrenergic agonists, which can stimulate the secretion of growth hormone acutely; inhibition of secretion can be produced by β-adrenergic agonists, free fatty acids, IGF-1, and growth hormone itself. Plasma glucose is also a powerful modulator of growth hormone secretion: hypoglycemia secondary to insulin administration or from other causes evokes a rapid rise in secretion; moreover, interference with the utilization of glucose by 2-deoxyglucose causes a similar response. Exercise, stress, emotional excitement, and ingestion of a protein-rich meal are all normal stimuli for enhanced secretion of growth hormone.

Based on these observations, several provocative tests have been devised to evaluate the capacity of the pituitary to secrete growth hormone (Abboud, 1986). The intravenous infusion of arginine in a dose of 30 g in 30 minutes in adults or 0.5 g/kg in children is safer and just as useful as the induction of hypoglycemia with insulin. The administration of levodopa, apomorphine, antagonists of 5-HT, and methylphenidate can also be used to evoke secretion of growth hormone, but the incidence of false-negative responses to these agents is relatively high. Obese subjects respond poorly to all of these stimuli, perhaps because of elevated plasma concentrations of free fatty acids.

Because the secretion of growth hormone is controlled by the CNS, each of the above tests assesses the integrity of the hypothalamic–pituitary axis. Although a deficiency in secretion of growth hormone can be detected, these tests cannot distinguish between hypothalamic or pituitary lesions as the cause. The use of GHRH for this purpose is discussed below.

Assays. The most definitive bioassays for growth hormone use young hypophysectomized rats. Gain in weight during 10 days of daily, subcutaneous injection is roughly proportional to the dose. In the tibia test, which is more sensitive, the increase in width of the epiphyseal cartilage is measured microscopically. The substances under test are injected subcutaneously daily for 4 days. The First International Standard of human growth hormone for bioassay was established in 1982, and has a specific activity of approximately 2.5 I.U./mg (Bangham *et al.,* 1985).

Immunoassays and radio-receptor assays for growth hormone are far more sensitive and rapid than bioassays, but they do not reflect the metabolic effects of the hormone or its stability in the circulation. The International Reference Preparation of human growth hormone *for immunoassay* was established in 1969 and has a specific activity of approximately 2.0 I.U./mg.

Absorption, Fate, and Excretion. Growth hormone is absorbed well after intramuscular or subcutaneous administration; maximal plasma concentrations are achieved 2 to 6 hours after injection. A small portion (20 to 25%) of the circulating hormone interacts with a binding protein in plasma that appears to be a secreted fragment of the growth hormone receptor (Leung *et al.,* 1987). The function of the binding protein is unknown, but it is unlikely to serve an important transport function because growth hormone is cleared with a half-life of 20 to 30 minutes. Several hours after the administration of growth hormone, IGF-1 appears in the plasma, where it is bound to carrier proteins. Peak plasma concentrations of IGF-1 are apparent approximately 20 hours after the injection of growth hormone. Because of the slow induction and clearance of IGF-1, the effects of growth hormone far outlast its survival in the circulation. Growth hormone is degraded primarily in the liver, kidney, and peripheral tissues, and little is excreted intact in the urine (Bennett and McMartin, 1979).

Preparations and Dosages. Until the middle of 1985, most of the growth hormone used in the United States was derived from human cadavers and was distributed by the National Hormone and Pituitary Program of the National Institutes of Health. However, this procedure was halted after it was determined that at least three individuals who had received human growth hormone in the 1960s and 1970s developed a fatal, degenerative neurological disease (Creutzfeldt-Jakob disease) (Brown *et al.,* 1985; Public Health Service, 1985). Since the Creutzfeldt-Jakob virus is difficult to detect, the potential contamination of any given preparation with small amounts of virus can neither be confirmed nor excluded completely.

The sudden lack of availability of pituitary growth hormone accelerated the approval of recombinant methionyl-growth hormone (somatrem) by the United States Food and Drug Administration in the autumn of 1985. Although somatrem is significantly more antigenic than pituitary-derived growth hormone, the potential development of neutralizing antibodies is less troubling than the alternatives of Creutzfeldt-Jakob disease or permanent dwarfism. The less immunogenic recombinant growth hormone (*somatropin*) was approved in early 1987. Both of these recombinant DNA-derived preparations are currently available in the United States.

Somatrem for injection (PROTROPIN), the analog containing an additional amino-terminal methionine residue, is supplied in vials containing 5 mg of lyophilized powder (approximately 10 I.U.) for solution. *Somatropin, recombinant, for injection*

(HUMATROPE) is supplied as a lyophilized powder for solution in vials containing 5 mg.

Growth hormone is administered intramuscularly in a dosage of 0.06 to 0.1 mg/kg three times weekly. Subcutaneous administration, however, is just as efficacious and facilitates self administration. Although a dose–response curve for growth hormone has been proposed (Frasier, 1983), the optimal schedule for treatment with growth hormone has not been established.

Therapeutic Uses. Growth hormone is approved for replacement therapy in growth hormone–deficient children. Until 1985, growth hormone therapy was usually reserved for those children with severe deficiency, characterized by short stature (below the third percentile of the Tanner growth chart), abnormally slow velocity of growth (4 cm per year or less), delayed bone age (75% of chronological age or less), abnormally low plasma concentrations of IGF-1, and poor responses to provocative tests for secretion of growth hormone. The majority of these children respond satisfactorily to growth hormone, increasing their rate of growth over many years of treatment until epiphyseal fusion (Frasier, 1983). Usually, the velocity of growth is greatest during the first year of treatment; thereafter, it declines toward the average velocity for a given chronological age. Thus, apart from the first year of rapid "catch up" growth, conventional treatment with growth hormone does not overcome the prognosis for a deficit in height that is present at diagnosis; only further loss of stature is halted (Bundak *et al.,* 1988). Whether larger doses of growth hormone can overcome this effect remains to be determined, but it is clear that early diagnosis of deficiency of growth hormone is important for the achievement of normal height. Although normal children and children with short stature from other causes are less sensitive to growth hormone than are those who are deficient, significant growth responses also can be achieved in these children, particularly with larger doses (Van Vliet *et al.,* 1983). Patients with partial deficiency and intermediate plasma concentrations of growth hormone may respond and are candidates for treatment (*see* Conference, 1988a).

To select those cases of short stature that are caused by deficient growth hormone, it is necessary to measure growth hormone in the plasma and to determine whether the response to a provocative stimulus is appropriate. The plasma concentration of IGF-1 should also be measured. Once initiated, therapy should be evaluated for 8 to 12 months for the expected acceleration of growth. An increase in the concentration of IGF-1 in plasma after 1 or 2 weeks of therapy may be indicative of a subsequent growth response (Rudman *et al.,* 1981). If growth hormone deficiency is the cause and therapy is successful, growth of 5 cm or more in 8 to 12 months can be expected. Evaluation of the growth response to shorter periods of therapy is frequently not possible. Treatment should ideally be continued throughout childhood, and sex hormones, if needed, should be given at the age of puberty to promote normal sexual development (*see* Chapters 58 and 59). The growth response to growth hormone decreases with increasing chronological age or bone age. Little or no growth response occurs in patients over 20 to 24 years of age. Interestingly, fatter children respond to therapy better than do thinner children (Frasier, 1983).

Investigational Uses. Although in clinical use for over 30 years, the limited supply of pituitary-derived human growth hormone was directed almost exclusively to the treatment of dwarfism. The development of recombinant growth hormone allows its evaluation in other disease states. On the basis of its anabolic activity, growth hormone is under investigation as an adjunct in the treatment of catabolic conditions produced by burn injuries, wounds, and malabsorption (Conference, 1988a). The retention of Ca^{2+} and osteogenesis produced by growth hormone may also be of use in the treatment of osteoporosis and nonhealing fractures. Because the metabolic actions of growth hormone are mediated by IGF-1, the latter hormone should be as effective in these conditions. Indeed, recombinant IGF-1 is also undergoing clinical study as an osteogenic agent.

Abuse. Recombinant growth hormone has great potential for misuse, primarily because of its real and perceived effects on body size and composition; enhanced athletic performance is the most commonly desired result. Although difficult to study ethically, normal children may respond to administration of growth hormone with a permanent increase in their build and stature—a potential competitive advantage in athletics. Growth hormone is useless for stimulating linear growth of adults because of epiphyseal closure. Yet it is anticipated that adult athletes will seek growth hormone to increase muscle mass and decrease body fat in a manner that is undetectable by current drug testing programs. Although these metabolic effects of growth hormone are seen during nutritional limitation, its effects on well-fed athletes whose endogenous production of growth hormone may be high (because of exercise) are unknown (Underwood, 1984; Council on Scientific Affairs, 1988).

Adverse Effects and Drug Interactions. Treatment of children with growth hormone has been associated with the development of hypothyroidism; this may be a result of the natural history of hypopituitarism. However, the development of deficiencies of additional pituitary hormones requires therapy. Pain and discomfort from growth hormone injections are minimal, but subcutaneous injection may lead to local lipoatrophy (Frasier, 1983, 1987). Antibodies to growth hormone are elicited in 30 to 40% and 7 to 20% of children treated with somatrem and somatropin, respectively (Marshak and Liu, 1988). However, resistance to treatment is rare and frequently can be overcome by increasing the dose of the hormone.

Administration of glucocorticoids to children can inhibit their growth (*see* Chapter 60). Although early reports suggested that concurrent glucocorticoid therapy could interfere with the actions of growth hormone, more recent trials have not confirmed this effect (Frasier, 1983). Nonetheless, it is recommended that daily doses of glucocorticoid (*e.g.*, hydrocortisone) not exceed 10 to 15 mg/m^2 during treatment with growth hormone.

Acromegaly. Over 90% of cases of acromegaly are caused by growth hormone–secreting adenomas (somatotropinomas) that can display a spectrum of independence from normal physiological and even pharmacological factors with respect to their secretion. Treatment of intrasellar somatotropinomas by irradiation or surgical removal is highly successful, and is the treatment of choice (Melmed, 1986). In cases where surgery fails or is not indicated, secretion of growth hormone can be suppressed with dopaminergic agonists such as bromocriptine (2-bromo-α-ergocryptine) (Wass *et al.*, 1977; Goldfine, 1978). This effect is paradoxical because dopaminergic agonists cause an *increased* secretion of growth hormone in normal individuals. Presumably, this reflects the clonal expansion of cells closely related to stem cells (somatomammotrophs) in such adenomas, which apparently express the inhibitory dopaminergic regulation of secretion that is characteristic of lactotrophs. Therapy with bromocriptine should be reserved for tumors without suprasellar extension and alterations in visual fields. Oral administration of 10 to 60 mg a day in divided doses is frequently effective. The initial dose of 1.25 to 2.5 mg per day of bromocriptine mesylate (PARLODEL) should be increased every few days, if necessary, to minimize side effects; these include nausea, vomiting, constipation, and perhaps hypotension. Failure of bromocriptine to lower concentrations of growth hormone in plasma acutely does not necessarily imply that the drug will not be effective during chronic administration. Withdrawal of the drug leads to a resurgence of growth hormone secretion.

Increased secretion of prolactin may also occur with acromegaly or other pituitary tumors, due to the removal of inhibitory control from the hypothalamus. Bromocriptine will effectively inhibit prolactin secretion, as discussed below. The dose required for suppression of prolactin is somewhat smaller. Bromocriptine is further discussed in Chapters 20 and 39.

Antagonists of 5-HT such as cyproheptadine and metergoline, as well as α-adrenergic antagonists (*e.g.*, phentolamine), can also inhibit the secretion of growth hormone in acromegaly, but their effects are weaker and inconsistent (Feldman *et al.*, 1976). Analogs of somatostatin are promising new agents in the management of acromegaly. Initial clinical studies with *octreotide* have demonstrated its effectiveness in relieving the signs and symptoms of acromegaly with surprisingly few side effects (Lamberts *et al.*, 1985). These agents may also be useful in controlling the rare case of acromegaly caused by ectopic secretion of GHRH from pancreatic islet-cell and carcinoid tumors (Frohman and Downs, 1987).

PROLACTIN

Although prolactin was discovered in 1928 and a wealth of information was obtained about its role in a wide variety of species, unequivocal evidence for the existence of the hormone in man was obtained only relatively recently. It is now appreciated, however, that prolactin plays an important role in normal human function and in certain pathophysiological states (Thorner, 1977).

History. The term *prolactin* was coined for the hormone responsible for the secretion of milk by the crop glands of the pigeon (Riddle *et al.*, 1933). In this bird there is a bilateral outpouching of the esophagus and, prompted by the psychological concomitants of brooding, a glandular structure grows within each pouch so that by the time of hatching a thick secretion (the crop milk), produced as a result of epithelial proliferation and desquamation, becomes available to each parent for regurgitating down the throats of the young. The response of the bird is a sensitive one; it is sufficient for one partner to see his mate sitting on the eggs for his pituitary to secrete prolactin and provoke the growth of the crop glands. In so naming the hormone, the tenuous analogy between the mammary gland and the crop sac was correctly drawn, because it later was clear that prolactin is also of importance in initiating secretion from the breast.

Chemistry. Prolactin is synthesized as a precursor of 227 amino acid residues (Truong *et al.*, 1984). After cleavage of its signal sequence, the mature hormone is secreted as a monomeric protein of 198 amino acid residues containing three disulfide bonds. Larger immunoreactive forms of prolactin are also identifiable in the circulation; they probably represent dimers and oligomers of monomeric prolactin, analogous to the aggregated forms of growth hormone described above. Unlike growth hormone, prolactin contains a consensus sequence for asparagine-linked glycosylation, and as much as 10 to 15% of pituitary prolactin contains carbohydrate. Although glycosylated prolactin is only 20 to 25% as potent as the unmodified hormone (Markoff *et al.*, 1988), glycosylation may stabilize the molecule to degradation; if so, the glycosylated hormone would accumulate in plasma. Although the amino acid sequences of growth hormone, prolactin, and placental lactogen are known for many species, the structural features that are responsible for selective binding to receptors for prolactin or growth hormone are not at all clear (Nicoll *et al.*, 1986).

Physiological Actions. *Breast.* The mammary gland is a site of immensely complex interactions; a number of hormones and the majority of endocrine organs participate vigorously during pregnancy to prepare the breast for secretion post partum. The hormones of the adrenal cortex, thyroid, and ovaries are all necessary, and their presence is dependent on the trophic hormones of the adenohypophysis. Insulin and perhaps growth hormone exert important anabolic influences. The vital participation of prolactin completes the contribution of the anterior pituitary, with all of its major secretions at work. The role of oxytocin is considered in Chapter 39.

The actions of prolactin on the mammary gland have been studied particularly in explanted rodent tissue. However, investigations of normal and aberrant prolactin secretion assure the existence of comparable functions in the human female. The increasing concentration of prolactin during pregnancy is required for growth and development of the breast in preparation for breast-feeding post partum. The high concentrations of estrogens and progestins that are present during pregnancy oppose some of the actions of prolactin. After delivery, the concentrations of the sex steroids decline markedly, and the actions of prolactin become unopposed. In systems *in vitro,* prolactin in the proper hormonal milieu binds to specific receptors and promotes proliferation and subsequent differentiation of mammary ductal and alveolar epithelium. There is a rapid increase in RNA synthesis and induction of the synthesis of milk proteins and of enzymes necessary for lactose synthesis (Bauman *et al.,* 1985). At the subcellular level, activation of the development of rough endoplasmic reticulum, Golgi apparatus, and secretory granules is prominent.

These "mammotrophic" actions of prolactin suggest a possible role of prolactin in mammary tumorigenesis (Smithline *et al.,* 1975). Prolonged prolactin administration, the grafting of extra pituitaries, or experimental lesions in the median eminence that cause increased prolactin secretion all result in a high percentage of mammary tumors in susceptible rats and mice. Furthermore, estrogen will not produce tumors in the absence of the pituitary; however, in rats treated with carcinogens, prolactin promotes tumorigenesis in the absence of estrogens or progestins. Moreover, drugs that enhance prolactin secretion (*e.g.,* reserpine, haloperidol—*see* below) facilitate experimental tumor growth, while those that inhibit secretion (*e.g.,* ergot derivatives) impede growth and reduce the incidence of spontaneous tumors in rodent models. Extrapolation between highly susceptible strains of rodents and man is obviously of questionable value, but these observations may provide additional explanations for the effectiveness of hormonal therapy of breast tumors. Most studies have shown normal concentrations of prolactin in patients with breast tumors, and there is thus little reason to believe that disorders of prolactin metabolism have etiological significance in mammary carcinogenesis in the human female (Kleinberg, 1987). However, prolactin may play only a permissive role in mammary growth, and recent evidence suggests that pituitary peptides unrelated to growth hormone or prolactin are capable of stimulating mammary mitogenesis directly (Newman *et al.,* 1987). The chemical nature of these factors and their role in breast cancer are under investigation.

Gonads. The effects of prolactin on the ovary are species dependent. Although the hormone was at one time also referred to as *luteotropin,* this description was based on observations on rats and mice, species in which prolactin prolongs the life of the corpus luteum. However, since prolactin does not stimulate progesterone biosynthesis by corpora lutea, it probably does not fulfill the role of a true luteotropic hormone in these species.

In human subjects prolactin may inhibit the secretion of gonadotropins or their effects on the gonads (Thorner, 1977). Suckling is a potent stimulus to prolactin secretion for several months post partum. The elevation of prolactin with breast-feeding and its inhibitory effects on ovarian function can explain the usual lack of ovulation and infertility during breast-feeding. This natural mechanism of contraception becomes ineffective several months post partum as the suckling stimulus to the secretion of prolactin declines. Prolactin-secreting tumors frequently lead to galactorrhea, amenorrhea, anovulatory cycles, and infertility in women, while hyperprolactinemia in men may cause loss of libido and impotence (Thorner, 1977). Paradoxically, prolactin may also directly stimulate testicular synthesis of testosterone (Rubin *et al.,* 1976).

Pregnancy. Although concentrations of prolactin increase 20- to 40-fold during human pregnancy, the hormone appears to have no role in maintenance of the pregnancy or the fetus. Normal pregnancies and deliveries have followed inhibition of prolactin secretion with bromocriptine or hypophysectomy (Melmed, 1986); however, failure of breast enlargement and lack of postpartum lactation are observed.

Other Effects. Sexual behavior of lower animals and birds is thought to be influenced by gonadotropins and steroids, while parental behavior involving the care, feeding, and protection of offspring may be regulated by prolactin. There is no evidence that similar functions of prolactin occur in man. Although prolactin has effects on salt and water metabolism in lower forms, the consensus is that comparable effects do not occur in man, despite several reports to the contrary; these discrepancies may be attributable to contaminants in the hormonal preparations used (Baumann and Loriaux, 1976).

Mechanism of Action. Prolactin binds to specific cell-surface receptors that are distributed widely in the body. They are similar in structure to receptors for growth hormone and are coupled to intracellular effectors by unknown mechanisms (Boutin *et al.,* 1988). It is also not known whether the effects of prolactin are mediated by factors analogous to the somatomedins. Both growth hormone and placental lactogen are potent agonists at prolactin receptors, which explains their lactogenic activities. In contrast, prolactin is incapable of binding to receptors for growth hormone and has no somatotrophic activity.

Prolactin Secretion. Prolactin is synthesized and stored in pituitary lactotrophs, which are probably derived from stem cells similar to those for somatotrophs. Human placental tissue can synthesize the hormone as well, and amniotic fluid has concentrations of prolactin that are considerably higher than those found in plasma.

Plasma prolactin concentrations are high in newborns but decrease to low levels until puberty, when they begin to increase in girls. Plasma concentrations of prolactin approximate 5 to 10 μg/l in the normal human adult and are somewhat less in males than in females. Prolactin concentrations rise markedly during pregnancy, reaching a maximum at term (values of about 200 μg/l). After delivery the concentrations of prolactin decline unless the mother breast-feeds. In nursing mothers prolactin secretion is critically controlled by the suckling stimulus or breast manipulation. Prolactin concentrations can rise 10- to 100-fold within 30 minutes of stimulation. This response becomes less prominent after several months of breast-feeding, and prolactin concentrations decline. Exceptions are noted in some primitive cultures where the response of prolactin to suckling may persist for longer times. In some normal menstruating women, but not in men, breast manipulation may produce small increases in the rate of secretion of prolactin.

Many of the physiological factors that influence the secretion of growth hormone have similar effects on prolactin; sleep, stress, hypoglycemia, fluctuations of the concentrations of estrogen, and exercise, all increase the secretion of both hormones. Prolactin shows a circadian rhythm, with peaks during sleep; superimposed on this pattern are minute-to-minute fluctuations caused by pulsatile secretion. The half-life of prolactin in plasma is 15 to 20 minutes. A variety of endogenous factors and drugs can alter the secretion of prolactin and are discussed below.

Secretion of prolactin by the pituitary is under predominantly negative control by the hypothalamus, and in this respect it is unique among the pituitary hormones. A prolactin release–inhibiting hormone (PRIH) is secreted by the hypothalamus and is carried by the hypothalamicoadenohypophyseal portal system to the adenohypophysis, where it inhibits prolactin secretion. There is considerable evidence that the release of prolactin is under dopaminergic control, and PRIH may in fact be dopamine (Leong *et al.,* 1983). Thus, the administration of levodopa *in vivo* inhibits prolactin secretion, and dopamine is a highly effective inhibitor when instilled into the third ventricle or when applied to the isolated pituitary *in vitro*. Predictably, the phenothiazine and butyrophenone antipsychotics (*e.g.,* chlorpromazine, haloperidol), which are dopamine antagonists, enhance prolactin secretion, as can metoclopramide and reserpine (*see* Chapter 18). The antipsychotic agents can cause significant galactorrhea associated with elevated concentrations of prolactin in plasma.

Dopamine, however, may not be the only hypothalamic PRIH. A potent peptide of 56 amino acid residues that is capable of inhibiting prolactin release *in vitro* exists in rats; it is synthesized along with gonadotropin-releasing hormone (GnRH) in a single precursor molecule (Nikolics *et al.,* 1985; Adelman *et al.,* 1986). The peptide has intrinsic GnRH activity as well, and its physiological role is under study.

Many hormones have been put forth as prolactin-releasing hormones, including opioid peptides and thyrotropin-releasing hormone (TRH) (Leong *et al.,* 1983). Although TRH can stimulate prolactin secretion, the physiological significance of this effect is not clear, and the secretion of thyrotropin and prolactin is dissociated during suckling. Nonetheless, a syndrome characterized by primary hypothyroidism, high plasma concentrations of prolactin, and galactorrhea suggests that stimulation of prolactin secretion by TRH is at least of pathophysiological importance. There is also some indirect evidence for the participation of endogenous opioids in the regulation of prolactin secretion. For example, female athletes engaged in vigorous training may become amenorrheic. In such circumstances, the opioid antagonist naloxone produces a prompt increase in the secretion of LH and FSH, and inhibits the exercise-induced release of prolactin and growth hormone (*see* Carr *et al.,* 1981; Mandenoff *et al.,* 1982).

Therapeutic Uses. Uses for prolactin have not been defined. Lactation in farm animals is not limited by the usual concentrations of circulating prolactin, and research has concentrated on growth hormone as a galactopoietic agent (Hart, 1987). Control of hyperprolactinemia is important for the maintenance of normal human reproductive function.

Hyperprolactinemia. This disorder may be associated with various drugs such as dopaminergic antagonists, infiltrative disorders of the hypothalamus or pituitary that interfere with regulation of prolactin secretion by PRIH, hypothyroidism with accompanying increases in TRH, and the use of oral contraceptives. Prolactin-secreting tumors are another cause, and may become apparent because of galactorrhea, amenorrhea, and infertility. These tumors, which account for at least 30% of all pituitary adenomas, can be treated with irradiation, surgical removal, or pharmacological agents (Melmed, 1986). When the tumors are microadenomata that are not associated with suprasellar extension or alterations in visual fields, pharmacological suppression of prolactin secretion is effective and should be considered. Suppression of galactorrhea by administration of levodopa has been attempted with variable success (Turkington, 1972). Some patients who respond initially become refractory to the drug. More promising clinical results have been achieved with ergot derivatives (Floss *et al.*, 1973). Certain of these compounds profoundly inhibit prolactin secretion *in vivo* and in isolated pituitary preparations *in vitro;* these effects can be antagonized by haloperidol. Hence it is likely that ergot alkaloids activate the dopaminergic receptors that inhibit prolactin release. The compound that is most useful is *bromocriptine* (PARLODEL), the dosage and side effects of which are discussed above with regard to its use in acromegaly. When bromocriptine is used to suppress prolactin secretion by functional tumors, the galactorrhea and amenorrhea usually cease within several weeks and pregnancy becomes possible. Pregnancies and offspring have been normal, but it is recommended that bromocriptine be discontinued during pregnancy. Generally galactorrhea, amenorrhea, and infertility will recur in the nonpregnant patient when the drug is stopped. Some prolactin-secreting tumors have decreased in size during administration of bromocriptine; the mechanism of tumor regression is unknown (Mehta and Tolis, 1981). The tumors recur when bromocriptine is discontinued.

Assays. The classical procedure for bioassay of prolactin is based on the original work of Riddle and associates (1933), namely, the increase in weight of the crop sacs of doves and pigeons. Other methods are based on the induction of secretory changes in the suitably prepared mammary glands of rodents. Most clinical measurements rely on immunoassays (Jeffcoate *et al.*, 1986).

Human Placental Lactogen. Preparations from the human placenta contain growth-promoting and lactogenic activity (*see* Fukushima, 1961); Josimovich and MacLaren (1962) showed that such extracts cross-reacted with antisera to human growth hormone. Purified preparations caused a local response in the crop sac of the pigeon and maintained the function of the corpora lutea of rats but caused little growth in hypophysectomized animals; the active principle was named *placental lactogen*. Friesen (1966) purified the protein to homogeneity and demonstrated that it was strikingly lactogenic in pseudopregnant rabbits.

In the early 1970s, the primary structure of human placental lactogen was elucidated in the laboratories of Niall and Li (Niall *et al.*, 1971; Li *et al.*, 1973). Its amino acid sequence proved to be 83% and 30% identical to that of growth hormone and prolactin, respectively. Because of its structural similarity to growth hormone, placental lactogen is also referred to as *chorionic somatomammotropin*. Placental lactogen is encoded by a cluster of four genes adjacent to the genes for growth hormone on chromosome 17. Only two of these genes are transcribed actively, however, and both encode the same sequence of 191 amino acids (Barrera-Saldaña *et al.*, 1983).

The functions of human placental lactogen have not been clearly defined. It is produced by the syncytiotrophoblasts of the placenta, yet is secreted almost exclusively into the maternal circulation. In addition to promoting growth and development of the mammary gland, it is luteotropic and may stimulate production of steroids by the corpus luteum during pregnancy (Porter, 1980).

GLYCOPROTEIN HORMONES

The family of human glycoprotein hormones consists of luteinizing hormone (LH), follicle-stimulating hormone (FSH), chorionic gonadotropin (CG), and thyroid-stimulating hormone (thyrotropin; TSH) (*see* Table 56–1). They each share a conserved subunit structure and a common mechanism of action. In addition, each glycoprotein hormone is useful clinically as a therapeutic or diagnostic agent.

Chemistry. The glycoprotein hormones have been purified and characterized, and the genes that encode them have been cloned from several species. The proteins exist as heterodimers of noncovalently linked subunits, designated α and β (Pierce and Parsons, 1981). The α subunits of each hormone are nearly identical and are encoded by the same gene, while the biological specificity resides in the distinct β subunits, which are encoded by separate genes (Fiddes and Talmadge, 1984). The β subunits of the different glycoprotein hormones are homologous. The closest evolutionary relationship is between the β subunits of CG and LH, where 82% of the first 115 amino acid residues are identical. The pairwise similarity between the other β subunits ranges from 25 to 40%.

Both the α and β subunits are derived from precursors containing a signal sequence that is typical of secreted proteins (von Heijne, 1983); they contain five (α subunit) or six (β subunit) internal disulfide bonds (Ryan *et al.*, 1988). The carbohydrate content of each of the glycoproteins is variable because of differences in the number and location of glycosylation sites (Baenziger and Green, 1988). The common α subunit of all four hormones contains two asparagine-linked oligosaccharide chains; the β subunits contain either one (LH and TSH) or two (FSH and CG) such chains. The β subunit of CG also contains four serine-linked carbohydrate moieties. Although covalently bound carbohydrate is not required for dimerization of α and β or for receptor binding, it is necessary for receptor activation (Sairam and Bhargavi, 1985). Each glycoprotein hormone is secreted as a heterogeneous mixture, the components differing in the amounts of sulfate and sialic acid linked to the different carbohydrate chains. The isoforms may differ in bioactivity, potency in immunoassays, or both.

GONADOTROPIC HORMONES

The gonadotropins—FSH, LH, and CG—are required for ovulation, spermatogenesis, and the biosynthesis of the sex steroids. Gonadotropin preparations of varying composition and purity have been used to promote fertility for over 30 years. The first use of gonadotropins to induce ovulation in hypogonadotropic women was accomplished by Gemzell in 1958 with human pituitary extracts. The difficulty and expense in obtaining human pituitaries, combined with the development of preparations of urinary gonadotropins, made this form of therapy short lived. The first human pregnancy that resulted from treatment with urinary gonadotropin was reported in 1962 by Lunenfeld.

Secretion and Physiological Actions. Despite an extraordinarily large number of experimental observations of the secretion and actions of gonadotropins, understanding of these areas is far from complete. Most studies have been carried out in species different from that of origin of the hormone, and in some instances impure preparations have been used, which may account for some anomalous responses. Observations on the responses of the normal human gonads to human gonadotropins are still relatively fragmentary.

Secretion. LH and FSH are produced and secreted by the same cell type in the pituitary, the gonadotroph. Secretion of LH and FSH is regulated through feedback inhibition by sex steroids in plasma. As discussed below, a single hypothalamic regulatory factor controls the secretion of both FSH and LH.

In infancy and prepuberty the concentrations of FSH and LH in plasma are measurable, but quite low. At puberty gonadotropin secretion increases about twofold, owing to an increase in the amplitude and frequency of pulses of GnRH (Marshall and Kelch, 1986; Stanhope and Brook, 1988). In men, plasma concentrations of FSH and LH are relatively constant, while rates of secretion in women are somewhat higher and vary according to the phase of the menstrual cycle. In normal women the daily rate of production of LH is about 500 to 1000 I.U.; this increases about three- to sixfold at ovulation and after menopause. In some gonadal disorders, concentrations of gonadotropins increase due to diminished concentrations of sex steroids and a resultant loss of their feedback inhibition on the pituitary. As with GnRH, gonadotropins are secreted in a pulsatile manner, which accounts for the minute-to-minute oscillations in plasma concentrations. Pituitary tumors may rarely secrete one or both gonadotropins (Snyder and Sterling, 1976).

Actions on the Ovary. During the follicular phase of the ovarian cycle successive groups of small follicles start to grow, and by the time ovulation is imminent follicles in all stages of development are found. This ovarian response represents the predominant action of FSH, and it is during this phase that estrogen is the main ovarian secretory product (*see* Figure 58–2, page 1388).

Shortly before ovulation is to take place, a series of ovarian changes follow in rapid succession, presumably mediated by a burst of FSH and LH secretion at this time; this burst is due to a positive feedback effect of estrogen on gonadotropin secretion. The largest follicles expand quickly; those in just the right stage of development to ovulate undergo cytological changes in the granulosa in the direction of luteinization and show intense hyperemia of the theca interna. One area on the surface of the dominant follicle thins and then undergoes dissolution, leaving an aperture through which the viscous follicular fluid oozes, carrying desquamated granulosa cells and the cumulus and its contained ovum with it. Those large follicles not destined to ovulate, perhaps for reasons of improper stage of development, remain avascular and begin to show regressive changes. While ovulation is in progress, widespread atresia involves all the other follicles that shortly before had been flourishing under the influence of FSH, and in certain species the atresic process extends also to the residual corpora lutea of antecedent cycles. It is tempting to attribute the regressive changes in the ovary, which parallel so closely ovulation and luteinization, to an action of LH.

The earliest stages of preovulatory follicular swelling are accompanied by evidence of the first secretion of progesterone. This has been shown in species that require the luteotropic action of prolactin as well as in those that do not. The critical influence is exerted by LH. LH maintains the corpus luteum until the secretion of estrogen and progesterone declines sufficiently to initiate menses, and a new cycle then begins. If pregnancy occurs, CG produced by the trophoblastic cells of the placenta maintains the corpus luteum.

Measurements of the gonadotropins in plasma throughout the menstrual cycle show that FSH is elevated during the follicular phase and slowly falls before it rises again at midcycle; it is lowest during the luteal phase. LH shows a striking peak at midcycle, usually on the same day that the FSH is highest (*see* Figure 58–2). This surge in the secretion of LH is an immediately preovulatory event (*see* Faiman and Ryan, 1967). (Further interactions between the gonadotropins and the sex steroids are discussed in Chapters 58 and 59.)

Actions on the Testis. Whereas in the ovary both gonadotropins are involved in the secretion of hormones, LH plays a predominant role in the testis. FSH is primarily a gametogenic hormone in males; it is responsible for the anatomical integrity of the seminiferous tubules and only under its influence are the complex stages of gametogenesis carried through to the production of spermatozoa. In the hypophysectomized animal, the major effect of FSH is stimulation of the seminiferous tubules. As the tubules make up the bulk of the testis, tubular growth is accurately reflected by an increase in testicular weight. Possible effects of FSH on testosterone secretion from the Leydig cells are controversial and are discussed in Chapter 59. LH stimulates the interstitial (Leydig) cells to secrete androgen, but the androgen, in turn, exerts a direct effect upon the tubules such that both components of the testis appear to be stimulated. These effects of LH have led to its alternate designation as interstitial cell–stimulating hormone (ICSH).

Mechanism of Action. Specific receptors for the gonadotropins exist only in gonadal tissues. In the ovary, LH binds to the surface of cells in the theca and corpus luteum as well as to the large follicle granulosa cells; it binds to Leydig cells in the testis. The receptor proteins have recently been purified, and their primary structures should be elucidated soon (Kusuda and Dufau, 1988). FSH binds to the surface of small follicle granulosa cells in the ovary and to Sertoli cells in the testis. The receptors for both LH and FSH are coupled to adenylyl cyclase by means of a guanine nucleotide-binding regulatory protein (G_s) (*see* Chapter 2). Elevation of intracellular cyclic AMP increases the amount of the mitochondrial enzyme complex that oxidatively cleaves the side chain of cholesterol; this reaction is the rate-limiting step in the conversion of cholesterol to pregnenolone (Trzeciak *et al.,* 1986). Although a similar effect occurs in the adrenal cortex in response to corticotropin, the overall rate of steroidogenesis is limited by the availability of free cholesterol in this tissue (*see* Chapter 60). It is not certain whether a similar mechanism for the regulation of the synthesis of sex steroids operates in the gonads. Although the mechanism by which gonadotropins stimulate gametogenesis is not known in entirety, it too is mediated by cyclic AMP.

Chorionic Gonadotropin (CG). CG is a hormone of human pregnancy; it is secreted by the syncytiotrophoblasts of fetal placenta as early as 7 days after ovulation, and it is absorbed into the blood in sufficient quantity to sustain luteal function and forestall the next menstrual period; the secretion of LH remains suppressed because of the rising concentrations of estrogen and progesterone.

CG is detectable in the urine by immunoassay several days before the first missed period, and this is the basis of the most commonly used test of pregnancy. The quantity excreted increases rapidly thereafter to a maximum about 6 weeks after ovulation. The urinary content then declines over the next month or so and stabilizes at a lower level for the remainder of pregnancy.

The changes in the corpus luteum in early pregnancy reflect the intense stimulation provided by the LH-like action of CG. Concentrations of placental lactogen increase progressively during pregnancy; it too is luteotropic and may play some role in concert with CG to stimulate steroid production by the corpus luteum. With the increasing secretion of estrogen and progesterone by the placenta during the third month, the ovaries and the corpus luteum become unessential to the maintenance of gestation, but the corpus luteum does not undergo a pronounced change at this time. Instead, there is a slow regression that, histologically, is not complete even at the time of delivery. In the presence of the flood of CG during pregnancy, the rest of the ovary remains quiescent.

Assays of CG and its subunits are also used to diagnose and to evaluate the treatment of trophoblastic tumors. Quantification of the secretion of the hormone by choriocarcinomas and hydatidiform moles can provide an accurate index of tumor regression or recurrence. This ability has contributed to the high rate of successful treatment of these tumors.

The action of CG on the testis can hardly be regarded as physiological, for the hormone gains access to the male only *in utero,* when it does cause minimal gonadal stimulation; otherwise the hormone is found in the male only in the rare event of a teratomatous tumor containing chorionic elements. Injected into men, however, CG stimulates the interstitial cells of the testis to secrete androgen. Activation of the seminiferous epithelium is minimal and may be mediated entirely by the androgen of Leydig-cell origin.

CG also has some thyrotropic activity, which is thought to be unimportant except in some trophoblastic tumors where the large amounts of hormone can lead to hyperthyroidism.

The mechanism of action of CG appears to be identical to that of LH.

Absorption, Fate, and Excretion. The gonadotropins of either pituitary or placental origin are effective only if given by injection, usually intramuscularly. The rate at which gonadotropins are cleared from plasma is difficult to measure accurately because of their structural heterogeneity and the background of pulsatile secretion of the endogenous hormones. Nonetheless, studies indicate that LH, FSH, and CG disappear from plasma with half-lives of 2.2, 2.9, and 5.6 hours, respectively (*see* Bennett and McMartin, 1979). The prolonged circulatory life of these glycoprotein hormones relative to many other peptide hormones is a result of their resistance to metabolic degradation in most tissue beds. Clearance of injected (and presumably of endogenous) glycoprotein hormones is by glomerular filtration, followed by degradation in the proximal renal tubule or excretion (unchanged) in the urine. Removal of the sialic acid residues results in their rapid and complete clearance by the hepatic reticuloendothelial system (Morell *et al.,* 1971). Thus, although sialic acid residues are not required for agonist activity at the appropriate receptor (*see* above), they are critical for biological activity *in vivo.*

Assays. Bioassay remains a necessary technique for evaluation of functional activity, which often bears no relationship to immunoreactivity. The gonadotropins pose a special problem because many responses to one hormone are modified by the concurrent action of others, and special conditions must be chosen to minimize this influence. References and descriptions of several techniques can be found in the *third* and *fourth editions* of this textbook.

For many purposes, particularly the measurement of gonadotropins in blood and urine, immunoassays are more accurate and far simpler than bioassays (Beastall *et al.,* 1987). While some polyclonal antibodies used in these immunoassays cross-react with the other gonadotropins, specific monoclonal antibodies against the β chain are available. Radioreceptor assays are also employed.

Preparations and Dosages. For certain purposes, quite crude preparations of gonadotropins from human pituitaries would be suitable, even though they contain both FSH and LH as well as other active principles. While purified human LH and FSH had been available for investigational uses from the National Hormone and Pituitary Program of the National Institutes of Health, distribution of all products derived from human pituitaries was discontinued because of possible contamination with Creutzfeldt-Jakob virus, as discussed above.

Menotropins for injection (PERGONAL) is a preparation of gonadotropins from the urine of postmenopausal women. While FSH and LH activities are present in equal unitage, CG is usually required in conjunction with menotropins to induce ovulation. The recommended initial dose is 75 I.U. of each gonadotropin intramuscularly daily for 7 to 12 days. This is followed by 10,000 I.U. of CG. If there is no evidence of ovulation, several treatment cycles may be necessary and the dosage may be increased. In some cases large quantities may be needed.

Chorionic gonadotropin for injection is a preparation derived from the urine of pregnant women, which is sold under various trade names (A.P.L., PREGNYL, others). It is given intramuscularly in a dosage of 500 to 4000 I.U. two or three times weekly for several weeks for the treatment of cryptorchism or hypogonadism in men, and in doses of 5000 to 10,000 I.U. one day following treatment with menotropins to evoke ovulation.

Urofollitropin for injection (METRODIN), a menotropin preparation with its LH component removed, is available as a powder for solution in ampules containing 75 I.U. of FSH. The dosage schedule for induction of ovulation is identical to that described above for the menotropins.

Gonadotropins require the correct complement of polysaccharides for full biological activity; this has complicated their production by recombinant DNA technology. Nevertheless, the expression of LH in a mammalian cell system has been accomplished, and the product is currently under investigation (Simon *et al.*, 1988).

Therapeutic Uses. The gonadotropins are used in therapy primarily for the treatment of infertility and cryptorchism.

Female Infertility. The gonadotropins are most useful for inducing ovulation in women who are infertile because of pituitary insufficiency. Extensive clinical experience with menotropins and human chorionic gonadotropin indicated the occurrence of ovulation in 90% of appropriately selected patients treated with the drugs (Kennedy and Adashi, 1987). Although ovulation is occasionally seen during administration of menotropins before CG is given, it usually takes place 36 to 48 hours after administration of the latter hormone. Pregnancy results in over 50% of the patients; of these, 20 to 30% result in spontaneous abortion, while approximately 30% result in multiple births. The male-to-female sex ratio has averaged 0.85 (James, 1985). The growth and development of children born of mothers receiving gonadotropin treatment have been normal (Hack *et al.*, 1970).

The chief complication reported for this therapy is excessive ovarian enlargement resulting from the maturation of many follicles; this, in turn, may lead to the release of multiple ova and to multiple births. Ovarian hyperstimulation may be seen several days after the administration of CG in a few percent of patients. In this condition the enlarged ovaries give rise to pain in the lower abdomen, and, if they bleed into the peritoneal cavity, the pain is severe. Under the latter circumstance, hospitalization and observation for ovarian rupture are required. Methods have been devised to avoid these complications (Kennedy and Adashi, 1987). For example, one can test ovarian responsiveness by measuring the excretion of estrogens in the urine in a preliminary trial and thereby be guided in the dosage appropriate for a therapeutic attempt. If the urinary estrogens exceed 150 μg/24 hours, CG should be withheld. Alternatively, several trials may be made with small doses before the larger recommended amounts are used.

It is remarkable how closely the experience with human gonadotropins parallels that following the use of clomiphene (*see* Chapter 58). Further experience will be needed to determine which types of ovarian disorders are best treated with gonadotropin and which with clomiphene or GnRH.

In-Vitro Fertilization. Gonadotropins alone or in combination with clomiphene or GnRH are used in procedures for fertilization *in vitro,* both to induce maturation of multiple oocytes and to induce ovulation at a specific time; this facilitates the retrieval of oocytes. Several treatment regimens have been developed for these purposes (Seibel, 1988).

Male Infertility. Although the use of human gonadotropins, either from the pituitary gland or from menopausal urine, to promote fertility in the male is a field that has not been extensively explored, men with hypopituitarism have been rendered fertile by this means (Luboshitzky *et al.*, 1981). As the process of germinal maturation in the tubules requires 10 weeks and the transit of the spermatozoa through the vas deferens several weeks more, investigation of this form of treatment is time consuming. The effectiveness of therapy with gonadotropins when more subtle forms of gametogenic failure are under study is more difficult to evaluate, and more extensive experience is required. Often, testicular failure appears to be due to an intrinsic fault of the testis itself, and additional gonadotropin would not be expected to be beneficial.

Cryptorchism. Failure of the descent of one testis or both is sometimes noted in childhood; it is most frequent in infancy and is less prevalent with advancing age until it becomes a rare finding in the adult. In the majority of cases, testes undescended in childhood assume their normal position at the time of puberty. In rare cases, cryptorchism denotes an abnormality of testicular development and in this event descent at puberty does not take place. There is also some indication that testicular development is quite normal if descent is achieved before age seven. This can often be accomplished by the administration of an androgen or CG. Such treatment is more effective when failure of testicular descent is bilateral, in contrast to the unilateral condition. CG is usually used and is customarily given intramuscularly in doses of 500 to 4000 I.U. two or three times weekly for several weeks, but therapy is stopped as soon as the desired result has been achieved. If such treatment is not successful, the undescended testis should be placed in the scrotum surgically or removed, since the incidence of testicular tumors is markedly increased in cryptorchism.

Contraception. Because of the importance of CG in early pregnancy, antagonism of its action is being explored as a means to achieve long-term contraception in females. The leading strategies are immunological, using fragments or epitopes of CG to produce a "vaccine" capable of eliciting the production of neutralizing anti-CG antibodies. Several such vaccines are in clinical trials (Stevens, 1986).

Adverse Effects. The administration of CG can elicit the production of anti-CG antibodies which, in rare cases, have sufficient affinity and binding capacity to cause resistance to treatment (Thau *et al.*, 1988). In these cases, success may still be obtainable by changing the treatment regimen to one that utilizes either GnRH or LH (if the patient's antibodies do not cross-react with LH).

THYROTROPIN (TSH)

The chemistry of TSH is discussed above and is summarized in Table 56–1; its physiological effects on the thyroid gland are discussed in Chapter 57.

Assays. A widely used bioassay is that described by McKenzie (1961). Thyroid stimulation is reflected in increased circulating radioactivity in mice with thyroids prelabeled with radioiodine. Immunoassays for human thyrotropin permit diagnostic studies of the circulating hormone. In primary hypothyroidism, the feedback inhibition of thyroid hormone to regulate the secretion of TSH is reduced or absent, resulting in increased secretion of the trophic hormone. Thus, hypothyroidism with elevated concentrations of TSH in plasma indicates thyroid failure, whereas the occurrence of low concentrations of both thyroid hormone and TSH points to a hypothalamic or pituitary defect. As discussed below and in Chapter 57, administration of thyrotropin-releasing hormone (TRH) is useful to distinguish between the latter two possibilities.

Preparation and Dosage. *Thyrotropin for injection* (THYTROPAR), a preparation of bovine TSH, is supplied as a sterile powder for solution in vials containing 10 I.U. of TSH. The usual intramuscular or subcutaneous dosage is 10 I.U. per day for 1 to 3 days.

Clinical Application. TSH is used to evaluate thyroid disorders in conjunction with the use of radioiodine. The hormone is administered to promote the uptake of radioiodine by differentiated thyroid carcinomas, metastases, and normal thyroid tissue in patients with a so-called toxic nodule. TSH was formerly used to distinguish hypopituitarism from primary myxedema, but the wide availability of sensitive and reliable immunoassays for TSH has made this use obsolete.

Autoimmune Thyroid Disease. Most patients suffering from Graves' disease (hyperthyroidism) have substances in their blood that exert a prolonged stimulatory action upon the thyroids of animals. These substances are called *long-acting thyroid stimulators* (LATS) and *long-acting thyroid stimulator-protector* (LATS-P), to distinguish them from TSH. These proteins are immunoglobulins of the IgG class that bind to antigenic sites on the plasma membrane of thyroid follicular cells. Presumably, the binding of these and perhaps other thyroid-stimulating antibodies can mimic the effects of TSH and produce hyperthyroidism (Bottazzo and Doniach, 1986). However, the precise role of thyroid-stimulating immunoglobulins in the pathogenesis of Graves' disease remains obscure. Their actions on the thyroid gland are essentially identical to those of TSH, and both TSH and LATS can stimulate the synthesis of cyclic AMP. The proteins evidently can traverse the placenta and thereby account for hyperthyroidism of the newborn infants of some hyperthyroid mothers.

CORTICOTROPIN AND RELATED PEPTIDES

The essential structural features of corticotropin (adrenocorticotropic hormone; ACTH) are summarized in Table 56–1 and Figure 60–1 (p. 1432). Although the biological properties of ACTH are discussed in Chapter 60, the hormone is related structurally to other peptide hormones that are discussed below and in Chapter 21.

ACTH is synthesized along with melanocyte-stimulating hormones (MSH), lipotropins (LPH), and β-endorphin as a precursor of 267 amino acid residues. After cleavage of the signal sequence, the precursor (termed *pro-opiomelanocortin; see* Figure 21–1, p. 487) is glycosylated and further cleaved at paired basic amino acid residues that are recognized by tissue-specific serine proteases. In the human pituitary, which unlike the pituitaries of lower mammals does not contain a discrete intermediate lobe, processing of pro-opiomelanocortin is limited to the synthesis of ACTH, β-LPH, a glycopeptide derived from the amino terminus of pro-opiomelanocortin (76 amino acids), and another peptide of unknown activity with 30 amino acid residues. In other tissues, such as brain and gut, these peptides are processed further: ACTH is cleaved to α-MSH and a corticotropin-like intermediate lobe peptide; β-LPH is hydrolyzed to γ-LPH and β-endorphin; and the amino-terminal peptide is proteolyzed to γ-MSH and other peptides of unknown function (*see* Figure 21–1). This organization of pro-opiomelanocortin is similar in teleost fishes, amphibians, and mammals (Martens *et al.*, 1985).

LIPOTROPINS AND MELANOCYTE-STIMULATING HORMONES

The definitive biological activities of ACTH, MSH, and LPH are stimulation of steroidogenesis in adrenal cortical cells, melanogenesis in pigment cells, and lipolysis in adipocytes, respectively. Yet each of these hormones possesses the full range of activities of the others *in vitro*, although their relative potencies vary markedly. For example, ACTH is 2% as potent as α-MSH in stimulating melanogenesis (in a frog skin bioassay), while α-MSH is only 0.2% as potent as ACTH in inducing adrenal steroidogenesis. The lipotropins are less potent than either ACTH or MSH in causing the darkening of amphibian skin or in stimulating lipolysis; they probably have no function in man.

The structural basis of these differences in bioactivity has been investigated in detail (*see* Inouye and Otsuka, 1987). ACTH, MSH, and LPH each contain a common tetrapeptide core (His-Phe-Arg-Trp) that is the minimum sequence required for biological activity; additional amino acid residues are required for maximal potency and selectivity. This situation is reminiscent of the opioid peptides, where a common pentapeptide consensus sequence (enkephalin) is required for binding to opioid receptors, and the remainder of the molecule serves to enhance or diminish selectivity of binding for the various types of opioid receptors.

A receptor analogous to the amphibian MSH receptor is apparently absent from man, and MSH is not secreted from the pituitary. All effects on skin pigmentation and adrenal steroidogenesis that emanate from the pituitary are mediated by ACTH, acting through ACTH receptors.

β-ENDORPHIN

Although the sequence of β-endorphin is contained within pro-opiomelanocortin, it does not share the consensus sequence of the ACTH–MSH–LPH hormones and is only a minor processing product in the human pituitary. β-Endorphin may have important functions as a neurotransmitter or neurohormone, and its relationship to the other opioid peptides is discussed in Chapters 12 and 21.

HYPOTHALAMIC CONTROL OF THE ANTERIOR PITUITARY

As a result of the pioneering studies of Harris, it is now well established that the influence of the central nervous system upon adenohypophyseal function is mediated by neurohumoral substances transported to the gland by the hypothalamico-adenohypophyseal-portal system from a capillary network in the region of the median eminence. These substances are referred to as either releasing hormones, releasing factors, or regulatory hormones. Many of these substances meet the commonly accepted definition of a hormone and influence both the synthesis and release of adenohypophyseal hormones.

The successful isolation and identification of these hormones have required herculean efforts. Tons of hypothalamic starting material containing hundreds of thousands of hypothalami have been required to purify milligram quantities of these substances. Six hypothalamic hormones with well characterized activity on the anterior pituitary are now recognized: gonadotropin-releasing hormone, growth hormone–releasing hormone, somatostatin, thyrotropin-releasing hormone, corticotropin-releasing hormone, and dopamine. Dopamine, which functions as a hormone that inhibits prolactin secretion, is discussed in Chapter 12.

GONADOTROPIN-RELEASING HORMONE

A single hypothalamic hormone, gonadotropin-releasing hormone (GnRH) (also known as luteinizing hormone–releasing hormone [LHRH]), is responsible for regulating the secretion of both FSH and LH in mammals. Endogenous human GnRH is cleaved from a protein with 92 amino acid residues that may also serve as a precursor of a peptide inhibitor of prolactin secretion (Adelman *et al.*, 1986). Mature GnRH is a decapeptide with blocked amino and carboxyl termini, and it is identical in all mammalian species studied to date. Thousands of GnRH analogs have been synthesized in the search for agonists and antagonists with useful pharmacokinetic properties; some of these are shown in Table 56–2.

Chemistry. Most of the GnRH agonists synthesized to date contain one or two substitutions in the peptide chain; hydrophobic D-amino acid residues replace glycine in position 6, while N-ethylamide replaces glycine-amide in position 10. These peptides are less susceptible to proteolysis and bind with greater affinity to GnRH receptors (and plasma proteins) than does natural GnRH. Their rates of clearance *in vivo* are thus reduced and their potency is enhanced (Karten and Rivier, 1986).

The structures of GnRH antagonists are more highly substituted; residues 1 to 3 are replaced with hydrophobic D-amino acids, and the substitutions

Table 56–2. CHEMICAL STRUCTURES OF NATIVE AND SYNTHETIC GnRH PEPTIDES

GnRH (Gonadorelin) * 5-Oxo-Pro-His-Trp-Ser-Tyr-Gly-Leu-Arg-Pro-Gly-NH_2
1 2 3 4 5 6 7 8 9 10

ANALOG	SUBSTITUTIONS	
	Residue 6	*Residue 10*
Buserelin	D-(t-butyl)-serine	ethylamide
Histrelin	D-(N-benzyl)-histidine	ethylamide
Leuprolide *	D-leucine	ethylamide
Nafarelin	D-3-(2-naphthyl)-alanine	—
Triptorelin	D-tryptophan	—

* Approved for clinical use in the United States.

described above for agonists are retained. Unfortunately, the GnRH antagonists also provoke histamine release and produce anaphylactoid reactions in animals. A new generation of GnRH antagonists with less potent histamine-releasing activity is under investigation (Bajusz *et al.*, 1988; Ljungqvist *et al.*, 1988).

Secretion. Endogenous GnRH is secreted from the hypothalamus in a pulsatile manner, and the frequency and amplitude of the pulses are critical for the control of gonadotropin secretion from the pituitary. A normal pulse frequency of 0.5 to 1 per hour is sufficient for proper maintenance of gametogenesis and steroidogenesis, and higher or lower frequencies result in suboptimal secretion of gonadotropins. GnRH secretion is under feedback control of the sex steroids and is also modulated by adrenergic and opioid peptide-mediated neuronal pathways (Marshall and Kelch, 1986).

Pharmacological Effects. Synthetic GnRH is highly active in man; a single intravenous dose of 10 to 100 μg elicits rapid elevation of the plasma concentrations of gonadotropins, leading to increased secretion of gonadal steroids. During the first week or two of long-term GnRH administration, concentrations of gonadotropins in plasma remain elevated. However, continued administration of GnRH over 2 to 4 weeks desensitizes the GnRH receptors on pituitary gonadotrophs, leading to a suppression of the secretion of both gonadotropins and gonadal steroids. The concentrations of estrogen and testosterone ultimately approach those seen in postmenopausal women and castrated men, respectively, and they remain suppressed for the duration of the administration of GnRH. The pharmacological oophorectomy or orchiectomy produced by prolonged treatment with GnRH is reversible, and normal steroidogenesis and gametogenesis return within 2 months of discontinuation of the drug (Peters and Walsh, 1987; Nafarelin Study Group, 1988). The effects of treatment with GnRH for periods longer than 6 months are unknown.

The *pulsatile* administration of GnRH or GnRH agonists does not desensitize the gonadotroph. Thus, chronic administration of such compounds in this fashion stimulates gonadotropin secretion effectively and produces normal menstrual cycles in women with GnRH deficiency (Reid *et al.*, 1988).

GnRH antagonists act as competitive inhibitors at GnRH receptors. Through blockade of the actions of endogenous GnRH, they also suppress secretion of gonadal steroids. In contrast to the effect of GnRH agonists, the hypogonadal state is produced without initial pituitary stimulation.

Mechanism of Action. Both GnRH agonists and antagonists bind to specific cell-surface receptors on pituitary gonadotrophs. These transmembrane glycoproteins have been purified, and their primary structures should be elucidated soon. The binding of GnRH stimulates both the synthesis and secretion of gonadotropin by effector mechanisms that involve the mobilization of intracellular Ca^{2+} and activation of protein kinase C (*see* Chapter 2). Gonadotropin synthesis is stimulated at the level of gene transcription. There is little evidence to support a direct action of GnRH on human gonads, although this may occur in other species. As mentioned, continuous exposure of gonadotrophs to GnRH results in their desensitization. Multiple processes appear to be involved, including the uncoupling of GnRH receptors from their effectors, intracellular sequestration of the receptors, and the depletion of stores of gonadotropins (Hazum and Conn, 1988; Huckle and Conn, 1988).

Absorption, Fate, and Excretion. Because GnRH agonists are absorbed very poorly after oral administration, they are given by intravenous, subcutaneous, or intranasal routes. The GnRH antagonists currently under investigation are more hydrophobic than native GnRH or its agonist analogs, and oral administration may become practical.

GnRH distributes into an apparent volume that approximates the extracellular space, from which it is cleared with a half-life of 2 to 8 minutes. Synthetic GnRH agonist analogs are cleared more slowly because of their relative resistance to tissue proteases and their binding to plasma proteins; leuprolide has a half-life in the circulation of 3 hours. The principal site of clearance is the kidney, where the hormone is partially degraded and excreted in the urine (Handelsman and Swerdloff, 1986).

Preparation, Dosage, and Therapeutic Uses. *Gonadorelin hydrochloride for injection* (FACTREL), a preparation of synthetic GnRH, is marketed as a lyophilized powder for subcutaneous or intravenous use. It is approved as an adjunct in the diagnosis of hypogonadism in either sex; GnRH (100 μg) is administered intravenously or subcutaneously and the concentration of LH in plasma is determined over a 2-hour period. Theoretically, the administration of GnRH should elicit a normal gonadotropic response in hypogonadotropic subjects with hypothalamic lesions and a weak or nonexistent response in subjects with pituitary disease. In practice, however, the long-term absence of GnRH can result in decreased responsiveness of the gonadotroph, which is restored only by repeated administration of GnRH ("priming") over several days. The differential diagnosis of hypogonadism is discussed by Abboud (1986).

The pulsatile administration of GnRH is under investigation for the treatment of delayed puberty, cryptorchism, and infertility secondary to congenital or acquired GnRH deficiency. Although steroidal feedback mechanisms are intact, the treatment of infertility with pulsatile GnRH results in multiple births (7%) and spontaneous abortions (20%) at frequencies that are similar to those seen with gonadotropins or clomiphene (Reid *et al.,* 1988).

Only one GnRH agonist preparation is currently marketed in the United States. *Leuprolide acetate injection* (LUPRON) is available as an aqueous solution (5 mg/ml) for subcutaneous injection; the recommended dose is 1 mg per day. A depot preparation (7.5 mg) is also available for intramuscular administration at monthly intervals; it has been approved as an alternative to orchiectomy for the palliative treatment of advanced prostatic cancer and can be used in conjunction with flutamide for this purpose (*see* Chapter 59). Leuprolide is about 30 times more active than natural GnRH and 100 times more active than gonadorelin. The indications for GnRH and its agonist analogs in the treatment of neoplastic disease are discussed in Chapter 52.

Various GnRH agonists are undergoing clinical trial for the treatment of endocrine disorders that respond to reductions in gonadal steroids, such as endometriosis (Nafarelin Study Group, 1988), uterine leiomyomas, and precocious puberty (Mansfield *et al.,* 1983). The use of GnRH agonists as contraceptive agents in men and women also is under investigation (Andreyko *et al.,* 1988). GnRH antagonists should prove as beneficial as agonists for these conditions.

Adverse Effects. Most adverse effects of chronic GnRH treatment stem from suppression of gonadal steroid synthesis; these are discussed in Chapters 52, 58, and 59. The chronic administration of GnRH can elicit the production of anti-GnRH antibodies which, in rare cases, have sufficient affinity and binding capacity to cause resistance to treatment (Meakin *et al.,* 1985). It is not known what effect these antibodies have on endogenous GnRH once treatment is withdrawn.

GROWTH HORMONE–RELEASING HORMONE

Growth hormone–releasing hormone (GHRH), along with somatostatin, directly controls the synthesis and release of growth hormone from pituitary somatotrophs. Characterized only in 1982, GHRH is a potentially useful agent in the diagnosis and treatment of growth hormone deficiency.

Human GHRH is synthesized as a precursor of 108 amino acid residues (Mayo *et al.,* 1985). The mature hormone contains 44 amino acid residues with an amidated carboxyl terminus, although additional proteolysis *in vivo* can yield peptides of 37 and 40 amino acids that possess full biological activity. In fact, synthetic peptides that contain only the first 29 residues of GHRH are fully efficacious and are nearly as potent as natural GHRH (Ling *et al.,* 1985). Although GHRH is a member of the glucagon-secretin peptide family (*see* Chapter 12), the latter hormones do not have GHRH activity.

GHRH stimulates the synthesis and secretion of growth hormone in somatotrophs by binding to specific cell-surface receptors that are coupled to adenylyl cyclase through G_s (Gelato and Merriam, 1986). The intravenous injection of 100 to 200 μg of synthetic GHRH into human subjects elicits the release of growth hormone within 5 minutes; maximal concentrations in plasma are observed 30 to 60 minutes later; there is little effect on other pituitary hormones (Thorner *et al.,* 1986). Few side effects are observed, and GHRH is eliminated with a half-life of 40 to 50 minutes. Unlike the effect of GnRH on gonadotrophs, long-term administration of GHRH results in only partial desensitization of somatotrophs. Thus, the secretion of growth hormone rises and remains pulsatile during long-term administration of GHRH; this may reflect the inhibitory activity of endogenous somatostatin, whose secretion is also pulsatile. Similar observations have been made in acromegalics with elevated plasma concentrations of GHRH owing to ectopic secretion (Thorner *et al.*, 1986).

Synthetic GHRH is under investigation as an adjunct in the assessment of growth hormone deficiency in children, where it may help distinguish deficient pituitary function from hypothalamic GHRH deficiency. Thus far, the experience with GHRH parallels that with GnRH. The chronic absence of GHRH arising from hypothalamic lesions can lead to atrophy of somatotrophs and poor responses to single injections of GHRH. In these cases, responsiveness can be restored by the long-term administration of GHRH, followed by repetition of the test.

GHRH may be useful as an alternative treatment for growth hormone–deficient children with hypothalamic lesions, although current therapy with growth hormone is effective in these cases. As many as 40 to 80% of growth hormone–deficient children respond to exogenous GHRH, suggesting that the defect in many of these children is, in fact, hypothalamic. Preliminary results indicate that properly selected, growth hormone–deficient children respond to GHRH with an increased velocity of growth; the optimal dosage and route of administration have not been determined (Gelato and Merriam, 1986).

SOMATOSTATIN

Although named for its activity as a growth hormone release–inhibiting hormone, somatostatin is distributed widely outside the hypothalamus, where it inhibits secretion in a variety of endocrine and exocrine glands. Thus, somatostatin is under investigation in the treatment of various hypersecretory syndromes that are secondary to neoplastic or gastrointestinal disease.

Human somatostatin is synthesized as a precursor of 116 amino acid residues that is processed proteolytically to peptides with 14 or 28 amino acids (Table 56–3). Biological activity resides within the ring formed by the disulfide bond that is common to both forms; this motif is incorporated into the many synthetic agonists under investigation (Cai *et al.*, 1986; Conference, 1988b). Immunoreactive somatostatin is found throughout the CNS, in D cells of the pancreatic islets, in gastric and duodenal mucosae, and in the circulation.

Not surprisingly, many of the effects of the administration of somatostatin are consistent with the syndrome associated with somatostatinomas (Vinik *et al.*, 1987). These tumors secrete somatostatin, elevating plasma concentrations of the peptide as much as 250-fold above normal. In the pituitary somatostatin inhibits secretion of growth hormone as evoked by GHRH, arginine, insulin, levodopa, exercise, or sleep. Secretion from thyrotrophs and lactotrophs is suppressed as well. In the endocrine pancreas, secretion of insulin and glucagon is inhibited, producing a transient hyperglycemia at low doses of somatostatin and diabetes mellitus at high doses. Most gastrointestinal secretions are suppressed, including those of gastrin, gastric acid, secretin, cholecystokinin, vasoactive intestinal peptide (VIP), digestive enzymes, and bicarbonate; this leads to malabsorption with steatorrhea, dyspepsia, hypochlorhydria, cholelithiasis, and a mild watery diarrhea. In the kidney, renal plasma flow is reduced, leading to a decreased glomerular filtration rate and a reduced urinary volume. Hepatic, splanchnic, and gastric mucosal blood flows are all reduced as well, as is production of saliva (Reichlin, 1983; Longnecker, 1988). At present, the dose of somatostatin required to elicit each of these responses is poorly defined.

Table 56–3. CHEMICAL STRUCTURES OF NATIVE AND SYNTHETIC SOMATOSTATIN PEPTIDES

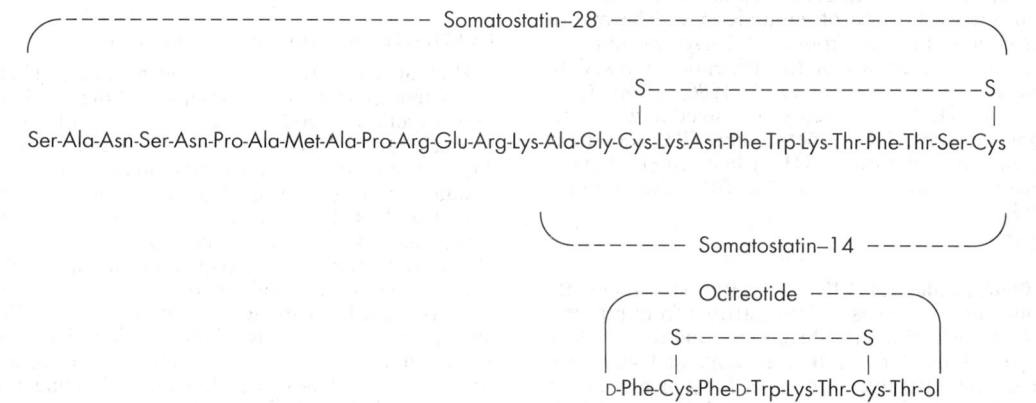

Somatostatin–28

Ser-Ala-Asn-Ser-Asn-Pro-Ala-Met-Ala-Pro-Arg-Glu-Arg-Lys-Ala-Gly-Cys-Lys-Asn-Phe-Trp-Lys-Thr-Phe-Thr-Ser-Cys (S—S bridge between the two Cys residues)

Somatostatin–14 (Ala-Gly-Cys-Lys-Asn-Phe-Trp-Lys-Thr-Phe-Thr-Ser-Cys)

Octreotide

D-Phe-Cys-Phe-D-Trp-Lys-Thr-Cys-Thr-ol (S—S bridge between the two Cys residues)

Somatostatin exerts these effects by binding to specific receptors on the surface of target cells; the liganded receptors interact with G proteins that mediate a number of intracellular events (*see* Chapter 2). Of these, the most thoroughly characterized is an inhibition of adenylyl cyclase activity and suppression of the accumulation of cyclic AMP. In some circumstances, enhanced K^+ conductance may be responsible for membrane hyperpolarization; this too may be directly mediated by G proteins. Either or both of these mechanisms could lead to decreased function of voltage-sensitive Ca^{2+} channels and could contribute to a decrease in the intracellular concentration of Ca^{2+} available to support secretion. Direct G protein–mediated inhibition of Ca^{2+} channels is an additional possibility.

The clinical use of somatostatin is limited by its short half-life (several minutes) and its lack of inhibitory selectivity. Fortunately, several agonists with superior pharmacokinetic properties are available for investigational use. In addition, one analog, *octreotide* (SANDOSTATIN) (*see* Table 56–3), is marketed in ampules containing 0.05, 0.10, or 0.5 mg/ml of the peptide. Octreotide has been approved for the management of secretory carcinoid tumors and VIP-secreting tumors. The drug is administered subcutaneously two to four times per day at total doses of 50 to 1500 μg per day; a usual dose is 450 μg per day or less.

Since somatostatin receptors in different tissues are pharmacologically heterogeneous, somatostatin agonists with greater selectivity may be forthcoming (Cai *et al.*, 1986). The antisecretory activity of somatostatin or somatostatin agonists may be useful in the palliative treatment of other hormone-secreting tumors (pancreatic islet-cell tumors, acromegaly, and others), hormone-dependent tumors (chondrosarcoma and osteosarcoma), cholera, and gastric acid-pepsin disorders. (For additional discussion, *see* Moreau and DeFeudis, 1987; Longnecker, 1988; Gordon *et al.*, 1989.)

THYROTROPIN-RELEASING HORMONE

Chemistry. Thyrotropin-releasing hormone (TRH) is a tripeptide with both terminal amino and carboxyl groups blocked: L-pyroglutamyl-L-histidyl-L-proline amide. Pyroglutamate is derived from the cyclization of glutamic acid. The mature hormone is derived from a precursor protein that contains five copies of the tripeptide flanked by dibasic residues (Lechan *et al.*, 1986). Many derivatives of TRH have been synthesized and studied. Some analogs, like 3-methyl-His-TRH, are more potent than natural TRH, while others have a longer duration of action (Griffiths and Bennett, 1983).

Pharmacological Effects. TRH stimulates the synthesis and release of thyrotropin from pituitary thyrotrophs. Human subjects respond to as little as 15 μg administered intravenously, and 400 μg is maximally effective. A dose of 5 mg or more is required orally because the peptide is poorly absorbed from the gut. In normal man, intravenous TRH provokes a maximal secretion of thyrotropin within 15 to 30 minutes. Plasma concentrations of thyrotropin remain elevated for 2 to 4 hours, although TRH is inactivated rapidly in human plasma and has a half-life *in vivo* of approximately 5 minutes (Bennett and McMartin, 1979). TRH also stimulates prolactin secretion from pituitary lactotrophs (*see* above).

TRH is distributed widely throughout the CNS, where it functions as a neurotransmitter. Administration of TRH to animals produces CNS-mediated effects on behavior, thermoregulation, autonomic tone, and cardiovascular function, including increases in blood pressure and heart rate (Horita *et al.*, 1987). These latter effects may be useful clinically. Indeed, TRH can improve cardiovascular performance in animal models of circulatory shock (McIntosh and Faden, 1986).

The actions of TRH are mediated by specific receptors in thyrotrophs and in various regions of the CNS that appear to have identical pharmacological properties. The stimulation of TRH receptors in the pituitary results in the increased hydrolysis of polyphosphoinositides and the synthesis of inositol trisphosphate (*see* Chapter 2). In some circumstances, TRH can enhance the accumulation of cyclic AMP in the presence of substances that stimulate the synthesis of this nucleotide (*see* Lamberts and MacLeod, 1990).

Preparations, Dosages, and Therapeutic Uses. The synthetic tripeptide (*protirelin*) is available for injection in 1-ml ampules that contain 0.5 mg (RELEFACT TRH, THYPINONE). TRH is used clinically in the diagnosis of thyroid disease; with TRH it can be determined whether secondary hypothyroidism is of pituitary or hypothalamic origin, and patients with primary and secondary hypothyroidism can also be distinguished. Patients with hyperthyroidism fail to respond. Testing involves the intravenous administration of protirelin in a dose of 200 to 500 μg, followed by serial determinations of thyroid hormones and of plasma thyrotropin by immunoassay (Jackson, 1982). Additional discussion of the use of TRH appears in Chapter 57.

CORTICOTROPIN-RELEASING HORMONE

Human corticotropin-releasing hormone (CRH) is a potent hypothalamic stimulator of the synthesis and secretion of ACTH (*i.e.*, pro-opiomelanocortin) in pituitary corticotrophs (Jones and Gillham, 1988). The mature hormone contains 41 amino acid residues; it is synthesized as a precursor of 196 amino acids that is expressed in a variety of tissues other than the hypothalamus (Shibahara *et al.*, 1983). The amino acid sequence of human CRH is very similar to that of the ovine hormone (83% identity), and both are active in man. Several CRH analogs are available for investigation, including some that behave as competitive antagonists (Rivier *et al.*, 1984). The human and ovine hormones are being studied as diagnostic agents. Although no clear indication for the administration of CRH has emerged, assay of this peptide in plasma and assessment of responses to its administration may help the clinician in the evaluation of adrenal or pituitary insufficiency. (For additional discussion, *see* Chapter 60; *see also* Taylor and Fishman, 1988.)

Regulation of Regulatory Hormones

Although any significant discussion of this important area of neuroendocrinology is beyond the scope of this text, a few points should be made. There is ample evidence to implicate important neural control of the secretion of regulatory hormones. Evidence exists for adrenergic, dopaminergic, and tryptaminergic mechanisms that regulate the formation and secretion of various hypothalamic releasing hormones. This has been discussed above in regard to the inhibitor of prolactin secretion. Similar evidence implicates adrenergic mechanisms in the secretion of growth hormone, thyrotropin, and gonadotropins. Drugs that alter central adrenergic mechanisms exert significant influences on the secretion of the adenohypophyseal hormones, and these are discussed under the individual agents involved.

Adelman, J. P.; Mason, A. J.; Hayflick, J. S.; and Seeburg, P. H. Isolation of the gene and hypothalamic cDNA for the common precursor of gonadotropin-releasing hormone and prolactin release-inhibiting factor in human and rat. *Proc. Natl. Acad. Sci. U.S.A.*, **1986**, *83*, 179–183.

Allen, B. M. Effects of extirpation of the anterior lobe of the hypophysis of *Rana pipiens*. *Biol. Bull. Mar. Biol. Lab., Woods Hole,* **1917**, *32*, 117–130.

Aschner, B. Demonstration von Hunden nach Extirpation der Hypophyse. *Wien. Klin. Wochenschr.*, **1909**, *22*, 1730–1731.

Bajusz, S.; Kovacs, M.; Gazdag, M.; Bokser, L.; Karashima, T.; Csernus, V. J.; Janaky, T.; Guoth, J.; and Schally, A. V. Highly potent antagonists of luteinizing hormone-releasing hormone free of edematogenic effects. *Proc. Natl. Acad. Sci. U.S.A.*, **1988**, *85*, 1637–1641.

Bangham, D. R.; Gaines Das, R. E.; and Schulster, D. The international standard for human growth hormone for bioassay: calibration and characterization by international collaborative study. *Mol. Cell. Endocrinol.*, **1985**, *42*, 269–282.

Barrera-Saldaña, H. A.; Seeburg, P. H.; and Saunders, G. F. Two structurally different genes produce the same secreted human placental lactogen hormone. *J. Biol. Chem.*, **1983**, *258*, 3787–3793.

Baumann, G., and Loriaux, D. L. Failure of endogenous prolactin to alter renal salt and water excretion and adrenal function in man. *J. Clin. Endocrinol. Metab.*, **1976**, *43*, 643–649.

Beastall, G. H.; Ferguson, K. M.; O'Reilly, D. St. J.; Seth, J.; and Sheridan, B. Assays for follicle stimulating hormone and luteinising hormone: guidelines for the provision of a clinical biochemistry service. *Ann. Clin. Biochem.*, **1987**, *24*, 246–262.

Boutin, J.-M.; Jolicoeur, C.; Okamura, H.; Gagnon, J.; Edery, M.; Shirota, M.; Banville, D.; Dusanter-Fourt, I.; Djiane, J.; and Kelly, P. A. Cloning and expression of the rat prolactin receptor, a member of the growth hormone/prolactin receptor gene family. *Cell,* **1988**, *53*, 69–77.

Brown, P.; Gajdusek, D. C.; Gibbs, C. J., Jr.; and Asher, D. M. Potential epidemic of Creutzfeldt-Jakob disease from human growth hormone therapy. *N. Engl. J. Med.*, **1985**, *313*, 728–731.

Bundak, R.; Hindmarsh, P. C.; Smith, P. J.; and Brook, C. G. D. Long-term auxologic effects of human growth hormone. *J. Pediatr.*, **1988**, *112*, 875–879.

Cai, R.-Z.; Szoke, B.; Lu, R.; Fu, D.; Redding, R. W.; and Schally, A. V. Synthesis and biological activity of highly potent octapeptide analogs of somatostatin. *Proc. Natl. Acad. Sci. U.S.A.*, **1986**, *83*, 1896–1900.

Carr, D. B.; Bullen, B. A.; Skrinar, G. S.; Arnold, M. A.; Rosenblatt, M.; Beitins, I. Z.; Martin, J. B.; and McArthur, J. W. Physical conditioning facilitates the exercise-induced secretion of beta-endorphin and beta-lipotropin in women, *N. Engl. J. Med.*, **1981**, *305*, 560–562.

Daughaday, W. H.; Salmon, W. D., Jr.; and Alexander, F. Sulfation factor activity of sera from patients with pituitary disorders. *J. Clin. Endocrinol. Metab.*, **1959**, *19*, 743–758.

Evans, H. M., and Long, J. A. The effect of the anterior lobe administered intraperitoneally upon growth, maturity, and oestrous cycles of the rat. *Anat. Rec.*, **1921**, *21*, 62–63.

Faiman, C., and Ryan, R. J. Serum follicle-stimulating hormone and luteinizing hormone concentrations during the menstrual cycle as determined by radioimmunoassays. *J. Clin. Endocrinol. Metab.*, **1967**, *27*, 1711–1716.

Feldman, J. M.; Plonk, J. W.; and Bivens, C. H. Inhibitory effect of serotonin antagonists on growth hormone release in acromegalic patients. *Clin. Endocrinol. (Oxf.)*, **1976**, *5*, 71–78.

Friesen, H. Lactation induced by human placental lactogen and cortisone acetate in rabbits. *Endocrinology,* **1966**, *79*, 212–215.

Fukushima, M. Studies on somatotropic hormone secretion in gynecology and obstetrics. *Tohoku J. Exp. Med.*, **1961**, *74*, 161–174.

Hack, M.; Brish, M.; Serr, D. M.; Inster, V.; and Lunenfeld, B. Outcome of pregnancies after induced ovulation. Follow-up of pregnancies and children born after gonadotropin therapy. *J.A.M.A.*, **1970**, *211*, 791–797.

Hirschberg, R., and Kopple, J. D. Evidence that insulin-like growth factor I increases renal plasma flow and glomerular filtration rate in fasted rats. *J. Clin. Invest.*, **1989**, *83*, 326–330.

James, W. H. The sex ratio of infants born after hormonal induction of ovulation. *Br. J. Obstet. Gynaecol.*, **1985**, *92*, 299–301.

Jeffcoate, S. L.; Bacon, R. R. A.; Beastall, G. H.; Diver, M. J.; Franks, S.; and Seth, J. Assays for prolactin: guidelines for the provision of a clinical biochemistry service. *Ann. Clin. Biochem.*, **1986**, *23*, 638–651.

Josimovich, J. B., and MacLaren, J. A. Presence in the human placenta and term serum of a highly lactogenic substance immunologically related to pituitary growth hormone. *Endocrinology,* **1962**, *71*, 209–220.

Kusuda, S., and Dufau, M. L. Characterization of ovarian gonadotropin receptor. *J. Biol. Chem.*, **1988**, *263*, 3046–3049.

Lamberts, S. W. J.; Uitterlinden, P.; Verschoor, L.; van Dongen, K. J.; and del Pozo, E. Long-term treatment of acromegaly with the somatostatin analogue SMS 201–995. *N. Engl. J. Med.*, **1985**, *313*, 1576–1580.

Laron, A.; Klinger, B.; Erster, B.; and Anin, S. Effect of acute administration of insulin-like growth factor I in patients with Laron-type dwarfism. *Lancet,* **1988**, *2*, 1170–1172.

Lechan, R. M.; Wu, P.; Jackson, I. M. D.; Wolf, H.; Cooperman, S.; Mandel, G.; and Goodman, R. H. Thyrotropin-releasing hormone precursor: characterization in rat brain. *Science,* **1986**, *231*, 159–161.

Leung, D. W.; Spencer, S. A.; Cachianes, G.; Hammonds, R. G.; Collins, C.; Henzel, W. J.; Barnard, R.; Waters, M. J.; and Wood, W. I. Growth hormone receptor and serum binding protein: purification, cloning and expression. *Nature,* **1987,** *330,* 537–543.

Li, C. H.; Dixon, J. S.; and Chung, D. Amino acid sequence of human chorionic somatomammotropin. *Arch. Biochem. Biophys.,* **1973,** *155,* 95–110.

Ljungqvist, A.; Feng, D.-M.; Hook, W.; Shen, Z.-X.; Bowers, C.; and Folkers, K. Antide and related antagonists of luteinizing hormone release with long action and oral activity. *Proc. Natl. Acad. Sci. U.S.A.,* **1988,** *85,* 8236–8240.

Luboshitzky, R.; Dickstein, G.; and Barzilai, D. Induction of spermatogenesis in isolated hypogonadotropic hypogonadism with exogenous human chorionic gonadotropin. *J. Endocrinol. Invest.,* **1981,** *4,* 217–219.

McKenzie, J. M. Studies on the thyroid activator of hyperthyroidism. *J. Clin. Endocrinol. Metab.,* **1961,** *21,* 635–647.

Mandenoff, A.; Fumeron, F.; Apfelbaum, M.; and Margules, D. L. Endogenous opiates and energy balance. *Science,* **1982,** *215,* 1536–1537.

Mansfield, M. J.; Beardworth, D. E.; Loughlin, J. S.; Crawford, J. D.; Bode, H. H.; Rivier, J.; Vale, W.; Kushner, D. C.; Crigler, J. F.; and Crowley, W. F. Long-term treatment of central precocious puberty with a long-acting analogue of luteinizing hormone–releasing hormone. *N. Engl. J. Med.,* **1983,** *309,* 1286–1290.

Markoff, E.; Sigel, M. B.; Lacour, N.; Seavey, B. K.; Friesen, H. G.; and Lewis, U. J. Glycosylation selectively alters the biological activity of prolactin. *Endocrinology,* **1988,** *123,* 1303–1306.

Marshall, J. C., and Kelch, R. P. Gonadotropin-releasing hormone: role of pulsatile secretion in the regulation of reproduction. *N. Engl. J. Med.,* **1986,** *315,* 1459–1468.

Martens, G. J. M.; Civelli, O.; and Herbert, E. Nucleotide sequence of cloned cDNA for pro-opiomelanocortin in the amphibian *Xenopus laevis. J. Biol. Chem.,* **1985,** *260,* 13685–13689.

Mayo, K. E.; Cerelli, G. M.; Lebo, R. V.; Bruce, B. D.; Rosenfeld, M. G.; and Evans, R. M. Gene encoding human growth hormone-releasing factor precursor: structure, sequence, and chromosomal assignment. *Proc. Natl. Acad. Sci. U.S.A.,* **1985,** *82,* 63–67.

Meakin, J. L.; Keogh, E. J.; and Martin, C. E. Human anti-luteinizing hormone releasing hormone antibodies in patients treated with synthetic luteinizing hormone-releasing hormone. *Fertil. Steril.,* **1985,** *43,* 811–813.

Morell, A. G.; Gregoriadis, G.; Scheinberg, I. H.; Hickman, J.; and Ashwell, G. The role of sialic acid in determining the survival of glycoproteins in the circulation. *J. Biol. Chem.,* **1971,** *246,* 1461–1467.

Nafarelin Study Group. Administration of nasal nafarelin as compared with oral danazol for endometriosis. *N. Engl. J. Med.,* **1988,** *318,* 485–489.

Newman, C. B.; Cosby, H.; Firesen, H. G.; Feldman, M.; Cooper, P.; De Crescito, V.; Pilon, M.; and Kleinberg, D. L. Evidence for a nonprolactin, non-growth-hormone mammary mitogen in the human pituitary gland. *Proc. Natl. Acad. Sci. U.S.A.,* **1987,** *84,* 8110–8114.

Niall, H. D.; Hogan, M. L.; Sauer, R.; Rosenblum, I. Y.; and Greenwood, F. C. Sequences of pituitary and placental lactogenic and growth hormones: evolution from a primordial peptide by gene reduplication. *Proc. Natl. Acad. Sci. U.S.A.,* **1971,** *68,* 866–869.

Nikolics, K.; Mason, A. J.; Szónyi, É.; Ramachandran, J.; and Seeburg, P. H. A prolactin-inhibiting factor within the precursor for human gonadotropin-releasing hormone. *Nature,* **1985,** *316,* 511–517.

Peters, C. A., and Walsh, P. C. The effect of nafarelin acetate, a luteinizing-hormone-releasing hormone agonist, on benign prostatic hyperplasia. *N. Engl. J. Med.,* **1987,** *317,* 599–604.

Public Health Service. Fatal degenerative neurological disease in patients who received pituitary-derived human growth hormone. *MMWR,* **1985,** *34,* 359–366.

Riddle, O.; Bates, R. W.; and Dykshorn, S. W. The preparation, identification and assay of prolactin—a hormone of the anterior pituitary. *Am. J. Physiol.,* **1933,** *105,* 191–216.

Rivier, J.; Rivier, C.; and Vale, W. Synthetic competitive antagonists of corticotropin-releasing factor: effect on ACTH secretion in the rat. *Science,* **1984,** *224,* 889–891.

Rose, S. R.; Ross, J. L.; Uriarte, M.; Barnes, K. M.; Cassorla, F. G.; and Cutler, G. B., Jr. The advantage of measuring stimulated as compared with spontaneous growth hormone levels in the diagnosis of growth hormone deficiency. *N. Engl. J. Med.,* **1988,** *319,* 201–207.

Rubin, R. T.; Poland, R. E.; and Tower, B. B. Prolactin-related testosterone secretion in normal adult man. *J. Clin. Endocrinol. Metab.,* **1976,** *42,* 112–116.

Rudman, D.; Kutner, M. H.; Blackston, R. D.; Cushman, R. A.; Bain, R. P.; and Patterson, J. H. Children with normal-variant short stature: treatment with human growth hormone for six months. *N. Engl. J. Med.,* **1981,** *305,* 123–131.

Sairam, M. R., and Bhargavi, G. N. A role for glycosylation of the α subunit in transduction of biological signal in glycoprotein hormones. *Science,* **1985,** *229,* 65–67.

Sheehan, H. L., and Summers, V. K. The syndrome of hypopituitarism. *Q. J. Med.,* **1949,** *18,* 319–379.

Shibahara, S.; Morimoto, Y.; Furutani, Y.; Notake, M.; Takahashi, H.; Shimizu, S.; Horikawa, S.; and Numa, S. Isolation and sequence analysis of the human corticotropin-releasing factor precursor gene. *EMBO J.,* **1983,** *2,* 775–779.

Simmonds, M. Über Hypophysisschwund mit tödlichen Ausgang. *Dtch. Med. Wochenschr.,* **1914,** *40,* 322–323.

Simon, J. A.; Danforth, D. R.; Hutchison, J. S.; and Hodgen, G. D. Characterization of recombinant DNA derived-human luteinizing hormone *in vitro* and *in vivo. J.A.M.A.,* **1988,** *259,* 3290–3295.

Smith, P. E. The disabilities caused by hypophysectomy and their repair. *J.A.M.A.,* **1927,** *88,* 158–161.

———. Hypophysectomy and a replacement therapy. *Am. J. Anat.,* **1930,** *45,* 205–256.

Snyder, P. J., and Sterling, F. H. Hypersecretion of LH and FSH by a pituitary adenoma. *J. Clin. Endocrinol. Metab.,* **1976,** *42,* 544–550.

Thau, R. B.; Goldstein, M.; Yamamoto, Y.; Burrow, G. N.; Phillips, D.; and Bardin, C. W. Failure of gonadotropin therapy secondary to chorionic gonadotropin-induced antibodies. *J. Clin. Endocrinol. Metab.,* **1988,** *66,* 862–867.

Truong, A. T.; Duez, C.; Belayew, A.; Renard, A.; Pictet, R.; Bell, G.; and Martial, J. A. Isolation and characterization of the human prolactin gene. *EMBO J.,* **1984,** *3,* 429–437.

Trzeciak, W. H.; Waterman, M. R.; and Simpson, E. R. Synthesis of the cholesterol side-chain cleavage enzymes in cultured rat ovarian granulosa cells: induction by follicle-stimulating hormone and dibutyryl adenosine 3′,5′-monophosphate. *Endocrinology,* **1986,** *119,* 323–330.

Turkington, R. W. Inhibition of prolactin secretion and successful therapy of the Forbes-Albright syndrome with L-dopa. *J. Clin. Endocrinol. Metab.,* **1972,** *34,* 306–311.

Van Vliet, G.; Styne, D. M.; Kaplan, S. L.; and Grumbach, M. M. Growth hormone treatment for short stature. *N. Engl. J. Med.,* **1983,** *309,* 1016–1022.

Wass, J. A. H.; Thorner, M. O.; Morris, D. V.; Rees, L. H.; Stuart, M. A.; Jones, A. E.; and Besser, G. M. Long-term treatment of acromegaly with bromocriptine. *Br. Med. J.*, **1977**, *1*, 875–878.

Monographs and Reviews

Abboud, C. F. Laboratory diagnosis of hypopituitarism. *Mayo Clin. Proc.*, **1986**, *61*, 35–48.

Andreyko, J. L.; Marshall, L. A.; Dumesic, D. A.; and Jaffe, R. J. Therapeutic uses of gonadotropin-releasing hormone analogs. *Obstet. Gynecol. Surv.*, **1988**, *42*, 1–21.

Baenziger, J. U., and Green, E. D. Pituitary glycoprotein hormone oligosaccharides: structure, synthesis and function of the asparagine-linked oligosaccharides on lutropin, follitropin and thyrotropin. *Biochim. Biophys. Acta*, **1988**, *947*, 287–306.

Bauman, D. E.; Eisemann, J. H.; and Currie, W. B. Hormonal effects on partitioning of nutrients for tissue growth: role of growth hormone and prolactin. *Fed. Proc.*, **1982**, *41*, 2538–2544.

Bauman, D. E.; Eppard, P. J.; De Geeter, M. J.; and Lanza, G. M. Responses of high producing dairy cows to long term treatment with pituitary somatotropin and recombinant somatotropin. *J. Dairy Sci.*, **1985**, *68*, 1352–1362.

Bennett, H. P. J., and McMartin, C. Peptide hormones and their analogues: distribution, clearance from the circulation, and inactivation *in vivo*. *Pharmacol. Rev.*, **1979**, *30*, 247–292.

Bottazzo, G. F., and Doniach, D. Autoimmune thyroid disease. *Annu. Rev. Med.*, **1986**, *37*, 353–359.

Brook, C. G. D.; Hindmarsh, P. C.; and Stanhope, R. Growth and growth hormone secretion. *J. Endocrinol.*, **1988**, *119*, 179–184.

Conference. Growth and growth disorders. *Acta Paediatr. Scand.*, **1988a**, *343*, Suppl., 3–246.

Conference. Somatostatin. Recent advances in basic research and clinical applications. *Horm. Res.*, **1988b**, *29*, 49–132.

Council on Scientific Affairs. Drug abuse in athletes. *J.A.M.A.*, **1988**, *259*, 1703–1705.

Daughaday, W. H. Hormonal regulation of growth by somatomedin and other tissue growth factors. *Clin. Endocrinol. Metab.*, **1977**, *6*, 117–135.

Davidson, M. B. Effect of growth hormone on carbohydrate and lipid metabolism. *Endocr. Rev.*, **1987**, *8*, 115–131.

Fiddes, J. C., and Talmadge, K. Structure, expression, and evolution of the genes for the human glycoprotein hormones. *Recent Prog. Horm. Res.*, **1984**, *40*, 43–74.

Floss, H. G.; Cassady, J. M.; and Robbers, J. E. Influence of ergot alkaloids on pituitary prolactin and prolactin-dependent processes. *J. Pharm. Sci.*, **1973**, *62*, 699–715.

Frasier, S. D. Human pituitary growth hormone (hGH) therapy in growth hormone deficiency. *Endocr. Rev.*, **1983**, *4*, 155–170.

———. Side effects of pituitary growth hormone therapy. In, *Pediatric and Adolescent Endocrinology*, Vol. 16. (Laron, Z.; Butenandt, O.; and Raiti, S.; eds.) S. Karger, Basel, **1987**, pp. 155–163.

Froesch, E. R.; Schmid, C.; Schwander, J.; and Zapf, J. Actions of insulin-like growth factors. *Annu. Rev. Physiol.*, **1985**, *47*, 443–467.

Frohman, L. A., and Downs, T. R. Ectopic GRH syndrome. In, *Acromegaly*. (Robbins, R., and Melmed, S., eds.) Plenum Press, New York, **1987**, pp. 115–126.

Gelato, M. C., and Merriam, G. R. Growth hormone releasing hormone. *Annu. Rev. Physiol.*, **1986**, *48*, 569–591.

Goldfine, I. D. Medical treatment of acromegaly. *Annu. Rev. Med.*, **1978**, *29*, 407–415.

Gordon, P.; Comi, R. J.; Maton, P. N.; and Vay Liang, W. G. Somatostatin and somatostatin analogue (SMS 201–995) in treatment of hormone-secreting tumors of the pituitary and gastrointestinal tract and non-neoplastic diseases of the gut. *Ann. Intern. Med.*, **1989**, *110*, 35–50.

Griffiths, E. C., and Bennett, G. W. (eds.). *Thyrotropin Releasing Hormone*. Raven Press, New York, **1983.**

Handelsman, D. J., and Swerdloff, R. S. Pharmacokinetics of gonadotropin-releasing hormone and its analogs. *Endocr. Rev.*, **1986**, *7*, 95–105.

Hart, I. C. Biotechnology and production-related hormones. *Proc. Nutr. Soc.*, **1987**, *46*, 393–405.

Hazum, E., and Conn, P. M. Molecular mechanism of gonadotropin releasing hormone (GnRH) action. I. The GnRH receptor. *Endocr. Rev.*, **1988**, *9*, 379–386.

Horita, A.; Carino, M. A.; and Lai, H. Pharmacology of thyrotropin-releasing hormone. *Annu. Rev. Pharmacol. Toxicol.*, **1987**, *26*, 311–332.

Huckle, W. R., and Conn, P. M. Molecular mechanism of gonadotropin releasing hormone action. II. The effector system. *Endocr. Rev.*, **1988**, *9*, 387–395.

Inouye, K., and Otsuka, H. ACTH: structure-function relationship. In, *Hormonal Proteins and Peptides*, Vol. XIII. (Li, C. H., ed.) Academic Press, Inc., New York, **1987**, pp. 1–29.

Isaksson, O. G. P.; Lindahl, A.; Nilsson, A.; and Isgaard, J. Mechanism of the stimulatory effect of growth hormone on longitudinal bone growth. *Endocr. Rev.*, **1987**, *8*, 426–438.

Jackson, I. Thyrotropin-releasing hormone. *N. Engl. J. Med.*, **1982**, *306*, 145–155.

Jones, M. T., and Gillham, B. Factors involved in the regulation of adrenocorticotropic hormone/β-lipotropic hormone. *Physiol. Rev.*, **1988**, *68*, 743–818.

Karten, M. J., and Rivier, J. E. Gonadotropin-releasing hormone analog design. Structure-function studies toward the development of agonists and antagonists: rationale and perspective. *Endocr. Rev.*, **1986**, *7*, 44–66.

Kennedy, J. L., and Adashi, E. Y. Ovulation induction. *Obstet. Gynecol. Clin. North Am.*, **1987**, *14*, 831–864.

Kleinberg, D. L. Prolactin and breast cancer. *N. Engl. J. Med.*, **1987**, *316*, 269–271.

Lamberts, S. W. J., and MacLeod, R. M. Prolactin: release and function. *Physiol. Rev.*, **1990**, In Press.

Leong, D. A.; Frawley, L. S.; and Neill, J. D. Neuroendocrine control of prolactin secretion. *Annu. Rev. Physiol.*, **1983**, *45*, 109–127.

Ling, N.; Zeytin, F.; Böhlen, P.; Esch, F.; Brazeau, P.; Wehrenberg, W. B.; Baird, A.; and Guillemin, R. Growth hormone releasing factors. *Annu. Rev. Biochem.*, **1985**, *54*, 403–423.

Longnecker, S. M. Somatostatin and octreotide: literature review and description of therapeutic activity in pancreatic neoplasia. *Drug Intell. Clin. Pharm.*, **1988**, *22*, 99–106.

McIntosh, T. K., and Faden, A. I. Thyrotropin-releasing hormone (TRH) and circulatory shock. *Circ. Shock*, **1986**, *18*, 241–258.

Marshak, D. R., and Liu, D. T. (eds.). *Banbury Report 29: Therapeutic Peptides and Proteins: Assessing the New Technologies*. Cold Spring Harbor Laboratory, New York, **1988.**

Mehta, A. D., and Tolis, G. Prolactin update. *Pathobiol. Annu.*, **1981**, *11*, 337–389.

Melmed, S. (moderator). Pituitary tumors secreting growth hormone and prolactin. *Ann. Intern. Med.*, **1986**, *105*, 238–253.

Moreau, J. P., and DeFeudis, F. V. Pharmacological studies of somatostatin and somatostatin-analogues:

therapeutic advances and perspectives. *Life Sci.*, **1987**, *40*, 419–437.

Müller, E. E. Neural control of somatotropic function. *Physiol. Rev.*, **1987**, *67*, 962–1053.

Nicoll, C. S.; Mayer, G. L.; and Russell, S. M. Structural features of prolactins and growth hormones that can be related to their biological properties. *Endocr. Rev.*, **1986**, *7*, 169–203.

Pierce, J. G., and Parsons, T. F. Glycoprotein hormones: structure and function. *Annu. Rev. Biochem.*, **1981**, *50*, 465–495.

Porter, D. G. Feto-maternal relationships: the actions and the control of certain placental hormones. *Placenta*, **1980**, *1*, 259–274.

Reichlin, S. Somatostatin. *N. Engl. J. Med.*, **1983**, *309*, 1495–1501, 1556–1563.

Reid, R. L.; Fretts, R.; and Van Vugt, D. A. The theory and practice of ovulation induction with gonadotropin-releasing hormone. *Am. J. Obstet. Gynecol.*, **1988**, *158*, 176–185.

Roth, R. A. Structure of the receptor for insulin-like growth factor II: the puzzle amplified. *Science*, **1988**, *239*, 1269–1271.

Ryan, R. J.; Charlesworth, M. C.; McCormick, D. J.; Milius, R. P.; and Keutmann, H. T. The glycoprotein hormones: recent studies of structure-function relationships. *FASEB J.*, **1988**, *2*, 2661–2669.

Seibel, M. M. A new era in reproductive technology: *in vitro* fertilization, gamete intrafallopian transfer, and donated gametes and embryos. *N. Engl. J. Med.*, **1988**, *318*, 828–834.

Smithline, F.; Sherman, L.; and Kolodny, H. D. Prolactin and breast carcinoma. *N. Engl. J. Med.*, **1975**, *292*, 784–792.

Stanhope, R., and Brook, C. G. D. An evaluation of hormonal changes at puberty in man. *J. Endocrinol.*, **1988**, *318*, 828–834.

Stevens, V. C. Current status of antifertility vaccines using gonadotropin immunogens. *Immunol. Today*, **1986**, *7*, 369–374.

Taylor, A. L., and Fishman, L. M. Corticotropin-releasing hormone. *N. Engl. J. Med.*, **1988**, *319*, 213–222.

Thorner, M. O. Prolactin. *Clin. Endocrinol. Metab.*, **1977**, *6*, 201–222.

Thorner, M. O., and others. Physiological and clinical studies of GRF and GH. *Recent Prog. Horm. Res.*, **1986**, *42*, 589–632.

Underwood, L. E. Report of the conference on uses and possible abuses of biosynthetic human growth hormone. *N. Engl. J. Med.*, **1984**, *311*, 606–608.

Vinik, A. I.; Strodel, W. E.; Eckhauser, F. E.; Moattari, A. R.; and Lloyd, R. Somatostatinomas, PPomas, neurotensinomas. *Semin. Oncol.*, **1987**, *14*, 263–281.

von Heijne, G. Patterns of amino acids near signal-sequence cleavage sites. *Eur. J. Biochem.*, **1983**, *133*, 17–21.

CHAPTER

57 THYROID AND ANTITHYROID DRUGS

Robert C. Haynes, Jr.

THYROID

The thyroid gland is the source of two fundamentally different types of hormones. Thyroxine and triiodothyronine are vital for normal growth and development and play an important role in energy metabolism. The other known glandular secretion, calcitonin, is considered in Chapter 62.

History. The thyroid gland was first described in 1656 by Wharton. Harington (1935) reviewed the many older opinions concerning the function of this gland. Wharton thought, for example, that the viscous fluid within the follicles lubricated the trachea. He also believed that the gland was larger in women to serve a cosmetic function in giving grace to the contour of the neck. Later observers, influenced by the liberal blood supply of the gland, believed that it provided a vascular shunt for the brain. With this function in mind, Rush in 1820 expressed the belief that the larger size of the gland in women was "necessary to guard the female system from the influence of the more numerous causes of irritation and vexation of mind to which they are exposed than the male sex." However, Hofrichter opposed this theory in the same year by pointing out that "If it were indeed true that the thyroid contains more blood at some times than at others, this effect would be visible to the naked eye; in this case women would certainly have long ceased to go about with bare necks, for husbands would have learned to recognize the swelling of this gland as a danger signal of threatening trouble from their better halves."

The thyroid was first recognized as an organ of importance when enlargement was observed to be associated with changes in the eyes and the heart in the condition we now call *hyperthyroidism*. It is of interest that this condition, the manifestations of which can on occasion be as striking as any in medicine, escaped description until Parry saw his first case in 1786. Parry's account was not published until 1825 (*see* Parry, 1895) and was followed in 1835 and 1840 by those of Graves and Basedow, whose names became applied to the disorder. In 1874 Gull first associated atrophy of the gland with the symptoms now known to be characteristic of thyroid deficiency, and hypofunction of the thyroid in adults is still known as *Gull's disease*. The term *myxedema* was applied to the clinical syndrome by Ord (1878) in the belief that the characteristic thickening of the subcutaneous tissues was due to excessive formation of mucus.

Extirpation experiments to elucidate the function of the thyroid were at first misinterpreted because of the simultaneous removal of the parathyroids. However, the pioneer research on the latter organs by Gley (1891) allowed the functional differentiation of these two endocrine glands. It was not until after calcitonin was discovered in 1961 that it was realized that the thyroid itself was also concerned with the regulation of Ca^{2+}. Murray (1891) was the first to treat a case of hypothyroidism by injecting an extract of the thyroid gland; in the following year, Howitz, Mackenzie, and Fox independently discovered that thyroid tissue was fully effective when given by mouth.

Magnus-Levy (1895) discovered the effect of the thyroid on metabolic rate; he found that Gull's disease was characterized by a low rate of metabolism and that the administration of thyroid to hypothyroid or normal individuals increased oxygen consumption.

Chemistry. The active principles of the thyroid gland are the iodine-containing amino acid derivatives of thyronine—*thyroxine* (T_4) and *triiodothyronine* (T_3) (Table 57–1). Thyroxine was first isolated in crystalline form from a hydrolysate of thyroid by Kendall (1915), who found that the crystalline product exerted the same physiological effects as the extract from which it was obtained. Eleven years later the structural formula of thyroxine was elucidated by Harington, and in the following year Harington and Barger (1927) synthesized the hormone.

Following the isolation and the chemical identification of thyroxine, it was generally believed that all the hormonal activity of thyroid tissue could be

Table 57–1. THE THYROID HORMONES

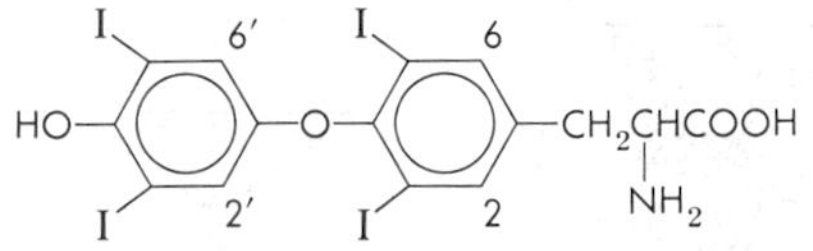

Thyroxine

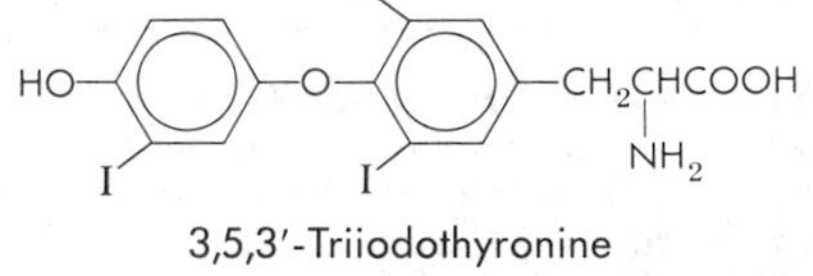

3,5,3′-Triiodothyronine

accounted for by its content of thyroxine. However, careful studies revealed that crude thyroid preparations possessed greater calorigenic activity than could be accounted for by their thyroxine content. The enigma was resolved with the detection, isolation, and synthesis of triiodothyronine (Gross and Pitt-Rivers, 1952; Roche *et al.*, 1952a, 1952b). Further studies revealed that triiodothyronine is qualitatively similar to thyroxine in its biological action but that it is much more potent on a molar basis (Gross and Pitt-Rivers, 1953a, 1953b).

Structure–Activity Relationship. A great many structural analogs of thyroxine have been synthesized in order to define the structure–activity relationship, to detect antagonists of thyroid hormones, or to find compounds exhibiting one desirable type of activity while not showing unwanted effects. The only significant success has been the partial separation of the cholesterol-lowering action of thyroxine analogs from their calorigenic or cardiac effects. The D isomer of thyroxine has had limited clinical use to lower the concentration of cholesterol in plasma, but cardiac side effects remain a significant problem. Newer analogs offer hope that more useful separation of these activities may yet be achievable (Underwood *et al.*, 1986).

The structural requirements for a significant degree of thyroid hormone activity have been defined (*see* Jorgensen, 1964 and *earlier editions* of this book). The 3′-monosubstituted compounds are more active than the 3′,5′-disubstituted molecules. Thus, triiodothyronine is four times more potent than thyroxine, while 3′-isopropyl-3,5-diiodothyronine has seven times the activity.

While the chemical nature of the 3, 5, 3′, and 5′ substituents is important, their effects on the conformation of the molecule are even more so. In thyronine, the two rings are angulated at about 120° at the ether oxygen and are free to rotate on their axes. As depicted schematically in Figure 57–1, when the 3,5 iodines are in place, rotation of the two rings is somewhat restricted, and they tend to take up positions perpendicular to one another. While not potent, even halogen-free derivatives possess some activity if the proper conformation is possible. In general, the affinity of iodothyronines for the thyroid hormone receptor parallels their biologic potency (Samuels *et al.*, 1988), but additional factors including affinity for plasma proteins, rate of entry into cell nuclei, and rate of metabolism can affect therapeutic potency.

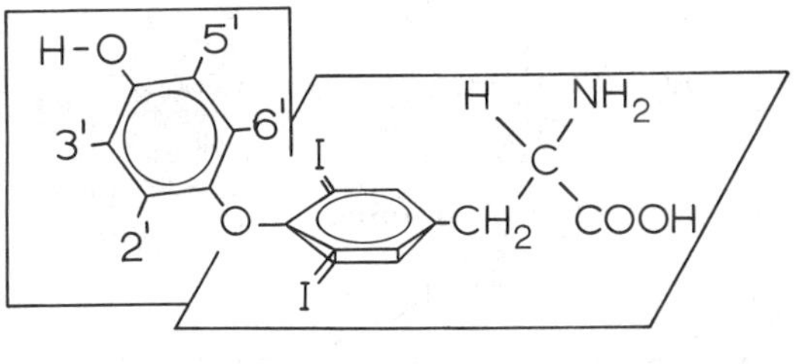

Figure 57–1. *Structural formula of 3,5-diiodothyronine, drawn to show the conformation in which the planes of the aromatic rings are perpendicular to each other.* (After Jorgensen, 1964. Courtesy of The Mayo Association. *See also* Cody and Duax, 1973.)

Synthesis of Thyroid Hormones. The synthesis of the thyroid hormones is unique, complex, and seemingly grossly inefficient. The thyroid hormones are synthesized and stored as amino acid residues of thyroglobulin, a protein constituting the vast majority of the thyroid follicular colloid. The thyroid gland is unique in storing great quantities of potential hormone in this way, and extracellular thyroglobulin can represent a large portion of the mass of the gland. Thyroglobulin is a complex glycoprotein made up of two apparently identical subunits, each with a molecular weight of 330,000. Interestingly, molecular cloning has revealed that thyroglobulin belongs to a superfamily of serine hydrolases, including acetylcholinesterase (*see* Chapter 7).

The major steps in the synthesis, storage, release, and interconversion of thyroid hormones are the following: (1) the uptake of iodide ion by the gland, (2) the oxidation of iodide and the iodination of tyrosyl groups of thyroglobulin, (3) the conversion of iodotyrosyl residues to iodothyronyl residues in this protein, (4) the proteolysis of thyroglobulin and the release of thyroxine and triiodothyronine into the blood, and (5) the conversion of thyroxine to triiodothyronine in peripheral tissues. These processes are summarized in Figure 57–2.

1. *Uptake of Iodide.* Iodine ingested in the diet reaches the circulation in the form of iodide. Under normal circumstances its concentration in the blood is very low (0.2 to 0.4 μg/dl; about 15 to 30 nM), but the thyroid efficiently and actively transports the ion. As a result, the ratio of thyroid to plasma iodide concentration is usually between 20 and 50 and can far exceed 100 when the gland is stimulated. The iodide transport mechanism is inhibited by a number of ions such as thiocyanate and perchlorate (*see* below). The transport system is stimulated by thyrotropin (thyroid-stimulating hormone [TSH]) (*see* below) and is also controlled by an autoregulatory mechanism. Thus, decreased stores of thyroid iodine enhance iodide uptake, and the administration of iodide can reverse this situation.

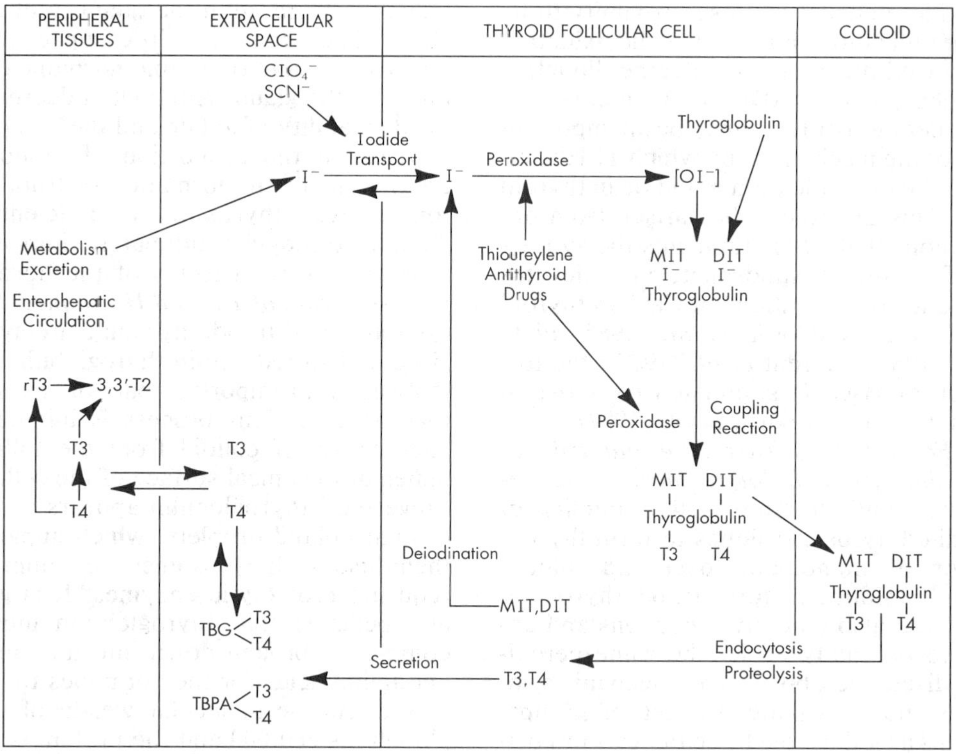

Figure 57–2. *The major pathways of iodine metabolism.*

Abbreviations are as follows: *T3* = triiodothyronine; *T4* = thyroxine; *rT3* = 3,3′,5′-triiodothyronine (reverse T_3); *3,3′-T2* = 3,3′-diiodothyronine; *MIT* = monoiodotyrosine; *DIT* = diiodotyrosine; *TBG* = thyroxine-binding globulin; *TBPA* = thyroxine-binding prealbumin.

If the further metabolism of iodide is blocked by antithyroid drugs, the iodide-concentrating mechanism can more easily be studied. Thus isolated, the mechanism resembles those found in other bodily structures that concentrate iodide, including the salivary glands, gastric mucosa, midportion of the small intestine, skin, mammary gland, and placenta, all of which maintain a concentration gradient of iodide some 10 to 50 times that of the blood. It has been suggested that the accumulation of iodide by the placenta and the mammary gland may be of importance in providing adequate supplies for the fetus and infant, but no obvious purpose is served by the accumulation of iodide at the other sites. It is evident that the iodide-accumulating system of the thyroid is not unique to the gland and does not account for the specific function of making thyroid hormone.

2. *Oxidation and Iodination.* Consistent with the conditions generally necessary for halogenation of aromatic rings, the iodination of tyrosine residues requires the iodinating species to be in a higher state of oxidation than is the anion. The exact nature of the iodinating species was uncertain for many years. However, Magnusson and coworkers (1984) have provided convincing evidence that it is hypoiodate, either as hypoiodous acid (HOI) or as an enzyme-linked species (E-OI).

The oxidation of iodide to its active form is accomplished by thyroid peroxidase, a heme-containing enzyme that utilizes H_2O_2 as the oxidant (Taurog *et al.*, 1970; Magnusson *et al.*, 1987). The peroxidase is membrane-bound and appears to be concentrated at or near the apical surface of the thyroid cell. The reaction results in the formation of monoiodotyrosyl and diiodotyrosyl residues in thyroglobulin just prior to its storage in the lumen of the thyroid follicle. It is thought that the formation of the H_2O_2 that serves as a substrate for the peroxidase occurs in close proximity to its site of utilization and involves the oxidation of reduced nicotinamide adenine dinucleotide phosphate (NADPH). An increase in the generation of H_2O_2 may be an important facet of the mechanism by which TSH stimulates the organification of iodide in thyroid cells. This hypothesis has arisen from observations that TSH stimulates the synthesis of inositol trisphosphate and elevates cytosolic concentrations of Ca^{2+} in thyroid follicular cells (Corda *et al.*, 1985; Field *et al.*, 1987; Laurent *et al.*, 1987); the formation of H_2O_2 is stimulated by a rise in cytosolic Ca^{2+} (Takasu *et al.*, 1987).

3. *Formation of Thyroxine and Triiodothyronine from Iodotyrosines.* The remaining synthetic step is the coupling of two diiodotyrosyl residues to form thyroxine or of monoiodotyrosyl and diiodotyrosyl residues to form triiodothyronine. These are also oxidative reactions and appear to be catalyzed by the same peroxidase discussed above. The mechanism involves the enzymatic transfer of groups, perhaps as iodotyrosyl free radicals or positively charged ions, within thyroglobulin. Although many other proteins can serve as substrates for the peroxidase, none is as efficient as thyroglobulin in yielding thyroxine. The configuration of the protein is thus presumed to be important in facilitating this coupling reaction. The sites of hormone synthesis within the structure of thyroglobulin have been determined recently (Dunn *et al.*, 1987). Thyroxine formation occurs primarily at a location near the amino terminus of the protein, while most of the triiodotyrosine is synthesized near the carboxyl terminus. The relative rates of synthetic activity at the various sites depend on the concentration of TSH and the availability of iodide. This may account, at least in part, for the long-known relationship between the proportion of thyroxine and triiodothyronine formed in the thyroid and the availability of iodide or the relative quantities of the two iodotyrosines. For example, when there is a deficiency of iodine in rat thyroid, the ratio of thyroxine to triiodothyronine decreases from 4:1 to 1:3 (Greer *et al.*, 1968). Since triiodothyronine is at least four times as active as thyroxine and contains only three fourths as much iodine, a decrease in the quantity of available iodine need have little impact on the effective amount of thyroid hormone elaborated by the gland. Although a decrease in the availability of iodide and the associated increase in the proportion of monoiodotyrosine favor the formation of triiodothyronine over thyroxine, a deficiency in diiodotyrosine can ultimately impair the formation of both forms of the hormone.

4. *Secretion of Thyroid Hormone.* Since thyroxine and triiodothyronine are synthesized and stored within thyroglobulin, proteolysis is an important part of the secretory process. This process is initiated by endocytosis of colloid from the follicular lumen at the apical surface of the cell. This "ingested" thyroglobulin appears as intracellular colloid droplets, which apparently then fuse with lysosomes containing the requisite proteolytic enzymes. It is generally believed that thyroglobulin must be completely broken down into its constituent amino acids for the hormones to be released. As the molecular weight of thyroglobulin is 660,000 and the protein is made up of about 300 carbohydrate residues and 5500 amino acid residues, only two to five of which are thyroxine, this is an extravagant process indeed. TSH appears to enhance the degradation of thyroglobulin by increasing the activity of several thiol endopeptidases of the lysosomes (Dunn and Dunn, 1988); the liberated hormones then exit from the cell, presumably at its basal membrane. When thyroglobulin is hydrolyzed, monoiodotyrosine and diiodotyrosine are also liberated, but they usually do not leave the thyroid. Instead, they are selectively metabolized, and the iodine, liberated in the form of iodide, is reincorporated into protein. Normally, all this iodide is reused; however, when proteolysis is activated intensely by TSH, some of the iodide reaches the circulation, at times accompanied by trace amounts of the iodotyrosines.

5. *Conversion of Thyroxine to Triiodothyronine.* The normal daily production of thyroxine has been estimated to range between 70 and 90 μg, while that of triiodothyronine is between 15 and 30 μg. Although triiodothyronine is secreted by the thyroid, the majority (approximately 80%) is synthesized by the metabolism of thyrox-

ine in peripheral tissues. Thus, when thyroxine is given to hypothyroid patients in doses that produce normal concentrations of thyroxine in plasma, the plasma concentration of triiodothyronine also reaches the normal range. This metabolic step has been demonstrated in preparations of a number of different tissues *in vitro;* the liver and kidney are the most active. The enzyme responsible for this reaction (5′-deiodinase) is inhibited by oxidizing agents and by the antithyroid drug propylthiouracil, which appears to form a complex with the enzyme. Methimazole, another antithyroid drug of the thioureylene group, does not inhibit the enzyme; in fact, it antagonizes the inhibition produced by propylthiouracil (Leonard and Rosenberg, 1978). Fasting and a number of acute and chronic illnesses decrease the activity of the 5′-deiodinase, such that the T_4:T_3 ratio of the plasma is increased (Braverman and Vagenakis, 1979). The clinical significance of the decreased plasma concentration of triiodothyronine in illness has been discussed by Utiger (1980). Estimation of the total amount of thyroxine eventually converted to triiodothyronine is difficult, but it has been calculated to be in the range of 35% (*see* Schimmel and Utiger, 1977).

The 5′-deiodinase that converts thyroxine to triiodothyronine exists in two forms. The type-I enzyme, found in liver and kidney, is the more significantly active quantitatively and is more sensitive to inhibition by propylthiouracil. This enzyme is responsible for synthesis of triiodothyronine for most peripheral tissues. The type-II enzyme of brown fat and pituitary has an extremely low Michaelis constant (K_m) for thyroxine (about 1 nM); the activity of this enzyme may be particularly important for acute regulation of the secretion of TSH by the pituitary, since it is strategically located to provide triiodothyronine to mediate this effect (Silva *et al.*, 1987). The deiodinase of brown fat is subject to complex stimulatory regulation by the sympathetic nervous system. Both α_1- and β-adrenergic receptors must be activated for a maximal response; there appear to be synergistic interactions between Ca^{2+}, cyclic AMP, and stimulators of protein kinase C, and protein synthesis is required (Raasmaja and Larsen, 1989).

Transport of Thyroid Hormone in the Blood. Iodine in the circulation is normally present in several forms, with 95% as organic iodine and approximately 5% as iodide. Most of the organic iodine is thyroxine (90 to 95%), while triiodothyronine represents a relatively minor fraction (about 5%). The thyroid hormones are transported in the blood in strong but noncovalent association with certain plasma proteins.

Thyroxine-binding globulin is the major carrier of thyroid hormones. It is an acidic glycoprotein with a molecular weight of approximately 63,000, and it binds one molecule of thyroxine per molecule of protein with a very high association constant (about 10^{10} M^{-1}). Triiodothyronine is bound less avidly. Thyroid hormones are also found associated with transthyretin (also called thyroxine-binding prealbumin). This protein is present in higher concentration than is the thyroxine-binding globulin, but it binds thyroxine and triiodothyronine with association constants near 10^7 M^{-1} and 10^6 M^{-1}, respectively. Despite the fact that transthyretin has four apparently identical subunits, it has a single high-affinity binding site. Albumin can also serve as a carrier for thyroxine when the more avid carriers are saturated. It is difficult, however, to estimate its quantitative or physiological importance.

Protein binding of thyroid hormones protects them from metabolism and excretion, resulting in their long half-life in the circulation. Only about 0.03% of the total thyroxine in plasma is free (*see* Utiger, 1974). Although triiodothyronine is much less firmly bound, the quantity that is free, 0.2 to 0.5%, is still a small percentage of the total. However, the unbound thyroid hormones constitute the fractions available for action, and their concentrations thus assume particular importance.

Certain drugs and a variety of pathological and physiological conditions can alter the binding of thyroid hormones to proteins or the amounts of these proteins. Thus, the total amounts of thyroid hormones in the plasma and the quantities of *free* hormones can vary somewhat independently. For example, pregnancy or the administration of estrogen causes elevation of the concentration of thyroxine-binding globulin. This leads to increased thyroxine binding and could lower the concentration of free hormone. Feedback mechanisms compensate, however, and increased thyroid secretion returns the concentration of free hormone to normal. The result is elevated total and bound thyroxine in plasma and a normal concentration of free thyroxine. Laboratory tests that measure only total thyroxine, therefore, would be subject to misinterpretation. Appropriate tests of thyroid function are discussed below.

Degradation and Excretion. Thyroxine is eliminated slowly from the body, with a half-life of 6 to 7 days. In hyperthyroidism the half-life is shortened to 3 or 4 days, whereas in myxedema it may be 9 to 10 days. These changes are presumably due to altered rates of metabolism of the hormone. In conditions associated with increased binding to the proteins of plasma, such as pregnancy, elimination is retarded; the reverse is observed when there is reduced protein in plasma, as in nephrosis or hepatic cirrhosis, or when binding to protein is inhibited by certain drugs, such as salicylate or dicumarol. Triiodothyronine, which is less avidly bound to protein, has a half-life of 2 days or less.

The liver is the major site of degradation of thyroid hormones; thyroxine and triiodothyronine are conjugated with glucuronic and sulfuric acids through the phenolic hydroxyl group and excreted in the bile. There is an enterohepatic circulation of the thyroid hormones, since they are liberated by hydrolysis in the intestine and reabsorbed. A portion of the conjugated material reaches the colon unchanged, is hydrolyzed there, and is eliminated as the free compounds in the feces. In man, approximately 20 to 40% of thyroxine is eliminated in the stool.

As discussed above, an important route of metabolism of thyroxine is to triiodothyronine. Another compound formed by peripheral metabolism of thyroxine is 3,3′,5′-triiodothyronine, often referred to as reverse T_3. Although the concentration of this inactive metabolite in plasma varies with diet and disease states, no significant clinical consequences of these changes have been demonstrated. Triiodothyronine and reverse T_3 are deiodinated to 3,3′-diiodothyronine, an inactive metabolite that is a normal constituent of human plasma. Additional metabolites in which the diphenyl ether linkage is either intact or cleaved have been detected both *in vitro* and *in vivo*.

Regulation of Thyroid Function. During the last century, it was appreciated that cellular changes occur in the anterior pituitary in association with endemic goiter or following thyroidectomy. The classical experimental observations of Cushing (1912) and the clinical observations of Simmonds (1914) established that ablation or disease of the pituitary causes thyroid hypoplasia. It was eventually determined that the anterior pituitary secretes the specific hormone, TSH (Chapter 56).

Although there was evidence that thyroid hormone or lack of it causes cellular changes in the pituitary, the control of secretion of TSH by the negative-feedback action of thyroid hormone was not appreciated fully until its central role in the pathogenesis of goiter was elucidated in the early 1940s. It is now recognized that the rate of secretion of TSH is delicately controlled by thyrotropin-releasing hormone (TRH) and the quantity of thyroid hormone in the circulation. If extra hormone is given, transcription of the thyrotropin gene is decreased (*see* Samuels *et al.,* 1988), the secretion of thyrotropin is suppressed, and the thyroid becomes inactive and regresses. Any decrease in the normal rate of secretion of the thyroid evokes an enhanced secretion of TSH and the thyroid is stimulated to increased growth and function. An additional mechanism of the effect of thyroid hormone on TSH secretion appears to be a reduction in the number of receptors for TRH on pituitary cells (Hinkle and Goh, 1982). The role of TRH is discussed in Chapter 56.

Actions of TSH on the Thyroid. When TSH is given to experimental animals, the first effect on thyroid hormone metabolism that can be measured is increased secretion. This can be monitored by prelabeling the hormone with radioactive iodine and measuring the radioactivity in blood leaving the gland. Under these circumstances, the response can be seen within minutes. All phases of hormone synthesis and release are eventually stimulated: iodide uptake and organification, hormone synthesis, endocytosis, and proteolysis of colloid. There is increased vascularity of the gland and hypertrophy and hyperplasia of thyroid cells.

A primary action of TSH is to activate thyroid adenylyl cyclase and to increase the glandular concentration of adenosine 3′,5′-monophosphate (cyclic AMP). Cyclic AMP, acting as the intracellular mediator of

TSH, appears to be able to reproduce the important actions of the hormone. Thus, iodide uptake and hormone synthesis are stimulated by the cyclic nucleotide, as are endocytosis and secretion of hormone. Protein and nucleic acid synthesis are increased; in fact, cyclic AMP has been shown to be goitrogenic. As noted above, recent evidence indicates that TSH can also enhance the production of diacylglycerol and inositol trisphosphate and induce a rise in cytosolic Ca^{2+}. The relationship between the activation of these two second messenger systems and their relative roles in mediating the actions of TSH have yet to be defined (*e.g., see* Manley *et al.,* 1988).

Relation of Iodine to Thyroid Function. Normal thyroid function obviously requires an adequate intake of iodine; without it, normal amounts of hormone cannot be made, TSH is secreted in excess, and the thyroid hypertrophies. The enlarged and stimulated thyroid becomes remarkably efficient at extracting the residual traces of iodide from the blood. The iodide-concentrating mechanism develops a gradient for the ion that may be ten times normal, and in extreme cases the vascularity may increase to the point that a bruit is heard over the gland. In this hypertrophied state the thyroid usually succeeds in making sufficient hormone, unless the iodine deficiency is severe.

In some areas of the world simple or nontoxic goiter is quite prevalent, because iodine is not abundant in most foods. The only rich natural sources commonly eaten are those derived from marine life. Sea fish contain 200 to 1000 μg/kg, shellfish a similar or slightly larger amount, and dried kelp 0.1 to 0.2%, but for those who do not eat marine fish the element can be scarce indeed. To ensure an adequate intake, which is usually taken to be about 100 μg daily, one would have to eat about 5 kg of vegetables or fruit, or 3 kg of meat or fresh-water fish. Milk and eggs are somewhat better sources, but most potable waters contain a negligible amount. However, unnatural sources of iodine in the environment are becoming prevalent and perhaps of concern. A slice of bread may contain 150 μg of iodate, added as a "conditioner" (London *et al.,* 1965). Other sources are as diverse as food colorings and automobile exhaust.

Iodine has been used empirically for the treatment of goiter for 150 years. However, its modern use was the outgrowth of the extensive studies of Marine, which culminated in the use of iodine to prevent goiter in school children in Akron, Ohio, a region where endemic goiter was prevalent (Marine and Kimball, 1917). The success of these experiments led to the adoption of this form of prophylaxis in many regions throughout the world where goiter is endemic; in some areas, injection of iodized oil has been used (Thilly *et al.,* 1973).

The most practicable method yet found for providing small supplements of iodine for large segments of the population is the addition of an iodide or iodate to table salt; iodate is now preferred. In some countries, the use of iodine in salt is required by law; in others, including the United States, the use is optional. In the United States, iodized salt provides 100 μg of iodine per gram.

Actions of Thyroid Hormones. The actions of the thyroid hormones are considered under the categories of (1) regulation of growth and development, (2) calorigenic effect, (3) cardiovascular effects, (4) metabolic effects, and (5) inhibition of the secretion of TSH by the pituitary. This last-named action on the pituitary is discussed above.

Growth and Development. It is generally believed that the thyroid hormones exert most if not all of their effects through control of DNA transcription and, ultimately, protein synthesis. This is certainly true for the actions of the hormones on the normal growth and development of the organism. Perhaps the most dramatic example is found in the tadpole, which is almost magically transformed into a frog by thyroxine. Not only does the animal grow limbs, lungs, and other terrestrial accoutrements, but the hormone also stimulates the synthesis of a host of enzymes and so influences the tail that it is digested away and used to build new tissue elsewhere.

Thyroid hormone has a critically important role in the development of the nervous system. Examination of the brain of hypothyroid animals reveals deficient development, particularly of axonal and dendritic networks. Myelinization is severely impaired, and several other deficits in biochemical development are also notable. It has thus been hypothesized that the effect of thyroid hormone is to initiate a series of reactions that lead to differentiation and to terminate the phase of cell proliferation (Hamburgh, 1969). Thus, for example, triiodothyronine stimulates the synthesis of mRNA for myelin basic protein, a major component of myelin (Shanker *et al.*, 1987). The effects of thyroid hormones on development of the brain are reviewed by Dussault and Ruel (1987).

The actions of thyroid hormones on protein synthesis and enzymatic activity are certainly not limited to the brain, and a large number of tissues are affected by the administration of thyroid hormone or by its deficiency. The extensive defects in growth and development that are found in cretins provide a vivid reminder of the pervasive effects of thyroid hormones in normal individuals.

Cretinism is usually classified as endemic or sporadic. *Endemic cretinism* is encountered in regions of endemic goiter and is usually due to extreme deficiency of iodine. Goiter may or may not be present. *Sporadic cretinism* is a consequence of failure of the thyroid to develop normally or the result of a defect in the synthesis of thyroid hormone. Goiter is present if a synthetic defect is at fault.

While detectable at birth, cretinism is often not recognized until 3 to 5 months of age. When untreated, the condition eventually leads to such gross changes as to be unmistakable. The child is dwarfed and the extremities are short, and the child is mentally retarded, inactive, uncomplaining, and listless. The face is puffy and expressionless, and the enlarged tongue may protrude through the thickened lips of the half-opened mouth. The skin may have a yellowish hue and feel doughy, and it is dry and cool to the touch. The heart rate is slow, the body temperature may be low, closure of the fontanels is delayed, and the teeth erupt late. Appetite is poor, feeding is slow and interrupted by choking, constipation is frequent, and there may be an umbilical hernia.

For treatment to be fully effective, the diagnosis must be made long before these obvious changes have come about. Screening of newborn infants for deficient function of the thyroid is established in the United States and in most industrialized countries. Concentrations of TSH and thyroxine are measured in blood from the umbilical cord or from a heel prick. The incidence of congenital dysfunction of the thyroid is about one per 6000 births (Fisher, 1977).

It is thus clear that thyroid hormones are important determinants of genetically coded developmental programs. While the precise biochemical mechanisms through which the thyroid controls growth and development are unknown, rapid progress is being made in understanding the control of gene expression by thyroid hormones. The thyroid hormones are bound to a limited number of high-affinity receptors in the nuclei of many cells. There is no convincing evidence that the hormones bind first to a cytoplasmic receptor. Both thyroxine and triiodothyronine are bound in nuclei (Galton, 1986), although thyroxine is bound with about tenfold lower affinity. Based on the assumption that binding of the hormones represents initiation of their action, it has been calculated that thyroxine accounts for only 15% or less of the total activity of the thyroid hormones. The nuclear binding of thyroid hormones in relation to their actions has been reviewed by Oppenheimer and colleagues (1987) and Samuels and coworkers (1988).

Recently, startling discoveries have been made related to the thyroid hormone receptor. First, it has been learned that the receptor is a member of a superfamily of related proteins that include the receptors for the different types of steroid hormones, vitamin D, and retinoids (*see* Chapter 2; *see also* Evans, 1988). Application of this knowledge has already led to the discovery of previously undetected, homologous molecules. Some of these are, in fact, distinct forms of the thyroid hormone receptor (*see* below). Furthermore, it has been shown that the thyroid hormone receptor is the protein product of the c-*erb*A protooncogene. This discovery spotlights the entire superfamily of receptors that are related in their DNA-binding sequences as possible factors in carcinogenesis.

The general model for transcriptional regulation of gene expression by members of this superfamily of receptors includes the following features: the receptor molecule, in its hormone-bound state, interacts with specific DNA sequences (hormone-response elements, or HREs) in the promoter regions of appropriate genes and modulates the initiation of their transcription. However, the thyroid hormone receptor may represent a significant variation on this theme. This receptor can suppress the activity of a responsive promoter in the *absence* of hormone. When hormone binds to the receptor-DNA complex, transcription is stimulated from the repressed level. The v-*erb*A oncogene, the oncogenic variant of the normal thyroid hormone receptor, contains an intact DNA-binding domain, but structural changes have resulted in a loss of thyroid hormone binding capacity. The v-*erb*A protein competes with the receptor for binding sites on DNA. Thus, in a sense, it acts as an antagonist of the receptor itself by repressing transcription in a manner that cannot be overcome by thyroid hormone (*see* Damm *et al.*, 1989).

Hybridization studies suggested the existence of multiple genes for thyroid hormone receptors, and complementary DNAs that encode distinct forms of the receptor have now been isolated (Thompson *et al.*, 1987; Hodin *et al.*, 1989). Certain of these receptors are products of distinct genes; others appear to arise from alternative splicing of mRNA. Although current information is relatively scanty, the ligand-binding properties of these receptors are distinct, as is their tissue distribution. One form of the receptor is apparently expressed exclusively in the anterior pituitary. These results clearly suggest that it may be possible to develop more selective analogs of the thyroid hormones.

Calorigenic Effect. Thyroid hormones increase the resting or basal metabolic rate of the whole organism, but only certain tissues seem to be affected when their oxygen consumption is measured *in vitro*. Heart, skeletal muscle, liver, and kidney are markedly stimulated by thyroxine, while the adult brain, spleen, and gonads are largely unresponsive. The calorigenic response is important in regulation of temperature in homeotherms, and thyroid secretion is stimulated by exposure to cold. The mechanism of the calorigenic effect of thyroid hormone is poorly understood, and the field is strewn with discarded hypotheses. For example, it was at one time erroneously believed that thyroid hormones act physiologically by uncoupling mitochondrial oxidative phosphorylation. In a review of the calorigenic effect of thyroid hormones, Sestoft (1980) suggested that approximately 15% of the increased oxygen consumption is a consequence of an enhanced futile cycle of lipolysis and synthesis of triglycerides in adipose tissue. He has also estimated that stimulation of the heart accounts for 30 to 40% of the increased energy utilized. If these estimates are correct, the explanation for a large fraction of the calorigenic effect still remains elusive.

Cardiovascular Effects. Changes in the cardiovascular system are prominent consequences of the action of thyroid hormones. These are most dramatically evident in the cardiac function of hyperthyroid patients (*see* below). Under the influence of thyroid hormones, the heart beats more rapidly and more forcefully, and cardiac output is thus increased. It would seem reasonable to assume that this represents an adaptation to the load placed on the cardiovascular system by the high rate of metabolism experienced by the body as a whole. To some degree this is certainly true, but a number of observations have indicated that the heart is a direct target of hormone action, rather than merely a passive responder to an increased demand. It has often been stated that the heart is hypersensitive to catecholamines in hyperthyroidism. In support of this it has been observed that the number of myocardial β-adrenergic receptors is increased, and β-adrenergic antagonists are of great value in the treatment of thyrotoxic patients. Furthermore, isolated rat atria exposed to triiodothyronine *in vitro* develop an enhanced chronotropic response to maximal doses of norepinephrine (Eiden and Ruth, 1981). Nevertheless, several other careful studies have failed to demonstrate an increased sensitivity to β-adrenergic agonists (*see* Morkin *et al.*, 1983). Decreased muscarinic control of the heart has also been ruled out as a mechanism (Cairoli and Crout, 1967).

A biochemical basis for at least a part of the inotropic effect of thyroid hormones has become apparent. Subsequent to the detection of an altered pattern of cardiac myosin isozymes by Flink and Morkin (1977) and by Hoh and colleagues (1978), it has been shown that thyroid hormones enhance the expression of the gene for the heavy chain of alpha myosin and decrease the expression of the gene for the heavy chain of beta myosin (Everett *et al.*, 1986). This change in isozyme composition enhances the Ca^{2+}-ATPase activity of the myosin, a reaction that is responsible for the generation of force in cardiac muscle (Morkin *et al.*, 1983).

Metabolic Effects. Thyroid hormones stimulate metabolism of cholesterol to bile acids, and hypercholesterolemia is a characteristic feature of hypothyroid states. Thyroid hormones have been shown to increase the specific binding of low density lipoprotein (LDL) by liver cells (Salter *et al.*, 1988), and the concentration of hepatic receptors for LDL is decreased in hypothyroidism (Scarabottolo *et al.*, 1986; Gross *et al.*, 1987). The number of LDL receptors available on the surface of hepatocytes is a strong determinant of the plasma cholesterol concentration (*see* Chapter 36).

Thyroid hormones enhance the lipolytic responses of fat cells to other hormones, for example, catecholamines, and elevated plasma free fatty acid concentrations are seen in hyperthyroidism. In contrast to other lipolytic hormones, thyroid hormones do not directly stimulate the accumulation of cyclic AMP. They may, however, regulate the capacity of other hormones to enhance the accumulation of the cyclic nucleotide by decreasing the activity of a microsomal phosphodiesterase that hydrolyzes cyclic AMP (Nunez and Correze, 1981). There is also evidence that thyroid hormones act to maintain normal coupling of the β-adrenergic receptor to the catalytic subunit of adenylyl cyclase in fat cells. Fat cells from hypothyroid rats have increased concentrations of guanine nucleotide–binding regulatory proteins (G proteins) that mediate the inhibitory control of adenylyl cyclase. This can account both for the decreased response to lipolytic hormones and the increased sensitivity to inhibitory regulators, such as adenosine, that are found in hypothyroidism (Ros *et al.*, 1988).

The effects of the thyroid hormones on carbohydrate metabolism are generally consistent with an accelerated utilization of carbohydrate, presumably secondary to increased caloric demand. The rate of intestinal absorption of glucose is increased, often resulting in higher concentrations of the sugar in plasma during the early phase of an *oral* glucose tolerance test. In contrast, the increased rate of metabolism of carbohydrate results in a flattened response to *intravenous* glucose.

In rats, thyroid hormones enhance the hepatic synthesis of glucose under certain conditions. The mechanism and significance of this action are not known (Muller and Seitz, 1984). Ahren (1986) has reviewed the effects of hyperthyroidism on glucose metabolism in man.

Thyroid Hyperfunction. Excessive secretion of thyroid hormones may lead to such striking changes that the diagnosis of hyperthyroidism is obvious to the casual observer, or the effects may cause distressing but subtle symptoms that give no clue to their origin. Two major forms of thyroid hyperfunction are recognized. Diffuse toxic goiter (Graves' disease), characterized by thyrotoxicosis and ophthalmopathy, occurs most commonly in young or middle-aged women. In this disease, which is now recognized as an autoimmune disorder, IgG antibodies to the TSH receptor are present. One group of these antibodies is able to bind to the receptor and activate it, thereby mimicking the acute and chronic effects of TSH (Burman and Baker, 1985; Bottazzo and Doniach, 1986). Other antibodies to the receptor are thought to be responsible for the characteristic exophthalmos and pretibial edema present in some patients with Graves' disease. The latter antibodies appear to be responses to epitopes on the TSH receptor that are shared by proteins in other tissues, and their interaction with target antigens in connective tissue cells is presumed to initiate the lesions of ophthalmopathy or pretibial edema (Rotella *et al.*, 1986). Toxic nodular goiter (Plummer's disease) occurs primarily in older patients and usually arises from long-standing nontoxic goiter; infiltrative ophthalmopathy is absent. At times, however, the distinction between these conditions can be difficult.

Most of the signs and symptoms of hyperthyroidism stem from the excessive production of heat and from increased motor activity and increased activity of the sympathetic nervous system. The skin is flushed, warm, and moist; the muscles are weak and tremulous; the heart rate is rapid, and the heart beat is forceful; and the arterial pulses are prominent and bounding. The increased expenditure of energy gives rise to increased appetite and, if intake is insufficient, to loss of weight. There may also be insomnia, difficulty in remaining still, anxiety and apprehension, intolerance to heat, and increased frequency of bowel movements. Angina, arrhythmias, and heart failure may be present in older patients. Some individuals may show extensive muscular wasting, suggestive of myopathy. Others have osteoporosis from excessive loss of Ca^{2+}.

Thyroid Hypofunction. Deficiency of thyroid hormone can be manifested at any age. In the adult, the condition is referred to simply as hypothyroidism or, when particularly severe, as myxedema. If the gland fails to develop or is congenitally incompetent, the deficiency may be noted soon after birth by signs of cretinism (*see* above). Later in childhood, failure of growth and development added to the features of the adult counterpart is recognized as juvenile myxedema.

Myxedema. In its fully developed, classical form, myxedema is associated with degeneration and atrophy of the thyroid gland. The same condition follows surgical removal of the thyroid or its destruction by radioactive iodine. Since it may also occur after Graves' disease, some have speculated that the condition can be the end stage of that disease. Indeed, it is now recognized that processes of cell-mediated immunity are operative in Graves' disease, and these may eventually lead to destruction of the gland (Volpe, 1987). Myxedema is sometimes associated with goiter when there is a severe defect in synthesis of thyroid hormone, when the gland is extensively involved in chronic thyroiditis (Hashimoto's disease), or when antithyroid drugs have been given. When the disease is mild, it may be subtle in its presentation. By the time it has become severe, however, all of the signs are overt. The appearance of the patient is pathognomonic. The face is quite expressionless, puffy, and pallid. The skin is cold and dry, the scalp is scaly, and the hair is coarse, brittle, and sparse. The fingernails are thickened and brittle, the subcutaneous tissue appears to be thickened, and there may be true edema. The voice is husky and low-pitched, speech is slow, hearing is often faulty, and mentality is impaired. The appetite is poor, the gastric juice contains little free hydrochloric acid, gastrointestinal activity is diminished, and abdominal distention and constipation are common. Atony of the urinary bladder suggests that the function of other smooth muscles may also be impaired. The voluntary muscles are weak and flabby, and deep-tendon reflexes are slowed. The heart is often dilated, and cardiac output is diminished. There may also be hydropericardium, hydrothorax, and ascites. Refractory anemia, occasionally hyperchromic and macrocytic in character, is often associated with the disease. Menstrual irregularities are prominent. The patient is prone to be drowsy and to sleep a great deal, and complains of the cold in winter but not of the heat in summer.

Thyroid Function Tests. The availability of protein-binding assays and radioimmunoassays for the thyroid hormones has greatly improved the laboratory diagnosis of thyroid disorders. These specific assays, together with the resin-triiodothyronine-uptake (RT_3U) test, which estimates the extent of saturation of thyroid-binding globulin, provide a valuable approach to an accurate diagnosis. Their use permits the estimation of the concentration of free thyroxine in plasma, an excellent index of the activity of the thyroid gland.

As mentioned above, the total concentration of thyroxine in plasma changes with alterations in the concentration of the thyroid-binding globulin, so that, for example, it is high in pregnancy and low in nephrosis even though the patient is euthyroid. From the estimates of the extent of saturation of the thyroid-binding globulin and the measurement of the total concentration of thyroxine in plasma, a free-thyroxine index can be calculated. The measurement of plasma triiodothyronine by radioimmunoassay is also useful for the diagnosis of hyperthyroidism.

The radioimmunoassay of TSH is the best and most sensitive test of thyroid function. Determination of an elevated concentration of this hormone in the plasma is usually diagnostic of failure of the thyroid gland. Patients with frank hypothyroidism who have normal or decreased concentrations of TSH in plasma are likely to have hypothyroidism secondary to pituitary or hypothalamic dysfunction. The response of plasma TSH to an injection of thyrotropin-releasing hormone may also be useful in this regard (*see* Chapter 56). Decreased plasma concentrations of TSH may also be found in hyperthyroidism and are of diagnostic value.

Measurement of the accumulation of radioactive iodine by the thyroid gland as a diagnostic technique is discussed below. Rock (1985) and Griffin (1985) have discussed the use of laboratory tests in the diagnosis of thyroid disease.

Preparations. *Thyroid* is a fine powder made from the thyroids of animals, usually pigs, by defatting and drying with acetone. The USP specifies that the content of iodine be between 0.17 and 0.23%, and, as most thyroid powders are stronger than this, they are diluted by an inert material. Although neither bioassay nor chemical analyses for thyroxine or triiodothyronine are specified, the product is remarkably uniform. *Thyroid tablets* (ARMOUR THYROID, THYRAR) are made from the compressed powder in numerous sizes from 16 to 325 mg. *Thyroglobulin* (PROLOID) is a purified extract of pig thyroid available in tablets containing from 32 to 200 mg. It conforms to the USP standard for iodine content and is subject to bioassay. Its potency is adjusted to be equivalent to thyroid powder. *Levothyroxine sodium* (SYNTHROID, LEVOTHROID, others) is the sodium salt of the natural isomer of thyroxine and is dispensed in the form of tablets containing 25 to 300 μg and as a powder for reconstitution for injection. *Liothyronine sodium* (CYTOMEL) is the somewhat uninformative designation for the salt of L-triiodothyronine. It is marketed as tablets containing 5, 25, and 50 μg. Mixtures of the sodium salts of levothyroxine and liothyronine in a ratio of 4:1 by weight are also marketed as *liotrix* (EUTHROID, THYROLAR). Their dubious advantage is replacement therapy with a pure mixture resembling the normal secretion of the gland.

Thyrotropin (THYTROPAR) is a preparation made from bovine pituitaries. It is available in vials containing 10 I.U. of powdered hormone to be reconstituted for injection. This is used only to test the ability of the thyroid to respond to exogenous stimulation. Synthetic *thyrotropin-releasing hormone* (*protirelin;* RELEFACT TRH, THYPINONE) is available in ampuls containing 500 μg in 1 ml.

Choice of Preparation. The pure compounds carry the attraction of single, reproducible substances of known and constant composition. There is evidence that absorption of levothyroxine sodium is variable and incomplete, as much as 30 to 40% being recoverable in the stool. Depending upon the form in which it is given, the proportion of a single oral dose absorbed may vary from 42 to 74%; this fraction is rapidly absorbed, while the rest traverses the intestine in a bound, unabsorbable form. Nevertheless, levothyroxine sodium has been extensively used with satisfaction and is widely held to be superior to thyroid because of better standardization and stability. Variability of absorption also occurs with desiccated thyroid.

Liothyronine sodium may occasionally be preferred to levothyroxine sodium when a quicker action is desired, for example, in the rare event of coma due to myxedema. It is perhaps less desirable than the other preparations for prolonged therapy because its briefer action might require more frequent dosing for steady response. Other disadvantages include altered normal values for thyroid function tests and higher cost.

Comparative Responses to Thyroid Preparations. There is no significant difference in the qualitative response of the patient with myxedema to triiodothyronine, thyroxine, or thyroid. However, there are obvious quantitative differences. Following the subcutaneous administration of a large experimental dose of L-triiodothyronine, a metabolic response can be detected within 4 to 6 hours, at which time the skin becomes detectably warmer and the pulse rate and temperature increase. With this dose, a metabolic rate of −40% can be raised to normal within 24 hours. The maximal response occurs in 2 days or less, and the effects subside with a half-time of about 8 days. The same single dose of thyroxine exerts much less effect. However, if thyroxine is given in approximately four times the dose of triiodothyronine, a comparable elevation in metabolic rate can be achieved. The peak effect of a single dose is evident in about 9 days, and this declines to half the maximum in 11 to 15 days. In both cases the effects outlast the presence of detectable amounts of hormone; these disappear from the blood with mean half-lives of approximately 2 and 6 days, respectively. Equivalent clinical responses are obtained from the daily administration of approximately 65 mg of thyroid, 65 mg of thyroglobulin, 100 μg of levothyroxine, or 25 μg of liothyronine.

Therapeutic Uses of Thyroid Hormone. The major indications for the therapeutic use of thyroid hormone are *hypothyroidism,* or *myxedema, cretinism,* and *simple goiter*. Inasmuch as they result from thyroid hypofunction, these uses represent true replacement therapy.

Hypothyroidism. It has been said that treatment of adult myxedema is as perfect a form of therapy as any known to medicine. The main objective is to arrive at the proper dose of a suitable thyroid preparation. The dose varies somewhat according to complications, especially those involving the heart. The object of therapy is to restore the patient to normal. However, replacement of thyroid hormone should be done gradually so as not to stress the patient and produce adverse cardiovascular effects. Often the patient may feel well when the astute observer can still see evidence of hypothyroidism. The reverse may also be true; the patient may feel ill, but the doctor does not recognize the insidious onset of the signs and symptoms of myxedema. Because long-standing hypothyroidism may have undesirable effects, including a predisposition to atherosclerosis, a full replacement dose should be given if possible.

A reasonable therapeutic regimen for adults is a daily dose of 50 μg of levothyroxine for 2 weeks, followed by a daily dose of 100 μg for the next 2 weeks. The optimal dose will usually be between 100 and 150 μg. This can be established by the clinical response and return of the plasma concentration of TSH to the normal range. Recent observations with sensitive assays for TSH indicate that many patients are overtreated with levothyroxine and have subclinical hyperthyroidism (Ross, 1988). Some individuals will require a dose as small as 50 μg while others need as much as 400 μg. Medication should be taken on an empty stomach to minimize irregular absorption. The patient should be carefully observed during the institution of treatment for untoward reactions such as cardiac pain or palpitations. If angina occurs, care should be exercised but therapy should not necessarily be withheld. Cardiac symptoms are the only serious complications of treatment. Arrhythmias have caused death during the initiation of thyroid therapy in myxedema.

Treatment of children is the same as for adults. In order to ensure normal growth and development, the dose should be adequate to correct the hypothyroidism without causing symptoms or failure to gain weight normally. A full adult dose is usually needed, and the schedule above can be used.

Myxedema Coma. A large number of dosage regimens have been advocated for this emergency, and the following serve as examples. Levothyroxine (200 to 500 μg, intravenously) or liothyronine (100 μg orally) is preferred initially. Treatment with adrenal steroids is also recommended because of the possibility of relative adrenal insufficiency either from the hypothyroidism or coexistent hypoadrenalism. Further therapy is dictated by the initial clinical response.

Cretinism. Success in the treatment of cretinism depends upon the age at which therapy is started. Unfortunately, many cases do not come to the attention of physicians until the retardation in development has become so obvious as to be alarming to the parents. In such cases, the detrimental effects of the deficiency on mental development will not be completely overcome. If, on the other hand, therapy is started soon after birth, normal physical and mental development may be achieved. Prognosis also depends on the age of onset of the deficiency. If no thyroid develops in the fetus, deficiency probably dates from the fetal age of 3 months, because little hormone is provided from the mother. It is believed, however, that the most critical need for thyroid hormone is during the period of myelination in the central nervous system (CNS) that occurs about the time of birth. Recommended daily doses of levothyroxine are 10 μg/kg for infants under 6 months of age, 8 μg/kg from 6 to 12 months, 6 μg/kg from 1 to 5 years, 4 μg/kg from 5 to 12 years, and 3 μg/kg in children over 12 years. Therapy is monitored by determination of the concentrations of thyroxine and TSH and, occasionally, triiodothyronine in the plasma. Intellectual and physical development are also guides for therapy in this condition, and error, if unavoidable, should be made on the side of higher dosage. Excessive dosage will, however, advance the bone age inappropriately.

Simple Goiter. In simple goiter, or thyroid enlargement without hyperthyroidism, a frequent underlying problem is deficient secretion of thyroid hormone, causing excessive secretion of TSH. The exceptions are unrecognized cases of subacute thyroiditis and autonomous thyroid tumors. In Hashimoto's thyroiditis, enlargement results from inflammation as well as from increased secretion of TSH. As the cause of the condition is frequently some defect in the production of thyroid hormone, treatment with thyroid can properly be regarded as replacement therapy.

The aim in treatment is to give full replacement doses of thyroid hormone so as to maintain plasma TSH in the low-normal range. Usually, this amounts to 100 to 200 μg of levothyroxine daily, but some patients may require 400 μg. The effectiveness of treatment can be judged both by the return of plasma concentrations of TSH to normal values and by the decrease in size of the goiter.

There have been wide differences in the experience of competent observers as to the proportion of cases of goiter that respond to treatment with a decrease in the size of the thyroid. Some have observed that only in a minority of cases is a worthwhile regression achieved. In several large series, however, an appreciable regression in the goiter was noted in about two thirds of the cases and a complete disappearance in half of these. In other series, almost every case showed some response. The degree of response is greatly affected by the duration of the goiter, its cause, the degree of nodularity, and the patient's age. In areas of endemic goiter where deficiency of iodine is the likely cause, thyroid medication has been shown to be prompt and effective unless the goiter has advanced to the stage of nodular degeneration. However, correction of the iodine deficiency is a more direct approach and is advocated for most cases.

Response to treatment with thyroid hormone of goiter commonly seen in the United States usually requires several weeks to become manifest, and the maximal response may not be seen for many months.

Nodular Goiter. The transition from diffuse to nodular goiter is much more important than simply the cosmetic aspect or the infrequent symptoms of compression with difficulty in swallowing. In some instances nodules may secrete hormone and cause hyperthyroidism (*toxic nodular goiter*); however, they are frequently not functional. Herein lies a controversial area of thyroid therapy, since it is necessary to determine whether the nonfunctional nodule is malignant. The choice of whether observation and treatment of the patient with thyroxine is continued or whether open surgical biopsy is undertaken is best made following the examination of a needle-biopsy sample and assessment of the clinical risks. Since there is some evidence that nonfunctional nodules are responsive to TSH, it is logical to continue the treatment with thyroxine; however, it is more difficult to shrink a nodule than to decrease the size of a diffusely enlarged gland.

ANTITHYROID DRUGS AND OTHER THYROID INHIBITORS

A large number of compounds are capable of interfering, directly or indirectly, with the synthesis of thyroid hormones. Several are of great clinical value for the temporary or extended control of hyperthyroid states. These will be discussed in detail. Others are primarily of research or toxicological interest and can only be mentioned briefly. The major inhibitors may be classified into four categories: (1) antithyroid drugs, which interfere directly with the synthesis of thyroid hormones; (2) ionic inhibitors, which block the iodide transport mechanism; (3) iodide itself, which in high concentrations suppresses the thyroid; and (4) radioactive iodine, which damages the gland with ionizing radiations. The antithyroid drugs have been reviewed by Cooper (1984).

ANTITHYROID DRUGS

The antithyroid drugs that have clinical utility are thioureylenes; propylthiouracil may be considered as the prototype.

History. Studies on the mechanism of the development of goiter began with the observation that rabbits fed a diet composed largely of cabbage often developed goiters. This result was probably due to the presence of precursors of the thiocyanate ion in cabbage leaves (*see* below). Later, two pure compounds were shown to produce goiter, sulfaguanidine and phenylthiourea.

Investigation of the effects of thiourea derivatives revealed that rats became hypothyroid despite hyperplastic changes in their thyroid glands that were characteristic of intense thyrotropic stimulation. After treatment was begun, no new hormone was made, and the goitrogen had no visible effect upon the thyroid gland following hypophysectomy or the administration of thyroid hormone. This suggested that the goiter was a compensatory change resulting from the induced state of hypothyroidism and that the primary action of the compounds was to inhibit the formation of thyroid hormone (Astwood, 1945). The therapeutic possibilities of such agents in hyperthyroidism were evident and the substances so used became known as *antithyroid drugs*.

Structure–Activity Relationship. The two goitrogens found in the early 1940s proved to be prototypes of two different classes of antithyroid drugs. These two, with one later addition, made up three general categories into which the majority of the agents can be assigned: (1) *thioureylenes* include all the compounds currently used clinically (Table 57–2); (2) *aniline derivatives*, of which the sulfonamides make up the largest number, embrace a few substances that have been found to inhibit the human thyroid; and (3) *polyhydric phenols*, such as resorcinol, which have caused goiter in man when applied to the abraded skin. A few other compounds, mentioned briefly below, do not fit into any of these categories.

Thiourea and its simpler aliphatic derivatives and heterocyclic compounds containing a thioureylene group make up the majority of the known antithyroid agents that are effective in man. Although most of them incorporate the entire thioureylene group, in some a nitrogen atom is replaced by oxygen or sulfur so that only the thioamide group is common to all. Among the heterocyclic compounds, the sulfur derivatives that are active are

Table 57–2. ANTITHYROID DRUGS OF THE THIOUREYLENE TYPE

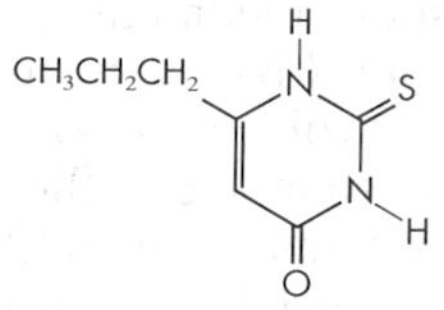

Propylthiouracil

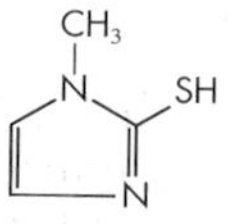

Methimazole

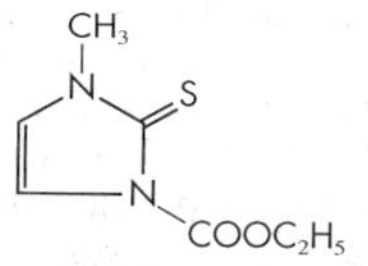

Carbimazole

representatives of imidazole, oxazole, hydantoin, thiazole, thiadiazole, uracil, and barbituric acid.

L-5-Vinyl-2-thiooxazolidone (goitrin) is responsible for the goiter that results from consuming turnips or the seeds or green parts of cruciferous plants. These plants are eaten by cows, and the compound is found in cow's milk in areas of endemic goiter in Finland; it is about as active as propylthiouracil in man. VanEtten (1969) has reviewed the chemistry of naturally occurring goitrogens.

As the result of industrial exposure, toxicological studies, or clinical trials for various purposes, several other compounds have been noted to possess antithyroid activity. Among compounds used clinically phenylbutazone and thiopental are weakly antithyroid in experimental animals. This is not significant at usual doses in man. However, antithyroid effects in man have been observed from dimercaprol, aminoglutethimide (McLaren and Alexander, 1979), and lithium salts (Schou *et al.*, 1968; Temple *et al.*, 1972). Amiodarone, used in management of arrhythmias, has complex effects on thyroid function and can produce hyperthyroidism or, more commonly, hypothyroidism. Some of these effects, which remain incompletely understood, may be due to iodine that is released from the drug during its metabolism (Editorial, 1987; Gammage and Franklyn, 1987).

Mechanism of Action. Antithyroid drugs inhibit the formation of thyroid hormones by interfering with the incorporation of iodine into tyrosyl residues of thyroglobulin; they also inhibit the coupling of these iodotyrosyl residues to form iodothyronines. This implies that they interfere with the oxidation of iodide ion and iodotyrosyl groups. Taurog (1976) proposed that the drugs inhibit the peroxidase enzyme, thereby preventing oxidation of iodide or iodotyrosyl groups to the required active state. Subsequent studies have confirmed that this is, indeed, the mechanism of action and that the antithyroid drugs bind to and inactivate the peroxidase only when the heme of the enzyme is in the oxidized state (Davidson *et al.*, 1978; Engler *et al.*, 1982). Over a period of time, the inhibition of hormone synthesis results in the depletion of stores of iodinated thyroglobulin as the protein is hydrolyzed and the hormones are released into the circulation. Only when the preformed hormone is depleted and the concentrations of circulating thyroid hormones begin to decline do clinical effects become noticeable.

There is some evidence that the coupling reaction may be more sensitive to an antithyroid drug, such as propylthiouracil, than is the iodination reaction (Taurog, 1970). This may explain why patients with hyperthyroidism respond well to doses of the drug that only partially suppress organification.

When Graves' disease is treated with antithyroid drugs, the concentration of thyroid-stimulating immunoglobulins in the circulation decreases. This has prompted some to propose that these agents act as immunosuppressants. Burman and Baker (1985) point out that perchlorate, which acts by an entirely different mechanism, also decreases thyroid-stimulating immunoglobulins, suggesting that improvement in hyperthyroidism may, itself, favorably affect the abnormal humoral immune state.

In addition to blocking hormone synthesis, propylthiouracil inhibits the peripheral deiodination of thyroxine to triiodothyronine. Methimazole does not have this effect and, as noted above, can antagonize the inhibition by propylthiouracil. Although the quantitative significance of this inhibition has not been established, it does provide a theoretical rationale for the choice of propylthiouracil over other antithyroid drugs in the treatment of thyroid storm. In this acute situation, a decreased rate of conversion of circulating thyroxine to triiodothyronine would be beneficial.

Absorption, Metabolism, and Excretion. Measurements of the course of organification of radioiodine by the thyroid show that absorption of *effective* amounts of propylthiouracil follows within 20 to 30 minutes of an oral dose. They also show that the duration of action of the compounds used clinically is brief. The effect of a dose of 100 mg of propylthiouracil begins to wane in 2 to 3 hours, and even a 500-mg dose is completely inhibitory for only 6 to 8 hours. As little as 0.5 mg of methimazole similarly stops the organification of radioiodine in the thyroid gland, but a single dose of 10 to 25 mg is needed to extend the inhibition to 24 hours.

The half-life of propylthiouracil in plasma is about 2 hours, while that for methimazole has been estimated to be between 6 and 13 hours. All the useful drugs appear to be concentrated in the thyroid, and methimazole, derived from the metabolism of carbimazole, accumulates after carbimazole is administered. Drugs and metabolites appear largely in the urine.

The antithyroid drugs cross the placenta and can also be found in milk. The use of these drugs during pregnancy is discussed below; women taking these agents should not breast-feed their infants.

Untoward Reactions. The incidence of side effects from propylthiouracil and methimazole as currently used is relatively low. The overall incidence as compiled from published cases by early investigators was 3% for propylthiouracil and 7% for methimazole, with 0.44 and 0.12% of cases, respectively, developing the most serious reaction, agranulocytosis. Further observations have found little, if any, difference in side effects between these two agents, and suggest that an incidence of agranulocytosis of 1 in 500 is a maximal figure. This reaction usually occurs during the first few weeks or months of therapy. Since agranulocytosis can develop rapidly, periodic white-cell counts are of little help. Patients should immediately report the development of sore throat or fever, which usually heralds the onset of this reaction. If the drug is discontinued rapidly, recovery is the rule. Mild granulocytopenia, if noted, may be due to thyrotoxicosis or may be the first sign of this dangerous drug reaction. Caution and frequent leukocyte counts are then required.

The most common reaction is a mild, sometimes purpuric, urticarial papular rash. It often subsides spontaneously without interrupting treatment but sometimes calls for changing to another drug, because cross-sensitivity is uncommon. Other less frequent complications are pain and stiffness in the joints, paresthesias, headache, nausea, and loss or depigmentation of the hair. Drug fever, hepatitis, and nephritis are very rare.

Preparations and Dosage. The compounds in current use are *propylthiouracil* (6-*n*-propylthiouracil), in the form of 50-mg tablets, and *methimazole* (1-methyl-2-mercaptoimidazole; TAPAZOLE), marketed in 5- and 10-mg tablets. *Methylthiouracil* is not available commercially in the United States at the present time. *Carbimazole* (NEO-MERCAZOLE) is a carbethoxy derivative of methimazole, which it closely resembles and into which it is converted in the body; it is widely used in Great Britain and elsewhere.

The usual dose of propylthiouracil for the treatment of hyperthyroidism is 100 mg every 8 hours. In some cases larger doses may be required. Failures of response to treatment with 300 mg daily are sometimes attributable to improper spacing of the doses, since the drug is fully effective for only a few hours. Delayed responses are also sometimes noted when the thyroid is unusually large and when iodine in any form has been given beforehand. When doses larger than 300 mg daily are needed, further subdivision of the time of administration of the daily dose into 4- or 6-hour intervals is perhaps advisable. After the patient is euthyroid, dosage can usually be reduced to one third for maintenance. In mild cases, good control can often be achieved with only one or two daily doses.

The corresponding initial dosage of methimazole or carbimazole for the majority of cases is 5 to 20 mg every 8 hours. Because the half-life of methimazole is 6 to 13 hours, this dosage regimen should produce an uninterrupted suppression of the thyroid gland. When a complete response has been achieved, the dose is reduced but the total daily dose is still subdivided. Only when very small amounts are needed is the frequency of dosage reduced to two or even one dose per day.

Therapeutic Uses. The antithyroid drugs are used in the treatment of *hyperthyroidism* in the following three ways: (1) as definitive treatment, to control the disorder in anticipation of a spontaneous remission; (2) in conjunction with radioiodine, to hasten recovery while awaiting the effects of radiation; and (3) to control the disorder in preparation for surgical treatment. There is no uniformity of opinion as to which form of treatment is the most desirable.

Response to Treatment. Hyperthyroidism may be of two kinds—Graves' disease and hyperthyroidism from one or more overfunctioning thyroid nodules; whichever the cause, the hyperthyroidism seems to respond to antithyroid drugs in the same way. After treatment is instituted, there is usually a latent period of a few days to 2 or more weeks before improvement is clearly manifest; however, in a few cases, and particularly when the hyperthyroidism is severe, definite improvement may be seen in 1 or 2 days. In patients with large goiters and particularly if they are nodular, the response may be slower. When iodine was commonly used for therapy, it was frequently observed that prior treatment with iodine delayed the response to antithyroid drugs for many weeks. Thus, the rate of response is determined by the quantity of stored hormone, the rate of turnover of hormone in the thyroid, the half-life of the hormone in the periphery, and the completeness of the block in synthesis imposed by the dosage given. When large doses are continued, and sometimes with the usual dose, recovery is followed by the development of hypothyroidism. The earliest signs of hypothyroidism call for a reduction in dose; if by chance they have advanced to the point of discomfort, thyroid hormone can be given to hasten recovery. A full dose of 100 to 150 μg daily of thyroxine or an equivalent dose of triiodothyronine for a week will usually suffice. The lower maintenance dose of antithyroid drug discussed above is instituted for continued suppression.

In most cases, treatment with an antithyroid drug requires medical attention only at monthly or bimonthly intervals and adjustment of dosage can be made entirely upon the basis of symptoms and simple clinical signs. If confirmatory tests are desirable, those reflecting the concentration of circulating hormones are the most helpful.

Control of the hyperthyroidism is not associated with further enlargement of the goiter unless hypothyroidism is induced. When this happens, the new enlargement is quickly reversed by giving thyroid hormone. The presumption is, therefore, that TSH is secreted in excessive amounts in response to the hypothyroidism and can be suppressed by thyroid hormone.

Remissions. The antithyroid drugs have been used in many patients to control the hyperthyroidism of Graves' disease until a remission occurs. Early investigators reported that 50% of patients so treated for 1 year remained well without further therapy for long periods, perhaps indefinitely. More recent reports have indicated that a much smaller percentage of patients sustain remissions after such treatment.

Unfortunately, there is no way of predicting before treatment is begun which patients will eventually achieve a lasting remission and which will relapse. It is clear that a favorable outcome is unlikely when the disorder is of long standing, the thyroid is quite large, and various forms of treatment have failed. To complicate the issue further, it is thought that remission and eventual hypothyroidism may represent the natural history of Graves' disease.

During treatment, a fairly certain sign that a remission may have taken place is a reduction in the size of the goiter. The persistence of goiter usually indicates failure, unless the patient becomes hypothyroid. Another favorable indication is continued freedom from all signs of hyperthyroidism when the maintenance dose is small.

The Therapeutic Choice. Because of the low rates of permanent remission of Graves' disease that can be achieved with antithyroid drugs, the majority of patients will eventually require surgery or treatment with radioactive iodine; a 1-year trial of antithyroid agents is not advisable. It may be worthwhile to try prolonged therapy with antithyroid drugs in patients who have minimal enlargement of the thyroid or very mild hyperthyroidism.

Radioiodine or surgery is indicated for definitive therapy in toxic nodular goiter, since spontaneous remissions are not characteristic of this condition.

There is considerable disagreement about the therapy of thyrotoxicosis during pregnancy. The antithyroid drugs cross the placenta and can cause fetal hypothyroidism and goiter. Knowledge of thyroid hormone transport to the fetus is poor. There are three choices of therapy; most specialists favor minimal doses of antithyroid drugs. The alternatives are full doses of antithyroid drugs with thyroid hormone supplementation, or surgery. Radioiodine is clearly contraindicated. McLaren and Alexander (1979) and Momotani and colleagues (1986) have discussed the use of antithyroid drugs in pregnancy and during the neonatal period.

Preoperative Preparation. An important use of antithyroid drugs is in the preparation of the hyperthyroid patient for subtotal thyroidectomy. It is possible to bring virtually 100% of patients to a euthyroid state; as a consequence, the operative mortality for a single-stage thyroidectomy in expert hands is very low. The treatment is continued until the patient is judged to be normal or nearly so, and then some physicians add iodide to the regimen for the 7 to 10 days immediately before the operation. Iodide reduces the vascularity of the gland and makes it less friable, which lessen the difficulties for the surgeon (*see* below).

Propranolol. This β-adrenergic antagonist does not inhibit the function of the thyroid, but it is useful for the temporary suppression of the signs and symptoms of thyrotoxicosis. As mentioned above, some of the cardiovascular manifestations of hyperthyroidism may be reinforced by the cardiac effects of catecholamines. β-Adrenergic antagonists also reduce the heart rate, tremor, and stare in hyperthyroidism and relieve palpitation, anxiety, and tension. The control of these manifestations is unmistakable and rapid. It is thus valuable in controlling symptoms while awaiting the response to antithyroid drugs or radioiodine, and it is very useful in the rare but potentially lethal complication, thyroid storm. A usual oral dosage of propranolol is 20 to 80 mg every 6 hours, but the amount should be adjusted according to the response. The heart rate is a reliable indicator, but it may be impossible to eliminate the tachycardia. Excessive β-adrenergic blockade can be dangerous if the patient has a cardiomyopathy.

IONIC INHIBITORS

The term *ionic inhibitors* serves to designate the substances that interfere with the concentration of iodide by the thyroid gland. The effective agents are themselves anions that in some ways resemble iodide; they are all monovalent, hydrated anions of a size similar to that of iodide. The most studied example, *thiocyanate,* differs from the others qualitatively; it is not concentrated by the thyroid gland, and in large amounts it inhibits the organification of iodine. Thiocyanate is produced following the enzymatic hydrolysis of certain plant glycosides. Thus, the eating of some foods (*e.g.,* cabbage) and cigarette smoking result in an increased concentration of thiocyanate in the blood and urine, as does the administration of sodium nitroprusside. Dietary precursors of thiocyanate may be a contributing factor in endemic goiter in certain parts of the world where the intake of iodine is very low (Delange and Ermans, 1971).

Among other anions, *perchlorate* (ClO_4^-) is ten times as active as thiocyanate. Although perchlorate can be used to control hyperthyroidism, it may cause fatal aplastic anemia and has been abandoned except in very unusual circumstances. Perchlorate can be used to "discharge" inorganic iodide from the thyroid gland in a diagnostic test of organification. Other ions, selected on the basis of their size, have also been found to be active; fluoborate (BF_4^-) is as effective as perchlorate. Li^+ affects the thyroid and can cause goiter when used therapeutically (*see* Chapter 18).

IODIDE

Iodide is the oldest remedy for disorders of the thyroid gland. Before the antithyroid drugs were used, it was the only substance available for control of the signs and symptoms of hyperthyroidism. Its use in this way is indeed paradoxical, and the explanation for this paradox is still incomplete.

Response to Iodide in Hyperthyroidism. The response to iodide of the patient with hyperthyroidism is often striking and rapid. The effect is usually discernible within 24 hours, and the basal metabolic rate may fall at a rate comparable to that following thyroidectomy. This provides evidence that the release of hormone into the circulation is quickly interrupted. The maximal effect is attained after 10 to 15 days of continuous therapy, when the signs and symptoms of hyperthyroidism may have greatly improved.

The changes in the thyroid gland have been studied in detail; vascularity is reduced, the gland becomes much firmer and even hard to the touch, the cells become smaller, colloid reaccumulates in the follicles, and the quantity of bound iodine increases. The changes are those that would be expected if the excessive stimulus to the gland had somehow been removed or antagonized.

Unfortunately, iodide therapy usually does not completely control the manifestations of hyperthyroidism, and after a variable period of time the beneficial effect disappears. With continued treatment, the hyperthyroidism may return in its initial intensity or may become even more severe than it was at first. It is for this reason that, when iodide was the only agent available for the treatment of hyperthyroidism, its use was usually restricted to preparation of the patient for thyroidectomy.

Mechanism of Action. High concentrations of iodide appear to influence all important aspects of iodine metabolism by the thyroid gland (*see* Ingbar, 1972). The capacity of iodide to limit its own transport has been mentioned above. Acute inhibition of the synthesis of iodotyrosine and iodothyronine by iodide is also well known (the *Wolff–Chaikoff effect*) (Wolff and Chaikoff, 1948). This inhibition is observed only above critical concentrations of iodide, and the intracellular rather than the extracellular concentration of the anion appears to be the major determinant. With time there is "escape" from this inhibition that is associated with an adaptive decrease in iodide transport and a lowered intracellular iodide concentration. The mechanism of the Wolff–Chaikoff effect is not understood. DeGroot and Niepomniszcze (1977) have reviewed the numerous hypotheses that have been proposed as explanations.

The most important clinical effect of high iodide concentration is an inhibition of the release of thyroid hormone. This action is rapid and efficacious in severe thyrotoxicosis. The effect is exerted directly on the thyroid gland, and it can be demonstrated in the euthyroid subject and experimental animals as well as in the hyperthyroid patient.

Iodide antagonizes the ability of both TSH and cyclic AMP to stimulate endocytosis of colloid, proteolysis, and hormone secretion (Pisarev *et al.*, 1971). Several groups of investigators have also reported that iodide attenuates the effect of TSH on the accumulation of cyclic AMP *in vivo* and in isolated tissues (Sherwin and Tong, 1975; Van Sande *et al.*, 1975). Because of the likelihood that cyclic AMP mediates many of the effects of TSH (and presumably the effects of the TSH-imitative immunoglobulins as well), this may help to explain the action of iodide.

Preparations and Dosage. The dosage or form in which iodide is administered bears little relationship to the response achieved in hyperthyroidism, provided not less than the minimal effective amount is given; this dosage is 6 mg per day in most, but not all, patients. *Strong iodine solution* (Lugol's solution) is widely used and consists of 5% iodine and 10% potassium iodide. The iodine is reduced to iodide in the intestine before absorption. While a dosage of 500 mg of iodide per day is often used, 50 to 150 mg per day seems more reasonable.

Therapeutic Uses. The uses of iodide in the treatment of hyperthyroidism are in the immediate preoperative period in preparation for thyroidectomy and, in conjunction with antithyroid drugs and propranolol, in the treatment of thyrotoxic crisis. Prior to surgery, iodide is sometimes employed alone, but more frequently it is used after the hyperthyroidism has been controlled by an antithyroid drug. It is then given during the 10 days immediately preceding the operation. Optimal control of hyperthyroidism is achieved if antithyroid drugs are first given alone. If iodine is also given from the beginning, variable responses are observed; sometimes the effect of iodide predominates, storage of hormone is promoted, and prolonged antithyroid treatment is required before the hyperthyroidism is controlled. These clinical observations may be explained by the ability of iodide to prevent the inactivation of thyroid peroxidase by antithyroid drugs (Davidson *et al.*, 1978).

Iodide salts are also useful expectorants when it is desired to liquefy tenacious bronchial secretions, for example, in the later stages of bronchitis, bronchiectasis, and asthma. Potassium iodide is commonly used in a dosage of 0.3 g in aqueous solution every 6 hours. Gastrointestinal irritation, anorexia, and vomiting are frequent side effects. The drug should not be administered longer than is actually necessary to "loosen" the cough. However, in some patients with chronic bronchitis or asthma, iodide may be prescribed more or less continuously if it appears to afford relief.

Iodide sometimes aids in the resolution of the granulomatous lesions of tuberculosis, leprosy, syphilis, and various fungal diseases. This does not depend on the effect of iodide on the responsible microorganism. With the advent of more efficacious drugs for the treatment of these diseases, iodide is rarely employed, except in the treatment of sporotrichosis (Utz and Shadomy, 1987). Another use of iodide is to protect the thyroid after accidental exposure to radioactive isotopes of the element, such as nuclear reactor accidents in which much of the contamination is from ^{131}I.

Untoward Reactions. Occasional individuals show marked sensitivity to iodide or to organic preparations that contain iodine when they are administered intravenously. The onset of an acute reaction may occur immediately or several hours after administration. Angioedema is the outstanding symptom, and swelling of the larynx may lead to suffocation. Multiple cutaneous hemorrhages may be present. Also, manifestations of the serum-sickness type of hypersensitivity, such as fever, arthralgia, lymph node enlargement, and eosinophilia, may appear. Thrombotic thrombocytopenic purpura and fatal periarteritis nodosa attributed to hypersensitivity to iodide have also been described.

The severity of symptoms of chronic intoxication with iodide (*iodism*) is related to the dose. The symptoms start with an unpleasant brassy taste and burning in the mouth and throat, as well as soreness of the teeth and gums. Increased salivation is noted. Coryza, sneezing, and irritation of the eyes with swelling of the eyelids are commonly observed. Mild iodism simulates a "head cold." The patient often complains of a severe headache that originates in the frontal sinuses. Irritation of the mucous glands of the respiratory tract causes a productive cough. Excess transudation into the bronchial tree may lead to pulmonary edema. In addition, the parotid and submaxillary glands may become enlarged and tender, and the syndrome may be mistaken for mumps parotitis. There also may be inflammation of the pharynx, larynx, and tonsils. Skin lesions are common, and vary in type and intensity. They usually are mildly acneform and distributed in the seborrheic areas. Rarely, severe and sometimes fatal eruptions (ioderma) may occur after the prolonged use of iodides. The lesions are bizarre, resemble those caused by bromide, and, as a rule, involute quickly when iodide is withdrawn. Symptoms of gastric irritation are common; and diarrhea, which is sometimes bloody, may occur. Fever is occasionally observed, and anorexia and depression may be present. The mechanisms involved in the production of these derangements remain unknown.

Fortunately, the symptoms of iodism disappear spontaneously within a few days after stopping the administration of iodide. The renal excretion of I^- can be increased by procedures that promote Cl^- excretion (*e.g.*, osmotic diuresis, chloruretic diuretics, and salt loading). These procedures may be useful when the symptoms of iodism are severe.

Iodide-Induced Goiter and Myxedema. In a small proportion of individuals given large doses of iodide for long periods, as in the treatment of asthma or chronic bronchitis, goiter and hypothyroidism supervene. The thyroid gland shows hyperplasia and is depleted of stores of iodine. Thyroid hormone corrects the hypothyroidism and causes the goiter to subside; the same result follows the withdrawal of the iodide.

RADIOACTIVE IODINE

Chemical and Physical Properties. While iodine has several radioactive isotopes, greatest use has been made of ^{131}I. It has a half-life of 8 days, and, therefore, over 99% of its radiant energy is expended within 56 days. Its radioactive emissions include both x-rays and β particles. The short-lived radionuclide of iodine, ^{123}I, emits x-rays with a half-life of only 13 hours. This permits relatively brief exposure to radiation during thyroid scans.

Effects on the Thyroid Gland. The chemical behavior of the radioactive isotopes of iodine is identical to that of the stable isotope, ^{127}I. ^{131}I is rapidly and efficiently trapped by the thyroid, incorporated into the iodoamino acids, and deposited in the colloid of the follicles, from which it is slowly liberated. Thus, the destructive beta rays originate within the follicle and act almost exclusively upon the parenchymal cells of the thyroid with little or no damage to surrounding tissue. The x-rays pass through the tissue and can be quantified by external detection. The effects of the radiation depend upon the dosage. When small tracer doses of ^{131}I are administered, thyroid function is not disturbed. However, when large amounts of radioactive iodine gain access to the gland, the characteristic cytotoxic actions of ionizing radiation are observed. Pyknosis and necrosis of the follicular cells are followed by disappearance of colloid and fibrosis of the gland. With properly selected doses of ^{131}I, it is possible to destroy the thyroid gland completely without detectable injury to adjacent tissues. After smaller doses, some of the follicles, usually in the periphery of the gland, retain their function.

Preparations. *Sodium iodide I 131* (IODOTOPE THERAPEUTIC) is available as a solution or in capsules containing ^{131}I suitable for oral administration. Sodium iodide I 131 is essentially carrier free. The information on the label includes the activity at a given hour and date. *Sodium iodide I 123* is available for scanning procedures.

Therapeutic Uses. Radioactive iodine finds its widest use in the treatment of hyperthyroidism and in the diagnosis of disorders of thyroid function. Discussion will be limited to the uses of ^{131}I.

Hyperthyroidism. Radioactive iodine is highly useful in the treatment of hyperthyroidism, and in many circumstances it is regarded as the therapeutic procedure of choice for this condition.

Dosage and Technique. ^{131}I is administered orally; the amount given is so small that it cannot be detected by taste or odor. The effective dose of ^{131}I differs for individual patients. It depends primarily upon the size of the thyroid, the iodine uptake of the gland, and the rate of release of radioactive iodine from the gland subsequent to its deposition in the colloid. To determine these variables insofar as possible, many investigators administer a tracer dose of ^{131}I and calculate the iodine accumulated by the gland and the rate of loss therefrom. The weight of the gland is estimated by palpation. From these data, the dose of isotope necessary to provide from 7000 to 10,000 rads per gram of thyroid tissue is determined. Even when dosage is controlled in this manner, it is difficult to predict the response of an individual to a given amount of the isotope. For these reasons, the optimal dose of ^{131}I, expressed in terms of microcuries taken up per gram of thyroid tissue, varies in different laboratories from 80 to 150 μCi. The usual total dose is 4 to 10 mCi. Lower-dosage ^{131}I therapy (80 μCi/g thyroid) has been advocated to reduce the incidence of subsequent hypothyroidism (Cevallos *et al.*, 1974). While the incidence of hypothyroidism in the early years after such therapy is lower, many patients with late hypothyroidism may go undetected, and the ultimate incidence of hypothyroidism is probably no less than with the larger doses (Glennon *et al.*, 1972).

Course of Disease. The course of Graves' disease in a patient who has received an optimal dose of ^{131}I is characterized by progressive recovery. It is very unusual for any tenderness to be noted in the thyroid region, and most observers have failed to detect any exacerbation of hyperthyroidism from loss of hormone from the damaged gland. Beginning a few weeks after treatment, the symptoms of hyperthyroidism gradually abate over a period of 2 to 3 months. If therapy has been inadequate, the necessity for further treatment is apparent within 3 months.

Depending to some extent upon the dosage schedule adopted, one half to two thirds of patients are cured by a single dose, one third to one fifth require two doses, and the remainder require three or more doses before the disorder is controlled. Although it is usual to allow only about 3 months to elapse before concluding that an incomplete response calls for another dose, late effects of the radiation make it desirable to wait much longer. But, again, this further delays the recovery.

Propranolol or antithyroid drugs or both can be used to hasten the control of hyperthyroidism while awaiting the full effects of the radioiodine. However, the antithyroid drugs should be withheld for a few days or a week before and after the therapeutic dose of ^{131}I.

Advantages. The advantages of radioactive iodine in the treatment of Graves' disease are many. No death as a direct result of the use of the isotope has been reported, and only by a gross miscalculation of dose could such an event conceivably occur. In the nonpregnant patient, no tissue other than the thyroid is exposed to sufficient ionizing radiation to be detectably altered. (Nevertheless, the continuing concern about potential effects of radiation on germ cells prompts many specialists to advocate antithyroid drugs or surgery in younger patients who are acceptable operative risks; *see* Dunn, 1984.) The patient is spared the risks and discomfort of surgery. The incidence of progressive exophthalmos appears to be no different than after surgical treatment. Finally, the cost is low, hospitalization usually is not required, and patients can indulge in their customary activities during the entire procedure.

Disadvantages. The chief disadvantage of the use of radioactive iodine is the high incidence of delayed hypothyroidism that is induced. Even when elaborate procedures are used to estimate iodine uptake and gland size, a certain percentage of patients will be overtreated. A distressing feature of this complication is its rising prevalence with the passage of time; the longer the interval after treatment, the higher the incidence. Several analyses of groups of patients treated 10 or more years previously suggest that the eventual rate may exceed 50%. However, it now appears that the incidence of hypothyroidism also increases progressively after subtotal thyroidectomy, and such failure of glandular function is probably part of the natural progression of Graves' disease, no matter what the therapy.

Although it is often said that hypothyroidism is not a serious complication because it can so easily be treated with thyroid hormone, its onset may be quite insidious and overlooked for some time. Also, once diagnosed it is difficult to ensure that patients who need the hormone actually take it. Hypothyroidism is obviously a serious complication deserving of painstaking care to make certain that optimal replacement therapy is provided.

Another disadvantage of radioiodine therapy is the long period of time that is sometimes required before the hyperthyroidism is controlled. When a single dose is effective, the response is most satisfactory; however, when multiple doses are needed, it may be many months or a year or more before the patient is well. This disadvantage can largely be overcome if the initial dose is sufficiently large.

Indications. The clearest indication for this form of treatment is hyperthyroidism in older patients and in those with heart disease. Radioiodine is also the best form of treatment when hyperthyroidism has persisted or recurred after subtotal thyroidectomy and when prolonged treatment with antithyroid drugs has not led to remission.

Contraindications. The risk of causing neoplastic changes in the gland has been constantly under consideration since radioiodine was first introduced, and only small numbers of children have been treated in this way. Indeed, many clinics have declined to treat younger patients for fear of causing cancer and have reserved radioiodine for patients over some arbitrary age, such as 25 or 30 years. Since experience with ^{131}I is now vast, these age limits are lower than they were in the past. There is no evidence that radioiodine therapy for Graves' disease has caused thyroid or any other form of cancer in adults, although the very large doses that are used to treat cancer (*see* below) may be associated with an increased incidence of leukemia. The use of radioiodine during pregnancy is contraindicated; after the first trimester the fetal thyroid would concentrate the isotope and thus suffer damage, but even during the first trimester radioiodine is best avoided because there may be adverse effects of radiation on fetal tissues.

Hyperthyroidism with Nodular Goiter. It is thought that the risk of inducing hypothyroidism is less in nodular goiter than in Graves' disease, perhaps because of the natural progression of the latter.

Metastatic Thyroid Cancer. Most thyroid carcinomas accumulate very little iodine. However, follicular carcinomas, which comprise 25% of thyroid malignancies, often do so, although they rarely synthesize sufficient hormone to cause thyrotoxicosis. Therapy with large doses of ^{131}I can shrink functional metastases (Leeper, 1973). In an attempt to stimulate uptake, TSH has been given or secretion of endogenous TSH has been evoked by inducing hypothyroidism by removal or radiation of the thyroid, or by prolonged treatment with antithyroid drugs. The increased uptake thus achieved is usually not large and may be negligible. Moreover, a number of observers have noted that these maneuvers may stimulate growth of the metastases, and have therefore questioned their advisability.

Papillary carcinoma is the most common type of thyroid cancer and may be partially dependent on TSH. Metastatic lesions occasionally regress when the secretion of TSH is suppressed by administration of thyroid hormone.

Diagnostic Uses. Tracer studies with radioiodine have found wide application in studies of disorders of the thyroid gland. Measurement of the thyroidal accumulation of a tracer dose is helpful in the diagnosis of hyperthyroidism, hypothyroidism, and goiter, and the response of the thyroid to TSH or to suppression by thyroid hormone can be evaluated in this way. Following the administration of a tracer dose, the pattern of localization in the thyroid gland can be depicted by a special scanning apparatus, and this technique is sometimes useful in defining thyroid nodules as functional ("hot") or nonfunctional ("cold") and in finding ectopic thyroid tissue and occasionally metastatic thyroid tumors.

Astwood, E. B. Chemotherapy of hyperthyroidism. *Harvey Lect.*, **1945**, *40*, 195–235.

Cairoli, V. J., and Crout, J. R. Role of the autonomic nervous system in the resting tachycardia of experimental hyperthyroidism. *J. Pharmacol. Exp. Ther.*, **1967**, *158*, 55–65.

Cevallos, J. L.; Hagen, G. A.; Maloof, F.; and Chapman, E. M. Low-dosage ^{131}I therapy of thyrotoxicosis (dif-

fuse goiters). A five-year follow-up study. *N. Engl. J. Med.*, **1974**, *290*, 141–143.
Cody, V., and Duax, W. L. Distal conformation of the thyroid hormone 3,5,3′-triiodo-L-thyronine. *Science*, **1973**, *181*, 757–758.
Corda, D.; Marcocci, C.; Kohn, L. D.; Axelrod, J.; and Luini, A. Association of the changes in cytosolic Ca^{++} and iodide efflux induced by thyrotropin and by stimulation of alpha adrenergic receptors in cultured rat thyroid cells. *J. Biol. Chem.*, **1985**, *260*, 9230–9236.
Cushing, H. *The Pituitary Body and Its Disorders*. J. B. Lippincott Co., Philadelphia, **1912.**
Damm, K.; Thompson, C. C.; and Evans, R. M. Protein encoded by v-*erb*A functions as a thyroid-hormone receptor antagonist. *Nature*, **1989**, *339*, 593–597.
Davidson, B.; Soodak, M.; Neary, J. T.; Strout, H. V.; Kieffer, J. D.; Mover, H.; and Maloof, F. The irreversible inactivation of thyroid peroxidase by methylmercaptoimidazole, thiouracil, and propylthiouracil *in vitro* and its relationship to *in vivo* findings. *Endocrinology*, **1978**, *103*, 871–882.
Delange, F., and Ermans, A. M. Role of a dietary goitrogen in the etiology of endemic goiter on Idjwi Island. *Am. J. Clin. Nutr.*, **1971**, *24*, 1354–1360.
Dunn, A. D., and Dunn, J. T. Cysteine proteinases from human thyroids and their actions on thyroglobulin. *Endocrinology*, **1988**, *123*, 1089–1097.
Dunn, J. T. Choice of therapy in young adults with hyperthyroidism of Graves' disease: a brief, case-directed poll of 54 thyroidologists. *Ann. Intern. Med.*, **1984**, *100*, 891–893.
Dunn, J. T.; Anderson, P. C.; Fox, J. W.; Fassler, C. A.; Dunn, A. D.; Hite, L. A.; and Moore, R. C. The sites of thyroid hormone formation in rabbit thyroglobulin. *J. Biol. Chem.*, **1987**, *262*, 16948–16952.
Eiden, L. E., and Ruth, J. A. Acute thyroid hormone increases noradrenergic responsiveness of rat atria *in vitro*. *Eur. J. Pharmacol.*, **1981**, *74*, 91–93.
Engler, H.; Taurog, A.; and Nakashima, T. Mechanism of inactivation of thyroid peroxidase by thioureylene drugs. *Biochem. Pharmacol.*, **1982**, *31*, 3801–3806.
Everett, A. W.; Umeda, P. K.; Sinha, A. M.; Rabinowitz, M.; and Zak, R. Expression of myosin heavy chains during thyroid hormone-induced cardiac growth. *Fed. Proc.*, **1986**, *45*, 2568–2572.
Field, J. B.; Ealey, P. A.; Marshall, N. J.; and Cockcroft, S. Thyroid-stimulating hormone stimulates increases in inositol phosphates as well as cyclic AMP in the FRTL-5 rat thyroid cell line. *Biochem. J.*, **1987**, *247*, 519–524.
Fisher, D. A. Screening for congenital hypothyroidism. *Hosp. Pract.*, **1977**, *12*, 73–78.
Flink, I. L., and Morkin, E. Evidence for a new cardiac myosin species in thyrotoxic rabbit. *FEBS Lett.*, **1977**, *81*, 391–394.
Galton, V. A. Thyroxine and 3,5,3′-triiodothyronine bind to the same putative receptor in hepatic nuclei of *Rana catesbeiana* tadpoles. *Endocrinology*, **1986**, *118*, 114–118.
Glennon, J. A.; Gordon, E. S.; and Sawin, C. T. Hypothyroidism after low-dose ^{131}I treatment of hyperthyroidism. *Ann. Intern. Med.*, **1972**, *76*, 721–723.
Gley, E. Sur les effets de l'extirpation du corps thyroide. *C. R. Soc. Biol. (Paris)*, **1891**, *43*, 551–554.
Greer, M. A.; Grimm, Y.; and Studer, H. Qualitative changes in the secretion of thyroid hormones induced by iodine deficiency. *Endocrinology*, **1968**, *83*, 1193–1198.
Griffin, J. E. The dilemma of abnormal thyroid function tests—is thyroid disease present or not? *Am. J. Med. Sci.*, **1985**, *289*, 76–88.
Gross, G.; Sykes, M.; Arellano, R.; Fong, B.; and Angel, A. HDL clearance and receptor-mediated catabolism of LDL are reduced in hypothyroid rats. *Atherosclerosis*, **1987**, *66*, 269–275.
Gross, J., and Pitt-Rivers, R. The identification of 3:5:3′-L-triiodothyronine in human plasma. *Lancet*, **1952**, *1*, 439–441.
———. 3:5:3′-Triiodothyronine. 1. Isolation from thyroid gland and synthesis. *Biochem. J.*, **1953a**, *53*, 645–652. 2. Physiological activity. *Ibid.*, **1953b**, *53*, 652–657.
Harington, C. R. Biochemical basis of thyroid function. *Lancet*, **1935**, *1*, 1199–1204, 1261–1266.
Harington, C. R., and Barger, G. Thyroxine. III. Constitution and synthesis of thyroxine. *Biochem. J.*, **1927**, *21*, 169–183.
Hinkle, P. M., and Goh, K. B. C. Regulation of thyrotropin-releasing hormone receptors and responses by L-triiodothyronine in dispersed rat pituitary cell cultures. *Endocrinology*, **1982**, *110*, 1725–1731.
Hodin, R. A.; Lazar, M. A.; Wintman, B. I.; Darling, D. S.; Koenig, R. J.; Larsen, P. R.; Moore, D. D.; and Chin, W. W. Identification of a thyroid hormone receptor that is pituitary-specific. *Science*, **1989**, *244*, 76–79.
Hoh, J. F. Y.; McGrath, P. A.; and Hale, P. T. Electrophoretic analysis of multiple forms of rat cardiac myosin: effects of hypophysectomy and thyroid replacement. *J. Mol. Cell. Cardiol.*, **1978**, *10*, 1053–1076.
Ingbar, S. H. Autoregulation of the thyroid response to iodide excess and depletion. *Mayo Clin. Proc.*, **1972**, *47*, 814–823.
Jorgensen, E. C. Stereochemistry of thyroxine and analogues. *Mayo Clin. Proc.*, **1964**, *39*, 560–568.
Kendall, E. C. The isolation in crystalline form of the compound containing iodine which occurs in the thyroid: its chemical nature and physiological activity. *Trans. Assoc. Am. Physicians*, **1915**, *30*, 420–449.
Laurent, E.; Mockel, J.; Van Sande, J.; Graff, I.; and Dumont, J. E. Dual activation by thyrotropin of the phospholipase C and cyclic AMP cascades in human thyroid. *Mol. Cell. Endocrinol.*, **1987**, *52*, 273–278.
Leeper, R. D. The effect of ^{131}I therapy on survival of patients with metastatic papillary or follicular thyroid carcinoma. *J. Clin. Endocrinol. Metab.*, **1973**, *36*, 1143–1152.
Leonard, J. L., and Rosenberg, I. N. Thyroxine 5′-deiodinase activity of rat kidney: observations on activation by thiols and inhibition by propylthiouracil. *Endocrinology*, **1978**, *103*, 2137–2144.
London, W. T.; Vought, R. L.; and Brown, F. A. Bread—a dietary source of large quantities of iodine. *N. Engl. J. Med.*, **1965**, *273*, 381.
Magnus-Levy, A. Über den respiratorischen Gaswechsel unter den Einfluss der Thyroidea sowie unter verschiedenden pathologischen Zustanden. *Berl. Klin. Wochenschr.*, **1895**, *32*, 650–652.
Magnusson, R. P.; Gestautas, J.; Taurog, A.; and Rappaport, B. Molecular cloning of the structural gene for porcine thyroid peroxidase. *J. Biol. Chem.*, **1987**, *262*, 13885–13888.
Magnusson, R. P.; Taurog, A.; and Dorris, M. L. Mechanisms of thyroid peroxidase- and lactoperoxidase-catalyzed reactions involving iodide. *J. Biol. Chem.*, **1984**, *259*, 13783–13790.
Manley, S. W.; Rose, D. S.; Huxham, G. J.; and Bourke, J. R. Role of calcium in the secretomotor response of the thyroid: effects of calcium ionophore A23187 on radioiodine turnover, membrane potential and fluid transport in cultured porcine thyroid cells. *J. Endocrinol.*, **1988**, *116*, 373–380.
Marine, D., and Kimball, O. P. The prevention of simple goiter in man: a survey of the incidence and types of thyroid enlargements in the schoolgirls of Akron, Ohio, from the 5th to the 12th grades, inclusive; the plan of prevention proposed. *J. Lab. Clin. Med.*, **1917**, *3*, 40–48.
Momotani, N.; Noh, J.; Oyanagi, H.; Ishikawa, N.; and Ito, K. Antithyroid drug therapy for Graves' disease during pregnancy. *N. Engl. J. Med.*, **1986**, *315*, 24–28.
Murray, G. R. Note on the treatment of myxedema by

hypodermic injection of an extract of the thyroid gland of a sheep. *Br. Med. J.*, **1891**, *2*, 796–797.
Nunez, J., and Correze, C. Interdependent effects of thyroid hormones and cAMP on lipolysis and lipogenesis in the fat cell. *Adv. Cyclic Nucleotide Res.*, **1981**, *14*, 539–554.
Ord, W. M. On myxoedema, a term proposed to be applied to an essential condition in the "cretinoid" affection occasionally observed in middle-aged women. *Med. Chir. Trans. (Lond.)*, **1878**, *61*, 57–78.
Parry, C. H. *Collections from the Unpublished Medical Writings of Dr. C. H. Parry*. Underwood, London, **1895.**
Pisarev, M. A.; DeGroot, L. J.; and Hati, R. KI and imidazole inhibition of TSH and c-AMP induced thyroidal iodine secretion. *Endocrinology*, **1971**, *88*, 1217–1221.
Raasmaja, A., and Larsen, P. R. Alpha$_1$- and β-adrenergic agents cause synergistic stimulation of the iodothyronine deiodinase in rat brown adipocytes. *Endocrinology*, **1989**, *125*, 2502–2509.
Roche, J.; Lissitzky, S.; and Michel, R. Sur la triiodothyronine, produit intermédiare de la transformation de la diiodothyronine en thyroxine. *C. R. Acad. Sci. [D] (Paris)*, **1952a**, *234*, 997–998.
———. Sur la présence de triiodothyronine dans la thyroglobuline. *Ibid.*, **1952b**, *234*, 1228–1230.
Rock, R. C. Interpreting thyroid tests in the elderly: updated guidelines. *Geriatrics*, **1985**, *40*, 61–68.
Ros, M.; Northup, J. K.; and Malbon, C. C. Steady-state levels of G-proteins and β-adrenergic receptors in rat fat cells. Permissive effects of thyroid hormones. *J. Biol. Chem.*, **1988**, *263*, 4362–4368.
Ross, D. S. Subclinical hypothyroidism: possible danger of overzealous thyroxine replacement therapy. *Mayo Clin. Proc.*, **1988**, *63*, 1223–1229.
Rotella, C. M.; Zonefrati, R.; Toccafondi, R.; Valente, W. A.; and Kohn, L. D. Ability of monoclonal antibodies to the thyrotropin receptor to increase collagen synthesis in human fibroblasts: an assay which appears to measure exophthalmogenic immunoglobulins in Graves' sera. *J. Clin. Endocrinol. Metab.*, **1986**, *62*, 357–367.
Salter, A. M.; Fisher, S. C.; and Brindley, D. N. Interactions of triiodothyronine, insulin, and dexamethasone on the binding of human LDL to rat hepatocytes in monolayer culture. *Atherosclerosis*, **1988**, *71*, 77–80.
Scarabottolo, L.; Trezzi, E.; Roma, P.; and Catapano, A. L. Experimental hypothyroidism modulates the expression of low density lipoprotein receptor by the liver. *Atherosclerosis*, **1986**, *59*, 329–333.
Schou, M.; Amdisen, A.; Jensen, S. E.; and Olsen, T. Occurrence of goitre during lithium treatment. *Br. Med. J.*, **1968**, *3*, 710–713.
Sestoft, L. Metabolic aspects of the calorigenic effect of thyroid hormones in mammals. *Clin. Endocrinol. (Oxf.)*, **1980**, *13*, 489–506.
Shanker, G.; Campagnoni, A. T.; and Pieringer, R. A. Investigations on myelinogenesis *in vitro*: developmental expression of myelin basic protein mRNA and its regulation by thyroid hormone in primary cerebral cell cultures from embryonic mice. *J. Neurosci. Res.*, **1987**, *17*, 220–224.
Sherwin, J. R., and Tong, W. Thyroidal autoregulation. Iodide-induced suppression of thyrotropin-stimulated cyclic AMP production and iodinating activity in thyroid cells. *Biochim. Biophys. Acta*, **1975**, *404*, 30–39.
Silva, J. E.; Mellen, S.; and Larsen, P. R. Comparison of kidney and brown adipose tissue iodothyronine 5′-deiodinases. *Endocrinology*, **1987**, *121*, 650–656.
Simmonds, M. Ueber Hypophysisschwund mit todlichem Ausang. *Dtsch. Med. Wochenschr.*, **1914**, *40*, 322–323.
Takasu, N.; Yamada, T.; and Shimizu, Y. Generation of H_2O_2 is regulated by cytoplasmic free calcium in cultured porcine thyroid cells. *Biochem. Biophys. Res. Commun.*, **1987**, *148*, 1527–1532.
Taurog, A. The mechanism of action of thioureylene antithyroid drugs. *Endocrinology*, **1976**, *98*, 1031–1046.
Taurog, A.; Lothrop, M. L.; and Estabrook, R. W. Improvements in the isolation procedure for thyroid peroxidase: nature of the heme prosthetic group. *Arch. Biochem. Biophys.*, **1970**, *139*, 221–229.
Temple, R.; Berman, M.; Carlson, H. E.; Robbins, J.; and Wolff, J. The use of lithium in Graves' disease. *Mayo Clin. Proc.*, **1972**, *47*, 872–878.
Thilly, C. H.; Delange, F.; Goldstein-Golaire, J.; and Ermans, A. M. Endemic goiter prevention of iodized oil: a reassessment. *J. Clin. Endocrinol. Metab.*, **1973**, *36*, 1196–1204.
Thompson, C. C.; Weinberger, C.; Lebo, R.; and Evans, R. M. Identification of a novel thyroid hormone receptor expressed in the mammalian central nervous system. *Science*, **1987**, *237*, 1610–1614.
Underwood, A. H.; Emmett, J. C.; Ellis, D.; Flynn, S. B.; Leeson, P. D.; Benson, G. M.; Novelli, R.; Pearce, N. J.; and Shah, V. P. A thyromimetic that decreases plasma cholesterol levels without increasing cardiac activity. *Nature*, **1986**, *324*, 425–429.
Utz, J. P., and Shadomy, H. J. Sporotrichosis. In, *Dermatology in General Medicine*, 3rd ed. (Fitzpatrick, T. B.; Eisen, A. Z.; Wolff, K.; Freedberg, I. M.; and Austen, K. F.; eds.) McGraw-Hill Book Co., New York, **1987**, pp. 2271–2272.
Van Sande, J.; Grenier, G.; Willems, C.; and Dumont, J. E. Inhibition by iodide of the activation of the thyroid cyclic 3′,5′-AMP system. *Endocrinology*, **1975**, *96*, 781–786.
Volpe, R. Immunoregulation in autoimmune thyroid disease. *N. Engl. J. Med.*, **1987**, *316*, 44–45.
Wolff, J., and Chaikoff, I. L. Plasma inorganic iodide as a homeostatic regulator of thyroid function. *J. Biol. Chem.*, **1948**, *174*, 555–564.

Monographs and Reviews

Ahren, B. Hyperthyroidism and glucose intolerance. *Acta Med. Scand.*, **1986**, *220*, 5–14.
Bottazzo, G. F., and Doniach, D. Autoimmune thyroid disease. *Annu. Rev. Med.*, **1986**, *37*, 353–359.
Braverman, L. E., and Vagenakis, A. G. The thyroid. *Clin. Endocrinol. Metab.*, **1979**, *8*, 621–639.
Burman, K. D., and Baker, J. R., Jr. Immune mechanisms in Graves' disease. *Endocr. Rev.*, **1985**, *6*, 183–232.
Cooper, D. S. Antithyroid drugs. *N. Engl. J. Med.*, **1984**, *311*, 1353–1362.
DeGroot, L. J., and Niepomniszcze, H. Biosynthesis of thyroid hormone: basic and clinical aspects. *Metabolism*, **1977**, *26*, 665–718.
Dussault, J. H., and Ruel, J. Thyroid hormones and brain development. *Annu. Rev. Physiol.*, **1987**, *49*, 321–334.
Editorial. Amiodarone and the thyroid: the Janus response. *Lancet*, **1987**, *2*, 24–25.
Evans, R. M. The steroid and thyroid hormone receptor superfamily. *Science*, **1988**, *240*, 889–895.
Gammage, M. D., and Franklyn, J. A. Amiodarone and the thyroid. *Q. J. Med.*, **1987**, *238*, 83–86.
Hamburgh, M. The role of thyroid and growth hormones in neurogenesis. *Curr. Top. Dev. Biol.*, **1969**, *4*, 109–148.
McLaren, E. H., and Alexander, W. D. Goitrogens. *Clin. Endocrinol. Metab.*, **1979**, *8*, 129–144.
Morkin, E.; Flink, I. L.; and Goldman, S. Biochemical and physiological effects of thyroid hormones on cardiac performance. *Prog. Cardiovasc. Dis.*, **1983**, *25*, 435–464.
Muller, M. J., and Seitz, H. J. Thyroid hormone action

on intermediary metabolism. *Klin. Wochenschr.*, **1984,** *62,* 11–18.
Oppenheimer, J. H.; Schwartz, H. L.; Mariash, C. N.; Kinlaw, W. B.; Wong, N. C. W.; and Freake, H. C. Advances in our understanding of the thyroid hormone action at the cellular level. *Endocr. Rev.*, **1987,** *8,* 288–308.
Samuels, H. H.; Forman, B. M.; Horowitz, Z. D.; and Ye, Z.-S. Regulation of gene expression by thyroid hormone. *J. Clin. Invest.*, **1988,** *81,* 957–967.
Schimmel, M., and Utiger, R. D. Thyroidal and peripheral production of thyroid hormones. *Ann. Intern. Med.*, **1977,** *87,* 760–768.
Taurog, A. Thyroid peroxidase and thyroxine biosynthesis. *Recent Prog. Horm. Res.*, **1970,** *26,* 189–241.
Utiger, R. D. Serum triiodothyronine in man. *Annu. Rev. Med.*, **1974,** *25,* 289–302.
———. Decreased extrathyroidal triiodothyronine production in nonthyroidal illness: benefit or harm? *Am. J. Med.*, **1980,** *69,* 807–810.
VanEtten, C. H. Goitrogens. In, *Toxic Constituents of Plant Foodstuffs.* (Liener, I. E., ed.) Academic Press, Inc., New York, **1969,** pp. 103–142.

CHAPTER

58 ESTROGENS AND PROGESTINS

Ferid Murad and Jeffrey A. Kuret

The controlled and cyclic formation of estrogens and progesterone is unique to the ovary. These hormones play a vital role in preparing the female reproductive tract for the reception of sperm and implantation of a fertilized ovum. Many features of the female habitus are also influenced by these agents. Current knowledge of the synthesis and action of the ovarian hormones has permitted rational therapeutic intervention in certain diseases. Much more clinical use, however, has been made of agents that can mimic or antagonize the effects of these hormones and that are used as contraceptives or for treatment of certain neoplasms.

History. It has long been known that removal of the ovaries results in uterine atrophy and a loss of sexual functions. The hormonal nature of the ovarian control of the female reproductive system was established in 1900 by Knauer when he found that ovarian transplants prevented the symptoms of gonadectomy. This observation was extended by Halban (1900), who showed that if the glands were transplanted, even in immature animals, normal sexual development and function were assured. In 1923, Allen and Doisy devised a simple bioassay for ovarian extracts based upon changes produced in the vaginal smear of the rat. Loewe (1925) first reported a female sex hormone in the blood of various species and, shortly thereafter, Frank and associates (1925) detected an active sex principle in the blood of sows in estrus. Of even greater significance was the discovery by Loewe and Lange (1926) of a female sex hormone in the urine of menstruating women and the observation that the concentration of the hormone in the urine varied with the phase of the menstrual cycle. The excretion of large amounts of estrogen in the urine during pregnancy was also reported (Zondek, 1928). This finding was a boon to the chemists, who soon isolated an active substance in crystalline form (Butenandt, 1929; Doisy *et al.*, 1929, 1930). A few years later its chemical structure was elucidated.

The results of early investigations indicated that the ovary secretes two substances. Beard (1897) had postulated that the corpus luteum serves a necessary function during pregnancy, and supporting evidence was offered by Fraenkel (1903), who showed that destruction of the corpora lutea in pregnant rabbits causes abortion. The contributions of Corner and Allen (1929) firmly established the hormonal function of the corpus luteum. These investigators showed that the abortion following extirpation of the corpora lutea in pregnant rabbits can be prevented by the injection of luteal extracts.

ESTROGENS

Chemistry. Estrogenic activity is shared by many steroidal and nonsteroidal compounds, some of which are shown in Table 58–1 and Figure 58–1. The most potent naturally occurring estrogens in humans are 17β-estradiol, followed by estrone and estriol. Each of these molecules is an 18-carbon steroid, containing a phenolic A ring (an aromatic ring with a hydroxyl group at carbon 3) and a β-hydroxyl group or ketone in position 17 of ring D. The phenolic A ring is the principal structural feature responsible for selective, high-affinity binding to estrogen receptors (Jordan *et al.*, 1985; Duax *et al.*, 1988). Most alkyl substitutions on the phenolic A ring impair such binding, but substitutions on ring C or D may be tolerated.

Certain chemical alterations of the natural estrogens render them effective by mouth, largely through protection from inactivation by the liver. One of the most highly potent estrogens known, ethinyl estradiol, is an example of this type wherein the elements of acetylene are attached at C 17. This estrogen and some of its derivatives are widely used and are also incorporated with progesterone-like compounds for regulation of the menstrual cycle and for the control of fertility.

Nonsteroidal compounds with estrogenic activity occur naturally in a variety of plants, including flavone, isoflavone, and coumestan derivatives (phytoestrogens). Many of these polycyclic compounds contain a phenolic ring that mimics the A ring of steroids. One of the first nonsteroidal estrogens to be synthesized (and still the most potent) was diethylstilbestrol (*see* Table 58–1). When viewed in its *trans* conformation, the structural similarity between diethylstilbestrol and estradiol is apparent. Although the estrogenic potency of diethylstilbestrol is dependent on species, it is as potent as estradiol in most bioassays. In contrast to the natural estrogens, it is highly active when given by mouth, and its duration of action after a single dose is longer; these properties are consistent with its slower rate of degradation in the body. The introduction of a cheap, plentiful, orally active estrogen at a time when the natural products were scarce was a milestone in the development of effective endocrine therapy.

Biosynthesis. Steroidal estrogens are formed ultimately from either androstenedione or testoster-

Table 58–1. STRUCTURAL FORMULAS OF SELECTED ESTROGENS

STEROIDAL ESTROGENS

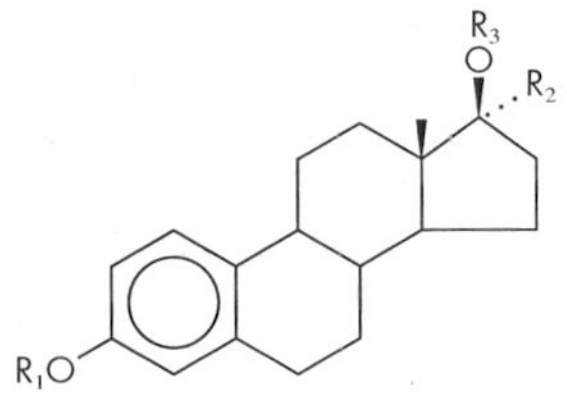

Derivative	R_1	R_2	R_3
Estradiol	—H	—H	—H
Estradiol valerate	—H	—H	$—\overset{O}{\overset{\Vert}{C}}(CH_2)_3CH_3$
Estradiol cypionate	—H	—H	$—\overset{O}{\overset{\Vert}{C}}(CH_2)_2—$ 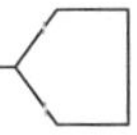
Ethinyl estradiol	—H	—C≡CH	—H
Mestranol	$—CH_3$	—C≡CH	—H
Quinestrol	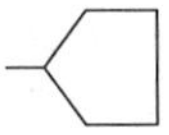	—C≡CH	—H

NONSTEROIDAL ESTROGENS

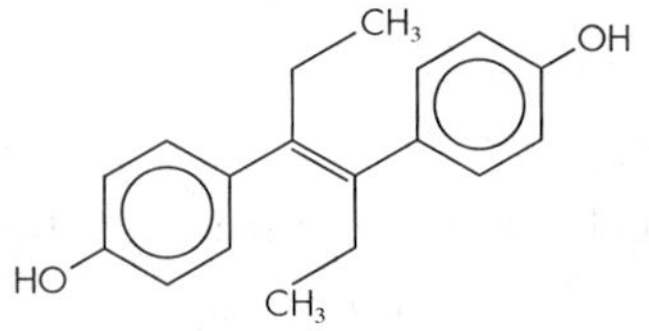

Diethylstilbestrol

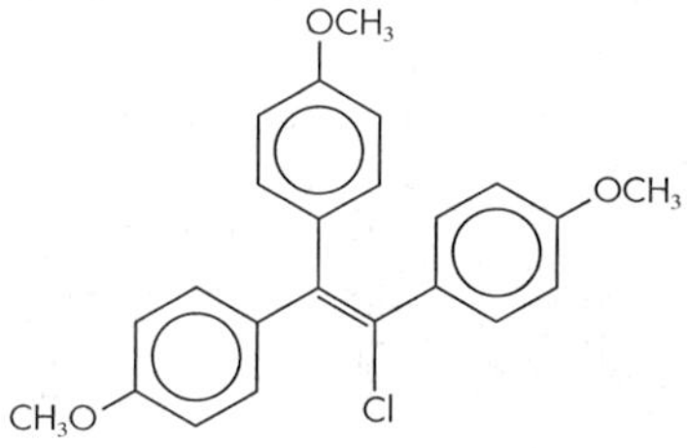

Chlorotrianisene

one as immediate precursors (*see* Figure 58–1). The reaction involves aromatization of the A ring, and it is catalyzed in three steps by a monooxygenase enzyme complex (aromatase) that uses NADPH and molecular oxygen as cosubstrates (Miller, 1988). In the first step of this reaction, C 19 (the angular methyl group residing on C 10 of the androgen precursor) is hydroxylated. A second hydroxylation results in the elimination of the newly formed C 19 hydroxymethyl group, and a final hydroxylation on C 2 results in the formation of an unstable intermediate that rearranges to form the phenolic A ring. The entire reaction consumes three molecules of oxygen and three molecules of NADPH.

Aromatase activity resides within a transmembrane glycoprotein ($P_{450,arom}$) that is homologous with the cytochrome P_{450} family of monooxygenases (Nebert and Gonzalez, 1987; Corbin *et al.*, 1988); also essential is a ubiquitous flavoprotein, NADPH-cytochrome P_{450} reductase. Both proteins are localized in the endoplasmic reticulum of ovarian granulosa cells, testicular Sertoli and Leydig cells, adipocytes, placental syncytiotrophoblasts, the preimplantation blastocyst, and various brain regions, including the hypothalamus.

The ovaries are the principal source of estrogen in premenopausal women. The major secretory product is estradiol, synthesized by granulosa cells from androgenic precursors provided by thecal cells. Here, as in other tissues, aromatase activity is induced by hormones such as gonadotropins that elevate intracellular concentrations of adenosine 3′,5′-monophosphate (cyclic AMP). Gonadotropins and cyclic AMP also increase the activity of the cholesterol side-chain cleavage enzyme and facilitate the transport of cholesterol (the precursor of all steroids) into the mitochondria of cells that synthesize steroids. Secreted estradiol is oxidized reversibly to estrone, and both of these estrogens can be converted to estriol (*see* Figure 58–1). These transformations take place mainly in the liver, where the interconversion between estrone and estradiol is catalyzed by 17-hydroxysteroid dehydrogenase. All three estrogens are excreted in the urine as glucuronides and sulfates, along with a host of related, minor products in water-soluble complexes.

In men and postmenopausal women, the principal source of estrogen is adipose tissue. In this and other peripheral tissues, estrone is synthesized from dehydroepiandrosterone, which is secreted by the adrenal cortex. Thus, the contribution of adipose tissue to the pool of estrogens is regulated in part by the availability of androgenic precursors (Mendelson and Simpson, 1987).

During pregnancy, large quantities of estrogens are synthesized by the placenta, which uses fetal dehydroepiandrosterone and its 16α-hydroxyl derivative to produce estrone and estriol, respectively. Thus, human urine of pregnancy is an abundant source of natural estrogens. The pregnant mare excretes over 100 mg daily, a record exceeded only by the stallion, who, despite clear manifestations of virility, excretes into his environment more estrogen than any other living creature.

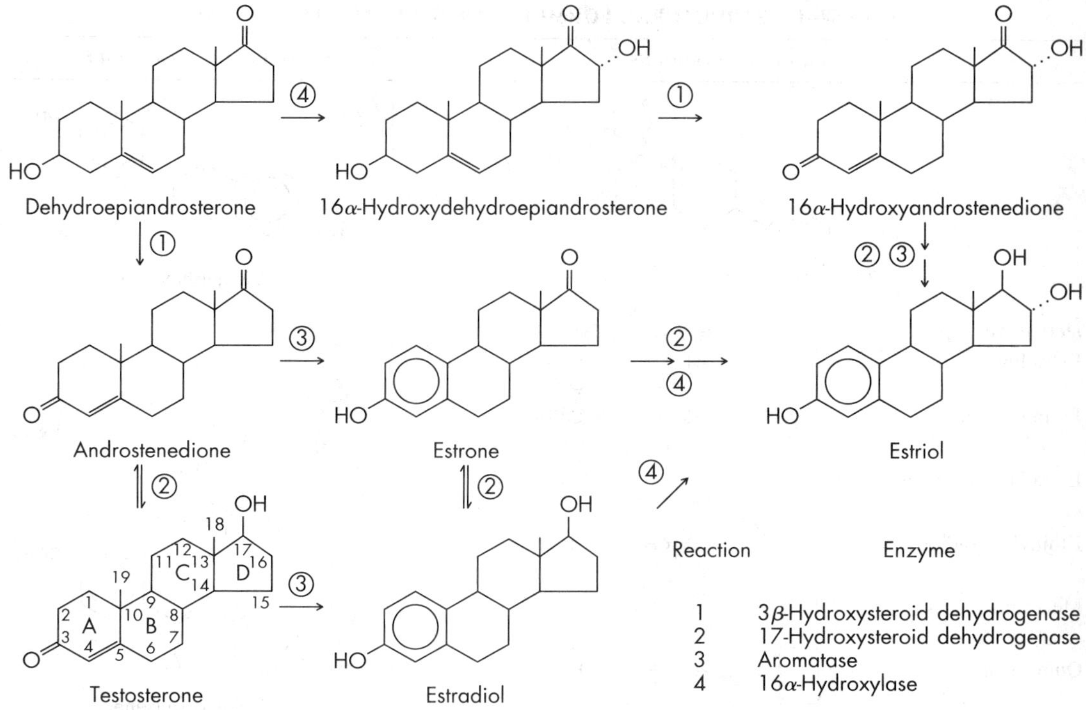

Figure 58–1. *The biosynthetic pathway for the estrogens.*

The 19-carbon precursors are synthesized primarily in the ovaries, testes, and adrenals, and their biosynthetic pathway is summarized in Figure 60–2 (page 1434). Steroid nomenclature and stereochemistry are summarized in Figure 60–4 (page 1447).

Physiological and Pharmacological Actions. The estrogens are largely responsible for the changes that take place at puberty in girls, and they go a long way toward accounting for the attributes of femininity. By a direct action, they cause growth and development of the vagina, uterus, and Fallopian tubes. They cause enlargement of the breasts through promotion of ductal growth, stromal development, and the accretion of fat, effects in which pituitary hormones also play a part. They also contribute in a poorly understood manner to molding the body contours, shaping the skeleton, and bringing about changes in the epiphyses of the long bones that condition the pubertal spurt in growth and its culmination by fusion of the epiphyses. Growth of axillary and pubic hair and regional pigmentation of the skin of the nipples and areolae and of the genital region are also effects of estrogen.

Psychological and emotional effects, so prominently displayed in lower animals in the form of sexual behavior, estrus, or heat, are partially obscured in human beings by other influences, but presumably estrogen conditions feminine behavior in important ways.

Superimposed upon the feminizing influences of the estrogens is the cyclical component in the intensity of their action, which is responsible for many features of the normal menstrual cycle. During the follicular phase of the cycle, there is proliferation of the vaginal and uterine mucosae, increased secretion of the glands of the uterine cervix, and noticeable fullness of the breasts. Decline in estrogenic activity at the end of the cycle can bring about menstruation. In the mature cycle with ovulation, progesterone further modifies the genital tract and mammary gland in the direction of pregnancy, and it is the cessation of secretion of progesterone that is the determinant of menstruation (Erickson, 1978; Naftolin and Tolis, 1978).

Androgens from the Ovary. A question

long of interest is whether the androgens secreted by the normal ovary are physiologically important. Measurements of steroids contained in venous ovarian blood indicate that both testosterone and androstenedione, precursors of estrogens, are normal ovarian secretions. The daily production rates of testosterone and androstenedione in women are about 0.5 and 1.5 mg, respectively. Furthermore, studies with rabbit ovary have demonstrated that luteinizing hormone (LH) increases ovarian synthesis and secretion of testosterone (Hilliard *et al.,* 1974).

The complete sexual development that can be brought about by the administration of estrogen alone and the reproduction of all the features of the menstrual cycle (except the ovarian changes) that can be achieved with estrogen and progesterone seem to leave little place for an androgen in the feminine economy. And yet certain features may be missing when estrogen–progestin therapy replaces ovarian function. The rapid rate of growth at puberty is hard to explain in view of the limited anabolic and growth-promoting properties of estrogen. The development of axillary and pubic hair under the influence of estrogen alone may not be as complete as it is in the normal girl, and it may be lacking altogether following therapy with estrogen in patients with hypopituitarism. When small doses of androgen are added to the estrogen, growth and distribution of hair on the body are normal even without the pituitary. Some aspects of sexual development in females are thus attributable to adrenal and ovarian androgens.

Acne, common during puberty in girls, is closely related to the growth and secretion of the sebaceous glands. The normal development and function of these structures cannot be brought about by estrogen or progesterone, but both can be induced by the administration of small amounts of androgen. Furthermore, while other treatments are preferred, acne can be effectively treated and the sebaceous glands caused to regress by suppressing gonadotropin secretion and ovarian function with estrogen or with a preparation of an estrogen and a progestin.

Although estrogen alone is effective replacement therapy in the menopause, a few observers believe that a more normal result is achieved when small amounts of androgen are given as well.

Actions on the Pituitary. The precise actions of estrogens on the secretory activity of the adenohypophysis have been very difficult to define. In the normal sexual cycle of mammals, the structural and the secretory changes in the ovary are brought about by the precisely timed and sequential secretion of gonadotropins from the hypophysis. The central mechanisms and events that lead to the cyclic secretion of gonadotropins and thereby initiate the onset of puberty and gonadal development are unknown.

One conceptual difficulty is that there appears to be but one gonadotropin-releasing hormone—LHRH/FSHRH, or GnRH; this hormone increases the pituitary secretion of both LH and FSH (*see* Chapter 56). The varying blood concentrations of each gonadotropin during the menstrual cycle (Figure 58–2) suggest that another regulatory hormone might exist to explain the apparent independence of their secretion. However, complex feedback effects of sex steroids and perhaps other gonadal factors on the pituitary and hypothalamus influence the secretion and action of GnRH, and this effect could explain the divergent patterns of release of each gonadotropin (*see* Schally, 1978).

While generalization is premature, certain interrelations seem definite. As the ovarian follicle grows under the influence of FSH, the increasing titer of estrogen that is produced decreases the release of GnRH and thereby suppresses FSH secretion. Under the influence of FSH the granulosa cells of the Graafian follicle may also secrete inhibin, which feeds back to decrease the secretion of FSH. Inhibin, first described in the testis, is a glycopeptide that is also produced by the ovaries and the placenta (*see* DeJong, 1988). It suppresses the secretion of FSH more than it does the secretion of LH (Ying, 1988). Although estrogens can decrease FSH secretion, they have a biphasic effect on LH. The rapid swelling of the follicle, culminating in ovulation, is brought about by the midcycle surge in LH (*see* Figure 58–2), probably due to increased GnRH release as well as to greater estrogen-induced sensitivity of the pituitary to the regulatory hormone. It is not known how just one of the many follicles that develop under the influence of FSH in primates is selected for rupture and ovulation.

Progesterone begins to be secreted during the formation of the corpus luteum, and secretion continues throughout its functional life. The control of the secretion of the corpus luteum is managed by various species in quite different ways. In women it is under the predominant control of LH.

The major mystery is the relatively precise cyclic and pulsatile nature of the pituitary secretion of gonadotropins and thus ovarian secretion of estrogens and progesterone. In addition to the more prolonged and larger oscillations in gonadotropins during the menstrual cycle, there are smaller, short-term variations in plasma concentrations of gonadotropins in normal women. The significance of the pulsatile secretion that causes these variations is not known.

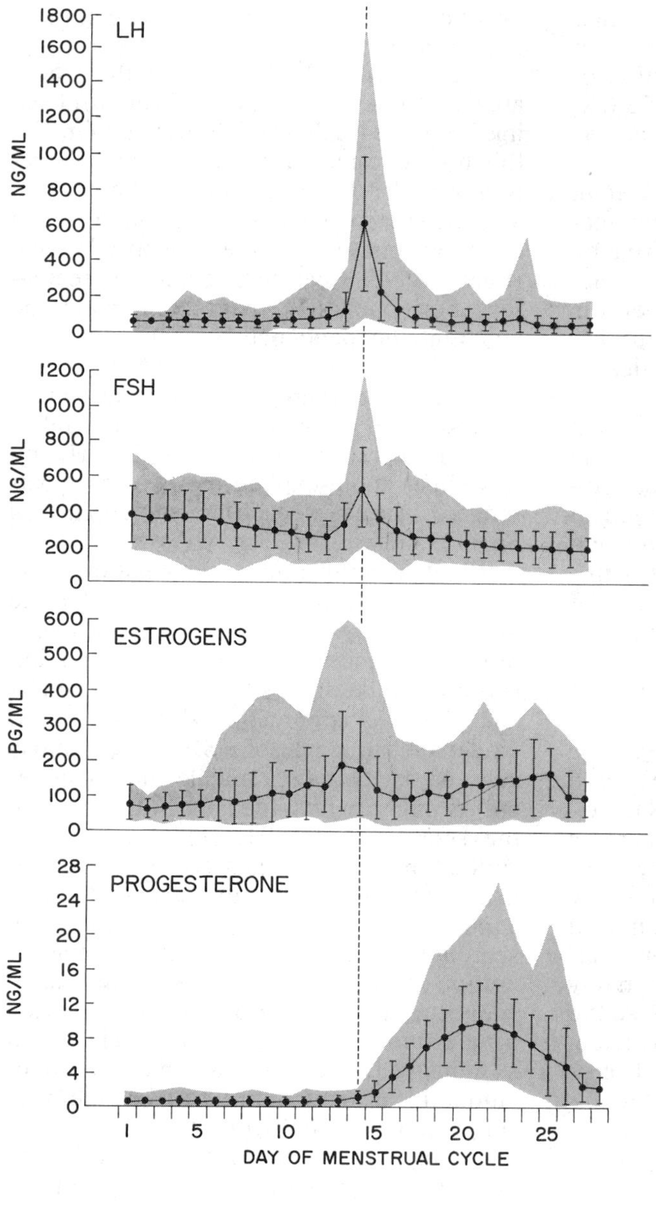

Figure 58–2. *Plasma concentrations of ovarian hormones and gonadotropins in women during normal menstrual cycles.*

Values are the mean ± standard deviation of 40 women. The shaded areas indicate the entire range of observations. Day 1 is the onset of menses. Ovulation on day 14 of the menstrual cycle occurs with the midcycle peak of LH, represented by the dashed line. (After Vande Wiele and Dyrenfurth, 1973. Courtesy of *Pharmacological Reviews*. © 1973 The Williams & Wilkins Co., Baltimore.)

In contrast, total daily secretion of gonadotropins in men is quite stable, while secretion during the course of the day is variable. In the male the secretion of both FSH and LH can be inhibited by estrogen and inhibin; as a result, spermatogenesis is arrested, the testicular tubules become atrophic, and the regressive changes in the genital tract show that the secretion of androgen is reduced (*see* Chapter 59).

When the ovaries or testes are removed or cease to function, there is overproduction of FSH and LH, which are excreted in the urine. Measurements of urinary or plasma gonadotropins are valuable clinical tests and can be used to assess pituitary function and to show the effectiveness of replacement doses of estrogen or testosterone, which, in amounts that might be considered physiological, specifically inhibit overproduction.

The regulation of gonadotropin secretion and the actions of FSH and LH are also discussed in Chapters 56 and 59.

Estrogens and Menstruation. When the ovaries are not functional or have been removed, menstrual flow can be induced by the administration and subsequent withdrawal of estrogen. Both the size of the dose and the duration of treatment are involved in determining whether bleeding will follow, and, within limits, the two determinants can be varied reciprocally with a similar outcome. Bleeding can be induced by a single large dose or by treatment for several weeks with a much smaller amount. When doses within a certain range are given, menstrual flow (breakthrough bleeding) may ensue even when the treatment is not interrupted. This has been referred to as the "threshold dose."

The action of progesterone upon the estrogen-treated uterus in causing menstruation is quite unrelated to its action in causing the secretory changes seen microscopically. When estrogen is given without interruption, brief treatment with progesterone is followed by menstruation a few days later; as little as 1 mg given in a single dose may be enough, whereas the histological changes in the endometrium require many days to develop.

Menstrual bleeding during continuous treatment with threshold doses of estrogen can be prevented by increasing the dose; however, when a brief treatment with progesterone is introduced, estrogen, even in large doses, will not prevent the ensuing menstruation.

Metabolic Actions. Estrogens are weaker anabolic agents than the androgens (*see* Chapter 59). Retention of salt and water to the point of causing edema is not a common feature of therapy with estrogen. However, edema may be troublesome when estrogen is given in large doses and particularly if an associated condition predisposes to retention of fluid. Although the edema responds well to diuretics, one should discontinue the estrogen if possible. The moderate fluid retention common in the latter half of the menstrual cycle is a result of the action of estrogen.

Estrogens can cause changes in circulating lipids. They decrease concentrations of low-density lipoprotein cholesterol and increase those of high-density lipoprotein (Burkman, 1988; Crook *et al.,* 1988). These changes may lower the risk of coronary artery disease and contribute to the lower incidence of myocardial infarction in premenopausal women. Use of estrogens in postmenopausal women has also been associated with a decreased incidence of coronary artery disease (Bush and Barrett-Connor, 1985; Gruchow *et al.,* 1988; Sullivan *et al.,* 1988). However, the data are not uniformly supportive of this notion (Porter *et al.,* 1987), and increased incidences of myocardial infarction and stroke have been observed in some studies (Henderson *et al.,* 1985; Wilson *et al.,* 1985).

Carcinogenic Action. In several mammalian species, the administration of estrogens is followed by the development of certain tumors. Since the early studies of Lacassagne (1936), it has been known that estrogens can induce tumors of the breast, uterus, testis, bone, kidney, and several other tissues in various animal species. These early studies disseminated a fear of cancer resulting from estrogen use. Until 1971, however, no evidence of a carcinogenic action of estrogens in human subjects had been reported. Since that time there have been many clinical reports of tumors that may be related to estrogens. In the earliest studies (Greenwald *et al.,* 1971; Herbst *et al.*, 1971), an increased incidence of vaginal and cervical adenocarcinoma was noted in female offspring of mothers who had taken diethylstilbestrol or other synthetic estrogens during the first trimester of pregnancy. This has been amply confirmed, and the incidence of clear-cell vaginal and cervical adenocarcinoma in women who were exposed to estrogens *in utero* is estimated to be 0.01 to 0.1% (*FDA Drug Bulletin*, 1985). Most of the affected women have been about 20 to 25 years of age at the time of detection of disease, but younger and older individuals have also been affected. Estrogen use during pregnancy can also cause vaginal adenosis (a nonmalignant proliferation of glandular tissue) in female offspring. Although males exposed to exogenous estrogens during intrauterine development may have an increased incidence of genital abnormalities, tumors have apparently not resulted from such exposure. Thus, pregnant patients should not be given estrogens, particularly during the first trimester—a time when the fetal reproductive tract is developing and may be influenced by exogenous estrogens.

Data from numerous studies have indicated that the use of estrogen by postmenopausal women is associated with the development of endometrial carcinoma (Shapiro *et al.*, 1985). The risk is estimated to be increased as much as 5- to 15-fold by estrogen and is related to dose and duration of use. The increased risk declines to normal several years after discontinuation of estrogen. Epidemiological studies indicate a lower incidence of endometrial carcinoma when low doses of estrogen are administered in a cyclical fashion or when a progestin is also given (Gambrell, 1985). Although earlier studies suggested that the use of oral contraceptives by premenopausal women was associated with the development of endometrial carcinoma (Silverberg and Makowski, 1975; Weiss and Sayvetz, 1980), more recent studies indicate that such use is associated with a decreased incidence of both endometrial and ovarian cancer (Centers for Disease Control, 1987a, 1987b).

Several reports have aroused the suspicion that estrogens or oral contraceptives may increase the incidence of breast tumors, a far more common problem than endometrial carcinoma (*see* Leis *et al.*, 1976; Kay, 1977). Although numerous factors are associated with an increased risk of breast cancer, some reports have suggested that use of estrogens or oral contraceptives can increase the risk two- to sixfold (Jick *et al.*, 1980; Ross *et al.*, 1980; Lawson *et al.*, 1981). Women who received diethylstilbestrol in pregnancy during the period from 1940 to 1960 were found to have a small increase in the incidence of carcinoma of the breast (Greenberg *et al.*, 1984; Hadjimichael *et al.*, 1984). A prospective (but not randomized or placebo-controlled) study of more than 20,000 Swedish women over the age of 35 indicated that use of estradiol nearly doubled the risk of breast cancer after 6 years of treatment. No increased risk was seen when conjugated estrogens or estriol was used, although the number of patients was smaller (Bergkvist *et al.*, 1989). The risk of breast cancer was highest among those who received a combination of an estrogen and a progestin. It should also be noted that many studies have not found an association between use of estrogens and breast cancer. Furthermore, evaluation of these issues is complex, particularly in view of the beneficial effects of estrogens on osteoporosis and, perhaps, cardiovascular disease (*see below; see also* Barrett-Connor, 1989).

After a report that the use of oral contraceptives by young women was associated with the occurrence of benign hepatomas (Baum *et al.*, 1973), a number of similar studies have confirmed this relationship.

Mechanism of Action. Estrogens, like other steroid hormones, act by regulating the transcription of a limited number of genes. The hormones diffuse passively through cell membranes, distribute themselves throughout the cell, and ultimately bind to the nuclear estrogen receptor. This protein, which is found in estrogen-responsive tissues (female reproductive tract, breast, pituitary, and hypothalamus), is a DNA-binding protein that is homologous with the receptors for other steroid hormones, vitamin D, retinoic acid, and the thyroid hormones (*see* Chapter 2). Once activated by ligand, the estrogen receptor binds to specific DNA sequences (hormone-response elements) that enhance the transcription of adjacent genes. The full number of proteins that are induced by estrogen is not known but is estimated to be 50 to 100 (*see* Gorski *et al.,* 1986; Evans, 1988; Beato, 1989).

Absorption, Fate, and Excretion. Estrogens used in therapy are, in general, readily absorbed through the skin, mucous membranes, and gastrointestinal tract. When they are applied for a local action, absorption is often sufficient to cause systemic effects. The absorption of most natural estrogens and their derivatives from the gastrointestinal tract is prompt and quite complete. Thus, the limited oral effectiveness of the natural estrogens and their esters is not due to poor absorption but to their hepatic metabolism, as discussed below.

The estrogens are practically insoluble in water. When dissolved in oil and injected, they are rapidly absorbed and quickly metabolized. The aryl and alkyl esters of estradiol become less polar as the size of the substituents increases; correspondingly, the rate of absorption of oily preparations is progressively slowed and the duration of action prolonged. Therapeutic doses of compounds such as estradiol valerate or estradiol cypionate are absorbed over several weeks after a single intramuscular injection.

The estrogens and their esters are handled in the body in much the same way as are the endogenous hormones. Inactivation of estrogen is carried out mainly in the liver. A certain proportion of the estrogen is excreted into the bile and then reabsorbed from the intestine. During this enterohepatic circulation, degradation of estrogen occurs through conversion to less active products such as estriol and numerous other estrogens, through oxidation to nonestrogenic substances, and through conjugation with sulfuric and glucuronic acids.

Ethinyl estradiol is active orally since its inactivation in the liver and other tissues is very slow. This accounts for the high intrinsic potency of the analog. Similarly, the nonsteroidal estrogens are degraded slowly.

The natural estrogens circulate in the blood in association with sex hormone–binding globulin and albumin (Heyns, 1977). A significant proportion of the estrogen is in the form of conjugates, particularly sulfate, which are excreted by the kidney.

In the normal menstrual cycle the mean daily excretion of estrogens at the midcycle ovulatory maximum is 25 to 100 μg; the second rise during the luteal phase is more prolonged, but the maximal rates of excretion are somewhat smaller (10 to 80 μg per day). After the menopause the average excretion of estrogens in normal women totals about 5 to 10 μg daily. As noted above, these estrogens are synthesized from androgenic precursors by nonovarian tissues. The values for normal men average 2 to 25 μg per day, quantities about equal to the urinary estrogens of women during the first week of the menstrual cycle. No estrogen is detectable in the urine of young children. During the first trimester of pregnancy the placenta becomes the primary source of the urinary estrogens, which continue to increase and reach levels of about 30 mg per day near term. Their serial determination can be used to assess placental and fetal function.

Preparations. Several widely used, orally active nonsteroidal estrogens are available. The most popular have been preparations of *diethylstilbestrol,* available in tablets containing from 0.1 to 5 mg. *Diethylstilbestrol diphosphate* (STILPHOSTROL) is available as an injection (50 mg/ml of the sodium salt) and in 50-mg tablets for use in prostatic carcinoma. Oral doses of 50 to 200 mg are taken three times daily (up to a maximum of 1 g per day) for this disorder. Intravenous infusions for induction and maintenance therapy in prostatic carcinoma range from 250 to 1000 mg daily or weekly (*see* Chapter 52).

Estradiol is available as 1- and 2-mg tablets of micronized estradiol (ESTRACE) and in the form of various esters. *Estradiol valerate* and *cypionate* are prepared in oil for slow release after intramuscular injection. These preparations contain 1 to 40 mg/ml and are sold under various trade names (*e.g.,* DELESTROGEN). Estradiol can also be administered as transcutaneous patches (ESTRADERM) that contain 4 or 8 mg of the hormone and are constructed to deliver 0.05 or 0.1 mg per day to the circulation. Patches should be changed twice weekly.

Estrone is the major component of many preparations. These include *estrone aqueous suspension* and *estrogenic substance* (aqueous suspensions) that contain 2 to 5 mg/ml for intramuscular injection. *Estropipate* is crystalline estrone sulfate stabilized with piperazine. It is marketed in tablets containing 0.625 to 5 mg (OGEN). *Conjugated estrogens* (PREMARIN, PROGENS) contain 50 to 65% estrone sodium sulfate and 20 to 35% sodium equilin (Δ^7-estrone) sulfate. They are available in oral (0.3 to 2.5 mg) and injectable preparations. *Esterified estrogens* (MENEST, ESTRATAB) contain 75 to

85% estrone sodium sulfate and 6 to 15% sodium equilin sulfate in tablets of 0.3 to 2.5 mg.

Ethinyl estradiol (ESTINYL, FEMINONE) is available in tablets that contain 0.02 to 0.5 mg. It is roughly 20 times as potent as diethylstilbestrol. The 3-methyl ether of ethinyl estradiol, *mestranol,* is inactive until it is converted to ethinyl estradiol in the body. Both of these estrogens are widely used in the combination oral contraceptives (*see* below). *Quinestrol* (ESTROVIS) is the 3-cyclopentyl ether of ethinyl estradiol. Since it is stored in fat and released slowly, it can be taken orally once per week in maintenance doses of 0.1 to 0.2 mg. It is available in 0.1-mg tablets.

Chlorotrianisene (TACE) is an oral preparation that is long acting because of sequestration in adipose tissue and, therefore, is not widely used. It is available in 12-, 25-, and 72-mg capsules and has about one eighth the activity of diethylstilbestrol.

A number of preparations in which estrogen is combined with another agent are also available. Oral contraceptives containing an estrogen and a progestin are discussed below. There are no compelling reasons to use formulations of estrogens combined with androgens or antianxiety preparations.

A variety of topical preparations with various estrogenic substances in creams are no longer widely used. However, senile vaginitis and kraurosis vulvae may be effectively treated with topical preparations for vaginal use. Many of the "over-the-counter" cosmetics and creams that contained estrogens have been removed from the United States market. While frequent and excessive topical use of estrogens can cause systemic effects, these are minimal when they are used as directed. Intravaginal use of some preparations can lead to significant concentrations of estrogen in blood, since the estrogen is readily absorbed and the initial circulation through the liver is bypassed with this route of administration (Rigg *et al.*, 1978).

Choice of Preparations. Claims have been made that some preparations of estrogen cause fewer side effects than others. However, prevailing information suggests that all estrogens cause the same spectrum of side effects. The following parenteral dosages of some estrogens are approximately equivalent: estradiol, 50 μg; ethinyl estradiol, 50 μg; mestranol, 80 μg; diethylstilbestrol, 5 mg; conjugated estrogens, 5 mg. The choice of preparation is largely determined by cost and convenience to the patient. Oral therapy is preferred; the action begins promptly, and treatment can be terminated at will. However, the relative potencies summarized above must be modified to account for diminished efficacy of some agents when given orally; such is the case with estradiol. With substances such as diethylstilbestrol or ethinyl estradiol, which are not quickly inactivated, a single dose each day is usually sufficient. Conjugated natural estrogens are less effective. The use of transdermal delivery of estrogens is increasing, but therapy by injection has little to recommend it. The long-acting esters given by injection may be useful for long-continued treatment with large doses in the therapy of patients with cancer. The esters are unsuitable in the management of menstrual disorders or as replacement therapy in menopause when cyclic therapy is desirable. Cyclic therapy with oral estrogens can be accomplished by interruption of dosage for 1 week per month. As noted below, a progestin may be added to the therapeutic regimen to diminish the incidence of endometrial carcinoma in postmenopausal women. However, the use of progestin may increase the risk of carcinoma of the breast and cause other side effects. In premenopausal women the addition of a progestin ensures a more normal menstrual period when estrogen and progestin are terminated together intermittently.

Untoward Responses. The most frequent unpleasant symptom attending the use of estrogen is nausea. With large doses there may also be anorexia, vomiting, and mild diarrhea. The nausea is of a peculiar type that seldom interferes with eating and does not cause a loss of weight; it may be noted at various times of the day but, like the "morning sickness" of early pregnancy, it is often troublesome at breakfast time. With continued treatment the symptom usually disappears, and only rarely is it so distressful that treatment must be stopped. Even when very large doses are given, as in the treatment of cancer of the breast, nausea is generally troublesome only for the first 1 or 2 weeks. The symptom can usually be avoided by starting with a small dose and gradually increasing it. Other liabilities to the use of estrogens have been discussed above and are discussed below, under oral contraceptives.

Therapeutic Uses. *Oral Contraception.* A major use of estrogens is in combination with progestins as oral contraceptives; such use is discussed in a separate section later in this chapter.

Menopause. The decline in the secretion of estrogen by the ovary is a slow and gradual process that continues for some years after menstruation has ceased (*see* Eskin, 1978). It is a frequent observation that menopausal symptoms are more severe following abrupt removal of estrogen, such as with oophorectomy, than with natural menopause. Sometimes hot flashes appear for the first time or become more intense if the ovaries are removed after menopause. The formation of small quantities of estrogens from androgenic precursors by nonovarian tissues may be important in slowing the estrogen withdrawal and the onset of menopausal symptoms in some patients.

The decline in ovarian function at menopause is associated with vasomotor symptoms in most women. The symptoms are clearly due to deficiency of estrogen. The characteristic hot flashes may alternate with chilly sensations, inappropriate sweating, and paresthesias. A variety of other symptoms often occur during menopause and include muscle cramps, myalgias, arthralgias, anxiety, overbreathing, palpitation, dizziness, faintness, and syncope. These and other symptoms may or may not be associated with estrogen deficiency. Some women feel genuinely miserable and lack vigor and initiative; many, obviously, tolerate the event quite well. The symptoms lessen and disappear with time. However, about 15 to 25% of menopausal women will seek medical advice or treatment.

Treatment with estrogen is specific and effective. Replacement therapy clearly relieves the hot flashes and other vasomotor symptoms and atrophic vaginitis (*see* Ryan, 1982; Ernster *et al.*, 1988). The lowest dose needed varies somewhat but can easily be determined by trial. The oral dose of diethylstilbestrol is about 0.2 to 1 mg once daily; 0.5 mg is seldom sufficient to cause withdrawal bleeding, 1 mg daily for several weeks sometimes causes bleeding when stopped, and 2 mg often does. Comparable doses of ethinyl estradiol are 0.01 to 0.05 mg; conjugated estrogens may be used in doses of 0.3 to 1.25 mg daily. Therapy with estrogen is best given in a cyclic manner, 3 weeks of treatment followed by 1 week without treatment. If withdrawal bleeding is going to occur, it will begin toward the end of the week of no treatment and the estrogen can be resumed before this induced menstrual period ceases. Menopausal symptoms usually do not return in full intensity during the week without treatment. Occasionally during cyclic therapy with estrogen alone uterine bleeding may continue in an irregular manner after estrogen is resumed. Larger doses of estrogen have been employed to control this bleeding, but the use of a progestin is more uniformly effective. Once a progesterone-withdrawal menstrual period has been induced, there may be no further trouble from the use of estrogen alone for many months. However, the use of a progestin in combination with an estrogen appears rational, since it can diminish the increased incidence of endometrial carcinoma observed in patients who take estrogens alone (Gambrell, 1985; Shapiro *et al.*, 1985; Centers for Disease Control, 1987a; Ernster *et al.*, 1988). Nevertheless, there is concern that a progestin may increase the incidence of carcinoma of the breast and that it might negate any beneficial cardiovascular effects that are bestowed by the estrogen (Barrett-Connor, 1989).

Senile or atrophic vaginitis, often associated with chronic infection of the atrophic structures, responds well to estrogen. Estrogens are more effective in preventing than in reversing atrophic changes of the vagina and the decrease in skin turgor (*see* Eskin, 1978). Kraurosis vulvae, a distressingly itchy condition due in part to deficiency in estrogen and in part to scratching and other as-yet-unknown factors, is favorably influenced by estrogen supplemented by local treatment, including the application of adrenocorticosteroids.

Some physicians are disinclined to prescribe estrogens in the menopause; others prescribe estrogens for periods of months or a few years only. Physicians with these views are undoubtedly concerned about the possible minor and serious side effects of estrogens in light of modest evidence to demonstrate their efficacy in preventing the more serious physical disorders accompanying menopause, such as atherosclerosis. However, indefinite systemic replacement in all menopausal patients, advocated by some, is certainly not necessary and may introduce more undesirable effects than the symptomatic improvement warrants. The major indication for replacement therapy is prevention of osteoporosis, as discussed below. Patients receiving estrogens should be examined every 6 to 12 months for possible side effects, and abnormal uterine bleeding should be investigated. Most agree that the risk-to-benefit ratio for estrogen therapy needs to be evaluated for each patient and should be reconsidered periodically; when used, estrogens should be administered in the lowest effective dose for the shortest possible time, and cyclic therapy is preferred, with or without concomitant use of a progestin.

Pregnancy. In the past, large doses of estrogens were given during pregnancy in attempts to prevent threatened or habitual abortion, among other reasons. There is no evidence that such uses are of any value. Because of this and the risk of producing vaginal tumors in female offspring and possible teratogenic effects in male offspring (*see* above), *the use of estrogens in pregnancy is not indicated.* The use of progestins in this condition is discussed below.

Dysmenorrhea. Dysmenorrhea can be relieved by inhibition of ovulation with estrogen. Cyclic therapy with an estrogen can often be used successfully if too long an interval is not permitted to elapse between courses. The additional use of an orally active progestin facilitates management. The disorder is probably due to uterine production of prostaglandins; nonsteroidal antiinflammatory agents are effective and are the preferred form of therapy (*see* Chapter 26).

The use of estrogens in the treatment of endometriosis is discussed below in connection with the therapeutic uses of progestins.

Dysfunctional Uterine Bleeding. This disorder usually occurs at the time of menarche or menopause and results from anovulatory cycles, with continuous secretion of estrogen and endometrial hyperplasia. Insufficient secretion of progesterone results in incomplete sloughing of the proliferative endometrium and excessive bleeding. Although estrogen can be used with some success, the cyclic use of a progestin is logically preferred (*see* below).

Failure of Ovarian Development. There are several unusual conditions in which the ovaries do not develop and, in consequence, puberty does not occur. In ovarian dysgenesis with dwarfism (Turner's syndrome), diagnosis can be made before the age of puberty by the associated congenital anomalies, the patient's stature, and from chromosomal studies. Therapy with estrogen at the appropriate time replicates the events of puberty, except for the spurt in growth and, of course, the changes in the ovary. The genital structures grow to normal size. The breasts develop, axillary and pubic hair grows, and the body assumes the normal feminine contour. Androgens have been used successfully to promote growth (*see* Chapter 59). It is common practice to start with small doses of estrogen, such as 0.2 to 0.5 mg of diethylstilbestrol or 0.02 mg of ethinyl estradiol, and then increase the dose slowly over a year or so before initiating menstrual periods by cyclic treatment with larger doses. There may be some merit in thus imitating the normal sequence of events at puberty.

Failure of ovarian development is also a part of the picture of hypopituitarism in childhood. Deficiency of the thyroid and the adrenal cortex is easily corrected with replacement therapy, and the failure of sexual development is treated with estrogen as outlined just above. Administration of human growth hormone permits achievement of a normal adult stature (*see* Chapter 56). Treatment with estrogen at the normal age of puberty can be expected to cause a small acceleration of growth, but the addition of small doses of androgen has a greater growth-promoting effect. While estrogens and androgens promote bone growth, they also accelerate epiphyseal fusion, and their premature use can thus result in a shorter ultimate height. Indeed, estrogens have been used in high doses to accelerate epiphyseal closure in tall girls; to be effective, estrogen must be given prior to menarche. This use of estrogen is rarely, if ever, indicated.

Acne. The common form of acne is a feature of puberty in both sexes, and androgens seem to be the essential factor, operating through stimulation of sebaceous glands. Treatment with estrogen is effective in both sexes by suppressing gonadotropins and gonadal androgen secretion, but its usefulness in the male is obviously limited. In young women estrogen is effective therapy in doses designed to suppress the ovary and may be continued with benefit for many months in a cyclic fashion. One of the combined oral contraceptive agents is more convenient. It may be given in the same manner as when used to prevent ovulation. However, tretinoin and antibiotics are preferred (*see* Melski and Arndt, 1980); isotretinoin is given orally for severe cystic acne (*see* Chapters 64 and 65).

Hirsutism. In most instances, excessive growth of body hair in women cannot be traced to an endocrine cause, but occasionally a mild androgenic influence of ovarian or adrenal origin is suspected. When suppression of the adrenal cortex by the administration of a corticosteroid is ineffectual, suppression of the ovary with an estrogen may be worthwhile. Concentrations of androgens in plasma should be measured and the response to treatment determined. If it is to be tried, suppression of the ovary for about a year with continuous therapy may be needed before it can be ascertained whether the maneuver is successful. Doses of about 2 mg daily of diethylstilbestrol or its equivalent are sufficient. Menstrual periods during this time can be evoked at intervals by cyclic use of an oral progestin, with preference for a progestin that has little androgenic activity. Antiandrogens may also be useful for severe hirsutism (*see* Chapter 59).

Prevention of Heart Attacks. In view of the favored position of women in the incidence of fatal myocardial infarction, estrogen therapy has been tried as a prophylactic measure in men. A large-scale study was conducted by the Coronary Drug Project Research Group. The administration of conjugated estrogens daily led to an *increased* incidence of cardiac and thromboembolic complications (Coronary Drug Project Research Group, 1970, 1973). The use of estrogen in the form of combination oral contraceptives may increase the incidence of morbidity and mortality from myocardial infarction in premenopausal women (*see* below). However, the administration of estrogen to postmenopausal women has not been associated with an increased incidence of complications from coronary artery disease (Rosenberg *et al.*, 1976; Weinstein, 1980; Ryan, 1982; Wilson *et al.*, 1985). Indeed, more recent studies have shown a *beneficial* effect of estrogen on the incidence of coronary artery disease in postmenopausal women (Bush and Barrett-Connor, 1985; Gruchow *et al.*, 1988). Some of the controversy rests with the amount of estrogen used and whether or not a progestin is used simultaneously. Estrogens and progestins have complex and usually opposite effects on plasma lipoproteins. Estrogens can decrease the concentrations of low-density lipoproteins (LDL) and increase high-density lipoproteins (HDL); progestins have the opposite effects (*see* below; Burkman, 1988). High concentrations of LDL and low levels of HDL are correlated with an increased incidence of atherosclerosis (*see* Chapter 36).

Osteoporosis. Osteoporosis is a disorder of the skeleton associated with the loss of both hydroxyapatite (calcium phosphate complexes) and protein matrix (colloid). The result is thinning and weakening of the bones and an increased incidence of fractures, particularly compression fractures of the vertebrae and fractures of the hip and wrist from minimal trauma. In older patients it is called *senile osteoporosis* and affects both sexes. Coming after menopause, this common disorder is referred to as *postmenopausal osteoporosis*. Unfortunately, substantial bone loss must occur before it can be detected with routine radiographic procedures. Many different methods of treatment have been tried with the aim of increasing bone density and substance. After several months of estrogen replacement in postmenopausal patients, Ca^{2+} balance becomes positive, bone resorption decreases to normal, and the incidence of hip fractures is decreased (Thalassinos *et al.*, 1982; Kiel *et al.*, 1987). The effects of estrogens in preventing postmenopausal bone loss are dose-related. Although the equivalent of 15 μg of ethinyl estradiol daily can prevent vasomotor symptoms in menopause, doses of 15 to 25 μg daily are required to prevent bone loss and 25 μg or more per day can result in a net increase in bone density (Horsman *et al.*, 1983). The positive effects of estrogen on Ca^{2+} balance and bone density are reversed rapidly when treatment is discontinued (Aloia *et al.*, 1985).

The prophylactic effect of estrogen in this condition appears greatest if hormone is given before significant osteoporosis occurs. The effects may also be greater when Ca^{2+} and/or fluoride are added to the therapeutic regimen (Riggs *et al.*, 1982; Conference, 1984; *Medical Letter*, 1987). However, since only 35% of postmenopausal patients develop significant osteoporosis and because exercise and increased intake of Ca^{2+} is also effective, the routine prophylactic use of estrogen is difficult to justify. In women who have undergone oophorectomy and hysterectomy, such use of an estrogen is more defensible, since one of the possible toxicities—endometrial carcinoma—is no longer an issue. Indeed, the risk-to-benefit ratio is most favorable in this situation (Weinstein, 1980; Richelson *et al.*, 1984). Androgens are less effective than estrogens in the treatment of postmenopausal osteoporosis, but they may be more effective in preventing osteoporosis induced by glucocorticoids. The use of androgens is discussed in Chapter 59, and the use of vitamin D, calcitonin, and fluoride is discussed in Chapter 62.

Breast Cancer. Many carcinomas of the breast are dependent upon the proper hormonal environment for their growth. About 50 to 65% of all breast cancers possess cytosolic estrogen receptors. Alteration of the hormonal environment can be used as a palliative measure in the therapy of metastatic breast cancer. Removal of estrogen by oophorectomy or the administration of antiestrogens (*see* below) or the administration of estrogens themselves can prolong both the quality and the duration of life. Favorable responses can be obtained in about 60 to 70% of patients if estrogen or progesterone receptors are present in the tumor, while such responses are observed in only 10 to 20% if receptors are absent (Clark *et al.*, 1983). This subject is discussed in more detail in Chapter 52.

Prostatic Carcinoma. Since the prostate is a target organ for the actions of androgens, the inhibition of androgen secretion can be used as palliative therapy in patients with metastatic prostatic carcinoma. This can be accomplished by orchiectomy and/or the administration of an estrogen such as diethylstilbestrol. Leuprolide (a synthetic GnRH analog) appears to be as effective as diethylstilbestrol, and administration of the peptide (1 mg subcutaneously, daily) is associated with fewer side effects (Leuprolide Study Group, 1984). This topic is discussed further in Chapter 52.

Suppression of Postpartum Lactation. Estrogens, progestins, and androgens have been used to decrease milk production in the postpartum period. However, their use for this purpose has decreased in recent years, since the incidence of painful engorgement is low and this condition is readily controlled with analgesics.

ANTIESTROGENS

The term *antiestrogen* can be applied to several classes of compounds that inhibit or modify the action of estrogen. These include competitive antagonists that act at the estrogen receptor, inhibitors of estrogen synthesis (*e.g.*, GnRH; aromatase inhibitors), and agents that exert opposing physiological actions (*e.g.*, progestins and androgens). Competitive estrogen antagonists are the most specific antiestrogens, and such drugs are used in the treatment of infertility and breast cancer. The pharmacology of clomiphene and tamoxifen, two compounds that are available for clinical use in the United States, are discussed below and in Chapter 52.

CLOMIPHENE AND TAMOXIFEN

History. Potent competitive antagonists of estrogen action came from an unexpected direction. It was found that the weakly estrogenic triarylethylene derivative chlorotrianisene (*see* Table 58–1) did not cause enlargement of the pituitary when given to rats in large doses. Estradiol normally causes pronounced enlargement of the pituitary, but when chlorotrianisene was given concurrently the effect was greatly reduced (Segal and Thompson, 1956). The related nonestrogenic triarylethylene ethamoxytriphetol was found to be strikingly antiestrogenic. It inhibited endogenous estrogen as well as estrogen given in the form of the natural compounds, diethylstilbestrol, or chlorotrianisene. The search for more potent derivatives culminated in the syntheses of clomiphene, tamoxifen, and nafoxidine in the late 1950s. Clomiphene became available for general use in the United States as a fertility agent in 1967.

Chemistry. The structures of enclomiphene and tamoxifen are as follows:

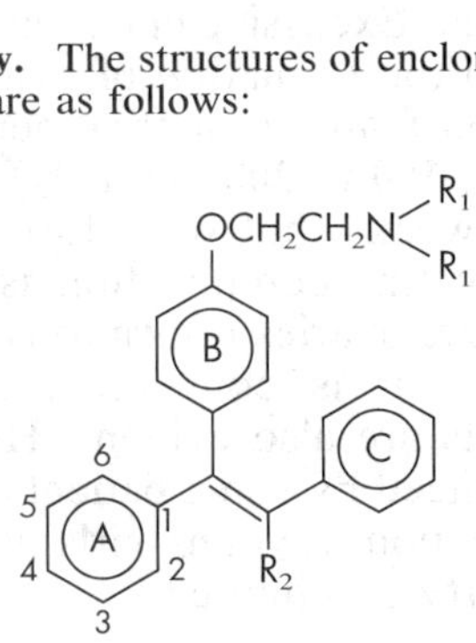

	Enclomiphene	Tamoxifen
R_1:	$—CH_2CH_3$	$—CH_3$
R_2:	—Cl	$—CH_2CH_3$

These triarylethylene antiestrogens are derived from the same stilbene nucleus as diethylstilbestrol (*see* Table 58–1), and they can display either agonist or antagonist activity depending on the orientation of the alkylaminoethoxy side chain. In the *trans* conformation (depicted above), these compounds are antiestrogens; in the *cis* conformation, they are agonists (Jordan *et al.*, 1985). In humans, both stereoisomers can be activated metabolically by hydroxylation at C 4 of the A ring, producing phenolic metabolites with affinities for the estrogen receptor that are 100-fold greater than those of the parent molecules. Although the stereoisomers of tamoxifen and clomiphene are relatively stable, their phenolic metabolites isomerize readily to produce racemic mixtures (Katzenellenbogen *et al.*, 1988). This may explain why antiestrogenic properties observed *in vivo* do not always agree with those detected *in vitro*. Tamoxifen is marketed as the pure *trans* isomer, whereas clomiphene is a racemic mixture of both the *cis* (zuclomiphene) and *trans* (enclomiphene) isomers. New phenolic antiestrogens with structures that cannot isomerize are under investigation (Miquel and Gilbert, 1988).

Pharmacological Effects. Initial animal tests with clomiphene showed very slight estrogenic activity and moderate antiestrogenic activity. The striking effect was inhibition of the pituitary's gonadotropic function. Thus, in both sexes the compound was a potent contraceptive. When given to women, however, the most prominent effect was impressive enlargement of the ovaries. Properly applied, the compound has proven to be a most remarkable and useful agent for the treatment of infertility. Greenblatt and coworkers (1962) found that ovulation can be induced in a high proportion of patients with amenorrhea, the Stein-Leventhal syndrome, and dysfunctional uterine bleeding with anovulatory cycles. Excessive enlargement of the ovaries and the formation of ovarian cysts are common features of treatment if large doses (*e.g.*, 100 to 200 mg daily) are given for 2 or 3 weeks, but with doses of 50 or 75 mg daily this complication is less frequent and the ovaries return to normal size after treatment is completed. Antiestrogenic effects are also evident. Hot flashes are experienced by some patients and vaginal cornification in young girls with precocious puberty is inhibited.

Mechanism of Action. Clomiphene acts as a competitive inhibitor at estrogen receptors, blocking their activation by endogenous estrogens (Jordan, 1984). In premenopausal women, blockade of the estrogen receptor in the anterior pituitary and hypothalamus disrupts normal feedback inhibition of GnRH and gonadotropin secretion, resulting in their enhanced secretion and ultimately in increased gametogenesis and steroidogenesis in the ovaries (*see* Chapter 56). Ovarian stimulation culminates in ovulation and, in some cases, the formation of large cystic ovaries. Not surprisingly, administration of clomiphene to postmenopausal women has little or no effect. The effect of clomiphene in men is similar to that in premenopausal women; augmented gametogenesis and steroidogenesis are observed in the testes.

Absorption, Fate, and Excretion. The pharmacokinetic properties of clomiphene and tamoxifen are very similar (*see* Chapter 52). Clomiphene is well absorbed after oral administration and is cleared slowly from the plasma ($t_{1/2}$ of 5 to 7 days), primarily because of high-affinity binding to plasma proteins, enterohepatic circulation, and accumulation in fatty tissues. Initial metabolism of clomiphene produces long-lived derivatives with antiestrogen activity; the potent activity of the *trans* 4-hydroxy derivative was mentioned above. Nonetheless, clomiphene and its metabolites are usually cleared from the circulation within 3 weeks of oral administration; they are found primarily in the feces (Geier *et al.*, 1987).

Preparations, Therapeutic Uses, and Toxicity. *Clomiphene citrate* (CLOMID, MILOPHENE, SEROPHENE) has been used clinically for the treatment of infertility in women in doses varying between 25 and 200 mg daily by mouth, for periods of a few days to a few weeks. It is available in 50-mg tablets. In view of the development of enlarged ovaries with higher doses, a dose of 50 mg daily for 5 days is recommended initially. This is started on the fifth day of the menstrual cycle except in patients who have not menstruated recently. In infertility and menstrual disorders, treatment has been repeated at monthly intervals with success. If ovulation and fertility are not achieved, the dose may be increased to 100 mg per day for 5 days. Ovulation is achieved in about 80% of patients whose pituitary and ovaries are capable of stimulated function, and pregnancy occurs in 30 to 40% of such women. The basis for the discrepancy between rates of ovulation and conception is not clear but is presumed to result from other causes of infertility (*e.g.*, hyperandrogenism, hyperprolactinemia).

The use of clomiphene can lead to ovarian hyperstimulation with formation of multiple cysts and a high incidence of multiple births (6 to 8%), 75% of which are twins. Although this frequency of multiple births is lower than that observed with gonadotropins (*see* Chapter 56), it is far higher than that observed in the general population (about 1%) (*see* Kennedy and Adashi, 1987). The effects of clomiphene on early gestation are not understood completely, and pregnancy should be ruled out before another course of clomiphene is prescribed.

In-Vitro Fertilization. Clomiphene is used in combination with gonadotropins to promote simultaneous maturation of multiple oocytes and to facilitate their retrieval by stimulation of ovulation at a specific time. Several treatment regimens have been developed for this purpose (Taymor *et al.*, 1985).

Male Infertility. Although some normogonadotropic men with oligozoospermia respond to treatment with clomiphene by improving the quality of semen, success is variable (Homonnai *et al.*, 1988). Criteria for selection of patients who will benefit from such treatment are not clear.

ESTROGEN SYNTHESIS INHIBITORS

Because of the importance of estrogens in metastatic breast cancer (*see* Chapter 52), agents capable of inhibiting estrogen biosynthesis are under investigation as antineoplastic agents.

Gonadotropin-Releasing Hormone (GnRH). The investigational use of GnRH analogs to inhibit ovarian secretion of estrogen is discussed in Chapter 56. These agents do not inhibit estrogen biosynthesis in adipose or other peripheral tissues that are not regulated by gonadotropins.

Aromatase Inhibitors. Inhibition of aromatase blocks the conversion of androgens to estrogens in all tissues; the use of aminoglutethimide for this purpose is discussed in Chapter 52. Unfortunately, aminoglutethimide also inhibits other cytochromes P_{450} that are involved in steroidogenesis (*see* Chapter 60). Several compounds with more selective ability to inhibit aromatase are under investigation, including 4-hydroxyandrostenedione (Dowsett *et al.*, 1987) and various imidazole derivatives (Schieweck *et al.*, 1988). Although these agents are expected to produce fewer side effects than does aminoglutethimide, their advantages over tamoxifen are not yet clear.

PROGESTINS

For some years after Corner and Allen had isolated progesterone from the corpora lutea of sows, the small amounts of the hormone available hampered experimental work and therapeutic application. With the introduction in the 1950s of new classes of progestational agents with prolonged activity and enhanced oral effectiveness, the structures associated with activity were found to be quite diverse. The number of progestins has proliferated, and some are employed widely as contraceptive agents.

Chemistry. Unlike the estrogen receptor, which requires a phenolic A ring for high-affinity binding, the progesterone receptor favors a Δ^4-3-one A ring structure in an inverted $1\beta,2\alpha$-conformation (Duax *et al.*, 1988). Other steroid hormone receptors also bind the Δ^4-3-one structure, although the optimal conformation differs from that for the progesterone receptor. Thus, many synthetic progestins also bind to receptors for glucocorticoids, androgens, and mineralocorticoids and possess a spectrum of activities that is largely dependent on substitutions on the D ring. The progestin analogs of greatest therapeutic interest are effective when given by mouth; some of these are illustrated in Table 58–2 and discussed below.

The first progestin that was reasonably effective orally was 17α-ethinyltestosterone (*ethisterone*). Derivatives of testosterone lacking the angular methyl group (C 19) attached to C 10—the 19-nortestosterones—were much more effective orally. The parent compound, 19-nortestosterone, is inactive, but a number of 17α-alkyl derivatives are effective. The 17α-methyl derivative is progestational and androgenic. 17α-Ethyl-19-nortestosterone (norethandrolone) is also progestational and androgenic and is used clinically as an anabolic agent. 17α-Ethinyl-19-nortestosterone, or norethindrone (norethisterone), is a potent oral progestin in man and is only mildly androgenic. Shift of the double bond in norethindrone yields the isomer norethynodrel, one of the first compounds to be widely used as a contraceptive. Reduction of the 3-keto group of norethindrone yields a partially reduced derivative of ethinyl estradiol termed *ethynodiol*, the diacetate of which is a particularly potent progestational agent. Removal of the oxygen function at position 3 gives rise to an interesting series of compounds, the estrenols, the biological activity of which is critically dependent upon the substituent grouping on C 17. Thus, ethinylestrenol is a powerful progestational agent free of androgenic and anabolic effects, allylestrenol has progestational and other actions, and ethylestrenol is used as an anabolic agent. The 13-ethyl analog of norethindrone, or 18-homonorethisterone (norgestrel), was found to be 100 times as progestational as norethindrone.

Another series of orally active progestins is typified by the compound chlormadinone acetate, which is 6α-chloro-Δ^6-17α-acetoxy progesterone, a purely progestational agent of high potency previously used in contraceptive formulations. The 6-methyl analog has similar properties and is referred to as megestrol.

Although 17α-hydroxyprogesterone, first isolated from the adrenal glands in 1940, is virtually inert, its esters are active and, when given by injection in oil, are long-acting. The caproate has been used extensively as a long-acting progestin, but it is virtually inactive when given by mouth. Other derivatives of 17α-hydroxyprogesterone are effective orally, and the one most widely studied is the

Table 58–2. STRUCTURAL RELATIONSHIP OF VARIOUS PROGESTINS TO PROGESTERONE

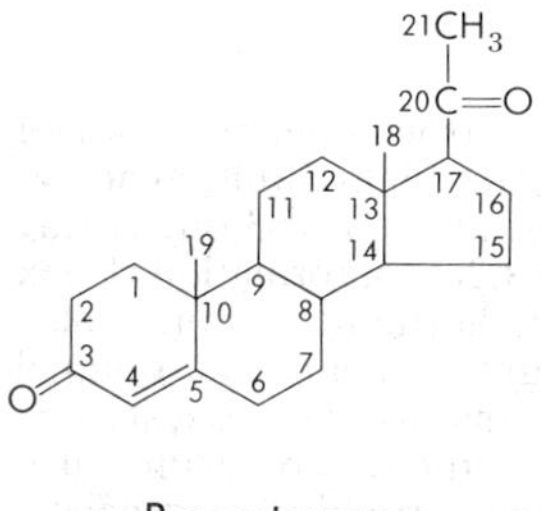

Progesterone

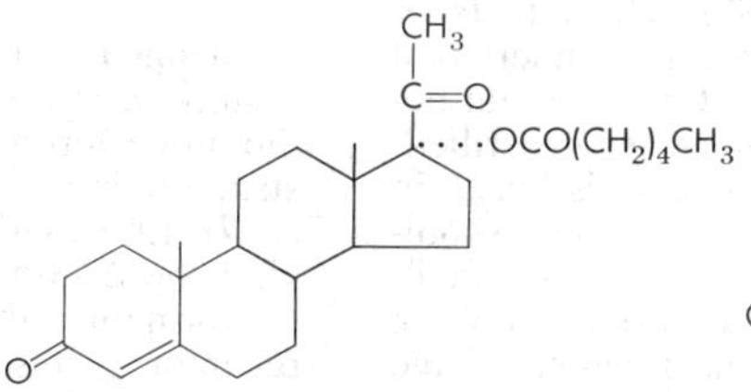

Hydroxyprogesterone Caproate

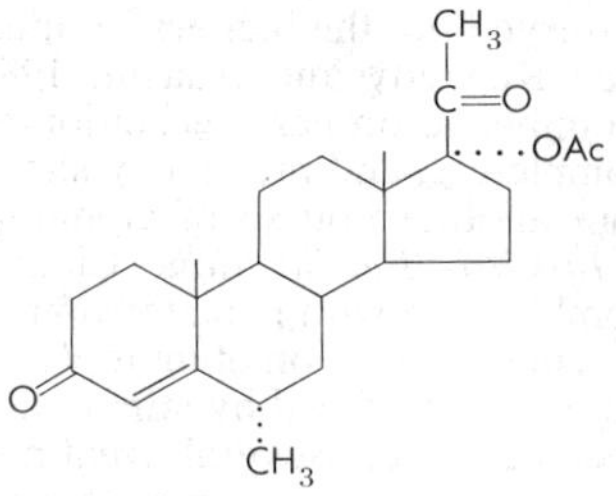

Medroxyprogesterone Acetate

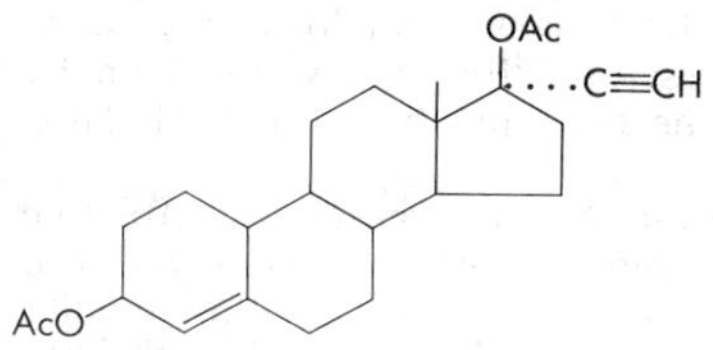

Ethynodiol Diacetate

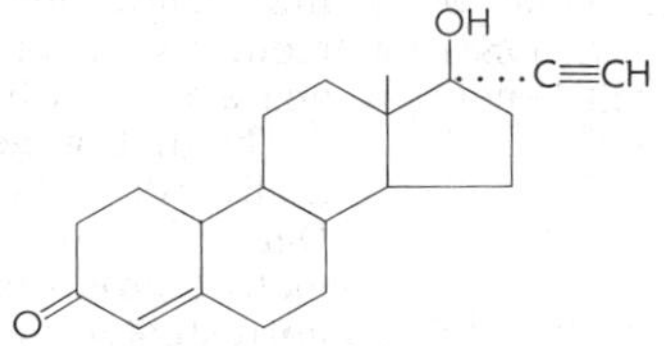

Norethindrone

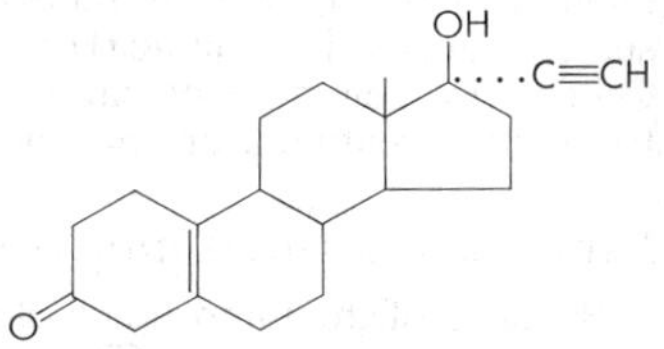

Norethynodrel

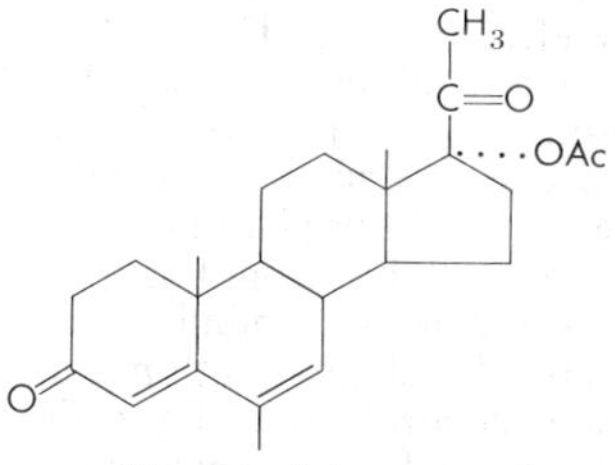

Megestrol Acetate

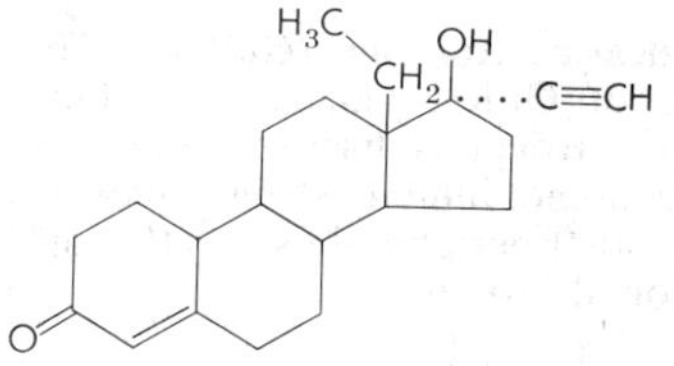

Norgestrel

6-methyl analog medroxyprogesterone acetate. The 16α, 17α-dihydroxy derivative of progesterone in the form of the acetophenone is moderately active when given by mouth but has the property of extremely long action when given parenterally.

Cyproterone acetate is a particularly potent progestin. However, it has had only limited use as a progestin, perhaps because of a greater interest in its use as an antiandrogen (Chapter 59).

Synthesis and Secretion. Progesterone is secreted by the ovary mainly from the corpus luteum during the second half of the menstrual cycle. Secretion actually begins just before ovulation from the follicle that is destined to release an ovum. The formation of progesterone from steroid precursors is summarized in Figure 60–2 (page 1434) and occurs in the ovary, testis, adrenal cortex, and placenta. The stimulatory effect of LH on progesterone synthesis and secretion by the corpus luteum is mediated by an increased synthesis of cyclic AMP.

If the ovum is fertilized, implantation takes place about 7 days later, and almost at once the developing trophoblast secretes its luteotropic hormone (chorionic gonadotropin) into the maternal circulation, thereby sustaining the functional life of the corpus luteum. Chorionic gonadotropin, detectable in urine several days before the expected time of the next menstrual period, is excreted in progressively increasing amounts for the next 5 weeks or so, and in reduced quantities thereafter throughout pregnancy. During the second or third month of pregnancy the developing placenta begins to secrete estrogen and progesterone in collaboration with the fetal adrenal glands, and thereafter the corpus luteum is not essential to continued gestation. Estrogen and progesterone continue to be secreted in large amounts by the placenta up to the time of delivery.

Measurements of the rate of secretion of progesterone suggest that, from a few milligrams a day secreted during the follicular phase of the cycle, the rate increases to 10 to 20 mg during the luteal phase and to several hundred milligrams during the latter part of pregnancy. Rates of from 1 to 5 mg per day have been measured in men, and are comparable to the values in women during the follicular phase of the cycle.

Physiological and Pharmacological Actions. Progesterone released during the luteal phase of the cycle leads to the development of a secretory endometrium. Abrupt decline in the release of progesterone from the corpus luteum at the end of the cycle is the main determinant of the onset of menstruation. If the duration of the luteal phase is artificially lengthened, either by sustaining luteal function or by treatment with progesterone, decidual changes in the endometrial stroma similar to those seen in early pregnancy can be induced. Under normal circumstances, estrogen antecedes and accompanies progesterone in its action upon the endometrium and is essential to the development of the normal pattern.

Progesterone also influences the endocervical glands, and the abundant watery secretion of the estrogen-stimulated structures is changed to a scant viscid material. When the estrogen-stimulated secretion dries on a glass slide, sodium chloride crystallizes to form a dendritic pattern called "ferning." Progestins inhibit this pattern.

The estrogen-induced maturation of the human vaginal epithelium is modified toward the condition of pregnancy by the action of progesterone, a change that can be detected in cytological alterations in the vaginal smear. If the quantity of estrogen concurrently acting is known to be adequate, or if it is assured by giving estrogen, the cytological response to a progestin can be used to evaluate its progestational potency.

Pregnancy. The increasing concentrations of progesterone that are present during the course of pregnancy have been discussed above. While progesterone is very important for the maintenance of pregnancy, in that it suppresses menstruation and uterine contractility, other effects may be equally important. The effects of progesterone to maintain pregnancy have led to the use of progestins to prevent threatened abortion. However, administration of progestins is of questionable benefit, probably because diminished progesterone is rarely the cause of spontaneous abortion (*see* below).

Mammary Gland. During pregnancy and to a minor degree during the luteal phase of the cycle, progesterone, acting with estrogen, brings about a proliferation of the acini of the mammary gland. Toward the end of pregnancy the acini fill with secretion and the vasculature of the gland is notably increased; however, only after the influences of estrogen and progesterone are withdrawn by the event of parturition does lactation begin. The action of estrogen or estrogen and progesterone, when used post partum for relieving the sensation of engorgement, is probably largely a direct one upon the mammary tissue to inhibit the effects of prolactin and the secretion of milk.

Thermogenic Action. If the body temperature is measured each day throughout the normal menstrual cycle, preferably at the same time before arising each morning, an increase of about 1° F may be noted at midcycle; this correlates with the event of ovulation. The temperature rise persists for the remainder of the cycle until the onset of menstrual flow. The phenomenon is caused by progesterone, as can be shown by its administration.

Mechanism of Action. Like other steroid hormones, progestins diffuse freely into the cell nucleus, where they bind to the progesterone receptor and ultimately influence the transcription of a limited set of genes (*see* Chapter 2). The progesterone receptor has the narrowest tissue distribution of any steroid hormone receptor, being expressed primarily in the female reproductive tract. The antiestrogenic action of progestins is mediated in part by the induction of 17-hydroxysteroid dehydrogenase (which catalyzes the oxidation of estradiol to the less potent estrone) and estrogen sulfotransferase (which catalyzes the sulfation and inactivation of estrogens); expression of estrogen receptors is also repressed. Progesterone promotes cell differentiation at the expense of growth, which is enhanced by estrogens.

Absorption, Fate, and Excretion. Administered orally, progesterone is relatively ineffective because of extensive first-pass metabolism in the liver. Progesterone injected in oily solution is also absorbed rapidly and metabolized quickly, but, if given daily in sufficient doses, is thoroughly effective. The half-life of progesterone in the circulation is only a few minutes, and many pregnane derivatives and isomers conjugated with glucuronide or sulfate are ultimately found in the urine. One of the major urinary products is the glucuronide of pregnane-3α,20α-diol. Pregnanediol is a specific product of progesterone metabolism, and its measurement in plasma or urine provides a valuable index of the secretion of endogenous progesterone. Approximately 1 mg per day is excreted during the follicular phase of the cycle, after menopause, and by men. During the luteal phase of the cycle 2- to 4-mg amounts are excreted daily, and during pregnancy the values increase to 50 to 70 mg before term.

Many analogs of progesterone that are less susceptible to hepatic metabolism are more effective than progesterone when given orally. The structures of these agents are shown in Table 58–2.

Preparations. Many orally active and parenteral preparations of progestational agents are available (*see* Table 58–2). Some of these substances when given in combination with estrogens are used widely as oral contraceptives, which are discussed below.

Progesterone injection (PROGESTAJECT, others) contains 25 to 100 mg of progesterone per milliliter of vegetable oil. Progesterone is peculiar among the commonly used steroids in being locally irritating, and not more than about 100 mg can be given intramuscularly in a single injection. Aqueous suspensions of progesterone are particularly painful and are seldom used. Progesterone is also available in a T-shaped intrauterine contraceptive device that provides continuous delivery of progesterone in the uterine cavity for 1 year. This is marketed under the name of PROGESTASERT and contains 38 mg of progesterone.

Medroxyprogesterone acetate (DEPO-PROVERA) contains 100 or 400 mg/ml in aqueous medium for intramuscular injection, and *medroxyprogesterone acetate tablets* (PROVERA, others) contain 2.5, 5, or 10 mg each.

Hydroxyprogesterone caproate injection (DURALUTIN, others) is provided as an oily solution of 125 mg/ml or 250 mg/ml for intramuscular injection.

Megestrol acetate (MEGACE) is available in 20- and 40-mg tablets.

Norethindrone (MICRONOR, NORLUTIN, NOR-QD) and *norethindrone acetate* (AYGESTIN, NORLUTATE) are available alone in 0.35- and 5-mg tablets and in combination with estrogens as oral contraceptives (*see* below).

Norgestrel (OVRETTE) is available in 0.075-mg tablets as an oral contraceptive; it and a variety of other oral progestin preparations are also combined with estrogens (ethinyl estradiol or mestranol) as oral contraceptives (*see* Table 58–3, page 1404).

It is not possible to give accurate values for the relative clinical effectiveness of the several compounds because careful comparisons are limited in number and different responses have been used in the published studies. In various tests in women, as with different bioassays in animals, the relative potencies of the progestins are not the same. Furthermore, some progestins possess more or less estrogenic and androgenic activities than do others.

Therapeutic Uses. Application of physiological principles in the management of ovarian disorders and contraception has made it possible to use these agents with notable therapeutic success.

Contraception. This represents the major use of these agents and is discussed later in this chapter.

Dysfunctional Uterine Bleeding. This is a common disorder, characterized by irregular cycles and episodes of prolonged hemorrhage. The condition may arise at any time during menstrual life, but is more frequent in young girls before regular ovulatory cycles are established and again with the approach of menopause. The condition usually results from the continuous action of estrogen, which causes endometrial hyperplasia, combined with an insufficient amount and poor cycling of progesterone. Other causes for uterine bleeding must be excluded before initiating cyclic therapy with progestins.

The immediate goal is to stop the bleeding, and the long-range aim is to regulate the cycle. It is best to give an orally active progestin in full doses to stop the bleeding. Five to 10 mg of norethindrone every 4 to 6 hours will usually be effective in 24 hours, and then 5 mg twice daily can be continued for 1 or 2 weeks to give a respite from bleeding. Withdrawal bleeding at the end of treatment will, in effect, be a normal menstrual flow, usually accompanied by cramps; however, it will be self-limited in duration and, if nothing further is done, there will be a free interval of several weeks. Other progestins may also be used, but those without inherent estrogenic activity are more effective if combined with an estrogen such as 0.1 mg of mestranol daily. To prevent a recurrence of bleeding, cyclic therapy is called for; an oral progestin, such as norethindrone, in a dose of 5 to 20 mg daily is given at monthly intervals from days 5 to 25 of the cycle. Regular menstrual periods can thus be induced for as long as one chooses.

Dysmenorrhea. Relief of dysmenorrhea by inhibiting ovulation is discussed in the section on estrogen. A progestin can be used to advantage either with the estrogen from days 5 to 25 of the cycle or added to the estrogen during the last 5 days. In either case menstruation is prompt, the treatment can be resumed 5 days later, and the cycle can be repeated indefinitely. Such cycles are quite physiological, lacking only the ovarian components and ovulation. As discussed earlier, nonsteroidal anti-inflammatory agents are the preferred method of therapy.

Premenstrual Syndrome. This is an ill-defined condition of uncertain etiology. Changes in concentrations of hormones and electrolytes are probably responsible for the irritability, breast tenderness, headache, and weight gain during the luteal phase of the cycle. Although progestins have been used, there is little or no evidence to suggest efficacy. Sometimes the symptoms are sufficiently distressing to warrant inhibition of ovulation with combined progestin-estrogen therapy.

Endometriosis. The severe dysmenorrhea of this condition is not completely understood. In many instances, suppression of ovulation with estrogen is followed by a painless, estrogen-withdrawal period; this suggests that the pain in the two conditions is of similar origin. Treatment of this form of endometriosis thus becomes the treatment of dysmenorrhea. In certain severe cases of endometriosis, the major problem is the development of painful extrauterine masses and infertility. Treatment is aimed at causing regression of the ectopic endometrial growths. Prolonged treatment, designed to prevent menstruation for many months, relieves a major difficulty by preventing bleeding into the endometrial masses or peritoneal cavity. Favorable effects have been achieved even with the continuous use of estrogen alone for this purpose. Better results have been described from the continuous use of oral progestins, and actual regression of the endometrial growths is observed. Norethindrone acetate may be used in oral doses of 5 mg daily for 2 weeks, after which the dose is increased in increments of 2.5 mg per day every 2 weeks until 15 mg per day is reached. Therapy may be continued for 6 to 9 months. Symptomatic relief can be expected in about 80% of patients and return of fertility in about 50% of patients. Danazol, which is a weak androgen, is also effective for the treatment of endometriosis (*see* Chapter 59).

Threatened and Habitual Abortion. Progestins have been used extensively in attempts to prevent abortion, but there is no evidence that the treatment is effective in the majority of patients. In addition, these agents may cause virilization and genital deformities of the fetus (Jacobson, 1962; Wentz, 1977; Aarskog, 1979).

There are thought to be a few patients who have an inadequate luteal response to gonadotropins with deficient secretion of progesterone; such women may benefit from treatment with a progestin during the first trimester of pregnancy. To identify such patients, plasma and urinary metabolites of progesterone must be determined to establish that a deficiency exists. The potential risks to the fetus must also be considered.

Suppression of Postpartum Lactation. While the administration of estrogens and/or progestins is effective in suppressing lactation in the immediate postpartum period, as mentioned above, their use for this purpose is not recommended. Significant reduction in milk secretion is seen with concentrations of estrogens and progestins achieved with use of some oral contraceptive preparations.

Carcinoma. Progestins may be used as a palliative measure in recurrent or metastatic endometrial carcinoma. When used in this manner, megestrol acetate may be given in divided oral doses of 40 to 320 mg daily for several months as a trial. Alternative therapy is the weekly intramuscular administration of 400 to 1000 mg of medroxyprogesterone acetate. Improvement can be expected in about one half of the patients treated (*see* Wentz, 1977). Progestins have also been used in the palliative treatment of renal carcinoma and breast carcinoma (*see* Chapter 52).

Hypoventilation. Progestins can stimulate respiration and have been used with some success in obese patients with hypoventilation (Pickwickian syndrome). However, other measures, particularly weight reduction and therapy for any pulmonary infection, should be stressed.

ANTIPROGESTINS

Antiprogestins are under investigation as contraceptive and contragestational agents. Efforts have concentrated on the development of competitive inhibitors that act at progesterone receptors (*e.g.*, mifepristone) and inhibitors of progesterone synthesis.

MIFEPRISTONE

Chemistry. Mifepristone (RU-486) is a potent competitive inhibitor that acts at both progesterone and glucocorticoid receptors. First synthesized in 1980 and undergoing clinical trials since 1982, it is an 11β-substituted derivative of norethindrone with the following structure:

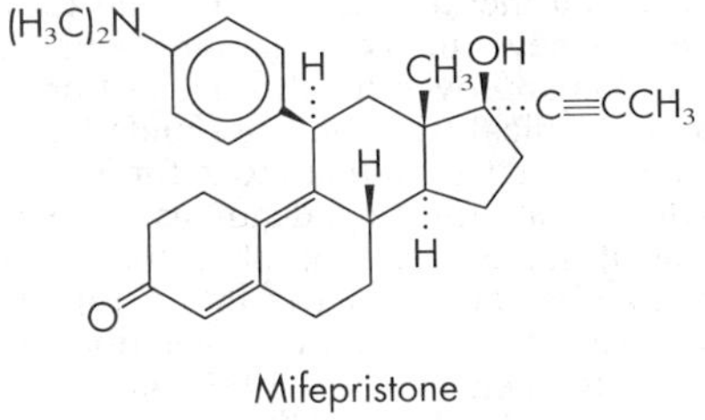

Mifepristone

Pharmacological Actions. Mifepristone is a weak partial agonist with predominantly antagonistic activity. When administered to normal women in the follicular phase of the menstrual cycle, the drug prevents ovulation by blocking progesterone at the level of the pituitary or hypothalamus; this suppresses the midcycle surge of gonadotropins and delays follicular development. During the luteal phase of the cycle, mifepristone acts directly on the uterus to block the action of progesterone, resulting in release of prostaglandins from the endometrium and subsequent menstrual bleeding. Similarly, mifepristone can terminate early pregnancy by facilitating luteolysis, menstruation, uterine motility, and detachment of the embryo. Other antiprogestational activities include softening of the cervix.

Mifepristone is also a glucocorticoid antagonist, and it binds to the rat glucocorticoid receptor with an affinity fourfold greater than that of dexamethasone. This blocks cortisol-mediated hypothalamic feedback inhibition, elicits the secretion of corticotropin-releasing hormone and corticotropin, and ultimately stimulates adrenal steroidogenesis.

Although mifepristone does not bind to receptors for estrogens or mineralocorticoids, it does bind to the rat prostate androgen receptor and possesses weak antiandrogenic activity.

Absorption, Fate, and Excretion. The oral bioavailability of mifepristone is about 25% and it is active by this route. Plasma levels peak about 2 to 3 hours after administration; the drug is then cleared slowly ($t_{1/2}$ of 20 hours) because of binding to plasma proteins (albumin and α_1-acid glycoprotein) and enterohepatic circulation. Mifepristone is inactivated by extensive metabolism in animals, and the metabolic products are found predominantly in the feces.

Therapeutic Prospects. Mifepristone is most promising as a therapeutic abortifacient for use in early pregnancy; in combination with prostaglandins, it is approved for this use in Europe and elsewhere. Clinical trials also are underway to establish the efficacy of mifepristone for induction of labor after intrauterine fetal death, as a cervical ripening agent in anticipation of second trimester abortion, and as an adjunct in the therapy of progesterone-sensitive tumors. (For additional discussion, *see* Baulieu *et al.*, 1987; Couzinet and Schaison, 1988; Baulieu, 1989a,b.)

PROGESTERONE SYNTHESIS INHIBITORS

Many such compounds are under investigation; they consist mostly of steroid derivatives that inhibit 3β-hydroxysteroid dehydrogenase (*see* Figure 60–2, page 1434; *see also* Ray and Sharma, 1987). Although these inhibitors are relatively selective *in vitro*, the role of progesterone as an intermediate in the biosynthesis of estrogens, androgens, glucocorticoids, and mineralocorticoids suggests that they are unlikely to be selective antiprogestins *in vivo*.

ORAL CONTRACEPTIVES

Of drugs requiring a prescription, oral contraceptives are among the most widely used agents. It is estimated that 10 million women in the United States and about 60 million worldwide are currently taking these agents.

History. The incredible growth of the world population stands out as one of the fundamental events of our era. The current world population of about 5 billion is expected to be 6 billion by the year 2000; most of the growth will be in underdeveloped countries. The Old Testament dictum "Be fruitful, and multiply" (Genesis 9:1) has been religiously followed by readers and nonreaders of the Bible alike. In 1798, Thomas Robert Malthus started a great controversy by opposing the prevailing view of unlimited progress for man by making two postulates and a conclusion. He postulated that "food is necessary to the existence of man," and that sexual attraction between woman and man is necessary and likely to persist, since "towards the extinction of the passion between the sexes, no progress whatever has hitherto been made," barring ". . . individual exceptions." Malthus concluded that "the power of population is infinitely greater than the power in the earth to produce subsistence for man," a "natural inequality" that would someday loom "insurmountable in the way to the perfectibility of society." Malthus' essay sparked great controversy and inquiry into the principle governing the growth of population. In seeking to discover the causes of population increase, T. R. Edmonds in 1832 suggested that "a deterioration in the condition of the English labourers . . . , the destruction of the feeling of self-respect" was such a great distress that "among the great body of the people . . . , sexual intercourse is the only gratification. . . . When they are better fed they will have other enjoyments at command than sexual intercourse, and their numbers . . . will not increase in the same proportion as at present." Today we realize that our sheer numbers have increased so much that they are straining Earth's capacity to supply food, energy, and raw materials. We also know, perhaps better than T. R. Edmonds, where some of the blame for this growth lies. Advances in medicine and public health have led to a significant decline in mortality and an increased life expectancy. Thus, medical science has begun to assume a portion of the responsibility for overpopulation. To this end, drugs in the form of hormones and their analogs have been developed to control human fertility.

As discussed below, oral contraceptives are very effective and are expected to play a major role in control of the world population explosion. The small but definite incidence of serious side effects that results from these agents must be weighed against some of the dire consequences of uncontrolled population growth. Furthermore, in underdeveloped nations the morbidity and mortality of pregnancy and delivery far exceed the incidence of adverse reactions from oral contraceptives. Indeed, in many countries oral contraceptives are available without a physician's prescription.

A comprehensive investigation of the inhibition of ovulation by the use of progestational agents was initiated by Rock, Pincus, and Garcia. The study showed that ovulation could be abolished at will for as long as desired and with great regularity (*see* Rock *et al.*, 1957; Pincus, 1960). The compounds used were derivatives of 19-nortestosterone, given by mouth from day 5 to day 25 of the menstrual cycle (the first day of menses is day 1). Extensive field studies of a combination of the progestin norethynodrel and the estrogen mestranol were started in San Juan, Puerto Rico, in 1955, under the direction of Pincus and associates at the Puerto Rico Family Planning Center. The success of these studies prompted many others, and the results of broad, almost worldwide, experience followed.

Among the first of the orally active steroids to be used in inhibiting ovulation, some had inherent estrogenic activity and some preparations of the progestins were later found to be contaminated with estrogen. In a way this was a happy chance, because it served to show that estrogen enhanced the suppressive effect of the progestin and led to the general use of a mixture of the two. As experience has been gained, the doses of progestin and estrogen have been decreased to minimize side effects while maintaining contraceptive efficacy.

Types of Oral Contraceptives. The most common type of oral contraceptive is the combination preparation, which contains both an estrogen and a progestin. Experience with these preparations shows them to be 99 to 100% effective. This method of reversible contraception is, then, the most effective yet devised. Other modifications of steroidal contraception have also been tried with success. Sequential preparations, in which an estrogen is taken for 14 to 16 days and a combination of an estrogen and a progestin is then taken for 5 or 6 days, have been about 98 to 99% successful as oral contraceptives. However, because of reports suggesting an increased incidence of endometrial tumors and a lower efficacy, sequential preparations of this type have been removed from the market. They have been replaced by products that contain estrogen and relatively low amounts of a progestin and with which the amount of progestin taken is varied during the monthly cycle. Biphasic and triphasic formulations of sequential preparations of oral contraceptives are listed in Table 58–3. These preparations have been developed in attempts to lower the total amounts of hormone given and thus to reduce the incidence and severity of side effects.

Single-entity preparations are also available. A progestin alone has come to be called the "minipill," while an estrogen alone is a postcoital or "morning-after pill." The "minipills" were introduced in order to eliminate the estrogen, the agent in combined preparations that was thought to be responsible for most of the side effects of oral contraceptives. Since the contraceptive efficacy of the "minipill" is about 97 to 98%, which is somewhat less than that of the combined preparations, and the menstrual cycles are more irregular, these preparations have been less popular. The intramuscular injection of medroxyprogesterone every few months has been effective but is not approved for use as a contraceptive in the United States because of the development of breast and uterine tumors in animals (*FDA Drug Bulletin*, 1978b). Diethylstilbestrol is effective as a postcoital contraceptive. Although its general use for this purpose is unpleasant and may be dangerous, postcoital contraception with an estrogen can be useful when the desirability of avoiding pregnancy is obvious, as in cases of rape or incest.

Preparations and Dosage. Some of the formulations used as oral contraceptives are listed in Table 58–3. The combined preparations contain 0.02 to 0.05 mg of ethinyl estradiol or mestranol and various amounts of a progestin, and are taken for 21 days. The next course is started 7 days after the last dose or 5 days after the onset of the menstrual flow. It should be noted that ethinyl estradiol is approximately twice as potent as mestranol.

Sequential preparations are formulated to be taken in two (biphasic) or three (triphasic) continuous phases. With biphasic preparations a fixed-dose combination of an estrogen and progestin is taken for 10 days, followed by a different fixed-dose combination of estrogen and progestin for 11 days. The pills are discontinued for 7 days before the cyclic administration is resumed. Triphasic preparations contain the same or different quantities of an estrogen and variable quantities of a progestin in three sets of tablets. Each set is taken for 5 to 10 days, depending upon the specific formulation. After 21 days of administration, the medication is discontinued for 7 days before the cycle is resumed.

Table 58–3. COMPOSITION AND DOSES OF SOME ORAL CONTRACEPTIVES

ESTROGEN (*mg*)	PROGESTIN [1] (*mg*)	REPRESENTATIVE TRADE NAME
Combinations [2]		
0.02 Ethinyl estradiol	1.0 Norethindrone acetate	LOESTRIN 1/20
0.03 Ethinyl estradiol	0.3 Norgestrel	LO/OVRAL
0.03 Ethinyl estradiol	1.5 Norethindrone acetate	LOESTRIN 1.5/30
0.03 Ethinyl estradiol	0.15 Levonorgestrel	NORDETTE
0.035 Ethinyl estradiol	0.4 Norethindrone	OVCON 35
0.035 Ethinyl estradiol	0.5 Norethindrone	BREVICON
0.035 Ethinyl estradiol	1.0 Ethynodiol diacetate	DEMULEN 1/35
0.035 Ethinyl estradiol	1.0 Norethindrone	ORTHO-NOVUM 1/35
0.05 Mestranol	1.0 Norethindrone	ORTHO-NOVUM 1/50
0.05 Ethinyl estradiol	0.5 Norgestrel	OVRAL
0.05 Ethinyl estradiol	1.0 Ethynodiol diacetate	DEMULEN 1/50
0.05 Ethinyl estradiol	1.0 Norethindrone	OVCON 50
0.05 Ethinyl estradiol	1.0 Norethindrone acetate	NORLESTRIN 1/50
0.05 Ethinyl estradiol	2.5 Norethindrone acetate	NORLESTRIN 2.5/50
Sequentials [3]		
0.03, 0.04, 0.03 Ethinyl estradiol	0.05, 0.075, 0.125 Levonorgestrel	TRI-LEVLEN
0.035 Ethinyl estradiol	0.5, 1.0, 0.5 Norethindrone	TRI-NORINYL
0.035 Ethinyl estradiol	0.5, 0.75, 1.0 Norethindrone	ORTHO-NOVUM 7/7/7
0.035 Ethinyl estradiol	0.5, 1.0 Norethindrone	ORTHO-NOVUM 10/11
"Minipills" [4]		
—	0.35 Norethindrone	MICRONOR
—	0.075 Norgestrel	OVRETTE
Postcoital [5]		
Diethylstilbestrol	—	—

[1] Of the progestins used, norgestrel is strongly androgenic, while the others have moderate androgenic activity.

[2] Combination tablets are taken for 21 days and are omitted for 7 days. These preparations are listed in order of increasing content of estrogen.

[3] These preparations include fixed-dose tablets with the same or different amounts of estrogen and variable amounts of progestin. With biphasic preparations, the first set of tablets is taken for 10 days and the second for 11 days, followed by 7 days of no medication. With triphasic preparations, each set of tablets is taken for 5 to 10 days in three sequential phases, followed by 7 days of no medication. (*See* text.)

[4] "Minipills" are taken daily continually.

[5] Diethylstilbestrol is taken in a dose of 25 mg twice daily for 5 days within 72 hours after sexual intercourse; *see* text for indications.

Many contraceptive preparations are dispensed in convenient calendar-like containers that help the user to count the days. Some obviate the need of counting by incorporating seven blank pills in the package to provide 3 weeks of treatment and 1 week of no treatment. A pill is taken every day, regardless of when menstruation starts or stops. Iron is included in the "blank" pills in some preparations.

The "minipills" (MICRONOR and NOR-QD, containing 0.35 mg of norethindrone, and OVRETTE, containing 75 μg of norgestrel) are taken daily continually. Since they are less effective and pregnancy is possible during their administration, patients should discontinue the "minipill" if they have amenorrhea for more than 45 to 60 days, and they should be examined for pregnancy. Likewise, if patients have missed one or more pills and have amenorrhea for more than 45 days, they should be similarly evaluated.

Medroxyprogesterone acetate (DEPO-PROVERA) is injected intramuscularly in a dose of 150 mg every 3 months (or 450 mg every 6 months) but should be used only if the possibility of permanent infertility is acceptable to the patient. An unpredictable duration of amenorrhea and anovulation can result from such therapy. Although long-acting preparations of a progestin are employed in a number of countries for contraception (*see* Vecchio, 1976), such use remains investigational in the United States.

The postcoital contraceptive diethylstilbestrol is started within 72 hours after sexual intercourse at a dose of 25 mg twice daily for 5 days. To be effective the tablets must be continued for 5 consecutive days in spite of nausea and vomiting, which commonly occur. Since estrogens are not advised in pregnancy because of the possibility of vaginal carcinoma in female offspring (*see* above), abortion should be performed if diethylstilbestrol is not effective.

Mechanism of Action. The administration of estrogen and a progestin could interfere with fertility in any of several ways. However, it is clear that, as currently used, the mixture inhibits ovulation. The effects of ovarian hormones upon the gonadotropic functions of the pituitary are discussed earlier in this chapter; the predominant effect of estrogen is to inhibit the secretion of FSH, while continued action of progesterone serves to inhibit the release of LH. It is clear that ovulation could be prevented either by inhibiting the ovulatory stimulus or by preventing the growth of follicles, and this accords with the experimental observations that follicular growth and ovulation can be prevented by either estrogen or progesterone given singly. The orally active progestins cannot be equated as a group with progesterone because some are inherently estrogenic, some are androgenic, and some are purely progestational; correspondingly, their ovulation-inhibiting potentialities may be mediated in somewhat different ways.

Measurements of circulating FSH and LH show that estrogen–progestin combinations suppress both hormones. The plasma concentrations of FSH and LH are stable; early follicular FSH and midcycle FSH and LH peaks are not seen (Swerdloff and Odell, 1969; Briggs, 1976).

One might reasonably conclude that the most widely used preparations to date owe their effectiveness in inhibiting ovulation to the estrogenic component and that the progestin serves the major purpose of ensuring that withdrawal bleeding will be prompt, brief, and essentially physiological.

Even if ovulation were not prevented, it is easy to imagine that the contraceptive agents could interfere with impregnation by their direct actions upon the genital tract. The endometrium must be in just the right stage of development under estrogen and progesterone for nidation to take place. It seems unlikely that implantation would be possible in the altered endometrium developed under the influence of most of the suppressants. Similarly, the abundant watery secretion of the cervix at the time of ovulation has always been regarded as essential to the well-being of the sperm, and the thick tenacious mucus secreted under the influence of progesterone to be a hostile environment. Although it can easily be imagined that estrogen–progestin mixtures could interfere with impregnation in these ways, there has been no opportunity to find out, because ovulation is almost always prevented when the agents are used in the usual way.

The fear that estrogen may have deleterious effects prompted the use of a progestin alone in various ways. Continuous administration of a progestin in sufficient dose abolishes the cycle for as long as it is given and leads to ovarian and endometrial atrophy. Very small doses may alter the structure of the endometrium and the consistency of the cervical mucus without disrupting the cycle or inhibiting ovulation. As currently administered, oral contraceptives that contain only a progestin cause variable suppression of FSH, LH, and ovulation, which may explain their lower degree of efficacy (*see* Briggs, 1976). With continued daily administration, menstruation occurs but the length of the cycle and the duration of bleeding are quite variable, factors that have influenced their popularity.

Long-acting progestins, given by intramuscular injection, are also effective, as noted above. For example, 150 mg of medroxyprogesterone acetate, administered every 3 months starting just after parturition, prevents pregnancy in all; irregular bleeding, troublesome at first, gives way to amenorrhea and an atrophic endometrium in most cases. Alternatively, an intrauterine device containing a reservoir of 38 mg of progesterone is available (*see* above) and releases progesterone continuously into the uterine cavity for 1 year. It is about as effective as other intrauterine devices (97 to 98%), and the side effects are also similar except that the incidence of ectopic pregnancies may be greater (*FDA Drug Bulletin,* 1978a).

The development of postcoital contraceptives is an intriguing subject. A vast number of hormones and other agents are effective in this regard in animals. It has long been known that the use of large doses of estrogen in women is effective in preventing implantation, but such doses are tolerated only in cases of single or very infrequent exposure. There is a rough correlation between the contraceptive potency of these substances and their estrogenic activity.

Large doses of estrogens used as postcoital contraceptives may act by inhibiting fertilization and nidation in several ways. The motility of the oviduct may be altered, the endometrium is changed, and withdrawal from the large doses of estrogens induces bleeding. The experimental use of progesterone antagonists such as mifepristone is discussed earlier in this chapter.

Undesirable Effects. A variety of major and minor side effects have been attributed to the use of oral contraceptives. In some instances the undesirable effects are well documented and their incidence has been determined. Of most concern are cardiovascular side effects and the induction or promotion of tumors. However, a number of possible side effects are not well substantiated. Most data on the undesirable effects of oral contraceptives have been gathered retrospectively and without appropriate controls. Furthermore, most studies utilized older preparations that contained higher amounts of estrogen and progestin than are currently in use. Since there are few well-controlled, prospective studies with the more modern preparations, current views of the undesirable effects of oral contraceptives are often extrapolations from older data. Furthermore, the incidence of some disorders is lowered by the use of oral contraceptives. An assessment of the risk-to-benefit ratio is essential for each patient in order to provide the most efficacious method of contraception with the least possible risk.

Cardiovascular Disorders. Clinical trials in sizable groups of women had been underway for 5 years or so before side effects of any consequence were described. Instances of thrombophlebitis, a rare disorder in healthy young women, then began to be noted, and several reports of thromboembolism appeared from England (Inman and Vessey, 1968; Vessey and Doll, 1968). In the latter report it was estimated that the incidence of thrombophlebitis in young women was increased six- to tenfold with oral contraceptives.

These retrospective (case–control) studies suffered from a statistical dilemma, because what was really studied was the incidence of medication among those with complications versus those without. Case–control studies are also generally criticized since cause-and-effect relationships cannot be established, the actual incidence of drug-associated illness cannot be determined, and biases are introduced owing to the means by which information is obtained (*see* Chapter 4).

Because of the British reports, numerous retrospective and prospective studies have since been conducted. The consensus of these reports is that the incidence of thrombophlebitis and thromboembolism is increased, and the incidence of thromboembolism is greater with preparations containing higher doses of estrogens. The Coronary Drug Project Research Group (1973) also found a twofold increase in the incidence of thrombophlebitis and pulmonary embolism in *men* who received conjugated estrogens daily for 4 to 5 years.

The increase in the incidence of thromboembolism is also supported by studies of various clotting factors and platelet aggregation (Bonnar, 1987; Huch *et al.*, 1987; Meade, 1988). Patients taking estrogens or combined oral contraceptives have increased platelet aggregation, accelerated blood clotting, altered blood concentrations of some clotting factors, and altered fibrinolytic activity. Venous thromboembolism appears to be attributable to the estrogen in these preparations, whereas arterial complications are probably due to both the estrogen and the progestin (Bonnar, 1987; Meade, 1988).

The incidence of cerebral and coronary thrombosis is also increased in "pill" users (Inman *et al.*, 1970). The Collaborative Group for the Study of Stroke in Young Women (1973, 1975) found an increased incidence of thrombotic and hemorrhagic strokes among women taking oral contraceptives. Similarly, in men with prostatic carcinoma the administration of diethylstilbestrol daily was associated with an increased incidence of myocardial infarction and strokes (Veterans Administration, 1967). Users of the "pill" appear to have a two- to fivefold greater incidence of nonfatal and fatal myocardial infarction and a two- to tenfold increase in the frequency of strokes (Kaplan, 1978; Vessey, 1980; Porter *et al.*, 1987; Shaw, 1987; Meade, 1988). The increased incidence of myocardial infarction is related to the duration of use of oral contraceptives, and the risk may remain elevated after the agent is discontinued (Slone *et al.,* 1981). The increased risk of myocardial infarction with use of oral contraceptives is additive to other risk factors, such as age, smoking, and hypertension (Woods, 1988); this information has been added to oral contraceptive package inserts.

Mild hypertension has been observed in many and significant hypertension in about 5% of those who use oral contraceptives (Weinberger, 1982; Woods, 1988). Although the increase in blood pressure is usually gradual, it may be quite severe. Generally the hypertension is reversible within several months of discontinuation of medication. These effects probably result from the capacity of both estrogen and progestin to facilitate retention of Na^+ and water secondary to increases in plasma renin activity and subsequent formation of angiotensin. However, the precise mechanism is not understood.

Most agree that the morbidity and mortality from cardiovascular diseases are increased with the use of combined oral contraceptives. The magnitude of the increased mortality is about two- to fourfold and is primarily from ischemic heart disease and cerebrovascular accidents (Royal College of General Practitioners' Oral Contraception Study, 1981; Slone *et al.,* 1981). However, thromboembolism and other cardiovascular disorders also contribute. The increased mortality is most apparent in women over 35 years of age and is greatest in women who smoke or have other risk factors for cardiovascular disorders. Mortality may increase as much as 15- to 18-fold in women over 45 years of age who smoke. Older women with risk factors for cardiovascular disease should be advised to consider other forms of contraception. The use of preparations with lower quantities of estrogen and progestin reduces the risks but does not eliminate them (*see* Speroff, 1982; Bonnar, 1987; Shaw, 1987; Meade, 1988; Woods, 1988).

The incidence of thrombophlebitis and other cardiovascular disorders rises during pregnancy and the postpartum period. Furthermore, increased mortality from various causes during pregnancy supports the view that the increased incidence of cardiovascular disorders with oral contraceptives is probably a comparatively minor and acceptable risk, since pregnancy is effectively prevented. Serious complications of pregnancy are perhaps so much more frequent than are those resulting from the use of oral contraceptives that the incidence of difficulties from unwanted pregnancies might be still higher if all couples switched to other methods of contraception, all of which are less effective.

Cancer. Because of the numerous animal and human studies that demonstrate an increased incidence of several different types of tumors with estrogen, there has been much concern that similar problems would occur in women taking oral contraceptives.

As discussed above, vaginal, uterine, and perhaps breast carcinomas have been caused by the use of estrogens (Shaw, 1987). In addition, a number of cases of benign and malignant hepatomas have been associated with the use of oral contraceptives. The primary danger of these benign tumors is rupture and hemorrhage due to their vascularity. The benign hepatomas usually regress when oral contraceptives are discontinued. An increased incidence of endometrial carcinoma and cervical neoplasia in premenopausal women receiving oral contraceptives has also been observed (*see* Shapiro *et al.,* 1985; Shaw, 1987). However, the increased incidence of endometrial carcinoma with use of estrogens is diminished when a progestin is also given (Gambrell, 1985). The incidence of ovarian cancer is decreased in users of oral contraceptives (Centers for Disease Control, 1987b). Studies discussed above have suggested that estrogens and progestins can increase the incidence of breast tumors, but most have found no association of this disease with the use of oral contraceptives (*see* Shaw, 1987). The relatively few incriminating reports, despite the vast use of these agents, may reflect the latent period needed for cellular transformation. Additional prospective studies are thus needed to establish whether oral contraceptives are associated with the development of these or other tumors.

Other Effects. The frequent, mild side effects—nausea, occasional vomiting, dizziness, headache, discomfort in the breasts, and weight gain—are manifestations of early pregnancy and are common symptoms with use of oral contraceptives. They are more frequent and may be more troublesome than the side effects in menopausal women given estrogen, probably because the contraceptives are not taken for the relief of symptoms. However, most of them are short lived or are noted only in the first cycle or two. Irregular menstrual bleeding—so-called breakthrough bleeding—is also more frequent at first; it seems to be less troublesome with the preparations containing larger doses of estrogen.

Oral contraceptives can cause intolerance to carbohydrates, with elevations in the concentrations of glucose and insulin in plasma (*see* Gaspard, 1987; Crook *et al.*, 1988). The changes tend to be small and are usually reversible. If notable aberrations of this type are seen, oral contraceptives should be discontinued and another form of contraception used. Oral contraceptives can also alter plasma concentrations of cholesterol and lipids. As discussed above, estrogens decrease LDL and increase HDL, while progestins have the opposite effect. The net effects of oral contraceptives are thus dependent upon the quantities of estrogen and progestin in the preparation and the antiestrogenic or androgenic activity of the progestin used (Gaspard, 1987; Burkman, 1988; Crook *et al.*, 1988).

Many other minor disturbances have been attributed to the oral contraceptives (Shaw, 1987; Meade, 1988). Some symptoms, including depression of mood, easy fatigue, and lack of initiative, have been attributed to the progestin in the tablets and are less troublesome or even unnoticed with the newer preparations containing smaller amounts. Gingivitis with hypertrophy and bleeding of the gums is sometimes observed. An increase in female-initiated sexual activity that is said to be present at the time of ovulation is suppressed or absent in women using oral contraceptives (Adams *et al.*, 1978).

Various ocular conditions have also been reported, including corneal sensitivity, retinal thrombosis, optic neuritis, diplopia, and others. However, it has not been determined that these are in fact related to oral contraceptives. Skin rashes, photosensitivity, alopecia, and hirsutism seldom occur, but chloasma (brownish macules on the face) may appear with prolonged use of most preparations. Cholestatic jaundice caused by the 17-alkyl-substituted steroids present in all of the preparations is rare. An increased incidence of gallbladder disease with estrogens has been reported by the Boston Collaborative Drug Surveillance Program (1974). Oral contraceptives increase the concentration of cholesterol in bile, which may provide the biochemical explanation for the increased incidence of cholelithiasis (Bennion *et al.*, 1976). Folate absorption may be decreased, but few patients develop anemia or other signs of deficiency (*see* Briggs, 1976). The resumption of spontaneous menses usually requires about 6 to 10 weeks after oral contraceptives have been discontinued. However, some patients have prolonged periods of anovulation and amenorrhea (sometimes associated with galactorrhea), requiring therapy with clomiphene, gonadotropin, or bromocriptine (*see* Chapter 56). The use of oral contraceptives may in some way provide a setting for the subsequent development of hyperprolactinemia and pituitary microadenomas when discontinued; however, the studies are incomplete (Shaw, 1987). The use of preparations with a low estrogen content may lead to breakthrough bleeding. Preparations with less than 30 to 35 μg of estrogen may also be less efficacious, particularly if the administration of other drugs increases hepatic metabolism of the estrogen. Continuation of intake of oral contraceptives during pregnancy may be associated with congenital limb deformation, masculinization, and cryptorchism in offspring (Janerich *et al.*, 1974; Koide and Ch'iu Lyle, 1975; Heinonen *et al.*, 1977; Rothman and Louik, 1978). However, some of these reports have not been adequately confirmed. Administration of oral contraceptives soon after delivery will decrease lactation and interfere with breast-feeding; the steroids are excreted in breast milk, and effects on nursing infants are unknown.

In view of these considerations, it seems highly prudent to continue to evaluate each patient and her need for oral contraceptives. The incidence of complications in patients under 30 years of age who do not have risk factors for cardiovascular disease appears to be small. A challenge to the physician is to evaluate the presence of such risk factors in older patients and, if present, to encourage the patient to consider other forms of contraception or to decrease or eliminate other risk factors. Clearly in some patients pregnancy is either very undesirable or contraindicated due to preexisting disease; the additional risks from oral contraceptives seem minor. However, in most patients the decision is more difficult. Many alternative means of contraception are available, but none is quite as effective as oral contraceptives. For extensive population control, these agents are extremely useful and a low incidence of complications is to be expected.

If oral contraceptives are prescribed, preparations with low estrogen and progestin content are preferred, and patients require periodic evaluation for side effects. The United States Food and Drug Administration exercises strict control over the labeling of estrogens and oral contraceptives. Contraindications to their use are thromboembolic and cardiovascular disorders or a past history of these conditions, markedly impaired hepatic function, known or suspected carcinoma of the breast or other estrogen-dependent neoplasia, pregnancy, and undiagnosed genital bleeding. In addition, various warnings and precautions, as well as the possible adverse reactions outlined above, must be listed. The extent to which these possible adverse reactions should be discussed with the patient at first was left to the discretion of the physician, but now a brief description of the hazards of this form of contraception is included in each package dispensed to the patient.

Aarskog, D. Maternal progestins as a possible cause of hypospadias. *N. Engl. J. Med.*, **1979**, *300*, 75–78.

Adams, D. B.; Gold, A. R.; and Burt, A. D. Rise in female-initiated sexual activity at ovulation and its suppression by oral contraceptives. *N. Engl. J. Med.*, **1978**, *299*, 1145–1150.

Allen, E., and Doisy, E. A. An ovarian hormone: a preliminary report on its localization, extraction, and partial purification, and action in test animals. *J.A.M.A.*, **1923**, *81*, 819–821.

Aloia, J. F.; Cohn, S. H.; Vaswani, A.; Yeh, J. K.; Yuen, K.; and Ellis, K. Risk factors for postmenopausal osteoporosis. *Am. J. Med.*, **1985**, *78*, 95–100.

Barrett-Connor, E. Postmenopausal estrogen replacement and breast cancer. *N. Engl. J. Med.*, **1989**, *321*, 319–320.

Baum, J. K.; Bookstein, J. J.; Holtz, F.; and Klein, E. W. Possible association between benign hepatomas and oral contraceptives. *Lancet*, **1973**, *2*, 926–929.

Beard, J. *The Span of Gestation and the Cause of Birth.* Gustav Fischer Verlag, Jena, **1897.**

Bennion, L. J.; Ginsberg, R. L.; Garnick, M. B.; and Bennett, P. H. Effects of oral contraceptives on the gallbladder bile of normal women. *N. Engl. J. Med.*, **1976**, *294*, 189–192.

Bergkvist, L.; Adami, H.-O.; Persson, I.; Hoover, R.; and Schairer, C. The risk of breast cancer after estrogen and estrogen-progestin replacement. *N. Engl. J. Med.*, **1989**, *321*, 293–297.

Bonnar, J. Coagulation effects of oral contraception. *Am. J. Obstet. Gynecol.*, **1987**, *157*, 1042–1048.

Boston Collaborative Drug Surveillance Program. Surgically confirmed gall bladder disease, venous thromboembolism, and breast tumors in relation to postmenopausal estrogen therapy. *N. Engl. J. Med.*, **1974**, *290*, 15–18.

Bush, T. L., and Barrett-Connor, E. Noncontraceptive estrogen use and cardiovascular disease. *Epidemiol. Rev.*, **1985**, *7*, 89–104.

Butenandt, A. Über "PROGYNON," ein crystallisiertes, weibliches Sexualhormon. *Naturwissenschaften*, **1929**, *17*, 879.

Centers for Disease Control. Combination oral contraceptive use and the risk of endometrial cancer. *J.A.M.A.*, **1987a**, *257*, 796–800.

———. The reduction in risk of ovarian cancer associated with oral contraceptive use. *N. Engl. J. Med.*, **1987b**, *316*, 650–655.

Clark, G. M.; McGuire, W. L.; Hubay, C. A.; Pearson, O. H.; and Marshall, J. S. Progesterone receptors as a prognostic factor in stage II breast cancer. *N. Engl. J. Med.*, **1983**, *309*, 1343–1347.

Collaborative Group for the Study of Stroke in Young Women. Oral contraception and increased risk of cerebral ischemia or thrombosis. *N. Engl. J. Med.*, **1973**, *288*, 871–878.

———. Oral contraceptives and stroke in young women; associated risk factors. *J.A.M.A.*, **1975**, *231*, 718–722.

Conference. Osteoporosis. *J.A.M.A.*, **1984**, *252*, 799–802.

Corbin, C. J.; Graham-Lorence, S.; McPhaul, M.; Mason, J. I.; Mendelson, C. R.; and Simpson, E. R. Isolation of a full-length cDNA encoding human aromatase system cytochrome P-450 and its expression in nonsteroidogenic cells. *Proc. Natl. Acad. Sci. U.S.A.*, **1988**, *85*, 8948–8952.

Corner, G. W., and Allen, W. M. Physiology of the corpus luteum. II. Production of a special uterine reaction (progestational proliferation) by extracts of the corpus luteum. *Am. J. Physiol.*, **1929**, *88*, 326–346.

Coronary Drug Project Research Group. The coronary drug project. Initial findings leading to modifications of its research protocol. *J.A.M.A.*, **1970**, *214*, 1303–1313.

———. The coronary drug project. Findings leading to discontinuation of the 2.5-mg/day estrogen group. *Ibid.*, **1973**, *226*, 652–657.

Crook, D.; Godsland, I. F.; and Wynn, V. Oral contraceptives and coronary heart disease: modulation of glucose tolerance and plasma lipid risk factors by progestins. *Am. J. Obstet. Gynecol.*, **1988**, *158*, 1612–1620.

Doisy, E. A.; Veler, C. D.; and Thayer, S. A. Folliculin from the urine of pregnant women. *Am. J. Physiol.*, **1929**, *90*, 329–330.

———. The preparation of the crystalline ovarian hormone from the urine of pregnant women. *J. Biol. Chem.*, **1930**, *86*, 499–509.

Dowsett, M.; Goss, P. E.; Powles, T. J.; Hutchinson, G.; Brodie, A. M. H.; Jeffcoate, S. L.; and Coombes, R. C.

Use of the aromatase inhibitor 4-hydroxyandrostenedione in postmenopausal breast cancer: optimization of therapeutic dose and route. *Cancer Res.*, **1987**, *47*, 1957–1961.

FDA Drug Bulletin. PROGESTASERT IUD and ectopic pregnancy. **1978a**, *8*, 10.

———. Approval of DEPO-PROVERA for contraception denied. **1978b**, *8*, 10–11.

———. Recommendations of DES Task Force. **1985**, *15*, 40–42.

Fraenkel, L. Die Funktion des Corpus Luteum. *Arch. Gynaekol.*, **1903**, *68*, 483–545.

Frank, R. T.; Frank, M. L.; Gustavson, R. G.; and Weyerts, W. W. Demonstration of the female sex hormone in the circulating blood. I. Preliminary report. *J.A.M.A.*, **1925**, *85*, 510.

Gambrell, R. D. Evidence supports estrogen-progestogen replacement therapy. *Postgrad. Med.*, **1985**, *78*, 35–38.

Gaspard, U. J. Metabolic effects of oral contraceptives. *Am. J. Obstet. Gynecol.*, **1987**, *157*, 1029–1041.

Geier, A.; Lunenfeld, B.; Pariente, C.; Koteveme, S.; Shadmi, A.; Kokie, E.; and Blankste, J. Estrogen receptor binding material in blood of patients after clomiphene citrate administration: determination by radioreceptor assay. *Fertil. Steril.*, **1987**, *47*, 778–784.

Greenberg, E. R.; Barnes, A. B.; Resseguie, L.; Barrett, J. A.; Burnside, S.; Lanza, L. L.; Neff, R. K.; Stevens, M.; Young, R. H.; and Colton, T. Breast cancer in mothers given diethylstilbestrol in pregnancy. *N. Engl. J. Med.*, **1984**, *311*, 1393–1398.

Greenblatt, R. B.; Roy, S.; Mahesh, V. B.; Barfield, W. E.; and Jungck, E. C. Induction of ovulation. *Am. J. Obstet. Gynecol.*, **1962**, *84*, 900–909.

Greenwald, P.; Barlow, J. J.; Nasca, P. C.; and Burnett, W. S. Vaginal cancer after maternal treatment with synthetic estrogens. *N. Engl. J. Med.*, **1971**, *285*, 390–392.

Gruchow, H. W.; Anderson, A. J.; Barboriak, J. J.; and Sobocinski, K. A. Postmenopausal use of estrogen and occlusion of coronary arteries. *Am. Heart J.*, **1988**, *115*, 954–963.

Hadjimichael, O. C.; Meigs, J. W.; Falcier, F. W.; Thompson, W. D.; and Flannery, J. T. Cancer risk among women exposed to exogenous estrogens during pregnancy. *J. Natl. Cancer Inst.*, **1984**, *73*, 831–834.

Halban, J. Ueber den Einfluss der Ovarien auf die Entwicklung des Genitales. *Monatsschr. Geburtshilfe Gynäkol.*, **1900**, *12*, 496–503.

Heinonen, O. P.; Slone, D.; Monson, R. R.; Hook, E. B.; and Shapiro, S. Cardiovascular birth defects and antenatal exposure to female sex hormones. *N. Engl. J. Med.*, **1977**, *296*, 67–70.

Henderson, B. E.; Ross, K. K.; and Paganini-Hiel, A. Estrogen use and cardiovascular disease. *J. Reprod. Med.*, **1985**, *30*, 814–820.

Herbst, A. L.; Ulfelder, H.; and Poskanzer, D. C. Adenocarcinoma of the vagina. Association of maternal stilbestrol therapy with tumor appearance in young women. *N. Engl. J. Med.*, **1971**, *284*, 878–881.

Hilliard, J.; Scaramuzzi, R. J.; Pang, C.-N.; Penardi, R.; and Sawyer, C. H. Testosterone secretion by rabbit ovary *in vivo*. *Endocrinology*, **1974**, *94*, 267–271.

Homonnai, Z. T.; Yavetz, H.; Yogev, L.; Rotem, R.; and Paz, G. F. Clomiphene citrate treatment in oligozoospermia: comparison between two regimens of low-dose treatment. *Fertil. Steril.*, **1988**, *50*, 801–804.

Horsman, A.; Jones, M.; Francis, R.; and Nordin, C. The effect of estrogen dose on postmenopausal bone loss. *N. Engl. J. Med.*, **1983**, *309*, 1405–1407.

Huch, K. M.; Elam, M. B.; and Chesney, C. M. Oral contraceptive steroid induced platelet coagulant hyperactivity: dissociation of *in vivo* and *in vitro* effects. *Thromb. Res.*, **1987**, *1*, 41–50.

Inman, W. H. W., and Vessey, M. P. Investigation of deaths from pulmonary, coronary and cerebral thrombosis and embolism in women of childbearing age. *Br. Med. J.*, **1968**, *2*, 193–199.

Inman, W. H. W.; Vessey, M. P.; Westerholm, B.; and Engelund, A. Thromboembolic disease and the steroidal content of oral contraceptives. *Br. Med. J.*, **1970**, *2*, 203–209.

Jacobson, B. D. Hazards of norethindrone therapy during pregnancy. *Am. J. Obstet. Gynecol.*, **1962**, *84*, 962–968.

Janerich, D. T.; Piper, J. M.; and Glebatis, D. M. Oral contraceptives and congenital limb-reduction defects. *N. Engl. J. Med.*, **1974**, *291*, 697–700.

Jick, H.; Walker, A. M.; Watkins, R. N.; D'ewart, D. C.; Hunter, J. R.; Danford, A.; Madsen, S.; Dinan, B. J.; and Rothman, K. J. Replacement estrogens and breast cancer. *Am. J. Epidemiol.*, **1980**, *112*, 586–594.

Katzenellenbogen, J. A.; Carlson, K. E.; and Katzenellenbogen, B. S. Facile geometric isomerization of phenolic non-steroidal estrogens and antiestrogens: limitations to the interpretation of experiments characterizing the activity of individual isomers. *J. Steroid Biochem.*, **1988**, *22*, 589–596.

Kiel, D. P.; Felson, D. T.; Anderson, J. J.; Wilson, P. W. F.; and Moskowitz, M. A. Hip fracture and the use of estrogen in postmenopausal women: the Framingham Study. *N. Engl. J. Med.*, **1987**, *317*, 1169–1174.

Knauer, E. Die Ovarien-Transplantation. *Arch. Gynaekol.*, **1900**, *60*, 322–376.

Lacassagne, A. Tumeurs malignes appareus au cours d'un traitement hormonal combiné, chez des souris appartenant a'des lignées réfractaires au cancer spontané. *C. R. Soc. Biol. (Paris)*, **1936**, *121*, 607–609.

Lawson, D. H.; Jick, H.; Hunter, J. R.; and Madsen, S. Exogenous estrogens and breast cancer. *Am. J. Epidemiol.*, **1981**, *114*, 710–713.

Leuprolide Study Group. Leuprolide versus diethylstilbestrol for metastatic prostate cancer. *N. Engl. J. Med.*, **1984**, *311*, 1281–1286.

Loewe, S. Nachweis brunsterzeugender Stoffe im weiblichen Blute. *Klin. Wochenschr.*, **1925**, *4*, 1407–1408.

Loewe, S., and Lange, F. Der Gehalt des Frauenharns an brunsterzeugenden Stoffen in Abhängigkeit von ovariellen Zyklus. *Klin. Wochenschr.*, **1926**, *5*, 1038–1039.

Medical Letter. Prevention and treatment of postmenopausal osteoporosis. **1987**, *29*, 75–77.

Pincus, G. Clinical effects of new progestational compounds. In, *Clinical Endocrinology I.* (Astwood, E. B., ed.) Grune & Stratton, Inc., New York, **1960**, pp. 526–531.

Porter, J. B.; Jick, H.; and Walker, A. M. Mortality among oral contraceptive users. *Obstet. Gynecol.*, **1987**, *70*, 29–32.

Richelson, L. S.; Wahner, H. W.; Melton, L. J., III; and Riggs, B. L. Relative contributions of aging and estrogen deficiency to postmenopausal bone loss. *N. Engl. J. Med.*, **1984**, *311*, 1273–1275.

Rigg, L. A.; Hermann, H.; and Yen, S. S. C. Absorption of estrogens from vaginal creams. *N. Engl. J. Med.*, **1978**, *298*, 195–197.

Riggs, B. L.; Seeman, E.; Hodgson, S. F.; Taves, D. R.; and O'Fallon, W. M. Effect of the fluoride/calcium regimen on vertebral fracture occurrence in postmenopausal osteoporosis. *N. Engl. J. Med.*, **1982**, *306*, 446–450.

Rosenberg, L.; Armstrong, B.; and Jick, H. Myocardial infarction and estrogen therapy in postmenopausal women. *N. Engl. J. Med.*, **1976**, *294*, 1256–1259.

Ross, R. K.; Paganini-Hill, A.; Gerkins, V. R.; Mack, T. M.; Pfeffer, R.; Arthur, M.; and Henderson, B. E. A case-control study of menopausal estrogen therapy and breast cancer. *J.A.M.A.*, **1980**, *243*, 1635–1639.

Rothman, K. J., and Louik, C. Oral contraceptives and birth defects. *N. Engl. J. Med.*, **1978**, *299*, 522–524.

Royal College of General Practitioners' Oral Contraception Study. Further analyses of mortality in oral contraceptive users. *Lancet*, **1981**, *1*, 541–546.

Schieweck, K.; Bhatnagar, A. S.; and Matter, A. CGS 16949A, a new nonsteroidal aromatase inhibitor: effects on hormone-dependent and -independent tumors *in vivo*. *Cancer Res.*, **1988**, *48*, 834–838.

Segal, S. J., and Thompson, C. R. Inhibition of estradiol-induced pituitary hypertrophy in rats. *Proc. Soc. Exp. Biol. Med.*, **1956**, *91*, 623–625.

Shapiro, S.; Kelly, J. P.; Rosenberg, L.; Kaufman, D. W.; Helmrich, S. P.; Rosenshein, N. B.; Lewis, J. L.; Knapp, R. C.; Stolley, P. D.; and Schottenfeld, D. Risk of localized and widespread endometrial cancer in relation to recent and discontinued use of conjugated estrogens. *N. Engl. J. Med.*, **1985**, *313*, 969–972.

Silverberg, S. G., and Makowski, E. L. Endometrial carcinoma in young women taking oral contraceptive agents. *Obstet. Gynecol.*, **1975**, *46*, 503–506.

Slone, D.; Shapiro, S.; Kaufman, D. W.; Rosenberg, L.; Miettinen, O. S.; and Stolley, P. D. Risk of myocardial infarction in relation to current and discontinued use of oral contraceptives. *N. Engl. J. Med.*, **1981**, *305*, 420–424.

Sullivan, J. M.; Vander Zwaag, R.; Lemp, G. F.; Hughes, J. P.; Maddock, V.; Kroetz, F. W.; Ramanathan, K. B.; and Mirvis, D. M. Postmenopausal estrogen use and coronary atherosclerosis. *Ann. Intern. Med.*, **1988**, *108*, 358–363.

Swerdloff, R. S., and Odell, W. D. Serum luteinizing and follicle stimulating hormone levels during sequential and nonsequential contraceptive treatment of eugonadal women. *J. Clin. Endocrinol. Metab.*, **1969**, *29*, 157–163.

Taymor, M. L.; Seibel, M.; Oskowitz, S. P.; Smith, D. M.; and Lee, G. *In vitro* fertilization and embryo transfer: an individualized approach to ovulation induction. *J. In Vitro Fert. Embryo Transfer*, **1985**, *2*, 162–165.

Thalassinos, N. C.; Gutteridge, D. H.; Joplin, G. F.; and Fraser, T. R. Calcium balance in osteoporotic patients on long-term oral calcium therapy with and without sex hormones. *Clin. Sci.*, **1982**, *62*, 221–226.

Vessey, M. P. Female hormones and vascular disease—an epidemiologic overview. *Br. J. Fam. Plann.*, **1980**, *6*, Suppl., 1–12.

Vessey, M. P., and Doll, R. Investigation of relation between use of oral contraceptives and thromboembolic disease. *Br. Med. J.*, **1968**, *2*, 199–205.

Veterans Administration. The Veterans Administration co-operative urological research group: treatment and survival of patients with cancer of the prostate. *Surg. Gynecol. Obstet.*, **1967**, *124*, 1011–1017.

Weinberger, M. H. Estrogens and hypertension. *Compr. Ther.*, **1982**, *8*, 71–75.

Weinstein, M. C. Estrogen use in postmenopausal women—costs, risks, and benefits. *N. Engl. J. Med.*, **1980**, *303*, 308–316.

Weiss, N. S., and Sayvetz, T. A. Incidence of endometrial cancer in relation to the use of oral contraceptives. *N. Engl. J. Med.*, **1980**, *302*, 551–554.

Wilson, P. W. F.; Garrison, R. J.; and Castelli, W. P. Postmenopausal estrogen use, cigarette smoking and cardiovascular morbidity in women over 50. *N. Engl. J. Med.*, **1985**, *313*, 1038–1043.

Woods, J. W. Oral contraceptives and hypertension. *Hypertension*, **1988**, *11*, Suppl. 11, 11–15.

Zondek, B. Darstellung des weiblichen Sexualhormon aus dem Harn, insbesondere dem Harn von Schwageren. *Klin. Wochenschr.*, **1928**, *7*, 485–486.

Monographs and Reviews

Baulieu, E. E. Contragestion and other clinical applications of RU 486, an antiprogesterone at the receptor. *Science*, **1989a**, *245*, 1351–1357.

Baulieu, E. E. RU-486 as an antiprogesterone steroid. *J.A.M.A.*, **1989b**, *262*; 1808–1814.

Baulieu, E. E.; Ulmann, A.; and Philibert, D. Contragestion by antiprogestin RU 486: a review. *Arch. Gynecol. Obstet.*, **1987**, *241*, 73–85.

Beato, M. Gene regulation by steroid hormones. *Cell*, **1989**, *56*, 335–344.

Briggs, M. Biochemical effects of oral contraceptives. *Adv. Steroid Biochem. Pharmacol.*, **1976**, *5*, 66–160.

Burkman, R. T. Lipid and lipoprotein changes in relation to oral contraception and hormonal replacement therapy. *Fertil. Steril.*, **1988**, *49*, 39S–50S.

Couzinet, B., and Schaison, G. Mifegyen (*mifepristone*), a new antiprogestagen with potential therapeutic use in human fertility control. *Drugs*, **1988**, *35*, 187–191.

DeJong, F. H. Inhibin. *Physiol. Rev.*, **1988**, *68*, 555–607.

Duax, W. L.; Griffin, J. F.; Weeks, C. M.; and Wawrzak, Z. The mechanism of action of steroid antagonists: insights from crystallographic studies. *J. Steroid Biochem.*, **1988**, *31*, 481–492.

Erickson, G. F. Normal ovarian function. *Clin. Obstet. Gynecol.*, **1978**, *21*, 31–52.

Ernster, V. L.; Huggins, G. R.; Hulka, B. S.; Kelsey, J. L.; and Schottenfeld, F. Benefits and risks of menopausal estrogen and/or progestin hormone use. *Prev. Med.*, **1988**, *17*, 201–223.

Eskin, B. A. Sex hormones and aging. *Adv. Exp. Med. Biol.*, **1978**, *97*, 207–224.

Evans, R. M. The steroid and thyroid hormone receptor superfamily. *Science*, **1988**, *240*, 889–895.

Gorski, J.; Welshons, W. V.; Sakai, D.; Hansen, J.; Walent, J.; Kassis, J.; Shull, J.; Stack, G.; and Campen, C. Evolution of a model of estrogen action. *Recent Prog. Horm. Res.*, **1986**, *42*, 297–329.

Heyns, W. The steroid-binding β-globulin of human plasma. *Adv. Steroid Biochem. Pharmacol.*, **1977**, *6*, 59–79.

Jordan, V. C. Biochemical pharmacology of antiestrogen action. *Pharmacol. Rev.*, **1984**, *36*, 245–276.

Jordan, V. C.; Mittal, S.; Gosden, B.; Koch, R.; and Lieberman, M. E. Structure-activity relationships of estrogens. *Environ. Health Perspect.*, **1985**, *61*, 97–110.

Kaplan, N. M. Cardiovascular complications of oral contraceptives. *Annu. Rev. Med.*, **1978**, *29*, 31–40.

Kay, C. R. Oral contraceptives—the clinical perspective. In, *Pharmacology of Steroid Contraceptive Drugs.* (Garattini, S., and Berendes, H. W., eds.) Raven Press, New York, **1977**, pp. 1–24.

Kennedy, J. L., and Adashi, E. Y. Ovulation induction. *Obstet. Gynecol. Clin. North Am.*, **1987**, *14*, 831–864.

Koide, S. S., and Ch'iu Lyle, K. Unusual signs and symptoms associated with oral contraceptive medication. *J. Reprod. Med.*, **1975**, *15*, 214–224.

Leis, H. P.; Black, M. M.; and Sall, S. The pill and the breast. *J. Reprod. Med.*, **1976**, *16*, 5–9.

Meade, T. W. Risks and mechanisms of cardiovascular events in users of oral contraceptives. *Am. J. Obstet. Gynecol.*, **1988**, *158*, 1646–1652.

Melski, J. W., and Arndt, K. A. Topical therapy for acne. *N. Engl. J. Med.*, **1980**, *302*, 503–506.

Mendelson, C. R., and Simpson, E. R. Regulation of estrogen biosynthesis by human adipose cells *in vitro*. *Mol. Cell Endocrinol.*, **1987**, *52*, 169–176.

Miller, W. L. Molecular biology of steroid hormone synthesis. *Endocr. Rev.*, **1988**, *9*, 295–318.

Miquel, J.-F., and Gilbert, J. A chemical classification of nonsteroidal antagonists of sex-steroid hormone action. *J. Steroid Biochem.*, **1988**, *31*, 525–544.

Naftolin, F., and Tolis, G. Neuroendocrine regulation of the menstrual cycle. *Clin. Obstet. Gynecol.*, **1978**, *21*, 17–29.

Nebert, D. W., and Gonzalez, F. J. P_{450} genes: structure, evolution, and regulation. *Annu. Rev. Biochem.*, **1987**, *56*, 945–993.

Ray, S., and Sharma, I. Development of progesterone antagonists as fertility regulating agents. *Pharmazie*, **1987**, *42*, 656–661.

Rock, J.; Garcia, C. M.; and Pincus, G. Synthetic progestins in the normal human menstrual cycle. *Recent Prog. Horm. Res.*, **1957**, *13*, 323–339.

Ryan, K. J. Postmenopausal estrogen use. *Annu. Rev. Med.*, **1982**, *33*, 171–181.

Schally, A. V. Aspects of hypothalamic regulation of the pituitary gland: its implications for the control of reproductive functions. *Science*, **1978**, *202*, 18–28.

Shaw, R. W. Adverse long-term effects of oral contraceptives: a review. *Br. J. Obstet. Gynecol.*, **1987**, *94*, 724–730.

Speroff, L. The formulation of oral contraceptives: does the amount of estrogen make any clinical difference? *Johns Hopkins Med. J.*, **1982**, *150*, 170–176.

Vande Wiele, R. L., and Dyrenfurth, I. Gonadotropin-steroid interrelationships. *Pharmacol. Rev.*, **1973**, *25*, 189–207.

Vecchio, T. J. Long-acting injectable contraceptives. *Adv. Steroid Biochem. Pharmacol.*, **1976**, *5*, 1–64.

Wentz, A. C. Assessment of estrogen and progestin therapy in gynecology and obstetrics. *Clin. Obstet. Gynecol.*, **1977**, *20*, 461–482.

Ying, S. Y. Inhibins, activins, and follistatins: gonadal proteins modulating the secretion of follicle-stimulating hormone. *Endocr. Rev.*, **1988**, *9*, 267–293.

CHAPTER

59 ANDROGENS

Jean D. Wilson

Testosterone, the principal androgen, is synthesized in the testis, the ovary, and the adrenal cortex. In the circulation, testosterone serves as a prohormone for the formation of two classes of steroids: 5α-reduced androgens, which act as the intracellular mediators of most androgen actions, and estrogens, which enhance some androgenic effects and block others. Thus, the net effect of the action of endogenous androgens is the sum of the effects of the secreted hormone (testosterone), its 5α-reduced metabolite (dihydrotestosterone), and its estrogenic derivative (estradiol) (*see* Table 59–1). Clear understanding of these interconversions is essential for the rational pharmacological use of these agents.

History. The observation that castration makes the eunuch, properly credited to primitive man, ushered in the dawn of endocrinology. The discovery that the testis is a gland of internal secretion is ascribed to Berthold, who in 1849 showed that the transplantation of gonads into castrated roosters prevents the typical signs of castration. This was the first published experimental evidence for the effect of an endocrine gland (Berthold, 1849). However, testosterone was one of the last steroid hormones to be isolated in pure form.

Chemistry. The elucidation of the chemistry of the male sex hormones was made possible by the development of methods of assay. The technique of Koch and coworkers for the determination of androgenic activity utilizing the growth response of the capon's comb was used in the first isolation of the urinary principle by Butenandt (1931), who by herculean effort obtained 15 mg of androsterone (5α-androstane-3α-ol-17-one) from 25,000 liters of male urine.

It soon became apparent, however, that androsterone could not account for the androgenic activity of testicular extracts, and attention was then focused on the testes as the source of male sex hormone. Active testicular extracts had been prepared as early as 1927 by Loewe, using the mammalian seminal vesicle for assay (*see* Loewe and Voss, 1930). The testicular hormone testosterone was isolated in crystalline form by Laqueur and associates (*see* David *et al.*, 1935); its chemical structure was soon elucidated, and the hormone was then synthesized (Ruzicka and Wettstein, 1935).

Testosterone is secreted by the testis and is the main androgen in the plasma of men. In women, small amounts of testosterone are synthesized by the ovary and adrenal. In many target tissues for androgens, testosterone is reduced at the 5α position to dihydrotestosterone, which serves as the intracellular mediator of most actions of the hormone. Dihydrotestosterone binds to the intracellular androgen receptor protein about ten times more tightly than does testosterone, and the dihydrotestosterone-receptor complex is more stable than the testosterone-receptor complex; its greater androgenic potency is thereby explained (*see* below; *see also* Kovacs *et al.*, 1984). A variety of other naturally occurring weak androgens have been described, including the testosterone precursor androstenedione, the adrenal androgen dehydroepiandrosterone, and the dihydrotestosterone metabolites 5α-androstane-3α,17β-diol and androsterone. However, these steroids bind so weakly to the androgen receptor that it is unlikely that they can act directly as androgens at physiological concentrations, and it is now believed that they are androgens only to the extent that they are converted to testosterone and/or dihydrotestosterone *in vivo*. Thus, the prior concept of weak androgens is now one of weak androgen precursors.

The major metabolites of androgens in urine are physiologically weak or inactive (either as free steroids or water-soluble conjugates); the predominant metabolites are etiocholanolone, a 5β-reduced metabolite of testosterone and of other Δ^4,3-keto androgens, and androsterone, a metabolite of dihydrotestosterone (Table 59–1).

Testosterone (but not dihydrotestosterone) can also be aromatized to estradiol in a variety of extraglandular tissues, a pathway that accounts for most estrogen synthesis in men and postmenopausal women (Siiteri and MacDonald, 1973). The role, if any, of the approximately 50 μg of estradiol synthesized each day in normal men has never been defined, but either relative or absolute excess of estrogen can cause feminization in men.

Soon after the identification of testosterone as the principal testicular androgen, it became apparent that the hormone cannot be given effectively by mouth or by parenteral injection. Oral administration of testosterone (or dihydrotestosterone) is followed by absorption into the portal blood and prompt degradation by the liver; insignificant amounts of hormone reach the systemic circulation. Parenteral administration is also followed by prompt metabolism. It is thus necessary to modify the androgen molecule to alter its properties or to devise means of administration that circumvent these problems.

Table 59–1. METABOLISM OF ANDROGENS

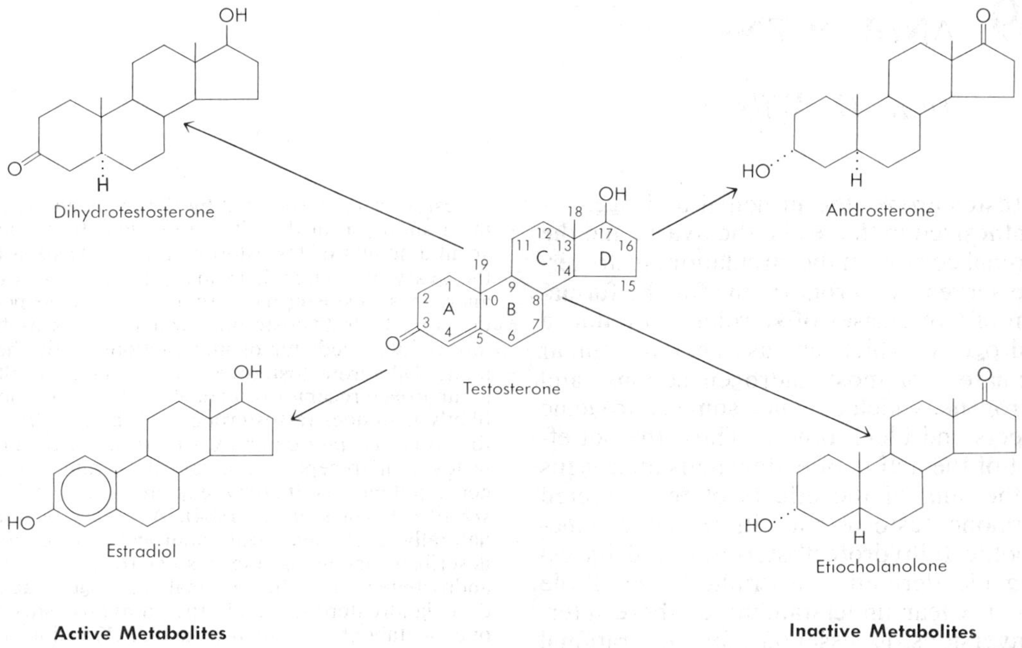

The aim of chemical modification is to retard the rate of catabolism or to enhance the androgenic potency of each molecule. Three general types of modification of androgens are clinically useful. (1) Esterification of the 17β-hydroxyl group with any of several carboxylic acids decreases the polarity of the molecule, makes it more soluble in the lipid vehicles used for injection, and hence slows release of the injected steroid into the circulation. The longer the carbon chain in the ester, the more lipid soluble the steroid becomes and the more prolonged the action. Such esters are hydrolyzed before the hormone acts, and the effectiveness of drug therapy can thus be monitored by assay of plasma concentrations of testosterone. Most esters must be injected, but two such compounds, methenolone acetate and testosterone undecanoate, have features that make oral administration possible. Testosterone undecanoate is absorbed via the intestinal lymphatic ducts rather than the portal system and hence gains direct access to the systemic circulation. The methyl group on the 1 position of methenolone acetate slows hepatic inactivation and hence allows effective concentrations to be achieved in blood. (2) Alkylation at the 17α position (as in methyltestosterone and fluoxymesterone) also allows androgens to be effective orally because the alkylated derivatives are slowly catabolized by the liver. The alkyl group is not removed metabolically, and, hence, the alkylated derivatives mediate the action of the hormone within cells. (3) Other alterations of the structure have been made empirically. In some instances the effect is to slow the rate of inactivation; in others the modification enhances the potency; and in still others it alters the pattern of its metabolism. For example, fluoxymesterone is a good androgen but a poor precursor of estrogen, whereas 19-nortestosterone, like dihydrotestosterone, binds more tightly to the androgen receptor. Most alkylated and altered steroids react poorly in the immunoassay for testosterone, and concentrations of these compounds in blood cannot be monitored in most clinical laboratories.

Synthesis and Secretion of Testosterone. The concentration of testosterone in the plasma of males is relatively high during three periods of life: the phase of embryonic development in which male phenotypic differentiation takes place, the neonatal period, and throughout adult sexual life. The concentration starts to rise in male embryos about the eighth week of development and declines prior to birth. It subsequently rises during the neonatal period and then falls to typical prepubertal values within a few months after birth. At the time of male puberty, the pituitary begins to secrete increased amounts of luteinizing hormone (LH) and follicle-stimulating hormone (FSH). Gonadotropins are secreted in a cyclic fashion that is initially synchronized with the sleep cycle. As puberty progresses, however, pulsatile secretion of gonadotropins occurs during both sleep and waking periods (Boyar, 1978). The hypothalamus and pituitary become less sensitive to feedback inhibition by sex hormones during puberty. The initiating event for these phenomena is unknown.

Prior to puberty, concentrations of testosterone in plasma are low (less than 20 ng/dl [0.7 nM]), although the immature testes are capable of synthesizing androgens if challenged with gonadotropin. In the adult male, plasma testosterone concentrations rise to 300 to 1000 ng/dl (10 to 35 nM), and the rate of production is 2.5 to 11 mg per day (Rosenfield, 1972). Pathways of androgen biosynthesis are shown in Figure 58–1 (page 1386). In plasma, about 44% of testosterone is bound to sex hormone–binding globulin and about 2% is free (unbound); the remainder is bound to albumin and other proteins. Protein-bound testosterone can dissociate within a capillary bed, such that the available fraction is actually about half of the total (*see* Pardridge, 1986).

Androgen–Gonadotropin Relationships. As mentioned, gonadotropins are secreted in a pulsatile manner. In adult men, the concentrations of LH, FSH, and testosterone in plasma fluctuate during the course of the day, although integrated daily values are relatively constant.

LH and FSH together regulate testicular growth, spermatogenesis, and steroidogenesis. Growth hormone may have a synergistic effect with LH on the testis, while estrogens can decrease the effects of LH on the secretion of testosterone. The actions of the gonadotropins are probably mediated through adenosine 3′,5′-monophosphate (cyclic AMP). LH, also called interstitial cell–stimulating hormone (ICSH), interacts with the interstitial (Leydig) cells of the testes to increase the synthesis of cyclic AMP and subsequently the conversion of cholesterol to androgens. Cyclic AMP enhances the activity of several enzymes in the steroidogenic pathway, including the cholesterol side chain cleavage enzyme, and it may also influence the availability of cholesterol to serve as substrate (*see* Miller, 1988). Although the major effects of FSH are thought to be on spermatogenesis in the seminiferous tubules and that of LH on testosterone synthesis by Leydig cells, complex interactions exist in the testis. FSH can also enhance testosterone synthesis and can augment the activity of LH (*see* Ewing and Robaire, 1978; Lipsett, 1980). Furthermore, testosterone is required for spermatogenesis and maturation of sperm. With immunohistochemical techniques, LH has been localized to Leydig and peritubular cells, and FSH to tubular Sertoli cells (Castro *et al.*, 1972). The Sertoli cells of the seminiferous tubules may also produce small amounts of testosterone in some species, and the seminiferous tubules can convert testosterone to dihydrotestosterone. Androgens released from the Leydig cell both act to promote spermatogenesis and gain access to the circulation (*see* Ritzen *et al.*, 1981). Both LH and FSH have growth-promoting effects on the testes. In the human testis the effects of human chorionic gonadotropin appear to be identical to those of LH.

Administration of testosterone to intact animals suppresses the secretion of LH and thereby causes atrophy of interstitial tissue. The administration of testosterone also suppresses the excessive secretion of FSH in eunuchism, but whether testosterone plays a major role in the physiological regulation of FSH secretion is not resolved. Implantation of testosterone in the median eminence of rats inhibits pituitary gonadotropin secretion by decreasing the concentration of gonadotropin-releasing hormone (GnRH) (Schally, 1978). Likewise, administration of testosterone to hypogonadal men causes a decrease in both the frequency and amplitude of pulses of LH secretion, presumably by inhibiting the release of GnRH (Matsumoto and Bremner, 1984).

In normal men, the concentration of estradiol in the spermatic vein exceeds that in peripheral plasma (Kelch *et al.*, 1972); about 15% of the estradiol in men is derived from the testes, probably the Leydig cells (*see* Lipsett, 1980). Estrogens are also synthesized from androgens in extraglandular tissue, including the brain (Siiteri and MacDonald, 1973; Marcus and Korenman, 1976). Estrogens formed locally in the brain from administered or endogenous androgen may be responsible in part for the regulation of gonadotropin secretion by testosterone.

Feedback inhibition of FSH secretion by testicular hormones involves peptides as well as steroids (Keogh *et al.,* 1976; Ramasharma and Sairam, 1982). Inhibin is a peptide hormone that contains both 20,000- and 15,000-dalton subunits (*see* McLachlan *et al.,* 1987). The protein is synthesized both by Sertoli cells and the ovary and is believed to regulate FSH secretion at the level of the pituitary (Duhey *et al.,* 1987).

Ovarian and Adrenal Androgens. Testosterone and other androgens are secreted by the ovary and the adrenal cortex as well as by the testis. Androstenedione and dehydroepiandrosterone, which are also produced by both the ovary and adrenal, can be converted to testosterone and estrogen in peripheral tissues. The daily rate of production of testosterone in women is about 0.25 mg, and about one half of this is derived from the metabolic conversion of androstenedione to testosterone at extraglandular sites (*see* Rosenfield, 1972; Givens, 1978). The synthesis and secretion of testosterone in rabbit ovary are enhanced by the administration of LH (Hilliard *et al.,* 1974).

Alterations in plasma concentrations of testosterone and androstenedione occur during the menstrual cycle. The concentration of testosterone in the plasma of women ranges from 15 to 65 ng/dl (0.5 to 2.3 nM). Two peaks of androgen concentration correspond to those of plasma estrogens at the preovulatory and luteal phases of the cycle (Judd and Yen, 1973). In some ovarian disorders, ovarian secretion of androgens may be increased, resulting in virilization.

In men, production of testosterone by the adrenal cortex is not sufficient to maintain spermatogenesis or secondary sexual features of the adult. In abnormal conditions such as congenital adrenal hyperplasia and adrenal tumors, the adrenal cortex can secrete large quantities of androgens and androgenic precursors.

Physiological and Pharmacological Actions. Androgens serve different functions at different stages of life. During embryonic life, they virilize the urogenital tract of the male embryo, and their action is thus central to the development of the male phenotype. The role of androgens, if any, during the neonatal surge of androgen secretion is not defined but may involve developmental functions within the central nervous system. At puberty, the hormones act to transform the boy into a man. Minimal androgen secretion from the prepubertal testis and adrenal cortex suppresses secretion of gonadotropins until, at a variable age, secretion of gonadotropins becomes less sensitive to feedback inhibition and the testes start to enlarge (*see* Franchimont, 1977; Boyar, 1978). Shortly thereafter the penis and scrotum begin to grow, and pubic hair appears. Early in puberty penile erections and masturbation become frequent in most boys. Almost simultaneously the growth-promoting property of androgen causes an increase in height and the development of the skeletal musculature, which contribute to a rapid increase in body weight. As the muscles grow physical vigor is increased. The testes reach adult proportions before all the changes of puberty are completed. As a result of the actions of androgens, the skin becomes thicker and tends to be oily owing to a proliferation of sebaceous glands; the latter are prone to plugging and infection, leading to acne in some individuals. Subcutaneous fat is lost, and the veins are prominent under the skin. Axillary hair grows, and hair on the trunk and limbs develops into a pattern typical of the male. Growth of the larynx causes difficulty at first in adjusting the tone of speech and later brings about a permanent deepening of the voice. Growth of beard and body hair lags behind the other events of puberty and is the last of the secondary sex characteristics to develop. Concurrently, those whose inheritance so dictates show the first signs of male pattern baldness, with recession of the hairline at the temples and thinning of the hair at the crown. At about this time the major spurt in growth comes to an end as the epiphyses of the larger long bones begin to close, and over the next few years only 1 to 2 cm of additional growth is usual.

Androgens may also be responsible in part for the aggressive and sexual behavior of males (*see* Lunde and Hamburg, 1972;

Wilson, 1982) and, in some species, for organizational effects in the brain during prenatal or early postnatal life (*see* Pardridge *et al.*, 1982). While this is a difficult matter to resolve, the differential behavior patterns of many male and female animals suggest that the role of sex hormones in sexual behavior is an important one. For example, the sexual behavior of female rats is changed to that characteristic of males after treatment with testosterone, either as neonates or as adults (Sachs *et al.*, 1973). However, psychopathic behavior in men is not associated with altered patterns of androgen metabolism.

When androgen is given before puberty or to a young eunuchoid man, the events of normal puberty are duplicated, and the time required for normal pubertal virilization (approximately 2 years) is not significantly shortened. Within 1 or 2 days of the start of treatment erections appear and may be embarrassingly inappropriate and frequent, even to the point of discomfort; with continued treatment at the same dose this response subsides. Increased physical vigor is noted within a few weeks, and a general feeling of well-being ensues. A distinct change in the voice can be noted, and soon thereafter the penis begins to grow and axillary and pubic hair become more luxuriant. The rapidity of skeletal growth is impressive in boys treated at or before the time of normal puberty; the height may increase 10 cm or more during the first year and continue at a diminished rate for 2 or 3 years. With continued treatment, development follows the course of normal puberty, with the growth of a beard as a late expression of therapy.

Failure of Puberty Owing to Hypogonadism. The normal actions of androgens are illustrated by the consequences of deficiency. If the testes fail to function or are removed in boyhood, puberty does not occur. Failure of the testicles to develop may result from a deficiency of gonadotropins or from a primary testicular defect. A boy so afflicted continues to grow and becomes abnormally tall; the hands and feet become especially large, and the limbs are unduly long. The childish appearance and demeanor are in striking contrast to the stature; the larynx does not grow, leaving the voice high-pitched. The skeletal musculature is underdeveloped and is made more inconspicuous by a layer of subcutaneous fat. Accumulation of fat is especially prominent around the shoulders and breasts and over the upper thighs, hips, and abdomen, the whole giving the mistaken impression of femininity. Male-pattern baldness does not appear, the beard is scant or nonexistent, the axillary and pubic hair is sparse, and the body hair is short and fine. The genitalia are those of a child, and there is no sex drive.

Hypogonadism after Puberty. Some of the sex characteristics developed during puberty are self-sustaining, while others must be supported by the continued action of androgen. Hypogonadism in the adult is typified by castration after puberty. The general bodily proportions remain the same, the penis does not shrink, the voice does not change, and the beard and body hair remain unchanged for a long time. Libido is greatly reduced or absent, and erectile potency is usually decreased. The prostate and seminal vesicles regress, and the volume of the semen is small or there is none at all.

Complete failure of the endocrine function of the testis in adult life is not common; a partial deficiency can originate from incomplete development at puberty, as in 47,XXY men with the Klinefelter syndrome, or from a disorder during adult life, such as pituitary failure or a viral infection of the testis (*see* Odell and Swerdloff, 1978). Testicular function commonly decreases slightly with age; generally this occurs at a slow rate after the sixth or seventh decade. However, the decrease in libido that often occurs in aging men usually cannot be attributed to altered testicular function.

Actions on the Testis and Accessory Structures. At about the eighth week of fetal life, testicular androgens begin to be secreted and express their important role in the differentiation and development of the male reproductive tract (Jost, 1971). Lack of androgens in the male fetus results in the development of a female external phenotype. The developing testes also produce a peptide hormone (Müllerian inhibiting substance) that causes degeneration of the Müllerian ducts of the fetus (*see* Donahoe *et al.*, 1984). Subsequently, under the influence of testosterone the Wolffian ducts differentiate into the epididymidis, vas deferens, and seminal vesicles. Dihydrotestosterone causes fusion of the labioscrotal fold to result in the development of the penis (male urethra) and the scrotum, and virilization of the urogenital sinus to form the prostate. During the latter part of gestation plasma concentrations of androgen in the male fetus begin to decline, and at birth they are essentially undetectable (*see* Rosenfield, 1972).

At puberty and thereafter androgens exert a direct effect upon the testis. Following hypophysectomy in the rat, shrinkage of the testis is slowed by the injection of androgen, and spermatogenesis is maintained for a long time. Likewise, the normal animal has a biphasic response to androgen; moderate doses produce atrophy of the testis through suppression of gonadotropins, while with larger doses the atrophy is less, possibly because of the direct sustaining effect of androgen upon the seminiferous tubules.

Androgens are required for spermatogenesis in the seminiferous tubules and for the maturation of sperm in their passage through the epididymis and vas deferens. These processes are highly ordered and complex, and the nature of the effects of testosterone thereon is unknown. Studies of these events are complicated by the fact that 10 weeks are required for completion of spermatogenesis and that several additional weeks are needed for passage of sperm through the vas deferens and for maturation of sperm.

In fetal, prepubertal, and pubertal life the actions of testosterone result in growth of the clitoris or penis. Androgens also control the growth and function of the seminal vesicle and prostate.

Anabolic Effects. The nitrogen-retaining effect of androgen was first demonstrated in castrated dogs injected with androgen-containing extracts from the urine of normal men (Kochakian and Murlin, 1935). Papanicolaou and Falk (1938) showed that certain skeletal muscles of male guinea pigs are larger than those of the female and that the difference is abolished by removal of the testes. Administration of testosterone to the female or the castrated male causes male muscle development; thus, male muscle development is a phenotypic characteristic dependent upon androgen for its expression. In man, the major difference in muscle development between the sexes is in the muscles of the shoulder girdle. The anabolic actions of androgens are mediated by the same receptor protein that mediates the actions of the hormone in other target tissues (*see* below; *see also* Saartok *et al.*, 1984).

The anabolic (nitrogen-retaining) effects of androgen in men were investigated by Kenyon and associates (*see* Knowlton *et al.*, 1942). The effects are more pronounced in hypogonadal men, in boys before puberty, and in women than in normal men. Indeed, normal men experience only a transient positive nitrogen balance of a slight degree when exogenous androgens are administered. A dose of 25 mg of testosterone propionate daily causes an average daily retention of nitrogen of 63 mg/kg of body weight in hypogonadal men. There is also retention of K^+, Na^+, Cl^-, phosphate, and sulfur, and a gain in weight, which can be accounted for largely by the water held in association with the retained electrolytes and protein. When the administration of androgen is stopped, Na^+, Cl^-, and water are quickly lost from the body, phosphate and K^+ are lost less rapidly and completely, and the stored nitrogen is retained for weeks.

Effects on Sebaceous Glands. Development of acne at puberty and during treatment with androgens is related to the growth and secretion of the sebaceous glands. Methyltestosterone is active in amounts as small as 5 mg daily, while a dose of 2.5 mg daily of fluoxymesterone has variable effects. However, these effects are not seen in adult men. When acne results from endogenous androgenic stimulation, estrogens will ameliorate this condition, probably by decreasing the secretion of gonadotropins and androgen (*see* Ebling, 1970).

Mechanism of Action. At many sites of action, testosterone is not the active form of the hormone. It is converted by a 5α-reductase in target tissues to the more active dihydrotestosterone (*see* Griffin and Wilson, 1989). In one form of male pseudohermaphroditism the target tissues are deficient in the reductase. In this disorder the genotypic male secretes normal amounts of testosterone from the testes, but the hormone is not converted to dihydrotestosterone and male external genitalia fail to develop; in contrast, virilization of the Wolffian ducts during embryogenesis is normal (*see* Griffin and Wilson, 1989). Another action of androgens that does not require the conversion of testosterone to dihydrotestosterone is the regulation of LH production by the hypothalamic-pituitary system (*see* Mainwaring, 1977; Odell and Swerdloff, 1978).

Testosterone or dihydrotestosterone binds to an intracellular protein receptor, and the hormone–receptor complex acts in the nucleus at specific binding sites on the chromosomes; increased RNA polymerase activity and increased synthesis of specific RNA and protein result. The human androgen receptor is a typical member of the superfamily of steroid and thyroid hormone receptors (*see* Evans, 1988; *see also* Chapter 2). It is encoded by a gene on the X chromosome and contains androgen-binding, DNA-binding, and functional domains (Chang *et al.,* 1988). In testicular feminization and other forms of androgen resistance that cause male pseudohermaphroditism, the genotypic male with normal amounts of testosterone develops a female phenotype because of the absence or defective function of the receptor protein for testosterone and dihydrotestosterone (*see* Griffin and Wilson, 1989).

Absorption, Metabolism, and Excretion. Testosterone injected as a solution in oil is so quickly absorbed, metabolized, and excreted that the androgenic effect is small. Testosterone given by mouth is readily absorbed but is even less effective, since most of the hormone is metabolized by the liver before reaching the systemic circulation. Alternate means of administering testosterone have been proposed to circumvent these difficulties. These include implantation of testosterone-filled Silastic capsules, oral administration of large amounts of the hormone in particulate form, administration by rectal suppositories or nasal drops, and transdermal administration in the form of creams or patches.

Testosterone esters are less polar than the free steroid and, when such esters are injected intramuscularly in oil, are absorbed more slowly. For example, testosterone propionate is more active than testosterone, even when each is injected every day. The cypionate and enanthate esters are fully effective when given at 1- to 3-week intervals in proportionately larger doses. Since these esters are hydrolyzed prior to action, the concentrations of testosterone in plasma can be monitored by conventional immunoassay. This greatly facilitates the administration of effective dosages for each patient (Caminos-Torres *et al.,* 1977).

Testosterone is inactivated primarily in the liver. Metabolism to androstenedione involves oxidation of the 17-OH group; 5α-reduction of ring A of androstenedione leads to formation of androstanedione, and the 3-keto group is reduced to form androsterone; alternatively, androstenedione can be reduced in the 5β position and can undergo 3-keto reduction to form etiocholanolone (*see* Table 59–1). Dihydrotestosterone itself is converted in the liver to androsterone, androstanedione, and androstanediol (*see* Fotherby and James, 1972). Alkylation of androgens at the 17 position markedly retards their hepatic metabolism and permits such analogs to be effective orally. Such alkylated androgens can cause hepatotoxicity (*see* below).

After the administration of radiolabelled testosterone, about 90% of the radioactivity appears in the urine; 6% appears in the feces after undergoing enterohepatic circulation. Urinary products include androsterone and etiocholanolone. Small amounts of androstanediol and estrogens are also excreted, largely as glucuronide and sulfate conjugates.

Androsterone and etiocholanolone, among many other compounds, are measured as urinary 17-ketosteroids in the usual clinical tests. However, the major fraction of the ketosteroids of urine consists of metabolic products of the adrenal steroids. Thus, measurement of the excretion of 17-ketosteroids is not a valid test for the functional activity of the testis. Low values may point to adrenal insufficiency rather than to hypogonadism, and high values almost always indicate adrenocortical hyperactivity or tumor. Without the testes, the human male is androgen deficient even though the urinary 17-ketosteroids may be within the normal range. Likewise, in women, measurement of the excretion of 17-ketosteroids is rarely helpful in elucidating whether an excess of androgen originates in the ovary or the adrenal.

The esters of testosterone are hydrolyzed to free testosterone and are subsequently metabolized in the same way as is testosterone itself, but other changes in the molecule (as in methyltestosterone and fluoxymesterone) alter the course of metabolic degradation. As a result, many synthetic androgens are metabolized less rapidly than is testosterone and have longer half-lives. Unaltered compounds, metabolites, and conjugates are excreted in the urine and feces (Fotherby and James, 1972).

Assays. Bioassay is used in the evaluation of androgenic potency of new compounds. The classical assay is based on the growth of the comb of the capon. Better correlation with clinical effectiveness is given by bioassays in mammals, and the most widely used test depends upon the growth of the seminal vesicles or ventral prostate of the castrated rat. The search for androgenic and anabolic steroids made use of a different series of bioassays, including assessment of the growth of the kidney or levator ani muscle of castrated rats. Another test for anabolic activity involves examination of nitrogen excretion and the nitrogen-retaining effects of agents given to animals on controlled diets (*see earlier editions* of this textbook for references). Unfortunately, none of these assays is totally satisfactory and able to predict the results obtained in clinical trials, and no pure anabolic steroid without androgenic effects has ever been described. The failure to separate the androgenic and anabolic effects is not surprising, since all known actions of the hormone are mediated by a single receptor protein.

Preparations and Dosage. Some of the parenteral and oral preparations of androgens available for clinical use are summarized in Tables 59–2 and 59–3.

Androgen therapy is used primarily in androgen-deficient men for the development or maintenance of secondary sex characteristics. When full replacement therapy with androgen is required, the intramuscular preparations are the most effective. Dosage should provide about 10 mg per day; with testosterone propionate this is met by giving 25 mg three times weekly. With the longer-acting esters, the dose is about 200 mg every 2 to 3 weeks. Long-term treatment with these doses ordinarily causes full masculine development, provided therapy is started sufficiently early in life. When androgen replacement is started late (over the age of 25) a variable degree of virilization is eventually attained, but it may be near normal.

A preparation of testosterone for transdermal use has been developed in which a testosterone-loaded film is applied each day to the scrotal skin. This preparation permits maintenance of plasma concentrations of testosterone within the normal male range, while circumventing the necessity for parenteral administration (Findley *et al.*, 1987; Bals-Pratsch *et al.*, 1988). Such therapy causes a disproportionate increase in the plasma concentration of dihydrotestosterone to a level that is 30 to 40% of that of testosterone, presumably because of conversion by the scrotal skin during absorption; however, dihydrotestosterone has no known deleterious effects at these concentrations.

Some preparations of androgens have been introduced primarily for use as anabolic agents, with the expectation that they would be relatively less androgenic than testosterone and its close relatives. However, none is free of androgenic activity.

Various mixtures of androgenic and anabolic steroids with estrogens, vitamins, and other agents are also available. However, the use of these fixed-dose combinations is to be discouraged. In particular, their prolonged use in postmenopausal women and geriatric patients is costly and usually irrational.

Untoward Effects. Three types of side effects of androgens can be recognized: (1) virilizing side effects are mediated by the androgen receptor and are inappropriate only when the recipient is not a hypogonadal adult man; (2) feminizing side effects are mediated by estrogenic metabolites of the administered steroid; and (3) toxic side effects are generally mediated by uncertain mechanisms.

Virilizing Effects. When used in women, all androgens carry the risk of causing masculinization. Among the undesirable manifestations are acne, the growth of facial hair, and coarsening of the voice. Menstrual irregularities occur if gonadotropin secretion is suppressed. If treatment is discontinued as soon as the initial symptoms are noticed, they slowly subside. With continued treatment, as in the long-term use of androgen in mammary carcinoma, male-pattern baldness, excessive body hair, prominent musculature, and hypertrophy of the clitoris may also develop. With prolonged treatment many of these effects, such as the deepening of the voice, are irreversible. During initial androgen-replacement therapy in hypogonadal males, sustained erections may be seen. This effect subsides with continued therapy at the same or lower doses of androgen.

Profound virilization and serious disturbances of growth and osseous development can occur when androgens are given to children. The capacity of androgens to enhance epiphyseal closure in children may persist for as long as several months after discontinuation of the drug. All androgens should be used with great care in children. Androgens should not be used during pregnancy, since they can cross the placenta and cause masculinization of the female fetus.

Although androgens are required for spermatogenesis and may maintain spermatogenesis for prolonged periods in animals after hypophysectomy, continued use of androgens in normal men may result in azoospermia owing to inhibition of gonadotropin secretion and conversion of androgens to estrogens. For example, administration of 25 mg of testosterone propionate daily for 6 weeks causes a decrease in spermatogenesis. Anabolic steroids may produce the same effect, and diminution in sperm count can sometimes persist for 12 weeks or more after the administration of anabolic steroids is stopped.

Feminizing Effects. Feminizing side effects, particularly gynecomastia, can occur in men who receive androgens. The patho-

Table 59–2. SOME PARENTERAL ANDROGENS USED IN THERAPY

NONPROPRIETARY NAME AND SOME TRADE NAMES	CHEMICAL STRUCTURE	DOSAGE FORMS AND USUAL DOSAGE FOR ANDROGEN DEFICIENCY *
Testosterone TESTOJECT-50	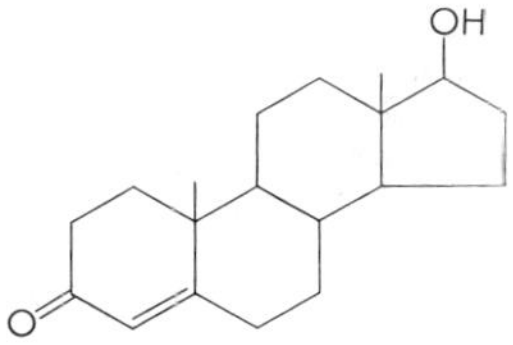	Aqueous suspension for i.m. use: 10 to 50 mg three times weekly
Testosterone propionate TESTEX	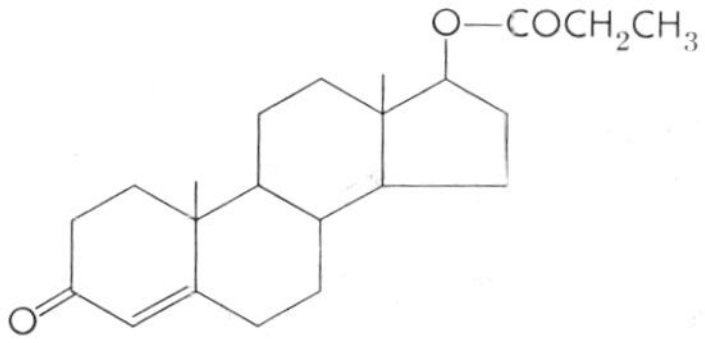	Oily solution for i.m. use: 10 to 25 mg two to three times weekly
Testosterone enanthate DELATESTRYL	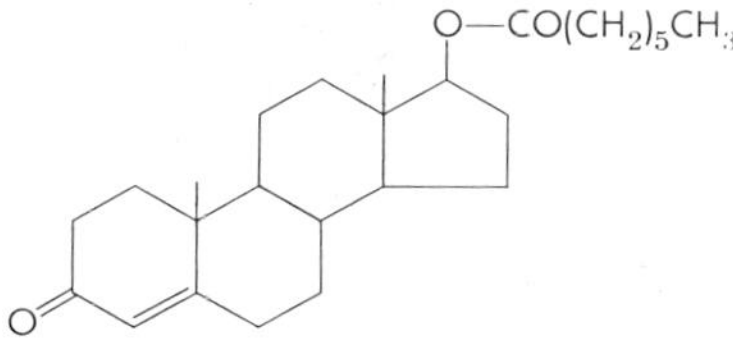	Oily solution for i.m. use: 50 to 400 mg every 2 to 4 weeks
Testosterone cypionate DEPO-TESTOSTERONE	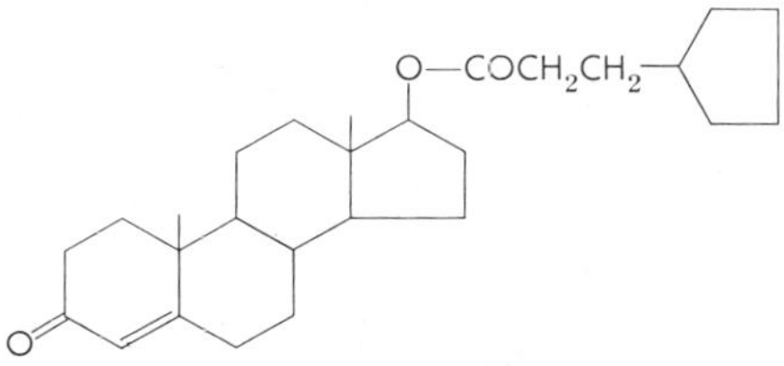	Oily solution for i.m. use: 50 to 400 mg every 2 to 4 weeks
Nandrolone decanoate DECA-DURABOLIN	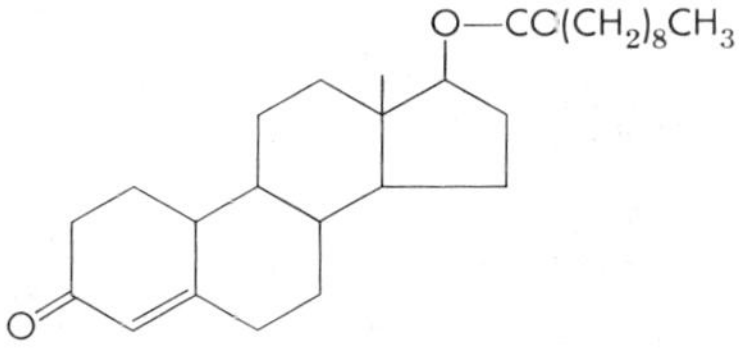	Oily solution for i.m. use: 50 to 100 mg every 3 to 4 weeks
Nandrolone phenpropionate DURABOLIN	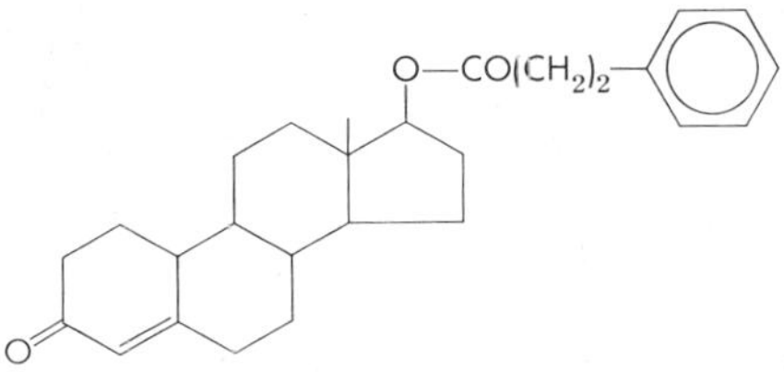	Oily solution for i.m. use: 50 to 100 mg weekly for breast carcinoma

* Dosage schedules for breast carcinoma in females are generally up to two to three times those for androgen replacement.

Table 59–3. SOME ORAL AND BUCCAL ANDROGENS USED IN THERAPY

NONPROPRIETARY NAME AND SOME TRADE NAMES	CHEMICAL STRUCTURE	DOSAGE FORMS AND USUAL DOSAGE
Danazol * DANOCRINE	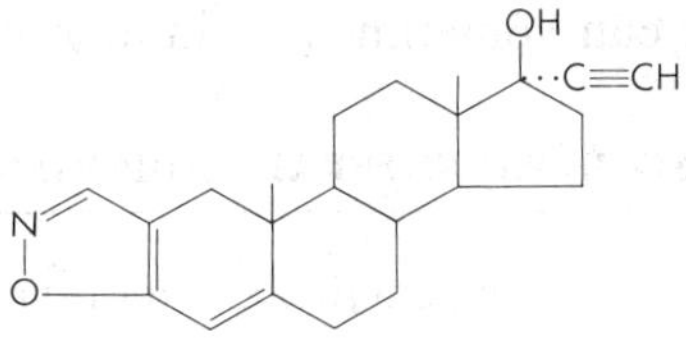	Capsules: 200 to 800 mg daily
Fluoxymesterone HALOTESTIN	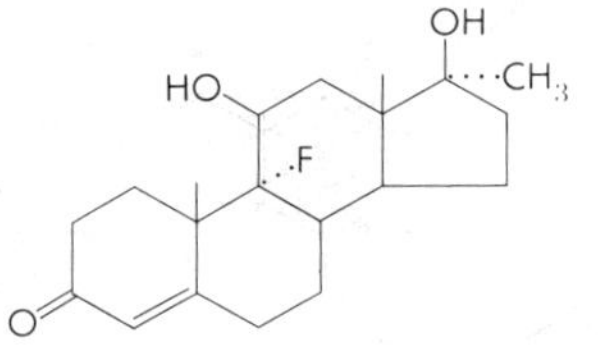	Tablets: 2.5 to 20 mg daily
Methandrostenolone DIANABOL	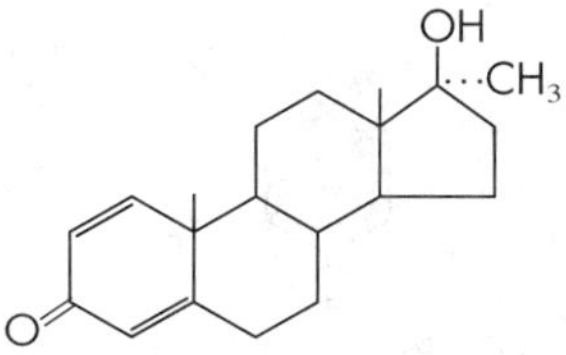	Tablets: 2.5 to 5 mg daily for osteoporosis
Methyltestosterone METANDREN, ORETON METHYL	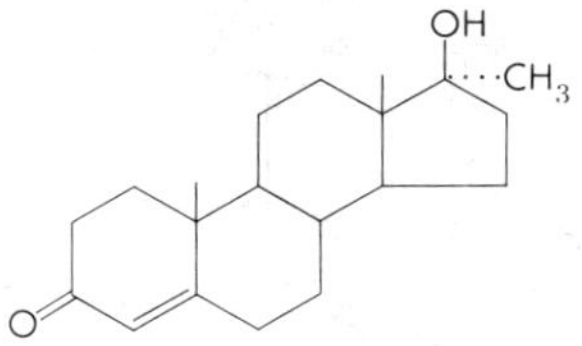	Tablets and capsules: 10 to 50 mg daily Buccal tablets: 5 to 25 mg daily
Oxandrolone ANAVAR	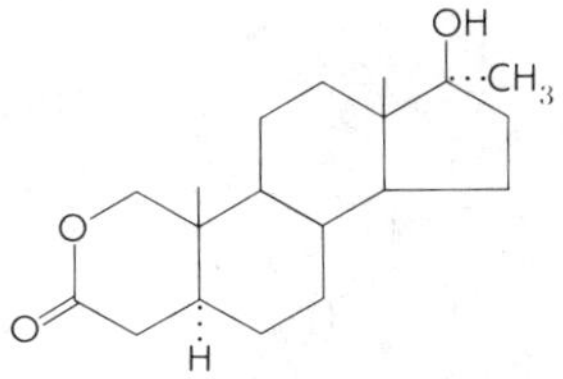	Tablets: 2.5 to 20 mg daily
Oxymetholone ANADROL-50	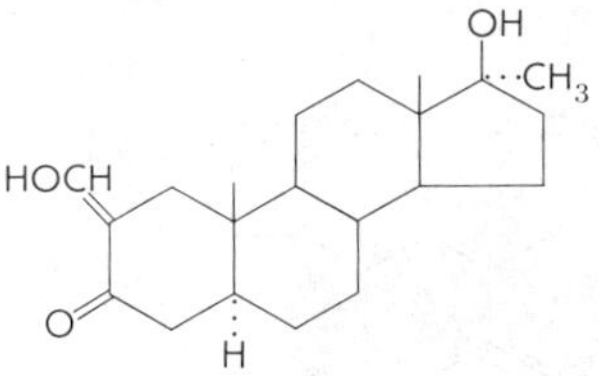	Tablets: 1 to 5 mg/kg daily for anemia
Stanozolol WINSTROL	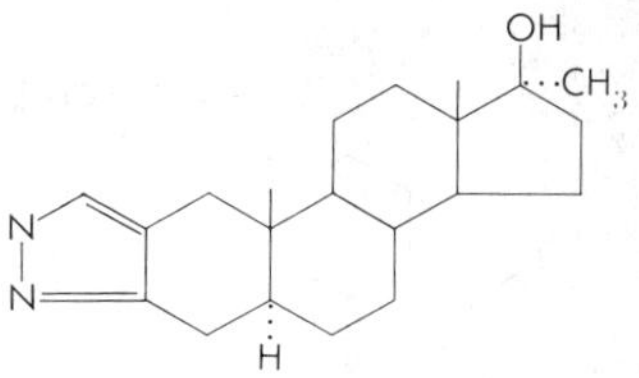	Tablets: 6 mg daily

* Used predominantly to suppress the pituitary and for the treatment of hereditary angioneurotic edema.

Table 59–3. SOME ORAL AND BUCCAL ANDROGENS USED IN THERAPY (Continued)

NONPROPRIETARY NAME AND SOME TRADE NAMES	CHEMICAL STRUCTURE	DOSAGE FORMS AND USUAL DOSAGE
Testolactone TESLAC	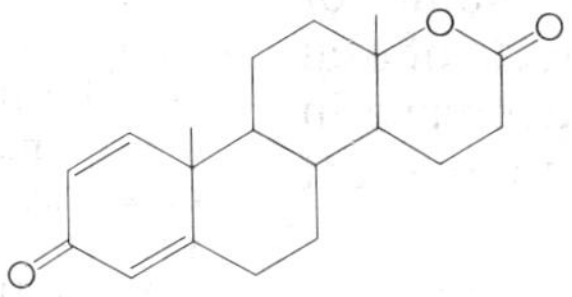	Tablets: 250 mg four times daily for breast carcinoma

genesis of this phenomenon is poorly understood. As stated above, androgens containing a Δ^4,3-keto configuration can be converted (aromatized) to estrogens in extraglandular tissues, and the administration of testosterone esters causes an increase in plasma concentrations of estrogen. The feminizing side effects are particularly severe in children (possibly because of their increased extraglandular aromatase activity compared with adults) and in men with liver disease (who have diminished rates of androgen clearance and hence shunt androgen substrate to extraglandular sites of aromatization).

Toxic Effects. Edema. Retention of water in association with sodium chloride appears to be a consistent effect of the administration of androgen and accounts for much of the gain in weight, at least in short-term treatment. In the doses used to treat hypogonadism, retention of fluid usually does not lead to detectable edema, but edema may become troublesome when large doses are given in the treatment of neoplastic diseases. Edema is also common in patients with congestive heart failure or renal insufficiency and in patients prone to edema from some other cause, such as cirrhosis of the liver or hypoproteinemia. Salt and water retention from androgens usually responds to the administration of natriuretics.

Jaundice. Methyltestosterone was the first of a number of androgens discovered to cause cholestatic hepatitis, and all androgens with 17α-alkyl substitutions can cause this complication. Disturbance of hepatic function has never been described with the parenteral use of testosterone esters. Jaundice is the prominent clinical feature, and the underlying disturbance is stasis and accumulation of bile in the biliary capillaries of the central portion of the hepatic lobules, without obstruction in the larger ducts (*see* Ishak, 1981). The hepatic cells usually exhibit only minor histological changes and remain viable. If jaundice occurs, it generally develops after 2 to 5 months of therapy. Alterations in various tests of hepatic function occur more commonly than jaundice and include increases in the concentration of bilirubin and the activities of aspartate aminotransferase and alkaline phosphatase in the plasma. The severity of the response is dependent on the dose and is particularly prominent when large amounts are given, as for palliation in neoplastic diseases. Because of these effects, testosterone esters should be administered instead of 17α-substituted steroids in virtually all clinical situations (except hereditary angioneurotic edema). In particular, the use of 17α-substituted esters should be avoided in patients with liver disease. Other forms of hepatic disease, such as peliosis hepatitis, are also rarely associated with the use of androgens (*see* Ishak, 1981).

Hepatic Carcinoma. Patients who have received 17α-alkyl substituted androgens for prolonged periods may develop hepatic adenocarcinoma. Most of the patients described received the derivatives for 1 to 7 years, and the complication may be more common in subjects with Fanconi's anemia (*see* Ishak, 1979).

Effects on Laboratory Tests. Androgens can decrease the concentration of thyroid-binding globulin in plasma and thereby influence thyroid function tests, increase the excretion of 17-ketosteroids, raise plasma LDL-cholesterol and lower plasma HDL-cholesterol concentrations, and increase the hematocrit. 17α-Alkyl-substituted steroids cause an increase in the hepatic synthesis and plasma concentrations of a variety of glycoproteins (Barbosa *et al.,* 1971). Alterations in tests of hepatic function are discussed above. Some of these agents also increase the effects of oral anticoagulants, necessitating a decrease in the dose of the anticoagulant to prevent bleeding.

Therapeutic Uses. The clearest therapeutic indication for androgens is deficient endocrine function of the testes. In addition, they have been tried in a variety of other situations in the hope that their effects on nongenital tissues would be beneficial. Testosterone esters are the preferred agents in all situations; the use of alkylated androgens should be restricted to hereditary angioneurotic edema (*see* below) or short-term therapy in patients with serious illnesses.

Hypogonadism. Failure of the testis to secrete androgen usually cannot be recognized in childhood and is first evident when the changes of puberty seem to be delayed. The age of onset of puberty varies widely among individuals, and when no evidence of maturation is seen by age 15 to 17, there may be great concern on the part of the patient and his parents. There is a good deal of debate about the use of androgen to hasten the changes of puberty in normal boys with delayed sexual maturation. Most physicians would agree that androgens should be withheld if parental pressures can be overcome.

Patients with delayed puberty should be evaluated for pituitary as well as gonadal dysfunction. Hypogonadism may be due to primary testicular failure or to diminished concentrations of gonadotropins. The latter could be due to hypopituitarism, as discussed below, or secondary to low concentrations of gonadotropin-releasing hormone. Some patients with the latter disorder have responded to long-term administration of leuprolide or gonadorelin (Hoffman and Crowley, 1982; Skarin *et al.,* 1982; Cutler *et al.,* 1985). The uses of gonadotropins and gonadotropin-releasing hormones for secondary hypogonadism are discussed in Chapter 56.

If an androgen is administered to boys with delayed puberty in the absence of an established diagnosis of hypogonadism, it can be given in courses of 4 to 6 months at a time and stopped for like periods to ascertain whether the testes are enlarging and development is progressing spontaneously. The secretion of gonadotropins must also be reevaluated after discontinuation of androgens.

When testicular failure is complete and puberty cannot occur, prolonged therapy is required. One of the long-acting esters of testosterone, such as the cypionate or the enanthate, may be given intramuscularly. It is recommended that initial doses of about one half of the eventual maintenance dose be given for 6 months to 1 year; the eventual maintenance dose of the long-acting esters of testosterone is about 200 mg every 2 weeks. Because of their effects on hepatic function, 17α-alkyl-substituted androgens should not be used for replacement therapy. Furthermore, the concentration of testosterone in plasma should be titrated to the normal range in all individuals (Caminos-Torres *et al.,* 1977).

When therapy is begun at the time of expected puberty in boys with either primary or secondary hypogonadism, the normal events of puberty proceed in the usual fashion. The normal growth spurt occurs, and penile development, deepening of the voice, and appearance of other secondary sex characteristics are apparent during the first year. Puberty in normal boys extends over several years, and treatment designed to replicate normal development cannot hasten the process greatly. Testosterone exerts its full action only in the presence of a balanced hormonal environment and specifically only in the presence of adequate concentrations of growth hormone. Consequently, prepubertal boys with coexisting deficiency of growth hormone exhibit a diminished response to androgens with regard to both growth and virilization unless growth hormone is given simultaneously.

If therapy is delayed until long after the usual time of puberty, the degree of virilization that can be achieved is variable. Many of these patients undergo a late but relatively complete anatomical and functional male maturation. If hypogonadism is primary and of long duration, suppression of plasma concentrations of LH to the normal range may not occur for months.

In postpubertal testicular failure, even of many years' duration, resumption of normal sexual activity is usual following adequate replacement. The major effect of androgen on sex drive appears to be on libido; the volume of the ejaculate and other secondary sex characteristics return to normal, and the effects of pubertal androgen on hemoglobin, nitrogen retention, and skeletal development are also reproduced. In contrast, administration of testosterone has no effect on libido in men with normal concentrations of the hormone in plasma.

Nitrogen Balance and Muscle Development. Effects of androgens on hypogonadal or castrated men include reduction in the urinary excretion of nitrogen, Na^+, K^+, and Cl^- and a gain in weight (*see* Wilson and Griffin, 1980). In contrast, in all situations other than hypogonadism, the positive nitrogen balance is short lived (probably lasting no more than 1 to 2 months).

Since androgens have significant effects on muscle mass and on body weight when administered to hypogonadal men, it was assumed, but never proven, that androgens in pharmacological doses could promote growth of muscle above the levels produced by the normal testicular secretion. This assumption was based on the belief that anabolic and androgenic actions are different, and a concerted effort was made to devise pure "anabolic" steroids that have no androgenic effects. In fact, androgenic and anabolic effects do not result from different actions of the same hormone but represent the same action in different tissues; androgen-responsive muscle contains the same receptor that mediates the action of the hormone in other target tissues (Saartok *et al.,* 1984). *All anabolic hormones tested to date are also androgenic.* In appropriate doses, most anabolic agents can be used for replacement of androgen. For example, methandrostenolone, which has a greater effect on nitrogen balance per unit weight than does methyltestosterone, is a potent androgen and has been used for replacement therapy in hypogonadal men. Nevertheless, androgens have been tried in a variety of clinical situations other than hypogonadism with the hope that improvement in nitrogen balance and muscle development would outweigh any deleterious side effects.

Catabolic States. Body protein is broken down more rapidly than it is formed following injury or surgery, and excess nitrogen is excreted in the urine as a consequence. During the subsequent recovery phase, nitrogen deficits are replaced. Anabolic steroids can improve the nitrogen balance during the first few days following relatively minor operations in well-nourished subjects, but the diminution in nitrogen loss is minimal and has not been shown to be of significant therapeutic benefit. Likewise, effects of androgens on weight in undernourished, debilitated, or elderly individuals are due predominantly to enhancement of appetite. In appropriately controlled studies, no consistent effects on weight or strength have been documented following treatment with androgen. These negative results are probably the consequence of several factors, including the dependence of anabolic effects on adequate nutrition and health, the paucity of effects of androgens in men with normal concentrations of testosterone, and the temporary nature of any positive nitrogen balance when it does occur. In short, androgens are ineffective in promoting anabolism in acute illness, severe trauma, and protein depletion associated with chronic illness (*see* Wilson and Griffin, 1980). Androgens are also of little value in the management of nitrogen accumulation in chronic renal failure; at best they induce a transient improvement in nitrogen balance that is of doubtful importance. In acute renal failure, androgens cause a decrease in the rate of production of urea and a consequent decrease in the frequency of dialysis required for some patients. Most of these patients do well without androgen therapy.

Athletic Performance. Androgens are sometimes used by athletes in the belief that athletic performance will be improved. Apparently, weight lifters and body builders began to use the drugs in the 1950s, and androgen abuse subsequently became widespread at all levels of athletic competition. Indeed, the problem continues to grow in magnitude and has received a great deal of attention in the press as a consequence of the disqualification of athletes at several international competitions. Most surveys suggest that about half of the athletes who abuse androgens obtain them through the "steroid underground" and that the others obtain them through physicians' prescriptions. The fact that any abusers obtain androgens from physicians is particularly worrisome because many aspects of androgen abuse are poorly understood.

First, androgens do promote muscle growth in boys and in women of all ages, and this phenomenon is mediated by the androgen receptor. However, it is not known whether androgens have any beneficial effects on muscle development, nitrogen balance, or athletic performance in sexually mature men. Two types of evidence do suggest that *massive* doses of androgen may enhance muscle development in men. After administration of 5 g or more of exogenous androgen, lean body mass increases (Forbes, 1985); pharmacological amounts of testosterone enanthate (3 mg/kg weekly) for 12 weeks cause an increase in muscle mass and whole body protein synthesis (Griggs *et al.,* 1989). Nevertheless, appropriately controlled studies of the effects of androgens on strength and performance in conditioned athletes have yielded inconclusive results. If androgens do have a beneficial effect it is not known how they work, since the androgen receptors in mature men appear to be functionally saturated. It is possible that high doses of androgens act at the level of the glucocorticoid receptor to inhibit the catabolic effects of glucocorticoids (for review, *see* Wilson, 1988).

Second, the question of the effect of androgens on athletic performance in men is not easy to resolve scientifically for several reasons. (1) The side effects of the drugs at doses taken by athletes are so pronounced as to preclude truly blinded studies of efficacy; (2) only a small subset of users may have a beneficial response, making it difficult to identify the rare responder; and (3) effects on athletic performance become more difficult to assess as the caliber of the athlete increases. For example, a 1% difference in power or speed might be difficult to document between groups but may make a very significant difference in the performance of an individual athlete. Regardless of the unresolved scientific issues, many athletes, coaches, and sports physicians believe that the agents do enhance athletic performance; as a consequence, the emphasis in organized sports has shifted from education to coercive drug testing.

Third, the side effects of androgens are still incompletely understood, in part because many of the agents that are used are either veterinary drugs or other unapproved derivatives for which no human safety data are available. In addition, certain side effects such as peliosis hepatitis may occur only in occasional patients. Finally, adequate long-term toxicity studies have not been performed for any of the agents. As stated above, the side effects of androgens can be separated into virilizing effects, feminizing effects, and toxic effects. All side effects are more common in women and children and hence preclude the use of androgens in these groups by all but a fanatic subset of women athletes. The feminizing and virilizing side effects in adult men are largely reversible, although some effects such as suppression of spermatogenesis may persist for months after the agents are discontinued. Certain long-term toxic effects such as impairment of hepatic function and suppression of high-density lipoprotein concentrations are probably mitigated by the usual pattern of intermittent use of the agents. On balance, however, the side effects in men are sufficiently severe to preclude their use for this purpose on medical grounds.

Stimulation of Erythropoiesis. The difference in the hematocrit between men and women is the result of a stimulatory effect of testosterone on the formation of erythropoietin. Castration of men results in a 10% decrease in the mass of red blood cells, a decrease in red-cell diameter, and an increase in osmotic fragility. Occasionally, the anemia may be severe. Administration of androgens to women increases erythropoiesis, and some women develop polycythemia during long-term administration of androgens, as in the treatment of carcinoma of the breast (Shahidi, 1973). In women treated with pharmacological doses of testosterone, the average concentration of hemoglobin increases by 43 g/l and the hematocrit increases by 0.11. The average increase in hemoglobin is about 10 g/l in normal men given pharmacological doses of testosterone esters. Because of these effects androgens have been used in the treatment of refractory anemias in both men and women (Shahidi, 1973). The capacity to enhance erythropoiesis is shared by all active androgens. Some erythropoietin is synthesized by tissues other than the kidney, and the presence of renal tissue is not an absolute requirement for stimulation of erythropoiesis by androgens.

Androgen therapy has also been tried in the anemias associated with failure of the bone marrow, myelofibrosis, and renal failure. Occasional dramatic increases in hemoglobin occur following the administration of androgens to subjects with bone-marrow failure (Azen and Shahidi, 1977). In large numbers of unselected patients treated with androgens, approximately half appear to respond, particularly when the bone marrow is hypoplastic or myelofibrotic. What is uncertain, however, is the frequency with which drug administration and therapeutic response is coincidental (Branda *et al.*, 1977; Camitta *et al.*, 1979). This is a particular problem with regard to acquired anemias, in which spontaneous remission can occur during the course of therapy. Additional randomized prospective studies are required before the role of androgens in the routine management of aplastic anemia can be defined. Until such evidence is available, trial with androgens (of limited duration) is probably warranted in selected subjects with aplastic anemia. When an apparent response occurs, the drug should be stopped temporarily to establish a cause-and-effect relationship between the drug and the apparent response.

Androgens have a minor role in treatment of the anemia of renal failure, particularly because of the availability of recombinant, human erythropoietin. Androgen-induced increases in concentrations of erythropoietin and hemoglobin are less marked in patients with renal failure than in normal subjects. In addition, the anemia of renal failure may undergo gradual improvement with time following the institution of an adequate dialysis program and correction of other coexisting causes of anemia. Nevertheless, most studies indicate that androgen therapy results in increases in hemoglobin (10 to 50 g/l) and in red-blood-cell volume (325 to 350 ml), provided dialysis is adequate and stores of iron and folate are normal (von Hartizsch *et al.*, 1977). Whether the benefits of such treatment outweigh the potential adverse effects is unclear.

Hereditary Angioneurotic Edema. In hereditary angioneurotic edema, an autosomal dominant disorder, the plasma contains either a nonfunctional inhibitor of the first component of complement or decreased concentrations of the inhibitor. Thus, there is unopposed activation of the complement cascade, which leads to the generation of factors that enhance the permeability of vessels and cause attacks of angioedema. A variety of 17α-alkylated steroids are efficacious in treating this condition. Such therapy not only increases the activity of the inhibitor in plasma but also restores the concentrations of the components of the complement system that are depleted secondarily. Orally active androgens are effective, and steroids such as danazol that are weak androgens appear to be as effective as or more effective than potent androgens. Furthermore, the response of men and women to such oral agents appears to be the same. 17α-Alkylated androgens (but not testosterone or testosterone esters) cause elevations of the concentrations of several plasma glycoproteins that are synthesized in the liver, including several clotting factors and the inhibitor of the first component of complement. The beneficial effect of oral androgens in this disorder is thus likely the result of a side effect of 17α-alkylated steroids on hepatic function rather than of androgen action *per se* (Barbosa *et al.*, 1971; Gralnick and Rick, 1983).

Short Stature. Androgens have been used for the management of growth retardation resulting from causes other than pituitary insufficiency. Their administration prior to epiphyseal closure results in an enhancement of linear growth, and the mean advance of height age may be more striking than is skeletal maturation (*see* Wilson and Griffin, 1980). Such therapy, when given for short periods (6 months or less), has no permanent effects on hypothalamic-pituitary or gonadal maturation. This acceleration of growth may be the result of both an increase in plasma concentration of growth hormone and a direct effect of androgens themselves (Clayton *et al.*, 1988). Whether such therapy has a beneficial effect on final adult height is not known. For example, in subjects with 45,X-gonadal dysgenesis, treatment with oral androgens causes a temporary acceleration of growth but has a relatively small effect on mean final height. Furthermore, administration of androgens to short children prior to the age of 9 years may actually have a deleterious effect on adult height (Bettman *et al.*, 1971). Thus, a role for androgens in the management of any form of short stature other than pituitary dwarfism has not been established.

Carcinoma of the Breast. Testosterone propionate has a palliative effect in some women with carcinoma of the breast. The mechanism of this effect is unknown, but the androgen may act as an antiestrogen. The response rates are equivalent to those induced by high doses of estrogen (where an antiestrogenic mechanism may also be operative). No androgen is more efficacious than testosterone, and structural changes in the testosterone molecule that decrease its androgenicity also diminish its effectiveness in breast cancer. Since remission rates are higher with conventional chemotherapy, androgens do not play a major role in the management of carcinoma of the breast (*see* Chapter 52).

Other Disorders. Androgen therapy is effective in treatment of the osteoporosis that complicates androgen deficiency; indeed, the histological response to hormonal replacement can be dramatic (Gordon, 1978). A role for androgens in the treatment of osteoporosis unassociated with male hypogonadism has not been established.

ANTIANDROGENS

Compounds that block the synthesis or action of androgens might be useful in the management of hyperplasia and carcinoma of the prostate, acne, male-pattern baldness, virilizing syndromes in women, and precocious puberty in boys and in the inhibition of sex drive in men who are sex offenders. The most effective inhibitor of testosterone synthesis is either gonadotropin-releasing hormone (GnRH) itself or an analog such as leuprolide; when such compounds are administered continuously, plasma concentrations of LH and testosterone fall such that the net consequence is the induction of a pharmacological (and reversible) castration (*see* Chapter 56). In general, two types of agents have been developed to block androgen action—drugs that compete for the binding of testosterone and dihydrotestosterone to the androgen receptor, and inhibitors of the 5α-reductase that converts testosterone to dihydrotestosterone.

Androgen-Receptor Antagonists. Several drugs, including spironolactone and cimetidine, have antiandrogenic side effects, but cyproterone acetate and flutamide are specific antagonists of the binding of androgen to its receptor.

Cyproterone Acetate. Progesterone itself is a weak antiandrogen, and in the search for orally active progestogens, cyproterone acetate was found to be a potent androgen antagonist (Table 59–4). Cyproterone acetate also possesses progestational activity and suppresses the secretion of gonadotropins (Neri, 1976; Neumann, 1982; Neumann and Töpert, 1986). The agent competes with dihydrotestosterone for binding to the androgen receptor (Brown *et al.*, 1981); when given in high doses to pregnant animals cyproterone acetate blocks the actions of androgen in the male fetus and hence induces a form of male pseudohermaphroditism similar to the testicular feminization syndrome (Hamada *et al.*, 1963). In the mature rat, the compound causes atrophy of the seminal vesicles, prostate, levator ani muscle, and other androgen-responsive tissues (Neumann, 1966). In the castrated animal about five times as much antagonist as testosterone reduces the androgenic response by about 50%; with larger doses of cyproterone acetate the antagonism is almost complete (Neumann *et al.*, 1970).

The administration of 100 mg per day of cyproterone acetate to normal young men causes a 50% decrease in plasma concentrations of LH and FSH and a 75% decrease in plasma testosterone; clinical actions of the drug thus result both from inhibition of testosterone production and from interference with androgen action (Knuth *et al.*, 1984). The agent has been used for the treatment of acne, male-pattern baldness, hirsutism, and virilizing syndromes (*see* Neri, 1976; Neumann, 1982; Neumann and Töpert, 1986). It has also been tried in the treatment of precocious puberty (Kauli *et al.*, 1976) and prostatic hypertrophy and carcinoma (*see* Namer, 1988) and to inhibit libido in men with severe deviations of sexual behavior (Laschet *et al.*, 1967). Although cyproterone acetate is still under investigation, the agent has orphan-drug status in the United States for the treatment of severe hirsutism.

Flutamide. Flutamide (*see* Table 59–4) is a nonsteroidal antiandrogen that is devoid of other hormonal activity; it probably acts after conversion *in vivo* to 2-hydroxyflutamide (*see* Neri, 1976). In the mature rat the agent causes regression of an-

Table 59–4. SOME ANTIANDROGENS

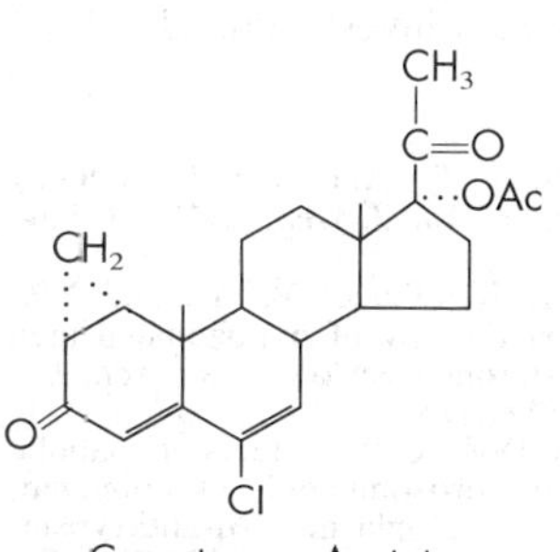

Cyproterone Acetate

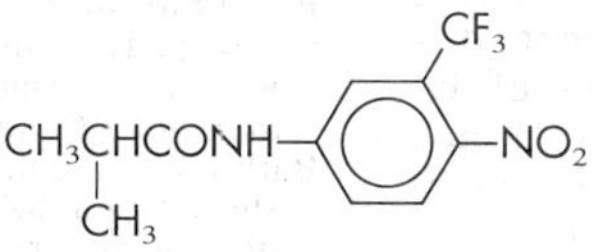

Flutamide

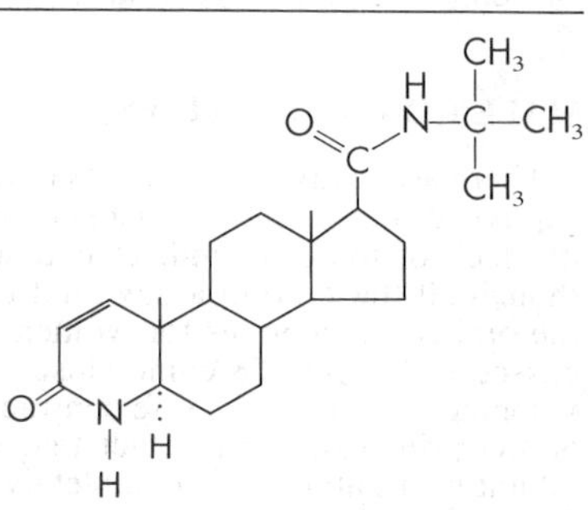

Finazteride

drogen target tissues such as the prostate and seminal vesicles, and, by blocking the inhibitory feedback of testosterone on LH production, results in a profound increase in plasma concentrations of LH and testosterone (Marchetti and Labrie, 1988). Similar effects have been observed in men treated with 750 mg of flutamide per day (Knuth *et al.*, 1984). The predominant effect of flutamide appears to be enhancement of the frequency of pulses of LH secretion (Urban *et al.*, 1988). Thus, while the drug is a pure antiandrogen, the rise in plasma testosterone serves to limit its antiandrogenic effects. As a consequence, flutamide is most useful to inhibit the action of adrenal androgens in castrated men or in men receiving GnRH continuously (GnRH blockade) or in situations in which LH production is not under predominant control of androgen (as in normal women).

The principal clinical application of flutamide to date is in the treatment of prostatic cancer, usually in conjunction with GnRH blockade or estrogen (*see* Geller *et al.*, 1988). Flutamide has also been used experimentally in combination with an oral contraceptive for the treatment of hirsutism in women (*see* Namer, 1988). If flutamide crosses the placenta, it would be expected to produce male pseudohermaphroditism, as is the case for cyproterone acetate.

Flutamide (EULEXIN) is available in 125-mg capsules. For the treatment of metastatic prostatic carcinoma, 250 mg of flutamide is taken three times daily in conjunction with a GnRH antagonist such as leuprolide.

5α-Reductase Inhibitors. Since the conversion of testosterone to dihydrotestosterone is essential for certain actions of androgens, inhibitors of 5α-reductase should selectively block androgen action in tissues such as the prostate where continuous production of dihydrotestosterone is essential. The azasteroid *finazteride* (*see* Table 59–4) is an orally active, competitive inhibitor of the 5α-reductase enzyme, and it causes a profound decrease in the concentrations of dihydrotestosterone in plasma (Vermeulen *et al.*, 1989) and in the prostate (McConnell *et al.*, 1989). The drug does not cause an increase in plasma concentrations of LH or testosterone and is under evaluation for the treatment of benign prostatic hyperplasia.

MALE CONTRACEPTIVES

There are many requirements of the ideal contraceptive drug: simplicity, acceptability, reversibility, lack of toxicity, and, of course, efficacy. Although all these criteria have not been attained in the oral contraceptives for women, the agents discussed in Chapter 58 come close. The lack of development of effective, safe contraceptives for men is due principally to the fact that it is difficult to inhibit spermatogenesis completely, and men have fathered children even when sperm counts are lowered by 99% (to values of approximately 1 million per milliliter) (*see* Diller and Hembree, 1977; Bialy and Patanelli, 1981; Reyes and Chavarria, 1981).

A variety of compounds, in addition to the antiandrogens discussed above, can inhibit spermatogenesis. They include antineoplastic agents, cadmium, nitrofuranes, α-chlorhydrin, and dinitropyrrole. However, the irreversible effects of some and the toxicity of many preclude their clinical use.

Gossypol, a phenolic compound extracted from the cotton plant of the genus *Gossypium,* reduces sperm density to less than 4 million/ml in 99.9% of men and impairs sperm motility. Normal sperm density is restored within several months of discontinuation of the drug (*see* Lawrence, 1981). Unfortunately, administration of gossypol causes hypokalemia and weakness; diarrhea, edema, dyspnea, neuritis, and paralysis are observed after higher doses are taken. These effects are also seen in cottonseed poisoning.

Gonadal steroids can suppress secretion of FSH and LH, which are required for spermatogenesis and the synthesis of testosterone by the testes (*see* Chapters 56 and 58). While estrogens and progestins are effective contraceptives in men, suppression of testosterone decreases both libido and potency; gynecomastia may also occur. Attempts have been made to overcome these unacceptable side effects by administration of exogenous androgens to inhibit secretion of gonadotropins and spermatogenesis. However, the treatment is not uniformly effective. The use of androgens alone is thus not encouraging.

Another approach has involved the dual administration of an androgen and progestin (Brenner *et al.*, 1975). The rationale for this combination was to enhance the suppression of gonadotropin secretion and spermatogenesis by testosterone with a progestogen and to prevent alteration of accessory sexual structures by the administration of testosterone (Bremner and DeKretser, 1976; Ewing and Robaire, 1978). Unfortunately, not all subjects develop azoospermia, and sperm counts are suppressed only after several months of treatment. A similar amount of time is required for the recovery of spermatogenesis when the drugs are stopped.

Potent agonists and antagonists of GnRH can inhibit secretion of gonadotropins and can be administered together with testosterone; however, this regimen does not result in uniform azoospermia (Heber and Swerdloff, 1980; Cutler *et al.*, 1985). All the methods described above for contraception in the male remain investigational.

Azen, E. A., and Shahidi, N. T. Androgen dependency in acquired aplastic anemia. *Am. J. Med.*, **1977**, *63*, 320–324.

Bals-Pratsch, M.; Larger, K.; Place, V. A.; and Nieschlag, E. Substitution therapy of hypogonadal men with transdermal testosterone over one year. *Acta Endocrinol. [Copenh.]*, **1988**, *118*, 7–13.

Barbosa, J.; Seal, H.; and Doe, R. P. Effects of anabolic steroids on haptoglobin, orosomucoid, plasminogen, fibrinogen, transferrin, ceruloplasmin, α-antitrypsin, β-glucuronidase, and total serum proteins. *J. Clin. Endocrinol.*, **1971**, *33*, 388–398.

Berthold, A. A. Transplantation der hoden. *Arch. Anat. Physiol. Wiss. Med.*, **1849**, *16*, 42–46.

Bettman, H. K.; Goldman, H. S.; Abramowicz, M.; and Sobel, E. H. Oxandrolone treatment of short stature: effect on predicted mature height. *J. Pediatr.*, **1971**, *79*, 1018–1023.

Bialy, G., and Patanelli, D. J. Potential use of male antifertility agents in developed countries. *Chemotherapy*, **1981**, *27*, 102–106.

Branda, R. F.; Amsden, T. W.; and Jacob, H. S. Randomized study of nandrolone therapy for anemias due to bone marrow failure. *Arch. Intern. Med.*, **1977**, *137*, 65–69.

Brenner, P. F.; Bernstein, G. S.; Roy, S.; Jeckt, E. W.; and Mischell, D. R. Administration of norethandrolone and testosterone as a contraceptive agent for men. *Contraception*, **1975**, *11*, 193–207.

Brown, T. R.; Rothwell, S. W.; Sultan, C.; and Migeon, C. J. Inhibition of androgen binding in human foreskin fibroblasts by antiandrogens. *Steroids*, **1981**, *37*, 635–648.

Butenandt, A. Über die chemische Untersuchung der Sexualhormons. *Z. Angew. Chem.*, **1931**, *44*, 905–908.

Caminos-Torres, R.; Ma, L.; and Snyder, P. J. Testosterone-induced inhibition of the LH and FSH responses to gonadotropin-releasing hormone occurs slowly. *J. Clin. Endocrinol.*, **1977**, *44*, 1142–1153.

Camitta, B. M.; Thomas, E. D.; and Nathan, D. G. A prospective study of androgens and bone marrow transplantation for treatment of severe aplastic anemia. *Blood*, **1979**, *53*, 504–514.

Castro, A. E.; Alonso, A.; and Mancini, R. E. Localization of follicle stimulating and luteinizing hormones in the rat testis using immunohistological tests. *J. Endocrinol.*, **1972**, *52*, 129–136.

Chang, C.; Kokontis, J.; and Liao, S. Molecular cloning of human and rat complementary DNA encoding androgen receptors. *Science*, **1988**, *240*, 324–328.

Clayton, P. E.; Shalet, S. M.; Price, D. A.; and Addison, G. M. Growth and growth hormone responses to oxandrolone in boys with constitutional delay of growth and puberty (CDGP). *Clin. Endocrinol. (Oxf.)*, **1988**, *29*, 123–130.

David, K.; Dingemanse, E.; Freud, J.; and Laqueur, E. Über krystallinisches männliches Hormon aus Hoden (Testosteron), wirksamer als aus Harn oder aus Cholesterin bereitetes Androsteron. *Hoppe Seylers Z. Physiol. Chem.*, **1935**, *233*, 281–282.

Diller, L., and Hembree, W. Male contraception and family planning: a social and historical review. *Fertil. Steril.*, **1977**, *28*, 1271–1279.

Duhey, A. K.; Zeleznik, A. J.; and Plant, T. M. In the rhesus monkey (*Macaca mulatta*) the negative feedback regulation of follicle-stimulating hormone secretion by an action of testosterone directly cannot be accounted for by either testosterone or estradiol. *Endocrinology*, **1987**, *121*, 2229–2237.

Findley, J. D.; Place, V. A.; and Snyder, P. J. Transdermal delivery of testosterone. *J. Clin. Endocrinol. Metab.*, **1987**, *64*, 266–268.

Forbes, G. The effect of anabolic steroids on lean body mass: the dose response curve. *Metabolism*, **1985**, *34*, 571–573.

Gralnick, H. R., and Rick, M. E. Danazol increases factor VIII and factor IX in classic hemophilia and Christmas disease. *N. Engl. J. Med.*, **1983**, *308*, 1393–1395.

Griggs, R. C.; Kingston, W.; Jozefowicz, R. F.; Herr, B. E.; Forbes, G.; and Halliday, D. Effect of testosterone on muscle mass and muscle protein synthesis. *J. Appl. Physiol.*, **1989**, *66*, 498–503.

Hamada, H.; Neumann, F.; and Junkmann, K. Intrauterine antimaskuline Beinflüssung von Rattenfeten durch ein stark Gestagen wirksames Steroid. *Acta Endocrinol. (Kbh.)*, **1963**, *44*, 380–388.

Heber, D., and Swerdloff, R. S. Male contraception: synergism of gonadotropin-releasing hormone analog and testosterone in suppressing gonadotropin. *Science*, **1980**, *209*, 936–938.

Hilliard, J.; Scaramuzzi, R. J.; Pang, C.-N.; Penardi, R.; and Sawyer, C. H. Testosterone secretion by rabbit ovary *in vivo*. *Endocrinology*, **1974**, *94*, 267–271.

Hoffman, A. R., and Crowley, W. F. Induction of puberty in men by long-term pulsatile administration of low-dose gonadotropin-releasing hormone. *N. Engl. J. Med.*, **1982**, *307*, 1237–1241.

Ishak, K. S. Hepatic neoplasms associated with contraceptive and anabolic steroids. *Recent Results Cancer Res.*, **1979**, *66*, 73–128.

Judd, H. L., and Yen, S. S. C. Serum adrenostenedione and testosterone levels during the menstrual cycle. *J. Clin. Endocrinol. Metab.*, **1973**, *36*, 475–481.

Kauli, R.; Pertzelan, A.; Prager-Lewin, R.; Grünebaum, M.; and Laron, Z. Cyproterone acetate in treatment of precocious puberty. *Arch. Dis. Child.*, **1976**, *51*, 202–208.

Kelch, R. P.; Jenner, M. R.; Weinstein, R.; Kaplan, S. L.; and Grumbach, M. M. Estradiol and testosterone secretion by human, simian, and canine testes in males with hypogonadism and in male pseudohermaphrodites with the feminizing testes syndrome. *J. Clin. Invest.*, **1972**, *51*, 824–830.

Keogh, E. J.; Lee, V. W. K.; Rennie, G. C.; Burger, H. G.; Hudson, B.; and DeKretser, D. M. Selective suppression of FSH by testicular extracts. *Endocrinology*, **1976**, *98*, 997–1004.

Knowlton, K.; Kenyon, A. T.; Sandiford, I.; Lotwin, G.; and Fricker, R. Comparative study of metabolic effects of estradiol benzoate and testosterone propionate in man. *J. Clin. Endocrinol. Metab.*, **1942**, *2*, 671–684.

Knuth, U. A.; Hano, R.; and Nieschlag, E. Effect of flutamide or cyproterone acetate on pituitary and testicular hormones in normal men. *J. Clin. Endocrinol. Metab.*, **1984**, *59*, 963–969.

Kochakian, C. D., and Murlin, J. R. The effect of male hormone on the protein and energy metabolism of castrate dogs. *J. Nutr.*, **1935**, *10*, 437–459.

Kovacs, W. J.; Griffin, J. E.; Weaver, D. D.; Carlson, B. R.; and Wilson, J. D. A mutation that causes lability of the androgen receptor under conditions that normally promote transformation to the DNA-binding state. *J. Clin. Invest.*, **1984**, *73*, 1095–1104.

Laschet, U.; Laschet, L.; Felzner, H.-R.; Glaesel, H.-U.; Mall, G.; and Naab, M. Results in the treatment of hyper- and abnormal sexuality of men with antiandrogens. *Acta Endocrinol. (Kbh.)*, **1967**, *56*, Suppl. 119, 54.

Loewe, S., and Voss, H. E. Der Stand der Erfassung des männlichen Sexualhormons (Androkinins). *Klin. Wochenschr.*, **1930**, *9*, 481–487.

McConnell, J. D.; Wilson, J. D.; George, F. W.; Geller, J.; Walsh, P. C.; Ewing, L. L.; Isaacs, J.; and Stoner, E. An inhibitor of 5α-reductase, MK-906, suppresses prostatic dihydrotestosterone in men with benign prostatic hyperplasia. *J. Urol.*, **1989**, *141*, 239A.

McLachlan, R. I.; Robertson, D. M.; and de Kretser, D. Inhibin—a non-steroidal regulator of pituitary follicle stimulating hormone. *Baillieres Clin. Endocrinol. Metab.*, **1987**, *1*, 89–112.

Marchetti, B., and Labrie, F. Characteristics of flutamide action on prostatic and testicular functions in the rat. *J. Steroid Biochem.*, **1988**, *29*, 691–698.

Matsumoto, A. M., and Bremner, W. J. Modulation of pulsatile gonadotropin secretion by testosterone in man. *J. Clin. Endocrinol. Metab.*, **1984**, *58*, 609–614.

Neumann, F. Auftreton von Kastrationszellen im Hypophysenvorderlappen männlicher Ratten nach Behandlung mit einem Antiandrogen. *Acta Endocrinol. (Kbh.)*, **1966**, *53*, 53–60.

Papanicolaou, G. N., and Falk, E. A. General muscular hypertrophy induced by androgenic hormones. *Science*, **1938**, *87*, 238–239.

Pardridge, W. M.; Gorski, R. A.; Lippe, B. M.; and Green, R. Androgens and sexual behavior. *Ann. Intern. Med.*, **1982**, *96*, 488–501.

Ramasharma, K., and Sairam, M. R. Isolation and characterization of inhibin from human seminal plasma. *Ann. N. Y. Acad. Sci.*, **1982**, *383*, 307–328.

Reyes, A., and Chavarria, M. E. Interference with epididymal physiology as possible site of male contraception. *Arch. Androl.*, **1981**, *7*, 159–168.

Ruzicka, L., and Wettstein, A. Synthetische Darstellung des Testishormons, Testosteron (Androsten-3-on-17-ol). *Helv. Chim. Acta*, **1935**, *18*, 1264–1275.

Saartok, T.; Dahlberg, E.; and Gustafsson, J. Relative binding affinity of anabolic-androgenic steroids: comparison of the binding to the androgen receptors in skeletal muscle and in prostate, as well as to sex hormone–binding globulin. *Endocrinology*, **1984**, *114*, 2100–2106.

Sachs, B. D.; Pollak, E. I.; Kreiger, M. S.; and Barfield, R. J. Sexual behavior: normal male patterning in androgenized female rats. *Science*, **1973**, *181*, 770–772.

Shahidi, N. T. Androgens and erythropoiesis. *N. Engl. J. Med.*, **1973**, *289*, 72–80.

Skarin, G.; Nillius, S. J.; Wibell, L.; and Wide, L. Chronic pulsatile low dose GnRH therapy for induction of testosterone production and spermatogenesis in a man with secondary hypogonadotropic hypogonadism. *J. Clin. Endocrinol. Metab.*, **1982**, *55*, 723–726.

Urban, R. J.; Davis, M. R.; Rogol, A. D.; Johnson, M. L.; and Veldhuis, J. D. Acute androgen receptor blockade increases luteinizing hormone secretory activity in men. *J. Clin. Endocrinol. Metab.*, **1988**, *67*, 1149–1155.

Vermeulen, A.; Giagulli, V. A.; De Schepper, P.; Buntinx, A.; and Stoner, E. Hormonal effects of an orally active 4-azasteroid inhibitor of 5α-reductase in humans. *Prostate*, **1989**, *14*, 45–53.

von Hartizsch, B.; Kerr, D. N. S.; and Morley, G. Androgens in the anemia of chronic renal failure. *Nephron*, **1977**, *18*, 13–20.

Monographs and Reviews

Boyar, R. M. Control of the onset of puberty. *Annu. Rev. Med.*, **1978**, *29*, 509–520.

Bremner, W. J., and DeKretser, D. M. The prospects for new reversible male contraceptives. *N. Engl. J. Med.*, **1976**, *295*, 1111–1116.

Cutler, G. B.; Hoffman, A. R.; Swerdloff, R. S.; Santen, J.; Meldrum, D. R.; and Comite, F. Therapeutic applications of luteinizing-hormone-releasing hormone and its analogs. *Ann. Intern. Med.*, **1985**, *102*, 643–657.

Donahoe, P. K.; Hutson, J. M.; Fallat, M. E.; Kamagata, S.; and Budzik, G. P. Mechanism of action of mullerian inhibiting substance. *Annu. Rev. Physiol.*, **1984**, *45*, 53–65.

Ebling, F. J. Steroids, hormones and sebaceous secretion. *Adv. Steroid Biochem. Pharmacol.*, **1970**, *2*, 1–39.

Evans, R. M. The steroid and thyroid hormone receptor superfamily. *Science*, **1988**, *240*, 889–895.

Ewing, L. L., and Robaire, B. Endogenous antispermatogenic agents: prospects for male contraception. *Annu. Rev. Pharmacol. Toxicol.*, **1978**, *18*, 167–187.

Fotherby, K., and James, F. Metabolism of synthetic steroids. *Adv. Steroid Biochem. Pharmacol.*, **1972**, *3*, 67–165.

Franchimont, P. Pituitary gonadotropins. *Clin. Endocrinol. Metab.*, **1977**, *6*, 101–116.

Geller, J.; Albert, J.; and Vik, A. Advantages of total androgen blockade in the treatment of advanced prostatic cancer. *Semin. Oncol.*, **1988**, *15*, Suppl. 1, 53–61.

Givens, J. R. Normal and abnormal androgen metabolism. *Clin. Obstet. Gynecol.*, **1978**, *21*, 115–123.

Gordon, G. S. Drug treatment of osteoporosis. *Annu. Rev. Pharmacol. Toxicol.*, **1978**, *18*, 253–268.

Griffin, J. E., and Wilson, J. D. The androgen resistance syndromes: 5α-reductase deficiency, testicular feminization, and related syndromes. In, *The Metabolic Basis of Inherited Disease*, 6th ed. (Scriver, C. R.; Beaudet, A. L.; Sly, W. S.; and Valle, D.; eds.) McGraw-Hill Book Company, New York, **1989**, pp. 1919–1944.

Ishak, K. G. Hepatic lesions caused by anabolic and contraceptive steroids. *Semin. Liver Dis.*, **1981**, *2*, 116–128.

Jost, A. Embryonic sexual differentiation. In, *Hermaphroditism, Genital Anomalies and Related Endocrine Disorders*, 2nd ed. (Jones, H. W., and Scott, W. W., eds.) The Williams & Wilkins Co., Baltimore, **1971**, pp. 16–64.

Lawrence, S. U. Gossypol: a potential male contraceptive? *Am. Pharm.*, **1981**, *21*, 57–59.

Lipsett, M. B. Physiology and pathology of the Leydig cell. *N. Engl. J. Med.*, **1980**, *303*, 682–688.

Lunde, D. T., and Hamburg, D. A. Techniques for assessing the effects of sex steroids on affect, arousal, and aggression in humans. *Recent Prog. Horm. Res.*, **1972**, *28*, 627–663.

Mainwaring, W. I. P. (ed.). The mechanism of action of androgens. *Monogr. Endocrinol.*, **1977**, *10*, 1–178.

Marcus, R., and Korenman, S. G. Estrogens and the human male. *Annu. Rev. Med.*, **1976**, *27*, 357–370.

Miller, W. L. Molecular biology of steroid hormone synthesis. *Endocr. Rev.*, **1988**, *9*, 295–318.

Namer, M. Clinical applications of antiandrogens. *J. Steroid Biochem.*, **1988**, *31*, 719–729.

Neri, R. O. Antiandrogens. *Adv. Sex Horm. Res.*, **1976**, *2*, 233–262.

Neumann, F. Pharmacology and clinical use of antiandrogens: a short review. *Ir. J. Med. Sci.*, **1982**, *15*, 61–70.

Neumann, F.; von Berswordt-Wallrabe, R.; Elger, W.; Steinbeck, H.; Hahn, J.; and Kramer, M. Aspects of androgen-dependent events as studied by antiandrogens. *Recent Prog. Horm. Res.*, **1970**, *26*, 337–405.

Neumann, F., and Töpert, M. Pharmacology of antiandrogens. *J. Steroid Biochem.*, **1986**, *25*, 885–895.

Odell, W. D., and Swerdloff, R. S. Abnormalities of gonadal function in men. *Clin. Endocrinol.* (*Oxf.*), **1978**, *8*, 149–180.

Pardridge, W. M. Serum bioavailability of sex steroid hormones. *Clin. Endocrinol. Metab.*, **1986**, *15*, 259–278.

Ritzen, E. M.; Hansson, V.; and French, S. The Sertoli cell. In, *The Testis*. (Burger, H., and DeKretser, D., eds.) Raven Press, New York, **1981**, pp. 171–194.

Rosenfield, R. L. Role of androgens in growth and development of the fetus, child, and adolescent. *Adv. Pediatr.*, **1972**, *19*, 172–213.

Schally, A. V. Aspects of hypothalamic regulation of the pituitary gland: its implications for the control of reproductive processes. *Science*, **1978**, *202*, 18–28.

Siiteri, P. K., and MacDonald, P. C. Role of extraglandular estrogen in human endocrinology. In, *Female Reproductive System*, Vol. 2, Pt. 1. Sect. 7, *Endocrinology. Handbook of Physiology*. (Greep, R. O., and Astwood, E. B., eds.) American Physiological Society, Washington, D. C., **1973**, pp. 615–629.

Wilson, J. D. Gonadal hormones and sexual behavior. In, *Clinical Neuroendocrinology*, Vol. II. (Martini, L., and Besser, G. M., eds.) Academic Press, Inc., New York, **1982**, pp. 1–19.

———. Androgen abuse by athletes. *Endocr. Rev.*, **1988**, *9*, 181–199.

Wilson, J. D., and Griffin, J. E. The use and misuse of androgens. *Metabolism*, **1980**, *29*, 1278–1295.

CHAPTER

60 ADRENOCORTICOTROPIC HORMONE; ADRENOCORTICAL STEROIDS AND THEIR SYNTHETIC ANALOGS; INHIBITORS OF THE SYNTHESIS AND ACTIONS OF ADRENOCORTICAL HORMONES

Robert C. Haynes, Jr.

Adrenocorticotropic hormone (ACTH, corticotropin) and the steroids of the adrenal cortex are considered together in this chapter because the primary physiological and pharmacological effects of ACTH result from the secretion of adrenocortical steroids. Biologically active synthetic analogs of the adrenocorticosteroids are also included, as are substances that alter the pattern of secretion of the adrenal cortex by inhibiting certain biosynthetic reactions. Synthetic steroids that inhibit the action of glucocorticoids are discussed here; agents that inhibit the action of aldosterone are presented in Chapter 28.

History. The physiological significance of the adrenals began to be appreciated when Addison (1855) described the clinical syndrome resulting from destructive disease of the adrenal glands. His observations interested the physiologist Brown-Séquard (1856), who did the pioneer experiments on the effects of adrenalectomy and concluded that the adrenal glands are essential to life.

By the third decade of this century it was generally recognized that the cortex rather than the medulla is the life-maintaining portion of the gland. The complex nature of adrenocortical deficiency was dramatized in the 1930s by the partisan character of research groups oriented to study either the imbalance of electrolytes or the defects in carbohydrate metabolism present in the deficient state. Renal loss of Na^+ was convincingly demonstrated to be a characteristic of adrenocortical insufficiency by Harrop and associates (1933) as well as by Loeb and coworkers (1933). Equally convincing was the demonstration of a depletion of carbohydrate stores (Cori and Cori, 1927). Furthermore, hypoglycemia could be corrected by adrenocortical extracts (Britton and Silvette, 1931). Glucose and glycogen, formed under the influence of the adrenal cortex during fasting, appeared to be derived from tissue protein (Long *et al.*, 1940). From these studies emerged the concepts of two types of adrenocortical hormones. The mineralocorticoids primarily regulate electrolyte homeostasis, and the glucocorticoids are hormones concerned with carbohydrate metabolism. This concept of the dichotomy of "salt" and "sugar" hormones (mineralocorticoids and glucocorticoids) has proved useful and survives at the present time in a modified form.

In 1932, the neurosurgeon Cushing described the syndrome of hypercorticism, which bears his name (Cushing, 1932). The cases Cushing described were those of "pituitary basophilism," recognized subsequently as being a condition characterized by hypersecretion of ACTH. The symptom complex is now known to result from excessive plasma concentrations of adrenocortical hormones, regardless of whether they originate endogenously or as the consequence of therapeutic intervention.

The preparation of adrenocortical extracts with a reasonable degree of activity was first accomplished in 1930. By 1942, organic chemists had isolated, crystallized, and elucidated the structures of 28 steroids from the adrenal cortex (Reichstein and Shoppee, 1943). Five of these compounds—cortisol (hydrocortisone), cortisone, corticosterone, 11-dehydrocorticosterone, and 11-desoxycorticosterone—were demonstrated to be biologically active. Another decade passed before the principal mineralocorticoid was discovered. Deming and Luetscher (1950) found that extracts of urine from patients with edema induced Na^+ retention and K^+ excretion in adrenalectomized rats. The definitive evidence for the source of the active material was provided by Tait and coworkers (1952), who purified the compound with this activity from adrenocortical extracts. The substance was crystallized, the structure was established, and the hormone named *aldosterone* (Simpson *et al.*, 1954).

In this same era the role of the adenohypophysis was being elucidated by other investigators. The classical studies of Foster and Smith (1926) established the fact that hypophysectomy results in atrophy of the adrenal cortex. By 1933, it had been demonstrated that cell-free extracts of the anterior pituitary had a stimulating effect upon the adrenal cortex of the hypophysectomized animal. Further chemical fractionation of such extracts led to the isolation of a hormone, ACTH, that acted selectively to cause chemical and morphological changes in the adrenal cortex (*see* Astwood *et al.*,

1952), and its structure was established by Bell and coworkers (1956). The rate of release of ACTH from the adenohypophysis was shown to be determined by the balance of the inhibitory effects of the hormones of the adrenal cortex (Ingle *et al.*, 1938) and the excitatory effects of the nervous system.

A detailed analysis of the morphology of the adrenal cortex had suggested to Swann (1940) and to Deane and Greep (1946) that the zona glomerulosa of the adrenal cortex functions relatively independently of the pituitary. Following hypophysectomy, the zona glomerulosa thickens, whereas the fasciculata shrinks markedly and the reticularis disappears almost entirely. These morphological observations, together with the fact that the hypophysectomized rat, in contrast to the adrenalectomized animal, can survive without salt therapy, prompted Swann as well as Deane and Greep to assign to the zona glomerulosa the specific function of autonomously elaborating a hormone regulating electrolyte balance. This hormone is now known to be aldosterone.

In 1949, Hench and coworkers announced the dramatic effects of cortisone and ACTH in the treatment of rheumatoid arthritis. As early as 1929, Hench had been impressed by the fact that arthritic patients, when pregnant or jaundiced, experienced a temporary remission; he believed that a metabolite was responsible for the remission. The possibility that the antirheumatic substance might be an adrenocortical hormone was entertained, and as soon as cortisone was available in sufficient quantity it was tested in a case of acute rheumatoid arthritis. Fortunately, an adequate dose was employed and the response was dramatic. Thereafter, the salutary effects of ACTH were also demonstrated (Hench *et al.*, 1949). Soon, therapeutic applications were extended to other diseases, with results to be presented later in this chapter. The impact upon the medical world can be appreciated from the fact that, in the year following the first published report of the efficacy of cortisone in the treatment of rheumatoid arthritis, the Nobel Prize in Medicine was jointly awarded to Kendall and Reichstein, who were responsible for much of the basic chemical research that led to the synthesis of the steroid, and to Hench, whose contribution has just been described.

ADRENOCORTICOTROPIC HORMONE

Chemistry. The structure of human ACTH, a peptide of 39 amino acid residues, is shown in Figure 60–1. Loss of one amino acid from the amino-terminal end of the molecule by hydrolytic cleavage results in complete loss of biological activity. In contrast, a number of amino acids may be split off the carboxyl-terminal end with no effect on potency. A 20-amino acid peptide (sequence 1 through 20, Figure 60–1) retains the activity of the parent hormone. The structure–activity relationship of ACTH has been reviewed by Otsuka and Inouye (1975). The structural relationships between ACTH, endorphins, lipotropins, and the melanocyte-stimulating hormones are discussed in Chapter 56.

Actions on the Adrenal Cortex. ACTH stimulates the human adrenal cortex to secrete cortisol, corticosterone, aldosterone, and a number of weakly androgenic substances. In the absence of the adenohypophysis, the adrenal cortex undergoes atrophy and the rates of secretion of cortisol and corticosterone, which are markedly reduced, do not respond to otherwise-effective stimuli. Although ACTH can stimulate secretion of aldosterone, the rate of secretion is relatively independent of the adenohypophysis, which explains the nearly normal electrolyte balance in the hypophysectomized animal. The zona glomerulosa is the least affected by atrophic changes that follow hypophysectomy, and it is the glomerulosa that is mainly responsible for the elaboration of aldosterone.

Prolonged administration of large doses of ACTH induces hyperplasia and hypertrophy of the adrenal cortex with continuous high output of cortisol, corticosterone, and androgens.

Mechanism of Action. ACTH acts to stimulate the synthesis of adrenocortical hormones. It is believed that the diffusion of preformed hormones from the cortical cells into the circulation is not affected by ACTH. ACTH, as do many other hormones, controls its target tissue through the agency of cyclic AMP. Thus, ACTH reacts with its specific receptor on the adrenal cell plasma membrane. The activity of adenylyl cyclase is stimulated and both the rate of formation and the concentration of cy-

Ser—Tyr—Ser—Met—Glu—His—Phe—Arg—Try—Gly—Lys—Pro—Val—Gly—Lys—Lys—Arg—Arg—Pro—Val—Lys—Val—
1 2 3 4 5 6 7 8 9 10 11 12 13 14 15 16 17 18 19 20 21 22

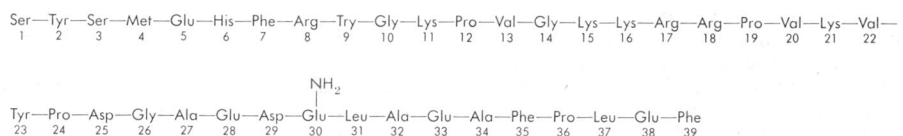

NH_2 (on Glu 30)

Tyr—Pro—Asp—Gly—Ala—Glu—Asp—Glu—Leu—Ala—Glu—Ala—Phe—Pro—Leu—Glu—Phe
23 24 25 26 27 28 29 30 31 32 33 34 35 36 37 38 39

Figure 60–1. *Amino acid sequence of human ACTH.*

Ovine, porcine, and bovine ACTHs differ from human ACTH only at amino acid positions 25, 31, and 33.

clic AMP is increased in adrenocortical cells. Cyclic AMP has been shown to stimulate steroidogenesis (Haynes *et al.*, 1959) and to maintain the weight of the adrenal gland after hypophysectomy (Ney, 1969). Therefore, it is believed that cyclic AMP mediates both the acute and long-term effects of ACTH on the adrenal cortex.

The principal metabolic site at which steroidogenesis is regulated by the cyclic nucleotide is the oxidative cleavage of the side chain of cholesterol, the reaction that results in the formation of pregnenolone (Figure 60–2). Although this step is rate-limiting in the sequence of reactions that leads to the formation of adrenal steroid hormones, it is now generally accepted that the availability of cholesterol is the factor that limits the rate in intact mitochondria (Kahnt *et al.*, 1974). The enzyme that catalyzes the cleavage of cholesterol's side chain is localized to the inner membrane of mitochondria in the adrenal, and ACTH acts in several ways to provide the substrate at this site. ACTH, via cyclic AMP–dependent phosphorylation, activates the cholesterol esterase that hydrolyzes esterified cholesterol within the cell (Beckett and Boyd, 1975; Pittman and Steinberg, 1977), and ACTH stimulates cholesterol uptake from plasma lipoproteins (Koper *et al.*, 1985). However, the most important mechanism is the facilitation of the transfer of cholesterol from the outer to the inner mitochondrial membrane. This transfer is thought to be mediated by a carrier protein that has an extremely short half-life, such that inhibitors of protein synthesis block steroidogenesis and its stimulation by ACTH almost immediately. The exact mechanism by which ACTH accelerates intramitochondrial transfer of cholesterol remains unknown.

The trophic effects of ACTH on the adrenal cortex are most evident in the induction of the enzymes of steroidogenesis. This effect results from the enhanced transcription of specific genes that encode the individual enzymes (Simpson and Waterman, 1988). The regulation of the adrenal cortex by ACTH has been reviewed by Privalle and colleagues (1987).

Extraadrenal Effects of ACTH. Large doses of ACTH given to adrenalectomized animals cause a number of metabolic changes, including ketosis, lipolysis, hypoglycemia (early after administration), and resistance to insulin (late after administration). These extraadrenal effects are of doubtful physiological significance, because of the large doses that are required.

Natural and synthetic corticotropins darken the isolated skin of the frog; this is not surprising since the amino acid sequence, 1 through 13, is identical with that of the melanocyte-stimulating hormone, α-MSH. Large doses of highly purified α-MSH and ACTH have been demonstrated to darken the skin of adrenalectomized human subjects. The hyperpigmentation of the skin that occurs in Addison's disease is thought to result from the high concentrations of ACTH that circulate in this condition (Thody, 1977; *see* Chapter 56).

Regulation of the Secretion of ACTH. The fluctuations in the rates of secretion of cortisol, corticosterone, and, to some extent, aldosterone are determined by the fluctuations in the release of ACTH from the adenohypophysis. The adenohypophysis, in turn, is under the influence of the nervous system and negative-feedback control exerted by corticosteroids (*see* Dallman *et al.*, 1987).

Nervous System: The Final Common Path. Stimuli that induce release of ACTH travel by neural paths converging on the median eminence of the hypothalamus. The functional link between the median eminence and the adenohypophysis, the final common path, is vascular. In response to an appropriate stimulus, corticotropin-releasing factor (CRF), a peptide of 41 amino acid residues, is elaborated at neuronal endings in the median eminence and transported in the hypophyseal-portal vessels to the adenohypophysis, where it stimulates the synthesis and secretion of ACTH. The effects of CRF are mediated by activation of adenylyl cyclase and the cyclic AMP–dependent protein kinase (Aquilera *et al.*, 1983). The isolation and synthesis of ovine CRF were reported by Vale and coworkers (1981), and the structure of human CRF was determined shortly thereafter (Shibahara *et al.*, 1983). CRF increases the concentrations of ACTH and cortisol in plasma when given intravenously to man. Intravenous injection of 100 μg of CRF results in an exaggerated response in patients with Cushing's syndrome caused by pituitary hyperfunction or ectopic CRF production. This test is thus useful in determining the cause of the disease and helps to rule out ectopic production of ACTH or functional tumors of the adrenal cortex as responsible (Müller *et al.*, 1987).

ACTH is synthesized in basophilic cells of the adenohypophysis and, like many other peptide hormones, it is derived from a larger precursor; the prohormone is a glycoprotein of about 30,000 molecular weight. The precursor of ACTH includes the sequences of MSH, the lipotropins, and the endorphins. In man, the role of these three groups of active peptides remains conjectural. The complex processing of the prohormone to ACTH, β-lipotropin, and other peptides has been studied extensively (*see* Imura, 1987).

Negative Feedback of the Corticosteroids (Cortisol and Corticosterone). Administration of certain corticosteroids suppresses the secretion of ACTH, reduces the store of ACTH in the adenohypophysis, and induces morphological changes (hyalinization of the basophilic cells) suggestive of functional impairment of the adenohypophysis. The adrenal cortex itself undergoes atrophy. In contrast, adrenalectomized animals and patients with Addison's disease have abnormally high concentrations of ACTH in the blood even under optimal

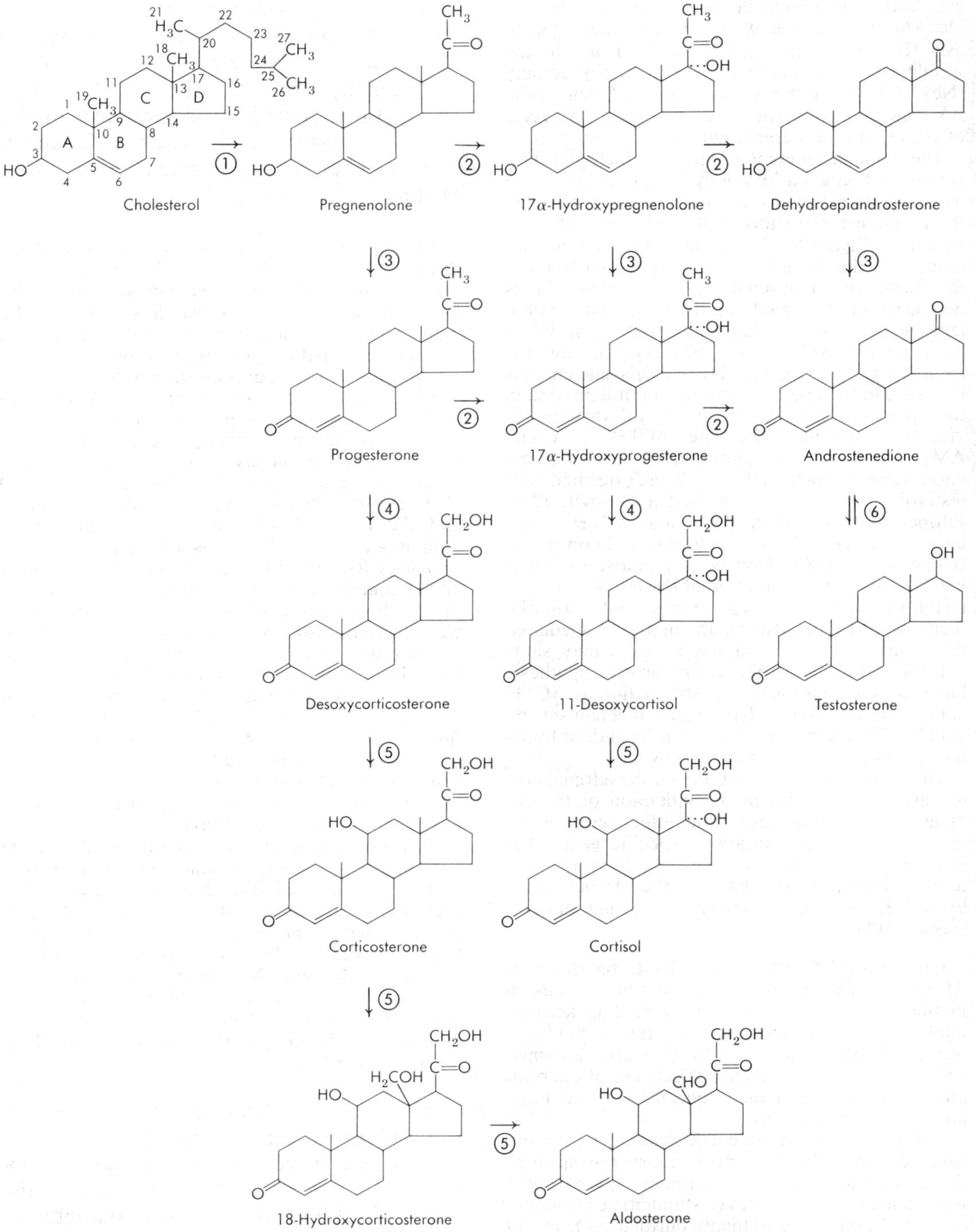

Figure 60–2. *Principal pathways for biosynthesis of adrenocorticosteroids and adrenal androgens.*

Reaction 1 is catalyzed by the cholesterol side chain–cleavage complex (cytochrome $P_{450,scc}$), reaction 2 by cytochrome $P_{450,C17}$, reaction 3 by 3β-hydroxysteroid dehydrogenase, reaction 4 by cytochrome $P_{450,C21}$, reaction 5 by cytochrome $P_{450,C11}$, and reaction 6 by 17-hydroxysteroid dehydrogenase.

environmental conditions. When a stimulus is applied to an adrenalectomized animal, the concentration of ACTH reaches even higher levels. These observations point out the important inhibitory role of the corticosteroids and clearly demonstrate that ACTH release remains under control of the nervous system in the absence of corticosteroid feedback. Secretion of ACTH at any instant is determined by the balance of neural excitatory and corticosteroid inhibitory effects.

Mechanism of Feedback by Corticosteroids. Binding of glucocorticoids has been detected in the pituitary, hypothalamus, and other areas of the brain (McEwen, 1979); however, the link between such binding and inhibition of secretion of ACTH has not been completely elucidated. There is evidence of control at both hypothalamic and hypophyseal sites. Nakanishi and coworkers (1977) demonstrated that glucocorticoids cause a decrease in the level of mRNA for ACTH in the pituitary, indicating that a degree of control is exerted at the level of transcription. Treatment of rats with glucocorticoids for a few days decreases the number of CRF receptors in the pituitary but not in the brain (Hauger *et al.*, 1987). This effect, together with inhibition of synthesis, may account in part for the "slow feedback" phase of glucocorticoid inhibition of ACTH secretion. It does not explain the "fast feedback" phase of inhibition that develops within seconds or minutes during a rise in circulating glucocorticoids. It is possible that these rapid effects are mediated by receptors for glucocorticoids on the surface of certain cells, analogous to those thought to mediate the actions of steroidal anesthetic agents (*see* Chapter 17). Feedback regulation of ACTH secretion has been reviewed by Keller-Wood and Dallman (1984).

Examples of Effective Stimuli of Secretion. A number of conditions have been demonstrated to stimulate adrenocortical secretion in man. These include the agonal state, severe infections, surgery, parturition, cold, exercise, and emotional stress. Stressful stimuli override the normal negative-feedback control mechanisms, and plasma concentrations of adrenocortical steroids can be elevated within a few minutes of the initiation of an appropriate stimulus.

Diurnal Cycles in Adrenocortical Activity. The rate of secretion of cortisol by the adrenal cortex of a normal human subject under optimal conditions is about 20 to 30 mg per day. However, the rate is not steady and exhibits rhythmic fluctuations; concentrations of adrenocortical steroids in plasma are relatively high in the early-morning hours, decline during the day, and reach a minimum during the evening. Plasma concentrations of ACTH are higher at 6 A.M. than at 6 P.M. The diurnal patterns of glucocorticoids and ACTH are not observed in patients with Cushing's disease, and this factor is considered in the diagnosis of the disorder.

Absorption and Fate. ACTH is readily absorbed from parenteral sites. The hormone rapidly disappears from the circulation following its intravenous administration; in man, the half-life in plasma is about 15 minutes because of rapid enzymatic hydrolysis.

Bioassay. The USP has adopted the Third International Standard for Corticotropin (Bangham *et al.*, 1962) as the reference standard in the United States. Potency is based on an assay in hypophysectomized rats in which depletion of adrenal ascorbic acid is measured after subcutaneous administration of the ACTH. Except for the synthetic product, cosyntropin, all commercial preparations are now described in these units only.

Preparations, Dosage, and Routes of Administration. *Corticotropin for injection* (ACTH) is available as a lyophilized powder (ACTHAR) for subcutaneous, intramuscular, or intravenous use. The preparation is derived from the pituitaries of mammals used for food. Maximal adrenocortical secretion is obtained in adults with a total dose of 25 USP units infused intravenously for 8 hours.

Repository corticotropin injection (H.P. ACTHAR GEL) is administered either intramuscularly or subcutaneously. It is a highly purified ACTH in gelatin solution. Typical doses are 40 to 80 units, given every 1 to 3 days. *Corticotropin zinc hydroxide suspension* (CORTROPHIN-ZINC) is a preparation of purified corticotropin adsorbed on zinc hydroxide, intended for intramuscular injection. Again, usual doses are 40 to 80 units every 1 to 3 days.

Cosyntropin (CORTROSYN) is a synthetic peptide corresponding to amino acid residues 1 to 24 of human ACTH. This preparation, approved for diagnostic purposes, is given intramuscularly or intravenously in a dose of 0.25 mg.

Therapeutic Uses and Diagnostic Applications of ACTH. At the present time, the most important use of ACTH is as a diagnostic agent in adrenal insufficiency. For this purpose, ACTH is administered and the concentration of cortisol in plasma is determined. A normal increase in plasma cortisol rules out primary adrenocortical failure. In the absence of an acute response, prolonged or repeated administration of ACTH may be required to stimulate an adrenal that has become atrophic because of lack of normal stimulation from ACTH. In cases of pituitary insufficiency, prolonged treatment can be expected to elicit a rise in plasma cortisol concentration.

Therapeutic uses of ACTH have included the treatment of secondary adrenocortical insufficiency and nonendocrine disorders that are responsive to glucocorticoids. However, therapy with ACTH is less predictable and much less convenient than is that with appropriate steroids. Furthermore, ACTH stimulates secretion of mineralocorticoids and, therefore, may cause acute retention of salt and water. ACTH would obviously be of no value in the treatment of primary adrenocortical failure. Furthermore, there is no substantial evidence that therapeutic goals can be attained with

ACTH in secondary adrenocortical insufficiency that cannot be attained with appropriate doses of currently available steroids. It must be kept in mind, however, that ACTH and corticosteroids are not pharmacologically equivalent. Treatment with ACTH exposes the tissues to a mixture of glucocorticoids, mineralocorticoids, and androgens, in contrast to the conventional, contemporary practice of administering a single glucocorticoid. It has been reported that patients treated for prolonged periods of time with ACTH do not develop dermal atrophy, in contrast to those treated with corticosteroids. This finding has been tentatively attributed to a protective action of androgens against the inhibitory effects of glucocorticoids on fibroblasts (Harvey and Grahame, 1973).

Clinical Toxicity of ACTH. The toxicity of ACTH, aside from rare hypersensitivity reactions, is entirely attributable to the increased rate of secretion of adrenocorticosteroids (*see* below). The synthetic ACTH peptides are thought to be less antigenic than is the parent molecule. ACTH, purified from pituitaries of animals, contains significant amounts of vasopressin, and life-threatening hyponatremia can result from its administration (Sheeler and Schumacher, 1979). For this reason cosyntropin, which contains no vasopressin, is preferred. ACTH causes more Na^+ retention, a greater degree of hypokalemic alkalosis, and more acne than do the synthetic congeners of cortisol.

ADRENOCORTICAL STEROIDS

The adrenal cortex synthesizes two classes of steroids: the corticosteroids (glucocorticoids and mineralocorticoids), with 21 carbon atoms, and the androgens, with 19. The major corticosteroids (cortisol, corticosterone, and aldosterone) are shown together with the androgens (dehydroepiandrosterone, androstenedione, and testosterone) in Figure 60–2.

Adrenocorticosteroid Biosynthesis. Cholesterol is an obligatory intermediate in the biosynthesis of corticosteroids. Although the adrenal cortex synthesizes cholesterol from acetate by processes similar to those occurring in liver, the greater part of the cholesterol (60 to 80%) utilized for corticosteroidogenesis comes from exogenous sources, both at rest and following administration of ACTH. Adrenocortical cells thus have large numbers of receptors that mediate the uptake of low-density lipoprotein, the predominant source of cholesterol (*see* Chapter 36). Cholesterol is enzymatically converted to 21-carbon corticosteroids and 19-carbon weak androgens by a series of steps presented in simplified form in Figure 60–2. Most of the reactions are catalyzed by mixed-function oxidases that contain cytochrome P_{450} and require NADPH and molecular oxygen.

In addition to other androgens, the adrenal cortex secretes testosterone; however, about half the plasma testosterone of normal women is derived from androstenedione at an extraadrenal site.

Table 60–1. TYPICAL RATES OF SECRETION AND PLASMA CONCENTRATIONS OF THE MAJOR BIOLOGICALLY ACTIVE CORTICOSTEROIDS IN MAN

		CORTISOL	ALDOSTERONE
Rate of secretion under optimal conditions, mg/day (μmol/day)		20 (55)	0.125 (0.35)
Concentrations in peripheral plasma of man, μg/dl (nM)	8 A.M.	16 (440)	0.01 (0.28)
	4 P.M.	4 (110)	

Adrenocorticosteroids are not stored in the adrenals. The amounts of corticosteroids found in adrenal tissue are insufficient to maintain normal rates of secretion for more than a few minutes in the absence of continuing biosynthesis. For this reason, the rate of biosynthesis is tantamount to the rate of secretion. Table 60–1 shows typical rates of secretion of the physiologically most important corticosteroids in man—cortisol and aldosterone—as well as their approximate concentrations in peripheral plasma. The mechanism of control of steroidogenesis by ACTH has been discussed above, and the regulation of aldosterone synthesis by renin and angiotensin is described in Chapter 31.

PHYSIOLOGICAL FUNCTIONS AND PHARMACOLOGICAL EFFECTS

The effects of the corticosteroids are numerous and widespread. They influence carbohydrate, protein, and lipid metabolism; electrolyte and water balance; and the functions of the cardiovascular system, the kidney, skeletal muscle, the nervous system, and other organs and tissues. Furthermore, the corticosteroids endow the organism with the capacity to resist many types of noxious stimuli and environmental changes. In the absence of the adrenal cortex, survival is possible but only under the most rigidly prescribed conditions; for example, food must be available regularly, sodium chloride ingested in relatively large quantities, and environmental temperature maintained within a suitably narrow range.

A given dose of corticosteroid may be physiological or pharmacological, depending on the environment and the activities of the organism. Under favorable conditions, a small dose of corticosteroid maintains the adrenalectomized animal in a state of wellbeing. Under adverse conditions a relatively large dose is needed if the animal is to survive. This same large dose given repetitively under optimal conditions induces hypercorticism—that is, signs of corticosteroid excess. The fluctuations in the secretory activity of a normal subject are presumed to reflect the body's varying requirements for corticosteroids.

The actions of corticosteroids are often complexly related to the functions of other hormones. For example, in the absence of lipolytic hormones, cortisol even in large concentrations has virtually no effect on the rate of lipolysis in adipose tissue *in vitro*. Likewise, a sympathomimetic amine has only a slight effect on the rate of lipolysis if there is a deficiency of glucocorticoids. However, if a necessary minimal amount of cortisol is added, the lipolytic effect of the sympathomimetic amine becomes evident. The necessary but not sufficient role of corticosteroids acting in concert with other regulatory forces has been termed "permissive."

Estimates of the potencies of naturally occurring and synthetic corticosteroids in the categories of Na^+ retention (reduction of Na^+ excretion by the kidney of the adrenalectomized animal); hepatic deposition of glycogen in fasted, adrenalectomized animals; and antiinflammatory effect (inhibition of the action of an agent that induces inflammation) are presented in Table 60–2. It should be noted that such values are not fixed ratios but vary considerably with the conditions of the bioassays used. Potencies of steroids as judged by their ability to sustain life in the adrenalectomized animal closely parallel those determined for Na^+ retention. Potencies based on deposition of liver glycogen, antiinflammatory effect, work capacity of skeletal muscle, and involution of lymphoid tissue closely parallel one another. Dissociations exist between potencies based on Na^+ retention and on hepatic glycogen deposition; traditionally, the corticosteroids have thus been classified into *mineralocorticoids* and *glucocorticoids,* according to potencies in the two categories. Desoxycorticosterone, the prototype of the mineralocorticoids, is highly potent in regard to Na^+ retention but without effect on hepatic glycogen deposition. Cortisol, the prototype of the glucocorticoids, is highly potent in regard to liver glycogen deposition but weak in regard to Na^+ retention. The naturally occurring corticosteroids cortisol and cortisone, as well as synthetic corticosteroids such as prednisolone and triamcinolone, are classified as glucocorticoids. However, corticosterone is a steroid that has modest but significant activities in both categories. In contrast, aldosterone is exceedingly potent with respect to Na^+ retention but has only modest potency for liver glycogen deposition. At rates secreted by the adrenal cortex or in doses that exert maximal effects on electrolyte balance, aldosterone has no significant effect on carbohydrate metabolism; it is thus classified as a mineralocorticoid.

Table 60–2. RELATIVE POTENCIES OF CORTICOSTEROIDS

	NA^+ RETENTION	HEPATIC GLYCOGEN DEPOSITION	ANTI-INFLAMMATORY EFFECT
Natural Steroids			
Cortisol	1 *	1	1
Cortisone	0.8 *	0.8	0.8
Corticosterone	15	0.35	0.3
11-Desoxycorticosterone	100	0	0
Aldosterone	3000	0.3	?
Synthetic Steroids			
Prednisolone	<1 *	4	4
Triamcinolone	0	5	5

* Promotes excretion of Na^+ under certain circumstances.

Mechanism of Action. Corticosteroids, like other steroid hormones, act by controlling the rate of synthesis of proteins. However, their nearly instantaneous inhibition of ACTH release (*see* above) is probably an exception. Corticosteroids react with receptor proteins in the cytoplasm of sensitive cells in many tissues to form a steroid-receptor complex. The complex undergoes a modification, as noted by an increase in the sedimentation constant, and then moves into the nucleus, where it binds to chromatin and regulates transcription of specific genes. In most known examples, transcription is enhanced, as manifest by increased amounts of specific mRNA. Nevertheless, glucocorticoids also decrease transcription of some genes, for example, the pro-opiomelanocortin gene that encodes ACTH.

It is now known that binding of corticosteroids by their receptor results in dissociation of a phosphorylated protein of approximately 90,000-dalton size from the receptor complex in the cytosol. This protein has been identified as a heat-shock protein (hsp90), one of a group of proteins synthesized by organisms as diverse as bacteria and mammals under conditions of heat or certain other types of stress. It is presumed that the release of this intriguing protein of, as yet, unknown function plays a major part in the transformation of the receptor, enabling the hormone-receptor complex to proceed to its nuclear destination or to interact fruitfully with DNA (*see* Pratt, 1987; Yamamoto *et al.*, 1988).

Molecular biological techniques have recently made the human glucocorticoid receptor available for study and have permitted manipulation of its structure by deletion or substitution of amino acid sequences. The receptor has a central domain that is responsible for binding to glucocorticoid-response elements (GREs)—short sequences of DNA in the promoter regions of genes whose transcription is controlled by glucocorticoids. This segment of the receptor contains a region that is similar to portions of receptors for the thyroid hormones as well as those for other steroids (*see* Chapter 2). The steroid-binding domain, located toward the carboxyl-terminal end of the protein, is now known to repress the functions of the DNA-binding segment. When a glucocorticoid associates with the receptor, DNA binding and enhancement of transcription are no longer inhibited; the effect of the glucocorticoid is thus to disinhibit the activity of the unliganded receptor (*see* Funder, 1987; Hollenberg *et al.*, 1987; Godowski *et al.*, 1988).

Carbohydrate and Protein Metabolism. The effects of adrenocortical hormones on carbohydrate and protein metabolism are epitomized in the teleological view that these steroids have evolved to protect glucose-dependent cerebral functions by stimulating the formation of glucose, diminishing its peripheral utilization, and promoting its storage as glycogen. Adrenalectomized animals exhibit no marked abnormality in carbohydrate metabolism if food is regularly available. Under such circumstances, normal concentrations of glucose in the plasma are maintained and glycogen is stored in the liver. However, a brief period of starvation rapidly depletes carbohydrate reserves. The concentration of glycogen in the liver, and to a lesser extent that in muscle, decreases and hypoglycemia develops. In light of these facts, it is not surprising that the adrenalectomized animal is hypersensitive to insulin. Patients with Addison's disease have similar abnormalities in carbohydrate metabolism.

Administration of a glucocorticoid such as cortisol corrects the defect in carbohydrate metabolism of the adrenalectomized animal; glycogen stores, particularly in the liver, are increased; concentrations of glucose in plasma remain normal during fasting; and sensitivity to insulin returns to normal. Increased excretion of nitrogen accompanies the increased production of glucose, indicating that protein is converted to carbohydrate. Prolonged exposure to large doses of glucocorticoids leads to an exaggeration of these changes in glucose metabolism, such that a diabetic-like state is produced: glucose in the plasma tends to be elevated in the fasting subject, resistance to insulin is increased, glucose tolerance is decreased, and glucosuria may be present.

The mechanism by which the glucocorticoids inhibit utilization of glucose in peripheral tissues is not yet understood. Decreased uptake of glucose has been demonstrated in adipose tissue, skin, fibroblasts, and thymocytes as a result of glucocorticoid action.

Glucocorticoids promote gluconeogenesis by both peripheral and hepatic actions. Peripherally these steroids act to mobilize amino acids from a number of tissues. This catabolic action is reflected in the atrophy of lymphatic tissues, reduced mass of muscle, osteoporosis (reduction in protein matrix of bone followed by calcium loss), thinning of the skin, and a negative nitrogen balance. Amino acids funnel into the liver, where they serve as substrates for enzymes involved in the production of glucose and glycogen.

In the liver the glucocorticoids induce *de-novo* synthesis of a number of enzymes involved in gluconeogenesis and amino acid metabolism. For example, the hepatic enzymes phosphoenolpyruvate carboxykinase, fructose-1,6-diphosphatase, and glucose-6-phosphatase, which catalyze reactions of glucose synthesis, are increased in concentration. However, induction of these enzymes requires a matter of hours and cannot account for the earliest effects of the hormones on gluconeogenesis. For example, when dexamethasone, a synthetic glucocorticoid, is added to isolated rat hepatocytes, gluconeogenesis is fully stimulated within 20 minutes, and this effect is not blocked by inhibition of protein synthesis with cycloheximide (Sistare and Haynes, 1985).

Prolonged, but not acute, treatment with glucocorticoids has been found to elevate the concentration of glucagon in the plasma (Marco *et al.*, 1973; Wise *et al.*, 1973). Inasmuch as glucagon itself stimulates gluconeogenesis, the rise in glucagon should also contribute to the enhanced synthesis of glucose. The deposition of glycogen in the liver found after treatment with glucocorticoids is thought to be the consequence of activation of hepatic glycogen synthase. This activation requires the presence of insulin but is not mediated by a rise in the concentration of insulin (*see* Hers, 1985). The effects of glucocorticoids on carbohydrate metabolism have been reviewed by McMahon and colleagues (1988).

Lipid Metabolism. Two effects of corticosteroids on lipid metabolism are firmly established. The first is the dramatic redistribution of body fat that occurs in the hypercorticoid state. The other is the facilitation of the effect of adipokinetic agents in eliciting lipolysis of the triglycerides of adipose tissue. In rare instances, prolonged exposure to excessive glucocorticoids produces an epidural lipomatosis that can result in neurological disability (Russell *et al.*, 1984). A number of other effects of corticosteroids on lipids have been reported, but in few, if any, instances have they turned out to be direct actions of the corticosteroids themselves.

Prolonged administration of large doses of glucocorticoids to human subjects or the hypersecretion of cortisol that occurs in Cushing's syndrome leads to a peculiar alteration in fat distribution. There is a gain of fat in depots in the back of the neck ("buffalo hump"), supraclavicular area, and face ("moon face") and a loss of fat from the extremities. One hypothesis to explain this phenomenon is that of Fain and Czech (1975), who proposed that the adipose tissue that hypertrophies in Cushing's syndrome responds preferentially to the lipogenic and antilipolytic actions of the elevated concentrations of insulin evoked by glucocorticoid-induced hyperglycemia. According to this hypothesis, adipocytes in the extremities, in contrast to those of the trunk, are less sensitive to insulin and more sensitive to the glucocorticoid-facilitated lipolytic effects of other hormones.

The mobilization of fat from peripheral fat depots by epinephrine, norepinephrine, or adipokinetic peptides of the adenohypophysis is markedly blunted in the absence of the adrenal cortex or the adenohypophysis. Cortisol acts in adipose tissue to facilitate the lipolytic response to cyclic AMP, rather than to enhance its accumulation. Hypophysectomy in rats has only a slight effect on the accumulation of cyclic AMP after exposure of adipose tissue to graded doses of epinephrine (Birnbaum and Goodman, 1973); however, hypophysectomy greatly decreases the lipolytic response of adipose tissue to the cyclic nucleotide. Treatment with cortisol restores the normal response to lipolytic hormones and to cyclic AMP (Goodman, 1968). Plasma lipids are not changed consistently in either hypocorticism or hypercorticism.

Electrolyte and Water Balance. Mineralocorticoids act on the distal tubules and collecting ducts of the kidney to enhance the reabsorption of Na^+ from the tubular fluid into the plasma; they increase the urinary excretion of both K^+ and H^+. The consequences of these three primary effects in concert with similar actions on cation transport in other tissues appear to account for the entire spectrum of physiological and pharmacological activities that are characteristic of the mineralocorticoids. Thus, the primary features of hypercorticism are positive Na^+ balance and expansion of the extracellular fluid volume, normal or slight increase in the concentration of Na^+ in the plasma, hypokalemia, and alkalosis. In contrast, those of the deficient state, hypocorticism, are Na^+ loss, hyponatremia, hyperkalemia, contraction of the extracellular fluid volume, and cellular hydration. A defect of major consequence in adrenocortical insufficiency is the renal loss of Na^+. The renal tubules normally reabsorb practically all the Na^+ filtered at the glomerulus. For example, on an ordinary diet, 99.5% may be reabsorbed to maintain Na^+ balance. Typically, in a patient with Addison's disease with a normal dietary intake, the maximal reabsorption attainable is 98.5%. Since approximately 24,000 mEq of Na^+ is filtered per day, the 1% difference between reabsorption in the normal subject and the patient with Addison's disease amounts to a loss of 240 mEq of Na^+ per day. The gravity of the situation is obvious when one considers that this amount of Na^+ is normally present in 1.7 liters of extracellular fluid. Proportionately more Na^+ than water is lost through the kidney and the concentration of extracellular Na^+ decreases; extracellular fluid becomes hypoosmotic, and water shifts from the extracellular into the intracellular compartment. This shift, together with the renal loss of water, results in a marked reduction in the volume of the extracellular fluid. Cells are hydrated, and the increase in the hematocrit value is due not only to a shrinkage of the plasma volume but also to the swelling of the erythrocytes. Hyperkalemia and the tendency toward acidosis are a result of impairments in the excretion of K^+ and H^+. Without administration of mineralocorticoids or sodium chloride solution or both, a rapid downhill course ensues in adrenocortical insufficiency. The shrinkage of extracellular fluid volume, the cellular hydration, and the hypodynamic state of the cardiovascular system combine to cause circulatory collapse, renal failure, and death.

In adrenocortical insufficiency, a basic defect in ion transport occurs in a variety of secretory cells. Not only the kidney but also the salivary glands, the sweat glands, the exocrine pancreas, and the mucosa of the gastrointestinal tract elaborate fluids abnormally high in the concentration of Na^+ and abnormally low in the concentration of K^+. In the patient with Addison's disease, sweating may contribute significantly to the negative balance of Na^+.

Aldosterone is by far the most potent of the naturally occurring corticosteroids with regard to electrolyte balance and plays an important role in the long-term regulation of Na^+ and K^+ balance. Evidence of this is the relatively normal electrolyte balance exhibited by the hypophysectomized animal as a result of continued secretion of aldosterone by the adrenal cortex, and the increased rate of secretion of aldosterone that occurs in man when dietary salt is severely limited. However, changes in the rate of secretion of aldosterone are not the cause of the rapid changes that may occur in Na^+ excretion. The latent period of action of the steroid is too long.

The intravenous administration of aldosterone to a normal subject is followed, after a delay of about an hour, by a decrease in the rate of renal Na^+ excretion and an increase in the rate of K^+ and H^+ excretion. If the administration of relatively large amounts of aldosterone is continued over a period of more than 10 to 14 days, Na^+ excretion again equals Na^+ intake. However, K^+ and H^+ excretion continues at an accelerated rate, resulting in hypokalemic alkalosis. The mechanism of "escape" from acute Na^+ retention is probably the result of the diuretic action of atrial natriuretic peptide, secreted in response to atrial distention. The effects of the mineralocorticoids have been reviewed by Mulrow and Forman (1972).

Aldosterone, like other steroids, acts to initiate transcription of mRNA that serves as template for the synthesis of specific proteins. One hypothetical "aldosterone-induced protein" is thought to facilitate the transport of Na^+ from the lumen of the distal tubules through the tubular cells and into the extracellular fluid. The most widely accepted model to describe the action of aldosterone was put forth by Marver (1980). The Na^+ of the tubular filtrate enters the cells of the distal tubules down a concentration gradient through the cell membrane facing the tubular lumen (apical or mucosal surface). Aldosterone and other mineralocorticoids facilitate this diffusion by increasing the permeability of the apical membrane to Na^+. Thus, Na^+ enters the cells at an accelerated rate and is pumped out into the extracellular space across the basolateral membrane by Na^+,K^+-activated adenosine triphosphatase (Na^+,K^+-ATPase) (Koeppen *et al.*, 1983). After aldosterone acts for a period of time, the amount of the Na^+, K^+-ATPase that is associated with the basolateral membrane increases (*see* Stanton, 1985).

The mechanisms of the enhanced excretion of K^+ and H^+ are less well understood. The exchange of Na^+ for K^+ by Na^+,K^+-ATPase tends to increase the concentration of K^+ in the tubular cells, from which it may escape either into the tubular lumen or back into the interstitial fluid. Diffusion into the tubular fluid results in the urinary excretion of K^+. For practical purposes one may visualize H^+ and K^+ as being "exchanged" for the additional Na^+ that is reabsorbed under the influence of the steroids, because the sum of the equivalents of the additional K^+ and H^+ excreted is equal to that of the additional Na^+ retained.

The glucocorticoids decrease the absorption of Ca^{2+} from the intestine and increase its renal excretion, thus producing a negative balance of the cation. These effects are considered to be the basis of the favorable therapeutic response to glucocorticoids seen in hypercalcemia (*see* Chapter 62).

Desoxycorticosterone is a natural mineralocorticoid of some historical interest for it was the first corticosteroid to be synthesized and made available for the treatment of Addison's disease. Desoxycorticosterone is practically devoid of glucocorticoid effects. Qualitatively, it is identical to aldosterone in its effects on electrolytes; quantitatively, it is about 3% as potent (*see* Table 60–2). Thus, despite the fact that the concentration of desoxycorticosterone in plasma is approximately the same as that of aldosterone, it apparently is of little physiological significance in the normal individual.

Cortisol induces Na^+ retention and K^+ excretion, but much less effectively than does aldosterone. In striking contrast to aldosterone, cortisol, under certain circumstances (especially Na^+ loading), enhances Na^+ excretion. This may be accounted for by the capacity of cortisol to increase the glomerular filtration rate (GFR). Aldosterone and desoxycorticosterone are ineffective in this regard. Furthermore, cortisol has a significant stimulatory influence on tubular secretory activity.

Impaired water diuresis in response to an administered water load, while not specific for adrenal insufficiency, has been used as a diagnostic criterion. In adrenal insufficiency, the GFR is reduced and the plasma concentration of antidiuretic hormone (ADH) is increased; these factors account for failure to excrete a water load (Ahmed *et al.*, 1967). Administration of cortisol, but not of aldosterone, increases the GFR and restores water diuresis (Gill *et al.*, 1962).

Hypercorticism caused by the administration of large doses of cortisol (or related glucocorticoids) or the excessive secretion of cortisol by the adrenals is sometimes associated with a hypokalemic alkalosis (*see* Chapter 27). However, the changes, particularly the degree of hypokalemia, are moderate in severity and reflect the relatively weak effect on electrolyte balance of cortisol as compared with aldosterone. Muscle weakness associated with glucocorticoid treatment is usually due to a loss of muscle mass rather than of K^+.

An important relationship between cortisol and aldosterone as mineralocorticoids has been discovered recently. The human mineralocorticoid receptor binds aldosterone and cortisol with similar affinity (Arriza *et al.*, 1987). Because the concentration of cortisol in plasma is hundreds of times that of aldosterone (*see* Table 60–1), it might be expected that the human organism would be in a constant state of hypermineralocorticism equivalent to clinical aldosteronism (*see* below). However, some tissues that contain mineralocorticoid receptors, in particular the kidney, colon, and salivary glands, also have a highly active 11-β-hydroxysteroid dehydrogenase that oxidizes cortisol to its inactive 11-keto derivative, cortisone. This reaction effectively shields the mineralocorticoid receptor from most of the cortisol; aldosterone is not a substrate for the dehydrogenase (Funder *et al.*, 1988). In licorice poisoning, the 11-β-dehydrogenase is inhibited by glycyrrhizic acid, a component of licorice. This allows excessive activation of the mineralocorticoid receptor by cortisol, thereby producing a state of hypermineralocorticism (Stewart *et al.*, 1987).

Cardiovascular System. The most striking effects of corticosteroids on the cardiovascular system are those that are the consequence of regulation of renal Na^+ excretion. These effects are seen most vividly in hypocorticism when reduction in blood volume accompanied by increased viscosity can lead to hypotension and cardiovascular collapse. However, the impairment of the cardiovascular system that occurs in patients with adrenocortical insufficiency obviously involves additional, poorly understood processes. The corticosteroids exert important actions on the various elements of the circulatory system, including the capillaries, the arterioles, and the myocardium. In the absence of the corticosteroids, there is increased capillary permeability, inadequate vasomotor response of the small vessels to catecholamines, and reduction in cardiac size and output.

An excess of mineralocorticoids occurs in its purest form in primary aldosteronism, the result of excessive secretion of this steroid. In this disease the major clinical findings are hypertension and hypokalemia. The hypokalemia is an obvious consequence of the renal effects of aldosterone, but the genesis of the hypertension has not been totally clarified. Development of hypertension requires a prolonged excess of mineralocorticoid and retention of Na^+ (Mulrow and Forman, 1972). Plasma renin activity is suppressed. Mineralocorticoid-induced hypertension can be treated by reduction of body stores of Na^+ with diuretics, implying that the hypertension is a result of Na^+ retention. Hypertension occurs in most cases of Cushing's syndrome and sometimes as the result of administration of synthetic glucocorticoids lacking mineralocorticoid activity. One hypothesis proposes that salt retention (or mineralocorticoids themselves) sensitizes blood vessels to pressor agents, in particular angiotensin and catecholamines (Brunner *et al.*, 1972; Yard and Kadowitz, 1972).

Glucocorticoid-induced hypertension has also not been well explained. With agents such as cortisol, retention of Na^+ may play a role. However, in contrast to primary aldosteronism, natriuresis is often not successful in normalizing blood pressure. In addition, plasma renin activity is normal or increased in glucocorticoid-induced hypertension and may have an effect (Krakoff *et al.*, 1975). There is also some evidence that ADH may be involved in the pathogenesis of the hypertension (Share and Crofton, 1982).

Skeletal Muscle. The maintenance of normal function of skeletal muscle requires adequate concentrations of corticosteroids, but excessive amounts of either mineralocorticoids or glucocorticoids lead to abnormalities.

It is well known that one of the outstanding signs of adrenocortical insufficiency is a diminished work capacity of striated muscle. In patients with Addison's disease this is manifested by weakness and fatigue. The most important single factor responsible for this dysfunction appears to be the inadequacy of the circulatory system. Abnormalities in electrolyte balance and carbohydrate metabolism in adrenocortical insufficiency contribute only in small measure to the impairment in skeletal muscle function.

Muscle weakness in primary aldosteronism is in large measure a result of the hypokalemia characteristic of this disease. Glucocorticoids given for prolonged periods in high doses or secreted in abnormal amounts in Cushing's syndrome tend to cause a wasting of skeletal muscle, the mechanism of which is not known. This steroid myopathy is responsible, at least in part, for the weakness and fatigue noted in the syndrome. Steroid-induced myopathy has been reviewed by Ellis (1985); acute myopathy is discussed by Knox and colleagues (1986).

Central Nervous System. The corticosteroids affect the central nervous system (CNS) in a number of indirect ways; in particular, they maintain normal concentrations of glucose in plasma, an adequate circulation, and the normal balance of electrolytes in the body. There is also an increasing recognition of direct effects of corticosteroids on the CNS as understanding of the distribution and function of steroid receptors in the brain has grown (McEwen *et al.,* 1986; Funder and Sheppard, 1987). An influence of the corticosteroids can be observed on mood, behavior, the electroencephalogram (EEG), and brain excitability.

Patients with Addison's disease exhibit apathy, depression, and irritability; some are frankly psychotic. Desoxycorticosterone is ineffective but cortisol is very effective in correcting these abnormalities of psyche and behavior. An array of reactions, varying in degree and kind, is seen in patients to whom glucocorticoids are administered for therapeutic purposes. Most patients respond with elevation in mood, which may be explained in part by the relief of the symptoms of the disease being treated. In some, more definite mood changes occur, characterized by euphoria, insomnia, restlessness, and increased motor activity. A smaller but significant percentage of patients treated with high doses of cortisol become anxious or depressed, and a still smaller percentage exhibit psychotic reactions. A high incidence of neuroses and psychoses has been noted among patients with Cushing's syndrome. The abnormalities of behavior usually disappear when the corticosteroids are withdrawn or the Cushing's syndrome is effectively treated (Lewis and Smith, 1983).

There is usually an increase in the excitability of neural tissue in hypocorticism and a decreased excitability in animals given large doses of desoxycorticosterone; these alterations appear to be related to changes in the concentrations of electrolytes in the brain. In contrast, administration of cortisol increases brain excitability without influencing the concentrations of Na^+ and K^+ in the brain. Thus, it has been concluded that the influence of desoxycorticosterone on excitability is mediated through its influence on Na^+ transport, whereas cortisol acts by a different mechanism, presumably mediated by cytoplasmic receptors (McEwen, 1979; Carpenter and Gruen, 1982).

Formed Elements of Blood. Glucocorticoids tend to increase the hemoglobin and red-cell content of the blood, as evidenced by the frequent occurrence of polycythemia in Cushing's syndrome and a mild, normochromic, normocytic anemia in Addison's disease. The capacity of these steroids to retard erythrophagocytosis may be a factor in the production of polycythemia.

The corticosteroids also affect circulating white cells. Addison was the first to observe the increase in mass of lymphoid tissue that accompanies adrenocortical insufficiency; lymphocytosis also occurs. In contrast, Cushing's syndrome is characterized by lymphocytopenia and decreased mass of lymphoid tissue. The administration of glucocorticoids leads to a decreased number of blood lymphocytes, eosinophils, monocytes, and basophils. A single dose of cortisol produces a decline of about 70% in circulating lymphocytes and a decline of over 90% in monocytes; this reaction occurs in 4 to 6 hours and lasts about 24 hours. The decrease in lymphocytes, monocytes, and eosinophils appears to result from the redistribution of cells rather than from their destruction. The cause of the fall in circulating basophils has not been established. In contrast, the administration of glucocorticoids causes an increase in the number of polymorphonuclear leukocytes in the blood as the result of their increased rate of entrance into the blood from the marrow, diminished rate of removal from the circulation, and increase in release from vascular walls.

After administration of a glucocorticoid, T lymphocytes are decreased proportionately more than are B cells. The profile of cellular responses of the lymphocytes remaining in the blood to various mitogens and antigens is also altered. These findings indicate that subpopulations of lymphocytes are differentially affected by the steroids (*see* Cupps and Fauci, 1982). The altered responsiveness of lymphocytes is an important facet of the antiinflammatory and immunosuppressive actions of the glucocorticoids (*see* below).

While glucocorticoids cause a rapid lysis of lymphatic tissue in rats and mice, evidence of a comparable effect in man is lacking. As noted above, the acute effects of steroids on circulating lymphocytes are due to sequestration from the blood, rather than to lymphocytolysis. However, acute lymphoblastic leukemia cells and, in some cases, cells of other lymphatic malignancies are destroyed by glucocorticoids in a manner presumed to be analogous to that which occurs in lymphoid tissue of rodents.

Antiinflammatory and Immunosuppressive Actions. Glucocorticoids have the capacity to prevent or suppress the development of the manifestations of inflammation. They inhibit the inflammatory response whether the inciting agent is radiant, mechanical, chemical, infectious, or immunological. Although the administration of corticosteroids for their antiinflammatory effects is palliative therapy because the underlying cause of the disease remains, the suppression of inflammation and its consequences has made these agents of great value clinically—indeed, at times lifesaving. The glucocorticoids are also of immense value in treating diseases that result from undesirable immune reactions. These diseases range from conditions that are predominantly the consequence of humoral immunity, such as urticaria, to those that are mediated by cellular immune mechanisms, such as rejection of transplanted organs. The immunosuppressive and antiinflammatory actions of the glucocorticoids are inextricably linked because they both result in large part from inhibition of specific functions of leukocytes. In several instances these effects on leukocytes are a consequence of glucocorticoid-induced inhibition of the elaboration and/or action of lymphokines.

Antiinflammatory Actions. The corticosteroids inhibit not only the early phenomena of the inflammatory process (edema, fibrin deposition, capillary dilatation, migration of leukocytes into the inflamed area, and phagocytic activity) but also the later manifestations (proliferation of capillaries and fibroblasts, deposition of collagen, and, still later, cicatrization). Although of great value in certain circumstances, the suppression of inflammatory manifestations by corticosteroids can invite potential disaster. The signs and symptoms of inflammation are expressions of the disease process that are often used by the physician in diagnosis and in evaluating the effectiveness of treatment. These may be missing in patients treated with glucocorticoids. For example, an infection may continue to progress while the patient superficially appears to improve, or a peptic ulcer may perforate without producing clinical signs.

A number of mechanisms are involved in the suppression of inflammation by the glucocorticoids, and many remain to be elucidated. The ability of glucocorticoids to inhibit the recruitment of leukocytes and monocyte-macrophages into affected areas has been thought for some time to be a very important factor in their antiinflammatory actions (Balow and Rosenthal, 1973; Parrillo and Fauci, 1979). Later investigations have confirmed this idea and have demonstrated that glucocorticoids inhibit the ability of these cells to elaborate a variety of chemotactic substances as well as factors that mediate increased capillary permeability, vasodilatation, and contraction of various nonvascular smooth muscles.

At present, the catalogue of substances whose synthesis and/or release is inhibited by glucocorticoids includes (1) arachidonic acid and its metabolites (*e.g.*, prostaglandins and leukotrienes), through glucocorticoid-induced synthesis of a protein or family of proteins (lipocortin or macrocortin) that inhibits the activity of phospholipase A_2 (DiRosa *et al.*, 1985); (2) platelet activating factor (PAF), apparently also mediated by the induction of lipocortin (Parente and Flower, 1985); (3) tumor necrosis factor (TNF, or cachectin), which incites many of the processes of inflammation and is normally released from phagocytic cells following their stimulation by bacterial endotoxins (Beutler and Cerami, 1987); and (4) interleukin-1 (IL-1), normally elaborated by monocyte-macrophages, which results from a glucocorticoid-induced decrease in the concentration of its mRNA (*see* Dinarello and Mier, 1986, 1987). IL-1 exerts a number of inflammatory actions, including stimulation of the production of PGE_2 and collagenase, activation of T lymphocytes, stimulation of fibroblast proliferation, and enhanced hepatic synthesis of "acute-phase" proteins; it also functions as a chemoattractant for leukocytes and causes neutrophilia (Lew *et al.*, 1988). Glucocorticoids also inhibit the formation of plasminogen activator by neutrophils. This enzyme converts plasminogen to plasmin (fibrinolysin), which is thought to facilitate the migration of leukocytes into sites of inflammation by hydrolyzing fibrin and other proteins (Granelli-Piperano *et al.*, 1977). In addition to inhibiting the release of mediators of inflammation, glucocorticoids can inhibit the actions of humoral regulators, such as PAF (Wallace and Whittle, 1988) and macrophage migration-inhibition factor (MIF), which normally causes the accumulation of nonsensitized macrophages at sites of inflammation (Balow and Rosenthal, 1973).

Immunosuppressive Actions. Although considered to be immunosuppressive, therapeutic doses of glucocorticoids do not significantly decrease the concentration of antibodies in the circulation. Furthermore, during glucocorticoid therapy, patients exhibit a nearly normal antibody response to antigenic challenge (Butler, 1975). Examination of the cellular immune system also produces seemingly anomalous observations. For example, although guinea pigs previously sensitized to tuberculin do not exhibit responses to tuberculin during treatment with steroids, the introduction of their lymphocytes into untreated recipient animals causes the recipient to become sensitive to intradermal tuberculin (Weston *et al.*, 1973). Thus, glucocorticoids eliminate neither humoral nor cellular hyperimmune states, but rather prevent their manifestations. Nevertheless, they do appear to inhibit early steps in the development of immunity. Thus far, most of the actions that have been elucidated involve disruptions of intercellular communication among leukocytes through interference with the production or function of lymphokines. Although researchers are not in complete agreement as to the sequence of events involved in the production of cell-mediated immunity, many of the current hypotheses are incorporated into the model schematically presented in Figure 60–3, which also includes probable sites of glucocorticoid action.

The immune response is initiated by the interaction of an antigen with macrophages and with surface antibodies on B lymphocytes. The macrophages ingest and process the antigen, which is then displayed on the cell surface of the macrophage together with a major histocompatibility antigen; they also secrete interleukin-1 (IL-1). Glucocorticoids interfere with the function of macrophages in several ways: (1) they inhibit the action of MIF, thereby promoting the egress of macrophages from affected areas; (2) they inhibit the processing and display of antigen by interfering with the facilitating actions of gamma interferon (Gerrard *et al.*, 1984; Mokoena and Gordon, 1985); and (3) they inhibit the synthesis and release of IL-1 (Lew *et al.*, 1988). Although IL-1 participates in the proliferation of B cells and their ultimate synthesis of antibody, glucocorticoids have little effect on antibody production (*see* above). More importantly, IL-1 participates in the activation of resting T lymphocytes when they come in contact with the processed antigen and histocompatibility antigen that is displayed on the surface of activated macrophages; hence, glucocorticoids suppress the activation of T cells by several mechanisms.

Activated T cells release a series of lymphokines, including interleukin-2 (IL-2), as well as gamma interferon and granulocyte-macrophage colony-stimulating factor. IL-2 directs activated T cells to proliferate, thereby expanding the population of clones of specific T cells; it also induces a particular group of lymphocytes to become cytotoxic ("killer") lymphocytes. Glucocorticoids suppress the amplification of cell-mediated immunity both by inhibiting the expression of the IL-2 gene in T cells and by interfering with the interaction of IL-2 with its receptors on T cells (Horst and Flad, 1987); there is some evidence that the effects on IL-2 synthesis are indirect and are mediated by suppression of the formation of leukotriene B_4 (Goodwin *et al.*, 1986). In addition to effects secondary to the suppression of IL-2 synthesis, glucocorticoids may interfere with the activation of cytotoxic lymphocytes by IL-2 as well as inhibit the function of natural killer lymphocytes (Gatti *et al.*, 1986; Papa *et al.*, 1986). The function of lymphokines in the generation of cell-mediated immunity has been reviewed by Dinarello and Mier (1987). (*See also* Chapter 53.)

Growth and Cell Division. Pharmacological doses of glucocorticoids retard or interrupt the growth of children, indicating an adverse effect on the epiphyseal cartilage. Inhibition of growth is a rather widespread effect of the glucocorticoids on tissues of laboratory animals. For example, glucocorticoids inhibit cell division or the synthesis of DNA in thymocytes; normal, developing, and regenerating liver; gastric mucosa; developing brain; developing lung; and human epidermis. Nevertheless, this effect is somewhat selective, and corticosteroids do not characteristically produce the bone-marrow depression or the enteritis that follows exposure to nonspecific antimitotic agents. How the steroids produce this effect is not known.

ABSORPTION, TRANSPORT, METABOLISM, AND EXCRETION

Absorption. Cortisol and numerous congeners, including synthetic analogs, are effective when given by mouth. Water-soluble esters of cortisol and its synthetic congeners are administered intravenously to achieve high concentrations in body fluids rapidly. More prolonged effects are obtained by intramuscular injection of suspensions of cortisol, its congeners, and its esters. Minor changes in chemical structure may result in large changes in the rate of absorption, time of onset of effect, and duration of action.

Glucocorticoids are absorbed from sites of local application such as synovial spaces, the conjunctival sac, and the skin. When administration is prolonged or when large areas of skin are involved, the absorption may be sufficient to cause systemic effects, including adrenocortical suppression.

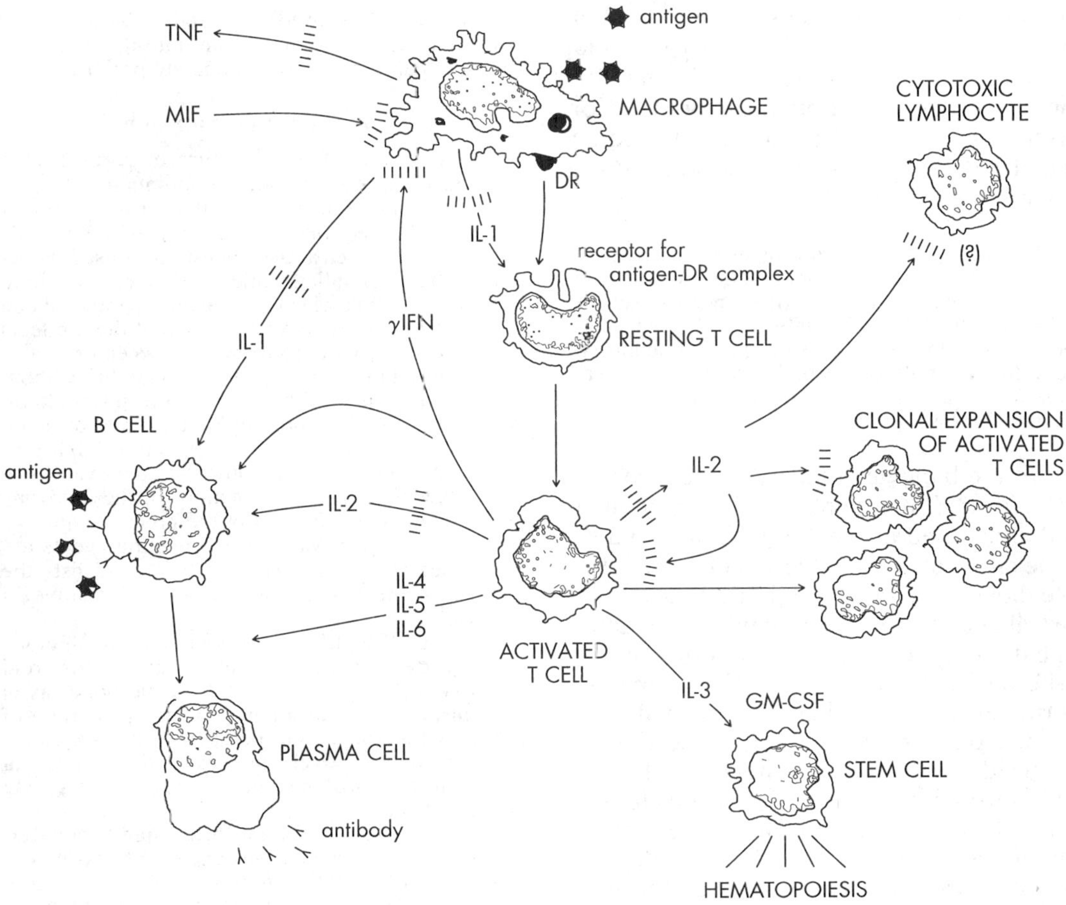

Figure 60–3. *Sites of action of glucocorticoids in the responses of leukocytes during antigenic challenge and inflammation.*

The humoral immune response is initiated by interaction of an antigen with surface antibodies on B cells; cell-mediated immunity begins with the ingestion and processing of an antigen by macrophages. The activated macrophages secrete interleukin-1 (IL-1) and tumor necrosis factor (TNF, cachectin) and display the processed antigen on the cell surface together with a major histocompatibility antigen (DR). Both IL-1 and TNF initiate a number of the processes involved in inflammation (*see* text). Under the influence of IL-1, resting T cells become activated following contact with processed antigen and DR and secrete a series of humoral factors (IL-2 through IL-6, gamma interferon [γIFN], and granulocyte-macrophage colony-stimulating factor [GM-CSF]). The cell-mediated response is amplified by γIFN, which enhances the processing of antigen by macrophages; by macrophage migration-inhibitory factor (MIF), which reduces the egress of wandering monocytes from affected areas; and by IL-2, which causes the clonal expansion of activated T cells. IL-2 also activates a particular group of cells to become cytotoxic (killer) lymphocytes. The inhibitory effects of glucocorticoids (represented by ||||||) are exerted on the release of IL-1 and TNF by activated macrophages, on the release of IL-2 by activated T cells, on the actions of MIF and γIFN on macrophages, and on the actions of IL-2 on activated T cells and perhaps on the precursors of killer lymphocytes. (Adapted from Dinarello and Mier, 1987.)

Transport, Metabolism, and Excretion. In the plasma, 90% or more of the cortisol is reversibly bound to protein under normal circumstances. The binding is accounted for by two proteins. One, corticosteroid-binding globulin, is a glycoprotein; the other is albumin. The globulin has high affinity but low total binding capacity, while albumin has low affinity but relatively large binding capacity. At low or normal concentrations of corticosteroids, most of the hormone is bound to globulin. Corticosteroids compete with each other for binding sites on the corticosteroid-binding globulin. Cortisol has high affinity; glucuronide-conjugated steroid metabolites and aldosterone have low affinities.

During pregnancy and during estrogen treatment in both sexes, corticosteroid-binding globulin, total plasma cortisol, and free cortisol increase severalfold. The physiological significance of these facts is not known. In contrast to the protein-bound steroid, the free hormone is biologically active, available for hepatic metabolism, and may be excreted by the kidney.

All the biologically active adrenocortical steroids and their synthetic congeners have a double bond in the 4,5 position and a ketone group at C 3. Reduction of the 4,5 double bond can occur at both hepatic and extrahepatic sites and yields an inactive substance. Subsequent reduction of the 3-ketone substituent to a 3-hydroxyl to form tetrahydrocortisol has been demonstrated only in liver. Most of the ring A–reduced metabolites are enzymatically coupled through the 3-hydroxyl with sulfate or with glucuronic acid to form water-soluble sulfate esters or glucuronides, and they are excreted as such. These conjugation reactions occur principally in liver and to some extent in kidney. Neither biliary nor fecal excretion is of quantitative importance in man.

Reversible oxidation of the 11-hydroxyl group has been demonstrated to occur slowly in a variety of tissues and rapidly in liver, kidney, colon, and parotid. As noted above, inactivation of cortisol by oxidation of the 11-hydroxyl group is thought to suppress the interaction of cortisol with the mineralocorticoid receptor in these organs (Funder *et al.*, 1988). Corticosteroids with an 11-ketone substituent require reduction to 11-hydroxyl compounds for their biological activity. Reduction of the 20-ketone group to a 20-hydroxyl configuration yields a substance having little, if any, biological activity. Corticosteroids with a hydroxyl group at C 17 undergo an oxidation that yields 17-ketosteroids and a two-carbon fragment. These 17-ketosteroids are totally lacking in corticosteroid activity but, in a few instances, have weak androgenic properties.

The metabolism of cortisol has been studied more extensively than that of all other corticosteroids, and it is generally assumed that the metabolism of its congeners and synthetic derivatives is qualitatively similar. Cortisol has a plasma half-life of about 1.5 hours. The metabolism of corticosteroids is greatly slowed by introduction of the 1,2 double bond or a fluorine atom into the molecule, and the half-life is correspondingly prolonged.

STRUCTURE–ACTIVITY RELATIONSHIP

Modifications of the structure of cortisol have led to increases in the ratio of antiinflammatory to Na^+-retaining potency, such that in a number of compounds electrolyte effects are of no serious consequence, even at the highest doses used. However, effects on inflammation and on carbohydrate and protein metabolism have always paralleled one another, and it seems very likely that these effects are mediated by the same type of receptor.

Changes in molecular structure may bring about changes in biological potency as a result of alterations in absorption, protein binding, rate of metabolic transformation, rate of excretion, ability to traverse membranes, and intrinsic effectiveness of the molecule at its site of action. In the following paragraphs, modifications of the pregnane nucleus that have been of value in therapeutic agents are described (*see* Figure 60–4). Table 60–3 lists the effects of the modifications discussed relative to cortisol.

Ring A. The 4,5 double bond and the 3-ketone are both necessary for typical adrenocorticosteroid activity. Introduction of a 1,2 double bond, as in prednisone or prednisolone, enhances the ratio of carbohydrate-regulating potency to Na^+-retaining potency by selectively increasing the former. In addition, prednisolone is metabolized more slowly than cortisol.

Ring B. 6α-Substitution has unpredictable effects. In the particular instance of cortisol, 6α-methylation increases antiinflammatory, nitrogen-wasting, and Na^+-retaining effects in man. In contrast, 6α-methylprednisolone has slightly greater antiinflammatory potency and less electrolyte-regulating potency than prednisolone. Fluorination in the 9α position enhances all biological activities of the corticosteroids, apparently by its electron-withdrawing effect on the 11β-hydroxy group.

Ring C. The presence of an oxygen function at C 11 is indispensable for significant antiinflammatory and carbohydrate-regulating potency (cortisol versus 11-desoxycortisol) but is not necessary for high Na^+-retaining potency, as demonstrated by desoxycorticosterone.

Ring D. 16-Methylation or hydroxylation eliminates the Na^+-retaining effect but only slightly modifies potency with respect to effects on metabolism and inflammation.

All presently used antiinflammatory steroids are 17α-hydroxy compounds. Although some carbohydrate-regulating and antiinflammatory effects may occur in 17-desoxy compounds (cortisol versus corticosterone), the fullest expression of these activities requires the presence of the 17α-hydroxy substituent.

All natural corticosteroids and most of the active synthetic analogs have a 21-hydroxy group. While some glycogenic and antiinflammatory activities may occur in its absence, its presence is required for significant Na^+-retaining activity.

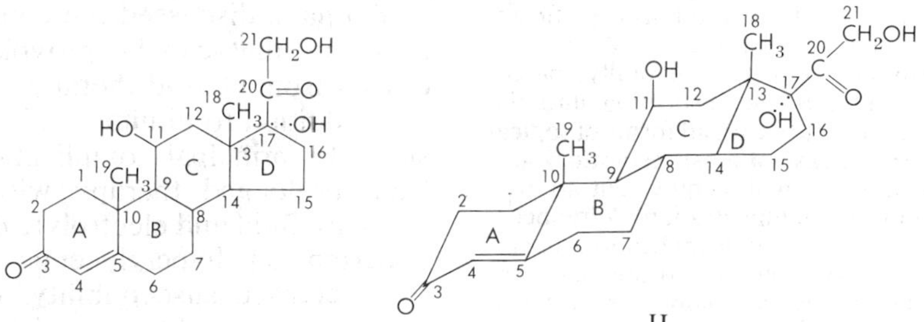

I II

Figure 60–4. *Structure, stereochemistry, and nomenclature of adrenocorticosteroids, as typified by cortisol (hydrocortisone).*

The four rings—A, B, C, and D—are not in a flat plane, as conventionally represented in I, but have the approximate configuration shown in II. (The planarity of the valence angles about the double bond between C 4 and C 5 prevents the chair form of ring A, as shown, from being an energetically probable conformational state. As a result, ring A is in a half-chair conformation, not easily represented in two dimensions.) Orientation of the groups attached to the steroid ring system is important for biological activity. The methyl groups at C 18 and C 19, the hydroxyl group at C 11, and the two-carbon ketol side chain at C 17 project above the plane of the steroid and are designated β. Their connection to the ring system is shown by full-line bonds. The hydroxy at C 17 projects below the plane and is designated α, and the connection to the ring is shown by a dotted bond.

PREPARATIONS AND ROUTES OF ADMINISTRATION

Organic chemists have synthesized a bewildering number of modified adrenocorticosteroids, many of which share the same properties and differ only with respect to absolute dosage. At the outset it should be reemphasized that, whereas a clear separation has been made between mineralocorticoids and glucocorticoids, there is no member of the latter group that is unique with respect to a separation of therapeutic and toxic effects. A working knowl-

Table 60–3. RELATIVE POTENCIES AND EQUIVALENT DOSES OF CORTICOSTEROIDS

COMPOUND	RELATIVE ANTI-INFLAMMATORY POTENCY	RELATIVE NA^+-RETAINING POTENCY	DURATION OF ACTION *	APPROXIMATE EQUIVALENT DOSE † (*mg*)
Cortisol (Hydrocortisone)	1	1	S	20
Tetrahydrocortisol	0	0	—	—
Prednisone (Δ^1-Cortisone)	4	0.8	I	5
Prednisolone (Δ^1-Cortisol)	4	0.8	I	5
6α-Methylprednisolone	5	0.5	I	4
Fludrocortisone (9α-Fluorocortisol)	10	125	S	—
11-Desoxycortisol	0	0	—	—
Cortisone (11-Dehydrocortisol)	0.8	0.8	S	25
Corticosterone	0.35	15	S	—
Triamcinolone (9α-Fluoro-16α-hydroxyprednisolone)	5	0	I	4
Paramethasone (6α-Fluoro-16α-methylprednisolone)	10	0	L	2
Betamethasone (9α-Fluoro-16β-methylprednisolone)	25	0	L	0.75
Dexamethasone (9α-Fluoro-16α-methylprednisolone)	25	0	L	0.75

* S = Short, or 8- to 12-hour biological half-life; I = intermediate, or 12- to 36-hour biological half-life; L = long, or 36- to 72-hour biological half-life.

† These dose relationships apply only to oral or intravenous administration; relative potencies may differ greatly when injected intramuscularly or into joint spaces.

edge of a small number of preparations is sufficient for nearly every clinical purpose.

Corticosteroids are administered orally, parenterally, and topically. Some absorption into the systemic circulation occurs with all forms of topical administration. In the case of most respiratory aerosols, absorption is virtually equivalent to that from parenteral or oral administration. Adrenocortical suppression can occur with applications of steroids to the conjunctival sac and to the skin. Absorption from the skin is especially marked when the steroid is applied under plastic film over a large surface area.

Information on available steroid preparations is presented in Table 60–4.

TOXICITY OF ADRENOCORTICAL STEROIDS

Two categories of toxic effects are observed in the therapeutic use of adrenocorticosteroids: those resulting from withdrawal and those resulting from continued use of large doses. Acute adrenal insufficiency results from too-rapid withdrawal of corticosteroids after prolonged therapy. Protocols for discontinuing corticosteroid therapy in patients who have been subjected to suppressive therapy for long periods have been described by Harter and associates (1963) and Byyny (1976). A characteristic corticosteroid withdrawal syndrome, consisting of fever, myalgia, arthralgia, and malaise, may be extremely difficult to distinguish from "reactivation" of rheumatoid arthritis or rheumatic fever (Amatruda *et al.*, 1960). Pseudotumor cerebri with papilledema is a rare reaction that follows reduction or withdrawal of corticosteroid therapy (Levine and Leopold, 1973).

The use of corticosteroids for days or a few weeks does not lead to adrenal insufficiency upon cessation of treatment, but prolonged therapy with corticosteroids may result in suppression of pituitary–adrenal function that can be slow in returning to normal. Graber and coworkers (1965) found that the processes of recovery of normal pituitary and adrenal function required 9 months in some patients. During this recovery period and for an additional 1 to 2 years, the patient may need to be protected during stressful situations, such as surgery or severe infections, by the administration of corticosteroids. Dixon and Christy (1980) have discussed the complex clinical problems that can be provoked by withdrawal from steroid therapy.

In addition to pituitary–adrenal suppression, the principal complications resulting from prolonged therapy with corticosteroids are fluid and electrolyte disturbances; hypertension; hyperglycemia and glycosuria; increased susceptibility to infections, including tuberculosis; peptic ulcers, which may bleed or perforate; osteoporosis; a characteristic myopathy; behavioral disturbances; posterior subcapsular cataracts; arrest of growth; and Cushing's habitus, consisting of "moon face," "buffalo hump," enlargement of supraclavicular fat pads, "central obesity," striae, ecchymoses, acne, and hirsutism.

Hypokalemic alkalosis and edema are rarely encountered in patients who are treated with synthetic corticosteroid congeners and almost never in patients taking the 16-substituted compounds. Glycosuria can usually be managed with diet and/or insulin, and its occurrence should not be an important factor in the decision to continue corticosteroid therapy or to initiate it in diabetic patients.

Increased susceptibility to infection in patients treated with corticosteroids is generally considered not to be specific for any particular bacterial or fungal pathogen. However, it should be noted that steroid-induced inhibition of phagocytic killing of *Aspergillus* spores and *Nocardia* is not reversed by gamma-interferon, although the killing of many other microorganisms is restored to normal by such treatment (Schaffner and Schaffner, 1987). If infection develops in a patient treated with corticosteroids, the dose may be maintained or increased and the best available treatment for the infection vigorously administered. Corticosteroid therapy may be initiated in patients having known infections of some consequence if effective, specific chemotherapy can be administered concomitantly with the hormones. However, in these circumstances the physician should be confident that the corticosteroid is needed, that the pathogen has been identified, and that chemotherapy will be effective.

Peptic ulceration is an occasional compli-

Table 60–4. PREPARATIONS OF ADRENOCORTICAL STEROIDS AND THEIR SYNTHETIC ANALOGS *

NONPROPRIETARY NAME (TRADE NAMES)	ORAL FORMS	INJECTABLE FORMS	OTHERS [1]
Fludrocortisone acetate [2] (FLORINEF ACETATE)	0.1 mg	—	—
Cortisol [3] (hydrocortisone) (CORTEF, HYDROCORTONE, others)	5–20 mg	25, 50 mg/ml (susp.)	TA: 0.25–2.5% 100-mg/60-ml enema 1% otic solution
Cortisol (hydrocortisone) acetate (HYDROCORTONE ACETATE, others)	—	25, 50 mg/ml (susp.)	TA: 0.5–1% 25-mg suppositories 10% rectal foam
Cortisol (hydrocortisone) cypionate (CORTEF)	2 mg/ml (susp.)	—	—
Cortisol (hydrocortisone) sodium phosphate (HYDROCORTONE PHOSPHATE)	—	50 mg/ml	—
Cortisol (hydrocortisone) sodium succinate (A-HYDROCORT, SOLU-CORTEF)	—	100–1000 mg (powder)	—
Beclomethasone dipropionate [4] (BECLOVENT, VANCERIL, others)	—	—	I: 42 μg per dose
Betamethasone [2] (CELESTONE)	0.6 mg 0.6 mg/5 ml (syrup)	—	—
Betamethasone benzoate (BENISONE, UTICORT)	—	—	TA: 0.025%
Betamethasone dipropionate (DIPROSONE, others)	—	—	TA: 0.05, 0.1%
Betamethasone sodium phosphate (CELESTONE PHOSPHATE, others)	—	4 mg/ml	—
Betamethasone sodium phosphate and acetate (CELESTONE SOLUSPAN)	—	6 mg/ml (susp.)	—
Betamethasone valerate (BETA-VAL, VALISONE, others)	—	—	TA: 0.01, 0.1%
Cortisone acetate [2] (CORTONE ACETATE)	5–25 mg	25, 50 mg/ml (susp.)	—
Dexamethasone [2] (DECADRON, others)	0.25–6.0 mg 0.5 mg/5 ml (elixir, soln.) 0.5 mg/0.5 ml (soln.)	—	TA: 0.01–0.1% O: 0.1%
Dexamethasone acetate (DECADRON-LA, others)	—	8, 16 mg/ml (susp.)	—
Dexamethasone sodium phosphate (DECADRON PHOSPHATE, HEXADROL PHOSPHATE, others)	—	4–24 mg/ml	TA: 0.1% O: 0.05, 0.1% I: 100 μg per dose
Flunisolide [4] (AEROBID, NASALIDE)	—	—	I: 25 μg per dose (nasal) 250 μg per dose (oral inhalation)

Table 60–4. PREPARATIONS OF ADRENOCORTICAL STEROIDS AND THEIR SYNTHETIC ANALOGS * (Continued)

NONPROPRIETARY NAME (TRADE NAMES)	ORAL FORMS	INJECTABLE FORMS	OTHERS [1]
Methylprednisolone [2] (MEDROL)	2–32 mg	—	—
Methylprednisolone acetate (DEPO-MEDROL, MEDROL ACETATE, others)	—	20–80 mg/ml (susp.)	TA: 0.25, 1%
Methylprednisolone sodium succinate (A-METHAPRED, SOLU-MEDROL)	—	40–2000 mg (powder)	—
Paramethasone acetate [2] (HALDRONE)	1, 2 mg	—	—
Prednisolone [2] (DELTA-CORTEF)	5 mg 3 mg/ml (syrup)	—	—
Prednisolone acetate (ECONOPRED, others)	—	25–100 mg/ml (susp.)	O: 0.12–1%
Prednisolone sodium phosphate (HYDELTRASOL, others)	1 mg/ml (liquid)	20 mg/ml	O: 0.125–1%
Prednisolone tebutate (HYDELTRA-T.B.A., others)	—	20 mg/ml (susp.)	—
Prednisone [2] (DELTASONE, others)	1–50 mg 1 mg/ml (syrup) 1, 5 mg/ml (soln.)	—	—
Triamcinolone [2] (ARISTOCORT, KENACORT)	1–8 mg	—	—
Triamcinolone acetonide (KENALOG, others)	—	3, 10, 40 mg/ml (susp.)	TA: 0.025–0.5% I: 100 μg per dose
Triamcinolone diacetate (ARISTOCORT, KENACORT DIACETATE, others)	2, 4 mg/5 ml (syrup)	25, 40 mg/ml (susp.)	—
Triamcinolone hexacetonide (ARISTOSPAN)	—	5, 20 mg/ml (susp.)	—
Alclometasone dipropionate [4] (ACLOVATE)	—	—	TA: 0.05%
Amcinonide [4] (CYCLOCORT)	—	—	TA: 0.1%
Clobetasol propionate [4] (TEMOVATE)	—	—	TA: 0.05%
Clocortolone pivalate [4] (CLODERM)	—	—	TA: 0.1%
Cortisol (hydrocortisone) butyrate (LOCOID)	—	—	TA: 0.1%
Cortisol (hydrocortisone) valerate (WESTCORT)	—	—	TA: 0.2%
Desonide [4] (DESOWEN, TRIDESILON)	—	—	TA: 0.05% 0.05% otic solution
Desoximetasone [4] (TOPICORT)	—	—	TA: 0.05, 0.25%

Table 60–4. PREPARATIONS OF ADRENOCORTICAL STEROIDS AND THEIR SYNTHETIC ANALOGS * (Continued)

NONPROPRIETARY NAME (TRADE NAMES)	ORAL FORMS	INJECTABLE FORMS	OTHERS [1]
Diflorasone diacetate [4] (FLORONE, MAXIFLOR)	—	—	TA: 0.05%
Fluocinolone acetonide [4] (FLUONID, SYNALAR, others)	—	—	TA: 0.01–0.2%
Fluocinonide [4] (LIDEX)	—	—	TA: 0.05%
Fluorometholone [4] (FLUOR-OP, FML)	—	—	O: 0.1, 0.25%
Flurandrenolide [4] (CORDRAN)	—	—	TA: 0.025, 0.05% 4 μg/sq cm tape
Halcinonide [4] (HALOG)	—	—	TA: 0.025, 0.1%
Medrysone [4] (HMS LIQUIFILM)	—	—	O: 1%
Mometasone furoate [4] (ELOCON)	—	—	TA: 0.1%

* The preparation above the double line is intended for use as a mineralocorticoid.

[1] TA = topical application to skin or mucous membranes in creams, solutions, ointments, gels, lotions, pastes (for oral lesions), or aerosols; O = ophthalmic solution, suspension, or ointment; I = nasal or oral inhalation.

[2] *See* Table 60–2 for chemical name.

[3] *See* Figure 60–2 for structure.

[4] Beclomethasone, 9α-chloro,16β-methylprednisolone,17,21-dipropionate; alclometasone dipropionate, 7α-chloro-11β,17,21-trihydroxy-16α-methylpregna-1,4-diene-3,20-dione 17,21-dipropionate; amcinonide, 9α-fluoro,16α-hydroxyprednisolone cyclic 16,17-acetal with cyclic pentanone,21-acetate; clobetasol propionate, 21-chloro-9-fluoro-11β,17-dihydroxy-16β-methylpregna-1,4-diene-3,20-dione 17-propionate; clocortolone, $\Delta^{1,2}$,6α-fluoro,9α-chloro,16α-methylcorticosterone 21-pivalate; desonide, 16α-hydroxyprednisolone, cyclic 16,17-acetal with acetone; desoximetasone, $\Delta^{1,2}$,9α-fluoro,16α-methylcorticosterone; diflorasone diacetate, 6α,9α-difluoro,16β-methylprednisolone, 17,21-diacetate; flunisolide, 6α-fluoro-11β,16α,17,21-tetrahydroxypregna-1,4-diene-3,20-dione cyclic 16,17-acetal with acetone, hemihydrate; fluocinolone, 6α,9α-difluoro, 16α-hydroxyprednisolone,16,17-acetal with acetone; fluocinonide, 6α,9α-difluoro,16α-hydroxyprednisolone,16,17-acetal with acetone,21-acetate; fluorometholone, $\Delta^{1,2}$,9α-fluoro,6α-methyl, 11β,17-dihydroxyprogesterone; flurandrenolide, 6α-fluoro,16α-hydroxycortisol, 16,17-acetal with acetone; halcinonide, 21-chloro,9α-fluoro,11β,16α,17-trihydroxypregn-4-ene-3,20-dione,16,17-acetal with acetone; medrysone, 11β-hydroxy,6α-methylprogesterone; mometasone, 9,21-dichloro-11β-17-dihydroxy-16α-methylpregna-1,4-diene-3,20-dione 17-(2-furoate).

cation of corticosteroid therapy. The high incidence of hemorrhage and perforation in these ulcers and the insidious nature of their development make them serious therapeutic problems. However, researchers disagree about the incidence of these ulcers, and some studies have concluded that the evidence does not support an association between peptic ulcers and treatment with glucocorticoids. It is also not known whether there is an interaction between glucocorticoids and nonsteroidal antiinflammatory drugs, such as aspirin, which, by themselves, can cause ulcers. Messer and associates (1983) concluded from a survey of the literature that steroid therapy approximately doubles the risk of ulcer (*see also* Spiro, 1983).

Myopathy, characterized by weakness of the proximal musculature of arms and legs and of their associated shoulder and pelvic muscles, is occasionally seen in patients taking large doses of corticosteroids. It may occur soon after treatment is begun and be sufficiently severe to prevent ambulation. It is not specific for synthetic corticosteroid congeners, for it is found in endogenous Cushing's syndrome. It is a serious complication and an indication for withdrawal of therapy. Recovery may be slow and incomplete (*see* Ellis, 1985; Knox *et al.*, 1986).

Behavioral disturbances may take various forms, including nervousness, insomnia, changes in mood or psyche, and psychopathies of the manic-depressive or schizophrenic type. Suicidal tendencies are not uncommon. It is no longer believed that previous psychiatric problems predispose to behavioral disturbances during therapy with glucocorticoids. Conversely, the absence of a history of psychiatric illness is no guarantee against the occurrence of psychosis during hormonal therapy. Psychiatric reactions to glucocorticoid therapy have been reviewed by Lewis and Smith (1983).

Posterior subcapsular cataracts have been reported in children receiving corticosteroid therapy. The majority of patients with rheumatoid arthritis who receive 20 mg of prednisone per day for 4 years develop cataracts (Levine and Leopold, 1973); it is possible that patients with this disease are particularly susceptible to this complication. The problem of corticosteroid-induced cataracts has been reviewed by Urban and Cotlier (1986).

Osteoporosis and vertebral compression fractures are frequent serious complications of corticosteroid therapy in patients of all ages. Ribs and vertebrae, bones with a high degree of trabecular structure, are generally the most severely affected. Glucocorticoids appear to inhibit the activities of osteoblasts directly, and, because of their inhibition of Ca^{2+} absorption by the intestine, glucocorticoids cause an increased secretion of parathyroid hormone (PTH). PTH stimulates the activity of osteoclasts; thus, both decreased formation and increased resorption of bone occur. As noted above, corticosteroids also increase Ca^{2+} excretion by the kidney. Osteoporosis is an indication for withdrawal of therapy and should be looked for regularly in radiographs of the spine in patients taking glucocorticoids for longer than a few months. Unfortunately, significant loss of bone must occur before it is apparent from radiography. The possibility of development of osteoporosis should be an important consideration when initiating and managing corticosteroid therapy, especially in postmenopausal women (*see* Baylink, 1983).

Aseptic necrosis of bone (osteonecrosis) may complicate long-term therapy with glucocorticoids and has also been reported following short courses with high doses. The femoral head is most often involved, but other large joints may be affected. Joint pain and stiffness may be the earliest symptoms, and the syndrome is not reversible. The mechanism of this reaction is not known (Zizic *et al.,* 1985).

Inhibition or arrest of growth can result from the administration of relatively small doses of glucocorticoids to children, and it cannot be overcome with exogenous human growth hormone. The widespread inhibitory effect of the glucocorticoids on DNA synthesis and cell division discussed above is apparently responsible.

THERAPEUTIC USES

With the exception of substitution therapy in deficiency states, the use of corticosteroids and their congeners in disease is largely empirical. From the experience accumulated since the introduction of glucocorticoids for clinical use, at least six therapeutic principles may be abstracted, as follows: (1) for any disease, in any patient, the appropriate dose to achieve a given therapeutic effect must be determined by trial and error and must be reevaluated from time to time as the stage and the activity of the disease change; (2) a single dose of corticosteroid, even a large one, is virtually without harmful effects; (3) a few days of corticosteroid therapy, in the absence of specific contraindications, is unlikely to produce harmful results except at the most extreme dosages; (4) as corticosteroid therapy is prolonged over periods of weeks or months, and to the extent that the dose exceeds the equivalent of substitution therapy, the incidence of disabling and potentially lethal effects increases; (5) except in adrenal insufficiency, the administration of corticosteroids is neither specific nor curative therapy but only palliative by virtue of their antiinflammatory and immunosuppressive effects; and (6) abrupt cessation of prolonged, high-dose corticosteroid therapy is associated with a significant risk of adrenal insufficiency of sufficient severity to be threatening to life.

Translated into the terms of clinical practice, these general principles are equivalent to the following rules. When corticosteroids are to be administered over long periods, the dose must be the smallest one that will achieve the desired effect. This dose must be found by trial and error. Where the goal of therapy is relief of painful or distressing symptoms not associated with an immediately life-threatening disease—for example, rheumatoid arthritis—the initial dose should be small and gradually increased until pain or distress has been reduced to tolerable levels. Complete relief is not sought. At frequent intervals the dose should be gradually reduced until the development of more severe symptoms signals that the minimally acceptable dose has been found. When therapy is directed at a state that is immediately life-threatening (*e.g.*, pemphigus), the initial dose should be a large one, estimated to achieve control of the crisis. If some benefit is not observed in a short time, the dose should be doubled or tripled. When potentially lethal disease is controlled by large amounts of corticosteroid, reduction of the dose should be carried out under conditions that permit frequent, accurate observations of the patient. Under these circumstances it is essential to assess constantly the relative dangers of therapy and of the disease being treated.

The apparently innocuous character of a single administration of corticosteroid in amounts within the conventional therapeutic range justifies its use without a definite diagnosis for crises in which there exists some probability that life is threatened by primary adrenal or pituitary insufficiency. If one of these conditions is present, a single intravenous injection of a soluble corticosteroid may prevent immediate death and allow time for diagnostic procedures.

Short courses of systemic corticosteroids in large doses may properly be given for diseases that do not threaten life, in the absence of specific contraindications. The general rule is that long courses of therapy at high dosage should be reserved for life-threatening disease. On occasion, and for definite cause, when the patient is threatened with permanent disability, this rule is justifiably violated.

It is not possible to define the precise dose of glucocorticoids that will produce pituitary and adrenocortical suppression in a given patient, since there is considerable variation. In general, the higher the dose and the more prolonged the therapy, the greater is the likelihood of suppression. Doses of short-acting glucocorticoids administered in the morning (upon waking) have less capacity to suppress the pituitary than do those given in the afternoon or evening; doses taken late in the day suppress the normal surge of ACTH that occurs during sleep.

Harter and associates (1963) suggested that some dissociation of therapeutic effects from certain undesirable metabolic effects can be achieved by the administration of a single large dose of corticosteroid every other day, in contrast to the usual daily multiple-dose schedule. A single dose every other day or at even longer intervals is acceptable therapy for some, but not all, patients with a variety of diseases modified by corticosteroid therapy. When this therapeutic regimen is possible, the degree of suppression of the pituitary and adrenal cortex can be minimized. However, long-acting steroids are not suitable for use by this dosage schedule.

Substitution Therapy. Insufficiency of secretion of the adrenal cortex results from structural or functional lesions of the adrenal cortex itself (primary adrenal insufficiency) or from structural or functional lesions of the anterior pituitary (secondary adrenal insufficiency). In either case, the patient may present with acute, catastrophic adrenal insufficiency (adrenal crisis) or chronic adrenal insufficiency. When the adrenal itself is the site of the lesion, all elements of normal adrenal secretion may be reduced or absent, or the deficiency may be selective for one or more components of secretion.

Acute Adrenal Insufficiency. This life-threatening disease is characterized by gastrointestinal symptoms, dehydration, hyponatremia, hyperkalemia, weakness, lethargy, and hypotension. It is usually associated with disorders of the adrenal, rather than the pituitary, although exceptions occur. It frequently follows abrupt withdrawal of high doses of corticosteroids.

The immediate needs of such patients are water, sodium chloride, glucose, cortisol, and appropriate therapy for precipitating causes, for example, infection, trauma, or hemorrhage. Inasmuch as these patients have a diminished capacity for a water diuresis and have often undergone some degree of cellular hydration, they are susceptible to water intoxication. The principal intravenous fluid should be isotonic sodium chloride solution. Glucose is required for nutrition and to prevent or treat hypoglycemia, but it should be given intravenously in isotonic sodium chloride solution. The total amount of intravenous fluid administered during the first 24 hours should not, in most instances, exceed 5% of ideal body weight. The patient should be monitored for evidence of rising venous pressure and pulmonary edema, because adrenocortical insufficiency reduces the functional capacity of the cardiovascular system. Cortisol (hydrocortisone) sodium succinate or cortisol sodium phosphate must be given intravenously at a rate of 100 mg every 8 hours, following an initial intravenous injection of 100 mg. This provides a quantity of cortisol that is equal to the maximal daily rate of secretion in response to stress. In the period of transition from intravenous fluid therapy to normal diet and activity, intramuscular cortisol sodium succinate or sodium phosphate may be used in a dose of 25 mg every 6 or 8 hours.

For the treatment of suspected but unconfirmed acute adrenal insufficiency, 4 mg of dexamethasone sodium phosphate should be substituted for cortisol (because dexamethasone does not interfere with measurements of plasma cortisol concentrations). In addition, cosyntropin (0.25 mg) should be given to test for adrenal responsiveness. Concentrations of cortisol and aldosterone in plasma are determined at the outset and after 30 and 60 minutes. A failure to obtain a response to cosyntropin (stimulation of steroid secretion) is diagnostic of primary adrenal insufficiency. A lack of response in terms of aldosterone indicates failure of the zona glomerulosa. An increase in plasma cortisol that requires prolonged infusion of cosyntropin indicates pituitary insufficiency with secondary adrenal atrophy.

Chronic Primary Adrenal Insufficiency. This disease results from adrenal surgery or destructive lesions of the adrenal cortex. It requires the administration of cortisol, 20 to 30 mg per day in divided doses. A common dose schedule is 20 mg on arising and 10 mg in the late afternoon. Most patients will also require a potent mineralocorticoid. The most convenient drug to use for this purpose is fludrocortisone acetate. The usual adult dose is 0.1 to 0.2 mg daily. Some patients do not need a mineralocorticoid and are adequately treated with cortisone and generous dietary salt. Therapy is guided by the patient's sense of well-being, alertness, appetite, weight, muscular strength, pigmentation, blood pressure, and freedom from orthostatic hypotension.

Adrenal Insufficiency Secondary to Anterior Pituitary Insufficiency. This condition is not usually associated with the dramatic signs and symptoms characteristic of adrenal insufficiency resulting from disease of the adrenal cortex unless there are complicating circumstances, for example, unusual fluid losses, trauma, or starvation. Hypoglycemia is the most frequent cause of symptoms. Quantitation of the electrolytes in plasma often reveals a dilutional hyponatremia. The administration of 20 mg of cortisol on arising and 10 mg in late afternoon is adequate replacement therapy for most patients with anterior pituitary insufficiency. This schedule mimics, to some extent, the normal diurnal cycle of adrenal secretion. Occasional patients require additional doses. When initiating treatment, it is customary to begin cortisol first and to add thyroid replacement therapy after adrenal insufficiency is under some degree of control, on the grounds that the administration of thyroid to a hypopituitary patient may precipitate acute adrenal insufficiency. Additional treatment is necessary during periods of stress. Cortisol, 300 to 400 mg per day, should be given to approximate the normal response to severe stress.

Congenital Adrenal Hyperplasia. This is a familial disorder in which activity of one of several enzymes required for biosynthesis of corticosteroids is deficient. With diminished or absent production of cortisol, aldosterone, or both, and consequent lack of inhibitory feedback, the adrenal cortex is stimulated to overproduce other hormonally active steroids. The clinical presentation, laboratory findings, and treatment depend on which of the six enzyme deficiencies thus far described is responsible. Only the syndrome of 21-hydroxylase deficiency will be described here.

About 90% of the patients with congenital adrenal hyperplasia have a deficiency of 21-hydroxylase activity. When the deficiency is only partial, the usual case, cortisol is secreted at normal rates as a result of continuous hypersecretion of ACTH, with consequent overproduction of adrenal androgens and their precursors. Aldosterone secretion is approximately normal. Female children undergo virilization (female pseudohermaphroditism) and male children show precocious development of secondary sex characteristics (macrogenitosomia). Linear growth is accelerated in childhood, but the height at maturity is reduced by premature closure of the epiphyses.

In about 30% of patients with 21-hydroxylase deficiency, the enzymatic defect is sufficiently severe to compromise increased aldosterone secretion in response to a hypovolemic stimulus. Such patients are unable to conserve Na^+ normally, in addition to manifesting androgenic effects (Bongiovanni *et al.*, 1967).

All patients with congenital adrenal hyperplasia resulting from a 21-hydroxylase deficiency require substitution therapy with cortisol or a suitable congener, and those with a salt-losing tendency require, in addition, a Na^+-retaining steroid. The usual oral dose of cortisol is about 0.6 mg/kg daily in two to four divided doses. The mineralocorticoid usually given is fludrocortisone acetate, 0.05 to 0.2 mg per day. Therapy is guided by gain in weight and height, by excretion of urinary 17-ketosteroids, and by blood pressure. Sudden spurts of linear growth may indicate inadequate pituitary suppression and excessive androgen secretion, whereas growth failure suggests overtreatment.

A number of rare forms of congenital adrenal hyperplasia are known in which enzyme deficiencies of the adrenal cortex, with similar defects of the gonads, result in clinical and laboratory findings very different from those described above for 21-hydroxylase deficiency. The types described thus far are "desmolase" deficiency (Camacho *et al.*, 1968), 3β-hydroxysteroid dehydrogenase deficiency (Bongiovanni *et al.*, 1967), 17α-hydroxylase deficiency (Goldsmith *et al.*, 1968), 11β-hydroxylase deficiency (Bongiovanni *et al.*, 1967), and 18-hydroxylase deficiency (David *et al.*, 1968). The clinical and laboratory findings and the treatment in these rare forms are quite different from those in 21-hydroxylase deficiency. The publications cited should be consulted for details.

Therapeutic Uses in Nonendocrine Diseases. Brief outlines of important uses of corticosteroids in diseases other than those involving the pituitary–adrenal complex are set forth below. The disorders discussed are not inclusive, but rather a representative list of the more common diseases for which the glucocorticoids are used.

The dosage of glucocorticoids varies greatly with the condition being treated. In the following discussion approximate doses of a representative corticosteroid congener, usually prednisone, are suggested. It is not meant to imply that prednisone has peculiar merit in general or for any particular disease over the other congeners. For a comparison of doses of glucocorticoids, *see* Table 60–3.

Arthritis. In rheumatoid arthritis, the criterion for initiating corticosteroid therapy is progressive disease with consequent disability, despite intensive treatment with rest, physical therapy, aspirin-like drugs, gold, and other agents. The decision to embark upon a program of hormone therapy must be made with due consideration for the fact that corticosteroid therapy, once started, may have to be continued for many years or for life, with the attendant risks of serious complications. The initial dose should be small and increased slowly until the desired degree of control is attained. The symptomatic effect of small reductions should be frequently tested to maintain the dose as low as possible. Complete relief is not sought. A regimen of rest, physical therapy, and aspirin-like drugs is continued. The usual initial dose is about 10 mg of prednisone (or equivalent) per day in divided doses. Optimal therapy for some patients with painful symptoms confined to one or a few joints may be intraarticular injection of the steroid into the affected joints. Typical doses are 5 to 20 mg of triamcinolone acetonide or its equivalent, depending upon the size of the joint cavity.

In osteoarthritis, intraarticular injection of corticosteroids is recommended for treatment of episodic manifestations of acute inflammation. Injections for this purpose should be infrequent because, in both rheumatoid arthritis and osteoarthritis, a significant incidence of painless destruction of the joint, reminiscent of Charcot's arthropathy, may be associated with repeated intraarticular injections of corticosteroids.

Rheumatic Carditis. Corticosteroids are reserved for patients failing to respond to salicylates and as initial therapy for patients severely ill with fever, acute congestive heart failure, arrhythmia, and pericarditis; acute manifestations are more rapidly suppressed by corticosteroids than by salicylates, a possibly lifesaving difference in a moribund patient. A dose of approximately 40 mg of prednisone or equivalent is usually given daily, in divided amounts, although much larger doses may on occasion be required. Reactivation of the disease occurs in a number of instances following withdrawal of steroid therapy. For this reason it has been suggested that salicylates be given concurrently with corticosteroids and be continued through and after the period of withdrawal of hormone therapy.

Renal Diseases. Corticosteroids do not modify the course of acute or chronic glomerulonephritis. However, patients with some forms of the nephrotic syndrome attributable to systemic lupus erythematosus or to primary renal disease (except renal amyloidosis) may be benefited by corticosteroid therapy. A typical therapeutic regimen consists in the daily administration, in divided doses, of 60 mg of prednisone or equivalent (2 mg/kg of edema-free body weight in children) for 3 or 4 weeks. If a remission with a diuresis and decreased proteinuria occurs during this period, maintenance treatment is continued for as long as a year. During maintenance therapy, the daily dose of prednisone is given only for the first 3 days of each week (Bacon and Spencer, 1973).

Collagen Diseases. The manifestations of most of the diseases in this group are controlled by glucocorticoids. An exception is scleroderma, which is generally considered refractory to these agents. It is important to distinguish between scleroderma and mixed connective tissue disease syndrome, which is responsive to steroids (Yount *et al.*, 1973). Polymyositis, polyarteritis nodosa, and the granulomatous-polyarteritis group (Wegener's granulomatosis, temporal-cranial arteritis, and polymyalgia rheumatica) are treated with daily doses of prednisone, approximately 1 mg/kg or equivalent, to induce a remission. The dose is then tapered down to the minimally effective level. Glucocorticoids decrease morbidity in all these diseases and prolong the survival times of patients with polyarteritis nodosa and Wegener's granulomatosis. In temporal (giant-cell) arteritis, adequate steroid therapy is necessary to prevent the blindness that occurs in about 20% of untreated cases. Fulminating systemic lupus erythematosus is a life-threatening condition, the manifestations of which should be suppressed by adrenocorticosteroid therapy with doses large enough to produce a prompt effect. Treatment usually consists of a 1-mg/kg daily dose of prednisone or equivalent. Within 48 hours, reduction of fever and improvement in the signs and symptoms of arthritis, pleuritis, or pericarditis should be observed. If not, the dose should be increased in 20-mg increments daily until a favorable response occurs. After the acute episode has been brought under control, corticosteroid therapy should be reduced by small steps, for example, 5 mg of prednisone per week, until signs or symptoms warn against further reductions. Salicylate or related drugs are then introduced and may permit a further reduction of corticosteroid dosage. A combination of glucocorticoids and antimetabolites, such as azathioprine, or the alkylating agent cyclophosphamide, has been used in selected patients with lupus erythematosus, particularly those with renal involvement. The concurrent use of these agents with steroids has been reviewed by Russell and Bretscher (1987).

Allergic Diseases. The manifestations of allergic disease that are of limited duration, such as hay fever, serum sickness, urticaria, contact dermatitis, drug reactions, bee stings, and angioneurotic edema, can, if necessary, be suppressed by adequate doses of glucocorticoids given as a supplement to the primary therapy. It must be emphasized, however, that the effects of the steroids require some time to develop, and severe reactions such as anaphylaxis and angioneurotic edema of the glottis require immediate therapy with epinephrine, 0.3 to 1.0 ml of a 1:1000 solution (0.3 to 1.0 mg) intramuscularly or subcutaneously. In life-threatening situations steroids may be given intravenously; dexamethasone sodium phosphate (8 to 12 mg or equivalent) is appropriate. In less severe diseases, such as serum sickness or hay fever, antihistaminic compounds are the drugs of first choice.

Bronchial Asthma. The corticosteroids should not be used routinely in the treatment of any asthmatic condition, acute or chronic, that can promptly be brought under moderate control with other measures. However, in status asthmaticus, glucocorticoids should be administered early and in large doses even though their effect is delayed (*see* Chapter 25). Intravenous administration of 60 to 120 mg of methylprednisolone sodium succinate every 6 hours is followed by daily oral doses of prednisone (40 to 60 mg) when the attack has subsided. The dose is then reduced in steps and withdrawal planned for about the tenth day after initiation of the prednisone therapy. Under favorable circumstances, patients can subsequently be managed once again with their prior medication.

Acute exacerbations of asthma are often treated with brief courses of oral corticosteroids. For example, 30 mg of prednisone (in children over 3 years of age) is administered twice daily for 5 days; an additional week of therapy at lower doses may be required. Upon restoration of adequate responses to other medications, the corticosteroid can usually be withdrawn abruptly; any suppression of adrenal function appears to dissipate within 1 or 2 weeks. In the treatment of severe chronic bronchial asthma (or less frequently, chronic obstructive pulmonary disease) that is not controlled by other measures, the administration of a corticosteroid may be necessary. As with other long-term uses of these agents, the lowest effective dose is utilized and care must be exercised when withdrawal is attempted; such therapy is never undertaken without the concurrent use of other medication, such as inhaled β_2-adrenergic agonists and/or oral theophylline.

The incorporation of inhaled corticosteroids in regimens for the treatment of bronchial asthma has increased substantially in recent years. In some patients, the use of inhaled solutions (most frequently beclomethasone dipropionate, triamcinolone acetonide, or flunisolide) can either reduce the duration of courses of oral corticosteroids or replace them entirely. In addition, many physicians recommend replacement of oral theophylline by inhaled glucocorticoids in the treatment of children with moderately severe asthma, in part because of the behavioral toxicity associated with long-term administration of theophylline. When inhaled, glucocorticoids are effective in reducing bronchial hyperreactivity and do not produce appreciable suppression of adrenal function when used at the recommended doses. Dysphonia or oropharyngeal candidiasis may develop, but the incidence of such side effects can be reduced substantially by maneuvers that reduce the deposition of drug in the oral cavity. The current status of glucocorticoids in the therapy of asthma has been reviewed by Cott and Cherniack (1988), and further discussion is presented in Chapter 25.

Ocular Diseases. Corticosteroids are frequently used to suppress inflammation in the eye, and used properly they are often responsible for preservation of sight. Levine and Leopold (1973) list 28 disorders of the eye that respond to corticosteroids. They are administered locally for disease of the outer eye and anterior segment. Both natural and synthetic corticosteroids attain therapeutic concentrations in the aqueous humor following instillation into the conjunctival cul-de-sac. For disease of the posterior segment, systemic administration is required.

A typical prescription is 0.1% dexamethasone sodium phosphate solution (ophthalmic), 2 drops in the conjunctival sac every 4 hours while awake, and 0.05% dexamethasone phosphate ointment (ophthalmic) at bedtime. For inflammations of the posterior segment of the eye, usual daily doses are approximately 30 mg of prednisone or equivalent, administered orally in divided doses.

It has been convincingly demonstrated that topical corticosteroid therapy frequently induces intraocular hypertension in normal eyes and further increases pressure in eyes with initially elevated pressure. The glaucoma has not always been reversible on cessation of corticosteroid treatment. It has been recommended that intraocular pressure be monitored when corticosteroids are applied to the eye for more than 2 weeks.

The local administration of corticosteroids to patients with bacterial, viral, or fungal conjunctivitis may mask evidence of progression of the infection until sight is lost. Corticosteroids are contraindicated in herpes simplex (dendritic keratitis) of the eye, because progression of the disease and irreversible clouding of the cornea may occur. Topical steroids should not be used in the treatment of mechanical lacerations and abrasions of the eye. They delay healing and promote the development and spread of infection. It is generally recommended that the ocular use of glucocorticoids be under the supervision of an ophthalmologist.

Skin Diseases. The development of corticosteroid preparations suitable for topical administration has revolutionized the therapy of the more common varieties of skin disease. Maibach and Stoughton (1973) have divided 20 dermatological disorders that respond to topical corticosteroids into those that are very responsive and those that require higher concentrations of steroids, occlusion of the drug under a plastic film, or intralesional administration. Attention must be paid to the concentration of steroid used; a large number of preparations of various concentrations are available for topical use (*see* Table 60–4). A typical prescription for an eczematous eruption is 1% cortisol ointment applied locally twice daily. Effectiveness is enhanced by application of the cream or ointment under a transparent plastic wrapping. Unfortunately, systemic absorption is also enhanced, occasionally sufficiently to suppress the pituitary–adrenal axis or to produce Cushing's syndrome. Adrenocorticosteroids are administered systemically for severe episodes of acute skin disorders and exacerbations of chronic disorders. The dose is usually 40 mg per day of prednisone or equivalent. Systemically administered corticosteroids may be lifesaving in pemphigus. Up to 120 mg of prednisone or equivalent per day may be required to control the disease. Further discussion of the treatment of skin disorders is presented in Chapter 65.

Diseases of the Intestinal Tract. Patients severely ill with untreated celiac sprue can often benefit from a course of glucocorticoid therapy given at the same time that management with a gluten-free diet is begun. Prednisolone, 30 mg per day or equivalent, is continued for 3 to 4 weeks. Patients who fail to respond to a gluten-free diet are helped by lower doses of prednisolone (7 to 12 mg per day or equivalent) for an indefinite period (Wall, 1973).

Corticosteroid therapy is indicated in selected patients with inflammatory bowel disease (chronic ulcerative colitis and Crohn's disease). Mildly ill patients with bowel symptoms but without disabling systemic symptoms usually can and should be managed with rest, diet, anticholinergic or other antidiarrheal agents, and sulfasalazine or metronidazole. However, patients who do not improve may benefit from corticosteroids. In mild ulcerative colitis, cortisol, 100 mg or equivalent, can be administered as a nightly retention enema in an attempt to induce remission. Alternate-day therapy may be effective. Patients with active Crohn's disease or ulcerative colitis may benefit from oral prednisone (10 to 30 mg daily). Severely ill patients with fever, anorexia, anemia, and malnutrition often improve dramatically when given systemic corticosteroid therapy. Large doses, 60 to 120 mg per day of prednisone or its equivalent, are recommended. Major complications of ulcerative colitis or Crohn's disease may occur despite corticosteroid therapy. Signs and symptoms of intestinal perforation and peritonitis may be difficult to detect during corticosteroid treatment (ReMine and McIlrath, 1980).

Cerebral Edema. Corticosteroids are of value in the reduction or prevention of cerebral edema associated with neoplasms, especially those that are metastatic. In spite of widespread use of glucocorticoids for treatment of the cerebral edema caused by trauma or cerebrovascular accidents, there is no convincing evidence of their value in these conditions (Nelson and Dick, 1975).

Malignancies. Glucocorticoids are used in the chemotherapy of acute lymphocytic leukemia and lymphomas because of their antilymphocytic effects. These diseases are treated in a complex fashion with rigidly scheduled sequences of combined drug therapy. Prednisone is commonly used in conjunction with an alkylating agent such as cyclophosphamide, an antimetabolite, and a vinca alkaloid (*see* Chapter 52).

Glucocorticoids can induce objective tumor regression in carcinoma of the breast in about 15% of patients; prednisolone (30 mg per day) has been the usual treatment. The presumed mechanism by which the corticosteroids act in this disease is through adrenocortical suppression, with an accompanying decrease in production of androgens, which are precursors of tumor-stimulating estrogens. A beneficial response should be expected only when the tumor has estrogen and/or progesterone receptors. Other forms of therapy are usually more effective.

Diseases of the Liver. The use of glucocorticoids in the treatment of hepatic diseases has been the subject of controversy. Careful studies have now indicated several diseases of the liver in which therapy with steroids significantly improves survival rates: subacute hepatic necrosis and chronic active hepatitis, alcoholic hepatitis, and nonalcoholic cirrhosis in women (Lesesne and Fallon, 1973; Copenhagen Study Group for Liver Diseases, 1974). Only certain patients with chronic active hepatitis should receive steroid therapy. Those who benefit have symptomatic disease, histological evidence of severe disease, and a negative reaction for hepatitis B surface antigen (Berk *et al.*, 1976). Treatment of subacute hepatic necrosis and chronic active hepatitis includes prednisolone, 60 to 100 mg per day; the dose is tapered as the disease improves. Treatment of alcoholic hepatitis with corticosteroids is reserved for patients who are severely ill, with evidence of hepatic encephalopathy. Prednisone (40 mg per day) is given for 1 month, followed by withdrawal over a period of 2 to 4 weeks (Carithers *et al.*, 1989). Nonalcoholic cirrhosis in women should be treated with glucocorticoids if the patient does not have ascites. Daily dosages average 15 to 20 mg of prednisone or equivalent when they are adjusted to the needs of the individual patients. The data indicate that steroid treatment lowers survival rates when ascites is present. Treatment of cirrhotic male patients with steroids has not been shown to be beneficial.

Shock. While corticosteroids are often administered to patients in shock, there is no convincing evidence to indicate that such therapy is efficacious.

Miscellaneous Diseases. Sarcoidosis is treated with prednisone, approximately 1 mg/kg per day or equivalent, to induce a remission. Maintenance doses, which are often required for long periods of time, may be 10 mg of prednisone per day or less. In this, as in other diseases treated by prolonged steroid therapy, patients with positive tuberculin reactions or other evidence of tuberculosis should receive prophylactic antituberculosis therapy. In thrombocytopenia, prednisone, 0.5 mg/kg or equivalent, is used to decrease the bleeding tendency. In severe cases and for initiation of treatment of idiopathic thrombocytopenia, daily doses of prednisone, 1 to 1.5 mg/kg, are employed. Hemolytic anemias with a positive Coombs' test are treated with prednisone, 1 mg/kg per day or equivalent. If hemolysis is severe, therapy is initiated with 100 mg of cortisol intravenously; as the disease improves, the dose is decreased. Small maintenance doses may be needed for several months if a positive response is obtained. In organ transplantation, high doses of prednisone (50 to 100 mg) are given at the time of the transplant surgery, usually in conjunction with immunosuppressive agents. Smaller maintenance doses (10 to 20 mg per day) are continued indefinitely, and the dosage is increased if rejection is threatened (*see* Chapter 53). Glucocorticoids have been used to treat aspiration of gastric contents, but no controlled studies have demonstrated their efficacy in this condition, and several uncontrolled studies suggest that steroids do not reduce morbidity or mortality.

DIAGNOSTIC APPLICATIONS OF ADRENOCORTICAL STEROIDS

Potent synthetic congeners of cortisol reduce urinary excretion of cortisol metabolites by inhibition of pituitary ACTH release. The dose required is so small, in gravimetric terms, that it contributes only negligibly to the urinary steroids. The administration of 0.5 mg of dexamethasone every 6 hours for a total of eight doses results in a marked suppression of excretion of cortisol metabolites in normal persons, but does not suppress urinary steroids in individuals with Cushing's syndrome. This test is useful in distinguishing persons with some nonspecific elevation of steroid excretion, for example, that due to obesity or stress, from patients with Cushing's syndrome. The administration of 2 mg of dexamethasone every 6 hours for a total of eight doses usually causes a suppression of cortisol secretion in most patients with pituitary-dependent hypercorticism, but ordinarily has little if any effect on the urinary steroids of patients with adrenal neoplasms or ectopic ACTH-producing tumors. However, "suppressible" tumors have been reported. The results of these tests are likely to be most definite if the urinary steroids are measured daily for 2 days before and for at least 2 days during administration of the suppressing agent. Variations of this procedure (shorter test period and measurement of plasma cortisol rather than urinary metabolites) have been described (Sawin *et al.*, 1968).

INHIBITORS OF THE BIOSYNTHESIS OF ADRENOCORTICAL STEROIDS

Five pharmacological agents have proved useful as inhibitors of adrenocortical secretion. Mitotane (*o,p'*-DDD), an adrenocorticolytic agent, is discussed in Chapter 52. Metyrapone, aminoglutethimide, ketoconazole, and trilostane are discussed here. The first three agents act by inhibiting those cytochrome P_{450}–containing enzymes that are involved in the synthesis of steroid hormones. As will be discussed below, there is considerable difference in susceptibility of the various reactions to these agents, thus providing some degree of specificity to their actions. Trilostane is a competitive inhibitor of the conversion of pregnenolone to progesterone.

Metyrapone. Metyrapone reduces cortisol production by inhibition of the 11β-hydroxylation reaction. It also inhibits 18-hydroxylation and side chain cleavage to some degree, but the latter effect is largely overcome when ACTH stimulates the gland. The biosynthetic process is terminated at 11-desoxycortisol (*see* Figure 60–2), a compound that has practically no inhibitory influence on the secretion of ACTH. In the normal person, a compensatory increase in ACTH secretion follows, and the secretion of 11-desoxycortisol, a "17-hydroxycorticoid," is markedly accelerated. Consequently, in normal persons, administration of metyrapone induces increases in the concentrations of ACTH and desoxycorticosterone in plasma and elevates the renal excretion of "17-hydroxycorticoids."

Metyrapone is used to test the capacity of the pituitary to respond to a decreased concentration of plasma cortisol. A response that is greater than normal is usually found in patients with Cushing's syndrome of pituitary origin, while in most cases of Cushing's syndrome caused by ectopic production of ACTH there is no response to the drug. Administration of metyrapone to patients with disease of the hypothalamico–pituitary complex who are unable to achieve a compensatory increase in the rate of secretion of ACTH is, of course, not followed by increased renal excretion of 17-hydroxycorticoids or increased plasma desoxycorticosterone.

The ability of the adrenal cortex to respond to ACTH should be demonstrated before metyrapone is employed, for two reasons: (1) administration of metyrapone can be used as a test for normal hypothalamico–pituitary function only if the adrenal glands are capable of responding to ACTH, and (2) the drug may induce acute adrenal insufficiency in patients with reduced adrenal secretory capacity. Metyrapone also inhibits synthesis of aldosterone, which, like cortisol, is an 11β-hydroxylated compound. However, metyrapone does not typically cause a deficiency of mineralocorticoids, with a consequent loss of Na^+ and retention of K^+, because the inhibition of the 11β-hydroxylation reaction results in an increased production of 11-desoxycorticosterone, a mineralocorticoid.

Metyrapone has been used successfully to treat the hypercortisolism that results either from adrenal neoplasms that function autonomously or from ectopic ACTH production by tumors. Its use in the treatment of Cushing's syndrome resulting from hypersecretion of ACTH by the pituitary is controversial (Orth, 1978; Gold, 1979). Long-term treatment with metyrapone can cause hypertension as the result of excessive secretion of desoxycorticosterone.

Metyrapone (METOPIRONE) is 2-methyl-1,2-di-3-pyridyl-1-propanone. The drug is marketed as 250-mg oral tablets. Following two 24-hour control periods, the drug is given orally at a dosage of 750 mg every 4 hours for six doses. Maximal urinary excretion of 17-hydroxycorticoids is observed on the next day.

Aminoglutethimide. This compound, α-ethyl-*p*-aminophenyl-glutarimide, primarily inhibits the conversion of cholesterol to 20α-hydroxycholesterol. This inhibition of the first reaction of steroidogenesis from cholesterol interrupts production of both cortisol and aldosterone.

Aminoglutethimide has been used successfully to decrease the hypersecretion of cortisol in autonomously functioning adrenal tumors and in hypersecretion resulting from ectopic production of ACTH. It has also been used in combination with metyrapone in the treatment of Cushing's syndrome that results from hypersecretion of ACTH by the pituitary (*see* Gold, 1979). Substitution of physiological doses of cortisol may be required to prevent adrenal insufficiency. It has also been used experimentally for treatment of prostatic and breast cancers (*see* Chapter 52).

Aminoglutethimide (CYTADREN) is marketed as 250-mg oral tablets. The suggested initial dosage is 250 mg every 6 hours. The dose is increased by 250 mg per day at 1- or 2-week intervals until the desired effect is achieved, side effects prohibit further increments, or a daily dose of 2 g is reached.

Ketoconazole. Ketoconazole is an antifungal agent, and this remains its most important role (*see* Chapter 50). In higher doses than those required for antimicrobial therapy, it is an effective inhibitor of steroid biosynthesis in the adrenal cortex and the testis. The most susceptible P_{450} system is apparently the C_{19-20} ligase of the testis, which accounts for its effectiveness in inhibiting the synthesis of testosterone. At higher doses, the drug inhibits the cholesterol side chain–cleavage enzyme system in the adrenal and effectively blocks the synthesis of adrenal hormones. Ketoconazole is a promising agent for management of Cushing's syndrome and carcinoma of the prostate, but the full metabolic consequences of its actions are not known. The use of ketoconazole as an inhibitor of hormone synthesis has been reviewed by Sonino (1987).

Trilostane. This compound ([2α,4α,5α,17β]-4,5-epoxy-17-hydroxy-3-oxoandrostane-2-carbonitrile) is a reversible inhibitor of 3β-hydroxysteroid dehydrogenase (*see* Figure 60–2). Trilostane reduces the synthesis of both cortisol and aldosterone and causes increased urinary excretion of 17-ketosteroids (primarily 3α-hydroxy-17-ketosteroids). The drug has been used in the treatment of Cushing's syndrome when more definitive therapy cannot be utilized. Experimentally, trilostane corrects the hypokalemia and lowers plasma concentrations of aldosterone and systemic blood pressure in patients with primary aldosteronism or in hypertensive patients who become hypokalemic during long-term therapy with diuretics (Winterberg *et al.*, 1985; Griffing and Melby, 1989). Although the drug is not likely to produce adrenocortical insufficiency, it may prevent an adequate response to ACTH during stress. Very few patients have been treated with trilostane for more than 3 months, and its place in long-term therapy has not been established.

Trilostane (MODRASTANE) is available in 30- and 60-mg capsules. Initial dosage is 30 mg four times a day; this is increased gradually at intervals of 3 to 4 days to a maximum daily dose of 480 mg.

ANTIGLUCOCORTICOIDS

A number of steroids have been shown to antagonize the effects of cortisol in systems *in vitro*. However, until recently, none of these agents displayed significant antiglucocorticoid effects *in vivo*. Mifepristone, (11β-4-dimethylaminophenyl)-17β-hydroxy-17α-(propyl-1-ynyl)estra-4,9-dien-3-one, was developed originally as a progesterone antagonist, but it also is a highly effective antagonist of the glucocorticoids. The role of mifepristone in the treatment of Cushing's syndrome caused by ectopic production of ACTH or autonomous corticosteroid secretion by adrenal tumors is currently being investigated. Glucocorticoid antagonists have been reviewed by Agarwal and associates (1987).

Addison, T. *On the Constitutional and Local Effects of Disease of the Suprarenal Capsules.* Samuel Highley, London, **1855.**

Ahmed, A. B. J.; George, B. C.; Gonzalez-Auvert, C.; and Dingman, J. F. Increased plasma arginine vasopressin in clinical adrenocortical insufficiency and its inhibition by glucosteroids. *J. Clin. Invest.*, **1967**, *46*, 111–123.

Amatruda, T. T., Jr.; Hollingsworth, D. R.; D'Esopo, N. D.; Upton, G. V.; and Bondy, P. K. A study of the mechanism of the steroid withdrawal syndrome. *J. Clin. Endocrinol. Metab.*, **1960**, *20*, 339–354.

Aquilera, G.; Harwood, J. P.; Wilson, J. X.; Morrell, J.; Brown, J. H.; and Catt, K. J. Mechanisms of action of corticotropin-releasing factor and other regulators of corticotropin release in rat pituitary cells. *J. Biol. Chem.*, **1983**, *258*, 8039–8045.

Arriza, J. L.; Weinberger, C.; Cerelli, G.; Glaser, T. M.; Handelin, B. L.; Housman, D. E.; and Evans, R. M. Cloning of human mineralocorticoid receptor complementary DNA: structure and functional kinship with the glucocorticoid receptor. *Science*, **1987**, *237*, 268–275.

Astwood, E. B.; Raben, M. S.; and Payne, R. W. Chemistry of corticotrophin. *Recent Prog. Horm. Res.*, **1952**, *7*, 1–57.

Bacon, G. E., and Spencer, M. L. Pediatric uses of steroids. *Med. Clin. North Am.*, **1973**, *57*, 1265–1276.

Balow, J. E., and Rosenthal, A. S. Glucocorticoid suppression of macrophage migration inhibitory factor. *J. Exp. Med.*, **1973**, *137*, 1031–1039.

Bangham, D. R.; Mussett, M. V.; and Stack-Dunne, M. P. The third international standard for corticotrophin. *Bull. WHO*, **1962**, *27*, 395–408.

Beckett, G. J., and Boyd, G. S. Evidence for the activation of bovine cholesterol ester hydrolase by a phosphorylation involving an adenosine 3′:5′-monophosphate-dependent protein kinase. *Biochem. Soc. Trans.*, **1975**, *3*, 892–894.

Bell, P. H.; Howard, K. S.; Shepherd, R. G.; Finn, B. M.; and Meisenhelder, J. H. Studies with corticotropin. II. Pepsin degradation of β-corticotropin. *J. Am. Chem. Soc.*, **1956**, *78*, 5059–5066.

Berk, P. D.; Jones, E. A.; Plotz, P. H.; Seeff, L. B.; and Wright, E. C. Corticosteroid therapy for chronic active hepatitis. *Ann. Intern. Med.*, **1976**, *85*, 523–525.

Beutler, B., and Cerami, A. Cachectin: more than a tumor necrosis factor. *N. Engl. J. Med.*, **1987**, *316*, 379–385.

Birnbaum, R. S., and Goodman, H. M. Effects of hypophysectomy on cyclic AMP accumulation and action in adipose tissue. *Fed. Proc.*, **1973**, *32*, 535.

Britton, S. W., and Silvette, H. Some effects of corticoadrenal extract and other substances on adrenalectomized animals. *Am. J. Physiol.*, **1931**, *99*, 15–32.

Brown-Séquard, C. E. Recherches expérimentales sur la physiologie et la pathologie des capsules surrenales. *C. R. Acad. Sci.* [*D*] (*Paris*), **1856**, *43*, 422–425.

Brunner, H. R.; Chang, P.; Wallace, R.; Sealey, J. E.; and Laragh, J. H. Angiotensin II vascular receptors. *J. Clin. Invest.*, **1972**, *51*, 58–67.

Butler, W. T. Corticosteroids and immunoglobulin synthesis. *Transplant. Proc.*, **1975**, *7*, 49–53.

Byyny, R. L. Withdrawal from glucocorticoid therapy. *N. Engl. J. Med.*, **1976**, *295*, 30–32.

Camacho, A. M.; Kowarski, A.; Migeon, C. J.; and Brough, A. J. Congenital adrenal hyperplasia due to a deficiency of one of the enzymes involved in the biosynthesis of pregnenolone. *J. Clin. Endocrinol. Metab.*, **1968**, *28*, 153–161.

Carithers, R. L., Jr.; Herlong, H. F.; Diehl, A. M.; Shaw, E. W.; Combes, B.; Fallon, H. F.; and Maddrey, W. C. Methylprednisolone therapy in patients with severe alcoholic hepatitis. A randomized multicenter trial. *Ann. Intern. Med.*, **1989**, *110*, 685–690.

Copenhagen Study Group for Liver Diseases. Sex, ascites, and alcoholism in survival of patients with cirrhosis. Effect of prednisone. *N. Engl. J. Med.*, **1974**, *293*, 271–273.

Cori, C. F., and Cori, G. T. The fate of sugar in the animal body. VII. The carbohydrate metabolism of adrenalectomized rats and mice. *J. Biol. Chem.*, **1927**, *74*, 473–494.

Cushing, H. The basophil adenomas of the pituitary body and their clinical manifestations. *Bull. Johns Hopkins Hosp.*, **1932**, *50*, 137–195.

David, R.; Golon, S.; and Drucker, W. Familial aldosterone deficiency: enzyme defect, diagnosis and clinical course. *Pediatrics*, **1968**, *41*, 403–414.

Deane, H., and Greep, R. O. A morphological and histochemical study of the rat's adrenal cortex after hypophysectomy, with comments on the liver. *Am. J. Anat.*, **1946**, *79*, 117–146.

Deming, Q. B., and Luetscher, J. A., Jr. Bioassay of desoxycorticosterone-like material in urine. *Proc. Soc. Exp. Biol. Med.*, **1950**, *73*, 171–175.

Dinarello, C. A., and Mier, J. W. Lymphokines. *N. Engl. J. Med.*, **1987**, *317*, 940–945.

DiRosa, M.; Calignano, A.; Carnuccio, R.; Ialenti, A.; and Sautebin, L. Multiple control of inflammation by glucocorticoids. *Agents Actions*, **1985**, *17*, 284–289.

Dixon, R. B., and Christy, N. P. On the various forms of corticosteroid withdrawal syndrome. *Am. J. Med.*, **1980**, *68*, 224–230.

Foster, G. L., and Smith, P. E. Hypophysectomy and replacement therapy in relation to basal metabolism and specific dynamic action in the rat. *J.A.M.A.*, **1926**, *87*, 2151–2153.

Funder, J. W. Adrenal steroids: new answers, new questions. *Science*, **1987**, *237*, 236–237.

Funder, J. W.; Pearce, P. T.; Smith, R.; and Smith, A. I. Mineralocorticoid action: target tissue specificity is enzyme, not receptor, mediated. *Science*, **1988**, *242*, 583–585.

Gatti, G.; Cavallo, R.; Sartori, M. L.; Marinone, C.; and Angeli, A. Cortisol at physiological concentrations and prostaglandin E_2 are active inhibitors of human natural killer cell activity. *Immunopharmacology*, **1986**, *11*, 119–128.

Gerrard, T. L.; Cupps, T. R.; Jurgensen, C. H.; and Fauci, A. S. Hydrocortisone-mediated inhibition of monocyte antigen presentation: dissociation of inhibitory effect and expression of DR antigens. *Cell. Immunol.*, **1984**, *85*, 330–339.

Gill, J. R., Jr.; Gann, D. S.; and Bartter, F. C. Restoration of water diuresis in Addisonian patients by expansion of the volume of extracellular fluid. *J. Clin. Invest.*, **1962**, *41*, 1078–1085.

Godowski, P. J.; Picard, D.; and Yamamoto, K. R. Signal transduction and transcriptional regulation by glucocorticoid receptor-LexA fusion proteins. *Science*, **1988**, *241*, 812–816.

Goldsmith, O.; Solomon, D. H.; and Horton, E. Hypogonadism and mineralocorticoid excess: the 17-hydroxylase deficiency syndrome. *N. Engl. J. Med.*, **1968**, *277*, 673–677.

Goodman, H. M. Endocrine control of lipolysis. In, *Progress in Endocrinology: Proceedings of the Third International Congress of Endocrinology, Mexico.* (Gual, C., and Ebling, F. J. G., eds.) Excerpta Medica, Amsterdam, **1968**, pp. 115–123.

Goodwin, J. S.; Atluru, D.; Sierakowski, S.; and Lianos, E. A. Mechanism of action of glucocorticoids. Inhibition of T cell proliferation and interleukin 2 production of hydrocortisone is reversed by leukotriene B. *J. Clin. Invest.*, **1986**, *77*, 1244–1250.

Graber, A. L.; Ney, R. E.; Nicholson, W. E.; Island, D. P.; and Liddle, G. W. Natural history of pituitary adrenal recovery following long term suppression with corticosteroids. *J. Clin. Endocrinol. Metab.*, **1965**, *25*, 11–16.

Granelli-Piperano, A.; Vassali, J. D.; and Reich, E. Secretion of plasminogen activator by human polymorphonuclear leukocytes. Modulation by glucocorticoids and other effectors. *J. Exp. Med.*, **1977**, *146*, 1693–1706.

Griffing, G. T., and Melby, J. D. Reversal of diuretic-induced secondary hyperaldosteronism and hypokalemia by trilostane, an inhibitor of adrenal steroidogenesis. *Metabolism*, **1989**, *38*, 353–356.

Harrop, G. A.; Soffer, L. J.; Ellsworth, R.; and Trescher, J. H. Studies on the suprarenal cortex. III. Plasma electrolytes and electrolyte excretion during suprarenal insufficiency in the dog. *J. Exp. Med.*, **1933**, *58*, 17–38.

Harter, J. G.; Reddy, W. J.; and Thorn, G. W. Studies on an intermittent corticosteroid dosage regimen. *N. Engl. J. Med.*, **1963**, *269*, 591–596.

Harvey, W., and Grahame, R. Effect of some adrenal steroid hormones on skin fibroblast replication *in vitro*. *Ann. Rheum. Dis.*, **1973**, *32*, 272.

Hauger, R. L.; Millan, M. A.; Catt, K. J.; and Aquilera, G. Differential regulation of brain and pituitary corticotropin-releasing factor receptors by corticosterone. *Endocrinology*, **1987**, *120*, 1527–1533.

Haynes, R. C., Jr.; Koritz, S. B.; and Péron, F. G. Influence of adenosine 3′,5′-monophosphate on corticoid production by rat adrenal glands. *J. Biol. Chem.*, **1959**, *234*, 1421–1423.

Hench, P. S.; Kendall, E. C.; Slocumb, C. H.; and Polley, H. F. The effect of a hormone of the adrenal cortex (17-hydroxy-11-dehydrocorticosterone; compound E) and of pituitary adrenocorticotropic hormone on rheumatoid arthritis. *Proc. Staff Meet. Mayo Clin.*, **1949**, *24*, 181–197.

Hollenberg, S. M.; Giguere, V.; Segui, P.; and Evans, R. M. Colocalization of DNA-binding and transcriptional activation functions in the human glucocorticoid receptor. *Cell*, **1987**, *49*, 39–46.

Horst, H.-J., and Flad, H. D. Corticosteroid-interleukin 2 interactions: inhibition of binding of interleukin 2 to interleukin 2 receptors. *Clin. Exp. Immunol.*, **1987**, *68*, 156–161.

Imura, H. Control of biosynthesis and secretion of ACTH. *Horm. Metab. Res. [Suppl.]*, **1987**, *16*, 1–6.

Ingle, D. J.; Higgins, G. M.; and Kendall, E. C. Atrophy of the adrenal cortex in the rat produced by administration of large amounts of cortin. *Anat. Rec.*, **1938**, *71*, 363–372.

Kahnt, F. W.; Milani, A.; Steffen, H.; and Neher, R. The rate-limiting step of adrenal steroidogenesis and adenosine 3′:5′-monophosphate. *Eur. J. Biochem.*, **1974**, *44*, 243–250.

Koeppen, B. M.; Biagi, B. A.; and Giebisch, G. H. Intracellular microelectrode characterization of the rabbit collecting duct. *Am. J. Physiol.*, **1983**, *244*, F35–F47.

Koper, W. J.; Cordle, S. R.; and Yeaman, S. J. Effect of high and low density lipoproteins on corticotropin-mediated cortisol synthesis by bovine zona fasiculata cells. *J. Steroid Biochem.*, **1985**, *23*, 369–371.

Knox, A. J.; Mascie-Taylor, B. H.; and Muers, M. F. Acute hydrocortisone myopathy in severe asthma. *Thorax*, **1986**, *41*, 411–412.

Krakoff, L.; Nicolis, G.; and Amsel, B. Pathogenesis of

hypertension in Cushing's syndrome. *Am. J. Med.*, **1975**, *58*, 216–220.

Lesesne, H. R., and Fallon, H. J. Treatment of liver disease with corticosteroids. *Med. Clin. North Am.*, **1973**, *57*, 1191–1201.

Levine, S. B., and Leopold, I. H. Advances in ocular corticosteroid therapy. *Med. Clin. North Am.*, **1973**, *57*, 1167–1177.

Lew, W.; Oppenheim, J. J.; and Matsushima, K. Analysis of the suppression of IL-1α and IL-1β production in human peripheral blood mononuclear adherent cells by a glucocorticoid hormone. *J. Immunol.*, **1988**, *140*, 1895–1902.

Loeb, R. F.; Atchley, D. W.; Benedict, E. M.; and Leland, J. Electrolyte balance studies in adrenalectomized dogs with particular reference to the excretion of sodium. *J. Exp. Med.*, **1933**, *57*, 775–792.

Long, C. N. H.; Katzin, B.; and Fry, E. G. Adrenal cortex and carbohydrate metabolism. *Endocrinology*, **1940**, *26*, 309–344.

McMahon, M.; Gerich, J.; and Rizza, R. Effects of glucocorticoids on carbohydrate metabolism. *Diabetes Metab. Rev.*, **1988**, *4*, 17–30.

Maibach, H. I., and Stoughton, R. B. Topical corticosteroids. *Med. Clin. North Am.*, **1973**, *57*, 1253–1264.

Marco, J.; Calle, C.; Román, D.; Diaz-Ferros, M.; Villanueva, M. L.; and Valverde, I. Hyperglucagonism induced by glucocorticoid treatment in man. *N. Engl. J. Med.*, **1973**, *288*, 128–131.

Messer, J.; Reitman, D.; Sacks, H. S.; Smith, H., Jr.; and Chalmers, T. C. Association of adrenocorticosteroid therapy and peptic ulcer disease. *N. Engl. J. Med.*, **1983**, *309*, 21–24.

Mokoena, T., and Gordon, S. Human macrophage activation. Modulation of mannosyl, fucosyl receptor activity *in vitro* by lymphokines, gamma and alpha interferons, and dexamethasone. *J. Clin. Invest.*, **1985**, *75*, 624–631.

Müller, O. A.; Stalla, G. K.; and von Werder, K. CRH in Cushing's syndrome. *Horm. Metab. Res. [Suppl.]*, **1987**, *16*, 51–58.

Nakanishi, S.; Kita, T.; Taii, S.; Imura, H.; and Numa, S. Glucocorticoid effect on the level of corticotropin messenger RNA activity in rat pituitary. *Proc. Natl. Acad. Sci. U.S.A.*, **1977**, *74*, 3283–3286.

Nelson, S. R., and Dick, A. R. Steroids in the treatment of brain edema. In, *Steroid Therapy*. (Azarnoff, D. L., ed.) W. B. Saunders Co., Philadelphia, **1975**, pp. 313–324.

Ney, R. L. Effects of dibutyryl cyclic AMP on adrenal growth and steroidogenic capacity. *Endocrinology*, **1969**, *84*, 168–170.

Orth, D. N. Metyrapone is useful only as adjunctive therapy in Cushing's disease. *Ann. Intern. Med.*, **1978**, *89*, 128–130.

Otsuka, H., and Inouye, L. K. Structure-activity relationships of adrenocorticotropin. *Pharmacol. Ther.* [*B*], **1975**, *1*, 501–527.

Papa, M. Z.; Vetto, J. T.; Ettinghausen, S. E.; Mule, J. J.; and Rosenberg, S. A. Effect of corticosteroid on the antitumor activity of lymphokine-activated killer cells and interleukin 2 in mice. *Cancer Res.*, **1986**, *46*, 5618–5623.

Parente, L., and Flower, R. J. Hydrocortisone and 'macrocortin' inhibit the zymosan-induced release of lyso-PAF from rat peritoneal leucocytes. *Life Sci.*, **1985**, *36*, 1225–1231.

Pittman, R. C., and Steinberg, D. Activatable cholesterol esterase and triacylglycerol lipase activities of rat adrenal and their relationship. *Biochim. Biophys. Acta*, **1977**, *487*, 431–444.

ReMine, S. G., and McIlrath, D. C. Bowel perforation in steroid-treated patients. *Ann. Surg.*, **1980**, *192*, 581–586.

Russell, A. S., and Bretscher, P. A. Immunosuppressive therapy in systemic lupus erythematosus. *J. Rheumatol.*, **1987**, Suppl. 13, 194–198.

Russell, N. A.; Belanger, G.; Benoit, B. G.; Latter, D. N.; Finestone, D. L.; and Armstrong, G. W. Spinal epidural lipomatosis: a complication of glucocorticoid therapy. *Can. J. Neurol. Sci.*, **1984**, *11*, 383–386.

Sawin, C. T.; Bray, G. A.; and Idelson, B. A. Overnight suppression test with dexamethasone in Cushing's syndrome. *J. Clin. Endocrinol. Metab.*, **1968**, *28*, 422–424.

Schaffner, A., and Schaffner, T. Glucocorticoid-induced impairment of macrophage antimicrobial activity: mechanisms and dependence on the state of activation. *Rev. Infect. Dis.*, **1987**, *9*, Suppl. 5, S620–S629.

Share, L., and Crofton, J. T. Contribution of vasopressin to hypertension. *Hypertension*, **1982**, *4*, Suppl. III, 85–92.

Sheeler, L. R., and Schumacher, O. P. Hyponatremia during ACTH infusions. *Ann. Intern. Med.*, **1979**, *90*, 798–799.

Shibahara, S.; Morimoto, Y.; Furutani, Y.; Notake, M.; Takahashi, H.; Shimizu, S.; Horikawa, S.; and Numa, S. Isolation and sequence analysis of the human corticotropin-releasing factor precursor gene. *EMBO J.*, **1983**, *2*, 775–779.

Simpson, E. R., and Waterman, M. R. Regulation of the synthesis of steroidogenic enzymes in adrenal cortical cells by ACTH. *Annu. Rev. Physiol.*, **1988**, *50*, 427–440.

Simpson, S. A.; Tait, J. F.; Wettstein, A.; Neher, R.; Euw, J. V.; Schindler, O.; and Reichstein, T. Konstitution des Aldosterons des neuen Mineralocorticoids. *Experientia*, **1954**, *10*, 132–133.

Sistare, F. D., and Haynes, R. C., Jr. Acute stimulation of glucocorticoids from lactate/pyruvate in isolated hepatocytes from adrenalectomized rats. *J. Biol. Chem.*, **1985**, *260*, 12754–12760.

Spiro, H. M. Is the steroid ulcer a myth? *N. Engl. J. Med.*, **1983**, *309*, 45–47.

Stanton, B. A. Role of adrenal hormones in regulating distal nephron structure and ion transport. *Fed. Proc.*, **1985**, *44*, 2717–2722.

Stewart, P. M.; Wallace, A. M.; Valentino, R.; Burt, D.; Shackleton, C. H. L.; and Edwards, C. R. W. Mineralocorticoid activity of liquorice: 11-beta-hydroxysteroid dehydrogenase comes of age. *Lancet*, **1987**, *2*, 821–824.

Swann, H. G. The pituitary-adrenocortical relationship. *Physiol. Rev.*, **1940**, *20*, 493–521.

Tait, J. F.; Simpson, S. A.; and Grundy, H. M. The effect of adrenal extract on mineral metabolism. *Lancet*, **1952**, *1*, 122–124.

Thody, A. J. The significance of melanocyte-stimulating hormone (MSH) and the control of its secretion in the mammal. *Adv. Drug Res.*, **1977**, *11*, 23–74.

Vale, W.; Spies, J.; Rivier, C.; and Rivier, J. Characterization of a 41-residue ovine hypothalamic peptide that stimulates secretion of corticotropin and β-endorphin. *Science*, **1981**, *213*, 1394–1397.

Wall, A. J. The use of glucocorticoids in intestinal disease. *Med. Clin. North Am.*, **1973**, *57*, 1241–1252.

Wallace, J. L., and Whittle, B. J. Gastrointestinal damage induced by platelet-activating factor. Inhibition by the corticoid, dexamethasone. *Dig. Dis. Sci.*, **1988**, *33*, 225–232.

Winterberg, B.; Vetter, W.; Groth, H.; Greminger, P.; and Vetter, H. Primary aldosteronism: treatment with trilostane. *Cardiology*, **1985**, *72*, Suppl. 1, 117–121.

Weston, W. L.; Mandel, M. J.; Yeckley, J. A.; Krueger, G. G.; and Claman, H. N. Mechanism of cortisol inhibition of adoptive transfer of tuberculin sensitivity. *J. Lab. Clin. Med.*, **1973**, *82*, 366–371.

Wise, J. K.; Hendler, R.; and Felig, P. Influence of glucocorticoids on glucagon secretion and plasma amino acid concentrations in man. *J. Clin. Invest.*, **1973**, *52*, 2774–2782.

Yamamoto, K. R.; Godowski, P. J.; and Picard, D. Ligand-regulated nonspecific inactivation of receptor function: a versatile mechanism for signal transduction. *Cold Spring Harbor Symp. Quant. Biol.*, **1988**, *LIII*, 803–811.
Yard, A. C., and Kadowitz, P. J. Studies on the mechanism of hydrocortisone potentiation of vasoconstrictor responses to epinephrine in the anesthetized animal. *Eur. J. Pharmacol.*, **1972**, *20*, 1–9.
Yount, W. J.; Utsinger, P. D.; Puritz, E. M.; and Ortbals, D. W. Corticosteroid therapy of the collagen vascular disorders. *Med. Clin. North Am.*, **1973**, *57*, 1343–1355.
Zizic, T. M.; Marcoux, C.; Hungerford, D. S.; Dansereau, J.-V.; and Stevens, M. B. Corticosteroid therapy associated with ischemic necrosis of bone in systemic lupus erythematosus. *Am. J. Med.*, **1985**, *79*, 596–604.

Monographs and Reviews

Agarwal, M. K.; Hainque, B.; Moustaid, N.; and Lazer, G. Glucocorticoid antagonists. *FEBS Lett.*, **1987**, *217*, 221–226.
Baylink, D. J. Glucocorticoid-induced osteoporosis. *N. Engl. J. Med.*, **1983**, *309*, 306–309.
Bongiovanni, A. M.; Eberlein, W. R.; Goldman, A. S.; and New, M. Disorders of adrenal steroid biogenesis. *Recent Prog. Horm. Res.*, **1967**, *23*, 375–449.
Carpenter, W. T., and Gruen, P. H. Cortisol's influence on human mental functioning. *J. Clin. Psychopharmacol.*, **1982**, *2*, 91–101.
Cott, G. R., and Cherniack, R. M. Steroids and "steroid-sparing" agents in asthma. *N. Engl. J. Med.*, **1988**, *318*, 634–636.
Cupps, T. R., and Fauci, A. S. Corticosteroid-mediated immunoregulation in man. *Immunol. Rev.*, **1982**, *65*, 133–154.
Dallman, M. F.; Akana, S. F.; Cascio, C. S.; Darlington, D. N.; Jacobson, L.; and Levin, N. Regulation of ACTH secretion: variations on a theme of B. *Recent Prog. Horm. Res.*, **1987**, *43*, 113–173.
Dinarello, C. A., and Mier, J. W. Interleukins. *Annu. Rev. Med.*, **1986**, *37*, 173–178.
Ellis, E. F. Steroid myopathy. *J. Allergy Clin. Immunol.*, **1985**, *76*, 431–432.
Fain, J. N., and Czech, M. P. Glucocorticoid effects on lipid mobilization and adipose tissue metabolism. In, *Adrenal Gland*, Vol. 6. Sect. 7, *Endocrinology. Handbook of Physiology*. (Blashko, H., ed.) American Physiological Society, Washington, D.C., **1975**, pp. 169–189.
Funder, J. W., and Sheppard, K. Adrenocortical steroids and the brain. *Annu. Rev. Physiol.*, **1987**, *49*, 397–411.
Gold, E. M. The Cushing's syndromes: changing views of diagnosis and treatment. *Ann. Intern. Med.*, **1979**, *90*, 829–844.
Hers, H. G. Effects of glucocorticoids on carbohydrate metabolism. *Agents Actions*, **1985**, *17*, 248–254.
Keller-Wood, M. E., and Dallman, M. F. Corticosteroid inhibition of ACTH secretion. *Endocr. Rev.*, **1984**, *5*, 1–24.
Lewis, D. A., and Smith, R. E. Steroid-induced psychiatric syndromes. *J. Affective Disord.*, **1983**, *5*, 319–332.
McEwen, B. S. Influences of adrenocortical hormones on pituitary and brain function. In, *Glucocorticoid Hormone Action*. (Baxter, J. D., and Rousseau, G. G., eds.) Springer-Verlag, New York, **1979**, pp. 467–492.
McEwen, B. S.; DeKloet, E. R.; and Rostene, W. Adrenal steroid receptors and actions in the nervous system. *Physiol. Rev.*, **1986**, *66*, 1121–1188.
Marver, D. Aldosterone action in target epithelia. *Vitam. Horm.*, **1980**, *38*, 57–117.
Mulrow, P. J., and Forman, B. H. The tissue effects of mineralocorticoids. *Am. J. Med.*, **1972**, *53*, 561–572.
Parrillo, J. E., and Fauci, A. S. Mechanisms of glucocorticoid action on immune processes. *Annu. Rev. Pharmacol. Toxicol.*, **1979**, *19*, 179–201.
Pratt, W. B. Transformation of glucocorticoid and progesterone receptors to the DNA-binding state. *J. Cell. Biochem.*, **1987**, *35*, 51–68.
Privalle, C. T.; McNamara, B. C.; Dhariwal, M. S.; and Jefcoate, C. R. ACTH control of cholesterol side-chain cleavage at adrenal mitochondrial cytochrome P-450_{scc}. Regulation of intramitochondrial cholesterol transfer. *Mol. Cell. Endocrinol.*, **1987**, *53*, 87–101.
Reichstein, T., and Shoppee, C. W. The hormones of the adrenal cortex. *Vitam. Horm.*, **1943**, *1*, 346–413.
Sonino, N. The use of ketoconazole as an inhibitor of steroid production. *N. Engl. J. Med.*, **1987**, *317*, 812–818.
Urban, R. C., Jr., and Cotlier, E. Corticosteroid-induced cataracts. *Surv. Opthalmol.*, **1986**, *31*, 102–110.

CHAPTER

61 INSULIN, ORAL HYPOGLYCEMIC AGENTS, AND THE PHARMACOLOGY OF THE ENDOCRINE PANCREAS

C. Ronald Kahn and Yoram Shechter

INSULIN

History. There are few events in the history of medicine more dramatic than the discovery of insulin. Although appropriately attributed to Banting and Best, there were several investigators and collaborators who provided important observations and techniques that made the discovery possible. In 1869, a German medical student, Paul Langerhans, noted that the pancreas contains two distinct groups of cells—the acinar cells, which secrete digestive enzymes, and cells that were clustered in islands, or islets, which he suggested served a second function. Direct evidence for this function came in 1889, when Oskar Minkowski and Joseph von Mering showed that pancreatectomized dogs exhibit a syndrome similar to diabetes mellitus in man (*see* Minkowski, 1989).

There were numerous attempts to extract the pancreatic substance responsible for regulation of blood glucose. In the early 1900s, Gurg Ludwig Zuelzer, an internist in Berlin, attempted to treat a dying diabetic patient with extracts of pancreas. Although the patient improved temporarily, he sank back into coma and died when the supply of extract was exhausted. E. L. Scott, a student at the University of Chicago, made another early attempt to isolate an active principle in 1911. Using alcoholic extracts of the pancreas (not so different from those eventually used by Banting and Best), Scott treated several diabetic dogs with encouraging results; however, he lacked clear measures of control of blood glucose concentrations, and his professor considered the experiments inconclusive at best. Between 1916 and 1920, the Romanian physiologist Nicolas Paulesco conducted a series of experiments in which he found that injections of pancreatic extracts reduced urinary sugar and ketones in diabetic dogs. Although he published the results of his experiments, their significance was fully appreciated only many years later.

Unaware of much of this previous work, in 1921 Frederick G. Banting, a young Canadian surgeon, convinced a professor of physiology in Toronto, J. J. R. Macleod, to allow him access to a laboratory to search for the antidiabetic principle of the pancreas. Banting assumed that the islet tissues secreted insulin, but that the hormone was destroyed by proteolytic digestion prior to or during extraction. Together with a fourth year medical student, Charles H. Best, he attempted to overcome the problem by tying the pancreatic ducts. The acinar tissue degenerated, leaving the islets undisturbed; the remaining tissue was then extracted with ethanol and acid. Banting and Best thus obtained a pancreatic extract that was effective in decreasing the concentration of blood glucose in diabetic dogs.

The first patient to receive the active extracts prepared by Banting and Best was Leonard Thompson, aged 14 (Banting *et al.*, 1922). He appeared at the Toronto General Hospital with a blood glucose of 500 mg/dl (28 mM), and he was excreting 3 to 5 liters of urine per day. Despite rigid control of diet (450 kcal per day), he continued to excrete large quantities of glucose, and, without insulin, the most likely outcome was death after a few months. The administration of Banting and Best's extracts induced a reduction in the concentration and excretion of blood glucose. Daily injections were then begun, and there was immediate improvement. The excretion of glucose was reduced from over 100 to as little as 7.5 g per day. Furthermore, "the boy became brighter, looked better and said he felt stronger." Thus, replacement therapy with the newly discovered hormone, insulin, had interrupted what was clearly an otherwise fatal metabolic disorder (Banting *et al.*, 1922). Banting and Best faced many trials and tribulations during the subsequent year. It was difficult to obtain active extracts reproducibly. This led to a greater involvement of Macleod, and Banting also sought help from J. B. Collip, a chemist with expertise in extraction and purification of epinephrine. Stable extracts were eventually obtained, and patients in many parts of North America were soon being treated with insulin. The Nobel Prize in Medicine or Physiology was awarded to Banting and Macleod with remarkable rapidity in 1923, and a furor over credit followed immediately. Banting announced that he would share half of his prize with Best; Macleod did the same with Collip. The early history of the discovery of insulin has been reviewed by Bliss (1982).

Chemistry. Insulin was purified and crystallized by Abel within a few years of the realization of the efficacy of pancreatic extracts in the treatment of diabetes. The amino acid sequence of the hormone was established by Sanger in 1960, and this led to the complete synthesis of the protein in 1963 (Katsoyannis *et al.*, 1963; Meienhofer *et al.*, 1963) and to the elucidation of its three-dimensional structure by Hodgkin and coworkers (*see* Hodgkin and Mercola, 1972). Insulin was the first hormone for which a radioimmunoassay was developed (Yalow, 1978).

The β cells of pancreatic islets synthesize insulin from a single chain precursor termed *proinsulin* (Figure 61–1). On conversion of human proinsulin to insulin, four basic amino acids and the remaining connector or C peptide are removed by proteolysis. This gives rise to the two peptide chains (A and B) of the insulin molecule, which contains one intrasubunit and two intersubunit disulfide bonds. The A chain is usually composed of 21 amino acid residues, and the B chain has 30; the molecular weight is thus about 5800. Although the amino acid sequence of insulin has been highly conserved in evolution, there are significant variations that account for differences in both biological potency and immunogenicity (Gammeltoft, 1984). There is a single insulin gene and a single protein product in most species. However, rats and mice have two genes that encode insulin, and they synthesize two molecules that differ from each other by two amino acid residues in the B chain.

The crystal structure reveals that the two chains of insulin form a highly ordered structure with several α-helical regions in both the A and B chains. The carboxyl-terminal portion of the B chain and the amino- and carboxyl-terminal residues of the A chain form the surface of the molecule that interacts with the receptor (Figure 61–2). The isolated chains of insulin are inactive. In solution, insulin can exist as a monomer or dimer or as a hexamer composed of a trimer of dimers. Two molecules of Zn^{2+} are coordinated in the hexamer, and this form of insulin is presumably stored in the granules of the pancreatic β cell. It is believed that Zn^{2+} has a functional role in the formation of crystals and that crystallization facilitates the conversion of proinsulin to insulin, as well as storage of the hormone. In the highly concentrated preparations used for therapy, insulin is hexameric. When the hormone is absorbed and the concentration falls to physiological levels (nanomolar), the hormone dissociates into monomers, and the monomer is most likely the biologically active form of insulin.

A great deal of information about the structure–activity relationship of insulin has been obtained by study of insulins purified from a wide variety of species and by modification of the molecule (*see* Gammeltoft, 1984). This work has contributed to the definition of the receptor-binding surface of insulin. In all cases there is a very close correlation between the affinity of an insulin for the insulin receptor and its potency for eliciting effects on glucose metabolism. Thus, interestingly, there are no partial agonists or competitive antagonists of insulin. There is, however, a range of potencies among natural insulins. When compared with human insulin, bovine and porcine insulins are equipotent; South American guinea pig insulin is much less potent, while certain avian insulins are significantly more so.

Insulin is a member of a family of related peptides, termed insulin-like growth factors (IGFs). Two IGFs (IGF-I and IGF-II) have been isolated

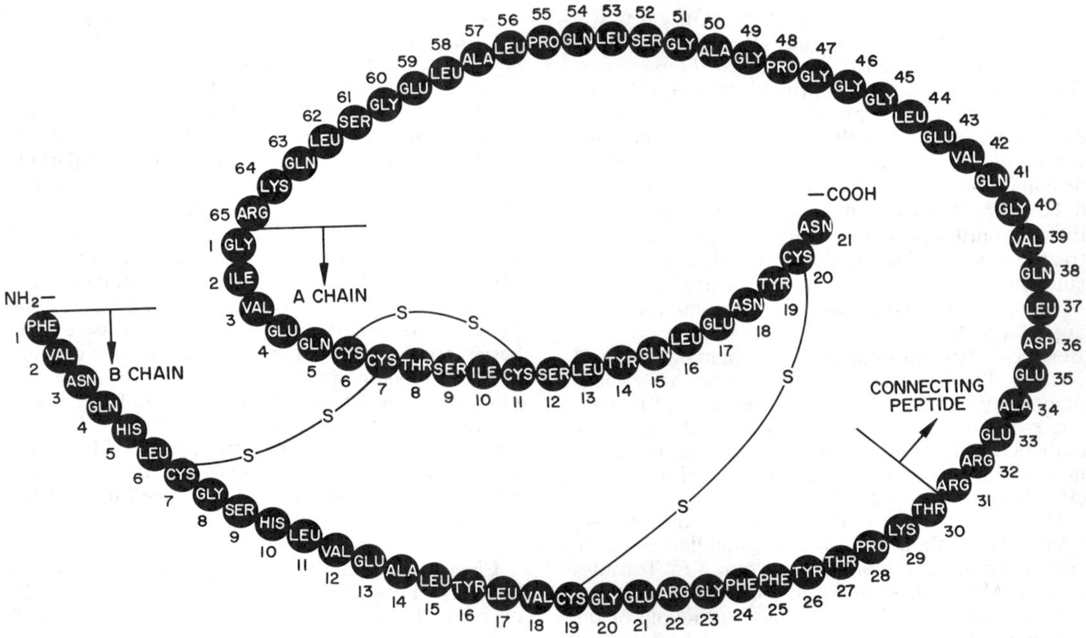

Figure 61–1. *Human proinsulin and its conversion to insulin.*

The amino acid sequence of human proinsulin is shown. By proteolytic cleavage, four basic amino acids (31, 32, 64, 65) and the connecting peptide are removed and proinsulin is converted to insulin. (For details, *see* the text.)

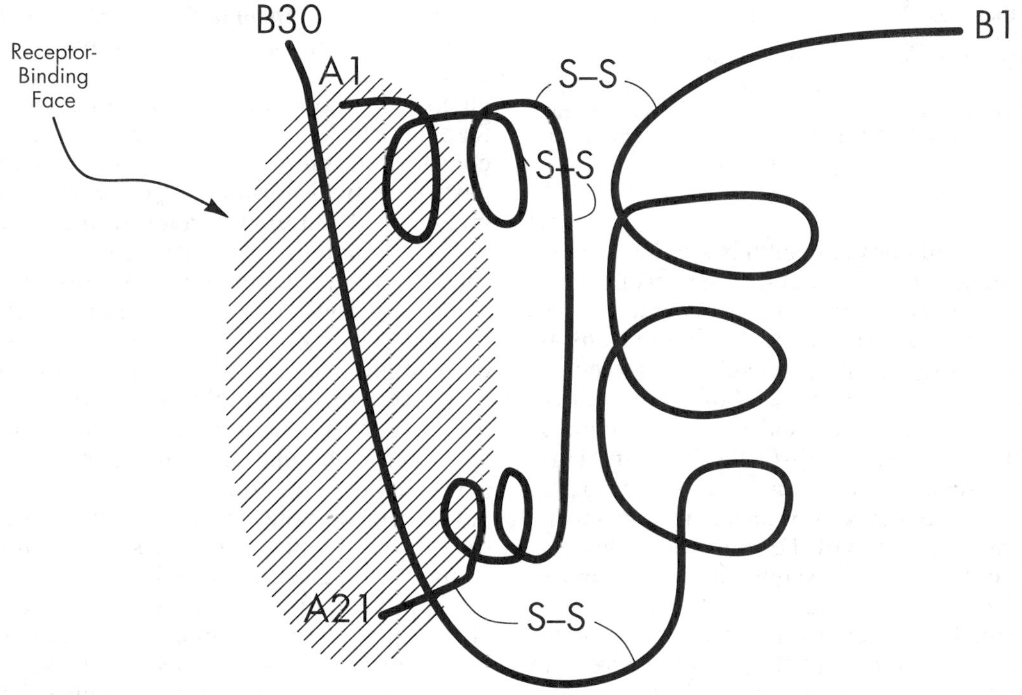

Figure 61–2. *Model of the three-dimensional structure of insulin.*

The shaded area indicates the receptor-binding face of the insulin molecule. (*See* Pullen *et al.*, 1976.)

from plasma and sequenced (Rinderknecht and Humbel, 1978a, 1978b). Both have molecular weights of about 7500 and structures that are homologous to that of proinsulin. However, the short equivalents of the C peptide in proinsulin are not removed from the IGFs. In contrast to insulin, the IGFs are produced in many tissues, and they may serve a more important function in regulation of growth than in regulation of metabolism. These peptides are the presumed mediators of the action of growth hormone, and they have also been termed *somatomedins* (*see* Daughaday and Rotwein, 1989; *see also* Chapter 56). The uterine hormone relaxin may also be a distant relative of this family of polypeptides (Blundell and Humbel, 1980).

The receptors for insulin and IGF-I are also closely related (Duronio and Jacobs, 1988). Thus, insulin can bind to the receptor for IGF-I with low affinity and vice versa. The growth-promoting actions of insulin appear to be mediated in part through the IGF-I receptor, and there may be discordance between the metabolic potency of an insulin analog and its ability to promote growth. For example, proinsulin has only 2% of the metabolic potency of insulin *in vitro*, but it is half as potent as insulin as a stimulator of mitogenesis (King and Kahn, 1981). This could be important in selecting insulins for therapy, since the mitogenic activity of insulin may contribute to an increased risk of atherosclerosis.

SYNTHESIS, SECRETION, DISTRIBUTION, AND DEGRADATION OF INSULIN

Insulin Production. The molecular and cellular events involved in the synthesis, storage, and secretion of insulin by the β cell and the ultimate degradation of the hormone by its target tissues have been studied in great detail and have served as a model for study of other cell types in the pancreatic islet (Orci, 1986). The islet of Langerhans is composed of four types of cells, each of which synthesizes and secretes a distinct polypeptide hormone: insulin in the β (B) cell, glucagon in the α (A) cell, somatostatin in the δ (D) cell, and pancreatic polypeptide in the PP or F cell. The β cells make up 60 to 80% of the islet and form its central core. The α, δ, and F cells form a discontinuous mantle, one to three cells thick, around this core.

The cells in the islet are connected by tight junctions that allow small molecules to pass and enable coordinated control of groups of cells (Orci, 1986). Arterioles enter the islets and branch into a glomerular-like capillary mass in the β-cell core. Capillaries then pass to the rim of the islet and coalesce into collecting venules (Bonner-Weir and Orci, 1982). Blood flows within the islet from the β cells to α and to δ cells (Samols *et al.*, 1986). Thus, the β cell is the primary glucose sensor for the islet, and the other cell types are presumably exposed to particularly high concentrations of insulin.

As noted above, insulin is synthesized as a single-chain precursor, proinsulin, in which the A and B chains are connected by the C peptide. However, the initial translation product is preproinsulin, a molecule that contains a sequence of 23 primarily hydrophobic amino acid residues attached to the amino terminus of the B chain. This signal sequence is required for the association and penetration of nascent preproinsulin into the lumen of the rough endoplasmic reticulum. This sequence is rapidly cleaved, and proinsulin is then transported in small vesicles to the Golgi complex. Here, proinsulin is packaged into secretory granules along with the enzyme(s) responsible for its conversion to insulin (Orci, 1986; Davidson *et al.*, 1988).

The conversion of proinsulin to insulin begins in the Golgi complex, continues within the secretory granules, and is nearly complete at the time of secretion. Thus, equimolar amounts of C peptide and insulin are released into the circulation. The C peptide has no known biological function, but it can serve as a useful index of insulin secretion (Polonsky and Rubenstein, 1986). Two distinct Ca^{2+}-dependent endopeptidases, which are found in the islet granules, are responsible for the conversion of proinsulin to insulin (Davidson *et al.*, 1988). Small quantities of proinsulin are also released from β cells. This presumably reflects either exocytosis of granules in which the conversion of proinsulin to insulin is not complete or secretion by another pathway (Gross *et al.*, 1989). Since the half-life of proinsulin in the circulation is much longer than that of insulin, up to 25% of immunoreactive insulin in plasma is, in reality, proinsulin. Mutant human proinsulin that lacks the Zn^{2+}-binding histidine residue (position B10) crystallizes less readily than does normal insulin (Gross *et al.*, 1989). This proinsulin is processed slowly in the β cell, with resultant hyperproinsulinemia.

Regulation of Insulin Secretion. Insulin secretion is a tightly regulated process, designed to provide stable concentrations of glucose in blood during both fasting and feeding. This regulation is achieved by the coordinated interplay of various nutrients, gastrointestinal hormones, pancreatic hormones, and autonomic neurotransmitters. Glucose, amino acids, fatty acids, and ketone bodies promote the secretion of insulin. The islets of Langerhans are richly innervated by both adrenergic and cholinergic nerves. Stimulation of α_2-adrenergic receptors inhibits insulin secretion, whereas β_2-adrenergic agonists and vagal nerve stimulation enhance release. In general, any condition that activates the autonomic nervous system (such as hypoxia, hypothermia, surgery, severe burns) suppresses the secretion of insulin by stimulation of α_2-adrenergic receptors. Predictably, α_2-adrenergic antagonists increase basal concentrations of insulin in plasma and β_2-adrenergic blockers decrease them (Porte and Halter, 1981; Shimazu and Ishikawa, 1981).

Glucose is the principal stimulus to insulin secretion in man and is an essential permissive factor for the actions of many other secretagogues (Meglasson and Matschinsky, 1986). The sugar is more effective in provoking insulin secretion when taken orally than when administered intravenously. This occurs because the ingestion of glucose (or food) induces the release of gastrointestinal hormones and stimulates vagal activity (Malaisse, 1986; Brelje and Sorenson, 1988). Several gastrointestinal hormones promote the secretion of insulin (*see* Ebert and Creutzfeld, 1987). The most potent of these are gastrointestinal inhibitory peptide and glucagon-like peptide-1 (Mojsov *et al.*, 1987). Insulin release is also stimulated by gastrin, secretin, cholecystokinin, vasoactive intestinal peptide, gastrin-releasing peptide, and enteroglucagon.

When evoked by glucose, insulin secretion is biphasic: the first phase reaches a peak after 1 to 2 minutes and is short lived, whereas the second phase has a delayed onset but a longer duration. The exact mechanism by which glucose and other secretagogues stimulate insulin release is not fully understood. Although some investigators have postulated the existence of a "glucoreceptor" on the β cell, most believe that stimulation of insulin release by glucose requires its entry into the β cell and metabolism (Meglasson and Matschinsky, 1986).

Glucose enters the β cell by facilitated transport, which is mediated by a specific subtype of glucose transporter (*see* below). The sugar is then phosphorylated by glucokinase. In contrast to hexokinase, which has a wide tissue distribution, expression of glucokinase is limited to pancreatic β cells and the liver. Its relatively high K_m (10 to 20 mM) gives it an important regulatory role at physiological concentrations of glucose. The capacity of sugars to undergo phosphorylation and subsequent glycolysis correlates closely with their ability to stimulate insulin release. This has led to the hypothesis that one or more glycolytic intermediates or enzyme cofactors is the actual stimulator of insulin secretion (Meglasson and Matschinsky, 1986).

Insulin secretion ultimately depends on the intracellular concentration of Ca^{2+} (Hellman, 1986; Wolf *et al.*, 1988), and glucose and its metabolites stimulate Ca^{2+} influx. The initial event seems to be a glucose- and ATP-dependent inhibition of an ATP-sensitive K^+ channel. This inhibition leads to depolarization and activation of a voltage-dependent Ca^{2+} channel. Ca^{2+} enters the β cell and activates phospholipase A_2 and phospholipase C, which results in the formation of arachidonic acid, inositol polyphosphates, and diacylglycerol (*see* Chapter 2). Inositol-1,4,5-trisphosphate mobilizes Ca^{2+} from the endoplasmic reticulum, further elevating the cytosolic concentration of the cation.

Elevation of free Ca^{2+} concentrations also occurs in response to stimulation of phospholipase C by acetylcholine and cholecystokinin and by hormones that increase intracellular concentrations of cyclic AMP (Ebert and Creutzfeld, 1987). Adenylyl cyclase, the enzyme that synthesizes cyclic AMP, is activated by glucagon, gastrointestinal inhibitory peptide, and glucagon-like peptide-1, and it is inhibited by somatostatin and α_2-adrenergic agonists (*see* Fleischer and Erlichman, 1989).

Most of the nutrients and hormones that stimulate insulin secretion also enhance the biosynthesis of the hormone (Gold *et al.*, 1982; Robbins *et al.*, 1984). Although there is a close correlation between the two processes, some factors affect one pathway but not the other. For example, lowering extracellular concentrations of Ca^{2+} inhibits secretion of insulin without affecting biosynthesis.

There is usually a reciprocal relationship between the rates of secretion of insulin and glucagon from the pancreatic islet (Unger and Orci, 1981; Unger, 1985a). In part this reflects the influence of insulin on the α cell (*see* below). In addition, somatostatin, a third islet-cell hormone, can modulate the secretion of both hormones (*see* below). Glucagon stimulates the release of somatostatin, and the latter may suppress the secretion of insulin. Glucose, amino acids, gastrointestinal hormones, and neurotransmitters also influence the secretion of somatostatin, which in turn can inhibit the secretion of glucagon (Unger, 1985b). Since the blood supply in the islet flows from the β cell core to the α and δ cells (Samols *et al.*, 1986), somatostatin must pass through the circulation to reach the α and β cells. Thus, while it is possible that insulin may act as a paracrine hormone to affect the secretion of glucagon and pancreatic polypeptide, somatostatin must be present in the systemic circulation in concentrations sufficient to influence the secretion of insulin.

Distribution and Degradation of Insulin. Insulin circulates in blood as the free monomer, and its volume of distribution approximates the volume of extracellular fluid. Under fasting conditions, the pancreas secretes about 40 μg (1 unit [U]) of insulin per hour into the portal vein to achieve a concentration of insulin in portal blood of 2 to 4 ng/ml (50 to 100 μU/ml) and in the peripheral circulation of 0.5 ng/ml (12 μU/ml) or about 0.1 nM. After ingestion of a meal there is a rapid rise in the concentration of insulin in portal blood, followed by a parallel but smaller rise in the peripheral circulation. A goal of insulin therapy is to mimic this pattern (Schade *et al.*, 1983).

The half-life of insulin in plasma is about 5 to 6 minutes in normal and uncomplicated diabetic subjects (Sodoyez *et al.*, 1983). This value may be increased in diabetics who develop anti-insulin antibodies (Hachiya *et al.*, 1987). The half-life of proinsulin is longer than that of insulin (about 17 minutes), and this protein usually accounts for 10 to 25% of the immunoreactive "insulin" in plasma (Robbins *et al.*, 1984). In patients with insulinoma, the percentage of proinsulin in the circulation is usually increased and may be as much as 80%. Since proinsulin is only about 2% as potent as insulin, the biologically effective concentration of insulin is somewhat lower than that estimated by immunoassay. C peptide is secreted in equimolar amounts with insulin; however, its molar concentration in plasma is higher because of its considerably longer half-life (about 30 minutes) (Robbins *et al.*, 1984).

Degradation of insulin occurs primarily in liver, kidney, and muscle (Duckworth, 1988). About 50% of the insulin that reaches the liver via the portal vein is destroyed and never reaches the general circulation. Insulin is filtered by the renal glomeruli and is reabsorbed by the tubules, which also degrade it. Severe impairment of renal function appears to affect the rate of disappearance of circulating insulin to a greater extent than does hepatic disease (Rabkin *et al.,* 1984). Hepatic degradation of insulin operates near its maximal capacity and cannot compensate for diminished renal breakdown of the hormone. The oral administration of glucose appears to reduce hepatic extraction of insulin (Hanks *et al.,* 1984); this effect may be mediated by intestinal hormones such as gastric inhibitory peptide. Arginine, cholecystokinin, and a high-protein diet have also been shown to alter hepatic extraction of insulin in animals (Duckworth, 1988). Peripheral tissues such as fat also inactivate insulin, but this is of less significance quantitatively.

Proteolytic degradation of insulin in the liver occurs primarily after internalization of the hormone and its receptor and, to a lesser extent, at the cell surface (Berman *et al.,* 1980). The primary pathway for internalization is receptor-mediated endocytosis. The complex of insulin and its receptor is internalized into small vesicles termed endosomes, where degradation is initiated (Duckworth, 1988). Some insulin is also delivered to lysosomes for degradation.

The extent to which internalized insulin is degraded by the cell varies considerably with the cell type. In hepatocytes, over 50% of the internalized insulin is degraded, whereas most internalized insulin is released intact from endothelial cells. In the latter case, this appears to be related to the role of these cells in transcytosis of insulin molecules from the intravascular to the extracellular space (King and Johnson, 1985). Transcytosis has an important role in the delivery of insulin to its target cells in tissues where endothelial cells form tight junctions, including skeletal muscle and adipose tissue.

Several enzymes have been implicated in insulin degradation. The primary insulin-degrading enzyme is a thiol metalloproteinase. It is primarily localized in hepatocytes (Shii and Roth, 1986), but immunologically related molecules have also been found in muscle, kidney, and brain (Duckworth, 1988). The major portion of insulin-degrading enzyme activity appears to be cytosolic, raising the question of how the internalized, vesicular insulin becomes associated with the degrading enzyme. Insulin-degrading enzyme may also have a role in the degradation of other hormones, including glucagon.

A glutathione-insulin transhydrogenase from liver may also have a role in insulin degradation (Varandani *et al.,* 1972). This enzyme, which is probably identical to protein disulfide isomerase, is capable of reducing the disulfide bonds of insulin and thus would inactivate the hormone. Subcutaneous degradation of insulin is a relatively minor problem in most diabetic patients, although several individuals have been described in which a presumed increase in subcutaneous destruction was associated with resistance to insulin (Schade and Duckworth, 1986). A few of these patients have been treated with protease inhibitors, such as aprotinin, with apparent improvement in sensitivity to insulin. The precise basis of this syndrome remains to be resolved.

MOLECULAR MECHANISMS OF INSULIN ACTION

Cellular Actions of Insulin. Insulin elicits a remarkable array of biological responses. The important target tissues for regulation of glucose homeostasis by insulin are liver, muscle, and fat, but insulin exerts potent regulatory effects on other cell types as well. One should bear in mind that insulin is the primary hormone responsible for controlling the storage and utilization of cellular nutrients. It activates the transport systems and the enzymes involved in intracellular utilization and storage of glucose, amino acids, and fatty acids, while it inhibits catabolic processes, such as the breakdown of glycogen, fat, and protein.

The actions of insulin are traditionally classified into three groups, based on their kinetics. The immediate or rapid effects of insulin occur within seconds or minutes and include activation of glucose and ion transport systems and the covalent modification (*i.e.,* phosphorylation and dephosphorylation) of enzymes. The intermediate effects, such as induction of ornithine decarboxylase and tyrosine aminotransferase, occur within 3 to 6 hours and result from regulation of gene expression. The long-term effects of insulin require many hours to several days and include stimulation of cell proliferation and differentiation. The diverse effects of insulin may result from several mechanistic pathways, and important actions may be exerted at receptors for both insulin and the IGFs.

The Insulin Receptor. The actions of insulin are initiated by binding to a cell-surface receptor, and such receptors are present in virtually all mammalian cells (Kahn and White, 1988). These include the classical targets for insulin action (liver, muscle, and fat) and such nonclassical targets as circulating blood cells, brain, and gonadal cells. The number of receptors varies from as few as 40 per cell on erythrocytes to 300,000 per cell on adipocytes and hepatocytes.

The insulin receptor is a large transmembrane glycoprotein, composed of two 135-kDa α subunits and two 95-kDa β subunits linked by disulfide bonds to form a β-α-α-β heterotetramer (Figure 61–3) (Czech, 1985; Ebina *et al.*, 1985; Ullrich *et al.*, 1985; Kahn and White, 1988). Both subunits are derived from a single-chain precursor molecule that contains the entire sequence of the α and β subunits, separated by a processing site consisting of four basic amino acid residues. These two subunits are specialized to perform the two functions of the receptor. The α subunits are entirely extracellular and contain the insulin-binding domain, while the β subunits are transmembrane proteins that possess tyrosine protein kinase activity. After insulin is bound, receptors aggregate and are rapidly internalized. Since bivalent (but not monovalent) anti-

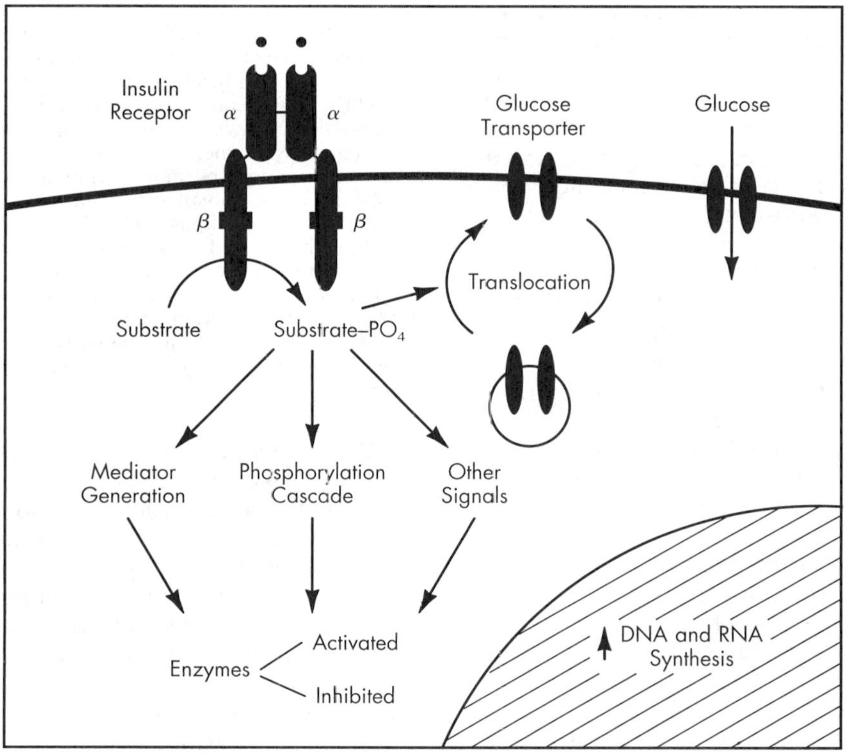

Figure 61–3. *Model of insulin action at the cellular and molecular level.*

Insulin binds to the α subunits of its receptor and stimulates the tyrosine kinase activity of the β subunits. This results in autophosphorylation of the insulin receptor on several tyrosine residues and further activation of kinase activity. Presumed consequences of these reactions include cascades of protein phosphorylation, the generation of putative mediators of insulin action, and other signals that ultimately result in insulin's characteristic effects on the metabolism of carbohydrates, lipids, and proteins.

insulin receptor antibodies cross-link adjacent receptors and mimic the rapid actions of insulin, it has been suggested that aggregation of the receptor is essential for signal transduction (Kahn *et al.*, 1978). After internalization, the receptor may be degraded or recycled back to the cell surface.

Tyrosine Phosphorylation in Insulin Action. The insulin receptor and the receptors for several other growth factors are ligand-activated tyrosine protein kinases (Kasuga *et al.*, 1982; Rosen, 1987; Kahn and White, 1988; *see* Chapter 2). Other growth factor receptors that exhibit such activity include those for epidermal growth factor, IGF-1, platelet-derived growth factor, and colony-stimulating factor 1 (*see* Yarden and Ullrich, 1988). In addition, several proteins (*e.g.*, src) that are encoded by retroviruses that cause cellular transformation are also tyrosine protein kinases.

Binding of hormone to the α subunits of the heterotetrameric insulin receptor leads to the rapid intramolecular autophosphorylation of several tyrosine residues in the β subunits (White *et al.*, 1988). Phosphorylation of the receptor is autocatalytic and results in substantial enhancement of the receptor's tyrosine kinase activity toward other substrates. In intact cells, the insulin receptor is also phosphorylated on serine and threonine residues, presumably by protein kinase C and cyclic AMP-dependent protein kinase. Such phosphorylation inhibits the tyrosine kinase activity of the insulin receptor (Roth and Beaudoin, 1987; Takayama *et al.*, 1988).

The tyrosine kinase activity of the insulin receptor appears to be required for signal transduction. Mutation of the insulin receptor to modify the ATP binding site or to replace the tyrosine residues at major sites of autophosphorylation results in a complete loss or a decrease of insulin-stimulated kinase activity and failure to initiate the cellular response to insulin (Ellis *et al.*, 1986; Chou *et al.*, 1987).

After activation of the receptor kinase, it is believed that the receptor catalyzes phosphorylation of cellular substrate proteins. The best characterized endogenous substrate is a cytosolic protein with a molecular weight of 185,000 (White *et al.*, 1985). Unfortunately, the function of this protein is unknown. Ultimately, many of the enzymes whose activities are modulated in the short term by insulin undergo phosphorylation or dephosphorylation on serine and/or threonine residues (Czech, 1985; Rosen, 1987). Acetyl-CoA carboxylase, ATP–citrate lyase, and ribosomal protein S6 exhibit increased activity caused by enhanced phosphorylation, whereas glycogen synthase and pyruvate dehydrogenase are activated by insulin as a result of dephosphorylation. Thus, a large number of insulin's actions are mediated by cascades of phosphorylation/dephosphorylation reactions that are also regulated by other hormones. Elucidation of the linkage between activation of the receptor tyrosine kinase and regulation of the activities of the serine/threonine kinases and phosphatases that control the ultimate targets of insulin action is crucial to the ultimate understanding of the mechanism of action of insulin.

Putative Mediators of Insulin Action. In addition to regulation of phosphorylation, insulin may also control the synthesis of second messengers that could mediate some of the hormone's actions on intracellular enzymes (Mato *et al.*, 1987; Low and Saltiel, 1988; Romero *et al.*, 1988). In this scheme of insulin action, hormonal stimulation causes activation of a phosphatidyl inositol (PI)–glycan specific phospholipase C. This phospholipase is thought to hydrolyze a membrane-associated substrate to produce the PI-glycan and 1,2-diacylglycerol, both of which could regulate intracellular enzymes. It is further suggested that the insulin mediator is released into the extracellular medium and is then taken up back into cells to exert its effects.

Regulation of Glucose Transport. Stimulation of glucose transport into muscle and adipose tissue is a crucial component of the physiological response to insulin. Activation of transport by insulin requires ATP and is rapid and independent of protein synthesis. Insulin does not stimulate glucose uptake into liver and several other tissues, despite the fact that these tissue possess insulin receptors and respond to the hormone in other ways.

Insulin stimulates glucose transport at least in part by promoting the energy-dependent translocation of intracellular vesicles that contain glucose transporters to the plasma membrane (Suzuki and Kono, 1980; Simpson and Cushman, 1986; James *et al.*, 1988; *see* Figure 61–3). This effect is reversible; the transporters return to the intracellular pool upon removal of insulin. In some tissues (*e.g.*, muscle) insulin may stimulate the intrinsic activity of the transporters in addition to facilitating their translocation (*see* Simpson and Cushman, 1986). Insulin can also regulate the synthesis of glucose transporters; this phenomenon may be particularly important when there is long-term insulin deficiency, as in patients with Type-I diabetes mellitus (Garvey *et al.*, 1989).

To date, complementary DNAs that encode seven distinct mammalian glucose transporters have been cloned and sequenced. Six of these are thought to be involved in Na^+-independent facilitated diffusion of glucose into cells; one is the Na^+/glucose cotransporter involved in active transport of glucose by intestinal epithelial and renal tubular cells. All of the facilitative glucose transporters are integral membrane glycoproteins with molecular weights of about 50,000. Each is thought to contain 12 membrane-spanning α-helical domains, with both the amino-terminus and the carboxyl-terminus in the cytoplasm. One transporter, the erythroid cell/brain glucose transporter, is present primarily in erythrocytes and in endothelial cells that form the blood–brain barrier (Mueckler *et al.*, 1985). Another, the liver glucose transporter, has a similar structure and is found mainly in hepatic plasma membranes and pancreatic β cells, where it may participate in glucose-stimulated insulin secretion (Fukumoto *et al.*, 1988; Thorens *et al.*, 1988). The transporter that is most responsive to insulin is the muscle glucose transporter-like protein. It is expressed predominantly in tissues in which glucose transport is sensitive to insulin, including skeletal muscle, cardiac muscle, and adipose tissue (Birnbaum, 1989; Charron *et al.*, 1989). Translocation of this transporter is stimulated by insulin (James *et al.*, 1988).

Diabetes Mellitus and the Physiological Effects of Insulin

Diabetes mellitus is a group of syndromes characterized by hyperglycemia; altered metabolism of lipids, carbohydrates, and proteins; and an increased risk of complications from vascular disease. Most patients can be classified clinically as having either insulin-dependent diabetes mellitus (IDDM or Type-I diabetes) or non-insulin-dependent diabetes mellitus (NIDDM or Type-II diabetes). Diabetes mellitus or carbohydrate intolerance is also associated with certain genetic syndromes, may be secondary to drug administration or other diseases (pancreatic disease, endocrinopathies, abnormalities of the insulin receptor), or may occur during pregnancy (gestational diabetes mellitus). The exact incidence of each type of diabetes varies widely throughout the world. In the United States, about 90% of diabetic patients have Type-II diabetes and most of the remainder have Type I, whereas in certain tropical countries, the most common cause of diabetes is chronic pancreatitis associated with nutritional or toxic factors (a form of secondary diabetes). On rare occasions, diabetes may also result from point mutations in the insulin gene (Tager, 1984; Chan *et al.*, 1987). Amino acid substitutions from such mutations may result in insulins with lower potency or alter the processing of proinsulin to insulin (*see* above).

There are genetic and environmental components to both Type-I and Type-II diabetes. Studies of identical twins show greater than 95% concordance for Type-II diabetes (Pyke, 1977); there is also a high prevalence of Type-II diabetes among first-degree relatives of those with the disease. However, the exact genetic mechanism in Type-II diabetes is poorly understood. It is likely that there is a primary defect in the sensitivity to insulin and that genetic factors also determine the individual's ability to maintain compensatory hyperinsulinemia. About 70% of Type-II diabetics in the United States are also obese, a factor that contributes significantly to insulin resistance.

With Type-I (insulin-dependent) diabetes, the concordance rate for identical twins is only 25 to 50%; this suggests that environmental, as well as genetic influences, have an important role in the disease. However, the genetic factors in Type-I diabetes are well characterized and relate to the genes that control the immune response. There is considerable evidence that Type-I diabetes is an autoimmune disease of the pancreatic β cell. Antibodies to components of islet cells are detected in up to 80% of Type-I patients early during the onset or prior to the onset of clinical disease. The antibodies are directed at both cytoplasmic and membrane-bound antigens, and in a significant fraction of patients, there are measurable titers of anti-insulin antibodies prior to initiation of treatment with insulin.

Individuals with Type-I diabetes tend to have antibodies directed toward other endocrine tissues, including the adrenal, parathyroid, and thyroid glands. They also have a higher than normal incidence of other autoimmune diseases.

There is an association of Type-I diabetes with specific human leukocyte antigen (HLA) types, especially at the B and Dr loci. Approximately 95% of patients with Type-I diabetes are positive for HLA-Dr3 and/or Dr4, as compared with only 40% of the general population (Nerup *et al.*, 1984). In contrast, the haplotype HLA-Dr2 appears to be negatively associated with the occurrence of the disease. A polymorphism of the HLA-DQβ chain at position 57 correlates even more closely with susceptibility to diabetes (Todd *et al.*, 1987). Type-I diabetes is associated with alleles coding for alanine, valine, or serine at position 57 in the DQβ chain, while aspartic acid in this position is negatively correlated with the disease in Caucasians (*see* Dotta and Eisenbarth, 1989). These findings implicate both humoral and cell-mediated immune mechanisms in the etiology of Type-I diabetes.

The trigger for the immune response remains unknown. Direct evidence exists for a viral cause of diabetes in animals, and there has been suggestive evidence in rare cases in man (Yoon *et al.*, 1979), but there is no clear diabetogenic virus in most patients with Type-I diabetes. The identification of triggering agents is difficult, since autoimmune destruction of pancreatic β cells may occur over a period of many months or several years before the onset of overt disease (Srikanta *et al.*, 1983). Whatever the causes, the final result in Type-I diabetes is an extensive and selective loss of pancreatic β cells and a state of hypoinsulinemia.

By contrast, there is no significant loss of β cells from the islets in Type-II diabetes. The mean plasma concentration of insulin over a 24-hour period is essentially normal or even elevated because of peripheral resistance to the action of the hormone (Genuth, 1973). Nevertheless, individuals with Type-II diabetes are relatively insulin-deficient. This is because a normal pancreatic β cell should be capable of secreting amounts of insulin that are considerably greater than normal when confronted with hyperglycemia, thus allowing an individual to maintain euglycemia in the face of moderate resistance to insulin (Weir *et al.*, 1986).

One defect commonly found in Type-II diabetes is an inability of the β cell to respond to a challenge with intravenous glucose; there is a loss of the first phase of insulin secretion. However, the responses to other secretagogues (*e.g.*, isoproterenol or arginine) are preserved, although there is less potentiation by glucose (Weir *et al.*, 1986). These abnormalities of the β cell in Type-II diabetes are most likely secondary to desensitization by a mild level of chronic hyperglycemia. Similar changes can be induced in animals by long-term infusions of low concentrations of glucose (Leahy *et al.*, 1987).

Virtually all forms of diabetes mellitus are due to either a decrease in the circulating concentration of insulin (insulin deficiency) or a decrease in the response of peripheral tissues to insulin (insulin resistance) in association with an excess of hormones with actions opposite to those of insulin (glucagon, growth hormone, cortisol, and catecholamines). These hormonal abnormalities lead to alterations in the metabolism of carbohydrates, lipids, ketones, and amino acids; the central feature of the syndrome is hyperglycemia (Figure 61–4).

Insulin lowers the concentration of glucose in blood by inhibiting hepatic glucose production (glycogenolysis and gluconeogenesis) and by stimulating the uptake and metabolism of glucose by muscle and adipose tissue. These two important effects occur at rather different concentrations of insulin. Production of glucose is inhibited half-maximally by an insulin concentration of about 20 to 30 μU/ml, while glucose utilization is stimulated half-maximally at about 100 μU/ml. Since the concentration of insulin in the portal vein is always higher than that in peripheral blood, this difference in response is accentuated further in normal individuals, such that hepatic glucose output is almost completely suppressed when glucose utilization is only minimally stimulated. In a Type-I diabetic patient who is receiving exogenous insulin, portal and peripheral concentrations of insulin are essentially identical; thus, as compared with a nondiabetic individual, insulin exerts a greater effect on peripheral glucose utilization than on hepatic glucose output. In patients with Type-II diabetes and some degree of insulin reserve, fasting concentrations of blood glucose may be normal because of the continued effect of insulin on the liver, despite a considerable degree of postprandial hyperglycemia. This almost never occurs in the truly insulin-deficient Type-I diabetic patient. In both types of diabetes, glucagon opposes the effect of insulin on the liver by stimulating glycogenolysis and gluconeogenesis, but it has relatively little effect on peripheral utilization of glucose. Thus, in the diabetic with insulin deficiency or insulin resistance and hyperglucagonemia, there is an increase in gluconeogenesis and glycogenolysis, a de-

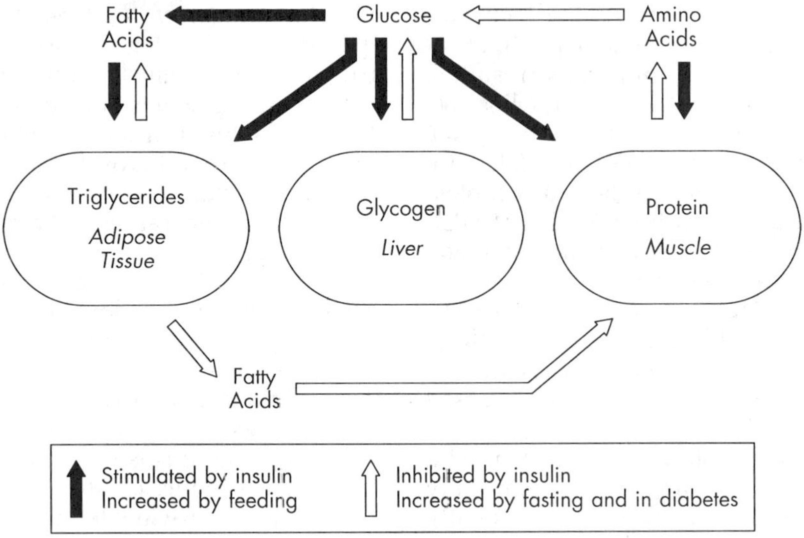

Figure 61–4. *Overview of insulin action.*

Insulin stimulates the storage of glucose in the liver as glycogen and in adipose tissue as triglycerides and the storage of amino acids in muscle as protein; it also promotes utilization of glucose in muscle for energy. These pathways, which are also enhanced by feeding, are indicated by the solid arrows. Insulin inhibits the breakdown of triglycerides, glycogen, and protein and the conversion of amino acids to glucose (gluconeogenesis), as indicated by the open arrows. These pathways are increased during fasting and in diabetic states. The conversions of amino acids to glucose and glucose to fatty acids occur primarily in the liver.

crease in peripheral glucose uptake, and a decrease in the conversion of glucose to glycogen in the liver (Schade *et al.*, 1983; Foster, 1984).

Alterations in secretion of insulin and glucagon also have profound effects on lipid, ketone, and protein metabolism. At concentrations below those required to stimulate glucose uptake, insulin inhibits the hormone-sensitive lipase in adipose tissue and thus inhibits the hydrolysis of triglycerides stored in the adipocyte. This counteracts the lipolytic action of catecholamines, glucagon, and other hormones and reduces the concentrations of glycerol (a substrate for gluconeogenesis) and free fatty acids (a substrate for production of ketone bodies). These actions of insulin are deficient in the diabetic patient, leading to increased gluconeogenesis and ketogenesis.

The liver produces ketone bodies by oxidation of free fatty acids to acetyl CoA, which is then converted to acetoacetate and β-hydroxybutyrate. The initial step in fatty acid oxidation is transport of the fatty acid into the mitochondria. This involves the interconversion of the CoA and carnitine esters of fatty acids by the enzyme acylcarnitine transferase (*see* Chapter 63). The activity of this enzyme is inhibited by intramitochondrial malonyl CoA, one of the products of fatty acid synthesis. Under normal conditions, insulin inhibits lipolysis, stimulates fatty acid synthesis (thereby increasing the concentration of malonyl CoA), and decreases the hepatic concentration of carnitine; all these factors decrease the production of ketone bodies. Conversely, glucagon stimulates ketone-body production by stimulating lipolysis, increasing fatty acid oxidation, and decreasing concentrations of malonyl CoA. In the diabetic patient, particularly with Type-I diabetes, the consequences of insulin deficiency and glucagon excess provide a hormonal milieu that favors ketogenesis and, in the absence of appropriate treatment, may lead to ketonemia and acidosis (*see* Foster, 1984).

Insulin also interacts with the capillary endothelium to activate lipoprotein lipase, the enzyme that hydrolyzes the triglycerides present in very-low-density lipoproteins (VLDL) and chylomicrons, resulting in release of intermediate-density lipoprotein (IDL) particles (Taskinen, 1987; *see also* Chapter 36). These IDL particles are converted by the liver to the more cholesterol-rich low-density lipoproteins (LDL). In the untreated or undertreated diabetic patient, hypertriglyceridemia may occur as a result of the decreased removal of VLDL secondary to the decreased activity of lipoprotein lipase. In addition, deficiency of insulin may be associated with increased production of VLDL.

The important role of insulin in protein metabolism is usually evident clinically only in diabetic patients with persistently poor control of their disease (Granner, 1987; Kimball and Jefferson, 1988). Insulin stimulates amino acid uptake and protein synthesis and inhibits protein degradation in muscle and other tissues; it thus causes a decrease in the circulating concentrations of most amino acids, except for alanine. With glutamine, alanine is a major amino acid precursor for gluconeogenesis. Insulin does not lower alanine concentrations, because it enhances the rate of transamination of pyruvate to alanine. In the diabetic, there is increased conversion of alanine to glucose, adding to the already enhanced rate of gluconeogenesis. The conversion of larger amounts of amino acids to glucose also results in increased production and excretion of urea and ammonia. In addition, there are increased circulating concentrations of the branched-chain amino acids as a result of increased proteolysis, decreased protein synthesis, and increased release of branched-chain amino acids from the liver.

An almost pathognomonic feature of diabetes mellitus is thickening of the capillary basement membrane and other vascular changes that occur during the course of the disease. The cumulative effect is progressive narrowing of the vessel lumina, causing inadequate perfusion of critical regions of certain organs. The matrix is expanded in many vessel walls, in the basement membrane of the retina (Kohner *et al.*, 1982), and in the mesangial cells of the renal glomerulus (Mauer *et al.*, 1984). Cellular proliferation in many large vessels further contributes to luminal narrowing. These pathological changes contribute to some of the major complications of diabetes, including premature atherosclerosis, intercapillary glomerulosclerosis, retinopathy, neuropathy, and ulceration and gangrene of the extremities.

It has been hypothesized that the factor responsible for the development of most complications of diabetes is the prolonged exposure of tissues to elevated concentrations of glucose (Pirart, 1978; Brownlee and Cerami, 1981). Although much data exists to suggest that this is the case, a controlled trial (the Diabetes Control and Complications Trial) to provide definitive evidence is currently under way. This hypothesis provides the rationale that underlies all attempts to exert rigid control over glucose concentrations in diabetic patients.

The toxic effects of hyperglycemia may be the result of accumulation of nonenzymatically glycosylated products and osmotically active sugar alcohols such as sorbitol in tissues; the effects of glucose on cellular metabolism may also be responsible. The covalent reaction of glucose with hemoglobin provides a convenient method to determine an integrated index of the glycemic state. Hemoglobin undergoes glycosylation on its amino terminal valine residue to form the glucosyl valine adduct of hemoglobin, termed *hemoglobin* A_{1c} (Higgins and Bunn, 1981; Garlick *et al.*, 1983; Bernstein, 1987). The half-life of the modified hemoglobin is equal to that of the erythrocyte (about 120 days). Since the amount of glycosylated protein formed is proportional to the glucose concentration and the time of exposure of the protein to glucose, the concentration of hemoglobin A_{1c} in the circulation reflects the severity of the glycemic state over an extended period (4 to 8 weeks) prior to sampling. Thus, a rise in hemoglobin A_{1c} from 5% to 10% suggests a prolonged doubling of the mean blood glucose concentration. Although this assay is applied widely, measurement of the glycosylation of proteins with somewhat shorter survival times (*e.g.*, albumin) has also proven useful.

Glycosylated products accumulate in tissues and may eventually form cross-linked proteins termed advanced glycosylation end products (Kent *et al.*, 1985; Brownlee *et al.*, 1988). It is possible that nonenzymatic glycosylation is directly responsible for expansion of the vascular matrix and the vascular complications of diabetes. Incubation of collagen with glucose causes cross-linking *in vitro*; circulating proteins also accumulate irreversibly in the basement membranes of retinal and glomerular arterioles of diabetic subjects (Cohn *et al.*, 1978; Michael and Brown, 1981; Brownlee *et al.*, 1988). The modified cellular proliferative activity in vascular lesions of diabetic patients might also be explained by this process, since macrophages appear to have receptors for advanced glycosylation end products. Binding of such proteins to macrophages in these lesions may stimulate the production of cytokines such as tumor necrosis factor and interleukin 1, which in turn induce degradative and proliferative cascades in mesenchymal and endothelial cells, respectively.

Other explanations for the toxic manifestations of hyperglycemia may exist. Intracellular glucose is reduced to its corresponding sugar alcohol, sorbitol, by the enzyme aldose reductase (Burg and Kador, 1988), and the rate of production of sorbitol is determined by the ambient glucose concentration. This is particularly true in tissues such as the lens, retina, arterial wall, and Schwann cells of peripheral nerves. In diabetic humans and rodents, these tissues have increased intracellular concentrations of sorbitol, which may contribute to an increased osmotic effect and tissue damage. Inhibitors of aldose reductase are currently being evaluated for treatment of diabetic neuropathy and retinopathy.

In neural tissue and perhaps in other tissues, glucose competes with myoinositol for transport into cells (Green *et al.*, 1987). Reduction of cellular concentrations of myoinositol may contribute to altered nerve function and neuropathy. Hyperglycemia may also enhance the *de-novo* synthesis of diacylglycerol, which could facilitate persistent activation of protein kinase C (Lee *et al.*, 1989).

INSULIN THERAPY

Preparations. Insulin is the mainstay for treatment of virtually all Type-I and many Type-II diabetic patients. When necessary, insulin may be administered intravenously or intramuscularly; however, long-term treatment relies on subcutaneous injection of the hormone. Subcutaneous administration of insulin differs from physiological secretion of insulin in at least two major ways: the kinetics of absorption are relatively slow and thus do not mimic the normal rapid rise and decline of insulin secretion in response to ingestion of nutrients, and the insulin diffuses into the peripheral circulation instead of being released into the portal circulation; the preferential effect of secreted insulin on hepatic metabolic processes is thus eliminated. Nonetheless, when performed carefully, considerable success is obviously achieved with such treatment.

Preparations of insulin can be classified according to their duration of action into short-, intermediate-, or long-acting, and by their species of origin—human, porcine, bovine, or a mixture of bovine and porcine. Human insulin is now widely available as a result of its production by recombinant DNA techniques; in theory it should be slightly less immunogenic than purified porcine insulin, which in turn should be less immunogenic than bovine insulin (Karam and Etzweiler, 1983; Owen, 1986). Bovine insulin differs from human insulin by three amino acid residues, whereas porcine differs from human insulin by only one amino acid at the carboxyl-terminus of the B chain. However, when highly purified, all three insulins have a relatively low, but measurable, capacity to stimulate the immune response. Currently, almost all insulin preparations contain less than 20 ppm of contaminating proteins (Skyler, 1988). Nonetheless, hypersensitivity is still a complication of treatment in a few patients. All preparations are now supplied at neutral pH, which improves stability and permits storage for long periods of time at room temperature.

For therapeutic purposes, doses and concentrations of insulin are expressed in units. This tradition dates to the time when preparations of the hormone were impure, and it was necessary to standardize them by bioassay. One unit of insulin is equal to the amount required to reduce the concentration of blood glucose in a fasting rabbit to 45 mg/dl (2.5 mM). The current international standard is a mixture of bovine and porcine insulins and contains 24 units (U)/mg. Homogeneous preparations of human insulin contain between 25 and 30 U/mg. Almost all commercial preparations of insulin are supplied in solution at a concentration of 100 U/ml. This solution contains about 3.6 mg of insulin/ml (0.6 mM). Insulin is also available in a more concentrated solution (500 U/ml) for patients who are resistant to the hormone. Table 61–1 provides a pharmacokinetic classification of commercial insulins. Preparations currently available in the United States are listed in Table 61–2.

Table 61–1. PROPERTIES OF INSULIN PREPARATIONS

TYPE	APPEARANCE	ADDED PROTEIN	ZINC CONTENT (MG/100 U)	BUFFER *	ACTION (HOURS) †		
					Onset	*Peak*	*Duration*
Rapid							
Regular (crystalline)	Clear	None	0.01–0.04	None	0.3–0.7	2–4	5–8
Semilente	Cloudy	None	0.2–0.25	Acetate	0.5–1.0	2–8	12–16
Intermediate							
NPH (Isophane)	Cloudy	Protamine	0.016–0.04	Phosphate	1–2	6–12	18–24
Lente	Cloudy	None	0.2–0.25	Acetate	1–2	6–12	18–24
Slow							
Ultralente	Cloudy	None	0.2–0.25	Acetate	4–6	16–18	20–36
Protamine zinc	Cloudy	Protamine	0.2–0.25	Phosphate	4–6	14–20	24–36

* At present, all insulin preparations are supplied at pH 7.2–7.4.

† These are approximate figures. There is considerable variation from patient to patient and from time to time in the same patient.

Classification of Insulins. Short- or *rapid-acting insulins* are simply solutions of *regular, crystalline zinc insulin* (*insulin injection*) dissolved in a buffer at neutral pH. These have the most rapid onset of action but the shortest duration (*see* Table 61–1). Short-acting insulin should usually be injected 30 to 45 minutes before meals (Dimitriadas and Gerich, 1983). Regular insulin may also be given intravenously or intramuscularly. After intravenous injection, there is a rapid fall in the blood glucose concentration, which usually reaches a nadir in 20 to 30 minutes. In the absence of a sustained infusion of insulin, the hormone is rapidly cleared and the glucose returns to baseline in about 2 to 3 hours. Intravenous infusions of insulin are useful in patients with ketoacidosis or when requirements for insulin may change rapidly, such as during the perioperative period, during labor and delivery, and in intensive-care situations (*see* below).

When metabolic conditions are stable, regular insulin is usually given subcutaneously in combination with an intermediate- or long-acting preparation. Short-acting insulin is the only form of the hormone that can be used in subcutaneous infusion pumps. Special formulations of regular insulin have been made for the latter purpose; these are less likely to crystallize in the tubing during the slow infusion associated with this type of therapy (Lougheed *et al.*, 1980).

The kinetics of absorption of *Semilente insulin* (*prompt insulin zinc suspension*) and regular insulin are similar, but Semilente insulin has a longer duration of action. It is available only as bovine and/or porcine insulins and is rarely used today.

Intermediate-acting insulins are formulated so

Table 61–2. INSULIN PREPARATIONS AVAILABLE IN THE UNITED STATES *

TYPE	HUMAN	BEEF/PORK	BEEF	PORK
Rapid				
Insulin injection (regular)	R, RB	S	P	P, C, S, PB
Prompt insulin zinc suspension (Semilente)	—	S	S	P
Intermediate				
Isophane insulin suspension (NPH)	R	S	S, P	P
Insulin zinc suspension (Lente)	R	S	S, P	P
Slow				
Extended insulin zinc suspension (Ultralente)	R	S	S, P	—
Protamine zinc insulin suspension (PZI)	—	S	P	P
Mixtures				
30% Regular/70% NPH	R	—	—	P

* S = standard insulins; P = purified insulins; C = purified concentrated insulin; R = recombinant or semisynthetic human insulins; RB = buffered human insulin; PB = purified, buffered insulin.

that they dissolve more gradually when administered subcutaneously; their durations of action are thus longer. The two preparations most frequently used are *neutral protamine Hagedorn (NPH) insulin* (*isophane insulin suspension*) and *Lente insulin* (*insulin zinc suspension*). NPH insulin is a suspension of insulin in a complex with zinc and protamine in a phosphate buffer. Lente insulin is a mixture of crystallized (Ultralente) and amorphous (Semilente) insulins in an acetate buffer, which minimizes the solubility of insulin. The preparations have similar pharmacokinetic profiles, although NPH insulin has a somewhat more rapid onset of action (*see* Table 61–1). For reasons that are not clear, the kinetics of action of human NPH and Lente insulins are slightly more rapid than those of the older mixtures of bovine and porcine insulins (Bilo *et al.*, 1987; Houtzagers *et al.*, 1988). This may create a problem with optimal timing for evening therapy; such preparations taken before dinner may not have a duration of action sufficient to prevent hyperglycemia by morning. Intermediate-acting insulins are usually given either once a day before breakfast or twice a day. In patients with Type-II diabetes, intermediate-acting insulin given at bedtime may help normalize fasting blood glucose (Riddle, 1985). When NPH or Lente insulin is mixed with regular insulin, some of the regular insulin may form a complex with the protamine or Zn^{2+} after several hours, and this may slow the absorption of the fast-acting insulin (Colagiuri and Villalobos, 1986).

Ultralente insulin (*extended insulin zinc suspension*) and *protamine zinc insulin suspension* are *long-acting insulins;* they have a very slow onset and a prolonged ("flat") peak of action. These insulins are advocated to provide a low basal concentration of insulin throughout the day. The long half-life of Ultralente insulin makes it difficult to determine the optimal dosage, since several days of treatment are required before a steady-state concentration of circulating insulin is achieved. As with the intermediate-acting insulins, beef–pork Ultralente insulin has an even more prolonged course of action than does human Ultralente insulin. When initiating therapy with this type of insulin, it is possible to give three times the normal daily dose as a loading dose (Holman and Turner, 1977). This is then followed by once- or twice-daily injections, which are adjusted according to the fasting blood glucose concentration. Protamine zinc insulin is rarely used today because of its very unpredictable and prolonged course of action.

The wide variability in the kinetics of insulin action between and even within individuals must be emphasized. The time to peak hypoglycemic effect can vary ± 50%. This is caused, at least in part, by large variations in the rate of subcutaneous absorption. This variability is more noticeable with the intermediate- and long-acting insulins. When this is coupled with normal variations in diet and exercise, it is sometimes surprising how many patients do achieve good control of blood glucose concentrations.

Indications and Goals for Therapy. Subcutaneous administration of insulin is the primary treatment for all patients with Type-I diabetes (IDDM), for Type-II diabetics who are not adequately controlled by diet and/or oral hypoglycemic agents, and for patients with postpancreatectomy diabetes or gestational diabetes (Frazier *et al.*, 1987; Skyler, 1988). In addition, insulin is critical for the management of diabetic ketoacidosis, and it has an important role in the treatment of hyperglycemic, nonketotic coma and in the perioperative management of both Type-I and Type-II diabetic patients. In all cases, the goal is the normalization not only of blood glucose but also of all aspects of metabolism; the latter is difficult to achieve. Optimal treatment requires a coordinated approach to diet, exercise, and the administration of insulin. A brief overview of the principles of therapy is given below. (For a more detailed description, *see* Schade *et al.*, 1983; Marble *et al.*, 1985.)

Near-normoglycemia can be attained in many patients with multiple daily doses of insulin or with so-called pump therapy. The goal is to achieve a fasting blood glucose concentration between 90 and 120 mg/dl (5 to 6.7 mM) and a two-hour postprandial value below 150 mg/dl (8.3 mM). In less disciplined patients or in those with defective responses of counterregulatory hormones, it may be necessary to accept higher fasting blood glucose concentrations (*e.g.*, 140 mg/dl [7.8 mM]) and two-hour postprandial concentrations (200 to 250 mg/dl [11.1 to 13.9 mM]). It is important to realize that euglycemia may be achieved without complete normalization of glucose metabolism in virtually all patients. This is so because insulin concentrations are equal in the portal and peripheral circulations when the hormone is supplied exogenously. Thus, as compared with normal individuals, the insulin-treated diabetic has an increased peripheral response to insulin relative to that occurring in the liver.

Daily Requirements. Insulin production by a normal, thin, healthy person is between 18 and 40 units per day or about 0.2 to 0.5 U/kg of body weight per day (Polonsky and Rubenstein, 1986). About half of this is secreted in the basal state and about half in response to meals. Thus, basal secretion is about 0.5 to 1 U per hour; after an oral glucose load, insulin secretion may increase to 6 U per hour (Waldhausl *et al.,* 1979). In nondiabetic, obese, insulin-resistant individuals, insulin secretion may be increased fourfold or more. Insulin is secreted into the portal circulation, and about 50% is destroyed by the liver before reaching the systemic circulation.

In a mixed population of Type-I diabetic patients, the average dose of insulin is usually 0.6 to 0.7 U/kg of body weight per day, with a range of 0.2 to 1 U/kg per day. Obese patients generally require more (about 2 U/kg per day) because of resistance of peripheral tissues to insulin. Patients who require less insulin than 0.5 U/kg per day may have some endogenous production of insulin or they are more sensitive to the hormone because of good physical conditioning. As in nondiabetics, the daily requirement for insulin can be divided into basal and postprandial needs. The basal dose suppresses hepatic output of glucose; it is usually 40 to 60% of the daily dose. The postprandial dose is necessary for disposition of nutrients after meals (Schade *et al.,* 1983). Insulin is often administered as a single daily dose of an intermediate-acting insulin, alone or in combination with regular insulin. This is rarely sufficient to achieve true euglycemia, and in view of the increasing evidence that hyperglycemia is a major determinant of the long-term complications of diabetes, more complex regimens that include combinations of intermediate- or long-acting insulins with regular insulin are used to reach this goal.

A number of commonly used dosage regimens that use mixtures of insulin given in two or three daily injections are depicted in Figure 61–5 (Schade *et al.,* 1983; Marble *et al.,* 1985). The most frequently used is the so-called "split-mixed" regimen, involving the pre-breakfast and pre-supper injection of a mixture of regular and intermediate-acting insulins (Figure 61–5, *A*). When the pre-supper NPH or Lente insulin is not sufficient to control hyperglycemia throughout the night, the evening dose may be divided into a pre-supper dose of regular insulin followed by NPH or Lente insulin at bedtime (Figure 61–5, *B*). Both normal and diabetic individuals have an increased requirement for insulin in the early morning; this has been termed the "dawn phenomenon" (Blackard *et al.,* 1989). It makes the kinetics and timing of the evening dose of insulin extremely important.

Another regimen, consists of a pre-breakfast dose of Ultralente and regular insulins, along with additional doses of regular insulin only at lunch and supper times (Figure 61–5, *C*). In this case, the Ultralente provides the basal requirement for insulin and the regular insulin meets the postprandial demand. To achieve more uniform basal concentrations of insulin, the dose of ultralente is sometimes divided in two—half given in the morning and half in the evening. This dosage regimen is very similar to the pattern of insulin administration achieved with a subcutaneous infusion pump (Figure 61–5, *D*), except that it is possible to control and vary the basal rate of insulin infusion more precisely with a pump (Kitabchi *et al.,* 1983). A less frequently used variation of this multidose regimen is the use of regular insulin at the time of meals, supplemented by a dose of NPH or Lente insulin (without Ultralente) at bedtime.

In all patients, the exact dose of insulin is chosen by monitoring therapeutic endpoints carefully. This is facilitated by the use of home glucose monitors and measurements of hemoglobin A_{1c} concentrations. Special care must be taken when the patient has other underlying diseases, deficiencies in other endocrine systems (*e.g.,* adrenocortical or pituitary failure), or substantial resistance to insulin.

Factors That Affect Insulin Absorption. The degree of control of plasma glucose concentrations may be modified by changes in insulin absorption, factors that alter insulin action, diet, exercise, and other factors, many of which are probably undefined. Factors that determine the rate of absorption of insulin after subcutaneous administration include the site of injection, subcutaneous blood flow, the volume and the concentration of the injected insulin, and the presence of circulating insulin antibodies. These variations should be minimized whenever possible.

Insulin is usually injected into the subcutaneous tissues of the abdomen, buttock, anterior thigh, or dorsal arm. Absorption is usually most rapid from the abdominal wall, followed by the arm, buttock, and thigh (Galloway *et al.,* 1981). Rotation of insulin injection sites has traditionally been advocated to avoid lipohypertrophy or lipoatrophy. This is less likely to occur with highly purified preparations of insulin, and injection into the same region (preferably to the abdominal wall) is currently favored to minimize day-to-day variability in the rate of absorption.

Several other factors may affect the absorption of insulin. Increased subcutaneous blood flow (brought about by massage, hot baths, and exercise) increases the rate of absorption. In the upright posture, subcutaneous blood flow diminishes considerably in the legs, and to a lesser extent in the abdominal wall. An altered volume or concentration of injected insulin affects the rate of absorption and the duration of action. When regular insulin is mixed with Lente insulin, some of the regular insulin becomes modified, causing a partial loss of the rapidly acting component (Galloway *et al.,* 1982; Forlani *et al.,* 1986). This problem is

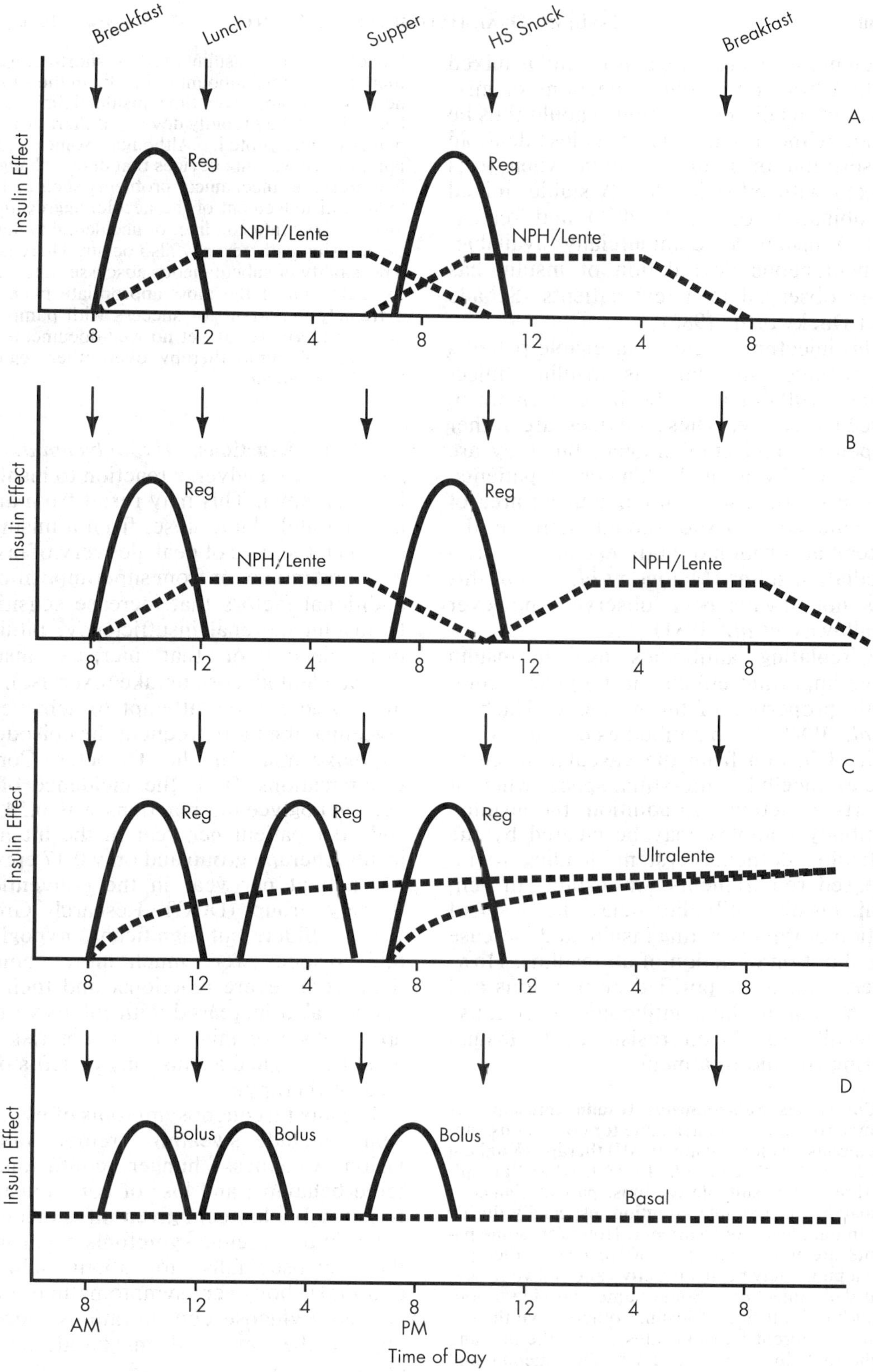

Figure 61–5. *Common multidose insulin regimens.*

A: A typical "split-mix" regimen, consisting of twice daily injections of a mixture of regular and intermediate-acting insulin. B: A variation in which the evening dose of intermediate-acting insulin is delayed until bedtime to increase the amount of insulin available the next morning. C: A regimen that incorporates Ultralente insulin. D: Patterns of insulin administration with a regimen of continuous subcutaneous insulin infusion.

even more severe if regular insulin is mixed with Ultralente insulin. Injections of mixtures of insulin preparations should thus be made without delay. There is less delay in absorption of regular insulin when it is mixed with NPH insulin. A stable, mixed combination of NPH (70%) and regular (30%) insulin is commercially available. Subcutaneous degradation of insulin has been observed in a few patients (Schade and Duckworth, 1986).

Jet injector systems that enable patients to receive subcutaneous insulin "injections" without a needle have been introduced recently. These devices are rather expensive and cumbersome, but they are preferred by a small number of patients. Dispersal of insulin throughout an area of subcutaneous tissue should increase the rate of absorption of both regular and intermediate insulins (Malone *et al.*, 1986); this has not always been observed, however (Galloway *et al.*, 1981).

Circulating antibodies against insulin have important effects on the pharmacokinetic properties of the hormone (Hachiya *et al.*, 1987). Such antibodies may delay the exit of insulin from the vascular space to the extracellular interstitial space, where it exerts its actions. In addition, the insulin–antibody complex may be cleared by the reticuloendothelial system, leading to increased requirements for insulin. In general, insulin antibodies delay the onset of action of rapidly acting insulin and increase the duration of action of all insulins. However, with more purified preparations and the human insulins, antibodies rarely cause clinically significant resistance to insulin during routine treatment.

Continuous Subcutaneous Insulin Infusion. A number of pumps are available for continuous subcutaneous insulin infusion (CSII) therapy (Kitabchi *et al.*, 1983; Schade *et al.*, 1983). CSII or "pump" therapy is not suitable for most patients, since it demands considerable attention, especially during the initial phases of treatment. However, some patients are interested in intensive insulin therapy, and a pump may be an attractive alternative to several daily injections. Some pumps provide a constant basal infusion of insulin; others have the option of different infusion rates during the day and night to help avoid the dawn phenomenon and bolus injections that are programmed according to the size and nature of a meal.

Pump therapy presents some unique problems. Since all of the insulin used is short-acting and there is a minimal amount of insulin in the subcutaneous pool at any given time, insulin deficiency and ketoacidosis may rapidly develop if therapy is accidentally interrupted. Although some modern pumps have warning devices that detect changes in line pressure, mechanical problems such as pump failure, dislodgement of the needle, aggregation of insulin in the infusion line, or accidental kinking of the infusion catheter may also occur. There is also a possibility of subcutaneous abscesses and cellulitis. Selection of the most appropriate patients is extremely important for success with pump therapy. Furthermore, as yet no well-documented advantages of pump therapy over other regimens have been shown.

Adverse Reactions. *Hypoglycemia.* The most common adverse reaction to insulin is hypoglycemia. This may result from an inappropriately large dose, from a mismatch between the time of peak delivery of insulin and food intake, or from superimposition of additional factors that increase sensitivity to insulin (adrenal insufficiency, pituitary insufficiency) or that increase insulin-independent glucose uptake (exercise). The more vigorous the attempt to achieve euglycemia, the more frequent the episodes of hypoglycemia. In the Diabetes Control Complications Trial, the incidence of severe hypoglycemic reactions was 0.54 episode per patient per year in the intensive insulin therapy group and only 0.17 episode per patient per year in the conventional therapy group (DCCT Research Group, 1988). Milder, but significant, hypoglycemic episodes were much more common than were severe reactions, and their frequency also increased with intensive therapy. Hypoglycemia is the major risk that must be weighed against any benefits of intensive therapy.

The most frequent symptoms of hypoglycemia include sweating, tremor, blurred vision, weakness, hunger, confusion, altered behavior, and loss of consciousness. In normal volunteers given infusions of insulin, hypoglycemic symptoms occur when the glucose falls to about 45 mg/dl (2.5 mM); however, symptoms may occur at higher glucose concentrations, depending on the rate and magnitude of the change.

With long-standing Type-I diabetes, the response of glucagon to hypoglycemia may be blunted or absent in a significant number of patients; a deficit in the epinephrine response may also occur (Gerich, 1988; Perriello *et al.,* 1988). Such patients are at high risk of developing severe, prolonged hypoglycemic reactions if subjected to intensive treatment protocols. All patients with longstanding diabetes should perhaps be given an insulin infusion test to evaluate their response to hypoglycemia before being considered for intensive treatment regimens.

With the ready availability of home glucose monitoring, hypoglycemia can be documented in most patients who experience suggestive symptoms. Hypoglycemia that occurs during sleep may be difficult to detect but should be suspected from a history of morning headaches, night sweats, or symptoms of hypothermia. Nocturnal hypoglycemia may also lead to rebound morning hyperglycemia, a syndrome known as the Somogyi phenomenon (Gerich, 1988); the treatment is to reduce the dose of insulin. This syndrome must be distinguished from hyperglycemia due to inadequate insulin dosage or the dawn phenomenon, where there is an indication to increase insulin dosage (Blackard *et al.,* 1989).

All diabetics who receive insulin should be aware of the symptoms of hypoglycemia, carry some form of easily ingested glucose, and carry an identification card or bracelet containing pertinent medical information. When possible, patients who suspect that they are experiencing hypoglycemia should document the glucose concentration with a measurement. Mild-to-moderate hypoglycemia may be treated simply by ingestion of glucose. When hypoglycemia is severe, it should be treated with intravenous glucose or an injection of glucagon (*see* below).

Insulin Allergy and Resistance. Although there has been a dramatic decrease in the incidence of resistance and allergic reactions to insulin with the use of human insulin or highly purified preparations of the hormone, these reactions still occur as a result of reactions to the small amounts of aggregated or denatured insulin in all preparations, to minor contaminants, or because of sensitivity to one of the components added to insulin in its formulation (protamine, Zn^{2+}, phenol, *etc.*). The most frequent allergic manifestations are IgE-mediated local cutaneous reactions, although on rare occasions patients may develop life-threatening systemic responses or insulin resistance due to IgG antibodies (Kahn and Rosenthal, 1979). Attempts should be made to identify the underlying cause of the hypersensitivity response by measuring insulin-specific IgG and IgE antibodies. Skin testing is also useful; however, many patients exhibit positive reactions to intradermal insulin without experiencing any adverse effects from subcutaneous insulin. If patients have allergic reactions to mixed beef–pork insulin, human insulin should be used. If allergy persists, desensitization may be attempted; it is successful in about 50% of cases. Antihistamines may provide relief in patients with cutaneous reactions, while glucocorticoids have been used in patients with resistance to insulin or more severe systemic reactions.

Lipoatrophy and Lipohypertrophy. Atrophy of subcutaneous fat at the site of insulin injection (lipoatrophy) is probably a variant of an immune response to insulin, whereas lipohypertrophy (enlargement of subcutaneous fat depots) has been ascribed to the lipogenic action of high local concentrations of insulin (Marble *et al.,* 1985). Both of these problems may be related to some contaminant in insulin, and they are rare with more purified preparations. When they occur, they may cause irregular absorption of insulin, as well as a cosmetic problem. The recommended treatment is to avoid the hypertrophic areas by use of other injection sites, and to inject insulin into the periphery of the atrophic sites in an attempt to restore the subcutaneous adipose tissue.

Insulin Edema. Some degree of edema, abdominal bloating, and blurred vision develop in many diabetic patients with severe hyperglycemia or ketoacidosis that is brought under control with insulin (Wheatly and Edwards, 1985). This is associated with a weight gain of 0.5 to 2.5 kg. The edema usually disappears spontaneously within several days to a week unless there is underlying cardiac or renal disease. Edema is attributed primarily to retention of Na^{+}, although increased capillary permeability associated with inadequate metabolic control may also contribute.

Insulin Treatment of Ketoacidosis and Other Special Situations. Acutely ill diabetic patients may have metabolic disturbances that are sufficiently severe or labile to justify intravenous administration of insulin. Such treatment is most appropriate in patients with ketoacidosis (Schade and Eaton, 1983; Kitabchi, 1989). Although there has been some controversy over appropriate dosage, infusion of a relatively low dose of insulin (0.1 U/kg per hour) will produce plasma concentrations of insulin of about 100 μU/ml—a level sufficient to inhibit lipolysis and gluconeogenesis completely and to produce near-maximal stimulation of glucose uptake in normal individuals. In most patients with ketoacidosis, blood glucose concentrations will fall by about 10% per hour; the acidosis is corrected more slowly. As treatment proceeds it may be necessary to administer glucose along with the insulin to prevent hypoglycemia but to allow clearance of all ketones. Some physicians prefer to initiate therapy with a loading dose of insulin, but this appears unnecessary since steady-state concentrations of the hormone are achieved within 30 minutes with a constant infusion. Patients with nonketotic, hyperglycemic coma are frequently more sensitive to insulin than are those with ketoacidosis. Appropriate replacement of fluid and electrolytes is an integral part of the therapy in both situations, since there is always a major deficit. Regardless of the exact insulin regimen used, the key to effective therapy is careful and frequent monitoring of the patient's clinical status, glucose, and electrolytes. A frequent error in the management of such patients is the failure to administer insulin subcutaneously at least 30 minutes before intravenous therapy is discontinued. This is necessary because of the very short half-life of insulin.

Intravenous administration of insulin is also well suited for the treatment of diabetic patients during the perioperative period and during childbirth. Several protocols have been proposed (Schade *et al.*, 1983). However, many physicians simply give patients half of their normal daily dose of insulin as intermediate-acting insulin subcutaneously on the morning before an operation, and then administer 5% dextrose infusions during surgery to maintain glucose concentrations. Although this may be satisfactory in most patients, use of an insulin with an intermediate duration of action provides less minute-to-minute control than is possible with an intravenous regimen. When insulin is given intravenously, only regular, crystalline insulin should be used.

Drug Interactions and Glucose Metabolism. A large number of drugs can cause hypoglycemia or hyperglycemia or may alter the response of diabetic patients to their existing therapeutic regimens (*see* Koffler *et al.*, 1989; Seltzer, 1989). A summary of drugs with hypoglycemic or hyperglycemic effects and their presumed sites of action is given in Table 61–3.

Aside from insulin and oral hypoglycemic drugs, the most common drug-induced hypoglycemic states are those caused by ethanol, β-adrenergic blockers, and salicylates. The primary action of ethanol is to inhibit gluconeogenesis. This effect is not an idiosyncratic reaction but is observed in all individuals. In diabetic patients, β-adrenergic blockers pose a risk of hypoglycemia because of their capacity to inhibit the effects of catecholamines on gluconeogenesis and glycogenolysis. These agents may also mask the sympathetically mediated symptoms associated with the fall in blood glucose (*e.g.*, tremor and palpitations). Salicylates, on the other hand, exert their hypoglycemic effect by enhancing β-cell sensitivity to glucose and potentiating insulin secretion. These agents also have a weak insulin-like action in the periphery. Pentamidine, an antiprotozoal agent now used frequently for the treatment of infections caused by *Pneumocystis carinii* can apparently cause both hypoglycemia and hyperglycemia. The hypoglycemic effect results from destruction of β cells and release of insulin; continuation of use may cause secondary hypoinsulinemia and hyperglycemia.

An equally large number of drugs may cause hyperglycemia in normal individuals or impair metabolic control in diabetic patients. Many of these are agents with direct effects on peripheral tissues that counter the actions of insulin; examples include epinephrine, glucocorticoids, and oral contraceptives. Other drugs cause hyperglycemia by inhibiting insulin secretion directly (phenytoin, clonidine, Ca^{2+}-channel blockers) or indirectly via depletion of K^+ (diuretics). A number of drugs have no direct hypoglycemic action but may potentiate the actions of sulfonylureas (*see* below). It is important to be aware of such interactions and to modify treatment regimens for diabetic patients accordingly.

Experimental Forms of Insulin Therapy. There are a number of experimental approaches to delivery of insulin, including the use of new insulins,

Table 61–3. DRUGS THAT CAUSE HYPOGLYCEMIA OR HYPERGLYCEMIA

DRUG	POSSIBLE SITE OF ACTION			
	Pancreas	*Liver*	*Periphery*	*Other*
Drugs with hypoglycemic effects				
β-Adrenergic antagonists		+	+	+
Salicylates	+			
Indomethacin *				
Naproxen *				
Ethanol		+		+
Clofibrate			+	
Converting-enzyme inhibitors			+	
Li^+		+	+	
Theophylline	+			
Ca^{2+}	+			
Bromocriptine			+	
Mebendazole	+			
Sulfonamides				+
Sulbactam/ampicillin *				
Tetracycline *				
Pyridoxine		+		
Pentamidine †	+			
Drugs with hyperglycemic effects				
Epinephrine	+	+	+	
Glucocorticosteroids		+	+	
Diuretics	+		+	
Diazoxide	+			
Oral contraceptives	+		+	
β_2-Adrenergic agonists	+	+	+	
Ca^{2+}-channel blockers	+			
Phenytoin	+			
Clonidine	+			+
H_2-receptor blockers	+			
Pentamidine †				+
Morphine	+			
Heparin				+
Nalidixic acid				?
Sulfinpyrazone *				
Marijuana				+
Nicotine *				

* Although these drugs are reported to have an effect on control of diabetes, there are no conclusive data about their effects on carbohydrate metabolism.
† Short-term effect is insulin release and hypoglycemia.
(Adapted from Koffler *et al.*, 1989.)

new routes of administration, intraperitoneal delivery devices, implantable pellets, the closed-loop artificial pancreas, islet-cell and pancreatic transplantation, and gene therapy.

Insulin Analogs. Recent development of insulin analogs that have altered rates of absorption have raised interest. Insulin with aspartate and glutamate substituted at positions B9 and B27, respectively, crystallizes poorly and has been termed "monomeric insulin" (Vora *et al.*, 1988). This insulin is absorbed more rapidly from subcutaneous depots and thus may be useful in meeting postprandial demands. By contrast, other insulin analogs tend to crystallize at the site of injection and are absorbed more slowly (Markussen *et al.*, 1988). Insulins with enhanced potency have been produced by substitution of aspartate for histidine at position B10 and by modification of the carboxyl-terminal residues of the B chain (Schwartz *et al.*, 1989).

New Routes of Delivery. Attempts have been made to administer insulin orally, nasally, rectally, and by subcutaneous implantation of pellets. The most promising of these is nasal delivery, which can be achieved by addition of various adjuvants such as fusidic acid to insulin to increase its absorption through the nasal mucosa (Salzman *et al.*, 1985; Longenecker *et al.*, 1987). The kinetics of absorption are rapid and approach the rate achieved with intravenous administration. Implantable pellets have been designed to release insulin slowly over days or weeks. Although oral delivery of insulin would be preferred by patients and would provide higher relative concentrations of insulin in the portal circulation, attempts to increase intestinal absorption of the hormone have met with only limited success. Efforts have focused on protection of insulin by encapsulation or incorporation into liposomes. Intraperitoneal infusion of insulin into the portal circulation has been used experimentally in human subjects for periods of several months (Schade *et al.*, 1983).

Transplantation and Gene Therapy. Transplantation and gene therapy are provocative approaches to replacement of insulin. Segmental pancreatic transplantation has been employed successfully in several hundred patients (Sutherland *et al.*, 1989). However, the surgery is technically complex and is usually considered only in patients with advanced disease and complications. Islet-cell transplants are theoretically less complicated. They have been accomplished in experimental rodent models of diabetes, but it is difficult to obtain adequate amounts of tissue for human transplantation. Introduction of an active insulin gene into cells such as fibroblasts, which can then be reintroduced into the host, has also been achieved in rodents.

ORAL HYPOGLYCEMIC AGENTS

History. In contrast to the systematic studies that led to the isolation of insulin, the sulfonylureas were discovered accidentally. In 1942, Janbon and colleagues noted that some sulfonamides caused hypoglycemia in experimental animals. These observations were soon extended, and 1-butyl-3-sulfonylurea (carbutamide) became the first clinically useful sulfonylurea for the treatment of diabetes. This compound was later withdrawn because of adverse effects on the bone marrow, but it led to the development of the entire class of sulfonylureas. Clinical trials of tolbutamide, the first widely used member of this group, were instituted in Type-II diabetic patients in the early 1950s. Since that time, approximately 20 different agents of this class have been in use worldwide.

Shortly after the introduction of the sulfonylureas, a second class of oral hypoglycemic agents, the biguanides, was discovered (Krall, 1985). However, phenformin, the primary drug in this group, was withdrawn from the market in the United States because of an increased frequency of lactic acidosis associated with its use. Newer agents of this type are currently being investigated.

SULFONYLUREAS

Chemistry. The sulfonylureas are traditionally divided into two groups or generations of agents. Their structural relationships are shown in Table 61–4. All members of this class of drugs are substituted arylsulfonylureas. They differ by substitutions at the *para* position on the benzene ring and at one nitrogen residue of the urea moiety. The first group of sulfonylureas includes tolbutamide, acetohexamide, tolazamide, and chlorpropamide. A second generation of hypoglycemic sulfonylureas has emerged. These drugs (glyburide [glibenclamide], glipizide, and gliclazide) are considerably more potent than the earlier agents.

Mechanism of Action. The sulfonylureas cause hypoglycemia by stimulating release of insulin from pancreatic β cells and by increasing the sensitivity of peripheral tissues to insulin. The predominant effect is on insulin secretion (Pfeifer *et al.*, 1981); sulfonylureas stimulate release of insulin from the isolated perfused pancreas, isolated islets, and insulinoma cells in culture (Hellman and Taljedal, 1975; Nelson *et al.*, 1987). The drugs are ineffective in pancreatectomized animals or patients and in diabetic patients who have no endogenous insulin. When given intravenously, the major effect is on the first phase of insulin secretion; however, the sulfonylureas are also effective in stimulating secretion of insulin throughout a meal (Kolterman *et al.*, 1984). Sulfonylureas also stimulate release of somatostatin, and they may suppress the secretion of glucagon slightly (Krall, 1985).

The effects of the sulfonylureas appear to be initiated by drug interaction with cell-surface receptors on the pancreatic β cell (Schmid-Anatomarchi *et al.*, 1987; Gaines *et al.*, 1988); this results in reduced conductance of an ATP-sensitive K^+ channel. The drugs thus resemble physiological secretagogues (*e.g.*, glucose, leucine), which also lower the conductance of this channel (Ribalet and Ciani, 1987; Boyd, 1988). Reduced K^+ conductance causes membrane depolarization and influx of Ca^{2+} through voltage-sensitive Ca^{2+} channels. It appears likely that the receptor for the sulfonylureas is the ATP-sensitive K^+ channel itself (Boyd, 1988).

Several studies suggest that there are also extrapancreatic sites of action of the sulfonylureas. During long-term treatment of diabetic patients with sulfonylureas, effects on plasma concentrations of insulin are inconsistent, despite a sustained reduction of plasma glucose concentrations. Fasting concentrations of insulin and C peptide do not change, but there is an increase in insulin secretion in response to stimuli such as food or glucose (Kolterman *et al.*, 1984). This may be indicative of an improved performance of β cells during treatment with sulfonylureas. Target tissues, especially the liver, may also become more sensitive to insulin (Kolterman, 1987). However, both phenomena may be secondary to the improved control of blood glucose concentrations; chronic hyperglycemia *per se* impairs insulin secretion and causes resistance to insulin in target tissues (Weir *et al.*, 1986).

The concentration of insulin receptors increases in the monocytes, adipocytes, and erythrocytes of Type-II diabetic patients who receive oral hypoglycemic agents (Olefsky and Reaven, 1976; Vigneri

Table 61–4. STRUCTURAL FORMULAS OF THE SULFONYLUREAS

General Formula

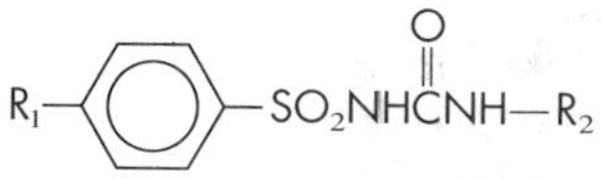

	R_1	R_2
First Generation		
Tolbutamide	$H_3C—$	$—C_4H_9$
Chlorpropamide	$Cl—$	$—C_3H_7$
Tolazamide	$H_3C—$	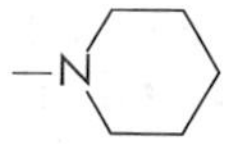
Acetohexamide	$H_3CCO—$	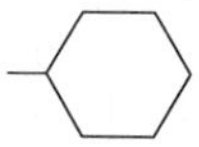
Second Generation		
Glyburide (Glibenclamide)	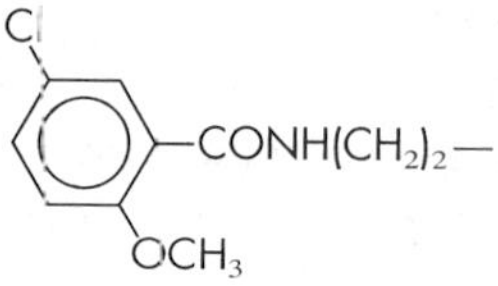	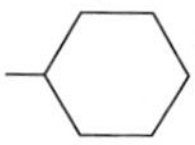
Glipizide	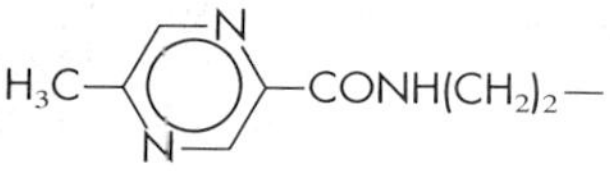	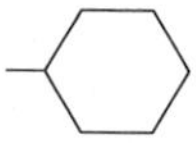
Gliclazide	$H_3C—$	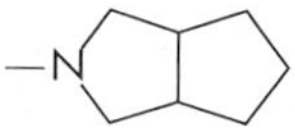

et al., 1982). Sulfonylureas enhance insulin action in cells in culture and stimulate the synthesis of glucose transporters (Jacobs *et al.*, 1989). Sulfonylureas have also been shown to suppress hepatic gluconeogenesis (Blumenthal, 1977); however, it is not clear if this is a direct effect of the drug or a reflection of increased sensitivity to insulin.

Absorption, Fate, and Excretion. The sulfonylureas have similar spectra of activities; thus, their pharmacokinetic properties are their most distinctive characteristics (Ferner, 1988; *see also* Appendix II). Although there are differences in the rates of absorption of the different sulfonylureas, all are effectively absorbed from the gastrointestinal tract. In view of the time required to reach an optimal concentration in plasma, some sulfonylureas may be more effective when given 30 minutes before eating. Sulfonylureas in plasma are largely (90 to 99%) bound to protein, especially albumin; plasma protein binding is least for chlorpropamide and greatest for glyburide. The volumes of distribution of most of the sulfonylureas are about 0.2 liter/kg.

The first-generation sulfonylureas vary

considerably in their half-lives and extents of metabolism. The half-life of acetohexamide is short, but it is reduced to an active compound with a half-life that is similar to those of tolbutamide and tolazamide (4 to 7 hours). It may be necessary to take these drugs in divided daily doses. Chlorpropamide has a long half-life (24 to 48 hours). The second-generation agents are approximately 100 times more potent than are those in the first group (Lebovitz and Feinglos, 1983). Their half-lives are short (1.5 to 5 hours). However, their hypoglycemic effects are evident for 12 to 24 hours, and it is often possible to administer these drugs once daily. The reason for the discrepancy between the half-life and duration of action of these drugs is not clear.

All of the sulfonylureas are metabolized by the liver, and the metabolites are excreted in the urine (Ferner, 1988). Metabolism of chlorpropamide is incomplete, and about 20% of the drug is excreted unchanged; this can create a problem for patients with impaired renal function.

Preparations and Dosage. Tolbutamide (ORAMIDE, ORINASE) is marketed as 250- and 500-mg tablets. Acetohexamide (DYMELOR) is available in 250- and 500-mg tablets. Tolazamide (TOLAMIDE, TOLINASE) is supplied in 100-, 250-, and 500-mg tablets. Chlorpropamide (DIABINESE) is marketed as 100- and 250-mg tablets. Glyburide (DIAβETA, MICRONASE) is available in 1.25-, 2.5-, and 5-mg tablets. Glipizide (GLUCOTROL) is marketed as 5- and 10-mg tablets. Gliclazide (DIAMICRON, others) is available in Europe and elsewhere, but it is not yet available in the United States.

The usual initial daily dose of tolbutamide is 500 mg, while 3000 mg is the maximally effective total dose; corresponding doses for acetohexamide are 250 and 1500 mg. Tolazamide and chlorpropamide are usually administered in a daily dose of 100 to 250 mg, while 750 to 1000 mg is maximal. Tolbutamide, acetohexamide, and tolazamide are often taken twice daily, 30 minutes before breakfast and dinner. The initial daily dose of glyburide is 2.5 to 5 mg, while daily doses of more than 20 mg are not recommended. Therapy with glipizide is usually initiated with 5 mg given once daily. The maximal recommended daily dose is 40 mg; daily doses of more than 15 mg should be divided. The starting dose of gliclazide is 40 to 80 mg per day, and the maximal daily dose is 320 mg. Treatment with the sulfonylureas must be guided by the individual patient's response, which must be monitored frequently.

Adverse Reactions. Adverse effects of the sulfonylureas are infrequent, occurring in about 4% of patients taking the first-generation drugs and perhaps slightly less often in patients receiving the second-generation agents (Paice *et al.*, 1985). Not unexpectedly, sulfonylureas may cause hypoglycemic reactions, including coma (Ferner and Neil, 1988; Seltzer, 1989). This is a particular problem in elderly patients with impaired hepatic or renal function who are taking longer-acting sulfonylureas. The relative risk of hypoglycemia is glyburide $\cong$ chlorpropamide $>$ glipizide $>$ tolbutamide (Berger *et al.*, 1986).

A number of other drugs may potentiate the effects of the sulfonylureas, particularly the first-generation agents, by inhibiting their metabolism or excretion. Some drugs also displace the sulfonylureas from binding proteins, thereby increasing the free concentration transiently (Seltzer, 1989). These include other sulfonamides, clofibrate, dicumarol, salicylates, and phenylbutazone. Other drugs, including ethanol, may enhance the action of sulfonylureas by causing hypoglycemia.

Other side effects of sulfonylureas include nausea and vomiting, cholestatic jaundice, agranulocytosis, aplastic and hemolytic anemias, generalized hypersensitivity reactions, and dermatological reactions. About 10 to 15% of patients who receive these drugs, particularly chlorpropamide, develop an alcohol-induced flush similar to that caused by disulfiram. Sulfonylureas, especially chlorpropamide, may also induce hyponatremia by potentiation of the effects of antidiuretic hormone on the renal collecting duct (Paice *et al.*, 1985). This undesirable side effect occurs in up to 5% of all patients; it is less frequent with tolbutamide and glipizide. This side effect has been used to therapeutic advantage in patients with mild forms of diabetes insipidus (*see* Chapter 29).

A major unresolved question is whether treatment with sulfonylureas is associated with increased cardiovascular mortality; this was suggested by a large multicenter trial (the University Group Diabetes Program or UGDP). The UGDP was designed to compare the effect of diet, oral agents (tolbutamide or phenformin), and fixed-dose insulin therapy on the development of vascular complications of Type-II diabetes.

During an 8-year period of observation, patients who received tolbutamide had a twofold increase in the rate of cardiovascular death as compared with placebo or insulin-treated patients (University Group Diabetes Program, 1970). A 10-year debate followed on the validity of this conclusion because the observation was unexpected, the study had not been designed to test this question, and all of the excess mortality occurred in only three centers. Although no comparable study has completely refuted this observation, most physicians continue to use oral hypoglycemic agents, since there are few therapeutic options other than insulin for the Type-II diabetic who has failed dietary therapy (American Diabetes Association, 1979).

Therapeutic Uses. Sulfonylureas are used to control hyperglycemia in Type-II diabetics who cannot achieve appropriate control with changes in diet alone. In all patients, however, continued dietary restrictions are essential to maximize the efficacy of the sulfonylureas. Some physicians still consider treatment with insulin to be the preferred approach in such patients. Patients with Type-II diabetes who are controlled with relatively low doses of insulin (less than 40 U per day) are more likely to respond to sulfonylureas, as are those who are obese and/or over 40 years of age. Contraindications to the use of these drugs include Type-I diabetes, pregnancy, lactation, and significant hepatic or renal insufficiency.

Between 50 and 80% of properly selected patients will respond initially to an oral hypoglycemic agent (Krall, 1985). All of the drugs appear to be equally efficacious. Concentrations of glucose are often lowered sufficiently to relieve symptoms of hyperglycemia, but they may not reach normal levels. To the extent that complications of diabetes may be related to hyperglycemia, the goal of treatment should be normalization of both fasting and postprandial glucose concentrations. However, since there are few therapeutic options, physicians frequently will continue treatment with a sulfonylurea in patients who have persistent, mild-to-moderate hyperglycemia. About 5 to 10% of patients per year who respond initially to a sulfonylurea become secondary failures, as defined by unacceptable levels of hyperglycemia. This may occur as a result of a change in drug metabolism, progression of β-cell failure, change in dietary compliance, or misdiagnosis of a patient with slow-onset Type-I diabetes. Changing to another oral agent will occasionally produce a satisfactory response, but most of these patients will eventually require insulin.

Combinations of insulin and oral agents have been used in some patients with Type-II diabetes (Simonson *et al.*, 1987; Lewitt *et al.*, 1989). The rationale for this treatment is based on the potential of sulfonylureas to increase tissue sensitivity to insulin. Most often, however, this combination does not produce a dramatic change in the dose of insulin needed and thus is of uncertain therapeutic advantage.

BIGUANIDES

Although their exact mechanism of action remains uncertain, the biguanides lower blood glucose concentrations by producing insulin-like effects on several tissues (Hermann, 1979). They suppress hepatic gluconeogenesis, stimulate glycolysis, and inhibit glucose absorption from the intestine (Jackson *et al.*, 1987). Although biguanides have no effect on the function of β cells, they are active only in patients with some endogenous insulin secretion. They are not effective in combination with insulin, but they have often been used in combination with sulfonylureas. The biguanides do not cause hypoglycemia in normal subjects, even when taken in excessive doses (Ferner, 1988).

Two biguanides have been used extensively in the clinic. Phenformin (phenethylbiguanide) was used in the United States until 1977 when it was withdrawn from the market because of an increased incidence of lactic acidosis. Metformin (dimethylbiguanide) and buformin (butylbiguanide) appear to be safer derivatives, and they are used widely in Europe and elsewhere. Metformin is only partially absorbed from the gastrointestinal tract. It has a half-life of 1.5 to 3 hours and is eliminated entirely by renal excretion (Hermann, 1979). It is contraindicated in patients with renal failure and in patients with severe hepatic or cardiovascular disease because of concern over lactic acidosis. When used in appropriate patients, the incidence of side effects from metformin is similar to those with the second-generation sulfonylureas. Metformin may produce nausea and diarrhea and should be taken with food.

OTHER ORAL HYPOGLYCEMIC AGENTS

Ciglitazone. Ciglitazone is a potent hypoglycemic agent in obese diabetic mice and in a Chinese hamster model of Type-II diabetes (Chang *et al.*, 1983; Diani *et al.*, 1984). Although it decreases the circulating concentration of insulin, the drug causes an increase in the basal rates of glucose metabolism and lipogenesis, apparently by increasing the concentration of insulin receptors (Diani *et al.*, 1984; Colca *et al.*, 1988). Ciglitazone also lowers food intake, but its effects on insulin and glucose occur without a change in body weight (Shargill *et al.*, 1986). This compound is currently undergoing clinical trials.

Glucosidase Inhibitors. α-Glucosidase inhibitors such as acarbose reduce gastrointestinal absorption of carbohydrates. For this reason this group of drugs has been known popularly as "starch blockers." They lower plasma glucose concentrations and tend to cause weight loss. A limiting side effect is flatulence. These agents might be of value in obese diabetic patients, but they are not indicated for individuals of normal weight because of their effects on nutrition.

GLUCAGON

History. Distinct populations of cells were identified in the islets of Langerhans before the discovery of insulin. Glucagon itself was discovered by Murlin and Kimball in 1923, less than 2 years after the discovery of insulin. In contrast to the excitement caused by the discovery of insulin, few were interested in glucagon, and it was not recognized as an important hormone for over 40 years. Glucagon is now known to have a significant physiological role in the regulation of glucose and ketone body metabolism, but it is only of minor therapeutic interest for the short-term management of hypoglycemia. It is also used in radiology for its inhibitory effects on intestinal smooth muscle.

Chemistry. Glucagon is a 29 amino acid, single-chain polypeptide (Figure 61–6). It shows significant homology with several other polypeptide hormones, including secretin, vasoactive intestinal peptide, and gastrointestinal inhibitory polypeptide. The primary sequence of glucagon is highly conserved in mammals, and it is identical in man, cattle, pigs, and rats.

Glucagon is synthesized from preproglucagon, a 180 amino acid precursor with five, separately processed domains (Bell *et al.*, 1983). An amino-terminal signal peptide is followed by glicentin-related pancreatic peptide, glucagon, glucagon-like peptide-1, and glucagon-like peptide-2. Processing of the protein is sequential and occurs in a tissue-specific fashion; this results in different secretory peptides in pancreatic α cells and intestinal α-like cells (termed L cells) (Mojsov *et al.*, 1986). Glicentin, a major processing intermediate, consists of glicentin-related pancreatic polypeptide at the amino terminus and glucagon at the carboxyl terminus with an arg–arg pair between. Enteroglucagon (or oxyntomodulin) consists of glucagon and a carboxyl-terminal hexapeptide linked by an arg–arg pair.

The biological roles of these precursor peptides are uncertain, but the highly controlled nature of the processing suggests that these peptides may have distinct biological functions. In the pancreatic α cell, the granule consists of a central core of glucagon surrounded by a halo of glicentin. Intestinal L cells contain only glicentin and presumably lack the enzyme required to process this precursor to glucagon. Enteroglucagon binds to hepatic glucagon receptors and stimulates adenylyl cyclase with 10 to 20% of the potency of glucagon. Glucagon-like peptide-1 is an extremely potent potentiator of insulin secretion (Mojsov *et al.*, 1987), although it apparently lacks significant hepatic actions. Glicentin, enteroglucagon, and the glucagon-like peptides are found predominantly in the intestine, and their secretion continues after total pancreatectomy.

Regulation of Secretion. The secretion of glucagon is regulated by dietary glucose, amino acids, and fatty acids (*see* Unger, 1985b); glucose is a potent inhibitor. As in insulin secretion, glucose is a more effective inhibitor of glucagon secretion when taken orally than when administered intravenously, suggesting a possible role for some gastrointestinal hormone in the response. The effect of glucose is lost in the untreated or undertreated Type-I diabetic patient and in isolated α cells, indicating that at least part of the effect is secondary to stimulation of insulin secretion. Somatostatin also inhibits glucagon secretion, as do free fatty acids and ketones.

Most amino acids stimulate the release of both glucagon and insulin. This coordinated response to amino acids may prevent insulin-induced hypoglycemia in individuals who ingest a meal of pure protein. Like glucose, amino acids are more potent when taken orally and thus may exert some of their effects via gastrointestinal hormones. Secretion of glucagon is also regulated by the autonomic innervation of the pancreatic islet. Stimulation of sympathetic nerves or administration of sympathomimetic amines increases glucagon secretion. Acetylcholine has a similar effect.

Glucagon in Diabetes Mellitus. Plasma concentrations of glucagon are elevated in poorly controlled Type-I and Type-II diabetic patients. In view of its capacity to enhance gluconeogenesis and glycogenolysis, glucagon exacerbates the hyperglycemia of diabetes. However, this abnormality of glucagon secretion appears to be secondary to the diabetic state and is corrected with improved control of the disease (Unger, 1985a). The importance of the hyperglucagonemia in diabetes has been evaluated by administration of somatostatin (Gerich *et al.*, 1975). Although somatostatin does not restore glucose metabolism to normal, it significantly slows the rate of development of hyperglycemia and ketonemia in the Type-I diabetic who is not receiving insulin.

Degradation. Glucagon is extensively degraded in liver, kidney, and plasma, as well as at its sites of action (Peterson *et al.*, 1982). Its half-life in plasma is approximately 3 to 6 minutes. Proteolytic removal of the amino-terminal histidine residue leads to loss of biological activity.

```
       NH2
        |
H—His—Ser—Glu—Gly—Thr—Phe—Thr—Ser—Asp—Tyr—Ser—Lys—Tyr—Leu—Asp—

                 NH2                   NH2                NH2
                  |                     |                  |
Ser—Arg—Arg—Ala—Glu—Asp—Phe—Val—Glu—Trp—Leu—Met—Asp—Thr—OH
```

Figure 61–6. *The structure of glucagon.*

Cellular and Physiological Actions. Glucagon interacts with a 60-kDa glycoprotein receptor on the plasma membrane of target cells (Sheetz and Tager, 1988). Although the exact structure of this receptor is not yet known, it interacts with the stimulatory guanine nucleotide-binding regulatory protein, G_s, that activates adenylyl cyclase (*see* Chapter 2). The primary effects of glucagon on the liver are mediated by cyclic AMP. In general, modifications of the amino-terminal region of glucagon (*e.g.*, [Phe^1]glucagon and des-His$_1$-[Glu^9]glucagon amide) result in molecules that behave as partial agonists—they retain some affinity for the glucagon receptor but have a marked reduction in capacity to stimulate adenylyl cyclase (Unson *et al.*, 1989).

Phosphorylase, the rate-limiting enzyme in glycogenolysis, is activated by glucagon as a result of cyclic AMP-stimulated phosphorylation, while concurrent phosphorylation of glycogen synthase inactivates the enzyme; glycogenolysis is enhanced and glycogen synthesis is inhibited. Cyclic AMP also stimulates transcription of the gene for phosphoenolpyruvate carboxykinase, a rate-limiting enzyme in gluconeogenesis (Granner *et al.*, 1986). These effects are normally opposed by insulin, and when maximal concentrations of both hormones are present, insulin is dominant.

Cyclic AMP also stimulates phosphorylation of the bifunctional enzyme, 6-phosphofructo 2-kinase/fructose 2,6-bisphosphatase (Pilkis *et al.*, 1981; Foster, 1984). This enzyme determines the cellular concentration of fructose-2, 6-bisphosphate, which acts as a potent regulator of gluconeogenesis and glycogenolysis. When the concentration of glucagon is high relative to that of insulin, this enzyme is phosphorylated and acts as a phosphatase, reducing the concentration of fructose-2,6-bisphosphate in the liver. When the concentration of insulin is high relative to that of glucagon, the enzyme is dephosphorylated and acts as a kinase, raising fructose-2,6-bisphosphate concentrations. Fructose-2,6-bisphosphate interacts allosterically with phosphofructokinase-1, the rate-limiting enzyme in glycolysis, increasing its activity. Thus, when glucagon concentrations are high, glycolysis is inhibited and gluconeogenesis is stimulated. This also leads to a decrease in the concentration of malonyl CoA, stimulation of fatty acid oxidation, and production of ketone bodies. Conversely, when insulin concentrations are high, glycolysis is stimulated and gluconeogenesis and ketogenesis are inhibited (*see* Foster, 1984).

Glucagon exerts effects on tissues other than liver, especially at higher concentrations. In adipose tissue, it stimulates adenylyl cyclase and increases lipolysis. In the heart, glucagon increases the force of contraction. Glucagon has relaxant effects on the gastrointestinal tract; this has been observed with analogs that apparently do not stimulate adenylyl cyclase. Some tissues (including liver) possess a second type of glucagon receptor that is linked to generation of inositol trisphosphate, diacylglycerol, and Ca^{2+} (Murphy *et al.*, 1987). The role of this receptor in regulation of metabolism remains uncertain.

Therapeutic Use and Preparations. Glucagon is used to treat severe hypoglycemia, particularly in diabetic patients when intravenous glucose is not available; it is also used by radiologists for its inhibitory effects on the gastrointestinal tract.

All glucagon used clinically is extracted from bovine and porcine pancreas; its sequence is identical to that of the human hormone. For hypoglycemic reactions, 1 mg is administered intravenously, intramuscularly, or subcutaneously. Either of the first two routes is preferred in an emergency. Clinical improvement is sought within 10 minutes to minimize the risk of neurological damage from hypoglycemia. The hyperglycemic action of glucagon is transient and may be inadequate if hepatic stores of glycogen are depleted. After the initial response to glucagon, patients should be given glucose or urged to eat to prevent recurrent hypoglycemia. Nausea and vomiting are the most frequent adverse effects.

Glucagon is also used to relax the intestinal tract to facilitate radiographic examination of the upper and lower gastrointestinal tract with barium and retrograde ileography (Monsein *et al.*, 1986) and in magnetic resonance imaging of the gastrointestinal tract (Goldberg and Thoeni, 1989). Glucagon has been used to treat the spasm associated with acute diverticulitis and disorders of the biliary tract and sphincter of Oddi, as an adjunct in basket retrieval of biliary calculi, and for impaction of the esophagus and intussusception (Friedland, 1983; Mortensson *et al.*, 1984; Kadir and Gadacz, 1987). It has been used for diagnostic purposes to distinguish obstructive from hepatocellular jaundice (Berstock *et al.*, 1982).

Glucagon releases catecholamines from a pheochromocytoma and has been used experimentally as a diagnostic test for this disorder. The hormone has also been used as a cardiac inotropic agent for the treatment of shock, particularly when prior administration of a β-adrenergic antagonist has rendered β-adrenergic agonists ineffective.

Glucagon is dispensed as a lyophilized powder in 1- or 10-mg vials; it is packaged with diluent to make solutions of 1 mg/ml.

SOMATOSTATIN

Somatostatin was first isolated and synthesized in 1973, following a search for hypothalamic factors that might regulate secretion of growth hormone from the pituitary gland (Brazeau *et al.*, 1973; *see also* Chapter 56). A potential physiological role for somatostatin in the islet was suggested by the observation that somatostatin inhibits secretion of insulin and glucagon (Alberti *et al.*, 1973; Gerich *et al.*, 1974). The peptide was subsequently identified in the D cells of the pancreatic islet, in similar cells of the gastrointestinal tract, and in the central nervous system (Dubois, 1975).

Somatostatin is secreted from pancreatic islets in response to many of the nutrients and hormones that stimulate insulin secretion, including glucose, arginine, leucine, glucagon, vasoactive intestinal polypeptide, cholecystokinin, and even tolbutamide (Ipp *et al.*, 1977; Weir *et al.*, 1979). Although it was initially suspected to act as a paracrine hormone in the islet, recent data suggest that the D or δ cell is the last to receive blood flow in the islet, that is, it is downstream from the β and α cells (Samols *et al.*, 1986). Thus, somatostatin may regulate the secretion of insulin and glucagon only via the systemic circulation.

The physiological role of somatostatin is uncertain. When administered in pharmacological concentrations, somatostatin inhibits the secretion of all of the hormones of the endocrine pancreas, growth hormone and TSH from the pituitary, and most gastrointestinal peptide hormones (Reichlin, 1983; Bloom and Polak, 1987). The α cell is about 50 times more sensitive to somatostatin than is the β cell, but inhibition of glucagon secretion is more transient. Somatostatin also inhibits nutrient absorption from the intestine, decreases intestinal motility, and reduces splanchnic blood flow. Patients with rare somatostatin-secreting islet-cell tumors often have diabetes mellitus because of suppression of insulin and glucagon secretion, malabsorption, steatorrhea, and a history of cholelithiasis. For additional information, *see* Chapter 56.

DIAZOXIDE

Diazoxide is an antihypertensive, antidiuretic benzothiadiazine derivative with potent hyperglycemic actions when given orally (*see* Chapter 33). Hyperglycemia results primarily from inhibition of insulin secretion (Levin *et al.*, 1975). Diazoxide interacts with an ATP-sensitive K^+ channel and either prevents its closing or prolongs the open time; this effect is opposite to that of the sulfonylureas (Misler *et al.*, 1989; Panteu *et al.*, 1989). The drug does not inhibit insulin synthesis, and thus there is an accumulation of insulin within the β cell. Diazoxide also has a modest capacity to inhibit peripheral glucose utilization by muscle and to stimulate hepatic gluconeogenesis.

Diazoxide (PROGLYCEM) has been used to treat patients with various forms of hypoglycemia (Grant *et al.*, 1986); it is available in 50-mg capsules and in an oral suspension. The usual oral dose is 3 to 8 mg/kg per day in adults and up to 20 mg/kg per day in children. The drug has a tendency to cause nausea and vomiting and thus is usually given in divided doses with meals. Diazoxide circulates largely bound to plasma proteins and has a half-life of about 48 hours. Thus, the patient should be maintained at any dosage for several days before evaluating the therapeutic result.

Diazoxide has a number of adverse effects that sometimes limit its use in the treatment of hypoglycemia (*see* Chapter 33). These include retention of Na^+ and fluid, hyperuricemia, hypertrichosis (especially in children), thrombocytopenia, and leukopenia. Despite these side effects, the drug may be quite useful in patients with inoperable insulinomas (Schein *et al.*, 1973) and in children with hyperinsulinism due to nesidioblastosis (Grant *et al.*, 1986).

Alberti, K. G. M. M.; Christensen, N. J.; Christensen, S. E.; Hanson, A. P.; Iversen, J.; Lindback, K.; Seyer-Hansen, K.; and Orskott, H. Inhibition of insulin secretion by somatostatin. *Lancet*, **1973**, *2*, 1299–1303.

American Diabetes Association. Policy Statement: the UGDP controversy. *Diabetes*, **1979**, *28*, 168–170.

Banting, F. G.; Best, C. H.; Collip, J. B.; Campbell, W. R.; and Fletcher, A. A. Pancreatic extracts in the treatment of diabetes mellitus. *Can. Med. Assoc. J.*, **1922**, *12*, 141–146.

Bell, G. I.; Sanchez-Pescador, R.; Laybourn, P. J.; and Najarian, R. C. Exon duplication and divergence on the human pre-proglucagon gene. *Nature*, **1983**, *304*, 368–371.

Berger, W.; Caduff, R.; Pasquel, M.; and Rump, A. Die relative Haufgkeit der Schweren Sulfonyl-harnstoft-hypoglykemie in den letzen 25 Jahnre in der Schweiz. *Schweiz. Med. Wochenschr.*, **1986**, *116*, 145–151.

Berman, M.; McGuire, E. A.; Roth, J.; and Zeleznik, A. J. Kinetic modeling of insulin binding to receptors and degradation *in vivo* in rabbits. *Diabetes*, **1980**, *29*, 50–59.

Berstock, D. A.; Wood, J. R.; and Williams, R. The glucagon test in obstructive and hepatocellular jaundice. *Postgrad. Med. J.*, **1982**, *58*, 485–486.

Bilo, H. J. G.; Heine, B. J.; Sikkenk, A. C.; Van Der Meer, J.; and Van Der Veen, E. A. Absorption kinetics and action profiles of intermediate acting human insulins. *Diabetes Res.*, **1987**, *4*, 39–43.

Birnbaum, M. J. Identification of a novel gene encoding an insulin-responsive glucose transporter protein. *Cell*, **1989**, *57*, 305–315.

Blackard, W. G.; Barlaseins, C. O.; Clore, J. N.; and Nestler, J. E. Morning insulin requirements: critique of dawn and meal phenomena. *Diabetes*, **1989**, *38*, 273–277.

Bloom, S. R., and Polak, J. M. Somatostatin. *Br. Med. J.*, **1987**, *295*, 288–290.

Blumenthal, S.A. Potentiation of the hepatic action of insulin by chlorpropamide. *Diabetes*, **1977**, *26*, 485–491.

Bonner-Weir, S., and Orci, L. New perspectives on the microvasculature of the islets of Langerhans in the rat. *Diabetes*, **1982**, *31*, 883–889.

Brazeau, P.; Vale, W.; Burgus, R.; Ling, N.; Butcher, M.; Rivier, J.; and Guillemin, R. Hypothalamic polypeptide that inhibits the secretion of immunoreactive pituitary growth hormone. *Science*, **1973**, *179*, 77–79.

Brelje, T. C., and Sorenson, R. L. Nutrient and hormonal regulation of glucose-stimulated insulin secretion in isolated rat pancreases. *Endocrinology*, **1988**, *123*, 1582–1590.

Chan, S. J.; Seino, S.; Grappuso, P. A.; Schwartz, R.; and Steiner, D. F. A mutation in the B chain coding region is associated with impaired proinsulin conversion in a family with hyperproinsulinemia. *Proc. Natl. Acad. Sci. U.S.A.*, **1987**, *84*, 2194–2197.

Chang, A. Y.; Wyse, B. M.; and Gilchrist, B. J. Ciglitazone, a new hypoglycemic agent. II. Effect on glucose and lipid metabolism and insulin binding in the adipose tissue of C57BL/6J-ob/ob and −+/? mice. *Diabetes*, **1983**, *32*, 839–845.

Charron, M. J.; Brosius, F. C., III; Alper, S. L.; and Lodish, H. F. A glucose transport protein expressed predominantly in insulin-responsive tissues. *Proc. Natl. Acad. Sci. U.S.A.*, **1989**, *86*, 2535–2539.

Chou, C. K.; Dull, T. J.; Russell, D. S.; Gherzi, R.; Lebwohl, D.; Ullrich, A.; and Rosen, O. M. Human insulin receptors mutated at the ATP-binding site lack protein tyrosine kinase activity and fail to mediate postreceptor effects of insulin. *J. Biol. Chem.*, **1987**, *262*, 1842–1847.

Cohn, R. A.; Mauer, S. M.; Barbosa, J.; and Michael, A. F. Immunofluorescence studies of skeletal muscle extracellular membranes in diabetes mellitus. *Lab. Invest.*, **1978,** *39,* 13–16.

Colagiuri, S., and Villalobos, S. Assessment of the effect of mixing insulins in subjects with diabetes mellitus using the glucose clamp technique. *Diabetes Care,* **1986,** *9,* 579–586.

Colca, J. R.; Wyse, B. M.; Sawada, G.; Jodelis, K. S.; Connell, C. L.; Fletcher-McGruder, B. L.; Palazuk, B. J.; and Diani, A. R. Ciglitazone, a hypoglycemic agent: early effects on pancreatic islets of ob/ob mice. *Metabolism,* **1988,** *37,* 276–280.

Davidson, H. W.; Rhodes, C. J.; and Hutton, J. C. Intraorganelle calcium and pH control proinsulin cleavage in the pancreatic β cell via two distinct site-specific endopeptidases. *Nature,* **1988,** *333,* 93–96.

DCCT Research Group. Are continuing studies of metabolic and microvascular complications in insulin dependent diabetes mellitus justified? *N. Engl. J. Med.,* **1988,** *318,* 246–247.

Diani, A. R.; Peterson, T.; Sawada, G. A.; Wyse, B. M.; Gilchrist, B. J.; Hearron, A. E.; and Chang, A. Y. Ciglitazone, a new hypoglycemic agent. 4. Effect on pancreatic islets of C57BL/6J-ob/ob and C57BL/KsJ-db/db mice. *Diabetologia,* **1984,** *27,* 225–234.

Dimitriadas, G. D., and Gerich, J. E. Importance of timing of preprandial subcutaneous insulin administration in the management of diabetes mellitus. *Diabetes Care,* **1983,** *6,* 374–377.

Dubois, M. P. Immunoreactive somatostatin is present in discrete cells of the endocrine pancreas. *Proc. Natl. Acad. Sci. U.S.A.,* **1975,** *72,* 1340–1344.

Ebina, Y.; Ellis, L.; Jarnagin, K.; Standring, D.; Beaudoin, J.; Roth, R. A.; and Rutter, W. J. The human insulin receptor cDNA: the structure basis for hormone-mediated transmembrane signalling. *Cell,* **1985,** *40,* 7447–7458.

Ellis, L.; Clauser, E.; Morgan, D. O.; Edery, M.; Roth, R. A.; and Rutter, W. J. Replacement of insulin receptor tyrosine residues 1162 and 1163 compromises insulin stimulated kinase activity and uptake of 2-deoxy glucose. *Cell,* **1986,** *45,* 721–732.

Ferner, R. E., and Neil, H. A. W. Sulfonylureas and hypoglycemia. *Br. Med. J.,* **1988,** *296,* 949–950.

Forlani, G.; Santacroce, G.; Ciavarella, A.; Capelli, M.; Mattioli, L.; and Vannini, P. Effects of mixing short and intermediate-acting insulins on absorption course and biological effect of short acting preparation. *Diabetes Care,* **1986,** *9,* 587–590.

Frazier, L. M.; Mulrow, C. D.; Alexander, L. T.; Harris, R. T.; Heise, K. R.; Brown, J. T.; and Feussner, J. R. Need for insulin therapy in type II diabetes mellitus: a randomized trial. *Arch. Intern. Med.,* **1987,** *147,* 1085–1089.

Friedland, G. W. The treatment of acute esophageal food impaction. *Radiology,* **1983,** *149,* 601–620.

Fukumoto, H.; Seino, S.; Imura, H.; Seino, Y.; Eddy, R. L.; Fukushima, Y.; Byers, M. G.; Shows, T. B.; and Bell, G. I. Sequence, tissue distribution and chromosomal localization of mRNA encoding a human glucose transporter-like protein. *Proc. Natl. Acad. Sci. U.S.A.,* **1988,** *85,* 5434–5438.

Gaines, K. L.; Hamilton, S.; and Boyd, A. E., III. Characterization of the sulfonylurea receptor on beta cell membranes. *J. Biol. Chem.,* **1988,** *263,* 2589–2592.

Galloway, J. A.; Spradlin, C. T.; Nelson, R. L.; Wentworth, S. M.; Davidson, J. A.; and Swarner, J. L. Factors influencing the absorption, serum insulin concentration, and blood glucose responses after injections of regular insulin and various insulin mixtures. *Diabetes Care,* **1981,** *4,* 366–376.

Garlick, R. L.; Mazer, J. S.; Higgins, P. J.; and Bunn, H. F. Characterization of glycosylated hemoglobins: relevance to monitoring of diabetic control and analysis of other proteins. *J. Clin. Invest.,* **1983,** *71,* 1062–1072.

Garvey, W. T.; Huckstеadt, T. P.; and Birnbaum, M. J. Pretranslational suppression of an insulin responsive glucose transporter in rats with diabetes mellitus. *Science,* **1989,** *245,* 60–63.

Genuth, S. Plasma insulin and glucose profiles in normal, obese, and diabetic persons. *Ann. Intern. Med.,* **1973,** *79,* 812–822.

Gerich, J. E.; Lorenzi, M.; Bier, D. M.; Schneider, V.; Tsalikian, E.; Karam, J. H.; and Forsham, P. H. Prevention of human diabetic ketoacidosis by somatostatin: evidence for an essential role of glucagon. *N. Engl. J. Med.,* **1975,** *292,* 985–989.

Gerich, J. E.; Lorenzi, M.; Schneider, V.; Kwan, C. W.; Karam, J. H.; Guillemin, R.; and Forsham, P. H. Inhibition of pancreatic glucagon secretion to arginine by somatostatin in normal man and in insulin-dependent diabetes. *Diabetes,* **1974,** *23,* 876–881.

Gold, G.; Gishizky, M. L.; and Grodsky, G. M. Evidence that glucose "marks" β cells resulting in preferential release of newly synthesized insulin. *Science,* **1982,** *218,* 56–58.

Grant, D. B.; Dunger, D. B.; and Burns, E. C. Long-term treatment with diazoxide in childhood hyperinsulinism. *Acta Endocrinol.* [*Suppl.*] (*Copenh.*), **1986,** *279,* 340–345.

Gross, D. J.; Halban, P. A.; Kahn, C. R.; Weir, C. G.; and Villa-Komaroff, L. Partial diversion of a mutant proinsulin (B10 aspartic acid) from the regulated to the constitutive pathway in transfected AET-20 cells. *Proc. Natl. Acad. Sci. U.S.A.,* **1989,** *86,* 4107–4111.

Hachiya, H. L.; Treves, S. T.; Kahn, C. R.; Sodoyez, J. C.; and Sodoyez-Goffaux, F. Altered insulin distribution and metabolism in Type I diabetics assessed by ^{123}I-insulin scanning. *J. Clin. Endocrinol. Metab.,* **1987,** *64,* 801–808.

Hanks, J. B.; Andersen, D. K.; Wise, J. E.; Putnam, W. J.; Meyers, W. C.; and Jones, R. S. The hepatic extraction of gastrointestinal inhibitory polypeptide and insulin. *Endocrinology,* **1984,** *115,* 1011–1018.

Higgins, P. J., and Bunn, H. F. Kinetic analysis of the nonenzymatic glycosylation of hemoglobin. *J. Biol. Chem.,* **1981,** *256,* 5204–5208.

Holman, R. R., and Turner, R. Diabetes: the quest for basal normoglycemia. *Lancet,* **1977,** *1,* 469–474.

Houtzagers, C. M. G. J.; Berntzen, P. A.; Vanderstap, H.; Heine, R. J.; and Van Der Veen, E. A. Absorption kinetics of short and intermediate-acting insulins after jet injection with Med-Jector II. *Diabetes Care,* **1988,** *11,* 739–745.

Ipp, E.; Dobb, R. E.; Arimura, A.; Vale, W.; Harris, V.; and Unger, R. H. Release of immunoreactive somatostatin from the pancreas in response to glucose, amino acids, pancreozymin–cholecystokinin, and tolbutamide. *J. Clin. Invest.,* **1977,** *60,* 760–767.

Jackson, R. A.; Hawa, M. I.; Jaspan, J. B.; Sim, B. M.; Silvio, D.; Featherbe, L.; and Kurtz, D. Mechanism of metformin action in non-insulin-dependent diabetes. *Diabetes,* **1987,** *36,* 632–640.

Jacobs, D. R.; Hayes, G. R.; and Lockwood, D. H. *In vitro* effects of sulfonylureas on glucose transport and translocation of glucose transporters in adipocytes from streptozotocin induced diabetic rats. *Diabetes,* **1989,** *38,* 205–211.

James, D. E.; Brown, R.; Navarro, J.; and Pilch, P. F. Insulin regulatable tissues express a unique insulin-sensitive glucose transport protein. *Nature,* **1988,** *333,* 183–185.

Kadir, S., and Gadacz, T. R. Adjuncts and modifications to basket retrieval of retained biliary calculi. *Cardiovasc. Intervent. Radiol.,* **1987,** *10,* 295–300.

Kahn, C. R.; Baird, K. L.; Jarrett, D. B.; and Flier, J. S. Direct demonstration that receptor cross-linking or aggregation is important in insulin action. *Proc. Natl. Acad. Sci. U.S.A.,* **1978,** *75,* 4209–4213.

Kasuga, M.; Karlsson, F. A.; and Kahn, C. R. Insulin stimulates the phosphorylation of the 95,000 dalton subunit of its own receptor. *Science,* **1982,** *215,* 185–187.
Katsoyannis, P. G.; Tometsko, A.; and Fukuda, K. Insulin peptides IX: the synthesis of the A-chain of insulin and its combination with natural B-chain to generate insulin activity. *J. Am. Chem. Soc.,* **1963,** *85,* 2863–2865.
Kent, M. J. C.; Light, N. D.; and Bailey, A. J. Evidence for glucose-mediated covalent cross-linking of collagen after glycosylation *in vitro. Biochem. J.,* **1985,** *225,* 745–752.
King, G. L., and Johnson, S. M. Receptor mediated transport of insulin across endothelial cells. *Science,* **1985,** *219,* 865–869.
King, G. L.; and Kahn, C. R. Non-parallel evolution of metabolic and growth promoting functions of insulin. *Nature,* **1981,** *292,* 644–646.
Kitabchi, A. E.; Fisher, J. N.; Matteri, R.; and Murphy, M. B. The use of continuous insulin delivery systems in treatment of diabetes mellitus. *Adv. Intern. Med.,* **1983,** *28,* 449–490.
Kohner, E. M.; McLeod, D.; and Marshall, J. Diabetic eye disease. In, *Complications of Diabetes,* 2nd ed. (Keen, H., and Jarrett, D., eds.) Edward Arnold, London, **1982,** pp. 19–102.
Kolterman, O. G.; Gray, R. S.; Shapiro, G.; Scarlett, J. A.; Griffin, J.; and Olefsky, J. M. The acute and chronic effects of sulfonylurea therapy in type II diabetic subjects. *Diabetes,* **1984,** *33,* 346–354.
Leahy, J. L.; Cooper, H. E.; Deal, D. A.; and Weir, G. C. Chronic hyperglycemia is associated with impaired glucose influence on insulin secretion: a study in normal rats using chronic *in vivo* glucose infusions. *J. Clin. Invest.,* **1987,** *77,* 908–915.
Lee, T.-S.; Saltsman, K. A.; Ohashi, H.; and King, G. L. Activation of protein kinase C by elevation of glucose concentration: proposal for a mechanism in the development of vascular complications. *Proc. Natl. Acad. Sci. U.S.A.,* **1989,** *86,* 5141–5145.
Levin, S. R.; Charles, M. A.; O'Connor, M.; and Grodsky, G. M. Use of diphenylhydantoin and diazoxide to investigate insulin secretory mechanisms. *Am. J. Physiol.,* **1975,** *229,* 49–54.
Lewitt, M. S.; Yu, V. K.; Rennie, G. C.; Carter, J. N.; Marel, G. M.; Yue, D. K.; and Hooper, M. J. Effects of combined insulin-sulfonylurea therapy in Type II patients. *Diabetes Care,* **1989,** *12,* 379–383.
Longenecker, J. P.; Moses, A. C.; Flier, J. S.; Silver, R. D.; Carey, M. C.; and Dobovi, E. J. Effects of sodium taurodihydrofusidate on nasal absorption of insulin in sheep. *J. Pharm. Sci.,* **1987,** *76,* 351–355.
Lougheed, W. D.; Woulfe-Flanagan, H.; Clement, J. R.; and Albisser, A. M. Insulin aggregation in artificial delivery systems. *Diabetologia,* **1980,** *19,* 1–9.
Malone, J. L.; Lowitt, S.; Grove, N. P.; and Shah, S. C. A comparison of insulin levels after injection by jet stream and the disposable insulin syringe. *Diabetes Care,* **1986,** *9,* 637–640.
Markussen, J.; Diers, I.; Hougaard, P.; Langkjaer, L.; Norris, K.; Snel, L.; Sorensen, A. R.; Sorensen, E.; and Voight, H. O. Soluble, prolonged-acting insulin derivatives. III. Degree of protraction, crystallizability and chemical stability of insulins substituted in positions A21, B13, B23, B27 and B30. *Protein Engr.,* **1988,** *2,* 157–166.
Mato, J. M.; Kelly, K. L.; Abler, A.; and Jarett, L. Identification of a novel insulin-sensitive glycophospholipid in H35 hepatoma cells. *J. Biol. Chem.,* **1987,** *262,* 2131–2137.
Mauer, S. M.; Steffes, M. W.; Ellis, E. N.; Sutherland, D. E. R.; Brown, D. M.; and Goetz, F. C. Structural-functional relationships in diabetic nephropathy. *J. Clin. Invest.,* **1984,** *74,* 1143–1155.
Meienhofer, J.; Schnabel, E.; Bremer, H.; Brinkoff, O.; Zabel, R.; Sroka, W.; Klostermeyer, H.; Brandenburg, D.; Okuda, T.; and Zahn, H. Synthese der Insulinketten and ihre Kombination zu insulinaktiven Präparaten. *Z. Naturforsch.* [*B*], **1963,** *18,* 1120–1121.
Michael, A. F., and Brown, D. M. Increased concentration of albumin in kidney basement membranes in diabetes mellitus. *Diabetes,* **1981,** *30,* 843–846.
Minkowski, O. Historical development of the theory of pancreatic diabetes. (Introduction and translation by R. Levine). *Diabetes,* **1989,** *38,* 1–6.
Misler, S.; Gee, W. M.; Gillis, K. D.; Sharp, D. W.; and Falke, L. C. Metabolite-regulated ATP-sensitive K^+ channel in human pancreatic islet cells. *Diabetes,* **1989,** *38,* 422–427.
Mojsov, S. G.; Heinrich, G.; Wilson, I. B.; Ravazzola, M.; Orci, L.; and Habener, J. F. Preproglucagon gene expression in pancreas and intestine diversifies at the level of post-transcriptional processing. *J. Biol. Chem.,* **1986,** *261,* 11880–11889.
Mojsov, S.; Weir, G. C.; and Habener, J. F. Insulinotropin glucagon-like peptide I (7–37) co-encoded in the glucagon gene is a potent stimulus of insulin release in the perfused rat pancreas. *J. Clin. Invest.,* **1987,** *79,* 616–619.
Monsein, L. H.; Halpert, R. D.; Harris, E. D.; and Feczko, P. J. Retrograde ileography: value of glucagon. *Radiology,* **1986,** *161,* 558–559.
Mortensson, W.; Eklof, O.; and Laurin, S. Hydrostatic reduction of childhood intussusception. The role of adjuvant "glucagon" medication. *Acta Radiol.* [*Diagn.*], **1984,** *25,* 2361–2364.
Mueckler, M.; Caruso, C.; Baldwin, S. A.; Panico, M.; Blench, I.; Morris, H. R.; Allard, W. J.; Lienhard, G. E.; and Lodish, H. F. Sequence and structure of a human glucose transporter. *Science,* **1985,** *229,* 941–945.
Murphy, G. J.; Hruby, V. J.; Trivedi, D.; Wakelan, O. N. J. O.; and Houslay, M. D. The rapid desensitization of glucagon-stimulated adenylate cyclase is a cyclic AMP-independent process that can be mimicked by hormones which stimulate inositol phospholipid metabolism. *Biochem. J.,* **1987,** *243,* 39–46.
Nelson, T. Y.; Gaines, K. L.; Rajan, A. S.; Berg, M.; and Boyd, A. E., III. Increased cytosolic calcium: a signal for sulfonylurea-stimulated insulin release from beta cells. *J. Biol. Chem.,* **1987,** *262,* 2608–2612.
Olefsky, J. M., and Reaven, G. M. Effects of sulfonylureas therapy on insulin binding to mononuclear leukocytes of diabetic patients. *Am. J. Med.,* **1976,** *60,* 89–95.
Panteu, U.; Burgfeld, J.; Goerke, F.; Rennicke, M.; Schwanstecher, M.; Wallasch, A.; Zunkler, B. J.; and Lenzen, S. Control of insulin secretion by sulfonylureas, meglitinide and diazoxide in relation to their binding to the sulfonylurea receptor in pancreatic islets. *Biochem. Pharmacol.,* **1989,** *38,* 1217–1219.
Perriello, G.; DeFeo, P.; and Torlone, E. The effect of asymptomatic nocturnal hypoglycemia on glycemic control in diabetes mellitus. *N. Engl. J. Med.,* **1988,** *319,* 1233–1236.
Peterson, D. R.; Carone, F. A.; Oparil, S.; and Christensen, E. I. Differences between renal tubular processing of glucagon and insulin. *Am. J. Physiol.,* **1982,** *242,* F112–F118.
Pfeifer, M. A.; Halter, J. B.; Beard, J. C.; and Porte, D. J. Differential effects of tolbutamide on first and second phase insulin secretion in non-insulin-dependent diabetes mellitus. *J. Clin. Endocrinol. Metab.,* **1981,** *53,* 1256–1262.
Pilkis, S. J.; El-Maghrabi, M. R.; Pilkis, J.; and Claus, T. H. Fructose-2,6-bisphosphate: a new activator of phosphofructokinase. *J. Biol. Chem.,* **1981,** *256,* 3171–3177.

Pirart, J. Diabetes mellitus and its degenerative complications: prospective study of 4,400 patients observed between 1947 and 1973. *Diabetes Care*, **1978**, *1*, 168–188, 252–263.
Pullen, R. A., and others. Receptor-binding region of insulin. *Nature*, **1976**, *259*, 369–373.
Pyke, D. A. Genetics of diabetes. *J. Clin. Endocrinol. Metab.*, **1977**, *6*, 285–303.
Rabkin, R.; Ryan, M. P.; and Duckworth, W. C. The renal metabolism of insulin. *Diabetologia*, **1984**, *27*, 351–357.
Ribalet, B., and Ciani, S. Regulation by cell metabolism and adenine nucleotides of a K^+ channel in insulin-secreting beta-cells (RIN M5F). *Proc. Natl. Acad. Sci. U.S.A.*, **1987**, *85*, 1721–1725.
Riddle, M. C. New tactics for Type II diabetes: regimens based on intermediate-acting insulin taken at bedtime. *Lancet*, **1985**, *1*, 192–195.
Rinderknecht, E., and Humbel, R. E. The amino acid sequence of human insulin-like growth factor I and its structural homology with proinsulin. *J. Biol. Chem.*, **1978a**, *253*, 2769–2773.
———. Primary structure of human insulin-like growth factor II. *FEBS Lett.*, **1978b**, *89*, 283–289.
Romero, G.; Luttrell, L.; Rogol, A.; Keller, K.; Hewlett, E.; and Larner, J. Phosphatidylinositol-glycan anchors of membrane proteins: potential precursors of insulin mediators. *Science*, **1988**, *240*, 509–511.
Roth, R. A., and Beaudoin, J. Phosphorylation of purified insulin receptors by cAMP kinase. *Diabetes*, **1987**, *36*, 123–126.
Salzman, R., and others. Intranasal aerosolized insulin: mixed meal studies and long-term use in Type I diabetes. *N. Engl. J. Med.*, **1985**, *312*, 1078–1082.
Samols, E.; Bonner-Weir, S.; and Weir, G. C. Intra-islet insulin-glucagon somatostatin relationships. *J. Clin. Endocrinol. Metab.*, **1986**, *15*, 53–58.
Schade, D. S., and Duckworth, W. C. In search of subcutaneous insulin resistance syndrome. *N. Engl. J. Med.*, **1986**, *315*, 147–153.
Schmid-Anatomarchi, H.; De Weile, J.; Fosset, M.; and Lazdunski, M. The receptor for the antidiabetic sulfonylureas controls the activity of the ATP-modulated K^+ channel. *J. Biol. Chem.*, **1987**, *262*, 15840–15844.
Schwartz, G. P.; Burke, G. T.; and Katsoyannis, P. G. A highly potent insulin: des(B26-B30)-[Asp^{B10}, Tyr^{B25}-NH_2]insulin (human). *Proc. Natl. Acad. Sci. U.S.A.*, **1989**, *86*, 458–461.
Shargill, N. S.; Tatoyan, A.; Fukushima, M.; Antwi, D.; Bray, G. A.; and Chan, T. M. Effect of ciglitazone on glucose uptake and insulin sensitivity in skeletal muscle of the obese (ob/ob) mouse: distinct insulin and glucocorticoid effects. *Metabolism*, **1986**, *35*, 64–70.
Sheetz, M. J., and Tager, H. S. Receptor-linked proteolysis of membrane-bound glucagon yields a membrane-associated hormone fragment. *J. Biol. Chem.*, **1988**, *263*, 8509–8514.
Shii, K., and Roth, R. A. Inhibition of insulin degradation by hepatoma cells after microinjections of monoclonal antibodies to a specific cytosolic protease. *Proc. Natl. Acad. Sci. U.S.A.*, **1986**, *83*, 4147–4151.
Shimazu, T., and Ishikawa, K. Modulation by the hypothalamus of glucagon and insulin secretion in rabbits: studies with electrical and chemical stimulations. *Endocrinology*, **1981**, *108*, 605–611.
Simonson, D. C.; Delprato, S.; Castellino, P.; Groop, L. and DeFronzo, R. A. Effect of glyburide on glycemic control, insulin requirements, and glucose metabolism in insulin-treated diabetic patients. *Diabetes*, **1987**, *36*, 136–142.
Sodoyez, J. C.; Sodoyez-Goffaux, F.; Guillaume, M.; and Merchie, G. ^{123}I-insulin metabolism in normal rats and humans: external detection by a scintillation camera. *Science*, **1983**, *219*, 865–868.
Srikanta, S.; Ganda, O. P.; Jackson, R. A.; Gleason, R. E.; Kaldany, A.; Garovoy, M. R.; Milford, E. L.; Carpenter, C. B.; Soeldner, J. S.; and Eisenbarth, G. S. Type I diabetes mellitus in monozygotic twins: chronic progressive beta cell dysfunction. *Ann. Intern. Med.*, **1983**, *99*, 320–326.
Sutherland, D. E. R.; Moudry, K. C.; and Fryd, D. S. Results of pancreas transplant registry. *Diabetes*, **1989**, *38*, Suppl. 1, 46–54.
Suzuki, K., and Kono, T. Evidence that insulin causes translocation of glucose transport activity of the plasma membrane from an intracellular storage site. *Proc. Natl. Acad. Sci. U.S.A.*, **1980**, *77*, 2542–2545.
Takayama, S.; White, M. F.; and Kahn, C. R. Phorbol ester induced serine phosphorylation of the insulin receptor decreases its tyrosine kinase activity. *J. Biol. Chem.*, **1988**, *263*, 3440–3447.
Thorens, B.; Sarker, H. K.; Kaback, H. R.; and Lodish, H. F. Cloning and functional expression in bacteria of a novel glucose transporter present in liver, intestine, kidney and β-pancreatic islet cells. *Cell*, **1988**, *55*, 281–291.
Todd, J. A.; Bell, J. F.; and McDevitt, H. O. HLA-DQ_β gene contributes to susceptibility and resistance to insulin-dependent diabetes mellitus. *Nature*, **1987**, *329*, 599–604.
Ullrich, A., and others. Human insulin receptor and its relationship to the tyrosine kinase family of oncogenes. *Nature*, **1985**, *313*, 756–761.
University Group Diabetes Program. A story of the effects of hypoglycemic agents on vascular complications in patients with adult-onset diabetes. II. Mortality results. *Diabetes*, **1970**, *19*, 789–830.
Unson, C. G. Gurzenda, E. M.; Iwasa, K.; and Merrifield, R. B. Glucagon antagonists: contributions to binding and activity of the amino terminal sequence 1–5, position 12, and the putative α-helical segment of 19–27. *J. Biol. Chem.*, **1989**, *264*, 789–794.
Varandani, P. T.; Shroyer, L. A.; and Nafz, M. A. Sequential degradation of insulin by rat liver homogenates. *Proc. Natl. Acad. Sci. U.S.A.*, **1972**, *69*, 1681–1685.
Vigneri, R.; Pezzino, V.; Wong, K. Y.; and Goldfine, I. D. Comparison of the *in vitro* effects of biguanides and sulfonylureas on insulin binding to its receptors in target cells. *J. Clin. Endocrinol. Metab.*, **1982**, *54*, 95–101.
Vora, J. P.; Owens, D. R.; Dolben, J.; Atiea, J. A.; Dean, J. D.; Kang, S.; Burch, A.; and Brange, J. Recombinant DNA derived monomeric insulin analogue: comparison with soluble human insulin in normal subjects. *Br. Med. J.*, **1988**, *297*, 1236–1239.
Waldhausl, W.; Bratusch-Marrain, P.; Gasic, S.; Korn, A.; and Nowotny, P. Insulin production rate following glucose ingestion estimated by splanchnic C-peptide output in normal man. *Diabetologia*, **1979**, *17*, 221–227.
Wheatly, T., and Edwards, O. M. Insulin edema and its clinical significance: metabolic studies in three cases. *Diabetic Med.*, **1985**, *2*, 400–406.
White, M. F.; Maron, R.; and Kahn, C. R. Insulin rapidly stimulates tyrosine phosphorylation of a Mr-185,000 protein in intact cells. *Nature*, **1985**, *318*, 183–186.
White M. F.; Shoelson, S. E.; Keutmann, H.; and Kahn, C. R. A cascade of tyrosine autophosphorylation in the β-subunit activates the phosphotransferase of the insulin receptor. *J. Biol. Chem.*, **1988**, *263*, 2969–2980.
Wolf, B. A.; Colca, J. R.; Turk, J.; Florholmen, J.; and McDaniel, M. L. Regulation of Ca^{2+} homeostasis by islet endoplasmic reticulum and its role in insulin secretion. *Am. J. Physiol.*, **1988**, *254*, E121–E136.
Yalow, R. S. Radioimmunoassay: a probe for the fine

structure of biological systems (Nobel lecture). *Science,* **1978,** *200,* 1236–1245.

Yoon, J. W.; Austin, M.; Onodera, T.; and Notkins, A. L. Virus-induced diabetes mellitus: isolation of a virus from the pancreas of a child with diabetic ketoacidosis. *N. Engl. J. Med.,* **1979,** *300,* 1173–1179.

Monographs and Reviews

Bernstein, R. E. Nonenzymatically glycosylated proteins. *Adv. Clin. Chem.,* **1987,** *26,* 1–78.

Bliss, M. *The Discovery of Insulin.* University of Chicago Press, Chicago, **1982.**

Blundell, T. L., and Humbel, R. E. Hormone families: pancreatic hormones and homologous growth factors. *Nature,* **1980,** *287,* 781–787.

Boyd, A. E., III. Sulfonylurea receptors, ion channels, and fruit flies. *Diabetes,* **1988,** *37,* 847–850.

Brownlee, M., and Cerami, A. The biochemistry of the complications of diabetes mellitus. *Annu. Rev. Biochem.,* **1981,** *50,* 385–432.

Brownlee, M.; Cerami, A.; and Vlassara, H. Advanced products of nonenzymatic glycosylation and the pathogenesis of diabetes vascular disease. *Diabetes Metab. Rev.,* **1988,** *4,* 437–451.

Burg, M. B., and Kador, P. F. Sorbitol, osmoregulation, and the complications of diabetes. *J. Clin. Invest.,* **1988,** *81,* 635–640.

Czech, M. P. The nature and regulation of the insulin receptor: structure and function. *Annu. Rev. Physiol.,* **1985,** *47,* 357–381.

Daughaday, W. H., and Rotwein, P. Insulin-like growth factors I and II. Peptide messenger ribonucleic acid and gene structures, serum and tissue concentrations. *Endocr. Rev.,* **1989,** *10,* 68–91.

Dotta, F., and Eisenbarth, G. S. Type I diabetes mellitus: a predictable autoimmune disease with interindividual variation in the rate of B cell destruction. *Clin. Immunol.,* **1989,** *50,* 585–595.

Duckworth, W. C. Insulin degradation: mechanisms, products and significance. *Endocr. Rev.,* **1988,** *9,* 319–345.

Duronio, V., and Jacobs, S. Comparison of insulin and IGF-I receptors. In, *Insulin Receptors.* Part B. *Clinical Assessment, Biological Responses and Comparison to the IGF-I Receptor.* (Kahn, C. R., and Harrison, L. C., eds.) Alan R. Liss, Inc., New York, **1988,** pp. 3–18.

Ebert, R., and Creutzfeld, W. Gastrointestinal peptides and insulin secretion. *Diabetes Metab. Rev.,* **1987,** *3,* 1–26.

Ferner, R. E. Oral hypoglycemic agents. *Med. Clin. North Am.,* **1988,** *72,* 1323–1335.

Fleischer, N., and Erlichman, J. Intracellular signals and protein phosphorylation: regulatory mechanisms in the control of insulin secretion from the pancreatic B cells. In, *Insulin Secretion,* Vol. I. (Draznin, B.; Melmed, S.; and LeRoith, D.; eds.) Alan R. Liss, Inc., New York, **1989,** pp. 107–116.

Foster, D. W. From glycogen to ketones and back. *Diabetes,* **1984,** *33,* 1188–1199.

Galloway, J. A.; Spradlin, C. T.; Jackson, R. L.; Ollo, D. C.; and Bechtel, L. D. Mixture of intermediate acting insulin (NPH and lente) with regular insulin: an update. In, *Insulin Update, 1982.* (Skyler, J. S., ed.) Proceedings of a Symposium. Excerpta Medica, Amsterdam, **1982,** pp. 111–119.

Gammeltoft, S. Insulin receptors: binding kinetics and structure–function relationship of insulin. *Physiol. Rev.,* **1984,** *64,* 1321–1378.

Gerich, J. E. Glucose counter-regulation and its impact on diabetes mellitus. *Diabetes,* **1988,** *37,* 1608–1617.

Goldberg, H. I., and Thoeni, R. F. MRI of the gastrointestinal tract. *Radiol. Clin. North Am.,* **1989,** *27,* 805–812.

Granner, D. K. The molecular biology of insulin action on protein synthesis. *Kidney Int.* [*Suppl.*], **1987,** *23,* 582–596.

Granner, D. K.; Sasaki, K.; and Chu, D. Multihormonal regulation of phosphoenolpyruvate carboxykinase gene transcription: the dominant role of insulin. *Ann. N.Y. Acad. Sci.,* **1986,** *478,* 175–190.

Green, D. A.; Lattimer, S. A.; and Sima, S. S. Sorbitol, phosphoinositides and sodium-potassium ATPase in the pathogenesis of diabetic complications. *N. Engl. J. Med.,* **1987,** *316,* 599–606.

Hellman, B. Calcium transport in the pancreatic β-cell: implications for glucose regulation of insulin release. *Diabetes Metab. Rev.,* **1986,** *2,* 215–242.

Hellman, B., and Taljedal, I. B. Effects of sulfonylurea derivatives in pancreatic β-cells. In, *Insulin II. Handbook of Experimental Pharmacology,* Vol. 32, Part 2. (Hasselblatt, A. V., and Bruchhausen, F. V., eds.) Springer Verlag, Berlin, **1975,** pp. 175–194.

Hermann, L. S. Metformin: a review of its pharmacological properties and therapeutic use. *Diabetic Metab.,* **1979,** *5,* 233–245.

Hodgkin, D. C., and Mercola, D. The secondary and tertiary structure of insulin. In, *Endocrine Pancreas.* Vol. 1, Sect. 7, *Endocrinology. Handbook of Physiology.* (Steiner, D. F., and Freinkel, N., eds.) American Physiological Society, Washington, D.C., **1972,** pp. 139–157.

Kahn, C. R., and Rosenthal, A. S. Immunologic reactions to insulin: insulin allergy, insulin resistance, and the autoimmune insulin syndrome. *Diabetes Care,* **1979,** *2,* 283–295.

Kahn, C. R., and White, M. F. The insulin receptor and the molecular mechanism of insulin action. *J. Clin. Invest.,* **1988,** *82,* 1151–1156.

Karam, J. H., and Etzweiler, D. D. (eds.). International Symposium on Human Insulin. *Diabetes Care,* **1983,** *6,* Suppl. 1, 1–68.

Kimball, S. R., and Jefferson, L. S. Cellular mechanisms involved in the action of insulin in protein synthesis. *Diabetes Metab. Rev.,* **1988,** *4,* 773–787.

Kitabchi, A. E. Low-dose insulin therapy in diabetic ketoacidosis: fact or fiction. *Diabetes Metab. Rev.,* **1989,** *5,* 337–363.

Koffler, M.; Ramirez, L. C.; and Raskin, P. The effect of many commonly used drugs on diabetic control. *Diabetes, Nutrition, and Metabolism,* **1989,** *2,* 75–93.

Kolterman, O. G. The impact of sulfonylureas on hepatic glucose metabolism in type II diabetics. *Diabetes Metab. Rev.,* **1987,** *3,* 399–414.

Krall, L. P. Oral hypoglycemic agents. In, *Joslin's Diabetes Mellitus,* 12th ed. (Marble, A.; Krall, L. P.; Bradley, R. F.; Christlieb, A. R.; and Soeldner, J. S.; eds.) Lea & Febiger, Philadelphia, **1985,** pp. 412–452.

Lebovitz, H. E., and Feinglos, M. N. The oral hypoglycemic agents. In, *Diabetes Mellitus, Theory and Practice,* 3rd ed. (Ellenberg, M., and Rifkin, H., eds.) Medical Examination Publishing, New Hyde Park, New York, **1983,** pp. 591–610.

Low, M. G., and Saltiel, A. R. Structural and functional roles of glycosyl-phosphatidylinositol in membranes. *Science,* **1988,** *239,* 268–275.

Malaisse, W. J. Stimulus-secretion coupling in the pancreatic B-cell: the cholinergic pathway for insulin release. *Diabetes Metab. Rev.,* **1986,** *2,* 243–259.

Marble, A.; Krall, L. P.; Bradley, R. F.; Christlieb, A. R.; and Soeldner, J. S. (eds.). *Joslin's Diabetes Mellitus,* 12th ed., Lea & Febiger, Philadelphia, **1985.**

Meglasson, M. D., and Matschinsky, F. M. Pancreatic islet glucose metabolism and regulation of insulin secretion. *Diabetes Metab. Rev.,* **1986,** *2,* 163–214.

Nerup, J.; Christy, M.; Patz, P.; Ryder, L. P.; and Suejgaard, A. Aspects of the genetics of insulin dependent diabetes mellitus. In, *Immunology in Diabetes.*

(Adreani, D.; Dimario, R.; Federlin, K. F.; and Hedings, L. G.; eds.) Medical Publications, Kimpton, London, **1984**, pp. 63–70.

Orci, L. The insulin cell: its cellular environment and how it processes (pro)insulin. *Diabetes Metab. Rev.*, **1986**, *2*, 71–106.

Owen, D. R. *Human Insulin*. MTP Press, Lancaster, England, **1986**.

Paice, B. J.; Patterson, K. R.; and Lawson, D. H. Undesired effects of sulfonylurea drugs. *Adverse Drug React. Acute Poisoning Rev.*, **1985**, *1*, 23–36.

Polonsky, K. S., and Rubenstein, A. H. Current approaches to measurement of insulin secretion. *Diabetes Metab. Rev.*, **1986**, *2*, 315–329.

Porte, D., Jr., and Halter, J. B. The endocrine pancreas and diabetes mellitus. In, *Textbook of Endocrinology*, 6th ed. (Williams, R. H., ed.) W. B. Saunders Co., Philadelphia, **1981**, pp. 716–843.

Reichlin, S. Somatostatin. (Parts I and II.) *N. Engl. J. Med.*, **1983**, *309*, 1495–1503, 1556–1563.

Robbins, D. C.; Tager, H. S.; and Rubenstein, A. H. Biologic and clinical importance of proinsulin. *N. Engl. J. Med.*, **1984**, *310*, 1165–1175.

Rosen, O. M. After insulin binds. *Science*, **1987**, *237*, 1452–1458.

Schade, D. S., and Eaton, R. P. Diabetic ketoacidosis—pathogenesis, prevention and therapy. *Clin. Endocrinol. Metab.*, **1983**, *12*, 321–338.

Schade, D. S.; Santiago, J. V.; Skyler, J. S.; and Rizza, R. A. *Intensive Insulin Therapy*. Medical Examination Publishing Co., Amsterdam, **1983**.

Schein, P. S.; DeLellis, R. A.; Kahn, C. R.; Gorden, P.; and Kraft, A. R. Islet cell tumors: current concepts and management. *Ann. Intern. Med.*, **1973**, *79*, 239–257.

Seltzer, H. S. Drug-induced hypoglycemia. *Endocrinol. Metab. Clin. North Am.*, **1989**, *18*, 163–183.

Simpson, I. A., and Cushman, S. W. Hormonal regulation of mammalian glucose transport. *Annu. Rev. Biochem.*, **1986**, *55*, 1059–1089.

Skyler, J. S. Insulin pharmacology. *Med. Clin North Am.*, **1988**, *72*, 1337–1354.

Tager, H. Abnormal products of the human insulin gene. *Diabetes*, **1984**, *33*, 693–699.

Taskinen, M. R. Lipoprotein lipase in diabetes. *Diabetes Metab. Rev.*, **1987**, *3*, 551–570.

Unger, R. H. Glucagon in diabetes. In, *Diabetes Annual*, Vol. I. (Alberti, K. G. M. M., and Krall, L. P., eds.) Elsevier Publishing Co., Amsterdam, **1985a**, pp. 480–491.

———. Glucagon physiology and pathophysiology in the light of new advances. *Diabetologia*, **1985b**, *28*, 574–578.

Unger, R. H., and Orci, L. Glucagon and the A cell (Parts I and II). *N. Engl. J. Med.*, **1981**, *304*, 1518–1524, 1575–1580.

Weir, G. C.; Leahy, J. L.; and Bonner-Weir, S. Experimental reduction of B-cell mass: implication for the pathogenesis of diabetes. *Diabetes Metab. Rev.*, **1986**, *2*, 125–161.

Weir, G. C.; Samols, E.; Loo, S.; Patel, Y. C.; and Gabbay, K. H. Somatostatin and pancreatic polypeptide secretion. Effects of glucagon, insulin and arginine. *Diabetes*, **1979**, *28*, 35–41.

Yarden, Y., and Ullrich, A. Growth factor receptor tyrosine kinases. *Annu. Rev. Biochem.*, **1988**, *57*, 443–478.

CHAPTER

62 AGENTS AFFECTING CALCIFICATION: CALCIUM, PARATHYROID HORMONE, CALCITONIN, VITAMIN D, AND OTHER COMPOUNDS

Robert C. Haynes, Jr.

CALCIUM

Calcium is the fifth most abundant element in the body, and the major portion is in bone. It is present in small quantities in the extracellular fluid and to a minor extent in the structure and cytoplasm of cells of soft tissues. Ca^{2+} plays important physiological roles, many of which are not completely understood. It is essential for the functional integrity of nerve and muscle, where it has a major influence on excitability and release of neurotransmitters. It is necessary for muscle contraction, cardiac function, maintenance of the integrity of membranes, and coagulation of the blood. In addition, Ca^{2+} mediates the intracellular actions of many hormones.

To carry out these various roles, Ca^{2+} must be available to the appropriate tissues in the proper concentration. As is the case for other essential constituents of the body, an endocrine control system has evolved that ordinarily keeps the plasma concentration of Ca^{2+} within narrow limits. This is accomplished by placing controls at the site of entry of Ca^{2+} into the system (intestinal absorption) and at a site of exit (the kidney), and by keeping a large store (the skeleton) accessible for deposits or withdrawals depending upon peripheral demand. Intracellular concentrations of Ca^{2+} are also strictly regulated by control of the exchange of the ion between the cell and its environment and between intracellular compartments. Drugs that affect organ function by blocking Ca^{2+} channels in the plasma membrane are discussed in Chapter 32.

This chapter will describe the roles of Ca^{2+} and three endocrine factors that control its metabolism: parathyroid hormone (PTH), calcitonin, and vitamin D. The actions of these hormones can be summarized as follows.

PTH is secreted in response to a fall in plasma Ca^{2+} concentration, and the hormone acts to restore Ca^{2+} to its normal concentration range by accelerating its transfer from the bone compartment, enhancing its intestinal absorption, and increasing its reabsorption by the kidney. In addition, PTH promotes phosphate excretion in the urine. The secretion of calcitonin can be stimulated by a rise in the concentration of Ca^{2+} in plasma; this hormone lowers plasma Ca^{2+} by decreasing bone resorption and by increasing renal excretion of the ion. Vitamin D, now recognized as a hormone, stimulates intestinal absorption of Ca^{2+} and phosphate and decreases their renal excretion; it also enhances resorption of bone.

Calcium Requirements and Body Stores. The Ca^{2+} intake varies from 200 to 2500 mg per day, and, in the United States, the predominant source is dairy products. Recommended daily dietary allowances (United States) are presented in Table XVI–1 (page 1525) (*see also* Nordin *et al.,* 1979). The skeleton contains more than 90% of the body's Ca^{2+} stores. The inorganic salts of bone resemble the mineral hydroxyapatite $[Ca_{10}(PO_4)_6(OH)_2]$. Bone crystals are not pure, however, and contain additional ions in the crystal lattice and in association with the crystals. These include Na^+, K^+, Mg^{2+}, CO_3^{2-}, and F^-. The steady-state content of Ca^{2+} in the skeleton is a consequence of the net effect of bone resorption and new-bone formation, and the Ca^{2+} of bone is in a constant exchange with that of the interstitial fluids. The rates of exchange can be modified by drugs, hormones, vitamins, and other factors that influence the level of Ca^{2+} in the interstitial fluids and also the forms in which the cation is present.

In plasma, Ca^{2+} is maintained at a fairly constant concentration of about 2.5 mM (5.0 mEq/l; 10 mg/dl). However, this represents the total of three different components: (1) about 40% of the plasma Ca^{2+} is bound to proteins, primarily albumin; (2) about 10% is diffusible but complexed with anions (*e.g.*, citrate and phosphate); and (3) the remaining fraction represents diffusible ionic calcium. The ionized calcium is the fraction that exerts physiological effects, and symptoms of hypocalcemia occur with its reduction. It is clear that hypocalcemia due to hypoproteinemia and a reduced concentration of protein-bound Ca^{2+} is not likely to be accompanied by the symptoms and signs of hypocalcemia unless the concentration of free Ca^{2+} is reduced as well. Hence, the interpretation of the significance of any given value of plasma Ca^{2+} is impossible without knowledge of the coincident concentration of plasma proteins, and nomograms are available for this purpose. As an approximation, an alteration in plasma albumin of 10 g/l (from a normal value of 40 to 44 g/l) can be expected to change total Ca^{2+} by 0.8 mg/dl (0.2 mM).

Absorption and Excretion. In general, the major portion of intestinal absorption takes place in the more proximal segments of the small bowel; in man, approximately one third of ingested Ca^{2+} is absorbed. Intestinal absorption involves the soluble ionized form of calcium and reflects at least two separate steps: (1) Ca^{2+} uptake at the mucosal pole and (2) efflux at the serosal pole of the intestinal epithelium. Mucosal uptake of Ca^{2+} is thought to be mediated either by Ca^{2+}-specific channels or by a carrier, but the mechanism has not been clarified. Ca^{2+} is extruded from the intestinal cells by a Ca^{2+}/Mg^{2+}-ATPase at the serosal membrane (Bronner, 1988).

The factors that clearly augment absorption of Ca^{2+}—vitamin D and PTH—are discussed below. It is also generally accepted that a diet low in Ca^{2+} results in increased fractional absorption of the ion.

Glucocorticoids and other factors depress Ca^{2+} transport across the small intestine. For example, phytate, oxalate, and probably phosphate in the bowel promote the formation of a complex or insoluble salt of Ca^{2+} that is not absorbed through the wall of the gut. Disease states such as steatorrhea may result in decreased absorption of the ion. Other diarrheas with chronic gastrointestinal malabsorption may promote increased fecal losses of Ca^{2+} as well.

Ca^{2+} is released into the gastrointestinal tract in saliva, bile, and pancreatic and intestinal secretions. This endogenous Ca^{2+} and the unabsorbed dietary Ca^{2+} constitute the sources of the cation excreted in the feces. Significant amounts of Ca^{2+} are lost in milk during lactation; sweat also accounts for daily losses.

The urinary excretion of Ca^{2+} is the net result of the quantity filtered and the amount reabsorbed. There is no evidence of renal tubular secretion of Ca^{2+}. The mechanisms for the renal reabsorption of Ca^{2+} are unknown, and for unexplained reasons there is, in general, a correlation between the urinary excretion of Na^{+} and Ca^{2+}. This is true when natriuresis is increased by loading with salt, and it also is noted with diuretics that act at the ascending limb of the loop of Henle. In animal studies approximately two thirds of the filtered Ca^{2+} is reabsorbed in the proximal convolution, 20 to 25% in the loop of Henle, and 10% in the distal convolution.

PTH stimulates renal reabsorption of Ca^{2+} apparently by means of an effect on the distal tubule. Although the active metabolites of vitamin D may stimulate proximal tubular reabsorption of Ca^{2+}, their principal effects on urinary excretion of Ca^{2+} appear to be indirect. Calcitonin inhibits the proximal tubular reabsorption of Ca^{2+}, thus facilitating excretion of the cation.

The influence of renal disease on urinary excretion of Ca^{2+} is variable. In chronic renal failure due primarily to glomerular disease, Ca^{2+} excretion diminishes as filtration rate falls. However, in those instances where filtration is only minimally depressed and the secretion of H^{+} is deficient due to an inability to attain a high concentration gradient for H^+ between tubular cell and lumen (renal tubular acidosis), the excretion of Ca^{2+} may be enhanced. This hypercalciuria may be diminished by the correction of the systemic acidosis. The renal excretion of Ca^{2+} has been reviewed by Peacock (1988).

PHYSIOLOGICAL AND PHARMACOLOGICAL ACTIONS

The cytoplasmic concentration of Ca^{2+} is normally maintained at very low values (~0.1 to 1 μM) by the extrusion of the ion from the cell and by its sequestration within cellular organelles, particularly the endoplasmic reticulum and, in muscle, the sarcoplasmic reticulum. The provocative hypothesis has been offered that the need for such transport systems arose in evolution when cells accumulated high concentrations of phosphate for use in energy metabolism (*see* Kretsinger, 1976). (The solubility product of calcium phosphate is very low.) Given the high gradient of Ca^{2+} between extracellular and intracellular compartments, use can be made of the ion in mechanisms for transmembrane signaling. Thus, in response to various electrical or chemical stimuli, Ca^{2+} influx across the plasma membrane or release from internal stores is triggered. This Ca^{2+} interacts with high-affinity binding sites on specific intracellular proteins (such as troponin or calmodulin) and thereby regulates a number of functional and metabolic processes of the cell.

Local Actions. Certain salts of Ca^{2+}, notably the chloride, are intensely irritating to tissue and will cause painful sloughing if injected subcutaneously. Therefore, whenever calcium chloride is administered parenterally, it must be given intravenously and every effort should be made to prevent extravasation.

Neuromuscular System. Moderate elevations of the concentration of Ca^{2+} in the extracellular fluid may have no clinically detectable influences on the neuromuscular apparatus. However, when hypercalcemia becomes extreme, the threshold for excitation of nerve and muscle is increased. This is manifested clinically by muscle weakness, lethargy, and eventually coma. In contrast, modest diminution in the concentration of Ca^{2+} may decrease the thresholds of excitation in a striking fashion, leading to positive Chvostek and Trousseau signs and tetanic seizures. The role played by Ca^{2+} in regulating the excitability of tissues is not completely understood. The influx of Ca^{2+} across the plasma membrane is thought to be by means of carrier-mediated facilitated diffusion and by exchange of Ca^{2+} for Na^+, which participates both in excitation and in the maintenance of the steady state. Several Ca^{2+} channels in cell membranes are regulated by hormones and other ligands as well as by membrane potential. However, in liver and skeletal muscle, the concentration of cytoplasmic Ca^{2+} is not controlled by cellular influx and efflux to nearly the same extent that it is by the endoplasmic reticulum and the sarcoplasmic reticulum, which sequester intracellular Ca^{2+}. Changes in extracellular Ca^{2+} cause relatively small changes in resting membrane potentials but modify the time–voltage relationships during the action potential in nerve and muscle. In addition, Ca^{2+} appears to play an important role in the regulation of cell-membrane permeability to Na^+ and K^+.

Ca^{2+} plays an important role in coupling excitation with muscle contraction. The action potential in muscle stimulates the release of Ca^{2+} from the sarcoplasmic reticulum, and the cation activates contraction. The binding of Ca^{2+} to troponin abolishes the inhibitory effect of troponin on the interaction of actin and myosin. Muscle relaxation occurs when Ca^{2+} is pumped back into the sarcoplasmic reticulum, restoring the inhibitory effect of troponin on actin and myosin.

Ca^{2+} is necessary for exocytosis and thus has an important role in stimulus–secretion coupling in most exocrine and endocrine glands. The release of catecholamines from the adrenal medulla, neurotransmitters at synapses, and certain autacoids (*e.g.*, histamine from mast cells) is dependent on Ca^{2+}.

There is an important interrelation between Ca^{2+} and K^+. A deficiency in K^+ coincident with hypocalcemia appears to protect against hypocalcemic tetany. Correction of the deficit of K^+ without attention to the level of Ca^{2+} may provoke tetany without a change in the concentration of Ca^{2+} in plasma.

Cardiovascular System. Ca^{2+} is essential for excitation–contraction coupling in cardiac muscle, as well as for the conduction of electrical impulses in certain regions of the heart, particularly through the AV node. Depolarization of myocardial fibers opens voltage-regulated Ca^{2+} channels and causes the "slow" inward current that occurs during the plateau of the action potential. This current allows the permeation of Ca^{2+} sufficient to trigger the release of additional Ca^{2+} from the sarcoplasmic reticulum, thereby causing contraction. The passage of Ca^{2+} through similar channels in tissues such as the AV node carries virtually all the inward (depolarizing) current during the action potential.

Ca^{2+} is responsible for the initiation of contraction in vascular and other smooth muscles, and it frequently carries an important fraction of depolarizing currents in these tissues. Hence Ca^{2+}-channel blockers have profound effects on the contractility of cardiac and vascular smooth muscle as well as on the conduction of impulses within the heart. These drugs have important uses in the treatment of angina, cardiac arrhythmias, and hypertension (*see* Chapters 32, 33, and 35).

Miscellaneous Effects. Ca^{2+} plays a role in maintaining the integrity of mucosal membranes, cell adhesion, and functions of individual cell membranes as well. The use of calcium salts to prevent effusions across capillary endothelial membranes is, however, without demonstrated benefit. Ca^{2+} is involved in blood coagulation, but the ion is not used to treat disorders of coagulation. Calcium chloride is an acidifying salt and will promote diuresis; however, ammonium salts are much more effective acidifying agents.

ABNORMALITIES OF CALCIUM METABOLISM

It should be clear from the discussion of some of the factors involved in maintaining Ca^{2+} homeostasis that there are many ways by which significant alterations in Ca^{2+} metabolism can occur. Some of these alterations may be accompanied by hypocalcemia, and others by hypercalcemia.

Hypocalcemic States. The prominent signs and symptoms of hypocalcemia include tetany and related phenomena such as paresthesias, increased neuromuscular excitability, laryngospasm, muscle cramps, and convulsions (usually tonic–clonic). Some causes of hypocalcemia are discussed below.

Deprivation of Ca^{2+} and vitamin D may readily promote hypocalcemia. This combination of events is observed in the various malabsorption states and also occurs from inadequate diets. When due to malabsorption, the hypocalcemia is accompanied by a depressed level of phosphate; total plasma proteins are usually low, and hypomagnesemia is common. During Mg^{2+} deficiency, hypocalcemia may be accentuated by diminished secretion and action of PTH (*see* below). Hypocalcemia stimulates the release of PTH, which causes the mobilization of Ca^{2+} from bone and demineralization. In infants with malabsorption or inadequate Ca^{2+} intake, Ca^{2+} concentrations are usually depressed, there is hypophosphatemia, and the resultant bone disease is rickets (*see* section on vitamin D).

Hypoparathyroidism may occur spontaneously as a result of a genetic disorder or as a consequence of thyroid or other neck surgery. In these disorders there is distinct hypocalcemia but *hyper*phosphatemia. Although other conditions of hypocalcemia may be associated with opacity of the lens, papilledema, and calcification of the basal ganglia, these conditions occur more commonly with hypoparathyroidism. Other changes include trophic alterations and fungal infections of the skin. Pseudohypoparathyroidism is a group of genetic diseases characterized by multiple structural defects and a failure to respond to exogenous PTH. The structural changes are manifested by a round face; short, thick figure; shortening of some of the metacarpal and metatarsal bones; and soft-tissue calcifications. As discussed below, at least one variety of this disease results from a deficiency of calcitriol (1,25-dihydroxycholecalciferol). In other individuals with pseudohypoparathyroidism there is a deficiency of the stimulatory guanine nucleotide–binding regulatory component of adenylyl cyclase. Pseudohypoparathyroidism has been reviewed recently by Hosking and Kerr (1988).

In the period (1 to 4 days) following removal of a parathyroid adenoma, hypocalcemia is not unusual, especially if bone disease is present.

Neonatal tetany may result from a temporary hypoparathyroidism that occurs in the newborn of mothers with hyperparathyroidism; indeed, it may be the infant's tetany that provides the clue to the mother's disorder. This problem is usually transient in the infant and disappears as soon as the infant's own parathyroid glands respond appropriately. Other situations in which neonatal hypocalcemia may supervene include hypernatremia and acute infections.

Hypocalcemia is frequently associated with advanced renal insufficiency accompanied by hyperphosphatemia. For reasons that are not clear, many patients with this condition do not develop tetany unless the severe accompanying acidosis is improved with treatment. High concentrations of phosphate in plasma appear to inhibit the conversion of 25-hydroxycholecalciferol to 1,25-dihydroxycholecalciferol (Haussler and McCain, 1977). Excessive use of potassium phosphate in the treatment of diabetic ketoacidosis can cause hypocalcemia and hypomagnesemia; potassium chloride is preferred.

Sodium fluoride forms an insoluble salt with Ca^{2+} and, if ingested in large enough quantities, may induce hypocalcemia and tetany (*see* below). Hypocalcemia can also occur following massive transfusions with citrated blood. The various etiologies and treatment of hypocalcemia have been reviewed by Zaloga and Chernow (1986).

Preparations and Routes of Administration in the Treatment of Hypocalcemia. Several preparations are available that can elevate systemic concentrations of Ca^{2+}. These differ in Ca^{2+} content and permissible routes of administration.

Calcium chloride ($CaCl_2 \cdot 2H_2O$) contains 27% Ca^{2+}; it is valuable in the treatment of hypocalcemic tetany. The salt can be given intravenously, but *it must never be injected into tissues*. It is somewhat irritating to the gastrointestinal tract. Injections of calcium chloride are accompanied by peripheral vasodilatation and a cutaneous burning sensation. The salt is usually given intravenously in a concentration of 10% (equivalent to 1.36 mEq Ca^{2+}/ml). The rate of injection should be slow (not over 1 ml per minute) to prevent a high concentration of Ca^{2+} from reaching the heart and causing syncope. A moderate fall in blood pressure due to vasodilatation may attend the injection. Since calcium chloride is an acidifying salt, it is usually undesirable in the treatment of the hypocalcemia caused by renal insufficiency.

Calcium gluceptate injection is a 22% solution (18 mg or 0.9 mEq Ca^{2+}/ml). It is administered intravenously in a dose of 5 to 20 ml for the treatment of severe hypocalcemic tetany; the injection may produce a transient tingling sensation. When the intravenous route is not possible, the injection may be given intramuscularly in a dose up to 5 ml, which may produce a mild local reaction.

Calcium gluconate ($[CH_2OH\{CHOH\}_4COO]_2Ca \cdot H_2O$) contains 9% Ca^{2+}. It is available as *cal-*

cium gluconate tablets, containing 500, 650, 975, or 1000 mg of the salt (equivalent to 2.3, 2.9, 4.4, or 4.5 mEq Ca^{2+}, respectively). It is nonirritating to the gastrointestinal tract. For intravenous injection, *calcium gluconate injection* is administered as a 10% solution (0.45 mEq Ca^{2+}/ml). It is a readily available source of Ca^{2+}, and the intravenous administration of this salt is the treatment of choice for severe hypocalcemic tetany. The intramuscular route should not be employed, since abscess formation at the site of injection may result.

Calcium lactate ($[CH_3CHOHCOO]_2Ca \cdot 5H_2O$) contains 13% Ca^{2+}. Its physical properties are similar to those of the gluconate. Tablets (325 mg or 650 mg) are available for oral administration. In the treatment of tetany, its absorption is apparently enhanced by the simultaneous administration of lactose.

Calcium carbonate is an insoluble powder containing 40% Ca^{2+}; it is available in tablets containing 350 mg to 1.5 g, capsules, and suspensions. After ingestion, it is converted to soluble Ca^{2+} salts in the bowel. Patients with achlorhydria may not solubilize Ca^{2+} from this preparation. It is also used as an antacid.

Dibasic calcium phosphate is a valuable source of Ca^{2+}, especially when it is desired to supply both Ca^{2+} and phosphate. It is an insoluble, tasteless powder that must be given orally.

Calcium levulinate contains 13% Ca^{2+}. It may be administered orally or parenterally.

Calcium glubionate contains 6.5% Ca^{2+} and is available as a syrup containing 1.8 g (115 mg of Ca^{2+}) per 5 ml.

Therapeutic Uses. Ca^{2+} is used in the treatment of deficiency states and as a dietary supplement when intake may be inadequate. Ca^{2+} salts are specific in the immediate treatment of low-Ca^{2+} tetany regardless of etiology. In severe manifest tetany, the symptoms are best brought under control by intravenous medication. Five to 20 ml of either 10% calcium gluconate or 22% calcium gluceptate solution is injected slowly. For the control of milder symptoms or latent tetany, oral medication suffices. Average doses are calcium gluconate, 15 g daily in divided doses; calcium lactate, 4 g, plus lactose, 8 g, with each meal; calcium carbonate or calcium phosphate, 1 to 2 g with meals.

The acute administration of Ca^{2+} may be lifesaving in patients with extreme hyperkalemia. Calcium gluconate (10 to 30 ml of a 10% solution) can reverse some of the cardiotoxic effects of hyperkalemia while other efforts are underway to lower the plasma concentration of K^+.

Hypercalcemic States. Hypercalcemia occurs in a number of diverse clinical conditions and requires differential diagnosis and appropriate corrective measures.

Ingestion of large quantities of a Ca^{2+} salt is unlikely by itself to cause hypercalcemia except in patients who have hypothyroidism; in this condition Ca^{2+} absorption is greater than normal (Benker *et al.*, 1988). Also, although now very uncommon, the hypercalcemic disorder known as the milk-alkali syndrome is caused by the ingestion of large quantities of milk and alkalinizing powders.

Hyperparathyroidism is classically associated with hypercalcemia accompanied by significant hypophosphatemia; the latter is due to the diminished ability of the renal tubules to reabsorb phosphate, owing to the excessive quantities of PTH. Some patients have renal calculi and peptic ulceration, and a few have mental aberrations with psychotic components. In more advanced stages, characteristic bone lesions are present and the condition can be diagnosed by radiography.

Benzothiadiazide diuretics produce a mild hypercalcemia in some individuals.

Vitamin D excess is a cause of hypercalcemia (*see* below).

Sarcoidosis is associated with about a 20% incidence of hypercalcemia. Increased intestinal absorption of Ca^{2+} is apparently due to excess production of calcitriol from calcifediol by the lymphatic cells of sarcoid lesions (*see* Reichel *et al.*, 1987).

Neoplasms with or without metastases to the bones may be accompanied by hypercalcemia. Some tumors secrete a peptide that resembles PTH at its amino terminus. This peptide can stimulate PTH receptors, but it does not cross-react with current antisera to PTH (Broadus *et al.*, 1988). Other tumors release prostaglandins that stimulate bone resorption. The hypercalcemia associated with such tumors is usually heralded by lethargy, weakness, nausea, and vomiting and not by renal stones or bone disease.

Occasionally, patients with hyperthyroidism have a mild hypercalcemia (Benker *et al.*, 1988). This is presumably due to an increased rate of bone resorption.

Disuse atrophy, as may occur when a patient must lie relatively immobile for a long time, may lead to hypercalcemia. This is most common after trauma that has involved large areas of the body and when extensive splinting with casts is necessary. Immobilization also often contributes to the hypercalcemia of patients with cancer.

Idiopathic hypercalcemia of infants is an unusual disease of unknown etiology. It has many similarities to intoxication with vitamin D.

Hypercalcemia is uncommonly noted in adrenocortical deficiency states, as in Addison's disease or during the period following operation for a hyperfunctioning tumor of the adrenal cortex or bilateral removal of hyperplastic adrenal glands.

Hypercalcemia occurs occasionally following successful renal transplantation, owing to secondary hyperparathyroidism resulting from the previous chronic renal failure.

The differential diagnosis of the various causes of hypercalcemia may be difficult. In contrast to former belief, hypophosphatemia is quite common with hypercalcemia of origins other than hyperparathyroidism. Many cases of hypercalcemia are discovered as a result of routine automated analyses of serum samples. The differential diagnosis of hypercalcemia entails the use of many tests, none of which is completely conclusive. Immunoassay of parathyroid hormone in plasma is quite useful, but it has limitations (*see* below). The excretion of adenosine 3′,5′-monophosphate (cyclic AMP) in the urine is increased in hyperparathyroidism, and evaluation of this parameter can facilitate diagnosis. Renal reabsorption of filtered phosphate is diminished in hyperparathyroidism, and this measurement can also be of diagnostic value.

Hypercalcemia of any etiology can have dire consequences. The predominant and most devastating lesion usually occurs in the kidney, with reduction of renal function. Pathological changes are prominent in the collecting ducts and distal tubules. Painful bone cysts, osteoporosis, and fractures may also occur if hypercalcemia is due to hyperparathyroidism.

On some occasions hypercalcemia is in itself a life-threatening situation. The use of agents that augment the excretion of Ca^{2+}, such as the administration of saline and loop diuretics, is the treatment of first choice. The employment of steroids to reduce hypercalcemia is of benefit in situations where the hypercalcemia is a consequence of diseases such as sarcoid or lymphoma or the excessive intake of vitamin D. Administration of calcitonin or plicamycin may be necessary and helpful (*see* below). Diphosphonates such as etidronate (discussed below) have also been utilized intravenously to lower plasma Ca^{2+} concentrations over a period of 48 to 72 hours. The use of sodium phosphate orally or intravenously does reduce the concentration of Ca^{2+} in plasma. However, the reduction results from plasma concentrations of phosphate that exceed the solubility product for calcium and phosphate ions. This causes precipitation of calcium phosphate in soft tissues throughout the body, a consequence that can be fatal. *The administration of sodium phosphate is therefore not recommended* (Vernava *et al.*, 1987).

Preparations Used for the Reduction of Hypercalcemia. As indicated above, infusions of saline with or without administration of diuretics such as furosemide are effective ways to promote the excretion of Ca^{2+}. This regimen constitutes the treatment of choice in most cases.

Prednisone and other steroids with similar characteristics are capable of reducing hypercalcemic concentrations to normal values, particularly when the abnormality is a consequence of sarcoid. Patients with nonmetastatic carcinomas or hyperparathyroidism are less responsive. Frequently, large doses (30 to 50 mg of prednisone a day) may be necessary initially. The response to glucocorticoid therapy is slow, and 1 to 2 weeks may be required before a fall in plasma Ca^{2+} occurs. A low-Ca^{2+} intake (virtual elimination of all milk and other dairy products) permits the use of the lowest dose of steroid possible to maintain normocalcemia. The complications of long-term use of steroids must be recalled, and the osteoporosis that results from prolonged administration of glucocorticoids can limit the duration of therapy.

Plicamycin (*mithramycin;* MITHRACIN) is a cytotoxic antibiotic that can be very useful in decreasing the plasma Ca^{2+} concentration in hypercalcemia (Perlia *et al.*, 1970). This agent probably acts directly on bone and blocks Ca^{2+} resorption. Reduction in the plasma Ca^{2+} concentration occurs within 24 to 48 hours with relatively low doses of this agent (25 μg/kg per day by intravenous infusion for 3 to 4 days), and its toxicity is thus less severe (*see* Chapter 52).

Calcitonin (CALCIMAR, MIACALCIN) may be useful for the treatment of hypercalcemia (*see* below).

Edetate disodium (disodium EDTA; ENDRATE, others) is a chelating agent that forms soluble complexes with Ca^{2+}. Chelation occurs in the blood and results in a rapid decrease in the concentration of Ca^{2+} in plasma before excretion of the complex occurs. Because of potential toxicities this agent is now used only rarely. Among the dangers of such therapy is the possibility that the concentration of Ca^{2+} may be reduced too quickly and reach hypocalcemic levels, thus resulting in tetany, convulsions, severe cardiac arrhythmias, and respiratory arrest.

PHOSPHATE

In addition to its role as a dynamic constituent of intermediary and energy metabolism, phosphate plays important roles in modifying concentrations of Ca^{2+} in tissues. Furthermore, phosphate ions are buffers of the intracellular fluid and play a primary role in the renal excretion of H^+.

Absorption, Distribution, and Excretion. Phosphate is absorbed from, and to a limited extent secreted into, the gastrointestinal tract. The transport of phosphate from the lumen of the gut is an active, energy-dependent process, and there are factors that appear to modify the degree of its intestinal absorption. The presence of large quantities of Ca^{2+} or Al^{3+} may lead to the formation of large amounts of insoluble phosphate and may therefore diminish the net absorption of phosphate from the bowel. Vitamin D stimulates phosphate absorption, and this effect has been reported to precede the action of the vitamin on transport of Ca^{2+} (Birge and Miller, 1977). In general, in adults, about two thirds of the ingested phosphate is absorbed from the bowel, and that which is absorbed from the gut is almost entirely excreted into the urine. In growing children, there is a positive balance of phosphate. Concentrations of phosphate in plasma are higher in children than in adults. This "hyperphosphatemia'' decreases the affinity of hemoglobin for oxygen and is hypothesized to explain the physiological ''anemia'' of childhood (Card and Brain, 1973).

Phosphate is present in plasma and extracellular fluid, in cell membranes and intracellular fluid, and in collagen and bone tissue. In the extracellular fluid, phosphate is primarily in inorganic form and only a small component of esterified phosphate is present. Plasma phosphate concentration is inversely related to the rate of renal hydroxylation of 25-hydroxycholecalciferol. A reduction of the plasma phosphate concentration permits the presence of more Ca^{2+} in the blood and inhibits deposition of new bone salt. An increased concentration of the phosphate anion in plasma facilitates the effect of calcitonin on deposition of Ca^{2+} in bone. The concentration of plasma inorganic phosphate may vary with age, and the range has been recorded in great detail by Greenberg and coworkers (1960). The ratio of disodium phosphate and monosodium phosphate in extracellular fluid is 4:1 at a pH of 7.40. This ratio varies, of course, with pH; however, due to its relatively low concentration, phosphate contributes relatively little to the buffering capacity of extracellular fluid.

The renal excretion of phosphate has been studied extensively. More than 90% of the phosphate in plasma is filterable, and the bulk is then actively reabsorbed by the initial segment of the proximal tubule. Phosphate reabsorption takes place to a smaller extent in the pars recta and/or loop of Henle, in the distal convoluted tubule, and possibly in the collecting duct (Kuntziger *et al.,* 1974; Lechene *et al.,* 1978). Expansion of plasma volume causes increased urinary phosphate excretion (Steele, 1970). Phosphate excreted in the urine probably represents the net difference between the amount filtered and that reabsorbed. There is little evidence for tubular secretion of phosphate in the mammalian kidney. Parathyroid hormone increases the urinary excretion of phosphate by blocking reabsorption in all segments proximal to the collecting duct (Lechene *et al.,* 1978). Vitamin D_3 and its metabolites directly stimulate proximal tubular reabsorption of phosphate (Puschett *et al.,* 1972).

Role of Phosphate in the Acidification of the Urine. The interrelations that exist between the rates of excretion of phosphate and titratable acid are referred to in Chapter 27 and in the Introduction to Section VI. Although the concentration of phosphate is low in the extracellular fluid, the anion is progressively concentrated in the renal tubule and represents the most abundant buffer system in the distal tubule. At this site, the secretion of H^+ by the tubular cell in exchange for Na^+ in the tubular urine converts disodium hydrogen phosphate to sodium dihydrogen phosphate. In this manner, large amounts of acid can be excreted without lowering the pH of the urine to a degree that would block H^+ transport by a high concentration gradient between the tubular cell and luminal fluid.

Actions of the Phosphate Ion. Once phosphate gains access to the body fluids and tissues, it exerts little pharmacological effect. If the ion is introduced into the gastrointestinal tract, the absorbed phosphate is rapidly excreted. If large amounts are given by this route, much of it may escape absorption. This property leads to a cathartic action, and, therefore, the phosphate salts are employed as mild laxatives. Inorganic phosphate poisoning following ingestion of laxatives that contain phosphate salts has been reported in adults and children (McConnell, 1971). The ingestion of large amounts of sodium dihydrogen phosphate lowers the pH of the urine. If excessive phosphate salts are introduced intravenously or orally, they may prove toxic (Vernava *et al.,* 1987). Toxicity results from reducing the concentration of Ca^{2+} in the circulation and from the precipitation of calcium phosphate in soft tissues.

Phosphate Depletion. There has been a question for some time concerning the possibility of clinical consequences of phosphate depletion. Familial hypophosphatemia is an X-linked dominant trait apparently due to defective intestinal absorption and/or renal reabsorption of inorganic phosphate that results in rickets and dwarfism. A report by Lichtman and coworkers (1969) describes a patient with striking hypophosphatemia who had a significant depression in the steady-state concentration of erythrocyte adenosine triphosphate (ATP). In addition to reduced ATP, hypophosphatemia causes a marked decrease in concentrations of 2,3-diphosphoglycerate in erythrocytes. Acute hemolytic anemia and impaired oxygenation of tissues can occur in severe hypophosphatemia (Jacob and Amsden, 1971). This raises the possibility that other cellular stores of ATP and other critical organic phosphate compounds may be depleted. These biochemical abnormalities, in turn, could well be responsible for certain features of the clinical syndrome.

In general, the phosphorus present in ordinary foods is an adequate source of the ion. The use of expensive preparations of organic phosphates as "tonics" has no validity.

Pathological Conditions Associated with a Disturbance in Phosphate Metabolism. A defect in phosphate metabolism occurs in a variety of diseases, as briefly mentioned below.

Osteoporosis. This condition is considered to be a primary disorder in the formation of bone matrix. There is no primary defect in phosphate metabolism, and plasma concentrations of phosphate are within usual limits.

Rickets. The consequences of deficiency of vitamin D with regard to the metabolism of both phosphate and calcium are described below, as are other forms of rickets. Familial hypophosphatemia is due to defective absorption and/or excretion of inorganic phosphate and has been mentioned above.

Osteomalacia. The loss of Ca^{2+} in stools (due to malabsorption) or the loss from body fluids by way of the kidney (essential hypercalciuria or renal tubular acidosis with augmented Ca^{2+} excretion) promotes a negative balance of Ca^{2+}. Such loss deprives the body of Ca^{2+} stores, and the concentration of Ca^{2+} in plasma falls slightly. This, in turn, stimulates the secretion of PTH, which restores the concentration of Ca^{2+} to normal but tends to promote some depression of plasma phosphate.

Osteitis Fibrosa Cystica. In this disorder, there is a primary increase in the secretion of PTH that is usually accompanied by an increase in plasma Ca^{2+}, some reduction of plasma phosphate, and decreased renal tubular reabsorption of phosphate.

Secondary Hyperparathyroidism. This condition may be seen in patients with chronic renal insufficiency. The sequence of events probably starts with a high plasma concentration of phosphate and a low value for Ca^{2+}; this situation stimulates parathyroid secretion. Since the elevated plasma phosphate is a consequence of renal insufficiency, it persists. The continuing hyperphosphatemia may be modified by the administration of aluminum hydroxide gel, which tends to inhibit the absorption of phosphate from the bowel because of the formation of insoluble aluminum phosphates. However, aluminum can be toxic in patients with renal insufficiency; hence, other phosphate-binding compounds are now recommended (*see* Chapter 37).

Hypoparathyroidism. In this disorder, characterized by deficient parathyroid secretion, there is a rise in plasma phosphate and a decreased concentration of Ca^{2+}. This condition can be readily treated with vitamin D with or without Ca^{2+} supplementation.

Preparations. Only certain of the preparations of inorganic phosphates are mentioned here; calcium phosphates are described elsewhere.

Phosphate (in the form of Na^{+} and/or K^{+} salts) is available in tablets, capsules (contents to be diluted with water), and powders for solution. It is also available as *sodium phosphates oral solution,* which is used as a laxative. *Potassium phosphate* and *sodium phosphate injections* are each available in solutions for intravenous administration that contain 3 mmol of phosphate per milliliter.

Therapeutic Uses. The phosphates are of limited therapeutic usefulness. Sodium phosphate has been employed to diminish hypercalcemia, but its use for this purpose is dangerous and is strongly discouraged (*see* above). The phosphates have a role in the management of the phosphate-depletion syndrome. Phosphate salts are also effective saline cathartics (*see* Chapter 38).

PARATHYROID HORMONE

History. Although there were many earlier references to the yellow glandular bodies attached to the thyroid, credit for the discovery of the parathyroid gland is usually given to Sandstrom, who in 1880 published an anatomical report that attracted little attention among physiologists. The glands were rediscovered a decade later by Gley, who determined the effects of their extirpation with the thyroid. Vassale and Generali then successfully removed the parathyroids without interfering with the thyroid and noted that tetany, convulsions, and death quickly followed. However, the symptoms following parathyroidectomy varied so greatly in different species that the importance of the organs was not appreciated, and controversies continued as to whether they were essential to life. The subsequent discovery of internal and accessory parathyroids accounted for the discrepancies in experimental results and paved the way to the elucidation of the important physiological role played by this endocrine gland.

MacCallum and Voegtlin (1909) first noted the effect of parathyroidectomy on the concentration of plasma Ca^{2+}. Since Howell and Loeb had previously established the physiological importance of Ca^{2+}, the relation of low plasma Ca^{2+} to parathyroprivic symptoms was quickly appreciated and a comprehensive picture of parathyroid function began to form. After various attempts to obtain active extracts of the gland, success was finally attained (Berman, 1924; Collip, 1925; Hanson, 1925). It was readily demonstrated that active extracts could alleviate hypocalcemic tetany in parathyroidectomized animals and raise the concentration of Ca^{2+} in the plasma of normal animals. For the first time, the relation of certain definite clinical abnormalities to parathyroid hyperfunction was appreciated.

While investigators in the United States, Canada, and England were utilizing the physiological approach to solve the problem of the function of the parathyroid glands, German and Austrian pathologists were associating the skeletal changes of osteitis fibrosa cystica with the presence of parathyroid tumors. In a delightful historical review, Albright (1948) traced the manner in which these two diverse types of investigations finally arrived at the same conclusion.

Chemistry. Human, bovine, and porcine parathyroid hormones are all single polypeptide chains of 84 amino acid residues. Their molecular weights are approximately 9500, and the entire amino acid sequence has been established for each. Biological activity is associated with the N-terminal portion of the peptide; residues 1 to 27 are required. Although derivatives lacking the first or second residue bind to PTH receptors, they are nearly inactive biologically (Aurbach, 1988). Bovine and porcine PTH differ by only seven amino acid residues, and the amino-terminal segment of the human hormone differs from the equivalent portion of the bovine and porcine molecules by only four and three amino acid residues, respectively. The three differ little in biological activity, but they are immunologically distinguishable; however, they cross-react with a single antibody, a feature that facilitates an immunoassay for PTH, as discussed below.

Synthesis, Secretion, and Immunoassay. PTH is synthesized initially in a prehormone form. The product of translation that is destined to become PTH is called preproparathyroid hormone, an unfortunate name that grew by accretion in an adaptation to new knowledge of PTH synthesis. This single-chain peptide of 115 amino acids is rapidly converted to proparathyroid hormone by cleavage of a 25 amino acid fragment from the amino terminus as the peptide is transferred to the intracisternal space of the endoplasmic reticulum. The proparathyroid hormone, which persists somewhat longer than its precursor (15 to 20 minutes, compared with 1 to 2 minutes), moves to the Golgi apparatus and is converted to PTH, again by the cleavage of an amino-terminal fragment of six predominantly basic amino acids. The PTH is enclosed within secretory granules, where it remains until secreted into the circulation. Normally, most of the PTH that is synthesized is degraded by proteolysis before it can be secreted. During periods of hypocalcemia, more PTH is secreted and a smaller fraction is hydrolyzed. This mechanism provides a supply of hormone that can be rapidly mobilized in response to acute needs without the delay entailed by increased synthesis of protein. In prolonged hypocalcemia, there is evidence of stimulation of PTH synthesis, and the gland hypertrophies. Neither preproparathyroid hormone nor proparathyroid hormone appears in plasma. The synthesis and processing of PTH have been reviewed by Cohn and associates (1986).

Intact PTH has a half-life in plasma of 2 to 5 minutes; removal by the liver and kidney accounts for about 90% of its clearance. Metabolism of PTH results in the production of fragments that circulate in the blood (Hruska *et al.*, 1981). Fragments are also released as a result of proteolysis of PTH within the parathyroid gland. A fragment of approximately 6000 daltons from the carboxyl terminus is the major circulating peptide that results from PTH metabolism. Although this peptide is not active biologically, it does react with antibodies prepared against the intact hormone. In contrast, the active region of PTH—residues 1 to 27—is poorly reactive immunologically, and fragments from this region tend not to be recognized as PTH by most antibodies. In spite of these problems, management of patients is generally satisfactory with immunoassays that recognize inactive peptides from the carboxyl terminus as well as the intact hormone. Ashby and Thakkar (1988) have discussed the limitations of these techniques. Recently, immunoassays have been developed that utilize antibodies directed against both the amino- and carboxyl-terminal regions; these assays are apparently specific for intact PTH (*see* Blind *et al.*, 1988). As noted, measurements of urinary concentrations of cyclic AMP can also provide a useful assessment of parathyroid function.

Physiological Functions. The primary function of PTH is to elicit the adaptive changes that serve to maintain a constant concentration of Ca^{2+} in the extracellular fluid. Processes that are regulated include the absorption of Ca^{2+} from the gastrointestinal tract, the deposition and mobilization of bone Ca^{2+}, and the excretion of the ion in urine, feces, sweat, and milk. There is evidence that PTH accomplishes its functions by directly or indirectly influencing all these mechanisms, but its most prominent effect is to promote the mobilization of Ca^{2+} from bone.

Regulation of Secretion. The concentration of Ca^{2+} in the blood (or, perhaps, the concentration of Ca^{2+} in parathyroid cells) is the primary factor that regulates the secretory activity of the parathyroid gland. When the concentration of Ca^{2+} is low, the secretion of PTH is increased, and hypertrophy and hyperplasia of the gland result if the hypocalcemia is sustained. If the concentration of Ca^{2+} is high, the secretion of PTH is decreased, and hypoplasia may result if the hypercalcemia is sustained. *In vitro* studies show that amino acid transport, nucleic acid and protein synthesis, cytoplasmic growth, and secretion of PTH are stimulated by exposure to low concentrations of Ca^{2+} and suppressed by exposure to high concentrations over an extended period of time. Thus, Ca^{2+} *per se* appears to regulate growth of the parathyroid gland and its synthesis and secretion of hormone (Roth and Raisz, 1964). Acutely, secretion of PTH can be elicited by hypocalcemia without alteration of the rate of synthesis of PTH (*see* above).

Although plasma Ca^{2+} is the most important regulator of PTH secretion, other effectors are active *in vitro*. Agents that stimulate adenylyl cyclase in parathyroid cells also increase secretion; these include β-adrenergic agonists, dopamine, secretin, and prostaglandins of the E series. Conversely, agents that inhibit adenylyl cyclase, such as α-adrenergic agonists and prostaglandin $F_{2\alpha}$, reduce the release of PTH. Although elevation of extracellular Ca^{2+} can lower the concentration of cyclic AMP in parathyroid cells, it is thought that this nucleotide plays no more than a minor role in the control of secretion by Ca^{2+}. Current evidence indicates that lowered extracellular concentrations of Ca^{2+} lead to the activation of protein kinase C in parathyroid cells, and that this, in turn, stimulates the secretory process (Brown *et al.*, 1987; Kobayashi *et al.*, 1988; Morrissey, 1988). Calcitriol (*see* below) inhibits secretion of PTH, but whether this is a direct effect of this vitamin D analog or the result of increased Ca^{2+} in plasma is not certain.

There appears to be no relation between extracellular concentrations of phosphate and the secretion of PTH, except indirectly as changes in phosphate values affect the concentration of Ca^{2+}. Both hypermagnesemia and hypomagnesemia can inhibit the secretion of PTH (Rude *et al.*, 1976).

Thus, the extracellular concentration of Ca^{2+} is controlled on a minute-to-minute basis by a feedback system, the afferent limb of which is sensitive to the concentration of Ca^{2+} and the efferent limb of which releases PTH. The hormone acts on various peripheral tissues to mobilize Ca^{2+} into the extracellular fluid and thus restores the concentration to normal.

Effects on Bone. PTH acts on bone to increase the rate of resorption of Ca^{2+} and phosphate. The site of the resorptive effect appears to be on the stable, older portion of bone mineral and not on the labile fraction.

Resorption of bone is brought about by osteolytic cells—osteoclasts and osteocytes. PTH stimulates the rate of bone resorption by these cells, increases the rate of conversion (differentiation) of mesenchymal cells to osteoclasts, and prolongs the half-life of these latter cells. Twenty minutes after the administration of PTH to some species, activation of osteoclasts is evident by the appearance of ruffled borders on the cells adjacent to bone surfaces (Miller, 1978). With prolonged action of PTH the number of bone-forming osteoblasts is also increased; thus, the rate of bone turnover and remodeling is enhanced. However, individual osteoblasts appear to be less active than normal, and PTH acts to inhibit their synthesis of collagen, a major component of bone matrix.

Biochemical correlates of PTH action have also been studied extensively in bone cultures. PTH causes resorption of cultured bone, and a number of biochemical effects of PTH have been described. A difficulty with this approach is that bone resorption *per se* leads to biochemical changes that may have no relation to specific actions of PTH. PTH stimulates the release of collagenase and other hydrolytic enzymes into the culture medium, stimulates glycolysis, and inhibits the oxidation of citrate—responses that may only reflect the breakdown of bone. Consequently, no satisfactory hypothesis has yet been offered to explain the action of PTH at the biochemical level. There is, however, evidence that PTH acts primarily on the osteoblasts in bone and causes the stimulation of adenylyl cyclase. It has been proposed that the activated osteoblasts induce osteoclasts to increase their resorption of bone through an unknown mechanism (Partridge *et al.*, 1981). There is also evidence to support the concept that the ultimate step in PTH-stimulated release of Ca^{2+} from bone involves Ca^{2+}–Na^{+} exchange (Krieger and Tashjian, 1980).

Effects on the Kidney. PTH acts on the kidney to increase tubular reabsorption of Ca^{2+} and to inhibit tubular reabsorption of phosphate. As a result, Ca^{2+} is retained and its concentration tends to increase in the plasma; phosphate is excreted and the plasma concentration tends to fall.

Calcium. PTH increases tubular reabsorption of Ca^{2+} at a distal site (Agus *et al.*, 1973). Therefore, when the plasma concentration of Ca^{2+} is in the normal range, extirpation of the gland decreases tubular reabsorption of Ca^{2+} and thereby increases Ca^{2+} excretion in the urine. When the plasma concentration falls significantly below 7 mg/dl (1.75 mM), a decrease in Ca^{2+} excretion occurs because the amount of Ca^{2+} filtered through the glomeruli is lowered to the point that the cation is almost completely reabsorbed despite the reduced tubular reabsorptive capacity. However, when parathyroidectomized animals are kept on a high-calcium diet and plasma Ca^{2+} remains higher than 7 mg/dl (1.75 mM), the hypercalciuria persists. If PTH is administered to such hypoparathyroid animals or man, tubular reabsorption of Ca^{2+} is increased and the excretion of Ca^{2-} initially decreases. This effect, along with mobilization of calcium from bone and increased absorption from the gut, results in an increased concentration of Ca^{2+} in plasma. When the value rises above normal, the increased glomerular filtration of

Ca^{2+} overwhelms the stimulatory effect of PTH on tubular reabsorption, and the hypercalciuria so characteristic of hyperparathyroidism ensues.

Phosphate. PTH increases the renal excretion of inorganic phosphate by decreasing the reabsorption of phosphate in all or most segments of the nephron proximal to the collecting duct (Lechene *et al.*, 1978).

Cyclic AMP mediates the effects of PTH on the kidney (*see* Aurbach, 1988). Adenylyl cyclase that is stimulated by PTH is located in the renal cortex, and cyclic AMP synthesized in response to the hormone affects tubular transport mechanisms. A portion of the cyclic nucleotide synthesized at this site escapes into the urine, and its assay serves as a measure of parathyroid activity (*see* below). Cyclic AMP may inhibit proximal tubular reabsorption of Ca^{2+}, phosphate, bicarbonate, and Na^+. The final effect on Ca^{2+} excretion is, however, inhibitory, since it stimulates distal Ca^{2+} reabsorption out of proportion to that of Na^+ (Agus *et al.*, 1973).

Other Ions. PTH also influences the excretion of other ions, most of which are constituents of bone. PTH reduces renal excretion of Mg^{2+}, and elevates the plasma concentration; in parathyroidectomized animals, Mg^{2+} excretion is usually increased and the plasma concentration is reduced. The hormonal effect on Mg^{2+} is probably due, as is true for Ca^{2+}, to both increased renal tubular reabsorption of Mg^{2+} and its mobilization from the exchangeable compartment of bone (MacIntyre *et al.*, 1963). PTH increases the excretion of water, amino acids, citrate, K^+, bicarbonate, Na^+, chloride, and sulfate, whereas it decreases the excretion of H^+. The increased excretion of bicarbonate appears to be mainly due to inhibition of proximal tubular reabsorption of this anion; this effect is antagonized by Ca^{2+}. Although the effects of PTH on regulation of acid–base metabolism by the kidney are similar to those of acetazolamide, they are independent of the carbonic anhydrase system. The effects of PTH on other ions involve actions on both proximal and distal tubules.

Effects on the Gastrointestinal Tract. PTH acts indirectly to increase intestinal absorption of Ca^{2+} and phosphate through the hormone's enhancement of the conversion of calcifediol to calcitriol in the kidney. PTH also acts directly and rapidly on the intestine to stimulate absorption of Ca^{2+}; the mechanism has not yet been elucidated (Nemere and Norman, 1986).

Miscellaneous Effects. PTH decreases the concentration of Ca^{2+} in milk and saliva. These effects are the opposite of those that would be expected from the concurrent changes in plasma Ca^{2+} concentration. It appears likely, therefore, that the hormone can conserve Ca^{2+} in the extracellular fluid not only by its effects on bone, kidney, and gut but also by reducing the rate of Ca^{2+} transport from extracellular fluid to milk and saliva.

PTH also reduces the Ca^{2+} concentration in the lens, a fact that explains the prevalence of cataracts in patients with hypoparathyroidism and the increased content of Ca^{2+} in the lens in hormone-deficient animals.

Hypoparathyroidism. Hypoparathyroidism is only one of the many causes of hypocalcemia; it occurs relatively rarely. The deficiency syndrome most commonly follows operative procedures on either the thyroid gland or the parathyroids themselves. Less frequently, disease of the parathyroids is the cause (idiopathic hypoparathyroidism). Also uncommon is a genetic disorder in which the target organs do not respond to PTH, despite adequate concentrations of the hormone (pseudohypoparathyroidism).

In all varieties of hypoparathyroidism, hypocalcemia and its associated symptoms are encountered clinically. The earliest prodromal symptoms of hypocalcemia are paresthesias in the extremities. Mechanical stimulation of peripheral nerves during physical examination usually produces contraction of the appropriate skeletal muscles. These signs and symptoms may be followed by manifest tetany, consisting of muscle spasms, especially carpopedal spasm and laryngospasm. Eventually, generalized convulsions and other central nervous system (CNS) manifestations occur. It is highly probable that smooth muscle is also affected. For example, hypocalcemia may be followed by spasm of the ciliary muscle, iris, esophagus, intestine, urinary bladder, and bronchi. ECG changes and a marked tachycardia indicate that the heart is involved. Vascular spasm in the fingers and toes is also commonly observed. In chronic hypoparathyroidism, ectodermal changes, consisting of loss of hair, grooved and brittle fingernails, defects of the dental enamel, and cataracts, are frequently encountered; calcification in the basal ganglia and perhaps other soft tissues also occurs. Psychiatric symptoms such as emotional lability, anxiety, depression, and delusions are often present.

Hypoparathyroidism is treated primarily with vitamin D (*see* below). Dietary supplementation with Ca^{2+} may also be necessary.

Hyperparathyroidism. Primary hyperparathyroidism results either from hypersecretion of the parathyroid glands (due to hyperplasia, adenoma, or, rarely, carcinoma) or from secretion of the PTH-like polypeptide from tumors arising at other sites (*see* above). Plasma concentrations of Ca^{2+} may be normal with primary hyperparathyroidism, but they are usually elevated, and plasma phosphate values are usually decreased. Hyperparathyroidism may also be secondary to conditions causing negative Ca^{2+} balance, such as malabsorption and renal disease; in these cases the concentration of Ca^{2+} in plasma is low and provides the stimulus for increased secretion of PTH. Hypersecretion of PTH from any cause may lead to a bone disorder known as osteitis fibrosa generalisata. However, only one third of cases of hyperparathyroidism exhibit advanced bone changes; another third show minor degrees of decalcification; and the remaining cases present no obvious skeletal abnormalities. However, metabolic studies indicate that resorption of bone is actively occurring in the last-named group; the Ca^{2+} intake may be sufficient to maintain balance. Symptoms of early decalcification are aching and pain in the bones and joints.

Uncomplicated primary hyperparathyroidism is invariably associated with hypercalciuria and hyperphosphaturia, and is sometimes accompanied by polyuria and polydipsia. The excretion of excessive amounts of Ca^{2+} and phosphate results in a high incidence of renal calculi, which often cause the presenting symptoms. An equally serious complication is a diffuse nephrocalcinosis, which may progress to a stage of extreme renal insufficiency. It is well to keep in mind that renal insufficiency secondary to nephrocalcinosis or to sequelae of urolithiasis may mask some of the cardinal biochemical features of hyperparathyroidism, namely, hyperphosphaturia, hypercalciuria, and hypophosphatemia.

Hypercalcemia *per se* can be the cause of some of the signs and symptoms of hyperparathyroidism. These include hypotonicity of muscle, with general skeletal muscle weakness and smooth muscle dysfunction leading to constipation, flatulence, anorexia, nausea, and vomiting. Occasionally, cardiac irregularities are observed. A higher-than-normal incidence of peptic ulcers and pancreatitis has been reported in patients with the disease. Neuropsychiatric manifestations also occur in many cases. Advanced cases of osteitis fibrosa generalisata may exhibit anemia and leukopenia.

In addition to laboratory study of Ca^{2+} and phosphate, there are more specific tests for hyperparathyroidism. The most widely used is the radioimmunoassay of PTH in plasma. However, only recently have these assays been able to distinguish between PTH and its inactive fragments (*see* above). Another method involves determination of the concentration of cyclic AMP in urine, which is elevated by the action of PTH on the kidney (Broadus and Rasmussen, 1981).

Treatment. Surgical resection of the hyperplastic or adenomatous glands is almost always required for the treatment of primary hyperparathyroidism. Surgery can return the patient to a euparathyroid state and prevent continued renal damage and bone dissolution. As discussed earlier, transient hypocalcemia often occurs following surgery, particularly when bone disease is present; this condition requires brief therapy with Ca^{2+}. If an excessive amount of parathyroid tissue is removed, permanent hypoparathyroidism may ensue. In this case vitamin D therapy and/or supplementation of the diet with Ca^{2+} is required. Long-term treatment consisting of a low-Ca^{2+} diet and liberal amounts of fluids is used to lower the plasma concentration of Ca^{2+} in selected patients in whom surgery is contraindicated.

Preparations. Parathyroid injection is not available commercially for clinical use. *Teriparatide* (*synthetic human parathyroid hormone*, residues 1 to 34) is available as PARATHAR.

Clinical Uses. PTH currently has no valid therapeutic uses; although it was formerly used to elevate the concentration of Ca^{2+} in plasma, this effect can be accomplished with greater safety by the administration of Ca^{2+} and/or vitamin D.

Teriparatide can be used diagnostically to distinguish between pseudohypoparathyroidism and hypoparathyroidism. Since the former disease is characterized by target-organ resistance to the hormone, patients with this condition fail to show an increased concentration of Ca^{2+} in plasma and fail to excrete increased amounts of phosphate and cyclic AMP in the urine after the administration of the peptide (200 units, intravenously) (*see* Chase *et al.*, 1969).

CALCITONIN

History and Source. A hypocalcemic hormone, the effects of which are generally opposite to those of the parathyroid hormone, was discovered and named *calcitonin* by Copp in 1962 (*see* Copp, 1964). It was demonstrated as a result of perfusion of dogs' parathyroid and thyroid glands with hypercalcemic blood. This procedure caused an immediate transitory hypocalcemic effect in the systemic blood that occurred significantly earlier than does the hypocalcemia observed after total parathyroidectomy. The observations led Copp to conclude that the parathyroid glands secreted calcitonin in response to hypercalcemia and in this way reduced the elevated plasma concentration of Ca^{2+} to normal. Munson and colleagues (Hirsch *et al.*, 1963) noted that parathyroidectomy in rats performed by cauterization caused more severe hypocalcemia than did thyroparathyroidectomy. They thus suspected the existence of a hypocalcemic principle in the thyroid gland. They found that extracts of thyroid produced a hypocalcemic response, and named the thyroid factor *thyrocalcitonin*. It is now known that the two factors are the same and that the hormone does originate from the thyroid; however, calcitonin is the name that is generally used.

The parafollicular C cells from the thyroid, which are embryologically derived from the ultimobranchial body, are the site of production and secretion of calcitonin. In nonmammalian vertebrates, calcitonin is found only in ultimobranchial bodies, which are separate organs from the thyroid gland. The hormone from both sources, thyroid and ultimobranchial bodies, is the same. In man, calcitonin is present in the thyroid, parathyroid, and thymus, an indication that the C cells are widely distributed.

Chemistry and Immunoreactivity. The amino acid sequence of calcitonin from several species including man, salmon, and pig, has been determined. In all cases, the hormone is a single-chain peptide of 32 amino acid residues. Eight of these residues are invariant, including a carboxyl-terminal prolinamide and a disulfide bridge between cysteines at positions 1 and 7. Both these structural features are essential for biological activity. The residues in the middle portion of the molecule (positions 10 to 27) are variable and appear to influence potency and/or duration of action. The calcitonins derived from the ultimobranchial bodies of salmon and eels are more potent than mammalian thyroidal calcitonins both *in vivo* and *in vitro*, and they differ from the human hormone by 13 and 16 amino acid residues, respectively. Therapeutically, salmon calcitonin appears to be more potent than human calcitonin, in part because it is cleared from the circulation more slowly.

Human calcitonin is processed proteolytically from a precursor polypeptide of 135 amino acid residues; two additional peptides are generated, but their biological significance is unknown. The calcitonin gene contains six exons; calcitonin itself is encoded by the fourth of these. In C cells, messenger RNA is processed such that exons 1 to 4 are represented in the final transcript. In neural tissue, however, the sequence corresponding to exon 4 is removed, and those for exons 1 to 3, 5, and 6 are included. Following translation and proteolytic processing of a precursor protein, a mature peptide of 37 amino acid residues is generated, the calcitonin gene–related peptide (CGRP). Although CGRP produces calcitonin-like effects in some species, it causes PTH-like effects in others and apparently acts upon receptors distinct from those that mediate the actions of calcitonin. Since little or no CGRP is produced by the C cells in the thyroid, it is unlikely that it functions significantly in Ca^{2+} homeostasis. CGRP and high-affinity binding sites for the peptide are widely distributed in the CNS, where CGRP is believed to serve as a neurotransmitter. In the periphery, CGRP is found in many bipolar neurons in sensory ganglia, and the peptide produces marked vasodilatation at low concentrations. The structure and synthesis of calcitonin and CGRP have been reviewed by MacIntyre and coworkers (1987) and by Zaidi and associates (1987).

Multiple forms of calcitonin are found in plasma, including molecules of high molecular weight that may represent aggregates or cross-linked products. This fact has impeded the development of useful immunoassays for calcitonin. However, a procedure that is specific for the entire peptide may soon be available (Motte *et al.*, 1988).

Regulation of Secretion. The secretion and biosynthesis of calcitonin are regulated by the concentration of Ca^{2+} in plasma. When the value is high, the amount of the hormone in plasma increases; when the concentration is low, the amount of the hormone decreases markedly and may be undetectable. Normal basal concentrations of calcitonin in plasma as measured by immunoassay are less than 100 pg/ml in more than 75% of subjects. Infusion of Ca^{2+} increases the basal concentration two- to threefold (Tashjian *et al.*, 1974). Most studies have reported that the mean concentration of calcitonin in the plasma of women is significantly lower than in men. Furthermore, the response to challenge with pentagastrin and Ca^{2+} is smaller in women than in men (Garcia-Ameijeiras *et al.*, 1987). The half-life of calcitonin is short (about 10 minutes); hence the hormone most likely is secreted at a fairly continuous rate when plasma concentrations of Ca^{2+} are normal.

While it is clear experimentally that calcitonin secretion can be stimulated by epinephrine, glucagon, gastrin, and cholecystokinin, presumably in a cyclic AMP–mediated fashion, the evidence for a physiological role of these hormones is not convincing. It is also not known to what extent normal physiological variations in secretion occur or whether calcitonin plays a significant role in Ca^{2+} homeostasis. High concentrations of calcitonin have been found in plasma, urine, and tumor tissue (50 to 5000 times normal) in patients with medullary carcinoma of the thyroid gland. The tumor cells originate from the parafollicular cells of the thyroid, and this disease represents a true calcitonin-excess syndrome. Measurement of the response of plasma calcitonin to an infusion of calcium gluconate and pentagastrin is a valuable procedure for detection of thyroid medullary carcinoma (Wells *et al.*, 1978). Because one form of this disease is inherited as a dominant trait, relatives of patients should be examined repeatedly (Tashjian *et al.*, 1974).

Mechanism of Action. Results from both short- and long-term experiments *in vivo* and culture of bone *in vitro* confirm that the hypocalcemic and hypophosphatemic effects of calcitonin are due predominately to direct inhibition of bone resorption by osteoclastic and osteocytic cells (*see* MacIntyre *et al.*, 1987). There is some evidence that calcitonin stimulates formation of bone by osteoblasts in addition to inhibiting bone resorption (Farley *et al.*, 1988).

Although calcitonin tends to negate the effects of PTH on osteolysis, it does not act as an antiparathyroid hormone. Thus, it does not block the activation of bone-cell adenylyl cyclase by PTH and does not inhibit the initial PTH-induced uptake of Ca^{2+} into bone. The actions of calcitonin are not blocked by inhibitors of RNA and protein synthesis. The hormone produces a decrease in the amount of ruffled border of osteoclasts, indicating their diminished activity in bone resorption. At least part of the effect of calcitonin appears to be mediated through increasing the cyclic AMP concentration in osteoclasts (Chambers *et al.*, 1985).

Calcitonin also antagonizes the inhibitory effects of PTH on pyrophosphatase activity in isolated Ehrlich ascites tumor cells. Pyrophosphate and pyrophosphatase are intimately involved in the processes of bone formation and resorption. Calcitonin decreases glucose utilization and lactate production in bone, effects opposite to those of PTH. As a result of depressed bone resorption, the urinary excretion of Ca^{2+}, Mg^{2+}, and hydroxyproline is decreased by calcitonin. Plasma phosphate concentration is also lowered, due mainly to decreased resorption of bone and also to increased urinary phosphate excretion. The direct effects of calcitonin on the kidney are dependent on the species. In man, calcitonin increases the excretion of Ca^{2+}, phosphate, and Na^{+}, effects also mediated in part by cyclic AMP (Murad *et al.*, 1970; Paillard *et al.*, 1972). Calcitonin probably does not affect absorption of Ca^{2+} from the intestinal tract.

Bioassay, Preparations, and Dosage. Bioassay of calcitonin preparations is performed by assessing their ability to lower the plasma concentration of Ca^{2+} in the rat.

Salmon, porcine, and human calcitonins have been studied experimentally. The hormone from salmon is considerably more potent in man than are the other two, perhaps in part because it is cleared from the circulation more slowly. Salmon calcitonin is available for clinical use as CALCIMAR or MIACALCIN, a synthetic preparation supplied in vials containing 100 or 200 I.U. per milliliter. The recommended dosage (administered subcutaneously or intramuscularly) is 4 to 8 units/kg every 6 to 12 hours for hypercalcemia; an initial dose of 100 units per day is used for Paget's disease (*see* below). Synthetic human calcitonin is available as CIBACALCIN in syringes that contain 0.5 mg. The initial daily dose for Paget's disease is 0.5 mg subcutaneously.

Therapeutic Uses. Calcitonin is effective in diminishing hypercalcemia and decreasing concentrations of phosphate in the plasma of patients with hyperparathyroidism, idiopathic hypercalcemia of infancy, vitamin D intoxication, and osteolytic bone metastases. The effect of a single dose lasts 6 to 10 hours. The decrease in plasma Ca^{2+} and phosphate is the result of their decreased resorption from bone. Although calcitonin is effective in the initial treatment of hypercalcemia from various causes, other measures are recommended and are generally more practical for long-term management (*see* section above on hypercalcemia).

Calcitonin is effective in diseases characterized by increased skeletal remodeling (increased bone resorption and bone formation), such as occurs in Paget's disease. In this disease, calcitonin given chronically produces symptomatic relief and reduction in alkaline phosphatase activity in plasma, urinary hydroxyproline, and blood flow through the affected area. However, patients may become resistant to therapy after several months. Development of antibodies to porcine or salmon calcitonin does occur with long-term therapy in many patients; this finding is more common with the porcine preparation and may explain the development of resistance. Favorable results are usually obtained with 100 MRC units of salmon calcitonin or 0.5 mg of human calcitonin given daily or three times a week by subcutaneous injection (Hosking, 1985). Side effects include nausea and swelling and tenderness of the hands; urticaria has also been observed. It is anticipated that human calcitonin will cause less resistance and allergic reactions.

Salmon calcitonin has also been approved for therapy of postmenopausal osteoporosis. A critical review of the use of calcitonin in this disease is provided by Fatourechi and Heath (1987).

SODIUM ETIDRONATE

This drug is available for the treatment of Paget's disease of bone. It is related to pyrophosphate, which may have a role in bone mineralization, and has the following structure:

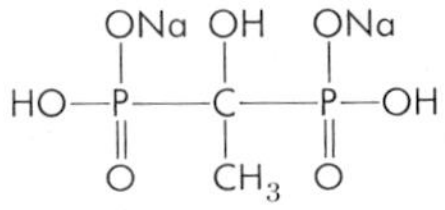

Sodium Etidronate

This compound (and other diphosphonates), when added to appropriate solutions and suspensions of calcium phosphate, slows the formation and dissolution of crystals of hydroxyapatite. Diphosphonates can protect experimental animals against calcification of soft tissues in vitamin D intoxication.

The physicochemical action of sodium etidronate on the dynamics of crystal formation and dissolution are thought to be responsible for its favorable effects in patients with Paget's disease. Paget's disease is associated with foci of increased turnover of bone; these lead to the characteristic alterations of bone structure, which in turn may produce secondary problems, including deafness, spinal cord injuries, high-output cardiac failure, and disabling pain. Sodium etidronate may decrease the elevated plasma alkaline phosphatase activity and the urinary excretion of hydroxyproline that are characteristic of this disease. Following treatment, most patients experience a decrease in bone pain, but worsening of bone pain has also been reported. There is an increase in the amount of nonmineralized osteoid, especially after treatment with higher doses; this effect may increase the risk of fractures. The drug is effective orally. It is excreted without metabolic alteration by the kidney; dosage must therefore be reduced in the presence of renal insufficiency.

Advantages of this agent over calcitonin include its oral efficacy, lower cost, and lack of antigenicity. Biochemical indices of the rate of bone turnover are more often normalized and control of Paget's disease may be better sustained when a combination of etidronate and calcitonin is used than when either is used alone (O'Donoghue and Hosking, 1987).

Etidronate and other diphosphonates have also been used successfully in the management of hypercalcemia associated with malignancy.

Etidronate disodium (DIDRONEL) is available in tablets containing 200 or 400 mg and in ampules containing 300 mg. The usual initial dose for Paget's disease is 5 mg/kg, given once daily in courses that should be given for no longer than 6 months. Such treatment may induce a remission of Paget's disease that can last years. If symptoms recur, additional courses of therapy may be effective. The drug is also used to reduce heterotropic ossification due to spinal cord injury or that which complicates total hip replacement.

When used for hypercalcemia of malignancy, etidronate is infused at a dose of 7.5 mg/kg in 250 ml of isotonic saline over at least 2 hours. The drug is usually given for 3 consecutive days, although some individuals require 5 to 7 days of treatment. Patients should be well hydrated, and a loop diuretic is also given to ensure an optimal response (Stevenson, 1988).

VITAMIN D

Traditionally, vitamin D was assigned a passive role in calcium metabolism in that its presence in adequate concentrations was thought to permit proper absorption of dietary Ca^{2+} and to allow full expression of the actions of parathyroid hormone. However, it is now known that vitamin D has a much more active role in the homeostatic mechanisms that control Ca^{2+} metabolism. Even though it is termed "vitamin" D, it is a hormone that, together with PTH and calcitonin, is a major regulator of the concentration of Ca^{2+} in plasma. The following characteristics of vitamin D are consistent with hormonal activity: vitamin D is synthesized in the skin and under ideal conditions probably is not required in the diet; it is transported by the blood to distant sites in the body, where it is activated; its active form then binds to specific receptors in target tissues, resulting ultimately in increased plasma Ca^{2+} concentration; and the conversion of vitamin D to its active form is a reaction that is regulated in a negative-feedback system by plasma Ca^{2+}. Moreover, it is now known that receptors for the activated form of vitamin D are expressed in many cells throughout the body, including hematopoietic cells, lymphocytes, epidermal cells, and neurons in the CNS, and mediate a variety of actions that are unrelated to Ca^{2+} homeostasis.

History. Vitamin D is the name applied to two related fat-soluble substances, cholecalciferol and calciferol, that have in common the ability to prevent or cure rickets. Prior to the discovery of vitamin D a high percentage of urban children, especially in the temperate zones, developed rickets. Some researchers believed that the disease was due to lack of fresh air and sunshine; others claimed a dietary factor caused the disease. The work of Mellanby (1919) and Huldschinsky (1919) showed both of these notions to be correct; the addition of cod liver oil to the diet or exposure to sunlight would either prevent or cure the disease. In 1924 it was found that irradiation of animal rations was as efficacious in curing rickets as was irradiation of the animal itself (Hess and Weinstock, 1924; Steenbock and Black, 1924). These observations led to the elucidation of the structures of cholecalciferol and calciferol and eventually to the discovery that these compounds are further metabolized in the body to active compounds. The discovery of metabolic activation is primarily attributable to studies conducted in the laboratories of DeLuca in the United States and Kodicek in England (*see* Kodicek, 1974; DeLuca and Schnoes, 1976).

Chemistry and Occurrence. Ultraviolet irradiation of a variety of animal and plant sterols results in their conversion to compounds with vitamin D (antirachitic) activity. Cleavage of the carbon-to-carbon bond between C 9 and C 10 is the essential alteration produced by the photochemical process, but not all sterols that undergo this cleavage possess antirachitic activity. The principal provitamin found in animal tissues is 7-dehydrocholesterol, which is synthesized in the skin. Exposure of the skin to sunlight converts 7-dehydrocholesterol to cholecalciferol (vitamin D_3) (*see* Figure 62–1). Holick and associates have found an intermediate in the photolysis reaction—previtamin D_3, a 6,7-*cis* isomer that accumulates in the skin after exposure to ultraviolet radiation (*see* Holick, 1981). This isomer slowly converts spontaneously to vitamin D_3 and may provide a sustained source of D_3 for some time after exposure to ultraviolet light.

Ergosterol, which is present in yeasts and fungi, is the provitamin for vitamin D_2 (calciferol). Ergosterol and vitamin D_2 differ from 7-dehydrocholesterol and vitamin D_3, respectively, only by each having a double bond between C 22 and C 23 and a methyl group at C 24. Vitamin D_2 is the active constituent in a number of commercial vitamin preparations as well as in irradiated bread and irradiated milk. The material historically designated as vitamin D_1 was later shown to be a mixture of antirachitic substances.

In some species the antirachitic potencies of vitamin D_2 and vitamin D_3 differ greatly from each other. In man there is no practical difference between the two, and in the following discussion vitamin D will be used as the collective term for vitamins D_2 and D_3.

METABOLIC ACTIVATION

Dietary vitamin D, or that which is synthesized intrinsically, requires metabolic activation to exert its characteristic actions on target tissues. It is now believed that the active form of the vitamin is calcitriol (1,25-$(OH)_2$ cholecalciferol), the product of two successive hydroxylations of D_3. The pathway of activation is shown in Figure 62–1. This subject has been reviewed by DeLuca and Schnoes (1983), and by Fraser (1988).

25-Hydroxylation of Vitamin D. In man the initial step in the activation of vitamin D_3 occurs predominantly in the liver, and the product is 25-hydroxycholecalciferol (or calcifediol). The hepatic enzyme system responsible for 25-hydroxylation of vitamin D has not been fully characterized, but it is associated with the microsomal and mitochondrial fractions of liver homogenates and requires NADPH and molecular oxygen for the hydroxylation reaction.

1-Hydroxylation of 25-OHD_3. After production in the liver, 25-OHD_3 enters the bloodstream, where it circulates in association with vitamin D–binding globulin. Final activation to calcitriol occurs primarily in the kidney, but it can also take place in the placenta and decidua (Weisman *et al.*, 1979) and in macrophages (Reichel *et al.*, 1987). The enzyme system responsible for 1-hydroxylation of 25-OHD_3 is associated with mitochondria in the proximal tubules of the kidney. It, too, is a mixed-function oxidase and requires molecular oxygen and NADPH as cofactors. Cytochrome P_{450}, a

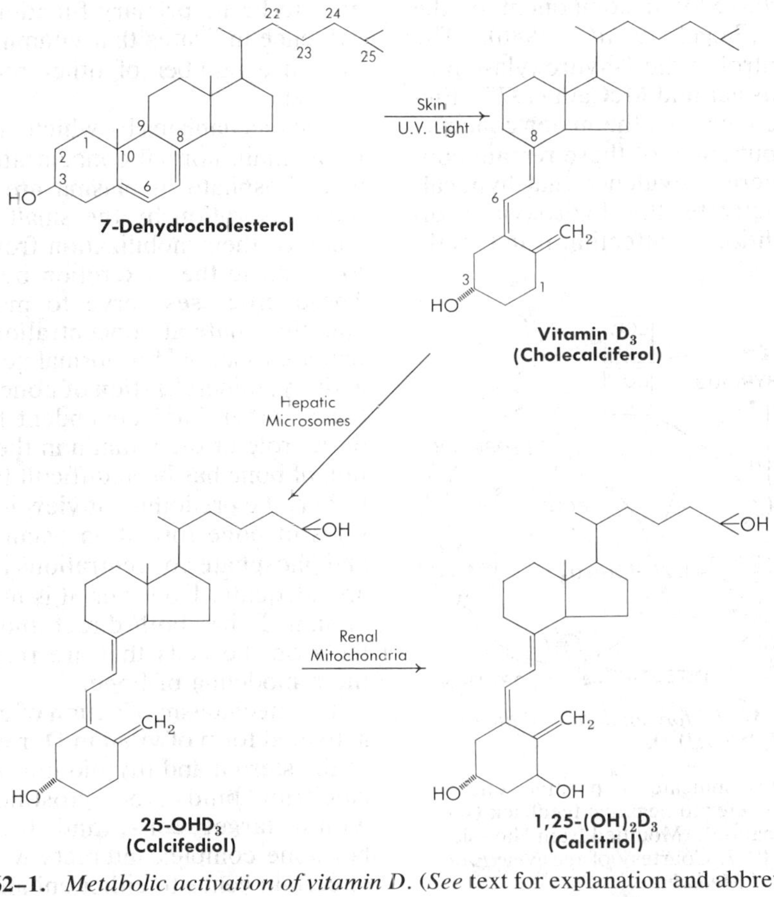

Figure 62–1. *Metabolic activation of vitamin D.* (*See* text for explanation and abbreviations.)

flavoprotein, and ferredoxin are components of the enzyme complex.

This enzyme is subject to dietary and endocrine regulations that result in changes in plasma concentrations of calcitriol appropriate for optimal Ca^{2+} homeostasis. Thus, the activity of the hydroxylase increases in dietary deficiencies of vitamin D, Ca^{2+}, and phosphate; it is also stimulated by PTH, prolactin, and estrogens. Conversely, its activity is suppressed by a high intake of vitamin D. The slowness of the responses to some of these agents and their sensitivity to metabolic inhibitors strongly suggest that the variations in enzymatic activity represent changes in the quantity of enzyme protein in the kidney. There is also evidence of an acute mechanism of control that can change the activity of the hydroxylase within a few minutes. In the case of PTH, this rapid effect is mediated by cyclic AMP, apparently through an indirect stimulation of a phosphoprotein phosphatase that acts on the ferredoxin component of the hydroxylase (Siegel *et al.,* 1986). The model for control of the 1-hydroxylase proposed by Haussler and McCain (1977) (Figure 62–2) encompasses the major concepts in this area, but some of these remain controversial. There is evidence that hypocalcemia can activate the hydroxylase directly, in addition to affecting it indirectly

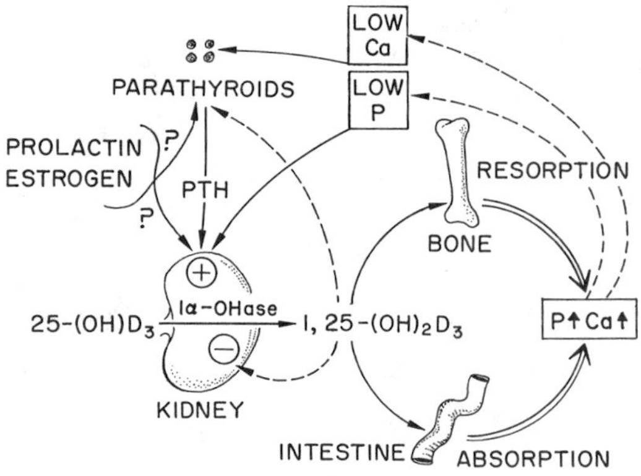

Figure 62–2. *Model for regulation of the biosynthesis of 1,25-(OH)$_2$D$_3$.*

Solid arrows indicate a positive effect; dashed arrows refer to negative feedback (*see* text for explanation). (Modified from Haussler and McCain, 1977. Courtesy of the *New England Journal of Medicine.*)

by eliciting secretion of PTH (*see* Fraser, 1980). Hypophosphatemia increases the activity of the hydroxylase, but it is not known whether this is a direct or indirect effect (Haussler and McCain, 1977; Fraser, 1980; Rosen and Chesney, 1983). Calcitriol exerts negative-feedback control of the enzyme that may be a consequence of a direct action on renal tissue or of inhibition of the secretion of PTH. The nature of the regulatory mechanisms of estrogens and prolactin on the 1α-hydroxylase is not known.

PHYSIOLOGICAL FUNCTIONS, MECHANISM OF ACTION, AND PHARMACOLOGICAL PROPERTIES

The physiological role of vitamin D is best characterized as that of a positive regulator in Ca^{2+} homeostasis. Phosphate metabolism is affected by the vitamin in a manner parallel to that of Ca^{2+}. Although regulation of Ca^{2+} homeostasis is considered to be its primary function, increasing evidence indicates that vitamin D is important in a number of other processes (*see* below).

The mechanisms by which vitamin D acts to maintain normal concentrations of Ca^{2+} and phosphate in plasma are to facilitate their absorption by the small intestine, to enhance their mobilization from bone, and to decrease their excretion by the kidney. These processes serve to maintain Ca^{2+} and phosphate at concentrations in plasma that are essential for normal neuromuscular activity, mineralization of bone, and a number of other Ca^{2+}-dependent functions. A direct role of the vitamin in the mineralization of bone has been difficult to document; rather, the predominant view is that normal rates of bone formation occur when Ca^{2+} and phosphate concentrations in the plasma are adequate. However, it is now clear that vitamin D has both direct and indirect effects on the cells that are responsible for the remodeling of bone.

The mechanism of action of calcitriol, the activated form of vitamin D, resembles that of the steroid and thyroid hormones. Thus, calcitriol binds to cytosolic receptors within target cells, and the receptor–hormone complex interacts with the DNA of certain genes to either enhance or inhibit their transcription. Structural analysis of the calcitriol receptor indicates that it belongs to the same supergene family as the steroid receptors (*see* Evans, 1988; Reichel *et al.*, 1989; *see also* Chapter 2). Calcitriol also appears to exert a few effects that occur too rapidly to be explained by genomic actions (*see,* for example, Barsony and Marx, 1988).

Intestinal Absorption of Calcium. A defect in intestinal absorption of Ca^{2+} in vitamin D–deficient rats was demonstrated over 50 years ago. Since then, numerous studies have demonstrated that treatment of such animals with the activated hormone leads within 2 to 4 hours to increased movement of Ca^{2+} from the mucosal to serosal surface of the intestine. However, the mechanisms underlying this action remain to be elucidated. One relatively early event is the induction of one of a family of small Ca^{2+}-binding proteins (CaBP); both an early increase in the rate of synthesis of mRNA for CaBP and a later decrease in its rate of degradation are involved (Theofan *et al.*, 1986; Dupret *et al.*, 1987). Although some investigators propose that CaBP acts to facilitate the passage of Ca^{2+} through the brush border and its diffusion to the basolateral membrane of mucosal cells (*see* Bronner, 1988), others contend that the accumulation of CaBP is poorly correlated with activation of Ca^{2+} transport (Nemere and Norman, 1988). Instead, it is proposed that calcitriol enhances the endocytotic uptake of Ca^{2+} from the intestinal lumen into vesicles within the brush border of mucosal cells. The endocytic vesicles fuse with lysosomes, which then deliver the Ca^{2+} to the basolateral membrane for extrusion (*see* Cancela *et al.*, 1988). The mechanisms by which calcitriol might promote such vesicle-mediated Ca^{2+} transport have not been defined. Although the time to onset of effects (2 to 3 hours) in vitamin D–deficient animals suggests the involvement of genomic mechanisms, calcitriol can also cause a rapid (within minutes), receptor-mediated stimulation of Ca^{2+} transport in vitamin D–replete animals (*see* Cancela *et al.*, 1988). It is not clear whether the extrusion of Ca^{2+} at the basolateral membrane is accomplished primarily by exocytosis or by a Ca^{2+}-Mg^{2+}-ATPase; however, there seems to be general agreement that the rates of uptake and translocation of Ca^{2+} determine the overall rate of absorption.

Mobilization of Bone Salts. Although vitamin D–deficient animals show obvious loss of bone minerals, there is little evidence that vitamin D directly promotes bone mineralization; thus, it is thought that normal deposition of minerals is sustained by the maintenance of optimal plasma concentrations of Ca^{2+} and phosphate through promotion of their intestinal absorption (*see* Stern, 1980). Indeed, children with an inherited form of rickets that is resistant to calcitriol have been treated successfully with intravenous infusions of Ca^{2+} and phosphate (*see* DeLuca, 1988). In contrast, it has been known for many years that physiological doses of vitamin D promote mobilization of Ca^{2+} from bone and that large doses cause an excessive amount of bone resorption. Although calcitriol-induced decalcification of bone may be reduced in parathyroidectomized animals, the response is restored when hyperphosphatemia is corrected (*see* Stern, 1980). Thus, both PTH and calcitriol act independently to enhance bone resorption.

The mechanisms responsible for mobilization of bone salts have been only partially defined, and the interaction of multiple factors appears to be involved (*see* Haussler, 1986; Reichel *et al.*, 1989). Paradoxically, the cells responsible for bone resorption (osteoclasts) are not directly acted upon by calcitriol and do not appear to contain calcitriol receptors. Instead, calcitriol causes an increase in the number of osteoclasts available to resorb bone; this may result from an action upon myeloid hematopoietic precursor cells that are induced to differentiate toward functional osteoclasts. The cells responsible for bone formation (osteoblasts) do contain receptors, and calcitriol causes them to elaborate several proteins, including osteocalcin, a vitamin K–dependent protein that contains γ-carboxyglutamic acid residues. The exact role of this protein is not known, but other unidentified substances are also elaborated that appear to stimulate the function of osteoclasts. In addition, calcitriol acts synergistically with gamma-interferon to increase the production of interleukin-1, a lymphokine that promotes bone resorption (Spear *et al.*, 1988). It has been suggested that patients with osteopetrosis, a disease in which resorption of bone is deficient, may have a genetic defect that prevents cellular differentiation of osteoclast precursors in response to agents such as calcitriol (Coccia, 1983; Key *et al.*, 1984).

Renal Retention of Calcium and Phosphate. The effects of vitamin D on renal handling of Ca^{2+} and phosphate have had relatively little study, and their quantitative importance is uncertain. Vitamin D has been shown to increase retention of Ca^{2+} independently of phosphate. There is evidence that vitamin D enhances the reabsorption of Ca^{2+} and phosphate by the proximal tubules.

Other Effects of Calcitriol. When calcitriol was first identified as the active form of vitamin D, it was generally considered to act only as a regulator of Ca^{2+} homeostasis. However, it has become evident that its effects are much broader and more complex. Receptors for calcitriol are distributed widely throughout the body (Braidman and Anderson, 1985); however, their function is largely unknown.

As noted above, calcitriol affects maturation and differentiation of mononuclear cells, as well as influencing lymphokine production. The effects of calcitriol on the immune system have been reviewed by Amento (1987). One thrust of current research is the potential therapeutic application of the ability of calcitriol to inhibit proliferation and to induce the differentiation of malignant cells (Braidman and Anderson, 1985; Haussler, 1986). The possibility of dissociating the hypercalcemic effect of calcitriol from its actions on cell differentiation has encouraged the search for analogs that might be useful for cancer therapy.

The relation of vitamin D to the function of skeletal muscle has been reviewed by Boland (1986), and possible effects of vitamin D in the brain have been reviewed by Luine and associates (1987).

Signs and Symptoms of Deficiency. A deficiency of vitamin D results in inadequate absorption of Ca^{2+} and phosphate. The consequent decrease in plasma Ca^{2+} stimulates PTH secretion, which acts to restore plasma Ca^{2+} at the expense of bone Ca^{2+}; plasma concentrations of phosphate remain subnormal. In infants and children, the result is a failure to mineralize newly formed osteoid tissue and cartilage matrix, causing the defect in bone growth known as rickets. As a consequence of inadequate calcification, the bones of individuals suffering from rickets are unusually soft, and the stress and strain of weight bearing give rise to the characteristic deformities of the disease.

In adults, vitamin D deficiency results in osteomalacia, or adult rickets, which is most likely to occur during times of increased need for Ca^{2+}, such as during pregnancy or lactation. The disease is characterized by a generalized decrease in bone density. Unlike osteoporosis, the remaining bone is abnormal in that it contains excessive amounts of uncalcified matrix. Gross deformities of bone occur only in advanced stages of the disease.

Hypervitaminosis. The acute or long-term administration of excessive amounts of vitamin D or enhanced responsiveness to normal amounts of the vitamin leads to a number of clinical syndromes that are the result of deranged Ca^{2+} metabolism. The physiological or pathological responses to vitamin D are a function of endogenous production of vitamin D, tissue reactivity to the vitamin, and particularly vitamin D intake. Some infants seem to be hyperreactive to relatively small doses of vitamin D. Certain cases of hypervitaminosis D in adults result from the administration of large doses of the vitamin in the attempt to treat conditions that have been wrongly purported to benefit from vitamin D therapy. Other cases are the consequence of excessive doses used in the treatment of hypoparathyroidism. More commonly, toxicity is seen in children as a result of accidental ingestion or excessive administration of the vitamin by parents.

The amount of vitamin D that causes hypervitaminosis varies widely among individuals. As a rough approximation, it may be stated that the continued ingestion of 60,000 units or more daily by a person with normal parathyroid function and normal sensitivity to vitamin D may result in poisoning. Hypercalcemia is particularly dangerous in patients who are receiving digitalis, because the toxic effects of the cardiac glycosides are enhanced (*see* Chapter 34).

Signs and Symptoms. The initial signs and symptoms of vitamin D toxicity are those associated with hypercalcemia and consist of weakness, fatigue, lassitude, headache, nausea, vomiting, and diarrhea. Obtundation and coma may develop. Early impairment of renal function from hypercalcemia is manifest by polyuria, polydipsia, nocturia, decreased urinary concentrating ability, and proteinuria. Some of these effects are due to failure of the kidney to develop sufficient hypertonicity in the interstitial fluid of the medulla. With prolonged hypercalcemia there may be deposition of Ca^{2+} salts in soft tissues, most significantly within the kidney; this results in nephrolithiasis, diffuse nephrocalcinosis, or both. Other sites of calcification may include blood vessels, heart, lungs, and skin. Some individuals exhibit hypertension. The characteristic changes in blood chemistry are elevated concentrations of Ca^{2+} and urea; phosphate concentrations are variable. Mobilization of Ca^{2+} from bone contributes to the hypercalcemia and is also responsible for the roentgenographic finding of localized or generalized osteoporosis in a significant percentage of cases of hypervitaminosis D.

In children, a single episode of moderately severe hypercalcemia may arrest growth completely for 6 months or more, and the deficit in height may never be fully corrected.

Vitamin D toxicity may be manifested in the fetus. There is a relationship between excess maternal vitamin D intake or extreme sensitivity to the vitamin and nonfamilial congenital supravalvular aortic stenosis. In infants, this anomaly is often found in association with other stigmata of hypercalcemia. Maternal hypercalcemia may also result in suppression of parathyroid function in the newborn, with resultant hypocalcemia, tetany, and seizures.

An occasional sequela resulting from an acute episode of hypercalcemia in patients treated for hypoparathyroidism is a marked increase in response to vitamin D after the disappearance of the hypercalcemia (Leeson and Fourman, 1966).

Treatment. The treatment of hypervitaminosis D consists of immediate withdrawal of the vitamin, a low-Ca^{2+} diet, administration of glucocorticoids, and a generous intake of fluid. With this regimen the plasma Ca^{2+} falls to normal and the Ca^{2+} in the soft tissue tends to be mobilized. A conspicuous improvement in renal function is often noted with return of the plasma Ca^{2+} to normal, but this may not occur if renal damage has been severe.

Absorption, Fate, and Excretion. Vitamin D is usually given by mouth, and gastrointestinal absorption is adequate under most conditions. Both vitamin D_2 and vitamin D_3 are absorbed from the small intestine, although vitamin D_3 may be absorbed more completely and more rapidly. The exact portion of the gut that is most effective in vitamin D absorption may be a function of the vehicle in which the vitamin is suspended or dissolved. Most of the vitamin appears first in lymph and primarily in the chylomicron fraction as a lipoprotein complex.

Bile is essential for adequate intestinal absorption of vitamin D; deoxycholic acid is the most important constituent of bile in this regard. Thus, hepatic or biliary dysfunction may seriously impair absorption of vitamin D. Likewise, other abnormalities of gastrointestinal function, especially those associated with steatorrhea, may interfere with proper absorption of orally administered vitamin D.

Absorbed vitamin D circulates in the blood in association with vitamin D–binding protein, which is a specific α-globulin. The vitamin disappears from plasma with a half-life of 19 to 25 hours, but it is stored in the body for prolonged periods (6 months or longer in the rat), apparently in fat deposits.

As discussed above, the liver is the site of conversion of vitamin D to its 25-hydroxy derivative, which also circulates in association with vitamin D–binding protein. In fact, calcifediol has a higher affinity for the binding protein than does the parent compound. The 25-hydroxy derivative has a biological half-life of 19 days and constitutes the major circulating form of vitamin D. The plasma half-life of calcitriol is estimated to be between 3 and 5 days in man, and 40% of an administered dose is excreted within 10 days (Mawer *et al.*, 1976). Calcitriol is hydroxylated to 1,24,25-$(OH)_3D_3$ by a renal hydroxylase that is induced by calcitriol and suppressed by those factors that stimulate the 25-OHD_3-1α-hydroxylase. This enzyme also hydroxylates calcifediol to form 24,25-$(OH)_2D_3$. Both 24-hydroxylated compounds are less active than calcitriol and presumably represent metabolites destined for excretion. Side chain oxidation of calcitriol also occurs.

The primary route of excretion of vitamin D is in the bile; only a small percentage of an administered dose is found in the urine.

An important interaction has been demonstrated between vitamin D and phenytoin or phenobarbital. Patients receiving the anticonvulsant agents for a prolonged time have a high incidence of rickets and osteomalacia. These agents also diminish the effects of vitamin D on intestinal absorption of Ca^{2+} and on bone resorption (*see* Habener and Mahaffey, 1978). Furthermore, these drugs protect rats against the toxic effects of high doses of vitamin D (Gascon-Barré and Côte, 1978). Plasma concentrations of calcifediol are decreased in patients receiving these drugs, and it was proposed that phenytoin and phenobarbital accelerate the metabolism of vitamin D to inactive products (Hahn *et al.*, 1972). However, concentrations of calcitriol in plasma are normal, despite the depression of the concentration of calcifediol, in patients receiving anticonvulsant therapy (Jubiz *et al.*, 1977). The drugs also accelerate the hepatic metabolism of vitamin K and reduce the synthesis of vitamin K–dependent proteins, such as osteocalcin (*see* Chapter 19).

Human Requirements and Unitage. An exhaustive and critical summary of the prophylactic requirements for vitamin D has been compiled by the Committee on Nutrition of the American Academy of Pediatrics (*see* Committee on Nutrition, 1963). In the more than 70 years that have elapsed since Mellanby demonstrated the efficacy of cod liver oil in the prevention of rickets, the disease has become a clinical rarity in the United States. Although sunlight provides adequate antirachitic prophylaxis in the equatorial belt, in the temperate climates insufficient cutaneous solar radiation in winter may necessitate dietary vitamin D supplementation.

Previously, the recommended allowance of vitamin D could be achieved only by the addition of oral vitamin D supplements to a normal diet. Since the advent of the addition of the vitamin to foodstuffs (especially milk, milk products, cereals, and candy), individuals of all ages receive variable and even excessive vitamin D without its special addition to the diet. Thus, the supplemental requirements vary not only with age, pregnancy, and lactation but also with the quality of the diet. Serious toxicity may result from excessive ingestion of the vitamin, and even as little as 1800 USP units per day in infants may lead to inhibition of growth. It is clear, therefore, that any recommendation for vitamin D supplementation must be made only after careful scrutiny of the diet.

In both the premature and the normal infant, a total of 400 units per day of vitamin D ensures full antirachitic prophylaxis and optimal growth. Whether this amount is obtained by way of the diet, by vitamin D supplementation, or by a combination of both is of no consequence. During adolescence and adulthood this amount is probably also sufficient. There is some evidence that vitamin D requirements are greater than normal during pregnancy and lactation, although a daily intake of 400 units is sufficient in these conditions as well (*see* Table XVI–1, page 1525).

The USP unit is identical with the international unit (I.U.) and is equivalent to the specific biological activity of 0.025 μg of vitamin D_3 (*i.e.*, 1 mg equals 40,000 units).

Bioassay procedures have been used in the past and depend upon evidence of alleviation of the rachitic state. They are still in use for experimental purposes.

Modified Forms of Vitamin D. Two derivatives of vitamin D are of considerable experimental and therapeutic interest.

Dihydrotachysterol (DHT) is an analog of vitamin D that may be regarded as the reduction product of vitamin D_2 (and is sometimes referred to as DHT_2); its structural formula is as follows:

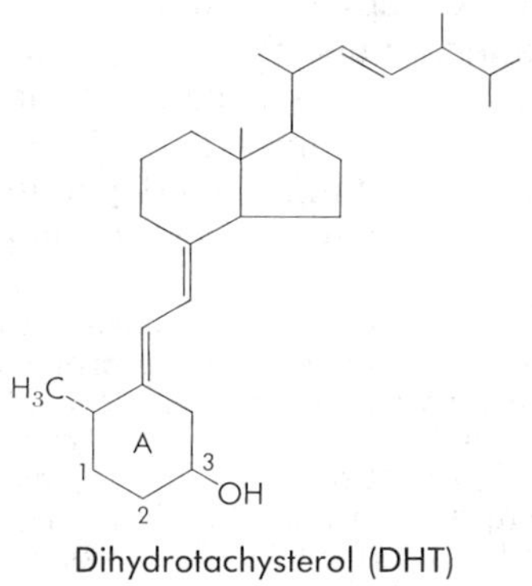

Dihydrotachysterol (DHT)

Although DHT is the compound available for therapeutic use, the corresponding derivative of vitamin D_3 (DHT_3) has been used in experimental studies. Presumably, DHT behaves in a manner analogous to that described for DHT_3. DHT is about 1/450 as active as vitamin D in the usual antirachitic assay, but at high doses it is much more effective than vitamin D in mobilizing Ca^{2+} from bone (Suda *et al.*, 1970). The latter effect is the basis for the use of DHT to maintain normal concentrations of Ca^{2+} in plasma in hypoparathyroidism.

Studies describing the metabolic activation of DHT_3 provide an explanation for the above findings. DHT_3 undergoes 25-hydroxylation to yield 25-hydroxydihydrotachysterol$_3$ (25-OHDHT$_3$), which appears to be the active form of DHT in both intestine and bone. Both DHT_3 and 25-OHDHT$_3$ are active in nephrectomized rats, indicating that DHT_3 does not require 1-hydroxylation in the kidney. A comparison of the structures of DHT and 1,25-$(OH)_2D_3$ shows that ring A of DHT is rotated so as to place its 3-hydroxyl group in approximately the same geometrical position as the 1-hydroxyl group of 1,25-$(OH)_2D_3$. It seems reasonable, therefore, to assume that 25-OHDHT$_3$ could interact with receptor sites for 1,25-$(OH)_2D_3$ without undergoing 1-hydroxylation in the kidney. Thus, DHT bypasses the renal mechanisms of metabolic control.

1α-Hydroxycholecalciferol (1-OHD$_3$) is a synthetic derivative of vitamin D_3 that is hydroxylated in the 1α position. It is readily hydroxylated in the 25 position by the hepatic microsomal system to form 1,25-$(OH)_2D_3$ and was therefore introduced as a substitute for this compound. In the chick assays for stimulation of intestinal absorption of Ca^{2+} and bone mineralization it is essentially equal in activity to calcitriol. Because it does not require renal hydroxylation it has been used to treat renal osteodystrophy. This drug is not available in the United States.

Preparations. Many preparations containing vitamin D are marketed. Those containing the vitamin as a single entity are listed below.

Ergocalciferol (*calciferol;* DRISDOL) is pure vitamin D_2. It is available in capsules or tablets that contain 1.25 mg (50,000 USP units) each. An oral solution (8000 units/ml) of the vitamin in propylene glycol is also available. An injection in oil (500,000 units/ml) is available for intramuscular administration.

Dihydrotachysterol (*DHT;* HYTAKEROL) is the pure crystalline compound obtained by reduction of vitamin D_2 and is available as tablets (0.125 to 0.4 mg), capsules (0.125 mg), an oral solution (0.2 mg/ml), and a solution in oil (0.25 mg/ml). These preparations are all for oral administration.

Calcifediol (*25-hydroxycholecalciferol;* CALDEROL) is available in capsules containing 20 or 50 μg. The recommended initial dose for hypocalcemia in patients who are receiving chronic renal dialysis is 300 to 350 μg per week, administered on a daily or alternate-day schedule.

Calcitriol (*1,25-dihydroxycholecalciferol;* CALCIJEX, ROCALTROL) is marketed in capsules for oral administration that contain 0.25 or 0.5 μg and as an injection (1 or 2 μg/ml). Dosage must be individualized but is often effective at 0.5 to 1 μg per day.

THERAPEUTIC USES

The major therapeutic uses of vitamin D may be divided into three categories: (1) prophylaxis and cure of nutritional rickets, (2) treatment of metabolic rickets and osteomalacia, particularly in the setting of chronic renal failure, and (3) treatment of hypoparathyroidism.

Nutritional Rickets. Nutritional rickets results from inadequate exposure to sunlight or a deficiency of vitamin D in the diet. The condition is extremely rare in the United States and other countries where milk and other foods contain added vitamin D. Infants and children receiving adequate amounts of vitamin D–fortified food do not require additional vitamin D; however, breast-fed infants or those fed unfortified formula should receive 400 units of vitamin D daily as a supplement. The usual practice is to administer vitamin A in combination with vitamin D. A number of well-balanced vitamin A and D preparations are available for this purpose. Premature infants are especially susceptible to rickets and may require supplemental vitamin D, since the fetus acquires more than 85% of its Ca^{2+} stores during the third trimester.

The curative dose of vitamin D for the treatment of fully developed rickets is larger than the prophylactic dose. One thousand units daily will produce normal Ca^{2+} and phosphate concentrations in plasma in approximately 10 days and roentgenographic evidence of healing within about 3 weeks. However, a daily dose of 3000 to 4000 units is often prescribed for more rapid healing; this is of particular importance in severe cases of thoracic rickets when respiration is embarrassed.

Certain conditions are known to lead to poor absorption of vitamin D. If untreated by vitamin supplementation, a frank deficiency may develop. Therefore, vitamin D may be of definite prophylactic value in such disorders as diarrhea, steatorrhea, biliary obstruction, and any other abnormality in gastrointestinal function in which absorption is appreciably diminished. Parenteral administration may be used in such cases.

Metabolic Rickets and Osteomalacia. This group of diseases, which presents as rickets in infants and children and osteomalacia in adults, is characterized by a failure to respond to physiological doses of vitamin D. Three types of metabolic rickets are discussed below, and the reader is referred to articles by Parfitt (1972), Smith (1972), and Scriver and coworkers (1978) for more complete discussions of other forms of the disease.

Hypophosphatemic vitamin D–resistant rickets is an X-linked inherited disorder of Ca^{2+} and phosphate metabolism. It is *not* characterized by a defect in vitamin D metabolism, but treatment with large doses of calcitriol in combination with phosphate salts may lead to clinical improvement (Brickman *et al.*, 1973).

Vitamin D–dependent rickets (pseudo-vitamin D deficiency rickets) is an inherited, autosomal recessive disease that appears to be due to an inborn error of vitamin D metabolism involving defective conversion of 25-OHD_3 to 1,25-$(OH)_2D_3$. The condition responds to physiological doses of calcitriol (Fraser *et al.*, 1973).

Renal osteodystrophy (renal rickets) is associated with chronic renal failure and is characterized by a decreased ability of the kidney to convert 25-OHD_3 to 1,25-$(OH)_2D_3$. Retention of phosphate results in decreased concentrations of Ca^{2+} in plasma, and there is secondary hyperparathyroidism. In addition, deficiency of 1,25-$(OH)_2D_3$ impairs intestinal absorption of Ca^{2+} and mobilization of Ca^{2+} from bone. Hypocalcemia is a common result (although some patients may actually become hypercalcemic because of severe hyperparathyroidism). Deposition of Al^{3+} in bone may also play a role in the genesis of renal osteodystrophy (*see* Chapter 37). Pathologically, the lesions are typical of hyperparathyroidism (osteitis fibrosa), deficiency of vitamin D (osteomalacia), or a mixture of both. In patients with chronic renal failure who are not receiving dialysis, the emphasis has been on treatment of hyperphosphatemia with phosphate binders and Ca^{2+} supplementation; these goals can be accomplished by the oral administration of calcium carbonate, combined with restriction of dietary phosphate (Coburn and Salusky, 1989). The use of vitamin D analogs in predialysis patients is still experimental, but these preparations are clearly useful in patients who are undergoing dialysis. The administration of calcitriol in this condition can raise the concentration of Ca^{2+} in plasma and lower the concentration of PTH, and it helps to maintain bone mineralization and growth in children (Berl *et al.*, 1978; Chesney *et al.*, 1978). Intravenous calcitriol may be effective in patients who are refractory to oral therapy (Andress *et al.*, 1989). DHT and 1-OHD_3 can also be used effectively, since renal hydroxylation is not required for their activity. Although calcifediol may also be effective, high doses must be utilized.

Hypoparathyroidism. Hypoparathyroidism is characterized by hypocalcemia and hyperphosphatemia (*see* above). Dihydrotachysterol has long been used to treat this condition, since it has a more rapid onset of action, a shorter duration of action, and, as noted above, a greater effect on mobilization of bone salts than does vitamin D. Calcitriol is effective in the management of hypoparathyroidism (Rosen *et al.*, 1977) and at least certain forms of pseudohypoparathyroidism in which an abnormally low concentration of calcitriol is present in plasma (Metz *et al.*, 1977). However, with the exception of the latter rare form of pseudohypoparathyroidism where the hydroxylase is deficient, most hypoparathyroid patients respond to any of the forms of vitamin D. Calcitriol may be the agent of choice for the temporary treatment of hypocalcemia while waiting for a slower-acting form of vitamin D to become effective.

Miscellaneous Uses of Vitamin D. Miscellaneous uses of vitamin D include treatment of the hypophosphatemia seen in the Fanconi syndrome. The use of large doses of vitamin D in patients with osteoporosis is of doubtful value and can be dangerous. Furthermore, the indiscriminate use of "over-the-counter" vitamin D preparations for conditions other than the aforementioned is irrational and can be dangerous.

FLUORIDE

Fluoride is of interest because of its toxic properties and its effect on dental enamel and bone. Fluoride is widely distributed in nature, and the soils of different regions of the world vary greatly in their fluoride content. The sources of atmospheric fluoride include the burning of soft coal and the manufacturing of superphosphate, aluminum, steel, lead, copper, and nickel. Man obtains fluoride in particular from the ingestion of plants and water.

Absorption, Distribution, and Excretion. Fluorides are absorbed from the gastrointestinal tract, the lungs, and the skin. The gastrointestinal tract is the major site of absorption. The degree of absorption of a fluoride compound is best correlated with its solubility. The relatively soluble compounds, such as cryolite (Na_3AlF_6) and the fluoride found absorbed, whereas relatively insoluble compounds, such as cryolite (Na_3AlF_6) and the fluoride found in bone meal (fluoroapatite), are poorly absorbed. The second most common route of absorption is by way of the lungs. Pulmonary inhalation of fluoride present in dusts and gases constitutes the major route of industrial exposure.

Fluoride has been detected in all organs and tissues, and it is concentrated in bone, thyroid, aorta, and perhaps kidney. Fluoride is preponderantly deposited in the skeleton and teeth, and the degree of skeletal storage is related to intake and age. Storage in bone is thought to be a function of the turnover rate of skeletal components, with growing bone showing a greater fluoride deposition than bone in mature animals. Prolonged periods of time are required for mobilization of fluoride from bone.

The major route of fluoride excretion is by way of the kidneys; however, fluoride is also excreted in small amounts by the sweat glands, the lactating breast, and the gastrointestinal tract. Under conditions of excessive sweating, the fraction of total fluoride excretion contributed by sweating can reach nearly one half. About 90% of the fluoride filtered by the glomerulus is reabsorbed by the renal tubules.

Pharmacological Actions. The pharmacological actions of fluoride, with the possible exception of its effect on bone and teeth, can be classified as toxic. Fluoride is an inhibitor of several enzyme systems and diminishes tissue respiration and anaerobic glycolysis. Fluoride is also a useful anticoagulant *in vitro* because of its binding of Ca^{2+}. It also inhibits the glycolytic utilization of glucose by erythrocytes, and for this reason is added to specimen tubes that receive blood for glucose determinations.

Fluoride has been used in treating Paget's disease of bone, but more effective therapeutic agents are now available. Several clinical studies have reported promising results in the treatment of osteoporosis with sodium fluoride, but its toxicity has been a limiting factor. A recent report indicates that fluoride, administered in a slow-release form together with supplemental Ca^{2+}, had no serious side effects and was effective in stimulating trabecular bone formation and decreasing vertebral fractures (Pak *et al.*, 1989). The radioactive nuclide ^{18}F has proven useful in bone imaging and the detection of bone metastases (Jones *et al.*, 1973).

Acute Poisoning. Acute fluoride poisoning is not rare. It usually results from the accidental ingestion of insecticides or rodenticides containing fluoride salts.

Initial symptoms are secondary to the local action of fluoride on the mucosa of the gastrointestinal tract. Salivation, nausea, abdominal pain, vomiting, and diarrhea are frequent. Systemic symptoms are varied and severe. There is increased irritability of the nervous system, consistent with the Ca^{2+}-binding effect of fluoride; both hypocalcemia and hypoglycemia are frequent. The blood pressure falls, presumably owing to central vasomotor depression as well as direct toxic action on cardiac muscle. Respiration is first stimulated and later depressed. Death usually results from either respiratory paralysis or cardiac failure. The lethal dose of sodium fluoride for man is about 5 g, although there is considerable variation. Treatment includes the intravenous administration of glucose in saline and gastric lavage with lime water (0.15% calcium hydroxide solution) or other Ca^{2+} salts to precipitate the fluoride. Calcium gluconate is given intravenously for tetany; urine volume is kept high with parenteral fluid.

Chronic Poisoning. In man, the major manifestations of chronic ingestion of excessive amounts of fluoride are osteosclerosis and mottled enamel. Long-term exposure to excess fluoride causes increased osteoblastic activity. Osteosclerosis is a phenomenon wherein the density and calcification of bone are increased; in the case of fluoride intoxication, it is thought to represent the replacement of hydroxyapatite by the denser fluoroapatite. However, the mechanism of its development remains unknown. The degree of skeletal involvement varies from changes that are barely detectable radiologically to marked thickening of the cortex of long bones, numerous exostoses scattered throughout the skeleton, and calcification of ligaments, tendons, and muscle attachments to bone. In its severest form it is a disabling disease and is designated as crippling fluorosis.

Mottled enamel or dental fluorosis is a well-recognized entity that was first described over 60 years ago. The gross changes in very mild mottling consist of small, opaque, paper-white areas scattered irregularly over the tooth surface. In severe cases, discrete or confluent, deep brown- to black-stained pits give the tooth a corroded appearance. Mottled enamel is the result of a partial failure of the enamel-forming cells properly to elaborate and lay down enamel. It is a nonspecific response to a variety of stimuli, one of which is the ingestion of excessive amounts of fluoride.

Since mottled enamel is a developmental injury, the ingestion of fluoride following the eruption of the tooth has no effect. Mottling is one of the first visible signs of an excessive intake of fluoride during childhood. Continuous use of water containing about 1.0 ppm of fluoride may result in the very mildest form of mottled enamel in 10% of children; at 4.0 to 6.0 ppm the incidence approaches 100%, with marked increase in severity.

Some concern has been expressed that fluoridation of public water supplies may result in an increased frequency of cancer or other diseases. Studies carried out by the National Cancer Institute and by the Bureau of Epidemiology of the United States Public Health Service indicate that mortality from cancer and mortality from all causes do not significantly differ between cities with fluoridated and those with nonfluoridated water (Hoover *et al.*, 1976; Erickson, 1978).

Fluoride and Dental Caries. Experiments in controlling the fluoride content of water took an unexpected and significant turn when it was observed that children born at Bauxite, Arkansas, after a new water supply had been obtained, showed a much higher incidence of caries than those who had been exposed to the former fluoride-containing water. This led to extensive studies on the part of the United States Public Health Service to ascertain whether fluoridation of water could be used as a practical measure to reduce the incidence of tooth decay. It has now been definitely established on the basis of large-scale studies in a number of communities that the fluoridation of water to a concentration of 1.0 ppm is a safe and practical public health measure that results in a substantial reduction in the incidence of caries in permanent teeth.

There are partial benefits for children who begin drinking fluoridated water at any age; however, optimal benefits are obtained at ages before permanent teeth erupt. Topical applications of fluoride solutions by dental personnel appear to be particularly effective on newly erupted teeth and can reduce the incidence of caries by 30 to 40%. The prescription of dietary fluoride supplements should be considered for children under 12 whose drinking water contains less than 0.7 ppm of fluoride. Conflicting results have been reported from studies of the effectiveness of fluoride-containing toothpastes.

Adequate incorporation of fluoride into teeth causes the outer layers of enamel to be harder and more resistant to demineralization. The deposition of fluoride ion appears to be an anion-exchange process with hydroxyl or citrate ions. Fluoride occupies the anionic spaces in the enamel apatite crystal surface. The mechanism of prevention of caries exerted by the deposition of minute amounts of fluoride in surface enamel is not completely understood. There is no convincing evidence that fluoride from any source reduces the development of caries after the permanent teeth are completely formed (usually about age 14).

Preparations and Uses. The fluoride salts usually employed in dentifrices are sodium fluoride and stannous fluoride. Sodium fluoride is also available in a variety of preparations for oral and topical use, including tablets, drops, rinses, and gels. Sodium fluoride, sodium fluosilicate (Na_2SiF_6), and cryolite are the salts commonly used in insecticides.

Agus, Z. S.; Gardner, L. B.; Beck, L. H.; and Goldberg, M. Effects of parathyroid hormone on renal tubular reabsorption of calcium, sodium, and phosphate. *Am. J. Physiol.*, **1973**, *224*, 1143–1148.

Amento, E. P. Vitamin D and the immune system. *Steroids*, **1987**, *49*, 55–72.

Andress, D. L.; Norris, K. C.; Coburn, J. W.; Slatopolsky, E. A.; and Sherrard, D. J. Intravenous calcitriol in the treatment of refractory osteitis fibrosa of chronic renal failure. *N. Engl. J. Med.*, **1989**, *321*, 274–279.

Ashby, J. P., and Thakkar, H. Diagnostic limitations of region-specific parathyroid hormone assays in the investigation of hypercalcemia. *Ann. Clin. Biochem.*, **1988**, *25*, 275–279.

Aurbach, G. D. Calcium-regulating hormones: parathyroid hormone and calcitonin. In, *Calcium in Human Biology*. (Nordin, B. E. C., ed.) Springer-Verlag, Berlin, **1988**, pp. 43–68.

Barsony, J., and Marx, S. J. Receptor-mediated rapid action of 1α; 25-dihydroxycholecalciferol: increase of intracellular cGMP in human fibroblasts. *Proc. Natl. Acad. Sci. U.S.A.*, **1988**, *85*, 1223–1226.

Benker, G.; Breuer, N.; Windeck, R.; and Reinwein, D. Calcium metabolism in thyroid disease. *J. Endocrinol. Invest.*, **1988**, *11*, 61–69.

Berl, T.; Berns, A. S.; Huffer, W. E.; Hammil, K.; Alfrey, A. C.; Arnaud, C. D.; and Schrier, R. W. 1,25-Dihydroxycholecalciferol effects in chronic dialysis. *Ann. Intern. Med.*, **1978**, *88*, 774–780.

Berman, L. A. Crystalline substance from the parathyroid glands that influences the calcium content of the blood. *Proc. Soc. Exp. Biol. Med.*, **1924**, *21*, 465.

Birge, S. J., and Miller, R. The role of phosphate in the action of vitamin D on the intestine. *J. Clin. Invest.*, **1977**, *60*, 980–988.

Blind, E.; Schmidt-Gayk, H.; Scharla, S.; Flentje, D.; Fischer, S.; Gohring, U.; and Hitzler, W. Two-site assay of intact parathyroid hormone in the investigation of primary hyperparathyroidism and other disorders of calcium metabolism compared with a midregion assay. *J. Clin. Endocrinol. Metab.*, **1988**, *67*, 353–360.

Brickman, A. S.; Coburn, J. W.; Kurokawa, K.; Bethune, J. E.; Harrison, H. E.; and Norman, A. W. Actions of 1,25-dihydroxycholecalciferol in patients with hypophosphatemic, vitamin-D-resistant rickets. *N. Engl. J. Med.*, **1973**, *289*, 495–498.

Broadus, A. E.; Mangin, M.; Ikeda, K.; Insogna, K. L.; Weir, E. C.; Burtis, W. J.; and Stewart, A. F. Humoral hypercalcemia of cancer. Identification of a novel parathyroid-like hormone peptide. *N. Engl. J. Med.*, **1988**, *319*, 556–563.

Cancela, L.; Nemere, I.; and Norman, A. W. 1α, $25(OH)_2$ vitamin D_3: a steroid hormone capable of producing pleiotropic receptor-mediated biological responses by both genomic and nongenomic mechanisms. *J. Steroid Biochem.*, **1988**, *30*, 33–39.

Card, R. T., and Brain, M. C. The "anemia" of childhood: evidence for a physiologic response to hyperphosphatemia. *N. Engl. J. Med.*, **1973**, *288*, 388–392.

Chambers, T. J.; McSheehy, P. M. J.; Thomson, B. M.; and Fuller, K. The effect of calcium-regulating hormones on bone resorption by isolated human osteoclastoma cells. *J. Pathol.*, **1985**, *145*, 297–305.

Chase, L. R.; Melson, G. L.; and Aurbach, G. D. Pseudohypoparathyroidism: defective excretion of 3′,5′-AMP in response to parathyroid hormone. *J. Clin. Invest.*, **1969**, *48*, 1823–1844.

Chesney, R. W.; Moorthy, A. V.; Eisman, J. A.; Jax, D. K.; Mazess, R. B.; and DeLuca, H. F. Increased growth after long-term oral 1α,25-vitamin D_3 in childhood renal osteodystrophy. *N. Engl. J. Med.*, **1978**, *298*, 238–242.

Coburn, J. W., and Salusky, I. B. Control of serum phosphorous in uremia. *N. Engl. J. Med.*, **1989**, *321*, 1140–1142.

Coccia, P. F. Cells that resorb bone. *N. Engl. J. Med.*, **1983**, *310*, 456–457.

Cohn, D. V.; Kumarasmy, R.; and Ramp, W. K. Intracellular processing and secretion of parathyroid gland proteins. *Vitam. Horm.*, **1986**, *43*, 283–316.

Collip, J. B. The extraction of a parathyroid hormone which will prevent or control parathyroid tetany and which regulates the level of blood calcium. *J. Biol. Chem.*, **1925**, *63*, 395–438.

Committee on Nutrition. The prophylactic requirement and toxicity of vitamin D. *Pediatrics*, **1963**, *31*, 512–523.

Dupret, J.-M.; Brun, P.; Perret, C.; Lomri, N.; Thomasset, M.; and Cuisinier-Gleizes, P. Transcriptional and post-transcriptional regulation of vitamin D–dependent calcium-binding protein gene expression in the rat duodenum by 1,25-dihydroxycholecalciferol. *J. Biol. Chem.*, **1987**, *262*, 16553–16557.

Erickson, J. D. Mortality in selected cities with fluoridated and non-fluoridated water supplies. *N. Engl. J. Med.*, **1978**, *298*, 1112–1116.

Farley, J. R.; Tarbaux, N. M.; Hall, S. L.; Linkhart, T. A.; and Baylink, D. J. The anti–bone-resorptive agent calcitonin also acts *in vitro* to directly increase bone formation and bone cell proliferation. *Endocrinology*, **1988**, *123*, 159–167.

Fraser, D. R. Calcium regulating hormones: vitamin D. In, *Calcium in Human Biology*. (Nordin, B. E. C., ed.) Springer-Verlag, Berlin, **1988**, pp. 27–41.

Fraser, D.; Kooh, S. W.; Kind, H. P.; Holick, M. F.; Tanaka, Y.; and DeLuca, H. F. Pathogenesis of hereditary vitamin-D–dependent rickets: an inborn error of vitamin D metabolism involving defective conversion of 25-hydroxyvitamin D to 1α,25-dihydroxyvitamin D. *N. Engl. J. Med.*, **1973**, *289*, 817–822.

Garcia-Ameijeiras, A.; De LaTorre, W.; Rodriguez-Espinosa, J.; Perez-Perez, A.; and De Leiva, A. Does testosterone influence the post-stimulatory levels of calcitonin in normal men? *Clin. Endocrinol. (Oxf.)*, **1987**, *27*, 545–552.

Gascon-Barré, M., and Côte, M. G. Effects of phenobarbital and diphenylhydantoin on acute vitamin D toxicity in the rat. *Toxicol. Appl. Pharmacol.*, **1978**, *43*, 125–135.

Greenberg, B. G.; Winters, R. W.; and Graham, J. B. The normal range of serum inorganic phosphorus and its utility as a discriminant in the diagnosis of congenital hypophosphatemia. *J. Clin. Endocrinol. Metab.*, **1960**, *20*, 364–379.

Hahn, T. J.; Hendin, B. A.; Scharp, C. R.; and Haddad, J. G., Jr. Effect of chronic anticonvulsant therapy on serum 25-hydroxycalciferol levels in adults. *N. Engl. J. Med.*, **1972**, *287*, 900–904.

Hanson, A. M. The hormone of the parathyroid gland. *Proc. Soc. Exp. Biol. Med.*, **1925**, *22*, 560–561.

Hess, A. F.; and Weinstock, M. Antirachitic properties imparted to inert fluids and to green vegetables by ultraviolet irradiation. *J. Biol. Chem.*, **1924**, *62*, 301–313.

Hirsch, P. F.; Gauthier, G. F.; and Munson, P. C. Thyroid hypocalcemic principle and recurrent laryngeal nerve injury as factors affecting the response to parathyroidectomy in rats. *Endocrinology*, **1963**, *73*, 244–252.

Holick, M. F. The cutaneous photosynthesis of previtamin D_3: a unique photoendocrine system. *J. Invest. Dermatol.*, **1981**, *76*, 51–58.

Hoover, R. N.; McKay, F. W.; and Fraumeni, J. F., Jr. Fluoridated drinking water and the occurrence of cancer. *J. Natl. Cancer Inst.*, **1976**, *57*, 757–768.

Hosking, D. J., and Kerr, D. Mechanisms of parathyroid hormone resistance in pseudohypoparathyroidism. *Clin. Sci.*, **1988**, *74*, 561–566.

Hruska, K. A.; Korkor, A.; Martin, K.; and Slatopolsky, E. Peripheral metabolism of intact parathyroid hormone. *J. Clin. Invest.*, **1981**, *67*, 885–892.

Huldschinsky, K. Heilung von Rachitis durch Kunstliche Hohensonne. *Dtsch. Med. Wochenschr.*, **1919**, *14*, 712–713.

Jacob, H. S., and Amsden, T. Acute hemolytic anemia with rigid red cells in hypophosphatemia. *N. Engl. J. Med.*, **1971**, *285*, 1446–1450.

Jones, A. E.; Ghaed, N.; Dunson, G. L.; and Hosain, F. Clinical evaluation of orally administered fluorine 18 for bone scanning. *Radiology*, **1973**, *107*, 129–131.

Jubiz, W.; Haussler, M. R.; McCain, T. A.; and Tolman, K. G. Plasma 1,25-dihydroxyvitamin D levels in patients receiving anticonvulsant drugs. *J. Clin. Endocrinol. Metab.*, **1977**, *44*, 617–621.

Key, L., and others. Treatment of congenital osteopetrosis with high-dose calcitriol. *N. Engl. J. Med.*, **1984**, *310*, 409–415.

Kobayashi, N.; Russell, J.; Lettieri, D.; and Sherwood, L. M. Regulation of protein kinase C by extracellular calcium in bovine parathyroid cells. *Proc. Natl. Acad. Sci. U.S.A.*, **1988**, *85*, 4857–4860.

Krieger, N. S., and Tashjian, A. H., Jr. Parathyroid hormone stimulates bone resorption via a Na-Ca exchange mechanism. *Nature*, **1980**, *287*, 843–845.

Kuntziger, H.; Amiel, C.; Roinel, N.; and Morel, F. Effect of parathyroidectomy and cyclic AMP on renal transport of phosphate, calcium, and magnesium. *Am. J. Physiol.*, **1974**, *227*, 905–911.

Lechene, C.; Colindres, R. E.; and Knox, F. G. Electron probe microanalysis of the renal effect of parathyroid hormone. In, *Endocrinology of Calcium Metabolism*. (Copp, D. H., and Talmage, R. V., eds.) Excerpta Medica, Amsterdam, **1978**, pp. 230–233.

Leeson, P. M., and Fourman, P. Increased sensitivity to vitamin D after vitamin D poisoning. *Lancet*, **1966**, *1*, 1182–1185.

Lichtman, M. A.; Miller, D. R.; and Freeman, R. B. Erythrocyte adenosine triphosphate depletion during hypophosphatemia. *N. Engl. J. Med.*, **1969**, *280*, 240–244.

Luine, V. N.; Sonnenberg, J.; and Christakos, S. Vitamin-D: is the brain a target? *Steroids*, **1987**, *49*, 133–153.

MacCallum, S. G., and Voegtlin, C. On the relation of tetany to the parathyroid glands and to calcium metabolism. *J. Exp. Med.*, **1909**, *11*, 118–151.

MacIntyre, I.; Alevizaki, M.; Bevis, P. J. R.; and Zaidi, M. Calcitonin and the peptides from the calcitonin gene. *Clin. Orthop.*, **1987**, *217*, 45–55.

MacIntyre, I.; Boss, S.; and Troughton, V. A. Parathyroid hormone and magnesium homeostasis. *Nature*, **1963**, *198*, 1058–1060.

McConnell, T. H. Fatal hypocalcemia from phosphate absorption from laxative preparations. *J.A.M.A.*, **1971**, *216*, 147–148.

Mawer, E. B.; Backhouse, J.; Davie, M.; Hill, C. F.; and Taylor, C. M. Metabolic fate of administered 1,25-dihydroxycholecalciferol in controls and in patients with hypoparathyroidism. *Lancet*, **1976**, *1*, 1203–1206.

Mellanby, E. An experimental investigation of rickets. *Lancet*, **1919**, *1*, 407–412.

Metz, S. A.; Baylink, D. J.; Hughes, M. R.; Haussler, M. R.; and Robertson, R. P. Selective deficiency of 1,25-dihydroxycholecalciferol. *N. Engl. J. Med.*, **1977**, *297*, 1084–1090.

Miller, S. C. Rapid activation of the medullary bone osteoclast cell surface by parathyroid hormone. *J. Cell Biol.*, **1978**, *76*, 615–618.

Morrissey, J. J. Effect of phorbol myristate acetate on

secretion of parathyroid hormone. *Am. J. Physiol.*, **1988**, *254*, E63–E70.
Motte, P.; Vauzelle, P.; Gardet, P.; Ghillani, P.; Caillou, B.; Parmentier, C.; Bohuon, C.; and Bellet, D. Construction and validation of a sensitive and specific assay for serum mature calcitonin using monoclonal anti-peptide antibodies. *Clin. Chim. Acta*, **1988**, *174*, 35–54.
Murad, F.; Brewer, H. B.; and Vaughan, M. Effect of thyrocalcitonin on adenosine 3′,5′-cyclic phosphate formation by rat kidney and bone. *Proc. Natl. Acad. Sci. U.S.A.*, **1970**, *65*, 446–453.
Nemere, I., and Norman, A. W. Parathyroid hormone stimulates calcium transport in perfused duodena from normal chicks: comparison with the rapid (transcalthachic) effect of 1,25-dihydroxyvitamin D_3. *Endocrinology*, **1986**, *119*, 1406–1408.
———. 1,25-Dihydroxyvitamin D_3–mediated vesicular transport of calcium in intestine: time course studies. *Ibid.*, **1988**, *122*, 2962–2969.
Nordin, B. E. C.; Horsman, A.; Marshall, D. H.; Simpson, M.; and Waterhouse, G. M. Calcium requirement and calcium therapy. *Clin. Orthop.*, **1979**, *140*, 216–239.
O'Donoghue, D. J., and Hosking, D. J. Biochemical response to combination of disodium etidronate with calcitonin in Paget's disease. *Bone*, **1987**, *8*, 219–225.
Paillard, F.; Ardaillou, R.; Malendin, H.; Fillastre, J. P.; and Prier, S. Renal effects on salmon calcitonin in man. *J. Lab. Clin. Med.*, **1972**, *80*, 200–216.
Pak, C. Y. C.; Sakhaee, K.; Zerwekh, J. E.; Parcel, C.; Peterson, R.; and Johnson, K. Safe and effective treatment of osteoporosis with intermittent slow release sodium fluoride: augmentation of vertebral bone mass and inhibition of fractures. *J. Clin. Endocrinol. Metab.*, **1989**, *68*, 150–159.
Parfitt, A. M. Hypophosphatemic vitamin D refractory rickets and osteomalacia. *Orthop. Clin. North Am.*, **1972**, *3*, 653–680.
Partridge, N. C.; Alcorn, D.; Michelangeli, V. P.; Kemp, B. E.; and Ryan, G. B. Functional properties of hormonally responsive cultured normal and malignant rat osteoblastic cells. *Endocrinology*, **1981**, *108*, 213–219.
Perlia, C. P.; Gubisch, N. J.; Wolter, J.; Edelberg, D.; Dederick, M. M.; and Taylor, S. G., III. Mithramycin treatment of hypercalcemia. *Cancer*, **1970**, *25*, 389–394.
Puschett, J. B.; Moranz, J.; and Kurnick, W. S. Evidence for a direct action of cholecalciferol and 25-hydroxycholecalciferol on the renal transport of phosphate, sodium, and calcium. *J. Clin. Invest.*, **1972**, *51*, 373–385.
Reichel, H.; Koeffler, H. P.; Barbers, R.; and Norman, A. W. Regulation of 1,25-dihydroxyvitamin D_3 production by cultured alveolar macrophages from normal human donors and from patients with pulmonary sarcoidosis. *J. Clin. Endocrinol. Metab.*, **1987**, *65*, 1201–1209.
Rosen, J. F., and Chesney, R. W. Circulating calcitriol concentrations in health and disease. *J. Pediatr.*, **1983**, *103*, 1–17.
Rosen, J. F.; Fleischman, A. R.; Finberg, L.; Eisman, J.; and DeLuca, H. F. 1,25-Dihydroxycholecalciferol: its use in the long-term management of idiopathic hypoparathyroidism in children. *J. Clin. Endocrinol. Metab.*, **1977**, *45*, 457–468.
Roth, S. I., and Raisz, L. G. Effect of calcium concentration on the ultrastructure of rat parathyroid in organ culture. *Lab. Invest.*, **1964**, *13*, 331–345.
Rude, R. K.; Oldham, S. B.; and Singer, F. R. Functional hypoparathyroidism and parathyroid hormone end-organ resistance in human magnesium deficiency. *Clin. Endocrinol.* (*Oxf.*), **1976**, *5*, 209–224.
Scriver, C. R.; Reade, T. M.; DeLuca, H. F.; and Hamstra, A. J. Serum 1,25-hydroxyvitamin D levels in normal subjects and in patients with hereditary rickets or bone disease. *N. Engl. J. Med.*, **1978**, *299*, 976–979.
Siegel, N.; Wongsurawat, N.; and Armbrecht, H. J. Parathyroid hormone stimulates dephosphorylation of the renoredoxin component of the 25-hydroxy D_3-1α-hydroxylase from rat renal cortex. *J. Biol. Chem.*, **1986**, *261*, 16998–17003.
Smith, R. The pathophysiology and management of rickets. *Orthop. Clin. North Am.*, **1972**, *3*, 601–621.
Spear, G. T.; Paulnock, D. M.; Helgeson, D. O.; and Borden, E. C. Requirement of differentiative signals of both interferon-γ and 1,25-dihydroxyvitamin D_3 for induction and secretion of interleukin-1 by HL-60 cells. *Cancer Res.*, **1988**, *48*, 1740–1744.
Steele, T. H. Increased urinary phosphate excretion following volume expansion in normal man. *Metabolism*, **1970**, *19*, 29–39.
Steenbock, H., and Black, A. Fat-soluble vitamins. XVII. The induction of growth-promoting and calcifying properties in a ration by exposure to ultraviolet light. *J. Biol. Chem.*, **1924**, *61*, 405–422.
Suda, T.; Hallick, R. B.; DeLuca, H. F.; and Schnoes, H. K. 25-Hydroxydihydrotachysterol$_3$. Synthesis and biological activity. *Biochemistry*, **1970**, *9*, 1651–1657.
Tashjian, A. H.; Wolfe, H. J.; and Voelkel, E. F. Human calcitonin. Immunologic assay, cytochemical localization and studies on medullary thyroid carcinoma. *Am. J. Med.*, **1974**, *56*, 840–849.
Theofan, G.; Nguyen, A. P.; and Norman, A. W. Regulation of calbindin-D_{28K} gene expression by 1,25-dihydroxyvitamin D_3 is correlated to receptor occupancy. *J. Biol. Chem.*, **1986**, *261*, 16943–16947.
Vernava, A. M., III; O'Neal, L. W.; and Palermo, V. Lethal hyperparathyroid crisis: hazards of phosphate administration. *Surgery*, **1987**, *102*, 941–948.
Weisman, Y.; Harell, A.; Edelstein, S.; David, M.; Spirer, Z.; and Golander, A. 1α-25-Dihydroxyvitamin D_3 and 24,25-dihydroxyvitamin D_3 *in vitro* synthesis by human decidua and placenta. *Nature*, **1979**, *281*, 317–319.
Wells, S. A., Jr.; Baylin, S. B.; Linehan, W. M.; Farrell, R. E.; Cox, E. G.; and Cooper, C. W. Provocative agents and the diagnosis of medullary carcinoma of the thyroid gland. *Ann. Surg.*, **1978**, *188*, 139–141.
Zaidi, M.; Breimer, L. H.; and MacIntyre, I. Biology of peptides from the calcitonin genes. *Q. J. Exp. Physiol.*, **1987**, *72*, 371–408.

Monographs and Reviews

Albright, F. A page out of the history of hyperparathyroidism. *J. Clin. Endocrinol. Metab.*, **1948**, *8*, 637–657.
Boland, R. Role of vitamin D in skeletal muscle function. *Endocr. Rev.*, **1986**, *7*, 434–448.
Braidman, I. P., and Anderson, D. C. Extra-endocrine functions of vitamin D. *Clin. Endocrinol.* (*Oxf.*), **1985**, *23*, 445–460.
Broadus, A. E., and Rasmussen, H. Clinical evaluation of parathyroid function. *Am. J. Med.*, **1981**, *70*, 475–478.
Bronner, F. Gastrointestinal absorption of calcium. In, *Calcium in Human Biology*. (Nordin, B. E. C., ed.) Springer-Verlag, Berlin, **1988**, pp. 93–123.
Brown, E. M.; LeBoff, M. S.; Oetting, M.; Posillico, J. T.; and Chen, C. Secretory control in normal and abnormal parathyroid tissue. *Recent Prog. Horm. Res.*, **1987**, *43*, 337–382.
Copp, D. H. Parathyroids, calcitonin, and control of plasma calcium. *Recent Prog. Horm. Res.*, **1964**, *20*, 59–88.
DeLuca, H. F. The vitamin D story: a collaborative effort of basic science and clinical medicine. *FASEB J.*, **1988**, *2*, 224–236.
DeLuca, H. F., and Schnoes, H. K. Metabolism and

mechanism of action of vitamin D. *Annu. Rev. Biochem.*, **1976**, *45*, 631–666.

———. Vitamin D: recent advances. *Ibid.*, **1983**, *52*, 411–439.

Evans, R. M. The steroid and thyroid hormone receptor superfamily. *Science*, **1988**, *240*, 889–895.

Fatourechi, V., and Heath, H., III. Salmon calcitonin in the treatment of postmenopausal osteoporosis. *Ann. Intern. Med.*, **1987**, *107*, 923–925.

Fraser, D. R. Regulation of the metabolism of vitamin D. *Physiol. Rev.*, **1980**, *60*, 551–613.

Habener, J. F., and Mahaffey, J. E. Osteomalacia and disorders of vitamin D metabolism. *Annu. Rev. Med.*, **1978**, *29*, 327–342.

Haussler, M. R. Vitamin D receptors: nature and function. *Annu. Rev. Nutr.*, **1986**, *6*, 527–562.

Haussler, M. R., and McCain, T. A. Basic and clinical concepts related to vitamin D metabolism and action. *N. Engl. J. Med.*, **1977**, *297*, 974–983.

Hosking, D. J. Paget's disease of the bone: an update on management. *Drugs*, **1985**, *30*, 156–173.

Kodicek, E. The story of vitamin D from vitamin to hormone. *Lancet*, **1974**, *1*, 325–329.

Kretsinger, R. H. Evolution and function of calcium-binding proteins. *Int. Rev. Cytol.*, **1976**, *46*, 323–393.

Peacock, M. Renal excretion of calcium. In, *Calcium in Human Biology*. (Nordin, B. E. C., ed.) Springer-Verlag, Berlin, **1988**, pp. 125–169.

Reichel, H.; Koeffler, H. P.; and Norman, A. W. The role of the vitamin D endocrine system in health and disease. *N. Engl. J. Med.*, **1989**, *320*, 980–991.

Stern, P. H. The D vitamins and bone. *Pharmacol. Rev.*, **1980**, *32*, 47–80.

Stevenson, J. C. Current management of malignant hypercalcaemia. *Drugs*, **1988**, *36*, 229–238.

Zaloga, G. P., and Chernow, B. Hypocalcemia in critical illness. *J.A.M.A.*, **1986**, *256*, 1924–1929.

SECTION

XVI The Vitamins

INTRODUCTION

Robert Marcus and Ann M. Coulston

The diet is the source of some 40 nutrients for man. These are classically divided into energy-yielding dietary components (carbohydrates, fats, and proteins), sources of essential and nonessential amino acids (proteins), essential unsaturated fatty acids (fats), minerals (including trace minerals), and vitamins (water-soluble and fat-soluble organic compounds) (*see* Shils and Young, 1988). In this section, the subject is vitamins.

Centuries ago, physicians described many of the diseases now recognized as vitamin deficiencies, notably night blindness (vitamin A deficiency), beriberi (thiamine deficiency), pellagra (niacin deficiency), scurvy (ascorbic acid deficiency), and rickets (vitamin D deficiency). Long before the era of vitamins, dietary factors were considered to be involved in all these conditions. However, the eventual identification of the active factor in the diet usually required reproduction of the disease in an experimental animal by feeding it a diet similar to that presumed to cause the condition in man, followed by prevention or cure of the disease by addition of certain foods or extracts of foods to the experimental diet. For example, beriberi, a form of polyneuritis, had been known for centuries to occur in populations eating polished (refined) rice. In 1897, Eijkman showed that fowl fed polished rice developed a polyneuritis similar to beriberi that could be cured by adding the husks or an extract of the husks back to the polished rice from which they had been derived. This animal model allowed Funk, in 1911, to isolate from the extract an antiberiberi substance, which he believed to be an amine. Because it was vital for life, he called the substance a *vitamine* and suggested that not only beriberi but also scurvy, pellagra, and possibly rickets were due to the lack of similar organic bases in the diet. The name was shortened to *vitamin* when it was subsequently recognized that dietary factors in this class are not necessarily amines and, indeed, have unrelated structures.

In the meantime, Osborne and Mendel (in 1911 to 1913) had demonstrated the presence in butter of a factor necessary for the growth of rats. In 1915, McCollum and Davis confirmed its presence in several dietary fats and named it *fat-soluble A,* which they distinguished from *water-soluble B,* another dietary factor necessary for the growth of rats; the latter was subsequently identified as Funk's antiberiberi factor. It soon became apparent that both the fat-soluble and the water-soluble factors (vitamins) consisted of several active components. Fats were shown to contain a factor (vitamin D) that prevented rickets and could be distinguished from the rat growth factor, vitamin A. Subsequent work has identified other fat-soluble factors (vitamins E and K) as essential dietary components. The water-soluble B fraction also proved to contain several components needed by man, namely thiamine, riboflavin, nicotinic acid, pyridoxine, pantothenic acid, biotin, folic acid, and cyanocobalamin. These were originally grouped together because they could be extracted in high concentration from certain foods, notably liver and yeast, in which the antiberiberi factor B had been identified. When active constituents were separately recognized in factor B, they were assigned the names vitamin B_1, vitamin B_2, and so forth; these have subsequently been replaced by chemical names. The members of the vitamin B complex are quite dissimilar in chemical structure, and they also differ in function. However, their continued classification together is justified by the similarity of their dietary sources and the consequent tendency for deficiency diseases to involve inadequate intakes of more than one member of the group. Discovered later, the water-soluble, antiscorbutic factor (ascorbic acid) was named vitamin C.

Although the individual vitamins differ widely in structure and function, some general statements do apply. Water-soluble vitamins are stored to only a limited extent, and frequent consumption is necessary to maintain saturation of tissues. Fat-soluble vitamins can be stored to massive degrees, and this property confers upon them a potential for serious toxicity that greatly exceeds that of the water-soluble group. As consumed, many vitamins are not biologically active and require processing *in vivo*. In the case of several water-soluble vitamins, activation includes phosphorylation (thiamine, riboflavin, niacin, pyridoxine) and may also require coupling to purine or pyridine nucleotides (riboflavin, niacin). In their major known actions water-soluble vitamins participate as cofactors for specific enzymes, whereas at least two fat-soluble vitamins, A and D, behave more like hormones and interact with specific intracellular receptors in their target tissues.

Definitions. Vitamins are thus a group of substances of diverse chemical composition. They can be defined as *organic* substances that must be provided in small quantities from the environment because either they cannot be synthesized *de novo* in man or their rate of synthesis is inadequate for the maintenance of health (*e.g.*, the production of niacin from tryptophan). In most cases, the environmental source is the diet, but an obvious exception to this general rule is the endogenous synthesis of vitamin D under the influence of ultraviolet light. This definition differentiates vitamins from essential trace minerals, which are *inorganic* nutrients needed in small quantities. It also excludes the essential amino acids, which are organic substances needed preformed in the diet in much larger quantities. The term *vitamin* is restricted here to include only organic substances required for the nutrition of mammals; substances required only by microorganisms and cells in culture should be defined as *growth factors,* in order to prevent scientifically unsound claims for their therapeutic benefit as vitamins for man. When the vitamin occurs in more than one chemical form (*e.g.*, pyridoxine, pyridoxal, pyridoxamine) or as a precursor (*e.g.*, carotene for vitamin A), these analogs are sometimes referred to as *vitamers.*

Vitamin Requirements. *Recommended Dietary Allowances.* In many countries throughout the world, scientific committees periodically assess the evidence about the requirements of the population for individual nutrients. In the United States, the National Academy of Sciences has a Food and Nutrition Board, one of whose functions is to recommend allowances of nutrients that will serve as a goal for good nutrition and will "encourage patterns of food consumption in the United States that will maintain and promote health" (Food and Nutrition Board, 1989). Recommended dietary allowances (RDA) for nutrients to ensure health were first published in 1941 and are periodically revised by the Dietary Allowances Committee of the Food and Nutrition Board to incorporate new knowledge. In 1989, the tenth edition of *Recommended Dietary Allowances* was issued. Its recommendations for males and females of different ages are summarized in Table XVI–1. These allowances are set at levels sufficiently high to cover the needs of almost all healthy individuals in that age and sex category. Levels are set high because the exact amounts of nutrients needed by each individual in the population are not known, and estimates are made from experiments on a limited number of subjects. If the upper limit of this range is taken as the recommended allowance, it is unlikely that a deficiency will occur in the population. Those with intakes below the recommended allowance will not necessarily develop a deficiency, but the risk of becoming deficient increases in proportion to the extent to which intake is less than the amount recommended.

It is important to remember that the RDA are subject to periodic reevaluation, and that

Table XVI–1. RECOMMENDED DAILY DIETARY ALLOWANCES [a]

							FAT-SOLUBLE VITAMINS				WATER-SOLUBLE VITAMINS							MINERALS						
		Weight		Height		Protein	Vitamin A	Vitamin D	Vitamin E	Vitamin K	Vitamin C	Thiamin	Riboflavin	Niacin	Vitamin B_6	Folate	Vitamin B_{12}	Calcium	Phosphorus	Magnesium	Iron	Zinc	Iodine	Selenium
Category	Age (years) or Condition	(kg)	(lb)	(cm)	(in)	(g)	(μg RE) [b]	(μg) [c]	(mg α-TE) [d]	(μg)	(mg)	(mg)	(mg)	(mg NE) [e]	(mg)	(μg)	(μg)	(mg)	(mg)	(mg)	(mg)	(mg)	(μg)	(μg)
Infants	0.0–0.5	6	13	60	24	13	375	7.5	3	5	30	0.3	0.4	5	0.3	25	0.3	400	300	40	6	5	40	10
	0.5–1.0	9	20	71	28	14	375	10	4	10	35	0.4	0.5	6	0.6	35	0.5	600	500	60	10	5	50	15
Children	1–3	13	29	90	35	16	400	10	6	15	40	0.7	0.8	9	1.0	50	0.7	800	800	80	10	10	70	20
	4–6	20	44	112	44	24	500	10	7	20	45	0.9	1.1	12	1.1	75	1.0	800	800	120	10	10	90	20
	7–10	28	62	132	52	28	700	10	7	30	45	1.0	1.2	13	1.4	100	1.4	800	800	170	10	10	120	30
Males	11–14	45	99	157	62	45	1,000	10	10	45	50	1.3	1.5	17	1.7	150	2.0	1,200	1,200	270	12	15	150	40
	15–18	66	145	176	69	59	1,000	10	10	65	60	1.5	1.8	20	2.0	200	2.0	1,200	1,200	400	12	15	150	50
	19–24	72	160	177	70	58	1,000	10	10	70	60	1.5	1.7	19	2.0	200	2.0	1,200	1,200	350	10	15	150	70
	25–50	79	174	176	70	63	1,000	5	10	80	60	1.5	1.7	19	2.0	200	2.0	800	800	350	10	15	150	70
	51+	77	170	173	68	63	1,000	5	10	80	60	1.2	1.4	15	2.0	200	2.0	800	800	350	10	15	150	70
Females	11–14	46	101	157	62	46	800	10	8	45	50	1.1	1.3	15	1.4	150	2.0	1,200	1,200	280	15	12	150	45
	15–18	55	120	163	64	44	800	10	8	55	60	1.1	1.3	15	1.5	180	2.0	1,200	1,200	300	15	12	150	50
	19–24	58	128	164	65	46	800	10	8	60	60	1.1	1.3	15	1.6	180	2.0	1,200	1,200	280	15	12	150	55
	25–50	63	138	163	64	50	800	5	8	65	60	1.1	1.3	15	1.6	180	2.0	800	800	280	15	12	150	55
	51+	65	143	160	63	50	800	5	8	65	60	1.0	1.2	13	1.6	180	2.0	800	800	280	10	12	150	55
Pregnant						60	800	10	10	65	70	1.5	1.6	17	2.2	400	2.2	1,200	1,200	320	30	15	175	65
Lactating	1st 6 months					65	1,300	10	12	65	95	1.6	1.8	20	2.1	280	2.6	1,200	1,200	355	15	19	200	75
	2nd 6 months					62	1,200	10	11	65	90	1.6	1.7	20	2.1	260	2.6	1,200	1,200	340	15	16	200	75

[a] The allowances, expressed as average daily intakes over time, are intended to provide for individual variations among most normal persons as they live in the United States under usual environmental stresses. Diets should be based on a variety of common foods in order to provide other nutrients for which human requirements have been less well defined.

[b] Retinol equivalents. 1 retinol equivalent = 1 μg retinol or 6 μg β-carotene. *See* text for calculation of vitamin A activity of diets as retinol equivalents.

[c] As cholecalciferol. 10 μg cholecalciferol = 400 IU of vitamin D.

[d] α-Tocopherol equivalents. 1 mg *d*-α tocopherol = 1 α-TE. *See* text for variation in allowances and calculation of vitamin E activity of the diet as α-tocopherol equivalents.

[e] 1 NE (niacin equivalent) is equal to 1 mg of niacin or 60 mg of dietary tryptophan.

(Modified from Food and Nutrition Board, National Research Council, 1989.)

changes do occur. As subgroups of the population are identified with unique requirements for one or more nutrients (*e.g.*, elderly women), one can anticipate further revisions of the RDA.

An additional feature of the tenth edition of *Recommended Dietary Allowances* is the inclusion of provisional allowances for some nutrients not given RDA. Table XVI–1 lists allowances for only 19 out of the 40 or so known essential nutrients consumed by man. In previous editions of the RDA a mixed diet was advised in order to include unrecognized nutritional needs and to ensure an adequate intake of essential nutrients for which no allowance could be provided. However, rising consumption of formulated foods, highly processed foods, and supplements of vitamins and trace elements has increased the risk of imbalances between nutrients, of deficiencies from underconsumption by some members of the population, and of toxicity from overdosage in others. The current RDA text therefore provides allowances for certain additional nutrients in the form of ranges within which adequate intakes are likely to be achieved (Table XVI–2). These provisional allowances include two water-soluble vitamins (biotin and pantothenic acid), as well as several trace elements (copper, manganese, fluoride, chromium, and molybdenum). Although these provisional allowances are presented as recommended ranges of intakes, it is to be emphasized that an intake at one end of the range should not be construed as more desirable than one at the other. Thus, all intakes within the recommended range are considered safe and effective, but consumption of greater or smaller amounts over extended periods of time will increase the risk of marginal toxicity or deficiency, respectively.

A number of other constituents in food have been claimed to be needed by man. As described in the RDA text, these substances fall into four classes: (1) those known to be essential for some animals but not shown to be needed by man, such as nickel, vanadium, and silicon; (2) substances that act as growth factors only for lower forms of life, such as paraaminobenzoic acid, carnitine, and pimelic acid; (3) substances in foods that are said to be vitamins but whose actions are probably pharmacological or nonexistent, such as rutin, for which unsubstantiated claims of antihemorrhagic and other actions have been made; and (4) substances for which scientific proof of a nutrient action has not been provided, such as pangamic acid (erroneously designated vitamin B_{15}), laetrile (misnamed vitamin B_{17}), and others promoted in the health-food literature and commercial outlets. Herbert (1979a, 1979b) has written detailed factual reviews of the controversies over laetrile and pangamic acid. The tenth edition of *Recommended Dietary Allowances* (Food and Nutrition Board, 1989) serves as a standard for the intelligent use of vitamin and mineral supplements.

Federal Regulations on Vitamins and Minerals. The United States Food and Drug Administration (FDA), under the authority of the Federal Food, Drug, and Cosmetic Act, regulates the labeling of vitamin and mineral products sold as foods or drugs. To facilitate the labeling of conventional foods with regard to nutrients, the FDA has designated an official U.S. RDA, which generally represents the highest daily allowance for each nutrient given in the seventh, 1968, edition of *Recommended Dietary Allowances*. Thus, the purchaser can determine what proportion of his daily allowance of each nutrient is provided by a given amount of the food. In addition, the U.S. RDA are used to label the amounts of vitamins and minerals relative to needs in supplements sold to the public. Although the FDA has only limited authority to control the nutrient content of supplements, except those intended for use by children under 12 years of age and by pregnant or lactating women, the label does provide the consumer with explicit information on content, thus permitting judgment of whether the product contains reasonable amounts, too little, or an excess of each nutrient relative to daily allowances. The FDA attempted in 1973 to classify *all* vitamin and mineral preparations in which the dosages exceeded 150% of the U.S. RDA as drugs rather than as special foods, but the regulation was struck by court order. That year also saw regulations developed that prevented sale to the public of vitamins A and D in doses ex-

Table XVI–2. ESTIMATED SAFE AND ADEQUATE DAILY DIETARY INTAKES OF ADDITIONAL SELECTED VITAMINS AND MINERALS *

		VITAMINS		TRACE ELEMENTS				
	Age (years)	*Biotin* (μg)	*Pantothenic Acid* (mg)	*Copper* (mg)	*Manganese* (mg)	*Fluoride* (mg)	*Chromium* (μg)	*Molybdenum* (μg)
Infants	0–0.5	10	2	0.4–0.6	0.3–0.6	0.1–0.5	10–40	15–30
	0.5–1	15	3	0.6–0.7	0.6–1.0	0.2–1.0	20–60	20–40
Children	1–3	20	3	0.7–1.0	1.0–1.5	0.5–1.5	20–80	25–50
and	4–6	25	3–4	1.0–1.5	1.5–2.0	1.0–2.5	30–120	30–75
Adolescents	7–10	30	4–5	1.0–2.0	2.0–3.0	1.5–2.5	50–200	50–150
	11+	30–100	4–7	1.5–2.5	2.0–5.0	1.5–2.5	50–200	75–250
Adults		30–100	4–7	1.5–3.0	2.0–5.0	1.5–4.0	50–200	75–250

* Because there is less information on which to base an allowance, these are not given in the main table of dietary allowances but are provided here in the form of ranges of recommended intakes. Since the toxic levels for many trace elements may be only several times usual intakes, the upper levels for the trace elements given in this table should not be habitually exceeded. (Modified from Food and Nutrition Board, National Research Council, 1989.)

ceeding 10,000 international units (I.U.) of the former and 400 I.U. of the latter without a prescription, because of the concern that higher doses of these fat-soluble vitamins can cause toxicity. The regulation was revoked in 1978 because of a court determination that dosages in excess of those amounts could not be *uniquely* classified as drugs by the FDA. Also, an amendment of the Federal Food, Drug, and Cosmetic Act passed by Congress in 1976 limits FDA control of supplements for adult use to cases of demonstrated toxicity but retains the FDA's authority over dietary supplements for children under 12 years and for pregnant or lactating women.

The uses of vitamins and other nutrients to treat disease come under FDA review, either as foods for special dietary use, including food supplements, or as "over-the-counter" or prescription drugs, depending on the purposes for which the product is intended and the claims made for it. Nutrient products designed specifically for special application in medical treatment, such as parenteral solutions for hyperalimentation and so-called medical foods (such as defined formula diets), are evaluated for safety and efficacy, as are "over-the-counter" drugs containing vitamins and minerals.

Range of Intakes of Vitamins and Minerals. Many millions of individuals living in the United States regularly ingest quantities of vitamins vastly in excess of the RDA. A recent survey (Stewart *et al.,* 1985) found that 40% of adults consume at least one vitamin-mineral supplement, reinforcing the concern that vast numbers of Americans hold inflated concepts regarding the benefits of taking supplemental vitamins and minerals. An important reason for taking vitamin supplements is the erroneous belief that such preparations provide extra energy and make one "feel better." This evidence of widespread nutritional self-medication, which is confirmed by other surveys, should be kept in mind when taking a medication history from a patient.

The use of vitamin supplements is medically advisable in a variety of circumstances where *vitamin deficiencies* are likely to occur. Such situations may arise from inadequate intake, malabsorption, increased tissue needs, or inborn errors of metabolism. In practice, these causes may overlap, as in the case of the alcoholic, who may have both inadequate food intake and impaired absorption.

While gross vitamin deficiencies due to inadequate intakes are encountered in underdeveloped areas of the world, few florid cases are seen in the United States. Ongoing surveillance of dietary intake is periodically conducted by the United States Government. The most recent survey (National Center for Health Statistics, 1983) indicated that mean intake consistently exceeds RDA for several major vitamins (A, thiamine, riboflavin, niacin, and ascorbic acid). Data from this and other surveys did show that individuals living below the poverty level, particularly the elderly and ethnic minorities, may have a substantially greater risk of inadequate intake of some vitamins, especially vitamins A and C. However, the data indicate *relative risks* for deficiency, and in no case was a significant incidence of overt vitamin deficiency observed. It should be kept in mind that data on intake of nutrients do not take into account such confounding factors as the relative bioavailability of nutrients in foods and losses of nutrients during food storage and preparation.

Certain individuals are exposed to deficient intakes of vitamins as a result of eccentric diets, such as food faddism, and the avoidance of food because of anorexia. Intakes of vitamins less than those recommended can also occur in subjects on reducing diets and among elderly people who eat little food for economic or social reasons. The consumption of excessive amounts of alcohol can also lead to inadequate intakes of vitamins and other nutrients.

Malabsorption of vitamins is also seen in various conditions. Examples include hepatobiliary and pancreatic diseases, prolonged diarrheal illness, hyperthyroidism, pernicious anemia, sprue, and intestinal bypass operations. Moreover, since a substantial proportion of vitamin K and biotin is synthesized by the bacteria of the gastrointestinal tract, treatment with antimicrobial agents that alter the intestinal bacterial flora inevitably leads to decreased availability of these vitamins.

Increased tissue requirements for vitamins may cause a nutritional deficiency to develop despite the ingestion of a diet that had previously been adequate. For example, requirements for some vitamins may be altered by the use of certain antivitamin drugs, such as the interference with the utilization of folic acid by trimethoprim (*see* Roe, 1981). Diseases associated with an increased metabolic rate, such as hyperthyroidism and conditions accompanied by fever or tissue wasting, also increase the body's requirements for vitamins.

Finally, an increasing number of cases are recorded in which genetic abnormalities lead to an increased need for a vitamin. This is usually due to an abnormality in the structure of an enzyme for which the vitamin provides a cofactor, leading to a decreased affinity of the abnormal enzyme protein for the cofactor (Scriver, 1973).

Role of Vitamins in Therapeutics. Oral supplements of vitamins are indicated in conditions associated with an increased risk for vitamin deficiency. In 1987, a task force of the American Dietetic Association issued a statement on vitamin and mineral supplementation with which the American Medical Association and American Institute of Nutrition agreed. The statement concludes that "the Recommended Dietary Allowances represent the best currently available assessment of safe and adequate intakes, and serve as the basis for the U.S. Recommended Daily Allowances shown on many product labels. There are no demonstrated benefits of self supplementation beyond these allowances" (Commentary, 1987). Nonetheless, it is recognized that many Americans take vitamin supplements. To minimize potential risks associated with this practice, the Council on Scientific Affairs of the American Medical Association has recommended that daily intake in healthy people should not exceed 150% of the U.S. RDA for any single vitamin (Council on Scientific Affairs, 1987).

For patients who cannot consume sufficient regular food for their needs, a number of specially defined formula diets are available. The vitamin content of these is regulated as *medical foods* by the FDA. Some patients require a complete supply of nutrients by the parenteral route. For this purpose, the dosage of water-soluble vitamins may have to be higher because of excessive urinary losses.

The impact of disease on requirements for nutrients may vary according to its phase and intensity. The need for therapy with vitamins may change throughout the course of the illness and, eventually, cure should be associated with cessation of this therapy; this point sometimes escapes the physician, who does not remind the patient to abandon the vitamin supplement.

Commentary. Recommendations concerning supplement usage: ADA statement. *J. Am. Diet. Assoc.*, **1987**, *87*, 1342–1343.

Council on Scientific Affairs. Vitamin preparations as dietary supplements and as therapeutic agents. *J.A.M.A.*, **1987**, *257*, 1929–1936.

Food and Nutrition Board, National Research Council. *Recommended Dietary Allowances*, 10th ed. National Academy of Sciences, Washington, D. C., **1989**.

Herbert, V. Laetrile: the cult of cyanide—promoting poison for profit. *Am. J. Clin. Nutr.*, **1979a**, *32*, 1121–1158.

———. Pangamic acid ("vitamin B_{15}"). *Ibid.*, **1979b**, *32*, 1534–1540.

National Center for Health Statistics; Carroll, M. D.; Abraham, S.; and Dress, C. M. Dietary intake source data: United States, 1976–80. *Vital Health Stat.* [*11*], No. 231. U.S. Government Printing Office, Washington, D.C., **1983**.

Roe, D. A. Drug interference with the assessment of nutritional status. *Clin. Lab. Med.*, **1981**, *1*, 647–664.

Scriver, C. R. Vitamin-responsive inborn error of metabolism. *Metabolism*, **1973**, *22*, 1319–1344.

Shils, M. E., and Young, V. R. (eds.). *Modern Nutrition in Health and Disease*, 7th ed. Lea & Febiger, Philadelphia, **1988**.

Stewart, M. L.; McDonald, J. T.; Levy, A. S.; Schucker, R. E.; and Henderson, D. P. Vitamin/mineral supplement use: a telephone survey of adults in the United States. *J. Am. Diet. Assoc.*, **1985**, *85*, 1585–1590.

CHAPTER

63 WATER-SOLUBLE VITAMINS

The Vitamin B Complex and Ascorbic Acid

Robert Marcus and Ann M. Coulston

The vitamin B complex comprises a large number of compounds that differ extensively in chemical structure and biological action. The reason for grouping them in a single class was their original isolation from the same sources, notably liver and yeast. Although the classical single-nutrient deficiency diseases were rampant in previous eras, it is far more common in contemporary Western society to see simultaneous deficiency of multiple nutrients.

There are traditionally 11 members of the vitamin B complex, namely, thiamine, riboflavin, nicotinic acid, pyridoxine, pantothenic acid, biotin, folic acid, cyanocobalamin, choline, inositol, and paraaminobenzoic acid. Although not a traditional member of the group, carnitine is considered here because of its biosynthetic relationship to choline and the recent recognition of deficiency states. Folic acid and cyanocobalamin are considered in Chapter 54 because of their special function in hematopoiesis. Paraaminobenzoic acid (PABA) is not a true vitamin for any mammalian species but is a growth factor for certain bacteria, where it is a precursor in the synthesis of folic acid. The vitamins of the B complex function in intermediary metabolism in many essential reactions; some of these functions are summarized in Figure 63–1, which serves to illustrate their prevalence and importance.

In addition to the vitamin B complex, this chapter also considers ascorbic acid (vitamin C). This water-soluble vitamin is especially concentrated in citrus fruits and is thus obtained mostly from sources differing from those of members of the vitamin B complex.

I. The Vitamin B Complex

THIAMINE

History. Thiamine was the first member of the vitamin B complex to be identified. Lack of thiamine produces a form of polyneuritis known as beriberi; this disease became widespread in East Asia in the nineteenth century due to the introduction of steam-powered rice mills, which produced polished rice lacking the vitamin-rich husk. A dietary cause for the disease was first indicated in 1880, when Admiral Takaki greatly reduced the incidence of beriberi in the Japanese Navy by adding fish, meat, barley, and vegetables to the sailors' diet of polished rice. In 1897, Eijkman, a Dutch physician working in Java where beriberi was also common, showed that fowl fed polished rice develop a polyneuritis similar to beriberi and that it could be cured by adding the rice polishings (husks) or an aqueous extract of the polishings back into the diet. He also demonstrated that rice polishings could cure beriberi in human beings.

In 1911, Funk isolated a highly concentrated form of the active factor and recognized that it belonged to a new class of food factors, which he called *vitamines,* later shortened to *vitamins.* The active factor was subsequently named vitamin B_1; in 1926 it was isolated in crystalline form by Jansen and Donath, and in 1936 its structure was determined by Williams. The Council on Pharmacy and Chemistry adopted the name *thiamine* to designate crystalline vitamin B_1.

Chemistry. Thiamine is an organic molecule containing a pyrimidine and a thiazole nucleus linked by a methylene bridge. Thiamine functions in the body in the form of the coenzyme thiamine pyrophosphate (TPP). The structures of thiamine and thiamine pyrophosphate are as follows:

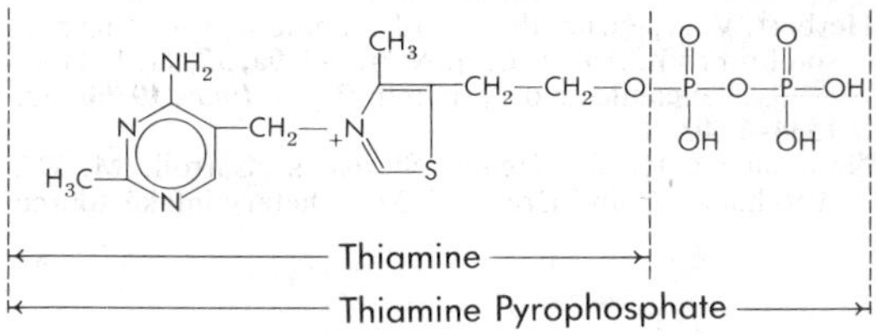

The conversion of thiamine to its coenzyme form is carried out by the enzyme *thiamine diphosphokinase,* with adenosine triphosphate (ATP) as the pyrophosphate (PP) donor. Antimetabolites to thiamine that inhibit this enzyme have been synthesized. The most important of these are neopyrithiamine (pyrithiamine) and oxythiamine.

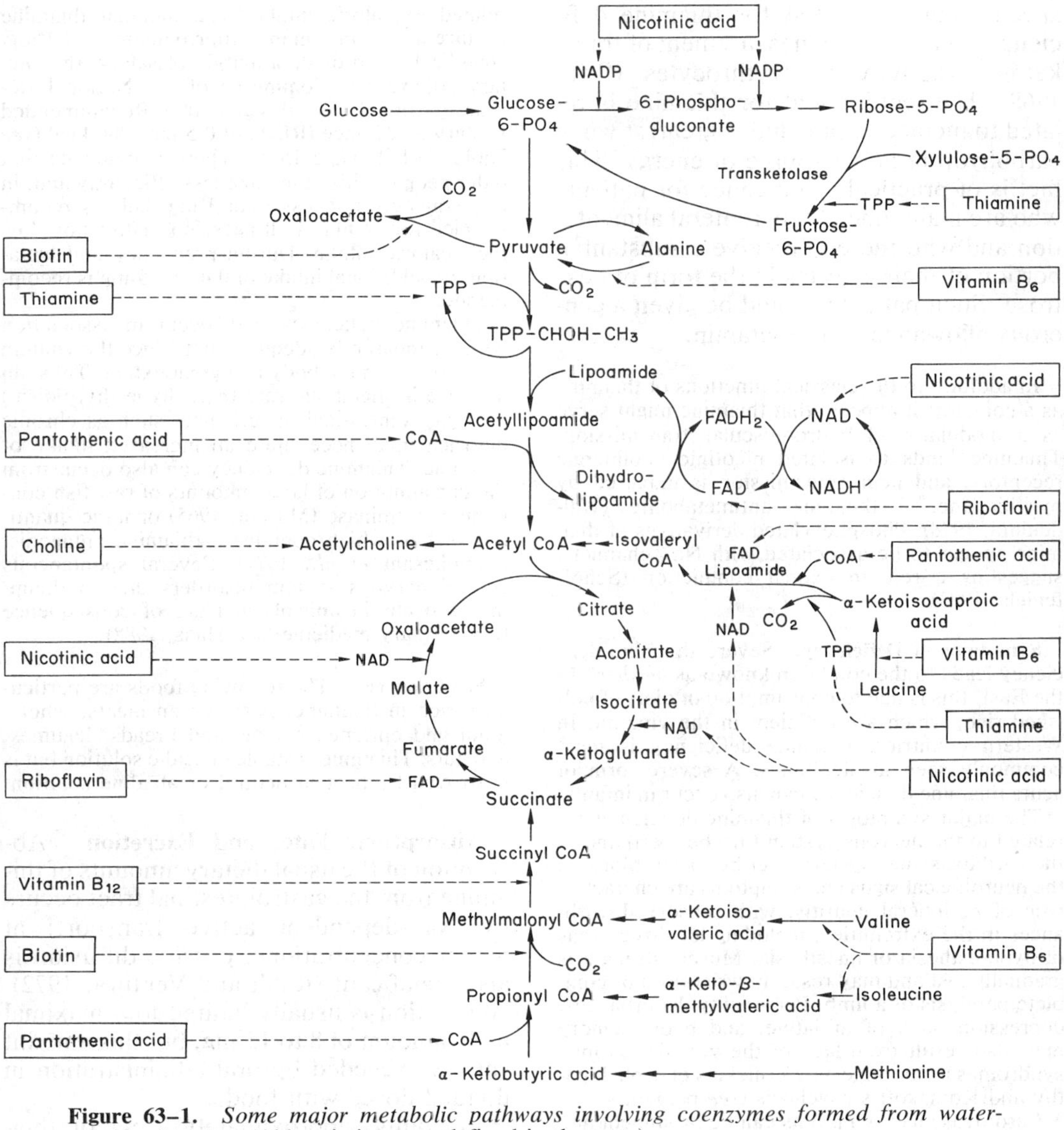

Figure 63–1. *Some major metabolic pathways involving coenzymes formed from water-soluble vitamins.* (Abbreviations are defined in the text.)

Pharmacological Actions. Thiamine is practically devoid of pharmacodynamic actions when given in usual therapeutic doses; even large doses produce no discernible effects. Isolated clinical reports of toxic reactions to the long-term parenteral administration of thiamine probably represent rare instances of hypersensitivity.

Physiological Functions. Thiamine pyrophosphate, the physiologically active form of thiamine, functions in carbohydrate metabolism as a coenzyme in the decarboxylation of α-keto acids such as pyruvate and α-ketoglutarate and in the utilization of pentose in the hexose monophosphate shunt; the latter function involves the thiamine pyrophosphate–dependent enzyme transketolase. Several metabolic changes of clinical importance can be related directly to the biochemical action of thiamine. In thiamine deficiency, the oxidation of α-keto acids is impaired, and an increase in the concentration of pyruvate in the blood has been used as one of the diagnostic signs of the deficiency state. A more specific diagnostic test for thiamine deficiency is based upon measurement of transketolase activity in erythrocytes (Brin, 1968). The requirement for thiamine is related to metabolic rate and is greatest when carbohydrate is the source of energy. This fact is of practical significance for patients who are maintained by parenteral alimentation and who thereby receive a substantial portion of their calories in the form of dextrose. Such patients should be given a generous allowance of the vitamin.

In addition to the classical functions of thiamine as a cofactor, it appears that thiamine might serve as a modulator of neuromuscular transmission. Thiamine binds to isolated nicotinic cholinergic receptors, and neurotransmission is impaired by pyrithiamine, a thiamine antimetabolite (Waldenlind, 1978). Phosphorylated derivatives of thiamine appear to be associated with Na^+ channels, suggesting a role in axonal conduction (Schoffeniels, 1983).

Symptoms of Deficiency. Severe thiamine deficiency leads to the condition known as *beriberi*. In the East, this is due to consumption of diets of polished rice, which are deficient in the vitamin. In Western countries, thiamine deficiency is most commonly seen in alcoholics. A severe form of acute thiamine deficiency can also occur in infants.

The major symptoms of thiamine deficiency are related to the nervous system (dry beriberi) and to the cardiovascular system (wet beriberi). Many of the neurological signs and symptoms are characteristic of peripheral neuritis, with sensory disturbances in the extremities, including localized areas of hyperesthesia or anesthesia. Muscle strength is gradually lost and may result in wrist-drop or complete paralysis of a limb. Personality disturbances, depression, lack of initiative, and poor memory may also result from lack of the vitamin, as may syndromes as extreme as Wernicke's encephalopathy and Korsakoff's psychosis (*see* below).

Cardiovascular symptoms can be prominent and include dyspnea on exertion, palpitation, tachycardia, and other cardiac abnormalities characterized by an abnormal ECG (chiefly low R-wave voltage, T-wave inversion, and prolongation of the Q–T interval) and cardiac failure of the high-output type. Such failure has been termed *wet beriberi;* there is extensive edema, largely as a result of hypoproteinemia from an inadequate intake of protein or concomitant liver disease together with failing ventricular function.

Symptoms referable to the gastrointestinal tract are also observed in severe cases of thiamine deficiency. Loss of appetite occurs early and is followed by constipation.

Human Requirements. Because thiamine is essential for energy metabolism, especially of carbohydrate, requirement for thiamine is commonly related to caloric intake. The minimal thiamine requirement in man approximates 0.3 mg/1000 kcal. To provide a margin of safety, the Dietary Allowances Committee of the National Research Council has designated a Recommended Dietary Allowance (RDA) of 0.5 mg/1000 kcal (*see* Table XVI–1, page 1525). There is evidence that older people utilize thiamine less efficiently and, in consequence, not less than 1 mg daily is recommended for adults of all ages, no matter how low their caloric intake. During pregnancy and lactation, an additional intake of 0.4 to 0.5 mg is recommended.

Thiamine deficiency may occur in association with an apparently adequate diet, since the vitamin is not stored in the body to a great extent. Thus, an increase in metabolic rate (*e.g.*, hyperthyroidism) or a gastrointestinal disturbance, such as chronic diarrhea, may necessitate an increased intake of thiamine. Thiamine deficiency can also occur from the consumption of large amounts of raw fish containing thiaminase (Murata, 1965) or large quantities of tea, which contains a thiamine antagonist (Vimokesant *et al.*, 1974). Several spontaneous central nervous system disorders due to thiaminases occur in animals and are of consequence to veterinary medicine (*see* Haas, 1988).

Food Sources. The following foods are particularly rich in thiamine: pork, organ meats, whole-grain and enriched cereals and breads, legumes, and nuts. Thiamine is stable in acidic solution but is destroyed by heat in neutral or alkaline solution.

Absorption, Fate, and Excretion. Absorption of the usual dietary amounts of thiamine from the gastrointestinal tract occurs by Na^+-dependent active transport; at higher concentrations, passive diffusion is also significant (Rindi and Ventura, 1972). Absorption is usually limited to a maximal daily amount of 8 to 15 mg, but this amount can be exceeded by oral administration in divided doses with food.

In adults, approximately 1 mg of thiamine per day is completely degraded by the tissues, and this is roughly the minimal daily requirement. When intake is at this low level, little or no thiamine is excreted in the urine. When intake exceeds the minimal requirement, tissue stores are first saturated. Thereafter, the excess appears quantitatively in the urine as intact thiamine or as pyrimidine, which arises from degradation of the thiamine molecule. As the intake of thiamine is further increased, more of the excess is excreted unchanged.

Preparations. Thiamine can be prescribed as the pure vitamin, in mixtures of pure vitamins, or in the form of vitamin-rich concentrates. Tablets of *thiamine hydrochloride* (*vitamin B_1 hydrochloride*) are available in amounts ranging from 5 to 500 mg each. *Thiamine hydrochloride injection* contains 100 or 200 mg/ml.

Therapeutic Uses. The only established therapeutic use of thiamine is in the treatment or the prophylaxis of thiamine deficiency. To correct the disorder as rapidly as possible, intravenous doses as large as 100 mg per liter of parenteral fluid are commonly used. Once thiamine deficiency has been corrected, there is no need for parenteral injection or the administration of amounts in excess of daily requirements except in instances when gastrointestinal disturbances preclude the ingestion or absorption of adequate amounts of vitamin.

The syndromes of thiamine deficiency seen clinically can range from beriberi through Wernicke's encephalopathy and Korsakoff's syndrome to alcoholic polyneuropathy. Because normal metabolism of carbohydrate results in consumption of thiamine, it has been observed repeatedly that administration of glucose may precipitate acute symptoms of thiamine deficiency in marginally nourished subjects. This has also been noted during the correction of endogenous hyperglycemia. *Thus, in any individual whose thiamine status may be suspect, the vitamin should be given before or along with dextrose-containing fluids; all alcoholic patients seen in an emergency room should routinely receive 50 to 100 mg of thiamine.* The clinical findings appear to depend on the amount of deprivation (McLaren, 1978). Encephalopathy and Korsakoff's syndrome result from severe deprivation, whereas beriberi heart disease occurs in less deficient subjects; polyneuritis is observed in milder deprivation. The following discussion describes briefly the varieties of thiamine deficiency and their treatment.

Alcoholic Neuritis. Alcoholism is the most common cause of thiamine deficiency in the United States. Alcoholic neuritis is basically a nutritional deficiency caused by an inadequate intake of thiamine. Two factors contribute to such inadequate intake in the chronic alcoholic: (1) appetite is usually poor, so food consumption drops; and (2) a large portion of the caloric intake is in the form of alcohol. The symptoms of neurological involvement in alcoholics are those of a polyneuritis with motor and sensory defects. Wernicke's syndrome is an additional serious consequence of alcoholism and thiamine deficiency. Certain characteristic signs of this disease, notably ophthalmoplegia, nystagmus, and ataxia, respond rapidly to the administration of thiamine but to no other vitamin. Wernicke's syndrome may be accompanied by an acute global confusional state that may also respond to thiamine. Left untreated, Wernicke's encephalopathy frequently leads to a chronic disorder in which learning and memory are impaired out of proportion to other cognitive functions in the otherwise-alert and responsive patient. This disorder (Korsakoff's psychosis) is characterized by confabulation, and it is less likely to be reversible once established (Victor *et al.,* 1971). It has been problematic that the thiamine stores of some patients with Wernicke's encephalopathy are similar to those in patients without neurological findings. It has been found that patients with Wernicke's encephalopathy have an abnormality in the thiamine-dependent enzyme transketolase (*see* Haas, 1988). In such instances, marginal concentrations of thiamine might produce serious neurological damage.

Chronic alcoholics with polyneuritis and motor or sensory defects should receive up to 40 mg of oral thiamine daily. The Wernicke–Korsakoff syndrome represents an acute emergency that should be treated with daily doses of at least 100 mg of the vitamin, intravenously.

Infantile Beriberi. Thiamine deficiency also occurs as an acute disease in infancy and may run a rapid and fulminating course. Although rare in western countries, infantile beriberi has been a common cause of infant death throughout this century in regions where rice consumption is high. It is still of significance in Third-World countries and is related to the low content of thiamine in breast milk of thiamine-deficient women. The onset consists in loss of appetite, vomiting, and greenish stools, followed by paroxysmal attacks of muscular rigidity. Aphonia due to loss of laryngeal nerve function is a diagnostic feature. Signs of cardiac involvement are prominent, and death may occur within 12 to 24 hours unless vigorous treatment is instituted. Infants with mild forms of this condition respond to oral therapy with 10 mg of thiamine daily. If acute collapse occurs, doses of 25 mg intravenously can be given cautiously, but the prognosis remains poor.

Subacute Necrotizing Encephalomyelopathy. This is a fatal inherited disease of children. Neuropathological features resemble those of the Wernicke–Korsakoff syndrome, and clinical features include difficulties with feeding and swallowing, vomiting, hypotonia, external ophthalmoplegia, peripheral neuropathy, and seizures. Although the syndrome may have multiple causes, the distribution of lesions and the elevated plasma concentrations of pyruvate and lactate suggest a pathogenetic relationship to thiamine; however, this remains unproven (*see* Haas, 1988). Some cases appear to be caused by a circulating inhibitor of the enzyme that synthesizes thiamine triphosphate from thiamine pyrophosphate in the nervous system (Pincus *et al.,* 1969). Metabolic abnormalities have also been found in liver and muscle tissue samples from affected infants. A urine test for the presence of the glycoprotein enzyme inhibitor has been described (Pincus *et al.*, 1974). When patients with this syndrome are treated daily with large doses of thiamine, marked temporary improvement is sometimes observed (Pincus *et al.*, 1973). Other inborn errors of metabolism that are sensitive to the administration of thiamine have also been described (*see* Scriver, 1973).

Cardiovascular Disease. Cardiovascular disease of nutritional origin is observed in chronic alcoholics, pregnant women, persons with gastrointestinal disorders, and those whose diet is deficient for other reasons. When the diagnosis of cardiovascular disease due to thiamine deficiency has been correctly made, the response to the administration of thiamine is striking. One of the pathognomonic features of the syndrome is an increased blood flow due to arteriolar dilatation. Within a few hours after the administration of thiamine, the cardiac output is reduced and the utilization of oxygen begins to return to normal. If edema is present and due to myocardial insufficiency, diuresis results after proper therapy. However, individuals suffering from a chronic deficiency may require protracted treatment. The usual dose of thiamine is 10 to 30 mg three times daily, given parenterally. The dosage can be reduced and the patient maintained on oral medication or by dietary management after signs of the deficiency state have been reversed. It is emphasized that administration of glucose may precipitate heart failure in individuals with marginal thiamine status. All patients potentially in this category should receive thiamine prophylactically; 100 mg is commonly given intramuscularly or added to the first few liters of intravenous fluid.

Gastrointestinal Disorders. In experimental and clinical beriberi, certain symptoms occur that are referable to the gastrointestinal tract. On this basis, thiamine has been used uncritically as a therapeutic agent for such unrelated conditions as ulcerative colitis, gastrointestinal hypotonia, and chronic diarrhea. Unless the disease being treated is the direct result of a deficiency of thiamine, the vitamin is not efficacious.

Neuritis of Pregnancy. Pregnancy increases the thiamine requirement slightly. The neuritis of pregnancy takes the form of multiple peripheral nerve involvement, and the signs and symptoms in well-developed cases resemble those described in patients with beriberi. The problem may occur because of poor intake of thiamine or in patients with hyperemesis gravidarum. Proof that the neuritis is due to thiamine deficiency is gained in those cases in which dramatic clinical improvement follows thiamine therapy. The dose employed is from 5 to 10 mg daily, given parenterally if vomiting is severe.

RIBOFLAVIN

History. At various times from 1879 onward, series of yellow pigmented compounds have been isolated from a variety of sources and designated as flavins, prefixed to indicate the source (*e.g.*, lacto-, ovo-, and hepato-). It was finally demonstrated that these various flavins are identical in chemical composition.

In the meantime, water-soluble vitamin B had been separated into a heat-labile antiberiberi factor (B_1) and a heat-stable growth-promoting factor (B_2), and it was eventually appreciated that concentrates of so-called vitamin B_2 had a yellow color. In 1932, Warburg and Christian described a yellow respiratory enzyme in yeast, and in 1933 the yellow pigment portion of the enzyme was identified as vitamin B_2. All doubt as to the identity of vitamin B_2 and the naturally occurring flavins was removed when lactoflavin was synthesized and the synthetic product was shown to possess full biological activity. The vitamin was designated as *riboflavin* because of the presence of ribose in its structure.

Chemistry. Riboflavin carries out its functions in the body in the form of one or the other of two coenzymes, riboflavin phosphate, commonly called flavin mononucleotide (FMN), and flavin adenine dinucleotide (FAD). The structures of riboflavin, FMN, and FAD are shown below. Riboflavin is converted to FMN and FAD by two enzyme-catalyzed reactions (McCormick, 1975):

$$\text{Riboflavin} + \text{ATP} \longrightarrow \text{FMN} + \text{ADP} \quad (1)$$
$$\text{FMN} + \text{ATP} \longrightarrow \text{FAD} + \text{PP} \quad (2)$$

Pharmacological Actions. No overt pharmacological effects follow the oral or parenteral administration of riboflavin.

Physiological Functions. FMN and FAD, the physiologically active forms of riboflavin, serve a vital role in metabolism as coenzymes for a wide variety of respiratory flavoproteins, some of which contain metals (*e.g.*, xanthine oxidase).

Symptoms of Deficiency. The signs and symptoms of spontaneous or experimentally produced riboflavin deficiency have been reviewed by Rivlin (1970) and by Lane and colleagues (1975). Sore throat and angular stomatitis generally appear first. Later, glossitis, cheilosis (red denuded lips), seborrheic dermatitis of the face, and dermatitis over the trunk and extremities occur, followed by anemia and neuropathy. In some subjects corneal vascularization and cataract formation are prominent.

The anemia that develops in riboflavin deficiency is normochromic and normocytic and is associated with reticulocytopenia; leukocytes and platelets are generally normal. Administration of riboflavin to deficient patients causes reticulocytosis, and the concentration of hemoglobin returns to normal. Anemia in patients with riboflavin deficiency may be related, at least in part, to disturbances in folic acid metabolism.

The problem in the clinical recognition of ribofla-

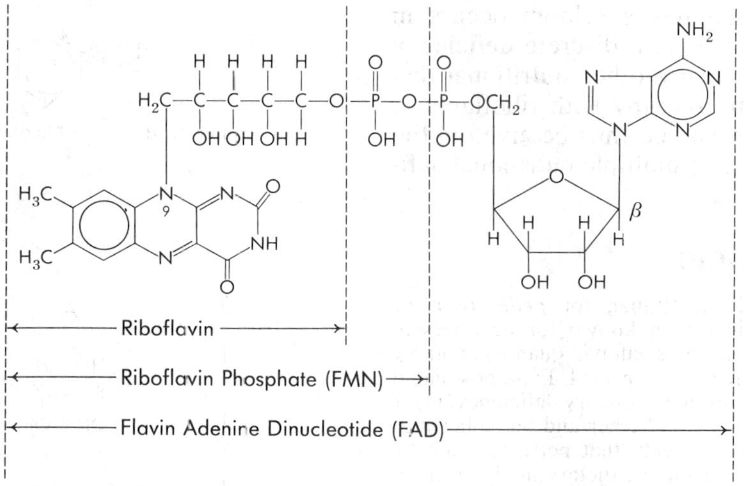

vin deficiency is that certain features, such as glossitis and dermatitis, are common signs, both in deficiencies of other vitamins and as manifestations of other diseases. Recognition of riboflavin deficiency is also difficult because it rarely occurs in isolation. In nutritional surveys of children in an urban area and of randomly selected hospitalized patients, deficiency of riboflavin was frequently observed, but almost invariably in conjunction with other vitamin deficiencies. Riboflavin deficiency has likewise been observed in association with deficiencies of other vitamins in a large proportion of urban alcoholics of low economic status (Rivlin, 1979). Biochemical evidence of riboflavin deficiency has been observed in newborn infants treated with ultraviolet light for hyperbilirubinemia. Breast-fed infants are most susceptible to this problem because of the relatively low riboflavin content in breast milk. Assessment of riboflavin status is made by correlating dietary history with clinical and laboratory findings. Biochemical tests include evaluation of urinary excretion of the vitamin (excretion of less than 50 μg of riboflavin daily is indicative of deficiency). Although concentrations of flavins in blood are not of diagnostic value, an enzyme activation assay that utilizes glutathione reductase from erythrocytes correlates well with riboflavin status (Prentice and Bates, 1981).

Human Requirements. The Dietary Allowances Committee of the National Research Council recommends a riboflavin intake of 0.6 mg/1000 kcal, which is equivalent to about 1.6 mg daily for young adult males and 1.2 mg daily for young adult females. It is recommended that intake for elderly adults should not be less than 1.2 mg daily, even when caloric intake falls below 2000 kcal. Turnover of riboflavin appears to be related to energy expenditure, and periods of increased physical activity are associated with a modest increase in requirement (Belko *et al.*, 1983).

Food Sources. Riboflavin is abundant in milk, cheese, organ meats, eggs, green leafy vegetables, and whole-grain and enriched cereals and breads.

Absorption, Fate, and Excretion. Riboflavin is readily absorbed from the upper gastrointestinal tract by a specific transport mechanism involving phosphorylation of the vitamin to FMN (Jusko and Levy, 1975). Here and in other tissues, riboflavin is converted to FMN by flavokinase, a reaction that is sensitive to thyroid-hormone status and inhibited by chlorpromazine and by tricyclic antidepressants (Rivlin, 1979); the antimalarial quinacrine also interferes with the utilization of riboflavin. Riboflavin is distributed to all tissues, but concentrations are uniformly low and little is stored. When riboflavin is ingested in amounts that approximate the minimal daily requirement, only about 9% appears in the urine. As the intake of riboflavin is increased above the minimal requirement, a larger proportion is excreted unchanged. Boric acid, a common household chemical, forms a complex with riboflavin and promotes its urinary excretion. Boric acid poisoning may therefore induce riboflavin deficiency.

Riboflavin is present in the feces. This probably represents vitamin synthesized by intestinal microorganisms, since, on low intakes of riboflavin, the amount excreted in the feces exceeds that ingested. There is no evidence that riboflavin synthesized by the bacteria in the colon can be absorbed.

Preparations. *Riboflavin (vitamin B_2) tablets* are available in amounts ranging from 5 to 250 mg.

Therapeutic Uses. The only established therapeutic application of riboflavin is to treat or prevent disease caused by deficiency. Ariboflavinosis seldom occurs in the United States as a discrete deficiency but may accompany other nutritional disorders. Specific therapy with riboflavin, 5 to 10 mg daily, should thus be given in the context of treating multiple nutritional deficiencies.

NICOTINIC ACID

History. Pellagra (Italian for *pelle agra,* or "rough skin") has been known for centuries in countries where maize is eaten in quantity, notably Italy and North America. In 1914, Funk postulated that the disease was due to dietary deficiency. Over the next few years Goldberger and his colleagues demonstrated conclusively that pellagra could be prevented by increasing the dietary intake of fresh meat, eggs, and milk. Goldberger subsequently produced an excellent animal model of human pellagra, "black tongue," by feeding deficient diets to dogs. Although initially thought to be a deficiency of essential amino acids, pellagra was soon found to be prevented by a distinct heat-resistant factor in "water-soluble B" vitamin preparations.

In 1935, Warburg and associates obtained nicotinic acid amide (nicotinamide) from a coenzyme isolated from the red blood cells of the horse, and this stimulated interest in the nutritional value of nicotinic acid. Since liver extracts were known to be highly effective in curing human pellagra and canine black tongue, Elvehjem and associates prepared highly active concentrates of liver; in 1937, they identified nicotinamide as the substance that was effective in the treatment of black tongue. Proof was established by the demonstration that synthetic nicotinic acid derivatives were also effective in alleviating the symptoms of black tongue and curing human pellagra. Goldberger and Tanner had previously shown that tryptophan could cure human pellagra; this effect was later determined to be due to the conversion of tryptophan to nicotinic acid. Goldsmith (1958) produced pellagra experimentally in man by feeding a diet deficient in nicotinic acid and tryptophan.

Nicotinic acid is also known as *niacin,* a term introduced to avoid confusion between the vitamin and the alkaloid nicotine. Pellagra is now quite uncommon in the United States, probably as a direct result of supplementation of flour with nicotinic acid since 1939.

Chemistry. Nicotinic acid functions in the body after conversion to either nicotinamide adenine dinucleotide (NAD) or nicotinamide adenine dinucleotide phosphate (NADP). It is to be noted that nicotinic acid occurs in these two nucleotides in the form of its amide, nicotinamide. The structures of nicotinic acid, nicotinamide, NAD, and NADP are shown below, where **R** = H in NAD and **R** = PO_3H_2 in NADP.

Synthetic analogs with antivitamin activity include pyridine-3-sulfonic acid and 3-acetyl pyridine.

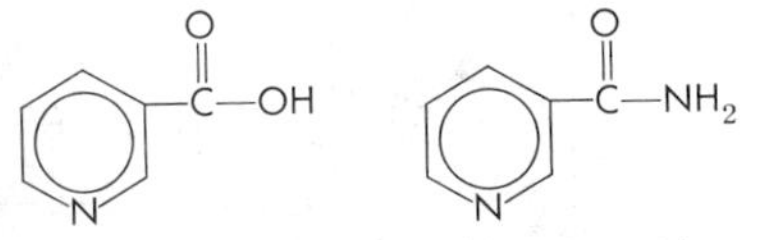

Nicotinic Acid Nicotinamide

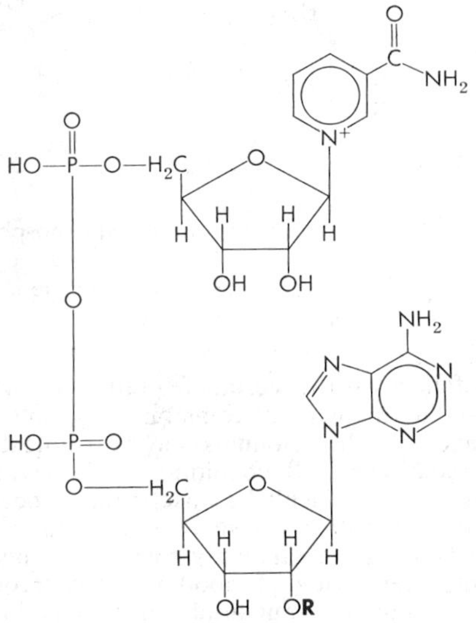

NAD and NADP

Pharmacological Actions. Nicotinic acid and nicotinamide are identical in their function as vitamins. However, they differ markedly as pharmacological agents. The pharmacological effects and toxicity of nicotinic acid in man include flushing, pruritus, gastrointestinal distress, hepatotoxicity, and activation of peptic ulcer disease. Large doses of nicotinic acid (2 to 6 g per day) are sometimes used in the treatment of hyperlipoproteinemia (*see* Chapter 36). The important toxic effects of nicotinic acid are generally seen only with these doses.

Physiological Functions. NAD and NADP, the physiologically active forms of nicotinic acid, serve a vital role in metabolism as coenzymes for a wide variety of proteins that catalyze oxidation-reduction reactions essential for tissue respiration. The coenzymes, bound to appropriate dehydrogenases, function as oxidants by accepting electrons and hydrogen from substrates and thus becoming reduced. The reduced pyridine nucleotides, in turn, are reoxidized by flavoproteins. NAD also participates as a substrate in the transfer of ADP-ribosyl moieties to proteins. For example, ADP-ribosylation is the mechanism by which cholera toxin (an ADP-ribosyl transferase) irreversibly activates the guanine nucleotide-binding regulatory protein that stimulates adenylyl cyclase (*see* Gilman, 1987).

The metabolic pathway for conversion of nicotinic acid to NAD has been elucidated for a variety of tissues, including human erythrocytes (*see* 1 to 3 below, where PRPP is 5-phosphoribosyl-1-pyrophosphate). NADP is synthesized from NAD according to reaction 4. The biosynthesis of NAD from tryptophan is more complicated. Tryptophan is converted to quinolinic acid by a series of enzymatic reactions; quinolinic acid is converted to nicotinic acid ribonucleotide, which enters the pathway at reaction 2.

Symptoms of Deficiency. A deficiency of nicotinic acid leads to the clinical condition known as pellagra. Pellagra is characterized by signs and symptoms referable especially to the skin, gastrointestinal tract, and central nervous system (CNS), a triad frequently referred to as dermatitis, diarrhea, and dementia, or the "three Ds." Pellagra now occurs most often in the setting of chronic alcoholism, protein-calorie malnutrition, and deficiencies of multiple vitamins (Spivak and Jackson, 1977). An erythematous eruption resembling sunburn first appears on the back of the hands. Other areas exposed to light (forehead, neck, and feet) are later involved, and eventually the lesions may be more widespread. The cutaneous manifestations are characteristically symmetrical and may darken, desquamate, and scar.

The chief symptoms referable to the digestive tract are stomatitis, enteritis, and diarrhea. The tongue becomes very red and swollen and may ulcerate. Salivary secretion is excessive, and the salivary glands may be enlarged. Nausea and vomiting are common. Steatorrhea may be present, even in the absence of diarrhea. When present, diarrhea is recurrent and stools may be watery and occasionally bloody.

Symptoms referable to the CNS are headache, dizziness, insomnia, depression, and impairment of memory. In severe cases, delusions, hallucinations, and dementia may appear. Motor and sensory disturbances of the peripheral nerves also occur. Common laboratory findings include macrocytic anemia, hypoalbuminemia, and hyperuricemia.

Biochemical assessment of deficiency is attempted by the measurement of urinary excretion of methylated metabolites of nicotinic acid (*e.g.*, N-methylnicotinamide). These tests do not provide unequivocal evidence of deficiency. The measurement of nicotinamide in blood and urine has not been shown to be useful in evaluating niacin status. In most cases, the diagnosis rests on a correlation of clinical findings with the response to supplemental nicotinamide.

Human Requirements. As indicated above, the dietary requirement for this vitamin can be satisfied not only by nicotinic acid but also by nicotinamide and the amino acid tryptophan. Therefore, the nicotinic acid requirement is influenced by the quantity and the quality of dietary protein. Administration of tryptophan to normal human subjects, as well as to patients with pellagra, and analysis of urinary metabolites indicate that an average of 60 mg of dietary tryptophan is equivalent to 1 mg of nicotinic acid. This conversion rate is reduced in women taking oral contraceptives. The minimal requirement of nicotinic acid (including that formed from tryptophan) to prevent pellagra averages 4.4 mg/1000 kcal. The recommended allowance of the Dietary Allowances Committee of the National Research Council, expressed in nicotinic acid equivalents, is 6.6 mg/1000 kcal (*see* Table XVI–1, page 1525). For people who consume few calories (*e.g.*, the elderly), daily intake should not fall below 13 mg of nicotinic acid or the equivalent.

The relationship between the nicotinic acid requirement and the intake of tryptophan has helped to explain the historical association between the incidence of pellagra and the presence of large amounts of corn in the diet. Corn protein is low in tryptophan, and the nicotinic acid in corn and other cereals is largely unavailable. When cornmeal provides the major portion of dietary protein, pellagra will develop at levels of intake of nicotinic acid that would be adequate if the dietary protein contained more tryptophan. Intake of animal protein is high among Americans; tryptophan thus helps significantly to meet the daily requirement for niacin.

Food Sources. Nicotinic acid is obtained from liver, meat, fish, poultry, whole-grain and enriched breads and cereals, nuts, and legumes. Tryptophan as a precursor is provided by animal protein in particular.

Absorption, Fate, and Excretion. Both nicotinic acid and nicotinamide are readily absorbed from all portions of the intestinal tract, and the vitamin is distributed to all tissues. When therapeutic doses of nico-

$$\text{Nicotinic Acid} + \text{PRPP} \longrightarrow \text{Nicotinic Acid Ribonucleotide} + \text{PP} \quad (1)$$

$$\text{Nicotinic Acid Ribonucleotide} + \text{ATP} \longrightarrow \text{Desamido-NAD} + \text{PP} \quad (2)$$

$$\text{Desamido-NAD} + \text{Glutamine} + \text{ATP} \longrightarrow \text{NAD} - \text{Glutamate} + \text{ADP} + \text{P} \quad (3)$$

$$\text{NAD} + \text{ATP} \longrightarrow \text{NADP} + \text{ADP} \quad (4)$$

tinic acid or its amide are administered, only small amounts of the unchanged vitamin appear in the urine. When extremely high doses of these vitamins are given, the unchanged vitamin represents the major urinary component. The principal route of metabolism of nicotinic acid and nicotinamide is by the formation of N-methylnicotinamide, which in turn is metabolized further.

Preparations. *Niacin* (*nicotinic acid, 3-pyridinecarboxylic acid*) is available in tablets and capsules that contain from 25 to 750 mg and in an elixir (50 mg/5 ml). *Niacin injection* contains 100 mg/ml. *Niacinamide* (*nicotinamide, nicotinic acid amide*) is available in tablets (50 to 1000 mg) and as an injection (100 mg/ml).

Therapeutic Uses. Nicotinic acid, nicotinamide, and their derivatives are used for prophylaxis and treatment of pellagra. In the acute exacerbations of the disease, therapy must be intensive. The recommended oral dose is 50 mg, given up to ten times daily. If oral medication is impossible, intravenous injection of 25 mg is given two or more times daily. Pellagra may occur in the course of two metabolic disorders. In Hartnup's disease intestinal and renal transport of tryptophan is defective. In some patients with carcinoid tumors large amounts of tryptophan are utilized by the tumor for the synthesis of 5-hydroxytryptophan and 5-hydroxytryptamine (serotonin).

The response to nicotinic acid or its derivatives is dramatic. Within 24 hours, the fiery redness and swelling of the tongue disappear and sialorrhea diminishes. Associated oral infections heal rapidly. Other infections of mucous membranes also disappear. Nausea, vomiting, and diarrhea may stop within 24 hours, and at the same time the patient is relieved of epigastric distress, abdominal pain, and distention. Appetite also improves. Mental symptoms are quickly relieved, sometimes overnight. Confused patients become mentally clear, and those who are delirious become calm, adjusted to their environment, and remember with insight the events of their psychotic state. So specific are nicotinic acid and its derivatives in this regard that they can be used as diagnostic agents in patients with frank psychoses but with questionable additional evidence of pellagra. Large doses of niacin are recommended, especially when the psychosis is associated with encephalopathy. The dermal lesions blanch and heal, but this occurs more slowly. The vitamin has less effect on cutaneous lesions that are moist, ulcerated, or pigmented. The porphyrinuria associated with pellagra also disappears.

Pellagra may be complicated by thiamine deficiency with associated peripheral neuritis. This complication does not respond to nicotinic acid or its congeners and must be treated with thiamine. Many pellagrins are also benefited by additional therapy with riboflavin and pyridoxine.

PYRIDOXINE

History. In 1926, dermatitis was produced in rats by feeding a diet deficient in vitamin B_2. However, in 1936 György distinguished the water-soluble factor whose deficiency was responsible for the dermatitis from vitamin B_2 and named it vitamin B_6. The structure of the vitamin was elucidated in 1939. Several related natural compounds (pyridoxine, pyridoxal, pyridoxamine) have been shown to possess the same biological properties, and therefore all should be called vitamin B_6. However, the Council on Pharmacy and Chemistry has assigned the name *pyridoxine* to the vitamin.

Chemistry. The structures of the three forms of vitamin B_6—that is, pyridoxine, pyridoxal, and pyridoxamine—are shown below.

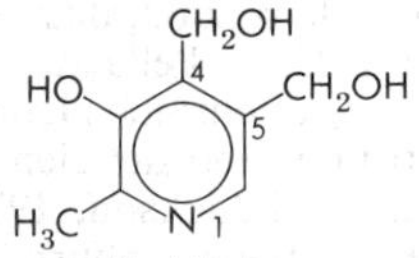

Pyridoxine

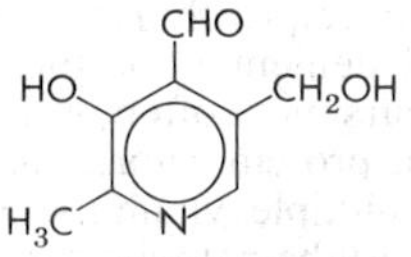

Pyridoxal

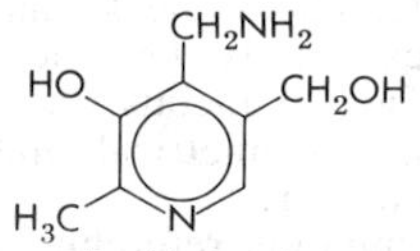

Pyridoxamine

The compounds differ in the nature of the substituent on the carbon atom in position 4 of the pyridine nucleus: pyridoxine is a primary alcohol, pyridoxal is the corresponding aldehyde, and pyridoxamine contains an aminomethyl group in this position. Each of these compounds can be readily utilized by mammals after conversion in the liver to pyridoxal 5′-phosphate, the active form of the vitamin.

Antimetabolites to pyridoxine have been synthesized and are capable of blocking the action of the vitamin and producing signs and symptoms of deficiency. The most active is 4-deoxypyridoxine, for which the antivitamin activity has been attributed to the formation *in vivo* of 4-deoxypyridoxine-5-phosphate, a competitive inhibitor of several pyridoxal phosphate–dependent enzymes.

Isonicotinic acid hydrazide (*isoniazid; see* Chapter 49), as well as other carbonyl compounds, combines with pyridoxal or pyridoxal phosphate to form hydrazones; as a result, it is a potent inhibitor of pyridoxal kinase. Enzymatic reactions in which pyridoxal phosphate participates as a coenzyme are also inhibited, but only by much greater concentrations than those required to inhibit the formation of pyridoxal phosphate. Isoniazid thus appears to exert its anti–vitamin B_6 effect primarily by inhibiting the formation of the coenzyme form of the vitamin.

Pharmacological Actions. Pyridoxine has low acute toxicity and elicits no outstanding pharmacodynamic actions after either oral or intravenous administration. However, recent evidence suggests that neurotoxicity may develop after prolonged ingestion of as little as 200 mg of pyridoxine per day (Schaumberg *et al.*, 1983; Parry and Bredesen, 1985). Symptoms of dependency have also been noted in adults given 200 mg daily followed by withdrawal (Canham *et al.*, 1964).

Physiological Functions. As a coenzyme, pyridoxal phosphate is involved in several metabolic transformations of amino acids, including decarboxylation, transamination, and racemization, as well as in enzymatic steps in the metabolism of sulfur-containing and hydroxy-amino acids. In the case of transamination, enzyme-bound pyridoxal phosphate is aminated to pyridoxamine phosphate by the donor amino acid, and the bound pyridoxamine phosphate is then deaminated to pyridoxal phosphate by the acceptor α-keto acid. Vitamin B_6 is also involved in the metabolism of tryptophan (Henderson and Hulse, 1978). A notable reaction is the conversion of tryptophan to 5-hydroxytryptamine. In vitamin B_6–deficient man and animals a number of metabolites of tryptophan are excreted in abnormally large quantities. The measurement of these urinary metabolites, particularly xanthurenic acid, following loading with tryptophan is used as a test of vitamin B_6 status. The conversion of methionine to cysteine is also dependent on the vitamin (Sturman, 1978). In addition to its classical cofactor functions, pyridoxine seems to modulate actions of steroid hormones *in vivo* by interacting with steroid receptor complexes (DiSorbo *et al.*, 1980; Müller *et al.*, 1980; Compton and Cidlowski, 1986). The significance of this interaction is uncertain.

Interactions with Drugs. Biochemical interactions occur between pyridoxal phosphate and certain drugs and toxins (Bauernfeind and Miller, 1978). The relationship with isoniazid has been discussed above. Prolonged use of penicillamine can cause deficiency of vitamin B_6. The drugs cycloserine and hydralazine are also antagonists of the vitamin, and its administration reduces the neurological side effects associated with the use of these compounds. Vitamin B_6 enhances the peripheral decarboxylation of levodopa and reduces its effectiveness for the treatment of Parkinson's disease (*see* Chapter 20).

Symptoms of Deficiency. Important features of pyridoxine deficiency involve the skin, the nervous system, and erythropoiesis.

Skin. In man, seborrhea-like skin lesions about the eyes, nose, and mouth accompanied by glossitis and stomatitis can be produced within a few weeks by feeding a diet poor in vitamin B complex plus daily doses of the vitamin antagonist 4-deoxypyridoxine. The lesions clear rapidly after the administration of pyridoxine but do not respond to other members of the B complex.

Nervous System. Convulsive seizures may occur when human subjects are maintained on a diet deficient in pyridoxine, and these seizures can be prevented by the vitamin. In the pig, degenerative changes in peripheral nerves, dorsal root ganglion cells, and posterior columns of the spinal cord have been described. In man, a peripheral neuritis associated with carpal synovial swelling and tenderness (*carpal tunnel syndrome*) has been attributed in some cases to deficiency of pyridoxine. However, earlier claims that high doses of pyridoxine reverse carpal tunnel syndrome have not been confirmed (Smith *et al.*, 1984).

The induction of convulsive seizures by pyridoxine deficiency may be the result of a lowered concentration of gamma-aminobutyric acid; glutamate decarboxylase, a pyridoxal phosphate–requiring enzyme, synthesizes this inhibitory CNS neurotransmitter. In addition, pyridoxine deficiency leads to decreased concentrations of the neurotransmitters norepinephrine and 5-hydroxytryptamine (Dakshinamurti, 1977).

Erythropoiesis. Although dietary deficiency of pyridoxine in man may rarely cause anemia, the usual pyridoxine-responsive anemia of man is apparently not due to inadequate supplies of this vitamin as judged by normal standards. This type of anemia is described in Chapter 54.

Human Requirements. The requirement for pyridoxine increases with the amount of protein in the diet (Linkswiler, 1978). The average adult minimal requirement for pyridoxine is about 1.5 mg per day in individuals ingesting 100 g of protein per day. To provide a reasonable margin of safety and to allow for daily intakes of more than 100 g of protein, the RDA for pyridoxine has been set at 2.0 mg per day for adult males and 1.6 mg per day for adult females (*see* Table XVI–1, page 1525).

Food Sources. Pyridoxine is supplied by meat, liver, whole-grain breads and cereals, soybeans, and vegetables. Substantial losses occur during cooking, and pyridoxine is sensitive to both ultraviolet light and oxidation.

Absorption, Fate, and Excretion. Pyridoxine, pyridoxal, and pyridoxamine are readily absorbed from the gastrointestinal tract following hydrolysis of their phosphorylated derivatives. Pyridoxal phosphate accounts for at least 60% of circulating vitamin B_6. Pyridoxal is thought to be the primary form that crosses cell membranes. The principal excretory product when any of the three forms of the vitamin is fed to man is 4-pyridoxic acid, formed by the action of hepatic aldehyde oxidase on free pyridoxal (*see* Brin, 1978; Leklem, 1988).

Preparations. *Pyridoxine hydrochloride* is available in tablets (10 to 500 mg) and as an injection (100 mg/ml).

Therapeutic Uses. Although there is no doubt that pyridoxine is essential in human nutrition, the clinical syndrome of simple pyridoxine deficiency is rare. Nevertheless, it may be presumed that an individual with a deficiency of other members of the B complex may also have a deficiency of pyridoxine. Therefore, pyridoxine should be a component of therapy for individuals suffering from a deficiency of other members of the B complex. On the basis that pyridoxine is essential in human nutrition, it is incorporated into many multivitamin preparations for prophylactic use. It has been pointed out that 30% or more of alcoholics have biochemically demonstrable deficiency of vitamin B_6 (Li, 1978).

As indicated above, vitamin B_6 influences the metabolism of certain drugs and vice versa. With considerable justification, vitamin B_6 is given prophylactically to patients receiving isoniazid to prevent the development of peripheral neuritis. In addition, pyridoxine is an antidote for the seizures and acidosis in patients who have ingested an overdose of isoniazid.

The concentration of pyridoxal phosphate is reduced in the blood of women who are pregnant or who are taking oral contraceptives. It has been suggested that 15 to 20% of women taking oral contraceptives have biochemical evidence of vitamin B_6 deficiency (Rose, 1978). However, the recommended intakes of vitamin B_6 appear to be sufficient to meet the requirements of such individuals (Bossé and Donald, 1979; Donald and Bossé, 1979). Moreover, although plasma concentrations of pyridoxal phosphate are lower in pregnant women, total circulating vitamin B_6 is not reduced, since the concentration of pyridoxal is markedly increased (Barnard *et al.*, 1987). Several reports have indicated that a subset of women who report symptoms of depression while taking oral contraceptive medication may be deficient in pyridoxine and respond favorably to a daily supplement of 50 mg of the vitamin (Adams *et al.*, 1973).

Pyridoxine-responsive anemia is a well-documented but uncommon condition. The use of the vitamin in this disease is discussed in Chapter 54. Such anemias in patients without apparent pyridoxine deficiency; a seizure disorder in infants that responds to the administration of pyridoxine; and those abnormalities characterized by xanthurenic aciduria, primary cystathioninuria, or homocystinuria all appear to constitute a group of genetically determined clinical states of "pyridoxine dependency," manifested by a requirement for large amounts of the vitamin (*see* Fowler, 1985).

PANTOTHENIC ACID

History. Pantothenic acid was first identified by Williams and associates in 1933 as a substance essential for the growth of yeast. Its name, derived from Greek words signifying "from everywhere," is indicative of the wide distribution of the vitamin in nature. The role of pantothenic acid in animal nutrition was first defined in chicks, in which a deficiency disease characterized by skin lesions was known to be cured by fractions prepared from liver extract. Although first thought to be a form of "chick pellagra," it was not cured by nicotinic acid. In 1939, Woolley and coworkers and also Jukes demonstrated that the chick antidermatitis factor was pantothenic acid. Elucidation of the biochemical function for the vitamin began in 1947 when Lipmann and coworkers showed that the acetylation of sulfanilamide required a cofactor that contained pantothenic acid.

Chemistry. Pantothenate consists of pantoic acid complexed to β-alanine. This is transformed in the body to 4′-phosphopantetheine by phosphorylation and linkage to cysteamine; this derivative is incorporated into either coenzyme A or acyl carrier protein, the functional forms of the vitamin. The chemical structures of pantothenic acid and coenzyme A are as follows:

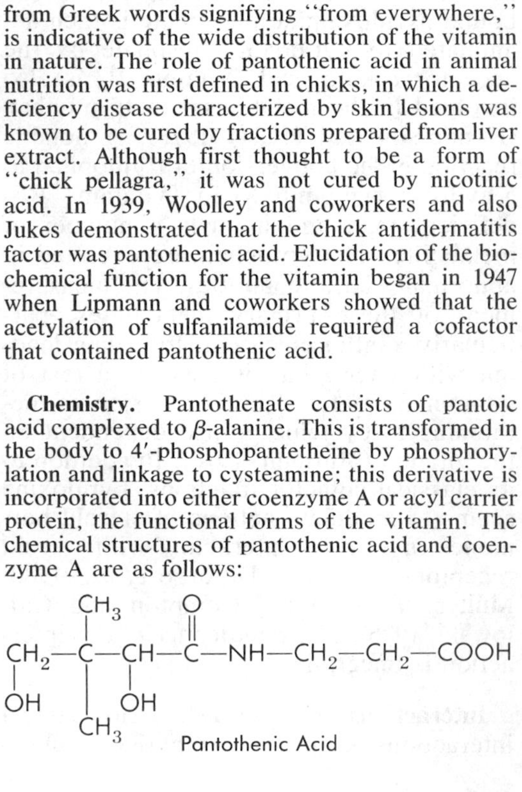

Pantothenic Acid

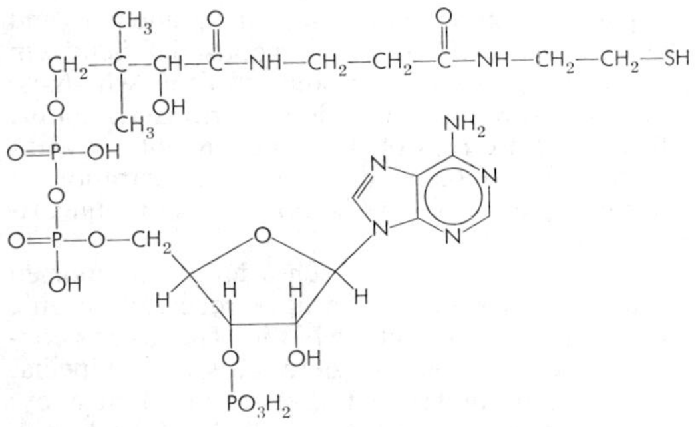

Coenzyme A

Many analogs of pantothenic acid have been studied in an attempt to find an antimetabolite. Although active antagonists have been synthesized (*e.g.*, ω-methyl pantothenate) and are of value as research tools, they are not therapeutic agents.

Pharmacological Actions. Pantothenic acid has no outstanding pharmacological actions when it is administered to experimental animals or normal man, even in large doses.

Physiological Functions. Coenzyme A serves as a cofactor for a variety of enzyme-catalyzed reactions involving transfer of acetyl (two-carbon) groups; the precursor fragments of various lengths are bound to the sulfhydryl group of coenzyme A. Such reactions are important in the oxidative metabolism of carbohydrates, gluconeogenesis, degradation of fatty acids, and the synthesis of sterols, steroid hormones, and porphyrins. As a component of acyl carrier protein, pantothenate participates in fatty acid synthesis. Recent evidence suggests that pantothenate also participates in the posttranslational modification of proteins, including N-terminal acetylation, acetylation of internal amino acids, and fatty acid acylation (*see* Plesofsky-Vig and Brambl, 1988). Such modifications influence the intracellular localization, stability, and activity of the proteins.

Symptoms of Deficiency. Deficiency of pantothenic acid is manifested by symptoms of neuromuscular degeneration and adrenocortical insufficiency. By administering a semisynthetic diet low in the vitamin together with ω-methylpantothenic acid, a syndrome in man is produced that is characterized by fatigue, headache, sleep disturbances, nausea, abdominal cramps, vomiting, and flatulence (Hodges *et al.*, 1959). The subjects complain of paresthesias in the extremities, muscle cramps, and impaired coordination. Fry and coworkers (1976) have produced the same syndrome by giving human subjects a diet devoid of pantothenic acid for 10 weeks. Pantothenic acid deficiency has not been recognized in man consuming a normal diet, presumably because of the ubiquitous occurrence of the vitamin in ordinary foods.

Human Requirements. Pantothenic acid is a required nutrient, but the magnitude of need is not precisely known. Accordingly, the Committee on Dietary Allowances provides provisional recommendations in the form of ranges of intakes (Table XVI–2, page 1527). For adults, this is 4 to 7 mg per day. Intakes for other groups are proportional to caloric consumption. In view of the widespread distribution of pantothenic acid in foods, dietary deficiency is very unlikely.

Food Sources. Pantothenic acid is ubiquitous. It is particularly abundant in organ meats, beef, and egg yolk. However, pantothenic acid is easily destroyed by heat and alkali.

Absorption, Fate, and Excretion. Pantothenic acid is readily absorbed from the gastrointestinal tract. It is present in all tissues, in concentrations ranging from 2 to 45 μg/g. Pantothenic acid apparently is not degraded in the human body since the intake and the excretion of the vitamin are approximately equal. About 70% of the absorbed pantothenic acid is excreted in the urine.

Preparations. *Calcium pantothenate* is available as tablets containing from 25 to 545 mg.

Therapeutic Uses. No clearly defined uses for pantothenic acid exist, although it is commonly included in multivitamin preparations and in products for enteral and parenteral alimentation.

BIOTIN

History. In 1916, Bateman observed that rats fed a diet containing raw egg white as the sole source of protein developed a syndrome characterized by neuromuscular disorders, severe dermatitis, and loss of hair. The syndrome could be prevented by cooking the protein or by administering yeast, liver, or extracts of these. In 1936, Kögl and Tönnis isolated from egg yolk a factor in crystalline form that was essential for growth of yeast, which they called *biotin*. It was then demonstrated that biotin and the factor that protected against egg-white toxicity were the same (György, 1940). In 1942, duVigneaud established the structural formula of biotin, and the vitamin was synthesized shortly thereafter.

In the meantime, the nature of the antagonist to

biotin in egg white received extensive study. The compound is a protein, first isolated by Eakin and associates in 1940 and called *avidin*. Avidin is a glycoprotein that binds biotin with great affinity and thus prevents its absorption.

Chemistry. Biotin has the following structural formula:

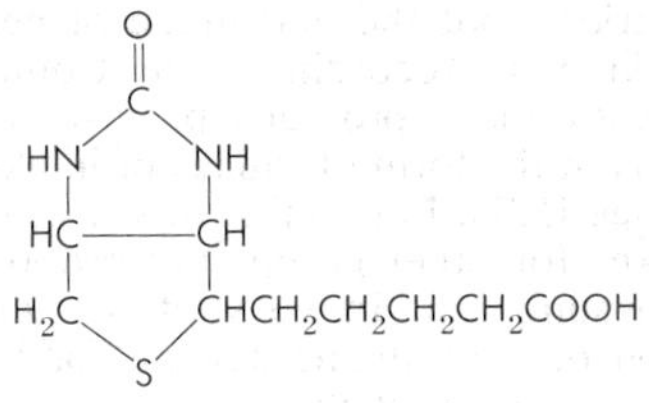

Biotin

Three forms of biotin, apart from free biotin itself, have been found in natural materials. These derivatives are biocytin (ε-biotinyl-L-lysine) and the D and L sulfoxides of biotin. Although the derived forms of biotin are active in supporting growth of some microorganisms, their efficacy as substitutes for biotin in human nutrition is unknown. Biocytin may represent a degradation product of a biotin–protein complex, since, in its role as a coenzyme, the vitamin is covalently linked to an ε-amino group of a lysine residue of the apoenzyme involved (*see* Dakshinamurti and Chauhan, 1988).

A number of compounds antagonize the actions of biotin. Among them are biotin sulfone, desthiobiotin, and certain imidazolidone carboxylic acids. The antagonism between avidin and biotin is described above.

Pharmacological Actions. Biotin toxicity has not been reported in man despite administration of large amounts for as long as 6 months (*see* Miller and Hayes, 1982).

Physiological Functions. In human tissues biotin is a cofactor for the enzymatic carboxylation of four substrates: pyruvate, acetyl coenzyme A (CoA), propionyl CoA, and β-methylcrotonyl CoA. As such, it plays an important role in both carbohydrate and fat metabolism. CO_2 fixation occurs in a two-step reaction, the first involving binding of CO_2 to the biotin moiety of the holoenzyme, and the second involving transfer of the biotin-bound CO_2 to an appropriate acceptor (*see* McCormick and Olson, 1984).

Symptoms of Deficiency. The ease of producing biotin deficiency varies with the animal species. In a few species, a deficiency state can be produced merely by feeding a synthetic diet deficient in this nutrient. In most, however, presumably owing to synthesis of the vitamin by intestinal bacteria, it is necessary to eliminate bacteria from the intestinal tract, feed raw egg white, or administer antimetabolites of biotin in order to produce the deficiency. In man, signs and symptoms of deficiency include dermatitis, atrophic glossitis, hyperesthesia, muscle pain, lassitude, anorexia, slight anemia, and changes in the ECG. Spontaneous deficiency in man has been observed in some subjects who have consumed raw eggs over long periods (Bonjour, 1977). Inborn errors of biotin-dependent enzymes are known and respond to the administration of massive doses of biotin (Bonjour, 1977; Baumgartner *et al.*, 1984).

Symptomatic biotin deficiency has been reported in children and adults who have received chronic parenteral nutrition lacking biotin. The lesions consist of severe exfoliative dermatitis and alopecia, and they are similar to those of zinc deficiency; however, they respond to small doses of biotin. These patients suffered from chronic inflammatory bowel disease, and inadequate synthesis of biotin by gut flora was a probable contributory factor. Few reports have provided biochemical validation of biotin deficiency, but in one case the correction by biotin of an elevated rate of urinary excretion of β-hydroxyisovaleric acid indicates defective function of the biotin-dependent β-methylcrotonyl CoA carboxylase (Gillis *et al.*, 1982).

Human Requirements. The daily requirement of adults for biotin has been assigned a provisional value of 30 to 100 μg by the Committee on Dietary Allowances (Table XVI–2, page 1527). The average American diet provides 100 to 300 μg of the vitamin. Part of the biotin synthesized by the bacterial flora is also available for absorption.

Food Sources. Organ meats, egg yolk, milk, fish, and nuts are rich sources of biotin. Biotin is stable to cooking, but less so in alkali.

Absorption, Fate, and Excretion. Ingested biotin is rapidly absorbed from the gastrointestinal tract and appears in the urine predominantly in the form of intact biotin and in lesser amounts as the metabolites *bis*-norbiotin and biotin sulfoxide. Mammals are unable to degrade the ring system of biotin.

Preparations. Although there is no official preparation of biotin, it is available commercially. It is also present in some multivitamin preparations.

Therapeutic Uses. Large doses of biotin (5 to 10 mg daily) are administered to babies with infantile seborrhea and to individuals with genetic alterations of biotin-dependent enzymes. Patients who receive long-term parenteral nutrition should be given vitamin formulations that contain biotin.

CHOLINE

Although choline is not a vitamin as defined above, sufficient ambiguity exists concerning a possible dietary requirement for this substance that it is customarily considered in discussions of water-soluble vitamins.

History. In 1932, Best and associates observed that pancreatectomized dogs maintained on insulin developed fatty livers; this could be prevented by inclusion in the diet of crude egg-yolk lecithin or beef pancreas. The substance responsible for this effect was shown to be choline. These studies marked the beginning of an extensive literature on the role of lipotropic substances, especially choline, in animal nutrition. Choline has other important functions in addition to those related to lipid metabolism. For example, it is a precursor of the neurochemical transmitter acetylcholine and of the autacoid, platelet-activating factor (PAF) (*see* Chapter 24).

Chemistry. Choline (trimethylethanolamine) has the following structural formula:

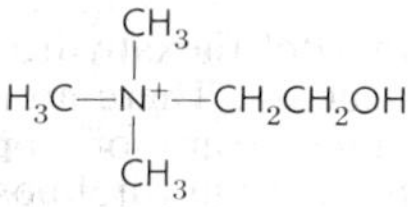

Choline

Pharmacological Actions. Qualitatively, choline has the same pharmacological actions as does acetylcholine, but it is far less active. Single oral doses of 10 g produce no obvious pharmacodynamic response.

Physiological Functions. Choline has several roles in the body. It is an important component of phospholipids, affects the mobilization of fat from the liver (lipotropic action), acts as a methyl donor, and is essential for the formation of the neurotransmitter acetylcholine and the autacoid PAF.

Phospholipid Constituent. Choline is a component of the major phospholipid, lecithin, and is also a constituent of plasmalogens, which are abundant in mitochondria, and sphingomyelin, which is found particularly in brain. Choline thus provides an essential structural component of many biological membranes and also of the plasma lipoproteins.

Lipotropic Action. As mentioned, the initial recognition of choline as a significant dietary factor depended on its capacity to reduce the fat content of the liver of diabetic dogs. Substances that stimulate removal of excess fat from the liver are known as lipotropic agents and include choline, inositol, methionine, vitamin B_{12}, and folic acid. Certain of these compounds appear to act by providing methyl groups for the synthesis of choline in the body. Formation of the lipid components of plasma lipoproteins is thus permitted, and this facilitates transport of fat from the liver.

Methyl Donor. Choline can donate methyl groups necessary for the synthesis of other compounds. The first step in transfer is the formation of betaine, which is the immediate donor of the methyl group. Thus, choline can transfer a methyl group to homocysteine to form methionine. The roles of cyanocobalamin and folic acid in the metabolism of one-carbon compounds are discussed in Chapter 54.

Acetylcholine Formation. Acetylcholine is synthesized from choline and acetyl CoA by choline acetyltransferase and is broken down by acetylcholinesterase (*see* Chapter 5). Choline is transported between the brain and the plasma by a bidirectional system localized in the endothelium of brain capillaries. This system operates by facilitated diffusion, and the amount of choline available to central neurons thus varies as a function of the concentration of choline in the plasma. When rats are given choline chloride, the concentrations of plasma choline, brain choline, and brain acetylcholine increase sequentially. Consumption of lecithin, which contains choline, also causes these changes (Growdon and Wurtman, 1979). These findings may be relevant to the treatment of diseases involving reduced capacity to synthesize acetylcholine (*see* below).

Synthesis of PAF. This autacoid is formed from a subset of choline-containing membrane phospholipids in which the moiety in position 1 of the glycerol backbone is an alkyl ether rather than a fatty acid ester. The phospholipid is acted upon by the hormonally regulated phospholipase A_2 to form 1-O-alkyl-lysophosphatidyl choline. This intermediate is converted to PAF through acetylation at the 2 position by acetyl CoA in a reaction catalyzed by lyso-PAF transacetylase. PAF has many important functions in inflammatory and other processes (*see* Chapter 24).

Symptoms of Deficiency. The effects of choline deficiency on animals are discussed in two reviews (Griffith and Nye, 1971; Kuksis and Mookerjea, 1978). The deficiency state is really one of available methyl groups, and consequently can only be produced as a result of a combined deficiency of choline and other methyl donors. In animals, the amount of choline needed is affected by growth rate, age, quantity of dietary fat, and quality of dietary protein, as well as by species differences in the capacity to synthesize choline from methyl donors. Some species, such as the guinea pig, have such a low capacity for synthesis that choline is a dietary essential. In such species it is possible to induce choline deficiency with a suitable diet. Not only is there accumulation of fat in the liver, followed by cirrhosis, but hemorrhagic renal lesions and motor incoordination from nerve degeneration have also been observed. Newberne and Chandra (1977) describe damage to the fetus, including atrophy of the thymus, when the pregnant rat is fed a diet with marginal contents of choline, methionine, folate, and vitamin B_{12}. None of these symptoms of deficiency has been identified in man (Kuksis and Mookerjea, 1978).

Human Requirements. The needs of the tissues for choline are met from both exogenous (dietary) and endogenous (metabolic) sources. Biosynthesis of choline occurs by transmethylation of ethanolamine with the methyl group of methionine or by a series of reactions requiring vitamin B_{12} and folate as cofactors (*see* Chapter 54). Thus, an adequate supply of methyl-group donors in the diet is desirable to protect against the hepatic accumulation of lipid. In addition, large amounts of choline appear to have a therapeutic effect on certain diseases of the nervous system, perhaps by stimulation of the synthesis of acetylcholine. However, none of the functions of choline justifies its classification as a vitamin. It has not been shown to act as a cofactor in any enzymatic reaction, and the doses needed to produce therapeutic effects (several grams) are much greater than those of any vitamin.

Because of the lack of evidence of a choline deficiency syndrome in human subjects, choline cannot be considered an essential dietary constituent for man. In addition, the American diet provides 400 to 900 mg per day of choline as a constituent of lecithin; it is thus difficult to consume a diet that is low in choline. Since human breast milk contains 7 mg choline/100 kcal, the Committee on Nutrition of the American Academy of Pediatrics (1976) recommends the fortification of infant formulas to this level.

Food Sources. Choline is found in egg yolk and in vegetable and animal fat, mostly as lecithin.

Absorption, Fate, and Excretion. Choline is absorbed from the diet as such or as lecithin. The latter is hydrolyzed by the intestinal mucosa to glycerophosphoryl choline, which either passes to the liver to liberate choline or to the peripheral tissues via the intestinal lymphatics. Free choline is not fully absorbed, especially after large doses, and intestinal bacteria metabolize choline to trimethylamine. Since this compound imparts a strong odor of decaying fish to the feces, lecithin is the clearly preferred oral vehicle for the administration of choline.

Preparations. Various preparations of *choline* are available in tablets containing 250 to 650 mg and as powders; it is also contained in some multivitamin preparations. In addition, preparations of lecithin are available, although many of them consist mainly of other phosphatides (Wurtman, 1979).

Therapeutic Uses. The use of choline to treat fatty liver and cirrhosis, usually alcoholic in etiology, has not proven to be effective (Griffith and Nye, 1971). Because of the synthesis of choline from other methyl donors, provision of a well-balanced diet is just as effective in alleviating the symptoms of hepatic damage.

The use of choline in large doses for the treatment of certain disorders of the nervous system has also been advocated (Growdon and Wurtman, 1979). Five such diseases are candidates for treatment with choline (Barbeau, 1978). They include tardive dyskinesia, a disease characterized by choreiform movements that are caused by chronic treatment with some neuroleptic drugs (*see* Growdon, 1978; *see also* Chapter 18). Some clinical improvement with choline treatment has also been reported in Huntington's chorea (Growdon, 1978), in which impaired mental function and involuntary muscle contractions are probably associated with reduced acetylcholine synthesis; in Gilles de la Tourette's disease; in Friedreich's ataxia; and in Alzheimer's disease (Barbeau, 1978). Doses of 150 to 300 mg/kg of choline chloride and of 350 mg/kg of lecithin have been administered in various studies. However, in none of these diseases has a role for choline as a therapeutic agent been established.

INOSITOL

History. Although inositol was identified more than 100 years ago in the urine of diabetic patients, a role for this substance in animal nutrition was not suspected until 1941, when Gavin and McHenry found that inositol had a lipotropic action in rats. Inositol was subsequently observed to cure alopecia induced in rats and mice by dietary means. A nutritional role for inositol was considerably strengthened when Eagle and colleagues showed in 1957 that this substance is essential for the growth of all human and other animal cells in tissue culture. However, its status as a vitamin for man remains uncertain, for reasons given below.

Chemistry. Inositol (hexahydroxycyclohexane) is an isomer of glucose. There are seven optically inactive and one pair of optically active stereoisomeric forms of inositol possible, of which only one, the optically inactive *myo*-inositol, is nutritionally active. It has the following structural formula:

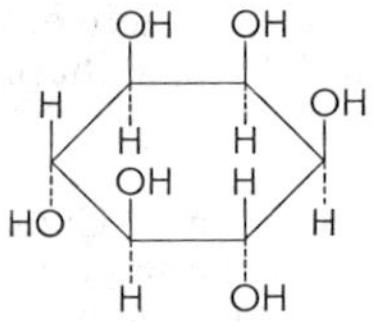

Myo-Inositol

Pharmacological Actions. Inositol possesses no significant pharmacological actions when given parenterally to human subjects in doses of 1 to 2 g.

Physiological Functions. The physiological role of inositol resembles that of choline in part. Thus, inositol is present in the form of phosphatidylinositol in the phospholipids of cell membranes and plasma lipoproteins. Polyphosphorylated derivatives of inositol (*e.g.*, inositol-1,4,5-trisphosphate) are released from such phospholipids in membranes in response to a variety of hormones, autacoids, and neurotransmitters. Inositol trisphosphate functions as an intracellular second messenger by stimulating the release of Ca^{2+} from intracellular stores (*see* Chapter 2; *see also* Berridge, 1984). In addition, inositol has a lipotropic action on fatty livers, and, in some species, will prevent fat accumulation in the intestine (Hegsted *et al.*, 1974). These effects on the transport of fat out of the cells of the liver and intestine appear to be dependent on the requirement for inositol to complete the assembly of fat-carrying lipoproteins in plasma.

Symptoms of Deficiency. Variable reserves of inositol, its production by gut bacteria, and possibly its synthesis in the cells of the body have made the demonstration of a dietary need for inositol difficult to achieve. However, certain animals can be made deficient; alopecia and fatty infiltration of the liver result. There has been no demonstration of a dietary need by man, but the studies of Eagle and colleagues (1957) showed that 18 human cell lines all needed *myo*-inositol for growth, probably because of its structural role in the formation of cell membranes. In view of the absence of a demonstrable human need for inositol, it may be synthesized in only a few organs, which then make it available for use by all cells. Rats can synthesize inositol, although this does not exclude a partial dependence on dietary sources.

Human Requirements. Although a human need for inositol has not been demonstrated, a high concentration is present in human milk (Committee on Nutrition, Academy of Pediatrics, 1976). As with choline, it may be desirable to add inositol to infant formulas to mimic more closely the content of human milk. The normal daily intake of inositol is about 1 g, mostly from plant sources. Inositol is present in cereals as the hexaphosphate, phytic acid. Inositol in this form is partly available for absorption because of hydrolysis in the intestinal mucosa. Inositol also occurs in vegetable and animal foods in other forms.

Food Sources. Inositol is provided by fruits, plants, and whole-grain cereals as phytic acid.

Absorption, Fate, and Excretion. Human consumption of inositol is about 1 g per day. The compound is easily absorbed from the gastrointestinal tract. Inositol is readily metabolized to glucose and is about one third as effective as glucose in alleviating starvation ketosis. The concentration of inositol in normal human plasma is about 5 mg/l (28 μM). Within the tissues, the concentration of inositol is particularly high in heart muscle, brain, and skeletal muscle (1.6, 0.9, and 0.4 g/100 g dry weight, respectively). Urine normally contains only small amounts of inositol, but in diabetic humans and animals the amount is markedly increased, probably because of competition between inositol and glucose for reabsorption by the renal tubule.

Preparations. *Inositol* is available in tablets containing 250 to 650 mg and as a powder; it is also contained in some multivitamin preparations.

Therapeutic Uses. Inositol has been given for the management of diseases associated with disturbances in the transport and metabolism of fat. There is no persuasive evidence that it has therapeutic efficacy. Peripheral nerves from diabetic animals and man contain elevated quantities of free sugars and a decreased level of *myo*-inositol; abnormal incorporation of *myo*-inositol into neural phospholipids has also been demonstrated. The effects of administration of *myo*-inositol on nerve function in human diabetes are unclear. However, improved sensory function has been shown after a few weeks of such treatment (Clements *et al.*, 1979).

CARNITINE

History. Carnitine was identified as a nitrogenous constituent of muscle in 1905. After its identification as a growth factor for meal worm larvae by Frankael and his colleagues, the role of carnitine in the oxidation of long-chain fatty acids in mammals was established in the laboratories of Fritz and Bremer in the late 1950s. The history and metabolic functions of carnitine have been reviewed by Rebouche and Paulson (1986) and by Bieber (1988).

Chemistry. Carnitine (β-hydroxy-γ-trimethylammonium butyrate) has the following structural formula:

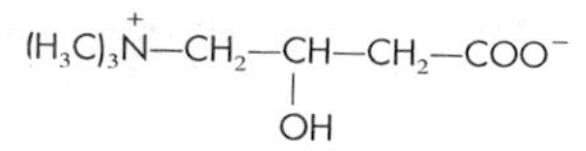

Carnitine

Only L-carnitine is synthesized in tissues and possesses biological activity.

Pharmacological Actions. The administration of L-carnitine to normal individuals is without appreciable effect, and oral doses of up to 15 g per day are usually well tolerated. By contrast, the administration of DL-carnitine can produce a syndrome that resembles myasthenia gravis, presumably because of the inhibitory effects of the D isomer on the transport and function of L-carnitine.

Physiological Functions. In general, carnitine is important for the oxidation of fatty acids; it also facilitates the aerobic metabolism of carbohydrate, enhances the rate of oxidative phosphorylation, and promotes the excretion of certain organic acids (*see* Bahl and Bressler, 1987; Bieber, 1988). These functions result from the following circumstances. (1) There exist a number of carnitine acyltransferases (CATs) that catalyze the interconversion of fatty acid esters of coenzyme A (CoA) and carnitine; these are strategically located in the cytosol and in mitochondrial membranes. (2) The esters of CoA and carnitine are thermodynamically equivalent, such that the net formation of either depends solely on the relative concentrations of reactants. (3) Specific translocases exist in mitochondrial and plasma membranes. The translocase in mitochondrial membranes readily transports both free carnitine and its esters in either direction, while that in the luminal plasma membrane of renal tubular cells transports only free carnitine *from* tubular urine almost exclusively. The properties of translocases in the plasma membranes of other cells are less well defined; nevertheless, free carnitine is actively transported into cells and acylcarnitines (particularly short-chain esters) are transported out of cells. (4) Fatty acid esters of CoA are formed almost exclusively in the cytosol and are not transported across membranes; they also inhibit enzymes of the Krebs cycle and those involved in oxidative phosphorylation. Hence, the oxidation of fatty acids requires the formation of acylcarnitines and their translocation into mitochondria, where the CoA esters are reformed and metabolized. If O_2 tension becomes limiting, carnitine serves to maintain a ratio of free to esterified CoA within mitochondria that is optimal for oxidative phosphorylation and for the consumption of acetyl CoA; in ischemic cardiac or skeletal muscle, this results in reduced formation of lactate and an increased capacity to perform mechanical work.

In the presence of a genetic deficiency of one of the acyl CoA dehydrogenases, carnitine serves to promote the removal of the corresponding organic acid from cells and the blood, since the acylcarnitine can be transported out of mitochondria and into the circulation but cannot be reabsorbed from renal tubules. Such removal of acylcarnitines from cells or blood carries the risk of producing a state of relative carnitine deficiency.

Symptoms of Deficiency. Primary carnitine deficiency is most clearly observed in a group of uncommon inherited disorders. Lipid metabolism is severely affected, resulting in storage of fat in muscle and functional abnormalities of cardiac and skeletal muscle. These conditions have been classified either as systemic or myopathic. Systemic disorders are manifest by low concentrations of carnitine in plasma, muscle, and liver. Symptoms are variable, but include muscle weakness, cardiomyopathy, abnormal hepatic function, impaired ketogenesis, and hypoglycemia during fasting. Myopathic disease is characterized primarily by muscle weakness. Fatty infiltration of muscle fibers is observed at biopsy, and the concentration of carnitine is low; however, plasma concentrations of carnitine are normal (20 to 70 μM). Defective transport of carnitine into muscle cells coupled with faulty renal reabsorption may underlie many cases of primary carnitine deficiency (Treem *et al.*, 1988).

Secondary forms of carnitine deficiency are also recognized. These include renal tubular disorders, in which excretion of carnitine may be excessive, and chronic renal failure, in which hemodialysis may promote excessive losses. Patients with inborn errors of metabolism associated with increased circulating concentrations of organic acids may also become deficient in carnitine. This consequence is not surprising in view of the role of carnitine in promoting the excretion of organic acids. Occasional patients receiving total parenteral alimentation with solutions lacking carnitine may also show biochemical and symptomatic evidence of carnitine deficiency that is reversed by supplementation.

Human Requirements. The need for carnitine is satisfied by dietary sources and by synthesis, primarily in the liver and kidney. Carnitine is synthesized from lysine residues in various proteins, beginning with formation of 6-N-trimethyllysine by a sequence of reactions involving S-adenosylmethionine (*see* Bieber, 1988). Four micronutrients are required for the various enzymatic steps, including ascorbic acid, niacin, pyridoxine, and iron. Although carnitine deficiency can be induced by administration of diets that are restricted to cereal grains and other vegetable sources of protein, formal nutritional requirements have not been established.

Food Sources. The primary sources of dietary carnitine are meat and dairy products. Cereal grains lack carnitine and may also be relatively deficient in lysine and methionine, its amino acid precursors.

Absorption, Fate, and Excretion. Dietary L-carnitine is almost completely absorbed from the intestine, largely by a saturable transport mechanism; hence, fractional absorption declines as the oral dose is increased. Carnitine is transported into most cells by an active mechanism; D-carnitine is also transported and can inhibit the uptake of L-carnitine. There is little metabolism of carnitine, and most of it is excreted in the urine as acylcarnitines; renal tubules usually reabsorb more than 90% of unesterified carnitine.

Preparations. Carnitine was approved by the Food and Drug Administration in 1986 as an orphan drug for treatment of primary carnitine deficiency. *Levocarnitine* (CARNITOR, VITACARN) is available as an enteral liquid (100 mg/ml) and in capsules and tablets. DL-carnitine, sold as "vitamin B_T" at health food stores, can actually produce symptoms of carnitine deficiency because of competitive inhibition of transport by the D-isomer.

Therapeutic Uses. Carnitine is indicated for the treatment of primary systemic and myopathic carnitine deficiency states. It may also be useful in the management of patients with conditions known to produce secondary carnitine deficiency. One to two grams per day in divided doses is adequate for most therapeutic purposes. Intravenous doses range from 40 to 100 mg/kg. For children, oral L-carnitine is given at 100 mg/kg per day (*see* Goa and Brogden, 1987).

Primary Carnitine Deficiency. The mainstay of treatment of systemic carnitine deficiency is a high-carbohydrate, low-fat diet. Carnitine supplementation of patients with both the myopathic and systemic disorders has been tried frequently, but results have been variable. Some patients report dramatic symptomatic and functional benefits following administration of up to 4 g per day, whereas others are not improved. The relationship of biochemical changes to symptomatic relief is not predictable. All patients with primary carnitine deficiency deserve a trial of supplemental oral carnitine.

Renal Disease. Patients receiving chronic hemodialysis can develop skeletal and possibly myocardial muscle carnitine deficiency. Treatment with oral L-carnitine may minimize the degree of deficiency and has been reported to improve symptoms such as muscle weakness and cramps (Bellinghieri *et al.*, 1983). Carnitine may also improve cardiac function in hemodialysis patients, but this use is more controversial (Fagher *et al.*, 1985).

Cardiomyopathies and Ischemic Cardiovascular Disease. The majority of myocardial energy needs are satisfied by fatty acid oxidation. In light of the critical role played by carnitine in normal cardiac energy metabolism and the development of cardiomyopathy in established carnitine deficiency states, the possibility that some individuals with primary cardiomyopathy may suffer carnitine deficiency has provoked great interest. Moreover, myocardial ischemia causes depletion of cardiac carnitine and accumulation of long-chain fatty acid esters of CoA and carnitine (*see* Corr *et al.*, 1987; DiPalma, 1988); the acylcarnitines may be important in the genesis of arrhythmias. The administration of carnitine appears to improve the exercise tolerance of patients with coronary artery disease (*see* DiPalma, 1988) and may benefit patients with congestive heart failure (Ghidini *et al.*, 1988). Ischemia in skeletal muscle causes similar disturbances in lipid and carnitine metabolism, and the administration of carnitine can increase the walking tolerance of patients who suffer from intermittent claudication (Brevetti *et al.*, 1988). Although these results are provocative, the therapeutic role of carnitine in these conditions remains to be established.

II. Ascorbic Acid (Vitamin C)

History. Scurvy, the deficiency disease caused by lack of vitamin C, has been known since the time of the Crusades, especially among Northern European populations who subsisted on diets lacking fresh fruits and vegetables over extensive periods of the year. The incidence of scurvy was reduced by the introduction of the potato (a source of vitamin C) to Europe in the seventeenth century. However, the long sea voyages of exploration in the sixteenth to eighteenth centuries, which were undertaken without a supply of fresh fruits and vegetables, resulted in large numbers of the crews dying from scurvy.

A dietary cause for scurvy had long been suspected. In 1535, Jacques Cartier learned from the Indians of Canada how to cure the scurvy in his crew by making a decoction from spruce leaves, and several subsequent ship captains prevented or cured scurvy by administration of lemon juice. However, a systematic study of the relationship of diet to scurvy had to wait until 1747 when Lind, a physician in the British Royal Navy, carried out a clinical trial on cases of frank scurvy who were given either cider, vitriol, vinegar, sea water, oranges and lemons, or garlic and mustard. Those who received citrus fruits recovered rapidly. The consequent introduction of lemon juice into the British Navy in 1800 resulted in a dramatic reduction in the incidence of scurvy; whereas the Royal Naval Hospital at Portsmouth admitted 1457 cases in 1780, only 2 cases were seen there in 1806.

The next significant episode in the history of vitamin C was the identification in 1907 of a suitable experimental animal by Holst and Fröhlich, who found that guinea pigs develop scurvy on a diet of oats and bran that is not supplemented with fresh vegetables. It was subsequently shown that most mammals synthesize ascorbic acid; man, nonhuman primates, the guinea pig, and Indian fruit bats are exceptions. The demonstration of scurvy in the guinea pig allowed testing of fractions from citrus fruits for antiscorbutic potency. In 1928, Szent-Györgyi isolated a reducing agent in pure form from cabbage and from adrenal glands; in 1932, Waugh and King identified Szent-Györgyi's compound as the active antiscorbutic factor in lemon juice. The chemical structure of this substance was then soon established in several laboratories, and the trivial chemical name *ascorbic acid* was assigned to designate its function in preventing scurvy. The term *vitamin C* should be used as a generic descriptor for all compounds that exhibit qualitatively the biological activity of ascorbic acid.

Chemistry. Ascorbic acid is a six-carbon ketolactone structurally related to glucose and other hexoses. It is reversibly oxidized in the body to dehydroascorbic acid. The latter compound possesses full vitamin C activity. The structural formulas of ascorbic acid and dehydroascorbic acid are as follows:

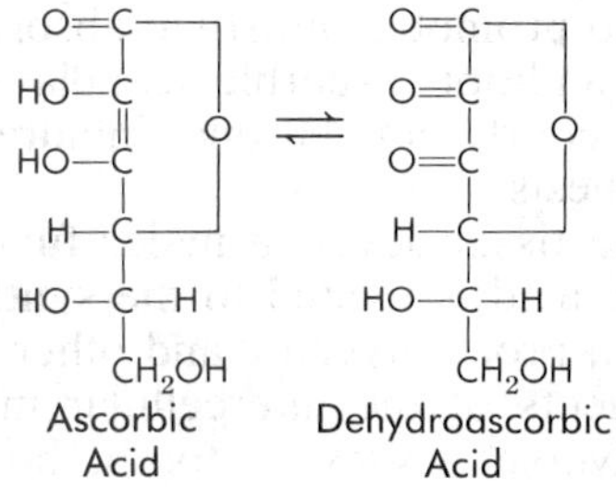

Ascorbic acid has an optically active carbon atom, and antiscorbutic activity resides almost totally in the L isomer. Another isomer, erythorbic acid (D-isoascorbic acid, D-araboascorbic acid), has very weak antiscorbutic action but has a similar redox potential. Both compounds have therefore been used to prevent nitrosoamine formation from nitrites in cured meats such as bacon. The reason for the lack of a stronger antiscorbutic action of erythorbic acid is probably the incapacity of the tissues to retain it in the quantities that ascorbic acid is stored (Hughes *et al.*, 1971). One consequence of the facile oxidation of ascorbic acid is the readiness with which it can be destroyed by exposure to air, especially in an alkaline medium and if copper is present as a catalyst.

Pharmacological Actions. Vitamin C possesses few pharmacological actions. Administration of the compound in amounts greatly in excess of the physiological requirements causes few demonstrable effects except in the scorbutic individual, whose symptoms are rapidly alleviated.

Physiological Functions. Ascorbic acid functions as a cofactor in a number of hydroxylation and amidation reactions by transferring electrons to enzymes that provide reducing equivalents (*see* Levine, 1986). Thus, it is required for or facilitates the conversion of certain proline and lysine residues in procollagen to hydroxyproline and hydroxylysine in the course of collagen synthesis, the oxidation of lysine side chains in proteins to provide hydroxytrimethyllysine for carnitine synthesis, the conversion of folic acid to folinic acid, microsomal drug metabolism, and the hydroxylation of dopamine to form norepinephrine. Ascorbic acid promotes the activity of an amidating enzyme thought to be involved in the processing of certain peptide hormones, such as oxytocin, antidiuretic hormone, and cholecystokinin (*see* Levine, 1986). By reducing nonheme ferric iron to the ferrous state in the stomach, ascorbic acid also promotes intestinal absorption of iron. In addition, ascorbic acid plays a role, albeit a poorly defined one, in adrenal steroidogenesis.

At the tissue level, a major function of ascorbic acid is related to the synthesis of collagen, proteoglycans, and other organic constituents of the intercellular matrix in such diverse tissues as tooth, bone, and capillary endothelium (Sebrell and Harris, 1967). Although the effect of ascorbic acid on collagen synthesis has been attributed to its role in the hydroxylation of proline, recent evidence also suggests that there is direct stimulation of collagen peptide synthesis (Murad *et al.,* 1981). Scurvy is associated with a defect in collagen synthesis that is apparent by the failure of wounds to heal, in defects in tooth formation, and in the rupture of capillaries, which leads to numerous petechiae and their coalescence to form ecchymoses. While this last has been attributed to leakage from capillaries because of inadequate adhesion of the endothelial cells, it is also thought that the pericapillary fibrous tissue is defective in scurvy, leading to inadequate support of the capillary and its rupture under pressure.

Absorption, Fate, and Excretion. Ascorbic acid is readily absorbed from the intestine, and absorption of dietary ascorbate is nearly complete (Kallner *et al.,* 1977). When vitamin C is given in a single oral dose, absorption decreases from 75% at 1 gram to 20% at 5 grams. Ascorbic acid is present in the plasma and is ubiquitously distributed in the cells of the body. Concentrations of the vitamin in leukocytes are sometimes taken to represent those in tissue and are less susceptible to depletion than is the plasma. The white blood cells of healthy adults have concentrations of about 27 μg of ascorbic acid per 10^8 cells. It should be noted that the amount of ascorbic acid in leukocytes may be inversely related to their number, and estimates of ascorbic acid status may be falsely low in patients with leukocytosis in whom white-cell ascorbate is measured (Vallance, 1979). Concentrations in plasma also vary with intake. Adequate ingestion is associated with concentrations over 0.5 mg/dl (28 μM), whereas concentrations of 0.15 mg/dl (8.5 μM) are seen in individuals with frank scurvy.

When the diet contains essentially no ascorbate, concentrations in plasma fall and, as mentioned, symptoms of scurvy are obvious when a value of 0.15 mg/dl (8.5 μM) is reached; the total body store of the vitamin at this time approximates 300 mg. When the intake of ascorbate is raised, the concentration in plasma also increases—at first linearly. The daily ingestion of 5 to 10 mg provides a total body store of 600 to 1000 mg of ascorbate. When 60 mg of vitamin C is consumed per day (the current adult RDA), the concentration in plasma reaches about 0.8 mg/dl (45 μM) and the body store is around 1500 mg. If intake is raised beyond 200 mg daily, the body store tends to level off at 2500 mg and the concentration in plasma at 2 mg/dl (110 μM). The renal threshold for ascorbic acid is about 1.5 mg/dl of plasma (85 μM), and increasing amounts of ingested ascorbic acid are excreted when the daily intake exceeds 100 mg.

Ascorbate is oxidized to CO_2 in rats and guinea pigs, but considerably less conversion can be detected in man. One route of metabolism of the vitamin in man involves its conversion to oxalate and eventual excretion in the urine; dehydroascorbate is presumably an intermediate. Ascorbic acid–2–sulfate has also been identified as a metabolite of vitamin C in human urine.

Biosynthesis of Ascorbic Acid. Man and other primates as well as the guinea pig and some bats are the only mammals known to be unable to synthesize ascorbic acid; consequently, they require dietary vitamin C for the prevention of scurvy. Typical of animals that do not require dietary vitamin C, the rat synthesizes ascorbic acid from glucose through the intermediate formation of D-glucuronic acid, L-gulonic acid, and L-gulonolactone. Man, monkey, and guinea pig lack the hepatic enzyme required to carry out the last reaction, that is, the conversion of L-gulonolactone to L-ascorbic acid.

Symptoms of Deficiency. A deficiency in the intake of vitamin C can lead to scurvy. Cases of scurvy are encountered among elderly people living alone, alcoholics, drug addicts, and others with inadequate diets, including infants.

Experimental scurvy has been produced in man in a number of studies (Crandon *et al.*, 1940; Krebs *et al.*, 1948; Hodges *et al.*, 1969). For example, the surgeon Crandon submitted himself to a diet devoid of vitamin C for 161 days; the concentration of ascorbic acid in his plasma fell to negligible values within 41 days, and the concentration in his white blood cells became undetectable after 121 days. Perifollicular hyperkeratosis (an accumulation of epidermal cells around the hair follicles) occurred at 120 days; hemorrhages appeared under his skin (petechiae and ecchymoses) at 161 days, and a wound made into the back failed to heal. In spontaneous cases of scurvy, there is usually loosening of the teeth, gingivitis, and anemia, which may be due to a specific function of ascorbic acid in hemoglobin synthesis. The picture of spontaneous scurvy in clinical practice is often complicated by insufficiencies of other nutrients as well.

Scurvy may occur in infants receiving formula diets prepared at home with inadequate concentrations of ascorbic acid. The infant is irritable and resents being touched because of pain. The pain is caused by hemorrhages under the periosteum of the long bones, and the resulting hematomas are often visible as swellings on the shafts of these bones.

Human Requirements. The daily intake of ascorbic acid must equal the amount that is excreted or destroyed by oxidation. Healthy adult human subjects lose 3 to 4% of their body store daily. To maintain a body store of 1500 mg of ascorbic acid or more in an adult man, it would thus be necessary to absorb approximately 60 mg daily. Values for vitamin C requirements of other age groups are based on similar reasoning (*see* Table XVI–1, page 1525).

Under special circumstances, more ascorbic acid appears to be required to achieve normal concentrations in the plasma. Thus, South African miners have been observed to require 200 to 250 mg of vitamin C daily to maintain a plasma concentration of 0.75 mg/dl (43 μM) (Visagie *et al.*, 1975). Concentrations of ascorbate in plasma are lowered by the use of cigarettes and of oral contraceptive agents, but the significance of these changes is unclear. Requirements can increase in certain diseases, particularly infectious diseases, and also following surgery (Irvin *et al.*, 1978).

Food Sources. Ascorbic acid is obtained from citrus fruits, tomatoes, strawberries, cabbage greens, and potatoes. Orange and lemon juices are outstanding sources and contain approximately 0.5 mg/ml (2.8 mM). Ascorbic acid is readily destroyed by heat, oxidation, and alkali.

Preparations. *Ascorbic acid* is available in a large number of preparations. Tablets contain from 50 to 1500 mg of the vitamin. Solutions for oral use are also available in various concentrations. *Calcium ascorbate* and *sodium ascorbate* are available as tablets or powders. *Ascorbic acid injection* contains from 100 to 500 mg/ml. *Sodium ascorbate injection* is also available and contains the equivalent of 222 or 500 mg/ml of ascorbic acid. Most multivitamin preparations contain ascorbic acid. The high vitamin content of fruit juices permits their use in therapy in place of pure preparations of the vitamin.

Apart from its role in nutrition, ascorbic acid is commonly used as an antioxidant to protect the natural flavor and color of many foods (*e.g.*, processed fruit, vegetables, and dairy products).

Routes of Administration. Vitamin C is usually administered orally; however, in conditions that prevent adequate absorption from the gastrointestinal tract, parenteral solutions may be given. In addition, ascorbic acid should be given to patients receiving parenteral hyperalimentation. Because of the loss of much of the infused ascorbic acid in the urine, daily doses of 200 mg are needed to maintain normal concentrations in plasma of about 1 mg/dl (60 μM) (Nichoalds *et al.*, 1977).

Therapeutic Uses. Vitamin C is used for the treatment of ascorbic acid deficiency, especially frank scurvy, which occurs rather infrequently in infants and in adults.

Human breast milk contains 30 to 55 mg of ascorbic acid per liter (about 200 μM), depending on the mother's intake. Consequently, the infant consuming 850 ml of breast milk will receive about 35 mg of ascorbic acid, which has been set as the recommended dietary allowance (*see* Table XVI–1, page 1525). Commercial formulas are usually fortified with ascorbic acid. Infants receiving formula based on cow's milk may be given orange juice to meet vitamin C requirements. In the rare cases of infantile scurvy, much larger therapeutic doses are used. Adults with scurvy should receive up to 1 g of ascorbic acid daily. This dose will cause a rapid disappearance of the subcutaneous hemorrhages.

The reducing properties of vitamin C have also been employed to control *idiopathic methemoglobinemia*, although it is less effective than methylene blue. Doses of at least 150 mg of ascorbic acid are needed to be effective in this condition.

In addition to these specific uses of vitamin C, extensive literature has appeared on the application of this vitamin to a wide variety of diseases. Many such claims are associated with megadosage practices, which are stated to prevent or cure viral respiratory infections (Pauling, 1970) and to be beneficial in cancer (Cameron and Pauling, 1978) and other diseases. However, beneficial effects were not observed when high doses of ascorbic acid were given to patients with advanced cancer (Creagan *et al.*, 1979; Moertel *et al.*, 1985). Anderson (1977) carried out a series of three carefully designed studies in Canada to test whether vitamin C plays any role in the prevention and treatment of the common cold. No obvious effect on the incidence of headcolds was seen from the administration of ascorbic acid, although there was a slight reduction in the number of days of missed work. Many other studies have yielded negative or inconsistent results (*see* Pitt and Costrini, 1979). Any benefit that might be derived from such use of ascorbic acid seems small when weighed against the expense and the risks of the megadosage treatment. The latter include formation of kidney stones resulting from the excessive excretion of oxalate, rebound scurvy in the offspring of mothers taking high doses (Herbert, 1975), and a similar phenomenon when subjects who are consuming large amounts of vitamin C suddenly stop. These rebound phenomena are presumably due to induction of pathways of ascorbic acid metabolism as a result of the preceding high dosage.

Adams, P. W.; Wynn, V.; Rose, D. P.; Seed, M.; Folkard, J.; and Strong, R. Effect of pyridoxine hydrochloride (vitamin B_6) upon depression with oral contraception. *Lancet,* **1973,** *1,* 897–904.

Anderson, T. W. Large scale studies with vitamin C. *Acta Vitaminol. Enzymol. (Milano),* **1977,** *31,* 43–50.

Barbeau, A. Emerging treatments: replacement therapy with choline or lecithin in neurological diseases. *Can. J. Neurol. Sci.,* **1978,** *5,* 157–160.

Barnard, H. C.; de Kock, J. J.; Vermaak, W. J. H.; and Potgieter, G. M. A new perspective in the assessment of vitamin B_6 nutritional status in humans. *J. Nutr.,* **1987,** *117,* 1303–1306.

Bauernfeind, J. C., and Miller, O. N. Vitamin B_6: nutritional and pharmaceutical usage, stability, bioavailability, antagonists, and safety. In, *Human Vitamin B_6 Requirements.* National Academy of Sciences, Washington, D. C., **1978,** pp. 78–110.

Baumgartner, E. R.; Suormala, T.; Wick, H.; and Bonjour, J. P. Biotin-responsive multiple carboxylase deficiency: deficient biotinidase activity. *J. Inherited Metab. Dis.,* **1984,** *7,* Suppl. 2, 123–125.

Belko, A. Z.; Obarzanek, E.; Kalkwarf, H. J.; Rotter, M. A.; Bogusz, B. S.; Miller, D.; Haas, J. D.; and Roe, D. A. Effects of exercise on riboflavin requirements of young women. *Am. J. Clin. Nutr.,* **1983,** *37,* 509–517.

Bellinghieri, L. G.; Savica, V.; Mallamace, A.; Di Stefano, C.; Consolo, F.; Spagnoli, L. G.; Villaschi, S.; Palmieri, G.; Corsi, M.; and Maccari, F. Correlation between increased serum and tissue L-carnitine levels and improved muscle symptoms in hemodialyzed patients. *Am. J. Clin. Nutr.,* **1983,** *38,* 523–531.

Berridge, M. J. Inositol triphosphate and diacylglycerol as second messengers. *Biochem. J.,* **1984,** *220,* 345–360.

Bonjour, J. P. Biotin in man's nutrition and therapy—a review. *Int. J. Vitam. Nutr. Res.,* **1977,** *47,* 107–118.

Bossé, T. R., and Donald, E. A. The vitamin B_6 requirement in oral contraceptive users. I. Assessment by pyridoxal level and transferase activity in erythrocytes. *Am. J. Clin. Nutr.,* **1979,** *32,* 1015–1023.

Brevetti, G.; Chiarello, M.; Ferulano, G.; Policicchio, A.; Nevola, E.; Rossini, A.; Attisano, T.; Ambrosio, G.; Siliprandi, N.; and Angelini, C. Increases in walking distance in patients with peripheral vascular disease treated with L-carnitine: a double-blind, cross-over study. *Circulation,* **1988,** *77,* 767–773.

Brin, M. Blood transketolase determination in the diagnosis of thiamine deficiency. *Heart Bull.,* **1968,** *17,* 86–89.

Cameron, E., and Pauling, L. Supplemental ascorbate in the supportive treatment of cancer: prolongation of survival times in terminal human cancer. *Proc. Natl. Acad. Sci. U. S. A.,* **1978,** *73,* 3685–3689.

Canham, J. E.; Nunes, W. T.; and Eberlin, E. W. Electroencephalographic and central nervous system manifestations of B_6 deficiency and induced B_6 dependency in normal human adults. In, *Proceedings of the Sixth International Congress of Nutrition.* E. & S. Livingstone, Ltd., Edinburgh, **1964,** p. 537.

Clements, R. S.; Vourganti, B.; Kuba, T.; Oh, S. J.; and Darnell, B. Dietary myoinositol intake and peripheral nerve function in diabetic neuropathy. *Metabolism,* **1979,** *28,* Suppl. 1, 477–483.

Committee on Nutrition, Academy of Pediatrics. Commentary on breast-feeding and infant formulas, including proposed standards for formulas. *Pediatrics,* **1976,** *57,* 278–285.

Crandon, J. H.; Lund, C. C.; and Dill, D. B. Experimental human scurvy. *N. Engl. J. Med.,* **1940,** *223,* 353–369.

Creagan, E. T.; Moertel, C. C.; O'Fallon, J. R.; Schutt, A. J.; O'Connell, M. J.; Rubin, J.; and Frytak, S. Failure of high-dose vitamin C to benefit patients with advanced cancer. *N. Engl. J. Med.,* **1979,** *301,* 687–690.

Dakshinamurti, K. B vitamins and nervous system function. In, *Nutrition and the Brain,* Vol. 1. (Wurtman, R. J., and Wurtman, J. J., eds.) Raven Press, New York, **1977,** pp. 249–318.

DiSorbo, D. M.; Phelps, D. S.; Ohl, V. S.; and Litwack, G. Pyridoxine deficiency influences the behavior of the glucocorticoid-receptor complex. *J. Biol. Chem.,* **1980,** *255,* 3866–3870.

Donald, E. A., and Bossé, T. R. The vitamin B_6 requirement in oral contraceptive users. II. Assessment by tryptophan metabolites, vitamin B_6, and pyridoxic acid levels in urine. *Am. J. Clin. Nutr.,* **1979,** *32,* 1024–1032.

Eagle, H.; Oyama, V.; Levy, M.; and Freeman, A. Myoinositol as an essential growth factor for normal and malignant human cells in tissue culture. *J. Biol. Chem.,* **1957,** *229,* 191–205.

Fagher, B.; Cederblad, G.; Monti, M.; Olsson, L.; Rasmussen, B.; and Thyseli, H. Carnitine and left ventricular function in haemodialysis patients. *Scand. J. Lab. Invest.,* **1985,** *45,* 193–198.

Fry, P. C.; Fox, H. M.; and Tao, H. G. Metabolic response to a pantothenic acid deficient diet in humans. *J. Nutr. Sci. Vitaminol. (Tokyo),* **1976,** *22,* 339–346.

Ghidini, O.; Azzurro, M.; Vita, G.; and Sartori, G. Evaluation of the therapeutic efficacy of L-carnitine in congestive heart failure. *Int. J. Clin. Pharmacol. Ther. Toxicol.,* **1988,** *26,* 217–220.

Gillis, J.; Murphy, F. R.; Boxall, L. B. H.; and Pencharg, P. B. Biotin deficiency in a child on long-term TPN. *J. P. E. N.,* **1982,** *6,* 308–310.

Goldsmith, G. A. Niacin-tryptophan relationship in man and niacin requirement. *Am. J. Clin. Nutr.,* **1958,** *6,* 479–486.

Growdon, J. H. Effects of choline on tardive dyskinesia and other movement disorders. *Psychopharmacol. Bull.,* **1978,** *14,* 55–56.

Growdon, J. H., and Wurtman, R. J. Dietary influences on the synthesis of neurotransmitters in the brain. *Nutr. Rev.,* **1979,** *37,* 129–136.

György, P. A further note on the identity of vitamin H with biotin. *Science,* **1940,** *92,* 609.

Hegsted, D. M.; Gallagher, A.; and Hanford, H. Inositol requirement of the gerbil. *J. Nutr.,* **1974,** *104,* 588–592.

Henderson, L. M., and Hulse, J. D. Vitamin B_6: relationship in tryptophan metabolism. In, *Human Vitamin B_6 Requirements.* National Academy of Sciences, Washington, D. C., **1978,** pp. 21–36.

Herbert, V. The rationale of massive-dose vitamin therapy. In, *Proceedings, Western Hemisphere Nutrition Congress IV.* Publishing Sciences Group, Inc., Acton, Mass., **1975,** pp. 84–91.

Hodges, R. E.; Baker, E. M.; Hood, J.; Sauberlich, H. E.; and March, S. C. Experimental scurvy in man. *Am. J. Clin. Nutr.*, **1969**, *22*, 535–548.

Hodges, R. E.; Bean, W. B.; Ohlson, M. A.; and Bleiler, R. Human pantothenic acid deficiency produced by omega-methyl pantothenic acid. *J. Clin. Invest.*, **1959**, *38*, 1421–1425.

Hughes, R. E.; Hurley, R. J.; and Jones, P. R. The retention of ascorbic acid by guinea-pig tissues. *Br. J. Nutr.*, **1971**, *26*, 433–438.

Irvin, T. T.; Chattopadhyay, D. K.; and Smythe, A. Ascorbic acid requirements in postoperative patients. *Surg. Gynecol. Obstet.*, **1978**, *147*, 49–55.

Jusko, W. J., and Levy, G. Absorption, protein binding, and elimination of riboflavin. In, *Riboflavin*. (Rivlin, R. S., ed.) Plenum Press, New York, **1975**, pp. 99–152.

Kallner, A.; Hartman, D.; and Hornig, D. On the absorption of ascorbic acid in man. *Int. J. Vitam. Nutr. Res.*, **1977**, *47*, 383–388.

Krebs, H. A.; Peters, R. A.; Coward, K. H.; Mapson, L. W.; Parsons, L. G.; Platt, B. S.; Spence, J. C.; and O'Brien, J. R. P. Vitamin-C requirement of human adults: experimental study of vitamin-C deprivation in man. *Lancet*, **1948**, *1*, 853–858.

Li, T. Factors influencing vitamin B_6 requirement in alcoholism. In, *Human Vitamin B_6 Requirements*. National Academy of Sciences, Washington, D. C., **1978**, pp. 210–225.

Linkswiler, H. M. Vitamin B_6 requirements of men. In, *Human Vitamin B_6 Requirements*. National Academy of Sciences, Washington, D. C., **1978**, pp. 279–290.

McCormick, D. B. Metabolism of riboflavin. In, *Riboflavin*. (Rivlin, R. S., ed.) Plenum Press, New York, **1975**, pp. 153–198.

McLaren, D. Metabolic disorders. In, *Current Therapy*. (Conn, H. F., ed.) W. B. Saunders Co., Philadelphia, **1978**, pp. 409–410.

Miller, D. R., and Hayes, K. C. Vitamin excess and toxicity. In, *Nutritional Toxicology*, Vol. 1. Academic Press, Inc., New York, **1982**, pp. 81–133.

Moertel, C. G.; Fleming, T. R.; Creagen, E. T.; Rubin, J.; O'Connell, M. J.; and Ames, M. M. High-dose vitamin C versus placebo in the treatment of patients with advanced cancer who have had no prior chemotherapy. *N. Engl. J. Med.*, **1985**, *312*, 137–141.

Müller, R. E.; Traish, A.; and Wotiz, H. J. Effects of pyridoxal 5′-phosphate on uterine estrogen receptor. *J. Biol. Chem.*, **1980**, *255*, 4062–4067.

Murad, S.; Grove, D.; Lindberg, K. A.; Reynolds, G.; Sivarajah, A.; and Pinnell, S. R. Regulation of collagen synthesis by ascorbic acid. *Proc. Natl Acad. Sci. U. S. A.*, **1981**, *78*, 2879–2882.

Murata, K. Thiaminase. In, *Review of Japanese Literature on Beriberi and Thiamine*. (Shimazono, N., and Katsura, E., eds.) Igaku Shoin, Ltd., Tokyo, **1965**, pp. 220–254.

Newberne, P. M., and Chandra, R. K. *Nutrition, Immunity and Infection: Mechanisms of Interactions*. Plenum Press, New York, **1977**.

Nichoalds, G. E.; Meng, H. C.; and Caldwell, M. D. Vitamin requirements in patients receiving total parenteral nutrition. *Arch. Surg.*, **1977**, *112*, 1061–1064.

Parry, G. J., and Bredesen, D. E. Sensory neuropathy with low-dose pyridoxine. *Neurology*, **1985**, *35*, 1466–1468.

Pauling, L. Evolution and the need for ascorbic acid. *Proc. Natl Acad. Sci. U. S. A.*, **1970**, *67*, 1643–1648.

Pincus, J. H.; Cooper, J. R.; Murphy, J. V.; Rabe, E. F.; Lonsdale, D.; and Dunn, H. G. Thiamine derivatives in subacute necrotizing encephalomyelopathy: a preliminary report. *Pediatrics*, **1973**, *51*, 716–721.

Pincus, H. J.; Cooper, J. R.; Piros, K.; and Turner, V. Specificity of the urine inhibitor test for Leigh's disease. *Neurology (Minneap.)*, **1974**, *24*, 885–890.

Pincus, H. J.; Itokawa, Y.; and Cooper, J. R. Enzyme inhibiting factors in subacute necrotizing encephalomyelopathy. *Neurology (Minneap.)*, **1969**, *19*, 841–845.

Pitt, H. A., and Costrini, A. M. Vitamin C prophylaxis in marine recruits. *J. A. M. A.*, **1979**, *241*, 908–911.

Prentice, A. M., and Bates, C. J. A biochemical evaluation of the erythrocyte glutathione reductase test for riboflavin status. *Br. J. Nutr.*, **1981**, *45*, 37–52.

Rindi, G., and Ventura, U. Thiamine intestinal transport. *Physiol. Rev.*, **1972**, *52*, 821–827.

Rivlin, R. S. Hormones, drugs and riboflavin. *Nutr. Rev.*, **1979**, *37*, 241–246.

Rose, D. P. Oral contraceptives and vitamin B_6. In, *Human Vitamin B_6 Requirements*. National Academy of Sciences, Washington, D. C., **1978**, pp. 193–201.

Schaumberg, J.; Kaplan, J.; Windebank, A.; Vick, N.; Rasmus, S.; Pleasure, D.; and Brown, M. J. Sensory neuropathy from pyridoxine abuse. A new megavitamin syndrome. *N. Engl. J. Med.*, **1983**, *309*, 445–448.

Schoffeniels, E. Thiamine phosphorylated derivatives and bioelectrogenesis. *Arch. Int. Physiol. Biochim.*, **1983**, *91*, 233–243.

Sebrell, W. H., and Harris, R. S. (eds.). *The Vitamins: Chemistry, Physiology, Pathology, Methods*, Vol. I. Academic Press, Inc., New York, **1967**.

Smith, G. P.; Rudge, P. J.; and Peters, T. J. Biochemical studies of pyridoxal and pyridoxal phosphate status and therapeutic trial of pyridoxine in patients with carpal tunnel syndrome. *Ann. Neurol.*, **1984**, *15*, 104–107.

Spivak, J. L., and Jackson, D. L. Pellagra: an analysis of 18 patients and a review of the literature. *Johns Hopkins Med. J.*, **1977**, *140*, 295–309.

Sturman, J. A. Vitamin B_6 and the metabolism of sulfur amino acids. In, *Human Vitamin B_6 Requirements*. National Academy of Sciences, Washington, D. C., **1978**, pp. 37–60.

Treem, W. R.; Stanley, C. A.; Finegold, D. N.; Hale, D. E.; and Coates, P. M. Primary carnitine deficiency due to a failure of carnitine transport in kidney, muscle, and fibroblasts. *N. Engl. J. Med.*, **1988**, *319*, 1331–1336.

Vallance, S. Leucocyte ascorbic acid and the leucocyte count. *Br. J. Nutr.*, **1979**, *41*, 409–411.

Victor, M.; Adams, R. D.; and Collins, G. H. *The Wernicke-Korsakoff Syndrome*. F. A. Davis Co., Philadelphia, **1971**, pp. 1–206.

Vimokesant, S. L.; Nakornchi, S.; Dhanamitta, S.; and Hilker, D. M. Effect of tea consumption on thiamine status in man. *Nutr. Rep. Int.*, **1974**, *9*, 371–374.

Visagie, M. E.; DuPlessis, J. P.; and Laubsher, N. Effect of vitamin C supplementation on black mine-workers. *S. Afr. Med. J.*, **1975**, *49*, 889–892.

Waldenlind, L. Studies on thiamine and neuromuscular transmission. *Acta Physiol. Scand.*, **1978**, Suppl., *459*, 1–35.

Wurtman, J. J. Sources of choline and lecithin in the diet. In, *Nutrition and the Brain*, Vol. 5. (Barbeau, A.; Growdon, J. H.; and Wurtman, R. J.; eds.) Raven Press, New York, **1979**, pp. 73–81.

Monographs and Reviews

Bahl, J. J., and Bressler, R. The pharmacology of carnitine. *Annu. Rev. Pharmacol. Toxicol.*, **1987**, *27*, 257–277.

Bieber, L. L. Carnitine. *Annu. Rev. Biochem.*, **1988**, *57*, 261–283.

Brin, M. Vitamin B_6: chemistry, absorption, metabolism, catabolism and toxicity. In, *Human Vitamin B_6 Requirements*. National Academy of Sciences, Washington, D. C., **1978**, pp. 1–20.

Compton, M. M., and Cidlowski, J. A. Vitamin B-6 and glucocorticoid actions. *Endocr. Rev.*, **1986**, *7*, 140–148.

Corr, P. B.; Saffitx, J. E.; and Sobel, B. E. Lysophospholipids, long chain acylcarnitines and membrane dys-

function in the ischaemic heart. *Basic Res. Cardiol.*, **1987**, *82*, Suppl. 1, 199–208.
Dakshinamurti, K., and Chauhan, J. Regulation of biotin enzymes. *Annu. Rev. Nutr.*, **1988**, *8*, 211–233.
DiPalma, J. R. Carnitine deficiency. *Am. Fam. Physician*, **1988**, *38*, 243–251.
Food and Nutrition Board, National Research Council. *Recommended Dietary Allowances*, 10th ed. National Academy of Sciences, Washington, D. C., **1989.**
Fowler, B. Recent advances in the mechanism of pyridoxine-responsive disorders. *J. Inherited Metab. Dis.*, **1985**, *8*, Suppl. 1, 76–83.
Gilman, A. G. G proteins: transducers of receptor-generated signals. *Annu. Rev. Biochem.*, **1987**, *56*, 615–649.
Goa, K. L., and Brogden, R. N. L-Carnitine. A preliminary review of its pharmacokinetics, and its therapeutic use in ischaemic cardiac disease and primary and secondary carnitine deficiencies in relationship to its role in fatty acid metabolism. *Drugs*, **1987**, *34*, 1–24.
Griffith, W. H., and Nye, J. F. Choline. In, *The Vitamins*, 2nd ed., Vol. III. (Sebrell, W. H., and Harris, R. S., eds.) Academic Press, Inc., New York, **1971**, pp. 3–154.
Haas, R. H. Thiamin and the brain. *Annu. Rev. Nutr.*, **1988**, *8*, 483–515.
Kuksis, A., and Mookerjea, S. Choline. *Nutr. Rev.*, **1978**, *36*, 201–207.
Lane, M.; Smith, F. E.; and Alfrey, C. P. Experimental dietary and antagonist-induced human riboflavin deficiency. In, *Riboflavin*. (Rivlin, R. S., ed.) Plenum Press, New York, **1975**, pp. 245–277.
Leklem, J. E. Vitamin B_6 metabolism and function in humans. In, *Clinical and Physiological Applications of Vitamin* B_6. (Leklem, J. E., and Reynolds, R. D., eds.) Alan R. Liss, Inc., New York, **1988**, pp. 3–28.
Levine, M. New concepts in the biology and biochemistry of ascorbic acid. *N. Engl. J. Med.*, **1986**, *314*, 892–899.
McCormick, D. B., and Olson, R. E. Biotin. In, *Present Knowledge in Nutrition*, 5th ed. (Olson, R. E.; Broquist, H. P.; Chichester, C. O.; Darby, W. J.; Kolbye, A. C.; and Stalvey, R. M.; eds.) The Nutrition Foundation, Inc., Washington, D. C., **1984**, pp. 365–376.
Plesofsky-Vig, N., and Brambl, R. Pantothenic acid and coenzyme A in cellular modification of proteins. *Annu. Rev. Nutr.*, **1988**, *8*, 461–482.
Rebouche, C. J., and Paulson, D. J. Carnitine metabolism and function in humans. *Annu. Rev. Nutr.*, **1986**, *6*, 41–66.
Rivlin, R. S. Riboflavin metabolism. *N. Engl. J. Med.*, **1970**, *283*, 463–472.
Scriver, C. R. Vitamin-responsive inborn errors of metabolism. *Metabolism*, **1973**, *22*, 1319–1344.
Shils, M. E., and Young, V. R. (eds.). *Modern Nutrition in Health and Disease*, 7th ed. Lea & Febiger, Philadelphia, **1988.**

CHAPTER

64 FAT-SOLUBLE VITAMINS

Vitamins A, K, and E

Robert Marcus and Ann M. Coulston

VITAMIN A

Although vitamin A must be supplied from the environment, most of its actions are exerted through hormone-like receptors, a property that it shares with vitamin D. Vitamin A has diverse actions in cellular regulation and differentiation that go far beyond its classically defined function in vision. In addition, because of its prominent effects on epithelia, analogs of vitamin A have found important therapeutic application in the treatment of a variety of dermatological conditions. The pharmacological properties of these vitamin A analogs are included in this chapter, while their therapeutic uses are discussed in Chapter 65.

History. Night blindness was apparently first described in Egypt around 1500 B.C. Although this disease was not then linked to dietary deficiency, topical treatment with roasted or fried liver was wisely recommended, and Hippocrates later suggested eating beef liver as a cure for the affliction. The relationship to nutritional deficiency was definitively recognized in the last century. Ophthalmia Brasiliana, a disease of the eyes that primarily afflicted poorly nourished slaves, was first described in 1865. In 1887, endemic night blindness was reported to occur among the orthodox Russian Catholics who fasted during the Lenten period. More pertinent was the observation that the nurslings of mothers who fasted were prone to develop spontaneous sloughing of the cornea. Many other reports of nutritional keratomalacia soon followed from all parts of the world, including the United States.

Experimental rather than clinical observations, however, led to the discovery of vitamin A. In 1913, two groups (McCollum and Davis; Osborne and Mendel) independently reported that animals fed artificial diets with lard as the sole source of fat developed a nutritional deficiency that could be corrected by the addition to the diet of a factor contained in butter, egg yolk, and cod liver oil. An outstanding symptom of this experimental nutritional deficiency was xerophthalmia (dryness and thickening of the conjunctiva). Clinical and experimental vitamin A deficiencies were recognized to be related during World War I, when it became apparent that xerophthalmia in human beings was a result of a decrease in the content of butterfat in the diet.

Terminology, Occurrence, and Chemistry. Although the term *vitamin A* has been used to denote specific chemical compounds, such as retinol or its esters, it now is used more as a generic descriptor for compounds that exhibit the biological properties of retinol. *Retinoid* refers to the chemical entity retinol or other closely related naturally occurring derivatives. Retinoids also include structurally related synthetic analogs, which need not have retinol-like (vitamin A) activity.

The simple observation of Steenbock (1919) that the vitamin A content of vegetables varies with the degree of pigmentation paved the way for the isolation and discovery of the chemical nature of the vitamin. Subsequently, it was demonstrated that the purified plant pigment carotene (provitamin A) is a remarkably potent source of vitamin A. β-Carotene, the most active carotenoid found in plants, has the structural formula shown below. In the United States, the average adult receives about half the daily intake of vitamin A as retinol or retinyl esters and the rest as carotenoids. Major dietary sources of vitamin A are liver, butter, cheese, whole milk, egg yolk, and fish. β-Carotene is present in various yellow or green fruits and vegetables. These foods also contain numerous carotenoids that cannot be converted to retinol. Nevertheless, many of these can function as antioxidants and may have useful health-promoting effects (*see* Symposium, 1989a).

Retinol (vitamin A_1), a primary alcohol, is present in esterified form in the tissues of animals and

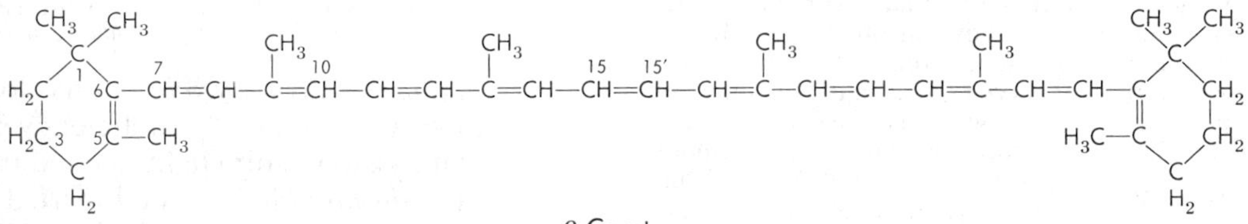

β-Carotene

salt-water fish, mainly in the liver. Its structural formula is as follows:

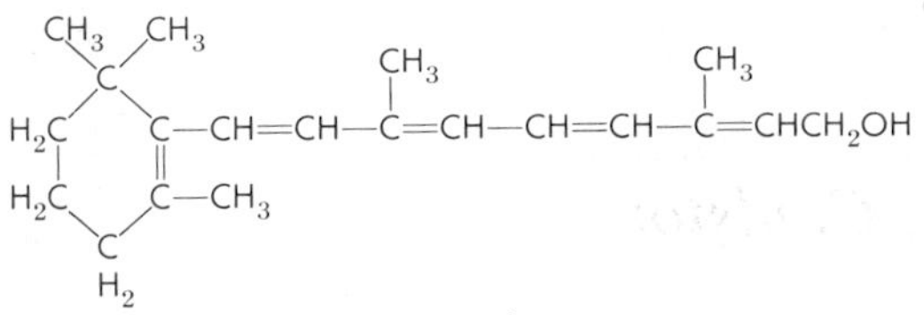

Retinol

A closely related compound, 3-dehydroretinol (vitamin A_2), is obtained from the tissues of fresh-water fish and usually occurs mixed with retinol.

A number of geometric isomers of retinol exist because of the possible *cis-trans* configurations around the double bonds in the side chain. Fish liver oils contain mixtures of the stereoisomers; synthetic retinol is the all-*trans* isomer. Interconversion between isomers readily takes place in the body. In the visual cycle, the reaction between retinal (vitamin A aldehyde) and opsin to form rhodopsin only occurs with the 11-*cis* isomer.

Ethers and esters derived from the alcohol also show activity *in vivo*. The ring structure of retinol (β-ionone), or the more unsaturated ring in 3-dehydroretinol (dehydro-β-ionone), is essential for activity; hydrogenation destroys biological activity. Of all known derivatives, all-*trans*-retinol and its aldehyde, retinal, exhibit the greatest biological potency *in vivo;* 3-dehydroretinol has about 40% the potency of all-*trans*-retinol.

Retinoic acid (vitamin A acid), in which the alcohol group has been oxidized, shares some but not all of the actions of retinol. Although retinoic acid is ineffective in restoring visual or reproductive function in certain species where retinol is effective, it is very potent in promoting growth and controlling differentiation and maintenance of epithelial tissue in vitamin A–deficient animals. Indeed, all-*trans*-retinoic acid (*tretinoin*) appears to be the active form of vitamin A in all tissues except the retina, and is 10- to 100-fold more potent than retinol in various systems *in vitro*. Isomerization of this compound in the body yields 13-*cis*-retinoic acid (*isotretinoin*), which is nearly as potent as tretinoin in many of its actions on epithelial tissues but may be as much as fivefold less potent in producing the toxic symptoms of hypervitaminosis A.

A large number of analogs of retinoic acid have been synthesized, including the prodrug, *etretinate*, which is the ethyl ester of the active compound, *acitretin*. These compounds are representative of the so-called "second-generation retinoids," in which the β-ionone ring is aromatized; they are more active than tretinoin in some systems but are less active in others. The highly potent "third-generation" retinoids feature two aromatic rings that serve to restrict the flexibility of the polyenoic side chain. This class of aromatic retinoids has been called *arotinoids*, and includes the carboxylic acid, Ro 13–7410, and the ethyl sulfone, Ro 15–1570. The structures of retinoic acids and certain aromatic retinoids are presented in Table 64–1. The structure–activity relationships of the synthetic retinoids have been reviewed in a recent symposium (1989b).

Physiological Functions and Pharmacological Actions. Vitamin A has a number of important functions in the body. It plays an essential role in the function of the retina. It is necessary for growth and differentiation of epithelial tissue and is required for growth of bone, reproduction, and embryonic development. Together with certain carotenoids, vitamin A appears to enhance the function of the immune system, to reduce the consequences of some infectious diseases, and to protect against the development of certain malignancies. As a result, there is considerable interest in the pharmacological use of retinoids for the prophylaxis of cancer and for the treatment of various premalignant conditions. Because of the effects of vitamin A on epithelial tissues, retinoids and their analogs are used in the treatment of a number of skin diseases, including some of the consequences of aging and prolonged exposure to the sun.

The functions of vitamin A are mediated by different forms of the molecule. In vision, the functional vitamin is retinal. Retinoic acid appears to be the active form in functions associated with growth, differentiation, and transformation. Although the administration of retinoic acid to vitamin A–deficient animals has not been observed to correct their reproductive disturbances, recent evidence suggests that pharmacokinetic, rather than pharmacodynamic, factors were responsible (Bagavandoss and Midgley, 1987, 1988). The major recognized reactions are as follows:

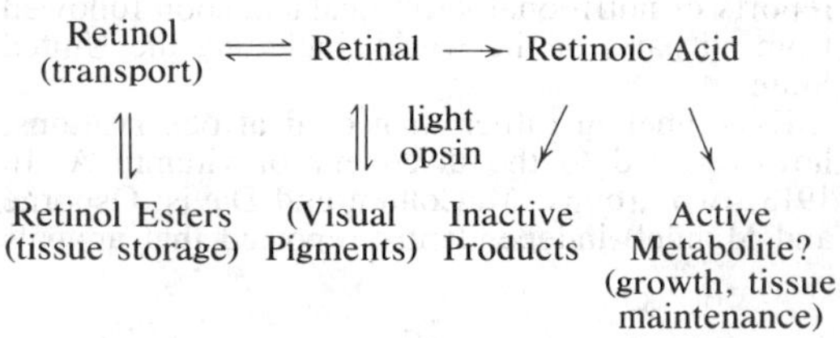

Retinal and the Visual Cycle. It has long been known that vitamin A deficiency interferes with vision in dim light, a condition known as *night blindness* (nyctalopia). The fundamental observations of Hecht (1937),

Table 64–1. STRUCTURES OF RETINOIC ACIDS AND VARIOUS RETINOIDS

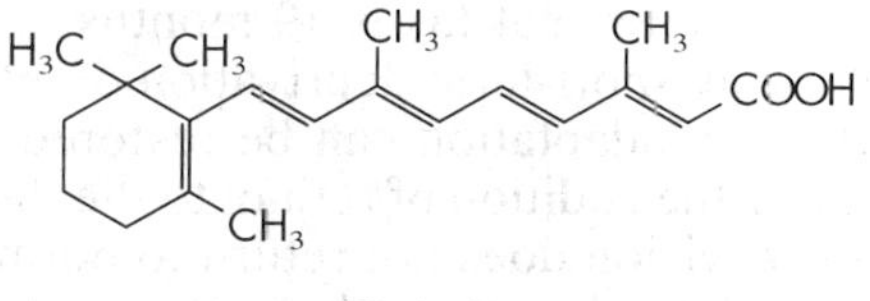

Tretinoin

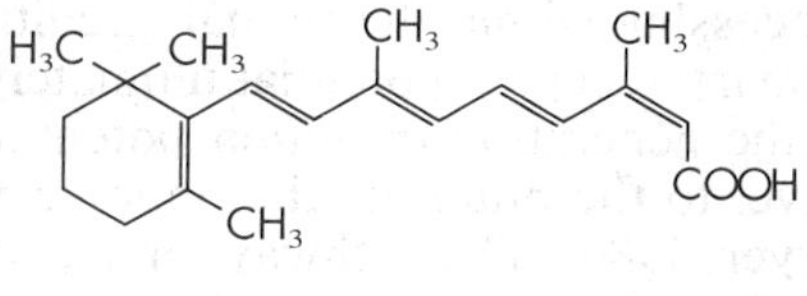

Isotretinoin

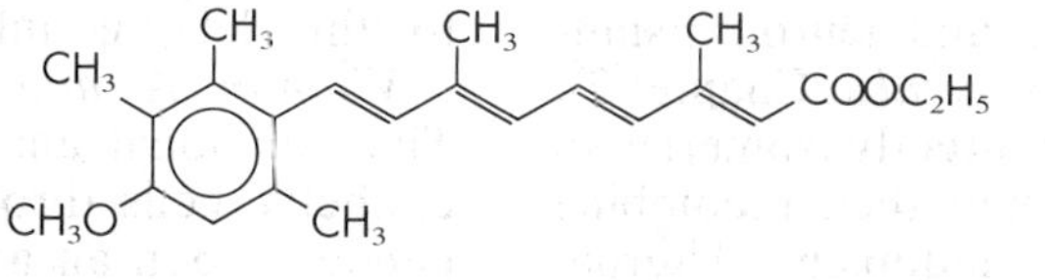

Etretinate

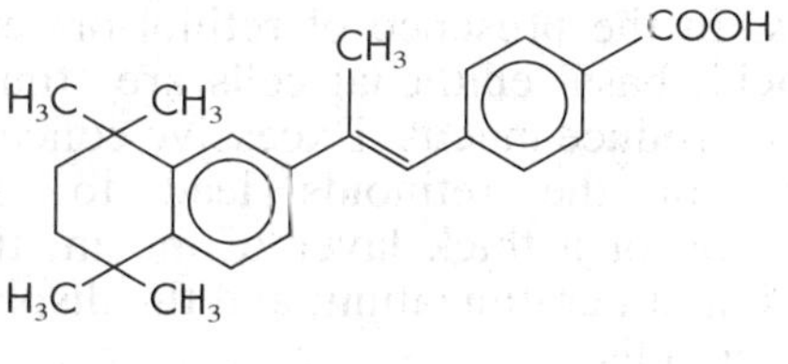

Ro 13-7410

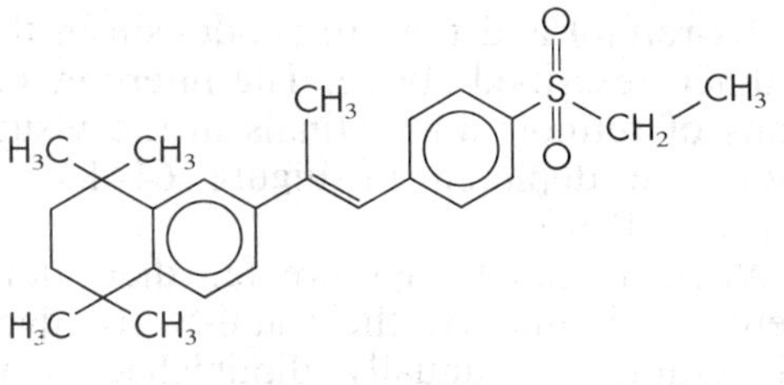

Ro 15-1570

Hubbard and colleagues (1965), and Wald and Brown (1965) contributed greatly to an understanding of this phenomenon (*see* Wald, 1968; Bridges, 1984).

Photoreception is accomplished by two types of specialized retinal cells, termed *rods* and *cones*. Rods are especially sensitive to light of low intensity; cones act as receptors of high-intensity light and are responsible for color vision. The initial step is the absorption of light by a chromophore attached to the receptor protein. The chromophore of both rods and cones is 11-*cis*-retinal. The holoreceptor in rods is termed *rhodopsin*—a combination of the protein opsin and 11-*cis*-retinal attached as a prosthetic group. The three different types of cone cells (red, green, and blue) contain individual related photoreceptor proteins and respond optimally to light of different wavelengths.

In the synthesis of rhodopsin, 11-*cis*-retinol is converted to 11-*cis*-retinal in a reversible reaction that requires pyridine nucleotides. 11-*Cis*-retinal then combines with the ϵ-amino group of a specific lysine residue in opsin to form rhodopsin. Most rhodopsin is located in the membranes of the discs situated in the outer segments of the rods. The polypeptide chain of the protein spans the membrane seven times. Thus, its structure is similar to those of the receptors described in Chapters 2 and 5 that interact with guanine nucleotide–binding regulatory proteins (G proteins), as is its mechanism of action.

The visual cycle is initiated by the absorption of a photon of light, followed by the photodecomposition, or bleaching, of rhodopsin through a cascade of unstable conformational states, leading ultimately to the isomerization of 11-*cis*-retinal to the all-*trans* form and dissociation of the opsin moiety. Activated rhodopsin interacts rapidly with another protein of the retinal rod outer segment, a G protein termed *transducin* or G_t. Transducin, in sequence, stimulates a guanosine 3′,5′-monophosphate–specific (cyclic GMP–specific) phosphodiesterase. The resultant decline in cyclic GMP concentration causes a decreased conductance of cyclic GMP–gated Na^+

channels in the plasma membrane and an increased transmembrane potential. After processing within the retinal circuitry, this primary receptor potential ultimately leads to the generation of action potentials that travel to the brain via the optic nerve (*see* Stryer, 1986). The pathway for signal transduction that starts with the receptor for photons (rhodopsin) is thus analogous to that for many hormones and neurotransmitters (*see* Gilman, 1987; *see also* Chapter 2).

All-*trans*-retinal can directly isomerize to 11-*cis*-retinal, which may then recombine with opsin to form rhodopsin. Alternatively, all-*trans*-retinal can be reduced to all-*trans*-retinol, which is first converted to 11-*cis*-retinol and then to rhodopsin in the manner described above. The interconversions of retinols and retinals in the visual cycle are depicted in Figure 64–1 (*see* Bridges, 1984).

When human beings are fed diets deficient in vitamin A, their ability for dark adaptation is gradually diminished. Rod vision is affected more than cone vision. Upon depletion of retinol from liver and blood, usually at plasma concentrations of retinol of less than 20 μg/dl (0.70 μM), the concentration of retinol and of rhodopsin in the retina falls. Unless the deficiency is overcome, opsin, lacking the stabilizing effect of retinal, decays and anatomical deterioration of the rods' outer segments takes place. In rats maintained on a vitamin A–deficient diet, irreversible ultrastructural changes leading to blindness then supervene, a process that takes 10 months.

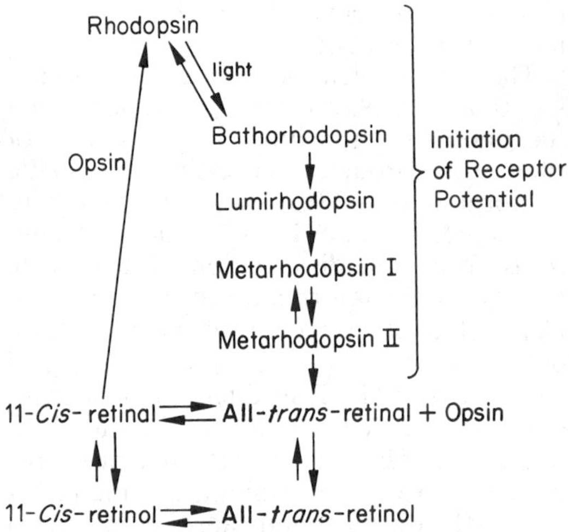

Figure 64–1. *The visual cycle.*

Following short-term deprivation of vitamin A, dark adaptation can be restored to normal by the addition of retinol to the diet. However, vision does not return to normal for several weeks after adequate amounts of retinol have been supplied. The reason for this delay is unknown.

Vitamin A and Epithelial Structures. The functional and structural integrity of epithelial cells throughout the body is dependent upon an adequate supply of vitamin A. The vitamin plays a major role in the induction and control of epithelial differentiation in mucus-secreting or keratinizing tissues. In the presence of retinol or retinoic acid, basal epithelial cells are stimulated to produce mucus. Excessive concentrations of the retinoids lead to the production of a thick layer of mucin, the inhibition of keratinization, and the display of goblet cells.

In the absence of vitamin A, goblet mucous cells disappear and are replaced by basal cells that have been stimulated to proliferate. These undermine and replace the original epithelium with a stratified, keratinizing epithelium. The suppression of normal secretions leads to irritation and infection. Reversal of these changes is achieved by the administration of retinol, retinoic acid, or other retinoids.

Mechanism of Action. In isolated fibroblasts or epithelial tissue, retinoids enhance the synthesis of some proteins (*e.g.*, fibronectin) and reduce the synthesis of others (*e.g.*, collagenase, certain species of keratin); such observations have frequently included evidence for action at the level of nuclear transcription (*see* Allen and Bloxham, in Symposium, 1989b). Retinoic acid appears to be considerably more potent than retinol in mediating these effects. In addition, retinoids can influence the expression of receptors for certain hormones and growth factors. For example, retinoic acid increases the synthesis of receptors for epidermal growth factor in fetal lung cells or fibroblasts, as well as those for interleukin-2 in activated thymocytes (Oberg *et al.*, 1988; Sidell and Ramsdell, 1988; Thompson and Rosner, 1989); by contrast, retinoic acid decreases the density of receptors for 1α,25-dihydroxyvitamin D_3 (calcitriol) in cells derived from fetal or neonatal calvaria (Petkovich *et al.*, 1987b). Thus retinoids can influence the growth, differentiation, and function of target cells by both direct and indirect actions.

Retinoic acid influences gene expression by combining with nuclear receptors whose structure is closely related to those of the thyroid hormone receptors (Giguere *et al.*, 1987; Petkovich *et al.*, 1987a). A second type of receptor with a tenfold higher affinity for retinoic acid has also been identified (Benbrook *et al.*, 1988; Brand *et al.*, 1988), but both molecules have about a 1000-fold lower affinity for retinol. The retinoic acid receptors belong to a "superfamily" that includes the receptors for steroids, thyroid hormone, and calcitriol (*see* Evans, 1988; *see also* Chapter 2). These proteins share a conserved DNA-binding domain and a common mechanism of action, in which binding of hormone facilitates interaction of the receptor with DNA and/or regulation of DNA transcription by the hormone–receptor complex. No comparable receptor for retinol has yet been detected, and it is possible that to produce its effects retinol must be oxidized to retinoic acid within target cells.

Vitamin A and Cancer. Because vitamin A has the ability to control cell differentiation and proliferation in epithelia, there has been considerable interest in the apparent ability of retinol and related compounds to interfere with carcinogenesis (*see* Moon and Itri, 1984, and related discussions in Sporn *et al.*, 1984). Deficiency of vitamin A appears to enhance susceptibility to carcinogenesis, even in man (Bjelke, 1975); the basal cells of various epithelia undergo marked hyperplasia and reduced cellular differentiation. The administration of retinol or other retinoids to animals reverses these changes in the epithelium of the respiratory tract, mammary gland, urinary bladder, and skin. Following the studies of Lasnitzki (1955), which demonstrated that treatment with retinoids caused replacement of atypical carcinogen-induced epithelial cells with more normal cells, it was shown that the compounds also prevent the development of epithelial cancer of the tissues mentioned. Thus, the progression of premalignant cells to cells with invasive, malignant characteristics is slowed, delayed, arrested, or even reversed in experimental animals (Hill and Grubbs, 1982). The antitumor effect is seen with chemically and virally induced malignancies, both of epithelial and mesenchymal origin, as well as with transformation induced with radiation or growth factors. Reversal of growth and metastasis of established tumors *in vivo* has been limited, as has prevention of the growth of transplantable neoplasms in animals.

The exact mechanism of the anticarcinogenic effect remains unclear, but obviously it is of enormous interest. The effect is observable even if the retinoid is administered many weeks after the exposure to a carcinogen, suggesting interference with the promotion or progression phase of carcinogenesis. A possible mechanism that may contribute to the antitumor effect is the induction of differentiation in malignant cells to form morphologically mature normal cells (Strickland and Mahdavi, 1978; Breitman *et al.*, 1980). For example, retinoids regulate the synthesis of specific proteins (*e.g.*, keratin) necessary for the differentiation of epithelial tissues (Fuchs and Green, 1981). Moreover, vitamin A appears to have a specific biochemical function in the synthesis of cell-surface glycoproteins and glycolipids that may be involved in cell adherence and communication. Conversion of retinol to retinyl phosphate in epithelial cells is followed by microsomal formation of mannosyl retinyl phosphate (Rosso *et al.*, 1975), a glycosylated retinol derivative that mediates the transfer of mannose to specific cell-surface glycoproteins. Formation of such proteins is sharply curtailed when vitamin A is deficient. Reactions of this type may explain the function of the vitamin in a number of processes that depend on the integrity of the cell surface, and might contribute to the suppression of the malignant phenotype previously induced by a carcinogen. The host's immune defense mechanisms may also be improved. In any event, a direct cytotoxic action appears unlikely.

Although numerous epidemiological studies have demonstrated an inverse relationship between the intake of dietary vitamin A and cancer morbidity and mortality (especially lung cancer), the correlation with the intake of retinol itself has been inconsistent (*see* De Vet, 1989; Ziegler, in Symposium, 1989a). As a result, attention is now being focused on biological effects of β-carotene and other carotenoids that are not shared by retinol (*see* Seifter *et al.*, 1988; Symposium, 1989a). One leading candidate is the capacity of β-carotene to act as a unique antioxidant, such that it can interfere with the mutagenic effects of certain carcinogens or of ionizing radiation; it can also promote the cytotoxic actions of activated polymorphonuclear leukocytes. These actions can also be produced by other dietary carotenoids (*e.g.*, canthaxanthin) that contain at least nine conjugated double bonds, even though these compounds cannot be converted to retinol or retinoic acid by mammalian tissues.

Symptoms of Deficiency. Tissue reserves of retinoids in the normal adult are sufficiently large to require long-term dietary deprivation in order to induce deficiency. Vitamin A deficiency occurs more commonly, therefore, in chronic diseases affecting fat absorption, such as biliary tract or pancreatic disease, sprue, colitis, and portal cirrhosis; following partial gastrectomy; or during extreme, chronic dietary inadequacy.

Vitamin A deficiency is one of the most serious nutritional deficiency diseases in the world today. It is widespread in Southeast Asia, the Middle East, Africa, and Central and South America, particularly in children, and is associated with general malnutrition. Deficiency of vitamin A may be fatal, especially in infants and young children suffering from kwashiorkor or marasmus. It has been estimated that more than one quarter million children in the world suffer irreversible blindness every year because of inadequate intake of vitamin A. Even mild xerophthalmia is associated with an increased risk of respiratory infections or diarrhea, as well as with an increased mortality due to these diseases or to measles (*see* Sommer, in Symposium, 1989a). In the United States, concentrations of retinol in plasma below the accepted lower limits of normal, 20 μg/dl (0.70 μM), are observed in about 3% of apparently healthy people. Most of these individuals are infants or children.

Signs and symptoms of mild vitamin A deficiency are easily overlooked. Skin lesions, such as follicular hyperkeratosis and infections, are among the earliest signs of deficiency, but the most recognizable manifestation is night blindness, even though its onset occurs only when vitamin A depletion is severe. Children may grow more slowly, although this may be recognized only after correction of deficiency. In general, rapidly proliferating tissues are more sensitive to vitamin A deficiency than are slowly growing tissues and may revert to an undifferentiated state more readily.

Eye. Keratomalacia, characterized by desiccation, ulceration, and xerosis of the cornea and conjunctiva, is occasionally seen as an acute symptom in the very young who are ingesting severely deficient diets. It is foreshadowed, usually, by night blindness, which appears as the earliest ocular sign of deficiency. Ultimately, severe visual impairment and even blindness result.

Bronchorespiratory Tract. Changes in the bronchorespiratory epithelium from mucus secretion to keratinization lead to increased incidence of respiratory infections in the deficiency state. There is also a decrease in elasticity of the lung and other tissues.

Skin. Keratinization and drying of the epidermis occur, and papular eruptions involving the pilosebaceous follicles may be found, especially on the extremities.

Genitourinary System. Urinary calculi are frequent concomitants of vitamin A deficiency. The epithelium of the urinary tract shares in the general pathological changes of all epithelial structures. Epithelial debris may thus provide the nidus around which a calculus is formed. Abnormalities of reproduction include impairment of spermatogenesis, degeneration of testes, abortion, resorption of fetuses, and production of malformed offspring.

Gastrointestinal Tract. The intestinal mucosa shows a reduction in the number of goblet cells but no keratinization. Alterations in intestinal epithelium and metaplasia of pancreatic ductal epithelium are common. They may be responsible for the diarrhea occasionally seen in vitamin A deficiency.

Sweat Glands. These glands may undergo atrophy and keratinizing squamous-cell metaplasia.

Bone. In animals, vitamin A deficiency is associated with faulty modeling of bone (with production of thick, cancellous bone instead of thinner, more compact bone).

Miscellaneous. Often both taste and smell are impaired in vitamin A–deficient individuals, undoubtedly a result of a keratinizing effect. Hearing may also be impaired. Vitamin A deficiency can interfere with erythropoiesis, which may be masked by abnormal losses of fluid. Nerve lesions, increased cerebrospinal fluid pressure, and hydrocephalus have been reported.

Hypervitaminosis A. An intake of retinoids greatly in excess of requirement results in a toxic syndrome known as hypervitaminosis A. Some 600 cases have been reported in the literature (*see* Kamm *et al.*, 1984; Bendich and Langseth, 1989). Some or all of the symptoms of hypervitaminosis A are also the major toxic effects that are manifest during the therapeutic use of natural and synthetic retinoids in the treatment of skin disorders (*see* Chapter 65).

Most frequently, high intakes in children are the result of overzealous prophylactic vitamin therapy on the part of parents. Toxicity in adults has resulted from extended self-medication or food fads, as well as from the use of retinoids for the therapy of acne or other skin lesions. The toxicity of retinol depends on the age of the patient, the dose, and the duration of administration. Although vitamin A toxicity is uncommon in adults who consume less than 30 mg of retinol per day, mild symptoms of chronic retinoid intoxication have been detected in individuals whose intake was about 10 mg per day for 6 months (*see* Bendich and Langseth, 1989). In infants, the daily consumption of as little as 7.5 to 15 mg of retinol for 30 days has induced toxicity. The acute consumption of more than 500 mg of retinol in an adult, 100 mg in a young child, or 30 mg in an infant frequently results in poisoning. Acute, sometimes fatal poisoning in man is also known to follow the ingestion of polar bear liver, which contains up to 12 mg of retinol per gram. The Food and Nutrition Board of the National Research Council (1980) has warned that the ingestion of more than 7.5 mg of retinol daily is ill advised. Nevertheless, almost 5% of users of vitamin A in the United States exceed that amount.

Early signs and symptoms of chronic retinoid intoxication include dry and pruritic skin, skin desquamation, erythematous dermatitis, disturbed hair growth, fissures of the lips, pain and tenderness of bones, hyperostosis, headache, papilledema, anorexia, edema, fatigue, irritability, and hemorrhage. Intracranial pressure may be increased, and neurological symptoms may mimic those of a brain tumor (pseudotumor cerebri). In infants, increased intracranial pressure, a bulging fontanel, and vomiting are seen early. In addition to hepatosplenomegaly, pathological changes in the liver include hypertrophy of fat-storing cells, fibrosis, sclerosis of central veins, and cirrhosis, with resultant portal hypertension and ascites. The activity of alkaline phosphatase in plasma rises because of the increased osteoblastic activity, and a number of cases of hypercalcemia have been reported in children. Elevations in plasma triglycerides and reductions in the cholesterol of high-density lipoprotein are also observed.

Signs and symptoms of acute poisoning include drowsiness, irritability or irresistible desire to sleep, severe headache due to increased intracranial pressure, dizziness, hepatomegaly, vomiting, papilledema, and, after 24 hours, generalized peeling of the skin.

Concentrations of retinol in plasma in excess of 100 μg/dl (3.5 μM) usually are diagnostic of hypervitaminosis A. Treatment consists in withdrawal of the retinoid. Most signs and symptoms disappear within a week, but the desquamation and hyperostoses remain evident for several months after clinical recovery, and in rare instances the bone malformations may be permanent. Long-term and sometimes irreversible damage to the liver may also occur.

The risk of hypervitaminosis A is increased in conditions that produce a decreased plasma concentration of retinol-binding protein (RBP) (*see* below). These include protein malnutrition and liver disease. Because vitamins A and D are often consumed together, some of the symptoms of hypervitaminosis A (*e.g.*, hypercalcemia) may actually be caused by overdosage with vitamin D. Indeed, large doses of vitamin A may protect against the adverse effects on bone metabolism of hypervitaminosis D. The hypoprothrombinemia of hypervitaminosis A may reflect antagonism of vitamin K. In experimental animals, the administration of vitamin E eliminates some of the toxic effects of large doses of vitamin A. Although similar observations in man have not been documented, small amounts of vitamin E are included in the preparations of vitamin A used in developing countries for intermittent high-level dosing (*see* Bendich and Langseth, 1989).

Congenital abnormalities can apparently occur in human infants whose mothers have consumed about 7.5 to 12 mg of retinol daily during the first trimester of pregnancy (Bernhardt and Dorsey, 1974). Obviously, pregnant women should not ingest quantities of retinoids in excess of those recommended. Moreover, women who have been treated with synthetic retinoids that accumulate in fat should practice contraception after discontinuing therapy until the drug has been eliminated from the body; after prolonged ingestion of etretinate, this may require 2 years or longer (*see* below).

Human Requirements. Human requirements for vitamin A have been approximated from studies that have attempted to correct experimentally produced deficiency states. The present recommendations of the Food and Nutrition Board of the National Research Council are based upon the amount of retinoid necessary to maintain normal dark adaptation plus an additional factor of safety to cover variations in absorption and utilization of retinol. The recommended daily allowances for the normal adult male and female are 1000 and 800 retinol equivalents per day, respectively (5000 and 4000 units, assuming that 50% of dietary vitamin A is derived from retinol and 50% from β-carotene). For the requirements of infants and children, *see* Table XVI–1 (page 1525) and below.

Absorption, Fate, and Excretion. *Retinol.* More than 90% of dietary retinol is in the form of esters, usually retinyl palmitate. As with triglycerides, most of the retinyl esters are hydrolyzed in the intestinal lumen by pancreatic enzymes and within the brush border of the intestinal epithelial cell before absorption. Although lipophilic, the uptake of retinol by intestinal cells apparently occurs by a carrier-mediated process and is facilitated by the presence of a cytosolic protein that specifically binds retinol with high affinity. This cellular retinol-binding protein (CRBP), which is closely related to the CRBP in numerous cells throughout the body (*see* below), is designated CRBP II. It occurs only in absorptive cells in the small intestine, where it constitutes about 1% of the total soluble protein (*see* Chytil and Ong, 1987). Most of the retinol is reesterified (mainly to palmitate) within these cells and is incorporated into chylomicrons; after large oral doses of retinol, significant amounts of retinyl esters also circulate in association with low-density lipoprotein. Appreciable quantities of retinol are also absorbed directly into the circulation where they are bound to the retinol-binding protein (RBP) in plasma.

When ingested in amounts that approximate daily requirements, the absorption of retinol is complete; however, some retinol escapes into the feces when large doses are taken. The concentration of esterified retinol reaches a peak in plasma about 4 hours after the ingestion of retinol. The absorption of retinol is reduced by abnormalities of fat digestion and absorption, such as occur in patients with pancreatic or hepatic disease, intestinal infections, and cystic fibrosis. Water-miscible preparations should be used in such patients.

Most of the absorbed retinyl esters are taken up by the liver through receptor-mediated internalization of chylomicron remnants. Until the hepatic stores of retinyl esters become saturated, the administration of retinol leads mainly to its accumulation in the liver rather than in blood. The median concentration of retinyl esters in human liver is about 100 to 300 μg/g, and the normal range of retinol in plasma is 30 to 70 μg/dl (1.1 to 2.4 μM). If an individual ingests a diet free of retinol or its precursors, plasma concentrations are maintained over many months at the expense of hepatic reserves; these decrease with a half-life of about 50 to 100 days. Blood concentrations, therefore, are not a sensitive guide to an individual's vitamin A status, but low plasma values imply that hepatic storage of the vitamin may be exhausted (*see* Underwood, 1984). Signs and symptoms of vitamin A deficiency appear when the plasma concentration falls below 10 to 20 μg/dl (0.35 to 0.70 μM) or when concentrations of retinoids in the liver are less than 5 to 20 μg/g. In alcoholic liver disease, hepatic concentrations of retinoids are severely depressed (Leo and Lieber, 1982).

Prior to entering the circulation from the liver, hepatic retinyl esters are hydrolyzed, and 90 to 95% of the retinol is associated with an α_1-globulin, which has a single binding site for the vitamin. This RBP is synthesized and secreted by the liver and then circulates in the blood complexed with and stabilized by transthyretin, a thyroxine-binding prealbumin. The formation of this complex protects the circulating RBP (and retinol) from metabolism and renal excretion.

More than 95% of plasma retinoids are normally bound to RBP. When hepatic stores of the vitamin and the RBP carrier system become saturated because of excessive intake of retinol or hepatic damage, up to 65% of the retinoids in plasma may be present as retinyl esters associated with lipoprotein. Similarly, after acute administration of alcohol, retinyl esters accumulate. Since retinol is biologically inert while bound to RBP, these retinyl esters, which are surfactants, may be responsible for much of the toxicity that is observed (Mallia *et al.*, 1975; Smith and Goodman, 1976).

Retinol bound to RBP reaches the cell membrane of the various target organs, where the complex binds to specific sites on the cell surface (Sivaprasadarao and Findlay, 1988a, 1988b). The retinol is transferred to a membrane-bound protein that appears to be closely related to the soluble CRBP and is converted to a retinyl ester (Ottonello *et al.*, 1987). The retinyl ester is then cleaved by a membrane-associated hydrolase, provided that unliganded cytosolic CRBP is available to accept the retinol. CRBP exists in virtually all tissues; exceptions include cardiac and skeletal muscle and the ileal mucosa, where the closely related CRBP II is found (*see* above; *see also* Chytil and Ong, 1987). In addition to its role in the uptake of retinol, CRBP functions as a reservoir for cellular retinol. It also delivers the vitamin to appropriate sites for its conversion to active compounds. In the retina, retinol is converted to 11-*cis*-retinal, which is incorporated into rhodopsin; a specific binding protein (distinct from CRBP) is also present. In other target tissues, retinol is apparently oxidized to retinoic acid, which is conveyed to receptors in the nucleus as a complex with the cellular retinoic acid-binding protein (CRABP). The tissue distribution of CRABP appears to be nearly identical with that of CRBP, with the possible exception of its absence from adult liver (*see* Chytil and Ong, 1987).

The concentration of RBP in plasma is crucial for the regulation of retinol in plasma and its transport to tissues. In vitamin A deficiency, the synthesis of RBP is maintained, the hepatic content of RBP rises, and its concentration in plasma falls, apparently because the secretion of RBP from the liver is blocked. Once retinol again becomes available, the liver rapidly releases RBP into the plasma for transport of retinol to the tissues. When there is protein deficiency (*e.g.*, caused by malnutrition, kwashiorkor, or parenchymal liver disease), the concentration of RBP becomes insufficient, and concentrations of retinol in plasma fall despite normal stores in the liver. Replenishment with calories and protein is then required. Deficiency of both RBP and retinol cannot be corrected by the administration of retinol alone.

Other pathological conditions also alter concentrations of retinol and RBP in plasma. In cystic fibrosis, alcohol-related cirrhosis, and other hepatic diseases, synthesis or release of RBP from the liver is depressed and plasma retinol concentrations are reduced. In proteinuria, febrile infections, or stress, the concentration of retinol in the blood may be reduced drastically, partially because of increased urinary excretion. In chronic renal disease, RBP catabolism is impaired, and concentrations of the protein and retinol are elevated.

Estrogens and oral contraceptives elevate the plasma concentrations of RBP, but the effects of pregnancy are complex. During the first trimester the mean content of retinol in plasma falls, followed by a slow rise and a return to normal at parturition. It is likely that the increased demands for retinol lead to its withdrawal from the blood at a rate exceeding that of its mobilization from liver. The placental barrier prevents the extensive transfer of retinol or carotenoids. Studies in animals suggest that transplacental transport of RBP occurs during early pregnancy; thereafter the fetus begins to synthesize its own RBP. The concentration of retinol in fetal blood is thus less than in maternal blood. Both colostrum and milk offer the newborn an adequate supply of retinol. The concentration of retinol in the milk is maintained at a fixed maximal concentration if the maternal dietary intake of retinol is adequate to permit storage in the liver.

Retinol is in part conjugated to form a β-glucuronide, which undergoes enterohepatic circulation and is oxidized to retinal and retinoic acid. Several other water-soluble metabolites are also excreted in the urine and feces. Normally, no retinol can be recovered unchanged from human urine.

Carotenoids. Unlike the extensive absorption of retinol, only about one third of β-carotene or other carotenoids is absorbed by man. The absorption of carotenoids takes place in a relatively nonspecific fashion and depends upon the presence of bile and absorbable fat in the intestinal tract; it is greatly decreased by steatorrhea and chronic diarrhea. A portion of the β-carotene is converted to retinol in the wall of the small intestine, principally by its initial cleavage at the 15,15′ double bond to form two molecules of retinal. Some of the retinal is further oxidized to retinoic acid; only one half is reduced to retinol, which is then esterified and transported in the lymph, as described above. Some β-carotene is absorbed as such and circulates in association with lipoproteins; it apparently partitions into body lipids and can be converted to vitamin A in numerous tissues, including the liver (*see* De Vet, 1989; Olson, in Symposium, 1989a). If very large amounts of carotene are ingested, very high concentrations may be achieved in blood (300 μg/dl; 5.6 μM), and the hypercarotenemia results in a reversible yellow discoloration of the skin; this can be distinguished from jaundice by the absence of scleral pigmentation. Hypervitaminosis does not develop, however, probably because of a limited conversion of carotene to retinol.

Retinoic Acid. Unlike retinol, relatively little all-*trans*-retinoic acid (tretinoin) is provided in the diet, and specific mechanisms for its absorption, transport in plasma, and storage in tissue do not exist. After oral administration, retinoic acid reaches the circulation by the portal vein and is transported in plasma as a complex with albumin; quantitative studies of its absorption by this route have not been performed in man. When applied to human skin, about 5% of the compound and its metabolites is recovered in the urine; little systemic toxicity is produced by this route. By contrast, attempts to treat dermatoses by oral administration of retinoic acid can produce severe symptoms of hypervitaminosis A.

Tretinoin is rapidly metabolized in the liver, and various conjugated forms and degradation products are secreted into bile and excreted in urine and feces. In addition to 13-*cis*-retinoic acid (isotretinoin), conjugates with glucuronic acid and taurine are formed; oxidation occurs at position 4 in the β-ionone ring (*see* Allen and Bloxham, in Symposium, 1989b).

Isotretinoin. After oral administration, peak concentrations of isotretinoin in plasma are reached in 2 to 4 hours. Its oral bioavailability in fasting subjects is estimated to be about 20%; the presence of food substantially increases the extent of systemic absorption. The drug is not effective topically. Isotretinoin is extensively bound to albumin in plasma, and its concentration in tissues is generally lower than that in the general circulation.

Isotretinoin and tretinoin are interconverted *in vivo*, and about 20 to 30% of a dose of isotretinoin is apparently metabolized by this route. With repeated administration, the major metabolite, 4-oxo-isotretinoin, accumulates in the blood. Excretion of metabolites and the parent compound in the bile occurs after conjugation with glucuronic acid. The half-life of isotretinoin in plasma ranges between 6 and 36 hours. With repeated administration, steady-state concentrations are established within 5 to 7 days. Several metabolites of isotretinoin are cleared from plasma rather slowly. Because of the general concern over the teratogenicity of retinoids, it is recommended that effective contraception be maintained for at least one month after treatment with isotretinoin is discontinued. The pharmacokinetics of isotretinoin have been reviewed by Allen and Bloxham (Symposium, 1989b).

Etretinate. Etretinate is the ethyl ester of acitretin, which is presumed to be the active form of the drug. The oral bioavailability of etretinate is about 50%, and absorption is enhanced in the presence of milk or fatty foods. After oral administration of single doses, the plasma concentrations of etretinate and acitretin are about equal and reach maximal values within 2 to 3 hours; thereafter, their concentrations decline with half-times of 7 to 9 hours. However, after continuous administration, etretinate and its active metabolites accumulate in fat and plasma, and their apparent half-lives increase as a function of the duration of treatment; values of 60 to 170 days may be observed after treatment for 1 year. As a result, it may be necessary for women to maintain effective contraception for at least 2 years after treatment is discontinued.

In addition to deesterification in the gut and liver, etretinate undergoes extensive metabolism and conjugation before excretion in the urine and bile. The metabolites of acitretin that have been identified include 13-*cis*-acitretin and demethylated products. The pharmacokinetic properties of etretinate have been reviewed by Allen and Bloxham (Symposium, 1989b).

Bioassay and Unitage. Most commercial preparations of vitamin A are synthetic retinyl esters. Preparations from animal sources must be assayed biologically to establish their activity. This assay depends upon the ability of retinol to support growth in vitamin-depleted rats. The concentration of suitably purified preparations can be determined spectrophotometrically. One I.U. of vitamin A is the specific biological activity of 0.3 μg of all-*trans*-retinol or 0.6 μg of β-carotene. Because of the relatively inefficient dietary utilization of β-carotene compared with retinol, the nomenclature is in terms of the retinol equivalent, which represents 1 μg of all-*trans*-retinol, 6 μg of dietary β-carotene, or 12 μg of other provitamin A carotenoids. One retinol equivalent equals 3.3 I.U. of vitamin A activity as supplied by retinol or 10 units of vitamin A activity as supplied by β-carotene (Bieri and McKenna, 1981). The methods for standardizing retinol and carotenoids have been reviewed (Simpson, 1983).

Preparations. There are many types of preparations that contain retinol. Absorption is greatest for aqueous preparations, intermediate for emulsions, and slowest for oil solutions. Whereas oil-soluble preparations may lead to greater hepatic storage of the vitamin, water-miscible preparations usually provide higher concentrations in plasma.

Vitamin A capsules contain 3 to 15 mg of retinol (10,000 to 50,000 I.U.) per capsule; oral drops are also available. A water-miscible preparation (15 mg/ml; 50,000 I.U./ml) can be given intramuscularly for individuals with malabsorption, nausea, vomiting, or severe ocular damage.

*Tretinoin (all-*trans*-retinoic acid*; RETIN-A) is available for topical use as a liquid (0.05%), a cream (0.025 to 0.1%), and a gel (0.025 and 0.01%). It is an irritant, causes skin peeling, and is used for the treatment of acne and other skin diseases.

*Isotretinoin (13-*cis*-retinoic acid;* ACCUTANE) is available for oral use as 10-, 20-, and 40-mg capsules. For the treatment of acne, the initial daily dose is usually 0.5 to 1 mg/kg in two divided doses up to a maximum of 2 mg/kg. A course of therapy is usually 15 to 20 weeks; if necessary, this may be repeated after an interval of 2 months. Lower doses may be equally effective, but relapses are more frequent. Isotretinoin has also been used in the treatment of various disorders of keratinization, but doses higher than usual may be required.

Etretinate (TEGISON) is available for oral use as 10- and 25-mg capsules. For the treatment of psoriasis, initial daily doses are usually 0.75 to 1 mg/kg up to a maximum of 1.5 mg/kg.

Therapeutic Uses. *Vitamin A Deficiency Diseases.* The normal requirement of vitamin A for adults is supplied by an adequate diet. The rational uses of retinol are in the treatment of vitamin A deficiency and as prophylaxis in high-risk subjects during periods of increased requirement, such as infancy, pregnancy, and lactation. Once a vitamin A deficiency has been diagnosed, intensive therapy should be instituted. The patient should then be maintained on a proper diet.

During pregnancy and lactation, it is advisable to increase the maternal intake of vitamin A by about 25%. Since the typical North American diet readily provides adequate intake of the vitamin, supplementation is not routinely indicated. Nevertheless, the administration of vitamin supplements to infants is a common practice in the United States. However, ingestion of 6 mg (20,000 I.U.) of retinol or more per day for 1 to 2 months by healthy infants or children on good diets is likely to produce signs and symptoms of toxicity.

Rarely, the absorption, mobilization, or storage of retinol may be adversely affected, and under such circumstances long-term therapy with retinol may be indicated, as, for example, in an individual with steatorrhea, severe biliary obstruction, or cirrhosis of the liver, or following a total gastrectomy. In other disease states where considerable retinol is lost from the body, replacement therapy may be necessary. In various infections in which mucous-cell turnover is accelerated and urinary excretion of retinol is increased, the need for retinol is further enhanced. There is no evidence, however, that an excessive intake of retinoids will influence the incidence of infections in an individual whose intake of retinoids is adequate. Although moderate amounts of vitamin A apparently do no harm, hepatotoxicity may be potentiated when such doses are taken by the chronic alcoholic. If vitamin A is prescribed as a dietary supplement, intake of 1.5 mg of retinol represents one and one-half times the recommended daily allowance. Long-term ingestion of much larger amounts may lead to hypervitaminosis.

In kwashiorkor and other severe vitamin A deficiencies in children, a single intramuscular injection of 30 mg of retinol as the water-miscible palmitate has been advocated, followed by intermittent oral treatment with retinoids. The World Health Organization treatment schedule for xerophthalmia in children older than 1 year includes 110 mg of retinyl palmitate orally or 55 mg intramuscularly, plus another 110 mg orally the following day and again prior to discharge (*see* Underwood, 1984). Vitamin E, 40 units, should be coadministered, since it apparently increases the efficacy of retinol. Pregnant women should receive only low doses of retinoids.

Dermatological Diseases. Vitamin A may be helpful in certain diseases of the skin, such as acne, psoriasis, Darier's disease, and ichthyosis. The use of other retinoids in these conditions has largely replaced that of retinol and is discussed in Chapter 65.

Other Uses. Because of toxicity, routine prophylactic use against cancer cannot be recommended. The potential value of retinoids in rheumatoid disease, and in the prevention of human tumors of the skin, bladder, breast, and other epithelial tissues is, however, currently under investigation.

VITAMIN K

History. Vitamin K is a dietary principle essential for the normal biosynthesis of several factors required for clotting of blood. In 1929, Dam observed that chickens fed inadequate diets developed a deficiency disease in which the outstanding symptom was spontaneous bleeding, apparently due to a low content of prothrombin in the blood. Subsequently, Dam and coworkers (1935, 1936) found that the condition could be rapidly alleviated by feeding an unidentified fat-soluble substance. To this substance Dam gave the name *vitamin K* (*Koagulation* vitamin). Independently, Almquist and Stokstad (1935) described the same hemorrhagic disease in chickens and the method for its prevention.

These investigations were reported at a time when the attention of several groups of workers was centered on the cause of the hemorrhagic tendency in patients with obstructive jaundice and diseases of the liver. For example, Quick and coworkers (1935) observed that the coagulation defect in jaundiced individuals was due to a decrease in the concentration of prothrombin in the blood. In the same year, Hawkins and Whipple reported that animals with biliary fistulas were likely to develop excessive bleeding. Hawkins and Brinkhous (1936) subsequently showed that this was due to a deficiency in prothrombin and that the condition could be relieved by the feeding of bile salts.

The culmination of these experimental studies came with the demonstration by Butt and coworkers (1938) as well as Warner and associates (1938) that combination therapy with vitamin K and bile salts was effective in the treatment of the hemorrhagic diathesis in cases of jaundice. Thus, the relationship between vitamin K, adequate hepatic function, and the physiological mechanisms operating in the normal clotting of blood was established.

Occurrence and Chemistry. The early investigations described above showed that vitamin K is a fat-soluble substance present in hog liver fat and in alfalfa. Subsequently, it has been demonstrated that the vitamin is concentrated in the chloroplasts of plant leaves and in many vegetable oils. The feces of most species of animals contain large amounts of the vitamin, which is synthesized by the bacteria in the intestinal tract (*see* Bentley and Meganathan, 1982).

Vitamin K activity is associated with at least two distinct natural substances, designated as vitamin K_1 and vitamin K_2. Vitamin K_1, or *phytonadione* (phylloquinone), is 2-methyl-3-phytyl-1,4-naphthoquinone; it is found in plants, and is the only natural vitamin K available for therapeutic use. Vitamin K_2 represents a series of compounds (the *menaquinones*) in which the phytyl side chain of phytonadione has been replaced by a side chain built up of 2 to 13 prenyl units. Considerable synthesis of menaquinones occurs in gram-positive bacteria. In animals, menaquinone-4 can be synthesized from the vitamin precursor, *menadione* (2-methyl-1,4-naphthoquinone), or vitamin K_3. Depending on the bioassay system used, menadione is at least as active on a molar basis as phytonadione.

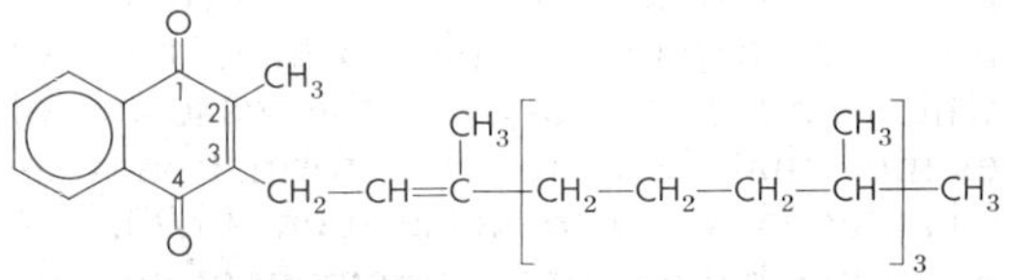

Phytonadione (Vitamin K_1; Phylloquinone)

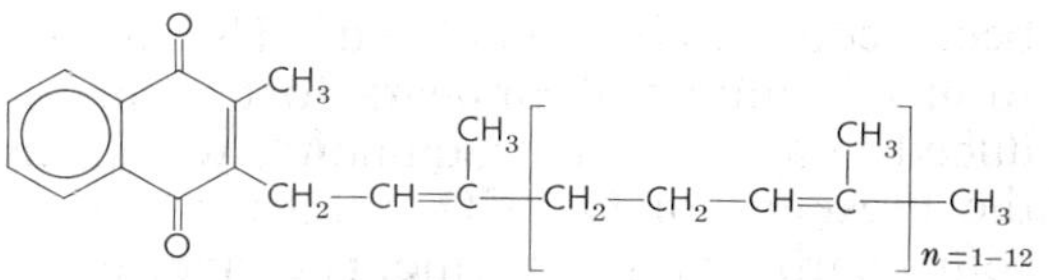

Menaquinone (Vitamin K_2) Series

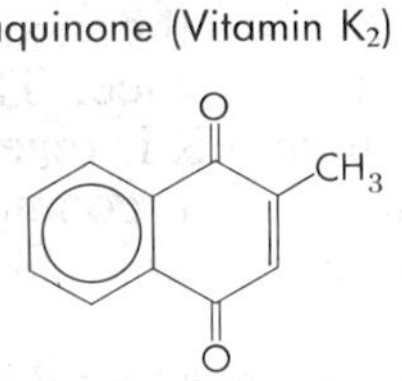

Menadione (Vitamin K_3)

The natural vitamins K and menadione are lipid soluble. It is possible to make active water-soluble derivatives of menadione by forming the sodium bisulfite salt or the tetrasodium salt of the diphosphoric acid ester. These compounds are converted in the body to menadione.

Physiological Functions and Pharmacological Actions. In normal animals and man, phytonadione and the menaquinones are virtually devoid of pharmacodynamic activity. In animals and man deficient in vitamin

K, the pharmacological action of vitamin K is identical to its normal physiological function, that is, to promote the hepatic biosynthesis of prothrombin (factor II), proconvertin (factor VII), plasma thromboplastin component (PTC, Christmas factor, factor IX), and the Stuart factor (factor X). The role of these factors in blood clotting is discussed in Chapter 55.

The vitamin K–dependent blood clotting factors, in the absence of vitamin K (or in the presence of the coumarin type of anticoagulant), are biologically inactive precursor proteins in the liver. Vitamin K functions as an essential cofactor for a microsomal enzyme system that activates these precursors by the conversion of multiple residues of glutamic acid near the amino terminus of each precursor to γ-carboxyglutamyl residues in the completed protein. The formation of this new amino acid, γ-carboxyglutamic acid, allows the protein to bind Ca^{2+} and in turn to be bound to a phospholipid surface, both of which are necessary in the cascade of events that lead to clot formation (*see* Chapter 55; *see also* Nelsestuen, 1978). The exact mechanism of involvement of vitamin K in this carboxylation reaction has not yet been completely elucidated. The active form of vitamin K appears to be the reduced vitamin K hydroquinone, which, in the presence of O_2, CO_2, and the microsomal carboxylase enzyme, is converted to its 2,3-epoxide at the same time γ-carboxylation takes place. The hydroquinone form of vitamin K is regenerated from the 2,3-epoxide by a coumarin-sensitive epoxide reductase (*see* Stenflo, 1978; Suttie, 1987).

Carboxyglutamate is found in a variety of proteins other than the vitamin K–dependent blood clotting factors (*see* Galloway *et al.*, 1980). One of these is osteocalcin in bone, which is a secretory product of osteoblasts. Its synthesis is regulated by calcitriol, the active form of vitamin D, and its concentration in plasma correlates with the turnover rate of bone. In blood, both protein S and protein C also contain carboxyglutamate; these proteins are involved in the inactivation of factor VIII and factor V (*see* Chapter 55).

Human Requirements. The human requirement of vitamin K has not been precisely defined; it appears to be extremely small. Frick and associates (1967) estimated the daily requirement, in patients made vitamin K deficient by a starvation diet and antibiotic therapy for 3 to 4 weeks, to be a minimum of 0.03 μg/kg of body weight; others place the daily requirement at 0.5 to 1 μg/kg, and the daily allowance recommended by the Food and Nutrition Board of the National Research Council approximates 1 μg/kg (*see* Table XVI–1, page 1525). These estimates have been based mainly on maintenance or restoration of the prothrombin time, which may not be sufficiently sensitive to detect subclinical deficiency of vitamin K (*see* Suttie, 1987). In the infant, 10 μg/kg of body weight of phytonadione is sufficient to prevent hypoprothrombinemia. Needs are satisfied by the average diet, and, in addition, the vitamin synthesized by intestinal bacteria is also available to the host.

Symptoms of Deficiency. The chief clinical manifestation of vitamin K deficiency is an increased tendency to bleed. Ecchymoses, epistaxis, hematuria, gastrointestinal bleeding, and postoperative hemorrhage are common; intracranial hemorrhage may occur. Hemoptysis is uncommon. A further discussion of hypoprothrombinemia is presented in the section on oral anticoagulants (Chapter 55). The discovery of a vitamin K–dependent protein in bone suggests that the fetal bone abnormalities associated with the administration of oral anticoagulants during the first trimester of pregnancy ("fetal warfarin syndrome") may be related to a deficiency of the vitamin.

Toxicity. Phytonadione and the menaquinones are nontoxic to animals, even when given in huge amounts. In man, intravenous administration of phytonadione has produced flushing, dyspnea, chest pains, cardiovascular collapse, and, rarely, death (*see* Barash *et al.*, 1976). Whether these reactions were due to the vitamin itself or to the agents used to disperse and emulsify the preparation is not clear.

In man, menadione is irritating to the skin and the respiratory tract. Its solutions have vesicant properties. Menadione and its derivatives have been implicated in producing hemolytic anemia, hyperbilirubinemia, and kernicterus in the newborn, especially in premature infants. Menadione also can induce hemolysis in individuals who are genetically deficient in glucose-6-phosphate dehydrogenase. In patients who have severe hepatic disease, the administration of large doses of menadione or phytonadione may further depress function of the liver (*see* below).

Absorption, Fate, and Excretion. The mechanism of intestinal absorption of compounds with vitamin K activity varies with their solubility. Phytonadione and the menaquinones are adequately absorbed from the gastrointestinal tract only if bile salts are present. Menadione and its water-soluble derivatives, however, are absorbed even in the absence of bile. Phytonadione and the menaquinones are absorbed almost entirely by way of the lymph; menadione and its water-soluble derivatives enter the bloodstream directly. Phytonadione is absorbed by an energy-dependent, saturable process in proximal portions of the small intestine; menaquinone and menadione are absorbed by diffusion in the distal portions of the small intestine and in the colon. Following intramuscular injection, both natural and synthetic vitamin K preparations are readily absorbed. After absorption, phytonadione is initially concentrated in the liver, but the concentration declines rapidly. Very little vitamin K accumulates in other tissues.

Phytonadione is rapidly metabolized to more polar metabolites, which are excreted in the bile and urine. The major urinary metabolites result from shortening of the side chain to five or seven carbon atoms, yielding carboxylic acids that are conjugated with glucuronate prior to excretion. Treatment with a coumarin-type anticoagulant results in a marked increase in the amount of phytonadione-2,3-epoxide in liver and blood. Such treatment also increases the urinary excretion of phytonadione metabolites, primarily degradative products of phytonadione-2,3-epoxide. The biliary metabolites of phytonadione have not been identified (*see* Shearer *et al.*, 1974). Menadione is apparently reduced to the diol (hydroquinone) form and excreted as glucuronide and sulfate conjugates.

Apparently there is little storage of vitamin K in the body. The limited stores of the vitamin present in tissue are slowly destroyed. Under circumstances where lack of bile interferes with absorption of vitamin K, hypoprothrombinemia develops slowly over a period of several weeks.

Assay and Unitage. Drugs with vitamin K activity may be chemically assayed and do not require bioassay. For the determination of the vitamin K content of foods, an assay based upon the ability of the preparation to increase the prothrombin level of deficient chicks is employed.

Preparations. *Phytonadione* (*vitamin K_1, phylloquinone;* AQUAMEPHYTON, KONAKION, MEPHYTON) is a viscous liquid that is insoluble in water. It is marketed in 5-mg tablets and in a dispersion of 2 or 10 mg/ml of phytonadione in a solution of buffered polysorbate and propylene glycol (KONAKION) or polyoxyethylated fatty acid derivatives and dextrose (AQUAMEPHYTON). KONAKION is administered only intramuscularly. AQUAMEPHYTON may be given by any parenteral route, although severe reactions resembling anaphylaxis have followed its intravenous injection; subcutaneous or intramuscular administration is preferred.

Menadione (*vitamin K_3*) is practically insoluble in water. *Menadiol sodium diphosphate* (SYNKAYVITE) is marketed for injection or as 5-mg tablets.

Therapeutic Uses. The rational therapeutic use of vitamin K is based on its ability to correct the bleeding tendency or hemorrhage associated with its deficiency. A deficiency of vitamin K and its attendant deficiency of prothrombin and related clotting factors can result from inadequate intake, absorption, or utilization of the vitamin, or as a consequence of the action of a vitamin K antagonist.

Inadequate Intake. After infancy, hypoprothrombinemia arising from a dietary deficiency of vitamin K is extremely rare, because not only is the vitamin present in many foods but also it is synthesized by intestinal bacteria. The combination of an inadequate diet and the prolonged use of drugs that inhibit intestinal bacterial growth may lead, however, to vitamin K deficiency (Frick *et al.*, 1967). Occasionally, the use of a broad-spectrum antibiotic may of itself produce a hypoprothrombinemia that responds readily to small doses of vitamin K and reestablishment of normal bowel flora. The use of such antibiotics in patients who have other causes for hypoprothrombinemia or a deficiency of vitamin K may have profound consequences. Hypoprothrombinemia can occur in patients receiving prolonged intravenous alimentation.

Hypoprothrombinemia of the Newborn. Healthy newborn infants show decreased plasma concentrations of vitamin K–dependent clotting factors for a few days after birth, the time required to obtain an adequate dietary intake of the vitamin and to establish a normal intestinal flora. Subsequently, levels begin to rise toward adult values. In premature infants and in infants with hemorrhagic disease of the newborn, the concentrations of clotting factors are particularly depressed (*see* Aballi and deLamerens, 1962). The degree to which these changes reflect true vitamin K deficiency is controversial. Using sensitive measurements of non-γ-carboxylated prothrombin, Shapiro and colleagues (1986) found evidence of vitamin K deficiency in about 3% of live births.

Hemorrhagic disease of the newborn has been associated with breast-feeding; human milk has low concentrations of vitamin K (*see* Haroon *et al.*, 1982), and, in addition, the intestinal flora of breast-fed infants apparently lacks microorganisms that synthesize the vitamin (Keenan *et al.*, 1971). The recent increase in incidence of hemorrhagic disease of the newborn is believed to be a consequence of an increased number of births outside of hospital and of an increase in breast-feeding (*see* O'Connor *et al.*, 1983).

Administration of vitamin K to the normal newborn infant prevents the decline in concentration of the clotting factors on the days following birth; it does not, however, raise these concentrations to the adult level. Premature infants usually display less of a response to the administration of vitamin K. In the infant with hemorrhagic disease of the newborn, the administration of vitamin K raises the concentration of these clotting factors to the level normal for the newborn infant and controls the bleeding tendency within about 6 hours (Wefring, 1962).

The routine prophylactic administration of a small dose of phytonadione to the newborn infant is recommended by the American Academy of Pediatrics (*see* Committee on Nutrition, 1961), since it appears to be nontoxic. A single dose of 0.5 to 1 mg should be administered parenterally to the infant immediately after delivery. This dose may have to be increased or repeated if the mother has received anticoagulant or anticonvulsant drug therapy, or if the infant develops bleeding tendencies. Alternatively, some clinicians treat mothers who are receiving anticonvulsants with oral vitamin K prior to delivery (20 mg per day for 2 weeks) (*see* Vert and Deblay, 1981).

Infants 1 to 5 months old seem to be vulnerable to vitamin K deficiency, especially if they have not received prophylactic administration of the vitamin at birth. The vitamin content of most commercial infant formulas satisfies the recommended intake if they are consumed in adequate amounts. However, inadequate consumption of such formulas may lead to a vitamin K deficiency in the presence of diarrhea, antibiotics that reduce intestinal flora, or any of the malabsorption syndromes (*see* below; *see also* Committee on Nutrition, 1971; Lukens, 1972).

Inadequate Absorption. Hypoprothrombinemia may be associated with either intrahepatic or extrahepatic biliary obstruction, because the lipid-soluble vitamin is poorly absorbed in the absence of bile. A severe defect in the intestinal absorption of fat from other causes can also interfere with absorption of the vitamin.

Biliary Obstruction or Fistula. Bleeding that accompanies obstructive jaundice or biliary fistula responds promptly to the administration of vitamin K. Oral phytonadione administered with bile salts is both safe and effective and should be used in the care of the jaundiced patient, both preoperatively and postoperatively. In the absence of significant hepatocellular disease, the prothrombin activity of the blood rapidly returns to normal. If for some reason oral administration is not feasible, a parenteral preparation should be used. The usual dose is 10 mg of vitamin K per day.

The treatment of a patient during hemorrhage requires transfusion of fresh blood or reconstituted fresh plasma. Vitamin K should also be given. If biliary obstruction has caused hepatic injury, the response to vitamin K may be poor.

Malabsorption Syndromes. Various disorders that result in inadequate absorption from the intestinal tract may lead to a deficiency of vitamin K and hypoprothrombinemia. These include mucoviscidosis, sprue, regional enteritis and enterocolitis, ulcerative colitis, dysentery, and extensive resection of bowel. Since drugs that greatly reduce the bacterial population of the bowel are frequently used in many of these disorders, the availability of the vitamin may be further reduced. Moreover, dietary restrictions may also limit the availability of the vitamin. For immediate correction of the deficiency, parenteral therapy should be given.

Inadequate Utilization. Hepatocellular Disease. Hypoprothrombinemia may accompany or follow hepatocellular disease. Hepatocellular damage may also be secondary to long-lasting biliary obstruction. In these conditions the damaged parenchymal cells may not be able to produce the vitamin K–dependent clotting factors, even if excess vitamin is available. However, in some instances an inadequate secretion of bile salts may contribute to the syndrome and some benefit may be obtained from the parenteral administration of 10 mg of phytonadione daily. Paradoxically, the administration of large doses of vitamin K or its analogs in an attempt to correct the hypoprothrombinemia associated with severe hepatitis or cirrhosis may actually result in a further depression of the concentration of prothrombin. The mechanism for this action is unknown.

Drug-Induced Hypoprothrombinemia. Anticoagulant drugs such as warfarin and its congeners act as competitive antagonists of vitamin K and interfere with the hepatic biosynthesis of prothrombin and factors VII, IX, and X. The mechanism of this antagonism has been discussed above and in Chapter 55. The treatment of bleeding caused by oral anticoagulants is also discussed in Chapter 55.

Vitamin K may be of help in combating the bleeding and hypoprothrombinemia that follow the bite of the tropical American pit viper or other species whose venom destroys or inactivates prothrombin.

VITAMIN E

In animals, the signs of deficiency of vitamin E include structural and functional abnormalities of many organs and organ systems. Attending these morphological alterations are biochemical defects that appear to involve fatty acid metabolism and numerous other enzyme systems. Notable is the fact that many signs and symptoms of vitamin E deficiency in animals superficially resemble disease states in humans; however, there is little unequivocal evidence that vitamin E is of nutritional significance in man.

History. The existence of vitamin E was first demonstrated in 1922 by Evans and Bishop, who found that female rats required a then-unrecognized dietary principle in order to sustain a normal pregnancy. Deficient animals were found to ovulate and conceive normally, but at some time during the period of gestation death and resorption of the fetuses occurred. Lesions in the testes were also described, and for a while vitamin E was referred to as the "antisterility vitamin." Further studies, however, revealed the more widespread effects of deficiency of the vitamin (*see* below).

Chemistry. The vitamin was isolated by Evans and coworkers (1936) from wheat germ oil. Eight naturally occurring tocopherols with vitamin E activity are now known. Alpha-tocopherol (5,7,8-trimethyl tocol) is considered to be the most important tocopherol since it comprises about 90% of the tocopherols in animal tissues and displays the greatest biological activity in most bioassay systems. Optical isomerism affects activity; *d* forms are more active than *l* forms.

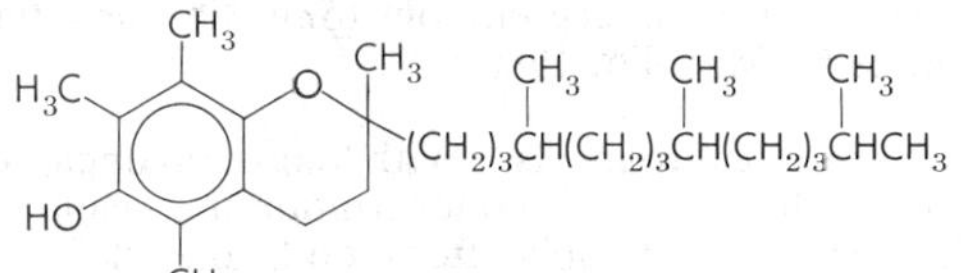

Alpha-tocopherol

Alpha-tocopherol bears a striking structural similarity to the 6-chromanol form of coenzyme Q_4, with which it shares biological activity in several systems.

One of the important chemical features of the tocopherols is that they are antioxidants, and this apparently is the basis for most, if not all, of the effects of vitamin E (*see* Machlin, 1980). The tocopherols deteriorate slowly when exposed to air or ultraviolet light.

Physiological Functions and Pharmacological Actions. Aside from relieving symptoms of its deficiency in animals, vitamin E displays no notable pharmacological effects or toxicity. Numerous contradictory findings and claims for the actions and mechanisms of action characterize the literature on vitamin E. In acting as an antioxidant, vitamin E presumably prevents oxidation of essential cellular constituents, such as ubiquinone (coenzyme Q), or prevents the formation of toxic oxidation products, such as the peroxidation products formed from unsaturated fatty acids that have been detected in its absence. Diets high in polyunsaturated fatty acids increase an animal's requirement for vitamin E (*see* Witting, 1972). However, other chemically unrelated substances, such as synthetic antioxidants, selenium, some sulfur-containing amino acids, and the coenzyme Q group, are able to prevent or reverse some of the symptoms of vitamin E deficiency in animal species (*see* Wasserman and Taylor, 1972). In animals, supplemental vitamin E also affords protection against various drugs, metals, and chemicals that can initiate free-radical formation. However, no such protection has been observed in man (*see* Bieri *et al.,* 1983). Some symptoms of vitamin E deficiency in animals are not relieved by other antioxidants, and it is presumed in these cases that the vitamin is acting in a more specific manner (*see* Green, 1972).

There appears to be a relationship between vitamins A and E. The intestinal absorption of vitamin A is enhanced by vitamin E, and hepatic and other cellular concentrations of vitamin A are elevated; this effect may be related to the protection of vitamin A by the antioxidant properties of vitamin E. In addition, vitamin E seems to protect against various effects of hypervitaminosis A (*see* Underwood, 1984).

Symptoms of Deficiency. Although manifestations of vitamin E deficiency in experimental animals are protean, various effects on the nervous, reproductive, muscular, cardiovascular, and hematopoietic systems are most important because they bear the closest resemblance to the clinical syndromes alleged to be benefited by vitamin E therapy.

Nervous System. In animals, particularly rats, vitamin E deficiency is associated with axonal dystrophy that involves degeneration in the posterior cord and in the gracile and cuneate nuclei. Observations in man suggest a relationship between vitamin E deficiency and a similar clinical syndrome. Patients with malabsorption syndromes that are associated with decreased absorption or transport of vitamin E develop similar neurological symptoms, including hyporeflexia, gait disturbances, decreased sensitivity to vibration and proprioception, and ophthalmoplegia. Visual impairment may result from a pigmented retinopathy. Neuropathological lesions, including axonal degeneration of the posterior cord and the gracilis nucleus, are comparable to those found in animals deficient in vitamin E. In some studies, treatment of patients with pharmacological doses of vitamin E prevented progression of the neurological abnormalities or caused improvement (*see* Bieri *et al.,* 1983; Sokol, 1988).

Reproductive System. Early evidence indicated that vitamin E is essential for normal reproduction in several mammalian species. Prolonged deficiency in the male rat produces irreversible sterility owing to degeneration of the germinal epithelium. In the vitamin E–deficient female, pregnancy terminates in about 10 days with fetal death. The fundamental mechanism by which vitamin E deficiency interferes with reproduction is apparently related to its antioxidant properties, since antioxidants incorporated into the diet can completely obviate the need for vitamin E for normal growth and reproduction in the rat (*see* Machlin, 1980).

On the basis of such animal studies, vitamin E has been used clinically for the treatment of recurrent abortion and for sterility in both men and women. It has also been used in toxemia of pregnancy, disorders of menstruation, vaginitis, and menopausal symptoms. There is no evidence that the vitamin is beneficial in any of these conditions.

Muscular System. In many species a vitamin E–deficient diet leads to the development of a necrotizing myopathy that resembles muscular dystrophy (Mason, 1973; Machlin, 1980). The anatomical and biochemical changes can be prevented, reversed, or ameliorated with alpha-tocopherol or other lipid-soluble antioxidants. The pathogenesis of the dystrophy is unknown. Although myopathic changes may occur in human subjects deprived of the vitamin, there is no evidence for vitamin E deficiency in the muscular dystrophies in man, and the administration of vitamin E is ineffective in these disorders (Berneske *et al.,* 1960).

Cardiovascular System. The lesions produced in skeletal muscle by a deficiency of vitamin E apparently are also found in cardiac muscle of several species, although involvement of the heart is generally less common and less severe. On this basis, vitamin E has been used in many types of cardiac disorders; carefully controlled clinical studies have failed to demonstrate any benefit (*see* Olsen, 1973).

Hematopoietic System. In several animal species a deficiency of vitamin E is associated with an anemia that has features of both abnormal hematopoiesis and decreased lifetime of erythrocytes. Erythrocytes from such animals have increased susceptibility to hemolysis by oxidizing agents. Indeed, in man this *in-vitro* laboratory test is the only consistent finding associated with low levels of tocopherol in plasma (*see* Leonard and Losowsky, 1967). Limited clinical studies in patients with hemolysis due to a genetic deficiency of glucose-6-phosphate dehydrogenase suggest that chronic treatment with large doses of vitamin E may improve survival of erythrocytes and the clinical condition (Corash *et al.,* 1980).

Four clinical situations have been reported to include alpha-tocopherol–responsive anemia (*see* Darby, 1968; Symposium, 1968). (1) A macrocytic, megaloblastic anemia observed in children with severe protein-calorie malnutrition, while unresponsive to treatment with iron, cyanocobalamin, folic acid, or ascorbic acid, was successfully reversed with large doses of alpha-tocopheryl acetate. However, subsequent controlled studies have attributed the defective hematopoiesis to deficiency of protein and/or iron rather than to vitamin E (*see* Bieri and Farrell, 1976). (2) Premature infants may develop a hemolytic anemia that is sometimes associated with increased erythrocyte susceptibility to peroxidative hemolysis and low concentrations of tocopherol in plasma. This anemia has been shown to develop only in infants who consume a diet rich in polyunsaturated fatty acids and fortified with iron (Williams *et al.,* 1975). Commercial formulas for premature infants have been modified, such that they now are very low in iron and have an appropriate ratio of vitamin E to fatty acids. It no longer appears to be necessary to administer vitamin E supplements to premature infants on a routine basis (*see* Bieri *et al.,* 1983; Zipursky *et al.,* 1987). (3) Erythrocytes that hemolyze spontaneously *in vitro* constitute one characteristic of the acanthocytosis syndrome. Patients with this rare genetic disease lack plasma β-lipoprotein and, therefore, have little or no circulating alpha-tocopherol. Further, they have impaired intestinal absorption of the vitamin. Parenteral administration of 100 mg of alpha-tocopheryl acetate can raise the plasma alpha-tocopherol concentration and apparently correct the autohemolytic feature of the disease for several weeks. (4) In malabsorption syndromes characterized by steatorrhea, alpha-tocopherol is not absorbed. Here, too, decreased erythrocyte lifetime and increased erythrocyte sensitivity to hydrogen peroxide are coincident with low concentrations of alpha-tocopherol in plasma and are responsive to administration of alpha-tocopherol. Adult human subjects, intentionally deprived of vitamin E over an extended period of time, have similar hematological lesions and respond to alpha-tocopherol (Horwitt *et al.,* 1963).

While the evidence outlined above seems to implicate vitamin E in normal hematopoiesis, other factors must also be considered. Patients with each of the above syndromes have multiple deficiencies. Furthermore, the ability of the coenzymes Q, selenium, other antioxidants, and the sulfur-amino acids to relieve "tocopherol-deficient" syndromes to varying degrees provides further complications for a definitive interpretation. (*See* Bieri and Farrell, 1976; Machlin, 1980.)

Human Requirements. With long-term depletion in man, the vitamin E concentration in plasma declines significantly only after months on a deficient diet (*see* Horwitt, 1962). It has been estimated that a daily intake of 10 to 30 mg of vitamin E is sufficient to maintain concentrations in blood within the normal range. Although some studies have suggested that diets containing large amounts of unsaturated fatty acids increase the daily requirement (Witting, 1972), it should be noted that dietary sources of these fats are also rich in vitamin E (*see* Bieri *et al.,* 1983). Diets containing selenium, sulfur-amino acids, chromenols, or antioxidants decrease the requirement.

The recommendations of the Food and Nutrition Board of the National Research Council include 10 mg of *d*-alpha-tocopherol per day for adult men and 8 mg of *d*-alpha-tocopherol per day for adult women. (*See* Table XVI–1, page 1525.) Human milk (in contrast to cows' milk) has sufficient alpha-tocopherol to meet normal requirements of infants. Tocopherols are present in adequate amounts in the normal adult diet. Indeed, vitamin E deficiency has not been detected as a primary deficiency disease in otherwise-healthy children or adults.

Absorption, Fate, and Excretion. Vitamin E is absorbed from the gastrointestinal tract by a mechanism probably similar to that for the other fat-soluble vitamins; bile is essential (MacMahon and Neale, 1970). When administered as an ester, hydrolysis takes place in the intestine. Vitamin E enters the bloodstream in chylomicrons by way of the lymph. It is taken up in chylomicron remnants by the liver, and is secreted in very-low-density lipoproteins; subsequently, it becomes associated with plasma β-lipoproteins. Vitamin E is distributed to all tissues. However, newborn infants have plasma tocopherol concentrations only about one fifth those of their mothers, suggesting poor placental transfer. Tissue stores (principally in the liver and adipose tissue) can provide a source of the vitamin for long periods of time, as evidenced by the long time animals must be kept on a vitamin E–deficient diet before signs of deficiency appear.

Seventy to 80% of an intravenously administered dose of radioactive vitamin E is excreted by the liver over a period of a week; the balance appears as metabolites in the urine. The urinary metabolites are glucuronides of tocopheronic acid and its γ-lactone. Several other metabolites with quinone structures have been found in tissues; dimer and trimer forms of the vitamin are believed to result from reaction with lipid peroxides (*see* Draper and Csallany, 1970).

Plasma concentrations vary widely among normal individuals and fluctuate with concentrations of lipids. As a result, measurement of the ratio of vitamin E to total lipids in plasma has been used to estimate vitamin E status; values below 0.8 mg/g are indicative of deficiency (*see* Horwitt *et al.*, 1972). In general, tocopherol concentrations in plasma appear to be related more closely to dietary intake and defects in intestinal absorption of fat than to the presence or absence of disease.

Assay and Unitage. The vitamin E activity of foods may be determined chemically or bioassayed. One international unit (I.U.) is equivalent to the activity of 1 mg of *dl*-alpha-tocopheryl acetate. *d*-Alpha-tocopheryl acetate has a potency of 1.36 I.U./mg; *d*-alpha-tocopherol, 1.49 I.U./mg; and *d*-alpha-tocopheryl succinate, 1.21 I.U./mg. The activity of 1 mg of *d*-alpha-tocopherol is equal to 1 alpha-tocopherol equivalent.

Preparations. *Vitamin E* (AQUASOL E, others) is a form of alpha-tocopherol that includes the *d* or the *d* and *l* isomers of alpha-tocopherol, alpha-tocopheryl acetate, or alpha-tocopheryl succinate. Tablets and capsules of many sizes are available (100 to 1000 I.U.), as are drops. For severe vitamin E deficiency in children, injectable *dl*-alpha-tocopherol (EPHYNAL, 50 mg/ml) is available from the manufacturer.

Therapeutic Uses. The lack of efficacy of vitamin E in treatment of those diseases in man that bear some resemblance to vitamin E deficiency in animals, namely, recurrent abortion, progressive muscular dystrophy, and cardiovascular disease, has been discussed. These are by no means the only disorders in which vitamin E therapy has been studied. The list extends from minor skin ailments to schizophrenia.

The use of vitamin E supplements may be indicated for patients at risk of developing deficiency of the vitamin in order to prevent or ameliorate the consequences of axonal dystrophy (*see* above). Children with cystic fibrosis, cholestatic liver disease, or other types of malabsorption syndromes are especially likely to develop vitamin E deficiency. There is also a rare congenital disorder that is characterized by vitamin E deficiency and neurological manifestations but without a disturbance of intestinal absorption (*see* Sokol, 1988). Correction of an established deficiency can usually be accomplished by the oral administration of high doses of vitamin E (50 to 200 I.U./kg per day). The dosage may be adjusted as the ratio of vitamin E to total lipids in plasma is altered. When oral therapy is unsuccessful, *dl*-alpha-tocopherol (1 to 2 mg/kg per day) may be administered intramuscularly (*see* Sokol, 1988). Pharmacological doses of vitamin E have also been used as an antioxidant in premature infants exposed to high concentrations of oxygen; thus, prophylactic use of an oral preparation (100 mg/kg per day) may reduce the incidence and severity of retrolental fibroplasia (*see* Hittner *et al.*, 1981). Only equivocal results have been obtained in the neonatal respiratory-distress syndrome.

Aballi, A. J., and deLamerens, S. Coagulation changes in the neonatal period and in early infancy. *Pediatr. Clin. North Am.*, **1962**, *9*, 785–815.

Almquist, H. J., and Stokstad, C. L. R. Hemorrhagic chick disease of dietary origin. *J. Biol. Chem.*, **1935**, *111*, 105–113.

Bagavandoss, P., and Midgley, A. R., Jr. Lack of difference between retinoic acid and retinol in stimulating progesterone production by luteinizing granulosa cells *in vitro*. *Endocrinology*, **1987**, *121*, 420–428.

———. Biphasic action of retinoids on gonadotropin receptor induction in rat granulosa cells *in vitro*. *Life Sci.*, **1988**, *43*, 1607–1614.

Barash, P.; Kitahata, L. M.; and Mandel, S. Acute cardiovascular collapse after intravenous phytonadione. *Anesth. Analg. Curr. Res.*, **1976**, *55*, 304–306.

Benbrook, D.; Lernhardt, E.; and Pfahl, M. A new retinoic acid receptor identified from a hepatocellular carcinoma. *Nature*, **1988**, *333*, 669–672.

Berneske, G. M.; Butson, A. R. C.; Gauld, E. N.; and Levy, D. Clinical trial of high dosage vitamin E in human muscular dystrophy. *Can. Med. Assoc. J.*, **1960**, *82*, 418–421.

Bernhardt, I. B., and Dorsey, D. J. Hypervitaminosis A and congenital renal anomalies in a human infant. *Obstet. Gynecol.*, **1974**, *43*, 750–755.

Bieri, J. G., and McKenna, M. C. Expressing dietary values for fat-soluble vitamins: changes in concepts and terminology. *Am. J. Clin. Nutr.*, **1981**, *34*, 289–295.

Bjelke, E. Dietary vitamin A and human lung cancer. *Int. J. Cancer*, **1975**, *15*, 561–565.

Brand, N.; Petkovich, M.; Krust, A.; Chambon, P.; de Thé, H.; Marchio, A.; Tiollais, P.; and Dejean, A. Identification of a second human retinoic acid receptor. *Nature*, **1988**, *332*, 850–853.

Breitman, T. R.; Selonick, S. E.; and Collin, S. J. Induction of differentiation of the human promyelocytic leukemia cell line (HL60) by retinoic acid. *Proc. Natl Acad. Sci. U. S. A.*, **1980**, *77*, 2936–2940.

Butt, H. R.; Snell, A. M.; and Osterberg, A. E. The use of vitamin K and bile in treatment of hemorrhagic diathesis in cases of jaundice. *Proc. Staff Meet. Mayo Clin.*, **1938**, *13*, 74–80.

Committee on Nutrition, American Academy of Pediatrics. Vitamin K compounds and the water-soluble analogues: use in therapy and prophylaxis in pediatrics. *Pediatrics*, **1961**, *28*, 501–506.

———. Vitamin K supplementation for infants receiving milk substitute infant formulas and for those with fat malabsorption. *Pediatrics,* **1971,** *48,* 483–487.

Corash, L.; Spielberg, S.; Bartsocas, C.; Boxer, L.; Steinherz, R.; Sheetz, M.; Egan, M.; Schlessleman, J.; and Schulman, J. D. Reduced chronic hemolysis during high-dose vitamin E administration in Mediterranean-type glucose-6-phosphate dehydrogenase deficiency. *N. Engl. J. Med.,* **1980,** *303,* 416–420.

Dam, H., and Schønheyder, F. The antihaemorrhagic vitamin of the chick. *Nature,* **1935,** *135,* 652–653.

Dam, H.; Schønheyder, F.; and Tage-Hansen, E. Studies on the mode of action of vitamin K. *Biochem. J.,* **1936,** *30,* 1075–1079.

Draper, H. H., and Csallany, A. S. Metabolism of vitamin E. In, *The Fat Soluble Vitamins.* (DeLuca, H. F., and Suttie, J. W., eds.) University of Wisconsin Press, Madison, **1970,** pp. 347–353.

Evans, H. M., and Bishop, K. S. On the relationship between fertility and nutrition. II. The ovulation rhythm in the rat on inadequate nutritional regimes. *J. Metab. Res.,* **1922,** *1,* 319–356.

Evans, H. M.; Emerson, O. H.; and Emerson, G. A. The isolation from wheat germ oil of an alcohol, α-tocopherol, having properties of vitamin E. *J. Biol. Chem.,* **1936,** *113,* 329–332.

Evans, R. M. The steroid and thyroid hormone receptor superfamily. *Science,* **1988,** *240,* 889–895.

Food and Nutrition Board, National Research Council. Fat-soluble vitamins. Vitamin A. In, *Recommended Dietary Allowances,* 9th ed. National Academy of Sciences, Washington, D. C., **1980,** pp. 55–60.

Frick, P. G.; Riedler, G.; and Brögli, H. Dose response and minimal daily requirement for vitamin K in man. *J. Appl. Physiol.,* **1967,** *23,* 387–389.

Fuchs, E., and Green, H. Regulation of terminal differentiation of cultured human keratinocytes by vitamin A. *Cell,* **1981,** *25,* 617–625.

Giguere, V.; Ong, E. S.; Segui, P.; and Evans, R. M. Identification of a receptor for the morphogen retinoic acid. *Nature,* **1987,** *330,* 624–629.

Green, J. Vitamin E and the biological antioxidant theory. *Ann. N. Y. Acad. Sci.,* **1972,** *203,* 29–44.

Haroon, Y.; Shearer, M. J.; Rabin, S.; Bunn, W. G.; McEnery, G.; and Barkhan, P. The content of phylloquinone (vitamin K_1) in human milk, cows' milk, and infant formula foods determined by high-performance liquid chromatography. *J. Nutr.,* **1982,** *112,* 1105–1117.

Hawkins, W. B., and Brinkhous, K. M. Prothrombin deficiency as the cause of bleeding in bile fistula dogs. *J. Exp. Med.,* **1936,** *63,* 795–801.

Hecht, S. Rods, cones, and the chemical basis of vision. *Physiol. Rev.,* **1937,** *17,* 239–290.

Hittner, H. M.; Godio, L. B.; Rudolph, A. J.; Adams, J. M.; Garcia-Prats, J. A.; Friedman, Z.; Kautz, J. A.; and Monaco, W. A. Retrolental fibroplasia: efficacy of vitamin E in a double-blind clinical study of preterm infants. *N. Engl. J. Med.,* **1981,** *305,* 1365–1371.

Horwitt, M. K. Interrelations between vitamin E and polyunsaturated fatty acids in adult men. *Vitam. Horm.,* **1962,** *20,* 541–558.

Horwitt, M. K.; Century, B.; and Zeman, A. A. Erythrocyte survival time and reticulocyte level after tocopherol depletion in man. *Am. J. Clin. Nutr.,* **1963,** *12,* 99–106.

Horwitt, M. K.; Harvey, C. C.; Dahm, C. H., Jr.; and Searcy, M. T. Relationship between tocopherol and serum lipid levels for determination of nutritional adequacy. *Ann. N. Y. Acad. Sci.,* **1972,** *203,* 223–236.

Hubbard, R.; Bownds, D.; and Yoshizawa, T. The chemistry of visual photoreception. *Cold Spring Harbor Symp. Quant. Biol.,* **1965,** *30,* 301–315.

Keenan, W. J.; Jewett, T.; and Glueck, H. I. Role of feeding and vitamin K in hypoprothrombinemia of the newborn. *Am. J. Dis. Child.,* **1971,** *121,* 271–277.

Lasnitzki, I. The influence of A hypervitaminosis on the effect of 20-methylcholanthrene on mouse prostate glands grown *in vitro. Br. J. Cancer,* **1955,** *9,* 434–441.

Leo, M. A., and Lieber, C. S. Hepatic vitamin A depletion in alcoholic liver injury. *N. Engl. J. Med.,* **1982,** *307,* 597–601.

Leonard, P. J., and Losowsky, M. S. Relationship between plasma vitamin E level and peroxide hemolysis test in human subjects. *Am. J. Clin. Nutr.,* **1967,** *20,* 795–798.

Lukens, J. H. Vitamin K and the older infant. *Am. J. Dis. Child.,* **1972,** *124,* 639–640.

MacMahon, M. T., and Neale, E. The absorption of α-tocopherol in control subjects and in patients with intestinal malabsorption. *Clin. Sci.,* **1970,** *38,* 197–210.

McCollum, E. V., and Davis, M. The necessity of certain lipids in the diet during growth. *J. Biol. Chem.,* **1913,** *15,* 167–175.

Mallia, A. K.; Smith, J. E.; and Goodman, D. S. Metabolism of retinol-binding protein and vitamin A during hypervitaminosis in the rat. *J. Lipid Res.,* **1975,** *16,* 180–188.

Nelsestuen, G. L. Interaction of vitamin K–dependent proteins with calcium ions and phospholipid membranes. *Fed. Proc.,* **1978,** *37,* 2621–2625.

Oberg, K. C.; Soderquist, A. M.; and Carpenter, G. Accumulation of epidermal growth factor receptors in retinoic acid-treated fetal rat lung cells is due to enhanced receptor synthesis. *Mol. Endocrinol.,* **1988,** *2,* 959–965.

O'Connor, M. E.; Livingstone, D. S.; Hennah, J.; and Wilkins, D. Vitamin K deficiency and breast-feeding. *Am. J. Dis. Child.,* **1983,** *137,* 601–602.

Olsen, R. E. Vitamin E and its relation to heart disease. *Circulation,* **1973,** *48,* 179–184.

Osborne, T. B., and Mendel, L. B. The relation of growth to the chemical constituents of the diet. *J. Biol. Chem.,* **1913,** *15,* 311–326.

Ottonello, S.; Petrucco, S.; and Maraini, G. Vitamin A uptake from retinol-binding protein in a cell-free system from pigment epithelial cells of bovine retina. *J. Biol. Chem.,* **1987,** *262,* 3975–3981.

Petkovich, M.; Brand, N. J.; Krust, A.; Chambon, P. A human retinoic acid receptor which belongs to the family of nuclear receptors. *Nature,* **1987a,** *330,* 444–450.

Petkovich, P. M.; Heersche, J. N. M.; Aubin, J. E.; Grigoriadis, A. E.; and Jones, G. Retinoic acid-induced changes in 1α,25-dihydroxyvitamin D_3 receptor levels in tumor and nontumor cells derived from rat bone. *J. Natl. Cancer Inst.,* **1987b,** *78,* 265–270.

Quick, A. J.; Stanley-Brown, M.; and Bancroft, F. W. A study of the coagulation defect in hemophilia and in jaundice. *Am. J. Med. Sci.,* **1935,** *190,* 501–511.

Rosso, G. C.; DeLuca, L.; Warren, C. D.; and Wolf, G. Enzymatic synthesis of mannosyl retinyl phosphate from retinyl phosphate and guanosine diphosphate mannose. *J. Lipid Res.,* **1975,** *16,* 235–243.

Seifter, E.; Mendecki, J.; Holtzman, S.; Kanofsky, J. D.; Friedenthal, E.; Davis, L.; and Weinzweig, J. Role of vitamin A and β carotene in radiation protection: relation to antioxidant properties. *Pharmacol. Ther.,* **1988,** *39,* 357–365.

Shapiro, A. D.; Jacobson, L. J.; Armon, M. E.; Manco-Johnson, M. J.; Hulac, P.; Lane, P. A.; and Hathaway, W. E. Vitamin K deficiency in the newborn infant: prevalence and perinatal risk factors. *J. Pediatr.,* **1986,** *109,* 675–680.

Sidell, N., and Ramsdell, F. Retinoic acid upregulates interleukin-2 receptors on activated human thymocytes. *Cell. Immunol.,* **1988,** *115,* 299–309.

Sivaprasadarao, A., and Findlay, J. B. C. The interaction of retinol-binding protein with its plasma-membrane receptor. *Biochem. J.,* **1988a,** *255,* 561–569.

———. The mechanism of uptake of retinol by plasma-membrane vesicles. *Ibid.,* **1988b,** *255,* 571–579.

Smith, F. R., and Goodman, D. S. Vitamin A transport in human vitamin A toxicity. *N. Engl. J. Med.*, **1976**, *294*, 805–808.
Steenbock, H. White corn vs. yellow corn, and a probable relation between the fat-soluble vitamin and yellow plant pigments. *Science*, **1919**, *50*, 352–353.
Strickland, S., and Mahdavi, V. The induction of differentiation in teratocarcinoma stem cells by retinoic acid. *Cell*, **1978**, *15*, 393–403.
Thompson, K. L., and Rosner, M. R. Regulation of epidermal growth factor receptor gene expression by retinoic acid and epidermal growth factor. *J. Biol. Chem.*, **1989**, *264*, 3230–3234.
Vert, P., and Deblay, M. F. Hemorrhagic disorders in infants of epileptic mothers. In, *Epilepsy, Pregnancy and the Child.* (Janz, D.; Bossi, L.; Daum, M.; Helge, H.; Richens, A.; and Schmidt, D.; eds.) Raven Press, New York, **1981**, pp. 387–388.
Wald, G. The molecular basis of visual excitation. *Nature*, **1968**, *219*, 800–807.
Wald, G., and Brown, P. K. Human color vision and color blindness. *Cold Spring Harbor Symp. Quant. Biol.*, **1965**, *30*, 345–361.
Warner, E. D.; Brinkhous, K. M.; and Smith, H. P. Bleeding tendency of obstructive jaundice: prothrombin deficiency and dietary factors. *Proc. Soc. Exp. Biol. Med.*, **1938**, *37*, 628–630.
Wefring, K. W. Hemorrhage in the newborn and vitamin K prophylaxis. *J. Pediatr.*, **1962**, *61*, 686–692.
Williams, M. L.; Shott, R. J.; O'Neal, P. L.; and Oski, F. A. Role of dietary iron and fat in vitamin E deficiency anemia of infancy. *N. Engl. J. Med.*, **1975**, *292*, 887–890.
Witting, L. A. The role of polyunsaturated fatty acids in determining vitamin E requirements. *Ann. N. Y. Acad. Sci.*, **1972**, *203*, 192–198.
Zipursky, A.; Brown, E. J.; Watts, J.; Milner, R.; Rand, C.; Blachette, V. S.; Bell, E. F.; Paes, B.; and Ling, E. Oral vitamin E supplementation for the prevention of anemia in premature infants: a controlled trial. *Pediatrics*, **1987**, *79*, 61–68.

Monographs and Reviews

Bendich, A., and Langseth, L. Safety of vitamin A. *Am. J. Clin. Nutr.*, **1989**, *49*, 358–371.
Bentley, R., and Meganathan, R. Biosynthesis of vitamin K (menaquinone) in bacteria. *Microbiol. Rev.*, **1982**, *46*, 241–280.
Bieri, J. G.; Corash, L.; and Hubbard, V. S. Medical uses of vitamin E. *N. Engl. J. Med.*, **1983**, *308*, 1063–1071.
Bieri, J. G., and Farrell, P. M. Vitamin E. *Vitam. Horm.*, **1976**, *34*, 31–75.
Bridges, C. D. B. Retinoids in photosensitive systems. In, *The Retinoids*, Vol. II. (Sporn, M. B.; Roberts, A. B.; and Goodman, DeW. S.; eds.) Academic Press, Inc., New York, **1984**, pp. 125–176.
Chytil, F., and Ong, D. E. Intracellular vitamin A-binding proteins. *Annu. Rev. Nutr.*, **1987**, *7*, 321–335.
Darby, W. J. Tocopherol-responsive anemias in man. *Vitam. Horm.*, **1968**, *26*, 685–699.
De Vet, H. C. W. The puzzling role of vitamin A in cancer prevention. *Anticancer Res.*, **1989**, *9*, 145–152.
Galloway, P. M.; Lian, J. B.; and Hauschka, P. V. Carboxylated calcium-binding proteins and vitamin K. *N. Engl. J. Med.*, **1980**, *302*, 1460–1466.
Gilman, A. G. G proteins: transducers of receptor-generated signals. *Annu. Rev. Biochem.*, **1987**, *56*, 615–649.
Hill, D. L., and Grubbs, C. J. Retinoids as chemopreventive and anticancer agents in intact animals. *Anticancer Res.*, **1982**, *2*, 111–124.
Kamm, J. J.; Ashenfelter, K. O.; and Ehmann, C. W. Preclinical and clinical toxicology of selected retinoids. In, *The Retinoids*, Vol. II. (Sporn, M. B.; Roberts, A. B.; and Goodman, DeW. S.; eds.) Academic Press, Inc., New York, **1984**, pp. 287–326.
Machlin, L. J. (ed.). *Vitamin E: A Comprehensive Treatise*. Marcel Dekker, Inc., New York, **1980.**
Mason, K. E. Effects of nutritional deficiencies on muscle. In, *The Structure and Function of Muscle*, 2nd ed., Vol. 4. (Bourne, G. H., ed.) Academic Press, Inc., New York, **1973**, pp. 155–206.
Moon, R. C., and Itri, L. M. Retinoids and cancer. In, *The Retinoids*, Vol. II. (Sporn, M. B.; Roberts, A. B.; and Goodman, DeW. S.; eds.) Academic Press, Inc., New York, **1984**, pp. 327–371.
Shearer, M. J.; McBurney, A.; and Barkhan, P. Studies on the absorption and metabolism of phylloquinone (vitamin K_1) in man. *Vitam. Horm.*, **1974**, *32*, 513–542.
Simpson, K. L. Relative value of carotenoids as precursors of vitamin A. *Proc. Nutr. Soc.*, **1983**, *42*, 7–17.
Sokol, R. J. Vitamin E deficiency and neurologic disease. *Annu. Rev. Nutr.*, **1988**, *8*, 351–373.
Sporn, M. B.; Roberts, A. B.; and Goodman, DeW. S. (eds.). *The Retinoids*, Vols. I and II. Academic Press, Inc., New York, **1984.**
Stenflo, J. Vitamin K, prothrombin, and gamma-carboxy glutamic acid. *Adv. Enzymol.*, **1978**, *46*, 1–31.
Stryer, L. Cyclic GMP cascade of vision. *Annu. Rev. Neurosci.*, **1986**, *9*, 87–119.
Suttie, J. W. Recent advances in hepatic vitamin K metabolism and function. *Hepatology*, **1987**, *7*, 367–376.
Symposium. (Various authors.) Hematological aspects of vitamin E. *Am. J. Clin. Nutr.*, **1968**, *21*, 1–56.
Symposium. (Various authors.) Biological actions of carotenoids. *J. Nutr.*, **1989a**, *119*, 94–136.
Symposium. (Various authors.) Retinoids. (MacKie, R. M., ed.) *Pharmacol. Ther.*, **1989b**, *40*, 1–169.
Underwood, B. A. Vitamin A in animal and human nutrition. In, *The Retinoids*, Vol. I. (Sporn, M. B.; Roberts, A. B.; and Goodman, DeW. S.; eds.) Academic Press, Inc., New York, **1984**, pp. 263–374.
Wasserman, R. H., and Taylor, A. N. Metabolic roles of fat-soluble vitamins D, E, and K. *Annu. Rev. Biochem.*, **1972**, *41*, 179–201.

SECTION

XVII Dermatology

CHAPTER

65 DERMATOLOGICAL PHARMACOLOGY

Mary-Margaret Chren and David R. Bickers

The pharmacological basis of therapeutics in dermatology is both unique and fascinating. Medical history is rich with accounts of man's attempts to minister to his skin; increased understanding of the pathophysiology of cutaneous disease now permits linkage of the considerable art of dermatology to a growing scientific base. Unique features of dermatopharmacology include the fact that the target tissue, skin, is also the route of administration of the drug. Skin can function as a reservoir for drugs and as a site of drug metabolism. The target is also itself an active immunological organ, and pharmacological manipulation of skin can have profound effects on systemic processes. And, of course, the target tissue is visible; effects of drugs can thus be monitored directly and continuously, although not always quantitatively.

The majority of drugs that are used to treat dermatological diseases are also employed systemically to treat disorders of other organ systems. The topical pharmacology and use of these drugs, as well as the unique aspects of their systemic use for diseases of the skin, are emphasized in this chapter. The basic features of the systemic pharmacology of these drugs are covered elsewhere in this textbook.

Skin as a Membrane. The primary role of the skin is to act as a barrier, and this role is well served by its structure—a multilayered epithelium of squamous cells. The outermost layer, the stratum corneum, is crucial for the relative impermeability of skin to chemical and physical agents. This layer consists of enucleated cells that evolve from keratinocytes in the basal epidermal layer. Each corneocyte is filled with filaments of α-keratin (a structural protein) embedded in an amorphous matrix that is rich in disulfide bonds. Each cell is surrounded by a thick envelope of involucrin, an intermediate filament protein, and the intercellular spaces are filled with strongly hydrophobic lamellar lipids. This structure of hydrophilic "bricks" in a hydrophobic lipid "mortar" is an efficient barrier to both hydrophilic and hydrophobic substances. There is ample proof that the stratum corneum is the primary barrier to drug absorption through the skin. For example, the rates of penetration of chemicals through live and dead skin are approximately equal, as are those through isolated stratum corneum and whole skin. Stripping the skin of its stratum corneum greatly enhances penetration by agents that are otherwise excluded (Wepierre and Marty, 1979).

The general impermeability of skin poses both disadvantages and advantages for the administration of drugs to achieve systemic effects. Absorption of drugs applied topically to the skin is both slow and incomplete; peak rates are not achieved for 12 to 24 hours (Franz, 1983). Thus, a large amount of drug cannot be given quickly. However, large fluctuations in plasma concentrations of drugs that result from rapid gastrointestinal absorption and metabolism can sometimes be avoided by transdermal administration, as can first-pass hepatic biotransformation. This may improve the therapeutic index of many compounds, and patient compliance may also be enhanced. These factors have contributed to recent interest in transdermal delivery systems for potent systemic drugs with low therapeutic indices and rapid rates of elimination. Examples include nitroglycerin, scopolamine, and clonidine.

Principles of Percutaneous Absorption. Although the permeability of the skin is generally low, some compounds are well absorbed. The rate of diffusion of a drug across the epidermal membrane is proportional to its concentration, the surface area of application, the diffusion constant of the drug in stratum corneum, and the partition coefficient of the drug between the stratum corneum and the vehicle. The diffusion constant is a measure of the mobility of the drug through the matrix of the barrier; increasing molecular size or altering the drug to enhance its interaction with the barrier decreases the diffusion constant (Franz, 1983). Increasing the lipid solubility of the drug usually increases its partition coefficient between the barrier and the vehicle and thus its permeability (Idson, 1983).

The skin is not an all-or-none barrier to drug absorption; it can also function as a reservoir for drugs, especially lipophilic drugs. For example, the application of a topical corticosteroid under occlusion for 24 hours establishes a reservoir that can persist for 2 weeks (Kligman, 1984).

Practical Considerations for Use of Drugs in Dermatological Therapy. *Vehicles.* Percutaneous absorption is affected in at least two ways by the vehicle in which the drug is dissolved. First, the vehicle may hydrate the stratum corneum by inhibiting transepidermal loss of water (*see* below). In general, the more occlusive the vehicle (water-in-oil emulsions, inert ointments), the greater the hydration and the greater the permeability (Idson, 1983).

Second, a change in vehicle can alter the partition coefficient of the drug between the barrier and the vehicle. For example, ethanol partitions more completely into the stratum corneum when dissolved in olive oil than in water, while the barrier:vehicle partition coefficient for octanol is greater if dissolved in water than in olive oil (Wepierre and Marty, 1979). However, a low solubility of the drug in a vehicle limits its concentration and this can reduce the rate of absorption.

Vehicles can have other therapeutic or unwanted effects. Short-term cutaneous inflammation may respond well to aqueous vehicles (*e.g.*, lotions), whereas long-term inflammation often improves with the hydration afforded by lipophilic vehicles (*e.g.*, creams and ointments) (Arndt, 1989). Conversely, vehicles can themselves behave as irritants or allergens.

Hydration of the Stratum Corneum. Drug absorption is enhanced as much as tenfold by hydration of the stratum corneum, mainly because of an increase in the diffusion constant; hydration swells the cells, decreases their density, and thereby decreases their resistance to diffusion (Idson, 1983). High ambient humidity increases hydration of the skin, as do certain vehicles. Occlusion under impermeable plastic film is another method of enhancing drug penetration by preventing transepidermal water loss and increasing epidermal hydration (Sulzberger and Witten, 1961).

Regional Anatomical Variations. Permeability is inversely proportional to the thickness of the stratum corneum, although in some areas where the skin is thicker (*e.g.*, the palms), differences in lipid composition may actually improve permeability. The face and intertriginous areas are sites of enhanced drug penetration (and often toxicity) because of the thinness of the stratum corneum. In addition, the orifices of skin appendages such as hair follicles and sweat ducts provide epidermal fenestrations that are limited but low-resistance shunts for drug penetration (Kligman, 1984).

Inflammation. The barrier function of the skin is compromised by damage or inflammation. For example, the permeability to hydrocortisone is significantly increased in children with severe dermatitis (Turpeinen, 1988).

Age. Children have an increased risk of systemic toxicity from topically applied drugs for at least two reasons. First, because of their greater surface-area-to-weight ratio, a given amount of applied drug represents a greater dose (in mg/kg) as compared with adults (Wester and Maibach, 1983). Second, at least in preterm neonates, the permeability of the skin is increased (Wester and Maibach, 1983). By contrast, the skin of elderly individuals may be less permeable to drugs, perhaps because of an altered lipid content (Roskos *et al.*, 1986).

Dosage. The amount of topical medication needed for a single application is an important factor in dermatological therapeutics. Covering the head, face, or hand requires about 2 g of a product, an arm 3 g, a leg 4 g, and the entire body 12 to 26 g or more (Arndt, 1989).

CORTICOSTEROIDS

TOPICAL AND INTRALESIONAL USE

The introduction of adrenocorticosteroids for topical use in the early 1950s revolutionized dermatological therapy. Structural modifications of hydrocortisone (cortisol) have yielded compounds with increased potency and diminished capacity to affect electrolyte balance. The general pharmacological properties of the adrenocorticosteroids are discussed in Chapter 60.

Chemistry. Although hydrocortisone is active when applied topically, it is not very potent. 9α-Fluoro derivatives such as dexamethasone offer no particular advantage over hydrocortisone. However, chemical modifications that increase the lipid solubility of the corticosteroids markedly increase their activity when used topically. Examples include the acetonide derivatives of certain fluorinated steroids (*e.g.*, triamcinolone acetonide) and several more hydrophobic esters (*e.g.*, betamethasone dipropionate and valerate) (*see* Chapter 60).

Pharmacological Effects and Bioassay. The pharmacological effects of corticosteroids applied topically are similar to those observed after systemic administration. These effects result from interaction of the steroids with cytoplasmic receptors, as described in Chapter 60; glucocorticoid receptors have been detected in both dermal and epidermal cells (Smith and Shuster, 1987). Glucocorticoids exert antiinflammatory, immunosuppressive, and catabolic effects on skin (Ashworth *et al.*, 1988). Dermal synthesis of collagen is specifically inhibited (Shull and Cutroneo, 1983). The mechanism of action of corticosteroids in proliferative states such as psoriasis is probably multifactorial and is probably not due to simple inhibition of cell replication.

A vasoconstriction bioassay is extremely useful to assess the potency and percutaneous absorption of topical corticosteroids (McKenzie and Stoughton, 1962; Stoughton, 1972). Although the basis of the effect remains to be defined, the degree of visible blanching at sites of application correlates with the antiinflammatory potency of topical corticosteroids. A solution of the corticosteroid is applied to the forearm, and the area is occluded for 16 hours prior to observation. The assay also measures penetration and clearance of the steroid (Bodor *et al.*, 1983).

Preparations and Doses. Several topical preparations of corticosteroids are listed according to their potency in Table 65–1. Many physicians find it useful to familiarize themselves with a limited number of drugs from the high-potency, medium-potency, and low-potency classes of agents. Vehicles contribute not only to potency but also to patient compliance; ointments are more soothing for chronic dermatoses, whereas lotions are better tolerated in hairy areas such as the scalp.

Although corticosteroids are often administered at frequent intervals, this may not be necessary in view of retention of these drugs as a reservoir in the skin (*see* above). Patients may become resistant to the effects of corticosteroids; this may not be prevented by alternate day application (du Vivier *et al.*, 1982).

Preparations of relatively insoluble analogs of triamcinolone are most often used when intralesional injections are given because of their longer duration of action (as compared with prednisolone or betamethasone) (Callen, 1981). Commonly used agents are triamcinolone diacetate, triamcinolone hexacetonide, triamcinolone acetonide, and betamethasone sodium phosphate and acetate. Injectable preparations of glucocorticoids are listed in Table 60–4 (page 1449).

Toxicity. Although relatively uncommon, systemic toxicity from corticosteroids administered topically is identical to that observed when these drugs are given systemically (*see* Chapter 60). Laboratory abnormalities that suggest suppression of the hypothalamic–pituitary–adrenal axis are fairly common, although they are not usually associated with symptoms. The risks of systemic toxicity are greatest if treatment is prolonged, if occlusion is used, if large and/or inflamed areas are treated (especially in children), and if the more potent preparations are employed (Bondi and Kligman, 1980). Retardation of growth is a particular concern in children.

By contrast, local cutaneous toxicity caused by corticosteroids is quite common. The most frequent adverse effects include atrophy and striae; these are usually not reversible. Other common side effects include telangiectasias, purpura, acneiform eruptions, perioral dermatitis, and steroid rosacea. Long-term application of corticosteroids around the eye may cause glaucoma or cataracts (Ticho and Ben-Dor, 1971). Infections with *Candida*, herpes simplex virus, or dermatophytes may be masked or aggravated (Bondi and Kligman, 1980). Again, risk factors for these untoward effects include long-term use of potent corticosteroids on diseased skin, application under occlusion, and use in naturally occluded epidermal areas such as intertriginous locations.

Table 65–1. POTENCY OF SELECTED TOPICAL CORTICOSTEROIDS *

CLASS †	DRUG	TRADE NAME
1	Betamethasone dipropionate cream, ointment 0.05%	DIPROLENE
	Clobetasol propionate cream, ointment 0.05%	TEMOVATE
	Diflorasone diacetate ointment 0.05%	PSORCON
2	Amcinonide ointment 0.1%	CYCLOCORT
	Desoximetasone cream or ointment 0.25%, gel 0.05%	TOPICORT
	Fluocinonide cream, ointment, gel 0.05%	LIDEX, LIDEX-E
	Halcinonide cream 0.1%	HALOG
3	Betamethasone valerate ointment 0.1%	VALISONE
	Diflorasone diacetate cream 0.05%	FLORONE, MAXIFLOR
	Triamcinolone acetonide ointment 0.1%, cream 0.5%	ARISTOCORT A
4	Amcinonide cream 0.1%	CYCLOCORT
	Desoximetasone cream 0.05%	TOPICORT LP
	Fluocinolone acetonide cream 0.2%	SYNALAR-HP
	Fluocinolone acetonide ointment 0.025%	SYNALAR
	Flurandrenolide ointment 0.05%	CORDRAN
	Hydrocortisone valerate ointment 0.2%	WESTCORT
5	Betamethasone dipropionate lotion 0.05%	DIPROSONE
	Betamethasone valerate cream, lotion 0.1%	VALISONE
	Fluocinolone acetonide cream 0.025%	SYNALAR
	Flurandrenolide cream 0.05%	CORDRAN SP
	Hydrocortisone butyrate cream 0.1%	LOCOID
	Hydrocortisone valerate cream 0.2%	WESTCORT
	Triamcinolone acetonide cream, lotion 0.1%	KENALOG
	Triamcinolone acetonide cream 0.025%	ARISTOCORT
6	Alclometasone dipropionate cream 0.05%	ACLOVATE
	Desonide cream 0.05%	TRIDESILON, DESOWEN
	Fluocinolone acetonide solution 0.01%	SYNALAR
7	Dexamethasone sodium phosphate cream 0.1%	DECADRON PHOSPHATE
	Hydrocortisone 0.5%, 1.0%, 2.5%	HYTONE
	Methylprednisolone acetate ointment 1%	MEDROL ACETATE

* Adapted from Arndt, 1989.
† Class 1 is most potent; class 7 is least potent.

Therapeutic Uses. Many dermatological diseases respond to topical or intralesional administration of glucocorticoids. The most common of these are listed in Tables 65–2 and 65–3. When potent topical corticosteroids are used, the patient should be switched to less potent agents before treatment is stopped, to minimize the risk of rebound flare of disease (Baker and Ryan, 1968).

SYSTEMIC USE IN DERMATOLOGICAL DISEASES

Corticosteroids are employed systemically, often in very high doses, for the management of life-threatening dermatoses such as pemphigus vulgaris and bullous pemphigoid; these drugs may be lifesaving in these entities. They are also useful for acute and self-limited but debilitating dermatoses such as severe allergic contact dermatitis. More problematic is the use of systemic corticosteroids for long-term illnesses that are not life threatening, such as eczematous dermatitis. As with nondermatological diseases, treatment must be individualized with considerable attention to relative risks and benefits.

The systemic use of corticosteroids to minimize or prevent the neuralgia that may follow herpes zoster (postherpetic neuralgia) is controversial. Many clinicians feel that administration of corticosteroids systemically for short periods minimizes the risk of this complication (Keczkes and Basheer, 1980); others feel that there is no clear evidence of efficacy (Esmann *et al.*, 1987).

Dosage. Single daily doses of prednisone are generally preferred to divided daily doses; compliance is improved and suppression of the hypothalamic–pituitary–adrenal axis is minimized. However, divided daily doses may be necessary for

Table 65–2. RESPONSIVENESS OF DERMATOLOGICAL DISORDERS TO TOPICAL CORTICOSTEROIDS

RELATIVELY RESPONSIVE	RELATIVELY NONRESPONSIVE
Atopic dermatitis	Pemphigus
Psoriasis	Pemphigoid
Eczematous dermatitis	Dermatitis herpetiformis
Contact dermatitis (chronic phase)	Herpes gestationis
	Epidermolysis bullosa
Irritant	Porphyria cutanea tarda
Allergic	Lupus erythematosus
Seborrheic dermatitis	Palmoplantar pustulosis
Stasis dermatitis	Noninfectious granulomas

Adapted from Bickers and associates (1984).

acute life-threatening dermatoses (*see* Bickers *et al.,* 1984). Although generally not as useful in the short term, alternate-day regimens are probably the safest way to administer corticosteroids for longer periods (Fine, 1979). So-called pulse therapy with very large daily doses of methylprednisolone sodium succinate given parenterally (*e.g.,* 1 g intravenously each day for 5 days) may be of value in the management of recalcitrant pyoderma gangrenosum and may be useful in selected patients with pemphigus and bullous pemphigoid (Johnson and Lazarus, 1982). Such treatment may cause cardiac arrhythmias, and appropriate monitoring should be employed when corticosteroids are administered in this manner (Belmonte *et al.,* 1986).

Toxicity. The untoward effects that follow the administration of corticosteroids are described in Chapter 60. Patients with skin diseases such as psoriasis may experience a rebound phenomenon (a flare in the intensity of disease) when a suppressive course of treatment with systemic or potent topical corticosteroids is stopped abruptly. In addition, the nature of the treated entity may change. For example, there may be a pustular flare of psoriasis after rapid discontinuation of suppressive treatment with corticosteroids (Baker and Ryan, 1968). This type of reaction must be considered when assessing the usefulness of systemic corticosteroids to treat relapses of chronic dermatological conditions.

RETINOIDS

Although night blindness has been known since antiquity, vitamin A was discovered only in the early part of the twentieth century; only then was it appreciated that this dietary factor is also an important regulator of the differentiation and proliferation of epithelial cells. When there is deficiency of vitamin A, mature differentiated epithelial cells are replaced with a hyperplastic growth of stratified, keratinizing epithelium (so-called phrynoderma or toad skin). In addition, experimental animals deficient in vitamin A have an increased incidence of certain malignancies (Mahrle, 1985). Selected retinoids enhance the differentiation of epithelial cells (Peck *et al.,* 1977), stimulate the production of mucin, inhibit keratinization, and inhibit the secretion of sebum (Stewart *et al.,* 1983). The synthesis of certain proteins is stimulated (*e.g.,* fibronectin), while that of others is inhibited (*e.g.,* collagenase, keratin). In addition, retinoids appear to function as morphogens—substances that are released by embryonic polarizing zones and that provoke responses in other cells, thereby altering their differentiation (Thaller and

Table 65–3. DERMATOLOGICAL DISORDERS THAT RESPOND TO INTRALESIONAL GLUCOCORTICOSTEROIDS

INFLAMMATORY	INFILTRATIVE	NONINFECTIOUS GRANULOMAS
Acne vulgaris	Keloids/hypertrophic scars	Granuloma annulare
Alopecia areata	Pretibial myxedema	Necrobiosis lipoidica diabeticorum
Eczema, localized		Sarcoidosis
Lichen planus		
Lupus erythematosus (discoid)		
Lymphocytic infiltrate of Jessner/Kanof		
Lymphocytoma cutis		
Psoriasis		
Pyoderma gangrenosum		

Adapted from Bickers and coworkers, 1984.

Eichele, 1987; Wood *et al.*, 1988). Thus, it is not surprising that these compounds have profound teratogenic effects when administered to pregnant women (Lammer *et al.*, 1985).

Vitamin A has been administered to treat a variety of disorders of keratinization. Interest in such therapy has been heightened by the more recent development of synthetic retinoids that have specific usefulness in certain dermatological conditions. Three such agents are currently available in the United States—isotretinoin (13-*cis*-retinoic acid), etretinate, and tretinoin (all-*trans*-retinoic acid). The pharmacological properties of vitamin A and other retinoids are discussed in Chapter 64.

Isotretinoin. Isotretinoin was released in the United States in 1982 for the oral treatment of recalcitrant severe nodulocystic acne vulgaris (Peck *et al.*, 1979). The drug decreases the size of sebaceous glands and alters keratinization of the glandular acroinfundibulum. The latter effect inhibits closure of the pore; such closure is associated with subsequent formation of cysts. The retinoids also inhibit release of arachidonic acid by macrophages, and this may contribute to their antiinflammatory effects (Fiedler-Nagy *et al.*, 1987). Of great importance is that the remissions that follow therapy may persist for months to years.

Other conditions in which isotretinoin may be useful include disorders of keratinization such as the ichthyoses and Darier's disease (keratosis follicularis). The drug may also be useful in the treatment or prevention of malignant skin disease in individuals who have an increased risk of cutaneous cancer; this group includes patients who have been exposed to arsenical insecticides, patients with multiple basal cell carcinomas because of the nevoid basal cell carcinoma syndrome, or individuals with xeroderma pigmentosum (in whom repair of DNA is impaired) (Peck, 1987; Kraemer *et al.*, 1988; Lippman *et al.*, 1988). Isotretinoin is not useful for psoriasis.

Isotretinoin (ACCUTANE) is available as 10-, 20-, and 40-mg capsules; the usual oral dose is 0.5 to 2 mg/kg per day. Daily doses as low as 0.1 mg/kg may work as well, but the remissions that result are generally of shorter duration (Strauss *et al.*, 1984). The usual course of treatment is 15 to 20 weeks; a second course is sometimes necessary after a rest period of at least 8 weeks. The pharmacokinetic properties of isotretinoin are discussed in Chapter 64.

Isotretinoin causes untoward effects with great frequency. The vast majority of patients complain of dermatological reactions, including xerosis, cheilitis, and conjunctival irritation. Hair loss and skin fragility are also frequent. Headache is common, and in some cases may be attributable to pseudotumor cerebri (Bigby and Stern, 1988). Other signs and symptoms of this reaction include papilledema, nausea, vomiting, and visual disturbances. About 25% of patients develop hypertriglyceridemia; a smaller number have decreased concentrations of high-density lipoproteins in plasma, raising questions about patients on long-term therapy developing cardiovascular disease (Bershad *et al.*, 1985). Hypertriglyceridemia is more common in obese patients and in those with diabetes mellitus (Bershad *et al.*, 1985). Although the changes in lipid concentrations are usually reversible, isotretinoin should be discontinued if triglyceride concentrations exceed 500 mg/dl because of the risk of pancreatitis.

Arthralgias are a common complaint, and may be associated with skeletal changes such as hyperostoses and tendinous calcifications (Pittsley and Yoder, 1983). In addition, premature epiphyseal closure and pathological fractures have been observed, usually in patients on long-term therapy.

The risk of teratogenicity is an extremely important factor in the appropriate use of isotretinoin. Major human fetal abnormalities have been associated with the use of this drug, including hydrocephalus, microcephalus, facial dysmorphia, cardiovascular abnormalities, and others (Lammer *et al.*, 1985). *Pregnancy is an absolute contraindication to the use of isotretinoin, and patients should not become pregnant for at least 1 month after the drug has been discontinued.* A negative *serum* pregnancy test should be obtained before such treatment is prescribed for any woman of childbearing age, and oral and written consent should be obtained from all such patients after the risks have been explained carefully. Two reliable forms of contraception should be used simultaneously.

Less common or less serious toxicities include reversible alterations of hepatic function tests, inflammatory bowel disease, decreased night vision, and corneal opacities (Orfanos *et al.,* 1987).

Etretinate. Etretinate, an aromatic retinoid, became available in the United States in 1986 for the treatment of severe, refractory psoriasis. Although the pharmacokinetic properties of etretinate are described in Chapter 64, to be noted is the fact that etretinate and its active metabolites accumulate in fat and plasma after continuous administration, and the half-time for their elimination approaches 100 days or more. The drug has been detected in plasma 3 years after its discontinuation (Orfanos *et al.,* 1987).

In contrast to isotretinoin, etretinate is useful for the treatment of psoriasis; the explanation for this differential effect is unknown. Conversely, etretinate does not have the potent sebosuppressive properties of isotretinoin, and it is thus of little use in acne. The efficacy of etretinate in psoriasis is thought to result from its effect on epidermal differentiation and keratinization, although decreased migration of neutrophils and monocytes has also been demonstrated in treated individuals (Dubertret *et al.,* 1982; Orfanos *et al.,* 1987).

Etretinate is approved only for the treatment of severe psoriasis where other less toxic methods have failed. The drug is especially useful in pustular psoriasis; in one study, 17 of 18 patients were cleared or virtually cleared of disease in 1.5 to 4.5 months of treatment (Wolska *et al.,* 1985). Etretinate is also useful in the erythrodermic variant of psoriasis, but it is less so for the plaque type of the disease. It may also be helpful in psoriatic arthritis and nail disease (Wolska *et al.,* 1983). Etretinate is often combined with psoralen-ultraviolet A (PUVA) photochemotherapy in a regimen known as RE-PUVA (*see* below); this seems to permit the use of fewer, shorter PUVA treatments, as well as lower doses of etretinate (Grupper and Berretti, 1981). Etretinate has also been used experimentally to treat neutrophilic pustular dermatoses, palmoplantar keratoses, the ichthyoses, and malignancies of the skin (Lippman *et al.,* 1988).

Etretinate (TEGISON) is available in 10- and 25-mg capsules for oral use. The recommended dose is 0.75 to 1.0 mg/kg per day initially, given in divided doses. After an initial response is obtained (usually 8 to 16 weeks), the dose is tapered to a maintenance dose of 0.5 to 0.75 mg/kg per day. The drug should be discontinued after the disease has cleared, but it may be necessary to reinstitute treatment (Wolska *et al.,* 1983).

The toxicity of etretinate is similar to that of isotretinoin with regard to mucocutaneous signs, hyperlipidemia (which appears to be reversible), and abnormal liver function tests. The majority of patients on long-term therapy (average, 60 months) developed tendinous and ligamentous calcifications, although hyperostoses were less common than with isotretinoin (DiGiovanna *et al.,* 1986). Etretinate is also teratogenic; 8 of 28 pregnancies in which the fetus was exposed to etretinate resulted in major fetal abnormalities (Orfanos *et al.,* 1987). Given its long elimination half-life, etretinate should not be prescribed for women of childbearing age unless there is no acceptable alternative and the patient is fully aware of the risk. *It is not known how long pregnancy should be avoided after etretinate is discontinued, and assurance on this subject cannot be given even after 2 or more years.*

Tretinoin. Tretinoin (all-*trans*-retinoic acid) is a topical preparation that was first used in the early 1960s for keratotic disorders. Its use for the treatment of comedogenic and papulo-pustular acne vulgaris is now well established.

Like isotretinoin, tretinoin normalizes acroinfundibular keratinization, and it promotes comedolysis (Lowe, 1986). Its effect on keratinization may also account for its usefulness in several other conditions, including molluscum contagiosum, flat warts, and some ichthyotic disorders (Haas and Arndt, 1986). Tretinoin may be effective in preventing or treating neoplasia, and it has been used for actinic keratoses (Orfanos *et al.,* 1987) and less commonly for dysplastic nevus syndrome or basal cell carcinoma (Lippman *et al.,* 1988).

Although not an approved indication, tretinoin is also said to be effective in reversing some of the signs of "photoaging." The drug reverses some of the dermal histological changes that are caused by high doses of ultraviolet radiation in the skin of hairless mice (Kligman, 1986). A randomized, double-blind vehicle-controlled study of 40 patients with photoaging showed improvement in some clinical signs (fine wrinkling) and histological signs of photoaging after treatment with tretinoin (Weiss *et al.*, 1988). The changes that were described were subtle, and these observations require confirmation. In addition, studies are needed to define the risk of toxicity that might result from long-term application of tretinoin to the skin of older individuals.

Tretinoin (RETIN-A) is usually applied once a day (at night, to minimize the enhanced irritability of the skin on exposure to sunlight); application every other day is used initially to decrease local side effects. Preparations include creams (0.025%, 0.05%, and 0.1%), gels (0.025% and 0.01%), and a liquid (0.05%).

Adverse effects of tretinoin include erythema and xerosis of the skin, which improve with continued therapy, and photosensitivity. No birth defects have been attributed to tretinoin. In mice, tretinoin may either potentiate or retard the development of ultraviolet radiation–induced skin cancers (Epstein and Grekin, 1981; Epstein, 1986a).

β-Carotene. β-Carotene is the most active carotenoid found in plants (*see* Chapter 64). *In vitro,* it can quench singlet oxygen and inhibit the formation of free radicals. Its major use in dermatology is to treat cutaneous photosensitivity, especially erythropoietic protoporphyria, in which it increases tolerance to sunlight, perhaps by protecting against porphyrin-induced formation of free radicals (Bickers *et al.*, 1984).

β-Carotene (SOLATENE, others) is available in 15- and 30-mg capsules; the usual daily dose for adults is 30 to 300 mg. The major untoward effect is a yellow-orange discoloration of the skin. Some patients may have occasional loose stools.

PHOTOCHEMOTHERAPY

The skin is exposed to many forms of electromagnetic radiation; of greatest interest to dermatologists is the photobiological action spectrum that includes visible light (wavelengths, 400 to 800 nm), long-wavelength ultraviolet light (UVA; wavelengths, 320 to 400 nm), and short-wavelength ultraviolet light (UVB; wavelengths, 290 to 320 nm). The terms *phototherapy* and *photochemotherapy* designate treatment methods in which light of an appropriate wavelength is used to induce a therapeutic response in the absence and presence of a photosensitizing drug, respectively. To produce its effect in either case, light must first be absorbed by a natural cutaneous chromophore or a photosensitizing drug (administered either topically or systemically). After absorption of photons, the chromophore becomes excited and undergoes chemical reactions that may cause biological effects.

History. Phototherapy is as ancient as the first discovery of the therapeutic effects of sunlight; photochemotherapy was employed as early as the fourteenth century B.C. in India, where plant extracts (psoralens) were used in combination with sunlight to treat the depigmented skin of individuals with vitiligo (Bickers *et al.*, 1984). Brocq first used crude coal tar as a skin photosensitizer in the nineteenth century, and the advent of electric light sources resulted in effective protocols for the management of psoriasis, most notably that described by Goeckerman (1925), who employed topical coal tar followed by exposure to UVB. Psoralens were shown to be useful for psoriasis in the 1950s, and Parrish and coworkers (1974) described the successful treatment of severe recalcitrant psoriasis with oral psoralen followed by UVA, a treatment method known as PUVA.

PSORALENS

Chemistry. Although psoralens occur naturally in many plants (*e.g.*, citrus fruits, parsley, celery, and figs), the drugs available for therapeutic use in the United States are synthetic compounds—methoxsalen and trioxsalen; their structural formulas are as follows:

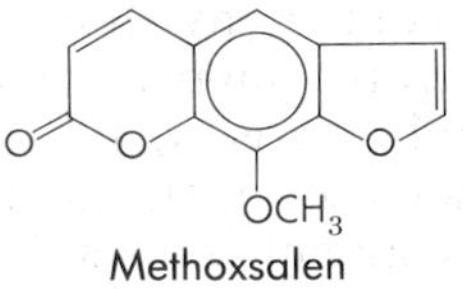

Methoxsalen

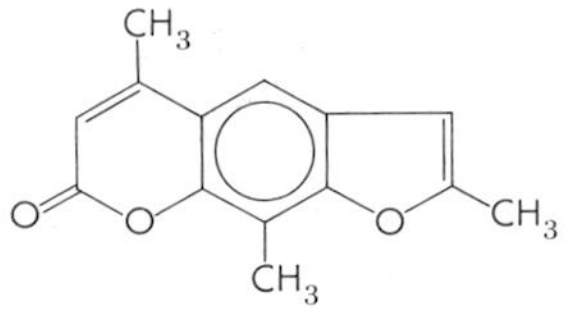

Trioxsalen

The psoralens are furocoumarins; they contain a furan ring fused to a double-ringed coumarin structure. Other derivatives such as isopsoralen and the angelicins (angulated psoralens), have not been approved for use in the United States; however, they may have certain therapeutic advantages (*see* Bickers *et al.,* 1984).

Mechanism of Action. Psoralens intercalate into DNA in the dark but do not form covalent bonds. When exposed to light of the appropriate wavelength (maximum absorption, 210 to 330 nm), the psoralen participates in two major types of photoreactions. The first is independent of oxygen and involves the formation of adducts with pyrimidine bases, either within one strand or between both strands of DNA. Interstrand adducts are most important for both the therapeutic and the toxic effects of the psoralens. In the second type of reaction energy is transferred from the psoralen to oxygen, creating reactive species such as singlet oxygen or superoxide anion. These species then mediate the ultimate effects of the photochemical reaction (Gupta and Anderson, 1987).

Pharmacological Effects. Psoralens inhibit DNA replication as a result of their formation of photochemical conjugates with the nucleic acid. This effect is believed to account for much of the beneficial effect of PUVA photochemotherapy in psoriasis, a disease characterized by epidermal hyperproliferation. However, other effects of such regimens may also contribute. PUVA is immunosuppressive. For example, such treatment alters the distribution and the function of circulating T lymphocytes and suppresses contact hypersensitivity reactions that involve suppressor lymphocytes (Kripke, 1984; Morison, 1984).

PUVA increases melanin pigmentation, and such treatment is useful in the treatment of vitiligo. This action depends on the presence of functional melanocytes. It may involve both activation of melanocyte proliferation and transfer of melanocytes from hair follicles to depigmented epidermis (Ortonne *et al.,* 1979). Studies in animals suggest that PUVA can also suppress degranulation of mast cells; this may explain the reported benefit of such treatment in cutaneous mast cell disease (Danno *et al.,* 1985).

Absorption, Fate, and Excretion. The psoralens are absorbed rapidly after oral administration; photosensitivity is maximal 1 to 2 hours after ingestion of methoxsalen and 2 hours after trioxsalen. The elimination half-lives of the drugs are about 2 hours, but the skin remains sensitive to light for 8 to 12 hours (Gupta and Anderson, 1987). Methoxsalen and trioxsalen are extensively metabolized and can induce the hepatic mixed-function oxidase system (Bickers and Pathak, 1984). When administered topically, psoralens penetrate the epidermis, and substantial absorption can occur. If 1% methoxsalen ointment is applied to half the body surface, plasma concentrations of drug are similar to those achieved after an oral dose of 0.5 mg/kg (Bickers *et al.,* 1984).

Preparations and Dosage. *Methoxsalen* is supplied in 10-mg capsules (OXSORALEN-ULTRA). The usual dose for treatment of psoriasis is 0.3 to 0.4 mg/kg administered 1.5 to 2 hours before exposure to UVA. *Trioxsalen* (TRISORALEN) is available in 5-mg tablets; the usual daily dose for treatment of vitiligo is 10 mg, which is taken 2 to 4 hours before exposure to UV light. A topical 1% lotion of methoxsalen (OXSORALEN) is also available for application to well-defined vitiliginous lesions.

Therapeutic Uses. PUVA is approved in the United States for the treatment of severe psoriasis. Large cooperative trials in both the United States and Europe have demonstrated that disease clears in about 90% of patients with psoriasis after an average of 20 treatments (Gupta and Anderson, 1987); weekly or biweekly maintenance therapy is then instituted.

PUVA is also useful in some patients with vitiligo; localized disease can be treated with topical PUVA, but generalized disease requires systemic therapy. Although some repigmentation occurs in many patients, it is complete in only a minority (Ortel *et al.,* 1986).

Early stage cutaneous T-cell lymphoma may

clear with PUVA treatment, and improvement of stage-II or more advanced disease has also been documented (Honigsmann *et al.,* 1984; Powell *et al.,* 1984). The use of psoralens in a unique therapeutic method known as extracorporeal photopheresis has been introduced recently for the management of cutaneous T-cell lymphoma (Edelson *et al.,* 1987). Blood containing a photosensitizing drug such as a psoralen is passed from one vein through a source of UVA light and then back to the patient through another vein. Depending upon the dose of drug and the intensity of light, lymphocytes may be damaged or destroyed (Gasparro *et al.,* 1986). It is believed that the return of damaged abnormal cells triggers an immune response directed against distinctive antigenic determinants on the abnormal lymphocytes. In one clinical trial, the majority of patients (73%) with otherwise resistant cutaneous T-cell lymphoma responded to this treatment (Edelson *et al.,* 1987); long-term follow-up is not yet available.

Other diseases in which PUVA has been employed successfully include atopic dermatitis (Soppi *et al.,* 1982), alopecia areata (Lassus *et al.,* 1984), dyshidrotic eczema (LeVine *et al.,* 1981), and polymorphous light eruption (Jansen *et al.,* 1982).

Toxicity. Short-term toxic reactions from PUVA therapy include nausea, which may be decreased by administration of the drug with milk, and pruritus (Gupta and Anderson, 1987). Painful erythema and blistering can occur 36 to 48 hours after treatment, although this is unlikely if the dose of UVA is monitored carefully and the patient avoids exposure to sunlight or other sources of UVA (Bickers *et al.,* 1984).

Long-term toxic reactions include changes in skin pigmentation, cataracts, and an increased incidence of skin cancer (but not melanoma) (Stern and Lange, 1988). From 20 to 40% of patients may develop pigmented macules (so-called PUVA lentigines), which appear to be related to dosage and duration of treatment. Although psoralens diffuse out of the eye after 12 to 24 hours, there is concern that the photoadducts may accumulate in the lens (Lerman *et al.,* 1980); animals given large doses of psoralens develop cataracts (Gupta and Anderson, 1987). However, in one large study there was no increase in the incidence of symptomatic cataracts in patients treated with PUVA over a 5-year period (Cox *et al.,* 1987). PUVA may increase the incidence of skin cancer, particularly basal cell and squamous cell carcinomas (Gupta *et al.,* 1988b; Stern and Lange, 1988). Previous exposure to cutaneous carcinogens (*e.g.,* ionizing radiation, arsenic, coal tar) may increase the risk of developing skin cancer after PUVA (Cox *et al.,* 1987).

Although there have been isolated reports of hepatotoxicity after PUVA, this complication appears to be uncommon (Pariser and Wyles, 1980; Freeman and Warin, 1984). Pregnancy is a contraindication to PUVA therapy.

COAL TAR

Topical preparations of coal tar continue to be used in dermatology, primarily to treat psoriasis and eczematous dermatitis. They are a complex mixture of organic compounds, rich in polycyclic hydrocarbons, and produced by the distillation of coal. The mechanism of action of coal tar is poorly understood, but it may relate to the fact that specific constituents such as benzo(a)pyrene are transformed into reactive species that bind to crucial cellular macromolecules (Koreeda *et al.,* 1978). Coal tar also contains photosensitizers that have absorption maxima in the range of UVA. It is possible that photochemical reactions inhibit DNA synthesis as described above for the psoralens (Walter *et al.,* 1978).

Little is known about the percutaneous absorption, fate, and excretion of coal tar, although epidermal metabolism of polyaromatic hydrocarbons does occur, and the urine of treated patients contains mutagenic substances that are probably derived from the applied material (Wheeler *et al.,* 1981).

The primary dermatologic use of coal tar is for the treatment of psoriasis or, more rarely, other inflammatory dermatoses. The Goeckerman regimen (Goeckerman, 1925)—topically applied coal tar that is partially removed before UVB therapy in gradually increasing doses—is a standard and effective treatment for psoriasis; however, the precise contribution of the coal tar to the success of such treatment remains to be defined (LeVine *et al.,* 1979). Many preparations of coal tar are available for topical use in a wide range of concentrations (0.5 to 30%).

Coal tar can cause a phototoxic (probably UVA-mediated) skin reaction known as "tarsmarts." More worrisome is the risk of oncogenesis from the long-term application of a heterogeneous mixture that is rich in polycyclic hydrocarbons. However, remarkably few cases of malignancy have been reported (Bickers, 1981).

HEMATOPORPHYRINS

So-called photodynamic therapy consists of the systemic administration of a synthetic photoactive porphyrin combined with exposure to visible light (Doiron and Keller, 1986). Porphyrins, which are potent photosensitizing agents, are thought to accumulate selectively in malignant cells. Such accumulation may be helpful in early diagnosis, and it may also provide a targeting advantage for photodynamic therapy.

The porphyrins that have been employed to date in these experimental regimens include a complex mixture called hematoporphyrin derivative (or photofrin I) and a more purified preparation called dihematoporphyrin ether (photofrin II). Visible light sources are used (including argon-pumped dye lasers), because the absorption maxima of these porphyrins are about 630 nm. Dougherty (1987) has reviewed the usefulness of such treatment of dermatological malignancies. Initial responses have been encouraging. A major problem has been the long elimination half-time of the porphyrins used, which renders treated patients exquisitely sensitive to light for as long as 4 to 8 weeks.

DAPSONE

Dapsone (4,4′-diaminodiphenylsulfone) is a sulfone that is used for the chemotherapy of leprosy, for prophylaxis against malaria, and in combination with trimethoprim to treat pneumonia caused by *Pneumocystis carinii*. It is also effective in a variety of noninfectious inflammatory dermatoses. Although the molecular basis of dapsone's action in cutaneous inflammation is not clear, it appears to be unrelated to the drug's capacity to interfere with the synthesis of folic acid in susceptible microorganisms. Major features of the pharmacology of dapsone are discussed in Chapter 49.

Many of the dermatological diseases in which dapsone is useful are characterized by infiltration with neutrophils; however, dapsone does not interfere with migration, phagocytosis, or release of lysosomal enzymes by neutrophils (Bernstein and Lorincz, 1981). Nevertheless, several cytopathic functions of neutrophils are inhibited by dapsone, and two hypotheses have been offered to explain its actions. Dapsone may inhibit the myeloperoxidase–based and hydrogen peroxide–based cytotoxic system of neutrophils (Fredenberg and Malkinson, 1987), or it may act as a scavenger of reactive oxygen species, thereby minimizing inflammation associated with their generation (Wozel and Barth, 1988).

Therapeutic Uses. Except for leprosy, dapsone is most widely used in dermatology for its steroid-sparing and antiinflammatory effects in autoimmune bullous diseases and a variety of other dermatoses. Of these, the drug is approved only for the treatment of dermatitis herpetiformis; failure of dapsone to relieve the pruritus of this disease promptly should lead to a reconsideration of the diagnosis. Clinical reports suggest that dapsone may also be useful for a variety of other eruptions, including linear IgA dermatosis (Leonard *et al.*, 1982), chronic bullous dermatosis of childhood (Marsden, 1982), subcorneal pustular dermatosis (Olsen *et al.*, 1979), generalized pustular psoriasis (Macmillan and Champion, 1973), necrotizing vasculitis (Fredenberg and Malkinson, 1987), erythema elevatum diutinum (Vollum, 1968), and granuloma faciale (Goldner and Sina, 1984), among others. In addition, some feel that dapsone is useful by itself or as an adjunct to treatment with antimalarials in certain forms of cutaneous lupus erythematosus (McCormack *et al.*, 1984; Lindskov and Reymann, 1986).

Treatment of dermatitis herpetiformis is begun with a daily dose of 50 mg for adults, and this is increased gradually over 2 to 3 weeks to 100 to 200 mg per day. Improvement should be apparent in 7 to 10 days. Reduction of dosage may then be possible, although there appears to be a threshold for recurrence. Adherence to a strict gluten-free diet may permit reduction of dosage (Fry *et al.*, 1982). Toxic effects of dapsone, which include significant hematological alterations, are described in Chapter 49.

ANTIMALARIALS

Although certain antimalarial drugs have been used to treat collagen vascular diseases since 1894, they were not regarded as acceptable therapeutic alternatives for discoid lupus erythematosus until 1951, when Page described the successful treatment of 18 patients with quinacrine. Aware of the usefulness of chloroquine in other photosensitivity diseases, London (1957) used chloroquine successfully to treat a patient with porphyria cutanea tarda. Subsequently, chloroquine was shown to have a direct effect on porphyrin-containing hepatocytes in such patients, forming drug–porphyrin complexes that augment the mobilization and excretion of the porphyrins (Scholnick *et al.*, 1973). Thus, these drugs are useful in dermatology in two different types of diseases—lupus erythematosus and photosensitivity diseases, especially porphyria cutanea tarda and severe polymorphous light eruption. Three antimalarial drugs are used for these conditions—chloroquine, hydroxychloroquine, and quinacrine. Their general pharmacological properties are discussed in Chapters 41 and 42.

Pharmacological Effects. Chloroquine, hydroxychloroquine, and quinacrine have a large number of effects on cellular physiology, and it is difficult to know which of those described, if any, accounts for their usefulness in dermatology. As weak bases, these drugs are concentrated in acidic cellular compartments. Thus, they interfere in particular with the functions of lysosomes. This impairs phagocytic activity in leukocytes; it also inhibits the recycling of cell membrane proteins to the cell surface after endocytosis. Chloroquine may also alter the structure of clathrin, a protein that coats certain endocytic vesicles (Mackenzie, 1983).

A number of potential antiinflammatory and immunosuppressive effects of chloroquine and its congeners have been described. For example, locomotion by neutrophils and chemotaxis by eosinophils are inhibited (Gauderer and Gleich, 1978; Ferrante *et al.*, 1986). The responsiveness of both macrophages and T lymphocytes to mitogens are diminished, and some complement-dependent antigen–antibody reactions are impaired (Isaacson *et al.*, 1982; Salmeron and Lipsky, 1983).

As mentioned, chloroquine and hydroxychloroquine form complexes with hepatic porphyrins. These complexes are more readily excreted in the urine than is free porphyrin, and this is believed by some to be the mechanism of action of these drugs in porphyria cutanea tarda (Isaacson *et al.*, 1982).

Chloroquine and hydroxychloroquine have a high affinity for melanin, and thus they are concentrated in the epidermis and in the choroid and ciliary body in the eye (Mackenzie, 1983). This may account for the retinal toxicity of these drugs (*see* below).

Therapeutic Uses. Although not drugs of first choice, chloroquine, hydroxychloroquine, and quinacrine are all useful in cutaneous (and rheumatological) lupus erythematosus; only hydroxychloroquine is approved for this purpose in the United States. These drugs are usually used in conjunction with topical corticosteroids and sunscreens. Most patients with chronic (discoid) lupus erythematosus will improve (Isaacson *et al.*, 1982). Hydroxychloroquine sulfate is usually given in a daily dose of 400 to 800 mg for 3 weeks; this is then tapered to a daily dose of 200 to 400 mg.

Phlebotomy is the preferred treatment for porphyria cutanea tarda. However, relatively low doses of chloroquine or hydroxychloroquine are useful in patients who have had an inadequate response to phlebotomy or in whom phlebotomy is contraindicated (Kordac and Semradova, 1974). A test dose of 125 mg of chloroquine or 100 mg of hydroxychloroquine is administered. If there is no untoward reaction (the "chloroquine reaction"; *see* below), treatment is continued with 125 mg of chloroquine or 100 mg of hydroxychloroquine given twice weekly until there is improvement (Isaacson *et al.*, 1982; Bickers and Merk, 1986). Treatment is continued until the 24-hour excretion of uroporphyrin in the urine falls below 100 μg; this usually takes 6 to 12 months (Fitzpatrick *et al.*, 1987).

Chloroquine and its congeners are also useful for the treatment of polymorphous light eruption in patients who are not controlled adequately by avoidance of the sun or the use of sunscreens (Epstein, 1986b). Treatment is usually necessary only during sunny months. The drugs have also been useful in some patients with solar urticaria (Epstein *et al.*, 1963; Willis and Epstein, 1974). The mechanism of these effects is unclear.

Toxicity. The toxic effects of chloroquine, hydroxychloroquine, and quinacrine are described in Chapters 41 and 42. It is notable that the dosages of these drugs used to treat dermatological conditions are significantly higher than those used for malaria, and toxic reactions are correspondingly more frequent and severe. Ocular toxicity including irreversible retinopathy is the most serious problem. This reaction is more common with chloroquine and hydroxychloroquine than with quinacrine. It is not clear if the extent of toxicity correlates more closely with the daily dose or the total dose of the drug taken. Some feel that chloroquine is relatively safe if given at doses less than or equal to 2 mg/kg per day (Isaacson *et al.*, 1982; *see also* Olansky, 1982; Portnoy and Callen, 1983). Exposure to these drugs should be minimized and ophthalmological examinations should be performed twice yearly.

A severe reaction to chloroquine may occur in patients with porphyria cutanea tarda. It consists of fever, nausea, abdominal pain, malaise, abnormal hepatocellular function, and massive uroporphyrinuria as a result of formation of drug–porphyrin complexes (Koranda, 1981).

ANTIMICROBIAL AGENTS

ANTIBACTERIAL AGENTS

Systemic Antibiotics. *Infections of the Skin.* Most skin and soft tissue infections are caused by *Streptococcus pyogenes* or *Staphylococcus aureus*. In general, systemic antibiotics such as penicillins, erythromycin, or cephalosporins are favored for all but the most localized infections, since deeper infections are beyond the reach of topical preparations. The microbiology of skin infections is changing, however, and there is an increasing incidence of infections caused by strains of *S. aureus* that are resistant to many antibiotics. The development of potent topical preparations such as mupirocin (*see* below) may change the traditional preference for systemic antibiotics in managing these disorders.

Noninfectious Diseases. Systemic antibiotics are also used to treat noninfectious dermatological diseases such as acne vulgaris. The predominant organisms that are cultured from pustules in acne vulgaris are nonpathogenic species such as *Staph. epidermidis,* anaerobic diphtheroids, and *Propionibacterium acnes* (Ad Hoc Committee Report, 1975). The traditional explanation for the effectiveness of tetracycline in acne vulgaris is that these bacteria elaborate lipases that cleave fatty acids from triglycerides in sebum (Puhvel and Reisner, 1972). These fatty acids are probably a major cause of inflammation, although their importance has been questioned (Weeks *et al.*, 1977).

Tetracycline is approved for systemic use in papulopustular acne vulgaris; erythromycin appears to be equally efficacious. Penicillins and sulfonamides are not effective, perhaps because they are not concentrated in sebum (Melski and Arndt, 1980). Common dosages of both tetracycline and erythromycin range from 250 mg to 1 g daily; higher doses are occasionally required. Patients who have failed to respond to one antibiotic may respond to the other; minocycline is an additional alternative. In general, these antibiotics are well tolerated during long-term use. Their pharmacological properties are discussed in detail in Chapter 48.

Additional uses for systemic antibiotics in noninfectious skin diseases include acne rosacea, exacerbations of atopic dermatitis colonized by staphylococci, and pityriasis lichenoides et varioliformis acuta (Bickers *et al.,* 1984).

Topical Antibacterial Agents. Topical antibacterial agents are probably of value in reducing the frequency of positive cultures from intravenous catheters (Leyden and Kligman, 1976; Hirschmann, 1988) and in the treatment of burns (Bickers *et al.,* 1984; *see also* Chapter 45). In addition, topical antibiotics are commonly used for localized impetigo contagiosa or other superficial skin infections, and they are of proven benefit in acne vulgaris.

Clindamycin, Erythromycin, and Tetracycline. Each of these antibiotics is effective when used topically to treat acne vulgaris (Dobson and Belknap, 1980; Stoughton *et al.,* 1980). Pseudomembranous colitis may occur rarely after topical use of clindamycin (Basler, 1976; Milstone *et al.,* 1981; *see also* Chapter 48). Colitis has also been induced in animals by the topical application of this antibiotic (Feingold *et al.,* 1979). It seems prudent to avoid using clindamycin to treat patients with inflammatory bowel disease, and the drug should be discontinued if diarrhea occurs (Arndt, 1989). Erythromycin is well tolerated. Tetracycline can color the skin yellow temporarily.

Clindamycin is available as CLEOCIN T in a 1% solution with 50% isopropyl alcohol and propylene glycol or as a gel or lotion. It is applied twice daily. *Erythromycin* is available as a 1.5% solution (STATICIN) or 2% solution (ERYDERM, others) in propylene glycol or polyethylene glycol and alcohol, as a 2% ointment (AKNE-MYCIN) or as a 2% gel (ERYGEL). These preparations are applied twice a day. *Tetracycline* (ACHROMYCIN) is available as a 3% ointment.

Benzoyl Peroxide. Benzoyl peroxide exerts antibacterial activity by virtue of its potent oxidizing properties. It is used most commonly for acne vulgaris, where it may also act as a sebosuppressant and comedolytic agent. It is converted in skin to benzoic acid; any drug that is absorbed is cleared rapidly by renal excretion, and systemic toxicity has never been observed. Local irritation and contact allergy occur in 10% of patients (Melski and Arndt, 1980; Yeung *et al.,* 1983). Benzoyl peroxide is available in a large number of over-the-counter and prescription preparations (2.5 to 10%) as creams, lotions, liquids, bars, and gels.

Mupirocin. Mupirocin (pseudomonic acid A) is produced by *Pseudomonas fluorescens.* It has a unique structure, as follows:

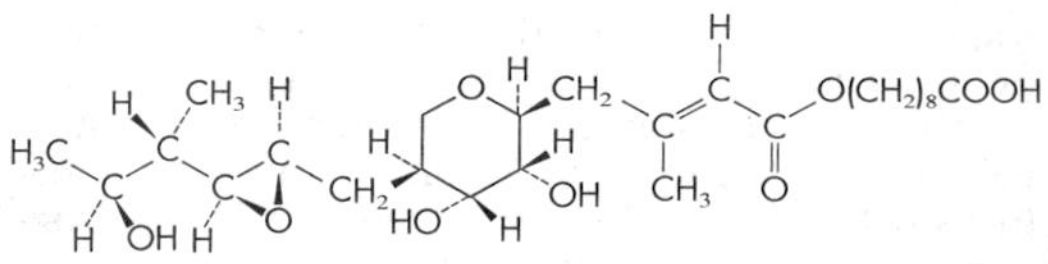

Mupirocin

Mupirocin blocks bacterial protein synthesis by binding reversibly to bacterial isoleucyl-tRNA synthase (Leyden, 1987). This mechanism differs from those of other commonly used antibiotics, and there is no cross resistance. Most gram-positive bacteria are susceptible to mupirocin, but many gram-negative microorganisms are resistant (with the exception of *Haemophilus influenzae, Neisseria meningitidis,* and *N. gonorrhoeae*). Few local side effects result from the use of mupirocin, and there is little to no systemic absorption. Unlike other topical antibiotics, mupirocin is effective for the treatment of impetigo caused by *Staph. aureus, Strep. pyogenes,* or other strains of streptococci. *Mupirocin* (BACTROBAN) is available in an ointment (2%) that is applied to the affected area three times daily.

Miscellaneous Antibiotics. Bacitracin, polymyxin B, and neomycin are available in a variety of topical preparations; many of these contain mixtures of antibiotics. These preparations are used for the prophylaxis or treatment of superficial infections.

ANTIFUNGAL AGENTS

Fungal infections of the hair, skin, and nails are a major source of morbidity throughout the world. It has been estimated that fungal infections account for about 5% of new outpatient referrals to dermatologists in temperate climates and as many as 20% in tropical climates (Hay, 1981). Most of these infections are caused either by dermatophytes or by yeasts, most commonly *Candida* species.

A crucial factor for the successful treatment of fungal infections of the skin is an understanding of the kinetics of turnover of epidermal cells. Microorganisms in glabrous (nonhairy) skin inhabit the stratum corneum, which is normally replaced every 2 to 3 weeks. Since the primary effect of most antifungal drugs is to prevent colonization of new tissue by the organisms, any agent should be used for a minimum of 4 weeks to eradicate the infection. Infections of hair begin at the root, which is 3 to 4 mm below the surface of the skin. Because scalp hair grows about 1 mm per week, treatment should be continued for 4 to 6 weeks to cure infected hair. Many fungal infections of the nails begin in the matrix, and cure thus consists of eradication of the organism from that protected site. This can take 6 to 12 months for fingernails and 12 to 24 months for toenails (where the success rate is probably less than 60%) (Artis *et al.*, 1981; Bickers *et al.*, 1984).

Systemic agents that are used for dermatological fungal infections include griseofulvin (for dermatophytes), ketoconazole (for dermatophytes and yeast), and potassium iodide (for *Sporothrix schenckii*). Topical agents include imidazoles and triazoles, nystatin, haloprogin, tolnaftate, ciclopirox olamine, and naftifine, as well as a variety of older remedies. The pharmacology of the antifungal drugs is presented in Chapter 50. Discussion here includes potassium iodide and older topical agents whose activity may not be directed primarily against the fungi.

Potassium Iodide. Potassium iodide is used to treat the lymphocutaneous form of sporotrichosis. It has no effect on the fungus *in vitro,* and its beneficial effect may be to enhance the tissue response to infection (Horio *et al.,* 1981). Iodide is readily absorbed orally and is excreted in the urine.

The usual oral dose of potassium iodide is 40 drops of a saturated solution (1 g/ml). This is taken three times daily for 1 month or more after inflammation has resolved. Other indications for potassium iodide include erythema nodosum and nodular vasculitis (Horio *et al.,* 1981, 1983). Toxic reactions include lacrimation, nausea, vomiting, metallic taste, swollen salivary glands, halogen acne, goiter, flares of pustular psoriasis, and erythema multiforme (Bickers *et al.,* 1984).

Older Topical Regimens. Castellani's paint (also called magenta paint or carbol-fuchsin topical) contains basic fuchsin, phenol, resorcinol (a keratolytic), acetone, and alcohol. It is mildly anesthetic as well as bactericidal and fungicidal, and it is soothing to moist macerated areas. The preparation is applied one to three times daily (Arndt, 1989). There is red discoloration of the skin; however, there is a similar colorless preparation that does not contain fuchsin.

Whitfield's ointment contains benzoic acid (a fungistatic) and salicylic acid (a keratolytic) in a 2:1 ratio, usually 6%:3%. It is most useful on the palms and soles. It can cause irritation or, rarely, salicylism if used over large areas (Lesher and Smith, 1987).

Gentian violet is hexamethylpararosaniline chloride; it is usually used in 0.5 to 2% concentrations for mucosal yeast infections. It causes deep purple staining.

Fatty acids or their salts are used primarily in combination preparations. The most common contains 2% undecylenic acid and 20% zinc undecylenate (DESENEX, others).

The 8-hydroxyquinolines (iodoquinol and clioquinol) have antifungal and antibacterial effects; they are available either alone or in combination with hydrocortisone for topical use. They may cause yellow staining of clothing.

Antiviral Agents

Antiviral agents such as acyclovir are used to treat serious viral infections that involve the skin, particularly those caused by the herpes simplex viruses and varicella–zoster virus. Interferon alfa-2b is given by intralesional injection to treat condylomata acuminata and nongenital warts. These drugs and their therapeutic uses are discussed in Chapter 51.

ANTIHISTAMINES

The primary use of histamine antagonists in dermatology is for relief of pruritus, particularly that associated with urticaria. The release of histamine and perhaps other vasoactive mediators from mast cells is felt to have an important causative role in chronic urticaria. Because sedation is a common side effect of many H_1 blockers, the nonsedating antihistamines such as terfenadine and astemizole are probably the drugs of choice for this condition (Monroe, 1988). Many studies have demonstrated their efficacy; astemizole is probably more effective than terfenadine.

Cutaneous blood vessels contain both H_1 and H_2 receptors; intradermal injection of an H_1 agonist such as 2-methylhistamine causes pruritus, whereas injection of an H_2 agonist such as 4-methylhistamine does not produce itching (Bickers *et al.,* 1984). However, total blockade of H_1 receptors in patients with chronic urticaria does not relieve itching totally, and some studies have shown that the combination of an H_1 and an H_2 blocker may be superior to an H_1 agent alone for the management of chronic urticaria (Bickers *et al.,* 1984; Aram, 1987) or symptomatic dermatographism (Matthews *et al.,* 1979).

H_2 antagonists such as cimetidine have also been used for other dermatological indications. Although these drugs can themselves cause pruritus, they have been useful for relief of itching associated with lymphoproliferative diseases such as polycythemia rubra vera and Hodgkin's disease (Aram, 1987). The pharmacology of the histamine antagonists is discussed in Chapters 23 and 37.

CYTOTOXIC AND IMMUNOSUPPRESSIVE AGENTS

Cytotoxic and immunosuppressive agents are used in dermatology for two broad categories of diseases—hyperproliferative disorders such as psoriasis, in which they act to inhibit the replication of keratinocytes, and immunological disorders such as bullous pemphigoid or leukocytoclastic vasculitis, in which they inhibit the replication and functions of lymphocytes (*see* Chapters 52 and 53; *see also* McDonald, 1985a, 1985b).

Antimetabolites. Methotrexate is used to treat severe, disabling psoriasis that is unresponsive to less toxic agents. The goal is to reduce the intensity of the disease with the smallest possible dose of the drug, not to attempt to eliminate disease. The drug is given orally, either as a single weekly dose or in three divided doses over a 24- or 36-hour period each week. These two regimens appear to be equally effective (Roenigk *et al.*, 1988). A parenteral test dose of 5 to 10 mg is given initially, and hematological studies are performed 1 week later to evaluate any unusual sensitivity. Methotrexate is also used to treat pityriasis rubra pilaris, sarcoidosis, Reiter's disease, and malignancies such as mycosis fungoides (Bickers *et al.*; 1984).

The toxicity of methotrexate is described in Chapter 52. Of special concern with the long-term, low-dose regimens used in dermatology are hepatic cirrhosis, aseptic pneumonitis, and unexpected pancytopenia. Hepatotoxicity appears to be correlated with the total (cumulative) dose of the drug and is uncommon with doses less than 1.5 g. The extent of damage to the liver is not predicted by the usual function tests, and biopsy appears to be necessary for evaluation (Jones *et al.*, 1986).

Azathioprine is used in dermatology to treat diseases presumed to have an autoimmune cause, including pemphigus vulgaris or bullous pemphigoid. It is usually given concurrently with a corticosteroid in order to minimize the dose of the steroid that must be used.

Fluorouracil is often used topically by dermatologists to treat actinic keratoses. This drug is also used for the treatment of superficial basal cell carcinomas when conventional treatments are impractical. A significant amount (5%) of fluorouracil may be absorbed after topical application. Nevertheless, concentrations in plasma remain low. The treated area becomes increasingly inflamed; this lasts for 2 to 4 weeks, and the lesion then heals. The most significant risk of this procedure is incomplete destruction of the tumor.

Alkylating Agents. Cyclophosphamide is approved for the treatment of advanced cutaneous T-cell lymphoma. It is also used in the management of presumed autoimmune diseases such as systemic lupus erythematosus, pemphigus vulgaris, and vasculitis. In these settings the drug is given orally at a dose of 2 to 3 mg/kg per day in three divided doses, and it is usually given concurrently with a corticosteroid.

Mechlorethamine is used topically for the early (and sometimes the later) stages of cutaneous T-cell lymphoma (Vonderheid *et al.*, 1989). Some believe that the major action of the drug in this condition is to induce allergic contact dermatitis. Toxicity consists of cutaneous reactions, postinflammatory changes, and an increased incidence of skin cancer (McDonald, 1985a).

Cyclosporine. The profound and unique immunosuppressive effects of cyclosporine have encouraged its experimental use in diseases such as resistant psoriasis, with some success (Biren and Barr, 1986). There are also scattered reports of its usefulness in dermatological conditions such as alopecia areata (Gupta *et al.*, 1988a), pyoderma gangrenosum (Shelley and Shelley, 1988), and atopic dermatitis (Logan and Camp, 1988). Topical preparations of cyclosporine are poorly absorbed, and the majority of patients who have been treated for psoriasis have received the drug orally.

Miscellaneous Agents. Vinblastine is used for the treatment of Kaposi's sarcoma and advanced stages of cutaneous T-cell lymphoma; both vinblastine and vincristine are used intralesionally for localized areas of Kaposi's sarcoma. Bleomycin is especially toxic to skin, since this tissue lacks bleomycin hydrolase. The antibiotic is used for the palliative treatment of squamous cell carcinomas and it is administered intralesionally for resistant verrucae vulgaris (Shumer and O'Keefe, 1983).

MISCELLANEOUS DRUGS

KERATOLYTIC AND DESTRUCTIVE AGENTS

Anthralin. Anthralin is a powerful reducing agent with the following structural formula:

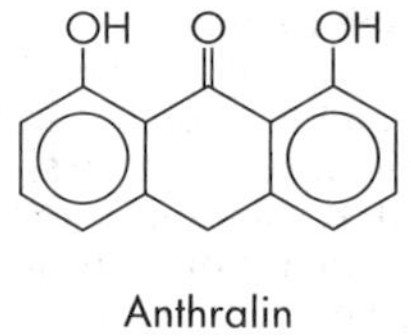

Anthralin

Anthralin is approved for topical use in psoriasis. Its mechanism of action is unknown, although it appears to damage mitochondria and it inhibits epidermal proliferation (Arndt, 1989).

Anthralin (ANTHRA-DERM, others) is available as an ointment or a cream in concentrations ranging from 0.1 to 1%. The major side effects of anthralin include discoloration of skin, hair, and nails and irritant dermatitis; the latter may be the mechanism for its reported beneficial effect in alopecia areata.

Salicylic Acid. This keratolytic agent dissolves the intercellular matrix and thereby softens hyperkeratotic areas by enhancing the shedding of scale (Arndt, 1989). It is available as a transdermal patch gel, ointment, liquid, cream, or plaster in concentrations of 2.5 to 60% for the treatment of psoriasis, warts, and other hyperkeratotic disorders.

Podophyllum Resin. Podophyllum resin (podophyllin) is a naturally occurring mixture of toxic chemicals derived from the roots of the American or Indian May apple plant. Podophyllotoxin is the primary cytotoxic ingredient; it binds to microtubules and causes mitotic arrest in metaphase. Advantage is taken of this local effect in the topical treatment of both condyloma acuminata and other warts; it is also used for multiple superficial epitheliomatosis and keratoses. Untoward effects include ulceration of the skin or severe neuropathy. The latter effect has followed the application of the drug to a large area, particularly including mucosal surfaces (Arndt, 1989). *Podophyllum resin* (PODOBEN, others) is supplied as a 25% liquid. It is also available in combination with cantharidin and salicylic acid.

Cantharidin. Cantharidin is a caustic chemical derived from the beetle *Cantharis vesicatoria*. It has a cytolytic action that does not extend beyond the epidermis, and thus there is no scarring from its application. It is applied topically to warts as a 0.7% liquid (CANTHARONE, VERR-CANTH).

SUNSCREENS

Solar ultraviolet radiation has both short- and long-term effects on the skin. Sunburn is predominantly caused by ultraviolet B radiation; both UVB and UVA probably contribute to aging and to skin cancer.

Sunscreens are chemical or physical agents that absorb or block ultraviolet radiation before it can be absorbed by chromophores in the skin. The most commonly used chemicals are aminobenzoic acid esters and benzophenones, often in combination with cinnamates, and salicylates (*Medical Letter,* 1988); these chemicals primarily absorb UVB. Butyl methoxydibenzoylmethane, used in combination with an ester of benzoic acid, has recently been shown to minimize the photochemical toxic response to UVA in psoralen-sensitized subjects (Lowe *et al.*, 1987). Sunblocks are physical agents that are opaque; they include titanium dioxide, talc, and zinc oxide.

The efficacy of a sunscreen is often defined by its sun protection factor (SPF). The SPF is the ratio of the time of ultraviolet exposure necessary to cause erythema with the sunscreen on to the time to erythema without the sunscreen. SPF values vary from 2 (minimal protection) to over 50. They are not accurate measures of protection from exposure to ultraviolet light because the values are determined under ideal conditions. Furthermore, to ensure efficiency of a sunscreen, reapplication is necessary after perspiration or exposure to water. It must also be realized that reapplication does not extend the "safe" period of exposure.

MINOXIDIL

Hypertrichosis develops in many patients treated with minoxidil (*see* Chapter 33). A topical solution of the drug is now available for the treatment of androgenic alopecia of the scalp vertex in males. The mechanism of action is not clear, although the drug enlarges vellus hair follicles and seems to maintain terminal follicles in the scalps of animals. After 4 months of treatment, approximately 25% of patients achieve minimal regrowth of hair, 7% moderate regrowth, and 0.7% dense regrowth. The response appears to be more favorable in men under the age of 40, in those who have been bald for less than 10 years, and when the balding area is less than 10 cm in diameter (Price, 1987).

Minoxidil is available as a 2% solution (ROGAINE), which is applied twice daily. No systemic effects have been documented, although small changes in hemodynamic parameters have been noted in patients using minoxidil topically. Local effects include cutaneous sensitivity to the drug or the vehicle.

CAPSAICIN

Cutaneous pain and other sensations of chronic inflammation may be mediated by substance P, an endogenous neuropeptide. Capsaicin, a natural product derived from plants of the Solanaceae family (*trans*-8-methyl-N-vanillyl-6-nonenamide), enhances the release of substance P from neurons and prevents its reaccumulation (Bernstein *et al.*, 1987). As a result of this effect, the drug is thought to render skin insensitive to pain by depleting substance P from peripheral sensory neurons. Capsaicin is approved for the relief of pain that follows herpes zoster infections (postherpetic neuralgia).

Capsaicin is available as a 0.025% cream (ZOSTRIX), which is applied three to four times per day to the affected skin after open lesions have healed. The only toxicity noted is occasional local burning.

Arndt, K. A. *Manual of Dermatologic Therapeutics with Essentials of Diagnosis*, 4th ed. Little, Brown & Co., Boston, **1989.**

Artis, W. M.; Odle, B. M.; and Jones, H. E. Griseofulvin-resistant dermatophytosis correlates with *in vitro* resistance. *Arch. Dermatol.*, **1981,** *117,* 16–19.

Ashworth, J.; Booker, J.; and Breathnach, S. M. Effects of topical corticosteroid therapy on Langerhans cell antigen presenting function in human skin. *Br. J. Dermatol.*, **1988,** *118,* 457–470.

Baker, H., and Ryan, T. J. Generalized pustular psoriasis: a clinical and epidemiological study of 104 cases. *Br. J. Dermatol.*, **1968,** *80,* 771–793.

Basler, R. S. Potential hazards of clindamycin in acne therapy. *Arch. Dermatol.*, **1976,** *112,* 383–385.

Belmonte, M. A.; Cequiere, A.; and Roig-Escofet, D. Severe ventricular arrhythmia after methylprednisolone pulse therapy in rheumatoid arthritis. *J. Rheumatol.*, **1986,** *13,* 477–479.

Bernstein, J. E.; Bickers, D. R.; Dahl, M. V.; and Roshal, J. Y. Treatment of chronic postherpetic neuralgia with topical capsaicin. *J. Am. Acad. Dermatol.*, **1987**, *17*, 93–96.

Bershad, S.; Rubinstein, A.; Paterniti, J. R.; Le, N.-A.; Poliak, S. C.; Heller, B.; Ginsberg, H. N.; Fleischmajer, R.; and Brown, W. V. Changes in plasma lipids and lipoproteins during isotretinoin therapy for acne. *N. Engl. J. Med.*, **1985**, *313*, 981–985.

Bickers, D. R. The carcinogenicity and mutagenicity of therapeutic coal tar—a perspective. *J. Invest. Dermatol.*, **1981**, *77*, 173–174.

Bickers, D. R.; Hazen, P. G.; and Lynch, W. S. *Clinical Pharmacology of Skin Disease*. Churchill Livingstone, New York, **1984**.

Bickers, D. R., and Merk, H. The treatment of porphyrias. *Semin. Dermatol.*, **1986**, *5*, 186–197.

Bodor, N.; Harget, A. J.; and Phillips, E. W. Structure-activity relationships in the antiinflammatory steroids: a pattern-recognition approach. *J. Med. Chem.*, **1983**, *26*, 318–328.

Bondi, E. E., and Kligman, A. M. Adverse effects of topical corticosteroids. *Prog. Dermatol.*, **1980**, *14*, 1–4.

Cox, N. H.; Jones, S. K.; Downey, J. D.; Tuyp, D. J.; Jay, J. L.; Moseley, H.; and Mackie, R. M. Cutaneous and ocular side-effects of oral photochemotherapy: results of an 8 year follow-up study. *Br. J. Dermatol.*, **1987**, *116*, 145–152.

Danno, K.; Toda, K.; and Horio, T. The effect of 8-methoxypsoralen plus long-wave ultraviolet (PUVA) radiation on mast cells: PUVA suppresses degranulation of mouse skin mast cells induced by compound 48/80 or concanavalin A. *J. Invest. Dermatol.*, **1985**, *85*, 110–114.

DiGiovanna, J. J.; Helfgott, R. K.; Gerber, L. H.; and Peck, G. L. Extraspinal tendon and ligament calcification associated with long-term therapy with etretinate. *N. Engl. J. Med.*, **1986**, *315*, 1177–1182.

Dobson, R. L., and Belknap, B. S. Topical erythromycin solution in acne. *J. Am. Acad. Dermatol.*, **1980**, *3*, 478–482.

Dubertret, L.; Lebreton, C.; and Touraine, R. Inhibition of neutrophil migration by etretinate and its main metabolite. *Br. J. Dermatol.*, **1982**, *107*, 681–685.

du Vivier, A.; Phillips, H.; and Hehir, M. Applications of glucocorticosteroids. The effects of twice-daily vs. once-every-other-day applications on mouse epidermal cell DNA synthesis. *Arch. Dermatol.*, **1982**, *118*, 305–308.

Edelson, R., and others. Treatment of cutaneous T cell lymphoma by extracorporeal photochemotherapy. *N. Engl. J. Med.*, **1987**, *316*, 297–303.

Epstein, J. H. All-*trans*-retinoic acid and cutaneous cancers. *J. Am. Acad. Dermatol.*, **1986a**, *15*, 772–778.

Epstein, J. H., and Grekin, D. A. Inhibition of ultraviolet-induced carcinogenesis by all-*trans*-retinoic acid. *J. Invest. Dermatol.*, **1981**, *76*, 178–180.

Esmann, V.; Kroon, S.; Peterslund, N. A.; Ronne-Rasmussen, J. O.; Geil, J. P.; Fogh, H.; Petersen, C. S.; and Danielsen, L. Prednisolone does not prevent post-herpetic neuralgia. *Lancet*, **1987**, *2*, 126–129.

Feingold, D. S.; Chen, W. C.; Chou, D. L.; and Chang, T. W. Induction of colitis in hamsters by topical application of antibiotics. *Arch. Dermatol.*, **1979**, *115*, 580–581.

Ferrante, A.; Rowan-Kelly, B.; Seow, W. K.; and Thong, Y. H. Depression of human polymorphonuclear leukocyte function by antimalarial drugs. *Immunology*, **1986**, *58*, 125–130.

Fiedler-Nagy, C.; Wittreich, B. H.; Georgiadis, A.; Hope, W. C.; Welton, A. F.; and Coffey, J. W. Comparative study of natural and synthetic retinoids as inhibitors of arachidonic acid release and metabolism in rat peritoneal macrophages. *Dermatologica*, **1987**, *175*, Suppl. 1, 81–92.

Fitzpatrick, T. B.; Eisen, A. Z.; Wolff, K.; Freedberg, I. M.; and Austen, K. F. (eds.). *Dermatology in General Medicine*, 3rd ed. McGraw-Hill, New York, **1987**.

Fredenberg, M. F., and Malkinson, F. D. Sulfone therapy in the treatment of leukocytoclastic vasculitis. *J. Am. Acad. Dermatol.*, **1987**, *16*, 772–778.

Freeman, K., and Warin, A. P. Deterioration of liver function during PUVA therapy. *Photodermatology*, **1984**, *1*, 147–148.

Fry, L.; Leonard, J. N.; Swain, F.; Tucker, W. F. G.; Haffenden, G.; Ring, N.; and McMinn, R. M. H. Long term follow-up of dermatitis herpatiformis with and without dietary gluten withdrawal. *Br. J. Dermatol.*, **1982**, *107*, 631–640.

Gasparro, F. P.; Song, J.; Knobler, R. M.; and Edelson, R. L. Quantitation of psoralen photoadducts in DNA isolated from lymphocytes treated with 8-methoxypsoralen and ultraviolet A radiation (extracorporeal photopheresis). *Curr. Probl. Dermatol.*, **1986**, *15*, 67–84.

Gauderer, C., and Gleich, G. J. Inhibition of eosinophilotaxis by chloroquine and corticosteroids. *Proc. Soc. Exp. Biol. Med.*, **1978**, *157*, 129–133.

Goeckerman, W. H. The treatment of psoriasis. *Northwest Medicine*, **1925**, *24*, 229–231.

Goldner, R., and Sina, B. Granuloma faciale: the role of dapsone and prior irradiation on the cause of the disease. *Cutis*, **1984**, *33*, 478–482.

Grupper, C., and Berretti, B. Treatment of psoriasis by oral PUVA therapy combined with aromatic retinoid (re-PUVA). In, *Retinoids: Advances in Basic Research and Therapy*. (Orfanos, C. E.; Braun-Falco, O.; Faber, E.; Grupper, C.; Polano, M. K.; and Schuppli, R.; eds.) Springer-Verlag, Berlin, **1981**, pp. 341–345.

Gupta, A. K.; Ellis, C. N.; Tellner, D. C.; and Voorhees, J. J. Cyclosporine A in the treatment of severe alopecia areata. *Transplant. Proc.*, **1988a**, *20*, 105–108.

Gupta, A. K.; Stern, R. S.; Swanson, N. A.; and Anderson, T. F. Cutaneous melanomas in patients treated with psoralens plus ultraviolet A. A case report and the experience of the PUVA follow-up study. *J. Am. Acad. Dermatol.*, **1988b**, *19*, 67–76.

Honigsmann, H.; Brenner, W.; Rauschmeier, W.; Konrad, K.; and Wolff, K. Photochemotherapy for cutaneous T-cell lymphoma: a follow-up study. *J. Am. Acad. Dermatol.*, **1984**, *10*, 238–245.

Horio, T.; Danno, K.; Okamoto, H.; Miyachi, Y.; and Imamura, S. Potassium iodide in erythema nodosum and other erythematous dermatoses. *J. Am. Acad. Dermatol.*, **1983**, *9*, 77–81.

Horio, T.; Imamura, S.; Danno, K.; and Ofugi, S. Potassium iodide in the treatment of erythema nodosum and nodular vasculitis. *Arch. Dermatol.*, **1981**, *117*, 29–31.

Jansen, C. T.; Karvonen, J.; and Malmiharju, T. PUVA therapy for polymorphous light eruptions: comparison of systemic methoxsalen and topical trioxsalen regimens and evaluation of local protective mechanisms. *Acta Derm. Venereol. (Stockh.)*, **1982**, *62*, 317–320.

Johnson, R. B., and Lazarus, G. S. Pulse therapy. Therapeutic efficacy in the treatment of pyoderma gangrenosum. *Arch. Dermatol.*, **1982**, *118*, 76–84.

Jones, S. K.; Aherne, W.; Campbell, M. J.; and White, J. E. Methotrexate pharmacokinetics in psoriatic patients developing hepatic fibrosis. *Arch. Dermatol.*, **1986**, *122*, 666–669.

Keczkes, K., and Basheer, A. M. Do corticosteroids prevent post-herpetic neuralgia? *Br. J. Dermatol.*, **1980**, *102*, 551–555.

Kligman, A. M. Skin permeability: dermatologic aspects of transdermal drug delivery. *Am. Heart J.*, **1984**, *108*, 200–206.

Kligman, L. H. Effects of all-*trans*-retinoic acid on the dermis of hairless mice. *J. Am. Acad. Dermatol.*, **1986**, *15*, 779–785.

Kordac, V., and Semradova, M. Treatment of porphyria cutanea tarda with chloroquine. *Br. J. Dermatol.*, **1974**, *90*, 95–100.

Koreeda, M.; Moore, P. D.; Wislocki, P. G.; Levin, W.; Conney, A. H.; Yagi, H.; and Jerina, D. M. Binding of benzo[a]pyrene 7,8-diol-9,10-epoxides to DNA, RNA, and protein of mouse skin occurs with high stereoselectivity. *Science*, **1978**, *199*, 778–781.

Kraemer, K. H.; DiGiovanna, J. J.; Moshell, A. N.; Tarone, R. E.; and Peck, G. L. Prevention of skin cancer in xeroderma pigmentosum with the use of oral isotretinoin. *N. Engl. J. Med.*, **1988**, *318*, 1633–1637.

Lammer, E. J., and others. Retinoic acid embryopathy. *N. Engl. J. Med.*, **1985**, *313*, 837–841.

Lassus, A.; Eskelinen, A.; and Johansson, E. Treatment of alopecia areata with three different PUVA modalities. *Photodermatol.*, **1984**, *1*, 141–144.

LeVine, M. J.; Parrish, J. A.; and Fitzpatrick, T. B. Oral methoxsalen photochemotherapy (PUVA) of dyshidrotic eczema. *Acta Derm. Venereol. (Stockh.)*, **1981**, *61*, 570–571.

LeVine, M. J.; White, H. A. D.; and Parrish, J. A. Components of the Goeckerman regimen. *J. Invest. Dermatol.*, **1979**, *73*, 170–173.

Leyden, J. J. Mupirocin: a new topical antibiotic. *Semin. Dermatol.*, **1987**, *6*, 48–54.

Leyden, J. J., and Kligman, A. M. The case for topical antibiotics. *Prog. Dermatol.*, **1976**, *10*, 13–16.

Lindskov, R., and Reymann, F. Dapsone in the treatment of cutaneous lupus erythematosus. *Dermatologica*, **1986**, *172*, 214–217.

Lippman, S. M.; Shimm, D. S.; and Meyskens, F. L. Non-surgical treatments for skin cancer: retinoids and alpha interferon. *J. Dermatol. Surg. Oncol.*, **1988**, *14*, 862–869.

Logan, R. A., and Camp, R. D. R. Severe atopic eczema: response to oral cyclosporin A. *J. R. Soc. Med.*, **1988**, *81*, 417–418.

London, I. Porphyria cutanea tarda. Report of a case successfully treated with chloroquine. *Arch. Dermatol.*, **1957**, *57*, 801–803.

Lowe, N. J. Topical retinoids: *in vivo* predictive assays. *J. Am. Acad. Dermatol.*, **1986**, *15*, 766–772.

Lowe, N. J.; Dromgoole, S. H.; Sefton, J.; Bourget, T.; and Weingarten, D. Indoor and outdoor efficacy testing of a broad spectrum sunscreen against ultraviolet A radiation in psoralen-sensitized subjects. *J. Am. Acad. Dermatol.*, **1987**, *17*, 224–230.

McCormack, L. S.; Elgart, M. L.; and Turner, M. L. C. Annular subacute cutaneous lupus erythematosus responsive to dapsone. *J. Am. Acad. Dermatol.*, **1984**, *11*, 397–401.

McKenzie, A. W., and Stoughton, R. B. Method for comparing percutaneous absorption of steroids. *Arch. Dermatol.*, **1962**, *86*, 608–610.

Macmillan, A. L., and Champion, R. H. Generalized pustular psoriasis treated with dapsone. *Br. J. Dermatol.*, **1973**, *88*, 183–185.

Marsden, R. A. The treatment of benign chronic bullous dermatosis of childhood, and dermatitis herpetiformis and bullous pemphigoid beginning in childhood. *Clin. Exp. Dermatol.*, **1982**, *7*, 653–663.

Matthews, C. N. A.; Boss, J. M.; Warin, R. P.; and Storari, F. The effect of H_1 and H_2 histamine antagonists on symptomatic dermographism. *Br. J. Dermatol.*, **1979**, *101*, 57–61.

Medical Letter. Sunscreens. **1988**, *30*, 61–63.

Milstone, E. B.; McDonald, A. J.; and Scholhamer, C. F. Pseudomembranous colitis after topical application of clindamycin. *Arch. Dermatol.*, **1981**, *117*, 154–155.

Olsen, T. G.; Wright, R. C.; and Lester, A. I. Subcorneal pustular dermatosis and crippling arthritis. *Arch. Dermatol.*, **1979**, *115*, 185–188.

Ortonne, J. P.; Macdonald, D. M.; Micoud, A.; and Thivolet, J. PUVA-induced repigmentation of vitiligo: a histochemical (split-DOPA) and ultrastructural study. *Br. J. Dermatol.*, **1979**, *101*, 1–12.

Pariser, D. M., and Wyles, R. J. Toxic hepatitis from oral methoxalen photochemotherapy (PUVA). *J. Am. Acad. Dermatol.*, **1980**, *3*, 248–250.

Parrish, J. A.; Fitzpatrick, T. B.; Tanenbaum, L.; and Pathak, M. A. Photochemotherapy of psoriasis with oral methoxsalen and longwave ultraviolet light. *N. Engl. J. Med.*, **1974**, *291*, 1207–1211.

Peck, G. L. Long-term retinoid therapy is needed for maintenance of cancer chemopreventive effect. *Dermatologica*, **1987**, *175*, Suppl. 1, 138–144.

Peck, G. L.; Elias, P. M.; and Wetzel, B. Effects of retinoic acid on embryonic chick skin. *J. Invest. Dermatol.*, **1977**, *69*, 463–476.

Peck, G. L.; Olsen, T. G.; Yoder, F. W.; Strauss, J. S.; Downing, D. T.; Pandya, M.; Butkus, D.; and Arnaud-Battandier, J. Prolonged remissions of cystic acne and conglobate acne with 13-*cis*-retinoic acid. *N. Engl. J. Med.*, **1979**, *300*, 329–333.

Pittsley, R. A., and Yoder, F. W. Retinoid hyperostosis. *N. Engl. J. Med.*, **1983**, *308*, 1012–1014.

Powell, F. C.; Spiegel, G. T.; and Muller, S. A. Treatment of parapsoriasis and mycosis fungoides: the role of psoralen and long-wave ultraviolet light A (PUVA). *Mayo Clin. Proc.*, **1984**, *59*, 538–546.

Puhvel, S. M., and Reisner, R. M. Effect of antibiotics on the lipases of *Corynebacterium acnes in vitro*. *Arch. Dermatol.*, **1972**, *106*, 45–49.

Roskos, K. V.; Guy, R. H.; and Maibach, H. I. Percutaneous absorption in the aged. *Dermatol. Clin.*, **1986**, *4*, 455–465.

Salmeron, G., and Lipsky, P. E. Immunosuppressive potential of antimalarials. *Am. J. Med.*, **1983**, *75*, Suppl. 1A, 19–24.

Scholnick, P. L.; Epstein J.; and Marver, H. S. The molecular basis of the action of chloroquine in porphyria cutanea tarda. *J. Invest. Dermatol.*, **1973**, *61*, 226–232.

Shelley, E. D., and Shelley, W. B. Cyclosporine therapy for pyoderma gangrenosum associated with sclerosing cholangitis and ulcerative colitis. *J. Am. Acad. Dermatol.*, **1988**, *18*, 1084–1088.

Shull, S., and Cutroneo, K. R. Glucocorticoids coordinately regulate procollagens Type I and Type II synthesis. *J. Biol. Chem.*, **1983**, *258*, 3364–3369.

Shumer, S. M., and O'Keefe, E. J. Bleomycin in the treatment of recalcitrant warts. *J. Am. Acad. Dermatol.*, **1983**, *9*, 91–96.

Smith, K., and Shuster, S. Characterization of the glucocorticoid receptor in human epidermis and dermis. *Clin. Exp. Dermatol.*, **1987**, *12*, 83–88.

Soppi, E.; Viander, M.; Soppi, A. M.; and Jansen, C. T. Cell-mediated immunity in untreated and PUVA treated atopic dermatitis. *J. Invest. Dermatol.*, **1982**, *79*, 213–217.

Stern, R. S., and Lange, R. Non-melanoma skin cancer occurring in patients treated with PUVA five to ten years after first treatment. *J. Invest. Dermatol.*, **1988**, *91*, 120–124.

Stewart, M. E.; Benoit, A. M.; Stranieri, A. M.; Rapini, R. P.; Strauss, J. S.; and Downing, D. T. Effect of oral 13-*cis*-retinoic acid at three dose levels on sustainable rates of sebum secretion and on acne. *J. Am. Acad. Dermatol.*, **1983**, *8*, 532–538.

Stoughton, R. B. Bioassay system for formulations of topically applied glucocorticosteroids. *Arch. Dermatol.*, **1972**, *106*, 825–827.

Stoughton, R. B.; Cornell, R. C.; Gange, R. W.; and Walter, J. F. Double-blind comparison of topical 1 percent clindamycin phosphate (CLEOCIN T) and oral tetracycline 500 mg/day in the treatment of acne vulgaris. *Cutis*, **1980**, *26*, 424–429.

Strauss, J. S.; Rapini, R. P.; Shalita, A. R.; Konecky, E.;

Pochi, P. E.; Comite, H.; and Exner, J. H. Isotretinoin therapy for acne: results of a multicenter dose-response study. *J. Am. Acad. Dermatol.*, **1984**, *10*, 490–496.

Sulzberger, M. B., and Witten, V. H. Thin pliable plastic films in topical dermatologic therapy. *Arch. Dermatol.*, **1961**, *84*, 1027–1028.

Thaller, C., and Eichele, G. Identification and spatial distribution of retinoids in the developing chick limb bud. *Nature*, **1987**, *327*, 625–628.

Ticho, U., and Ben-Dor, D. Developmental glaucoma aggravated by topical steroids. *Ann. Ophthalmol.*, **1971**, *3*, 1257–1259.

Turpeinen, M. Influence of age and severity of dermatitis on the percutaneous absorption of hydrocortisone in children. *Br. J. Dermatol.*, **1988**, *118*, 517–522.

Vollum, D. I. Erythema elevatum diutinum-vesicular lesions and sulphone response. *Br. J. Dermatol.*, **1968**, *80*, 178–183.

Vonderheid, E. C.; Tan, E. T.; Kantor, A. F.; Shrager, L.; Micaily, B.; and Van Scott, E. J. Long term efficacy, curature potential, and carcinogenicity of topical mechlorethamine chemotherapy in cutaneous T cell lymphoma. *J. Am. Acad. Dermatol.*, **1989**, *20*, 416–428.

Walter, J. F.; Stoughton, R. B.; and DeQuoy, P. R. Suppression of epidermal proliferation by ultraviolet light, coal tar, and anthralin. *Br. J. Dermatol.*, **1978**, *99*, 89–96.

Weeks, J. G.; McCarty, L.; Black, T.; and Fulton, J. E. The inability of a bacterial lipase inhibitor to control acne vulgaris. *J. Invest. Dermatol.*, **1977**, *69*, 236–243.

Weiss, J. S.; Ellis, C. N.; Headington, J. T.; Tincoff, T.; Hamilton, T. A.; and Voorhees, J. J. Topical tretinoin improves photoaged skin. *J.A.M.A.*, **1988**, *259*, 527–532.

Wheeler, L. A.; Saperstein, M. D.; and Lowe, N. J. Mutagenicity of urine from psoriatic patients undergoing treatment with coal tar and ultraviolet light. *J. Invest. Dermatol.*, **1981**, *77*, 181–185.

Willis, I., and Epstein, J. H. Solar- vs. heat-induced urticaria. *Arch. Dermatol.*, **1974**, *110*, 389–392.

Wolska, H.; Jablonska, S.; and Bounameaux, Y. Etretinate in severe psoriasis. Results of double-blind study and maintenance therapy in pustular psoriasis. *J. Am. Acad. Dermatol.*, **1983**, *9*, 883–889.

Wolska, H.; Jablonska, S.; Langner, A.; and Fraczykowska, M. Etretinate therapy in generalized pustular psoriasis (Zumbusch Type). Immediate and long-term results. *Dermatologica*, **1985**, *171*, 297–304.

Yeung, D.; Nacht, S.; Bucks, D.; and Maibach, H. I. Benzoyl peroxide: percutaneous penetration and metabolic disposition. II. Effect of concentration. *J. Am. Acad. Dermatol.*, **1983**, *9*, 920–924.

Monographs and Reviews

Ad Hoc Committee Report on the Use of Antibiotics in Dermatology. Systemic antibiotics for treatment of acne vulgaris. Efficacy and safety. *Arch. Dermatol.*, **1975**, *111*, 1630–1636.

Aram, H. Cimetidine in dermatology. *Int. J. Dermatol.*, **1987**, *26*, 161–166.

Bernstein, J. E., and Lorincz, A. L. Sulfonamides and sulfones in dermatologic therapy. *Int. J. Dermatol.*, **1981**, *20*, 81–88.

Bickers, D. R., and Pathak, M. A. Psoralen pharmacology: studies on metabolism and enzyme induction. In, *Photobiologic, Toxicologic, and Pharmacologic Aspects of Psoralens*. (Pathak, M. A., and Dunnick, J. K., eds.) National Cancer Institute Monograph, Vol. 66., U.S. Department of Health and Human Services, Bethesda, Md., **1984**, pp. 77–84.

Bigby, M., and Stern, R. S. Adverse reactions to isotretinoin. *J. Am. Acad. Dermatol.*, **1988**, *18*, 543–553.

Biren, C. A., and Barr, R. J. Dermatologic applications of cyclosporine. *Arch. Dermatol.*, **1986**, *122*, 1028–1032.

Callen, J. P. Intralesional corticosteroids. *J. Am. Acad. Dermatol.*, **1981**, *4*, 149–151.

Doiron, D. R., and Keller, G. S. Porphyrin photodynamic therapy: principles and clinical applications. *Curr. Probl. Dermatol.*, **1986**, *15*, 85–93.

Dougherty, T. J. Photosensitizers: therapy and detection of malignant tumors. *Photochem. Photobiol.*, **1987**, *45*, 879–889.

Epstein, J. H. Polymorphous light eruption. *Dermatol. Clin.*, **1986b**, *4*, 243–251.

Epstein, J. H.; Vandenberg, J. J.; and Wright, W. L. Solar urticaria. *Arch. Dermatol.*, **1963**, *88*, 135–141.

Fine, R. M. The systemic use of corticosteroids in dermatology. *Prog. Dermatol.*, **1979**, *13*, 1–4.

Franz, T. J. Kinetics of cutaneous drug penetration. *Int. J. Dermatol.*, **1983**, *22*, 499–505.

Gupta, A. K., and Anderson, T. F. Psoralen photochemotherapy. *J. Am. Acad. Dermatol.*, **1987**, *17*, 703–734.

Haas, A., and Arndt, K. A. Selected therapeutic applications of topical tretinoin. *J. Am. Acad. Dermatol.*, **1986**, *15*, 870–877.

Hay, R. J. Treatment of superficial fungal infections. *Clin. Exp. Dermatol.*, **1981**, *6*, 509–513.

Hirschmann, J. V. Topical antibiotics in dermatology. *Arch. Dermatol.*, **1988**, *124*, 1691–1700.

Idson, B. Vehicle effects in percutaneous absorption. *Drug Metab. Rev.*, **1983**, *14*, 207–222.

Isaacson, D.; Elgart, M.; and Turner, M. L. Antimalarials in dermatology. *Int. J. Dermatol.*, **1982**, *21*, 379–395.

Koranda, F. C. Antimalarials. *J. Am. Acad. Dermatol.*, **1981**, *4*, 650–655.

Kripke, M. L. Effects of methoxsalen plus near-ultraviolet radiation or mid-ultraviolet radiation on immunologic mechanisms. In, *Photobiologic, Toxicologic, and Pharmacologic Aspects of Psoralens*. (Pathak, M. A., and Dunnick, J. K., eds.) National Cancer Institute Monograph, Vol. 66, U.S. Department of Health and Human Services, Bethesda, Md., **1984**, pp. 247–251.

Leonard, J. N., and others. Linear IgA disease in adults. *Br. J. Dermatol.*, **1982**, *107*, 301–316.

Lerman, S.; Megaw, J.; and Willis, I. Potential ocular complications from PUVA therapy and their prevention. *J. Invest. Dermatol.*, **1980**, *74*, 197–199.

Lesher, J. L., and Smith, J. G. Antifungal agents in dermatology. *J. Am. Acad. Dermatol.*, **1987**, *17*, 383–394.

McDonald, C. J. Cytotoxic agents for use in dermatology. I. *J. Am. Acad. Dermatol.*, **1985a**, *12*, 753–775.

———. Use of cytotoxic drugs in dermatologic diseases. II. *J. Am. Acad. Dermatol.*, **1985b**, *12*, 965–975.

Mackenzie, A. H. Pharmacologic actions of 4-aminoquinoline compounds. *Am. J. Med.*, **1983**, *75*, Suppl. 1A, 40–45.

Mahrle, G. Retinoids in oncology. *Curr. Probl. Dermatol.*, **1985**, *13*, 128–163.

Melski, J. W., and Arndt, K. A. Topical therapy for acne. *N. Engl. J. Med.*, **1980**, *302*, 503–506.

Monroe, E. W. Chronic urticaria: review of nonsedating H_1 antihistamines in treatment. *J. Am. Acad. Dermatol.*, **1988**, *19*, 842–849.

Morison, W. L. *In vivo* effects of psoralens plus long-wave ultraviolet radiation on immunity. In, *Photobiologic, Toxicologic, and Pharmacologic Aspects of Psoralens*. (Pathak, M. A., and Dunnick, J. K., eds.) National Cancer Institute Monograph, Vol. 66, U.S. Department of Health and Human Services, Bethesda, Md., **1984**, pp. 243–246.

Olansky, A. J. Antimalarials and ophthalmologic safety. *J. Am. Acad. Dermatol.*, **1982**, *6*, 19–23.

Orfanos, C. E.; Ehlert, R.; and Gollnick, H. The retinoids. A review of their clinical pharmacology and therapeutic use. *Drugs*, **1987**, *34*, 459–503.

Ortel, B.; Tanew, A.; and Honigsmann, H. Vitiligo treatment. *Curr. Probl. Dermatol.*, **1986**, *15*, 265–271.

Portnoy, J. Z., and Callen, J. P. Ophthalmologic aspects of chloroquine and hydroxychloroquine therapy. *Int. J. Dermatol.*, **1983**, *22*, 273–278.

Price, V. H. Summary. ROGAINE (topical minoxidil 2%) in the management of male pattern baldness and alopecia areata. Proceedings of a symposium. *J. Am. Acad. Dermatol.*, **1987**, *16*, 749–750.

Roenigk, H. H.; Auerbach, R.; Maibach, H. I.; and Weinstein, G. D. Methotrexate in psoriasis: revised guidelines. *J. Am. Acad. Dermatol.*, **1988**, *19*, 145–156.

Wepierre, J., and Marty, J. P. Percutaneous absorption of drugs. *Trends Pharmacol. Sci.*, **1979**, *1*, 23–26.

Wester, R. C., and Maibach, H. I. Cutaneous pharmacokinetics: 10 steps to percutaneous absorption. *Drug Metab. Rev.*, **1983**, *14*, 169–205.

Wood, E. J.; Raxworthy, M. J.; and Holland, D. B. Retinoids and the epidermis. *Biochem. Soc. Trans.*, **1988**, *16*, 668–671.

Wozel, G., and Barth, J. Current aspects of modes of action of dapsone. *J. Invest. Dermatol.*, **1988**, *27*, 547–552.

SECTION XVIII Toxicology

CHAPTER 66 HEAVY METALS AND HEAVY-METAL ANTAGONISTS

Curtis D. Klaassen

People have always been exposed to heavy metals in the environment. In areas with high concentrations, metallic contamination of food and water probably led to the first poisonings. Metals leached from eating utensils and cookware have also contributed to inadvertent poisonings. The emergence of the industrial age and large-scale mining brought occupational diseases caused by various toxic metals. Metallic constituents of pesticides and therapeutic agents (*e.g.*, antimicrobials) were additional sources of hazardous exposure. The burning of fossil fuels containing heavy metals, the addition of tetraethyllead to gasoline, and the increase in industrial applications of metals have now made environmental pollution the major source of heavy-metal poisoning.

Heavy metals, which, of course, cannot be metabolized, persist in the body and exert their toxic effects by combining with one or more reactive groups (ligands) essential for normal physiological functions. Heavy-metal antagonists (chelating agents) are designed specifically to compete with these groups for the metals, and thereby prevent or reverse toxic effects and enhance the excretion of metals. Heavy metals, particularly those in the transition series, may react with O-, S-, and N-containing ligands, which in the body take the form of —OH, —COO^-, —OPO_3H^-, >C=O, —SH, —S—S—, —NH_2, and >NH. The resultant metal complex (or coordination compound) is formed by a coordinate bond—one in which both electrons are contributed by the ligand.

The heavy-metal antagonists discussed in this chapter possess the common property of forming complexes with heavy metals, thereby preventing or reversing the binding of metallic cations to body ligands. These drugs are referred to as *chelating agents*. A *chelate* is a complex formed between a metal and a compound that contains two or more potential ligands. The product of such a reaction is a heterocyclic ring. Five- and six-membered chelate rings are the most stable, and a polydentate (multiligand) chelator is typically designed to form such a highly stable complex. Formation of a polydentate chelate results in a far more stable compound than when the metal is combined with only one ligand atom.

The stability of chelates varies with the metal and the ligand atoms. For example, lead and mercury have greater affinities for sulfur and nitrogen than for oxygen ligands; calcium behaves in the opposite manner. These differences in affinity serve as the basis of selectivity of action of a chelating agent in the body.

The effectiveness of a chelating agent for the treatment of poisoning by a heavy metal depends on several factors. These include the relative affinity of the chelator for the heavy metal as compared to essential body metals, the distribution of the chelator in the body as compared with the distribution of the metal, and the ability of the chelator to mobilize the metal from the body once chelated.

An ideal chelating agent would have the following properties: high solubility in water, resistance to biotransformation, ability to reach sites of metal storage, capacity to form nontoxic complexes with toxic metals, ability to retain chelating activity at the pH of body fluids, and ready excretion of the chelate. A low affinity for Ca^{2+} is also desirable, because Ca^{2+} in plasma is readily available for chelation and a drug might produce hypocalcemia despite high affinity for heavy metals. The most important property is greater affinity for the metal than that possessed by the endogenous ligands. The large number of available ligands in the body is a formidable barrier to the effectiveness of a chelating agent. Observations *in vitro* on chelator–metal interactions provide only a rough guide to the treatment of heavy-metal poisoning. Empirical observations *in vivo* are necessary to determine the clinical utility of a chelating agent.

LEAD

Lead is virtually ubiquitous in the environment as a result of its natural occurrence and its industrial use. The use of lesser amounts of lead (*e.g.*, tetraethyllead) in gasoline during the past decade has resulted in a decrease in blood lead concentrations in man (Annest *et al.*, 1983). Overall, human exposure to lead is primarily from food. The average daily intake of lead for an adult in the United States ranges from 0.1 to 2 mg. However, most of the overt toxicity from lead results from environmental and industrial exposure.

Acidic foods and beverages, including tomato juice, fruit juice, cola drinks, cider, and pickles, can dissolve the lead in improperly glazed containers. Food and beverage thus contaminated have caused fatal human lead poisoning. Lead is also a common contaminant of illicitly distilled whisky ("moonshine") made in the United States because automobile radiators are frequently used as condensers and other components are connected by lead solder. Lead poisoning in children is a fairly common result of their ingestion of paint chips from old buildings. Paints applied to dwellings before World War II, when lead carbonate (white) and lead oxide (red) were common constituents of both interior and exterior house paint, are primarily responsible. In such paint, lead may constitute 5 to 40% of dried solids. Young children are poisoned most often by nibbling lead-painted windowsills and frames. The American Standards Association specified in 1955 that paints for toys, furniture, and the interior of dwellings should not contain more than 1% lead in the final dried solids of fresh paint (National Academy of Sciences, 1972). Lead poisoning from the use of discarded automobile-battery casings made of wood and vulcanite and used as fuel during times of economic distress has been reported. Sporadic cases of lead poisoning have been traced to miscellaneous sources such as lead toys, lead dust in shooting galleries, drinking water that is conveyed through lead pipes, artists' paint pigments, ashes and fumes of painted wood, jewelers' wastes, home battery manufacture, and lead type.

Occupational exposure to lead has decreased markedly over the past 50 years because of appropriate regulations and programs of medical surveillance. Workers in lead smelters have the highest potential for exposure, since fumes are generated and dust containing lead oxide is deposited in their environment. Workers in storage-battery factories face similar risks.

Absorption, Distribution, and Excretion. The major routes of absorption of lead are from the gastrointestinal tract and the respiratory system. Gastrointestinal absorption of lead varies with age; adults absorb approximately 10% of ingested lead, while children absorb up to 40%. Little is known about lead transport across the gastrointestinal mucosa. It has been speculated that Pb^{2+} and Ca^{2+} may compete for a common transport mechanism, since there is a reciprocal relationship between the dietary content of calcium and lead absorption. Iron deficiency has also been shown to enhance intestinal absorption of lead. Absorption of inhaled lead varies with the form (vapor versus particle), as well as with concentration. Approximately 90% of inhaled lead particles from ambient air are absorbed (Goyer, 1985).

After absorption, inorganic lead is distributed initially in the soft tissues, particularly the tubular epithelium of the kidney and in the liver. In time, lead is redistributed and deposited in bone, teeth, and hair. About 95% of the body burden of the metal is eventually found in bone. Only small quantities of inorganic lead accumulate in the brain, with most of that in gray matter and the basal ganglia (Task Group on Metal Accumulation, 1973). Nearly all circulating inorganic lead is associated with erythrocytes; only when lead is present in relatively high concentrations does a significant portion remain in the plasma.

The deposition of lead in bone closely resembles that of calcium, but it is deposited as tertiary lead phosphate. Lead in the bone salts does not contribute to toxicity. After a recent exposure, the concentration of lead is often higher in the flat bones than in the long bones (Kehoe, 1961a, 1961b), although, as a general rule, the long bones contain more lead. In the early period of deposition, the concentration of lead is highest in the epiphyseal portion of the long bones. This is especially true in growing bones, where deposits may be detected by x-ray examination as rings of increased density in the ossification centers of the epiphyseal cartilage and as a series of transverse lines in the diaphyses, so-called lead lines. Such findings are of diagnostic significance in children.

Factors that affect the distribution of calcium similarly affect that of lead. Thus, a high intake of phosphate favors skeletal storage of lead and a lower concentration in soft tissues. Conversely, a low phosphate intake mobilizes lead in bone and elevates its content in soft tissues. High intake of calcium in the absence of elevated intake of phosphate has a similar effect, owing to competition with lead for available phosphate. Vitamin D tends to promote the deposition of lead in bone if a sufficient amount of phosphate is available; otherwise, deposition of calcium preempts that of lead. Parathyroid hormone and dihydrotachysterol mobilize lead from the skeleton and augment the concentration of lead in blood and the rate of its excretion in urine.

In experimental animals, lead is excreted into bile, and much more lead is excreted into feces than into urine (Gregus and Klaassen, 1986). In man, urinary excretion is a more important route (Kehoe, 1987), and the concentration of lead in urine is directly proportional to that in plasma. However, because most lead in blood is in the erythrocytes, very little is filtered. Lead is also excreted in milk and sweat and is deposited in hair and nails. Placental transfer of lead is also known to occur.

The half-life of lead in blood is 1 to 2 months, and a steady state is thus achieved in about 6 months. After establishment of a steady state early in human life, the daily intake of lead approximates the output, under normal conditions, and concentrations of lead in soft tissues change little. However, the concentration of lead in bone appears to increase (Gross *et al.*, 1975), and its half-life in bone has been estimated to be 20 to 30 years. Because the rate of excretion of lead is limited, even a slight increase in daily intake may produce a positive lead balance. The average daily intake of lead is approximately 0.3 mg, while positive lead balance begins at a daily intake of about 0.6 mg. This amount will not ordinarily produce overt toxicity within a lifetime. However, the time to accumulate toxic amounts shortens disproportionately as the amount ingested increases. For example, a daily intake of 2.5 mg of lead requires nearly 4 years for the accumulation of a toxic burden, whereas a daily intake of 3.5 mg requires but a few months, since deposition in bone is too slow to protect the soft tissues during rapid accumulation.

Acute Lead Poisoning. Acute lead poisoning is relatively infrequent and occurs from ingestion of acid-soluble lead compounds or inhalation of lead vapors. Local actions in the mouth produce marked astringency, thirst, and a metallic taste. Nausea, abdominal pain, and vomiting ensue. The vomitus may be milky from the presence of lead chloride. Although the abdominal pain is severe, it is unlike that of chronic poisoning. Stools may be black from lead sulfide, and there may be diarrhea or constipation. If large amounts of lead are absorbed rapidly, a shock syndrome may develop as the result of massive gastrointestinal loss of fluid. Acute central nervous system (CNS) symptoms include paresthesias, pain, and muscle weakness. An acute hemolytic crisis sometimes occurs and causes severe anemia and hemoglobinuria. The kidneys are damaged, and oliguria and urinary changes are evident. Death may occur in 1 or 2 days. If the patient survives the acute episode, characteristic signs and symptoms of chronic lead poisoning are likely to appear.

Chronic Lead Poisoning. Signs and symptoms of chronic lead poisoning (plumbism) can be divided into six categories: gastrointestinal, neuromuscular, CNS, hematological, renal, and other. They may occur separately or in combination. The neuromuscular and CNS syndromes usually result from intense exposure, while the abdominal syndrome is a more common manifestation of a very slowly and insidiously developing intoxication. The CNS syndrome is usually more common among children, while the gastrointestinal syndrome is more prevalent in adults.

Gastrointestinal Effects. Lead affects the smooth muscle of the gut, producing intestinal symptoms that are an important, early sign of exposure to the metal. The abdominal syndrome often begins with vague symptoms, such as anorexia, muscle discomfort, malaise, and headache. Constipation is usually an early sign, especially in adults, but diarrhea occasionally occurs. A persistent metallic taste appears early in the course of the syndrome. As intoxication advances, anorexia and constipation become more marked. Intestinal spasm, which causes severe abdominal pain, or *lead colic,* is the most distressing feature of the advanced abdominal syndrome. The attacks are paroxysmal and generally excruciating (Janin *et al.,* 1985). The abdominal muscles become rigid, and tenderness is especially manifested in the region of the umbilicus. In cases where colic is not severe, removal of the patient from the environment in which he was exposed may be sufficient for relief of symptoms. Calcium gluconate administered intravenously is recommended for relief of pain and is usually more effective than morphine.

Neuromuscular Effects. The neuromuscular syndrome, or *lead palsy,* is now rare in the United States. It is a manifestation of advanced subacute poisoning. Muscle weakness and easy fatigue occur long before actual paralysis and may be the only symptoms. Weakness or palsy may not become evident until after extended muscle activity. The muscle groups involved are usually the most active ones (extensors of the forearm, wrist, and fingers and extraocular muscles), and the palsy often occurs only on the dominant side. Wrist-drop and, to a lesser extent, foot-drop with the appropriate history of exposure have been considered almost pathognomonic for lead poisoning. There is usually no sensory involvement. Degenerative changes in the motoneurons and their axons have been described.

CNS Effects. The CNS syndrome has been termed *lead encephalopathy*. It is the most serious manifestation of lead poisoning, and is much more common in children than in adults. The early signs of the syndrome may be clumsiness, vertigo, ataxia, falling, headache, insomnia, restlessness, and irritability. As the encephalopathy develops, the patient may first become excited and confused; delirium with repetitive tonic–clonic convulsions or lethargy and coma follow. Vomiting, a common sign, is usually projectile. Visual disturbances are also present. Although the signs and symptoms are characteristic of increased intracranial pressure, flap craniotomy to relieve intracranial pressure is not beneficial. However, treatment for cerebral edema may become necessary. There may be a proliferative meningitis, intense edema, punctate hemorrhages, gliosis, and areas of focal necrosis. Demyelination has been observed in nonhuman primates. The mortality rate among patients who develop cerebral involvement is about 25%. When chelation therapy is begun after the symptoms of acute encephalopathy appear, approximately 40% of survivors have neurological sequelae, such as mental retardation, electroencephalographic abnormalities or frank seizures, cerebral palsy, optic atrophy, or dystonia musculorum deformans (Smith *et al.,* 1963; Chisolm and Barltrop, 1979).

Exposure to lead occasionally produces clear-cut, progressive mental deterioration in children. The history of these children indicates normal development during the first 12 to 18 months of life or longer, followed by a steady loss of motor skills and speech. They may have severe hyperkinetic and aggressive behavior disorders and a poorly controlled convulsive disorder. The lack of sensory perception severely impairs learning. Concentrations of lead in blood exceed 60 μg/dl (2.9 μM) of whole blood, and x-rays may show heavy, multiple bands of increased density in the growing long bones (*see* above). Until recently it was thought that such exposure to lead was largely restricted to children in inner-city slums. However, all children are exposed chronically to low levels of lead in their diets, in the air they breathe, and in the dirt and dust in their play areas. This is reflected in elevated concentrations of lead in blood of many children and may be a cause of subtle CNS toxicity. An increased incidence of hyperkinetic behavior and a statistically significant, although modest, decrease in IQ have been shown in children with blood lead concentrations of 30 to 50 μg/dl (1.4 to 2.4 μM) (Needleman *et al.,* 1979; Needleman and Leviton, 1982; Smith, 1985). As a result, workers at the Centers for Disease Control consider a blood lead concentration of 25 μg/dl (1.2 μM) or above to be indicative of excessive absorption of lead in children and to constitute grounds for intervention (American Academy of Pediatrics, 1987). Recent data suggest that the fetal brain may be even more sensitive to the toxic effects of lead (Bellinger *et al.,* 1987; Davis and Svendsgaard, 1987).

Hematological Effects. When the blood lead concentration is near 80 μg/dl (3.9 μM) or greater, basophilic stippling (the aggregation of ribonucleic acid) occurs in erythrocytes. This is thought to result from the inhibitory effect of lead on the enzyme pyrimidine-5′-nucleotidase. Basophilic stippling is not, however, pathognomonic of lead poisoning.

A more common hematological result of chronic lead intoxication is a hypochromic microcytic anemia, which is more frequently observed in children and is morphologically similar to that which results from iron deficiency. The anemia is thought to result from two factors: a decreased life span of the erythrocytes and an inhibition of heme synthesis.

Very low concentrations of lead influence the synthesis of heme. The enzymes necessary for heme synthesis are widely distributed in mammalian tissues, and it is highly probable that each cell synthesizes its own heme for incorporation into such proteins as hemoglobin, myoglobin, cytochromes, and catalases. Lead inhibits heme formation at several points, as shown in Figure 66–1. Inhibition of δ-aminolevulinate (δ-ALA) dehydratase and ferrochelatase, which are sulfhydryl-dependent enzymes, is well documented. Lead poisoning in both man and experimental animals is characterized by accumulation of protoporphyrin IX and nonheme iron in red blood cells, by accumulation of δ-ALA in plasma, and by increased urinary excretion of δ-ALA. There is also increased urinary excretion of coproporphyrin III (the oxidation product of coproporphyrinogen III), but it is not clear whether this is due to inhibition of enzymatic activity or to other factors. Increased excretion of porphobilinogen and uroporphyrin has been reported only in severe cases. The pattern of excretion of pyrroles found in lead poisoning differs from that characteristic of symptomatic episodes of acute intermittent porphyria and other hepatocellular disorders, as shown in Table 66–1. The increase

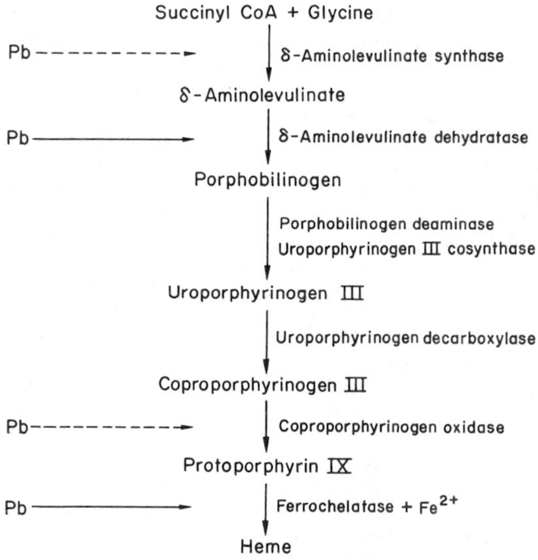

Figure 66–1. *Lead interferes with the biosynthesis of heme at several enzymatic steps.*

Steps that are definitely inhibited by lead are indicated by ——►; steps at which lead is thought to act but evidence is inconclusive are indicated by – – ►.

in δ-ALA synthase activity is due to the reduction of the cellular concentration of heme, which regulates the synthesis of δ-ALA synthase by feedback inhibition.

Measurement of heme precursors provides a sensitive index of recent absorption of inorganic lead salts. δ-ALA dehydratase activity in hemolysates and δ-ALA in urine are sensitive indicators of exposure to lead, and abnormalities of these parameters precede the appearance of symptoms (National Academy of Sciences, 1972). Because they are early signs of abnormal exposure to lead and can be detected by relatively simple laboratory procedures, these measurements are used routinely in diagnosis.

Renal Effects. Although the renal effects of lead are less dramatic than those in the CNS and gastrointestinal tract, nephropathy does occur. Renal toxicity occurs in two forms (Goyer, 1985): a reversible renal tubular disorder (usually seen after acute exposure of children to lead) and an irreversible interstitial nephropathy (more commonly observed in long-term industrial lead exposure). Clinically, a Fanconi-like syndrome is seen with proteinuria, hematuria, and casts in the urine (Craswell, 1987; Bernard and Becker, 1988). Hyperuricemia with gout occurs more frequently in the presence of chronic lead nephropathy than in any other type of chronic renal disease. Histologically, lead nephropathy is revealed by a characteristic nuclear inclusion body, composed of a lead-protein complex; this appears early and resolves after chelation therapy. Such inclusion bodies have been reported in the urine sediment of workers exposed to lead in an industrial setting (Schumann *et al.,* 1980).

Other Effects. Other signs and symptoms of plumbism are an ashen color of the face and pallor of the lips; retinal stippling; appearance of "premature aging," with stooped posture, poor muscle tone, and emaciation; and a black or grayish so-called lead line along the gingival margin. The lead line, a result of periodontal deposition of lead sulfide, may be removed by good dental hygiene. Similar pigmentation may result from the absorption of mercury, bismuth, silver, thallium, or iron. There is a relationship between the concentration of lead in blood and blood pressure, and it has been suggested that this may be due to subtle changes in calcium metabolism or renal function (Pirkle *et al.,* 1985; Sharp *et al.,* 1987). Lead also interferes with vitamin D metabolism (Rosen *et al.,* 1980; Mahaffey *et al.,* 1982). The carcinogenicity of lead in man is not well established, but it has been suggested (Cooper and Gaffey, 1975), and several case reports of renal adenocarcinoma in lead workers have been published (Baker *et al.,* 1980; Kazantzis, 1986).

Diagnosis of Lead Poisoning. In the absence of a positive history of abnormal exposure to lead, the diagnosis of lead poisoning is easily missed. Furthermore, the signs and symptoms of lead poisoning are shared by other diseases. For example, the signs of encephalopathy may resemble those of various degenerative conditions. Physical examination does not easily distinguish lead colic from

Table 66–1. PATTERNS OF INCREASED EXCRETION OF PYRROLES IN URINE OF ACUTELY SYMPTOMATIC PATIENTS *

DISEASE	PYRROLES †			
	ALA	*PBG*	*URO*	*COPRO*
Lead poisoning	+++	0	±	+++
Acute intermittent porphyria	++++	++++	+ to ++++	+ to +++
Acute hepatitis	0	0	0	+ to +++
Acute alcoholism	0	0	±	+ to +++

* Modified from Chisolm, 1967.

† 0 = normal; + to ++++ = degree of increase; ALA = δ-aminolevulinic acid; PBG = porphobilinogen; URO = uroporphyrin; COPRO = coproporphyrin.

other abdominal disorders. Clinical suspicion should be confirmed by determinations of the concentration of lead in blood and protoporphyrin in erythrocytes.

The concentration of lead in blood is one indication of recent absorption of the metal, but measurement of erythrocyte protoporphyrin alone is more cost effective (Berwick and Komaroff, 1982). In normal children and adults, blood lead values are about 10 to 20 μg/dl of whole blood (0.5 to 1.0 μM). Children with concentrations of lead in blood above 25 μg/dl (1.2 μM) are at risk of developmental disabilities. Adults with concentrations of 40 to 60 μg/dl (1.9 to 2.9 μM) exhibit no known functional injury or symptoms; however, they will have a definite decrease in δ-ALA dehydratase activity, a slight increase in urinary excretion of δ-ALA, and an increase in erythrocyte protoporphyrin. Patients with a blood lead concentration of 60 to 80 μg/dl (2.9 to 3.9 μM) have all of the above laboratory abnormalities and, usually, nonspecific, mild symptoms of lead poisoning. Clear symptoms of lead poisoning are associated with concentrations that exceed 80 μg/dl of whole blood (3.9 μM) (Kehoe, 1961a, 1961b), and lead encephalopathy is usually apparent when lead concentrations are greater than 120 μg/dl (5.8 μM) (National Academy of Sciences, 1972). In persons with moderate-to-severe anemia, interpretation of the significance of concentrations of lead in blood is improved by correcting the observed value to approximate that which would be expected if the patient's hematocrit were within the normal range.

Urinary excretion of lead in normal adults is generally less than 80 μg/l (0.4 μM) (Kehoe, 1961a, 1961b; Goldwater and Hoover, 1967). Most patients with lead poisoning show concentrations of lead in urine of 150 to 300 μg/l (0.7 to 1.4 μM). However, in persons with chronic lead nephropathy or other forms of renal insufficiency, urinary excretion of lead may be within the normal range.

Because the onset of lead poisoning is usually insidious, it is often desirable to estimate the body burden of lead in individuals who are exposed to an environment that is contaminated with the metal. Use of the edetate calcium disodium ($CaNa_2EDTA$) mobilization test helps determine whether there is an increased body burden of lead in those in whom exposure occurred much earlier (Emmerson, 1963). This test is performed by intravenous administration of a single dose of $CaNa_2EDTA$ (50 mg/kg). Urine is collected for 8 hours. The test is positive for children when the lead excretion ratio (micrograms of lead excreted in the urine per milligram of $CaNa_2EDTA$ administered) is greater than 0.6. This test is not used in symptomatic patients or in those whose concentration of lead in blood is greater than 100 μg/dl (4.8 μM), because these patients require the proper therapeutic regimen with chelating agents (*see* below). In an experimental model of chronic low-level exposure to lead in rats, administration of $CaNa_2EDTA$ doubles the brain concentrations of lead; this brings the safety of the diagnostic test into question (Cory-Slechta *et al.*, 1987).

In summary, the diagnosis of lead poisoning is usually based on the patient's history and clinical presentation and is easily confirmed by laboratory determinations. Other diagnostic information includes characteristic lead lines in the long bones of children, unabsorbed lead seen radiographically in the gastrointestinal tract in a child with recent ingestion, basophilic stippling of erythrocytes associated with anemia, renal dysfunction, and neurological lesions.

Organic Lead Poisoning. Tetraethyllead and tetramethyllead are lipid-soluble compounds and are readily absorbed from the skin, gastrointestinal tract, and lungs. The toxicity of tetraethyllead is believed to be due to its metabolic conversion to triethyllead and inorganic lead.

The major symptoms of intoxication with tetraethyllead are referable to the CNS (Seshia *et al.*, 1978). The victim suffers from insomnia, nightmares, anorexia, nausea and vomiting, diarrhea, headache, muscular weakness, and emotional instability. Subjective CNS symptoms such as irritability, restlessness, and anxiety are next evident. At this time there is usually hypothermia, bradycardia, and hypotension. With continued exposure, or in the case of intense short-term exposure, CNS manifestations progress to delusions, ataxia, exaggerated muscular movements, and, finally, a maniacal state.

The diagnosis of poisoning by tetraethyllead is established by relating these signs and symptoms to a history of exposure. The urinary excretion of lead may increase markedly, but the concentration of lead in blood remains nearly normal. Anemia and basophilic stippling of erythrocytes are uncommon in organic lead poisoning. There is little effect on the metabolism of porphyrins, and erythrocyte protoporphyrin concentrations are inconsistently elevated (Garrettson, 1983). In the case of severe exposure, death may occur within a few hours or may be delayed for several weeks. If the patient survives the acute phase of organic lead poisoning, recovery is usually complete; however, instances of residual CNS damage have been reported.

Treatment of Lead Poisoning. Initial treatment of the acute phase of lead intoxication involves supportive measures. Prevention of further exposure is important. Seizures are treated with diazepam (Chapter 19); fluid and electrolyte balances must be maintained; cerebral edema is treated with mannitol and dexamethasone. The concentration of lead in blood should be determined prior to initiation of chelation therapy.

Chelation therapy is indicated in symptomatic patients or in patients with a blood lead concentration in excess of 50 to 60 μg/dl (about 2.5 μM). Three chelators are commonly employed in the treatment of lead intoxication: edetate calcium disodium ($CaNa_2EDTA$), dimercaprol (British anti-Lewisite; BAL), and D-penicillamine. $CaNa_2EDTA$ and dimercaprol are usually used in combination for lead encephalopathy.

$CaNa_2EDTA$ is employed at a dose of 50 to 75 mg/kg per day in two divided doses, either by deep intramuscular injection or slow intravenous infusion for up to 5 consecutive days. The first dose of $CaNa_2EDTA$ should be delayed until 4 hours after the first dose of dimercaprol. An additional course of $CaNa_2EDTA$ may be given after an interruption of 2 days. Each course of therapy with $CaNa_2EDTA$ should not exceed a total dose of 500 mg/kg. Urine output must be monitored, because the chelator–lead complex is believed to be nephrotoxic. Treatment with $CaNa_2EDTA$ can alleviate symptoms quickly. Colic may disappear within 2 hours; paresthesia and tremor cease after 4 or 5 days; coproporphyrinuria, stippled erythrocytes, and gingival lead lines tend to decrease in 4 to 9 days. Urinary elimination of lead is usually greatest during the initial infusion.

Dimercaprol is given intramuscularly at a dose of 4 mg/kg every 4 hours for 48 hours, then every 6 hours for 48 hours, and finally every 6 to 12 hours for an additional 7 days. The combination of dimercaprol and $CaNa_2EDTA$ is more effective than is either chelator alone (Chisolm, 1973).

In contrast to $CaNa_2EDTA$ and dimercaprol, penicillamine is effective orally and may be included in the regimen at a dosage of 250 mg given four times daily for 5 days. During chronic therapy with penicillamine, the dose should not exceed 40 mg/kg per day.

Lead poisoning in children is more dangerous than in adults, primarily because of the greater incidence of encephalopathy. The mortality rate of untreated, severe lead encephalopathy may approach 65%, and neurological sequelae are common in survivors. Hospitalization is recommended for any symptomatic child or any child with a blood lead concentration of 80 μg/dl (3.9 μM) or greater. Exposure is thereby terminated, and careful monitoring and supportive measures are essential.

Long-term chelation therapy for patients with residual encephalopathy or with blood lead concentrations exceeding 60 μg/dl (2.9 μM) and with prominent radiographic evidence of lead deposition in bone is most easily accomplished with oral penicillamine (40 mg/kg per day, maximum). One must remember that the oral chelator may promote absorption of lead from the gastrointestinal tract. Avoidance of continued exposure to lead is thus very important.

Treatment of organic lead poisoning is symptomatic. Chelation therapy will promote the excretion of the inorganic lead produced from the metabolism of organic lead, but the increase is not dramatic (Boyd, 1957).

MERCURY

Mercury was an important constituent of drugs for centuries—as an ingredient in many diuretics, antibacterials, antiseptics, skin ointments, and laxatives. More specific and effective modes of therapy have largely replaced the mercurials in recent decades, and drug-induced signs of mercury poisoning have become rare. However, mercury poisoning from environmental pollution has become an area of concern. There have been epidemics of mercury poisoning among wildlife and human populations in many countries. With very few exceptions and for numerous reasons, such outbreaks were misdiagnosed for months or even years. Reasons for these tragic delays included the insidious onset of the affliction, vagueness of early clinical signs, and the medical profession's unfamiliarity with the disease (Gerstner and Huff, 1977).

Chemical Forms and Sources of Mercury. With regard to the toxicity of mercury, three major chemical forms of the metal must be distinguished: mercury vapor (elemental mercury), salts of mercury, and organic mercurials.

Elemental mercury is the most volatile of the inorganic forms of the metal. Human exposure to mercury vapor is mainly occupational and has been known since antiquity. Chronic exposure to mercury in ambient air after inadvertent spills in poorly ventilated rooms, often scientific laboratories, can produce toxic effects. Mercury vapor can also be released from silver-amalgam dental restorations, but the amount of mercury released does not appear to be of significance for human health (Enwonwu, 1987).

Salts of mercury exist in two states of oxidation—as monovalent mercurous salts or as divalent mercuric salts. Mercurous chloride or calomel, the best-known mercurous compound, was used in some skin creams as an antiseptic and was employed as a diuretic and cathartic. Mercuric salts are the most irritating and acutely toxic form of the metal. Mercuric nitrate was a common industrial hazard in the felt-hat industry more than 400 years ago. Occupational exposure produced neurological and behavioral changes depicted by the Mad Hatter in Lewis Carroll's *Alice's Adventures in Wonderland*. Mercuric chloride, once a widely used antiseptic, was also commonly used for suicidal purposes. Mercuric salts are still widely employed in industry, and industrial discharge into rivers has introduced mercury into the environment in many parts of the world. The main industrial uses of inorganic mercury today are in chloralkali production and in electronics. Other uses of the metal include the manufacturing of plastics, fungicides, and germicides and the formulation of amalgams in dentistry.

The organomercurials in use today contain mercury with one covalent bond to a carbon atom. This is a heterogeneous group of compounds, and its members have varying abilities to produce toxic effects. The alkylmercury salts are by far the most dangerous of these compounds; methylmercury is the most common. Alkylmercury salts have been widely used as fungicides and, as such, have produced toxic effects in man. Major incidents of human poisoning from the inadvertent consumption of mercury-treated seed grain have occurred in Iraq, Pakistan, Ghana, and Guatemala. The most catastrophic outbreak occurred in Iraq in 1972. During the fall of 1971, Iraq imported large quantities of seed (wheat and barley) treated with methylmercury and distributed the grain for spring planting. Despite official warnings, the grain was ground into flour and made into bread. As a result, 6530 victims were hospitalized and 500 died (Bakir *et al.*, 1973, 1980).

Minamata disease was also due to methylmercury. Minamata is a small town in Japan, and its major industry is a chemical plant that empties its effluent directly into Minamata Bay. The chemical plant used inorganic mercury as a catalyst, and some of it was methylated before it entered the bay. In addition, microorganisms convert inorganic mercury to methylmercury; the compound is then taken up rapidly by plankton algae and is concentrated in fish via the food chain. Residents of Minamata who consumed fish as a large portion of their diet were the first to be poisoned. Eventually 121 persons were poisoned and 46 died (McAlpine and Shukuro, 1958; Smith and Smith, 1975; Tamashiro *et al.*, 1985). In the United States, human poisonings have resulted from ingestion of meat from pigs fed grain treated with an organomercurial fungicide.

Chemistry and Mechanism of Action. Mercury readily forms covalent bonds with sulfur, and it is this property that accounts for most of the biological properties of the metal. When the sulfur is in the form of sulfhydryl groups, divalent mercury replaces the hydrogen atom to form mercaptides, X—Hg—SR and $Hg(SR)_2$, where X is an electronegative radical and R is protein. Organic mercurials form mercaptides of the type RHg—SR′. Even in low concentrations mercurials are capable of inactivating sulfhydryl enzymes and thus interfering with cellular metabolism and function. The affinity of mercury for thiols provides the basis for treatment of mercury poisoning with such agents as dimercaprol and penicillamine. Mercury also combines with other ligands of physiological importance, such as phosphoryl, carboxyl, amide, and amine groups.

The various therapeutic and toxic actions of the mercurials are associated with chemical substituents that affect solubility, dissociation, relative affinity for various cellular receptors, distribution, and excretion.

Absorption, Biotransformation, Distribution, and Excretion. *Elemental Mercury.* Elemental mercury is not particularly toxic when ingested because of very low absorption from the gastrointestinal tract; this is due to the formation of droplets and because the metal in this form cannot react with biologically important molecules. However, inhaled mercury vapor is completely absorbed by the lung and is then oxidized to the divalent mercuric cation by catalase in the erythrocytes (Magos *et al.*, 1978). Within a few hours the deposition of inhaled mercury vapor resembles that after ingestion of mercuric salts, with one important difference. Because mercury vapor crosses membranes much more readily than does divalent mercury, a significant amount of the vapor enters the brain before it is oxidized. CNS toxicity is thus more prominent after exposure to mercury vapor than to divalent forms of the metal.

Inorganic Salts of Mercury. The soluble inorganic mercuric salts (Hg^{2+}) gain access to the circulation when taken orally. Gastrointestinal absorption is approximately 10% of that ingested, and a considerable portion of the Hg^{2+} may remain bound to the alimentary mucosa and the intestinal contents. Insoluble inorganic mercurous compounds, such as calomel (Hg_2Cl_2), may undergo some oxidation to soluble compounds that are more readily absorbed. Inorganic mercury has a markedly nonuniform distribution after absorption. The highest concentration of Hg^{2+} is found in the kidneys, where the metal is retained longer than in other tissues. Concentrations of inorganic mercury are similar in whole blood and plasma. Inorganic mercurials do not readily pass the blood–brain barrier or the placenta. The metal is excreted in the urine and feces with a half-life of about 60 days (Friberg and Vostal, 1972); studies in laboratory animals indicate that fecal excretion is quantitatively more important (Klaassen, 1975).

Organic Mercurials. Organic mercurials are more completely absorbed from the gastrointestinal tract than are the inorganic salts because they are more lipid soluble and less corrosive to the intestinal mucosa. Over 90% of methylmercury is absorbed from the human gastrointestinal tract. The organic mercurials cross the blood–brain barrier and the placenta and thus produce more neurological and teratogenic effects than do the inorganic salts. Organic mercurials are more uniformly distributed to the various tissues than are the inorganic salts (Klaassen, 1975). A significant portion of the body burden of organic mercurials is in the red blood cells. The ratio of the concentration of organomercurial in erythrocytes to that in plasma varies with the compound; for methylmercury, it approximates 20:1 (Kershaw *et al.*, 1980). The carbon–mercury bond of some organic mercurials is cleaved after absorption; with methylmercury the cleavage is quite slow and the inorganic mercury formed is not thought to play a major role in methylmercury toxicity. Aryl mercurials, like mercurophen, usually contain a labile mercury–carbon bond, and the toxicity of these compounds is similar to that of inorganic mercury. Excretion of methylmercury by man is mainly in the feces; less than 10% of a dose appears in urine. The biological half-life of methylmercury in man is about 65 days (Bakir *et al.*, 1973).

Toxicity. *Elemental Mercury.* Short-term exposure to elemental mercury vapor may produce symptoms within several hours; these include weakness, chills, metallic taste, nausea, vomiting, diarrhea, dyspnea, cough, and a feeling of tightness in the chest. Pulmonary toxicity may progress to an interstitial pneumonitis with severe compromise of respiratory function. Recovery, although usually complete, may be complicated by residual interstitial fibrosis.

Chronic exposure to mercury vapor produces a more insidious form of toxicity that is dominated by neurological effects (Friberg and Vostal, 1972). The syndrome is referred to as the *asthenic vegetative syndrome* and consists of neurasthenic symptoms in addition to three or more of the following findings (Goyer, 1985): goiter, increased uptake of radioiodine by the thyroid, tachycardia, labile pulse, gingivitis, dermographia, and increased mercury in the urine. With continued exposure, tremor becomes quite noticeable and psychological changes consist of depression, irritability, excessive shyness, insomnia, emotional instability, forgetfulness, confusion, and vasomotor disturbances (such as excessive perspiration and uncontrolled blushing, which together are referred to as *erethism*). Common features of intoxication from mercury vapor are severe salivation and gingivitis. The triad of increased excitability, tremors, and gingivitis has been recognized historically as the major manifestation of exposure to mercury vapor when mercury nitrate was used in the fur, felt, and hat industries. Renal dysfunction has also been reported to result from long-term industrial exposure to mercury vapor.

Inorganic Salts of Mercury. Inorganic, ionic mercury (*e.g.*, mercuric chloride) can produce severe acute toxicity. Precipitation of mucous membrane proteins by mercuric salts results in an ashen-gray appearance of the mucosa of the mouth, pharynx, and intestine and also causes intense pain, which may be accompanied by vomiting. The vomiting is protective, since it removes unabsorbed mercury from the stomach, and should not be inhibited (assuming the patient is awake and alert). The local, corrosive effect of ionic inorganic mercury on the gastrointestinal mucosa results in severe hematochezia with evidence of mucosal sloughing in the stool. Hypovolemic shock and death usually result in the absence of proper treatment. However, these local effects can be overcome readily with prompt corrective treatment. Systemic toxicity may begin within a few hours after exposure to mercury and last for days. A strong metallic taste is followed by stomatitis with gingival irritation, foul breath, and loosening of the teeth. The most serious and, unfortunately, the most frequently encountered systemic effect of inorganic mercury is renal toxicity. Renal tubular necrosis occurs after short-term exposure, leading to oliguria or anuria. Renal injury also follows long-term exposure to inorganic mercury; however, glomerular injury predominates. This is the result of both direct effects on the glomerular basement membrane and a later indirect effect mediated by immune complexes (Goyer, 1985).

The symptom complex of acrodynia (pink disease) also commonly follows chronic exposure to inorganic mercury ions. Acrodynia is an erythema of the extremities, chest, and face with photophobia, diaphoresis, anorexia, tachycardia, and either constipation or diarrhea. This symptom complex is seen almost exclusively after ingestion of mercury and is believed to be the result of a hypersensitivity reaction to mercury (Matherson *et al.*, 1980).

Organic Mercurials. Most human toxicological data about organic mercury concern methylmercury and have been collected as the unfortunate result of several large-scale accidental exposures. Symptoms of exposure to methylmercury are mainly neurological in origin and consist of visual disturbance (scotoma and visual-field constriction), ataxia, paresthesias, neurasthenia, hearing loss, dysarthria, mental deterioration, muscle tremor, movement disorders, and with severe exposure, paralysis and death (Table 66–2). Certain regions of the brain have been found to be particularly sensitive to the toxic effects of methylmercury, namely, the cerebral cortex (especially the visual cortex) and the granular layer of the cerebellum. Effects of methylmercury on the fetus can occur even when the mother is asymptomatic; mental retardation and neuromuscular deficits have been observed.

Diagnosis of Mercury Poisoning. A history of exposure to mercury, either industrial or environmental, is obviously valuable in making the diagnosis of mercury poisoning. Without such a history, clinical suspicions can be confirmed by laboratory analysis. The upper limit of a normal concentration of mercury in blood is generally considered to be 3 to 4 μg/dl (0.15 to 0.20 μM). A concentration of mercury in blood in excess of 4 μg/dl (0.20 μM) should be considered abnormal in adults. Because

Table 66–2. FREQUENCY OF SYMPTOMS OF METHYLMERCURY POISONING IN RELATION TO CONCENTRATION OF MERCURY IN BLOOD *

CONCENTRATION OF MERCURY IN BLOOD *µg/ml (µM)*	CASES WITH SYMPTOMS (%)					
	Paresthesias	*Ataxia*	*Visual Defects*	*Dysarthria*	*Hearing Defects*	*Death*
0.1–0.5 (0.5–2.5)	5	0	0	5	0	0
0.5–1.0 (2.5–5.0)	42	11	21	5	5	0
1–2 (5–10)	60	47	53	24	5	0
2–3 (10–15)	79	60	56	25	13	0
3–4 (15–20)	82	100	58	75	36	17
4–5 (20–25)	100	100	83	85	66	28

* Based on data in Bakir *et al.*, 1973.

methylmercury is concentrated in erythrocytes and inorganic mercury is not, the distribution of total mercury between red blood cells and plasma may indicate whether the patient has been poisoned with inorganic or organic mercury. Measurement of total mercury in red blood cells gives a better estimate of the body burden of methylmercury than it does for inorganic mercury. The relationship between concentrations of mercury in blood and the frequency of symptoms that result from exposure to methylmercury is shown in Table 66–2; however, this is only a rough guide. Concentrations of mercury in plasma provide a better index of the body burden of inorganic mercury; however, the relationship between body burden and the concentration of inorganic mercury in plasma is not well documented. The relationship between the concentration of inorganic mercury in blood and toxicity depends on the form of exposure. For example, exposure to vapor results in concentrations in brain about 10 times higher than those that follow an equivalent dose of inorganic mercuric salts.

The concentration of mercury in the urine has also been used as a measure of the body burden of the metal. The upper limit for excretion of mercury into urine in the normal population is 25 μg/l (0.12 μM). There is a linear relationship between plasma concentration and urinary excretion of mercury after exposure to vapor; workers in a chloralkali plant exhibited tremors when the concentrations of mercury in urine reached 500 μg/l (2.5 μM) (Langolf *et al.*, 1977). In contrast, the excretion of mercury in urine is a poor indicator of the amount of methylmercury in the blood, since it is eliminated mainly in feces (Bakir *et al.*, 1973).

Hair is rich in sulfhydryl groups, and the concentration of mercury in hair is about 300 times that in blood. Furthermore, the most recent growth of hair reflects a fairly current concentration of mercury in blood. Human hair grows about 20 cm a year, and a history of exposure may be obtained by analysis of different segments of hair.

Treatment of Mercury Poisoning. Measurement of the concentration of mercury in blood should be performed as soon as possible after poisoning with any form of the metal.

Elemental Mercury Vapor. Therapeutic measures include immediate termination of exposure and close monitoring of pulmonary status. Short-term respiratory support may be necessary. Chelation therapy, as described below for inorganic mercury, should be initiated immediately and continued as indicated by the clinical condition and the concentrations of mercury in blood and urine.

Inorganic Mercury. Prompt attention to fluid and electrolyte balance and hematological status is of critical importance in moderate-to-severe oral exposures. Emesis should be induced if the patient is awake and alert. Alternatively, gastric lavage may be performed to remove mercury from the gastrointestinal tract. Activated charcoal and a magnesium cathartic should then be administered to limit further absorption.

Chelation therapy with dimercaprol (for high-level exposures or symptomatic patients) or penicillamine (for low-level exposures or asymptomatic patients) is routinely used to treat poisoning with either inorganic or elemental mercury. Recommended treatment includes dimercaprol, 5 mg/kg intramuscularly initially, followed by 2.5 mg/kg intramuscularly every 12 to 24 hours for 10 days. Penicillamine (250 mg orally every 6 hours) may be used alone or following treatment with dimercaprol. The duration of chelation therapy will vary, and progress can be monitored by following concentrations of mercury in urine and blood. Two newer derivatives of dimercaprol succimer (2,3-dimercaptosuccinic acid; DMSA) and 2,3-dimercaptopropane-1-sulfonate (DMPS), appear promising for the treatment of inorganic mercury poisoning (Magos, 1976; Campbell *et al.*, 1986). Similarly, a derivative of penicillamine, N-acetyl-D-penicillamine (NAP), is also effective for treatment of mercury poisoning (Kark *et al.*, 1971).

The dimercaprol–mercury chelate is excreted into both bile and urine, whereas the penicillamine–mercury chelate is excreted only into urine. Thus, penicillamine should be used with extreme caution when renal function is impaired. In fact, hemodialysis may be necessary in the poisoned patient whose renal function declines. Chelators may still be used, because the dimercaprol–mercury complex is removed by dialysis (Giunta *et al.*, 1983).

Organic Mercury. The short-chain organic mercurials, especially methylmercury, are the most difficult forms of mercury to mobilize from the body, presumably due to their poor reactivity with chelating agents. Dimercaprol is contraindicated in methylmercury poisoning because it increases brain concentrations of methylmercury in experimental animals. Although penicillamine facilitates the removal of methylmercury from the body, its clinical efficacy in the treatment of intoxication with methylmercury is not impressive (Bakir *et al.*, 1976, 1980). The dose of penicillamine normally used in the treatment of poisoning with inorganic mercury (1 g per day) produces only a small reduction in the concentration of methylmercury in blood; larger doses (2 g per day) are needed. During the initial 1 to 3 days of administration of penicillamine the concentration of mercury in the blood increases before it decreases. This is probably due to the mobilization of metal from tissues to blood at a rate more rapid than that for excretion of mercury into urine and feces.

Methylmercury compounds undergo extensive enterohepatic recirculation in experimental animals. Therefore, introduction of a nonabsorbable mercury-binding substance into the intestinal tract should facilitate their removal from the body. A polythiol resin has been used for this purpose in man and appears to be effective (Bakir *et al.*, 1973). The resin has certain advantages over penicillamine. It does not cause redistribution of mercury in the body with a subsequent increase in the concentration of mercury in blood, and it has fewer adverse effects than do sulfhydryl agents that are absorbed. Clinical experience with various treatments for methylmercury poisoning in Iraq indicates that penicillamine, N-acetyl-D-penicillamine, and an oral nonabsorbable thiol resin can all reduce blood concentrations of mercury; however, clinical improvement was not clearly related to reduction of the body burden of methylmercury (Bakir *et al.*, 1980).

Conventional hemodialysis is of little value in the treatment of methylmercury poisoning because methylmercury concentrates in erythrocytes and little is contained in the plasma. However, it has been shown that L-cysteine can be infused into the arterial blood entering the dialyzer to convert methylmercury into a diffusible form. Both free cysteine and the methylmercury–cysteine complex formed in the blood then diffuse across the membrane into the dialysate. This method has been shown to be effective in man (Al-Abbasi *et al.*, 1978). Studies in animals indicate that succimer may be more effective than cysteine in this regard (Kostyniak, 1982).

ARSENIC

Arsenic was used more than 2400 years ago in Greece and Rome as a therapeutic agent and as a poison. The history and folklore of arsenic prompted intensive studies by early pharmacologists. Indeed, the foundations of many modern concepts of chemotherapy derive from Ehrlich's early work with organic arsenicals, and such drugs were once a mainstay of chemotherapy. In current therapeutics, arsenicals are important only in the treatment of certain tropical diseases, such as African trypanosomiasis (*see* Chapter 43). In the United States the impact of arsenic on health is predominantly from industrial and environmental exposures. (For reviews, *see* Winship, 1984, and Hindmarsh and McCurdy, 1986.)

Arsenic is found in soil, water, and air as a common environmental toxicant. Well water in sections of Argentina, Chile, and Taiwan has especially high concentrations of arsenic, which results in widespread poisoning. The element is usually not mined as such but is recovered as a by-product from the smelting of copper, lead, zinc, and other ores. This can result in the release of arsenic into the environment. Mineral-spring waters and the effluent from geothermal power plants leach arsenic from soils and rocks containing high concentrations of the metal. It is also present in coal at variable concentrations and is released into the environment during combustion. Application of pesticides and herbicides containing arsenic has increased its environmental dispersion. Fruits and vegetables sprayed with arsenicals may also be a source of this element, and it is concentrated in many species of fish and shellfish. Arsenicals are sometimes added to the feed of poultry and other livestock to promote growth. The major source of occupational exposure to arsenic-containing compounds is from the manufacture of arsenical herbicides and pesticides (Landrigan, 1981). Arsenic as gallium arsenide is also widely used in the electronics industry to make semiconductors. The average daily human intake of arsenic is about 300 μg. Almost all of this is ingested with food and water.

Chemical Forms of Arsenic. The arsenic atom exists in the elemental form and in trivalent and pentavalent oxidation states. The toxicity of a given arsenical is related to the rate of its clearance from the body and therefore to its degree of accumulation in tissues. In general, toxicity increases in the sequence of organic arsenicals $< As^{5+} < As^{3+} <$ arsine (AsH_3).

The organic arsenicals contain arsenic linked to a carbon atom by a covalent bond, where arsenic exists in the trivalent or pentavalent state. Arsphenamine contains trivalent arsenic; sodium arsanilate contains arsenic in the pentavalent form.

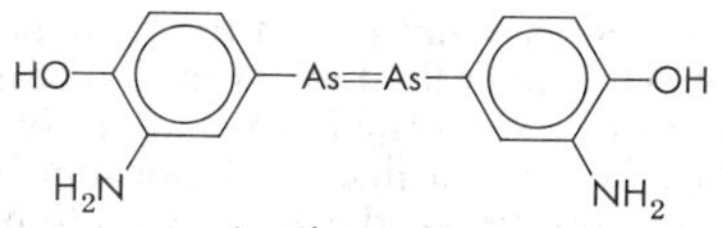

Arsphenamine

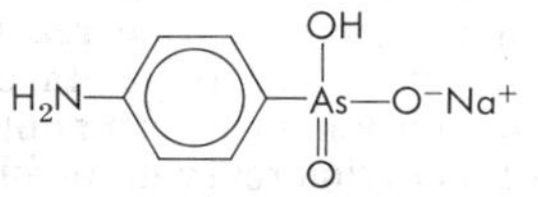

Sodium Arsanilate

The organic arsenicals are usually excreted more rapidly than are the inorganic forms.

The pentavalent oxidation state is found in arsenates (such as lead arsenate, $PbHAsO_4$), which are salts of arsenic acid, H_3AsO_4. The pentavalent arsenicals have very low affinity for thiol groups, in contrast to the trivalent compounds, and are much less toxic. The arsenites (for example, potassium arsenite [$KAsO_2$]), and salts of arsenious acid contain trivalent arsenic. Arsine (AsH_3) is a gaseous hydride of trivalent arsenic; it produces toxic effects that are distinct from those of the other arsenic compounds.

Mechanism of Action. Arsenate (pentavalent) is a well-known uncoupler of mitochondrial oxidative phosphorylation. The mechanism is thought to be related to competitive substitution of arsenate for inorganic phosphate in the formation of adenosine triphosphate, with subsequent formation of an unstable arsenate ester that is rapidly hydrolyzed. This process is termed *arsenolysis*.

Trivalent arsenicals, including inorganic arsenite, are regarded primarily as sulfhydryl reagents. As such, trivalent arsenicals inhibit many enzymes by reacting with biological ligands containing available —SH groups. The pyruvate dehydrogenase system is especially sensitive to trivalent arsenicals because of their interaction with two sulfhydryl groups of lipoic acid to form a stable six-membered ring, as shown below.

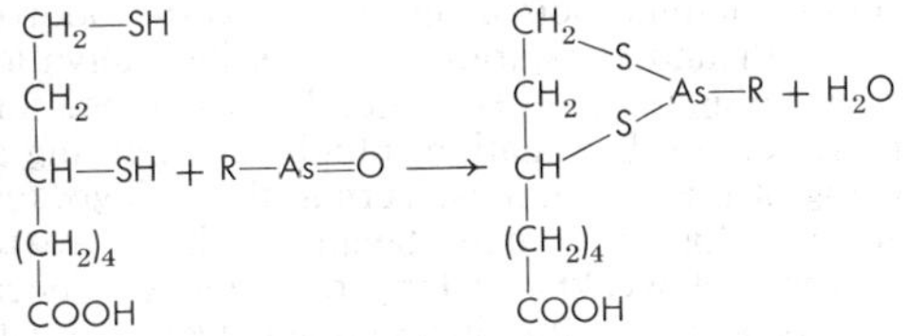

Absorption, Distribution, and Excretion. The absorption of poorly water-soluble arsenicals, such as As_2O_3, greatly depends on the physical state of the compound. Coarsely powdered material is less toxic because it can be eliminated in feces before it dissolves. The arsenite salts are more soluble in water and are better absorbed than the oxide. Experimental evidence has shown a high degree of gastrointestinal absorption of both trivalent and pentavalent forms of arsenic (Tam *et al.*, 1979).

The distribution of arsenic depends upon the duration of administration and the particular arsenical involved. Arsenic is stored mainly in liver, kidney, heart, and lung. Much smaller amounts are found in muscle and neural tissue. Because of the high sulfhydryl content of keratin, high concentrations of arsenic are found in hair and nails. Deposition in hair starts within 2 weeks after administration, and arsenic stays fixed at this site for years. Because of its chemical similarity to phosphorus, it is deposited in bone and teeth and is retained there for long periods. Arsenic readily crosses the placental barrier, and fetal damage has been reported. Concentrations of arsenic in human umbilical-cord blood are equivalent to those in the maternal circulation.

Little is known about the biotransformations of arsenicals in man. Some pentavalent arsenicals are partly reduced *in vivo* to the trivalent form. However, the redox equilibria *in vivo* favor the oxidized form, and trivalent arsenic is slowly oxidized in the body to the pentavalent state. The low toxicity and high recovery of pentavalent arsenicals in urine and excreta indicate that very little reduction takes place. It appears that both trivalent and pentavalent forms are methylated in man, because dimethylarsenic acid is a major form of arsenic excreted in urine. Arsenic is eliminated by many routes (feces, urine, sweat, milk, hair, skin, lungs), although most is excreted in urine in man. The half-life for the urinary excretion of arsenic is 3 to 5 days.

Pharmacological and Toxicological Effects of Arsenic. Arsenicals have varied effects on many organ systems. These are summarized below.

Cardiovascular System. Small doses of inorganic arsenic induce mild vasodilatation. This may lead to an occult edema, particularly facial, which has been mistaken for a healthy weight gain and misinterpreted as a "tonic" effect of arsenic. Larger doses evoke capillary dilatation; increased capillary permeability may occur in all capillary beds, but it is most pronounced in the splanchnic area. Transudation of plasma may also occur, and the decrease in intravascular volume may be significant. Long-term exposure results in gangrene of the extremities, especially of the feet, and thus is often referred to as blackfoot disease. Myocardial damage and hypotension may also become evident after more prolonged exposure to arsenic. Electrocardiographic abnormalities (prolongation of the Q–T interval and abnormal T waves) can persist for months after recovery from short-term intoxication.

Gastrointestinal Tract. Small doses of inorganic arsenicals, especially the trivalent compounds, cause mild splanchnic hyperemia. Capillary transudation of plasma, resulting from larger doses, produces vesicles under the gastrointestinal mucosa. These eventually rupture, epithelial fragments slough off, and plasma is discharged into the lumen of the intestine, where it coagulates. Tissue damage and the bulk cathartic action of the increased fluid in the lumen lead to increased peristalsis and characteristic watery diarrhea ("rice-water stools"). Normal proliferation of the epithelium is suppressed, which accentuates the damage. Soon the feces become bloody. Damage to the upper gastrointestinal tract usually results in hematemesis. Stomatitis may also be evident. The onset of gastrointestinal symptoms may be so gradual that the possibility of arsenic poisoning may be overlooked.

Kidneys. The action of arsenic on the renal capillaries, tubules, and glomeruli may cause severe renal damage. Initially, the glomeruli are affected and proteinuria results. Varying degrees of tubular necrosis and degeneration occur later. Oliguria with proteinuria, hematuria, and casts frequently results from exposure to arsenic.

Skin. In the short term, many arsenicals have a vesicant effect on the skin that results in necrosis and sloughing. Long-term ingestion of low doses of inorganic arsenicals causes cutaneous vasodilatation and a "milk and roses" complexion. Prolonged use of arsenic, however, also causes hyperkeratosis, particularly of the palms and soles, and hyperpigmentation over the trunk and extremities. Eventually these actions proceed to atrophy and degeneration, and possibly to cancer.

Nervous System. Both short- and long-term exposure to arsenic can cause encephalopathy; however, the most common arsenic-induced neurological lesion is a peripheral neuropathy with a "stocking-glove" distribution of dysesthesia. The syndrome is similar to acute inflammatory demyelinating polyradiculoneuropathy (Guillain–Barré syndrome) (Donofrio *et al.*, 1987). This is followed by muscular weakness in the extremities, and, with continued exposure, deep-tendon reflexes diminish and muscular atrophy follows. The cerebral lesions are mainly vascular in origin and occur in both the gray and white matter; characteristic multiple, symmetrical foci of hemorrhagic necrosis occur.

Blood. Inorganic arsenicals affect the bone marrow and alter the cellular composition of the blood. Hematological evaluation usually reveals anemia with slight-to-moderate leukopenia; eosinophilia may also be present. Anisocytosis becomes evident with increasing exposure to arsenic. The vascularity of the bone marrow is increased. Some of the chronic hematological effects may result from impaired absorption of folic acid. Serious, irreversible blood and bone-marrow disturbances from organic arsenicals are rare.

Liver. Inorganic arsenicals and a number of now-obsolete organic arsenicals are particularly toxic to the liver and produce fatty infiltration, central necrosis, and cirrhosis. The damage may be mild or so severe that death may ensue. The injury is generally to the hepatic parenchyma, but in some cases the clinical picture may closely resemble occlusion of the common bile duct, the principle lesions being pericholangitis and bile thrombi in the finer biliary radicles.

Carcinogenesis and Teratogenesis. There is overwhelming epidemiological evidence that long-term ingestion of arsenic in drinking water or long-term exposure from the use of inorganic arsenicals in sheep-dip or vineyard sprays predisposes to intraepidermal squamous-cell and superficial basal-cell carcinomas of the skin (Jackson and Grainge, 1975). In addition to skin cancer, arsenic is also known to produce lung cancer and is suspected to cause liver cancer (Pershagen, 1981).

Acute Arsenic Poisoning. Federal restrictions on the allowable content of arsenic in food and in the occupational environment not only have improved safety procedures and decreased the number of intoxications but also have decreased the amount of arsenic in use; only the annual production of arsenic-containing herbicides is increasing.

The incidence of accidental, homicidal, and suicidal arsenic poisoning has greatly diminished in recent decades. Arsenic in the form of As_2O_3 used to be a common cause of poisoning because it is readily available, is practically tasteless, and has the appearance of sugar.

Gastrointestinal discomfort is usually experienced within an hour after intake of an arsenical, although it may be delayed as much as 12 hours after oral ingestion if food is in the stomach. Burning lips, constriction of the throat, and difficulty in swallowing may be the first symptoms, followed by excruciating gastric pain, projectile vomiting, and severe diarrhea. Oliguria with proteinuria and hematuria is usually present; eventually anuria may occur. The patient often complains of marked skeletal muscle cramps and severe thirst. As the loss of fluid proceeds, symptoms of shock appear. Hypoxic convulsions may occur terminally, and coma and death ensue. In severe poisoning, death can occur within an hour, but the usual interval is 24 hours. With prompt application of corrective therapy, patients may survive the acute phase of the toxicity only to develop neuropathies and other disorders. In a series of 57 such patients, 37 had peripheral neuropathy and 5 had encephalopathy. The motor system appears to be spared only in the mildest cases; severe crippling is common (Jenkins, 1966).

Chronic Arsenic Poisoning. The most common early signs of chronic arsenic poisoning are muscle weakness and aching, skin pigmentation (especially of the neck, eyelids, nipples, and axillae), hyperkeratosis, and edema. Gastrointestinal involvement is less prominent in long-term exposures. Other signs and symptoms that should arouse suspicion of arsenic poisoning include garlic odor of the breath and perspiration, excessive salivation and sweating, stomatitis, generalized itching, sore throat, coryza, lacrimation, numbness, burning or tingling of the extremities, dermatitis, vitiligo, and alopecia. Poisoning may begin insidiously with symptoms of weakness, languor, anorexia, occasional nausea and vomiting, and diarrhea or constipation. Subsequent symptoms may simulate acute coryza. Dermatitis and keratosis of the palms and soles are common features. Mee's lines are characteristically found in the fingernails (white transverse lines of deposited arsenic that usually appear 6 weeks after exposure). Because the fingernail grows at a rate of 0.1 mm per day, the approximate time of exposure may be determined. Desquamation and scaling of the skin may initiate an exfoliative process involving many epithelial structures of the body. The liver may enlarge, and obstruction of the bile ducts may result in jaundice. Eventually cirrhosis may occur from the hepatotoxic action. Renal dysfunction may also be encountered. As intoxication advances, encephalopathy may develop. Peripheral neuritis results in motor and sensory paralysis of the extremities; usually the legs are more severely affected than the arms, in contrast to lead palsy. The bone marrow is seriously injured by arsenic. With severe exposure, all hematological elements may be affected.

Treatment of Arsenic Poisoning. After short-term exposure to arsenic, routine measures are taken to stabilize the patient and prevent further absorption of the poison. In particular, attention is directed to the status of the intravascular volume, since the effects of arsenic on the gastrointestinal tract can result in fatal hypovolemic shock. Hypotension requires fluid replacement and may necessitate pharmacological support of blood pressure with pressor agents such as dopamine.

Chelation therapy is often begun with dimercaprol (3 mg/kg intramuscularly every 4 hours) until abdominal symptoms subside and charcoal (if given initially) is passed in the feces. Oral treatment with penicillamine may then be substituted for dimercaprol and continued for 4 days. Penicillamine should be given in four divided doses to a maximum of 1 g per day. If symptoms recur after cessation of chelation therapy, a second course of penicillamine may be instituted. Succimer (2,3-dimercaptosuccinic acid), a derivative of dimercaprol, appears to be an extremely promising agent for the treatment of arsenic poisoning (Graziano *et al.,* 1978a; Lenz *et al.,* 1981).

After long-term exposure to arsenic, treatment with dimercaprol and penicillamine may also be used, but oral penicillamine alone is usually sufficient. The duration of therapy is determined by the clinical condition of the patient, and the decision is aided by periodic determinations of urinary arsenic concentrations. Adverse effects of the chelating agents may limit the usefulness of therapy (*see* below). Dialysis may become necessary with severe arsenic-induced nephropathy; successful removal of arsenic by dialysis has been reported (Vaziri *et al.*, 1980).

Arsine. Arsine gas, generated by electrolytic or metallic reduction of arsenic in nonferrous metal products, is a rare cause of industrial intoxication. Rapid and often fatal hemolysis is a unique characteristic of arsine poisoning and probably results from arsine combining with hemoglobin and then reacting with oxygen to cause hemolysis. A few hours after exposure, headache, anorexia, vomiting, paresthesia, abdominal pain, chills, hemoglobinuria, bilirubinemia, and anuria occur. Jaundice appears after 24 hours. A coppery skin pigmentation is frequently observed and is thought to be due to methemoglobin. Kidneys of persons poisoned by arsine characteristically contain casts of hemoglobin, and there is cloudy swelling and necrosis of the cells of the proximal tubule. If the patient survives the severe hemolysis, death often results from renal failure. Treatment consists of exchange transfusions and forced alkaline diuresis. Dimercaprol has no effect on the hemolysis, and beneficial effects on renal function have not been established; it is thus not recommended.

CADMIUM

Cadmium ranks close to lead and mercury as a metal of current toxicological concern. It occurs in nature in association with zinc and lead, and extraction and processing of these metals thus often lead to environmental contamination with cadmium. The element was discovered in 1817 but was seldom used until its valuable metallurgical properties were discovered approximately 50 years ago. A high resistance to corrosion, valuable electrochemical properties, and other useful chemical properties account for cadmium's wide applications in electroplating and galvanization and its use in plastics, paint pigments (cadmium yellow), and nickel-cadmium batteries. Applications for and production of cadmium will continue to increase. Because less than 5% of the metal is recycled, environmental pollution is an important consideration. Coal and other fossil fuels contain cadmium, and their combustion releases the element into the environment.

Workers in smelters and other metal-processing plants may be exposed to high concentrations of cadmium in the air; however, for most of the population, exposure from contamination of food is most important. Uncontaminated foodstuffs contain less than 0.05 μg of cadmium per gram wet weight, and the average daily intake is about 50 μg. Drinking water normally does not contribute significantly to cadmium intake, but cigarette smoking does. One cigarette contains 1 to 2 μg of cadmium, and, with even 10% pulmonary absorption (Elinder *et al.*, 1983), the smoking of one pack of cigarettes per day results in a dose of approximately 1 mg of cadmium per year from smoking alone. Shellfish and animal liver and kidney are among foods that can have concentrations of cadmium higher than 0.05 μg/g, even under normal circumstances. When foods such as rice and wheat are contaminated by cadmium in soil and water, the concentration of the metal may increase considerably (1 μg/g).

In Fuchu, Japan, shortly after World War II, a large number of people complained of rheumatic and myalgic pains; the disease was named *itai-itai* ("ouch-ouch"). It was determined that cadmium had washed into the local rice fields from the effluent from a lead–zinc processing plant.

Absorption, Distribution, and Excretion. Cadmium occurs only in one valency state, 2+, and does not form stabile alkyl compounds or other organometallic compounds of known toxicological significance.

Cadmium is poorly absorbed from the gastrointestinal tract. Studies in laboratory animals indicate the extent of absorption to be only about 1.5% (Engstrom and Nordberg, 1979), and limited studies in man indicate a value of about 5% (Rahola *et al.*, 1972). Absorption from the respiratory tract appears to be more complete; cigarette smokers may absorb 10 to 40% of inhaled cadmium (Friberg *et al.*, 1974).

After absorption, cadmium is transported in blood, bound mainly to blood cells and albumin. After distribution, approximately 50% of the total body burden is found in the liver and kidney. These organs also contain metallothionein, a low-molecular-weight protein with high affinity for metals such as cadmium and zinc. One third of the amino acid residues in metallothionein are cysteine. Metallothionein is inducible by exposure to cadmium, and elevated concentrations of this metal-binding protein may be protective by preventing the interaction of cadmium with other functional macromolecules (Goering and Klaassen, 1983, 1984).

The half-life of cadmium in the body is 10 to 30 years. Consequently, with continuous environmental exposure, concentrations of the metal in tissues increase throughout life. The body burden of cadmium in a 50-year-old adult in the United States is about 30 mg (Friberg *et al.*, 1974). Its extremely long biological half-life renders cadmium an environmental poison very prone to accumulation. After a single intravenous injection of cadmium into laboratory animals, the biliary route of excretion is quantitatively more important than the urinary route (Klaassen and Kotsonis, 1977). After multiple exposures the biliary excretion of cadmium is almost abolished because of binding to metallothionein (Klaassen, 1978). Overall, fecal elimination is quantitatively more important than urinary excretion of the metal. Urinary excretion of cadmium becomes significant only after substantial renal toxicity has occurred.

Acute Cadmium Poisoning. Acute poisoning usually results from inhalation of cadmium dusts and fumes (usually cadmium oxide) and from the ingestion of cadmium salts. The early toxic effects are due to local irritation. In the case of oral intake, these include nausea, vomiting, salivation, diarrhea, and abdominal cramps. In the short term, cadmium is more toxic when inhaled. Signs and symptoms, which appear within a few hours, include irritation of the upper respiratory tract, chest pains, nausea, dizziness, and diarrhea. Toxicity may progress to include fatal pulmonary edema or residual emphysema with peribronchial and perivascular fibrosis (Zavon and Meadow, 1970).

Chronic Cadmium Poisoning. The toxic effects of long-term exposure to cadmium differ somewhat with the route of exposure. The kidney is affected following either pulmonary or gastrointestinal exposure; marked effects are observed in the lungs only after exposure by inhalation.

Kidney. When the concentration of cadmium in the kidney reaches a level of 200 μg/g, there is renal injury. It seems probable that binding of the metal by metallothionein protects the organ when concentrations are lower. Proteinuria is due to proximal tubular injury (Lauwerys *et al.*, 1979). The quantitation of β_2-microglobulin in urine appears to be the most sensitive index of cadmium-induced nephrotoxicity (Piscator and Pettersson, 1977). With more severe exposure, glomerular injury occurs, filtration is decreased, and there is aminoaciduria, glycosuria, and proteinuria. The nature of the glomerular injury is unknown but may involve an autoimmune component (Lauwerys *et al.*, 1984).

Lung. The consequence of excessive inhalation of cadmium fumes and dusts is loss of ventilatory capacity, with a corresponding increase in residual lung volume. Dyspnea is the most frequent complaint of patients with cadmium-induced lung disease. The pathogenesis of cadmium-induced emphysema and pulmonary fibrosis is not well understood (Davison *et al.*, 1988); however, cadmium specifically inhibits the synthesis of plasma α_1-antitrypsin (Chowdhury and Louria, 1976), and there is an association between severe α_1-antitrypsin deficiency of genetic origin and emphysema in men.

Cardiovascular System. Perhaps the most controversial issue concerning the effects of cadmium on man is the suggestion that the metal plays a significant role in the cause of hypertension (Schroeder, 1965). The initial study was epidemiological. People dying from hypertension were found to have significantly higher concentrations of cadmium and higher cadmium-to-zinc ratios in their kidneys than people dying of other causes. Others have found similar correlations (Thind and Fischer, 1976). However, consistent effects of cadmium on the blood pressure of experimental animals have not been observed, and hypertension is not prominent in industrial cadmium poisoning.

Bone. One of the hallmarks of itai-itai was osteomalacia. However, studies in Sweden and the United Kingdom failed to corroborate this effect of cadmium poisoning (Kazantzis *et al.*, 1963; Adams *et al.*, 1969). The intake of calcium and fat-soluble vitamins such as vitamin D is much higher in these countries than in Japan. The Japanese victims were mostly multiparous, postmenopausal women. Thus, there may be an interaction between cadmium, nutrition, and bone disease. Body stores of calcium have been found to be decreased in subjects exposed to cadmium occupationally (Scott *et al.*, 1980). This presumed effect of cadmium may be due to interference with renal regulation of calcium and phosphate balance.

Testis. Testicular necrosis, a common characteristic of short-term exposure to cadmium in experimental animals, is uncommon with long-term, low-level exposure (Kotsonis and Klaassen, 1978). Cadmium-induced testicular necrosis has not been observed in men.

Treatment of Cadmium Poisoning. Effective therapy for cadmium poisoning has been difficult to achieve. After short-term inhalation the patient must be removed from the source, and pulmonary ventilation should be monitored carefully. Respiratory support and steroid therapy may become necessary.

Chelation therapy with $CaNa_2EDTA$ is recommended, although there is no clearly proven benefit. The dosage of $CaNa_2EDTA$ should be 75 mg/kg per day in three to six divided doses for 5 days. After a minimum of 2 days without treatment, a second 5-day course may be given. The total dose of $CaNa_2EDTA$ per 5-day course should not exceed 500 mg/kg. Dimercaprol is contraindicated because it increases nephrotoxicity.

Although data for man are not available, experimental data in animals have shown that polycarboxylic acid chelators, such as $CaNa_2EDTA$ and calcium trisodium diethylenetriaminepentaacetate (pentetate calcium trisodium; $CaNa_3DTPA$), can be effective when administered immediately after exposure to cadmium (Cantilena and Klaassen, 1982a). Unfortunately, there is a rapid decrease in the effectiveness of such chelation therapy with time, due to distribution of the metal to sites that are not reached by the chelators (Waalkes *et al.*, 1983). Therefore, chelation therapy must be instituted as soon as possible after exposure to the metal.

IRON

Although iron is not an environmental poison, accidental intoxication with ferrous salts used to treat iron-deficiency anemias has made iron a frequently encountered source of poisoning in young children. Iron poisoning is discussed in Chapter 54 (*see also* below).

RADIOACTIVE HEAVY METALS

The widespread production and use of radioactive heavy metals for nuclear generation of electricity, nuclear weapons, laboratory research, manufacturing, and medical diagnosis have generated unique problems in dealing with accidental poisoning by such metals. Since the toxicity of radioactive metals is almost entirely a consequence of ionizing radiation, the therapeutic objective following exposure is not just the chelation of the metals but their removal from the body as rapidly and completely as possible.

Treatment of the acute radiation syndrome is largely symptomatic. Attempts have been made to investigate the effectiveness of organic reducing agents (such as mercaptamine [cysteamine]), administered to prevent the formation of free radicals. Success has been limited.

Major products of a nuclear accident or the use of nuclear weapons include ^{239}Pu, ^{137}Cs, ^{144}Ce, and ^{90}Sr. Isotopes of strontium and radium have proven to be extremely difficult to remove from the body with chelating agents. Several factors are involved in the relative resistance of radioactive metals to chelation therapy; these include the affinity of these particular metals for individual chelators and the observation that radiation from Sr and Ra in bone destroys nearby capillaries. Blood flow in bone is thereby decreased and the radioisotopes become imprisoned. Many chelating agents have been used experimentally, including $CaNa_3DTPA$, which has been shown to be effective against ^{239}Pu (Jones *et al.*, 1986). One gram of $CaNa_3DTPA$, administered by slow intravenous drip on alternate days, three times per week, has enhanced excretion 50- to 100-fold in animals and in human subjects exposed in accidents. As is commonly seen with heavy-metal poisoning, effectiveness of treatment diminishes very rapidly with an increasing delay between exposure and the initiation of therapy.

HEAVY-METAL ANTAGONISTS

EDETATE CALCIUM DISODIUM

Ethylenediaminetetraacetic acid (EDTA), its sodium salt (edetate disodium, Na_2EDTA), and a number of closely related compounds have been used for many years as industrial and analytical reagents because they chelate many divalent and trivalent metals. The cation used to make a water-soluble salt of EDTA has an important role in the toxicity of the chelator. Na_2EDTA causes hypocalcemic tetany. However, edetate calcium disodium ($CaNa_2EDTA$) can be used for treatment of poisoning by metals that have higher affinity for the chelating agent than does Ca^{2+}.

Chemistry and Mechanism of Action. The structure of $CaNa_2EDTA$ is as follows:

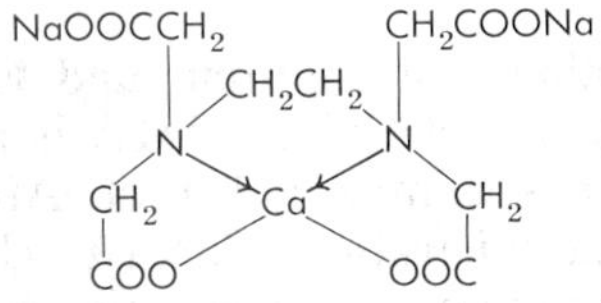

Edetate Calcium Disodium

The pharmacological effects of $CaNa_2EDTA$ result from formation of chelates with divalent and trivalent metals in the body. Accessible metal ions (both exogenous and endogenous) with a higher affinity for $CaNa_2EDTA$ than Ca^{2+} will be chelated, mobilized, and usually excreted. Experimental studies in mice have shown that administration of $CaNa_2EDTA$ mobilizes several endogenous metallic cations, including those of zinc, manganese, and iron (Cantilena and Klaassen, 1982b). The main therapeutic use of $CaNa_2EDTA$ is in the treatment of metal intoxications, especially lead intoxication.

The successful use of $CaNa_2EDTA$ in the treatment of lead poisoning is due, in part, to the capacity of lead to displace calcium from the chelate. Enhanced mobilization and excretion of lead indicate that the metal is accessible to EDTA. Mercury poisoning, by contrast, does not respond to the drug, despite the fact that mercury displaces calcium from $CaNa_2EDTA$ *in vitro*. Mercury is unavailable to the chelate, perhaps because it is too tightly bound by body ligands (—SH) or sequestered in body compartments that are not penetrated by $CaNa_2EDTA$. Because of its ionic character, it is unlikely that $CaNa_2EDTA$ penetrates cells significantly and the volume of distribution of $CaNa_2EDTA$ is approximately equal to that of extracellular fluid.

Bone provides the primary source of lead that is chelated by $CaNa_2EDTA$ (Hammond, 1971). After such chelation, lead is redistributed from soft tissues to the skeleton.

Chelation therapy with $CaNa_2EDTA$ has been advocated by some and heralded in the lay press for the treatment of atherosclerosis. The premise is the presence of calcium deposits in atherosclerotic plaques. There is no reasonable rationale for such therapy and, more importantly, no evidence that it is efficacious (Rathmann and Golightly, 1984).

Absorption, Distribution, and Excretion. Less than 5% of $CaNa_2EDTA$ is absorbed from the gastrointestinal tract. After intravenous administration, $CaNa_2EDTA$ disappears from the circulation with a half-life of 20 to 60 minutes. In blood, all of the drug is found in plasma. About 50% is excreted in the urine in 1 hour and over 95% in 24 hours. For this reason, adequate renal function is necessary for successful therapy. Renal clearance of the compound in dogs equals that of inulin, and glomerular filtration accounts entirely for urinary excretion. Altering either the pH or the rate of flow of urine has no effect on the rate of excretion. There is very little metabolic degradation of EDTA. The drug is distributed mainly in the extracellular fluids, but very little gains access to the spinal fluid (5% of the plasma concentration).

Toxicity. Rapid intravenous administration of Na_2EDTA causes hypocalcemic tetany. However, a slow infusion (less than 15 mg per minute) administered to a normal individual elicits no symptoms of hypocalcemia because of the ready availability of extracirculatory stores of Ca^{2+}. In contrast, $CaNa_2EDTA$ can be administered intravenously in relatively large quantities with no untoward effects because the change in the concentration of Ca^{2+} in the plasma and total body is negligible.

The principal toxic effect of $CaNa_2EDTA$ is on the kidney. Repeated large doses of the drug cause hydropic vacuolization of the proximal tubule, loss of the brush border, and, eventually, degeneration of proximal tubular cells (Catsch and Harmuth-Hoene, 1979). Changes in distal tubules and glomeruli are less conspicuous. The early renal effects are usually reversible, and urinary abnormalities disappear rapidly upon cessation of treatment.

Renal toxicity may be related to the large amounts of chelated metals that pass through the renal tubule in a relatively short period during drug therapy. Some dissociation of chelates may occur because of competition for the metal by physiological ligands or because of pH changes in the cell or the lumen of the tubule. However, a more likely mechanism of toxicity may be the interaction between the chelator and endogenous metals in proximal tubular cells.

Other less serious side effects have been reported with use of $CaNa_2EDTA$, including malaise, fatigue, and excessive thirst, followed by the sudden appearance of chills and fever. This may, in turn, be followed by severe myalgia, frontal headache, anorexia, occasional nausea and vomiting, and, rarely, increased urinary frequency and urgency. Other possible undesirable effects include sneezing, nasal congestion, and lacrimation; glycosuria; anemia; dermatitis, with lesions strikingly similar to those of vitamin B_6 deficiency; transitory lowering of systolic and diastolic blood pressures; prolonged prothrombin time; and inversion of the T wave of the electrocardiogram.

Preparations, Routes of Administration, and Dosage. $CaNa_2EDTA$ is available as *edetate calcium disodium* (CALCIUM DISODIUM VERSENATE). For parenteral use, an injection containing 200 mg/ml is employed. Intramuscular administration of $CaNa_2EDTA$ results in good absorption, but pain occurs at the injection site. For intravenous use, $CaNa_2EDTA$ is diluted in either 5% dextrose or 0.9% saline and is administered slowly by intravenous drip over at least a 1-hour period. A dilute solution is necessary to avoid thrombophlebitis. Regimens for the treatment of intoxications with specific metals are described above. For children, the maximal daily dosage is 75 mg/kg of body weight, divided into two or three doses. To minimize nephrotoxicity, adequate urine production should be established prior to and during treatment with $CaNa_2EDTA$. However, in patients with lead encephalopathy and increased intracranial pressure, excess fluids must be avoided. In such cases, conservative replacement of fluid is advised and intramuscular administration of $CaNa_2EDTA$ is recommended.

Edetate disodium injection is used for the emergency treatment of hypercalcemia (*see* Chapter 62).

Therapeutic Uses. The uses of $CaNa_2EDTA$ for the treatment of intoxication with various metals are described above under each metal.

PENTETIC ACID (DIETHYLENETRIAMINEPENTAACETIC ACID; DTPA)

DTPA, like EDTA, is a polycarboxylic acid chelator, but it has somewhat greater affinity for most heavy metals. Many investigations in animals have shown that the spectrum of clinical effectiveness of DTPA is similar to that of EDTA. Because of its relatively greater affinity for metals, DTPA has been tried in cases of heavy-metal poisoning that do not respond to EDTA, particularly poisoning by radioactive metals. Unfortunately, success has been limited, probably because DTPA also has limited access to intracellular sites of metal storage. Since DTPA rapidly binds Ca^{2+}, $CaNa_3DTPA$ is employed. The use of DTPA is investigational.

DIMERCAPROL

History. During World War II, an intensive effort was made to develop an antidote to lewisite, a vesicant arsenical war gas. Knowing that arsenicals reacted with SH-containing molecules, Stocken and Thompson, at Oxford University, initiated a systematic study of thiol compounds to find one that would successfully compete with the tissue SH groups for the arsenicals. Their investigations indicated that the arsenicals would form a very stable and relatively nontoxic chelate ring with the dithiol compound, dimercaprol (2,3-dimercaptopropanol). When scientists in the United States joined their British colleagues in these studies, they designated dimercaprol as British anti-Lewisite (BAL). Pharmacological investigators revealed that this compound would protect against the toxic effects of other heavy metals as well.

Chemistry. Dimercaprol has the following structure:

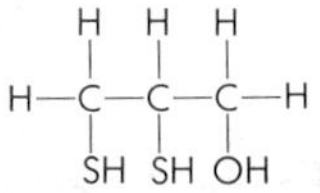

Dimercaprol

It is an oily fluid with a pungent, disagreeable odor typical of mercaptans. Because of its instability in aqueous solutions, peanut oil is the solvent employed in pharmaceutical preparations. Dimercaprol and related thiols are readily oxidized.

Mechanism of Action. The pharmacological actions of dimercaprol are the result of formation of chelation complexes between its sulfhydryl groups and metals. The molecular properties of the dimercaprol–metal chelate have considerable practical significance. With metals such as mercury, gold, and arsenic, the strategy is to attain a stable complex to promote elimination of the metal. Dissociation of the complex and oxidation of dimercaprol can occur *in vivo*. Furthermore, the sulfur–metal bond may be labile in the acidic tubular urine, which may increase delivery of metal to renal tissue and increase toxicity. The dosage regimen is therefore designed to maintain a concentration of dimercaprol in plasma adequate to favor the continuous formation of the more stable 2:1 (BAL:metal) complex and its rapid excretion. However, because of pronounced and dose-related side effects, excessive plasma concentrations must be avoided. The concentration in plasma must therefore be maintained by repeated fractional dosage until the offending metal can be excreted.

Dimercaprol is much more effective when given as soon as possible after exposure to the metal, because it is more effective in preventing inhibition of sulfhydryl enzymes than in reactivating them. This therapeutic principle applies to the use of all chelating agents.

Dimercaprol antagonizes the biological actions of metals that form mercaptides with essential cellular sulfhydryl groups, principally arsenic, gold, and mercury. It is also used in combination with $CaNa_2EDTA$ to treat lead poisoning. Intoxication by selenites, which oxidize sulfhydryl enzymes, is not influenced by dimercaprol.

Absorption, Distribution, and Excretion. Dimercaprol cannot be administered orally; it is given by deep intramuscular injection as a 10% solution in oil. Peak concentrations in blood are attained in 30 to 60 minutes. The half-life is short, and metabolic degradation and excretion are essentially complete within 4 hours.

Toxicity. In man, the administration of dimercaprol produces a variety of side effects that are usually more alarming than serious. Reactions to dimercaprol occur in approximately 50% of subjects receiving 5 mg/kg intramuscularly. The effects of repeated administration of this dose are not cumulative if an interval of at least 4 hours elapses between injections. One of the most consistent responses to dimercaprol is a rise in systolic and diastolic arterial pressures, accompanied by tachycardia. The rise in pressure may be as great as 50 mm Hg in response to the second of two doses (5 mg/kg) given 2 hours apart. The pressure rises immediately but returns to normal within 2 hours.

Other signs and symptoms, many of which tend to parallel the change in blood pressure in time and intensity, are the following, listed in approximate order of frequency: nausea and vomiting; headache; a burning sensation in the lips, mouth, and throat and a feeling of constriction, sometimes pain, in the throat, chest, or hands; conjunctivitis, blepharospasm, lacrimation, rhinorrhea, and salivation; tingling of the hands; a burning sensation in the penis; sweating of the forehead, hands, and other areas; abdominal pain; and occasional appearance of painful sterile abscesses at the injection site. Symptoms are often accompanied by a feeling of anxiety and unrest. Because the dimercaprol–metal complex breaks down easily in an acidic medium, production of an alkaline urine protects the kidney during therapy. Children react as do adults, although approximately 30% may also experience a fever that disappears upon withdrawal of the drug. A transient reduction of the percentage of polymorphonuclear leukocytes may also be observed. Dimercaprol may also cause hemolytic anemia in patients deficient in glucose-6-phosphate dehydrogenase. Dimercaprol is contraindicated in patients with hepatic insufficiency, except when this is a result of arsenic poisoning.

Preparation. *Dimercaprol (2,3-dimercaptopropanol)* is available for injection as a solution in peanut oil (100 mg/ml). Treatment regimens are described above for the individual metals.

SUCCIMER (2,3-DIMERCAPTOSUCCINIC ACID)

Succimer has the following structure:

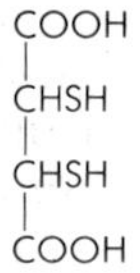

Succimer

It is a disulfhydryl compound and is thus similar to dimercaprol. However, it is much less toxic than dimercaprol and is effective orally (Aposhian, 1983). Succimer is a promising, orally effective, relatively nontoxic chelator for the treatment of not only mercury poisoning (Friedheim and Corvi, 1975) but also poisoning with arsenic (Graziano *et al.*, 1978a) and lead (Friedheim *et al.*, 1976; Graziano *et al.*, 1978b, 1985, 1988).

PENICILLAMINE

History. Penicillamine was first isolated in 1953 from the urine of patients with liver disease who were receiving penicillin. Discovery of its chelating properties led to its use in patients with Wilson's disease and heavy-metal intoxications.

Chemistry. Penicillamine is D-β,β-dimethylcysteine. Its structure is as follows:

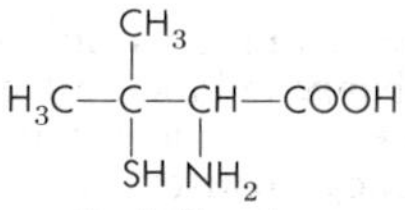

Penicillamine

The D isomer is used clinically, although the L isomer also forms chelation complexes. Penicillamine is an effective chelator of copper, mercury, zinc, and lead and promotes the excretion of these metals in the urine.

Absorption, Distribution, and Excretion. Penicillamine is well absorbed (40 to 70%) from the gastrointestinal tract and, therefore, has a decided advantage over other chelating agents. Food, antacids, and iron reduce its absorption. Peak concentrations in blood are obtained between 1 and 3 hours after administration (Bannwarth *et al.*, 1987). Unlike cysteine, its nonmethylated parent compound, penicillamine is somewhat resistant to attack by cysteine desulfhydrase or L-amino acid oxidase. As a result, penicillamine is relatively stable *in vivo*. N-acetylpenicillamine is more effective than penicillamine in protecting against the toxic effects of mercury (Aposhian and Aposhian, 1959), presumably because it is even more resistant to metabolism. Hepatic biotransformation is responsible for most of the degradation of penicillamine, and very little is excreted unchanged. Metabolites are found in both urine and feces (Perrett, 1981).

Therapeutic Uses. In addition to its use as a chelating agent for the treatment of copper, mercury, and lead poisoning, penicillamine is used in Wilson's disease (hepatolenticular degeneration due to an excess of copper), cystinuria, and rheumatoid arthritis. The rationale for its use in cystinuria is that penicillamine forms a relatively soluble disulfide compound with cysteine through a disulfide interchange mechanism and thereby decreases the formation of cystine-containing renal stones.

The mechanism of action of penicillamine in rheumatoid arthritis remains uncertain, although suppression of the disease may result from marked reduction in concentrations of IgM rheumatoid factor (Wernick *et al.*, 1983). Uniquely, this decrease is not accompanied by reductions of the concentrations of immunoglobulins in plasma. Other experimental uses of penicillamine include the treatment of primary biliary cirrhosis and scleroderma. The mechanism of action of penicillamine in these diseases may also involve effects on immunoglobulins and immune complexes (Epstein *et al.*, 1979).

Toxicity. The main disadvantage of penicillamine for short-term use as a chelating agent is the concern that it might cause anaphylactic reactions in patients allergic to penicillin (Bell and Graziano, 1983). However, preparations of the drug no longer contain trace amounts of penicillin. With long-term use, penicillamine induces several cutaneous lesions, including urticaria, macular or papular reactions, pemphigoid lesions, lupus erythematosus, dermatomyositis, adverse effects on collagen, and other less serious reactions, such as dryness and scaling. Cross-reactivity with penicillin may be responsible for some episodes of urticarial or maculopapular reactions with generalized edema, pruritus, and fever that occur in as many as one third of patients taking penicillamine (*see* Bell and Graziano, 1983). For a detailed review of the adverse dermatological effects of penicillamine, *see* Levy and coworkers (1983).

The hematological system may also be affected severely; reactions include leukopenia, aplastic anemia, and agranulocytosis. These may occur at any time during therapy, and they may be fatal. Patients must obviously be monitored carefully.

Renal toxicity induced by penicillamine is usually manifested as reversible proteinuria and hematuria, but it may progress to the nephrotic syndrome with membranous glomerulopathy. More rarely, fatalities have been reported from Goodpasture's syndrome (Hill, 1979).

Toxicity to the pulmonary system is uncommon, but severe dyspnea has been reported from penicillamine-induced bronchoalveolitis. Myasthenia gravis has also been induced by long-term therapy with penicillamine (Gordon and Burnside, 1977). Less serious side effects include nausea, vomiting, diarrhea, dyspepsia, anorexia, and a transient loss of taste for sweet and salt, which is relieved by supplementation of the diet with copper. Contraindications to penicillamine therapy include pregnancy, a previous history of penicillamine-induced agranulocytosis or aplastic anemia, or the presence of renal insufficiency.

Preparations and Dosage. *Penicillamine* is available in capsules containing 125 or 250 mg (CUPRIMINE) or as 250-mg tablets (DEPEN). The drug should be given on an empty stomach to avoid interference by metals in food. For chelation therapy, the usual dose is 500 mg to 1.5 g per day in four divided doses (*see* sections under individual metals). In cystinuria, the urinary excretion of cystine is used to adjust dosage, although 2 g per day in four divided doses is usually employed. Various dosage regimens have been studied for the treatment of rheumatoid arthritis. A single daily dose of 125 to 250 mg is usually used to initiate therapy. Dosage is increased at intervals of 1 to 3 months as necessary. Two or three months may be required before improvement is evident. Many patients eventually respond to 500 to 750 mg per day or less. For the treatment of Wilson's disease, four daily doses are taken, and 1 to 2 g per day is usually employed. The urinary excretion of copper should be monitored to determine if the dosage of penicillamine is adequate.

TRIENTINE

Penicillamine is the drug of choice for treatment of Wilson's disease. However, the drug produces undesirable effects, as discussed above, and some patients become intolerant. For these individuals, trientine (triethylenetetramine dehydrochloride [CUPRID]) is an acceptable alternative. Trientine is an effective cupriuretic agent in patients with Wilson's disease, although it may be less potent than penicillamine. The drug is effective orally. Maximal daily doses of 2 g for adults or 1.5 g for children are taken in two to four divided portions on an empty stomach. Trientine may cause iron deficiency; this can be overcome with short courses of iron therapy, but iron and trientine should not be ingested within 2 hours of each other.

DEFEROXAMINE

The structure of deferoxamine is shown below. It is isolated as the iron chelate from *Streptomyces pilosus* and is treated chemically to obtain the metal-free ligand. Deferoxamine has the desirable properties of a remarkably high affinity for ferric iron ($K_a = 10^{31}$) coupled with a very low affinity for calcium ($K_a = 10^2$). Studies *in vitro* have shown that it removes iron from hemosiderin and ferritin and, to a lesser extent, from transferrin. Iron in hemoglobin or cytochromes is not removed by deferoxamine.

Deferoxamine is poorly absorbed after oral administration, and parenteral administration is required in most cases. Deferoxamine is metabolized principally by plasma enzymes, but the pathways have not yet been defined. The drug is also readily excreted in the urine.

Deferoxamine causes a number of aller-

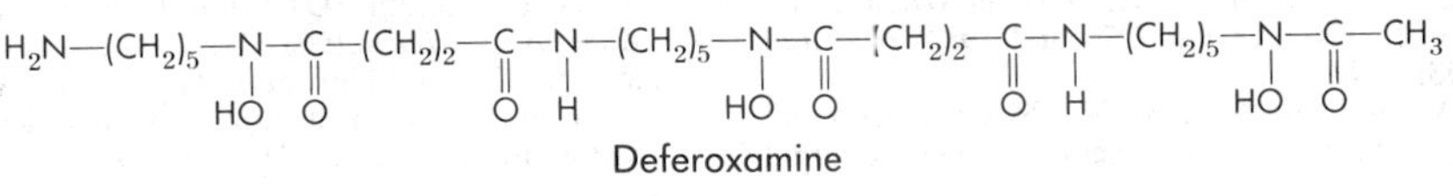

Deferoxamine

gic reactions, including pruritus, wheals, rash, and anaphylaxis. Other adverse effects include dysuria, abdominal discomfort, diarrhea, fever, leg cramps, and tachycardia. Occasional cases of cataract formation have been reported. Deferoxamine may cause neurotoxicity during long-term, high-dose therapy for transfusion-dependent thalassemia major; both visual and auditory changes have been described (Olivieri *et al.*, 1986). Contraindications to the use of deferoxamine include renal insufficiency and anuria; during pregnancy, the drug should be used only if clearly indicated.

Preparation, Dosage, and Uses. *Deferoxamine mesylate* (DESFERAL MESYLATE) is available in vials containing 500 mg of the drug. In acute iron poisoning the intramuscular route is preferred, unless the patient is in shock. Initially, for adults and children, 1 g is given, followed by 500 mg every 4 hours for two doses. The 500-mg injections may be continued at 4- or 12-hour intervals, depending on the clinical response, but the total amount of drug administered should not exceed 6 g in 24 hours. The intravenous route is required when a patient is in shock. The dosage schedule and limitations are the same as those indicated for the intramuscular route. However, the infusion rate must never exceed 15 mg/kg per hour. As soon as the clinical situation permits, intravenous administration should be discontinued and the drug given intramuscularly. Other aspects of the treatment of acute iron poisoning are discussed in Chapter 54.

For chronic iron intoxication (*e.g.*, thalassemia), an intramuscular dose of 0.5 to 1.0 g per day is recommended, although continuous subcutaneous administration (1 to 2 g per day) is almost as effective as intravenous administration (Propper *et al.*, 1977). When blood is being transfused to patients with thalassemia, 2.0 g of deferoxamine (per unit of blood) should be given by slow intravenous infusion (rate not to exceed 15 mg/kg per hour) during the transfusion, but not by the same intravenous line. Deferoxamine is not recommended in primary hemochromatosis; phlebotomy is the treatment of choice. Deferoxamine has also been used for the chelation of aluminum in dialysis patients (Swartz, 1985).

Adams, R. G.; Harrison, J. F.; and Scott, P. The development of cadmium-induced proteinuria, impaired renal function and osteomalacia in alkaline battery workers. *Q. J. Med.*, **1969**, *38*, 425–443.

Al-Abbasi, A. H.; Kostyniak, P. J.; and Clarkson, T. W. An extracorporeal complexing hemodialysis system for the treatment of methylmercury poisoning. III. Clinical applications. *J. Pharmacol. Exp. Ther.*, **1978**, *207*, 249–254.

Annest, J. L.; Pirkle, J. L.; Makuc, D.; Neese, J. W.; Bayse, D. D.; and Kovar, M. G. Chronological trend in blood lead levels between 1976 and 1980. *N. Engl. J. Med.*, **1983**, *308*, 1373–1377.

Aposhian, H. V., and Aposhian, M. M. N-acetyl-DL-penicillamine, a new oral protective agent against the lethal effects of mercuric chloride. *J. Pharmacol. Exp. Ther.*, **1959**, *126*, 131–135.

Baker, E. L.; Goyer, R. A.; Fowler, B. A.; Khettry, U.; Bernard, O. B.; Adler, S.; White, R.; Babyor, R.; and Feldman, R. G. Occupational lead exposure, nephropathy and renal cancer. *Am. J. Industr. Med.*, **1980**, *1*, 139–148.

Bakir, F.; Al-Khalidi, A.; Clarkson, T. W.; and Greenwood, R. Clinical observations on treatment of alkylmercury poisoning in hospital patients. *Bull. W.H.O.*, **1976**, *53*, Suppl., 87–92.

Bakir, F.; Damluji, S. F.; Amin-Zaki, L.; Mortadha, M.; Khalidi, A.; Al-Rawi, N. Y.; Tikriti, S.; Dhahir, H. I.; Clarkson, T. W.; Smith, J. C.; and Doherty, R. A. Methylmercury poisoning in Iraq. An interuniversity report. *Science*, **1973**, *181*, 230–241.

Bakir, F.; Rustin, H.; Tikriti, S.; Al-Damluji, S. F.; and Shihristani, H. Clinical and epidemiological aspects of methylmercury poisoning. *Postgrad. Med. J.*, **1980**, *56*, 1–10.

Bannwarth, B.; Pere, P.; and Nicolas, A. Clinical pharmacokinetics of D-penicillamine. *Pharmacokinet.*, **1987**, *13*, 317–333.

Bell, C. L., and Graziano, F. M. The safety of administration of penicillamine to penicillin-sensitive individuals. *Arthritis Rheum.*, **1983**, *26*, 801–803.

Bellinger, D.; Leviton, A.; Waternaux, C.; Needleman, H.; and Rabinowitz, M. Longitudinal analyses of prenatal and postnatal lead exposure and early cognitive development. *N. Engl. J. Med.*, **1987**, *316*, 1037–1043.

Berwick, D. M., and Komaroff, A. L. Cost effectiveness of lead screening. *N. Engl. J. Med.*, **1982**, *306*, 1392–1398.

Boyd, P. R. The treatment of tetraethyl lead poisoning. *Lancet*, **1957**, *1*, 181–185.

Campbell, J. R.; Clarkson, T. W.; and Omar, M. D. The therapeutic use of 2,3-dimercaptopropane-1-sulfonate in two cases of inorganic mercury poisoning. *J.A.M.A.*, **1986**, *256*, 3127–3130.

Cantilena, L. R., and Klaassen, C. D. Decreased effectiveness of chelation therapy for Cd poisoning with time. *Toxicol. Appl. Pharmacol.*, **1982a**, *63*, 173–180.

———. The effect of chelating agents on the excretion of endogenous metals. *Ibid.*, **1982b**, *63*, 344–350.

Chisolm, J. J. Management of increased lead absorption and lead poisoning in children. *N. Engl. J. Med.*, **1973**, *289*, 1016–1018.

Chisolm, J. J., and Barltrop, D. Recognition and management of children with increased lead absorption. *Arch. Dis. Child.*, **1979**, *54*, 249–262.

Chowdhury, P., and Louria, D. B. Influence of cadmium and other trace metals on human α_1-antitrypsin: an *in vitro* study. *Science*, **1976**, *191*, 480–481.

Cooper. W. C., and Gaffey, W. R. Mortality of lead workers. *J. Occup. Med.*, **1975**, *17*, 100–107.

Cory-Slechta, D. A.; Weiss, B.; and Cox, C. Mobilization and redistribution of lead over the course of calcium disodium ethylenediamine tetraacetate chelation therapy. *J. Pharmacol. Exp. Ther.*, **1987**, *243*, 804–813.

Davison, A. G., and others. Cadmium fume inhalation and emphysema. *Lancet*, **1988**, *1*, 663–667.

Donofrio, P. D.; Wilbourn, A. J.; Albers, J. W.; Rogers, L.; Salanga, V.; and Greenberg, H. S. Acute arsenic intoxication presenting as Guillain-Barré-like syndrome. *Muscle Nerve*, **1987**, *10*, 114–120.

Elinder, C. G.; Kjellstrom, T.; Lind, B.; Linnman, L.; Piscator, M.; and Sundstedt, K. Cadmium exposure from smoking cigarettes. Variations with time and country where purchased. *Environ. Res.*, **1983**, *32*, 220–227.

Emmerson, B. T. Chronic lead neuropathy: the diagnostic use of calcium EDTA and the association with gout. *Aust. Ann. Med.*, **1963**, *12*, 310–324.

Engstrom, B., and Nordberg, G. F. Dose dependence of gastrointestinal absorption and biological half-time of cadmium in mice. *Toxicology*, **1979**, *13*, 215–222.

Epstein, O.; De Villiers, D.; Jain, S.; Potter, B. J.; Thomas, H. C.; and Sherlock, S. Reduction of immune complexes and immunoglobulin induced by D-penicillamine in primary biliary cirrhosis. *N. Engl. J. Med.*, **1979**, *300*, 274–278.

Friedheim, E., and Corvi, C. Meso-dimercaptosuccinic acid: a chelating agent for the treatment of mercury poisoning. *J. Pharm. Pharmacol.*, **1975**, *27*, 624–626.

Friedheim, E.; Corvi, C.; and Walker, C. J. Meso-dimercaptosuccinic acid: a chelating agent for the treatment of mercury and lead poisoning. *J. Pharm. Pharmacol.*, **1976**, *28*, 711–712.

Gerstner, H., and Huff, J. Clinical toxicology of mercury. *J. Toxicol. Environ. Health*, **1977**, *2*, 491–526.

Giunta, F.; DiLandro, D.; and Chiarmda, M. Severe acute poisoning from the ingestion of a permanent wave solution of mercuric chloride. *Hum. Toxicol.*, **1983**, *2*, 243–246.

Goering, P. L., and Klaassen, C. D. Altered subcellular distribution of cadmium following cadmium pretreatment: possible mechanism of tolerance to cadmium-induced lethality. *Toxicol. Appl. Pharmacol.*, **1983**, *70*, 195–203.

———. Tolerance to cadmium-induced hepatotoxicity following cadmium pretreatment. *Ibid.*, **1984**, *74*, 308–313.

Goldwater, L. J., and Hoover, A. W. An international study of "normal" levels of lead in blood and urine. *Arch. Environ. Health*, **1967**, *15*, 60–63.

Gordon, R. A., and Burnside, J. W. Penicillamine induced myasthenia gravis in rheumatoid arthritis. *Ann. Intern. Med.*, **1977**, *87*, 578–579.

Graziano, J. H.; Cuccia, D.; and Friedheim, E. Potential usefulness of 2,3-dimercaptosuccinic acid for the treatment of arsenic poisoning. *J. Pharmacol. Exp. Ther.*, **1978a**, *207*, 1051–1055.

Graziano, J. H.; Leong, J. K.; and Friedheim, E. 2,3-Dimercaptosuccinic acid: a new agent for the treatment of lead poisoning. *Ibid.*, **1978b**, *206*, 696–700.

Graziano, J. H.; Lolacono, N. J.; and Meyer, P. Dose-response study of oral 2,3-dimercaptosuccinic acid in children with elevated blood lead concentrations. *J. Pediatr.*, **1988**, *113*, 751–757.

Graziano, J. H.; Siris, E. S.; Lolacono, N.; Silverberg, S. J.; and Turgeon, L. 2,3-Dimercaptosuccinic acid as an antidote for lead intoxication. *Clin. Pharmacol. Ther.*, **1985**, *37*, 431–438.

Gregus, Z., and Klaassen, C. D. Disposition of metals in rats: a comparative study of fecal, urinary, and biliary excretion and tissue distribution of eighteen metals. *Toxicol. Appl. Pharmacol.*, **1986**, *85*, 24–38.

Gross, S. B.; Pfitzer, E. A.; Yeager, D. W.; and Kehoe, R. A. Lead in human tissues. *Toxicol. Appl. Pharmacol.*, **1975**, *32*, 638–651.

Hammond, P. B. The effects of chelating agents on the tissue distribution and excretion of lead. *Toxicol. Appl. Pharmacol.*, **1971**, *18*, 296–310.

Hill, H. F. H. Penicillamine in rheumatoid arthritis. Adverse effects. *Scand. J. Rheumatol.* [*Suppl.*], **1979**, *28*, 94–99.

Jackson, R., and Grainge, J. W. Arsenic and cancer. *Can. Med. Assoc. J.*, **1975**, *113*, 396–401.

Jenkins, R. B. Inorganic arsenic and the nervous system. *Brain*, **1966**, *89*, 479–498.

Jones, C. W.; Mays, C. W.; Taylor, G. N.; Lloyd, R. D.; and Packer, S. M. Reducing the cancer risk of ^{239}Pu by chelation therapy. *Radiat. Res.*, **1986**, *107*, 296–306.

Kark, R. A. P.; Poskanzer, D. C.; Bullock, J. D.; and Boylen, G. Mercury poisoning and its treatment with *N*-acetyl-D,L-penicillamine. *N. Engl. J. Med.*, **1971**, *285*, 10–16.

Kazantzis, G.; Flynn, F. V.; Spowage, J.; and Trott, D. G. Renal tubular malfunction and pulmonary emphysema in cadmium pigment workers. *Q. J. Med.*, **1963**, *32*, 165–192.

Kehoe, R. A. The metabolism of lead in man in health and disease. *Arch. Environ. Health*, **1961a**, *2*, 418–422.

———. The metabolism of lead in man in health and disease: The Harben Lectures, 1960. *J. R. Inst. Public Health Hyg.*, **1961b**, *24*, 81–97, 101–120, 129–143.

———. Studies of lead administration and elimination in adult volunteers under natural and experimentally induced conditions over extended periods of time. *Food Chem. Toxicol.*, **1987**, *25*, 421–493.

Kershaw, T. G.; Dhahir, P. H.; and Clarkson, T. W. The relationship between blood levels and dose of methylmercury in man. *Arch. Environ. Health*, **1980**, *35*, 28–36.

Klaassen, C. D. Biliary excretion of mercury compounds. *Toxicol. Appl. Pharmacol.*, **1975**, *33*, 356–365.

———. Effect of metallothionein on the hepatic disposition of metals. *Am. J. Physiol.*, **1978**, *234*, E47–E53.

Klaassen, C. D., and Kotsonis, F. N. Biliary excretion of cadmium in the rat, rabbit and dog. *Toxicol. Appl. Pharmacol.*, **1977**, *41*, 101–112.

Kostyniak, P. J. Mobilization and removal of methylmercury in the dog during extracorporeal complexing hemodialysis with 2,3-dimercaptosuccinic acid (DMSA). *J. Pharmacol. Exp. Ther.*, **1982**, *221*, 63–68.

Kotsonis, F. N., and Klaassen, C. D. The relationship of metallothionein to the toxicity of cadmium after prolonged oral administration to rats. *Toxicol. Appl. Pharmacol.*, **1978**, *46*, 39–54.

Landrigan, P. Arsenic—state of the art. *Am. J. Industr. Med.*, **1981**, *2*, 5–14.

Langolf, G. D.; Chaffin, D. B.; Whittle, H. P.; and Henderson, R. Effects of industrial mercury exposure on urinary mercury, EMG and psychomotor functions. In, *Clinical Chemistry and Chemical Toxicology of Metals.* (Brown, S. S., ed.) Elsevier/North Holland Biomedical Press, Amsterdam, **1977**, pp. 213–220.

Lauwerys, R. R.; Bernard, A.; Roels, H. A.; Buchet, J.-P.; and Viau, C. Characterization of cadmium proteinuria in man and rat. *Environ. Health Perspect.*, **1984**, *54*, 147–152.

Lauwerys, R. R.; Roels, H. A.; Buchet, J.-P.; Bernard, A.; and Stanesca, D. Investigations on the lung and kidney function in workers exposed to cadmium. *Environ. Health Perspect.*, **1979**, *28*, 137–146.

Lenz, K.; Hruby, K.; Druml, W.; Eder, A.; Gazner, A.; Kleinberger, G.; Pichler, M.; and Weiser, M. 2,3-Dimercaptosuccinic acid in human arsenic poisoning. *Arch. Toxicol.*, **1981**, *47*, 241–243.

Levy, R. S.; Fisher, M.; and Alter, J. N. Penicillamine: review of cutaneous manifestations. *J. Am. Acad. Dermatol.*, **1983**, *8*, 548–558.

McAlpine, D., and Shukuro, A. Minimata disease. An unusual neurological disorder caused by contaminated fish. *Lancet*, **1958**, *2*, 629–631.

Magos, L. The effects of dimercaptosuccinic acid on the excretion and distribution of mercury in rats and mice treated with mercuric chloride and methylmercury chloride. *Br. J. Pharmacol.*, **1976**, *56*, 479–484.

Magos, L.; Halbach, S.; and Clarkson, T. W. Role of catalase in the oxidation of mercury vapor. *Biochem. Pharmacol.*, **1978**, *27*, 1373–1377.

Mahaffey, K. R.; Rosen, J. F.; Chesney, R. W.; Peeler, J. T.; Smith, C. M.; and DeLuca, H. F. Association between age, blood lead concentration, and serum 1,25-dehydroxycholecalciferol levels in children. *Am. J. Clin. Nutr.*, **1982**, *35*, 1327–1331.

Matherson, D. S.; Clarkson, T. W.; and Gelfand, E. W. Mercury toxicity (acradynia) induced by long term injection of gammaglobulin. *J. Pediatr.*, **1980**, *97*, 153–155.

Needleman, H. L.; Gunne, C.; Leviton, A.; Reed, R.; Peresie, H.; Maher, C.; and Barrett, P. Defects in psychologic and classroom performance in children with elevated dentine lead levels. *N. Engl. J. Med.*, **1979**, *300*, 689–695.

Needleman, H. L., and Leviton, A. Lead associated intellectual defect. *N. Engl. J. Med.*, **1982**, *306*, 367.

Olivieri, N. F., and others. Visual and auditory neurotoxicity in patients receiving subcutaneous deferoxamine infusions. *N. Engl. J. Med.*, **1986**, *314*, 869–873.

Perrett, D. The metabolism and pharmacology of D-penicillamine in man. *J. Rheumatol.* [*Suppl.*], **1981**, *8*, 51–55.

Pershagen, G. The carcinogenicity of arsenic. *Environ. Health Perspect.*, **1981**, *40*, 93–100.

Pirkle, J. L.; Schwartz, J.; Landis, R.; and Harlan, W. R. The relationship between blood lead levels and blood pressure and its cardiovascular risk implications. *Am. J. Epidemiol.*, **1985**, *121*, 246–258.

Piscator, M., and Pettersson, B. Chronic cadmium poisoning: diagnosis and prevention. In, *Clinical Chemistry and Chemical Toxicology of Metals*. (Brown, S. S., ed.) Elsevier/North Holland Biomedical Press, Amsterdam, **1977**, pp. 143–155.

Propper, R. D.; Cooper, B.; Rufo, R. R.; Nienhuis, A. W.; Anderson, W. F.; Bunn, H. F.; Rosenthal, A.; and Nathan, D. G. Continuous subcutaneous administration of deferoxamine in patients with iron overload. *N. Engl. J. Med.*, **1977**, *297*, 418–423.

Rahola, T.; Aaran, R. K.; and Mietinen, J. K. Half-time studies of mercury and cadmium by whole body counting. International Atomic Energy Agency symposium on the assessment of radioactive organ and body burdens. In, *Assessment of Radioactive Contamination in Man*. The Agency, Vienna, **1972.**

Rathmann, K. L., and Golightly, L. K. Chelation therapy of atherosclerosis. *Drug Intell. Clin. Pharm.*, **1984**, *18*, 1000–1003.

Rosen, J. F.; Chesney, R. W.; Hamstra, A.; DeLuca, H. F.; and Mahaffey, K. R. Reduction in 1,25-dihydroxyvitamin D in children with increased lead absorption. *N. Engl. J. Med.*, **1980**, *302*, 1128–1131.

Schroeder, H. A. Cadmium as a factor in hypertension. *J. Chronic Dis.*, **1965**, *18*, 217–228.

Schumann, G. B.; Lerner, S. I.; Weiss, M. A.; Gawronski, L.; and Lohiya, G. K. Inclusion-bearing cells in industrial workers exposed to lead. *Am. J. Clin. Pathol.*, **1980**, *74*, 192–196.

Scott, R.; Haywood, J. K.; Broddy, K.; Williams, E. D.; Harvey, I.; and Paterson, P. J. Whole body calcium deficit in cadmium exposed workers with hypercalciuria. *Urology*, **1980**, *15*, 356–359.

Seshia, S. S.; Rajani, K. R.; Boeckx, R. L.; and Chow, P. N. The neurological manifestations of chronic inhalation of leaded gasoline. *Dev. Med. Child Neurol.*, **1978**, *20*, 323–334.

Smith, H. D.; Boehner, R. L.; Carney, T.; and Majors, W. J. The sequelae of pica with and without lead poisoning. *Am. J. Dis. Child.*, **1963**, *105*, 609–616.

Swartz, R. D. Deferoxamine and aluminum removal. *Am. J. Kidney Dis.*, **1985**, *6*, 358–364.

Tam, G. K. H.; Charbenneau, S. M.; Bryce, F.; Pomroy, C.; and Sandi, E. Metabolism of inorganic arsenic (^{74}As) in humans following oral ingestion. *Toxicol. Appl. Pharmacol.*, **1979**, *50*, 319–322.

Tamashiro, H.; Arakaki, M.; Akagi, H.; Futatsuka, M.; and Roht, L. H. Mortality and survival for Minamata disease. *Int. J. Epidemiol.*, **1985**, *14*, 582–588.

Thind, G. S., and Fischer, G. Plasma cadmium and zinc in human hypertension. *Clin. Sci. Mol. Med.*, **1976**, *51*, 483–486.

Vaziri, N. D.; Upham, T.; and Barton, C. H. Hemodialysis clearance of arsenic. *Clin. Toxicol.*, **1980**, *17*, 451–456.

Waalkes, M. P.; Watkins, J. B.; and Klaassen, C. D. Minimal role of metallothionein in decreased chelator efficacy for cadmium. *Toxicol. Appl. Pharmacol.*, **1983**, *68*, 392–398.

Wernick, R.; Merryman, P.; Jaffe, I.; and Ziff, M. IgG and IgM rheumatoid factors in rheumatoid arthritis. *Arthritis Rheum.*, **1983**, *26*, 593–598.

Zavon, M. R., and Meadow, C. D. Vascular sequelae to cadmium fume exposure. *Am. Ind. Hyg. Assoc. J.*, **1970**, *31*, 180–182.

Monographs and Reviews

American Academy of Pediatrics. Statement on childhood lead poisoning. *Pediatrics*, **1987**, *79*, 457–465.

Aposhian, H. V. DMSA and DMPS—water soluble antidotes for heavy metal poisoning. *Annu. Rev. Pharmacol. Toxicol.*, **1983**, *23*, 193–215.

Bernard, B. P., and Becker, C. E. Environmental lead exposure and the kidney. *J. Toxicol. Clin. Toxicol.*, **1988**, *26*, 1–34.

Catsch, A., and Harmuth-Hoene, A.-E. Pharmacology and therapeutic applications of agents used in heavy metal poisoning. In, *The Chelation of Heavy Metals*. (Levine, W. G., ed.) Pergamon Press, New York, **1979**, pp. 116–124.

Chisolm, J. J., Jr. Treatment of lead poisoning. *Mod. Treat.*, **1967**, *4*, 710–727.

Craswell, P. W. Chronic lead nephropathy. *Annu. Rev. Med.*, **1987**, *38*, 169–173.

Davis, J. M., and Svendsgaard, D. J. Lead and child development. *Nature*, **1987**, *329*, 297–300.

Enwonwu, C. O. Potential health hazard of use of mercury in dentistry: critical review of the literature. *Environ. Res.*, **1987**, *42*, 257–274.

Friberg, L.; Piscator, M.; Nordberg, G. F.; and Kjellstrom, T. *Cadmium in the Environment*, 2nd ed. CRC Press, Inc., Cleveland, **1974.**

Friberg, L., and Vostal, J. *Mercury in the Environment: An Epidemiological and Toxicological Appraisal*. CRC Press, Inc., Cleveland, **1972.**

Garrettson, L. K. Lead. In, *Clinical Management of Poisoning and Drug Overdose*. (Haddad, L. M., and Winchester, J. F., eds.) W. B. Saunders Co., Philadelphia, **1983**, pp. 649–655.

Goyer, R. A. Toxic effects of metals. In, *Casarett and Doull's Toxicology: The Basic Science of Poisons*, 3rd ed. (Klaassen, C. D.; Amdur, M. O.; and Doull, J.; eds.) Macmillan Publishing Co., New York, **1985**, pp. 582–635.

Hindmarsh, J. T., and McCurdy, R. F. Clinical and environmental aspects of arsenic toxicity. *C.R.C. Crit. Rev. Clin. Lab. Sci.*, **1986**, *23*, 315–347.

Janin, Y.; Couinaud, C.; Stone, A.; and Wise, L. The "lead induced colic" syndrome in lead intoxication. *Surg. Annu.*, **1985**, *17*, 287–307.

Kazantzis, G. Lead: sources, exposure and possible carcinogenicity. *IARC Sci. Publ.*, **1986**, *71*, 103–111.

National Academy of Sciences. *Lead: Airborne Lead in Perspective*. National Research Council, Washington, D. C., **1972.**

Sharp, D. S.; Becker, C. E.; and Smith, A. H. Chronic low-level lead exposure. Its role in the pathogenesis of hypertension. *Med. Toxicol.*, **1987**, *2*, 210–232.

Smith, M. Recent work on low-level lead exposure and its impact on behavior, intelligence, and learning: a review. *J. Am. Acad. Child Psychiatry*, **1985**, *24*, 24–32.

Smith, W. E., and Smith, A. M. *Minamata*. Holt, Rinehart & Winston, New York, **1975.**

Task Group on Metal Accumulation. Accumulation of toxic metals with specific reference to their absorption, excretion, and biological half-times. *Environ. Physiol. Biochem.*, **1973**, *3*, 65–107.

Winship, K. A. Toxicity of inorganic arsenic salts. *Adverse Drug React. Acute Poisoning Rev.*, **1984**, *3*, 129–160.

CHAPTER

67 NONMETALLIC ENVIRONMENTAL TOXICANTS: AIR POLLUTANTS, SOLVENTS AND VAPORS, AND PESTICIDES

Curtis D. Klaassen

Environmental pollution, an undesired spin-off of human activity, was relatively insignificant until urbanization. People dug coal from the ground, used it to heat homes, and thus created an atmosphere of sulfurous smoke above the cities. From the thirteenth century onward, periodic efforts were made to forbid the burning of coal in London, but, on the whole, people have accepted a polluted atmosphere as part of urban life. Power plants burn fossil fuels to generate electricity; steel mills have grown along river banks and lake shores; oil refineries have risen near ports and oil fields; smelters roast and refine metals near great mineral deposits; the automobile is all-prevalent. All these operations pollute the air, water, and soil around them.

When synthetic materials came of age, factories were built to produce them. Little thought was given to the toxicity of chemicals not intended for use in man. Relatively few of the three million known chemicals have been tested for toxic effects; many have been indiscriminately disseminated throughout the environment.

AIR POLLUTION

Air pollutants enter the body predominantly through the lungs. Some of these chemicals are absorbed into the blood, whereas the lungs eliminate substances that are not absorbed.

Absorption and Deposition of Toxicants by the Lungs

The site of deposition of aerosols in the respiratory tract depends on the size of the particle. Particles of 5 μm or larger in diameter are usually deposited in the upper airway. Those deposited in the unciliated anterior portion of the nose remain until removed by wiping, blowing, or sneezing. In the posterior portion of the nose, a mucus blanket propelled by cilia carries insoluble particles to the pharynx in minutes. These particles are swallowed and pass to the gastrointestinal tract. Soluble particles dissolved in the mucus may be carried to the pharynx or absorbed through the epithelium into the blood.

Particles of 1 to 5 μm are deposited in the tracheobronchial tree and cleared by the cilia's upward movement of mucus. Although the rate of ciliary movement varies in different parts of the respiratory tract, it is rapid and efficient. Rates of transport are between 0.1 and 1 mm per minute, resulting in half-lives for the particles that range from 30 to 300 minutes. Coughing and sneezing move mucus and particles rapidly toward the glottis. The particles may also be swallowed.

Particles less than 1 μm in diameter remain suspended in the inhaled air and reach the alveolar zone of the lung, where they may be readily absorbed. The surface area is large (50 to 100 m^2); the rate of blood flow is high; and the blood is in close proximity to the alveolar air (10 μm). The factors that govern the rate of absorption of gases are discussed in Chapter 13. Liquid aerosols cross the alveolar cell membranes by passive diffusion in proportion to their lipid solubility. Mechanisms for removal or absorption of particulate matter (usually less than 1 μm in diameter) from the alveolus are less clearly defined and are less efficient than those that remove particles from the tracheobronchial tree. Three processes are apparently operative. The first is physical removal; particles deposited on the fluid layer of the alveoli are believed to be aspirated onto the mucociliary escalator of the tracheobronchial tree. The second is phagocytosis, usually by mononuclear phagocytes or alveolar macrophages. The third is by absorption into the lymphatic system. Particles can remain in lymphatic tissue for long periods, and, for this reason, the lymphatic tissue has been called the dust store of the lungs.

Overall, removal of particulates from the alveolus is relatively inefficient. Only about 20% of such matter is removed during the first day after deposition; that which remains longer than 24 hours is often removed very slowly. The rate of this clearance can be predicted from the solubility of the substance in lung fluids. The least soluble compounds are removed at a slower rate. Such removal is apparently largely due to dissolution and absorption into the blood. Some particles may remain in the alveoli indefinitely if the cells that phagocytize them proliferate and join the reticular network to form an alveolar dust plaque or nodule.

Types and Sources of Air Pollutants

Five pollutants account for nearly 98% of air pollution. These are carbon monoxide (52%), sulfur oxides (18%), hydrocarbons (12%), particulate matter (10%), and nitrogen oxides (6%) (Amdur, 1985). A distinction is often made between two kinds of pollution. The first is characterized by sulfur dioxide and smoke from incomplete combustion of coal and by conditions of fog and cool temperatures. Because of its chemical nature, it is termed a *reducing type of pollution*. The second is characterized by hydrocarbons, oxides of nitrogen, and photochemical oxidants. It is caused by automobile exhaust and occurs especially in areas such as the Los Angeles basin, where intense sunlight causes photochemical reactions in polluted air masses that are trapped by a meteorological inversion layer. Because of its nature, it is described as an *oxidizing type of pollution* or *photochemical air pollution*.

Five major sources account for 90% of the tons of pollutants that are emitted annually (Amdur, 1985): transportation (particularly automobiles) (60%), industry (18%), electric-power generation (13%), space heating (6%), and refuse disposal (3%).

Health Effects of Air Pollution

Episodes of high pollution cause mortality and morbidity. There are three classical examples: 65 people died in the Meuse Valley, Belgium, in 1930; 20 people died in Donora, Pennsylvania, in 1948; 4000 people died in London in 1952. Each of these incidents occurred during an atmospheric temperature inversion that lasted 3 to 4 days. During this time the concentration of pollutants surpassed the usual levels for these already heavily polluted areas; because coal was the main fuel, the pollution was the reducing kind. Most of the people who became ill or died were elderly; some had either cardiac or respiratory diseases or both; none could cope with the added stress of breathing heavily polluted air.

Acute effects on health are thus clearly associated with the reducing type of pollution. While there is less evidence to associate photochemical oxidant pollution with such effects on human health, there are significant correlations between levels of oxidants in the air and hospital admissions for allergic disorders, inflammatory disease of the eye, acute upper respiratory infections, influenza, and bronchitis.

Toxicology of Air Pollutants

Sulfur Dioxide. Sulfur dioxide gas is generated primarily by the burning of fossil fuels that contain sulfur. The concentration of sulfur dioxide required to kill laboratory animals is so high that it has little relevance to problems of air pollution. However, daily exposure of rats to 10 ppm of sulfur dioxide for 1 to 2 months thickens the mucus layer in the trachea about fivefold. Although the cilia beat with normal frequency, the thick mucus retards clearance. The abnormal mucus layer is caused by increased numbers of mucus-secreting cells in the main bronchi, where such cells are common, and in the peripheral airways, where they are normally absent (Hirsch *et al.,* 1975).

A basic physiological response to inhalation of sulfur dioxide is a mild degree of bronchial constriction that is dependent on intact parasympathetic innervation. When exposed to 5 ppm of sulfur dioxide for 10 minutes, most human subjects show increased resistance to the flow of air. Asthmatics have an increased sensitivity to sulfur dioxide; bronchoconstriction may occur at concentrations as low as 0.25 ppm (Sheppard *et al.,* 1981).

It appears that an increase in the concentration of atmospheric sulfur oxides, which is generally accompanied by an elevation in the level of particulate matter, significantly affects morbidity and mortality. In heavily polluted cities (London, New York, Cracow), exposure for 24 hours to sulfur dioxide concentrations of 0.11 to 0.15 ppm and total particulate concentrations of 500 to 600 $\mu g/m^3$ results in increased morbidity and mortality, and a temporary decrease in pulmonary function is observed at about 0.1 ppm of sulfur dioxide and 250 $\mu g/m^3$ of particulate matter (Ware *et al.*, 1981).

Sulfuric Acid. A portion of sulfur dioxide in the atmosphere is converted to sulfuric acid, ammonium sulfate, and other sulfates. The conversion to sulfuric acid can be initiated by soot or by trace metals such as vanadium or manganese. Stable sulfite complexes may be formed in the presence of metals such as copper or iron.

Sulfuric acid increases airway resistance in relation to both concentration and particle size (Amdur *et al.*, 1978). Particles of 1 μm (1 mg/m^3) produce a rapid and marked increase in resistance to flow, whereas particles of 7 μm produce only a slight increase because they cannot penetrate beyond the upper respiratory tract. Sulfuric acid produces a greater increase in resistance to flow than does sulfur dioxide after either a short- or long-term exposure.

Particulate Sulfates. Sulfates vary greatly in their effects on respiration, and the sulfate ion *per se* does not alter respiratory function. Zinc ammonium sulfate, a reported constituent of the Donora fog, increases respiratory resistance at a concentration of 0.25 mg/m^3; it produces a greater increase in resistance to flow than does sulfur dioxide.

Ozone. The oxidant found in the highest concentrations in polluted atmosphere is ozone (O_3). Several miles above the earth's surface there is sufficient short-wave ultraviolet light to convert O_2 to O_3 by direct absorption. Of the major atmospheric pollutants, nitrogen dioxide is the most efficient in absorbing ultraviolet light. Such absorption leads to a complex series of reactions, which may be simplified as follows:

$$NO_2 \xrightarrow{UV} NO + O$$
$$O + O_2 \longrightarrow O_3$$
$$O_3 + NO \longrightarrow NO_2 + O_2$$

Because NO_2 is regenerated by the reaction of NO with O_3, the result is cyclical. Simultaneously, oxygen atoms react with hydrocarbons in the atmosphere, especially olefins and substituted aromatics, resulting in oxidized compounds and free radicals that react with NO to produce more NO_2. The result is accumulation of NO_2 and O_3, while concentrations of NO are depleted.

Ozone is a lung irritant that is capable of causing death from pulmonary edema. Gross pulmonary edema is evident in mice exposed to concentrations above 2 ppm. Ozone causes desquamation of the epithelium throughout the ciliated airways and produces degenerative changes in type-I cells and swelling or rupture of the capillary endothelium in the alveoli. The type-I cells are later replaced by type-II cells; this type-II cell proliferation is a hallmark of ozone toxicity (Menzel, 1984). It is important to note that pulmonary toxicity has been observed in experimental animals after relatively short exposures to concentrations of ozone that occasionally exist for short periods in polluted urban areas.

Long-term exposure to ozone may cause thickening of the terminal respiratory bronchioles. Chronic bronchitis, fibrosis, and emphysematous changes are observed in a variety of species exposed to ozone at concentrations slightly above 1 ppm (Amdur, 1985).

Ozone at concentrations of 0.25 to 0.75 ppm causes shallow, rapid breathing, a decrease in pulmonary compliance, and subjective symptoms, such as cough, tightness in the chest, and dryness of the throat. Such concentrations of ozone may be present during long, high-altitude flights (Folinsbee, 1983). Ozone also increases the sensitivity of the lung to bronchoconstrictors such as histamine, acetylcholine, and allergens. It increases the incidence of infection in laboratory animals exposed to an aerosol of infectious microorganisms, probably through inhibition of clearance mechanisms (Gardner, 1984). However, epidemiological studies have failed to detect an increased incidence of ozone-induced respiratory infections in man.

The biochemical mechanism of pulmonary injury produced by ozone may be due to the formation of reactive free-radical intermediates (Menzel, 1970). Ozone-induced free radicals may be derived from interaction with sulfhydryl groups, from oxidative decomposition of unsaturated fatty acids, or both. Several lines of evidence indicate that one of the biological actions of ozone is reaction with unsaturated fatty acids. The ozonization of these fatty acids is essentially equivalent to lipid peroxidation. Sulfhydryl compounds and antioxidants (such as ascorbic acid and α-tocopherol) protect against ozone toxicity in laboratory animals but have not been shown to have protective effects in man (Menzel, 1984).

Nitrogen Dioxide. Nitrogen dioxide, like ozone, is a lung irritant that is capable of causing pulmonary edema. This pollutant is a particular risk to farmers, because sufficient amounts of nitrogen dioxide can be liberated from ensilage to produce the symptoms of pulmonary damage known as silo-filler's disease. The LC_{50} for a 4-hour exposure to nitrogen dioxide is about 90 ppm. As with ozone, nitrogen dioxide damages type-I cells of the alveoli. Chronic exposure of animals to nitrogen dioxide results in emphysematous lesions (Freeman *et al.*, 1972).

Experimental exposure of animals or man to nitrogen dioxide causes measurable alterations in pulmonary function. The pattern of changes resembles that produced by ozone—increased respiratory frequency and decreased compliance. Pulmonary resistance to air flow is minimally altered. The changes in pulmonary function occur when healthy subjects are exposed to 2 to 3 ppm and may happen at far lower concentrations in some asthmatic subjects (Orehek *et al.*, 1976).

Aldehydes. Aldehydes are formed by oxidation of hydrocarbons by sunlight and by incomplete combustion (automobile exhaust, forest fires); they are released from formaldehyde-containing resins (such as those in plywood, particle board, and urea-formaldehyde foam insulation). The high reactivity of aldehydes results in rather short half-lives of a few hours in the atmosphere. The concentration of aldehydes is 0.0005 to 0.002 ppm in a clean atmosphere, 0.004 to 0.05 ppm in ambient urban air, and up to 0.8 ppm in indoor environments where formaldehyde-emitting materials are found (Committee on Aldehydes, 1981; Woodbury and Zenz, 1983). About 50% of the total aldehyde in polluted air is formaldehyde (H_2CO), and about 5% is acrolein ($H_2C{=}CHCHO$). These materials probably contribute to the odor of photochemical smog and the ocular irritation that it causes.

Formaldehyde irritates mucous membranes of the nose, upper respiratory tract, and eyes. Concentrations of 0.5 to 1 ppm are detectable by odor, 2 to 3 ppm produce mild irritation, and 4 to 5 ppm are intolerable to most people. The concentration of formaldehyde may approach 1 ppm in the air of newly built homes, especially mobile homes. A significant correlation was found between the formaldehyde concentration in home air and the incidence of ocular irritation. Other symptoms (*e.g.*, runny nose, sore throat, headache, and cough) are also more frequent in people living in indoor environments with high levels of formaldehyde (Woodbury and Zenz, 1983). The overall pattern of respiratory response to formaldehyde resembles that to sulfur dioxide. Formaldehyde can provoke skin reactions in sensitized subjects, not only by contact but also by inhalation (Maibach, 1983). Occupational exposure to formaldehyde can also cause asthma (Nordman *et al.*, 1985). Inhalation of formaldehyde (6 to 15 ppm) for 2 years induces squamous-cell carcinomas in the nasal cavity of mice and rats (Kerns *et al.*, 1983). However, there is no evidence that exposure to formaldehyde produces human malignancies (U.A.R.E.P., 1988).

Acrolein is much more irritating than formaldehyde. Acrolein is a major contributor to the irritative quality of cigarette smoke and photochemical smog. The occupational threshold limit value (TLV) for acrolein is 0.1 ppm; 1 ppm causes lacrimation in less than 5 minutes (Committee on Aldehydes, 1981). Acrolein increases airway resistance and tidal volume and decreases respiratory frequency. Aldehydes increase resistance to air flow at concentrations below those that decrease respiratory frequency.

Carbon Monoxide. Carbon monoxide (CO) is a colorless, odorless, tasteless, and nonirritating gas resulting from incomplete combustion of organic matter. CO is the most abundant pollutant found in the lower atmosphere, and a large number of accidental and suicidal deaths occur yearly from its inhalation.

The average concentration of CO in the atmosphere is about 0.1 ppm. Natural sources, such as atmospheric oxidation of methane, forest fires, terpine oxidation, and the ocean (where microorganisms produce CO), are responsible for about 90% of the atmospheric CO; human activity produces about 10%.

Inadequate venting of furnaces and automobiles results in many deaths each year. Most victims of fires die from acute CO poisoning rather than from burns. The automobile is the greatest source of CO; concentrations can reach 115 ppm in heavy traffic, 75 ppm in vehicles on expressways, and 23 ppm in residential areas. In underground garages and tunnels, CO levels have been found to exceed 100 ppm for extended periods. The installation of pollution-control devices, including catalytic converters in automobile exhaust systems, has reduced CO emissions from about 90 to 3.4 g per mile of automobile travel and should decrease concentrations of CO in urban atmospheres (National Research Council, 1977).

The average concentration of CO in the atmosphere appears to be stabilized by efficient natural means of removal (sinks). The most important sink seems to be the reaction of CO with ambient hydroxyl radicals to form carbon dioxide; the upper atmosphere and the soil also are sinks.

Another source of exposure to CO is smoking. Goldsmith and Landaw (1968) reported a median carboxyhemoglobin (COHb) level of 5.9% in heavy smokers (two packs of cigarettes per day) who inhale.

Reaction of CO with Hemoglobin. Toxicity from CO is due to its combination with hemoglobin to form COHb. Hemoglobin in this form cannot carry oxygen, since both gases react with the same group in the hemoglobin molecule. Because the affinity of hemoglobin for CO is approximately 220 times greater than for oxygen, CO is dangerous even at very low concentrations. Since air contains 21% oxygen by volume, exposure to a gas mixture of 0.1% CO (1000 ppm) in air would result in approximately 50% carboxyhemoglobinemia.

The reduction in the oxygen-carrying capacity of blood is proportional to the amount of COHb present. However, the amount of oxygen available to the tissues is reduced further by the inhibitory influence of COHb on the dissociation of any oxyhemoglobin (O_2Hb) still available. This can be understood best by comparing an anemic individual having a hemoglobin value of 80 g per liter with a person having a hemoglobin value of 160 g per liter but with half of it in the form of COHb (Figure 67–1). In each instance the oxygen-carrying capacity is the same. The anemic individual may show few, if any, symptoms whereas the person suffering from CO poisoning will be near collapse.

The toxicity of CO is not due solely to the interference of CO with the delivery of O_2 by the blood. CO also exerts a direct toxic effect by binding to cellular cytochromes, such as those contained in

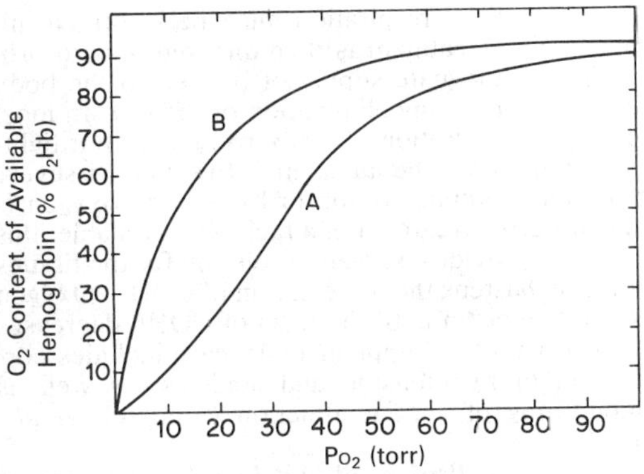

Figure 67–1. *The effect of carboxyhemoglobin (COHb) on the dissociation curve of oxyhemoglobin.*

Curve A represents the normal oxygen dissociation curve, which is unaffected by the presence of anemia (*e.g.*, 80 g/l of hemoglobin in the blood). Curve B represents the situation when there is 50% COHb and a normal concentration of hemoglobin (160 g/l of hemoglobin in the blood and half of the binding sites occupied by CO). The oxygen-carrying capacity is the same in both cases; however, when COHb is present, oxygen dissociates from hemoglobin at lower values of Po_2. This effect results from interactions between binding sites for O_2 or CO; there are four such sites per molecule of hemoglobin.

respiratory enzymes and myoglobin (Gutierrez, 1982).

Factors Governing CO Toxicity. Factors that govern the toxicity of CO include the concentration of the gas in inspired air, the duration of exposure, the respiratory minute volume, the cardiac output, the oxygen demand of the tissues, and the concentration of hemoglobin in the blood. Anemic persons are more susceptible to CO poisoning than are individuals with normal amounts of hemoglobin. Increased metabolic rate enhances the severity of symptoms in CO poisoning; this is why children succumb earlier than adults when exposed to a given concentration of the gas.

Change in barometric pressure does not affect the relative affinities of hemoglobin for O_2 and CO. However, at high altitudes and in other situations where oxygen tension is low, the effects of a given concentration of CO will be correspondingly more severe.

Signs and Symptoms of CO Toxicity. The signs and symptoms of CO poisoning are characteristic of hypoxia. They have been correlated with the COHb content of the blood. The relation between symptomatology and COHb concentration is shown in Table 67–1. It should not be inferred that all these symptoms are experienced by any one individual. Although inhalation of a high concentration may produce warning signs (transient weakness and dizziness) before consciousness is lost, there may be no warning at all.

Moderate concentrations of COHb have little effect on vital functions in the human subject at rest. As mentioned previously, the presence of COHb reduces the oxygen-carrying capacity but not the Po_2 of arterial blood. As a result, there is no stimulation of respiration by the carotid and aortic chemoreceptor mechanism. Cardiac rate, on the other hand, increases in all subjects when COHb reaches 30%, probably to compensate for peripheral vasodilatation caused by hypoxia, and lactic acidosis results from tissue hypoxia.

The clinical findings in patients acutely poisoned by CO are varied. Many patients exhibit symptoms not usually associated with CO poisoning: skin lesions, excessive sweating, hepatic enlargement, bleeding tendency, pyrexia, leukocytosis, albuminuria, and glycosuria.

Pathology of Acute CO Poisoning. The tissues most affected are those most sensitive to oxygen deprivation, such as the brain and the heart, and the lesions are predominantly hemorrhagic. The severe headache following exposure to CO is believed to be caused by cerebral edema and increased intracranial pressure resulting from excessive transudation across hypoxic capillaries. Finck (1966) has catalogued the gross pathological changes observed in 351 fatal cases of accidental CO poisoning. Rapidly fatal cases of CO poisoning are characterized by congestion and hemorrhages in all organs. In longer-term, eventually fatal cases, the hypoxic lesions observed are related to the duration of posthypoxic unconsciousness.

Bokonjić (1963) has shown that the maximal period of CO-induced posthypoxic unconsciousness compatible with complete neurological recovery is

Table 67–1. CORRELATION BETWEEN COHb CONCENTRATION AND SIGNS AND SYMPTOMS OF CARBON MONOXIDE POISONING *

% OF BLOOD SATURATION	SIGNS AND SYMPTOMS
0–10	No symptoms
10–20	Tightness across forehead; possibly slight headache; dilatation of cutaneous blood vessels
20–30	Headache; throbbing in temples
30–40	Severe headache; weakness; dizziness; dimness of vision; nausea and vomiting; collapse
40–50	Same as previous item with greater possibility of collapse or syncope; increased respiration and pulse
50–60	Syncope; increased respiration and pulse; coma with intermittent convulsions; Cheyne–Stokes respiration
60–70	Coma with intermittent convulsions; depressed cardiac function and respiration; possible death
70–80	Weak pulse and slowed respiration; respiratory failure and death

* Modified from Sayers and Davenport, 1930.

21 hours in patients under 48 years of age and 11 hours in older patients. Complete recovery of mental function was not observed when the CO-induced unconsciousness exceeded 15 hours in the older group or 64 hours in the younger group. Perhaps the most insidious effect of CO poisoning is the delayed development of neuropsychiatric impairment, which is manifested as inappropriate euphoria and impairment of judgment, abstract thinking, and concentration. The heart is also sensitive to hypoxia and may be permanently damaged by the presence of COHb in the blood. Evidence of ischemic changes and subendocardial infarction may be observed. Severe CO poisoning can produce skin lesions varying from areas of erythema and edema to marked blister and bulla formation. Rhabdomyolysis, presumably caused by the direct toxic effect of CO on myoglobin, and myoglobinuria with renal failure may also occur.

Diagnosis of Acute CO Poisoning. The presumptive diagnosis of acute CO poisoning is usually facilitated by circumstantial evidence, since the victim is commonly found under circumstances that leave little doubt as to the cause of the condition. COHb is cherry-red in color, and its presence in high concentrations in capillary blood may impart an abnormal red color to the skin, mucous membranes, and fingernails. However, the living patient is commonly cyanotic and pale, and "cherry-red cyanosis" is seen only at autopsy. A final diagnosis depends upon the demonstration of COHb in the blood. Therapy is not delayed to perform such a test in a severely poisoned individual, but the demonstration of COHb often has a forensic significance. If a person succumbs in an atmosphere containing CO, a postmortem blood sample usually contains 60% COHb; however, death sometimes occurs at lower concentrations. If the patient is removed from such an atmosphere while still breathing, the concentration of COHb rapidly declines, and, if respiratory exchange continues to be adequate, the blood is freed of this form of hemoglobin over a course of hours.

Fate and Excretion of CO. COHb is fully dissociable and, once acute exposure is terminated, the CO will be excreted via the lungs. Only a very small amount is oxidized to CO_2.

CO cannot be excreted without active respiration. Furthermore, COHb is extremely stable and is little affected by putrefaction. Therefore, valid measurements of COHb concentrations in the body can be made long after death. Conversely, little or no CO is absorbed post mortem and analysis of the blood in the heart provides an accurate measurement of the concentration of COHb in the blood at death. These factors have medicolegal importance.

When room air is breathed by a resting subject, the CO content of blood decreases with a half-time of 320 minutes. If 100% oxygen is substituted for air, this value is reduced to 80 minutes; under hyperbaric conditions, the half-time may be less than 25 minutes (Peterson and Stewart, 1970). These facts provide the basic principles for treatment of CO poisoning.

Treatment of CO Poisoning. It is first essential to transfer the patient to fresh air. If respiration has failed, artificial respiration must be instituted immediately. Treatment is then directed toward providing an adequate supply of oxygen to the body cells and hastening elimination of the CO. In most cases administration of 100% oxygen with a tight-fitting mask will be adequate. However, in severe poisoning, administration of hyperbaric oxygen is the preferred treatment if a facility is available; this not only provides oxygen in solution for the tissues but also hastens the dissociation of COHb. Oxygen should be given until the level of COHb decreases to at least 10%. Supplementary care includes correction of hypotension and acidosis, as well as monitoring of cardiac function (Tintinalli *et al.*, 1983).

Toxicity of Prolonged and Low-Level Exposure to CO. The cardiovascular system, particularly the heart, is susceptible to adverse effects of low concentrations of COHb. At 6 to 12% COHb metabolism shifts from aerobic to anaerobic (Ayres *et al.*, 1970). Experimental and clinical studies have suggested that long-term exposure to CO can facilitate the development of atherosclerosis (Thomsen, 1974). CO also seems to affect human behavior. Performance on tests of vigilance is impaired when COHb is as low as 2 to 5%. However, these low levels of COHb probably have no effect on other behaviors, such as driving, reaction time, temporal discriminations, coordination, sensory processes, and complex intellectual tasks (National Research Council, 1977).

The fetus may be extremely susceptible to effects of CO, and the gas readily crosses the placenta. Infants born to women who have survived short-term exposure to a high concentration of the gas while pregnant often display neurological sequelae, and there may be gross damage to the brain (Longo, 1977). Persistent low levels of COHb in the fetus of a woman who has smoked during pregnancy may also have effects on the development of the central nervous system (CNS).

Polycythemia develops in the course of long-term exposure to CO. Other compensatory mechanisms are likely, but they have not been demonstrated. Healthy human subjects are exquisitely responsive to any hypoxic stress; they immediately compensate by increasing cardiac output and flow to critical organs. Those with significant cardiovascular disease are more vulnerable to the toxicity of CO because they may be unable to compensate for the hypoxia (*see* Stewart, 1975).

Particulate Material. Pneumoconiosis is a category of disease caused by inhalation of dusts. The most common condition of this type is silicosis. Next to oxygen, silicon is the most abundant element found on Earth. Approximately 60% of the rocks in the earth's crust contain silica, and silica dusts are prevalent in many industries, particularly in the mining of gold, iron, and coal; in stonework; and in sandblasting. Particles larger than 10 μm are of little clinical significance, because they seldom reach the alveoli. Particles less than 2 to 3 μm are phagocytized by alveolar macrophages, and these cells are eventually destroyed. Other macrophages proliferate and migrate to sites of reaction. The silicotic nodules that result from such reactions are scattered uniformly throughout both lungs. The disease usually requires 10 to 25 years to develop. As the mass of fibrotic tissue increases, vital capacity decreases and the afflicted individual experiences shortness of breath.

Other pulmonary diseases develop concurrently with silicosis, and silica may facilitate their pathogenesis. Long known to enhance susceptibility to tuberculosis, silicosis also increases the risk of infection by other microorganisms.

Asbestosis results from long-term inhalation of asbestos dust. Asbestos is a fibrous substance composed of hydrated silicate minerals. It is widely used in industry because it is nonflammable, flexible, and resistant to acids and alkalies and has high tensile strength, low density, and high electrical resistivity. Although asbestos is often used for insulation, brake linings, shingles, and other purposes, regulations to eliminate such use have been proposed in the United States.

Asbestosis (a form of pulmonary fibrosis) develops first in areas adjacent to the bronchioles, where there seems to be preferential deposition of longer asbestos fibers. There is also a fibrous pleuritis in which the pleural membrane thickens to encase the lung in a rigid fibrous capsule. Clinical symptoms of asbestosis resemble those of silicosis: dyspnea, tachypnea, and cough. However, tuberculosis is not a prominent complication.

Bronchial cancer associated with inhalation of asbestos occurs some 20 to 30 years after initial exposure. Inhalation of asbestos combined with cigarette smoking significantly increases the incidence of lung cancer over that caused by exposure to either factor alone (Selikoff and Hammond, 1979). Mesothelioma, a rapidly fatal malignancy, is also associated with exposure to asbestos fibers. It may appear in the pleura or the peritoneum, usually 25 to 40 years after initial exposure (Selikoff and Hammond, 1979). A high incidence of mesothelioma has been attributed to fibrous tremolite in household stucco and whitewash in Turkey. It thus appears that mesothelioma is not a specific reaction to asbestos, but that any natural or synthetic fibrous material with similar fiber dimensions might be carcinogenic (Elmes, 1980). However, except for long-term inhalation of fibrous matter and the strong suspicion of an increase in risk for persons living adjacent to emissions containing arsenic, there is as yet little convincing evidence that environmental air pollution contributes to the risk of cancer (Kaplan and Morgan, 1981).

Many other occupational pulmonary diseases are caused by long-term inhalation of dusts containing minerals or organic matter. These include coal workers' pneumoconiosis (black lung disease), aluminosis (bauxite lung), baritosis (from barium), beryllium disease, byssinosis (from cotton), and others (*see* Speizer, 1983).

SOLVENTS AND VAPORS

Organic solvents and their vapors are a common part of our environment. Short, incidental exposures to low concentrations of solvent vapors, such as gasoline, lighter fluids, aerosol sprays, and spot removers, may be relatively harmless; however, exposures to paint removers, floor and tile cleaners, and other solvents in home or industry may be dangerous. In addition, disposal of many of these chemicals has been improper; as a result there is leakage from toxic dump sites and contamination of drinking water. Because so many industrial workers are exposed to toxic solvents and vapors, considerable effort has gone into determining safe levels of exposure. Threshold limit values (TLV) or maximum allowable concentrations (MAC) have been established for the airborne poisons; a TLV represents the concentration to which most workers may safely be exposed for an 8-hour period.

A variety of anesthetic gases, solvents, and fluorohydrocarbons (used as propellants in aerosol products) cause subjective effects when inhaled and are frequently abused in this way. This dangerous practice, which has caused many deaths, is discussed in Chapter 22.

ALIPHATIC HYDROCARBONS

C_1–C_4 Aliphatic Hydrocarbons. The straight-chain hydrocarbons with four or fewer carbon atoms are present in natural gas (methane, ethane) and in bottled gas (propane, butane). Methane and ethane produce no general systemic effects. They are "simple asphyxiants"; effects are observed only when their concentration in the air is so high that it decreases the amount of oxygen.

C_5–C_8 Aliphatic Hydrocarbons. The higher-molecular-weight aliphatic hydrocarbons, like most organic solvents, depress the central nervous system (CNS) and cause dizziness and incoordination. However, polyneuropathy is the primary toxic reaction to *n*-hexane, a widely used solvent (USEPA, 1988b). This was observed first in Japan, where 93 workers engaged in the production of sandals were afflicted when using a glue that contained at least 60% *n*-hexane (Iida *et al.,* 1973). 2-Hexanone (methyl *n*-butyl ketone) produces neurological changes similar to those of *n*-hexane. Clinical symptoms include symmetrical sensory dysfunction of the distal portions of the extremities, which progresses to muscle weakness in toes and fingers and loss of deep sensory reflexes. A decrease in nerve conduction velocity precedes the onset of symptoms (Seppäläinen, 1982). The prognosis for recovery is generally good, except for severely injured patients, but the recovery is slow (Graham *et al.,* 1987). The cytochrome P_{450}–mediated biotransformation of *n*-hexane and 2-hexanone to 2,5-hexadione appears to be responsible for the peripheral neuropathy associated with exposure to these solvents (Couri and Milks, 1982).

Gasoline and Kerosene. Gasoline and kerosene, petroleum distillates prepared by the fractionation of crude petroleum oil, contain aliphatic, aromatic, and a variety of branched and unsaturated hydrocarbons. They are used as illuminating fuels, heating fuels, motor fuels, vehicles for many pesticides, cleaning agents, and paint thinners. Because they often are stored in containers previously used for beverages, they are a common cause of accidental poisoning in children.

Intoxication by ingestion of gasoline and kerosene resembles that from ethyl alcohol. Signs and symptoms include incoordination, restlessness, excitement, confusion, disorientation, ataxia, delirium, and finally coma, which may last a few hours or several days. Inhalation of high concentrations of gasoline vapors, as by workmen cleaning storage tanks, can cause immediate death. Gasoline vapors sensitize the myocardium such that small amounts of circulating epinephrine may precipitate ventricular fibrillation; many hydrocarbons have this action. High concentrations of gasoline vapor may also lead to rapid depression of the CNS and death from respiratory failure.

Poisoning from these hydrocarbons results either from inhalation of the vapors or from ingestion of the liquid. Ingestion is more hazardous, because the liquids have a low surface tension and can easily be aspirated into the respiratory tract by vomiting or eructation. Morbidity is attributed to aspiration, whether it occurs at the time of ingestion or during treatment. Pulmonary damage does not result from gastrointestinal absorption of gasoline or kerosene. Chemical pneumonitis, complicated by secondary bacterial pneumonia and pulmonary edema, is the most serious sequel to aspiration. Death caused by hemorrhagic pulmonary edema usually occurs in 16 to 18 hours and seldom later than 24 hours after aspiration.

Examination of tissues from fatal cases reveals heavy, edematous, and hemorrhagic lungs. The alveoli are filled with an exudate that is rich in proteins, cells, and fibrin, often in a pattern resembling that of hyaline membrane disease. Alveolar walls are weakened and may rupture, leading to less frequent sequelae, such as emphysema and pneumothorax. Pulmonary lymph nodes are inflamed, and bronchopneumonia and atelectasis have been noted.

Symptomatic and supportive care is probably the best treatment for intoxication by gasoline or kerosene (Ervin, 1983; Gosselin *et al.*, 1984). Because of the danger of aspiration, emesis or gastric lavage should not be employed unless the risks are justified by the presence of additional toxic substances in the petroleum. Catharsis may be induced with magnesium or sodium sulfate. Antibiotics are used if there is a specific indication, such as bacterial pneumonitis. Epinephrine and related substances should be avoided because they may induce cardiac arrhythmias. Treatment should include correction of imbalances of fluid and electrolytes.

Long-term exposure to gasoline has become a concern because numerous underground gasoline storage tanks leak, and their contents may eventually enter the drinking water (Scala, 1988). The primary concern is the potential for the development of leukemia, since gasoline contains about 2% benzene (*see* below).

HALOGENATED HYDROCARBONS

The excellent solvent properties and low flammability of halogenated hydrocarbons have placed them among the most widely used industrial solvents. Several low-molecular-weight hydrocarbons are found in drinking water. Some of these, such as chloroform, bromodichloromethane, dibromochloromethane, and bromoform, are produced from naturally occurring precursors during chlorination of water; others, such as carbon tetrachloride, dichloromethane, and 1,2-dichloroethane, do not appear to arise from such treatment. Filtration or treatment of water with charcoal prior to chlorination effectively reduces formation of chlorinated hydrocarbons. However, the halogenated hydrocarbons are common at toxic waste sites, and thus they all have the potential to enter the supply of drinking water. Because some of these compounds have been shown to be carcinogenic in animals and because correlations have been reported between the chlorination of water and the incidence of cancer of the colon, rectum, and breast, there is a cause for concern about the exposure of a very large percentage of the population to these chemicals in drinking water (*see* Menzer and Nelson, 1985). Since the halogenated hydrocarbons are extremely soluble in lipid, they are readily absorbed after inhalation or ingestion. Like most other organic solvents, halogenated hydrocarbons depress the CNS.

Carbon Tetrachloride. Carbon tetrachloride (CCl_4) has been used for medical purposes and was once commonly employed as a spot remover and carpet cleaner; however, its use has now been abandoned because safer alternatives are available.

Transient exposure to toxic concentrations of CCl_4 vapor results in the following symptoms: irritation of the eyes, nose, and throat; nausea and vomiting; a sense of fullness in the head; dizziness; and headache. If the exposure is soon terminated, symptoms usually disappear within a few hours. Continued exposure or absorption of larger quantities of the chemical may cause stupor, convulsions, coma, or death from CNS depression. Sudden death may occur from ventricular fibrillation or depression of vital medullary centers.

Delayed toxic effects of CCl_4 include nausea, vomiting, abdominal pain, diarrhea, and hematemesis. The most serious delayed toxic effects of CCl_4 result from its hepatotoxic and nephrotoxic actions. Signs and symptoms of hepatic injury may appear after a delay of several hours or 2 to 3 days and may occur in the absence of earlier severe effects on the CNS. Biochemical evidence of hepatic injury often includes greatly elevated activities of transaminases and a variety of other hepatic enzymes in plasma. Alkaline phosphatase activity is, however, only slightly elevated. The chief histological abnormalities include hepatic steatosis and hepatic centrilobular necrosis.

The mechanism of CCl_4-induced hepatic injury has interested many investigators (*see* Kalf *et al.*, 1987), and the compound has become the reference substance for all hepatotoxic compounds. Injury produced by CCl_4 seems to be mediated by a reactive metabolite—trichloromethyl free radical ($\cdot CCl_3$)—formed by the homolytic cleavage of CCl_4, or by an even more reactive species—trichloromethylperoxy free radical ($Cl_3COO\cdot$)—formed by the reaction of $\cdot CCl_3$ with O_2 (Slater, 1982). This biotransformation is catalyzed by a cytochrome P_{450}–dependent monooxygenase. Thus, agents such as DDT and phenobarbital, which induce such enzymes, strikingly enhance the hepatotoxic effects of CCl_4. Conversely, agents that inhibit the drug-metabolizing activity diminish the hepatotoxicity of CCl_4. Biotransformation of CCl_4 to the reactive intermediate is a reductive rather than an oxidative reaction. As a result, it is slower at high oxygen tensions. Rats poisoned with CCl_4 show less hepatic injury if treated with hyperbaric oxygen (Burk *et al.*, 1986).

The toxicity produced by CCl_4 is thought to be due to the reaction of free radicals ($\cdot CCl_3$ or $Cl_3COO\cdot$) with lipids and proteins; however, the relative importance of interactions with various tissue constituents in producing injury is controversial. Recknagel and Glende (1973) proposed that the free radical causes the peroxidation of the polyenoic lipids of the endoplasmic reticulum and the generation of secondary free radicals derived from these lipids—a chain reaction. This destructive lipid peroxidation leads to breakdown of membrane structure and function, and, if a sufficient quantity of CCl_4 has been consumed, damage extends to all cellular membranes (*see* Recknagel and Glende, 1973; Zimmerman, 1978; Plaa, 1985; Kalf *et al.*, 1987).

Individuals recovering from acute ingestion of ethanol seem more susceptible to the hepatotoxic properties of halogenated hydrocarbons. Other alcohols, such as isopropanol, have an even greater ability to potentiate such effects of CCl_4 (Plaa, 1985). This interaction between isopropanol and CCl_4 was highlighted by an industrial accident in an isopropanol-packaging plant, where workers exposed to both agents were adversely affected (Folland *et al.*, 1976).

As hepatic injury develops, signs of renal damage may also be observed and may dominate the clinical picture. Experimental studies in rats indicate that CCl_4 produces an early, reversible lesion of the proximal tubule; initial changes occur in the mitochondria and are followed by cellular swelling, proliferation of the smooth endoplasmic reticulum, and a simultaneous increase in the excretion of sodium salts and water (Striker *et al.*, 1968). Mild poisoning in man may be characterized by a reversible oliguria lasting only a few days. In nonfatal poisoning, recovery of renal function occurs in three phases. In the first, after 1 to 3 days, oliguria stops but concentrations of creatinine and urea in plasma remain elevated. The second phase starts with a rapid decline in these concentrations. In the third phase, about 1 month after the initial injury, renal blood flow and glomerular filtration begin to improve, and renal function is recovered after 100 to 200 days.

Emergency treatment of CCl_4 poisoning should be initiated promptly in any person suspected of having absorbed toxic quantities of the compound. The individual exposed to toxic vapor should be moved to fresh air. If the patient is seen shortly after oral ingestion of CCl_4, the stomach should be emptied immediately, by inducing vomiting if the patient is conscious or by gastric lavage, and a saline laxative should be administered to minimize absorption. If the patient is first seen in the stage of advanced CNS depression, every effort should be made to prevent hypoxia. Under no circumstances should sympathomimetic drugs be used because of the danger of producing serious arrhythmias in the sensitized myocardium.

Treatment of the acute hepatic and renal insufficiency caused by CCl_4 is difficult. Although hepatic insufficiency is a prominent feature of CCl_4 poisoning, renal failure is the most frequent cause of death. Even though the presenting signs and symptoms may be associated with functional impairment of the liver, renal function should be observed closely and oliguria or anuria anticipated.

Other Halogenated Hydrocarbons. Chloroform, dichloromethane (methylene chloride), trichloroethylene, tetrachloroethylene (perchlorethylene), 1,1,1-trichloroethane, and 1,1,2-trichloroethane produce many of the same toxic effects as does CCl_4 (Von Oettingen, 1964). All these compounds produce CNS depression, and some have been used as inhalational anesthetics. They also have the potential to sensitize the heart to arrhythmias produced by catecholamines. The hepatotoxic potential is highest with chloroform and 1,1,2-trichloroethane, and least with trichloroethylene, tetrachloroethylene, 1,1,1-trichloroethane, and dichloromethane; chloroform may be hepatotoxic because it is metabolized to phosgene (Krishna *et al.*, 1978). Chloroform, 1,1,2-trichloroethane, and tetrachloroethylene are also nephrotoxic. Because they produce less organ damage than do CCl_4 and chloroform, 1,1,1-trichloroethane, tetrachloroethylene, and trichloroethylene are widely used as dry-cleaning agents and industrial solvents, and dichloromethane is used as a paint stripper. Dichloromethane has an additional toxic effect because it is metabolized to CO by cytochrome P_{450} (Kubic and Anders, 1975). Many of these chlorinated hydrocarbon solvents produce hepatic cancer in mice; this effect has not been demonstrated in man (Williams and Weisburger, 1985).

Between 1961 and 1980, Great Britain reported 330 poisonings and 17 deaths caused by inhalation of trichloroethylene, tetrachloroethylene, and 1,1,1-trichloroethane, the three most commonly used solvents in industry (McCarthy and Jones, 1983). Deaths were due to deep narcosis, aspiration of vomitus during anesthesia, or cardiac arrhythmias (Jones and Winter, 1983). Signs of hepatotoxicity were not observed. Exposure to high concentrations of trichloroethylene has been associated with trigeminal neuropathy (Annau, 1981); long-term exposure of workers to halogenated hydrocarbon solvents has resulted in behavioral alterations (Annau, 1981; Lindstrom, 1982).

ALIPHATIC ALCOHOLS

Ethanol is discussed in Chapter 17.

Methanol. Methanol (methyl alcohol or wood alcohol) is a common industrial solvent. It is also used as an antifreeze fluid, a solvent for shellac and some paints and varnishes, and a component of paint removers. Solid, canned fuels contain methanol. As an adulterant, it renders unpotable and tax free the ethanol that is used for cleaning, paint removal, and other purposes.

The absorption and distribution of methanol and ethanol are similar. In addition, methanol is metabolized in man by the same enzymes that metabolize ethanol—alcohol dehydrogenase and aldehyde dehydrogenase—to formaldehyde and formic acid (Tephly *et al.*, 1974, 1979). Oxidation of methanol, like that of ethanol, proceeds at a rate that is independent of its concentration in the blood. However, this rate is only one seventh that of ethanol, and complete oxidation and excretion thus usually require several days.

Methanol causes less inebriation than ethanol; indeed, inebriation is not a prominent symptom of methanol intoxication unless a very large amount is consumed or ethanol is also ingested. An asymptomatic latent period of 8 to 36 hours may precede the onset of symptoms of intoxication. If ethanol is imbibed simultaneously in sufficient amounts, signs and symptoms of methanol poisoning may be considerably delayed or, on occasion, even averted. In such cases ethanol intoxication is prominent, and ingestion of methanol may not be suspected.

Signs and symptoms of methanol poisoning include headache, vertigo, vomiting, severe upper abdominal pain, back pain, dyspnea, motor restlessness, cold clammy extremities, blurring of vision, and hyperemia of the optic disc. Blood pressure is usually unaffected. The pulse is slow in severely ill patients.

The most pronounced laboratory finding is severe metabolic acidosis—the result of oxidation of methanol to formic acid, which accumulates (McMartin *et al.*, 1977; Jacobson and McMartin, 1986). Moderate ketonemia and acetonuria are also evident. Despite the severe acidosis, Kussmaul respiration is not common because of respiratory depression caused by the intoxication. Coma can develop with amazing rapidity in relatively asymptomatic subjects. In moribund patients the respiration is slow, shallow, gasping, and "fish-mouth." Death, which usually is due to respiratory failure, may be sudden or it may occur after many hours of coma.

Pancreatic necrosis has been observed at autopsy, and pancreatic injury is believed to cause the severe abdominal pain that frequently accompanies methanol intoxication (Kaplan, 1962).

Visual disturbances, the most distinctive aspect of methanol poisoning in man, become evident soon after the onset of acidosis. Dilated, unreactive pupils and dim vision are characteristic. The ocular lesion, which involves chiefly the ganglion cells of the retina, is a destructive inflammation followed by atrophy. In the short term, the retina is congested and edematous, and the edges of the optic disc may be blurred (Gosselin *et al.*, 1984). The final result is bilateral blindness, which is usually permanent. Ocular toxicity appears to be caused specifically by elevated concentrations of formic acid and is probably not due to acidosis *per se* (Tephly *et al.*, 1979). Death from methanol is nearly always preceded by blindness. As little as 15 ml of methanol has caused blindness; ingestion of 70 to 100 ml usually is fatal unless the patient is treated.

The severity of most symptoms of methanol poisoning is thought to be proportional to the acidosis, and correction of acidosis is thus a keystone of proper therapy (*see* Chapter 27). In addition, inhibition of methanol metabolism decreases the concentrations of formaldehyde and formic acid in the blood and thereby decreases toxicity. This is accomplished with ethanol, acting as a competitive substrate. Since ethanol has about a 100-fold greater affinity for alcohol dehydrogenase than does methanol, competition by ethanol is effective. In practice, a blood ethanol concentration of 1 g per liter is optimal. A loading dose of ethanol (0.6 g/kg) should be administered as soon as the diagnosis of a significant ingestion has been made, and an infusion of ethanol (about 10 g per hour in an adult) is begun to maintain the desired concentration. Hemodialysis should be initiated as soon as possible after the administration of ethanol in patients with acidosis or who have blood methanol concentrations in excess of 500 mg per liter. Dialysis removes the methanol and corrects the acidosis that may be resistant to administration of bicarbonate. Because ethanol will also be removed by dialysis, the rate of its infusion should be increased by about 6 g per hour. 4-Methylpyrazole is a specific inhibitor of alcohol dehydrogenase and has been used as an antidote in experimental animals (McMartin *et al.*, 1980). Folate has also been used in an attempt to enhance the rate of metabolism of formate (Noker *et al.*, 1980). Neurological damage, characterized by permanent motor dysfunction, may follow methanol poisoning; levodopa may relieve the rigidity and hypokinesis (Guggenheim *et al.*, 1971).

Isopropanol. Isopropanol, used for rubbing alcohol, in hand lotions, and in deicing and antifreeze preparations, is occasionally the cause of accidental poisoning. Like ethanol and methanol, isopropanol is a CNS depressant, but it does not produce retinal damage or acidosis as does methanol.

In adults, the probable lethal dose of isopropanol is about 250 ml; it is thus more toxic than ethanol. While the signs and symptoms of isopropanol toxicity resemble those of ethanol toxicity, there are notable differences. Isopropanol produces a more prominent gastritis, with pain, nausea, vomiting, and hemorrhage. Vomiting with aspiration is a serious threat and dangerous complication. Isopropanol intoxication lasts longer because the compound is oxidized more slowly than ethanol (Gosselin *et al.*, 1984) and because its major metabolite, acetone, is also a CNS depressant. Ketoacidosis and ketones in urine (without glucosuria) support the diagnosis. As with the other alcohols, hemodialysis is useful for removing isopropanol from the body (King *et al.*, 1970).

GLYCOLS

In addition to their use as heat exchangers, antifreeze formulations, hydraulic fluids, or chemical intermediates, glycols are also used as solvents for pharmaceuticals, food additives, cosmetics, and lacquers.

Ethylene Glycol. Ethylene glycol ($HOCH_2$-CH_2OH) is widely used as antifreeze for automobile radiators, and such products are the usual cause of ethylene glycol poisonings. Like ethanol, ethylene glycol produces CNS depression. Patients who ingest large quantities develop narcosis, which may lead to coma and death. In addition to the CNS depression, ethylene glycol produces severe renal injury; most victims experience acute renal failure. Those who die from uremia exhibit marked renal disease, including destruction of epithelial cells, interstitial edema, focal hemorrhagic necrosis in the cortex, extensive hydropic degeneration, numerous cellular casts, and oxalate crystals in the convoluted tubules (Gosselin *et al.*, 1984).

The initial step in the oxidation of ethylene glycol to the monoaldehyde (glycoaldehyde) is mediated by alcohol dehydrogenase; oxidation of glycoaldehyde to the major acidic metabolite, glycolic acid, is catalyzed by aldehyde dehydrogenase. Both of these oxidative steps produce NADH from NAD, thus shifting the redox potential and favoring the production of lactate from pyruvate. Glycolic acid is further metabolized to glyoxylic acid and then to oxalic acid (HOOCCOOH). The ethylene glycol probably causes the initial CNS depression; oxalate and the other intermediates seem to be responsible for nephrotoxicity. Typical crystals of calcium oxalate are often seen in the urine and may be an early clue to the diagnosis of ethylene glycol poisoning. Glycolic acid and lactic acid are responsible for most of the metabolic acidosis (Gabow *et al.*, 1986).

The specific treatment of poisoning with ethylene glycol is similar to that for methanol poisoning (Gosselin *et al.*, 1984). Metabolic acidosis is treated with sodium bicarbonate. Ethanol is used as a competitive substrate for alcohol dehydrogenase to decrease the rate of formation of toxic metabolites. 4-Methylpyrazole, a more effective experimental inhibitor of alcohol dehydrogenase, may be superior to ethanol (Baud *et al.*, 1988). Hemodialysis is effective in removing unmetabolized ethylene glycol and in correcting the acidosis. Parenteral administration of Ca^{2+} is recommended for muscle spasms, which may develop because of chelation of Ca^{2+} by the oxalate formed in the biotransformation of ethylene glycol.

Diethylene Glycol. Diethylene glycol ($HOCH_2$-$CH_2OCH_2CH_2OH$) is used in lacquer, cosmetics, antifreeze, and lubricants, and as a softening agent and plasticizer. Its toxicity was a major problem only when the compound was used in the 1930s as a solvent in a preparation of sulfanilamide. In that incident, 105 of 353 children who ingested the sulfanilamide–diethylene glycol preparation died of renal damage. Effects of diethylene glycol resemble those of ethylene glycol, and intoxication should be treated similarly.

Propylene Glycol. The physical properties of propylene glycol ($CH_3CHOHCH_2OH$) are similar to those of ethylene glycol, but it is much less toxic. For this reason propylene glycol is used as a solvent for drugs, cosmetics, lotions, and ointments; in food materials; as a plasticizer; in antifreeze formulations; as a heat exchanger; and in hydraulic fluids. Like ethanol, its primary pharmacological action is to produce CNS depression; however, its elimination is slower and its actions are thus prolonged.

Glycol Ethers. Prolonged inhalation of ethylene glycol monomethyl ether and ethylene glycol monoethyl ether by male mice, rats, and rabbits can induce testicular atrophy and infertility (Miller *et al.*, 1983; Andrews and Snyder, 1985). In addition, these glycol ethers are teratogenic in rats and rabbits. Both ethylene glycol ethers are metabolized by alcohol dehydrogenase to alkoxyacids. Because methoxyacetic acid also produces testicular toxicity in male rats, it appears that alkoxyacids are responsible for this toxic effect. In contrast, propylene glycol monomethyl ether, which is a poor substrate for alcohol dehydrogenase, does not produce testicular atrophy.

AROMATIC HYDROCARBONS

Benzene. Benzene is an excellent solvent. It is widely used for chemical syntheses and is a natural constituent of automobile fuels. However, benzene is very toxic.

After a short exposure to a large amount of benzene, by ingestion or by breathing concentrated vapors, the major toxic effect is on the CNS. Symptoms from mild exposure include dizziness, weakness, euphoria, headache, nausea, vomiting, tightness in the chest, and staggering. If exposure is more severe, symptoms progress to blurred vision, tremors, shallow and rapid respiration, ventricular irregularities, paralysis, and unconsciousness.

Long-term exposure to benzene is usually due to inhalation of vapor. Signs and symptoms include effects on the CNS and the gastrointestinal tract (headache, loss of appetite, drowsiness, nervousness, and pallor), but the major manifestation of toxicity is aplastic anemia. Bone-marrow cells in early stages of development are the most sensitive to benzene (Snyder *et al.*, 1977), and arrest of maturation leads to gradual depletion of circulating cells.

A major concern is the relationship between long-term exposure to benzene and leukemia

(Aksoy, 1985; Rinsky *et al.*, 1987). Epidemiological studies have been conducted on workers in the tire industry and in shoe factories, where benzene is used extensively. Among workers who died of exposure to benzene, death was caused by either leukemia or aplastic anemia, in approximately equal proportions.

The first product of the metabolic oxidation of benzene is postulated to be a highly unstable compound, benzene oxide (Jerina and Daley, 1974). Benzene oxide, formed by introduction of oxygen into the molecule by the cytochrome P_{450} system, rearranges to form phenol. The sulfate ester of phenol is the major metabolite in the urine, and the level of exposure of workers to benzene can be estimated by determination of the increase in organic sulfate excreted in the urine. Further hydroxylations of phenol result in the formation of hydroquinone and 1,2,4-benzenetriol. When oxidized, these polyphenols form potentially toxic, covalently binding intermediates that may be responsible for the toxic effects of benzene on the bone marrow (Kalf *et al.*, 1987).

Toluene. Toluene ($C_6H_5CH_3$) is widely used as a solvent in paints, varnishes, glues, enamels, and lacquers and as a chemical intermediate in the synthesis of organic compounds. Toluene is a CNS depressant, and low concentrations produce fatigue, weakness, and confusion. It is for the CNS effects of solvents such as toluene that "glue sniffers" inhale the vapors of glue. Unlike benzene, toluene produces neither aplastic anemia nor leukemia. However, the solvents in glue are often mixed, and the "glue sniffer" is usually exposed to other solvents in addition to toluene.

PESTICIDES

Pesticide is a general classification that includes insecticides, rodenticides, fungicides, herbicides, and fumigants. These compounds are manufactured for the sole purpose of destroying some form of life. Selective toxicity of pesticides is extremely desirable; however, all can produce at least some toxicity in man.

INSECTICIDES

The use of insecticides in agriculture has grown tremendously since World War II, and the potential is great for occupational exposure to these chemicals, both in production and in use. However, exposure to insecticides is not limited to occupational incidents; residues often remain on produce, and man is exposed to low levels of the chemicals in food. Numerous incidents of acute poisoning from pesticides have resulted from eating food that was grossly contaminated during storage or shipping. Insecticides used in homes and gardens have caused accidental poisoning in young children.

Organochlorine Insecticides. Organochlorine insecticides include chlorinated ethane derivatives, of which DDT is the best known; cyclodienes, including chlordane, aldrin, dieldrin, heptachlor, and endrin; and other hydrocarbons, including such hexachlorocyclohexanes as lindane, toxaphene, mirex, and chlordecone (KEPONE). From the mid-1940s to the mid-1960s, organochlorine insecticides were widely used in agriculture and in programs for the control of malaria.

DDT. DDT, the most common of the chlorinated ethane derivatives, is also known as *chlorophenothane*.

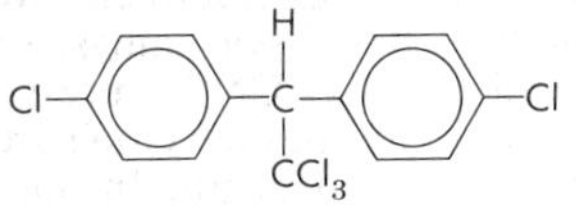

DDT

Prior to placement of major restrictions on its use in many countries, DDT was the best known, least expensive, and probably one of the most effective synthetic insecticides. It was thus widely used after its introduction in the mid-1940s.

DDT has extremely low solubility in water and very high solubility in fat. It is readily absorbed when dissolved in oils, fats, or lipid solvents but is poorly absorbed as a dry powder or an aqueous suspension. Once absorbed, DDT concentrates in adipose tissue. Storage of DDT in the fat is protective, because it decreases the amount of the chemical at its site of toxic action—the brain. DDT crosses the placenta and its concentration in umbilical cord blood is in the same range as that in the blood of the exposed mother (Saxena *et al.*, 1981).

Because DDT is degraded very slowly in the environment and is stored in the fat of animals, it is a prime candidate for biomagnification; that is, a series of organisms in a food chain accumulate increasingly greater quantities in their fat at each higher trophic level. Ultimately, a species at the top of a food chain is adversely affected. For example, the population of fish-eating birds has declined. The decline is attributed to thinning of the eggshell, a demonstrated result of ingesting DDT and related chlorinated hydrocarbon insecticides.

Because of the ubiquity of DDT, everyone born since the mid-1940s has had a lifetime of exposure to this insecticide and storage of it in fatty tissues. At a constant rate of intake, the concentration of DDT in adipose tissue reaches a steady-state value and remains relatively constant. The concentration of DDT and its metabolites in the fat of man is about 3 ppm, which is less than half the value determined in the mid 1970s. The concentration of DDT in the blood of people living downstream from a defunct manufacturing plant was 0.076 ppm, more than five times higher than the average in the United States (Kreiss *et al.*, 1981). When exposure ceases, DDT is eliminated from the body slowly. Elimination has been estimated to occur at a rate of approximately 1% of stored DDT excreted per day. Prior to excretion it is slowly dehalogenated and oxidized by cytochrome P_{450}–dependent monooxygenases; one of the major excretory products is DDA (*bis*[*p*-chlorophenyl] acetic acid).

DDT has a wide margin of safety and, despite its widespread use and availability, there is no documented, unequivocal report of a fatal human poisoning from DDT. The few human deaths associated with excess exposure to DDT probably resulted from the kerosene solvent rather than the insecticide. The most prominent short-term effect of DDT is stimulation of the CNS. In rats, there is a good correlation between concentrations of DDT in brain and signs of toxicity.

Signs and symptoms of poisoning from high doses of DDT in man include paresthesias of the tongue, lips, and face; apprehension; hypersusceptibility to stimuli; irritability; dizziness; tremor; and tonic and clonic convulsions (Murphy, 1985). The mechanism of action of DDT on the CNS is not completely known. The compound is capable of altering the transport of Na^+ and K^+ across axonal membranes, resulting in an increased negative afterpotential, prolonged action potentials, repetitive firing after a single stimulus, and spontaneous trains of action potentials. Specifically, DDT seems to inhibit the inactivation of Na^+ channels and the activation of K^+ conductance (Narahashi, 1979, 1983).

In laboratory animals, intravenous administration of DDT causes death by ventricular fibrillation. Apparently, DDT shares with other chlorinated hydrocarbons a tendency to sensitize the myocardium, and, through its action on the CNS and adrenal medulla, it may produce the stimulus necessary for ventricular fibrillation.

Relatively low doses of DDT induce the mixed-function oxidase system of the hepatic endoplasmic reticulum. This effect has also been demonstrated in exterminators (Kolmodin *et al.*, 1969) and in workers in a DDT factory (Poland *et al.*, 1970). The result is altered metabolism of drugs, xenobiotics, and steroid hormones. It is perhaps also responsible for the increased frequency of breakage of eggs and the status of the breeding population in certain birds (*e.g.*, *see* Radcliffe, 1967). Induction of cytochrome P_{450} by DDT seems to increase metabolism of estrogens in the birds. The resulting endocrine imbalance probably affects calcium metabolism, egg laying, and nesting in such a way that total reproductive success and survival of the young may be reduced (Lundholm, 1987). To compound the problem, DDT also exerts an estrogenic effect (Kupfer and Bulger, 1982) and inhibits a Ca^{2+}-ATPase that is necessary for the calcification of egg shells (Miller and Kinter, 1976).

Human volunteers have consumed 35 mg of DDT daily, about 1000 times higher than the average human intake, for as long as 25 months without obvious ill effects (Hayes, 1963). However, there is concern that DDT might be carcinogenic following exposure to small amounts of the chemical over a long period (IARC, 1974a). Extensive use of DDT in industrial countries has not been associated with increased hepatic cancer in man. In a survey of the mortality of over 3800 licensed pest-control workers, no significant elevation in their standardized mortality ratio was found, but there were excess deaths from leukemia, particularly myeloid leukemia, and from cancers of the brain and lungs (Blair *et al.*, 1983).

DDT was banned in the United States in 1972 for all but essential public health use and for a few minor uses to protect crops for which no effective alternatives were available. The decision was prompted by the prospect of ecological imbalance from continued use of DDT, the uncertainty of the effect, if any, of continued prolonged exposure and storage of low concentrations of DDT in man, and the development of resistant strains of insects. Several other countries have taken similar action. As a result, other pesticides have replaced DDT, but many of them are more toxic to man.

Methoxychlor. The structural formula of methoxychlor, a chlorinated ethane derivative, is as follows:

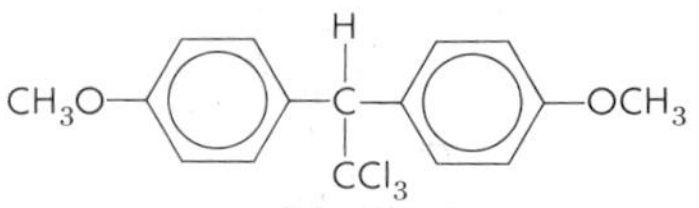

Methoxychlor

The compound is used increasingly as a replacement for DDT. The attractiveness of methoxychlor is that it is much less toxic to mammals than DDT (LD_{50} in rats is 6000 mg/kg, as compared with 250 mg/kg for DDT), it is not carcinogenic, and it does not persist in the body for as long. Methoxychlor is stored in adipose tissue to about 0.2% of the extent of DDT, and its half-life in rats is only about 2 weeks, as compared with 6 months for DDT (Murphy, 1985). The shorter half-life is a reflection of more rapid metabolism by O-demethylation (Kapoor *et al.*, 1970); it is then conjugated and excreted in the urine.

Chlorinated Cyclodienes. Structures of the more commonly used chlorinated cyclodienes are shown in Table 67–2. These compounds stimulate the CNS, and many signs and symptoms of poisoning thus resemble those of DDT. Unlike DDT, however, these compounds tend to produce convulsions before other, less serious signs of illness have appeared. Persons poisoned by cyclodiene insecticides have reported headache and nausea, vomiting, dizziness, and mild clonic jerking, but some patients have convulsions without warning symptoms (Hayes, 1963). Unlike DDT, cyclodiene insecticides have caused numerous fatalities as a result of acute poisoning.

An important difference between DDT and the chlorinated cyclodienes is that the latter are readily absorbed from intact skin. Cyclodienes may not pose an appreciably greater risk than DDT to the general population exposed to small quantities in food, but manipulation of concentrated solutions of a cyclodiene is more hazardous.

Like DDT, chlorinated cyclodiene insecticides are highly soluble in lipid and are stored in adipose tissue; they induce the mixed-function oxidase system of the liver, are degraded slowly, persist

Table 67–2. CHEMICAL STRUCTURES OF SOME CHLORINATED CYCLODIENES

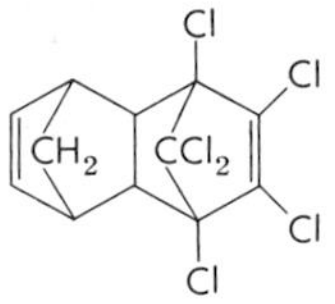

Aldrin

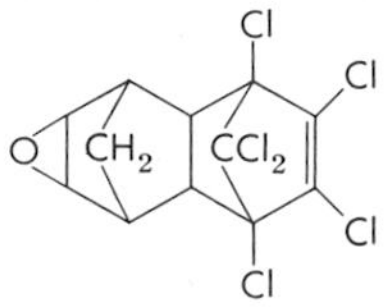

Dieldrin *

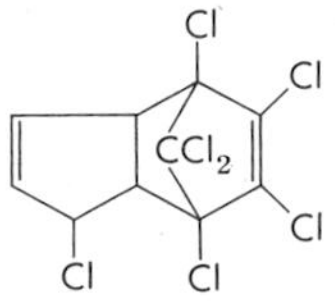

Heptachlor

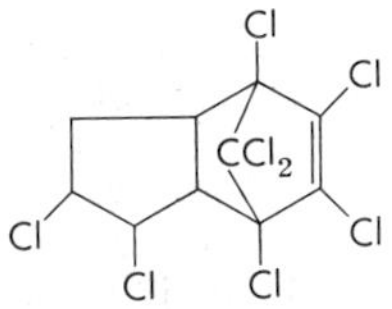

Chlordane

* Endrin is a stereoisomer of dieldrin.

in the environment, and undergo biomagnification through the food chain of animals. This class of insecticides has produced dose-related hepatomas in mice and has the greatest carcinogenic potential among the insecticides (National Academy of Sciences, 1977). For these reasons aldrin and dieldrin were banned in the United States in 1974, and the use of chlordane and heptachlor for agricultural crops was suspended in 1976.

Other Chlorinated Hydrocarbons. This group of insecticides includes lindane, toxaphene, mirex, and chlordecone. These chemicals share many properties with DDT. While they do not modify axonal conduction, they do act on presynaptic nerve terminals in the CNS and enhance the release of neurotransmitters (Shankland, 1982).

Benzene Hexachloride (BHC) and Lindane. Benzene hexachloride (more properly called hexachlorocyclohexane) has the following structural formula:

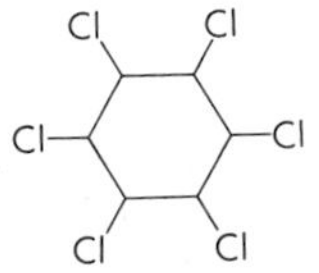

Benzene Hexachloride

It is a mixture of eight isomers, and the γ isomer is referred to as *lindane*. The γ isomer is the most toxic, and virtually all insecticidal activity of BHC resides in lindane. The compound is used clinically as an ectoparasiticide (*see* below). Lindane causes signs of poisoning that resemble those produced by DDT: tremors, ataxia, convulsions, and prostration. Violent tonic and clonic convulsions occur in severe cases of acute poisoning. The α and γ isomers are CNS stimulants, but the β and δ isomers are depressants. CNS stimulation appears to be due to blockade of the effects of gamma-aminobutyric acid (GABA) (Matsumura and Ghiasuddin, 1979). Lindane induces hepatic microsomal enzymes. Lindane and BHC have been implicated in numerous cases of aplastic anemia (West, 1967); however, a study of 60 cases of aplastic anemia failed to demonstrate an association between the incidence of aplastic anemia and occupational exposure to pesticides (Wang and Grufferman, 1981). A number of the isomers of BHC, including lindane, have been shown to produce hepatomas in rodents (Cueto, 1980).

Biotransformation of the isomers of BHC involves the formation of chlorophenols. Compared with DDT, lindane has a relatively low persistence in the environment.

Toxaphene. Toxaphene is a complex mixture of more than 175 C_{10} polychlorinated hydrocarbons, of which only a few are known (*e.g.*, heptachlorobornane) (Turner *et al.*, 1977). Like the other chlorinated hydrocarbon insecticides, the major toxicity of toxaphene is stimulation of the CNS. Toxaphene seems to be metabolized quite readily and thus has a shorter half-life than most of the other chlorinated hydrocarbon insecticides. Toxaphene has been shown to induce hepatic tumors in mice and to produce mutations (Hooper *et al.*, 1979). These observations have resulted in a dramatic reduction in the use of toxaphene.

Mirex and Chlordecone. Mirex and chlordecone (KEPONE) are extremely persistent chlorinated hydrocarbon insecticides, and they are concentrated several thousandfold in the food chain (Waters *et al.*, 1977). Their structural formulas are as follows:

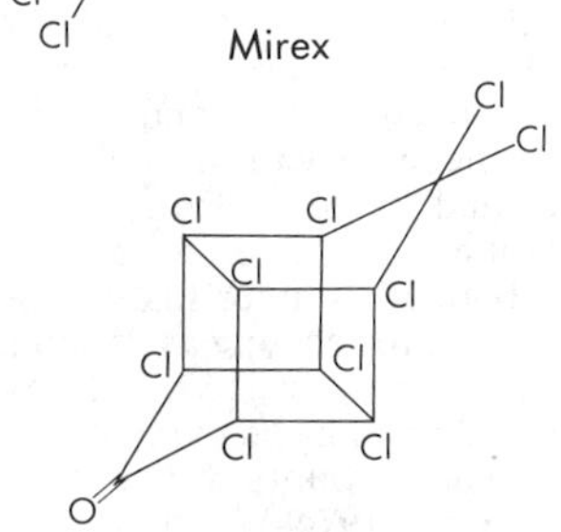

Mirex

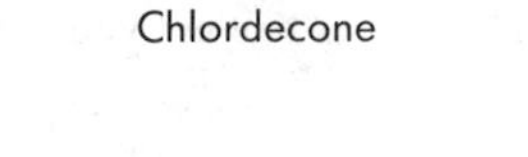

Chlordecone

Like the other chlorinated hydrocarbon insecticides, mirex and chlordecone produce stimulation of the CNS, hepatic injury, and induction of the cytochrome P_{450} system. Inhibition of mitochondrial and synaptosomal ATPases has been suggested to be the basis of neurotoxicity (Desaiah, 1981) and hepatobiliary dysfunction (Mehendale, 1979). Testicular atrophy and reduced sperm production may be due to a direct estrogenic action of chlordecone (Eroschenko, 1981). Mirex and chlordecone are carcinogenic in laboratory animals (Cueto *et al.*, 1976; Waters *et al.*, 1977).

Gross negligence in industrial hygiene resulted in the poisoning of 76 of 148 exposed workers engaged in the manufacture of chlordecone in Hopewell, Virginia (Taylor *et al.*, 1978). These workers suffered neurological effects, characterized by tremors, ocular flutter (opsoclonus), hepatomegaly, splenomegaly, rashes, mental changes, and widened gaits. Laboratory tests showed reduced sperm counts and reduced motility of sperm. Contamination of the area surrounding the manufacturing plant resulted in curtailment of fishing and the procurement of shellfish in the James River and threatened portions of the Chesapeake Bay.

Mirex is probably oxidized to chlordecone (Carlson *et al.*, 1976). The main metabolite of chlordecone is chlordecone alcohol, which appears in human bile as glucuronic acid conjugates (Guzelian, 1982). The major route of elimination of chlordecone is in the stool. Cholestyramine (*see* Chapter 36) administered to poisoned patients increases the fecal excretion of chlordecone 3- to 18-fold, shortens its half-life in blood from 140 to 80 days, and enhances the rate of recovery from toxic manifestations (Cohn *et al.*, 1978). Fecal chlordecone originates from both biliary and intestinal excretion (Guzelian, 1982). In man, only 5 to 10% of the chlordecone excreted into bile appears in the stool, which indicates extensive intestinal reabsorption of the chemical (Cohn *et al.*, 1978); bile appears to enhance such reabsorption greatly (Boylan *et al.*, 1979). Thus, cholestyramine may enhance intestinal excretion of chlordecone by binding constituents of bile in the intestinal lumen. Chlordecone has been detected in the milk of women, cows, and rats (Guzelian, 1982). Milk from contaminated cows can be a source of human exposure.

Organophosphorus Insecticides. Organophosphorus insecticides have largely replaced the chlorinated hydrocarbons. The organophosphates do not persist in the environment and have an extremely low carcinogenic potential; however, they have a much higher acute toxicity in man. In fact, parathion is the pesticide most frequently involved in fatal poisoning. The pharmacology and toxicology of these agents are discussed in Chapter 7.

Carbamate Insecticides. The carbamate insecticides resemble the organophosphates in many ways. The most common of these agents is carbaril; since carbaril and related compounds are inhibitors of cholinesterase, they too are discussed in Chapter 7.

Botanical Insecticides. Pyrethrums are obtained from flowers of the pyrethrum plant, *Chrysanthemum cincerariaefolium.* The insecticidal activity and toxicity of this group of chemicals reside in a number of structurally similar compounds, and the greatest insecticidal activity resides in pyrethrin I. Its structural formula is as follows:

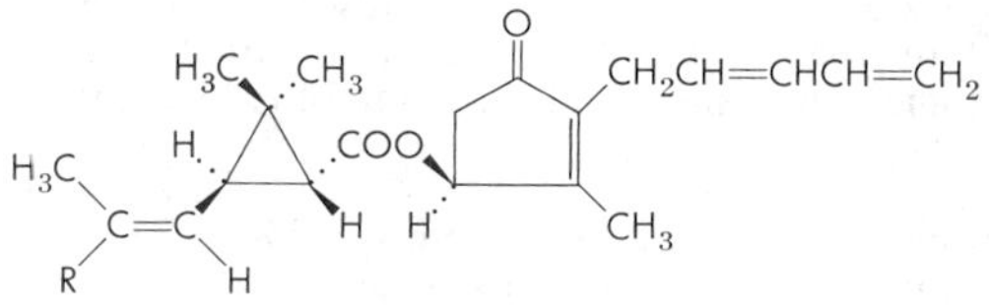

Pyrethrin I

Pyrethrum and synthetic pyrethrin derivatives (pyrethroids) are used in many household insecticides because of their rapid action. Their mechanism of action on neuronal membranes resembles that of DDT (Narahashi, 1983). Pyrethrum is generally rated as the safest insecticide because its primary toxicity is low. The low toxicity of pyrethroids in mammals is due largely to their rapid biotransformation by ester hydrolysis and/or hydroxylation (Aldridge, 1983). The slow biotransformation of pyrethrum in insects is further decreased by its formulation with piperonyl butoxide (which inhibits cytochrome P_{450}), which increases insecticidal efficacy. Unlike mammals, aquatic organisms are extremely sensitive to pyrethroids (Khan, 1983).

The allergenic properties of pyrethroids are marked in comparison with other pesticides. Many cases of contact dermatitis and respiratory allergy have been reported. Persons sensitive to ragweed pollen are particularly prone to such reactions. Preparations containing synthetic pyrethroids are less likely to cause allergic reactions than are the preparations made from pyrethrum powder.

Rotenone is obtained from the roots of plants such as *Derris* and *Lonchocarpus*. It was first used to paralyze fish before being used as an insecticide. Rotenone has the following structural formula:

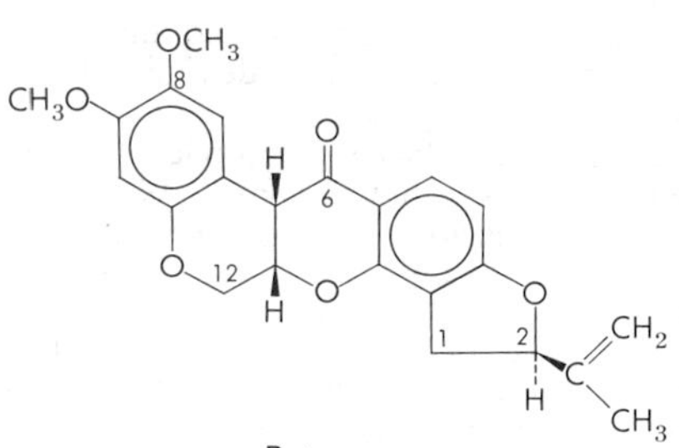

Rotenone

Human poisoning by rotenone is rare. The compound has been applied directly to treat head lice, scabies, and other ectoparasites. Local effects include conjunctivitis, dermatitis, pharyngitis, and rhinitis. Oral ingestion of rotenone produces gastrointestinal irritation, nausea, and vomiting. Inhalation of the dust is more hazardous; it can cause respiratory stimulation followed by depression and convulsions. Rotenone inhibits the oxidation of NADH to NAD. Consequently, it blocks the oxidation by NAD of substrates such as glutamate, α-ketoglutarate, and pyruvate.

Nicotine is one of the most toxic insecticides (*see* Chapter 9). Poisoning is followed by salivation and vomiting (from ganglionic stimulation), muscular weakness (from stimulation followed by depression at the neuromuscular junction), and, ultimately, clonic convulsions and cessation of respiration (effects on the CNS).

Insecticides Used as Ectoparasiticides. The term *ectoparasiticides* denotes drugs that are used against animal parasites. In man, these are primarily pediculocides and miticides.

Lindane (*gamma benzene hexachloride;* KWELL, SCABENE, others) (*see* above) is a miticide used for the treatment of scabies. It is employed in 1% concentration in a cream, lotion, or shampoo. The mixture is applied in a thin layer over the entire cutaneous surface (from the neck down) (30 g of cream for an adult) and is not removed for 8 to 12 hours. Pruritus is usually relieved within 24 hours, and the great majority of patients do not require a second treatment. If necessary, however, second and third applications can be made at weekly intervals.

The drug is also a very active pediculocide and is effective in the treatment of pediculosis pubis, capitis, and corporis. A single application of the 1% cream, lotion, or shampoo usually suffices to eradicate the ectoparasite. Lindane is also used to treat infestation by *Phthirus pubis* (crab lice).

Malathion is an organophosphate insecticide. The general pharmacology of the anticholinesterases is discussed in Chapter 7. Malathion is rapidly pediculocidal and niticidal; lice and their eggs (nits) are killed within 3 seconds by 0.003% and 0.06% malathion in acetone, respectively. The pharmaceutical preparation contains 78% isopropanol.

Malathion (PRIODERM) is available as a lotion, liquid, and shampoo outside of the United States for the treatment of head lice and nits. It is gently rubbed onto the scalp and left on for 8 to 12 hours, after which the hair is shampooed and combed. A second application may be made after 7 to 9 days if necessary.

Pyrethrins (*see* above) are moderately effective as pediculocides. They are available as a gel, a shampoo, and various liquids. Preparations should be kept away from the eyes and mucous membranes.

Benzyl benzoate is a relatively harmless substance that in high concentration is toxic to *Acarus scabiei*. The compound has been widely used in the treatment of scabies and is also useful in the treatment of pediculosis. Benzyl benzoate is used as a 26 to 30% lotion. In the treatment of scabies, the lotion is applied to the entire body from the neck down after thorough cleansing. When the first application is dry, a second coat is applied. The residue is washed off after 24 hours.

Crotamiton (N-ethyl-*o*-crotonotoluidide; EURAX) is an effective scabicide. It is available as a cream or lotion containing 10% crotamiton. It occasionally causes irritation, especially on inflamed skin or when applied over a prolonged period of time. It can cause sensitization. Paradoxically, the preparations also have antipruritic properties.

An emulsion of 31% tetrahydronaphthalene and 0.03% copper oleate is promoted as a pediculocide and niticide, but its true efficacy remains to be determined.

Thiabendazole can be applied to the skin as a 10% suspension in the treatment of cutaneous larva migrans (*see* Chapter 40). It has scabicidal activity, for which it is used outside the United States. It is also reputed to be mildly antifungal.

FUMIGANTS

Fumigants are used to control insects, rodents, and soil nematodes. They exert pesticidal action in gaseous form and are used because they can penetrate otherwise-inaccessible areas. Agents used to protect stored foodstuffs include hydrogen cyanide, acrylonitrile (an organic cyanide, $CH_2{=}CHCN$), carbon disulfide, carbon tetrachloride, chloropicrin, ethylene dibromide, ethylene oxide, methyl bromide, and phosphine.

Cyanide. Cyanide (hydrocyanic acid [HCN], prussic acid) is one of the most rapidly acting poisons. Victims may die within minutes of exposure. Hydrogen cyanide gas is used to fumigate ships and buildings and to sterilize soil. Because of its ability to form complexes with metals, cyanide is used in metallurgy, electroplating, and metal cleaning. In the home, cyanides are present in silver polish, insecticides, rodenticides, and fruit seeds. The major toxicity of laetrile is due to its cyanogenic glycoside. Cytochrome P_{450}–dependent monooxygenases liberate cyanide from organic nitriles (Willhite and Smith, 1981), as do glutathione S-transferases from organic thiocyanates (Ohkawa and Casida, 1971); cyanide is also a metabolite of nitroprusside (Cottrell *et al.*, 1978). Combustion of nitrogen-containing plastics may result in release of HCN. Fire on board airplanes killed 119 passengers in Paris in 1973 and 303 pilgrims in Riyadh, Saudi Arabia, in 1980 due to combustion of plastic material that produced HCN (Weger, 1983). Cyanide is also used for executions in so-called gas chambers and was used for more than 900 religious "suicide-murders" in Guyana in 1978.

Cyanide has a very high affinity for iron in the ferric state. When absorbed, it reacts readily with the trivalent iron of cytochrome oxidase in mitochondria; cellular respiration is thus inhibited, resulting in lactic acidosis and cytotoxic hypoxia. Since utilization of oxygen is blocked, venous blood is oxygenated and is almost as bright red as arterial blood. Respiration is stimulated because chemoreceptive cells respond as they do to decreased oxygen. A transient stage of CNS stimulation with hyperpnea and headache is observed; finally hypoxic convulsions occur, and death is due to respiratory arrest.

Treatment of cyanide poisoning must be rapid to

be effective. Diagnosis may be aided by the characteristic odor of cyanide (oil of bitter almonds). Because toxicity results from binding to the ferric form of cytochrome oxidase, treatment is aimed at prevention or reversal of such binding by providing a large pool of ferric iron to compete for cyanide. An effective mechanism is to administer substances, such as nitrite, that oxidize hemoglobin to methemoglobin. Amyl nitrite is usually administered by inhalation, while a solution of sodium nitrite is prepared for intravenous administration (10 ml of a 3% solution). Methemoglobin competes with cytochrome oxidase for the cyanide ion; the reaction favors methemoglobin because of mass action. Cyanmethemoglobin is formed, and cytochrome oxidase is restored. Alternatively, 4-dimethylaminophenol, which also oxidizes hemoglobin to methemoglobin, can be used in a dose of 3 mg/kg intravenously (Weger, 1983). Cobalt compounds have a high affinity for cyanide (Way, 1984), and Co_2EDTA has been used successfully in treatment of cyanide poisoning in man (Cottrell *et al.*, 1978; Weger, 1983). Similarly, hydroxocobalamin can be used to treat cyanide toxicity, since it combines with cyanide to form cyanocobalamin (vitamin B_{12}).

The major mechanism for removing cyanide from the body is its enzymatic conversion, by the mitochondrial enzyme rhodanese (transsulfurase), to thiocyanate, which is relatively nontoxic. To accelerate detoxication, sodium thiosulfate is administered intravenously (50 ml of a 25% aqueous solution), and the thiocyanate formed is readily excreted in the urine.

$$Na_2S_2O_3 + CN^- \xrightarrow{\text{Rhodanese}} SCN^- + Na_2SO_3$$

Way and associates (1972) demonstrated that nitrite increases the LD_{50} of potassium cyanide in mice from 11 mg/kg to 21 mg/kg; administration of thiosulfate increases the value to 35 mg/kg, while nitrite followed by thiosulfate increases the LD_{50} to 52 mg/kg. Many cases of acute cyanide poisoning in man have been treated successfully with such therapy.

Oxygen alone, even at hyperbaric pressures, has only a slight protective effect in cyanide poisoning; however, it dramatically potentiates the protective effects of thiosulfate or of nitrite and thiosulfate (Way *et al.*, 1972). The mechanism for this action is not clear, but the intracellular oxygen tension may be high enough to cause nonenzymatic oxidation of reduced cytochromes, or oxygen may displace cyanide from cytochrome oxidase by mass action.

If cyanide has been ingested, gastric lavage should follow, not precede, initiation of more specific treatment.

Methyl Bromide. Methyl bromide is used as an insecticidal fumigant and in some fire extinguishers. It is said to have been responsible for more deaths in California in the 1960s among occupationally exposed persons than all the organophosphate insecticides (Hine, 1969). Because methyl bromide is so toxic, chloropicrin (CCl_3NO_2), a powerful stimulator of lacrimation, is added as a warning.

Major signs and symptoms of intoxication with methyl bromide are referable to the CNS. These include malaise, headache, visual disturbances, nausea, and vomiting. Death usually occurs during a convulsion. After severe respiratory exposure, pulmonary edema may prove fatal. The high affinity of methyl bromide for sulfhydryl groups may have a role in its toxic action. Sulfhydryl agents may thus be beneficial as antidotes in poisoning with methyl bromide.

Dibromochloropropane and Ethylene Dibromide. Dibromochloropropane ($ClCH_2CHBrCH_2Br$) and ethylene dibromide (1,2-dibromoethane) are soil fumigants used to control nematodes. In man, they produce moderate depression of the CNS and pulmonary congestion after exposure by inhalation, and they cause acute gastrointestinal distress and pulmonary edema after ingestion. Both agents cause gastric carcinoma in rats and mice (Powers *et al.*, 1975; IARC, 1977). Dibromochloropropane causes sterility and/or abnormally low sperm counts in workmen engaged in its manufacture. Use of both agents is being decreased because of their carcinogenicity and their adverse effects on reproductive function.

Phosphine. Phosphine (PH_3) is a fumigant for grain; it is released gradually, in the presence of atmospheric moisture, from tablets of aluminum phosphide. Phosphine is more toxic than methyl bromide; however, since less is required to fumigate a given volume of grain, it has proven to be safer. Severe pulmonary irritation and pulmonary edema are the main toxic effects of phosphine; hepatic and myocardial injury is also observed.

RODENTICIDES

Some rodenticides are quite toxic to man, but the toxicity of others is more selective. In some cases, selectivity is based on a unique aspect of the physiology of rodents; in others, advantage is taken of the habits of these animals. Since rodenticides can be used in baits and placed in inaccessible places, the likelihood of their contaminating the environment is much less than that of other pesticides. The toxicological problem posed by rodenticides, therefore, is primarily one of accidental or suicidal ingestion.

Warfarin. Warfarin, one of the most frequently used rodenticides, is considered safe because its toxicity depends on repeated ingestion. However, daily intake by man of 1 to 2 mg/kg for 6 days has produced severe illness in an attempted suicide. Warfarin, an oral anticoagulant, is discussed in Chapter 55.

Red Squill. The bulbs of red squill (*Urginea maritima*) have been used for many years as a relatively safe rodenticide. The active principles are scillaren glycosides. These glycosides, like the digitalis glycosides, have cardiotonic actions (*see*

Chapter 34). Signs and symptoms associated with ingestion of large doses of red squill include vomiting and abdominal pain, blurred vision, cardiac irregularities, convulsions, and death from ventricular fibrillation. The selective rodenticidal usefulness of squill is due to the inability of rats to vomit (Lisella *et al.*, 1971). Treatment of ingestion in man, if indicated, is the same as for overdosage of digitalis (*see* Chapter 34).

Sodium Fluoroacetate. Sodium fluoroacetate and fluoroacetamide are among the most potent rodenticides. Because they are also highly toxic to other animals, their use is restricted to licensed pest-control operators. Fluoroacetate produces its toxic action by inhibiting the citric acid cycle. The compound is incorporated into fluoroacetyl coenzyme A, which condenses with oxaloacetate to form fluorocitrate. Fluorocitrate inhibits the enzyme aconitase and thereby inhibits conversion of citrate to isocitrate. As might be expected, the heart and CNS are the tissues most critically involved by a general inhibition of oxidative energy metabolism. Thus, the signs and symptoms of fluoroacetate poisoning, in addition to nonspecific signs of nausea and vomiting, include cardiac irregularities, cyanosis, generalized convulsions, and death from ventricular fibrillation or respiratory failure. Provision of large quantities of acetate appears to antagonize fluoroacetate in a competitive manner; monkeys have been successfully protected from fluoroacetate poisoning by the administration of glycerol monoacetate.

Strychnine. Strychnine is the principal alkaloid present in nux vomica, the seeds of a tree native to India, *Strychnos nuxvomica*. Nux vomica was introduced into Germany in the sixteenth century as a poison for rats and other animal pests. Its use as a pesticide persists to this day and is a source of accidental strychnine poisoning of children. The structural formula of strychnine is as follows:

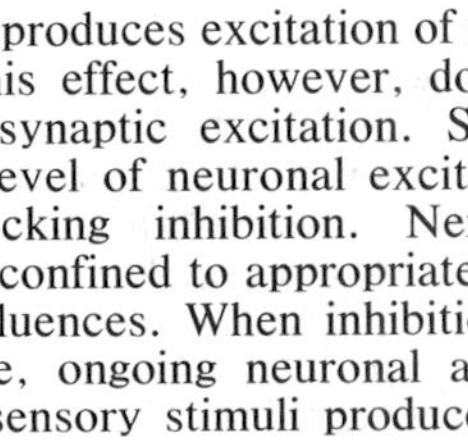

Strychnine

Strychnine produces excitation of all portions of the CNS. This effect, however, does not result from direct synaptic excitation. Strychnine increases the level of neuronal excitability by selectively blocking inhibition. Nerve impulses are normally confined to appropriate pathways by inhibitory influences. When inhibition is blocked by strychnine, ongoing neuronal activity is enhanced and sensory stimuli produce exaggerated reflex effects.

Strychnine is a powerful convulsant, and the convulsion has a characteristic motor pattern. Inasmuch as strychnine reduces inhibition, including the reciprocal inhibition existing between antagonistic muscles, the pattern of convulsion is determined by the most powerful muscles acting at a given joint. In most laboratory animals, this convulsion is characterized by tonic extension of the body and of all limbs. Tonic extension is preceded and followed during the phase of postictal depression by phasic symmetrical extensor thrusts that may be initiated by any modality of sensory stimulus.

The convulsant action of strychnine is due to interference with postsynaptic inhibition that is mediated by glycine. Glycine is an important inhibitory transmitter to motoneurons and interneurons in the spinal cord, and strychnine acts as a selective, competitive antagonist to block the inhibitory effects of glycine at all glycine receptors (*see* Chapter 12). Well-known examples of this type of postsynaptic inhibition are the inhibitory influences existing between the motoneurons of antagonistic muscle groups and recurrent spinal inhibition mediated by the Renshaw cell. Renshaw cells are excited by intraspinal collaterals of motoneuron axons that liberate acetylcholine. Strychnine blocks recurrent inhibition at the Renshaw cell–motoneuron synapse by antagonizing the action of glycine released by the Renshaw cell. Strychnine-sensitive postsynaptic inhibition in higher centers of the CNS is also mediated by glycine.

The effects of strychnine in man closely resemble those described above for laboratory animals. The first effect that is noticed is stiffness of the face and neck muscles. Heightened reflex excitability soon becomes evident. Any sensory stimulus may produce a violent motor response. In the early stages this response is a coordinated extensor thrust, and in the later stages it may be a full tetanic convulsion. In this convulsion, the body is arched in hyperextension (opisthotonos) so that only the crown of the head and the heels may be touching the ground. All voluntary muscles, including those of the face, are in full contraction. Respiration ceases owing to the contraction of the diaphragm and the thoracic and abdominal muscles. Convulsive episodes may recur repeatedly with intermittent periods of depression; sensory stimulation increases the frequency and severity of the convulsions. Death results from medullary paralysis, which is due primarily to the hypoxia resulting from the periods of impaired respiration. In the early stages the patient not only is conscious but also is acutely perceptive to all stimuli. The muscle contractions are quite painful and the patient is extremely apprehensive and fearful of impending death. If untreated, death from strychnine often occurs after the second to fifth full convulsion, but the first may be fatal if it is sustained. The combination of impaired respiration and intense muscular contractions can produce severe respiratory and metabolic acidosis.

The most urgent objectives in the treatment of strychnine poisoning are the prevention of convulsions and the support of respiration. Diazepam is the most useful agent for this purpose. It antagonizes the convulsions without potentiating postictal depression (Gosselin *et al.*, 1984). Anesthesia or neuromuscular blockade may be necessary to control resistant convulsions in severely intoxicated patients. All forms of sensory stimulation should be minimized. If adequate respiratory ventilation is not restored by the termination of convulsions, intubation and mechanical assistance are essential.

Phosphorus. White or yellow elemental phosphorus has poisoned man when it was spread in paste on bread to bait rodents. Shortly after ingestion, phosphorus produces severe gastrointestinal irritation, and, if the dose is sufficient, hemorrhage and cardiovascular failure may prove fatal within 24 hours. The vomitus is luminescent and has a characteristic garlic odor. If the patient survives the initial phase of gastrointestinal injury, secondary systemic poisoning and hepatic necrosis may ensue. Severe acute yellow atrophy of the liver is a delayed sequela that may prove fatal.

Long-term poisoning from phosphorus is characterized by cachexia, anemia, bronchitis, and necrosis of the mandible, the so-called phossy jaw.

Zinc Phosphide. Zinc phosphide reacts with water and HCl in the gastrointestinal tract to produce the gas phosphine (PH_3), which causes severe gastrointestinal irritation. Apparent insensitivity of dogs and cats has been attributed to the emetic qualities of zinc in animals other than rodents. Later phases of toxicity resemble poisoning by yellow elemental phosphorus.

***α*-Naphthylthiourea.** The structural formula of *α*-naphthylthiourea is as follows:

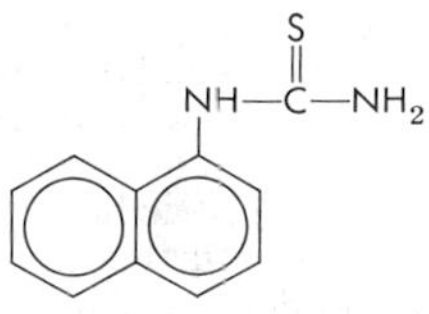

α-Naphthylthiourea

Its selective rodenticidal properties are due to different susceptibilities of various species. The LD_{50} in rats is about 3 mg/kg, in dogs 10 mg/kg, in guinea pigs 400 mg/kg, and in monkeys 4 g/kg. The principal toxic effect in susceptible species is massive pulmonary edema and pleural effusion, apparently the result of an action on pulmonary capillaries. Microsomes from rat liver and lung release atomic sulfur from *α*-naphthylthiourea (Lee *et al.*, 1980). Pulmonary toxicity may result, at least in part, from binding of atomic sulfur to tissue macromolecules. Sulfhydryl blocking agents are effective antidotes for rats in some experimental conditions (Koch and Schwarze, 1956).

Thallium. Thallium sulfate is very hazardous. Since it is not selectively toxic for rodents and many people have been poisoned by thallium, its use is now strictly regulated in many countries. Acute poisoning is accompanied by gastrointestinal irritation, motor paralysis, and death from respiratory failure. Sublethal doses taken over a period of time redden the skin and cause alopecia, characteristic signs of thallium poisoning. Pathological changes include perivascular cuffing and degenerative changes in the brain, liver, and kidney. Neurological symptoms are prominent and include tremors, leg pains, paresthesias of the hands and feet, and polyneuritis, especially in the legs. Psychoses, delirium, convulsions, and other types of encephalopathy may also be noted. Treatment of thallium intoxication involves the oral administration of ferric ferrocyanide (Prussian blue), hemodialysis, and forced diuresis. Prussian blue binds thallium in the intestine and enhances its fecal excretion. Administration of systemic chelating agents should be avoided, because they may increase uptake of thallium into the brain (Hayes, 1982).

HERBICIDES

The production and use of chemicals for destruction of noxious weeds have increased markedly in the past two decades. Herbicides now exceed insecticides in quantities used and values of sales. Although some herbicidal compounds have very low toxicity in mammals, others are highly toxic and have caused human fatalities.

Chlorophenoxy Compounds. The compounds 2,4-dichlorophenoxyacetic acid (2,4-D) and 2,4,5-trichlorophenoxyacetic acid (2,4,5-T), as their salts and esters, are probably the most familiar herbicides. Their structural formulas are as follows:

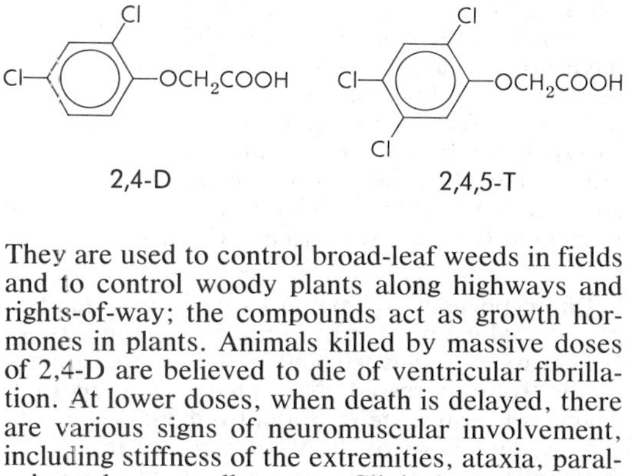

2,4-D 2,4,5-T

They are used to control broad-leaf weeds in fields and to control woody plants along highways and rights-of-way; the compounds act as growth hormones in plants. Animals killed by massive doses of 2,4-D are believed to die of ventricular fibrillation. At lower doses, when death is delayed, there are various signs of neuromuscular involvement, including stiffness of the extremities, ataxia, paralysis, and, eventually, coma. Clinical reports of poisoning from chlorophenoxy herbicides are rare.

These herbicides do not accumulate in animals. They are not extensively metabolized but are actively excreted into the urine (Berndt and Koschier, 1973). Their plasma half-life in man is about 1 day (Gehring *et al.*, 1973).

Chlorophenoxy herbicides have produced contact dermatitis in man, and a rather severe type of dermatitis, chloracne, has been observed in workers involved in the manufacture of 2,4,5-T (Poland *et al.*, 1971). The dermatitis seems due primarily to the action of a contaminant, 2,3,7,8-tetrachlorodibenzo-*p*-dioxin (TCDD), the structure of which is as follows:

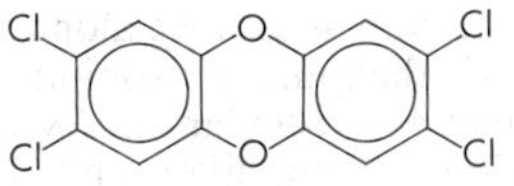

TCDD

TCDD is particularly toxic for some species. It has an LD_{50} of 0.6 μg/kg in guinea pigs, but this value is 10,000 times higher in hamsters. The mechanism of death is not known; morphological changes in the liver, thymus, and reproductive organs are observed but are not sufficiently severe to account for death. TCDD shows no toxic effect on cell cultures. TCDD is a potent inducer of aryl hydrocarbon hydroxylase, a microsomal cytochrome P_{450}–dependent monooxygenase (Poland and Glover, 1974). It is also a very potent teratogen (Neubert *et al.*, 1973) and has been demonstrated to be a carcinogen in laboratory animals (Van Miller *et al.*, 1977; Kociba *et al.*, 1978). Hence, 2,4,5-T has been banned in the United States and its production has been halted.

Accidental human exposures indicate that TCDD has low toxicity for man as compared with that for certain species (*e.g.*, guinea pig) (Holmstedt, 1980). Effects of TCDD poisoning in exposed persons include chloracne, porphyria, hypercholesterolemia, and psychiatric disturbances (Hayes, 1982). Epidemiological studies do not support the hypothesis that TCDD is a teratogen or carcinogen in man at existing levels of exposure. During the Vietnam War, Agent Orange, a mixture of 2,4-D and 2,4,5-T (which was contaminated with TCDD) was sprayed over large jungle areas, and many soldiers were presumed to have been exposed to the compounds. Although controversial, epidemiological studies have not revealed any TCDD-related adverse effects on health in Vietnam veterans. There appears to be no difference in the plasma concentration of TCDD in Vietnam veterans and non-Vietnam veterans, indicating that exposure of United States soldiers in Vietnam to TCDD was much less than suspected (Centers for Disease Control, 1988).

Dinitrophenols. Several substituted dinitrophenols, alone or as salts of aliphatic amines or alkalies, are used in weed control. Human poisonings by dinitroorthocresol (DNOC) have been reported. The short-term toxicity of dinitrophenols is due to the uncoupling of oxidative phosphorylation. The metabolic rate of the poisoned individual can increase markedly, and the body temperature is elevated. Signs and symptoms of acute poisoning in man include nausea, restlessness, flushed skin, sweating, rapid respiration, tachycardia, fever, cyanosis, and, finally, collapse and coma. The illness runs a rapid course; death or recovery occurs within 24 to 48 hours. If production of heat exceeds the capacity for its dissipation, fatal hyperthermia may result. Specific treatment consists of ice baths to reduce fever, administration of oxygen, and correction of fluid and electrolyte imbalances.

Bipyridyl Compounds. Paraquat is the most important compound in this class of herbicides from a toxicological viewpoint. The structural formula of paraquat is as follows:

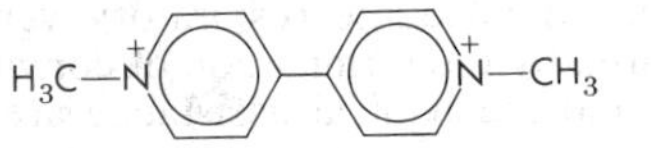

Paraquat

Several hundred cases of accidental or suicidal fatalities from paraquat poisoning have been reported during the past decade. Pathological changes observed at autopsy are indicative of damage to the lungs, liver, and kidneys; myocarditis is sometimes present. The most striking pathological change is a widespread proliferation of fibroblastic cells in the lungs, an effect that is not dependent on the route of administration. Although ingestion of paraquat causes gastrointestinal upset within a few hours, the onset of respiratory symptoms and eventual death by respiratory distress may be delayed for several days.

A biochemical mechanism for paraquat-induced pulmonary injury has been proposed (Bus *et al.*, 1976; Smith, 1988). Paraquat is believed to undergo a single-electron cyclic reduction–oxidation, with subsequent formation of superoxide anion radical (O_2^-). Superoxide anion radical is nonenzymatically transformed to singlet oxygen, which attacks polyunsaturated lipids associated with cell membranes to form lipid hydroperoxides. The lipid hydroperoxides are unstable in the presence of trace amounts of transition metal ions and decompose to lipid-free radicals. The chain reaction of lipid peroxidation thus initiated is somewhat similar to that described above for CCl_4.

Because of the serious, delayed pulmonary toxicity produced by paraquat, prompt treatment is important. This involves removal of paraquat from the alimentary tract by gastric lavage and the use of cathartics, prevention of further absorption by oral administration of Fuller's earth, and removal of absorbed paraquat by hemodialysis or hemoperfusion (Cavalli and Fletcher, 1977; Davies *et al.*, 1977).

A survey found that 21% of marijuana samples from the Southwestern United States and 3.6% of the samples collected from the entire country were contaminated with paraquat. The source of contamination was an aerial spraying program in Mexico. It was projected that marijuana smokers could be exposed to 0.5 mg or more of paraquat per year by inhalation. However, much of the paraquat is probably pyrolyzed as the leaves burn. No clinical case of paraquat poisoning has been recognized among marijuana smokers, although no systematic search for such cases has been undertaken (Landrigan *et al.*, 1983).

Other Herbicides. There are a large number of other herbicides that, for the most part, have relatively low acute toxicities for mammals. These include carbamates (*e.g.*, propham and barban), substituted ureas (*e.g.*, monuron and diuron), triazines (*e.g.*, atrazine and the related compound aminotriazole), aniline derivatives (*e.g.*, alachlor, propachlor, and propanil), dinitroaniline derivatives (*e.g.*, trifluralin), and benzoic acid derivatives (*e.g.*, amiben).

FUNGICIDES

Fungicides, like other classes of pesticides, comprise a heterogeneous group of chemical compounds. With few exceptions, the fungicides have not been the subject of detailed toxicological research. Although many compounds used to control fungal diseases on plants, seeds, and produce are rather nontoxic in the short term, there are some notable exceptions; the mercury-containing fungicides have caused the greatest concern. They have been responsible for many deaths or permanent neurological disabilities resulting from the misdirection of treated seed grains into human and animal food. The toxicities of mercury and its compounds are discussed in Chapter 66.

Dithiocarbamates. Fungicides of this group are commonly used in agriculture. They have a low order of acute toxicity, and values of the oral LD_{50} in rats range from several hundred milligrams to several grams per kilogram. Except for contact dermatitis induced by dithiocarbamate (Fisher, 1983), there is little evidence of human injury from exposure to these compounds. However, they may have some teratogenic and/or carcinogenic potential (World Health Organization, 1975). Two groups of dithiocarbamates that have been used, the dimethyldithiocarbamates and the ethylenebisdithiocarbamates, have the following general formulas:

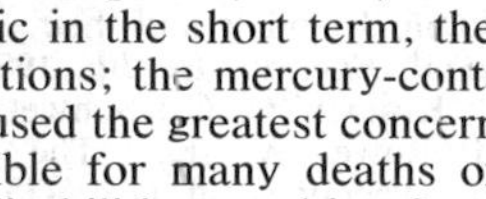

Dimethyldithiocarbamates

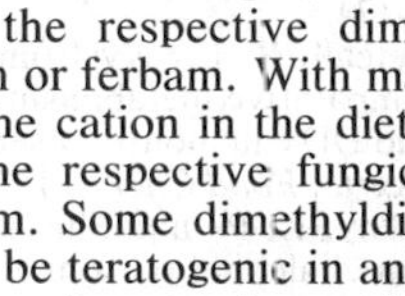

Ethylenebisdithiocarbamates

The names of the fungicides are derived from the metallic cations. For example, when the cation is zinc or iron, the respective dimethyldithiocarbamate is ziram or ferbam. With manganese, zinc, or sodium as the cation in the diethyldithiocarbamate series, the respective fungicide is maneb, zineb, or nabam. Some dimethyldithiocarbamates are reported to be teratogenic in animals, and they can form nitrosamines *in vitro* and *in vivo* (IARC, 1974b; World Health Organization, 1975). The ethylenebisdithiocarbamates are also reported to be teratogenic. Furthermore, this group of compounds breaks down to form ethylenethiourea (ETU) *in vivo,* in the environment, and during cooking of foods containing their residues. ETU is carcinogenic, mutagenic, and teratogenic, as well as being an antithyroid agent (IARC, 1974b, 1976). Dithiocarbamate fungicides are analogs of disulfiram, and they can produce a disulfiram-like response when ethanol is ingested (*see* Chapter 17).

Hexachlorobenzene. Exposure to hexachlorobenzene results in an increase in hepatic weight, in the quantity of smooth endoplasmic reticulum, and in the activities of cytochrome P_{450}–dependent monooxygenases (Carlson and Tardiff, 1976). Between 1955 and 1959, more than 300 human poisonings occurred in Turkey as a result of the use of hexachlorobenzene-treated wheat (Schmid, 1960). Some deaths resulted; the major syndrome was cutaneous porphyria with skin lesions, porphyrinuria, and photosensitization. Hexachlorobenzene is eliminated from the body predominantly in the feces as a result of intestinal excretion. This process can be enhanced fivefold in rhesus monkeys by the oral administration of mineral oil (Rozman *et al.*, 1983).

Pentachlorophenol. Pentachlorophenol is used as an insecticide and a herbicide, as well as a fungicide, with major application as a wood preservative. Several cases of human poisoning have been associated with its use. The acute toxic action of pentachlorophenol in man and experimental animals resembles that of the nitrophenolic herbicides—a marked increase in metabolic rate as the result of uncoupling of oxidative phosphorylation. Pentachlorophenol is readily absorbed through the skin. Two cases of fatal poisonings and several nonfatal cases occurred in a hospital nursery; pentachlorophenol had been used as a fungicide in the laundry room and ultimately came in contact with infants through their diapers (Armstrong *et al.*, 1969).

In recent years it has become apparent that many commercial samples of pentachlorophenol are contaminated with polychlorinated dibenzodioxins and dibenzofurans (Buser, 1975). These contaminants are generally less toxic than the tetrachlorodioxin contaminant (TCDD) in 2,4,5-T. Although pentachlorophenol is highly toxic in its own right, some studies suggest that the contaminants may be responsible for some of the untoward effects of the technical-grade product (Johnson *et al.*, 1973; Goldstein *et al.*, 1976). Treatment of intoxication with pentachlorophenol is similar to that for poisoning with dinitrophenols. Fecal excretion of pentachlorophenol can be enhanced by cholestyramine, which interrupts the enterohepatic circulation of the chemical (Rozman *et al.*, 1982).

Aksoy, M. Benzene as a leukemogenic and carcinogenic agent. *Am. J. Ind. Med.*, **1985**, *8*, 9–20.

Amdur, M. O.; Dubriel, M.; and Creasia, D. A. Respiratory response of guinea pigs to low levels of sulfuric acid. *Environ. Res.*, **1978**, *15*, 418–423.

Armstrong, R. W.; Eichner, E. R.; Klein, D. E.; Barthel, W. F.; Bennett, J. V.; Jonsson, V.; Bruce, H.; and Loveless, L. E. Pentachlorophenol poisoning in a nursery for newborn infants. II. Epidemiological and toxicologic studies. *J. Pediatr.*, **1969**, *75*, 317–325.

Ayres, S. M.; Giammelli, S., Jr.; and Mueller, H. Effects

of low concentrations of carbon monoxide. Part IV. Myocardial and systemic responses to carboxyhemoglobin. *Ann. N.Y. Acad. Sci.*, **1970**, *174*, 268–293.

Baud, F. J.; Galliot, M.; Astier, A.; Bien, D. V.; Garnier, R.; Likforman, J.; and Bismuth, C. Treatment of ethylene glycol poisoning with intravenous 4-methylpyrazole. *N. Engl. J. Med.*, **1988**, *319*, 97–100.

Berndt, W. O., and Koschier, F. *In vitro* uptake of 2,4-dichlorophenoxyacetic acid (2,4,-D) and 2,4,5-trichlorophenoxyacetic acid (2,4,5-T) by renal cortical tissue of rabbits and rats. *Toxicol. Appl. Pharmacol.*, **1973**, *26*, 1114–1117.

Blair, A.; Grauman, D. J.; Lubin, J. H.; and Fraumeni, J. F. Lung cancer and other causes of death among licensed pesticide applicators. *J. Natl. Cancer Inst.*, **1983**, *71*, 31–37.

Bokonjić, N. Stagnant anoxia and carbon monoxide poisoning. *Electroencephalogr. Clin. Neurophysiol.*, **1963**, Suppl. 21, 1–102.

Boylan, J. J.; Cohn, W. J.; Egle, J. L.; Blanke, R. V.; and Guzelian, P. S. Excretion of chlordecone by the gastrointestinal tract: evidence for a nonbiliary mechanism. *Clin. Pharmacol. Ther.*, **1979**, *25*, 579–585.

Burk, R. F.; Rieter, R.; and Lane, J. M. Hyperbaric oxygen protection against carbon tetrachloride hepatotoxicity in the rat. *Gastroenterology*, **1986**, *90*, 812–818.

Bus, J. S.; Cagen, S. Z.; Olgaard, M.; and Gibson, J. E. A mechanism of paraquat toxicity in mice and rats. *Toxicol. Appl. Pharmacol.*, **1976**, *35*, 501–513.

Buser, H. R. Analysis of polychlorinated dibenzo-*p*-dioxins and dibenzofurans in chlorinated phenols by mass fragmentography. *J. Chromatogr.*, **1975**, *107*, 295–310.

Carlson, D. A.; Konyhu, K. D.; Wheeler, W. B.; Marshall, G. P.; and Zaylskie, R. G. Mirex in the environment: its degradation to KEPONE and related compounds. *Science*, **1976**, *94*, 939–941.

Carlson, G. P., and Tardiff, R. G. Effect of chlorinated benzenes on the metabolism of foreign organic compounds. *Toxicol. Appl. Pharmacol.*, **1976**, *36*, 383–394.

Cavalli, R. D., and Fletcher, K. An effective treatment for paraquat poisoning. In, *Biochemical Mechanism of Paraquat Toxicity.* (Autor, A. P., ed.) Academic Press, Inc., New York, **1977**, pp. 213–228.

Centers for Disease Control Veterans Health Studies. Serum 2,3,7,8-tetrachlorodibenzo-*p*-dioxin levels in U.S. army Vietnam-era veterans. *J.A.M.A.*, **1988**, *260*, 1249–1254.

Cohn, W. J.; Boylan, J. J.; Blanke, R. V.; Furiss, M. W.; Howell, J. R.; and Guzelian, P. S. Treatment of chlordecone (KEPONE) toxicity with cholestyramine. *N. Engl. J. Med.*, **1978**, *298*, 243–248.

Cottrell, J. E.; Casthely, P.; Brodie, J. B.; Pathel, K.; Klein, A.; and Turndorf, H. Cyanide toxicity with nitroprusside infusions. *N. Engl. J. Med.*, **1978**, *298*, 809–811.

Cueto, C. Consideration of the possible carcinogenicity of some pesticides. *J. Environ. Sci. Health* [B], **1980**, *15*, 949–975.

Cueto, C.; Page, N.; and Saffiott, V. *Report of Carcinogenesis, Bioassay of Technical Grade Chlordecone* (KEPONE). National Cancer Institute, Bethesda, Md., **1976**.

Davies, D. S.; Hawksworth, G. M.; and Bennett, P. N. Paraquat poisoning. *Proc. Eur. Soc. Toxicol.*, **1977**, *18*, 21–26.

Desaiah, D. Interaction of chlordecone with biological membranes. *J. Toxicol. Environ. Health*, **1981**, *8*, 719–730.

Elmes, P. C. Mesotheliomas, minerals and man-made mineral fibres. *Thorax*, **1980**, *35*, 561–563.

Eroschenko, V. P. Estrogenic activity of the insecticide chlordecone in the reproductive tract of birds and mammals. *J. Toxicol. Environ. Health*, **1981**, *8*, 731–742.

Folland, D. S.; Schaffner, W.; Grinn, H. E.; Crofford, O. B.; and McMurray, D. R. Carbon tetrachloride toxicity potentiated by isopropyl alcohol. *J.A.M.A.*, **1976**, *236*, 1853–1856.

Freeman, G.; Crane, S. C.; Furiosi, N. J.; Stephens, R. J.; Evans, M. J.; and Moore, W. D. Covert reduction in ventilatory surface in rats during prolonged exposure to subacute nitrogen dioxide. *Am. Rev. Respir. Dis.*, **1972**, *106*, 563–579.

Gabow, P. A.; Clay, K.; Sullivan, J. B.; and Lepoff, R. Organic acids in ethylene glycol intoxication. *Ann. Intern. Med.*, **1986**, *105*, 16–20.

Gardner, D. E. Oxidant-induced enhanced sensitivity to infection in animal models and their extrapolations to man. *J. Toxicol. Environ. Health*, **1984**, *13*, 423–439.

Gehring, P. J.; Kramer, C. G.; Schwetz, B. A.; Rose, J. Q.; and Rowe, V. K. The fate of 2,4,5-trichlorophenoxyacetic acid (2,4,5-T) following oral administration to man. *Toxicol. Appl. Pharmacol.*, **1973**, *26*, 352–361.

Goldsmith, J. R., and Landaw, S. A. Carbon monoxide and human health. *Science*, **1968**, *162*, 1352–1359.

Goldstein, J. A.; Linder, R. E.; Hickman, P.; and Bergman, H. Effects of pentachlorophenol on hepatic drug metabolism and porphyria related to contamination with chlorinated dibenzo-*p*-dioxins. *Toxicol. Appl. Pharmacol.*, **1976**, *37*, 145–146.

Guggenheim, M. A.; Couch, J. R.; and Weinberg, W. Motor dysfunction as a permanent complication of methanol ingestion. *Arch. Neurol.*, **1971**, *24*, 550–554.

Hine, C. H. Methyl bromide poisoning: a review of ten cases. *J. Occup. Med.*, **1969**, *11*, 1–10.

Hirsch, J. A.; Swenson, E. W.; and Wanner, A. Tracheal mucous transport in beagles after long-term exposure to 1 ppm sulfur dioxide. *Arch. Environ. Health*, **1975**, *30*, 249–253.

Hooper, N. K.; Ames, B. N.; Salek, M. A.; and Casida, J. E. Toxophane, a complex mixture of polychloroterpenes and a major insecticide, is mutagenic. *Science*, **1979**, *205*, 591–593.

Iida, M.; Yamamoto, H.; and Sobue, I. Prognosis of *n*-hexane polyneuropathy: follow-up studies on mass outbreak in F district of Mie prefecture. *Igaku No Ayumi*, **1973**, *84*, 199–201.

Jacobson, D., and McMartin, K. E. Methanol and ethylene glycol poisonings: mechanism of toxicity, clinical course, diagnosis and treatment. *Med. Toxicol.*, **1986**, *1*, 309–334.

Jerina, D. M., and Daley, J. R. Arene oxides: a new aspect of drug metabolism. *Science*, **1974**, *185*, 573–582.

Johnson, R. L.; Gehring, P. J.; Kociba, R. J.; and Schwetz, B. A. Chlorinated dibenzodioxins and pentachlorophenol. *Environ. Health Perspect.*, **1973**, *5*, 171–175.

Jones, R. D., and Winter, D. P. Two case reports of deaths on industrial premises attributed to 1,1,1-trichloroethane. *Arch. Environ. Health*, **1983**, *38*, 59–61.

Kaplan, K. Methyl alcohol poisoning. *Am. J. Med. Sci.*, **1962**, *244*, 170–174.

Kapoor, I. P.; Metcalf, R. L.; Nystrom, R. F.; and Sangha, G. H. Comparative metabolism of methoxychlor, methiochlor, and DDT in mouse, insects and in a model ecosystem. *J. Agric. Food Chem.*, **1970**, *18*, 1145–1152.

King, L. H.; Bradley, K. P.; and Shires, D. L. Hemodialysis for isopropyl alcohol poisoning. *J.A.M.A.*, **1970**, *211*, 1855.

Koch, R., and Schwarze, W. Die Hemmung der α-Naphthylthioharnstoffvergiftung durch Cysteamin und seine Derivate. (Zugleich ein Beitrag zur Toxikologie und Strahlenschutzwirkung dieser Sulfhydrylkorper). *Naunyn Schmiedebergs Arch. Exp. Pathol. Pharmakol.*, **1956**, *29*, 428–441.

Kociba, R. J., and others. Result of a 2-year chronic toxicity and oncogenicity study of 2,3,7,8-tetrachlorodibenzo-*p*-dioxin in rats. *Toxicol. Appl. Pharmacol.*, **1978**, *46*, 279–303.

Kolmodin, B.; Azarnoff, D. L.; and Sjoqvist, F. Effect of environmental factors on drug metabolism: decreased plasma half-life of antipyrine in workers exposed to chlorinated hydrocarbon insecticides. *Clin. Pharmacol. Ther.*, **1969**, *10*, 638–642.

Kreiss, K.; Zack, M.; Kimbrough, R. D.; Needham, L. L.; Smreak, A. L.; and Jones, B. T. Cross-study of a community with exceptional exposure to DDT. *J.A.M.A.*, **1981**, *245*, 1926–1930.

Krishna, G.; Pohl, L. R.; and Bhooshan, B. Mechanism of the metabolic activation of chloroform. *Toxicol. Appl. Pharmacol.*, **1978**, *45*, 238.

Kubic, V., and Anders, M. Metabolism of dihalomethanes to carbon monoxide. II. *In vitro* studies. *Drug Metab. Dispos.*, **1975**, *3*, 104–112.

Landrigan, P. J.; Powell, K. E.; James, L. M.; and Taylor, P. R. Paraquat and marijuana: epidemiological risk assessment. *Am. J. Public Health*, **1983**, *73*, 784–788.

Lee, P. W.; Arnau, T.; and Neal, R. A. Metabolism of α-naphthylthiourea by rat liver and rat lung microsomes. *Toxicol. Appl. Pharmacol.*, **1980**, *53*, 164–173.

Lindstrom, K. Behavioral effects of long-term exposure to organic solvents. *Acta Neurol. Scand.*, **1982**, *66*, 131–141.

Lisella, F. S.; Long, K. R.; and Scott, H. G. Toxicology of rodenticides and their relation to human health. *J. Environ. Health*, **1971**, *33*, 231–237, 361–365.

Longo, L. D. The biological effects of carbon monoxide on the pregnant woman, fetus, and newborn infant. *Am. J. Obstet. Gynecol.*, **1977**, *129*, 69–103.

McCarthy, T. B., and Jones, R. D. Industrial gassing poisonings due to trichlorethylene, perchlorethylene, and 1,1,1-trichloroethane, 1961–80. *Br. J. Ind. Med.*, **1983**, *40*, 450–455.

McMartin, K. E.; Hedström, K.-G.; Tolf, B.-R.; Östling-Wintzell, H.; and Blomstrand, R. Studies on the metabolic interactions between 4-methylpyrazole and methanol using the monkeys as an animal model. *Arch. Biochem. Biophys.*, **1980**, *199*, 606–614.

McMartin, K. E.; Martin-Amat, G.; Makar, A. B.; and Tephly, T. R. Methanol poisoning. V. Role of formate metabolism in the monkey. *J. Pharmacol. Exp. Ther.*, **1977**, *201*, 564–572.

Miller, D. S., and Kinter, W. B. Enzymatic basis for DDE-induced eggshell thinning in a sensitive bird. *Nature*, **1976**, *259*, 122–124.

Miller, R. R.; Ayres, J. A.; Young, J. T.; and McKenna, M. J. Ethylene glycol monoethyl ether. 1. Subchronic vapor inhalation study with rats and rabbits. *Fundam. Appl. Toxicol.*, **1983**, *3*, 49–54.

National Academy of Sciences. *Drinking Water and Health*. The Academy, Washington, D.C., **1977**, p. 939.

Neubert, D.; Zens, P.; Rothenwallner, A.; and Merker, H. J. A survey of the embryotoxic effects of TCDD in mammalian species. *Environ. Health Perspect.*, **1973**, *5*, 67–79.

Noker, P. E.; Eells, J. T.; and Tephly, T. R. Methanol toxicity: treatment with folic acid and 5-formyl tetrahydrofolic acid. *Alcohol. Clin. Exp. Res.*, **1980**, *4*, 378–383.

Nordman, H.; Keskinen, H.; and Tuppurainen, M. Formaldehyde asthma—rare or overlooked? *J. Allergy Clin. Immunol.*, **1985**, *75*, 91–99.

Ohkawa, H., and Casida, J. E. Glutathione S-transferases liberate hydrogen cyanide from organic thiocyanates. *Biochem. Pharmacol.*, **1971**, *20*, 1708–1711.

Orehek, J.; Massar, J. P.; Gayrard, P.; Grimaud, C.; and Charpin, J. Effect of short-term, low-level nitrogen dioxide exposure on bronchial sensitivity of asthmatic patients. *J. Clin. Invest.*, **1976**, *57*, 301–307.

Peterson, J. E., and Stewart, R. D. Absorption and elimination of carbon monoxide by inactive young men. *Arch. Environ. Health*, **1970**, *21*, 165–171.

Poland, A. P., and Glover, E. Comparison of 2,3,7,8-tetrachlorodibenzo-*p*-dioxin, a potent inducer of aryl hydrocarbon hydroxylase, with 3-methylcholanthrene. *Mol. Pharmacol.*, **1974**, *10*, 349–359.

Poland, A. P.; Smith, D.; Kuntzman, R.; Jacobson, M.; and Conney, A. H. Effect of extensive occupational exposure to DDT on phenylbutazone and cortisol metabolism in human beings. *Clin. Pharmacol. Ther.*, **1970**, *11*, 724–732.

Poland, A. P.; Smith, D.; Metter, G.; and Possiek, P. A health survey of workers in a 2,4-D and 2,4,5-T plant with special attention to chloracne, porphyria cutanea tarda and psychologic parameters. *Arch. Environ. Health*, **1971**, *22*, 759–768.

Powers, M. B.; Voelker, R. W.; Page, N. P.; Weisburger, E. K.; and Kraybill, H. F. Carcinogenicity of ethylene dibromide (EDB) and 1,2-dibromo-3 chloropropane (DBCP) after oral administration in rats and mice. *Toxicol. Appl. Pharmacol.*, **1975**, *33*, 171–172.

Radcliffe, D. A. Decrease in eggshell weight in certain birds of prey. *Nature*, **1967**, *215*, 208–210.

Rinsky, R. A.; Smith, A. B.; Hornung, R.; Filloon, T. G.; Young, R. J.; Okun, A. H.; and Landrigan, P. J. Benzene and leukemia: an epidemiologic risk assessment. *N. Engl. J. Med.*, **1987**, *316*, 1044–1050.

Rozman, K.; Rozman, T.; and Greim, H. Stimulation of nonbiliary, intestinal excretion of hexachlorobenzene in rhesus monkeys by mineral oil. *Toxicol. Appl. Pharmacol.*, **1983**, *70*, 255–261.

Rozman, T.; Ballhorn, L.; Rozman, K.; Klaassen, C.; and Greim, H. Effect of cholestyramine on the disposition of pentachlorophenol in rhesus monkeys. *J. Toxicol. Environ. Health*, **1982**, *10*, 277–283.

Saxena, M. C.; Siddiqui, M. K. J.; Bhargava, A. K.; Murti, C. R. K.; and Kutty, D. Placental transfer of pesticides in humans. *Arch. Toxicol.*, **1981**, *48*, 127–134.

Scala, R. A. Motor gasoline toxicity. *Fundam. Appl. Toxicol.*, **1988**, *10*, 553–562.

Schmid, R. Cutaneous porphyria in Turkey. *N. Engl. J. Med.*, **1960**, *263*, 397–398.

Selikoff, I. J., and Hammond, E. C. Asbestos and smoking. *J.A.M.A.*, **1979**, *242*, 458–459.

Seppäläinen, A. M. Neurophysiological findings among workers exposed to organic solvents. *Acta Neurol. Scand.*, **1982**, *66*, 109–116.

Shankland, D. L. Neurotoxic action of chlorinated hydrocarbon insecticides. *Neurobehav. Toxicol. Teratol.*, **1982**, *4*, 805–811.

Sheppard, D. A.; Saisho, A.; Nadel, J. A.; and Boushey, H. A. Exercise increases sulfur dioxide induced bronchoconstriction in asthmatic subjects. *Am. Rev. Respir. Dis.*, **1981**, *123*, 486–491.

Snyder, R.; Lee, E. W.; Kocsis, J. J.; and Witmer, C. M. Bone marrow depressant and leukemogenic actions of benzene. *Life Sci.*, **1977**, *21*, 1709–1722.

Striker, G. E.; Smuckler, E. A.; Kohnen, P. W.; and Nagle, R. B. Structural and functional changes in rat kidney during CCl_4 intoxication. *Am. J. Pathol.*, **1968**, *53*, 769–789.

Taylor, J. R.; Selhorst, J. B.; Houff, S. A.; and Martinez, A. J. Chlordecone intoxication in man. 1. Clinical observations. *Neurology (Minneap.)*, **1978**, *28*, 626–635.

Thomsen, H. K. Carbon monoxide–induced atherosclerosis in primates. An electron-microscopic study on the coronary arteries of *Macaca irus* monkeys. *Atherosclerosis*, **1974**, *20*, 233–240.

Turner, W. V.; Engel, J. L.; and Casida, J. E. Toxaphene components and related compounds: preparation and toxicity of some hepta-, octa-, and nonachlorobornanes, hexa-, and heptachlorobornenes and a hexachlorobornadiene. *J. Agric. Food Chem.*, **1977**, *25*, 1394–1401.

Van Miller, J. P.; Lalich, J. J.; and Allen, J. R. Increased incidence of neoplasms in rats exposed to low levels of 2,3,7,8-tetrachlorodibenzo-*o*-dioxin. *Chemosphere*, **1977**, *9*, 537–544.

Wang, H. H., and Grufferman, S. Aplastic anemia and occupational pesticide exposure: a case-control study. *J. Occup. Med.*, **1981**, *23*, 364–366.

Ware, F. H.; Thibodeau, L. A.; Speizer, F. E.; Colome, S.; and Ferris, B. G. Assessment of the health effects of atmospheric sulfur oxides and particulate matter: evidence from observational studies. *Environ. Health Perspect.*, **1981**, *41*, 255–276.

Waters, E. M.; Huff, J. E.; and Gerstner, H. B. Mirex, an overview. *Environ. Res.*, **1977**, *14*, 212–222.

Way, J. L.; End, E.; Sheehy, M. H.; DeMiranda, P.; Feitknecht, O. F.; Bachand, R.; Gibbson, S. L.; and Burrows, G. E. Effects of oxygen on cyanide intoxication. IV. Hyperbaric oxygen. *Toxicol. Appl. Pharmacol.*, **1972**, *22*, 415–421.

West, I. Lindane and hematologic reactions. *Arch. Environ. Health*, **1967**, *15*, 97–101.

Willhite, C. C., and Smith, R. P. The role of cyanide liberation on acute toxicity of aliphatic nitriles. *Toxicol. Appl. Pharmacol.*, **1981**, *59*, 589–602.

Monographs and Reviews

Aldridge, W. N. Toxicology of pyrethroids. In, *Pesticide Chemistry: Human Welfare and the Environment*, Vol. 3. (Miyamoto, J., and Kearney, P. C., eds.) Pergamon Press, Ltd., Oxford, **1983**, pp. 485–490.

Amdur, M. O. Air pollutants. In, *Casarett and Doull's Toxicology: The Basic Science of Poisons*, 3rd ed. (Klaassen, C. D.; Amdur, M. O.; and Doull, J.; eds.) Macmillan Publishing Co., New York, **1985**, pp. 801–824.

Andrews, L. S., and Snyder, R. Toxic effects of solvents and vapors. In, *Casarett and Doull's Toxicology: The Basic Science of Poisons*, 3rd ed. (Klaassen, C. D.; Amdur, M. O.; and Doull, J.; eds.) Macmillan Publishing Co., New York, **1985**, pp. 636–668.

Annau, Z. The neurobehavioral toxicity of trichloroethylene. *Neurobehav. Toxicol. Teratol.*, **1981**, *3*, 417–424.

Committee on Aldehydes. *Formaldehyde and Other Aldehydes*. National Academy Press, Washington, D.C., **1981**.

Couri, D., and Milks, M. Toxicity and metabolism of the neurotoxic hexacarbons *n*-hexane, 2-hexanone, and 2,5-hexadione. *Annu. Rev. Pharmacol. Toxicol.*, **1982**, *22*, 145–166.

Ervin, M. E. Petroleum distillates and turpentine. In, *Clinical Management of Poisoning and Drug Overdose*. (Haddad, L. M., and Winchester, J. F., eds.) W. B. Saunders Co., Philadelphia, **1983**, pp. 771–779.

Finck, P. A. Exposure to carbon monoxide: review of the literature and 567 autopsies. *Milit. Med.*, **1966**, *131*, 1513–1539.

Fisher, H. A. Occupational contact dermatitis from pesticides: patch testing procedures. *Cutis*, **1983**, *31*, 483–508.

Folinsbee, L. J. Effects of ozone exposure on lung function in man: a review. *Rev. Environ. Health*, **1983**, *3*, 211–240.

Gosselin, R. E.; Smith, R. P.; and Hodge, H. C. *Clinical Toxicology of Commercial Products*, 5th ed. The Williams & Wilkins Co., Baltimore, **1984**.

Graham, D. G.; Genter, M. B.; and Lowndes, H. E. n-Hexane. In, *Ethel Browning's Toxicity and Metabolism of Industrial Solvents*, 2nd ed., Vol. 1. (Snyder, R., ed.) Elsevier-North Holland, Inc., New York, **1987**, pp. 327–335.

Gutierrez, G. Carbon monoxide toxicity. In, *Air Pollution—Physiological Effects*. (McGrath, J. J., and Barnes, C. D., eds.) Academic Press, Inc., New York, **1982**, pp. 127–147.

Guzelian, P. S. Comparative toxicology of chlordecone (KEPONE) in humans and experimental animals. *Annu. Rev. Pharmacol. Toxicol.*, **1982**, *22*, 89–113.

Hayes, W. J., Jr. *Clinical Handbook on Economic Poisons*. Public Health Service Publication No. 476, U.S. Government Printing Office, Washington, D.C., **1963**.

———. *Pesticides Studied in Man*. The Williams & Wilkins Co., Baltimore, **1982**.

Holmstedt, B. Prolegomena to Seveso. *Arch. Toxicol.*, **1980**, *44*, 211–230.

IARC. *Monographs on the Evaluation of the Carcinogenic Risk of Chemicals to Man*. Vol. 5, *Some Organochlorine Pesticides*. International Agency for Research on Cancer, Lyon, France, **1974a**.

———. *Monographs on the Evaluation of the Carcinogenic Risk of Chemicals to Man*. Vol. 7, *Some Antithyroid and Related Substances, Nitrofurans and Industrial Chemicals*. International Agency for Research on Cancer, Lyon, France, **1974b**.

———. *Monographs on the Evaluation of Carcinogenic Risk of Chemicals to Man*. Vol. 12, *Some Carbamates, Thiocarbamates and Carbazides*. International Agency for Research on Cancer, Lyon, France, **1976**.

———. *Monographs on the Evaluation of the Carcinogenic Risk of Chemicals to Man*. Vol. 15, *Some Fumigants, the Herbicides 2,4-D and 2,4,5-T, Chlorinated Dibenzodioxins and Miscellaneous Industrial Chemicals*. International Agency for Research on Cancer, Lyon, France, **1977**.

Kalf, G. F.; Post, G. B.; and Snyder, R. Solvent toxicology: recent advances in the toxicology of benzene, the glycol ethers, and carbon tetrachloride. *Annu. Rev. Pharmacol. Toxicol.*, **1987**, *27*, 399–427.

Kaplan, S. D., and Morgan, R. W. Airborne carcinogens and human cancer. *Rev. Environ. Health*, **1981**, *3*, 329–368.

Kerns, W. D.; Donofrio, D. J.; and Pavkov, K. L. The chronic effects of formaldehyde inhalation in rats and mice: a preliminary report. In, *Formaldehyde Toxicity*. (Gibson, J. E., ed.) Hemisphere Publishing Corp., Washington, D.C., **1983**, pp. 111–131.

Khan, N. Y. An assessment of the hazard of synthetic pyrethroid insecticides to fish and fish habitat. In, *Pesticide Chemistry: Human Welfare and the Environment*, Vol. 3. (Miyamoto, J., and Kearney, P. C., eds.) Pergamon Press, Ltd., Oxford, **1983**, pp. 115–121.

Kupfer, D., and Bulger, W. H. Estrogenic actions of chlorinated hydrocarbons. In, *Effects of Chronic Exposures to Pesticides on Animal Systems*. (Chambers, J. E., and Yarbrough, J. D., eds.) Raven Press, New York, **1982**, pp. 121–146.

Lundholm, E. Thinning of eggshells in birds by DDE: mode of action on the eggshell gland. *Comp. Biochem. Physiol.* [*C*], **1987**, *88*, 1–22.

Maibach, H. Formaldehyde: effects on animal and human skin. In, *Formaldehyde Toxicity*. (Gibson, J. E., ed.) Hemisphere Publishing Corp., Washington, D.C., **1983**, pp. 166–174.

Matsumura, F., and Ghiasuddin, S. M. DDT-sensitive Ca-ATPase in the axonic membrane. In, *Neurotoxicology of Insecticides and Pheromones*. (Narahashi, T., ed.) Plenum Press, New York, **1979**, pp. 245–257.

Mehendale, H. M. Modification of hepatobiliary function by toxic chemicals. *Fed. Proc.*, **1979**, *38*, 2240–2245.

Menzel, D. B. Toxicity of ozone, oxygen, and radiation. *Annu. Rev. Pharmacol.*, **1970**, *10*, 379–394.

———. Ozone: an overview of its toxicity in man and animals. *J. Toxicol. Environ. Health*, **1984**, *13*, 183–204.

Menzer, R. E., and Nelson, J. O. Water and soil pollutants. In, *Casarett and Doull's Toxicology: The Basic Science of Poisons*, 3rd ed. (Klaassen, C. D.; Amdur, M. O.; and Doull, J.; eds.) Macmillan Publishing Co., New York, **1985**, pp. 825–856.

Murphy, S. D. Toxic effects of pesticides. In, *Casarett*

and Doull's Toxicology: The Basic Science of Poisons, 3rd ed. (Klaassen, C. D.; Amdur, M. O.; and Doull, J.; eds.) Macmillan Publishing Co., Inc., New York, **1985**, pp. 519–581.

Narahashi, T. Nerve membrane ionic channels as the target of insecticides. In, *Neurotoxicology of Insecticides and Pheromones*. (Narahashi, T., ed.) Plenum Press, New York, **1979**, pp. 211–243.

———. Interaction of pyrethroids and DDT-like compounds with the sodium channels in the nerve membrane. In, *Pesticide Chemistry: Human Welfare and the Environment*, Vol. 3. (Miyamoto, J., and Kearney, P. C., eds.) Pergamon Press, Ltd., Oxford, **1983**, pp. 109–114.

National Research Council. Committee on Medical and Biologic Effects of Environmental Pollutants. *Carbon Monoxide*. National Academy of Sciences, Washington, D.C., **1977**.

Plaa, G. L. Toxic responses of the liver. In, *Casarett and Doull's Toxicology: The Basic Science of Poisons*, 3rd ed. (Klaassen, C. D.; Amdur, M. O.; and Doull, J.; eds.) Macmillan Publishing Co., New York, **1985**, pp. 286–309.

Recknagel, R. O., and Glende, E. H., Jr. Carbon tetrachloride hepatotoxicity: an example of lethal cleavage. *CRC Crit. Rev. Toxicol.*, **1973**, *2*, 263–297.

Sayers, P. R., and Davenport, S. J. *Review of Carbon Monoxide Poisoning*. Public Health Bulletin No. 195, U.S. Government Printing Office, Washington, D.C., **1930**.

Slater, T. F. Free radicals as reactive intermediates in tissue injury. In, *Biological Reactive Intermediates II: Chemical Mechanisms and Biological Effects*. (Snyder, R.; Parke, D. V.; Kocsis, J. J.; Jollow, D. J.; Gibson, G. G.; and Witmer, C. M.; eds.) Plenum Press, New York, **1982**, pp. 575–589.

Smith, L. L. The toxicity of paraquat. *Adverse Drug React. Acute Poisoning Rev.*, **1988**, *7*, 1–17.

Speizer, F. E. Environmental lung diseases. In, *Harrison's Principles of Internal Medicine*, 10th ed. (Petersdorf, R. G.; Adams, R. D.; Braunwald, E.; Isselbacher, K. J.; Martin, J. B.; and Wilson, J.; eds.) McGraw-Hill Book Co., New York, **1983**, pp. 1524–1532.

Stewart, R. D. The effects of carbon monoxide on humans. *Annu. Rev. Pharmacol.*, **1975**, *15*, 409–423.

Tephly, T.; Watkins, W. D.; and Goodman, J. I. The biochemical toxicology of methanol. In, *Essays in Toxicology*, Vol. 5. (Hayes, W. J., Jr., ed.) Academic Press, Inc., New York, **1974**, pp. 149–177.

Tephly, T. R.; Makar, A. B.; McMartin, K. E.; Hayreh, S. S.; and Martin-Amat, G. Methanol: its metabolism and toxicity. In, *Biochemistry and Pharmacology of Ethanol*, Vol. 1. (Majchrowicz, E., and Noble, E. P., eds.) Plenum Press, New York, **1979**, pp. 145–164.

Tintinalli, J. E.; Rominger, M.; and Kittleson, K. Carbon monoxide. In, *Clinical Management of Poisoning and Drug Overdose*. (Haddad, L. M., and Winchester, J. F., eds.) W. B. Saunders Co., Philadelphia, **1983**, pp. 748–753.

U.A.R.E.P. (Universities Associated for Research and Education in Pathology, Inc.) Epidemiology of chronic occupational exposure to formaldehyde: report of the ad hoc panel on health aspects of formaldehyde. *Toxicol. Ind. Health*, **1988**, *4*, 77–90.

USEPA. (United States Environmental Protection Agency Office of Drinking Water Health Advisories.) *Rev. Environ. Contam. Toxicol.*, **1988a**, *104*, 1–225.

———. (United States Environmental Protection Agency Office of Drinking Water Health Advisories.) *Rev. Environ. Contam. Toxicol.*, **1988b**, *106*, 1–221.

Von Oettingen, W. F. *The Halogenated Hydrocarbons of Industrial and Toxicological Significance*. Elsevier Publishing Co., New York, **1964**.

Way, J. L. Cyanide intoxication and its mechanism of antagonism. *Annu. Rev. Pharmacol. Toxicol.*, **1984**, *24*, 451–481.

Weger, N. P. Treatment of cyanide poisoning with 4-dimethylaminophenol (DMAP)-experimental and clinical overview. *Fundam. Appl. Toxicol.*, **1983**, *3*, 387–396.

Williams, G. M., and Weisburger, J. H. Chemical carcinogens. In, *Casarett and Doull's Toxicology: The Basic Science of Poisons*, 3rd ed. (Klaassen, C. D.; Amdur, M. O.; and Doull, J.; eds.) Macmillan Publishing Co., New York, **1985**, pp. 99–173.

Woodbury, M. A., and Zenz, C. Formaldehyde in the home environment: prenatal and infant exposures. In, *Formaldehyde Toxicity*. (Gibson, J. E., ed.) Hemisphere Publishing Corp., Washington, D.C., **1983**, pp. 203–211.

World Health Organization. *1974 Evaluations of Some Pesticide Residue in Food*. World Health Organization Pesticide Residue Series, No. 4, Geneva, Switzerland, **1975**, pp. 261–263.

Zimmerman, H. J. *Hepatotoxicity: The Adverse Effects of Drugs and Other Chemicals on the Liver*. Appleton-Century-Crofts, New York, **1978**.

APPENDIX

I PRINCIPLES OF PRESCRIPTION ORDER WRITING AND PATIENT COMPLIANCE INSTRUCTIONS

Leslie Z. Benet

The prescription order is an important therapeutic transaction between physician and patient. It brings into focus the diagnostic acumen and therapeutic proficiency of the physician with instructions for palliation or restoration of the patient's health. The most carefully conceived prescription order may become therapeutically useless, however, unless it communicates clearly with the pharmacist and adequately instructs the patient on how to take the prescribed medication.

PRESCRIPTION ORDER WRITING

The practice of writing complex prescription orders containing many active ingredients, adjuvants, correctives, and elegant vehicles has been abandoned in favor of single drugs and mixtures of drugs compounded by pharmaceutical companies. Even when two or more active ingredients are desired for oral administration, it is often preferable and rational to prescribe each separately so that the physician may adjust the dose of each ingredient to the individual requirements of the patient. A recent audit of prescriptions reveals that 99% of all orders in the United States are for precompounded drugs. Only 1% (but still 140 million per year) requires compounding. The availability of precompounded drugs is desirable in the great majority of instances, but simplicity has its drawbacks. Many physicians rely upon fixed-dose combinations rather than adjust the doses of the agents to the particular needs of the patient. For example, the prescription audit referred to above shows that 55 of the 200 most frequently prescribed drugs are combination products.

Proficiency at writing a prescription order accurately and speedily requires practice. The prescription order should be written legibly. It is convenient and the accepted form to have one's name, address, telephone number, office hours, and Drug Enforcement Administration (DEA) registry number printed on the prescription order blank. Because prescription orders are medicolegal documents, they should be written in ink; this practice is compulsory for controlled substances in schedule II. It is also an excellent custom, too infrequently followed, for the doctor to keep a copy for the files. This protects the physician and serves to complete the record of treatment.

Choice of Drug Name. Most drugs can be prescribed by their official names (*United States Pharmacopeia;* USP), by their nonproprietary names (United States Adopted Names; USAN), or by the manufacturers' proprietary (brand) names. The nonproprietary name is often referred to as the generic name (*see* Chapter 4).

There is much discussion concerning the relative advantages of prescribing by nonproprietary versus proprietary name. Arguments in favor of the use of nonproprietary names are based, for the most part, on the elimination of duplication of drug products and the possibility of an economic benefit to the patient. Arguments against such practice usually include concerns about the quality of generic drugs and the possibility of therapeutic inequivalence when patients are switched from one product (proprietary or not) to another (*see* Chapters 1 and 4); in addition, many nonproprietary names are difficult to remember and spell. Virtually all states have adopted laws that allow the pharmacist to substitute the product of one company for the same formulation from a different manufacturer under specified circumstances. Such laws also speak to mechanisms whereby the clinician can facilitate or prevent such substitution. Clinicians and pharmacists must be familiar with the laws of their own state. The United States Food and Drug Administration (FDA) has prepared a monograph that identifies currently marketed prescription drug products and that contains evaluations of therapeutic equivalence for the multisource approved drug products (Food and Drug Administration, 1988). Ideally, this information should minimize the uncertainty associated with prescribing and dispensing generic drugs. In general, as discussed in Chapters 1 and 4, documented cases of nonequivalence in terms of the bioavailability of approved drug products are now very uncommon. However, certain patients do exhibit changes in response when they are switched from one manufacturer's product to another. Such changes may be due in part to placebo effects. However, they may also be observed in individual patients who are taking drugs with low therapeutic indices, where a small change in drug concentration can lead to dramatic undesirable effects (*e.g.*, drugs for epilepsy). In these cases the physician can prevent substitution by writing "dispense as written" on the prescription order or by verbal communication to the pharmacist that only the product requested is to be dispensed.

Nonproprietary or generic names are now selected by the United States Adopted Name (USAN) Council. The USAN Council is sponsored jointly by the American Medical Association, the United States Pharmacopeial Convention, Inc., and the American Pharmaceutical Association. The Council includes a liaison representative of the United States Food and Drug Administration.

In writing prescription orders it is best to use the nonproprietary name followed by the name of the manufacturer in parentheses if a specific manufacturer's product has distinct advantages or if the physician wishes to prevent a change of product on subsequent refills. This not only eliminates the necessity for memorizing multiple drug names but also assures the physician that the product of a particular manufacturer will be dispensed.

Choice of a System of Weights and Measures. Prescription orders should always be written in the metric system. It is necessary only to designate amounts of drug by numbers and to indicate the metric unit of weight or volume desired.

Apothecaries' System. Since doses in older publications may appear in units of the apothecaries' system, metric and apothecaries' equivalents are presented in Table A–I–1.

Household Measures. Unfortunately, the drugs prescribed so carefully by the physician in milligrams and milliliters are usually measured by the patient with convenient kitchen utensils. The "drop," which varies in size, presents a special problem. Its size depends on the particular fluid being dropped—its specific gravity, temperature, and viscosity—as well as on the orifice of the dropper and the angle at which the dropper is held. When accuracy of dosage is important, a dropper that has been calibrated especially for the preparation with which it is supplied should be used; this is the case for most commercial products. The size of the household teaspoon also varies considerably. For household purposes, an American Standard Teaspoon has been established by the American National Standards Institute, containing 4.93 ± 0.24 ml. The USP specifies that this teaspoon may be regarded as containing 5 ml. A tablespoon is said to contain 15 ml.

Other devices, such as molded plastic cylinders and measuring caps, have been developed for measuring and administering liquid medications. A novel oral syringe may be used to measure and administer drugs to children; these syringes are available in a variety of sizes to assure accurate administration of drugs. Such devices have been strongly recommended by the Committee on Drugs, American Academy of Pediatrics (1975), to replace the usual household utensils.

Table A–I–1. METRIC AND APOTHECARIES' EQUIVALENTS

1 milligram	=	1/65	grain
1 gram	=	15.43	grains
1 kilogram	=	2.20	pounds
1 milliliter	=	16.23	minims
1 grain	=	0.065	gram
1 ounce	=	31.1	grams
1 minim	=	0.062	ml
1 fluid ounce	=	29.57	ml
1 pint	=	473.2	ml
1 quart	=	946.4	ml

Construction of the Prescription Order. Traditionally, a prescription order follows a definite pattern that facilitates its interpretation. This pattern is essentially the same whether the prescription order is for a single drug or a mixture of two or more drugs. Only one prescription should be written on an order blank. The major elements of a model order are illustrated in example No. 1. The numbers at the left call attention to the several parts of a prescription order, which are explained below.

1. *Date.* The date when the prescription order is written is important. Federal law requires that prescription orders for drugs listed in schedules II, III, and IV of the Controlled Substances Act of 1970 be dated; orders for substances in schedules III and IV cannot be filled or refilled more than 6 months after date of issuance.

2. *Name, Address, and Age of the Patient.* These are necessary in order to expedite the handling of the prescription order and to avoid possible confusion with medications intended for someone else. Moreover, the pharmacist should verify the patient's name and age; otherwise it is impossible to monitor the prescribed dose. The pharmacist should place the name of the patient on the bottle or container exactly as the doctor has written it. Prescription orders for schedule-II drugs are required to contain the full name and address of the patient.

3. The symbol ℞ (not "Rx") is an abbreviation for *recipe*, the Latin for "take thou."

(No. 1)

1. July 3, 1990
2. Dee Fleming, Age 6
817 Woodhaven Dr.
Dallas, TX 75248
3. ℞
4. Ampicillin Oral Suspension 250 mg/5 ml
5. Dispense 200 ml (with oral syringe).
6. Label: Take 5 ml orally at 8 A.M., 12 noon, 4 P.M., and 8 P.M. daily for 10 days for infection.
Ampicillin 250 mg/5 ml. 200 ml.
7. Do not refill.
8. Jane P. Rall, M.D.
DEA No. AB1234321
1407 Colgate
Dallas, TX 75248

4. *Drug, Strength, and Inert Additives.* The body of the prescription order contains the name and strength (dose) of the desired drug. Drugs are prescribed in the United States by official English names. Abbreviations should be avoided since their use frequently results in error. When two or more drugs are desired in the same prescription order, the name and amount of each drug are placed together on a line directly under the preceding one. If the formulation has more than one ingredient, the principal drug (which gives the prescription its chief action) goes first and the vehicle, the solvent for a solution, or the bulking agent for a capsule goes last.

5. *Directions to the Pharmacist.* In prescription orders for a single drug this usually consists of "Dispense 10 tablets," "Dispense 200 ml," "Dispense with oral syringe," and so forth; in the case of prescription orders for two or more drugs it is usually either a short sentence such as "Make a solution," or "Mix and place into 10 capsules," or a word such as "Mix."

6. *Directions to the Patient.* The directions to the patient should always be written in English. The use of Latin abbreviations serves no useful purpose. The directions to the patient contain instructions as to the amount of drug to be taken, the time and frequency of the dose, and other factors such as dilution and route of administration. If a device is involved in the administration of the medication, the physician and/or pharmacist should either demonstrate how it is used or review the instructions with the patient. If the drug is to be used externally only, or to be shaken well before using, or if it is a poison, such facts are included.

Expressions such as "take as directed" and "take as necessary" are never satisfactory and should be avoided. If the drug is to be taken at a specific time of day or if it is to be taken three or four times a day, the exact time or times should be specified on the label; patients are often confused by directions such as "every 8 hours." However, if it is therapeutically important to take the drug at an 8-hour interval, this should be emphasized and explained to the patient. The physician should be particularly sensitive to the needs of aged, ill, and handicapped patients, as well as those with language difficulties. The directions for these individuals should also be written in greater detail on a separate instruction sheet and left with the patient. To avoid possible error, the first word of the directions to the patient should serve as a reminder of the correct route of administration. Thus, the directions for a preparation for internal use should start with the word *take;* for an ointment or lotion, the word *apply;* for suppositories, the word *insert;* and for drops to be placed in the conjunctival sac, external auditory canal, or nostril, the word *place*. The directions to the patient should also be employed as a reminder of the intended purpose of the prescription, by including such phrases as "for relief of pain," "for relief of headache," or "to relieve itching." However, directions that would be embarrassing to the patient if placed on the prescription order or label should be given in private.

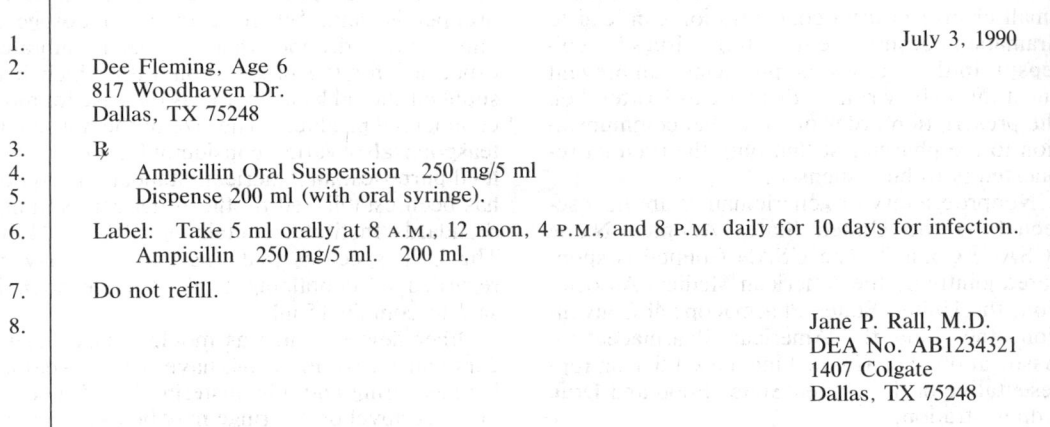

There are many cogent reasons why the prescription medication and the quantity dispensed should be identified on the label. For example, the rapid identification of a drug and a quick estimate of the amount consumed can help with the initiation of appropriate therapy in the case of adverse drug reactions, or accidental or deliberate overdosage. Therefore, many states require that the name, strength, and quantity of drug dispensed be indicated on the label. When appropriate, the pharmacist should also indicate the expiration date and special storage instructions on the prescription label.

The pharmacist always should be on the alert to detect overdoses of potent drugs in the prescriptions he dispenses. This serves as an added check for the safety of the patient. If it is desirable to administer a drug in a larger amount than is customarily employed, it is best for the prescriber to underline the dose, and to write "correct amount" or "correct dose" and his or her initials at the side.

7. *Refill Information.* Under the Durham–Humphrey Amendment to the Federal Food, Drug, and Cosmetic Act (*see* page 1646), prescription orders for drugs that bear the caution legend, "Federal law prohibits dispensing without prescription," may not be refilled without the consent of the prescriber. Under the Drug Abuse Control Amendments to the above act (*see* page 1646), prescription orders for schedule-III and schedule-IV drugs cannot be refilled more than five times and the prescription order is invalid 6 months from the date of issue. These restrictions are intended to control the overuse and abuse of prescription medications. For these reasons, the physician should indicate his wishes with respect to refills on each original prescription order, irrespective of whether it is for a controlled substance. This may be indicated by instruction to refill a certain number of times or not to refill. Statements such as "Refill prn" and "Refill ad lib" are never appropriate. Such information need not be written on narcotic prescription orders for schedule-II substances, since by law these cannot be refilled.

8. *Signature.* The prescription order is completed by the practitioner signing the bottom of the blank, with the appropriate professional degree following it. Federal law requires that the physician's address and DEA registry number also appear on every prescription order for controlled drugs and that such an order be signed (last name in full) with ink.

Classes of Prescription Orders. On the basis of the availability of the prescribed medication, prescription orders may be divided into two classes: precompounded and extemporaneous. A *precompounded* prescription order is one that calls for a drug or mixture of drugs supplied by the pharmaceutical company by its official or proprietary name and in a form that the pharmacist dispenses without pharmaceutical alteration. An *extemporaneous* prescription order, also called *compounded,* is the type in which the physician selects the drugs, doses, and pharmaceutical form desired and the pharmacist prepares the medication. Examples of prescription orders for precompounded and extemporaneous preparations are given below and will serve to illustrate the principles of prescription order writing.

Examples of Prescription Orders for Precompounded Preparations. When writing a prescription order for a precompounded preparation, it is necessary to know the name of the preparation desired, the pharmaceutical form in which it is available (*i.e.*, ointment, tablet, *etc.*), the single dose, the route and frequency of administration, and the approximate number of days of therapy. Suppose one wishes to renew a prescription order for a 3-month supply of digoxin for an adult with congestive heart failure, who is well stabilized and has been thoroughly instructed regarding compliance. Since digoxin is marketed by several manufacturers, it is good practice to prescribe the drug by its USAN, but to indicate a manufacturer's product that will ensure adequate, dependable bioavailability, as shown below.

(No. 2)

Digoxin Tablets
(Burroughs Wellcome Co.) 0.25 mg

Dispense 100 tablets.

Label: Take 1 tablet at 9:00 A.M. each morning.
Digoxin, 0.25 mg. 100 tablets.

Precompounded prescription orders for orally administered liquid preparations are constructed in a similar manner. It is necessary, however, to know the concentration of the active ingredient(s) in the preparation. Suppose one desires to prescribe ampicillin suspension (250 mg/5 ml) for a child with otitis media in a dose of 250 mg to be given four times daily. A prescription order providing 7 days of medication may be written as follows:

(No. 3)

Ampicillin suspension, 250 mg/5 ml

Dispense 150 ml.

Label: Give one teaspoonful at 7 A.M.,
12 noon, 5 P.M., and 10 P.M.
for 7 days.

Ampicillin suspension, 250 mg/5 ml. 150 ml

Do not refill.

Prescription orders for orally administered precompounded remedies, such as solutions, syrups, suspensions, and tinctures, are written as illustrated in the previous example, as are those for preparations that are intended for local application. If special instructions to the pharmacist are necessary, these may be indicated. For example, physicians should remember that the 1970 Poison Prevention Packaging Act was extended in 1974 to require child-resistant containers for all oral prescriptions, although several exceptions are permitted (*e.g.*, oral contraceptives). Many patients have difficulty in using the special containers. In such cases the prescriber or patient may request the use of a conventional container.

Examples of Prescription Orders for Extemporaneous Preparations. In writing prescription orders for an extemporaneous preparation for oral administration, it is of course necessary to know the single dose of each ingredient, the number of doses to be taken each day, and the number of days of medication. This knowledge allows the calculation of the total dosage of each ingredient in the prescription. Suppose it is desired to prescribe an antitussive–expectorant mixture to be taken orally every 4 hours. This means that at least four doses will be taken daily. If teaspoonful doses (5 ml) are used and enough medicine is dispensed to last 6 days, 24 doses, or a 120-ml total volume, will be needed. The total amounts of codeine phosphate (antitussive) and ammonium chloride (expectorant) are calculated as the per-dose amounts (10 mg codeine phosphate and 0.3 g ammonium chloride) multiplied by 24, with the addition of sufficient volume of the vehicle (aromatic elixir) to make 120 ml.

(No. 4)

Codeine Phosphate	0.24 g
Ammonium Chloride	7.2 g
Aromatic Elixir, to make 120 ml	

Extemporaneous prescription orders for other liquid preparations for oral or local administration are constructed similarly.

The principles of calculation of dosage illustrated above apply also to prescription orders for dry forms of medication to be taken internally. Since pharmacists are not equipped to compound compressed tablets, dry forms of medication are commonly prescribed in capsules. Whereas it is fairly easy to ingest liquid medicines, it may be difficult to swallow capsules that are too large. Therefore, capsules are limited to approximately 0.5 g in bulk (for adults) for most medicines. If a larger amount is required for the single dose, then the drug must be divided into 2 or more capsules for each dose. If the ingredients make too small a bulk to be dispensed conveniently in solid form, an inert powder may be added. There are many such powders and excipients (*e.g.*, lactose), and the pharmacist often selects and adds them at his own discretion.

Suppose it is desired to prescribe in capsule form an analgesic mixture containing aspirin (300 mg), acetaminophen (300 mg), and amobarbital (50 mg) for a patient with painful myositis. The medicine is to be taken every 4 hours during waking hours (*i.e.*, four doses per day) and enough is to be prescribed to last 5 days, *i.e.*, 20 doses. The prescription order is as follows:

(No. 5)

July 9, 1990

Theodore Apse, Age 44
601 King Street
Charlottesville, VA 22901

Aspirin	6.0 g
Acetaminophen	6.0 g
Amobarbital	1.0 g

Mix and divide into 40 capsules.

Label: Take 2 capsules at 8:00 A.M., 12 noon, 4:00 P.M., and 8:00 P.M. for muscle pain. Aspirin 300 mg, Acetaminophen 300 mg, and Amobarbital 50 mg. 40 capsules.

Do not refill.

Prescription orders for medicines to be taken internally may also be written by the single-dose method. The pharmacist is then instructed to prepare a given number of doses. For example, prescription order No. 5, if written by the single-dose method, would appear as follows:

(No. 6)

Aspirin	300 mg
Acetaminophen	300 mg
Amobarbital	50 mg

Make 20 such doses and place in 40 capsules.

Label: *etc.*

Most compounded ointments today are prescribed by dermatologists who have found particular ingredients to be effective for specialized conditions. Prescription No. 7 (below) prescribed for rosacea contains hydrocortisone as the primary active ingredient; precipitated sulfur, a keratolytic; and coal tar solution, which is often used in the treatment of chronic skin diseases. These ingredients are contained in a commercial ointment base that is described as restoring and maintaining the protective acidity of the skin.

The therapeutic efficacy of an ointment is achieved only if the active ingredients are incorporated into the proper ointment base. The ideal ointment base should be compatible with the skin, stable, permanent, smooth and pliable, nonirritating, nonsensitizing, and inert, and should readily release incorporated medication. Four classes of ointment bases are recognized: absorption, emulsion, oleaginous, and water soluble. Unless the physician becomes familiar with the physical properties of the various bases, the help of a pharmacist should be sought in the selection of an appropriate base. As in prescription order No. 7, the ingredients of an ointment are expressed on a weight/weight percentage basis.

(No. 7)

Hydrocortisone Acetate	1%
Precipitated Sulfur	2%
Coal Tar Solution	3%
Acid Mantle Creme amount to make 60 g	

Make an ointment.

Label: Apply a thin film to affected areas on face night and morning.

1% Hydrocortisone Ointment, 60 g.

A prescription order for a lotion for external use on the skin is similar in construction to that for an ointment in that only the percentages of the ingredients and not absolute doses need be ordered.

Prescription orders for many liquid preparations for local administration, such as ophthalmic solutions, nasal sprays, inhalants, gargles, and douches, are constructed similarly to those cited above. Aqueous solutions prepared for use in the eye are less irritating if they are adjusted to isotonicity with the lacrimal fluid. If it is desired to prescribe an isotonic ophthalmic solution, this fact can be indicated by inserting the phrase, "Sodium chloride, to make isotonic." Solutions to be used in the nose can also be used with much greater comfort if made approximately isotonic.

Dosage. Instructions about dosage are an extremely important part of prescription order writing. The number of days for which medication is contemplated, the number of doses per day, and the size of each dose determine the bulk of the prescription. The total quantity of prescribed medication has no minimal limit, and as little as a single dose may be ordered. On the other hand, a maximal limit is indicated for most prescriptions, even when medication is to continue for an indefinite period; this limit is influenced by the stability and cost of the drug and the possible necessity for alteration of the treatment. A major factor that should be a determinant of the quantity of the drug dispensed is the mental state of the patient and the potential toxicity of the drug. *If a patient is depressed or potentially suicidal, do not prescribe total quantities of drug that would prove lethal if taken all at one time.* In the absence of such problems, a convenient rule of thumb is to prescribe only enough medication for 7 to 14 days unless the patient will be taking the drug for an extended period of time. Storage of unused portions of a prescription and sharing of prescriptions with others who were not intended to receive them should be explicitly discussed with any patient who receives an important prescription. Blackwell (1972) reported that 9 of 75 patients used drugs that were prescribed for other individuals.

Size and Form of Medication. The upper limit for adults of the weight of a single capsule or tablet is usually about 0.5 g. However, this arbitrary limit based on what the patient can comfortably swallow may be exceeded when the drug product is dense. Conversely, even a smaller unit dosage may be indicated for light, bulky medication or for certain patients, especially the very young or old.

Many drugs are commercially available only in a limited variety of dose forms (*e.g.*, only capsules of a single weight). For obvious reasons of convenience and economy, these "standard" forms of medication should be preferred, except under unusual circumstances. Until knowledge of the dosage forms available for the various drugs is acquired through experience, the physician is well advised to rely upon the pharmacist for this information. Other useful sources of information include the sections on preparations in this textbook; *Facts and Comparisons; Drug Evaluations,* a publication of the American Medical Association; *Drug Information for the Health Care Professional* (*USP–DI*); *American Hospital Formulary Service Drug Information,* published by the American Society of Hospital Pharmacists; and the *Physicians' Desk Reference* (*PDR*).

Usual Doses. The physician should consult the above-mentioned references (especially the *USP–DI* or *Facts and Comparisons*) or the package insert for guidance on the recommended *Usual Adult Doses* and *Usual Pediatric Doses.* These represent the doses that should produce the recognized therapeutic effects in adults and children following oral administration unless otherwise specified. The *Usual Dose* is intended to serve only as a guide to the physician, who very frequently must give more or less than what is usual in order to optimize therapy. Some of the above references also give the *Usual Adult Prescribing Limits,* intended primarily to guide the pharmacist with respect to confirmation of prescription orders calling for unusually large dosages.

Prescription Refills. Prescription drugs were formerly controlled by several federal laws, including the Federal Food, Drug, and Cosmetic Act; the Federal Narcotic–Internal Revenue Regulations (historically known as the Harrison Narcotic Act); and the Federal Marihuana Regulations. On May 1, 1971, the Comprehensive

Drug Abuse Prevention and Control Act of 1970 became fully effective and, except for the Durham–Humphrey Amendment (Section 503B), repealed all the aforementioned laws controlling prescription drugs.

The Durham–Humphrey Amendment defines certain types of drugs that may be sold by the pharmacist only on the prescription order of a practitioner licensed by law to administer such drugs. These drugs are required to bear the label, *"Caution: Federal law prohibits dispensing without a prescription."* Under the Durham–Humphrey Amendment, a prescription order cannot be refilled unless authorized by the prescriber. The prescriber may indicate the number of times a prescription order may be refilled in the blank space in the statement, "Refill ________ times"; this statement may be printed on the prescription order blank.

The Comprehensive Drug Abuse Prevention and Control Act, commonly referred to as the Controlled Substances Act (*see* below), is designed to control the distribution of all depressant and stimulant drugs (*e.g.*, opioids, barbiturates, and amphetamines) and other drugs with abuse potential as designated by the Drug Enforcement Administration, Department of Justice. This act requires the pharmacist to keep a record of the receipt and the disposition of all controlled substances. The records must be maintained for a period of at least 2 years and be available for inspection by authorized persons. Prescription orders for controlled substances in schedule II must be typewritten or written in ink and signed by the practitioner; such prescription orders cannot be refilled. The physician must write a new prescription if administration of the drug is to be continued. Prescription orders for drugs covered by schedule III or IV may be issued either orally or in writing by a practitioner and may be refilled, if so authorized, not more than five times and may not be filled or refilled more than 6 months after date of issue. After five refills or after 6 months, the prescribing practitioner may write or authorize a new prescription order. Drugs in schedule V may be prescribed the same as drugs in schedules III and IV, and, under certain conditions, may be dispensed without a prescription.

Physicians should do all they can to prevent abuses of prescription orders. It is a good practice to write out the number of refills desired during a specific time period on every prescription order; Arabic numerals may easily be altered and, if not indicated, instructions may easily be forged. Furthermore, when an authorization for refill is not given on the prescription order, it cannot be refilled without personal authorization by the prescriber.

Controlled Substances Act. Various federal, state, and city laws exist to control the standard of purity of drugs and their manufacture, sale, and dispensing. These laws must be known and observed by the practitioner. The most stringent law takes precedence, whether it be federal, state, or local. The most important laws are embodied in the Controlled Substances Act (Title II of the Comprehensive Drug Abuse Prevention and Control Act of 1970) and the amendments of 1984. Selected portions of the regulations of most concern to practitioners and students may be found in the *United States Pharmacopeia XXII National Formulary XVII* (1990). This act divides opioids and other drugs into five schedules.

Schedule I. Drugs in this schedule have a high potential for abuse and *no* currently accepted medical use in the United States. Such drugs include 55 opiates (*e.g.*, levomoramide); 23 opium derivatives (*e.g.*, codeine methylbromide and heroin); 17 hallucinogenic substances (*e.g.*, lysergic acid diethylamide, marihuana, mescaline, peyote, psilocybin); 4 depressants and stimulants (*e.g.*, methaqualone and N-ethylamphetamine); and a temporary list of substances subject to emergency listing. Substances listed in this schedule are not for prescription use but may be obtained for research and instructional use or for chemical analysis by application to the Drug Enforcement Administration, Department of Justice (Form 225), supported by a protocol of the proposed use.

Schedule II. Drugs in this schedule have a high potential for abuse with severe liability to cause psychic or physical dependence. Schedule-II controlled substances consist of certain opioid drugs and drugs containing amphetamines or methamphetamines as the single active ingredient or in combination with each other. Examples of substances included in this schedule are opium, morphine, codeine, hydromorphone, methadone, meperidine, cocaine, oxycodone, oxymorphone, dextroamphetamine, and methamphetamine. Also included in schedule II are phenmetrazine, methylphenidate, amobarbital, pentobarbital, secobarbital, etorphine hydrochloride, and diphenoxylate.

Schedule III. The drugs in this schedule have a potential for abuse that is less than for those in schedules I and II; their abuse may lead to moderate or low physical dependence or high psychological dependence. This schedule includes compounds containing limited quantities of certain opioid drugs and also certain nonopioid drugs, such as chlorhexadol, glutethimide, methyprylon, sulfondiethylmethane, sulfonmethane, nalorphine, benzphetamine, chlorphentermine, clortermine, phendimetrazine, and certain barbiturates (except those listed in another schedule).

Schedule IV. The drugs in this schedule have a low potential for abuse that leads only to limited physical dependence or psychological dependence relative to drugs in schedule III. In this schedule are barbital, phenobarbital, methylphenobarbital, chloral hydrate, ethchlorvynol, ethinamate, meprobamate, paraldehyde, methohexital, fenfluramine, diethylpropion, phentermine, approximately 35 benzodiazepines, and propoxyphene.

Schedule V. The drugs in this schedule have a potential for abuse that is less than those listed in schedule IV. Drugs in this schedule consist of preparations containing moderate quantities of certain opioid drugs, generally for antitussive or antidiarrheal purposes, which may be distributed without a prescription order. Substances in this schedule may also be prescribed as are those in schedules III and IV. In addition, drugs in schedule V may be dispensed without a prescription order provided (1) such distribution is made only by a pharmacist; (2) not more than 240 ml of any schedule-V substance containing opium, nor more than 120 ml or more than 24 solid dosage units of any other controlled substance, is sold to the same consumer in any given 48-hour period without a valid prescription order; (3) the retail purchaser is at least 18 years of age; (4) the pharmacist obtains suitable identification; (5) a record book is maintained that contains the name and address of the purchaser, name and quantity of Controlled Substance purchased, date of sale, and initials of the pharmacist; and (6) other federal, state, or local law does not require a prescription order.

The label of any controlled substance in schedule II, III, or IV, when dispensed to or for a patient pursuant to a prescription order, must contain the following warning; *"Caution: Federal law prohibits the transfer of this drug to any person other than the patient for whom it was prescribed."*

In order to prescribe controlled substances, a physician must register with the Drug Enforcement Administration, Registration Unit, Department of Justice. If physicians have more than one office in which they administer and/or dispense any of the drugs listed in the five schedules, they then are required to register at each office. The registration must be renewed annually. The number on the certificate of registration must be indicated on all prescription orders for controlled substances. Physicians must also take an inventory of the controlled substances on hand every 2 years; file a revised form if the practice location is changed; keep a record of controlled substances listed in schedules II through V that they dispense, if they regularly charge patients either separately or together with professional services for such medication; and order supplies of controlled substances listed in schedule II for dispensing or administering on special order forms, obtainable from the Drug Enforcement Administration, Registration Unit, P.O. Box 28083, Central Station, Washington, DC 20005.

Both the physician and the pharmacist are legally responsible for the proper prescribing and dispensing of drugs covered by the Controlled Substances Act. There are many technical details in the regulations and, as a result, the physician may innocently violate the law in his professional use of controlled substances, especially as related to the use of opioids for patients with incurable diseases or in the management of drug addiction. An outline of the Controlled Substances Act of 1970, entitled *A Manual for the Medical Practitioner,* is especially informative on these problems. Copies may be obtained from the Drug Enforcement Administration at the address indicated in the previous paragraph.

PATIENT COMPLIANCE INSTRUCTIONS

Most physicians assume that once the diagnosis is made and the prescription order is written the patient will benefit from his diagnostic and therapeutic acumen. Unfortunately, drug treatment of any kind is often compromised by lack of full compliance by the patient. Common errors of compliance to a regimen by a patient may be of omission, purpose (taking medicines for the wrong reasons), dosage, timing or sequence, adding medications not prescribed, or premature termination of drug therapy. In addition, from 3 to 18% of patients fail to have their prescription orders "filled" within 10 days (Boyd *et al.,* 1974). A recent study that used microelectronic monitoring of patients' drug-taking habits during long-term therapy yielded the following results: 49% of patients made only minor mistakes in the timing of doses; 40% of patients made major omissions in dosing; 10% of patients frequently overdosed; and only 1% of patients made no mistakes (at least within 1 month) (Kass *et al.,* 1987). Urquhart (1987) reported that hidden among the dose omissions is a special pattern: a drug "holiday" of 3 or more days in which the patient takes no drug at all. One patient in five takes at least one such "holiday" each month. Observations of this kind suggest that attention should be directed to some of the basic principles of instruction of the patient about the importance of compliance.

Factors Associated with Noncompliance. The drug defaulter, like the placebo reactor, is not a readily identifiable individual (Roth and Caron, 1978; Solomon, 1980). Patients who are unreliable under one treatment regimen may not be so under another. Solutions to the problem of noncompliance are not readily forthcoming, although increased communication with patients by physicians and pharmacists is generally helpful. A number of factors are briefly reviewed here to indicate some of the steps that clinicians can take to improve patient compliance. For a more detailed analysis, the reader is referred to several excellent articles and reviews (Blackwell, 1979; Haynes *et al.*, 1979; Sackett, 1980; Solomon, 1980; Leventhal *et al.*, 1984).

The Patient's Illness. After the prescription order has been written, the physician should make sure that the patient understands the nature and prognosis of the illness and what to expect from the medication (both acceptable and unacceptable unwanted effects, as well as signs of efficacy that may help to enforce compliance). The physician should explain how the medication alters the disease process. Patients frequently discontinue taking a medication such as penicillin for streptococcal pharyngitis because they have not been told the necessity for continuing the drug after the acute symptoms have subsided. Similarly, patients taking antidepressant medication frequently discontinue treatment because the physician failed to mention the untoward effects that might appear or to advise the patient that weeks may elapse before any improvement is noticeable. Patients with chronic illnesses are prone to lapse in compliance, especially if the treatment is prophylactic or suppressive, the condition is associated with only mild or no symptoms, or the consequences of missing a dose or two are not immediate. In contrast, when relapse is immediate or severe, the patient is much less likely to deviate from the prescribed regimen.

The Patient. Errors and noncompliance occur more frequently at the extremes of age and in patients who live alone. Geriatric patients present problems because of lapses in memory or self-neglect. Poor compliance among children is related to problems of taste and swallowing, although the mother's impression of the severity of the illness has a marked influence on compliance in pediatric patients. The physician must explore the patient's eating, sleeping, and working habits. Otherwise, he might prescribe a drug to be taken three times a day with meals for a patient who either eats only twice a day or sleeps all day and works at night. Educational, economic, ethnic, and personality factors may also influence patient compliance. In the United States the problem is severe with patients whose primary language is not English, and who may require carefully worded written and oral instructions in that language.

The Physician. Physicians are notoriously unable to predict poor compliance or to recognize it by interview (Pullar *et al.*, 1988). Furthermore, studies by Mazzullo and associates (1974) suggest that physicians who do not explain the reasons for their decisions may be a major determinant of the patient's noncompliance. The physician's relationship with the patient and how clearly the treatment regimen is explained have a powerful impact on compliance. Thus, the physician–patient relationship should be viewed as a process of instruction and motivation for both parties as they enter into a health-related contract. The effectiveness of physician–patient communication is inversely related to the error rate in the taking of drugs. Directions on prescription orders should include all the details necessary for a patient to know how, with what, when, and for how long to take the medication.

The Medication Prescribed. Multiple medications, frequent-dose regimens, and the physical features of the medication itself often foster poor compliance. Patients taking three or more medications are less likely to use them as directed. Likewise, when a medication is directed to be taken more frequently than twice a day, it is less likely it will be taken as prescribed (Pullar *et al.*, 1988). Considerable confusion may also develop when multiple drugs of similar appearance are prescribed for the same patient. It is helpful to provide the patient with an identifying name for each medication prescribed, for example, "heart pill" or "water pill," assuming the patient has been told what each medication is designed to accomplish. The color plates in the *Physicians' Desk Reference* can be used to show patients what their medication will look like.

Patients frequently discontinue medication upon the appearance of minor untoward effects because they have not been told that such reactions are common and not to be feared. Special instruction should be given to the patient relative to symptoms that indicate overdosage, such as dizziness from antihypertensive agents. Before instruction is given, however, the doctor should determine (by taking a nonleading history) whether the patient already has the symptoms that could later be misinterpreted as drug related. Such a misunderstanding could lead to an unjustifiable discontinuation of a very useful drug.

The Treatment Environment. The setting in which the prescribed medication is to be taken has a marked influence on compliance. A series of studies in the same psychiatric hospital revealed that noncompliance increased progressively from 19% in inpatients to 37% in day patients and 48% in outpatients (Hare and Wilcox, 1967). This finding emphasizes the need to teach the principles of self-medication before the patient leaves the hospital as well as the added responsibility the physician must assume to achieve satisfactory compliance with patients seen in clinics and private offices.

Consequences of Noncompliance. The consequences of noncompliance, although quite apparent, are often not fully appreciated by either the physician or the patient. Underutilization of the prescribed drug deprives the patient of the intended therapeutic benefits. This may result in a recurrence or worsening of the illness, emergence of antibiotic-resistant microorganisms, or the prescribing of a larger dose or a more potent agent that could lead to toxicity if compliance is improved. Before a patient is judged to be unresponsive or not optimally controlled with initial therapy, some effort should be made to determine whether the medication is being taken according to instructions. Overutilization of the prescribed drug places the patient at increased risk of adverse reactions. Such problems may develop rather innocently; frequently the patient either forgets a dose and hence doubles the next one or adopts an attitude that if one tablet is good, two must be better.

The prevalence of noncompliance has raised questions relative to the effect of this variable on clinical trials of new drugs. Although numerous controls are built into such studies, the difficulties associated with noncompliance must, to some extent, compromise the ability to establish true rates of efficacy and toxicity of any given agent.

The Pharmacist and Patient Compliance. The pharmacist is usually the last professional to be in contact with the ambulatory private patient (or representative) before medication is started. Pharmacists can effectively cooperate with the physician in education about compliance and can counsel the patient on how to take the medication. Cooperation between physician and pharmacist is in the interest of optimal drug therapy, especially with patients who are likely to make errors in taking drugs. Unfortunately, in certain states such cooperation may be in conflict with laws designed to prevent collusion between pharmacists and physicians.

American Hospital Formulary Service Drug Information. American Society of Hospital Pharmacists, Bethesda, Md., **1989.**

Blackwell, B. The drug defaulter. *Clin. Pharmacol. Ther.*, **1972,** *13,* 841–848.

———. The drug regime and treatment compliance. In, *Compliance in Health Care*. (Haynes, R. B.; Taylor, D. W.; and Sackett, D.; eds.) Johns Hopkins University Press, Baltimore, **1979.**

Boyd, J. R.; Covington, T. R.; Stanaszck, W. F.; and Coussons, R. T. Drug defaulting—Part II: Analysis of noncompliance patterns. *Am. J. Hosp. Pharm.*, **1974,** *31,* 485–491.

Committee on Drugs, American Academy of Pediatrics. Inaccuracies in administering liquid medication. *Pediatrics*, **1975,** *56,* 327–328.

Drug Evaluations, 6th ed. American Medical Association, Chicago, **1986.**

Drug Information for the Health Care Professional (USP DI), 9th ed. The United States Pharmacopeial Convention, Inc., Rockville, Md., **1989.**

Facts and Comparisons. Facts and Comparisons Division of J. B. Lippencott Co., St. Louis. Updated monthly.

Food and Drug Administration. *Approved Prescription Drug Products with Therapeutic Equivalence Evaluations*, 8th ed. U.S. Department of Health and Human Services, Washington, D. C., **1988.**

Hare, E. H., and Wilcox, D. R. C. Do psychiatric inpatients take their pills? *Br. J. Psychiatry*, **1967,** *113,* 1435–1439.

Haynes, R. B.; Taylor, D. W.; and Sackett, D. L. (eds.). *Compliance in Health Care*. Johns Hopkins University Press, Baltimore, **1979.**

Kass, M. A.; Gordon, M.; Morley, R. E.; Meltzer, D. W.; and Goldberg, J. J. Compliance with topical timolol treatment. *Am. J. Ophthalmol.*, **1987,** *103,* 188–193.

Leventhal, H.; Zimmerman, R.; and Gutmann, M. Compliance: a topic for behavioral medicine research. In, *Handbook of Behavioral Medicine*. (Gentry, D., ed.) Guilford Press, New York, **1984.**

Mazzullo, J.; Cohn, K.; Lasagna, L.; and Griner, P. Variations in interpretation of prescription instructions. *J.A.M.A.*, **1974,** *227,* 929–931.

Physicians' Desk Reference, 43rd ed. Medical Economics Co., Inc., Oradell, NJ, **1989.**

Pullar, T.; Birtwell, A. J.; Wiles, P. G.; Hay, A.; and Feely, M. P. Use of a pharmacologic indicator to compare compliance with tablets prescribed to be taken once, twice, or three times daily. *Clin. Pharmacol. Ther.*, **1988,** *44,* 540–545.

Roth, H. P., and Caron, H. S. Accuracy of doctors' estimates and patient statements on adherence to a drug regimen. *Clin. Pharmacol. Ther.*, **1978,** *23,* 361–370.

Sackett, D. L. Is there a patient compliance problem? If so, what do we do about it? In, *Controversies in Therapeutics*. (Lasagna, L., ed.) W. B. Saunders Co., Philadelphia, **1980,** pp. 552–558.

Solomon, H. S. How to improve patient compliance. In, *Controversies in Therapeutics*. (Lasagna, L., ed.) W. B. Saunders Co., Philadelphia, **1980,** pp. 567–572.

United States Pharmacopeia XXII National Formulary XVII. United States Pharmacopeial Convention, Inc., Rockville, Md., **1990,** pp. 1629–1665.

USAN and the USP Dictionary of Drug Names, 27th ed. (Heller, W. M., ed.) United States Pharmacopeial Convention, Inc., Rockville, Md., **1990.**

Urquhart, J. A call for a new discipline. *Pharm. Technol.*, **1987,** *11,* 16–17.

APPENDIX

II DESIGN AND OPTIMIZATION OF DOSAGE REGIMENS; PHARMACOKINETIC DATA

Leslie Z. Benet and Roger L. Williams

The objective of this appendix is to present pharmacokinetic data in a format that allows the clinician to make rational choices of doses of drugs. Table A–II–1 (pages 1655–1735) contains quantitative information about the absorption, distribution, and elimination of drugs and the effects of disease states on these processes, as well as information about the correlation of efficacy and toxicity with measured concentrations of drugs in plasma. The general principles that are used to select the appropriate maintenance dose and dosing interval (and, where appropriate, the loading dose) for the average patient are described in Chapter 1. Discussion of individualization of these variables for a particular patient is presented here.

To use the data that are presented, one must understand clearance concepts and their application for the computation of drug-dosage regimens. One must also know average values of clearance, as well as some measures of the extent and kinetics of drug absorption and distribution. The text below defines the eight basic parameters that are listed in the tabular material for each drug, as well as some factors that influence these values in both normal subjects and in patients with particular diseases.

It would obviously be most useful if there was a consensus about the correct value for a given pharmacokinetic parameter, rather than being faced with 10 or 20 separate (and often disparate) estimates of that parameter. Unfortunately, a consensus has been reached for only a very limited number of drugs. In Table A–II–1, single values for each parameter and for its variability (standard deviation) in the population have been selected from the literature, based on the scientific judgment of the authors. Values in the tables are those determined in healthy normal adults, unless otherwise indicated in footnotes. The direction of change for these values in particular disease states is noted next to the average value. One or two important references are provided for each drug at the end of the table. In most cases, at least one of these references represents a recent review of the clinical pharmacokinetic properties of the drug. Further information can usually be found in monographs that detail the effects of disease and altered physiological states on pharmacokinetic parameters (Benet *et al.*, 1984; Evans *et al.*, 1986; Ritschel, 1986; Bass and Williams, 1988; Bennett, 1988; Vozeh *et al.*, 1988).

TABULATED PHARMACOKINETIC PARAMETERS

Each of the eight parameters presented in Table A–II–1 has been discussed in detail in Chapter 1. The following discussion focuses on the format in which the values are presented, as well as on factors (physiological or pathological) that influence the parameters.

Availability. The extent of availability of the drug after oral administration is expressed as a percentage of the dose. This value represents the percentage of an oral dose that is available to produce pharmacological actions—the fraction of the oral dose that reaches the arterial blood in an active form. *Fractional availability* (F) is a similar parameter used elsewhere in this appendix; this value varies from 0 to 1. Measures of the *rate* of availability are not provided in Table A–II–1. Since pharmacokinetic concepts are most useful in the design of multiple dosage regimens, the *extent* rather than the rate of availability is more critical to obtain an appropriate concentration of drug in the body (*see* Chapter 1).

It is important to keep in mind that poor patient compliance may be mistaken for decreased bioavailability. A true decrease in bioavailability may result from a poorly formulated dosage form that fails to disintegrate or dissolve in the gastrointestinal fluids, interactions between drugs in the gastrointestinal tract, metabolism of the drug in the gastrointestinal tract, and/or first-pass hepatic metabolism or biliary excretion (*see* Chapters 1 and 4). Hepatic disease in particular may cause increased availability because hepatic metabolic capacity decreases and/or because of the development of vascular shunts around the liver.

Urinary Excretion of Unchanged Drug. The second parameter in Table A–II–1 is the amount of drug eventually excreted unchanged in the urine, expressed as a percentage of the administered dose. Values represent the percentage expected in a healthy young adult (creatinine clearance greater than 100 ml/min). When possible, the value listed is that determined after bolus intravenous administration of the drug, at which time availability is assumed to be 100%. If the drug is given orally, this parameter may also reflect loss of drug because of low availability; such values are indicated in a footnote.

Renal disease is the primary factor that causes changes in this parameter. This is especially true when alternate pathways of elimination are available; thus, as renal function decreases, a greater fraction of the dose is available for elimination by other routes. Since renal function generally decreases as a function of age, the percentage of drug excreted unchanged also usually decreases with age when alternate pathways of elimination are available. For a number of acidic and basic drugs with values of pK_a in the range of the usual pH of urine, changes in the latter will affect the rate or extent of urinary excretion (*see* Chapter 1).

Binding to Plasma Proteins. The tabulated value is the percentage of drug in the plasma that is bound to plasma proteins at concentrations of the drug that are achieved clinically. In almost all cases the values are from measurements performed *in vitro* (rather than from measurements of binding to the proteins in plasma that was obtained from patients to whom the drug had been administered). When a single mean value is presented, there is no apparent change in this percentage over the range of concentrations normally found in patients taking the drug. In cases in which saturation of binding is approached at usual plasma concentrations, values are provided at concentrations that correspond to the lower and upper limits of the usual range.

Plasma protein binding is primarily affected by disease states (such as hepatic disease) that alter the concentration of albumin or other proteins in plasma that bind drugs. Some metabolic states and conditions such as uremia also change the affinity of binding for some drugs. Such changes in protein binding as a function of disease can dramatically affect the volume of distribution of a drug.

Clearance. Total systemic clearance of drug from plasma (*see* equation 3, Chapter 1) is given in Table A–II–1; values are usually reported in units of ml · min^{-1} · kg^{-1}. In some cases, separate values for renal and nonrenal clearance are also provided. For some drugs, particularly those that are predominantly excreted unchanged in the urine, equations are given that relate total or renal clearance to creatinine clearance (also expressed as ml · min^{-1} · kg^{-1}). For drugs that exhibit saturation kinetics, K_m and V_m are given and represent, respectively, the plasma concentration at which half of the maximal rate of elimination is reached (in units of mass/volume) and the maximal rate of elimination (in units of mass · time^{-1} · kg of body weight^{-1}). The concentration of the drug in plasma (C_p) must, of course, be in the same units as K_m.

As discussed in Chapter 1, intrinsic clearance from blood is the maximal possible clearance by the organ responsible for elimination when blood flow (delivery) of drug is not limiting. Intrinsic clearance is tabulated for a few drugs. Note that intrinsic clearance is defined in terms of the concentration of drug in *blood*. If one wishes to relate changes in elimination of drug to pathological changes either in the organ itself or to blood flow to the organ, it is necessary to express clearance with respect to concentrations of drug in blood rather than those in plasma. This requires measurement of concentrations in whole blood or knowledge of the distribution of drug between plasma and red blood cells; such information is currently limited. Clearances from plasma are presented in Table A–II–1, since these are most useful to relate dosage of drug to concentrations of drugs in plasma that have been determined previously to be effective or toxic.

Clearance can be determined only when the fractional availability F of the drug is known. Therefore, to be accurate, clearances must be determined after intravenous dosage. When such data are not available, the ratio of CL/F is given; values of this kind are indicated in a footnote.

Clearance varies as a function of body size and, therefore, is presented in the table in units of ml · min^{-1} · kg of body weight^{-1}. Although normalization to measures of size other than weight may sometimes be appropriate, weight is so convenient that this offsets any small loss in accuracy, especially in adults.

Volume of Distribution. The total body volume of distribution at steady state (V_{ss}) is given in Table A–II–1 and is expressed in units of liters/kg.

When estimates of V_{ss} are not available, values for V_{area} are provided (*see* Chapter 1). These values are obtained by dividing clearance by the terminal rate constant for elimination. V_{area} is a convenient and easily calculated parameter. However, unlike V_{ss}, this volume term varies when the rate constant for drug elimination changes, even though there has been no change in the distribution space. Since the clinician may wish to know whether a particular disease state influences either clearance or the distribution of the drug within the body independently, it is preferable to define volume in terms of V_{ss}, a parameter that is theoretically independent of changes in the rate of elimination.

As is the case for clearance, V_{ss} is usually defined in the table in terms of concentration in plasma, rather than in blood. If data were not obtained after intravenous administration of the drug, a footnote will make clear that the parameter determined, V_{ss}/F, contains a measure of availability.

Volume of distribution is primarily a function of body size, and values in the table are given in liters/kg. As mentioned for clearance, normalization to measures of size other than weight may sometimes be appropriate.

Half-life. The time required for one half of the amount of drug in the body to be eliminated is provided. However, drug concentrations in plasma often follow a multiexponential pattern of decline when this value is measured as a function of time. The single number listed in each component of the table corresponds to the rate of elimination that describes the major fraction of total clearance of drug from the body. In many cases this half-life may correspond to the terminal log-linear rate of elimination. For some drugs, however, a more prolonged half-life may be observed at very low plasma concentrations when extremely sensitive assay techniques are used. If this component accounts for only 10% of drug clearance, predictions of steady-state concentrations of drug in plasma will be in error by only 10% if this longer half-life is ignored, no matter how large its value. This is true because half-life is a function of both elimination and distribution, as discussed in Chapter 1.

Half-life is usually independent of body size, since it is a function of the ratio of two parameters, clearance and volume of distribution, each of which is proportional to body size.

Effective and Toxic Concentrations. There is no general agreement about the best way to describe the relationship between the concentration of drug in plasma and its effect. Many different kinds of data are presented in the literature, and extraction of a single parameter or even a set of parameters is difficult. Furthermore, there may not be agreement as to which measures are most relevant. Footnotes are common in Table A–II–1 to indicate the meaning and relevance of these values; in many cases reference is made to a chapter in the text for discussion. This is particularly true for antimicrobial agents, since the effective concentration depends on the identity of the microorganism causing the infection.

The relationships between the concentration of drug in plasma and the effect of the drug are imperfect, as might be expected (*see* Chapters 2 and 4). Little information is available about the variation between individuals of receptor number or affinity or subsequent coupling to a response, or about the effects of disease states on these factors. For many drugs, the form of the relationship between effect and plasma concentration is unknown. Because the concentration of free drug determines the degree of effect, changes in protein binding due to disease may be expected to cause changes in the *total* concentration of drug associated with a desired or an unwanted effect. It is also important to realize that concentration–effect relationships are only meaningful at steady state or during the terminal log-linear phase of the concentration-versus-time curve, when the ratio of the drug concentration at sites of action to that in the plasma can be expected to remain constant over time. Thus, when attempting to correlate pharmacokinetics with pharmacodynamics, the time of distribution of drug to its site of action must be taken into account (Verotta *et al.,* 1989).

ALTERATIONS OF PARAMETERS IN THE INDIVIDUAL PATIENT

The values in Table A–II–1 represent mean values for populations of normal adults, and it may be necessary to modify them for calculation of dosage regimens for individual patients. The fraction of free drug (α) in a given patient must be known in order to compute a desired steady-state concentration. The fraction available (F) and clearance must also be estimated to compute a maintenance dose. To calculate the loading dose and to estimate half-life and dosing interval, knowledge of the volume of distribution is needed. The figures in the table and the adjustments apply only to adults unless specifically designated otherwise. Although the values may sometimes, with caution, be applied to children who weigh more than about 30 kg (after proper adjustment for size; *see* below), it is best to consult a textbook of pediatrics or other source for definitive advice.

For each drug, changes in the parameters occasioned by certain disease states are noted within the eight segments of the table. In most cases, a qualitative direction of changes is noted, such as "↓ Hep," which indicates a significant decrease in the parameter in a patient with hepatitis. A reasonable quantitative translation is to multiply the value of the parameter by 0.5 for each applicable condition that is noted to decrease the parameter and to multiply it by 2 for each condition that is noted to increase the parameter. Such an adjustment can only be approximate; yet, since reliable data are limited, no better approach may be possible. The relevant literature should be consulted for more definitive quantitative information.

Protein Binding. Most acidic drugs that are extensively bound to plasma proteins are bound to albumin. Basic drugs, such as propranolol, are often bound to other plasma proteins (*e.g.*, α_1-acid glycoprotein). The degree of drug binding to proteins will differ in states that cause changes in the concentration of the binding proteins. Unfortunately, among binding proteins only albumin is commonly measured. For drugs that are bound to albumin (*alb*), a patient's fraction of free drug (α_{pt}) can be approximated from the following relationship:

$$\alpha_{pt} = 1 \Big/ \left[\left(\frac{alb_{pt}}{alb_{nl}} \right) \left(\frac{1 - \alpha_{nl}}{\alpha_{nl}} \right) + 1 \right] \tag{1}$$

where alb_{nl} and α_{nl} refer to values of the concentration of albumin in plasma and the fraction of free drug in normal individuals, respectively. Use of this equation assumes that the molar concentration of drug is far less than that of albumin, that only one type of drug binding site is present on albumin, and that there are no cooperative binding interactions. Therefore, it cannot be exact. However, it is a reasonable approximation and, in the absence of actual measurement of the patient's fraction of free drug, can prove quite useful.

Clearance. Clearance must often be adjusted for alterations in renal function. The quantities required for this adjustment are the fraction of normal renal function remaining and the fraction of drug usually excreted unchanged in the urine. The latter quantity appears in the table; the former can be estimated as the ratio of the patient's creatinine clearance to a normal value (120 ml/min per 70 kg). If creatinine clearance has not been measured, it may be estimated from measurements of the concentration of creatinine in serum, using a number of different equations or nomograms. One such method is to estimate the fraction of normal renal function present (*rfx*) as the reciprocal of the patient's serum creatinine concentration, minus 0.01 for each year of age over 40. This is a crude estimate, but more accurate ones are seldom justified or necessary, since the whole process of adjustment of clearance is already approximate because of considerable unpredictable interindividual variation in clearance, which is independent of renal function. The following equation for adjustment of clearance uses the quantities just discussed:

$$rf_{pt} = 1 - fe_{nl}(1 - rfx_{pt}) \tag{2}$$

where fe_{nl} is the fraction of drug excreted unchanged in normal individuals (*see* table). The renal factor (rf_{pt}) is the value that, when multiplied by normal total clearance, gives the total clearance of the drug adjusted for disturbances of renal function.

Example. Clearance of terbutaline in a patient with depressed renal function (creatinine clearance = 40 ml · min^{-1} · 70 kg^{-1}) may be estimated as follows:

$$\begin{aligned}
rfx_{pt} &= 40 \text{ ml/min} \div 120 \text{ ml/min} = 0.33 \\
fe_{nl} &= 0.56 \ (\textit{see} \text{ listing for terbutaline}) \\
rf_{pt} &= 1\text{–}0.56\ (1\text{–}0.33) = 0.62 \\
CL_{pt} &= CL_{nl} \cdot rf_{pt} \\
CL_{pt} &= (3.4 \text{ ml} \cdot \text{min}^{-1} \cdot \text{kg}^{-1})\ (0.62) \\
&= 2.1 \text{ ml} \cdot \text{min}^{-1} \cdot \text{kg}^{-1}
\end{aligned}$$

Clearance must also be adjusted for the size of the patient. For convenience, the figures in the table are normalized to weight. However, clearance of drug often varies in proportion to metabolic rate, which is best related to weight to the 0.75 power. To take this into account, the clearance figure in the table can be multiplied by the factor *wf*, instead of by weight:

$$wf = Wt_{nl}(Wt_{pt}/Wt_{nl})^{0.75} \tag{3}$$

which for weight in kg (where Wt_{nl} = 70 kg) becomes:

$$wf = 2.9(Wt_{pt})^{0.75} \tag{4}$$

Calculation of the weight factor seldom pays for itself by yielding significantly more accurate estimates. It should be done, however, for patients at extremes of size, especially the very obese.

If drug elimination is proportional to the free (rather than the total) concentration of drug in plasma, clearance is then further adjusted by multiplying it by the ratio of the normal free fraction to the free fraction of the patient, calculated as indicated previously.

All the adjustments to clearance should be applied simultaneously. That is, the figure in the table is multiplied by a weight factor (usually weight itself), *and* multiplied by the binding correction, if applicable, *and* multiplied by the renal correction factor, if applicable, *and,* finally, multiplied by the appropriate values of 0.5 and/or 2 for other factors that are present and qualitatively indicated to modify clearance. Obviously, if a quantitative correction is made for renal function, a qualitative one (multiplication by 0.5) should not also be made for this same factor.

Volume of Distribution. Volume of distribution should be adjusted for the modifying factors indicated in Table A–II–1, as well as for size. The figures in the table are normalized to weight. Unlike clearance, volume of distribution is probably most often proportional to weight itself. Whether or not this is so, however, depends on the actual sites of distribution of drug, and no absolute rule applies.

Whether to adjust volume of distribution for changes in binding to plasma proteins cannot be decided in general, since the decision critically depends on whether the factors that alter binding to plasma proteins also alter binding to tissues. In such cases the qualitative changes in volume of distribution are indicated in the table. Again, each adjustment to volume of distribution should be made independently of any other, and the final estimate should reflect all adjustments simultaneously.

Half-life. Finally, half-life may be estimated from the adjusted estimates of clearance and volume of distribution:

$$t_{1/2} = 0.693\ V_{pt}/CL_{pt} \tag{5}$$

Since, historically, half-life has been the parameter most often measured, qualitative changes for this parameter are almost always given in the table.

INDIVIDUALIZATION OF DOSAGE

By using the parameters for the individual patient, calculated as described above, initial dosing regimens may be chosen. The maintenance dose may be calculated with equation 17, Chapter 1, and the estimated values for *CL* and *F* for the individual patient. The target concentration may need to be adjusted for changes in protein binding in the patient, as described above. The loading dose may be calculated by use of equation 21 in Chapter 1 and the estimated parameters for V_{ss} and *F*. A particular dosing interval may be chosen; the maximal and minimal steady-state concentrations can be calculated by using equations 19 and 20 in Chapter 1, and these can be compared with the efficacious and toxic concentrations listed for the drug. As with the target concentration, these values may need to be adjusted for changes in the extent of protein binding. Use of equations 19 and 20 also requires estimates of values for *F*, V_{ss}, and *k* ($k = 0.693/t_{1/2}$) for the individual patient.

Note that these adjustments of the pharmacokinetic parameters for an individual patient are suggested for the rational choice of initial dosing regimen. As emphasized in Chapter 1, measurements of drug concentrations in the patient can then be used to adjust the dosage regimen to achieve the desired range of concentrations.

Bass, N. M., and Williams, R. L. Guide to drug dosage in hepatic disease. *Clin. Pharmacokinet.*, **1988**, *15*, 396–420.

Benet, L. Z.; Massoud, N.; and Gambertoglio, J. G. (eds.). *Pharmacokinetic Basis for Drug Treatment.* Raven Press, New York, **1984.**

Bennett, W. M. Guide to drug dosage in renal failure. *Clin. Pharmacokinet.*, **1988**, *15*, 326–354.

Evans, W. E.; Schentag, J. J.; and Jusko, W. J. (eds.). *Applied Pharmacokinetics: Principles of Therapeutic Drug Monitoring*, 2nd ed. Applied Therapeutics, Spokane, Wash., **1986.**

Ritschel, W. A. *Handbook of Basic Pharmacokinetics, Including Clinical Applications*, 3rd ed. Drug Intelligence Publications, Hamilton, Ill., **1986.**

Verotta, D.; Beal, S. L.; and Sheiner, L. B. Semiparametric approach to pharmacokinetic-pharmacodynamic data. *Am J. Physiol.*, **1989**, *256*, R1005–R1010.

Vozeh, S.; Schmidlin, O.; and Taeschner, W. Pharmacokinetic drug data. *Clin. Pharmacokinet.*, **1988**, *15*, 254–282.

Table A–II–1. PHARMACOKINETIC DATA

AVAILABILITY (ORAL) (%)	URINARY EXCRETION (%)	BOUND IN PLASMA (%)	CLEARANCE ($ml \cdot min^{-1} \cdot kg^{-1}$)	VOL. DIST. (*liters/kg*)	HALF-LIFE (*hours*)	EFFECTIVE CONCENTRATIONS	TOXIC CONCENTRATIONS
ACEBUTOLOL [a] (Chapters 11, 35)							
37 ± 12 [b]	40 ± 11	26 ± 3	6.8 ± 0.8 ⟷ Urem [c]	1.2 ± 0.3	2.7 ± 0.4 ⟷ Urem [c]	[a]	—

[a] An acetylated metabolite, diacetolol, which may have pharmacological activity, is present at steady state at concentrations 2.7 times those of acebutolol.
[b] Some increase in availability (perhaps to 50%) occurs at higher doses and at steady state.
[c] Prolonged half-life and decreased clearance of diacetolol in uremia.

AVAILABILITY (ORAL) (%)	URINARY EXCRETION (%)	BOUND IN PLASMA (%)	CLEARANCE ($ml \cdot min^{-1} \cdot kg^{-1}$)	VOL. DIST. (*liters/kg*)	HALF-LIFE (*hours*)	EFFECTIVE CONCENTRATIONS	TOXIC CONCENTRATIONS
ACETAMINOPHEN [a] (Chapter 26)							
88 ± 15 ⟷ Child	3 ± 1 ⟷ Neo, Child	0 at < 60 ng/ml	5.0 ± 1.4 [b] ↓ Hep [c] ⟷ Aged, Child ↑ Obes, HTh, Preg	0.95 ± 0.12 [b] ⟷ Aged, Hep [c], LTh, HTh, Child	2.0 ± 0.4 ⟷ Urem, Obes, Child ↑ Neo, Hep [c] ↓ HTh, Preg	10–20 μg/ml [d]	>300 μg/ml [e]

[a] Values reported are for a linear kinetic model for doses less than 2 g; drug exhibits dose-dependent kinetics above this dose.
[b] Assuming 70-kg weight; reported range, 65–72 kg.
[c] Acetaminophen-induced hepatic damage or acute viral hepatitis.
[d] Analgesia, antipyresis.
[e] Hepatic toxicity for these concentrations 4 hours after ingestion; no hepatic toxicity if concentrations < 120 μg/ml 4 hours after ingestion.

AVAILABILITY (ORAL) (%)	URINARY EXCRETION (%)	BOUND IN PLASMA (%)	CLEARANCE ($ml \cdot min^{-1} \cdot kg^{-1}$)	VOL. DIST. (*liters/kg*)	HALF-LIFE (*hours*)	EFFECTIVE CONCENTRATIONS	TOXIC CONCENTRATIONS
N-ACETYLPROCAINAMIDE (Chapter 35)							
83 ± 12	81 ± 1	10 ± 9	3.1 ± 0.4 ↓ Urem, Aged, CAD, Obes	1.4 ± 0.2 ⟷ Urem, Aged, CAD	6.0 ± 0.2 ↑ Urem, Aged, CAD	21 μg/ml [a] (12–35 μg/ml)	—

[a] 70% reduction in mean frequency of premature ventricular contractions during long-term therapy.

Key: Adult = adults; Aged = aged; Alb = hypoalbuminemia; Arth = arthritis; Atr Fib = atrial fibrillation; AVH = acute viral hepatitis; Burn = burn patients; CAD = coronary artery disease; Celiac = celiac disease; CF = cystic fibrosis; CHF = congestive heart failure; Child = children; Cirr = cirrhosis; COPD = chronic obstructive pulmonary disease; CP = cor pulmonale; CPBS = cardiopulmonary bypass surgery; CRI = chronic respiratory insufficiency; Crohn = Crohn's disease; Cush = Cushing's syndrome; Epilep = epileptic; Fem = female; Hep = Hepatitis; HL = hyperlipoproteinemia; HTh = hyperthyroid; Inflam = inflammation; LTh = hypothyroid; MI = myocardial infarction; Neo = neonate; NS = nephrotic syndrome; Obes = obese; Pneu = pneumonia; Preg = pregnant; Prem = premature; RA = rheumatoid arthritis; Smk = smoking; Tach = ventricular tachycardia; Ulcer = ulcer patients; Urem = uremia

References: *See* end of table.

Table A–II–1. PHARMACOKINETIC DATA (Continued)

AVAILABILITY (ORAL) (%)	URINARY EXCRETION (%)	BOUND IN PLASMA (%)	CLEARANCE ($ml \cdot min^{-1} \cdot kg^{-1}$)	VOL. DIST. (*liters/kg*)	HALF-LIFE (*hours*)	EFFECTIVE CONCENTRATIONS	TOXIC CONCENTRATIONS
ACETYLSALICYLIC ACID [a] (Chapter 26)							
68 ± 3 ⟷ Aged, Cirr	1.4 ± 1.2	49 ↓ Urem	9.3 ± 1.1 ⟷ Aged, Cirr	0.15 ± 0.03	0.25 ± 0.03 ⟷ Hep	*See* Salicylic Acid	*See* Salicylic Acid

[a] Values given are for unchanged acetylsalicylic acid. Acetylsalicylic acid is converted to salicylic acid during and after absorption. *See* Salicylic Acid for parameters for that compound.

AVAILABILITY (ORAL) (%)	URINARY EXCRETION (%)	BOUND IN PLASMA (%)	CLEARANCE ($ml \cdot min^{-1} \cdot kg^{-1}$)	VOL. DIST. (*liters/kg*)	HALF-LIFE (*hours*)	EFFECTIVE CONCENTRATIONS	TOXIC CONCENTRATIONS
ACYCLOVIR (Chapter 51)							
15–30 [a]	75 ± 10	15 ± 4	$CL = 3.37\ CL_{cr} + 0.41$ ↓ Neo ⟷ Child	0.69 ± 0.19 ↓ Neo ⟷ Urem	2.4 ± 0.7 ↑ Urem, Neo ⟷ Child	*See* Chapter 51	—

[a] Decreases with increasing dose.

AVAILABILITY (ORAL) (%)	URINARY EXCRETION (%)	BOUND IN PLASMA (%)	CLEARANCE ($ml \cdot min^{-1} \cdot kg^{-1}$)	VOL. DIST. (*liters/kg*)	HALF-LIFE (*hours*)	EFFECTIVE CONCENTRATIONS	TOXIC CONCENTRATIONS
ALFENTANIL (Chapters 14, 21)							
—	<1	92 ± 2 ↓ Cirr	6.7 ± 2.4 [a] ↓ Aged, Cirr ⟷ CPBS	0.8 ± 0.3 ⟷ Aged ↑ CPBS ↓ Cirr	1.6 ± 0.2 ↑ Aged, Cirr, CPBS	100–200 ng/ml [b] 310–340 ng/ml [c]	—

[a] Blood-to-plasma ratio = 0.63 ± 0.02.
[b] Adequate anesthesia for superficial surgery.
[c] Adequate anesthesia for abdominal surgery.

AVAILABILITY (ORAL) (%)	URINARY EXCRETION (%)	BOUND IN PLASMA (%)	CLEARANCE ($ml \cdot min^{-1} \cdot kg^{-1}$)	VOL. DIST. (*liters/kg*)	HALF-LIFE (*hours*)	EFFECTIVE CONCENTRATIONS	TOXIC CONCENTRATIONS
ALPRAZOLAM (Chapters 17, 18)							
92 ± 17	20	71 ± 3 ↑ Cirr ⟷ Obes, Aged	0.74 ± 0.14 ↓ Obes, Cirr, Aged [a] ⟷ Urem	0.72 ± 0.12 ⟷ Obes, Cirr, Aged	12 ± 2 ↑ Obes, Cirr, Aged [a] ⟷ Urem	—	—

[a] In males only.

AVAILABILITY (ORAL) (%)	URINARY EXCRETION (%)	BOUND IN PLASMA (%)	CLEARANCE ($ml \cdot min^{-1} \cdot kg^{-1}$)	VOL. DIST. (*liters/kg*)	HALF-LIFE (*hours*)	EFFECTIVE CONCENTRATIONS	TOXIC CONCENTRATIONS
ALTEPLASE (t-PA) (Chapter 55)							
—	Low	—	9.8 ± 0.9	0.10 ± 0.01	0.05 ± 0.006 [a]	—	—

[a] Initial half-life is dominant; terminal half-life is 0.43 ± 0.17 hours.

AMANTADINE (Chapter 51)							
50–90 [a]	50–90 [a]	67	4.8 ± 0.8 ↓ Aged, Urem	6.6 ± 1.5 ↓ Aged ⟷ Urem	16 ± 3.4 ↑ Aged, Urem	300 ng/ml [b]	>1 μg/ml [c]

[a] Drug is not metabolized; oral bioavailability equals percent excreted unchanged.
[b] Trough concentration for prophylaxis of influenza A.
[c] Psychosis.

AMIKACIN (Chapter 47)							
—	98	4 ± 8 [a]	1.3 ± 0.6 $CL = 0.6\ CL_{cr} + 0.14$ ↓ Obes ↑ CF	0.27 ± 0.06 ⟷ Aged, Child, CF ↓ Obes ↑ Neo	2.3 ± 0.4 ↑ Urem ⟷ Obes ↓ Burn, Child, CF	*See* Chapter 47	*See* Chapter 47

[a] At serum concentration of 15 μg/ml.

AMILORIDE (Chapter 28)							
[a]	49 ± 10 ↑ Hep ↓ Urem	40	9.7 ± 1.9 [b] ↓ Aged, Hep, Urem	17 ± 4 [b] ↓ Urem ⟷ Hep, Aged	21 ± 3 ↑ Aged, Hep, Urem	—	—

[a] Greater than or equal to percent excreted unchanged.
[b] CL/F and V_{area}/F, assuming 70-kg weight.

AMIODARONE [a] (Chapter 35)							
46 ± 22	0	99.98 ± 0.01	1.9 ± 0.4 [b]	66 ± 44	25 ± 12 days [c]	0.5–2.5 μg/ml [d]	>2.5 μg/ml [d]

[a] Significant concentrations of an active desethyl metabolite are found (ratio of drug/metabolite ~1); $t_{1/2}$ = 61 days.
[b] Blood-to-plasma ratio = 0.73 ± 0.06.
[c] Longer half-lives noted in patients (53 ± 24 days); all half-lives may be underestimated because of insufficient sampling.
[d] Suggested upper limit; no definitive data.

Key: Adult = adults; Aged = aged; Alb = hypoalbuminemia; Arth = arthritis; Atr Fib = atrial fibrillation; AVH = acute viral hepatitis; Burn = burn patients; CAD = coronary artery disease; Celiac = celiac disease; CF = cystic fibrosis; CHF = congestive heart failure; Child = children; Cirr = cirrhosis; COPD = chronic obstructive pulmonary disease; CP = cor pulmonale; CPBS = cardiopulmonary bypass surgery; CRI = chronic respiratory insufficiency; Crohn = Crohn's disease; Cush = Cushing's syndrome; Epilep = epileptic; Fem = female; Hep = Hepatitis; HL = hyperlipoproteinemia; HTh = hyperthyroid; Inflam = inflammation; LTh = hypothyroid; MI = myocardial infarction; Neo = neonate; NS = nephrotic syndrome; Obes = obese; Pneu = pneumonia; Preg = pregnant; Prem = premature; RA = rheumatoid arthritis; Smk = smoking; Tach = ventricular tachycardia; Ulcer = ulcer patients; Urem = uremia

References: *See* end of table.

Table A–II–1. PHARMACOKINETIC DATA (Continued)

AVAILABILITY (ORAL) (%)	URINARY EXCRETION (%)	BOUND IN PLASMA (%)	CLEARANCE ($ml \cdot min^{-1} \cdot kg^{-1}$)	VOL. DIST. (*liters/kg*)	HALF-LIFE (*hours*)	EFFECTIVE CONCENTRATIONS	TOXIC CONCENTRATIONS
AMITRIPTYLINE [a] (Chapter 18)							
48 ± 11 ⟷ Aged	<2	94.8 ± 0.8 ⟷ Aged ↑ HL	11.5 ± 3.4 [b] ⟷ Aged, Smk	15 ± 3 [b] ↑ Aged	21 ± 5 ↑ Aged	60–220 ng/ml [c]	>1 μg/ml [d]
[a] Active metabolite is nortriptyline. [b] Blood *CL* and V_{ss}; blood-to-plasma concentration ratio = 0.86 ± 0.13. [c] Optimal range of amitriptyline plus nortriptyline. [d] Combined data for toxic effects of tricyclic antidepressants.							
AMOXICILLIN (Chapter 46)							
93 ± 10 [a]	86 ± 8	18	2.6 ± 0.4 ⟷ Child ↓ Urem, Aged [b]	0.21 ± 0.03 ⟷ Urem, Aged	1.7 ± 0.3 ⟷ Child ↑ Urem, Aged [b]	*See* Chapter 46	*See* Chapter 46
[a] Dose dependent; value shown is for 375 mg; decreases to about 50% at 3000 mg. [b] No change if renal function not decreased.							
AMPHOTERICIN B (Chapter 50)							
—	2–5	>90	0.46 ± 0.20 [a] ⟷ Urem, Prem	0.76 ± 0.52 [b]	18 ± 7 [c]	*See* Chapter 50	—
[a] Data for eight children (aged 8 months to 14 years) yield a linear regression with *CL* decreasing with age: *CL* = −0.046 · Age (yr) + 0.86. [b] Volume of central compartment. [c] A terminal elimination phase ($t_{1/2}$ = 15 ± 2 days) observed in two adults after cessation of treatment.							
AMPICILLIN (Chapter 46)							
62 ± 17	82 ± 10	18 ± 2 ↓ Neo	$CL = 1.7\ CL_{cr} + 0.21$ ⟷ Cirr, Preg	0.28 ± 0.07 ⟷ Urem, Preg ↑ Cirr	1.3 ± 0.2 ↑ Urem, Cirr, Neo ⟷ Preg	*See* Chapter 46	*See* Chapter 46

AMRINONE (Chapter 34)

93 ± 12	25 ± 10	35–49	4.0 ± 1.6 [a] 8.9 ± 2.7 [b] ↓ CHF, Neo	1.3 ± 0.3 [a,b] ⟷ Neo	4.4 ± 1.4 [a] 2.0 ± 0.6 [b] ↑ CHF, Neo	3.7 μg/ml [c]	>2.5 μg/ml [d]

[a] Slow acetylators.
[b] Fast acetylators.
[c] 50% increase in cardiac index in patients with CHF.
[d] Thrombocytopenia.

ATENOLOL [a] (Chapter 11)

56 ± 30 ⟷ Aged, Preg	94 ± 8	<5	2.4 ± 0.2 [b] ↓ Age, Urem ⟷ Child	0.95 ± 0.15 ⟷ Aged, Child, Urem	6.1 ± 2.0 ⟷ Preg, HTh, Child ↑ Urem, Aged	1.0 μg/ml [c]	—

[a] Racemic mixture; (−)-enantiomer active. Renal clearance and $t_{1/2}$ of enantiomers do not differ.
[b] Blood-to-plasma ratio = 1.07 ± 0.25.
[c] To achieve a 30% reduction in exercise-induced cardioacceleration.

ATRACURIUM (Chapter 9)

—	<1	—	5.5 ± 1.0 ↑ Burn ↓ CPBS ⟷ Urem	0.16 ± 0.02 [a] ⟷ Urem	0.33 ± 0.04 ⟷ Urem	0.65 μg/ml [b] 1.3 μg/ml [c]	—

[a] V_{area}.
[b] To achieve 50% depression of twitch tension.
[c] To achieve 95% depression of twitch tension.

ATROPINE [a] (Chapter 8)

50	57 ± 8	14–22 ⟷ Aged	5.9 ± 3.6 [b] ↓ Aged	1.7 ± 0.7 [b,c] ↑ Child [d]	4.3 ± 1.7 [b] ↑ Aged, Child [d]	—	—

[a] Racemic mixture of active S-(−)-hyoscyamine and inactive R-(+)-hyoscyamine.
[b] Values for active S-(−)-enantiomer.
[c] V_{area}.
[d] Less than 2 years of age.

Key: Adult = adults; Aged = aged; Alb = hypoalbuminemia; Arth = arthritis; Atr Fib = atrial fibrillation; AVH = acute viral hepatitis; Burn = burn patients; CAD = coronary artery disease; Celiac = celiac disease; CF = cystic fibrosis; CHF = congestive heart failure; Child = children; Cirr = cirrhosis; COPD = chronic obstructive pulmonary disease; CP = cor pulmonale; CPBS = cardiopulmonary bypass surgery; CRI = chronic respiratory insufficiency; Crohn = Crohn's disease; Cush = Cushing's syndrome; Epilep = epileptic; Fem = female; Hep = Hepatitis; HL = hyperlipoproteinemia; HTh = hyperthyroid; Inflam = inflammation; LTh = hypothyroid; MI = myocardial infarction; Neo = neonate; NS = nephrotic syndrome; Obes = obese; Pneu = pneumonia; Preg = pregnant; Prem = premature; RA = rheumatoid arthritis; Smk = smoking; Tach = ventricular tachycardia; Ulcer = ulcer patients; Urem = uremia

References: *See* end of table.

Table A–II–1. PHARMACOKINETIC DATA (Continued)

AVAILABILITY (ORAL) (%)	URINARY EXCRETION (%)	BOUND IN PLASMA (%)	CLEARANCE ($ml \cdot min^{-1} \cdot kg^{-1}$)	VOL. DIST. (*liters/kg*)	HALF-LIFE (*hours*)	EFFECTIVE CONCENTRATIONS	TOXIC CONCENTRATIONS
AURANOFIN [a] (Chapter 26)							
15–25	15	60	0.025 ± 0.016 [b]	0.045 [b]	17–25 days [c] 80 days [d]	0.5–0.7 μg/ml [e]	—

[a] Values refer to gold.
[b] CL/F and V_{area}/F, assuming 70-kg weight.
[c] Plasma measurements.
[d] $T_{1/2}$ calculated for whole body.
[e] Steady-state concentration range with 6-mg daily dose.

AVAILABILITY (ORAL) (%)	URINARY EXCRETION (%)	BOUND IN PLASMA (%)	CLEARANCE ($ml \cdot min^{-1} \cdot kg^{-1}$)	VOL. DIST. (*liters/kg*)	HALF-LIFE (*hours*)	EFFECTIVE CONCENTRATIONS	TOXIC CONCENTRATIONS
AZATHIOPRINE [a] (Chapter 53)							
60 ± 31 [b]	<2	—	57 ± 31 [c]	0.81 ± 0.65 [c]	0.16 ± 0.07 [c] ⟷ Urem	—	—

[a] Values given are for azathioprine. Azathioprine is metabolized to mercaptopurine. *See* Mercaptopurine for parameters for that compound.
[b] Determined by the availability of mercaptopurine.
[c] In kidney transplant patients.

AVAILABILITY (ORAL) (%)	URINARY EXCRETION (%)	BOUND IN PLASMA (%)	CLEARANCE ($ml \cdot min^{-1} \cdot kg^{-1}$)	VOL. DIST. (*liters/kg*)	HALF-LIFE (*hours*)	EFFECTIVE CONCENTRATIONS	TOXIC CONCENTRATIONS
AZLOCILLIN (Chapter 46)							
—	65 ± 9	28 ± 6 ⟷ Urem	Dose-dependent [a] ↓ Urem ⟷ CF	0.22 ± 0.06 ⟷ Urem, CF	1.4 ± 0.2 ↑ Urem, Neo, Prem ⟷ CF	*See* Chapter 46	—

[a] For 30-mg/kg dose, $CL = 3.1 \pm 0.7$ ml · min^{-1} · kg^{-1}; for 80-mg/kg dose, $CL = 2.2 \pm 0.4$ ml · min^{-1} · kg^{-1}.

AVAILABILITY (ORAL) (%)	URINARY EXCRETION (%)	BOUND IN PLASMA (%)	CLEARANCE ($ml \cdot min^{-1} \cdot kg^{-1}$)	VOL. DIST. (*liters/kg*)	HALF-LIFE (*hours*)	EFFECTIVE CONCENTRATIONS	TOXIC CONCENTRATIONS
BETAMETHASONE (Chapter 60)							
72 [a]	4.8 ± 1.4 ⟷ Preg	64 ± 6 [b] ⟷ Preg	2.9 ± 0.9 ⟷ Preg [c]	1.4 ± 0.3 [d] ⟷ Preg	5.6 ± 0.8 ⟷ Preg	—	—

[a] Calculated from separate studies of intravenous and oral administration. Predictions based on hepatic first-pass metabolism suggest availability <87%.
[b] Blood-to-plasma ratio = 1.1 ± 0.1.
[c] Increase in CL reported, but values not corrected for body weight of pregnant subjects.
[d] V_{area}.

BLEOMYCIN (Chapter 52)

—	68 ± 9	—	1.1 ± 0.3 ↓ Urem ⟷ Child	0.27 ± 0.09 ⟷ Child	3.1 ± 1.7 ↑ Urem ⟷ Child	—	—

BRETYLIUM (Chapter 35)

23 ± 9	77 ± 15	0–8	10.2 ± 1.9 ↓ Urem	5.9 ± 0.8	8.9 ± 1.8 ↑ Urem	—	—

BUMETANIDE (Chapter 28)

81 ± 18 ⟷ CHF	62 ± 20 ⟷ CHF	99 ± 0.3 ↓ Urem ⟷ CHF	2.6 ± 0.5 ↓ Urem, Cirr ⟷ CHF	0.13 ± 0.03 ↑ Urem	0.8 ± 0.2 ↑ CHF, Urem, Cirr	—	—

BUPIVACAINE (Chapter 15)

—	2 ± 2	95 ± 1 [a] ↓ Neo	7.1 ± 2.8 [b] ↑ Child ↓ Aged	0.9 ± 0.4 [b] ↑ Child	2.4 ± 1.2 ⟷ Aged, Child	—	>1.6 μg/ml

[a] Increased postoperatively with increased concentration of α_1-acid glycoprotein.

[b] Blood *CL* and V_{ss}; blood-to-plasma concentration ratio = 0.73 ± 0.05.

BUSULFAN (Chapter 52)

—	1	—	4.5 ± 0.9 [a]	0.99 ± 0.23 [a]	2.6 ± 0.5	—	—

[a] Oral administration; values are *CL/F* and V_{area}/F.

Key: Adult = adults; Aged = aged; Alb = hypoalbuminemia; Arth = arthritis; Atr Fib = atrial fibrillation; AVH = acute viral hepatitis; Burn = burn patients; CAD = coronary artery disease; Celiac = celiac disease; CF = cystic fibrosis; CHF = congestive heart failure; Child = children; Cirr = cirrhosis; COPD = chronic obstructive pulmonary disease; CP = cor pulmonale; CPBS = cardiopulmonary bypass surgery; CRI = chronic respiratory insufficiency; Crohn = Crohn's disease; Cush = Cushing's syndrome; Epilep = epileptic; Fem = female; Hep = Hepatitis; HL = hyperlipoproteinemia; HTh = hyperthyroid; Inflam = inflammation; LTh = hypothyroid; MI = myocardial infarction; Neo = neonate; NS = nephrotic syndrome; Obes = obese; Pneu = pneumonia; Preg = pregnant; Prem = premature; RA = rheumatoid arthritis; Smk = smoking; Tach = ventricular tachycardia; Ulcer = ulcer patients; Urem = uremia

References: *See* end of table.

Table A–II–1. PHARMACOKINETIC DATA (Continued)

AVAILABILITY (ORAL) (%)	URINARY EXCRETION (%)	BOUND IN PLASMA (%)	CLEARANCE ($ml \cdot min^{-1} \cdot kg^{-1}$)	VOL. DIST. (*liters/kg*)	HALF-LIFE (*hours*)	EFFECTIVE CONCENTRATIONS	TOXIC CONCENTRATIONS
CAFFEINE (Chapter 25)							
100 ± 13	1.1 ± 0.5	36 ± 7	1.4 ± 0.5 ↓ Neo ↑ Smk	0.61 ± 0.02	4.9 ± 1.8 ↑ Neo, Preg, Cirr ↓ Smk	—	—
CAPTOPRIL (Chapter 31)							
65	38 ± 11	30 ± 6 ↓ Urem ⟷ Aged	12.0 ± 1.4 ↓ Urem ⟷ Aged, CHF	0.81 ± 0.18 ↑ CHF	2.2 ± 0.5 ↑ Urem, CHF ⟷ Aged	50 ng/ml [a]	—

[a] Complete inhibition of converting enzyme.

AVAILABILITY (ORAL) (%)	URINARY EXCRETION (%)	BOUND IN PLASMA (%)	CLEARANCE ($ml \cdot min^{-1} \cdot kg^{-1}$)	VOL. DIST. (*liters/kg*)	HALF-LIFE (*hours*)	EFFECTIVE CONCENTRATIONS	TOXIC CONCENTRATIONS
CARBAMAZEPINE [a] (Chapter 19)							
>70	<1	74 ± 3 ⟷ Urem, Hep, Cirr, Epilep, Preg	1.3 ± 0.5 [b,c] ↑ Preg ⟷ Child, Aged, Smk	1.4 ± 0.4 [b] ⟷ Child, Neo, Smk	15 ± 5 [b,c] ⟷ Child, Neo, Aged	4–10 μg/ml [a] 6.5 ± 3.0 μg/ml [a,d]	>9 μg/ml [a,e]

[a] A metabolite, the 10,11-epoxide, is equipotent in animal studies; *see also* data for Carbamazepine-10,11-epoxide.
[b] Data from oral, multiple-dose regimen; values are CL/F and V_{area}/F.
[c] Data from multiple-dose regimen. Carbamazepine induces its own metabolism; for a single dose, $CL/F = 0.36 \pm 0.07$ ml · min^{-1} · kg^{-1} and half-life = 36 ± 5 hours.
[d] To achieve control of psychomotor seizures.
[e] Threshold concentration for prominent side effects, such as distinct drowsiness, ataxia, and diplopia.

AVAILABILITY (ORAL) (%)	URINARY EXCRETION (%)	BOUND IN PLASMA (%)	CLEARANCE ($ml \cdot min^{-1} \cdot kg^{-1}$)	VOL. DIST. (*liters/kg*)	HALF-LIFE (*hours*)	EFFECTIVE CONCENTRATIONS	TOXIC CONCENTRATIONS
CARBAMAZEPINE-10,11-EPOXIDE [a] (Chapter 19)							
90 ± 11 [b]	<1	50	1.7 ± 0.3 [c]	1.1 ± 0.2 [c]	7.4 ± 1.8 [c]	[d]	[d]

[a] Active metabolite of carbamazepine.
[b] Estimated.
[c] Data from single oral doses (100–200 mg); values are CL/F and V_{area}/F.
[d] Assumed to be equipotent with carbamazepine. In patients receiving only carbamazepine, ratio of plasma concentrations of epoxide to carbamazepine = 0.12; in patients also receiving phenytoin, primidone, phenobarbital, or valproic acid, ratio ~0.2.

CARBENICILLIN (Chapter 46)							
—	82 ± 9	50	$CL = 0.68\ CL_{cr} + 0.15$	0.18 [a]	1.0 ± 0.2 ↑ Urem, Hep [b], Prem, Neo	*See* Chapter 46	*See* Chapter 46

[a] Assuming 70-kg body weight.

[b] Half-life is markedly prolonged in oliguric patients with concomitant hepatic dysfunction.

CARMUSTINE (BCNU) (Chapter 52)							
—	—	—	56 ± 56	3.3 ± 1.7	1.5 ± 2.0	—	—

CEFACLOR (Chapter 46)							
[a]	52 ± 17	25	6.1 ± 1.5 [b] ↑ Child ↓ Urem	0.36 [b] ↑ Child	0.67 ± 0.33 ↑ Urem ⟷ Child	*See* Chapter 46	—

[a] At least equivalent to percent urinary excretion.

[b] CL/F and V_{area}/F.

CEFADROXIL (Chapter 46)							
100	93 ± 4	20	2.6 ± 0.6 [a] ↓ Urem	0.22 ± 0.05 [a] ⟷ Urem	1.1 ± 0.2 ↑ Urem	*See* Chapter 46	—

[a] CL/F and V_{area}/F.

Key: Adult = adults; Aged = aged; Alb = hypoalbuminemia; Arth = arthritis; Atr Fib = atrial fibrillation; AVH = acute viral hepatitis; Burn = burn patients; CAD = coronary artery disease; Celiac = celiac disease; CF = cystic fibrosis; CHF = congestive heart failure; Child = children; Cirr = cirrhosis; COPD = chronic obstructive pulmonary disease; CP = cor pulmonale; CPBS = cardiopulmonary bypass surgery; CRI = chronic respiratory insufficiency; Crohn = Crohn's disease; Cush = Cushing's syndrome; Epilep = epileptic; Fem = female; Hep = Hepatitis; HL = hyperlipoproteinemia; HTh = hyperthyroid; Inflam = inflammation; LTh = hypothyroid; MI = myocardial infarction; Neo = neonate; NS = nephrotic syndrome; Obes = obese; Pneu = pneumonia; Preg = pregnant; Prem = premature; RA = rheumatoid arthritis; Smk = smoking; Tach = ventricular tachycardia; Ulcer = ulcer patients; Urem = uremia

References: *See* end of table.

Table A–II–1. PHARMACOKINETIC DATA (Continued)

AVAILABILITY (ORAL) (%)	URINARY EXCRETION (%)	BOUND IN PLASMA (%)	CLEARANCE ($ml \cdot min^{-1} \cdot kg^{-1}$)	VOL. DIST. (*liters/kg*)	HALF-LIFE (*hours*)	EFFECTIVE CONCENTRATIONS	TOXIC CONCENTRATIONS
CEFAMANDOLE (Chapter 46)							
—	96 ± 3	74 ⟷ Urem [a]	2.8 ± 1.0 ↓ Urem	0.16 ± 0.05 ⟷ Urem, CPBS	0.78 ± 0.10 ↑ Urem, Neo, CPBS	*See* Chapter 46	—

[a] No difference observed between patients with normal and impaired renal function, but percent bound reported as 32% (range, 17–58%).

AVAILABILITY (ORAL) (%)	URINARY EXCRETION (%)	BOUND IN PLASMA (%)	CLEARANCE ($ml \cdot min^{-1} \cdot kg^{-1}$)	VOL. DIST. (*liters/kg*)	HALF-LIFE (*hours*)	EFFECTIVE CONCENTRATIONS	TOXIC CONCENTRATIONS
CEFAZOLIN (Chapter 46)							
—	80 ± 16	89 ± 2 ↓ Urem, CPBS, Neo, Child	0.95 ± 0.17 [a] ↓ Urem, CPBS ↑ Preg ⟷ Neo, Obes, Child	0.12 ± 0.03 [a] ↑ Urem, Neo ⟷ Preg, Obes, Child	1.8 ± 0.4 ↑ Urem, Neo, CPBS ↓ Preg ⟷ Obes, Child	*See* Chapter 46	—

[a] Assuming 70-kg weight.

AVAILABILITY (ORAL) (%)	URINARY EXCRETION (%)	BOUND IN PLASMA (%)	CLEARANCE ($ml \cdot min^{-1} \cdot kg^{-1}$)	VOL. DIST. (*liters/kg*)	HALF-LIFE (*hours*)	EFFECTIVE CONCENTRATIONS	TOXIC CONCENTRATIONS
CEFONICID (Chapter 46)							
—	88 ± 6 ⟷ Child	98	0.32 ± 0.06 ↓ Urem ↑ Child	0.11 ± 0.01 ⟷ Urem ↑ Child	4.4 ± 0.8 ↑ Urem ⟷ Child	*See* Chapter 46	—
CEFOPERAZONE (Chapter 46)							
—	29 ± 4 ↑ Cirr	89–93 [a]	1.2 ± 0.1 ⟷ Cirr, Urem ↓ Hep	0.09 ± 0.01 [b] ↑ Cirr ⟷ Urem, Hep	2.1 ± 0.3 ↑ Cirr, Hep, Aged ⟷ Urem	*See* Chapter 46	—

[a] Nonlinear binding; value decreases from 93% at 25 μg/ml to 89% at 250 μg/ml.

[b] V_{area} is about 50% larger than V_{ss} given here.

AVAILABILITY (ORAL) (%)	URINARY EXCRETION (%)	BOUND IN PLASMA (%)	CLEARANCE ($ml \cdot min^{-1} \cdot kg^{-1}$)	VOL. DIST. (*liters/kg*)	HALF-LIFE (*hours*)	EFFECTIVE CONCENTRATIONS	TOXIC CONCENTRATIONS
CEFORANIDE (Chapter 46)							
—	84 ± 3	80–82	$CL = 0.26\ CL_{cr} + 0.07$	0.14 ± 0.04 ⟷ Urem	2.6 ± 0.5 ↑ Urem	*See* Chapter 46	—

CEFOTAXIME [a] (Chapter 46)							
—	50 ± 5	36 ⟷ Cirr [b]	3.7 ± 0.6 ↓ Urem [c], Cirr [b], Fem ⟷ Obes	0.23 ± 0.06 ⟷ Urem, Obes ↑ Cirr [b]	1.1 ± 0.3 ↑ Urem, Cirr [b] ⟷ Obes	*See* Chapter 46	—

[a] Active metabolite, desacetylcefotaxime, accounts for 16 ± 4% of dose excreted; $t_{1/2}$ = 2.2 ± 0.3 hours.

[b] Cirrhotic patients with ascites.

[c] Nonrenal clearance also decreased in end-stage renal disease.

CEFOTETAN (Chapter 46)							
—	61 ± 1	88 ± 3	0.42 ± 0.05 ↓ Urem	0.13 ± 0.02 ⟷ Urem	3.5 ± 1.1 ↑ Urem	*See* Chapter 46	—

CEFOXITIN (Chapter 46)							
—	78	73	$CL = 3.3\ CL_{cr} + 0.19$	0.31 ± 0.12 ↑ Neo ⟷ Child, Urem	0.65 ± 0.09 ↑ Neo, Urem ↓ Child	*See* Chapter 46	—

CEFTAZIDIME (Chapter 46)							
—	84 ± 4 ⟷ CF	21 ± 6	$CL = 1.05\ CL_{cr} + 0.12$ ⟷ CF, Burn	0.23 ± 0.02 ⟷ Urem, CF ↑ Aged, Burn	1.6 ± 0.1 ↑ Urem, Prem, Neo, Aged ⟷ CF	*See* Chapter 46	—

Key: Adult = adults; Aged = aged; Alb = hypoalbuminemia; Arth = arthritis; Atr Fib = atrial fibrillation; AVH = acute viral hepatitis; Burn = burn patients; CAD = coronary artery disease; Celiac = celiac disease; CF = cystic fibrosis; CHF = congestive heart failure; Child = children; Cirr = cirrhosis; COPD = chronic obstructive pulmonary disease; CP = cor pulmonale; CPBS = cardiopulmonary bypass surgery; CRI = chronic respiratory insufficiency; Crohn = Crohn's disease; Cush = Cushing's syndrome; Epilep = epileptic; Fem = female; Hep = Hepatitis; HL = hyperlipoproteinemia; HTh = hyperthyroid; Inflam = inflammation; LTh = hypothyroid; MI = myocardial infarction; Neo = neonate; NS = nephrotic syndrome; Obes = obese; Pneu = pneumonia; Preg = pregnant; Prem = premature; RA = rheumatoid arthritis; Smk = smoking; Tach = ventricular tachycardia; Ulcer = ulcer patients; Urem = uremia

References: *See* end of table.

Table A–II–1. PHARMACOKINETIC DATA (Continued)

AVAILABILITY (ORAL) (%)	URINARY EXCRETION (%)	BOUND IN PLASMA (%)	CLEARANCE ($ml \cdot min^{-1} \cdot kg^{-1}$)	VOL. DIST. (*liters/kg*)	HALF-LIFE (*hours*)	EFFECTIVE CONCENTRATIONS	TOXIC CONCENTRATIONS
CEFTIZOXIME (Chapter 46)							
—	93 ± 8	28 ± 5 [a]	$CL = 1.1\ CL_{cr} + 0.07$	0.36 ± 0.19 ⟷ Urem	1.8 ± 0.7 ↑ Urem	*See* Chapter 46	—

[a] Values ranging between 28 and 65% have been reported.

AVAILABILITY (ORAL) (%)	URINARY EXCRETION (%)	BOUND IN PLASMA (%)	CLEARANCE ($ml \cdot min^{-1} \cdot kg^{-1}$)	VOL. DIST. (*liters/kg*)	HALF-LIFE (*hours*)	EFFECTIVE CONCENTRATIONS	TOXIC CONCENTRATIONS
CEFTRIAXONE (Chapter 46)							
—	46 ± 7 [a] ↑ Neo, Child	90–95 [b] ↓ Cirr, Neo, Child ⟷ Aged	0.24 ± 0.06 ↓ Urem, Neo [c], Aged [c] ↑ Cirr, CF ⟷ CPBS	0.16 ± 0.03 [d] ↑ Neo, Cirr, CF, CPBS ⟷ Urem, Aged	7.3 ± 1.6 ↑ Urem [e], Aged, Neo, CPBS ⟷ Cirr	*See* Chapter 46	—

[a] Remainder via biliary excretion.
[b] Saturable binding (5% unbound at plasma concentration of 70 μg/ml; >40% unbound at 600 μg/ml); lower binding increases plasma clearance.
[c] Clearance of free drug.
[d] V_{area}.
[e] Usually minor, but can increase to 50 hours in end-stage renal disease.

AVAILABILITY (ORAL) (%)	URINARY EXCRETION (%)	BOUND IN PLASMA (%)	CLEARANCE ($ml \cdot min^{-1} \cdot kg^{-1}$)	VOL. DIST. (*liters/kg*)	HALF-LIFE (*hours*)	EFFECTIVE CONCENTRATIONS	TOXIC CONCENTRATIONS
CEFUROXIME (Chapter 46)							
—	96 ± 10	33 ± 6	$CL = 0.94\ CL_{cr} + 0.28$	0.19 ± 0.04 ⟷ Urem, Aged	1.7 ± 0.6 ↑ Urem	*See* Chapter 46	—
CEPHALEXIN (Chapter 46)							
90 ± 9	91 ± 18	14 ± 3	4.3 ± 1.1 [a] ↓ Urem	0.26 ± 0.03 [a] ⟷ Urem	0.90 ± 0.18 ↑ Urem	*See* Chapter 46	—

[a] Assuming 70-kg weight.

AVAILABILITY (ORAL) (%)	URINARY EXCRETION (%)	BOUND IN PLASMA (%)	CLEARANCE ($ml \cdot min^{-1} \cdot kg^{-1}$)	VOL. DIST. (*liters/kg*)	HALF-LIFE (*hours*)	EFFECTIVE CONCENTRATIONS	TOXIC CONCENTRATIONS
CEPHALOTHIN (Chapter 46)							
—	52	71 ± 3	6.7 ± 1.7 [a] ↓ Urem, CPBS	0.26 ± 0.11 [a] ↑ Child	0.57 ± 0.32 ↑ Urem, CPBS	*See* Chapter 46	—

[a] Assuming 70-kg weight; one-compartment model.

CEPHAPIRIN (Chapter 46)							
—	48 ± 7	62 ± 4	6.9 ± 2.0 ↓ Urem	0.21 ± 0.06	0.72 ± 0.18 ↑ Urem	*See* Chapter 46	—
CEPHRADINE (Chapter 46)							
>90 ⟷ Preg	86 ± 10 [a]	14 ± 3	5.1 ± 1.2 [b] ↓ Urem ↑ Preg	0.25 ± 0.01 [b] ⟷ Preg	0.77 ± 0.30 ↑ Urem ↓ Preg	*See* Chapter 46	—

[a] Oral dose.

[b] Assuming 70-kg weight.

CHLORAMBUCIL [a] (Chapter 52)							
87 ± 20	<1 [b]	99	2.6 ± 0.9 [c]	0.29 ± 0.21 [c,d]	1.3 ± 0.9	—	—

[a] Active metabolite, phenylacetic acid mustard. AUC (following chlorambucil) about 25% greater than parent drug; $t_{1/2}$ = 2.0 ± 1.1 hours.

[b] Drug and active metabolite.

[c] Assuming 70-kg weight.

[d] V_{area}.

CHLORAMPHENICOL (Chapter 48)							
75–90 69 ± 13 [a]	25 ± 15 [a]	53 ± 5 ↓ Cirr, Prem, Neo ⟷ Urem	2.4 ± 0.2 ↓ Cirr, Prem, Neo ⟷ Urem	0.94 ± 0.06 ⟷ Cirr	4.0 ± 2.0 [b] ↑ Cirr, Prem, Neo ⟷ Urem	*See* Chapter 48	*See* Chapter 48

[a] After intravenous administration of succinate ester; 27 ± 11% excreted as the ester.

[b] Shorter half-life reported previously due to substantial elimination of the succinate ester. Value given here is for parent drug (*i.e.*, chloramphenicol) only.

Key: Adult = adults; Aged = aged; Alb = hypoalbuminemia; Arth = arthritis; Atr Fib = atrial fibrillation; AVH = acute viral hepatitis; Burn = burn patients; CAD = coronary artery disease; Celiac = celiac disease; CF = cystic fibrosis; CHF = congestive heart failure; Child = children; Cirr = cirrhosis; COPD = chronic obstructive pulmonary disease; CP = cor pulmonale; CPBS = cardiopulmonary bypass surgery; CRI = chronic respiratory insufficiency; Crohn = Crohn's disease; Cush = Cushing's syndrome; Epilep = epileptic; Fem = female; Hep = Hepatitis; HL = hyperlipoproteinemia; HTh = hyperthyroid; Inflam = inflammation; LTh = hypothyroid; MI = myocardial infarction; Neo = neonate; NS = nephrotic syndrome; Obes = obese; Pneu = pneumonia; Preg = pregnant; Prem = premature; RA = rheumatoid arthritis; Smk = smoking; Tach = ventricular tachycardia; Ulcer = ulcer patients; Urem = uremia

References: *See* end of table.

Table A–II–1. PHARMACOKINETIC DATA (Continued)

AVAILABILITY (ORAL) (%)	URINARY EXCRETION (%)	BOUND IN PLASMA (%)	CLEARANCE (*ml* · *min*$^{-1}$ · *kg*$^{-1}$)	VOL. DIST. (*liters/kg*)	HALF-LIFE (*hours*)	EFFECTIVE CONCENTRATIONS	TOXIC CONCENTRATIONS
CHLORDIAZEPOXIDE [a] (Chapters 17, 18)							
100	<1	96.5 ± 1.8 ↓ AVH, Cirr ⟷ Aged	0.54 ± 0.49 ↓ Aged, AVH, Cirr ↑ Fem ⟷ Smk	0.30 ± 0.03 ↑ Aged, Fem, AVH [b], Cirr [b]	10.0 ± 3.4 ↑ Aged, AVH, Cirr	>0.7 μg/ml [c]	—

[a] Active metabolites: desmethylchlordiazepoxide, demoxepam, desmethyldiazepam, and oxazepam.
[b] Because of decreased binding to plasma protein; V_{ss} for free drug is unchanged. Other data suggest no change in V_{area} in patients with cirrhosis.
[c] Decrease in anxiety and hostility; reduction in anxiety correlates with steady-state concentrations of metabolites (desmethylchlordiazepoxide and demoxepam) but not with that of chlordiazepoxide.

AVAILABILITY (ORAL) (%)	URINARY EXCRETION (%)	BOUND IN PLASMA (%)	CLEARANCE (*ml* · *min*$^{-1}$ · *kg*$^{-1}$)	VOL. DIST. (*liters/kg*)	HALF-LIFE (*hours*)	EFFECTIVE CONCENTRATIONS	TOXIC CONCENTRATIONS
CHLOROQUINE [a] (Chapter 41)							
89 ± 16	61 ± 4	61 ± 9 ⟷ RA	1.8 ± 0.4 [b]	115 ± 61 [b]	41 ± 14 days [b,c]	15 ng/ml [d] 30 ng/ml [e]	0.25 μg/ml [f]

[a] Active metabolite, desethylchloroquine, accounts for 20 ± 3% of urinary excretion; $t_{1/2}$ = 15 ± 6 days.
[b] Blood *CL/F*, V_{ss}/F, and $t_{1/2}$; blood-to-plasma ratio = 9.
[c] Shorter half-lives reported previously when sampling stopped after 1 month.
[d] *Plasmodium vivax.*
[e] *P. falciparum.*
[f] Diplopia; dizziness.

AVAILABILITY (ORAL) (%)	URINARY EXCRETION (%)	BOUND IN PLASMA (%)	CLEARANCE (*ml* · *min*$^{-1}$ · *kg*$^{-1}$)	VOL. DIST. (*liters/kg*)	HALF-LIFE (*hours*)	EFFECTIVE CONCENTRATIONS	TOXIC CONCENTRATIONS
CHLOROTHIAZIDE (Chapter 28)							
Dose-dependent [a]	92 ± 5	94.6 ± 1.3	4.5 ± 1.7 ↓ Urem	0.20 ± 0.08	1.5 ± 0.2 ↑ Urem, CHF [b]	—	—

[a] Ranges from 56% for 50-mg dose to 9% for 1-g dose.
[b] May reflect decreased renal function in elderly patients, rather than CHF.

AVAILABILITY (ORAL) (%)	URINARY EXCRETION (%)	BOUND IN PLASMA (%)	CLEARANCE (*ml* · *min*$^{-1}$ · *kg*$^{-1}$)	VOL. DIST. (*liters/kg*)	HALF-LIFE (*hours*)	EFFECTIVE CONCENTRATIONS	TOXIC CONCENTRATIONS
CHLORPHENIRAMINE [a] (Chapter 23)							
41 ± 16	0.3–26 [b]	70 ± 3	1.7 ± 0.1 ↑ Child	3.2 ± 0.3 ⟷ Child	20 ± 5 ↓ Child	—	—

[a] Administered as racemic mixture; parameters are for racemic drug. Activity predominantly from S-(+)-enantiomer, which has 60% longer $t_{1/2}$ than R-(−)-enantiomer.
[b] Renal elimination increases with increased urine flow and lower pH.

CHLORPROMAZINE [a] (Chapter 18)							
32 ± 19 [b]	<1	95–98 ⟷ Urem	8.6 ± 2.9 [c] ↓ Child [d] ⟷ Cirr	21 ± 9 [c]	30 ± 7	30–350 ng/ml [e] Children: 40–80 ng/ml	750–1000 ng/ml [f]

[a] Active metabolites: 7-hydroxychlorpromazine ($t_{1/2}$ = 25 ± 15 hours) and possibly chlorpromazine N-oxide ($t_{1/2}$ = 6.7 ± 1.4 hours) yield AUCs comparable to the parent drug (single doses).
[b] After single dose. Availability may decrease to about 20% with repeated administration.
[c] $CL/F_{intramuscular}$ and $V_{area,\ intramuscular}$.
[d] CL/F_{oral}; there may be induction of metabolism and dose-dependent kinetics.
[e] Values are controversial because of several active and inactive metabolites.
[f] Neurotoxicity (tremors and convulsions).

CHLORPROPAMIDE (Chapter 61)							
>90 [a]	20 ± 18 [b]	96 ± 0.6	0.030 ± 0.005 [c,d]	0.097 ± 0.011 [c]	33 ± 6 [e]	—	—

[a] Predicted.
[b] Dependent on urinary pH; acidic urine, 1.4 ± 0.5%, basic urine, 85 ± 11%.
[c] CL/F and V_{area}/F.
[d] Acidic urine, 0.018 ± 0.006 $ml \cdot min^{-1} \cdot kg^{-1}$; basic urine, 0.086 ± 0.013 $ml \cdot min^{-1} \cdot kg^{-1}$.
[e] Acidic urine, 69 ± 26 hours; basic urine, 13 ± 3 hours.

CHLORTHALIDONE (Chapter 28)							
64 ± 10	65 ± 9 [a]	75 ± 1 [b]	1.6 ± 0.3 ↓ Aged	3.9 ± 0.8	44 ± 10 [c] ↑ Aged	—	—

[a] Value is for 50- and 100-mg doses; renal clearance is decreased at an oral dose of 200 mg, and there is a concomitant decrease in the percentage excreted unchanged.
[b] Blood-to-plasma ratio = 72.5.
[c] Chlorthalidone is sequestered in erythrocytes; the half-life is longer if blood, rather than plasma, is analyzed.

CIMETIDINE (Chapter 37)							
62 ± 6 [a]	62 ± 20 ⟷ Cirr, CF	19	8.3 ± 2.0 ↓ Urem, Aged ⟷ Ulcer, Cirr ↑ Burn, CF	1.0 ± 0.2 ⟷ Urem, Cirr, Ulcer, Burn ↑ CF	2.0 ± 0.3 ↑ Urem ⟷ Ulcer, Cirr, CF ↓ Burn	0.78 μg/ml 3.9 μg/ml [b]	—

[a] Oral liquid and tablets are equivalent; value is the same in patients with ulcers.
[b] Concentrations to inhibit gastric acid secretion by 50% and 90%, respectively.

Key: Adult = adults; Aged = aged; Alb = hypoalbuminemia; Arth = arthritis; Atr Fib = atrial fibrillation; AVH = acute viral hepatitis; Burn = burn patients; CAD = coronary artery disease; Celiac = celiac disease; CF = cystic fibrosis; CHF = congestive heart failure; Child = children; Cirr = cirrhosis; COPD = chronic obstructive pulmonary disease; CP = cor pulmonale; CPBS = cardiopulmonary bypass surgery; CRI = chronic respiratory insufficiency; Crohn = Crohn's disease; Cush = Cushing's syndrome; Epilep = epileptic; Fem = female; Hep = Hepatitis; HL = hyperlipoproteinemia; HTh = hyperthyroid; Inflam = inflammation; LTh = hypothyroid; MI = myocardial infarction; Neo = neonate; NS = nephrotic syndrome; Obes = obese; Pneu = pneumonia; Preg = pregnant; Prem = premature; RA = rheumatoid arthritis; Smk = smoking; Tach = ventricular tachycardia; Ulcer = ulcer patients; Urem = uremia

References: *See* end of table.

Table A–II–1. PHARMACOKINETIC DATA (Continued)

AVAILABILITY (ORAL) (%)	URINARY EXCRETION (%)	BOUND IN PLASMA (%)	CLEARANCE ($ml \cdot min^{-1} \cdot kg^{-1}$)	VOL. DIST. (*liters/kg*)	HALF-LIFE (*hours*)	EFFECTIVE CONCENTRATIONS	TOXIC CONCENTRATIONS
CINOXACIN (Chapter 45)							
[a]	60–85 [a]	63	2.5	0.33 [b]	2.1	*See* Chapter 45	—
[a] Bioavailability at least equal to percent excreted unchanged after oral administration.				[b] V_{area}.			
CIPROFLOXACIN (Chapter 45)							
60 ± 12	65 ± 12	40	6.0 ± 1.2 ↓ Urem, Aged ↑ CF	1.8 ± 0.4 ↓ Aged ⟷ CF	4.1 ± 0.9 ↑ Urem ⟷ Aged ↓ CF	*See* Chapter 45	—
CISPLATIN [a] (Chapter 52)							
—	23 ± 9	—	6.3 ± 1.2	0.28 ± 0.07	0.53 ± 0.10	—	—
[a] Early studies measured total platinum, rather than the parent compound; values reported here are for cisplatin in seven patients with ovarian cancer; mean CL_{cr} = 66 ± 27 ml/min.							
CLAVULANIC ACID [a] (Chapter 46)							
75 ± 21	43 ± 14	9	3.6 ± 1.0 [b] ↓ Urem ⟷ Child	0.21 ± 0.05 [b] ⟷ Urem, Child	0.9 ± 0.1 ↑ Neo, Urem ⟷ Child	—	—
[a] Kinetic parameters do not change appreciably in presence of amoxicillin or ticarcillin.				[b] Assuming 70-kg weight.			
CLINDAMYCIN (Chapter 48)							
~87 [a] Topical: 2	13	93.6 ± 0.2	4.7 ± 1.3 ⟷ Child	1.1 ± 0.3 [b] ⟷ Urem, Child	2.9 ± 0.7 ⟷ Child, Urem, Preg ↑ Prem	*See* Chapter 48	—
[a] Clindamycin hydrochloride.				[b] V_{area}.			

CLOFIBRATE [a] (Chapter 36)

95 ± 10	5.7 ± 2.1 [b]	96.5 ± 0.3 [c] ↓ NS, Cirr, Urem ⟷ AVH	0.12 ± 0.01 [b] ↑ NS ↓ Urem [d] ⟷ AVH, Cirr	0.11 ± 0.02 [b] ↑ Cirr, Urem	13 ± 3 ↑ Urem [d]	—	—

[a] Clofibrate is the ethyl ester of *p*-chlorophenoxyisobutyric acid (CPIB). All values are for CPIB, since clofibrate is rapidly deesterified upon absorption.
[b] Oral dosage; *CL/F* and V_{area}/F.
[c] Binding may decrease at high concentrations of CPIB (>200 μg/ml).
[d] Due to accumulation of glucuronide metabolite, which is hydrolyzed back to parent drug.

CLONAZEPAM (Chapters 17, 19)

98 ± 31	<1	86 ± 0.5 ↓ Neo	1.55 ± 0.28 [a]	3.2 ± 1.1	23 ± 5	5–70 ng/ml [b]	[c]

[a] *CL/F*; this value is consistent for a number of studies, but it is higher than the clearance determined in a single study of intravenous administration.
[b] Most patients, including children, whose seizures are controlled by clonazepam have concentrations of the drug in plasma in this range. However, patients who do not respond and those with side effects display similar values.
[c] Occurrence of side effects is apparently not correlated with concentrations of clonazepam or its 7-amino metabolite.

CLONIDINE (Chapters 10, 33)

95	62 ± 11	20	3.1 ± 1.2 ↓ Urem	2.1 ± 0.4	12 ± 7 ↑ Urem	0.2–2 ng/ml [a]	1 ng/ml [b]

[a] Reduction in blood pressure.
[b] Sedation, dry mouth.

CLORAZEPATE [a] (Chapters 17, 18, 19)

—	<1	—	1.8 ± 0.2 [b] ↑ Preg	0.33 ± 0.17 [b] ⟷ Preg	2.0 ± 0.9 ↓ Preg	—	—

[a] Clorazepate is essentially a prodrug for desmethyldiazepam; *see also* listing for that compound. Values presented here are for clorazepate.
[b] *CL/F* and V_{area}/F.

Key: Adult = adults; Aged = aged; Alb = hypoalbuminemia; Arth = arthritis; Atr Fib = atrial fibrillation; AVH = acute viral hepatitis; Burn = burn patients; CAD = coronary artery disease; Celiac = celiac disease; CF = cystic fibrosis; CHF = congestive heart failure; Child = children; Cirr = cirrhosis; COPD = chronic obstructive pulmonary disease; CP = cor pulmonale; CPBS = cardiopulmonary bypass surgery; CRI = chronic respiratory insufficiency; Crohn = Crohn's disease; Cush = Cushing's syndrome; Epilep = epileptic; Fem = female; Hep = Hepatitis; HL = hyperlipoproteinemia; HTh = hyperthyroid; Inflam = inflammation; LTh = hypothyroid; MI = myocardial infarction; Neo = neonate; NS = nephrotic syndrome; Obes = obese; Pneu = pneumonia; Preg = pregnant; Prem = premature; RA = rheumatoid arthritis; Smk = smoking; Tach = ventricular tachycardia; Ulcer = ulcer patients; Urem = uremia

References: *See* end of table.

Table A–II–1. PHARMACOKINETIC DATA (Continued)

AVAILABILITY (ORAL) (%)	URINARY EXCRETION (%)	BOUND IN PLASMA (%)	CLEARANCE ($ml \cdot min^{-1} \cdot kg^{-1}$)	VOL. DIST. (*liters/kg*)	HALF-LIFE (*hours*)	EFFECTIVE CONCENTRATIONS	TOXIC CONCENTRATIONS
CLOXACILLIN (Chapter 46)							
43 ± 16 ↑ Urem ⟷ CF	75 ± 14	94.6 ± 0.6 ⟷ CF	2.2 ± 0.5 [a] ↓ Urem ↑ CF	0.094 ± 0.015 [a] ↑ CF, Urem	0.55 ± 0.07 ↑ Urem	*See* Chapter 46	—

[a] Assuming 70-kg weight.

COCAINE (Chapters 15, 22)							
57 ± 19 [a]	<2	91	32 ± 6 [b]	2.0 ± 0.2	0.8 ± 0.2	—	—

[a] Intranasal; 100-mg total dose. Smoking ~70%.
[b] Blood-to-plasma ratio ~1.0.

CODEINE [a] (Chapter 21)							
50 ± 7 [b]	Negligible	7	11 ± 2 [c]	2.6 ± 0.3 [c]	2.9 ± 0.7	65 ng/ml	—

[a] Active metabolite, morphine.
[b] Oral/intramuscular availability.
[c] *CL/F* and V_{area}/F for intramuscular dose.

CYCLOPHOSPHAMIDE [a] (Chapter 52)							
74 ± 22	6.5 ± 4.3	13	1.3 ± 0.5 ↑ Child ↓ Cirr ⟷ Urem	0.78 ± 0.57 ⟷ Child	7.5 ± 4.0 ↓ Child ↑ Cirr	—	—

[a] Cyclophosphamide is activated by hepatic metabolism (*see* Chapter 52); kinetic parameters are for cyclophosphamide itself. Active metabolites include phosphoramide mustard ($t_{1/2}$ = 9 hours) and nornitrogen mustard ($t_{1/2}$ = 3.3 hours).

CYCLOSPORINE [a] (Chapter 53)							
23 ± 7 [b]	<1	93 ± 2	5.9 ± 1.0 [b] ↓ Hep, Cirr, Aged ⟷ Urem ↑ Child	1.2 ± 0.2 [b] ↓ Aged ↑ Child	5.6 ± 2 [b] ↓ Child ⟷ Aged	*See* Chapter 53	*See* Chapter 53

[a] Active metabolites, but relevance uncertain.
[b] Measurements in blood with a specific assay.

CYTARABINE (Chapter 52)

20	11 ± 8	13	13 ± 4	3.0 ± 1.9	2.6 ± 0.6	—	—

DAPSONE (Chapter 49)

93 ± 8 [a]	15 [b]	73 ± 1 ⟷ Urem	0.60 ± 0.17	1.0 ± 0.1	22 ± 6	—	—

[a] Decreased in severe leprosy.
[b] Urine pH = 6–7.

DESIPRAMINE (Chapter 18)

38 ± 13	2	82 ± 2 ⟷ Urem	10 ± 2 [a,b] ↓ Aged	20 ± 3 [c]	22 ± 5 ↑ Aged	40–160 ng/ml	>1 μg/ml [d]

[a] Blood-to-plasma ratio = 0.96 ± 0.08.
[b] Significantly lower in a Chinese population and higher in alcoholics.
[c] V_{area}.
[d] Combined data for toxic effects of tricyclic antidepressants.

DESMETHYLDIAZEPAM (NORDAZEPAM) [a] (Chapters 17, 18, 19)

99 ± 6	<1	97.5 ↓ Urem ⟷ Obes, Aged	0.14 ± 0.05 [b] ↑ Smk ↓ Hep, Cirr, Obes, Aged [c] ⟷ Preg	0.78 ± 0.12 [d] ↑ Obes, Preg ⟷ Hep, Cirr, Aged	73 ± 33 [b] ↑ Obes, Preg, Aged [c] ↓ Hep, Cirr, Smk	—	—

[a] Desmethyldiazepam is the active species delivered after oral administration of clorazepate and prazepam. It is an active metabolite of diazepam and is itself metabolized to oxazepam.
[b] Genetic variability in clearance related to hydroxylation phenotype.
[c] In males only.
[d] V_{area}.

Key: Adult = adults; Aged = aged; Alb = hypoalbuminemia; Arth = arthritis; Atr Fib = atrial fibrillation; AVH = acute viral hepatitis; Burn = burn patients; CAD = coronary artery disease; Celiac = celiac disease; CF = cystic fibrosis; CHF = congestive heart failure; Child = children; Cirr = cirrhosis; COPD = chronic obstructive pulmonary disease; CP = cor pulmonale; CPBS = cardiopulmonary bypass surgery; CRI = chronic respiratory insufficiency; Crohn = Crohn's disease; Cush = Cushing's syndrome; Epilep = epileptic; Fem = female; Hep = Hepatitis; HL = hyperlipoproteinemia; HTh = hyperthyroid; Inflam = inflammation; LTh = hypothyroid; MI = myocardial infarction; Neo = neonate; NS = nephrotic syndrome; Obes = obese; Pneu = pneumonia; Preg = pregnant; Prem = premature; RA = rheumatoid arthritis; Smk = smoking; Tach = ventricular tachycardia; Ulcer = ulcer patients; Urem = uremia

References: *See* end of table.

Table A–II–1. PHARMACOKINETIC DATA (Continued)

AVAILABILITY (ORAL) (%)	URINARY EXCRETION (%)	BOUND IN PLASMA (%)	CLEARANCE ($ml \cdot min^{-1} \cdot kg^{-1}$)	VOL. DIST. (*liters/kg*)	HALF-LIFE (*hours*)	EFFECTIVE CONCENTRATIONS	TOXIC CONCENTRATIONS
DEXAMETHASONE (Chapter 60)							
78 ± 14 ⟷ Smk	2.6 ± 0.6	68 ± 3 ⟷ Preg	3.7 ± 0.9 ↑ Preg ⟷ Smk	0.82 ± 0.22 ⟷ Smk, Preg	3.0 ± 0.8 ⟷ Smk, Preg	—	—
DIAZEPAM [a] (Chapters 17, 18, 19)							
100 ± 14	<1	98.7 ± 0.2 ↓ Urem, Cirr, NS, Preg, Neo, Alb [b], Burn ⟷ Aged, HTh	0.38 ± 0.06 [a] ↑ Alb, Epilep [c] ↓ Cirr, Hep ⟷ Aged, Smk, HTh	1.1 ± 0.3 ↑ Cirr, Aged, Alb ⟷ Urem, HTh	43 ± 13 [a] ↑ Aged, Cirr, Hep ↓ Epilep [c] ⟷ HTh	300–400 ng/ml [d] >600 ng/ml [e]	—

[a] Active metabolites, desmethyldiazepam and oxazepam; *see also* listings for those compounds. Genetic variability in clearance related to hydroxylation phenotype.
[b] Alcoholics.
[c] Due to administration of other drugs that induce metabolic enzymes.
[d] Anxiolytic.
[e] For control of seizures.

AVAILABILITY (ORAL) (%)	URINARY EXCRETION (%)	BOUND IN PLASMA (%)	CLEARANCE ($ml \cdot min^{-1} \cdot kg^{-1}$)	VOL. DIST. (*liters/kg*)	HALF-LIFE (*hours*)	EFFECTIVE CONCENTRATIONS	TOXIC CONCENTRATIONS
DIAZOXIDE (Chapters 33, 61)							
86–96	20–50	94 ± 14 [a] ↓ Urem	0.06 ± 0.02	0.21 ± 0.02	48 ± 12	35 μg/ml [b]	—

[a] Decreased at higher concentrations (*e.g.*, 84% at 250 μg/ml).
[b] 20% reduction in mean arterial pressure.

AVAILABILITY (ORAL) (%)	URINARY EXCRETION (%)	BOUND IN PLASMA (%)	CLEARANCE ($ml \cdot min^{-1} \cdot kg^{-1}$)	VOL. DIST. (*liters/kg*)	HALF-LIFE (*hours*)	EFFECTIVE CONCENTRATIONS	TOXIC CONCENTRATIONS
DICLOFENAC (Chapter 26)							
54 ± 2	<1	>99.5	4.2 ± 0.9 ↓ Aged ⟷ Urem, Cirr, RA	0.17 ± 0.11 ↑ RA	1.1 ± 0.2 ⟷ RA	—	—
DICLOXACILLIN (Chapter 46)							
50–85	60 ± 7	95.8 ± 0.2 ↓ Urem ⟷ CF	1.6 ± 0.3 [a,b] ↓ Urem ↑ CF [c]	0.086 ± 0.017 [a] ↑ Urem, CF	0.70 ± 0.07 ↑ Urem ⟷ CF	*See* Chapter 46	—

[a] Assuming 70-kg weight.
[b] Possible saturation of renal clearance at doses of 1–2 g.
[c] Concomitant increase in clearance of both drug and creatinine.

DIFLUNISAL (Chapter 26)							
~90	6 ± 3	99.9 ± 0.01 [a] ↓ Urem	0.10 ± 0.02 [b,c] ↓ Urem [d] ⟷ Aged, RA	0.10 ± 0.01 [b] ↑ Urem ⟷ Aged, RA	11 ± 2 [b,c] ↑ Urem [d] ⟷ Aged, RA	—	—

[a] Decreases at concentrations >100 μg/ml.
[b] Values at 500-mg dose, assuming F = 90%.
[c] Like salicylic acid, kinetic parameters of diflunisal are dependent on drug concentration; CL decreases and $t_{1/2}$ increases at higher concentrations.
[d] Because of accumulation of acyl glucuronide, which is hydrolyzed back to parent drug.

DIGITOXIN [a] (Chapter 34)							
>90 ⟷ Urem, Child	32 ± 15	97 ± 0.5 ↓ NS, Urem ⟷ Child	0.055 ± 0.018 ↑ NS, Child ⟷ Aged, Urem	0.54 ± 0.14 ↑ Child ⟷ Aged, Urem	6.7 ± 1.7 days ↓ NS ⟷ Aged, Urem, Child	>10 ng/ml	29, 39, 48 ng/ml [b]

[a] Values for unchanged drug and cardioactive metabolites.
[b] Concentrations causing arrhythmias or other abnormal conduction in 10, 50, and 90% of patients, respectively.

DIGOXIN (Chapter 34)							
70 ± 13 [a] ⟷ Urem, MI, CHF, LTh, HTh, Aged	60 ± 11	25 ± 5 ↓ Urem	CL = (0.88 CL_{cr} + 0.33) ± 52% [b,c] ↓ LTh ↑ HTh, Neo, Child, Preg	V = (3.12 CL_{cr} + 3.84) ± 30% ↓ LTh ↑ HTh ⟷ CHF	39 ± 13 ↓ HTh ↑ Urem, CHF, Aged, LTh ⟷ Obes	>0.8 ng/ml [d]	1.7, 2.5, 3.3 ng/ml [e] ↑ Child

[a] LANOXIN tablets; digoxin solutions, elixirs, and capsules may be absorbed more completely.
[b] Equation applies to patients with some degree of heart failure. If heart failure is not present, the coefficient of CL_{cr} is 1.0. Units of CL_{cr} must be $ml \cdot min^{-1} \cdot kg^{-1}$.
[c] Occasional individuals metabolize digoxin very rapidly to an inactive metabolite, dihydrodigoxin.
[d] Inotropic effect.
[e] Concentrations at which the probability of digoxin-induced arrhythmias are 10, 50, and 90%, respectively.

Key: Adult = adults; Aged = aged; Alb = hypoalbuminemia; Arth = arthritis; Atr Fib = atrial fibrillation; AVH = acute viral hepatitis; Burn = burn patients; CAD = coronary artery disease; Celiac = celiac disease; CF = cystic fibrosis; CHF = congestive heart failure; Child = children; Cirr = cirrhosis; COPD = chronic obstructive pulmonary disease; CP = cor pulmonale; CPBS = cardiopulmonary bypass surgery; CRI = chronic respiratory insufficiency; Crohn = Crohn's disease; Cush = Cushing's syndrome; Epilep = epileptic; Fem = female; Hep = Hepatitis; HL = hyperlipoproteinemia; HTh = hyperthyroid; Inflam = inflammation; LTh = hypothyroid; MI = myocardial infarction; Neo = neonate; NS = nephrotic syndrome; Obes = obese; Pneu = pneumonia; Preg = pregnant; Prem = premature; RA = rheumatoid arthritis; Smk = smoking; Tach = ventricular tachycardia; Ulcer = ulcer patients; Urem = uremia

References: *See* end of table.

Table A–II–1. PHARMACOKINETIC DATA (Continued)

AVAILABILITY (ORAL) (%)	URINARY EXCRETION (%)	BOUND IN PLASMA (%)	CLEARANCE ($ml \cdot min^{-1} \cdot kg^{-1}$)	VOL. DIST. (*liters/kg*)	HALF-LIFE (*hours*)	EFFECTIVE CONCENTRATIONS	TOXIC CONCENTRATIONS
DILTIAZEM [a] (Chapters 32, 35)							
44 ± 10	<4	78 ± 3	12 ± 4 [b,c] ⟷ Urem, Aged	3.1 ± 1.2 ⟷ Aged	3.7 ± 1.2 [d] ⟷ Urem, Aged	—	—

[a] Active metabolites, desacetyldiltiazem ($t_{1/2}$ = 9 ± 2 hours) and N-demethyldiltiazem ($t_{1/2}$ = 7.5 ± 1 hours).
[b] More than a twofold decrease with multiple dosing.
[c] Blood-to-plasma ratio 1.0 ± 0.1.
[d] $T_{1/2}$ for oral dosage 5–6 hours; does not change with multiple dosing.

DIPHENHYDRAMINE (Chapter 23)							
72 ± 25	1.9 ± 0.8 ⟷ Cirr	78 ± 3 ↓ Cirr	6.2 ± 1.7 [a] ⟷ Cirr	4.5 ± 2.8 [a,b] ⟷ Cirr	8.5 ± 3.2 ↑ Cirr	>25 ng/ml [c] 30–40 ng/ml [d]	>60 ng/ml [e]

[a] Increased *CL*, decreased *V*, and no change in half-life in Orientals, presumably due to decreased protein binding.
[b] V_{area}.
[c] Antihistaminic effect.
[d] Drowsiness.
[e] Mental impairment.

DISOPYRAMIDE [a] (Chapter 35)							
83 ± 11 ⟷ MI, CHF	55 ± 6	Dose-dependent [b] ↓ Neo, NS, Cirr ↑ Aged, MI, Urem	1.2 ± 0.4 [c] ↓ MI, Tach, CHF [d], Urem, Cirr [d] ⟷ Smk	0.59 ± 0.15 [c] ↓ Cirr [d] ⟷ CHF [d], Urem, Smk	6.0 ± 1.0 ↑ Urem, CHF [d] ⟷ MI, Smk	>1.5 μg/ml [e]	—

[a] Racemic mixture; S-(+)-enantiomer has greater anticholinergic activity; relative antiarrhythmic activity not known.
[b] 89% at 0.38 μg/ml and 68% at 3.8 μg/ml.
[c] Unbound clearance, 5.4 ± 2.8 $ml \cdot min^{-1} \cdot kg^{-1}$; unbound V_{ss}, 1.7 ± 0.8 liters/kg.
[d] Comparison of unbound parameters.
[e] Free concentration.

DOBUTAMINE (Chapter 10)							
—	—	—	59 ± 22 [a]	0.20 ± 0.08 [a]	2.4 ± 0.7 min [a]	—	—

[a] Values for patients with CHF; *V*, for example, is lower when less edema is present. Values likely represent distribution, rather than elimination.

DOXEPIN [a] (Chapter 18)							
27 ± 10 [b]	~0	—	14 ± 3 [c]	20 ± 8 [c,d]	17 ± 6	30–150 ng/ml [e]	—

[a] Active metabolite desmethyldoxepin has a longer half-life (37 ± 15 hours).
[b] Calculated from results of oral administration only, assuming complete absorption, elimination only by the liver, hepatic blood flow of 1500 ml per minute, and equal partition between plasma and erythrocytes.
[c] Calculated assuming $F = 0.27$.
[d] V_{area}.
[e] Doxepin + desmethyldoxepin; optimal concentrations have not been defined.

DOXORUBICIN [a] (Chapter 52)							
5	<15	79–85	17 ± 3 ↑ Child	25	30 ± 14 [b] ⟷ Cirr, Urem	—	—

[a] Active metabolites.
[b] Prolonged when bilirubin concentration elevated.

DOXYCYCLINE (Chapter 48)							
93	41 ± 19	88 ± 5 ↓ Urem [a]	0.53 ± 0.18 ↓ HL, Aged ⟷ Urem	0.75 ± 0.32 ↓ HL, Aged	16 ± 6 ⟷ Urem, HL, Aged	*See* Chapter 48	—

[a] Changes in plasma protein binding and erythrocyte partitioning yield decrease from 88 ± 5% bound in blood of normals to 71 ± 3% in patients with uremia.

EDROPHONIUM (Chapter 7)							
—	—	—	9.6 ± 2.7	1.1 ± 0.2	1.8 ± 0.6	<0.15 μg/ml [a]	—

[a] 80% reversal of 95% blockade due to tubocurarine.

Key: Adult = adults; Aged = aged; Alb = hypoalbuminemia; Arth = arthritis; Atr Fib = atrial fibrillation; AVH = acute viral hepatitis; Burn = burn patients; CAD = coronary artery disease; Celiac = celiac disease; CF = cystic fibrosis; CHF = congestive heart failure; Child = children; Cirr = cirrhosis; COPD = chronic obstructive pulmonary disease; CP = cor pulmonale; CPBS = cardiopulmonary bypass surgery; CRI = chronic respiratory insufficiency; Crohn = Crohn's disease; Cush = Cushing's syndrome; Epilep = epileptic; Fem = female; Hep = Hepatitis; HL = hyperlipoproteinemia; HTh = hyperthyroid; Inflam = inflammation; LTh = hypothyroid; MI = myocardial infarction; Neo = neonate; NS = nephrotic syndrome; Obes = obese; Pneu = pneumonia; Preg = pregnant; Prem = premature; RA = rheumatoid arthritis; Smk = smoking; Tach = ventricular tachycardia; Ulcer = ulcer patients; Urem = uremia

References: *See* end of table.

Table A–II–1. PHARMACOKINETIC DATA (Continued)

AVAILABILITY (ORAL) (%)	URINARY EXCRETION (%)	BOUND IN PLASMA (%)	CLEARANCE ($ml \cdot min^{-1} \cdot kg^{-1}$)	VOL. DIST. (*liters/kg*)	HALF-LIFE (*hours*)	EFFECTIVE CONCENTRATIONS	TOXIC CONCENTRATIONS
ENALAPRIL [a] (Chapter 31)							
41 ± 15 ↓ Cirr	88 ± 7 [b] ↓ Cirr	<50	4.9 ± 1.5 [c] ↓ Urem, Aged, CHF	1.7 ± 0.7 [c]	11 [d] ↑ Urem, Cirr	—	—

[a] Hydrolyzed to active compound, enalaprilic acid (enalaprilat); values and disease comparisons are for enalaprilat, following oral administration of enalapril.
[b] For intravenous enalaprilat.
[c] *CL/F* and V_{ss}/F after multiple oral doses of enalapril. Values after single intravenous dose of enalaprilat are misleading, since binding to converting enzyme leads to a prolonged $t_{1/2}$, which does not represent a significant fraction of the clearance upon multiple dosing.
[d] Estimated from the approach to steady state during multiple dosing.

AVAILABILITY (ORAL) (%)	URINARY EXCRETION (%)	BOUND IN PLASMA (%)	CLEARANCE ($ml \cdot min^{-1} \cdot kg^{-1}$)	VOL. DIST. (*liters/kg*)	HALF-LIFE (*hours*)	EFFECTIVE CONCENTRATIONS	TOXIC CONCENTRATIONS
ENCAINIDE [a] (Chapter 35)							
30 ± 19 ↑ Cirr, Urem 83 ± 19 [b]	5 ± 2 [c] ↑ Cirr [c] 39 ± 6 [b]	70 ± 6 [c] ↑ Urem [c] ⟷ Cirr [c] 78 ± 1 [b]	25 ± 8 ↓ Cirr [d] ⟷ Urem 2.6 ± 0.6 [b]	3.6 ± 1.0 ⟷ Urem, Cirr 2.5 [b,e]	2.3 ± 1.0 ↑ Cirr ⟷ Urem 11.3 ± 0.6 [b]	250 ng/ml [f]	—

[a] Metabolites O-desmethylencainide (ODE) and 3-methoxy-O-desmethylencainide (MODE) have activity at least equal to that of encainide; formation of metabolites is subject to hydroxylation polymorphism (93% of U.S. population extensive metabolizers and 7% poor metabolizers). Values are for multiple doses of encainide in extensive metabolizers unless otherwise noted. Pharmacokinetic parameters for ODE and MODE are presented elsewhere (*see* Encainide Active Metabolites).
[b] Poor metabolizers; multiple doses.
[c] Single-dose studies.
[d] Clearance is reduced in cirrhosis, but concentrations of metabolites do not change and dosage adjustment probably not necessary.
[e] V_{area}.
[f] Suppression of arrhythmias.

AVAILABILITY (ORAL) (%)	URINARY EXCRETION (%)	BOUND IN PLASMA (%)	CLEARANCE ($ml \cdot min^{-1} \cdot kg^{-1}$)	VOL. DIST. (*liters/kg*)	HALF-LIFE (*hours*)	EFFECTIVE CONCENTRATIONS	TOXIC CONCENTRATIONS
ENCAINIDE ACTIVE METABOLITES [a] (Chapter 35)							
ODE —	11 ± 3 [b] ⟷ Cirr [b]	—	13 ± 4 [c] ↓ Urem 5.3 ± 1.3 [c,d]	2.6 ± 0.8 [c,e] 2.0 ± 0.3 [c,d,e]	3.5 ± 1.2 ↑ Cirr [b] 6.7 ± 2.5 [d]	30 ng/ml [f]	—
MODE —	4 ± 3 [b] ⟷ Cirr [b]	—	4.1 ± 1.2 [c] ↓ Urem 2.7 ± 2.2 [c,d]	1.3 ± 0.8 [c,e] 1.3 ± 0.4 [c,d,e]	6.4 ± 5.1 ↑ Cirr [b] 4–24 [d]	100 ng/ml [f]	—

[a] *See* Encainide. In extensive metabolizers of encainide, ODE and MODE account for the activity of encainide. Values are for extensive metabolizers, unless otherwise noted.
[b] Following administration of encainide.
[c] Assuming 70-kg weight.
[d] Poor metabolizers; two subjects.
[e] V_{area}.
[f] Suppression of arrhythmias.

ERYTHROMYCIN (Chapter 48)							
35 ± 25 [a] ↓ Preg [b]	12 ± 7	84 ± 3 [c] ⟷ Urem	9.1 ± 4.1 ⟷ Urem	0.78 ± 0.44 ↑ Urem	1.6 ± 0.7 ↑ Cirr ⟷ Urem	*See* Chapter 48	—

[a] Value for enteric-coated erythromycin base.
[b] Decreased concentrations in pregnancy possibly due to decreased availability (or to increased clearance).
[c] Erythromycin base. Values for the propionate ester range from 90 to 99%.

ESMOLOL (Chapters 11, 35)							
—	<1	55	170 ± 70 ⟷ Urem, Cirr	1.9 ± 1.3 [a] ⟷ Urem, Cirr	0.13 ± 0.07 ⟷ Urem, Cirr	—	—

[a] V_{area}.

ETHAMBUTOL (Chapter 49)							
77 ± 8	79 ± 3	<5	8.6 ± 0.8	1.6 ± 0.2	3.1 ± 0.4 ↑ Urem	—	>10 μg/ml [a]

[a] Estimated from kinetics and dosage at which visual toxicity occurs.

ETHANOL (Chapter 17)							
80 [a]	<3	—	V_m = 124 ± 10 mg · kg^{-1} · hr^{-1} K_m = 82 ± 29 mg/l [b] *CL* ↑ Smk	0.54 ± 0.05	0.24 ± 0.08 [b]	—	800–1500 mg/l [c]

[a] Bioavailability predicted for an 11.25-g dose absorbed over 20 min; *F* increases with increasing dose.
[b] Ethanol is eliminated by a saturable (Michaelis–Menten) process; the half-life is the fastest possible—that theoretically present at zero concentration.
[c] Legal basis for intoxication in many states of the United States.

Key: Adult = adults; Aged = aged; Alb = hypoalbuminemia; Arth = arthritis; Atr Fib = atrial fibrillation; AVH = acute viral hepatitis; Burn = burn patients; CAD = coronary artery disease; Celiac = celiac disease; CF = cystic fibrosis; CHF = congestive heart failure; Child = children; Cirr = cirrhosis; COPD = chronic obstructive pulmonary disease; CP = cor pulmonale; CPBS = cardiopulmonary bypass surgery; CRI = chronic respiratory insufficiency; Crohn = Crohn's disease; Cush = Cushing's syndrome; Epilep = epileptic; Fem = female; Hep = Hepatitis; HL = hyperlipoproteinemia; HTh = hyperthyroid; Inflam = inflammation; LTh = hypothyroid; MI = myocardial infarction; Neo = neonate; NS = nephrotic syndrome; Obes = obese; Pneu = pneumonia; Preg = pregnant; Prem = premature; RA = rheumatoid arthritis; Smk = smoking; Tach = ventricular tachycardia; Ulcer = ulcer patients; Urem = uremia

References: *See* end of table.

Table A–II–1. PHARMACOKINETIC DATA (Continued)

AVAILABILITY (ORAL) (%)	URINARY EXCRETION (%)	BOUND IN PLASMA (%)	CLEARANCE ($ml \cdot min^{-1} \cdot kg^{-1}$)	VOL. DIST. (*liters/kg*)	HALF-LIFE (*hours*)	EFFECTIVE CONCENTRATIONS	TOXIC CONCENTRATIONS
ETHOSUXIMIDE (Chapter 19)							
—	25 ± 15	0	0.19 ± 0.04 [a,b] ↑ Child	0.72 ± 0.16 [a] ⟷ Child	45 ± 8 [a] ↓ Child ⟷ Neo	40–100 μg/ml	—
ETOPOSIDE (Chapter 52)							
52 ± 17 [a]	35 ± 5	96 ± 0.4 [b] ↓ Alb	0.68 ± 0.23 ⟷ Child, Cirr ↓ Urem	0.36 ± 0.15 ⟷ Child, Cirr	8.1 ± 4.3 ↑ Urem ⟷ Child, Cirr	—	—
FAMOTIDINE (Chapter 37)							
45 ± 14	67 ± 15	17 ± 7	7.1 ± 1.7 ↓ Urem, Aged	1.3 ± 0.2 ⟷ Urem	2.6 ± 1.0 ↑ Urem, Aged	13 ng/ml [a]	—
FENTANYL (Chapters 14, 21)							
—	8	84 ± 2	13 ± 2 [a] ↓ Aged ⟷ Cirr	4.0 ± 0.4	3.7 ± 0.4 ↑ CPBS, Aged	1 ng/ml [b] 3 ng/ml [c]	>0.7 ng/ml [d]
FLECAINIDE [a] (Chapter 35)							
70 ± 11	43 ± 3	61 ± 10 ↓ MI	5.6 ± 1.3 ↓ Urem, Cirr ↑ Child	4.9 ± 0.4 ↑ Cirr [b]	11 ± 3 ↑ Urem, Cirr, CHF ↓ Child	0.4–0.8 μg/ml	>1 μg/ml

Ethosuximide notes:
[a] Data from oral, multiple-dose regimen; values are *CL/F* and V_{area}/F.
[b] *CL/F* decreases 15% from single dose and may be nonlinear with increasing dose.

Etoposide notes:
[a] Decreases at oral doses greater than 200 mg.
[b] Decreases with hyperbilirubinemia.

Famotidine notes:
[a] To inhibit gastric acid secretion by 50%.

Fentanyl notes:
[a] Blood-to-plasma ratio = 0.97 ± 0.06.
[b] Postoperative analgesia.
[c] Intraoperative analgesia.
[d] Respiratory depression.

Flecainide notes:
[a] Racemate; enantiomers appear to exert similar electrophysiological effects.
[b] V_{area}.

FLUCYTOSINE (Chapter 50)

84 ± 6 ⟷ Urem	99 ± 7	4	$CL = CL_{cr}$	0.68 ± 0.04 ⟷ Urem	4.2 ± 0.3 ↑ Urem	35–70 μg/ml	>100 μg/ml

FLUNITRAZEPAM [a] (Chapter 17)

~85	<1	77–79	3.5 ± 0.4 [b]	3.3 ± 0.6 [b]	15 ± 5	—	—

[a] Active metabolite, desmethylflunitrazepam.
[b] CL/F and V_{ss}/F.

FLUOROURACIL (Chapter 52)

28 [a]	<10	8–12	16 ± 7	0.25 ± 0.12	11 ± 4 min [b]	—	—

[a] Higher F with rapid absorption and lower F with slower absorption due to saturable first-pass effect.
[b] A longer (~20 hour) half-life is seen at very low concentrations of drug.

FLUOXETINE [a] (Chapter 18)

>60	<2.5	94 ⟷ Cirr, Urem	9.6 ± 6.9 [b,c] ⟷ Urem, Aged ↓ Cirr	35 ± 21 [d] ⟷ Urem, Cirr	53 ± 41 [e] ↑ Cirr ⟷ Urem, Aged	—	—

[a] Active metabolite, norfluoxetine; $t_{1/2}$ of norfluoxetine is 6.4 ± 2.5 days (12 ± 2 days in cirrhosis).
[b] Lower with repetitive dosing and with increasing doses between 40 and 80 mg.
[c] CL/F.
[d] V_{area}/F.
[e] Higher with repetitive dosing and with increasing doses.

FLURAZEPAM [a] (Chapter 17)

—	<1	96.6	4.5 ± 2.3 [b] ↓ Fem	22 ± 7 [b]	74 ± 24 ↑ Aged [c]	—	—

[a] Flurazepam is essentially a prodrug for desalkylflurazepam; values presented are for the active metabolite.
[b] CL/F and V_{area}/F.
[c] Males.

Key: Adult = adults; Aged = aged; Alb = hypoalbuminemia; Arth = arthritis; Atr Fib = atrial fibrillation; AVH = acute viral hepatitis; Burn = burn patients; CAD = coronary artery disease; Celiac = celiac disease; CF = cystic fibrosis; CHF = congestive heart failure; Child = children; Cirr = cirrhosis; COPD = chronic obstructive pulmonary disease; CP = cor pulmonale; CPBS = cardiopulmonary bypass surgery; CRI = chronic respiratory insufficiency; Crohn = Crohn's disease; Cush = Cushing's syndrome; Epilep = epileptic; Fem = female; Hep = Hepatitis; HL = hyperlipoproteinemia; HTh = hyperthyroid; Inflam = inflammation; LTh = hypothyroid; MI = myocardial infarction; Neo = neonate; NS = nephrotic syndrome; Obes = obese; Pneu = pneumonia; Preg = pregnant; Prem = premature; RA = rheumatoid arthritis; Smk = smoking; Tach = ventricular tachycardia; Ulcer = ulcer patients; Urem = uremia

References: *See* end of table.

Table A–II–1. PHARMACOKINETIC DATA (Continued)

AVAILABILITY (ORAL) (%)	URINARY EXCRETION (%)	BOUND IN PLASMA (%)	CLEARANCE ($ml \cdot min^{-1} \cdot kg^{-1}$)	VOL. DIST. (*liters/kg*)	HALF-LIFE (*hours*)	EFFECTIVE CONCENTRATIONS	TOXIC CONCENTRATIONS
FUROSEMIDE (Chapter 28)							
61 ± 17 ⟷ CHF, Cirr, CRI	66 ± 7 ↓ CF ⟷ Aged	98.8 ± 0.2 ↓ Urem, NS, Cirr, Alb, Aged ⟷ CHF, Smk	2.0 ± 0.4 ↓ Urem, CHF, Prem, Neo, Aged ⟷ Cirr ↑ CF	0.11 ± 0.02 ↑ NS, Neo, Prem, Cirr ⟷ Urem, CHF, Aged, Smk	92 ± 7 min ↑ Urem, CHF, Prem, Neo, Cirr, Aged ⟷ NS	[a]	25 μg/ml [b]

[a] Efficacy better correlated with concentration of drug in urine.
[b] Ototoxicity.

AVAILABILITY (ORAL) (%)	URINARY EXCRETION (%)	BOUND IN PLASMA (%)	CLEARANCE ($ml \cdot min^{-1} \cdot kg^{-1}$)	VOL. DIST. (*liters/kg*)	HALF-LIFE (*hours*)	EFFECTIVE CONCENTRATIONS	TOXIC CONCENTRATIONS
GENTAMICIN (Chapter 47)							
—	>90	<10	$CL = 0.82\ CL_{cr} + 0.11$ ↓ Obes	0.31 ± 0.10 ⟷ Urem, Aged, CF, Child ↓ Obes ↑ Neo	2–3 53 ± 25 [a] ↑ Urem ⟷ Obes ↓ Burn	*See* Chapter 47	*See* Chapter 47

[a] Gentamicin has a very long terminal half-life, which accounts for urinary excretion for up to 3 weeks.

AVAILABILITY (ORAL) (%)	URINARY EXCRETION (%)	BOUND IN PLASMA (%)	CLEARANCE ($ml \cdot min^{-1} \cdot kg^{-1}$)	VOL. DIST. (*liters/kg*)	HALF-LIFE (*hours*)	EFFECTIVE CONCENTRATIONS	TOXIC CONCENTRATIONS
GLIPIZIDE (Chapter 61)							
95	<5	98.4	0.52 ± 0.18 ⟷ Urem, Aged	0.17 ± 0.02 ⟷ Aged	3.4 ± 0.7 ⟷ Urem, Aged	—	—
GOLD SODIUM THIOMALATE [a] (Chapter 26)							
—	70	95	7.0 ± 0.6 [b]	0.26 ± 0.05 [b,c]	25 ± 5 days	—	—

[a] Values refer to gold.
[b] Intramuscular dose.
[c] V_{area}.

HALOPERIDOL [a] (Chapter 18)

60 ± 18	1	92 ± 2 ↑ Cirr ⟷ Aged, Child	11.8 ± 2.9 ↑ Child; Smk ↓ Aged	18 ± 7	18 ± 5 [a] ↓ Child	4 – 20 ng/ml	—

[a] Reversible metabolism to and from less active reduced haloperidol, which has $CL = 10 \pm 5$ ml · min^{-1} · kg^{-1} and $t_{1/2} = 67 \pm 51$ hours. Slow conversion from reduced haloperidol to parent compound probably responsible for prolonged (70-hour) $t_{1/2}$ for haloperidol observed with 7-day sampling.

HEPARIN (Chapter 55)

—	Negligible	Extensive	1/(0.65 + 0.008D) ± 0.1[a]	0.058 ± 0.011 [b]	(26 + 0.323D) ± 12 min [a]	*See* Chapter 55	—

[a] D is dose in I.U./kg. Half-life and clearance are dose dependent, perhaps due to saturable metabolism with end-product inhibition.

[b] V_{area}.

HEXOBARBITAL [a] (Chapter 17)

>90	<1	42–52 ⟷ Cirr	3.9 ± 0.7 ↓ Cirr, AVH	1.2 ± 0.3 ⟷ Cirr, AVH	3.7 ± 0.9 ↑ Cirr, AVH	—	—

[a] Racemic mixture; elimination of active *d*-hexobarbital ($CL = 1.9 \pm 0.5$ ml · min^{-1} · kg^{-1}; $V_{area} = 0.97 \pm 0.26$ liters/kg; $t_{1/2} = 5.6 \pm 1.5$ hours) is significantly slower than that of inactive *l*-enantiomer. Decreased clearance of *l*-hexobarbital with aging has no effect on elimination of *d*-enantiomer.

HYDRALAZINE (Chapter 33)

16 ± 6 [a,b] 35 ± 4 [c] ⟷ CHF	1–15	87	56 ± 13 [d,e] ↓ CHF	1.5 ± 1.0 [d,e] ⟷ CHF	0.96 ± 0.28 [d] ↑ CHF	100 ng/ml [f]	—

[a] Rapid acetylator.
[b] Availability may increase with large doses that saturate first-pass metabolism.
[c] Slow acetylator.
[d] Same for rapid and slow acetylators after intravenous administration because of other pathways of metabolic alteration.
[e] Blood CL and V_{ss}. Blood-to-plasma concentration ratio = 1.65.
[f] Decrease in mean arterial pressure of 10–20 mm Hg.

Key: Adult = adults; Aged = aged; Alb = hypoalbuminemia; Arth = arthritis; Atr Fib = atrial fibrillation; AVH = acute viral hepatitis; Burn = burn patients; CAD = coronary artery disease; Celiac = celiac disease; CF = cystic fibrosis; CHF = congestive heart failure; Child = children; Cirr = cirrhosis; COPD = chronic obstructive pulmonary disease; CP = cor pulmonale; CPBS = cardiopulmonary bypass surgery; CRI = chronic respiratory insufficiency; Crohn = Crohn's disease; Cush = Cushing's syndrome; Epilep = epileptic; Fem = female; Hep = Hepatitis; HL = hyperlipoproteinemia; HTh = hyperthyroid; Inflam = inflammation; LTh = hypothyroid; MI = myocardial infarction; Neo = neonate; NS = nephrotic syndrome; Obes = obese; Pneu = pneumonia; Preg = pregnant; Prem = premature; RA = rheumatoid arthritis; Smk = smoking; Tach = ventricular tachycardia; Ulcer = ulcer patients; Urem = uremia

References: *See* end of table.

Table A–II–1. PHARMACOKINETIC DATA (Continued)

AVAILABILITY (ORAL) (%)	URINARY EXCRETION (%)	BOUND IN PLASMA (%)	CLEARANCE ($ml \cdot min^{-1} \cdot kg^{-1}$)	VOL. DIST. (*liters/kg*)	HALF-LIFE (*hours*)	EFFECTIVE CONCENTRATIONS	TOXIC CONCENTRATIONS
HYDROCHLOROTHIAZIDE (Chapter 28)							
71 ± 15	>95	58 ± 17	4.9 ± 1.1 [a] ↓ Urem, CHF [b], Aged	0.83 ± 0.31 [c] ↓ Aged	2.5 ± 0.2 ↑ Urem, CHF [b], Aged	—	—

[a] Renal clearance, which should approximate total plasma clearance; calculated assuming 70-kg weight.
[b] Changes may reflect decreased renal function.
[c] Calculated from individual values of renal clearance, terminal half-life, and fraction of drug excreted unchanged; 70-kg weight assumed.

AVAILABILITY (ORAL) (%)	URINARY EXCRETION (%)	BOUND IN PLASMA (%)	CLEARANCE ($ml \cdot min^{-1} \cdot kg^{-1}$)	VOL. DIST. (*liters/kg*)	HALF-LIFE (*hours*)	EFFECTIVE CONCENTRATIONS	TOXIC CONCENTRATIONS
IBUPROFEN [a] (Chapter 26)							
>80	<1	>99 [b] ⟷ RA, Alb	0.75 ± 0.20 [b,c] ↑ CF ⟷ Child, RA	0.15 ± 0.02 [c] ↑ CF	2 ± 0.5 [b] ⟷ RA, CF, Child	10 μg/ml [d]	—

[a] Racemic mixture. Kinetic parameters (CL/F, V_{ss}/F, $t_{1/2}$) for active (S-(+)-enantiomer do not differ from those for inactive R-(−) enantiomer when administered separately; 63 ± 6% of R-(−)-enantiomer is inverted to active species.
[b] Unbound percent of S-(+)-ibuprofen (0.77 ± 0.20%) significantly greater than that of R-(−)-ibuprofen (0.45 ± 0.06%). Binding of each enantiomer is concentration dependent and is influenced by presence of optical antipode, leading to nonlinear kinetics.
[c] CL/F and V_{ss}/F.
[d] Antipyresis in febrile children.

AVAILABILITY (ORAL) (%)	URINARY EXCRETION (%)	BOUND IN PLASMA (%)	CLEARANCE ($ml \cdot min^{-1} \cdot kg^{-1}$)	VOL. DIST. (*liters/kg*)	HALF-LIFE (*hours*)	EFFECTIVE CONCENTRATIONS	TOXIC CONCENTRATIONS
IMIPENEM/CILASTATIN [a] (Chapter 46)							
IMIPENEM —	69 ± 15 ↓ Neo, Inflam ⟷ Child, CF	<20	2.9 ± 0.3 ↑ Child ↓ Urem ⟷ CF, Inflam, Neo, Aged	0.23 ± 0.05 ↑ Neo, Child ⟷ CF, Urem, Aged	0.9 ± 0.1 ↑ Neo, Urem ⟷ CF, Child, Aged	*See* Chapter 46	—
CILASTATIN —	70 ± 3 ↓ Neo ⟷ CF	~ 35	3.0 ± 0.3 ↑ Child ↓ Neo, Urem ⟷ CF, Aged	0.20 ± 0.03 ⟷ Neo, Urem, CF, Aged	0.8 ± 0.1 ↑ Neo ⟷ CF, Aged		

[a] Cilastatin inhibits metabolism of imipenem by the kidney, increasing concentrations of imipenem in the urine; cilastatin does not change plasma concentrations of imipenem appreciably. Values are for simultaneous administration.

IMIPRAMINE [a] (Chapter 18)

40 ± 12	<2	90.1 ± 1.4 ↑ HL, MI, Burn ⟷ RA	15 ± 4 [b] ↓ Aged ↑ Smk	23 ± 8 [c]	18 ± 7	100–300 ng/ml [d]	>1 μg/ml [e]

[a] Active metabolite, desipramine.
[b] Blood-to-plasma ratio = 1.1 ± 0.1.
[c] V_{area}.
[d] Antidepressant effect; combination of imipramine and desipramine.
[e] Concentration of imipramine and desipramine; combined data for toxic effects of tricyclic antidepressants.

INDOMETHACIN [a] (Chapter 26)

98	15 ± 8	90 ⟷ Alb, Prem, Neo	2.0 ± 0.4 [b] ↓ Prem, Neo	0.26 ± 0.07 [b]	2.4 ± 0.4 [a] ⟷ RA, Urem ↑ Neo, Prem	0.3–3 μg/ml	>5 μg/ml

[a] There is significant enterohepatic recycling (~50% after an intravenous dose), which may contribute to low plasma concentrations of the drug for prolonged periods of time.
[b] Assuming 70-kg weight.

INTERFERON ALFA (Chapters 51, 52)

Intramuscular: 100 Subcutaneous: 93	—	—	2.8 ± 0.6	0.40 ± 0.19	0.67 [a]	—	—

[a] A terminal $t_{1/2}$ of 5.1 ± 1.6 hours accounts for 23% of clearance.

Key: Adult = adults; Aged = aged; Alb = hypoalbuminemia; Arth = arthritis; Atr Fib = atrial fibrillation; AVH = acute viral hepatitis; Burn = burn patients; CAD = coronary artery disease; Celiac = celiac disease; CF = cystic fibrosis; CHF = congestive heart failure; Child = children; Cirr = cirrhosis; COPD = chronic obstructive pulmonary disease; CP = cor pulmonale; CPBS = cardiopulmonary bypass surgery; CRI = chronic respiratory insufficiency; Crohn = Crohn's disease; Cush = Cushing's syndrome; Epilep = epileptic; Fem = female; Hep = Hepatitis; HL = hyperlipoproteinemia; HTh = hyperthyroid; Inflam = inflammation; LTh = hypothyroid; MI = myocardial infarction; Neo = neonate; NS = nephrotic syndrome; Obes = obese; Pneu = pneumonia; Preg = pregnant; Prem = premature; RA = rheumatoid arthritis; Smk = smoking; Tach = ventricular tachycardia; Ulcer = ulcer patients; Urem = uremia

References: *See* end of table.

Table A–II–1. PHARMACOKINETIC DATA (Continued)

AVAILABILITY (ORAL) (%)	URINARY EXCRETION (%)	BOUND IN PLASMA (%)	CLEARANCE ($ml \cdot min^{-1} \cdot kg^{-1}$)	VOL. DIST. (*liters/kg*)	HALF-LIFE (*hours*)	EFFECTIVE CONCENTRATIONS	TOXIC CONCENTRATIONS
ISONIAZID (Chapter 49)							
[a]	29 ± 5 [b,c] 7 ± 2 [b,d]	~ 0	3.7 ± 1.1 [c] 7.4 ± 2.0 [d] ⟷ Aged	0.67 ± 0.15 ⟷ Aged	1.1 ± 0.1 [d] 3.1 ± 1.1 [c] ↑ AVH, Cirr, Neo, Urem [e] ⟷ Aged, Obes, Child, HTh	*See* Chapter 49	—

[a] It is usually stated that isoniazid is completely absorbed; however, good estimates of possible loss due to first-pass metabolism are not available. Absorption is decreased in the presence of food or antacids.
[b] After oral administration; assay includes unchanged drug and its acid-labile hydrazones. Higher percentages have been noted after intravenous administration, suggesting significant first-pass metabolism.
[c] Slow acetylators.
[d] Fast acetylators.
[e] No apparent correlation with degree of renal impairment.

AVAILABILITY (ORAL) (%)	URINARY EXCRETION (%)	BOUND IN PLASMA (%)	CLEARANCE ($ml \cdot min^{-1} \cdot kg^{-1}$)	VOL. DIST. (*liters/kg*)	HALF-LIFE (*hours*)	EFFECTIVE CONCENTRATIONS	TOXIC CONCENTRATIONS
ISOSORBIDE DINITRATE [a] (Chapter 32)							
Oral: 22 ± 14 [b] Sublingual: 30 ± 8 [b] Percutaneous: 33 ± 17 [b]	<1	28 ± 12	45 ± 20 ↓ Cirr ⟷ Smk, Urem	1.5 ± 0.8	0.8 ± 0.4 ⟷ Urem	—	—

[a] Isosorbide dinitrate is metabolized to the 2- and 5-mononitrates. Both metabolites and the parent compound are thought to be active. Values above are for the dinitrate. *See also* listings for isosorbide mononitrates.
[b] Availability calculations from single doses, since systemic clearance may be decreased after long-term use.

AVAILABILITY (ORAL) (%)	URINARY EXCRETION (%)	BOUND IN PLASMA (%)	CLEARANCE ($ml \cdot min^{-1} \cdot kg^{-1}$)	VOL. DIST. (*liters/kg*)	HALF-LIFE (*hours*)	EFFECTIVE CONCENTRATIONS	TOXIC CONCENTRATIONS
ISOSORBIDE-2-MONONITRATE [a] (Chapter 32)							
100	—	—	5.8 ± 1.6	0.82 ± 0.34	1.9 ± 0.5 ⟷ CHF, Urem	—	—

[a] Active metabolite of isosorbide dinitrate.

AVAILABILITY (ORAL) (%)	URINARY EXCRETION (%)	BOUND IN PLASMA (%)	CLEARANCE ($ml \cdot min^{-1} \cdot kg^{-1}$)	VOL. DIST. (*liters/kg*)	HALF-LIFE (*hours*)	EFFECTIVE CONCENTRATIONS	TOXIC CONCENTRATIONS
ISOSORBIDE-5-MONONITRATE [a] **(ISOSORBIDE NITRATE)** (Chapter 32)							
93 ± 13 ⟷ Cirr, Urem	<5	0	1.81 ± 0.26 ⟷ Cirr, Urem	0.79 ± 0.13 ⟷ Cirr	4.4 ± 0.5 ⟷ Cirr, Urem, MI	100 ng/ml	—

[a] Active metabolite of isosorbide dinitrate.

ISOTRETINOIN [a] (Chapters 64, 65)							
—	<1	99.9	5.5 ± 2.8 [b]	7 [b]	14 ± 5	—	—

[a] Linear kinetics after oral doses of 80–240 mg.
[b] CL/F and V_{area}/F.

KANAMYCIN (Chapter 47)							
—	90	0	1.4 ± 0.2 [a] $CL = 0.62\ CL_{cr} + 0.03$ ↑ Burn	0.26 ± 0.05	2.1 ± 0.2 ↑ Urem, Neo, Prem ↓ Burn	*See* Chapter 47	*See* Chapter 47

[a] Values reported per 1.73 m^2; calculated assuming 70-kg weight.

KETAMINE [a] (Chapter 14)							
20 ± 7	4 ± 3	12	15 ± 5	1.8 ± 0.7	2.3 ± 0.5	100–150 ng/ml	—

[a] Racemic mixture. No significant differences in pharmacokinetic parameters between more potent S-(+)-ketamine, less potent R-(−)-ketamine, and racemic mixture.

KETOCONAZOLE (Chapter 50)							
[a]	<1	99.0 ± 0.1	8.4 ± 4.1 [b]	2.4 ± 1.6 [b]	3.3 ± 10 [b,c]	—	—

[a] Unknown because of lack of intravenous formulation. Diminished with hypochlorhydria (antacids, H_2 blockers, some AIDS patients).
[b] CL/F, V_{area}/F, and $t_{1/2}$ with 200-mg daily doses for more than 1 month. With single dose, CL/F, and V_{area}/F lower; $t_{1/2}$ about 8 hours.
[c] Conflicting data in normal subjects suggests increasing $t_{1/2}$ with increasing dose and repeated dosage.

KETOPROFEN (Chapter 26)							
~100	<1	99.2 ± 0.1 ⟷ Cirr, Aged	1.2 ± 0.3 ↓ Aged, Urem [a] ⟷ Cirr, RA	0.15 ± 0.03	1.8 ± 0.3 ↑ Aged, Urem [a] ⟷ Cirr	—	—

[a] Owing to accumulation of glucuronide metabolite, which is hydrolyzed to parent drug.

Key: Adult = adults; Aged = aged; Alb = hypoalbuminemia; Arth = arthritis; Atr Fib = atrial fibrillation; AVH = acute viral hepatitis; Burn = burn patients; CAD = coronary artery disease; Celiac = celiac disease; CF = cystic fibrosis; CHF = congestive heart failure; Child = children; Cirr = cirrhosis; COPD = chronic obstructive pulmonary disease; CP = cor pulmonale; CPBS = cardiopulmonary bypass surgery; CRI = chronic respiratory insufficiency; Crohn = Crohn's disease; Cush = Cushing's syndrome; Epilep = epileptic; Fem = female; Hep = Hepatitis; HL = hyperlipoproteinemia; HTh = hyperthyroid; Inflam = inflammation; LTh = hypothyroid; MI = myocardial infarction; Neo = neonate; NS = nephrotic syndrome; Obes = obese; Pneu = pneumonia; Preg = pregnant; Prem = premature; RA = rheumatoid arthritis; Smk = smoking; Tach = ventricular tachycardia; Ulcer = ulcer patients; Urem = uremia

References: *See* end of table.

Table A–II–1. PHARMACOKINETIC DATA (Continued)

AVAILABILITY (ORAL) (%)	URINARY EXCRETION (%)	BOUND IN PLASMA (%)	CLEARANCE ($ml \cdot min^{-1} \cdot kg^{-1}$)	VOL. DIST. (*liters/kg*)	HALF-LIFE (*hours*)	EFFECTIVE CONCENTRATIONS	TOXIC CONCENTRATIONS
LABETALOL (Chapter 11)							
18 ± 5 ↑ Aged, Cirr	<5	50	25 ± 10 [a,b] ⟷ Urem, Preg, Cirr ↓ Aged	9.4 ± 3.4 [b]	4.9 ± 2.0 [b] ⟷ Cirr, Urem, Preg ↑ Aged	—	—

[a] Blood-to-plasma ratio = 1.4.

[b] *CL* significantly lower in young hypertensive patients (20 ± 8). Disease effects are compared with values in young patients.

AVAILABILITY (ORAL) (%)	URINARY EXCRETION (%)	BOUND IN PLASMA (%)	CLEARANCE ($ml \cdot min^{-1} \cdot kg^{-1}$)	VOL. DIST. (*liters/kg*)	HALF-LIFE (*hours*)	EFFECTIVE CONCENTRATIONS	TOXIC CONCENTRATIONS
LEUCOVORIN [a] (Chapter 54)							
25 mg: 97 [a] 50 mg: 75 [a] 100 mg: 37 [a] 25 mg: 100 [b] 25 mg: 28 [c]	10 [b] 100 [c] 31 [d]	35–45 [b]	3.9 ± 0.8 [a]	3.2 ± 1.2 [a,e]	9.3 ± 2.8 [a] 0.5 ± 0.1 [b] 7.5 ± 1.1 [c] 3.8 ± 2.0 [d]	—	—

[a] Racemic mixture.
[b] Active (−)-isomer
[c] Inactive (+)-isomer.
[d] Active metabolite
[e] V_{area}.

AVAILABILITY (ORAL) (%)	URINARY EXCRETION (%)	BOUND IN PLASMA (%)	CLEARANCE ($ml \cdot min^{-1} \cdot kg^{-1}$)	VOL. DIST. (*liters/kg*)	HALF-LIFE (*hours*)	EFFECTIVE CONCENTRATIONS	TOXIC CONCENTRATIONS
LIDOCAINE [a] (Chapter 35)							
35 ± 11 [b] ↑ Cirr, Aged	2 ± 1 ↑ Neo	70 ± 5 ↓ Neo ↑ MI, CPBS, Aged, Urem ⟷ NS, Smk, Child	9.2 ± 2.4 ↓ CHF, Cirr, CPBS [c], Obes ↑ Smk ⟷ Urem, AVH [d], Neo, Aged [e]	1.1 ± 0.4 ↓ CHF, CPBS [c] ↑ Cirr, Neo ⟷ Urem, Aged, Obes	1.8 ± 0.4 ↑ Cirr, MI [f], Neo, Obes ⟷ Urem, CPBS, CHF [g]	1.5–6 μg/ml	Occasional: 6–10 μg/ml Frequent: >10 μg/ml

[a] Active metabolite, monoethylglycylxylidide is 60–80% as potent as lidocaine; concentrations reach 36 ± 26% of those of parent drug (15 ± 3% protein bound).
[b] Commercial preparations are for parenteral administration.
[c] Decrease (~40%) on day 3 after surgery; return toward normal on day 7.
[d] During acute phase, blood clearance was 13 ± 4 $ml \cdot min^{-1} \cdot kg^{-1}$, which increased to 20 ± 4 $ml \cdot min^{-1} \cdot kg^{-1}$ after recovery.
[e] Decreased *CL* with increasing age noted in patients with MI.
[f] Half-life increased when infusion longer than 24 hours, probably related to increased plasma binding.
[g] Short term, no change; long term, marked increase possibly related to increased binding.

LITHIUM (Chapter 18)							
100	95 ± 15	0	0.35 ± 0.11 [a] ↓ Urem, Aged ↑ Preg	0.79 ± 0.34 [b]	22 ± 8 [c] ↑ Urem, Aged	0.5–1.25 mEq/l	>2.0 mEq/l

[a] Renal clearance of Li^+ parallels that of Na^+. The ratio of clearances of Li^+ and creatinine is about 0.2 ± 0.03.
[b] V_{area}.
[c] A shorter half-life of 5.6 ± 0.5 hours is due to distribution; this influences drug concentrations for at least 12 hours.

LORAZEPAM (Chapters 17, 18, 19)							
93 ± 10	<1	91 ± 2 ↓ Cirr ⟷ Aged, Burn	1.1 ± 0.4 ⟷ Aged, Cirr, AVH, Smk ↑ Burn	1.3 ± 0.2 [a] ↑ Cirr, Burn ⟷ Aged	14 ± 5 ↑ Cirr, Neo ⟷ Aged, Urem, CPBS ↓ Burn	—	—

[a] V_{area}.

LORCAINIDE [a] (Chapter 35)							
Dose-dependent [b]	<2	85 ± 5 ⟷ Cirr, Urem	17.5 ± 2.8 [c] ↓ Cirr ⟷ Aged, Urem	6.4 ± 2.4 ↑ Aged ⟷ Cirr, Urem	7.6 ± 2.2 [d] ↑ Cirr, CHF, Aged ⟷ Urem	100 ng/ml [e]	—

[a] Active metabolite, N-dealkyl lorcainide (norlorcainide).
[b] Saturable first-pass metabolism. F = 1–4% for 100-mg dose; 35–65% for 200-mg dose.
[c] Blood-to-plasma ratio = 0.70 (0.80 in alcoholic cirrhosis).
[d] Norlorcainide, half-life = 27 ± 8 hours. Steady-state ratio of norlorcainide to lorcainide = 2.2 ± 0.9.
[e] 75% suppression of premature ventricular contractions.

MELPHALAN (Chapter 52)							
71 ± 23	12 ± 7	90 ± 5 [a]	5.2 ± 2.9 [b] ⟷ Child	0.45 ± 0.15 ⟷ Child	1.4 ± 0.2 [c] ⟷ Child	—	—

[a] Decreases to 80 ± 5% after high doses (180 mg/m^2).
[b] Blood-to-plasma ratio = 0.96 ± 0.25.
[c] Approximately equal to half-life of melphalan *in vitro* in human plasma at 37°C.

Key: Adult = adults; Aged = aged; Alb = hypoalbuminemia; Arth = arthritis; Atr Fib = atrial fibrillation; AVH = acute viral hepatitis; Burn = burn patients; CAD = coronary artery disease; Celiac = celiac disease; CF = cystic fibrosis; CHF = congestive heart failure; Child = children; Cirr = cirrhosis; COPD = chronic obstructive pulmonary disease; CP = cor pulmonale; CPBS = cardiopulmonary bypass surgery; CRI = chronic respiratory insufficiency; Crohn = Crohn's disease; Cush = Cushing's syndrome; Epilep = epileptic; Fem = female; Hep = Hepatitis; HL = hyperlipoproteinemia; HTh = hyperthyroid; Inflam = inflammation; LTh = hypothyroid; MI = myocardial infarction; Neo = neonate; NS = nephrotic syndrome; Obes = obese; Pneu = pneumonia; Preg = pregnant; Prem = premature; RA = rheumatoid arthritis; Smk = smoking; Tach = ventricular tachycardia; Ulcer = ulcer patients; Urem = uremia

References: *See* end of table.

Table A–II–1. PHARMACOKINETIC DATA (Continued)

AVAILABILITY (ORAL) (%)	URINARY EXCRETION (%)	BOUND IN PLASMA (%)	CLEARANCE ($ml \cdot min^{-1} \cdot kg^{-1}$)	VOL. DIST. (*liters/kg*)	HALF-LIFE (*hours*)	EFFECTIVE CONCENTRATIONS	TOXIC CONCENTRATIONS
MEPERIDINE (Chapter 21)							
52 ± 3 ↑ Cirr	1–25 [a]	58 ± 9 [b] ↓ Aged, Urem ⟷ Cirr	17 ± 5 ↓ AVH, Cirr, Urem ⟷ Aged, Preg, Smk	4.4 ± 0.9 ↑ Aged ⟷ Cirr, Preg, Urem	3.2 ± 0.8 [c] ↑ AVH, Cirr, Aged, Urem ⟷ Preg	0.4–0.7 μg/ml [d]	—

[a] Meperidine is a weak acid ($pK_a = 9.6$) and is excreted to a greater extent in the urine at low urinary pH and to a lesser extent at high pH.
[b] Correlates with the concentration of α_1-acid glycoprotein.
[c] A longer half-life (7 hours) is also observed.
[d] Postoperative analgesia.

AVAILABILITY (ORAL) (%)	URINARY EXCRETION (%)	BOUND IN PLASMA (%)	CLEARANCE ($ml \cdot min^{-1} \cdot kg^{-1}$)	VOL. DIST. (*liters/kg*)	HALF-LIFE (*hours*)	EFFECTIVE CONCENTRATIONS	TOXIC CONCENTRATIONS
MERCAPTOPURINE (Chapter 52)							
12 ± 7 [a]	22 ± 12	19	11 ± 4 [b]	0.56 ± 0.38	0.90 ± 0.37	—	—

[a] Increases to 60% when first-pass metabolism inhibited by allopurinol (100 mg three times daily).
[b] Despite inhibition of intrinsic clearance by allopurinol, hepatic metabolism is limited by blood flow, and clearance is thus little changed by allopurinol.

AVAILABILITY (ORAL) (%)	URINARY EXCRETION (%)	BOUND IN PLASMA (%)	CLEARANCE ($ml \cdot min^{-1} \cdot kg^{-1}$)	VOL. DIST. (*liters/kg*)	HALF-LIFE (*hours*)	EFFECTIVE CONCENTRATIONS	TOXIC CONCENTRATIONS
METHADONE (Chapter 21)							
92 ± 21	24 ± 10 [a]	89 ± 1.4	1.4 ± 0.5 [a,b]	3.8 ± 0.6 [c]	35 ± 12 [c]	>100 ng/ml [d]	—

[a] Inversely correlated with urine pH.
[b] Blood-to-plasma ratio = 0.75 ± 0.03
[c] Directly correlated with urine pH.
[d] Prevention of withdrawal symptoms.

AVAILABILITY (ORAL) (%)	URINARY EXCRETION (%)	BOUND IN PLASMA (%)	CLEARANCE ($ml \cdot min^{-1} \cdot kg^{-1}$)	VOL. DIST. (*liters/kg*)	HALF-LIFE (*hours*)	EFFECTIVE CONCENTRATIONS	TOXIC CONCENTRATIONS
METHICILLIN (Chapter 46)							
—	88 ± 17	39 ± 2	6.1 ± 1.3 ↓ Urem ↑ CF	0.43 ± 0.10	0.85 ± 0.23 ↑ Urem, Prem, Neo	*See* Chapter 46	—
METHOHEXITAL (Chapters 14, 17)							
—	<1	—	10.9 ± 3.0	2.2 ± 0.7	3.9 ± 2.1	3.5–11 μg/ml	—

METHOTREXATE (Chapter 52)							
70 ± 27 [a]	48 ± 18 [b]	34 ± 8	2.1 ± 0.8 ↓ Urem ↑, ⟷ Child	0.55 ± 0.19 ⟷ Child	7.2 ± 2.1 [c]	—	10 μM [d]

[a] *F* may be as low as 20% when doses exceed 80 mg/m^2.
[b] For 10 mg/m^2; increased to 85 ± 11% at high doses.
[c] A faster half-life (2 hours) is seen initially.
[d] Bone-marrow toxicity correlated with concentrations greater than 10 μM at 24 hours, greater than 1 μM at 48 hours, or greater than 0.1 μM at 72 hours.

METHYLDOPA (Chapter 33)							
25 ± 16	28 ± 9 ↓ Crohn [a]	1–16 ⟷ Crohn	3.1 ± 0.9 ↓ Urem [b]	0.37 ± 0.10	1.8 ± 0.2 ↑ Urem, Neo ⟷ Crohn	—	—

[a] Interpreted as a decrease in absorption in Crohn's disease.
[b] Clearances of unchanged drug and active metabolites are reduced.

METHYLPREDNISOLONE (Chapter 60)							
82 ± 13 [a]	4.9 ± 2.3	78 ± 3	6.2 ± 0.9 ⟷ NS, RA, CRI	1.2 ± 0.2 ⟷ NS, RA, CRI	2.3 ± 0.5 ⟷ NS, Urem, RA, CRI	—	—

[a] May be decreased to 50–60% at high doses.

METOCLOPRAMIDE (Chapter 38)							
76 ± 38 ⟷ Aged	20 ± 9	40 ± 4 ⟷ Urem	6.2 ± 1.3 ↓ Urem ⟷ Aged	3.4 ± 1.3 ⟷ Urem, Aged	5.0 ± 1.4 ↑ Urem ⟷ Aged	—	—

Key: Adult = adults; Aged = aged; Alb = hypoalbuminemia; Arth = arthritis; Atr Fib = atrial fibrillation; AVH = acute viral hepatitis; Burn = burn patients; CAD = coronary artery disease; Celiac = celiac disease; CF = cystic fibrosis; CHF = congestive heart failure; Child = children; Cirr = cirrhosis; COPD = chronic obstructive pulmonary disease; CP = cor pulmonale; CPBS = cardiopulmonary bypass surgery; CRI = chronic respiratory insufficiency; Crohn = Crohn's disease; Cush = Cushing's syndrome; Epilep = epileptic; Fem = female; Hep = Hepatitis; HL = hyperlipoproteinemia; HTh = hyperthyroid; Inflam = inflammation; LTh = hypothyroid; MI = myocardial infarction; Neo = neonate; NS = nephrotic syndrome; Obes = obese; Pneu = pneumonia; Preg = pregnant; Prem = premature; RA = rheumatoid arthritis; Smk = smoking; Tach = ventricular tachycardia; Ulcer = ulcer patients; Urem = uremia

References: *See* end of table.

Table A–II–1. PHARMACOKINETIC DATA (Continued)

AVAILABILITY (ORAL) (%)	URINARY EXCRETION (%)	BOUND IN PLASMA (%)	CLEARANCE (*ml · min⁻¹ · kg⁻¹*)	VOL. DIST. (*liters/kg*)	HALF-LIFE (*hours*)	EFFECTIVE CONCENTRATIONS	TOXIC CONCENTRATIONS
METOCURINE (Chapter 9)							
—	50	35 ± 6	1.3 ± 0.3 ↓ Urem, Aged ⟷ CPBS	0.35 ± 0.04 ⟷ Urem, Aged, CPBS	4.7 ± 0.9 ↑ Urem, Aged ⟷ CPBS	0.23 μg/ml [a] 0.63 μg/ml [b] ↑ Burn, Urem ⟷ Aged, CPBS	—
[a] 50% depression of twitch tension.				[b] 95% depression of twitch tension.			
METOPROLOL [a] (Chapter 11)							
38 ± 14 ↑ Cirr ↓ Preg	10 ± 3	11 ± 1 ⟷ Preg	15 ± 3 [b] ↑ HTh, Preg ⟷ Aged, Smk	4.2 ± 0.7 ↑ Preg	3.2 ± 0.2 ↑ Cirr, Neo ⟷ Aged, HTh, Preg, Smk	25 ng/ml [c]	—
[a] Racemic mixture. Metabolism of less active R-(+)-enantiomer (CL/F = 28 ml · min⁻¹ · kg⁻¹; V_{area}/F = 7.6 liters/kg; $t_{1/2}$ = 2.7 hours) is faster than that of more active S-(−)-enantiomer (CL/F = 20 ml · min⁻¹ · kg⁻¹; V_{area}/F = 5.5 liters/kg; $t_{1/2}$ = 3 hours). Small fraction of population metabolizes metoprolol slowly; F is increased in such individuals.				[b] Blood-to-plasma ratio = 1. [c] To achieve a 10% decrease in resting heart rate.			
METRONIDAZOLE [a] (Chapter 42)							
99 ± 8 ⟷ Crohn	10 ± 2	10	1.3 ± 0.3 ↓ Cirr, Neo ⟷ Preg, Urem, Crohn	0.74 ± 0.10 ⟷ Urem, Crohn, Cirr	8.5 ± 2.9 ↑ Neo, Cirr ⟷ Preg, Urem [a], Crohn, Child	3–6 μg/ml	—
[a] Active hydroxylated metabolite, which accumulates in renal failure.							
MEXILETINE (Chapter 35)							
87 ± 13	4–15 [a]	63 ± 3 ⟷ MI	6.3 ± 2.7 ↓ MI, Urem [b] ⟷ CHF, Aged	4.9 ± 0.5 ⟷ MI	9.2 ± 2.1 ↑ MI, CHF, Urem [b] ⟷ Aged	0.7–2.0 μg/ml	>2.0 μg/ml
[a] Dependent on urinary pH.				[b] Only in patients with CL_{cr} < 10 ml/min.			

MEZLOCILLIN (Chapter 46)							
—	45 ± 6	16–42	$CL = 1.44\ CL_{cr} + 0.23$ [a] ↓ Neo, Prem, Aged ⟷ Child	Dose-dependent [b] ↑ Prem, Neo, Aged ⟷ Urem, Child	1.3 ± 0.4 ↑ Urem, Prem, Neo ⟷ Child, Aged	—	—

[a] For 5-g dose. For 1-g dose, $CL = 2.07\ CL_{cr} + 0.97$.

[b] $V_{ss} = 0.20 \pm 0.06$ for 1-g dose and 0.14 ± 0.05 for 5-g dose.

MIDAZOLAM (Chapters 14, 17)							
44 ± 17 ↑ Cirr	56 ± 26 ⟷ Smk, Aged	95 ± 2 ↓ Aged, Urem ⟷ Smk, Cirr	6.6 ± 1.8 ↑ Urem [a] ↓ Cirr ⟷ Obes, Smk	1.1 ± 0.6 ↑ Obes ⟷ Cirr	1.9 ± 0.6 ↑ Aged, Obes, Cirr ⟷ Smk	—	—

[a] Owing to increased free fraction; unbound clearance is unchanged.

MINOCYCLINE (Chapter 48)							
95–100	11 ± 2	76	1.0 ± 0.3 ⟷, ↑ Urem [a] ↓ HL	1.3 ± 0.2 [b] ↑ Urem ↓ HL	16 ± 2 ⟷ Urem, Cirr, HL	—	—

[a] In patients with reduced CL_{cr}, single-dose infusion studies indicate that clearance is increased, which is consistent with the increased V and unchanged $t_{1/2}$. However, there is no accumulation of drug beyond that seen in normal subjects during repeated administration of minocycline to patients with CL_{cr} between 18 and 45 ml/min.

[b] V_{area}.

MINOXIDIL (Chapter 33)							
[a]	20 ± 6	0	24 ± 6 [b]	2.7 ± 0.7 [b]	3.1 ± 0.6 [c]	—	—

[a] Previous reports indicate complete absorption. However, high value of CL/F suggests that bioavailability is decreased.

[b] CL/F and V_{area}/F.

[c] Value in hypertensive patients. In healthy young normal subjects, $t_{1/2} = 1.3$ hours, consistent with CL/F and V_{area}/F.

Key: Adult = adults; Aged = aged; Alb = hypoalbuminemia; Arth = arthritis; Atr Fib = atrial fibrillation; AVH = acute viral hepatitis; Burn = burn patients; CAD = coronary artery disease; Celiac = celiac disease; CF = cystic fibrosis; CHF = congestive heart failure; Child = children; Cirr = cirrhosis; COPD = chronic obstructive pulmonary disease; CP = cor pulmonale; CPBS = cardiopulmonary bypass surgery; CRI = chronic respiratory insufficiency; Crohn = Crohn's disease; Cush = Cushing's syndrome; Epilep = epileptic; Fem = female; Hep = Hepatitis; HL = hyperlipoproteinemia; HTh = hyperthyroid; Inflam = inflammation; LTh = hypothyroid; MI = myocardial infarction; Neo = neonate; NS = nephrotic syndrome; Obes = obese; Pneu = pneumonia; Preg = pregnant; Prem = premature; RA = rheumatoid arthritis; Smk = smoking; Tach = ventricular tachycardia; Ulcer = ulcer patients; Urem = uremia

References: *See* end of table.

Table A–II–1. PHARMACOKINETIC DATA (Continued)

AVAILABILITY (ORAL) (%)	URINARY EXCRETION (%)	BOUND IN PLASMA (%)	CLEARANCE ($ml \cdot min^{-1} \cdot kg^{-1}$)	VOL. DIST. (*liters/kg*)	HALF-LIFE (*hours*)	EFFECTIVE CONCENTRATIONS	TOXIC CONCENTRATIONS
MORPHINE [a] (Chapter 21)							
24 ± 12	6–10	35 ± 2 ↓ AVH, Cirr, Alb	24 ± 10 ⟷ Aged, Cirr, Urem, Child ↓ Neo	3.3 ± 0.9 ⟷ Cirr, Urem	1.9 ± 0.5 ⟷ Cirr, Urem, Child ↑ Neo	65 ± 80 ng/ml [b]	—

[a] Active metabolite, morphine-6-glucuronide; $t_{1/2}$ = 4.0 ± 1.5 hours (50 ± 37 hours in uremia).
[b] To achieve surgical analgesia.

AVAILABILITY (ORAL) (%)	URINARY EXCRETION (%)	BOUND IN PLASMA (%)	CLEARANCE ($ml \cdot min^{-1} \cdot kg^{-1}$)	VOL. DIST. (*liters/kg*)	HALF-LIFE (*hours*)	EFFECTIVE CONCENTRATIONS	TOXIC CONCENTRATIONS
MOXALACTAM [a] (Chapter 46)							
70–100 [b]	76 ± 12	[a]	$CL = 1.0\ CL_{cr} + 0.071$	0.25 ± 0.08 ⟷ Urem, Aged, Neo, Child	2.1 ± 0.7 ↑ Urem, Neo ⟷ Child, Preg	—	—

[a] Racemic mixture. More active R-epimer is cleared more rapidly than S-epimer, probably because it is less extensively bound to plasma proteins (53 vs. 67%).
[b] Intramuscular.

AVAILABILITY (ORAL) (%)	URINARY EXCRETION (%)	BOUND IN PLASMA (%)	CLEARANCE ($ml \cdot min^{-1} \cdot kg^{-1}$)	VOL. DIST. (*liters/kg*)	HALF-LIFE (*hours*)	EFFECTIVE CONCENTRATIONS	TOXIC CONCENTRATIONS
NADOLOL (Chapter 11)							
34 ± 5	73 ± 4	20 ± 4	2.9 ± 0.6 ↓ Urem	1.9 ± 0.2	16 ± 2 ↑ Urem	—	—
NAFCILLIN (Chapter 46)							
36 [a]	27 ± 5 ↑ Cirr [b]	89.4 ± 0.2 ↓ Neo	7.5 ± 1.9 ↓ Cirr [c]	0.35 ± 0.09 ↓ Cirr [c]	1.0 ± 0.2 ⟷ Cirr [b], Urem	*See* Chapter 46	—

[a] Calculated from mean values of excretion after oral versus intramuscular administration.
[b] Significant increase noted for patients with extrahepatic biliary obstruction.
[c] Significant decrease also noted for patients with extrahepatic biliary obstruction.

AVAILABILITY (ORAL) (%)	URINARY EXCRETION (%)	BOUND IN PLASMA (%)	CLEARANCE ($ml \cdot min^{-1} \cdot kg^{-1}$)	VOL. DIST. (*liters/kg*)	HALF-LIFE (*hours*)	EFFECTIVE CONCENTRATIONS	TOXIC CONCENTRATIONS
NALBUPHINE (Chapter 21)							
16 ± 8 ↑ Aged	4 ± 2 ⟷ Aged	—	22 ± 5 ↑ Child ⟷ Aged	3.8 ± 1.1 ⟷ Aged, Child	2.3 ± 1.2 ↓ Child ⟷ Aged	—	—

NALOXONE (Chapter 21)							
~2 [a]	Negligible	—	22 ↑ Neo ⟷ Urem	2.1 ↑ Neo	1.1 ± 0.6 ⟷ Neo	—	—

[a] Absorption is relatively complete (91%), but most of the drug is subject to hepatic first-pass metabolism.

NALTREXONE [a] (Chapter 21)							
5–40	<1	20	48 ± 6 [b]	19 ± 5 [b,c]	2.7 ± 1.0	—	—

[a] Weakly active metabolite, 6-naltrexol; $t_{1/2}$ = 8.8 hours.
[b] Assuming 70-kg weight.
[c] V_{area}.

NAPROXEN (Chapter 26)							
99 [a]	<1	99.7 ± 0.1 [b] ↑ Urem, Aged [c], Cirr ↓ RA, Alb	0.13 ± 0.02 [d] ↓ Urem ⟷ Aged [c], Cirr [c] ↑ RA	0.16 ± 0.02 [e] ↑ Urem, Cirr, RA ⟷ Aged	14 ± 1 ⟷ Urem, RA	>50 μg/ml [f]	—

[a] Estimated.
[b] Saturable protein binding yields apparent nonlinear kinetics.
[c] No change in total clearance, but significant (50%) decrease in clearance of unbound drug; it is thus suggested that dosing rate be decreased. A second study in elderly patients found decreased *CL* and increased $t_{1/2}$ with no change in percent bound.
[d] *CL/F*.
[e] V_{area}/F.
[f] 76% of patients with rheumatoid arthritis responded with trough concentrations in plasma above this value.

NEOSTIGMINE (Chapter 7)							
[a]	67	—	8.4 ± 2.7 ↓ Urem	0.7 ± 0.3	1.3 ± 0.8 ↑ Urem	—	—

[a] Absorption is presumed to be less than complete, since oral dosage must greatly exceed intravenous to achieve a similar effect.

Key: Adult = adults; Aged = aged; Alb = hypoalbuminemia; Arth = arthritis; Atr Fib = atrial fibrillation; AVH = acute viral hepatitis; Burn = burn patients; CAD = coronary artery disease; Celiac = celiac disease; CF = cystic fibrosis; CHF = congestive heart failure; Child = children; Cirr = cirrhosis; COPD = chronic obstructive pulmonary disease; CP = cor pulmonale; CPBS = cardiopulmonary bypass surgery; CRI = chronic respiratory insufficiency; Crohn = Crohn's disease; Cush = Cushing's syndrome; Epilep = epileptic; Fem = female; Hep = Hepatitis; HL = hyperlipoproteinemia; HTh = hyperthyroid; Inflam = inflammation; LTh = hypothyroid; MI = myocardial infarction; Neo = neonate; NS = nephrotic syndrome; Obes = obese; Pneu = pneumonia; Preg = pregnant; Prem = premature; RA = rheumatoid arthritis; Smk = smoking; Tach = ventricular tachycardia; Ulcer = ulcer patients; Urem = uremia

References: *See* end of table.

Table A–II–1. PHARMACOKINETIC DATA (Continued)

AVAILABILITY (ORAL) (%)	URINARY EXCRETION (%)	BOUND IN PLASMA (%)	CLEARANCE ($ml \cdot min^{-1} \cdot kg^{-1}$)	VOL. DIST. (*liters/kg*)	HALF-LIFE (*hours*)	EFFECTIVE CONCENTRATIONS	TOXIC CONCENTRATIONS
NETILMICIN (Chapter 47)							
—	80–90 [a]	<10	1.3 ± 0.2 ↓ Urem, Neo, Prem ⟷ Child, CPBS, Cirr ↑ CF	0.20 ± 0.02 ⟷ Urem, CPBS ↑ Prem	2.3 ± 0.7 37 ± 6 [b] ↑ Urem, Neo, Prem ↓ CF ⟷ Child, Cirr	*See* Chapter 47	*See* Chapter 47

[a] Possibly higher, since drug persists in tissues for a long time.
[b] Netilmicin has a long terminal half-life, which accounts for prolonged urinary excretion.

AVAILABILITY (ORAL) (%)	URINARY EXCRETION (%)	BOUND IN PLASMA (%)	CLEARANCE ($ml \cdot min^{-1} \cdot kg^{-1}$)	VOL. DIST. (*liters/kg*)	HALF-LIFE (*hours*)	EFFECTIVE CONCENTRATIONS	TOXIC CONCENTRATIONS
NICARDIPINE (Chapter 32)							
19–38 [a]	<1	89–99.5	13.4 ± 4.0 ⟷ Urem	1.1 ± 0.3	1.3 ± 0.3 ⟷ Urem	—	—

[a] Saturable metabolism after oral administration; *F* increases at higher doses.

AVAILABILITY (ORAL) (%)	URINARY EXCRETION (%)	BOUND IN PLASMA (%)	CLEARANCE ($ml \cdot min^{-1} \cdot kg^{-1}$)	VOL. DIST. (*liters/kg*)	HALF-LIFE (*hours*)	EFFECTIVE CONCENTRATIONS	TOXIC CONCENTRATIONS
NICOTINE (Chapters 9, 22)							
Oral: 30 Smoking: 90 [a]	16.7 ± 8.6	4.9 ± 2.8	18.5 ± 5.4	2.6 ± 0.9	2.0 ± 0.7	—	—

[a] Habitual smokers.

AVAILABILITY (ORAL) (%)	URINARY EXCRETION (%)	BOUND IN PLASMA (%)	CLEARANCE ($ml \cdot min^{-1} \cdot kg^{-1}$)	VOL. DIST. (*liters/kg*)	HALF-LIFE (*hours*)	EFFECTIVE CONCENTRATIONS	TOXIC CONCENTRATIONS
NIFEDIPINE (Chapter 32)							
50 ± 13 ↑ Cirr, Aged ⟷ Urem	~ 0	96 ± 1 ↓ Cirr, Urem	7.0 ± 1.8 ↓ Cirr, Aged ⟷ Urem, Smk	0.78 ± 0.22 ↑ Cirr, Urem ⟷ Aged	1.8 ± 0.4 [a] ↑ Cirr, Urem, Aged ⟷ Smk	47 ± 20 ng/ml [b] ↓ Cirr [c], Urem [c]	—

[a] Longer $t_{1/2}$ after oral administration (2.5 ± 1.3 hours).
[b] To decrease diastolic blood pressure in hypertensive patients.
[c] No difference when free concentration compared.

AVAILABILITY (ORAL) (%)	URINARY EXCRETION (%)	BOUND IN PLASMA (%)	CLEARANCE ($ml \cdot min^{-1} \cdot kg^{-1}$)	VOL. DIST. (*liters/kg*)	HALF-LIFE (*hours*)	EFFECTIVE CONCENTRATIONS	TOXIC CONCENTRATIONS
NITRAZEPAM (Chapters 17, 19)							
78 ± 16	<1	87 ± 1 ↓ Cirr ⟷ Aged	0.86 ± 0.12 ⟷ Aged, Cirr, Obes	1.9 ± 0.3 ↑ Aged ⟷ Cirr, Obes	26 ± 3 ↑ Aged, Obes ⟷ Cirr	—	>200 ng/ml [a]

[a] Sedation and drowsiness.

NITROGLYCERIN [a] (Chapter 32)							
Oral: <1 Sublingual: 38 ± 26 [b] Topical: 72 ± 20	<1	—	230 ± 90 [c]	3.3 ± 1.2 [d]	2.3 ± 0.6 min	1.2–11 ng/ml [e]	—

[a] Active dinitrate metabolites have weak activity compared to nitroglycerin (<10%), but, because of prolonged half-life (~40 min), they may accumulate during administration of sustained-release preparations to yield concentrations in plasma 10–20 times greater than the parent drug.

[b] Sublingual dose rinsed out of the mouth after 8 min. Rinse contained 31 ± 19% of the dose.

[c] Following a prolonged infusion.

[d] V_{area}.

[e] 25% fall in capillary wedge pressure in patients with CHF.

NIZATIDINE (Chapter 37)							
90	61 ± 3	35 ± 3	10.0 ± 3.3 ↓ Urem, Aged [a]	1.2 ± 0.5	1.3 ± 0.3 ↑ Urem, Aged [a] ⟷ Cirr	0.7 μg/ml [b]	—

[a] Related to changing renal function.

[b] To inhibit gastric acid secretion by 50%.

NORFLOXACIN (Chapter 45)							
30–40	26–32 [a]	15–20	7.2 ± 3.0 [b]	3.2 ± 1.4 [b]	5.0 ± 0.7 ↑ Urem	—	—

[a] Oral dose.

[b] CL/F and V_{area}/F, assuming 70-kg weight.

NORTRIPTYLINE [a] (Chapter 18)							
51 ± 5	2 ± 1	92 ± 2 ↑ HL	7.2 ± 1.8 ↓ Aged, Inflam ⟷ Smk, Urem	18 ± 4 [b]	31 ± 13 ↑ Aged ⟷ Urem	50–140 ng/ml [c]	—

[a] Active metabolite, 10-hydroxynortriptyline, accumulates to twice the concentration of nortriptyline.

[b] V_{area}.

[c] At concentrations in plasma above 140 ng/ml, the antidepressant effect appears to be less.

Key: Adult = adults; Aged = aged; Alb = hypoalbuminemia; Arth = arthritis; Atr Fib = atrial fibrillation; AVH = acute viral hepatitis; Burn = burn patients; CAD = coronary artery disease; Celiac = celiac disease; CF = cystic fibrosis; CHF = congestive heart failure; Child = children; Cirr = cirrhosis; COPD = chronic obstructive pulmonary disease; CP = cor pulmonale; CPBS = cardiopulmonary bypass surgery; CRI = chronic respiratory insufficiency; Crohn = Crohn's disease; Cush = Cushing's syndrome; Epilep = epileptic; Fem = female; Hep = Hepatitis; HL = hyperlipoproteinemia; HTh = hyperthyroid; Inflam = inflammation; LTh = hypothyroid; MI = myocardial infarction; Neo = neonate; NS = nephrotic syndrome; Obes = obese; Pneu = pneumonia; Preg = pregnant; Prem = premature; RA = rheumatoid arthritis; Smk = smoking; Tach = ventricular tachycardia; Ulcer = ulcer patients; Urem = uremia

References: *See* end of table.

Table A–II–1. PHARMACOKINETIC DATA (Continued)

AVAILABILITY (ORAL) (%)	URINARY EXCRETION (%)	BOUND IN PLASMA (%)	CLEARANCE ($ml \cdot min^{-1} \cdot kg^{-1}$)	VOL. DIST. (*liters/kg*)	HALF-LIFE (*hours*)	EFFECTIVE CONCENTRATIONS	TOXIC CONCENTRATIONS
OXACILLIN (Chapter 46)							
33	46 ± 4	92.2 ± 0.6	6.1 ± 1.7	0.33 ± 0.09 [a]	0.4–0.7 ↑ Urem	*See* Chapter 46	—
[a] V_{area}.							
OXAZEPAM (Chapters 17, 18)							
97 ± 11	<1	97.8 ± 2.3 ↑ Urem ⟷ Aged, Alb, AVH, Cirr	1.05 ± 0.36 ↑ HTh, Smk, Urem [a] ⟷ LTh, Aged, AVH, Cirr	0.60 ± 0.20 ↑ Urem ⟷ Aged, AVH, Cirr	6.8 ± 1.3 ↑ Urem, Neo ↓ HTh ⟷ Aged, AVH, Cirr, LTh, Preg	—	—
[a] *CL/F* of unbound drug is unchanged in uremia.							
PANCURONIUM (Chapter 9)							
—	67 ± 18	29 ± 9	1.8 ± 0.4 ↓ Aged, Urem, CPBS ⟷ Cirr	0.26 ± 0.07 ⟷ Aged, Urem ↑ Cirr	2.3 ± 0.4 ↑ Aged, Urem, Cirr	0.25 ± 0.07 μg/ml [a] 0.40 μg/ml [b]	—
[a] 50% decrease in twitch tension.				[b] 95% decrease in twitch tension.			
PENTAMIDINE (Chapter 43)							
Negligible	<5	—	113 ± 23 [a] ⟷ Urem	16 ± 9 [a]	6.2 ± 1.2 [a,b] ⟷ Urem	—	—
[a] Determined from first intravenous dose in patients with AIDS.				[b] A prolonged $t_{1/2}$ of 5–9 days is observed in urine after multiple doses; this is consistent with values of *CL* and V_{ss}.			
PENTAZOCINE (Chapter 21)							
47 ± 15	15 ± 7	65	17 ± 5 [a]	7.1 ± 1.4 [a]	4.6 ± 1.0	—	—
[a] *CL/F* and V_{area}/F for intramuscular dose, assuming 70-kg weight.							

PENTOXIFYLLINE [a] (Chapter 25)							
19 ± 13	0	0	19 ± 13 [b] ↓ Aged	2.4 ± 1.2 [b,c]	1.6 ± 0.8 ↑ Aged	—	—

[a] High concentrations of active metabolite (5-hydroxypentoxifylline) accumulate after oral administration because of extensive first-pass metabolism; concentrations of metabolite decline in parallel with those of parent drug.

[b] Assuming 70-kg weight.

[c] V_{area}.

PHENOBARBITAL (Chapters 17, 19)							
100 ± 11	24 ± 5 [a] ⟷ Cirr, AVH	51 ± 3 ↓ Neo ⟷ Preg, Aged	0.062 ± 0.013 [b] ↑ Preg, Child, Neo ⟷ Epilep, Smk	0.54 ± 0.03 ⟷ Epilep ↑ Neo	99 ± 18 ↑ Cirr, Aged ↓ Child ⟷ Epilep, Neo	10–25 μg/ml [c] 15 μg/ml [d]	>30 μg/ml 65–117 μg/ml [e] 100–134 μg/ml [f]

[a] Increased when urine is alkaline; decreased with decreased urine flow.

[b] Blood-to-plasma ratio = 1.12 ± 0.08.

[c] Tonic–clonic seizures.

[d] Febrile convulsions in children.

[e] Stage III—comatose, reflexes present.

[f] Stage IV—no deep-tendon reflexes.

PHENYLBUTAZONE [a] (Chapter 26)							
80–100 [b]	~ 1	96.1 ± 1.1 ↓ Cirr, AVH, Urem, Hep, Aged ⟷ Smk	0.023 ± 0.003 [c] ↑ Smk	0.097 ± 0.005 [c] ↑ Urem ⟷ Smk	56 ± 8 ↓ Child, Smk ⟷ Aged, RA, Cirr, Urem	50–150 μg/ml	—

[a] Active metabolites, oxyphenbutazone and γ-hydroxyphenylbutazone.

[b] Estimate.

[c] CL/F and V_{area}/F.

Key: Adult = adults; Aged = aged; Alb = hypoalbuminemia; Arth = arthritis; Atr Fib = atrial fibrillation; AVH = acute viral hepatitis; Burn = burn patients; CAD = coronary artery disease; Celiac = celiac disease; CF = cystic fibrosis; CHF = congestive heart failure; Child = children; Cirr = cirrhosis; COPD = chronic obstructive pulmonary disease; CP = cor pulmonale; CPBS = cardiopulmonary bypass surgery; CRI = chronic respiratory insufficiency; Crohn = Crohn's disease; Cush = Cushing's syndrome; Epilep = epileptic; Fem = female; Hep = Hepatitis; HL = hyperlipoproteinemia; HTh = hyperthyroid; Inflam = inflammation; LTh = hypothyroid; MI = myocardial infarction; Neo = neonate; NS = nephrotic syndrome; Obes = obese; Pneu = pneumonia; Preg = pregnant; Prem = premature; RA = rheumatoid arthritis; Smk = smoking; Tach = ventricular tachycardia; Ulcer = ulcer patients; Urem = uremia

References: *See* end of table.

Table A–II–1. PHARMACOKINETIC DATA (Continued)

AVAILABILITY (ORAL) (%)	URINARY EXCRETION (%)	BOUND IN PLASMA (%)	CLEARANCE ($ml \cdot min^{-1} \cdot kg^{-1}$)	VOL. DIST. (*liters/kg*)	HALF-LIFE (*hours*)	EFFECTIVE CONCENTRATIONS	TOXIC CONCENTRATIONS
PHENYLETHYLMALONAMIDE [a] (Chapter 19)							
91 ± 4	79 ± 5 [b]	8 ± 1	0.52 ± 0.11 ↓ Urem ⟷ Epilep	0.69 ± 0.10 ⟷ Epilep	16 ± 3 ↑ Urem, Neo ⟷ Epilep	[c]	—

[a] One of the two major metabolites of primidone.
[b] After oral dose.
[c] Antiepileptic efficacy not established; active in rats.

AVAILABILITY (ORAL) (%)	URINARY EXCRETION (%)	BOUND IN PLASMA (%)	CLEARANCE ($ml \cdot min^{-1} \cdot kg^{-1}$)	VOL. DIST. (*liters/kg*)	HALF-LIFE (*hours*)	EFFECTIVE CONCENTRATIONS	TOXIC CONCENTRATIONS
PHENYTOIN (Chapters 19, 35)							
90 ± 3	2 ± 8	89 ± 23 ↓ Urem, Hep, Alb, Neo, AVH, Cirr, NS, Preg, Epilep, Burn ⟷ Obes, Smk, Aged	V_m = 5.9 ± 1.2 mg · kg^{-1} · day^{-1} ↓ Aged; ↑ Child K_m = 5.7 ± 2.9 mg/l [a] ⟷ Aged; ↓ Child ↑ [b] NS, Urem ↓ [b] Prem ⟷ [b] AVH, LTh, HTh, Smk	0.64 ± 0.04 [c] ↑ Neo, NS, Urem ⟷ AVH, LTh, HTh	6–24 [d] ↑ [b] Prem ↓ [b] Urem ⟷ [b] AVH, LTh, HTh, Smk	>10 μg/ml [e]	>20 μg/ml [f]

[a] Significantly decreased in Japanese.
[b] Comparison of clearances and half-lives with similar doses in normal subjects and patients; nonlinear kinetics not considered.
[c] V_{area}.
[d] Apparent half-life is dependent on plasma concentration.
[e] Suppression of tonic–clonic convulsions.
[f] Nystagmus; ataxia may not occur until concentrations exceed 30 μg/ml.

AVAILABILITY (ORAL) (%)	URINARY EXCRETION (%)	BOUND IN PLASMA (%)	CLEARANCE ($ml \cdot min^{-1} \cdot kg^{-1}$)	VOL. DIST. (*liters/kg*)	HALF-LIFE (*hours*)	EFFECTIVE CONCENTRATIONS	TOXIC CONCENTRATIONS
PIMOZIDE (Chapter 18)							
<50 [a]	—	99	4.1 ± 3.8 [b] 3.5 ± 2.1 [b,c]	28 ± 18 [d] 20 ± 15 [c,d]	111 ± 57 [e] 66 ± 49 [c]	—	—

[a] About 50–60% is absorbed.
[b] *CL/F*.
[c] Children 6 to 13 years old.
[d] V_{ss}/F.
[e] Previous reports of $t_{1/2}$ = 53 ± 3 hours in schizophrenic adults.

PINDOLOL (Chapter 11)

75 ± 9 ↓ Urem	54 ± 9	51 ± 3 [a] ↑ RA	8.3 ± 1.8 ↓ Urem, Cirr	2.3 ± 0.9 ⟷ Urem	3.6 ± 0.6 ↑ Urem, Cirr ⟷ Smk	4.5 ng/ml [b]	—

[a] Blood-to-plasma ratio = 0.69 ± 0.08.

[b] 50% decrease in exercise-induced cardioacceleration.

PIPERACILLIN (Chapter 46)

—	71 ± 14	16, 48 [a]	2.6 ± 0.7 $CL = 1.36\ CL_{cr} + 1.50$ ↓ Child ↑ CF	0.18 ± 0.03 ↓ CF ⟷ Urem, Child	0.93 ± 0.12 ↑ Urem ↓ Child, CF	—	—

[a] Different studies report 16, 21, and 48%.

PIROXICAM (Chapter 26)

[a]	<5	99.3 ± 0.2 ↓ Alb ⟷ Aged	0.036 ± 0.008 [b] ↓ Cirr [c] ⟷ Aged [d], Urem, RA	0.15 ± 0.03 [e] ↑ Alb ⟷ Aged	48 ± 8 ⟷ Aged [d], Urem, RA	—	—

[a] Good absorption and low hepatic clearance suggest that F is high.
[b] CL/F.
[c] Severe disease only.

[d] CL decreased and $t_{1/2}$ increased in eldery women.
[e] V_{area}/F.

PRAZEPAM [a] (Chapters 17, 18)

[b]	0	—	140 ± 100 [c]	14.4 ± 5.1 [c]	1.3 ± 0.7	—	—

[a] Prazepam is essentially a prodrug for desmethyldiazepam; *see also* listing for that compound. Values above are for prazepam.

[b] Availability of desmethyldiazepam from prazepam is 51 ± 5% of that from clorazepate.
[c] CL/F and V_{area}/F.

Key: Adult = adults; Aged = aged; Alb = hypoalbuminemia; Arth = arthritis; Atr Fib = atrial fibrillation; AVH = acute viral hepatitis; Burn = burn patients; CAD = coronary artery disease; Celiac = celiac disease; CF = cystic fibrosis; CHF = congestive heart failure; Child = children; Cirr = cirrhosis; COPD = chronic obstructive pulmonary disease; CP = cor pulmonale; CPBS = cardiopulmonary bypass surgery; CRI = chronic respiratory insufficiency; Crohn = Crohn's disease; Cush = Cushing's syndrome; Epilep = epileptic; Fem = female; Hep = Hepatitis; HL = hyperlipoproteinemia; HTh = hyperthyroid; Inflam = inflammation; LTh = hypothyroid; MI = myocardial infarction; Neo = neonate; NS = nephrotic syndrome; Obes = obese; Pneu = pneumonia; Preg = pregnant; Prem = premature; RA = rheumatoid arthritis; Smk = smoking; Tach = ventricular tachycardia; Ulcer = ulcer patients; Urem = uremia

References: *See* end of table.

Table A–II–1. PHARMACOKINETIC DATA (Continued)

AVAILABILITY (ORAL) (%)	URINARY EXCRETION (%)	BOUND IN PLASMA (%)	CLEARANCE ($ml \cdot min^{-1} \cdot kg^{-1}$)	VOL. DIST. (*liters/kg*)	HALF-LIFE (*hours*)	EFFECTIVE CONCENTRATIONS	TOXIC CONCENTRATIONS
PRAZOSIN (Chapter 11, 33)							
68 ± 17	<1	95 ± 1 ↓ Cirr, Alb, Urem ⟷ CHF	3.0 ± 0.3 [a] ↓ CHF, Preg ⟷ Aged, Urem	0.60 ± 0.13 [a] ↑ Aged	2.9 ± 0.8 ↑ CHF, Aged, Preg ⟷ Urem	—	—

[a] Assuming 70-kg weight.

AVAILABILITY (ORAL) (%)	URINARY EXCRETION (%)	BOUND IN PLASMA (%)	CLEARANCE ($ml \cdot min^{-1} \cdot kg^{-1}$)	VOL. DIST. (*liters/kg*)	HALF-LIFE (*hours*)	EFFECTIVE CONCENTRATIONS	TOXIC CONCENTRATIONS
PREDNISOLONE (Chapter 60)							
82 ± 13 ⟷ Hep, Cush, Urem, Crohn, Celiac, Smk, Aged ↓ HTh	26 ± 9 [a] ↓ Aged, HTh	90–95 (<200 ng/ml) [b] ~70 (>1 μg/ml) ↓ Alb, NS, Aged, HTh, Cirr ⟷ Hep	8.7 ± 1.6 [c,d] ⟷ Hep, Cush, Smk, CRI, NS [c], HTh [c] ↓ Aged [c], Cirr [c]	1.5 ± 0.2 [c,e] ⟷ Hep, Cush, Smk, CRI, NS [c] ↓ HTh [c], Aged [c]	2.2 ± 0.5 ⟷ Hep, Cush, Smk, Urem, CRI, NS [c] ↓ HTh ↑ Aged	—	—

[a] An additional 3 ± 2% is excreted as prednisone.
[b] Extent of binding to plasma proteins is dependent on concentration over range encountered.
[c] Values for unbound drug.
[d] Clearance of unbound drug increases slightly but significantly with increasing dose. Total clearance increases markedly as protein binding is saturated.
[e] Independent of dose. When total drug concentration is measured, *V* increases due to saturable protein binding.

AVAILABILITY (ORAL) (%)	URINARY EXCRETION (%)	BOUND IN PLASMA (%)	CLEARANCE ($ml \cdot min^{-1} \cdot kg^{-1}$)	VOL. DIST. (*liters/kg*)	HALF-LIFE (*hours*)	EFFECTIVE CONCENTRATIONS	TOXIC CONCENTRATIONS
PREDNISONE (Chapter 60)							
80 ± 11 [a] ⟷ Hep, Cush, Urem, Crohn, Celiac, Smk, Aged	3 ± 2 [b] ⟷ HTh	75 ± 2 [c]	3.6 ± 0.8 [d] ⟷ Hep	0.97 ± 0.11 [d] ⟷ Hep	3.6 ± 0.4 ⟷ Smk, Hep	—	—

[a] Measured relative to equivalent intravenous dose of prednisolone.
[b] An additional 15 ± 5% excreted as prednisolone.
[c] In contrast to prednisolone, no dependence on concentration.
[d] Kinetic values for prednisone are often reported in terms of the values for prednisolone, with which it is interconverted. However, the values above were obtained by measurement of prednisone after the intravenous administration of prednisone.

PRIMIDONE [a] (Chapter 19)

92 ± 18 [b,c]	42 ± 15 [b]	19 [d]	0.94 ± 0.35 [e] ↓ Urem, Preg ⟷ Child	0.59 ± 0.47 [b,e]	8.0 ± 4.8 ↑ Neo, Urem ⟷ Child	5–10 μg/ml [f]	>10 μg/ml 70–80 μg/ml [g]

[a] Primidone is metabolized to phenobarbital and phenylethylmalonamide; *see also* listings for these compounds.
[b] Children.
[c] Based on percentage of dose recovered in urine as primidone and its two primary metabolites.
[d] Based on ratio of drug concentrations in cerebrospinal fluid and plasma. Blood-to-plasma ratio = 0.97 ± 0.12.
[e] Data from oral, multiple-dose regimen; values are CL/F and V_{area}/F.
[f] Concentrations observed in patients with seizures who are improved or controlled by primidone. Concentrations of phenobarbital are considered to be more relevant.
[g] Crystalluria.

PROBENECID (Chapter 30)

100	1.2 ± 0.2	[a]	$V_m = 23 \pm 5$ $\mu g \cdot kg^{-1} \cdot min^{-1}$ [b] $K_m = 3.0 \pm 0.6$ $\mu g \cdot ml^{-1}$ [b]	0.17 ± 0.03 [c]	Dose-dependent [d]	—	—

[a] Nonlinear; percent unbound = 26 · $C/(140 + C)$, where C = total concentration in μg/ml.
[b] Values for calculation of clearance of free drug, using concentrations of free drug.
[c] V_{area} for total drug concentration.
[d] Below saturation (*e.g.*, 0.5-g dose), $t_{1/2} = 4.5 \pm 0.6$ hours. At 200 μg/ml (the peak concentration after a 2 g oral dose), parameters given here predict $t_{1/2} = 11.8$ hours.

PROCAINAMIDE [a] (Chapter 35)

83 ± 16	67 ± 8 ↓ CHF, COPD, CP, Cirr	16 ± 5	$CL = 2.7\ CL_{cr} + 1.7$ + 3.2 (fast) [b] or + 1.1 (slow) [b] ↑ Child ↓ MI ⟷ CHF, Tach	1.9 ± 0.3 ↓ CHF, Obes ⟷ Urem, Child, Tach	3.0 ± 0.6 ↑ Urem, MI ↓ Child ⟷ Obes, Tach	3–14 μg/ml	>14 μg/ml

[a] Active metabolite; *see also* data for N-acetylprocainamide.
[b] Clearance depends on acetylation phenotype. Use a mean value of 2.2 if phenotype unknown.

Key: Adult = adults; Aged = aged; Alb = hypoalbuminemia; Arth = arthritis; Atr Fib = atrial fibrillation; AVH = acute viral hepatitis; Burn = burn patients; CAD = coronary artery disease; Celiac = celiac disease; CF = cystic fibrosis; CHF = congestive heart failure; Child = children; Cirr = cirrhosis; COPD = chronic obstructive pulmonary disease; CP = cor pulmonale; CPBS = cardiopulmonary bypass surgery; CRI = chronic respiratory insufficiency; Crohn = Crohn's disease; Cush = Cushing's syndrome; Epilep = epileptic; Fem = female; Hep = Hepatitis; HL = hyperlipoproteinemia; HTh = hyperthyroid; Inflam = inflammation; LTh = hypothyroid; MI = myocardial infarction; Neo = neonate; NS = nephrotic syndrome; Obes = obese; Pneu = pneumonia; Preg = pregnant; Prem = premature; RA = rheumatoid arthritis; Smk = smoking; Tach = ventricular tachycardia; Ulcer = ulcer patients; Urem = uremia

References: *See* end of table.

Table A–II–1. PHARMACOKINETIC DATA (Continued)

AVAILABILITY (ORAL) (%)	URINARY EXCRETION (%)	BOUND IN PLASMA (%)	CLEARANCE ($ml \cdot min^{-1} \cdot kg^{-1}$)	VOL. DIST. (*liters/kg*)	HALF-LIFE (*hours*)	EFFECTIVE CONCENTRATIONS	TOXIC CONCENTRATIONS
PROPRANOLOL [a] (Chapters 11, 32, 33, 35)							
26 ± 10 ↑ Cirr	<0.5	87 ± 6 [b] ↑ Inflam, Crohn, Preg, Obes ⟷ Urem, Fem, Aged ↓ Cirr	16 ± 5 [c] ↑ Smk, HTh ↓ Hep, Cirr, Obes ⟷ Aged, Urem, Fem	4.3 ± 0.6 [c] ↑ Hep, HTh, Cirr ↓ Crohn ⟷ Aged, Urem, Obes, Fem	3.9 ± 0.4 [c] ↑ Hep, Cirr, Obes ⟷ Aged, Urem, Smk, Fem	20 ng/ml [d]	—

[a] Racemic mixture. For S-(−)-enantiomer (100-fold more active) compared to R-(+)-enantiomer, *CL* is 19% lower and V_{area} is 15% lower because of a higher degree of protein binding (18% less free drug); no difference in $t_{1/2}$s between enantiomers. Active metabolite, 4-hydroxypropranolol.

[b] Drug bound primarily to α_1-acid glycoprotein, which is elevated in a number of inflammatory conditions; blood-to-plasma ratio = 0.89 ± 0.03.

[c] Blood measurements.

[d] To achieve a 50% decrease in exercise-induced cardioacceleration. Antianginal effects are manifest at 15–90 ng/ml. Concentrations up to 1000 ng/ml may be required to control resistant ventricular arrhythmias.

AVAILABILITY (ORAL) (%)	URINARY EXCRETION (%)	BOUND IN PLASMA (%)	CLEARANCE ($ml \cdot min^{-1} \cdot kg^{-1}$)	VOL. DIST. (*liters/kg*)	HALF-LIFE (*hours*)	EFFECTIVE CONCENTRATIONS	TOXIC CONCENTRATIONS
PROTRIPTYLINE (Chapter 18)							
77–93 [a]	—	92 ± 0.6 [b]	3.6 ± 0.6 [c]	22 ± 1 [d]	78 ± 11	100–200 ng/ml	—

[a] Estimated from reported values of *CL/F*, assuming erythrocyte-to-plasma ratio ranges from 0 to 2, complete absorption, hepatic blood flow of 1500 ml/min, and hematocrit of 0.45.

[b] Determined at 24–26°C in heparinized plasma.

[c] *CL/F*.

[d] V_{area}/F.

AVAILABILITY (ORAL) (%)	URINARY EXCRETION (%)	BOUND IN PLASMA (%)	CLEARANCE ($ml \cdot min^{-1} \cdot kg^{-1}$)	VOL. DIST. (*liters/kg*)	HALF-LIFE (*hours*)	EFFECTIVE CONCENTRATIONS	TOXIC CONCENTRATIONS
PYRIDOSTIGMINE (Chapter 7)							
14 ± 3	80–90	—	8.5 ± 1.7 ↓ Urem	1.1 ± 0.3 ⟷ Urem	1.9 ± 0.2 (intravenous) 3.7 ± 1.0 (oral) ↑ Urem	50–100 ng/ml [a]	—

[a] Restoration of neuromuscular transmission in patients with myasthenia gravis.

AVAILABILITY (ORAL) (%)	URINARY EXCRETION (%)	BOUND IN PLASMA (%)	CLEARANCE ($ml \cdot min^{-1} \cdot kg^{-1}$)	VOL. DIST. (*liters/kg*)	HALF-LIFE (*hours*)	EFFECTIVE CONCENTRATIONS	TOXIC CONCENTRATIONS
PYRIMETHAMINE (Chapter 41)							
[a]	65 [b]	87 ± 1	0.41 ± 0.06 [c]	2.9 ± 0.5 [c]	83 ± 14	—	—

[a] Reported to be well absorbed. Since *CL* is low, availability is presumably high.

[b] Estimated.

[c] *CL/F* and V_{area}/F.

QUINIDINE [a] (Chapter 35)							
Sulfate: 80 ± 15 Gluconate: 71 ± 17	18 ± 5 ⟷ CHF	87 ± 3 ↓ Cirr, Hep, Neo, Preg ⟷ Urem, CRI, HL, Aged	4.7 ± 1.8 ↓ CHF, Aged ⟷ Cirr, Smk	2.7 ± 1.2 ↓ CHF ↑ Cirr ⟷ Aged	6.2 ± 1.8 ↑ Aged, Cirr ⟷ CHF, Urem	2–6 μg/ml [b]	6, 9, 14 μg/ml [c]

[a] Active metabolite, 3-hydroxyquinidine ($t_{1/2}$ = 12 ± 3 hours; percent bound in plasma = 60 ± 10).

[b] Specific assay methods for quinidine show >75% reduction in frequency of premature ventricular contractions at concentrations of 0.7–5.9 μg/ml, but active metabolites were not measured. Older, less specific assays of both active and inactive metabolites suggested a range of 2–7 μg/ml.

[c] Nonspecific assay; concentrations that cause toxic effects in 10, 30, and 50% of patients, respectively.

QUININE (Chapter 41)							
~90	12	93 ± 3 ↓ Neo, Preg	1.9 ± 0.5 ⟷ Preg [a], Child, Urem [a]	1.8 ± 0.4 ↓ Preg [a], Child ⟷ Urem [a]	11 ± 2 ↓ Preg [a], Child ⟷ Urem [a]	—	—

[a] Malaria patients.

RANITIDINE (Chapter 37)							
52 ± 11 ↑ Cirr ⟷ Urem	69 ± 6 ↓ Urem	15 ± 3	10.4 ± 1.1 ↓ Urem	1.3 ± 0.4 ⟷ Cirr, Urem	2.1 ± 0.2 ↑ Urem, Cirr	100 ng/ml [a]	—

[a] IC50 for inhibition of gastric acid secretion.

Key: Adult = adults; Aged = aged; Alb = hypoalbuminemia; Arth = arthritis; Atr Fib = atrial fibrillation; AVH = acute viral hepatitis; Burn = burn patients; CAD = coronary artery disease; Celiac = celiac disease; CF = cystic fibrosis; CHF = congestive heart failure; Child = children; Cirr = cirrhosis; COPD = chronic obstructive pulmonary disease; CP = cor pulmonale; CPBS = cardiopulmonary bypass surgery; CRI = chronic respiratory insufficiency; Crohn = Crohn's disease; Cush = Cushing's syndrome; Epilep = epileptic; Fem = female; Hep = Hepatitis; HL = hyperlipoproteinemia; HTh = hyperthyroid; Inflam = inflammation; LTh = hypothyroid; MI = myocardial infarction; Neo = neonate; NS = nephrotic syndrome; Obes = obese; Pneu = pneumonia; Preg = pregnant; Prem = premature; RA = rheumatoid arthritis; Smk = smoking; Tach = ventricular tachycardia; Ulcer = ulcer patients; Urem = uremia

References: *See* end of table.

Table A–II–1. PHARMACOKINETIC DATA (Continued)

AVAILABILITY (ORAL) (%)	URINARY EXCRETION (%)	BOUND IN PLASMA (%)	CLEARANCE ($ml \cdot min^{-1} \cdot kg^{-1}$)	VOL. DIST. (*liters/kg*)	HALF-LIFE (*hours*)	EFFECTIVE CONCENTRATIONS	TOXIC CONCENTRATIONS
RIFAMPIN [a] (Chapter 49)							
[b]	7 ± 3 ↑ Neo	89 ± 1	3.5 ± 1.6 ↑ Neo ↓ Urem [c] ⟷ Aged	0.97 ± 0.36 ↑ Neo ⟷ Aged	3.5 ± 0.8 [d] ↑ Hep, Cirr, AVH, Urem [c] ⟷ Child, Aged	—	—

[a] Active desacetyl metabolite.
[b] Although some studies indicate complete absorption, data are insufficient. Such reports presumably refer to rifampin plus its desacetyl metabolite, since considerable first-pass metabolism would be expected.
[c] Not observed with 300-mg doses, but pronounced differences with 900-mg doses.
[d] Half-life is longer with high single doses and is shorter after repeated administration.

AVAILABILITY (ORAL) (%)	URINARY EXCRETION (%)	BOUND IN PLASMA (%)	CLEARANCE ($ml \cdot min^{-1} \cdot kg^{-1}$)	VOL. DIST. (*liters/kg*)	HALF-LIFE (*hours*)	EFFECTIVE CONCENTRATIONS	TOXIC CONCENTRATIONS
SALICYLIC ACID [a] (Chapter 26)							
100	2–30 [b] ⟷ Aged, Cirr, RA	Dose-dependent [c] ↓ Urem, Alb, Neo, Preg ⟷ RA	0.88 ± 0.16 at 11–16 μg/ml 0.20 ± 0.01 at 134–157 μg/ml 0.18 ± 0.02 at 254–312 μg/ml [d] ↓ Neo, Hep ⟷ Aged, RA	0.17 ± 0.03 [e] ⟷ Cirr, RA	Dose-dependent [f] ⟷ Cirr, RA ↑ Hep	150–300 μg/ml [g]	>200 μg/ml [h]

[a] Drug displays dose-dependent kinetics.
[b] Dependent on dose and pH of urine.
[c] 95% at 14 μg/ml; 80% at 300 μg/ml; decreases further at higher concentrations.
[d] Note that total clearance does not change over therapeutic range in steady-state studies in normals (urine pH < 6) because of inversely related changes in protein binding and clearance of unbound drug.
[e] At a dose of 1.2 g per day, *V* increases with increasing dose due to changes in protein binding.
[f] Ranges from 2.4 hours at 300-mg dose to 19 hours and longer when there is intoxication.
[g] Anti-inflammatory effects.
[h] Tinnitus.

AVAILABILITY (ORAL) (%)	URINARY EXCRETION (%)	BOUND IN PLASMA (%)	CLEARANCE ($ml \cdot min^{-1} \cdot kg^{-1}$)	VOL. DIST. (*liters/kg*)	HALF-LIFE (*hours*)	EFFECTIVE CONCENTRATIONS	TOXIC CONCENTRATIONS
SCOPOLAMINE (Chapter 8)							
27 ± 12	6 ± 4	—	16 ± 13 [a]	1.4 ± 0.7 [b]	2.9 ± 1.2	40 pg/ml [c]	—

[a] Assuming 70-kg weight.
[b] V_{area}.
[c] Prevention of motion sickness.

SPIRONOLACTONE [a] (Chapter 28)							
Unknown [b] 25 ± 9 [c]	<1 [b,c]	>90 [b,c]	100 ± 19 [b,d] 4.2 ± 1.7 [c] ↓ Aged [c]	14 ± 4 [b,d] 1.8 [c]	1.6 ± 0.3 [b] 4.9 ± 1.8 [c] ↑ Aged [c]	—	—

[a] Extensive first-pass metabolism produces several metabolites after oral administration; activity is attributable to parent drug and at least two metabolites, canrenone and 7-α-thiomethyl spironolactone.
[b] Values for spironolactone after oral administration with meals.
[c] Values for canrenone after intravenous administration of canrenone (CL, V_{area}, $t_{1/2}$) or oral administration of spironolactone (F).
[d] CL/F and V_{area}/F.

STREPTOKINASE (Chapter 55)							
—	0	—	0.15 ± 0.12 [a]	0.016 ± 0.010 [b]	1.4 ± 0.4	—	—

[a] Clearance and thrombolytic activity appear to decline with continuous infusion; assuming 70-kg weight.
[b] V_{area}, assuming 70-kg weight.

STREPTOMYCIN (Chapter 47)							
—	50–60	48 ± 14	1.2 ± 0.3 [a] ↓ Urem	0.25 ± 0.02 [a,b]	2.6 ± 0.4 [a] ↑ Urem, Neo	—	—

[a] Values for children with tuberculosis.
[b] V_{area}.

SUFENTANIL (Chapters 14, 21)							
—	6	93 ± 1 ⟷ Cirr	12.7 ± 2.5 [a] ⟷ Cirr, Urem, Child, Aged ↓ Neo	1.7 ± 0.6 ↑ Neo, Aged ⟷ Urem	2.7 ± 1.2 ↑ Neo, Aged ⟷ Cirr, Urem, Child	—	—

[a]Blood-to-plasma ratio = 0.74 ± 0.05.

Key: Adult = adults; Aged = aged; Alb = hypoalbuminemia; Arth = arthritis; Atr Fib = atrial fibrillation; AVH = acute viral hepatitis; Burn = burn patients; CAD = coronary artery disease; Celiac = celiac disease; CF = cystic fibrosis; CHF = congestive heart failure; Child = children; Cirr = cirrhosis; COPD = chronic obstructive pulmonary disease; CP = cor pulmonale; CPBS = cardiopulmonary bypass surgery; CRI = chronic respiratory insufficiency; Crohn = Crohn's disease; Cush = Cushing's syndrome; Epilep = epileptic; Fem = female; Hep = Hepatitis; HL = hyperlipoproteinemia; HTh = hyperthyroid; Inflam = inflammation; LTh = hypothyroid; MI = myocardial infarction; Neo = neonate; NS = nephrotic syndrome; Obes = obese; Pneu = pneumonia; Preg = pregnant; Prem = premature; RA = rheumatoid arthritis; Smk = smoking; Tach = ventricular tachycardia; Ulcer = ulcer patients; Urem = uremia

References: *See* end of table.

Table A–II–1. PHARMACOKINETIC DATA (Continued)

AVAILABILITY (ORAL) (%)	URINARY EXCRETION (%)	BOUND IN PLASMA (%)	CLEARANCE ($ml \cdot min^{-1} \cdot kg^{-1}$)	VOL. DIST. (*liters/kg*)	HALF-LIFE (*hours*)	EFFECTIVE CONCENTRATIONS	TOXIC CONCENTRATIONS
SULFADIAZINE (Chapter 45)							
~100	57 ± 14 [a]	54 ± 4 ⟷ Aged	0.55 ± 0.17 [a]	0.29 ± 0.04 [a]	9.9 ± 4.3 [a]	—	—

[a] Study included concurrent administration of trimethoprim.

AVAILABILITY (ORAL) (%)	URINARY EXCRETION (%)	BOUND IN PLASMA (%)	CLEARANCE ($ml \cdot min^{-1} \cdot kg^{-1}$)	VOL. DIST. (*liters/kg*)	HALF-LIFE (*hours*)	EFFECTIVE CONCENTRATIONS	TOXIC CONCENTRATIONS
SULFAMETHOXAZOLE (Chapter 45)							
~100	14 ± 2	62 ± 5 ↓ Urem, Alb ⟷ Aged	0.32 ± 0.04 [a,b] ⟷ Urem ↑ CF	0.21 ± 0.02 [a,b] ↑ Urem ⟷ Child, CF	10.1 ± 4.6 [b] ↑ Urem ⟷ Child ↓ CF	*See* Chapter 45	—

[a] Assuming 70-kg weight.
[b] Studies included concurrent administration of trimethoprim and variation in urinary pH; these factors had no marked effect on the clearance of sulfamethoxazole.

AVAILABILITY (ORAL) (%)	URINARY EXCRETION (%)	BOUND IN PLASMA (%)	CLEARANCE ($ml \cdot min^{-1} \cdot kg^{-1}$)	VOL. DIST. (*liters/kg*)	HALF-LIFE (*hours*)	EFFECTIVE CONCENTRATIONS	TOXIC CONCENTRATIONS
SULFINPYRAZONE [a] (Chapters 30, 55)							
100	39 ± 9	98.3 ± 0.5 [b]	2.4 ± 0.6 [b] ⟷ MI, Crohn	0.74 ± 0.23 [b]	4.0 ± 1.2 [b] ⟷ MI [c], Crohn [c]	—	—

[a] Antiplatelet activity attributed primarily to sulfide metabolite, which is formed by colonic bacteria; $t_{1/2}$ = 14 ± 5 hours.
[b] Data for oral multiple-dose regimen. For a single oral dose: percent bound = 98.8 ± 0.2; CL = 0.96 ± 0.32 ml · min^{-1} · kg^{-1}; V_{ss} = 0.29 ± 0.10 liters/kg; $t_{1/2}$ = 3.8 ± 0.9 hours.
[c] For parent drug and sulfide metabolite.

AVAILABILITY (ORAL) (%)	URINARY EXCRETION (%)	BOUND IN PLASMA (%)	CLEARANCE ($ml \cdot min^{-1} \cdot kg^{-1}$)	VOL. DIST. (*liters/kg*)	HALF-LIFE (*hours*)	EFFECTIVE CONCENTRATIONS	TOXIC CONCENTRATIONS
SULFISOXAZOLE (Chapter 45)							
96 ± 14	49 ± 8 [a]	91.4 ± 1.2 ↓ Urem, Preg, Cirr	0.33 ± 0.01 ↑ Cirr [b]	0.15 ± 0.02 ↑ Cirr [b]	6.6 ± 0.7 ↑ Urem ⟷ Cirr	*See* Chapter 45	*See* Chapter 45

[a] Dependent on rate of urine formation and pH.
[b] Changes due to differences in protein binding.

SULINDAC [a] (Chapter 26)							
—	Negligible	99.4 ± 0.1 ↓ Urem	1.5 ± 0.9 [b] ↓ Aged, Urem [c]	2 [d]	15 ± 4 ↑ Aged	—	—

[a] Reduced reversibly to active metabolite, sulindac sulfide, in part by gut flora after biliary excretion of parent drug; data are for sulindac sulfide.
[b] *CL/F* (*F* is composite of fraction absorbed and fraction converted to sulindac sulfide).
[c] AUC of sulindac sulfide significantly decreased but formation impaired in end-stage renal disease.
[d] V_{area}/F.

TEMAZEPAM (Chapter 17)							
>80	<1 ⟷ Cirr	97.6 ⟷ Aged ↓ Urem, Cirr	0.87 ± 0.18 [a] ⟷ Aged, Cirr	1.06 ± 0.31 [a] ⟷ Aged, Cirr	13 ± 3 ⟷ Aged, Urem, Cirr	—	—

[a] *CL/F* and V_{area}/F.

TERAZOSIN (Chapters 11, 33)							
90 ⟷ CHF, Aged	12 ± 3	90–94	1.1 ± 0.2 [a] ⟷ Urem, Aged, CHF	0.80 ± 0.18 [a] ⟷ Urem	12 ± 3 ⟷ Urem, Aged CHF	—	—

[a] Assuming 70-kg weight.

TERBUTALINE [a] (Chapter 10)							
14 ± 2 [b]	56 ± 4	20	3.4 ± 0.6 [b] ↑ Preg ⟷ Child	1.8 ± 0.2 [b] ⟷ Preg, Child	14 ± 2 [b] ⟷ Child	2.3 ± 1.8 ng/ml [c]	—

[a] Racemic mixture; only (−)-enantiomer active.
[b] Values for (−)-enantiomer: *F* = 15 ± 2%; $CL = 2.1 \pm 0.5$ ml · min^{-1} · kg^{-1}; $V_{ss} = 1.8 \pm 0.4$ liters/kg; $t_{1/2} = 15 \pm 2$ hours.
[c] 50% increase in FEV_1 in asthmatic patients.

Key: Adult = adults; Aged = aged; Alb = hypoalbuminemia; Arth = arthritis; Atr Fib = atrial fibrillation; AVH = acute viral hepatitis; Burn = burn patients; CAD = coronary artery disease; Celiac = celiac disease; CF = cystic fibrosis; CHF = congestive heart failure; Child = children; Cirr = cirrhosis; COPD = chronic obstructive pulmonary disease; CP = cor pulmonale; CPBS = cardiopulmonary bypass surgery; CRI = chronic respiratory insufficiency; Crohn = Crohn's disease; Cush = Cushing's syndrome; Epilep = epileptic; Fem = female; Hep = Hepatitis; HL = hyperlipoproteinemia; HTh = hyperthyroid; Inflam = inflammation; LTh = hypothyroid; MI = myocardial infarction; Neo = neonate; NS = nephrotic syndrome; Obes = obese; Pneu = pneumonia; Preg = pregnant; Prem = premature; RA = rheumatoid arthritis; Smk = smoking; Tach = ventricular tachycardia; Ulcer = ulcer patients; Urem = uremia

References: *See* end of table.

Table A–II–1. PHARMACOKINETIC DATA (Continued)

AVAILABILITY (ORAL) (%)	URINARY EXCRETION (%)	BOUND IN PLASMA (%)	CLEARANCE (*ml · min⁻¹ · kg⁻¹*)	VOL. DIST. (*liters/kg*)	HALF-LIFE (*hours*)	EFFECTIVE CONCENTRATIONS	TOXIC CONCENTRATIONS
TETRACYCLINE (Chapter 48)							
77	58 ± 8	65 ± 3	1.67 ± 0.24	1.5 ± 0.08 [a]	10.6 ± 1.5	*See* Chapter 48	—

[a] V_{area}.

AVAILABILITY (ORAL) (%)	URINARY EXCRETION (%)	BOUND IN PLASMA (%)	CLEARANCE (*ml · min⁻¹ · kg⁻¹*)	VOL. DIST. (*liters/kg*)	HALF-LIFE (*hours*)	EFFECTIVE CONCENTRATIONS	TOXIC CONCENTRATIONS
TETRAHYDROCANNABINOL [a] **(DRONABINOL)** (Chapters 22, 38)							
Oral: 4–12 Smoking: 2–50	<1	95	3.5 ± 0.9	8.9 ± 4.2	32 ± 12 [b]	—	—

[a] Equipotent hydroxylated metabolite achieves significant concentrations after oral administration but not after smoking or intravenous administration.

[b] Effects more closely parallel initial phase of distribution.

AVAILABILITY (ORAL) (%)	URINARY EXCRETION (%)	BOUND IN PLASMA (%)	CLEARANCE (*ml · min⁻¹ · kg⁻¹*)	VOL. DIST. (*liters/kg*)	HALF-LIFE (*hours*)	EFFECTIVE CONCENTRATIONS	TOXIC CONCENTRATIONS
THEOPHYLLINE (Chapter 25)							
96 ± 8	18 ± 3 ↑ Neo, Prem ⟷ CF, Aged	56 ± 4 ↓ Aged, Cirr, Neo, Preg, Obes	0.65 ± 0.20 [a] ↓ Neo, Prem, Cirr, CHF, CP, Hep, LTh, Obes, Pneu ↑ Smk, CF, HTh, Epilep [b] ⟷ Aged, Preg, Urem	0.50 ± 0.16 ↓ Obes ↑ Prem, CF ⟷ Aged, Preg, Cirr, Epilep, HTh, LTh, Urem	9.0 ± 2.1 ↓ Smk, CF, Epilep [b], HTh ↑ Prem, Neo, Cirr, CHF, Hep, CP, LTh ⟷ Aged, Urem	10 μg/ml	20 μg/ml

[a] Nonlinear kinetics due to saturable metabolism, especially in children at steady state. Ratio of percent increase in steady-state concentration to percent increase in dose was >1.5 in 15% of children changed to a higher dose.

[b] Owing to enzyme induction by antiepileptic drugs.

AVAILABILITY (ORAL) (%)	URINARY EXCRETION (%)	BOUND IN PLASMA (%)	CLEARANCE (*ml · min⁻¹ · kg⁻¹*)	VOL. DIST. (*liters/kg*)	HALF-LIFE (*hours*)	EFFECTIVE CONCENTRATIONS	TOXIC CONCENTRATIONS
THIOPENTAL (Chapters 14, 17)							
—	<1	85 ± 4 ↓ Aged [a], Cirr, CPBS	3.9 ± 1.2 ⟷ Cirr, Aged, Obes CL_{int} = 28 ± 9 ↓ Cirr	2.3 ± 0.5 ↑ Aged [a], Obes	9.0 ± 1.6 ↑ Aged [a], Cirr, Obes, Neo	19 ± 7 μg/ml [b]	—

[a] Females only.

[b] Concentration to cause 50% of maximal EEG slowing.

TICARCILLIN (Chapter 46)							
—	92 ± 2	65	2.0 ± 0.2 ↓ Urem ⟷ CF	0.21 ± 0.03 ⟷ CF	1.3 ± 0.1 ↑ Urem ⟷ CF	*See* Chapter 46	—

TIMOLOL [a] (Chapter 11)							
50	15	60 ± 3 ↑ RA	7.3 ± 3.3 ⟷ MI, Aged	2.1 ± 0.8 ⟷ MI	4.1 ± 1.1 ⟷ MI, Urem	15 ng/ml [b]	—

[a] Values for extensive metabolizers. In poor metabolizers, AUC after oral administration is four fold greater; $t_{1/2}$ = 7.5 hours.

[b] 50% decrease in exercise-induced cardioacceleration.

TOBRAMYCIN (Chapter 47)							
—	90 [a]	<10	$CL = 0.98\ CL_{cr} \pm 32\%$ ↓ Obes ↑ CF	0.33 ± 0.08 [b] ↓ Obes ⟷ Urem, Aged, Burn ↑ CF, Neo	2.2 ± 0.1 100 ± 57 [c] ↑ Urem, Neo, Prem ⟷ Obes, CF ↓ Burn	*See* Chapter 47	*See* Chapter 47

[a] Possibly higher, since drug persists in tissues for long periods of time.
[b] Volume of central compartment.

[c] Tobramycin has a very long terminal half-life, which accounts for prolonged urinary excretion.

TOCAINIDE [a] (Chapter 35)							
89 ± 5	38 ± 7	10 ± 15	2.6 ± 0.5 ↓ CHF, Urem, NS ⟷ MI	3.0 ± 0.2 ↓ CHF ⟷ MI, Urem	13.5 ± 2.3 ↑ Urem, NS ⟷ MI, CHF	6–15 μg/ml	—

[a] Racemic mixture; relative activity of two enantiomers not known. S-(−)-enantiomer ($t_{1/2}$ = 10 ± 4 hours) cleared 1.8 times more rapidly than R-(+)-enantiomer ($t_{1/2}$ = 17 ± 6 hours); V_{ss} the same for the two enantiomers.

Key: Adult = adults; Aged = aged; Alb = hypoalbuminemia; Arth = arthritis; Atr Fib = atrial fibrillation; AVH = acute viral hepatitis; Burn = burn patients; CAD = coronary artery disease; Celiac = celiac disease; CF = cystic fibrosis; CHF = congestive heart failure; Child = children; Cirr = cirrhosis; COPD = chronic obstructive pulmonary disease; CP = cor pulmonale; CPBS = cardiopulmonary bypass surgery; CRI = chronic respiratory insufficiency; Crohn = Crohn's disease; Cush = Cushing's syndrome; Epilep = epileptic; Fem = female; Hep = Hepatitis; HL = hyperlipoproteinemia; HTh = hyperthyroid; Inflam = inflammation; LTh = hypothyroid; MI = myocardial infarction; Neo = neonate; NS = nephrotic syndrome; Obes = obese; Pneu = pneumonia; Preg = pregnant; Prem = premature; RA = rheumatoid arthritis; Smk = smoking; Tach = ventricular tachycardia; Ulcer = ulcer patients; Urem = uremia

References: *See* end of table.

Table A–II–1. PHARMACOKINETIC DATA (Continued)

AVAILABILITY (ORAL) (%)	URINARY EXCRETION (%)	BOUND IN PLASMA (%)	CLEARANCE ($ml \cdot min^{-1} \cdot kg^{-1}$)	VOL. DIST. (*liters/kg*)	HALF-LIFE (*hours*)	EFFECTIVE CONCENTRATIONS	TOXIC CONCENTRATIONS
TOLBUTAMIDE (Chapter 61)							
93 ± 10	0	96 ± 1 ↓ AVH, Aged	0.24 ± 0.04 ↑ AVH	0.10 ± 0.02 ⟷ AVH	5.9 ± 1.4 ↓ AVH, CRI ⟷ Aged, Urem	80–240 μg/ml [a]	—

[a] Decrease in blood glucose concentration of greater than 25%.

AVAILABILITY (ORAL) (%)	URINARY EXCRETION (%)	BOUND IN PLASMA (%)	CLEARANCE ($ml \cdot min^{-1} \cdot kg^{-1}$)	VOL. DIST. (*liters/kg*)	HALF-LIFE (*hours*)	EFFECTIVE CONCENTRATIONS	TOXIC CONCENTRATIONS
TOLMETIN (Chapter 26)							
[a]	7 ± 3 [b]	99.6 ± 0.1 ↓ Urem ⟷ RA, Aged	1.3 ± 0.3 [c] ⟷ RA, Aged	0.54 ± 0.07 [d] ⟷ RA, Aged	4.9 ± 0.3 ⟷ Aged	—	—

[a] Completely absorbed; availability probably >90%.
[b] Oral dosage.
[c] *CL/F*.
[d] V_{area}/F.

AVAILABILITY (ORAL) (%)	URINARY EXCRETION (%)	BOUND IN PLASMA (%)	CLEARANCE ($ml \cdot min^{-1} \cdot kg^{-1}$)	VOL. DIST. (*liters/kg*)	HALF-LIFE (*hours*)	EFFECTIVE CONCENTRATIONS	TOXIC CONCENTRATIONS
TRAZODONE [a] (Chapter 18)							
81 ± 29 ⟷ Aged, Obes	<1	93	2.1 ± 0.6 ↓ Aged [b], Obes [c]	1.0 ± 0.3 [d] ↑ Aged, Obes	5.9 ± 1.9 ↑ Aged, Obes	—	—

[a] Active metabolite, *m*-chlorophenylpiperazine, is a tryptaminergic agonist.
[b] Males.
[c] No difference when clearance is normalized to ideal body weight.
[d] V_{area}.

AVAILABILITY (ORAL) (%)	URINARY EXCRETION (%)	BOUND IN PLASMA (%)	CLEARANCE ($ml \cdot min^{-1} \cdot kg^{-1}$)	VOL. DIST. (*liters/kg*)	HALF-LIFE (*hours*)	EFFECTIVE CONCENTRATIONS	TOXIC CONCENTRATIONS
TRIAMTERENE [a] (Chapter 28)							
54 ± 12 [b]	52 ± 10 [b] ↓ Cirr [c] ⟷ Aged [b]	61 ± 2 [d] ↑ HL ↓ Urem, Alb, Cirr [e]	63 ± 20 [f] ↓ Cirr, Urem [e], Aged [e]	13.4 ± 4.9 [f]	4.2 ± 0.7 [g] ↑ Urem [e]	—	—

[a] Active metabolite, hydroxytriamterene sulfuric acid ester.
[b] Triamterene plus active metabolite.
[c] Decreased active metabolite; increased parent drug.
[d] For metabolite, percent bound = 90.4 ± 1.3.
[e] Active metabolite.
[f] Since triamterene is predominantly present in plasma as the active metabolite, these values are deceptively high. $CL_{renal} = 3.6 \pm 0.7$ for triamterene and 2.3 ± 0.6 for the metabolite.
[g] Metabolite $t_{1/2} = 3.1 \pm 1.2$ hours.

TRIAZOLAM (Chapter 17)

Oral: 44 Sublingual: 53	2	90.1 ± 1.5 ⟷ Urem, Alb, Obes, Aged, Smk	5.6 ± 2.0 [a] ↓ Obes, Aged, Cirr	1.1 ± 0.4 [a] ⟷ Obes, Aged	2.9 ± 1.0 [b] ↑ Obes, Cirr ⟷ Aged, Urem	—	—

[a] CL/F and V_{area}/F.

[b] Prolonged absorption and elimination half-lives at night.

TRIMETHOPRIM (Chapter 45)

~100	69 ± 17	44 ⟷ Urem, Alb	2.2 ± 0.6 [a,b,c] ↓ Urem ↑ CF, Child	1.8 ± 0.2 [a,b] ⟷ Urem, CF ↑ Neo ↓ Child	11 ± 1.4 [b] ↑ Urem ↓ Child, CF	*See* Chapter 45	—

[a] Assuming 70-kg weight.

[b] Studies included concurrent administration of sulfamethoxazole and variation in urinary pH; these factors had no marked effect on the clearance of trimethoprim.

[c] Blood-to-plasma ratio = 1.0.

TUBOCURARINE (Chapter 9)

—	63 ± 35	50 ± 8 ↑ Burn ⟷ Urem, Cirr	1.9 ± 0.6 ↓ Urem, CPBS, Burn, Aged	0.39 ± 0.14 ↑ Child ↓ Burn, Aged ⟷ CPBS	2.0 ± 1.1 [a] ↑ Urem, Child, CPBS ⟷ Burn, Aged	0.6 ± 0.2 μg/ml [b] 1.2 μg/ml [c] ↓ Child ↑ Burn ⟷ CPBS, Urem, Aged	—

[a] Calculated from two-compartment analysis. Three-compartment analysis suggests a terminal half-life of 3.9 hours.

[b] 50% reduction in twitch tension. Effective concentration is less in the presence of halothane (0.5–0.7% end tidal) and greater in the presence of enflurane (1.3–1.4% end tidal).

[c] 95% reduction in twitch tension.

Key: Adult = adults; Aged = aged; Alb = hypoalbuminemia; Arth = arthritis; Atr Fib = atrial fibrillation; AVH = acute viral hepatitis; Burn = burn patients; CAD = coronary artery disease; Celiac = celiac disease; CF = cystic fibrosis; CHF = congestive heart failure; Child = children; Cirr = cirrhosis; COPD = chronic obstructive pulmonary disease; CP = cor pulmonale; CPBS = cardiopulmonary bypass surgery; CRI = chronic respiratory insufficiency; Crohn = Crohn's disease; Cush = Cushing's syndrome; Epilep = epileptic; Fem = female; Hep = Hepatitis; HL = hyperlipoproteinemia; HTh = hyperthyroid; Inflam = inflammation; LTh = hypothyroid; MI = myocardial infarction; Neo = neonate; NS = nephrotic syndrome; Obes = obese; Pneu = pneumonia; Preg = pregnant; Prem = premature; RA = rheumatoid arthritis; Smk = smoking; Tach = ventricular tachycardia; Ulcer = ulcer patients; Urem = uremia

References: *See* end of table.

Table A–II–1. PHARMACOKINETIC DATA (Continued)

AVAILABILITY (ORAL) (%)	URINARY EXCRETION (%)	BOUND IN PLASMA (%)	CLEARANCE (*ml · min⁻¹ · kg⁻¹*)	VOL. DIST. (*liters/kg*)	HALF-LIFE (*hours*)	EFFECTIVE CONCENTRATIONS	TOXIC CONCENTRATIONS
VALPROIC ACID [a] (Chapter 19)							
100 ± 10	1.8 ± 2.4	93 ± 1 [b] ↓ Urem, Cirr, Preg, Aged, Neo, Burn, Alb	0.11 ± 0.02 [c] ↑ Epilep [d], Child [d] ⟷ Cirr, Aged	0.22 ± 0.07 ↑ Cirr, Child, Neo ⟷ Aged	14 ± 3 [c] ↑ Cirr, Neo ↓ Epilep [d], Child [d] ⟷ Aged	30–100 μg/ml [e]	—

[a] Active metabolites.
[b] Dose dependent; value shown for doses of 250 and 500 mg/day. At 1000 mg/day, % bound = 90 ± 2. Blood-to-plasma ratio = 0.64.
[c] Multiple dosing (500 mg/day). Single-dose value: 0.14 ± 0.04 ml · min^{-1} · kg^{-1}; $t_{1/2}$ = 9.8 ± 2.6 hours. Total clearance the same at 1000 mg per day, although clearance of free drug increases.
[d] Increased clearance possibly due to enzyme induction due to concomitant administration of other antiepileptic drugs.
[e] For control of seizures; value questionable because of active metabolites.

AVAILABILITY (ORAL) (%)	URINARY EXCRETION (%)	BOUND IN PLASMA (%)	CLEARANCE	VOL. DIST.	HALF-LIFE	EFFECTIVE CONCENTRATIONS	TOXIC CONCENTRATIONS
VANCOMYCIN (Chapter 48)							
—	79 ± 11	30 ± 10 ⟷ Urem	1.4 ± 0.1 $CL = 0.79\ CL_{cr} + 0.22$ ↓ Urem, Aged ⟷ Obes, CPBS	0.39 ± 0.06 ↓ Obes ⟷ Urem, CPBS	5.6 ± 1.8 ↑ Urem, Aged ↓ Obes	*See* Chapter 48	>80 μg/ml [a]

[a] Ototoxicity.

AVAILABILITY (ORAL) (%)	URINARY EXCRETION (%)	BOUND IN PLASMA (%)	CLEARANCE	VOL. DIST.	HALF-LIFE	EFFECTIVE CONCENTRATIONS	TOXIC CONCENTRATIONS
VECURONIUM (Chapter 9)							
—	18 ± 5	30 ± 9	3.0 ± 0.1 ↓ Cirr, Aged ⟷ Child, Urem	0.21 ± 0.08 ↓ Aged ⟷ Child, Cirr, Urem	1.5 ± 0.7 ↑ Cirr ⟷ Child, Aged, Urem	0.2 μg/ml [a] 0.37 μg/ml [b]	—

[a] 50% reduction of twitch tension.
[b] 95% reduction of twitch tension.

VERAPAMIL [a,b] (Chapters 32, 35)

22 ± 8 ↑ Cirr	<3	90 ± 2 ↓ Cirr ⟷ Urem, Atr Fib	15 ± 6 [c] ↓ Cirr, Aged ↓ , ⟷ Atr Fib ⟷ Urem, Child	5.0 ± 2.1 ↑ Cirr ↓ , ⟷ Atr Fib ⟷ Urem, Aged	4.0 ± 1.5 [c] ↑ Cirr, Aged ↑ , ⟷ Atr Fib ⟷ Urem, Child	120 ± 20 ng/ml [d] 120 ± 40 ng/ml [e]	—

[a] Racemic mixture; (−)-enantiomer more active. Bioavailability of (+)-verapamil is 2.5-fold greater than that for (−)-enantiomer because of lower *CL* (10 ± 2 versus 18 ± 3 ml · min^{-1} · kg^{-1}). Relative concentrations of enantiomers change as a function of route of administration.

[b] Active metabolite, norverapamil, is a vasodilator but has no direct effect on heart rate or P–R interval. At steady state (oral administration), AUC equivalent to parent drug ($t_{1/2}$ = 9 ± 3 hours).

[c] Multiple dosing causes greater than twofold decrease in *CL/F* and prolongation of half-life in some studies, but no change of $t_{1/2}$ in others.

[d] EC_{50} for prolongation of P–R interval after oral administration of racemate; value for intravenous administration of racemate is 40 ± 25 ng/ml. After oral administration, racemate concentrations above 100 ng/ml cause more than 25% reduction in heart rate in atrial fibrillation, more than 10% prolongation of P–R interval, and more than 50% increase in duration of exercise in angina patients.

[e] To terminate reentrant supraventricular tachycardias after intravenous administration.

WARFARIN [a] (Chapter 55)

93 ± 8	<2	99 ± 1 [b] ↓ Urem ⟷ Preg	0.045 ± 0.024 [c,d] ⟷ Aged, AVH	0.14 ± 0.06 [b,d] ⟷ Aged, AVH	37 ± 15 [e] ⟷ Aged, AVH	2.2 ± 0.4 μg/ml	—

[a] Values are for racemic warfarin; the S-(−)-enantiomer is three to five times more potent than the R-(+)-enantiomer.

[b] No difference between enantiomers in binding or V_{area}.

[c] The clearance of the R-(+) form is about 70% of that of the S-(−)-enantiomer (0.043 vs. 0.059 ml · min^{-1} · kg^{-1}).

[d] Conditions leading to decreased binding (*e.g.*, uremia) presumably increase clearance and volume of distribution.

[e] Half-life of the R-(+)-enantiomer is longer than that of the S-(−) form (43 ± 14 vs. 32 ± 12 hours).

ZIDOVUDINE (Chapter 51)

63 ± 13	18 ± 5	<25	26 ± 6 ↓ Urem [a] ⟷ Child	1.4 ± 0.4 ↓ Urem [a] ⟷ Child	1.1 ± 0.2 ⟷ Urem	—	—

[a] *CL/F* and V_{area}/F.

Key: Adult = adults; Aged = aged; Alb = hypoalbuminemia; Arth = arthritis; Atr Fib = atrial fibrillation; AVH = acute viral hepatitis; Burn = burn patients; CAD = coronary artery disease; Celiac = celiac disease; CF = cystic fibrosis; CHF = congestive heart failure; Child = children; Cirr = cirrhosis; COPD = chronic obstructive pulmonary disease; CP = cor pulmonale; CPBS = cardiopulmonary bypass surgery; CRI = chronic respiratory insufficiency; Crohn = Crohn's disease; Cush = Cushing's syndrome; Epilep = epileptic; Fem = female; Hep = Hepatitis; HL = hyperlipoproteinemia; HTh = hyperthyroid; Inflam = inflammation; LTh = hypothyroid; MI = myocardial infarction; Neo = neonate; NS = nephrotic syndrome; Obes = obese; Pneu = pneumonia; Preg = pregnant; Prem = premature; RA = rheumatoid arthritis; Smk = smoking; Tach = ventricular tachycardia; Ulcer = ulcer patients; Urem = uremia

References: *See* end of table.

Table A–II–1. PHARMACOKINETIC DATA (Continued)

ACEBUTOLOL

Singh, B. N.; Thoden, W. R.; and Wahl, J. Acebutolol: a review of its pharmacology, pharmacokinetics, clinical uses, and adverse effects. *Pharmacotherapy*, **1986**, *6*, 45–63.

ACETAMINOPHEN

Forrest, J. A. H.; Clements, J. A.; and Prescott, L. F. Clinical pharmacokinetics of paracetamol. *Clin. Pharmacokinet.*, **1982**, *7*, 93–107.

Rawlins, M. D.; Henderson, D. B.; and Hijab, A. R. Pharmacokinetics of paracetamol (acetaminophen) after intravenous and oral administration. *Eur. J. Clin. Pharmacol.*, **1977**, *11*, 283–286.

N-ACETYLPROCAINAMIDE

Atkinson, A. J., Jr.; Ruo, T. I.; Piergies, A. A.; Breiter, H. C.; Connelly, T. J.; Sedek, G. S.; Juan, D.; Hubler, G. L.; and Hsieh, A.-M. Pharmacokinetics of N-acetylprocainamide in patients profiled with a stable isotope method. *Clin. Pharmacol. Ther.*, **1989**, *46*, 182–189.

Connolly, S. J., and Kates, R. E. Clinical pharmacokinetics of N-acetylprocainamide. *Clin. Pharmacokinet.*, **1982**, *7*, 206–220.

ACETYLSALICYLIC ACID

Roberts, M. S.; Rumble, R. H.; Wanwimolruk, S.; Thomas, D.; and Brooks, P. M. Pharmacokinetics of aspirin and salicylate in elderly subjects and in patients with alcoholic liver disease. *Eur. J. Clin. Pharmacol.*, **1983**, *25*, 253–261.

Rowland, M., and Riegelman, S. Pharmacokinetics of acetylsalicylic acid and salicylic acid after intravenous administration in man. *J. Pharm. Sci.*, **1968**, *57*, 1313–1319.

ACYCLOVIR

Blum, M. R.; Liao, S. H. T.; and de Miranda, P. Overview of acyclovir pharmacokinetic disposition in adults and children. *Am. J. Med.*, **1982**, *73*, Suppl., 186–192.

Laskin, O. L. Clinical pharmacokinetics of acyclovir. *Clin. Pharmacokinet.*, **1983**, *8*, 187–201.

ALFENTANIL

Bodenham, A., and Park, G. R. Alfentanil infusions in patients requiring intensive care. *Clin. Pharmacokinet.*, **1988**, *15*, 216–226.

ALPRAZOLAM

Garzone, P. D., and Kroboth, P. D. Pharmacokinetics of the newer benzodiazepines. *Clin. Pharmacokinet.*, **1989**, *16*, 337–364.

ALTEPLASE

Seifried, E.; Tanswell, P.; Rijken, D. C.; Barrett-Bergshoeff, M. M.; Su, C. A. P. F.; and Kluft, D. Pharmacokinetics of antigen and activity of recombinant tissue type plasminogen activator and infusion in healthy volunteers. *Arzneimittelforschung*, **1988**, *38*, 418–422.

Zeller, F. P., and Spinler, S. A. Alteplase: a tissue plasminogen activator for acute myocardial infarction. *Drug Intell. Clin. Pharm.*, **1988**, *22*, 6–14.

AMANTADINE

Aoki, F. Y., and Sitar, D. S. Clinical pharmacokinetics of amantadine hydrochloride. *Clin. Pharmacokinet.*, **1988**, *14*, 35–51.

AMIKACIN

Bauer, L. A., and Blouin, R. A. Influence of age on amikacin pharmacokinetics in patients without renal disease. Comparison with gentamicin and tobramycin. *Eur. J. Clin. Pharmacol.*, **1983**, *24*, 639–642.

Pechere, J. C., and Dugal, R. Clinical pharmacokinetics of aminoglycoside antibiotics. *Clin. Pharmacokinet.*, **1979**, *4*, 170–199.

AMILORIDE

Sabanathan, K.; Castleden, C. M.; Adam, H. K.; Ryan, J.; and Fitzsimons, T. J. A comparative study of the pharmacokinetics and pharmacodynamics of atenolol, hydrochlorothiazide and amiloride in normal young and elderly subjects and elderly hypertensive patients. *Eur. J. Clin. Pharmacol.*, **1987**, *32*, 53–60.

Spahn, H.; Reuter, K.; Mutschler, E.; Gerok, W.; and Knauf, H. Pharmacokinetics of amiloride in renal and hepatic disease. *Eur. J. Clin. Pharmacol.*, **1987**, *33*, 493–498.

AMIODARONE

Somani, P. Basic and clinical pharmacology of amiodarone: relationship of antiarrhythmic effects, dose and drug concentrations to intracellular inclusion bodies. *J. Clin. Pharmacol.*, **1989**, *29*, 405–412.

Veronese, M. E.; McLean, S.; and Hendriks, R. Plasma protein binding of amiodarone in a patient population: measurement by erythrocyte partitioning and a novel glass-binding method. *Br. J. Clin. Pharmacol.*, **1988**, *26*, 721–731.

AMITRIPTYLINE

Schulz, P.; Dick, P.; Blaschke, T. F.; and Hollister, L. Discrepancies between pharmacokinetic studies of amitriptyline. *Clin. Pharmacokinet.*, **1985**, *10*, 257–268.

AMOXICILLIN

Sjövall, J.; Alván, G.; and Huitfeld, B. Intra- and inter-individual variation in pharmacokinetics of intravenously infused amoxycillin and ampicillin to elderly volunteers. *Br. J. Clin. Pharmacol.*, **1986**, ***21***, 171–181.

Sjövall, J.; Alván, G.; and Westerlund, D. Dose-dependent absorption of amoxycillin and bacampicillin. *Clin. Pharmacol. Ther.*, **1985**, ***38***, 241–250.

AMPHOTERICIN B

Benson, J. M., and Nahata, M. C. Pharmacokinetics of amphotericin B in children. *Antimicrob. Agents Chemother.*, **1989**, *33*, 1989–1993.

AMPICILLIN

Ehrnebo, M.; Nilsson, S.-O.; and Boreus, L. O. Pharmacokinetics of ampicillin and its prodrugs, bacampicillin and pivampicillin, in man. *J. Pharmacokinet. Biopharm.*, **1979**, *7*, 429–451.

Lewis, G. P., and Jusko, W. J. Pharmacokinetics of ampicillin in cirrhosis. *Clin. Pharmacol. Ther.*, **1975**, *18*, 475–484.

AMRINONE

Hamilton, R. A.; Kowalsky, S. F.; Wright, E. M.; Cernak, P.; Benziger, D. P.; Stroshane, R. M.; and Edelson, J. Effect of the acetylator phenotype on amrinone pharmacokinetics. *Clin. Pharmacol. Ther.*, **1986**, ***40***, 615–619.

Park, G. B.; Kershner, R. P.; Angellotti, J.; Williams, R. L.; Benet, L. Z.; and Edelson, J. Oral bioavailability and intravenous pharmacokinetics of amrinone in humans. *J. Pharm. Sci.*, **1983**, *72*, 817–819.

ATENOLOL

Boyd, R. A.; Chin, S. K.; Don-Pedro, O.; Williams, R. L.; and Giacomini, K. M. The pharmacokinetics of the enantiomers of atenolol. *Clin. Pharmacol. Ther.*, **1989**, ***45***, 403–410.

Kirch, W., and Görg, K. G. Clinical pharmacokinetics of atenolol—a review. *Eur. J. Drug Metab. Pharmacokinet.*, **1982**, *7*, 81–91.

ATRACURIUM

Shanks, C. A. Pharmacokinetics of the nondepolarizing neuromuscular relaxants applied to calculation of bolus and infusion dosage regimens. *Anesthesiology*, **1986**, ***64***, 72–86.

ATROPINE

Kanto, J., and Klotz, U. Pharmacokinetic implications for the clinical use of atropine, scopolamine and glycopyrrolate. *Acta Anaesthesiol. Scand.*, **1988**, ***32***, 69–78.

AURANOFIN

Blocka, K. L. N.; Paulus, H. E.; and Furst, D. E. Clinical pharmacokinetics of oral and injectable gold compounds. *Clin. Pharmacokinet.*, **1986**, ***11***, 133–144.

AZATHIOPRINE

Ding, T. L.; Gambertoglio, J. G.; Amend, W. J. C.; Birnbaum, J.; and Benet, L. Z. Azathioprine (AZA) bioavailability and pharmacokinetics in kidney transplant patients. *Clin. Pharmacol. Ther.*, **1980**, *27*, 250.

Lin, S.-N.; Jessup, K.; Floyd, M.; Wang, T.-P. F.; Van Buren, C. T.; Caprioli, R. M.; and Kahan, B. D. Quantitation of plasma azathioprine and 6-mercaptopurine levels in renal transplant patients. *Transplantation*, **1980**, *29*, 290–294.

AZLOCILLIN

Lander, R. D.; Henderson, R. P.; and Pyszczynski, D. R. Pharmacokinetic comparison of 5g of azlocillin every 8h and 4g every 6h in healthy volunteers. *Antimicrob. Agents Chemother.*, **1989**, ***33***, 710–713.

BETAMETHASONE

Loo, J. C. K.; McGilveray, I. J.; Jordan, N.; and Brien, R. Pharmacokinetic evaluation of betamethasone and its water soluble phosphate ester in humans. *Biopharm. Drug Dispos.*, **1981**, *2*, 265–272.

Petersen, M. C.; Nation, R. L.; McBride, W. G.; Ashley, J. J.; and Moore, R. G. Pharmacokinetics of betamethasone in healthy adults after intravenous administration. *Eur. J. Clin. Pharmacol.*, **1983**, *25*, 643–650.

BLEOMYCIN

Kramer, W. G.; Feldman, S.; Broughton, A.; Strong, J. E.; Hall, S. W.; and Holoye, P. Y. The pharmacokinetics of bleomycin in man. *J. Clin. Pharmacol.*, **1978**, *18*, 346–352.

Yee, G. C.; Crom, W. R.; Lee, F. H.; Smyth, R. D.; and Evans, W. E. Bleomycin disposition in children with cancer. *Clin. Pharmacol. Ther.*, **1983**, *33*, 668–673.

BRETYLIUM

Rapeport, W. G. Clinical pharmacokinetics of bretylium. *Clin. Pharmacokinet.*, **1985**, ***10***, 248–256.

Table A–II–1. PHARMACOKINETIC DATA (Continued)

BUMETANIDE

Cook, J. A.; Smith, D. E.; Cornish, L. A.; Tankanow, R. M.; Nicklas, J. M.; and Hyneck, M. L. Kinetics, dynamics, and bioavailability of bumetanide in healthy subjects and patients with congestive heart failure. *Clin. Pharmacol. Ther.*, **1988**, *44*, 487–499.

Ward, A., and Heel, R. C. Bumetanide: a review of its pharmacodynamic and pharmacokinetic properties and therapeutic use. *Drugs*, **1984**, *28*, 426–464.

BUPIVACAINE

Burm, A. G. L. Clinical pharmacokinetics of epidural and spinal anesthesia. *Clin. Pharmacokinet.*, **1989**, *16*, 283–311.

BUSULFAN

Ehrsson, H.; Hassan, M.; Ehrnebo, M.; and Beran, M. Busulfan kinetics. *Clin. Pharmacol. Ther.*, **1983**, *34*, 86–89.

CAFFEINE

Blanchard, J., and Sawers, S. J. A. Comparative pharmacokinetics of caffeine in young and elderly men. *J. Pharmacokinet. Biopharm.*, **1983**, *11*, 109–126.

Busto, U.; Bendayan, R.; and Sellers, E. M. Clinical pharmacokinetics of non-opiate abused drugs. *Clin. Pharmacokinet.*, **1989**, *16*, 1–26.

CAPTOPRIL

Creasey, W. A.; Morrison, R. A.; Singhvi, S. M.; and Willard, D. A. Pharmacokinetics of intravenous captopril in healthy men. *Eur. J. Clin. Pharmacol.*, **1988**, *35*, 367–370.

Duchin, K. L.; McKinstry, D. N.; Cohen, A. I.; and Migdalof, B. H. Pharmacokinetics of captopril in healthy subjects and in patients with cardiovascular diseases. *Clin. Pharmacokinet.*, **1988**, *14*, 241–259.

CARBAMAZEPINE

Bertilsson, L., and Tomson, T. Clinical pharmacokinetics and pharmacological effects of carbamazepine and carbamazepine-10, 11-epoxide. *Clin. Pharmacokinet.*, **1986**, *11*, 177–198.

CARBAMAZEPINE-10,11-EPOXIDE

Bertilsson, L., and Tomson, T. Clinical pharmacokinetics and pharmacological effects of carbamazepine and carbamazepine-10, 11-epoxide. *Clin. Pharmacokinet.*, **1986**, *11*, 177–198.

Spina, E.; Tomson, T.; Svensson, J.-O.; Faighe, J. W.; and Bertilsson, L. Single-dose kinetics of an enteric-coated formulation of carbamazepine-10, 11-epoxide, an active metabolite of carbamazepine. *Ther. Drug Monit.*, **1988**, *10*, 382–385.

CARBENICILLIN

Latos, D. L.; Bryan, C. S.; and Stone, W. J. Carbenicillin therapy in patients with normal and impaired renal function. *Clin. Pharmacol. Ther.*, **1975**, *17*, 692–700.

Libke, R. D.; Clarke, J. T.; Ralph, E. D.; Luthy, R. P.; and Kirby, W. M. M. Ticarcillin vs carbenicillin: clinical pharmacokinetics. *Clin. Pharmacol. Ther.*, **1975**, *17*, 441–446.

CARMUSTINE (BCNU)

Levin, V. A.; Hoffman, W.; and Weinkam, R. J. Pharmacokinetics of BCNU in man: a preliminary study of 20 patients. *Cancer Treat. Rep.*, **1978**, *62*, 1305–1312.

CEFACLOR

Sides, G. D.; Franson, T. R.; DeSante, K. A.; and Black, H. R. A comprehensive review of the clinical pharmacology and pharmacokinetics of cefaclor. *Clin. Ther.*, **1988**, *11*, Suppl. A, 5–19.

CEFADROXIL

Humbert, G.; Leroy, A.; Fillastre, J. P.; and Godin, M. Pharmacokinetics of cefadroxil in normal subjects and in patients with renal insufficiency. *Chemotherapy*, **1979**, *25*, 189–195.

Welling, P. G.; Selen, A.; Pearson, J. G.; Kwok, F.; Rogge, M. C.; Ifan, A.; Marrero, D.; Craig, W. A.; and Johnson, C. A. A pharmacokinetic comparison of cephalexin and cefadroxil using HPLC assay procedures. *Biopharm. Drug Dispos.*, **1985**, *6*, 147–157.

CEFAMANDOLE

Aziz, N. S.; Gambertoglio, J. G.; Lin, E. T.; Grausz, H.; and Benet, L. Z. Pharmacokinetics of cefamandole using a HPLC assay. *J. Pharmacokinet. Biopharm.*, **1978**, *6*, 153–164.

Neu, H. C., and Srinivasan, S. Pharmacology of ceftizoxime compared with that of cefamandole. *Antimicrob. Agents Chemother.*, **1981**, *20*, 366–369.

CEFAZOLIN

Deguchi, Y.; Koshida, R.; Nakashima, E.; Watanabe, R.; Taniguchi, N.; Ichimura, R.; and Tsuji, A. Interindividual changes in volume of distribution of cefazolin in newborn infants and its prediction based on physiological pharmacokinetic concepts. *J. Pharm. Sci.*, **1988**, *77*, 674–678.

Scheld, W. M.; Spyker, D. A.; Donowitz, G. R.; Bolton, W. K.; and Sande, M. A. Moxalactam and cefazolin: comparative pharmacokinetics in normal subjects. *Antimicrob. Agents Chemother.*, **1981**, *19*, 613–619.

CEFONICID

Dudley, M. N.; Quintiliani, R.; and Nightingale, C. H. Review of cefonicid, a long-acting cephalosporin. *Clin. Pharm.*, **1984**, *3*, 23–32.

Furlanut, M.; D'Elia, R.; Riva, E.; and Pasinelli, F. Pharmacokinetics of cefonicid in children. *Eur. J. Clin. Pharmacol.*, **1989**, *36*, 79–82.

CEFOPERAZONE

Barriere, S. L., and Flaherty, J. F. Third-generation cephalosporins: a critical review. *Clin. Pharm.*, **1984**, *3*, 351–373.

CEFORANIDE

Estey, E. H.; Weaver, S. S.; LeBlanc, B. M.; Brown, N.; Ho, D. H.; and Bodey, G. P. Ceforanide kinetics. *Clin. Pharmacol. Ther.*, **1981**, *30*, 398–403.

Hawkins, S. S.; Alford, R. H.; Stone, W. J.; Smyth, R. D.; and Pfeffer, M. Ceforanide kinetics in renal insufficiency. *Clin. Pharmacol. Ther.*, **1981**, *30*, 468–474.

CEFOTAXIME

Hary, L.; Andrejak, M.; Leleu, S.; Orfila, J.; and Capron, J. P. The pharmacokinetics of ceftriazone and cefotaxime in cirrhotic patients with ascites. *Eur. J. Clin. Pharmacol.*, **1989**, *36*, 613–616.

Rondini, L. C.; Flaherty, J. F.; Schoenfeld, P.; Barriere, S. L.; and Gambertoglio, J. G. Influence of coadministration on the pharmacokinetics of mezlocillin and cefotaxime in healthy volunteers and in patients with renal failure. *Clin. Pharmacol. Ther.*, **1989**, *45*, 527–534.

CEFOTETAN

Ward, A., and Richards, D. M. Cefotetan: a review of its antibacterial activity, pharmacokinetic properties and therapeutic use. *Drugs*, **1985**, *30*, 382–426.

Zimmerman, J.; Cohen, A.; and Thyrom, P. Absolute bioavailability and noncompartmental analysis of intravenous and intramuscular cefotan (cefotetan) in normal volunteers. *J. Clin. Pharmacol.*, **1989**, *29*, 151–157.

CEFOXITIN

Kampf, D.; Schurig, R.; Korsukewitz, I.; and Brückner, O. Cefoxitin pharmacokinetics: relation to three different renal clearance studies in patients with various degrees of renal insufficiency. *Antimicrob. Agents Chemother.*, **1981**, *20*, 741–746.

Regazzi, M. B.; Chirico, G.; Cristiani, D.; Rondini, G.; and Rondanelli, R. Cefoxitin in newborn infants. *Eur. J. Clin. Pharmacol.*, **1983**, *25*, 507–509.

CEFTAZIDIME

Balant, L.; Dayer, P.; and Auckenthaler, R. Clinical pharmacokinetics of the third generation cephalosporines. *Clin. Pharmacokinet.*, **1985**, *10*, 141–143.

Hedman, A.; Adan-Abdi, Y.; Alvan, G.; Strandvik, B.; and Arvidsson, A. Influence of glomerular filtration rate on renal clearance of ceftazidime in cystic fibrosis. *Clin. Pharmacokinet.*, **1988**, *15*, 57–65.

CEFTIZOXIME

Barriere, S. L., and Flaherty, J. F. Third-generation cephalosporins: a critical evaluation. *Clin. Pharm.*, **1984**, *3*, 351–373.

Cutler, R. E.; Blair, A. D.; Burgess, E. D.; and Parks, D. Pharmacokinetics of ceftizoxime. *J. Antimicrob. Chemother.*, **1982**, *10*, Suppl. C, 91–97.

CEFTRIAXONE

Hayton, W. L., and Stoeckel, K. Age-associated changes in ceftriaxone pharmacokinetics. *Clin. Pharmacokinet.*, **1986**, *11*, 76–86.

Yuk, J. H.; Nightingale, C. H.; and Quintiliani, R. Clinical pharmacokinetics of ceftriaxone. *Clin. Pharmacokinet.*, **1989**, *17*, 223–235.

CEFUROXIME

Bundtzen, R. W.; Toothaker, R. D.; Nielson, O. S.; Madsen, P. O.; Welling, P. G.; and Craig, W. A. Pharmacokinetics of cefuroxime in normal and impaired renal function: comparison of high-pressure liquid chromatography and microbiological assays. *Antimicrob. Agents Chemother.*, **1981**, *19*, 443–449.

Foord, R. D. Cefuroxime: human pharmacokinetics. *Antimicrob. Agents Chemother.*, **1976**, *9*, 741–747.

CEPHALEXIN

Finkelstein, E.; Quintiliani, R.; Lee, R.; Bracci, A.; and Nightingale, C. H. Pharmacokinetics of oral cephalosporins: cephradine and cephalexin. *J. Pharm. Sci.*, **1978**, *67*, 1447–1450.

Spyker, D. A.; Thomas, B. L.; Sande, M. A.; and Bolton, W. K. Pharmacokinetics of cefaclor and cephalexin: dosage nomograms for impaired renal function. *Antimicrob. Agents Chemother.*, **1978**, *14*, 172–177.

CEPHALOTHIN

Kirby, W. M. M.; DeMaine, J. B.; and Serril, W. S. Pharmacokinetics of the cephalosporins in healthy volunteers and uremic patients. *Postgrad. Med. J.*, **1971**, *47*, Suppl., 41–46.

Nightingale, C. H.; Greene, D. S.; and Quintiliani, R. Pharmacokinetics and clinical use of cephalosporin antibiotics. *J. Pharm. Sci.*, **1975**, *64*, 1899–1927.

CEPHAPIRIN

Bergan, T. Comparative pharmacokinetics of cefazolin, cephalothin, cephacetrile, and cephapirin after intravenous administration. *Chemotherapy*, **1977**, *23*, 389–404.

Nightingale, C. H.; Greene, D. S.; and Quintiliani, R. Pharmacokinetics and clinical use of cephalosporin antibiotics. *J. Pharm. Sci.*, **1975**, *64*, 1899–1927.

CEPHRADINE

Finkelstein, E.; Quintiliani, R.; Lee, R.; Bracci, A.; and Nightingale, C. H. Pharmacokinetics of oral cephalosporins: cephradine and cephalexin. *J. Pharm. Sci.*, **1978**, *67*, 1447–1450.

Philpson, A.; Stiernstedt, G.; and Ehrnebo, M. Comparison of the pharmacokinetics of cephradine and cefazolin in pregnant and nonpregnant women. *Clin. Pharmacokinet.*, **1987**, *12*, 136–144.

CHLORAMBUCIL

Newell, D. R.; Calvert, A. H.; Harrap, K. R.; and McElwain, T. J. Studies on the pharmacokinetics of chlorambucil and prednimustine in man. *Br. J. Clin. Pharmacol.*, **1983**, *15*, 253–258.

Oppitz, M. M.; Musch, E.; Malek, M.; Rüb, H. P.; von Unruh, G. E.; and Loos, U. Studies on the pharmacokinetics of chlorambucil and prednimustine in patients using a new high-performance liquid chromatographic assay. *Cancer Chemother. Pharmacol.*, **1989**, *23*, 208–212.

CHLORAMPHENICOL

Ambrose, P. J. Clinical pharmacokinetics of chloramphenicol and chloramphenicol succinate. *Clin. Pharmacokinet.*, **1984**, *9*, 222–238.

Nahata, M. C., and Powell, D. A. Bioavailability and clearance of chloramphenicol after intravenous chloramphenicol succinate. *Clin. Pharmacol. Ther.*, **1981**, *30*, 368–372.

CHLORDIAZEPOXIDE

Boxenbaum, H. G.; Greitner, K. A.; Jack, M. L.; Dixon, W. R.; Speigel, H. E.; Symington, J.; Christian, R.; Moore, J. D.; Weissman, L.; and Kaplan, S. A. Pharmacokinetic and biopharmaceutic profile of chlordiazepoxide HCl in healthy subjects: single-dose studies by the intravenous, intramuscular, and oral routes. *J. Pharmacokinet. Biopharm.*, **1977**, *5*, 3–23.

Greenblatt, D. J.; Shader, R. I.; MacLeod, S. M.; and Sellers, E. M. Clinical pharmacokinetics of chlordiazepoxide. *Clin. Pharmacokinet.*, **1978**, *3*, 381–394.

CHLOROQUINE

Frisk-Holmberg, M.; Bergqvist, Y.; Termond, E.; and Domeij-Nyberg, B. The single-dose kinetics of chloroquine and its major metabolite desmethylchloroquine in healthy subjects. *Eur. J. Clin. Pharmacol.*, **1984**, *26*, 521–530.

White, N. J. Clinical pharmacokinetics of antimalarial drugs. *Clin. Pharmacokinet.*, **1985**, *10*, 187–215.

CHLOROTHIAZIDE

Gee, W. L.; Lin, E. T.; Brater, D. C.; Gustafson, H. J.; and Benet, L. Z. Chlorothiazide pharmacokinetics following oral and i.v. dosing in man. Presented to Academy of Pharmaceutical Sciences, Anaheim, Calif., April, **1979**, Abstract P-52.

Osman, M. A.; Patel, R. B.; Irwin, D. S.; Craig, W. A.; and Welling, P. G. Bioavailability of chlorothiazide from 50, 100, and 250 mg solution doses. *Biopharm. Drug Dispos.*, **1982**, *3*, 89–94.

CHLORPHENIRAMINE

Rumore, M. M. Clinical pharmacokinetics of chlorpheniramine. *Drug Intell. Clin. Pharm.*, **1984**, *18*, 701–707.

CHLORPROMAZINE

Dahl, S. G., and Strandjord, R. E. Pharmacokinetics of chlorpromazine after single and chronic dosage. *Clin. Pharmacol. Ther.*, **1977**, *21*, 437–448.

Rivera-Calimlim, L.; Masrallah, H.; Strass, J.; and Lasagna, L. Clinical response and plasma levels: effect of dose, dosage schedules, and drug interactions on plasma chlorpromazine levels. *Am. J. Psychiatry*, **1976**, *133*, 646–652.

CHLORPROPAMIDE

Balant, L. Clinical pharmacokinetics of sulphonylurea-hypoglycaemic agents. *Clin. Pharmacokinet.*, **1981**, *6*, 215–241.

Neuvonen, P. J., and Kärkkäinen, S. Effects of charcoal, sodium bicarbonate, and ammonium chloride on chlorpropamide kinetics. *Clin. Pharmacol. Ther.*, **1983**, *33*, 386–393.

CHLORTHALIDONE

Beermann, B., and Groschinsky-Grind, M. Clinical pharmacokinetics of diuretics. *Clin. Pharmacokinet.*, **1980**, *5*, 221–245.

Fleuren, H. L. J.; Thien, T. A.; Verwey-van Wissen, C. P. W.; and van Rossum, J. M. Absolute bioavailability of chlorthalidone in man: a cross-over study after intravenous and oral administration. *Eur. J. Clin. Pharmacol.*, **1979**, *15*, 35–50.

CIMETIDINE

Chin, T. W. F.; Spino, M.; MacLeod, S. M.; Mahon, W. A.; and Soldin, S. J. Pharmacokinetics of cimetidine after subchronic administration. *Eur. J. Clin. Pharmacol.*, **1986**, *30*, 741–744.
Schentag, J. J.; Cerra, F. B.; Calleri, G. M.; Leising, M. E.; French, M. A.; and Bernhard, H. Age, disease, and cimetidine disposition in healthy subjects and chronically ill patients. *Clin. Pharmacol. Ther.*, **1981**, *29*, 737–743.

CINOXACIN

Brogard, J. M.; Comte, F.; and Lavillaureix, J. Comparative pharmacokinetic profiles of cinoxacin and pipemidic acid in humans. *Eur. J. Drug Metab. Pharmacokinet.*, **1983**, *8*, 251–259.
Sisca, T. S.; Heel, R. C.; and Romankiewicz, J. A. Cinoxacin: a review of its pharmacological properties and therapeutic efficacy in the treatment of urinary tract infections. *Drugs*, **1983**, *25*, 544–569.

CIPROFLOXACIN

Drusano, G. L.; Plaisance, K. I.; Forrest, A.; and Standiford, H. C. Dose ranging study and constant infusion evaluation of ciprofloxacin. *Antimicrob. Agents Chemother.*, **1986**, *30*, 440–443.
Sörgel, F.; Jaehde, U.; Naber, K.; and Stephan, U. Pharmacokinetic disposition of quinolones in human body fluids and tissues. *Clin. Pharmacokinet.*, **1989**, *16*, Suppl. 1, 5–24.

CISPLATIN

Reece, P. A.; Stafford, I.; Davy, M.; and Freeman, S. Disposition of unchanged cisplatin in patients with ovarian cancer. *Clin. Pharmacol. Ther.*, **1987**, *42*, 320–325.

CLAVULANIC ACID

Watson, I. D.; Stewart, M. J.; and Platt, D. J. Clinical pharmacokinetics of enzyme inhibitors in antimicrobial chemotherapy. *Clin. Pharmacokinet.*, **1988**, *15*, 133–164.

CLINDAMYCIN

Eller, M. G.; Smith, R. B.; and Phillips, J. P. Absorption kinetics of topical clindamycin preparations. *Biopharm. Drug Dispos.*, **1989**, *10*, 505–512.
Plaisance, K. I.; Drusano, G. L.; Forrest, A.; Townsend, R. J.; and Standiford, H. C. Pharmacokinetic evaluation of two dosage regimens of clindamycin phosphate. *Antimicrob. Agents Chemother.*, **1989**, *33*, 618–620.

CLOFIBRATE

Gugler, R.; Kurten, J. W.; Jensen, C. J.; Klehr, U.; and Hartlapp, J. Clofibrate disposition in renal failure and acute and chronic liver disease. *Eur. J. Clin. Pharmacol.*, **1979**, *15*, 341–347.
Veenendaal, J. R.; Brooks, P. M.; and Meffin, P. J. Probenecid–clofibrate interaction. *Clin. Pharmacol. Ther.*, **1981**, *29*, 351–358.

CLONAZEPAM

Berlin, A., and Dahlstrom, H. Pharmacokinetics of the anticonvulsant drug clonazepam evaluated from single oral and intravenous doses and by repeated oral administration. *Eur. J. Clin. Pharmacol.*, **1975**, *9*, 155–159.
Khoo, K.-C.; Mendels, J.; Rothbart, M.; Garland, W. A.; Colburn, W. A.; Min, B. H.; Lucek, R.; Carbone, J. J.; Boxenbaum, H. G.; and Kaplan, S. A. Influence of phenytoin and phenobarbital on the disposition of a single oral dose of clonazepam. *Clin. Pharmacol. Ther.*, **1980**, *28*, 368–375.

CLONIDINE

Lowenthal, D. T.; Matzek, K. M.; and MacGregor, T. R. Clinical pharmacokinetics of clonidine. *Clin. Pharmacokinet.*, **1988**, *14*, 287–310.

CLORAZEPATE

Rey, E.; d'Athis, P.; Giraux, P.; de Lauture, D.; Turquais, J. M.; Chavinie, J.; and Olive, G. Pharmacokinetics of clorazepate in pregnant and nonpregnant women. *Eur. J. Clin. Pharmacol.*, **1979**, *15*, 175–180.

CLOXACILLIN

Nauta, E. H., and Mattie, H. Dicloxacillin and cloxacillin: pharmacokinetics in healthy and hemodialysis subjects. *Clin. Pharmacol. Ther.*, **1976**, *20*, 98–108.
Spino, M.; Chai, R. P.; Isles, A. F.; Thiessen, J. J.; Tesoro, A.; Gold, R.; and MacLeod, S. M. Cloxacillin absorption and disposition in cystic fibrosis. *J. Pediatr.*, **1984**, *105*, 829–835.

COCAINE

Busto, U.; Bendayan, R.; and Sellers, E. M. Clinical pharmacokinetics of non-opiate abused drugs. *Clin. Pharmacokinet.*, **1989**, *16*, 1–26.
Jeffcoat, A. R.; Perez-Reyes, M.; Hill, J. M.; Sadler, B. M.; and Cook, E. C. Cocaine disposition in humans after intravenous injection, nasal insufflation (snorting), or smoking. *Drug Metab. Dispos.*, **1989**, *17*, 153–159.

Table A–II–1. PHARMACOKINETIC DATA (Continued)

CODEINE

Quiding, H.; Anderson, P.; Bondesson, U.; Boreus, L. O.; and Hynning, P. A. Plasma concentrations of codeine and its metabolite, morphine, after single and repeated oral administration. *Eur. J. Clin. Pharmacol.*, **1986**, *30*, 673–677.

Rogers, J. F.; Findlay, J. W. A.; Hull, J. H.; Butz, R. F.; Jones, E. C.; Bustrack, J. A.; and Welch, R. M. Codeine disposition in smokers and nonsmokers. *Clin. Pharmacol. Ther.*, **1982**, *32*, 218–227.

CYCLOPHOSPHAMIDE

Grochow, L. B., and Colvin, M. Clinical pharmacokinetics of cyclophosphamide. *Clin. Pharmacokinet.*, **1979**, *4*, 380–394.

Wiebe, V. J.; Benz, C. C.; and DeGregorio, M. W. Clinical pharmacokinetics of drugs used in the treatment of breast cancer. *Clin. Pharmacokinet.*, **1988**, *15*, 180–193.

CYCLOSPORINE

Gupta, S. K.; Manfro, R. C.; Tomlanovich, S. J.; Gambertoglio, J. G.; Garovoy, M. R.; and Benet, L. Z. Effect of food on the pharmacokinetics of cyclosporine in healthy subjects following oral and intravenous administrations. *J. Clin. Pharmacol.*, **1990**, *30*, In press.

Rodighiero, V. Therapeutic drug monitoring of cyclosporine. *Clin. Pharmacokinet.*, **1989**, *16*, 27–37.

CYTARABINE

Balis, F. M.; Holcenberg, J. S.; and Bleyer, W. A. Clinical pharmacokinetics of commonly used anticancer drugs. *Clin. Pharmacokinet.*, **1983**, *8*, 202–232.

Wan, S. H.; Huffman, D. H.; Azarnoff, D. L.; Hoogstraten, B.; and Larsen, W. E. Pharmacokinetics of 1-β-D-arabinofuranosylcytosine in humans. *Cancer Res.*, **1974**, *34*, 392–397.

DAPSONE

Venkatesan, K. Clinical pharmacokinetic considerations in the treatment of patients with leprosy. *Clin. Pharmacokinet.*, **1989**, *16*, 365–386.

DESIPRAMINE

Ciraulo, D. A.; Barnhill, J. A.; and Jaffe, J. H. Clinical pharmacokinetics of imipramine and desipramine in alcoholics and normal volunteers. *Clin. Pharmacol. Ther.*, **1988**, *43*, 509–518.

Rudorfer, M. V.; Lane, E. A.; Chang, W.-H.; Zhang, M.; and Potter, W. Z. Desipramine pharmacokinetics in Chinese and Caucasian volunteers. *Br. J. Clin. Pharmacol.*, **1984**, *17*, 433–440.

DESMETHYLDIAZEPAM (NORDAZEPAM)

Bertilsson, L.; Henthorn, T. K.; Sanz, E.; Tybring, G.; Säwe, J.; and Villén, T. Importance of genetic factors in the regulation of diazepam metabolism: relationship of S-mephenytoin, but not debrisoquin, hydroxylation phenotype. *Clin. Pharmacol. Ther.*, **1989**, *45*, 348–355.

Greenblatt, D. J.; Divoll, M. K.; Soong, M. H.; Boxenbaum, H. G.; Harmatz, J. S.; and Shader, R. I. Desmethyldiazepam pharmacokinetics: studies following intravenous and oral desmethyldiazepam, oral clorazepate, and intravenous diazepam. *J. Clin. Pharmacol.*, **1988**, *28*, 853–859.

DEXAMETHASONE

Gustavson, L. E., and Benet, L. Z. Pharmacokinetics of natural and synthetic glucocorticoids. In, *Butterworth's International Medical Reviews in Endocrinology.* Vol. 4, *The Adrenal Cortex.* (Anderson, D. C., and Winter, J. S. D., eds.) Butterworth & Co., London, **1985**, pp. 235–281.

Tsuei, S. E.; Moore, R. G.; Ashley, J. J.; and McBride, W. G. Disposition of synthetic glucocorticoids. I. Pharmacokinetics of dexamethasone in healthy adults. *J. Pharmacokinet. Biopharm.*, **1979**, *7*, 249–264.

DIAZEPAM

Bertilsson, L.; Henthorn, T. K.; Sanz, E.; Tybring, G.; Säwe, J.; and Villén, T. Importance of genetic factors in the regulation of diazepam metabolism: relationship to S-mephenytoin, but not debrisoquin, hydroxylation phenotype. *Clin. Pharmacol. Ther.*, **1989**, *45*, 348–355.

Greenblatt, D. J.; Allen, M. D.; Harmatz, J. S.; and Shader, R. I. Diazepam disposition determinants. *Clin. Pharmacol. Ther.*, **1980**, *27*, 301–312.

DIAZOXIDE

Pearson, R. M. Pharmacokinetics and response to diazoxide in renal failure. *Clin. Pharmacokinet.*, **1977**, *2*, 198–204.

Pearson, R. M., and Breckenridge, A. M. Renal function, protein binding and pharmacological response to diazoxide. *Br. J. Clin. Pharmacol.*, **1976**, *3*, 169–175.

DICLOFENAC

Todd, P. A., and Sorkin, E. J. Diclofenac sodium: a reappraisal of its pharmacodynamic and pharmacokinetic properties and therapeutic efficacy. *Drugs*, **1988**, *35*, 244–285.

Willis, J. V.; Kendall, M. J.; Flinn, R. M.; Thornhill, D. P.; and Welling, P. G. The pharmacokinetics of diclofenac sodium following intravenous and oral administration. *Eur. J. Clin. Pharmacol.*, **1979**, *16*, 405–410.

DICLOXACILLIN

Jusko, W. J.; Mosovich, L. L.; Gerbracht, L. M.; Mattar, M. E.; and Yaffe, S. J. Enhanced renal excretion of dicloxacillin in patients with cystic fibrosis. *Pediatrics*, **1975**, *56*, 1038–1044.

Nauta, E. H., and Mattie, H. Dicloxacillin and cloxacillin: pharmacokinetics in healthy and hemodialysis subjects. *Clin. Pharmacol. Ther.*, **1976**, *20*, 98–108.

DIFLUNISAL

Eriksson, L. O.; Wåhlin-Boll, E.; Odar-Cederlöf, I.; Lindholm, L.; and Melander, A. Influence of renal failure, rheumatoid arthritis and old age on the pharmacokinetics of diflunisal. *Br. J. Clin. Pharmacol.*, **1989**, *36*, 165–174.

Loewen, G. R.; Herman, R. J.; Ross, S. G.; and Verbeeck, R. K. Effect of dose on the glucuronidation and sulphation kinetics of diflunisal in man: single dose studies. *Eur. J. Clin. Pharmacol.*, **1988**, *26*, 31–39.

DIGITOXIN

Mooradian, A. D. Digitalis: an update of clinical pharmacokinetics, therapeutic monitoring techniques, and treatment recommendations. *Clin. Pharmacokinet.*, **1988**, *15*, 165–179.

Sheiner, L. B.; Benet, L. Z.; and Pagliaro, L. A. A standard approach to compiling clinical pharmacokinetic data. *J. Pharmacokinet. Biopharm.*, **1981**, *9*, 59–127.

DIGOXIN

Mooradian, A. D. Digitalis: an update of clinical pharmacokinetics, therapeutic monitoring techniques, and treatment recommendations. *Clin. Pharmacokinet.*, **1988**, *15*, 165–179.

Sheiner, L. B.; Rosenberg, B. G.; and Marathe, V. V. Estimation of population characteristics of pharmacokinetic parameters from routine clinical data. *J. Pharmacokinet. Biopharm.*, **1977**, *5*, 445–479.

DILTIAZEM

Echizen, H., and Eichelbaum, M. Clinical pharmacokinetics of verapamil, nifedipine and diltiazem. *Clin. Pharmacokinet.*, **1986**, *11*, 425–449.

Montamat, S. C., and Abernethy, D. R. Calcium antagonists in geriatric patients: diltiazem in elderly persons with hypertension. *Clin. Pharmacol. Ther.*, **1989**, *45*, 682–691.

DIPHENHYDRAMINE

Blyden, G. T.; Greenblatt, D. J.; Scavone, J. M.; and Shader, R. I. Pharmacokinetics of diphenhydramine and a demethylated metabolite following intravenous and oral administration. *J. Clin. Pharmacol.*, **1986**, *26*, 529–533.

Gengo, F.; Gabos, C.; and Miller, J. K. The pharmacodynamics of diphenhydramine-induced drowsiness and changes in mental performance. *Clin. Pharmacol. Ther.*, **1989**, *45*, 15–21.

DISOPYRAMIDE

Le Corre, P.; Gibassier, D.; Sado, P.; and Le Verge, R. Stereoselective metabolism and pharmacokinetics of disopyramide enantiomers in humans. *Drug Metab. Dispos.*, **1988**, *16*, 858–864.

Siddoway, L. A., and Woosley, R. L. Clinical pharmacokinetics of disopyramide. *Clin. Pharmacokinet.*, **1986**, *11*, 214–222.

DOBUTAMINE

Kates, R. E., and Leier, C. V. Dobutamine pharmacokinetics in severe heart failure. *Clin. Pharmacol. Ther.*, **1978**, *24*, 537–541.

DOXEPIN

Faulkner, R. D.; Pitts, W. M.; Lee, C. S.; Lewis, W. A.; and Fann, W. E. Multiple-dose doxepin kinetics in depressed patients. *Clin. Pharmacol. Ther.*, **1983**, *34*, 509–515.

DOXORUBICIN

Speth, P. A. J.; Van Hoesel, Q. G. C. M.; and Haanen, C. Clinical pharmacokinetics of doxorubicin. *Clin. Pharmacokinet.*, **1988**, *15*, 15–31.

DOXYCYCLINE

Saivin, S., and Hovin, G. Clinical pharmacokinetics of doxycycline and minocycline. *Clin. Pharmacokinet.*, **1988**, *15*, 355–366.

EDROPHONIUM

Morris, R. B.; Cronnelly, R.; Miller, R. D.; Stanski, D. R.; and Fahey, M. R. Pharmacokinetics of edrophonium and neostigmine when antagonizing *d*-tubocurarine neuromuscular blockade in man. *Anesthesiology*, **1981**, *54*, 399–402.

ENALAPRIL

Lees, K. R., and Reid, J. L. Age and the pharmacokinetics and pharmacodynamics of chronic enalapril treatment. *Clin. Pharmacol. Ther.*, **1987**, *41*, 597–602.

Till, A. E.; Gomez, H. J.; Hichens, M.; and Bolognese, J. A. Pharmacokinetics of repeated single oral doses of enalapril maleate (MK-421) in normal volunteers. *Biopharm. Drug Dispos.*, **1984**, *5*, 273–280.

Table A–II–1. PHARMACOKINETIC DATA (Continued)

ENCAINIDE

Roden, D. M., and Woosley, R. L. Clinical pharmacokinetics of encainide. *Clin. Pharmacokinet.*, **1988**, ***14***, 141–147.

ENCAINIDE ACTIVE METABOLITES

Barbey, J. T.; Thompson, K. A.; Echt, D. S.; Woosley, R. L.; and Roden, D. M. Antiarrhythmic activity, electrocardiographic effects and pharmacokinetics of the encainide metabolites O-desmethyl-encainide and 3-methoxy-O-desmethyl encainide in man. *Circulation*, **1988**, ***77***, 380–391.

ERYTHROMYCIN

Periti, P.; Mazzei, T.; Mini, E.; and Novelli, A. Clinical pharmacokinetics of the macrolide antibiotics. *Clin. Pharmacokinet.*, **1989**, ***16***, 193–214.

ESMOLOL

Benfield, P., and Sorkin, E. M. Esmolol: a preliminary review of its pharmacodynamic and pharmacokinetic properties and therapeutic efficacy. *Drugs*, **1987**, ***33***, 392–412.
Flaherty, J. R.; Wong, B.; La Follette, G.; Warnock, D. G.; Hulse, J. D.; and Gambertoglio, J. G. Pharmacokinetics of esmolol and ASL-8123 in renal failure. *Clin. Pharmacol. Ther.*, **1989**, ***45***, 321–327.

ETHAMBUTOL

Holdiness, M. R. Clinical pharmacokinetics of the antituberculosis drugs. *Clin. Pharmacokinet.*, **1984**, *9*, 511–544.
Lee, C. S.; Brater, D. C.; Gambertoglio, J. G.; and Benet, L. Z. Disposition kinetics of ethambutol. *J. Pharmacokinet. Biopharm.*, **1980**, *8*, 335–346.

ETHANOL

Holford, N. H. G. Clinical pharmacokinetics of ethanol. *Clin. Pharmacokinet.*, **1987**, *13*, 273–292.
Wilkinson, P. K.; Sedman, A. J.; Sakmar, E.; Earhart, R. H.; Weidler, D. J.; and Wagner, J. G. Blood ethanol concentrations during and following constant-rate intravenous infusion of alcohol. *Clin. Pharmacol. Ther.*, **1976**, *19*, 213–223.
Wilkinson, P. K.; Sedman, A. J.; Sakmar, E.; Kay, D. R.; and Wagner, J. G. Pharmacokinetics of ethanol after oral administration in the fasting state. *J. Pharmacokinet. Biopharm.*, **1977**, *5*, 207–224.

ETHOSUXIMIDE

Bauer, L. A.; Harris, C.; Wilensky, A. J.; Raisys, V. A.; and Levy, R. H. Ethosuximide kinetics: possible interaction with valproic acid. *Clin. Pharmacol. Ther.*, **1982**, *31*, 741–745.

ETOPOSIDE

Clark, P. I., and Slevin, J. L. The clinical pharmacology of etoposide and teniposide. *Clin. Pharmacokinet.*, **1987**, ***12***, 223–253.
Fleming, R. A.; Miller, A. A.; and Stewart, C. F. Etoposide: an update. *Clin. Pharm.*, **1989**, ***8***, 274–293.

FAMOTIDINE

Krishna, D. R., and Klotz, U. Newer H_2-receptor antagonists. Clinical pharmacokinetics and drug interaction potential. *Clin. Pharmacokinet.*, **1988**, ***15***, 205–215.

FENTANYL

Mather, L. E. Clinical pharmacokinetics of fentanyl and its newer derivatives. *Clin. Pharmacokinet.*, **1983**, *8*, 422–446.

FLECAINIDE

McQuinn, R. L.; Pentikäinen, P. J.; Chang, S. F.; and Conrad, G. J. Pharmacokinetics of flecainide in patients with cirrhosis of the liver. *Clin. Pharmacol. Ther.*, **1988**, ***44***, 566–572.
Tjandra-Maga, T. B.; Verbessent, R.; Van Hecken, A.; Mullie, A.; and DeSchepper, P. J. Flecainide: single and multiple oral dose kinetics, absolute bioavailability and effect of food and antacid in man. *Br. J. Clin. Pharmacol.*, **1986**, **22**, 309–316.

FLUCYTOSINE

Cutler, R. E.; Blair, A. D.; and Kelly, M. R. Flucytosine kinetics in subjects with normal and impaired renal function. *Clin. Pharmacol. Ther.*, **1978**, *24*, 333–342.
Daneshmend, T. K., and Warnock, D. W. Clinical pharmacokinetics of systemic antifungal drugs. *Clin. Pharmacokinet.*, **1983**, *8*, 17–42.

FLUNITRAZEPAM

Boxenbaum, H. G.; Posmanter, H. N.; Macasieb, T.; Geitner, K. A.; Weinfeld, R. E.; Moore, J. D.; Darragh, A.; O'Kelly, D. A.; Weissman, L.; and Kaplan, S. A. Pharmacokinetics of flunitrazepam following single- and multiple-dose oral administration to healthy human subjects. *J. Pharmacokinet. Biopharm.*, **1978**, *6*, 283–293.

FLUOROURACIL

Diasio, R. B., and Harris, B. E. Clinical pharmacology of 5-fluorouracil. *Clin. Pharmacokinet.*, **1989**, *16*, 215–237.

FLUOXETINE

Schenker, S.; Bergstrom, R. F.; Wolen, R. L.; and Lemberger, L. Fluoxetine disposition and elimination in cirrhosis. *Clin. Pharmacol. Ther.*, **1988**, *44*, 353–359.

Sommi, R. W.; Crismon, M. L.; and Bowden, C. L. Fluoxetine: a serotonin-specific second-generation antidepressant. *Pharmacotherapy*, **1987**, *7*, 1–15.

FLURAZEPAM

Greenblatt, D. J.; Divoll, M.; Harmatz, J. S.; MacLaughlin, D. S.; and Shader, R. I. Kinetics and clinical effects of flurazepam in young and elderly noninsomniacs. *Clin. Pharmacol. Ther.*, **1981**, *30*, 475–486.

Kaplan, S. A.; deSilva, J. A. F.; Jack, M. L.; Alexander, K.; Strojny, N.; Weinfeld, R. E.; Puglisi, C. V.; and Weissman, L. Blood level profile in man following chronic oral administration of flurazepam hydrochloride. *J. Pharm. Sci.*, **1973**, *62*, 1932–1935.

FUROSEMIDE

Hammarlund-Udenaes, M., and Benet, L. Z. Furosemide pharmacokinetics and pharmacodynamics in health and disease—an update. *J. Pharmacokinet. Biopharm.*, **1989**, *17*, 1–46.

GENTAMICIN

Keller, F. Gentamicin volume of distribution as a power function of body weight. *Br. J. Clin. Pharmacol.*, **1989**, *28*, 479–481.

Matzke, G. R.; Millikin, S. P.; and Kovarik, J. M. Variability in pharmacokinetic values for gentamicin, tobramycin, and netilmicin in patients with renal insufficiency. *Clin. Pharm.*, **1989**, *8*, 800–806.

GLIPIZIDE

Kobayashi, K. A.; Bauer, L. A.; Horn, J. R.; Opheim, K.; Wood, F.; and Kradjan, W. A. Glipizide pharmacokinetics in young and elderly volunteers. *Clin. Pharmacokinet.*, **1988**, *7*, 224–228.

Lebovitz, H. E. Glipizide: a second-generation sulfonylurea hypoglycemic agent. *Pharmacotherapy*, **1985**, *5*, 63–67.

GOLD SODIUM THIOMALATE

Blocka, K. L. N.; Paulus, H. E.; and Furst, D. E. Clinical pharmacokinetics of oral and injectable gold compounds. *Clin. Pharmacokinet.*, **1986**, *11*, 133–144.

Massarella, J. W.; Waller, E. S.; Crout, J. E.; and Yakatan, G. J. The pharmacokinetics of intramuscular gold sodium thiomalate in normal volunteers. *Biopharm. Drug Dispos.*, **1984**, *5*, 101–107.

HALOPERIDOL

Froemming, J. S.; Lam, Y. W. F.; Jann, M. W.; and Davis, C. M. Pharmacokinetics of haloperidol. *Clin. Pharmacokinet.*, **1989**, *17*, 396–423.

HEPARIN

Bjornsson, T. D.; Wolfram, K. M.; and Kitchell, B. B. Heparin kinetics determined by three assay methods. *Clin. Pharmacol. Ther.*, **1982**, *31*, 104–113.

Estes, J. W. Clinical pharmacokinetics of heparin. *Clin. Pharmacokinet.*, **1980**, *5*, 204–220.

HEXOBARBITAL

Chandler, M. H. H.; Scott, S. R.; and Blouin, R. A. Age-associated stereoselective alterations in hexobarbital metabolism. *Clin. Pharmacol. Ther.*, **1988**, *43*, 436–441.

Vermeulen, N. P. E.; Rietveld, C. T.; and Breimer, D. D. Disposition of hexobarbitone in healthy man: kinetics of parent drug and metabolites following oral administration. *Br. J. Clin. Pharmacol.*, **1983**, *15*, 459–464.

HYDRALAZINE

Ludden, T. M.; McNay, J. L., Jr.; Shepherd, A. M. M.; and Lin, M.-S. Clinical pharmacokinetics of hydralazine. *Clin. Pharmacokinet.*, **1982**, *7*, 185–205.

Mulrow, J. P., and Crawford, M. H. Clinical pharmacokinetics and therapeutic use of hydralazine in congestive heart failure. *Clin. Pharmacokinet.*, **1989**, *16*, 86–99.

HYDROCHLOROTHIAZIDE

Beermann, B., and Groschinsky-Grind, M. Pharmacokinetics of hydrochlorothiazide in man. *Eur. J. Clin. Pharmacol.*, **1977**, *12*, 297–303.

Sabanathan, K.; Castleden, C. M.; Adam, H. K.; Ryan, J.; and Fitzsimons, T. J. A comparative study of the pharmacokinetics and pharmacodynamics of atenolol, hydrochlorothiazide and amiloride in normal young and elderly subjects and elderly hypertensive patients. *Eur. J. Clin. Pharmacol.*, **1987**, *32*, 53–60.

Table A–II–1. PHARMACOKINETIC DATA (Continued)

IBUPROFEN

Evans, A. M.; Nation, R. L.; Sansom, L. N.; Bochner, F.; and Somogyi, A. A. Stereoselective plasma protein binding of ibuprofen enantiomers. *Eur. J. Clin. Pharmacol.*, **1989**, *36*, 283–290.

Lee, E. J. D.; Williams, K.; Day, R.; Graham, G.; and Champion, D. Stereoselective disposition of ibuprofen enantiomers in man. *Br. J. Clin. Pharmacol.*, **1985**, *19*, 669–674.

IMIPENEM/CILASTATIN

Drusano, G. L.; Standiford, H. C.; Bustamante, C.; Forrest, A.; Rivera, G.; Leslie, J.; Tatem, B.; Delaportas, D.; MacGregor, R. R.; and Schimpff, S. C. Multiple-dose pharmacokinetics of imipenem-cilastatin. *Antimicrob. Agents Chemother.*, **1984**, *26*, 715–721.

IMIPRAMINE

Abernethy, D. R.; Greenblatt, D. J.; and Shader, R. I. Imipramine-cimetidine interaction: impairment of clearance and enhanced absolute bioavailability. *J. Pharmacol. Exp. Ther.*, **1984**, *229*, 702–705.

Brøsen, K., and Gram, L. F. First-pass metabolism of imipramine and desipramine: impact of the sparteine oxidation phenotype. *Clin. Pharmacol. Ther.*, **1988**, *43*, 400–406.

Ciraulo, D. A.; Barnhill, J. A.; and Jaffe, J. H. Clinical pharmacokinetics of imipramine and desipramine in alcoholics and normal volunteers. *Clin. Pharmacol. Ther.*, **1988**, *43*, 509–518.

INDOMETHACIN

Helleberg, L. Clinical pharmacokinetics of indomethacin. *Clin. Pharmacokinet.*, **1981**, *6*, 245–258.

Kwan, K. C.; Breault, G. O.; Davis, R. L.; Lei, B. W.; Czerwinski, A. W.; Besselaar, G. H.; and Duggan, D. E. Effects of concomitant aspirin administration on the pharmacokinetics of indomethacin in man. *J. Pharmacokinet. Biopharm.*, **1978**, *6*, 451–476.

INTERFERON ALFA

Wills, R. J.; Dennis, S.; Spiegel, H. E.; Gibson, D. M.; and Nadler, P. I. Interferon kinetics and adverse reactions after intravenous, intramuscular, and subcutaneous injection. *Clin. Pharmacol. Ther.*, **1984**, *35*, 722–727.

Wills, R. J., and Smith, R. A. Pharmacokinetics of interferons. In, *Interferon Treatment of Neurologic Disorders.* (Smith, R. A., ed.) Marcel Dekker, New York, **1988**, pp. 103–133.

ISONIAZID

Holdiness, M. R. Clinical pharmacokinetics of the antituberculosis drugs. *Clin. Pharmacokinet.*, **1984**, *9*, 511–544.

Kergueris, M. F.; Bourin, M.; and Larousse, C. Pharmacokinetics of isoniazid: influence of age. *Eur. J. Clin. Pharmacol.*, **1986**, *30*, 335–340.

ISOSORBIDE DINITRATE

Morrison, R. A.; Wiegand, U.-W.; Jähnchen, E.; Höhmann, D.; Bechtold, H.; Meinertz, T.; and Fung, H.-L. Isosorbide dinitrate kinetics and dynamics after intravenous, sublingual, and percutaneous dosing in angina. *Clin. Pharmacol. Ther.*, **1983**, *33*, 747–756.

Straehl, P., and Galeazzi, R. L. Isosorbide dinitrate bioavailability, kinetics, and metabolism. *Clin. Pharmacol. Ther.*, **1985**, *38*, 140–149.

ISOSORBIDE-2-MONONITRATE

Bogaert, M. G.; Rosseel, M. T.; Boelaert, J.; and Daneels, R. Fate of isosorbide dinitrate and mononitrates in patients with renal failure. *Eur. J. Clin. Pharmacol.*, **1981**, *21*, 73–76.

Straehl, P.; Galeazzi, R. L.; and Soliva, M. Isosorbide 5-mononitrate and isosorbide 2-mononitrate kinetics after intravenous and oral dosing. *Clin. Pharmacol. Ther.*, **1984**, *36*, 485–492.

ISOSORBIDE-5-MONONITRATE (ISOSORBIDE NITRATE)

Major, R. M.; Taylor, T.; Chasseaud, L. F.; Darragh, A.; and Lambe, R. F. Isosorbide 5-mononitrate kinetics. *Clin. Pharmacol. Ther.*, **1984**, *35*, 653–659.

Straehl, P.; Galeazzi, R. L.; and Soliva, M. Isosorbide 5-mononitrate and isosorbide 2-mononitrate kinetics after intravenous and oral dosing. *Clin. Pharmacol. Ther.*, **1984**, *36*, 485–492.

ISOTRETINOIN

Allan, J. G., and Bloxham, D. P. The pharmacology and pharmacokinetics of the retinoids. *Pharmacol. Ther.*, **1989**, *40*, 1–27.

Lucek, R. W., and Colburn, W. A. Clinical pharmacokinetics of the retinoids. *Clin. Pharmacokinet.*, **1985**, *10*, 38–62.

KANAMYCIN

Clarke, J. T.; Libke, R. K.; Regamey, C.; and Kirby, W. M. M. Comparative pharmacokinetics of amikacin and kanamycin. *Clin. Pharmacol. Ther.*, **1974**, *15*, 610–616.

Holdiness, M. R. Clinical pharmacokinetics of the antituberculosis drugs. *Clin. Pharmacokinet.*, **1984**, *9*, 511–544.

KETAMINE

Grant, I. S.; Nimmo, W. S.; and Clements, J. A. Pharmacokinetics and analgesic effects of i.m. and oral ketamine. *Br. J. Anaesth.*, **1981**, *53*, 805–809.

White, P. F.; Schüttler, J.; Shafer, A.; Stanski, D. R.; Horai, Y.; and Trevor, A. J. Comparative pharmacology of the ketamine isomers. *Br. J. Anaesth.*, **1985**, *57*, 197–203.

KETOCONAZOLE

Badcock, N. R.; Bartholomeusz, F. D.; Frewin, D. B.; Sansom, L. N.; and Reid, J. G. The pharmacokinetics of ketoconazole after chronic administration in adults. *Eur. J. Clin. Pharmacol.*, **1987**, *33*, 531–534.

KETOPROFEN

Williams, R. L., and Upton, R. A. The clinical pharmacology of ketoprofen. *J. Clin. Pharmacol.*, **1988**, *28*, S13–S22.

LABETALOL

Goa, K. L.; Benfield, P.; and Sorkin, E. M. Labetalol: a reappraisal of its pharmacology, pharmacokinetics and therapeutic use in hypertension and ischaemic heart disease. *Drugs*, **1989**, *37*, 583–627.

McNeil, J. J., and Louis, W. J. Clinical pharmacokinetics of labetalol. *Clin. Pharmacokinet.*, **1984**, *9*, 157–167.

LEUCOVORIN

McGuire, B. W.; Sia, L. L.; Leese, P. T.; Gutierrez, M. L.; and Stokstad, E. L. R. Pharmacokinetics of leucovorin calcium after intravenous, intramuscular, and oral administration. *Clin. Pharm.*, **1988**, *7*, 52–58.

Straw, J. A.; Szapary, D.; and Wynn, W. T. Pharmacokinetics of the diastereoisomers of leucovorin after intravenous and oral administration to normal subjects. *Cancer Res.*, **1984**, *44*, 3114–3119.

LIDOCAINE

Cusack, B.; O'Malley, K.; Lavan, J.; Noel, J.; and Kelly, J. G. Protein binding and disposition of lignocaine in the elderly. *Eur. J. Clin. Pharmacol.*, **1985**, *29*, 323–329.

Nattel, S.; Gagne, G.; and Pineau, M. The pharmacokinetics of lignocaine and β-adrenoceptor antagonists in patients with acute myocardial infarction. *Clin. Pharmacokinet.*, **1987**, *13*, 293–316.

LITHIUM

Hunter, R. Steady-state pharmacokinetics of lithium carbonate in healthy subjects. *Br. J. Clin. Pharmacol.*, **1988**, *25*, 375–380.

Mason, R. W.; McQueen, E. G.; Keary, P. J.; and James, N. McL. Pharmacokinetics of lithium: elimination half-time, renal clearance and apparent volume of distribution in schizophrenia. *Clin. Pharmacokinet.*, **1978**, *3*, 241–246.

LORAZEPAM

Greenblatt, D. J. Clinical pharmacokinetics of oxazepam and lorazepam. *Clin. Pharmacokinet.*, **1981**, *6*, 89–105.

Martyn, J., and Greenblatt, D. J. Lorazepam conjugation is unimpaired in burn trauma. *Clin. Pharmacol. Ther.*, **1988**, *43*, 250–255.

LORCAINIDE

Gillis, A. M., and Kates, R. E. Clinical pharmacokinetics of the newer antiarrhythmic agents. *Clin. Pharmacokinet.*, **1984**, *9*, 375–403.

Somani, P.; Fraker, T. D., Jr.; and Temesy-Armos, P. N. Pharmacokinetic implications of lorcainide therapy in patients with normal and depressed cardiac function. *J. Clin. Pharmacol.*, **1987**, *27*, 122–132.

MELPHALAN

Loos, U.; Musch, E.; Engel, M.; Hartlapp, J. H.; Hügl, E.; and Dengler, H. J. The pharmacokinetics of melphalan during intermittent therapy of multiple myeloma. *Eur. J. Clin. Pharmacol.*, **1988**, *35*, 187–193.

MEPERIDINE

Chan, K.; Tse, J.; Jennings, F.; and Orma, M. L'E. Pharmacokinetics of low dose intravenous pethidine in patients with renal dysfunction. *J. Clin. Pharmacol.*, **1987**, *27*, 516–522.

Edwards, D. J.; Svensson, C. K.; Visco, J. P.; and Lalka, D. Clinical pharmacokinetics of pethidine: 1982. *Clin. Pharmacokinet.*, **1982**, *7*, 421–433.

MERCAPTOPURINE

Arndt, C. A. S.; Balis, F. M.; McCully, C. L.; Jeffries, S. L.; Doherty, K.; Murphy, R.; and Poplack, D. G. Bioavailability of low-dose vs high-dose 6-mercaptopurine. *Clin. Pharmacol. Ther.*, **1988**, *43*, 588–591.

Zimm, S.; Collins, J. M.; O'Neill, D.; Chabner, B. A.; and Poplack, D. G. Inhibition of first-pass metabolism in cancer chemotherapy: interaction of 6-mercaptopurine and allopurinol. *Clin. Pharmacol. Ther.*, **1983**, *34*, 810–817.

METHADONE

Inturrisi, C. E.; Colburn, W. A.; Kaiko, R. F.; Houde, R. W.; and Foley, K. M. Pharmacokinetics and pharmacodynamics of methadone in patients with chronic pain. *Clin. Pharmacol. Ther.*, **1987**, *41*, 392–401.

Säwe, J. High-dose morphine and methadone in cancer patients. Clinical pharmacokinetic considerations of oral treatment. *Clin. Pharmacokinet.*, **1986**, *11*, 87–106.

Table A–II–1. PHARMACOKINETIC DATA (Continued)

METHICILLIN

Bulger, R. J.; Lindholm, D. D.; Murray, J. S.; and Kirby, W. M. M. Effect of uremia on methicillin and oxacillin blood levels. *J.A.M.A.*, **1964**, *187*, 319–322.

Yaffe, S. J.; Gerbracht, L. M.; Mosovich, L. L.; Mattar, M. E.; Danish, M.; and Jusko, W. J. Pharmacokinetics of methicillin in patients with cystic fibrosis. *J. Infect. Dis.*, **1977**, *135*, 828–831.

METHOHEXITAL

Hudson, R. J.; Stanski, D. R.; and Burch, P. G. Pharmacokinetics of methohexital and thiopental in surgical patients. *Anesthesiology*, **1983**, *59*, 215–219.

Lauven, P. M.; Schwilden, H.; and Stoeckel, H. Threshold hypnotic concentration of methohexitone. *Eur. J. Clin. Pharmacol.*, **1987**, *33*, 261–265.

METHOTREXATE

Crom, W. R.; Glynn-Barnhart, A. M.; Rodman, J. H.; Teresi, M. E.; Kavanagh, R. E.; Christensen, M. L.; Relling, M. V.; and Evans, W. E. Pharmacokinetics of anticancer drugs in children. *Clin. Pharmacokinet.*, **1987**, *12*, 168–213.

Herman, R. A.; Veng-Pedersen, P.; Hoffman, J.; Koehnke, R.; and Furst, D. E. Pharmacokinetics of low-dose methotrexate in rheumatoid arthritis patients. *J. Pharm. Sci.*, **1989**, *78*, 165–171.

METHYLDOPA

Myhre, E.; Rugstad, H. E.; and Hansen, T. Clinical pharmacokinetics of methyldopa. *Clin. Pharmacokinet.*, **1982**, *7*, 221–223.

Renwick, A. G.; Higgins, V.; Powers, K.; Smith, C. L.; and George, C. F. The absorption and conjugation of methyldopa in patients with coeliac and Crohn's diseases during treatment. *Br. J. Clin. Pharmacol.*, **1983**, *16*, 77–83.

METHYLPREDNISOLONE

Gustavson, L. E., and Benet, L. Z. Pharmacokinetics of natural and synthetic glucocorticoids. In, *Butterworth's International Medical Reviews in Endocrinology*. Vol. 4, *The Adrenal Cortex*. (Anderson, D. C., and Winter, J. S. D., eds.) Butterworth & Co., London, **1985**, pp. 235–281.

Kong, A.-N.; Ludwig, E. A.; Slaughter, R. L.; DiStefano, P. M.; DeMasi, J.; Middleton, E., Jr.; and Jusko, W. J. Pharmacokinetics and pharmacodynamic modeling of direct suppression effects of methylprednisolone on serum cortisol and blood histamine in human subjects. *Clin. Pharmacol. Ther.*, **1989**, *46*, 616–628.

METOCLOPRAMIDE

Wright, M. R.; Axelson, J. E.; Rurak, D. W.; McErlane, B.; McMorland, G. H.; Ongley, R. C.; Tam, Y. K.; and Price, J. D. E. Linearity of metoclopramide kinetics at doses of 5–20 mg. *Br. J. Clin. Pharmacol.*, **1988**, *26*, 469–473.

———. Effect of haemodialysis on metoclopramide kinetics in patients with severe renal failure. *Ibid.*, **1988**, *26*, 474–477.

METOCURINE

Avram, M. J.; Shanks, C. A.; Henthorn, T. K.; Ronai, A. K.; Kinzer, J.; and Wilkinson, C. J. Metocurine kinetics in patients undergoing operations requiring cardiopulmonary bypass. *Clin. Pharmacol. Ther.*, **1987**, *42*, 576–581,

Shanks, C. A. Pharmacokinetics of the nondepolarizing neuromuscular relaxants applied to calculation of bolus and infusion dosage regimens. *Anesthesiology*, **1986**, *64*, 72–86.

METOPROLOL

Dayer, P.; Leemann, T.; Marmy, A.; and Rosenthaler, J. Interindividual variation of beta-adrenoceptor blocking drugs, plasma concentration and effect: influence of genetic status on behaviour of atenolol, bopindolol and metoprolol. *Eur. J. Clin. Pharmacol.*, **1985**, *28*, 149–153.

Toon, S.; Davidson, E. M.; Garstang, F. M.; Batra, H.; Bowes, R. J.; and Rowland, M. The racemic metoprolol H_2-antagonist interaction. *Clin. Pharmacol. Ther.*, **1988**, *43*, 283–289.

METRONIDAZOLE

Loft, S.; Poulsen, H. E.; Sonne, J.; and Døssing, M. Metronidazole clearance: a one-sample method and influencing factors. *Clin. Pharmacol. Ther.*, **1988**, *43*, 420–428.

Ralph, E. D. Clinical pharmacokinetics of metronidazole. *Clin. Pharmacokinet.*, **1983**, *8*, 43–62.

MEXILETINE

Brockmeyer, N. H.; Breithaupt, H.; Ferdinand, W.; von Hattingberg, M.; and Ohnhaus, E. E. Kinetics of oral and intravenous mexiletine: lack of effect of cimetidine and ranitidine. *Eur. J. Clin. Pharmacol.*, **1989**, *36*, 375–378.

Gillis, A. M., and Kates, R. E. Clinical pharmacokinetics of the newer antiarrhythmic agents. *Clin. Pharmacokinet.*, **1984**, *9*, 375–403.

MEZLOCILLIN

Deeter, R. G.; Barriere, S. L.; and Fekety, R. Pharmacokinetic and pharmacodynamic comparison of mezlocillin and ticarcillin. *Clin. Pharm.*, **1988**, *7*, 380–384.

Mangione, A.; Boudinot, F. D.; Schultz, R. M.; and Jusko, W. J. Dose-dependent pharmacokinetics of mezlocillin in relation to renal impairment. *Antimicrob. Agents Chemother.*, **1982**, *21*, 428–435.

MIDAZOLAM

Garzone, P. D., and Kroboth, P. D. Pharmacokinetics of the newer benzodiazepines. *Clin. Pharmacokinet.*, **1989**, *16*, 337–364.

MINOCYCLINE

Saivin, S., and Hovin, G. Clinical pharmacokinetics of doxycycline and minocycline. *Clin. Pharmacokinet.*, **1988**, *15*, 355–366.

MINOXIDIL

Fleishaker, J. C.; Andreadis, N. A.; Welshman, I. R.; and Wright, C. E. The pharmacokinetics of 2.5- to 10-mg oral doses of minoxidil in healthy volunteers. *J. Clin. Pharmacol.*, **1989**, *29*, 162–167.

MORPHINE

Choonara, I. A.; McKay, P.; Hain, R.; and Rane, A. Morphine metabolism in children. *Br. J. Clin. Pharmacol.*, **1989**, *28*, 599–604.

Hoskin, P. J.; Hanks, G. W.; Aherne, G. W.; Chapman, D.; Littleton, P.; and Filshie, J. The bioavailability and pharmacokinetics of morphine after intravenous, oral and buccal administration in healthy volunteers. *Br. J. Clin. Pharmacol.*, **1989**, *27*, 499–505.

MOXALACTAM

Barriere, S. L., and Flaherty, J. F. Third-generation cephalosporins: a critical review. *Clin. Pharm.*, **1984**, *3*, 351–373.

Nahata, M. C.; Durrell, D. E.; and Barson, W. J. Moxalactam epimer kinetics in children. *Clin. Pharmacol. Ther.*, **1982**, *31*, 528–532.

NADOLOL

Dreyfuss, J.; Brannick, L. J.; Vukovich, R. A.; Shaw, J. M.; and Willard, D. A. Metabolic studies in patients with nadolol: oral and intravenous administration. *J. Clin. Pharmacol.*, **1977**, *17*, 300–307.

Morrison, R. A.; Singhvi, S. M.; Creasey, W. A.; and Willard, D. A. Dose proportionality of nadolol pharmacokinetics after intravenous administration to healthy subjects. *Eur. J. Clin. Pharmacol.*, **1988**, *33*, 625–628.

NAFCILLIN

Marshall, J. P.; Salt, W. B.; Elam, R. O.; Wilkinson, G. R.; and Schenker, S. Disposition of nafcillin in patients with cirrhosis and extrahepatic biliary obstruction. *Gastroenterology*, **1977**, *73*, 1388–1392.

Rudnick, M.; Morrison, G.; Walker, B.; and Singer, I. Renal failure, hemodialysis, and nafcillin kinetics. *Clin. Pharmacol. Ther.*, **1976**, *20*, 413–423.

NALBUPHINE

Aitkenhead, A. R.; Lin, E. S.; and Achola, K. J. The pharmacokinetics of oral and intravenous nalbuphine in healthy volunteers. *Br. J. Clin. Pharmacol.*, **1988**, *25*, 264–268.

Jaillon, P.; Gardin, M. E.; Lecocq, B.; Ricard, M. O.; Meignan, S.; Blondel, Y.; Grippat, J. C.; Begnieres, J.; and Vergnoux, O. Pharmacokinetics of nalbuphine in infants, young healthy volunteers, and elderly patients. *Clin. Pharmacol. Ther.*, **1989**, *46*, 226–233.

NALOXONE

Handal, K. A.; Schauben, J. L.; and Salamone, F. R. Naloxone. *Ann. Emerg. Med.*, **1983**, *12*, 438–445.

Stile, I. L.; Fort, M.; Wurzburger, R. J.; Rodvold, K. A.; Spector, S.; Hiatt, I. M.; and Hegyi, T. The pharmacokinetics of naloxone in the premature newborn. *Dev. Pharmacol. Ther.*, **1987**, *10*, 454–459.

NALTREXONE

Gonzalez, J. P., and Brogden, R. N. Naltrexone: a review of its pharmacodynamic and pharmacokinetic properties and therapeutic efficacy in the management of opioid dependence. *Drugs*, **1988**, *35*, 192–213.

Wall, M. E.; Brine, D. R.; and Perez-Reyes, M. Metabolism and disposition of naltrexone in man after oral and intravenous administration. *Drug Metab. Dispos.*, **1981**, *9*, 369–375.

NAPROXEN

van den Ouweland, F. A.; Gribnau, F. W. J.; van Ginneken, C. A. M.; Tan, Y.; and van de Putte, L. B. A. Naproxen kinetics and disease activity in rheumatoid arthritis: a within-patient study. *Clin. Pharmacol. Ther.*, **1988**, *43*, 79–85.

Verbeeck, R. K.; Blackburn, J. L.; and Loewen, G. R. Clinical pharmacokinetics of non-steroidal anti-inflammatory drugs. *Clin. Pharmacokinet.*, **1983**, *8*, 297–331.

NEOSTIGMINE

Cronnelly, R.; Stanski, D. R.; Miller, R. D.; Sheiner, L. B.; and Sohn, Y. J. Renal function and the pharmacokinetics of neostigmine in anesthetized man. *Anesthesiology*, **1979**, *51*, 222–226.

Nowell, P. T.; Scott, C. A.; and Wilson, A. Determination of neostigmine and pyridostigmine in the urine of patients with myasthenia gravis. *Br. J. Pharmacol.*, **1962**, *18*, 617–624.

Table A–II–1. PHARMACOKINETIC DATA (Continued)

NETILMICIN

Campoli-Richards, D. M.; Chaplin, S.; Sayce, R. H.; and Goa, K. L. Netilmicin: a review of its antibacterial activity, pharmacokinetic properties and therapeutic use. *Drugs*, **1989**, *5*, 703–756.

Craig, W. A.; Gudmundsson, S.; and Reich, R. M. Netilmicin sulfate: a comparative evaluation of antimicrobial activity, pharmacokinetics, adverse reactions and clinical efficacy. *Pharmacotherapy*, **1983**, *3*, 305–315.

NICARDIPINE

Guerret, M.; Cheymol, G.; Hubert, M.; Julien-Larose, C.; and Lavene, D. Simultaneous study of the pharmacokinetics of intravenous and oral nicardipine using a stable isotope. *Eur. J. Clin. Pharmacol.*, **1989**, *37*, 381–385.

Wagner, J. G.; Ling, T.-L.; Mroszczak, E. J.; Freedman, D.; Wu, A.; Huang, B.; Massey, I. J.; and Roe, R. R. Single intravenous dose and steady-state oral dose pharmacokinetics of nicardipine in healthy subjects. *Biopharm. Drug Dispos.*, **1987**, *8*, 133–148.

NICOTINE

Benowitz, N. L.; Jacob, P., III; Jones, R. T.; and Rosenberg, J. Interindividual variability in the metabolism and cardiovascular effects of nicotine in man. *J. Pharmacol. Exp. Ther.*, **1982**, *221*, 368–372.

Busto, U.; Bendayan, R.; and Sellers, E. M. Clinical pharmacokinetics of non-opiate abused drugs. *Clin. Pharmacokinet.*, **1989**, *16*, 1–26.

NIFEDIPINE

Echizen, H., and Eichelbaum, M. Clinical pharmacokinetics of verapamil, nifedipine and diltiazem. *Clin. Pharmacokinet.*, **1986**, *11*, 425–449.

Kleinbloesem, C. H.; von Brummelen, P.; and Breimer, D. D. Nifedipine: relationship between pharmacokinetics and pharmacodynamics. *Clin. Pharmacokinet.*, **1987**, *12*, 12–29.

NITRAZEPAM

Abernethy, D. R.; Greenblatt, D. J.; Locniskar, A.; Ochs, H. R.; Harmatz, J. S.; and Shader, R. I. Obesity effects on nitrazepam disposition. *Br. J. Clin. Pharmacol.*, **1986**, *22*, 551–557.

Kangas, L., and Breimer, D. D. Clinical pharmacokinetics of nitrazepam. *Clin. Pharmacokinet.*, **1981**, *6*, 346–366.

NITROGLYCERIN

Thadani, U., and Whitsett, T. Relationship of pharmacokinetic and pharmacodynamic properties of the organic nitrates. *Clin. Pharmacokinet.*, **1988**, *15*, 32–43.

NIZATIDINE

Krishna, D. R., and Klotz, U. Newer H_2-receptor antagonists: clinical pharmacokinetics and drug interaction potential. *Clin. Pharmacokinet.*, **1988**, *15*, 205–215.

NORFLOXACIN

Sörgel, F.; Jaehde, U.; Naber, K.; and Stephan, U. Pharmacokinetic disposition of quinolones in human body fluids and tissues. *Clin. Pharmacokinet.*, **1989**, *16*, Suppl. 1, 5–24.

NORTRIPTYLINE

Dahl-Puustinen, M-L.; Perry, T. L.; Dumont, E.; von Bahr, C.; Nordin, C.; and Bertilsson, L. Stereoselective disposition of racemic E-10-hydroxynortriptyline in human beings. *Clin. Pharmacol. Ther.*, **1989**, *45*, 650–656.

Nordin, C.; Siwers, B.; Benitez, J.; and Bertilsson, L. Plasma concentrations of nortriptyline and its 10-hydroxy metabolite in depressed patients - relationship to the debrisoquine hydroxylation metabolic ratio. *Br. J. Clin. Pharmacol.*, **1985**, *19*, 832–835.

OXACILLIN

Dittert, L. W.; Griffen, W. O.; La Piana, J. C.; Shainfeld, F. J.; and Doluisio, J. T. Pharmacokinetic interpretation of penicillin levels in serum and urine after intravenous administration. *Antimicrob. Agents Chemother.*, **1969**, *9*, 42–48.

Wirth, K.; Hengstmann, J. H.; Langebartels, F. H.; and Träger, S. Zur Kinetik von Ampicillin, Oxacillin und Carbenicillin nach intravenöser Kurzinfusion beim Menschen. *Arzneimittelforschung*, **1976**, *26*, 1709–1715.

OXAZEPAM

Greenblatt, D. J. Clinical pharmacokinetics of oxazepam and lorazepam. *Clin. Pharmacokinet.*, **1981**, *6*, 89–105.

Sonne, J.; Loft, S.; Døssing, M.; Vollmer-Larsen, A.; Olesen, K. L.; Victor, M.; Andreasen, F.; and Andreasen, P. B. Bioavailability and pharmacokinetics of oxazepam. *Eur. J. Clin. Pharmacol.*, **1988**, *35*, 385–389.

PANCURONIUM

Shanks, C. A. Pharmacokinetics of the nondepolarizing neuromuscular relaxants applied to calculation of bolus and infusion dosage regimens. *Anesthesiology*, **1986**, *64*, 72–86.

PENTAMIDINE

Conte, J. E.; Upton, R. A.; and Lin, E. T. Pentamidine pharmacokinetics in patients with AIDS with impaired renal function. *J. Infect. Dis.*, **1987**, *156*, 885–890.

PENTAZOCINE

Beckett, A. H.; Taylor, J. F.; and Kourounakis, P. The absorption, distribution and excretion of pentazocine in man after oral and intravenous administration. *J. Pharm. Pharmacol.*, **1970**, *22*, 123–128.

Yeh, S. Y.; Todd, G. D.; Johnson, R. E.; Gorodetzky, C. W.; and Lange, W. R. The pharmacokinetics of pentazocine and tripelennamine. *Clin. Pharmacol. Ther.*, **1986**, *39*, 669–676.

PENTOXIFYLLINE

Beermann, B.; Ings, R.; Mansby, J.; Chamberlain, J.; and McDonald, A. Kinetics of intravenous and oral pentoxifylline in healthy subjects. *Clin. Pharmacol. Ther.*, **1985**, *37*, 25–28.

Ward, A., and Clissold, S. P. Pentoxifylline: a review of its pharmacodynamic and pharmacokinetic properties, and its therapeutic efficacy. *Drugs*, **1987**, *34*, 50–97.

PHENOBARBITAL

Browne, T. R.; Evans, J. E.; Szabo, G. K.; Evans, B. A.; and Greenblatt, D. J. Studies with stable isotopes II: phenobarbital pharmacokinetics during monotherapy. *J. Clin. Pharmacol.*, **1985**, *25*, 51–58.

Buchthal, F., and Lennox-Buchthal, M. A. Phenobarbital. Relation of serum concentration to control of seizures. In, *Antiepileptic Drugs*. (Woodbury, D. M.; Penry, J. K.; and Schmidt, R. P.; eds.) Raven Press, New York, **1972**, pp. 335–343.

PHENYLBUTAZONE

Aarbakke, J. Clinical pharmacokinetics of phenylbutazone. *Clin. Pharmacokinet.*, **1978**, *3*, 369–380.

Verbeeck, R. K.; Blackburn, J. L.; and Loewen, G. R. Clinical pharmacokinetics of non-steroidal anti-inflammatory drugs. *Clin. Pharmacokinet.*, **1983**, *8*, 297–331.

PHENYLETHYLMALONAMIDE

Pisani, F., and Richens, A. Pharmacokinetics of phenylethylmalonamide (PEMA) after oral and intravenous administration. *Clin. Pharmacokinet.*, **1983**, *8*, 272–276.

Streete, J. M.; Berry, D. J.; Newberry, J. E.; and Crome, P. Pharmacokinetics of phenylethylmalonamide (PEMA) in elderly men. *Eur. J. Clin. Pharmacol.*, **1987**, *33*, 431–434.

PHENYTOIN

Crowley, J. J.; Koup, J. R.; Cusack, B. J.; Ludden, T. M.; and Vestal, R. E. Evaluation of a proposed method for phenytoin maintenance dose prediction following an intravenous loading dose. *Eur. J. Clin. Pharmacol.*, **1987**, *32*, 141–148.

Grasela, T. H., and others. Steady-state pharmacokinetics of phenytoin from routinely collected patient data. *Clin. Pharmacokinet.*, **1983**, *8*, 355–364.

PIMOZIDE

Sallee, R. F.; Pollock, B. G.; Stiller, R. L.; Stull, S.; Everett, G.; and Perel, J. M. Pharmacokinetics of pimozide in adults and children with Tourette's syndrome. *J. Clin. Pharmacol.*, **1987**, *27*, 776–781.

PINDOLOL

Guerret, M.; Cheymol, G.; Aubry, J. P.; Cheymol, A.; Lavene, D.; and Kiechel, J. R. Estimation of the absolute oral bioavailability of pindolol by two analytical methods. *Eur. J. Clin. Pharmacol.*, **1983**, *25*, 357–359.

Lavene, D.; Weiss, Y. A.; Safar, M. E.; Loria, Y.; Agorus, N.; Georges, D.; and Milliez, P. L. Pharmacokinetics and hepatic extraction ratio of pindolol in hypertensive patients with normal and impaired renal function. *J. Clin. Pharmacol.*, **1979**, *17*, 501–508.

Regårdh, C. G. Pharmacokinetic aspects of some β-adrenoceptor blocking drugs. *Acta Med. Scand.*, **1982**, *665*, Suppl., 49–60.

PIPERACILLIN

Tartaglione, T. A.; Nye, L.; Vishniavsky, N.; Poynor, W.; and Polk, R. E. Multiple-dose pharmacokinetics of piperacillin and azlocillin in 12 healthy volunteers. *Clin. Pharm.*, **1986**, *5*, 911–916.

Welling, P. G.; Craig, W. A.; Bundtzen, R. W.; Kwok, F. W.; Gerber, A. U.; and Madsen, P. O. Pharmacokinetics of piperacillin in subjects with various degrees of renal function. *Antimicrob. Agents Chemother.*, **1983**, *23*, 881–887.

PIROXICAM

Brogden, R. N.; Heel, R. C.; Speight, T. M.; and Avery, G. S. Piroxicam: a reappraisal of its pharmacology and therapeutic efficacy. *Drugs*, **1984**, *28*, 292–323.

Verbeeck, R. K.; Richardson, C. J.; and Blocka, K. L. N. Clinical pharmacokinetics of piroxicam. *J. Rheumatol.*, **1986**, *13*, 789–796.

PRAZEPAM

Ochs, H. R.; Greenblatt, D. J.; Verburg-Ochs, B.; and Locniskar, A. Comparative single-dose kinetics of oxazolam, prazepam and clorazepate: three precursors of desmethyldiazepam. *J. Clin. Pharmacol.*, **1984**, *24*, 446–451.
Smith, M. T.; Evan, L. E. J.; Eadie, M. J.; and Tyrer, J. H. Pharmacokinetics of prazepam in man. *Eur. J. Clin. Pharmacol.*, **1979**, *16*, 141–147.

PRAZOSIN

Lameire, N., and Gordts, J. A pharmacokinetic study of prazosin in patients with varying degrees of chronic renal failure. *Eur. J. Clin. Pharmacol.*, **1986**, *31*, 333–337.
Vincent, J.; Meredith, P. A.; Reid, J. L.; Elliott, H. L.; and Rubin, P. C. Clinical pharmacokinetics of prazosin—1985. *Clin. Pharmacokinet.*, **1985**, *10*, 144–154.

PREDNISOLONE

Frey, F. J.; Horber, F. F.; and Frey, B. M. Altered metabolism and decreased efficacy of prednisolone and prednisone in patients with hyperthyroidism. *Clin. Pharmacol. Ther.*, **1988**, *44*, 510–521.
Gustavson, L. E., and Benet, L. Z. Pharmacokinetics of natural and synthetic glucocorticoids. In, *Butterworth's International Medical Reviews in Endocrinology*. Vol. 4, *The Adrenal Cortex*. (Anderson, D. C., and Winter, J. S. D., eds.) Butterworth & Co., London, **1985**, pp. 235–281.

PREDNISONE

Gustavson, L. E., and Benet, L. Z. Pharmacokinetics of natural and synthetic glucocorticoids. In, *Butterworth's International Medical Reviews in Endocrinology*. Vol. 4, *The Adrenal Cortex*. (Anderson, D. C., and Winter, J. S. D., eds.) Butterworth & Co., London, **1985**, pp. 235–281.
Schalm, S. W.; Summerskill, W. H. J.; and Go, V. L. W. Prednisone for chronic active liver disease: pharmacokinetics, including conversion to prednisolone. *Gastroenterology*, **1977**, *72*, 910–913.

PRIMIDONE

Gallagher, B. B.; Baumel, I. P.; and Mattson, R. H. Metabolic disposition of primidone and its metabolites in epileptic subjects after single and repeated administration. *Neurology (Minneap.)*, **1972**, *22*, 1186–1192.
Kauffman, R. E.; Habersang, R.; and Lansky, L. Kinetics of primidone metabolism and excretion in children. *Clin. Pharmacol. Ther.*, **1977**, *22*, 200–205.

PROBENECID

Emanuelsson, B.-M.; Beermann, B.; and Paalzow, L. K. Non-linear elimination and protein binding of probenecid. *Eur. J. Clin. Pharmacol.*, **1987**, *32*, 395–401.

PROCAINAMIDE

Benet, L. Z., and Ding, R. W. Die renale Elimination von Procainamide: Pharmakokinetik bei Niereninsuffizienz. In, *Die Behandlung von Herzrhythmusstörungen bei Nierenkranken*. (Braun, J.; Pilgrim, R.; Gessler, U.; and Seybold, D.; eds.) S. Karger, Basel, **1984**, pp. 96–111.
Follath, F.; Ganzinger, U.; and Schuetz, E. Reliability of antiarrhythmic drug plasma concentration monitoring. *Clin. Pharmacokinet.*, **1983**, *8*, 63–82.

PROPRANOLOL

Riddell, J. G.; Harron, D. W. G.; and Shanks, R. G. Clinical pharmacokinetics of β-adrenoceptor antagonists: an update. *Clin. Pharmacokinet.*, **1987**, *12*, 305–320.
Ward, S. A.; Walle, T.; Walle, U. K.; Wilkinson, G. R.; and Branch, R. A. Propranolol's metabolism is determined by both mephenytoin and debrisoquin hydroxylase activities. *Clin. Pharmacol. Ther.*, **1989**, *45*, 72–79.

PROTRIPTYLINE

Baldessarini, R. J. Status of psychotropic drug blood level assays and other biochemical measurements in clinical practice. *Am. J. Psychiatry*, **1979**, *136*, 1177–1180.
Moody, J. P.; Whyte, S. F.; MacDonald, A. J.; and Naylor, G. J. Pharmacokinetic aspects of protriptyline plasma levels. *Eur. J. Clin. Pharmacol.*, **1977**, *11*, 51–56.

PYRIDOSTIGMINE

Breyer-Pfaff, U.; Maier, U.; Brinkmann, A. M.; and Schumm, F. Pyridostigmine kinetics in healthy subjects and patients with myasthenia gravis. *Clin. Pharmacol. Ther.*, **1985**, *37*, 495–501.
Cronnelly, R.; Stanski, D. R.; Miller, R. D.; and Sheiner, L. B. Pyridostigmine kinetics with and without renal function. *Clin. Pharmacol. Ther.*, **1980**, *28*, 78–81.

PYRIMETHAMINE

Ahmad, R. A., and Rogers, H. J. Pharmacokinetics and protein binding interactions of dapsone and pyrimethamine. *Br. J. Clin. Pharmacol.*, **1980**, *10*, 519–524.
White, N. J. Clinical pharmacokinetics of antimalarial drugs. *Clin. Pharmacokinet.*, **1985**, *10*, 187–215.

QUINIDINE

Ochs, H. R.; Greenblatt, D. J.; and Woo, E. Clinical pharmacokinetics of quinidine. *Clin. Pharmacokinet.*, **1980**, *5*, 150–168.

Wooding-Scott, R. A.; Smalley, J.; Visco, J.; and Slaughter, R. L. The pharmacokinetics and pharmacodynamics of quinidine and 3-hydroxyquinidine. *Br. J. Clin. Pharmacol.*, **1988**, *26*, 415–421.

QUININE

White, N. J. Clinical pharmacokinetics of antimalarial drugs. *Clin. Pharmacokinet.*, **1985**, *10*, 187–215.

RANITIDINE

Grant, S. M.; Langtry, H. D.; and Brogden, R. N. Ranitidine: an updated review of its pharmacodynamic and pharmacokinetic properties and therapeutic use in peptic ulcer disease and other allied diseases. *Drugs*, **1989**, *37*, 801–870.

RIFAMPIN

Holdiness, M. R. Clinical pharmacokinetics of the antituberculosis drugs. *Clin. Pharmacokinet.*, **1984**, *9*, 511–544.

Israili, Z. H.; Rogers, C. M.; and El-Attar, H. Pharmacokinetics of antituberculosis drugs in patients. *J. Clin. Pharmacol.*, **1987**, *27*, 78–83.

SALICYLIC ACID

Furst, D. E.; Tozer, T. N.; and Melmon, K. L. Salicylate clearance, the resultant of protein binding and metabolism. *Clin. Pharmacol. Ther.*, **1979**, *26*, 380–389.

Owen, S. G.; Roberts, M. S.; Friesen, W. T.; and Francis, H. W. Salicylate pharmacokinetics in patients with rheumatoid arthritis. *Br. J. Clin. Pharmacol.*, **1989**, *28*, 449–461.

SCOPOLAMINE

Kanto, J., and Klotz, U. Pharmacokinetic implications for the clinical use of atropine, scopolamine and glycopyrrolate. *Acta Anaesthesiol. Scand.*, **1988**, *32*, 69–78.

Putcha, L.; Cintrón, N. M.; Tsui, J.; Vanderploeg, J. M.; and Kramer, W. G. Pharmacokinetics and oral bioavailability of scopolamine in normal subjects. *Pharm. Res.*, **1989**, *6*, 481–485.

SPIRONOLACTONE

Krause, W.; Karras, J.; and Seifert, W. Pharmacokinetics of canrenone after oral administration of spironolactone and intravenous injection of canrenoate-K in healthy man. *Eur. J. Clin. Pharmacol.*, **1983**, *25*, 449–453.

Overdiek, H. W., and Merkus, F. W. The metabolism and biopharmaceutics of spironolactone in man. *Rev. Drug Metab. Drug Interact.*, **1987**, *5*, 273–302.

STREPTOKINASE

Grierson, D. S., and Bjornsson, T. D. Pharmacokinetics of streptokinase in patients based on amidolytic activator complex activity. *Clin. Pharmacol. Ther.*, **1987**, *41*, 304–313.

STREPTOMYCIN

Bolme, P.; Eriksson, M.; Habte, D.; and Paalzow, L. Pharmacokinetics of streptomycin in Ethiopian children with tuberculosis and of different nutritional status. *Eur. J. Clin. Pharmacol.*, **1988**, *33*, 647–649.

Holdiness, M. R. Clinical pharmacokinetics of the antituberculosis drugs. *Clin. Pharmacokinet.*, **1984**, *9*, 511–544.

SUFENTANIL

Bovill, J. G.; Sebel, P. S.; Blackburn, C. L.; Oei-Lim, V.; and Heykants, J. J. The pharmacokinetics of sufentanil in surgical patients. *Anesthesiology*, **1984**, *61*, 502–506.

Chauvin, M.; Ferrier, C.; Haberer, J. P.; Spielvogel, C.; Lebrault, C.; Levron, J. C.; and Duvaldestin, P. Sufentanil pharmacokinetics in patients with cirrhosis. *Anesth. Analg.*, **1989**, *68*, 1–4.

SULFADIAZINE

Bergan, T.; Örtengren, B.; and Westerlund, D. Clinical pharmacokinetics of co-trimazine. *Clin. Pharmacokinet.*, **1986**, *11*, 372–386.

Männistö, P. T.; Mäntylä, R.; Mattila, J.; Nykänen, S.; and Lamminsivu, U. Comparison of the pharmacokinetics of sulphadiazine and sulphamethoxazole after intravenous infusion. *J. Antimicrob. Chemother.*, **1982**, *9*, 461–470.

SULFAMETHOXAZOLE

Bergan, T.; Örtengren, B.; and Westerlund, D. Clinical pharmacokinetics of co-trimazine. *Clin. Pharmacokinet.*, **1986**, *11*, 372–386.

Patel, R. B., and Welling, P. G. Clinical pharmacokinetics of co-trimoxazole. *Clin. Pharmacokinet.*, **1980**, *5*, 405–423.

SULFINPYRAZONE

Schlicht, F.; Staiger, Ch.; Gundert-Remy, U.; Hildebrandt, R.; Harenberg, J.; Wang, N. S.; and Weber, E. Pharmacokinetics of sulphinpyrazone and its major metabolites after a single dose and during chronic treatment. *Eur. J. Clin. Pharmacol.*, **1985**, *28*, 97–103.

Strong, H. A.; Angus, R.; Oates, J.; Sembi, J.; Howarth, P.; Renwick, A. G.; and George, C. F. Effects of ischaemic heart disease, Crohn's disease and antimicrobial therapy on the pharmacokinetics of sulphinpyrazone. *Clin. Pharmacokinet.*, **1986**, *11*, 402–410.

Table A–II–1. PHARMACOKINETIC DATA (Continued)

SULFISOXAZOLE

Cello, J. P., and Øie, S. Binding and disposition of sulfisoxazole in alcoholic cirrhosis. *J. Pharmacokinet. Biopharm.*, **1985**, *13*, 1–12.
Øie, S.; Gambertoglio, J. G.; and Fleckenstein, L. Comparison of the disposition of total and unbound sulfisoxazole after single and multiple dosing. *J. Pharmacokinet. Biopharm.*, **1982**, *10*, 157–172.

SULINDAC

Gibson, T. P.; Dobrinska, M. R.; Lin, J. H.; Entwistle, L. A.; and Davies, R. O. Biotransformation of sulindac in end-stage renal disease. *Clin. Pharmacol. Ther.*, **1987**, *42*, 82–88.
Matilla, J.; Mantyla, R.; Vuorela, A.; Lamminsivu, U.; and Mannisto, P. Pharmacokinetics of graded oral doses of sulindac in man. *Arzneimittelforschung*, **1984**, *34*, 226–229.

TEMAZEPAM

Ghabrial, H.; Desmond, P. V.; Watson, K. J. R.; Gijsbers, A. J.; Harman, P. J.; Breen, K. J.; and Mashford, M. L. The effects of age and chronic liver disease on the elimination of temazepam. *Eur. J. Clin. Pharmacol.*, **1986**, *30*, 93–97.
Greenblatt, D. J.; Divoll, M.; Abernethy, D. R.; Ochs, H. R.; and Shader, R. I. Clinical pharmacokinetics of the newer benzodiazepines. *Clin. Pharmacokinet.*, **1983**, *8*, 233–252.

TERAZOSIN

Titmarsh, S., and Monk, J. P. Terazosin: a review of its pharmacodynamic and pharmacokinetic properties and therapeutic efficacy in essential hypertension. *Drugs*, **1987**, *33*, 461–477.

TERBUTALINE

Borgström, L.; Nyberg, L.; Jönsson, S.; Lindberg, C.; and Paulson, J. Pharmacokinetic evaluation in man of terbutaline given as separate enantiomers and as the racemate. *Br. J. Clin. Pharmacol.*, **1989**, *27*, 49–56.

TETRACYCLINE

Jaffe, J. M.; Colaizzi, J. L.; Poust, R. I.; and McDonald, R. H. Effect of altered urinary pH on tetracycline and doxycycline excretion in humans. *J. Pharmacokinet. Biopharm.*, **1973**, *1*, 267–282.
Raghuram, T. C., and Krishnaswamy, K. Pharmacokinetics of tetracycline in nutritional oedema. *Chemotherapy*, **1982**, *28*, 428–433.

TETRAHYDROCANNABINOL (DRONABINOL)

Busto, U.; Bendayan, R.; and Sellers, E. M. Clinical pharmacokinetics of non-opiate abused drugs. *Clin. Pharmacokinet.*, **1989**, *16*, 1–26.

THEOPHYLLINE

Bierman, C. W., and Williams, P. V. Therapeutic monitoring of theophylline: rationale and current status. *Clin. Pharmacokinet.*, **1989**, *17*, 377–384.
Driscoll, M. S.; Ludden, T. M.; Casto, D. T.; and Littlefield, L. C. Evaluation of theophylline pharmacokinetics in a pediatric population using mixed effects models. *J. Pharmacokinet. Biopharm.*, **1989**, *17*, 141–168.

THIOPENTAL

Homer, T. D., and Stanski, D. R. The effect of increasing age on thiopental disposition and anesthetic requirement. *Anesthesiology*, **1985**, *62*, 714–724.

TICARCILLIN

Davies, B. E.; Humphrey, M. J.; Langley, P. F.; Lees, L.; Legg, B.; and Wadds, G. A. Pharmacokinetics of ticarcillin in man. *Eur. J. Clin. Pharmacol.*, **1982**, *23*, 167–172.
de Groot, R., and Smith, A. L. Antibiotic pharmacokinetics in cystic fibrosis. *Clin. Pharmacokinet.*, **1987**, *13*, 228–253.

TIMOLOL

McGourty, J. C.; Silas, J. H.; Fleming, J. J.; McBurney, A.; and Ward, J. W. Pharmacokinetics and beta-blocking effects of timolol in poor and extensive metabolizers of debrisoquin. *Clin. Pharmacol. Ther.*, **1985**, *38*, 409–413.
Vedin, J. A.; Kristianson, J. K.; and Wilhelmsson, C.-E. Pharmacokinetics of intravenous timolol in patients with acute myocardial infarction and in healthy volunteers. *Eur. J. Clin. Pharmacol.*, **1982**, *23*, 43–47.

TOBRAMYCIN

Aarons, L.; Vozeh, S.; Wenk, M.; Weiss, Ph.; and Follath, F. Population pharmacokinetics of tobramycin. *Br. J. Clin. Pharmacol.*, **1989**, *28*, 305–314.

TOCAINIDE

Gillis, A. M., and Kates, R. E. Clinical pharmacokinetics of the newer antiarrhythmic agents. *Clin. Pharmacokinet.*, **1984**, *9*, 375–403.
Thomson, A. H.; Murdoch, G.; Pottage, A.; Kelman, A. W.; Whiting, B.; and Hillis, W. S. The pharmacokinetics of R- and S-tocainide in patients with acute ventricular arrhythmias. *Br. J. Clin. Pharmacol.*, **1986**, *21*, 149–154.

TOLBUTAMIDE

Balant, L. Clinical pharmacokinetics of sulphonylurea-hypoglycaemic agents. *Clin. Pharmacokinet.*, **1981**, *6*, 215–241.

Robson, R. A.; Miners, J. O.; Whitehead, A. G.; and Birkett, D. J. Specificity of the inhibitory effect of dextropropoxyphene on oxidative drug metabolism in man: effects on theophylline and tolbutamide disposition. *Br. J. Clin. Pharmacol.*, **1987**, *23*, 772–775.

TOLMETIN

Furst, D. E.; Dromgoole, S. H.; Desiraju, R. K.; and Paulus, H. E. Clinical pharmacology of tolmetin: comparisons in rheumatoid arthritis patients and normal volunteers. *J. Clin. Pharmacol.*, **1983**, *23*, 329–335.

Hyneck, M. L.; Smith, P. C.; Munafo, A.; McDonagh, A. F.; and Benet, L. Z. Disposition and irreversible plasma protein binding of tolmetin in humans. *Clin. Pharmacol. Ther.*, **1988**, *44*, 107–114.

TRAZODONE

Greenblatt, D. J.; Friedman, H.; Burstein, E. S.; Scavone, J. M.; Blyden, G. T.; Ochs, H. R.; Miller, L. G.; Harmatz, J. S.; and Shader, R. I. Trazodone kinetics: effect of age, gender and obesity. *Clin. Pharmacol. Ther.*, **1987**, *42*, 193–200.

TRIAMTERENE

Gilfrich, H. J.; Kremer, G.; Möhrke, W.; Mutschler, E.; and Völger, K.-D. Pharmacokinetics of triamterene after i.v. administration to man: determination of bioavailability. *Eur. J. Clin. Pharmacol.*, **1983**, *25*, 237–241.

Williams, R. L.; Thornhill, M. D.; Upton, R. A.; Blume, C.; Clark, T. S.; Lin, E.; and Benet, L. Z. Absorption and disposition of two combination formulations of hydrochlorothiazide and triamterene: influence of age and renal function. *Clin. Pharmacol. Ther.*, **1986**, *40*, 226–232.

TRIAZOLAM

Garzone, P. D., and Kroboth, P. D. Pharmacokinetics of the newer benzodiazepines. *Clin. Pharmacokinet.*, **1989**, *16*, 337–364.

TRIMETHOPRIM

Bergan, T.; Örtengren, B.; and Westerlund, D. Clinical pharmacokinetics of co-trimazine. *Clin. Pharmacokinet.*, **1986**, *11*, 372–386.

Hoppu, K. Age differences in trimethoprim pharmacokinetics: need for revised dosing in children? *Clin. Pharmacol. Ther.*, **1987**, *41*, 336–343.

TUBOCURARINE

Fisher, D. M.; O'Keeffe, C.; Stanski, D. R.; Cronnelly, R.; Miller, R. D.; and Gregory, G. A. Pharmacokinetics and pharmacodynamics of *d*-tubocurarine in infants, children, and adults. *Anesthesiology*, **1982**, *57*, 203–208.

Shanks, C. A. Pharmacokinetics of the nondepolarizing neuromuscular relaxants applied to calculation of bolus and infusion dosage regimens. *Anesthesiology*, **1986**, *64*, 72–86.

VALPROIC ACID

Zaccara, G.; Messori, A.; and Moroni, F. Clinical pharmacokinetics of valproic acid—1988. *Clin. Pharmacokinet.*, **1988**, *15*, 367–389.

VANCOMYCIN

Boeckh, M.; Lode, H.; Borner, K.; Höffken, G.; Wagner, J.; and Koeppe, P. Pharmacokinetics and serum bactericidal activity of vancomycin alone and in combination with ceftazidime in healthy volunteers. *Antimicrob. Agents Chemother.*, **1988**, *32*, 92–95.

Rodvold, K. A.; Blum, R. A.; Fischer, J. H.; Zokufa, H. Z.; Rotschafer, J. C.; Crossley, K. B.; and Riff, L. J. Vancomycin pharmacokinetics in patients with various degrees of renal function. *Antimicrob. Agents Chemother.*, **1988**, *32*, 848–852.

VECURONIUM

Shanks, C. A. Pharmacokinetics of the nondepolarizing neuromuscular relaxants applied to calculation of bolus and infusion dosage regimens. *Anesthesiology*, **1986**, *64*, 72–86.

Shanks, C. A.; Avram, M. J.; Fragen, R. J.; and O'Hara, D. A. Pharmacokinetics and pharmacodynamics of vecuronium administered by bolus and infusion during halothane or balanced anesthesia. *Clin. Pharmacol. Ther.*, **1987**, *42*, 459–464.

VERAPAMIL

Echizen, H., and Eichelbaum, M. Clinical pharmacokinetics of verapamil, nifedipine and diltiazem. *Clin. Pharmacokinet.*, **1986**, *11*, 425–449.

McTavish, D., and Sorkin, E. M. Verapamil: an updated review of its pharmacodynamic and pharmacokinetic properties and therapeutic use in hypertension. *Drugs*, **1989**, *38*, 19–76.

WARFARIN

Holford, N. H. G. Clinical pharmacokinetics and pharmacodynamics of warfarin: understanding the dose-effect relationship. *Clin. Pharmacokinet.*, **1986**, *11*, 483–504.

Toon, S.; Hopkins, K. J.; Garstang, F. M.; and Rowland, M. Comparative effects of ranitidine and cimetidine on the pharmacokinetics and pharmacodynamics of warfarin in man. *Eur. J. Clin. Pharmacol.*, **1987**, *32*, 165–172.

ZIDOVUDINE

Collins, J. M., and Unadkat, J. D. Clinical pharmacokinetics of zidovudine. *Clin. Pharmacokinet.*, **1989**, *17*, 1–9.

INDEX